DRUG INFORMATION HANDBOOK for DENTISTRY

Including Oral Medicine for Medically-Compromised Patients & Specific Oral Conditions

Richard L. Wynn, BSPharm, PhD
Timothy F. Meiller, DDS, PhD
Harold L. Crossley, DDS, PhD

th Edition

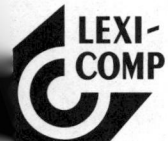

LEXI-COMP

DRUG
INFORMATION
HANDBOOK
for DENTISTRY

Including Oral Medicine for
Medically-Compromised Patients
& Specific Oral Conditions

Richard L. Wynn, BSPharm, PhD
Timothy F. Meiller, DDS, PhD
Harold L. Crossley, DDS, PhD

Edition

LEXI-COMP

NOTES

NOTES

DRUG INFORMATION HANDBOOK for DENTISTRY

Including Oral Medicine for Medically-Compromised Patients & Specific Oral Conditions

Richard L. Wynn, BSPharm, PhD
Professor of Pharmacology
Baltimore College of Dental Surgery
Dental School
University of Maryland Baltimore
Baltimore, Maryland

Timothy F. Meiller, DDS, PhD
Professor
Diagnostic Sciences and Pathology
Baltimore College of Dental Surgery
Professor of Oncology
Greenebaum Cancer Center
University of Maryland Baltimore
Baltimore, Maryland

Harold L. Crossley, DDS, PhD
Professor Emeritus
Baltimore College of Dental Surgery
Dental School
University of Maryland Baltimore
Baltimore, Maryland

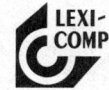

LEXI-COMP

NOTICE

This handbook is intended to serve the user as a handy reference and not as a complete drug information resource. It does not include information on every therapeutic agent available. The publication covers a combination of commonly used drugs in dentistry and medicine and is specifically designed to present important aspects of drug data in a more concise format than is typically found in medical literature, exhaustive drug compendia, or product material supplied by manufacturers.

Drug information is constantly evolving because of ongoing research and clinical experience and is often subject to interpretation. While great care has been taken to ensure the accuracy of the information presented, the reader is advised that the authors, editors, reviewers, contributors, and publishers cannot be responsible for the continued currency of the information or for any errors, omissions, or the application of this information, or for any consequences arising therefrom. Therefore, the author(s) and/or the publisher shall have no liability to any person or entity with regard to claims, loss, or damage caused, or alleged to be caused, directly or indirectly, by the use of information contained herein. Because of the dynamic nature of drug information, readers are advised that decisions regarding drug therapy must be based on the independent judgment of the clinician, changing information about a drug (eg, as reflected in the literature and manufacturer's most current product information), and changing medical practices. The editors are not responsible for any inaccuracy of quotation or for any false or misleading implication that may arise due to the text or formulas as used or due to the quotation of revisions no longer official.

The editors, authors, and contributors have written this book in their private capacities. No official support or endorsement by any federal or state agency or pharmaceutical company is intended or inferred.

The publishers have made every effort to trace the copyright holders for borrowed material. If they have inadvertently overlooked any, they will be pleased to make the necessary arrangements at the first opportunity.

If you have any suggestions or questions regarding any information presented in this handbook, please contact our drug information pharmacist at (330) 650-6506.

This manual was produced using Lexi-Comp's Information Management System™ (LIMS) — a complete publishing service of Lexi-Comp, Inc.

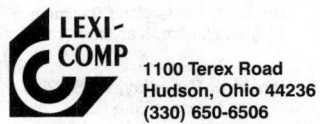

LEXI-COMP

1100 Terex Road
Hudson, Ohio 44236
(330) 650-6506

ISBN 978-1-59195-217-6

TABLE OF CONTENTS

TABLE OF CONTENTS *(Continued)*

ABOUT THE AUTHORS

Richard L. Wynn, BSPharm, PhD

Richard L. Wynn, PhD, is Professor of Pharmacology at the Baltimore College of Dental Surgery, Dental School, University of Maryland Baltimore. Dr Wynn has served as a dental educator, researcher, and teacher of dental pharmacology and dental hygiene pharmacology for his entire professional career. He holds a BS (pharmacy; registered pharmacist, Maryland), an MS (physiology) and a PhD (pharmacology) from the University of Maryland. Dr Wynn chaired the Department of Pharmacology at the University of Maryland Dental School from 1980 to 1995. Previously, he chaired the Department of Oral Biology at the University of Kentucky College of Dentistry.

Dr Wynn has to his credit over 300 publications including original research articles, textbooks, textbook chapters, monographs, and articles in continuing education journals. He has given over 500 continuing education seminars to dental professionals in the U.S., Canada, and Europe. Dr Wynn has been a consultant to the drug industry for 25 years and his research laboratories have contributed to the development of new analgesics and anesthetics. He is a consultant to the Academy of General Dentistry, the American Dental Association, and a former consultant to the Council on Dental Education, Commission on Accreditation. He is a featured columnist and his drug review articles, entitled *Pharmacology Today*, appear in each issue of *General Dentistry*, a journal published by the Academy. One of his primary interests continues to be keeping dental professionals informed on all aspects of drug use in dental practice.

Timothy F. Meiller, DDS, PhD

Dr Meiller is Professor of Diagnostic Sciences and Pathology at the Baltimore College of Dental Surgery and Professor of Oncology in the Program of Oncology at the Greenebaum Cancer Center, University of Maryland Baltimore. He has held his position in Diagnostic Sciences at the Dental School for 30 years and serves as an attending faculty at the Greenebaum Cancer Center.

Dr Meiller is a Diplomate of the American Board of Oral Medicine and a graduate of Johns Hopkins University and the University of Maryland Dental and Graduate Schools, holding a DDS and a PhD in Immunology/Virology. He has over 200 publications to his credit, maintains an active general dental practice, and is a consultant to the National Institutes of Health. He is currently engaged in ongoing investigations into cellular immune dysfunction in oral diseases associated with AIDS, in cancer patients, and in other medically-compromised patients.

Harold L. Crossley, DDS, PhD

Dr Crossley is Professor Emeritus at the University of Maryland Dental School. A native of Rhode Island, Dr Crossley received a Bachelor of Science degree in Pharmacy from the University of Rhode Island in 1964. He later was awarded the Master of Science (1970) and Doctorate degrees (1972) in Pharmacology. The University of Maryland Dental School in Baltimore awarded Dr Crossley the DDS degree in 1980. The liaison between the classroom and his dental practice, which he mentored on a part-time basis in the Dental School Intramural Faculty Practice, produced a practical approach to understanding the pharmacology of drugs used in the dental office.

Dr Crossley has coauthored a number of articles and four books dealing with a variety of topics within the field of pharmacology. Other areas of expertise include the pharmacology of street drugs and chemical dependency. He serves on the Maryland State Dental Association's Well-Being Committee, was a member of the University Interdisciplinary Committee for Drug Abuse Education, and served on the Governor's Commission on Prescription Drug Abuse. He is an active member of Phi Kappa Phi, Omicron Kappa Upsilon Honorary Dental Society, the American College of Dentists, and International College of Dentists. He has been a consultant for the United States Drug Enforcement Administration and other law enforcement agencies since 1974. Drawing on this unique background, Dr Crossley has become nationally and internationally recognized as an expert on street drugs and chemical dependency as well as the clinical pharmacology of dental drugs.

Laura Cummings, PharmD, BCPS
Clinical Pharmacy Specialist, Pediatrics
The Children's Hospital at MetroHealth
Cleveland, Ohio

Andrew J. Donnelly, PharmD, MBA
Director of Pharmacy
and
Clinical Professor of Pharmacy Practice
University of Illinois Medical Center at Chicago
Chicago, Illinois

Julie A. Dopheide, PharmD, BCPP
Associate Professor of Clinical Pharmacy,
Psychiatry and the Behavioral Sciences
University of Southern California
Schools of Pharmacy and Medicine
Los Angeles, California

Michael S. Edwards, PharmD, MBA
Assistant Director, Weinberg Pharmacy
Johns Hopkins Hospital
Baltimore, Maryland

Vicki L. Ellingrod, PharmD, BCPP
Associate Professor
University of Iowa
Iowa City, Iowa

Kelley K. Engle, BSPharm
Pharmacotherapy Specialist
Lexi-Comp, Inc
Hudson, Ohio

Margaret A. Fitzgerald, MS, APRN, BC, NP-C, FAANP
President
Fitzgerald Health Education Associates, Inc.
North Andover, Massachusetts
Family Nurse Practitioner
Greater Lawrence Family Health Center
Lawrence, Massachusetts

Lawrence A. Frazee, PharmD
Pharmacotherapy Specialist in Internal Medicine
Akron General Medical Center
Akron, Ohio

Matthew A. Fuller, PharmD, BCPS, BCPP, FASHP
Clinical Pharmacy Specialist, Psychiatry
Cleveland Department of Veterans Affairs Medical Center
Brecksville, Ohio
Associate Clinical Professor of Psychiatry
Clinical Instructor of Psychology
Case Western Reserve University
Cleveland, Ohio
Adjunct Associate Professor of Clinical Pharmacy
University of Toledo
Toledo, Ohio

Morton P. Goldman, PharmD
Director of Pharmacotherapy Services
The Cleveland Clinic Foundation
Cleveland, Ohio

Julie A. Golembiewski, PharmD
Clinical Associate Professor
Colleges of Pharmacy and Medicine
Clinical Pharmacist, Anesthesia/Pain
University of Illinois
Chicago, Illinois

Jeffrey P. Gonzales, PharmD, BCPS
Critical Care Clinical Pharmacy Specialist
University of Maryland Medical Center
Baltimore, Maryland

Roland Grad, MDCM, MSc, CCFP, FCFP
Department of Family Medicine
McGill University
Montreal, Quebec, Canada

EDITORIAL ADVISORY PANEL *(Continued)*

Charles Lacy, RPh, PharmD, FCSHP
Vice President, Information Technologies
Professor, Pharmacy Practice
Professor, Business Leadership
University of Southern Nevada
Las Vegas, Nevada

Brenda R. Lance, RN, MSN
Program Development Director
Northcoast HealthCare Management Company
Northcoast Infusion Therapies
Oakwood Village, Ohio

Leonard L. Lance, RPh, BSPharm
Clinical Pharmacist
Lexi-Comp Inc
Hudson, Ohio

Jerrold B. Leikin, MD, FACP, FACEP, FACMT, FAACT
Director, Medical Toxicology
Evanston Northwestern Healthcare-OMEGA
Glenbrook Hospital
Glenview, Illinois
Associate Director
Toxikon Consortium at Cook County Hospital
Chicago, Illinois
Professor of Medicine
Pharmacology and Health Systems Management
Rush Medical College
Chicago, Ilinois
Professor of Medicine
Feinberg School of Medicine
Northwestern University
Chicago, Ilinois

Jeffrey D. Lewis, PharmD
Pharmacotherapy Specialist
Lexi-Comp, Inc
Hudson, Ohio

Laurie S. Mauro, BS, PharmD
Professor of Clinical Pharmacy
College of Pharmacy
Adjunct Associate Professor of Medicine
College of Medicine
The University of Toledo
Toledo, Ohio

Vincent F. Mauro, BS, PharmD, FCCP
Professor of Clinical Pharmacy
College of Pharmacy
Adjunct Professor of Medicine
College of Medicine
The University of Toledo
Toledo, Ohio

Barrie McCombs, MD, FCFP
Medical Information Service Coordinator
The Alberta Rural Physician Action Plan
Calgary, Alberta, Canada

Timothy F. Meiller, DDS, PhD
Professor
Diagnostic Sciences and Pathology
Baltimore College of Dental Surgery
Professor of Oncology
Greenebaum Cancer Center
University of Maryland Baltimore
Baltimore, Maryland

Michael A. Militello, PharmD, BCPS
Clinical Cardiology Specialist
Department of Pharmacy
The Cleveland Clinic Foundation
Cleveland, Ohio

Julie Miller, PharmD
Pharmacy Clinical Specialist, Cardiology
Columbus Children's Hospital
Columbus, Ohio

7

EDITORIAL ADVISORY PANEL *(Continued)*

Mary Temple, PharmD
Pediatric Clinical Research Specialist
Hillcrest Hospital
Mayfield Heights, Ohio

Elizabeth A. Tomsik, PharmD, BCPS
Pharmacotherapy Specialist
Lexi-Comp, Inc
Hudson, Ohio

Jennifer Trofe, PharmD
Clinical Transplant Pharmacist
Hospital of The University of Pennsylvania
Philadelphia, Pennsylvania

Beatrice B. Turkoski, RN, PhD
Associate Professor, Graduate Faculty
Advanced Pharmacology
College of Nursing
Kent State University
Kent, Ohio

Amy VanOrman, PharmD
Pharmacotherapy Specialist
Lexi-Comp, Inc
Hudson, Ohio

David M. Weinstein, PhD, RPh
Pharmacotherapy Specialist
Lexi-Comp, Inc.
Hudson, Ohio

Anne Marie Whelan, PharmD
College of Pharmacy
Dalhousie University
Halifax, Nova Scotia

Richard L. Wynn, PhD
Professor of Pharmacology
Baltimore College of Dental Surgery
Dental School
University of Maryland Baltimore
Baltimore, Maryland

PREFACE TO THE THIRTEENTH EDITION

The *Drug Information Handbook for Dentistry* continues to receive indicators of success and the authors are extremely gratified in this regard. We wish to thank each practitioner and student who has made all of the previous editions so widely accepted in the field of dentistry. In this new 13th edition, we have continued, as always, to respond to all of the comments and creative suggestions that come from our readership each year.

The authors of the 13th edition of the *Drug Information Handbook for Dentistry* are extremely proud that the book remains as popular and as successful as its readers have affirmed. We are confident that the dental practitioners and dental hygienists who utilize the text have found it to be easy to navigate and their knowledge regarding pharmacotherapeutics and oral medicine questions has been enhanced by its use. The complete cross-referencing of generic and brand names along with the foreign brands, makes the text the complete drug reference guide for dental practice.

We know that our text remains an excellent companion to oral medicine and medical reference libraries that every clinician has available in their office. We hope that the active general dentist, the specialist, the dental hygienist, and the advanced student of dentistry remain better prepared for patient care while using this new 13th edition.

Recently the American Heart Association and the American Dental Association released in the journal *Circulation* the latest recommendations for preprocedural antibiotics to prevent infective endocarditis. The authors have completely revised the appropriate section and the example prescriptions related to these latest changes.

The monographs now include over 1,500 drugs and these have been updated in the 13th edition with the fields easier to read and identify for all of the drugs. The drugs most commonly used in dentistry have the added fields regarding specific use considerations in dentistry. Important medical drugs also include dosing and dose formulation information. In addition, the adverse reaction section and the important uses and effects on dental treatment for all drugs have been updated throughout the text. As in each previous edition, the Oral Medicine section has been updated offering a selection of drug possibilities for management of common conditions often seen in the oral cavity. Example prescriptions are now in a stand-alone section for quicker reference. Prescribing information options are outlined and are available for easy cross reference for the dental practitioner. A new subsection for nonsurgical management of periodontal conditions has been added with appropriate prescription examples.

The alphabetical index at the back of the text guides the reader through the text, as does the alphabetical listing of all drug names (both generic and brand names) throughout the monograph sections. The natural products section, drug synonyms, and U.S., Canadian, and Mexican brand names have all been updated.

Richard L. Wynn
Timothy F. Meiller
Harold L. Crossley

ACKNOWLEDGMENTS

This handbook exists in its present form as a result of the concerted efforts of many individuals, including Jack D. Bolinski, DDS, and Brad F. Bolinski, who recognized the need for a comprehensive dental and medical drug compendium; Robert D. Kerscher, publisher and chief executive officer of Lexi-Comp, Inc; Steven Kerscher, president and chief operating officer; Mark F. Bonfiglio, BS, PharmD, RPh, chief content officer; Stacy S. Robinson, editorial manager; Ginger S. Stein, project manager; David C. Marcus, chief information officer; Leslie Jo Hoppes, pharmacology database manager; Tracey J. Henterly, senior graphic designer; Alexandra Hart, composition specialist; and Brad F. Bolinski, director, dentistry.

Much of the material contained in this book was a result of contributions by pharmacists throughout the United States and Canada. Lexi-Comp has assisted many medical institutions in developing hospital-specific formulary manuals that contain clinical drug information, as well as dosing. Working with these clinical pharmacists, hospital pharmacy and therapeutics committees, and hospital drug information centers, Lexi-Comp has developed an evolutionary drug database that reflects the practice of pharmacy in these major institutions.

Special acknowledgment goes out to all Lexi-Comp staff members for their contributions to this handbook. In addition, the authors wish to thank their families, friends, and colleagues who supported them in their efforts to complete this handbook.

DESCRIPTION OF SECTIONS AND FIELDS

The *Drug Information Handbook for Dentistry, 13th Edition* is organized into six sections: Introductory text; alphabetical listing of drug monographs; natural products; oral medicine topics; appendix; and indexes which include pharmacologic categories and alphabetical listings containing generic product names and index terms, as well as U.S., Canadian, and Mexican brand names.

INTRODUCTORY TEXT

Helpful guides to understanding the organization and format of the information in this handbook.

DRUG MONOGRAPHS

This alphabetical listing of drugs contains comprehensive monographs for medications commonly prescribed in dentistry and concise monographs for other popular drugs which dental patients may be taking. Monographs may contain the following fields:

Generic Name	U.S. adopted name
Pronunciation	Phonetic pronunciation guide
Related Information	Cross-reference(s) to pertinent information in other sections of this handbook
Related Sample Prescriptions	Cross-reference(s) to sample prescriptions.
U.S. Brand Names	Trade name(s) (manufacturer-specific) found in the United States. The symbol [DSC] appears after trade names that have been recently discontinued.
Canadian Brand Names	Trade name(s) found in Canada
Mexican Brand Names	Trade name(s) found in Mexico
Generic Available	Indicated by a "yes" or "no" if information available
Index Terms	Includes names or accepted abbreviations of the generic drug; may include common brand names no longer available; this field is used to create cross-references to monographs
Pharmacologic Category	Indicates one or more systematic classifications of the drug
Dental Use	Information in the **Dental Use** field indicates when a drug has an established use specific to dentistry and/or oral medicine. In some cases, these uses are considered to be unlabeled, as they are not included in the FDA-approved product labeling. (see Description of Dental Use)
Use	Statements under the **Use** field reflect the approved labeling by the FDA based on accepted clinical evaluation on safety and efficacy of the drug as submitted in the New Drug Application (NDA). The "gold standard" of clinical testing of a new drug requires a randomly-selected cohort of subjects, using a double-blind and placebo controlled protocol and an acceptable method of assessment to test differences between test compound and placebo. It is assumed that by their approval of the labeling, the FDA considers the new drug "safe and effective" for treating a particular condition in a given patient population.
Unlabeled/Investigational Use	Statements under the **Unlabeled/Investigational** use field refer to other conditions, dosages, or routes of administration which are decided by the prescriber, where such uses have not been officially approved by the FDA. Such "off label" use usually occurs in response to published studies supporting a drug's effectiveness in a new use and/or alternative dosing strategy. It is important to note that individual reports do not necessarily indicate in and of themselves that the safety and effectiveness of the drug in question has been established for the new use. If an individual report is one of many studies, the clinician is encouraged to read and critically review all of the studies in order to arrive at a decision on the safety and efficacy for the "off label" use.
Local Anesthetic/Vasoconstrictor Precautions	Specific information to prevent potential drug interactions related to anesthesia
Effects on Dental Treatment	Includes significant side effects of drug therapy which may directly or indirectly affect dental treatment or diagnosis; may also contain suggested management approaches and patient handling or care.

Significant Adverse Effects	Side effects are grouped by percentage of incidence (if known) and/or body system; in the interest of saving space, <1% effects are grouped only by percentage **Note:** For nondental-specific drugs, this field includes only the most common adverse effects and does not include <1% effects.
Restrictions	The controlled substance classification from the Drug Enforcement Agency (DEA). U.S. schedules are I-V. Schedules vary by country and sometimes state (ie, Massachusetts uses I-VI)
Dental Usual Dosing	The amount of the drug to be typically given or taken during dental treatment for children and adults
Dosage	The amount of the drug to be typically given or taken during therapy for children and adults; also includes any dosing adjustment/comments for renal impairment or hepatic failure
Mechanism of Action	How the drug works in the body to elicit a response
Contraindications	Information pertaining to inappropriate use of the drug
Warnings/Precautions	Precautionary considerations, hazardous conditions related to use of the drug, and disease states or patient populations in which the drug should be cautiously used
Drug Interactions	If a drug has demonstrated involvement with cytochrome P450 enzymes, the initial line of this field will identify the drug as an inhibitor, inducer, or substrate of specific isoenzymes (ie, CYP1A2). Isoenzymes are identified as substrates (minor or major), inhibitors (weak or moderate or strong), and inducers (weak or strong). A summary of this information can also be found in a tabular format within the introductory section. The remainder of the field presents a description of the interaction between the drug listed in the monograph and other drugs or drug classes. May include possible mechanisms and effect of combined therapy. May also include a strategy to manage the patient on combined therapy (ie, quinidine). **Note:** For nondental-specific drugs, the Drug Interactions field is abbreviated and broken down into 3 subcategories: **Cytochrome P450 Effect, Increased Effect/Toxicity, and Decreased Effect**
Ethanol/Nutrition/Herb Interactions	Information regarding potential interactions with food, nutritionals, herbal products, vitamins, or ethanol
Dietary Considerations	Includes information on how the medication should be taken relative to meals or food
Pharmacodynamics/Kinetics	The magnitude of a drug's effect depends on the drug concentration at the site of action. The pharmacodynamics are expressed in terms of onset of action and duration of action. Pharmacokinetics are expressed in terms of absorption, distribution (including appearance in breast milk and crossing of the placenta), protein binding, metabolism, bioavailability, half-life, time to peak serum concentration, and elimination.
Pregnancy Risk Factor	Five categories established by the FDA to indicate the potential of a systemically absorbed drug for causing birth defects
Lactation	Information describing characteristics of using the drug listed in the monograph while breast-feeding (where recommendation of American Academy of Pediatrics differs, notation is made).
Breast-Feeding Considerations	Further information relating to taking the drug while nursing
Dosage Forms	Information with regard to form, strength, and availability of the drug. **Note:** Please consult individual product labeling for additional formulation information (eg, excipients, preservatives).
Dental Comment	Pharmacology-related comments and considerations relevant to the dental professional
Selected Readings	Sources and literature where the user may find additional information

13

DESCRIPTION OF SECTIONS AND FIELDS *(Continued)*

NATURAL PRODUCTS: HERBAL AND DIETARY SUPPLEMENTS

This section is divided into three parts. First, is a brief introduction to popular natural products, followed by an alphabetical listing of herbal and dietary supplements commonly purchased over-the-counter which patients may be taking. Monographs may contain the following:

NATURAL PRODUCT MONOGRAPHS

Name	Common name
Related Information	Cross-reference(s) to related monographs
Index Terms	Other names (scientific or slang) and accepted abbreviations
Pharmacologic Category	Indicates one or more systematic classifications of the drug
Use	Information pertaining to appropriate medical indications for the product; some include recommendations from Commission E.
Local Anesthetic/Vasoconstrictor Precautions	Specific information to prevent potential interactions related to anesthesia
Effects on Bleeding	How the product affects bleeding during dental procedures
Warnings/Precautions	Cautions and hazardous conditions related to use

ORAL MEDICINE TOPICS

This section is divided into three major parts and contains text on Oral Medicine topics. In each subsection, the systemic condition or the oral disease state is described briefly, followed by the pharmacologic considerations with which the dentist must be familiar.

Part I: **Dental Management and Therapeutic Considerations in Medically-Compromised Patients:** Focuses on common medical conditions and their associated drug therapies with which the dentist must be familiar. Patient profiles with commonly associated drug regimens are described.

Part II: **Dental Management and Therapeutic Considerations in Patients With Specific Oral Conditions:** Focuses on therapies the dentist may choose to prescribe for patients suffering from oral disease or who are in need of special care. Some overlap between these sections has resulted from systemic conditions that have oral manifestations and vice-versa. Cross-references to the descriptions and the monographs for individual drugs described elsewhere in this handbook allow for easy retrieval of information. Example prescriptions for drugs commonly used in the treatment of each condition are presented so that the clinician can evaluate alternate approaches to treatment. Seldom is there a single drug of choice.

Note: Prescriptions listed represent prototype drugs and popular prescriptions and are examples only. The pharmacologic category index is available for cross-referencing if alternatives or additional drugs are sought.

Part III: **Sample Prescriptions:** Examples provided for prototype drugs and popular prescriptions. Prescriptions included for the following uses: Bacterial endocarditis (prevention), prosthetic joint late infections (prevention), oral pain, bacterial infections and periodontal diseases, sinus infection treatment, antimicrobial rinses, fungal infections, viral infections, ulcerative and erosive disorders, sedation (prior to dental treatment)

APPENDIX

The appendix is broken down into various sections for easy use and offers a compilation of tables and guidelines which can often be helpful when considering patient care. It includes descriptions of most over-the-counter oral care products and dental drug interactions, in addition to, infectious disease information and the top 200 drugs prescribed in 2006.

INDEXES

This section includes a pharmacologic category index with an easy-to-use classification system in alphabetical order and an alphabetical index which provides a quick reference for generic names, index terms, U.S., Canadian, and Mexican brand names. From this index, the reader can cross-reference to the monographs.

DESCRIPTION OF DENTAL USE

UNLABELED USE AND ROUTES OF ADMINISTRATION IN DENTISTRY AND ORAL MEDICINE

The off-label use of a medication may involve differences in either the intended purpose or the route of administration of a particular medication. In dentistry, there are some situations which are common (clindamycin for endocarditis prophylaxis), and uncommon (application of Kenalog® cream to the oral mucosa) which may be termed "unlabeled use". Depending on the degree of familiarity, the prescription of a drug for an off-label purpose may create concern on the part of healthcare professionals who are less familiar with the dental use of these medications. For example, a pharmacist may note the statement "for external use only" on the label of a tube of topical cream and question whether the drug should be applied to the oral mucosa. Usually, reinforcement of the use of a drug as well as an analysis of the likely systemic exposure/toxicity, can address these concerns.

The dentist who prescribes a drug bears the responsibility for deciding on the purpose of the prescription and the detail of the dosing regimen. These professional decisions are based on information from a variety of sources, including (but not limited to) the official labeling, sound scientific evidence, expert medical judgment, or published literature. In selected situations, these sources may justify the use of a drug in an off-label manner. Accepted professional standards indicate off-label use of a drug must be initiated in good faith, serve the best interest of the patient, and must be undertaken without fraudulent intent. Healthcare providers should recognize that the approved labeling is not intended to limit the practitioners in the exercise of his or her best professional judgment in serving the interest of patients. In addition, the purpose of labeling is not intended to impose liability for off-label use. However, it should be noted that a practitioner may be accountable for the negligent use in a civil action regardless of whether the FDA has approved the use of the drug in question. Based on these assertions, at least one medical organization (the American Academy of Pediatrics) has published in an official policy statement that the practice of medicine may actually require a practitioner to use drugs in an off-label manner in order to provide the most appropriate treatment for a given patient. Off-label use in dentistry and oral medicine is a frequently encountered issue. A discussion of the off-label use of drugs in dentistry appears in the *ADA Guide to Dental Therapeutics*, 3rd Edition, edited by Sebastian G. Ciancio, DDS in cooperation with the ADA Council on Scientific Affairs.

CONTROLLED SUBSTANCES

Schedule I = C-I

The drugs and other substances in this schedule have no legal medical uses except research. They have a **high** potential for abuse. They include selected opiates such as heroin, opium derivatives, and hallucinogens.

Schedule II = C-II

The drugs and other substances in this schedule have legal medical uses and a **high** abuse potential which may lead to severe dependence. They include former "Class A" narcotics, amphetamines, barbiturates, and other drugs.

Schedule III = C-III

The drugs and other substances in this schedule have legal medical uses and a **lesser** degree of abuse potential which may lead to **moderate** dependence. They include former "Class B" narcotics and other drugs.

Schedule IV = C-IV

The drugs and other substances in this schedule have legal medial uses and **low** abuse potential which may lead to **moderate** dependence. They include barbiturates, benzodiazepines, propoxyphenes, and other drugs.

Schedule V = C-V

The drugs and other substances in this schedule have legal medical uses and **low** abuse potential which may lead to **moderate** dependence. They include narcotic cough preparations, diarrhea preparations, and other drugs.

Note: These are federal classifications. Your individual state may place a substance into a more restricted category. When this occurs, the more restricted category applies. Consult your state law.

FDA PREGNANCY CATEGORIES

Throughout this book there is a field labeled Pregnancy Risk Factor (PRF) and the letter A, B, C, D, or X immediately following which signifies a category. The FDA has established these five categories to indicate the potential of a systemically absorbed drug for causing birth defects. The key differentiation among the categories rests upon the reliability of documentation and the risk:benefit ratio. Pregnancy Category X is particularly notable in that if any data exists that may implicate a drug as a teratogen and the risk:benefit ratio is clearly negative, the drug is contraindicated during pregnancy.

These categories are summarized as follows:

A	Controlled studies in pregnant women fail to demonstrate a risk to the fetus in the first trimester with no evidence of risk in later trimesters. The possibility of fetal harm appears remote.
B	Either animal-reproduction studies have not demonstrated a fetal risk but there are no controlled studies in pregnant women, or animal-reproduction studies have shown an adverse effect (other than a decrease in fertility) that was not confirmed in controlled studies in women in the first trimester and there is no evidence of a risk in later trimesters.
C	Either studies in animals have revealed adverse effects on the fetus (teratogenic or embryocidal effects or other) and there are no controlled studies in women, or studies in women and animals are not available. Drugs should be given only if the potential benefits justify the potential risk to the fetus.
D	There is positive evidence of human fetal risk, but the benefits from use in pregnant women may be acceptable despite the risk (eg, if the drug is needed in a life-threatening situation or for a serious disease for which safer drugs cannot be used or are ineffective).
X	Studies in animals or human beings have demonstrated fetal abnormalities or there is evidence of fetal risk based on human experience, or both, and the risk of the use of the drug in pregnant women clearly outweighs any possible benefit. The drug is contraindicated in women who are or may become pregnant.

FDA NAME DIFFERENTIATION PROJECT: THE USE OF TALL-MAN LETTERS

Confusion between similar drug names is an important cause of medication errors. For years, The Institute For Safe Medication Practices (ISMP), has urged generic manufacturers to use a combination of large and small letters as well as bolding (ie, chlorpro**MA-ZINE** and chlorpro**PAMIDE**) to help distinguish drugs with look-alike names, especially when they share similar strengths. Recently the FDA's Division of Generic Drugs began to issue recommendation letters to manufacturers suggesting this novel way to label their products to help reduce this drug name confusion. Although this project has had marginal success, the method has successfully eliminated problems with products such as diphenhydr**AMINE** and dimenhy**DRINATE**. Hospitals should also follow suit by making similar changes in their own labels, preprinted order forms, computer screens and printouts, and drug storage location labels.

The following is a list of product names and recommended FDA revisions you will find in this book:

Drug Product	Recommended Revision
acetazolamide	aceta**ZOLAMIDE**
acetohexamide	aceto**HEXAMIDE**
bupropion	bu**PROP**ion
buspirone	bus**PIR**one
chlorpromazine	chlorpro**MAZINE**
chlorpropamide	chlorpro**PAMIDE**
clomiphene	clomi**PHENE**
clomipramine	clomi**PRAMINE**
cycloserine	cyclo**SERINE**
cyclosporine	cyclo**SPORINE**
daunorubicin	**DAUNO**rubicin
dimenhydrinate	dimenhy**DRINATE**
diphenhydramine	diphenhydr**AMINE**
dobutamine	**DOBUT**amine
dopamine	**DOP**amine
doxorubicin	**DOXO**rubicin
glipizide	glipi**ZIDE**
glyburide	gly**BURIDE**
hydralazine	hydr**ALAZINE**
hydroxyzine	hydr**OXY**zine
medroxyprogesterone	medroxy**PROGESTER**one
methylprednisolone	methyl**PREDNIS**olone
methyltestosterone	methyl**TESTOSTER**one
nicardipine	ni**CAR**dipine
nifedipine	**NIFE**dipine
prednisolone	predniso**LONE**
prednisone	predni**SONE**
sulfadiazine	sulfa**DIAZINE**
sulfisoxazole	sulfi**SOXAZOLE**
tolazamide	**TOLAZ**amide
tolbutamide	**TOLBUT**amide
vinblastine	vin**BLAS**tine
vincristine	vin**CRIS**tine

Institute for Safe Medication Practices. "New Tall-Man Lettering Will Reduce Mix-Ups Due to Generic Drug Name Confusion," *ISMP Medication Safety Alert*, September 19, 2001. Available at: http://www.ismp.org.

Institute for Safe Medication Practices. "Prescription Mapping, Can Improve Efficiency While Minimizing Errors With Look-Alike Products," *ISMP Medication Safety Alert*, October 6, 1999. Available at: http://www.ismp.org.

U.S. Pharmacopeia, "USP Quality Review: Use Caution-Avoid Confusion," March 2001, No. 76. Available at: http://www.usp.org.

PRESCRIPTION WRITING

Doctor's Name
Address
Phone Number

Patient's Name/Date

Patient's Address/Age

Rx

Drug Name/Dosage Size

Disp: Number of tablets, capsules, ounces to be dispensed (roman numerals added as precaution for abused drugs)

Sig: Direction on how drug is to be taken

Doctor's signature

State license number

DEA number (if required)

PRESCRIPTION REQUIREMENTS

1. Date
2. Full name and address of patient
3. Name and address of prescriber
4. Signature of prescriber

If Class II drug, Drug Enforcement Agency (DEA) number necessary.

If Class II and Class III narcotic, a triplicate prescription form (in the state of California) is necessary and it must be handwritten by the prescriber.

Please turn to appropriate oral medicine chapters for examples of prescriptions.

SAFE WRITING PRACTICES

Health professionals and their support personnel frequently produce handwritten copies of information they see in print; therefore, such information is subjected to even greater possibilities for error or misinterpretation on the part of others. Thus, particular care must be given to how drug names and strengths are expressed when creating written health-care documents.

The following are a few examples of safe writing rules suggested by the Institute for Safe Medication Practices, Inc.*

1. There should be a space between a number and its units as it is easier to read. There should be no periods after the abbreviations mg or mL.

Correct	Incorrect
10 mg	10mg
100 mg	100mg

2. Never place a decimal and a zero after a whole number (2 mg is correct and 2.0 mg is **incorrect**). If the decimal point is not seen because it falls on a line or because individuals are working from copies where the decimal point is not seen, this causes a tenfold overdose.

3. Just the opposite is true for numbers less than one. Always place a zero before a naked decimal (0.5 mL is correct, .5 mL is **incorrect**).

4. Never abbreviate the word unit. The handwritten U or u, looks like a 0 (zero), and may cause a tenfold overdose error to be made.

5. IU is not a safe abbreviation for international units. The handwritten IU looks like IV. Write out international units or use int. units.

6. Q.D. is not a safe abbreviation for once daily, as when the Q is followed by a sloppy dot, it looks like QID which means four times daily.

7. O.D. is not a safe abbreviation for once daily, as it is properly interpreted as meaning "right eye" and has caused liquid medications such as saturated solution of potassium iodide and Lugol's solution to be administered incorrectly. There is no safe abbreviation for once daily. It must be written out in full.

8. Do not use chemical names such as 6-mercaptopurine or 6-thioguanine, as sixfold overdoses have been given when these were not recognized as chemical names. The proper names of these drugs are mercaptopurine or thioguanine.

9. Do not abbreviate drug names (5FC, 6MP, 5-ASA, MTX, HCTZ, CPZ, PBZ, etc) as they are misinterpreted and cause error.

10. Do not use the apothecary system or symbols.

11. Do not abbreviate microgram as µg; instead use mcg as there is less likelihood of misinterpretation.

12. When writing an outpatient prescription, write a complete prescription. A complete prescription can prevent the prescriber, the pharmacist, and/or the patient from making a mistake and can eliminate the need for further clarification. The legible prescriptions should contain:

a. patient's full name

b. for pediatric or geriatric patients: their age (or weight where applicable)

c. drug name, dosage form and strength; if a drug is new or rarely prescribed, print this information

d. number or amount to be dispensed

e. complete instructions for the patient, including the purpose of the medication

f. when there are recognized contraindications for a prescribed drug, indicate to the pharmacist that you are aware of this fact (ie, when prescribing a potassium salt for a patient receiving an ACE inhibitor, write "K serum leveling being monitored")

*From "Safe Writing" by Davis NM, PharmD and Cohen MR, MS, Lecturers and Consultants for Safe Medication Practices, 1143 Wright Drive, Huntington Valley, PA 19006. Phone: (215) 947-7566.

ALPHABETICAL LISTING OF DRUGS

ABACAVIR

1370-999-397 *see* Anagrelide *on page 127*

A₁-PI *see* A₁-Proteinase Inhibitor *on page 74*

A200® Lice [OTC] *see* Permethrin *on page 1284*

A-200® Maximum Strength [OTC] *see* Pyrethrins and Piperonyl Butoxide *on page 1388*

A and D® Original [OTC] *see* Vitamin A and Vitamin D *on page 1663*

Abacavir (a BAK a veer)

Related Information
   HIV Infection and AIDS *on page 1753*

U.S. Brand Names Ziagen®

Canadian Brand Names Ziagen®

Mexican Brand Names Ziagenavir

Generic Available No

Index Terms Abacavir Sulfate; ABC

Pharmacologic Category Antiretroviral Agent, Reverse Transcriptase Inhibitor (Nucleoside)

Use Treatment of HIV infections in combination with other antiretroviral agents

Local Anesthetic/Vasoconstrictor Precautions No information available to require special precautions

Effects on Dental Treatment No significant effects or complications reported

Common Adverse Effects Hypersensitivity reactions (which may be fatal) occur in ~5% of patients. Symptoms may include anaphylaxis, fever, rash (including erythema multiforme), fatigue, diarrhea, abdominal pain; respiratory symptoms (eg, pharyngitis, dyspnea, cough, adult respiratory distress syndrome, or respiratory failure); headache, malaise, lethargy, myalgia, myolysis, arthralgia, edema, paresthesia, nausea and vomiting, mouth ulcerations, conjunctivitis, lymphadenopathy, hepatic failure, and renal failure.

Note: Rates of adverse reactions were defined during combination therapy with other antiretrovirals (lamivudine and efavirenz **or** lamivudine and zidovudine). Only reactions which occurred at a higher frequency in adults (except where noted) than in the comparator group are noted. Adverse reaction rates attributable to abacavir alone are not available.

>10%:
   Central nervous system: Headache (7% to 13%)
   Gastrointestinal: Nausea (7% to 19%, children 9%)

1% to 10%:
   Central nervous system: Depression (6%), fever/chills (6%, children 9%), anxiety (5%)
   Dermatologic: Rash (5% to 6%, children 7%)
   Endocrine & metabolic: Triglycerides increased (2% to 6%)
   Gastrointestinal: Diarrhea (7%), vomiting (children 9%), amylase increased (2%)
   Hematologic: Thrombocytopenia (1%)
   Hepatic: AST increased (6%)
   Neuromuscular and skeletal: Musculoskeletal pain (5% to 6%)
   Miscellaneous: Hypersensitivity reactions (2% to 9%; may include reactions to other components of antiretroviral regimen), infection (EENT 5%)

Restrictions An FDA-approved medication guide and warning card (summarizing symptoms of hypersensitivity) must be distributed when dispensing an outpatient prescription (new or refill) where this medication is to be used without direct supervision of a healthcare provider. Medication guides are available at http://www.fda.gov/cder/Offices/ODS/medication_guides.htm.

Mechanism of Action Nucleoside reverse transcriptase inhibitor. Abacavir is a guanosine analogue which is phosphorylated to carbovir triphosphate which interferes with HIV viral RNA-dependent DNA polymerase resulting in inhibition of viral replication.

Drug Interactions
   Increased Effect/Toxicity: Ganciclovir/valganciclovir may increase the adverse/toxic effects of nucleoside reverse transcriptase inhibitors. Concomitant use of ribavirin with or without interferon alfa and nucleoside analogues may increase the risk of developing hepatic decompensation or other signs of mitochondrial toxicity, including pancreatitis or lactic acidosis.

Pharmacodynamics/Kinetics
   Absorption: Rapid and extensive absorption
   Distribution: V_d: 0.86 L/kg
   Protein binding: 50%
   Metabolism: Hepatic via alcohol dehydrogenase and glucuronyl transferase to inactive carboxylate and glucuronide metabolites
   Bioavailability: 83%

Half-life elimination: 1.5 hours
Time to peak: 0.7-1.7 hours
Excretion: Primarily urine (as metabolites, 1.2% as unchanged drug); feces (16% total dose)
Pregnancy Risk Factor C

Abacavir and Lamivudine (a BAK a veer & la MI vyoo deen)

Related Information
Abacavir on page 22
Lamivudine on page 944
U.S. Brand Names Epzicom™
Canadian Brand Names Kivexa™
Generic Available No
Index Terms Abacavir Sulfate and Lamivudine; Lamivudine and Abacavir
Pharmacologic Category Antiretroviral Agent, Reverse Transcriptase Inhibitor (Nucleoside)
Use Treatment of HIV infections in combination with other antiretroviral agents
Local Anesthetic/Vasoconstrictor Precautions No information available to require special precautions
Effects on Dental Treatment No significant effects or complications reported
Common Adverse Effects See individual agents.
Restrictions An FDA-approved medication guide and warning card (summarizing symptoms of hypersensitivity) must be distributed when dispensing an outpatient prescription (new or refill) where this medication is to be used without direct supervision of a healthcare provider. Medication guides are available at http://www.fda.gov/cder/Offices/ODS/medication_guides.htm.
Mechanism of Action Nucleoside reverse transcriptase inhibitor combination.

Abacavir is a guanosine analogue which is phosphorylated to carbovir triphosphate which interferes with HIV viral RNA-dependent DNA polymerase resulting in inhibition of viral replication.

Lamivudine is a cytosine analog. After lamivudine is triphosphorylated, the principle mode of action is inhibition of HIV reverse transcription via viral DNA chain termination; inhibits RNA-dependent DNA polymerase activities of reverse transcriptase.

Drug Interactions
Increased Effect/Toxicity: See individual agents.
Decreased Effect: See individual agents.
Pharmacodynamics/Kinetics See individual agents.
Pregnancy Risk Factor C

Abacavir, Lamivudine, and Zidovudine
(a BAK a veer, la MI vyoo deen, & zye DOE vyoo deen)

Related Information
Abacavir on page 22
Lamivudine on page 944
Zidovudine on page 1680
U.S. Brand Names Trizivir®
Mexican Brand Names Trizivir
Generic Available No
Index Terms Azidothymidine, Abacavir, and Lamivudine; AZT, Abacavir, and Lamivudine; Compound S, Abacavir, and Lamivudine; Lamivudine, Abacavir, and Zidovudine; 3TC, Abacavir, and Zidovudine; ZDV, Abacavir, and Lamivudine; Zidovudine, Abacavir, and Lamivudine
Pharmacologic Category Antiretroviral Agent, Reverse Transcriptase Inhibitor (Nucleoside)
Use Treatment of HIV infection (either alone or in combination with other antiretroviral agents) in patients whose regimen would otherwise contain the components of Trizivir®
Local Anesthetic/Vasoconstrictor Precautions No information available to require special precautions
Effects on Dental Treatment No significant effects or complications reported
Common Adverse Effects Fatal hypersensitivity reactions have occurred in patients taking abacavir (in Trizivir®). If Trizivir® is to be restarted following an interruption in therapy, first evaluate the patient for previously unsuspected symptoms of hypersensitivity. Do not restart if hypersensitivity is suspected or if hypersensitivity cannot be ruled out.
(Continued)

Abacavir, Lamivudine, and Zidovudine *(Continued)*

The following information is based on CNA3005 study data concerning effects noted in patients receiving abacavir, lamivudine, and zidovudine. See individual agents for additional information.

>10%:
Central nervous system: Headache (13%), malaise (12%), fatigue (12%)
Gastrointestinal: Nausea (19%)

1% to 10%:
Central nervous system: Fever/chills (6%), depression (6%), anxiety (5%)
Dermatologic: Rash (5%)
Endocrine & metabolic: Triglycerides increased (2% grade 3-4)
Gastrointestinal: Nausea and vomiting (10%), diarrhea (7%), amylase increased (2%)
Hematologic: Neutropenia (5%)
Hepatic: ALT increased (6%)
Neuromuscular & skeletal: CPK increased (7%)
Otic: Ear infection (5%)
Respiratory: Nose/throat infection (5%)
Miscellaneous: Hypersensitivity (2% to 9% based on abacavir component), viral infection (5%)
Other (frequency unknown): Pancreatitis, GGT increased, fat redistribution, immune reconstitution syndrome

Restrictions An FDA-approved medication guide and warning card (summarizing symptoms of hypersensitivity) must be distributed when dispensing an outpatient prescription (new or refill) where this medication is to be used without direct supervision of a healthcare provider. Medication guides are available at http://www.fda.gov/cder/Offices/ODS/medication_guides.htm.

Mechanism of Action The combination of abacavir, lamivudine, and zidovudine is believed to act synergistically to inhibit reverse transcriptase via DNA chain termination after incorporation of the nucleoside analogue as well as to delay the emergence of mutations conferring resistance.

Drug Interactions
Increased Effect/Toxicity: See individual agents.
Decreased Effect: See individual agents.

Pharmacodynamics/Kinetics Bioavailability studies of Trizivir® show no difference in AUC or C_{max} when compared to abacavir, lamivudine, and zidovudine given together as individual agents. See individual agents.

Pregnancy Risk Factor C

Abacavir Sulfate *see* Abacavir *on page 22*
Abacavir Sulfate and Lamivudine *see* Abacavir and Lamivudine *on page 23*

Abarelix *(a ba REL iks)*

U.S. Brand Names Plenaxis™ [DSC]
Generic Available No
Index Terms PPI-149; R-3827
Pharmacologic Category Gonadotropin Releasing Hormone Antagonist
Use Palliative treatment of advanced prostate cancer; treatment is limited to men who are not candidates for LHRH therapy, refuse surgical castration, and have one or more of the following complications due to metastases or local encroachment: 1) risk of neurological compromise, 2) ureteral or bladder outlet obstruction, or 3) severe bone pain (persisting despite narcotic analgesia)

Local Anesthetic/Vasoconstrictor Precautions Abarelix is one of the drugs confirmed to prolong the QT interval and is accepted as having a risk of causing torsade de pointes. The risk of drug-induced torsade de pointes is extremely low when a single QT interval prolonging drug is prescribed. In terms of epinephrine, it is not known what effect vasoconstrictors in the local anesthetic regimen will have in patients with a known history of congenital prolonged QT interval or in patients taking any medication that prolongs the QT interval. Until more information is obtained, it is suggested that the clinician consult with the physician prior to the use of a vasoconstrictor in suspected patients, and that the vasoconstrictor (epinephrine, levonordefrin [Neo-Cobefrin®]) be used with caution.

Effects on Dental Treatment No significant effects or complications reported
Common Adverse Effects
>10%:
Cardiovascular: Hot flushes (79%), peripheral edema (15%)
Central nervous system: Sleep disturbance (44%), pain (31%), dizziness (12%), headache (12%)
Endocrine & metabolic: Breast enlargement (30%), nipple discharge/tenderness (20%)

Gastrointestinal: Constipation (15%), diarrhea (11%)
Neuromuscular & skeletal: Back pain (17%)
Respiratory: Upper respiratory infection (12%)
1% to 10%:
Central nervous system: Fatigue (10%)
Endocrine & metabolic: Serum triglycerides increased (10%)
Gastrointestinal: Nausea (10%)
Genitourinary: Dysuria (10%), micturition frequency (10%), urinary retention (10%), urinary tract infection (10%)
Hepatic: Transaminases increased (2% to 8%)
Miscellaneous: Allergic reactions (urticaria, pruritus, syncope, hypotension); risk increases with prolonged treatment

Restrictions Abarelix is not distributed through retail pharmacies. Prior to its discontinuation, prescribing and distribution of abarelix was limited to physicians and hospital pharmacies participating in the Plenaxis™ PLUS program. Additional information may be obtained by calling 1-877-772-3247 or 1-866-753-2947.

Mechanism of Action Competes with naturally-occurring GnRH for binding on receptors of the pituitary. Suppresses LH and FSH, resulting in decreased testosterone.

Drug Interactions
Increased Effect/Toxicity: When used with other QT_c-prolonging agents, additive QT_c prolongation may occur. Life-threatening ventricular arrhythmias may result; example drugs include class Ia and class III antiarrhythmics, cisapride, selected quinolones, erythromycin, pimozide, mesoridazine, and thioridazine.

Pharmacodynamics/Kinetics
Distribution: V_d: 4040 L (± 1607)
Metabolism: Hepatic, via peptide hydrolysis
Half-life elimination: 13 days
Time to peak, serum: 3 days (following I.M. administration)
Excretion: Urine (13% as unchanged drug)
Pregnancy Risk Factor X

Abatacept (ab a TA sept)

U.S. Brand Names Orencia®
Generic Available No
Index Terms CTLA-4Ig
Pharmacologic Category Antirheumatic, Disease Modifying
Use Treatment of rheumatoid arthritis not responsive to other disease-modifying antirheumatic drugs (DMARD); may be used as monotherapy or in combination with other DMARDs (**not** in combination with anakinra or TNF-blocking agents)
Local Anesthetic/Vasoconstrictor Precautions No information available to require special precautions
Effects on Dental Treatment No significant effects or complications reported
Common Adverse Effects Note: Percentages not always reported; COPD patients experienced a higher frequency of COPD-related adverse reactions (COPD exacerbation, cough, dyspnea, pneumonia, rhonchi)

>10%:
Central nervous system: Headache (18%)
Gastrointestinal: Nausea
Respiratory: Nasopharyngitis (12%), upper respiratory tract infection
Miscellaneous: Infection (54%)
1% to 10%:
Cardiovascular: Hypertension (7%)
Central nervous system: Dizziness (9%)
Dermatologic: Rash (4%)
Gastrointestinal: Dyspepsia (6%)
Genitourinary: Urinary tract infection (6%)
Neuromuscular & skeletal: Back pain (7%), limb pain (3%)
Respiratory: Cough (8%), bronchitis, pneumonia, rhinitis, sinusitis
Miscellaneous: Infusion-related reactions (9%), herpes simplex, influenza

Mechanism of Action Selective costimulation modulator; inhibits T-cell (T-lymphocyte) activation by binding to CD80 and CD86 on antigen presenting cells (APC), thus blocking the required CD28 interaction between APCs and T cells. Activated T lymphocytes are found in the synovium of rheumatoid arthritis patients.

Drug Interactions
Increased Effect/Toxicity: Abatacept may increase the risk of infections associated with vaccines (live organism). TNF-blocking agents used in combination with abatacept is contraindicated (may increase risk of infections).
(Continued)

Abatacept *(Continued)*

Decreased Effect: Abatacept may decrease the efficacy of immune response to vaccines (dead and live organism).

Pharmacodynamics/Kinetics
Distribution: V_{ss}: 0.02-0.13 L/kg
Half-life elimination: 8-25 days

Pregnancy Risk Factor C

Abbott-43818 *see* Leuprolide *on page 958*

ABC *see* Abacavir *on page 22*

ABCD *see* Amphotericin B Cholesteryl Sulfate Complex *on page 114*

Abciximab *(ab SIK si mab)*

Related Information
Cardiovascular Diseases *on page 1726*

U.S. Brand Names ReoPro®

Canadian Brand Names Reopro®

Mexican Brand Names ReoPro

Generic Available No

Index Terms C7E3; 7E3

Pharmacologic Category Antiplatelet Agent, Glycoprotein IIb/IIIa Inhibitor

Use Prevention of acute cardiac ischemic complications in patients at high risk for abrupt closure of the treated coronary vessel and patients at risk of restenosis; an adjunct with heparin to prevent cardiac ischemic complications in patients with unstable angina not responding to conventional therapy when a percutaneous coronary intervention (PCI) is scheduled within 24 hours

Unlabeled/Investigational Use Acute MI - combination regimen of abciximab (full dose), tenecteplase (half dose), and heparin (unlabeled dose)

Local Anesthetic/Vasoconstrictor Precautions No information available to require special precautions

Effects on Dental Treatment Key adverse event(s) related to dental treatment: As with all anticoagulants, bleeding is a potential adverse effect of abciximab during dental surgery; risk is dependent on multiple variables, including the intensity of anticoagulation and patient susceptibility. Medical consult is suggested. It is unlikely that ambulatory patients presenting for dental treatment will be taking intravenous anticoagulant therapy.

Common Adverse Effects As with all drugs which may affect hemostasis, bleeding is associated with abciximab. Hemorrhage may occur at virtually any site. Risk is dependent on multiple variables, including the concurrent use of multiple agents which alter hemostasis and patient susceptibility.

>10%:
Cardiovascular: Hypotension (14%), chest pain (11%)
Gastrointestinal: Nausea (14%)
Hematologic: Minor bleeding (4% to 17%)
Neuromuscular & skeletal: Back pain (18%)

1% to 10%:
Cardiovascular: Bradycardia (5%), peripheral edema (2%)
Central nervous system: Headache (7%)
Gastrointestinal: Vomiting (7%), abdominal pain (3%)
Hematologic: Major bleeding (1% to 14%), thrombocytopenia: <100,000 cells/mm³ (3% to 6%); <50,000 cells/mm³ (0.4% to 2%)
Local: Injection site pain (4%)

Mechanism of Action Fab antibody fragment of the chimeric human-murine monoclonal antibody 7E3; this agent binds to platelet IIb/IIIa receptors, resulting in steric hindrance, thus inhibiting platelet aggregation

Drug Interactions
Increased Effect/Toxicity: The risk of bleeding is increased when abciximab is given with heparin, other anticoagulants, thrombolytics, or antiplatelet drugs. However, aspirin and heparin were used concurrently in the majority of patients in the major clinical studies of abciximab. Allergic reactions may be increased in patients who have received diagnostic or therapeutic monoclonal antibodies due to the presence of HACA antibodies. Concomitant use of other glycoprotein IIb/IIIa antagonists is contraindicated.

Pharmacodynamics/Kinetics Half-life elimination: ~30 minutes

Pregnancy Risk Factor C

Abelcet® *see* Amphotericin B (Lipid Complex) *on page 117*

ABI-007 *see* Paclitaxel (Protein Bound) *on page 1241*

Abilify® *see* Aripiprazole *on page 141*

Abilify® Discmelt™ *see* Aripiprazole *on page 141*

ABLC *see* Amphotericin B (Lipid Complex) *on page 117*

A/B Otic *see* Antipyrine and Benzocaine *on page 133*

Abraxane® *see* Paclitaxel (Protein Bound) *on page 1241*

Abreva® [OTC] *see* Docosanol *on page 522*

Absorbable Cotton *see* Cellulose (Oxidized/Regenerated) *on page 316*

Absorbable Gelatin Sponge *see* Gelatin (Absorbable) *on page 770*

ABX-EGF *see* Panitumumab *on page 1248*

9-AC *see* Aminocamptothecin *on page 87*

AC 2993 *see* Exenatide *on page 663*

Acamprosate (a kam PROE sate)

U.S. Brand Names Campral®

Canadian Brand Names Campral®

Generic Available No

Index Terms Acamprosate Calcium; Calcium Acetylhomotaurinate

Pharmacologic Category GABA Agonist/Glutamate Antagonist

Use Maintenance of alcohol abstinence

Local Anesthetic/Vasoconstrictor Precautions No information available to require special precautions

Effects on Dental Treatment Key adverse event(s) related to dental treatment: Xerostomia and changes in salivation (normal salivary flow resumes upon discontinuation) and taste perversion.

Common Adverse Effects

Note: Many adverse effects associated with treatment may be related to alcohol abstinence; reported frequency range may overlap with placebo.

>10%: Gastrointestinal: Diarrhea (10% to 17%)

1% to 10%:

Cardiovascular: Syncope, palpitation, edema (peripheral)

Central nervous system: Insomnia (6% to 9%), anxiety (5% to 8%), depression (4% to 8%), dizziness (3% to 4%), pain (2% to 4%), paresthesia (2% to 3%), headache, somnolence, amnesia, tremor, chills

Dermatologic: Pruritus (3% to 4%), rash

Endocrine and metabolic: Weight gain, libido decreased

Gastrointestinal: Anorexia (2% to 5%), flatulence (1% to 3%), nausea (3% to 4%), abdominal pain, dry mouth (1% to 3%), vomiting, dyspepsia, constipation, appetite increased, taste perversion

Genitourinary: Impotence

Neuromuscular & skeletal: Weakness (5% to 7%), back pain, myalgia, arthralgia

Ocular: Abnormal vision

Respiratory: Rhinitis, dyspnea, pharyngitis, bronchitis

Miscellaneous: Diaphoresis (2% to 3%), suicide attempt

Mechanism of Action Mechanism not fully defined. Structurally similar to gamma-amino butyric acid (GABA), acamprosate appears to increase the activity of the GABA-ergic system, and decreases activity of glutamate within the CNS, including a decrease in activity at N-methyl D-aspartate (NMDA) receptors; may also affect CNS calcium channels. Restores balance to GABA and glutamate activities which appear to be disrupted in alcohol dependence. During therapeutic use, reduces alcohol intake, but does not cause a disulfiram-like reaction following alcohol ingestion.

Drug Interactions

Decreased Effect: No clinically-significant drug-to-drug interactions have been identified.

Pharmacodynamics/Kinetics

Distribution: V_d: 1 L/kg

Protein binding: Negligible

Metabolism: Not metabolized

Bioavailability: 11%

Half-life elimination: 20-33 hours

Excretion: Urine (as unchanged drug)

Pregnancy Risk Factor C

Acamprosate Calcium *see* Acamprosate *on page 27*

Acarbose (AY car bose)

Related Information

Endocrine Disorders and Pregnancy *on page 1750*

(Continued)

Acarbose *(Continued)*

U.S. Brand Names Precose®
Canadian Brand Names Prandase®
Mexican Brand Names Glucobay
Generic Available No
Pharmacologic Category Antidiabetic Agent, Alpha-Glucosidase Inhibitor
Use
  Monotherapy, as indicated as an adjunct to diet to lower blood glucose in patients with type 2 diabetes mellitus (noninsulin dependent, NIDDM) whose hyperglycemia cannot be managed on diet alone
  Combination with a sulfonylurea, metformin, or insulin in patients with type 2 diabetes mellitus (noninsulin dependent, NIDDM) when diet plus acarbose do not result in adequate glycemic control. The effect of acarbose to enhance glycemic control is additive to that of other hypoglycemic agents when used in combination.
Local Anesthetic/Vasoconstrictor Precautions No information available to require special precautions
Effects on Dental Treatment No significant effects or complications reported
Common Adverse Effects >10%:
  Gastrointestinal: Abdominal pain (21%) and diarrhea (33%) tend to return to pretreatment levels over time, and the frequency and intensity of flatulence (77%) tend to abate with time
  Hepatic: Transaminases increased
Mechanism of Action Competitive inhibitor of pancreatic α-amylase and intestinal brush border α-glucosidases, resulting in delayed hydrolysis of ingested complex carbohydrates and disaccharides and absorption of glucose; dose-dependent reduction in postprandial serum insulin and glucose peaks; inhibits the metabolism of sucrose to glucose and fructose
Drug Interactions
  Increased Effect/Toxicity: Acarbose may increase the risk of hypoglycemia when used with oral hypoglycemics.
  Decreased Effect: The effect of acarbose is antagonized/decreased by thiazide and related diuretics, corticosteroids, phenothiazines, thyroid products, estrogens, oral contraceptives, phenytoin, nicotinic acid, sympathomimetics, calcium channel-blocking drugs, isoniazid, intestinal adsorbents (eg, charcoal), and digestive enzyme preparations (eg, amylase, pancreatin). Acarbose decreases the absorption/serum concentration of digoxin.
Pharmacodynamics/Kinetics
  Absorption: <2% as active drug
  Metabolism: Exclusively via GI tract, principally by intestinal bacteria and digestive enzymes; 13 metabolites identified
  Bioavailability: Low systemic bioavailability of parent compound; acts locally in GI tract
  Excretion: Urine (~34%)
Pregnancy Risk Factor B

Acebutolol *(a se BYOO toe lole)*

Related Information
  Cardiovascular Diseases *on page 1726*
U.S. Brand Names Sectral®
Canadian Brand Names Apo-Acebutolol®; Gen-Acebutolol; Monitan®; Novo-Acebutolol; Nu-Acebutolol; Rhotral; Rhoxal-acebutolol; Sandoz-Acebutolol; Sectral®
Generic Available Yes
Index Terms Acebutolol Hydrochloride
Pharmacologic Category Antiarrhythmic Agent, Class II; Beta Blocker With Intrinsic Sympathomimetic Activity
Use Treatment of hypertension, ventricular arrhythmias, angina
Local Anesthetic/Vasoconstrictor Precautions No information available to require special precautions

Effects on Dental Treatment Acebutolol is a cardioselective beta-blocker. Local anesthetic with vasoconstrictor can be safely used in patients medicated with acebutolol. Nonselective beta-blockers (ie, propranolol, nadolol) enhance the pressor response to epinephrine, resulting in hypertension and bradycardia; this has not been reported for acebutolol. Many nonsteroidal anti-inflammatory drugs, such as ibuprofen and indomethacin, can reduce the hypotensive effect of beta-blockers after 3 or more weeks of therapy with the NSAID. Short-term NSAID use (ie, 3 days) requires no special precautions in patients taking beta-blockers.

Common Adverse Effects

>10%: Central nervous system: Fatigue (11%)

1% to 10%:

Cardiovascular: Chest pain (2%), edema (2%), bradycardia, hypotension, CHF

Central nervous system: Headache (6%), dizziness (6%), insomnia (3%), depression (2%), abnormal dreams (2%), anxiety, hyperesthesia, hypoesthesia, impotence

Dermatologic: Rash (2%), pruritus

Gastrointestinal: Constipation (4%), diarrhea (4%), dyspepsia (4%), nausea (4%), flatulence (3%), vomiting, abdominal pain

Genitourinary: Micturition frequency (3%), dysuria, nocturia, impotence (2%)

Neuromuscular & skeletal: Arthralgia (2%), myalgia (2%), back pain, joint pain

Ocular: Abnormal vision (2%), conjunctivitis, dry eyes, eye pain

Respiratory: Dyspnea (4%), rhinitis (2%), cough (1%), pharyngitis, wheezing

Potential adverse effects (based on experience with other beta-blocking agents) include reversible mental depression, disorientation, catatonia, short-term memory loss, emotional lability, slightly clouded sensorium, laryngospasm, respiratory distress, allergic reactions, erythematous rash, agranulocytosis, purpura, thrombocytopenia, mesenteric artery thrombosis, ischemic colitis, alopecia, Peyronie's disease, claudication

Mechanism of Action Competitively blocks $beta_1$-adrenergic receptors with little or no effect on $beta_2$-receptors except at high doses; exhibits membrane stabilizing and intrinsic sympathomimetic activity

Drug Interactions

Cytochrome P450 Effect: Inhibits CYP2D6 (weak)

Increased Effect/Toxicity: Acebutolol may increase the effects of other drugs which slow AV conduction (digoxin, verapamil, diltiazem), alpha-blockers (prazosin, terazosin), and alpha-adrenergic stimulants (epinephrine, phenylephrine). Acebutolol may mask the tachycardia from hypoglycemia caused by insulin and oral hypoglycemics. In patients receiving concurrent therapy, the risk of hypertensive crisis is increased when either clonidine or the beta-blocker is withdrawn. Reserpine has been shown to enhance the effect of acebutolol. Beta-blockers may increase the action or levels of ethanol, disopyramide, nondepolarizing muscle relaxants, and theophylline although the effects are difficult to predict.

Decreased Effect: Decreased effect of acebutolol with aluminum salts, barbiturates, calcium salts, cholestyramine, colestipol, NSAIDs, penicillins (ampicillin), rifampin, and salicylates due to decreased bioavailability and plasma levels. The effect of sulfonylureas may be decreased by beta-blockers; however, the decreased effect has not been shown with tolbutamide.

Pharmacodynamics/Kinetics

Onset of action: 1-2 hours

Duration: 12-24 hours

Absorption: Oral: 40%

Protein binding: 5% to 15%

Metabolism: Extensive first-pass effect

Half-life elimination: 6-7 hours

Time to peak: 2-4 hours

Excretion: Feces (~55%); urine (35%)

Pregnancy Risk Factor B (manufacturer); D (2nd and 3rd trimesters - expert analysis)

Acebutolol Hydrochloride *see* Acebutolol *on page 28*

Acenocoumarin *see* Acenocoumarol *on page 29*

Acenocoumarol (a see no KOOM a rol)

Canadian Brand Names Sintrom®
Generic Available No
(Continued)

Acenocoumarol (Continued)

Index Terms Acenocoumarin; Nicoumalone

Pharmacologic Category Anticoagulant, Coumarin Derivative

Use Prophylaxis and treatment of venous thrombosis, pulmonary embolism, and thromboembolic disorders; atrial fibrillation with risk of embolism; adjunct in the prophylaxis of coronary occlusion and transient ischemic attacks

Local Anesthetic/Vasoconstrictor Precautions No information available to require special precautions

Effects on Dental Treatment Signs of acenocoumarol overdose may first appear as bleeding from gingival tissue; consultation with prescribing physician is advisable prior to surgery to determine temporary dose reduction or withdrawal of medication.

Common Adverse Effects As with all anticoagulants, bleeding is the major adverse effect of acenocoumarol. Hemorrhage may occur at virtually any site. Risk is dependent on multiple variables, including the intensity of anticoagulation and patient susceptibility.

Frequency not defined.

Cardiovascular: Hemorrhagic shock

Central nervous system: Fever, headache, stroke (hemorrhagic)

Dermatologic: Rash, urticaria, skin necrosis

Skin necrosis/gangrene, due to paradoxical local thrombosis, is a known but rare risk of oral anticoagulant therapy. Its onset is usually within the first few days of therapy and is frequently localized to the limbs, breast, or penis. The risk of this effect is increased in patients with protein C or S deficiency.

Additional adverse reactions associated with warfarin, but likely to also occur with indanediones, include priapism and skin necrosis ("purple toe" syndrome or cutaneous gangrene).

Gastrointestinal: Gastrointestinal bleeding, melena

Genitourinary: Hematuria

Hematologic: Hemorrhage, retroperitoneal hematoma, unrecognized bleeding sites (eg, colon cancer) may be uncovered by anticoagulation. Other hematologic reactions reported with coumarin derivatives include agranulocytosis, red cell aplasia, anemia, thrombocytopenia, eosinophilia.

Hepatic: Hepatitis, hepatotoxicity, hematobilia

Ocular: Ocular hemorrhage

Respiratory: Epistaxis, hemoptysis, pulmonary hemorrhage

Miscellaneous: Hypersensitivity/allergic reactions

Restrictions Not available in U.S.

Dosage Note: Dosage must be individualized. The following information is based on the manufacturer's labeling in Canada. Adults:

Oral: Initial: 8-12 mg on day 1, followed by 4-8 mg on day 2. Subsequent dosage should be based on PT/INR measurements. Usual range of maintenance doses: 1-10 mg/day. Tapering of dosage is recommended prior to discontinuation.

Mechanism of Action Interferes with hepatic synthesis of vitamin K-dependent coagulation factors (II, VII, IX, X)

Contraindications Hypersensitivity to acenocoumarol or any component of the formulation; hemorrhagic tendencies; hemophilia; thrombocytopenia purpura; leukemia; recent or potential surgery of the eye or CNS; major regional lumbar block anesthesia or surgery resulting in large, open surfaces; bleeding from the GI, respiratory, or GU tract; threatened abortion; aneurysm; prolonged dietary insufficiencies (vitamin K deficiency); ascorbic acid deficiency; history of bleeding diathesis; prostatectomy; continuous tube drainage of the small intestine; polyarthritis; diverticulitis; emaciation; malnutrition; cerebrovascular hemorrhage; eclampsia/pre-eclampsia; blood dyscrasias; severe uncontrolled or malignant hypertension; severe hepatic disease; pericarditis or pericardial effusion; subacute bacterial endocarditis; visceral carcinoma; following spinal puncture and other diagnostic or therapeutic procedures with potential for significant bleeding; history of warfarin-induced necrosis; an unreliable, noncompliant patient; alcoholism; patient who has a history of falls or is a significant fall risk; pregnancy

Warnings/Precautions Use care in the selection of patients appropriate for this treatment. Use with caution in trauma, acute infection (antibiotics and fever may alter affects), renal insufficiency, moderate-severe hypertension, polycythemia vera, vasculitis, open wound, active TB, history of PUD, anaphylactic disorders, indwelling catheters, severe diabetes, thyroid disease, and menstruating and postpartum women. Necrosis or gangrene of the skin and other tissues can occur (rarely) due to early hypercoagulability; risk is increased in patients with protein C deficiency. "Purple toe" syndrome, due to cholesterol microembolization, has been described with coumarin-type anticoagulants. Women may be at risk of developing ovarian hemorrhage at the time of ovulation.

Hemorrhage is the most serious risk of therapy. Risk factors for bleeding include high intensity anticoagulation (INR >4), age (>65 years), variable INRs, history of GI bleeding, hypertension, cerebrovascular disease, serious heart disease, anemia, severe diabetes, malignancy, trauma, renal insufficiency, polycythemia vera, vasculitis, open wound, history of PUD, indwelling catheters, menstruating and postpartum women, drug-drug interactions and long duration of therapy. Patient must be instructed to report bleeding, accidents, or falls. Patient must also report any new or discontinued medications, herbal or alternative products used, significant changes in smoking or dietary habits. Ensure patient cooperation especially from the alcoholic, illicit drug user, demented, or psychotic patient. The elderly may be more sensitive to anticoagulant therapy. Safety and efficacy have not been established in children.

Drug Interactions
Cytochrome P450 Effect: Substrate of CYP1A2 (major), 2C9 (major), 2C19 (minor)

Increased Effect/Toxicity: The following agents may increase the levels and/or effects of acenocoumarol: Acetaminophen, amiodarone, anticoagulants, antiplatelet agents, CYP1A2 inhibitors (example inhibitors include ciprofloxacin, fluvoxamine, ketoconazole, norfloxacin, ofloxacin, and rofecoxib), CYP2C9 inhibitors (example inhibitors include delavirdine, fluconazole, gemfibrozil, ketoconazole, nicardipine, pioglitazone, and sulfonamides), miconazole, NSAIDs, salicylates, sulfamethoxazole, sulfinpyrazone, tetracycline antibiotics, and trimethoprim.

Decreased Effect: CYP1A2 and/or 2C9 inducers may decrease the levels/effects of acenocoumarol; example inducers of these enzymes include aminoglutethimide, carbamazepine, phenobarbital, phenytoin, rifampin, rifapentine, and secobarbital.

Ethanol/Nutrition/Herb Interactions
Ethanol: Avoid ethanol. Acute ethanol ingestion (binge drinking) decreases the metabolism of oral anticoagulants and increases PT/INR. Chronic daily ethanol use increases the metabolism of oral anticoagulants and decreases PT/INR.

Food: The anticoagulant effects of acenocoumarol may be decreased if taken with foods rich in vitamin K. Vitamin E may increase anticoagulant effect.

Herb/Nutraceutical: St John's wort may decrease oral anticoagulant levels. Alfalfa contains large amounts of vitamin K as do many enteral products. Coenzyme Q_{10} may decrease response to oral anticoagulants. Avoid cat's claw, dong quai, evening primrose, feverfew, red clover, horse chestnut, garlic, green tea, ginseng, and ginkgo (all have additional antiplatelet activity).

Dietary Considerations
Foods high in vitamin K (eg, beef liver, pork liver, green tea, and leafy green vegetables) inhibit anticoagulant effect. Do not change dietary habits once stabilized on acenocoumarol therapy. A balanced diet with a consistent intake of vitamin K is essential. Avoid large amounts of alfalfa, asparagus, broccoli, Brussels sprouts, cabbage, cauliflower, green teas, kale, lettuce, spinach, turnip greens, watercress; these decrease efficacy of oral anticoagulants. It is recommended that the diet contain a CONSISTENT vitamin K content of 70-140 mcg/day. Check with healthcare provider before changing diet. Avoid using multivitamins that contain vitamin K.

Pharmacodynamics/Kinetics
Onset of action: Peak anticoagulant effect: Oral: 36-48 hours

Absorption: Oral: 60%

Protein binding: 99%

Metabolism: Hepatic, via oxidation (possibly by CYP1A2, 2C9, and 2C19) to inactive metabolites

Half-life elimination: 8-11 hours

Time to peak, plasma: 1-3 hours

Excretion: Urine (60%) and feces (29%) as metabolites

Dosage Forms [CAN] = Canadian brand name
Tablet:
Sintrom® [CAN]: 1 mg, 4 mg [not available in the U.S.]

Acetaminophen (a seet a MIN oh fen)

Related Information
Oral Pain *on page 1788*

Related Sample Prescriptions
Mild/Moderate Oral Pain *on page 1834*

(Continued)

Acetaminophen *(Continued)*

U.S. Brand Names Acephen™ [OTC]; Apra Children's [OTC]; Aspirin Free Anacin® Maximum Strength [OTC]; Cetafen® [OTC]; Cetafen Extra® [OTC]; Comtrex® Sore Throat Maximum Strength [OTC]; FeverALL® [OTC]; Genapap™ [OTC]; Genapap™ Children [OTC]; Genapap™ Extra Strength [OTC]; Genapap™ Infant [OTC]; Genebs [OTC]; Genebs Extra Strength [OTC]; Infantaire [OTC]; Mapap [OTC]; Mapap Children's [OTC]; Mapap Extra Strength [OTC]; Mapap Infants [OTC]; Nortemp Children's [OTC]; Pain Eze [OTC]; Silapap® Children's [OTC]; Silapap® Infants [OTC]; Tycolene [OTC]; Tycolene Maximum Strength [OTC]; Tylenol® [OTC]; Tylenol® 8 Hour [OTC]; Tylenol® Arthritis Pain [OTC]; Tylenol® Children's [OTC]; Tylenol® Children's with Flavor Creator [OTC]; Tylenol® Extra Strength [OTC]; Tylenol® Infants [OTC]; Tylenol® Junior [OTC]; Valorin [OTC]; Valorin Extra [OTC]

Canadian Brand Names Abenol®; Apo-Acetaminophen®; Atasol®; Novo-Gesic; Pediatrix; Tempra®; Tylenol®

Mexican Brand Names Dismifen; Dolotemp; Temzzard; Tylenol

Generic Available Yes: Excludes extended release products

Index Terms APAP; N-Acetyl-P-Aminophenol; Paracetamol

Pharmacologic Category Analgesic, Miscellaneous

Dental Use Treatment of postoperative pain

Use Treatment of mild-to-moderate pain and fever (antipyretic/analgesic); does not have antirheumatic or anti-inflammatory effects

Local Anesthetic/Vasoconstrictor Precautions No information available to require special precautions

Effects on Dental Treatment No significant effects or complications reported (see Dental Comment)

Significant Adverse Effects Frequency not defined.

Dermatologic: Rash

Endocrine & metabolic: May increase chloride, uric acid, glucose; may decrease sodium, bicarbonate, calcium

Hematologic: Anemia, blood dyscrasias (neutropenia, pancytopenia, leukopenia)

Hepatic: Bilirubin increased, alkaline phosphatase increased

Renal: Ammonia increased, nephrotoxicity with chronic overdose, analgesic nephropathy

Miscellaneous: Hypersensitivity reactions (rare)

Dental Usual Dosing Postoperative pain: Oral, rectal:

Children <12 years: 10-15 mg/kg/dose every 4-6 hours as needed; do **not** exceed 5 doses (2.6 g) in 24 hours; alternatively, the following age-based doses may be used

Adults: 325-650 mg every 4-6 hours or 1000 mg 3-4 times/day; do **not** exceed 4 g/day

Dosage Oral, rectal:

Children <12 years: 10-15 mg/kg/dose every 4-6 hours as needed; do **not** exceed 5 doses (2.6 g) in 24 hours; alternatively, the following age-based doses may be used; see table.

Acetaminophen Dosing

Age	Dosage (mg)	Age	Dosage (mg)
0-3 mo	40	4-5 y	240
4-11 mo	80	6-8 y	320
1-2 y	120	9-10 y	400
2-3 y	160	11 y	480

Note: Higher rectal doses have been studied for use in preoperative pain control in children. However, specific guidelines are not available and dosing may be product dependent. The safety and efficacy of alternating acetaminophen and ibuprofen dosing has not been established.

Adults: 325-650 mg every 4-6 hours or 1000 mg 3-4 times/day; do **not** exceed 4 g/day

Dosing interval in renal impairment:

Cl_{cr} 10-50 mL/minute: Administer every 6 hours

Cl_{cr} <10 mL/minute: Administer every 8 hours (metabolites accumulate)

Hemodialysis: Moderately dialyzable (20% to 50%)

Dosing adjustment/comments in hepatic impairment: Use with caution. Limited, low-dose therapy is usually well tolerated in hepatic disease/cirrhosis. However, cases of hepatotoxicity at daily acetaminophen dosages <4 g/day have been reported. Avoid chronic use in hepatic impairment.

Mechanism of Action Inhibits the synthesis of prostaglandins in the central nervous system and peripherally blocks pain impulse generation; produces antipyresis from inhibition of hypothalamic heat-regulating center

Contraindications Hypersensitivity to acetaminophen or any component of the formulation

Warnings/Precautions Limit dose to <4 g/day. May cause severe hepatic toxicity on acute overdose; in addition, chronic daily dosing in adults has resulted in liver damage in some patients. Use with caution in patients with alcoholic liver disease; consuming ≥3 alcoholic drinks/day may increase the risk of liver damage. Use caution in patients with known G6PD deficiency.

OTC labeling: When used for self-medication, patients should be instructed to contact healthcare provider if used for fever lasting >3 days or for pain lasting >10 days in adults or >5 days in children.

Drug Interactions Substrate (minor) of CYP1A2, 2A6, 2C9, 2D6, 2E1, 3A4; **Inhibits** CYP3A4 (weak)

Decreased effect: Barbiturates, carbamazepine, hydantoins, rifampin, sulfinpyrazone may decrease the analgesic effect of acetaminophen. Cholestyramine may decrease acetaminophen absorption (separate dosing by at least 1 hour).

Increased toxicity: Barbiturates, carbamazepine, hydantoins, isoniazid, rifampin, sulfinpyrazone may increase the hepatotoxic potential of acetaminophen. Chronic ethanol abuse increases risk for acetaminophen toxicity; effect of warfarin may be enhanced.

Ethanol/Nutrition/Herb Interactions

Ethanol: Excessive intake of ethanol may increase the risk of acetaminophen-induced hepatotoxicity. Avoid ethanol or limit to <3 drinks/day.

Food: Rate of absorption may be decreased when given with food.

Herb/Nutraceutical: St John's wort may decrease acetaminophen levels.

Dietary Considerations Chewable tablets may contain phenylalanine (amount varies, ranges between 3-12 mg/tablet); consult individual product labeling.

Pharmacodynamics/Kinetics

Onset of action: <1 hour

Duration: 4-6 hours

Absorption: Incomplete; varies by dosage form

Protein binding: 8% to 43% at toxic doses

Metabolism: At normal therapeutic dosages, hepatic to sulfate and glucuronide metabolites, while a small amount is metabolized by CYP to a highly reactive intermediate (acetylimidoquinone) which is conjugated with glutathione and inactivated; at toxic doses (as little as 4 g daily) glutathione conjugation becomes insufficient to meet the metabolic demand causing an increase in acetylimidoquinone concentration, which may cause hepatic cell necrosis

Half-life elimination: Prolonged following toxic doses

Neonates: 2-5 hours

Adults: 1-3 hours (may be increased in elderly; however, this should not affect dosing)

Time to peak, serum: Oral: 10-60 minutes; may be delayed in acute overdoses

Excretion: Urine (2% to 5% unchanged; 55% as glucuronide metabolites; 30% as sulphate metabolites)

Pregnancy Risk Factor B

Lactation Enters breast milk/compatible

Dosage Forms Excipient information presented when available (limited, particularly for generics); consult specific product labeling. [DSC] = Discontinued product

Caplet: 500 mg

Cetafen Extra® Strength, Genapap™ Extra Strength, Genebs Extra Strength, Mapap Extra Strength, Tycolene Maximum Strength, Tylenol® Extra Strength: 500 mg

Caplet, extended release:

Tylenol® 8 Hour, Tylenol® Arthritis Pain: 650 mg

Capsule: 500 mg

Elixir: 160 mg/5 mL (120 mL, 480 mL, 3780 mL)

Apra Children's: 160 mg/5 mL (120 mL, 480 mL, 3780 mL) [alcohol free; contains benzoic acid; cherry and grape flavors]

Mapap Children's: 160 mg/5 mL (120 mL) [alcohol free; contains benzoic acid and sodium benzoate; cherry flavor]

Gelcap:

Mapap Extra Strength, Tylenol® Extra Strength: 500 mg

Geltab:

Tylenol® Extra Strength: 500 mg

Geltab, extended release:

Tylenol® 8 Hour: 650 mg [DSC]

Liquid, oral: 500 mg/15 mL (240 mL)

(Continued)

Acetaminophen (Continued)

Comtrex® Sore Throat Maximum Strength: 500 mg/15 mL (240 mL) [contains sodium benzoate; honey lemon flavor]

Genapap™ Children: 160 mg/5 mL (120 mL) [contains sodium benzoate; cherry and grape flavors]

Silapap®: 160 mg/5 mL (120 mL, 240 mL, 480 mL) [sugar free; contains sodium benzoate; cherry flavor]

Tylenol® Extra Strength: 500 mg/15 mL (240 mL) [contains sodium benzoate; cherry flavor]

Solution, oral: 160 mg/5 mL (120 mL, 480 mL)

Solution, oral [drops]: 80 mg/0.8 mL (15 mL) [droppers are marked at 0.4 mL (40 mg) and at 0.8 mL (80 mg)]

Genapap™ Infant: 80 mg/0.8 mL (15 mL) [fruit flavor]

Infantaire: 80 mg/0.8mL (15 mL, 30 mL)

Silapap® Infant's: 80 mg/0.8 mL (15 mL, 30 mL) [contains sodium benzoate; cherry flavor]

Suppository, rectal: 120 mg, 325 mg, 650 mg

Acephen™: 120 mg, 325 mg, 650 mg

FeverALL®: 80 mg, 120 mg, 325 mg, 650 mg

Mapap: 125 mg, 650 mg

Suspension, oral:

Mapap Children's: 160 mg/5 mL (120 mL) [contains sodium benzoate; cherry flavor]

Nortemp Children's: 160 mg/5 mL (120 mL) [alcohol free; contains sodium benzoate; cotton candy flavor]

Tylenol® Children's: 160 mg/5 mL (120 mL, 240 mL) [contains sodium benzoate; bubble gum yum, cherry blast, dye free cherry, grape splash, and very berry strawberry flavors]

Tylenol® Children's with Flavor Creator: 160 mg/5 mL (120 mL) [contains sodium 2 mg/5 mL and sodium benzoate; cherry blast flavor; packaged with apple (4), bubblegum (8), chocolate (4), & strawberry (4) sugar free flavor packets]

Suspension, oral [drops]:

Mapap Infants: 80 mg/0.8 mL (15 mL, 30 mL) [contains sodium benzoate; cherry flavor]

Tylenol® Infants: 80 mg/0.8 mL (15 mL, 30 mL) [contains sodium benzoate; cherry, dye free cherry, and grape flavors]

Tablet: 325 mg, 500 mg

Aspirin Free Anacin® Extra Strength, Genapap™ Extra Strength, Genebs Extra Strength, Mapap Extra Strength, Pain Eze, Tylenol® Extra Strength, Valorin Extra: 500 mg

Cetafen®, Genapap™, Genebs, Mapap, Tycolene, Tylenol®, Valorin: 325 mg

Tablet, chewable: 80 mg

Genapap™ Children: 80 mg [contains phenylalanine 6 mg/tablet; fruit and grape flavors]

Mapap Children's: 80 mg [contains phenylalanine 3 mg/tablet; bubble gum, fruit, and grape flavors]

Mapap Junior Strength: 160 mg [contains phenylalanine 12 mg/tablet; grape flavor]

Tablet, orally disintegrating: 80 mg, 160 mg

Tylenol® Children's Meltaways: 80 mg [bubble gum, grape, and watermelon flavors]

Tylenol® Junior Meltaways: 160 mg [bubble gum and grape flavors]

Dental Comment Hepatotoxicity caused by acetaminophen is potentiated by chronic ethanol consumption. People who consume ethanol at the same time that they use acetaminophen, even in therapeutic doses, are at risk of developing hepatotoxicity.

A study by Hylek, et al, suggested that the combination of acetaminophen with warfarin (Coumadin®) may cause enhanced anticoagulation. The following recommendations have been made by Hylek, et al, and supported by an editorial in *JAMA* by Bell.

Dose and duration of acetaminophen should be as low as possible, individualized, and monitored.

The study by Hylek reported that for patients who reported taking the equivalent of at least 4 regular strength (325 mg) tablets for longer than a week, the odds of having an INR >6.0 were increased 10-fold above those not taking acetaminophen. Risk decreased with lower intakes of acetaminophen reaching a background level of risk at a dose of 6 or fewer 325 mg tablets per week.

Selected Readings

Ahmad N, Grad HA, Haas DA, et al, "The Efficacy of Nonopioid Analgesics for Postoperative Dental Pain: A Meta-Analysis," *Anesth Prog*, 1997, 44(4):119-26.

Bell WR, "Acetaminophen and Warfarin: Undesirable Synergy," *JAMA*, 1998, 279(9):702-3.

Botting RM, "Mechanism of Action of Acetaminophen: Is There a Cyclooxygenase 3?" *Clin Infect Dis*, 2000, Suppl 5:S202-10.

Chandrasekharan NV, Dai H, Roos KL, et al, "COX-3, a Cyclooxygenase-1 Variant Inhibited by Acetaminophen and Other Analgesic/Antipyretic Drugs: Cloning, Structure, and Expression," *Proc Natl Acad Sci U S A*, 2002, 99(21):13926-31.

Dart RC, Kuffner EK, and Rumack BH, "Treatment of Pain or Fever With Paracetamol (Acetaminophen) in the Alcoholic Patient: A Systematic Review," *Am J Ther*, 2000, 7(2):123-34.

Dionne R, "Additive Analgesia Without Opioid Side Effects," *Compend Contin Educ Dent*, 2000, 21(7):572-4, 576-7.

Dionne RA and Berthold CW, "Therapeutic Uses of Nonsteroidal Anti-inflammatory Drugs in Dentistry," *Crit Rev Oral Biol Med*, 2001, 12(4):315-30.

Graham GG and Scott KF, "Mechanisms of Action of Paracetamol and Related Analgesics," *Inflammopharmacology*, 2003, 11(4):401-13.

Grant JA and Weiler JM, "A Report of a Rare Immediate Reaction After Ingestion of Acetaminophen," *Ann Allergy Asthma Immunol*, 2001, 87(3):227-9.

Hylek EM, Heiman H, Skates SJ, et al, "Acetaminophen and Other Risk Factors for Excessive Warfarin Anticoagulation," *JAMA*, 1998, 279(9):657-62.

Kwan D, Bartle WR, and Walker SE, "The Effects of Acetaminophen on Pharmacokinetics and Pharmacodynamics of Warfarin," *J Clin Pharmacol*, 1999, 39(1):68-75.

Lee WM, "Drug-Induced Hepatotoxicity," *N Engl J Med*, 1995, 333(17):1118-27.

Licht H, Seeff LB, and Zimmerman HJ, "Apparent Potentiation of Acetaminophen Hepatotoxicity by Alcohol," *Ann Intern Med*, 1980, 92(4):511.

McClain CJ, Price S, Barve S, et al, "Acetaminophen Hepatotoxicity: An Update," *Curr Gastroenterol Rep*, 1999, 1(1):42-9.

Nguyen AM, Graham DY, Gage T, et al, "Nonsteroidal Anti-Inflammatory Drug Use in Dentistry: Gastrointestinal Implications," *Gen Dent*, 1999, 47(6):590-6.

Schwab JM, Schluesener HJ, and Laufer S, "COX-3: Just Another COX or the Solitary Elusive Target of Paracetamol?" *Lancet*, 2003, 361(9362):981-2.

Shek KL, Chan LN, and Nutescu E, "Warfarin-Acetaminophen Drug Interaction Revisited," *Pharmacotherapy*, 1999, 19(10):1153-8.

Tanaka E, Yamazaki K, and Misawa S, "Update: The Clinical Importance of Acetaminophen Hepatotoxicity in Nonalcoholic and Alcoholic Subjects," *J Clin Pharm Ther*, 2000, 25(5):325-32.

Wynn RL, "Update on Nonprescription Pain Relievers for Dental Pain," *Gen Dent*, 2004, 52(2):94-8.

Acetaminophen and Chlorpheniramine see Chlorpheniramine and Acetaminophen on page 339

Acetaminophen and Codeine (a seet a MIN oh fen & KOE deen)

Related Information
Acetaminophen *on page 31*
Codeine *on page 404*

Related Sample Prescriptions
Moderate/Moderately Severe Oral Pain *on page 1834*

U.S. Brand Names Capital® and Codeine; Tylenol® With Codeine

Canadian Brand Names ratio-Emtec; ratio-Lenoltec; Triatec-8; Triatec-8 Strong; Triatec-30; Tylenol Elixir with Codeine; Tylenol No. 1; Tylenol No. 1 Forte; Tylenol No. 2 with Codeine; Tylenol No. 3 with Codeine; Tylenol No. 4 with Codeine

Mexican Brand Names Tylex CD

Generic Available Yes

Index Terms Codeine and Acetaminophen

Pharmacologic Category Analgesic, Opioid

Dental Use Treatment of postoperative pain

Use Relief of mild-to-moderate pain

Local Anesthetic/Vasoconstrictor Precautions No information available to require special precautions

Effects on Dental Treatment No significant effects or complications reported (see Dental Comment)

Significant Adverse Effects
>10%:
Central nervous system: Lightheadedness, dizziness, sedation
Gastrointestinal: Nausea, vomiting
Respiratory: Dyspnea
1% to 10%:
Central nervous system: Euphoria, dysphoria
Dermatologic: Pruritus
Gastrointestinal: Constipation, abdominal pain
Miscellaneous: Histamine release
<1% (Limited to important or life-threatening): Antidiuretic hormone release, biliary tract spasm, bradycardia, hypotension, intracranial pressure increased, physical and psychological dependence, respiratory depression, urinary retention

Restrictions C-III; C-V
Note: In countries outside of the U.S., some formulations of Tylenol® with Codeine (eg, Tylenol® No. 3) include caffeine.

Dental Usual Dosing Postoperative pain: Adults: Analgesic: Based on codeine (30-60 mg/dose) every 4-6 hours (maximum: 4000 mg/24 hours based on acetaminophen component)
(Continued)

Acetaminophen and Codeine *(Continued)*

Dosage Doses should be adjusted according to severity of pain and response of the patient. Adult doses ≥60 mg codeine fail to give commensurate relief of pain but merely prolong analgesia and are associated with an appreciably increased incidence of side effects. Oral:

Children: Analgesic:

Codeine: 0.5-1 mg codeine/kg/dose every 4-6 hours

Acetaminophen: 10-15 mg/kg/dose every 4 hours up to a maximum of 2.6 g/ 24 hours for children <12 years; **alternatively, the following can be used:**

3-6 years: 5 mL 3-4 times/day as needed of elixir

7-12 years: 10 mL 3-4 times/day as needed of elixir

>12 years: 15 mL every 4 hours as needed of elixir

Adults:

Antitussive: Based on codeine (15-30 mg/dose) every 4-6 hours (maximum: 360 mg/24 hours based on codeine component)

Analgesic: Based on codeine (30-60 mg/dose) every 4-6 hours (maximum: 4000 mg/24 hours based on acetaminophen component)

Dosing adjustment in renal impairment: See individual agents.

Dosing adjustment in hepatic impairment: Use with caution. Limited, low-dose therapy is usually well tolerated in hepatic disease/cirrhosis; however, cases of hepatotoxicity at daily acetaminophen dosages <4 g/day have been reported. Avoid chronic use in hepatic impairment.

Mechanism of Action Inhibits the synthesis of prostaglandins in the central nervous system and peripherally blocks pain impulse generation; produces antipyresis from inhibition of hypothalamic heat-regulating center; binds to opiate receptors in the CNS, causing inhibition of ascending pain pathways, altering the perception of and response to pain; causes cough supression by direct central action in the medulla; produces generalized CNS depression. Caffeine (contained in some non-U.S. formulations) is a CNS stimulant; use with acetaminophen and codeine increases the level of analgesia provided by each agent.

Contraindications Hypersensitivity to acetaminophen, codeine, or any component of the formulation; significant respiratory depression (in unmonitored settings); acute or severe bronchial asthma; hypercapnia; paralytic ileus

Warnings/Precautions Use with caution in patients with hypersensitivity reactions to other phenanthrene-derivative opioid agonists (morphine, hydrocodone, hydromorphone, levorphanol, oxycodone, oxymorphone); tablets contain metabisulfite which may cause allergic reactions. Tolerance or drug dependence may result from extended use.

Limit total acetaminophen dose to <4 g/day. May cause severe hepatic toxicity on acute overdose; in addition, chronic daily dosing in adults has resulted in liver damage in some patients. Use with caution in patients with alcoholic liver disease; consuming 3 alcoholic drinks/day may increase the risk of liver damage. Use caution in patients with known G6PD deficiency.

This combination should be used with caution in elderly or debilitated patients, hypotension, adrenocortical insufficiency, abdominal conditions, hepatic impairment, renal impairment, respiratory disease, thyroid disorders, prostatic hyperplasia, urethral stricture, seizure disorder, CNS depression, head injury or increased intracranial pressure. Causes sedation; caution must be used in performing tasks which require alertness (eg, operating machinery or driving). Safety and efficacy in pediatric patients have not been established. Effects may be potentiated when used with other sedative drugs or ethanol.

Note: Some non-U.S. formulations (including most Canadian formulations) may contain caffeine as an additional ingredient. Caffeine may cause CNS and cardiovascular stimulation, as well as GI irritation in high doses. Use with caution in patients with a history of peptic ulcer or GERD; avoid in patients with symptomatic cardiac arrhythmias.

Drug Interactions Acetaminophen: **Substrate** (minor) of CYP1A2, 2A6, 2C9, 2D6, 2E1, 3A4; **Inhibits** CYP3A4 (weak)

Increased toxicity: CNS depressants, phenothiazines, tricyclic antidepressants, guanabenz, MAO inhibitors (may also decrease blood pressure); effect of warfarin may be enhanced.

Ethanol/Nutrition/Herb Interactions Ethanol: Excessive intake of ethanol may increase the risk of acetaminophen-induced hepatotoxicity. Avoid ethanol or limit to <3 drinks/day.

Dietary Considerations May be taken with food.

Pharmacodynamics/Kinetics See individual agents.

Pregnancy Risk Factor C

Lactation Enters breast milk/use caution

Dosage Forms Excipient information presented when available (limited, particularly for generics); consult specific product labeling. [DSC] = Discontinued product; [CAN] = Canadian brand name

Caplet:

ratio-Lenoltec No. 1 [CAN], Tylenol No. 1 [CAN]: Acetaminophen 300 mg, codeine phosphate 8 mg, and caffeine 15 mg [not available in the U.S.]

Tylenol No. 1 Forte [CAN]: Acetaminophen 500 mg, codeine phosphate 8 mg, and caffeine 15 mg [not available in the U.S.]

Elixir, oral [C-V]: Acetaminophen 120 mg and codeine phosphate 12 mg per 5 mL (5 mL, 10 mL, 12.5 mL, 15 mL, 120 mL, 480 mL) [contains alcohol 7%]

Tylenol® with Codeine [DSC]: Acetaminophen 120 mg and codeine phosphate 12 mg per 5 mL (480 mL) [contains alcohol 7%; cherry flavor]

Tylenol Elixir with Codeine [CAN]: Acetaminophen 160 mg and codeine phosphate 8 mg per 5 mL (500 mL) [contains alcohol 7%, sucrose 31%; cherry flavor; not available in the U.S.]

Suspension, oral [C-V] (Capital® and Codeine): Acetaminophen 120 mg and codeine phosphate 12 mg per 5 mL (480 mL) [alcohol free; fruit punch flavor]

Tablet [C-III]: Acetaminophen 300 mg and codeine phosphate 15 mg; acetaminophen 300 mg and codeine phosphate 30 mg; acetaminophen 300 mg and codeine phosphate 60 mg

ratio-Emtec [CAN], Triatec-30 [CAN]: Acetaminophen 300 mg and codeine phosphate 30 mg [not available in the U.S.]

ratio-Lenoltec No. 1 [CAN]: Acetaminophen 300 mg, codeine phosphate 8 mg, and caffeine 15 mg [not available in the U.S.]

ratio-Lenoltec No. 2 [CAN], Tylenol No. 2 with Codeine [CAN]: Acetaminophen 300 mg, codeine phosphate 15 mg, and caffeine 15 mg [not available in the U.S.]

ratio-Lenoltec No. 3 [CAN], Tylenol No. 3 with Codeine [CAN]: Acetaminophen 300 mg, codeine phosphate 30 mg, and caffeine 15 mg [not available in the U.S.]

ratio-Lenoltec No. 4 [CAN], Tylenol No. 4 with Codeine [CAN]: Acetaminophen 300 mg and codeine phosphate 60 mg [not available in the U.S.]

Triatec-8 [CAN]: Acetaminophen 325 mg, codeine phosphate 8 mg, and caffeine 30 mg [not available in the U.S.]

Triatec-8 Strong [CAN]: Acetaminophen 500 mg, codeine phosphate 8 mg, and caffeine 30 mg [not available in the U.S.]

Tylenol® with Codeine No. 3: Acetaminophen 300 mg and codeine phosphate 30 mg [contains sodium metabisulfite]

Tylenol® with Codeine No. 4: Acetaminophen 300 mg and codeine phosphate 60 mg [contains sodium metabisulfite]

Dental Comment Codeine products, as with other narcotic analgesics, are recommended only for acute dosing (ie, 3 days or less). The most common adverse effect you will see in your dental patients from codeine is nausea, followed by sedation and constipation. Codeine has narcotic addiction liability, especially when given long-term. Because of the acetaminophen component, this product should be used with caution in patients with alcoholic liver disease.

A study by Hylek, et al, suggested that the combination of acetaminophen with warfarin (Coumadin®) may cause enhanced anticoagulation. The following recommendations have been made by Hylek, et al, and are supported by an editorial in *JAMA* by Bell.

Dose and duration of acetaminophen should be as low as possible, individualized, and monitored.

The study by Hylek reported that for patients who reported taking the equivalent of at least 4 regular strength (325 mg) tablets for longer than a week, the odds of having an INR >6.0 were increased 10-fold above those not taking acetaminophen. Risk decreased with lower intakes of acetaminophen reaching a background level of risk at a dose of 6 or fewer 325 mg tablets per week.

Selected Readings

Change DJ, Fricke JR, Bird SR, et al, "Rofecoxib Versus Codeine/Acetaminophen in Postoperative Dental Pain: A Double-Blind, Randomized, Placebo- and Active Comparator-Controlled Clinical Trial," *Clin Ther*, 2001, 23(9):1446-55.

Dionne RA, "New Approaches to Preventing and Treating Postoperative Pain," *J Am Dent Assoc*, 1992, 123(6):26-34.

Forbes JA, Butterworth GA, Burchfield WH, et al, "Evaluation of Ketorolac, Aspirin, and an Acetaminophen-Codeine Combination in Postoperative Oral Surgery Pain," *Pharmacotherapy*, 1990, 10(6 Pt 2):77S-93S.

Gobetti JP, "Controlling Dental Pain," *J Am Dent Assoc*, 1992, 123(6):47-52.

Mullican WS and Lacy JR, "Tramadol/Acetaminophen Combination Tablets and Codeine/Acetaminophen Combination Capsules for the Management of Chronic Pain: A Comparative Trial," *Clin Ther*, 2001, 23(9):1429-45.

Wynn RL, "Narcotic Analgesics for Dental Pain: Available Products, Strengths, and Formulations," *Gen Dent*, 2001, 49(2):126-8, 130, 132 passim.

Acetaminophen and Diphenhydramine
(a seet a MIN oh fen & dye fen HYE dra meen)

Related Information
Acetaminophen *on page 31*
DiphenhydrAMINE *on page 510*
U.S. Brand Names Excedrin® P.M. [OTC]; Goody's PM® [OTC]; Legatrin PM® [OTC]; Percogesic® Extra Strength [OTC]; Tylenol® PM [OTC]; Tylenol® Severe Allergy [OTC]
Generic Available Yes: Excludes gelcap, powder, and liquid
Index Terms Diphenhydramine and Acetaminophen
Pharmacologic Category Analgesic, Miscellaneous
Use Aid in the relief of insomnia accompanied by minor pain
Local Anesthetic/Vasoconstrictor Precautions No information available to require special precautions
Effects on Dental Treatment Key adverse event(s) related to dental treatment: Xerostomia (normal salivary flow resumes upon discontinuation)
Common Adverse Effects See individual agents.
Drug Interactions
Cytochrome P450 Effect:
Acetaminophen: **Substrate** (minor) of CYP1A2, 2A6, 2C9, 2D6, 2E1, 3A4; **Inhibits** CYP3A4 (weak)
Diphenhydramine: **Inhibits** CYP2D6 (moderate)
Increased Effect/Toxicity: See individual agents.
Decreased Effect: See individual agents.
Pharmacodynamics/Kinetics See individual agents.

Acetaminophen and Hydrocodone *see* Hydrocodone and Acetaminophen *on page 822*

Acetaminophen and Oxycodone *see* Oxycodone and Acetaminophen *on page 1228*

Acetaminophen and Pentazocine *see* Pentazocine and Acetaminophen *on page 1275*

Acetaminophen and Phenyltoloxamine
(a seet a MIN oh fen & fen il to LOKS a meen)

Related Information
Acetaminophen *on page 31*
U.S. Brand Names Aceta-Gesic [OTC]; Alpain; Dologesic®; Flextra 650; Flextra-DS; Genasec™ [OTC]; Hyflex-DS®; Lagesic™; Percogesic® [OTC]; Phenagesic [OTC]; Phenylgesic [OTC]; RhinoFlex™; RhinoFlex 650; Staflex
Generic Available Yes: Tablet
Index Terms Phenyltoloxamine Citrate and Acetaminophen
Pharmacologic Category Analgesic, Miscellaneous
Use Relief of mild pain
Local Anesthetic/Vasoconstrictor Precautions No information available to require special precautions
Effects on Dental Treatment No significant effects or complications reported
Mechanism of Action Acetaminophen inhibits the synthesis of prostaglandins in the central nervous system and peripherally blocks pain impulse generation; produces antipyresis from inhibition of hypothalamic heat-regulating center. Phenyltoloxamine is an antihistamine (H₁-blocking agent) which acts primarily to inhibit secretions in the nose, mouth, and pharynx, as well as causing CNS depression.
Drug Interactions
Cytochrome P450 Effect: Acetaminophen: **Substrate** (minor) of CYP1A2, 2A6, 2C9, 2D6, 2E1, 3A4; **Inhibits** CYP3A4 (weak)
Increased Effect/Toxicity:
Refer to Acetaminophen monograph.
Pregnancy Risk Factor C

Acetaminophen and Propoxyphene *see* Propoxyphene and Acetaminophen *on page 1369*

Acetaminophen and Pseudoephedrine
(a seet a MIN oh fen & soo doe e FED rin)

Related Information
Acetaminophen *on page 31*
Pseudoephedrine *on page 1381*

U.S. Brand Names Allerest® Allergy and Sinus Relief [OTC]; Genapap™ Sinus Maximum Strength [OTC]; Mapap Sinus Maximum Strength [OTC]; Medi-Synal [OTC]; Oranyl Plus [OTC]; Ornex® [OTC]; Ornex® Maximum Strength [OTC]; Sinus-Relief [OTC] [DSC]; Sudafed® Multi-Symptom Sinus and Cold [OTC]; Tylenol® Cold Daytime, Children's [OTC]; Tylenol® Cold, Infants [OTC]; Tylenol® Sinus Daytime [OTC]

Canadian Brand Names Contac® Cold and Sore Throat, Non Drowsy, Extra Strength; Dristan® N.D.; Dristan® N.D., Extra Strength; Sinutab® Non Drowsy; Sudafed® Head Cold and Sinus Extra Strength; Tylenol® Decongestant; Tylenol® Sinus

Generic Available Yes

Index Terms Pseudoephedrine and Acetaminophen

Pharmacologic Category Alpha/Beta Agonist; Analgesic, Miscellaneous

Use Relief of mild-to-moderate pain; relief of congestion

Local Anesthetic/Vasoconstrictor Precautions Use with caution since pseudoephedrine is a sympathomimetic amine which could interact with epinephrine to cause a pressor response

Effects on Dental Treatment Key adverse event(s) related to dental treatment: Pseudoephedrine: Xerostomia (normal salivary flow resumes upon discontinuation).

Common Adverse Effects See individual agents.

Drug Interactions
Cytochrome P450 Effect: Acetaminophen: **Substrate** (minor) of CYP1A2, 2A6, 2C9, 2D6, 2E1, 3A4; **Inhibits** CYP3A4 (weak)
Increased Effect/Toxicity: See individual agents.
Decreased Effect: See individual agents.

Pharmacodynamics/Kinetics See individual agents.

Acetaminophen and Tramadol
(a seet a MIN oh fen & TRA ma dole)

Related Information
Acetaminophen *on page 31*
Oral Pain *on page 1788*
Tramadol *on page 1595*

Related Sample Prescriptions
Moderate/Moderately Severe Oral Pain *on page 1834*

U.S. Brand Names Ultracet™

Canadian Brand Names Tramacet

Mexican Brand Names Tramacet; Zaldiar

Generic Available Yes

Index Terms APAP and Tramadol; Tramadol Hydrochloride and Acetaminophen

Pharmacologic Category Analgesic, Miscellaneous; Analgesic, Nonopioid

Dental Use Treatment of postoperative pain (≤5 days)

Use Short-term (≤5 days) management of acute pain

Local Anesthetic/Vasoconstrictor Precautions No information available to require special precautions

Effects on Dental Treatment Key adverse event(s) related to dental treatment: Xerostomia and changes in salivation (normal salivary flow resumes upon discontinuation)

Significant Adverse Effects
1% to 10%:
Central nervous system: Somnolence (6%), dizziness (3%), insomnia (2%), anxiety, confusion, euphoria, fatigue, headache, nervousness, tremor
Dermatologic: Pruritus (2%), rash
Endocrine & metabolic: Hot flashes
Gastrointestinal: Constipation (6%), anorexia (3%), diarrhea (3%), nausea (3%), dry mouth (2%), abdominal pain, dyspepsia, flatulence, vomiting
Genitourinary: Prostatic disorder (2%)
Neuromuscular & skeletal: Weakness
Miscellaneous: Diaphoresis increased (4%)
<1% (Limited to important or life-threatening): Allergic reactions, amnesia, anaphylactoid reactions, anaphylaxis, arrhythmia, coma, depersonalization, drug abuse, dysphagia, dyspnea, emotional lability, hallucination, hepatitis, hypertonia, impotence, liver failure, migraine, muscle contractions (involuntary), oliguria, paresthesia, paroniria, pulmonary edema, rigors, seizure, serotonin syndrome, shivering, Stevens-Johnson syndrome, suicidal tendency, stupor, syncope, tinnitus, tongue edema, toxic epidermal necrolysis, urinary retention, urticaria, vertigo
A withdrawal syndrome may occur with abrupt discontinuation; includes anxiety, diarrhea, hallucinations (rare), nausea, pain, piloerection, rigors, sweating, (Continued)

Acetaminophen and Tramadol *(Continued)*

and tremor. Uncommon discontinuation symptoms may include severe anxiety, panic attacks, or paresthesia.

Dental Usual Dosing Acute postoperative pain (≤5 days): Adults: Oral: Two tablets every 4-6 hours as needed for pain relief (maximum: 8 tablets/day); treatment should not exceed 5 days

Dosage Oral: Adults: Acute pain: Two tablets every 4-6 hours as needed for pain relief (maximum: 8 tablets/day); treatment should not exceed 5 days

Dosage adjustment in renal impairment: Cl$_{cr}$ <30 mL/minute: Maximum of 2 tablets every 12 hours; treatment should not exceed 5 days

Dosage adjustment in hepatic impairment: Use is not recommended.

Mechanism of Action

Based on **acetaminophen** component: Inhibits the synthesis of prostaglandins in the central nervous system and peripherally blocks pain impulse generation; produces antipyresis from inhibition of hypothalamic heat-regulating center

Based on **tramadol** component: Binds to μ-opiate receptors in the CNS causing inhibition of ascending pain pathways, altering the perception of and response to pain; also inhibits the reuptake of norepinephrine and serotonin, which also modifies the ascending pain pathway

Contraindications Hypersensitivity to acetaminophen, tramadol, opioids, or any component of the formulation; opioid-dependent patients; acute intoxication with ethanol, hypnotics, narcotics, centrally-acting analgesics, opioids, or psychotropic drugs; hepatic dysfunction

Warnings/Precautions May cause CNS depression, which may impair physical or mental abilities; patients must be cautioned about performing tasks which require mental alertness (eg, operating machinery or driving). Should be used only with extreme caution in patients receiving MAO inhibitors. Use with caution and reduce dosage when administering to patients receiving other CNS depressants. Seizures may occur when taken within the recommended dosage; risk is increased in patients receiving serotonin reuptake inhibitors (SSRIs or anorectics), tricyclic antidepressants, other cyclic compounds (including cyclobenzaprine, promethazine), neuroleptics, MAO inhibitors, or drugs which may lower seizure threshold. Patients with a history of seizures, or with a risk of seizures (head trauma, metabolic disorders, CNS infection, malignancy, or during alcohol/drug withdrawal) are also at increased risk.

Limit acetaminophen to <4 g/day. May cause severe hepatic toxicity in acute overdose; in addition, chronic daily dosing in adults has resulted in liver damage in some patients. Use with caution in patients with alcoholic liver disease; consuming ≥3 alcoholic drinks/day may increase the risk of liver damage. Use caution in patients with known G6PD deficiency.

Elderly, debilitated patients and patients with chronic respiratory disorders may be at greater risk of adverse events. Use with caution in patients with increased intracranial pressure or head injury. May obscure diagnosis or clinical course of patients with acute abdominal conditions. Use tramadol with caution and reduce dosage in patients with renal dysfunction. Tolerance or drug dependence may result from extended use (withdrawal symptoms have been reported); abrupt discontinuation should be avoided. Tapering of dose at the time of discontinuation limits the risk of withdrawal symptoms. Safety and efficacy in pediatric patients have not been established.

Drug Interactions

Acetaminophen: **Substrate** (minor) of CYP1A2, 2A6, 2C9, 2D6, 2E1, 3A4; **Inhibits** CYP3A4 (weak)

Tramadol: **Substrate** of CYP2D6 (major), 3A4 (minor)

Amphetamines: May increase the risk of seizures with tramadol.

Anesthetic agents: May increase risk of CNS and respiratory depression; use together with caution and in reduced dosage.

Barbiturates: Barbiturates may increase the hepatotoxic effects of acetaminophen; in addition, acetaminophen levels may be lowered.

Carbamazepine: Carbamazepine decreases half-life of tramadol by 33% to 50%; also have increased risk of seizures; in addition, carbamazepine may increase the hepatotoxic effects and lower serum levels of acetaminophen; concomitant use is not recommended.

CYP2D6 inhibitors: May decrease the effects of tramadol. Example inhibitors include chlorpromazine, delavirdine, fluoxetine, miconazole, paroxetine, pergolide, quinidine, quinine, ritonavir, and ropinirole.

Digoxin: Rare reports of digoxin toxicity with concomitant tramadol use.

Hydantoin anticonvulsants: Phenytoin may increase the hepatotoxic effects of acetaminophen; in addition, acetaminophen levels may be lowered.

MAO inhibitors: May increase the risk of seizures. Use extreme caution.

Naloxone: May increase the risk of seizures (if administered in tramadol overdose).

Neuroleptic agents: May increase the risk of tramadol-associated seizures and may have additive CNS depressant effects.

Narcotics: May increase risk of CNS and respiratory depression; use together with caution and in reduced dosage.

Opioids: May increase the risk of seizures, and may have additive CNS depressant effects. Use together with caution and in reduced dosage.

Phenothiazines: May increase risk of CNS and respiratory depression; use together with caution and in reduced dosage.

Rifampin: Rifampin may increase the clearance of acetaminophen.

Quinidine: May increase the tramadol serum concentrations by inhibiting CYP metabolism.

SSRIs: May increase the risk of seizures with tramadol by inhibiting CYP metabolism (citalopram, fluoxetine, paroxetine, sertraline).

Sulfinpyrazone: Sulfinpyrazone may increase the hepatotoxic effects of acetaminophen; in addition, acetaminophen levels may be lowered.

Tricyclic antidepressants: May increase the risk of seizures.

Warfarin: Acetaminophen and tramadol may lead to an elevation of prothrombin times; monitor.

Ethanol/Nutrition/Herb Interactions
Ethanol: Avoid ethanol (increased liver toxicity with concomitant use).

Food: May delay time to peak plasma levels, however, the extent of absorption is not affected.

Herb/Nutraceutical:

Acetaminophen: Avoid St John's wort (may decrease acetaminophen levels).

Tramadol: Avoid valerian, St John's wort, kava kava, gotu kola (may increase CNS depression).

Dietary Considerations May be taken with or without food. Avoid use of ethanol and ethanol-containing products.

Pharmacodynamics/Kinetics See individual agents.

Pregnancy Risk Factor C

Lactation Tramadol: Enters breast milk/contraindicated

Breast-Feeding Considerations Not recommended for postdelivery analgesia in nursing mothers.

Dosage Forms Excipient information presented when available (limited, particularly for generics); consult specific product labeling.

Tablet: Acetaminophen 325 mg and tramadol hydrochloride 37.5 mg

Selected Readings
Fricke JR Jr, Hewitt DJ, Jordan DM, et al, "A Double-Blind Placebo-Controlled Comparison of Tramadol/Acetaminophen and Tramadol in Patients With Postoperative Dental Pain," *Pain*, 2004, 109(3):250-7.

Fricke JR Jr, Karim R, Jordan D, et al, "A Double-Blind, Single-Dose Comparison of the Analgesic Efficacy of Tramadol/Acetaminophen Combination Tablets, Hydrocodone/Acetaminophen Combination Tablets, and Placebo After Oral Surgery," *Clin Ther*, 2002, 24(6):953-68.

Hiller B and Rosenberg M, "Ultracet: A New Combination Analgesic," *J Mass Dent Soc*, 2003, 52(2):38-40.

Medve RA, Wang J, and Karim R, "Tramadol and Acetaminophen Tablets for Dental Pain," *Anesth Prog*, 2001, 48(3):79-81.

Smith AB, Ravikumar TS, Kamin M, et al, "Combination Tramadol Plus Acetaminophen for Postsurgical Pain," *Am J Surg*, 2004, 187(4):521-7.

Wynn RL, "NSAIDS and Cardiovascular Effects, Celecoxib for Dental Pain, and a New Analgesic - Tramadol with Acetaminophen," *Gen Dent*, 2002, 50(3):218-222.

Acetaminophen, Aspirin, and Caffeine
(a seet a MIN oh fen, AS pir in, & KAF een)

Related Information
Acetaminophen *on page 31*
Aspirin *on page 149*
Caffeine *on page 255*

U.S. Brand Names Excedrin® Extra Strength [OTC]; Excedrin® Migraine [OTC]; Fem-Prin® [OTC]; Genaced™ [OTC]; Goody's® Extra Strength Headache Powder [OTC]; Goody's® Extra Strength Pain Relief [OTC]; Pain-Off [OTC]; Vanquish® Extra Strength Pain Reliever [OTC]

Generic Available Yes

Index Terms Aspirin, Acetaminophen, and Caffeine; Aspirin, Caffeine and Acetaminophen; Caffeine, Acetaminophen, and Aspirin; Caffeine, Aspirin, and Acetaminophen

Pharmacologic Category Analgesic, Miscellaneous

Use Relief of mild-to-moderate pain; mild-to-moderate pain associated with migraine headache

Local Anesthetic/Vasoconstrictor Precautions No information available to require special precautions

Effects on Dental Treatment No significant effects or complications reported

Common Adverse Effects See individual agents.

(Continued)

Acetaminophen, Aspirin, and Caffeine (Continued)

Drug Interactions

Cytochrome P450 Effect:

Acetaminophen: **Substrate** (minor) of CYP1A2, 2A6, 2C9, 2D6, 2E1, 3A4; **Inhibits** CYP3A4 (weak)

Aspirin: **Substrate** (minor) of CYP2C9

Caffeine: **Substrate** of CYP1A2 (major), 2C9 (minor), 2D6 (minor), 2E1 (minor), 3A4 (minor); **Inhibits** CYP1A2 (weak), 3A4 (moderate)

Increased Effect/Toxicity: See individual agents.

Decreased Effect: See individual agents.

Pharmacodynamics/Kinetics See individual agents.

Pregnancy Risk Factor D

Acetaminophen, Butalbital, and Caffeine see Butalbital, Acetaminophen, and Caffeine on page 247

Acetaminophen, Caffeine, and Dihydrocodeine
(a seet a MIN oh fen, KAF een, & dye hye droe KOE deen)

Related Information

Acetaminophen on page 31
Caffeine on page 255

U.S. Brand Names Panlor® DC; Panlor® SS; ZerLor™

Generic Available Yes: Tablet

Index Terms Caffeine, Dihydrocodeine, and Acetaminophen; Dihydrocodeine Bitartrate, Acetaminophen, and Caffeine

Pharmacologic Category Analgesic Combination (Opioid)

Dental Use Relief of moderate to moderately-severe dental pain

Use Relief of moderate to moderately-severe pain

Local Anesthetic/Vasoconstrictor Precautions No information available to require special precautions

Effects on Dental Treatment No significant effects or complications reported

Significant Adverse Effects Frequency not defined. Most common reactions with this combination include:

Central nervous system: Dizziness, drowsiness, lightheadedness, sedation
Dermatologic: Pruritus, skin reactions
Gastrointestinal: Constipation, nausea, vomiting

Restrictions C-III

Dental Usual Dosing Relief of moderate-to-moderately severe dental pain: Adults: Oral:

Panlor® DC: 2 capsules every 4 hours as needed; adjust dose based on severity of pain (maximum dose: 10 capsules/24 hours)

Panlor® SS: 1 tablet every 4 hours as needed; adjust dose based on severity of pain (maximum dose: 5 tablets/24 hours)

Dosage Oral: Adults: Relief of pain:

Panlor® DC: 2 capsules every 4 hours as needed; adjust dose based on severity of pain (maximum dose: 10 capsules/24 hours)

Panlor® SS, ZerLor™: 1 tablet every 4 hours as needed; adjust dose based on severity of pain (maximum dose: 5 tablets/24 hours)

Mechanism of Action

Acetaminophen inhibits the synthesis of prostaglandins in the central nervous system and peripherally blocks pain impulse generation; produces antipyresis from inhibition of hypothalamic heat-regulating center.

Caffeine is a CNS stimulant; use with acetaminophen and dihydrocodeine increases the level of analgesia provided by each agent.

Dihydrocodeine binds to opiate receptors in the CNS, causing inhibition of ascending pain pathways, altering the perception of and response to pain; produces generalized CNS depression.

Contraindications Hypersensitivity to acetaminophen, caffeine, dihydrocodeine, codeine, or any component of the formulation; significant respiratory depression (in unmonitored settings); acute or severe bronchial asthma; hypercapnia; paralytic ileus

Warnings/Precautions Acetaminophen may cause severe hepatotoxicity in acute overdose; limit acetaminophen to <4 g/day; in addition, chronic daily dosing in adults has resulted in liver damage in some patients. Use with caution in patients with alcoholic liver disease; consuming ≥3 alcoholic drinks/day may increase the risk of liver damage. Use caution in patients with known G6PD deficiency. Caffeine may cause CNS and cardiovascular stimulation as well as GI irritation in high doses. Dihydrocodeine should be used with caution in patients with hypersensitivity reactions to other phenanthrene-derivative opioid agonists (morphine, hydrocodone, hydromorphone, levorphanol, oxycodone, oxymorphone), respiratory diseases including asthma, emphysema, COPD, history of drug abuse or severe hepatic or renal insufficiency. Use caution with MAO inhibitors.

This combination should be used with caution in elderly or debilitated patients, hypotension, adrenocortical insufficiency, thyroid disorders, prostatic hyperplasia, urethral stricture, seizure disorder, CNS depression, head injury or increased intracranial pressure. Causes sedation; caution must be used in performing tasks which require alertness (eg, operating machinery or driving). Safety and efficacy in pediatric patients have not been established.

Drug Interactions

Acetaminophen: **Substrate** (minor) of CYP1A2, 2A6, 2C9, 2D6, 2E1, 3A4; **Inhibits** CYP3A4 (weak)

Caffeine: **Substrate** of CYP1A2 (major), 2C9 (minor), 2D6 (minor), 2E1 (minor), 3A4 (minor); **Inhibits** CYP1A2 (weak), 3A4 (moderate)

Dihydrocodeine: **Substrate** of CYP2D6 (major)

Acetaminophen: See individual agents for associated interactions.

Caffeine:

CYP1A2 inhibitors: May increase the levels/effects of caffeine. Example inhibitors include amiodarone, fluvoxamine, ketoconazole, and rofecoxib.

CYP3A4 substrates: Caffeine may increase the levels/effects of CYP3A4 substrates. Example substrates include benzodiazepines, calcium channel blockers, ergot derivatives, mirtazapine, nateglinide, nefazodone, tacrolimus, and venlafaxine.

Quinolone antibiotics (specifically ciprofloxacin, norfloxacin, ofloxacin): Quinolones may increase the level/effects of caffeine.

Dihydrocodeine:

CYP2D6 inhibitors: May decrease the effects of dihydrocodeine. Example inhibitors include chlorpromazine, delavirdine, fluoxetine, miconazole, paroxetine, pergolide, quinidine, quinine, ritonavir, and ropinirole.

Quinidine: Quinidine may decrease the effects of dihydrocodeine.

Ethanol/Nutrition/Herb Interactions

Ethanol: Excessive intake of ethanol may increase the risk of acetaminophen-induced toxicity. Ethanol may also increase CNS depression.

Pregnancy Risk Factor C

Lactation Enters breast milk/not recommended

Breast-Feeding Considerations Acetaminophen and caffeine are both excreted in breast milk. Specific information for dihydrocodeine is not available; however, similar agents (eg, codeine, morphine) are excreted in breast milk.

Dosage Forms Excipient information presented when available (limited, particularly for generics); consult specific product labeling.

Capsule:

Panlor® DC: Acetaminophen 356.4 mg, caffeine 30 mg, and dihydrocodeine bitartrate 16 mg

Tablet:

Panlor® SS, ZerLor™: Acetaminophen 712.8 mg, caffeine 60 mg, and dihydrocodeine bitartrate 32 mg

Acetaminophen, Caffeine, Codeine, and Butalbital see Butalbital, Acetaminophen, Caffeine, and Codeine on page 248

Acetaminophen, Caffeine, Hydrocodone, Chlorpheniramine, and Phenylephrine see Hydrocodone, Chlorpheniramine, Phenylephrine, Acetaminophen, and Caffeine on page 833

Acetaminophen, Chlorpheniramine, and Pseudoephedrine

(a seet a MIN oh fen, klor fen IR a meen, & soo doe e FED rin)

Related Information

Acetaminophen on page 31
Chlorpheniramine on page 338
Pseudoephedrine on page 1381

U.S. Brand Names Actifed® Cold and Sinus [OTC]; Alka-Seltzer® Plus Cold Liqui-Gels® [OTC]; Comtrex® Flu Therapy Day/Night [OTC]; Comtrex® Flu Therapy Nighttime [OTC]; Drinex [OTC]; Kolephrin® [OTC]; Sinutab® Sinus Allergy Maximum Strength [OTC]; Tylenol® Allergy Complete [OTC] [DSC]; Tylenol® Children's Plus Cold Nighttime [OTC]

Canadian Brand Names Sinutab® Sinus & Allergy; Tylenol® Allergy Sinus

Generic Available Yes

Index Terms Acetaminophen, Pseudoephedrine, and Chlorpheniramine; Chlorpheniramine, Acetaminophen, and Pseudoephedrine; Chlorpheniramine, Pseudoephedrine, and Acetaminophen; Pseudoephedrine, Acetaminophen, and Chlorpheniramine; Pseudoephedrine, Chlorpheniramine, and Acetaminophen

(Continued)

Acetaminophen, Chlorpheniramine, and Pseudoephedrine *(Continued)*

Pharmacologic Category Analgesic, Miscellaneous; Antihistamine

Use Temporary relief of sinus symptoms

Local Anesthetic/Vasoconstrictor Precautions Use with caution since pseudoephedrine is a sympathomimetic amine which could interact with epinephrine to cause a pressor response

Effects on Dental Treatment Key adverse event(s) related to dental treatment:

Chlorpheniramine: Significant xerostomia with prolonged use (normal salivary flow resumes upon discontinuation).

Pseudoephedrine: Xerostomia (normal salivary flow resumes upon discontinuation).

Common Adverse Effects See individual agents.

Drug Interactions

Cytochrome P450 Effect:

Acetaminophen: **Substrate** (minor) of CYP1A2, 2A6, 2C9, 2D6, 2E1, 3A4; **Inhibits** CYP3A4 (weak)

Chlorpheniramine: **Substrate** of CYP2D6 (minor), 3A4 (major); **Inhibits** CYP2D6 (weak)

Increased Effect/Toxicity: See individual agents.

Decreased Effect: See individual agents.

Pharmacodynamics/Kinetics See individual agents.

Pregnancy Risk Factor B

Acetaminophen, Dextromethorphan, and Pseudoephedrine

(a seet a MIN oh fen, deks troe meth OR fan, & soo doe e FED rin)

Related Information

Acetaminophen *on page 31*

Dextromethorphan *on page 477*

Pseudoephedrine *on page 1381*

U.S. Brand Names Comtrex® Non-Drowsy Cold and Cough Relief [OTC] [DSC]; Infants' Tylenol® Cold Plus Cough Concentrated Drops [OTC] [DSC]; Sudafed® Severe Cold [OTC]; Triaminic® Cough and Sore Throat Formula [OTC] [DSC]; Tylenol® Cold Day Non-Drowsy [OTC]; Tylenol® Flu Non-Drowsy Maximum Strength [OTC]; Vicks® DayQuil® Multi-Symptom Cold and Flu [OTC] [DSC]

Canadian Brand Names Contac® Complete; Contac® Cough, Cold and Flu Day & Night™; Sudafed® Cold & Cough Extra Strength; Tylenol® Cold Daytime

Generic Available No

Index Terms Dextromethorphan, Acetaminophen, and Pseudoephedrine; Pseudoephedrine, Acetaminophen, and Dextromethorphan; Pseudoephedrine, Dextromethorphan, and Acetaminophen

Pharmacologic Category Antihistamine; Antitussive

Use Treatment of mild-to-moderate pain and fever; symptomatic relief of cough and congestion

Local Anesthetic/Vasoconstrictor Precautions Use with caution since pseudoephedrine is a sympathomimetic amine which could interact with epinephrine to cause a pressor response

Effects on Dental Treatment Key adverse event(s) related to dental treatment: Pseudoephedrine: Xerostomia (normal salivary flow resumes upon discontinuation)

Common Adverse Effects See individual agents.

Drug Interactions

Cytochrome P450 Effect:

Acetaminophen: **Substrate** (minor) of CYP1A2, 2A6, 2C9, 2D6, 2E1, 3A4; **Inhibits** CYP3A4 (weak)

Dextromethorphan: **Substrate** of CYP2B6 (minor), 2C9 (minor), 2C19 (minor), 2D6 (major), 2E1 (minor), 3A4 (minor); **Inhibits** CYP2D6 (weak)

Increased Effect/Toxicity: See individual agents.

Decreased Effect: See individual agents.

Pharmacodynamics/Kinetics See individual agents.

Acetaminophen, Dichloralphenazone, and Isometheptene *see* Acetaminophen, Isometheptene, and Dichloralphenazone *on page 45*

Acetaminophen, Isometheptene, and Dichloralphenazone

(a seet a MIN oh fen, eye soe me THEP teen, & dye KLOR al FEN a zone)

Related Information
Acetaminophen *on page 31*
U.S. Brand Names Amidrine [DSC]; Duradrin®; Midrin®; Migquin; Migratine; Migrazone®; Migrin-A
Generic Available Yes
Index Terms Acetaminophen, Dichloralphenazone, and Isometheptene; Dichloralphenazone, Acetaminophen, and Isometheptene; Dichloralphenazone, Isometheptene, and Acetaminophen; Isometheptene, Acetaminophen, and Dichloralphenazone; Isometheptene, Dichloralphenazone, and Acetaminophen
Pharmacologic Category Analgesic, Miscellaneous
Use Relief of migraine and tension headache
Local Anesthetic/Vasoconstrictor Precautions No information available to require special precautions
Effects on Dental Treatment No significant effects or complications reported
Common Adverse Effects Frequency not defined.
Central nervous system: Transient dizziness
Dermatological: Rash
Restrictions C-IV
Drug Interactions
Cytochrome P450 Effect: Acetaminophen: **Substrate** (minor) of CYP1A2, 2A6, 2C9, 2D6, 2E1, 3A4; **Inhibits** CYP3A4 (weak)
Increased Effect/Toxicity: See individual agents.
Decreased Effect: See individual agents.

Acetaminophen, Pseudoephedrine, and Chlorpheniramine *see* Acetaminophen, Chlorpheniramine, and Pseudoephedrine *on page 43*

Acetasol® HC *see* Acetic Acid, Propylene Glycol Diacetate, and Hydrocortisone *on page 45*

AcetaZOLAMIDE (a set a ZOLE a mide)

U.S. Brand Names Diamox® Sequels®
Canadian Brand Names Apo-Acetazolamide®; Diamox®
Mexican Brand Names Acetadiazol; Diamox
Generic Available Yes: Injection, tablet
Pharmacologic Category Anticonvulsant, Miscellaneous; Carbonic Anhydrase Inhibitor; Diuretic, Carbonic Anhydrase Inhibitor; Ophthalmic Agent, Antiglaucoma
Use Treatment of glaucoma (chronic simple open-angle, secondary glaucoma, preoperatively in acute angle-closure); drug-induced edema or edema due to congestive heart failure (adjunctive therapy); centrencephalic epilepsies (immediate release dosage form); prevention or amelioration of symptoms associated with acute mountain sickness
Unlabeled/Investigational Use Urine alkalinization; respiratory stimulant in COPD; metabolic alkalosis
Local Anesthetic/Vasoconstrictor Precautions No information available to require special precautions
Effects on Dental Treatment Key adverse event(s) related to dental treatment: Metallic taste (resolves upon discontinuation)
Mechanism of Action Reversible inhibition of the enzyme carbonic anhydrase resulting in reduction of hydrogen ion secretion at renal tubule and an increased renal excretion of sodium, potassium, bicarbonate, and water to decrease production of aqueous humor; also inhibits carbonic anhydrase in central nervous system to retard abnormal and excessive discharge from CNS neurons
Pregnancy Risk Factor C

Acetic Acid, Hydrocortisone, and Propylene Glycol Diacetate *see* Acetic Acid, Propylene Glycol Diacetate, and Hydrocortisone *on page 45*

Acetic Acid, Propylene Glycol Diacetate, and Hydrocortisone

(a SEE tik AS id, PRO pa leen GLY kole dye AS e tate, & hye droe KOR ti sone)

Related Information
Hydrocortisone *on page 836*
(Continued)

Acetic Acid, Propylene Glycol Diacetate, and Hydrocortisone *(Continued)*

U.S. Brand Names Acetasol® HC; VoSol® HC

Generic Available Yes

Index Terms Acetic Acid, Hydrocortisone, and Propylene Glycol Diacetate; Hydrocortisone, Acetic Acid, and Propylene Glycol Diacetate; Propylene Glycol Diacetate, Acetic Acid, and Hydrocortisone

Pharmacologic Category Otic Agent, Anti-infective

Use Treatment of superficial infections of the external auditory canal caused by organisms susceptible to the action of the antimicrobial, complicated by swelling

Local Anesthetic/Vasoconstrictor Precautions No information available to require special precautions

Effects on Dental Treatment No significant effects or complications reported

---

Acetohydroxamic Acid *(a SEE toe hye droks am ik AS id)*

U.S. Brand Names Lithostat®

Canadian Brand Names Lithostat®

Generic Available No

Index Terms AHA

Pharmacologic Category Urinary Tract Product

Use Adjunctive therapy in chronic urea-splitting urinary infection

Local Anesthetic/Vasoconstrictor Precautions No information available to require special precautions

Effects on Dental Treatment No significant effects or complications reported

Common Adverse Effects Frequency not defined.

Cardiovascular: Deep vein thrombosis (rare), embolism, palpitation, phlebitis

Central nervous system: Anorexia, anxiety, depression, headache, malaise, nervousness, tremor

Dermatologic: Flushing (with ethanol consumption), rash (nonpruritic, macular)

Gastrointestinal: Nausea, vomiting

Hematologic: Hemolytic anemia (15% with laboratory evidence; ~3% severe requiring discontinuation; may be accompanied by GI symptoms or systemic complaints of malaise and/or fatigue); hyperbilirubinemia

Respiratory: Pulmonary embolism (rare)

Mechanism of Action Acetohydroxamic acid inhibits bacterial urease enzymes, decreasing the formation of ammonia in the urine by urea-splitting organisms. A reduction in urinary ammonia may increase the antibacterial activity of some antibiotic agents.

Drug Interactions

Decreased Effect: Acetohydroxamic acid may chelate divalent metals, decreasing the absorption of both agents; avoid concurrent use. Orally-administered iron may be chelated by acetohydroxamic acid, decreasing the absorption of both agents (parenteral iron should be used to treat hypochromic anemia).

Pregnancy Risk Factor X

Acetoxymethylprogesterone *see* MedroxyPROGESTERone *on page 1026*

Acetylcholine *(a se teel KOE leen)*

U.S. Brand Names Miochol®-E

Canadian Brand Names Miochol®-E

Generic Available No

Index Terms Acetylcholine Chloride

Pharmacologic Category Cholinergic Agonist; Ophthalmic Agent, Miotic

Use Produces complete miosis in cataract surgery, keratoplasty, iridectomy, and other anterior segment surgery where rapid miosis is required

Local Anesthetic/Vasoconstrictor Precautions No information available to require special precautions

Effects on Dental Treatment No significant effects or complications reported

Mechanism of Action Causes contraction of the sphincter muscles of the iris, resulting in miosis and contraction of the ciliary muscle, leading to accommodation spasm

Pregnancy Risk Factor C

Acetylcholine Chloride *see* Acetylcholine *on page 46*

Acetylcysteine (a se teel SIS teen)

U.S. Brand Names Acetadote®
Canadian Brand Names Acetylcysteine Solution; Mucomyst®; Parvolex®
Mexican Brand Names ACC
Generic Available Yes: Solution for inhalation
Index Terms Acetylcysteine Sodium; Mercapturic Acid; Mucomyst; NAC; N-Acetylcysteine; N-Acetyl-L-cysteine
Pharmacologic Category Antidote; Mucolytic Agent
Use Adjunctive mucolytic therapy in patients with abnormal or viscid mucous secretions in acute and chronic bronchopulmonary diseases; pulmonary complications of surgery and cystic fibrosis; diagnostic bronchial studies; antidote for acute acetaminophen toxicity
Unlabeled/Investigational Use Prevention of radiocontrast-induced renal dysfunction (oral, I.V.); distal intestinal obstruction syndrome (DIOS, previously referred to as meconium ileus equivalent)
Local Anesthetic/Vasoconstrictor Precautions No information available to require special precautions
Effects on Dental Treatment Key adverse event(s) related to dental treatment: Stomatitis, drowsiness, fever, vomiting, nausea, bronchospasm, rhinorrhea, hemoptysis, and dizziness
Common Adverse Effects
  Inhalation: Frequency not defined.
    Central nervous system: Drowsiness, chills, fever
    Gastrointestinal: Vomiting, nausea, stomatitis
    Local: Irritation, stickiness on face following nebulization
    Respiratory: Bronchospasm, rhinorrhea, hemoptysis
    Miscellaneous: Acquired sensitization (rare), clamminess, unpleasant odor during administration
  Intravenous:
  >10%: Miscellaneous: Anaphylactoid reaction (~17%; reported as severe in 1% or moderate in 10% of patients within 15 minutes of first infusion; severe in 1% or mild to moderate in 6% to 7% of patients after 60-minute infusion)
  1% to 10%:
    Cardiovascular: Angioedema (2% to 8%), vasodilation (1% to 6%), hypotension (1% to 4%), tachycardia (1% to 4%), syncope (1% to 3%), chest tightness (1%), flushing (1%)
    Central nervous system: Dysphoria (<1% to 2%)
    Dermatologic: Urticaria (2% to 7%), rash (1% to 5%), facial erythema (≤1%), palmar erythema (≤1%), pruritus (≤1% to 3%), pruritus with rash and vasodilation (2% to 9%)
    Gastrointestinal: Vomiting (<1% to 10%), nausea (1% to 10%), dyspepsia (≤1%)
    Neuromuscular & skeletal: Gait disturbance (<1% to 2%)
    Ocular: Eye pain (<1% to 3%)
    Otic: Ear pain (1%)
    Respiratory: Bronchospasm (1% to 6%), cough (1% to 4%), dyspnea (<1% to 3%), pharyngitis (1%), rhinorrhea (1%), rhonchi (1%), throat tightness (1%)
    Miscellaneous: Diaphoresis (≤1%)
Mechanism of Action Exerts mucolytic action through its free sulfhydryl group which opens up the disulfide bonds in the mucoproteins thus lowering mucous viscosity. The exact mechanism of action in acetaminophen toxicity is unknown; thought to act by providing substrate for conjugation with the toxic metabolite.
Drug Interactions
  Decreased Effect: Adsorbed by activated charcoal; clinical significance is minimal, though, once a pure acetaminophen ingestion requiring N-acetylcysteine is established; further charcoal dosing is unnecessary once the appropriate initial charcoal dose is achieved (5-10 g:g acetaminophen)
Pharmacodynamics/Kinetics
  Onset of action: Inhalation: 5-10 minutes
  Duration: Inhalation: >1 hour
  Distribution: 0.47 L/kg
  Protein binding, plasma: 83%
  Half-life elimination:
    Reduced acetylcysteine: 2 hours
    Total acetylcysteine: Adults: 5.5 hours; Newborns: 11 hours
  Time to peak, plasma: Oral: 1-2 hours
  Excretion: Urine
Pregnancy Risk Factor B

Acetylcysteine Sodium see Acetylcysteine on page 47
Acetylsalicylic Acid see Aspirin on page 149

Acrivastine and Pseudoephedrine
(AK ri vas teen & soo doe e FED rin)

Related Information
Pseudoephedrine *on page 1381*

U.S. Brand Names Semprex®-D

Generic Available No

Index Terms Pseudoephedrine Hydrochloride and Acrivastine

Pharmacologic Category Antihistamine

Use Temporary relief of nasal congestion, decongest sinus openings, running nose, itching of nose or throat, and itchy, watery eyes due to hay fever or other upper respiratory allergies

Local Anesthetic/Vasoconstrictor Precautions Use with caution since pseudoephedrine is a sympathomimetic amine which could interact with epinephrine to cause a pressor response

Effects on Dental Treatment Key adverse event(s) related to dental treatment: Pseudoephedrine: Xerostomia (normal salivary flow resumes upon discontinuation).

Common Adverse Effects
>10%: Central nervous system: Drowsiness, headache

1% to 10%:
Cardiovascular: Tachycardia, palpitation
Central nervous system: Nervousness, dizziness, insomnia, vertigo, lightheadedness, fatigue
Gastrointestinal: Nausea, vomiting, xerostomia, diarrhea
Genitourinary: Dysuria
Neuromuscular & skeletal: Weakness
Respiratory: Pharyngitis, cough increased
Miscellaneous: Diaphoresis

Mechanism of Action Refer to Pseudoephedrine; acrivastine is an analogue of triprolidine and it is considered to be relatively less sedating than traditional antihistamines; believed to involve competitive blockade of H_1-receptor sites resulting in the inability of histamine to combine with its receptor sites and exert its usual effects on target cells

Drug Interactions
Increased Effect/Toxicity: Increased risk of hypertensive crisis when acrivastine and pseudoephedrine are given with MAO inhibitors or sympathomimetics. Increased risk of severe CNS depression when given with CNS depressants and ethanol.

Decreased Effect: Decreased effect of guanethidine, reserpine, methyldopa, and beta-blockers when given in conjunction with acrivastine and pseudoephedrine.

Pharmacodynamics/Kinetics
Pseudoephedrine: See Pseudoephedrine.
Acrivastine:
Metabolism: Minimally hepatic
Time to peak: ~1.1 hours
Excretion: Urine (84%); feces (13%)

Pregnancy Risk Factor B

Acticin® *see* Permethrin *on page 1284*

Actidose-Aqua® [OTC] *see* Charcoal, Activated *on page 327*

Actidose® with Sorbitol [OTC] *see* Charcoal, Activated *on page 327*

Actifed® Cold and Allergy [OTC] [DSC] *see* Triprolidine and Pseudoephedrine *on page 1624*

Actifed® Cold and Sinus [OTC] *see* Acetaminophen, Chlorpheniramine, and Pseudoephedrine *on page 43*

Actigall® *see* Ursodiol *on page 1634*

Actimmune® *see* Interferon Gamma-1b *on page 899*

Actinomycin *see* Dactinomycin *on page 437*

Actinomycin D *see* Dactinomycin *on page 437*

Actinomycin Cl *see* Dactinomycin *on page 437*

Actiq® *see* Fentanyl *on page 679*

Activase® *see* Alteplase *on page 78*

Activated Carbon *see* Charcoal, Activated *on page 327*

Activated Charcoal *see* Charcoal, Activated *on page 327*

Activated Dimethicone *see* Simethicone *on page 1472*

Activated Ergosterol *see* Ergocalciferol *on page 583*

Activated Methylpolysiloxane *see* Simethicone *on page 1472*

Activated Protein C, Human, Recombinant *see* Drotrecogin Alfa *on page 548*

Activella® *see* Estradiol and Norethindrone *on page 603*

Actonel® *see* Risedronate *on page 1428*

Actonel® and Calcium *see* Risedronate and Calcium *on page 1431*

Actoplus Met™ *see* Pioglitazone and Metformin *on page 1309*

Actos® *see* Pioglitazone *on page 1307*

ACT® Plus [OTC] *see* Fluoride *on page 710*

ACT® x2™ [OTC] *see* Fluoride *on page 710*

Acular® *see* Ketorolac *on page 934*

Acular LS™ *see* Ketorolac *on page 934*

Acular® PF *see* Ketorolac *on page 934*

ACV *see* Acyclovir *on page 49*

Acycloguanosine *see* Acyclovir *on page 49*

Acyclovir (ay SYE kloe veer)

Related Information
Systemic Viral Diseases *on page 1767*
Treatment of Sexually-Transmitted Infections *on page 1920*
Valacyclovir *on page 1635*
Viral Infections *on page 1806*

Related Sample Prescriptions
Herpes Simplex (Primary) *on page 1843*
Shingles (Varicella-Zoster Virus) *on page 1843*

U.S. Brand Names Zovirax®

Canadian Brand Names Apo-Acyclovir®; Gen-Acyclovir; Nu-Acyclovir; ratio-Acyclovir; Zovirax®

Mexican Brand Names Cicloferon; Laciken; Olvit; Opthavir; Zetavir; Zovirax

Generic Available Yes: Excludes cream, ointment

Index Terms Aciclovir; ACV; Acycloguanosine

Pharmacologic Category Antiviral Agent

Dental Use Treatment of initial and prophylaxis of recurrent mucosal and cutaneous herpes simplex (HSV-1 and HSV-2) infections in immunocompromised patients

Use Treatment of genital herpes simplex virus (HSV), herpes labialis (cold sores), herpes zoster (shingles), HSV encephalitis, neonatal HSV, mucocutaneous HSV in immunocompromised patients, varicella-zoster (chickenpox)

Unlabeled/Investigational Use Prevention of HSV reactivation in HIV-positive patients; prevention of HSV reactivation in hematopoietic stem-cell transplant (HSCT); prevention of HSV reactivation during periods of neutropenia in patients with acute leukemia

Local Anesthetic/Vasoconstrictor Precautions No information available to require special precautions

Effects on Dental Treatment Key adverse event(s) related to dental treatment: Topical (Zovirax® cream): Dry/cracked lips and dry/flaky skin were reported in fewer than 1 in 100 patients in clinical studies.

Significant Adverse Effects
Systemic: Oral:
>10%: Central nervous system: Malaise (12%)
(Continued)

Acyclovir *(Continued)*

1% to 10%:
  Central nervous system: Headache (2%)
  Gastrointestinal: Nausea (2% to 5%), vomiting (3%), diarrhea (2% to 3%)

Systemic: Parenteral:

1% to 10%:
  Dermatologic: Hives (2%), itching (2%), rash (2%)
  Gastrointestinal: Nausea/vomiting (7%)
  Hepatic: Liver function tests increased (1% to 2%)
  Local: Inflammation at injection site or phlebitis (9%)
  Renal: BUN increased (5% to 10%), creatinine increased (5% to 10%), acute renal failure

Topical:

>10%: Dermatologic: Mild pain, burning, or stinging (ointment 30%)

1% to 10%: Dermatologic: Pruritus (ointment 4%), itching

All forms: <1% (Limited to important or life-threatening): Abdominal pain, aggression, agitation, alopecia, anaphylaxis, anemia, angioedema, anorexia, ataxia, coma, confusion, consciousness decreased, delirium, desquamation, diarrhea, disseminated intravascular coagulopathy (DIC), dizziness, dry lips, dysarthria, encephalopathy, erythema multiforme, fatigue, fever, gastrointestinal distress, hallucinations, hematuria, hemolysis, hepatitis, hyperbilirubinemia, hypotension, insomnia, jaundice, leukocytoclastic vasculitis, leukocytosis, leukopenia, local tissue necrosis (following extravasation), lymphadenopathy, mental depression, myalgia, neutrophilia, paresthesia, peripheral edema, photosensitization, pruritus, psychosis, renal failure, seizure, somnolence, sore throat, Stevens-Johnson syndrome, thrombocytopenia, thrombocytopenic purpura/hemolytic uremic syndrome (TTP/HUS), thrombocytosis, toxic epidermal necrolysis, tremor, urticaria, visual disturbances

Dental Usual Dosing

Herpes labialis (cold sores): Children ≥12 years and Adults: Topical: Cream: Apply 5 times/day for 4 days

Mucocutaneous HSV: Adults:
  Immunocompromised (unlabeled use): Oral: 400 mg 5 times a day for 7-14 days
  Nonlife-threatening, immunocompromised: Topical: Ointment: 1/2" ribbon of ointment for a 4" square surface area every 3 hours (6 times/day) for 7 days

Dosage Note: Obese patients should be dosed using ideal body weight

Genital HSV:

I.V.: Children ≥12 years and Adults (immunocompetent): Initial episode, severe: 5 mg/kg every 8 hours for 5-7 days

Oral:
  Children:
    Initial episode (unlabeled use): 40-80 mg/kg/day divided into 3-4 doses for 5-10 days (maximum: 1 g/day)
    Chronic suppression (unlabeled use; limited data): 80 mg/kg/day in 3 divided doses (maximum: 1 g/day), re-evaluate after 12 months of treatment
  Adults:
    Initial episode: 200 mg every 4 hours while awake (5 times/day) for 10 days (per manufacturer's labeling); 400 mg 3 times/day for 5-10 days has also been reported
    Recurrence: 200 mg every 4 hours while awake (5 times/day) for 5 days (per manufacturer's labeling); begin at earliest signs of disease); 400 mg 3 times/day for 5 days has also been reported
    Chronic suppression: 400 mg twice daily or 200 mg 3-5 times/day, for up to 12 months followed by re-evaluation (per manufacturer's labeling); 400-1200 mg/day in 2-3 divided doses has also been reported

Topical: Adults (immunocompromised): Ointment: Initial episode: 1/2" ribbon of ointment for a 4" square surface area every 3 hours (6 times/day) for 7 days

Herpes labialis (cold sores): Topical: Children ≥12 years and Adults: Cream: Apply 5 times/day for 4 days

Herpes zoster (shingles):

Oral: Adults (immunocompetent): 800 mg every 4 hours (5 times/day) for 7-10 days

I.V.:
  Children <12 years (immunocompromised): 20 mg/kg/dose every 8 hours for 7 days
  Children ≥12 years and Adults (immunocompromised): 10 mg/kg/dose or 500 mg/m^2/dose every 8 hours for 7 days

HSV encephalitis: I.V.:

Children 3 months to 12 years: 20 mg/kg/dose every 8 hours for 10 days (per manufacturer's labeling); dosing for 14-21 days also reported

Children ≥12 years and Adults: 10 mg/kg/dose every 8 hours for 10 days (per manufacturer's labeling); 10-15 mg/kg/dose every 8 hours for 14-21 days also reported

Mucocutaneous HSV:

I.V.:

Children <12 years (immunocompromised): 10 mg/kg/dose every 8 hours for 7 days

Children ≥12 years and Adults (immunocompromised): 5 mg/kg/dose every 8 hours for 7 days (per manufacturer's labeling); dosing for up to 14 days also reported

Oral: Adults (immunocompromised, unlabeled use): 400 mg 5 times a day for 7-14 days

Topical: Ointment: Adults (nonlife-threatening, immunocompromised): 1/2" ribbon of ointment for a 4" square surface area every 3 hours (6 times/day) for 7 days

Neonatal HSV: I.V.: Neonate: Birth to 3 months: 10 mg/kg/dose every 8 hours for 10 days (manufacturer's labeling); 15 mg/kg/dose or 20 mg/kg/dose every 8 hours for 14-21 days has also been reported

Varicella-zoster (chickenpox): Begin treatment within the first 24 hours of rash onset:

Oral:

Children ≥2 years and ≤40 kg (immunocompetent): 20 mg/kg/dose (up to 800 mg/dose) 4 times/day for 5 days

Children >40 kg and Adults (immunocompetent): 800 mg/dose 4 times a day for 5 days

I.V.:

Children <1 year (immunocompromised, unlabeled use): 10 mg/kg/dose every 8 hours for 7-10 days

Children ≥1 year and Adults (immunocompromised, unlabeled use): 1500 mg/m^2/day divided every 8 hours or 10 mg/kg/dose every 8 hours for 7-10 days

Prevention of HSV reactivation in HIV-positive patients, for use only when recurrences are frequent or severe (unlabeled use): Oral:

Children: 80 mg/kg/day in 3-4 divided doses

Adults: 200 mg 3 times/day or 400 mg 2 times/day

Prevention of HSV reactivation in HSCT (unlabeled use): Note: Start at the beginning of conditioning therapy and continue until engraftment or until mucositis resolves (~30 days)

Oral: Adults: 200 mg 3 times/day

I.V.:

Children: 250 mg/m^2/dose every 8 hours or 125 mg/m^2/dose every 6 hours

Adults: 250 mg/m^2/dose every 12 hours

Bone marrow transplant recipients (unlabeled use): I.V.: Children and Adults: Allogeneic patients who are HSV and CMV seropositive: 500 mg/m^2/dose (10 mg/kg) every 8 hours; for clinically-symptomatic CMV infection, consider replacing acyclovir with ganciclovir

Dosing adjustment in renal impairment:

Oral:

Cl_{cr} 10-25 mL/minute/1.73 m^2: Normal dosing regimen 800 mg every 4 hours: Administer 800 mg every 8 hours

Cl_{cr} <10 mL/minute/1.73 m^2:

Normal dosing regimen 200 mg every 4 hours, 200 mg every 8 hours, or 400 mg every 12 hours: Administer 200 mg every 12 hours

Normal dosing regimen 800 mg every 4 hours: Administer 800 mg every 12 hours

I.V.:

Cl_{cr} 25-50 mL/minute/1.73 m^2: Administer recommended dose every 12 hours

Cl_{cr} 10-25 mL/minute/1.73 m^2: Administer recommended dose every 24 hours

Cl_{cr} <10 mL/minute/1.73 m^2: Administer 50% of recommended dose every 24 hours

Hemodialysis: Administer dose after dialysis

Peritoneal dialysis: No supplemental dose needed

CAVH: 3.5 mg/kg/day

CVVHD/CVVH: Adjust dose based upon Cl_{cr} 30 mL/minute

Mechanism of Action Acyclovir is converted to acyclovir monophosphate by virus-specific thymidine kinase then further converted to acyclovir triphosphate by other cellular enzymes. Acyclovir triphosphate inhibits DNA synthesis and (Continued)

Acyclovir *(Continued)*

viral replication by competing with deoxyguanosine triphosphate for viral DNA polymerase and being incorporated into viral DNA.

Contraindications Hypersensitivity to acyclovir, valacyclovir, or any component of the formulation

Warnings/Precautions Use with caution in immunocompromised patients; thrombocytopenic purpura/hemolytic uremic syndrome (TTP/HUS) has been reported. Use caution in the elderly, pre-existing renal disease, or in those receiving other nephrotoxic drugs. Renal failure (sometimes fatal) has been reported. Maintain adequate hydration during oral or intravenous therapy. Use I.V. preparation with caution in patients with underlying neurologic abnormalities, serious hepatic or electrolyte abnormalities, or substantial hypoxia.

Safety and efficacy of oral formulations have not been established in pediatric patients <2 years of age.

Chickenpox: Treatment should begin within 24 hours of appearance of rash; oral route not recommended for routine use in otherwise healthy children with varicella, but may be effective in patients at increased risk of moderate to severe infection (>12 years of age, chronic cutaneous or pulmonary disorders, long-term salicylate therapy, corticosteroid therapy).

Genital herpes: Physical contact should be avoided when lesions are present; transmission may also occur in the absence of symptoms. Treatment should begin with the first signs or symptoms.

Herpes labialis: For external use only to the lips and face; do not apply to eye or inside the mouth or nose. Treatment should begin with the first signs or symptoms.

Herpes zoster: Acyclovir should be started within 72 hours of appearance of rash to be effective.

Ethanol/Nutrition/Herb Interactions Food: Does not affect absorption of oral acyclovir.

Dietary Considerations May be taken with or without food. Acyclovir 500 mg injection contains sodium ~50 mg (~2 mEq).

Pharmacodynamics/Kinetics
Absorption: Oral: 15% to 30%
Distribution: V_d: 0.8 L/kg (63.6 L): Widely (eg, brain, kidney, lungs, liver, spleen, muscle, uterus, vagina, CSF)
Protein binding: 9% to 33%
Metabolism: Converted by viral enzymes to acyclovir monophosphate, and further converted to diphosphate then triphosphate (active form) by cellular enzymes
Bioavailability: Oral: 10% to 20% with normal renal function (bioavailability decreases with increased dose)
Half-life elimination: Terminal: Neonates: 4 hours; Children 1-12 years: 2-3 hours; Adults: 3 hours
Time to peak, serum: Oral: Within 1.5-2 hours
Excretion: Urine (62% to 90% as unchanged drug and metabolite)

Pregnancy Risk Factor B

Lactation Enters breast milk/use with caution (AAP rates "compatible")

Breast-Feeding Considerations Nursing mothers with herpetic lesions near or on the breast should avoid breast-feeding. Limited data suggest exposure to the nursing infant of ~0.3 mg/kg/day following oral administration of acyclovir to the mother.

Dosage Forms Excipient information presented when available (limited, particularly for generics); consult specific product labeling. [DSC] = Discontinued product
Capsule: 200 mg
 Zovirax®: 200 mg
Cream, topical:
 Zovirax®: 5% (2 g, 5 g)
Injection, powder for reconstitution, as sodium: 500 mg, 1000 mg
 Zovirax®: 500 mg [DSC]
Injection, solution, as sodium [preservative free]: 25 mg/mL (20 mL, 40 mL); 50 mg/mL (10 mL, 20 mL)
Ointment, topical:
 Zovirax®: 5% (15 g)
Suspension, oral: 200 mg/5 mL (480 mL)
 Zovirax®: 200 mg/5 mL (480 mL) [banana flavor]
Tablet: 400 mg, 800 mg
 Zovirax®: 400 mg, 800 mg

Aczone™ *see* Dapsone *on page 441*
AD3L *see* Valrubicin *on page 1642*

Adagen® *see* Pegademase Bovine *on page 1259*
Adalat® CC *see* NIFEdipine *on page 1173*

Adalimumab (a da LIM yoo mab)

Related Information
Rheumatoid Arthritis, Osteoarthritis, and Osteoporosis *on page 1759*
U.S. Brand Names Humira®
Canadian Brand Names Humira®
Mexican Brand Names Humira
Generic Available No
Index Terms Antitumor Necrosis Factor Apha (Human); D2E7; Human Antitumor Necrosis Factor Alpha
Pharmacologic Category Antirheumatic, Disease Modifying; Monoclonal Antibody; Tumor Necrosis Factor (TNF) Blocking Agent
Use
Treatment of active rheumatoid arthritis, active psoriatic arthritis (moderate-to-severe), or ankylosing spondylitis; may be used alone or in combination with disease-modifying antirheumatic drugs (DMARDs).
Treatment of moderate-to-severe active Crohn's disease which has inadequate response to conventional treatment, or which has lost response to or is intolerant of infliximab
Local Anesthetic/Vasoconstrictor Precautions No information available to require special precautions
Effects on Dental Treatment No significant effects or complications reported
Common Adverse Effects Frequency > placebo in rheumatoid arthritis studies:
>10%:
Central nervous system: Headache (12%)
Dermatologic: Rash (12%)
Local: Injection site reaction (12% to 20%; includes erythema, itching, hemorrhage, pain, swelling)
Respiratory: Upper respiratory tract infection (17%), sinusitis (11%)
5% to 10%:
Cardiovascular: Hypertension (5%)
Endocrine & metabolic: Hyperlipidemia (7%), hypercholesterolemia (6%)
Gastrointestinal: Nausea (9%), abdominal pain (7%)
Genitourinary: Urinary tract infection (8%)
Hepatic: Alkaline phosphatase increased (5%)
Local: Injection site reaction (8%; other than erythema, itching, hemorrhage, pain, swelling)
Neuromuscular & skeletal: Back pain (6%)
Renal: Hematuria (5%)
Miscellaneous: Accidental injury (10%), flu-like syndrome (7%)
<5%:
Cardiovascular: Arrhythmia, atrial fibrillation, chest pain, CHF, coronary artery disorder, heart arrest, MI, palpitation, pericardial effusion, pericarditis, peripheral edema, syncope, tachycardia, thrombosis (leg), vascular disorder
Central nervous system: Confusion, fever, hypertensive encephalopathy, multiple sclerosis, subdural hematoma
Dermatologic: Cellulitis, erysipelas
Endocrine & metabolic: Dehydration, menstrual disorder, parathyroid disorder
Gastrointestinal: Diverticulitis, esophagitis, gastroenteritis, gastrointestinal hemorrhage, vomiting
Genitourinary: Cystitis, pelvic pain
Hematologic: Agranulocytosis, granulocytopenia, leukopenia, pancytopenia, paraproteinemia, polycythemia
Hepatic: Cholecystitis, cholelithiasis, hepatic necrosis
Neuromuscular & skeletal: Arthritis, bone fracture, bone necrosis, joint disorder, muscle cramps, myasthenia, pain in extremity, paresthesia, pyogenic arthritis, synovitis, tendon disorder, tremor
Ocular: Cataract
Renal: Kidney calculus, pyelonephritis
Respiratory: Asthma, bronchospasm, dyspnea, lung function decreased, pleural effusion, pneumonia
Miscellaneous: Adenoma, allergic reactions (1%), carcinoma (including breast, gastrointestinal, skin, urogenital), healing abnormality, herpes zoster, ketosis, lupus erythematosus syndrome, lymphoma, melanoma, postsurgical infection, sepsis, tuberculosis (reactivation of latent infection; miliary, lymphatic, peritoneal and pulmonary)
Mechanism of Action Adalimumab is a recombinant monoclonal antibody that binds to human tumor necrosis factor alpha (TNF-alpha), thereby interfering (Continued)

Adalimumab (Continued)

with binding to TNFα receptor sites and subsequent cytokine-driven inflammatory processes. Elevated TNF levels in the synovial fluid are involved in the pathologic pain and joint destruction in immune-mediated arthritis. Adalimumab decreases signs and symptoms of psoriatic arthritis, rheumatoid arthritis, and ankylosing spondylitis. It inhibits progression of structural damage of rheumatoid and psoriatic arthritis.

Drug Interactions

Increased Effect/Toxicity: Concomitant use with abatacept or anakinra may increase risk of infections; not recommended. Allergic reactions to abciximab may be increased in patients who received therapeutic or diagnostic monoclonal antibodies.

Decreased Effect: Concomitant use with vaccines (live) has not been studied; due to potential for vaccinal infection, concurrent use is not recommended. The response to vaccines (dead organism) may be diminished in patients receiving adalimumab; monitor closely.

Pharmacodynamics/Kinetics
Distribution: V$_d$: 4.7-6 L; Synovial fluid concentrations: 31% to 96% of serum
Bioavailability: Absolute: 64%
Half-life elimination: Terminal: ~2 weeks (range 10-20 days)
Time to peak, serum: SubQ: 131 ± 56 hours
Excretion: Clearance increased in the presence of antiadalimumab antibodies; decreased in patients 40 years and older

Pregnancy Risk Factor B

Adamantanamine Hydrochloride *see* Amantadine *on page 83*

Adapalene (a DAP a leen)

U.S. Brand Names Differin®
Canadian Brand Names Differin®; Differin® XP
Mexican Brand Names Adaferin
Generic Available No
Pharmacologic Category Acne Products; Topical Skin Product, Acne
Use Treatment of acne vulgaris
Local Anesthetic/Vasoconstrictor Precautions No information available to require special precautions
Effects on Dental Treatment No significant effects or complications reported
Common Adverse Effects >10%: Dermatologic: Erythema, scaling, dryness, pruritus, burning, pruritus or burning immediately after application
Mechanism of Action Retinoid-like compound which is a modulator of cellular differentiation, keratinization, and inflammatory processes, all of which represent important features in the pathology of acne vulgaris
Pharmacodynamics/Kinetics
Absorption: Topical: Minimal
Excretion: Bile
Pregnancy Risk Factor C

Adderall® *see* Dextroamphetamine and Amphetamine *on page 474*
Adderall XR® *see* Dextroamphetamine and Amphetamine *on page 474*

Adefovir (a DEF o veer)

Related Information
HIV Infection and AIDS *on page 1753*
U.S. Brand Names Hepsera™
Canadian Brand Names Hepsera™
Generic Available No
Index Terms Adefovir Dipivoxil
Pharmacologic Category Antiretroviral Agent, Reverse Transcriptase Inhibitor (Nucleoside)
Use Treatment of chronic hepatitis B with evidence of active viral replication (based on persistent elevation of ALT/AST or histologic evidence), including patients with lamivudine-resistant hepatitis B
Local Anesthetic/Vasoconstrictor Precautions No information available to require special precautions
Effects on Dental Treatment No significant effects or complications reported
Common Adverse Effects For a majority of adverse reactions, the incidence in adefovir-receiving patients was similar to or less than that observed with placebo treatment.

>10%:
  Hepatic: ALT increased (>5 x ULN: 20%)
  Neuromuscular & skeletal: Weakness (13%)
  Renal: Hematuria (grade ≥3: 11%)
1% to 10%:
  Central nervous system: Headache (9%)
  Dermatologic: Rash, pruritus
  Endocrine & metabolic: Hypophosphatemia (1% to 2%)
  Gastrointestinal: Abdominal pain (9%), nausea (5%), amylase increased (grade ≥3: 4%), flatulence (4%), diarrhea (3%), dyspepsia (3%), vomiting
  Hepatic: AST increased (>5 x ULN: 8%), abnormal liver function, hepatic failure
  Neuromuscular & skeletal: Creatine kinase increased (7%)
  Renal: Serum creatinine increased (2% to 3%), glycosuria (grade ≥3: 1%), renal failure, renal insufficiency
    Note: In liver transplant patients with baseline renal dysfunction, frequency of increased serum creatinine has been observed to be as high as 32% to 53% at 48 and 96 weeks post-transplantation, respectively; considering the concomitant use of other potentially nephrotoxic medications, baseline renal insufficiency, and predisposing comorbidities, the role of adefovir in these changes could not be established.

Mechanism of Action Acyclic nucleotide reverse transcriptase inhibitor (adenosine analog) which interferes with HBV viral RNA-dependent DNA polymerase resulting in inhibition of viral replication.

Drug Interactions
  Increased Effect/Toxicity: Concurrent use of nephrotoxic agents (including aminoglycosides, cyclosporine, NSAIDs, tacrolimus, vancomycin) may increase the risk of nephrotoxicity. Use of ganciclovir (valganciclovir) may increase the incidence of adverse effects/toxicity of adefovir. Concomitant use of ribavirin with or without interferon alfa and nucleoside analogues may increase the risk of developing hepatic decompensation or other signs of mitochondrial toxicity, including pancreatitis or lactic acidosis.

Pharmacodynamics/Kinetics
  Distribution: 0.35-0.39 L/kg
  Protein binding: ≤4%
  Metabolism: Prodrug; rapidly converted to adefovir (active metabolite) in intestine
  Bioavailability: 59%
  Half-life elimination: 7.5 hours; prolonged in renal impairment
  Time to peak: 1.75 hours
  Excretion: Urine (45% as active metabolite within 24 hours)

Pregnancy Risk Factor C

Adefovir Dipivoxil *see* Adefovir *on page 54*

Adenocard® *see* Adenosine *on page 55*

Adenoscan® *see* Adenosine *on page 55*

Adenosine (a DEN oh seen)

U.S. Brand Names Adenocard®; Adenoscan®
Canadian Brand Names Adenocard®; Adenoscan®; Adenosine Injection, USP
Mexican Brand Names Krenosin
Generic Available Yes
Index Terms 9-Beta-D-Ribofuranosyladenine
Pharmacologic Category Antiarrhythmic Agent, Class IV; Diagnostic Agent
Use
  Adenocard®: Treatment of paroxysmal supraventricular tachycardia (PSVT) including that associated with accessory bypass tracts (Wolff-Parkinson-White syndrome); when clinically advisable, appropriate vagal maneuvers should be attempted prior to adenosine administration; **not effective in atrial flutter, atrial fibrillation, or ventricular tachycardia**
  Adenoscan®: Pharmacologic stress agent used in myocardial perfusion thallium-201 scintigraphy
Unlabeled/Investigational Use Adenoscan®: Acute vasodilator testing in pulmonary artery hypertension
Local Anesthetic/Vasoconstrictor Precautions No information available to require special precautions
Effects on Dental Treatment No significant effects or complications reported
Mechanism of Action Slows conduction time through the AV node, interrupting the re-entry pathways through the AV node, restoring normal sinus rhythm
Pregnancy Risk Factor C

Adept® *see* Icodextrin *on page 859*

ADH *see* Vasopressin *on page 1650*

Adipex-P® *see* Phentermine *on page 1291*

Adoxa™ *see* Doxycycline (Systemic) *on page 541*

Adrenalin® *see* Epinephrine *on page 572*

Adrenaline *see* Epinephrine *on page 572*

Adrenocorticotropic Hormone *see* Corticotropin *on page 415*

ADR (error-prone abbreviation) *see* DOXOrubicin *on page 536*

Adria *see* DOXOrubicin *on page 536*

Adriamycin PFS® *see* DOXOrubicin *on page 536*

Adriamycin RDF® *see* DOXOrubicin *on page 536*

Adrucil® *see* Fluorouracil *on page 713*

Adsorbent Charcoal *see* Charcoal, Activated *on page 327*

Advair Diskus® *see* Fluticasone and Salmeterol *on page 729*

Advair® HFA *see* Fluticasone and Salmeterol *on page 729*

Advantage-S™ [OTC] *see* Nonoxynol 9 *on page 1185*

Advate *see* Antihemophilic Factor (Recombinant) *on page 132*

Advicor® *see* Niacin and Lovastatin *on page 1167*

Advil® [OTC] *see* Ibuprofen *on page 853*

Advil® Children's [OTC] *see* Ibuprofen *on page 853*

Advil® Cold, Children's [OTC] *see* Pseudoephedrine and Ibuprofen *on page 1384*

Advil® Cold & Sinus [OTC] *see* Pseudoephedrine and Ibuprofen *on page 1384*

Advil® Infants' [OTC] *see* Ibuprofen *on page 853*

Advil® Junior [OTC] *see* Ibuprofen *on page 853*

Advil® Migraine [OTC] *see* Ibuprofen *on page 853*

AeroBid® *see* Flunisolide *on page 705*

AeroBid®-M *see* Flunisolide *on page 705*

aeroKid™ *see* Chlorpheniramine, Phenylephrine, and Methscopolamine *on page 342*

Aerospan™ *see* Flunisolide *on page 705*

Afeditab™ CR *see* NIFEdipine *on page 1173*

Afrin® Extra Moisturizing [OTC] *see* Oxymetazoline *on page 1236*

Afrin® Original [OTC] *see* Oxymetazoline *on page 1236*

Afrin® Severe Congestion [OTC] *see* Oxymetazoline *on page 1236*

Afrin® Sinus [OTC] *see* Oxymetazoline *on page 1236*

AG *see* Aminoglutethimide *on page 89*

Agalsidase Beta (aye GAL si days BAY ta)

U.S. Brand Names Fabrazyme®
Canadian Brand Names Fabrazyme®
Generic Available No
Index Terms Alpha-Galactosidase-A (Human, Recombinant); r-h α-GAL
Pharmacologic Category Enzyme
Use Replacement therapy for Fabry disease
Local Anesthetic/Vasoconstrictor Precautions No information available to require special precautions
Effects on Dental Treatment No significant effects or complications reported
Common Adverse Effects Note: The most common and serious adverse reactions are infusion reactions (symptoms may include fever, tachycardia, hypertension, throat tightness, dyspnea, chills, abdominal pain, pruritus, urticaria, vomiting).

>10%:
  Cardiovascular: Edema (21%), chest pain (17%), hypotension (14%)
  Central nervous system: Fever (48%), headache (45%), anxiety (28%), pain (21%), dizziness (14%), paresthesia (14%)
  Dermatologic: Pallor (14%)
  Gastrointestinal: Nausea (28%)
  Neuromuscular & skeletal: Rigors (52%), skeletal pain (21%)
  Respiratory: Rhinitis (38%), pharyngitis (28%)
  Miscellaneous: Infusion reactions (alteration of temperature sensation 17%)
1% to 10%:
  Cardiovascular: Cardiomegaly (10%), hypertension (10%)
  Central nervous system: Depression (10%)
  Gastrointestinal: Dyspepsia (10%)
  Genitourinary: Testicular pain (7%)
  Neuromuscular & skeletal: Arthrosis (10%)

Respiratory: Bronchitis (10%), bronchospasm (7%), laryngitis (7%), sinusitis (7%)

Other reported severe reactions (frequency not established): Arrhythmia, ataxia, bradycardia, cardiac arrest, cardiac output decreased, nephritic syndrome, stroke, vertigo

Mechanism of Action Agalsidase beta is a recombinant form of the enzyme alpha-galactosidase-A, which is required for the hydrolysis of GL-3 and other glycosphingolipids. The compounds may accumulate (over many years) within the tissues of patients with Fabry disease, leading to renal and cardiovascular complications. In clinical trials of limited duration, agalsidase been noted to reduce tissue inclusions of a key sphingolipid (GL-3). It is believed that long-term enzyme replacement may reduce clinical manifestations of renal failure, cardiomyopathy, and stroke. However, the relationship to a reduction in clinical manifestations has not been established.

Pharmacodynamics/Kinetics Half-life elimination: 42-102 minutes (nonlinear)

Pregnancy Risk Factor B

Albendazole (al BEN da zole)

U.S. Brand Names Albenza®

Mexican Brand Names Bendapar; Eskazole; Gascop; Loveral; Vermin Plus; Zentel

Generic Available No

Pharmacologic Category Anthelmintic

Use Treatment of parenchymal neurocysticercosis caused by *Taenia solium* and cystic hydatid disease of the liver, lung, and peritoneum caused by *Echinococcus granulosus*

Unlabeled/Investigational Use Albendazole has activity against *Ascaris lumbricoides* (roundworm); *Ancylostoma caninum*; *Ancylostoma duodenale* and *Necator americanus* (hookworms); cutaneous larva migrans; *Enterobius* (Continued)

57

Albendazole *(Continued)*

vermicularis (pinworm); *Gnathostoma spinigerum*; *Gongylonema* sp; *Hymenolepis nana* sp (tapeworms); *Mansonella perstans* (filariasis); *Opisthorchis sinensis* and *Opisthorchis viverrini* (liver flukes); *Strongyloides stercoralis* and *Trichuris trichiura* (whipworm); visceral larva migrans (toxocariasis); activity has also been shown against the liver fluke *Clonorchis sinensis, Giardia lamblia, Cysticercus cellulosae,* and *Echinococcus multilocularis.* Albendazole has also been used for the treatment of intestinal microsporidiosis (*Encephalitozoon intestinalis*), disseminated microsporidiosis (*E. hellem, E. cuniculi, E. intestinalis, Pleistophora* sp, *Trachipleistophora* sp, *Brachiola vesicularum*), and ocular microsporidiosis (*E. hellem, E. cuniculi, Vittaforma corneae*).

Local Anesthetic/Vasoconstrictor Precautions No information available to require special precautions

Effects on Dental Treatment No significant effects or complications reported

Common Adverse Effects

N = Neurocysticercosis; H = Hydatid disease

>10%:
    Central nervous system: Headache (11% - N; 1% - H)
    Hepatic: LFTs increased (~15% - H; <1% - N)
1% to 10%:
    Central nervous system: Dizziness, vertigo, fever (≤1%), intracranial pressure increased (1% - N), meningeal signs (1% - N)
    Dermatologic: Alopecia (2% - H; <1% - N)
    Gastrointestinal: Abdominal pain (6% - H; 0% - N), nausea/vomiting (3% to 6%)
    Hematologic: Leukopenia (reversible) (<1%)
    Miscellaneous: Allergic reactions (<1%)

Mechanism of Action Active metabolite, albendazole, causes selective degeneration of cytoplasmic microtubules in intestinal and tegmental cells of intestinal helminths and larvae; glycogen is depleted, glucose uptake and cholinesterase secretion are impaired, and desecratory substances accumulate intracellulary. ATP production decreases causing energy depletion, immobilization, and worm death.

Drug Interactions

Cytochrome P450 Effect: Substrate (minor) of CYP1A2, 3A4; **Inhibits** CYP1A2 (weak)

Pharmacodynamics/Kinetics

Absorption: <5%; may increase up to 4-5 times when administered with a fatty meal

Distribution: Well inside hydatid cysts and CSF

Protein binding: 70%

Metabolism: Hepatic; extensive first-pass effect; pathways include rapid sulfoxidation (major), hydrolysis, and oxidation

Half-life elimination: 8-12 hours

Time to peak, serum: 2-2.4 hours

Excretion: Urine (<1% as active metabolite); feces

Pregnancy Risk Factor C

Albenza® *see* Albendazole *on page 57*

Albumin-Bound Paclitaxel *see* Paclitaxel (Protein Bound) *on page 1241*

Albuterol *(al BYOO ter ole)*

Related Information
    Respiratory Diseases *on page 1747*

U.S. Brand Names AccuNeb®; ProAir™ HFA; Proventil®; Proventil® HFA; Ventolin® HFA; VoSpire ER®

Canadian Brand Names Airomir; Alti-Salbutamol; Apo-Salvent®; Apo-Salvent® CFC Free; Apo-Salvent® Respirator Solution; Apo-Salvent® Sterules; Gen-Salbutamol; PMS-Salbutamol; ratio-Inspra-Sal; ratio-Salbutamol; Rhoxal-salbutamol; Salbu-2; Salbu-4; Ventolin®; Ventolin® Diskus; Ventolin® HFA; Ventrodisk

Mexican Brand Names Assal; Salbutalan; Ventolin; Zibil

Generic Available Yes

Index Terms Albuterol Sulfate; Salbutamol

Pharmacologic Category Beta₂-Adrenergic Agonist

Use Bronchodilator in reversible airway obstruction due to asthma or COPD; prevention of exercise-induced bronchospasm

Local Anesthetic/Vasoconstrictor Precautions No information available to require special precautions

Effects on Dental Treatment Key adverse event(s) related to dental treatment: Xerostomia (normal salivary flow resumes upon discontinuation)

Common Adverse Effects Incidence of adverse effects is depen
age of patient, dose, and route of administration.

Cardiovascular: Angina, atrial fibrillation, chest discomfort, extras
flushing, hypertension, palpitation, tachycardia

Central nervous system: CNS stimulation, dizziness, drowsiness hea
insomnia, irritability, lightheadedness, migraine, nervousness, ightn
restlessness, sleeplessness, tremor

Dermatologic: Angioedema, erythema multiforme, rash, Stevens John
syndrome, urticaria

Endocrine & metabolic: Hypokalemia, serum glucose increased, serul pota
sium decreased

Gastrointestinal: Diarrhea, dry mouth, gastroenteritis, nausea, unusua ste,
vomiting, tooth discoloration

Genitourinary: Micturition difficulty

Neuromuscular & skeletal: Muscle cramps, weakness

Otic: Otitis media, vertigo

Respiratory: Asthma exacerbation, bronchospasm, cough, epistaxis, laryngit
oropharyngeal drying/irritation, oropharyngeal edema

Miscellaneous: Allergic reaction, lymphadenopathy

Dosage

Oral:

Children: Bronchospasm (treatment):

2-6 years: 0.1-0.2 mg/kg/dose 3 times/day; maximum dose not to exceed 12 mg/day (divided doses)

6-12 years: 2 mg/dose 3-4 times/day; maximum dose not to exceed 24 mg/day (divided doses)

Extended release: 4 mg every 12 hours; maximum dose not to exceed 24 mg/day (divided doses)

Children >12 years and Adults: Bronchospasm (treatment): 2-4 mg/dose 3-4 times/day; maximum dose not to exceed 32 mg/day (divided doses)

Extended release: 8 mg every 12 hours; maximum dose not to exceed 32 mg/day (divided doses). A 4 mg dose every 12 hours may be sufficient in some patients, such as adults of low body weight.

Elderly: Bronchospasm (treatment): 2 mg 3-4 times/day; maximum: 8 mg 4 times/day

Inhalation: MDI 90 mcg/puff:

Children ≤12 years:

Bronchospasm (acute): 4-8 puffs every 20 minutes for 3 doses, then every 1-4 hours; spacer/holding-chamber device should be used

Exercise-induced bronchospasm (prophylaxis): 1-2 puffs 5 minutes prior to exercise

Children >12 years and Adults:

Bronchospasm (acute): 4-8 puffs every 20 minutes for up to 4 hours, then every 1-4 hours as needed

Exercise-induced bronchospasm (prophylaxis): 2 puffs 5-30 minutes prior to exercise

Children ≥4 years and Adults: Bronchospasm (chronic treatment): 1-2 inhalations every 4-6 hours; maximum: 12 inhalations/day

NIH guidelines: 2 puffs 3-4 times a day as needed; may double dose for mild exacerbations

Nebulization:

Children ≤12 years:

Bronchospasm (treatment): 0.05 mg/kg every 4-6 hours; minimum dose: 1.25 mg, maximum dose: 2.5 mg

2-12 years: AccuNeb®: 0.63 mg or 1.25 mg 3-4 times/day, as needed, delivered over 5-15 minutes

Children >40 kg, patients with more severe asthma, or children 11-12 years: May respond better with a 1.25 mg dose

Bronchospasm (acute): Solution 0.5%: 0.15 mg/kg (minimum dose: 2.5 mg) every 20 minutes for 3 doses, then 0.15-0.3 mg/kg (up to 10 mg) every 1-4 hours as needed; may also use 0.5 mg/kg/hour by continuous infusion. Continuous nebulized albuterol at 0.3 mg/kg/hour has been used safely in the treatment of severe status asthmaticus in children; continuous nebulized doses of 3 mg/kg/hour ± 2.2 mg/kg/hour in children whose mean age was 20.7 months resulted in no cardiac toxicity; the optimal dosage for continuous nebulization remains to be determined.

Note: Use of the 0.5% solution should be used for bronchospasm (acute or treatment) in children <15 kg. AccuNeb® has not been studied for the treatment of acute bronchospasm; use of the 0.5% concentrated solution may be more appropriate.

Children >12 years and Adults:

Bronchospasm (treatment): 2.5 mg, diluted to a total of 3 mL, 3-4 times/day over 5-15 minutes

NIH guidelines: 1.25-5 mg every 4-8 hours

(Continued)

59

Albuterol (Continued)

Bronchospasm (acute) in intensive care patients: 2.5-5 mg every 20 minutes for 3 doses, then 2.5-10 mg every 1-4 hours as needed, **or** 10-15 mg/hour continuously

Hemodialysis: Not removed

Peritoneal dialysis: Significant drug removal is unlikely based on physiochemical characteristics

Mechanism of Action Relaxes bronchial smooth muscle by action on β_2-receptors with little effect on heart rate

Contraindications Hypersensitivity to albuterol, adrenergic amines, or any component of the formulation

Warnings/Precautions Optimize anti-inflammatory treatment before initiating maintenance treatment with albuterol. Do not use as a component of chronic therapy without an anti-inflammatory agent. Only the mildest forms of asthma (Step 1 and/or exercise-induced) would not require concurrent use based upon asthma guidelines. Patient must be instructed to seek medical attention in cases where acute symptoms are not relieved or a previous level of response is diminished. The need to increase frequency of use may indicate deterioration of asthma, and treatment must not be delayed.

Use caution in patients with cardiovascular disease (arrhythmia or hypertension or CHF), convulsive disorders, diabetes, glaucoma, hyperthyroidism, or hypokalemia. Beta-agonists may cause elevation in blood pressure, heart rate, and result in CNS stimulation/excitation. Beta$_2$-agonists may increase risk of arrhythmia, increase serum glucose, or decrease serum potassium.

Immediate hypersensitivity reactions (urticaria, angioedema, rash, bronchospasm) have been reported. Do not exceed recommended dose; serious adverse events, including fatalities, have been associated with excessive use of inhaled sympathomimetics. Rarely, paradoxical bronchospasm may occur with use of inhaled bronchodilating agents; this should be distinguished from inadequate response. All patients should utilize a spacer device when using a metered-dose inhaler; in addition, face masks should be used in children <4 years of age.

Because of its minimal effect on beta$_1$-receptors and its relatively long duration of action, albuterol is a rational choice in the elderly when an inhaled beta-agonist is indicated. Oral use should be avoided in the elderly due to adverse effects. Patient response may vary between inhalers that contain chlorofluorocarbons and those which are chlorofluorocarbon-free.

Drug Interactions

Cytochrome P450 Effect: **Substrate** of CYP3A4 (major)

Increased Effect/Toxicity: When used with inhaled ipratropium, an increased duration of bronchodilation may occur. Cardiovascular effects are potentiated in patients also receiving MAO inhibitors, tricyclic antidepressants, and sympathomimetic agents (eg, amphetamine, dopamine, dobutamine). Albuterol may increase the risk of malignant arrhythmias with inhaled anesthetics (eg, enflurane, halothane).

Decreased Effect: When used with nonselective beta-adrenergic blockers (eg, propranolol) the effect of albuterol is decreased. Levels/effects of albuterol may be decreased by aminoglutethimide, carbamazepine, nafcillin, nevirapine, phenobarbital, phenytoin, rifamycins, and other CYP3A4 inducers.

Ethanol/Nutrition/Herb Interactions

Food: Avoid or limit caffeine (may cause CNS stimulation).

Herb/Nutraceutical: Avoid ephedra, yohimbe (may cause CNS stimulation).

Dietary Considerations Oral forms should be administered with water 1 hour before or 2 hours after meals.

Pharmacodynamics/Kinetics

Onset of action: Peak effect:

Nebulization/oral inhalation: 0.5-2 hours

CFC-propelled albuterol: 10 minutes

Ventolin® HFA: 25 minutes

Oral: 2-3 hours

Duration: Nebulization/oral inhalation: 3-4 hours; Oral: 4-6 hours

Metabolism: Hepatic to an inactive sulfate

Half-life elimination: Inhalation: 3.8 hours; Oral: 3.7-5 hours

Excretion: Urine (30% as unchanged drug)

Pregnancy Risk Factor C

Dosage Forms

Aerosol, for oral inhalation [contains chlorofluorocarbon]: 90 mcg/metered inhalation (17 g)

Proventil®: 90 mcg/metered inhalation (17 g)

Aerosol, for oral inhalation [chlorofluorocarbon free]: 90 mcg/metered inhalation (8.5 g)
 ProAir™ HFA: 90 mcg/metered inhalation (8.5 g)
 Proventil® HFA: 90 mcg/metered inhalation (6.7 g)
 Ventolin® HFA: 90 mcg/metered inhalation (18 g)
Solution for nebulization: 0.042% (3 mL); 0.083% (3 mL); 0.5% (0.5 mL, 20 mL)
 AccuNeb® [preservative free]: 0.63 mg/3 mL (3 mL) [0.021%]; 1.25 mg/3 mL (3 mL) [0.042%]
 Proventil®: 0.083% (3 mL) [preservative free]; 0.5% (20 mL) [contains benzalkonium chloride]
Syrup: 2 mg/5 mL
Tablet: 2 mg, 4 mg
Tablet, extended release: 4 mg, 8 mg
 VoSpire ER™: 4 mg, 8 mg

Alclometasone (al kloe MET a sone)

U.S. Brand Names Aclovate®
Generic Available Yes
Index Terms Alclometasone Dipropionate
Pharmacologic Category Corticosteroid, Topical
Dental Use Treatment of inflammation of corticosteroid-responsive dermatosis (low potency topical corticosteroid)
Use Treatment of inflammation of corticosteroid-responsive dermatosis (low potency topical corticosteroid)
Local Anesthetic/Vasoconstrictor Precautions No information available to require special precautions
Effects on Dental Treatment No significant effects or complications reported
Significant Adverse Effects Frequency not defined.
 Dermatologic: Acne, allergic dermatitis, hypopigmentation, maceration of the skin, skin atrophy, striae, miliaria, telangiectasia
 Endocrine & metabolic: HPA suppression, Cushing's syndrome, growth retardation
 Local: Burning, erythema, itching, irritation, dryness, folliculitis, hypertrichosis
 Systemic: HPA axis suppression, Cushing's syndrome, hyperglycemia; these reactions occur more frequently with occlusive dressings
 Miscellaneous: Secondary infection
Dosage Topical: Apply a thin film to the affected area 2-3 times/day. Therapy should be discontinued when control is achieved; if no improvement is seen, reassessment of diagnosis may be necessary.
Mechanism of Action Stimulates the synthesis of enzymes needed to decrease inflammation, suppress mitotic activity, and cause vasoconstriction
Contraindications Hypersensitivity to alclometasone or any component of the formulation; viral, fungal, or tubercular skin lesions
Warnings/Precautions Systemic absorption of topical corticosteroids may cause hypothalamic-pituitary-adrenal (HPA) axis suppression (reversible) particularly in younger children. HPA axis suppression may lead to adrenal crisis. Risk is increased when used over large surface areas, for prolonged periods, or with occlusive dressings. Adverse systemic effects including hyperglycemia, glycosuria, fluid and electrolyte changes, and HPA suppression may occur when used on large surface areas, for prolonged periods, or with an occlusive dressing. Prolonged treatment with corticosteroids has been associated with the development of Kaposi's sarcoma (case reports); if noted, discontinuation of therapy should be considered. Allergic contact dermatitis can occur, it is usually diagnosed by failure to heal rather than clinical exacerbation. Safety and efficacy have not been established in children <1 year of age. Chronic use of corticosteroids in children may interfere with growth and development.
Drug Interactions No data reported
Pregnancy Risk Factor C
Dosage Forms Excipient information presented when available (limited, particularly for generics); consult specific product labeling.
 Cream, as dipropionate: 0.05% (15 g, 45 g, 60 g)
 Ointment, as dipropionate: 0.05% (15 g, 45 g, 60 g)

Aldara™ *see* Imiquimod *on page 867*

Aldesleukin (al des LOO kin)

U.S. Brand Names Proleukin®
Canadian Brand Names Proleukin®
Mexican Brand Names Proleukin
Generic Available No
Index Terms Epidermal Thymocyte Activating Factor; ETAF; IL-2; Interleukin-2; Lymphocyte Mitogenic Factor; NSC-373364; T-Cell Growth Factor; TCGF; Thymocyte Stimulating Factor
Pharmacologic Category Biological Response Modulator
Use Treatment of metastatic renal cell cancer, melanoma
Unlabeled/Investigational Use Investigational: Multiple myeloma, HIV infection, and AIDS; may be used in conjunction with lymphokine-activated killer (LAK) cells, tumor-infiltrating lymphocyte (TIL) cells, interleukin-1, and interferons; colorectal cancer; non-Hodgkin's lymphoma
Local Anesthetic/Vasoconstrictor Precautions No information available to require special precautions
Effects on Dental Treatment Key adverse event(s) related to dental treatment: Stomatitis
Common Adverse Effects
>10%:
   Cardiovascular: Hypotension (85%), dose-limiting, possibly fatal; sinus tachycardia (70%); arrhythmia (22%); edema (47%); angina
   Central nervous system: Mental status changes (transient memory loss, confusion, drowsiness) (73%); dizziness (17%); cognitive changes, fatigue, malaise, somnolence, and disorientation (25%); headaches; insomnia; paranoid delusion
   Dermatologic: Macular erythematous rash (100% of patients on high-dose therapy), pruritus (48%), erythema (41%), rash (26%), exfoliative dermatitis (14%), dry skin (15%)
   Endocrine & metabolic: Fever and chills (89%), electrolyte levels decreased (magnesium, calcium, phosphate, potassium, sodium) (1% to 15%)
   Gastrointestinal: Nausea and vomiting (87%), diarrhea (76%), stomatitis (32%), GI bleeding (13%), weight gain (23%), anorexia (27%)
   Hematologic: Anemia (77%), thrombocytopenia (64%), leukopenia (34%) - may be dose-limiting, coagulation disorders (10%)
   Hepatic: Transient elevations of bilirubin (64%) and enzymes (56%), jaundice (11%)
   Neuromuscular & skeletal: Weakness; rigors - respond to acetaminophen, diphenhydramine, an NSAID, or meperidine
   Renal: Oliguria/anuria (63%, severe in 5% to 6%); proteinuria (12%); renal failure (dose-limiting toxicity) manifested as oliguria noted within 24-48 hours of initiation of therapy; marked fluid retention, azotemia, and increased serum creatinine seen, which may return to baseline within 7 days of discontinuation of therapy; hypophosphatemia
   Respiratory: Congestion (54%), dyspnea (27% to 52%)
   Miscellaneous: Pain (54%), infection (including sepsis and endocarditis) due to neutrophil impairment (23%)
1% to 10%:
   Cardiovascular: Capillary leak syndrome, including peripheral edema, ascites, pulmonary infiltration, and pleural effusion (2% to 4%), may be dose-limiting and potentially fatal; MI (2%)
   Central nervous system: Seizures (1%)
   Endocrine & metabolic: Hypo- and hyperglycemia (2%), electrolyte levels increased (magnesium, calcium, phosphate, potassium, sodium) (1%), hypothyroidism
   Hepatic: Ascites (4%)
   Neuromuscular & skeletal: Arthralgia (6%), myalgia (6%)
   Renal: Hematuria (9%), creatinine increased (5%)
   Respiratory: Pleural effusions, edema (10%)
Mechanism of Action Aldesleukin promotes proliferation, differentiation, and recruitment of T and B cells, natural killer (NK) cells, and thymocytes; causes cytolytic activity in a subset of lymphocytes and subsequent interactions between the immune system and malignant cells; can stimulate lymphokine-activated killer (LAK) cells and tumor-infiltrating lymphocytes (TIL) cells.
Drug Interactions
   Increased Effect/Toxicity: Aldesleukin may affect central nervous function; therefore, interactions could occur following concomitant administration of psychotropic drugs (eg, narcotics, analgesics, antiemetics, sedatives, tranquilizers).

Concomitant administration of drugs possessing nephrotoxic (eg, aminoglycosides, indomethacin), myelotoxic (eg, cytotoxic chemotherapy), cardiotoxic (eg, doxorubicin), or hepatotoxic effects with aldesleukin may increase toxicity in these organ systems.

Beta-blockers and other antihypertensives may potentiate the hypotension seen with aldesleukin.

Decreased Effect: Corticosteroids have been shown to decrease toxicity of aldesleukin, but may reduce the efficacy of the lymphokine.

Pharmacodynamics/Kinetics
Distribution: V_d: 4-7 L; primarily in plasma and then in the lymphocytes
Bioavailability: I.M.: 37%
Half-life elimination: Initial: 6-13 minutes; Terminal: 80-120 minutes

Pregnancy Risk Factor C

Aldex™ *see* Guaifenesin and Phenylephrine *on page 797*

Aldomet *see* Methyldopa *on page 1077*

Aldoril® *see* Methyldopa and Hydrochlorothiazide *on page 1078*

Aldroxicon I [OTC] *see* Aluminum Hydroxide, Magnesium Hydroxide, and Simethicone *on page 82*

Aldroxicon II [OTC] *see* Aluminum Hydroxide, Magnesium Hydroxide, and Simethicone *on page 82*

Aldurazyme® *see* Laronidase *on page 951*

Alefacept (a LE fa sept)

U.S. Brand Names Amevive®
Canadian Brand Names Amevive®
Generic Available No
Index Terms B 9273; BG 9273; Human LFA-3/IgG(1) Fusion Protein; LFA-3/IgG(1) Fusion Protein, Human
Pharmacologic Category Monoclonal Antibody
Use Treatment of moderate to severe chronic plaque psoriasis in adults who are candidates for systemic therapy or phototherapy
Local Anesthetic/Vasoconstrictor Precautions No information available to require special precautions
Effects on Dental Treatment No significant effects or complications reported
Common Adverse Effects
≥10%:
 Hematologic: Lymphopenia (up to 10% of patients required temporary discontinuation, up to 17% during a second course of therapy)
 Local: Injection site reactions (up to 16% of patients; includes pain, inflammation, bleeding, edema, or other reaction)
1% to 10%:
 Central nervous system: Chills (6%; primarily during intravenous administration), dizziness (≥2%)
 Dermatologic: Pruritus (≥2%)
 Gastrointestinal: Nausea (≥2%)
 Neuromuscular & skeletal: Myalgia (≥2%)
 Respiratory: Pharyngitis (≥2%), cough increased (≥2%)
 Miscellaneous: Malignancies (1% vs 0.5% in placebo), antibodies to alefacept (3%; significance unknown), infection (1% requiring hospitalization)
Restrictions Alefacept will be distributed directly to physician offices or to a specialty pharmacy; injections are intended to be administered in the physician's office
Mechanism of Action Binds to CD2, a receptor on the surface of lymphocytes, inhibiting their interaction with leukocyte functional antigen 3 (LFA-3). Interaction between CD2 and LFA-3 is important for the activation of T lymphocytes in psoriasis. Activated T lymphocytes secrete a number of inflammatory mediators, including interferon gamma, which are involved in psoriasis. Since CD2 is primarily expressed on T lymphocytes, treatment results in a reduction in $CD4^+$ and $CD8^+$ T lymphocytes, with lesser effects on other cell populations (NK and B lymphocytes).
Drug Interactions
Increased Effect/Toxicity: No formal drug interaction studies have been completed.
Decreased Effect: No formal drug interaction studies have been completed.
Pharmacodynamics/Kinetics
Distribution: V_d: 0.094 L/kg
Bioavailability: 63% (following I.M. administration)
Half-life: 270 hours (following I.V. administration)
Excretion: Clearance: 0.25 mL/hour/kg
Pregnancy Risk Factor B

Alemtuzumab (ay lem TU zoo mab)

U.S. Brand Names Campath®
Canadian Brand Names MabCampath®
Generic Available No
Index Terms C1H; Campath-1H; DNA-Derived Humanized Monoclonal Antibody; Humanized IgG1 Anti-CD52 Monoclonal Antibody; NSC-715969
Pharmacologic Category Antineoplastic Agent, Monoclonal Antibody
Use Treatment of B-cell chronic lymphocytic leukemia (B-CLL)
Unlabeled/Investigational Use Treatment of refractory T-cell prolymphocytic leukemia (T-PLL); rheumatoid arthritis; graft-versus-host disease; multiple myeloma; preconditioning regimen for stem-cell transplantation and renal and liver transplantation; post-transplant rejection (renal); treatment of autoimmune cytopenias
Local Anesthetic/Vasoconstrictor Precautions No information available to require special precautions
Effects on Dental Treatment Key adverse event(s) related to dental treatment: Stomatitis and mucositis.
Common Adverse Effects
>10%:
  Cardiovascular: Hypotension (15% to 32%), peripheral edema (13%), hypertension (11% to 15%), tachycardia/SVT (11%)
  Central nervous system: Fever (83% to 85%), fatigue (22% to 34%), headache (13% to 24%), dysthesias (15%), dizziness (12%)
  Dermatologic: Rash (30% to 40%), urticaria (22% to 30%), pruritus (14% to 24%)
  Gastrointestinal: Nausea (47% to 54%), vomiting (33% to 41%), anorexia (20%), diarrhea (13% to 22%), stomatitis/mucositis (14%), abdominal pain (11%)
  Hematologic: Neutropenia (85%; grade 3/4: 64% to 70%; median duration: 28 days), anemia (80%; grade 3/4: 38% to 47%), thrombocytopenia (72%; grade 3/4: 50% to 52%; median duration: 21 days)
  Local: Injection site reaction (SubQ administration: 90%)
  Neuromuscular & skeletal: Rigors (86% to 89%), skeletal pain (24%), weakness (13%), myalgia (11%)
  Respiratory: Dyspnea (17% to 26%), cough (25%), bronchitis/pneumonitis (21%), pneumonia (16%), pharyngitis (12%)
  Miscellaneous: Infection (43% to 66%; grades 3/4: 37%; incidence is lower if prophylactic anti-infectives are utilized), diaphoresis (19%), sepsis (15%), herpes viral infections (1% to 11%)
1% to 10%:
  Cardiovascular: Chest pain (10%)
  Central nervous system: Insomnia (10%), malaise (9%), depression (7%), temperature change sensation (5%), somnolence (5%)
  Dermatologic: Purpura (8%)
  Gastrointestinal: Dyspepsia (10%), constipation (9%)
  Hematologic: Neutropenic fever (10%), pancytopenia/marrow hypoplasia (5% to 6%; grade 3/4: 3%), positive Coombs' test without hemolysis (2%), autoimmune thrombocytopenia (2%), autoimmune hemolytic anemia (1%)
  Neuromuscular & skeletal: Back pain (10%), tremor (7%)
  Respiratory: Bronchospasm (9%), epistaxis (7%), rhinitis (7%)
  Miscellaneous: Moniliasis (8%)
Mechanism of Action Binds to CD52, a nonmodulating antigen present on the surface of B and T lymphocytes, a majority of monocytes, macrophages, NK cells, and a subpopulation of granulocytes. After binding to $CD52^+$ cells, an antibody-dependent lysis of leukemic cells occurs.
Drug Interactions
  Increased Effect/Toxicity: Monoclonal antibodies (eg, abciximab, infliximab, and rituximab) may increase the risk for allergic reactions to alemtuzumab due to the presence of HACA antibodies. Alemtuzumab may enhance the adverse/toxic effects of vaccines (live organisms); vaccinal infections may develop.
  Decreased Effect:
  Alemtuzumab may decrease the effect of vaccines (dead organisms).
Pharmacodynamics/Kinetics
  Distribution: V_d: 0.18 L/kg
  Metabolism: Clearance decreases with repeated dosing (due to loss of CD52 receptors in periphery), resulting in a sevenfold increase in AUC.
  Half-life elimination: 11 hours (following first 30 mg dose); 6 days (following the last 30 mg dose)
Pregnancy Risk Factor C

Alendronate (a LEN droe nate)

Related Information
Rheumatoid Arthritis, Osteoarthritis, and Osteoporosis *on page 1759*
U.S. Brand Names Fosamax®
Canadian Brand Names Apo-Alendronate®; CO Alendronate; Fosamax®; Gen-Alendronate; Novo-Alendronate; PMS-Alendronate; ratio-Alendronate; Riva-Alendronate; Sandoz Alendronate
Mexican Brand Names Fosamax
Generic Available No
Index Terms Alendronate Sodium
Pharmacologic Category Bisphosphonate Derivative
Use Treatment and prevention of osteoporosis in postmenopausal females; treatment of osteoporosis in males; Paget's disease of the bone in patients who are symptomatic, at risk for future complications, or with alkaline phosphatase ≥2 times the upper limit of normal; treatment of glucocorticoid-induced osteoporosis in males and females with low bone mineral density who are receiving a daily dosage ≥7.5 mg of prednisone (or equivalent)
Local Anesthetic/Vasoconstrictor Precautions No information available to require special precautions
Effects on Dental Treatment Osteonecrosis of the jaw (ONJ), generally associated with local infection and/or tooth extraction and often with delayed healing, has been reported in patients taking bisphosphonates. Symptoms included nonhealing extraction socket or an exposed jawbone. Most reported cases of bisphosphonate-associated osteonecrosis have been in cancer patients treated with intravenous bisphosphonates. However, some have occurred in patients with postmenopausal osteoporosis taking oral bisphosphonates. Dental surgery may exacerbate ONJ. For patients requiring dental procedures, there are no data available to suggest whether discontinuation of bisphosphonate treatment reduces the risk of ONJ. Patients who develop ONJ while on bisphosphonate therapy should receive care by an oral surgeon. See Dental Comment.
Common Adverse Effects Note: Incidence of adverse effects (mostly GI) increases significantly in patients treated for Paget's disease at 40 mg/day.

>10%: Endocrine & metabolic: Hypocalcemia (transient, mild, 18%); hypophosphatemia (transient, mild, 10%)
1% to 10%:
Central nervous system: Headache (up to 3%)
Gastrointestinal: Abdominal pain (1% to 7%), acid reflux (1% to 4%), dyspepsia (1% to 4%), nausea (1% to 4%), flatulence (up to 4%), diarrhea (1% to 3%), gastroesophageal reflux disease (1% to 3%), constipation (up to 3%), esophageal ulcer (up to 2%), abdominal distension (up to 1%), gastritis (up to 1%), vomiting (up to 1%), dysphagia (up to 1%), gastric ulcer (1%), melena (1%)
Neuromuscular & skeletal: Musculoskeletal pain (up to 6%), muscle cramps (up to 1%)
Dosage Oral: Adults: **Note:** Patients treated with glucocorticoids and those with Paget's disease should receive adequate amounts of calcium and vitamin D.
Osteoporosis in postmenopausal females:
Prophylaxis: 5 mg once daily **or** 35 mg once weekly
Treatment: 10 mg once daily **or** 70 mg once weekly
Osteoporosis in males: 10 mg once daily **or** 70 mg once weekly
Osteoporosis secondary to glucocorticoids in males and females: Treatment: 5 mg once daily; a dose of 10 mg once daily should be used in postmenopausal females who are not receiving estrogen.
Paget's disease of bone in males and females: 40 mg once daily for 6 months
Retreatment: Relapses during the 12 months following therapy occurred in 9% of patients who responded to treatment. Specific retreatment data are not available. Following a 6-month post-treatment evaluation period, retreatment with alendronate may be considered in patients who have relapsed based on increases in serum alkaline phosphatase, which should be measured periodically. Retreatment may also be considered in those who failed to normalize their serum alkaline phosphatase.
Elderly: No dosage adjustment is necessary
Dosage adjustment in renal impairment:
Cl_{cr} 35-60 mL/minute: None necessary
Cl_{cr} <35 mL/minute: Alendronate is not recommended due to lack of experience
Dosage adjustment in hepatic impairment: None necessary
Mechanism of Action A bisphosphonate which inhibits bone resorption via actions on osteoclasts or on osteoclast precursors; decreases the rate of bone resorption, leading to an indirect increase in bone mineral density. In Paget's
(Continued)

Alendronate *(Continued)*

disease, characterized by disordered resorption and formation of bone, inhibition of resorption leads to an indirect decrease in bone formation; but the newly-formed bone has a more normal architecture.

Contraindications Hypersensitivity to alendronate, other bisphosphonates, or any component of the formulation; hypocalcemia; abnormalities of the esophagus which delay esophageal emptying such as stricture or achalasia; inability to stand or sit upright for at least 30 minutes; oral solution should not be used in patients at risk of aspiration

Warnings/Precautions Use caution in patients with renal impairment (not recommended for use in patients with Cl_{cr} <35 mL/minute); hypocalcemia must be corrected before therapy initiation; ensure adequate calcium and vitamin D intake. May cause irritation to upper gastrointestinal mucosa. Esophagitis, esophageal ulcers, esophageal erosions, and esophageal stricture (rare) have been reported; risk increases in patients unable to comply with dosing instructions. Use with caution in patients with dysphagia, esophageal disease, gastritis, duodenitis, or ulcers (may worsen underlying condition).

Bisphosphonate therapy has been associated with osteonecrosis, primarily of the jaw; this has been observed mostly in cancer patients, but also in patients with postmenopausal osteoporosis and other diagnoses. Dental exams and preventative dentistry should be performed prior to placing patients with risk factors on chronic bisphosphonate therapy. Invasive dental procedures should be avoided during treatment.

Infrequently, severe (and occasionally debilitating) bone, joint, and/or muscle pain have been reported during bisphosphonate treatment. The onset of pain ranged from a single day to several months. Symptoms usually resolve upon discontinuation. Some patients experienced recurrence when rechallenged with same drug or another bisphosphonate; avoid use in patients with a history of these symptoms in association with bisphosphonate therapy.

Safety and efficacy in children have not been established.

Drug Interactions
Increased Effect/Toxicity: Aminoglycosides may lower serum calcium levels with prolonged administration; concomitant use may have an additive hypocalcemic effect. Aspirin and NSAIDs may enhance the gastrointestinal adverse/toxic effects (increased incidence of GI ulcers) of bisphosphonate derivatives. Bisphosphonate derivatives may enhance the hypocalcemic effect of phosphate supplements.
Decreased Effect: The following agents may decrease the absorption of oral bisphosphonate derivatives: Antacids (aluminum, calcium, magnesium), oral calcium salts, oral iron salts, and oral magnesium salts.

Ethanol/Nutrition/Herb Interactions
Ethanol: Avoid ethanol (may increase risk of osteoporosis and gastric irritation).
Food: All food and beverages interfere with absorption. Coadministration with caffeine may reduce alendronate efficacy. Coadministration with dairy products may decrease alendronate absorption. Beverages (especially orange juice and coffee) and food may reduce the absorption of alendronate as much as 60%.

Dietary Considerations Ensure adequate calcium and vitamin D intake; however, wait at least 30 minutes after taking alendronate before taking any supplement. Alendronate must be taken with plain water first thing in the morning and at least 30 minutes before the first food or beverage of the day.

Pharmacodynamics/Kinetics
Distribution: 28 L (exclusive of bone)
Protein binding: ~78%
Metabolism: None
Bioavailability: Fasting: 0.6%; reduced 60% with food or drink
Half-life elimination: Exceeds 10 years
Excretion: Urine; feces (as unabsorbed drug)

Pregnancy Risk Factor C

Dosage Forms Note: Strength expressed as free acid
Solution, oral:
Fosamax®: 70 mg/75 mL
Tablet:
Fosamax®: 5 mg, 10 mg, 35 mg, 40 mg, 70 mg

Dental Comment A report by the Council of Scientific Affairs of the American Dental Association (accessed at: http://www.ada.org/prof/resources/topics/osteonecrosis.asp) as of July 2006 gave an estimated incidence of 0.7 cases for every 100,000 person-years of exposure to alendronate (Fosamax®). This translates to one case for every 142,857 person-years exposure. This figure from the ADA report was based on information received from Merck & Co citing 170 worldwide cases for alendronate (Fosamax®). In addition, Procter &

Gamble Pharmaceuticals has cited 20 cases for risedronate (Actonel®) and Roche Laboratories has cited one case for ibandronate (Boniva®).

Consumer Reports On Health stated that the risk of jaw bone osteoporosis due to alendronate (Fosamax®), risedronate (Actonel®), or ibandronate (Boniva®) taken to prevent osteoporosis is very low and is estimated to be one out of every 20,000 users. That report mentioned that tooth extraction or implants increase the risk of developing osteonecrosis in patients taking any of these drugs for osteoporosis. The report also recommended that patients should stop taking any of these oral drugs 1-2 months before and after such dental treatment. No evidence was presented to support this statement.

In terms of length of exposure to oral bisphosphonates prior to onset of ONJ, data from large population studies or controlled studies is lacking. A report by Marx et al, observed that of three cases of ONJ associated with Fosamax® exposure, one patient had been taking 10 mg/day by mouth for 6 years and the other two patients 10 mg/day by mouth for 3 and 2 years respectively. In contrast, they observed that in cancer patients receiving intravenous bisphosphonates, the time period between the first doses of the bisphosphonate to first recognition of exposed bone either by the patients or by the clinician, was 9.4 months for zoledronate (Zometa®), 14.3 months for pamidronate (Aredia®), and 12.1 months for pamidronate then to zoledronate.

Information on Fosamax® use in Australia and the incidence of ONJ has been reported. A survey form was sent to all of the Australian members of the Australian and New Zealand Association of Oral and Maxillofacial Surgeons requesting cases that they had identified as ONJ in 2004 and 2005. The definition of ONJ for the survey was an area of exposed bone in the jawbones that failed to heal within 6 weeks in patients taking bisphosphonates for bone disease. The frequency of ONJ in osteoporotic patients mainly on weekly oral alendronate was 1 in 8470 to 1 in 2260 (0.01% to 0.04%) patients. If extractions were carried out, the calculated frequency was 1 in 1130 to 1 in 296 (0.09% to 0.34%) patients. The minimum values in these cases were determined from the survey whereas the maximum values were obtained from the extrapolation to the entire Australia of the South Australian survey data. The median time to onset of ONJ in alendronate patients was 24 months.

Selected Readings

Author Unknown, "Safety Update: Bone-Building Drugs: Risks Explained," *Consumer Reports on Health*, 2006, 18(5):3.

Marx RE, Sawatari Y, Fortin M, et al, "Bisphosphonate-Induced Exposed Bone (Osteonecrosis/Osteopetrosis) of the Jaws: Risk Factors, Recognition, Prevention, and Treatment," *J Oral Maxillofac Surg*, 2005, 63(11):1567-75.

Mavrokokki T, Cheng A, Stein B, et al, "Nature and Frequency of Bisphosphonate-Associated Osteonecrosis of the Jaws in Australia," *J Oral Maxillofac Surg*, 2007, 65(3):415-23.

Alendronate and Cholecalciferol
(a LEN droe nate & kole e kal SI fer ole)

U.S. Brand Names Fosamax Plus D™
Canadian Brand Names Fosavance
Mexican Brand Names Fosamax Plus
Generic Available No
Index Terms Alendronate Sodium and Cholecalciferol; Cholecalciferol and Alendronate; Vitamin D₃
Pharmacologic Category Bisphosphonate Derivative; Vitamin D Analog
Use Treatment of osteoporosis in postmenopausal females; increase bone mass in males with osteoporosis
Local Anesthetic/Vasoconstrictor Precautions No information available to require special precautions
Effects on Dental Treatment Osteonecrosis of the jaw (ONJ), generally associated with local infection and/or tooth extraction and often with delayed healing, has been reported in patients taking bisphosphonates. Symptoms included nonhealing extraction socket or an exposed jawbone. Most reported cases of bisphosphonate-associated osteonecrosis have been in cancer patients treated with intravenous bisphosphonates. However, some have occurred in patients with postmenopausal osteoporosis taking oral bisphosphonates. Dental surgery may exacerbate ONJ. For patients requiring dental procedures, there are no data available to suggest whether discontinuation of bisphosphonate treatment reduces the risk of ONJ. Patients who develop ONJ while on bisphosphonate therapy should receive care by an oral surgeon. See Dental Comment in Alendronate monograph.
Common Adverse Effects See individual agents.
Mechanism of Action See individual agents.
(Continued)

Alendronate and Cholecalciferol *(Continued)*

Drug Interactions
  Increased Effect/Toxicity: See individual agents.
  Decreased Effect: See individual agents.
Pregnancy Risk Factor C
Dental Comment See Alendronate monograph.

Alendronate Sodium *see* Alendronate *on page 65*
Alendronate Sodium and Cholecalciferol *see* Alendronate and Cholecalciferol *on page 67*
Alenic Alka [OTC] *see* Aluminum Hydroxide and Magnesium Carbonate *on page 81*
Alenic Alka Tablet [OTC] *see* Aluminum Hydroxide and Magnesium Trisilicate *on page 82*
Aler-Cap [OTC] *see* DiphenhydrAMINE *on page 510*
Aler-Dryl [OTC] *see* DiphenhydrAMINE *on page 510*
Aler-Tab [OTC] *see* DiphenhydrAMINE *on page 510*
Alesse® *see* Ethinyl Estradiol and Levonorgestrel *on page 633*
Aleve® [OTC] *see* Naproxen *on page 1148*
Aleve® Cold & Sinus [OTC] *see* Naproxen and Pseudoephedrine *on page 1151*
Aleve® Sinus & Headache [OTC] *see* Naproxen and Pseudoephedrine *on page 1151*
Alfenta® *see* Alfentanil *on page 68*

Alfentanil *(al FEN ta nil)*

U.S. Brand Names Alfenta®
Canadian Brand Names Alfenta®; Alfentanil Injection, USP
Generic Available Yes
Index Terms Alfentanil Hydrochloride
Pharmacologic Category Analgesic, Opioid
Use Analgesic adjunct given by continuous infusion or in incremental doses in maintenance of anesthesia with barbiturate or N_2O or a primary anesthetic agent for the induction of anesthesia in patients undergoing general surgery in which endotracheal intubation and mechanical ventilation are required
Local Anesthetic/Vasoconstrictor Precautions No information available to require special precautions
Effects on Dental Treatment Key adverse event(s) related to dental treatment: Orthostatic hypotension.
  Erythromycin inhibits the liver metabolism of alfentanil resulting in increased sedation and prolonged respiratory depression. Clarithromycin may act similarly.
Common Adverse Effects
  >10%:
    Cardiovascular: Bradycardia, peripheral vasodilation
    Central nervous system: Drowsiness, sedation, intracranial pressure increased
    Gastrointestinal: Nausea, vomiting, constipation
    Endocrine & metabolic: Antidiuretic hormone release
    Ocular: Miosis
  1% to 10%:
    Cardiovascular: Cardiac arrhythmia, orthostatic hypotension
    Central nervous system: Confusion, CNS depression
    Ocular: Blurred vision
Restrictions C-II
Mechanism of Action Binds with stereospecific receptors at many sites within the CNS, increases pain threshold, alters pain perception, inhibits ascending pain pathways; is an ultra short-acting narcotic
Drug Interactions
  Cytochrome P450 Effect: Substrate of CYP3A4 (major)
  Increased Effect/Toxicity: Dextroamphetamine may enhance the analgesic effect of morphine and other opiate agonists. CNS depressants (eg, benzodiazepines, barbiturates, tricyclic antidepressants), erythromycin, reserpine, beta-blockers may increase the toxic effects of alfentanil. Alfentanil levels/effects may be increased by azole antifungals, clarithromycin, diclofenac, doxycycline, erythromycin, imatinib, isoniazid, nefazodone, nicardipine, propofol, protease inhibitors, quinidine, verapamil, telithromycin, and other inhibitors of CYP3A4.
Pharmacodynamics/Kinetics
  Onset of action: Rapid
  Duration (dose dependent): 30-60 minutes

Distribution: V_d: Newborns, premature: 1 L/kg; Children: 0.163-0.48 L/kg; Adults: 0.46 L/kg

Half-life elimination: Newborns, premature: 5.33-8.75 hours; Children: 40-60 minutes; Adults: 83-97 minutes

Pregnancy Risk Factor C

Alfentanil Hydrochloride *see* Alfentanil *on page 68*

Alferon® N *see* Interferon Alfa-n3 *on page 896*

Alfuzosin (al FYOO zoe sin)

U.S. Brand Names Uroxatral®
Canadian Brand Names Xatral
Mexican Brand Names Xatral OD
Generic Available No
Index Terms Alfuzosin Hydrochloride
Pharmacologic Category Alpha$_1$ Blocker
Use Treatment of the functional symptoms of benign prostatic hyperplasia (BPH)
Local Anesthetic/Vasoconstrictor Precautions No information available to require special precautions
Effects on Dental Treatment No significant effects or complications reported
Common Adverse Effects 1% to 10%:
Central nervous system: Dizziness (6%), fatigue (3%), headache (3%), pain (1% to 2%)
Gastrointestinal: Abdominal pain (1% to 2%), constipation (1% to 2%), dyspepsia (1% to 2%), nausea (1% to 2%)
Genitourinary: Impotence (1% to 2%)
Respiratory: Upper respiratory tract infection (3%), bronchitis (1% to 2%), pharyngitis (1% to 2%), sinusitis (1% to 2%)
Mechanism of Action An antagonist of alpha$_1$-adrenoreceptors in the lower urinary tract. Smooth muscle tone is mediated by the sympathetic nervous stimulation of alpha$_1$-adrenoreceptors, which are abundant in the prostate, prostatic capsule, prostatic urethra, and bladder neck. Blockade of these adrenoreceptors can cause smooth muscles in the bladder neck and prostate to relax, resulting in an improvement in urine flow rate and a reduction in symptoms of BPH.
Drug Interactions
Cytochrome P450 Effect: Substrate of CYP3A4 (major)
Increased Effect/Toxicity: Alfuzosin levels/effects may be increased by azole antifungals, clarithromycin, diclofenac, doxycycline, erythromycin, imatinib, isoniazid, nefazodone, nicardipine, propofol, protease inhibitors, quinidine, verapamil, telithromycin, and other CYP3A4 inhibitors. Concurrent use of itraconazole, ketoconazole, or ritonavir is contraindicated.
Decreased Effect: Levels/effects of alfuzosin may be decreased by aminoglutethimide, carbamazepine, nafcillin, nevirapine, phenobarbital, phenytoin, rifamycins, and other CYP3A4 inducers.
Pharmacodynamics/Kinetics
Absorption: Decreased 50% under fasting conditions
Distribution: V_d: 3.2 L/kg
Protein binding: 82% to 90%
Metabolism: Hepatic, primarily via CYP3A4; metabolism includes oxidation, O-demethylation, and N-dealkylation; forms metabolites (inactive)
Bioavailability: 49% following a meal
Half-life elimination: 10 hours
Time to peak, plasma: 8 hours following a meal
Excretion: Feces (69%); urine (24%)
Pregnancy Risk Factor B

Alfuzosin Hydrochloride *see* Alfuzosin *on page 69*

Alglucerase (al GLOO ser ase)

U.S. Brand Names Ceredase®
Generic Available No
Index Terms Glucocerebrosidase
Pharmacologic Category Enzyme
Use Replacement therapy for Gaucher's disease (type 1)
Local Anesthetic/Vasoconstrictor Precautions No information available to require special precautions
Effects on Dental Treatment No significant effects or complications reported
Common Adverse Effects Frequency not defined.
Cardiovascular: Peripheral edema
(Continued)

Alglucerase (Continued)

Central nervous system: Chills, fatigue, fever, headache, lightheadedness

Endocrine & metabolic: Hot flashes, menstrual abnormalities

Gastrointestinal: Abdominal discomfort, diarrhea, nausea, oral ulcerations, vomiting

Local: Injection site: Abscess, burning, discomfort, pruritus, swelling

Neuromuscular & skeletal: Backache, weakness

Miscellaneous: Dysosmia; hypersensitivity reactions (abdominal cramping, angioedema, chest discomfort, flushing, hypotension, nausea, pruritus, respiratory symptoms, urticaria); IgG antibody formation (~13%)

Mechanism of Action Alglucerase is a modified form of glucocerebrosidase; it is prepared from human placental tissue. Glucocerebrosidase is an enzyme deficient in Gaucher's disease. It is needed to catalyze the hydrolysis of glucocerebroside to glucose and ceramide.

Pharmacodynamics/Kinetics Half-life elimination: ~3-11 minutes

Pregnancy Risk Factor C

Alimta® see Pemetrexed on page 1264

Alinia® see Nitazoxanide on page 1178

Aliskiren (a lis KYE ren)

U.S. Brand Names Tekturna®

Generic Available No

Index Terms Aliskiren Hemifumarate; SPP100

Pharmacologic Category Renin Inhibitor

Use Treatment of hypertension, alone or in combination with other antihypertensive agents

Local Anesthetic/Vasoconstrictor Precautions No information available to require special precautions

Effects on Dental Treatment No significant effects or complications required

Common Adverse Effects 1% to 10%:

Central nervous system: Dizziness (2%)

Dermatologic: Rash (1%)

Endocrine and metabolic: Hyperkalemia (monotherapy ≤1%; concurrent with ACE inhibitor in diabetic patients 6%)

Gastrointestinal: Diarrhea (1% to 2%)

Hematologic: Creatine kinase increased (>300%: 1%)

Renal: BUN increased (≤7%), serum creatinine increased (≤7%)

Respiratory: Cough (1% to 5%)

Mechanism of Action Aliskerin is a direct renin inhibitor, resulting in blockade of the conversion of angiotensinogen to angiotensin I. Angiotensin I suppression decreases the formation of angiotensin II (Ang II), a potent blood pressure-elevating peptide (via direct vasoconstriction, aldosterone release, and sodium retention). Ang II also functions within the Renin-Angiotensin-Aldosterone System (RAAS) as a negative inhibitory feedback mediator within the renal parenchyma to suppress the further release of renin. Thus, reductions in Ang II levels suppress this feedback loop, leading to further increased plasma renin concentrations (PRC) and subsequent activity (PRA). This disinhibition effect can be potentially problematic for ACE inhibitor and ARB therapy, as increased PRA could partially overcome the pharmacologic inhibition of the RAAS. As aliskerin is a direct inhibitor of renin activity, blunting of PRA despite the increased PRC (from loss of the negative feedback) may be clinically advantageous.

Drug Interactions

Cytochrome P450 Effect: Substrate of CYP3A4 (minor)

Increased Effect/Toxicity: Atorvastatin and ketoconazole may increase the level/effect of aliskiren.

Decreased Effect: Aliskiren may decrease the level/effect of furosemide.

Pharmacodynamics/Kinetics

Onset of action: Maximum antihypertensive effect: Within 2 weeks

Absorption: Poor; absorption decreased by high-fat meal

Metabolism: Extent of metabolism unknown; in vitro studies indicate metabolism via CYP3A4

Bioavailability: ~3%

Half-life elimination: ~24 hours (range: 16-32 hours)

Time to peak, plasma: 1-3 hours

Excretion: Urine (~25% of absorbed dose excreted unchanged in urine); feces (unchanged via biliary excretion)

Pregnancy Risk Factor C (1st trimester)/D (2nd and 3rd trimesters)

Aliskiren Hemifumarate see Aliskiren on page 70

Alitretinoin (a li TRET i noyn)

U.S. Brand Names Panretin®
Canadian Brand Names Panretin®
Generic Available No
Pharmacologic Category Antineoplastic Agent, Miscellaneous
Use Orphan drug: Topical treatment of cutaneous lesions in AIDS-related Kaposi's sarcoma
Unlabeled/Investigational Use Cutaneous T-cell lymphomas
Local Anesthetic/Vasoconstrictor Precautions No information available to require special precautions
Effects on Dental Treatment No significant effects or complications reported
Common Adverse Effects
>10%:
Central nervous system: Pain (0% to 34%)
Dermatologic: Rash (25% to 77%), pruritus (8% to 11%)
Neuromuscular & skeletal: Paresthesia (3% to 22%)
5% to 10%:
Cardiovascular: Edema (3% to 8%)
Dermatologic: Exfoliative dermatitis (3% to 9%), skin disorder (0% to 8%)
Mechanism of Action Binds to retinoid receptors to inhibit growth of Kaposi's sarcoma
Drug Interactions
Increased Effect/Toxicity: Increased toxicity of DEET may occur if products containing this compound are used concurrently with alitretinoin. Due to limited absorption after topical application, interaction with systemic medications is unlikely.
Pharmacodynamics/Kinetics Absorption: Not extensive
Pregnancy Risk Factor D

Allopurinol (al oh PURE i nole)

U.S. Brand Names Aloprim™; Zyloprim®
Canadian Brand Names Alloprin®; Apo-Allopurinol®; Novo-Purol; Zyloprim®
Mexican Brand Names Atisuril; Etindrax; Zyloric
Generic Available Yes
(Continued)

Allopurinol *(Continued)*

Index Terms Allopurinol Sodium

Pharmacologic Category Xanthine Oxidase Inhibitor

Use

Oral: Prevention of attack of gouty arthritis and nephropathy; treatment of secondary hyperuricemia which may occur during treatment of tumors or leukemia; prevention of recurrent calcium oxalate calculi

I.V.: Treatment of elevated serum and urinary uric acid levels when oral therapy is not tolerated in patients with leukemia, lymphoma, and solid tumor malignancies who are receiving cancer chemotherapy

Local Anesthetic/Vasoconstrictor Precautions No information available to require special precautions

Effects on Dental Treatment No significant effects or complications reported

Common Adverse Effects >1%:

Dermatologic: Rash (increased with ampicillin or amoxicillin use, 1.5% per manufacturer, >10% in some reports)

Gastrointestinal: Nausea (1.3%), vomiting (1.2%)

Renal: Renal failure/impairment (1.2%)

Mechanism of Action Allopurinol inhibits xanthine oxidase, the enzyme responsible for the conversion of hypoxanthine to xanthine to uric acid. Allopurinol is metabolized to oxypurinol which is also an inhibitor of xanthine oxidase; allopurinol acts on purine catabolism, reducing the production of uric acid without disrupting the biosynthesis of vital purines.

Drug Interactions

Increased Effect/Toxicity: Allopurinol may increase the effects of azathioprine, chlorpropamide, mercaptopurine, theophylline, and oral anticoagulants. An increased risk of bone marrow suppression may occur when given with myelosuppressive agents (cyclophosphamide, possibly other alkylating agents). Amoxicillin/ampicillin, ACE inhibitors, and thiazide diuretics have been associated with hypersensitivity reactions when combined with allopurinol (rare), and the incidence of rash may be increased with penicillins (ampicillin, amoxicillin). Urinary acidification with large amounts of vitamin C may increase kidney stone formation.

Decreased Effect: Ethanol decreases effectiveness.

Pharmacodynamics/Kinetics

Onset of action: Peak effect: 1-2 weeks

Absorption: Oral: ~80%; Rectal: Poor and erratic

Distribution: V_d: ~1.6 L/kg; V_{ss}: 0.84-0.87 L/kg; enters breast milk

Protein binding: <1%

Metabolism: ~75% to active metabolites, chiefly oxypurinol

Bioavailability: 49% to 53%

Half-life elimination:

Normal renal function: Parent drug: 1-3 hours; Oxypurinol: 18-30 hours

End-stage renal disease: Prolonged

Time to peak, plasma: Oral: 30-120 minutes

Excretion: Urine (76% as oxypurinol, 12% as unchanged drug)

Allopurinol and oxypurinol are dialyzable

Pregnancy Risk Factor C

Almotriptan *(al moh TRIP tan)*

Related Information

Temporomandibular Dysfunction (TMD) *on page 1822*

U.S. Brand Names Axert™

Canadian Brand Names Axert™

Generic Available No

Index Terms Almotriptan Malate

Pharmacologic Category Antimigraine Agent; Serotonin 5-HT$_{1B, 1D}$ Receptor Agonist

Use Acute treatment of migraine with or without aura

Local Anesthetic/Vasoconstrictor Precautions No information available to require special precautions

Effects on Dental Treatment Key adverse effect(s) related to dental treatment: Xerostomia (normal salivary flow resumes upon discontinuation)

Common Adverse Effects 1% to 10%:
  Central nervous system: Headache (>1%), dizziness (>1%), somnolence (>1%)
  Gastrointestinal: Nausea (1% to 2%), xerostomia (1%)
  Neuromuscular & skeletal: Paresthesia (1%)
Dosage Oral: Adults: Migraine: Initial: 6.25-12.5 mg in a single dose; if the headache returns, repeat the dose after 2 hours; no more than 2 doses in 24-hour period
  Note: If the first dose is ineffective, diagnosis needs to be re-evaluated. Safety of treating more than 4 migraines/month has not been established.
  Dosage adjustment in renal impairment: Initial: 6.25 mg in a single dose; maximum daily dose: ≤12.5 mg
  Dosage adjustment in hepatic impairment: Initial: 6.25 mg in a single dose; maximum daily dose: ≤12.5 mg
Mechanism of Action Selective agonist for serotonin (5-HT$_{1B}$, 5-HT$_{1D}$, 5-HT$_{1F}$ receptors) in cranial arteries; causes vasoconstriction and reduce sterile inflammation associated with antidromic neuronal transmission correlating with relief of migraine
Contraindications Hypersensitivity to almotriptan or any component of the formulation; use as prophylactic therapy for migraine; hemiplegic or basilar migraine; cluster headache; known or suspected ischemic heart disease (angina pectoris, MI, documented silent ischemia, coronary artery vasospasm, Prinzmetal's variant angina); peripheral vascular syndromes (including ischemic bowel disease); uncontrolled hypertension; use within 24 hours of another 5-HT$_1$ agonist; use within 24 hours of ergotamine derivative; concurrent administration or within 2 weeks of discontinuing an MAO inhibitor (specifically MAO type A inhibitors)
Warnings/Precautions Almotriptan is indicated only in patients ≥18 years of age with a clear diagnosis of migraine headache. If a patient does not respond to the first dose, the diagnosis of migraine should be reconsidered. Do not give to patients with risk factors for CAD until a cardiovascular evaluation has been performed; if evaluation is satisfactory, the healthcare provider should administer the first dose and cardiovascular status should be periodically re-evaluated. Cardiac events (coronary artery vasospasm, transient ischemia, myocardial infarction, ventricular tachycardia/fibrillation, cardiac arrest, and death), cerebral/subarachnoid hemorrhage, stroke, peripheral vascular ischemia, and colonic ischemia have been reported with 5-HT$_1$ agonist administration. Significant elevation in blood pressure, including hypertensive crisis, has also been reported on rare occasions in patients with and without a history of hypertension. Use with caution in liver or renal dysfunction. Symptoms of agitation, confusion, hallucinations, hyper-reflexia, myoclonus, shivering, and tachycardia (serotonin syndrome) may occur with concomitant proserotonergic drugs (ie, SSRIs/SNRIs or triptans) or agents which reduce almotriptan's metabolism. Safety and efficacy in pediatric patients have not been established.
Drug Interactions
  Cytochrome P450 Effect: Substrate (minor) of CYP2D6, 3A4
  Increased Effect/Toxicity: Ergot-containing drugs prolong vasospastic reactions; ketoconazole increases almotriptan serum concentration; SSRIs/SNRIs or other serotonin agonists may increase symptoms of hyper-reflexia, weakness, and incoordination; MAO inhibitors may increase toxicity
Dietary Considerations May be taken without regard to meals
Pharmacodynamics/Kinetics
  Absorption: Well absorbed
  Distribution: V$_d$: 180-200 L
  Protein binding: ~35%
  Metabolism: MAO type A oxidative deamination (~27% of dose); via CYP3A4 and 2D6 (~12% of dose) to inactive metabolites
  Bioavailability: 70%
  Half-life elimination: 3-4 hours
  Time to peak: 1-3 hours
  Excretion: Urine (40% as unchanged drug); feces (13% unchanged and metabolized)
Pregnancy Risk Factor C
Dosage Forms
  Tablet:
    Axert™: 6.25 mg, 12.5 mg

Alosetron (a LOE se tron)

U.S. Brand Names Lotronex®
Generic Available No
Pharmacologic Category Selective 5-HT$_3$ Receptor Antagonist
Use Treatment of women with severe diarrhea-predominant irritable bowel syndrome (IBS) who have failed to respond to conventional therapy
Local Anesthetic/Vasoconstrictor Precautions No information available to require special precautions
Effects on Dental Treatment No significant effects or complications reported
Common Adverse Effects
>10%: Gastrointestinal: Constipation (dose related) (29%)
1% to 10%: Gastrointestinal: Abdominal discomfort and pain (7%), nausea (6%), gastrointestinal discomfort and pain (6%), abdominal distention (2%), hemorrhoids (2%), regurgitation and reflux (2%)
Restrictions Only physicians enrolled in GlaxoSmithKline's Prescribing Program for Lotronex® may prescribe this medication. Program stickers must be affixed to all prescriptions; no phone, fax, or computerized prescriptions are permitted with this program.
An FDA-approved medication guide must be distributed when dispensing an outpatient prescription (new or refill) where this medication is to be used without direct supervision of a healthcare provider. Medication guides are available at http://www.fda.gov/cder/Offices/ODS/medication_guides.htm.
Mechanism of Action Alosetron is a potent and selective antagonist of a subtype of the serotonin 5-HT$_3$ receptor. 5-HT$_3$ receptors are ligand-gated ion channels extensively distributed on enteric neurons in the human gastrointestinal tract, as well as other peripheral and central locations. Activation of these channels affect the regulation of visceral pain, colonic transit, and gastrointestinal secretions. In patients with irritable bowel syndrome, blockade of these channels may reduce pain, abdominal discomfort, urgency, and diarrhea.
Drug Interactions
Cytochrome P450 Effect: Substrate of CYP1A2 (major), 2C9 (minor), 3A4 (minor); **Inhibits** CYP1A2 (weak), 2E1 (weak)
Increased Effect/Toxicity: CYP1A2 inhibitors may increase the levels/effects of alosetron; example inhibitors include ciprofloxacin, fluvoxamine (contraindicated), ketoconazole, norfloxacin, ofloxacin, and rofecoxib.
Pharmacodynamics/Kinetics
Distribution: V$_d$: 65-95 L
Protein binding: 82%
Metabolism: Extensive hepatic metabolism. Alosetron is metabolized by CYP2C9, 3A4, and 1A2. Thirteen metabolites have been detected in the urine. Biological activity of these metabolites in unknown.
Bioavailability: Mean: 50% to 60% (range: 30% to >90%); decreased with food (25%)
Half-life elimination: 1.5 hours for alosetron
Time to peak: 1 hour after oral administration
Excretion: Urine (73%) and feces (24%); 7% as unchanged drug (1% feces, 6% urine)
Pregnancy Risk Factor B

Alpha$_1$-Proteinase Inhibitor (al fa won PRO tee in ase in HI bi tor)

U.S. Brand Names Aralast; Prolastin®; Zemaira®
Canadian Brand Names Prolastin®
Generic Available No
Index Terms Alpha$_1$-Antitrypsin; α_1-PI; Alpha$_1$-Proteinase Inhibitor, Human; A$_1$-PI

Pharmacologic Category Antitrypsin Deficiency Agent

Use Replacement therapy in congenital alpha$_1$-antitrypsin deficiency with clinical emphysema

Local Anesthetic/Vasoconstrictor Precautions No information available to require special precautions

Effects on Dental Treatment Key adverse event(s) related to dental treatment: Pharyngitis

Common Adverse Effects

>10%: Hepatic: ALT/AST increased (11%; ~4 times ULN)

1% to 10%: Respiratory: Pharyngitis (2%)

Mechanism of Action Alpha$_1$-antitrypsin (AAT) is the principle protease inhibitor in serum. Its major physiologic role is to render proteolytic enzymes (secreted during inflammation) inactive. A decrease in AAT, as seen in congenital AAT deficiency, leads to increased elastic damage in the lung, causing emphysema.

Pharmacodynamics/Kinetics

Half-life elimination: Metabolic: 5.9 days (Aralast™)

Time to peak, serum: Threshold levels achieved after 3 weeks

Pregnancy Risk Factor C

Alph-E [OTC] *see* Vitamin E *on page 1664*

Alph-E-Mixed [OTC] *see* Vitamin E *on page 1664*

Alprazolam (al PRAY zoe lam)

Related Information

Sedation *on page 1825*

Temporomandibular Dysfunction (TMD) *on page 1822*

Related Sample Prescriptions

Sedation (Prior to Dental Treatment) *on page 1846*

U.S. Brand Names Alprazolam Intensol®; Niravam™; Xanax®; Xanax XR®

Canadian Brand Names Alti-Alprazolam; Apo-Alpraz®; Apo-Alpraz® TS; Gen-Alprazolam; Novo-Alprazol; Nu-Alprax; Xanax®; Xanax TS™

Mexican Brand Names Neupax; Tafil

Generic Available Yes: Extended release tablet, immediate release tablet

Pharmacologic Category Benzodiazepine

Dental Use Preoperative sedation

Use Treatment of anxiety disorder (GAD); panic disorder, with or without agoraphobia; anxiety associated with depression

Unlabeled/Investigational Use Anxiety in children

Local Anesthetic/Vasoconstrictor Precautions No information available to require special precautions

Effects on Dental Treatment Key adverse event(s) related to dental treatment: Significant xerostomia and changes in salivation (normal salivary flow resumes upon discontinuation)

Significant Adverse Effects

>10%:

Central nervous system: Abnormal coordination, cognitive disorder, depression, drowsiness, fatigue, irritability, lightheadedness, memory impairment, sedation, somnolence

Gastrointestinal: Appetite increased/decreased, constipation, salivation decreased, weight gain/loss, xerostomia

Genitourinary: Micturition difficulty

Neuromuscular & skeletal: Dysarthria

1% to 10%:

Cardiovascular: Hypotension

Central nervous system: Agitation, attention disturbance, confusion, depersonalization, derealization, disorientation, disinhibition, dizziness, dream abnormalities, fear, hallucinations, hypersomnia, nightmares, seizure, talkativeness

Dermatologic: Dermatitis, pruritus, rash

Endocrine & metabolic: Libido decreased/increased, menstrual disorders

Gastrointestinal: Salivation increased

Genitourinary: Incontinence

Hepatic: Bilirubin increased, jaundice, liver enzymes increased

Neuromuscular & skeletal: Arthralgia, ataxia, myalgia, paresthesia

Ocular: Diplopia

Respiratory: Allergic rhinitis, dyspnea

<1% (Limited to important or life-threatening): Amnesia, falls, galactorrhea, gynecomastia, hepatic failure, hepatitis, hyperprolactinemia, Stevens-Johnson syndrome

Restrictions C-IV

(Continued)

Alprazolam *(Continued)*

Dental Usual Dosing Preoperative sedation: Adults: Oral: 0.5 mg in evening at bedtime and 0.5 mg 1 hour before procedure

Dosage Oral: **Note:** Treatment >4 months should be re-evaluated to determine the patient's continued need for the drug

Children: Anxiety (unlabeled use): Immediate release: Initial: 0.005 mg/kg/dose or 0.125 mg/dose 3 times/day; increase in increments of 0.125-0.25 mg, up to a maximum of 0.02 mg/kg/dose or 0.06 mg/kg/day (0.375-3 mg/day)

Adults:

Anxiety: Immediate release: Effective doses are 0.5-4 mg/day in divided doses; the manufacturer recommends starting at 0.25-0.5 mg 3 times/day; titrate dose upward; usual maximum: 4 mg/day. Patients requiring doses >4 mg/day should be increased cautiously. Periodic reassessment and consideration of dosage reduction is recommended.

Anxiety associated with depression: Immediate release: Average dose required: 2.5-3 mg/day in divided doses

Ethanol withdrawal (unlabeled use): Immediate release: Usual dose: 2-2.5 mg/day in divided doses

Panic disorder:

Immediate release: Initial: 0.5 mg 3 times/day; dose may be increased every 3-4 days in increments ≤1 mg/day. Mean effective dosage: 5-6 mg/day; many patients obtain relief at 2 mg/day, as much as 10 mg/day may be required

Extended release: 0.5-1 mg once daily; may increase dose every 3-4 days in increments ≤1 mg/day (range: 3-6 mg/day)

Switching from immediate release to extended release: Patients may be switched to extended release tablets by taking the total daily dose of the immediate release tablets and giving it once daily using the extended release preparation.

Preoperative sedation: 0.5 mg in evening at bedtime and 0.5 mg 1 hour before procedure

Dose reduction: Abrupt discontinuation should be avoided. Daily dose may be decreased by 0.5 mg every 3 days, however, some patients may require a slower reduction. If withdrawal symptoms occur, resume previous dose and discontinue on a less rapid schedule.

Elderly: Initial: 0.125-0.25 mg twice daily; increase by 0.125 mg/day as needed. The smallest effective dose should be used. **Note:** Elderly patients may be more sensitive to the effects of alprazolam including ataxia and oversedation. The elderly may also have impaired renal function leading to decreased clearance. Titrate gradually, if needed.

Immediate release: Initial: 0.25 mg 2-3 times/day

Extended release: Initial: 0.5 mg once daily

Dosing adjustment in renal impairment: No guidelines for adjustment; use caution

Dosing adjustment in hepatic impairment: Reduce dose by 50% to 60% or avoid in cirrhosis

Mechanism of Action Binds to stereospecific benzodiazepine receptors on the postsynaptic GABA neuron at several sites within the central nervous system, including the limbic system, reticular formation. Enhancement of the inhibitory effect of GABA on neuronal excitability results by increased neuronal membrane permeability to chloride ions. This shift in chloride ions results in hyperpolarization (a less excitable state) and stabilization.

Contraindications Hypersensitivity to alprazolam or any component of the formulation (cross-sensitivity with other benzodiazepines may exist); narrow-angle glaucoma; concurrent use with ketoconazole or itraconazole; pregnancy

Warnings/Precautions Rebound or withdrawal symptoms, including seizures, may occur 18 hours to 3 days following abrupt discontinuation or large decreases in dose (more common in patients receiving >4 mg/day or prolonged treatment). Breakthrough anxiety may occur at the end of dosing interval. Use with caution in patients receiving concurrent CYP3A4 inhibitors. Use with caution in renal impairment or predisposition to urate nephropathy. Use with caution in elderly or debilitated patients, patients with hepatic disease (including alcoholics), renal impairment, or obese patients.

Causes CNS depression (dose related) which may impair physical and mental capabilities. Patients must be cautioned about performing tasks that require mental alertness (eg, operating machinery or driving). Effects with other sedative drugs or ethanol may be potentiated. Benzodiazepines have been associated with falls and traumatic injury and should be used with extreme caution in patients who are at risk of these events (especially the elderly). Use with caution in patients with respiratory disease or impaired gag reflex.

Use caution in patients with depression, particularly if suicidal risk may be present. Episodes of mania or hypomania have occurred in depressed patients treated with alprazolam. May cause physical or psychological dependence. Acute withdrawal may be precipitated in patients after administration of flumazenil.

Benzodiazepines have been associated with anterograde amnesia. Paradoxical reactions have been reported with benzodiazepines, particularly in adolescent/pediatric or psychiatric patients. Does not have analgesic, antidepressant, or antipsychotic properties.

Drug Interactions Substrate of CYP3A4 (major)

CNS depressants: Sedative effects and/or respiratory depression may be additive with CNS depressants. Includes ethanol, barbiturates, opioid analgesics, and other sedative agents; monitor for increased effect.

CYP3A4 inducers: CYP3A4 inducers may decrease the levels/effects of alprazolam. Example inducers include aminoglutethimide, carbamazepine, nafcillin, nevirapine, phenobarbital, phenytoin, and rifamycins.

CYP3A4 inhibitors: May increase the levels/effects of alprazolam. Example inhibitors include azole antifungals, clarithromycin, diclofenac, doxycycline, erythromycin, imatinib, isoniazid, nefazodone, nicardipine, propofol, protease inhibitors, quinidine, telithromycin, and verapamil. Contraindicated with itraconazole and ketoconazole.

Fluoxetine: May increase plasma concentrations/effects of alprazolam.

Oral contraceptives: May increase serum levels/effects of alprazolam.

Theophylline: May partially antagonize some of the effects of benzodiazepines; monitor for decreased response; may require higher doses for sedation.

Tricyclic antidepressants: Plasma concentrations of imipramine and desipramine have been reported to be increased 31% and 20%, respectively, by concomitant administration; monitor.

Ethanol/Nutrition/Herb Interactions

Cigarette smoking: May decrease alprazolam concentrations up to 50%.

Ethanol: Avoid ethanol (may increase CNS depression).

Food: Alprazolam serum concentration is unlikely to be increased by grapefruit juice because of alprazolam's high oral bioavailability. The C_{max} of the extended release formulation is increased by 25% when a high-fat meal is given 2 hours before dosing. T_{max} is decreased 30% when food is given immediately prior to dose. T_{max} is increased by 30% when food is given ≥1 hour after dose.

Herb/Nutraceutical: St John's wort may decrease alprazolam levels. Avoid valerian, St John's wort, kava kava, gotu kola (may increase CNS depression).

Pharmacodynamics/Kinetics

Distribution: V_d: 0.9-1.2 L/kg; enters breast milk

Protein binding: 80%

Metabolism: Hepatic via CYP3A4; forms two active metabolites (4-hydroxyalprazolam and α-hydroxyalprazolam)

Bioavailability: 90%

Half-life elimination:

Adults: 11.2 hours (range: 6.3-26.9)

Elderly: 16.3 hours (range: 9-26.9 hours)

Alcoholic liver disease: 19.7 hours (range: 5.8-65.3 hours)

Obesity: 21.8 hours (range: 9.9-40.4 hours)

Time to peak, serum: 1-2 hours

Excretion: Urine (as unchanged drug and metabolites)

Pregnancy Risk Factor D

Lactation Enters breast milk/not recommended (AAP rates "of concern")

Breast-Feeding Considerations Symptoms of withdrawal, lethargy, and loss of body weight have been reported in infants exposed to alprazolam and/or benzodiazepines while nursing. Breast-feeding is not recommended.

Dosage Forms Excipient information presented when available (limited, particularly for generics); consult specific product labeling.

Solution, oral [concentrate]:

Alprazolam Intensol®: 1 mg/mL (30 mL)

Tablet: 0.25 mg, 0.5 mg, 1 mg, 2 mg

Xanax®: 0.25 mg, 0.5 mg, 1 mg, 2 mg

Tablet, extended release: 0.5 mg, 1 mg, 2 mg, 3 mg

Xanax XR®: 0.5 mg, 1 mg, 2 mg, 3 mg

Tablet, orally disintegrating [scored]:

Niravam™: 0.25 mg, 0.5 mg, 1 mg, 2 mg [orange flavor]

Alprazolam Intensol® see Alprazolam on page 75

Alprostadil (al PROS ta dill)

U.S. Brand Names Caverject®; Caverject Impulse®; Edex®; Muse®; Prostin VR Pediatric®

Canadian Brand Names Caverject®; Muse® Pellet; Prostin® VR

Mexican Brand Names Caverject

Generic Available Yes: Solution for injection

Index Terms PGE$_1$; Prostaglandin E$_1$

Pharmacologic Category Prostaglandin

Use

Prostin VR Pediatric®: Temporary maintenance of patency of ductus arteriosus in neonates with ductal-dependent congenital heart disease until surgery can be performed. These defects include cyanotic (eg, pulmonary atresia, pulmonary stenosis, tricuspid atresia, Fallot's tetralogy, transposition of the great vessels) and acyanotic (eg, interruption of aortic arch, coarctation of aorta, hypoplastic left ventricle) heart disease.

Caverject®: Treatment of erectile dysfunction of vasculogenic, psychogenic, or neurogenic etiology; adjunct in the diagnosis of erectile dysfunction

Edex®, Muse®: Treatment of erectile dysfunction of vasculogenic, psychogenic, or neurogenic etiology

Unlabeled/Investigational Use Investigational: Treatment of pulmonary hypertension in infants and children with congenital heart defects with left-to-right shunts

Local Anesthetic/Vasoconstrictor Precautions No information available to require special precautions

Effects on Dental Treatment No significant effects or complications reported

Mechanism of Action Causes vasodilation by means of direct effect on vascular and ductus arteriosus smooth muscle; relaxes trabecular smooth muscle by dilation of cavernosal arteries when injected along the penile shaft, allowing blood flow to and entrapment in the lacunar spaces of the penis (ie, corporeal veno-occlusive mechanism)

Pregnancy Risk Factor X/C (Muse®)

Alrex® see Loteprednol on page 1006

Altabax™ see Retapamulin on page 1417

Altace® see Ramipril on page 1406

Altachlore [OTC] see Sodium Chloride on page 1480

Altafrin see Phenylephrine on page 1293

Altamist [OTC] see Sodium Chloride on page 1480

Altarussin DM [OTC] see Guaifenesin and Dextromethorphan on page 796

Altaryl [OTC] see DiphenhydrAMINE on page 510

Alteplase (AL te plase)

Related Information

Cardiovascular Diseases on page 1726

U.S. Brand Names Activase®; Cathflo® Activase®

Canadian Brand Names Activase® rt-PA; Cathflo® Activase®

Mexican Brand Names Actilyse

Generic Available No

Index Terms Alteplase, Recombinant; Alteplase, Tissue Plasminogen Activator, Recombinant; tPA

Pharmacologic Category Thrombolytic Agent

Use Management of acute myocardial infarction for the lysis of thrombi in coronary arteries; management of acute ischemic stroke

Acute myocardial infarction (AMI): Chest pain ≥20 minutes, ≤12-24 hours; S-T elevation ≥0.1 mV in at least two ECG leads

Acute pulmonary embolism (APE): Age ≤75 years: Documented massive pulmonary embolism by pulmonary angiography or echocardiography or high probability lung scan with clinical shock

Cathflo® Activase®: Restoration of central venous catheter function

Unlabeled/Investigational Use Acute peripheral arterial occlusive disease

Local Anesthetic/Vasoconstrictor Precautions No information available to require special precautions

Effects on Dental Treatment Key adverse event(s) related to dental treatment: As with all drugs which may affect hemostasis, bleeding is the major adverse effect associated with alteplase. Hemorrhage may occur at virtually any site; risk is dependent on multiple variables, including the dosage administered, concurrent use of multiple agents which alter hemostasis, and patient predisposition. Rapid lysis of coronary artery thrombi by thrombolytic agents may be associated with reperfusion-related atrial and/or ventricular arrhythmias.

Common Adverse Effects As with all drugs which may affect hemostasis, bleeding is the major adverse effect associated with alteplase. Hemorrhage may occur at virtually any site. Risk is dependent on multiple variables, including the dosage administered, concurrent use of multiple agents which alter hemostasis, and patient predisposition. Rapid lysis of coronary artery thrombi by thrombolytic agents may be associated with reperfusion-related atrial and/or ventricular arrhythmia. **Note:** Lowest rate of bleeding complications expected with dose used to restore catheter function.

1% to 10%:
  Cardiovascular: Hypotension
  Central nervous system: Fever
  Dermatologic: Bruising (1%)
  Gastrointestinal: GI hemorrhage (5%), nausea, vomiting
  Genitourinary: GU hemorrhage (4%)
  Hematologic: Bleeding (0.5% major, 7% minor: GUSTO trial)
  Local: Bleeding at catheter puncture site (15.3%, accelerated administration)

Additional cardiovascular events associated **with use in MI:** AV block, cardiogenic shock, heart failure, cardiac arrest, recurrent ischemia/infarction, myocardial rupture, electromechanical dissociation, pericardial effusion, pericarditis, mitral regurgitation, cardiac tamponade, thromboembolism, pulmonary edema, asystole, ventricular tachycardia, bradycardia, ruptured intracranial AV malformation, seizure, hemorrhagic bursitis, cholesterol crystal embolization

Additional events associated **with use in pulmonary embolism:** Pulmonary re-embolization, pulmonary edema, pleural effusion, thromboembolism

Additional events associated **with use in stroke:** Cerebral edema, cerebral herniation, seizure, new ischemic stroke

Mechanism of Action Initiates local fibrinolysis by binding to fibrin in a thrombus (clot) and converts entrapped plasminogen to plasmin

Drug Interactions
  Increased Effect/Toxicity: The potential for hemorrhage with alteplase is increased by oral anticoagulants (warfarin), heparin, low molecular weight heparins, and drugs which affect platelet function (eg, NSAIDs, dipyridamole, ticlopidine, clopidogrel, IIb/IIIa antagonists). Concurrent use with aspirin and heparin may increase the risk of bleeding. However, aspirin and heparin were used concomitantly with alteplase in the majority of patients in clinical studies.

  Decreased Effect: Aminocaproic acid (an antifibrinolytic agent) may decrease the effectiveness of thrombolytic therapy. Nitroglycerin may increase the hepatic clearance of alteplase, potentially reducing lytic activity (limited clinical information).

Pharmacodynamics/Kinetics
  Duration: >50% present in plasma cleared ~5 minutes after infusion terminated, ~80% cleared within 10 minutes
  Excretion: Clearance: Rapidly from circulating plasma (550-650 mL/minute), primarily hepatic; >50% present in plasma is cleared within 5 minutes after the infusion is terminated, ~80% cleared within 10 minutes

Pregnancy Risk Factor C

Altretamine (al TRET a meen)

U.S. Brand Names Hexalen®
Canadian Brand Names Hexalen®
Generic Available No
Index Terms Hexamethylmelamine; HEXM; HMM; HXM; NSC-13875
Pharmacologic Category Antineoplastic Agent, Miscellaneous
Use Palliative treatment of persistent or recurrent ovarian cancer
Local Anesthetic/Vasoconstrictor Precautions No information available to require special precautions
Effects on Dental Treatment No significant effects or complications reported
(Continued)

Altretamine *(Continued)*

Common Adverse Effects

>10%:

Central nervous system: Peripheral sensory neuropathy (31%; moderate-to-severe 9%), neurotoxicity (21%; may be progressive and dose-limiting)

Gastrointestinal: Nausea/vomiting (33% to 70%; severe 1%), diarrhea (48%)

Hematologic: Anemia (33%), leukopenia (5% to 15%; grade 4: 1%), neutropenia

1% to 10%:

Central nervous system: Fatigue (1%), seizure (1%)

Gastrointestinal: Stomach cramps, anorexia (1%)

Hematologic: Thrombocytopenia (9%)

Hepatic: Alkaline phosphatase increased (9%)

Mechanism of Action Although altretamine's clinical antitumor spectrum resembles that of alkylating agents, the drug has demonstrated activity in alkylator-resistant patients. The drug selectively inhibits the incorporation of radioactive thymidine and uridine into DNA and RNA, inhibiting DNA and RNA synthesis; reactive intermediates covalently bind to microsomal proteins and DNA; can spontaneously degrade to demethylated melamines and formaldehyde which are also cytotoxic.

Drug Interactions

Increased Effect/Toxicity: Altretamine may enhance the hypotensive effects of MAO inhibitors and tricyclic antidepressants.

Decreased Effect: Pyridoxine may diminish the effect of altretamine.

Pharmacodynamics/Kinetics

Absorption: Well absorbed (75% to 89%)

Distribution: Highly concentrated hepatically and renally; low in other organs

Protein binding: 50% to 94%

Metabolism: Hepatic; rapid and extensive demethylation to active metabolites (pentamethylmelamine and tetramethylmelamine)

Half-life elimination: 13 hours

Time to peak, plasma: 0.5-3 hours

Excretion: Urine (90%, <1% as unchanged drug)

Pregnancy Risk Factor D

Aluminum Chloride *(a LOO mi num KLOR ide)*

U.S. Brand Names Hemodent™

Generic Available No

Pharmacologic Category Astringent; Hemostatic Agent

Dental Use Hemostatic; gingival retraction; to control bleeding created during a dental procedure

Use Hemostatic

Local Anesthetic/Vasoconstrictor Precautions No information available to require special precautions

Effects on Dental Treatment No significant effects or complications reported

Significant Adverse Effects No data reported.

Dental Usual Dosing Control of dental bleeding: Apply retraction cord as directed

Dosage Control of bleeding: Apply retraction cord as directed

Mechanism of Action Precipitates tissue and blood proteins causing a mechanical obstruction to hemorrhage from injured blood vessels

Contraindications No data reported

Warnings/Precautions Since large amounts of astringents may cause tissue irritation and possible damage, only small amounts should be applied.

Drug Interactions No data reported

Dosage Forms Excipient information presented when available (limited, particularly for generics); consult specific product labeling.

Liquid:

Hemodent™: 21% (10 mL, 20 mL, 40 mL)

Retraction cord [impregnated with 21% solution]:

Hemodent™: Braided cord, thin (7 ft); braided cord medium thin (7 ft); twisted cord #3 (7 ft); twisted cord #9 (7ft)

Aluminum Hydroxide *(a LOO mi num hye DROKS ide)*

U.S. Brand Names ALternaGel® [OTC]; Dermagran® [OTC]

Canadian Brand Names Amphojel®; Basaljel®

Generic Available Yes: Suspension

Pharmacologic Category Antacid; Antidote; Protectant, Topical

Use Treatment of hyperacidity; hyperphosphatemia; temporary protection of minor cuts, scrapes, and burns

Local Anesthetic/Vasoconstrictor Precautions No information available to require special precautions

Effects on Dental Treatment Key adverse event(s) related to dental treatment: Chalky taste. Aluminum and magnesium ions prevent GI absorption of tetracycline by forming a large ionized chelated molecule with the aluminum ion and tetracyclines in the stomach. Aluminum hydroxide prevents GI absorption of ketoconazole and itraconazole by increasing the pH in the GI tract. Any of these drugs should be administered at least 1 hour before $Al(OH)_3$.

Common Adverse Effects Frequency not defined.

Gastrointestinal: Constipation, stomach cramps, fecal impaction, nausea, vomiting, discoloration of feces (white speckles)

Endocrine & metabolic: Hypophosphatemia, hypomagnesemia

Mechanism of Action Neutralizes hydrochloride in stomach to form Al $(Cl)_3$ salt + H_2O

Drug Interactions

Decreased Effect: Aluminum hydroxide may decrease the absorption of allopurinol, antibiotics (tetracyclines, quinolones, some cephalosporins), bisphosphonate derivatives, corticosteroids, cyclosporine, delavirdine, iron salts, imidazole antifungals, isoniazid, mycophenolate, penicillamine, phosphate supplements, phenytoin, phenothiazines, trientine. Absorption of aluminum hydroxide may be decreased by citric acid derivatives.

Pregnancy Risk Factor C

Aluminum Hydroxide and Magnesium Carbonate

(a LOO mi num hye DROKS ide & mag NEE zhum KAR bun nate)

Related Information

Aluminum Hydroxide *on page 80*

U.S. Brand Names Acid Gone [OTC]; Acid Gone Extra Strength [OTC]; Alenic Alka [OTC]; Gaviscon® Extra Strength [OTC]; Gaviscon® Liquid [OTC]; Genaton™ [OTC]

Generic Available Yes

Index Terms Magnesium Carbonate and Aluminum Hydroxide

Pharmacologic Category Antacid

Use Temporary relief of symptoms associated with gastric acidity

Local Anesthetic/Vasoconstrictor Precautions No information available to require special precautions

Effects on Dental Treatment Key adverse event(s) related to dental treatment: Chalky taste. Aluminum and magnesium ions prevent GI absorption of tetracycline by forming a large ionized chelated molecule with the tetracyclines in the stomach. Aluminum hydroxide prevents GI absorption of ketoconazole and itraconazole by increasing the pH in the GI tract. Any of these drugs should be administered at least 1 hour before aluminum hydroxide.

Common Adverse Effects 1% to 10%:

Endocrine & metabolic: Hypermagnesemia, aluminum intoxication (prolonged use and concomitant renal failure), hypophosphatemia

Gastrointestinal: Constipation, diarrhea

Neuromuscular & skeletal: Osteomalacia

Drug Interactions

Decreased Effect: Tetracyclines, digoxin, indomethacin, iron salts, isoniazid, allopurinol, benzodiazepines, corticosteroids, penicillamine, phenothiazines, ranitidine, ketoconazole, itraconazole

---

Aluminum Hydroxide and Magnesium Hydroxide

(a LOO mi num hye DROKS ide & mag NEE zhum hye DROK side)

Related Information

Aluminum Hydroxide *on page 80*

Magnesium Hydroxide *on page 1014*

U.S. Brand Names Alamag [OTC]; Rulox [OTC]; Rulox No. 1 [DSC]

Canadian Brand Names Diovol®; Diovol® Ex; Gelusil® Extra Strength; Mylanta™

Generic Available Yes

Index Terms Magnesium Hydroxide and Aluminum Hydroxide

Pharmacologic Category Antacid

Use Antacid, hyperphosphatemia in renal failure

Local Anesthetic/Vasoconstrictor Precautions No information available to require special precautions

(Continued)

Aluminum Hydroxide and Magnesium Hydroxide
(Continued)

Effects on Dental Treatment Key adverse event(s) related to dental treatment: Chalky taste. Aluminum and magnesium ions prevent GI absorption of tetracycline by forming a large ionized chelated molecule with the tetracyclines in the stomach. Aluminum hydroxide prevents GI absorption of ketoconazole and itraconazole by increasing the pH in the GI tract. Any of these drugs should be administered at least 1 hour before aluminum hydroxide.

Common Adverse Effects
>10%: Gastrointestinal: Constipation, chalky taste, stomach cramps, fecal impaction

1% to 10%: Gastrointestinal: Nausea, vomiting, discoloration of feces (white speckles)

Drug Interactions
Decreased Effect: Tetracyclines, digoxin, indomethacin, iron salts, isoniazid, allopurinol, benzodiazepines, corticosteroids, penicillamine, phenothiazines, ranitidine, ketoconazole, itraconazole

Pregnancy Risk Factor C

Aluminum Hydroxide and Magnesium Trisilicate
(a LOO mi num hye DROKS ide & mag NEE zhum trye SIL i kate)

Related Information
Aluminum Hydroxide *on page 80*

U.S. Brand Names Alenic Alka Tablet [OTC]; Gaviscon® Tablet [OTC]; Genaton Tablet [OTC]

Generic Available Yes

Index Terms Magnesium Trisilicate and Aluminum Hydroxide

Pharmacologic Category Antacid

Use Temporary relief of hyperacidity

Local Anesthetic/Vasoconstrictor Precautions No information available to require special precautions

Effects on Dental Treatment Key adverse event(s) related to dental treatment: Chalky taste. Aluminum and magnesium ions prevent GI absorption of tetracycline by forming a large ionized chelated molecule with the tetracyclines in the stomach. Aluminum hydroxide prevents GI absorption of ketoconazole and itraconazole by increasing the pH in the GI tract. Any of these drugs should be administered at least 1 hour before aluminum hydroxide.

Drug Interactions
Decreased Effect: Tetracyclines, digoxin, indomethacin, iron salts, isoniazid, allopurinol, benzodiazepines, corticosteroids, penicillamine, phenothiazines, ranitidine, ketoconazole, itraconazole

Pregnancy Risk Factor C

Aluminum Hydroxide, Magnesium Hydroxide, and Simethicone
(a LOO mi num hye DROKS ide, mag NEE zhum hye DROKS ide, & sye METH i kone)

Related Information
Aluminum Hydroxide *on page 80*
Magnesium Hydroxide *on page 1014*
Simethicone *on page 1472*

U.S. Brand Names Alamag Plus [OTC]; Aldroxicon I [OTC]; Aldroxicon II [OTC]; Almacone® [OTC]; Almacone Double Strength® [OTC]; Gelusil® [OTC]; Maalox® [OTC]; Maalox® Max [OTC]; Mi-Acid [OTC]; Mi-Acid Maximum Strength [OTC]; Mintox Extra Strength [OTC]; Mintox Plus [OTC]; Mylanta® Liquid [OTC]; Mylanta® Maximum Strength Liquid [OTC]

Canadian Brand Names Diovol Plus®; Gelusil®; Mylanta® Double Strength; Mylanta® Extra Strength; Mylanta® Regular Strength

Generic Available Yes

Index Terms Magnesium Hydroxide, Aluminum Hydroxide, and Simethicone; Simethicone, Aluminum Hydroxide, and Magnesium Hydroxide

Pharmacologic Category Antacid; Antiflatulent

Use Temporary relief of hyperacidity associated with gas; may also be used for indications associated with other antacids

Local Anesthetic/Vasoconstrictor Precautions No information available to require special precautions

Effects on Dental Treatment Key adverse event(s) related to dental treatment: Chalky taste. Aluminum and magnesium ions prevent GI absorption of tetracycline by forming a large ionized chelated molecule with the tetracyclines in the stomach. Aluminum hydroxide prevents GI absorption of ketoconazole and itraconazole by increasing the pH in the GI tract. Any of these drugs should be administered at least 1 hour before aluminum hydroxide.

Common Adverse Effects
>10%: Gastrointestinal: Chalky taste, stomach cramps, constipation, bowel motility decreased, fecal impaction, hemorrhoids

1% to 10%: Gastrointestinal: Nausea, vomiting, discoloration of feces (white speckles)

Drug Interactions
Decreased Effect: Tetracyclines, digoxin, indomethacin, iron salts, isoniazid, allopurinol, benzodiazepines, corticosteroids, penicillamine, phenothiazines, ranitidine, ketoconazole, itraconazole

Pregnancy Risk Factor C

Aluminum Potassium Sulfate and Epinephrine (Racemic) (Dental) *see* Epinephrine (Racemic) and Aluminum Potassium Sulfate *on page 576*

Aluminum Sucrose Sulfate, Basic *see* Sucralfate *on page 1499*

Aluminum Sulfate and Calcium Acetate
(a LOO mi num SUL fate & KAL see um AS e tate)

Related Information
Calcium Acetate *on page 259*

U.S. Brand Names Domeboro® [OTC]; Gordon Boro-Packs [OTC]; Pedi-Boro® [OTC]

Generic Available No

Index Terms Calcium Acetate and Aluminum Sulfate

Pharmacologic Category Topical Skin Product

Use Astringent wet dressing for relief of inflammatory conditions of the skin; reduce weeping that may occur in dermatitis

Local Anesthetic/Vasoconstrictor Precautions No information available to require special precautions

Effects on Dental Treatment No significant effects or complications reported

Alupent® *see* Metaproterenol *on page 1055*

Amantadine (a MAN ta deen)

Related Information
Respiratory Diseases *on page 1747*
Systemic Viral Diseases *on page 1767*

U.S. Brand Names Symmetrel®

Canadian Brand Names Endantadine®; PMS-Amantadine; Symmetrel®

Generic Available Yes

Index Terms Adamantanamine Hydrochloride; Amantadine Hydrochloride

Pharmacologic Category Anti-Parkinson's Agent, Dopamine Agonist; Antiviral Agent, Adamantane

Use Prophylaxis and treatment of influenza A viral infection (per manufacturer labeling; also refer to current CDC guidelines for recommendations during current flu season); treatment of parkinsonism; treatment of drug-induced extrapyramidal symptoms

Local Anesthetic/Vasoconstrictor Precautions No information available to require special precautions

Effects on Dental Treatment Key adverse event(s) related to dental treatment: Xerostomia (prolonged use may cause significant xerostomia; normal salivary flow resumes upon discontinuation) and orthostatic hypotension.

Common Adverse Effects 1% to 10%:
Cardiovascular: Orthostatic hypotension, peripheral edema
Central nervous system: Agitation, anxiety, ataxia, confusion, delirium, depression, dizziness, dream abnormality, fatigue, hallucinations, headache, insomnia, irritability, nervousness, somnolence
Dermatologic: Livedo reticularis
Gastrointestinal: Anorexia, constipation, diarrhea, nausea, xerostomia
Respiratory: Dry nose

Mechanism of Action As an antiviral, blocks the uncoating of influenza A virus preventing penetration of virus into host; antiparkinsonian activity may be due to its blocking the reuptake of dopamine into presynaptic neurons or by increasing dopamine release from presynaptic fibers
(Continued)

Amantadine *(Continued)*

Drug Interactions

Increased Effect/Toxicity: Anticholinergics (benztropine and trihexyphenidyl) may potentiate CNS side effects of amantadine. Triamterene may increase toxicity of amantadine; monitor for altered response.

Decreased Effect: Antipsychotics (typical) may reduce the anti-Parkinsonian effects of amantadine. The live, attenuated form of influenza vaccine (administered intranasally) should not be administered within 2 weeks before or 48 hours after amantadine (unless medically indicated). Inactivated vaccine (trivalent) may be administered without concern to patients receiving amantadine.

Pharmacodynamics/Kinetics

Onset of action: Antidyskinetic: Within 48 hours

Absorption: Well absorbed

Distribution: V_d: Normal: 1.5-6.1 L/kg; Renal failure: 5.1 ± 0.2 L/kg; in saliva, tear film, and nasal secretions; in animals, tissue (especially lung) concentrations higher than serum concentrations; crosses blood-brain barrier

Protein binding: Normal renal function: ~67%; Hemodialysis: ~59%

Metabolism: Not appreciable; small amounts of an acetyl metabolite identified

Bioavailability: 86% to 90%

Half-life elimination: Normal renal function: 16 ± 6 hours (9-31 hours); End-stage renal disease: 7-10 days

Excretion: Urine (80% to 90% unchanged) by glomerular filtration and tubular secretion

Total clearance: 2.5-10.5 L/hour

Pregnancy Risk Factor C

Amantadine Hydrochloride *see* Amantadine *on page 83*

Amaryl® *see* Glimepiride *on page 780*

Ambenonium *(am be NOE nee um)*

U.S. Brand Names Mytelase®
Canadian Brand Names Mytelase®
Generic Available No
Index Terms Ambenonium Chloride
Pharmacologic Category Cholinergic Agonist
Use Treatment of myasthenia gravis
Local Anesthetic/Vasoconstrictor Precautions No information available to require special precautions
Effects on Dental Treatment No significant effects or complications reported
Pregnancy Risk Factor C

Ambenonium Chloride *see* Ambenonium *on page 84*

Ambien® *see* Zolpidem *on page 1689*

Ambien CR™ *see* Zolpidem *on page 1689*

Ambifed-G *see* Guaifenesin and Pseudoephedrine *on page 798*

Ambifed-G DM *see* Guaifenesin, Pseudoephedrine, and Dextromethorphan *on page 800*

AmBisome® *see* Amphotericin B (Liposomal) *on page 118*

Amcinonide *(am SIN oh nide)*

U.S. Brand Names Cyclocort® [DSC]
Canadian Brand Names Amcort®; Cyclocort®; ratio-Amcinonide; Taro-Amcinonide
Generic Available Yes
Pharmacologic Category Corticosteroid, Topical
Use Relief of the inflammatory and pruritic manifestations of corticosteroid-responsive dermatoses (high potency corticosteroid)
Local Anesthetic/Vasoconstrictor Precautions No information available to require special precautions
Effects on Dental Treatment No significant effects or complications reported
Common Adverse Effects Frequency not defined.

Dermatologic: Acne, hypopigmentation, allergic dermatitis, maceration of the skin, skin atrophy, striae, miliaria, telangiectasia

Endocrine & metabolic: Cushing's syndrome, growth retardation (long-term use), HPA suppression, hyperglycemia; these reactions occur more frequently with occlusive dressings

Local: Burning, itching, irritation, dryness, folliculitis, hypertrichosis

Miscellaneous: Secondary infection

Mechanism of Action Stimulates the synthesis of enzymes needed to decrease inflammation, suppress mitotic activity, and cause vasoconstriction

Pharmacodynamics/Kinetics

Absorption: Adequate through intact skin; increases with skin inflammation or occlusion

Metabolism: Hepatic

Excretion: Urine and feces

Pregnancy Risk Factor C

Amdry-D *see* Pseudoephedrine and Methscopolamine *on page 1384*

Amerge® *see* Naratriptan *on page 1152*

Americaine® [OTC] *see* Benzocaine *on page 195*

Americaine® Hemorrhoidal [OTC] *see* Benzocaine *on page 195*

A-Methapred *see* MethylPREDNISolone *on page 1083*

Amethocaine Hydrochloride *see* Tetracaine *on page 1546*

Amethopterin *see* Methotrexate *on page 1068*

Amevive® *see* Alefacept *on page 63*

Amfepramone *see* Diethylpropion *on page 493*

AMG 073 *see* Cinacalcet *on page 359*

Amibid DM [DSC] *see* Guaifenesin and Dextromethorphan *on page 796*

Amicar® *see* Aminocaproic Acid *on page 88*

Amidal [DSC] *see* Guaifenesin and Phenylephrine *on page 797*

Amidate® *see* Etomidate *on page 659*

Amidrine [DSC] *see* Acetaminophen, Isometheptene, and Dichloralphenazone *on page 45*

Amifostine (am i FOS teen)

U.S. Brand Names Ethyol®

Canadian Brand Names Ethyol®

Mexican Brand Names Ethyol

Generic Available No

Index Terms Ethiofos; Gammaphos; WR-2721; YM-08310

Pharmacologic Category Adjuvant, Chemoprotective Agent (Cytoprotective); Antidote

Use Reduce the incidence of moderate to severe xerostomia in patients undergoing postoperative radiation treatment for head and neck cancer, where the radiation port includes a substantial portion of the parotid glands; reduce the cumulative renal toxicity associated with repeated administration of cisplatin

Local Anesthetic/Vasoconstrictor Precautions No information available to require special precautions

Effects on Dental Treatment No significant effects or complications reported

Common Adverse Effects >10%:

Cardiovascular: Hypotension (15% to 62%; grades 3/4: 3% to 8%; dose dependent)

Gastrointestinal: Nausea/vomiting (53% to 96%; grades 3/4: 8% to 30%; dose dependent)

Mechanism of Action Prodrug that is dephosphorylated by alkaline phosphatase in tissues to a pharmacologically-active free thiol metabolite. The free thiol is available to bind to, and detoxify, reactive metabolites of cisplatin; and can also act as a scavenger of free radicals that may be generated in tissues.

Drug Interactions

Increased Effect/Toxicity: Antihypertensives may potentiate the hypotensive effects of amifostine.

Pharmacodynamics/Kinetics

Distribution: V_d: 3.5 L

Metabolism: Hepatic dephosphorylation to two metabolites (active-free thiol and disulfide)

Half-life elimination: 8-9 minutes

Excretion: Urine

Clearance, plasma: 2.17 L/minute

Pregnancy Risk Factor C

Amigesic® *see* Salsalate *on page 1454*

Amikacin (am i KAY sin)

U.S. Brand Names Amikin®

Canadian Brand Names Amikacin Sulfate Injection, USP; Amikin®

Mexican Brand Names Amikafur; Amikayect; Amikin; Gamikal; Yectamid

Generic Available Yes

(Continued)

Amikacin (Continued)

Index Terms Amikacin Sulfate

Pharmacologic Category Antibiotic, Aminoglycoside

Use Treatment of serious infections (bone infections, respiratory tract infections, endocarditis, and septicemia) due to organisms resistant to gentamicin and tobramycin, including *Pseudomonas*, *Proteus*, *Serratia*, and other gram-negative bacilli; documented infection of mycobacterial organisms susceptible to amikacin

Local Anesthetic/Vasoconstrictor Precautions No information available to require special precautions

Effects on Dental Treatment No significant effects or complications reported

Common Adverse Effects 1% to 10%:
Central nervous system: Neurotoxicity
Otic: Ototoxicity (auditory), ototoxicity (vestibular)
Renal: Nephrotoxicity

Mechanism of Action Inhibits protein synthesis in susceptible bacteria by binding to 30S ribosomal subunits

Drug Interactions
Increased Effect/Toxicity: Amikacin may increase or prolong the effect of neuromuscular blocking agents. Concurrent use of amphotericin (or other nephrotoxic drugs) may increase the risk of amikacin-induced nephrotoxicity. The risk of ototoxicity from amikacin may be increased with other ototoxic drugs.

Pharmacodynamics/Kinetics
Absorption:
I.M.: Rapid
Oral: Poorly absorbed
Distribution: Primarily into extracellular fluid (highly hydrophilic); penetrates blood-brain barrier when meninges inflamed
Relative diffusion of antimicrobial agents from blood into CSF: Good only with inflammation (exceeds usual MICs)
CSF:blood level ratio: Normal meninges: 10% to 20%; Inflamed meninges: 15% to 24%
Protein-binding: 0% to 11%
Half-life elimination (renal function and age dependent):
Infants: Low birth weight (1-3 days): 7-9 hours; Full-term >7 days: 4-5 hours
Children: 1.6-2.5 hours
Adults: Normal renal function: 1.4-2.3 hours; Anuria/end-stage renal disease: 28-86 hours
Time to peak, serum: I.M.: 45-120 minutes
Excretion: Urine (94% to 98%)

Pregnancy Risk Factor D

Amikacin Sulfate *see* Amikacin *on page 85*

Amikin® *see* Amikacin *on page 85*

Amiloride (a MIL oh ride)

Related Information
Cardiovascular Diseases *on page 1726*

U.S. Brand Names Midamor® [DSC]

Canadian Brand Names Apo-Amiloride®

Generic Available Yes

Index Terms Amiloride Hydrochloride

Pharmacologic Category Diuretic, Potassium-Sparing

Use Counteracts potassium loss induced by other diuretics in the treatment of hypertension or edematous conditions including CHF, hepatic cirrhosis, and hypoaldosteronism; usually used in conjunction with more potent diuretics such as thiazides or loop diuretics

Unlabeled/Investigational Use Investigational: Cystic fibrosis; reduction of lithium-induced polyuria; pediatric hypertension

Local Anesthetic/Vasoconstrictor Precautions No information available to require special precautions

Effects on Dental Treatment No significant effects or complications reported

Common Adverse Effects 1% to 10%:
Central nervous system: Headache, fatigue, dizziness
Endocrine & metabolic: Hyperkalemia (up to 10%; risk reduced in patients receiving kaliuretic diuretics), hyperchloremic metabolic acidosis, dehydration, hyponatremia, gynecomastia
Gastrointestinal: Nausea, diarrhea, vomiting, abdominal pain, gas pain, appetite changes, constipation
Genitourinary: Impotence

Neuromuscular & skeletal: Muscle cramps, weakness
Respiratory: Cough, dyspnea
Mechanism of Action Interferes with potassium/sodium exchange (active transport) in the distal tubule, cortical collecting tubule, and collecting duct by inhibiting sodium, potassium-ATPase; decreases calcium excretion; increases magnesium loss

Drug Interactions
Increased Effect/Toxicity: Increased risk of amiloride-associated hyperkalemia with triamterene, spironolactone, ACE inhibitors or angiotensin receptor antagonists, potassium preparations, cyclosporine, tacrolimus, and indomethacin. Amiloride may increase the toxicity of amantadine and lithium by reduction of renal excretion. Quinidine and amiloride together may increase risk of malignant arrhythmias.
Decreased Effect: Decreased effect of amiloride with use of NSAIDs. Amoxicillin's absorption may be reduced with concurrent use.

Pharmacodynamics/Kinetics
Onset of action: 2 hours
Duration: 24 hours
Absorption: ~15% to 25%
Distribution: V_d: 350-380 L
Protein binding: 23%
Metabolism: No active metabolites
Half-life elimination: Normal renal function: 6-9 hours; End-stage renal disease: 8-144 hours
Time to peak, serum: 6-10 hours
Excretion: Urine and feces (equal amounts as unchanged drug)
Pregnancy Risk Factor B

Amiloride and Hydrochlorothiazide
(a MIL oh ride & hye droe klor oh THYE a zide)

Related Information
Amiloride *on page 86*
Hydrochlorothiazide *on page 819*
Canadian Brand Names Apo-Amilzide®; Gen-Amilazide; Moduret; Novamilor; Nu-Amilzide
Mexican Brand Names Moduretic
Generic Available Yes
Index Terms Hydrochlorothiazide and Amiloride
Pharmacologic Category Diuretic, Combination
Use Potassium-sparing diuretic; antihypertensive
Local Anesthetic/Vasoconstrictor Precautions No information available to require special precautions
Effects on Dental Treatment No significant effects or complications reported
Common Adverse Effects See individual agents.
Drug Interactions
Increased Effect/Toxicity: See individual agents.
Decreased Effect: See individual agents.
Pharmacodynamics/Kinetics See individual agents.
Pregnancy Risk Factor B

Amiloride Hydrochloride *see* Amiloride *on page 86*
2-Amino-6-Mercaptopurine *see* Thioguanine *on page 1557*
2-Amino-6-Methoxypurine Arabinoside *see* Nelarabine *on page 1157*
2-Amino-6-Trifluoromethoxy-benzothiazole *see* Riluzole *on page 1427*
Aminobenzylpenicillin *see* Ampicillin *on page 119*

Aminocamptothecin (a min o camp to THE sin)

Generic Available No
Index Terms 9-AC; 9-Aminocamptothecin; NSC-603071
Pharmacologic Category Antineoplastic Agent, DNA Binding Agent; Enzyme Inhibitor, Topoisomerase I Inhibitor
Unlabeled/Investigational Use Phase II trials: Relapsed lymphoma, refractory breast cancer, nonsmall cell lung cancer, untreated colorectal carcinoma
Local Anesthetic/Vasoconstrictor Precautions No information available to require special precautions
Effects on Dental Treatment Key adverse event(s) related to dental treatment: Mucositis
Common Adverse Effects Frequency not defined.
Central nervous system: Fatigue
(Continued)

Aminocamptothecin *(Continued)*

Dermatologic: Alopecia

Gastrointestinal: Nausea, vomiting, diarrhea, mucositis, anorexia

Hematologic: Neutropenia (may be dose limiting), thrombocytopenia (reversible, but may be dose limiting), anemia

Restrictions Not available in U.S./Investigational

Mechanism of Action Aminocamptothecin binds to topoisomerase I, stabilizing the cleavable DNA-topoisomerase I complex, resulting in arrest of the replication fork and inhibition of DNA synthesis.

Drug Interactions

Decreased Effect: Anticonvulsants may decrease aminocamptothecin levels.

Pharmacodynamics/Kinetics Ratio of lactone to total drug is 8.7% ± 4.7% because of instability of aminocamptothecin lactone in plasma.

Distribution: V_d: 46-92 L

Metabolism: None identified

Half-life elimination: Terminal: 8-17 hours for total aminocamptothecin

Excretion: Urine (32% of total drug delivered)

9-Aminocamptothecin *see* Aminocamptothecin *on page 87*

Aminocaproic Acid *(a mee noe ka PROE ik AS id)*

U.S. Brand Names Amicar®

Generic Available Yes

Index Terms Epsilon Aminocaproic Acid

Pharmacologic Category Hemostatic Agent

Use Treatment of excessive bleeding from fibrinolysis

Unlabeled/Investigational Use Treatment of traumatic hyphema; control bleeding in thrombocytopenia; control oral bleeding in congenital and acquired coagulation disorders

Local Anesthetic/Vasoconstrictor Precautions No information available to require special precautions

Effects on Dental Treatment No significant effects or complications reported (see Dental Comment)

Common Adverse Effects Frequency not defined.

Cardiovascular: Arrhythmia, bradycardia, hypotension, peripheral ischemia, syncope, thrombosis

Central nervous system: Confusion, delirium, dizziness, fatigue, hallucinations, headache, intracranial hypertension, malaise, seizure, stroke

Dermatologic: Rash, pruritus

Gastrointestinal: Abdominal pain, anorexia, cramps, diarrhea, GI irritation, nausea

Genitourinary: Dry ejaculation

Hematologic: Agranulocytosis, bleeding time increased, leukopenia, thrombocytopenia

Neuromuscular & skeletal: CPK increased, myalgia, myositis, myopathy, rhabdomyolysis (rare), weakness

Ophthalmic: Watery eyes, vision decreased

Otic: Tinnitus

Renal: Failure (rare), myoglobinuria (rare)

Respiratory: Dyspnea, nasal congestion, pulmonary embolism

Mechanism of Action Competitively inhibits activation of plasminogen to plasmin, also, a lesser antiplasmin effect

Drug Interactions

Increased Effect/Toxicity: Increased risk of hypercoagulability with oral contraceptives, estrogens. Should not be administered with factor IX complex concentrate or anti-inhibitor complex concentrates due to an increased risk of thrombosis.

Pharmacodynamics/Kinetics

Onset of action: ~1-72 hours

Distribution: Widely through intravascular and extravascular compartments

V_d: Oral: 23 L, I.V.: 30 L

Metabolism: Minimally hepatic

Half-life elimination: 2 hours

Time to peak: Oral: Within 2 hours

Excretion: Urine (65% as unchanged drug, 11% as metabolite)

Pregnancy Risk Factor C

Dental Comment Antifibrinolytic drugs are useful to control bleeding after dental extractions in patients with hemophilia. A clinical trial reported that aminocaproic acid or tranexamic acid reduces both recurrent bleeding and the amount of clotting factor replacement therapy required. In adults, the oral dose was 50-60 mg aminocaproic acid per kg every 4 hours until dental sockets were completely healed.

Extemporaneous solutions incorporating 100 mg aminocaproic acid per 5 mL of oral solution have been used as an oral rinse with some success. Use, however, must be carefully considered since it may not show efficacy in all patients with either drug-induced or hereditary coagulation problems. Studies are ongoing and commercial products may be available in the future.

Amino-Cerv™ *see* Urea *on page 1632*

Aminoglutethimide (a mee noe gloo TETH i mide)

U.S. Brand Names Cytadren®
Generic Available No
Index Terms AG; AGT; BA-16038; Elipten
Pharmacologic Category Antineoplastic Agent, Aromatase Inhibitor; Enzyme Inhibitor; Hormone Antagonist, Anti-Adrenal; Nonsteroidal Aromatase Inhibitor
Use Suppression of adrenal function in selected patients with Cushing's syndrome
Unlabeled/Investigational Use Treatment of breast and prostate cancer (androgen synthesis inhibitor)
Local Anesthetic/Vasoconstrictor Precautions No information available to require special precautions
Effects on Dental Treatment Key adverse event(s) related to dental treatment: Nausea and orthostatic hypotension
Common Adverse Effects Most adverse effects will diminish in incidence and severity after the first 2-6 weeks

>10%:
  Central nervous system: Headache, dizziness, drowsiness, lethargy, clumsiness
  Dermatologic: Skin rash
  Gastrointestinal: Nausea, anorexia
  Hepatic: Cholestatic jaundice
  Neuromuscular & skeletal: Myalgia
  Renal: Nephrotoxicity
  Respiratory: Pulmonary alveolar damage
1% to 10%:
  Cardiovascular: Hypotension, tachycardia, orthostasis
  Dermatologic: Hirsutism, pruritus
  Endocrine & metabolic: Adrenocortical insufficiency
  Gastrointestinal: Vomiting

Mechanism of Action Blocks the enzymatic conversion of cholesterol to delta-5-pregnenolone, thereby reducing the synthesis of adrenal glucocorticoids, mineralocorticoids, estrogens, aldosterone, and androgens
Drug Interactions
  Cytochrome P450 Effect: Induces CYP1A2 (strong), 2C19 (strong), 3A4 (strong)
  Decreased Effect: Aminoglutethimide may decrease therapeutic effect of dexamethasone, warfarin, medroxyprogesterone, megestrol, and tamoxifen. Aminoglutethimide may decrease the levels/effects of aminophylline, benzodiazepines, calcium channel blockers, citalopram, clarithromycin, cyclosporine, diazepam, erythromycin, estrogens, fluvoxamine, methsuximide, mirtazapine, nateglinide, nefazodone, nevirapine, phenytoin, proton pump inhibitors, protease inhibitors, ropinirole, sertraline, tacrolimus, theophylline, venlafaxine, voriconazole, and other drugs metabolized by CYP1A2, 2C19, or 3A4.
Pharmacodynamics/Kinetics
  Onset of action: Adrenal suppression: 3-5 days; following withdrawal of therapy, adrenal function returns within 72 hours
  Absorption: 90%
  Protein binding, plasma: 20% to 25%
  Metabolism: Major metabolite is N-acetylaminoglutethimide; induces its own metabolism
  Half-life elimination: 7-15 hours; shorter following multiple doses
  Excretion: Urine (34% to 50% as unchanged drug, 25% as metabolites)
Pregnancy Risk Factor D

Aminolevulinic Acid (a MEE noh lev yoo lin ik AS id)

U.S. Brand Names Levulan® Kerastick®
Canadian Brand Names Levulan®
Generic Available No
(Continued)

89

Aminolevulinic Acid *(Continued)*

Index Terms Aminolevulinic Acid Hydrochloride

Pharmacologic Category Photosensitizing Agent, Topical; Topical Skin Product

Use Treatment of minimally to moderately thick actinic keratoses (grade 1 or 2) of the face or scalp; to be used in conjunction with blue light illumination

Local Anesthetic/Vasoconstrictor Precautions No information available to require special precautions

Effects on Dental Treatment Key adverse event(s) related to dental treatment: Bleeding/hemorrhage.

Common Adverse Effects Transient stinging, burning, itching, erythema, and edema result from the photosensitizing properties of this agent. Symptoms subside between 1 minute and 24 hours after turning off the blue light illuminator. Severe stinging or burning was reported in at least 50% of patients from at least 1 lesional site treatment.

>10%: Dermatologic: Severe stinging or burning (50%), scaling of the skin/crusted skin (64% to 71%), hyper-/hypopigmentation (22% to 36%), itching (14% to 25%), erosion (2% to 14%)

1% to 10%:

Central nervous system: Dysesthesia (up to 2%)

Dermatologic: Skin ulceration (2% to 4%), vesiculation (4% to 5%), pustular drug eruption (up to 4%), skin disorder (5% to 12%)

Hematologic: Bleeding/hemorrhage (2% to 4%)

Local: Wheal/flare (2% to 7%), local pain (1%), tenderness (1% to 2%), edema (1%), scabbing (up to 2%), ulceration (2% to 4%), excoriation (1%)

Mechanism of Action Aminolevulinic acid is a metabolic precursor of protoporphyrin IX (PpIX), which is a photosensitizer. Photosensitization following application of aminolevulinic acid topical solution occurs through the metabolic conversion to PpIX. When exposed to light of appropriate wavelength and energy, accumulated PpIX produces a photodynamic reaction.

Drug Interactions

Increased Effect/Toxicity: Photosensitizing agents such as griseofulvin, thiazide diuretics, sulfonamides, sulfonylureas, phenothiazines, and tetracyclines theoretically may increase the photosensitizing potential of aminolevulinic acid.

Pharmacodynamics/Kinetics

PpIX:

Peak fluorescence intensity: 11 hours ± 1 hour

Half-life, mean clearance for lesions: 30 ± 10 hours

Pregnancy Risk Factor C

Aminolevulinic Acid Hydrochloride *see* Aminolevulinic Acid *on page 89*

Aminophylline *(am in OFF i lin)*

Related Information

Respiratory Diseases *on page 1747*
Theophylline *on page 1554*

Canadian Brand Names Phyllocontin®; Phyllocontin®-350

Mexican Brand Names Drafilyn "Z"

Generic Available Yes

Index Terms Theophylline Ethylenediamine

Pharmacologic Category Theophylline Derivative

Use Bronchodilator in reversible airway obstruction due to asthma or COPD; increase diaphragmatic contractility

Local Anesthetic/Vasoconstrictor Precautions No information available to require special precautions

Effects on Dental Treatment Prescribe erythromycin products with caution to patients taking theophylline products. Erythromycin will delay the normal metabolic inactivation of theophyllines leading to increased blood levels; this has resulted in nausea, vomiting, and CNS restlessness.

Common Adverse Effects

Uncommon at serum theophylline concentrations ≤15 mcg/mL

1% to 10%:

Cardiovascular: Tachycardia

Central nervous system: Nervousness, restlessness

Gastrointestinal: Nausea, vomiting

Mechanism of Action Causes bronchodilatation, diuresis, CNS and cardiac stimulation, and gastric acid secretion by blocking phosphodiesterase which increases tissue concentrations of cyclic adenine monophosphate (cAMP) which in turn promote catecholamine stimulation of lipolysis, glycogenolysis, and gluconeogenesis and induce release of epinephrine from adrenal medulla cells

Drug Interactions

Cytochrome P450 Effect: Substrate of CYP1A2 (major), 2E1 (minor), 3A4 (minor)

Increased Effect/Toxicity: Levels/effects of aminophylline may be increased by ciprofloxacin, fluvoxamine, ketoconazole, norfloxacin, ofloxacin, rofecoxib, and other CYP1A2 inhibitors.

Decreased Effect: Levels/effects of aminophylline may be decreased by aminoglutethimide, carbamazepine, phenobarbital, rifampin, and other CYP1A2 inducers.

Pharmacodynamics/Kinetics

Theophylline:

Absorption: Oral: Dosage form dependent

Distribution: 0.45 L/kg based on ideal body weight

Protein binding: 40%, primarily to albumin

Metabolism: Children >1 year and Adults: Hepatic; involves CYP1A2, 2E1, and 3A4; forms active metabolites (caffeine and 3-methylxanthine)

Half-life elimination: Highly variable and dependent upon age, liver function, cardiac function, lung disease, and smoking history

Time to peak, serum:

Oral: Immediate release: 1-2 hours

I.V.: Within 30 minutes

Excretion: Children >3 months and Adults: Urine (10% as unchanged drug)

Pregnancy Risk Factor C

Aminosalicylate Sodium *see Aminosalicylic Acid on page 91*

Aminosalicylic Acid (a mee noe sal i SIL ik AS id)

Related Information

Rheumatoid Arthritis, Osteoarthritis, and Osteoporosis *on page 1759*

Tuberculosis *on page 1765*

U.S. Brand Names Paser®

Generic Available No

Index Terms Aminosalicylate Sodium; 4-Aminosalicylic Acid; Para-Amino-salicylate Sodium; PAS; Sodium PAS

Pharmacologic Category Salicylate

Use Adjunctive treatment of tuberculosis used in combination with other anti-tubercular agents

Unlabeled/Investigational Use Crohn's disease

Local Anesthetic/Vasoconstrictor Precautions No information available to require special precautions

Effects on Dental Treatment NSAID formulations are known to reversibly decrease platelet aggregation via mechanisms different than observed with aspirin. The dentist should be aware of the potential of abnormal coagulation. Caution should also be exercised in the use of NSAIDs in patients already on anticoagulant therapy with drugs such as warfarin (Coumadin®).

Common Adverse Effects Frequency not defined.

Cardiovascular: Pericarditis, vasculitis

Central nervous system: Encephalopathy, fever

Dermatologic: Skin eruptions

Endocrine & metabolic: Goiter (with or without myxedema), hypoglycemia

Gastrointestinal: Abdominal pain, diarrhea, nausea, vomiting

Hematologic: Agranulocytosis, anemia (hemolytic), leukopenia, thrombocytopenia

Hepatic: Hepatitis, jaundice

Ocular: Optic neuritis

Respiratory: Eosinophilic pneumonia

Mechanism of Action Aminosalicylic acid (PAS) is a highly-specific bacteriostatic agent active against *M. tuberculosis*. Structurally related to para-aminobenzoic acid (PABA) and its mechanism of action is thought to be similar to the sulfonamides, a competitive antagonism with PABA; disrupts plate biosynthesis in sensitive organisms.

Drug Interactions

Decreased Effect: Aminosalicylic acid may decrease serum levels of digoxin and vitamin B_{12}.

Pharmacodynamics/Kinetics

Absorption: Readily, >90%

Protein binding: 50% to 60%

Metabolism: Hepatic (>50%) via acetylation

Half-life elimination: Reduced with renal impairment

Time to peak, serum: 6 hours

(Continued)

Aminosalicylic Acid *(Continued)*

Excretion: Urine (>80% as unchanged drug and metabolites)
Pregnancy Risk Factor C

4-Aminosalicylic Acid *see* Aminosalicylic Acid *on page 91*
5-Aminosalicylic Acid *see* Mesalamine *on page 1052*
Aminoxin® [OTC] *see* Pyridoxine *on page 1389*

Amiodarone (a MEE oh da rone)

Related Information
Cardiovascular Diseases *on page 1726*
U.S. Brand Names Cordarone®; Pacerone®
Canadian Brand Names Alti-Amiodarone; Amiodarone Hydrochloride for Injection®; Apo-Amiodarone®; Cordarone®; Gen-Amiodarone; Novo-Amiodarone; PMS-Amiodarone; Rhoxal-amiodarone; Sandoz-Amiodarone
Mexican Brand Names Braxan; Cordarone; Forken
Generic Available Yes
Index Terms Amiodarone Hydrochloride
Pharmacologic Category Antiarrhythmic Agent, Class III
Use Management of life-threatening recurrent ventricular fibrillation (VF) or hemodynamically-unstable ventricular tachycardia (VT) refractory to other antiarrhythmic agents or in patients intolerant of other agents used for these conditions
Unlabeled/Investigational Use
Cardiac arrest with persistent ventricular tachycardia (VT) or ventricular fibrillation (VF) if defibrillation, CPR, and vasopressor administration have failed (ACLS/PALS guidelines)
Control of hemodynamically-stable VT, polymorphic VT with a normal QT interval, or wide-complex tachycardia of uncertain origin (ACLS/PALS guidelines)
Control of rapid ventricular rate due to accessory pathway conduction in pre-excited atrial arrhythmias (ACLS guidelines)
Heart rate control in patients with atrial fibrillation and heart failure [no accessory pathway] (ACC/AHA/ESC Practice Guidelines)
Paroxysmal supraventricular tachycardia (SVT)
Prevention of postoperative atrial fibrillation during cardiothoracic surgery
Pharmacologic adjunct to ICD therapy to suppress symptomatic ventricular tachyarrhythmias in otherwise optimally-treated patients with heart failure (ACC/AHA/ESC Practice Guidelines)
Pharmacologic conversion of atrial fibrillation to normal sinus rhythm; maintenance of normal sinus rhythm
Local Anesthetic/Vasoconstrictor Precautions Amiodarone is one of the drugs confirmed to prolong the QT interval and is accepted as having a risk of causing torsade de pointes. The risk of drug-induced torsade de pointes is extremely low when a single QT interval prolonging drug is prescribed. In terms of epinephrine, it is not known what effect vasoconstrictors in the local anesthetic regimen will have in patients with a known history of congenital prolonged QT interval or in patients taking any medication that prolongs the QT interval. Until more information is obtained, it is suggested that the clinician consult with the physician prior to the use of a vasoconstrictor in suspected patients, and that the vasoconstrictor (epinephrine, levonordefrin [Neo-Cobefrin®]) be used with caution.
Effects on Dental Treatment Key adverse event(s) related to dental treatment: Oral: Abnormal salivation and taste
Common Adverse Effects In a recent meta-analysis, patients taking lower doses of amiodarone (152-330 mg daily for at least 12 months) were more likely to develop thyroid, neurologic, skin, ocular, and bradycardic abnormalities than those taking placebo (Vorperian, 1997). Pulmonary toxicity was similar in both the low dose amiodarone group and the placebo group but there was a trend towards increased toxicity in the amiodarone group. Gastrointestinal and hepatic events were seen to a similar extent in both the low dose amiodarone group and placebo group. As the frequency of adverse events varies considerably across studies as a function of route and dose, a consolidation of adverse event rates is provided by Goldschlager, 2000.

Cardiovascular: Hypotension (I.V. 16%, refractory in rare cases)
Central nervous system (3% to 40%): Abnormal gait/ataxia, dizziness, fatigue, headache, malaise, impaired memory, involuntary movement, insomnia, poor coordination, peripheral neuropathy, sleep disturbances, tremor
Dermatologic: Photosensitivity (10% to 75%)
Endocrine & Metabolic: Hypothyroidism (1% to 22%)

Gastrointestinal: Nausea, vomiting, anorexia, and constipation (10% to 33%)

Hepatic: AST or ALT level >2x normal (15% to 50%)

Ocular: Corneal microdeposits (>90%; causes visual disturbance in <10%)

1% to 10%:

Cardiovascular: CHF (3%), bradycardia (3% to 5%), AV block (5%), conduction abnormalities, SA node dysfunction (1% to 3%), cardiac arrhythmia, flushing, edema. Additional effects associated with I.V. administration include asystole, cardiac arrest, electromechanical dissociation, ventricular tachycardia, and cardiogenic shock.

Dermatologic: Slate blue skin discoloration (<10%)

Endocrine & metabolic: Hyperthyroidism (3% to 10%; more common in iodine-deficient regions of the world), libido decreased

Gastrointestinal: Abdominal pain, abnormal salivation, abnormal taste (oral)

Hematologic: Coagulation abnormalities

Hepatic: Hepatitis and cirrhosis (<3%)

Local: Phlebitis (I.V., with concentrations >3 mg/mL)

Ocular: Visual disturbances (2% to 9%), halo vision (<5% occurring especially at night), optic neuritis (1%)

Respiratory: Pulmonary toxicity has been estimated to occur at a frequency between 2% and 7% of patients (some reports indicate a frequency as high as 17%). Toxicity may present as hypersensitivity pneumonitis; pulmonary fibrosis (cough, fever, malaise); pulmonary inflammation; interstitial pneumonitis; or alveolar pneumonitis. ARDS has been reported in up to 2% of patients receiving amiodarone, and postoperatively in patients receiving oral amiodarone.

Miscellaneous: Abnormal smell (oral)

Restrictions An FDA-approved medication guide must be distributed when dispensing an outpatient prescription (new or refill) where this medication is to be used without direct supervision of a healthcare provider. Medication guides are available at http://www.fda.gov/cder/Offices/ODS/medication_guides.htm.

Mechanism of Action Class III antiarrhythmic agent which inhibits adrenergic stimulation (alpha- and beta-blocking properties), affects sodium, potassium, and calcium channels, prolongs the action potential and refractory period in myocardial tissue; decreases AV conduction and sinus node function

Drug Interactions

Cytochrome P450 Effect: Substrate of CYP1A2 (minor), 2C8 (major at low concentration), 2C19 (minor), 2D6 (minor), 3A4 (major); **Inhibits** CYP1A2 (weak), 2A6 (moderate), 2B6 (weak), 2C9 (moderate), 2C19 (weak), 2D6 (moderate), 3A4 (moderate)

Increased Effect/Toxicity: The effect of drugs which prolong the QT interval, including amitriptyline, azole antifungals, bepridil, cisapride, clarithromycin, disopyramide, erythromycin, gatifloxacin, haloperidol, imipramine, moxifloxacin, quinidine, pimozide, procainamide, sotalol, sparfloxacin, theophylline, and thioridazine may be increased. Cisapride and sparfloxacin are contraindicated. Use of amiodarone with diltiazem, verapamil, digoxin, beta-blockers, and other drugs which delay AV conduction may cause excessive AV block (amiodarone may also decrease the metabolism of some of these agents - see below).

Amiodarone may increase the levels of digoxin (reduce dose by 50% on initiation), flecainide (decrease dose up to 33%), phenothiazines, procainamide (reduce dose), and quinidine. Amiodarone may increase the levels/effects of aminophylline, amphetamines, selected benzodiazepines, selected beta-blockers, calcium channel blockers, cyclosporine, dexmedetomidine, dextromethorphan, fluoxetine, fluvoxamine, glimepiride, glipizide, ifosfamide, imatinib, isoniazid, lidocaine, mexiletine, mirtazapine, nateglinide, nefazodone, paroxetine, phenytoin, pioglitazone, risperidone, ritonavir, ropinirole, rosiglitazone, sildenafil (and other PDE-5 inhibitors), sertraline, tacrolimus, telithromycin, theophylline, thioridazine, trazodone, tricyclic antidepressants, trifluoperazine, venlafaxine, warfarin, and other CYP2A6, 2C9, CYP2D6, and/or CYP3A4 substrates. Selected benzodiazepines (midazolam, triazolam), cisapride, ergot alkaloids, selected HMG-CoA reductase inhibitors (lovastatin and simvastatin), mesoridazine, pimozide, and thioridazine are generally contraindicated with strong CYP3A4 inhibitors; example CYP3A4 inhibitors include azole antifungals, clarithromycin, diclofenac, doxycycline, erythromycin, imatinib, isoniazid, nefazodone, nicardipine, propofol, protease inhibitors, quinidine, telithromycin, and verapamil. When used with strong CYP3A4 inhibitors, dosage adjustment/limits are recommended for sildenafil and other PDE-5 inhibitors; consult individual monographs.

The levels/effects of amiodarone may be increased by atazanavir, gemfibrozil, ritonavir, and other CYP2C8 inhibitors.

Concurrent use of fentanyl may lead to bradycardia, sinus arrest, and hypotension. Amiodarone may alter thyroid function and response to thyroid

(Continued)

Amiodarone *(Continued)*

supplements. Amiodarone enhances the myocardial depressant and conduction effects of inhalation anesthetics (monitor).

Decreased Effect: Levels/effects of amiodarone may be decreased by aminoglutethimide, carbamazepine, nafcillin, nevirapine, phenobarbital, phenytoin, rifampin, rifapentine, secobarbital, and other CYP2C8 inducers and CYP3A4 inducers. Amiodarone may decrease the levels/effects of codeine, hydrocodone, oxycodone, tramadol, and other prodrug substrates of CYP2D6. Amiodarone may alter thyroid function and response to thyroid supplements; monitor closely.

Pharmacodynamics/Kinetics

Onset of action: Oral: 2 days to 3 weeks; I.V.: May be more rapid

Peak effect: 1 week to 5 months

Duration after discontinuing therapy: 7-50 days

Note: Mean onset of effect and duration after discontinuation may be shorter in children than adults

Distribution: V_d: 66 L/kg (range: 18-148 L/kg); crosses placenta; enters breast milk in concentrations higher than maternal plasma concentrations

Protein binding: 96%

Metabolism: Hepatic via CYP2C8 and 3A4 to active N-desethylamiodarone metabolite; possible enterohepatic recirculation

Bioavailability: Oral: ~50%

Half-life elimination: Terminal: 40-55 days (range: 26-107 days); shorter in children than adults

Excretion: Feces; urine (<1% as unchanged drug)

Pregnancy Risk Factor D

Amiodarone Hydrochloride see Amiodarone on page 92

Ami-Tex LA [DSC] see Guaifenesin and Phenylephrine on page 797

Amitiza™ see Lubiprostone on page 1010

Amitriptyline *(a mee TRIP ti leen)*

Related Information

Temporomandibular Dysfunction (TMD) *on page 1822*

Canadian Brand Names Apo-Amitriptyline®; Levate®; Novo-Triptyn; PMS-Amitriptyline

Mexican Brand Names Anapsique; Tryptanol

Generic Available Yes

Index Terms Amitriptyline Hydrochloride; Elavil

Pharmacologic Category Antidepressant, Tricyclic (Tertiary Amine)

Dental Use Management of chronic neuropathic pain in temporomandibular dysfunction (TMD)

Use Relief of symptoms of depression

Unlabeled/Investigational Use Analgesic for certain chronic and neuropathic pain; prophylaxis against migraine headaches; treatment of depressive disorders in children

Local Anesthetic/Vasoconstrictor Precautions Amitriptyline is one of the drugs confirmed to prolong the QT interval and is accepted as having a risk of causing torsade de pointes. In terms of epinephrine, it is not known what effect vasoconstrictors in the local anesthetic regimen will have in patients with a known history of congenital prolonged QT interval or in patients taking any medication that prolongs the QT interval. Until more information is obtained, it is suggested that the clinician consult with the physician prior to the use of a vasoconstrictor in suspected patients, and that the vasoconstrictor (epinephrine, levonordefrin [Neo-Cobefrin®]) be used with caution. See Dental Comment.

Effects on Dental Treatment Key adverse event(s) related to dental treatment: Xerostomia and changes in salivation (normal salivary flow resumes upon discontinuation), orthostatic hypotension, stomatitis, peculiar taste, and black tongue. Amitriptyline is the most anticholinergic and sedating of the antidepressants; has pronounced effects on the cardiovascular system. Long-term treatment with TCAs such as amitriptyline increases the risk of caries by reducing salivation and salivary buffer capacity. In a study by Rundergren, et al, pathological alterations were observed in the oral mucosa of 72% of 58 patients; 55% had new carious lesions after taking TCAs for a median of $5^1/_2$ years. Current research is investigating the use of the salivary stimulant pilocarpine (Salagen®) to overcome the xerostomia from amitriptyline.

Significant Adverse Effects Anticholinergic effects may be pronounced; moderate to marked sedation can occur (tolerance to these effects usually occurs).

Frequency not defined.

Cardiovascular: Orthostatic hypotension, tachycardia, ECG changes (nonspecific), AV conduction changes, cardiomyopathy (rare), MI, stroke, heart block, arrhythmia, syncope, hypertension, palpitation

Central nervous system: Restlessness, dizziness, insomnia, sedation, fatigue, anxiety, cognitive function impaired, seizure, extrapyramidal symptoms, coma, hallucinations, confusion, disorientation, coordination impaired, ataxia, headache, nightmares, hyperpyrexia

Dermatologic: Allergic rash, urticaria, photosensitivity, alopecia

Endocrine & metabolic: Syndrome of inappropriate ADH secretion

Gastrointestinal: Weight gain, xerostomia, constipation, paralytic ileus, nausea, vomiting, anorexia, stomatitis, peculiar taste, diarrhea, black tongue

Genitourinary: Urinary retention

Hematologic: Bone marrow depression, purpura, eosinophilia

Neuromuscular & skeletal: Numbness, paresthesia, peripheral neuropathy, tremor, weakness

Ocular: Blurred vision, mydriasis, ocular pressure increased

Otic: Tinnitus

Miscellaneous: Diaphoresis, withdrawal reactions (nausea, headache, malaise)

Postmarketing and/or case reports: Neuroleptic malignant syndrome (rare), serotonin syndrome (rare)

Restrictions An FDA-approved medication guide concerning the use of antidepressants in children, adolescents, and young adults must be distributed when dispensing an outpatient prescription (new or refill) where this medication is to be used without direct supervision of a healthcare provider. Medication guides are available at http://www.fda.gov/cder/Offices/ODS/medication_guides.htm. Dispense to parents or guardians of children and adolescents receiving this medication.

Dental Usual Dosing

Chronic neuropathic pain in temporomandibular dysfunction (TMD) (unlabeled use): Adults: Oral: Initial: 25 mg at bedtime; may increase as tolerated to 100 mg/day

Dosage

Children:

Chronic pain management (unlabeled use): Oral: Initial: 0.1 mg/kg at bedtime, may advance as tolerated over 2-3 weeks to 0.5-2 mg/kg at bedtime

Depressive disorders (unlabeled use): Oral: Initial doses of 1 mg/kg/day given in 3 divided doses with increases to 1.5 mg/kg/day have been reported in a small number of children (n=9) 9-12 years of age; clinically, doses up to 3 mg/kg/day (5 mg/kg/day if monitored closely) have been proposed

Migraine prophylaxis (unlabeled use): Oral: Initial: 0.25 mg/kg/day, given at bedtime; increase dose by 0.25 mg/kg/day to maximum 1 mg/kg/day. Reported dosing ranges: 0.1-2 mg/kg/day; maximum suggested dose: 10 mg.

Adolescents: Depressive disorders: Oral: Initial: 25-50 mg/day; may administer in divided doses; increase gradually to 100 mg/day in divided doses

Adults:

Depression:

Oral: 50-150 mg/day single dose at bedtime or in divided doses; dose may be gradually increased up to 300 mg/day

Migraine prophylaxis (unlabeled use): Oral: Initial: 10-25 mg at bedtime; usual dose: 150 mg; reported dosing ranges: 10-400 mg/day

Pain management (unlabeled use): Oral: Initial: 25 mg at bedtime; may increase as tolerated to 100 mg/day

Elderly: Depression: Oral: Initial: 10-25 mg at bedtime; dose should be increased in 10-25 mg increments every week if tolerated; dose range: 25-150 mg/day

Dosing interval in hepatic impairment: Use with caution and monitor plasma levels and patient response

Hemodialysis: Nondialyzable

Mechanism of Action Increases the synaptic concentration of serotonin and/or norepinephrine in the central nervous system by inhibition of their reuptake by the presynaptic neuronal membrane

Contraindications Hypersensitivity to amitriptyline or any component of the formulation (cross-sensitivity with other tricyclics may occur); use of MAO inhibitors within past 14 days; acute recovery phase following myocardial infarction; concurrent use of cisapride

Warnings/Precautions [U.S. Boxed Warning]: Antidepressants increase the risk of suicidal thinking and behavior in children, adolescents, and young adults (18-24 years of age) with major depressive disorder (MDD) and other psychiatric disorders; consider risk prior to prescribing. Short-term studies did not show an increased risk in patients >24 years of age and showed a decreased risk in patients ≥65 years. Closely monitor for clinical worsening, suicidality, or unusual changes in behavior; the patient's family or caregiver

(Continued)

Amitriptyline *(Continued)*

should be instructed to closely observe the patient and communicate condition with healthcare provider. Such observation would generally include at least weekly face-to-face contact with patients or their family members or caregivers during the first 4 weeks of treatment, then every other week visits for the next 4 weeks, then at 12 weeks, and as clinically indicated beyond 12 weeks. Additional contact by telephone may be appropriate between face-to-face visits. Adults treated with antidepressants should be observed similarly for clinical worsening and suicidality, especially during the initial few months of a course of drug therapy, or at times of dose changes, either increases or decreases. A medication guide should be dispensed with each prescription. **Amitriptyline is not FDA-approved for use in children <12 years of age.**

The possibility of a suicide attempt is inherent in major depression and may persist until remission occurs. Monitor for worsening of depression or suicidality, especially during initiation of therapy (generally first 1-2 months) or with dose increases or decreases. Worsening depression and severe abrupt suicidality that are not part of the presenting symptoms may require discontinuation or modification of drug therapy. The patient's family or caregiver should be alerted to monitor patients for the emergence of suicidality and associated behaviors (such as agitation, irritability, hostility, impulsivity, and hypomania) and notify healthcare provider.

May worsen psychosis in some patients or precipitate a shift to mania or hypomania in patients with bipolar disorder. Patients presenting with depressive symptoms should be screened for bipolar disorder. Monotherapy in patients with bipolar disorder should be avoided. **Amitriptyline is not FDA approved for bipolar depression.**

The degree of sedation, anticholinergic effects, orthostasis, and conduction abnormalities are high relative to other antidepressants. Amitriptyline often causes drowsiness/sedation, resulting in impaired performance of tasks requiring alertness (eg, operating machinery or driving). Sedative effects may be additive with other CNS depressants and/or ethanol. Use with caution in patients with a history of cardiovascular disease (including previous MI, stroke, tachycardia, or conduction abnormalities). Use with caution in patients with urinary retention, benign prostatic hyperplasia, narrow-angle glaucoma, xerostomia, visual problems, constipation, or a history of bowel obstruction.

May alter glucose control - use with caution in patients with diabetes. May cause hyponatremia/SIADH. Consider discontinuing, when possible, prior to elective surgery. Therapy should not be abruptly discontinued in patients receiving high doses for prolonged periods. May lower seizure threshold - use caution in patients with a previous seizure disorder or condition predisposing to seizures such as brain damage, alcoholism, or concurrent therapy with other drugs which lower the seizure threshold. May increase the risks associated with electroconvulsive therapy. Use with caution in hyperthyroid patients or those receiving thyroid supplementation. Use with caution in patients with hepatic or renal dysfunction and in elderly patients.

Drug Interactions Substrate of CYP1A2 (minor), 2B6 (minor), 2C9 (minor), 2C19 (minor), 2D6 (major), 3A4 (minor); **Inhibits** CYP1A2 (weak), 2C9 (weak), 2C19 (weak), 2D6 (weak), 2E1 (weak)

Altretamine: Concurrent use may cause orthostatic hypertension.

Amphetamines: TCAs may enhance the effect of amphetamines; monitor for adverse CV effects.

Anticholinergics: Combined use with TCAs may produce additive anticholinergic effects.

Antihypertensives: Amitriptyline inhibits the antihypertensive response to bethanidine, clonidine, debrisoquin, guanadrel, guanethidine, guanabenz, guanfacine; monitor BP; consider alternate antihypertensive agent.

Beta-agonists: When combined with TCAs may predispose patients to cardiac arrhythmias.

Bupropion: May increase the levels of tricyclic antidepressants; based on limited information, monitor response.

Carbamazepine: Tricyclic antidepressants may increase carbamazepine levels; monitor.

Cholestyramine and colestipol: May bind TCAs and reduce their absorption; monitor for altered response.

Cisapride: May increase the risk of QT_c prolongation and/or arrhythmia; concurrent use is contraindicated.

Clonidine: Abrupt discontinuation of clonidine may cause hypertensive crisis; amitriptyline may enhance the response (also see note on antihypertensives).

CNS depressants: Sedative effects may be additive with TCAs; monitor for increased effect; includes benzodiazepines, barbiturates, antipsychotics, ethanol, and other sedative medications.

CYP2D6 inhibitors: May increase the levels/effects of amitriptyline; example inhibitors include chlorpromazine, delavirdine, fluoxetine, miconazole, paroxetine, pergolide, quinidine, quinine, ritonavir, and ropinirole.

Epinephrine (and other direct alpha-agonists): Pressor response to I.V. epinephrine, norepinephrine, and phenylephrine may be enhanced in patients receiving TCAs. (**Note:** Effect is unlikely with epinephrine or levonordefrin dosages typically administered as infiltration in combination with local anesthetics.)

Fenfluramine: May increase tricyclic antidepressant levels/effects.

Hypoglycemic agents (including insulin): TCAs may enhance the hypoglycemic effects of tolazamide, chlorpropamide, or insulin; monitor for changes in blood glucose levels; reported with chlorpropamide, tolazamide, and insulin.

Levodopa: Tricyclic antidepressants may decrease the absorption (bioavailability) of levodopa; rare hypertensive episodes have also been attributed to this combination.

Linezolid: Hyperpyrexia, hypertension, tachycardia, confusion, seizures, and **deaths have been reported** with agents which inhibit MAO (serotonin syndrome); this combination should be avoided.

Lithium: Concurrent use with a TCA may increase the risk for neurotoxicity.

MAO inhibitors: Hyperpyrexia, hypertension, tachycardia, confusion, seizures, and **deaths have been reported** (serotonin syndrome); this combination should be avoided.

Methylphenidate: Metabolism of amitriptyline may be decreased.

Phenothiazines: Serum concentrations of some TCAs may be increased; in addition, TCAs may increase concentration of phenothiazines; monitor for altered clinical response.

QT_c prolonging agents: Concurrent use of tricyclic agents with other drugs which may prolong QT_c interval may increase the risk of potentially fatal arrhythmias; includes type Ia and type III antiarrhythmics agents, selected quinolones (sparfloxacin, gatifloxacin, moxifloxacin, grepafloxacin), cisapride, and other agents.

Ritonavir: Combined use of high-dose tricyclic antidepressants with ritonavir may cause serotonin syndrome in HIV-positive patients; monitor.

Sucralfate: Absorption of tricyclic antidepressants may be reduced with coadministration.

Sympathomimetics, indirect-acting: Tricyclic antidepressants may result in a decreased sensitivity to indirect-acting sympathomimetics; includes dopamine and ephedrine; also see interaction with epinephrine (and direct-acting sympathomimetics).

Tramadol: Tramadol's risk of seizures may be increased with TCAs.

Valproic acid: May increase serum concentrations/adverse effects of some tricyclic antidepressants.

Warfarin (and other oral anticoagulants): Amitriptyline may increase the anticoagulant effect in patients stabilized on warfarin; monitor INR.

Ethanol/Nutrition/Herb Interactions

Ethanol: Avoid ethanol (may increase CNS depression).

Food: Grapefruit juice may inhibit the metabolism of some TCAs and clinical toxicity may result.

Herb/Nutraceutical: St John's wort may decrease amitriptyline levels. Avoid valerian, St John's wort, kava kava, gotu kola (may increase CNS depression).

Pharmacodynamics/Kinetics

Onset of action: Migraine prophylaxis: 6 weeks, higher dosage may be required in heavy smokers because of increased metabolism; Depression: 4-6 weeks, reduce dosage to lowest effective level

Distribution: Crosses placenta; enters breast milk

Metabolism: Hepatic to nortriptyline (active), hydroxy and conjugated derivatives; may be impaired in the elderly

Half-life elimination: Adults: 9-27 hours (average: 15 hours)

Time to peak, serum: ~4 hours

Excretion: Urine (18% as unchanged drug); feces (small amounts)

Pregnancy Risk Factor C

Lactation Enters breast milk/not recommended (AAP rates "of concern")

Breast-Feeding Considerations Generally, it is not recommended to breast-feed if taking antidepressants because of the long half-life, active metabolites, and the potential for side effects in the infant.

Dosage Forms Excipient information presented when available (limited, particularly for generics); consult specific product labeling.

Tablet, as hydrochloride: 10 mg, 25 mg, 50 mg, 75 mg, 100 mg, 150 mg

Dental Comment Amitriptyline is known to prolong the QT interval. The QT interval is measured as the time and distance between the Q point of the QRS complex and the end of the T wave in the ECG tracing. After adjustment for heart rate, the QT interval is defined as prolonged if it is more than 450 msec in (Continued)

Amitriptyline *(Continued)*

men and 460 msec in women. A long QT syndrome was first described in the 1950s and 60s as a congenital syndrome involving QT interval prolongation and syncope and sudden death. Some of the congenital long QT syndromes were characterized by a peculiar electrocardiographic appearance of the QRS complex involving a premature atria beat followed by a pause, then a subsequent sinus beat showing marked QT prolongation and deformity. This type of cardiac arrhythmia was originally termed "torsade de pointes" (translated from the French as "twisting of the points").

Prolongation of the QT interval is thought to result from delayed ventricular repolarization. The repolarization process within the myocardial cell is due to the efflux of intracellular potassium. The channels associated with this current can be blocked by many drugs and predispose the electrical propagation cycle to torsade de pointes.

Amitriptyline is considered as having a risk of causing torsade de pointes. The risk of drug-induced torsade de pointes is extremely low when a single QT interval prolonging drug is prescribed. It is not known what effect vasoconstrictors in the local anesthetic regimen will have in patients with a known history of congenital prolonged QT interval or in patients taking any medication that prolongs the QT interval. Until more information is obtained, it is suggested that the clinician consult with the physician prior to the use of a vasoconstrictor in suspected patients, and that the vasoconstrictor (epinephrine, levonordefrin [Neo-Cobefrin®]) be used with caution.

Selected Readings

Boakes AJ, Laurence DR, Teoh PC, et al, "Interactions Between Sympathomimetic Amines and Antidepressant Agents in Man," *Br Med J*, 1973, 1(849):311-5.

Friedlander AH and Mahler ME, "Major Depressive Disorder. Psychopathology, Medical Management, and Dental Implications," *J Am Dent Assoc*, 2001, 132(5):629-38.

Ganzberg S, "Psychoactive Drugs," *ADA Guide to Dental Therapeutics*, 2nd ed, Chicago, IL: ADA Publishing, a Division of ADA Business Enterprises, Inc, 2000, 376-405.

Jastak JT and Yagiela JA, "Vasoconstrictors and Local Anesthesia: A Review and Rationale for Use," *J Am Dent Assoc*, 1983, 107(4):623-30.

Rundegren J, van Dijken J, Mörnstad H, et al, "Oral Conditions in Patients Receiving Long-Term Treatment With Cyclic Antidepressant Drugs," *Swed Dent J*, 1985, 9(2):55-64.

Yagiela JA, "Adverse Drug Interactions in Dental Practice: Interactions Associated With Vasoconstrictors. Part V of a Series," *J Am Dent Assoc*, 1999, 130(5):701-9.

Amitriptyline and Chlordiazepoxide
(a mee TRIP ti leen & klor dye az e POKS ide)

Related Information
Amitriptyline *on page 94*
Chlordiazepoxide *on page 331*

U.S. Brand Names Limbitrol®; Limbitrol® DS

Canadian Brand Names Limbitrol®

Generic Available Yes

Index Terms Chlordiazepoxide and Amitriptyline Hydrochloride

Pharmacologic Category Antidepressant, Tricyclic (Tertiary Amine); Benzodiazepine

Use Treatment of moderate to severe anxiety and/or agitation and depression

Local Anesthetic/Vasoconstrictor Precautions Use with caution; epinephrine and levonordefrin have been shown to have an increased pressor response in combination with TCAs

Effects on Dental Treatment Key adverse event(s) related to dental treatment:

Amitriptyline: Xerostomia and changes in salivation (normal salivary flow resumes upon discontinuation), orthostatic hypotension, stomatitis, peculiar taste, and black tongue. Amitriptyline is the most anticholinergic and sedating of the antidepressants; has pronounced effects on the cardiovascular system. Long-term treatment with TCAs such as amitriptyline increases the risk of caries by reducing salivation and salivary buffer capacity. In a study by Rundergren, et al, pathological alterations were observed in the oral mucosa of 72% of 58 patients; 55% had new carious lesions after taking TCAs for a median of 5½ years. Current research is investigating the use of the salivary stimulant pilocarpine (Salagen®) to overcome the xerostomia from amitriptyline.

Chlordiazepoxide: Over 10% of patients will experience xerostomia which disappears with cessation of drug therapy.

Common Adverse Effects See individual agents.

Restrictions C-IV

An FDA-approved medication guide concerning the use of antidepressants in children, adolescents, and young adults must be distributed when dispensing an outpatient prescription (new or refill) where this medication is to be used without direct supervision of a healthcare provider. Medication guides are available at http://www.fda.gov/cder/Offices/ODS/medication_guides.htm. Dispense to parents or guardians of children and adolescents receiving this medication.

Mechanism of Action See individual agents.

Drug Interactions

Cytochrome P450 Effect:

Amitriptyline: **Substrate** of CYP1A2 (minor), 2B6 (minor), 2C9 (minor), 2C19 (minor), 2D6 (major), 3A4 (minor); **Inhibits** CYP1A2 (weak), 2C9 (weak), 2C19 (weak), 2D6 (weak), 2E1 (weak)

Chlordiazepoxide: **Substrate** of CYP3A4 (major)

Increased Effect/Toxicity: See individual agents.

Decreased Effect: See individual agents.

Pharmacodynamics/Kinetics See individual agents.

Pregnancy Risk Factor D

Amitriptyline and Perphenazine
(a mee TRIP ti leen & per FEN a zeen)

Related Information
Amitriptyline on page 94
Perphenazine on page 1284

Canadian Brand Names Etrafon®

Generic Available Yes

Index Terms Perphenazine and Amitriptyline Hydrochloride

Pharmacologic Category Antidepressant, Tricyclic (Tertiary Amine); Antipsychotic Agent, Typical, Phenothiazine

Use Treatment of patients with moderate to severe anxiety and depression

Unlabeled/Investigational Use Depression with psychotic features

Local Anesthetic/Vasoconstrictor Precautions
Amitriptyline: Use with caution; epinephrine and levonordefrin have been shown to have an increased pressor response in combination with TCAs
Perphenazine: No information available to require special precautions

Effects on Dental Treatment Key adverse event(s) related to dental treatment:
Amitriptyline: Xerostomia and changes in salivation (normal salivary flow resumes upon discontinuation), orthostatic hypotension, stomatitis, peculiar taste, and black tongue. Amitriptyline is the most anticholinergic and sedating of the antidepressants; has pronounced effects on the cardiovascular system. Long-term treatment with TCAs such as amitriptyline increases the risk of caries by reducing salivation and salivary buffer capacity. In a study by Rundergren, et al, pathological alterations were observed in the oral mucosa of 72% of 58 patients; 55% had new carious lesions after taking TCAs for a median of 5½ years. Current research is investigating the use of the salivary stimulant pilocarpine (Salagen®) to overcome the xerostomia from amitriptyline.

Perphenazine: Extrapyramidal symptoms (pseudoparkinsonism, akathisia, dystonias, tardive dyskinesia), dizziness, seizures, headache, drowsiness, paradoxical excitement, restlessness, and hyperactivity.

Tardive dyskinesia: Prevalence rate may be 40% in elderly; development of the syndrome and the irreversible nature are proportional to duration and total cumulative dose over time. Extrapyramidal reactions are more common in elderly with up to 50% developing these reactions after 60 years of age. Drug-induced Parkinson's syndrome occurs often; akathisia is the most common extrapyramidal reaction in elderly.

Increased confusion, memory loss, psychotic behavior, and agitation frequently occur as a consequence of anticholinergic effects. Antipsychotic associated sedation in nonpsychotic patients is extremely unpleasant due to feelings of depersonalization, derealization, and dysphoria.

Common Adverse Effects Frequency not defined.
Based on **amitriptyline** component: Anticholinergic effects may be pronounced; moderate to marked sedation can occur (tolerance to these effects usually occurs).
Cardiovascular: Orthostatic hypotension, tachycardia, ECG changes (nonspecific), AV conduction changes
Central nervous system: Restlessness, dizziness, insomnia, sedation, fatigue, anxiety, cognitive function impaired, seizure, extrapyramidal symptoms
Dermatologic: Allergic rash, urticaria, photosensitivity
Gastrointestinal: Weight gain, xerostomia, constipation
Genitourinary: Urinary retention
Ocular: Blurred vision, mydriasis
Miscellaneous: Diaphoresis
(Continued)

Amitriptyline and Perphenazine *(Continued)*

Based on **perphenazine** component:
Cardiovascular: Hyper-/hypotension, orthostatic hypotension, tachycardia, bradycardia, dizziness, cardiac arrest

Central nervous system: Extrapyramidal symptoms (pseudoparkinsonism, akathisia, dystonias, tardive dyskinesia), dizziness, cerebral edema, seizure, headache, drowsiness, paradoxical excitement, restlessness, hyperactivity, insomnia, neuroleptic malignant syndrome (NMS), impairment of temperature regulation

Dermatologic: Sun sensitivity increased, rash, discoloration of skin (blue-gray)

Endocrine & metabolic: Hypoglycemia, hyperglycemia, galactorrhea, lactation, breast enlargement, gynecomastia, menstrual irregularity, amenorrhea, SIADH, libido changes

Gastrointestinal: Constipation, weight gain, vomiting, stomach pain, nausea, xerostomia, salivation, diarrhea, anorexia, ileus

Genitourinary: Difficulty in urination, ejaculatory disturbances, incontinence, polyuria, ejaculating dysfunction, priapism

Hematologic: Agranulocytosis, leukopenia, eosinophilia, hemolytic anemia, thrombocytopenic purpura, pancytopenia

Hepatic: Cholestatic jaundice, hepatotoxicity

Neuromuscular & skeletal: Tremor

Ocular: Pigmentary retinopathy, blurred vision, cornea and lens changes

Respiratory: Nasal congestion

Miscellaneous: Diaphoresis

Restrictions An FDA-approved medication guide concerning the use of antidepressants in children, adolescents, and young adults must be distributed when dispensing an outpatient prescription (new or refill) where this medication is to be used without direct supervision of a healthcare provider. Medication guides are available at http://www.fda.gov/cder/Offices/ODS/medication_guides.htm. Dispense to parents or guardians of children and adolescents receiving this medication.

Mechanism of Action

Amitriptyline increases the synaptic concentration of serotonin and/or norepinephrine in the central nervous system by inhibition of their reuptake by the presynaptic neuronal membrane.

Perphenazine is a piperazine phenothiazine antipsychotic which blocks postsynaptic mesolimbic dopaminergic receptors in the brain; exhibits alpha-adrenergic blocking effect and depresses the release of hypothalamic and hypophyseal hormones.

Drug Interactions

Cytochrome P450 Effect:

Amitriptyline: **Substrate** of CYP1A2 (minor), 2B6 (minor), 2C9 (minor), 2C19 (minor), 2D6 (major), 3A4 (minor); **Inhibits** CYP1A2 (weak), 2C9 (weak), 2C19 (weak), 2D6 (weak), 2E1 (weak)

Perphenazine: **Substrate** of CYP1A2 (minor), 2C9 (minor), 2C19 (minor), 2D6 (major), 3A4 (minor); **Inhibits** CYP1A2 (weak), 2D6 (weak)

Increased Effect/Toxicity: See individual agents.

Decreased Effect: See individual agents.

Pharmacodynamics/Kinetics See individual agents.

Pregnancy Risk Factor D

Amitriptyline Hydrochloride *see* Amitriptyline *on page 94*

AMJ 9701 *see* Palifermin *on page 1242*

AmLactin® [OTC] *see* Lactic Acid and Ammonium Hydroxide *on page 941*

Amlexanox *(am LEKS an oks)*

Related Information

Ulcerative and Erosive Disorders *on page 1809*

Related Sample Prescriptions

Recurrent Aphthous Stomatitis *on page 1844*

U.S. Brand Names Aphthasol®

Generic Available No

Pharmacologic Category Anti-inflammatory, Locally Applied

Dental Use Treatment of aphthous ulcers (ie, canker sores)

Use Treatment of aphthous ulcers (ie, canker sores)

Unlabeled/Investigational Use Allergic disorders

Local Anesthetic/Vasoconstrictor Precautions No information available to require special precautions

Effects on Dental Treatment Key adverse event(s) related to dental treatment: Allergic contact dermatitis and oral irritation. Discontinue therapy if rash or contact mucositis develops (see Dental Comment).

Significant Adverse Effects
1% to 2%:
- Dermatologic: Allergic contact dermatitis
- Gastrointestinal: Oral irritation

<1% (Limited to important or life-threatening): Contact mucositis

Dosage Topical: Administer (0.5 cm - $1/4$") directly on ulcers 4 times/day following oral hygiene, after meals, and at bedtime

Mechanism of Action As a benzopyrano-bipyridine carboxylic acid derivative, amlexanox has anti-inflammatory and antiallergic properties; it inhibits chemical mediatory release of the slow-reacting substance of anaphylaxis (SRS-A) and may have antagonistic effects on interleukin-3

Contraindications Hypersensitivity to amlexanox or any component of the formulation

Warnings/Precautions Discontinue therapy if rash or contact mucositis develops.

Pharmacodynamics/Kinetics
Absorption: Some from swallowed paste
Metabolism: Hydroxylated and conjugated metabolites
Half-life elimination: 3.5 hours
Time to peak, serum: 2 hours
Excretion: Urine (17% as unchanged drug)

Pregnancy Risk Factor B

Lactation Excretion in breast milk unknown/use caution

Dosage Forms Excipient information presented when available (limited, particularly for generics); consult specific product labeling.
Paste: 5% (5 g) [contains benzyl alcohol]

Dental Comment Treatment of canker sores with amlexanox showed a 76% median reduction in ulcer size compared to a 40% reduction with placebo. Greer, et al, reported an overall mean reduction in ulcer size of 1.82 mm^2 for patients treated with 5% amlexanox versus an average reduction of 0.52 mm^2 for the control group. Recent studies in over thousands of patients have confirmed that amlexanox accelerates the resolution of pain and healing of aphthous ulcers more significantly than vehicle and no treatment.

Selected Readings
Barrons RW, "Treatment Strategies for Recurrent Oral Aphthous Ulcers," *Am J Health Syst Pharm*, 2001, 58(1):41-50.

Binnie WH, Curro FA, Khandwala A, et al, "Amlexanox Oral Paste: A Novel Treatment That Accelerates the Healing of Aphthous Ulcers," *Compend Contin Educ Dent*, 1997, 18(11):1116-8, 1120-2, 1124.

Eisen D and Lynch DP, "Selecting Topical and Systemic Agents for Recurrent Aphthous Stomatitis," *Cutis*, 2001, 68(3):201-6.

Greer RO Jr, Lindenmuth JE, Juarez T, et al, "A Double-Blind Study of Topically Applied 5% Amlexanox in the Treatment of Aphthous Ulcers," *J Oral Maxillofac Surg*, 1993, 51(3):243-8.

Khandwala A, Van Inwegen RG, and Alfano MC, "5% Amlexanox Oral Paste, A New Treatment for Recurrent Minor Aphthous Ulcers: I. Clinical Demonstration of Acceleration of Healing and Resolution of Pain," *Oral Surg Oral Med Oral Pathol Oral Radiol Endod*, 1997, 83(2):222-30.

Khandwala A, Van Inwegen RG, Charney MR, et al, "5% Amlexanox Oral Paste, A New Treatment for Recurrent Minor Aphthous Ulcers: II. Pharmacokinetics and Demonstration of Clinical Safety," *Oral Surg Oral Med Oral Pathol Oral Radiol Endod*, 1997, 83(2):231-8.

Amlodipine (am LOE di peen)

Related Information
Cardiovascular Diseases *on page 1726*

U.S. Brand Names Norvasc®

Canadian Brand Names Norvasc®

Mexican Brand Names Norvas

Generic Available Yes

Index Terms Amlodipine Besylate

Pharmacologic Category Calcium Channel Blocker

Use Treatment of hypertension; treatment of symptomatic chronic stable angina, vasospastic (Prinzmetal's) angina (confirmed or suspected); prevention of hospitalization due to angina with documented CAD (limited to patients without heart failure or ejection fraction <40%)

Local Anesthetic/Vasoconstrictor Precautions No information available to require special precautions

Effects on Dental Treatment Fewer reports of gingival hyperplasia with amlodipine than with other CCBs (usually resolves upon discontinuation); consultation with physician is suggested.

Common Adverse Effects
>10%: Cardiovascular: Peripheral edema (2% to 15% dose related)
1% to 10%:
- Cardiovascular: Flushing (1% to 3%), palpitation (1% to 4%)
- Central nervous system: Headache (7%; similar to placebo 8%), dizziness (1% to 3%), fatigue (4%), somnolence (1% to 2%)

(Continued)

Amlodipine *(Continued)*

Dermatologic: Rash (1% to 2%), pruritus (1% to 2%)

Endocrine & metabolic: Male sexual dysfunction (1% to 2%)

Gastrointestinal: Nausea (3%), abdominal pain (1% to 2%), dyspepsia (1% to 2%), gingival hyperplasia

Neuromuscular & skeletal: Muscle cramps (1% to 2%), weakness (1% to 2%)

Respiratory: Dyspnea (1% to 2%), pulmonary edema (15% from PRAISE trial, CHF population)

Dosage Oral:

Children 6-17 years: Hypertension: 2.5-5 mg once daily

Adults:

Hypertension: Initial dose: 5 mg once daily; maximum dose: 10 mg once daily. In general, titrate in 2.5 mg increments over 7-14 days. Usual dosage range (JNC 7): 2.5-10 mg once daily.

Angina: Usual dose: 5-10 mg; lower dose suggested in elderly or hepatic impairment; most patients require 10 mg for adequate effect

Elderly: Dosing should start at the lower end of dosing range due to possible increased incidence of hepatic, renal, or cardiac impairment. Elderly patients also show decreased clearance of amlodipine.

Hypertension: 2.5 mg once daily

Angina: 5 mg once daily

Dialysis: Hemodialysis and peritoneal dialysis does not enhance elimination. Supplemental dose is not necessary.

Dosage adjustment in hepatic impairment:

Angina: Administer 5 mg once daily.

Hypertension: Administer 2.5 mg once daily.

Mechanism of Action Inhibits calcium ion from entering the "slow channels" or select voltage-sensitive areas of vascular smooth muscle and myocardium during depolarization, producing a relaxation of coronary vascular smooth muscle and coronary vasodilation; increases myocardial oxygen delivery in patients with vasospastic angina

Contraindications Hypersensitivity to amlodipine or any component of the formulation

Warnings/Precautions Increased angina and/or MI has occurred with initiation or dosage titration of calcium channel blockers. Symptomatic hypotension with or without syncope can rarely occur; blood pressure must be lowered at a rate appropriate for the patient's clinical condition. Use caution in severe aortic stenosis and/or hypertrophic cardiomyopathy. Use caution in patients with hepatic impairment. The most common side effect is peripheral edema; occurs within 2-3 weeks of starting therapy. Reflex tachycardia may occur with use. Dosage titration should occur after 7-14 days on a given dose. Initiate at a lower dose in the elderly. Safety and efficacy have not been established in children <6 years of age.

Drug Interactions

Cytochrome P450 Effect: Substrate of CYP3A4 (major); **Inhibits** CYP1A2 (moderate), 2A6 (weak), 2B6 (weak), 2C8 (weak), 2C9 (weak), 2D6 (weak), 3A4 (weak)

Increased Effect/Toxicity: Amlodipine may increase the levels/effects of aminophylline, fluvoxamine, mexiletine, mirtazapine, ropinirole, theophylline, trifluoperazine and other CYP1A2 substrates. Levels/effects of amlodipine may be increased by azole antifungals, clarithromycin, diclofenac, doxycycline, erythromycin, imatinib, isoniazid, nefazodone, nicardipine, propofol, protease inhibitors, quinidine, telithromycin, verapamil, and other CYP3A4 inhibitors. Cyclosporine levels may be increased by amlodipine. Blood pressure-lowering effects of sildenafil, tadalafil, and vardenafil are additive with amlodipine (use caution).

Decreased Effect: Calcium may reduce the calcium channel blocker's hypotensive effects. Levels/effects of amlodipine may be decreased by aminoglutethimide, carbamazepine, nafcillin, nevirapine, phenobarbital, phenytoin, rifamycins, and other CYP3A4 inducers.

Ethanol/Nutrition/Herb Interactions

Food: Grapefruit juice may modestly increase amlodipine levels.

Herb/Nutraceutical: St John's wort may decrease amlodipine levels. Avoid dong quai if using for hypertension (has estrogenic activity). Avoid ephedra, yohimbe, ginseng (may worsen hypertension). Avoid garlic (may have increased antihypertensive effects).

Dietary Considerations May be taken without regard to meals.

Pharmacodynamics/Kinetics

Onset of action: Antihypertensive: 30-50 minutes

Duration of antihypertensive effect: 24 hours

Absorption: Oral: Well absorbed

Distribution: V_d: 21 L/kg

Protein binding: 93% to 98%
Metabolism: Hepatic (>90%) to inactive metabolite
Bioavailability: 64% to 90%
Half-life elimination: 30-50 hours; increased with hepatic dysfunction
Time to peak, plasma: 6-12 hours
Excretion: Urine (10% as parent, 60% as metabolite)

Pregnancy Risk Factor C

Dosage Forms
    Tablet: 2.5 mg, 5 mg, 10 mg
       Norvasc®: 2.5 mg, 5 mg, 10 mg

Selected Readings
    Jorgensen MG, "Prevalence of Amlodipine-Related Gingival Hyperplasia," *J Periodontol*, 1997, 68(7):676-8.
    Wynn RL, "An Update on Calcium Channel Blocker-Induced Gingival Hyperplasia," *Gen Dent*, 1995, 43(3):218-22.
    Wynn RL, "Calcium Channel Blockers and Gingival Hyperplasia," *Gen Dent*, 1991, 39(4):240-3.

Amlodipine and Atorvastatin
(am LOW di peen & a TORE va sta tin)

Related Information
    Amlodipine *on page 101*
    Atorvastatin *on page 162*

U.S. Brand Names Caduet®
Canadian Brand Names Caduet®
Mexican Brand Names Caduet
Generic Available No
Index Terms Atorvastatin Calcium and Amlodipine Besylate
Pharmacologic Category Antilipemic Agent, HMG-CoA Reductase Inhibitor; Calcium Channel Blocker
Use For use when treatment with both amlodipine and atorvastatin is appropriate:
    Amlodipine: Treatment of hypertension; treatment of symptomatic chronic stable angina, vasospastic (Prinzmetal's) angina (confirmed or suspected); prevention of hospitalization due to angina with documented CAD (limited to patients without heart failure or ejection fraction <40%)
    Atorvastatin: Treatment of dyslipidemias or primary prevention of cardiovascular disease (atherosclerotic) as detailed here:
        Primary prevention of cardiovascular disease (high-risk for CVD): To reduce the risk of MI or stroke in patients without evidence of heart disease who have multiple CVD risk factors or type 2 diabetes. Treatment reduces the risk for angina or revascularization procedures in patients with multiple risk factors.
        Treatment of dyslipidemias: To reduce elevations in total cholesterol, LDL-C, apolipoprotein B, and triglycerides in patients with elevations of one or more components, and/or to increase HDL-C as present in heterozygous hypercholesterolemia (Fredrickson type IIa hyperlipidemias); treatment of primary dysbetalipoproteinemia (Fredrickson type III), elevated serum TG levels (Fredrickson type IV), and homozygous familial hypercholesterolemia
        Treatment of heterozygous familial hypercholesterolemia (HeFH) in adolescent patients (10-17 years of age, females >1 year postmenarche) having LDL-C ≥190 mg/dL or LDL-C ≥160 mg/dL with positive family history of premature cardiovascular disease (CVD) or with two or more CVD risk factors.
Local Anesthetic/Vasoconstrictor Precautions No information available to require special precautions
Effects on Dental Treatment No significant effects or complications reported
Common Adverse Effects See individual agents.
Mechanism of Action
    Amlodipine: Inhibits calcium ion from entering the "slow channels" or select voltage-sensitive areas of vascular smooth muscle and myocardium during depolarization, producing a relaxation of coronary vascular smooth muscle and coronary vasodilation; increases myocardial oxygen delivery in patients with vasospastic angina
    Atorvastatin: Inhibitor of 3-hydroxy-3-methylglutaryl coenzyme A (HMG-CoA) reductase, the rate limiting enzyme in cholesterol synthesis (reduces the production of mevalonic acid from HMG-CoA); this then results in a compensatory increase in the expression of LDL receptors on hepatocyte membranes and a stimulation of LDL catabolism
Drug Interactions
    Cytochrome P450 Effect:
        Amlodipine: **Substrate** of CYP3A4 (major); **Inhibits** CYP1A2 (moderate), 2A6 (weak), 2B6 (weak), 2C8 (weak), 2C9 (weak), 2D6 (weak), 3A4 (weak)
        Atorvastatin: **Substrate** of CYP3A4 (major); **Inhibits** CYP3A4 (weak)
(Continued)

Amlodipine and Atorvastatin *(Continued)*

Pharmacodynamics/Kinetics See individual agents.

Pregnancy Risk Factor X

Amlodipine and Benazepril *(am LOE di peen & ben AY ze pril)*

Related Information
Amlodipine *on page 101*
Benazepril *on page 191*

U.S. Brand Names Lotrel®

Generic Available No

Index Terms Benazepril Hydrochloride and Amlodipine Besylate

Pharmacologic Category Antihypertensive Agent, Combination

Use Treatment of hypertension

Local Anesthetic/Vasoconstrictor Precautions No information available to require special precautions

Effects on Dental Treatment Fewer reports of gingival hyperplasia with amlodipine than with other CCBs (usually resolves upon discontinuation); consultation with physician is suggested.

Common Adverse Effects See individual agents.

Dosage Oral:

Adults: 2.5-10 mg (amlodipine) and 10-40 mg (benazepril) once daily; maximum: Amlodipine: 10 mg/day; benazepril: 40 mg/day

Elderly: Initial dose: 2.5 mg based on amlodipine component

Dosage adjustment in renal impairment: Cl_{cr} ≤30 mL/minute: Use of combination product is not recommended.

Dosage adjustment in hepatic impairment: Initial dose: 2.5 mg based on amlodipine component

Mechanism of Action The mechanism through which benazepril lowers blood pressure is believed to be primarily suppression of the renin-angiotensin-aldosterone system; benazepril has an antihypertensive effect even in patients with low-renin hypertension; amlodipine is a dihydropyridine calcium antagonist that inhibits the transmembrane influx of calcium ions into vascular smooth muscle and cardiac muscle; amlodipine is a peripheral arterial vasodilator that acts directly on vascular smooth muscle to cause a reduction in peripheral vascular resistance and reduction in blood pressure

Contraindications Hypersensitivity to amlodipine, benazepril, other ACE inhibitors, or any component of the formulation; pregnancy (2nd and 3rd trimesters)

Warnings/Precautions Used as a replacement for separate dosing of components or combination therapy when response to single agent is suboptimal. The fixed combination is not indicated for initial treatment of hypertension. See individual agents for additional warnings/precautions.

Drug Interactions

Cytochrome P450 Effect: Amlodipine: **Substrate** of CYP3A4 (major); **Inhibits** CYP1A2 (moderate), 2A6 (weak), 2B6 (weak), 2C8 (weak), 2C9 (weak), 2D6 (weak), 3A4 (weak)

Increased Effect/Toxicity: See individual agents.

Decreased Effect: See individual agents.

Pharmacodynamics/Kinetics See individual agents.

Pregnancy Risk Factor C/D (2nd and 3rd trimesters)

Dosage Forms

Capsule:

Lotrel®:

2.5/10: Amlodipine 2.5 mg and benazepril 10 mg

5/10: Amlodipine 5 mg and benazepril 10 mg

5/20: Amlodipine 5 mg and benazepril 20 mg

5/40: Amlodipine 5 mg and benazepril 40 mg

10/20: Amlodipine 10 mg and benazepril 20 mg

10/40: Amlodipine 10 mg and benazepril 40 mg

Selected Readings

Wynn RL, "An Update on Calcium Channel Blocker-Induced Gingival Hyperplasia," *Gen Dent*, 1995, 43(3):218-22.

Wynn RL, "Calcium Channel Blockers and Gingival Hyperplasia," *Gen Dent*, 1991, 39(4):240-3.

Amlodipine Besylate *see* Amlodipine *on page 101*

Ammens® Medicated Deodorant [OTC] *see* Zinc Oxide *on page 1683*

Ammonapse *see* Sodium Phenylbutyrate *on page 1483*

Ammonia Spirit (Aromatic)
(a MOE nee ah SPEAR it, air oh MAT ik)

Generic Available Yes
Index Terms Smelling Salts
Pharmacologic Category Respiratory Stimulant
Dental Use Emergency use in syncope
Use Respiratory and circulatory stimulant; treatment of fainting
Local Anesthetic/Vasoconstrictor Precautions No information available to require special precautions
Effects on Dental Treatment No significant effects or complications reported
Significant Adverse Effects 1% to 10%:
Gastrointestinal: Nausea, vomiting
Respiratory: Irritation to nasal mucosa, cough
Dosage Used as "smelling salts" to treat or prevent fainting
Contraindications Hypersensitivity to ammonia or any component of the formulation
Drug Interactions No data reported
Pregnancy Risk Factor C
Dosage Forms Excipient information presented when available (limited, particularly for generics); consult specific product labeling.
Solution for inhalation [ampul]: 1.7% to 2.1% (0.33 mL)

Ammonium Chloride (a MOE nee um KLOR ide)

Generic Available Yes
Pharmacologic Category Electrolyte Supplement, Parenteral
Use Treatment of hypochloremic states or metabolic alkalosis
Local Anesthetic/Vasoconstrictor Precautions No information available to require special precautions
Effects on Dental Treatment No significant effects or complications reported
Common Adverse Effects Frequency not defined.
Central nervous system: Headache, coma, drowsiness, EEG abnormalities, mental confusion, seizure
Dermatologic: Rash
Endocrine & metabolic: Calcium-deficient tetany, hyperchloremia, hypokalemia, metabolic acidosis, potassium and sodium may be decreased
Gastrointestinal: Abdominal pain, gastric irritation, nausea, vomiting
Hepatic: Ammonia may be increased
Local: Pain at site of injection
Neuromuscular & skeletal: Twitching
Respiratory: Hyperventilation
Mechanism of Action Increases acidity by increasing free hydrogen ion concentration
Pharmacodynamics/Kinetics
Metabolism: Hepatic; forms urea and hydrochloric acid
Excretion: Urine
Pregnancy Risk Factor C

Ammonium Lactate see Lactic Acid and Ammonium Hydroxide on page 941
Amnesteem™ see Isotretinoin on page 918

Amobarbital (am oh BAR bi tal)

U.S. Brand Names Amytal®
Canadian Brand Names Amytal®
Generic Available No
Index Terms Amobarbital Sodium; Amylobarbitone
Pharmacologic Category Barbiturate
Use Hypnotic in short-term treatment of insomnia; reduce anxiety and provide sedation preoperatively
Unlabeled/Investigational Use Therapeutic or diagnostic "Amytal® Interviewing"; Wada test
Local Anesthetic/Vasoconstrictor Precautions No information available to require special precautions
Effects on Dental Treatment No significant effects or complications reported
Mechanism of Action Interferes with transmission of impulses from the thalamus to the cortex of the brain resulting in an imbalance in central inhibitory and facilitatory mechanisms
Pregnancy Risk Factor D

Amobarbital and Secobarbital
(am oh BAR bi tal & see koe BAR bi tal)

Related Information
Amobarbital *on page 105*
Secobarbital *on page 1459*
U.S. Brand Names Tuinal® [DSC]
Generic Available No
Index Terms Amobarbital Sodium and Secobarbital Sodium; Secobarbital and Amobarbital
Pharmacologic Category Barbiturate
Use Short-term treatment of insomnia
Local Anesthetic/Vasoconstrictor Precautions No information available to require special precautions
Effects on Dental Treatment No significant effects or complications reported
Pregnancy Risk Factor D

Amobarbital Sodium *see* Amobarbital *on page 105*

Amobarbital Sodium and Secobarbital Sodium *see* Amobarbital and Secobarbital *on page 106*

Amoclan *see* Amoxicillin and Clavulanate Potassium *on page 110*

Amonafide (a MON a fide)

Generic Available No
Index Terms Amonafide Hydrochloride; Benzisoquinolinedione; BIDA; M-FA-142; Nafidimide; NSC-308847
Pharmacologic Category Antineoplastic Agent, DNA Binding Agent; Enzyme Inhibitor, Topoisomerase II Inhibitor
Unlabeled/Investigational Use Investigational: Breast, prostate, renal cell, ovarian, pancreatic, and nonsmall cell lung cancers
Local Anesthetic/Vasoconstrictor Precautions No information available to require special precautions
Effects on Dental Treatment No significant effects or complications reported
Common Adverse Effects
>10%:
Gastrointestinal: Nausea and vomiting (mild)
Hematologic: Granulocytopenia, possibly dose-limiting; nadir occurs at days 12-15, recovery by day 21
1% to 10%:
Cardiovascular: Chest pain
Central nervous system: Dizziness, fatigue, headache
Dermatologic: Skin rash, exfoliative dermatitis, alopecia
Local: Inflammatory reactions
Otic: Tinnitus
Neuromuscular & skeletal: Myoclonic jerking, weakness
Mechanism of Action Amonafide acts as a DNA intercalator, stabilizing DNA to thermal denaturation and producing single-strand DNA breaks.
Pharmacodynamics/Kinetics
Distribution: V_d: 370-530 L/m^2
Protein binding: High
Half-life:
Elimination: 3.5-11 hours
Terminal: 3-6 hours
Metabolism: Hepatic, primarily by oxidation and N-acetylation. N-acetylamonafide (active) and amonafide-N′-oxide are the major metabolites. Clearance depends on whether the patient is a fast or slow acetylator. Fast acetylators may experience greater toxicity from the drug.
Excretion: Urine (3% to 22% as unchanged drug)

Amonafide Hydrochloride *see* Amonafide *on page 106*

Amoxapine (a MOKS a peen)

Generic Available Yes
Index Terms Asendin [DSC]
Pharmacologic Category Antidepressant, Tricyclic (Secondary Amine)
Use Treatment of depression, psychotic depression, depression accompanied by anxiety or agitation
Local Anesthetic/Vasoconstrictor Precautions Use with caution; epinephrine and levonordefrin have been shown to have an increased pressor response

in combination with TCAs. Amoxapine is one of the drugs confirmed to prolong the QT interval and is accepted as having a risk of causing torsade de pointes. The risk of drug-induced torsade de pointes is extremely low when a single QT interval prolonging drug is prescribed. In terms of epinephrine, it is not known what effect vasoconstrictors in the local anesthetic regimen will have in patients with a known history of congenital prolonged QT interval or in patients taking any medication that prolongs the QT interval. Until more information is obtained, it is suggested that the clinician consult with the physician prior to the use of a vasoconstrictor in suspected patients, and that the vasoconstrictor (epinephrine, levonordefrin [Neo-Cobefrin®]) be used with caution.

Effects on Dental Treatment Key adverse event(s) related to dental treatment: Xerostomia and changes in salivation (normal salivary flow resumes upon discontinuation). Long-term treatment with TCAs, such as amoxapine, increases the risk of caries by reducing salivation and salivary buffer capacity.

Common Adverse Effects

>10%:
   Central nervous system: Drowsiness
   Gastrointestinal: Xerostomia, constipation

1% to 10%:
   Central nervous system: Dizziness, headache, confusion, nervousness, restlessness, insomnia, ataxia, excitement, anxiety
   Dermatologic: Edema, skin rash
   Endocrine: Prolactin levels increased
   Gastrointestinal: Nausea
   Neuromuscular & skeletal: Tremor, weakness
   Ocular: Blurred vision
   Miscellaneous: Diaphoresis

Restrictions An FDA-approved medication guide concerning the use of antidepressants in children, adolescents, and young adults must be distributed when dispensing an outpatient prescription (new or refill) where this medication is to be used without direct supervision of a healthcare provider. Medication guides are available at http://www.fda.gov/cder/Offices/ODS/medication_guides.htm. Dispense to parents or guardians of children and adolescents receiving this medication.

Mechanism of Action Reduces the reuptake of serotonin and norepinephrine. The metabolite, 7-OH-amoxapine has significant dopamine receptor blocking activity similar to haloperidol.

Drug Interactions

Cytochrome P450 Effect: Substrate of CYP2D6 (major)

Increased Effect/Toxicity: Amoxapine increases the effects of amphetamines, anticholinergics, other CNS depressants (sedatives, hypnotics, or ethanol), chlorpropamide, tolazamide, and warfarin. When used with MAO inhibitors, hyperpyrexia, hypertension, tachycardia, confusion, seizures, and **deaths have been reported** (serotonin syndrome). Serotonin syndrome has also been reported with ritonavir (rare). CYP2D6 inhibitors may increase the levels/effects of amoxapine; example inhibitors include chlorpromazine, delavirdine, fluoxetine, miconazole, paroxetine, pergolide, quinidine, quinine, ritonavir, and ropinirole. Use of lithium with a TCA may increase the risk for neurotoxicity. Phenothiazines may increase concentration of some TCAs and TCAs may increase the concentration of phenothiazines. Pressor response to I.V. epinephrine, norepinephrine, and phenylephrine may be enhanced in patients receiving TCAs (**Note:** Effect is unlikely with epinephrine or levonordefrin dosages typically administered as infiltration in combination with local anesthetics). Combined use of beta-agonists or drugs which prolong QT_c (including quinidine, procainamide, disopyramide, cisapride, sparfloxacin, gatifloxacin, moxifloxacin) with TCAs may predispose patients to cardiac arrhythmias.

Decreased Effect: Amoxapine inhibits the antihypertensive effects of bethanidine, clonidine, debrisoquin, guanadrel, guanethidine, guanabenz, or guanfacine. Cholestyramine and colestipol may bind TCAs and reduce their absorption.

Pharmacodynamics/Kinetics

Onset of antidepressant effect: Usually occurs after 1-2 weeks, but may require 4-6 weeks
Absorption: Rapid and well absorbed
Distribution: V_d: 0.9-1.2 L/kg; enters breast milk
Protein binding: 80%
Metabolism: Primarily hepatic
Half-life elimination: Parent drug: 11-16 hours; Active metabolite (8-hydroxy): Adults: 30 hours
Time to peak, serum: 1-2 hours
Excretion: Urine (as unchanged drug and metabolites)

Pregnancy Risk Factor C

Amoxicillin (a moks i SIL in)

Related Information
Antibiotic Prophylaxis *on page 1772*
Bacterial Infections *on page 1793*
Gastrointestinal Disorders *on page 1745*
Periodontal Diseases *on page 1801*
Sexually-Transmitted Diseases *on page 1766*

Related Sample Prescriptions
Bacterial Infections and Periodontal Diseases *on page 1837*
Infective Endocarditis (Prevention) *on page 1832*
Prosthetic Joint Late Infections (Prevention) *on page 1833*

U.S. Brand Names Amoxil®

Canadian Brand Names Apo-Amoxi®; Gen-Amoxicillin; Lin-Amox; Novamoxin®; Nu-Amoxi; PHL-Amoxicillin; PMS-Amoxicillin

Mexican Brand Names Acimox; Amoxil; Amoxisol; Amoxivet; Gimalxina; Hidramox; Penamox

Generic Available Yes: Excludes drops

Index Terms Amoxicillin Trihydrate; Amoxycillin; *p*-Hydroxyampicillin

Pharmacologic Category Antibiotic, Penicillin

Dental Use Antibiotic for standard prophylactic regimen for dental patients who are at risk for infective endocarditis; prophylaxis in total joint replacement patients undergoing dental procedures which produce bacteremia; antibiotic used to treat orofacial infections

Use Treatment of otitis media, sinusitis, and infections caused by susceptible organisms involving the respiratory tract, skin, and urinary tract; prophylaxis of bacterial endocarditis in patients undergoing surgical or dental procedures; as part of a multidrug regimen for *H. pylori* eradication

Unlabeled/Investigational Use Postexposure prophylaxis for anthrax exposure with documented susceptible organisms

Local Anesthetic/Vasoconstrictor Precautions No information available to require special precautions

Effects on Dental Treatment Prolonged use of penicillins may lead to development of oral candidiasis

Significant Adverse Effects Frequency not defined.
Central nervous system: Hyperactivity, agitation, anxiety, insomnia, confusion, convulsions, behavioral changes, dizziness
Dermatologic: Acute exanthematous pustulosis, erythematous maculopapular rash, erythema multiforme, Stevens-Johnson syndrome, exfoliative dermatitis, toxic epidermal necrolysis, hypersensitivity vasculitis, urticaria
Gastrointestinal: Nausea, vomiting, diarrhea, hemorrhagic colitis, pseudomembranous colitis, tooth discoloration (brown, yellow, or gray; rare)
Hematologic: Anemia, hemolytic anemia, thrombocytopenia, thrombocytopenia purpura, eosinophilia, leukopenia, agranulocytosis
Hepatic: AST and ALT increased, cholestatic jaundice, hepatic cholestasis, acute cytolytic hepatitis
Renal: Crystalluria

Dental Usual Dosing Oral:
Children >3 months and <40 kg: Infective endocarditis prophylaxis: 50 mg/kg 30-60 minutes before procedure
Adults:
Infective endocarditis prophylaxis: 2 g 30-60 minutes before procedure
Orofacial infection: 250-500 mg every 8 hours or 500-875 mg twice daily
Prophylaxis in total joint replacement patients undergoing dental procedures which produce bacteremia: 2 g 1 hour prior to procedure

Dosage
Usual dosage range:
Children ≤3 months: Oral: 20-30 mg/kg/day divided every 12 hours
Children >3 months and <40 kg: Oral: 20-50 mg/kg/day in divided doses every 8-12 hours
Adults: Oral: 250-500 mg every 8 hours or 500-875 mg twice daily
Indication-specific dosing:
Children >3 months and <40 kg: Oral:
Acute otitis media: 80-90 mg/kg/day divided every 12 hours
Anthrax exposure (CDC guidelines): Note: Postexposure prophylaxis only with documented susceptible organisms: 80 mg/kg/day in divided doses every 8 hours (maximum: 500 mg/dose)
Community-acquired pneumonia:
4 months to <5 years: 80-100 mg/kg/day divided every 8 hours
5-15 years: 100 mg/kg/day divided every 8 hours; **Note:** Treatment with a macrolide or doxycycline (if age >8 years) is preferred due to higher prevalence of atypical pathogens in this age group

Ear, nose, throat, genitourinary tract, or skin/skin structure infections:
> *Mild to moderate:* 25 mg/kg/day in divided doses every 12 hours **or** 20 mg/kg/day in divided doses every 8 hours
>
> *Severe:* 45 mg/kg/day in divided doses every 12 hours **or** 40 mg/kg/day in divided doses every 8 hours

Endocarditis (subacute bacterial) prophylaxis: 50 mg/kg 1 hour before procedure

Lower respiratory tract infections: 45 mg/kg/day in divided doses every 12 hours **or** 40 mg/kg/day in divided doses every 8 hours

Lyme disease: 25-50 mg/kg/day divided every 8 hours (maximum: 500 mg)

Adults: Oral:

Anthrax exposure (CDC guidelines): Note: Postexposure prophylaxis in pregnant or nursing women only with documented susceptible organisms: 500 mg every 8 hours

Ear, nose, throat, genitourinary tract, or skin/skin structure infections:
> *Mild to moderate:* 500 mg every 12 hours **or** 250 mg every 8 hours
>
> *Severe:* 875 mg every 12 hours **or** 500 mg every 8 hours

Endocarditis prophylaxis: 2 g 1 hour before procedure

Helicobacter pylori **eradication:** 1000 mg twice daily; requires combination therapy with at least one other antibiotic and an acid-suppressing agent (proton pump inhibitor or H_2 blocker)

Lower respiratory tract infections: 875 mg every 12 hours **or** 500 mg every 8 hours

Lyme disease: 500 mg every 6-8 hours (depending on size of patient) for 21-30 days

Dosing interval in renal impairment: The 875 mg tablet should not be used in patients with Cl_{cr} <30 mL/minute.

Cl_{cr} 10-30 mL/minute: 250-500 mg every 12 hours

Cl_{cr} <10 mL/minute: 250-500 mg every 24 hours

Dialysis: Moderately dialyzable (20% to 50%) by hemo- or peritoneal dialysis; approximately 50 mg of amoxicillin per liter of filtrate is removed by continuous arteriovenous or venovenous hemofiltration; dose as per Cl_{cr} <10 mL/minute guidelines

Mechanism of Action Inhibits bacterial cell wall synthesis by binding to one or more of the penicillin-binding proteins (PBPs) which in turn inhibits the final transpeptidation step of peptidoglycan synthesis in bacterial cell walls, thus inhibiting cell wall biosynthesis. Bacteria eventually lyse due to ongoing activity of cell wall autolytic enzymes (autolysins and murein hydrolases) while cell wall assembly is arrested.

Contraindications Hypersensitivity to amoxicillin, penicillin, or any component of the formulation

Warnings/Precautions In patients with renal impairment, doses and/or frequency of administration should be modified in response to the degree of renal impairment. A high percentage of patients with infectious mononucleosis have developed skin rash during therapy with amoxicillin. Serious and occasionally severe or fatal hypersensitivity (anaphylactoid) reactions have been reported in patients on penicillin therapy, especially with a history of beta-lactam hypersensitivity, history of sensitivity to multiple allergens, or previous IgE-mediated reactions (eg, anaphylaxis, angioedema, urticaria). Use with caution in asthmatic patients. Prolonged use may result in fungal or bacterial superinfection, including *C. difficile*-associated diarrhea and pseudomembranous colitis. Chewable tablets contain phenylalanine.

Drug Interactions

Allopurinol: Theoretically has an additive potential for amoxicillin rash.

Aminoglycosides: May be synergistic against selected organisms.

Methotrexate: Penicillins may increase the exposure to methotrexate during concurrent therapy; monitor.

Oral contraceptives: Anecdotal reports suggesting decreased contraceptive efficacy with penicillins have been refuted by more rigorous scientific and clinical data.

Probenecid, disulfiram: May increase levels of penicillins (amoxicillin).

Warfarin: Effects of warfarin may be increased.

Dietary Considerations May be taken with food. Amoxil® chewable contains phenylalanine 1.82 mg per 200 mg tablet, phenylalanine 3.64 mg per 400 mg tablet.

Pharmacodynamics/Kinetics

Absorption: Oral: Rapid and nearly complete; food does not interfere

Distribution: Widely to most body fluids and bone; poor penetration into cells, eyes, and across normal meninges

> Pleural fluids, lungs, and peritoneal fluid; high urine concentrations are attained; also into synovial fluid, liver, prostate, muscle, and gallbladder; penetrates into middle ear effusions, maxillary sinus secretions, tonsils,

(Continued)

Amoxicillin *(Continued)*

sputum, and bronchial secretions; crosses placenta; low concentrations enter breast milk

CSF:blood level ratio: Normal meninges: <1%; Inflamed meninges: 8% to 90%

Protein binding: 17% to 20%

Metabolism: Partially hepatic

Half-life elimination:

Neonates, full-term: 3.7 hours

Infants and Children: 1-2 hours

Adults: Normal renal function: 0.7-1.4 hours

Cl_{cr} <10 mL/minute: 7-21 hours

Time to peak: Capsule: 2 hours; Suspension: 1 hour

Excretion: Urine (80% as unchanged drug); lower in neonates

Pregnancy Risk Factor B

Lactation Enters breast milk/compatible

Dosage Forms Excipient information presented when available (limited, particularly for generics); consult specific product labeling.

Capsule: 250 mg, 500 mg

Amoxil®: 500 mg

Powder for oral suspension: 125 mg/5 mL (80 mL, 100 mL, 150 mL); 200 mg/5 mL (50 mL, 75 mL, 100 mL); 250 mg/5 mL (80 mL, 100 mL, 150 mL); 400 mg/5 mL (50 mL, 75 mL, 100 mL)

Amoxil®: 200 mg/5 mL (50 mL, 75 mL, 100 mL) [contains sodium benzoate; bubble gum flavor]; 250 mg/5 mL (100 mL, 150 mL) [contains sodium benzoate; bubble gum flavor]; 400 mg/5 mL (5 mL, 50 mL, 75 mL, 100 mL) [contains sodium benzoate; bubble gum flavor]

Powder for oral suspension [drops]:

Amoxil®: 50 mg/mL (30 mL) [contains sodium benzoate; bubble gum flavor]

Tablet: 500 mg, 875 mg

Amoxil®: 500 mg, 875 mg

Tablet, chewable: 125 mg, 200 mg, 250 mg, 400 mg

Amoxil®: 200 mg [contains phenylalanine 1.82 mg/tablet; cherry banana peppermint flavor]; 400 mg [contains phenylalanine 3.64 mg/tablet; cherry banana peppermint flavor]

Selected Readings

ADA Division of Legal Affairs, "A Legal Perspective on Antibiotic Prophylaxis," *J Am Dent Assoc*, 2003, 134(9):1260.

American Dental Association; American Academy of Orthopedic Surgeons, "Antibiotic Prophylaxis for Dental Patients With Total Joint Replacements," *J Am Dent Assoc*, 2003, 134(7):895-9.

American Dental Association Council on Scientific Affairs, "Combating Antibiotic Resistance," *J Am Dent Assoc*, 2004, 135(4):484-7.

Dajani AS, Taubert KA, Wilson W, et al, "Prevention of Bacterial Endocarditis. Recommendations by the American Heart Association," *JAMA*, 1997, 277(22):1794-801.

Dajani AS, Taubert KA, Wilson W, et al, "Prevention of Bacterial Endocarditis: Recommendations by the American Heart Association," *J Am Dent Assoc*, 1997, 128(8):1142-51.

Wynn RL, Bergman SA, Meiller TF, et al, "Antibiotics in Treating Oral-Facial Infections of Odontogenic Origin: An Update", *Gen Dent*, 2001, 49(3):238-40, 242, 244 passim.

Amoxicillin and Clavulanate Potassium

(a moks i SIL in & klav yoo LAN ate poe TASS ee um)

Related Information

Amoxicillin *on page 108*

Bacterial Infections *on page 1793*

Related Sample Prescriptions

Bacterial Infections and Periodontal Diseases *on page 1837*

U.S. Brand Names Amoclan; Augmentin®; Augmentin ES-600®; Augmentin XR®

Canadian Brand Names Alti-Amoxi-Clav; Apo-Amoxi-Clav®; Augmentin®; Clavulin®; Novo-Clavamoxin; ratio-Aclavulanate

Mexican Brand Names Amoxiclav; Amoxiclav-BID; Clamoxin

Generic Available Yes: Excludes extended release

Index Terms Amoxicillin and Clavulanic Acid; Clavulanic Acid and Amoxicillin

Pharmacologic Category Antibiotic, Penicillin

Dental Use Treatment of orofacial infections when beta-lactamase-producing staphylococci and beta-lactamase-producing *Bacteroides* are present

Use Treatment of otitis media, sinusitis, and infections caused by susceptible organisms involving the lower respiratory tract, skin and skin structure, and urinary tract; spectrum same as amoxicillin with additional coverage of beta-lactamase producing *B. catarrhalis*, *H. influenzae*, *N. gonorrhoeae*, and *S. aureus* (not MRSA). The expanded coverage of this combination makes it a useful alternative when amoxicillin resistance is present and patients cannot tolerate alternative treatments.

Local Anesthetic/Vasoconstrictor Precautions No information available to require special precautions

Effects on Dental Treatment Prolonged use of penicillins may lead to development of oral candidiasis (see Dental Comment)

Significant Adverse Effects

>10%: Gastrointestinal: Diarrhea (3% to 34%; incidence varies upon dose and regimen used)

1% to 10%:

Dermatologic: Diaper rash, skin rash, urticaria

Gastrointestinal: Abdominal discomfort, loose stools, nausea, vomiting

Genitourinary: Vaginitis, vaginal mycosis

Miscellaneous: Moniliasis

<1% (Limited to important or life-threatening): Cholestatic jaundice, flatulence, headache, hepatic dysfunction, prothrombin time increased, thrombocytosis

Additional adverse reactions seen with **ampicillin-class antibiotics:** Agitation, agranulocytosis, alkaline phosphatase increased, anaphylaxis, anemia, angioedema, anxiety, behavioral changes, bilirubin increased, black "hairy" tongue, confusion, convulsions, crystalluria, dizziness, enterocolitis, eosinophilia, erythema multiforme, exanthematous pustulosis, exfoliative dermatitis, gastritis, glossitis, hematuria, hemolytic anemia, hemorrhagic colitis, indigestion, insomnia, hyperactivity, interstitial nephritis, leukopenia, mucocutaneous candidiasis, pruritus, pseudomembranous colitis, serum sickness-like reaction, Stevens-Johnson syndrome, stomatitis, transaminases increased, thrombocytopenia, thrombocytopenic purpura, tooth discoloration, toxic epidermal necrolysis

Dental Usual Dosing Orofacial infections: Children >40 kg and Adults: Oral: 250-500 mg every 8 hours or 875 mg every 12 hours

Dosage Note: Dose is based on the amoxicillin component; see "Augmentin® Product-Specific Considerations" table on next page.

Usual dosage range:

Infants <3 months: Oral: 30 mg/kg/day divided every 12 hours using the 125 mg/5 mL suspension

Children ≥3 months and <40 kg: Oral: 20-90 mg/kg/day divided every 8-12 hours

Children >40 kg and Adults: Oral: 250-500 mg every 8 hours or 875 mg every 12 hours

Indication-specific dosing:

Children ≥3 months and <40 kg: Oral:

Lower respiratory tract infections, severe infections, sinusitis: 45 mg/kg/day divided every 12 hours **or** 40 mg/kg/day divided every 8 hours

Mild-to-moderate infections: 25 mg/kg/day divided every 12 hours or 20 mg/kg/day divided every 8 hours

Otitis media (Augmentin® ES-600): 90 mg/kg/day divided every 12 hours for 10 days in children with severe illness and when coverage for β-lactamase-positive *H. influenzae* and *M. catarrhalis* is needed.

Children ≥16 years and Adults: Oral:

Acute bacterial sinusitis: Extended release tablet: Two 1000 mg tablets every 12 hours for 10 days

Bite wounds (animal/human): 875 mg every 12 hours **or** 500 mg every 8 hours

Chronic obstructive pulmonary disease: 875 mg every 12 hours **or** 500 mg every 8 hours

Diabetic foot: Extended release tablet: Two 1000 mg tablets every 12 hours for 7-14 days

Diverticulitis, perirectal abscess: Extended release tablet: Two 1000 mg tablets every 12 hours for 7-10 days

Erysipelas: 875 mg every 12 hours **or** 500 mg every 8 hours

Febrile neutropenia: 875 mg every 12 hours

Pneumonia:

Aspiration: 875 mg every 12 hours

Community-acquired: Extended release tablet: Two 1000 mg tablets every 12 hours for 7-10 days

Pyelonephritis (acute, uncomplicated): 875 mg every 12 hours **or** 500 mg every 8 hours

Skin abscess: 875 mg every 12 hours

Dosing interval in renal impairment:

Cl_{cr} <30 mL/minute: Do not use 875 mg tablet or extended release tablets

Cl_{cr} 10-30 mL/minute: 250-500 mg every 12 hours

Cl_{cr} <10 mL/minute: 250-500 every 24 hours

Hemodialysis: Moderately dialyzable (20% to 50%)

250-500 mg every 24 hours; administer dose during and after dialysis. Do not use extended release tablets.

Peritoneal dialysis: Moderately dialyzable (20% to 50%)

(Continued)

Amoxicillin and Clavulanate Potassium *(Continued)*

Amoxicillin: Administer 250 mg every 12 hours

Clavulanic acid: Dose for Cl_{cr} <10 mL/minute

Continuous arteriovenous or venovenous hemofiltration effects:

Amoxicillin: ~50 mg of amoxicillin/L of filtrate is removed

Clavulanic acid: Dose for Cl_{cr} <10 mL/minute

Augmentin® Product-Specific Considerations

Strength	Form	Consideration
125 mg	CT, S	q8h dosing
	S	For adults having difficulty swallowing tablets, 125 mg/5 mL suspension may be substituted for 500 mg tablet.
200 mg	CT, S	q12h dosing
	CT	Contains phenylalanine
	S	For adults having difficulty swallowing tablets, 200 mg/5 mL suspension may be substituted for 875 mg tablet.
250 mg	CT, S, T	q8h dosing
	CT	Contains phenylalanine
	T	Not for use in patients <40 kg
	CT, T	Tablet and chewable tablet are not interchangeable due to differences in clavulanic acid.
	S	For adults having difficulty swallowing tablets, 250 mg/5 mL suspension may be substituted for 500 mg tablet.
400 mg	CT, S	q12h dosing
	CT	Contains phenylalanine
	S	For adults having difficulty swallowing tablets, 400 mg/5 mL suspension may be substituted for 875 mg tablet.
500 mg	T	q8h or q12h dosing
600 mg	S	q12h dosing
		Contains phenylalanine
		Not for use in adults or children ≥40 kg
		600 mg/5 mL suspension is not equivalent to or interchangeable with 200 mg/5 mL or 400 mg/5 mL due to differences in clavulanic acid.
875 mg	T	q12h dosing; not for use in Cl_{cr} <30 mL/minute
1000 mg	XR	q12h dosing
		Not for use in children <16 years of age
		Not interchangeable with two 500 mg tablets
		Not for use if Cl_{cr} <30 mL/minute or hemodialysis

Legend: CT = chewable tablet, S = suspension, T = tablet, XR = extended release.

Mechanism of Action Clavulanic acid binds and inhibits beta-lactamases that inactivate amoxicillin resulting in amoxicillin having an expanded spectrum of activity. Amoxicillin inhibits bacterial cell wall synthesis by binding to one or more of the penicillin-binding proteins (PBPs) which in turn inhibits the final transpeptidation step of peptidoglycan synthesis in bacterial cell walls, thus inhibiting cell wall biosynthesis. Bacteria eventually lyse due to ongoing activity of cell wall autolytic enzymes (autolysins and murein hydrolases) while cell wall assembly is arrested.

Contraindications Hypersensitivity to amoxicillin, clavulanic acid, penicillin, or any component of the formulation; history of cholestatic jaundice or hepatic dysfunction with amoxicillin/clavulanate potassium therapy; Augmentin XR™: severe renal impairment (Cl_{cr} <30 mL/minute) and hemodialysis patients

Warnings/Precautions Hypersensitivity reactions, including anaphylaxis (some fatal), have been reported. Prolonged use may result in fungal or bacterial superinfection, including *C. difficile*-associated diarrhea and pseudomembranous colitis. In patients with renal impairment, doses and/or frequency of administration should be modified in response to the degree of renal impairment. High percentage of patients with infectious mononucleosis have developed rash during therapy. Incidence of diarrhea is higher than with amoxicillin alone. Use caution in patients with hepatic dysfunction. Hepatic dysfunction, although rare, is more common in elderly and/or males, and occurs more frequently with prolonged treatment, and may occur after therapy is complete. Due to differing content of clavulanic acid, not all formulations are interchangeable. Low incidence of cross-allergy with cephalosporins exists. Some products contain phenylalanine.

Drug Interactions

Allopurinol: Additive potential for amoxicillin rash.

Aminoglycosides: May be synergistic against selected organisms.

Methotrexate: Penicillins may increase the exposure to methotrexate during concurrent therapy; monitor.

Oral contraceptives: Anecdotal reports suggesting decreased contraceptive efficacy with penicillins have been refuted by more rigorous scientific and clinical data.

Probenecid: May increase levels of penicillins (amoxicillin); concomitant use not recommended.

Warfarin: Effects of warfarin may be increased.

Dietary Considerations May be taken with meals or on an empty stomach; take with meals to increase absorption and decrease GI intolerance; may mix with milk, formula, or juice. Extended release tablets should be taken with food. Some products contain phenylalanine. If you have phenylketonuria or PKU, avoid use. All dosage forms contain potassium.

Pharmacodynamics/Kinetics Amoxicillin pharmacokinetics are not affected by clavulanic acid.

Amoxicillin: See Amoxicillin.

Clavulanic acid:

Metabolism: Hepatic

Excretion: Urine (30% to 40% as unchanged drug)

Pregnancy Risk Factor B

Lactation Enters breast milk/use caution (AAP rates "compatible")

Breast-Feeding Considerations The AAP considers amoxicillin to be "compatible" with breast-feeding.

Dosage Forms Excipient information presented when available (limited, particularly for generics); consult specific product labeling.

Powder for oral suspension: 200: Amoxicillin 200 mg and clavulanate potassium 28.5 mg per 5 mL (50 mL, 75 mL, 100 mL) [contains phenylalanine]; 400: Amoxicillin 400 mg and clavulanate potassium 57 mg per 5 mL (50 mL, 75 mL, 100 mL) [contains phenylalanine]; 600: Amoxicillin 600 mg and clavulanic potassium 42.9 mg per 5 mL (75 mL, 125 mL, 200 mL) [contains phenylalanine]

Amoclan:

200: Amoxicillin 200 mg and clavulanate potassium 28.5 mg per 5 mL (50 mL, 75 mL, 100 mL) [contains phenylalanine 7 mg/5 mL and potassium 0.14 mEq/5 mL; fruit flavor]

400: Amoxicillin 400 mg and clavulanate potassium 57 mg per 5 mL (50 mL, 75 mL, 100 mL) [contains phenylalanine 7 mg/5 mL and potassium 0.29 mEq/5 mL; fruit flavor]

Augmentin®:

125: Amoxicillin 125 mg and clavulanate potassium 31.25 mg per 5 mL (75 mL, 100 mL, 150 mL) [contains potassium 0.16 mEq/5 mL; banana flavor]

200: Amoxicillin 200 mg and clavulanate potassium 28.5 mg per 5 mL (50 mL, 75 mL, 100 mL) [contains phenylalanine 7 mg/5 mL and potassium 0.14 mEq/5 mL; orange flavor]

250: Amoxicillin 250 mg and clavulanate potassium 62.5 mg per 5 mL (75 mL, 100 mL, 150 mL) [contains potassium 0.32 mEq/5 mL; orange flavor]

400: Amoxicillin 400 mg and clavulanate potassium 57 mg per 5 mL (50 mL, 75 mL, 100 mL) [contains phenylalanine 7 mg/5 mL and potassium 0.29 mEq/5 mL; orange flavor]

Augmentin ES-600®: Amoxicillin 600 mg and clavulanic potassium 42.9 mg per 5 mL (75 mL, 125 mL, 200 mL) [contains phenylalanine 7 mg/5 mL and potassium 0.23 mEq/5 mL; strawberry cream flavor]

Tablet: 250: Amoxicillin 250 mg and clavulanate potassium 125 mg; 500: Amoxicillin 500 mg and clavulanate potassium 125 mg; 875: Amoxicillin 875 mg and clavulanate potassium 125 mg

Augmentin®:

250: Amoxicillin 250 mg and clavulanate potassium 125 mg [contains potassium 0.63 mEq/tablet]

500: Amoxicillin 500 mg and clavulanate potassium 125 mg [contains potassium 0.63 mEq/tablet]

875: Amoxicillin 875 mg and clavulanate potassium 125 mg [contains potassium 0.63 mEq/tablet]

Tablet, chewable: 200: Amoxicillin 200 mg and clavulanate potassium 28.5 mg [contains phenylalanine]; 400: Amoxicillin 400 mg and clavulanate potassium 57 mg [contains phenylalanine]

Augmentin®:

125: Amoxicillin 125 mg and clavulanate potassium 31.25 mg [contains potassium 0.16 mEq/tablet; lemon-lime flavor]

200: Amoxicillin 200 mg and clavulanate potassium 28.5 mg [contains phenylalanine 2.1 mg/tablet and potassium 0.14 mEq/tablet; cherry-banana flavor]

250: Amoxicillin 250 mg and clavulanate potassium 62.5 mg [contains potassium 0.32 mEq/tablet; lemon-lime flavor]

(Continued)

Amoxicillin and Clavulanate Potassium *(Continued)*

400: Amoxicillin 400 mg and clavulanate potassium 57 mg [contains phenyl-alanine 4.2 mg/tablet and potassium 0.29 mEq/tablet; cherry-banana flavor]

Tablet, extended release:

Augmentin XR®: Amoxicillin 1000 mg and clavulanic acid 62.5 mg [contains potassium 29.3 mg (1.27 mEq) and sodium 12.6 mg (0.32 mEq) per tablet; packaged in either a 7-day or 10-day package]

Dental Comment In maxillary sinus, anterior nasal cavity, and deep neck infections, beta-lactamase-producing staphylococci and beta-lactamase-producing *Bacteroides* usually are present. In these situations, antibiotics that resist the beta-lactamase enzyme are indicated. Amoxicillin and clavulanic acid is administered orally for moderate infections. Ampicillin sodium and sulbactam sodium (Unasyn®) is administered parenterally for more severe infections.

Selected Readings

American Dental Association Council on Scientific Affairs, "Combating Antibiotic Resistance," *J Am Dent Assoc*, 2004, 135(4):484-7.

Wynn RL, Bergman SA, Meiller TF, et al, "Antibiotics in Treating Oral-Facial Infections of Odontogenic Origin: An Update," *Gen Dent*, 2001, 49(3):238-40, 242, 244 passim.

Amoxicillin and Clavulanic Acid *see* Amoxicillin and Clavulanate Potassium *on page 110*

Amoxicillin, Lansoprazole, and Clarithromycin *see* Lansoprazole, Amoxicillin, and Clarithromycin *on page 948*

Amoxicillin Trihydrate *see* Amoxicillin *on page 108*

Amoxil® *see* Amoxicillin *on page 108*

Amoxycillin *see* Amoxicillin *on page 108*

Amphadase™ *see* Hyaluronidase *on page 817*

Amphetamine and Dextroamphetamine *see* Dextroamphetamine and Amphetamine *on page 474*

Amphocin® [DSC] *see* Amphotericin B (Conventional) *on page 115*

Amphotec® *see* Amphotericin B Cholesteryl Sulfate Complex *on page 114*

Amphotericin B Cholesteryl Sulfate Complex

(am foe TER i sin bee kole LES te ril SUL fate KOM plecks)

U.S. Brand Names Amphotec®

Canadian Brand Names Amphotec®

Mexican Brand Names Amphocil

Generic Available No

Index Terms ABCD; Amphotericin B Colloidal Dispersion

Pharmacologic Category Antifungal Agent, Parenteral

Use Treatment of invasive aspergillosis in patients who have failed amphotericin B deoxycholate treatment, or who have renal impairment or experience unacceptable toxicity which precludes treatment with amphotericin B deoxycholate in effective doses.

Unlabeled/Investigational Use Effective in patients with serious *Candida* species infections

Local Anesthetic/Vasoconstrictor Precautions No information available to require special precautions

Effects on Dental Treatment No significant effects or complications reported

Common Adverse Effects

>10%: Central nervous system: Chills, fever

1% to 10%:

Cardiovascular: Hypotension, tachycardia

Central nervous system: Headache

Dermatologic: Rash

Endocrine & metabolic: Hypokalemia, hypomagnesemia

Gastrointestinal: Nausea, diarrhea, abdominal pain

Hematologic: Thrombocytopenia

Hepatic: LFT change

Neuromuscular & skeletal: Rigors

Renal: Creatinine increased

Respiratory: Dyspnea

Note: Amphotericin B colloidal dispersion has an improved therapeutic index compared to conventional amphotericin B, and has been used safely in patients with amphotericin B-related nephrotoxicity; however, continued decline of renal function has occurred in some patients.

Mechanism of Action Binds to ergosterol altering cell membrane permeability in susceptible fungi and causing leakage of cell components with subsequent cell death. Proposed mechanism suggests that amphotericin causes an oxidation-dependent stimulation of macrophages (Lyman, 1992).

Drug Interactions
Increased Effect/Toxicity: Toxic effect with other nephrotoxic drugs (eg, cyclosporine and aminoglycosides) may be additive. Corticosteroids may increase potassium depletion caused by amphotericin. Amphotericin B may predispose patients receiving digitalis glycosides or neuromuscular blocking agents to toxicity secondary to hypokalemia.

Decreased Effect: Pharmacologic antagonism may occur with azole antifungals (eg, ketoconazole, miconazole).

Pharmacodynamics/Kinetics
Distribution: V_d: Total volume increases with higher doses, reflects increasing uptake by tissues (with 4 mg/kg/day = 4 L/kg); predominantly distributed in the liver; concentrations in kidneys and other tissues are lower than observed with conventional amphotericin B

Half-life elimination: 28-29 hours; prolonged with higher doses

Pregnancy Risk Factor B

Amphotericin B Colloidal Dispersion *see* Amphotericin B Cholesteryl Sulfate Complex *on page 114*

Amphotericin B (Conventional)
(am foe TER i sin bee con VEN sha nal)

Related Information
Fungal Infections *on page 1804*

U.S. Brand Names Amphocin® [DSC]

Canadian Brand Names Fungizone®

Generic Available Yes

Index Terms Amphotericin B Desoxycholate

Pharmacologic Category Antifungal Agent, Parenteral

Use Treatment of severe systemic and central nervous system infections caused by susceptible fungi such as *Candida* species, *Histoplasma capsulatum*, *Cryptococcus neoformans*, *Aspergillus* species, *Blastomyces dermatitidis*, *Torulopsis glabrata*, and *Coccidioides immitis*; fungal peritonitis; irrigant for bladder fungal infections; used in fungal infection in patients with bone marrow transplantation, amebic meningoencephalitis, ocular aspergillosis (intraocular injection), candidal cystitis (bladder irrigation), chemoprophylaxis (low-dose I.V.), immunocompromised patients at risk of aspergillosis (intranasal/nebulized), refractory meningitis (intrathecal), coccidioidal arthritis (intra-articular/I.M.).

Low-dose amphotericin B has been administered after bone marrow transplantation to reduce the risk of invasive fungal disease.

Local Anesthetic/Vasoconstrictor Precautions No information available to require special precautions

Effects on Dental Treatment No significant effects or complications reported

Common Adverse Effects
>10%:
Central nervous system: Fever, chills, headache, malaise, generalized pain
Endocrine & metabolic: Hypokalemia, hypomagnesemia
Gastrointestinal: Anorexia
Hematologic: Anemia
Renal: Nephrotoxicity

1% to 10%:
Cardiovascular: Hypotension, hypertension, flushing
Central nervous system: Delirium, arachnoiditis, pain along lumbar nerves
Gastrointestinal: Nausea, vomiting
Genitourinary: Urinary retention
Hematologic: Leukocytosis
Local: Thrombophlebitis
Neuromuscular & skeletal: Paresthesia (especially with I.T. therapy)
Renal: Renal tubular acidosis, renal failure

Dosage
Premedication: For patients who experience infusion-related immediate reactions, premedicate with the following drugs 30-60 minutes prior to drug administration: NSAID (with or without diphenhydramine) **or** acetaminophen with diphenhydramine **or** hydrocortisone 50-100 mg. If the patient experiences rigors during the infusion, meperidine may be administered.

Infants and Children: I.V.:
Test dose: 0.1 mg/kg/dose to a maximum of 1 mg; infuse over 30-60 minutes. Many clinicians believe a test dose is unnecessary.
Maintenance dose: 0.25-1 mg/kg/day given once daily; infuse over 2-6 hours. Once therapy has been established, amphotericin B can be administered on an every-other-day basis at 1-1.5 mg/kg/dose; cumulative dose: 1.5-2 g over 6-10 weeks.

(Continued)

Amphotericin B (Conventional) *(Continued)*

Adults: I.V.:
Test dose: 1 mg infused over 20-30 minutes. Many clinicians believe a test dose is unnecessary.

Maintenance dose: Usual: 0.25-1.5 mg/kg/day; 1-1.5 mg/kg over 4-6 hours every other day may be given once therapy is established; aspergillosis, mucormycosis, rhinocerebral phycomycosis often require 1-1.5 mg/kg/day; do not exceed 1.5 mg/kg/day

Duration of therapy varies with nature of infection: Usual duration is 4-12 weeks or cumulative dose of 1-4 g

Meningitis, coccidioidal or cryptococcal: I.T.:
Children.: 25-100 mcg every 48-72 hours; increase to 500 mcg as tolerated

Adults: Initial: 25-300 mcg every 48-72 hours; increase to 500 mcg to 1 mg as tolerated; maximum total dose: 15 mg has been suggested

Bone marrow transplantation (prophylaxis): Adults: I.V.: Low-dose amphotericin B 0.1-0.25 mg/kg/day has been administered after bone marrow transplantation to reduce the risk of invasive fungal disease.

Bladder irrigation: Candidal cystitis: Irrigate with 50 mcg/mL solution instilled periodically or continuously for 5-10 days or until cultures are clear

Note: Alternative routes of administration and extemporaneous preparations have been used when standard antifungal therapy is not available (eg, inhalation, intraocular injection, subconjunctival application, intracavitary administration into various joints and the pleural space).

Dosing adjustment in renal impairment: If renal dysfunction is due to the drug, the daily total can be decreased by 50% or the dose can be given every other day; I.V. therapy may take several months

Dialysis: Poorly dialyzed; no supplemental dosage necessary when using hemo- or peritoneal dialysis or continuous arteriovenous or venovenous hemodiafiltration effects

Administration in dialysate: Children and Adults: 1-2 mg/L of peritoneal dialysis fluid either with or without low-dose I.V. amphotericin B (a total dose of 2-10 mg/kg given over 7-14 days). Precipitate may form in ionic dialysate solutions.

Mechanism of Action Binds to ergosterol altering cell membrane permeability in susceptible fungi and causing leakage of cell components with subsequent cell death. Proposed mechanism suggests that amphotericin causes an oxidation-dependent stimulation of macrophages (Lyman, 1992).

Contraindications Hypersensitivity to amphotericin or any component of the formulation

Warnings/Precautions Anaphylaxis has been reported with amphotericin B-containing drugs. During the initial dosing, the drug should be administered under close clinical observation. Avoid use with other nephrotoxic drugs; drug-induced renal toxicity usually improves with interrupting therapy, decreasing dosage, or increasing dosing interval. Infusion reactions are most common 1-3 hours after starting the infusion and diminish with continued therapy. Use amphotericin B with caution in patients with decreased renal function.

Drug Interactions

Increased Effect/Toxicity: Use of amphotericin with other nephrotoxic drugs (eg, cyclosporine and aminoglycosides) may result in additive toxicity. Amphotericin may increase the toxicity of flucytosine. Antineoplastic agents may increase the risk of amphotericin-induced nephrotoxicity, bronchospasms, and hypotension. Corticosteroids may increase potassium depletion caused by amphotericin. Amphotericin B may predispose patients receiving digitalis glycosides or neuromuscular-blocking agents to toxicity secondary to hypokalemia.

Decreased Effect: Pharmacologic antagonism may occur with azole antifungal agents (ketoconazole, miconazole).

Pharmacodynamics/Kinetics

Distribution: Minimal amounts enter the aqueous humor, bile, CSF (inflamed or noninflamed meninges), amniotic fluid, pericardial fluid, pleural fluid, and synovial fluid

Protein binding, plasma: 90%

Half-life elimination: Biphasic: Initial: 15-48 hours; Terminal: 15 days

Time to peak: Within 1 hour following a 4- to 6-hour dose

Excretion: Urine (2% to 5% as biologically active form); ~40% eliminated over a 7-day period and may be detected in urine for at least 7 weeks after discontinued use

Pregnancy Risk Factor B

Dosage Forms

Injection, powder for reconstitution: 50 mg

Selected Readings

Anderson RP and Clark DA, "Amphotericin B Toxicity Reduced by Administration in Fat Emulsion," *Ann Pharmacother*, 1995, 29(5):496-500.

Arning M, Heer-Sonderhoff A, and Schneider W, "Cardiopulmonary Toxicity After Liposomal Amphotericin B (AmBisome®) in Neutropenic Patients With Acute Leukemia," *Onkologie*, 1994, 17:4.

Arsura EL, Ismail Y, Freedman S, et al, "Amphotericin B-Induced Dilated Cardiomyopathy," *Am J Med*, 1994, 97(6):560-2.

Benson JM and Nahata MC, "Clinical Use of Systemic Antifungal Agents," *Clin Pharm*, 1988, 7(6):424-38.

Benson JM and Nahata MC, "Pharmacokinetics of Amphotericin B in Children," *Antimicrob Agents Chemother*, 1989, 33(11):1989-93.

Bianco JA, Almgren J, Kern DL, et al, "Evidence That Oral Pentoxifylline Reverses Acute Renal Dysfunction in Bone Marrow Transplant Recipients Receiving Amphotericin B and Cyclosporine," *Transplantation*, 1991, 51(4):925-7.

Branch RA, "Prevention of Amphotericin B-Induced Renal Impairment. A Review on the Use of Sodium Supplementation," *Arch Intern Med*, 1988, 148(11):2389-94.

Brent J, Hunt M, Kulig K, et al, "Amphotericin B Overdoses in Infants: Is There a Role for Exchange Transfusion?" *Vet Hum Toxicol*, 1990, 32(2):124-5.

Cruz JM, Peacock JE Jr, Loomer L, et al, "Rapid Intravenous Infusion of Amphotericin B: A Pilot Study," *Am J Med*, 1992, 93:123-30.

Devuyst O, Goffin E, and Van Ypersele de Strihou C, "Recurrent Hemiparesis Under Amphotericin B for *Candida albicans* Peritonitis," *Nephrol Dial Transplant*, 1995, 10(5):699-701.

Edwards JE Jr, Bodey GP, Bowden RA, et al, "International Conference for the Development of a Consensus on the Management and Prevention of Severe Candidal Infections," *Clin Infect Dis*, 1997, 25(1):43-59.

Eggimann P, Francioli P, Bille J, et al, "Fluconazole Prophylaxis Prevents Intra-Abdominal Candidiasis in High-Risk Surgical Patients," *Crit Care Med*, 1999, 27(6):1066-72.

Gales MA and Gales BJ, "Rapid Infusion of Amphotericin B in Dextrose," *Ann Pharmacother*, 1995, 29(5):523-9.

Gallis HA, Drew RH, and Pickard WW, "Amphotericin B: 30 Years of Clinical Experience," *Rev Infect Dis*, 1990, 12(2):308-29.

Goodwin SD, Cleary JD, Walawander CA, et al, "Pretreatment Regimens for Adverse Events Related to Infusion of Amphotericin B," *Clin Infect Dis*, 1995, 20(4):755-61.

Jeffery GM, Beard ME, Ikram RB, et al, "Intranasal Amphotericin B Reduces the Frequency of Invasive Aspergillosis in Neutropenic Patients," *Am J Med*, 1991, 90(6):685-92.

Jones RS, Barman A, Suh B, et al, "Successful Treatment of *Aspergillus vertebral* Osteomyelitis With Amphotericin B Lipid Complex," *Infect Dis Clin Pract*, 1995, 4:237-9.

Kauffman CA and Carver PL, "Antifungal Agents in the 1990s. Current Status and Future Developments," *Drugs*, 1997, 53(4):539-49.

Kintzel PE and Smith GH, "Practical Guidelines for Preparing and Administering Amphotericin B," *Am J Hosp Pharm*, 1992, 49(5):1156-64.

Koren G, Lau A, Klein J, et al, "Pharmacokinetics and Adverse Effects of Amphotericin B in Infants and Children," *J Pediatr*, 1988, 113(3):559-63.

Levy M, Domaratzki J, and Koren G, "Amphotericin-Induced Heart Rate Decrease in Children," *Clin Pediatr (Phila)*, 1995, 34(7):358-64.

Lyman CA and Walsh TJ, "Systemically Administered Antifungal Agents. A Review of Their Clinical Pharmacology and Therapeutic Applications," *Drugs*, 1992, 44(1):9-35.

Patel R, "Antifungal Agents. Part I. Amphotericin B Preparations and Flucytosine," *Mayo Clin Proc*, 1998, 73(12):1205-25.

Rex JH, Bennett JE, Sugar AM, "A Randomized Trial Comparing Fluconazole With Amphotericin B for the Treatment of Candidemia in Patients Without Neutropenia. Candidemia Study Group and the National Institute," *N Engl J Med*, 1994, 331(20):1325-30.

Rex JH, Walsh TJ, Sobel JD, et al, "Practice Guidelines for the Treatment of Candidiasis. Infectious Diseases Society of America, *Clin Infect Dis*, 2000, 30(4):662-78.

Slain D, "Lipid-Based Amphotericin B for the Treatment of Fungal Infections," *Pharmacotherapy*, 1999, 19(3):306-23.

The Ad Hoc Advisory Panel on Peritonitis Management. "Continuous Ambulatory Peritoneal Dialysis (CAPD) Peritonitis Treatment Recommendations: 1989 Update," *Perit Dial Int*, 1989, 9(4):247-56.

Wong-Beringer A, Beringer PM, and Rho JP, "Focus on Amphotericin B Lipid Complex," *Formulary*, 1996, 13(3):169-85.

Amphotericin B Desoxycholate *see* Amphotericin B (Conventional) *on page 115*

Amphotericin B (Lipid Complex)
(am foe TER i sin bee LIP id KOM pleks)

U.S. Brand Names Abelcet®

Canadian Brand Names Abelcet®; Amphotec®

Generic Available No

Index Terms ABLC

Pharmacologic Category Antifungal Agent, Parenteral

Use Treatment of aspergillosis or any type of progressive fungal infection in patients who are refractory to or intolerant of conventional amphotericin B therapy

Unlabeled/Investigational Use Effective in patients with serious *Candida* species infections

Local Anesthetic/Vasoconstrictor Precautions No information available to require special precautions

Effects on Dental Treatment No significant effects or complications reported

Common Adverse Effects Nephrotoxicity and infusion-related hyperpyrexia, rigor, and chilling are reduced relative to amphotericin deoxycholate.

>10%:
Central nervous system: Chills, fever
Renal: Serum creatinine increased
(Continued)

Amphotericin B (Lipid Complex) *(Continued)*

Miscellaneous: Multiple organ failure

1% to 10%:

Cardiovascular: Hypotension, cardiac arrest

Central nervous system: Headache, pain

Dermatologic: Rash

Endocrine & metabolic: Bilirubinemia, hypokalemia, acidosis

Gastrointestinal: Nausea, vomiting, diarrhea, gastrointestinal hemorrhage, abdominal pain

Renal: Renal failure

Respiratory: Respiratory failure, dyspnea, pneumonia

Mechanism of Action Binds to ergosterol altering cell membrane permeability in susceptible fungi and causing leakage of cell components with subsequent cell death. Proposed mechanism suggests that amphotericin causes an oxidation-dependent stimulation of macrophages.

Drug Interactions

Increased Effect/Toxicity: See Drug Interactions - Increased Effect/Toxicity in Amphotericin B (Conventional).

Decreased Effect: See Drug Interactions - Decreased Effect in Amphotericin B (Conventional).

Pharmacodynamics/Kinetics

Distribution: V_d: Increases with higher doses; reflects increased uptake by tissues (131 L/kg with 5 mg/kg/day)

Half-life elimination: ~24 hours

Excretion: Clearance: Increases with higher doses (5 mg/kg/day): 400 mL/hour/kg

Pregnancy Risk Factor B

Amphotericin B (Liposomal) (am foe TER i sin bee lye po SO mal)

U.S. Brand Names AmBisome®

Canadian Brand Names AmBisome®

Generic Available No

Index Terms L-AmB

Pharmacologic Category Antifungal Agent, Parenteral

Use Empirical therapy for presumed fungal infection in febrile, neutropenic patients; treatment of patients with *Aspergillus* species, *Candida* species, and/or *Cryptococcus* species infections refractory to amphotericin B desoxycholate, or in patients where renal impairment or unacceptable toxicity precludes the use of amphotericin B desoxycholate; treatment of cryptococcal meningitis in HIV-infected patients; treatment of visceral leishmaniasis

Unlabeled/Investigational Use Effective in patients with serious *Candida* species infections

Local Anesthetic/Vasoconstrictor Precautions No information available to require special precautions

Effects on Dental Treatment Key adverse event(s) related to dental treatment: Facial swelling, postural hypotension, mucositis, stomatitis, and ulcerative stomatitis (see Dental Comment)

Common Adverse Effects Percentage of adverse reactions is dependent upon population studied and may vary with respect to premedications and underlying illness. Incidence of decreased renal function and infusion-related events are lower than rates observed with amphotericin B deoxycholate.

>10%:

Cardiovascular: Peripheral edema (15%), edema (12% to 14%), tachycardia (9% to 18%), hypotension (7% to 14%), hypertension (8% to 20%), chest pain (8% to 12%), hypervolemia (8% to 12%)

Central nervous system: Chills (29% to 48%), insomnia (17% to 22%), headache (9% to 20%), anxiety (7% to 14%), pain (14%), confusion (9% to 13%)

Dermatologic: Rash (5% to 25%), pruritus (11%)

Endocrine & metabolic: Hypokalemia (31% to 51%), hypomagnesemia (15% to 50%), hyperglycemia (8% to 23%), hypocalcemia (5% to 18%), hyponatremia (8% to 12%)

Gastrointestinal: Nausea (16% to 40%), vomiting (10% to 32%), diarrhea (11% to 30%), abdominal pain (7% to 20%), constipation (15%), anorexia (10% to 14%)

Hematologic: Anemia (27% to 48%), blood transfusion reaction (9% to 18%), leukopenia (15% to 17%), thrombocytopenia (6% to 13%)

Hepatic: Alkaline phosphatase increased (7% to 22%), BUN increased (7% to 21%), bilirubinemia (9% to 18%), ALT increased (15%), AST increased (13%), liver function tests abnormal (not specified) (4% to 13%)

Local: Phlebitis (9% to 11%)

Neuromuscular & skeletal: Weakness (6% to 13%), back pain (12%)

Renal: Creatinine increased (18% to 40%), hematuria (14%)

Respiratory: Dyspnea (18% to 23%), lung disorder (14% to 18%), cough increased (2% to 18%), epistaxis (8% to 15%), pleural effusion (12%), rhinitis (11%)

Miscellaneous: Sepsis (7% to 14%), infection (11% to 12%)

2% to 10%:

Cardiovascular: Arrhythmia, atrial fibrillation, bradycardia, cardiac arrest, cardiomegaly, facial swelling, flushing, postural hypotension, valvular heart disease, vascular disorder

Central nervous system: Agitation, abnormal thinking, coma, convulsion, depression, dysesthesia, dizziness (7% to 8%), hallucinations, malaise, nervousness, somnolence

Dermatologic: Alopecia, bruising, cellulitis, dry skin, maculopapular rash, petechia, purpura, skin discoloration, skin disorder, skin ulcer, urticaria, vesiculobullous rash

Endocrine & metabolic: Acidosis, fluid overload, hypernatremia (4%), hyperchloremia, hyperkalemia, hypermagnesemia, hyperphosphatemia, hypophosphatemia, hypoproteinemia, lactate dehydrogenase increased, nonprotein nitrogen increased

Gastrointestinal: Constipation, dry mouth, dyspepsia, abdomen enlarged, amylase increased, eructation, fecal incontinence, flatulence, gastrointestinal hemorrhage (10%), hematemesis, hemorrhoids, gum/oral hemorrhage, ileus, mucositis, rectal disorder, stomatitis, ulcerative stomatitis

Genitourinary: Vaginal hemorrhage

Hematologic: Coagulation disorder, hemorrhage, decreased prothrombin, thrombocytopenia

Hepatic: Hepatocellular damage, hepatomegaly, veno-occlusive liver disease

Local: Injection site inflammation

Neuromuscular & skeletal: Arthralgia, bone pain, dystonia, myalgia, neck pain, paresthesia, rigors, tremor

Ocular: Conjunctivitis, dry eyes, eye hemorrhage

Renal: Abnormal renal function, acute kidney failure, dysuria, kidney failure, toxic nephropathy, urinary incontinence

Respiratory: Asthma, atelectasis, cough, dry nose, hemoptysis, hyperventilation, lung edema, pharyngitis, pneumonia, respiratory alkalosis, respiratory insufficiency, respiratory failure, sinusitis, hypoxia (6% to 8%)

Miscellaneous: Allergic reaction, cell-mediated immunological reaction, flu-like syndrome, graft-versus-host disease, herpes simplex, hiccup, procedural complication (8% to 10%), diaphoresis (7%)

Mechanism of Action Binds to ergosterol altering cell membrane permeability in susceptible fungi and causing leakage of cell components with subsequent cell death. Proposed mechanism suggests that amphotericin causes an oxidation-dependent stimulation of macrophages (Lyman, 1992).

Drug Interactions

Increased Effect/Toxicity: Drug interactions have not been studied in a controlled manner; however, drugs that interact with conventional amphotericin B may also interact with amphotericin B liposome for injection. See Drug Interactions - Increased Effect/Toxicity in Amphotericin B (Conventional) monograph.

Pharmacodynamics/Kinetics

Distribution: V_d: 131 L/kg

Half-life elimination: Terminal: 174 hours

Pregnancy Risk Factor B

Dental Comment Amphotericin B, liposomal is a true single bilayer liposomal drug delivery system. Liposomes are closed, spherical vesicles created by mixing specific proportions of amphophilic substances such as phospholipids and cholesterol so that they arrange themselves into multiple concentric bilayer membranes when hydrated in aqueous solutions. Single bilayer liposomes are then formed by microemulsification of multilamellar vesicles using a homogenizer. Amphotericin B, liposomal consists of these unilamellar bilayer liposomes with amphotericin B intercalated within the membrane. Due to the nature and quantity of amphophilic substances used, and the lipophilic moiety in the amphotericin B molecule, the drug is an integral part of the overall structure of the amphotericin B liposomes. Amphotericin B, liposomal contains true liposomes that are <100 nm in diameter.

Ampicillin (am pi SIL in)

Related Information

Antibiotic Prophylaxis *on page 1772*

(Continued)

Ampicillin *(Continued)*

Canadian Brand Names Apo-Ampi®; Novo-Ampicillin; Nu-Ampi

Mexican Brand Names Amsapen; Anglopen; Binotal; Diferin; Omnipen; Penbritin

Generic Available Yes

Index Terms Aminobenzylpenicillin; Ampicillin Sodium; Ampicillin Trihydrate

Pharmacologic Category Antibiotic, Penicillin

Dental Use I.V. or I.M. administration for the prevention of infective bacterial endocarditis in patients not allergic to penicillin and unable to take oral amoxicillin; I.V. or I.M. administration for prophylaxis in total joint replacement patients not allergic to penicillin and unable to take oral medications undergoing dental procedures which produce bacteremia

Use Treatment of susceptible bacterial infections (nonbeta-lactamase-producing organisms); susceptible bacterial infections caused by streptococci, pneumococci, nonpenicillinase-producing staphylococci, *Listeria*, meningococci; some strains of *H. influenzae*, *Salmonella*, *Shigella*, *E. coli*, *Enterobacter*, and *Klebsiella*

Local Anesthetic/Vasoconstrictor Precautions No information available to require special precautions

Effects on Dental Treatment Key adverse event(s) related to dental treatment: Oral candidiasis, black hairy tongue, glossitis, sore mouth or tongue, and stomatitis.

Significant Adverse Effects Frequency not defined.

Central nervous system: Fever, penicillin encephalopathy, seizure

Dermatologic: Erythema multiforme, exfoliative dermatitis, rash, urticaria

> **Note:** Appearance of a rash should be carefully evaluated to differentiate (if possible) nonallergic ampicillin rash from hypersensitivity reaction. Incidence is higher in patients with viral infection, *Salmonella* infection, lymphocytic leukemia, or patients that have hyperuricemia.

Gastrointestinal: Black hairy tongue, diarrhea, enterocolitis, glossitis, nausea, pseudomembranous colitis, sore mouth or tongue, stomatitis, vomiting, oral candidiasis

Hematologic: Agranulocytosis, anemia, hemolytic anemia, eosinophilia, leukopenia, thrombocytopenia purpura

Hepatic: AST increased

Renal: Interstitial nephritis (rare)

Respiratory: Laryngeal stridor

Miscellaneous: Anaphylaxis, serum sickness-like reaction

Dental Usual Dosing

Infective endocarditis prophylaxis: I.M., I.V.: Dental, oral, respiratory tract, or esophageal procedures:

Infants and Children: 50 mg/kg within 30-60 minutes prior to procedure in patients not allergic to penicillin and unable to take oral amoxicillin

Adults: 2 g within 30-60 minutes prior to procedure in patients not allergic to penicillin and unable to take oral amoxicillin. **Note:** Intramuscular injections should be avoided in patients who are receiving anticoagulant therapy. In these circumstances, orally administered regimens should be given whenever possible. Intravenously administered antibiotics should be used for patients who are unable to tolerate or absorb oral medications.

Prophylaxis in total joint replacement patient: Adults: I.M., I.V.: 2 g 1 hour prior to the procedure

Dosage

Usual dosage range:

Infants and Children:

Oral: 50-100 mg/kg/day in doses divided every 6 hours (maximum: 2-4 g/day)

I.M., I.V.: 100-400 mg/kg/day in divided doses every 6 hours (maximum: 12 g/day)

Adults: Oral, I.M., I.V.: 250-500 mg every 6 hours

Indication-specific dosing:

Infants and Children:

Endocarditis prophylaxis:

Dental, oral, respiratory tract, or esophageal procedures: I.M., I.V.: 50 mg/kg within 30 minutes prior to procedure in patients unable to take oral amoxicillin

Genitourinary and gastrointestinal tract (except esophageal) procedures: I.M., I.V.:

High-risk patients: 50 mg/kg (maximum: 2 g) within 30 minutes prior to procedure, followed by ampicillin 25 mg/kg (or amoxicillin 25 mg/kg orally) 6 hours later; must be used in combination with gentamicin.

Moderate-risk patients: 50 mg/kg within 30 minutes prior to procedure

Mild-to-moderate infections:
Oral: 50-100 mg/kg/day in doses divided every 6 hours (maximum: 2-4 g/day)
I.M., I.V.: 100-150 mg/kg/day in divided doses every 6 hours (maximum: 2-4 g/day)
Severe infections, meningitis: I.M., I.V.: 200-400 mg/kg/day in divided doses every 6 hours (maximum: 6-12 g/day)
Adults:
Actinomycosis: I.V.: 50 mg/kg/day for 4-6 weeks then oral amoxicillin
Cholangitis (acute): I.V.: 2 g every 4 hours with gentamicin
Diverticulitis: I.M., I.V.: 2 g every 6 hours with metronidazole
Endocarditis:
Infective: I.V.: 12 g/day via continuous infusion or divided every 4 hours
Prophylaxis: Dental, oral, respiratory tract, or esophageal procedures: I.M., I.V.: 2 g within 30 minutes prior to procedure in patients unable to take oral amoxicillin
Genitourinary and gastrointestinal tract (except esophageal) procedures:
High-risk patients: I.M., I.V.: 2 g within 30 minutes prior to procedure, followed by ampicillin 1 g (or amoxicillin 1g orally) 6 hours later; must be used in combination with gentamicin.
Moderate-risk patients: I.M., I.V.: 2 g within 30 minutes prior to procedure
Group B strep prophylaxis (intrapartum): I.V.: 2 g initial dose, then 1 g every 4 hours until delivery
Listeria **infections:** I.V.: 200 mg/kg/day divided every 6 hours
Sepsis/meningitis: I.M., I.V.: 150-250 mg/kg/day divided every 3-4 hours (range: 6-12 g/day)
Urinary tract infections (enterococcus suspected): I.V.: 1-2 g every 6 hours with gentamicin
Dosing interval in renal impairment:
Cl_{cr} >50 mL/minute: Administer every 6 hours
Cl_{cr} 10-50 mL/minute: Administer every 6-12 hours
Cl_{cr} <10 mL/minute: Administer every 12-24 hours
Hemodialysis: Moderately dialyzable (20% to 50%); administer dose after dialysis
Peritoneal dialysis: Moderately dialyzable (20% to 50%)
Administer 250 mg every 12 hours
Continuous arteriovenous or venovenous hemofiltration effects: Dose as for Cl_{cr} 10-50 mL/minute; ~50 mg of ampicillin per liter of filtrate is removed

Mechanism of Action Inhibits bacterial cell wall synthesis by binding to one or more of the penicillin-binding proteins (PBPs) which in turn inhibits the final transpeptidation step of peptidoglycan synthesis in bacterial cell walls, thus inhibiting cell wall biosynthesis. Bacteria eventually lyse due to ongoing activity of cell wall autolytic enzymes (autolysins and murein hydrolases) while cell wall assembly is arrested.

Contraindications Hypersensitivity to ampicillin, any component of the formulation, or other penicillins

Warnings/Precautions Dosage adjustment may be necessary in patients with renal impairment. Serious and occasionally severe or fatal hypersensitivity (anaphylactoid) reactions have been reported in patients on penicillin therapy, especially with a history of beta-lactam hypersensitivity, history of sensitivity to multiple allergens, or previous IgE-mediated reactions (eg, anaphylaxis, angioedema, urticaria). Use with caution in asthmatic patients. High percentage of patients with infectious mononucleosis have developed rash during therapy with ampicillin. Appearance of a rash should be carefully evaluated to differentiate a nonallergic ampicillin rash from a hypersensitivity reaction. Ampicillin rash is a generalized dull red, maculopapular rash, generally appearing 3-14 days after the start of therapy. It normally begins on the trunk and spreads over most of the body. It may be most intense at pressure areas, elbows, and knees. Prolonged use may result in fungal or bacterial superinfection, including *C. difficile*-associated diarrhea and pseudomembranous colitis.

Drug Interactions
Allopurinol: Theoretically has an additive potential for ampicillin/amoxicillin rash.
Aminoglycosides: May be synergistic against selected organisms.
Methotrexate: Penicillins may increase the exposure to methotrexate during concurrent therapy; monitor.
Oral contraceptives: Anecdotal reports suggesting decreased contraceptive efficacy with penicillins have been refuted by more rigorous scientific and clinical data.
Probenecid, disulfiram: May increase levels of penicillins (ampicillin).
Warfarin: Effects of warfarin may be increased.

Ethanol/Nutrition/Herb Interactions Food: Food decreases ampicillin absorption rate; may decrease ampicillin serum concentration.
(Continued)

Ampicillin *(Continued)*

Dietary Considerations Take on an empty stomach 1 hour before or 2 hours after meals.

Sodium content of 5 mL suspension (250 mg/5 mL): 10 mg (0.4 mEq)
Sodium content of 1 g: 66.7 mg (3 mEq)

Pharmacodynamics/Kinetics

Absorption: Oral: 50%

Distribution: Bile, blister, and tissue fluids; penetration into CSF occurs with inflamed meninges only, good only with inflammation (exceeds usual MICs)
Normal meninges: Nil; Inflamed meninges: 5% to 10%

Protein binding: 15% to 25%

Half-life elimination:
Children and Adults: 1-1.8 hours
Anuria/end-stage renal disease: 7-20 hours

Time to peak: Oral: Within 1-2 hours

Excretion: Urine (~90% as unchanged drug) within 24 hours

Pregnancy Risk Factor B

Lactation Enters breast milk/use caution

Dosage Forms Excipient information presented when available (limited, particularly for generics); consult specific product labeling.

Capsule: 250 mg, 500 mg

Injection, powder for reconstitution, as sodium: 125 mg, 250 mg, 500 mg, 1 g, 2 g, 10 g

Powder for oral suspension: 125 mg/5 mL (100 mL, 200 mL); 250 mg/5 mL (100 mL, 200 mL)

Selected Readings

ADA Division of Legal Affairs, "A Legal Perspective on Antibiotic Prophylaxis," *J Am Dent Assoc*, 2003, 134(9):1260.

American Dental Association; American Academy of Orthopedic Surgeons, "Antibiotic Prophylaxis for Dental Patients With Total Joint Replacements," *J Am Dent Assoc*, 2003, 134(7):895-9.

American Dental Association Council on Scientific Affairs, "Combating Antibiotic Resistance," *J Am Dent Assoc*, 2004, 135(4):484-7.

Dajani AS, Taubert KA, Wilson W, et al, "Prevention of Bacterial Endocarditis. Recommendations by the American Heart Association," *JAMA*, 1997, 277(22):1794-801.

Dajani AS, Taubert KA, Wilson W, et al, "Prevention of Bacterial Endocarditis: Recommendations by the American Heart Association," *J Am Dent Assoc*, 1997, 128(8):1142-51.

Wynn RL, Bergman SA, Meiller TF, et al, "Antibiotics in Treating Oral-Facial Infections of Odontogenic Origin: An Update", *Gen Dent*, 2001, 49(3):238-40, 242, 244 passim.

Ampicillin and Sulbactam *(am pi SIL in & SUL bak tam)*

Related Information
Ampicillin *on page 119*
Sexually-Transmitted Diseases *on page 1766*

U.S. Brand Names Unasyn®

Canadian Brand Names Unasyn®

Mexican Brand Names Unasyna

Generic Available Yes

Index Terms Sulbactam and Ampicillin

Pharmacologic Category Antibiotic, Penicillin

Dental Use Parenteral beta-lactamase-resistant antibiotic combination to treat more severe orofacial infections where beta-lactamase-producing staphylococci and beta-lactamase-producing *Bacteroides* are present

Use Treatment of susceptible bacterial infections involved with skin and skin structure, intra-abdominal infections, gynecological infections; spectrum is that of ampicillin plus organisms producing beta-lactamases such as *S. aureus*, *H. influenzae*, *E. coli*, *Klebsiella*, *Acinetobacter*, *Enterobacter*, and anaerobes

Local Anesthetic/Vasoconstrictor Precautions No information available to require special precautions

Effects on Dental Treatment Prolonged use of penicillins may lead to development of oral candidiasis (see Dental Comment)

Significant Adverse Effects Also see Ampicillin.

>10%: Local: Pain at injection site (I.M.)

1% to 10%:
Dermatologic: Rash
Gastrointestinal: Diarrhea
Local: Pain at injection site (I.V.), thrombophlebitis
Miscellaneous: Allergic reaction (may include serum sickness, urticaria, bronchospasm, hypotension, etc)

<1% (Limited to important or life-threatening): Abdominal distension, candidiasis, chest pain, chills, dysuria, edema, epistaxis, erythema, facial swelling, fatigue, flatulence, glossitis, hairy tongue, headache, interstitial nephritis,

itching, liver enzymes increased, malaise, mucosal bleeding, nausea, pseudomembranous colitis, seizure, substernal pain, throat tightness, thrombocytopenia, urine retention, vomiting

Dental Usual Dosing Severe orofacial infections: Adults: I.M., I.V.: 1-2 g ampicillin (1.5-3 g Unasyn®) every 6 hours (maximum: 8 g ampicillin/day, 12 g Unasyn®)

Dosage Note: Unasyn® (ampicillin/sulbactam) is a combination product. Dosage recommendations for Unasyn® are based on the ampicillin component.

Usual dosage range:
Children ≥1 year: I.V.: 100-400 mg ampicillin/kg/day divided every 6 hours (maximum: 8 g ampicillin/day, 12 g Unasyn®). **Note:** The American Academy of Pediatrics recommends a dose of up to 300 mg/kg/day for severe infection in infants >1 month of age.

Adults: I.M., I.V.: 1-2 g ampicillin (1.5-3 g Unasyn®) every 6 hours (maximum: 8 g ampicillin/day, 12 g Unasyn®)

Indication-specific dosing:
Children:
Epiglottitis: I.V.: 100-200 mg ampicillin/kg/day divided in 4 doses
Mild-to-moderate infections: I.M., I.V.: 100-200 mg ampicillin/kg/day (150-300 mg Unasyn®) divided every 6 hours (maximum: 8 g ampicillin/day, 12 g Unasyn®)
Peritonsillar and retropharyngeal abscess: I.V.: 50 mg ampicillin/kg/dose every 6 hours
Severe infections: I.M., I.V.: 200-400 mg ampicillin/kg/day divided every 6 hours (maximum: 8 g ampicillin/day, 12 g Unasyn®)
Adults: Doses expressed as ampicillin/sulbactam combination:
Amnionitis, cholangitis, diverticulitis, endometritis, endophthalmitis, epididymitis/orchitis, liver abscess, osteomyelitis (diabetic foot), peritonitis: I.V.: 3 g every 6 hours
Endocarditis: I.V.: 3 g every 6 hours with gentamicin or vancomycin for 4-6 weeks
Orbital cellulitis: I.V.: 1.5 g every 6 hours
Parapharyngeal space infections: I.V.: 3 g every 6 hours
***Pasteurella multocida* (human, canine/feline bites):** I.V.: 1.5-3 g every 6 hours
Pelvic inflammatory disease: I.V.: 3 g every 6 hours with doxycycline
Peritonitis (CAPD): Intraperitoneal:
Anuric, intermittent: 3 g every 12 hours
Anuric, continuous: Loading dose: 1.5 g; maintenance dose: 150 mg
Pneumonia:
Aspiration, community-acquired: I.V.: 1.5-3 g every 6 hours
Hospital-acquired: I.V.: 3 g every 6 hours
Urinary tract infections, pyelonephritis: I.V.: 3 g every 6 hours for 14 days
Dosing interval in renal impairment:
Cl$_{cr}$ 15-29 mL/minute: Administer every 12 hours
Cl$_{cr}$ 5-14 mL/minute: Administer every 24 hours

Mechanism of Action The addition of sulbactam, a beta-lactamase inhibitor, to ampicillin extends the spectrum of ampicillin to include some beta-lactamase-producing organisms; inhibits bacterial cell wall synthesis by binding to one or more of the penicillin-binding proteins (PBPs) which in turn inhibits the final transpeptidation step of peptidoglycan synthesis in bacterial cell walls, thus inhibiting cell wall biosynthesis. Bacteria eventually lyse due to ongoing activity of cell wall autolytic enzymes (autolysins and murein hydrolases) while cell wall assembly is arrested.

Contraindications Hypersensitivity to ampicillin, sulbactam, penicillins, or any component of the formulations

Warnings/Precautions Dosage adjustment may be necessary in patients with renal impairment. Serious and occasionally severe or fatal hypersensitivity (anaphylactoid) reactions have been reported in patients on penicillin therapy, especially with a history of beta-lactam hypersensitivity, history of sensitivity to multiple allergens, or previous IgE-mediated reactions (eg, anaphylaxis, angioedema, urticaria). Use with caution in asthmatic patients. A high percentage of patients with infectious mononucleosis have developed rash during therapy with ampicillin. Appearance of a rash should be carefully evaluated to differentiate a nonallergic ampicillin rash from a hypersensitivity reaction. Prolonged use may result in fungal or bacterial superinfection, including *C. difficile*-associated diarrhea and pseudomembranous colitis. Safety and efficacy have not been established in children <1 year of age.

Drug Interactions
Allopurinol: Theoretically has an additive potential for ampicillin/amoxicillin rash.
Aminoglycosides: May be synergistic against selected organisms.
(Continued)

Ampicillin and Sulbactam *(Continued)*

Methotrexate: Penicillins may increase the exposure to methotrexate during concurrent therapy; monitor.

Oral contraceptives: Anecdotal reports suggesting decreased contraceptive efficacy with penicillins have been refuted by more rigorous scientific and clinical data.

Probenecid, disulfiram: May increase levels of penicillins (ampicillin).

Warfarin: Effects of warfarin may be increased.

Dietary Considerations Sodium content of 1.5 g injection: 115 mg (5 mEq)

Pharmacodynamics/Kinetics

Ampicillin: See Ampicillin.

Sulbactam:

Distribution: Bile, blister, and tissue fluids

Protein binding: 38%

Half-life elimination: Normal renal function: 1-1.3 hours

Excretion: Urine (~75% to 85% as unchanged drug) within 8 hours

Pregnancy Risk Factor B

Lactation Enters breast milk/use caution

Dosage Forms Excipient information presented when available (limited, particularly for generics); consult specific product labeling.

Injection, powder for reconstitution: 1.5 g: Ampicillin 1 g and sulbactam 0.5 g [contains sodium 115 mg (5 mEq)/1.5 g)]; 3 g: Ampicillin 2 g and sulbactam 1 g [contains sodium 115 mg (5 mEq)/1.5 g)]; 15 g: Ampicillin 10 g and sulbactam 5 g [bulk package; contains sodium 115 mg (5 mEq)/1.5 g)]

Unasyn®:

1.5 g: Ampicillin 1 g and sulbactam 0.5 g [contains sodium 115 mg (5 mEq)/ 1.5 g)]

3 g: Ampicillin 2 g and sulbactam 1 g [contains sodium 115 mg (5 mEq)/1.5 g)]

15 g: Ampicillin 10 g and sulbactam 5 g [bulk package; contains sodium 115 mg (5 mEq)/1.5 g)]

Dental Comment In maxillary sinus, anterior nasal cavity, and deep neck infections, beta-lactamase-producing staphylococci and beta-lactamase-producing *Bacteroides* usually are present. In these situations, antibiotics that resist the beta-lactamase enzyme should be administered. Amoxicillin and clavulanic acid is administered orally for moderate infections. Ampicillin sodium and sulbactam sodium (Unasyn®) is administered parenterally for more severe infections.

Ampicillin Sodium *see* Ampicillin *on page 119*
Ampicillin Trihydrate *see* Ampicillin *on page 119*

Amprenavir *(am PREN a veer)*

Related Information

HIV Infection and AIDS *on page 1753*
Tuberculosis Treatment *on page 1909*

U.S. Brand Names Agenerase®

Canadian Brand Names Agenerase®

Mexican Brand Names Agenerase

Generic Available No

Pharmacologic Category Antiretroviral Agent, Protease Inhibitor

Use Treatment of HIV infections in combination with at least two other antiretroviral agents; oral solution should only be used when capsules or other protease inhibitors are not therapeutic options

Local Anesthetic/Vasoconstrictor Precautions No information available to require special precautions

Effects on Dental Treatment Key adverse event(s) related to dental treatment: Perioral tingling/numbness and taste disorder

Common Adverse Effects

>10%:

Central nervous system: Depression/mood disorder (9% to 16%), paresthesia (peripheral 10% to 14%)

Dermatologic: Rash (20% to 27%)

Endocrine & metabolic: Hyperglycemia (>160 mg/dL: 37% to 41%), hypertriglyceridemia (>399 mg/dL: 36% to 47%; >750 mg/dL: 8% to 13%)

Gastrointestinal: Nausea (43% to 74%), vomiting (24% to 34%), diarrhea (39% to 60%), abdominal symptoms

Miscellaneous: Perioral tingling/numbness (26% to 31%)

1% to 10%:

Central nervous system: Headache, fatigue

Dermatologic: Stevens-Johnson syndrome (1% of total, 4% of patients who develop a rash)

Endocrine & metabolic: Hypercholesterolemia (>260 mg/dL: 4% to 9%), hyperglycemia (>251 mg/dL: 2% to 3%), fat redistribution

Gastrointestinal: Taste disorders (2% to 10%), amylase increased (3% to 4%)

Hepatic: AST increased (3% to 5%), ALT increased (4%)

Mechanism of Action Binds to the protease activity site and inhibits the activity of the enzyme. HIV protease is required for the cleavage of viral polyprotein precursors into individual functional proteins found in infectious HIV. Inhibition prevents cleavage of these polyproteins, resulting in the formation of immature, noninfectious viral particles.

Drug Interactions

Cytochrome P450 Effect: Substrate of CYP2C9 (minor), 3A4 (major); **Inhibits** CYP2C19 (weak), 3A4 (strong)

Increased Effect/Toxicity: Concurrent use of cisapride, midazolam, pimozide, quinidine, or triazolam is contraindicated. Concurrent use of ergot alkaloids (dihydroergotamine, ergotamine, ergonovine, methylergonovine) with amprenavir is also contraindicated (may cause vasospasm and peripheral ischemia). Concurrent use of oral solution with disulfiram or metronidazole is contraindicated, due to the risk of propylene glycol toxicity.

Serum concentrations of amiodarone, bepridil, lidocaine, quinidine, and other antiarrhythmics may be increased, potentially leading to toxicity; when amprenavir is coadministered with ritonavir, flecainide and propafenone are contraindicated. HMG-CoA reductase inhibitors serum concentrations may be increased by amprenavir, increasing the risk of myopathy/rhabdomyolysis; lovastatin and simvastatin are not recommended; fluvastatin and pravastatin may be safer alternatives.

Amprenavir may increase the levels/effects of selected benzodiazepines (midazolam and triazolam are contraindicated), calcium channel blockers, cyclosporine, mirtazapine, nateglinide, nefazodone, quinidine, sildenafil (and other PDE-5 inhibitors), tacrolimus, venlafaxine, and other CYP3A4 substrates. Amprenavir may increase the levels/effects of trazodone (monitor for signs of hypotension/syncope); reduce dose of trazodone. When used with strong CYP3A4 inhibitors, dosage adjustment/limits are recommended for sildenafil and other PDE-5 inhibitors; refer to individual monographs. Amprenavir may increase the levels/effects of inhaled corticosteroids; monitor for adrenal suppression, Cushing's syndrome; concomitant use of fluticasone with amprenavir/ritonavir is not recommended.

Concurrent therapy with ritonavir may result in increased serum concentrations: dosage adjustment is recommended; avoid concurrent use of amprenavir and ritonavir oral solutions due to metabolic competition between formulation components. Clarithromycin, indinavir, nelfinavir may increase serum concentrations of amprenavir.

Decreased Effect: Serum concentrations of estrogen (oral contraceptives) may be decreased, use alternative (nonhormonal) forms of contraception. Serum concentrations of delavirdine may be decreased; may lead to loss of virologic response and possible resistance to delavirdine; concomitant use is not recommended. Efavirenz and nevirapine may decrease serum concentrations of amprenavir (dosing for combinations not established). Avoid St John's wort (may lead to subtherapeutic concentrations of amprenavir). Effect of amprenavir may be diminished when administered with methadone (consider alternative antiretroviral); in addition, effect of methadone may be reduced (dosage increase may be required). The levels/effects of amprenavir may be decreased by include aminoglutethimide, carbamazepine, nafcillin, nevirapine, phenobarbital, phenytoin, rifamycins, and other CYP3A4 inducers. The administration of antacids and didanosine (buffered formulation) should be separated from amprenavir by 1 hour to limit interaction between formulations.

Pharmacodynamics/Kinetics

Absorption: 63%

Distribution: 430 L

Protein binding: 90%

Metabolism: Hepatic via CYP (primarily CYP3A4)

Bioavailability: Not established; increased sixfold with high-fat meal; oral solution: 86% relative to capsule formulation (14% less bioavailable than capsule)

Half-life elimination: 7.1-10.6 hours

Time to peak: 1-2 hours

Excretion: Feces (75%, ~68% as metabolites); urine (14% as metabolites)

Pregnancy Risk Factor C

AMPT *see* Metyrosine *on page 1094*

Amrinone Lactate *see* Inamrinone *on page 874*

AMSA *see* Amsacrine *on page 126*

Amsacrine (AM sah kreen)

Canadian Brand Names Amsa P-D

Generic Available No

Index Terms 4-(9-Acridinylamino) Methanesulfon-m-Anisidide; Acridinyl Anisididide; AMSA; m-AMSA; NSC-249992

Pharmacologic Category Antineoplastic Agent

Unlabeled/Investigational Use Investigational: Refractory acute lymphocytic and nonlymphocytic leukemias, Hodgkin's disease, and non-Hodgkin's lymphomas; head and neck tumors

Local Anesthetic/Vasoconstrictor Precautions No information available to require special precautions

Effects on Dental Treatment Key adverse event(s) related to dental treatment: Oral ulcerations and stomatitis

Common Adverse Effects

>10%:

Cardiovascular: ECG changes (T-wave flattening, S-T wave alterations) consistent with anterolateral ischemia, ventricular fibrillation, ventricular extrasystoles, atrial tachycardia and fibrillation, CHF, cardiac arrest. Patients with hypokalemia, who have received >400 mg/m^2 of doxorubicin or daunorubicin (or the equivalent), >200 mg/m^2 of amsacrine within 48 hours, or a total dose of anthracycline + amsacrine >900 mg/m^2 have an increased risk of cardiac toxicity.

Dermatologic: Alopecia

Gastrointestinal: Nausea and vomiting (30%), diarrhea (30%), stomatitis (dose-limiting - 32%), oral ulceration (10%)

Genitourinary: Orange-red discoloration of the urine

Hematologic: Leukopenia (nadir at 10 days); thrombocytopenia (nadir at 12-14 days), with recovery at 21-25 days

Hepatic: Hyperbilirubinemia (30%), liver enzymes increased (10%)

Local: Phlebitis

1% to 10%:

Central nervous system: Headache, dizziness, confusion, convulsions

Hematologic: Anemia

Neuromuscular & skeletal: Paresthesias

Ocular: Blurred vision

Restrictions Not available in U.S./Investigational

Mechanism of Action Amsacrine has been shown to inhibit DNA synthesis by binding to, and intercalating with, DNA; inhibits topoisomerase II activity.

Pharmacodynamics/Kinetics

Distribution: V_d: 1.67 L/kg; minimal CNS penetration

Protein binding: 96% to 98%

Metabolism: Hepatic, to inactive metabolites (major metabolite is 5' glutathione conjugate)

Half-life elimination: 1.4-5 hours; Terminal: 5.6-7.8 hours

Excretion: Bile; urine (2% to 10% as unchanged drug)

Amyl Nitrite (AM il NYE trite)

Generic Available Yes

Index Terms Isoamyl Nitrite

Pharmacologic Category Antidote; Vasodilator

Use Coronary vasodilator in angina pectoris; adjunct in treatment of cyanide poisoning; produce changes in the intensity of heart murmurs

Local Anesthetic/Vasoconstrictor Precautions No information available to require special precautions

Effects on Dental Treatment Key adverse event(s) related to dental treatment: Postural hypotension

Common Adverse Effects 1% to 10%:

Cardiovascular: Postural hypotension; cutaneous flushing of head, neck, and clavicular area; tachycardia

Central nervous system: Headache, restlessness

Gastrointestinal: Nausea, vomiting

Mechanism of Action Relaxes vascular smooth muscle; decreased venous ratios and arterial blood pressure; reduces left ventricular work; decreases myocardial O_2 consumption; in cyanide poisoning, amyl nitrite converts hemoglobin to methemoglobin that binds with cyanide to form cyanate hemoglobin

Drug Interactions

Increased Effect/Toxicity: Ethanol taken with amyl nitrite may have additive side effects. Avoid concurrent use of sildenafil - severe reactions may result.

Pharmacodynamics/Kinetics
Onset of action: Angina: Within 30 seconds
Duration: 3-15 minutes
Pregnancy Risk Factor C

Amylobarbitone *see* Amobarbital *on page 105*

Amytal® *see* Amobarbital *on page 105*

AN100226 *see* Natalizumab *on page 1153*

Anadrol® *see* Oxymetholone *on page 1237*

Anafranil® *see* ClomiPRAMINE *on page 388*

Anagrelide *(an AG gre lide)*

U.S. Brand Names Agrylin®
Canadian Brand Names Agrylin®; Gen-Anagrelide; PMS-Anagrelide; Rhoxal-anagrelide; Sandoz-Anagrelide
Generic Available Yes
Index Terms 1370-999-397; Anagrelide Hydrochloride; BL4162A; 6,7-Dichloro-1,5-Dihydroimidazo [2,1b] quinazolin-2(3H)-one Monohydrochloride
Pharmacologic Category Phospholipase A_2 Inhibitor
Use Treatment of essential thrombocythemia (ET) and thrombocythemia associated with chronic myelogenous leukemia (CML), polycythemia vera, and other myeloproliferative disorders
Local Anesthetic/Vasoconstrictor Precautions No information available to require special precautions
Effects on Dental Treatment Key adverse event(s) related to dental treatment: Orthostatic hypotension
Common Adverse Effects
>10%:
Cardiovascular: Palpitation (27%), edema (other than peripheral: 21%)
Central nervous system: Headache (44%), dizziness (15%), pain (15%)
Gastrointestinal: Diarrhea (26%), nausea (17%), abdominal pain (16%)
Neuromuscular & skeletal: Weakness (23%)
Respiratory: Dyspnea (12%)
1% to 10%:
Cardiovascular: Angina, arrhythmias, cardiovascular disease, chest pain (8%), CHF, hypertension, orthostatic hypotension, peripheral edema (9%), syncope, tachycardia (7%), thrombosis, vasodilatation
Central nervous system: Amnesia, chills, confusion, depression, fever (9%), insomnia, malaise (6%), migraine, nervousness, somnolence
Dermatologic: Alopecia, photosensitivity, pruritus (6%), rash (8%), urticaria
Endocrine & skeletal: Dehydration
Gastrointestinal: Anorexia (8%), aphthous stomatitis, constipation, dyspepsia (5%), eructation, flatulence (10%), gastritis, GI distress, GI hemorrhage, melena, vomiting (10%)
Hematologic: Anemia, ecchymosis, hemorrhage, lymphadenoma, thrombocytopenia
Hepatic: Liver enzymes increased
Neuromuscular & skeletal: Arthralgia, back pain (6%), leg cramps, myalgia, paresthesia (6%)
Ocular: Amblyopia, diplopia, tinnitus, visual field abnormality
Renal: Dysuria, hematuria, renal failure
Respiratory: Asthma, bronchitis, cough (6%), epistaxis, pharyngitis (7%), pneumonia, rhinitis, sinusitis
Miscellaneous: Flu-like syndrome
Frequency not defined: Atrial fibrillation, cardiomegaly, cardiomyopathy, cerebrovascular accident, complete heart block, gastric/duodenal ulceration, leukocyte count increased, MI, pancreatitis, pericarditis, pericardial effusion, pleural effusion, pulmonary fibrosis, pulmonary infiltrates, pulmonary hypertension, seizure
Mechanism of Action Anagrelide appears to inhibit cyclic nucleotide phosphodiesterase and the release of arachidonic acid from phospholipase, possibly by inhibiting phospholipase A_2. It also causes a dose-related reduction in platelet production, which results from decreased megakaryocyte hypermaturation. The drug disrupts the postmitotic phase of maturation.
Drug Interactions
Cytochrome P450 Effect: Substrate of CYP1A2 (minor)
Increased Effect/Toxicity: Antiplatelet agents may enhance the adverse/toxic effects of drotrecogin alfa. Concurrent use of NSAIDs, salicylates, or treprostinil may enhance the adverse/toxic effects of antiplatelet agents.
(Continued)

Anagrelide *(Continued)*

Pharmacodynamics/Kinetics
Duration: 6-24 hours
Metabolism: Hepatic
Half-life elimination, plasma: 1.3 hours
Time to peak, serum: 1 hour
Excretion: Urine (<1% as unchanged drug)
Pregnancy Risk Factor C

Anagrelide Hydrochloride see Anagrelide on page 127

Anakinra *(an a KIN ra)*

U.S. Brand Names Kineret®
Canadian Brand Names Kineret®
Generic Available No
Index Terms IL-1Ra; Interleukin-1 Receptor Antagonist
Pharmacologic Category Antirheumatic, Disease Modifying; Interleukin-1 Receptor Antagonist
Use Treatment of moderately- to severely-active rheumatoid arthritis in adult patients who have failed one or more disease-modifying antirheumatic drugs (DMARDs); may be used alone or in combination with DMARDs (other than tumor necrosis factor-blocking agents)
Local Anesthetic/Vasoconstrictor Precautions No information available to require special precautions
Effects on Dental Treatment No significant effects or complications reported
Common Adverse Effects
>10%:
  Central nervous system: Headache (12%)
  Local: Injection site reaction (majority mild, typically lasting 14-28 days, characterized by erythema, ecchymosis, inflammation, and pain; up to 71%)
  Miscellaneous: Infection (39% versus 37% in placebo; serious infection 2% to 3%)
1% to 10%:
  Gastrointestinal: Nausea (8%), diarrhea (7%), abdominal pain (5%)
  Hematologic: Neutropenia (8%; grades 3/4: 0.4%)
  Respiratory: Sinusitis (7%)
  Miscellaneous: Flu-like syndrome (6%)
Mechanism of Action Antagonist of the interleukin-1 (IL-1) receptor. Endogenous IL-1 is induced by inflammatory stimuli and mediates a variety of immunological responses, including degradation of cartilage (loss of proteoglycans) and stimulation of bone resorption.
Drug Interactions
Increased Effect/Toxicity: Anti-TNF agents (adalimumab, etanercept, infliximab, lenalidomide, thalidomide) may increase risk of serious infection during concomitant use (has been reported with etanercept). Anakinra may increase the risk of secondary infection from live (organism) vaccines.
Pharmacodynamics/Kinetics
Bioavailability: SubQ: 95%
Half-life elimination: Terminal: 4-6 hours
Time to peak: SubQ: 3-7 hours
Pregnancy Risk Factor B

Ana-Kit® see Epinephrine and Chlorpheniramine on page 575
Analpram-HC® see Pramoxine and Hydrocortisone on page 1335
AnaMantle® HC see Lidocaine and Hydrocortisone on page 980
Anaprox® see Naproxen on page 1148
Anaprox® DS see Naproxen on page 1148
Anaspaz® see Hyoscyamine on page 847

Anastrozole *(an AS troe zole)*

U.S. Brand Names Arimidex®
Canadian Brand Names Arimidex®
Mexican Brand Names Arimidex
Generic Available No
Index Terms ICI-D1033; NSC-719344; ZD1033
Pharmacologic Category Antineoplastic Agent, Aromatase Inhibitor
Use Treatment of locally-advanced or metastatic breast cancer (ER-positive or hormone receptor unknown) in postmenopausal women; treatment of advanced breast cancer in postmenopausal women with disease progression following

tamoxifen therapy; adjuvant treatment of early ER-positive breast cancer in postmenopausal women

Local Anesthetic/Vasoconstrictor Precautions No information available to require special precautions

Effects on Dental Treatment Key adverse event(s) related to dental treatment: Xerostomia (normal salivary flow resumes upon discontinuation).

Common Adverse Effects
>10%:
Cardiovascular: Vasodilatation (25% to 36%), hypertension (2% to 13%)
Central nervous system: Mood disturbance (19%), fatigue (19%), pain (11% to 17%), headache (9% to 13%), depression (5% to 13%)
Dermatologic: Rash (6% to 11%)
Endocrine & metabolic: Hot flashes (12% to 36%)
Gastrointestinal: Nausea (11% to 19%), vomiting (8% to 13%)
Neuromuscular & skeletal: Weakness (16% to 19%), arthritis (17%), arthralgia (2% to 15%), back pain (10% to 12%), bone pain (6% to 11%), osteoporosis (11%)
Respiratory: Pharyngitis (6% to 14%), cough increased (8% to 11%)
1% to 10%:
Cardiovascular: Peripheral edema (5% to 10%), chest pain (5% to 7%), ischemic cardiovascular disease (4%), venous thromboembolic events (3% to 4%), ischemic cerebrovascular events (2%), angina (2%)
Central nervous system: Insomnia (2% to 10%), dizziness (6% to 8%), anxiety (2% to 6%), fever (2% to 5%), malaise (2% to 5%), confusion (2% to 5%), nervousness (2% to 5%), somnolence (2% to 5%), lethargy (1%)
Dermatologic: Alopecia (2% to 5%), pruritus (2% to 5%)
Endocrine & metabolic: Hypercholesterolemia (9%), breast pain (2% to 8%)
Gastrointestinal: Constipation (7% to 9%), abdominal pain (7% to 9%), diarrhea (8% to 9%), anorexia (5% to 7%), xerostomia (6%), dyspepsia (7%), weight gain (2% to 9%), weight loss (2% to 5%)
Genitourinary: Urinary tract infection (2% to 8%), vulvovaginitis (6%), pelvic pain (5%), vaginal bleeding (1% to 5%), vaginitis (4%), vaginal discharge (4%), vaginal hemorrhage (2% to 4%), leukorrhea (2% to 3%), vaginal dryness (2%)
Hematologic: Anemia (2% to 5%), leukopenia (2% to 5%)
Hepatic: Liver function tests increased (2% to 5%), alkaline phosphatase increased (2% to 5%), gamma GT increased (2% to 5%)
Local: Thrombophlebitis (2% to 5%)
Neuromuscular & skeletal: Fracture (2% to 10%), arthrosis (7%), paresthesia (5% to 7%), joint disorder (6%), myalgia (2% to 6%), neck pain (2% to 5%), hypertonia (3%)
Ocular: Cataracts (6%)
Respiratory: Dyspnea (8% to 10%), sinusitis (2% to 6%), bronchitis (2% to 5%), rhinitis (2% to 5%)
Miscellaneous: Lymph edema (10%), infection (2% to 9%), flu-like syndrome (2% to 7%), diaphoresis (2% to 5%), cyst (5%), tumor flare (3%)

Mechanism of Action Potent and selective nonsteroidal aromatase inhibitor. By inhibiting aromatase, the conversion of androstenedione to estrone, and testosterone to estradiol, is prevented. Anastrozole causes an 85% decrease in estrone sulfate levels.

Drug Interactions
Cytochrome P450 Effect: Inhibits CYP1A2 (weak), 2C8 (weak), 2C9 (weak), 3A4 (weak)
Decreased Effect: Estrogen derivatives and tamoxifen may decrease the levels/effects of anastrozole.

Pharmacodynamics/Kinetics
Onset of estradiol reduction: 70% reduction after 24 hours; 80% after 2 weeks therapy
Duration of estradiol reduction: 6 days
Absorption: Well absorbed; not affected by food
Protein binding, plasma: 40%
Metabolism: Extensively hepatic (~85%) via N-dealkylation, hydroxylation, and glucuronidation; primary metabolite inactive
Half-life elimination: ~50 hours
Excretion: Urine (10% as unchanged drug; 60% as metabolites)

Pregnancy Risk Factor D

Ancobon® *see* Flucytosine *on page 699*

Andehist DM NR Drops [DSC] *see* Carbinoxamine, Pseudoephedrine, and Dextromethorphan *on page 282*

Andehist NR Drops [DSC] *see* Carbinoxamine and Pseudoephedrine *on page 282*

Andehist NR Syrup *see* Brompheniramine and Pseudoephedrine *on page 231*

Androderm® *see* Testosterone *on page 1543*

AndroGel® *see* Testosterone *on page 1543*

Android® *see* MethylTESTOSTERone *on page 1085*

Anestacon® *see* Lidocaine *on page 972*

Aneurine Hydrochloride *see* Thiamine *on page 1556*

Anexsia® *see* Hydrocodone and Acetaminophen *on page 822*

Anextuss *see* Guaifenesin, Dextromethorphan, and Phenylephrine *on page 798*

Angeliq® *see* Drospirenone and Estradiol *on page 547*

Angiomax® *see* Bivalirudin *on page 220*

Anhydrous Glucose *see* Dextrose *on page 478*

Anidulafungin (ay nid yoo la FUN jin)

U.S. Brand Names Eraxis™
Generic Available No
Index Terms LY303366
Pharmacologic Category Antifungal Agent, Parenteral; Echinocandin
Use Treatment of candidemia and other forms of *Candida* infections (including those of intra-abdominal, peritoneal, and esophageal locus)
Local Anesthetic/Vasoconstrictor Precautions No information available to require special precautions
Effects on Dental Treatment No significant effects or complications reported
Common Adverse Effects 2% to 10%:
Endocrine & metabolic: Hypokalemia (3%)
Gastrointestinal: Diarrhea (3%)
Hepatic: Transaminase increased (<1% to 2%)
Mechanism of Action Noncompetitive inhibitor of 1,3-beta-D-glucan synthase resulting in reduced formation of 1,3-beta-D-glucan, an essential polysaccharide comprising 30% to 60% of *Candida* cell walls (absent in mammalian cells); decreased glucan content leads to osmotic instability and cellular lysis
Pharmacodynamics/Kinetics
Distribution: 30-50 L
Protein binding: 84%
Metabolism: No hepatic metabolism observed; undergoes slow chemical hydrolysis to open-ring peptide-lacking antifungal activity
Half-life elimination: 27 hours
Excretion: Feces (30%, 10% as unchanged drug); urine (<1%)
Pregnancy Risk Factor C

Anolor 300 *see* Butalbital, Acetaminophen, and Caffeine *on page 247*

Ansaid® [DSC] *see* Flurbiprofen *on page 722*

Ansamycin *see* Rifabutin *on page 1422*

Antabuse® *see* Disulfiram *on page 519*

Antara™ *see* Fenofibrate *on page 674*

Anthralin (AN thra lin)

U.S. Brand Names Dritho-Scalp®; Psoriatec™
Canadian Brand Names Anthraforte®; Anthranol®; Anthrascalp®; Micanol®
Generic Available No
Index Terms Dithranol
Pharmacologic Category Antipsoriatic Agent; Keratolytic Agent
Use Treatment of psoriasis (quiescent or chronic psoriasis)
Local Anesthetic/Vasoconstrictor Precautions No information available to require special precautions
Effects on Dental Treatment No significant effects or complications reported
Mechanism of Action Reduction of the mitotic rate and proliferation of epidermal cells in psoriasis by inhibiting synthesis of nucleic protein from inhibition of DNA synthesis to affected areas
Pregnancy Risk Factor C

Anthrax Vaccine (Adsorbed) (AN thraks vak SEEN ad SORBED)

Related Information
  Immunizations (Vaccines) *on page 1886*
U.S. Brand Names BioThrax™
Generic Available No
Index Terms AVA
Pharmacologic Category Vaccine
Use Immunization against *Bacillus anthracis*. Recommended for individuals who may come in contact with animal products which come from anthrax endemic areas and may be contaminated with *Bacillus anthracis* spores; recommended for high-risk persons such as veterinarians and other handling potentially infected animals. Routine immunization for the general population is not recommended.

The Department of Defense is implementing an anthrax vaccination program against the biological warfare agent anthrax, which will be administered to all active duty and reserve personnel.
Unlabeled/Investigational Use Postexposure prophylaxis in combination with antibiotics
Local Anesthetic/Vasoconstrictor Precautions No information available to require special precautions
Effects on Dental Treatment No significant effects or complications reported
Common Adverse Effects (Includes pre- and postlicensure data; systemic reactions reported more often in women than in men)

>10%:
  Central nervous system: Malaise (4% to 11%)
  Local: Tenderness (58% to 71%), erythema (12% to 43%), subcutaneous nodule (4% to 39%), induration (8% to 21%), warmth (11% to 19%), local pruritus (7% to 19%)
  Neuromuscular & skeletal: Arm motion limitation (7% to 12%)
1% to 10%:
  Central nervous system: Headache (4% to 7%), fever (<1% to 7%)
  Gastrointestinal: Anorexia (4%), vomiting (4%), nausea (<1% to 4%)
  Local: Mild local reactions (edema/induration <30 mm) (9%), edema (8%)
  Neuromuscular & skeletal: Myalgia (4% to 7%)
  Respiratory: Respiratory difficulty (4%)
Restrictions Not commercially available in the U.S.; presently, all anthrax vaccine lots are owned by the U.S. Department of Defense. The Centers for Disease Control (CDC) does not currently recommend routine vaccination of the general public.
Mechanism of Action Active immunization against *Bacillus anthracis*. The vaccine is prepared from a cell-free filtrate of *B. anthracis*, but no dead or live bacteria.
Drug Interactions
  Decreased Effect: Effect of vaccine may be decreased with chemotherapy, corticosteroids (high doses, ≥14 days), immunosuppressant agents, and radiation therapy; consider waiting at least 3 months between discontinuing therapy and administering vaccine.
  Pharmacodynamics/Kinetics Duration: Unknown; may be 1-2 years following two inoculations based on animal data
Pregnancy Risk Factor D

Anti-4 Alpha Integrin *see* Natalizumab *on page 1153*
Anti-CD11a *see* Efalizumab *on page 557*
Anti-CD20 Monoclonal Antibody *see* Rituximab *on page 1437*
Antidigoxin Fab Fragments, Ovine *see* Digoxin Immune Fab *on page 500*
Antidiuretic Hormone *see* Vasopressin *on page 1650*

Antihemophilic Factor (Human)
  (an tee hee moe FIL ik FAK tor HYU man)

U.S. Brand Names Hemofil M; Koāte®-DVI; Monarc-M™; Monoclate-P®
Canadian Brand Names Hemofil M
Generic Available Yes
Index Terms AHF (Human); Factor VIII (Human)
Pharmacologic Category Antihemophilic Agent; Blood Product Derivative
Use Prevention and treatment of hemorrhagic episodes in patients with hemophilia A (classic hemophilia); perioperative management of hemophilia A; can be of significant therapeutic value in patients with acquired factor VIII inhibitors not exceeding 10 Bethesda units/mL
(Continued)

131

Antihemophilic Factor (Human) *(Continued)*

Local Anesthetic/Vasoconstrictor Precautions No information available to require special precautions

Effects on Dental Treatment No significant effects or complications reported

Mechanism of Action Protein (factor VIII) in normal plasma which is necessary for clot formation and maintenance of hemostasis; activates factor X in conjunction with activated factor IX; activated factor X converts prothrombin to thrombin, which converts fibrinogen to fibrin, and with factor XIII forms a stable clot

Pharmacodynamics/Kinetics Half-life elimination: Mean: 8-27 hours

Pregnancy Risk Factor C

Antihemophilic Factor (Recombinant)

(an tee hee moe FIL ik FAK tor ree KOM be nant)

U.S. Brand Names Advate; Helixate® FS; Kogenate® FS; Recombinate; ReFacto®

Canadian Brand Names Helixate® FS; Kogenate®; Kogenate® FS; Recombinate; ReFacto®

Mexican Brand Names Koate DVI

Generic Available No

Index Terms AHF (Recombinant); Factor VIII (Recombinant); rAHF

Pharmacologic Category Antihemophilic Agent

Use Prevention and treatment of hemorrhagic episodes in patients with hemophilia A (classic hemophilia); perioperative management of hemophilia A; can be of significant therapeutic value in patients with acquired factor VIII inhibitors ≤10 Bethesda units/mL

Local Anesthetic/Vasoconstrictor Precautions No information available to require special precautions

Effects on Dental Treatment Key adverse event(s) related to dental treatment: Taste perversion.

Common Adverse Effects Actual frequency may vary by product.

>1%:

Central nervous system: Chills, dizziness, fever, headache, pain

Dermatologic: Pruritus

Gastrointestinal: Nausea, taste perversion

Hematologic: Hemorrhage

Local: Injection site pain

Neuromuscular & skeletal: Arthralgia, weakness

Respiratory: Dyspnea, nasopharyngitis, pharyngolaryngeal pain

Miscellaneous: Catheter thrombosis, factor VIII inhibitor formation

Mechanism of Action Factor VIII replacement, necessary for clot formation and maintenance of hemostasis. It activates factor X in conjunction with activated factor IX; activated factor X converts prothrombin to thrombin, which converts fibrinogen to fibrin, and with factor XIII forms a stable clot.

Pharmacodynamics/Kinetics Half-life elimination: Mean: 9-19 hours

Pregnancy Risk Factor C

Antihemophilic Factor/von Willebrand Factor Complex (Human)

(an tee hee moe FIL ik FAK tor von WILL le brand FAK tor KOM plex HYU man)

U.S. Brand Names Alphanate®; Humate-P®

Canadian Brand Names Humate-P®

Generic Available No

Index Terms AHF (Human); Factor VIII (Human); FVIII/vWF; vWF:RCof

Pharmacologic Category Antihemophilic Agent; Blood Product Derivative

Use

Prevention and treatment of hemorrhagic episodes in patients with hemophilia A (classical hemophilia) (Alphanate®, Humate-P®) or acquired factor VIII deficiency (Alphanate®)

Treatment of spontaneous bleeding in patients with von Willebrand disease (vWD) (mild, moderate, or severe) where use of desmopressin is known or suspected to be inadequate (Humate-P®)

Prophylaxis with surgical and/or invasive procedures in patients with vWD when desmopressin is either ineffective or contraindicated (Alphanate®)

Local Anesthetic/Vasoconstrictor Precautions No information available to require special precautions

Effects on Dental Treatment No significant effects or complications reported

Common Adverse Effects Frequency not defined.

Cardiovascular: Cardiorespiratory arrest, chest tightness, edema, femoral venous thrombosis, flushing, hypervolemia, orthostatic hypotension, shock, thromboembolic events, vasodilation

Central nervous system: Chills, dizziness, fever, headache, lethargy, pain, seizure, somnolence

Dermatologic: Itching, pruritus, rash, urticaria

Endocrine & metabolic: Parotid gland swelling

Gastrointestinal: Nausea, vomiting

Hematologic: Hematocrit decreased (moderate), hemorrhage, hemolysis, pseudothrombocytopenia (severe)

Hepatic: ALT increased

Local: Injection site stinging, phlebitis

Neuromuscular & skeletal: Extremity pain, joint pain, paresthesia, rigors

Respiratory: Dyspnea, pharyngitis, pulmonary embolus (large doses)

Miscellaneous: Allergic reactions, anaphylactic reactions, factor VIII inhibitor formation

Mechanism of Action Factor VIII and von Willebrand factor (vWF), obtained from pooled human plasma, are use to replace endogenous factor VIII and vWF in patients with hemophilia or vWD. Factor VIII in conjunction with activated factor IX, activates factor X which converts prothrombin to thrombin and fibrinogen to fibrin. vWF promotes platelet aggregation and adhesion to damaged vascular endothelium and acts as a stabilizing carrier protein for factor VIII. [Circulating levels of functional vWF are measured as ristocetin cofactor activity (vWF:RCof)]

Pharmacodynamics/Kinetics

Duration: vWD: Shortening of bleeding time sustained 22-26 hours postinfusion

Half-life elimination:

FVIII:C: 8-27 hours in patients with hemophilia A

vWF:RCof: 4-16 hours in patients with vWD

Pregnancy Risk Factor C

Anti-inhibitor Coagulant Complex
(an tee-in HI bi tor coe AG yoo lant KOM pleks)

U.S. Brand Names Autoplex® T [DSC]; Feiba VH

Canadian Brand Names Feiba VH Immuno

Generic Available No

Index Terms AICC; Coagulant Complex Inhibitor

Pharmacologic Category Activated Prothrombin Complex Concentrate (aPCC); Antihemophilic Agent; Blood Product Derivative

Use Hemophilia A & B patients with factor VIII inhibitors who are to undergo surgery or those who are bleeding

Local Anesthetic/Vasoconstrictor Precautions No information available to require special precautions

Effects on Dental Treatment No significant effects or complications reported

Common Adverse Effects Frequency not defined.

Cardiovascular: Blood pressure changes, flushing, MI, pulse rate changes

Central nervous system: Headache, lethargy

Dermatologic: Rash, urticaria

Gastrointestinal: Nausea

Hematologic: DIC

Miscellaneous: Allergic reaction, anamnestic response, infusion-related reactions (fever, chills)

Drug Interactions

Increased Effect/Toxicity: Coadministration of aminocaproic acid or tranexamic acid may increase risk of thrombosis.

Pregnancy Risk Factor C

Antipyrine and Benzocaine (an tee PYE reen & BEN zoe kane)

Related Information

Benzocaine *on page 195*

U.S. Brand Names A/B Otic; Allergen®; Aurodex

Canadian Brand Names Auralgan®

Generic Available Yes

Index Terms Benzocaine and Antipyrine

Pharmacologic Category Otic Agent, Analgesic; Otic Agent, Cerumenolytic

Use Temporary relief of pain and reduction of swelling associated with acute congestive and serous otitis media, swimmer's ear, otitis externa; facilitates ear wax removal

(Continued)

Antipyrine and Benzocaine *(Continued)*

Local Anesthetic/Vasoconstrictor Precautions No information available to require special precautions

Effects on Dental Treatment No significant effects or complications reported

Pregnancy Risk Factor C

Antiseptic Mouthwash *see* Mouthwash (Antiseptic) *on page 1128*

Antithrombin III (an tee THROM bin three)

U.S. Brand Names Thrombate III®
Canadian Brand Names Thrombate III®
Mexican Brand Names Atend
Generic Available No
Index Terms AT-III; Heparin Cofactor I
Pharmacologic Category Anticoagulant; Blood Product Derivative
Use Treatment of hereditary antithrombin III deficiency in connection with surgical procedures, obstetrical procedures, or thromboembolism
Unlabeled/Investigational Use Acquired antithrombin III deficiencies related to disseminated intravascular coagulation (DIC)
Local Anesthetic/Vasoconstrictor Precautions No information available to require special precautions
Effects on Dental Treatment No significant effects or complications reported
Common Adverse Effects 1% to 10%: Central nervous system: Dizziness (2%)
Mechanism of Action Antithrombin III is the primary physiologic inhibitor of *in vivo* coagulation. It is an alpha$_2$-globulin. Its principal actions are the inactivation of thrombin, plasmin, and other active serine proteases of coagulation, including factors IXa, Xa, XIa, and XIIa. The inactivation of proteases is a major step in the normal clotting process. The strong activation of clotting enzymes at the site of every bleeding injury facilitates fibrin formation and maintains normal hemostasis. Thrombosis in the circulation would be caused by active serine proteases if they were not inhibited by antithrombin III after the localized clotting process.
Drug Interactions
Increased Effect/Toxicity: Heparin's anticoagulant effects are potentiated by antithrombin III (half-life of antithrombin III is decreased by heparin). Risk of hemorrhage with antithrombin III may be increased by drotrecogin alfa, thrombolytic agents, oral anticoagulants (warfarin), treprostinil, and drugs which affect platelet function (eg, aspirin, NSAIDs, dipyridamole, ticlopidine, clopidogrel, and IIb/IIIa antagonists).
Pharmacodynamics/Kinetics Half-life elimination: Biologic: 2.5 days (immunologic assay); 3.8 days (functional AT-III assay). Half-life may be decreased following surgery, with hemorrhage, acute thrombosis, and/or during heparin administration.
Pregnancy Risk Factor B

Antithymocyte Globulin (Equine) (an te THY moe site GLOB yu lin, E kwine)

U.S. Brand Names Atgam®
Canadian Brand Names Atgam®
Generic Available No
Index Terms Antithymocyte Immunoglobulin; ATG; Horse Antihuman Thymocyte Gamma Globulin; Lymphocyte Immune Globulin
Pharmacologic Category Immune Globulin; Immunosuppressant Agent
Use Prevention and treatment of acute renal allograft rejection; treatment of moderate to severe aplastic anemia in patients not considered suitable candidates for bone marrow transplantation
Unlabeled/Investigational Use Prevention and treatment of other solid organ allograft rejection; prevention of graft-versus-host disease following bone marrow transplantation
Local Anesthetic/Vasoconstrictor Precautions No information available to require special precautions
Effects on Dental Treatment Key adverse event(s) related to dental treatment: Stomatitis
Common Adverse Effects
>10%:
Central nervous system: Fever, chills
Dermatologic: Pruritus, rash, urticaria
Hematologic: Leukopenia, thrombocytopenia

1% to 10%:

Cardiovascular: Bradycardia, chest pain, CHF, edema, encephalitis, hyper-/hypotension, myocarditis, tachycardia

Central nervous system: Agitation, headache, lethargy, lightheadedness, listlessness, seizure

Gastrointestinal: Diarrhea, nausea, stomatitis, vomiting

Hepatic: Hepatosplenomegaly, liver function tests abnormal

Local: Pain at injection site, phlebitis, thrombophlebitis, burning soles/palms

Neuromuscular & skeletal: Myalgia, back pain, arthralgia

Ocular: Periorbital edema

Renal: Abnormal renal function tests

Respiratory: Dyspnea, respiratory distress

Miscellaneous: Anaphylaxis, serum sickness, viral infection, night sweats, diaphoresis, lymphadenopathy

Mechanism of Action May involve elimination of antigen-reactive T lymphocytes (killer cells) in peripheral blood or alteration of T-cell function

Pharmacodynamics/Kinetics

Distribution: Poorly into lymphoid tissues; binds to circulating lymphocytes, granulocytes, platelets, bone marrow cells

Half-life elimination, plasma: 1.5-12 days

Excretion: Urine (~1%)

Pregnancy Risk Factor C

Antithymocyte Immunoglobulin *see* Antithymocyte Globulin (Equine) *on page 134*

Antitumor Necrosis Factor Apha (Human) *see* Adalimumab *on page 53*

Anti-VEGF Monoclonal Antibody *see* Bevacizumab *on page 212*

Antivert® *see* Meclizine *on page 1024*

Antizol® *see* Fomepizole *on page 739*

Anucort-HC® *see* Hydrocortisone *on page 836*

Anu-Med [OTC] *see* Phenylephrine *on page 1293*

Anusol-HC® *see* Hydrocortisone *on page 836*

Anusol® HC-1 [OTC] *see* Hydrocortisone *on page 836*

Anusol® Ointment [OTC] *see* Pramoxine *on page 1334*

Anzemet® *see* Dolasetron *on page 525*

APAP *see* Acetaminophen *on page 31*

APAP and Tramadol *see* Acetaminophen and Tramadol *on page 39*

Apatate® [OTC] *see* Vitamin B Complex Combinations *on page 1664*

ApexiCon™ *see* Diflorasone *on page 494*

ApexiCon™ E *see* Diflorasone *on page 494*

Aphrodyne® *see* Yohimbine *on page 1674*

Aphthasol® *see* Amlexanox *on page 100*

Apidra® *see* Insulin Glulisine *on page 885*

Aplisol® *see* Tuberculin Tests *on page 1628*

Aplonidine *see* Apraclonidine *on page 136*

Apokyn® *see* Apomorphine *on page 135*

Apomorphine (a poe MOR feen)

U.S. Brand Names Apokyn®

Generic Available No

Index Terms Apomorphine Hydrochloride; Apomorphine Hydrochloride Hemihydrate

Pharmacologic Category Anti-Parkinson's Agent, Dopamine Agonist

Use Treatment of hypomobility, "off" episodes with Parkinson's disease

Unlabeled/Investigational Use Treatment of erectile dysfunction

Local Anesthetic/Vasoconstrictor Precautions Apomorphine is one of the drugs confirmed to prolong the QT interval and is accepted as having a risk of causing torsade de pointes. The risk of drug-induced torsade de pointes is extremely low when a single QT interval prolonging drug is prescribed. In terms of epinephrine, it is not known what effect vasoconstrictors in the local anesthetic regimen will have in patients with a known history of congenital prolonged QT interval or in patients taking any medication that prolongs the QT interval. Until more information is obtained, it is suggested that the clinician consult with the physician prior to the use of a vasoconstrictor in suspected patients, and that the vasoconstrictor (epinephrine, levonordefrin [Neo-Cobefrin®]) be used with caution.

Effects on Dental Treatment Key adverse event(s) related to dental treatment: Orthostatic hypotension has been reported in significant numbers of patients.

(Continued)

Apomorphine *(Continued)*

Common Adverse Effects

>10%:

Cardiovascular: Chest pain/pressure or angina (15%)

Central nervous system: Drowsiness or somnolence (35%), dizziness or orthostatic hypotension (20%)

Gastrointestinal: Nausea and/or vomiting (30%)

Neuromuscular & skeletal: Falls (30%), dyskinesias (24% to 35%)

Respiratory: Yawning (40%), rhinorrhea (20%)

1% to 10%:

Cardiovascular: Edema (10%), vasodilation (3%), hypotension (2%), syncope (2%), CHF

Central nervous system: Hallucinations or confusion (10%), anxiety, depression, fatigue, headache, insomnia, pain

Dermatologic: Bruising

Endocrine & metabolic: Dehydration

Gastrointestinal: Constipation, diarrhea

Local: Injection site reactions

Neuromuscular & skeletal: Arthralgias, weakness

Miscellaneous: Diaphoresis increased

Mechanism of Action Stimulates postsynaptic D2-type receptors within the caudate putamen in the brain.

Drug Interactions

Cytochrome P450 Effect: Substrate (minor) of CYP1A2, 3A4, 2C19; **Inhibits** CYP1A2 (weak), 3A (weak), 2C19 (weak)

Increased Effect/Toxicity: Antihypertensives, vasodilators, and $5HT_3$ antagonists may increase risk of hypotension. QT_c prolongation may rarely occur with concurrent use of QT_c-prolonging agents. Effects of concomitant levodopa may be increased.

Decreased Effect: Typical antipsychotics may decrease the efficacy of apomorphine.

Pharmacodynamics/Kinetics

Onset: SubQ: Rapid

Distribution: V_d: Mean: 218 L

Metabolism: Not established; potential routes of metabolism include sulfation, N-demethylation, glucuronidation, and oxidation; catechol-O methyltransferase and nonenzymatic oxidation. CYP isoenzymes do not appear to play a significant role.

Half-life elimination: Terminal: 40 minutes

Time to peak, plasma: Improved motor scores: 20 minutes

Excretion: Urine 93% (as metabolites); feces 16%

Pregnancy Risk Factor C

Apomorphine Hydrochloride *see* Apomorphine *on page 135*

Apomorphine Hydrochloride Hemihydrate *see* Apomorphine *on page 135*

APPG *see* Penicillin G Procaine *on page 1270*

Apra Children's [OTC] *see* Acetaminophen *on page 31*

Apraclonidine *(a pra KLOE ni deen)*

U.S. Brand Names Iopidine®

Canadian Brand Names Iopidine®

Generic Available No

Index Terms Aplonidine; Apraclonidine Hydrochloride; p-Aminoclonidine

Pharmacologic Category Alpha₂ Agonist, Ophthalmic

Use Prevention and treatment of postsurgical intraocular pressure (IOP) elevation; short-term, adjunctive therapy in patients who require additional reduction of IOP

Local Anesthetic/Vasoconstrictor Precautions No information available to require special precautions

Effects on Dental Treatment Key adverse event(s) related to dental treatment: Xerostomia (normal salivary flow resumes upon discontinuation)

Mechanism of Action Apraclonidine is a potent alpha-adrenergic agent similar to clonidine; relatively selective for alpha₂-receptors but does retain some binding to alpha₁-receptors; appears to result in reduction of aqueous humor formation; its penetration through the blood-brain barrier is more polar than clonidine which reduces its penetration through the blood-brain barrier and suggests that its pharmacological profile is characterized by peripheral rather than central effects.

Pregnancy Risk Factor C

Apraclonidine Hydrochloride *see* Apraclonidine *on page 136*

Aprepitant (ap RE pi tant)

U.S. Brand Names Emend®
Generic Available No
Index Terms L 754030; MK 869
Pharmacologic Category Antiemetic; Substance P/Neurokinin 1 Receptor Antagonist
Use Prevention of acute and delayed nausea and vomiting associated with moderately- and highly-emetogenic chemotherapy in combination with a corticosteroid and 5-HT$_3$ receptor antagonist; prevention of postoperative nausea and vomiting (PONV)
Local Anesthetic/Vasoconstrictor Precautions No information available to require special precautions
Effects on Dental Treatment Key adverse event(s) related to dental treatment: Hiccups, stomatitis, and mucous membrane disorder.
Common Adverse Effects Note: Adverse reactions reported as part of a combination chemotherapy regimen or with general anesthesia.

>10%:
  Central nervous system: Fatigue (18% to 22%)
  Gastrointestinal: Nausea (7% to 13%), constipation (9% to 12%)
  Neuromuscular & skeletal: Weakness (3% to 18%)
  Miscellaneous: Hiccups (11%)
1% to 10%:
  Cardiovascular: Hypotension (6%), bradycardia (4%)
  Central nervous system: Dizziness (>0.5% to 7%)
  Endocrine & metabolic: Dehydration (6%), hot flushing (3%)
  Gastrointestinal: Diarrhea (6% to 10%), dyspepsia (8%), abdominal pain (5%), stomatitis (5%), epigastric discomfort (4%), gastritis (4%), mucous membrane disorder (3%), throat pain (3%), vomiting (3%)
  Hematologic: Neutropenia (3% to 9%), leukopenia (9%), hemoglobin decreased (2% to 5%)
  Hepatic: ALT increased (1% to 6%), AST increased (3%)
  Renal: BUN increased (5%), proteinuria (7%), serum creatinine increased (4%)
Mechanism of Action Prevents acute and delayed vomiting at the substance P/neurokinin 1 (NK$_1$) receptor; augments the antiemetic activity of the 5-HT$_3$ receptor antagonist and corticosteroid activity and inhibits both acute and delayed phases of cisplatin-induced emesis.
Drug Interactions
  Cytochrome P450 Effect: Substrate of CYP1A2 (minor), 2C19 (minor), 3A4 (major); **Inhibits** CYP2C9 (weak), 2C19 (weak), 3A4 (moderate); **Induces** CYP2C9 (weak), 3A4 (weak)
  Increased Effect/Toxicity: Use with cisapride or pimozide is contraindicated. CYP3A4 inhibitors may increase the levels/effects of aprepitant; example inhibitors include azole antifungals, clarithromycin, diclofenac, diltiazem, doxycycline, erythromycin, imatinib, isoniazid, nefazodone, nicardipine, propofol, protease inhibitors, quinidine, telithromycin, and verapamil. Aprepitant may increase the bioavailability of corticosteroids; dose adjustment of dexamethasone and methylprednisolone is needed. Aprepitant may increase the levels/effects of CYP3A4 substrates; example substrates include benzodiazepines, calcium channel blockers, ergot derivatives, mirtazapine, nateglinide, nefazodone, tacrolimus, and venlafaxine. Aprepitant may increase the levels/effects of pimecrolimus.
  Decreased Effect: CYP3A4 inducers may decrease the levels/effects of aprepitant; example inducers include aminoglutethimide, carbamazepine, nafcillin, nevirapine, phenobarbital, phenytoin, and rifamycins. Metabolism of warfarin may be induced; monitor INR following the start of each cycle. Efficacy of hormone-containing contraceptives (estrogens) may be decreased (plasma levels of ethinyl estradiol and norethindrone decreased with concomitant use).
Pharmacodynamics/Kinetics
  Distribution: V$_d$: 70 L; crosses the blood brain barrier
  Protein binding: >95%
  Metabolism: Extensively hepatic via CYP3A4 (major); CYP1A2 and CYP2C19 (minor); forms seven metabolites (weakly active)
  Bioavailability: 60% to 65%
  Half-life elimination: Terminal: 9-13 hours
  Time to peak, plasma: 4 hours
Pregnancy Risk Factor B

Apresazide [DSC] *see* Hydralazine and Hydrochlorothiazide *on page 818*
Apresoline [DSC] *see* HydrALAZINE *on page 817*

Apri® *see* Ethinyl Estradiol and Desogestrel *on page 621*
Aprodine® [OTC] *see* Triprolidine and Pseudoephedrine *on page 1624*

Aprotinin (a proe TYE nin)

U.S. Brand Names Trasylol®
Canadian Brand Names Trasylol®
Mexican Brand Names Protinin; Trasylol
Generic Available No
Pharmacologic Category Blood Product Derivative; Hemostatic Agent
Use Prevention of perioperative blood loss in patients who are at increased risk for blood loss and blood transfusions in association with cardiopulmonary bypass in coronary artery bypass graft surgery
Local Anesthetic/Vasoconstrictor Precautions No information available to require special precautions
Effects on Dental Treatment No significant effects or complications reported
Common Adverse Effects
>10%:
Central nervous system: Fever (15%)
Gastrointestinal: Nausea (11%)
1% to 10%:
Cardiovascular: Atrial flutter (6%), ventricular extrasystoles (6%), ventricular tachycardia (1% to 5%), heart failure (1% to 5%), arrhythmia (4%), supraventricular tachycardia (4%), bradycardia (1% to 2%), thrombosis (1% to 2%), bundle branch block (1% to 2%), cardiac arrest (1% to 2%), heart block (1% to 2%), hemorrhage (1% to 2%), myocardial ischemia (1% to 2%), pericardial effusion (1% to 2%), ventricular fibrillation (1% to 2%), shock (<1% to 2%)
Central nervous system: Agitation (1% to 2%), anxiety (1% to 2%), dizziness (1% to 2%), seizure (1% to 2%)
Endocrine & metabolic: Creatinine phosphokinase increase (2%), acidosis (1% to 2%), hyperglycemia (1% to 2%), hypervolemia (1% to 2%), hypokalemia
Gastrointestinal: Diarrhea (3%), dyspepsia (1% to 2%), gastrointestinal hemorrhage (1% to 2%)
Hematologic: Disseminated intravascular coagulation (DIC), leukocytosis (1% to 2%), prothrombin decreased (1% to 2%), thrombocytopenia (1% to 2%)
Hepatic: Jaundice (1% to 2%), hepatic failure (1% to 2%)
Neuromuscular & skeletal: Arthralgia (1% to 2%)
Renal: Serum creatinine increase of >0.5 mg/dL above baseline (high dose: 9%), oliguria (1% to 2%), tubular necrosis (1% to 2%), kidney failure (1%)
Respiratory: Hypoxia (2%), pulmonary hypertension (1% to 2%), pneumonia (1% to 2%), apnea (1% to 2%), cough increased (1% to 2%)
Miscellaneous: Sepsis (1% to 2%), multisystem organ failure (1% to 2%)
Mechanism of Action Bleeding from CABG surgery is thought to result from a systemic inflammatory response induced by the procedure. Contact of blood cells with the cardiopulmonary bypass (CPB) equipment leads to deregulated activation of the coagulation and fibrinolysis systems, with concurrent upregulation of proinflammatory cytokines. Aprotinin is a broad spectrum serine protease inhibitor that attenuates the coagulation, fibrinolytic and inflammatory pathways by interfering with the chemical mediators (thrombin, plasmin, kallikrein). Additionally, it protects platelet-expressed glycoproteins from mechanical shear forces. This preserves normal hemostatic activity through protease receptor-independent mechanisms (eg, via ADP, IIb/IIIa), while blocking CPB-induced thrombin-mediated aggregation.
Drug Interactions
Decreased Effect: Aprotinin decreases the effects of thrombolytics. The antihypertensive effects of captopril (and other ACE inhibitors) may be blocked.
Pharmacodynamics/Kinetics
Distribution: Extracellular space; renal phagolysosomes
Metabolism: Aprotinin is slowly degraded by lysosomal enzymes.
Half-life elimination: 2.5 hours (plasma); terminal: 10 hours
Excretion: Urine (25% to 40%; <10% as unchanged drug)
Pregnancy Risk Factor B

Aptivus® *see* Tipranavir *on page 1575*
Aquacare® [OTC] *see* Urea *on page 1632*
Aquachloral® Suprettes® *see* Chloral Hydrate *on page 327*
AquaLase™ *see* Balanced Salt Solution *on page 183*
Aquanil™ HC [OTC] *see* Hydrocortisone *on page 836*
Aquaphilic® With Carbamide [OTC] *see* Urea *on page 1632*
AquaSite® [OTC] *see* Artificial Tears *on page 147*

Arformoterol (ar for MOE ter ol)

U.S. Brand Names Brovana™
Generic Available No
Index Terms Arformoterol Tartrate; (R,R)-Formoterol L-Tartrate
Pharmacologic Category Beta₂-Adrenergic Agonist
Use Long-term maintenance treatment of bronchoconstriction in chronic obstructive pulmonary disease (COPD), including chronic bronchitis and emphysema
Local Anesthetic/Vasoconstrictor Precautions No information available to require special precautions
Effects on Dental Treatment No significant effects or complications reported
Common Adverse Effects 2% to 10%:
Cardiovascular: Chest pain (7%), peripheral edema (3%)
Central nervous system: Pain (8%)
Dermatologic: Rash (4%)
Gastrointestinal: Diarrhea (6%)
Neuromuscular & skeletal: Back pain (6%), leg cramps (4%)
Respiratory: Dyspnea (4%), sinusitis (5%), congestive conditions (2%)
Miscellaneous: Flu-like syndrome (3%)
Restrictions An FDA-approved medication guide must be distributed when dispensing an outpatient prescription (new or refill) where this medication is to be used without direct supervision of a healthcare provider. Medication guides are available at http://www.fda.gov/cder/Offices/ODS/medication_guides.htm.
Mechanism of Action Arformoterol, the (R,R)-enantiomer of the racemic formoterol, is a long-acting beta₂-agonist that relaxes bronchial smooth muscle by selective action on beta₂-receptors with little effect on cardiovascular system.
Drug Interactions
Cytochrome P450 Effect: Substrate of CY2D6 (minor) and CYP2C19 (minor)
Increased Effect/Toxicity: Atomoxetine may enhance the tachycardia effect of beta₂-agonists. Sympathomimetics may enhance the toxic/adverse effects of arformoterol.
Decreased Effect: Beta₂-agonists may diminish the bradycardia effect of beta-blockers (beta₁ selective). Alpha-/beta-blockers, beta-blockers (nonselective), and betahistine may diminish the therapeutic effect of beta₂-agonists.
Pharmacodynamics/Kinetics
Onset of action: 7-20 minutes
Peak effect: 1-3 hours
Absorption: A portion of inhaled dose is absorbed into systemic circulation
Protein binding: 52% to 65%
Metabolism: Hepatic via direct glucuronidation and secondarily via O-demethylation; CYP2D6 and CYP2C19 (to a lesser extent) involved in O-demethylation
Half-life elimination: 26 hours
Time to peak: 0.5-3 hours
Pregnancy Risk Factor C

Arformoterol Tartrate see Arformoterol on page 139

Argatroban (ar GA troh ban)

Related Information
Cardiovascular Diseases on page 1726
Generic Available No
(Continued)

Argatroban *(Continued)*

Pharmacologic Category Anticoagulant, Thrombin Inhibitor

Use Prophylaxis or treatment of thrombosis in adults with heparin-induced thrombocytopenia; adjunct to percutaneous coronary intervention (PCI) in patients who have or are at risk of thrombosis associated with heparin-induced thrombocytopenia

Local Anesthetic/Vasoconstrictor Precautions No information available to require special precautions

Effects on Dental Treatment Key adverse event(s) related to dental treatment: As with all anticoagulants, bleeding is a potential adverse effect of argatroban during dental surgery; risk is dependent on multiple variables, including the intensity of anticoagulation and patient susceptibility. Medical consult is suggested. It is unlikely that ambulatory patients presenting for dental treatment will be taking intravenous anticoagulant therapy.

Common Adverse Effects As with all anticoagulants, bleeding is the major adverse effect of argatroban. Hemorrhage may occur at virtually any site. Risk is dependent on multiple variables, including the intensity of anticoagulation and patient susceptibility.

>10%:

Cardiovascular: Chest pain (<1% to 15%), hypotension (7% to 11%)

Gastrointestinal: Gastrointestinal bleed (minor, 3% to 14%)

Genitourinary: Genitourinary bleed and hematuria (minor, 2% to 12%)

1% to 10%:

Cardiovascular: Cardiac arrest (6%), ventricular tachycardia (5%), bradycardia (5%), myocardial infarction (PCI: 4%), atrial fibrillation (3%), angina (2%), CABG-related bleeding (minor, 2%), myocardial ischemia (2%), cerebrovascular disorder (<1% to 2%), thrombosis (<1% to 2%)

Central nervous system: Fever (<1% to 7%), headache (5%), pain (5%), intracranial bleeding (1% to 4%)

Gastrointestinal: Nausea (5% to 7%), diarrhea (6%), vomiting (4% to 6%), abdominal pain (3% to 4%), bleeding (major, <1% to 2%)

Genitourinary: Urinary tract infection (5%)

Hematologic: Hemoglobin (<2 g/dL) and hematocrit (minor, 2% to 10%) decreased

Local: Bleeding at injection or access site (minor, 2% to 5%)

Neuromuscular & skeletal: Back pain (8%)

Renal: Abnormal renal function (3%)

Respiratory: Dyspnea (8% to 10%), cough (3% to 10%), hemoptysis (minor, <1% to 3%), pneumonia (3%)

Miscellaneous: Sepsis (6%), infection (4%)

Mechanism of Action A direct, highly-selective thrombin inhibitor. Reversibly binds to the active thrombin site of free and clot-associated thrombin. Inhibits fibrin formation; activation of coagulation factors V, VIII, and XIII; protein C; and platelet aggregation.

Drug Interactions

Cytochrome P450 Effect: Substrate of CYP3A4 (minor)

Increased Effect/Toxicity:

Drugs which affect platelet function (eg, aspirin, NSAIDs, dipyridamole, ticlopidine, clopidogrel), anticoagulants, or thrombolytics may potentiate the risk of hemorrhage. Sufficient time must pass after heparin therapy is discontinued; allow heparin's effect on the aPTT to decrease.

Concomitant use of argatroban with warfarin increases PT and INR greater than that of warfarin alone. Argatroban is commonly continued during the initiation of warfarin therapy to assure anticoagulation and to protect against possible transient hypercoagulability.

Pharmacodynamics/Kinetics

Onset of action: Immediate

Distribution: 174 mL/kg

Protein binding: Albumin: 20%; α_1-acid glycoprotein: 35%

Metabolism: Hepatic via hydroxylation and aromatization. Metabolism via CYP3A4/5 to four known metabolites plays a minor role. Unchanged argatroban is the major plasma component. Plasma concentration of metabolite M1 is 0% to 20% of the parent drug and is three- to fivefold weaker.

Half-life elimination: 39-51 minutes; Hepatic impairment: ≤181 minutes

Time to peak: Steady-state: 1-3 hours

Excretion: Feces (65%); urine (22%); low quantities of metabolites M2-4 in urine

Pregnancy Risk Factor B

Arginine (AR ji neen)

U.S. Brand Names R-Gene®
Generic Available No
Index Terms Arginine Hydrochloride
Pharmacologic Category Diagnostic Agent
Use Pituitary function test (growth hormone)
Unlabeled/Investigational Use Management of severe, uncompensated, metabolic alkalosis (pH ≥7.55) **after** optimizing therapy with sodium and potassium supplements
Local Anesthetic/Vasoconstrictor Precautions No information available to require special precautions
Effects on Dental Treatment No significant effects or complications reported
Mechanism of Action Stimulates pituitary release of growth hormone and prolactin through origins in the hypothalamus; patients with impaired pituitary function have lower or no increase in plasma concentrations of growth hormone after administration of arginine. Arginine hydrochloride has been used for severe metabolic alkalosis due to its high chloride content.

Arginine hydrochloride has been used investigationally to treat metabolic alkalosis. Arginine contains 475 mEq of hydrogen ions and 475 mEq of chloride ions/L. Arginine is metabolized by the liver to produce hydrogen ions. It may be used in patients with relative hepatic insufficiency because arginine combines with ammonia in the body to produce urea.
Pregnancy Risk Factor B

Arginine Hydrochloride *see* Arginine *on page 141*
8-Arginine Vasopressin *see* Vasopressin *on page 1650*
Aricept® *see* Donepezil *on page 526*
Aricept® ODT *see* Donepezil *on page 526*
Arimidex® *see* Anastrozole *on page 128*

Aripiprazole (ay ri PIP ray zole)

U.S. Brand Names Abilify®; Abilify® Discmelt™
Mexican Brand Names Abilify
Generic Available No
Index Terms BMS 337039; OPC-14597
Pharmacologic Category Antipsychotic Agent, Atypical
Use Treatment of schizophrenia; stabilization and maintenance therapy of bipolar disorder (with acute manic or mixed episodes); agitation associated with schizophrenia or bipolar mania
Unlabeled/Investigational Use Depression with psychotic features; aggression (children); bipolar disorder (children); conduct disorder (children); Tourette syndrome (children)
Local Anesthetic/Vasoconstrictor Precautions No information available to require special precautions
Effects on Dental Treatment Key adverse event(s) related to dental treatment: Extrapyramidal symptoms (similar to placebo) (see Dental Comment); xerostomia and changes in salivation (normal salivary flow resumes upon discontinuation).
Common Adverse Effects Unless otherwise noted, frequency of adverse reactions is shown as reported for oral administration.
>10%:
  Central nervous system: Headache (31%; injection 12%), agitation (25%), anxiety (20%), insomnia (20%), extrapyramidal symptoms (6% to 17%), somnolence (12% to 15%, dose related; injection 7%), akathisia (12% to 15%; injection 2%), lightheadedness (11%)
  Gastrointestinal: Nausea (16%; injection 9%), dyspepsia (15%; injection 1%), constipation (11% to 13%), vomiting (11%; injection 3%), weight gain (8% to 30%, highest frequency in patients with BMI <23)
1% to 10%:
  Cardiovascular: Edema (peripheral 2%), hypertension (2%), tachycardia, hypotension, bradycardia, chest pain
  Central nervous system: Abnormal dreams, confusion, delusion, depression, fever, hallucination, hostility, mania, nervousness, paranoid reaction, schizophrenic reaction, suicidal thought
  Dermatologic: Bruising, dry skin, skin ulcer
  Endocrine & metabolic: Dehydration
  Gastrointestinal: Salivation increased (3%), xerostomia (injection 1%), weight loss
  Genitourinary: Urinary incontinence, pelvic pain
(Continued)

Aripiprazole *(Continued)*

Hematologic: Anemia

Neuromuscular & skeletal: Tremor (4% to 9%), weakness (8%), myalgia (4%), neck pain, neck rigidity, muscle cramp, CPK increased, abnormal gait

Ocular: Blurred vision (3%), conjunctivitis

Respiratory: Rhinitis (4%), pharyngitis (4%), cough (3%), asthma, dyspnea, pneumonia, sinusitis

Miscellaneous: Accidental injury (5% to 6%), flu-like syndrome, diaphoresis

Mechanism of Action Aripiprazole is a quinolinone antipsychotic which exhibits high affinity for D_2, D_3, 5-HT_{1A}, and 5-HT_{2A} receptors; moderate affinity for D_4, 5-HT_{2C}, 5-HT_7, alpha$_1$ adrenergic, and H_1 receptors. It also possesses moderate affinity for the serotonin reuptake transporter; has no affinity for muscarinic (cholinergic) receptors. Aripiprazole functions as a partial agonist at the D_2 and 5-HT_{1A} receptors, and as an antagonist at the 5-HT_{2A} receptor.

Drug Interactions

Cytochrome P450 Effect: Substrate (major) of CYP2D6, 3A4

Increased Effect/Toxicity: CYP2D6 inhibitors may increase the levels/effects of aripiprazole; example inhibitors include chlorpromazine, delavirdine, fluoxetine, miconazole, paroxetine, pergolide, quinidine, quinine, ritonavir, and ropinirole. CYP3A4 inhibitors may increase the levels/effects of aripiprazole; example inhibitors include azole antifungals, clarithromycin, diclofenac, doxycycline, erythromycin, imatinib, isoniazid, nefazodone, nicardipine, propofol, protease inhibitors, quinidine, telithromycin, and verapamil. Manufacturer recommends a 50% reduction in dose during concurrent ketoconazole therapy. Similar reductions in dose may be required with other potent inhibitors. CNS depressants may increase adverse effects/toxicity of aripiprazole. Acetylcholinesterase inhibitors (central) may increase the risk of antipsychotic-related extrapyramidal symptoms. Lithium may increase neurotoxicity of antipsychotics.

Decreased Effect: CYP3A4 inducers may decrease the levels/effects of aripiprazole; example inducers include aminoglutethimide, carbamazepine, nafcillin, nevirapine, phenobarbital, phenytoin, and rifamycins. Manufacturer recommends a doubling of the aripiprazole dose when carbamazepine is added. Similar increases may be required with other inducers.

Pharmacodynamics/Kinetics

Onset: Initial: 1-3 weeks

Absorption: Well absorbed

Distribution: V_d: 4.9 L/kg

Protein binding: ≥99%, primarily to albumin

Metabolism: Hepatic, via CYP2D6, CYP3A4 (dehydro-aripiprazole metabolite has affinity for D_2 receptors similar to the parent drug and represents 40% of the parent drug exposure in plasma)

Bioavailability: I.M.: 100%; Tablet: 87%

Half-life elimination: Aripiprazole: 75 hours; dehydro-aripiprazole: 94 hours CYP2D6 poor metabolizers: Aripiprazole: 146 hours

Time to peak, plasma: I.M.: 1-3 hours; Tablet: 3-5 hours

With high-fat meal: Aripiprazole: Delayed by 3 hours; dehydro-aripiprazole: Delayed by 12 hours

Excretion: Feces (55%, ~18% unchanged drug); urine (25%, <1% unchanged drug)

Pregnancy Risk Factor C

Dental Comment Aripiprazole works differently from the classic antipsychotics, such as chlorpromazine, in that it does not appear to block central dopaminergic receptors, but rather seems to be a stabilizer of dopamine-serotonin central systems. The risk of extrapyramidal reactions such as pseudoparkinsonism, acute dystonic reactions, akathisia, and tardive dyskinesia are low and the frequencies reported are similar to placebo. Aripiprazole may be associated with neuroleptic malignant syndrome (NMS).

Aristocort® [DSC] *see* Triamcinolone *on page 1608*

Aristocort® A [DSC] *see* Triamcinolone *on page 1608*

Aristospan® *see* Triamcinolone *on page 1608*

Arixtra® *see* Fondaparinux *on page 741*

A.R.M® [OTC] *see* Chlorpheniramine and Pseudoephedrine *on page 340*

Armour® Thyroid *see* Thyroid *on page 1562*

Aromasin® *see* Exemestane *on page 662*

Arranon® *see* Nelarabine *on page 1157*

Artane *see* Trihexyphenidyl *on page 1619*

ArthriCare® for Women Extra Moisturizing [OTC] [DSC] *see* Capsaicin *on page 268*

ArthriCare® for Women Multi-Action [OTC] [DSC] *see* Capsaicin *on page 268*

ArthriCare® for Women Silky Dry [OTC] [DSC] *see* Capsaicin *on page 268*
ArthriCare® for Women Ultra Strength [OTC] [DSC] *see* Capsaicin *on page 268*
Arthrotec® *see* Diclofenac and Misoprostol *on page 489*

Articaine and Epinephrine (AR ti kane & ep i NEF rin)

Related Information
Epinephrine *on page 572*
Oral Pain *on page 1788*

U.S. Brand Names Septocaine® with epinephrine 1:100,000; Septocaine® with epinephrine 1:200,000; Zorcaine™

Canadian Brand Names Astracaine® with epinephrine 1:200,000; Astracaine® with epinephrine forte 1:100,000; Septanest® N; Septanest® SP; Ultracaine® D-S; Ultracaine® D-S Forte; Zorcaine™

Generic Available No

Index Terms Epinephrine and Articaine Hydrochloride

Pharmacologic Category Local Anesthetic

Dental Use Local, infiltrative, or conductive anesthesia in both simple and complex dental and periodontal procedures

Local Anesthetic/Vasoconstrictor Precautions No information available to require special precautions (see Dental Comment)

Effects on Dental Treatment No significant effects or complications reported

Significant Adverse Effects Adverse reactions to Septocaine™ are characteristic of those associated with other amide-type local anesthetics; adverse reactions to this group of drugs may also result from excessive plasma levels which may be due to overdosage, unintentional intravascular injection, or slow metabolic degradation.

≥1% (in controlled trial of 882 patients):
  Central nervous system: Headache (4%), paresthesia (1%)
  Gastrointestinal: Gingivitis (1%)
  Miscellaneous: Pain (body as a whole 13%), facial edema (1%)
<1% (adverse and intercurrent events recorded in 1 or more patients in controlled trials, occurring at an overall rate of <1%, and considered clinically significant): Abdominal pain, accidental injury, arthralgia, asthenia, back pain, constipation, diarrhea, dizziness, dry mouth, dysmenorrhea, dyspepsia, ear pain, ecchymosis, edema, facial paralysis, glossitis, gum hemorrhage, hemorrhage, hyperesthesia, lymphadenopathy, malaise, methemoglobinemia, migraine, mouth ulceration, myalgia, nausea, neck pain, nervousness, neuropathy, osteomyelitis, pharyngitis, pruritus, rhinitis, salivation increased, skin disorder, somnolence, stomatitis, syncope, tachycardia, taste perversion, thirst, tongue edema, tooth disorder, vomiting
Additional adverse reactions reported with articaine and epinephrine: Arrhythmia, myocardial depression, asthma, convulsions, allergic reactions, injection site reactions, tissue necrosis

Dental Usual Dosing Adults:
Infiltration: Injection volume of 4% solution: 0.5-2.5 mL; total dose: 20-100 mg
Nerve block: Injection volume of 4% solution: 0.5-3.4 mL; total dose: 20-136 mg
Oral surgery: Injection volume of 4% solution: 1-5.1 mL; total dose: 40-204 mg
Note: These dosages are guides only; other dosages may be used; however, do not exceed maximum recommended dose

Special populations: The clinician is reminded that these doses serve only as a guide to the amount of anesthetic required for most routine procedures. The actual volumes to be used depend upon a number of factors, such as type and extent of surgical procedure, depth of anesthesia, degree of muscular relaxation, and condition of the patient. In all cases, the smallest dose that will produce the desired result should be given. Dosages should be reduced for pediatric patients, elderly patients, and patients with cardiac and/or liver disease.

Dosage Summary of recommended volumes and concentrations for various types of anesthetic procedures; dosages (administered by submucosal injection and/or nerve block) apply to normal healthy adults:

Infiltration: Injection volume of 4% solution: 0.5-2.5 mL; total dose: 20-100 mg
Nerve block: Injection volume of 4% solution: 0.5-3.4 mL; total dose: 20-136 mg
Oral surgery: Injection volume of 4% solution: 1-5.1 mL; total dose: 40-204 mg
Note: These dosages are guides only; other dosages may be used; however, do not exceed maximum recommended dose

Special populations: The clinician is reminded that these doses serve only as a guide to the amount of anesthetic required for most routine procedures. The actual volumes to be used depend upon a number of factors, such as type and
(Continued)

Articaine and Epinephrine *(Continued)*

extent of surgical procedure, depth of anesthesia, degree of muscular relaxation, and condition of the patient. In all cases, the smallest dose that will produce the desired result should be given. Dosages should be reduced for pediatric patients, elderly patients, and patients with cardiac and/or liver disease.

Children <4 years: Safety and efficacy have not been established

Children 4-16 years (dosages in a clinical trial of 61 patients):

Simple procedures: 0.76-5.65 mg/kg (0.9-5.1 mL) was administered safely to 51 patients

Complex procedures: 0.37-7.48 mg/kg (0.7-3.9 mL) was administered safely to 10 patients

Note: Approximately 13% of the pediatric patients required additional injections for complete anesthesia

Geriatric patients (dosages in a clinical trial):

65-75 years:

Simple procedures: 0.43-4.76 mg/kg (0.9-11.9 mL) was administered safely to 35 patients

Complex procedures: 1.05-4.27 mg/kg (1.3-6.8 mL) was administered safely to 19 patients

≥75 years:

Simple procedures: 0.78-4.76 mg/kg (1.3-11.9 mL) was administered safely to 7 patients

Complex procedures: 1.12-2.17 mg/kg (1.3-5.1 mL) was administered safely to 4 patients

Note: Approximately 6% of the patients 65-75 years of age (none of the patients ≥75 years of age) required additional injections for complete anesthesia, compared to 11% of the patients 17-65 years of age who required additional injections.

Maximum recommended dosages:

Children (use in pediatric patients <4 years is not recommended): Not to exceed 7 mg/kg (0.175 mL/kg) **or** 3.2 mg/lb (0.0795 mL/lb) of body weight

Adults (normal, healthy): Submucosal infiltration and/or nerve block: Not to exceed 7 mg/kg (0.175 mL/kg) **or** 3.2 mg/lb (0.0795 mL/lb) of body weight

The following numbers of dental cartridges (1.7 mL) provide the indicated amounts of articaine hydrochloride 4% and epinephrine 1:100,000:

1 cartridge provides 68 mg articaine HCl (4%) and 0.017 mg vasoconstrictor (epinephrine 1:100,000)

2 cartridges provides 136 mg articaine HCl (4%) and 0.034 mg vasoconstrictor (epinephrine 1:100,000)

3 cartridges provides 204 mg articaine HCl (4%) and 0.051 mg vasoconstrictor (epinephrine 1:100,000)

4 cartridges provides 272 mg articaine HCl (4%) and 0.068 mg vasoconstrictor (epinephrine 1:100,000)

5 cartridges provides 340 mg articaine HCl (4%) and 0.085 mg vasoconstrictor (epinephrine 1:100,000)

6 cartridges provides 408 mg articaine HCl (4%) and 0.102 mg vasoconstrictor (epinephrine 1:100,000)

7 cartridges provides 476 mg articaine HCl (4%) and 0.119 mg vasoconstrictor (epinephrine 1:100,000)

8 cartridges provides 544 mg articaine HCl (4%) and 0.136 mg vasoconstrictor (epinephrine 1:100,000)

The following numbers of dental cartridges (1.7 mL) provide the indicated amounts of articaine hydrochloride 4% and epinephrine 1:200,000:

1 cartridge provides 68 mg articaine HCl (4%) and 0.0085 mg vasoconstrictor (epinephrine 1:200,000)

2 cartridges provides 136 mg articaine HCl (4%) and 0.017 mg vasoconstrictor (epinephrine 1:200,000)

3 cartridges provides 204 mg articaine HCl (4%) and 0.026 mg vasoconstrictor (epinephrine 1:200,000)

4 cartridges provides 272 mg articaine HCl (4%) and 0.034 mg vasoconstrictor (epinephrine 1:200,000)

5 cartridges provides 340 mg articaine HCl (4%) and 0.043 mg vasoconstrictor (epinephrine 1:200,000)

6 cartridges provides 408 mg articaine HCl (4%) and 0.051 mg vasoconstrictor (epinephrine 1:200,000)

7 cartridges provides 476 mg articaine HCl (4%) and 0.060 mg vasoconstrictor (epinephrine 1:200,000)

8 cartridges provides 544 mg articaine HCl (4%) and 0.068 mg vasoconstrictor (epinephrine 1:200,000)

Mechanism of Action Local anesthetics block the generation and conduction of nerve impulses, presumably by increasing the threshold for electrical excitation in the nerve, by slowing the propagation of the nerve impulse, and by reducing the rate of rise of the action potential. In general, the progression of anesthesia is related to the diameter, myelination, and conduction velocity of the affected nerve fibers. Clinically, the order of loss of nerve function is as follows: 1) pain, 2) temperature, 3) touch, 4) proprioception, and 5) skeletal muscle tone.

Contraindications Hypersensitivity to local anesthetics of the amide type or any component of the formulation

Warnings/Precautions Intravascular injections should be avoided; aspiration should be performed prior to administration; the needle must be repositioned until no return of blood can be elicited by aspiration; however, absence of blood in the syringe does not guarantee that intravascular injection has been avoided. **Accidental intravascular injection may be associated with convulsions, followed by CNS or cardiorespiratory depression and coma, ultimately progressing to respiratory arrest.** Dental practitioners and/or clinicians using local anesthetic agents should be well trained in diagnosis and management of emergencies that may arise from the use of these agents. Resuscitative equipment, oxygen, and other resuscitative drugs should be available for immediate use.

Contains epinephrine, which can cause local tissue necrosis or systemic toxicity, usual precautions for epinephrine administration should be observed. Administration of articaine HCl with epinephrine results in a three- to fivefold increase in plasma epinephrine concentrations compared to baseline; however, in healthy adults, it does not appear to be associated with marked increases in blood pressure or heart rate, except in the case of accidental intravascular injection.

Products may contain sodium metabisulfite, which may cause allergic-type reactions (including anaphylactic symptoms, and life-threatening or less severe asthmatic episodes) in certain susceptible patients. The overall prevalence of the sulfite sensitivity in the general population is unknown, and is seen more frequently in asthmatic than in nonasthmatic persons.

To avoid serious adverse effects and high plasma levels, the lowest dosage resulting in effective anesthesia should be administered. Repeated doses may cause significant increases in blood levels with each repeated dose due to the possibility of accumulation of the drug or its metabolites. Tolerance to elevated blood levels varies with patient status. Reduced dosages, commensurate with age and physical condition, should be given to debilitated patients, elderly patients, acutely-ill patients, and pediatric patients. Use caution in patients with heart block.

Local anesthetic solutions containing a vasoconstrictor should be used cautiously. Patients with peripheral vascular disease or hypertensive vascular disease may exhibit exaggerated vasoconstrictor response, possibly resulting in ischemic injury or necrosis. It should also be used cautiously in patients during or following the administration of a potent general anesthetic agent, since cardiac arrhythmias may occur under these conditions.

Systemic absorption of local anesthetics may produce CNS and cardiovascular effects. Changes in cardiac conduction, excitability, refractoriness, contractility, and peripheral vascular resistance are minimal at blood concentrations produced by therapeutic doses. However, toxic blood concentrations depress cardiac conduction and excitability, which may lead to AV block, ventricular arrhythmias, and cardiac arrest (sometimes resulting in death). In addition, myocardial contractility is depressed and peripheral vasodilation occurs, leading to decreased cardiac output and arterial blood pressure.

Careful and constant monitoring of cardiovascular and respiratory (adequacy of ventilation) vital signs and the patient's state of consciousness should be done following each local anesthetic injection; at such times, restlessness, anxiety, tinnitus, dizziness, blurred vision, tremors, depression, or drowsiness may be early warning signs of CNS toxicity. Methemoglobinemia has been reported with articaine. Treatment is primarily symptomatic and supportive. Methemoglobinemia may be treated with methylene blue, 1-2 mg/kg I.V. infused over several minutes.

In vitro studies show that ~5% to 10% of articaine is metabolized by the human liver microsomal P450 isoenzyme system; however, no studies have been performed in patient with liver dysfunction, and caution should be used in patients with severe hepatic disease. Use with caution in patients with impaired cardiovascular function, since they may be less able to compensate for function changes associated with prolonged AV conduction produced by these drugs. (Continued)

Articaine and Epinephrine *(Continued)*

Small doses of local anesthetics injected into dental blocks may produce adverse reactions similar to systemic toxicity seen in unintentional intravascular injections at larger doses. Confusion, convulsions, respiratory depression and/ or respiratory arrest, and cardiovascular stimulation or depression have been reported. These reactions may be due to intra-arterial injection of the local anesthetic with retrograde flow to the cerebral circulation. Patients receiving such blocks should be observed constantly with resuscitative equipment and personnel trained in treatment of adverse reactions immediately available. Dosage recommendations should not be exceeded.

Drug Interactions

MAO inhibitors: Administration of local anesthetic solutions containing epinephrine may produce severe, prolonged hypertension.

Phenothiazines, butyrophenones: May reduce or reverse the pressor effects of epinephrine; concurrent use of these agents should be avoided; in situations when concurrent therapy is necessary, careful patient monitoring is essential.

Tricyclic antidepressants: Pressor response to I.V. epinephrine, norepinephrine, and phenylephrine may be enhanced in patients receiving TCAs (**Note:** Effect is unlikely with epinephrine or levonordefrin dosages typically administered as infiltration in combination with local anesthetics).

Pharmacodynamics/Kinetics

Onset of action: 1-6 minutes

Duration: Complete anesthesia: ~1 hour

Metabolism: Hepatic via plasma carboxyesterase to articainic acid (inactive)

Half-life elimination: Articaine: 1.8 hours; Articainic acid: 1.5 hours

Excretion: Urine (primarily as metabolites)

Pregnancy Risk Factor C

Lactation Excretion in breast milk unknown/use caution

Breast-Feeding Considerations It is not known whether articaine is excreted in human milk.

Dosage Forms Excipient information presented when available (limited, particularly for generics); consult specific product labeling.

Excipient information presented when available (limited, particularly for generics); consult specific product labeling. [CAN] = Canadian brand name

Injection, solution:

Astracaine® with epinephrine 1:200,000 [CAN]: Articaine 4% and epinephrine 1:200,000 (1.8 mL) [not available in the U.S.]

Astracaine® Forte with epinephrine forte 1:100,000 [CAN]: Articaine 4% and epinephrine 1:100,000 (1.8 mL) [not available in the U.S.]

Septanest® N [CAN]: Articaine 4% and epinephrine 1:200,000 (1.7 mL) [not available in the U.S.]

Septanest® SP [CAN]: Articaine 4% and epinephrine 1:100,000 (1.7 mL) [not available in the U.S.]

Septocaine® with epinephrine 1:100,000: Articaine hydrochloride 4% and epinephrine bitartrate 1:100,000 (1.7 mL) [contains sodium metabisulfite]

Septocaine® with epinephrine 1:200,000: Articaine hydrochloride 4% and epinephrine bitartrate 1:200,000 (1.7 mL) [contains sodium metabisulfite]

Ultracaine DS® [CAN]: Articaine hydrochloride 4% and epinephrine 1:200,000 (1.7 mL) [contains sodium metabisulfite; not available in the U.S.]

Ultracaine DS Forte® [CAN]: Articaine hydrochloride 4% and epinephrine 1:100,000 (1.7 mL) [contains sodium metabisulfite; not available in the U.S.]

Zorcaine™: Articaine hydrochloride 4% and epinephrine bitartrate 1:100,000 (1.7 mL) [contains sodium metabisulfite]

Dental Comment

Septocaine™ (articaine hydrochloride 4% and epinephrine 1:100,000) is the first FDA approval in 30 years of a new local dental anesthetic providing complete pulpal anesthesia for approximately 1 hour. Chemically, articaine contains both an amide linkage and an ester linkage, making it chemically unique in the class of local anesthetics. Since it contains the ester linkage, articaine HCl is rapidly metabolized by plasma carboxyesterase to its primary metabolite, articainic acid, which is an inactive product of this metabolism. According to the manufacturer, *in vitro* studies show that the human liver microsomal P450 isoenzyme system metabolizes approximately 5% to 10% of available articaine with nearly quantitative conversion to articainic acid. The elimination half-life of articaine is about 1.8 hours, and that of articainic acid is about 1.5 hours. Articaine is excreted primarily through urine with 53% to 57% of the administered dose eliminated in the first 24 hours following submucosal administration. Articainic acid is the primary metabolite in urine. A minor metabolite, articainic acid glucuronide, is also excreted in the urine. Articaine constitutes only 2% of the total dose excreted in urine.

The anesthetic efficacy of the articaine 4% with 1:200,000 epinephrine (A/200) was compared to that of articaine 4% with 1:100,000 (A/100) using electric pulp tester to assess anesthesia using 63 subjects after either maxillary infiltration (Moore, 2006) or inferior alveolar block (Hersh, 2006).

After maxillary infiltration of 1 mL of each formula, the onset times to anesthesia were 3.1 ± 2.3 minutes for articaine 4% and 1:200,000 epinephrine (A/200), 3 ± 2.1 minutes for articaine 4% and 1:100,000 epinephrine (A/100), 3 ± 2 minutes for articaine 4% with no epinephrine (A/no). These three mean times of onset were not statistically different. Durations of anesthesia were 41.6 ± 21.1 minutes A/200, 45 ± 23.6 minutes A/100, 13.3 ± 6.8 minutes for A/no. There was no statistically significant difference between the durations elicited by the A/200 and A/100 formulations (Moore, 2006). In the second trial of the study, also using 63 subjects, the investigators administered an inferior alveolar nerve block injection of one cartridge (1.7 mL) using a standard intra-oral injection technique for inferior alveolar block anesthesia. Pulpal anesthesia was measured again using the pulp tester.

The onset times to anesthesia were 4.7 ± 2.6 minutes A/200, 4.2 ± 2.8 minutes A/100, and 4.3 ± 2.5 minutes for A/no. There were no statistically significant differences in these times to onset. Durations of anesthesia were 51.2 ± 55.9 minutes A/200, 61.8 ± 59 minutes A/100, and 49.7 ± 44.6 minutes for A/no. There were no statistically significant differences in the duration between A/200, A/100, and A/no formulations (Hersh, 2006).

Selected Readings

Budenz AW, "Local Anesthetics in Dentistry: Then and Now," *J Calif Dent Assoc*, 2003, 31(5):388-96.

Dower JS Jr, "A Review of Paresthesia in Association With Administration of Local Anesthesia," *Dent Today*, 2003, 22(2):64-9.

Finder RL and Moore PA, "Adverse Drug Reactions to Local Anesthesia," *Dent Clin North Am*, 2002, 46(4):747-57, x.

Haas DA, "An Update on Local Anesthetics in Dentistry," *J Can Dent Assoc*, 2002, 68(9):546-51.

Hawkins JM and Moore PA, "Local Anesthesia: Advances in Agents and Techniques," *Dent Clin North Am*, 2002, 46(4):719-32, ix.

Hersh EV, Giannakopoulos H, Levin LM, et al, "The Pharmacokinetics and Cardiovascular Effects of High-Dose Articaine With 1:100,000 and 1:200,000 Epinephrine," *J Am Dent Assoc*, 2006, 137(11):1562-71.

"Injectable Local Anesthetics," *J Am Dent Assoc*, 2003, 134(5):628-9.

Malamed SF, Gagnon S, Leblanc D, "A Comparison Between Articaine HCl and Lidocaine HCl in Pediatric Dental Patients," *Pediatr Dent*, 2000, 22(4):307-11.

Malamed SF, "Allergy and Toxic Reactions to Local Anesthetics," *Dent Today*, 2003, 22(4):114-6, 118-21.

Malamed SF, Gagnon S, Leblanc D, "Articaine Hydrochloride: A Study of the Safety of a New Amide Local Anesthetic," *J Am Dent Assoc*, 2001, 132(2):177-85.

Malamed SF, Gagnon S, Leblanc D, "Efficacy of Articaine: A New Amide Local Anesthetic," *J Am Dent Assoc*, 2000, 131(5):635-42.

Moore PA, Boynes SG, Hersh EV, et al, "The Anesthetic Efficacy of 4 Percent Articaine 1:200,000 Epinephrine: Two Controlled Clinical Trials," *J Am Dent Assoc*, 2006, 137(11):1562-71.

Schertzer ER Jr, "Articaine vs lidocaine," *J Am Dent Assoc*, 2000, 131(9):1248, 1250.

Weaver JM, "Articaine, A New Local Anesthetic for American Dentists: Will It Supersede Lidocaine?" *Anesth Prog*, 1999, 46(4):111-2.

Wynn RL, Bergman SA, and Meiller TF, "Paresthesia Associated With Local Anesthetics: A Perspective on Articaine," *Gen Dent*, 2003, 51(6):498-501.

Artificial Tears (ar ti FISH il tears)

U.S. Brand Names Akwa Tears® [OTC]; AquaSite® [OTC]; Bion® Tears [OTC]; HypoTears [OTC]; HypoTears PF [OTC]; Liquifilm® Tears [OTC]; Moisture® Eyes [OTC]; Moisture® Eyes PM [OTC]; Murine® Tears [OTC]; Murocel® [OTC]; Nature's Tears® [OTC]; Nu-Tears® [OTC]; Nu-Tears® II [OTC]; OcuCoat® [OTC]; OcuCoat® PF [OTC]; Puralube® Tears [OTC]; Refresh® [OTC]; Refresh Plus® [OTC]; Refresh Tears® [OTC]; Soothe® [OTC]; Systane® [OTC]; Systane® Free [OTC]; Teargen® [OTC]; Teargen® II [OTC]; Tearisol® [OTC]; Tears Again® [OTC]; Tears Naturale® [OTC]; Tears Naturale® Free [OTC]; Tears Naturale® II [OTC]; Tears Plus® [OTC]; Tears Renewed® [OTC]; Ultra Tears® [OTC]; Viva-Drops® [OTC]

Canadian Brand Names Teardrops®

Generic Available Yes

Index Terms Hydroxyethylcellulose; Polyvinyl Alcohol

Pharmacologic Category Ophthalmic Agent, Miscellaneous

Use Ophthalmic lubricant; for relief of dry eyes and eye irritation

Local Anesthetic/Vasoconstrictor Precautions No information available to require special precautions

Effects on Dental Treatment No significant effects or complications reported

Pregnancy Risk Factor C

Ascorbic Acid (a SKOR bik AS id)

U.S. Brand Names C-500-GR™ [OTC]; Cecon® [OTC]; Cevi-Bid® [OTC]; C-Gram [OTC]; Dull-C® [OTC]; Vita-C® [OTC]
Canadian Brand Names Proflavanol C™; Revitalose C-1000®
Mexican Brand Names Cevalin; Redoxon Forte
Generic Available Yes
Index Terms Vitamin C
Pharmacologic Category Vitamin, Water Soluble
Use Prevention and treatment of scurvy; acidify the urine
Unlabeled/Investigational Use Investigational: In large doses, to decrease the severity of "colds"; dietary supplementation; a 20-year study was recently completed involving 730 individuals which indicates a possible decreased risk of death by stroke when ascorbic acid at doses ≥45 mg/day was administered
Local Anesthetic/Vasoconstrictor Precautions No information available to require special precautions
Effects on Dental Treatment No significant effects or complications reported
Common Adverse Effects 1% to 10%: Renal: Hyperoxaluria with large doses
Mechanism of Action Not fully understood; necessary for collagen formation and tissue repair; involved in some oxidation-reduction reactions as well as other metabolic pathways, such as synthesis of carnitine, steroids, and catecholamines and conversion of folic acid to folinic acid
Drug Interactions
Increased Effect/Toxicity: Ascorbic acid enhances iron absorption from the GI tract. Concomitant ascorbic acid taken with oral contraceptives may increase contraceptive effect.
Decreased Effect: Ascorbic acid and fluphenazine may decrease fluphenazine levels. Ascorbic acid and warfarin may decrease anticoagulant effect. Changes in dose of ascorbic acid when taken with oral contraceptives may reduce the contraceptive effect.
Pharmacodynamics/Kinetics
Absorption: Oral: Readily absorbed; an active process thought to be dose dependent
Distribution: Large
Metabolism: Hepatic via oxidation and sulfation
Excretion: Urine (with high blood levels)
Pregnancy Risk Factor A/C (dose exceeding RDA recommendation)

Ascorbic Acid and Ferrous Sulfate see Ferrous Sulfate and Ascorbic Acid on page 688
Ascriptin® [OTC] see Aspirin on page 149
Ascriptin® Maximum Strength [OTC] see Aspirin on page 149
Asendin [DSC] see Amoxapine on page 106
Asmanex® Twisthaler® see Mometasone Furoate on page 1118

Asparaginase (a SPEAR a ji nase)

U.S. Brand Names Elspar®
Canadian Brand Names Elspar®; Kidrolase®
Generic Available No
Index Terms E. coli Asparaginase; Erwinia Asparaginase; L-asparaginase; NSC-106977 (Erwinia); NSC-109229 (E. coli)
Pharmacologic Category Antineoplastic Agent, Miscellaneous
Use Treatment of acute lymphocytic leukemia
Unlabeled/Investigational Use Treatment of lymphoma
Local Anesthetic/Vasoconstrictor Precautions No information available to require special precautions
Effects on Dental Treatment Key adverse event(s) related to dental treatment: Stomatitis
Common Adverse Effects Note: Immediate effects: Fever, chills, nausea, and vomiting occur in 50% to 60% of patients.

>10%:
Central nervous system: Fatigue, fever, chills, depression, agitation, seizure (10% to 60%), somnolence, stupor, confusion, coma (25%)
Endocrine & metabolic: Hyperglycemia (10%)
Gastrointestinal: Nausea, vomiting (50% to 60%), anorexia, abdominal cramps (70%), acute pancreatitis (15%, may be severe in some patients)
Hematologic: Hypofibrinogenemia and depression of clotting factors V and VIII, variable decrease in factors VII and IX, severe protein C deficiency and decrease in antithrombin III (may be dose limiting or fatal)

Hepatic: Transaminases, bilirubin, and alkaline phosphatase increased (transient)

Hypersensitivity: Acute allergic reactions (fever, rash, urticaria, arthralgia, hypotension, angioedema, bronchospasm, anaphylaxis (15% to 35%); may be dose limiting in some patients, may be fatal)

Renal: Azotemia (66%)

1% to 10%:

Endocrine & metabolic: Hyperuricemia

Gastrointestinal: Stomatitis

Mechanism of Action Asparaginase inhibits protein synthesis by hydrolyzing asparagine to aspartic acid and ammonia. Leukemia cells, especially lymphoblasts, require exogenous asparagine; normal cells can synthesize asparagine. Asparaginase is cycle-specific for the G_1 phase.

Drug Interactions

Increased Effect/Toxicity: Asparaginase (I.V.) may increase the toxicity of vincristine and prednisone.

Decreased Effect: Asparaginase may diminish the effects of methotrexate.

Pharmacodynamics/Kinetics

Absorption: I.M.: Produces peak blood levels 50% lower than those from I.V. administration

Distribution: V_d: 4-5 L/kg; 70% to 80% of plasma volume; <1% CSF penetration

Metabolism: Systemically degraded

Half-life elimination: I.M.: 39-49 hours; I.V.: 8-30 hours

Time to peak, plasma: I.M.: 14-24 hours

Pregnancy Risk Factor C

Aspart Insulin *see* Insulin Aspart *on page 883*

Aspercin [OTC] *see* Aspirin *on page 149*

Aspercreme® [OTC] *see* Triethanolamine Salicylate *on page 1617*

Aspergum® [OTC] *see* Aspirin *on page 149*

Aspirin (AS pir in)

Related Information

Cardiovascular Diseases *on page 1726*

Oral Pain *on page 1788*

Rheumatoid Arthritis, Osteoarthritis, and Osteoporosis *on page 1759*

U.S. Brand Names Ascriptin® [OTC]; Ascriptin® Maximum Strength [OTC]; Aspercin [OTC]; Aspergum® [OTC]; Aspirtab [OTC]; Bayer® Aspirin Extra Strength [OTC]; Bayer® Aspirin Regimen Adult Low Dose [OTC]; Bayer® Aspirin Regimen Children's [OTC]; Bayer® Aspirin Regimen Regular Strength [OTC]; Bayer® Genuine Aspirin [OTC]; Bayer® Plus Extra Strength [OTC]; Bayer® Women's Aspirin Plus Calcium [OTC]; Buffasal [OTC]; Bufferin® [OTC]; Bufferin® Extra Strength [OTC]; Buffinol [OTC]; Easprin®; Ecotrin® [OTC]; Ecotrin® Low Strength [OTC]; Ecotrin® Maximum Strength [OTC]; Genacote™ [OTC]; Halfprin® [OTC]; St. Joseph® Adult Aspirin [OTC]; ZORprin®

Canadian Brand Names Asaphen; Asaphen E.C.; Entrophen®; Novasen

Mexican Brand Names Adiro; Ecotrin

Generic Available Yes: Excludes gum

Index Terms Acetylsalicylic Acid; ASA

Pharmacologic Category Salicylate

Dental Use Treatment of postoperative pain

Use Treatment of mild-to-moderate pain, inflammation, and fever; may be used as prophylaxis of myocardial infarction; prophylaxis of stroke and/or transient ischemic episodes; management of rheumatoid arthritis, rheumatic fever, osteoarthritis, and gout (high dose); adjunctive therapy in revascularization procedures (coronary artery bypass graft [CABG], percutaneous transluminal coronary angioplasty [PTCA], carotid endarterectomy), stent implantation

Unlabeled/Investigational Use Low doses have been used in the prevention of pre-eclampsia, complications associated with autoimmune disorders such as lupus or antiphospholipid syndrome

Local Anesthetic/Vasoconstrictor Precautions No information available to require special precautions

Effects on Dental Treatment Key adverse event(s) related to dental treatment: As with all drugs which may affect hemostasis, bleeding is associated with aspirin. Hemorrhage may occur at virtually any site; risk is dependent on multiple variables including dosage, concurrent use of multiple agents which alter hemostasis, and patient susceptibility. Many adverse effects of aspirin are dose related, and are rare at low dosages. Other serious reactions are idiosyncratic, related to allergy or individual sensitivity (see Dental Comment).

Aspirin and clopidogrel (Plavix®) in combination is the primary prevention strategy against stent thrombosis after placement of drug-eluting metal stents (Continued)

Aspirin *(Continued)*

in coronary patients. Premature discontinuation of this combination antiplatelet therapy strongly increases the risk of a catastrophic event of stent thrombosis leading to myocardial infarction and/or death, so says a science advisory issued in January 2007 from the American Heart Association in collaboration with the American Dental Association and other professional healthcare organizations. The advisory stresses a 12-month therapy of aspirin and Plavix® combination after placement of a drug-eluting stent in order to prevent thrombosis at the stent site. Any elective surgery should be postponed for 1 year after stent implantation, and if surgery must be performed, consideration should be given to continuing the antiplatelet therapy during the perioperative period in high-risk patients with drug-eluting stents.

This advisory was issued from a science panel made up of representatives from the American Heart Association (AHA), the American College of Cardiology, the Society for Cardiovascular Angiography and Interventions, the American College of Surgeons, the American Dental Association (ADA), and the American College of Physicians (Grines, 2007).

Significant Adverse Effects As with all drugs which may affect hemostasis, bleeding is associated with aspirin. Hemorrhage may occur at virtually any site. Risk is dependent on multiple variables including dosage, concurrent use of multiple agents which alter hemostasis, and patient susceptibility. Many adverse effects of aspirin are dose related, and are extremely rare at low dosages. Other serious reactions are idiosyncratic, related to allergy or individual sensitivity. Accurate estimation of frequencies is not possible.

Cardiovascular: Hypotension, tachycardia, dysrhythmias, edema

Central nervous system: Fatigue, insomnia, nervousness, agitation, confusion, dizziness, headache, lethargy, cerebral edema, hyperthermia, coma

Dermatologic: Rash, angioedema, urticaria

Endocrine & metabolic: Acidosis, hyperkalemia, dehydration, hypoglycemia (children), hyperglycemia, hypernatremia (buffered forms)

Gastrointestinal: Nausea, vomiting, dyspepsia, epigastric discomfort, heartburn, stomach pain, gastrointestinal ulceration (6% to 31%), gastric erosions, gastric erythema, duodenal ulcers

Hematologic: Anemia, disseminated intravascular coagulation (DIC), prothrombin times prolonged, coagulopathy, thrombocytopenia, hemolytic anemia, bleeding, iron-deficiency anemia

Hepatic: Hepatotoxicity, transaminases increased, hepatitis (reversible)

Neuromuscular & skeletal: Rhabdomyolysis, weakness, acetabular bone destruction (OA)

Otic: Hearing loss, tinnitus

Renal: Interstitial nephritis, papillary necrosis, proteinuria, renal failure (including cases caused by rhabdomyolysis), BUN increased, serum creatinine increased

Respiratory: Asthma, bronchospasm, dyspnea, laryngeal edema, hyperpnea, tachypnea, respiratory alkalosis, noncardiogenic pulmonary edema

Miscellaneous: Anaphylaxis, prolonged pregnancy and labor, stillbirths, low birth weight, peripartum bleeding, Reye's syndrome

Postmarketing and/or case reports: Colonic ulceration, esophageal stricture, esophagitis with esophageal ulcer, esophageal hematoma, oral mucosal ulcers (aspirin-containing chewing gum), coronary artery spasm, conduction defect and atrial fibrillation (toxicity), delirium, ischemic brain infarction, colitis, rectal stenosis (suppository), cholestatic jaundice, periorbital edema, rhinosinusitis

Dental Usual Dosing Postoperative pain:

Analgesic and antipyretic: Oral, rectal:

Children: 10-15 mg/kg/dose every 4-6 hours, up to a total of 4 g/day

Adults: 325-650 mg every 4-6 hours up to 4 g/day

Anti-inflammatory: Oral: Initial:

Children: 60-90 mg/kg/day in divided doses; usual maintenance: 80-100 mg/kg/day divided every 6-8 hours; monitor serum concentrations

Adults: 2.4-3.6 g/day in divided doses; usual maintenance: 3.6-5.4 g/day; monitor serum concentrations

Dosage

Children:

Analgesic and antipyretic: Oral, rectal: 10-15 mg/kg/dose every 4-6 hours, up to a total of 4 g/day

Anti-inflammatory: Oral: Initial: 60-90 mg/kg/day in divided doses; usual maintenance: 80-100 mg/kg/day divided every 6-8 hours; monitor serum concentrations

Antiplatelet effects: Adequate pediatric studies have not been performed; pediatric dosage is derived from adult studies and clinical experience and is not well established; suggested doses have ranged from 3-5 mg/kg/day to

5-10 mg/kg/day given as a single daily dose. Doses are rounded to a convenient amount (eg, $\frac{1}{2}$ of 80 mg tablet).

Mechanical prosthetic heart valves: 6-20 mg/kg/day given as a single daily dose (used in combination with an oral anticoagulant in children who have systemic embolism despite adequate oral anticoagulation therapy (INR 2.5-3.5) and used in combination with low-dose anticoagulation (INR 2-3) and dipyridamole when full-dose oral anticoagulation is contraindicated)

Blalock-Taussig shunts: 3-5 mg/kg/day given as a single daily dose

Kawasaki disease: Oral: 80-100 mg/kg/day divided every 6 hours; monitor serum concentrations; after fever resolves: 3-5 mg/kg/day once daily; in patients without coronary artery abnormalities, give lower dose for at least 6-8 weeks or until ESR and platelet count are normal; in patients with coronary artery abnormalities, low-dose aspirin should be continued indefinitely

Antirheumatic: Oral: 60-100 mg/kg/day in divided doses every 4 hours

Adults:

Analgesic and antipyretic: Oral, rectal: 325-650 mg every 4-6 hours up to 4 g/day

Anti-inflammatory: Oral: Initial: 2.4-3.6 g/day in divided doses; usual maintenance: 3.6-5.4 g/day; monitor serum concentrations

Myocardial infarction prophylaxis: 75-325 mg/day; use of a lower aspirin dosage has been recommended in patients receiving ACE inhibitors

Acute myocardial infarction: 160-325 mg/day (have patient chew tablet if not taking aspirin before presentation)

CABG: 75-325 mg/day starting 6 hours following procedure; if bleeding prevents administration at 6 hours after CABG, initiate as soon as possible

PTCA: Initial: 80-325 mg/day starting 2 hours before procedure; longer pretreatment durations (up to 24 hours) should be considered if lower dosages (80-100 mg) are used

Stent implantation: Oral: 325 mg 2 hours prior to implantation and 160-325 mg daily thereafter

Carotid endarterectomy: 81-325 mg/day preoperatively and daily thereafter

Acute stroke: 160-325 mg/day, initiated within 48 hours (in patients who are not candidates for thrombolytics and are not receiving systemic anticoagulation)

Stroke prevention/TIA: 30-325 mg/day (dosages up to 1300 mg/day in 2-4 divided doses have been used in clinical trials)

Pre-eclampsia prevention (unlabeled use): 60-80 mg/day during gestational weeks 13-26 (patient selection criteria not established)

Dosing adjustment in renal impairment: Cl_{cr} <10 mL/minute: Avoid use.
Hemodialysis: Dialyzable (50% to 100%)

Dosing adjustment in hepatic disease: Avoid use in severe liver disease.

Mechanism of Action Inhibits prostaglandin synthesis, acts on the hypothalamus heat-regulating center to reduce fever, blocks prostaglandin synthetase action which prevents formation of the platelet-aggregating substance thromboxane A_2

Contraindications Hypersensitivity to salicylates, other NSAIDs, or any component of the formulation; asthma; rhinitis; nasal polyps; inherited or acquired bleeding disorders (including factor VII and factor IX deficiency); do not use in children (<16 years of age) for viral infections (chickenpox or flu symptoms), with or without fever, due to a potential association with Reye's syndrome; pregnancy (3rd trimester especially)

Warnings/Precautions Use with caution in patients with platelet and bleeding disorders, renal dysfunction, dehydration, erosive gastritis, or peptic ulcer disease. Heavy ethanol use (>3 drinks/day) can increase bleeding risks. Avoid use in severe renal failure or in severe hepatic failure. Discontinue use if tinnitus or impaired hearing occurs. Caution in mild-to-moderate renal failure (only at high dosages). Patients with sensitivity to tartrazine dyes, nasal polyps, and asthma may have an increased risk of salicylate sensitivity. Surgical patients should avoid ASA if possible, for 1-2 weeks prior to surgery, to reduce the risk of excessive bleeding (except in patients with cardiac stents that have not completed their full course of dual antiplatelet therapy [aspirin, clopidogrel]; patient-specific situations need to be discussed with cardiologist; AHA/ACC/SCAI/ACS/ADA Science Advisory provides recommendations).

When used for self-medication (OTC labeling): Children and teenagers who have or are recovering from chickenpox or flu-like symptoms should not use this product. Changes in behavior (along with nausea and vomiting) may be an early sign of Reye's syndrome; patients should be instructed to contact their healthcare provider if these occur.

Drug Interactions Substrate of CYP2C9 (minor)

ACE inhibitors: The effects of ACE inhibitors may be blunted by aspirin administration, particularly at higher dosages.

Buspirone increases aspirin's free % *in vitro*.

(Continued)

Aspirin (Continued)

Carbonic anhydrase inhibitors and corticosteroids have been associated with alteration in salicylate serum concentrations.

Heparin and low molecular weight heparins: Concurrent use may increase the risk of bleeding.

Methotrexate serum levels may be increased; consider discontinuing aspirin 2-3 days before high-dose methotrexate treatment or avoid concurrent use.

NSAIDs may increase the risk of gastrointestinal adverse effects and bleeding. Serum concentrations of some NSAIDs may be decreased by aspirin. Ibuprofen, and possibly other COX-1 inhibitors, may reduce the cardioprotective effects of aspirin. Avoid giving prior to aspirin therapy or on a regular basis in patients with CAD.

Platelet inhibitors (IIb/IIIa antagonists): Risk of bleeding may be increased.

Probenecid effects may be antagonized by aspirin.

Sulfonylureas: The effects of older sulfonylurea agents (tolazamide, tolbutamide) may be potentiated due to displacement from plasma proteins. This effect does not appear to be clinically significant for newer sulfonylurea agents (glyburide, glipizide, glimepiride).

Valproic acid may be displaced from its binding sites which can result in toxicity.

Verapamil may potentiate the prolongation of bleeding time associated with aspirin.

Warfarin and oral anticoagulants may increase the risk of bleeding.

Ethanol/Nutrition/Herb Interactions

Ethanol: Avoid ethanol (may enhance gastric mucosal damage).

Food: Food may decrease the rate but not the extent of oral absorption.

Folic acid: Hyperexcretion of folate; folic acid deficiency may result, leading to macrocytic anemia.

Iron: With chronic aspirin use and at doses of 3-4 g/day, iron-deficiency anemia may result.

Sodium: Hypernatremia resulting from buffered aspirin solutions or sodium salicylate containing high sodium content. Avoid or use with caution in CHF or any condition where hypernatremia would be detrimental.

Benedictine liqueur, prunes, raisins, tea, and gherkins: Potential salicylate accumulation.

Fresh fruits containing vitamin C: Displace drug from binding sites, resulting in increased urinary excretion of aspirin.

Herb/Nutraceutical: Avoid cat's claw, dong quai, evening primrose, feverfew, garlic, ginger, ginkgo, red clover, horse chestnut, green tea, ginseng (all have additional antiplatelet activity). Limit curry powder, paprika, licorice; may cause salicylate accumulation. These foods contain 6 mg salicylate/100 g. An ordinarily American diet contains 10-200 mg/day of salicylate.

Dietary Considerations Take with food or large volume of water or milk to minimize GI upset.

Pharmacodynamics/Kinetics

Duration: 4-6 hours

Absorption: Rapid

Distribution: V_d: 10 L; readily into most body fluids and tissues

Metabolism: Hydrolyzed to salicylate (active) by esterases in GI mucosa, red blood cells, synovial fluid, and blood; metabolism of salicylate occurs primarily by hepatic conjugation; metabolic pathways are saturable

Bioavailability: 50% to 75% reaches systemic circulation

Half-life elimination: Parent drug: 15-20 minutes; Salicylates (dose dependent): 3 hours at lower doses (300-600 mg), 5-6 hours (after 1 g), 10 hours with higher doses

Time to peak, serum: ~1-2 hours

Excretion: Urine (75% as salicyluric acid, 10% as salicylic acid)

Pregnancy Risk Factor C/D (full-dose aspirin in 3rd trimester - expert analysis)

Lactation Enters breast milk/use caution

Breast-Feeding Considerations Low amounts of aspirin can be found in breast milk. Milk/plasma ratios ranging from 0.03-0.3 have been reported. Peak levels in breast milk are reported to be at ~9 hours after a dose. Metabolic acidosis was reported in one infant following an aspirin dose of 3.9 g/day in the mother. The AAP states that aspirin should be used with caution while breast-feeding. The WHO considers occasional doses of aspirin to be compatible with breast-feeding, but to avoid long-term therapy and consider monitoring the infant for adverse effects. Other sources suggest avoiding aspirin while breast-feeding due to the theoretical risk of Reye's syndrome.

Dosage Forms Excipient information presented when available (limited, particularly for generics); consult specific product labeling. [DSC] = Discontinued product

Caplet:

Bayer® Aspirin Extra Strength: 500 mg

Bayer® Aspirin Regimen Regular Strength: 325 mg

Bayer® Genuine Aspirin: 325 mg

Bayer® Plus Extra Strength: 500 mg [contains calcium carbonate]

Bayer® Women's Aspirin Plus Calcium: 81 mg [contains elemental calcium 300 mg]

Caplet, buffered:

Ascriptin® Maximum Strength: 500 mg [contains aluminum hydroxide, calcium carbonate, and magnesium hydroxide]

Gelcap:

Bayer® Aspirin Extra Strength: 500 mg [DSC]

Gum:

Aspergum®: 227 mg [cherry or orange flavor]

Suppository, rectal: 300 mg, 600 mg

Tablet: 325 mg

Aspercin, Aspirtab: 325 mg

Bayer® Genuine Aspirin: 325 mg

Tablet, buffered: 325 mg

Ascriptin®: 325 mg [contains aluminum hydroxide, calcium carbonate, and magnesium hydroxide]

Buffasal: 325 mg [contains magnesium oxide]

Bufferin®: 325 mg [contains calcium carbonate, magnesium oxide, and magnesium carbonate; contains calcium 65 mg/tablet, magnesium 50 mg/tablet]

Bufferin® Extra Strength: 500 mg [contains calcium carbonate, magnesium oxide, and magnesium carbonate; contains calcium 90 mg/tablet, magnesium 70 mg/tablet]

Buffinol: 325 mg [contains magnesium oxide]

Tablet, chewable: 81 mg

Bayer® Aspirin Regimen Children's: 81 mg [cherry or orange flavor]

St. Joseph® Adult Aspirin: 81 mg [orange flavor]

Tablet, controlled release (ZORprin®): 800 mg

Tablet, enteric coated: 81 mg, 325 mg, 500 mg, 650 mg, 975 mg

Bayer® Aspirin Regimen Adult Low Dose, Ecotrin® Low Strength, St. Joseph Adult Aspirin: 81 mg

Easprin®: 975 mg

Ecotrin®, Genacote™: 325 mg

Ecotrin® Maximum Strength: 500 mg

Halfprin®: 81 mg, 162 mg

Dental Comment There is no scientific evidence to warrant discontinuance of aspirin prior to dental surgery. Patients taking one aspirin tablet daily as an antithrombotic and who require dental surgery should be given special consideration in consultation with the physician before removal of the aspirin relative to prevention of postoperative bleeding.

The Food and Drug Administration (FDA), has issued a letter updating information and considerations regarding the use of ibuprofen (400 mg doses) in patients who are taking low dose aspirin (81 mg, immediate release; not enteric coated) for cardioprotection and stroke prevention. Ibuprofen, at these doses, may interfere with aspirin's antiplatelet effect depending upon when it is administered. Patients initiated on aspirin first (for ~1 week) then ibuprofen (400 mg tid for 10 days) seem to maintain aspirin's platelet effect (Cryer B, 2005). Ibuprofen has the greatest impact on aspirin if administered less than 8 hours before aspirin (Catella-Lawson F, 2001).

Patients may require counseling about the appropriate timing of ibuprofen dosing in relationship to aspirin therapy. With occasional use of ibuprofen, a clinically-significant interaction with aspirin in unlikely. To avoid interference during chronic dosing, a single dose of ibuprofen should be taken 30-120 minutes after aspirin ingestion or at least 8 hours should elapse after ibuprofen dosing before giving aspirin (FDA, 2006; Catella-Lawson F, 2001).

The clinical implications of the interaction are unclear. There have not been any clinical endpoint studies conducted at this time. Avoidance of this interaction is potentially important because aspirin's vascular protection could be decreased or negated.

Other nonselective NSAIDs may have potential for a similar interaction with aspirin. Such has been described with naproxen (Capone ML, 2005). Acetaminophen does not appear to interfere with the antiplatelet effect of aspirin. Other clinical scenarios (use of smaller ibuprofen doses, other aspirin products, other doses of aspirin) have not been evaluated.

Additional information is available at: http://www.fda.gov/cder/drug/infopage/aspirin/default.htm.

Selected Readings

Daniel NG, Goulet J, Bergeron M, et al, "Antiplatelet Drugs: Is There a Surgical Risk?" *J Can Dent Assoc*, 2002, 68(11):683-7.

(Continued)

Aspirin *(Continued)*

Forbes JA, Butterworth GA, Burchfield WH, et al, "Evaluation of Ketorolac, Aspirin, and an Aceta-minophen-Codeine Combination in Postoperative Oral Surgery Pain," *Pharmacotherapy*, 1990, 10(6 Pt 2):77S-93S.

Grines CL, Bonow RO, Casey DE, et al, "AHA/ACC/SCAI/ACS/ADA Science Advisory, Prevention of Premature Discontinuation of Dual Antiplatelet Therapy in Patients With Coronary Artery Stents. A Science Advisory From the American Heart Association, American College of Cardiology, Society of Cardiovascular Angiography and Interventions, American College of Surgeons, and American Dental Association With Representation From The Amercian College Of Physicians," *Circulation*, 2007, 115(6):813-8. Available at http://www.acc.org/qualityandscience/clinical/pdfs/Final_Dual_Antiplatelet_Statement_010507.pdf.

Hurlen M, Erikssen J, Smith P, et al, "Comparison of Bleeding Complications of Warfarin and Warfarin Plus Acetylsalicylic Acid: A Study in 3166 Outpatients," *J Intern Med*, 1994, 236(3):299-304.

Jeske AH, Suchko GD, ADA Council on Scientific Affairs and Division of Science, et al, "Lack of a Scientific Basis for Routine Discontinuation of Oral Anticoagulation Therapy Before Dental Treatment," *J Am Dent Assoc*, 2003, 134(11):1492-7.

Little JW, Miller CS, Henry RG, et al, "Antithrombotic Agents: Implications in Dentistry," *Oral Surg Oral Med Oral Pathol Oral Radiol Endod*, 2002, 93(5):544-51.

Schrodi J, Recio L, Fiorellini J, et al, "The Effect of Aspirin on the Periodontal Parameter Bleeding on Probing," *J Periodontol*, 2002, 73(8):871-6.

Scully C and Wolff A, "Oral Surgery in Patients on Anticoagulant Therapy," *Oral Surg Oral Med Oral Pathol Oral Radiol Endod*, 2002, 94(1):57-64.

Aspirin, Acetaminophen, and Caffeine *see* Acetaminophen, Aspirin, and Caffeine *on page 41*

Aspirin and Carisoprodol *see* Carisoprodol and Aspirin *on page 286*

Aspirin and Dipyridamole *(AS pir in & dye peer ID a mole)*

Related Information
Aspirin *on page 149*
Cardiovascular Diseases *on page 1726*
Dipyridamole *on page 516*

U.S. Brand Names Aggrenox®
Canadian Brand Names Aggrenox®
Generic Available No
Index Terms Aspirin and Extended-Release Dipyridamole; Dipyridamole and Aspirin
Pharmacologic Category Antiplatelet Agent
Use Reduction in the risk of stroke in patients who have had transient ischemia of the brain or completed ischemic stroke due to thrombosis

Local Anesthetic/Vasoconstrictor Precautions No information available to require special precautions

Effects on Dental Treatment Key adverse event(s) related to dental treatment: As with all drugs which may affect hemostasis, bleeding is associated with aspirin. Hemorrhage may occur at virtually any site; risk is dependent on multiple variables including dosage, concurrent use of multiple agents which alter hemostasis, and patient susceptibility. Many adverse effects of aspirin are dose related, and are rare at low dosages. Other serious reactions are idiosyncratic, related to allergy or individual sensitivity (see Dental Comment).

Common Adverse Effects
>10%:
  Central nervous system: Headache (38%; tolerance usually develops)
  Gastrointestinal: Dyspepsia, abdominal pain (18%), nausea (16%), diarrhea (13%)
1% to 10%:
  Cardiovascular: Cardiac failure (2%), syncope (1%)
  Central nervous system: Pain (6%), seizure (2%), fatigue (6%), malaise (2%), amnesia (2%), confusion (1%), somnolence (1%)
  Dermatologic: Purpura (1%)
  Gastrointestinal: Vomiting (8%), bleeding (4%), rectal bleeding (2%), hemorrhoids (1%), hemorrhage (1%), anorexia (1%)
  Hematologic: Anemia (2%)
  Neuromuscular & skeletal: Back pain (5%), weakness (2%), arthralgia (6%), arthritis (2%), arthrosis (1%), myalgia (1%)
  Respiratory: Cough (2%), upper respiratory tract infection (1%), epistaxis (2%)

Mechanism of Action The antithrombotic action results from additive antiplatelet effects. Dipyridamole inhibits the uptake of adenosine into platelets, endothelial cells, and erythrocytes. Aspirin inhibits platelet aggregation by irreversible inhibition of platelet cyclooxygenase and thus inhibits the generation of thromboxane A_2.

Drug Interactions

Cytochrome P450 Effect: Aspirin: **Substrate** of CYP2C9 (minor)

Increased Effect/Toxicity: See individual agents.

Decreased Effect: See individual agents.

Pharmacodynamics/Kinetics See individual agents.

Pregnancy Risk Factor D

Dental Comment There is no scientific evidence to warrant discontinuance of aspirin prior to dental surgery. Patients taking one aspirin tablet daily as an antithrombotic and who require dental surgery should be given special consideration in consultation with the physician before removal of the aspirin relative to prevention of postoperative bleeding.

The Food and Drug Administration (FDA), has issued a letter updating information and considerations regarding the use of ibuprofen (400 mg doses) in patients who are taking low dose aspirin (81 mg, immediate release; not enteric coated) for cardioprotection and stroke prevention. Ibuprofen, at these doses, may interfere with aspirin's antiplatelet effect depending upon when it is administered. Patients initiated on aspirin first (for ~1 week) then ibuprofen (400 mg tid for 10 days) seem to maintain aspirin's platelet effect (Cryer B, 2005). Ibuprofen has the greatest impact on aspirin if administered less than 8 hours before aspirin (Catella-Lawson F, 2001).

Patients may require counseling about the appropriate timing of ibuprofen dosing in relationship to aspirin therapy. With occasional use of ibuprofen, a clinically-significant interaction with aspirin in unlikely. To avoid interference during chronic dosing, a single dose of ibuprofen should be taken 30-120 minutes after aspirin ingestion or at least 8 hours should elapse after ibuprofen dosing before giving aspirin (FDA, 2006; Catella-Lawson F, 2001).

The clinical implications of the interaction are unclear. There have not been any clinical endpoint studies conducted at this time. Avoidance of this interaction is potentially important because aspirin's vascular protection could be decreased or negated.

Other nonselective NSAIDs may have potential for a similar interaction with aspirin. Such has been described with naproxen (Capone ML, 2005). Acetaminophen does not appear to interfere with the antiplatelet effect of aspirin. Other clinical scenarios (use of smaller ibuprofen doses, other aspirin products, other doses of aspirin) have not been evaluated.

Additional information is available at: http://www.fda.gov/cder/drug/infopage/aspirin/default.htm.

Aspirin and Extended-Release Dipyridamole *see* Aspirin and Dipyridamole *on page 154*

Aspirin and Hydrocodone *see* Hydrocodone and Aspirin *on page 825*

Aspirin and Meprobamate *see* Meprobamate and Aspirin *on page 1049*

Aspirin and Oxycodone *see* Oxycodone and Aspirin *on page 1231*

Aspirin and Pravastatin (AS pir in & PRA va stat in)

Related Information

Aspirin *on page 149*

Pravastatin *on page 1335*

U.S. Brand Names Pravigard™ PAC [DSC]

Canadian Brand Names PravASA

Generic Available No

Index Terms Buffered Aspirin and Pravastatin Sodium; Pravastatin and Aspirin

Pharmacologic Category Antilipemic Agent, HMG-CoA Reductase Inhibitor; Salicylate

Use Combination therapy in patients who need treatment with aspirin and pravastatin to reduce the incidence of cardiovascular events, including myocardial infarction, stroke, and death

Local Anesthetic/Vasoconstrictor Precautions No information available to require special precautions

Effects on Dental Treatment Key adverse event(s) related to dental treatment: Aspirin: As with all drugs which may affect hemostasis, bleeding is associated with aspirin. Hemorrhage may occur at virtually any site; risk is dependent on multiple variables including dosage, concurrent use of multiple agents which alter hemostasis, and patient susceptibility. Many adverse effects of aspirin are dose related, and are rare at low dosages. Other serious reactions are idiosyncratic, related to allergy or individual sensitivity (see Dental Comment).

Common Adverse Effects Clinical studies of this combination product have not been conducted. See individual agents.

(Continued)

Aspirin and Pravastatin *(Continued)*

Mechanism of Action
Aspirin: Inhibits prostaglandin synthesis, acts on the hypothalamus heat-regulating center to reduce fever, blocks prostaglandin synthetase action which prevents formation of the platelet-aggregating substance thromboxane A_2

Pravastatin: Competitive inhibitor of 3-hydroxy-3-methylglutaryl coenzyme A (HMG-CoA) reductase, which is the rate-limiting enzyme involved in *de novo* cholesterol synthesis.

Drug Interactions
Cytochrome P450 Effect:
Aspirin: **Substrate** of CYP2C9 (minor)
Pravastatin: **Substrate** of CYP3A4 (minor); **Inhibits** CYP2C9 (weak), 2D6 (weak), 3A4 (weak)
Increased Effect/Toxicity: See individual agents.
Decreased Effect: See individual agents.
Pharmacodynamics/Kinetics See individual agents.

Pregnancy Risk Factor X

Dental Comment Aspirin: There is no scientific evidence to warrant discontinuance of aspirin prior to dental surgery. Patients taking one aspirin tablet daily as an antithrombotic and who require dental surgery should be given special consideration in consultation with the physician before removal of the aspirin relative to prevention of postoperative bleeding.

Aspirin, Caffeine and Acetaminophen *see* Acetaminophen, Aspirin, and Caffeine *on page 41*

Aspirin, Caffeine, and Butalbital *see* Butalbital, Aspirin, and Caffeine *on page 250*

Aspirin, Caffeine, and Propoxyphene *see* Propoxyphene, Aspirin, and Caffeine *on page 1371*

Aspirin, Caffeine, Codeine, and Butalbital *see* Butalbital, Aspirin, Caffeine, and Codeine *on page 251*

Aspirin, Carisoprodol, and Codeine *see* Carisoprodol, Aspirin, and Codeine *on page 287*

Aspirin Free Anacin® Maximum Strength [OTC] *see* Acetaminophen *on page 31*

Aspirin, Orphenadrine, and Caffeine *see* Orphenadrine, Aspirin, and Caffeine *on page 1213*

Aspirtab [OTC] *see* Aspirin *on page 149*

Astelin® *see* Azelastine *on page 175*

AsthmaNefrin® *see* Epinephrine (Racemic) *on page 576*

Astramorph/PF™ *see* Morphine Sulfate *on page 1123*

AT-III *see* Antithrombin III *on page 134*

Atacand® *see* Candesartan *on page 264*

Atacand HCT™ *see* Candesartan and Hydrochlorothiazide *on page 265*

Atazanavir *(a ta za NA veer)*

U.S. Brand Names Reyataz®
Canadian Brand Names Reyataz®
Mexican Brand Names Reyataz
Generic Available No
Index Terms Atazanavir Sulfate; BMS-232632
Pharmacologic Category Antiretroviral Agent, Protease Inhibitor
Use Treatment of HIV-1 infections in combination with at least two other antiretroviral agents
Note: In patients with prior virologic failure, coadministration with ritonavir is recommended.
Local Anesthetic/Vasoconstrictor Precautions No information available to require special precautions
Effects on Dental Treatment No significant effects or complications reported
Common Adverse Effects Includes data from both treatment-naive and treatment-experienced patients.

>10%:
Dermatologic: Rash (21%; median onset 8 weeks)
Endocrine & metabolic: Cholesterol increased (≥240 mg/dL: 6% to 25%)
Gastrointestinal: Nausea (6% to 14%), amylase increased (up to 14%)
Hepatic: Bilirubin increased (≥2.6 times ULN: 35% to 49%)
Neuromuscular & skeletal: CPK increased (6% to 11%)
2% to 10%:
Cardiovascular: AV block (1st degree: 6%)

Central nervous system: Headache (1% to 6%), peripheral neuropathy (<1% to 4%), insomnia (<1% to 3%), depression (2%), fever (2%), dizziness (<1% to 2%)

Endocrine & metabolic: Triglycerides increased (<1% to 8%), hyperglycemia (≥251 mg/dL: up to 5%)

Gastrointestinal: Lipase increased (<1% to 5%), abdominal pain (4%), vomiting (3% to 4%), diarrhea (1% to 3%)

Hematologic: Neutropenia (3% to 7%), hemoglobin decreased (<1% to 5%), thrombocytopenia (up to 2%)

Hepatic: ALT increased (≥5 times ULN: 4% to 9%; 15% to 25% in patients seropositive for hepatitis B and/or C), AST increased (≥5 times ULN: 2% to 7%; 9% to 10% in patients seropositive for hepatitis B and/or C), jaundice (7% to 9%)

Neuromuscular & skeletal: Myalgia (4%)

Mechanism of Action Inhibits the HIV-1 protease; inhibition of the viral protease prevents cleavage of the gag-pol polyprotein resulting in the production of immature, noninfectious virus

Drug Interactions

Cytochrome P450 Effect: Substrate of CYP3A4 (major); **Inhibits** CYP1A2 (weak), 2C8 (strong), 2C9 (weak), 3A4 (strong)

Increased Effect/Toxicity: Serum concentrations of medications significantly metabolized by CYP2C8, CYP3A4, or UGT1A1 may be elevated by atazanavir. Concurrent therapy with cisapride, ergot derivatives (dihydroergotamine, ergonovine, ergotamine, methylergonovine), indinavir, irinotecan, lovastatin, midazolam, pimozide, simvastatin, or triazolam is contraindicated (or not recommended, per manufacturer).

Atazanavir may increase the levels/effects of selected benzodiazepines, calcium channel blockers, cyclosporine, delavirdine, eplerenone, fentanyl, mirtazapine, nateglinide, nefazodone, quinidine, sildenafil (and other PDE-5 inhibitors), tacrolimus, telithromycin, tenofovir, venlafaxine, and other CYP3A4 substrates. When used with strong CYP3A4 inhibitors, dosage adjustment/limits are recommended for sildenafil and other PDE-5 inhibitors; consult individual monographs. Serum concentrations of antiarrhythmics (amiodarone, lidocaine, and quinidine) may be increased; monitor serum concentrations of these agents. Serum concentrations/effects of trazodone may be increased; use caution and reduce trazodone dose.

The levels/effects of atazanavir may be increased by azole antifungals, clarithromycin, delavirdine, diclofenac, doxycycline, erythromycin, imatinib, isoniazid, nefazodone, nicardipine, propofol, protease inhibitors, quinidine, telithromycin, verapamil, and other CYP3A4 inhibitors. Serum concentrations of atazanavir are increased by ritonavir; specific dosing adjustment of atazanavir in combination with ritonavir and efavirenz has been established. Serum concentrations of saquinavir may be increased by atazanavir; dosing recommendations for the combination have not been established. Tenofovir concentrations are increased by atazanavir. Concurrent use of indinavir may increase the risk of hyperbilirubinemia; concomitant administration is not recommended. Serum concentrations of orally inhaled corticosteroids (fluticasone, budesonide) may be increased by atazanavir (with or without ritonavir) resulting in decreased serum cortisol, HPA axis suppression; concurrent use with atazanavir plus ritonavir not recommended.

Atazanavir may increase serum concentrations of clarithromycin, potentially increasing the risk of QT_c prolongation. A 50% reduction in clarithromycin dose or an alternative agent (except in *M. avium* complex infections) should be considered. An increase in rifabutin plasma AUC (>200%) has been observed when coadministered with atazanavir (decrease rifabutin's dose by up to 75%).

Decreased Effect: Concurrent use of proton pump inhibitors may reduce atazanavir absorption; avoid concurrent use. Antacids and buffered formulations (eg, didanosine pediatric oral solution) may reduce the serum concentrations of atazanavir. Administer atazanavir 2 hours before or 1 hour after these medications. H_2 antagonists may reduce the absorption of atazanavir; avoid concurrent use or administer H_2 antagonist at least 10 hours before or 2 hours after atazanavir. Serum levels/effects of enteric-coated didanosine may be decreased by atazanavir

The levels/effects of atazanavir may be decreased by aminoglutethimide, carbamazepine, nafcillin, nevirapine, phenobarbital, phenytoin, rifamycins, and other CYP3A4 inducers. Rifampin decreases bioavailability of protease inhibitors by ~90%; loss of virologic response and resistance may occur; the two drugs should not be administered together. St John's wort (*Hypericum perforatum*) decreases serum concentrations of protease inhibitors and may lead to treatment failures; concurrent use is contraindicated. Tenofovir may decrease serum concentrations of atazanavir, resulting in a loss of virologic

(Continued)

Atazanavir *(Continued)*

response (specific atazanavir dosing recommendations provided by manufacturer).

Pharmacodynamics/Kinetics
Absorption: Rapid; enhanced with food
Protein binding: 86%
Metabolism: Hepatic, via multiple pathways including CYP3A4; forms two metabolites (inactive)
Half-life elimination: Unboosted therapy: 7-8 hours; Boosted therapy (with ritonavir): 9-18 hours
Time to peak, plasma: 2-3 hours
Excretion: Feces (79%, 20% as unchanged drug); urine (13%, 7% as unchanged drug)

Pregnancy Risk Factor B

Atazanavir Sulfate *see* Atazanavir *on page 156*

Atenolol *(a TEN oh lole)*

Related Information
Cardiovascular Diseases *on page 1726*

U.S. Brand Names Tenormin®

Canadian Brand Names Apo-Atenol®; Gen-Atenolol; Novo-Atenol; Nu-Atenol; PMS-Atenolol; RAN™-Atenolol; Rhoxal-atenolol; Riva-Atenolol; Sandoz-Atenolol; Tenolin; Tenormin®

Mexican Brand Names Blotex; Tenormin

Generic Available Yes: Tablet

Pharmacologic Category Beta Blocker, Beta$_1$ Selective

Use Treatment of hypertension, alone or in combination with other agents; management of angina pectoris, postmyocardial infarction patients

Unlabeled/Investigational Use Acute ethanol withdrawal, supraventricular and ventricular arrhythmias, and migraine headache prophylaxis

Local Anesthetic/Vasoconstrictor Precautions No information available to require special precautions

Effects on Dental Treatment Atenolol is a cardioselective beta-blocker. Local anesthetic with vasoconstrictor can be safely used in patients medicated with atenolol. Nonselective beta-blockers (ie, propranolol, nadolol) enhance the pressor response to epinephrine, resulting in hypertension and bradycardia; this has not been reported for atenolol. Many nonsteroidal anti-inflammatory drugs, such as ibuprofen and indomethacin, can reduce the hypotensive effect of beta-blockers after 3 or more weeks of therapy with the NSAID. Short-term NSAID use (ie, 3 days) requires no special precautions in patients taking beta-blockers.

Common Adverse Effects 1% to 10%:
Cardiovascular: Persistent bradycardia, hypotension, chest pain, edema, heart failure, second- or third-degree AV block, Raynaud's phenomenon
Central nervous system: Dizziness, fatigue, insomnia, lethargy, confusion, mental impairment, depression, headache, nightmares
Gastrointestinal: Constipation, diarrhea, nausea
Genitourinary: Impotence
Miscellaneous: Cold extremities

Dosage
Oral:
Children: Hypertension: 0.5-1 mg/kg/dose given daily; range of 0.5-1.5 mg/kg/day; maximum dose: 2 mg/kg/day up to 100 mg/day
Adults:
Hypertension: 25-50 mg once daily, may increase to 100 mg/day. Doses >100 mg are unlikely to produce any further benefit.
Angina pectoris: 50 mg once daily, may increase to 100 mg/day. Some patients may require 200 mg/day.
Postmyocardial infarction: Follow I.V. dose with 100 mg/day or 50 mg twice daily for 6-9 days postmyocardial infarction.
I.V.:
Hypertension: Dosages of 1.25-5 mg every 6-12 hours have been used in short-term management of patients unable to take oral enteral beta-blockers
Postmyocardial infarction: Early treatment: 5 mg slow I.V. over 5 minutes; may repeat in 10 minutes. If both doses are tolerated, may start oral atenolol 50 mg every 12 hours or 100 mg/day for 6-9 days postmyocardial infarction.
Dosing interval for oral atenolol in renal impairment:
Cl$_{cr}$ 15-35 mL/minute: Administer 50 mg/day maximum.
Cl$_{cr}$ <15 mL/minute: Administer 50 mg every other day maximum.

Hemodialysis: Moderately dialyzable (20% to 50%) via hemodialysis; administer dose postdialysis or administer 25-50 mg supplemental dose.

Peritoneal dialysis: Elimination is not enhanced; supplemental dose is not necessary.

Mechanism of Action Competitively blocks response to beta-adrenergic stimulation, selectively blocks $beta_1$-receptors with little or no effect on $beta_2$-receptors except at high doses

Contraindications Hypersensitivity to atenolol or any component of the formulation; sinus bradycardia; sinus node dysfunction; heart block greater than first-degree (except in patients with a functioning artificial pacemaker); cardiogenic shock; uncompensated cardiac failure; pulmonary edema; pregnancy

Warnings/Precautions Consider pre-existing conditions such as sick sinus syndrome before initiating. Administer cautiously in compensated heart failure and monitor for a worsening of the condition (efficacy of atenolol in heart failure has not been established). Beta-blocker therapy should not be withdrawn abruptly (particularly in patients with CAD), but gradually tapered to avoid acute tachycardia, hypertension, and/or ischemia. Use caution with concurrent use of beta-blockers and either verapamil or diltiazem; bradycardia or heart block can occur. Avoid concurrent I.V. use of both agents. Beta-blockers should be avoided in patients with bronchospastic disease (asthma). Atenolol, with B_1 selectivity, has been used cautiously in bronchospastic disease with close monitoring. Use cautiously in peripheral arterial disease, especially if severe disease is present. Use cautiously in patients with diabetes - may mask hypoglycemic symptoms. Use cautiously in the renally impaired (dosage adjustment required). Use care with anesthetic agents which decrease myocardial function. Caution in myasthenia gravis or psychiatric disease (may cause CNS depression). Adequate alpha-blockade is required prior to use of any beta-blocker for patients with untreated pheochromocytoma. Safety and efficacy have not been established in children.

Drug Interactions

Increased Effect/Toxicity: Atenolol may increase the effects of other drugs which slow AV conduction (digoxin, verapamil, diltiazem), alpha-blockers (prazosin, terazosin), and alpha-adrenergic stimulants (epinephrine, phenylephrine). Atenolol may mask the tachycardia from hypoglycemia caused by insulin and oral hypoglycemics. In patients receiving concurrent therapy, the risk of hypertensive crisis is increased when either clonidine or the beta-blocker is withdrawn. Reserpine has been shown to enhance the effect of atenolol. Beta-blockers may increase the action or levels of ethanol, disopyramide, nondepolarizing muscle relaxants, and theophylline although the effects are difficult to predict.

Decreased Effect: Decreased effect of atenolol with aluminum salts, barbiturates, calcium salts, cholestyramine, colestipol, NSAIDs, penicillins (ampicillin), rifampin, salicylates, and sulfinpyrazone due to decreased bioavailability and plasma levels. Beta-blockers may decrease the effect of sulfonylureas.

Ethanol/Nutrition/Herb Interactions

Food: Atenolol serum concentrations may be decreased if taken with food.

Herb/Nutraceutical: Avoid dong quai if using for hypertension (has estrogenic activity). Avoid ephedra, yohimbe, ginseng (may worsen hypertension). Avoid garlic (may have increased antihypertensive effect).

Dietary Considerations May be taken without regard to meals.

Pharmacodynamics/Kinetics

Onset of action: Peak effect: Oral: 2-4 hours

Duration: Normal renal function: 12-24 hours

Absorption: Incomplete

Distribution: Low lipophilicity; does not cross blood-brain barrier

Protein binding: 3% to 15%

Metabolism: Limited hepatic

Half-life elimination: Beta:

Neonates: ≤35 hours; Mean: 16 hours

Children: 4.6 hours; children >10 years may have longer half-life (>5 hours) compared to children 5-10 years (<5 hours)

Adults: Normal renal function: 6-9 hours, prolonged with renal impairment; End-stage renal disease: 15-35 hours

Excretion: Feces (50%); urine (40% as unchanged drug)

Pregnancy Risk Factor D

Dosage Forms

Injection, solution:

Tenormin®: 0.5 mg/mL (10 mL)

Tablet: 25 mg, 50 mg, 100 mg

Tenormin®: 25 mg, 50 mg, 100 mg

(Continued)

Atenolol *(Continued)*

Selected Readings

Foster CA and Aston SJ, "Propranolol-Epinephrine Interaction: A Potential Disaster," *Plast Reconstr Surg*, 1983, 72(1):74-8.

Wong DG, Spence JD, Lamki L, et al, "Effect of Nonsteroidal Anti-inflammatory Drugs on Control of Hypertension of Beta-Blockers and Diuretics," *Lancet*, 1986, 1(8488):997-1001.

Wynn RL, "Dental Nonsteroidal Anti-inflammatory Drugs and Prostaglandin-Based Drug Interactions-Part Two," *Gen Dent*, 1992, 40(2):104, 106, 108.

Wynn RL, "Epinephrine Interactions With Beta-Blockers," *Gen Dent*, 1994, 42(1):16, 18.

Atenolol and Chlorthalidone (a TEN oh lole & klor THAL i done)

Related Information
Atenolol *on page 158*
Chlorthalidone *on page 347*

U.S. Brand Names Tenoretic®

Canadian Brand Names Apo-Atenidone®; Tenoretic®

Mexican Brand Names Tenoretic

Generic Available Yes

Index Terms Chlorthalidone and Atenolol

Pharmacologic Category Antihypertensive Agent, Combination

Use Treatment of hypertension with a cardioselective beta-blocker and a diuretic

Local Anesthetic/Vasoconstrictor Precautions No information available to require special precautions

Effects on Dental Treatment Atenolol is a cardioselective beta-blocker. Local anesthetic with vasoconstrictor can be safely used in patients medicated with atenolol. Nonselective beta-blockers (ie, propranolol, nadolol) enhance the pressor response to epinephrine, resulting in hypertension and bradycardia; this has not been reported for atenolol. Many nonsteroidal anti-inflammatory drugs, such as ibuprofen and indomethacin, can reduce the hypotensive effect of beta-blockers after 3 or more weeks of therapy with the NSAID. Short-term NSAID use (ie, 3 days) requires no special precautions in patients taking beta-blockers.

Common Adverse Effects See individual agents.

Drug Interactions
  Increased Effect/Toxicity: See individual agents.
  Decreased Effect: See individual agents.

Pharmacodynamics/Kinetics See individual agents.

Pregnancy Risk Factor D

ATG *see* Antithymocyte Globulin (Equine) *on page 134*

Atgam® *see* Antithymocyte Globulin (Equine) *on page 134*

Ativan® *see* Lorazepam *on page 1001*

Atomoxetine (AT oh mox e teen)

U.S. Brand Names Strattera®

Canadian Brand Names Strattera®

Mexican Brand Names Strattera

Generic Available No

Index Terms Atomoxetine Hydrochloride; LY139603; Methylphenoxy-Benzene Propanamine; Tomoxetine

Pharmacologic Category Norepinephrine Reuptake Inhibitor, Selective

Use Treatment of attention deficit/hyperactivity disorder (ADHD)

Local Anesthetic/Vasoconstrictor Precautions Use vasoconstrictor with caution. Atomoxetine may increase heart rate or blood pressure in the presence of pressor agents. Pressor agents include the vasoconstrictors epinephrine and levonordefrin (Neo-Cobefrin®)

Effects on Dental Treatment Key adverse event(s) related to dental treatment: Xerostomia (normal salivary flow resumes upon discontinuation)

Common Adverse Effects Percentages as reported in children and adults; some adverse reactions may be increased in "poor metabolizers" (CYP2D6).

>10%:
  Central nervous system: Headache (17% to 27%), insomnia (16%)
  Gastrointestinal: Xerostomia (4% to 21%), abdominal pain (20%), vomiting (11% to 15%), appetite decreased (10% to 14%), nausea (12%)
  Respiratory: Cough (11%)
1% to 10%:
  Cardiovascular: Palpitation (4%), diastolic pressure increased (<1% to 5%), systolic blood pressure increased (2% to 9%), orthostatic hypotension (2%), tachycardia (2% to 3%)

Central nervous system: Fatigue/lethargy (7% to 9%), irritability (≤8%), somnolence (7%), dizziness (6%), mood swings (2% to 5%), abnormal dreams (4%), sleep disturbance (4%), pyrexia (3%), rigors (3%), crying (2%), flushing (<2%), tearfulness (<2%)

Dermatologic: Dermatitis (2% to 4%)

Endocrine & metabolic: Dysmenorrhea (7%), libido decreased (6%), menstruation disturbance (2% to 3%), hot flashes (3%), orgasm abnormal (2%)

Gastrointestinal: Dyspepsia (4% to 6%), diarrhea (4%), flatulence (2%), constipation (3% to 10%), weight loss (2%), anorexia (<2%)

Genitourinary: Urinary hesitation/retention (8%), erectile disturbance (7%), ejaculatory disturbance (5%), prostatitis (3%), impotence (3%)

Neuromuscular & skeletal: Paresthesia (4%), myalgia (3%)

Ocular: Mydriasis (<2%)

Otic: Ear infection (3%)

Respiratory: Sinusitis (6%), rhinorrhea (4%), sinus headache (3%)

Miscellaneous: Diaphoresis increased (4%), influenza (≤3%)

Restrictions An FDA-approved medication guide must be distributed when dispensing an outpatient prescription (new or refill) for this medication. Medication guides are available at http://www.fda.gov/cder/drug/infopage/ADHD/default.htm. Dispense to all patients or parents or guardians of children and teenagers receiving this medication.

Dosage Oral: **Note:** Atomoxetine may be discontinued without the need for tapering dose.

Children and Adolescents ≤70 kg: ADHD: Initial: 0.5 mg/kg/day, increase after minimum of 3 days to ~1.2 mg/kg/day; may administer as either a single daily dose or 2 evenly divided doses in morning and late afternoon/early evening. Maximum daily dose: 1.4 mg/kg or 100 mg, whichever is less.

Dosage adjustment in patients receiving strong CYP2D6 inhibitors (eg, paroxetine, fluoxetine, quinidine): Do not exceed 1.2 mg/kg/day; dose adjustments should occur only after 4 weeks.

Children and Adolescents >70 kg and Adults: ADHD: Initial: 40 mg/day, increased after minimum of 3 days to ~80 mg/day; may administer as either a single daily dose or two evenly divided doses in morning and late afternoon/early evening. May increase to 100 mg in 2-4 additional weeks to achieve optimal response.

Dosage adjustment in patients receiving strong CYP2D6 inhibitors (eg, paroxetine, fluoxetine, quinidine): Do not exceed 80 mg/day; dose adjustments should occur only after 4 weeks.

Elderly: Use has not been evaluated in the elderly

Dosage adjustment in renal impairment: No adjustment needed

Dosage adjustment in hepatic impairment:

Moderate hepatic insufficiency (Child-Pugh class B): All doses should be reduced to 50% of normal

Severe hepatic insufficiency (Child-Pugh class C): All doses should be reduced to 25% of normal

Mechanism of Action Selectively inhibits the reuptake of norepinephrine (Ki 4.5nM) with little to no activity at the other neuronal reuptake pumps or receptor sites.

Contraindications Hypersensitivity to atomoxetine or any component of the formulation; use with or within 14 days of MAO inhibitors; narrow-angle glaucoma

Warnings/Precautions [U.S. Boxed Warning]: Use caution in pediatric patients; may be an increased risk of suicidal ideation. Closely monitor for clinical worsening, suicidality, or unusual changes in behavior; the child's family or caregiver should be instructed to closely observe the patient and communicate condition with healthcare provider. Patients should be observed for, especially during the initial few months of a course of drug therapy, or at times of dose changes, either increases or decreases. New or worsening symptoms of hostility or aggressive behaviors have been associated with atomoxetine, particularly with the initiation of therapy. Use caution in patients with a history of psychotic illness or bipolar disorder; therapy may induce mixed/manic disorder or psychotic symptoms. Atomoxetine is not approved for major depressive disorder. Patients presenting with depressive symptoms should be screened for bipolar disorder. Recommended to be used as part of a comprehensive treatment program for attention deficit disorders. A medication guide should be dispensed with each prescription.

Use caution with hepatic (dosage adjustments necessary in hepatic impairment). Use may be associated with rare but severe hepatotoxicity; discontinue and do not restart if signs or symptoms of hepatotoxic reaction (eg, jaundice, pruritus, flu-like symptoms) are noted. Use caution in patients who are poor metabolizers of CYP2D6 metabolized drugs ("poor metabolizers"), bioavailability increases.

(Continued)

Atomoxetine *(Continued)*

CNS stimulant use has been associated with serious cardiovascular events including sudden death in patients with pre-existing structural cardiac abnormalities or other serious heart problems (sudden death in children and adolescents; sudden death, stroke, and MI in adults). These products should be avoided in patients with known serious structural cardiac abnormalities, cardiomyopathy, serious heart rhythm abnormalities, or other serious cardiac problems that could increase the risk of sudden death that these conditions alone carry. Patients should be carefully evaluated for cardiac disease prior to initiation of therapy. May cause increased heart rate or blood pressure; use caution with hypertension or other cardiovascular disease. Use caution with renal impairment. May cause urinary retention/hesitancy; use caution in patients with history of urinary retention or bladder outlet obstruction. Allergic reactions (including angioneurotic edema, urticaria, and rash) may occur.

Growth should be monitored during treatment. Height and weight gain may be reduced during the first 9-12 months of treatment, but should recover by 3 years of therapy. Safety and efficacy of long-term use of atomoxetine have not been evaluated. Safety and efficacy have not been evaluated in pediatric patients <6 years of age.

Drug Interactions

Cytochrome P450 Effect: Substrate of CYP2C19 (minor), 2D6 (major)

Increased Effect/Toxicity: MAO inhibitors may increase risk of CNS toxicity (combined use is contraindicated). CNS depressants may enhance the adverse/toxic effect of atomoxetine. CYP2D6 inhibitors may increase the levels/effects of atomoxetine (dose adjustment may be needed in patients who are extensive metabolizers of CYP2D6); example inhibitors include chlorpromazine, delavirdine, fluoxetine, miconazole, paroxetine, pergolide, quinidine, quinine, ritonavir, and ropinirole. Albuterol may increase risk of cardiovascular toxicity.

Ethanol/Nutrition/Herb Interactions Ethanol: Avoid ethanol (may increase CNS depression).

Dietary Considerations May be taken with or without food.

Pharmacodynamics/Kinetics

Absorption: Rapid

Distribution: V_d: I.V.: 0.85 L/kg

Protein binding: 98%, primarily albumin

Metabolism: Hepatic, via CYP2D6 and CYP2C19; forms metabolites (4-hydroxyatomoxetine, active, equipotent to atomoxetine; N-desmethylatomoxetine in poor metabolizers, limited activity)

Bioavailability: 63% in extensive metabolizers; 94% in poor metabolizers

Half-life elimination: Atomoxetine: 5 hours (up to 24 hours in poor metabolizers); Active metabolites: 4-hydroxyatomoxetine: 6-8 hours; N-desmethylatomoxetine: 6-8 hours (34-40 hours in poor metabolizers)

Time to peak, plasma: 1-2 hours

Excretion: Urine (80%, as conjugated 4-hydroxy metabolite); feces (17%)

Pregnancy Risk Factor C

Dosage Forms

Capsule:

Strattera®: 10 mg, 18 mg, 25 mg, 40 mg, 60 mg, 80 mg, 100 mg

Atomoxetine Hydrochloride *see* Atomoxetine *on page 160*

Atorvastatin *(a TORE va sta tin)*

Related Information

Cardiovascular Diseases *on page 1726*

U.S. Brand Names Lipitor®

Canadian Brand Names Lipitor®

Mexican Brand Names Lipitor

Generic Available No

Pharmacologic Category Antilipemic Agent, HMG-CoA Reductase Inhibitor

Use Treatment of dyslipidemias or primary prevention of cardiovascular disease (atherosclerotic) as detailed below:

Primary prevention of cardiovascular disease (high-risk for CVD): To reduce the risk of MI or stroke in patients without evidence of heart disease who have multiple CVD risk factors or type 2 diabetes. Treatment reduces the risk for angina or revascularization procedures in patients with multiple risk factors.

Secondary prevention of cardiovascular disease: To reduce the risk of MI, stroke, revascularization procedures, and angina in patients with evidence of heart disease. To reduce the risk of hospitalization for heart failure.

Treatment of dyslipidemias: To reduce elevations in total cholesterol, LDL-C, apolipoprotein B, and triglycerides in patients with elevations of one or more components, and/or to increase HDL-C as present in Fredrickson type IIa, IIb, III, and IV hyperlipidemias; treatment of primary dysbetalipoproteinemia, homozygous familial hypercholesterolemia

Treatment of heterozygous familial hypercholesterolemia (HeFH) in adolescent patients (10-17 years of age, females >1 year postmenarche) having LDL-C ≥190 mg/dL or LDL-C ≥160 mg/dL with positive family history of premature cardiovascular disease (CVD) or with two or more CVD risk factors.

Local Anesthetic/Vasoconstrictor Precautions No information available to require special precautions

Effects on Dental Treatment No significant effects or complications reported

Common Adverse Effects
>10%: Central nervous system: Headache (3% to 17%)
2% to 10%:
Cardiovascular: Chest pain, peripheral edema
Central nervous system: Insomnia, dizziness
Dermatologic: Rash (1% to 4%)
Gastrointestinal: Abdominal pain (up to 4%), constipation (up to 3%), diarrhea (up to 4%), dyspepsia (1% to 3%), flatulence (1% to 3%), nausea
Genitourinary: Urinary tract infection
Hepatic: Transaminases increased (2% to 3% with 80 mg/day dosing)
Neuromuscular & skeletal: Arthralgia (up to 5%), arthritis, back pain (up to 4%), myalgia (up to 6%), weakness (up to 4%)
Respiratory: Sinusitis (up to 6%), pharyngitis (up to 3%), bronchitis, rhinitis
Miscellaneous: Infection (3% to 10%), flu-like syndrome (up to 3%), allergic reaction (up to 3%)
Additional class-related events or case reports (not necessarily reported with atorvastatin therapy): Alkaline phosphatase increased, cataracts, cirrhosis, CPK increased (>10x normal), dermatomyositis, eosinophilia, erectile dysfunction, extraocular muscle movement impaired, fulminant hepatic necrosis, gynecomastia, hemolytic anemia, memory loss, ophthalmoplegia, peripheral nerve palsy, polymyalgia rheumatica, positive ANA, renal failure (secondary to rhabdomyolysis), systemic lupus erythematosus-like syndrome, thyroid dysfunction, tremor, vasculitis, vertigo

Dosage Oral: **Note:** Doses should be individualized according to the baseline LDL-cholesterol levels, the recommended goal of therapy, and patient response; adjustments should be made at intervals of 2-4 weeks
Children 10-17 years (females >1 year postmenarche): Heterozygous familial hypercholesterolemia (HeFH): 10 mg once daily (maximum: 20 mg/day)
Adults:
Hyperlipidemias: Initial: 10-20 mg once daily; patients requiring >45% reduction in LDL-C may be started at 40 mg once daily; range: 10-80 mg once daily
Primary prevention of CVD: 10 mg once daily
Dosing adjustment in renal impairment: No dosage adjustment is necessary.
Dosing adjustment in hepatic impairment: Do not use in active liver disease.

Mechanism of Action Inhibitor of 3-hydroxy-3-methylglutaryl coenzyme A (HMG-CoA) reductase, the rate-limiting enzyme in cholesterol synthesis (reduces the production of mevalonic acid from HMG-CoA); this then results in a compensatory increase in the expression of LDL receptors on hepatocyte membranes and a stimulation of LDL catabolism

Contraindications Hypersensitivity to atorvastatin or any component of the formulation; active liver disease; unexplained persistent elevations of serum transaminases; pregnancy

Warnings/Precautions Secondary causes of hyperlipidemia should be ruled out prior to therapy. Liver function must be monitored by periodic laboratory assessment. May cause hepatic dysfunction. Use with caution in patients who consume large amounts of ethanol or have a history of liver disease. Monitoring is recommended. Patients with a history of hemorrhagic stroke may be at increased risk for another with use.

Rhabdomyolysis with acute renal failure has occurred. Risk is dose related and is increased with concurrent use of lipid-lowering agents which may cause rhabdomyolysis (gemfibrozil, fibric acid derivatives, or niacin at doses ≥1 g/day) or during concurrent use with potent CYP3A4 inhibitors (including amiodarone, clarithromycin, cyclosporine, erythromycin, itraconazole, ketoconazole, nefazodone, grapefruit juice in large quantities, verapamil, or protease inhibitors such as indinavir, nelfinavir, or ritonavir). Weigh the risk versus benefit when combining any of these drugs with atorvastatin. Discontinue in any patient experiencing an acute or serious condition predisposing to renal failure secondary to rhabdomyolysis. Use with caution in patients with advanced age, these patients are predisposed to myopathy. Safety and efficacy have not been established in patients <10 years of age or in premenarcheal girls.
(Continued)

Atorvastatin *(Continued)*

Drug Interactions

Cytochrome P450 Effect: Substrate of CYP3A4 (major); **Inhibits** CYP3A4 (weak)

Increased Effect/Toxicity: CYP3A4 inhibitors may increase the levels/effects of atorvastatin; example inhibitors include azole antifungals, clarithromycin, diclofenac, doxycycline, erythromycin, imatinib, isoniazid, nefazodone, nicardipine, propofol, protease inhibitors, quinidine, telithromycin, and verapamil. The risk of myopathy and rhabdomyolysis due to concurrent use of a CYP3A4 inhibitor with atorvastatin is probably less than lovastatin or simvastatin. Cyclosporine, clofibrate, diltiazem, fenofibrate, gemfibrozil, and niacin may also increase the risk of myopathy and rhabdomyolysis. The effect/toxicity of levothyroxine may be increased by atorvastatin. Levels of digoxin and ethinyl estradiol may be increased by atorvastatin.

Decreased Effect: Colestipol, antacids decreased plasma concentrations but effect on LDL-cholesterol was not altered. Cholestyramine may decrease absorption of atorvastatin when administered concurrently.

Ethanol/Nutrition/Herb Interactions

Ethanol: Avoid excessive ethanol consumption (due to potential hepatic effects).

Food: Atorvastatin serum concentrations may be increased by grapefruit juice; avoid concurrent intake of large quantities (>1 quart/day). Red yeast rice contains an estimated 2.4 mg lovastatin per 600 mg rice.

Herb/Nutraceutical: St John's wort may decrease atorvastatin levels.

Dietary Considerations May take with food if desired; may take without regard to time of day. Before initiation of therapy, patients should be placed on a standard cholesterol-lowering diet for 3-6 months and the diet should be continued during drug therapy. Red yeast rice contains an estimated 2.4 mg lovastatin per 600 mg rice.

Pharmacodynamics/Kinetics

Onset of action: Initial changes: 3-5 days; Maximal reduction in plasma cholesterol and triglycerides: 2 weeks

Absorption: Rapid

Distribution: V_d: 318 L

Protein binding: ≥98%

Metabolism: Hepatic; forms active ortho- and parahydroxylated derivates and an inactive beta-oxidation product

Half-life elimination: Parent drug: 14 hours

Time to peak, serum: 1-2 hours

Excretion: Bile; urine (2% as unchanged drug)

Pregnancy Risk Factor X

Dosage Forms

Tablet:

Lipitor®: 10 mg, 20 mg, 40 mg, 80 mg

Selected Readings

Siedlik PH, Olson, SC, Yang BB, et al, "Erythromycin Coadministration Increases Plasma Atorvastatin Concentrations," *J Clin Pharmacol*, 1999, 39(5):501-4.

Atorvastatin Calcium and Amlodipine Besylate *see* Amlodipine and Atorvastatin on page 103

Atovaquone *(a TOE va kwone)*

Related Information

Systemic Viral Diseases on page 1767

U.S. Brand Names Mepron®

Canadian Brand Names Mepron®

Generic Available No

Pharmacologic Category Antiprotozoal

Use Acute oral treatment of mild-to-moderate *Pneumocystis carinii* pneumonia (PCP) in patients who are intolerant to co-trimoxazole; prophylaxis of PCP in patients intolerant to co-trimoxazole; treatment/suppression of *Toxoplasma gondii* encephalitis; primary prophylaxis of HIV-infected persons at high risk for developing *Toxoplasma gondii* encephalitis

Local Anesthetic/Vasoconstrictor Precautions No information available to require special precautions

Effects on Dental Treatment Key adverse event(s) related to dental treatment: Oral moniliasis

Common Adverse Effects Note: Adverse reaction statistics have been compiled from studies including patients with advanced HIV disease; consequently, it is difficult to distinguish reactions attributed to atovaquone from those caused by the underlying disease or a combination thereof.

>10%:
    Central nervous system: Headache, fever, insomnia, anxiety
    Dermatologic: Rash
    Gastrointestinal: Nausea, diarrhea, vomiting
    Respiratory: Cough
1% to 10%:
    Central nervous system: Dizziness
    Dermatologic: Pruritus
    Endocrine & metabolic: Hypoglycemia, hyponatremia
    Gastrointestinal: Abdominal pain, constipation, anorexia, dyspepsia, amylase increased
    Hematologic: Anemia, neutropenia, leukopenia
    Hepatic: Liver enzymes increased
    Neuromuscular & skeletal: Weakness
    Renal: BUN/creatinine increased
    Miscellaneous: Oral moniliasis

Mechanism of Action Has not been fully elucidated; may inhibit electron transport in mitochondria inhibiting metabolic enzymes

Drug Interactions
    Increased Effect/Toxicity: Possible increased toxicity with other highly protein-bound drugs.
    Decreased Effect: Rifamycins (rifampin) used concurrently decrease the steady-state plasma concentrations of atovaquone.

Pharmacodynamics/Kinetics
    Absorption: Significantly increased with a high-fat meal
    Distribution: 3.5 L/kg
    Protein binding: >99%
    Metabolism: Undergoes enterohepatic recirculation
    Bioavailability: Tablet: 23%; Suspension: 47%
    Half-life elimination: 2-3 days
    Excretion: Feces (94% as unchanged drug)

Pregnancy Risk Factor C

Atovaquone and Proguanil (a TOE va kwone & pro GWA nil)

Related Information
    Atovaquone *on page 164*
U.S. Brand Names Malarone®
Canadian Brand Names Malarone®; Malarone® Pediatric
Generic Available No
Index Terms Proguanil and Atovaquone
Pharmacologic Category Antimalarial Agent
Use Prevention or treatment of acute, uncomplicated *P. falciparum* malaria
Local Anesthetic/Vasoconstrictor Precautions No information available to require special precautions
Effects on Dental Treatment No significant effects or complications reported
Common Adverse Effects The following adverse reactions were reported in patients being treated for malaria. When used for prophylaxis, reactions are similar to those seen with placebo.

>10%: Gastrointestinal: Abdominal pain (17%), nausea (12%), vomiting (children 10% to 13%, adults 12%)
1% to 10%:
    Central nervous system: Headache (10%), dizziness (5%)
    Dermatologic: Pruritus (children 6%)
    Gastrointestinal: Diarrhea (children 6%, adults 8%), anorexia (5%)
    Neuromuscular & skeletal: Weakness (8%)

Mechanism of Action
    Atovaquone: Selectively inhibits parasite mitochondrial electron transport.
    Proguanil: The metabolite cycloguanil inhibits dihydrofolate reductase, disrupting deoxythymidylate synthesis. Together, atovaquone/cycloguanil affect the erythrocytic and exoerythrocytic stages of development.

Drug Interactions
    Cytochrome P450 Effect: Proguanil: **Substrate** (minor) of 1A2, 2C19, 3A4
    Decreased Effect: Metoclopramide decreases bioavailability of atovaquone. Rifabutin decreases atovaquone levels by 34%. Rifampin decreases atovaquone levels by 50%. Tetracycline decreases plasma concentrations of atovaquone by 40%.

Pharmacodynamics/Kinetics
    Atovaquone: See Atovaquone.
    Proguanil:
        Absorption: Extensive
        Distribution: 42 L/kg
(Continued)

Atovaquone and Proguanil (Continued)

Protein binding: 75%

Metabolism: Hepatic to active metabolites, cycloguanil (via CYP2C19) and 4-chlorophenylbiguanide

Half-life elimination: 12-21 hours

Excretion: Urine (40% to 60%)

Pregnancy Risk Factor C

ATRA see Tretinoin (Oral) on page 1606

Atridox™ see Doxycycline Hyclate (Periodontal) on page 539

Atripla™ see Efavirenz, Emtricitabine, and Tenofovir on page 559

AtroPen® see Atropine on page 166

Atropine (A troe peen)

U.S. Brand Names AtroPen®; Atropine-Care®; Isopto® Atropine; Sal-Tropine™

Canadian Brand Names Dioptic's Atropine Solution; Isopto® Atropine

Generic Available Yes: Excludes tablet

Index Terms Atropine Sulfate

Pharmacologic Category Anticholinergic Agent; Anticholinergic Agent, Ophthalmic; Antidote; Antispasmodic Agent, Gastrointestinal; Ophthalmic Agent, Mydriatic

Dental Use Reduction of salivation and bronchial secretions

Use

Injection: Preoperative medication to inhibit salivation and secretions; treatment of symptomatic sinus bradycardia; AV block (nodal level); ventricular asystole; antidote for organophosphate pesticide poisoning

Ophthalmic: Produce mydriasis and cycloplegia for examination of the retina and optic disc and accurate measurement of refractive errors; uveitis

Oral: Inhibit salivation and secretions

Unlabeled/Investigational Use Pulseless electric activity, asystole, neuromuscular blockade reversal; treatment of nerve agent toxicity (chemical warfare) in combination with pralidoxime

Local Anesthetic/Vasoconstrictor Precautions No information available to require special precautions

Effects on Dental Treatment Key adverse event(s) related to dental treatment: Xerostomia and changes in salivation (normal salivary flow resumes upon discontinuation), dry throat, and nasal dryness

Significant Adverse Effects Severity and frequency of adverse reactions are dose related and vary greatly; listed reactions are limited to significant and/or life-threatening.

Cardiovascular: Arrhythmia, flushing, hypotension, palpitation, tachycardia

Central nervous system: Ataxia, coma, delirium, disorientation, dizziness, drowsiness, excitement, fever, hallucinations, headache, insomnia, nervousness

Dermatologic: Anhidrosis, urticaria, rash, scarlatiniform rash

Gastrointestinal: Bloating, constipation, delayed gastric emptying, loss of taste, nausea, paralytic ileus, vomiting, xerostomia, dry throat, nasal dryness

Genitourinary: Urinary hesitancy, urinary retention

Neuromuscular & skeletal: Weakness

Ocular: Angle-closure glaucoma, blurred vision, cycloplegia, dry eyes, mydriasis, ocular tension increased

Respiratory: Dyspnea, laryngospasm, pulmonary edema

Miscellaneous: Anaphylaxis

Restrictions The AtroPen® formulation is available for use primarily by the Department of Defense.

Dental Usual Dosing Inhibit salivation and secretions (preanesthesia): Adults (doses <0.5 mg have been associated with paradoxical bradycardia):

I.M., I.V., SubQ: 0.4-0.6 mg 30-60 minutes preop and repeat every 4-6 hours as needed

Oral: 0.4 mg; may repeat in 4 hours if necessary; 0.4 mg initial dose may be exceeded in certain cases and may repeat in 4 hours if necessary (see Dental Comment)

Dosage

Neonates, Infants, and Children: Doses <0.1 mg have been associated with paradoxical bradycardia.

Inhibit salivation and secretions (preanesthesia): Oral, I.M., I.V., SubQ:

<5 kg: 0.02 mg/kg/dose 30-60 minutes preop then every 4-6 hours as needed. Use of a minimum dosage of 0.1 mg in neonates <5 kg will result in dosages >0.02 mg/kg. There is no documented minimum dosage in this age group.

>5 kg: 0.01-0.02 mg/kg/dose to a maximum 0.4 mg/dose 30-60 minutes preop; minimum dose: 0.1 mg

Alternate dosing:
3-7 kg (7-16 lb): 0.1 mg
8-11 kg (17-24 lb): 0.15 mg
11-18 kg (24-40 lb): 0.2 mg
18-29 kg (40-65 lb): 0.3 mg
>30 kg (>65 lb): 0.4 mg

Bradycardia: I.V., intratracheal: 0.02 mg/kg, minimum dose 0.1 mg, maximum single dose: 0.5 mg in children and 1 mg in adolescents; may repeat in 5-minute intervals to a maximum total dose of 1 mg in children or 2 mg in adolescents. (**Note:** For intratracheal administration, the dosage must be diluted with normal saline to a total volume of 1-5 mL). When treating bradycardia in neonates, reserve use for those patients unresponsive to improved oxygenation and epinephrine.

Infants and Children: Nerve agent toxicity management (unlabeled use): See **Note** under adult dosing.

Prehospital ("in the field"): I.M.:
Birth to <2 years: Mild-to-moderate symptoms: 0.05 mg/kg; severe symptoms: 0.1 mg/kg
2-10 years: Mild-to-moderate symptoms: 1 mg; severe symptoms: 2 mg
>10 years: Mild-to-moderate symptoms: 2 mg; severe symptoms: 4 mg

Hospital/emergency department: I.M.:
Birth to <2 years: Mild-to-moderate symptoms: 0.05 mg/kg I.M. **or** 0.02 mg/kg I.V.; severe symptoms: 0.1 mg/kg I.M. **or** 0.02 mg/kg I.V.
2-10 years: Mild-to-moderate symptoms: 1 mg; severe symptoms: 2 mg
>10 years: Mild-to-moderate symptoms: 2 mg; severe symptoms: 4 mg

Note: Pralidoxime is a component of the management of nerve agent toxicity; consult Pralidoxime for specific route and dose. For prehospital ("in the field") management, repeat atropine I.M. (children: 0.05-0.1 mg/kg) at 5-10 minute intervals until secretions have diminished and breathing is comfortable or airway resistance has returned to near normal. For hospital management, repeat atropine I.M. (infants 1 mg; all others: 2 mg) at 5-10 minute intervals until secretions have diminished and breathing is comfortable or airway resistance has returned to near normal.

Children: Organophosphate or carbamate poisoning:
I.V.: 0.03-0.05 mg/kg every 10-20 minutes until atropine effect, then every 1-4 hours for at least 24 hours
I.M. (AtroPen®): Mild symptoms: Administer dose listed below as soon as exposure is known or suspected. If severe symptoms develop after first dose, 2 additional doses should be repeated in 10 minutes; do not administer more than 3 doses. Severe symptoms: Immediately administer 3 doses as follows:
<6.8 kg (15 lb): Use of **AtroPen® formulation not recommended;** administer atropine 0.05 mg/kg
6.8-18 kg (15-40 lb): 0.5 mg/dose
18-41 kg (40-90 lb): 1 mg/dose
>41 kg (>90 lb): 2 mg/dose

Adults (doses <0.5 mg have been associated with paradoxical bradycardia):
Asystole or pulseless electrical activity:
I.V.: 1 mg; repeat in 3-5 minutes if asystole persists; total dose of 0.04 mg/kg.
Intratracheal: Administer 2-2.5 times the recommended I.V. dose; dilute in 10 mL NS or distilled water. **Note:** Absorption is greater with distilled water, but causes more adverse effects on PaO₂.
Inhibit salivation and secretions (preanesthesia):
I.M., I.V., SubQ: 0.4-0.6 mg 30-60 minutes preop and repeat every 4-6 hours as needed
Oral: 0.4 mg; may repeat in 4 hours if necessary; 0.4 mg initial dose may be exceeded in certain cases and may repeat in 4 hours if necessary
Bradycardia: I.V.: 0.5-1 mg every 5 minutes, not to exceed a total of 3 mg or 0.04 mg/kg; may give intratracheally in 10 mL NS (intratracheal dose should be 2-2.5 times the I.V. dose)
Neuromuscular blockade reversal: I.V.: 25-30 mcg/kg 30-60 seconds before neostigmine or 7-10 mcg/kg 30-60 seconds before edrophonium
Organophosphate or carbamate poisoning:
I.V.: 2 mg, followed by 2 mg every 5-60 minutes until adequate atropinization has occurred; initial doses of up to 6 mg may be used in life-threatening cases
I.M. (AtroPen®): Mild symptoms: Administer 2 mg as soon as exposure is known or suspected. If severe symptoms develop after first dose, 2 additional doses should be repeated in 10 minutes; do not administer more than 3 doses. Severe symptoms: Immediately administer three 2 mg doses.

(Continued)

Atropine *(Continued)*

Nerve agent toxicity management (unlabeled use): I.M.: See **Note**. Prehospital ("in the field") or hospital/emergency department: Mild-to-moderate symptoms: 2-4 mg; severe symptoms: 6 mg

Note: Pralidoxime is a component of the management of nerve agent toxicity; consult Pralidoxime for specific route and dose. For prehospital ("in the field") management, repeat atropine I.M. (2 mg) at 5-10 minute intervals until secretions have diminished and breathing is comfortable or airway resistance has returned to near normal. For hospital management, repeat atropine I.M. (2 mg) at 5-10 minute intervals until secretions have diminished and breathing is comfortable or airway resistance has returned to near normal.

Mydriasis, cycloplegia (preprocedure): Ophthalmic (1% solution): Instill 1-2 drops 1 hour before procedure.

Uveitis: Ophthalmic:

1% solution: Instill 1-2 drops 4 times/day

Ointment: Apply a small amount in the conjunctival sac up to 3 times/day; compress the lacrimal sac by digital pressure for 1-3 minutes after instillation

Elderly, frail patients: Nerve agent toxicity management (unlabeled use): I.M.: See **Note** under adult dosing.

Prehospital ("in the field"): Mild-to-moderate symptoms: 1 mg; severe symptoms: 2-4 mg

Hospital/emergency department: Mild-to-moderate symptoms: 1 mg; severe symptoms: 2 mg

Mechanism of Action Blocks the action of acetylcholine at parasympathetic sites in smooth muscle, secretory glands, and the CNS; increases cardiac output, dries secretions, antagonizes histamine and serotonin

Contraindications Hypersensitivity to atropine or any component of the formulation; narrow-angle glaucoma; adhesions between the iris and lens; tachycardia; obstructive GI disease; paralytic ileus; intestinal atony of the elderly or debilitated patient; severe ulcerative colitis; toxic megacolon complicating ulcerative colitis; hepatic disease; obstructive uropathy; renal disease; myasthenia gravis (unless used to treat side effects of acetylcholinesterase inhibitor); asthma; thyrotoxicosis; Mobitz type II block

Warnings/Precautions Heat prostration can occur in the presence of a high environmental temperature. Psychosis can occur in sensitive individuals. The elderly may be sensitive to side effects. Use caution in patients with myocardial ischemia. Use caution in hyperthyroidism, autonomic neuropathy, BPH, CHF, tachyarrhythmias, hypertension, and hiatal hernia associated with reflux esophagitis. Use with caution in children with spastic paralysis.

AtroPen®: There are no absolute contraindications for the use of atropine in severe organophosphate poisonings, however in mild poisonings, use caution in those patients where the use of atropine would be otherwise contraindicated. Formulation for use by trained personnel only.

Drug Interactions

Drugs with anticholinergic activity (including phenothiazines and TCAs) may increase anticholinergic effects when used concurrently.

Sympathomimetic amines may cause tachyarrhythmias; avoid concurrent use.

Pharmacodynamics/Kinetics

Onset of action: I.V.: Rapid

Absorption: Complete

Distribution: Widely throughout the body; crosses placenta; trace amounts enter breast milk; crosses blood-brain barrier

Metabolism: Hepatic

Half-life elimination: 2-3 hours

Excretion: Urine (30% to 50% as unchanged drug and metabolites)

Pregnancy Risk Factor C

Lactation Enters breast milk (trace amounts)/use caution (AAP rates "compatible")

Breast-Feeding Considerations Anticholinergic agents may suppress lactation.

Dosage Forms Excipient information presented when available (limited, particularly for generics); consult specific product labeling.

Injection, solution, as sulfate: 0.05 mg/mL (5 mL); 0.1 mg/mL (5 mL, 10 mL); 0.4 mg/0.5 mL (0.5 mL); 0.4 mg/mL (0.5 mL, 1 mL, 20 mL); 1 mg/mL (1 mL)

AtroPen® [prefilled autoinjector]: 0.5 mg/0.7 mL (0.7 mL); 1 mg/0.7 mL (0.7 mL); 2 mg/0.7 mL (0.7 mL)

Ointment, ophthalmic, as sulfate: 1% (3.5 g)

Solution, ophthalmic, as sulfate: 1% (2 mL, 5 mL, 15 mL)

Atropine-Care®: 1% (2 mL) [contains benzalkonium chloride]

Isopto® Atropine: 1% (5 mL, 15 mL) [contains benzalkonium chloride]

Tablet, as sulfate (Sal-Tropine™): 0.4 mg

Dental Comment The possibility of the need for an initial dose in excess of 0.4 mg has been confirmed by the American Dental Association in its recommendation on the use of this medication to reduce salivation during dental procedures.

Atropine and Difenoxin *see* Difenoxin and Atropine *on page 494*

Atropine and Diphenoxylate *see* Diphenoxylate and Atropine *on page 514*

Atropine-Care® *see* Atropine *on page 166*

Atropine, Hyoscyamine, Scopolamine, and Phenobarbital *see* Hyoscyamine, Atropine, Scopolamine, and Phenobarbital *on page 848*

Atropine Sulfate *see* Atropine *on page 166*

Atropine Sulfate and Edrophonium Chloride *see* Edrophonium and Atropine *on page 556*

Atropine Sulfate (Dental Tablets)
(A troe peen SUL fate DEN tal TAB lets)

Related Information
Atropine *on page 166*
Dentin Hypersensitivity, High Caries Index, and Xerostomia *on page 1812*
U.S. Brand Names Sal-Tropine™
Generic Available No
Dental Use Reduction of salivation and bronchial secretions
Use Treatment of GI disorders (eg, peptic ulcer disease, irritable bowel syndrome, hypermotility of colon)
Local Anesthetic/Vasoconstrictor Precautions No information available to require special precautions
Effects on Dental Treatment
Key adverse event(s) related to dental treatment:
Doses <0.1 mg have been associated with paradoxical bradycardia
Children: May produce fever (by inhibiting heat loss by evaporation), scarlitiniform rash
Causes significant xerostomia when used in therapeutic doses (normal salivary flow resumes upon discontinuation):
0.5 mg: Slight dryness of nose and mouth; bradycardia
1 mg: Increased dryness of nose and mouth; thirst; slowing then acceleration of heart rate; mydriasis
2 mg: Significant xerostomia; tachycardia with palpitations; mydriasis; slight blurring of vision; flushing, dry skin
5 mg: Increase in above symptoms plus disturbance of speech; difficulty swallowing; headache; hot, dry skin; restlessness with asthenia
10 mg: Above symptoms to extreme degree plus ataxia, excitement, disorientation, hallucinations, delirium, coma
Dental Usual Dosing Inhibition of salivation and secretions (preanesthesia): Oral:
Neonates, Infants, and Children (no documented minimum dosage):
3-7 kg (7-16 lb): 0.1 mg
8-11 kg (17-24 lb): 0.15 mg
11-18 kg (24-40 lb): 0.2 mg
18-29 kg (40-65 lb): 0.3 mg
>30 kg (>65 lb): 0.4 mg
Adults: 0.4 mg; may repeat in 4 hours, if necessary.
Dosage
Inhibition of salivation and secretions (preanesthesia): Oral:
Neonates, Infants, and Children (no documented minimum dosage):
3-7 kg (7-16 lb): 0.1 mg
8-11 kg (17-24 lb): 0.15 mg
11-18 kg (24-40 lb): 0.2 mg
18-29 kg (40-65 lb): 0.3 mg
>30 kg (>65 lb): 0.4 mg
Adults: 0.4 mg; may repeat in 4 hours, if necessary.
Mechanism of Action Refer to Atropine monograph.
Contraindications Refer to Atropine monograph.
Warnings/Precautions Lower doses (<0.5 mg) may have vagalmimetic effects (ie, increase vagal tone causing paradoxical bradycardia). A total dose of 3 mg (0.04 mg/kg) results in full vagal blockade in humans. Doses of 0.5-1 mg of atropine are mildly stimulating to the CNS. Geriatric patients may be sensitive to side effects; anticholinergic agents are generally not well tolerated in the elderly and their use should be avoided when possible. Larger doses may produce mental disturbances; psychosis can occur in sensitive individuals. Heat prostration can occur in the presence of a high environmental temperature. Use caution in CHF, tachyarrhythmias, hypertension, and hiatal hernia associated with reflux esophagitis. Lower doses (<0.5 mg) may have vagalmimetic effects
(Continued)

Atropine Sulfate (Dental Tablets) *(Continued)*

(ie, increase vagal tone causing paradoxical bradycardia). A total dose of 3 mg (0.04 mg/kg) results in full vagal blockade in humans.

Drug Interactions

Increased Effect: Atropine-induced mouth dryness may be increased if it is given with other drugs that have anticholinergic actions, such as tricyclic antidepressants, antipsychotics, some antihistamines, and antiparkinsonism drugs.

Decreased Effect: May interfere with absorption of other medications.

Breast-Feeding Considerations Although atropine enters breast milk (trace amounts), the AAP rates this drug as "compatible" with breast-feeding; should be used with caution; anticholinergic agents may suppress lactation

Dosage Forms Tablet, as sulfate (Sal-Tropine™): 0.4 mg

Atrovent® *see Ipratropium on page 905*

Atrovent® HFA *see Ipratropium on page 905*

Attapulgite *(at a PULL gite)*

Related Information
Ulcerative and Erosive Disorders *on page 1809*

U.S. Brand Names Children's Kaopectate® [OTC] [DSC]; Diasorb® [OTC]; Kaopectate® Advanced Formula [OTC] [DSC]; Kaopectate® Maximum Strength Caplets [OTC] [DSC]

Canadian Brand Names Kaopectate®

Generic Available Yes

Pharmacologic Category Antidiarrheal

Use Symptomatic treatment of diarrhea

Local Anesthetic/Vasoconstrictor Precautions No information available to require special precautions

Effects on Dental Treatment No significant effects or complications reported

Mechanism of Action Controls diarrhea because of its absorbent action

Pregnancy Risk Factor B

Attenuvax® *see Measles Virus Vaccine (Live) on page 1021*

Atuss® HX *see Hydrocodone and Guaifenesin on page 828*

Augmentin® *see Amoxicillin and Clavulanate Potassium on page 110*

Augmentin ES-600® *see Amoxicillin and Clavulanate Potassium on page 110*

Augmentin XR® *see Amoxicillin and Clavulanate Potassium on page 110*

Auranofin *(au RANE oh fin)*

Related Information
Rheumatoid Arthritis, Osteoarthritis, and Osteoporosis *on page 1759*

U.S. Brand Names Ridaura®

Canadian Brand Names Ridaura®

Generic Available No

Pharmacologic Category Gold Compound

Use Management of active stage of classic or definite rheumatoid arthritis in patients who do not respond to or tolerate other agents; psoriatic arthritis; adjunctive or alternative therapy for pemphigus

Local Anesthetic/Vasoconstrictor Precautions No information available to require special precautions

Effects on Dental Treatment Key adverse event(s) related to dental treatment: Glossitis and stomatitis.

Common Adverse Effects
>10%:
Dermatologic: Itching, rash
Gastrointestinal: Stomatitis
Ocular: Conjunctivitis
Renal: Proteinuria
1% to 10%:
Dermatologic: Urticaria, alopecia
Gastrointestinal: Glossitis
Hematologic: Eosinophilia, leukopenia, thrombocytopenia
Renal: Hematuria

Mechanism of Action The exact mechanism of action of gold is unknown; gold is taken up by macrophages which results in inhibition of phagocytosis and lysosomal membrane stabilization; other actions observed are decreased serum rheumatoid factor and alterations in immunoglobulins. Additionally, complement activation is decreased, prostaglandin synthesis is inhibited, and lysosomal enzyme activity is decreased.

Drug Interactions

Increased Effect/Toxicity: Toxicity of penicillamine, antimalarials, hydroxychloroquine, cytotoxic agents, and immunosuppressants may be increased.

Pharmacodynamics/Kinetics

Onset of action: Delayed; therapeutic response may require as long as 3-4 months

Duration: Prolonged

Absorption: Oral: ~20% gold in dose is absorbed

Protein binding: 60%

Half-life elimination (single or multiple dose dependent): 21-31 days

Time to peak, serum: ~2 hours

Excretion: Urine (60% of absorbed gold); remainder in feces

Pregnancy Risk Factor C

Azacitidine (ay za SYE ti deen)

U.S. Brand Names Vidaza®

Generic Available No

Index Terms AZA-CR; Azacytidine; 5-Azacytidine; 5-AZC; Ladakamycin; NSC-102816

Pharmacologic Category Antineoplastic Agent, DNA Methylation Inhibitor

Use Treatment of myelodysplastic syndrome (MDS)

Unlabeled/Investigational Use Investigational: Refractory acute lymphocytic and myelogenous leukemia

Local Anesthetic/Vasoconstrictor Precautions No information available to require special precautions

Effects on Dental Treatment Key adverse event(s) related to dental treatment: Mucositis, gingival bleeding, oral mucosal petechiae, stomatitis, oral hemorrhage, and tongue ulceration.

(Continued)

171

Azacitidine *(Continued)*

Common Adverse Effects

>10%:

Cardiovascular: Peripheral edema (7% to 19%), chest pain (16%), pallor (16%), pitting edema (15%)

Central nervous system: Fever (52%), fatigue (13% to 36%), headache (22%), dizziness (19%), anxiety (13%), depression (12%), insomnia (11%), malaise (11%), pain (11%)

Dermatologic: Bruising (19% to 31%), petechiae (24%), erythema (17%), skin lesion (15%), rash (14%), pruritus (12%)

Endocrine & metabolic: Hypokalemia (13%)

Gastrointestinal: Nausea (71%), vomiting (54%), diarrhea (36%), constipation (34%), anorexia (13% to 21%), weight loss (16%), abdominal pain (11% to 16%), abdominal tenderness (12%)

Hematologic: Anemia (70%), thrombocytopenia (66%), leukopenia (48%), neutropenia (32%), febrile neutropenia (16%), myelosuppression (nadir: days 10-17; recovery: days 28-31)

Hepatic: Hepatic enzymes increased (I.V. 37%)

Local: Injection site: Erythema (35%; more common with I.V. administration), pain (23%; more common with I.V. administration), bruising (14%)

Neuromuscular & skeletal: Weakness (29%), rigors (26%), arthralgia (22%), limb pain (20%), back pain (19%), myalgia (16%)

Respiratory: Cough (11% to 30%), dyspnea (5% to 29%), pharyngitis (20%), epistaxis (16%), nasopharyngitis (15%), upper respiratory tract infection (13%), pneumonia (11%), crackles (11%)

Miscellaneous: Diaphoresis (11%)

5% to 10%:

Cardiovascular: Cardiac murmur (10%), tachycardia (9%), hypotension (7%), syncope (6%), chest wall pain (5%)

Central nervous system: Lethargy (8%), hypoesthesia (5%), postprocedural pain (5%)

Dermatologic: Cellulitis (8%), urticaria (6%), dry skin (5%), skin nodule (5%)

Gastrointestinal: Gingival bleeding (10%), oral mucosal petechiae (8%), stomatitis (8%), dyspepsia (7%), hemorrhoids (7%), abdominal distension (6%), loose stools (6%), dysphagia (5%), oral hemorrhage (5%), tongue ulceration (5%)

Genitourinary: Dysuria (8%), urinary tract infection (8%)

Hematologic: Hematoma (9%), postprocedural hemorrhage (6%)

Local: Injection site: Pruritus (7%), granuloma (5%), pigmentation change (5%), swelling (5%)

Neuromuscular & skeletal: Muscle cramps (6%)

Respiratory: Rhinorrhea (10%), rales (9%), wheezing (9%), breath sounds decreased (8%), pleural effusion (6%), postnasal drip (6%), rhonchi (6%), nasal congestion (6%), atelectasis (5%), sinusitis (5%)

Miscellaneous: Lymphadenopathy (10%), herpes simplex (9%), night sweats (9%), transfusion reaction (7%), mouth hemorrhage (5%)

Mechanism of Action Antineoplastic effects may be a result of azacitidine's ability to promote hypomethylation of DNA leading to direct toxicity of abnormal hematopoietic cells in the bone marrow.

Pharmacodynamics/Kinetics

Absorption: SubQ: Rapid and complete

Distribution: V_d: I.V.: 76 ± 26 L; does not cross blood-brain barrier

Metabolism: Hepatic; hydrolysis to several metabolites

Bioavailability: SubQ: 89%

Half-life elimination: I.V., SubQ: ~4 hours

Time to peak, plasma: SubQ: 30 minutes

Excretion: Urine (50% to 85%); feces (minor)

Pregnancy Risk Factor D

AZA-CR *see* Azacitidine *on page 171*

Azactam® *see* Aztreonam *on page 180*

Azacytidine *see* Azacitidine *on page 171*

5-Azacytidine *see* Azacitidine *on page 171*

Azasan® *see* Azathioprine *on page 172*

Azathioprine *(ay za THYE oh preen)*

U.S. Brand Names Azasan®; Imuran®

Canadian Brand Names Alti-Azathioprine; Apo-Azathioprine®; Gen-Azathioprine; Imuran®; Novo-Azathioprine

Mexican Brand Names Azatrilem; Imuran

Generic Available Yes

Index Terms Azathioprine Sodium

Pharmacologic Category Immunosuppressant Agent

Dental Use Adjunct with prednisone for managing severe erosive lichen planus, major aphthous stomatitis, erythema multiforme, and benign mucous membrane pemphigoid

Use Adjunctive therapy in prevention of rejection of kidney transplants; active rheumatoid arthritis

Unlabeled/Investigational Use Adjunct in prevention of rejection of solid organ (nonrenal) transplants; steroid-sparing agent for corticosteroid-dependent Crohn's disease (CD) and ulcerative colitis (UC); maintenance of remission in CD; fistulizing Crohn's disease

Local Anesthetic/Vasoconstrictor Precautions No information available to require special precautions

Effects on Dental Treatment No significant effects or complications reported

Significant Adverse Effects Frequency not defined; dependent upon dose, duration, and concomitant therapy.

Central nervous system: Chills, fever, malaise
Dermatologic: Alopecia, rash (erythematous or maculopapular)
Gastrointestinal: Diarrhea, nausea, pancreatitis, vomiting
Hematologic: Bleeding, leukopenia, macrocytic anemia, pancytopenia, thrombocytopenia
Hepatic: Hepatotoxicity, hepatic veno-occlusive disease, steatorrhea
Neuromuscular & skeletal: Arthralgia, myalgia
Respiratory: Interstitial pneumonitis
Miscellaneous: Hypersensitivity reactions (rare), infection secondary to immunosuppression, neoplasia

Dental Usual Dosing Adjunctive management of severe recurrent aphthous stomatitis (unlabeled use): Adults: Oral: 50 mg once daily in conjunction with prednisone

Dosage I.V. dose is equivalent to oral dose (dosing should be based on ideal body weight):

Children (unlabeled) and Adults:
Renal transplantation: Oral, I.V.: Initial: 3-5 mg/kg/day usually given as a single daily dose, then 1-3 mg/kg/day maintenance
Rheumatoid arthritis: Oral:
Initial: 1 mg/kg/day given once daily or divided twice daily for 6-8 weeks; increase by 0.5 mg/kg every 4 weeks until response or up to 2.5 mg/kg/day; an adequate trial should be a minimum of 12 weeks
Maintenance dose: Reduce dose by 0.5 mg/kg every 4 weeks until lowest effective dose is reached; optimum duration of therapy not specified; may be discontinued abruptly

Adults: Oral:
Adjunctive management of severe recurrent aphthous stomatitis (unlabeled use): 50 mg once daily in conjunction with prednisone
Reduction of steroid use in CD or UC, maintenance of remission in CD or fistulizing disease (unlabeled uses): Initial: 50 mg daily; may increase by 25 mg/day every 1-2 weeks as tolerated to target dose of 2-3 mg/kg/day

Dosing adjustment in renal impairment:
Cl_{cr} 10-50 mL/minute: Administer 75% of normal dose daily
Cl_{cr} <10 mL/minute: Administer 50% of normal dose daily
Hemodialysis: Dialyzable (~45% removed in 8 hours)
Administer dose posthemodialysis: CAPD effects: Unknown; CAVH effects: Unknown

Mechanism of Action Azathioprine is an imidazolyl derivative of mercaptopurine; antagonizes purine metabolism and may inhibit synthesis of DNA, RNA, and proteins; may also interfere with cellular metabolism and inhibit mitosis. The 6-thioguanine nucleotides appear to mediate the majority of azathioprine's immunosuppressive and toxic effects.

Contraindications Hypersensitivity to azathioprine or any component of the formulation; pregnancy

Warnings/Precautions [U.S. Boxed Warning]: **Chronic immunosuppression increases the risk of neoplasia and serious infections.** Azathioprine has mutagenic potential to both men and women and with possible hematologic toxicities; hematologic toxicities are dose-related and may be more severe with renal transplants undergoing rejection. Gastrointestinal toxicity may occur within the first several weeks of therapy and is reversible. Symptoms may include severe nausea, vomiting, diarrhea, rash, fever, malaise, myalgia, hypotension, and liver enzyme abnormalities. Use with caution in patients with liver disease, renal impairment; monitor hematologic function closely. Patients with genetic deficiency of thiopurine methyltransferase (TPMT) or concurrent therapy with drugs which may inhibit TPMT may be sensitive to myelosuppressive effects. Azathioprine is metabolized to mercaptopurine; concomitant use may result in profound myelosuppression and should be avoided.
(Continued)

Azathioprine *(Continued)*

Drug Interactions

ACE inhibitors: Concomitant therapy may induce anemia and severe leukopenia.

Allopurinol: May increase serum levels of azathioprine's active metabolite (mercaptopurine). Decrease azathioprine dose to $1/3$ to $1/4$ of normal dose.

Aminosalicylates (olsalazine, mesalamine, sulfasalazine): May inhibit TPMT, increasing toxicity/myelosuppression of azathioprine. Use caution.

Mercaptopurine: Azathioprine is metabolized to mercaptopurine; concomitant use may result in profound myelosuppression and should be avoided.

Warfarin: Effect may be decreased by azathioprine.

Ethanol/Nutrition/Herb Interactions Herb/Nutraceutical: Avoid cat's claw, echinacea (have immunostimulant properties).

Dietary Considerations May be taken with food.

Pharmacodynamics/Kinetics

Distribution: Crosses placenta

Protein binding: ~30%

Metabolism: Hepatic, to 6-mercaptopurine (6-MP), possibly by glutathione S-transferase (GST). Further metabolism of 6-MP (in the liver and GI tract), via three major pathways: Hypoxanthine guanine phosphoribosyltransferase (to 6-thioguanine-nucleotides, or 6-TGN), xanthine oxidase (to 6-thiouric acid), and thiopurine methyltransferase (TPMT), which forms 6-methylmercaptopurine (6-MMP).

Half-life elimination: Parent drug: 12 minutes; mercaptopurine: 0.7-3 hours; End-stage renal disease: Slightly prolonged

Time to peak, plasma: 1-2 hours (including metabolites)

Excretion: Urine (primarily as metabolites)

Pregnancy Risk Factor D

Lactation Enters breast milk/not recommended

Breast-Feeding Considerations Due to risk of immunosuppression, breast-feeding is not recommended.

Dosage Forms Excipient information presented when available (limited, particularly for generics); consult specific product labeling.

Injection, powder for reconstitution: 100 mg

Tablet [scored]: 50 mg

Azasan®: 75 mg, 100 mg

Imuran®: 50 mg

Azathioprine Sodium see Azathioprine on page 172

5-AZC see Azacitidine on page 171

Azelaic Acid *(a zeh LAY ik AS id)*

U.S. Brand Names Azelex®; Finacea®

Canadian Brand Names Finacea®

Mexican Brand Names Cutacelan

Generic Available No

Pharmacologic Category Topical Skin Product, Acne

Use Topical treatment of inflammatory papules and pustules of mild-to-moderate rosacea; mild-to-moderate inflammatory acne vulgaris

Finacea®: Not FDA-approved for the treatment of acne

Local Anesthetic/Vasoconstrictor Precautions No information available to require special precautions

Effects on Dental Treatment No significant effects or complications reported

Common Adverse Effects

>5%: Dermatologic: Pruritus (1% to 6%), burning/stinging/itching (1% to 6%)

1% to 5%:

Dermatologic: Acne (<1% to 1%), edema, erythema, rash, peeling, dermatitis, contact dermatitis, irritation, scaling/dry skin/xerosis

Neuromuscular & skeletal: Paresthesia

Mechanism of Action Azelaic acid is a dietary constituent normally found in whole grain cereals; can be formed endogenously. Exact mechanism is not known. *In vitro*, azelaic acid possesses antimicrobial activity against *Propionibacterium acnes* and *Staphylococcus epidermidis*. May decrease microcomedo formation.

Pharmacodynamics/Kinetics

Absorption: Cream: ~3% to 5% penetrates stratum corneum; up to 10% found in epidermis and dermis; 4% systemic

Half-life elimination: Topical: Healthy subjects: 12 hours

Excretion: Urine (as unchanged drug)

Pregnancy Risk Factor B

Azelastine (a ZEL as teen)

U.S. Brand Names Astelin®; Optivar®
Canadian Brand Names Astelin®
Mexican Brand Names Astelin
Generic Available No
Index Terms Azelastine Hydrochloride
Pharmacologic Category Antihistamine
Use

Nasal spray: Treatment of the symptoms of seasonal allergic rhinitis such as rhinorrhea, sneezing, and nasal pruritus in children ≥5 years of age and adults; treatment of the symptoms of vasomotor rhinitis in children ≥12 years of age and adults

Ophthalmic: Treatment of itching of the eye associated with seasonal allergic conjunctivitis in children ≥3 years of age and adults

Local Anesthetic/Vasoconstrictor Precautions No information available to require special precautions

Effects on Dental Treatment Key adverse event(s) related to dental treatment: Bitter taste, xerostomia (normal salivary flow resumes upon discontinuation), aphthous stomatitis, glossitis, and burning sensation in throat. Chronic use of antihistamines will inhibit salivary flow, particularly in elderly patients. May contribute to periodontal disease and oral discomfort.

Common Adverse Effects
Nasal spray:
>10%:

Central nervous system: Headache (8% to 15%), somnolence (<1% to 12%)
Gastrointestinal: Bitter taste (8% to 20%)
Respiratory: Cold symptoms/rhinitis (2% to 17%), cough (11%)

2% to 10%:

Central nervous system: Dysesthesia (8%), dizziness (2%), fatigue (2%)
Gastrointestinal: Nausea (3%), weight gain (2%), dry mouth (3%)
Ocular: Conjunctivitis (<2% to 5%)
Respiratory: Asthma (5%), nasal burning (4%), pharyngitis (4%), paroxysmal sneezing (3%), sinusitis (3%), epistaxis (2% to 3%)

<2%:

Cardiovascular: Flushing, hypertension, tachycardia
Central nervous system: Abnormal thinking, anxiety, depersonalization, depression, drowsiness, fever, hypoesthesia, malaise, nervousness, sleep disorder, vertigo
Dermatologic: Contact dermatitis, eczema, furunculosis, hair and follicle infection
Endocrine & metabolic: Amenorrhea, breast pain
Gastrointestinal: Abdominal pain, ALT increased, aphthous stomatitis, appetite increased, constipation, diarrhea, gastroenteritis, glossitis, ulcerative stomatitis, toothache, vomiting
Genitourinary: Albuminuria, hematuria, polyuria
Hepatic: Liver enzymes increased
Neuromuscular & skeletal: Back pain, extremity pain, hyperkinesia, myalgia, rheumatoid arthritis, temporomandibular dislocation
Ocular: Eye pain, watery eyes
Respiratory: Bronchitis, bronchospasm, laryngitis, nasal congestion, nocturnal dyspnea, postnasal drip, sinus hypersecretion, throat burning
Miscellaneous: Allergic reactions, viral infection

<1%, postmarketing, and/or case reports: Anaphylactoid reaction, chest pain, nasal congestion, confusion, diarrhea, dyspnea, facial edema, involuntary muscle contractions, paresthesia, parosmia, pruritus, rash, skin irritation, tolerance, urinary retention, visual abnormalities, xerophthalmia

Ophthalmic:
>10%:

Central nervous system: Headache (15%)
Ocular: Transient burning/stinging (30%)

1% to 10%:

Central nervous system: Fatigue
Gastrointestinal: Bitter taste (10%)
Ocular: Conjunctivitis, eye pain, blurred vision (temporary)
Respiratory: Asthma, dyspnea, pharyngitis
Miscellaneous: Flu-like syndrome

Mechanism of Action Competes with histamine for H_1-receptor sites on effector cells and inhibits the release of histamine and other mediators involved in the allergic response; when used intranasally, reduces hyper-reactivity of the airways; increases the motility of bronchial epithelial cilia, improving mucociliary transport
(Continued)

Azelastine (Continued)

Drug Interactions

Cytochrome P450 Effect: Substrate (minor) of CYP1A2, 2C19, 2D6, 3A4; **Inhibits** CYP2B6 (weak), 2C9 (weak), 2C19 (weak), 2D6 (weak), 3A4 (weak)

Increased Effect/Toxicity: Azelastine may increase the CNS effects of ethanol and the arrhythmogenic effects of antipsychotics agents (phenothiazines). Other anticholinergics, cimetidine, CNS depressants and pramlintide may enhance the effects of azelastine.

Decreased Effect: Acetylcholinesterase inhibitors (central) may decreased the effects of azelastine; azelastine may diminish the effects of acetylcholinesterase inhibitors.

Pharmacodynamics/Kinetics

Onset of action: Peak effect: Nasal spray: 3 hours; Ophthalmic solution: 3 minutes

Duration: Nasal spray: 12 hours; Ophthalmic solution: 8 hours

Protein binding: 88%

Metabolism: Hepatic via CYP; active metabolite, desmethylazelastine

Bioavailability: Intranasal: 40%

Half-life elimination: 22 hours

Time to peak, serum: 2-3 hours

Pregnancy Risk Factor C

Azelastine Hydrochloride *see* Azelastine *on page 175*

Azelex® *see* Azelaic Acid *on page 174*

Azidothymidine *see* Zidovudine *on page 1680*

Azidothymidine, Abacavir, and Lamivudine *see* Abacavir, Lamivudine, and Zidovudine *on page 23*

Azilect® *see* Rasagiline *on page 1412*

Azithromycin (az ith roe MYE sin)

Related Information

Antibiotic Prophylaxis *on page 1772*
Bacterial Infections *on page 1793*
Periodontal Diseases *on page 1801*
Treatment of Sexually-Transmitted Infections *on page 1920*

Related Sample Prescriptions

Bacterial Infections and Periodontal Diseases *on page 1837*
Infective Endocarditis (Prevention) *on page 1832*

U.S. Brand Names Zithromax®; Zmax™

Canadian Brand Names Apo-Azithromycin®; CO Azithromycin; Dom-Azithromycin; GMD-Azithromycin; Novo-Azithromycin; PHL-Azithromycin; PMS-Azithromycin; ratio-Azithromycin; Sandoz-Azithromycin; Zithromax®

Mexican Brand Names Azitrocin

Generic Available Yes: Injection, powder for oral suspension, tablet

Index Terms Azithromycin Dihydrate; Zithromax® TRI-PAK™; Zithromax® Z-PAK®

Pharmacologic Category Antibiotic, Macrolide

Dental Use Alternate oral antibiotic for prevention of infective endocarditis in individuals allergic to penicillins or ampicillin, when amoxicillin cannot be used; alternate antibiotic in the treatment of common orofacial infections caused by aerobic gram-positive cocci and susceptible anaerobes

Use Treatment of acute otitis media due to *H. influenzae, M. catarrhalis,* or *S. pneumoniae;* pharyngitis/tonsillitis due to *S. pyogenes;* treatment of mild-to-moderate upper and lower respiratory tract infections, infections of the skin and skin structure, community-acquired pneumonia, pelvic inflammatory disease (PID), sexually-transmitted diseases (urethritis/cervicitis), pharyngitis/tonsillitis (alternative to first-line therapy), and genital ulcer disease (chancroid) due to susceptible strains of *C. trachomatis, M. catarrhalis, H. influenzae, S. aureus, S. pneumoniae, Mycoplasma pneumoniae,* and *C. psittaci;* acute bacterial exacerbations of chronic obstructive pulmonary disease (COPD) due to *H. influenzae, M. catarrhalis,* or *S. pneumoniae;* acute bacterial sinusitis

Unlabeled/Investigational Use Prevention of (or to delay onset of) or treatment of MAC in patients with advanced HIV infection; prophylaxis of bacterial endocarditis in patients who are allergic to penicillin and undergoing surgical or dental procedures; pertussis

Local Anesthetic/Vasoconstrictor Precautions No information available to require special precautions

Effects on Dental Treatment No significant effects or complications reported

Significant Adverse Effects

>10%: Gastrointestinal: Diarrhea (4% to 11%)

1% to 10%:

Central nervous system: Headache

Gastrointestinal: Nausea, abdominal pain, cramping, vomiting (especially with high single-dose regimens)

<1% (Limited to important or life-threatening): Acute renal failure, allergic reaction, aggressive behavior, anaphylaxis, angioedema, arrhythmia (including ventricular tachycardia), cholestatic jaundice, constipation, convulsion, deafness, dehydration, enteritis, erythema multiforme (rare), hearing loss, hepatic necrosis (rare), hepatitis, hypertrophic pyloric stenosis, hypotension, interstitial nephritis, leukopenia, LFTs increased, neutropenia, oral candidiasis, oral moniliasis, palpitation, pancreatitis, paresthesia, pruritus, pseudomembranous colitis, QT_c prolongation (rare), seizure, somnolence, Stevens-Johnson syndrome (rare), syncope, taste perversion, thrombocytopenia, tinnitus, tongue discoloration (rare), torsade de pointes (rare), urticaria, vertigo

Dental Usual Dosing

Infective endocarditis prophylaxis: Oral:

Children: 15 mg/kg 30-60 minutes before procedure

Adolescents ≥16 years and Adults: 500 mg 30-60 minutes prior to the procedure

Bacterial sinusitis: Oral:

Children ≥6 months: 10 mg/kg once daily for 3 days (maximum: 500 mg/day)

Adolescents ≥16 years and Adults: 500 mg/day for a total of 3 days

Extended release suspension (Zmax™): 2 g as a single dose

Orofacial infections: Adolescents ≥16 years and Adults: Oral: 500 mg/day, then 250 mg days 2-5

Treatment of periodontal disease: 500 mg once daily for 4-7 days

Dosage Note: Extended release suspension (Zmax™) is not interchangeable with immediate release formulations. Use should be limited to approved indications. All doses are expressed as immediate release azithromycin unless otherwise specified.

Usual dosage range:

Children ≥6 months: Oral: 5-12 mg/kg given once daily (maximum: 500 mg/day) **or** 30 mg/kg as a single dose (maximum: 1500 mg)

Adolescents ≥16 years and Adults:

Oral: 250-600 mg once daily **or** 1-2 g as a single dose

I.V.: 250-500 mg once daily

Indication-specific dosing:

Children: Oral:

Bacterial sinusitis: 10 mg/kg once daily for 3 days (maximum: 500 mg/day)

Cat scratch disease (unlabeled use): <45.5 kg: 10 mg/kg as a single dose, then 5 mg/kg once daily for 4 days

Community-acquired pneumonia: 10 mg/kg on day 1 (maximum: 500 mg/day) followed by 5 mg/kg/day once daily on days 2-5 (maximum: 250 mg/day)

Disseminated _M. avium_ (unlabeled use):

HIV-infected patients: 5 mg/kg/day once daily (maximum: 250 mg/day) or 20 mg/kg (maximum: 1200 mg) once weekly given alone or in combination with rifabutin

Treatment and secondary prevention in HIV-negative patients: 5 mg/kg/day once daily (maximum: 250 mg/day) in combination with ethambutol, with or without rifabutin

Endocarditis, prophylaxis (unlabeled use): 15 mg/kg 1 hour before procedure (maximum: 500 mg)

Otitis media:

1-day regimen: 30 mg/kg as a single dose (maximum: 1500 mg)

3-day regimen: 10 mg/kg once daily for 3 days (maximum: 500 mg/day)

5-day regimen: 10 mg/kg on day 1 (maximum: 500 mg/day) followed by 5 mg/kg/day once daily on days 2-5 (maximum: 250 mg/day)

Pharyngitis, tonsillitis: Children ≥2 years: 12 mg/kg/day once daily for 5 days (maximum: 500 mg/day)

Pertussis (CDC guidelines):

Children <6 months: 10 mg/kg/day for 5 days

Children ≥6 months: 10 mg/kg on day 1 (maximum: 500 mg/day) followed by 5 mg/kg/day once daily on days 2-5 (maximum: 250 mg/day)

Uncomplicated chlamydial urethritis or cervicitis (unlabeled use): Children ≥45 kg: 1 g as a single dose

Adolescents ≥16 years and Adults:

Bacterial sinusitis: Oral: 500 mg/day for a total of 3 days

Extended release suspension (Zmax™): 2 g as a single dose

Cat scratch disease (unlabeled use): Oral: >45.5 kg: 500 mg as a single dose, then 250 mg once daily for 4 days

Chancroid due to _H. ducreyi_: Oral: 1 g as a single dose

(Continued)

Azithromycin *(Continued)*

Community-acquired pneumonia:
Oral (Zmax™): 2 g as a single dose
I.V.: 500 mg as a single dose for at least 2 days, follow I.V. therapy by the oral route with a single daily dose of 500 mg to complete a 7- to 10-day course of therapy.

Disseminated *M. avium* complex disease in patients with advanced HIV infection (unlabeled use): Oral:
Prophylaxis: 1200 mg once weekly (may be combined with rifabutin)
Treatment: 600 mg daily (in combination with ethambutol 15 mg/kg)

Endocarditis, prophylaxis (unlabeled use): Oral: 500 mg 1 hour prior to the procedure

Mild-to-moderate respiratory tract, skin, and soft tissue infections:
Oral: 500 mg in a single loading dose on day 1 followed by 250 mg/day as a single dose on days 2-5
Alternative regimen: Bacterial exacerbation of COPD: 500 mg/day for a total of 3 days

Pelvic inflammatory disease (PID): I.V.: 500 mg as a single dose for 1-2 days, follow I.V. therapy by the oral route with a single daily dose of 250 mg to complete a 7-day course of therapy

Pertussis (CDC guidelines): Oral: 500 mg on day 1 followed by 250 mg/day on days 2-5 (maximum: 500 mg/day)

Urethritis/cervicitis: Oral:
Due to C. trachomatis: 1 g as a single dose
Due to N. gonorrhoeae: 2 g as a single dose

Dosage adjustment in renal impairment: Use caution in patients with Cl_{cr} <10 mL/minute

Dosage adjustment in hepatic impairment: Use with caution due to potential for hepatotoxicity (rare). Specific guidelines for dosing in hepatic impairment have not been established.

Mechanism of Action Inhibits RNA-dependent protein synthesis at the chain elongation step; binds to the 50S ribosomal subunit resulting in blockage of transpeptidation

Contraindications Hypersensitivity to azithromycin, other macrolide antibiotics, or any component of the formulation

Warnings/Precautions Use with caution in patients with pre-existing liver disease; hepatic impairment, including hepatocellular and/or cholestatic hepatitis, with or without jaundice, has been observed. Discontinue if symptoms of malaise, nausea, vomiting, abdominal colic, and fever. May mask or delay symptoms of incubating gonorrhea or syphilis, so appropriate culture and susceptibility tests should be performed prior to initiating azithromycin. Prolonged use may result in fungal or bacterial superinfection, including *C. difficile*-associated diarrhea and pseudomembranous colitis. Use caution with renal dysfunction. Prolongation of the QT_c interval has been reported with macrolide antibiotics; use caution in patients at risk of prolonged cardiac repolarization. Safety and efficacy have not been established in children <6 months of age with acute otitis media, acute bacterial sinusitis, or community-acquired pneumonia, or in children <2 years of age with pharyngitis/tonsillitis. Suspensions (immediate release and extended release) are not interchangeable.

Drug Interactions Substrate of CYP3A4 (minor); **Inhibits** CYP3A4 (weak)
Cardiac glycosides: Macrolides may increase the serum concentrations of cardiac glycosides; monitor.
Colchicine: Macrolides may increase the adverse/toxic effects of colchicine.
Nelfinavir: May increase azithromycin serum levels; monitor for adverse effects.
Warfarin: Azithromycin and other macrolides may decrease metabolism, via CYP isoenzymes, of warfarin. Monitor for increased effects.

Ethanol/Nutrition/Herb Interactions Food: Rate and extent of GI absorption may be altered depending upon the formulation. Azithromycin suspension, not tablet form, has significantly increased absorption (46%) with food.

Dietary Considerations
Oral suspension, immediate release, may be administered with or without food.
Oral suspension, extended release, should be taken on an empty stomach (at least 1 hour before or 2 hours following a meal).
Tablet may be administered with food to decrease GI effects.
Sodium content:
Injection: 114 mg (4.96 mEq) per vial
Oral suspension, immediate release: 3.7 mg per 100 mg/5 mL of constituted suspension; 7.4 mg per 200 mg/5 mL of constituted suspension; 37 mg per 1 g single-dose packet
Oral suspension, extended release: 148 mg per 2 g constituted suspension
Tablet: 0.9 mg/250 mg tablet; 1.8 mg/500 mg tablet; 2.1 mg/600 mg tablet

Pharmacodynamics/Kinetics

Absorption: Rapid

Distribution: Extensive tissue; distributes well into skin, lungs, sputum, tonsils, and cervix; penetration into CSF is poor; I.V.: 33.3 L/kg; Oral: 31.1 L/kg

Protein binding (concentration dependent): 7% to 51%

Metabolism: Hepatic

Bioavailability: 38%, decreased by 17% with extended release suspension; variable effect with food (increased with immediate or delayed release oral suspension, unchanged with tablet)

Half-life elimination: Terminal: Immediate release: 68-72 hours; Extended release: 59 hours

Time to peak, serum: Immediate release: 2-3 hours; Extended release: 5 hours

Excretion: Biliary (major route); urine (6%)

Pregnancy Risk Factor B

Lactation Enters breast milk/use caution

Breast-Feeding Considerations Azithromycin is excreted in low amounts into breast milk. The manufacturer recommends that caution be exercised when administering azithromycin to nursing women.

Compared to erythromycin, azithromycin achieves higher tissue concentrations when compared to serum concentrations. Since serum concentrations determine infant exposure, azithromycin may achieve treatment results in the mother with less exposure to the breast-feeding infant. Nondose-related effects could include modification of bowel flora.

Based on available data, azithromycin is generally considered compatible (low risk to infant) while breast-feeding [human data].

Dosage Forms Excipient information presented when available (limited, particularly for generics); consult specific product labeling.

Note: Strength expressed as base

Injection, powder for reconstitution, as dihydrate: 500 mg
Zithromax®: 500 mg [contains sodium 114 mg (4.96 mEq) per vial]

Injection, powder for reconstitution, as monohydrate: 500 mg

Microspheres for oral suspension, extended release, as dihydrate:
Zmax™: 2 g [single-dose bottle; contains sodium 148 mg per bottle; cherry and banana flavor]

Injection, powder for reconstitution, as monohydrate: 500 mg

Powder for oral suspension, as monohydrate: 100 mg/5 mL (15 mL); 200 mg/5 mL (15 mL, 22.5 mL, 30 mL)

Powder for oral suspension, immediate release, as dihydrate:
Zithromax®: 100 mg/5 mL (15 mL) [contains sodium 3.7 mg/ 5 mL; cherry creme de vanilla and banana flavor]; 200 mg/5 mL (15 mL, 22.5 mL, 30 mL) [contains sodium 7.4 mg/5 mL; cherry creme de vanilla and banana flavor]; 1 g [single-dose packet; contains sodium 37 mg per packet; cherry creme de vanilla and banana flavor]

Tablet, as dihydrate:
Zithromax®: 250 mg [contains sodium 0.9 mg per tablet]; 500 mg [contains sodium 1.8 mg per tablet]; 600 mg [contains sodium 2.1 mg per tablet]
Zithromax® TRI-PAK™ [unit-dose pack]: 500 mg (3s) [contains sodium 1.8 mg per tablet]
Zithromax® Z-PAK® [unit-dose pack]: 250 mg (6s) [contains sodium 0.9 mg per tablet]

Tablet, as monohydrate: 250 mg, 500 mg, 600 mg

Selected Readings

ADA Division of Legal Affairs, "A Legal Perspective on Antibiotic Prophylaxis," *J Am Dent Assoc*, 2003, 134(9):1260.

American Dental Association Council on Scientific Affairs, "Combating Antibiotic Resistance," *J Am Dent Assoc*, 2004, 135(4):484-7.

Cotter CJ and Bierne JC, "Azithromycin for Odontogenic Infection," *J Oral Maxillofac Surg*, 2003, 61(10):1238.

Dajani AS, Taubert KA, Wilson W, et al, "Prevention of Bacterial Endocarditis. Recommendations by the American Heart Association," *JAMA*, 1997, 277(22):1794-801.

Dajani AS, Taubert KA, Wilson W, et al, "Prevention of Bacterial Endocarditis: Recommendations by the American Heart Association," *J Am Dent Assoc*, 1997, 128(8):1142-51.

Moore PA, "Dental Therapeutic Indications for the Newer Long-Acting Macrolide Antibiotics," *J Am Dent Assoc*, 1999, 130(9):1341-3.

Williams JD, Maskell JP, Shain H, et al, "Comparative *In Vitro* Activity of Azithromycin, Macrolides (Erythromycin, Clarithromycin and Spiramycin) and Streptogramin RP 59500 Against Oral Organisms," *J Antimicrob Chemother*, 1992, 30(1):27-37.

Wynn RL, Bergman SA, Meiller TF, et al, "Antibiotics in Treating Oral-Facial Infections of Odontogenic Origin: An Update," *Gen Dent*, 2001, 49(3):238-40, 242, 244 passim.

Wynn RL, "New Erythromycins," *Gen Dent*, 1996, 44(4):304-7.

AZTREONAM

Aztreonam (AZ tree oh nam)

U.S. Brand Names Azactam®
Canadian Brand Names Azactam®
Generic Available No
Index Terms Azthreonam
Pharmacologic Category Antibiotic, Miscellaneous
Use Treatment of patients with urinary tract infections, lower respiratory tract infections, septicemia, skin/skin structure infections, intra-abdominal infections, and gynecological infections caused by susceptible gram-negative bacilli
Local Anesthetic/Vasoconstrictor Precautions No information available to require special precautions
Effects on Dental Treatment No significant effects or complications reported
Common Adverse Effects As reported in adults: 1% to 10%:
   Dermatologic: Rash
   Gastrointestinal: Diarrhea, nausea, vomiting
   Local: Thrombophlebitis, pain at injection site
Mechanism of Action Inhibits bacterial cell wall synthesis by binding to one or more of the penicillin binding proteins (PBPs) which in turn inhibits the final transpeptidation step of peptidoglycan synthesis in bacterial cell walls, thus inhibiting cell wall biosynthesis. Bacteria eventually lyse due to ongoing activity of cell wall autolytic enzymes (autolysins and murein hydrolases) while cell wall assembly is arrested. Monobactam structure makes cross-allergenicity with beta-lactams unlikely.
Drug Interactions
   Decreased Effect: Avoid antibiotics that induce beta-lactamase production (cefoxitin, imipenem).
Pharmacodynamics/Kinetics
   Absorption: I.M.: Well absorbed; I.M. and I.V. doses produce comparable serum concentrations
   Distribution: Widely to most body fluids and tissues; crosses placenta; enters breast milk
      V_d: Children: 0.2-0.29 L/kg; Adults: 0.2 L/kg
      Relative diffusion of antimicrobial agents from blood into CSF: Good only with inflammation (exceeds usual MICs)
      CSF:blood level ratio: Meninges: Inflamed: 8% to 40%; Normal: ~1%
   Protein binding: 56%
   Metabolism: Hepatic (minor %)
   Half-life elimination:
      Children 2 months to 12 years: 1.7 hours
      Adults: Normal renal function: 1.7-2.9 hours
      End-stage renal disease: 6-8 hours
   Time to peak: I.M., I.V. push: Within 60 minutes; I.V. infusion: 1.5 hours
   Excretion: Urine (60% to 70% as unchanged drug); feces (~13% to 15%)
Pregnancy Risk Factor B

Bacitracin (bas i TRAY sin)

U.S. Brand Names AK-Tracin® [DSC]; Baciguent® [OTC]; BaciiM®
Canadian Brand Names Baciguent®; Baciject®
Generic Available Yes

Pharmacologic Category Antibiotic, Miscellaneous; Antibiotic, Ophthalmic; Antibiotic, Topical

Use Treatment of susceptible bacterial infections mainly; has activity against gram-positive bacilli; due to toxicity risks, systemic and irrigant uses of bacitracin should be limited to situations where less toxic alternatives would not be effective

Unlabeled/Investigational Use Oral administration: Successful in antibiotic-associated colitis; has been used for enteric eradication of vancomycin-resistant enterococci (VRE)

Local Anesthetic/Vasoconstrictor Precautions No information available to require special precautions

Effects on Dental Treatment No significant effects or complications reported

Common Adverse Effects 1% to 10%:
Cardiovascular: Hypotension, edema of the face/lips, chest tightness
Central nervous system: Pain
Dermatologic: Rash, itching
Gastrointestinal: Anorexia, nausea, vomiting, diarrhea, rectal itching
Hematologic: Blood dyscrasias
Miscellaneous: Diaphoresis

<1%: Rare cases of anaphylaxis have been reported in association with topical and intraoperative exposures.

Mechanism of Action Inhibits bacterial cell wall synthesis by preventing transfer of mucopeptides into the growing cell wall

Drug Interactions
Increased Effect/Toxicity: Nephrotoxic drugs, neuromuscular blocking agents, and anesthetics (increased neuromuscular blockade).

Pharmacodynamics/Kinetics
Duration: 6-8 hours
Absorption: Poor from mucous membranes and intact or denuded skin; rapidly following I.M. administration; not absorbed by bladder irrigation, but absorption can occur from peritoneal or mediastinal lavage
Distribution: CSF: Nil even with inflammation
Protein binding, plasma: Minimal
Time to peak, serum: I.M.: 1-2 hours
Excretion: Urine (10% to 40%) within 24 hours

Pregnancy Risk Factor C

Bacitracin and Polymyxin B (bas i TRAY sin & pol i MIKS in bee)

Related Information
Bacitracin *on page 180*
Polymyxin B *on page 1322*

U.S. Brand Names AK-Poly-Bac™; Betadine® First Aid Antibiotics + Moisturizer [OTC] [DSC]; Polysporin® [OTC]

Canadian Brand Names LID-Pack®; Optimyxin®

Generic Available Yes

Index Terms Polymyxin B and Bacitracin

Pharmacologic Category Antibiotic, Ophthalmic; Antibiotic, Topical

Use Treatment of superficial infections caused by susceptible organisms

Local Anesthetic/Vasoconstrictor Precautions No information available to require special precautions

Effects on Dental Treatment No significant effects or complications reported

Common Adverse Effects 1% to 10%: Local: Rash, itching, burning, anaphylactoid reactions, swelling, conjunctival erythema

Mechanism of Action See individual agents.

Pharmacodynamics/Kinetics See individual agents.

Pregnancy Risk Factor C

Bacitracin, Neomycin, and Polymyxin B
(bas i TRAY sin, nee oh MYE sin, & pol i MIKS in bee)

Related Information
Bacitracin *on page 180*
Neomycin *on page 1160*
Polymyxin B *on page 1322*

U.S. Brand Names Neosporin® Neo To Go® [OTC]; Neosporin® Ophthalmic Ointment [DSC]; Neosporin® Topical [OTC]

Canadian Brand Names Neosporin® Ophthalmic Ointment

Mexican Brand Names Neosporin Dermico; Polixin Ungena; Tribiot

Generic Available Yes

(Continued)

Bacitracin, Neomycin, and Polymyxin B *(Continued)*

Index Terms Neomycin, Bacitracin, and Polymyxin B; Polymyxin B, Bacitracin, and Neomycin; Triple Antibiotic

Pharmacologic Category Antibiotic, Ophthalmic; Antibiotic, Topical

Use Helps prevent infection in minor cuts, scrapes, and burns; short-term treatment of superficial external ocular infections caused by susceptible organisms

Local Anesthetic/Vasoconstrictor Precautions No information available to require special precautions

Effects on Dental Treatment No significant effects or complications reported

Common Adverse Effects Frequency not defined.
Dermatologic: Reddening, allergic contact dermatitis
Local: Itching, failure to heal, swelling, irritation
Ophthalmic: Conjunctival edema
Miscellaneous: Anaphylaxis

Mechanism of Action Refer to individual agents, Bacitracin *on page 180*, Neomycin *on page 1160*, and Polymyxin B *on page 1322*.

Pharmacodynamics/Kinetics See individual agents.

Pregnancy Risk Factor C

Bacitracin, Neomycin, Polymyxin B, and Hydrocortisone

(bas i TRAY sin, nee oh MYE sin, pol i MIKS in bee, & hye droe KOR ti sone)

Related Information
Bacitracin *on page 180*
Hydrocortisone *on page 836*
Neomycin *on page 1160*
Polymyxin B *on page 1322*

U.S. Brand Names Cortisporin® Ointment

Canadian Brand Names Cortisporin® Topical Ointment

Generic Available Yes: Ophthalmic ointment

Index Terms Hydrocortisone, Bacitracin, Neomycin, and Polymyxin B; Neomycin, Bacitracin, Polymyxin B, and Hydrocortisone; Polymyxin B, Bacitracin, Neomycin, and Hydrocortisone

Pharmacologic Category Antibiotic, Ophthalmic; Antibiotic, Otic; Antibiotic, Topical; Corticosteroid, Ophthalmic; Corticosteroid, Otic; Corticosteroid, Topical

Use Prevention and treatment of susceptible inflammatory conditions where bacterial infection (or risk of infection) is present

Local Anesthetic/Vasoconstrictor Precautions No information available to require special precautions

Effects on Dental Treatment No significant effects or complications reported

Common Adverse Effects Frequency not defined.
Dermatologic: Rash, generalized itching
Ocular: Irritation
Respiratory: Apnea
Miscellaneous: Secondary infection

Mechanism of Action Refer to individual agents, Bacitracin *on page 180*, Neomycin *on page 1160*, Polymyxin B *on page 1322*, and Hydrocortisone *on page 836*.

Drug Interactions
Cytochrome P450 Effect: Hydrocortisone: **Substrate** of CYP3A4 (minor); **Induces** CYP3A4 (weak)

Pharmacodynamics/Kinetics See individual agents.

Pregnancy Risk Factor C

Bacitracin, Neomycin, Polymyxin B, and Pramoxine

(bas i TRAY sin, nee oh MYE sin, pol i MIKS in bee, & pra MOKS een)

Related Information
Bacitracin *on page 180*
Neomycin *on page 1160*
Polymyxin B *on page 1322*
Pramoxine *on page 1334*

U.S. Brand Names Neosporin® + Pain Relief Ointment [OTC]; Spectrocin Plus™ [OTC] [DSC]; Tri Biozene [OTC]

Generic Available Yes

Index Terms Neomycin, Bacitracin, Polymyxin B, and Pramoxine; Polymyxin B, Neomycin, Bacitracin, and Pramoxine; Pramoxine, Neomycin, Bacitracin, and Polymyxin B

Pharmacologic Category Antibiotic, Topical

Use Prevention and treatment of susceptible superficial topical infections and provide temporary relief of pain or discomfort

Local Anesthetic/Vasoconstrictor Precautions No information available to require special precautions

Effects on Dental Treatment No significant effects or complications reported

Baclofen (BAK loe fen)

U.S. Brand Names Lioresal®

Canadian Brand Names Apo-Baclofen®; Gen-Baclofen; Lioresal®; Liotec; Nu-Baclo; PMS-Baclofen

Generic Available Yes: Tablets only

Pharmacologic Category Skeletal Muscle Relaxant

Use Treatment of reversible spasticity associated with multiple sclerosis or spinal cord lesions

    Orphan drug: Intrathecal: Treatment of intractable spasticity caused by spinal cord injury, multiple sclerosis, and other spinal disease (spinal ischemia or tumor, transverse myelitis, cervical spondylosis, degenerative myelopathy)

Unlabeled/Investigational Use Intractable hiccups, intractable pain relief, bladder spasticity, trigeminal neuralgia, cerebral palsy, Huntington's chorea

Local Anesthetic/Vasoconstrictor Precautions No information available to require special precautions

Effects on Dental Treatment No significant effects or complications reported

Common Adverse Effects

    >10%:

        Central nervous system: Drowsiness, vertigo, psychiatric disturbances, insomnia, slurred speech, ataxia, hypotonia

        Neuromuscular & skeletal: Weakness

    1% to 10%:

        Cardiovascular: Hypotension

        Central nervous system: Fatigue, confusion, headache

        Dermatologic: Rash

        Gastrointestinal: Nausea, constipation

        Genitourinary: Polyuria

Mechanism of Action Inhibits the transmission of both monosynaptic and polysynaptic reflexes at the spinal cord level, possibly by hyperpolarization of primary afferent fiber terminals, with resultant relief of muscle spasticity

Drug Interactions

    Increased Effect/Toxicity: Effects may be additive with CNS depressants.

Pharmacodynamics/Kinetics

    Onset of action: 3-4 days

        Peak effect: 5-10 days

    Absorption (dose dependent): Oral: Rapid

    Protein binding: 30%

    Metabolism: Hepatic (15% of dose)

    Half-life elimination: 3.5 hours

    Time to peak, serum: Oral: Within 2-3 hours

    Excretion: Urine and feces (85% as unchanged drug)

Pregnancy Risk Factor C

BactoShield® CHG [OTC] *see* Chlorhexidine Gluconate *on page 332*

Bactrim™ *see* Sulfamethoxazole and Trimethoprim *on page 1504*

Bactrim™ DS *see* Sulfamethoxazole and Trimethoprim *on page 1504*

Bactroban® *see* Mupirocin *on page 1132*

Bactroban® Nasal *see* Mupirocin *on page 1132*

Baking Soda *see* Sodium Bicarbonate *on page 1480*

BAL *see* Dimercaprol *on page 508*

Balacet 325™ *see* Propoxyphene and Acetaminophen *on page 1369*

Balanced Salt Solution (BAL anced salt soe LOO shun)

U.S. Brand Names AquaLase™; BSS®; BSS Plus®

Canadian Brand Names BSS®; BSS Plus®; Eye-Stream®

Generic Available Yes

Pharmacologic Category Irrigating Solution; Ophthalmic Agent, Miscellaneous

(Continued)

Balanced Salt Solution *(Continued)*

Use
Irrigation solution for ophthalmic surgery:
    AquaLase™, BSS®: Intraocular or extraocular irrigating solution
    BSS® Plus: Intraocular irrigating solution
Irrigation solution for eyes, ears, nose, or throat

Local Anesthetic/Vasoconstrictor Precautions No information available to require special precautions

Effects on Dental Treatment No significant effects or complications reported

BAL in Oil® *see* Dimercaprol *on page 508*

Balmex® [OTC] *see* Zinc Oxide *on page 1683*

Balnetar® [OTC] *see* Coal Tar *on page 402*

Balsalazide (bal SAL a zide)

U.S. Brand Names Colazal®
Generic Available No
Index Terms Balsalazide Disodium
Pharmacologic Category 5-Aminosalicylic Acid Derivative; Anti-inflammatory Agent
Use Treatment of mild-to-moderate active ulcerative colitis
Local Anesthetic/Vasoconstrictor Precautions No information available to require special precautions
Effects on Dental Treatment No significant effects or complications reported
Common Adverse Effects
>10%:
    Central nervous system: Headache (children 15%; adults 8%)
    Gastrointestinal: Abdominal pain (children 12% to 13%; adults 6%)
1% to 10%:
    Central nervous system: Insomnia (adults 2%), fatigue (children 4%; adults2%), fever (children 6%; adults 2%)
    Endocrine & metabolic: Dysmenorrhea (children 3%)
    Gastrointestinal: Diarrhea (children 9%; adults 5%), ulcerative colitis exacerbation (children 6%; adults 1%), nausea (children 4%; adults 5%), vomiting (children 10%; adults 4%), hematochezia (children 4%), stomatitis (children 3%), anorexia (adults 2%), dyspepsia (adults 2%), flatulence (adults 2%), cramps (adults 1%), constipation (adults 1%), dry mouth (adults 1%)
    Genitourinary: Urinary tract infection (adults 1%)
    Neuromuscular & skeletal: Arthralgia (adults 4%), back pain (adults 2%), myalgia (adults 1%)
    Respiratory: Respiratory infection (adults 4%), cough (children 3%; adults 2%), pharyngitis (children 6%; adults 2%), pharyngolaryngeal pain (children 3%), rhinitis (adults 2%)
    Miscellaneous: Flu-like syndrome (children 4%; adults 1%)
Mechanism of Action Balsalazide is a prodrug, converted by bacterial azoreduction to 5-aminosalicylic acid (mesalamine, active), 4-aminobenzoyl-β-alanine (inert), and their metabolites. 5-aminosalicylic acid may decrease inflammation by blocking the production of arachidonic acid metabolites topically in the colon mucosa.
Drug Interactions
    Increased Effect/Toxicity: 5-ASA derivatives may decrease the metabolism of azathioprine, mercaptopurine, thioguanine
    Decreased Effect: 5-ASA derivatives may decrease the absorption of digoxin.
Pharmacodynamics/Kinetics
    Onset of action: Delayed; may require several days to weeks
    Absorption: Very low and variable
    Protein binding: Balsalazide: ≥99%
    Metabolism: Azoreduced in the colon to 5-aminosalicylic acid (active), 4-aminobenzoyl-β-alanine (inert), and N-acetylated metabolites
    Half-life elimination: Primary effect is topical (colonic mucosa); systemic half-life not determined
    Time to peak: Balsalazide: 1-2 hours
    Excretion: Feces (65% as 5-aminosalicylic acid, 4-aminobenzoyl-β-alanine, and N-acetylated metabolites); urine (25% as N-acetylated metabolites); Parent drug: Urine or feces (<1%)
Pregnancy Risk Factor B

Balsalazide Disodium *see* Balsalazide *on page 184*

Balsam Peru, Trypsin, and Castor Oil *see* Trypsin, Balsam Peru, and Castor Oil *on page 1628*

Baltussin *see* Dihydrocodeine, Chlorpheniramine, and Phenylephrine *on page 502*

Band-Aid® Hurt-Free™ Antiseptic Wash [OTC] *see* Lidocaine *on page 972*

Banophen® [OTC] *see* DiphenhydrAMINE *on page 510*

Banophen® Anti-Itch [OTC] *see* DiphenhydrAMINE *on page 510*

Baraclude™ *see* Entecavir *on page 570*

Baricon™ *see* Barium *on page 185*

Baridium® [OTC] *see* Phenazopyridine *on page 1286*

Barium (BA ree um)

U.S. Brand Names Anatrast; Baricon™; Barobag®; Baro-Cat®; Barosperse®; Bar-Test; CheeTah®; Enhancer; Entero Vu™; Entrobar®; EntroEase®; Esopho-Cat®; E-Z-Cat®; E-Z-Cat® Dry; E-Z-Disk™; HD 200® Plus; Intropaste; Liqui-Coat HD®; Liquid Barosperse®; Medebar® Plus; Prepcat; Readi-Cat®; Readi-Cat® 2; Tomocat®; Tomocat® 1000; Tonojug; Tonopaque; Varibar® Honey; Varibar® Nectar; Varibar® Pudding; Varibar® Thin Honey; Varibar® Thin Liquid; VoLumen™

Generic Available No

Index Terms Barium Sulfate

Pharmacologic Category Radiopaque Agents

Use Diagnostic aid for computed tomography or x-ray examinations of the GI tract

Local Anesthetic/Vasoconstrictor Precautions No information available to require special precautions

Effects on Dental Treatment No significant effects or complications reported

Barium Sulfate *see* Barium *on page 185*

Barobag® *see* Barium *on page 185*

Baro-Cat® *see* Barium *on page 185*

Barosperse® *see* Barium *on page 185*

Bar-Test *see* Barium *on page 185*

Base Ointment *see* Zinc Oxide *on page 1683*

Basiliximab (ba si LIK si mab)

U.S. Brand Names Simulect®

Canadian Brand Names Simulect®

Mexican Brand Names Simulect

Generic Available No

Pharmacologic Category Monoclonal Antibody

Use Prophylaxis of acute organ rejection in renal transplantation

Local Anesthetic/Vasoconstrictor Precautions No information available to require special precautions

Effects on Dental Treatment Key adverse event(s) related to dental treatment: Facial edema and ulcerative stomatitis. Causes gingival hypertrophy (GH) similar to that caused by cyclosporine; early reports indicate that frequency/incidence of basiliximab-induced GH not as high as cyclosporine-induced GH.

Common Adverse Effects Administration of basiliximab did not appear to increase the incidence or severity of adverse effects in clinical trials. Adverse events were reported in 96% of both the placebo and basiliximab groups.

>10%:
  Cardiovascular: Hypertension, peripheral edema
  Central nervous system: Fever, headache, insomnia, pain
  Dermatologic: Acne, wound complications
  Endocrine & metabolic: Hypercholesterolemia, hyperglycemia, hyper-/hypo-kalemia, hyperuricemia, hypophosphatemia
  Gastrointestinal: Abdominal pain, constipation, diarrhea, dyspepsia, nausea, vomiting
  Genitourinary: Urinary tract infection
  Hematologic: Anemia
  Neuromuscular & skeletal: Tremor
  Respiratory: Dyspnea, infection (upper respiratory)
  Miscellaneous: Viral infection
3% to 10%:
  Cardiovascular: Abnormal heart sounds, angina pectoris, arrhythmia, atrial fibrillation, cardiac failure, chest pain, generalized edema, hypotension, tachycardia
  Central nervous system: Agitation, anxiety, depression, dizziness, fatigue, hypoesthesia, malaise, neuropathy, rigors
(Continued)

Basiliximab (Continued)

Dermatologic: Cyst, hypertrichosis, pruritus, rash, skin disorder, skin ulceration

Endocrine & metabolic: Acidosis, dehydration, diabetes mellitus, fluid overload, hyper-/hypocalcemia, hyperlipidemia, hypertriglyceridemia, hypoglycemia, hypomagnesemia, hyponatremia

Gastrointestinal: Abdomen enlarged, esophagitis, flatulence, gastroenteritis, GI hemorrhage, gingival hyperplasia, melena, moniliasis, stomatitis (including ulcerative), weight gain

Genitourinary: Albuminuria, bladder disorder, dysuria, genital edema, hematuria, impotence, oliguria, renal function abnormal, renal tubular necrosis, ureteral disorder, urinary frequency, urinary retention

Hematologic: Hematoma, hemorrhage, leukopenia, polycythemia, purpura, thrombocytopenia, thrombosis

Neuromuscular & skeletal: Arthralgia, arthropathy, back pain, cramps, fracture, hernia, leg pain, myalgia, paresthesia, weakness

Ocular: Abnormal vision, cataract, conjunctivitis

Respiratory: Bronchitis, bronchospasm, cough, pharyngitis, pneumonia, pulmonary edema, sinusitis, rhinitis

Miscellaneous: Accidental trauma, facial edema, glucocorticoids increased, herpes infection, sepsis

Mechanism of Action Chimeric (murine/human) monoclonal antibody which blocks the alpha-chain of the interleukin-2 (IL-2) receptor complex; this receptor is expressed on activated T lymphocytes and is a critical pathway for activating cell-mediated allograft rejection

Drug Interactions

Increased Effect/Toxicity: Allergic reactions may be increased in patients who have received diagnostic or therapeutic monoclonal antibodies due to the presence of human antichimeric antibody (HACA). Basiliximab may increase the risk of vaccinial infection with live organism vaccine administration.

Decreased Effect: Basiliximab may decrease the effect of vaccines (dead organisms).

Pharmacodynamics/Kinetics

Duration: Mean: 36 days (determined by IL-2R alpha saturation)

Distribution: Mean: V_d: Children 1-11 years: 4.8 ± 2.1 L; Adolescents 12-16 years: 7.8 ± 5.1 L; Adults: 8.6 ± 4.1 L

Half-life elimination: Children 1-11 years: 9.5 days; Adolescents 12-16 years: 9.1 days; Adults: Mean: 7.2 days

Excretion: Clearance: Children 1-11 years: 17 mL/hour; Adolescents 12-16 years: 31 mL/hour; Adults: Mean: 41 mL/hour

Pregnancy Risk Factor B (manufacturer)

BCG Vaccine (bee see jee vak SEEN)

Related Information

Immunizations (Vaccines) on page 1886

U.S. Brand Names TheraCys®; TICE® BCG

Canadian Brand Names ImmuCyst®; Oncotice™; Pacis™

Mexican Brand Names OncoTICE

Generic Available No

Index Terms Bacillus Calmette-Guérin (BCG) Live; BCG, Live; BCG Vaccine U.S.P. (percutaneous use product)

Pharmacologic Category Biological Response Modulator; Vaccine

Use Immunization against tuberculosis and immunotherapy for cancer; treatment and prophylaxis of carcinoma *in situ* of the bladder; prophylaxis of primary or recurrent superficial papillary tumors following transurethral resection

Local Anesthetic/Vasoconstrictor Precautions No information available to require special precautions

Effects on Dental Treatment No significant effects or complications reported

Common Adverse Effects All serious adverse reactions must be reported to the U.S. Department of Health and Human Services (DHHS) Vaccine Adverse Event Reporting System (VAERS) 1-800-822-7967.

Adverse reactions associated with **intravesicular administration**:

>10%:

Central nervous system: Malaise (7% to 40%), fever (20% to 38%), chills (34%)

Gastrointestinal: Nausea/vomiting (3% to 16%), anorexia/weight loss (2% to 11%)

Genitourinary: Dysuria (52% to 60%), bladder irritation (50% to 60%), polyuria (40% to 42%), hematuria (26% to 39%), cystitis (6% to 29%), urinary urgency (6% to 18%), urinary tract infection (2% to 18%)

Hematological: Anemia (<1% to 21%)

Miscellaneous: Flu-like syndrome (33%)

1% to 10%:

Central nervous system: Fatigue (7%), headache/dizziness (2%)

Dermatologic: Rash (2%)

Gastrointestinal: Diarrhea (6%), abdominal pain (2% to 3%)

Genitourinary: Genital pain (10%), bladder cramps/pain (6%), urinary incontinence (2% to 6%), bladder spasm (5%), nocturia (5%), urinary debris (2%), genital inflammation/abscess (2%)

Hematological: Leukopenia (5%), coagulopathy (3%)

Neuromuscular & skeletal: Arthralgia/myalgia (3% to 7%), cramps/pain (4% to 6%), rigors (3%)

Renal: Renal toxicity (10%)

Respiratory: Pulmonary infection (3%)

Miscellaneous: Infection (3%), allergy (2%)

Adverse reactions associated with **BCG vaccination**: Axillary lymphadenopathy, cervical lymphadenopathy, disseminated BCG infection (BCG osteomyelitis), local reactions (induration, itching, lesions, lymphadenitis, pustule, tenderness, ulceration). Local reactions may persist for up to 3 months; more severe manifestations may occur up to 5 months after vaccination and persist for several weeks.

Mechanism of Action BCG live is an attenuated strain of bacillus Calmette-Guérin (*Mycobacterium bovis*) used as a biological response modifier. BCG live, when used intravesicularly for treatment of bladder carcinoma *in situ*, is thought to cause a local, chronic inflammatory response involving macrophage and leukocyte infiltration of the bladder. By a mechanism not fully understood, this local inflammatory response leads to destruction of superficial tumor cells of the urothelium. BCG is active immunotherapy which stimulates the host's immune mechanism to reject the tumor. Evidence of systemic immune response is also commonly seen, manifested by a positive PPD tuberculin skin test reaction, however, its relationship to clinical efficacy is not well-established.

Drug Interactions

Increased Effect/Toxicity: The following agents may decrease the effectiveness of BCG vaccine: Antimicrobials, immune globulins, immunosuppressants, and other live organism vaccines. Antimicrobials may interfere with the effectiveness of intravesicular BCG.

Decreased Effect: Immunosuppressants may increase the risk of vaccinal infections. BCG vaccination results in a reactive tuberculin skin test.

Pregnancy Risk Factor C

BCG Vaccine U.S.P. *(percutaneous use product) see* BCG Vaccine *on page 186*

BCNU *see* Carmustine *on page 288*

B Complex Combinations *see* Vitamin B Complex Combinations *on page 1664*

Bebulin® VH *see* Factor IX Complex (Human) *on page 667*

Becaplermin (be KAP ler min)

U.S. Brand Names Regranex®

Canadian Brand Names Regranex®

Mexican Brand Names Regranex

Generic Available No

(Continued)

Becaplermin *(Continued)*

Index Terms Recombinant Human Platelet-Derived Growth Factor B; rPDGF-BB

Pharmacologic Category Growth Factor, Platelet-Derived; Topical Skin Product

Use Debridement adjunct for the treatment of diabetic ulcers that occur on the lower limbs and feet

Local Anesthetic/Vasoconstrictor Precautions No information available to require special precautions

Effects on Dental Treatment No significant effects or complications reported

Mechanism of Action Recombinant B-isoform homodimer of human platelet-derived growth factor (rPDGF-BB) which enhances formation of new granulation tissue, induces fibroblast proliferation and differentiation to promote wound healing

Pharmacodynamics/Kinetics

Onset of action: Complete healing: 15% of patients within 8 weeks, 25% at 10 weeks

Absorption: Minimal

Distribution: Binds to PDGF beta-receptors in normal skin and granulation tissue

Pregnancy Risk Factor C

Beclomethasone *(be kloe METH a sone)*

Related Information

Respiratory Diseases *on page 1747*

U.S. Brand Names Beconase® AQ; QVAR®

Canadian Brand Names Apo-Beclomethasone®; Gen-Beclo; Nu-Beclomethasone; Propaderm®; QVAR®; Rivanase AQ; Vanceril® AEM

Mexican Brand Names Beconase

Generic Available No

Index Terms Beclomethasone Dipropionate

Pharmacologic Category Corticosteroid, Inhalant (Oral); Corticosteroid, Nasal

Use

Oral inhalation: Maintenance and prophylactic treatment of asthma; includes those who require corticosteroids and those who may benefit from a dose reduction/elimination of systemically-administered corticosteroids. Not for relief of acute bronchospasm.

Nasal aerosol: Symptomatic treatment of seasonal or perennial rhinitis; prevent recurrence of nasal polyps following surgery.

Local Anesthetic/Vasoconstrictor Precautions No information available to require special precautions

Effects on Dental Treatment Key adverse event(s) related to dental treatment: Oral candidiasis, xerostomia (normal salivary flow resumes upon discontinuation), nasal dryness, and dry throat. Localized infections with *Candida albicans* or *Aspergillus niger* occur frequently in the mouth and pharynx with repetitive use of an oral inhaler; may require treatment with appropriate antifungal therapy or discontinuance of inhaler use.

Significant Adverse Effects Frequency not defined.

Central nervous system: Agitation, depression, dizziness, dysphonia, headache, lightheadedness, mental disturbances

Dermatologic: Acneiform lesions, angioedema, atrophy, bruising, pruritus, purpura, striae, rash, urticaria

Endocrine & metabolic: Cushingoid features, growth velocity reduction in children and adolescents, HPA function suppression

Gastrointestinal: Dry/irritated nose, throat and mouth, hoarseness, localized *Candida* or *Aspergillus* infection, loss of smell, loss of taste, nausea, unpleasant smell, unpleasant taste, vomiting, weight gain

Local: Nasal spray: Burning, epistaxis, localized *Candida* infection, nasal septum perforation (rare), nasal stuffiness, nosebleeds, rhinorrhea, sneezing, transient irritation, ulceration of nasal mucosa (rare)

Ocular: Cataracts, glaucoma, intraocular pressure increased

Respiratory: Cough, paradoxical bronchospasm, pharyngitis, sinusitis, wheezing

Miscellaneous: Anaphylactic/anaphylactoid reactions, death (due to adrenal insufficiency, reported during and after transfer from systemic corticosteroids to aerosol in asthmatic patients), immediate and delayed hypersensitivity reactions

Dosage Nasal inhalation and oral inhalation dosage forms are not to be used interchangeably

Inhalation, nasal: Rhinitis, nasal polyps (Beconase® AQ): Children ≥6 years and Adults: 1-2 inhalations each nostril twice daily; total dose 168-336 mcg/day

Inhalation, oral: Asthma (doses should be titrated to the lowest effective dose once asthma is controlled) (QVAR®):

Children 5-11 years: Initial: 40 mcg twice daily; maximum dose: 80 mcg twice daily

Children ≥12 years and Adults:

Patients previously on bronchodilators only: Initial dose 40-80 mcg twice daily; maximum dose: 320 mcg twice day

Patients previously on inhaled corticosteroids: Initial dose 40-160 mcg twice daily; maximum dose: 320 mcg twice daily

NIH Asthma Guidelines (NAEPP, 2002; NIH, 1997): HFA formulation (eg, QVAR®): Administer in divided doses:

Children ≤12 years:

"Low" dose: 80-160 mcg/day

"Medium" dose: 160-320 mcg/day

"High" dose: >320 mcg/day

Children >12 years and Adults:

"Low" dose: 80-240 mcg/day

"Medium" dose: 240-480 mcg/day

"High" dose: >480 mcg/day

Mechanism of Action Controls the rate of protein synthesis; depresses the migration of polymorphonuclear leukocytes, fibroblasts; reverses capillary permeability and lysosomal stabilization at the cellular level to prevent or control inflammation

Contraindications Hypersensitivity to beclomethasone or any component of the formulation; status asthmaticus

Warnings/Precautions May cause hypercorticism or suppression of hypothalamic-pituitary-adrenal (HPA) axis, particularly in younger children or in patients receiving high doses for prolonged periods. HPA axis suppression may lead to adrenal crisis. Withdrawal and discontinuation of a corticosteroid should be done slowly and carefully. Particular care is required when patients are transferred from systemic corticosteroids to inhaled products due to possible adrenal insufficiency or withdrawal from steroids, including an increase in allergic symptoms. Patients receiving >20 mg per day of prednisone (or equivalent) may be most susceptible. Fatalities have occurred due to adrenal insufficiency in asthmatic patients during and after transfer from systemic corticosteroids to aerosol steroids; aerosol steroids do not provide the systemic steroid needed to treat patients having trauma, surgery, or infections.

Bronchospasm may occur with wheezing after inhalation; if this occurs stop steroid and treat with a fast-acting bronchodilator. Supplemental steroids (oral or parenteral) may be needed during stress or severe asthma attacks. Not to be used in status asthmaticus or for the relief of acute bronchospasm. Corticosteroid use may cause psychiatric disturbances, including depression, euphoria, insomnia, mood swings, and personality changes. Pre-existing psychiatric conditions may be exacerbated by corticosteroid use. Prolonged use of corticosteroids may also increase the incidence of secondary infection, mask acute infection (including fungal infections), prolong or exacerbate viral infections, or limit response to vaccines. Exposure to chickenpox should be avoided; corticosteroids should not be used to treat ocular herpes simplex. Corticosteroids should not be used for cerebral malaria. Close observation is required in patients with latent tuberculosis and/or TB reactivity; restrict use in active TB (only in conjunction with antituberculosis treatment). Prolonged treatment with corticosteroids has been associated with the development of Kaposi's sarcoma (case reports); if noted, discontinuation of therapy should be considered.

Use with caution in patients with thyroid disease, hepatic impairment, renal impairment, cardiovascular disease, diabetes, glaucoma, cataracts, myasthenia gravis, patients at risk for osteoporosis, patients at risk for seizures, or GI diseases (diverticulitis, peptic ulcer, ulcerative colitis) due to perforation risk. Use caution following acute MI (corticosteroids have been associated with myocardial rupture). Because of the risk of adverse effects, systemic corticosteroids should be used cautiously in the elderly in the smallest possible effective dose for the shortest duration. Avoid nasal corticosteroid use in patients with recent nasal septal ulcers, nasal surgery or nasal trauma until healing has occurred.

Orally-inhaled and intranasal corticosteroids may cause a reduction in growth velocity in pediatric patients (~1 centimeter per year [range 0.3-1.8 cm per year] and related to dose and duration of exposure). To minimize the systemic effects of orally-inhaled and intranasal corticosteroids, each patient should be titrated to the lowest effective dose. Growth should be routinely monitored in pediatric patients. Safety and efficacy have not been established in children <5 years of age. There have been reports of systemic corticosteroid withdrawal symptoms (Continued)

Beclomethasone *(Continued)*

(eg, joint/muscle pain, lassitude, depression) when withdrawing oral inhalation therapy.

Drug Interactions Salmeterol: The addition of salmeterol has been demonstrated to improve response to inhaled corticosteroids (as compared to increasing steroid dosage).

Pharmacodynamics/Kinetics

Onset of action: Therapeutic effect: 1-4 weeks

Absorption: Readily; quickly hydrolyzed by pulmonary esterases prior to absorption

Distribution: Beclomethasone: 20 L; active metabolite: 424 L

Protein binding: 87%

Metabolism: Hepatic via CYP3A4 to active metabolites

Bioavailability: Of active metabolite, 44% following nasal inhalation (43% from swallowed portion)

Half-life elimination: Initial: 3 hours

Excretion: Feces (60%); urine (12%)

Pregnancy Risk Factor C

Lactation Excretion in breast milk unknown/use caution

Breast-Feeding Considerations Other corticosteroids have been found in breast milk; however, information for beclomethasone is not available. Inhaled corticosteroids are recommended for the treatment of asthma (most information available using budesonide) while breast-feeding.

Dosage Forms Excipient information presented when available (limited, particularly for generics); consult specific product labeling.

Aerosol for oral inhalation, as dipropionate:

QVAR®: 40 mcg/inhalation [100 metered actuations] (7.3 g); 80 mcg/inhalation [100 metered actuations] (7.3 g)

Suspension, intranasal, as dipropionate [aqueous spray]:

Beconase® AQ: 42 mcg/inhalation [180 metered sprays] (25 g)

Beclomethasone Dipropionate *see* Beclomethasone *on page 188*

Beconase® AQ *see* Beclomethasone *on page 188*

Behenyl Alcohol *see* Docosanol *on page 522*

Belladonna Alkaloids With Phenobarbital *see* Hyoscyamine, Atropine, Scopolamine, and Phenobarbital *on page 848*

Belladonna and Opium *(bel a DON a & OH pee um)*

Related Information

Opium Tincture *on page 1210*

U.S. Brand Names B&O Supprettes®

Generic Available Yes

Index Terms Opium and Belladonna

Pharmacologic Category Analgesic Combination (Opioid); Antispasmodic Agent, Urinary

Use Relief of moderate-to-severe pain associated with ureteral spasms not responsive to nonopioid analgesics and to space intervals between injections of opiates

Local Anesthetic/Vasoconstrictor Precautions No information available to require special precautions

Effects on Dental Treatment Key adverse event(s) related to dental treatment: Xerostomia and changes in salivation (normal salivary flow resumes upon discontinuation), and dry throat and nose.

Mechanism of Action The pharmacologically active agents present in the belladonna component are atropine and scopolamine. Atropine blocks the action of acetylcholine at parasympathetic sites in smooth muscle, secretory glands, and the CNS causing a relaxation of smooth muscle and drying of secretions. The principle agent in opium is morphine. Morphine binds to opiate receptors in the CNS, causing inhibition of ascending pain pathways, altering the perception of and response to pain.

Pregnancy Risk Factor C

Belladonna, Phenobarbital, and Ergotamine
(bel a DON a, fee noe BAR bi tal, & er GOT a meen)

Related Information

Ergotamine *on page 585*

Phenobarbital *on page 1288*

U.S. Brand Names Bellamine S; Bel-Tabs [DSC]; Eperbel-S; Spastrin®
Canadian Brand Names Bellergal® Spacetabs®
Generic Available Yes
Index Terms Ergotamine Tartrate, Belladonna, and Phenobarbital; Phenobarbital, Belladonna, and Ergotamine Tartrate
Pharmacologic Category Ergot Derivative
Use Management and treatment of menopausal disorders, GI disorders, and recurrent throbbing headache
Local Anesthetic/Vasoconstrictor Precautions No information available to require special precautions
Effects on Dental Treatment Key adverse event(s) related to dental treatment: Xerostomia (normal salivary flow resumes upon discontinuation), dry throat, nasal dryness, and difficulty swallowing.
Pregnancy Risk Factor X

Bellamine S *see* Belladonna, Phenobarbital, and Ergotamine *on page 190*

Bel-Tabs [DSC] *see* Belladonna, Phenobarbital, and Ergotamine *on page 190*

Benadryl-D™ Allergy and Sinus Fastmelt™ [OTC] *see* Diphenhydramine and Pseudoephedrine *on page 514*

Benadryl-D™ Children's Allergy and Sinus [OTC] *see* Diphenhydramine and Pseudoephedrine *on page 514*

Benadryl® Allergy [OTC] *see* DiphenhydrAMINE *on page 510*

Benadryl® Children's Allergy [OTC] *see* DiphenhydrAMINE *on page 510*

Benadryl® Children's Allergy and Cold Fastmelt™ [OTC] *see* Diphenhydramine and Pseudoephedrine *on page 514*

Benadryl® Children's Allergy Fastmelt® [OTC] *see* DiphenhydrAMINE *on page 510*

Benadryl® Dye-Free Allergy [OTC] *see* DiphenhydrAMINE *on page 510*

Benadryl® Injection *see* DiphenhydrAMINE *on page 510*

Benadryl® Itch Stopping [OTC] *see* DiphenhydrAMINE *on page 510*

Benadryl® Itch Stopping Extra Strength [OTC] *see* DiphenhydrAMINE *on page 510*

Benazepril (ben AY ze pril)

Related Information
Cardiovascular Diseases *on page 1726*
U.S. Brand Names Lotensin®
Canadian Brand Names Apo-Benazepril®; Lotensin®
Mexican Brand Names Lotensin
Generic Available Yes
Index Terms Benazepril Hydrochloride
Pharmacologic Category Angiotensin-Converting Enzyme (ACE) Inhibitor
Use Treatment of hypertension, either alone or in combination with other antihypertensive agents
Local Anesthetic/Vasoconstrictor Precautions No information available to require special precautions
Effects on Dental Treatment No significant effects or complications reported
Common Adverse Effects 1% to 10%:
Cardiovascular: Postural dizziness (2%)
Central nervous system: Headache (6%), dizziness (4%), fatigue (3%), somnolence (2%)
Endocrine & metabolic: Hyperkalemia (1%), uric acid increased
Gastrointestinal: Nausea (2%)
Renal: Serum creatinine increased (2%), worsening of renal function may occur in patients with bilateral renal artery stenosis or hypovolemia
Respiratory: Cough (1% to 10%)
Eosinophilic pneumonitis, neutropenia, anaphylaxis, renal insufficiency, and renal failure have been reported with other ACE inhibitors. In addition, a syndrome including fever, myalgia, arthralgia, interstitial nephritis, vasculitis, rash, eosinophilia, and elevated ESR has been reported to be associated with ACE inhibitors.
Dosage Oral: Hypertension:
Children ≥6 years: Initial: 0.2 mg/kg/day (up to 10 mg/day) as monotherapy; dosing range: 0.1-0.6 mg/kg/day (maximum dose: 40 mg/day)
Adults: Initial: 10 mg/day in patients not receiving a diuretic; 20-40 mg/day as a single dose or 2 divided doses; the need for twice-daily dosing should be assessed by monitoring peak (2-6 hours after dosing) and trough responses.
Note: Patients taking diuretics should have them discontinued 2-3 days prior to starting benazepril. If they cannot be discontinued, then initial dose should be 5 mg; restart after blood pressure is stabilized if needed.
(Continued)

Benazepril *(Continued)*

Elderly: Oral: Initial: 5-10 mg/day in single or divided doses; usual range: 20-40 mg/day; adjust for renal function; also see **Note** in adult dosing.

Dosing interval in renal impairment: Cl_{cr} <30 mL/minute:

Children: Use is not recommended.

Adults: Administer 5 mg/day initially; maximum daily dose: 40 mg.

Hemodialysis: Moderately dialyzable (20% to 50%); administer dose postdialysis or administer 25% to 35% supplemental dose.

Peritoneal dialysis: Supplemental dose is not necessary.

Mechanism of Action Competitive inhibition of angiotensin I being converted to angiotensin II, a potent vasoconstrictor, through the angiotensin I-converting enzyme (ACE) activity, with resultant lower levels of angiotensin II which causes an increase in plasma renin activity and a reduction in aldosterone secretion

Contraindications Hypersensitivity to benazepril or any component of the formulation; angioedema or serious hypersensitivity related to previous treatment with an ACE inhibitor; bilateral renal artery stenosis; patients with idiopathic or hereditary angioedema; pregnancy (2nd and 3rd trimesters)

Warnings/Precautions Anaphylactic reactions can occur. Angioedema can occur at any time during treatment (especially following first dose). Angioedema can occur at any time during treatment (especially following first dose). It may involve head and neck (potentially affecting the airway) or the intestine (presenting with abdominal pain). Prolonged monitoring may be required especially if tongue, glottis, or larynx are involved as they are associated with airway obstruction. Those with a history of airway surgery in this situation have a higher risk. Careful blood pressure monitoring with first dose (hypotension can occur especially in volume-depleted patients). **[U.S. Boxed Warning]: Based on human data, ACEIs can cause injury and death to the developing fetus when used in the second and third trimesters. ACEIs should be discontinued as soon as possible once pregnancy is detected.** Dosage adjustment needed in renal impairment. Use with caution in hypovolemia; collagen vascular diseases; valvular stenosis (particularly aortic stenosis); hyperkalemia; or before, during, or immediately after anesthesia. Hyperkalemia may occur. Avoid rapid dosage escalation which may lead to renal insufficiency. Rare toxicities associated with ACE inhibitors include cholestatic jaundice (which may progress to hepatic necrosis) and neutropenia/agranulocytosis with myeloid hyperplasia. Hypersensitivity reactions may be seen during hemodialysis with high-flux dialysis membranes (eg, AN69). May be associated with deterioration of renal function and/or increases in serum creatinine, particularly in patients dependent on renin-angiotensin-aldosterone system. Use with caution in unilateral renal artery stenosis and pre-existing renal insufficiency; if patient has renal impairment then a baseline WBC with differential and serum creatinine should be evaluated and monitored closely during the first 3 months of therapy. Safety and efficacy have not been established in children <6 years of age.

Drug Interactions

Increased Effect/Toxicity: Potassium supplements, co-trimoxazole (high dose), angiotensin II receptor antagonists (eg, candesartan, losartan, irbesartan), or potassium-sparing diuretics (amiloride, spironolactone, triamterene) may result in elevated serum potassium levels when combined with benazepril. ACE inhibitor effects may be increased by phenothiazines or probenecid (increases levels of captopril). ACE inhibitors may increase serum concentrations/effects of lithium. Diuretics have additive hypotensive effects with ACE inhibitors, and hypovolemia increases the potential for adverse renal effects of ACE inhibitors. In patients with compromised renal function, coadministration with NSAIDs may result in further deterioration of renal function. Allopurinol and ACE inhibitors may cause a higher risk of hypersensitivity reaction when taken concurrently. ACE inhibitors may enhance the adverse/toxic effects (nitritoid reaction) of gold sodium thiomalate.

Decreased Effect: Aspirin (high dose) may reduce the therapeutic effects of ACE inhibitors; at low dosages this does not appear to be significant. Rifampin may decrease the effect of ACE inhibitors. Antacids may decrease the bioavailability of ACE inhibitors (may be more likely to occur with captopril); separate administration times by 1-2 hours. NSAIDs, specifically indomethacin, may reduce the hypotensive effects of ACE inhibitors.

Ethanol/Nutrition/Herb Interactions Herb/Nutraceutical: Avoid dong quai if using for hypertension (has estrogenic activity). Avoid ephedra, yohimbe, ginseng (may worsen hypertension). Avoid garlic (may have increased antihypertensive effect).

Pharmacodynamics/Kinetics

Reduction in plasma angiotensin-converting enzyme (ACE) activity:

Onset of action: Peak effect: 1-2 hours after 2-20 mg dose

Duration: >90% inhibition for 24 hours after 5-20 mg dose

Reduction in blood pressure:

Peak effect: Single dose: 2-4 hours; Continuous therapy: 2 weeks

Absorption: Rapid (37%); food does not alter significantly; metabolite (benazeprilat) itself unsuitable for oral administration due to poor absorption

Distribution: V_d: ~8.7 L

Metabolism: Rapidly and extensively hepatic to its active metabolite, benazeprilat, via enzymatic hydrolysis; extensive first-pass effect

Half-life elimination: Benazeprilat: Effective: 10-11 hours; Terminal: Children: 5 hours, Adults: 22 hours

Time to peak: Parent drug: 0.5-1 hour

Excretion: Clearance: Nonrenal clearance (ie, biliary, metabolic) appears to contribute to the elimination of benazeprilat (11% to 12%), particularly patients with severe renal impairment; hepatic clearance is the main elimination route of unchanged benazepril

Dialysis: ~6% of metabolite removed within 4 hours of dialysis following 10 mg of benazepril administered 2 hours prior to procedure; parent compound not found in dialysate

Pregnancy Risk Factor C (1st trimester)/D (2nd and 3rd trimesters)

Dosage Forms
Tablet: 5 mg, 10 mg, 20 mg, 40 mg
Lotensin®: 5 mg, 10 mg, 20 mg, 40 mg

Benazepril and Hydrochlorothiazide
(ben AY ze pril & hye droe klor oh THYE a zide)

Related Information
Benazepril on page 191
Hydrochlorothiazide on page 819
U.S. Brand Names Lotensin® HCT
Generic Available Yes
Index Terms Hydrochlorothiazide and Benazepril
Pharmacologic Category Antihypertensive Agent, Combination
Use Treatment of hypertension
Local Anesthetic/Vasoconstrictor Precautions No information available to require special precautions
Effects on Dental Treatment No significant effects or complications reported
Common Adverse Effects See individual agents.
Drug Interactions
Increased Effect/Toxicity: See individual agents.
Decreased Effect: See individual agents.
Pharmacodynamics/Kinetics See individual agents.
Pregnancy Risk Factor C/D (2nd and 3rd trimesters)

Benazepril Hydrochloride see Benazepril on page 191

Benazepril Hydrochloride and Amlodipine Besylate see Amlodipine and Benazepril on page 104

Bendroflumethiazide and Nadolol see Nadolol and Bendroflumethiazide on page 1140

BeneFix® see Factor IX on page 667

Benemid [DSC] see Probenecid on page 1354

Benicar® see Olmesartan on page 1203

Benicar HCT® see Olmesartan and Hydrochlorothiazide on page 1204

Benoquin® see Monobenzone on page 1120

Ben-Tann see DiphenhydrAMINE on page 510

Bentoquatam (BEN toe kwa tam)

U.S. Brand Names IvyBlock® [OTC]
Generic Available No
Index Terms Quaternium-18 Bentonite
Pharmacologic Category Topical Skin Product
Use Skin protectant for the prevention of allergic contact dermatitis to poison oak, ivy, and sumac
Local Anesthetic/Vasoconstrictor Precautions No information available to require special precautions
Effects on Dental Treatment No significant effects or complications reported
Mechanism of Action An organoclay substance which is capable of absorbing or binding to urushiol, the active principle in poison oak, ivy, and sumac. Bentoquatam serves as a barrier, blocking urushiol skin contact/absorption.

Bentyl® see Dicyclomine on page 491

Benzac® AC see Benzoyl Peroxide on page 200

Benzac® AC Wash see Benzoyl Peroxide on page 200

BenzaClin® *see* Clindamycin and Benzoyl Peroxide *on page 381*
Benzac® W [DSC] *see* Benzoyl Peroxide *on page 200*
Benzac® W Wash *see* Benzoyl Peroxide *on page 200*
Benzagel® *see* Benzoyl Peroxide *on page 200*
Benzagel® Wash [DSC] *see* Benzoyl Peroxide *on page 200*

Benzalkonium Chloride (benz al KOE nee um KLOR ide)

Related Information
Periodontal Diseases *on page 1801*
U.S. Brand Names HandClens® [OTC]; 3M™ Cavilon™ Skin Cleanser [OTC] [DSC]; Pedi-Pro®; Pronto® Plus Lice Egg Remover Kit [OTC]; Zephiran® [OTC]
Generic Available No
Index Terms BAC
Pharmacologic Category Antibiotic, Topical
Dental Use Surface antiseptic and germicidal preservative
Use Surface antiseptic and germicidal preservative
Local Anesthetic/Vasoconstrictor Precautions No information available to require special precautions
Effects on Dental Treatment No significant effects or complications reported
Significant Adverse Effects 1% to 10%: Hypersensitivity
Dosage Thoroughly rinse anionic detergents and soaps from the skin or other areas prior to use of solutions because they reduce the antibacterial activity of BAC. To protect metal instruments stored in BAC solution, add crushed Anti-Rust Tablets, 4 tablets/quart, to antiseptic solution. Change solution at least once weekly. Not to be used for storage of aluminum or zinc instruments, instruments with lenses fastened by cement, lacquered catheters, or some synthetic rubber goods.
Contraindications Hypersensitivity to benzalkonium or any component of the formulation
Pregnancy Risk Factor C
Dosage Forms Excipient information presented when available (limited, particularly for generics); consult specific product labeling. [DSC] = Discontinued product
Lotion, topical [foam]:
HandClens®: 0.13% (50 mL, 240 mL, 1800 mL)
Lotion, topical [spray]:
HandClens®: 0.13% (15 mL)
Powder, topical:
Pedi-Pro®: 1% (60 g)
Solution, topical:
Pronto® Plus Lice Egg Remover Kit: 0.1% (60 mL)
Zephiran®: 1:750 (240 mL, 3840 mL) [aqueous]
Solution, topical [spray]:
3M™ Cavilon™ Skin Cleanser: 0.11% (240 mL) [DSC]

Benzalkonium Chloride and Isopropyl Alcohol
(benz al KOE nee um KLOR ide & eye so PRO pil AL koe hol)

Related Information
Benzalkonium Chloride *on page 194*
Viral Infections *on page 1806*
Related Sample Prescriptions
Herpes Simplex (Recurrent) *on page 1843*
U.S. Brand Names Viroxyn® [OTC]
Generic Available No
Index Terms Isopropyl Alcohol Tincture of Benzylkonium Chloride
Pharmacologic Category Antiseptic, Topical
Dental Use Topical: Germicidal for the treatment of cold sores/fever blisters
Local Anesthetic/Vasoconstrictor Precautions No information available to require special precautions
Effects on Dental Treatment No significant effects or complications reported (see Dental Comment)
Significant Adverse Effects Frequency not defined
Ocular: Irritation (following inadvertent contact)
Respiratory: Vapors may cause cough, dyspnea
Dosage Topical: One single application treatment to affected area. Secondary events (new viral load in the initial lesion, which may occur 12-72 hours after initial symptoms) or additional sore presentations will require additional treatment with a new vial. See Dental Comment for application instructions.

Manufacturer states medication should not be used >3 times/day; however, instructions indicate that a single application is generally effective if instructions are followed.

Mechanism of Action Germicidal due to disruption of the viral capsid coat by the quaternary ammonium benzalkonium chloride ingredient.

Contraindications Hypersensitivity to benzalkonium chloride, isopropyl alcohol, or any component of the formulation

Warnings/Precautions For topical use only; ingestion may lead to gastric irritation or distress. Avoid contact with eyes; flush with eye bath if inadvertent contact occurs. Avoid use of anionic cleansers or acidic products for at least 1 hour following application (active ingredient will be neutralized). Avoid the use of soap, toothpaste, cleansers, or drinks containing citric acid (including lemonade and orange juice). Should not be used >3 times/day. Avoid use in pregnant or lactating women. Avoid use in children <2 years of age. Formulation in isopropyl alcohol is flammable; avoid use near sparks, flames, or high temperatures.

Drug Interactions No specific drug interactions have been reported.

Dietary Considerations Avoid citric acid-containing beverages (eg, lemonade or orange juice) for at least 1 hour following application.

Dosage Forms Excipient information presented when available (limited, particularly for generics); consult specific product labeling.

Solution, topical: Benzalkonium 0.13% in isopropyl alcohol [kit includes 3 single-dose applicators]

Dental Comment Use this product according to the following directions from the manufacturer. 1) Prior to treatment, clean area to be treated of all other preparations (ointments, treatments, lipstick). Do not use soap or other cleansers. A dry wipe may be sufficient, or you may use water or alcohol if necessary. 2) Remove cap from vial and replace on the other end over the clear plastic tube. Hold vial between thumb and index finger, applicator end up. Pinch vial in the center at top of cap until the inner ampoule of medication breaks. 3) Hold white applicator down and allow medication to saturate the swab. If necessary, pinch vial gently until a drop of medication just appears. 4) Place the applicator against the area of skin to be treated so that the tip of the applicator is held flat against the skin. The key is to massage medication into the sore and the surrounding area by rubbing. Do not rub so hard that you cause damage to the skin. For best results, the patient should massage drug into the sore by rubbing. The rubbing should proceed for about 10 minutes or until all the drug has been massaged into the sore. The application may sting. This is normal and should subside quickly. For best results, medication must penetrate the subepidermal layers of the skin to site of infection. The ingredients facilitate penetration, but mechanical action is critical. Simply dabbing the drug onto the sore is not likely to give best results. 5) If treating at prodrome (tingling sensation before lesion erupts), a more vigorous rubbing is easily tolerated and gives best results. If the lesion has progressed to vesicle or ulcerated lesion, the patient may prefer to rub less vigorously but for a longer time period. 6) Keep applicator saturated at all times. If necessary, pause and hold vial so as to allow medication to flow into applicator. When finished recap vial. Dispose of immediately. Do not disassemble. Store at room temperature. Flammable; do not expose to high heat or flame. Keep out of reach of children.

Benzamycin® see Erythromycin and Benzoyl Peroxide on page 595
Benzamycin® Pak see Erythromycin and Benzoyl Peroxide on page 595
BenzaShave® see Benzoyl Peroxide on page 200
Benzathine Benzylpenicillin see Penicillin G Benzathine on page 1268
Benzathine Penicillin G see Penicillin G Benzathine on page 1268
Benzazoline Hydrochloride see Tolazoline on page 1582
Benzedrex® [OTC] see Propylhexedrine on page 1377
Benzene Hexachloride see Lindane on page 985
Benzhexol Hydrochloride see Trihexyphenidyl on page 1619
Benziq™ see Benzoyl Peroxide on page 200
Benziq™ LS see Benzoyl Peroxide on page 200
Benzisoquinolinedione see Amonafide on page 106
Benzmethyzin see Procarbazine on page 1355

Benzocaine (BEN zoe kane)

Related Information
Mouth Pain, Cold Sore, and Canker Sore Products on page 1938
Oral Pain on page 1788

Related Sample Prescriptions
Recurrent Aphthous Stomatitis on page 1844

U.S. Brand Names Americaine® [OTC]; Americaine® Hemorrhoidal [OTC]; Anbesol® [OTC]; Anbesol® Baby [OTC]; Anbesol® Cold Sore Therapy [OTC]; (Continued)

Benzocaine *(Continued)*

Anbesol® Jr. [OTC]; Anbesol® Maximum Strength [OTC]; Benzodent® [OTC]; Cepacol® Sore Throat [OTC]; Chiggerex® [OTC]; Chiggertox® [OTC]; Cylex® [OTC]; Dentapaine® [OTC]; Dent's Extra Strength Toothache [OTC]; Dent's Maxi-Strength Toothache [OTC]; Dermoplast® Antibacterial [OTC]; Dermoplast® Pain Relieving [OTC]; Detane® [OTC]; Foille® [OTC]; HDA® Toothache [OTC]; Hurricaine® [OTC]; Ivy-Rid® [OTC]; Kanka® Soft Brush™ [OTC]; Lanacane® [OTC]; Lanacane® Maximum Strength [OTC]; Mycinettes® [OTC]; Orabase® with Benzocaine [OTC]; Orajel® Baby Daytime and Nighttime [OTC]; Orajel® Baby Teething [OTC]; Orajel® Baby Teething Nighttime [OTC]; Orajel® Denture Plus [OTC]; Orajel® Maximum Strength [OTC]; Orajel® Medicated Toothache [OTC]; Orajel® Mouth Sore [OTC]; Orajel® Multi-Action Cold Sore [OTC]; Orajel PM® [OTC]; Orajel® Ultra Mouth Sore [OTC]; Oticaine; Otocaine™; Outgro® [OTC]; Red Cross™ Canker Sore [OTC]; Rid-A-Pain Dental Drops [OTC]; Skeeter Stik [OTC]; Sting-Kill [OTC]; Tanac® [OTC]; Thorets [OTC]; Trocaine® [OTC]; Zilactin®-B [OTC]; Zilactin Toothache and Gum Pain® [OTC]

Canadian Brand Names Anbesol® Baby; Zilactin-B®; Zilactin Baby®

Mexican Brand Names Auralyt

Generic Available Yes: Lozenge, otic drops

Index Terms Ethyl Aminobenzoate

Pharmacologic Category Local Anesthetic

Dental Use Ester-type topical local anesthetic for temporary relief of pain associated with toothache, minor sore throat pain, and canker sore

Use Temporary relief of pain associated with pruritic dermatosis, pruritus, minor burns, acute congestive and serous otitis media, swimmer's ear, otitis externa, bee stings, insect bites; mouth and gum irritations (toothache, minor sore throat pain, canker sores, dentures, orthodontia, teething, mucositis, stomatitis); sunburn; hemorrhoids; anesthetic lubricant for passage of catheters and endoscopic tubes

Local Anesthetic/Vasoconstrictor Precautions No information available to require special precautions

Effects on Dental Treatment No significant effects or complications reported

Significant Adverse Effects Frequency not defined.

Hematologic: Methemoglobinemia

Local: Burning, contact dermatitis, edema, erythema, pruritus, rash, stinging, tenderness, urticaria

Miscellaneous: Hypersensitivity

Dental Usual Dosing Relief of pain (toothache, minor sore throat pain, and canker sore): Children ≥2 years and Adults: Topical (oral): 10% to 20%: Apply thin layer to affected area up to 4 times daily

Dosage Note: These are general dosing guidelines; refer to specific product labeling for dosing instructions.

Children ≥4 months: Topical (oral): Teething pain: 7.5% to 10%: Apply to affected gum area up to 4 times daily

Children ≥2 years and Adults:

Topical:

Bee stings, insect bites, minor burns, sunburn: 5% to 20%: Apply to affected area 3-4 times a day as needed. In cases of bee stings, remove stinger before treatment.

Lubricant for passage of catheters and instruments: 20%: Apply evenly to exterior of instrument prior to use

Topical (oral): Mouth and gum irritation: 10% to 20%: Apply thin layer to affected area up to 4 times daily

Children ≥5 years and Adults: Oral: Sore throat: Allow one lozenge (10-15 mg) to dissolve slowly in mouth; may repeat every 2 hours as needed

Children ≥12 years and Adults: Rectal: Hemorrhoids: 5% to 20%: Apply externally to affected area up to 6 times daily

Adults: Otic: 20%: Instill 4-5 drops into external auditory canal; may repeat in 1-2 hours if needed

Mechanism of Action Ester local anesthetic blocks both the initiation and conduction of nerve impulses by decreasing the neuronal membrane's permeability to sodium ions, which results in inhibition of depolarization with resultant blockade of conduction

Contraindications Hypersensitivity to benzocaine, other ester-type local anesthetics, or any component of the formulation; secondary bacterial infection of area; ophthalmic use; otic preparations are also contraindicated in the presence of perforated tympanic membrane

Warnings/Precautions Methemoglobinemia has been reported following topical use (rare), particularly with higher concentration (14% to 20%) spray formulations applied to the mouth or mucous membranes. When applied as a spray to the mouth or throat, multiple sprays (or sprays of longer than indicated duration) are not recommended. Use caution with breathing problems (asthma, bronchitis, emphysema, in smokers), inflamed/damaged mucosa, heart disease, children <6 months of age, and hemoglobin or enzyme abnormalities (glucose-6-phosphodiesterase deficiency, hemoglobin-M disease, NADH-methemoglobin reductase deficiency, pyruvate-kinase deficiency). Alternatives to benzocaine sprays, such as topical lidocaine preparations, should be considered for patients at higher risk of this reaction.

The classical clinical finding of methemoglobinemia is chocolate brown-colored arterial blood. However, suspected cases should be confirmed by co-oximetry, which yields a direct and accurate measure of methemoglobin levels. Standard pulse oximetry readings or arterial blood gas values are not reliable. Clinically significant methemoglobinemia requires immediate treatment.

When used for self-medication (OTC), notify healthcare provider if condition worsens or does not improve within 7 days, or if swelling, rash, or fever develops. Do not use on open wounds. Avoid contact with the eyes.

Drug Interactions May antagonize actions of sulfonamides

Pharmacodynamics/Kinetics

Absorption: Topical: Poor to intact skin; well absorbed from mucous membranes and traumatized skin

Metabolism: Hepatic (to a lesser extent) and plasma via hydrolysis by cholinesterase

Excretion: Urine (as metabolites)

Pregnancy Risk Factor C

Lactation Excretion in breast milk unknown/use caution

Dosage Forms Excipient information presented when available (limited, particularly for generics); consult specific product labeling.

Aerosol, oral spray (Hurricaine®): 20% (60 mL) [dye free; cherry flavor]

Aerosol, topical spray:

Americaine®: 20% (60 mL)

Dermoplast® Antibacterial: 20% (83 mL) [contains aloe vera, benzethonium chloride, menthol]

Dermoplast® Pain Relieving: 20% (60 mL, 83 mL) [contains menthol]

Foille®: 5% (92 g) [contains chloroxylenol 0.63% and corn oil]

Ivy-Rid®: 2% (83 mL)

Lanacane® Maximum Strength: 20% (120 mL) [contains alcohol]

Solarcaine®: 20% (120 mL) [contains triclosan 0.13%, alcohol 35%]

Combination package (Orajel® Baby Daytime and Nighttime):

Gel, oral [Daytime Regular Formula]: 7.5% (5.3 g)

Gel, oral [Nighttime Formula]: 10% (5.3 g)

Cream, oral:

Benzodent®: 20% (7.5 g, 30 g)

Orajel PM®: 20% (5.3 g, 7 g)

Cream, topical:

Lanacane®: 6% (30 g, 60 g)

Lanacane® Maximum Strength: 20% (30 g)

Gel, oral:

Anbesol®: 10% (7.5 g) [contains benzyl alcohol; cool mint flavor]

Anbesol® Baby: 7.5% (7.5 g) [contains benzoic acid; grape flavor]

Anbesol® Jr.: 10% (7 g) [contains benzyl alcohol; bubble gum flavor]

Anbesol® Maximum Strength: 20% (7.5 g, 10 g) [contains benzyl alcohol]

Dentapaine: 20% (11 g) [contains clove oil]

HDA® Toothache: 6.5% (15 mL) [contains benzyl alcohol]

Hurricaine®: 20% (5 g) [dye free; wild cherry flavor]; (30 g) [dye free; mint, pina colada, watermelon, and wild cherry flavors]

Kanka® Soft Brush™: 20% (2 mL) [packaged in applicator with brush tip]

Orabase® with Benzocaine®: 20% (7 g) [contains ethyl alcohol 48%; mild mint flavor]

Orajel®: 10% (5.3 g, 7 g, 9.4 g)

Orajel® Baby Teething: 7.5% (9.4 g, 11.9 g) [cherry flavor]

Orajel® Baby Teething Nighttime: 10% (5.3 g)

Orajel® Denture Plus: 15% (9 g) [contains menthol 2%, ethyl alcohol 66.7%]

Orajel® Maximum Strength: 20% (5.3 g, 7 g, 9.4 g, 11.9 g)

Orajel® Mouth Sore: 20% (5.3 g, 9.4 g, 11.9 g) [contains benzalkonium chloride 0.02%, zinc chloride 0.1%]

Orajel® Multi-Action Cold Sore: 20% (9.4 g) [contains allantoin 0.5%, camphor 3%, dimethicone 2%]

Orajel® Ultra Mouth Sore: 15% (9.4 g) [contains ethyl alcohol 66.7%, menthol 2%]

Zilactin®-B: 10% (7.5 g)

Gel, topical (Detane®): 7.5% (15 g)

Liquid, oral:

Anbesol®: 10% (9 mL) [cool mint flavor]

Anbesol® Maximum Strength: 20% (9 mL) [contains benzyl alcohol]

Hurricaine®: 20% (30 mL) [pina colada and wild cherry flavors]

(Continued)

Benzocaine *(Continued)*

Orajel® Baby Teething: 7.5% (13 mL) [very berry flavor]
Orajel® Maximum Strength: 20% (13 mL) [contains ethyl alcohol 44%, tartrazine]

Liquid, oral drop:
Dent's Maxi-Strength Toothache: 20% (3.7 mL) [contains alcohol 74%]
Rid-A-Pain Dental Drops: 6.3% (30 mL) [contains alcohol 70%]

Liquid, topical:
Chiggertox®: 2% (30 mL)
Outgro®: 20% (9 mL)
Skeeter Stik: 5% (14 mL) [contains menthol]
Tanac®: 10% (13 mL) [contains benzalkonium chloride]

Lozenge: 6 mg (18s) [contains menthol]; 15 mg (10s)
Cepacol® Sore Throat: 10 mg (18s) [contains cetylpyridinium, menthol; cherry, citrus, honey lemon, and menthol flavors]
Cepacol® Sore Throat: 10 mg (16s) [sugar free; contains cetylpyridinium, menthol; cherry and menthol flavors]
Cylex®: 15 mg [sugar free; contains cetylpyridinium chloride 5 mg; cherry flavor]
Mycinettes®: 15 mg (12s) [sugar free; contains sodium 9 mg; cherry or regular flavor]
Thorets: 18 mg (500s) [sugar free]
Trocaine®: 10 mg (40s, 400s)

Ointment, oral:
Anbesol® Cold Sore Therapy: 20% (7.1 g) [contains benzyl alcohol, allantoin, aloe, camphor, menthol, vitamin E]
Red Cross™ Canker Sore: 20% (7.5 g) [contains coconut oil]

Ointment, rectal (Americaine® Hemorrhoidal): 20% (30 g)

Ointment, topical:
Chiggerex®: 2% (50 g) [contains aloe vera]
Foille®: 5% (3.5 g, 14 g, 28 g) [contains chloroxylenol 0.1%, benzyl alcohol; corn oil base]

Pads, topical (Sting-Kill): 20% (8s) [contains menthol and tartrazine]
Paste, oral (Orabase® with Benzocaine): 20% (6 g)
Solution, otic drops (Oticaine, Otocaine™): 20% (15 mL)

Swabs, oral:
Hurricaine®: 20% (6s, 100s) [dye free; wild cherry flavor]
Orajel® Baby Teething: 7.5% (12s) [berry flavor]
Orajel® Medicated Mouth Sore, Orajel® Medicated Toothache: 20% (8s, 12s) [contains tartrazine]
Zilactin® Toothache and Gum Pain: 20% (8s) [grape flavor]

Swabs, topical (Sting-Kill): 20% (5s) [contains menthol and tartrazine]
Wax, oral (Dent's Extra Strength Toothache Gum): 20% (1 g)

Dental Comment Health Canada has issued a reminder to healthcare professionals that benzocaine sprays must be used judiciously to minimize the risk of methemoglobinemia. Almost all reported cases have been associated with higher concentration (14% to 20% benzocaine) spray products used in the mouth and on other mucous membranes. Alternatives to benzocaine sprays, such as topical lidocaine preparations, should be considered for patients at higher risk of this reaction.

Benzocaine and Antipyrine *see* Antipyrine and Benzocaine *on page 133*

Benzocaine and Cetylpyridinium Chloride *see* Cetylpyridinium and Benzocaine *on page 325*

Benzocaine, Butamben, and Tetracaine
(BEN zoe kane, byoo TAM ben, & TET ra kane)

Related Information
Benzocaine *on page 195*
Tetracaine *on page 1546*

U.S. Brand Names Cetacaine®; Exactacain™

Generic Available No

Index Terms Benzocaine, Butamben, and Tetracaine Hydrochloride; Benzocaine, Butyl Aminobenzoate, and Tetracaine; Butamben, Tetracaine, and Benzocaine; Tetracaine, Benzocaine, and Butamben

Pharmacologic Category Local Anesthetic

Dental Use Topical anesthetic for accessible mucous membranes

Use Topical anesthetic to control pain in surgical or endoscopic procedures; anesthetic for accessible mucous membranes except for the eyes

Local Anesthetic/Vasoconstrictor Precautions No information available to require special precautions

Effects on Dental Treatment Key adverse event(s) related to dental treatment: A patient history of allergy to ester-type local anesthetics contraindicates the use of this product.

Significant Adverse Effects Frequency not defined. Also see individual monograph for Benzocaine.

Dermatologic: Contact dermatitis (eg, erythema, pruritus, vesiculation, oozing); dehydration of the epithelium; escharotic effect

Miscellaneous: Hypersensitivity/anaphylaxis reaction (rare)

Dental Usual Dosing Topical anesthetic (Exactacain™): Adults: 3 metered sprays (maximum dose: 6 metered sprays); each metered spray delivers 9.3 mg benzocaine, 1.3 mg butamben, 1.3 mg tetracaine

Dosage Topical anesthetic: **Note:** Decrease dose in the acutely-ill patient:

Children: Dose has not been established; dose reduction is suggested

Adults:

Cetacaine®:

Aerosol: Apply for ≤1 second; use of sprays >2 seconds is contraindicated

Gel: Apply ~0.5 inch (13 mm) x 3/16 inch (5 mm); application of >1 inch (26 cm) x 3/16 inch (5 mm) is contraindicated

Liquid: Apply 6-7 drops (0.2 mL); application of >12-14 drops (0.4 mL) is contraindicated

Exactacain™: 3 metered sprays (use of >6 metered sprays is contraindicated)

Elderly: Dose reduction is suggested

Mechanism of Action Reversible blockage of initiation and conduction of nerve impulses by deceasing the neuronal membrane's permeability to sodium ions

Contraindications Hypersensitivity to benzocaine, butamben, tetracaine, or any component of the formulation; ophthalmic use; cholinesterase deficiencies; large areas of denuded or inflamed tissue; administration in excess of product labeling

Warnings/Precautions For topical use only. Methemoglobinemia has been reported following topical benzocaine use (rare), particularly with higher concentration (14% to 20%) spray formulations applied to the mouth or mucous membranes. The classical clinical finding of methemoglobinemia is chocolate brown-colored arterial blood. However, suspected cases should be confirmed by co-oximetry, which yields a direct and accurate measure of methemoglobin levels. Standard pulse oximetry readings or arterial blood gas values are not reliable. Clinically-significant methemoglobinemia requires immediate treatment.

Use caution with breathing problems (asthma, bronchitis, emphysema, in smokers), inflamed/damaged mucosa, heart disease, children <6 months of age, and hemoglobin or enzyme abnormalities (glucose-6-phosphodiesterase deficiency, hemoglobin-M disease, NADH-methemoglobin reductase deficiency, pyruvate-kinase deficiency). Alternatives to benzocaine sprays, such as topical lidocaine preparations, should be considered for patients at higher risk of this reaction.

Use caution in debilitated, elderly, acutely ill, and very young patients; dose adjustment is suggested. Do not use under dentures or cotton rolls; retention of active ingredients may cause escharotic effect.

Pharmacodynamics/Kinetics Also see individual monograph for Benzocaine.

Onset of action: ~30 seconds

Duration: 30-60 minutes

Metabolism: Plasma via hydrolysis by cholinesterase to inactive metabolites

Excretion: Urine (as inactive metabolites)

Dosage Forms Excipient information presented when available (limited, particularly for generics); consult specific product labeling.

Aerosol, topical [spray]:

Cetacaine®: Benzocaine 14%, butamben 2%, and tetracaine hydrochloride 2% (56 g) [delivers benzocaine 28 mg, butamben 4 mg, and tetracaine hydrochloride 4 mg per second; contains benzalkonium chloride and CFCs; packaged with cannula]

Exactacain™: Benzocaine 14%, butamben 2%, and tetracaine hydrochloride 2% (60 g) [delivers benzocaine 9.3 mg, butamben 1.3 mg, and tetracaine 1.3 mg per metered spray; contains benzalkonium chloride; cherry flavor; packaged with 100 disposable applicators]

Gel, topical:

Cetacaine®: Benzocaine 14%, butamben 2%, and tetracaine hydrochloride 2% (29 g) [provides benzocaine 28 mg, butamben 4 mg and tetracaine hydrochloride 4 mg per 0.5 inch (13 mm) x 3/16 inch (5 mm) application; contains benzalkonium chloride]

Liquid, topical:

Cetacaine®: Benzocaine 14%, butamben 2%, and tetracaine hydrochloride 2% (56 g) [provides benzocaine 28 mg, butamben 4 mg, and tetracaine hydrochloride 4 mg per 6-7 drops (0.2 mL); contains benzalkonium chloride]

(Continued)

Benzocaine, Butamben, and Tetracaine *(Continued)*

Dental Comment Manufacturer indication for use is suppression of gag reflex for gastroenterological procedures.

Health Canada has issued a reminder to healthcare professionals that benzocaine sprays must be used judiciously to minimize the risk of methemoglobinemia. Almost all reported cases have been associated with higher concentration (14% to 20% benzocaine) spray products used in the mouth and on other mucous membranes. Alternatives to benzocaine sprays, such as topical lidocaine preparations, should be considered for patients at higher risk of this reaction.

Benzocaine, Butamben, and Tetracaine Hydrochloride *see* Benzocaine, Butamben, and Tetracaine *on page 198*

Benzocaine, Butyl Aminobenzoate, and Tetracaine *see* Benzocaine, Butamben, and Tetracaine *on page 198*

Benzodent® [OTC] *see* Benzocaine *on page 195*

Benzoin (BEN zoin)

U.S. Brand Names TinBen® [OTC] [DSC]
Generic Available Yes
Index Terms Gum Benjamin
Pharmacologic Category Antibiotic, Topical; Topical Skin Product
Use Protective application for irritations of the skin; sometimes used in boiling water as steam inhalants for its expectorant and soothing action
Local Anesthetic/Vasoconstrictor Precautions No information available to require special precautions
Effects on Dental Treatment No significant effects or complications reported

Benzonatate (ben ZOE na tate)

Related Information
Management of Patients Undergoing Cancer Therapy *on page 1826*
U.S. Brand Names Tessalon®
Canadian Brand Names Tessalon®
Mexican Brand Names Tusitato
Generic Available Yes
Pharmacologic Category Antitussive
Use Symptomatic relief of nonproductive cough
Local Anesthetic/Vasoconstrictor Precautions No information available to require special precautions
Effects on Dental Treatment No significant effects or complications reported
Common Adverse Effects 1% to 10%:
Central nervous system: Sedation, headache, dizziness
Dermatologic: Rash
Gastrointestinal: GI upset
Neuromuscular & skeletal: Chest numbness
Ocular: Burning sensation in eyes
Respiratory: Nasal congestion
Dosage Children >10 years and Adults: Oral: 100 mg 3 times/day or every 4 hours up to 600 mg/day
Mechanism of Action Tetracaine congener with antitussive properties; suppresses cough by topical anesthetic action on the respiratory stretch receptors
Contraindications Hypersensitivity to benzonatate, related compounds (such as tetracaine), or any component of the formulation
Pharmacodynamics/Kinetics
Onset of action: Therapeutic: 15-20 minutes
Duration: 3-8 hours
Pregnancy Risk Factor C
Dosage Forms
Capsule, softgel: 100 mg, 200 mg
Tessalon®: 100 mg, 200 mg

Benzoyl Peroxide (BEN zoe il peer OKS ide)

U.S. Brand Names Benzac® AC; Benzac® AC Wash; Benzac® W [DSC]; Benzac® W Wash; Benzagel®; Benzagel® Wash [DSC]; BenzaShave®; Benziq™; Benziq™ LS; Brevoxyl®; Brevoxyl® Cleansing; Brevoxyl® Wash; Clearplex [OTC]; Clinac™ BPO; Del Aqua®; Desquam-E™; Desquam-X®; Exact®

Acne Medication [OTC]; Fostex® 10% BPO [OTC]; Loroxide® [OTC]; Neutrogena® Acne Mask [OTC]; Neutrogena® On The Spot® Acne Treatment [OTC]; Oxy 10® Balanced Medicated Face Wash [OTC]; Oxy 10® Balance Spot Treatment [OTC]; Palmer's® Skin Success Acne [OTC]; PanOxyl®; PanOxyl®-AQ; PanOxyl® Aqua Gel; PanOxyl® Bar [OTC]; Seba-Gel™; Triaz®; Triaz® Cleanser; Zapzyt® [OTC]; Zoderm®

Canadian Brand Names Acetoxyl®; Benoxyl®; Benzac AC®; Benzac W® Gel; Benzac W® Wash; Desquam-X®; Oxyderm™; PanOxyl®; Solugel®

Mexican Brand Names Benoxyl AQ AL; Benzac AC; Benzac W; Panoxyl Wash Lotion

Generic Available Yes: Excludes cream, pads, and soap

Pharmacologic Category Acne Products; Topical Skin Product; Topical Skin Product, Acne

Use Adjunctive treatment of mild-to-moderate acne vulgaris and acne rosacea

Local Anesthetic/Vasoconstrictor Precautions No information available to require special precautions

Effects on Dental Treatment No significant effects or complications reported

Common Adverse Effects 1% to 10%: Dermatologic: Irritation, contact dermatitis, dryness, erythema, peeling, stinging

Mechanism of Action Releases free-radical oxygen which oxidizes bacterial proteins in the sebaceous follicles decreasing the number of anaerobic bacteria and decreasing irritating-type free fatty acids

Drug Interactions
Increased Effect/Toxicity: Increased toxicity: Benzoyl peroxide potentiates adverse reactions seen with tretinoin

Pharmacodynamics/Kinetics
Absorption: ~5% via skin; gel more penetrating than cream
Metabolism: Converted to benzoic acid in skin

Pregnancy Risk Factor C

Benzoyl Peroxide and Clindamycin *see* Clindamycin and Benzoyl Peroxide *on page 381*

Benzoyl Peroxide and Erythromycin *see* Erythromycin and Benzoyl Peroxide *on page 595*

Benzoyl Peroxide and Hydrocortisone
(BEN zoe il peer OKS ide & hye droe KOR ti sone)

Related Information
Benzoyl Peroxide *on page 200*
Hydrocortisone *on page 836*

U.S. Brand Names Vanoxide-HC®

Canadian Brand Names Vanoxide-HC®

Generic Available No

Index Terms Hydrocortisone and Benzoyl Peroxide

Pharmacologic Category Acne Products; Topical Skin Product; Topical Skin Product, Acne

Use Treatment of acne vulgaris and oily skin

Local Anesthetic/Vasoconstrictor Precautions No information available to require special precautions

Effects on Dental Treatment No significant effects or complications reported

Common Adverse Effects See individual agents.

Drug Interactions
Cytochrome P450 Effect: Hydrocortisone: **Substrate** of CYP3A4 (minor); **Induces** CYP3A4 (weak)

Pharmacodynamics/Kinetics See individual agents.

Pregnancy Risk Factor C

Benzphetamine (benz FET a meen)

U.S. Brand Names Didrex®

Canadian Brand Names Didrex®

Generic Available No

Index Terms Benzphetamine Hydrochloride

Pharmacologic Category Anorexiant; Sympathomimetic

Use Short-term (few weeks) adjunct in exogenous obesity

Local Anesthetic/Vasoconstrictor Precautions Use with caution since amphetamines have actions similar to epinephrine and norepinephrine

Effects on Dental Treatment Key adverse event(s) related to dental treatment: Xerostomia (normal salivary flow resumes upon discontinuation) and metallic taste.
(Continued)

Benzphetamine *(Continued)*

Common Adverse Effects Frequency not defined.

Cardiovascular: Cardiomyopathy (with chronic amphetamine use), hypertension, palpitation, tachycardia

Central nervous system: Depression (with withdrawal), dizziness, headache, insomnia, nervousness, psychosis, restlessness

Dermatologic: Urticaria

Endocrine & metabolic: Libido changes

Gastrointestinal: Diarrhea, nausea, unpleasant taste, xerostomia

Neuromuscular & skeletal: Tremor

Ocular: Mydriasis

Miscellaneous: Diaphoresis, tachyphylaxis

Restrictions C-III

Pharmacotherapy for weight loss is recommended only for obese patients with a body mass index $\geq$30 kg/m^2, or $\geq$27 kg/m^2 in the presence of other risk factors such as hypertension, diabetes, and/or dyslipidemia or a high waist circumference; therapy should be used in conjunction with a comprehensive weight management program. Rule out organic causes of obesity (eg, untreated hypothyroidism) prior to use.

Note: Benzphetamine is not approved for long-term use. The limited usefulness of medications in this class should be weighed against possible risks associated with their use. Consult weight loss guidelines for current pharmacotherapy recommendations.

Mechanism of Action Benzphetamine is a sympathomimetic amine with pharmacologic properties similar to the amphetamines. The mechanism of action in reducing appetite appears to be secondary to CNS effects, including stimulation of the hypothalamus to release norepinephrine.

Drug Interactions

Cytochrome P450 Effect: Substrate of CYP2B6 (minor), 3A4 (major)

Increased Effect/Toxicity: Antacids and carbonic anhydrase inhibitors may decrease the excretion of benzphetamine. Severe hypertensive episodes have occurred with amphetamine when used in patients receiving MAO inhibitors; concurrent use or use within 14 days is contraindicated. Due to MAO inhibition, use with linezolid should generally be avoided. Concomitant use with another sympathomimetic agent may increase the risk of related adverse effects, especially on the cardiovascular system (eg, increased blood pressure, tachycardia). Concomitant use with other CNS stimulants is contraindicated. CYP3A4 inhibitors may increase the levels/effects of benzphetamine; example inhibitors include azole antifungals, clarithromycin, diclofenac, doxycycline, erythromycin, imatinib, isoniazid, nefazodone, nicardipine, propofol, protease inhibitors, quinidine, telithromycin, and verapamil.

Decreased Effect: CYP3A4 inducers may decrease the levels/effects of benzphetamine; example inducers include aminoglutethimide, carbamazepine, nafcillin, nevirapine, phenobarbital, phenytoin, and rifamycins.

Pregnancy Risk Factor X

Benzphetamine Hydrochloride *see* Benzphetamine *on page 201*

Benztropine *(BENZ troe peen)*

U.S. Brand Names Cogentin®

Canadian Brand Names Apo-Benztropine®

Generic Available Yes: Tablet

Index Terms Benztropine Mesylate

Pharmacologic Category Anti-Parkinson's Agent, Anticholinergic; Anticholinergic Agent

Use Adjunctive treatment of Parkinson's disease; treatment of drug-induced extrapyramidal symptoms (except tardive dyskinesia)

Local Anesthetic/Vasoconstrictor Precautions No information available to require special precautions

Effects on Dental Treatment Key adverse event(s) related to dental treatment: Xerostomia and changes in salivation (normal salivary flow resumes upon discontinuation), dry throat, and nasal dryness (very prevalent).

Common Adverse Effects Frequency not defined.

Cardiovascular: Tachycardia

Central nervous system: Confusion, disorientation, memory impairment, toxic psychosis, visual hallucinations

Dermatologic: Rash

Endocrine & metabolic: Heat stroke, hyperthermia

Gastrointestinal: Constipation, dry throat, ileus, nasal dryness, nausea, vomiting, xerostomia

Genitourinary: Urinary retention, dysuria
Ocular: Blurred vision, mydriasis
Miscellaneous: Fever

Mechanism of Action Possesses both anticholinergic and antihistaminic effects. *In vitro* anticholinergic activity approximates that of atropine; *in vivo* it is only about half as active as atropine. Animal data suggest its antihistaminic activity and duration of action approach that of pyrilamine maleate. May also inhibit the reuptake and storage of dopamine, thereby prolonging the action of dopamine.

Drug Interactions
Cytochrome P450 Effect: Substrate of CYP2D6 (minor)
Increased Effect/Toxicity: Central and/or peripheral anticholinergic syndrome can occur when benztropine is administered with amantadine, rimantadine, opioid analgesics, phenothiazines and other antipsychotics (especially with high anticholinergic activity), tricyclic antidepressants, quinidine and some other antiarrhythmics, and antihistamines. Benztropine may increase the absorption of digoxin.
Decreased Effect: May increase gastric degradation of levodopa and decrease the amount of levodopa absorbed by delaying gastric emptying. Therapeutic effects of cholinergic agents (tacrine, donepezil) and neuroleptics may be antagonized.

Pharmacodynamics/Kinetics
Onset of action: Oral: Within 1 hour; Parenteral: Within 15 minutes
Duration: 6-48 hours
Metabolism: Hepatic (N-oxidation, N-dealkylation, and ring hydroxylation)
Bioavailability: 29%
Pregnancy Risk Factor C

Benztropine Mesylate see Benztropine on page 202

Benzydamine (ben ZID a meen)

Canadian Brand Names Apo-Benzydamine®; Dom-Benzydamine; Novo-Benzydamine; PMS-Benzydamine; ratio-Benzydamine; Sun-Benz®; Tantum®
Generic Available Yes
Index Terms Benzydamine Hydrochloride
Pharmacologic Category Local Anesthetic, Oral
Dental Use Symptomatic treatment of pain associated with acute pharyngitis; treatment of pain associated with radiation-induced oropharyngeal mucositis
Use Symptomatic treatment of pain associated with acute pharyngitis; treatment of pain associated with radiation-induced oropharyngeal mucositis
Local Anesthetic/Vasoconstrictor Precautions No information available to require special precautions
Effects on Dental Treatment Key adverse event(s) related to dental treatment: Numbness, burning/stinging sensation, and xerostomia (normal salivary flow resumes upon discontinuation).
Significant Adverse Effects
Central nervous system: Drowsiness, headache
Gastrointestinal: Nausea and/or vomiting (2%), dry mouth
Local: Numbness (10%), burning/stinging sensation (8%)
Respiratory: Pharyngeal irritation, cough
Restrictions Not available in U.S.
Dental Usual Dosing
Acute pharyngitis: Adults: Oral rinse: Gargle with 15 mL every 1½-3 hours until symptoms resolve. Patient should expel solution from mouth following use; solution should not be swallowed.
Radiation-associated mucositis: Adults: Oral rinse: 15 mL as a gargle or rinse 3-4 times/day; contact between the liquid and the oral mucosa should be maintained for at least 30 seconds, followed by expulsion from the mouth. Clinical studies maintained contact for ~2 minutes, up to 8 times/day. Patient should not swallow the liquid. Begin treatment 1 day prior to initiation of radiation therapy and continue daily during treatment. Continue oral rinse treatments after the completion of radiation therapy until desired result/healing is achieved.
Dosage Oral rinse: Adults:
Acute pharyngitis: Gargle with 15 mL of undiluted solution every 1½-3 hours until symptoms resolve. Patient should expel solution from mouth following use; solution should not be swallowed.
Mucositis: 15 mL of undiluted solution as a gargle or rinse 3-4 times/day; contact should be maintained for at least 30 seconds, followed by expulsion from the mouth. Clinical studies maintained contact for ~2 minutes, up to 8 times/day. Patient should not swallow the liquid. Begin treatment 1 day prior to
(Continued)

203

Benzydamine *(Continued)*

initiation of radiation therapy and continue daily during treatment. Continue oral rinse treatments after the completion of radiation therapy until desired result/healing is achieved.

Dosage adjustment in renal impairment: No adjustment required.

Mechanism of Action Local anesthetic and anti-inflammatory, reduces local pain and inflammation. Does not interfere with arachidonic acid metabolism.

Contraindications Hypersensitivity to benzydamine or any component of the formulation

Warnings/Precautions May cause local irritation and/or burning sensation in patients with altered mucosal integrity. Dilution (1:1 in warm water) may attenuate this effect. Use caution in renal impairment. Safety and efficacy have not been established in children ≤5 years of age.

Drug Interactions Substrate (minor) of CYP1A2, 2C19, 2D6, 3A4

No drug interactions established.

Pharmacodynamics/Kinetics

Absorption: Oral rinse may be absorbed, at least in part, through the oral mucosa

Excretion: Urine (primarily as unchanged drug)

Lactation Excretion in breast milk unknown/use caution

Dosage Forms Excipient information presented when available (limited, particularly for generics); consult specific product labeling. [CAN] = Canadian brand name

Oral rinse: 0.15% (100 mL, 250 mL) [not available in the U.S.]

Benzydamine Hydrochloride *see* Benzydamine *on page 203*
Benzylpenicillin Benzathine *see* Penicillin G Benzathine *on page 1268*
Benzylpenicillin Potassium *see* Penicillin G (Parenteral/Aqueous) *on page 1269*
Benzylpenicillin Sodium *see* Penicillin G (Parenteral/Aqueous) *on page 1269*

Benzylpenicilloyl-polylysine *(BEN zil pen i SIL oyl pol i LIE seen)*

U.S. Brand Names Pre-Pen® [DSC]
Generic Available No
Index Terms Penicilloyl-polylysine; PPL
Pharmacologic Category Diagnostic Agent
Use Adjunct in assessing the risk of administering penicillin (penicillin or benzylpenicillin) in adults with a history of clinical penicillin hypersensitivity
Local Anesthetic/Vasoconstrictor Precautions No information available to require special precautions
Effects on Dental Treatment No significant effects or complications reported
Common Adverse Effects Frequency not defined.

Cardiovascular: Hypotension
Dermatologic: Angioneurotic edema, pruritus, erythema, urticaria
Local: Intense local inflammatory response at skin test site, wheal (locally)
Respiratory: Dyspnea
Miscellaneous: Systemic allergic reactions occur rarely

Mechanism of Action Elicits IgE antibodies which produce type I accelerate urticarial reactions to penicillins

Drug Interactions

Decreased Effect: Corticosteroids and other immunosuppressive agents may inhibit the immune response to the skin test.

Pregnancy Risk Factor C

Beractant *(ber AKT ant)*

U.S. Brand Names Survanta®
Canadian Brand Names Survanta®
Mexican Brand Names Survanta
Generic Available No
Index Terms Bovine Lung Surfactant; Natural Lung Surfactant
Pharmacologic Category Lung Surfactant
Use Prevention and treatment of respiratory distress syndrome (RDS) in premature infants

Prophylactic therapy: Body weight <1250 g in infants at risk for developing, or with evidence of, surfactant deficiency (administer within 15 minutes of birth)

Rescue therapy: Treatment of infants with RDS confirmed by x-ray and requiring mechanical ventilation (administer as soon as possible - within 8 hours of age)

Local Anesthetic/Vasoconstrictor Precautions No information available to require special precautions

Effects on Dental Treatment No significant effects or complications reported

Common Adverse Effects During the dosing procedure:

>10%: Cardiovascular: Transient bradycardia

1% to 10%: Respiratory: Oxygen desaturation

Mechanism of Action Replaces deficient or ineffective endogenous lung surfactant in neonates with respiratory distress syndrome (RDS) or in neonates at risk of developing RDS. Surfactant prevents the alveoli from collapsing during expiration by lowering surface tension between air and alveolar surfaces.

Drug Interactions

Increased Effect/Toxicity: No data reported

Decreased Effect: No data reported

Pharmacodynamics/Kinetics Excretion: Clearance: Alveolar clearance is rapid

9-Beta-D-Ribofuranosyladenine *see* Adenosine *on page 55*

Beta-Carotene (BAY ta KARE oh teen)

U.S. Brand Names A-Caro-25; B-Caro-T™; Lumitene™

Generic Available Yes

Pharmacologic Category Vitamin, Fat Soluble

Unlabeled/Investigational Use Prophylaxis and treatment of polymorphous light eruption; prophylaxis against photosensitivity reactions in erythropoietic protoporphyria

Local Anesthetic/Vasoconstrictor Precautions No information available to require special precautions

Effects on Dental Treatment No significant effects or complications reported

Common Adverse Effects >10%: Dermatologic: Carotenodermia (yellowing of palms, hands, or soles of feet, and to a lesser extent the face)

Mechanism of Action The exact mechanism of action in erythropoietic protoporphyria has not as yet been elucidated; although patient must become carotenemic before effects are observed, there appears to be more than a simple internal light screen responsible for the drug's action. A protective effect was achieved when beta-carotene was added to blood samples. The concentrations of solutions used were similar to those achieved in treated patients. Topically applied beta-carotene is considerably less effective than systemic therapy.

Pharmacodynamics/Kinetics

Metabolism: Prior to absorption, converted to vitamin A in the wall of the small intestine, then oxidized to retinoic acid and retinol in the presence of fat and bile acids; small amounts are then stored in the liver; retinol (active) is conjugated with glucuronic acid

Excretion: Urine and feces

Pregnancy Risk Factor C

Betadine® [OTC] *see* Povidone-Iodine *on page 1332*

Betadine® First Aid Antibiotics + Moisturizer [OTC] [DSC] *see* Bacitracin and Polymyxin B *on page 181*

Betadine® Ophthalmic *see* Povidone-Iodine *on page 1332*

Betagan® *see* Levobunolol *on page 961*

Beta-HC® *see* Hydrocortisone *on page 836*

Betaine (BAY ta een)

U.S. Brand Names Cystadane®

Canadian Brand Names Cystadane®

Generic Available No

Index Terms Betaine Anhydrous

Pharmacologic Category Homocystinuria, Treatment Agent

Use Treatment of homocystinuria (eg, deficiencies or defects in cystathionine beta-synthase [CBS], 5,10-methylene tetrahydrofolate reductase [MTHFR], and cobalamin cofactor metabolism [CBL])

Local Anesthetic/Vasoconstrictor Precautions No information available to require special precautions

Effects on Dental Treatment No significant effects or complications reported

Common Adverse Effects

Frequency not defined: Gastrointestinal: Diarrhea, GI distress, nausea

Postmarketing and/or case reports: Cerebral edema (associated with hypermethioninemia)

(Continued)

Betaine *(Continued)*

Mechanism of Action Betaine acts as a methyl group donor in the remethylation of homocysteine to methionine. Homocystinuria is an inborn error of metabolism in which elevated plasma homocysteine levels can lead to mental retardation, ocular abnormalities, osteoporosis, premature atherosclerosis and thromboembolic disease. Remethylation is one of the two divergent pathways in the metabolism of homocysteine. The second pathway involves transsulfuration of homocysteine to produce cysteine. A number of enzymes and cofactors are also involved in these pathways.

Pregnancy Risk Factor C

Betaine Anhydrous *see* Betaine *on page 205*

BetaMed [OTC] *see* Pyrithione Zinc *on page 1391*

Betamethasone (bay ta METH a sone)

Related Information
Respiratory Diseases *on page 1747*

Related Sample Prescriptions
Recurrent Aphthous Stomatitis *on page 1844*

U.S. Brand Names Beta-Val®; Celestone®; Celestone® Soluspan®; Diprolene®; Diprolene® AF; Luxiq®

Canadian Brand Names Betaderm; Betaject™; Betnesol®; Betnovate®; Celestone® Soluspan®; Diprolene® Glycol; Diprosone®; Ectosone; Prevex® B; Taro-Sone®; Topilene®; Topisone®; Valisone® Scalp Lotion

Mexican Brand Names Betnovate; Celestoderm V; Celestone (500 mcg); Celestone-Soluspan; Diprosone

Generic Available Yes: Excludes aerosol, injection, solution

Index Terms Betamethasone Dipropionate; Betamethasone Dipropionate, Augmented; Betamethasone Sodium Phosphate; Betamethasone Valerate; Flubenisolone

Pharmacologic Category Corticosteroid, Systemic; Corticosteroid, Topical

Dental Use Treatment of a variety of oral diseases of allergic, inflammatory, or autoimmune origin

Use Inflammatory dermatoses such as seborrheic or atopic dermatitis, neurodermatitis, anogenital pruritus, psoriasis, inflammatory phase of xerosis

Local Anesthetic/Vasoconstrictor Precautions No information available to require special precautions

Effects on Dental Treatment No significant effects or complications reported

Significant Adverse Effects

Systemic:

Cardiovascular: Congestive heart failure, edema, hyper-/hypotension

Central nervous system: Dizziness, headache, insomnia, intracranial pressure increased, lightheadedness, nervousness, pseudotumor cerebri, seizure, vertigo

Dermatologic: Ecchymoses, facial erythema, fragile skin, hirsutism, hyper-/hypopigmentation, perioral dermatitis (oral), petechiae, striae, wound healing impaired

Endocrine & metabolic: Amenorrhea, Cushing's syndrome, diabetes mellitus, growth suppression, hyperglycemia, hypokalemia, menstrual irregularities, pituitary-adrenal axis suppression, protein catabolism, sodium retention, water retention

Gastrointestinal: Abdominal distention, appetite increased, hiccups, indigestion, peptic ulcer, pancreatitis, ulcerative esophagitis

Local: Injection site reactions (intra-articular use), sterile abscess

Neuromuscular & skeletal: Arthralgia, muscle atrophy, fractures, muscle weakness, myopathy, osteoporosis, necrosis (femoral and humeral heads)

Ocular: Cataracts, glaucoma, intraocular pressure increased

Miscellaneous: Anaphylactoid reaction, diaphoresis, hypersensitivity, secondary infection

Topical:

Dermatologic: Acneiform eruptions, allergic dermatitis, burning, dry skin, erythema, folliculitis, hypertrichosis, irritation, miliaria, pruritus, skin atrophy, striae, vesiculation

Endocrine and metabolic effects have occasionally been reported with topical use.

Dental Usual Dosing Allergic or inflammatory diseases: Topical: Gel: Apply small quantity with Q-tip to affected area 3-4 times/day

Dosage Base dosage on severity of disease and patient response

Children: Use lowest dose listed as initial dose for adrenocortical insufficiency (physiologic replacement)

I.M.: 0.0175-0.125 mg base/kg/day divided every 6-12 hours **or** 0.5-7.5 mg base/m^2/day divided every 6-12 hours

Oral: 0.0175-0.25 mg/kg/day divided every 6-8 hours **or** 0.5-7.5 mg/m^2/day divided every 6-8 hours

Topical:
≤12 years: Use is not recommended.
≥13 years: Use minimal amount for shortest period of time to avoid HPA axis suppression

Gel, augmented formulation: Apply once or twice daily; rub in gently. **Note:** Do not exceed 2 weeks of treatment or 50 g/week.

Lotion: Apply a few drops twice daily
Augmented formulation: Apply a few drops once or twice daily; rub in gently. **Note:** Do not exceed 2 weeks of treatment or 50 mL/week.

Cream/ointment: Apply once or twice daily.
Augmented formulation: Apply once or twice daily. **Note:** Do not exceed 2 weeks of treatment or 45 g/week.

Adolescents and Adults:
Oral: 2.4-4.8 mg/day in 2-4 doses; range: 0.6-7.2 mg/day
I.M.: Betamethasone sodium phosphate and betamethasone acetate: 0.6-9 mg/day (generally, $^1/_3$ to $^1/_2$ of oral dose) divided every 12-24 hours

Adults:
Intrabursal, intra-articular, intradermal: 0.25-2 mL
Intralesional: Rheumatoid arthritis/osteoarthritis:
Very large joints: 1-2 mL
Large joints: 1 mL
Medium joints: 0.5-1 mL
Small joints: 0.25-0.5 mL

Topical:
Foam: Apply to the scalp twice daily, once in the morning and once at night
Gel, augmented formulation: Apply once or twice daily; rub in gently. **Note:** Do not exceed 2 weeks of treatment or 50 g/week.

Lotion: Apply a few drops twice daily
Augmented formulation: Apply a few drops once or twice daily; rub in gently. **Note:** Do not exceed 2 weeks of treatment or 50 mL/week.

Cream/ointment: Apply once or twice daily
Augmented formulation: Apply once or twice daily. **Note:** Do not exceed 2 weeks of treatment or 45 g/week.

Dosing adjustment in hepatic impairment: Adjustments may be necessary in patients with liver failure because betamethasone is extensively metabolized in the liver

Mechanism of Action Controls the rate of protein synthesis; depresses the migration of polymorphonuclear leukocytes, fibroblasts; reverses capillary permeability and lysosomal stabilization at the cellular level to prevent or control inflammation

Contraindications Hypersensitivity to betamethasone, other corticosteroids, or any component of the formulation; systemic fungal infections

Warnings/Precautions Very high potency topical products are not for treatment of rosacea, perioral dermatitis; not for use on face, groin, or axillae; not for use in a diapered area. Avoid concurrent use of other corticosteroids.

May cause hypercorticism or suppression of hypothalamic-pituitary-adrenal (HPA) axis, particularly in younger children or in patients receiving high doses for prolonged periods. HPA axis suppression may lead to adrenal crisis. Withdrawal and discontinuation of a corticosteroid should be done slowly and carefully. Particular care is required when patients are transferred from systemic corticosteroids to inhaled products due to possible adrenal insufficiency or withdrawal from steroids, including an increase in allergic symptoms. Patients receiving >20 mg per day of prednisone (or equivalent) may be most susceptible. Fatalities have occurred due to adrenal insufficiency in asthmatic patients during and after transfer from systemic corticosteroids to aerosol steroids; aerosol steroids do not provide the systemic steroid needed to treat patients having trauma, surgery, or infections. In stressful situations, HPA axis-suppressed patients should receive adequate supplementation with natural glucocorticoids (hydrocortisone or cortisone) rather than betamethasone (due to lack of mineralocorticoid activity).

Acute myopathy has been reported with high dose corticosteroids, usually in patients with neuromuscular transmission disorders; may involve ocular and/or respiratory muscles; monitor creatine kinase; recovery may be delayed. Corticosteroid use may cause psychiatric disturbances, including depression, euphoria, insomnia, mood swings, and personality changes. Pre-existing psychiatric conditions may be exacerbated by corticosteroid use. Prolonged use of corticosteroids may also increase the incidence of secondary infection, mask acute infection (including fungal infections), prolong or exacerbate viral infections, or
(Continued)

Betamethasone *(Continued)*

limit response to vaccines. Exposure to chickenpox should be avoided; cortico-steroids should not be used to treat ocular herpes simplex. Corticosteroids should not be used for cerebral malaria. Close observation is required in patients with latent tuberculosis and/or TB reactivity; restrict use in active TB (only in conjunction with antituberculosis treatment). Prolonged treatment with corticosteroids has been associated with the development of Kaposi's sarcoma (case reports); if noted, discontinuation of therapy should be considered.

Use with caution in patients with thyroid disease, hepatic impairment, renal impairment, cardiovascular disease, diabetes, glaucoma, cataracts, myasthenia gravis, patients at risk for osteoporosis, patients at risk for seizures, or GI diseases (diverticulitis, peptic ulcer, ulcerative colitis) due to perforation risk. Use caution following acute MI (corticosteroids have been associated with myocardial rupture). Because of the risk of adverse effects, systemic corticoste-roids should be used cautiously in the elderly in the smallest possible effective dose for the shortest duration. Do not use occlusive dressings on weeping or exudative lesions and general caution with occlusive dressings should be observed; adverse effects may be increased. Discontinue if skin irritation or contact dermatitis should occur; do not use in patients with decreased skin circulation. Withdraw therapy with gradual tapering of dose. May affect growth velocity; growth should be routinely monitored in pediatric patients. Topical use in patients ≤12 years of age is not recommended.

Drug Interactions Inhibits CYP3A4 (weak)

Phenytoin, phenobarbital, rifampin increase clearance of betamethasone.

Potassium-depleting diuretics increase potassium loss.

Skin test antigens, immunizations: Betamethasone may decrease response and increase potential infections.

Insulin or oral hypoglycemics: Betamethasone may increase blood glucose.

Ethanol/Nutrition/Herb Interactions

Ethanol: Avoid ethanol (may enhance gastric mucosal irritation).

Food: Betamethasone interferes with calcium absorption.

Herb/Nutraceutical: Avoid cat's claw, echinacea (have immunostimulant proper-ties).

Dietary Considerations May be taken with food to decrease GI distress.

Pharmacodynamics/Kinetics

Protein binding: 64%

Metabolism: Hepatic

Half-life elimination: 6.5 hours

Time to peak, serum: I.V.: 10-36 minutes

Excretion: Urine (<5% as unchanged drug)

Pregnancy Risk Factor C

Lactation Excretion in breast milk unknown/use caution

Breast-Feeding Considerations Systemic corticosteroids are excreted in human milk. The extent of topical absorption is variable. Use with caution while breast-feeding; do not apply to nipples.

Dosage Forms Excipient information presented when available (limited, particu-larly for generics); consult specific product labeling.

Note: Potency expressed as betamethasone base.

Aerosol, topical, as valerate [foam]:

Luxiq®: 0.12% (50 g, 100 g, 150 g) [strength expressed as salt; contains ethanol 60.4%]

Cream, topical, as dipropionate: 0.05% (15 g, 45 g)

Cream, topical, as dipropionate augmented: 0.05% (15 g, 50 g)

Diprolene® AF: 0.05% (15 g, 50 g)

Cream, topical, as valerate (Beta-Val®): 0.1% (15 g, 45 g)

Beta-Val®: 0.1% (15 g, 45 g)

Gel, topical, as dipropionate augmented: 0.05% (15 g, 50 g)

Injection, suspension:

Celestone® Soluspan®: Betamethasone sodium phosphate 3 mg/mL and betamethasone acetate 3 mg per mL (5 mL) [6 mg/mL]

Lotion, topical, as dipropionate: 0.05% (60 mL)

Lotion, topical, as dipropionate augmented:

Diprolene®: 0.05% (30 mL, 60 mL)

Lotion, topical, as valerate: 0.1% (60 mL)

Beta-Val®: 0.1% (60 mL)

Ointment, topical, as dipropionate: 0.05% (15 g, 45 g)

Ointment, topical, as dipropionate augmented: 0.05% (15 g, 50 g)

Diprolene®: 0.05% (15 g, 50 g)

Ointment, topical, as valerate: 0.1% (15 g, 45 g)

Solution, as base:

Celestone®: 0.6 mg/5 mL (118 mL) [contains alcohol and sodium benzoate; cherry-orange flavor]

Betamethasone and Clotrimazole
(bay ta METH a sone & kloe TRIM a zole)

Related Information
Betamethasone *on page 206*
Clotrimazole *on page 398*
U.S. Brand Names Lotrisone®
Canadian Brand Names Lotriderm®
Mexican Brand Names Lotriderm
Generic Available Yes
Index Terms Clotrimazole and Betamethasone
Pharmacologic Category Antifungal Agent, Topical; Corticosteroid, Topical
Dental Use Treatment of a variety of oral diseases of allergic, inflammatory, or autoimmune origin
Use Topical treatment of various dermal fungal infections (including tinea pedis, cruris, and corpora in patients ≥17 years of age)
Local Anesthetic/Vasoconstrictor Precautions No information available to require special precautions
Effects on Dental Treatment No significant effects or complications reported
Significant Adverse Effects Also see individual agents.
1% to 10%:
Dermatologic: Dry skin (2%)
Local: Burning (2%)
Neuromuscular & skeletal: Paresthesia (2%)
<1% (Limited to important or life-threatening): Cushing's syndrome, edema, glycosuria, HPA axis suppression (higher in children), hyperglycemia, rash, secondary infection, stinging. Growth suppression, intracranial hypertension, and striae have also been reported with use in children.
Dental Usual Dosing Allergic or inflammatory diseases: Children ≥17 years and Adults: Topical: Apply to affected area twice daily, morning and evening
Dosage
Children <17 years: Do not use
Children ≥17 years and Adults:
Allergic or inflammatory diseases: Topical: Apply to affected area twice daily, morning and evening
Tinea corporis, tinea cruris: Topical: Massage into affected area twice daily, morning and evening; do not use for longer than 2 weeks; re-evaluate after 1 week if no clinical improvement; do not exceed 45 g cream/week or 45 mL lotion/week
Tinea pedis: Topical: Massage into affected area twice daily, morning and evening; do not use for longer than 4 weeks; re-evaluate after 2 weeks if no clinical improvement; do not exceed 45 g cream/week or 45 mL lotion/week
Elderly: Use with caution; skin atrophy and skin ulceration (rare) have been reported in patients with thinning skin; do not use for diaper dermatitis or under occlusive dressings
Mechanism of Action Betamethasone dipropionate is a corticosteroid. Clotrimazole is an antifungal agent.
Contraindications Hypersensitivity to betamethasone, clotrimazole, other corticosteroids or imidazoles, or any component of the formulation
Warnings/Precautions Systemic absorption of topical corticosteroids may cause hypothalamic-pituitary-adrenal (HPA) axis suppression (reversible) particularly in younger children. HPA axis suppression may lead to adrenal crisis. Risk is increased when used over large surface areas, for prolonged periods, or with occlusive dressings. Adverse systemic effects including hyperglycemia, glycosuria, fluid and electrolyte changes, and HPA suppression may occur when used on large surface areas, for prolonged periods, or with an occlusive dressing. Prolonged treatment with corticosteroids has been associated with the development of Kaposi's sarcoma (case reports); if noted, discontinuation of therapy should be considered. Not for use in pediatric patients <17 years of age. Do not use for diaper dermatitis.
Drug Interactions
Betamethasone: **Inhibits** CYP3A4 (weak)
Clotrimazole: **Inhibits** CYP1A2 (weak), 2A6 (weak), 2B6 (weak), 2C8/9 (weak), 2C19 (weak), 2D6 (weak), 2E1 (weak), 3A4 (moderate)
Also see individual agents.
Pharmacodynamics/Kinetics See individual agents.
Pregnancy Risk Factor C
Lactation Excretion in breast milk unknown/use caution
Breast-Feeding Considerations Betamethasone: Systemic corticosteroids are excreted in human milk. The extent of topical absorption is variable. Use with caution while breast-feeding; do not apply to nipples.
(Continued)

Betamethasone and Clotrimazole *(Continued)*

Dosage Forms Excipient information presented when available (limited, particularly for generics); consult specific product labeling.

Cream: Betamethasone dipropionate 0.05% (base) and clotrimazole 1% (15 g, 45 g) [contains benzyl alcohol]

Lotrisone®: Betamethasone dipropionate 0.05% (base) and clotrimazole 1% (15 g, 45 g) [contains benzyl alcohol]

Lotion: Betamethasone dipropionate 0.05% (base) and clotrimazole 1% (30 mL) [contains benzyl alcohol]

Lotrisone®: Betamethasone dipropionate 0.05% (base) and clotrimazole 1% (30 mL) [contains benzyl alcohol]

Betaxolol *(be TAKS oh lol)*

Related Information
Cardiovascular Diseases *on page 1726*

U.S. Brand Names Betoptic® S; Kerlone®

Canadian Brand Names Betoptic® S; Sandoz-Betaxolol

Mexican Brand Names Betoptic S

Generic Available Yes: Solution, tablet

Index Terms Betaxolol Hydrochloride

Pharmacologic Category Beta Blocker, Beta₁ Selective

Use Treatment of chronic open-angle glaucoma and ocular hypertension; management of hypertension

Local Anesthetic/Vasoconstrictor Precautions No information available to require special precautions

Effects on Dental Treatment Betaxolol is a cardioselective beta-blocker. Local anesthetic with vasoconstrictor can be safely used in patients medicated with betaxolol. Nonselective beta-blockers (ie, propranolol, nadolol) enhance the pressor response to epinephrine, resulting in hypertension and bradycardia; this has not been reported for betaxolol. Many nonsteroidal anti-inflammatory drugs, such as ibuprofen and indomethacin, can reduce the hypotensive effect of beta-blockers after 3 or more weeks of therapy with the NSAID. Short-term NSAID use (ie, 3 days) requires no special precautions in patients taking beta-blockers.

Common Adverse Effects
Ophthalmic:

>10%: Ocular: Short-term discomfort (25%)

Frequency not defined: Ocular: Anisocoria, blurred vision, corneal sensitivity decreased, corneal staining, crusty lashes, discharge, dry eyes, edema, erythema, foreign body sensation, inflammation, itching sensation, keratitis, photophobia, tearing, visual acuity decreased

Systemic:

>10%:

Central nervous system: Drowsiness, insomnia

Endocrine & metabolic: Sexual ability decreased

1% to 10%:

Cardiovascular: Bradycardia, palpitation, edema, CHF, peripheral circulation reduced

Central nervous system: Mental depression

Gastrointestinal: Diarrhea or constipation, nausea, vomiting, stomach discomfort

Respiratory: Bronchospasm

Miscellaneous: Cold extremities

Mechanism of Action Competitively blocks beta₁-receptors, with little or no effect on beta₂-receptors; ophthalmic reduces intraocular pressure by reducing the production of aqueous humor

Drug Interactions
Cytochrome P450 Effect: Substrate (major) of CYP1A2, 2D6; **Inhibits** CYP2D6 (weak)

Increased Effect/Toxicity: Acetylcholinesterase inhibitors, amiodarone, cardiac glycosides, dipyridamole, disopyramide, and SSRIs may enhance the bradycardic effects of beta-blockers. Beta-blockers may enhance the vasopressor effects of alpha-/beta-agonists, the orthostatic effects of alpha$_1$-agonists, and the rebound hypertensive effect of alpha$_2$-agonists after abrupt withdrawal. Aminoquinolones (amtimalarial), antipsychotic agents, calcium channel blockers, CYP1A2 inhibitors, 2D6 inhibitors, and propoxyphene may increase the effects of beta-blockers. Beta-blockers may enhance the effects of insulin(hypoglycemia), lidocaine, and sulfonylureas (hypoglycemia).

Decreased Effect: Barbiturates, CYP1A2 inducers, NSAIDs, and rifamycin derivatives may decrease the effects of beta-blockers. Beta$_2$-agonists may decrease the bradycardic effect of beta-blockers. Beta-blockers may decrease the bronchodilatory effect of theophylline.

Pharmacodynamics/Kinetics
Onset of action: Ophthalmic: 30 minutes; Oral: 1-1.5 hours
Duration: Ophthalmic: ≥12 hours
Absorption: Ophthalmic: Some systemic; Oral: ~100%
Metabolism: Hepatic to multiple metabolites
Protein binding: Oral: 50%
Bioavailability: Oral: 89%
Half-life elimination: Oral: 12-22 hours
Time to peak: Ophthalmic: ~2 hours; Oral: 1.5-6 hours
Excretion: Urine

Pregnancy Risk Factor C (manufacturer); D (2nd and 3rd trimesters - expert analysis)

Betaxolol Hydrochloride *see* Betaxolol *on page 210*

Bethanechol (be THAN e kole)

U.S. Brand Names Urecholine®
Canadian Brand Names Duvoid®; Myotonachol®; PMS-Bethanechol
Generic Available Yes
Index Terms Bethanechol Chloride
Pharmacologic Category Cholinergic Agonist
Use Nonobstructive urinary retention and retention due to neurogenic bladder
Unlabeled/Investigational Use Treatment and prevention of bladder dysfunction caused by phenothiazines; diagnosis of flaccid or atonic neurogenic bladder; gastroesophageal reflux
Local Anesthetic/Vasoconstrictor Precautions No information available to require special precautions
Effects on Dental Treatment This is a cholinergic agent similar to pilocarpine; expect to see salivation and sweating in patients.
Common Adverse Effects Frequency not defined.
Cardiovascular: Hypotension, tachycardia, flushed skin
Central nervous system: Headache, malaise
Gastrointestinal: Abdominal cramps, diarrhea, nausea, vomiting, salivation, eructation
Genitourinary: Urinary urgency
Ocular: Lacrimation, miosis
Respiratory: Asthmatic attacks, bronchial constriction
Miscellaneous: Diaphoresis
Mechanism of Action Stimulates cholinergic receptors in the smooth muscle of the urinary bladder and gastrointestinal tract resulting in increased peristalsis, increased GI and pancreatic secretions, bladder muscle contraction, and increased ureteral peristaltic waves
Drug Interactions
Increased Effect/Toxicity: Bethanechol and ganglionic blockers may cause a critical fall in blood pressure. Cholinergic drugs or anticholinesterase agents may have additive effects with bethanechol.
Decreased Effect: Procainamide, quinidine may decrease the effects of bethanechol. Anticholinergic agents (atropine, antihistamines, TCAs, phenothiazines) may decrease effects.
Pharmacodynamics/Kinetics
Onset of action: 30-90 minutes
Duration: Up to 6 hours
Absorption: Variable
Pregnancy Risk Factor C

Bethanechol Chloride *see* Bethanechol *on page 211*
Betimol® *see* Timolol *on page 1570*
Betoptic® S *see* Betaxolol *on page 210*

Bevacizumab (be vuh SIZ uh mab)

U.S. Brand Names Avastin®
Canadian Brand Names Avastin®
Mexican Brand Names Avastin
Generic Available No
Index Terms Anti-VEGF Monoclonal Antibody; NSC-704865; rhuMAb-VEGF
Pharmacologic Category Antineoplastic Agent, Monoclonal Antibody; Vascular Endothelial Growth Factor (VEGF) Inhibitor
Use Treatment of metastatic colorectal cancer; treatment of nonsquamous, nonsmall cell lung cancer
Unlabeled/Investigational Use Breast cancer, malignant mesothelioma, prostate cancer, ovarian cancer (early stage), renal cell cancer, age-related macular degeneration (AMD)
Local Anesthetic/Vasoconstrictor Precautions No information available to require special precautions
Effects on Dental Treatment Key adverse event(s) related to dental treatment: Xerostomia (normal salivary flow resumes upon discontinuation), stomatitis, taste disorder, and gingival bleeding.
Common Adverse Effects Percentages reported as part of combination chemotherapy regimens.
>10%:
   Cardiovascular: Hypertension (8% to 67%; grades 3/4: 8% to 18%), thromboembolism (18%); hypotension (7% to 15%)
   Central nervous system: Pain (61% to 62%), headache (2% to 26%), dizziness (19% to 26%), fatigue (5% to 19%), sensory neuropathy (1% to 17%)
   Dermatologic: Alopecia (6% to 32%), dry skin (7% to 20%), exfoliative dermatitis (3% to 19%), skin discoloration (2% to 16%)
   Endocrine & metabolic: Weight loss (15% to 16%), hypokalemia (12% to 16%)
   Gastrointestinal: Abdominal pain (8% to 61%), diarrhea (2% to 18%; grades 3/4: 34%), vomiting (6% to 52%), anorexia (35% to 43%), constipation (29% to 40%), stomatitis (30% to 32%), gastrointestinal hemorrhage (19% to 24%), dyspepsia (17% to 24%), taste disorder (14% to 21%), flatulence (11% to 19%), nausea (6% to 12%)
   Hematologic: Leukopenia (grades 3/4: 37%), neutropenia (grades 3/4: 21% to 27%)
   Neuromuscular & skeletal: Weakness (73% to 74%), myalgia (8% to 15%)
   Ocular: Tearing increased (6% to 18%)
   Renal: Proteinuria (36%)
   Respiratory: Upper respiratory infection (40% to 47%), epistaxis (32% to 35%), dyspnea (25% to 26%)
   Miscellaneous: Infection (serious: 14%; pneumonia, catheter, or wound infections)
1% to 10%:
   Cardiovascular: DVT (6% to 9%; grades 3/4: 9%); arterial thrombosis (3% to 4%), syncope (grades 3/4: 3%), intra-abdominal venous thrombosis (grades 3/4: 3%), cardio-/cerebrovascular arterial thrombotic event (2% to 4%), CHF (2%)
   Central nervous system: Confusion (1% to 6%), abnormal gait (1% to 5%)
   Dermatologic: Nail disorder (2% to 8%), skin ulcer (6%), wound dehiscence (1%)
   Endocrine & metabolic: Dehydration (6% to 10%)
   Gastrointestinal: Xerostomia (4% to 7%), colitis (1% to 6%), ileus (4% to 5%), gingival bleeding (2%), fistula (1%), gastrointestinal perforation (<1% to 4%), intra-abdominal abscess (1%)
   Genitourinary: Polyuria/urgency (3% to 6%), vaginal hemorrhage (4%)
   Hematologic: Neutropenic fever (5%), thrombocytopenia (5%), hemorrhage (4% to 5%)
   Hepatic: Bilirubinemia (1% to 6%)
   Respiratory: Voice alteration (6% to 9%), hemoptysis (nonsquamous histology 2%)
   Miscellaneous: Infusion reactions (<3%)
Mechanism of Action Bevacizumab is a recombinant, humanized monoclonal antibody which binds to, and neutralizes, vascular endothelial growth factor (VEGF), preventing its association with endothelial receptors. VEGF binding initiates angiogenesis (endothelial proliferation and the formation of new blood vessels). The inhibition of microvascular growth is believed to retard the growth of all tissues (including metastatic tissue).

Drug Interactions
Increased Effect/Toxicity: Bevacizumab may potentiate the cardiotoxic effects of anthracyclines. Serum concentrations of irinotecan's active metabolite may be increased by bevacizumab; an approximate 33% increase has been observed.
Pharmacodynamics/Kinetics
Distribution: V_d: 46 mL/kg
Half-life elimination: 20 days (range: 11-50 days)
Excretion: Clearance: 2.75-5 mL/kg/day
Pregnancy Risk Factor C

Bexarotene (beks AIR oh teen)

U.S. Brand Names Targretin®
Canadian Brand Names Targretin®
Generic Available No
Pharmacologic Category Antineoplastic Agent, Miscellaneous
Use
Oral: Treatment of cutaneous manifestations of cutaneous T-cell lymphoma in patients who are refractory to at least one prior systemic therapy
Topical: Treatment of cutaneous lesions in patients with refractory cutaneous T-cell lymphoma (stage 1A and 1B) or who have not tolerated other therapies
Local Anesthetic/Vasoconstrictor Precautions No information available to require special precautions
Effects on Dental Treatment Key adverse event(s) related to dental treatment: Xerostomia (normal salivary flow resumes upon discontinuation) and gingivitis.
Common Adverse Effects First percentage is at a dose of 300 mg/m²/day; the second percentage is at a dose >300 mg/m²/day.

Oral:
>10%:
Cardiovascular: Peripheral edema (13% to 11%)
Central nervous system: Headache (30% to 42%), chills (10% to 13%)
Dermatologic: Rash (17% to 23%), exfoliative dermatitis (10% to 28%)
Endocrine & metabolic: Hyperlipidemia (about 79% in both dosing ranges), hypercholesteremia (32% to 62%), hypothyroidism (29% to 53%)
Hematologic: Leukopenia (17% to 47%)
Neuromuscular & skeletal: Weakness (20% to 45%)
Miscellaneous: Infection (13% to 23%)
<10%:
Cardiovascular: Hemorrhage, hypertension, angina pectoris, right heart failure, tachycardia, cerebrovascular accident
Central nervous system: Fever (5% to 17%), insomnia (5% to 11%), subdural hematoma, syncope, depression, agitation, ataxia, confusion, dizziness, hyperesthesia
Dermatologic: Dry skin (about 10% for both dosing ranges), alopecia (4% to 11%), skin ulceration, acne, skin nodule, maculopapular rash, serous drainage, vesicular bullous rash, cheilitis
Endocrine & metabolic: Hypoproteinemia, hyperglycemia, weight loss/gain, breast pain
Gastrointestinal: Abdominal pain (11% to 4%), nausea (16% to 8%), diarrhea (7% to 42%), vomiting (4% to 13%), anorexia (2% to 23%), constipation, xerostomia, flatulence, colitis, dyspepsia, gastroenteritis, gingivitis, melena, pancreatitis, serum amylase increased
Genitourinary: Albuminuria, hematuria, urinary incontinence, urinary tract infection, urinary urgency, dysuria, kidney function abnormality
Hematologic: Hypochromic anemia (4% to 13%), anemia (6% to 25%), eosinophilia, thrombocythemia, coagulation time increased, lymphocytosis, thrombocytopenia
Hepatic: LDH increase (7% to 13%), hepatic failure
Neuromuscular & skeletal: Back pain (2% to 11%), arthralgia, myalgia, bone pain, myasthenia, arthrosis, neuropathy
Ocular: Dry eyes, conjunctivitis, blepharitis, corneal lesion, visual field defects, keratitis
Otic: Ear pain, otitis externa
Renal: Creatinine increased
Respiratory: Pharyngitis, rhinitis, dyspnea, pleural effusion, bronchitis, cough increased, lung edema, hemoptysis, hypoxia
Miscellaneous: Flu-like syndrome (4% to 13%), bacterial infection (1% to 13%)
Topical:
Cardiovascular: Edema (10%)
(Continued)

Bexarotene (Continued)

Central nervous system: Headache (14%), weakness (6%), pain (30%)
Dermatologic: Rash (14% to 72%), pruritus (6% to 40%), contact dermatitis (14%), exfoliative dermatitis (6%)
Hematologic: Leukopenia (6%), lymphadenopathy (6%)
Neuromuscular & skeletal: Paresthesia (6%)
Respiratory: Cough (6%), pharyngitis (6%)
Miscellaneous: Diaphoresis (6%), infection (18%)

Mechanism of Action The exact mechanism is unknown. Binds and activates retinoid X receptor subtypes. Once activated, these receptors function as transcription factors that regulate the expression of genes which control cellular differentiation and proliferation. Bexarotene inhibits the growth *in vitro* of some tumor cell lines of hematopoietic and squamous cell origin.

Drug Interactions

Cytochrome P450 Effect: Substrate of CYP3A4 (minor); **Induces** CYP3A4 (weak)

Increased Effect/Toxicity: Bexarotene plasma concentrations may be increased by gemfibrozil. Bexarotene may increase the toxicity of DEET.

Decreased Effect: Bexarotene may decrease the plasma levels of hormonal contraceptives and tamoxifen.

Pharmacodynamics/Kinetics

Absorption: Significantly improved by a fat-containing meal
Protein binding: >99%
Metabolism: Hepatic via CYP3A4 isoenzyme; four metabolites identified; further metabolized by glucuronidation
Half-life elimination: 7 hours
Time to peak: 2 hours
Excretion: Primarily feces; urine (<1% as unchanged drug and metabolites)

Pregnancy Risk Factor X

BG 9273 *see* Alefacept *on page 63*
Biaxin® *see* Clarithromycin *on page 371*
Biaxin® XL *see* Clarithromycin *on page 371*

Bicalutamide (bye ka LOO ta mide)

U.S. Brand Names Casodex®
Canadian Brand Names Casodex®; CO Bicalutamide; Novo-Bicalutamide; PMS-Bicalutamide; ratio-Bicalutamide; Sandoz-Bicalutamide
Mexican Brand Names Casodex
Generic Available No
Index Terms CDX; ICI-176334; NC-722665
Pharmacologic Category Antineoplastic Agent, Antiandrogen
Use In combination therapy with LHRH agonist analogues in treatment of metastatic prostate cancer
Unlabeled/Investigational Use Monotherapy for locally-advanced prostate cancer
Local Anesthetic/Vasoconstrictor Precautions No information available to require special precautions
Effects on Dental Treatment Key adverse event(s) related to dental treatment: Xerostomia (normal salivary flow resumes upon discontinuation).
Common Adverse Effects Adverse reaction percentages reported as part of combination regimen with an LHRH analogue.

>10%:
Cardiovascular: Peripheral edema (13%)
Central nervous system: Pain (35%)
Endocrine & metabolic: Hot flashes (53%)
Gastrointestinal: Constipation (22%), nausea (15%), diarrhea (12%), abdominal pain (11%)
Genitourinary: Pelvic pain (21%), nocturia (12%), hematuria (12%)
Hematologic: Anemia (11%)
Neuromuscular & skeletal: Back pain (25%), weakness (22%)
Respiratory: Dyspnea (13%)
Miscellaneous: Infection (18%)

≥2% to 10%:
Cardiovascular: Chest pain (8%), hypertension (8%), angina pectoris (2% to <5%), CHF (2% to <5%), edema (2% to <5%), MI (2% to <5%), coronary artery disorder (2% to <5%), syncope (2% to <5%)
Central nervous system: Dizziness (10%), headache (7%), insomnia (7%), anxiety (5%), depression (4%), chills (2% to <5%), confusion (2% to <5%), fever (2% to <5%), nervousness (2% to <5%), somnolence (2% to <5%)

Dermatologic: Rash (9%), alopecia (2% to <5%), dry skin (2% to <5%), pruritus (2% to <5%), skin carcinoma (2% to <5%)

Endocrine & metabolic: Gynecomastia (9%), breast pain (6%; up to 39% as monotherapy), hyperglycemia (6%), dehydration (2% to <5%), gout (2% to <5%), hypercholesterolemia (2% to <5%), libido decreased (2% to <5%)

Gastrointestinal: Dyspepsia (7%), weight loss (7%), anorexia (6%), flatulence (6%), vomiting (6%), weight gain (5%), dysphagia (2% to <5%), gastrointestinal carcinoma (2% to <5%), melena (2% to <5%), periodontal abscess (2% to <5%), rectal hemorrhage (2% to <5%), xerostomia (2% to <5%)

Genitourinary: Urinary tract infection (9%), impotence (7%), polyuria (6%), urinary retention (5%), urinary impairment (5%), urinary incontinence (4%), dysuria (2% to <5%), urinary urgency (2% to <5%)

Hepatic: LFTs increased (7%), alkaline phosphatase increased (5%)

Neuromuscular & skeletal: Bone pain (9%), paresthesia (8%), myasthenia (7%), arthritis (5%), pathological fracture (4%), hypertonia (2% to <5%), leg cramps (2% to <5%), myalgia (2% to <5%), neck pain (2% to <5%), neuropathy (2% to <5%)

Ocular: Cataract (2% to <5%)

Renal: BUN increased, creatinine increased, hydronephrosis

Respiratory: Cough (8%), pharyngitis (8%), bronchitis (6%), pneumonia (4%), rhinitis (4%), asthma (2% to <5%), epistaxis (2% to <5%), sinusitis (2% to <5%)

Miscellaneous: Flu syndrome (7%), diaphoresis (6%), cyst (2% to <5%), hernia (2% to <5%), herpes zoster (2% to <5%), sepsis (2% to <5%)

Mechanism of Action Pure nonsteroidal antiandrogen that binds to androgen receptors; specifically a competitive inhibitor for the binding of dihydrotestosterone and testosterone; prevents testosterone stimulation of cell growth in prostate cancer

Pharmacodynamics/Kinetics

Absorption: Rapid and complete

Protein binding: 96%

Metabolism: Extensively hepatic; glucuronidation and oxidation of the R (active) enantiomer to inactive metabolites

Half-life elimination: Active enantiomer ~6 days, ~10 days in severe liver disease

Time to peak, plasma: 31 hours

Excretion: Urine (36%, as inactive metabolites); feces (42%, as unchanged drug and inactive metabolites)

Pregnancy Risk Factor X

Bicillin® L-A see Penicillin G Benzathine on page 1268

Bicillin® C-R see Penicillin G Benzathine and Penicillin G Procaine on page 1269

Bicillin® C-R 900/300 see Penicillin G Benzathine and Penicillin G Procaine on page 1269

Bicitra® see Sodium Citrate and Citric Acid on page 1481

BiCNU® see Carmustine on page 288

BIDA see Amonafide on page 106

Bidhist see Brompheniramine on page 230

BiDil® see Isosorbide Dinitrate and Hydralazine on page 915

Biltricide® see Praziquantel on page 1337

Bimatoprost (bi MAT oh prost)

U.S. Brand Names Lumigan®

Canadian Brand Names Lumigan®

Mexican Brand Names Lumigan

Generic Available No

Pharmacologic Category Ophthalmic Agent, Antiglaucoma; Prostaglandin, Ophthalmic

Use Reduction of intraocular pressure (IOP) in patients with open-angle glaucoma or ocular hypertension

Local Anesthetic/Vasoconstrictor Precautions No information available to require special precautions

Effects on Dental Treatment No significant effects or complications reported

Mechanism of Action As a synthetic analog of prostaglandin with ocular hypotensive activity, bimatoprost decreases intraocular pressure by increasing the outflow of aqueous humor.

Pregnancy Risk Factor C

Biocef® see Cephalexin on page 317

Biolon™ [DSC] see Hyaluronate and Derivatives on page 816

Bion® Tears [OTC] see Artificial Tears on page 147

Bio-Statin® *see* Nystatin *on page 1194*
BioThrax™ *see* Anthrax Vaccine (Adsorbed) *on page 131*

Biperiden (bye PER i den)

U.S. Brand Names Akineton®
Canadian Brand Names Akineton®
Mexican Brand Names Akineton; Akineton Retard; Kinex
Generic Available No
Index Terms Biperiden Hydrochloride; Biperiden Lactate
Pharmacologic Category Anti-Parkinson's Agent, Anticholinergic; Anticholinergic Agent
Use Adjunct in the therapy of all forms of Parkinsonism; control of extrapyramidal symptoms secondary to antipsychotics
Local Anesthetic/Vasoconstrictor Precautions No information available to require special precautions
Effects on Dental Treatment Key adverse event(s) related to dental treatment: Xerostomia (normal salivary flow resumes upon discontinuation), nasal dryness, dry throat (very prevalent), and orthostatic hypotension.
Common Adverse Effects Frequency not defined.
  Cardiovascular: Orthostatic hypotension, bradycardia
  Central nervous system: Drowsiness, euphoria, disorientation, agitation, sleep disorder (decreased REM sleep and increased REM latency)
  Gastrointestinal: Constipation, xerostomia, dry throat, nasal dryness
  Genitourinary: Urinary retention
  Neuromuscular & skeletal: Choreic movements
  Ocular: Blurred vision
Mechanism of Action Biperiden is a weak peripheral anticholinergic agent with nicotinolytic activity. The beneficial effects in Parkinson's disease and neuroleptic-induced extrapyramidal symptoms are believed to be due to the inhibition of striatal cholinergic receptors.
Drug Interactions
  Cytochrome P450 Effect: Inhibits CYP2D6 (weak)
  Increased Effect/Toxicity: Central and/or peripheral anticholinergic syndrome can occur when administered with amantadine (or rimantadine), opioid analgesics, phenothiazines and other antipsychotics (especially with high anticholinergic activity), tricyclic antidepressants, quinidine and some other antiarrhythmics, and antihistamines. Anticholinergics may increase the bioavailability of atenolol (and possibly other beta-blockers). Anticholinergics may decrease gastric degradation and increase the amount of digoxin or levodopa absorbed by delaying gastric emptying.
  Decreased Effect: Anticholinergics may antagonize the therapeutic effect of neuroleptics and cholinergic agents (includes tacrine and donepezil).
Pharmacodynamics/Kinetics
  Bioavailability: 29%
  Half-life elimination, serum: 18.4-24.3 hours
  Time to peak, serum: 1-1.5 hours
Pregnancy Risk Factor C

Biperiden Hydrochloride *see* Biperiden *on page 216*
Biperiden Lactate *see* Biperiden *on page 216*
Bird Flu Vaccine *see* Influenza Virus Vaccine (H5N1) *on page 882*
Bisac-Evac™ [OTC] *see* Bisacodyl *on page 216*

Bisacodyl (bis a KOE dil)

U.S. Brand Names Alophen® [OTC]; Bisac-Evac™ [OTC]; Bisacodyl Uniserts® [OTC] [DSC]; Bisolax™ [OTC]; Correctol® Tablets [OTC]; Dacodyl™ [OTC]; Doxidan® [OTC]; Dulcolax® [OTC]; ex-lax® Ultra [OTC]; Fematrol [OTC]; Femilax™ [OTC]; Fleet® Bisacodyl [OTC]; Fleet® Stimulant Laxative [OTC]; Veracolate [OTC]
Canadian Brand Names Apo-Bisacodyl®; Carter's Little Pills®; Dulcolax®; Gentlax®
Generic Available Yes: Excludes enema
Pharmacologic Category Laxative, Stimulant
Use Treatment of constipation; colonic evacuation prior to procedures or examination
Local Anesthetic/Vasoconstrictor Precautions No information available to require special precautions
Effects on Dental Treatment No significant effects or complications reported

Mechanism of Action Stimulates peristalsis by directly irritating the smooth muscle of the intestine, possibly the colonic intramural plexus; alters water and electrolyte secretion producing net intestinal fluid accumulation and laxation

Drug Interactions

Decreased Effect: Milk or antacids may decrease the effect of bisacodyl. Bisacodyl may decrease the effect of warfarin.

Pharmacodynamics/Kinetics

Onset of action: Oral: 6-10 hours; Rectal: 0.25-1 hour

Absorption: Oral, rectal: Systemic, <5%

Pregnancy Risk Factor C

Bisacodyl Uniserts® [OTC] [DSC] see Bisacodyl on page 216

bis-chloronitrosourea see Carmustine on page 288

Bismatrol see Bismuth on page 217

Bismatrol [OTC] see Bismuth on page 217

Bismatrol Maximum Strength [OTC] see Bismuth on page 217

Bismuth (BIZ muth)

Related Information

Gastrointestinal Disorders on page 1745

U.S. Brand Names Bismatrol [OTC]; Bismatrol Maximum Strength [OTC]; Diotame® [OTC]; Kaopectate® [OTC]; Kaopectate® Extra Strength [OTC]; Kao-Tin [OTC]; Kapectolin [OTC]; Maalox® Total Stomach Relief® [OTC]; Pepto-Bismol® [OTC]; Pepto-Bismol® Maximum Strength [OTC]

Generic Available Yes

Index Terms Bismatrol; Bismuth Subgallate; Bismuth Subsalicylate; Pink Bismuth

Pharmacologic Category Antidiarrheal

Use

Subsalicylate formulation: Symptomatic treatment of mild, nonspecific diarrhea; control of traveler's diarrhea (enterotoxigenic *Escherichia coli*); as part of a multidrug regimen for *H. pylori* eradication to reduce the risk of duodenal ulcer recurrence

Subgallate formulation: An aid to reduce fecal odors from a colostomy or ileostomy

Local Anesthetic/Vasoconstrictor Precautions No information available to require special precautions

Effects on Dental Treatment Key adverse event(s) related to dental treatment: Darkening of tongue.

Common Adverse Effects Frequency not defined; subsalicylate formulation:

Central nervous system: Anxiety, confusion, headache, mental depression, slurred speech

Gastrointestinal: Discoloration of the tongue (darkening), grayish black stools, impaction may occur in infants and debilitated patients

Neuromuscular & skeletal: Muscle spasms, weakness

Ocular: Hearing loss, tinnitus

Mechanism of Action Bismuth subsalicylate exhibits both antisecretory and antimicrobial action. This agent may provide some anti-inflammatory action as well. The salicylate moiety provides antisecretory effect and the bismuth exhibits antimicrobial directly against bacterial and viral gastrointestinal pathogens.

Drug Interactions

Increased Effect/Toxicity: Toxicity of aspirin, warfarin, and/or hypoglycemics may be increased.

Decreased Effect: The effects of tetracyclines and uricosurics may be decreased.

Pharmacodynamics/Kinetics

Absorption: Bismuth: <1%; Subsalicylate: >90%

Metabolism: Bismuth subsalicylate is converted to salicylic acid and insoluble bismuth salts in the GI tract.

Half-life elimination: Terminal: Bismuth: Highly variable

Excretion: Bismuth: Urine and feces; Salicylate: Urine

Pregnancy Risk Factor C/D (3rd trimester)

Bismuth Subgallate see Bismuth on page 217

Bismuth Subsalicylate see Bismuth on page 217

Bismuth Subsalicylate, Metronidazole, and Tetracycline
(BIZ muth sub sa LIS i late, me troe NI da zole, & tet ra SYE kleen)

Related Information
Bismuth *on page 217*
Metronidazole *on page 1091*
Tetracycline *on page 1548*
U.S. Brand Names Helidac®
Generic Available No
Index Terms Bismuth Subsalicylate, Tetracycline, and Metronidazole; Metronidazole, Bismuth Subsalicylate, and Tetracycline; Tetracycline, Metronidazole, and Bismuth Subsalicylate
Pharmacologic Category Antibiotic, Tetracycline Derivative; Antidiarrheal
Use In combination with an H_2 antagonist, as part of a multidrug regimen for *H. pylori* eradication to reduce the risk of duodenal ulcer recurrence
Local Anesthetic/Vasoconstrictor Precautions No information available to require special precautions
Effects on Dental Treatment Tetracyclines are not recommended for use during pregnancy since they can cause enamel hypoplasia and permanent teeth discoloration; long-term use associated with oral candidiasis.
Common Adverse Effects See individual agents.
>1%:
Central nervous system: Dizziness
Gastrointestinal: Nausea, diarrhea, abdominal pain, vomiting, anal discomfort, anorexia
Neuromuscular & skeletal: Paresthesia
Mechanism of Action Bismuth subsalicylate, metronidazole, and tetracycline individually have demonstrated *in vitro* activity against most susceptible strains of *H. pylori* isolated from patients with duodenal ulcers. Resistance to metronidazole is increasing in the U.S.; an alternative regimen, not containing metronidazole, if *H. pylori* is not eradicated follow therapy.
Drug Interactions
Cytochrome P450 Effect:
Metronidazole: **Inhibits** CYP2C8/9 (weak), 3A4 (moderate)
Tetracycline: **Substrate** of CYP3A4 (major); **Inhibits** CYP3A4 (moderate)
Increased Effect/Toxicity: See individual agents.
Decreased Effect: See individual agents.
Pharmacodynamics/Kinetics See individual agents.
Pregnancy Risk Factor D (tetracycline); B (metronidazole)

Bismuth Subsalicylate, Tetracycline, and Metronidazole *see* Bismuth Subsalicylate, Metronidazole, and Tetracycline *on page 218*

Bisolax™ [OTC] *see* Bisacodyl *on page 216*

Bisoprolol (bis OH proe lol)

Related Information
Cardiovascular Diseases *on page 1726*
U.S. Brand Names Zebeta®
Canadian Brand Names Apo-Bisoprolol®; Monocor®; Novo-Bisoprolol; Sandoz-Bisoprolol; Zebeta®
Mexican Brand Names Concor
Generic Available Yes
Index Terms Bisoprolol Fumarate
Pharmacologic Category Beta Blocker, Beta₁ Selective
Use Treatment of hypertension, alone or in combination with other agents
Unlabeled/Investigational Use Angina pectoris, supraventricular arrhythmias, PVCs, CHF
Local Anesthetic/Vasoconstrictor Precautions No information available to require special precautions
Effects on Dental Treatment Bisoprolol is a cardioselective beta-blocker. Local anesthetic with vasoconstrictor can be safely used in patients medicated with bisoprolol. Nonselective beta-blockers (ie, propranolol, nadolol) enhance the pressor response to epinephrine, resulting in hypertension and bradycardia; this has not been reported for bisoprolol. Many nonsteroidal anti-inflammatory drugs, such as ibuprofen and indomethacin, can reduce the hypotensive effect of beta-blockers after 3 or more weeks of therapy with the NSAID. Short-term NSAID use (ie, 3 days) requires no special precautions in patients taking beta-blockers.

Common Adverse Effects

>10%:

Central nervous system: Drowsiness, insomnia

Endocrine & metabolic: Sexual ability decreased

1% to 10%:

Cardiovascular: Bradycardia, palpitation, edema, CHF, peripheral circulation reduced

Central nervous system: Mental depression

Gastrointestinal: Diarrhea, constipation, nausea, vomiting, stomach discomfort

Ocular: Mild ocular stinging and discomfort, tearing, photophobia, corneal sensitivity decreased, keratitis

Respiratory: Bronchospasm

Miscellaneous: Cold extremities

Mechanism of Action Selective inhibitor of beta$_1$-adrenergic receptors; competitively blocks beta$_1$-receptors, with little or no effect on beta$_2$-receptors at doses <10 mg

Drug Interactions

Cytochrome P450 Effect: Substrate of CYP2D6 (minor), 3A4 (major)

Increased Effect/Toxicity: Bisoprolol may increase the effects of other drugs which slow AV conduction (digoxin, verapamil, diltiazem), alpha-blockers (prazosin, terazosin), and alpha-adrenergic stimulants (epinephrine, phenylephrine). Bisoprolol may mask the tachycardia from hypoglycemia caused by insulin and oral hypoglycemics. In patients receiving concurrent therapy, the risk of hypertensive crisis is increased when either clonidine or the beta-blocker is withdrawn. Reserpine has been shown to enhance the effect of beta-blockers. Beta-blockers may increase the action or levels of ethanol, disopyramide, nondepolarizing muscle relaxants, and theophylline although the effects are difficult to predict. CYP3A4 inhibitors may increase the levels/effects of bisoprolol; example inhibitors include azole antifungals, clarithromycin, diclofenac, doxycycline, erythromycin, imatinib, isoniazid, nefazodone, nicardipine, propofol, protease inhibitors, quinidine, telithromycin, and verapamil.

Decreased Effect: Decreased effect of bisoprolol with aluminum salts, calcium salts, cholestyramine, colestipol, NSAIDs, penicillins (ampicillin), and salicylates due to decreased bioavailability and plasma levels. The effect of sulfonylureas may be decreased by beta-blockers. CYP3A4 inducers may decrease the levels/effects of bisoprolol; example inducers include aminoglutethimide, carbamazepine, nafcillin, nevirapine, phenobarbital, phenytoin, and rifamycins.

Pharmacodynamics/Kinetics

Onset of action: 1-2 hours

Absorption: Rapid and almost complete

Distribution: Widely; highest concentrations in heart, liver, lungs, and saliva; crosses blood-brain barrier; enters breast milk

Protein binding: 26% to 33%

Metabolism: Extensively hepatic; significant first-pass effect

Half-life elimination: 9-12 hours

Time to peak: 1.7-3 hours

Excretion: Urine (3% to 10% as unchanged drug); feces (<2%)

Pregnancy Risk Factor C (manufacturer); D (2nd and 3rd trimesters - expert analysis)

Bisoprolol and Hydrochlorothiazide

(bis OH proe lol & hye droe klor oh THYE a zide)

Related Information

Bisoprolol *on page 218*

Hydrochlorothiazide *on page 819*

U.S. Brand Names Ziac®

Canadian Brand Names Ziac®

Mexican Brand Names Biconcor

Generic Available Yes

Index Terms Hydrochlorothiazide and Bisoprolol

Pharmacologic Category Antihypertensive Agent, Combination

Use Treatment of hypertension

Unlabeled/Investigational Use Pediatric hypertension

Local Anesthetic/Vasoconstrictor Precautions No information available to require special precautions

Effects on Dental Treatment Bisoprolol is a cardioselective beta-blocker. Local anesthetic with vasoconstrictor can be safely used in patients medicated with bisoprolol. Nonselective beta-blockers (ie, propranolol, nadolol) enhance (Continued)

Bisoprolol and Hydrochlorothiazide *(Continued)*

the pressor response to epinephrine, resulting in hypertension and bradycardia; this has not been reported for bisoprolol. Many nonsteroidal anti-inflammatory drugs, such as ibuprofen and indomethacin, can reduce the hypotensive effect of beta-blockers after 3 or more weeks of therapy with the NSAID. Short-term NSAID use (ie, 3 days) requires no special precautions in patients taking beta-blockers.

Common Adverse Effects

>10%: Central nervous system: Fatigue

1% to 10%:

Cardiovascular: Chest pain, edema, bradycardia, hypotension

Central nervous system: Headache, dizziness, depression, abnormal dreams, insomnia

Dermatologic: Rash, photosensitivity

Endocrine & metabolic: Hypokalemia, fluid and electrolyte imbalances (hypocalcemia, hypomagnesemia, hyponatremia), hyperglycemia

Gastrointestinal: Constipation, diarrhea, dyspepsia, nausea, flatulence

Genitourinary: Micturition (frequency)

Hematologic: Rarely blood dyscrasias

Neuromuscular & skeletal: Arthralgia, myalgia

Ocular: Abnormal vision

Renal: Prerenal azotemia

Respiratory: Rhinitis, cough, dyspnea

Drug Interactions

Cytochrome P450 Effect: Bisoprolol: Substrate of CYP2D6 (minor), 3A4 (major)

Increased Effect/Toxicity: See individual agents.

Decreased Effect: See individual agents.

Pharmacodynamics/Kinetics See individual agents.

Pregnancy Risk Factor C/D (2nd and 3rd trimesters)

Bisoprolol Fumarate *see* Bisoprolol *on page 218*

Bistropamide *see* Tropicamide *on page 1627*

Bivalirudin *(bye VAL i roo din)*

U.S. Brand Names Angiomax®

Canadian Brand Names Angiomax®

Generic Available No

Index Terms Hirulog

Pharmacologic Category Anticoagulant, Thrombin Inhibitor

Use Anticoagulant used in conjunction with aspirin for patients with unstable angina undergoing percutaneous transluminal coronary angioplasty (PTCA) or percutaneous coronary intervention (PCI) with provisional glycoprotein IIb/IIIa inhibitor; anticoagulant used in patients undergoing PCI with (or at risk of) heparin-induced thrombocytopenia (HIT) / thrombosis syndrome (HITTS)

Local Anesthetic/Vasoconstrictor Precautions No information available to require special precautions

Effects on Dental Treatment Key adverse event(s) related to dental treatment: As with all anticoagulants, bleeding is the major adverse effect of bivalirudin. Hemorrhage may occur at virtually any site. Risk is dependent on multiple variables, including the intensity of anticoagulation and patient susceptibility. Additional adverse effects are often related to idiosyncratic reactions, and the frequency is difficult to estimate. Adverse reactions reported were generally less than those seen with heparin.

Common Adverse Effects As with all anticoagulants, bleeding is the major adverse effect of bivalirudin. Hemorrhage may occur at virtually any site. Risk is dependent on multiple variables, including the intensity of anticoagulation and patient susceptibility. Additional adverse effects are often related to idiosyncratic reactions, and the frequency is difficult to estimate. Adverse reactions reported were generally less than those seen with heparin.

>10%:

Cardiovascular: Hypotension (3% to 12%)

Central nervous system: Pain (15%), headache (3% to 12%)

Gastrointestinal: Nausea (3% to 15%)

Neuromuscular & skeletal: Back pain (9% to 42%)

1% to 10%:

Cardiovascular: Hypertension (6%), bradycardia (5%), angina (up to 5%)

Central nervous system: Insomnia (7%), anxiety (6%), fever (5%), nervousness (5%)

Gastrointestinal: Vomiting (6%), dyspepsia (5%), abdominal pain (5%)

Genitourinary: Urinary retention (4%)

Hematologic: Major hemorrhage (2% to 4%, compared to 4% to 9% with heparin); transfusion required (1% to 2%, compared to 2% to 6% with heparin), thrombocytopenia (<1% to 4%)

Local: Injection site pain (3% to 8%)

Neuromuscular & skeletal: Pelvic pain (6%)

Mechanism of Action Bivalirudin acts as a specific and reversible direct thrombin inhibitor; it binds to the catalytic and anionic exosite of both circulating and clot-bound thrombin. Catalytic binding site occupation functionally inhibits coagulant effects by preventing thrombin-mediated cleavage of fibrinogen to fibrin monomers, and activation of factors V, VIII, and XIII. Shows linear dose- and concentration-dependent prolongation of ACT, aPTT, PT, and TT.

Drug Interactions

Increased Effect/Toxicity: Aspirin may increase anticoagulant effect of bivalirudin (**Note:** All clinical trials included coadministration of aspirin). Other anticoagulants may increase the risk of bleeding complications (monitor).Treprostinil may increase risk of bleeding.

Pharmacodynamics/Kinetics

Onset of action: Immediate

Duration: Coagulation times return to baseline ~1 hour following discontinuation of infusion

Distribution: 0.2 L/kg

Protein binding, plasma: Does not bind other than thrombin

Half-life elimination: Normal renal function: 25 minutes; Cl_{cr} 10-29 mL/minute: 57 minutes

Excretion: Urine, proteolytic cleavage

Pregnancy Risk Factor B

BL4162A *see* Anagrelide *on page 127*

Black-Draught Tablets [OTC] *see* Senna *on page 1462*

Blenoxane® *see* Bleomycin *on page 221*

Bleo *see* Bleomycin *on page 221*

Bleomycin (blee oh MYE sin)

U.S. Brand Names Blenoxane®

Canadian Brand Names Blenoxane®; Bleomycin Injection, USP

Mexican Brand Names Blanoxan; Bleolem

Generic Available Yes

Index Terms Bleo; Bleomycin Sulfate; BLM; NSC-125066

Pharmacologic Category Antineoplastic Agent, Antibiotic

Use Treatment of squamous cell carcinomas, melanomas, sarcomas, testicular carcinoma, Hodgkin's lymphoma, and non-Hodgkin's lymphoma; sclerosing agent for malignant pleural effusion

Local Anesthetic/Vasoconstrictor Precautions No information available to require special precautions

Effects on Dental Treatment Key adverse event(s) related to dental treatment: Stomatitis and mucositis.

Common Adverse Effects

>10%:

Dermatologic: Pain at the tumor site, phlebitis. About 50% of patients develop erythema, rash, striae, induration, hyperkeratosis, vesiculation, and peeling of the skin, particularly on the palmar and plantar surfaces of the hands and feet. Hyperpigmentation (50%), alopecia, nailbed changes may also occur. These effects appear dose related and reversible with discontinuation.

Gastrointestinal: Stomatitis and mucositis (30%), anorexia, weight loss

Respiratory: Tachypnea, rales, acute or chronic interstitial pneumonitis, and pulmonary fibrosis (5% to 10%); hypoxia and death (1%). Symptoms include cough, dyspnea, and bilateral pulmonary infiltrates. The pathogenesis is not certain, but may be due to damage of pulmonary, vascular, or connective tissue. Response to steroid therapy is variable and somewhat controversial.

Miscellaneous: Acute febrile reactions (25% to 50%)

1% to 10%:

Dermatologic: Skin thickening, diffuse scleroderma, onycholysis, pruritus

Miscellaneous: Anaphylactoid-like reactions (characterized by hypotension, confusion, fever, chills, and wheezing; onset may be immediate or delayed for several hours); idiosyncratic reactions (1% in lymphoma patients)

Mechanism of Action Inhibits synthesis of DNA; binds to DNA leading to single- and double-strand breaks

(Continued)

Bleomycin (Continued)

Drug Interactions
Increased Effect/Toxicity: Cisplatin may decrease bleomycin elimination.

Decreased Effect: Bleomycin may decrease plasma levels of digoxin. Concomitant therapy with phenytoin results in decreased phenytoin levels.

Pharmacodynamics/Kinetics
Absorption: I.M. and intrapleural administration: 30% to 50% of I.V. serum concentrations; intraperitoneal and SubQ routes produce serum concentrations equal to those of I.V.

Distribution: V_d: 22 L/m^2; highest concentrations in skin, kidney, lung, heart tissues; lowest in testes and GI tract; does not cross blood-brain barrier

Protein binding: 1%

Metabolism: Via several tissues including hepatic, GI tract, skin, pulmonary, renal, and serum

Half-life elimination: Biphasic (renal function dependent):
  Normal renal function: Initial: 1.3 hours; Terminal: 9 hours
  End-stage renal disease: Initial: 2 hours; Terminal: 30 hours

Time to peak, serum: I.M.: Within 30 minutes

Excretion: Urine (50% to 70% as active drug)

Pregnancy Risk Factor D

Bortezomib (bore TEZ oh mib)

U.S. Brand Names Velcade®
Canadian Brand Names Velcade®
Mexican Brand Names Velcade
Generic Available No
Index Terms LDP-341; MLN341; NSC-681239; PS-341
Pharmacologic Category Antineoplastic Agent; Proteasome Inhibitor
Use Treatment of relapsed or refractory multiple myeloma; relapsed or refractory mantle cell lymphoma
Unlabeled/Investigational Use Treatment of non-Hodgkin's lymphomas (other than mantle cell lymphoma)
Local Anesthetic/Vasoconstrictor Precautions No information available to require special precautions
Effects on Dental Treatment Key adverse event(s) related to dental treatment: Abnormal taste and stomatitis.
Common Adverse Effects
>10%:
  Cardiovascular: Edema (11% to 28%), hypotension (12% to 15%; grades 3/4: 3%)
  Central nervous system: Fever (19% to 37%), psychiatric disturbance (35%), headache (17% to 26%), dysesthesia (9% to 27%), insomnia (18% to 21%), dizziness (14% to 23%; excludes vertigo), anxiety (5% to 11%)
  Dermatologic: Rash (17% to 28%), pruritus (10% to 18%)
  Endocrine & metabolic: Dehydration (7% to 11%)
  Gastrointestinal: Diarrhea (47% to 57%), nausea (44% to 57%), constipation (40% to 50%), anorexia (34% to 39%), vomiting (27% to 35%), abdominal pain (14% to 16%), abnormal taste (13%), dyspepsia (13%)
  Hematologic: Thrombocytopenia (21% to 38%; grade 4: 4%; nadir: Day 11; recovery: days 12-21), anemia (17% to 30%; grade 4: <1%), neutropenia (6% to 19%; grade 4: 2%)
  Neuromuscular & skeletal: Weakness (61% to 72%; grades 3/4: 12% to 19%), peripheral neuropathy (36% to 55%; grades 3/4: 7% to 13%), paresthesia (9% to 27%), arthralgia (13% to 18%), limb pain (5% to 17%), bone pain (2% to 16%), back pain (<1 % to 15%), myalgia (10% to 12%), muscle cramps (5% to 12%), rigors (11%)

Ocular: Blurred vision (11%)

Respiratory: Dyspnea (20% to 23%), cough (19% to 21%), lower respiratory infection (15%), upper respiratory tract infection (11% to 15%), nasopharyngitis (8% to 14%), pneumonia (9% to 12%)

Miscellaneous: Herpesvirus infections (7% to 13%)

1% to 10%:

Cardiovascular: Syncope (2%)

Endocrine & metabolic: Hypercalcemia (grade 4: 2%)

Frequency not defined (including postmarketing and/or case reports; limited to important or life-threatening): Acute diffuse infiltrative pulmonary disease, acute respiratory distress syndrome, allergic reaction, anaphylaxis, angina, angioedema, ascites, aspergillosis, atelectasis, atrial fibrillation, atrial flutter, AV block, bacteremia, bradycardia, cardiac amyloidosis, cardiac arrest, cardiac tamponade, cardiogenic shock, cerebral hemorrhage, cerebrovascular accident, CHF, cholestasis, coma, confusion, cranial palsy, deafness, deep venous thrombosis, diplopia, disseminated intravascular coagulation (DIC), duodenitis (hemorrhagic), dysautonomia, dysphagia, edema (facial), encephalopathy, embolism, epistaxis, fecal impaction, fracture, gastritis (hemorrhagic), gastroenteritis, glomerular nephritis, hematemesis, hematuria, hemoptysis, hemorrhagic cystitis, hepatic failure, hepatic hemorrhage, hepatitis, herpes meningoencephalitis, hyperbilirubinemia, hyper-/hypoglycemia, hyper-/hypokalemia, hyper-/hyponatremia, hypersensitivity, hyperuricemia, hypocalcemia, hypoxia, immune complex hypersensitivity, injection site reaction, intestinal obstruction, intestinal perforation, ischemic colitis, laryngeal edema, leukocytoclastic vasculitis, leukopenia, listeriosis, lymphopenia, melena, MI, myocardial ischemia, neuralgia, neutropenic fever, oral candidiasis, pancreatitis, paralytic ileus, paraplegia, pericardial effusion, pericarditis, peritonitis, pleural effusion, pneumonia, pneumonitis, portal vein thrombosis, proliferative glomerular nephritis, pulmonary edema, pulmonary embolism, pulmonary hypertension, psychosis, QT_c prolongation, renal calculus, renal failure, respiratory insufficiency, reversible posterior leukoencephalopathy syndrome (RPLS), seizure, septic shock, sepsis, sinus arrest, spinal cord compression, stomatitis, stroke (hemorrhagic), stroke, subdural hematoma, suicidal ideation, torsade de pointes, toxic epidermal necrolysis, toxoplasmosis, transient ischemic attack, tumor lysis syndrome, urinary incontinence, urinary retention, urinary tract infection, urticaria, ventricular tachycardia

Mechanism of Action Bortezomib inhibits proteasomes, enzyme complexes which regulate protein homeostasis within the cell. Specifically, it reversibly inhibits chymotrypsin-like activity at the 26S proteasome, leading to activation of signaling cascades, cell-cycle arrest, and apoptosis.

Drug Interactions

Cytochrome P450 Effect: Substrate of CYP1A2 (minor), 2C9 (minor), 2C19 (major), 2D6 (minor), 3A4 (major); **Inhibits** CYP1A2 (weak), 2C9 (weak), 2C19 (moderate), 2D6 (weak), 3A4 (weak)

Increased Effect/Toxicity: Bortezomib may increase the levels/effects citalopram, diazepam, methsuximide, phenytoin, propranolol, sertraline, and other CYP2C19 substrates. Levels/effects of bortezomib may be increased by azole antifungals, clarithromycin, delavirdine, diclofenac, doxycycline, erythromycin, fluconazole, fluvoxamine, gemfibrozil, imatinib, isoniazid, nefazodone, nicardipine, omeprazole, propofol, protease inhibitors, quinidine, telithromycin, ticlopidine, verapamil, and other CYP2C19 and CYP3A4 inhibitors.

Decreased Effect: Levels/effects of bortezomib may be decreased by aminoglutethimide, carbamazepine, nafcillin, nevirapine, phenobarbital, phenytoin, rifamycins, rifapentine, and other CYP2C19 and CYP3A4 inducers.

Pharmacodynamics/Kinetics

Distribution: 498-1884 L/m^2

Protein binding: ~83%

Metabolism: Hepatic primarily via CYP2C19 and 3A4 and to a lesser extent CYP1A2; forms metabolites (inactive) via deboronization followed by hydroxylation

Half-life elimination: Single dose: 9-15 hours; multiple dosing: 1 mg/m^2: 40-193 hours; 1.3 mg/m^2: 76-108 hours

Pregnancy Risk Factor D

Bosentan (boe SEN tan)

U.S. Brand Names Tracleer®
Canadian Brand Names Tracleer®
Generic Available No
(Continued)

Bosentan *(Continued)*

Pharmacologic Category Endothelin Antagonist

Use Treatment of pulmonary artery hypertension (PAH) (WHO Group I) in patients with World Health Organization (WHO) Class III or IV symptoms to improve exercise capacity and decrease the rate of clinical deterioration

Local Anesthetic/Vasoconstrictor Precautions No information available to require special precautions

Effects on Dental Treatment No significant effects or complications reported

Common Adverse Effects

>10%:
Central nervous system: Headache (16% to 22%)
Hematologic: Hemoglobin decreased (≥1 g/dL in up to 57%; <11 g/dL: 3% to 6%; typically in first 6 weeks of therapy)
Hepatic: Transaminases increased (>3 times upper limit of normal; up to 12%; dose-related)
Respiratory: Nasopharyngitis (11%)

1% to 10%:
Cardiovascular: Flushing (7% to 9%), edema (lower limb, 5% to 8%; generalized 4%), hypotension (7%), palpitation (5%)
Central nervous system: Fatigue (4%)
Dermatologic: Pruritus (4%)
Gastrointestinal: Dyspepsia (4%)
Hematologic: Anemia (3%)
Hepatic: Abnormal hepatic function (6% to 8%)

Restrictions Bosentan (Tracleer®) is available only through a limited distribution program directly from the manufacturer (Actelion Pharmaceuticals 1-866-228-3546). It will not be available through wholesalers or individual pharmacies. An FDA-approved medication guide must be distributed when dispensing an outpatient prescription (new or refill) where this medication is to be used without direct supervision of a healthcare provider. Medication guides are available at http://www.fda.gov/cder/Offices/ODS/medication_guides.htm.

Mechanism of Action Blocks endothelin receptors on vascular endothelium and smooth muscle. Stimulation of these receptors is associated with vasoconstriction. Although bosentan blocks both ET_A and ET_B receptors, the affinity is higher for the A subtype. Improvement in symptoms of pulmonary artery hypertension and a decrease in the rate of clinical deterioration have been demonstrated in clinical trials.

Drug Interactions

Cytochrome P450 Effect: Substrate (major) of CYP2C9, 3A4; **Induces** CYP2C9 (strong), 3A4 (strong)

Increased Effect/Toxicity: An increased risk of serum transaminase elevations was observed during concurrent therapy with glyburide; concurrent use is contraindicated. Cyclosporine increases serum concentrations of bosentan (approximately 3-4 times baseline). Concurrent use of cyclosporine is contraindicated.

CYP2C9 inhibitors may increase the levels/effects of bosentan; example inhibitors include delavirdine, fluconazole, gemfibrozil, ketoconazole, nicardipine, NSAIDs, pioglitazone, and sulfonamides. CYP3A4 inhibitors may increase the levels/effects of bosentan; example inhibitors include azole antifungals, clarithromycin, diclofenac, doxycycline, erythromycin, imatinib, isoniazid, nefazodone, nicardipine, propofol, protease inhibitors, quinidine, telithromycin, and verapamil. Sildenafil may increase the serum concentration of bosentan.

Decreased Effect: Bosentan may enhance the metabolism of cyclosporine, decreasing its serum concentrations by ~50%; effect on sirolimus and/or tacrolimus has not been specifically evaluated, but may be similar. Concurrent use of cyclosporine is contraindicated. CYP2C9 inducers may decrease the levels/effects of bosentan; example inducers include carbamazepine, phenobarbital, phenytoin, rifampin, rifapentine, and secobarbital. Bosentan may decrease the levels/effects of CYP2C9 substrates; example substrates include celecoxib, dapsone, fluoxetine, glimepiride, glipizide, losartan, montelukast, nateglinide, paclitaxel, phenytoin, sulfonamides, trimethoprim, warfarin, and zafirlukast. Bosentan may increase the metabolism, via CYP isoenzymes, of sildenafil.

CYP3A4 inducers may decrease the levels/effects of bosentan; example inducers include aminoglutethimide, carbamazepine, nafcillin, nevirapine, phenobarbital, phenytoin, and rifamycins. Bosentan may enhance the metabolism of methadone resulting in methadone withdrawal. Bosentan may decrease the levels/effects of CYP3A4 substrates; example substrates include benzodiazepines, calcium channel blockers, ergot derivatives, mirtazapine, nateglinide, nefazodone, tacrolimus, and venlafaxine. Bosentan may decrease levels of hormonal contraceptives; additional methods of contraception are recommended.

Pharmacodynamics/Kinetics

Distribution: V_d: 18 L

Protein binding, plasma: >98% primarily to albumin

Metabolism: Hepatic via CYP2C9 and 3A4 to three primary metabolites (one contributing ~10% to 20% pharmacologic activity)

Bioavailability: 50%

Half-life elimination: 5 hours; prolonged with heart failure, possibly in PAH

Time to peak, plasma: 3-5 hours

Excretion: Feces (as metabolites); urine (<3% as unchanged drug)

Pregnancy Risk Factor X

B&O Supprettes® *see* Belladonna and Opium *on page 190*

Botox® *see* Botulinum Toxin Type A *on page 225*

Botox® Cosmetic *see* Botulinum Toxin Type A *on page 225*

Botulinum Toxin Type A (BOT yoo lin num TOKS in type aye)

U.S. Brand Names Botox®; Botox® Cosmetic

Canadian Brand Names Botox®; Botox® Cosmetic

Generic Available No

Index Terms BTX-A

Pharmacologic Category Neuromuscular Blocker Agent, Toxin; Ophthalmic Agent, Toxin

Use Treatment of strabismus and blepharospasm associated with dystonia (including benign essential blepharospasm or VII nerve disorders in patients ≥12 years of age); cervical dystonia (spasmodic torticollis) in patients ≥16 years of age; temporary improvement in the appearance of lines/wrinkles of the face (moderate to severe glabellar lines associated with corrugator and/or procerus muscle activity) in adult patients ≤65 years of age; treatment of severe primary axillary hyperhidrosis in adults not adequately controlled with topical treatments

Orphan drug: Treatment of dynamic muscle contracture in pediatric cerebral palsy patients

Unlabeled/Investigational Use Treatment of oromandibular dystonia, spasmodic dysphonia (laryngeal dystonia) and other dystonias (ie, writer's cramp, focal task-specific dystonias); migraine treatment and prophylaxis

Local Anesthetic/Vasoconstrictor Precautions No information available to require special precautions

Effects on Dental Treatment Key adverse event(s) related to dental treatment: Xerostomia (normal salivary flow resumes upon discontinuation), facial pain, and facial weakness. Affects occur in ~1 week and may last up to several months.

Common Adverse Effects Adverse effects usually occur in 1 week and may last up to several months

>10%:

Central nervous system: Headache (cervical dystonia up to 11%, reduction of glabellar lines up to 13%; can occur with other uses)

Gastrointestinal: Dysphagia (cervical dystonia 19%)

Neuromuscular & skeletal: Neck pain (cervical dystonia 11%)

Ocular: Ptosis (blepharospasm 10% to 40%, strabismus 1% to 38%, reduction of glabellar lines 1% to 5%), vertical deviation (strabismus 17%)

Respiratory: Upper respiratory infection (cervical dystonia 12%)

2% to 10%:

Central nervous system: Anxiety (primary axillary hyperhydrosis), dizziness (cervical dystonia, reduction of glabellar lines), drowsiness (cervical dystonia), fever (cervical dystonia, primary axillary hyperhydrosis), speech disorder (cervical dystonia)

Dermatologic: Nonaxillary sweating (primary axillary hyperhydrosis), pruritus (primary axillary hyperhydrosis)

Gastrointestinal: Xerostomia (cervical dystonia), nausea (cervical dystonia, reduction of glabellar lines)

Local: Injection site reaction

Neuromuscular & skeletal: Back pain (cervical dystonia), facial pain (reduction of glabellar lines), hypertonia (cervical dystonia), weakness (cervical dystonia, reduction of glabellar lines)

Ocular: Dry eyes (blepharospasm 6%), superficial punctate keratitis (blepharospasm 6%)

Respiratory: Cough (cervical dystonia), infection (reduction of glabellar lines, primary axillary hyperhydrosis), pharyngitis (primary axillary hyperhydrosis), rhinitis (cervical dystonia)

(Continued)

Botulinum Toxin Type A *(Continued)*

Miscellaneous: Flu syndrome (cervical dystonia, reduction of glabellar lines, primary axillary hyperhydrosis)

Mechanism of Action Botulinum A toxin is a neurotoxin produced by *Clostridium botulinum*, spore-forming anaerobic bacillus, which appears to affect only the presynaptic membrane of the neuromuscular junction in humans, where it prevents calcium-dependent release of acetylcholine and produces a state of denervation. Muscle inactivation persists until new fibrils grow from the nerve and form junction plates on new areas of the muscle-cell walls.

Drug Interactions

Increased Effect/Toxicity: Aminoglycosides, neuromuscular-blocking agents, and other agents which may block neuromuscular transmission.

Pharmacodynamics/Kinetics

Onset of action (improvement):

Blepharospasm: ~3 days

Cervical dystonia: ~2 weeks

Strabismus: ~1-2 days

Reduction of glabellar lines (Botox® Cosmetic): 1-2 days, increasing in intensity during first week

Duration:

Blepharospasm: ~3 months

Cervical dystonia: <3 months

Strabismus: ~2-6 weeks

Primary axillary hyperhydrosis: 201 days (mean)

Reduction of glabellar lines (Botox® Cosmetic): Up to 3 months

Absorption: Not expected to be present in peripheral blood at recommended doses

Time to peak:

Blepharospasm: 1-2 weeks

Cervical dystonia: ~6 weeks

Strabismus: Within first week

Pregnancy Risk Factor C (manufacturer)

Botulinum Toxin Type B (BOT yoo lin num TOKS in type bee)

U.S. Brand Names Myobloc®

Generic Available No

Pharmacologic Category Neuromuscular Blocker Agent, Toxin

Use Treatment of cervical dystonia (spasmodic torticollis)

Unlabeled/Investigational Use Treatment of cervical dystonia in patients who have developed resistance to botulinum toxin type A

Local Anesthetic/Vasoconstrictor Precautions No information available to require special precautions

Effects on Dental Treatment Key adverse event(s) related to dental treatment: Xerostomia (normal salivary flow resumes upon discontinuation), stomatitis, and abnormal taste.

Common Adverse Effects

>10%:

Central nervous system: Headache (10% to 16%), pain (6% to 13%; placebo 10%)

Gastrointestinal: Dysphagia (10% to 25%), xerostomia (3% to 34%)

Local: Injection site pain (12% to 16%)

Neuromuscular & skeletal: Neck pain (up to 17%; placebo: 16%)

Miscellaneous: Infection (13% to 19%; placebo: 15%)

1% to 10%:

Cardiovascular: Chest pain, vasodilation, peripheral edema

Central nervous system: Dizziness (3% to 6%), fever, malaise, migraine, anxiety, tremor, hyperesthesia, somnolence, confusion, vertigo

Dermatologic: Pruritus, bruising

Gastrointestinal: Nausea (3% to 10%; placebo: 5%), dyspepsia (up to 10%; placebo: 5%), vomiting, stomatitis, taste perversion

Genitourinary: Urinary tract infection, cystitis, vaginal moniliasis

Hematologic: Serum neutralizing activity

Neuromuscular & skeletal: Torticollis (up to 8%; placebo: 7%), arthralgia (up to 7%; placebo: 5%), back pain (3% to 7%; placebo: 3%), myasthenia (3% to 6%; placebo: 3%), weakness (up to 6%; placebo: 4%), arthritis

Ocular: Amblyopia, abnormal vision

Otic: Otitis media, tinnitus

Respiratory: Cough (3% to 7%; placebo: 3%), rhinitis (1% to 5%; placebo: 6%), dyspnea, pneumonia

Miscellaneous: Flu-syndrome (6% to 9%), allergic reaction, viral infection, abscess, cyst

Mechanism of Action Botulinum B toxin is a neurotoxin produced by *Clostridium botulinum*, spore-forming anaerobic bacillus. It cleaves synaptic Vesicle Association Membrane Protein (VAMP; synaptobrevin) which is a component of the protein complex responsible for docking and fusion of the synaptic vesicle to the presynaptic membrane. By blocking neurotransmitter release, botulinum B toxin paralyzes the muscle.

Drug Interactions

Increased Effect/Toxicity: Aminoglycosides, neuromuscular-blocking agents, botulinum toxin type A, and other agents which may block neuromuscular transmission

Pharmacodynamics/Kinetics

Duration: 12-16 weeks

Absorption: Not expected to be present in peripheral blood at recommended doses

Pregnancy Risk Factor C (manufacturer)

Boudreaux's® Butt Paste [OTC] *see* Zinc Oxide *on page 1683*

Bovine Lung Surfactant *see* Beractant *on page 204*

Bravelle® *see* Urofollitropin *on page 1633*

Breathe Right® Saline [OTC] *see* Sodium Chloride *on page 1480*

Brethaire [DSC] *see* Terbutaline *on page 1540*

Brevibloc® *see* Esmolol *on page 598*

Brevicon® *see* Ethinyl Estradiol and Norethindrone *on page 640*

Brevital® Sodium *see* Methohexital *on page 1066*

Brevoxyl® *see* Benzoyl Peroxide *on page 200*

Brevoxyl® Cleansing *see* Benzoyl Peroxide *on page 200*

Brevoxyl® Wash *see* Benzoyl Peroxide *on page 200*

Bricanyl [DSC] *see* Terbutaline *on page 1540*

Brimonidine (bri MOE ni deen)

U.S. Brand Names Alphagan® P

Canadian Brand Names Alphagan®; Apo-Brimonidine®; PMS-Brimonidine Tartrate; ratio-Brimonidine

Mexican Brand Names Alphagan

Generic Available Yes

Index Terms Brimonidine Tartrate

Pharmacologic Category Alpha$_2$ Agonist, Ophthalmic; Ophthalmic Agent, Antiglaucoma

Use Lowering of intraocular pressure (IOP) in patients with open-angle glaucoma or ocular hypertension

Local Anesthetic/Vasoconstrictor Precautions No information available to require special precautions

Effects on Dental Treatment Key adverse event(s) related to dental treatment: Xerostomia (normal salivary flow resumes upon discontinuation).

Mechanism of Action Selective agonism for alpha$_2$-receptors; causes reduction of aqueous humor formation and increased uveoscleral outflow

Pregnancy Risk Factor B

Brimonidine Tartrate *see* Brimonidine *on page 227*

Brinzolamide (brin ZOH la mide)

U.S. Brand Names Azopt®

Canadian Brand Names Azopt®

Mexican Brand Names Azopt

Generic Available No

Pharmacologic Category Carbonic Anhydrase Inhibitor; Ophthalmic Agent, Antiglaucoma

Use Lowers intraocular pressure in patients with ocular hypertension or open-angle glaucoma

Local Anesthetic/Vasoconstrictor Precautions No information available to require special precautions

Effects on Dental Treatment Key adverse event(s) related to dental treatment: Taste disturbances.

Mechanism of Action Brinzolamide inhibits carbonic anhydrase, leading to decreased aqueous humor secretion. This results in a reduction of intraocular pressure.

Pregnancy Risk Factor C

Brioschi® [OTC] *see* Sodium Bicarbonate *on page 1480*

British Anti-Lewisite *see* Dimercaprol *on page 508*

BRL 43694 *see* Granisetron *on page 793*

Bromaline® [OTC] *see* Brompheniramine and Pseudoephedrine *on page 231*

Bromaxefed RF [DSC] *see* Brompheniramine and Pseudoephedrine *on page 231*

Bromazepam (broe MA ze pam)

Canadian Brand Names Apo-Bromazepam®; Gen-Bromazepam; Lectopam®; Novo-Bromazepam; Nu-Bromazepam

Generic Available Yes

Pharmacologic Category Benzodiazepine

Use Short-term, symptomatic treatment of anxiety

Local Anesthetic/Vasoconstrictor Precautions No information available to require special precautions

Effects on Dental Treatment Key adverse event(s) related to dental treatment: Xerostomia (normal salivary flow resumes upon discontinuation).

Common Adverse Effects Frequency not defined.

Cardiovascular: Hypotension, palpitation, tachycardia

Central nervous system: Drowsiness, ataxia, dizziness, confusion, depression, euphoria, lethargy, slurred speech, stupor, headache, seizure, anterograde amnesia. In addition, paradoxical reactions (including excitation, agitation, hallucinations, and psychosis) are known to occur with benzodiazepines.

Dermatologic: Rash, pruritus

Endocrine & metabolic: Hyperglycemia, hypoglycemia

Gastrointestinal: Xerostomia, nausea, vomiting

Genitourinary: Incontinence, libido decreased

Hematologic: Hemoglobin decreased, hematocrit decreased, WBCs increased/decreased

Hepatic: Transaminases increased, alkaline phosphatase increased, bilirubin increased

Neuromuscular & skeletal: Weakness, muscle spasm

Ocular: Blurred vision, depth perception decreased

Restrictions CDSA IV; Not available in U.S.

Mechanism of Action Binds to stereospecific benzodiazepine receptors on the postsynaptic GABA neuron at several sites within the central nervous system, including the limbic system, reticular formation. Enhancement of the inhibitory effect of GABA on neuronal excitability results by increased neuronal membrane permeability to chloride ions. This shift in chloride ions results in hyperpolarization (a less excitable state) and stabilization.

Drug Interactions

Cytochrome P450 Effect: Substrate of CYP3A4 (major); **Inhibits** CYP2E1 (weak)

Increased Effect/Toxicity: Benzodiazepines potentiate the CNS depressant effects of narcotic analgesics, barbiturates, phenothiazines, ethanol, antihistamines, MAO inhibitors, sedative-hypnotics, and cyclic antidepressants. CYP3A4 inhibitors may increase the levels/effects of bromazepam; example inhibitors include azole antifungals, clarithromycin, diclofenac, doxycycline, erythromycin, imatinib, isoniazid, nefazodone, nicardipine, propofol, protease inhibitors, quinidine, telithromycin, and verapamil.

Decreased Effect: CYP3A4 inducers may decrease the levels/effects of bromazepam; example inducers include aminoglutethimide, carbamazepine, nafcillin, nevirapine, phenobarbital, phenytoin, and rifamycins.

Pharmacodynamics/Kinetics

Protein binding: 70%

Metabolism: Hepatic

Bioavailability: 60%

Half-life elimination: 20 hours

Excretion: Urine (69%), as metabolites

Pregnancy Risk Factor D (based on other benzodiazepines)

Bromfenac (BROME fen ak)

U.S. Brand Names Xibrom™

Generic Available No

Index Terms Bromfenac Sodium

Pharmacologic Category Nonsteroidal Anti-inflammatory Drug (NSAID), Ophthalmic

Use Treatment of postoperative inflammation and reduction in ocular pain following cataract removal

Local Anesthetic/Vasoconstrictor Precautions No information available to require special precautions

Effects on Dental Treatment No significant effects or complications reported

Common Adverse Effects 2% to 7%:
Central nervous system: Headache
Ocular: Abnormal vision, abnormal sensation, conjunctival hyperemia, eye pain, iritis, pruritus

Mechanism of Action Inhibits prostaglandin synthesis by decreasing the activity of the enzyme, cyclooxygenase, which results in decreased formation of prostaglandin precursors.

Drug Interactions
Increased Effect/Toxicity: Concurrent use of ophthalmic corticosteroids may increase the risk of healing problems.
Decreased Effect: Bromfenac may decrease the reduction in IOP produced by latanoprost.

Pharmacodynamics/Kinetics
Absorption: Theoretically, systemic absorption may occur following ophthalmic use (not characterized); anticipated levels are below the limits of assay detection
Metabolism: Hepatic
Half-life elimination: 0.5-4 hours (following oral administration)

Pregnancy Risk Factor C/D (3rd trimester)

Bromfenac Sodium *see* Bromfenac *on page 228*

Bromfenex® *see* Brompheniramine and Pseudoephedrine *on page 231*

Bromfenex® PD *see* Brompheniramine and Pseudoephedrine *on page 231*

Bromhist-NR *see* Brompheniramine and Pseudoephedrine *on page 231*

Bromhist Pediatric *see* Brompheniramine and Pseudoephedrine *on page 231*

Bromocriptine (broe moe KRIP teen)

U.S. Brand Names Parlodel®; Parlodel® SnapTabs®
Canadian Brand Names Apo-Bromocriptine®; Parlodel®; PMS-Bromocriptine
Mexican Brand Names Diken; Parlodel; Serocryptin
Generic Available Yes
Index Terms Bromocriptine Mesylate
Pharmacologic Category Anti-Parkinson's Agent, Dopamine Agonist; Ergot Derivative
Use Treatment of hyperprolactinemia associated with amenorrhea with or without galactorrhea, infertility, or hypogonadism; treatment of prolactin-secreting adenomas; treatment of acromegaly; treatment of Parkinson's disease
Unlabeled/Investigational Use Neuroleptic malignant syndrome
Local Anesthetic/Vasoconstrictor Precautions No information available to require special precautions
Effects on Dental Treatment Key adverse event(s) related to dental treatment: Orthostatic hypotension.
Common Adverse Effects Note: Frequency of adverse effects may vary by dose and/or indication.

>10%:
Cardiovascular: Hypotension (up to 30%)
Central nervous system: Headache, dizziness
Gastrointestinal: Nausea, constipation
1% to 10%:
Cardiovascular: Orthostasis, vasospasm (cold-sensitive), Raynaud's syndrome, syncope
Central nervous system: Fatigue, lightheadedness, drowsiness
Gastrointestinal: Anorexia, vomiting, abdominal cramps, diarrhea, dyspepsia, GI bleeding, xerostomia
Respiratory: Nasal congestion
Withdrawal reactions: Abrupt discontinuation has resulted in rare cases of a withdrawal reaction with symptoms similar to neuroleptic malignant syndrome.

Mechanism of Action Semisynthetic ergot alkaloid derivative and a dopamine receptor agonist which activates postsynaptic dopamine receptors in the tubero-infundibular (inhibiting pituitary prolactin secretion) and nigrostriatal pathways (enhancing coordinated motor control).

Drug Interactions
Cytochrome P450 Effect: Substrate of CYP3A4 (major); **Inhibits** CYP1A2 (weak), 3A4 (weak)
Increased Effect/Toxicity: Effect/toxiicty of bromocriptine may be increased by alpha agonists/sympathomimetics, antifungals (azole derivatives), macrolide antibiotics, protease inhibitors, and MAO inhibitors. Bromocriptine
(Continued)

Bromocriptine *(Continued)*

may increase the effects of sibutramine and other serotonin agonists (serotonin syndrome). CYP3A4 inhibitors may increase the levels/effects of bromocriptine; example inhibitors include azole antifungals, clarithromycin, diclofenac, doxycycline, erythromycin, imatinib, isoniazid, nefazodone, nicardipine, propofol, protease inhibitors, quinidine, telithromycin, and verapamil. Concurrent use of bromocriptine with antihypertensive agents may increase the risk of hypotension. Concurrent use of levodopa may increase the risk of hallucinations (dose-dependant).

Decreased Effect: Effects of bromocriptine may be diminished by antipsychotics, metoclopramide.

Pharmacodynamics/Kinetics

Bioavailability: 28%

Protein binding: 90% to 96%

Metabolism: Primarily hepatic

Half-life elimination: Biphasic: Initial: 6-8 hours; Terminal: 50 hours

Time to peak, serum: 1-2 hours

Excretion: Feces; urine (2% to 6% as unchanged drug)

Pregnancy Risk Factor B

Bromocriptine Mesylate *see* Bromocriptine *on page 229*

Brompheniramine *(brome fen IR a meen)*

U.S. Brand Names Bidhist; BroveX™; BroveX™ CT; B-Vex; Lodrane® 12 Hour; Lodrane® 24; Lodrane® XR; LoHist-12; TanaCof-XR

Generic Available Yes: Excludes chewable tablet

Index Terms Brompheniramine Maleate; Brompheniramine Tannate

Pharmacologic Category Antihistamine

Use Symptomatic relief of perennial and seasonal allergic rhinitis, vasomotor rhinitis, and other respiratory allergies

Local Anesthetic/Vasoconstrictor Precautions No information available to require special precautions

Effects on Dental Treatment Key adverse event(s) related to dental treatment: Xerostomia (normal salivary flow resumes upon discontinuation). Chronic use of antihistamines will inhibit salivary flow, particularly in elderly patients; this may contribute to periodontal disease and oral discomfort.

Common Adverse Effects Frequency not defined.

Cardiovascular: Angina, blood pressure increased, circulatory collapse, extrasystoles, hypotension, palpitation, tachycardia

Central nervous system: Anxiety, chills, confusion, coordination impaired, dizziness, drowsiness, euphoria, excitation, fatigue, headache, hysteria, insomnia, irritability, nervousness, neuritis, restlessness, sedation, seizure, sleepiness, stimulation, tension, vertigo

Dermatologic: Photosensitivity, rash, urticaria

Endocrine & metabolic: Early menses

Gastrointestinal: Abdominal cramps, anorexia, constipation, diarrhea, dry throat, epigastric distress, nausea, vomiting, xerostomia

Genitourinary: Dysuria, polyuria, urinary retention

Hematologic: Agranulocytosis, hemolytic anemia, hypoplastic anemia, thrombocytopenia

Neuromuscular & skeletal: Paresthesia, tremor, weakness

Ocular: Blurred vision, diplopia, mydriasis

Otic: Labyrinthitis (acute), tinnitus

Respiratory: Dry nose, nasal congestion, thickening of bronchial secretions, wheezing

Miscellaneous: Anaphylactic shock, diaphoresis

Mechanism of Action Competes with histamine for H_1-receptor sites on effector cells

Drug Interactions

Increased Effect/Toxicity: Brompheniramine may increase CNS depressant effects of barbiturates, CNS depressants, and tricyclic antidepressants. MAO inhibitors and tricyclic antidepressants may increase anticholinergic effects of brompheniramine.

Pharmacodynamics/Kinetics

Metabolism: Hepatic

Excretion: Urine

Pregnancy Risk Factor C

Brompheniramine and Pseudoephedrine
(brome fen IR a meen & soo doe e FED rin)

Related Information
Pseudoephedrine *on page 1381*

U.S. Brand Names AccuHist®; Andehist NR Syrup; Bromaline® [OTC]; Bromaxefed RF [DSC]; Bromfenex®; Bromfenex® PD; Bromhist-NR; Bromhist Pediatric; Brotapp; Brovex SR; Children's Dimetapp® Elixir Cold & Allergy [OTC] [DSC]; Dimaphen [OTC]; Histex™ SR; Lodrane®; Lodrane® 12D; Lodrane® 24D; Lodrane® D; LoHist 12D; LoHist LQ; LoHist PD; Sildec Syrup; Touro® Allergy

Generic Available Yes

Index Terms Brompheniramine Maleate and Pseudoephedrine Hydrochloride; Brompheniramine Maleate and Pseudoephedrine Sulfate; Pseudoephedrine and Brompheniramine

Pharmacologic Category Antihistamine/Decongestant Combination

Use Temporary relief of symptoms of seasonal and perennial allergic rhinitis, and vasomotor rhinitis, including nasal obstruction

Local Anesthetic/Vasoconstrictor Precautions Use with caution since pseudoephedrine is a sympathomimetic amine which could interact with epinephrine to cause a pressor response

Effects on Dental Treatment Key adverse event(s) related to dental treatment:
Brompheniramine: Prolonged use may decrease salivary flow.
Pseudoephedrine: Xerostomia (normal salivary flow resumes upon discontinuation).

Common Adverse Effects Frequency not defined.
Cardiovascular: Arrhythmias, flushing, hypertension, pallor, palpitation, tachycardia
Central nervous system: Convulsions, CNS stimulation, dizziness, excitability (children; rare), giddiness, hallucinations, headache, insomnia, irritability, lassitude, nervousness, sedation
Gastrointestinal: Anorexia, diarrhea, dyspepsia, nausea, vomiting, xerostomia
Neuromuscular skeletal: Tremors, weakness
Ocular: Diplopia
Renal: Dysuria, polyuria, urinary retention (with BPH)
Respiratory: Respiratory difficulty

Mechanism of Action Brompheniramine maleate is an antihistamine with H_1-receptor activity; pseudoephedrine, a sympathomimetic amine and isomer of ephedrine, acts as a decongestant in respiratory tract mucous membranes with less vasoconstrictor action than ephedrine in normotensive individuals.

Pharmacodynamics/Kinetics
See Pseudoephedrine.
Brompheniramine:
Metabolism: Hepatic
Time to peak: Syrup: 5 hours
Excretion: Urine

Pregnancy Risk Factor C

Budesonide (byoo DES oh nide)

U.S. Brand Names Entocort® EC; Pulmicort Flexhaler®; Pulmicort Respules®; Pulmicort Turbuhaler®; Rhinocort® Aqua®

Canadian Brand Names Entocort®; Gen-Budesonide AQ; Pulmicort®; Rhinocort® Turbuhaler®

Mexican Brand Names Entocort; Numark; Pulmicort; Rhinocort

Generic Available No

Pharmacologic Category Corticosteroid, Inhalant (Oral); Corticosteroid, Nasal; Corticosteroid, Systemic

Use

Intranasal: Management of symptoms of seasonal or perennial rhinitis

Nebulization: Maintenance and prophylactic treatment of asthma

Oral capsule: Treatment of active Crohn's disease (mild-to-moderate) involving the ileum and/or ascending colon; maintenance of remission (for up to 3 months) of Crohn's disease (mild-to-moderate) involving the ileum and/or ascending colon

Oral inhalation: Maintenance and prophylactic treatment of asthma; includes patients who require corticosteroids and those who may benefit from systemic dose reduction/elimination

Local Anesthetic/Vasoconstrictor Precautions No information available to require special precautions

Effects on Dental Treatment Key adverse event(s) related to dental treatment: Xerostomia (normal salivary flow resumes upon discontinuation), dry throat, abnormal taste, and herpes simplex. Localized infections with *Candida albicans* or *Aspergillus niger* have occurred frequently in the mouth and pharynx with repetitive use of oral inhaler of corticosteroids. These infections may require treatment with appropriate antifungal therapy or discontinuance of treatment with corticosteroid inhaler.

Common Adverse Effects Reaction severity varies by dose and duration; not all adverse reactions have been reported with each dosage form.

>10%:

Central nervous system: Headache (up to 21%)

Gastrointestinal: Nausea (up to 11%)

Respiratory: Respiratory infection, rhinitis

Miscellaneous: Symptoms of HPA axis suppression and/or hypercorticism may occur in >10% of patients following administration of dosage forms which result in higher systemic exposure (ie, oral capsule), but may be less frequent than rates observed with comparator drugs (prednisolone). These symptoms may be rare (<1%) following administration via methods which result in lower exposures (topical).

1% to 10%:

Cardiovascular: Chest pain, edema, flushing, hypertension, palpitation, syncope, tachycardia

Central nervous system: Dizziness, dysphonia, emotional lability, fatigue, fever, insomnia, migraine, nervousness, pain, vertigo

Dermatologic: Acne, alopecia, bruising, contact dermatitis, eczema, hirsutism, pruritus, pustular rash, rash, striae

Endocrine & metabolic: Adrenal insufficiency, hypokalemia, menstrual disorder

Gastrointestinal: Abdominal pain, anorexia, diarrhea, dry mouth, dyspepsia, flatulence, gastroenteritis, oral candidiasis, taste perversion, vomiting, weight gain

Genitourinary: Dysuria, hematuria, nocturia, pyuria

Hematologic: Cervical lymphadenopathy, leukocytosis, purpura

Hepatic: Alkaline phosphatase increased

Neuromuscular & skeletal: Arthralgia, back pain, fracture, hyperkinesis, hypertonia, myalgia, neck pain, weakness, paresthesia

Ocular: Conjunctivitis, eye infection

Otic: Earache, ear infection, external ear infection

Respiratory: Bronchitis, bronchospasm, cough, epistaxis, nasal irritation, pharyngitis, sinusitis, stridor

Miscellaneous: Abscess, allergic reaction, C-reactive protein increased, erythrocyte sedimentation rate increased, fat distribution (moon face, buffalo hump), flu-like syndrome, herpes simplex, infection, moniliasis, viral infection, voice alteration

Dosage

Nasal inhalation: (Rhinocort® Aqua®): Children ≥6 years and Adults: 64 mcg/day as a single 32 mcg spray in each nostril. Some patients who do not achieve adequate control may benefit from increased dosage. A reduced dosage may be effective after initial control is achieved.

Maximum dose: Children <12 years: 128 mcg/day; Adults: 256 mcg/day

Nebulization: Children 12 months to 8 years: Pulmicort Respules®: Titrate to lowest effective dose once patient is stable; start at 0.25 mg/day or use as follows:

Previous therapy of bronchodilators alone: 0.5 mg/day administered as a single dose or divided twice daily (maximum daily dose: 0.5 mg)

Previous therapy of inhaled corticosteroids: 0.5 mg/day administered as a single dose or divided twice daily (maximum daily dose: 1 mg)

Previous therapy of oral corticosteroids: 1 mg/day administered as a single dose or divided twice daily (maximum daily dose: 1 mg)

Oral inhalation:

Children ≥6 years:

Pulmicort® Turbuhaler®:

Previous therapy of bronchodilators alone: 200 mcg twice initially which may be increased up to 400 mcg twice daily

Previous therapy of inhaled corticosteroids: 200 mcg twice initially which may be increased up to 400 mcg twice daily

Previous therapy of oral corticosteroids: The highest recommended dose in children is 400 mcg twice daily

Pulmicort® Flexhaler®: Initial: 180 mcg twice daily (some patients may be initiated at 360 mcg twice daily); maximum 360 mcg twice daily

Adults:

Pulmicort® Turbuhaler®:

Previous therapy of bronchodilators alone: 200-400 mcg twice initially which may be increased up to 400 mcg twice daily

Previous therapy of inhaled corticosteroids: 200-400 mcg twice initially which may be increased up to 800 mcg twice daily

Previous therapy of oral corticosteroids: 400-800 mcg twice daily which may be increased up to 800 mcg twice daily

Pulmicort® Flexhaler®: Initial: 360 mcg twice daily (selected patients may be initiated at 180 mcg twice daily); maximum 720 mcg twice daily

NIH Guidelines (NIH, 1997) (give in divided doses twice daily):

Children:

"Low" dose: 100-200 mcg/day

"Medium" dose: 200-400 mcg/day (1-2 inhalations/day)

"High" dose: >400 mcg/day (>2 inhalation/day)

Adults:

"Low" dose: 200-400 mcg/day (1-2 inhalations/day)

"Medium" dose: 400-600 mcg/day (2-3 inhalations/day)

"High" dose: >600 mcg/day (>3 inhalation/day)

Oral: Adults: Crohn's disease (active): 9 mg once daily in the morning for up to 8 weeks; recurring episodes may be treated with a repeat 8-week course of treatment

Note: Patients receiving CYP3A4 inhibitors should be monitored closely for signs and symptoms of hypercorticism; dosage reduction may be required. If switching from oral prednisolone, prednisolone dosage should be tapered while budesonide (Entocort™ EC) treatment is initiated.

Maintenance of remission: Following treatment of active disease (control of symptoms with CDAI <150), treatment may be continued at a dosage of 6 mg once daily for up to 3 months. If symptom control is maintained for 3 months, tapering of the dosage to complete cessation is recommended. Continued dosing beyond 3 months has not been demonstrated to result in substantial benefit.

Dosage adjustment in hepatic impairment: Monitor closely for signs and symptoms of hypercorticism; dosage reduction may be required.

Mechanism of Action Controls the rate of protein synthesis; depresses the migration of polymorphonuclear leukocytes, fibroblasts; reverses capillary permeability and lysosomal stabilization at the cellular level to prevent or control inflammation

Contraindications Hypersensitivity to budesonide or any component of the formulation

Inhalation: Contraindicated in primary treatment of status asthmaticus, acute episodes of asthma; not for relief of acute bronchospasm

Warnings/Precautions May cause hypercorticism or suppression of hypothalamic-pituitary-adrenal (HPA) axis, particularly in younger children or in patients receiving high doses for prolonged periods. HPA axis suppression may lead to adrenal crisis. Withdrawal and discontinuation of a corticosteroid should be done slowly and carefully. Particular care is required when patients are transferred from systemic corticosteroids to inhaled products due to possible adrenal insufficiency or withdrawal from steroids, including an increase in allergic symptoms. Patients receiving >20 mg per day of prednisone (or equivalent) may be most susceptible. Fatalities have occurred due to adrenal insufficiency in asthmatic patients during and after transfer from systemic corticosteroids to aerosol (Continued)

Budesonide *(Continued)*

steroids; aerosol steroids do not provide the systemic steroid needed to treat patients having trauma, surgery, or infections. Do not use this product to transfer patients from oral corticosteroid therapy.

Bronchospasm may occur with wheezing after inhalation; if this occurs stop steroid and treat with a fast-acting bronchodilator. Supplemental steroids (oral or parenteral) may be needed during stress or severe asthma attacks. Not to be used in status asthmaticus or for the relief of acute bronchospasm. Acute myopathy has been reported with high dose corticosteroids, usually in patients with neuromuscular transmission disorders; may involve ocular and/or respiratory muscles; monitor creatine kinase; recovery may be delayed. Corticosteroid use may cause psychiatric disturbances, including depression, euphoria, insomnia, mood swings, and personality changes. Pre-existing psychiatric conditions may be exacerbated by corticosteroid use. Prolonged use of corticosteroids may also increase the incidence of secondary infection, mask acute infection (including fungal infections), prolong or exacerbate viral infections, or limit response to vaccines. Exposure to chickenpox should be avoided; corticosteroids should not be used to treat ocular herpes simplex. Corticosteroids should not be used for cerebral malaria. Close observation is required in patients with latent tuberculosis and/or TB reactivity; restrict use in active TB (only in conjunction with antituberculosis treatment). Prolonged treatment with corticosteroids has been associated with the development of Kaposi's sarcoma (case reports); if noted, discontinuation of therapy should be considered.

Use with caution in patients with thyroid disease, hepatic impairment, renal impairment, cardiovascular disease, diabetes, glaucoma, cataracts, myasthenia gravis, patients at risk for osteoporosis, patients at risk for seizures, or GI diseases (diverticulitis, peptic ulcer, ulcerative colitis) due to perforation risk. Use caution following acute MI (corticosteroids have been associated with myocardial rupture). Because of the risk of adverse effects, systemic corticosteroids should be used cautiously in the elderly in the smallest possible effective dose for the shortest duration. Avoid nasal corticosteroid use in patients with recent nasal septal ulcers, nasal surgery or nasal trauma until healing has occurred.

Orally-inhaled and intranasal corticosteroids may cause a reduction in growth velocity in pediatric patients (~1 centimeter per year [range 0.3-1.8 cm per year] and related to dose and duration of exposure). To minimize the systemic effects of orally-inhaled and intranasal corticosteroids, each patient should be titrated to the lowest effective dose. Growth should be routinely monitored in pediatric patients. Withdraw systemic therapy with gradual tapering of dose. There have been reports of systemic corticosteroid withdrawal symptoms (eg, joint/muscle pain, lassitude, depression) when withdrawing oral inhalation therapy. Enteric-coated capsules should not be crushed or chewed.

Drug Interactions
Cytochrome P450 Effect: Substrate of CYP3A4 (major)

Increased Effect/Toxicity: Cimetidine may decrease the clearance and increase the bioavailability of budesonide, increasing its serum concentrations. In addition, CYP3A4 inhibitors may increase the serum level and/or toxicity of budesonide this effect was shown with ketoconazole, but not erythromycin. Other potential inhibitors include amiodarone, cimetidine, clarithromycin, delavirdine, diltiazem, dirithromycin, disulfiram, fluoxetine, fluvoxamine, grapefruit juice, indinavir, itraconazole, ketoconazole, nefazodone, nevirapine, propoxyphene, quinupristin-dalfopristin, ritonavir, saquinavir, telithromycin, verapamil, zafirlukast, and zileuton. The addition of salmeterol has been demonstrated to improve response to inhaled corticosteroids (as compared to increasing steroid dosage).

Decreased Effect: Theoretically, proton pump inhibitors (omeprazole, pantoprazole) alter gastric pH and may affect the rate of dissolution of enteric-coated capsules. Administration with omeprazole did not alter kinetics of budesonide capsules.

Ethanol/Nutrition/Herb Interactions
Food: Grapefruit juice may double systemic exposure of orally-administered budesonide. Administration of capsules with a high-fat meal delays peak concentration, but does not alter the extent of absorption.

Herb/Nutraceutical: St John's wort may decrease budesonide levels.

Dietary Considerations Avoid grapefruit juice when using oral capsules.

Pharmacodynamics/Kinetics
Onset of action: Respules®: 2-8 days; Rhinocort® Aqua®: ~10 hours; Inhalation: 24 hours

Peak effect: Respules®: 4-6 weeks; Rhinocort® Aqua®: ~2 weeks; Inhalation: 1-2 weeks

Distribution: 2.2-3.9 L/kg

Protein binding: 85% to 90%

Metabolism: Hepatic via CYP3A4 to two metabolites: 16 alpha-hydroxy-prednisolone and 6 beta-hydroxybudesonide; minor activity

Bioavailability: Limited by high first-pass effect; Capsule: 9% to 21%; Respules®: 6%; Inhalation: 6% to 13%; Nasal: 34%

Half-life elimination: 2-3.6 hours

Time to peak: Capsule: 0.5-10 hours (variable in Crohn's disease); Respules®: 10-30 minutes; Inhalation: 1-2 hours; Nasal: 1 hour

Excretion: Urine (60%) and feces as metabolites

Pregnancy Risk Factor C/B (Pulmicort Respules®, Flexhaler®, and Turbuhaler®; Rhinocort® Aqua®)

Dosage Forms [CAN] = Canadian brand name

Capsule, enteric coated:
Entocort® EC: 3 mg

Powder for oral inhalation:
Pulmicort Flexhaler®: 90 mcg/inhalation (165 mg)
Pulmicort Flexhaler®: 180 mcg/inhalation (225 mg)
Pulmicort Turbuhaler®: 200 mcg/inhalation (104 g)
Pulmicort Turbuhaler® [CAN]: 100 mcg/inhalation, 200 mcg/inhalation, 400 mcg/inhalation [not available in the U.S.]

Suspension, intranasal [spray]:
Rhinocort® Aqua®: 32 mcg/inhalation (8.6 g)

Suspension for nebulization:
Pulmicort Respules®: 0.25 mg/2 mL, 0.5 mg/2 mL

Buffasal [OTC] see Aspirin on page 149

Buffered Aspirin and Pravastatin Sodium see Aspirin and Pravastatin on page 155

Bufferin® [OTC] see Aspirin on page 149

Bufferin® Extra Strength [OTC] see Aspirin on page 149

Buffinol [OTC] see Aspirin on page 149

Bumetanide (byoo MET a nide)

Related Information
Cardiovascular Diseases on page 1726
U.S. Brand Names Bumex®
Canadian Brand Names Bumex®; Burinex®
Mexican Brand Names Bumedyl; Drenural; Miccil
Generic Available Yes
Pharmacologic Category Diuretic, Loop
Use Management of edema secondary to congestive heart failure or hepatic or renal disease including nephrotic syndrome; may be used alone or in combination with antihypertensives in the treatment of hypertension; can be used in furosemide-allergic patients

Local Anesthetic/Vasoconstrictor Precautions No information available to require special precautions

Effects on Dental Treatment No significant effects or complications reported

Common Adverse Effects
>10%:
Endocrine & metabolic: Hyperuricemia (18%), hypochloremia (15%), hypokalemia (15%)
Renal: Azotemia (11%)
1% to 10%:
Central nervous system: Dizziness (1%)
Endocrine & metabolic: Hyponatremia (9%); hyperglycemia (7%); variations in phosphorus (5%), CO_2 content (4%), bicarbonate (3%), and calcium (2%)
Neuromuscular & skeletal: Muscle cramps (1%)
Otic: Ototoxicity (1%)
Renal: Serum creatinine increased (7%)

Mechanism of Action Inhibits reabsorption of sodium and chloride in the ascending loop of Henle and proximal renal tubule, interfering with the chloride-binding cotransport system, thus causing increased excretion of water, sodium, chloride, magnesium, phosphate, and calcium; it does not appear to act on the distal tubule

Drug Interactions
Increased Effect/Toxicity: Bumetanide-induced hypokalemia may predispose to digoxin toxicity and may increase the risk of arrhythmia with drugs which may prolong QT interval, including type Ia and type III antiarrhythmic agents, cisapride, and some quinolones (sparfloxacin, gatifloxacin, and moxifloxacin). The risk of toxicity from lithium and salicylates (high dose) may be increased by loop diuretics. Hypotensive effects and/or adverse renal
(Continued)

Bumetanide *(Continued)*

effects of ACE inhibitors and NSAIDs are potentiated by bumetanide-induced hypovolemia. The effects of peripheral adrenergic-blocking drugs or ganglionic blockers may be increased by bumetanide.

Bumetanide may increase the risk of ototoxicity with other ototoxic agents (aminoglycosides, cis-platinum), especially in patients with renal dysfunction. Synergistic diuretic effects occur with thiazide-type diuretics. Diuretics tend to be synergistic with other antihypertensive agents, and hypotension may occur.

Decreased Effect: Glucose tolerance may be decreased by loop diuretics, requiring adjustment of hypoglycemic agents. Cholestyramine or colestipol may reduce bioavailability of bumetanide. Indomethacin (and other NSAIDs) may reduce natriuretic and hypotensive effects of diuretics. Hypokalemia may reduce the efficacy of some antiarrhythmics.

Pharmacodynamics/Kinetics
Onset of action: Oral, I.M.: 0.5-1 hour; I.V.: 2-3 minutes
Duration: 4-6 hours
Distribution: V_d: 13-25 L/kg
Protein binding: 95%
Metabolism: Partially hepatic
Half-life elimination: Neonates: ~6 hours; Infants (1 month): ~2.4 hours; Adults: 1-1.5 hours
Excretion: Primarily urine (as unchanged drug and metabolites)

Pregnancy Risk Factor C (manufacturer); D (expert analysis)

Bumex® *see* Bumetanide *on page 235*

Bupap *see* Butalbital and Acetaminophen *on page 249*

Buphenyl® *see* Sodium Phenylbutyrate *on page 1483*

Bupivacaine *(byoo PIV a kane)*

Related Information
Oral Pain *on page 1788*

U.S. Brand Names Marcaine®; Marcaine® Spinal; Sensorcaine®; Sensorcaine®-MPF; Sensorcaine®-MPF Spinal

Canadian Brand Names Marcaine®; Sensorcaine®

Generic Available Yes

Index Terms Bupivacaine Hydrochloride

Pharmacologic Category Local Anesthetic

Dental Use None; not to be confused with bupivacaine and epinephrine dental anesthetic. Refer to Bupivacaine and Epinephrine.

Use Local anesthetic (injectable) for peripheral nerve block, infiltration, sympathetic block, caudal or epidural block, retrobulbar block

Local Anesthetic/Vasoconstrictor Precautions No information available to require special precautions

Effects on Dental Treatment No significant effects or complications reported

Common Adverse Effects Note: Incidence of adverse reactions is difficult to define. Most effects are dose related, and are often due to accelerated absorption from the injection site, unintentional intravascular injection, or slow metabolic degradation. The development of any central nervous system symptoms may be an early indication of more significant toxicity (seizure).

Cardiovascular: Hypotension, bradycardia, palpitation, heart block, ventricular arrhythmia, cardiac arrest

Central nervous system: Restlessness, anxiety, dizziness, seizure (0.1%); rare symptoms (usually associated with unintentional subarachnoid injection during high spinal anesthesia) include persistent anesthesia, paresthesia, paralysis, headache, septic meningitis, and cranial nerve palsies

Gastrointestinal: Nausea, vomiting; rare symptoms (usually associated with unintentional subarachnoid injection during high spinal anesthesia) include fecal incontinence and loss of sphincter control

Genitourinary: Rare symptoms (usually associated with unintentional subarachnoid injection during high spinal anesthesia) include urinary incontinence, loss of perineal sensation, and loss of sexual function

Neuromuscular & skeletal: Weakness

Ocular: Blurred vision, pupillary constriction

Otic: Tinnitus

Respiratory: Apnea, hypoventilation (usually associated with unintentional subarachnoid injection during high spinal anesthesia)

Miscellaneous: Allergic reactions (urticaria, pruritus, angioedema), anaphylactoid reactions

Mechanism of Action Blocks both the initiation and conduction of nerve impulses by decreasing the neuronal membrane's permeability to sodium ions, which results in inhibition of depolarization with resultant blockade of conduction

Drug Interactions

  Cytochrome P450 Effect: Substrate (minor) of CYP1A2, 2C19, 2D6, 3A4

Pharmacodynamics/Kinetics

  Onset of action: Anesthesia (route and dose dependent): 1-17 minutes

  Duration (route and dose dependent): 2-9 hours

  Protein binding: ~95%

  Metabolism: Hepatic; forms metabolite (PPX)

  Half-life elimination (age dependent): Neonates: 8.1 hours; Adults: 1.5-5.5 hours

  Excretion: Urine (~6% unchanged)

Pregnancy Risk Factor C

Bupivacaine and Epinephrine (byoo PIV a kane & ep i NEF rin)

Related Information

  Bupivacaine *on page 236*

  Epinephrine *on page 572*

  Oral Pain *on page 1788*

U.S. Brand Names Marcaine® with Epinephrine; Sensorcaine®-MPF with Epinephrine; Sensorcaine® with Epinephrine

Canadian Brand Names Sensorcaine® with Epinephrine

Generic Available Yes

Index Terms Epinephrine Bitartrate and Bupivacaine Hydrochloride

Pharmacologic Category Local Anesthetic

Dental Use Local anesthesia

Use Local anesthetic (injectable) for peripheral nerve block, infiltration, sympathetic block, caudal or epidural block, retrobulbar block

Local Anesthetic/Vasoconstrictor Precautions No information available to require special precautions

Effects on Dental Treatment It is common to misinterpret psychogenic responses to local anesthetic injection as an allergic reaction. Intraoral injections are perceived by many patients as a stressful procedure in dentistry. Common symptoms to this stress are diaphoresis, palpitations, and hyperventilation. Patients may exhibit hypersensitivity to bisulfites contained in local anesthetic solution to prevent oxidation of epinephrine. In general, patients reacting to bisulfites have a history of asthma and their airways are hyper-reactive to asthmatic syndrome.

Degree of adverse effects in the CNS and cardiovascular system is directly related to the blood levels of bupivacaine: Bradycardia, hypersensitivity reactions (rare; may be manifest as dermatologic reactions and edema at injection site), asthmatic syndromes.

High blood levels: Anxiety, restlessness, disorientation, confusion, dizziness, tremors, seizures, CNS depression (resulting in somnolence, unconsciousness and possible respiratory arrest), nausea, and vomiting.

Significant Adverse Effects See individual agents.

Dental Usual Dosing

  Infiltration and nerve block in maxillary and mandibular area: Children >12 years and Adults: 9 mg (1.8 mL) of bupivacaine as a 0.5% solution with epinephrine 1:200,000 per injection site. A second dose may be administered if necessary to produce adequate anesthesia after allowing up to 10 minutes for onset. Up to a maximum of 90 mg of bupivacaine hydrochloride per dental appointment. The effective anesthetic dose varies with procedure, intensity of anesthesia needed, duration of anesthesia required, and physical condition of the patient; always use the lowest effective dose along with careful aspiration.

# of Cartridges (1.8 mL)	mg Bupivacaine (0.5%)	mg Vasoconstrictor (Epinephrine 1:200,000)
1	9	0.009
2	18	0.018
3	27	0.027
4	36	0.036
5	45	0.045
6	54	0.054
7	63	0.063
8	72	0.072
9	81	0.081
10	90	0.090

(Continued)

Bupivacaine and Epinephrine *(Continued)*

The following numbers of dental carpules (1.8 mL) provide the indicated amounts of bupivacaine hydrochloride 0.5% and vasoconstrictor (epinephrine 1:200,000). See table on previous page.

Note: Adult and children doses of bupivacaine hydrochloride with epinephrine cited from USP Dispensing Information (USP DI), 17th ed, The United States Pharmacopeial Convention, Inc, Rockville, MD, 1997, 134.

Dosage Dose varies with procedure, depth of anesthesia, vascularity of tissues, duration of anesthesia, and condition of patient. Do not use solutions containing preservatives for caudal or epidural block.

Children >12 years and Adults:

Caudal block (preservative free): 15-30 mL of 0.25% or 0.5%

Epidural block (other than caudal block, preservative free): 10-20 mL of 0.25% or 0.5%. Administer in 3-5 mL increments, allowing sufficient time to detect toxic manifestations of inadvertent I.V. or I.T. administration.

Surgical procedures requiring a high degree of muscle relaxation and prolonged effects only: 10-20 mL of 0.75% (**Note:** Not to be used in obstetrical cases)

Local anesthesia: Infiltration: 0.25% infiltrated locally (maximum: 175 mg of bupivacaine)

Peripheral nerve block: 5 mL of 0.25 or 0.5% (maximum: 400 mg/day of bupivacaine)

Retrobulbar anesthesia: 2-4 mL of 0.75%

Sympathetic nerve block: 20-50 mL of 0.25%

Infiltration and nerve block in maxillary and mandibular area: 9 mg (1.8 mL) of bupivacaine as a 0.5% solution with epinephrine 1:200,000 per injection site. A second dose may be administered if necessary to produce adequate anesthesia after allowing up to 10 minutes for onset. Up to a maximum of 90 mg of bupivacaine hydrochloride per dental appointment. The effective anesthetic dose varies with procedure, intensity of anesthesia needed, duration of anesthesia required, and physical condition of the patient; always use the lowest effective dose along with careful aspiration.

Note: Adult and children doses of bupivacaine hydrochloride with epinephrine cited from USP Dispensing Information (USP DI), 17th ed, The United States Pharmacopeial Convention, Inc, Rockville, MD, 1997, 134.

Mechanism of Action Local anesthetics bind selectively to the intracellular surface of sodium channels to block influx of sodium into the axon. As a result, depolarization necessary for action potential propagation and subsequent nerve function is prevented. The block at the sodium channel is reversible. When drug diffuses away from the axon, sodium channel function is restored and nerve propagation returns.

Epinephrine prolongs the duration of the anesthetic actions of bupivacaine by causing vasoconstriction (alpha-adrenergic receptor agonist) of the vasculature surrounding the nerve axons. This prevents the diffusion of bupivacaine away from the nerves resulting in a longer retention in the axon

Contraindications Hypersensitivity to bupivacaine, epinephrine, amide-type local anesthetics, or any component of the formulation

Warnings/Precautions Some commercially available formulations contain sodium metabisulfite, which may cause allergic-type reactions. Do not use solutions containing preservatives for caudal or epidural block. Local anesthetics have been associated with rare occurrences of sudden respiratory arrest. Convulsions due to systemic toxicity leading to cardiac arrest have also been reported, presumably following unintentional intravascular injection. The 0.75% is not recommended for obstetrical anesthesia. A test dose is recommended prior to epidural administration and all reinforcing doses with continuous catheter technique. Use caution with cardiovascular dysfunction, hepatic impairment, or patients with compromised blood supply. Use caution in debilitated, elderly, or acutely ill patients; dose reduction may be required. Not recommended for use in children <12 years of age.

Drug Interactions Bupivacaine: **Substrate** (minor) of CYP1A2, 2C19, 2D6, 3A4 Also see individual agents.

Pharmacodynamics/Kinetics Refer to Bupivacaine; epinephrine reduces the rate of absorption and peak plasma concentration of bupivacaine

Pregnancy Risk Factor C

Lactation Enters breast milk/not recommended

Dosage Forms Excipient information presented when available (limited, particularly for generics); consult specific product labeling.

Injection, solution [preservative free]: Bupivacaine hydrochloride 0.25% and epinephrine bitartrate 1:200,000 (10 mL, 30 mL); bupivacaine hydrochloride 0.5% and epinephrine bitartrate 1:200,000 (1.8 mL, 10 mL, 30 mL)

Marcaine® with Epinephrine Preservative Free: Bupivacaine hydrochloride 0.25% and epinephrine bitartrate 1:200,000 (10 mL, 30 mL) [contains sodium metabisulfite]; bupivacaine hydrochloride 0.5% and epinephrine bitartrate 1:200,000 (1.8 mL, 3 mL, 10 mL, 30 mL) [contains sodium metabisulfite]; bupivacaine hydrochloride 0.75% and epinephrine bitartrate 1:200,000 (30 mL) [contains sodium metabisulfite]

Sensorcaine® MPF with Epinephrine: Bupivacaine hydrochloride 0.25% and epinephrine bitartrate 1:200,000 (10 mL, 30 mL) [contains sodium metabisulfite]; bupivacaine hydrochloride 0.5% and epinephrine bitartrate 1:200,000 (10 mL, 30 mL) [contains sodium metabisulfite]

Injection, solution: Bupivacaine hydrochloride 0.25% and epinephrine bitartrate 1:200,000 (50 mL); bupivacaine hydrochloride 0.5% and epinephrine bitartrate 1:200,000 (50 mL)

Marcaine® with Epinephrine, Sensorcaine® with Epinephrine: Bupivacaine hydrochloride 0.25% and epinephrine bitartrate 1:200,000 (50 mL) [contains methylparaben]; bupivacaine hydrochloride 0.5% and epinephrine bitartrate 1:200,000 (50 mL) [contains methylparaben]

Selected Readings

Ayoub ST and Coleman AE, "A Review of Local Anesthetics," *Gen Dent*, 1992, 40(4):285-7, 289-90.

Budenz AW, "Local Anesthetics in Dentistry: Then and Now," *J Calif Dent Assoc*, 2003, 31(5):388-96.

Dower JS Jr, "A Review of Paresthesia in Association With Administration of Local Anesthesia," *Dent Today*, 2003, 22(2):64-9.

Finder RL and Moore PA, "Adverse Drug Reactions to Local Anesthesia," *Dent Clin North Am*, 2002, 46(4):747-57, x.

Haas DA, "An Update on Local Anesthetics in Dentistry," *J Can Dent Assoc*, 2002, 68(9):546-51.

Hawkins JM and Moore PA, "Local Anesthesia: Advances in Agents and Techniques," *Dent Clin North Am*, 2002, 46(4):719-32, ix.

"Injectable Local Anesthetics," *J Am Dent Assoc*, 2003, 134(5):628-9.

Jastak JT and Yagiela JA, "Vasoconstrictors and Local Anesthesia: A Review and Rationale for Use," *J Am Dent Assoc*, 1983, 107(4):623-30.

MacKenzie TA and Young ER, "Local Anesthetic Update," *Anesth Prog*, 1993, 40(2):29-34.

Malamed SF, "Allergy and Toxic Reactions to Local Anesthetics," *Dent Today*, 2003, 22(4):114-6, 118-21.

Wahl MJ, Schmitt MM, Overton DA, et al, "Injection Pain of Bupivacaine With Epinephrine vs. Prilocaine Plain," *J Am Dent Assoc*, 2002, 133(12):1652-6.

Wynn RL, "Epinephrine Interactions With Beta-Blockers," *Gen Dent*, 1994, 42(1):16, 18.

Yagiela JA, "Local Anesthetics," *Anesth Prog*, 1991, 38(4-5):128-41.

Bupivacaine and Lidocaine see Lidocaine and Bupivacaine on page 976

Bupivacaine Hydrochloride see Bupivacaine on page 236

Buprenex® see Buprenorphine on page 239

Buprenorphine (byoo pre NOR feen)

U.S. Brand Names Buprenex®; Subutex®
Canadian Brand Names Buprenex®; Subutex®
Mexican Brand Names Temgesic
Generic Available Yes: Injection
Index Terms Buprenorphine Hydrochloride
Pharmacologic Category Analgesic, Opioid
Use
Injection: Management of moderate to severe pain
Tablet: Treatment of opioid dependence
Unlabeled/Investigational Use Injection: Heroin and opioid withdrawal
Local Anesthetic/Vasoconstrictor Precautions No information available to require special precautions
Effects on Dental Treatment No significant effects or complications reported
Common Adverse Effects
Injection:
>10%: Central nervous system: Sedation
1% to 10%:
Cardiovascular: Hypotension
Central nervous system: Respiratory depression, dizziness, headache
Gastrointestinal: Vomiting, nausea
Ocular: Miosis
Otic: Vertigo
Miscellaneous: Diaphoresis
Tablet:
>10%:
Central nervous system: Headache (30%), pain (24%), insomnia (21% to 25%), Oralety (12%), depression (11%)
(Continued)

Buprenorphine *(Continued)*

Gastrointestinal: Nausea (10% to 14%), abdominal pain (12%), constipation (8% to 11%)

Neuromuscular & skeletal: Back pain (14%), weakness (14%)

Respiratory: Rhinitis (11%)

Miscellaneous: Withdrawal syndrome (19%; placebo 37%), infection (12% to 20%), diaphoresis (12% to 13%)

1% to 10%:

Central nervous system: Chills (6%), nervousness (6%), somnolence (5%), dizziness (4%), fever (3%)

Gastrointestinal: Vomiting (5% to 8%), diarrhea (5%), dyspepsia (3%)

Ocular: Lacrimation (5%)

Respiratory: Cough (4%), pharyngitis (4%)

Miscellaneous: Flu-like syndrome (6%)

Restrictions Injection: C-V/C-III; Tablet: C-III

Prescribing of tablets for opioid dependence is limited to physicians who have met the qualification criteria and have received a DEA number specific to prescribing this product. Tablets will be available through pharmacies and wholesalers which normally provide controlled substances.

Mechanism of Action Buprenorphine exerts its analgesic effect via high affinity binding to μ opiate receptors in the CNS; displays both agonist and antagonist activity

Drug Interactions

Cytochrome P450 Effect: Substrate of CYP3A4 (major); **Inhibits** CYP1A2 (weak), 2A6 (weak), 2C19 (weak), 2D6 (weak)

Increased Effect/Toxicity: Barbiturate anesthetics and other CNS depressants may produce additive respiratory and CNS depression. Respiratory and CV collapse was reported in a patient who received diazepam and buprenorphine. Effects may be additive with other CNS depressants. CYP3A4 inhibitors may increase the levels/effects of buprenorphine; example inhibitors include azole antifungals, clarithromycin, diclofenac, doxycycline, erythromycin, imatinib, isoniazid, nefazodone, nicardipine, propofol, protease inhibitors, quinidine, and verapamil.

Decreased Effect: CYP3A4 inducers may decrease the levels/effects of buprenorphine; example inducers include aminoglutethimide, carbamazepine, nafcillin, nevirapine, phenobarbital, phenytoin, and rifamycins. Naltrexone may antagonize the effect of opioid analgesics; concurrent use or use within 7-10 days of injection for pain relief is contraindicated.

Pharmacodynamics/Kinetics

Onset of action: Analgesic: 10-30 minutes

Duration: 6-8 hours

Absorption: I.M., SubQ: 30% to 40%

Distribution: V_d: 97-187 L/kg

Protein binding: High

Metabolism: Primarily hepatic; extensive first-pass effect

Half-life elimination: 2.2-3 hours

Excretion: Feces (70%); urine (20% as unchanged drug)

Pregnancy Risk Factor C

Buprenorphine and Naloxone
(byoo pre NOR feen & nal OKS one)

Related Information

Buprenorphine *on page 239*

Naloxone *on page 1144*

U.S. Brand Names Suboxone®

Generic Available No

Index Terms Buprenorphine Hydrochloride and Naloxone Hydrochloride Dihydrate; Naloxone and Buprenorphine; Naloxone Hydrochloride Dihydrate and Buprenorphine Hydrochloride

Pharmacologic Category Analgesic, Opioid

Use Treatment of opioid dependence

Local Anesthetic/Vasoconstrictor Precautions No information available to require special precautions

Effects on Dental Treatment No significant effects or complications reported

Common Adverse Effects Also see individual agents.

>10%:

Central nervous system: Headache (36%), pain (22%)

Gastrointestinal: Nausea (15%), constipation (12%), abdominal pain (11%)

Miscellaneous: Withdrawal syndrome (25%; placebo 37%), diaphoresis (14%)

1% to 10%:
  Cardiovascular: Vasodilation (9%)
  Gastrointestinal: Vomiting (7%)
Restrictions C-III; Prescribing of tablets for opioid dependence is limited to physicians who have met the qualification criteria and have received a DEA number specific to prescribing this product. Tablets will be available through pharmacies and wholesalers which normally provide controlled substances.
Mechanism of Action See individual agents.
Drug Interactions
  Decreased Effect: See individual agents.
Pharmacodynamics/Kinetics See individual agents.
  Absorption: Absorption of the combination product is variable among patients following sublingual use, but variability within each individual patient is low.
Pregnancy Risk Factor C

Buprenorphine Hydrochloride *see* Buprenorphine *on page 239*

Buprenorphine Hydrochloride and Naloxone Hydrochloride Dihydrate *see* Buprenorphine and Naloxone *on page 240*

Buproban™ *see* BuPROPion *on page 241*

BuPROPion (byoo PROE pee on)

U.S. Brand Names Budeprion™ SR; Buproban™; Wellbutrin®; Wellbutrin SR®; Wellbutrin XL™; Zyban®
Canadian Brand Names Novo-Bupropion SR; Wellbutrin®; Wellbutrin XL™; Zyban®
Mexican Brand Names Wellbutrin
Generic Available Yes: Excludes Wellbutrin XL™
Pharmacologic Category Antidepressant, Dopamine-Reuptake Inhibitor; Smoking Cessation Aid
Use Treatment of major depressive disorder, including seasonal affective disorder (SAD); adjunct in smoking cessation
Unlabeled/Investigational Use Attention-deficit/hyperactivity disorder (ADHD); depression associated with bipolar disorder
Local Anesthetic/Vasoconstrictor Precautions Part of the mechanism of bupropion is to block reuptake of norepinephrine along with dopamine. Because of the potential for norepinephrine elevation within CNS synapses, it is suggested that vasoconstrictor be administered with caution and to monitor vital signs in dental patients taking antidepressants that affect norepinephrine in this way.
Effects on Dental Treatment Key adverse event(s) related to dental treatment: Abnormal taste, significant xerostomia (normal salivary flow resumes with discontinuation).
Common Adverse Effects Frequencies, when reported, reflect highest incidence reported with sustained release product.

>10%:
  Cardiovascular: Tachycardia (11%)
  Central nervous system: Headache (25% to 34%), insomnia (11% to 20%), dizziness (6% to 11%)
  Gastrointestinal: Xerostomia (17% to 26%), weight loss (14% to 23%), nausea (1% to 18%)
  Respiratory: Pharyngitis (3% to 13%)
1% to 10%:
  Cardiovascular: Palpitation (2% to 6%), arrhythmias (5%), chest pain (3% to 4%), hypertension (2% to 4%, may be severe), flushing (1% to 4%), hypotension (3%)
  Central nervous system: Agitation (2% to 9%), confusion (8%), anxiety (5% to 7%), hostility (6%), nervousness (3% to 5%), sleep disturbance (4%), sensory disturbance (4%), migraine (1% to 4%), abnormal dreams (3%), irritability (2% to 3%), somnolence (2% to 3%), pain (2% to 3%), memory decreased (up to 3%), fever (1% to 2%), CNS stimulation (1% to 2%), depression
  Dermatologic: Rash (1% to 5%), pruritus (2% to 4%), urticaria (1% to 2%)
  Endocrine & metabolic: Menstrual complaints (2% to 5%), hot flashes (1% to 3%), libido decreased (3%)
  Gastrointestinal: Constipation (5% to 10%), abdominal pain (2% to 9%), diarrhea (5% to 7%), flatulence (6%), anorexia (3% to 5%), appetite increased (4%), taste perversion (2% to 4%), vomiting (2% to 4%), dyspepsia (3%), dysphagia (up to 2%)
  Genitourinary: Urinary frequency (2% to 5%), urinary urgency (up to 2%), vaginal hemorrhage (up to 2%), UTI (up to 1%)
(Continued)

BuPROPion *(Continued)*

Neuromuscular & skeletal: Tremor (3% to 6%), myalgia (2% to 6%), weakness (2% to 4%), arthralgia (1% to 4%), arthritis (2%), akathisia (2%), paresthesia (1% to 2%), twitching (1% to 2%), neck pain

Ocular: Amblyopia (2%), blurred vision (2% to 3%)

Otic: Tinnitus (3% to 6%), auditory disturbance (5%)

Respiratory: Upper respiratory infection (9%), cough increased (1% to 4%), sinusitis (1% to 5%)

Miscellaneous: Infection (8% to 9%), diaphoresis increased (5% to 6%), allergic reaction (including anaphylaxis, pruritus, urticaria)

Restrictions An FDA-approved medication guide concerning the use of antidepressants in children, adolescents, and young adults must be distributed when dispensing an outpatient prescription (new or refill) where this medication is to be used without direct supervision of a healthcare provider. Medication guides are available at http://www.fda.gov/cder/Offices/ODS/medication_guides.htm. Dispense to parents or guardians of children and adolescents receiving this medication.

Dosage Oral:

Children and Adolescents: ADHD (unlabeled use): 1.4-6 mg/kg/day

Adults:

Depression:

Immediate release: 100 mg 3 times/day; begin at 100 mg twice daily; may increase to a maximum dose of 450 mg/day

Sustained release: Initial: 150 mg/day in the morning; may increase to 150 mg twice daily by day 4 if tolerated; target dose: 300 mg/day given as 150 mg twice daily; maximum dose: 400 mg/day given as 200 mg twice daily

Extended release: Initial: 150 mg/day in the morning; may increase as early as day 4 of dosing to 300 mg/day; maximum dose: 450 mg/day

SAD (Wellbutrin XL™): Initial: 150 mg/day in the morning; if tolerated, may increase after 1 week to 300 mg/day

Note: Prophylactic treatment should be reserved for those patients with frequent depressive episodes and/or significant impairment. Initiate treatment in the Autumn prior to symptom onset, and discontinue in early Spring with dose tapering to 150 mg/day for 2 weeks

Smoking cessation (Zyban®): Initiate with 150 mg once daily for 3 days; increase to 150 mg twice daily; treatment should continue for 7-12 weeks

Elderly: Depression: 50-100 mg/day, increase by 50-100 mg every 3-4 days as tolerated; there is evidence that the elderly respond at 150 mg/day in divided doses, but some may require a higher dose

Dosing conversion between immediate, sustained, and extended release products: Convert using same total daily dose (up to the maximum recommended dose for a given dosage form), but adjust frequency as indicated for sustained (twice daily) or extended (once daily) release products

Dosing adjustment/comments in renal impairment: Per the manufacturer, the elimination of hydroxybupropion and threohydrobupropion are reduced in patients with end-stage renal failure. Other research has noted a reduction in bupropion clearance (Turpeinen, 2007). Consider a reduction in frequency and/or dosage in this patient population.

Dosing adjustment in hepatic impairment:

Note: The mean AUC increased by ~1.5-fold for hydroxybupropion and ~2.5-fold for erythro/threohydrobupropion; median T_{max} was observed 19 hours later for hydroxybupropion, 31 hours later for erythro/threohydrobupropion; mean half-life for hydroxybupropion increased fivefold, and increased twofold for erythro/threohydrobupropion in patients with severe hepatic cirrhosis compared to healthy volunteers.

Mild-to-moderate hepatic impairment: Use with caution and/or reduced dose/frequency

Severe hepatic cirrhosis: Use with extreme caution; maximum dose:

Wellbutrin®: 75 mg/day

Wellbutrin SR®: 100 mg/day or 150 mg every other day

Wellbutrin XL™: 150 mg every other day

Zyban®: 150 mg every other day

Mechanism of Action Aminoketone antidepressant structurally different from all other marketed antidepressants; like other antidepressants the mechanism of bupropion's activity is not fully understood. Bupropion is a relatively weak inhibitor of the neuronal uptake of norepinephrine and dopamine, and does not inhibit monoamine oxidase or the reuptake of serotonin. Metabolite inhibits the reuptake of norepinephrine. The primary mechanism of action is thought to be dopaminergic and/or noradrenergic.

Contraindications Hypersensitivity to bupropion or any component of the formulation; seizure disorder; anorexia/bulimia; use of MAO inhibitors within 14 days; patients undergoing abrupt discontinuation of ethanol or sedatives (including benzodiazepines); patients receiving other dosage forms of bupropion

Warnings/Precautions [U.S. Boxed Warning]: Antidepressants increase the risk of suicidal thinking and behavior in children, adolescents, and young adults (18-24 years of age) with major depressive disorder (MDD) and other psychiatric disorders; consider risk prior to prescribing. Short-term studies did not show an increased risk in patients >24 years of age and showed a decreased risk in patients ≥65 years. All patients must be closely monitored for clinical worsening, suicidality, or unusual changes in behavior, especially during the initiation of therapy (generally first 1-2 months) or following an increase or decrease in dosage. The patient's family or caregiver should be instructed to closely observe the patient and communicate condition with healthcare provider. A medication guide should be dispensed with each prescription. **Bupropion is not FDA approved for use in children.**

The possibility of a suicide attempt is inherent in major depression and may persist until remission occurs. Use caution in high-risk patients. Worsening depression and severe abrupt suicidality that are not part of the presenting symptoms may require discontinuation or modification of drug therapy. The patient's family or caregiver should be alerted to monitor patients for the emergence of suicidality and associated behaviors (such as agitation, irritability, hostility, impulsivity, and hypomania) and notify the healthcare provider.

May worsen psychosis in some patients or precipitate a shift to mania or hypomania in patients with bipolar disorder. Patients presenting with depressive symptoms should be screened for bipolar disorder. Monotherapy in patients with bipolar disorder should be avoided. **Bupropion is not FDA approved for bipolar depression.**

The risk of seizures is dose-dependent and increased in patients with a history of seizures, anorexia/bulimia, head trauma, CNS tumor, severe hepatic cirrhosis, abrupt discontinuation of sedative-hypnotics or ethanol, medications which lower seizure threshold (antipsychotics, antidepressants, theophyllines, systemic steroids), stimulants, or hypoglycemic agents. Discontinue and do not restart in patients experiencing a seizure. May cause CNS stimulation (restlessness, anxiety, insomnia) or anorexia. May increase the risks associated with electroconvulsive therapy. Consider discontinuing, when possible, prior to elective surgery. May cause weight loss; use caution in patients where weight loss is not desirable. The incidence of sexual dysfunction with bupropion is generally lower than with SSRIs.

Use caution in patients with cardiovascular disease, history of hypertension, or coronary artery disease; treatment-emergent hypertension (including some severe cases) has been reported, both with bupropion alone and in combination with nicotine transdermal systems. Use with caution in patients with hepatic or renal dysfunction and in elderly patients; reduced dose recommended. Elderly patients may be at greater risk of accumulation during chronic dosing. May cause motor or cognitive impairment in some patients; use with caution if tasks requiring alertness such as operating machinery or driving are undertaken. Arthralgia, myalgia, and fever with rash and other symptoms suggestive of delayed hypersensitivity resembling serum sickness have been reported.

Extended release tablet: Insoluble tablet shell may remain intact and be visible in the stool.

Drug Interactions

Cytochrome P450 Effect: Substrate of CYP1A2 (minor), 2A6 (minor), 2B6 (major), 2C9 (minor), 2D6 (minor), 2E1 (minor), 3A4 (minor); **Inhibits** CYP2D6 (weak)

Increased Effect/Toxicity: Treatment-emergent hypertension may occur in patients treated with bupropion and nicotine patch. Toxicity of bupropion is enhanced by levodopa and phenelzine (MAO inhibitors). Risk of seizures may be increased with agents that may lower seizure threshold (antipsychotics, antidepressants, theophylline, abrupt discontinuation of benzodiazepines, systemic steroids). Effect of warfarin may be altered by bupropion. Concomitant therapy with metoprolol may result in bradycardia. Concurrent use with amantadine or CNS depressants appears to result in a higher incidence of adverse effects; use caution. CYP2B6 inhibitors may increase the levels/effects of bupropion; example inhibitors include desipramine, paroxetine, and sertraline. Combined use of CYP2B6 inhibitors (orphenadrine, thiotepa, cyclophosphamide) with bupropion may increase serum concentrations and may result in seizures.

Decreased Effect: CYP2B6 inducers may decrease the levels/effects of bupropion; example inducers include carbamazepine, nevirapine, phenobarbital, phenytoin, and rifampin.

Ethanol/Nutrition/Herb Interactions

Ethanol: Avoid ethanol (may increase CNS depression).

(Continued)

BuPROPion *(Continued)*

Herb/Nutraceutical: Avoid valerian, St John's wort, SAMe, gotu kola, kava kava (may increase CNS depression).

Pharmacodynamics/Kinetics

Absorption: Rapid

Distribution: V_d: 19-21 L/kg

Protein binding: 82% to 88%

Metabolism: Extensively hepatic via CYP2B6 to hydroxybupropion; non-CYP-mediated metabolism to erythrohydrobupropion and threohydrobupropion. Metabolite activity ranges from 20% to 50% potency of bupropion.

Bioavailability: 5% to 20% in animals

Half-life:

Distribution: 3-4 hours

Elimination: 21 ± 9 hours; Metabolites: Hydroxybupropion: 20 ± 5 hours; Erythrohydrobupropion: 33 ± 10 hours; Threohydrobupropion: 37 ± 13 hours (metabolite accumulation has been noted in ESRD).

Time to peak, serum: Bupropion: ~3 hours; bupropion extended release: ~5 hours

Metabolites: Hydroxybupropion, erythrohydrobupropion, threohydrobupropion: 6 hours

Excretion: Urine (87%); feces (10%)

Pregnancy Risk Factor C

Dosage Forms

Tablet: 75 mg, 100 mg

Wellbutrin®: 75 mg, 100 mg

Tablet, extended release: 100 mg, 150 mg

Budeprion™ SR: 100 mg [equivalent to Wellbutrin® SR], 150 mg [equivalent to Wellbutrin® SR]

Buproban™: 150 mg [equivalent to Zyban®]

Wellbutrin XL™: 150 mg, 300 mg

Tablet, sustained release: 100 mg, 150 mg [equivalent to Wellbutrin® SR], 150 mg [equivalent to Zyban®]

Wellbutrin® SR: 100 mg, 150 mg, 200 mg

Zyban®: 150 mg

Selected Readings

Tonstad S and Johnston JA, "Does Bupropion Have Advantages Over Other Medical Therapies in the Cessation of Smoking?" *Expert Opin Pharmacother,* 2004, 5(4):727-34.

Burnamycin [OTC] *see* Lidocaine *on page 972*

Burn Jel [OTC] *see* Lidocaine *on page 972*

Burn-O-Jel [OTC] *see* Lidocaine *on page 972*

BuSpar® *see* BusPIRone *on page 244*

BusPIRone *(byoo SPYE rone)*

Related Information

Sedation *on page 1825*

U.S. Brand Names BuSpar®

Canadian Brand Names Apo-Buspirone®; BuSpar®; Buspirex; Bustab®; Gen-Buspirone; Lin-Buspirone; Novo-Buspirone; Nu-Buspirone; PMS-Buspirone

Mexican Brand Names Buspar

Generic Available Yes

Index Terms Buspirone Hydrochloride

Pharmacologic Category Antianxiety Agent, Miscellaneous

Use Management of generalized anxiety disorder (GAD)

Unlabeled/Investigational Use Management of aggression in mental retardation and secondary mental disorders; major depression; potential augmenting agent for antidepressants; premenstrual syndrome

Local Anesthetic/Vasoconstrictor Precautions No information available to require special precautions

Effects on Dental Treatment Key adverse event(s) related to dental treatment: Xerostomia (normal salivary flow resumes upon discontinuation).

Common Adverse Effects

>10%: Central nervous system: Dizziness

1% to 10%:

Central nervous system: Drowsiness, EPS, serotonin syndrome, confusion, nervousness, lightheadedness, excitement, anger, hostility, headache

Dermatologic: Rash

Gastrointestinal: Diarrhea, nausea

Neuromuscular & skeletal: Muscle weakness, numbness, paresthesia, incoordination, tremor

Ocular: Blurred vision, tunnel vision

Miscellaneous: Diaphoresis, allergic reactions

Dosage Oral:

Generalized anxiety disorder:

Children and Adolescents: Initial: 5 mg daily; increase in increments of 5 mg/day at weekly intervals as needed, to a maximum dose of 60 mg/day divided into 2-3 doses

Adults: 15 mg/day (7.5 mg twice daily); may increase in increments of 5 mg/day every 2-4 days to a maximum of 60 mg/day; target dose for most people is 30 mg/day (15 mg twice daily)

Elderly: Initial: 5 mg twice daily, increase by 5 mg/day every 2-3 days as needed up to 20-30 mg/day; maximum daily dose: 60 mg/day.

Dosing adjustment in renal or hepatic impairment: Buspirone is metabolized by the liver and excreted by the kidneys. Patients with impaired hepatic or renal function demonstrated increased plasma levels and a prolonged half-life of buspirone. Therefore, use in patients with severe hepatic or renal impairment cannot be recommended.

Mechanism of Action The mechanism of action of buspirone is unknown. Buspirone has a high affinity for serotonin $5-HT_{1A}$ and $5-HT_2$ receptors, without affecting benzodiazepine-GABA receptors. Buspirone has moderate affinity for dopamine D_2 receptors.

Contraindications Hypersensitivity to buspirone or any component of the formulation

Warnings/Precautions Use in hepatic or renal impairment is not recommended; does not prevent or treat withdrawal from benzodiazepines. Low potential for cognitive or motor impairment. Use with MAO inhibitors may result in hypertensive reactions.

Drug Interactions

Cytochrome P450 Effect: Substrate of CYP2D6 (minor), 3A4 (major)

Increased Effect/Toxicity: Concurrent use of buspirone with SSRIs or trazodone may cause serotonin syndrome. Buspirone should not be used concurrently with an MAO inhibitor due to reports of increased blood pressure; theoretically, a selective MAO type B inhibitors (selegiline) has a lower risk of this reaction. Concurrent use of buspirone with nefazodone may increase risk of CNS adverse events; limit buspirone initial dose (eg, 2.5 mg/day). CYP3A4 inhibitors may increase the levels/effects of buspirone; example inhibitors include azole antifungals, clarithromycin, diclofenac, doxycycline, erythromycin, imatinib, isoniazid, nefazodone, nicardipine, propofol, protease inhibitors, quinidine, telithromycin, and verapamil.

Decreased Effect: CYP3A4 inducers may decrease the levels/effects of buspirone; example inducers include aminoglutethimide, carbamazepine, nafcillin, nevirapine, phenobarbital, phenytoin, and rifamycins.

Ethanol/Nutrition/Herb Interactions

Ethanol: Ethanol (may increase CNS depression).

Food: Food may decrease the absorption of buspirone, but it may also decrease the first-pass metabolism, thereby increasing the bioavailability of buspirone. Grapefruit juice may cause increased buspirone concentrations; avoid concurrent use.

Herb/Nutraceutical: St John's wort may decrease buspirone levels or increase CNS depression. Avoid valerian, gotu kola, kava kava (may increase CNS depression).

Pharmacodynamics/Kinetics

Absorption: Oral: ~100%

Distribution: V_d: 5.3 L/kg

Protein binding: 95%

Metabolism: Hepatic via oxidation; extensive first-pass effect

Bioavailability: ~4%

Half-life elimination: Mean: 2.4 hours (range: 2-11 hours)

Time to peak, serum: Within 0.7-1.5 hours

Excretion: Urine: 65%; feces: 35%; ~1% dose excreted unchanged

Pregnancy Risk Factor B

Dosage Forms

Tablet: 5 mg, 7.5 mg, 10 mg, 15 mg, 30 mg

BuSpar®: 5 mg, 10 mg, 15 mg, 30 mg

Buspirone Hydrochloride *see* BusPIRone *on page 244*

Busulfan (byoo SUL fan)

U.S. Brand Names Busulfex®; Myleran®
Canadian Brand Names Busulfex®; Myleran®
Mexican Brand Names Myleran
Generic Available No
Index Terms NSC-750
Pharmacologic Category Antineoplastic Agent, Alkylating Agent
Use
  Oral: Chronic myelogenous leukemia; conditioning regimens for bone marrow transplantation
  I.V.: Combination therapy with cyclophosphamide as a conditioning regimen prior to allogeneic hematopoietic progenitor cell transplantation for chronic myelogenous leukemia
Unlabeled/Investigational Use Oral: Bone marrow disorders, such as polycythemia vera and myeloid metaplasia; thrombocytosis
Local Anesthetic/Vasoconstrictor Precautions No information available to require special precautions
Effects on Dental Treatment Key adverse event(s) related to dental treatment: Xerostomia (normal salivary flow resumes upon discontinuation), mucositis/stomatitis.
Common Adverse Effects Frequency not always defined.
  Cardiovascular: Arrhythmia, atrial fibrillation, chest pain, edema, hyper-/hypotension, hypervolemia, tachycardia, tamponade (children with thalassemia: 2%), third-degree heart block, thrombosis, vasodilation, ventricular extrasystoles
  Central nervous system: Anxiety, chills, depression, dizziness, fever, headache, insomnia, pain, seizure (2%)
  Dermatologic: Alopecia, erythema, hyperpigmentation of skin (busulfan tan 5% to 10%), pruritus, rash, urticaria
  Endocrine & metabolic: Amenorrhea, hyperglycemia, hypocalcemia, hypokalemia, hypomagnesemia
  Gastrointestinal: Abdominal fullness, abdominal pain, anorexia, constipation, diarrhea, dyspepsia, hematemesis, ileus, mucositis/stomatitis, nausea, pancreatitis, vomiting, weight gain, xerostomia
  Hematologic: Anemia (I.V.: 69%), bone marrow suppression, leukopenia, lymphopenia, neutropenia (I.V.: ≤100%; onset: 4 days; recovery: 9-22 days), severe pancytopenia, thrombocytopenia (I.V.: ≤98%; onset 5-6 days)
  Hepatic: ALT increased, hyperbilirubinemia, veno-occlusive disease (stem cell transplantation: 8% to 12%)
  Local: Injection site pain and inflammation
  Neuromuscular & skeletal: Back pain, weakness
  Renal: Creatinine increased
  Respiratory: Cough, dyspnea, epistaxis, lung disorder, pneumonia, rhinitis
  Miscellaneous: Allergic reaction, infection
Mechanism of Action Reacts with N-7 position of guanosine and interferes with DNA replication and transcription of RNA. Busulfan has a more marked effect on myeloid cells than on lymphoid cells. The drug is also very toxic to hematopoietic stem cells. Busulfan exhibits little immunosuppressive activity. Interferes with the normal function of DNA by alkylation and cross-linking the strands of DNA.
Drug Interactions
  Cytochrome P450 Effect: Substrate of CYP3A4 (major)
  Increased Effect/Toxicity: CYP3A4 inhibitors may increase the levels/effects of busulfan; example inhibitors include azole antifungals, clarithromycin, diclofenac, doxycycline, erythromycin, imatinib, isoniazid, nefazodone, nicardipine, propofol, protease inhibitors, quinidine, telithromycin, and verapamil. Metronidazole may increase busulfan plasma levels. Pulmonary toxicity of other cytotoxic agents may be additive.
  Decreased Effect: CYP3A4 inducers may decrease the levels/effects of busulfan; example inducers include aminoglutethimide, carbamazepine, nafcillin, nevirapine, phenobarbital, phenytoin, and rifamycins.
Pharmacodynamics/Kinetics
  Duration: 28 days
  Absorption: Rapid and complete
  Distribution: V_d: ~1 L/kg; into CSF and saliva with levels similar to plasma
  Protein binding: ~14% to 32%
  Metabolism: Extensively hepatic (may increase with multiple doses); glutathione conjugation followed by oxidation
  Half-life elimination: After first dose: 3.4 hours; After last dose: 2.3 hours
  Time to peak, serum: Oral: Within 4 hours; I.V.: Within 5 minutes

Excretion: Urine (10% to 50% as metabolites) within 24 hours (<2% as unchanged drug)
Pregnancy Risk Factor D

Busulfex® *see* Busulfan *on page 246*

Butabarbital (byoo ta BAR bi tal)

U.S. Brand Names Butisol Sodium®
Generic Available No
Pharmacologic Category Barbiturate
Use Sedative; hypnotic
Local Anesthetic/Vasoconstrictor Precautions No information available to require special precautions
Effects on Dental Treatment No significant effects or complications reported
Common Adverse Effects
>10%: Central nervous system: Dizziness, lightheadedness, drowsiness, "hangover" effect
1% to 10%:
Central nervous system: Confusion, mental depression, unusual excitement, nervousness, faint feeling, headache, insomnia, nightmares
Gastrointestinal: Constipation, nausea, vomiting
Restrictions C-III
Mechanism of Action Interferes with transmission of impulses from the thalamus to the cortex of the brain resulting in an imbalance in central inhibitory and facilitatory mechanisms
Drug Interactions
Increased Effect/Toxicity: When butabarbital is combined with other CNS depressants, ethanol, opioid analgesics, antidepressants, or benzodiazepines, additive respiratory and CNS depression may occur. Barbiturates may enhance the hepatotoxic potential of acetaminophen overdoses. Chloramphenicol, MAO inhibitors, valproic acid, and felbamate may inhibit barbiturate metabolism. Barbiturates may impair the absorption of griseofulvin, and may enhance the nephrotoxic effects of methoxyflurane.
Decreased Effect: Barbiturates, such as butabarbital, are hepatic enzyme inducers, and may increase the metabolism of antipsychotics, some beta-blockers (unlikely with atenolol and nadolol), calcium channel blockers, chloramphenicol, cimetidine, corticosteroids, cyclosporine, disopyramide, doxycycline, ethosuximide, felbamate, furosemide, griseofulvin, lamotrigine, phenytoin, propafenone, quinidine, tacrolimus, TCAs, and theophylline. Barbiturates may increase the metabolism of estrogens and reduce the efficacy of oral contraceptives; an alternative method of contraception should be considered. Barbiturates inhibit the hypoprothrombinemic effects of oral anticoagulants via increased metabolism. Barbiturates may enhance the metabolism of methadone resulting in methadone withdrawal.
Pharmacodynamics/Kinetics
Distribution: V_d: 0.8 L/kg
Protein binding: 26%
Metabolism: Hepatic
Half-life elimination: 1.6 days to 5.8 days
Time to peak, serum: 40-60 minutes
Excretion: Urine (as metabolites)
Pregnancy Risk Factor D

Butalbital, Acetaminophen, and Caffeine
(byoo TAL bi tal, a seet a MIN oh fen, & KAF een)

Related Information
Acetaminophen *on page 31*
Caffeine *on page 255*
U.S. Brand Names Anolor 300; Dolgic® LQ; Dolgic® Plus; Esgic®; Esgic-Plus™; Fioricet®; Medigesic®; Repan®; Zebutal™
Generic Available Yes: Excludes elixir
Index Terms Acetaminophen, Butalbital, and Caffeine
Pharmacologic Category Barbiturate
Use Relief of the symptomatic complex of tension or muscle contraction headache
Local Anesthetic/Vasoconstrictor Precautions No information available to require special precautions
Effects on Dental Treatment No significant effects or complications reported
(Continued)

Butalbital, Acetaminophen, and Caffeine *(Continued)*

Common Adverse Effects Note: Specific percentages not reported.
Frequently observed:
Central nervous system: Dizziness, drowsiness, lightheadedness, sedation
Gastrointestinal: Abdominal pain, nausea, vomiting
Respiratory: Dyspnea
Miscellaneous: Intoxicated feeling

Mechanism of Action
Butalbital is a short- to intermediate-acting barbiturate. Barbiturates depress the sensory cortex, decrease motor activity, alter cerebellar function, and produce drowsiness, sedation, hypnosis, and dose-dependent respiratory depression.
Acetaminophen inhibits the synthesis of prostaglandins in the central nervous system and peripherally blocks pain impulse generation; produces antipyresis from inhibition of hypothalamic heat-regulating center
Caffeine increases levels of 3'5' cyclic AMP by inhibiting phosphodiesterase; CNS stimulant which increases medullary respiratory center sensitivity to carbon dioxide, stimulates central inspiratory drive, and improves skeletal muscle contraction (diaphragmatic contractility)

Drug Interactions
Cytochrome P450 Effect:
Acetaminophen: **Substrate** (minor) of CYP1A2, 2A6, 2C9, 2D6, 2E1, 3A4; **Inhibits** CYP3A4 (weak)
Caffeine: **Substrate** of CYP1A2 (major), 2C9 (minor), 2D6 (minor), 2E1 (minor), 3A4 (minor); **Inhibits** CYP1A2 (weak), 3A4 (moderate)
Increased Effect/Toxicity: See Acetaminophen and Caffeine. For butalbital, refer to Phenobarbital.

Pharmacodynamics/Kinetics Also see Acetaminophen and Caffeine.
Absorption: Butalbital: Well absorbed
Protein binding: Butalbital: 45%
Half-life elimination: Butalbital: 35 hours
Excretion: Butalbital: Urine (59% to 88% as unchanged drug and metabolites)
Pregnancy Risk Factor C

Butalbital, Acetaminophen, Caffeine, and Codeine
(byoo TAL bi tal, a seet a MIN oh fen, KAF een, & KOE deen)

Related Information
Acetaminophen *on page 31*
Caffeine *on page 255*
Codeine *on page 404*
U.S. Brand Names Fioricet® with Codeine
Generic Available Yes
Index Terms Acetaminophen, Caffeine, Codeine, and Butalbital; Caffeine, Acetaminophen, Butalbital, and Codeine; Codeine, Acetaminophen, Butalbital, and Caffeine
Pharmacologic Category Analgesic Combination (Opioid); Barbiturate
Use Relief of symptoms of complex tension (muscle contraction) headache
Local Anesthetic/Vasoconstrictor Precautions No information available to require special precautions
Effects on Dental Treatment Key adverse event(s) related to dental treatment: Xerostomia (normal salivary flow resumes upon discontinuation).
Significant Adverse Effects Frequency not defined.
Cardiovascular: Tachycardia, palpitation, hypotension, edema, syncope
Central nervous system: Drowsiness, fatigue, mental confusion, disorientation, nervousness, hallucination, euphoria, depression, seizure, headache, agitation, fainting, excitement, fever
Dermatologic: Rash, erythema, pruritus, urticaria, erythema multiforme, exfoliative dermatitis, toxic epidermal necrolysis
Gastrointestinal: Nausea, xerostomia, constipation, gastrointestinal spasm, heartburn, flatulence
Genitourinary: Urinary retention, diuresis
Neuromuscular & skeletal: Leg pain, weakness, numbness
Otic: Tinnitus
Miscellaneous: Allergic reaction, anaphylaxis
Note: Potential reactions associated with components of Fioricet® with Codeine include agranulocytosis, irritability, nausea, thrombocytopenia, tremor, vomiting
Restrictions C-III
Dosage Oral: Adults: 1-2 capsules every 4 hours. Total daily dosage should not exceed 6 capsules.

Dosing adjustment/comments in hepatic impairment: Use with caution. Limited, low-dose therapy usually well tolerated in hepatic disease/cirrhosis. However, cases of hepatotoxicity at daily acetaminophen dosages <4 g/day have been reported. Avoid chronic use in hepatic impairment.

Mechanism of Action Combination product for the treatment of tension headache. Contains codeine (narcotic analgesic), butalbital (barbiturate), caffeine (CNS stimulant), and acetaminophen (nonopiate, nonsalicylate analgesic).

Contraindications Hypersensitivity to butalbital, codeine, caffeine, acetaminophen, or any component of the formulation; porphyria; known G6PD deficiency; pregnancy (prolonged use or high doses at term)

Warnings/Precautions May cause CNS depression, which may impair physical or mental abilities; patients must be cautioned about performing tasks which require mental alertness (eg, operating machinery or driving). Limit acetaminophen to <4 g/day. Use with caution in patients with alcoholic liver disease; consuming ≥3 alcoholic drinks/day may increase the risk of liver damage. Effects may be potentiated when used with other sedative drugs or ethanol. May cause severe hepatic toxicity in acute overdose. In addition, chronic daily dosing in adults has resulted in liver damage in some patients. Use with caution in patients with hypersensitivity reactions to other phenanthrene-derivative opioid agonists (eg, morphine, hydrocodone, oxycodone). Use caution with Addison's disease, known G6PD deficiency, severe renal or hepatic impairment. Use caution in patients with head injury or other intracranial lesions, acute abdominal conditions, urethral stricture of BPH, or in patients with respiratory diseases. Elderly (not recommended for use) and/or debilitated patients may be more susceptible to CNS depressants, as well as constipating effects of narcotics. Tolerance or drug dependence may result from extended use. Caffeine may cause CNS and cardiovascular stimulation, as well as GI irritation in high doses. Use with caution in patients with a history of peptic ulcer or GERD; avoid in patients with symptomatic cardiac arrhythmias. Safety and efficacy in pediatric patients have not been established.

Drug Interactions
Acetaminophen: **Substrate** of (minor) CYP1A2, 2A6, 2C9, 2D6, 2E1, 3A4; **Inhibits** CYP3A4 (weak)
Caffeine: **Substrate** of CYP1A2 (major), 2C9 (minor), 2D6 (minor), 2E1 (minor), 3A4 (minor); **Inhibits** CYP1A2 (weak), 3A4 (moderate)
Butalbital: Refer to Phenobarbital.
See also Acetaminophen, Caffeine, and Codeine.

Ethanol/Nutrition/Herb Interactions Ethanol: Avoid ethanol (may increase CNS depression).

Pregnancy Risk Factor C (per manufacturer); D (prolonged use or high doses at term)

Lactation Enters breast milk/not recommended

Breast-Feeding Considerations Codeine, caffeine, barbiturates, and acetaminophen are excreted in breast milk in small amounts. Discontinuation of breast-feeding or discontinuation of the drug should be considered.

Dosage Forms Excipient information presented when available (limited, particularly for generics); consult specific product labeling.
Capsule: Butalbital 50 mg, caffeine 40 mg, acetaminophen 325 mg, and codeine phosphate 30 mg
  Fioricet® with Codeine: Butalbital 50 mg, caffeine 40 mg, acetaminophen 325 mg, and codeine phosphate 30 mg [may contain benzyl alcohol]
  Phrenilin® with Caffeine and Codeine: Butalbital 50 mg, caffeine 40 mg, acetaminophen 325 mg, and codeine phosphate 30 mg [contains benzyl alcohol and lactose]

Selected Readings
Botting RM, "Mechanism of Action of Acetaminophen: Is There a Cyclooxygenase 3?" *Clin Infect Dis*, 2000, Suppl 5:S202-10.
Dart RC, Kuffner EK, and Rumack BH, "Treatment of Pain or Fever With Paracetamol (Acetaminophen) in the Alcoholic Patient: A Systematic Review," *Am J Ther*, 2000, 7(2):123-34.
Grant JA and Weiler JM, "A Report of a Rare Immediate Reaction After Ingestion of Acetaminophen," *Ann Allergy Asthma Immunol*, 2001, 87(3):227-9.
Kwan D, Bartle WR, and Walker SE, "The Effects of Acetaminophen on Pharmacokinetics and Pharmacodynamics of Warfarin," *J Clin Pharmacol*, 1999, 39(1):68-75.
McClain CJ, Price S, Barve S, et al, "Acetaminophen Hepatotoxicity: An Update," *Curr Gastroenterol Rep*, 1999, 1(1):42-9.
Shek KL, Chan LN, and Nutescu E, "Warfarin-Acetaminophen Drug Interaction Revisited," *Pharmacotherapy*, 1999, 19(10):1153-8.
Tanaka E, Yamazaki K, and Misawa S, "Update: The Clinical Importance of Acetaminophen Hepatotoxicity in Nonalcoholic and Alcoholic Subjects," *J Clin Pharm Ther*, 2000, 25(5):325-32.

Butalbital and Acetaminophen
(byoo TAL bi tal & a seet a MIN oh fen)

Related Information
Acetaminophen *on page 31*
(Continued)

Butalbital and Acetaminophen *(Continued)*

Phenobarbital *on page 1288*

U.S. Brand Names Bupap; Cephadyn; Phrenilin®; Phrenilin® Forte; Promacet; Sedapap®

Generic Available Yes

Index Terms Butalbital and Acetaminophen

Pharmacologic Category Analgesic, Miscellaneous; Barbiturate

Use Relief of the symptomatic complex of tension or muscle contraction headache

Local Anesthetic/Vasoconstrictor Precautions No information available to require special precautions

Effects on Dental Treatment No significant effects or complications reported

Common Adverse Effects

Frequently observed:

Central nervous system: Dizziness, drowsiness, lightheadedness, sedation

Gastrointestinal: Abdominal pain, nausea, vomiting

Respiratory: Dyspnea

Miscellaneous: Intoxicated feeling

Infrequently observed:

Cardiovascular: Tachycardia

Central nervous system: Agitation, confusion, depression, euphoria, excitement, faintness, fever, headache, seizure

Dermatologic: Hyperhidrosis, pruritus

Endocrine & metabolic: Hot spells

Gastrointestinal: Constipation, dysphagia, heartburn, flatulence, xerostomia

Neuromuscular & skeletal: Leg pain, muscle fatigue, numbness, paresthesia

Ocular: Heavy eyelids

Otic: Earache, tinnitus

Renal: Diuresis

Respiratory: Nasal congestion

Miscellaneous: Allergic reaction, high energy, shaky feeling, sluggishness

Mechanism of Action

Butalbital is a short- to intermediate-acting barbiturate. Barbiturates depress the sensory cortex, decrease motor activity, alter cerebellar function, and produce drowsiness, sedation, hypnosis, and dose-dependent respiratory depression.

Acetaminophen inhibits the synthesis of prostaglandins in the central nervous system and peripherally blocks pain impulse generation; produces antipyresis from inhibition of hypothalamic heat-regulating center.

Drug Interactions

Cytochrome P450 Effect:

Acetaminophen: **Substrate** (minor) of CYP1A2, 2A6, 2C9, 2D6, 2E1, 3A4; **Inhibits** CYP3A4 (weak)

Butalbital: See Phenobarbital monograph

Increased Effect/Toxicity: Monoamine oxidase inhibitors (MAOIs) may enhance the CNS effects of butalbital.

Pharmacodynamics/Kinetics Also see Acetaminophen monograph.

Absorption: Butalbital: Well absorbed

Protein binding: Butalbital: 45%

Half-life elimination: Butalbital: 35 hours

Excretion: Butalbital: Urine (59% to 88% as unchanged drug or metabolites)

Pregnancy Risk Factor C

Butalbital and Acetaminophen see Butalbital and Acetaminophen on page 249

Butalbital, Aspirin, and Caffeine

(byoo TAL bi tal, AS pir in, & KAF een)

Related Information

Aspirin *on page 149*

Caffeine *on page 255*

U.S. Brand Names Fiorinal®

Canadian Brand Names Fiorinal®

Generic Available Yes

Index Terms Aspirin, Caffeine, and Butalbital; Butalbital Compound

Pharmacologic Category Barbiturate

Use Relief of the symptomatic complex of tension or muscle contraction headache

Local Anesthetic/Vasoconstrictor Precautions No information available to require special precautions

Effects on Dental Treatment Key adverse event(s) related to dental treatment: Aspirin: As with all drugs which may affect hemostasis, bleeding is associated with aspirin. Hemorrhage may occur at virtually any site; risk is dependent on multiple variables including dosage, concurrent use of multiple agents which alter hemostasis, and patient susceptibility. Many adverse effects of aspirin are dose related, and are rare at low dosages. Other serious reactions are idiosyncratic, related to allergy or individual sensitivity (see Dental Comment).

Common Adverse Effects

>10%:

Central nervous system: Dizziness, lightheadedness, drowsiness, "hangover" effect

Gastrointestinal: Heartburn, stomach pain, dyspepsia, epigastric discomfort, nausea

1% to 10%:

Central nervous system: Confusion, mental depression, unusual excitement, nervousness, faint feeling, headache, insomnia, nightmares, fatigue

Dermatologic: Skin rash

Gastrointestinal: Constipation, vomiting, gastrointestinal ulceration

Hematologic: Hemolytic anemia

Neuromuscular & skeletal: Weakness

Respiratory: Troubled breathing

Miscellaneous: Anaphylactic shock

Restrictions C-III

Drug Interactions

Cytochrome P450 Effect:

Aspirin: **Substrate** of CYP2C9 (minor)

Caffeine: **Substrate** of CYP1A2 (major), 2C9 (minor), 2D6 (minor), 2E1 (minor), 3A4 (minor); **Inhibits** CYP1A2 (weak), 3A4 (moderate)

Increased Effect/Toxicity: Enhanced effect/toxicity with oral anticoagulants (warfarin), oral antidiabetic agents, insulin, mercaptopurine, methotrexate, NSAIDs, narcotic analgesics (propoxyphene, meperidine, etc), benzodiazepines, sedative-hypnotics, other CNS depressants. The CNS effects of butalbital may be enhanced by MAO inhibitors.

Decreased Effect: May decrease the effect of uricosuric agents (probenecid and sulfinpyrazone) reducing their effect on gout.

Pregnancy Risk Factor C/D (prolonged use or high doses at term)

Dental Comment There is no scientific evidence to warrant discontinuance of aspirin prior to dental surgery. Patients taking one aspirin tablet daily as an antithrombotic and who require dental surgery should be given special consideration in consultation with the physician before removal of the aspirin relative to prevention of postoperative bleeding.

The Food and Drug Administration (FDA), has issued a letter updating information and considerations regarding the use of ibuprofen (400 mg doses) in patients who are taking low dose aspirin (81 mg, immediate release; not enteric coated) for cardioprotection and stroke prevention. Ibuprofen, at these doses, may interfere with aspirin's antiplatelet effect depending upon when it is administered. Patients initiated on aspirin first (for ~1 week) then ibuprofen (400 mg tid for 10 days) seem to maintain aspirin's platelet effect (Cryer B, 2005). Ibuprofen has the greatest impact on aspirin if administered less than 8 hours before aspirin (Catella-Lawson F, 2001).

Patients may require counseling about the appropriate timing of ibuprofen dosing in relationship to aspirin therapy. With occasional use of ibuprofen, a clinically-significant interaction with aspirin in unlikely. To avoid interference during chronic dosing, a single dose of ibuprofen should be taken 30-120 minutes after aspirin ingestion or at least 8 hours should elapse after ibuprofen dosing before giving aspirin (FDA, 2006; Catella-Lawson F, 2001).

The clinical implications of the interaction are unclear. There have not been any clinical endpoint studies conducted at this time. Avoidance of this interaction is potentially important because aspirin's vascular protection could be decreased or negated.

Other nonselective NSAIDs may have potential for a similar interaction with aspirin. Such has been described with naproxen (Capone ML, 2005). Acetaminophen does not appear to interfere with the antiplatelet effect of aspirin. Other clinical scenarios (use of smaller ibuprofen doses, other aspirin products, other doses of aspirin) have not been evaluated.

Additional information is available at: http://www.fda.gov/cder/drug/infopage/aspirin/default.htm.

Butalbital, Aspirin, Caffeine, and Codeine

(byoo TAL bi tal, AS pir in, KAF een, & KOE deen)

Related Information

Aspirin on page 149

(Continued)

Butalbital, Aspirin, Caffeine, and Codeine *(Continued)*

Caffeine *on page 255*

Codeine *on page 404*

U.S. Brand Names Fiorinal® With Codeine

Canadian Brand Names Fiorinal®-C 1/2; Fiorinal®-C 1/4; Tecnal C 1/2; Tecnal C 1/4

Generic Available Yes

Index Terms Aspirin, Caffeine, Codeine, and Butalbital; Butalbital Compound and Codeine; Codeine and Butalbital Compound; Codeine, Butalbital, Aspirin, and Caffeine

Pharmacologic Category Analgesic Combination (Opioid); Barbiturate

Use Mild-to-moderate pain when sedation is needed

Local Anesthetic/Vasoconstrictor Precautions No information available to require special precautions

Effects on Dental Treatment Key adverse event(s) related to dental treatment: Aspirin: As with all drugs which may affect hemostasis, bleeding is associated with aspirin. Hemorrhage may occur at virtually any site; risk is dependent on multiple variables including dosage, concurrent use of multiple agents which alter hemostasis, and patient susceptibility. Many adverse effects of aspirin are dose related, and are rare at low dosages. Other serious reactions are idiosyncratic, related to allergy or individual sensitivity (see Dental Comment).

Common Adverse Effects

>10%:

Central nervous system: Dizziness, lightheadedness, drowsiness

Gastrointestinal: Nausea, heartburn, stomach pain, dyspepsia, epigastric discomfort

1% to 10%:

Central nervous system: Confusion, mental depression, unusual excitement, nervousness, faint feeling, insomnia, nightmares, intoxicated feeling

Dermatologic: Rash

Gastrointestinal: Constipation, GI ulceration

Restrictions C-III

Drug Interactions

Cytochrome P450 Effect:

Aspirin: **Substrate** of CYP2C9 (minor)

Caffeine: **Substrate** of CYP1A2 (major), 2C9 (minor), 2D6 (minor), 2E1 (minor), 3A4 (minor); **Inhibits** CYP1A2 (weak), 3A4 (moderate)

Increased Effect/Toxicity: MAO inhibitors may enhance the CNS effects of butalbital. In patients receiving concomitant corticosteroids during the chronic use of ASA, withdrawal of corticosteroids may result in salicylism. Butalbital compound and codeine may enhance effects of oral anticoagulants. Increased effect with oral antidiabetic agents and insulin, mercaptopurine and methotrexate, NSAIDs, other narcotic analgesics, ethanol, general anesthetics, tranquilizers such as chlordiazepoxide, sedative hypnotics, or other CNS depressants.

Decreased Effect: Aspirin, butalbital, caffeine, and codeine may diminish effects of uricosuric agents such as probenecid and sulfinpyrazone.

Pregnancy Risk Factor C/D (prolonged use or high doses at term)

Dental Comment There is no scientific evidence to warrant discontinuance of aspirin prior to dental surgery. Patients taking one aspirin tablet daily as an antithrombotic and who require dental surgery should be given special consideration in consultation with the physician before removal of the aspirin relative to prevention of postoperative bleeding.

The Food and Drug Administration (FDA), has issued a letter updating information and considerations regarding the use of ibuprofen (400 mg doses) in patients who are taking low dose aspirin (81 mg, immediate release; not enteric coated) for cardioprotection and stroke prevention. Ibuprofen, at these doses, may interfere with aspirin's antiplatelet effect depending upon when it is administered. Patients initiated on aspirin first (for ~1 week) then ibuprofen (400 mg tid for 10 days) seem to maintain aspirin's platelet effect (Cryer B, 2005). Ibuprofen has the greatest impact on aspirin if administered less than 8 hours before aspirin (Catella-Lawson F, 2001).

Patients may require counseling about the appropriate timing of ibuprofen dosing in relationship to aspirin therapy. With occasional use of ibuprofen, a clinically-significant interaction with aspirin in unlikely. To avoid interference during chronic dosing, a single dose of ibuprofen should be taken 30-120 minutes after aspirin ingestion or at least 8 hours should elapse after ibuprofen dosing before giving aspirin (FDA, 2006; Catella-Lawson F, 2001).

The clinical implications of the interaction are unclear. There have not been any clinical endpoint studies conducted at this time. Avoidance of this interaction is potentially important because aspirin's vascular protection could be decreased or negated.

Other nonselective NSAIDs may have potential for a similar interaction with aspirin. Such has been described with naproxen (Capone ML, 2005). Acetaminophen does not appear to interfere with the antiplatelet effect of aspirin. Other clinical scenarios (use of smaller ibuprofen doses, other aspirin products, other doses of aspirin) have not been evaluated.

Additional information is available at: http://www.fda.gov/cder/drug/infopage/aspirin/default.htm.

Butalbital Compound see Butalbital, Aspirin, and Caffeine on page 250

Butalbital Compound and Codeine see Butalbital, Aspirin, Caffeine, and Codeine on page 251

Butamben, Tetracaine, and Benzocaine see Benzocaine, Butamben, and Tetracaine on page 198

Butenafine (byoo TEN a feen)

U.S. Brand Names Lotrimin® Ultra™ [OTC]; Mentax®
Generic Available No
Index Terms Butenafine Hydrochloride
Pharmacologic Category Antifungal Agent, Topical
Use Topical treatment of tinea pedis (athlete's foot), tinea cruris (jock itch), tinea corporis (ringworm), and tinea versicolor
Local Anesthetic/Vasoconstrictor Precautions No information available to require special precautions
Effects on Dental Treatment No significant effects or complications reported
Common Adverse Effects >1%: Dermatologic: Burning, stinging, irritation, erythema, pruritus (2%)
Mechanism of Action Butenafine exerts antifungal activity by blocking squalene epoxidation, resulting in inhibition of ergosterol synthesis (antidermatophyte and *Sporothrix schenckii* activity). In higher concentrations, the drug disrupts fungal cell membranes (anticandidal activity).
Pharmacodynamics/Kinetics
 Absorption: Minimal systemic
 Metabolism: Hepatic via hydroxylation
 Half-life elimination: 35 hours
 Time to peak, serum: 6 hours
Pregnancy Risk Factor B

Butenafine Hydrochloride see Butenafine on page 253

Butisol Sodium® see Butabarbital on page 247

Butoconazole (byoo toe KOE na zole)

Related Information
 Treatment of Sexually-Transmitted Infections on page 1920
U.S. Brand Names Gynazole-1®
Canadian Brand Names Femstat® One; Gynazole-1®
Generic Available No
Index Terms Butoconazole Nitrate
Pharmacologic Category Antifungal Agent, Vaginal
Use Local treatment of vulvovaginal candidiasis
Local Anesthetic/Vasoconstrictor Precautions No information available to require special precautions
Effects on Dental Treatment No significant effects or complications reported
Common Adverse Effects Frequency not defined.
 Gastrointestinal: Abdominal pain or cramping
 Genitourinary: Pelvic pain; vulvar/vaginal burning, itching, soreness, and swelling
Mechanism of Action Increases cell membrane permeability in susceptible fungi (*Candida*)
Pharmacodynamics/Kinetics
 Absorption: 2%
 Metabolism: Not reported
 Time to peak: 12-24 hours
Pregnancy Risk Factor C (use only in 2nd or 3rd trimester)

Butoconazole Nitrate see Butoconazole on page 253

Butorphanol (byoo TOR fa nole)

U.S. Brand Names Stadol®
Canadian Brand Names Apo-Butorphanol®; PMS-Butorphanol
Generic Available Yes
Index Terms Butorphanol Tartrate
Pharmacologic Category Analgesic, Opioid
Use
Parenteral: Management of moderate-to-severe pain; preoperative medication; supplement to balanced anesthesia; management of pain during labor
Nasal spray: Management of moderate-to-severe pain, including migraine headache pain

Local Anesthetic/Vasoconstrictor Precautions No information available to require special precautions
Effects on Dental Treatment Key adverse event(s) related to dental treatment: Xerostomia (normal salivary flow resumes upon discontinuation) and unpleasant aftertaste

Common Adverse Effects
>10%:
Central nervous system: Drowsiness (43%), dizziness (19%), insomnia (Stadol® NS)
Gastrointestinal: Nausea/vomiting (13%)
Respiratory: Nasal congestion (Stadol® NS)
1% to 10%:
Cardiovascular: Vasodilation, palpitation
Central nervous system: Lightheadedness, headache, lethargy, anxiety, confusion, euphoria, somnolence
Dermatologic: Pruritus
Gastrointestinal: Anorexia, constipation, xerostomia, stomach pain, unpleasant aftertaste
Neuromuscular & skeletal: Tremor, paresthesia, weakness
Ocular: Blurred vision
Otic: Ear pain, tinnitus
Respiratory: Bronchitis, cough, dyspnea, epistaxis, nasal irritation, pharyngitis, rhinitis, sinus congestion, sinusitis, upper respiratory infection
Miscellaneous: Diaphoresis increased

Restrictions C-IV
Mechanism of Action Mixed narcotic agonist-antagonist with central analgesic actions; binds to opiate receptors in the CNS, causing inhibition of ascending pain pathways, altering the perception of and response to pain; produces generalized CNS depression

Drug Interactions
Increased Effect/Toxicity: Increased toxicity with CNS depressants, phenothiazines, barbiturates, skeletal muscle relaxants, alfentanil, guanabenz, and MAO inhibitors.

Pharmacodynamics/Kinetics
Onset of action: I.M.: 5-10 minutes; I.V.: <10 minutes; Nasal: Within 15 minutes
Peak effect: I.M.: 0.5-1 hour; I.V.: 4-5 minutes
Duration: I.M., I.V.: 3-4 hours; Nasal: 4-5 hours
Absorption: Rapid and well absorbed
Protein binding: 80%
Metabolism: Hepatic
Bioavailability: Nasal: 60% to 70%
Half-life elimination: 2.5-4 hours
Excretion: Primarily urine

Pregnancy Risk Factor C/D (prolonged use or high doses at term)

Cabergoline (ca BER goe leen)

U.S. Brand Names Dostinex®
Canadian Brand Names Dostinex®
Mexican Brand Names Dostinex
Generic Available Yes
Pharmacologic Category Ergot Derivative
Use Treatment of hyperprolactinemic disorders, either idiopathic or due to pituitary adenomas
Local Anesthetic/Vasoconstrictor Precautions No information available to require special precautions
Effects on Dental Treatment Key adverse event(s) related to dental treatment: Xerostomia (normal salivary flow resumes upon discontinuation), throat irritation, and toothache.
Common Adverse Effects
>10%:
  Central nervous system: Headache (26%), dizziness (15% to 17%)
  Gastrointestinal: Nausea (27% to 29%)
1% to 10%:
  Cardiovascular: Postural hypotension (4%), hypotension (1%), dependent edema (1%), edema (peripheral 1%), palpitation (1%), syncope (1%)
  Central nervous system: Fatigue (5% to 7%), vertigo (1% to 4%), depression (3%), somnolence (2% to 5%), nervousness (1% to 2%), anxiety (1%), insomnia (1%), concentration impaired (1%), malaise (1%)
  Dermatologic: Acne (1%), pruritus (1%)
  Endocrine: Hot flashes (1% to 3%), breast pain (1% to 2%), dysmenorrhea (1%)
  Gastrointestinal: Constipation (7% to 10%), abdominal pain (5%), dyspepsia (2% to 5%), vomiting (2% to 4%), xerostomia (2% to 4%), diarrhea (2%), flatulence (2%), anorexia (1%), throat irritation (1%), toothache (1%)
  Neuromuscular & skeletal: Weakness (6% to 9%), pain (2%), paresthesia (1% to 2%), arthralgia (1%)
  Ocular: Abnormal vision (1%), periorbital edema (1%)
  Respiratory: Rhinitis (1%)
  Miscellaneous: Flu-like syndrome (1%)
Mechanism of Action Cabergoline is a long acting dopamine receptor agonist with a high affinity for D_2 receptors; prolactin secretion by the anterior pituitary is predominantly under hypothalamic inhibitory control exerted through the release of dopamine. It is a potent $5\text{-}HT_{2B}$-receptor agonist, which may contribute to observed fibrotic/valvulopathic events.
Drug Interactions
  Increased Effect/Toxicity: Cabergoline may increase the effects of sibutramine and other serotonin modulators (serotonin syndrome). Ergot derivatives may enhance the vasoconstriction effect of dopamine.
  Decreased Effect: Effects of cabergoline may be diminished by antipsychotics, nitroglycerin.
Pharmacodynamics/Kinetics
  Distribution: Extensive, particularly to the pituitary
  Protein binding: 40% to 42%
  Metabolism: Extensively hepatic via hydrolysis; minimal CYP mediated metabolism
  Half-life elimination: 63-69 hours
  Time to peak: 2-3 hours
  Excretion: Primarily feces (60%); urine (20%, <4% as unchanged drug)
Pregnancy Risk Factor B

Ca-DTPA see Diethylene Triamine Penta-Acetic Acid on page 493
Caduet® see Amlodipine and Atorvastatin on page 103
CaEDTA see Edetate Calcium Disodium on page 554
Cafcit® see Caffeine on page 255
Cafergot® see Ergotamine and Caffeine on page 586

Caffeine (KAF een)

U.S. Brand Names Cafcit®; Enerjets [OTC]; No Doz® Maximum Strength [OTC]; Vivarin® [OTC]
Generic Available Yes: Tablet, caffeine and sodium benzoate injection
Index Terms Caffeine and Sodium Benzoate; Caffeine Citrate; Sodium Benzoate and Caffeine
(Continued)

Caffeine *(Continued)*

Pharmacologic Category Stimulant

Use

Caffeine citrate: Treatment of idiopathic apnea of prematurity

Caffeine and sodium benzoate: Treatment of acute respiratory depression (not a preferred agent)

Caffeine [OTC labeling]: Restore mental alertness or wakefulness when experiencing fatigue

Unlabeled/Investigational Use Caffeine and sodium benzoate: Treatment of spinal puncture headache; CNS stimulant; diuretic

Local Anesthetic/Vasoconstrictor Precautions No information available to require special precautions

Effects on Dental Treatment No significant effects or complications reported

Common Adverse Effects Frequency not specified; primarily serum-concentration related.

Cardiovascular: Angina, arrhythmia (ventricular), chest pain, flushing, palpitation, sinus tachycardia, tachycardia (supraventricular), vasodilation

Central nervous system: Agitation, delirium, dizziness, hallucinations, headache, insomnia, irritability, psychosis, restlessness

Dermatologic: Urticaria

Gastrointestinal: Esophageal sphincter tone decreased, gastritis

Neuromuscular & skeletal: Fasciculations

Ocular: Intraocular pressure increased (>180 mg caffeine), miosis

Renal: Diuresis

Mechanism of Action Increases levels of 3'5' cyclic AMP by inhibiting phosphodiesterase; CNS stimulant which increases medullary respiratory center sensitivity to carbon dioxide, stimulates central inspiratory drive, and improves skeletal muscle contraction (diaphragmatic contractility); prevention of apnea may occur by competitive inhibition of adenosine

Drug Interactions

Cytochrome P450 Effect: Substrate of CYP1A2 (major), 2C9 (minor), 2D6 (minor), 2E1 (minor), 3A4 (minor); **Inhibits** CYP1A2 (weak), 3A4 (moderate)

Increased Effect/Toxicity: Quinolones (specifically ciprofloxacin, norfloxacin, ofloxacin) and CYP1A2 inhibitors may increase the levels/effects of caffeine; example inhibitors include fluvoxamine, ketoconazole, and rofecoxib

Decreased Effect: Caffeine may diminish the sedative or anxiolytic effects of benzodiazepines. CYP1A2 inducers may decrease the levels/effects of caffeine; example inducers include aminoglutethimide, carbamazepine, phenobarbital, and rifampin.

Pharmacodynamics/Kinetics

Distribution: V_d:

Neonates: 0.8-0.9 L/kg

Children >9 months to Adults: 0.6 L/kg

Protein binding: 17% (children) to 36% (adults)

Metabolism: Hepatic, via demethylation by CYP1A2. **Note:** In neonates, interconversion between caffeine and theophylline has been reported (caffeine levels are ~25% of measured theophylline after theophylline administration and ~3% to 8% of caffeine would be expected to be converted to theophylline)

Half-life elimination:

Neonates: 72-96 hours (range: 40-230 hours)

Children >9 months and Adults: 5 hours

Time to peak, serum: Oral: Within 30 minutes to 2 hours

Excretion:

Neonates ≤1 month: 86% excreted unchanged in urine

Infants >1 month and Adults: In urine, as metabolites

Pregnancy Risk Factor C

Caffeine, Acetaminophen, and Aspirin *see* Acetaminophen, Aspirin, and Caffeine *on page 41*

Caffeine, Acetaminophen, Butalbital, and Codeine *see* Butalbital, Acetaminophen, Caffeine, and Codeine *on page 248*

Caffeine and Ergotamine *see* Ergotamine and Caffeine *on page 586*

Caffeine and Sodium Benzoate *see* Caffeine *on page 255*

Caffeine, Aspirin, and Acetaminophen *see* Acetaminophen, Aspirin, and Caffeine *on page 41*

Caffeine Citrate *see* Caffeine *on page 255*

Caffeine, Dihydrocodeine, and Acetaminophen *see* Acetaminophen, Caffeine, and Dihydrocodeine *on page 42*

Caffeine, Hydrocodone, Chlorpheniramine, Phenylephrine, and Acetaminophen *see* Hydrocodone, Chlorpheniramine, Phenylephrine, Acetaminophen, and Caffeine *on page 833*

Calcipotriene (kal si POE try een)

U.S. Brand Names Dovonex®
Mexican Brand Names Daivonex
Generic Available No
Pharmacologic Category Topical Skin Product; Vitamin D Analog
Use Treatment of plaque psoriasis
Local Anesthetic/Vasoconstrictor Precautions No information available to require special precautions
Effects on Dental Treatment No significant effects or complications reported
Common Adverse Effects Frequency may vary with site of application.
>10%: Dermatologic: Burning, itching, rash, skin irritation, stinging, tingling
1% to 10%: Dermatologic: Dermatitis, dry skin, erythema, peeling, worsening of psoriasis
Note: Skin atrophy, hyperpigmentation, folliculitis, and hypercalcemia are potential adverse effects of calcipotriene.
Mechanism of Action Synthetic vitamin D_3 analog which regulates skin cell production and proliferation
Drug Interactions
  Increased Effect/Toxicity: No data reported
  Decreased Effect: No data reported
Pharmacodynamics/Kinetics
  Onset of action: Improvement begins after 2 weeks; marked improvement seen after 8 weeks
  Absorption: When applied to psoriasis plaques: Cream, ointment: ~6%; Solution: <1%
  Metabolism: Converted in the skin to inactive metabolites
Pregnancy Risk Factor C

Calcitonin (kal si TOE nin)

Related Information
  Rheumatoid Arthritis, Osteoarthritis, and Osteoporosis *on page 1759*
U.S. Brand Names Fortical®; Miacalcin®
Canadian Brand Names Apo-Calcitonin®; Calcimar®; Caltine®; Miacalcin® NS
Mexican Brand Names Miacalcic; Oseum
Generic Available No
Index Terms Calcitonin (Salmon)
Pharmacologic Category Antidote; Hormone
Use Calcitonin (salmon): Treatment of Paget's disease of bone (osteitis deformans); adjunctive therapy for hypercalcemia; treatment of postmenopausal osteoporosis
Local Anesthetic/Vasoconstrictor Precautions No information available to require special precautions
Effects on Dental Treatment No significant effects or complications reported
Common Adverse Effects Unless otherwise noted, frequencies reported are with nasal spray.

>10%: Respiratory: Rhinitis (12%)
1% to 10%:
  Cardiovascular: Flushing (nasal spray: <1%; injection: 2% to 5%), angina (1% to 3%), hypertension (1% to 3%)
  Central nervous system: Depression (1% to 3%), dizziness (1% to 3%), fatigue (1% to 3%)
(Continued)

Calcitonin *(Continued)*

Dermatologic: Erythematous rash (1% to 3%)

Gastrointestinal: Abdominal pain (1% to 3%), constipation (1% to 3%), diarrhea (1% to 3%), dyspepsia (1% to 3%), nausea (injection: 10%; nasal spray: 1% to 3%)

Genitourinary: Cystitis (1% to 3%)

Local: Injection site reactions (injection: 10%)

Neuromuscular & skeletal: Back pain (5%), arthrosis (1% to 3%), myalgia (1% to 3%), paresthesia (1% to 3%)

Ocular: Conjunctivitis (1% to 3%), lacrimation abnormality (1% to 3%)

Respiratory: Bronchospasm (1% to 3%), sinusitis (1% to 3%), upper respiratory tract infection (1% to 3%)

Miscellaneous: Flu-like syndrome (1% to 3%), infection (1% to 3%), lymphadenopathy (1% to 3%)

Mechanism of Action Peptide sequence similar to human calcitonin; functionally antagonizes the effects of parathyroid hormone. Directly inhibits osteoclastic bone resorption; promotes the renal excretion of calcium, phosphate, sodium, magnesium, and potassium by decreasing tubular reabsorption; increases the jejunal secretion of water, sodium, potassium, and chloride

Pharmacodynamics/Kinetics

Hypercalcemia: I.M. or SubQ:

Onset of action: ~2 hours

Duration: 6-8 hours

Absorption: Nasal: ~3% of I.M. level (range: 0.3% to 31%)

Distribution: Does not cross placenta

Half-life elimination: SubQ: 1.2 hours; Nasal: 43 minutes

Time to peak: Nasal: ~30-40 minutes

Excretion: Urine (as inactive metabolites)

Pregnancy Risk Factor C

Calcitonin (Salmon) *see* Calcitonin *on page 257*

Cal-Citrate® 250 [OTC] *see* Calcium Citrate *on page 262*

Calcitriol *(kal si TRYE ole)*

U.S. Brand Names Calcijex®; Rocaltrol®

Canadian Brand Names Calcijex®; Rocaltrol®

Mexican Brand Names Lemytriol; Rocaltrol; Tirocal

Generic Available Yes

Index Terms 1,25 Dihydroxycholecalciferol

Pharmacologic Category Vitamin D Analog

Use Management of hypocalcemia in patients on chronic renal dialysis; management of secondary hyperparathyroidism in moderate-to-severe chronic renal failure; management of hypocalcemia in hypoparathyroidism and pseudohypoparathyroidism

Unlabeled/Investigational Use Decrease severity of psoriatic lesions in psoriatic vulgaris; vitamin D-resistant rickets

Local Anesthetic/Vasoconstrictor Precautions No information available to require special precautions

Effects on Dental Treatment Key adverse event(s) related to dental treatment: Metallic taste and xerostomia (normal salivary flow resumes upon discontinuation).

Common Adverse Effects

>1%: Endocrine & metabolic: Hypercalcemia (33%)

Frequency not defined:

Cardiovascular: Cardiac arrhythmia, hyper-/hypotension

Central nervous system: Headache, irritability, seizure (rare), somnolence, psychosis

Dermatologic: Pruritus, erythema multiforme

Endocrine & metabolic: Hypermagnesemia, hyperphosphatemia, polydipsia

Gastrointestinal: Anorexia, constipation, metallic taste, nausea, pancreatitis, vomiting, xerostomia

Hepatic: LFTs increased

Neuromuscular & skeletal: Bone pain, myalgia, dystrophy, soft tissue calcification

Ocular: Conjunctivitis, photophobia

Renal: Polyuria

Mechanism of Action Promotes absorption of calcium in the intestines and retention at the kidneys thereby increasing calcium levels in the serum; decreases excessive serum phosphatase levels, parathyroid hormone levels, and decreases bone resorption; increases renal tubule phosphate resorption

Drug Interactions

Cytochrome P450 Effect: Induces CYP3A4 (weak)

Increased Effect/Toxicity: Risk of hypercalcemia with thiazide diuretics. Risk of hypermagnesemia with magnesium-containing antacids. Risk of digoxin toxicity may be increased (if hypercalcemia occurs).

Decreased Effect: Cholestyramine and colestipol decrease absorption/effect of calcitriol. Thiazide diuretics and corticosteroids may reduce the effect of calcitriol.

Pharmacodynamics/Kinetics

Onset of action: ~2-6 hours

Duration: 3-5 days

Absorption: Oral: Rapid

Protein binding: 99.9%

Metabolism: Primarily to 1,24,25-trihydroxycholecalciferol and 1,24,25-trihydroxy ergocalciferol

Half-life elimination: 3-8 hours

Excretion: Primarily feces; urine (4% to 6%)

Pregnancy Risk Factor C (manufacturer); A/D (dose exceeding RDA recommendation) (expert analysis)

Calcium Acetate (KAL see um AS e tate)

Related Information

Rheumatoid Arthritis, Osteoarthritis, and Osteoporosis *on page 1759*

U.S. Brand Names PhosLo®

Canadian Brand Names PhosLo®

Generic Available Yes: Solution for injection

Pharmacologic Category Antidote; Calcium Salt; Phosphate Binder

Use

Oral: Control of hyperphosphatemia in end-stage renal failure; does not promote aluminum absorption

I.V.: Calcium supplementation in parenteral nutrition therapy

Local Anesthetic/Vasoconstrictor Precautions No information available to require special precautions

Effects on Dental Treatment No significant effects or complications reported

Mechanism of Action Combines with dietary phosphate to form insoluble calcium phosphate which is excreted in feces

Pregnancy Risk Factor C

Calcium Acetate and Aluminum Sulfate *see* Aluminum Sulfate and Calcium Acetate *on page 83*

Calcium Acetylhomotaurinate *see* Acamprosate *on page 27*

Calcium and Risedronate *see* Risedronate and Calcium *on page 1431*

Calcium and Vitamin D (KAL see um & VYE ta min dee)

U.S. Brand Names Cal-CYUM [OTC]; Caltrate® 600+D [OTC]; Caltrate® 600+Soy™ [OTC]; Caltrate® ColonHealth™ [OTC]; Chew-Cal [OTC]; Liqua-Cal [OTC]; Os-Cal® 500+D [OTC]; Oysco 500+D [OTC]; Oysco D [OTC]; Oyst-Cal-D [OTC]; Oyst-Cal-D 500 [OTC]

Generic Available Yes

Index Terms Vitamin D and Calcium Carbonate

Pharmacologic Category Calcium Salt; Electrolyte Supplement, Oral; Vitamin, Fat Soluble

Use Dietary supplement, antacid

Local Anesthetic/Vasoconstrictor Precautions No information available to require special precautions

Effects on Dental Treatment No significant effects or complications reported

Common Adverse Effects Frequency not defined; also see individual agents

Central nervous system: Headache

Endocrine & metabolic: Hypercalcemia, hypercalciuria

Gastrointestinal: Gastrointestinal discomfort

Dosage Oral: Adults: Refer to individual monographs for dietary reference intake.

Dosage adjustment in renal impairment: Use caution in severe renal impairment

Contraindications Hypersensitivity to any component of the formulation; hypophosphatemia, hypercalcemia, evidence of vitamin D toxicity; history of kidney stones

Warnings/Precautions Calcium carbonate absorption is impaired in achlorhydria Administration is followed by increased gastric acid secretion within 2 hours of administration. While hypercalcemia and hypercalciuria may result when

(Continued)

Calcium and Vitamin D (Continued)

therapeutic replacement amounts are given for prolonged periods, they are most likely to occur in hypoparathyroid patients receiving high doses of vitamin D. Use with caution in renal failure; monitoring of serum calcium may be necessary. Use with caution in patients who may be at risk of cardiac arrhythmias.

Some products may contain soy, tartrazine, or phenylalanine, or may be derived from shellfish.

Drug Interactions

Increased Effect/Toxicity: Thiazide diuretics can cause hypercalcemia (milk-alkali syndrome); monitor response. Calcium supplementation may potentiate digoxin toxicity.

Decreased Effect: Calcium channel blockers (eg, verapamil) effects may be diminished. The absorption of fluoroquinolones, tetracyclines, atenolol (and potentially other beta-blockers), iron, bisphosphonates, sodium fluoride, and zinc may be significantly reduced; space administration times. Calcium carbonate (and possibly other calcium salts) may decrease T_4 absorption; separate dose from levothyroxine by at least 4 hours. The potassium-binding ability of polystyrene sulfonate is reduced; avoid concurrent use.

Ethanol/Nutrition/Herb Interactions

Ethanol: Avoid ethanol (may increase risk of osteoporosis).

Food: Food may increase calcium absorption. Calcium may decrease iron absorption. Bran, foods high in oxalates, or whole grain cereals may decrease calcium absorption.

Dietary Considerations Take with food to minimize GI upset. Some products may contain phenylalanine (avoid use in phenylketonurics), tartrazine, gluten, and/or soy.

Dosage Forms

Capsule, softgel: Calcium 500 mg and vitamin D 500 int. units; calcium 600 mg and vitamin D 100 int. units; calcium 600 mg and vitamin D 200 int. units

Liqua-Cal: Calcium 600 mg and vitamin D 200 int. units

Tablet: Calcium 250 mg and vitamin D 125 int. units; calcium 500 mg and vitamin D 125 int. units; calcium 500 mg and vitamin D 200 int. units; calcium 600 mg and vitamin D 125 int. units; calcium 600 mg and vitamin D 200 int. units

Caltrate® 600+D: Calcium 600 mg and vitamin D 200 int. units

Caltrate® 600+ Soy™: Calcium 600 mg and vitamin D 200 int. units

Caltrate® ColonHealth™: Calcium 600 mg and vitamin D 200 int. units

Oysco D: Calcium 250 mg and vitamin D 125 int. units

Oysco 500+D: Calcium 500 mg and vitamin D 200 int. units

Oyst-Cal-D: Calcium 250 mg and vitamin D 125 int. units

Oyst-Cal-D 500: Calcium 500 mg and vitamin D 200 int. units

Tablet, chewable: Calcium 500 mg and vitamin D 100 int. units; calcium 600 mg and vitamin D 400 int. units

Os-Cal® 500+D: Calcium 500 mg and vitamin D 400 int. units

Wafer, chewable:

Cal-CYUM: Calcium 519 mg and vitamin D 150 int. units (50s)

Chew-Cal: Calcium 333 mg and vitamin D 40 int. units (100s, 250s)

Calcium Carbonate (KAL see um KAR bun ate)

Related Information

Rheumatoid Arthritis, Osteoarthritis, and Osteoporosis *on page 1759*

U.S. Brand Names Alcalak [OTC]; Alka-Mints® [OTC]; Calcarb 600 [OTC]; Calci-Chew® [OTC]; Calci-Mix® [OTC]; Cal-Gest [OTC]; Cal-Mint [OTC]; Caltrate® 600 [OTC]; Children's Pepto [OTC]; Chooz® [OTC]; Florical® [OTC]; Maalox® Regular Chewable [OTC]; Mylanta® Children's [OTC]; Nephro-Calci® [OTC]; Nutralox® [OTC]; Os-Cal® 500 [OTC] [DSC]; Oysco 500 [OTC]; Oyst-Cal 500 [OTC]; Rolaids® Softchews [OTC]; Titralac™ [OTC]; Tums® [OTC]; Tums® E-X [OTC]; Tums® Extra Strength Sugar Free [OTC]; Tums® Smoothies™ [OTC]; Tums® Ultra [OTC]

Canadian Brand Names Apo-Cal®; Calcite-500; Caltrate®; Caltrate® Select; Os-Cal®

Mexican Brand Names Calsan; Caltrate; Osteomin; Tums

Generic Available Yes

Pharmacologic Category Antacid; Antidote; Calcium Salt; Electrolyte Supplement, Oral

Use As an antacid; treatment and prevention of calcium deficiency or hyperphosphatemia (eg, osteoporosis, osteomalacia, mild/moderate renal insufficiency, hypoparathyroidism, postmenopausal osteoporosis, rickets); has been used to bind phosphate

Local Anesthetic/Vasoconstrictor Precautions No information available to require special precautions

Effects on Dental Treatment Key adverse event(s) related to dental treatment: Xerostomia (normal salivary flow resumes upon discontinuation).

Mechanism of Action As dietary supplement, used to prevent or treat negative calcium balance; in osteoporosis, it helps to prevent or decrease the rate of bone loss. The calcium in calcium salts moderates nerve and muscle performance and allows normal cardiac function. Also used to treat hyperphosphatemia in patients with advanced renal insufficiency by combining with dietary phosphate to form insoluble calcium phosphate, which is excreted in feces. Calcium salts as antacids neutralize gastric acidity resulting in increased gastric and duodenal bulb pH; they additionally inhibit proteolytic activity of peptic if the pH is increased >4 and increase lower esophageal sphincter tone.

Calcium Carbonate and Etidronate Disodium *see* Etidronate and Calcium *on page 654*

Calcium Carbonate and Magnesium Hydroxide
(KAL see um KAR bun ate & mag NEE zhum hye DROKS ide)

Related Information
Calcium Carbonate *on page 260*
Magnesium Hydroxide *on page 1014*

U.S. Brand Names Mi-Acid™ Double Strength [OTC]; Mylanta® Gelcaps® [OTC]; Mylanta® Supreme [OTC]; Mylanta® Ultra [OTC]; Rolaids® [OTC]; Rolaids® Extra Strength [OTC]

Generic Available Yes: Chewable tablet

Index Terms Magnesium Hydroxide and Calcium Carbonate

Pharmacologic Category Antacid

Use Hyperacidity

Local Anesthetic/Vasoconstrictor Precautions No information available to require special precautions

Effects on Dental Treatment No significant effects or complications reported

Calcium Carbonate and Simethicone
(KAL see um KAR bun ate & sye METH i kone)

Related Information
Calcium Carbonate *on page 260*
Simethicone *on page 1472*

U.S. Brand Names Gas Ban™ [OTC]; Titralac® Plus [OTC]

Generic Available No

Index Terms Simethicone and Calcium Carbonate

Pharmacologic Category Antacid; Antiflatulent

Use Relief of acid indigestion, heartburn

Local Anesthetic/Vasoconstrictor Precautions No information available to require special precautions

Effects on Dental Treatment Do not give tetracyclines concomitantly.

Pharmacodynamics/Kinetics See individual agents.

Pregnancy Risk Factor C

Calcium Carbonate, Magnesium Hydroxide, and Famotidine *see* Famotidine, Calcium Carbonate, and Magnesium Hydroxide *on page 671*

Calcium Chloride (KAL see um KLOR ide)

Generic Available Yes

Pharmacologic Category Calcium Salt; Electrolyte Supplement, Parenteral

Use Cardiac resuscitation when epinephrine fails to improve myocardial contractions, cardiac disturbances of hyperkalemia, hypocalcemia; emergent treatment of hypocalcemic tetany; treatment of hypermagnesemia

Unlabeled/Investigational Use Calcium channel blocker overdose

Local Anesthetic/Vasoconstrictor Precautions No information available to require special precautions

Effects on Dental Treatment No significant effects or complications reported

Mechanism of Action Moderates nerve and muscle performance via action potential excitation threshold regulation

Pregnancy Risk Factor C

Calcium Citrate (KAL see um SIT rate)

Related Information
Rheumatoid Arthritis, Osteoarthritis, and Osteoporosis *on page 1759*
U.S. Brand Names Cal-Citrate® 250 [OTC]; Citracal® [OTC]
Canadian Brand Names Osteocit®
Generic Available Yes
Pharmacologic Category Calcium Salt
Use Antacid; treatment and prevention of calcium deficiency or hyperphosphatemia (eg, osteoporosis, osteomalacia, mild/moderate renal insufficiency, hypoparathyroidism, postmenopausal osteoporosis, rickets)
Local Anesthetic/Vasoconstrictor Precautions No information available to require special precautions
Effects on Dental Treatment No significant effects or complications reported
Mechanism of Action Moderates nerve and muscle performance via action potential excitation threshold regulation
Pregnancy Risk Factor C

Calcium Disodium Edetate *see* Edetate Calcium Disodium *on page 554*
Calcium Disodium Versenate® *see* Edetate Calcium Disodium *on page 554*
Calcium EDTA *see* Edetate Calcium Disodium *on page 554*

Calcium Glubionate (KAL see um gloo BYE oh nate)

Related Information
Rheumatoid Arthritis, Osteoarthritis, and Osteoporosis *on page 1759*
U.S. Brand Names Calcionate [OTC]
Generic Available Yes
Pharmacologic Category Calcium Salt
Use Dietary supplement
Local Anesthetic/Vasoconstrictor Precautions No information available to require special precautions
Effects on Dental Treatment No significant effects or complications reported
Mechanism of Action As dietary supplement, used to prevent or treat negative calcium balance. The calcium in calcium salts moderates nerve and muscle performance and allows normal cardiac function.

Calcium Gluconate (KAL see um GLOO koe nate)

Related Information
Rheumatoid Arthritis, Osteoarthritis, and Osteoporosis *on page 1759*
Generic Available Yes
Pharmacologic Category Calcium Salt; Electrolyte Supplement, Oral; Electrolyte Supplement, Parenteral
Use Treatment and prevention of hypocalcemia; treatment of tetany; cardiac disturbances of hyperkalemia, cardiac resuscitation when epinephrine fails to improve myocardial contractions, hypocalcemia; calcium supplementation
Unlabeled/Investigational Use Hydrofluoric acid (HF) burns; calcium channel blocker overdose
Local Anesthetic/Vasoconstrictor Precautions No information available to require special precautions
Effects on Dental Treatment No significant effects or complications reported
Mechanism of Action As dietary supplement, used to prevent or treat negative calcium balance; in osteoporosis, it helps to prevent or decrease the rate of bone loss. The calcium in calcium salts moderates nerve and muscle performance and allows normal cardiac function.
Pregnancy Risk Factor C

Calcium Lactate (KAL see um LAK tate)

Related Information
Rheumatoid Arthritis, Osteoarthritis, and Osteoporosis *on page 1759*
Generic Available Yes
Pharmacologic Category Calcium Salt
Use Adjunct in prevention of postmenopausal osteoporosis; treatment and prevention of calcium depletion
Local Anesthetic/Vasoconstrictor Precautions No information available to require special precautions
Effects on Dental Treatment No significant effects or complications reported

Mechanism of Action As dietary supplement, used to prevent or treat negative calcium balance; in osteoporosis, it helps to prevent or decrease the rate of bone loss. The calcium in calcium salts moderates nerve and muscle performance and allows normal cardiac function.

Pregnancy Risk Factor C

Calcium Leucovorin *see* Leucovorin *on page 957*

Calcium Pantothenate *see* Pantothenic Acid *on page 1251*

Calcium Phosphate (Tribasic) (KAL see um FOS fate tri BAY sik)

Related Information
Rheumatoid Arthritis, Osteoarthritis, and Osteoporosis *on page 1759*
U.S. Brand Names Posture® [OTC]
Generic Available No
Index Terms Tricalcium Phosphate
Pharmacologic Category Calcium Salt
Use Dietary supplement
Local Anesthetic/Vasoconstrictor Precautions No information available to require special precautions
Effects on Dental Treatment No significant effects or complications reported
Mechanism of Action As dietary supplement, used to prevent or treat negative calcium balance; in osteoporosis, it helps to prevent or decrease the rate of bone loss. The calcium in calcium salts moderates nerve and muscle performance and allows normal cardiac function.

Cal-CYUM [OTC] *see* Calcium and Vitamin D *on page 259*

Caldecort® [OTC] *see* Hydrocortisone *on page 836*

Calfactant (kaf AKT ant)

U.S. Brand Names Infasurf®
Generic Available No
Pharmacologic Category Lung Surfactant
Use Prevention of respiratory distress syndrome (RDS) in premature infants at high risk for RDS and for the treatment ("rescue") of premature infants who develop RDS

Prophylaxis: Therapy at birth with calfactant is indicated for premature infants <29 weeks of gestational age at significant risk for RDS. Should be administered as soon as possible, preferably within 30 minutes after birth.

Treatment: For infants ≤72 hours of age with RDS (confirmed by clinical and radiologic findings) and requiring endotracheal intubation.

Local Anesthetic/Vasoconstrictor Precautions No information available to require special precautions
Effects on Dental Treatment No significant effects or complications reported
Common Adverse Effects
Cardiovascular: Bradycardia (34%), cyanosis (65%)
Respiratory: Airway obstruction (39%), reflux (21%), requirement for manual ventilation (16%), reintubation (1% to 10%)
Mechanism of Action Endogenous lung surfactant is essential for effective ventilation because it modifies alveolar surface tension, thereby stabilizing the alveoli. Lung surfactant deficiency is the cause of respiratory distress syndrome (RDS) in premature infants and lung surfactant restores surface activity to the lungs of these infants.
Pharmacodynamics/Kinetics No human studies of absorption, biotransformation, or excretion have been performed

Cal-Gest [OTC] *see* Calcium Carbonate *on page 260*

Callergy Clear [OTC] *see* Pramoxine *on page 1334*

Cal-Mint [OTC] *see* Calcium Carbonate *on page 260*

Caltrate® 600 [OTC] *see* Calcium Carbonate *on page 260*

Caltrate® 600+D [OTC] *see* Calcium and Vitamin D *on page 259*

Caltrate® 600+ Soy™ [OTC] *see* Calcium and Vitamin D *on page 259*

Caltrate® ColonHealth™ [OTC] *see* Calcium and Vitamin D *on page 259*

Camila™ *see* Norethindrone *on page 1186*

Campath® *see* Alemtuzumab *on page 64*

Campath-1H *see* Alemtuzumab *on page 64*

Campho-Phenique® [OTC] *see* Camphor and Phenol *on page 264*

Camphor and Phenol (KAM for & FEE nole)

Related Information
Phenol *on page 1290*
U.S. Brand Names Campho-Phenique® [OTC]
Generic Available Yes: Liquid
Index Terms Phenol and Camphor
Pharmacologic Category Topical Skin Product
Use Relief of pain and itching associated with minor burns, sunburn, minor cuts, insect bites, minor skin irritation; temporary relief of pain from cold sores
Local Anesthetic/Vasoconstrictor Precautions No information available to require special precautions
Effects on Dental Treatment No significant effects or complications reported
Pregnancy Risk Factor C

Camphorated Tincture of Opium (error-prone synonym) *see* Paregoric *on page 1253*

Campral® *see* Acamprosate *on page 27*

Camptosar® *see* Irinotecan *on page 909*

Camptothecin-11 *see* Irinotecan *on page 909*

Canasa™ *see* Mesalamine *on page 1052*

Cancidas® *see* Caspofungin *on page 294*

Candesartan (kan de SAR tan)

Related Information
Cardiovascular Diseases *on page 1726*
U.S. Brand Names Atacand®
Canadian Brand Names Atacand®
Mexican Brand Names Atacand; Blopress
Generic Available No
Index Terms Candesartan Cilexetil
Pharmacologic Category Angiotensin II Receptor Blocker
Use Alone or in combination with other antihypertensive agents in treating essential hypertension; treatment of heart failure (NYHA class II-IV)
Local Anesthetic/Vasoconstrictor Precautions No information available to require special precautions
Effects on Dental Treatment No significant effects or complications reported
Common Adverse Effects
Cardiovascular: Angina, hypotension (CHF 19%), MI, palpitation, tachycardia
Central nervous system: Dizziness, lightheadedness, drowsiness, headache, vertigo, anxiety, depression, somnolence, fever
Dermatologic: Angioedema, rash
Endocrine & metabolic: Hyperglycemia, hyperkalemia (CHF <1% to 6%), hypertriglyceridemia, hyperuricemia
Gastrointestinal: Dyspepsia, gastroenteritis
Genitourinary: Hematuria
Neuromuscular & skeletal: Back pain, CPK increased, myalgia, paresthesia, weakness
Renal: Serum creatinine increased (up to 13% in patients with CHF with drug discontinuation required in 6%)
Respiratory: Dyspnea, epistaxis, pharyngitis, rhinitis, upper respiratory tract infection
Miscellaneous: Diaphoresis increased
Dosage Adults: Oral:
Hypertension: Usual dose is 4-32 mg once daily; dosage must be individualized. Blood pressure response is dose related over the range of 2-32 mg. The usual recommended starting dose of 16 mg once daily when it is used as monotherapy in patients who are not volume depleted. It can be administered once or twice daily with total daily doses ranging from 8-32 mg. Larger doses do not appear to have a greater effect and there is relatively little experience with such doses.
Congestive heart failure: Initial: 4 mg once daily; double the dose at 2-week intervals, as tolerated; target dose: 32 mg
Note: In selected cases, concurrent therapy with an ACE inhibitor may provide additional benefit.
Elderly: No initial dosage adjustment is necessary for elderly patients (although higher concentrations (C_{max}) and AUC were observed in these populations), for patients with mildly impaired renal function, or for patients with mildly impaired hepatic function.

Dosage adjustment in hepatic impairment: No initial dosage adjustment required in mild hepatic impairment. Consider initiation at lower dosages in moderate hepatic impairment (AUC increased by 145%). No data available concerning dosing in severe hepatic impairment.

Mechanism of Action
Candesartan is an angiotensin receptor antagonist. Angiotensin II acts as a vasoconstrictor. In addition to causing direct vasoconstriction, angiotensin II also stimulates the release of aldosterone. Once aldosterone is released, sodium as well as water are reabsorbed. The end result is an elevation in blood pressure. Candesartan binds to the AT1 angiotensin II receptor. This binding prevents angiotensin II from binding to the receptor thereby blocking the vasoconstriction and the aldosterone secreting effects of angiotensin II.

Contraindications
Hypersensitivity to candesartan or any component of the formulation; hypersensitivity to other A-II receptor antagonists; bilateral renal artery stenosis; pregnancy

Warnings/Precautions
[U.S. Boxed Warning]: Based on human data, drugs that act on the angiotensin system can cause injury and death to the developing fetus when used in the second and third trimesters. Angiotensin receptor blockers should be discontinued as soon as possible once pregnancy is detected. May cause hyperkalemia; avoid potassium supplementation unless specifically required by healthcare provider. Avoid use or use a smaller dose in patients who are volume depleted; correct depletion first. May be associated with deterioration of renal function and/or increases in serum creatinine, particularly in patients dependent on renin-angiotensin-aldosterone system. Use with caution in unilateral renal artery stenosis, hepatic dysfunction, pre-existing renal insufficiency, or significant aortic/mitral stenosis. Use caution when initiating in heart failure; may need to adjust dose, and/or concurrent diuretic therapy, because of candesartan-induced hypotension. Hypotension may occur during major surgery and anesthesia; use cautiously before, during, and immediately after such interventions. Although some properties may be shared between these agents, concurrent therapy with ACE inhibitor may be rational in selected patients. Safety and efficacy have not been established in children.

Drug Interactions
Cytochrome P450 Effect: Substrate of CYP2C9 (minor); **Inhibits** CYP2C8 (weak), 2C9 (weak)

Increased Effect/Toxicity: The risk of lithium toxicity may be increased by candesartan; monitor lithium levels. Concurrent use with potassium-sparing diuretics (amiloride, spironolactone, triamterene), potassium supplements, or trimethoprim (high-dose) may increase the risk of hyperkalemia.

Ethanol/Nutrition/Herb Interactions
Food: Food reduces the time to maximal concentration and increases the C_{max}.

Herb/Nutraceutical: Avoid dong quai if using for hypertension (has estrogenic activity). Avoid ephedra, yohimbe, ginseng (may worsen hypertension). Avoid garlic (may have increased antihypertensive effect).

Pharmacodynamics/Kinetics
Onset of action: 2-3 hours
  Peak effect: 6-8 hours
Duration: >24 hours
Distribution: V_d: 0.13 L/kg
Protein binding: 99%
Metabolism: To candesartan by the intestinal wall cells
Bioavailability: 15%
Half-life elimination (dose dependent): 5-9 hours
Time to peak: 3-4 hours
Excretion: Urine (26%)
  Clearance: Total body: 0.37 mL/kg/minute; Renal: 0.19 mL/kg/minute

Pregnancy Risk Factor
C/D (2nd and 3rd trimesters)

Dosage Forms
Tablet:
  Atacand®: 4 mg, 8 mg, 16 mg, 32 mg

Candesartan and Hydrochlorothiazide
(kan de SAR tan & hye droe klor oh THYE a zide)

Related Information
Candesartan *on page 264*
Cardiovascular Diseases *on page 1726*
Hydrochlorothiazide *on page 819*
(Continued)

Candesartan and Hydrochlorothiazide *(Continued)*

U.S. Brand Names Atacand HCT™
Canadian Brand Names Atacand® Plus
Mexican Brand Names Atacand Plus
Generic Available No
Index Terms Candesartan Cilexetil and Hydrochlorothiazide
Pharmacologic Category Angiotensin II Receptor Blocker Combination; Antihypertensive Agent, Combination; Diuretic, Thiazide
Use Treatment of hypertension; combination product should not be used for initial therapy
Local Anesthetic/Vasoconstrictor Precautions No information available to require special precautions
Effects on Dental Treatment No significant effects or complications reported
Common Adverse Effects Reactions which follow have been reported with the combination product; see individual drug agents for additional adverse reactions that may be expected from each agent.

1% to 10%:
Central nervous system: Dizziness (3%), headache (3%, placebo 5%)
Neuromuscular & skeletal: Back pain (3%)
Respiratory: Upper respiratory tract infection (4%)
Miscellaneous: Flu-like syndrome (2%)

Mechanism of Action
Candesartan: Candesartan is an angiotensin receptor antagonist. Angiotensin II acts as a vasoconstrictor. In addition to causing direct vasoconstriction, angiotensin II also stimulates the release of aldosterone. Once aldosterone is released, sodium as well as water are reabsorbed. The end result is an elevation in blood pressure. Candesartan binds to the AT1 angiotensin II receptor. This binding prevents angiotensin II from binding to the receptor, thereby blocking the vasoconstriction and the aldosterone-secreting effects of angiotensin II.

Hydrochlorothiazide: Inhibits sodium reabsorption in the distal tubules causing increased excretion of sodium and water as well as potassium and hydrogen ions

Drug Interactions
Cytochrome P450 Effect: Candesartan: **Substrate** of CYP2C9 (minor); **Inhibits** CYP2C8 (weak), 2C9 (weak)
Increased Effect/Toxicity: See individual agents.
Decreased Effect: See individual agents.
Pharmacodynamics/Kinetics See individual agents.
Pregnancy Risk Factor C/D (2nd and 3rd trimesters)

Candesartan Cilexetil *see* Candesartan *on page 264*

Candesartan Cilexetil and Hydrochlorothiazide *see* Candesartan and Hydrochlorothiazide *on page 265*

Cankaid® [OTC] *see* Carbamide Peroxide *on page 276*

Cannabidiol and Tetrahydrocannabinol *see* Tetrahydrocannabinol and Cannabidiol *on page 1550*

Cantharidin *(kan THAR e din)*

Canadian Brand Names Canthacur®; Cantharone®
Generic Available No
Pharmacologic Category Keratolytic Agent
Use Removal of ordinary and periungual warts
Local Anesthetic/Vasoconstrictor Precautions No information available to require special precautions
Effects on Dental Treatment No significant effects or complications reported
Common Adverse Effects 1% to 10%:
Cardiovascular: Syncope
Central nervous system: Delirium, ataxia
Dermatologic: Dermal irritation, dermal burns, acantholysis
Gastrointestinal: GI hemorrhage, rectal bleeding, dysphagia
Genitourinary: Priapism
Hepatic: Fatty degeneration
Neuromuscular & skeletal: Hyper-reflexia
Ocular: Conjunctivitis, iritis, keratitis
Renal: Proteinuria, hematuria
Respiratory: Burning of oropharynx
Pregnancy Risk Factor C

Cantil® [DSC] *see* Mepenzolate *on page 1038*

Capastat® Sulfate *see* Capreomycin *on page 268*

Capecitabine (ka pe SITE a been)

Related Information
Fluorouracil *on page 713*
U.S. Brand Names Xeloda®
Canadian Brand Names Xeloda®
Mexican Brand Names Xeloda
Generic Available No
Index Terms NSC-712807
Pharmacologic Category Antineoplastic Agent, Antimetabolite; Antineoplastic Agent, Antimetabolite (Pyrimidine Antagonist)
Use Treatment of metastatic colorectal cancer; adjuvant therapy of Dukes' C colon cancer; treatment of metastatic breast cancer
Local Anesthetic/Vasoconstrictor Precautions No information available to require special precautions
Effects on Dental Treatment Key adverse event(s) related to dental treatment: Stomatitis, abnormal taste, and taste disturbance.
Common Adverse Effects Frequency listed derived from monotherapy trials.

>10%:
Cardiovascular: Edema (9% to 15%)
Central nervous system: Fatigue (16% to 42%), fever (7% to 18%), pain (12%)
Dermatologic: Palmar-plantar erythrodysesthesia (hand-and-foot syndrome) (54% to 60%; grade 3: 11% to 17%; may be dose limiting), dermatitis (27% to 37%)
Gastrointestinal: Diarrhea (47% to 57%; may be dose limiting; grade 3: 12% to 13%; grade 4: 2% to 3%), nausea (34% to 53%), vomiting (15% to 37%), abdominal pain (7% to 35%), stomatitis (22% to 25%), appetite decreased (26%), anorexia (9% to 23%), constipation (9% to 15%)
Hematologic: Lymphopenia (94%; grade 4: 14%), anemia (72% to 80%; grade 4: <1% to 1%), neutropenia (2% to 26%; grade 4: 2%), thrombocytopenia (24%; grade 4: 1%)
Hepatic: Bilirubin increased (22% to 48%; grades 3/4: 11% to 23%)
Neuromuscular & skeletal: Paresthesia (21%)
Ocular: Eye irritation (13% to 15%)
Respiratory: Dyspnea (14%)
5% to 10%:
Cardiovascular: Venous thrombosis (8%), chest pain (6%)
Central nervous system: Headache (5% to 10%), lethargy (10%), dizziness (6% to 8%), insomnia (7% to 8%), mood alteration (5%), depression (5%)
Dermatologic: Nail disorder (7%), rash (7%), skin discoloration (7%), alopecia (6%), erythema (6%)
Endocrine & metabolic: Dehydration (7%)
Gastrointestinal: Motility disorder (10%), oral discomfort (10%), dyspepsia (6% to 8%), upper GI inflammatory disorders (colorectal cancer: 8%), hemorrhage (6%), ileus (6%), taste perversion (colorectal cancer: 6%)
Neuromuscular & skeletal: Back pain (10%), weakness (10%), neuropathy (10%), myalgia (9%), arthralgia (8%), limb pain (6%)
Ocular: Abnormal vision (colorectal cancer: 5%), conjunctivitis (5%)
Respiratory: Cough (7%)
Miscellaneous: Viral infection (colorectal cancer: 5%)
Mechanism of Action Capecitabine is a prodrug of fluorouracil. It undergoes hydrolysis in the liver and tissues to form fluorouracil which is the active moiety. Fluorouracil is a fluorinated pyrimidine antimetabolite that inhibits thymidylate synthetase, blocking the methylation of deoxyuridylic acid to thymidylic acid, interfering with DNA, and to a lesser degree, RNA synthesis. Fluorouracil appears to be phase specific for the G_1 and S phases of the cell cycle.
Drug Interactions
Increased Effect/Toxicity: Phenytoin and warfarin levels or effects may be increased.
Pharmacodynamics/Kinetics
Absorption: Rapid and extensive
Protein binding: <60%; ~35% to albumin
Metabolism:
Hepatic: Inactive metabolites: 5'-deoxy-5-fluorocytidine, 5'-deoxy-5-fluorouridine
Tissue: Active metabolite: Fluorouracil
Half-life elimination: 0.5-1 hour
Time to peak: 1.5 hours; Fluorouracil: 2 hours
Excretion: Urine (96%, 57% as α-fluoro-β-alanine); feces (<3%)
Pregnancy Risk Factor D

Capex™ *see* Fluocinolone *on page 706*

Caphasol *see* Saliva Substitute *on page 1452*

Capital® and Codeine *see* Acetaminophen and Codeine *on page 35*

Capitrol® [DSC] *see* Chloroxine *on page 338*

Capoten® *see* Captopril *on page 269*

Capozide® *see* Captopril and Hydrochlorothiazide *on page 271*

Capreomycin (kap ree oh MYE sin)

Related Information
Tuberculosis *on page 1765*
U.S. Brand Names Capastat® Sulfate
Generic Available No
Index Terms Capreomycin Sulfate
Pharmacologic Category Antibiotic, Miscellaneous; Antitubercular Agent
Use Treatment of tuberculosis in conjunction with at least one other anti-tuberculosis agent
Local Anesthetic/Vasoconstrictor Precautions No information available to require special precautions
Effects on Dental Treatment No significant effects or complications reported
Common Adverse Effects
>10%:
   Otic: Ototoxicity [subclinical hearing loss (11%), clinical loss (3%)], tinnitus
   Renal: Nephrotoxicity (36%, increased BUN)
1% to 10%: Hematologic: Eosinophilia (dose related, mild)
Mechanism of Action Capreomycin is a cyclic polypeptide antimicrobial. It is administered as a mixture of capreomycin IA and capreomycin IB. The mechanism of action of capreomycin is not well understood. Mycobacterial species that have become resistant to other agents are usually still sensitive to the action of capreomycin. However, significant cross-resistance with viomycin, kanamycin, and neomycin occurs.
Drug Interactions
Increased Effect/Toxicity: May increase effect/duration of nondepolarizing neuromuscular blocking agents. Additive toxicity (nephrotoxicity and ototoxicity), respiratory paralysis may occur with aminoglycosides (eg, streptomycin).
Pharmacodynamics/Kinetics
Half-life elimination: Normal renal function: 4-6 hours
Time to peak, serum: I.M.: ~1 hour
Excretion: Urine (as unchanged drug)
Pregnancy Risk Factor C

Capreomycin Sulfate *see* Capreomycin *on page 268*

Capsagel® [OTC] *see* Capsaicin *on page 268*

Capsaicin (kap SAY sin)

Related Information
Cayenne *on page 1704*
U.S. Brand Names ArthriCare® for Women Extra Moisturizing [OTC] [DSC]; ArthriCare® for Women Multi-Action [OTC] [DSC]; ArthriCare® for Women Silky Dry [OTC] [DSC]; ArthriCare® for Women Ultra Strength [OTC] [DSC]; Capsagel® [OTC]; Capzasin-HP® [OTC]; Capzasin-P® [OTC]; Zostrix® [OTC]; Zostrix®-HP [OTC]
Canadian Brand Names Zostrix®; Zostrix® H.P.
Mexican Brand Names Capsidol
Generic Available Yes: Cream
Pharmacologic Category Analgesic, Topical; Topical Skin Product
Use Topical treatment of pain associated with postherpetic neuralgia, rheumatoid arthritis, osteoarthritis, diabetic neuropathy; postsurgical pain
Unlabeled/Investigational Use Treatment of pain associated with psoriasis, chronic neuralgias unresponsive to other forms of therapy, and intractable pruritus
Local Anesthetic/Vasoconstrictor Precautions No information available to require special precautions
Effects on Dental Treatment No significant effects or complications reported
Common Adverse Effects Frequency not defined.
Dermatologic: Itching, stinging sensation, erythema

Local: Transient burning on application which usually diminishes with repeated use

Respiratory: Cough

Mechanism of Action Induces release of substance P, the principal chemomediator of pain impulses from the periphery to the CNS, from peripheral sensory neurons; after repeated application, capsaicin depletes the neuron of substance P and prevents reaccumulation

Drug Interactions
Cytochrome P450 Effect: Substrate of CYP2E1 (minor)

Pharmacodynamics/Kinetics
Onset of action: 14-28 days
Peak effect: 4-6 weeks of continuous therapy
Duration: Several hours

Pregnancy Risk Factor C

Captopril (KAP toe pril)

Related Information
Cardiovascular Diseases *on page 1726*

U.S. Brand Names Capoten®

Canadian Brand Names Alti-Captopril; Apo-Capto®; Capoten™; Gen-Captopril; Novo-Captopril; Nu-Capto; PMS-Captopril

Mexican Brand Names Capotena; Captral; Cardipril; Ecaten; Midrat; Toprilem

Generic Available Yes

Index Terms ACE

Pharmacologic Category Angiotensin-Converting Enzyme (ACE) Inhibitor

Use Management of hypertension; treatment of congestive heart failure, left ventricular dysfunction after myocardial infarction, diabetic nephropathy

Unlabeled/Investigational Use Treatment of hypertensive crisis, rheumatoid arthritis; diagnosis of anatomic renal artery stenosis, hypertension secondary to scleroderma renal crisis; diagnosis of aldosteronism, idiopathic edema, Bartter's syndrome, postmyocardial infarction for prevention of ventricular failure; increase circulation in Raynaud's phenomenon, hypertension secondary to Takayasu's disease

Local Anesthetic/Vasoconstrictor Precautions No information available to require special precautions

Effects on Dental Treatment Key adverse event(s) related to dental treatment: Loss or diminished perception of taste and orthostatic hypotension.

Common Adverse Effects
1% to 10%:
Cardiovascular: Hypotension (1% to 3%), tachycardia (1%), chest pain (1%), palpitation (1%)
Dermatologic: Rash (maculopapular or urticarial) (4% to 7%), pruritus (2%); in patients with rash, a positive ANA and/or eosinophilia has been noted in 7% to 10%.
Endocrine & metabolic: Hyperkalemia (1% to 11%)
Hematologic: Neutropenia may occur in up to 4% of patients with renal insufficiency or collagen-vascular disease.
Renal: Proteinuria (1%), serum creatinine increased, worsening of renal function (may occur in patients with bilateral renal artery stenosis or hypovolemia)
Respiratory: Cough (<1% to 2%)
Miscellaneous: Hypersensitivity reactions (rash, pruritus, fever, arthralgia, and eosinophilia) have occurred in 4% to 7% of patients (depending on dose and renal function); dysgeusia - loss of taste or diminished perception (2% to 4%)
Frequency not defined:
Cardiovascular: Angioedema, cardiac arrest, cerebrovascular insufficiency, rhythm disturbances, orthostatic hypotension, syncope, flushing, pallor, angina, MI, Raynaud's syndrome, CHF
Central nervous system: Ataxia, confusion, depression, nervousness, somnolence
Dermatologic: Bullous pemphigus, erythema multiforme, Stevens-Johnson syndrome, exfoliative dermatitis
Endocrine & metabolic: Alkaline phosphatase increased, bilirubin increased, gynecomastia
Gastrointestinal: Pancreatitis, glossitis, dyspepsia
Genitourinary: Urinary frequency, impotence
Hematologic: Anemia, thrombocytopenia, pancytopenia, agranulocytosis, anemia
Hepatic: Jaundice, hepatitis, hepatic necrosis (rare), cholestasis, hyponatremia (symptomatic), transaminases increased
(Continued)

Captopril *(Continued)*

Neuromuscular & skeletal: Asthenia, myalgia, myasthenia
Ocular: Blurred vision
Renal: Renal insufficiency, renal failure, nephrotic syndrome, polyuria, oliguria
Respiratory: Bronchospasm, eosinophilic pneumonitis, rhinitis
Miscellaneous: Anaphylactoid reactions

Dosage Note: Titrate dose according to patient's response; use lowest effective dose. Oral:

Infants: Initial: 0.15-0.3 mg/kg/dose; titrate dose upward to maximum of 6 mg/kg/day in 1-4 divided doses; usual required dose: 2.5-6 mg/kg/day

Children: Initial: 0.5 mg/kg/dose; titrate upward to maximum of 6 mg/kg/day in 2-4 divided doses

Older Children: Initial: 6.25-12.5 mg/dose every 12-24 hours; titrate upward to maximum of 6 mg/kg/day

Adolescents: Initial: 12.5-25 mg/dose given every 8-12 hours; increase by 25 mg/dose to maximum of 450 mg/day

Adults:

Acute hypertension (urgency/emergency): 12.5-25 mg, may repeat as needed (may be given sublingually, but no therapeutic advantage demonstrated)

Hypertension:

Initial dose: 12.5-25 mg 2-3 times/day; may increase by 12.5-25 mg/dose at 1- to 2-week intervals up to 50 mg 3 times/day; maximum dose: 150 mg 3 times/day; add diuretic before further dosage increases

Usual dose range (JNC 7): 25-100 mg/day in 2 divided doses

Congestive heart failure:

Initial dose: 6.25-12.5 mg 3 times/day in conjunction with cardiac glycoside and diuretic therapy; initial dose depends upon patient's fluid/electrolyte status

Target dose: 50 mg 3 times/day

LVD after MI: Initial dose: 6.25 mg followed by 12.5 mg 3 times/day; then increase to 25 mg 3 times/day during next several days and then over next several weeks to target dose of 50 mg 3 times/day

Diabetic nephropathy: 25 mg 3 times/day; other antihypertensives often given concurrently

Dosing adjustment in renal impairment:

Cl_{cr} 10-50 mL/minute: Administer at 75% of normal dose.

Cl_{cr} <10 mL/minute: Administer at 50% of normal dose.

Note: Smaller dosages given every 8-12 hours are indicated in patients with renal dysfunction; renal function and leukocyte count should be carefully monitored during therapy.

Hemodialysis: Moderately dialyzable (20% to 50%); administer dose postdialysis or administer 25% to 35% supplemental dose.

Peritoneal dialysis: Supplemental dose is not necessary.

Mechanism of Action Competitive inhibitor of angiotensin-converting enzyme (ACE); prevents conversion of angiotensin I to angiotensin II, a potent vasoconstrictor; results in lower levels of angiotensin II which causes an increase in plasma renin activity and a reduction in aldosterone secretion

Contraindications Hypersensitivity to captopril or any component of the formulation; angioedema related to previous treatment with an ACE inhibitor; idiopathic or hereditary angioedema; bilateral renal artery stenosis; pregnancy (2nd or 3rd trimester)

Warnings/Precautions Anaphylactic reactions can occur. Angioedema can occur at any time during treatment (especially following first dose). It may involve head and neck (potentially affecting the airway) or the intestine (presenting with abdominal pain). Prolonged monitoring may be required especially if tongue, glottis, or larynx are involved as they are associated with airway obstruction. Those with a history of airway surgery in this situation have a higher risk. Careful blood pressure monitoring with first dose (hypotension can occur especially in volume-depleted patients). **[U.S. Boxed Warning]: Based on human data, ACEIs can cause injury and death to the developing fetus when used in the second and third trimesters. ACEIs should be discontinued as soon as possible once pregnancy is detected.** Use with caution in collagen vascular diseases; valvular stenosis (particularly aortic stenosis); hyperkalemia; or before, during, or immediately after anesthesia. Avoid rapid dosage escalation which may lead to renal insufficiency. Hyperkalemia may rarely occur. Rare toxicities associated with ACE inhibitors include cholestatic jaundice (which may progress to hepatic necrosis) and neutropenia/agranulocytosis with myeloid hyperplasia. May be associated with deterioration of renal function and/or increases in serum creatinine, particularly in patients dependent on renin-angiotensin-aldosterone system. Use with caution in unilateral renal artery stenosis and pre-existing renal insufficiency; if patient has renal impairment then a baseline WBC with differential and serum creatinine should be evaluated and monitored closely during the first 3 months of therapy. Hypersensitivity reactions may be seen during hemodialysis with high-flux dialysis membranes (eg, AN69).

Use with caution and decrease dosage in patients with renal impairment (especially renal artery stenosis), severe CHF, or with coadministered diuretic therapy; experience in children is limited. Severe hypotension may occur in patients who are sodium and/or volume depleted; initiate lower doses and monitor closely when starting therapy in these patients. ACE inhibitors may be preferred agents in elderly patients with CHF and diabetes mellitus (diabetic proteinuria is reduced, minimal CNS effects, and enhanced insulin sensitivity); however, due to decreased renal function, tolerance must be carefully monitored.

Drug Interactions
Cytochrome P450 Effect: Substrate of CYP2D6 (major)

Increased Effect/Toxicity: Potassium supplements, co-trimoxazole (high dose), angiotensin II receptor antagonists (candesartan, losartan, irbesartan, etc), or potassium-sparing diuretics (amiloride, spironolactone, triamterene) may result in elevated serum potassium levels when combined with captopril. CYP2D6 inhibitors may increase the levels/effects of captopril; example inhibitors include chlorpromazine, delavirdine, fluoxetine, miconazole, paroxetine, pergolide, quinidine, quinine, ritonavir, and ropinirole. ACE inhibitor effects may be increased by phenothiazines or probenecid (increases levels of captopril). ACE inhibitors may increase serum concentrations/effects of lithium. ACE inhibitors may enhance the adverse/toxic effects (nitritoid reaction) of gold sodium thiomalate.

Diuretics have additive hypotensive effects with ACE inhibitors, and hypovolemia increases the potential for adverse renal effects of ACE inhibitors. In patients with compromised renal function, coadministration with NSAIDs may result in further deterioration of renal function. Allopurinol and ACE inhibitors may cause a higher risk of hypersensitivity reaction when taken concurrently.

Decreased Effect: Aspirin (high dose) may reduce the therapeutic effects of ACE inhibitors; at low dosages this does not appear to be significant. Rifampin may decrease the effect of ACE inhibitors. Antacids may decrease the bioavailability of ACE inhibitors (may be more likely to occur with captopril); separate administration times by 1-2 hours. NSAIDs, specifically indomethacin, may reduce the hypotensive effects of ACE inhibitors. More likely to occur in low renin or volume-dependent hypertensive patients.

Ethanol/Nutrition/Herb Interactions
Food: Captopril serum concentrations may be decreased if taken with food. Long-term use of captopril may result in a zinc deficiency which can result in a decrease in taste perception.

Herb/Nutraceutical: Avoid dong quai if using for hypertension (has estrogenic activity). Avoid ephedra, yohimbe, ginseng (may worsen hypertension). Avoid garlic (may have increased antihypertensive effect).

Dietary Considerations Should be taken at least 1 hour before or 2 hours after eating.

Pharmacodynamics/Kinetics
Onset of action: Peak effect: Blood pressure reduction: 1-1.5 hours after dose

Duration: Dose related, may require several weeks of therapy before full hypotensive effect

Absorption: 60% to 75%; reduced 30% to 40% by food

Protein binding: 25% to 30%

Metabolism: 50%

Half-life elimination (renal and cardiac function dependent):
Adults, healthy volunteers: 1.9 hours; Congestive heart failure: 2.06 hours; Anuria: 20-40 hours

Excretion: Urine (95%) within 24 hours

Pregnancy Risk Factor C (1st trimester)/D (2nd and 3rd trimesters)

Dosage Forms
Tablet: 12.5 mg, 25 mg, 50 mg, 100 mg
Capoten®: 12.5 mg, 25 mg, 50 mg, 100 mg

Captopril and Hydrochlorothiazide
(KAP toe pril & hye droe klor oh THYE a zide)

Related Information
Captopril on page 269
Cardiovascular Diseases on page 1726
Hydrochlorothiazide on page 819
(Continued)

Captopril and Hydrochlorothiazide *(Continued)*

U.S. Brand Names Capozide®
Canadian Brand Names Capozide®
Mexican Brand Names Capozide
Generic Available Yes
Index Terms Hydrochlorothiazide and Captopril
Pharmacologic Category Antihypertensive Agent, Combination
Use Management of hypertension and treatment of congestive heart failure
Local Anesthetic/Vasoconstrictor Precautions No information available to require special precautions
Effects on Dental Treatment No significant effects or complications reported
Common Adverse Effects See individual agents.
Mechanism of Action Captopril is a competitive inhibitor of angiotensin-converting enzyme (ACE); prevents conversion of angiotensin I to angiotensin II, a potent vasoconstrictor. This results in lower levels of angiotensin II which causes an increase in plasma renin activity and a reduction in aldosterone secretion. Hydrochlorothiazide inhibits sodium reabsorption in the distal tubules causing increased excretion of sodium and water as well as potassium and hydrogen ions.
Drug Interactions
  Cytochrome P450 Effect: Captopril: **Substrate** of CYP2D6 (major)
  Increased Effect/Toxicity: See individual agents.
  Decreased Effect: See individual agents.
Pharmacodynamics/Kinetics See individual agents.
Pregnancy Risk Factor C/D (2nd and 3rd trimesters)

Capzasin-HP® [OTC] *see* Capsaicin *on page 268*
Capzasin-P® [OTC] *see* Capsaicin *on page 268*
Carac™ *see* Fluorouracil *on page 713*
Carafate® *see* Sucralfate *on page 1499*

Carbachol *(KAR ba kole)*

U.S. Brand Names Carbastat® [DSC]; Isopto® Carbachol; Miostat®
Canadian Brand Names Isopto® Carbachol; Miostat®
Generic Available No
Index Terms Carbacholine; Carbamylcholine Chloride
Pharmacologic Category Cholinergic Agonist; Ophthalmic Agent, Antiglaucoma; Ophthalmic Agent, Miotic
Use Lowers intraocular pressure in the treatment of glaucoma; cause miosis during surgery
Local Anesthetic/Vasoconstrictor Precautions No information available to require special precautions
Effects on Dental Treatment Key adverse event(s) related to dental treatment: Increased salivation.
Mechanism of Action Synthetic direct-acting cholinergic agent that causes miosis by stimulating muscarinic receptors in the eye
Pregnancy Risk Factor C

Carbacholine *see* Carbachol *on page 272*

Carbamazepine *(kar ba MAZ e peen)*

Related Information
  Temporomandibular Dysfunction (TMD) *on page 1822*
U.S. Brand Names Carbatrol®; Epitol®; Equetro™; Tegretol®; Tegretol®-XR
Canadian Brand Names Apo-Carbamazepine®; Gen-Carbamazepine CR; Mapezine®; Novo-Carbamaz; Nu-Carbamazepine; PMS-Carbamazepine; Taro-Carbamazepine Chewable; Tegretol®
Mexican Brand Names Carbazep; Carbazina; Clostedal; Neugeron; Nordotol; Tegretol
Generic Available Yes: Excludes capsule (extended release), tablet (extended release)
Index Terms CBZ; SPD417
Pharmacologic Category Anticonvulsant, Miscellaneous
Dental Use Pain relief of trigeminal or glossopharyngeal neuralgia
Use
  Carbatrol®, Tegretol®, Tegretol®-XR: Partial seizures with complex symptomatology (psychomotor, temporal lobe), generalized tonic-clonic seizures (grand mal), mixed seizure patterns, trigeminal neuralgia
  Equetro™: Acute manic and mixed episodes associated with bipolar 1 disorder

Unlabeled/Investigational Use Treatment of resistant schizophrenia, ethanol withdrawal, restless leg syndrome, psychotic behavior associated with dementia, post-traumatic stress disorders

Local Anesthetic/Vasoconstrictor Precautions No information available to require special precautions

Effects on Dental Treatment Key adverse event(s) related to dental treatment: Xerostomia (normal salivary flow resumes upon discontinuation).

Significant Adverse Effects Frequency not defined, unless otherwise specified.

Cardiovascular: Arrhythmias, AV block, bradycardia, chest pain (bipolar use), CHF, edema, hyper-/hypotension, lymphadenopathy, syncope, thromboembolism, thrombophlebitis

Central nervous system: Amnesia (bipolar use), anxiety (bipolar use), aseptic meningitis (case report), ataxia (bipolar use 15%), confusion, depression (bipolar use), dizziness (bipolar use 44%), fatigue, headache (bipolar use 22%), sedation, slurred speech, somnolence (bipolar use 32%)

Dermatologic: Alopecia, alterations in skin pigmentation, erythema multiforme, exfoliative dermatitis, photosensitivity reaction, pruritus (bipolar use 8%), purpura, rash, Stevens-Johnson syndrome, toxic epidermal necrolysis, urticaria

Endocrine & metabolic: Chills, fever, hyponatremia, syndrome of inappropriate ADH secretion (SIADH)

Gastrointestinal: Abdominal pain, anorexia, constipation, diarrhea, dyspepsia (bipolar use), gastric distress, nausea (bipolar use 29%), pancreatitis, vomiting (bipolar use 18%), xerostomia (bipolar use)

Genitourinary: Azotemia, impotence, renal failure, urinary frequency, urinary retention

Hematologic: Acute intermittent porphyria, agranulocytosis, aplastic anemia, bone marrow suppression, eosinophilia, leukocytosis, leukopenia, pancytopenia, thrombocytopenia

Hepatic: Abnormal liver function tests, hepatic failure, hepatitis, jaundice

Neuromuscular & skeletal: Back pain, pain (bipolar use 12%), peripheral neuritis, weakness

Ocular: Blurred vision, conjunctivitis, lens opacities, nystagmus

Otic: Hyperacusis, tinnitus

Miscellaneous: Diaphoresis, hypersensitivity (including multiorgan reactions, may include disorders mimicking lymphoma, eosinophilia, hepatosplenomegaly, vasculitis); infection (bipolar use 12%)

Dental Usual Dosing Trigeminal or glossopharyngeal neuralgia: Oral:

Adults: Initial: 100 mg twice daily with food, gradually increasing in increments of 100 mg twice daily as needed

Maintenance: Usual: 400-800 mg daily in 2 divided doses; maximum dose: 1200 mg/day

Dosage Dosage must be adjusted according to patient's response and serum concentrations. Administer tablets (chewable or conventional) in 2-3 divided doses daily and suspension in 4 divided doses daily. Oral:

Epilepsy:

Children:

<6 years: Initial: 10-20 mg/kg/day divided twice or 3 times daily as tablets or 4 times/day as suspension; increase dose every week until optimal response and therapeutic levels are achieved

Maintenance dose: Divide into 3-4 doses daily (tablets or suspension); maximum recommended dose: 35 mg/kg/day

6-12 years: Initial: 100 mg twice daily (tablets or extended release tablets) or 50 mg of suspension 4 times/day (200 mg/day); increase by up to 100 mg/day at weekly intervals using a twice daily regimen of extended release tablets or 3-4 times daily regimen of other formulations until optimal response and therapeutic levels are achieved

Maintenance: Usual: 400-800 mg/day; maximum recommended dose: 1000 mg/day

Note: Children <12 years who receive ≥400 mg/day of carbamazepine may be converted to extended release capsules (Carbatrol®) using the same total daily dosage divided twice daily

Children >12 years and Adults: Initial: 200 mg twice daily (tablets, extended release tablets, or extended release capsules) or 100 mg of suspension 4 times/day (400 mg daily); increase by up to 200 mg/day at weekly intervals using a twice daily regimen of extended release tablets or capsules, or a 3-4 times/day regimen of other formulations until optimal response and therapeutic levels are achieved; usual dose: 800-1200 mg/day

Maximum recommended doses:

Children 12-15 years: 1000 mg/day

Children >15 years: 1200 mg/day

(Continued)

Carbamazepine *(Continued)*

Adults: 1600 mg/day; however, some patients have required up to 1.6-2.4 g/day

Trigeminal or glossopharyngeal neuralgia: Adults: Initial: 100 mg twice daily with food, gradually increasing in increments of 100 mg twice daily as needed

Maintenance: Usual: 400-800 mg daily in 2 divided doses; maximum dose: 1200 mg/day

Bipolar disorder: Adults: Initial: 400 mg/day in divided doses, twice daily; may adjust by 200 mg daily increments; maximum dose: 1600 mg/day.

Note: Equetro™ is the only formulation specifically approved by the FDA for the managment of bipolar disorder.

Mechanism of Action In addition to anticonvulsant effects, carbamazepine has anticholinergic, antineuralgic, antidiuretic, muscle relaxant, antimanic, antidepressive, and antiarrhythmic properties; may depress activity in the nucleus ventralis of the thalamus or decrease synaptic transmission or decrease summation of temporal stimulation leading to neural discharge by limiting influx of sodium ions across cell membrane or other unknown mechanisms; stimulates the release of ADH and potentiates its action in promoting reabsorption of water; chemically related to tricyclic antidepressants

Contraindications Hypersensitivity to carbamazepine, tricyclic antidepressants, or any component of the formulation; bone marrow depression; with or within 14 days of MAO inhibitor use

Warnings/Precautions [U.S. Boxed Warning]: Potentially fatal blood cell abnormalities have been reported. Patients with a previous history of adverse hematologic reaction to any drug may be at increased risk. Administer carbamazepine with caution to patients with history of cardiac damage, hepatic or renal disease. When used to treat bipolar disorder, the smallest effective dose is suggested to reduce the risk for overdose/suicide; high-risk patients should be monitored. Prescription should be written for the smallest quantity consistent with good patient care. Actuation of latent psychosis is possible. Potentially serious, sometimes fatal multiorgan hypersensitivity reactions have been reported with some antiepileptic drugs; monitor for signs and symptoms of possible disparate manifestations associated with lymphatic, hepatic, renal, and/or hematologic organ systems; gradual discontinuation and conversion to alternate therapy may be required.

Carbamazepine is not effective in absence, myoclonic, or akinetic seizures; exacerbation of certain seizure types have been seen after initiation of carbamazepine therapy in children with mixed seizure disorders. Abrupt discontinuation is not recommended in patients being treated for seizures. Dizziness or drowsiness may occur; caution should be used when performing tasks which require alertness until the effects are known. Effects with other sedative drugs or ethanol may be potentiated. Coadministration of carbamazepine and delavirdine may lead to loss of virologic response and possible resistance. Elderly may have increased risk of SIADH-like syndrome. Carbamazepine has mild anticholinergic activity; use with caution in patients with increased intraocular pressure, or sensitivity to anticholinergic effects. Severe dermatologic reactions, including toxic epidermal necrolysis and Stevens-Johnson syndrome, although rarely reported, have resulted in fatalities. Discontinue if there are any signs of hypersensitivity.

Drug Interactions Substrate of CYP2C8 (minor), 3A4 (major); **Induces** CYP1A2 (strong), 2B6 (strong), 2C8 (strong), 2C9 (strong), 2C19 (strong), 3A4 (strong)

Acetaminophen: Carbamazepine may enhance hepatotoxic potential of acetaminophen; risk is greater in acetaminophen overdose.

Antimalarial drugs (chloroquine, mefloquine): Concomitant use with carbamazepine may reduce seizure control by lowering plasma levels; monitor.

Antipsychotics: Carbamazepine may decrease the serum levels/effects of antipsychotics (typical and atypical); monitor for altered response; dose adjustment may be needed.

Barbiturates: May reduce serum concentrations of carbamazepine; monitor.

Benzodiazepines: Serum concentrations and effect of benzodiazepines may be reduced by carbamazepine; monitor for decreased effect.

Calcium channel blockers: Diltiazem and verapamil may increase carbamazepine levels, due to enzyme inhibition (see below); other calcium channel blockers (felodipine) may be decreased by carbamazepine due to enzyme induction.

Chlorpromazine: **Note:** Carbamazepine suspension is incompatible with chlorpromazine solution. Schedule carbamazepine suspension at least 1-2 hours apart from other liquid medicinals.

Corticosteroids: Metabolism may be increased by carbamazepine.

Cyclosporine (and other immunosuppressants): Carbamazepine may enhance the metabolism of immunosuppressants, decreasing its clinical effect; includes both cyclosporine and tacrolimus.

CYP1A2 substrates: Carbamazepine may decrease the levels/effects of CYP1A2 substrates. Example substrates include aminophylline, estrogens, fluvoxamine, mirtazapine, ropinirole, and theophylline.

CYP2B6 substrates: Carbamazepine may decrease the levels/effects of CYP2B6 substrates. Example substrates include bupropion, efavirenz, promethazine, selegiline, and sertraline.

CYP2C8 substrates: Carbamazepine may decrease the levels/effects of CYP2C8 substrates. Example substrates include amiodarone, paclitaxel, pioglitazone, repaglinide, and rosiglitazone.

CYP2C9 substrates: Carbamazepine may decrease the levels/effects of CYP2C9 substrates. Example substrates include bosentan, celecoxib, dapsone, fluoxetine, glimepiride, glipizide, losartan, montelukast, nateglinide, paclitaxel, phenytoin, sulfonamides, trimethoprim, warfarin, and zafirlukast.

CYP2C19 substrates: Carbamazepine may decrease the levels/effects of CYP2C19 substrates. Example substrates include citalopram, diazepam, methsuximide, phenytoin, propranolol, proton pump inhibitors, sertraline, and voriconazole.

CYP3A4 inducers: CYP3A4 inducers may decrease the levels/effects of carbamazepine. Example inducers include aminoglutethimide, nafcillin, nevirapine, phenobarbital, phenytoin, and rifamycins. Carbamazepine may induce its own metabolism.

CYP3A4 inhibitors: May increase the levels/effects of carbamazepine. Example inhibitors include azole antifungals, clarithromycin, diclofenac, doxycycline, erythromycin, imatinib, isoniazid, nefazodone, nicardipine, propofol, protease inhibitors, quinidine, telithromycin, and verapamil.

CYP3A4 substrates: Carbamazepine may decrease the levels/effects of CYP3A4 substrates. Example substrates include benzodiazepines, calcium channel blockers, clarithromycin, cyclosporine, erythromycin, estrogens, mirtazapine, nateglinide, nefazodone, nevirapine, protease inhibitors, tacrolimus, and venlafaxine.

Danazol: May increase serum concentrations of carbamazepine; monitor.

Delavirdine: May lead to loss of virologic response and possible resistance.

Doxycycline: Carbamazepine may enhance the metabolism of doxycycline, decreasing its clinical effect.

Ethosuximide: Serum levels may be reduced by carbamazepine.

Felbamate: May increase carbamazepine levels and toxicity (increased epoxide metabolite concentrations); carbamazepine may decrease felbamate levels due to enzyme induction.

Immunosuppressants: Carbamazepine may enhance the metabolism of immunosuppressants, decreasing its clinical effect; includes both cyclosporine and tacrolimus.

Isoniazid: May increase the serum concentrations and toxicity of carbamazepine; in addition, carbamazepine may increase the hepatic toxicity of isoniazid (INH).

Isotretinoin: May decrease the effect of carbamazepine.

Lamotrigine: Increases the epoxide metabolite of carbamazepine resulting in toxicity; carbamazepine increases the metabolism of lamotrigine.

Lithium: Neurotoxicity may result in patients receiving concurrent carbamazepine.

Loxapine: May increase concentrations of epoxide metabolite and toxicity of carbamazepine.

Methadone: Carbamazepine may enhance the metabolism of methadone resulting in methadone withdrawal.

Methylphenidate: concurrent use of carbamazepine may reduce the therapeutic effect of methylphenidate; limited documentation; monitor for decreased effect.

Neuromuscular blocking agents, nondepolarizing: Effects may be of shorter duration when administered to patients receiving carbamazepine.

Oral contraceptives: Metabolism may be increased by carbamazepine, resulting in a loss of efficacy.

Phenytoin: Carbamazepine levels may be decreased by phenytoin. Metabolism of phenytoin may be altered by carbamazepine; phenytoin levels may be increased or decreased.

SSRIs: Metabolism may be increased by carbamazepine (due to enzyme induction).

Theophylline: Serum levels may be reduced by carbamazepine.

Thioridazine: **Note:** Carbamazepine suspension is incompatible with thioridazine liquid. Schedule carbamazepine suspension at least 1-2 hours apart from other liquid medicinals.

Thyroid: Serum levels may be reduced by carbamazepine.

(Continued)

Carbamazepine *(Continued)*

Tiagabine: Carbamazepine may reduce the serum concentrations of tiagabine; monitor.

Topiramate: Carbamazepine may reduce the serum concentrations of topiramate; monitor.

Tramadol: Tramadol's risk of seizures may be increased with TCAs (carbamazepine may be associated with similar risk due to chemical similarity to TCAs).

Trazodone: Serum concentrations may be reduced by carbamazepine; monitor.

Tricyclic antidepressants: May increase serum concentrations of carbamazepine; carbamazepine may decrease concentrations of tricyclics due to enzyme induction. The serum concentrations of clomipramine are increased by carbamazepine.

Valproic acid: Serum levels may be reduced by carbamazepine; carbamazepine levels may also be altered by valproic acid.

Warfarin: Carbamazepine may inhibit the hypoprothrombinemic effects of oral anticoagulants via increased metabolism; this combination should generally be avoided.

Zonisamide: Carbamazepine may reduce the serum concentrations of zonisamide; monitor.

Ethanol/Nutrition/Herb Interactions

Ethanol: Avoid ethanol (may increase CNS depression).

Food: Carbamazepine serum levels may be increased if taken with food. Carbamazepine serum concentration may be increased if taken with grapefruit juice; avoid concurrent use.

Herb/Nutraceutical: Avoid evening primrose (seizure threshold decreased). Avoid valerian, St John's wort, kava kava, gotu kola (may increase CNS depression).

Dietary Considerations Drug may cause GI upset, take with large amount of water or food to decrease GI upset. May need to split doses to avoid GI upset.

Pharmacodynamics/Kinetics

Absorption: Slow

Distribution: V_d: Neonates: 1.5 L/kg; Children: 1.9 L/kg; Adults: 0.59-2 L/kg

Protein binding: Carbamazepine: 75% to 90%, may be decreased in newborns; Epoxide metabolite: 50%

Metabolism: Hepatic via CYP3A4 to active epoxide metabolite; induces hepatic enzymes to increase metabolism

Bioavailability: 85%

Half-life elimination:

Carbamazepine: Initial: 18-55 hours; Multiple doses: Children: 8-14 hours; Adults: 12-17 hours

Epoxide metabolite: Initial: 25-43 hours

Time to peak, serum: Unpredictable:

Immediate release: Suspension: 1.5 hour; tablet: 4-5 hours

Extended release: Carbatrol®, Equetro™: 12-26 hours (single dose), 4-8 hours (multiple doses); Tegretol®-XR: 3-12 hours

Excretion: Urine 72% (1% to 3% as unchanged drug); feces (28%)

Pregnancy Risk Factor D

Lactation Enters breast milk/not recommended (AAP rates "compatible")

Breast-Feeding Considerations Carbamazepine and its metabolites are found in breast milk. The manufacturer does not recommend use while breast-feeding. However, AAP rates this medication "compatible" in breast-feeding.

Dosage Forms Excipient information presented when available (limited, particularly for generics); consult specific product labeling.

Capsule, extended release:

Carbatrol®, Equetro™: 100 mg, 200 mg, 300 mg

Suspension, oral: 100 mg/5 mL (10 mL, 450 mL)

Tegretol®: 100 mg/5 mL (450 mL) [citrus vanilla flavor]

Tablet: 200 mg

Epitol®, Tegretol®: 200 mg

Tablet, chewable: 100 mg

Tegretol®: 100 mg

Tablet, extended release:

Tegretol®-XR: 100 mg, 200 mg, 400 mg

Carbamide *see* Urea *on page 1632*

Carbamide Peroxide *(KAR ba mide per OKS ide)*

Related Information

Oral Rinse Products *on page 1941*

U.S. Brand Names Cankaid® [OTC]; Debrox® [OTC]; Dent's Ear Wax [OTC]; E•R•O [OTC]; Gly-Oxide® [OTC]; Murine® Ear Wax Removal System [OTC]; Orajel® Perioseptic® Spot Treatment [OTC]

Generic Available Yes

Index Terms Urea Peroxide

Pharmacologic Category Anti-inflammatory, Locally Applied; Otic Agent, Cerumenolytic

Dental Use Relief of minor inflammation of gums, oral mucosal surfaces, and lips (including canker sores and dental irritation)

Use Relief of minor inflammation of gums, oral mucosal surfaces, and lips including canker sores and dental irritation; emulsify and disperse ear wax

Local Anesthetic/Vasoconstrictor Precautions No information available to require special precautions

Effects on Dental Treatment No significant effects or complications reported

Significant Adverse Effects Frequency not defined.
Dermatologic: Rash
Local: Irritation, redness
Miscellaneous: Superinfection

Dental Usual Dosing Minor inflammation of gums, oral mucosal surfaces and lips: Children and Adults: Topical: Oral solution (should not be used for >7 days): Apply several drops undiluted on affected area 4 times/day after meals and at bedtime; expectorate after 2-3 minutes **or** place 10 drops onto tongue, mix with saliva, swish for several minutes, expectorate

Dosage Children and Adults:
Oral: Inflammation/dental irritation: Solution (should not be used for >7 days): Oral preparation should not be used in children <2 years of age; apply several drops undiluted on affected area 4 times/day after meals and at bedtime; expectorate after 2-3 minutes **or** place 10 drops onto tongue, mix with saliva, swish for several minutes, expectorate

Otic:
Children <12 years: Tilt head sideways and individualize the dose according to patient size; 3 drops (range: 1-5 drops) twice daily for up to 4 days, tip of applicator should not enter ear canal; keep drops in ear for several minutes by keeping head tilted and placing cotton in ear

Children ≥12 years and Adults: Tilt head sideways and instill 5-10 drops twice daily up to 4 days, tip of applicator should not enter ear canal; keep drops in ear for several minutes by keeping head tilted and placing cotton in ear

Mechanism of Action Carbamide peroxide releases hydrogen peroxide which serves as a source of nascent oxygen upon contact with catalase; deodorant action is probably due to inhibition of odor-causing bacteria; softens impacted cerumen due to its foaming action

Contraindications Hypersensitivity to carbamide peroxide or any component of the formulation; otic preparation should not be used in patients with a perforated tympanic membrane; ear drainage, ear pain, or rash in the ear

Warnings/Precautions
Oral: With prolonged use of oral carbamide peroxide, there is a potential for overgrowth of opportunistic organisms, damage to periodontal tissues, and delayed wound healing; should not be used for longer than 7 days. Not for OTC use in children <2 years of age.
Otic: Do not use if ear drainage or discharge, ear pain, irritation, or rash in ear. Should not be used for longer than 4 days. Not for OTC use in children <12 years of age.

Drug Interactions No data reported

Pharmacodynamics/Kinetics Onset of action: ~24 hours

Pregnancy Risk Factor C

Dosage Forms Excipient information presented when available (limited, particularly for generics); consult specific product labeling.
Solution, oral: 10% (60 mL)
Cankaid®: 10% (22 mL) [in anhydrous glycerol]
Gly-Oxide®: 10% (15 mL, 60 mL) [contains glycerin]
Orajel® Perioseptic® Spot Treatment: 15% (13.3 mL) [contains anhydrous glycerin]
Solution, otic: 6.5% (15 mL)
Debrox®: 6.5% (15 mL, 30 mL) [contains propylene glycol]
Dent's Ear Wax: 6.5% (3.7 mL) [contains glycerin]
E•R•O: 6.5% (15 mL)
Murine® Ear Wax Removal System: 6.5% (15 mL) [contains alcohol 6.3% and glycerin]

Carbaxefed DM RF [DSC] *see* Carbinoxamine, Pseudoephedrine, and Dextromethorphan *on page 282*

Carbaxefed RF [DSC] *see* Carbinoxamine and Pseudoephedrine *on page 282*

Carbenicillin (kar ben i SIL in)

U.S. Brand Names Geocillin®

Generic Available No

Index Terms Carbenicillin Indanyl Sodium; Carindacillin

Pharmacologic Category Antibiotic, Penicillin

Use Treatment of serious urinary tract infections and prostatitis caused by susceptible gram-negative aerobic bacilli

Local Anesthetic/Vasoconstrictor Precautions No information available to require special precautions

Effects on Dental Treatment Key adverse event(s) related to dental treatment: Unpleasant taste and glossitis. Prolonged use of penicillins may lead to development of oral candidiasis.

Common Adverse Effects

>10%: Gastrointestinal: Diarrhea

1% to 10%: Gastrointestinal: Nausea, bad taste, vomiting, flatulence, glossitis

Mechanism of Action Inhibits bacterial cell wall synthesis by binding to one or more of the penicillin-binding proteins (PBPs) which in turn inhibits the final transpeptidation step of peptidoglycan synthesis in bacterial cell walls, thus inhibiting cell wall biosynthesis. Bacteria eventually lyse due to ongoing activity of cell wall autolytic enzymes (autolysins and murein hydrolases) while cell wall assembly is arrested.

Drug Interactions

Increased Effect/Toxicity: Increased bleeding effects if taken with high doses of heparin or oral anticoagulants. Aminoglycosides may be synergistic against selected organisms. Penicillins may increase the exposure to methotrexate during concurrent therapy; monitor. Probenecid and disulfiram may increase levels of penicillins (carbenicillin).

Decreased Effect: Decreased effectiveness with tetracyclines. Although anecdotal reports suggest oral contraceptive efficacy could be reduced by penicillins, this has been refuted by more rigorous scientific and clinical data.

Pharmacodynamics/Kinetics

Absorption: 30% to 40%

Distribution: Crosses placenta; small amounts enter breast milk; distributes into bile; low concentrations attained in CSF

Protein binding: ~50%

Half-life elimination: Children: 0.8-1.8 hours; Adults: 1-1.5 hours, prolonged to 10-20 hours with renal insufficiency

Time to peak, serum: Normal renal function: 0.5-2 hours; concentrations are inadequate for treatment of systemic infections

Excretion: Urine (~80% to 99% as unchanged drug)

Pregnancy Risk Factor B

Carbenicillin Indanyl Sodium *see* Carbenicillin *on page 278*

Carbetapentane and Chlorpheniramine (kar bay ta PEN tane & klor fen IR a meen)

Related Information

Chlorpheniramine *on page 338*

U.S. Brand Names Tannate 12 S; Tannic-12; Tannic-12 S; Tannihist-12 RF; Tussi12®; Tussi-12 S™; Tussizone-12 RF™

Generic Available Yes

Index Terms Carbetapentane Tannate and Chlorpheniramine Tannate; Chlorpheniramine and Carbetapentane

Pharmacologic Category Antihistamine/Antitussive

Use Symptomatic relief of cough associated with upper respiratory tract conditions, such as the common cold, bronchitis, bronchial asthma

Local Anesthetic/Vasoconstrictor Precautions No information available to require special precautions

Effects on Dental Treatment Key adverse event(s) related to dental treatment: Dry mucous membranes. Chronic use of antihistamines will inhibit salivary flow, particularly in elderly patients; this may contribute to periodontal disease and oral discomfort.

Common Adverse Effects Frequency not defined.

Central nervous system: Drowsiness, excitation (children), sedation

Gastrointestinal: GI motility decreased, dry mucous membranes

Mechanism of Action Carbetapentane is a nonopioid cough suppressant; chlorpheniramine is an H$_1$-receptor antagonist

Drug Interactions

Increased Effect/Toxicity: Sedative effects of CNS depressants may be potentiated. MAO inhibitors may increase and prolong anticholinergic effects. Avoid use with and within 14 days of treatment with MAO. inhibitors

Pharmacodynamics/Kinetics

Carbetapentane: Data not available

Chlorpheniramine: See individual agents

Pregnancy Risk Factor C

Carbetapentane and Phenylephrine
(kar bay ta PEN tane & fen il EF rin)

U.S. Brand Names L-All 12

Generic Available No

Index Terms Phenylephrine Tannate and Carbetapentane Tannate

Pharmacologic Category Antitussive; Antitussive/Decongestant; Sympathomimetic

Use Symptomatic relief of upper respiratory tract conditions such as the common cold, bronchial asthma, and bronchitis (acute and chronic)

Local Anesthetic/Vasoconstrictor Precautions Use with caution since phenylephrine is a sympathomimetic amine which could interact with epinephrine to cause a pressor response

Effects on Dental Treatment Key adverse event(s) related to dental treatment: Phenylephrine: Tachycardia, palpitations (use vasoconstrictor with caution), and xerostomia (normal salivary flow resumes upon discontinuation).

Common Adverse Effects Also see Phenylephrine monograph. Frequency not defined.

Central nervous system: Drowsiness, sedation

Gastrointestinal: Xerostomia

Mechanism of Action Carbetapentane is a nonopioid cough suppressant; phenylephrine is a sympathomimetic agent (primarily alpha), decongestant

Drug Interactions

Increased Effect/Toxicity: Sedative effects of CNS depressants may be potentiated. Anticholinergic and sympathomimetic effects of MAO inhibitors may be increased and prolonged; avoid use with and within 14 days of treatment with MAO inhibitors. Alpha-/Beta-Agonists may enhance the arrhythmogenic effect of phenothiazines; thioridazine is of most concern. Concurrent use of other sympathomimetics may lead to increased stimulatory and cardiovascular effects; includes methylphenidate and dextroamphetamine.

Decreased Effect: The effects of antihypertensive drugs may be decreased.

Pregnancy Risk Factor C

Carbetapentane, Ephedrine, Phenylephrine, and Chlorpheniramine *see* Chlorpheniramine, Ephedrine, Phenylephrine, and Carbetapentane *on page 341*

Carbetapentane, Guaifenesin, and Phenylephrine
(kar bay ta PEN tane, gwye FEN e sin, & fen il EF rin)

U.S. Brand Names Carbetaplex; Gentex LQ; Levall™; Phencarb GG

Generic Available Yes

Index Terms Guaifenesin, Carbetapentane Citrate, and Phenylephrine Hydrochloride; Phenylephrine Hydrochloride, Carbetapentane Citrate, and Guaifenesin

Pharmacologic Category Antitussive; Expectorant; Expectorant/Decongestant/Antitussive; Sympathomimetic

Use Relief of nonproductive cough accompanying respiratory tract congestion associated with the common cold, influenza, sinusitis, and bronchitis

Local Anesthetic/Vasoconstrictor Precautions Use with caution since phenylephrine is a sympathomimetic amine which could interact with epinephrine to cause a pressor response

Effects on Dental Treatment Key adverse event(s) related to dental treatment:

Guaifenesin: No significant effects or complications reported

Phenylephrine: Tachycardia, palpitations (use vasoconstrictor with caution)

Common Adverse Effects Frequency not defined. Also see individual agents.

Central nervous system: Dizziness, drowsiness, excitability, headache, insomnia, nervousness, mild stimulation, restlessness, weakness

Gastrointestinal: Nausea, vomiting

(Continued)

Carbetapentane, Guaifenesin, and Phenylephrine
(Continued)

Mechanism of Action
Carbetapentane is a centrally-acting nonopioid cough suppressant.
Guaifenesin is an expectorant.
Phenylephrine hydrochloride is a sympathomimetic agent (primarily alpha), decongestant.

Drug Interactions
Increased Effect/Toxicity: When used with MAO inhibitors, sympathomimetic effect may be increased.
Decreased Effect: Effects of antihypertensive agents may be decreased.

Pregnancy Risk Factor C

Carbetapentane, Phenylephrine, and Pyrilamine
(kar bay ta PEN tane, fen il EF rin, & peer II a meen)

Related Information
Phenylephrine *on page 1293*
U.S. Brand Names Tussi-12® D; Tussi-12® DS
Generic Available Yes: Suspension
Index Terms Phenylephrine Tannate, Carbetapentane Tannate, and Pyrilamine Tannate; Pyrilamine, Phenylephrine, and Carbetapentane
Pharmacologic Category Antihistamine; Antihistamine/Decongestant/Antitussive; Antitussive; Decongestant
Use Symptomatic relief of cough associated with respiratory tract conditions such as the common cold, bronchial asthma, acute and chronic bronchitis
Local Anesthetic/Vasoconstrictor Precautions Use with caution since phenylephrine is a sympathomimetic amine which could interact with epinephrine to cause a pressor response
Effects on Dental Treatment Key adverse event(s) related to dental treatment: Tachycardia, palpitations (use vasoconstrictor with caution), and xerostomia (normal salivary flow resumes upon discontinuation).
Mechanism of Action
Carbetapentane is a nonopioid cough suppressant
Phenylephrine hydrochloride is a sympathomimetic agent (primarily alpha), decongestant.
Pyrilamine is an H_1-receptor antagonist.
Pregnancy Risk Factor C

Carbetapentane Tannate and Chlorpheniramine Tannate *see* Carbetapentane and Chlorpheniramine *on page 278*

Carbetaplex *see* Carbetapentane, Guaifenesin, and Phenylephrine *on page 279*

Carbidopa (kar bi DOE pa)

U.S. Brand Names Lodosyn®
Generic Available No
Pharmacologic Category Anti-Parkinson's Agent, Dopamine Agonist
Use Given with levodopa in the treatment of parkinsonism to enable a lower dosage of levodopa to be used and a more rapid response to be obtained and to decrease side effects; for details of administration and dosage, see Levodopa; has no effect without levodopa
Local Anesthetic/Vasoconstrictor Precautions No information available to require special precautions
Effects on Dental Treatment Key adverse event(s) related to dental treatment: Orthostatic hypotension. Dopaminergic therapy in Parkinson's disease includes the use of carbidopa in combination with levodopa. Carbidopa/levodopa combination is associated with orthostatic hypotension. Patients medicated with this drug combination should be carefully assisted from the chair and observed for signs of orthostatic hypotension.

Common Adverse Effects Adverse reactions are associated with concomitant administration with levodopa

>10%: Central nervous system: Anxiety, confusion, nervousness, mental depression
1% to 10%:
Cardiovascular: Orthostatic hypotension, palpitation, cardiac arrhythmia
Central nervous system: Memory loss, insomnia, fatigue, hallucinations, ataxia, dystonic movements
Gastrointestinal: Nausea, vomiting, GI bleeding
Ocular: Blurred vision

Mechanism of Action Carbidopa is a peripheral decarboxylase inhibitor with little or no pharmacological activity when given alone in usual doses. It inhibits the peripheral decarboxylation of levodopa to dopamine; and as it does not cross the blood-brain barrier, unlike levodopa, effective brain concentrations of dopamine are produced with lower doses of levodopa. At the same time, reduced peripheral formation of dopamine reduces peripheral side-effects, notably nausea and vomiting, and cardiac arrhythmias, although the dyskinesias and adverse mental effects associated with levodopa therapy tend to develop earlier.

Pharmacodynamics/Kinetics

Absorption: 40% to 70%

Distribution: Does not cross the blood-brain barrier; in rats, reported to cross placenta and be excreted in milk

Protein binding: 36%

Half-life elimination: 1-2 hours

Excretion: Urine (as unchanged drug and metabolites)

Pregnancy Risk Factor C

Carbidopa and Levodopa *see* Levodopa and Carbidopa *on page 964*

Carbidopa, Levodopa, and Entacapone *see* Levodopa, Carbidopa, and Entacapone *on page 965*

Carbinoxamine (kar bi NOKS a meen)

U.S. Brand Names Palgic®

Generic Available No

Index Terms Carbinoxamine Maleate

Pharmacologic Category Antihistamine

Use Seasonal and perennial allergic rhinitis; vasomotor rhinitis; urticaria; decrease severity of other allergic reactions

Local Anesthetic/Vasoconstrictor Precautions No information available to require special precautions

Effects on Dental Treatment Key adverse event(s) related to dental treatment: Xerostomia (normal salivary flow resumes upon discontinuation).

Common Adverse Effects Frequency not defined.

Cardiovascular: Extrasystoles, hypotension, palpitation, tachycardia

Central nervous system: Chills, confusion, coordination impaired (most frequent), dizziness (most frequent), euphoria, excitability (children), fatigue, headache, insomnia, irritability, nervousness, neuritis, restlessness, sedation (most frequent), seizure, sleepiness (most frequent), vertigo

Dermatologic: Photosensitivity, rash, urticaria

Endocrine & metabolic: Early menses

Gastrointestinal: Anorexia, constipation, diarrhea, epigastric distress (most frequent), heartburn, nausea, vomiting, xerostomia

Genitourinary: Difficult urination, urinary frequency, urinary retention

Hematologic: Agranulocytosis, hemolytic anemia, thrombocytopenia

Neuromuscular & skeletal: Paresthesia, tremor, weakness

Ocular: Blurred vision, diplopia

Renal: Polyuria

Respiratory: Bronchial secretions thickening (most frequent), chest tightness, nasal congestion, nasopharyngeal dryness, wheezing

Miscellaneous: Hypersensitivity reactions (including anaphylactic shock), diaphoresis

Mechanism of Action Carbinoxamine competes with histamine for H_1-receptor sites on effector cells in the gastrointestinal tract, blood vessels, and respiratory tract.

Drug Interactions

Increased Effect/Toxicity: Antihistamines may increase arrhythmogenic effects of antipsychotics (phenothiazines). CNS depressants may increase the adverse/toxic effect of carbinoxamine. MAO inhibitors may increase the anticholinergic effects of carbinoxamine. Pramlintide may increase the anticholinergic effects (in the GI tract) of carbinoxamine.

Decreased Effect: Acetylcholinesterase inhibitors (central) may decrease the effect of carbinoxamine. Carbinoxamine may decrease the effect of acetylcholinesterase inhibitors (central).

Pharmacodynamics/Kinetics Half-life elimination: 10-20 hours

Pregnancy Risk Factor C

Carbinoxamine and Pseudoephedrine
(kar bi NOKS a meen & soo doe e FED rin)

Related Information
Carbinoxamine *on page 281*
Pseudoephedrine *on page 1381*

U.S. Brand Names Andehist NR Drops [DSC]; Carbaxefed RF [DSC]; Carboxine-PSE [DSC]; Cordron-D NR [DSC]; Hydro-Tussin™-CBX; Palgic®-D [DSC]; Palgic®-DS [DSC]; Pediatex™-D [DSC]; Sildec [DSC]

Generic Available Yes

Index Terms Pseudoephedrine and Carbinoxamine

Pharmacologic Category Adrenergic Agonist Agent; Antihistamine, H₁ Blocker; Decongestant

Use Seasonal and perennial allergic rhinitis; vasomotor rhinitis

Local Anesthetic/Vasoconstrictor Precautions Use with caution since pseudoephedrine is a sympathomimetic amine which could interact with epinephrine to cause a pressor response

Effects on Dental Treatment Key adverse event(s) related to dental treatment: Pseudoephedrine: Xerostomia (normal salivary flow resumes upon discontinuation).

Common Adverse Effects Frequency not defined.
Cardiovascular: Arrhythmias, cardiovascular collapse, hypertension, pallor, tachycardia
Central nervous system: Anxiety, convulsions, CNS stimulation, dizziness, excitability (children; rare), fear, hallucinations, headache, insomnia, nervousness, restlessness, sedation
Gastrointestinal: Anorexia, diarrhea, dyspepsia, nausea, vomiting, xerostomia
Neuromuscular skeletal: Tremors, weakness
Ocular: Diplopia
Renal: Dysuria, polyuria, urinary retention (with BPH)
Respiratory: Respiratory difficulty

Mechanism of Action Carbinoxamine competes with histamine for H₁-receptor sites on effector cells in the gastrointestinal tract, blood vessels, and respiratory tract; pseudoephedrine, a sympathomimetic amine and isomer of ephedrine, acts as a decongestant in respiratory tract mucous membranes with less vasoconstrictor action than ephedrine in normotensive individuals

Drug Interactions
Increased Effect/Toxicity: Increased sedation/CNS depression with barbiturates and other CNS depressants. Anticholinergic effects may be increased by MAO inhibitors, tricyclic antidepressants.
Decreased Effect: May decrease effects of antihypertensive agents.

Pregnancy Risk Factor C

Carbinoxamine, Dextromethorphan, and Pseudoephedrine *see* Carbinoxamine, Pseudoephedrine, and Dextromethorphan *on page 282*

Carbinoxamine Maleate *see* Carbinoxamine *on page 281*

Carbinoxamine, Pseudoephedrine, and Dextromethorphan
(kar bi NOKS a meen, soo doe e FED rin, & deks troe meth OR fan)

Related Information
Carbinoxamine *on page 281*
Dextromethorphan *on page 477*
Pseudoephedrine *on page 1381*

U.S. Brand Names Andehist DM NR Drops [DSC]; Carbaxefed DM RF [DSC]; Cordron-DM NR [DSC]; Pediatex™ DM [DSC]; Sildec-DM [DSC]; Tussafed® [DSC]

Generic Available Yes

Index Terms Carbinoxamine, Dextromethorphan, and Pseudoephedrine; Dextromethorphan, Carbinoxamine, and Pseudoephedrine; Dextromethorphan, Pseudoephedrine, and Carbinoxamine; Pseudoephedrine, Carbinoxamine, and Dextromethorphan; Pseudoephedrine, Dextromethorphan, and Carbinoxamine

Pharmacologic Category Antihistamine/Decongestant/Antitussive

Use Relief of coughs and upper respiratory symptoms, including nasal congestion, associated with allergy or the common cold

Local Anesthetic/Vasoconstrictor Precautions Use with caution since pseudoephedrine is a sympathomimetic amine which could interact with epinephrine to cause a pressor response

Effects on Dental Treatment Key adverse event(s) related to dental treatment: Pseudoephedrine: Xerostomia (normal salivary flow resumes upon discontinuation).

Common Adverse Effects Frequency not defined.

Cardiovascular: Arrhythmias, cardiovascular collapse, hypertension, pallor, tachycardia

Central nervous system: Anxiety, convulsions, CNS stimulation, dizziness, drowsiness, excitability (children; rare), fear, hallucinations, headache, insomnia, nervousness, restlessness, sedation

Gastrointestinal: Anorexia, diarrhea, dyspepsia, GI upset, nausea, vomiting, xerostomia

Neuromuscular skeletal: Tremors, weakness

Ocular: Diplopia

Renal: Dysuria, polyuria, urinary retention (with BPH)

Respiratory: Respiratory difficulty

Mechanism of Action Carbinoxamine competes with histamine for H_1-receptor sites on effector cells in the gastrointestinal tract, blood vessels, and respiratory tract; pseudoephedrine, a sympathomimetic amine and isomer of ephedrine, acts as a decongestant in respiratory tract mucous membranes with less vaso-constrictor action than ephedrine in normotensive individuals; dextromethorphan, a non-narcotic antitussive, increases cough threshold by its activity on the medulla oblongata.

Drug Interactions

Cytochrome P450 Effect: Dextromethorphan: **Substrate** of CYP2B6 (minor), 2C9 (minor), 2C19 (minor), 2D6 (major), 2E1 (minor), 3A4 (minor); **Inhibits** CYP2D6 (weak)

Pregnancy Risk Factor C

Carbinoxamine, Pseudoephedrine, and Hydrocodone see Hydrocodone, Carbinoxamine, and Pseudoephedrine on page 832

Carbocaine® see Mepivacaine on page 1042

Carbocaine® see Mepivacaine (Dental Anesthetic) on page 1044

Carbocaine® 2% with Neo-Cobefrin® see Mepivacaine and Levonordefrin on page 1045

Carbolic Acid see Phenol on page 1290

Carboplatin (KAR boe pla tin)

U.S. Brand Names Paraplatin® [DSC]

Canadian Brand Names Paraplatin-AQ

Mexican Brand Names Blastocarb; Carbotec; Ifacap; Paraplatin

Generic Available Yes

Index Terms CBDCA; NSC-241240

Pharmacologic Category Antineoplastic Agent, Alkylating Agent

Use Treatment of ovarian cancer

Unlabeled/Investigational Use Lung cancer, head and neck cancer, endometrial cancer, esophageal cancer, bladder cancer, breast cancer, cervical cancer, CNS tumors, germ cell tumors, osteogenic sarcoma, and high-dose therapy with stem cell/bone marrow support

Local Anesthetic/Vasoconstrictor Precautions No information available to require special precautions

Effects on Dental Treatment Key adverse event(s) related to dental treatment: Stomatitis, mucositis, and taste dysgeusia.

Common Adverse Effects Percentages reported with single-agent therapy.

>10%:

Central nervous system: Pain (23%)

Endocrine & metabolic: Hyponatremia (29% to 47%), hypomagnesemia (29% to 43%), hypocalcemia(22% to 31%), hypokalemia (20% to 28%)

Gastrointestinal: Vomiting (65% to 81%), abdominal pain (17%), nausea (10% to 15%)

Hematologic: Myelosuppression (dose related and dose limiting; nadir at ~21 days; recovery by ~28 days), leukopenia (85%; grades 3/4: 15% to 26%), anemia (71% to 90%; grades 3/4: 21%), neutropenia (67%; grades 3/4: 16% to 21%), thrombocytopenia (62%; grades 3/4: 25% to 35%)

Hepatic: Alkaline phosphatase increased (24% to 37%), AST increased (15% to 19%)

Neuromuscular & skeletal: Weakness (11%)

Renal: Creatinine clearance decreased (27%), BUN increased (14% to 22%)

1% to 10%:

Central nervous system: Neurotoxicity (5%)

Dermatologic: Alopecia (2% to 3%)

(Continued)

Carboplatin (Continued)

Gastrointestinal: Constipation (5%), diarrhea (6%), stomatitis/mucositis (1%), taste dysgeusia (1%)

Hematologic: Hemorrhagic complications (5%)

Hepatic: Bilirubin increased (5%)

Local: Pain at injection site

Neuromuscular & skeletal: Peripheral neuropathy (4% to 6%; up to 10% in older and/or previously-treated patients)

Ocular: Visual disturbance (1%)

Otic: Ototoxicity (1%)

Renal: Creatinine increased (6% to 10%)

Miscellaneous: Infection (5%), hypersensitivity (2%)

Mechanism of Action Carboplatin is an alkylating agent which covalently binds to DNA; possible cross-linking and interference with the function of DNA

Drug Interactions

Increased Effect/Toxicity: Aminoglycosides increase risk of ototoxicity and/or nephrotoxicity. When administered as sequential infusions, observational studies indicate a potential for increased toxicity when platinum derivatives (carboplatin, cisplatin) are administered before taxane derivatives (docetaxel, paclitaxel).

Pharmacodynamics/Kinetics

Distribution: V_d: 16 L/kg; into liver, kidney, skin, and tumor tissue

Protein binding: 0%; platinum is 30% irreversibly bound

Metabolism: Minimally hepatic to aquated and hydroxylated compounds

Half-life elimination: Terminal: 22-40 hours; Cl_{cr} >60 mL/minute: 2.5-5.9 hours

Excretion: Urine (~60% to 90%) within 24 hours

Pregnancy Risk Factor D

Carboprost see Carboprost Tromethamine on page 284

Carboprost Tromethamine (KAR boe prost tro METH a meen)

U.S. Brand Names Hemabate®
Canadian Brand Names Hemabate®
Generic Available No
Index Terms Carboprost; Prostaglandin F_2
Pharmacologic Category Abortifacient; Prostaglandin
Use Termination of pregnancy; treatment of refractory postpartum uterine bleeding
Unlabeled/Investigational Use Investigational: Hemorrhagic cystitis
Local Anesthetic/Vasoconstrictor Precautions No information available to require special precautions
Effects on Dental Treatment No significant effects or complications reported
Common Adverse Effects Frequency not defined. Effects due to increased smooth muscle contractility are most common.

Cardiovascular: Chest pain, flushing, hypertension, syncope, palpitation, tachycardia, tightness of chest

Central nervous system: Anxiety, chills/shivering, dizziness, drowsiness, dystonia, faintness, headache, lethargy, lightheadedness, nervousness, sleep disturbance, temperature elevation (may be drug induced or due to postabortion endometritis), vasovagal syndrome, vertigo

Dermatologic: Rash

Endocrine & metabolic: Breast tenderness, dysmenorrhea-like pain, endometritis, hot flashes, thyroid storm

Gastrointestinal: Choking sensation, diarrhea (~2/3 patients), dry throat, epigastric pain, gagging/retching, hematemesis, nausea (~1/3 patients), taste alteration, thirst, throat fullness, vomiting (~2/3 patients), xerostomia

Genitourinary: Perforated uterus, posterior cervical perforation, urinary tract infection, uterine bleeding (excessive), uterine rupture, uterine sacculation

Local: Injection site pain

Neuromuscular & skeletal: Backache, leg cramps, muscular pain, paresthesia, torticollis, weakness

Ocular: Blurred vision, eye pain, eyelid twitching

Otic: Tinnitus

Respiratory: Asthma, cough, bronchospasm, dyspnea, epistaxis, hyperventilation, pulmonary edema, respiratory distress, upper respiratory tract infection, wheezing

Miscellaneous: Diaphoresis, hiccups, retained placental fragment, septic shock

Mechanism of Action Carboprost tromethamine is a prostaglandin similar to prostaglandin F_2 alpha (dinoprost) except for the addition of a methyl group at the C-15 position. This substitution produces longer duration of activity than dinoprost; carboprost stimulates uterine contractility which usually results in expulsion of the products of conception and is used to induce abortion between 13-20 weeks of pregnancy. Hemostasis at the placentation site is achieved through the myometrial contractions produced by carboprost.

Drug Interactions

Increased Effect/Toxicity: May augment activity of other oxytocic agents (concomitant use is not recommended).

Pharmacodynamics/Kinetics Excretion: Urine

Pregnancy Risk Factor C

Carboxymethylcellulose (kar boks ee meth il SEL yoo lose)

U.S. Brand Names Refresh Liquigel™ [OTC]; Refresh Plus® [OTC]; Refresh Tears® [OTC]; Tears Again® Gel Drops™ [OTC]; Tears Again® Night and Day™ [OTC]; Theratears®

Canadian Brand Names Celluvisc™; Refresh Plus®; Refresh Tears®

Generic Available Yes

Index Terms Carbose D; Carboxymethylcellulose Sodium

Pharmacologic Category Ophthalmic Agent, Miscellaneous

Use Artificial tear substitute

Local Anesthetic/Vasoconstrictor Precautions No information available to require special precautions

Effects on Dental Treatment No significant effects or complications reported

Carisoprodol (kar eye soe PROE dole)

U.S. Brand Names Soma®

Canadian Brand Names Soma®

Generic Available Yes

Index Terms Carisoprodate; Isobamate

Pharmacologic Category Skeletal Muscle Relaxant

Dental Use Treatment of muscle spasms and pain associated with acute temporomandibular joint (TMJ) pain

Use Relief of discomfort associated with skeletal muscle condition

Local Anesthetic/Vasoconstrictor Precautions No information available to require special precautions

Effects on Dental Treatment No significant effects or complications reported

Significant Adverse Effects Frequency not defined.

Cardiovascular: Flushing of face, hypotension (postural), syncope, tachycardia, tightness in chest

Central nervous system: Agitation, allergic fever, ataxia, depression, dizziness, drowsiness, dysarthria, headache, insomnia, irritability, lightheadedness, paradoxical CNS stimulation, seizure, vertigo

Dermatologic: Angioedema, dermatitis (allergic), erythema multiforme, fixed drug reaction, pruritus, rash, urticaria

Gastrointestinal: Nausea, epigastric distress, vomiting

Hematologic: Aplastic anemia, eosinophilia, leukopenia

Neuromuscular & skeletal: Tremor

Ocular: Blurred vision, burning eyes

Respiratory: Dyspnea

Miscellaneous: Anaphylaxis, hiccups, hypersensitivity reaction, idiosyncratic reaction (symptoms may include ataxia, dysarthria, temporary vision loss, extreme weakness, agitation, euphoria, transient quadriplegia, confusion, and/or disorientation); withdrawal symptoms (abdominal cramps, headache, nausea, seizure) may occur upon abrupt discontinuation

(Continued)

Carisoprodol *(Continued)*

Dental Usual Dosing Treatment of muscle spasms and pain associated with acute TMJ pain: Adults: Oral: 350 mg 3-4 times/day; take last dose at bedtime; compound: 1-2 tablets 4 times/day

Dosage Oral: Adults: 350 mg 3-4 times/day; take last dose at bedtime

Mechanism of Action Precise mechanism is not yet clear, but many effects have been ascribed to its central depressant actions

Contraindications Hypersensitivity to carisoprodol, meprobamate, or any component of the formulation; acute intermittent porphyria

Warnings/Precautions May cause CNS depression, which may impair physical or mental abilities. Effects with other sedative drugs or ethanol may be potentiated. Use with caution in patients with hepatic/renal dysfunction. Tolerance or drug dependence may result from extended use. Limit to 2-3 weeks; use caution in patients who may be prone to addiction. Idiosyncratic reactions and/or severe allergic reactions may occur. Idiosyncratic reactions occur following the initial dose and may include severe weakness, transient quadriplegia, euphoria, or vision loss (temporary). Has been associated (rarely) with seizures in patients with and without seizure history. Safety and efficacy in children <12 years of age have not been established.

Drug Interactions Substrate of CYP2C19 (major)

CNS depressants (includes CNS depressants, benzodiazepines, and phenothiazines): Sedation may be increased; avoid concurrent use.

CYP2C19 inhibitors: May increase the levels/effects of carisoprodol. Example inhibitors include delavirdine, fluconazole, fluvoxamine, gemfibrozil, isoniazid, omeprazole, and ticlopidine.

Ethanol/Nutrition/Herb Interactions Ethanol: Avoid ethanol (may increase CNS depression).

Pharmacodynamics/Kinetics

Onset of action: ~30 minutes

Duration: 4-6 hours

Distribution: Crosses placenta; high concentrations enter breast milk

Metabolism: Hepatic, via CYP2C19 to active metabolite (meprobamate)

Half-life elimination: 2.4 hours; Meprobamate: 10 hours

Excretion: Urine, as metabolite

Pregnancy Risk Factor C

Lactation Enters breast milk (high concentrations)/not recommended

Breast-Feeding Considerations Carisoprodol levels in breast milk are 2-4 times that of maternal plasma levels.

Dosage Forms Excipient information presented when available (limited, particularly for generics); consult specific product labeling.

Tablet: 350 mg

Soma®: 350 mg

Carisoprodol and Aspirin *(kar eye soe PROE dole & AS pir in)*

Related Information

Aspirin *on page 149*

Carisoprodol *on page 285*

U.S. Brand Names Soma® Compound

Generic Available Yes

Index Terms Aspirin and Carisoprodol

Pharmacologic Category Skeletal Muscle Relaxant

Dental Use Treatment of muscle spasms and pain associated with acute temporomandibular joint pain (TMJ)

Use Skeletal muscle relaxant

Local Anesthetic/Vasoconstrictor Precautions No information available to require special precautions

Effects on Dental Treatment Key adverse event(s) related to dental treatment: Elderly are a high-risk population for adverse effects from nonsteroidal anti-inflammatory agents. As many as 60% of elderly patients with GI complications from NSAIDs can develop peptic ulceration and/or hemorrhage asymptomatically. Concomitant disease and drug use contribute to the risk of GI adverse effects. Use lowest effective dose for shortest period possible. Consider renal function decline with age.

Aspirin: As with all drugs which may affect hemostasis, bleeding is associated with aspirin. Hemorrhage may occur at virtually any site; risk is dependent on multiple variables including dosage, concurrent use of multiple agents which alter hemostasis, and patient susceptibility. Many adverse effects of aspirin are dose related, and are rare at low dosages. Other serious reactions are idiosyncratic, related to allergy or individual sensitivity (see Dental Comment).

Dental Usual Dosing Treatment of muscle spasms and pain associated with acute TMJ pain: Adults: Oral: 1-2 tablets 4 times/day

Dosage Oral: Adults: 1-2 tablets 4 times/day

Drug Interactions
Carisoprodol: **Substrate** of CYP2C19 (major)
Aspirin: **Substrate** of CYP2C9 (minor)
Also see individual agents.

Ethanol/Nutrition/Herb Interactions Ethanol: Avoid ethanol (may increase CNS depression).

Pharmacodynamics/Kinetics See individual agents.

Pregnancy Risk Factor C/D (full-dose aspirin in 3rd trimester)

Lactation Enters breast milk/contraindicated

Dosage Forms Excipient information presented when available (limited, particularly for generics); consult specific product labeling.
Tablet: Carisoprodol 200 mg and aspirin 325 mg

Dental Comment There is no scientific evidence to warrant discontinuance of aspirin prior to dental surgery. Patients taking one aspirin tablet daily as an antithrombotic and who require dental surgery should be given special consideration in consultation with the physician before removal of the aspirin relative to prevention of postoperative bleeding.

The Food and Drug Administration (FDA), has issued a letter updating information and considerations regarding the use of ibuprofen (400 mg doses) in patients who are taking low dose aspirin (81 mg, immediate release; not enteric coated) for cardioprotection and stroke prevention. Ibuprofen, at these doses, may interfere with aspirin's antiplatelet effect depending upon when it is administered. Patients initiated on aspirin first (for ~1 week) then ibuprofen (400 mg tid for 10 days) seem to maintain aspirin's platelet effect (Cryer B, 2005). Ibuprofen has the greatest impact on aspirin if administered less than 8 hours before aspirin (Catella-Lawson F, 2001).

Patients may require counseling about the appropriate timing of ibuprofen dosing in relationship to aspirin therapy. With occasional use of ibuprofen, a clinically-significant interaction with aspirin in unlikely. To avoid interference during chronic dosing, a single dose of ibuprofen should be taken 30-120 minutes after aspirin ingestion or at least 8 hours should elapse after ibuprofen dosing before giving aspirin (FDA, 2006; Catella-Lawson F, 2001).

The clinical implications of the interaction are unclear. There have not been any clinical endpoint studies conducted at this time. Avoidance of this interaction is potentially important because aspirin's vascular protection could be decreased or negated.

Other nonselective NSAIDs may have potential for a similar interaction with aspirin. Such has been described with naproxen (Capone ML, 2005). Acetaminophen does not appear to interfere with the antiplatelet effect of aspirin. Other clinical scenarios (use of smaller ibuprofen doses, other aspirin products, other doses of aspirin) have not been evaluated.

Additional information is available at: http://www.fda.gov/cder/drug/infopage/aspirin/default.htm.

Carisoprodol, Aspirin, and Codeine
(kar eye soe PROE dole, AS pir in, and KOE deen)

Related Information
Aspirin *on page 149*
Carisoprodol *on page 285*
Codeine *on page 404*

U.S. Brand Names Soma® Compound w/Codeine

Generic Available Yes

Index Terms Aspirin, Carisoprodol, and Codeine; Codeine, Aspirin, and Carisoprodol

Pharmacologic Category Skeletal Muscle Relaxant

Dental Use Treatment of muscle spasms and pain associated with acute temporomandibular joint pain (TMJ)

Use Skeletal muscle relaxant

Local Anesthetic/Vasoconstrictor Precautions No information available to require special precautions

Effects on Dental Treatment Key adverse event(s) related to dental treatment: Elderly are a high-risk population for adverse effects from nonsteroidal anti-inflammatory agents. As many as 60% of elderly patients with GI complications from NSAIDs can develop peptic ulceration and/or hemorrhage asymptomatically. Concomitant disease and drug use contribute to the risk of GI (Continued)

Carisoprodol, Aspirin, and Codeine *(Continued)*

adverse effects. Use lowest effective dose for shortest period possible. Consider renal function decline with age.

Aspirin: As with all drugs which may affect hemostasis, bleeding is associated with aspirin. Hemorrhage may occur at virtually any site; risk is dependent on multiple variables including dosage, concurrent use of multiple agents which alter hemostasis, and patient susceptibility. Many adverse effects of aspirin are dose related, and are rare at low dosages. Other serious reactions are idiosyncratic, related to allergy or individual sensitivity (see Dental Comment).

Restrictions C-III

Dental Usual Dosing Treatment of muscle spasms and pain associated with acute TMJ pain: Adults: Oral: 1 or 2 tablets 4 times/day

Dosage Oral: Adults: 1 or 2 tablets 4 times/day

Drug Interactions

Carisoprodol: **Substrate** of CYP2C19 (major)

Aspirin: **Substrate** of CYP2C9 (minor)

Also see individual agents.

Ethanol/Nutrition/Herb Interactions Ethanol: Avoid ethanol (may increase CNS depression).

Pharmacodynamics/Kinetics See individual agents.

Pregnancy Risk Factor C/D (full-dose aspirin in 3rd trimester)

Lactation Enters breast milk/contraindicated

Dosage Forms Excipient information presented when available (limited, particularly for generics); consult specific product labeling.

Tablet: Carisoprodol 200 mg, aspirin 325 mg, and codeine phosphate 16 mg

Dental Comment There is no scientific evidence to warrant discontinuance of aspirin prior to dental surgery. Patients taking one aspirin tablet daily as an antithrombotic and who require dental surgery should be given special consideration in consultation with the physician before removal of the aspirin relative to prevention of postoperative bleeding.

The Food and Drug Administration (FDA), has issued a letter updating information and considerations regarding the use of ibuprofen (400 mg doses) in patients who are taking low dose aspirin (81 mg, immediate release; not enteric coated) for cardioprotection and stroke prevention. Ibuprofen, at these doses, may interfere with aspirin's antiplatelet effect depending upon when it is administered. Patients initiated on aspirin first (for ~1 week) then ibuprofen (400 mg tid for 10 days) seem to maintain aspirin's platelet effect (Cryer B, 2005). Ibuprofen has the greatest impact on aspirin if administered less than 8 hours before aspirin (Catella-Lawson F, 2001).

Patients may require counseling about the appropriate timing of ibuprofen dosing in relationship to aspirin therapy. With occasional use of ibuprofen, a clinically-significant interaction with aspirin in unlikely. To avoid interference during chronic dosing, a single dose of ibuprofen should be taken 30-120 minutes after aspirin ingestion or at least 8 hours should elapse after ibuprofen dosing before giving aspirin (FDA, 2006; Catella-Lawson F, 2001).

The clinical implications of the interaction are unclear. There have not been any clinical endpoint studies conducted at this time. Avoidance of this interaction is potentially important because aspirin's vascular protection could be decreased or negated.

Other nonselective NSAIDs may have potential for a similar interaction with aspirin. Such has been described with naproxen (Capone ML, 2005). Acetaminophen does not appear to interfere with the antiplatelet effect of aspirin. Other clinical scenarios (use of smaller ibuprofen doses, other aspirin products, other doses of aspirin) have not been evaluated.

Additional information is available at: http://www.fda.gov/cder/drug/infopage/aspirin/default.htm.

Carmol® 10 [OTC] *see* Urea *on page 1632*

Carmol® 20 [OTC] *see* Urea *on page 1632*

Carmol® 40 *see* Urea *on page 1632*

Carmol® Deep Cleaning *see* Urea *on page 1632*

Carmol-HC® *see* Urea and Hydrocortisone *on page 1633*

Carmol® Scalp *see* Sulfacetamide *on page 1502*

Carmustine *(kar MUS teen)*

U.S. Brand Names BiCNU®; Gliadel®

Canadian Brand Names BiCNU®; Gliadel Wafer®

Mexican Brand Names BiCNU

Generic Available No

Index Terms BCNU; bis-chloronitrosourea; Carmustinum; NSC-409962; WR-139021

Pharmacologic Category Antineoplastic Agent; Antineoplastic Agent, Alkylating Agent (Nitrosourea); Antineoplastic Agent, DNA Adduct-Forming Agent; Antineoplastic Agent, DNA Binding Agent

Use

Injection: Treatment of brain tumors (glioblastoma, brainstem glioma, medulloblastoma, astrocytoma, ependymoma, and metastatic brain tumors), multiple myeloma, Hodgkin's disease (relapsed or refractory), non-Hodgkin's lymphomas (relapsed or refractory),

Wafer (implant): Adjunct to surgery in patients with recurrent glioblastoma multiforme; adjunct to surgery and radiation in patients with high-grade malignant glioma

Unlabeled/Investigational Use Melanoma

Local Anesthetic/Vasoconstrictor Precautions No information available to require special precautions

Effects on Dental Treatment Key adverse event(s) related to dental treatment: Stomatitis.

Common Adverse Effects

>10%:

Cardiovascular: Hypotension (with high-dose I.V. therapy, due to the alcohol content of the diluent)

Central nervous system: Ataxia, dizziness

Postoperatively: Seizure (wafer 5% to 54%), brain edema (wafer 4% to 23%)

Dermatologic: Burning (with skin contact), hyperpigmentation of skin (with skin contact)

Gastrointestinal: Severe nausea and vomiting, usually begins within 2-4 hours of drug administration and lasts for 4-6 hours; dose related. Patients should receive a prophylactic antiemetic regimen.

Hematologic: Myelosuppression (cumulative, dose related, delayed, and dose limiting), thrombocytopenia (onset: 28 days; recovery: 35-42 days), leukopenia (onset: 35-42 days; recovery: 42-56 days)

Hepatic: Reversible increases in bilirubin, alkaline phosphatase, and AST occur in 20% to 25% of patients

Local: Pain and burning at injection site, phlebitis

Neuromuscular & skeletal: Weakness (wafer 22%)

Ocular: Ocular toxicities (transient conjunctival flushing and blurred vision), retinal hemorrhages

Respiratory: Interstitial fibrosis occurs in up to 50% of patients receiving a cumulative dose >1400 mg/m^2, or bone marrow transplantation doses; may be delayed up to 3 years; rare in patients receiving lower doses. A history of lung disease or concomitant bleomycin therapy may increase the risk of this reaction. Patients with forced vital capacity (FVC) or carbon monoxide diffusing capacity of the lungs (DLCO) <70% of predicted are at higher risk.

Miscellaneous: Disease progression/performance deterioration (wafer 82%)

1% to 10%:

Cardiovascular: Chest pain, deep thrombophlebitis (wafer), facial edema (wafer), peripheral edema (wafer)

Central nervous system: Wafer: Amnesia, anxiety, aphasia, ataxia, brain abscess, confusion, convulsion, CSF leaks, depression, diplopia, dizziness, facial paralysis, headache, hemiplegia, hydrocephalus, hypoesthesia, insomnia, intracranial hypertension, meningitis, somnolence, speech disorder, stupor

Dermatologic: Facial flushing, probably due to the alcohol diluent; alopecia, rash (wafer), wound healing abnormal (wafer)

Gastrointestinal: Abdominal pain, anorexia, constipation, diarrhea, stomatitis

Hematologic: Anemia, hemorrhage (wafer)

Local: Abscess (wafer)

Neuromuscular & skeletal: Back pain

Mechanism of Action Interferes with the normal function of DNA and RNA by alkylation and cross-linking the strands of DNA and RNA, and by possible protein modification; may also inhibit enzyme processes by carbamylation of amino acids in protein

Drug Interactions

Increased Effect/Toxicity: Cimetidine may increase the bone marrow toxicity of carmustine

Decreased Effect:

Carmustine may decrease the absorption of digoxin tablets.

Pharmacodynamics/Kinetics

Distribution: 3.3 L/kg; readily crosses blood-brain barrier producing CSF levels equal to >50% of blood plasma levels; highly lipid soluble

Metabolism: Rapidly hepatic; forms active metabolites

(Continued)

Carmustine *(Continued)*

Half-life elimination: Biphasic: Initial: 1.4 minutes; Secondary: 20 minutes (active metabolites: plasma half-life of 67 hours)

Excretion: Urine (~60% to 70%) within 96 hours; lungs (6% to 10% as CO_2)

Pregnancy Risk Factor D

Carmustinum *see* Carmustine *on page 288*

Carnitor® *see* Levocarnitine *on page 963*

Carnitor® SF *see* Levocarnitine *on page 963*

Carrington Antifungal [OTC] *see* Miconazole *on page 1097*

Carteolol *(KAR tee oh lole)*

Related Information

Cardiovascular Diseases *on page 1726*

U.S. Brand Names Cartrol®; Ocupress® [DSC]

Canadian Brand Names Cartrol® Oral; Ocupress® Ophthalmic

Generic Available Yes: Ophthalmic solution

Index Terms Carteolol Hydrochloride

Pharmacologic Category Beta Blocker With Intrinsic Sympathomimetic Activity; Ophthalmic Agent, Antiglaucoma

Use Management of hypertension; treatment of chronic open-angle glaucoma and intraocular hypertension

Local Anesthetic/Vasoconstrictor Precautions No information available to require special precautions

Effects on Dental Treatment Carteolol is a nonselective beta-blocker and may enhance the pressor response to epinephrine, resulting in hypertension and bradycardia. Many nonsteroidal anti-inflammatory drugs, such as ibuprofen and indomethacin, can reduce the hypotensive effect of beta-blockers after 3 or more weeks of therapy with the NSAID. Short-term NSAID use (ie, 3 days) requires no special precautions in patients taking beta-blockers.

Common Adverse Effects

Ophthalmic:

>10%: Ocular: Conjunctival hyperemia

1% to 10%: Ocular: Anisocoria, corneal punctate keratitis, corneal sensitivity decreased, corneal staining, eye pain, vision disturbances

Systemic:

>10%:

Central nervous system: Drowsiness, insomnia

Endocrine & metabolic: Sexual ability decreased

1% to 10%:

Cardiovascular: Bradycardia, palpitation, edema, CHF, peripheral circulation reduced

Central nervous system: Mental depression

Gastrointestinal: Constipation, diarrhea, nausea, vomiting, stomach discomfort

Respiratory: Bronchospasm

Miscellaneous: Cold extremities

Mechanism of Action Blocks both beta$_1$- and beta$_2$-receptors and has mild intrinsic sympathomimetic activity; has negative inotropic and chronotropic effects and can significantly slow AV nodal conduction

Drug Interactions

Cytochrome P450 Effect: Substrate of CYP2D6 (minor)

Increased Effect/Toxicity: Carteolol may increase the effects of other drugs which slow AV conduction (digoxin, verapamil, diltiazem), alpha-blockers (prazosin, terazosin), and alpha-adrenergic stimulants (epinephrine, phenylephrine). Carteolol may mask the tachycardia from hypoglycemia caused by insulin and oral hypoglycemics. In patients receiving concurrent therapy, the risk of hypertensive crisis is increased when either clonidine or the beta-blocker is withdrawn. Reserpine has been shown to enhance the effect of beta-blockers. Beta-blockers may increase the action or levels of ethanol, disopyramide, nondepolarizing muscle relaxants, and theophylline although the effects are difficult to predict.

Decreased Effect: Decreased effect of beta-blockers with aluminum salts, barbiturates, calcium salts, cholestyramine, colestipol, NSAIDs, penicillins (ampicillin), rifampin, salicylates, and sulfinpyrazone due to decreased bioavailability and plasma levels. Beta-blockers may decrease the effect of sulfonylureas (possibly hyperglycemia). Nonselective beta-blockers blunt the effect of beta-2 adrenergic agonists (albuterol).

Pharmacodynamics/Kinetics

Onset of action: Oral: 1-1.5 hours

Peak effect: 2 hours

Duration: 12 hours
Absorption: Oral: 80%
Protein binding: 23% to 30%
Metabolism: 30% to 50%
Half-life elimination: 6 hours
Excretion: Urine (as metabolites)

Pregnancy Risk Factor C (manufacturer); D (2nd and 3rd trimesters - expert analysis)

Carteolol Hydrochloride *see* Carteolol *on page 290*

Cartia XT™ *see* Diltiazem *on page 505*

Cartrol® *see* Carteolol *on page 290*

Carvedilol (KAR ve dil ole)

Related Information
Cardiovascular Diseases *on page 1726*

U.S. Brand Names Coreg®; Coreg CR™

Canadian Brand Names Apo-Carvedilol®; Coreg®; Novo-Carvedilol; PMS-Carvedilol; RAN™-Carvedilol; ratio-Carvedilol

Mexican Brand Names Dilatrend

Generic Available No

Pharmacologic Category Beta Blocker With Alpha-Blocking Activity

Use Mild-to-severe heart failure of ischemic or cardiomyopathic origin (usually in addition to standardized therapy); left ventricular dysfunction following myocardial infarction (MI) (clinically stable with LVEF ≤40%); management of hypertension

Unlabeled/Investigational Use Angina pectoris

Local Anesthetic/Vasoconstrictor Precautions No information available to require special precautions

Effects on Dental Treatment Key adverse event(s) related to dental treatment: Postural hypotension and periodontitis. Many nonsteroidal anti-inflammatory drugs, such as ibuprofen and indomethacin, can reduce the hypotensive effect of beta-blockers after 3 or more weeks of therapy with the NSAID. Short-term NSAID use (ie, 3 days) requires no special precautions in patients taking beta-blockers.

Common Adverse Effects Note: Frequency ranges include data from hypertension and heart failure trials. Higher rates of adverse reactions have generally been noted in patients with CHF. However, the frequency of adverse effects associated with placebo is also increased in this population. Events occurring at a frequency > placebo in clinical trials.

>10%:
Cardiovascular: Hypotension (9% to 20%)
Central nervous system: Dizziness (2% to 32%), fatigue (4% to 24%)
Endocrine & metabolic: Hyperglycemia (5% to 12%), weight gain (10% to 12%)
Gastrointestinal: Diarrhea (1% to 12%)
Neuromuscular & skeletal: Weakness (11%)

1% to 10%:
Cardiovascular: Bradycardia (2% to 10%), syncope (3% to 8%), peripheral edema (1% to 7%), generalized edema (5% to 6%), angina (2% to 6%), dependent edema (4%), AV block (3%), hypertension (3%), postural hypotension (2%), palpitation
Central nervous system: Headache (5% to 8%), fever (3%), somnolence (2%), insomnia (1% to 2%), malaise, hypoesthesia, vertigo
Endocrine & metabolic: Alkaline phosphatase increased, gout (6%), hypercholesterolemia (4%), dehydration (2%), hyperkalemia (3%), hypervolemia (2%), hypertriglyceridemia (1%), hyperuricemia, hypoglycemia, hyponatremia
Gastrointestinal: Nausea (2% to 9%), vomiting (6%), melena, periodontitis
Genitourinary: Hematuria (3%), impotence
Hematologic: Thrombocytopenia (1% to 2%), prothrombin decreased, purpura
Hepatic: Transaminases increased
Neuromuscular & skeletal: Back pain (2% to 7%), arthralgia (6%), myalgia (3%), muscle cramps, paresthesia (1%)
Ocular: Blurred vision (3% to 5%), lacrimation
Renal: BUN increased (6%), creatinine increased (3%), renal function abnormal, albuminuria, glycosuria, kidney failure
Respiratory: Cough increased (5%), nasopharyngitis (4%), rhinitis (2%), nasal congestion (1%), sinus congestion (1%)
Miscellaneous: Injury (3% to 6%), allergy, sudden death

Dosage Oral: Adults: Reduce dosage if heart rate drops to <55 beats/minute.
(Continued)

Carvedilol *(Continued)*

Hypertension:

Immediate release: 6.25 mg twice daily; if tolerated, dose should be maintained for 1-2 weeks, then increased to 12.5 mg twice daily. Dosage may be increased to a maximum of 25 mg twice daily after 1-2 weeks; maximum dose: 50 mg/day.

Extended release: Initial: 20 mg once daily, if tolerated, dose should be maintained for 1-2 weeks then increased to 40 mg once daily if necessary; maximum dose: 80 mg once daily

Congestive heart failure:

Immediate release: 3.125 mg twice daily for 2 weeks; if this dose is tolerated, may increase to 6.25 mg twice daily. Double the dose every 2 weeks to the highest dose tolerated by patient. (Prior to initiating therapy, other heart failure medications should be stabilized and fluid retention minimized.)

Maximum recommended dose:

Mild-to-moderate heart failure:

<85 kg: 25 mg twice daily

>85 kg: 50 mg twice daily

Severe heart failure: 25 mg twice daily

Extended release: Initial: 10 mg once daily for 2 weeks; if the dose is tolerated, increase dose to 20 mg, 40 mg, and 80 mg over successive intervals of at least 2 weeks. Maintain on lower dose if higher dose is not tolerated.

Left ventricular dysfunction following MI: **Note:** Should be initiated only after patient is hemodynamically stable and fluid retention has been minimized.

Immediate release: Initial 3.125-6.25 mg twice daily; increase dosage incrementally (ie, from 6.25-12.5 mg twice daily) at intervals of 3-10 days, based on tolerance, to a target dose of 25 mg twice daily.

Extended release: Initial: 20 mg once daily; increase dosage incrementally at intervals of 3-10 days. Target dose: 80 mg once daily.

Angina pectoris (unlabeled use): Immediate release: 25-50 mg twice daily

Conversion from immediate release to extended release (Coreg CR™):

Current dose immediate release tablets 3.125 mg twice daily: Convert to extended release capsules 10 mg once daily

Current dose immediate release tablets 6.25 mg twice daily: Convert to extended release capsules 20 mg once daily

Current dose immediate release tablets 12.5 mg twice daily: Convert to extended release capsules 40 mg once daily

Current dose immediate release tablets 25 mg twice daily: Convert to extended release capsules 80 mg once daily

Dosing adjustment in renal impairment: None necessary

Dosing adjustment in hepatic impairment: Use is contraindicated in severe liver dysfunction.

Mechanism of Action As a racemic mixture, carvedilol has nonselective beta-adrenoreceptor and alpha-adrenergic blocking activity. No intrinsic sympathomimetic activity has been documented. Associated effects in hypertensive patients include reduction of cardiac output, exercise- or beta-agonist-induced tachycardia, reduction of reflex orthostatic tachycardia, vasodilation, decreased peripheral vascular resistance (especially in standing position), decreased renal vascular resistance, reduced plasma renin activity, and increased levels of atrial natriuretic peptide. In CHF, associated effects include decreased pulmonary capillary wedge pressure, decreased pulmonary artery pressure, decreased heart rate, decreased systemic vascular resistance, increased stroke volume index, and decreased right arterial pressure (RAP).

Contraindications Hypersensitivity to carvedilol or any component of the formulation; decompensated cardiac failure requiring intravenous inotropic therapy; bronchial asthma or related bronchospastic conditions; second- or third-degree AV block, sick sinus syndrome, and severe bradycardia (except in patients with a functioning artificial pacemaker); cardiogenic shock; severe hepatic impairment; pregnancy (2nd and 3rd trimesters)

Warnings/Precautions Consider pre-existing conditions such as sick sinus syndrome before initiating. Initiate cautiously and monitor for possible deterioration in patient status (including symptoms of CHF). Adjustment of other medications (ACE inhibitors and/or diuretics) may be required. In severe chronic heart failure, trial patients were excluded if they had cardiac-related rales, ascites, or a serum creatinine >2.8 mg/dL. Congestive heart failure patients may experience a worsening of renal function; risks include ischemic disease, diffuse vascular disease, underlying renal dysfunction; systolic BP <100 mm Hg. Patients should be advised to avoid driving or other hazardous tasks during initiation of therapy due to the risk of syncope. Beta-blocker therapy should not be withdrawn abruptly (particularly in patients with CAD), but gradually tapered to avoid acute tachycardia, hypertension, and/or ischemia.

Manufacturer recommends discontinuation of therapy if liver injury occurs (confirmed by laboratory testing). In general, patients with bronchospastic disease should not receive beta-blockers; if used at all, should be used cautiously with close monitoring. Use caution in patients with PVD (can aggravate arterial insufficiency). Use caution with concurrent use of verapamil or diltiazem; bradycardia or heart block can occur. Use cautiously in diabetics because it can mask prominent hypoglycemic symptoms. Use with caution in patients with myasthenia gravis or psychiatric disease (may cause CNS depression). Use with caution in patients with mild-to-moderate hepatic impairment. Adequate alpha-blockade is required prior to use of any beta-blocker for patients with untreated pheochromocytoma. Use care with anesthetic agents that decrease myocardial function. Safety and efficacy in children <18 years of age have not been established.

Drug Interactions

Cytochrome P450 Effect: Substrate of CYP1A2 (minor), 2C9 (major), 2D6 (major), 2E1 (minor), 3A4 (minor)

Increased Effect/Toxicity: CYP2C9 Inhibitors may increase the levels/effects of carvedilol; example inhibitors include delavirdine, fluconazole, gemfibrozil, ketoconazole, nicardipine, NSAIDs, sulfonamides, and tolbutamide. CYP2D6 inhibitors may increase the levels/effects of carvedilol; example inhibitors include chlorpromazine, delavirdine, fluoxetine, miconazole, paroxetine, pergolide, quinidine, quinine, ritonavir, and ropinirole. Cimetidine increase the serum levels and effects of carvedilol. Carvedilol may increase the effects of other drugs which slow AV conduction (digoxin, verapamil, diltiazem) and alpha-blockers (prazosin, terazosin). Carvedilol may mask the tachycardia from hypoglycemia caused by insulin and oral hypoglycemics. SSRIs may decrease the metabolism of carvedilol.

Decreased Effect: CYP2C9 inducers may decrease the levels/effects of carvedilol; example inducers include carbamazepine, phenobarbital, phenytoin, rifampin, rifapentine, and secobarbital. Decreased antihypertensive effect of beta-blockers has occurred with concurrent NSAID or salicylate use. Beta-blockers may alter the effect of sulfonylureas. Disopyramide may exacerbate heart failure or enhance bradycardic effect of beta-blockers. Beta-blockers may counteract desired effects of beta-agonists.

Ethanol/Nutrition/Herb Interactions

Ethanol: Coreg CR™: Avoid ethanol (including prescription and over the counter medications containing ethanol). Ethanol may affect extended release properties causing a faster release; separate by at least 2 hours.

Food: Food decreases rate but not extent of absorption. Administration with food minimizes risks of orthostatic hypotension.

Herb/Nutraceutical: Avoid dong quai if using for hypertension (has estrogenic activity). Avoid ephedra, yohimbe, ginseng (may worsen hypertension). Avoid garlic (may have increased antihypertensive effect).

Dietary Considerations Should be taken with food to minimize the risk of orthostatic hypotension.

Pharmacodynamics/Kinetics

Onset of action: 1-2 hours

Peak antihypertensive effect: ~1-2 hours

Absorption: Rapid

Distribution: V_d: 115 L

Protein binding: >98%, primarily to albumin

Metabolism: Extensively hepatic, via CYP2C9, 2D6, 3A4, and 2C19 (2% excreted unchanged); three active metabolites (4-hydroxyphenyl metabolite is 13 times more potent than parent drug for beta-blockade); first-pass effect; plasma concentrations in the elderly and those with cirrhotic liver disease are 50% and 4-7 times higher, respectively

Bioavailability: Immediate release: 25% to 35%; Extended release: 85% of immediate release

Half-life elimination: 7-10 hours

Excretion: Primarily feces

Pregnancy Risk Factor C (manufacturer); D (2nd and 3rd trimesters - expert analysis)

Dosage Forms

Capsule, extended release:

Coreg CR™: 10 mg, 20 mg, 40 mg, 80 mg

Tablet:

Coreg®: 3.125 mg, 6.25 mg, 12.5 mg, 25 mg

Selected Readings

Foster CA and Aston SJ, "Propranolol-Epinephrine Interaction: A Potential Disaster," *Plast Reconstr Surg*, 1983, 72(1):74-8.

Wong DG, Spence JD, Lamki L, et al, "Effect of Nonsteroidal Anti-inflammatory Drugs on Control of Hypertension by Beta-Blockers and Diuretics," *Lancet*, 1986, 1(8488):997-1001.

Wynn RL, "Dental Nonsteroidal Anti-inflammatory Drugs and Prostaglandin-Based Drug Interactions, Part Two," *Gen Dent*, 1992, 40(2):104, 106, 108.

Wynn RL, "Epinephrine Interactions With Beta-Blockers," *Gen Dent*, 1994, 42(1):16, 18.

Casodex® *see* Bicalutamide *on page 214*

Caspofungin (kas poe FUN jin)

Related Information
Fungal Infections *on page 1804*
U.S. Brand Names Cancidas®
Canadian Brand Names Cancidas®
Mexican Brand Names Cancidas
Generic Available No
Index Terms Caspofungin Acetate
Pharmacologic Category Antifungal Agent, Parenteral; Echinocandin
Dental Use Management of angular cheilitis
Use Treatment of invasive *Aspergillus* infections in patients who are refractory or intolerant of other therapy; treatment of candidemia and other *Candida* infections (intra-abdominal abscesses, esophageal, peritonitis, pleural space); empirical treatment for presumed fungal infections in febrile neutropenic patient
Local Anesthetic/Vasoconstrictor Precautions No information available to require special precautions
Effects on Dental Treatment No significant effects or complications reported
Common Adverse Effects
>10%:
Central nervous system: Headache (up to 11%), fever (3% to 26%), chills (up to 14%)
Endocrine & metabolic: Hypokalemia (4% to 11%)
Hematologic: Hemoglobin decreased (1% to 12%)
Hepatic: Serum alkaline phosphatase increased (3% to 11%), transaminases increased (up to 13%)
Local: Infusion site reactions (2% to 12%), phlebitis/thrombophlebitis (up to 16%)
1% to 10%:
Cardiovascular: Flushing (2% to 3%), facial edema (up to 3%), hypertension (1% to 2%), tachycardia (1% to 2%), hypotension (1%)
Central nervous system: Dizziness (2%), pain (1% to 5%), insomnia (1%)
Dermatologic: Rash (<1% to 6%), pruritus (1% to 3%), erythema (1% to 2%)
Gastrointestinal: Nausea (2% to 6%), vomiting (1% to 4%), abdominal pain (1% to 4%), diarrhea (1% to 4%), anorexia (1%)
Hematologic: Eosinophils increased (3%), neutrophils decreased (2% to 3%), WBC decreased (5% to 6%), anemia (up to 4%), platelet count decreased (2% to 3%)
Hepatic: Bilirubin increased (3%)
Local: Induration (up to 3%)
Neuromuscular & skeletal: Myalgia (up to 3%), paresthesia (1% to 3%), tremor (≤2%)
Renal: Nephrotoxicity (8%)*, proteinuria (5%), hematuria (2%), serum creatinine increased (<1% to 4%), urinary WBCs increased (up to 8%), urinary RBCs increased (1% to 4%), blood urea nitrogen increased (1%)
*Nephrotoxicity defined as serum creatinine ≥2x baseline value or ≥1 mg/dL in patients with serum creatinine above ULN range (patients with Cl_{cr} <30 mL/minute were excluded)
Miscellaneous: Flu-like syndrome (3%), diaphoresis (up to 3%)
Mechanism of Action Inhibits synthesis of β(1,3)-D-glucan, an essential component of the cell wall of susceptible fungi. Highest activity in regions of active cell growth. Mammalian cells do not require β(1,3)-D-glucan, limiting potential toxicity.
Drug Interactions
Increased Effect/Toxicity: Concurrent administration of cyclosporine may increase caspofungin concentrations; hepatic serum transaminases may be observed.
Decreased Effect: Caspofungin may decrease blood concentrations of tacrolimus. Dosage adjustment of caspofungin to 70 mg is required for patients on rifampin.
Pharmacodynamics/Kinetics
Protein binding: 97% to albumin
Metabolism: Slowly, via hydrolysis and N-acetylation as well as by spontaneous degradation, with subsequent metabolism to component amino acids. Overall metabolism is extensive.
Half-life elimination: Beta (distribution): 9-11 hours; Terminal: 40-50 hours
Excretion: Urine (41% as metabolites, 1% to 9% unchanged) and feces (35% as metabolites)
Pregnancy Risk Factor C

Castor Oil (KAS tor oyl)

U.S. Brand Names Emulsoil® [OTC] [DSC]; Purge® [OTC]
Generic Available Yes: Oil
Index Terms Oleum Ricini
Pharmacologic Category Laxative, Miscellaneous
Use Preparation for rectal or bowel examination or surgery; rarely used to relieve constipation; also applied to skin as emollient and protectant
Local Anesthetic/Vasoconstrictor Precautions No information available to require special precautions
Effects on Dental Treatment No significant effects or complications reported
Mechanism of Action Acts primarily in the small intestine; hydrolyzed to ricinoleic acid which reduces net absorption of fluid and electrolytes and stimulates peristalsis
Pregnancy Risk Factor X

Cefaclor (SEF a klor)

Related Information
Bacterial Infections *on page 1793*
U.S. Brand Names Raniclor™
Canadian Brand Names Apo-Cefaclor®; Ceclor®; Novo-Cefaclor; Nu-Cefaclor; PMS-Cefaclor
Mexican Brand Names Ceclor; Cefalan; Serviclor; Teraclox
Generic Available Yes: Excludes chewable tablet
Pharmacologic Category Antibiotic, Cephalosporin (Second Generation)
Dental Use Alternative antibiotic for treatment of orofacial infections in patients allergic to penicillins; susceptible bacteria including aerobic gram-positive bacteria and anaerobes
Use Treatment of susceptible bacterial infections including otitis media, lower respiratory tract infections, acute exacerbations of chronic bronchitis, pharyngitis and tonsillitis, urinary tract infections, skin and skin structure infections
Local Anesthetic/Vasoconstrictor Precautions No information available to require special precautions
Effects on Dental Treatment No significant effects or complications reported (see Dental Comment)
Significant Adverse Effects
1% to 10%:
  Dermatologic: Rash (maculopapular, erythematous, or morbilliform) (1% to 2%)
  Gastrointestinal: Diarrhea (3%)
(Continued)

Cefaclor *(Continued)*

    Genitourinary: Vaginitis (2%)
    Hematologic: Eosinophilia (2%)
    Hepatic: Transaminases increased (3%)
    Miscellaneous: Moniliasis (2%)
  <1% (Limited to important or life-threatening): Agitation, agranulocytosis, anaphylaxis, angioedema, aplastic anemia, arthralgia, cholestatic jaundice, CNS irritability, confusion, dizziness, hallucinations, hemolytic anemia, hepatitis, hyperactivity, insomnia, interstitial nephritis, nausea, nervousness, neutropenia, paresthesia, PT prolonged, pruritus, pseudomembranous colitis, seizure, serum-sickness, somnolence, Stevens-Johnson syndrome, thrombocytopenia, toxic epidermal necrolysis, urticaria, vomiting

  Reactions reported with other cephalosporins: Abdominal pain, cholestasis, fever, hemorrhage, renal dysfunction, superinfection, toxic nephropathy

Dental Usual Dosing Orofacial infections: Adults: Oral: Dosing range: 250-500 mg every 8 hours

Dosage
  Usual dosage range:
    Children >1 month: Oral: 20-40 mg/kg/day divided every 8-12 hours (maximum dose: 1 g/day)
    Adults: Oral: 250-500 mg every 8 hours
  Indication-specific dosing:
    Children: Oral:
      Otitis media: 40 mg/kg/day divided every 12 hours
      Pharyngitis: 20 mg/kg/day divided every 12 hours
  Dosing adjustment in renal impairment:
    Cl_{cr} 10-50 mL/minute: Administer 50% to 100% of dose
    Cl_{cr} <10 mL/minute: Administer 50% of dose
    Hemodialysis: Moderately dialyzable (20% to 50%)

Mechanism of Action Inhibits bacterial cell wall synthesis by binding to one or more of the penicillin-binding proteins (PBPs) which in turn inhibits the final transpeptidation step of peptidoglycan synthesis in bacterial cell walls, thus inhibiting cell wall biosynthesis. Bacteria eventually lyse due to ongoing activity of cell wall autolytic enzymes (autolysins and murein hydrolases) while cell wall assembly is arrested.

Contraindications Hypersensitivity to cefaclor, any component of the formulation, or other cephalosporins

Warnings/Precautions Modify dosage in patients with severe renal impairment. Prolonged use may result in fungal or bacterial superinfection, including *C. difficile*-associated diarrhea and pseudomembranous colitis. Use with caution in patients with a history of penicillin allergy, especially IgE-mediated reactions (eg, anaphylaxis, urticaria). Beta-lactamase-negative, ampicillin-resistant (BLNAR) strains of *H. influenzae* should be considered resistant to cefaclor. Extended release tablets are not approved for use in children <16 years of age. Some products may contain phenylalanine.

Drug Interactions
  Aminoglycosides: May be additive to nephrotoxicity.
  Furosemide: May be additive to nephrotoxicity.
  Probenecid: May decrease cephalosporin elimination.

Ethanol/Nutrition/Herb Interactions
  Food: Cefaclor serum levels may be decreased slightly if taken with food. The bioavailability of cefaclor extended release tablets is decreased 23% and the maximum concentration is decreased 67% when taken on an empty stomach.

Dietary Considerations Capsule, chewable tablet, and suspension may be taken with or without food. Raniclor™ contains phenylalanine 2.8 mg/cefaclor 125 mg.

Pharmacodynamics/Kinetics
  Absorption: Well absorbed, acid stable
  Distribution: Widely throughout the body and reaches therapeutic concentration in most tissues and body fluids, including synovial, pericardial, pleural, peritoneal fluids; bile, sputum, and urine; bone, myocardium, gallbladder, skin and soft tissue; crosses placenta; enters breast milk
  Protein binding: 25%
  Metabolism: Partially hepatic
  Half-life elimination: 0.5-1 hour; prolonged with renal impairment
  Time to peak: Capsule: 60 minutes; Suspension: 45 minutes
  Excretion: Urine (80% as unchanged drug)

Pregnancy Risk Factor B

Lactation Enters breast milk/use caution

Breast-Feeding Considerations Theoretically, drug absorbed by nursing infant may change bowel flora or affect fever work-up result. Small amounts can be detected in breast milk (trace amounts after 1 hour, increasing to 0.16 mcg/mL at 5 hours). **Note:** As a class, cephalosporins are used to treat bacterial infections in infants.

Dosage Forms Excipient information presented when available (limited, particularly for generics); consult specific product labeling.

Capsule: 250 mg, 500 mg

Powder for oral suspension: 125 mg/5 mL (75 mL, 150 mL); 250 mg/5 mL (75 mL, 150 mL); 375 mg/5 mL (50 mL, 100 mL)

Tablet, chewable:

Raniclor™: 250 mg [contains phenylalanine 5.6 mg/tablet and tartrazine; fruity flavor]; 375 mg [contains phenylalanine 8.4 mg/tablet and tartrazine; fruity flavor]

Tablet, extended release: 500 mg

Dental Comment Patients allergic to penicillins can use a cephalosporin; the incidence of cross-reactivity between penicillins and cephalosporins is 1% when the allergic reaction to penicillin is delayed. Cefaclor is effective against anaerobic bacteria, but the sensitivity of alpha-hemolytic *Streptococcus* varies; approximately 10% of strains are resistant. Nearly 70% are intermediately sensitive. If the patient has a history of immediate reaction to penicillin, the incidence of cross-reactivity is 20%; cephalosporins are contraindicated in these patients.

Cefadroxil (sef a DROKS il)

Related Information
Bacterial Infections *on page 1793*
U.S. Brand Names Duricef®
Canadian Brand Names Apo-Cefadroxil®; Duricef®; Novo-Cefadroxil
Mexican Brand Names Cefamox; Cepotec; Duracef; Teroxina
Generic Available Yes
Index Terms Cefadroxil Monohydrate
Pharmacologic Category Antibiotic, Cephalosporin (First Generation)
Use Treatment of susceptible bacterial infections, including those caused by group A beta-hemolytic *Streptococcus*; prophylaxis against bacterial endocarditis in patients who are allergic to penicillin and undergoing surgical or dental procedures
Local Anesthetic/Vasoconstrictor Precautions No information available to require special precautions
Effects on Dental Treatment No significant effects or complications reported
Common Adverse Effects
1% to 10%: Gastrointestinal: Diarrhea
Reactions reported with other cephalosporins: Toxic epidermal necrolysis, abdominal pain, superinfection, renal dysfunction, toxic nephropathy, aplastic anemia, hemolytic anemia, hemorrhage, prothrombin time prolonged, BUN increased, creatinine increased, eosinophilia, pancytopenia, seizure
Mechanism of Action Inhibits bacterial cell wall synthesis by binding to one or more of the penicillin-binding proteins (PBPs) which in turn inhibits the final transpeptidation step of peptidoglycan synthesis in bacterial cell walls, thus inhibiting cell wall biosynthesis. Bacteria eventually lyse due to ongoing activity of cell wall autolytic enzymes (autolysins and murein hydrolases) while cell wall assembly is arrested.
Drug Interactions
Increased Effect/Toxicity: Bleeding may occur when administered with anticoagulants. Probenecid may decrease cephalosporin elimination.
Pharmacodynamics/Kinetics
Absorption: Rapid and well absorbed
Distribution: Widely throughout the body and reaches therapeutic concentrations in most tissues and body fluids, including synovial, pericardial, pleural, and peritoneal fluids; bile, sputum, and urine; bone, myocardium, gallbladder, skin and soft tissue; crosses placenta; enters breast milk
Protein binding: 20%
Half-life elimination: 1-2 hours; Renal failure: 20-24 hours
Time to peak, serum: 70-90 minutes
Excretion: Urine (>90% as unchanged drug)
Pregnancy Risk Factor B
Cefadroxil Monohydrate *see* Cefadroxil *on page 297*

Cefazolin (sef A zoe lin)

Related Information
Antibiotic Prophylaxis *on page 1772*
Generic Available Yes
(Continued)

Cefazolin *(Continued)*

Index Terms Cefazolin Sodium

Pharmacologic Category Antibiotic, Cephalosporin (First Generation)

Dental Use Alternative antibiotic for prevention of bacterial endocarditis when parenteral administration is needed. Individuals allergic to amoxicillin (penicillins) may receive cefazolin provided they have not had an immediate, local, or systemic IgE-mediated anaphylactic allergic reaction to penicillin. Alternate antibiotic for premedication in patients not allergic to penicillin who may be at potential increased risk of hematogenous total joint infection when parenteral administration is needed.

Use Treatment of respiratory tract, skin and skin structure, genital, urinary tract, biliary tract, bone and joint infections, and septicemia due to susceptible gram-positive cocci (except enterococcus); some gram-negative bacilli including *E. coli*, *Proteus*, and *Klebsiella* may be susceptible; perioperative prophylaxis

Unlabeled/Investigational Use Prophylaxis against bacterial endocarditis

Local Anesthetic/Vasoconstrictor Precautions No information available to require special precautions

Effects on Dental Treatment No significant effects or complications reported

Significant Adverse Effects Frequency not defined.

Central nervous system: Fever, seizure

Dermatologic: Rash, pruritus, Stevens-Johnson syndrome

Gastrointestinal: Diarrhea, nausea, vomiting, abdominal cramps, anorexia, pseudomembranous colitis, oral candidiasis

Genitourinary: Vaginitis

Hepatic: Transaminases increased, hepatitis

Hematologic: Eosinophilia, neutropenia, leukopenia, thrombocytopenia, thrombocytosis

Local: Pain at injection site, phlebitis

Renal: BUN increased, serum creatinine increased, renal failure

Miscellaneous: Anaphylaxis

Reactions reported with other cephalosporins: Toxic epidermal necrolysis, abdominal pain, cholestasis, superinfection, toxic nephropathy, aplastic anemia, hemolytic anemia, hemorrhage, prothrombin time prolonged, pancytopenia

Dental Usual Dosing

Infective endocarditis prophylaxis: I.M., I.V.:

Infants and Children: 50 mg/kg 30-60 minutes before procedure; maximum dose: 1 g

Adults: 1 g 30-60 minutes before procedure. **Note:** Intramuscular injections should be avoided in patients who are receiving anticoagulant therapy. In these circumstances, orally administered regimens should be given whenever possible. Intravenously administered antibiotics should be used for patients who are unable to tolerate or absorb oral medications.

Prophylaxis in total joint replacement patient: I.M., I.V.: Adults: 1 g 1 hour prior to the procedure

Dosage

Usual dosage range: I.M., I.V.:

Children >1 month: 25-100 mg/kg/day divided every 6-8 hours; maximum: 6 g/day

Adults: 250 mg to 2 g every 6-12 (usually 8) hours, depending on severity of infection; maximum dose: 12 g/day

Indication-specific dosing:

Prophylaxis against bacterial endocarditis (unlabeled use):

Infants and Children: 25 mg/kg 30 minutes before procedure; maximum dose: 1 g

Adults: 1 g 30 minutes before procedure

Mild-to-moderate infections: Adults: 500 mg to 1 g every 6-8 hours

Mild infection with gram-positive cocci: Adults: 250-500 mg every 8 hours

Perioperative prophylaxis: Adults: 1 g given 30 minutes prior to surgery (repeat with 500 mg to 1 g during prolonged surgery); followed by 500 mg to 1 g every 6-9 hours for 24 hours postop

Pneumococcal pneumonia: Adults: 500 mg every 12 hours

Severe infection: Adults: 1-2 g every 6 hours

Prophylaxis against bacterial endocarditis (unlabeled use): Adults: 1 g 30 minutes before procedure

UTI (uncomplicated): Adults: 1 g every 12 hours

Dosing adjustment in renal impairment:

Cl_{cr} 10-30 mL/minute: Administer every 12 hours

Cl_{cr} <10 mL/minute: Administer every 24 hours

Hemodialysis: Moderately dialyzable (20% to 50%); administer dose postdialysis or administer supplemental dose of 0.5-1 g after dialysis

Peritoneal dialysis: Administer 0.5 g every 12 hours

Continuous arteriovenous or venovenous hemofiltration: Dose as for Cl_{cr} 10-30 mL/minute; removes 30 mg of cefazolin per liter of filtrate per day

Mechanism of Action Inhibits bacterial cell wall synthesis by binding to one or more of the penicillin-binding proteins (PBPs) which in turn inhibits the final transpeptidation step of peptidoglycan synthesis in bacterial cell walls, thus inhibiting cell wall biosynthesis. Bacteria eventually lyse due to ongoing activity of cell wall autolytic enzymes (autolysins and murein hydrolases) while cell wall assembly is arrested.

Contraindications Hypersensitivity to cefazolin sodium, any component of the formulation, or other cephalosporins

Warnings/Precautions Modify dosage in patients with severe renal impairment. Use with caution in patients with a history of penicillin allergy, especially IgE-mediated reactions (eg, anaphylaxis, angioedema, urticaria). Prolonged use may result in fungal or bacterial superinfection, including *C. difficile*-associated diarrhea and pseudomembranous colitis. May be associated with increased INR, especially in nutritionally-deficient patients, prolonged treatment, hepatic or renal disease. Use with caution in patients with a history of seizure disorder; high levels, particularly in the presence of renal impairment, may increase risk of seizures.

Drug Interactions

Aminoglycosides: Aminoglycosides increase nephrotoxic potential.

Probenecid: High-dose probenecid decreases clearance.

Warfarin: Cefazolin may increase the hypothrombinemic response to warfarin (due to alteration of GI microbial flora).

Dietary Considerations Sodium content of 1 g: 48 mg (2 mEq)

Pharmacodynamics/Kinetics

Distribution: Widely into most body tissues and fluids including gallbladder, liver, kidneys, bone, sputum, bile, pleural, and synovial; CSF penetration is poor; crosses placenta; enters breast milk

Protein binding: 74% to 86%

Metabolism: Minimally hepatic

Half-life elimination: 90-150 minutes; prolonged with renal impairment

Time to peak, serum: I.M.: 0.5-2 hours

Excretion: Urine (80% to 100% as unchanged drug)

Pregnancy Risk Factor B

Lactation Enters breast milk (small amounts)/use caution (AAP rates "compatible")

Breast-Feeding Considerations Theoretically, drug absorbed by nursing infant may change bowel flora or affect fever work-up result. **Note:** As a class, cephalosporins are used to treat infections in infants.

Dosage Forms Excipient information presented when available (limited, particularly for generics); consult specific product labeling.

Infusion [premixed in D_5W]: 1 g (50 mL)

Injection, powder for reconstitution: 500 mg, 1 g, 10 g, 20 g

Selected Readings

ADA Division of Legal Affairs, "A Legal Perspective on Antibiotic Prophylaxis," *J Am Dent Assoc*, 2003, 134(9):1260.

"Advisory Statement. Antibiotic Prophylaxis for Dental Patients With Total Joint Replacements. American Dental Association; American Academy of Orthopedic Surgeons," *J Am Dent Assoc*, 1997, 128(7):1004-8.

American Dental Association; American Academy of Orthopedic Surgeons, "Antibiotic Prophylaxis for Dental Patients With Total Joint Replacements," *J Am Dent Assoc*, 2003, 134(7):895-9.

American Dental Association Council on Scientific Affairs, "Combating Antibiotic Resistance," *J Am Dent Assoc*, 2004, 135(4):484-7.

Dajani AS, Taubert KA, Wilson W, et al, "Prevention of Bacterial Endocarditis. Recommendations by the American Heart Association," *JAMA*, 1997, 277(22):1794-801.

Dajani AS, Taubert KA, Wilson W, et al, "Prevention of Bacterial Endocarditis: Recommendations by the American Heart Association," *J Am Dent Assoc*, 1997, 128(8):1142-51.

Donowitz GR and Mandell GL, "Drug Therapy. Beta-Lactam Antibiotics (1)," *N Engl J Med*, 1988, 318(7):419-26.

Donowitz GR and Mandell GL, "Drug Therapy. Beta-Lactam Antibiotics (2)," *N Engl J Med*, 1988, 318(8):490-500.

Gustaferro CA and Steckelberg JM, "Cephalosporin Antimicrobial Agents and Related Compounds," *Mayo Clin Proc*, 1991, 66(10):1064-73.

Cefazolin Sodium *see* Cefazolin *on page 297*

Cefdinir (SEF di ner)

U.S. Brand Names Omnicef®
Canadian Brand Names Omnicef®
Generic Available No

(Continued)

Cefdinir *(Continued)*

Index Terms CFDN

Pharmacologic Category Antibiotic, Cephalosporin (Third Generation)

Use Treatment of community-acquired pneumonia, acute exacerbations of chronic bronchitis, acute bacterial otitis media, acute maxillary sinusitis, pharyngitis/tonsillitis, and uncomplicated skin and skin structure infections.

Local Anesthetic/Vasoconstrictor Precautions No information available to require special precautions

Effects on Dental Treatment No significant effects or complications reported

Common Adverse Effects

>10%: Gastrointestinal: Diarrhea (8% to 15%)

1% to 10%:

Central nervous system: Headache (2%)

Dermatologic: Rash (≤3%)

Gastrointestinal: Nausea (≤3%), abdominal pain (≤1%), vomiting (≤1%)

Genitourinary: Vaginal moniliasis (≤4%), urine leukocytes increased (2%), urine protein increased (1% to 2%), vaginitis (≤1%)

Hematologic: Eosinophils increased (1%)

Hepatic: Alkaline phosphatase increased (≤1%), platelets increased (1%)

Renal: Microhematuria (1%)

Miscellaneous: Lymphocytes increased (≤2%), GGT increased (1%), lactate dehydrogenase increased (≤1%), bicarbonate decreased (≤1%), lymphocytes decreased (≤1%), PMN changes (≤1%)

Reactions reported with other cephalosporins: Dizziness, fever, encephalopathy, asterixis, neuromuscular excitability, seizure, aplastic anemia, interstitial nephritis, toxic nephropathy, angioedema, hemorrhage, PT prolonged, and superinfection

Mechanism of Action Inhibits bacterial cell wall synthesis by binding to one or more of the penicillin-binding proteins (PBPs) which in turn inhibits the final transpeptidation step of peptidoglycan synthesis in bacterial cell walls, thus inhibiting cell wall biosynthesis. Bacteria eventually lyse due to ongoing activity of cell wall autolytic enzymes (autolysins and murein hydrolases) while cell wall assembly is arrested.

Drug Interactions

Increased Effect/Toxicity: Probenecid may increase the effects of cefdinir by decreasing renal elimination (peak plasma levels of cefdinir are increased by 54% and half-life is prolonged by 50%).

Decreased Effect: Coadministration with iron or antacids reduces the rate and extent of cefdinir absorption.

Pharmacodynamics/Kinetics

Distribution: V_d:

Children 6 months to 12 years: 0.29-1.05 L/kg

Adults: 0.06-0.64 L/kg

Protein binding: 60% to 70%

Metabolism: Minimally hepatic

Bioavailability: Capsule: 16% to 21%; suspension 25%

Half-life elimination: 100 minutes

Excretion: Primarily urine

Pregnancy Risk Factor B

Cefditoren *(sef de TOR en)*

Related Information

Bacterial Infections *on page 1793*

U.S. Brand Names Spectracef™

Generic Available No

Index Terms Cefditoren Pivoxil

Pharmacologic Category Antibiotic, Cephalosporin

Dental Use Bactericidal antibiotic for infections due to susceptible organisms

Use Treatment of acute bacterial exacerbation of chronic bronchitis or community-acquired pneumonia (due to susceptible organisms including *Haemophilus influenzae*, *Haemophilus parainfluenzae*, *Streptococcus pneumoniae*-penicillin susceptible only, *Moraxella catarrhalis*); pharyngitis or tonsillitis (*Streptococcus pyogenes*); and uncomplicated skin and skin-structure infections (*Staphylococcus aureus* - not MRSA, *Streptococcus pyogenes*)

Local Anesthetic/Vasoconstrictor Precautions No information available to require special precautions

Effects on Dental Treatment No significant effects or complications reported

Significant Adverse Effects

>10%: Gastrointestinal: Diarrhea (11% to 15%)

1% to 10%:
 Central nervous system: Headache (2% to 3%)
 Endocrine & metabolic: Glucose increased (1% to 2%)
 Gastrointestinal: Nausea (4% to 6%), abdominal pain (2%), dyspepsia (1% to 2%), vomiting (1%)
 Genitourinary: Vaginal moniliasis (3% to 6%)
 Hematologic: Hematocrit decreased (2%)
 Renal: Hematuria (3%), urinary white blood cells increased (2%)
<1% (Limited to important or life-threatening): Acute renal failure, albumin decreased, allergic reaction, arthralgia, asthma, BUN increased, calcium decreased, eosinophilic pneumonia, coagulation time increased, erythema multiforme, fungal infection, hyperglycemia, interstitial pneumonia, leukopenia, leukorrhea, positive direct Coombs' test, potassium increased, pseudomembranous colitis, rash, sodium decreased, Stevens-Johnson syndrome, thrombocythemia, thrombocytopenia, toxic epidermal necrolysis, white blood cells increased/decreased
Reactions reported with other cephalosporins: Anaphylaxis, aplastic anemia, cholestasis, hemorrhage, hemolytic anemia, renal dysfunction, reversible hyperactivity, serum sickness-like reaction, toxic nephropathy

Dental Usual Dosing Dental infections (unlabeled use): Children ≥12 years and Adults: Oral: 400 mg twice daily for 10 days

Dosage
 Usual dosage range:
 Children ≥12 years and Adults: Oral: 200-400 mg twice daily
 Indication-specific dosing:
 Children ≥12 years and Adults: Oral:
  Acute bacterial exacerbation of chronic bronchitis: 400 mg twice daily for 10 days
  Dental infections (unlabeled use): 400 mg twice daily for 10 days
  Community-acquired pneumonia: 400 mg twice daily for 14 days
  Pharyngitis, tonsillitis, uncomplicated skin and skin structure infections: 200 mg twice daily for 10 days
 Dosage adjustment in renal impairment:
  Cl_{cr} 30-49 mL/minute/1.73 m^2: Maximum dose: 200 mg twice daily
  Cl_{cr} <30 mL/minute/1.73 m^2: Maximum dose: 200 mg once daily
  End-stage renal disease: Appropriate dosing not established
 Dosage adjustment in hepatic impairment:
  Mild-to-moderate impairment: Adjustment not required
  Severe impairment (Child-Pugh Class C): Specific guidelines not available

Mechanism of Action Inhibits bacterial cell wall synthesis by binding to one or more of the penicillin binding proteins (PBPs) which in turn inhibits the final transpeptidation step of peptidoglycan synthesis in bacterial cell walls, thus inhibiting cell wall biosynthesis. Bacteria eventually lyse due to ongoing activity of cell wall autolytic enzymes (autolysins and murein hydrolases) while cell wall assembly is arrested.

Contraindications Hypersensitivity to cefditoren, any component of the formulation, other cephalosporins, or milk protein; carnitine deficiency

Warnings/Precautions Use with caution in patients with a history of penicillin allergy, especially IgE-mediated reactions (eg, anaphylaxis, urticaria). Prolonged use may result in fungal or bacterial superinfection, including *C. difficile*-associated diarrhea and pseudomembranous colitis. Caution in individuals with seizure disorders; high levels, particularly in the presence of renal impairment, may increase risk of seizures. Use caution in patients with renal or hepatic impairment; modify dosage in patients with severe renal impairment. Cefditoren causes renal excretion of carnitine; do not use in patients with carnitine deficiency; not for long-term therapy due to the possible development of carnitine deficiency over time. May prolong prothrombin time; use with caution in patients with a history of bleeding disorder. Cefditoren tablets contain sodium caseinate, which may cause hypersensitivity reactions in patients with milk protein hypersensitivity; this does not affect patients with lactose intolerance. Safety and efficacy have not been established in children <12 years of age.

Drug Interactions
 Probenecid: Serum concentration of cefditoren may be increased.
 Warfarin: Prothrombin time may be prolonged by cefditoren; monitor.

Ethanol/Nutrition/Herb Interactions Food: Moderate- to high-fat meals increase bioavailability and maximum plasma concentration.

Dietary Considerations Cefditoren should be taken with meals. Plasma carnitine levels are decreased during therapy (39% with 200 mg dosing, 63% with 400 mg dosing); normal concentrations return within 7-10 days after treatment is discontinued.

Pharmacodynamics/Kinetics
 Distribution: 9.3 ± 1.6 L
 (Continued)

Cefditoren *(Continued)*

Protein binding: 88% (*in vitro*), primarily to albumin
Metabolism: Cefditoren pivoxil is hydrolyzed to cefditoren (active) and pivalate
Bioavailability: ~14% to 16%, increased by moderate to high-fat meal
Half-life elimination: 1.6 ± 0.4 hours
Time to peak: 1.5-3 hours
Excretion: Urine (as cefditoren and pivaloylcarnitine)

Pregnancy Risk Factor B

Lactation Excretion in breast milk unknown/use caution

Dosage Forms Excipient information presented when available (limited, particularly for generics); consult specific product labeling.
Tablet, as pivoxil: 200 mg [equivalent to cefditoren; contains sodium caseinate]

Cefditoren Pivoxil *see* Cefditoren *on page 300*

Cefepime *(SEF e pim)*

U.S. Brand Names Maxipime®
Canadian Brand Names Maxipime®
Mexican Brand Names Maxipime
Generic Available No
Index Terms Cefepime Hydrochloride
Pharmacologic Category Antibiotic, Cephalosporin (Fourth Generation)
Use Treatment of uncomplicated and complicated urinary tract infections, including pyelonephritis caused by typical urinary tract pathogens; monotherapy for febrile neutropenia; uncomplicated skin and skin structure infections caused by *Streptococcus pyogenes*; moderate-to-severe pneumonia caused by pneumococcus, *Pseudomonas aeruginosa*, and other gram-negative organisms; complicated intra-abdominal infections (in combination with metronidazole). Also active against methicillin-susceptible staphylococci, *Enterobacter* sp, and many other gram-negative bacilli.

Children 2 months to 16 years: Empiric therapy of febrile neutropenia patients, uncomplicated skin/soft tissue infections, pneumonia, and uncomplicated/complicated urinary tract infections.

Local Anesthetic/Vasoconstrictor Precautions No information available to require special precautions

Effects on Dental Treatment No significant effects or complications reported

Common Adverse Effects
>10%: Hematologic: Positive Coombs' test without hemolysis
1% to 10%:
Central nervous system: Fever (1%), headache (1%)
Dermatologic: Rash, pruritus
Gastrointestinal: Diarrhea, nausea, vomiting
Local: Erythema at injection site, pain
Reactions reported with other cephalosporins: Aplastic anemia, erythema multiforme, hemolytic anemia, hemorrhage, pancytopenia, PT prolonged, renal dysfunction, Stevens-Johnson syndrome, superinfection, toxic epidermal necrolysis, toxic nephropathy, vaginitis

Mechanism of Action Inhibits bacterial cell wall synthesis by binding to one or more of the penicillin-binding proteins (PBPs) which in turn inhibits the final transpeptidation step of peptidoglycan synthesis in bacterial cell walls, thus inhibiting cell wall biosynthesis. Bacteria eventually lyse due to ongoing activity of cell wall autolytic enzymes (autolysis and murein hydrolases) while cell wall assembly is arrested.

Drug Interactions
Increased Effect/Toxicity: High-dose probenecid decreases clearance and increases effect of cefepime. Aminoglycosides increase nephrotoxic potential when taken with cefepime.

Pharmacodynamics/Kinetics
Absorption: I.M.: Rapid and complete
Distribution: V_d: Adults: 14-20 L; penetrates into inflammatory fluid at concentrations ~80% of serum levels and into bronchial mucosa at levels ~60% of those reached in the plasma; crosses blood-brain barrier
Protein binding, plasma: 16% to 19%
Metabolism: Minimally hepatic
Half-life elimination: 2 hours
Time to peak: 0.5-1.5 hours
Excretion: Urine (85% as unchanged drug)

Pregnancy Risk Factor B

Cefepime Hydrochloride *see* Cefepime *on page 302*

Cefixime (sef IKS eem)

Related Information
Sexually-Transmitted Diseases *on page 1766*
U.S. Brand Names Suprax®
Canadian Brand Names Suprax®
Mexican Brand Names Denvar
Generic Available No
Index Terms Cefixime Trihydrate
Pharmacologic Category Antibiotic, Cephalosporin (Third Generation)
Use Treatment of urinary tract infections, otitis media, respiratory infections due to susceptible organisms including *S. pneumoniae* and *S. pyogenes*, *H. influenzae*, and many Enterobacteriaceae; uncomplicated cervical/urethral gonorrhea due to *N. gonorrhoeae*
Local Anesthetic/Vasoconstrictor Precautions No information available to require special precautions
Effects on Dental Treatment No significant effects or complications reported
Common Adverse Effects
>10%: Gastrointestinal: Diarrhea (16%)
2% to 10%: Gastrointestinal: Abdominal pain, nausea, dyspepsia, flatulence, loose stools
Reactions reported with other cephalosporins: Interstitial nephritis, aplastic anemia, hemolytic anemia, hemorrhage, pancytopenia, agranulocytosis, colitis, superinfection
Mechanism of Action Inhibits bacterial cell wall synthesis by binding to one or more of the penicillin binding proteins (PBPs); which in turn inhibits the final transpeptidation step of peptidoglycan synthesis in bacterial cell walls, thus inhibiting cell wall biosynthesis. Bacteria eventually lyse due to ongoing activity of cell wall autolytic enzymes (autolysins and murein hydrolases) while cell wall assembly is arrested.
Drug Interactions
Increased Effect/Toxicity: Aminoglycosides and furosemide may be possible additives to nephrotoxicity. Probenecid increases cefixime concentration. Cefixime may increase carbamazepine. Cefixime may increase prothrombin time when administered with warfarin.
Pharmacodynamics/Kinetics
Absorption: 40% to 50%
Distribution: Widely throughout the body and reaches therapeutic concentration in most tissues and body fluids, including synovial, pericardial, pleural, peritoneal; bile, sputum, and urine; bone, myocardium, gallbladder, and skin and soft tissue
Protein binding: 65%
Half-life elimination: Normal renal function: 3-4 hours; Renal failure: Up to 11.5 hours
Time to peak, serum: 2-6 hours; delayed with food
Excretion: Urine (50% of absorbed dose as active drug); feces (10%)
Pregnancy Risk Factor B

Cefixime Trihydrate *see* Cefixime *on page 303*
Cefizox® *see* Ceftizoxime *on page 309*
Cefotan® [DSC] *see* Cefotetan *on page 304*

Cefotaxime (sef oh TAKS eem)

Related Information
Sexually-Transmitted Diseases *on page 1766*
U.S. Brand Names Claforan®
Canadian Brand Names Claforan®
Mexican Brand Names Benaxima; Biosint; Cefoclin; Sepsilem; Taporin; Tirotax; Viken
Generic Available Yes: Powder
Index Terms Cefotaxime Sodium
Pharmacologic Category Antibiotic, Cephalosporin (Third Generation)
Use Treatment of susceptible infection in respiratory tract, skin and skin structure, bone and joint, urinary tract, gynecologic as well as septicemia, and documented or suspected meningitis. Active against most gram-negative bacilli (not *Pseudomonas*) and gram-positive cocci (not enterococcus). Active against many penicillin-resistant pneumococci.
Local Anesthetic/Vasoconstrictor Precautions No information available to require special precautions
Effects on Dental Treatment No significant effects or complications reported
(Continued)

Cefotaxime *(Continued)*

Common Adverse Effects
1% to 10%:
Dermatologic: Rash, pruritus
Gastrointestinal: Diarrhea, nausea, vomiting, colitis
Local: Pain at injection site
Reactions reported with other cephalosporins: Agranulocytosis, aplastic anemia, cholestasis, hemolytic anemia, hemorrhage, nephropathy, pancytopenia, renal dysfunction, seizure, superinfection.

Mechanism of Action
Inhibits bacterial cell wall synthesis by binding to one or more of the penicillin-binding proteins (PBPs) which in turn inhibits the final transpeptidation step of peptidoglycan synthesis in bacterial cell walls, thus inhibiting cell wall biosynthesis. Bacteria eventually lyse due to ongoing activity of cell wall autolytic enzymes (autolysins and murein hydrolases) while cell wall assembly is arrested.

Drug Interactions
Increased Effect/Toxicity: Probenecid may decrease cephalosporin elimination resulting in increased levels. Furosemide, aminoglycosides in combination with cefotaxime may result in additive nephrotoxicity.

Pharmacodynamics/Kinetics
Distribution: Widely to body tissues and fluids including aqueous humor, ascitic and prostatic fluids, bone; penetrates CSF best when meninges are inflamed; crosses placenta; enters breast milk
Metabolism: Partially hepatic to active metabolite, desacetylcefotaxime
Half-life elimination:
Cefotaxime: Premature neonates <1 week: 5-6 hours; Full-term neonates <1 week: 2-3.4 hours; Adults: 1-1.5 hours; prolonged with renal and/or hepatic impairment
Desacetylcefotaxime: 1.5-1.9 hours; prolonged with renal impairment
Time to peak, serum: I.M.: Within 30 minutes
Excretion: Urine (as unchanged drug and metabolites)

Pregnancy Risk Factor B

Cefotaxime Sodium *see* Cefotaxime *on page 303*

Cefotetan *(SEF oh tee tan)*

U.S. Brand Names Cefotan® [DSC]
Canadian Brand Names Cefotan®
Generic Available No
Index Terms Cefotetan Disodium
Pharmacologic Category Antibiotic, Cephalosporin (Second Generation)
Use Surgical prophylaxis; intra-abdominal infections and other mixed infections; respiratory tract, skin and skin structure, bone and joint, urinary tract and gynecologic as well as septicemia; active against gram-negative enteric bacilli including *E. coli*, *Klebsiella*, and *Proteus*; less active against staphylococci and streptococci than first generation cephalosporins, but active against anaerobes including *Bacteroides fragilis*
Local Anesthetic/Vasoconstrictor Precautions No information available to require special precautions
Effects on Dental Treatment No significant effects or complications reported

Common Adverse Effects
1% to 10%:
Gastrointestinal: Diarrhea (1%)
Hepatic: Transaminases increased (1%)
Miscellaneous: Hypersensitivity reactions (1%)
Reactions reported with other cephalosporins: Seizure, Stevens-Johnson syndrome, toxic epidermal necrolysis, renal dysfunction, toxic nephropathy, cholestasis, aplastic anemia, hemolytic anemia, hemorrhage, pancytopenia, agranulocytosis, colitis, superinfection

Mechanism of Action
Inhibits bacterial cell wall synthesis by binding to one or more of the penicillin-binding proteins (PBPs) which in turn inhibits the final transpeptidation step of peptidoglycan synthesis in bacterial cell walls, thus inhibiting cell wall biosynthesis. Bacteria eventually lyse due to ongoing activity of cell wall autolytic enzymes (autolysins and murein hydrolases) while cell wall assembly is arrested.

Drug Interactions
Increased Effect/Toxicity: Disulfiram-like reaction may occur if ethanol is consumed by a patient taking cefotetan. Probenecid may increase cefotetan plasma levels. Cefotetan may increase risk of bleeding in patients receiving warfarin.

Pharmacodynamics/Kinetics

Distribution: Widely to body tissues and fluids including bile, sputum, prostatic, peritoneal; low concentrations enter CSF; crosses placenta; enters breast milk

Protein binding: 76% to 90%

Half-life elimination: 3-5 hours

Time to peak, serum: I.M.: 1.5-3 hours

Excretion: Primarily urine (as unchanged drug); feces (20%)

Pregnancy Risk Factor B

Cefotetan Disodium *see* Cefotetan *on page 304*

Cefoxitin (se FOKS i tin)

Related Information

Sexually-Transmitted Diseases *on page 1766*

U.S. Brand Names Mefoxin®

Canadian Brand Names Apo-Cefoxitin®

Generic Available Yes: Powder for injection

Index Terms Cefoxitin Sodium

Pharmacologic Category Antibiotic, Cephalosporin (Second Generation)

Use Less active against staphylococci and streptococci than first generation cephalosporins, but active against anaerobes including *Bacteroides fragilis*; active against gram-negative enteric bacilli including *E. coli*, *Klebsiella*, and *Proteus*; used predominantly for respiratory tract, skin and skin structure, bone and joint, urinary tract and gynecologic as well as septicemia; surgical prophylaxis; intra-abdominal infections and other mixed infections; indicated for bacterial *Eikenella corrodens* infections

Local Anesthetic/Vasoconstrictor Precautions No information available to require special precautions

Effects on Dental Treatment No significant effects or complications reported

Common Adverse Effects

1% to 10%: Gastrointestinal: Diarrhea

Reactions reported with other cephalosporins: Agranulocytosis, aplastic anemia, cholestasis, colitis, erythema multiforme, hemolytic anemia, hemorrhage, pancytopenia, renal dysfunction, serum-sickness reactions, seizure, Stevens-Johnson syndrome, superinfection, toxic nephropathy, vaginitis

Mechanism of Action Inhibits bacterial cell wall synthesis by binding to one or more of the penicillin-binding proteins (PBPs) which in turn inhibits the final transpeptidation step of peptidoglycan synthesis in bacterial cell walls, thus inhibiting cell wall biosynthesis. Bacteria eventually lyse due to ongoing activity of cell wall autolytic enzymes (autolysins and murein hydrolases) while cell wall assembly is arrested.

Drug Interactions

Increased Effect/Toxicity: Probenecid may decrease cephalosporin elimination. Furosemide, aminoglycosides in combination with cefoxitin may result in additive nephrotoxicity.

Pharmacodynamics/Kinetics

Distribution: Widely to body tissues and fluids including pleural, synovial, ascitic, bile; poorly penetrates into CSF even with inflammation of the meninges; crosses placenta; small amounts enter breast milk

Protein binding: 65% to 79%

Half-life elimination: 45-60 minutes; significantly prolonged with renal impairment

Time to peak, serum: I.M.: 20-30 minutes

Excretion: Urine (85% as unchanged drug)

Pregnancy Risk Factor B

Cefoxitin Sodium *see* Cefoxitin *on page 305*

Cefpodoxime (sef pode OKS eem)

U.S. Brand Names Vantin®

Canadian Brand Names Vantin®

Generic Available Yes: Tablet

Index Terms Cefpodoxime Proxetil

Pharmacologic Category Antibiotic, Cephalosporin (Third Generation)

Use Treatment of susceptible acute, community-acquired pneumonia caused by *S. pneumoniae* or nonbeta-lactamase producing *H. influenzae*; acute uncomplicated gonorrhea caused by *N. gonorrhoeae*; uncomplicated skin and skin structure infections caused by *S. aureus* or *S. pyogenes*; acute otitis media caused by *S. pneumoniae*, *H. influenzae*, or *M. catarrhalis*; pharyngitis or tonsillitis; and uncomplicated urinary tract infections caused by *E. coli*, *Klebsiella*, and *Proteus*

(Continued)

Cefpodoxime *(Continued)*

Local Anesthetic/Vasoconstrictor Precautions No information available to require special precautions

Effects on Dental Treatment No significant effects or complications reported

Common Adverse Effects

>10%:
  Dermatologic: Diaper rash (12%)
  Gastrointestinal: Diarrhea in infants and toddlers (15%)

1% to 10%:
  Central nervous system: Headache (1%)
  Dermatologic: Rash (1%)
  Gastrointestinal: Diarrhea (7%), nausea (4%), abdominal pain (2%), vomiting (1% to 2%)
  Genitourinary: Vaginal infection (3%)

Reactions reported with other cephalosporins: Seizure, Stevens-Johnson syndrome, toxic epidermal necrolysis, erythema multiforme, urticaria, serum-sickness reactions, renal dysfunction, interstitial nephritis toxic nephropathy, cholestasis, aplastic anemia, hemolytic anemia, hemorrhage, pancytopenia, agranulocytosis, colitis, vaginitis, superinfection

Mechanism of Action Inhibits bacterial cell wall synthesis by binding to one or more of the penicillin-binding proteins (PBPs) which in turn inhibits the final transpeptidation step of peptidoglycan synthesis in bacterial cell walls, thus inhibiting cell wall biosynthesis. Bacteria eventually lyse due to ongoing activity of cell wall autolytic enzymes (autolysins and murein hydrolases) while cell wall assembly is arrested.

Drug Interactions

Increased Effect/Toxicity: Probenecid may decrease cephalosporin elimination. Furosemide, aminoglycosides in combination with cefpodoxime may result in additive nephrotoxicity.

Decreased Effect: Antacids and H$_2$-receptor antagonists reduce absorption and serum concentration of cefpodoxime.

Pharmacodynamics/Kinetics

Absorption: Rapid and well absorbed (50%), acid stable; enhanced in the presence of food or low gastric pH

Distribution: Good tissue penetration, including lung and tonsils; penetrates into pleural fluid

Protein binding: 18% to 23%

Metabolism: De-esterified in GI tract to active metabolite, cefpodoxime

Half-life elimination: 2.2 hours; prolonged with renal impairment

Time to peak: Within 1 hour

Excretion: Urine (80% as unchanged drug) in 24 hours

Pregnancy Risk Factor B

Cefpodoxime Proxetil *see* Cefpodoxime *on page 305*

Cefprozil *(sef PROE zil)*

U.S. Brand Names Cefzil®

Canadian Brand Names Apo-Cefprozil®; Cefzil®

Mexican Brand Names Procef

Generic Available Yes

Pharmacologic Category Antibiotic, Cephalosporin (Second Generation)

Use Treatment of otitis media and infections involving the respiratory tract and skin and skin structure; active against methicillin-sensitive staphylococci, many streptococci, and various gram-negative bacilli including *E. coli*, some *Klebsiella*, *P. mirabilis*, *H. influenzae*, and *Moraxella*.

Local Anesthetic/Vasoconstrictor Precautions No information available to require special precautions

Effects on Dental Treatment No significant effects or complications reported

Common Adverse Effects

1% to 10%:
  Central nervous system: Dizziness (1%)
  Dermatologic: Diaper rash (2%)
  Gastrointestinal: Diarrhea (3%), nausea (4%), vomiting (1%), abdominal pain (1%)
  Genitourinary: Vaginitis, genital pruritus (2%)
  Hepatic: Transaminases increased (2%)
  Miscellaneous: Superinfection

Reactions reported with other cephalosporins: Seizure, toxic epidermal necrolysis, renal dysfunction, interstitial nephritis, toxic nephropathy, aplastic anemia, hemolytic anemia, hemorrhage, pancytopenia, agranulocytosis, colitis, vaginitis, superinfection

Mechanism of Action Inhibits bacterial cell wall synthesis by binding to one or more of the penicillin-binding proteins (PBPs) which in turn inhibits the final transpeptidation step of peptidoglycan synthesis in bacterial cell walls, thus inhibiting cell wall biosynthesis. Bacteria eventually lyse due to ongoing activity of cell wall autolytic enzymes (autolysins and murein hydrolases) while cell wall assembly is arrested.

Drug Interactions
Increased Effect/Toxicity: Probenecid may decrease cephalosporin elimination. Furosemide, aminoglycosides in combination with cefprozil may result in additive nephrotoxicity.

Pharmacodynamics/Kinetics
Absorption: Well absorbed (94%)
Distribution: Low amounts enter breast milk
Protein binding: 35% to 45%
Half-life elimination: Normal renal function: 1.3 hours
Time to peak, serum: Fasting: 1.5 hours
Excretion: Urine (61% as unchanged drug)

Pregnancy Risk Factor B

Ceftazidime (SEF tay zi deem)

U.S. Brand Names Ceptaz® [DSC]; Fortaz®; Tazicef®
Canadian Brand Names Fortaz®
Mexican Brand Names Fortum; Tagal; Waytrax; Zadolina
Generic Available No
Pharmacologic Category Antibiotic, Cephalosporin (Third Generation)
Use Treatment of documented susceptible *Pseudomonas aeruginosa* infection and infections due to other susceptible aerobic gram-negative organisms; empiric therapy of a febrile, granulocytopenic patient
Local Anesthetic/Vasoconstrictor Precautions No information available to require special precautions
Effects on Dental Treatment No significant effects or complications reported
Common Adverse Effects
1% to 10%:
Gastrointestinal: Diarrhea (1%)
Local: Pain at injection site (1%)
Miscellaneous: Hypersensitivity reactions (2%)
Reactions reported with other cephalosporins: Seizure, urticaria, serum-sickness reactions, renal dysfunction, interstitial nephritis, toxic nephropathy, BUN increased, creatinine increased, cholestasis, aplastic anemia, hemolytic anemia, pancytopenia, agranulocytosis, colitis, prolonged PT, hemorrhage, superinfection

Mechanism of Action Inhibits bacterial cell wall synthesis by binding to one or more of the penicillin-binding proteins (PBPs) which in turn inhibits the final transpeptidation step of peptidoglycan synthesis in bacterial cell walls, thus inhibiting cell wall biosynthesis. Bacteria eventually lyse due to ongoing activity of cell wall autolytic enzymes (autolysins and murein hydrolases) while cell wall assembly is arrested.

Drug Interactions
Increased Effect/Toxicity: Probenecid may decrease cephalosporin elimination. Cephalosporins may increase the anticoagulant effect of coumarin derivatives. When combined with aminoglycosides, *in vitro* studies indicate additive or synergistic effect against some strains of Enterobacteriaceae and *Pseudomonas aeruginosa.*

Pharmacodynamics/Kinetics
Distribution: Widely throughout the body including bone, bile, skin, CSF (higher concentrations achieved when meninges are inflamed), endometrium, heart, pleural and lymphatic fluids
Protein binding: 17%
Half-life elimination: 1-2 hours, prolonged with renal impairment; Neonates <23 days: 2.2-4.7 hours
Time to peak, serum: I.M.: ~1 hour
Excretion: Urine (80% to 90% as unchanged drug)

Pregnancy Risk Factor B

Ceftibuten (sef TYE byoo ten)

Related Information
Bacterial Infections *on page 1793*
(Continued)

Ceftibuten (Continued)

U.S. Brand Names Cedax®

Mexican Brand Names Cedax

Generic Available No

Pharmacologic Category Antibiotic, Cephalosporin (Third Generation)

Use Oral cephalosporin for treatment of bronchitis, otitis media, and pharyngitis/tonsillitis due to *H. influenzae* and *M. catarrhalis*, both beta-lactamase-producing and nonproducing strains, as well as *S. pneumoniae* (weak) and *S. pyogenes*

Local Anesthetic/Vasoconstrictor Precautions No information available to require special precautions

Effects on Dental Treatment No significant effects or complications reported

Common Adverse Effects

1% to 10%:

Central nervous system: Headache (3%), dizziness (1%)

Gastrointestinal: Nausea (4%), diarrhea (3%), dyspepsia (2%), vomiting (1%), abdominal pain (1%)

Hematologic: Eosinophils increased (3%), hemoglobin decreased (2%), thrombocytosis

Hepatic: ALT increased (1%), bilirubin increased (1%)

Renal: BUN increased (4%)

Reactions reported with other cephalosporins: Anaphylaxis, fever, paresthesia, pruritus, Stevens-Johnson syndrome, toxic epidermal necrolysis, erythema multiforme, angioedema, pseudomembranous colitis, hemolytic anemia, candidiasis, vaginitis, encephalopathy, asterixis, neuromuscular excitability, seizure, serum-sickness reactions, renal dysfunction, interstitial nephritis, toxic nephropathy, cholestasis, aplastic anemia, hemolytic anemia, pancytopenia, agranulocytosis, colitis, prolonged PT, hemorrhage, superinfection

Dosage

Usual dosage range:

Children <12 years: Oral: 9 mg/kg/day for 10 days (maximum dose: 400 mg/day)

Children ≥12 years and Adults: Oral: 400 mg once daily for 10 days (maximum dose: 400 mg/day)

Dosage adjustment in renal impairment:

Cl_{cr} 30-49 mL/minute: Administer 4.5 mg/kg or 200 mg every 24 hours

Cl_{cr} 5-29 mL/minute: Administer 2.25 mg/kg or 100 mg every 24 hours.

Hemodialysis: Administer 400 mg or 9 mg/kg (maximum: 400 mg) after hemodialysis

Mechanism of Action Inhibits bacterial cell wall synthesis by binding to one or more of the penicillin-binding proteins (PBPs) which in turn inhibits the final transpeptidation step of peptidoglycan synthesis in bacterial cell walls, thus inhibiting cell wall biosynthesis. Bacteria eventually lyse due to ongoing activity of cell wall autolytic enzymes (autolysins and murein hydrolases) while cell wall assembly is arrested.

Contraindications Hypersensitivity to ceftibuten, any component of the formulation, or other cephalosporins

Warnings/Precautions Modify dosage in patients with severe renal impairment. Prolonged use may result in fungal or bacterial superinfection, including *C. difficile*-associated diarrhea and pseudomembranous colitis. Use with caution in patients with a history of penicillin allergy, especially IgE-mediated reactions (eg, anaphylaxis, urticaria).

Drug Interactions

Increased Effect/Toxicity: High-dose probenecid decreases clearance. Aminoglycosides in combination with ceftibuten may increase nephrotoxic potential.

Dietary Considerations

Capsule: Take without regard to food.

Suspension: Take 2 hours before or 1 hour after meals; contains 1 g of sucrose per 5 mL

Pharmacodynamics/Kinetics

Absorption: Rapid; food decreases peak concentrations, delays T_{max}, and lowers AUC

Distribution: V_d: Children: 0.5 L/kg; Adults: 0.21 L/kg

Half-life elimination: 2 hours

Time to peak: 2-3 hours

Excretion: Urine

Pregnancy Risk Factor B

Dosage Forms

Capsule:

Cedax®: 400 mg

Powder for oral suspension:

Cedax®: 90 mg/5 mL

Ceftin® *see* Cefuroxime *on page 310*

Ceftizoxime (sef ti ZOKS eem)

Related Information
Treatment of Sexually-Transmitted Infections *on page 1920*
U.S. Brand Names Cefizox®
Canadian Brand Names Cefizox®
Generic Available No
Index Terms Ceftizoxime Sodium
Pharmacologic Category Antibiotic, Cephalosporin (Third Generation)
Use Treatment of susceptible bacterial infections, mainly respiratory tract, skin and skin structure, bone and joint, urinary tract and gynecologic, as well as septicemia; active against many gram-negative bacilli (not *Pseudomonas*), some gram-positive cocci (not *Enterococcus*), and some anaerobes
Local Anesthetic/Vasoconstrictor Precautions No information available to require special precautions
Effects on Dental Treatment No significant effects or complications reported
Common Adverse Effects
1% to 10%:
Central nervous system: Fever
Dermatologic: Rash, pruritus
Hematologic: Eosinophilia, thrombocytosis
Hepatic: Alkaline phosphatase increased, transaminases increased
Local: Pain, burning at injection site
Reactions reported with other cephalosporins: Stevens-Johnson syndrome, toxic epidermal necrolysis, erythema multiforme, pseudomembranous colitis, angioedema, hemolytic anemia, candidiasis, encephalopathy, asterixis, neuromuscular excitability, seizure, serum-sickness reactions, renal dysfunction, interstitial nephritis, toxic nephropathy, cholestasis, aplastic anemia, hemolytic anemia, pancytopenia, agranulocytosis, colitis, prolonged PT, hemorrhage, superinfection
Mechanism of Action Inhibits bacterial cell wall synthesis by binding to one or more of the penicillin-binding proteins (PBPs) which in turn inhibits the final transpeptidation step of peptidoglycan synthesis in bacterial cell walls, thus inhibiting cell wall biosynthesis. Bacteria eventually lyse due to ongoing activity of cell wall autolytic enzymes (autolysins and murein hydrolases) while cell wall assembly is arrested.
Drug Interactions
Increased Effect/Toxicity: Probenecid may decrease cephalosporin elimination. Furosemide, aminoglycosides in combination with ceftizoxime may result in additive nephrotoxicity.
Pharmacodynamics/Kinetics
Distribution: V_d: 0.35-0.5 L/kg; widely into most body tissues and fluids including gallbladder, liver, kidneys, bone, sputum, bile, pleural and synovial fluids; has good CSF penetration; crosses placenta; small amounts enter breast milk
Protein binding: 30%
Half-life elimination: 1.6 hours; Cl_{cr} <10 mL/minute: 25 hours
Time to peak, serum: I.M.: 0.5-1 hour
Excretion: Urine (as unchanged drug)
Pregnancy Risk Factor B

Ceftizoxime Sodium *see* Ceftizoxime *on page 309*

Ceftriaxone (sef trye AKS one)

Related Information
Antibiotic Prophylaxis *on page 1772*
Sexually-Transmitted Diseases *on page 1766*
U.S. Brand Names Rocephin®
Canadian Brand Names Rocephin®
Mexican Brand Names Benaxona; Cefaxona; Ceftrex; Ceftrilem; Megion; Rocephin; Tacex; Triaken
Generic Available Yes
Index Terms Ceftriaxone Sodium
Pharmacologic Category Antibiotic, Cephalosporin (Third Generation)
Dental Use Alternative antibiotic for prevention of infective endocarditis when parenteral administration is needed. Individuals allergic to amoxicillin (penicillins) may receive ceftriaxone provided they have not had an immediate, local, or systemic IgE-mediated anaphylactic allergic reaction to penicillin.
(Continued)

Ceftriaxone *(Continued)*

Use Treatment of lower respiratory tract infections, acute bacterial otitis media, skin and skin structure infections, bone and joint infections, intra-abdominal and urinary tract infections, pelvic inflammatory disease (PID), uncomplicated gonorrhea, bacterial septicemia, and meningitis; used in surgical prophylaxis

Unlabeled/Investigational Use Treatment of chancroid, epididymitis, complicated gonococcal infections; sexually-transmitted diseases (STD); periorbital or buccal cellulitis; salmonellosis or shigellosis; atypical community-acquired pneumonia; Lyme disease; used in chemoprophylaxis for high-risk contacts and persons with invasive meningococcal disease; sexual assault

Local Anesthetic/Vasoconstrictor Precautions No information available to require special precautions

Effects on Dental Treatment No significant effects or complications reported

Common Adverse Effects

1% to 10%:
Dermatologic: Rash (2%)
Gastrointestinal: Diarrhea (3%)
Hematologic: Eosinophilia (6%), thrombocytosis (5%), leukopenia (2%)
Hepatic: Transaminases increased (3.1% to 3.3%)
Local: Pain, induration at injection site (I.V. 1%); warmth, tightness, induration (5% to 17%) following I.M. injection
Renal: BUN increased (1%)

Reactions reported with other cephalosporins: Angioedema, aplastic anemia, asterixis, cholestasis, encephalopathy, erythema multiforme, hemorrhage, interstitial nephritis, neuromuscular excitability, pancytopenia, paresthesia, renal dysfunction, Stevens-Johnson syndrome, superinfection, toxic epidermal necrolysis, toxic nephropathy

Mechanism of Action Inhibits bacterial cell wall synthesis by binding to one or more of the penicillin-binding proteins (PBPs) which in turn inhibits the final transpeptidation step of peptidoglycan synthesis in bacterial cell walls, thus inhibiting cell wall biosynthesis. Bacteria eventually lyse due to ongoing activity of cell wall autolytic enzymes (autolysins and murein hydrolases) while cell wall assembly is arrested.

Drug Interactions

Increased Effect/Toxicity: Cephalosporins may increase the anticoagulant effect of coumarin derivatives (eg, dicumarol, warfarin).

Decreased Effect: Uricosuric agents (eg, probenecid, sulfinpyrazone) may decrease the excretion of cephalosporin; monitor for toxic effects.

Pharmacodynamics/Kinetics

Absorption: I.M.: Well absorbed
Distribution: Widely throughout the body including gallbladder, lungs, bone, bile, CSF (higher concentrations achieved when meninges are inflamed); crosses placenta; enters amniotic fluid and breast milk
Protein binding: 85% to 95%
Half-life elimination: Normal renal and hepatic function: 5-9 hours
Time to peak, serum: I.M.: 1-2 hours
Excretion: Urine (33% to 65% as unchanged drug); feces

Pregnancy Risk Factor B

Ceftriaxone Sodium see Ceftriaxone on page 309

Cefuroxime *(se fyoor OKS eem)*

Related Information
Bacterial Infections *on page 1793*

U.S. Brand Names Ceftin®; Zinacef®

Canadian Brand Names Apo-Cefuroxime®; Ceftin®; ratio-Cefuroxime; Zinacef®

Mexican Brand Names Cetoxil; Froxal; Zinnat

Generic Available Yes: Excludes powder for oral suspension

Index Terms Cefuroxime Axetil; Cefuroxime Sodium

Pharmacologic Category Antibiotic, Cephalosporin (Second Generation)

Use Treatment of infections caused by staphylococci, group B streptococci, *H. influenzae* (type A and B), *E. coli*, *Enterobacter*, *Salmonella*, and *Klebsiella*; treatment of susceptible infections of the lower respiratory tract, otitis media, urinary tract, skin and soft tissue, bone and joint, sepsis and gonorrhea

Local Anesthetic/Vasoconstrictor Precautions No information available to require special precautions

Effects on Dental Treatment No significant effects or complications reported

Common Adverse Effects

1% to 10%:
Endocrine & metabolic: Alkaline phosphatase increased (2%)

Hematologic: Eosinophilia (7%), hemoglobin and hematocrit decreased (10%)

Hepatic: Transaminases increased (4%)

Local: Thrombophlebitis (2%)

Reactions reported with other cephalosporins: Agranulocytosis, aplastic anemia, asterixis, encephalopathy, hemorrhage, neuromuscular excitability, serum-sickness reactions, superinfection, toxic nephropathy

Mechanism of Action Inhibits bacterial cell wall synthesis by binding to one or more of the penicillin-binding proteins (PBPs) which in turn inhibits the final transpeptidation step of peptidoglycan synthesis in bacterial cell walls, thus inhibiting cell wall biosynthesis. Bacteria eventually lyse due to ongoing activity of cell wall autolytic enzymes (autolysins and murein hydrolases) while cell wall assembly is arrested.

Drug Interactions

Increased Effect/Toxicity: High-dose probenecid decreases clearance. Aminoglycosides in combination with cefuroxime may result in additive nephrotoxicity.

Pharmacodynamics/Kinetics

Absorption: Oral (cefuroxime axetil): Increases with food

Distribution: Widely to body tissues and fluids; crosses blood-brain barrier; therapeutic concentrations achieved in CSF even when meninges are not inflamed; crosses placenta; enters breast milk

Protein binding: 33% to 50%

Bioavailability: Tablet: Fasting: 37%; Following food: 52%

Half-life elimination: Adults: 1-2 hours; prolonged with renal impairment

Time to peak, serum: I.M.: ~15-60 minutes; I.V.: 2-3 minutes

Excretion: Urine (66% to 100% as unchanged drug)

Pregnancy Risk Factor B

Cefuroxime Axetil *see* Cefuroxime *on page 310*

Cefuroxime Sodium *see* Cefuroxime *on page 310*

Cefzil® *see* Cefprozil *on page 306*

Celebrex® *see* Celecoxib *on page 311*

Celecoxib (se le KOKS ib)

Related Information

Oral Pain *on page 1788*

Rheumatoid Arthritis, Osteoarthritis, and Osteoporosis *on page 1759*

U.S. Brand Names Celebrex®

Canadian Brand Names Celebrex®; GD-Celecoxib

Mexican Brand Names Celebrex

Generic Available No

Pharmacologic Category Nonsteroidal Anti-inflammatory Drug (NSAID), COX-2 Selective

Dental Use Management of acute dental pain

Use Relief of the signs and symptoms of osteoarthritis, ankylosing spondylitis, juvenile rheumatoid arthritis (JRA), and rheumatoid arthritis; management of acute pain; treatment of primary dysmenorrhea; decreasing intestinal polyps in familial adenomatous polyposis (FAP).

Canadian note: Celecoxib is only indicated for relief of symptoms of rheumatoid arthritis, osteoarthritis, and relief of acute pain in adults

Local Anesthetic/Vasoconstrictor Precautions No information available to require special precautions

Effects on Dental Treatment Key adverse event(s) related to dental treatment: Stomatitis, abnormal taste, xerostomia (normal salivary flow resumes upon discontinuation), and tooth disorder. Nonselective NSAIDs are known to reversibly decrease platelet aggregation via mechanisms different than observed with aspirin. According to the manufacturer, celecoxib, at single doses up to 800 mg and multiple doses of 600 mg twice daily, had no effect on platelet aggregation or bleeding time. Comparative NSAIDs (naproxen 500 mg twice daily, ibuprofen 800 mg three times daily, or diclofenac 75 mg twice daily) significantly reduced platelet aggregation and prolonged the bleeding times. See Dental Comment.

Significant Adverse Effects Note: Percentages noted in adults.

>10%: Central nervous system: Headache (15.8%)

2% to 10%:

Cardiovascular: Peripheral edema (2.1%)

Central nervous system: Insomnia (2.3%), dizziness (2%)

Dermatologic: Skin rash (2.2%)

Gastrointestinal: Dyspepsia (8.8%), diarrhea (5.6%), abdominal pain (4.1%), nausea (3.5%), flatulence (2.2%)

Neuromuscular & skeletal: Back pain (2.8%)

(Continued)

Celecoxib *(Continued)*

Respiratory: Upper respiratory tract infection (8.1%), sinusitis (5%), pharyngitis (2.3%), rhinitis (2%)

Miscellaneous: Accidental injury (2.9%)

<2%, postmarketing, and/or case reports (limited to important or life-threatening): Acute renal failure, agranulocytosis, albuminuria, allergic reactions, alopecia, anaphylactoid reactions, angioedema, aplastic anemia, arthralgia, aseptic meningitis, ataxia, bronchospasm, cerebrovascular accident, CHF, colitis, conjunctivitis, cystitis, deafness, diabetes mellitus, DVT, dyspnea, dysuria, ecchymosis, erythema multiforme, esophageal perforation, esophagitis, exfoliative dermatitis, flu-like syndrome, gangrene, gastroenteritis, gastroesophageal reflux, gastrointestinal bleeding, glaucoma, hematuria, hepatic failure, hepatitis, hypertension, hypoglycemia, hypokalemia, hyponatremia, interstitial nephritis, intestinal perforation, intracranial hemorrhage, jaundice, leukopenia, melena, migraine, myalgia, MI, neuralgia, neuropathy, pancreatitis, pancytopenia, paresthesia, photosensitivity, prostate disorder, pulmonary embolism, rash, renal calculi, sepsis, Stevens-Johnson syndrome, stomatitis, sudden death, syncope, thrombophlebitis, tinnitus, toxic epidermal necrolysis, urticaria, vaginal bleeding, vaginitis, vasculitis, ventricular fibrillation, vertigo, vomiting

Restrictions An FDA-approved medication guide must be distributed when dispensing an oral outpatient prescription (new or refill) where this medication is to be used without direct supervision of a healthcare provider. Medication guides are available at http://www.fda.gov/cder/Offices/ODS/medication_guides.htm.

Dental Usual Dosing Acute dental pain: Adults: Oral: 400 mg, followed by an additional 200 mg if needed on day 1; maintenance dose: 200 mg twice daily as needed

Dosage Note: Use the lowest effective dose for the shortest duration of time, consistent with individual patient goals. Oral:

Children ≥2 years: JRA
    ≥10 kg to ≤25 kg: 50 mg twice daily
    >25 kg: 100 mg twice daily

Adults:
Acute pain or primary dysmenorrhea: Initial dose: 400 mg, followed by an additional 200 mg if needed on day 1; maintenance dose: 200 mg twice daily as needed

Ankylosing spondylitis: 200 mg/day as a single dose or in divided doses twice daily; if no effect after 6 weeks, may increase to 400 mg/day. If no response following 6 weeks of treatment with 400 mg/day, consider discontinuation and alternative treatment.

Familial adenomatous polyposis: 400 mg twice daily

Osteoarthritis: 200 mg/day as a single dose or in divided dose twice daily

Rheumatoid arthritis: 100-200 mg twice daily

Elderly: No specific adjustment based on age is recommended. However, the AUC in elderly patients may be increased by 50% as compared to younger subjects. Use the lowest recommended dose in patients weighing <50 kg.

Dosing adjustment in renal impairment: No specific dosage adjustment is recommended; not recommended in patients with severe renal dysfunction

Dosing adjustment in hepatic impairment: Reduced dosage is recommended (AUC may be increased by 40% to 180%); decrease dose by 50% in patients with moderate hepatic impairment (Child-Pugh class B). Not recommended for use with severe impairment.

Mechanism of Action Inhibits prostaglandin synthesis by decreasing the activity of the enzyme, cyclooxygenase-2 (COX-2), which results in decreased formation of prostaglandin precursors. Celecoxib does not inhibit cyclooxygenase-1 (COX-1) at therapeutic concentrations. Celecoxib has no effect on platelets. In FAP, celecoxib reduces the number of colorectal polyps.

Contraindications Hypersensitivity to celecoxib, sulfonamides, aspirin, other NSAIDs, or any component of the formulation; perioperative pain in the setting of coronary artery bypass surgery (CABG); pregnancy (3rd trimester)

Warnings/Precautions [U.S. Boxed Warning]: NSAIDs are associated with an increased risk of adverse cardiovascular events, including MI, and new onset or worsening of pre-existing hypertension. Risk may be increased with duration of use or pre-existing cardiovascular risk factors or disease. Carefully evaluate individual cardiovascular risk profiles prior to prescribing. Use caution with fluid retention, CHF, cerebrovascular disease, ischemic heart disease, or hypertension. Long-term cardiovascular risk in children has not been evaluated.

[U.S. Boxed Warning]: Celecoxib is contraindicated for treatment of perioperative pain in the setting of coronary artery bypass surgery (CABG). Risk of MI and stroke may be increased with use following CABG surgery.

[U.S. Boxed Warning]: NSAIDs may increase risk of gastrointestinal irritation, ulceration, bleeding, and perforation. These events may occur at any time during therapy and without warning. Use caution with a history of GI disease (bleeding or ulcers), concurrent therapy with aspirin, anticoagulants and/or corticosteroids, smoking, use of alcohol, the elderly or debilitated patients.

Use the lowest effective dose for the shortest duration of time, consistent with individual patient goals, to reduce risk of cardiovascular or GI adverse events. Alternate therapies should be considered for patients at high risk.

NSAIDs may cause serious skin adverse events including exfoliative dermatitis, Stevens-Johnson syndrome (SJS), and toxic epidermal necrolysis (TEN). Anaphylactoid reactions may occur, even without prior exposure; patients with "aspirin triad" (bronchial asthma, aspirin intolerance, rhinitis) may be at increased risk. Do not use in patients who experience bronchospasm, asthma, rhinitis, or urticaria with NSAID or aspirin therapy. Use caution in other forms of asthma.

Use with caution in patients with decreased hepatic or renal function. Closely monitor patients with any abnormal LFT. Severe hepatic reactions (eg, fulminant hepatitis, liver failure) have occurred with NSAID use, rarely; discontinue if signs or symptoms of liver disease develop, or if systemic manifestations occur. Use of NSAIDs can compromise existing renal function. Renal toxicity can occur in patients with impaired renal function, dehydration, heart failure, liver dysfunction, those taking diuretics and ACE inhibitors, and the elderly. Rehydrate patient before starting therapy; monitor renal function closely. Not recommended for use in patients with advanced renal disease.

Anaphylactoid reactions may occur, even with no prior exposure to celecoxib. Use caution in patients with known or suspected deficiency of cytochrome P450 isoenzyme 2C9.

When used for the treatment of FAP, routine monitoring and care should be continued. When used for JRA, safety and efficacy have not been established in children <2 years of age or in children <10 kg. Use caution with systemic onset JRA. Safety and efficacy have not been established for use in children for indications other than JRA.

Drug Interactions **Substrate** of CYP2C9 (major), 3A4 (minor); **Inhibits** CYP2C8 (moderate), 2D6 (weak)

ACE inhibitors: Antihypertensive effect may be diminished by celecoxib.

Aminoglycosides: Celecoxib may decrease excretion; monitor levels.

Anticoagulants: Celecoxib may enhance the anticoagulant effect of anticoagulants; monitor.

Antiplatelet agents: Celecoxib may enhance the adverse/toxic effect of antiplatelet agents. An increased risk of bleeding may occur.

Aspirin: Low-dose aspirin may be used with celecoxib, however, monitor for GI complications.

Beta-blockers: Antihypertensive effect may be diminished by celecoxib.

Bile acid sequestrants: May decrease absorption of NSAIDs.

CYP2C8 substrates: Celecoxib may increase the levels/effects of CYP2C8 substrates. Example substrates include amiodarone, paclitaxel, pioglitazone, repaglinide, and rosiglitazone.

CYP2C9 inducers: May decrease the levels/effects of celecoxib. Example inducers include carbamazepine, phenobarbital, phenytoin, rifampin, rifapentine, and secobarbital.

CYP2C9 inhibitors: May increase the levels/effects of celecoxib. Example inhibitors include delavirdine, fluconazole, gemfibrozil, ketoconazole, nicardipine, NSAIDs, pioglitazone, and sulfonamides.

Cyclosporine: NSAIDs may increase levels/nephrotoxicity of cyclosporine.

Fluconazole: Fluconazole increases celecoxib concentrations twofold. Lowest dose of celecoxib should be used.

Hydralazine: Antihypertensive effect may be diminished by celecoxib.

Lithium: Plasma levels of lithium are increased by ~17% when used with celecoxib. Monitor lithium levels closely when treatment with celecoxib is started or withdrawn.

Loop diuretics (bumetanide, furosemide, torsemide): Natriuretic effect of furosemide and other loop diuretics may be decreased by celecoxib.

Methotrexate: Severe bone marrow suppression, aplastic anemia, and GI toxicity have been reported with concomitant NSAID therapy. Selective COX-2 inhibitors appear to have a lower risk of this toxicity, however, caution is warranted.

Probenecid: Probenecid may increase the serum concentration of celecoxib; monitor.

Quinolone antibiotics: Celecoxib may enhance the neuroexcitatory and/or seizure-potentiating effect of quinolone antibiotics.

(Continued)

Celecoxib (Continued)

Thiazide diuretics: Natriuretic effects of thiazide diuretics may be decreased by celecoxib.

Treprostinil: Treprostinil may enhance the adverse/toxic effect of celecoxib. Bleeding may occur; monitor.

Vancomycin: Celecoxib may decrease excretion; monitor levels.

Ethanol/Nutrition/Herb Interactions

Ethanol: Avoid ethanol (increased GI irritation).

Food: Peak concentrations are delayed and AUC is increased by 10% to 20% when taken with a high-fat meal.

Herb/Nutraceutical: Avoid concomitant use with herbs possessing anticoagulation/antiplatelet properties, including alfalfa, anise, bilberry, bladderwrack, bromelain, cat's claw, celery, chamomile, coleus, cordyceps, dong quai, evening primrose oil, fenugreek, feverfew, garlic, ginger, ginkgo biloba, ginseng, grapeseed, green tea, guggul, horse chestnut seed, horseradish, licorice, prickly ash, red clover, reishi, SAMe, sweet clover, turmeric, white willow

Dietary Considerations Lower doses (200 mg twice daily) may be taken without regard to meals. Larger doses should be taken with food to improve absorption.

Pharmacodynamics/Kinetics

Distribution: V_d (apparent): 400 L

Protein binding: 97% primarily to albumin

Metabolism: Hepatic via CYP2C9; forms inactive metabolites

Bioavailability: Absolute: Unknown

Half-life elimination: 11 hours (fasted)

Time to peak: 3 hours

Excretion: Urine (27% as metabolites, <3% as unchanged drug); feces (57%)

Pregnancy Risk Factor C/D (3rd trimester)

Lactation Enters breast milk/not recommended

Breast-Feeding Considerations Based on limited data, celecoxib has been found to be excreted in milk; a decision should be made whether to discontinue nursing or discontinue the drug, taking into account the importance of the drug to the mother.

Dosage Forms Excipient information presented when available (limited, particularly for generics); consult specific product labeling.

Capsule:

Celebrex®: 50 mg, 100 mg, 200 mg, 400 mg

Dental Comment The Food and Drug Administration (FDA) has announced product labeling changes for all NSAIDs, including COX-2 selective and over-the-counter (OTC) medications. These changes are the result of the Arthritis and Drug Safety and Risk Management Advisory Committee meeting held in February, 2005.

The FDA has asked that all labels be revised to include information related to the potential for increased risk of cardiovascular (CV) events and gastrointestinal (GI) bleeding associated with their use. In addition, prescription nonselective NSAIDs are being asked to add a contraindication for use in patients who have recently undergone coronary artery bypass graft (CABG) surgery and a boxed warning concerning the CV and GI events. Medication guides will be required for all prescription products. Manufacturers of OTC products are being asked to include a warning about potential skin reactions, which is already included in prescription labeling. The FDA will be working with manufacturers to conduct long-term clinical trials to assess the safety of these agents.

Pfizer, Inc, the manufacturer of celecoxib (Celebrex®) has reported an increased risk of cardiovascular events in one clinical trial during an interim analysis. The increased risk was observed in a trial evaluating celecoxib in patients at risk of colon cancer, prompting the National Cancer Institute to end the study. Other similar clinical studies (which were subjected to analysis by data monitoring committees) are continuing, since an interim analysis of these trials did not reveal an increased risk of cardiovascular events. Further analysis of risk factors related to cardiovascular risk appear warranted. A notice posted by the Food and Drug Administration (FDA) states that the agency "will obtain all available data on these and other ongoing Celebrex® trials as soon as possible and will determine the appropriate regulatory action."

The FDA further notes that these new findings for celecoxib are similar to results with other drugs in this class. Increased cardiovascular risk noted in a study of rofecoxib (Vioxx®) led to a voluntary withdrawal of the product by Merck. In addition, another drug in this class, valdecoxib (Bextra®) demonstrated an increased risk for cardiovascular events in patients following cardiovascular surgery. Valdecoxib (Bextra®) was withdrawn from the market in May 2005.

In their statement, the FDA encourages physicians to consider this developing information in risk-to-benefit evaluations as they consider the use of celecoxib in individual patients. In addition, the FDA advises an evaluation of alternative therapy. If physicians determine that continued use is appropriate for individual patients, the lowest effective dose of celecoxib should be prescribed. Pfizer has not announced a decision to withdraw celecoxib from the market as of December 20, 2004.

The association between selective COX-2 inhibitors and increased cardiovascular risk has been noted previously and prompted by publication of a meta-analysis entitled "Risk of Cardiovascular Events Associated With Selective COX-2 Inhibitors" in the August 22, 2001, edition of the *Journal of the American Medical Association (JAMA)*. The researchers reanalyzed four previously published trials, assessing cardiovascular events in patients receiving either celecoxib or rofecoxib. They found an association between the use of COX-2 inhibitors and cardiovascular events (including MI and ischemic stroke). The annualized MI rate was found to be significantly higher in patients receiving celecoxib or rofecoxib than in the control (placebo) group from a recent meta-analysis of primary prevention trials. Although cause and effect cannot be established (these trials were originally designed to assess GI effects, not cardiovascular ones), the authors believe the available data raise a cautionary flag concerning the risk of cardiovascular events with the use of COX-2 inhibitors. The manufacturers of these agents, as well as other healthcare professionals, dispute the methods and validity of the study's conclusions. To date, the FDA has not required any change in the labeling of these agents. Further study is required before any potential risk may be defined.

Cross-reactivity, including bronchospasm, between aspirin and other NSAIDs has been reported in aspirin-sensitive patients. The manufacturer suggests that celecoxib should not be administered to patients with this type of aspirin sensitivity and should be used with caution in patients with pre-existing asthma.

The manufacturer studied the effect of celecoxib on the anticoagulant effect of warfarin and found no alteration of anticoagulant effect, as determined by prothrombin time, in patients taking 2 mg to 5 mg daily. However, the manufacturer has issued a caution when using celecoxib with warfarin since those patients are at increased risk of bleeding complications.

Selected Readings

Dionne R, "COX-2 Inhibitors: Better Than Ibuprofen for Dental Pain?" *Compend Contin Educ Dent*, 1999, 20(6):518-20, 522-4.

Doyle G, Jayawardena S, Ashraf E, et al, "Efficacy and Tolerability of Nonprescription Ibuprofen Versus Celecoxib for Dental Pain," *J Clin Pharmacol*, 2002, 42(8):912-9.

Everts B, Wahrborg P, and Hedner T, "COX-2 Specific Inhibitors - The Emergence of a New Class of Analgesic and Anti-inflammatory Drugs," *Clin Rheumatol*, 2000, 19(5):331-43.

Geis GS, et al, "Efficacy and Safety of Celecoxib, A Specific COX-2 Inhibitor, in Patients With Rheumatoid Arthritis," *Arthritis Rheum*, 1998, 41(9 Suppl):316:1699.

Jeske AH, "COX-2 Inhibitors and Dental Pain Control," *J Gt Houst Dent Soc*, 1999, 71(4):39-40.

Jeske AH, "Selecting New Drugs for Pain Control: Evidence-Based Decisions or Clinical Impressions?" *J Am Dent Assoc*, 2002, 133(8):1052-6.

Jouzeau JY, Terlain B, Abid A, et al, "Cyclo-oxygenase Isoenzymes. How Recent Findings Affect Thinking About Nonsteroidal Anti-inflammatory Drugs," *Drugs*, 1997, 53(4):563-82.

Kaplan-Machlis B and Klostermeyer BS, "The Cyclo-oxygenase-2 Inhibitors: Safety and Effectiveness," *Ann Pharmacother*, 1999, 33(9):979-88.

Karim A, et al, "Celecoxib, A Specific COX-2 Inhibitor, Lacks Significant Drug-Drug Interactions With Methotrexate or Warfarin," *Arthritis Rheum*, 1998, 41(9 Suppl):315:1698.

Kellstein D, Ott D, Jayawardene S, et al, "Analgesic Efficacy of a Single Dose of Lumiracoxib Compared With Rofecoxib, Celecoxib and Placebo in the Treatment of Post-Operative Dental Pain," *Int J Clin Pract*, 2004, 58(3):244-50.

Kurumbail RG, Stevens AM, Gierse JK, et al, "Structural Basis for Selective Inhibition of Cyclo-oxygenase-2 By Anti-inflammatory Agents," *Nature*, 1996, 384(6610):644-8.

Lane NE, "Pain Management in Osteoarthritis: The Role of COX-2 Inhibitors," *J Rheumatol*, 1997, 24(Suppl 49):20-4.

Lipsky PE and Isakson PC, "Outcome of Specific COX-2 Inhibition in Rheumatoid Arthritis," *J Rheumatol*, 1997, 24(Suppl 49):9-14.

Malmstrom K, Daniels S, Kotey P, et al, "Comparison of Rofecoxib and Celecoxib, Two Cyclooxygenase-2 Inhibitors, in Postoperative Dental Pain: A Randomized Placebo- and Active-Comparator-Controlled Clinical Trial," *Clin Ther*, 1999, 21(10):1653-63.

McAdam BF, Catella-Lawson F, Mardini IA, et al, "Systemic Biosynthesis of Prostacyclin by Cyclo-oxygenase (COX)-2: The Human Pharmacology of a Selective Inhibitor of COX-2," *Proc Natl Acad Sci U S A*, 1999, 96(1):272-7.

Mengle-Gaw L, et al, "A Study of the Platelet Effects of SC-58635, A Novel COX-2 Selective Inhibitor," *Arthritis Rheum*, 1998, 41(9 Suppl):93-374.

Moore PA and Hersh EV, "Celecoxib and Rofecoxib. The Role of COX-2 Inhibitors in Dental Practice," *J Am Dent Assoc*, 2001, 132(4):451-6.

Needleman P and Isakson PC, "The Discovery and Function of COX-2," *J Rheumatol*, 1997, 24(S49):6-8.

Simon LS, et al, "Preliminary Study of the Safety and Efficacy of SC-58635, A Novel Cyclo-oxygenase 2 Inhibitor: Efficacy and Safety in Two Placebo-Controlled Trials in Osteoarthritis and Rheumatoid Arthritis, and Studies of Gastrointestinal and Platelet Effects," *Arthritis Rheum*, 1998, 41:1591-1602.

Whelton A, Maurath CJ, Verburg KM, et al, "Renal Safety and Tolerability of Celecoxib, a Novel Cyclo-oxygenase-2 Inhibitor," *Am J Ther*, 2000, 7(3):159-75.

Wynn RL, "The New COX-2 Inhibitors: Celecoxib and Rofecoxib," *Home Health Care Consultant*, 2001, 8(10):24-31.

(Continued)

Celecoxib *(Continued)*

Wynn RL, "The New COX-2 Inhibitors: Rofecoxib (Vioxx®) and Celecoxib (Celebrex™)," *Gen Dent*, 2000, 48(1):16-20.

Wynn RL, "NSAIDS and Cardiovascular Effects, Celecoxib for Dental Pain, and a New Analgesic - Tramadol With Acetaminophen," *Gen Dent*, 2002, 50(3):218-22.

Celestone® *see* Betamethasone *on page 206*

Celestone® Soluspan® *see* Betamethasone *on page 206*

Celexa® *see* Citalopram *on page 367*

CellCept® *see* Mycophenolate *on page 1134*

Cellugel® *see* Hydroxypropyl Methylcellulose *on page 844*

Cellulose (Oxidized/Regenerated)

(SEL yoo lose, OKS i dyzed re JEN er aye ted)

U.S. Brand Names Surgicel®; Surgicel® Fibrillar; Surgicel® NuKnit

Generic Available No

Index Terms Absorbable Cotton; Oxidized Regenerated Cellulose

Pharmacologic Category Hemostatic Agent

Dental Use To control bleeding created during a dental procedure

Use Hemostatic; temporary packing for the control of capillary, venous, or small arterial hemorrhage

Local Anesthetic/Vasoconstrictor Precautions No information available to require special precautions

Effects on Dental Treatment No significant effects or complications reported

Significant Adverse Effects Frequency not defined.

Central nervous system: Headache

Respiratory: Nasal burning or stinging, sneezing (rhinological procedures)

Miscellaneous: Encapsulation of fluid, foreign body reactions (with or without) infection

Postmarketing and/or case reports: Numbness, pain, paralysis

Dental Usual Dosing Control bleeding created during a dental procedure: Topical: Minimal amounts of the fabric strip are laid on the bleeding site or held firmly against the tissues until hemostasis occurs; remove excess material

Dosage Minimal amounts of the fabric strip are laid on the bleeding site or held firmly against the tissues until hemostasis occurs; remove excess material

Mechanism of Action Cellulose, oxidized regenerated is saturated with blood at the bleeding site and swells into a brownish or black gelatinous mass which aids in the formation of a clot. When used in small amounts, it is absorbed from the sites of implantation with little or no tissue reaction. In addition to providing hemostasis, oxidized regenerated cellulose also has been shown *in vitro* to have bactericidal properties.

Contraindications Hypersensitivity to any component of the formulation; implantation into bone defects; hemorrhage from large arteries; nonhemorrhagic oozing; use as an adhesion product

Warnings/Precautions Pain, numbness, or paralysis have been reported if used near a bony or neural space and left inside patient; use minimum amount necessary to achieve hemostasis. Remove as much of agent as possible after hemostasis is achieved. Do not leave in a contaminated or infected space. Always remove completely following hemostasis if applied in proximity to foramina in bone, areas of bony confine, the spinal cord or optic nerve and chasm; product may swell and exert unwanted pressure. The material should not be moistened before insertion since the hemostatic effect is greater when applied dry. The material should not be impregnated with anti-infective agents. Its hemostatic effect is not enhanced by the addition of thrombin.

Drug Interactions No data reported

Pharmacodynamics/Kinetics Absorption: 7-14 days

Pregnancy Risk Factor No data reported

Dosage Forms Excipient information presented when available (limited, particularly for generics); consult specific product labeling.

Fabric, fibrous (Surgicel® Fibrillar):

1" x 2" (10s)

2" x 4" (10s)

4" x 4" (10s)

Fabric, knitted (Surgicel® NuKnit):

1" x 1" (24s)

1" x 3½" (10s)

3" x 4" (24s)

6" x 9" (10s)

Fabric, sheer weave (Surgicel®):

½" x 2" (24s)

2" x 3" (24s)

2" x 14" (24s)

4" x 8" (24s)

Cellulose Sodium Phosphate
(sel yoo lose SOW dee um FOS fate)

U.S. Brand Names Calcibind®
Canadian Brand Names Calcibind®
Generic Available No
Index Terms CSP; Sodium Cellulose Phosphate
Pharmacologic Category Urinary Tract Product
Use Adjunct to dietary restriction to reduce renal calculi formation in absorptive hypercalciuria type I
Local Anesthetic/Vasoconstrictor Precautions No information available to require special precautions
Effects on Dental Treatment No significant effects or complications reported
Pregnancy Risk Factor C

Celontin® *see* Methsuximide *on page 1076*

Cenestin® *see* Estrogens (Conjugated A/Synthetic) *on page 606*

Centany™ *see* Mupirocin *on page 1132*

Centrum® [OTC] *see* Vitamins (Multiple/Oral) *on page 1665*

Centrum® Performance™ [OTC] *see* Vitamins (Multiple/Oral) *on page 1665*

Centrum® Silver® [OTC] *see* Vitamins (Multiple/Oral) *on page 1665*

Cepacol® Antibacterial Mouthwash [OTC] *see* Cetylpyridinium *on page 324*

Cepacol® Antibacterial Mouthwash Gold [OTC] *see* Cetylpyridinium *on page 324*

Cepacol® Sore Throat [OTC] *see* Benzocaine *on page 195*

Cepastat® [OTC] *see* Phenol *on page 1290*

Cepastat® Extra Strength [OTC] *see* Phenol *on page 1290*

Cephadyn *see* Butalbital and Acetaminophen *on page 249*

Cephalexin (sef a LEKS in)

Related Information
Antibiotic Prophylaxis *on page 1772*
Bacterial Infections *on page 1793*
Related Sample Prescriptions
Bacterial Infections and Periodontal Diseases *on page 1837*
Infective Endocarditis (Prevention) *on page 1832*
Prosthetic Joint Late Infections (Prevention) *on page 1833*
U.S. Brand Names Biocef®; Keflex®; Panixine DisperDose™ [DSC]
Canadian Brand Names Apo-Cephalex®; Keftab®; Novo-Lexin; Nu-Cephalex
Mexican Brand Names Ceporex; Keflex; Paferxin; Servicef
Generic Available Yes: Excludes tablet for oral suspension
Index Terms Cephalexin Monohydrate
Pharmacologic Category Antibiotic, Cephalosporin (First Generation)
Dental Use Prophylaxis in total joint replacement patients undergoing dental procedures which produce bacteremia; alternative oral antibiotic for prevention of infective endocarditis in individuals allergic to penicillins or ampicillin
  Note: Individuals allergic to amoxicillin (penicillins) may receive cephalexin provided they have not had an immediate, local, or systemic IgE-mediated anaphylactic allergic reaction to penicillin.
Use Treatment of susceptible bacterial infections including respiratory tract infections, otitis media, skin and skin structure infections, bone infections, and genitourinary tract infections, including acute prostatitis; alternative therapy for acute bacterial endocarditis prophylaxis
Local Anesthetic/Vasoconstrictor Precautions No information available to require special precautions
Effects on Dental Treatment No significant effects or complications reported (see Dental Comment)
Significant Adverse Effects Frequency not defined.
Central nervous system: Agitation, confusion, dizziness, fatigue, hallucinations, headache
Dermatologic: Angioedema, erythema multiforme (rare), rash, Stevens-Johnson syndrome (rare), toxic epidermal necrolysis (rare), urticaria
Gastrointestinal: Abdominal pain, diarrhea, dyspepsia, gastritis, nausea (rare), pseudomembranous colitis, vomiting (rare)
Genitourinary: Genital pruritus, genital moniliasis, vaginitis, vaginal discharge
Hematologic: Eosinophilia, hemolytic anemia, neutropenia, thrombocytopenia
(Continued)

317

Cephalexin *(Continued)*

Hepatic: AST/ALT increased, cholestatic jaundice (rare), transient hepatitis (rare)

Neuromuscular & skeletal: Arthralgia, arthritis, joint disorder

Renal: Interstitial nephritis (rare)

Miscellaneous: Allergic reactions, anaphylaxis

Dental Usual Dosing

Infective endocarditis prophylaxis (dental, oral, respiratory tract, or esophageal procedures): Oral:

Children >1 year: 50 mg/kg 30-60 minutes prior to procedure; maximum: 2 g

Children >15 years and Adults: 2 g 30-60 minutes prior to procedure

Prophylaxis in total joint replacement patients undergoing dental procedures which produce bacteremia: Oral: Adults: 2 g 1 hour prior to procedure

Dosage

Usual dosage range:

Children >1 year: Oral: 25-100 mg/kg/day every 6-8 hours (maximum: 4 g/day)

Adults: Oral: 250-1000 mg every 6 hours; maximum: 4 g/day

Indication-specific dosing:

Children >1 year: Oral:

Furunculosis: 25-50 mg/kg/day in 4 divided doses

Impetigo: 25 mg/kg/day in 4 divided doses

Otitis media: 75-100 mg/kg/day in 4 divided doses

Prophylaxis of bacterial endocarditis (dental, oral, respiratory tract, or esophageal procedures): 50 mg/kg 1 hour prior to procedure (maximum: 2 g)

Severe infections: 50-100 mg/kg/day in divided doses every 6-8 hours

Skin abscess: 50 mg/kg/day in 4 divided doses (maximum: 4 g)

Streptococcal pharyngitis, skin and skin structure infections: 25-50 mg/kg/day divided every 12 hours

Children >15 years and Adults: Oral:

Cellulitis and mastitis: 500 mg every 6 hours

Furunculosis/skin abscess: 250 mg 4 times/day

Prophylaxis of bacterial endocarditis (dental, oral, respiratory tract, or esophageal procedures): 2 g 1 hour prior to procedure

Streptococcal pharyngitis, skin and skin structure infections: 500 mg every 12 hours

Uncomplicated cystitis: 500 mg every 12 hours for 7-14 days

Dosing adjustment in renal impairment: Adults:

Cl_{cr} 10-50 mL/minute: 500 mg every 8-12 hours

Cl_{cr} <10: 250-500 mg every 12-24 hours

Hemodialysis: 250 mg every 12-24 hours; moderately dialyzable (20% to 50%); give dose after dialysis session

Mechanism of Action Inhibits bacterial cell wall synthesis by binding to one or more of the penicillin-binding proteins (PBPs) which in turn inhibits the final transpeptidation step of peptidoglycan synthesis in bacterial cell walls, thus inhibiting cell wall biosynthesis. Bacteria eventually lyse due to ongoing activity of cell wall autolytic enzymes (autolysins and murein hydrolases) while cell wall assembly is arrested.

Contraindications Hypersensitivity to cephalexin, any component of the formulation, or other cephalosporins

Warnings/Precautions Modify dosage in patients with severe renal impairment. Use with caution in patients with a history of penicillin allergy, especially IgE-mediated reactions (eg, anaphylaxis, urticaria). Prolonged use may result in fungal or bacterial superinfection, including *C. difficile*-associated diarrhea and pseudomembranous colitis. May be associated with increased INR, especially in nutritionally-deficient patients, prolonged treatment, hepatic or renal disease.

Drug Interactions

Aminoglycosides: Increase nephrotoxic potential.

Probenecid: High-dose probenecid decreases clearance of cephalexin.

Typhoid vaccine: Antibiotics may diminish the efficacy of the live, attenuated Ty21a strain vaccine.

Ethanol/Nutrition/Herb Interactions Food: Peak antibiotic serum concentration is lowered and delayed, but total drug absorbed is not affected. Cephalexin serum levels may be decreased if taken with food.

Dietary Considerations Take without regard to food. If GI distress, take with food. Panixine DisperDose™ contains phenylalanine 2.8 mg/cephalexin 125 mg.

Pharmacodynamics/Kinetics

Absorption: Delayed in young children

Distribution: Widely into most body tissues and fluids, including gallbladder, liver, kidneys, bone, sputum, bile, and pleural and synovial fluids; CSF penetration is poor; crosses placenta; enters breast milk

Protein binding: 6% to 15%
Half-life elimination: Adults: 0.5-1.2 hours; prolonged with renal impairment
Time to peak, serum: ~1 hour
Excretion: Urine (80% to 100% as unchanged drug) within 8 hours
Pregnancy Risk Factor B
Lactation Enters breast milk (small amounts)/use caution
Breast-Feeding Considerations Theoretically, drug absorbed by nursing infant may change bowel flora or affect fever work-up result. Cephalexin levels can be detected in breast milk, reaching a maximum concentration 4 hours after a single oral dose and gradually decreasing by 8 hours after administration. **Note:** As a class, cephalosporins are used to treat bacterial infections in infants.
Dosage Forms Excipient information presented when available (limited, particularly for generics); consult specific product labeling. [DSC] = Discontinued product
Capsule: 250 mg, 500 mg
Biocef®: 500 mg
Keflex®: 250 mg, 333 mg [DSC], 500 mg, 750 mg
Powder for oral suspension: 125 mg/5 mL (100 mL, 200 mL); 250 mg/5 mL (100 mL, 200 mL)
Biocef®: 125 mg/5 mL (100 mL); 250 mg/5 mL (100 mL)
Keflex®: 125 mg/5 mL (100 mL, 200 mL); 250 mg/5 mL (100 mL, 200 mL)
Tablet, for oral suspension (Panixine DisperDose™): 125 mg [contains phenylalanine 2.8 mg; peppermint flavor], 250 mg [contains phenylalanine 5.6 mg; peppermint flavor] [DSC]
Dental Comment Cephalexin is effective against anaerobic bacteria, but the sensitivity of alpha-hemolytic *Streptococcus* vary; approximately 10% of strains are resistant. Nearly 70% are intermediately sensitive. Patients allergic to penicillins can use a cephalosporin; the incidence of cross-reactivity between penicillins and cephalosporins is 1% when the allergic reaction to penicillin is delayed. If the patient has a history of immediate reaction to penicillin, the incidence of cross-reactivity is 20%; cephalosporins are contraindicated in these patients.
Selected Readings

ADA Division of Legal Affairs, "A Legal Perspective on Antibiotic Prophylaxis," *J Am Dent Assoc*, 2003, 134(9):1260.
"Advisory Statement. Antibiotic Prophylaxis for Dental Patients With Total Joint Replacements. American Dental Association; American Academy of Orthopedic Surgeons," *J Am Dent Assoc*, 1997, 128(7):1004-8.
American Dental Association; American Academy of Orthopedic Surgeons, "Antibiotic Prophylaxis for Dental Patients With Total Joint Replacements," *J Am Dent Assoc*, 2003, 134(7):895-9.
American Dental Association Council on Scientific Affairs, "Combating Antibiotic Resistance," *J Am Dent Assoc*, 2004, 135(4):484-7.
Dajani AS, Taubert KA, Wilson W, et al, "Prevention of Bacterial Endocarditis. Recommendations by the American Heart Association," *JAMA*, 1997, 277(22):1794-801.
Dajani AS, Taubert KA, Wilson W, et al, "Prevention of Bacterial Endocarditis: Recommendations by the American Heart Association," *J Am Dent Assoc*, 1997, 128(8):1142-51.
Saxon A, Beall GN, Rohr AS, et al, "Immediate Hypersensitivity Reactions to Beta-Lactam Antibiotics," *Ann Intern Med*, 1987, 107(2):204-15.
Wynn RL, Bergman SA, Meiller TF, et al, "Antibiotics in Treating Oral-Facial Infections of Odontogenic Origin: An Update," *Gen Dent*, 2001, 49(3):238-40, 242, 244 passim.

Cephalexin Monohydrate *see* Cephalexin *on page 317*

Cephradine (SEF ra deen)

Related Information
Antibiotic Prophylaxis *on page 1772*
Bacterial Infections *on page 1793*
U.S. Brand Names Velosef®
Mexican Brand Names Veracef
Generic Available No
Pharmacologic Category Antibiotic, Cephalosporin (First Generation)
Dental Use Prophylaxis in total joint replacement patients undergoing dental procedures which produce bacteremia
Use Treatment of infections when caused by susceptible strains in respiratory, genitourinary, gastrointestinal, skin and soft tissue, bone and joint infections; treatment of susceptible gram-positive bacilli and cocci (never enterococcus); some gram-negative bacilli including *E. coli*, *Proteus*, and *Klebsiella* may be susceptible
Local Anesthetic/Vasoconstrictor Precautions No information available to require special precautions
Effects on Dental Treatment No significant effects or complications reported
Significant Adverse Effects Frequency not defined.
Central nervous system: Dizziness
Dermatologic: Rash, pruritus
Gastrointestinal: Diarrhea, nausea, vomiting, pseudomembranous colitis
(Continued)

Cephradine *(Continued)*

Hematologic: Leukopenia, neutropenia, eosinophilia

Neuromuscular & skeletal: Joint pain

Renal: BUN increased, creatinine increased

Reactions reported with other cephalosporins include anaphylaxis, erythema multiforme, toxic epidermal necrolysis, Stevens-Johnson syndrome, fever, headache, encephalopathy, asterixis, neuromuscular excitability, seizure, agranulocytosis, pancytopenia, aplastic anemia, hemolytic anemia, interstitial nephritis, toxic nephropathy, vaginitis, angioedema, cholestasis, hemorrhage, prolonged PT, serum-sickness reactions, superinfection

Dental Usual Dosing Prophylaxis in total joint replacement patients undergoing dental procedures which produce bacteremia: Adults: Oral: 2 g 1 hour prior to procedure

Dosage

Usual dosage range:

Children ≥9 months: Oral: 25-100 mg/kg/day in divided doses every 6 or 12 hours (maximum: 4 g/day)

Adults: Oral: 250-500 mg every 6-12 hours

Indication-specific dosing:

Children ≥9 months: Oral:

Otitis media: 75-100 mg/kg/day in divided doses every 6 or 12 hours (maximum: 4 g/day)

Dosing adjustment in renal impairment: Adults:

Cl_{cr} 10-50 mL/minute: 250 mg every 6 hours

Cl_{cr} <10 mL/minute: 125 mg every 6 hours

Mechanism of Action Inhibits bacterial cell wall synthesis by binding to one or more of the penicillin-binding proteins (PBPs) which in turn inhibits the final transpeptidation step of peptidoglycan synthesis in bacterial cell walls, thus inhibiting cell wall biosynthesis. Bacteria eventually lyse due to ongoing activity of cell wall autolytic enzymes (autolysins and murein hydrolases) while cell wall assembly is arrested.

Contraindications Hypersensitivity to cephradine, any component of the formulation, or cephalosporins

Warnings/Precautions Use caution with renal impairment; dose adjustment required; use with caution in patients with a history of penicillin allergy, especially IgE-mediated reactions (eg, anaphylaxis, urticaria). Prolonged use may result in fungal or bacterial superinfection, including *C. difficile*-associated diarrhea and pseudomembranous colitis.

Drug Interactions

Increased effect: High-dose probenecid decreases clearance.

Increased toxicity: Aminoglycosides may increase nephrotoxic potential.

Ethanol/Nutrition/Herb Interactions Food: Food delays cephradine absorption but does not decrease extent.

Dietary Considerations May administer with food to decrease GI distress.

Pharmacodynamics/Kinetics

Absorption: Well absorbed

Distribution: Widely into most body tissues and fluids including gallbladder, liver, kidneys, bone, sputum, bile, and pleural and synovial fluids; CSF penetration is poor; crosses placenta; enters breast milk

Protein binding: 18% to 20%

Half-life elimination: 1-2 hours; prolonged with renal impairment

Time to peak, serum: 1-2 hours

Excretion: Urine (~80% to 90% as unchanged drug) within 6 hours

Pregnancy Risk Factor B

Lactation Enters breast milk/use caution

Breast-Feeding Considerations Theoretically, drug absorbed by nursing infant may change bowel flora or affect fever work-up result. **Note:** As a class, cephalosporins are used to treat infections in infants.

Dosage Forms Excipient information presented when available (limited, particularly for generics); consult specific product labeling. [DSC] = Discontinued product

Capsule: 250 mg, 500 mg [DSC]

Powder for oral suspension: 250 mg/5 mL (100 mL) [fruit flavor]

Selected Readings

ADA Division of Legal Affairs, "A Legal Perspective on Antibiotic Prophylaxis," *J Am Dent Assoc*, 2003, 134(9):1260.

"Advisory Statement. Antibiotic Prophylaxis for Dental Patients With Total Joint Replacements. American Dental Association; American Academy of Orthopedic Surgeons," *J Am Dent Assoc*, 1997, 128(7):1004-8.

American Dental Association; American Academy of Orthopedic Surgeons, "Antibiotic Prophylaxis for Dental Patients With Total Joint Replacements," *J Am Dent Assoc*, 2003, 134(7):895-9.

American Dental Association Council on Scientific Affairs, "Combating Antibiotic Resistance," *J Am Dent Assoc*, 2004, 135(4):484-7.

Donowitz GR and Mandell GL, "Drug Therapy. Beta-Lactam Antibiotics (1)," *N Engl J Med*, 1988, 318(7):419-26.

Donowitz GR and Mandell GL, "Drug Therapy. Beta-Lactam Antibiotics (2)," *N Engl J Med*, 1988, 318(8):490-500.

Gustaferro CA and Steckelberg JM, "Cephalosporin Antimicrobial Agents and Related Compounds," *Mayo Clin Proc*, 1991, 66(10):1064-73.

Ceprotin *see* Protein C Concentrate (Human) *on page 1378*

Ceptaz® [DSC] *see* Ceftazidime *on page 307*

Cerebyx® *see* Fosphenytoin *on page 751*

Ceredase® *see* Alglucerase *on page 69*

Cerezyme® *see* Imiglucerase *on page 865*

Ceron *see* Chlorpheniramine and Phenylephrine *on page 340*

Ceron-DM *see* Chlorpheniramine, Phenylephrine, and Dextromethorphan *on page 342*

Cerovel™ *see* Urea *on page 1632*

Certuss-D® *see* Guaifenesin, Dextromethorphan, and Phenylephrine *on page 798*

Cerubidine® *see* DAUNOrubicin Hydrochloride *on page 450*

Cerumenex® [DSC] *see* Triethanolamine Polypeptide Oleate-Condensate *on page 1617*

Cervidil® *see* Dinoprostone *on page 509*

C.E.S. *see* Estrogens (Conjugated/Equine) *on page 609*

Cesia™ *see* Ethinyl Estradiol and Desogestrel *on page 621*

Cetacaine® *see* Benzocaine, Butamben, and Tetracaine *on page 198*

Cetacort® *see* Hydrocortisone *on page 836*

Cetafen® [OTC] *see* Acetaminophen *on page 31*

Cetafen Extra® [OTC] *see* Acetaminophen *on page 31*

Ceta-Plus® *see* Hydrocodone and Acetaminophen *on page 822*

Cetirizine (se TI ra zeen)

U.S. Brand Names Zyrtec®
Canadian Brand Names Apo-Cetirizine®; Reactine™
Mexican Brand Names Virlix; Zyrtec
Generic Available No
Index Terms Cetirizine Hydrochloride; P-071; UCB-P071
Pharmacologic Category Antihistamine
Use Perennial and seasonal allergic rhinitis and other allergic symptoms including urticaria; chronic idiopathic urticaria
Local Anesthetic/Vasoconstrictor Precautions No information available to require special precautions
Effects on Dental Treatment Key adverse event(s) related to dental treatment: Xerostomia and increased salivation (normal salivary flow resumes upon discontinuation).
Common Adverse Effects
>10%: Central nervous system: Headache (children 11% to 14%, placebo 12%), somnolence (adults 14%, children 2% to 4%)
2% to 10%:
Central nervous system: Insomnia (children 9%, adults <2%), fatigue (adults 6%), malaise (4%), dizziness (adults 2%)
Gastrointestinal: Abdominal pain (children 4% to 6%), dry mouth (adults 5%), diarrhea (children 2% to 3%), nausea (children 2% to 3%, placebo 2%), vomiting (children 2% to 3%)
Respiratory: Epistaxis (children 2% to 4%, placebo 3%), pharyngitis (children 3% to 6%, placebo 3%), bronchospasm (children 2% to 3%, placebo 2%)
Dosage Oral:
Children:
6-12 months: Chronic urticaria, perennial allergic rhinitis: 2.5 mg once daily
12 months to <2 years: Chronic urticaria, perennial allergic rhinitis: 2.5 mg once daily; may increase to 2.5 mg every 12 hours if needed
2-5 years: Chronic urticaria, perennial or seasonal allergic rhinitis: Initial: 2.5 mg once daily; may be increased to 2.5 mg every 12 hours **or** 5 mg once daily
Children ≥6 years and Adults: Chronic urticaria, perennial or seasonal allergic rhinitis: 5-10 mg once daily, depending upon symptom severity
Elderly: Initial: 5 mg once daily; may increase to 10 mg/day. **Note:** Manufacturer recommends 5 mg/day in patients ≥77 years of age.
Dosage adjustment in renal/hepatic impairment:
Children <6 years: Cetirizine use not recommended
Children 6-11 years: <2.5 mg once daily
(Continued)

Cetirizine *(Continued)*

Children ≥12 and Adults:

Cl_{cr} 11-31 mL/minute, hemodialysis, or hepatic impairment: Administer 5 mg once daily

Cl_{cr} <11 mL/minute, not on dialysis: Cetirizine use not recommended

Mechanism of Action Competes with histamine for H_1-receptor sites on effector cells in the gastrointestinal tract, blood vessels, and respiratory tract

Contraindications Hypersensitivity to cetirizine, hydroxyzine, or any component of the formulation

Warnings/Precautions Cetirizine should be used cautiously in patients with hepatic or renal dysfunction, the elderly and in nursing mothers. May cause drowsiness; use caution performing tasks which require alertness (eg, operating machinery or driving). Safety and efficacy in pediatric patients <6 months of age have not been established.

Drug Interactions

Cytochrome P450 Effect: Substrate of CYP3A4 (minor)

Increased Effect/Toxicity: Increased toxicity with CNS depressants and anticholinergics.

Ethanol/Nutrition/Herb Interactions Ethanol: Avoid ethanol (may increase CNS depression).

Dietary Considerations May be taken with or without food.

Pharmacodynamics/Kinetics

Onset of action: 15-30 minutes

Absorption: Rapid

Protein binding, plasma: Mean: 93%

Metabolism: Limited hepatic

Half-life elimination: 8 hours

Time to peak, serum: 1 hour

Excretion: Urine (70%); feces (10%)

Pregnancy Risk Factor B

Dosage Forms

Syrup:

Zyrtec®: 5 mg/5 mL

Tablet:

Zyrtec®: 5 mg, 10 mg

Tablet, chewable:

Zyrtec®: 5 mg, 10 mg

Cetirizine and Pseudoephedrine
(se TI ra zeen & soo doe e FED rin)

Related Information

Cetirizine *on page 321*
Pseudoephedrine *on page 1381*

U.S. Brand Names Zyrtec-D 12 Hour™

Canadian Brand Names Reactine® Allergy and Sinus

Mexican Brand Names Cipan; Virlix D; Zyrtec-D

Generic Available No

Index Terms Cetirizine Hydrochloride and Pseudoephedrine Hydrochloride; Pseudoephedrine Hydrochloride and Cetirizine Hydrochloride

Pharmacologic Category Antihistamine/Decongestant Combination

Use Treatment of symptoms of seasonal or perennial allergic rhinitis

Local Anesthetic/Vasoconstrictor Precautions Use with caution since pseudoephedrine is a sympathomimetic amine which could interact with epinephrine to cause a pressor response

Effects on Dental Treatment Key adverse event(s) related to dental treatment: Pseudoephedrine: Xerostomia (normal salivary flow resumes upon discontinuation).

Common Adverse Effects Percentages reported with combination product. Additional adverse effects reported; refer to individual agents.

1% to 10%:

Central nervous system: Insomnia (4%), fatigue (2%), somnolence (2%), dizziness (1%)

Gastrointestinal: Xerostomia (4%)

Respiratory: Pharyngitis (2%), epistaxis (1%)

Mechanism of Action Cetirizine is an antihistamine; exhibits selective inhibition of H_1 receptors. Pseudoephedrine is a sympathomimetic and exerts a decongestant action on nasal mucosa.

Drug Interactions
Cytochrome P450 Effect: Cetirizine: **Substrate** of CYP3A4 (minor)
Increased Effect/Toxicity: See individual agents.
Decreased Effect: See individual agents.
Pharmacodynamics/Kinetics
Zyrtec-D 12 Hour™:
Half-life elimination: Cetirizine: 7.9 hours; Pseudoephedrine: 6 hours
Time to peak: Cetirizine: 2.2 hours; Pseudoephedrine: 4.4 hours
Excretion: Urine (70%); feces (10%)
See individual agents.
Pregnancy Risk Factor C

Cetirizine Hydrochloride *see* Cetirizine *on page 321*

Cetirizine Hydrochloride and Pseudoephedrine Hydrochloride *see* Cetirizine and Pseudoephedrine *on page 322*

Cetrorelix (set roe REL iks)

U.S. Brand Names Cetrotide®
Canadian Brand Names Cetrotide®
Mexican Brand Names Cetrotide
Generic Available No
Index Terms Cetrorelix Acetate
Pharmacologic Category Gonadotropin Releasing Hormone Antagonist
Use Inhibits premature luteinizing hormone (LH) surges in women undergoing controlled ovarian stimulation
Local Anesthetic/Vasoconstrictor Precautions No information available to require special precautions
Effects on Dental Treatment No significant effects or complications reported
Common Adverse Effects 1% to 10%:
Central nervous system: Headache (1%)
Endocrine & metabolic: Ovarian hyperstimulation syndrome, WHO grade II or III (4%)
Gastrointestinal: Nausea (1%)
Hepatic: ALT, AST, GGT, and alkaline phosphatase increased (1% to 2%)
Mechanism of Action Competes with naturally-occurring GnRH for binding on receptors of the pituitary. This delays luteinizing hormone surge, preventing ovulation until the follicles are of adequate size.
Drug Interactions
Increased Effect/Toxicity: No formal studies have been performed.
Decreased Effect: No formal studies have been performed.
Pharmacodynamics/Kinetics
Onset of action: 0.25 mg dose: 2 hours; 3 mg dose: 1 hour
Duration: 3 mg dose (single dose): 4 days
Absorption: Rapid
Protein binding: 86%
Metabolism: Transformed by peptidases; cetrorelix and peptides (1-9), (1-7), (1-6), and (1-4) are found in the bile; peptide (1-4) is the predominant metabolite
Bioavailability: 85%
Half-life elimination: 0.25 mg dose: 5 hours; 0.25 mg multiple doses: 20.6 hours; 3 mg dose: 62.8 hours
Time to peak: 0.25 mg dose: 1 hour; 3 mg dose: 1.5 hours
Excretion: Feces (5% to 10% as unchanged drug and metabolites); urine (2% to 4% as unchanged drug); within 24 hours
Pregnancy Risk Factor X

Cetrorelix Acetate *see* Cetrorelix *on page 323*

Cetrotide® *see* Cetrorelix *on page 323*

Cetuximab (se TUK see mab)

U.S. Brand Names Erbitux®
Canadian Brand Names Erbitux®
Generic Available No
Index Terms C225; IMC-C225; NSC-714692
Pharmacologic Category Antineoplastic Agent, Monoclonal Antibody; Epidermal Growth Factor Receptor (EGFR) Inhibitor
Use Treatment of metastatic colorectal cancer; treatment of squamous cell cancer of the head and neck
Unlabeled/Investigational Use Breast cancer, tumors overexpressing EGFR
(Continued)

Cetuximab (Continued)

Local Anesthetic/Vasoconstrictor Precautions No information available to require special precautions

Effects on Dental Treatment No significant effects or complications reported

Common Adverse Effects Except where noted, percentages reported for cetuximab monotherapy.

>10%:

Central nervous system: Malaise (48%), pain (17% to 28%), fever (5% to 27%), headache (26%)

Dermatologic: Acneform rash (76% to 90%; grades 3/4: 1% to 8%), nail disorder (16%), pruritus (11%)

Endocrine & metabolic: Hypomagnesemia (50%; grades 3/4: 10% to 15%)

Gastrointestinal: Nausea (mild to moderate 29%), weight loss (7% to 27%), constipation (26%), abdominal pain (26%), diarrhea (25%), vomiting (25%), anorexia (23%)

Neuromuscular & skeletal: Weakness (45% to 48%)

Respiratory: Dyspnea (17%), cough (11%)

Miscellaneous: Infusion reaction (19% to 21%; grades 3/4: 2% to 4%; 90% with first infusion), infection (14%)

1% to 10%:

Cardiovascular: Peripheral edema (10%), cardiopulmonary arrest (2%; with radiation therapy)

Central nervous system: Insomnia (10%), depression (7%)

Dermatologic: Alopecia (4%), skin disorder (4%)

Endocrine & metabolic: Dehydration (2% to 10%)

Gastrointestinal: Stomatitis (10%), dyspepsia (6%)

Hematologic: Anemia (9%)

Hepatic: Alkaline phosphatase increased (5% to 10%), transaminases increased (5% to 10%)

Neuromuscular & skeletal: Back pain (10%)

Ocular: Conjunctivitis (7%)

Renal: Kidney failure (2%)

Respiratory: Pulmonary embolus (1%)

Miscellaneous: Sepsis (3%)

Mechanism of Action Recombinant human/mouse chimeric monoclonal antibody which binds specifically to the epidermal growth factor receptor (EGFR, HER1, c-ErbB-1) and competitively inhibits the binding of epidermal growth factor (EGF) and other ligands. Binding to the EGFR blocks phosphorylation and activation of receptor-associated kinases, resulting in inhibition of cell growth, induction of apoptosis, and decreased matrix metalloproteinase and vascular endothelial growth factor production.

Drug Interactions

Increased Effect/Toxicity: Interactions have not been evaluated in clinical trials.

Pharmacodynamics/Kinetics

Distribution: V_d: ~2-3 L/m^2

Half-life elimination: 112 hours (range: 63-230 hours)

Pregnancy Risk Factor C

Cetylpyridinium (SEE til peer i DI nee um)

U.S. Brand Names Cepacol® Antibacterial Mouthwash [OTC]; Cepacol® Antibacterial Mouthwash Gold [OTC]; DiabetAid Gingivitis Mouth Rinse [OTC]

Generic Available No

Index Terms Cetylpyridinium Chloride; CPC

Pharmacologic Category Antiseptic, Oral Mouthwash

Dental Use Antiseptic to aid in the prevention and reduction of plaque and gingivitis, and to freshen breath

Use Antiseptic to aid in the prevention and reduction of plaque and gingivitis, and to freshen breath

Local Anesthetic/Vasoconstrictor Precautions No information available to require special precautions

Effects on Dental Treatment Key adverse event(s) related to dental treatment: Tooth and tongue staining and oral irritation.

Significant Adverse Effects Frequency not defined: Gastrointestinal: Tooth and tongue staining, oral irritation

Dental Usual Dosing Prevention and reduction of plaque and gingivitis, and to freshen breath: Children ≥6 years and Adults: Oral (OTC labeling): Rinse or gargle as directed; may be used before or after brushing (2-3 times/day)

Dosage Children ≥6 years and Adults: Oral (OTC labeling): Rinse or gargle to freshen mouth; may be used before or after brushing

Contraindications Hypersensitivity to cetylpyridinium or any component of the formulation

Warnings/Precautions Not labeled for OTC use in children <6 years of age.

Pregnancy Risk Factor C

Dosage Forms Excipient information presented when available (limited, particularly for generics); consult specific product labeling.

Liquid, as chloride, oral [mouthwash/gargle]:

Cepacol® Antibacterial Mouthwash Gold: 0.05% (120 mL, 360 mL, 720 mL, 960 mL) [contains alcohol 14% and tartrazine; original flavor]

Cepacol® Antibacterial Mouthwash: 0.05% (120 mL, 360 mL, 720 mL, 960 mL) [contains alcohol 14% and tartrazine; mint flavor]

DiabetAid Gingivitis Mouth Rinse: 0.1% (480 mL) [sugar free]

Cetylpyridinium and Benzocaine
(SEE til peer i DI nee um & BEN zoe kane)

Related Information
Benzocaine *on page 195*
Cetylpyridinium *on page 324*

Canadian Brand Names Cepacol®; Kank-A®

Index Terms Benzocaine and Cetylpyridinium Chloride; Cetylpyridinium Chloride and Benzocaine

Pharmacologic Category Local Anesthetic

Dental Use Antiseptic/anesthetic for oral cavity

Use Symptomatic relief of sore throat

Local Anesthetic/Vasoconstrictor Precautions No information available to require special precautions

Effects on Dental Treatment No significant effects or complications reported

Restrictions Not available in U.S.

Dosage Antiseptic/anesthetic: Oral: Dissolve in mouth as needed for sore throat

Drug Interactions See individual agents.

Pregnancy Risk Factor C

Dosage Forms Excipient information presented when available (limited, particularly for generics); consult specific product labeling.

Cetylpyridinium Chloride *see* Cetylpyridinium *on page 324*

Cetylpyridinium Chloride and Benzocaine *see* Cetylpyridinium and Benzocaine *on page 325*

Cevi-Bid® [OTC] *see* Ascorbic Acid *on page 148*

Cevimeline (se vi ME leen)

Related Information
Management of Patients Undergoing Cancer Therapy *on page 1826*

U.S. Brand Names Evoxac®

Canadian Brand Names Evoxac®

Generic Available No

Index Terms Cevimeline Hydrochloride

Pharmacologic Category Cholinergic Agonist

Dental Use Treatment of symptoms of dry mouth in patients with Sjögren's syndrome

Use Treatment of symptoms of dry mouth in patients with Sjögren's syndrome

Local Anesthetic/Vasoconstrictor Precautions No information available to require special precautions

Effects on Dental Treatment Key adverse event(s) related to dental treatment: Excessive salivation, salivary gland pain, xerostomia (normal salivary flow resumes upon discontinuation), ulcerative stomatitis, and tooth disorder.

Significant Adverse Effects
>10%:

Central nervous system: Headache (14%; placebo 20%)

Gastrointestinal: Nausea (14%), diarrhea (10%)

Respiratory: Rhinitis (11%), sinusitis (12%), upper respiratory infection (11%)

Miscellaneous: Diaphoresis increased (19%)

1% to 10%:

Cardiovascular: Peripheral edema, chest pain, edema, palpitation

Central nervous system: Dizziness (4%), fatigue (3%), pain (3%), insomnia (2%), anxiety (1%), fever, depression, migraine, hypoesthesia, vertigo

Dermatologic: Rash (4%; placebo 6%), pruritus, skin disorder, erythematous rash

Endocrine & metabolic: Hot flashes (2%)

Gastrointestinal: Dyspepsia (8%; placebo 9%), abdominal pain (8%), vomiting (5%), excessive salivation (2%), constipation, salivary gland pain, dry

(Continued)

Cevimeline (Continued)

mouth, sialoadenitis, gastroesophageal reflux, flatulence, ulcerative stomatitis, eructation, amylase increased, anorexia, tooth disorder

Genitourinary: Urinary tract infection (6%), vaginitis, cystitis

Hematologic: Anemia

Local: Abscess

Neuromuscular & skeletal: Back pain (5%), arthralgia (4%), skeletal pain (3%), rigors (1%), hypertonia, tremor, myalgia, hyporeflexia, leg cramps

Ocular: Conjunctivitis (4%), abnormal vision, eye pain, eye abnormality, xerophthalmia

Otic: Earache, otitis media

Respiratory: Coughing (6%), bronchitis (4%), pneumonia, epistaxis

Miscellaneous: Flu-like syndrome, infection, fungal infection, allergy, hiccups

<1% (Limited to important or life-threatening): Aggravated multiple sclerosis, aggressive behavior, alopecia, angina, anterior chamber hemorrhage, aphasia, apnea, arrhythmia, arthropathy, avascular necrosis (femoral head), bronchospasm, bullous eruption, bundle branch block, cholecystitis, cholelithiasis, cholinergic syndrome, coma, deafness, delirium, dementia, depersonalization, dyskinesia, eosinophilia, esophageal stricture, esophagitis, fall, gastric ulcer, gastrointestinal hemorrhage, gingival hyperplasia, glaucoma, granulocytopenia, hallucination, hematuria, hypothyroidism, ileus, impotence, intestinal obstruction, leukopenia, lymphocytosis, manic reaction, MI, neuropathy, paralysis, paranoia, paresthesia, peptic ulcer, pericarditis, peripheral ischemia, photosensitivity reaction, pleural effusion, pulmonary embolism, pulmonary fibrosis, renal calculus, seizure, sepsis, somnolence, syncope, systemic lupus erythematosus, tenosynovitis, thrombocytopenia, thrombocytopenic purpura, thrombophlebitis, T-wave inversion, urinary retention, vasculitis

Dental Usual Dosing Dry mouth (in Sjögren's syndrome): Adults: Oral: 30 mg 3 times/day

Dosage Adults: Oral: 30 mg 3 times/day

Dosage adjustment in renal/hepatic impairment: Not studied; no specific dosage adjustment is recommended

Elderly: No specific dosage adjustment is recommended; however, use caution when initiating due to potential for increased sensitivity

Mechanism of Action Binds to muscarinic (cholinergic) receptors, causing an increase in secretion of exocrine glands (including salivary glands)

Contraindications Hypersensitivity to cevimeline or any component of the formulation; uncontrolled asthma; narrow-angle glaucoma; acute iritis; other conditions where miosis is undesirable

Warnings/Precautions May alter cardiac conduction and/or heart rate; use caution in patients with significant cardiovascular disease, including angina, myocardial infarction, or conduction disturbances. Use with caution in patients with controlled asthma, COPD, or chronic bronchitis. May cause decreased visual acuity (particularly at night and in patients with central lens changes) and impaired depth perception. May cause a variety of parasympathomimetic effects, which may be particularly dangerous in elderly patients; excessive sweating may lead to dehydration in some patients.

Use with caution in patients with a history of biliary stones or nephrolithiasis; cevimeline may precipitate cholangitis, cholecystitis, biliary obstruction, renal colic, or ureteral reflux in susceptible patients. Patients with a known or suspected deficiency of CYP2D6 may be at higher risk of adverse effects. Safety and efficacy have not been established in pediatric patients.

Drug Interactions Substrate (minor) of CYP2D6, CYP3A4

Increased effect: The effects of other cholinergic agents may be increased during concurrent administration with cevimeline. Concurrent use of cevimeline and beta-blockers may increase the potential for conduction disturbances.

Decreased effect: Anticholinergic agents (atropine, TCAs, phenothiazines) may antagonize the effects of cevimeline.

Dietary Considerations Take with or without food.

Pharmacodynamics/Kinetics

Distribution: V_d: 6 L/kg

Protein binding: <20%

Metabolism: Hepatic via CYP2D6 and CYP3A4

Half-life elimination: 5 hours

Time to peak: 1.5-2 hours

Excretion: Urine (as metabolites and unchanged drug)

Pregnancy Risk Factor C

Lactation Excretion in breast milk unknown/not recommended

Dosage Forms Excipient information presented when available (limited, particularly for generics); consult specific product labeling.

Capsule, as hydrochloride: 30 mg

Cevimeline Hydrochloride *see* Cevimeline *on page 325*

CFDN *see* Cefdinir *on page 299*

CG *see* Chorionic Gonadotropin (Human) *on page 352*

CGP-42446 *see* Zoledronic Acid *on page 1685*

CGP-57148B *see* Imatinib *on page 863*

C-Gram [OTC] *see* Ascorbic Acid *on page 148*

CGS-20267 *see* Letrozole *on page 956*

Chantix™ *see* Varenicline *on page 1649*

Char-Caps [OTC] *see* Charcoal, Activated *on page 327*

Charcoal, Activated (CHAR kole AK tiv ay ted)

U.S. Brand Names Actidose-Aqua® [OTC]; Actidose® with Sorbitol [OTC]; Char-Caps [OTC]; Charcoal Plus® DS [OTC]; Charcocaps® [OTC]; EZ-Char™ [OTC]; Kerr Insta-Char® [OTC]

Canadian Brand Names Charcadole®; Charcadole®, Aqueous; Charcadole® TFS

Generic Available Yes: Powder

Index Terms Activated Carbon; Activated Charcoal; Adsorbent Charcoal; Liquid Antidote; Medicinal Carbon; Medicinal Charcoal

Pharmacologic Category Antidote

Use Emergency treatment in poisoning by drugs and chemicals; aids the elimination of certain drugs and improves decontamination of excessive ingestions of sustained-release products or in the presence of bezoars; repetitive doses have proven useful to enhance the elimination of certain drugs (eg, theophylline, phenobarbital, and aspirin); repetitive doses for gastric dialysis in uremia to adsorb various waste products; dietary supplement (digestive aid)

Local Anesthetic/Vasoconstrictor Precautions No information available to require special precautions

Effects on Dental Treatment No significant effects or complications reported

Mechanism of Action Adsorbs toxic substances or irritants, thus inhibiting GI absorption; adsorbs intestinal gas; the addition of sorbitol results in hyperosmotic laxative action causing catharsis

Pregnancy Risk Factor C

Charcoal Plus® DS [OTC] *see* Charcoal, Activated *on page 327*

Charcocaps® [OTC] *see* Charcoal, Activated *on page 327*

CheeTah® *see* Barium *on page 185*

Cheracol® *see* Guaifenesin and Codeine *on page 795*

Cheracol® [OTC] *see* Phenol *on page 1290*

Cheracol® D [OTC] *see* Guaifenesin and Dextromethorphan *on page 796*

Cheracol® Plus [OTC] *see* Guaifenesin and Dextromethorphan *on page 796*

Chew-Cal [OTC] *see* Calcium and Vitamin D *on page 259*

CHG *see* Chlorhexidine Gluconate *on page 332*

Chiggerex® [OTC] *see* Benzocaine *on page 195*

Chiggertox® [OTC] *see* Benzocaine *on page 195*

Children's Dimetapp® Elixir Cold & Allergy [OTC] [DSC] *see* Brompheniramine and Pseudoephedrine *on page 231*

Children's Kaopectate® [OTC] [DSC] *see* Attapulgite *on page 170*

Children's Pepto [OTC] *see* Calcium Carbonate *on page 260*

ChiRhoStim™ *see* Secretin *on page 1459*

Chirocaine® [DSC] *see* Levobupivacaine *on page 961*

Chloral *see* Chloral Hydrate *on page 327*

Chloral Hydrate (KLOR al HYE drate)

U.S. Brand Names Aquachloral® Supprettes®; Somnote™

Canadian Brand Names PMS-Chloral Hydrate

Generic Available Yes: Syrup

Index Terms Chloral; Hydrated Chloral; Trichloroacetaldehyde Monohydrate

Pharmacologic Category Hypnotic, Nonbenzodiazepine

Dental Use Short-term sedative/hypnotic for dental procedures

Use Short-term sedative and hypnotic (<2 weeks); sedative/hypnotic for diagnostic procedures; sedative prior to EEG evaluations

Local Anesthetic/Vasoconstrictor Precautions No information available to require special precautions

Effects on Dental Treatment No significant effects or complications reported

Significant Adverse Effects Frequency not defined.

(Continued)

Chloral Hydrate *(Continued)*

Central nervous system: Ataxia, disorientation, sedation, excitement (paradoxical), dizziness, fever, headache, confusion, lightheadedness, nightmares, hallucinations, drowsiness, "hangover" effect

Dermatologic: Rash, urticaria

Gastrointestinal: Gastric irritation, nausea, vomiting, diarrhea, flatulence

Hematologic: Leukopenia, eosinophilia, acute intermittent porphyria

Miscellaneous: Physical and psychological dependence may occur with prolonged use of large doses

Restrictions C-IV

Dental Usual Dosing

Conscious sedation: Children: Oral: 50-75 mg/kg/dose 30-60 minutes prior to procedure; may repeat 30 minutes after initial dose if needed, to a total maximum dose of 120 mg/kg or 1 g total

Hypnotic: Adults: Oral, rectal: 500-1000 mg at bedtime or 30 minutes prior to procedure, not to exceed 2 g/24 hours

Sedation, anxiety: Oral, rectal:

Children: 5-15 mg/kg/dose every 8 hours (maximum: 500 mg/dose)

Adults: 250 mg 3 times/day

Dosage

Children:

Sedation or anxiety: Oral, rectal: 5-15 mg/kg/dose every 8 hours (maximum: 500 mg/dose)

Prior to EEG: Oral, rectal: 20-25 mg/kg/dose, 30-60 minutes prior to EEG; may repeat in 30 minutes to maximum of 100 mg/kg or 2 g total

Hypnotic: Oral, rectal: 20-40 mg/kg/dose up to a maximum of 50 mg/kg/24 hours or 1 g/dose or 2 g/24 hours

Conscious sedation: Oral: 50-75 mg/kg/dose 30-60 minutes prior to procedure; may repeat 30 minutes after initial dose if needed, to a total maximum dose of 120 mg/kg or 1 g total

Adults: Oral, rectal:

Sedation, anxiety: 250 mg 3 times/day

Hypnotic: 500-1000 mg at bedtime or 30 minutes prior to procedure, not to exceed 2 g/24 hours

Discontinuation: Withdraw gradually over 2 weeks if patient has been maintained on high doses for prolonged period of time. Do not stop drug abruptly; sudden withdrawal may result in delirium.

Dosing adjustment/comments in renal impairment: Cl_{cr} <50 mL/minute: Avoid use

Hemodialysis: Dialyzable (50% to 100%); supplemental dose is not necessary

Dosing adjustment/comments in hepatic impairment: Avoid use in patients with severe hepatic impairment

Mechanism of Action Central nervous system depressant effects are due to its active metabolite trichloroethanol, mechanism unknown

Contraindications Hypersensitivity to chloral hydrate or any component of the formulation; hepatic or renal impairment; gastritis or ulcers; severe cardiac disease

Warnings/Precautions Use with caution in patients with porphyria. Use with caution in neonates. Drug may accumulate with repeated use; prolonged use in neonates associated with hyperbilirubinemia. Tolerance to hypnotic effect develops, therefore, not recommended for use longer than 2 weeks. Taper dosage to avoid withdrawal with prolonged use. Trichloroethanol (TCE), a metabolite of chloral hydrate, is a carcinogen in mice; there is no data in humans. Chloral hydrate is considered a second line hypnotic agent in the elderly. Recent interpretive guidelines from the Centers for Medicare and Medicaid Services (CMS) discourage the use of chloral hydrate in residents of long-term care facilities.

Drug Interactions

CNS depressants: Sedative effects and/or respiratory depression with chloral hydrate may be additive with other CNS depressants; monitor for increased effect; includes ethanol, sedatives, antidepressants, opioid analgesics, and benzodiazepines.

Furosemide: Diaphoresis, flushing, and hypertension have occurred in patients who received I.V. furosemide within 24 hours after administration of chloral hydrate; consider using a benzodiazepine.

Phenytoin: Half-life may be decreased by chloral hydrate; limited documentation (small, single-dose study); monitor.

Warfarin: Effect of oral anticoagulants may be increased by chloral hydrate; monitor INR; warfarin dosage may require adjustment. Chloral hydrate's metabolite may displace warfarin from its protein binding sites resulting in an increase in the hypoprothrombinemic response to warfarin.

Ethanol/Nutrition/Herb Interactions

Ethanol: Avoid ethanol (may increase CNS depression).

Herb/Nutraceutical: Avoid valerian, St John's wort, kava kava, gotu kola (may increase CNS depression).

Pharmacodynamics/Kinetics

Onset of action: Peak effect: 0.5-1 hour

Duration: 4-8 hours

Absorption: Oral, rectal: Well absorbed

Distribution: Crosses placenta; negligible amounts enter breast milk

Metabolism: Rapidly hepatic to trichloroethanol (active metabolite); variable amounts hepatically and renally to trichloroacetic acid (inactive)

Half-life elimination: Active metabolite: 8-11 hours

Excretion: Urine (as metabolites); feces (small amounts)

Pregnancy Risk Factor C

Lactation Enters breast milk/compatible

Dosage Forms Excipient information presented when available (limited, particularly for generics); consult specific product labeling.

Capsule (Somnote™): 500 mg

Suppository, rectal (Aquachloral® Supprettes®): 325 mg [contains tartrazine], 650 mg

Syrup: 500 mg/5 mL (480 mL) [contains sodium benzoate]

Chlorambucil (klor AM byoo sil)

U.S. Brand Names Leukeran®

Canadian Brand Names Leukeran®

Mexican Brand Names Leukeran

Generic Available No

Index Terms CB-1348; Chlorambucilum; Chloraminophene; Chlorbutinum; NSC-3088; WR-139013

Pharmacologic Category Antineoplastic Agent, Alkylating Agent

Use Management of chronic lymphocytic leukemia (CLL), Hodgkin's lymphoma, non-Hodgkin's lymphoma (NHL)

Unlabeled/Investigational Use Nephrotic syndrome, Waldenström's macroglobulinemia

Local Anesthetic/Vasoconstrictor Precautions No information available to require special precautions

Effects on Dental Treatment Key adverse event(s) related to dental treatment: Stomatitis.

Common Adverse Effects Frequency not always defined.

Central nervous system: Agitation (rare), ataxia (rare), confusion (rare), drug fever, focal/generalized seizures (rare), hallucinations (rare)

Dermatologic: Angioneurotic edema, erythema multiforme (rare), rash, skin hypersensitivity, Stevens-Johnson syndrome (rare), toxic epidermal necrolysis (rare), urticaria

Endocrine & metabolic: Amenorrhea, infertility, SIADH (rare)

Gastrointestinal: Diarrhea (infrequent), nausea (infrequent), oral ulceration (infrequent), vomiting (infrequent)

Genitourinary: Azoospermia, cystitis (sterile)

Hematologic: Neutropenia (25%; dose- and duration-related; onset: 3 weeks; recovery: 10 days after last dose), bone marrow failure (irreversible), bone marrow suppression, anemia, leukemia (secondary), leukopenia, lymphopenia, pancytopenia, thrombocytopenia

Hepatic: Hepatotoxicity, jaundice

Neuromuscular & skeletal: Flaccid paresis (rare), muscular twitching (rare), myoclonia (rare), peripheral neuropathy, tremor (rare)

Respiratory: Interstitial pneumonia, pulmonary fibrosis

Miscellaneous: Allergic reactions, malignancies (secondary)

Mechanism of Action Interferes with DNA replication and RNA transcription by alkylation and cross-linking the strands of DNA

Drug Interactions

Increased Effect/Toxicity: Vaccines (live organism): Avoid the administration of live vaccines during chlorambucil treatment.

Pharmacodynamics/Kinetics

Absorption: Rapid and complete

Distribution: V_d: 0.14-0.24 L/kg

Protein binding: ~99%

Metabolism: Hepatic; forms a major active metabolite (phenylacetic acid mustard) and inactive metabolites

Bioavailability: Reduced 10% to 20% with food

Half-life elimination: ~1.5 hours; Phenylacetic acid mustard: ~1.8 hours

Time to peak, plasma: Within 1 hour; Phenylacetic acid mustard: 1.2-2.6 hours

Excretion: Urine (15% to 60% primarily as inactive metabolites, <1% as unchanged drug or phenylacetic acid mustard)

Pregnancy Risk Factor D

Chlorambucilum *see* Chlorambucil *on page 329*

Chloraminophene *see* Chlorambucil *on page 329*

Chloramphenicol (klor am FEN i kole)

U.S. Brand Names Chloromycetin® Sodium Succinate
Canadian Brand Names Chloromycetin®; Chloromycetin® Succinate; Diochloram®; Pentamycetin®
Mexican Brand Names Cetina; Chloromycetin (MX, MX); Cloramfeni Ofteno; Cloramfeni Ungena; Quemicetina; Quemicitina
Generic Available Yes
Pharmacologic Category Antibiotic, Miscellaneous
Use Treatment of serious infections due to organisms resistant to other less toxic antibiotics or when its penetrability into the site of infection is clinically superior to other antibiotics to which the organism is sensitive; useful in infections caused by *Bacteroides*, *H. influenzae*, *Neisseria meningitidis*, *Salmonella*, and *Rickettsia*; active against many vancomycin-resistant enterococci
Local Anesthetic/Vasoconstrictor Precautions No information available to require special precautions
Effects on Dental Treatment Key adverse event(s) related to dental treatment: Glossitis and stomatitis.
Common Adverse Effects
Three (3) major toxicities associated with chloramphenicol include:
Aplastic anemia, an idiosyncratic reaction which can occur with any route of administration; usually occurs 3 weeks to 12 months after initial exposure to chloramphenicol.
Bone marrow suppression is thought to be dose related with serum concentrations >25 mcg/mL and reversible once chloramphenicol is discontinued; anemia and neutropenia may occur during the first week of therapy.
Gray syndrome is characterized by circulatory collapse, cyanosis, acidosis, abdominal distention, myocardial depression, coma, and death. Reaction appears to be associated with serum levels ≥50 mcg/mL. May result from drug accumulation in patients with impaired hepatic or renal function.
Additional adverse reactions, frequency not defined:
Central nervous system: Confusion, delirium, depression, fever, headache
Dermatologic: Angioedema, rash, urticaria
Gastrointestinal: Diarrhea, enterocolitis, glossitis, nausea, stomatitis, vomiting
Hematologic: Granulocytopenia, hypoplastic anemia, pancytopenia, thrombocytopenia
Ocular: Optic neuritis
Miscellaneous: Anaphylaxis, hypersensitivity reactions
Mechanism of Action Reversibly binds to 50S ribosomal subunits of susceptible organisms preventing amino acids from being transferred to growing peptide chains thus inhibiting protein synthesis
Drug Interactions
Cytochrome P450 Effect: Inhibits CYP2C9 (weak), 3A4 (weak)
Increased Effect/Toxicity: Chloramphenicol increases serum concentrations of chlorpropamide, phenytoin, and oral anticoagulants.
Decreased Effect: Phenobarbital and rifampin may decrease serum concentrations of chloramphenicol.
Pharmacodynamics/Kinetics
Distribution: To most tissues and body fluids; readily crosses placenta; enters breast milk
CSF:blood level ratio: Normal meninges: 66%; Inflamed meninges: >66%
Protein binding: 60%
Metabolism: Extensively hepatic (90%) to inactive metabolites, principally by glucuronidation; chloramphenicol sodium succinate is hydrolyzed by esterases to active base
Half-life elimination:
. Normal renal function: 1.6-3.3 hours
End-stage renal disease: 3-7 hours
Cirrhosis: 10-12 hours
Excretion: Urine (5% to 15%)
Pregnancy Risk Factor C

ChloraPrep® [OTC] *see* Chlorhexidine Gluconate *on page 332*

Chloraseptic® Gargle [OTC] *see* Phenol *on page 1290*

Chloraseptic® Mouth Pain [OTC] *see* Phenol *on page 1290*

Chloraseptic® Pocket Pump [OTC] *see* Phenol *on page 1290*

Chloraseptic® Spray [OTC] see Phenol on page 1290
Chloraseptic® Spray for Kids [OTC] see Phenol on page 1290
Chlorbutinum see Chlorambucil on page 329

Chlordiazepoxide (klor dye az e POKS ide)

U.S. Brand Names Librium®
Canadian Brand Names Apo-Chlordiazepoxide®
Generic Available Yes: Capsule
Index Terms Methaminodiazepoxide Hydrochloride
Pharmacologic Category Benzodiazepine
Use Management of anxiety disorder or for the short-term relief of symptoms of anxiety; withdrawal symptoms of acute alcoholism; preoperative apprehension and anxiety
Local Anesthetic/Vasoconstrictor Precautions No information available to require special precautions
Effects on Dental Treatment Key adverse event(s) related to dental treatment: Xerostomia (normal salivary flow resumes upon discontinuation).
Common Adverse Effects
>10%:
Central nervous system: Drowsiness, fatigue, ataxia, lightheadedness, memory impairment, dysarthria, irritability
Dermatologic: Rash
Endocrine & metabolic: Libido decreased, menstrual disorders
Gastrointestinal: Xerostomia, salivation decreased, appetite increased or decreased, weight gain/loss
Genitourinary: Micturition difficulties
1% to 10%:
Cardiovascular: Hypotension
Central nervous system: Confusion, dizziness, disinhibition, akathisia
Dermatologic: Dermatitis
Endocrine & metabolic: Libido increased
Gastrointestinal: Salivation increased
Genitourinary: Sexual dysfunction, incontinence
Neuromuscular & skeletal: Rigidity, tremor, muscle cramps
Otic: Tinnitus
Respiratory: Nasal congestion
Restrictions C-IV
Mechanism of Action Binds to stereospecific benzodiazepine receptors on the postsynaptic GABA neuron at several sites within the central nervous system, including the limbic system, reticular formation. Enhancement of the inhibitory effect of GABA on neuronal excitability results by increased neuronal membrane permeability to chloride ions. This shift in chloride ions results in hyperpolarization (a less excitable state) and stabilization.
Drug Interactions
Cytochrome P450 Effect: Substrate of CYP3A4 (major)
Increased Effect/Toxicity: Chlordiazepoxide potentiates the CNS depressant effects of opioid analgesics, barbiturates, phenothiazines, ethanol, antihistamines, MAO inhibitors, sedative-hypnotics, and cyclic antidepressants. CYP3A4 inhibitors may increase the levels/effects of chlordiazepoxide; example inhibitors include azole antifungals, clarithromycin, diclofenac, doxycycline, erythromycin, imatinib, isoniazid, nefazodone, nicardipine, propofol, protease inhibitors, quinidine, telithromycin, and verapamil.
Decreased Effect: CYP3A4 inducers may decrease the levels/effects of chlordiazepoxide; example inducers include aminoglutethimide, carbamazepine, nafcillin, nevirapine, phenobarbital, phenytoin, and rifamycins.
Pharmacodynamics/Kinetics
Distribution: V_d: 3.3 L/kg; crosses placenta; enters breast milk
Protein binding: 90% to 98%
Metabolism: Extensively hepatic to desmethyldiazepam (active and long-acting)
Half-life elimination: 6.6-25 hours; End-stage renal disease: 5-30 hours; Cirrhosis: 30-63 hours
Time to peak, serum: Oral: Within 2 hours; I.M.: Results in lower peak plasma levels than oral
Excretion: Urine (minimal as unchanged drug)
Pregnancy Risk Factor D

Chlordiazepoxide and Amitriptyline Hydrochloride see Amitriptyline and Chlordiazepoxide on page 98
Chlordiazepoxide and Clidinium see Clidinium and Chlordiazepoxide on page 377

Chlordiazepoxide and Methscopolamine
(klor dye az e POKS ide & meth skoe POL a meen)

U.S. Brand Names Librax® *[reformulation]* [DSC]
Generic Available No
Index Terms Methscopolamine Nitrate and Chlordiazepoxide Hydrochloride
Pharmacologic Category Anticholinergic Agent; Benzodiazepine
Use Adjunctive treatment of peptic ulcer; treatment of irritable bowel syndrome, acute enterocolitis
Local Anesthetic/Vasoconstrictor Precautions No information available to require special precautions
Effects on Dental Treatment Key adverse event(s) related to dental treatment: Xerostomia and changes in salivation (normal salivary flow resumes upon discontinuation).
Common Adverse Effects See individual agents.
Restrictions C-IV
Mechanism of Action Chlordiazepoxide binds to stereospecific benzodiazepine (BZD) binding sites on GABA (A) receptor complexes at several sites within the central nervous system, including the limbic system and reticular formation. BZDs enhance GABA-mediated chloride influx through GABA receptor channels, causing membrane hyperpolarization. The net neuroinhibitory effects result in the observed sedative, hypnotic, anxiolytic, and muscle relaxant properties.
Methscopolamine is a peripheral anticholinergic agent with limited ability to cross the blood-brain barrier and provides a peripheral blockade of muscarinic receptors. This agent reduces the volume and the total acid content of gastric secretions, inhibits salivation, and reduces gastrointestinal motility.
Pharmacodynamics/Kinetics See individual agents.
Pregnancy Risk Factor C

Chlorhexidine Gluconate (klor HEKS i deen GLOO koe nate)

Related Information
Bacterial Infections *on page 1793*
Dentin Hypersensitivity, High Caries Index, and Xerostomia *on page 1812*
Management of Patients Undergoing Cancer Therapy *on page 1826*
Periodontal Diseases *on page 1801*
Ulcerative and Erosive Disorders *on page 1809*
Related Sample Prescriptions
Antimicrobial Oral Rinse *on page 1840*
U.S. Brand Names Avagard™ [OTC]; BactoShield® CHG [OTC]; Betasept® [OTC]; ChloraPrep® [OTC]; Dyna-Hex® [OTC]; Hibiclens® [OTC]; Hibistat® [OTC]; Operand® Chlorhexidine Gluconate [OTC]; Peridex®; PerioChip®; Perio-Gard®
Canadian Brand Names Hibidil® 1:2000; ORO-Clense
Mexican Brand Names Perioxidin
Generic Available Yes: Oral liquid
Index Terms CHG; 3M™ Avagard™ [OTC]
Pharmacologic Category Antibiotic, Oral Rinse; Antibiotic, Topical
Dental Use
Antibacterial dental rinse; chlorhexidine is active against gram-positive and gram-negative organisms, facultative anaerobes, aerobes, and yeast
Chip, for periodontal pocket insertion: Indicated as an adjunct to scaling and root planing procedures for reduction of pocket depth in patients with adult periodontitis; may be used as part of a periodontal maintenance program
Use Skin cleanser for surgical scrub, cleanser for skin wounds, preoperative skin preparation, germicidal hand rinse, and as antibacterial dental rinse. Chlorhexidine is active against gram-positive and gram-negative organisms, facultative anaerobes, aerobes, and yeast.
Orphan drug: Peridex®: Oral mucositis with cytoreductive therapy when used for patients undergoing bone marrow transplant
Local Anesthetic/Vasoconstrictor Precautions No information available to require special precautions
Effects on Dental Treatment Key adverse event(s) related to dental treatment: Increased tartar on teeth, altered taste perception, staining of oral surfaces (mucosa, teeth, dorsum of tongue), and oral/tongue irritation. Staining may be visible as soon as 1 week after therapy begins and is more pronounced when there is a heavy accumulation of unremoved plaque and when teeth fillings have rough surfaces. Stain does not have a clinically adverse effect but because removal may not be possible, patient with frontal restoration should be advised of the potential permanency of the stain.

Significant Adverse Effects

Oral:

>10%: Tartar on teeth increased, taste changes. Staining of oral surfaces (mucosa, teeth, dorsum of tongue) may be visible as soon as 1 week after therapy begins and is more pronounced when there is a heavy accumulation of unremoved plaque and when teeth fillings have rough surfaces. Stain does not have a clinically adverse effect but because removal may not be possible, patient with frontal restoration should be advised of the potential permanency of the stain.

1% to 10%: Gastrointestinal: Tongue irritation, oral irritation

<1% (Limited to important or life-threatening): Dyspnea, facial edema, nasal congestion

Topical: Skin erythema and roughness, dryness, sensitization, allergic reactions

Dental Usual Dosing Adults:

Oral rinse (Peridex®, PerioGard®):

Floss and brush teeth, completely rinse toothpaste from mouth and swish 15 mL (one capful) undiluted oral rinse around in mouth for 30 seconds, then expectorate. Caution patient not to swallow the medicine and instruct not to eat for 2-3 hours after treatment. (Cap on bottle measures 15 mL.)

Treatment of gingivitis: Oral prophylaxis: Swish for 30 seconds with 15 mL chlorhexidine, then expectorate; repeat twice daily (morning and evening). Patient should have a re-evaluation followed by a dental prophylaxis every 6 months.

Periodontal chip: One chip is inserted into a periodontal pocket with a probing pocket depth ≥5 mm. Up to 8 chips may be inserted in a single visit. Treatment is recommended every 3 months in pockets with a remaining depth ≥5 mm. If dislodgment occurs 7 days or more after placement, the subject is considered to have had the full course of treatment. If dislodgment occurs within 48 hours, a new chip should be inserted. The chip biodegrades completely and does not need to be removed. Patients should avoid dental floss at the site of PerioChip® insertion for 10 days after placement because flossing might dislodge the chip.

Insertion of periodontal chip: Pocket should be isolated and surrounding area dried prior to chip insertion. The chip should be grasped using forceps with the rounded edges away from the forceps. The chip should be inserted into the periodontal pocket to its maximum depth. It may be maneuvered into position using the tips of the forceps or a flat instrument.

Dosage Adults:

Oral rinse (Peridex®, PerioGard®):

Floss and brush teeth, completely rinse toothpaste from mouth and swish 15 mL (one capful) undiluted oral rinse around in mouth for 30 seconds, then expectorate. Caution patient not to swallow the medicine and instruct not to eat for 2-3 hours after treatment. (Cap on bottle measures 15 mL.)

Treatment of gingivitis: Oral prophylaxis: Swish for 30 seconds with 15 mL chlorhexidine, then expectorate; repeat twice daily (morning and evening). Patient should have a re-evaluation followed by a dental prophylaxis every 6 months.

Periodontal chip: One chip is inserted into a periodontal pocket with a probing pocket depth ≥5 mm. Up to 8 chips may be inserted in a single visit. Treatment is recommended every 3 months in pockets with a remaining depth ≥5 mm. If dislodgment occurs 7 days or more after placement, the subject is considered to have had the full course of treatment. If dislodgment occurs within 48 hours, a new chip should be inserted. The chip biodegrades completely and does not need to be removed. Patients should avoid dental floss at the site of PerioChip® insertion for 10 days after placement because flossing might dislodge the chip.

Insertion of periodontal chip: Pocket should be isolated and surrounding area dried prior to chip insertion. The chip should be grasped using forceps with the rounded edges away from the forceps. The chip should be inserted into the periodontal pocket to its maximum depth. It may be maneuvered into position using the tips of the forceps or a flat instrument.

Cleanser:

Surgical scrub: Scrub 3 minutes and rinse thoroughly, wash for an additional 3 minutes

Hand sanitizer (Avagard™): Dispense 1 pumpful in palm of one hand; dip fingertips of opposite hand into solution and work it under nails. Spread remainder evenly over hand and just above elbow, covering all surfaces. Repeat on other hand. Dispense another pumpful in each hand and reapply to each hand up to the wrist. Allow to dry before gloving.

Hand wash: Wash for 15 seconds and rinse

Hand rinse: Rub 15 seconds and rinse

Mechanism of Action The bactericidal effect of chlorhexidine is a result of the binding of this cationic molecule to negatively charged bacterial cell walls and extramicrobial complexes. At low concentrations, this causes an alteration of
(Continued)

Chlorhexidine Gluconate *(Continued)*

bacterial cell osmotic equilibrium and leakage of potassium and phosphorous resulting in a bacteriostatic effect. At high concentrations of chlorhexidine, the cytoplasmic contents of the bacterial cell precipitate and result in cell death.

Contraindications Hypersensitivity to chlorhexidine gluconate or any component of the formulation

Warnings/Precautions

Oral: Staining of oral surfaces (mucosa, teeth, tooth restorations, dorsum of tongue) may occur; may be visible as soon as 1 week after therapy begins and is more pronounced when there is a heavy accumulation of unremoved plaque and when teeth fillings have rough surfaces. Stain does not have a clinically adverse effect, but because removal may not be possible, patient with frontal restoration should be advised of the potential permanency of the stain.

Topical: For topical use only. Avoid application over large surfaces or into open wounds. Keep out of eyes and ears. May stain fabric. There have been case reports of anaphylaxis following chlorhexidine disinfection. Not for preoperative preparation of face or head; avoid contact with meninges (do not use on lumbar puncture sites). Solutions may be flammable (contain isopropyl alcohol); avoid exposure to open flame and/or ignition source (eg, electrocautery) until completely dry; avoid application to hairy areas which may significantly delay drying time. Avoid use in children <2 months of age due to increased absorption and/or irritation.

Drug Interactions No data reported

Pharmacodynamics/Kinetics

Topical hand sanitizer (Avagard™): Duration of antimicrobial protection: 6 hours

Oral rinse (Peridex®, PerioGard®):

Absorption: ~30% retained in the oral cavity following rinsing and slowly released into oral fluids; poorly absorbed

Time to peak, plasma: Oral rinse: Detectable levels not present after 12 hours

Excretion: Feces (~90%); urine (<1%)

Pregnancy Risk Factor B

Dosage Forms Excipient information presented when available (limited, particularly for generics); consult specific product labeling.

Chip, for periodontal pocket insertion:

PerioChip®: 2.5 mg

Liquid, topical [surgical scrub]:

Avagard™: 1% (500 mL) [contains ethyl alcohol and moisturizers]

BactoShield® CHG: 2% (120 mL, 480 mL, 750 mL, 1000 mL, 3800 mL); 4% (120 mL, 480 mL, 750 mL, 1000 mL, 3800 mL) [contains isopropyl alcohol]

Betasept®: 4% (120 mL, 240 mL, 480 mL, 960 mL, 3840 mL) [contains isopropyl alcohol]

ChloraPrep®: 2% (0.67 mL, 1.5 mL, 3 mL, 10.5 mL) [contains isopropyl alcohol 70%; prefilled applicator]

Dyna-Hex®: 2% (120 mL, 960 mL, 3840 mL); 4% (120 mL, 960 mL, 3840 mL)

Hibiclens®: 4% (15 mL, 120 mL, 240 mL, 480 mL, 960 mL, 3840 mL) [contains isopropyl alcohol]

Operand® Chlorhexidine Gluconate: 2% (120 mL); 4% (120 mL, 240 mL, 480 mL, 960 mL, 3840 mL) [contains isopropyl alcohol]

Liquid, oral rinse: 0.12% (480 mL)

Peridex®: 0.12% (480 mL) [contains alcohol 11.6%]

PerioGard®: 0.12% (480 mL) [contains alcohol 11.6%; mint flavor]

Pad [prep pad] (Hibistat®): 0.5% (50s) [contains isopropyl alcohol]

Sponge/Brush (BactoShield® CHG): 4% per sponge/brush [contains isopropyl alcohol]

Selected Readings

al-Tannir MA and Goodman HS, "A Review of Chlorhexidine and Its Use in Special Populations," *Spec Care Dentist*, 1994, 14(3):116-22.

Ercan E, Ozekinci T, Atakul F, et al, "Antibacterial Activity of 2% Chlorhexidine Gluconate and 5.25% Sodium Hypochlorite in Infected Root Canal: *In Vivo* Study," *J Endod*, 2004, 30(2):84-7.

Ferretti GA, Brown AT, Raybould TP, et al, "Oral Antimicrobial Agents - Chlorhexidine," *NCI Monogr*, 1990, 9:51-5.

Greenstein G, Berman C, and Jaffin R, "Chlorhexidine. An Adjunct to Periodontal Therapy," *J Periodontol*, 1986, 57(6):370-7.

Johnson BT, "Uses of Chlorhexidine in Dentistry," *Gen Dent*, 1995, 43(2):126-32, 134-40.

Noiri Y, Okami Y, Narimatsu M, et al, "Effects of Chlorhexidine, Minocycline, and Metronidazole on Porphyromonas Gingivalis Strain 381 in Biofilms," *J Periodontol*, 2003, 74(11):1647-51.

Reddy MS, Jeffcoat MK, Geurs NC, et al, "Efficacy of Controlled-Release Subgingival Chlorhexidine to Enhance Periodontal Regeneration," *J Periodontol*, 2003, 74(4):411-9.

Soskolne WA, Proskin HM, and Stabholz A, "Probing Depth Changes Following 2 Years of Periodontal Maintenance Therapy Including Adjunctive Controlled Release of Chlorhexidine," *J Periodontol*, 2003, 74(4):420-7.

Yusof ZA, "Chlorhexidine Mouthwash: A Review of Its Pharmacological Activity, Clinical Effects, Uses and Abuses," *Dent J Malays*, 1988, 10(1):9-16.

Chlormeprazine *see* Prochlorperazine *on page 1356*

Chlor-Mes-D *see* Chlorpheniramine, Phenylephrine, and Methscopolamine *on page 342*

2-Chlorodeoxyadenosine *see* Cladribine *on page 371*

Chloroethane *see* Ethyl Chloride *on page 653*

Chloromag® *see* Magnesium Chloride *on page 1013*

Chloromycetin® Sodium Succinate *see* Chloramphenicol *on page 330*

Chlorophyll (KLOR oh fil)

U.S. Brand Names Nullo® [OTC]
Generic Available No
Index Terms Chlorophyllin
Pharmacologic Category Gastrointestinal Agent, Miscellaneous
Use Control fecal odors in colostomy or ileostomy
Local Anesthetic/Vasoconstrictor Precautions No information available to require special precautions
Effects on Dental Treatment No significant effects or complications reported
Common Adverse Effects Frequency not defined: Gastrointestinal: Diarrhea, green stools, abdominal cramping

Chlorophyllin *see* Chlorophyll *on page 335*

Chlorophyllin Copper Complex Sodium, Papain, and Urea *see* Chlorophyllin, Papain, and Urea *on page 335*

Chlorophyllin, Papain, and Urea
(KLOR oh fil in, pa PAY in, & yoor EE a)

U.S. Brand Names Allanfil 405; Allanfil Spray; Panafil®; Panafil® SE; Ziox™ [DSC]; Ziox 405™
Generic Available Yes: Ointment, solution
Index Terms Chlorophyllin Copper Complex Sodium, Papain, and Urea; Papain, Urea, and Chlorophyllin; Urea, Chlorophyllin, and Papain
Pharmacologic Category Enzyme, Topical Debridement
Use Treatment of acute and chronic lesions, such as varicose, diabetic decubitus ulcers, burns, postoperative wounds, pilonidal cyst wounds, carbuncles, and miscellaneous traumatic or infected wounds
Local Anesthetic/Vasoconstrictor Precautions No information available to require special precautions
Effects on Dental Treatment No significant effects or complications reported
Common Adverse Effects Local: Burning sensation, skin irritation
Mechanism of Action
Papain: Potent digestant of nonviable protein matter; harmless to viable tissue. Requires activation to exert its function.
Urea: Exposes papain activators (sulfhydryl groups) and denatures nonviable protein matter making it more susceptible to enzymatic digestion.
Chlorophyllin copper complex sodium: Inhibits the hemagglutinating and inflammatory properties of protein degradation products in the wound; the resulting healthy granulation, decreased local inflammation, and decreased wound odor promotes wound healing.
Drug Interactions
Decreased Effect: Heavy metals, hydrogen peroxide

Chloroprocaine (klor oh PROE kane)

Related Information
Oral Pain *on page 1788*
U.S. Brand Names Nesacaine®; Nesacaine®-MPF
Canadian Brand Names Nesacaine®-CE
Generic Available Yes
Index Terms Chloroprocaine Hydrochloride
Pharmacologic Category Local Anesthetic
Use Infiltration anesthesia and peripheral and epidural anesthesia
Local Anesthetic/Vasoconstrictor Precautions No information available to require special precautions
Effects on Dental Treatment No significant effects or complications reported
Common Adverse Effects Frequency not defined.
Cardiovascular: Bradycardia, cardiac arrest, hypotension, ventricular arrhythmia
Central nervous system: Anxiety, dizziness, restlessness, tinnitus, unconsciousness
Dermatologic: Angioneurotic edema, erythema, pruritus, urticaria
Ocular: Blurred vision
(Continued)

Chloroprocaine *(Continued)*

Respiratory: Respiratory arrest

Miscellaneous: Allergic reactions, anaphylactoid reactions

Mechanism of Action Chloroprocaine HCl is benzoic acid, 4-amino-2-chloro-2-(diethylamino) ethyl ester monohydrochloride. Chloroprocaine is an ester-type local anesthetic, which stabilizes the neuronal membranes and prevents initiation and transmission of nerve impulses thereby affecting local anesthetic actions. Local anesthetics including chloroprocaine, reversibly prevent generation and conduction of electrical impulses in neurons by decreasing the transient increase in permeability to sodium. The differential sensitivity generally depends on the size of the fiber; small fibers are more sensitive than larger fibers and require a longer period for recovery. Sensory pain fibers are usually blocked first, followed by fibers that transmit sensations of temperature, touch, and deep pressure. High concentrations block sympathetic somatic sensory and somatic motor fibers. The spread of anesthesia depends upon the distribution of the solution. This is primarily dependent on the volume of drug injected.

Drug Interactions

Decreased Effect: The para-aminobenzoic acid metabolite of chloroprocaine may decrease the efficacy of sulfonamide antibiotics.

Pharmacodynamics/Kinetics

Onset of action: 6-12 minutes

Duration: 30-60 minutes

Distribution: V_d: Depends upon route of administration; high concentrations found in highly perfused organs such as liver, lungs, heart, and brain

Metabolism: Plasma cholinesterases

Excretion: Urine

Pregnancy Risk Factor C

Chloroprocaine Hydrochloride *see* Chloroprocaine *on page 335*

Chloroquine *(KLOR oh kwin)*

U.S. Brand Names Aralen®

Canadian Brand Names Aralen®; Novo-Chloroquine

Mexican Brand Names Aralen Phosphate

Generic Available Yes

Index Terms Chloroquine Phosphate

Pharmacologic Category Aminoquinoline (Antimalarial)

Use Suppression or chemoprophylaxis of malaria; treatment of uncomplicated or mild-to-moderate malaria; extraintestinal amebiasis

Unlabeled/Investigational Use Rheumatoid arthritis; discoid lupus erythematosus

Local Anesthetic/Vasoconstrictor Precautions No information available to require special precautions

Effects on Dental Treatment Key adverse event(s) related to dental treatment: Stomatitis.

Common Adverse Effects Frequency not defined.

Cardiovascular: Hypotension (rare), ECG changes (rare; including T-wave inversion), cardiomyopathy

Central nervous system: Fatigue, personality changes, headache, psychosis, seizure, delirium, depression

Dermatologic: Pruritus, hair bleaching, pleomorphic skin eruptions, alopecia, lichen planus eruptions, alopecia, mucosal pigmentary changes (blue-black), photosensitivity

Gastrointestinal: Nausea, diarrhea, vomiting, anorexia, stomatitis, abdominal cramps

Hematologic: Aplastic anemia, agranulocytosis (reversible), neutropenia, thrombocytopenia

Neuromuscular & skeletal: Rare cases of myopathy, neuromyopathy, proximal muscle atrophy, and depression of deep tendon reflexes have been reported

Ocular: Retinopathy (including irreversible changes in some patients long-term or high-dose therapy), blurred vision

Otic: Nerve deafness, tinnitus, hearing reduced (risk increased in patients with pre-existing auditory damage)

Mechanism of Action Binds to and inhibits DNA and RNA polymerase; interferes with metabolism and hemoglobin utilization by parasites; inhibits prostaglandin effects; chloroquine concentrates within parasite acid vesicles and raises internal pH resulting in inhibition of parasite growth; may involve aggregates of ferriprotoporphyrin IX acting as chloroquine receptors causing membrane damage; may also interfere with nucleoprotein synthesis

Drug Interactions

Cytochrome P450 Effect: Substrate (major) of CYP2D6, 3A4; **Inhibits** CYP2D6 (moderate)

Increased Effect/Toxicity: Chloroquine may increase the levels/effects of dextromethorphan, fluoxetine, lidocaine, mirtazapine, nefazodone, paroxetine, risperidone, ritonavir, thioridazine, tricyclic antidepressants, venlafaxine, and other CYP2D6 substrates. Chloroquine may increase the levels/effects of cyclosporine. The levels/effects of chloroquine may be increased by azole antifungals, chlorpromazine, cimetidine, clarithromycin, delavirdine, diclofenac, doxycycline, erythromycin, fluoxetine, imatinib, isoniazid, miconazole, nefazodone, nicardipine, paroxetine, pergolide, propofol, protease inhibitors, quinidine, quinine, ritonavir, ropinirole, telithromycin, verapamil, and other CYP2D6 or 3A4 inhibitors.

Decreased Effect: Chloroquine levels may be decreased by antacids or kaolin. Chloroquine may decrease ampicillin and/or praziquantel levels. Chloroquine may decrease the levels/effects of CYP2D6 prodrug substrates; example prodrug substrates include codeine, hydrocodone, oxycodone, and tramadol. The levels/effects of chloroquine may be decreased by aminoglutethimide, carbamazepine, nafcillin, nevirapine, phenobarbital, phenytoin, rifamycins, and other CYP3A4 inducers.

Pharmacodynamics/Kinetics

Duration: Small amounts may be present in urine months following discontinuation of therapy

Absorption: Oral: Rapid (~89%)

Distribution: Widely in body tissues (eg, eyes, heart, kidneys, liver, lungs) where retention prolonged; crosses placenta; enters breast milk

Metabolism: Partially hepatic

Half-life elimination: 3-5 days

Time to peak, serum: 1-2 hours

Excretion: Urine (~70% as unchanged drug); acidification of urine increases elimination

Pregnancy Risk Factor C

Chloroquine Phosphate see Chloroquine on page 336

Chlorothiazide (klor oh THYE a zide)

Related Information

Cardiovascular Diseases on page 1726

U.S. Brand Names Diuril®

Canadian Brand Names Diuril®

Generic Available Yes: Tablet

Pharmacologic Category Diuretic, Thiazide

Use Management of mild-to-moderate hypertension; adjunctive treatment of edema

Local Anesthetic/Vasoconstrictor Precautions No information available to require special precautions

Effects on Dental Treatment Key adverse event(s) related to dental treatment: Orthostatic hypotension.

Common Adverse Effects Frequency not defined.

Cardiovascular: Hypotension, orthostatic hypotension, necrotizing angiitis

Central nervous system: Dizziness, headache, restlessness, vertigo

Dermatologic: Alopecia, erythema multiforme, exfoliative dermatitis, photosensitivity, Stevens-Johnson syndrome, toxic epidermal necrolysis

Endocrine & metabolic: Cholesterol increased, hypokalemia, hypomagnesemia, triglycerides increased

Gastrointestinal: Abdominal cramping, anorexia, constipation, diarrhea, gastric irritation, nausea, pancreatitis, sialadenitis, vomiting

Genitourinary: Impotence

Hematologic: Agranulocytosis, aplastic anemia, hemolytic anemia, leukopenia, thrombocytopenia

Hepatic: Jaundice

Neuromuscular & skeletal: Muscle spasm, paresthesia, weakness

Ocular: Blurred vision, xanthopsia

Renal: Azotemia, hematuria, interstitial nephritis, renal failure, renal dysfunction

Respiratory: Pneumonitis, pulmonary edema, respiratory distress

Miscellaneous: Anaphylactic reactions, systemic lupus erythematosus

Mechanism of Action Inhibits sodium reabsorption in the distal tubules causing increased excretion of sodium and water as well as potassium and hydrogen ions, magnesium, phosphate, calcium

Drug Interactions

Increased Effect/Toxicity: Increased effect of chlorothiazide with furosemide and other loop diuretics. Increased hypotension and/or renal adverse

(Continued)

Chlorothiazide (Continued)

effects of ACE inhibitors may result in aggressively diuresed patients. Beta-blockers increase hyperglycemic effects of thiazides in Type 2 diabetes mellitus. Cyclosporine and thiazides can increase the risk of gout or renal toxicity. Digoxin toxicity can be exacerbated if a thiazide induces hypokalemia or hypomagnesemia. Lithium toxicity can occur with thiazides due to reduced renal excretion of lithium. Thiazides may prolong the duration of action with neuromuscular-blocking agents. Corticosteroids may increase electrolyte-depletion effects of chlorothiazide.

Decreased Effect: Effects of oral hypoglycemics may be decreased. Decreased absorption of chlorothiazide with cholestyramine and colestipol. NSAIDs can decrease the efficacy of thiazides, reducing the diuretic and antihypertensive effects.

Pharmacodynamics/Kinetics
Onset of action: Diuresis: Oral: 2 hours; I.V.: 15 minutes
Duration of diuretic action: Oral: 6-12 hours; I.V.: ~2 hours
Absorption: Oral: Poor
Half-life elimination: 1-2 hours
Time to peak, serum: Oral: ~4 hours; I.V.: 30 minutes
Excretion: Urine (as unchanged drug)
Pregnancy Risk Factor C (manufacturer); D (expert analysis)

Chloroxine (klor OKS een)

U.S. Brand Names Capitrol® [DSC]
Canadian Brand Names Capitrol®
Generic Available No
Pharmacologic Category Topical Skin Product
Use Treatment of dandruff or seborrheic dermatitis of the scalp
Local Anesthetic/Vasoconstrictor Precautions No information available to require special precautions
Effects on Dental Treatment No significant effects or complications reported
Pregnancy Risk Factor C

Chlorphen [OTC] see Chlorpheniramine on page 338

Chlorpheniramine (klor fen IR a meen)

Related Information
Bacterial Infections on page 1793
Related Sample Prescriptions
Sinus Infection Treatment on page 1839
U.S. Brand Names Ahist™; Aller-Chlor® [OTC]; Chlorphen [OTC]; Chlor-Trimeton® [OTC]; Diabetic Tussin® Allergy Relief [OTC]; PediaTan™; QDALL® AR; Teldrin® HBP [OTC]
Canadian Brand Names Chlor-Tripolon®; Novo-Pheniram
Mexican Brand Names Cloro-Trimeton; Trimeton Repetabs
Generic Available Yes: Syrup, tablet
Index Terms Chlorpheniramine Maleate; CTM
Pharmacologic Category Antihistamine
Dental Use Treatment of histamine-induced allergic symptoms
Use Perennial and seasonal allergic rhinitis and other allergic symptoms including urticaria
Local Anesthetic/Vasoconstrictor Precautions No information available to require special precautions
Effects on Dental Treatment Key adverse event(s) related to dental treatment: Xerostomia (normal salivary flow resumes upon discontinuation). Chronic use of antihistamines will inhibit salivary flow, particularly in elderly patients; this may contribute to periodontal disease and oral discomfort.
Significant Adverse Effects
>10%:
Central nervous system: Slight to moderate drowsiness
Respiratory: Thickening of bronchial secretions
1% to 10%:
Central nervous system: Headache, excitability, fatigue, nervousness, dizziness
Gastrointestinal: Nausea, xerostomia, diarrhea, abdominal pain, appetite increase, weight gain
Genitourinary: Urinary retention
Neuromuscular & skeletal: Arthralgia, weakness
Ocular: Diplopia

Renal: Polyuria

Respiratory: Pharyngitis

Dosage

Children: Oral: 0.35 mg/kg/day in divided doses every 4-6 hours

2-6 years: 1 mg every 4-6 hours, not to exceed 6 mg in 24 hours

6-12 years: 2 mg every 4-6 hours, not to exceed 12 mg/day or sustained release 8 mg at bedtime

Children >12 years and Adults: Oral: 4 mg every 4-6 hours, not to exceed 24 mg/day or sustained release 8-12 mg every 8-12 hours, not to exceed 24 mg/day

Elderly: Oral: 4 mg once or twice daily. **Note:** Duration of action may be 36 hours or more when serum concentrations are low.

Hemodialysis: Supplemental dose is not necessary

Mechanism of Action Competes with histamine for H₁-receptor sites on effector cells in the gastrointestinal tract, blood vessels, and respiratory tract

Contraindications Hypersensitivity to chlorpheniramine maleate or any component of the formulation; narrow-angle glaucoma; bladder neck obstruction; symptomatic prostate hypertrophy; during acute asthmatic attacks; stenosing peptic ulcer; pyloroduodenal obstruction. Avoid use in premature and term newborns due to possible association with SIDS.

Warnings/Precautions Causes sedation, caution must be used in performing tasks which require alertness (eg, operating machinery or driving). Sedative effects of CNS depressants or ethanol are potentiated. Use with caution in patients with angle-closure glaucoma, pyloroduodenal obstruction (including stenotic peptic ulcer), urinary tract obstruction (including bladder neck obstruction and symptomatic prostatic hyperplasia), hyperthyroidism, increased intraocular pressure, and cardiovascular disease (including hypertension and tachycardia). High sedative and anticholinergic properties, therefore may not be considered the antihistamine of choice for prolonged use in the elderly. May cause paradoxical excitation in pediatric patients, and can result in hallucinations, coma, and death in overdose.

Drug Interactions Substrate of CYP2D6 (minor), 3A4 (major); **Inhibits** CYP2D6 (weak)

Increased toxicity (CNS depression): CNS depressants, MAO inhibitors, tricyclic antidepressants, phenothiazines

CYP3A4 inhibitors: May increase the levels/effects of chlorpheniramine. Example inhibitors include azole antifungals, clarithromycin, diclofenac, doxycycline, erythromycin, imatinib, isoniazid, nefazodone, nicardipine, propofol, protease inhibitors, quinidine, telithromycin, and verapamil.

Ethanol/Nutrition/Herb Interactions Ethanol: Avoid ethanol (may increase CNS depression).

Dietary Considerations May be taken with food or water.

Pharmacodynamics/Kinetics Half-life elimination, serum: 20-24 hours

Pregnancy Risk Factor B

Dosage Forms Excipient information presented when available (limited, particularly for generics); consult specific product labeling.

Capsule, variable release, as maleate:

QDALL® AR: Chlorpheniramine 12 mg [immediate release and sustained release]

Suspension, as tannate:

PediaTan™: 8 mg/5 mL (480 mL) [sugar free; contains sodium benzoate; bubble gum flavor]

Syrup, as maleate:

Aller-Chlor®: 2 mg/5 mL (120 mL) [contains alcohol 5%]

Diabetic Tussin® Allergy Relief: 2 mg/5 mL (120 mL) [alcohol free, dye free, sugar free]

Tablet, as maleate: 4 mg

Aller-Chlor®, Chlor-Trimeton®, Chlorphen, Teldrin® HBP: 4 mg

Tablet, extended release, as maleate:

Chlor-Trimeton®: 12 mg

Tablet, long acting, as tannate [scored]:

Ahist™: 12 mg

Chlorpheniramine, Acetaminophen, and Pseudoephedrine *see* Acetaminophen, Chlorpheniramine, and Pseudoephedrine *on page 43*

Chlorpheniramine and Acetaminophen

(klor fen IR a meen & a seet a MIN oh fen)

Related Information

Acetaminophen *on page 31*

Chlorpheniramine *on page 338*

(Continued)

Chlorpheniramine and Acetaminophen *(Continued)*

U.S. Brand Names Coricidin HBP® Cold and Flu [OTC]
Generic Available No
Index Terms Acetaminophen and Chlorpheniramine
Pharmacologic Category Antihistamine/Analgesic
Use Symptomatic relief of congestion, headache, aches and pains of colds and flu
Local Anesthetic/Vasoconstrictor Precautions No information available to require special precautions
Effects on Dental Treatment Key adverse event(s) related to dental treatment: Chronic use of antihistamines will inhibit salivary flow, particularly in elderly patients; this may contribute to periodontal disease and oral discomfort.
Common Adverse Effects See individual agents.
Drug Interactions
Cytochrome P450 Effect:
Acetaminophen: **Substrate** (minor) of CYP1A2, 2A6, 2C9, 2D6, 2E1, 3A4; **Inhibits** CYP3A4 (weak)
Chlorpheniramine: **Substrate** of CYP2D6 (minor), 3A4 (major); **Inhibits** CYP2D6 (weak)
Pharmacodynamics/Kinetics See individual agents.

Chlorpheniramine and Carbetapentane *see* Carbetapentane and Chlorpheniramine *on page 278*

Chlorpheniramine and Phenylephrine
(klor fen IR a meen & fen il EF rin)

Related Information
Chlorpheniramine *on page 338*
Phenylephrine *on page 1293*
U.S. Brand Names Acitfed® Cold and Allergy [OTC] *[reformulation]*; AllanTan Pediatric; AlleRx™ Suspension; Ceron; C-Phen; Dallergy-JR®; Dec-Chlorphen; Ed A-Hist®; NoHist; PD-Hist-D; PediaTan™D; Phenabid®; Relera; Rescon-Jr; Rondec®; R-Tanna; Rynatan®; Rynatan® Pediatric Suspension; Sildec PE
Generic Available Yes
Index Terms Chlorpheniramine Maleate and Phenylephrine Hydrochloride; Chlorpheniramine Tannate and Phenylephrine Tannate; Phenylephrine and Chlorpheniramine
Pharmacologic Category Antihistamine/Decongestant Combination
Use Temporary relief of upper respiratory conditions such as nasal congestion, runny nose, and sneezing due to the common cold, hay fever, or allergic or vasomotor rhinitis
Local Anesthetic/Vasoconstrictor Precautions Use with caution since phenylephrine is a sympathomimetic amine which could interact with epinephrine to cause a pressor response
Effects on Dental Treatment Key adverse event(s) related to dental treatment:

Chlorpheniramine: Prolonged use will cause significant xerostomia (normal salivary flow resumes upon discontinuation).
Phenylephrine: Up to 10% of patients could experience tachycardia, palpitations, and xerostomia (prolonged use worsens); use vasoconstrictor with caution.
Common Adverse Effects See individual agents.
Drug Interactions
Cytochrome P450 Effect: Chlorpheniramine: **Substrate** of CYP2D6 (minor), 3A4 (major); **Inhibits** CYP2D6 (weak)
Increased Effect/Toxicity: See individual agents.
Decreased Effect: See individual agents.
Pharmacodynamics/Kinetics See individual agents.
Pregnancy Risk Factor C

Chlorpheniramine and Pseudoephedrine
(klor fen IR a meen & soo doe e FED rin)

Related Information
Chlorpheniramine *on page 338*
Pseudoephedrine *on page 1381*
U.S. Brand Names Allerest® Maximum Strength Allergy and Hay Fever [OTC]; A.R.M® [OTC]; Chlor-Trimeton® Allergy D [OTC] [DSC]; Deconamine®; Deconamine® SR; Dicel™; Dynahist-ER Pediatric®; Histade™; Histex™; Kronofed-A®; Kronofed-A®-Jr; LoHist-D; PediaCare® Cold and Allergy [OTC] [DSC]; QDALL®;

Sudafed® Sinus & Allergy [OTC]; Sudal® 12; Triaminic® Cold and Allergy [OTC]
[DSC]

Canadian Brand Names Triaminic® Cold & Allergy

Generic Available Yes: Tablet, extended release capsule, suspension

Index Terms Chlorpheniramine Maleate and Pseudoephedrine Hydrochloride;
Chlorpheniramine Tannate and Pseudoephedrine Tannate; Pseudoephedrine
and Chlorpheniramine

Pharmacologic Category Alpha/Beta Agonist; Antihistamine

Use Relief of nasal congestion associated with the common cold, hay fever, and
other allergies, sinusitis, eustachian tube blockage, and vasomotor and allergic
rhinitis

Local Anesthetic/Vasoconstrictor Precautions Use with caution since
pseudoephedrine is a sympathomimetic amine which could interact with
epinephrine to cause a pressor response

Effects on Dental Treatment Key adverse event(s) related to dental treatment:

Chlorpheniramine: Prolonged use will cause significant xerostomia (normal salivary flow resumes upon discontinuation).

Pseudoephedrine: Xerostomia (prolonged use worsens; normal salivary flow
resumes upon discontinuation).

Common Adverse Effects See individual agents.

Mechanism of Action

Chlorpheniramine competes with histamine for H_1-receptor sites on effector
cells in the gastrointestinal tract, blood vessels, and respiratory tract.

Pseudoephedrine is a sympathomimetic amine and isomer of ephedrine; acts
as a decongestant in respiratory tract mucous membranes with less vasoconstrictor action than ephedrine in normotensive individuals.

Drug Interactions

Cytochrome P450 Effect: Chlorpheniramine: **Substrate** of CYP2D6 (minor),
3A4 (major); **Inhibits** CYP2D6 (weak)

Increased Effect/Toxicity: See individual agents.

Decreased Effect: See individual agents.

Pharmacodynamics/Kinetics See individual agents.

Pregnancy Risk Factor C

Chlorpheniramine, Ephedrine, Phenylephrine, and Carbetapentane

(klor fen IR a meen, e FED rin, fen il EF rin, & kar bay ta PEN tane)

Related Information

Chlorpheniramine *on page 338*
Ephedrine *on page 571*
Phenylephrine *on page 1293*

U.S. Brand Names Rynatuss®; Rynatuss® Pediatric [DSC]; Tetra Tannate Pediatric

Generic Available Yes: Suspension

Index Terms Carbetapentane, Ephedrine, Phenylephrine, and Chlorpheniramine; Ephedrine, Chlorpheniramine, Phenylephrine, and Carbetapentane;
Phenylephrine, Ephedrine, Chlorpheniramine, and Carbetapentane

Pharmacologic Category Antihistamine/Decongestant/Antitussive

Use Symptomatic relief of cough with a decongestant and an antihistamine

Local Anesthetic/Vasoconstrictor Precautions

Ephedrine: Use vasoconstrictor with caution since ephedrine may enhance
cardiostimulation and vasopressor effects of sympathomimetics

Phenylephrine: Use with caution since phenylephrine is a sympathomimetic
amine which could interact with epinephrine to cause a pressor response

Effects on Dental Treatment Key adverse event(s) related to dental treatment:

Chlorpheniramine: Prolonged use will cause significant xerostomia (normal salivary flow resumes upon discontinuation).

Ephedrine: No significant effects or complications reported.

Phenylephrine: Up to 10% of patients could experience tachycardia, palpitations, and xerostomia; use vasoconstrictor with caution.

Drug Interactions

Cytochrome P450 Effect: Chlorpheniramine: **Substrate** of CYP2D6 (minor),
3A4 (major); **Inhibits** CYP2D6 (weak)

Increased Effect/Toxicity: See individual agents.

Decreased Effect: See individual agents.

Pregnancy Risk Factor C

Chlorpheniramine, Phenylephrine, and Dextromethorphan

(klor fen IR a meen, fen il EF rin, & deks troe meth OR fan)

Related Information
Chlorpheniramine *on page 338*
Dextromethorphan *on page 477*
Phenylephrine *on page 1293*

U.S. Brand Names Ceron-DM; Coldtuss DR [DSC]; Corfen DM; C-Phen DM; Dec-Chlorphen DM; De-Chlor DM; De-Chlor DR; Dex PC; Neo DM; PD-Cof; Phenabid DM®; Rondec®-DM; Sildec PE-DM; Statuss™ DM; Tri-Vent™ DPC

Generic Available Yes: Excludes timed release tablet

Index Terms Dextromethorphan, Chlorpheniramine, and Phenylephrine; Phenylephrine, Chlorpheniramine, and Dextromethorphan

Pharmacologic Category Antihistamine/Decongestant/Antitussive

Use Temporary relief of cough and upper respiratory symptoms associated with allergies or the common cold

Local Anesthetic/Vasoconstrictor Precautions

Chlorpheniramine, Dextromethorphan: No information available to require special precautions

Phenylephrine: Use with caution since phenylephrine is a sympathomimetic amine which could interact with epinephrine to cause a pressor response

Effects on Dental Treatment Key adverse event(s) related to dental treatment:

Chlorpheniramine: Prolonged use will cause significant xerostomia (normal salivary flow resumes upon discontinuation).

Dextromethorphan: No significant effects or complications reported

Phenylephrine: Up to 10% of patients could experience tachycardia, palpitations, and xerostomia (prolonged use worsens); use vasoconstrictor with caution.

Common Adverse Effects See individual agents.

Drug Interactions

Cytochrome P450 Effect:

Chlorpheniramine: **Substrate** of CYP2D6 (minor), 3A4 (major); **Inhibits** CYP2D6 (weak)

Dextromethorphan: **Substrate** of CYP2B6 (minor), 2C9 (minor), 2C19 (minor), 2D6 (major), 2E1 (minor), 3A4 (minor); **Inhibits** CYP2D6 (weak)

Increased Effect/Toxicity: See individual agents.

Decreased Effect: See individual agents.

Pharmacodynamics/Kinetics See individual agents.

Pregnancy Risk Factor C

Chlorpheniramine, Phenylephrine, and Methscopolamine

(klor fen IR a meen, fen il EF rin, & meth skoe POL a meen)

Related Information
Chlorpheniramine *on page 338*
Methscopolamine *on page 1075*
Phenylephrine *on page 1293*

U.S. Brand Names aeroKid™; Ah-Chew®; Ah-Chew® II; Chlor-Mes-D; Dallergy®; Dehistine; Duradryl®; Durahist™ PE; Extendryl; Extendryl JR; Extendryl SR; Hista-Vent® DA; OMNIhist® II L.A.; PCM; PCM Allergy; Phenylephrine CM; Ralix; Rescon®; Rescon® MX

Generic Available Yes: Excludes capsule, suspension

Index Terms Methscopolamine Nitrate, Chlorpheniramine Maleate, and Phenylephrine Hydrochloride; Phenylephrine Tannate, Chlorpheniramine Tannate, and Methscopolamine Nitrate

Pharmacologic Category Antihistamine/Decongestant/Anticholinergic

Use Treatment of upper respiratory symptoms such as respiratory congestion, allergic rhinitis, vasomotor rhinitis, sinusitis, and allergic skin reactions of urticaria and angioedema

Local Anesthetic/Vasoconstrictor Precautions Use with caution since phenylephrine is a sympathomimetic amine which could interact with epinephrine to cause a pressor response

Effects on Dental Treatment Key adverse event(s) related to dental treatment:

Chlorpheniramine: Significant xerostomia with prolonged use (normal salivary flow resumes upon discontinuation).

Methscopolamine: Anticholinergic side effects can cause a reduction of saliva production or secretion contributes to discomfort and dental disease (ie, caries, oral candidiasis and periodontal disease).

Phenylephrine: Tachycardia, palpitations, and xerostomia; use vasoconstrictor with caution.

Common Adverse Effects Frequency not defined.

Cardiovascular: Arrhythmias, bradycardia, cardiovascular collapse, flushing, hypotension, pallor, palpitation, tachycardia

Central nervous system: Anxiety, convulsions, CNS depression, dizziness, drowsiness, excitability, fear, giddiness, hallucinations, headache, insomnia, irritability, lassitude, restlessness, tenseness, tremor

Gastrointestinal: Constipation, dysphagia, gastric irritation, nausea, xerostomia

Genitourinary: Dysuria, urinary retention

Neuromuscular & skeletal: Weakness

Ocular: Blurred vision, mydriasis

Respiratory: Dry nose, dry throat, respiratory difficulty

Mechanism of Action

Chlorpheniramine maleate: Antihistamine

Phenylephrine hydrochloride: Sympathomimetic agent (primarily alpha), decongestant

Methscopolamine nitrate: Derivative of scopolamine, antisecretory effects

Drug Interactions

Cytochrome P450 Effect: Chlorpheniramine: **Substrate** of CYP2D6 (minor), 3A4 (major); **Inhibits** CYP2D6 (weak)

Increased Effect/Toxicity: See individual agents.

Pharmacodynamics/Kinetics See individual agents.

Pregnancy Risk Factor C

Chlorpheniramine, Phenylephrine, and Phenyltoloxamine

(klor fen IR a meen, fen il EF rin, & fen il tole LOKS a meen)

Related Information

Chlorpheniramine on page 338

Phenylephrine on page 1293

U.S. Brand Names Comhist®; Nalex®-A

Generic Available Yes: Liquid, prolonged release tablet

Index Terms Phenylephrine, Chlorpheniramine, and Phenyltoloxamine; Phenyltoloxamine, Chlorpheniramine, and Phenylephrine

Pharmacologic Category Antihistamine/Decongestant Combination

Use Symptomatic relief of rhinitis and nasal congestion due to colds or allergy

Local Anesthetic/Vasoconstrictor Precautions Use with caution since phenylephrine is a sympathomimetic amine which could interact with epinephrine to cause a pressor response

Effects on Dental Treatment Key adverse event(s) related to dental treatment:

Chlorpheniramine: Prolonged use will cause significant xerostomia (normal salivary flow resumes upon discontinuation).

Phenylephrine: Up to 10% of patients could experience tachycardia, palpitations, and xerostomia; use vasoconstrictor with caution.

Common Adverse Effects Frequency not defined.

Cardiovascular: Hypotension, palpitation

Central nervous system: Headache, dizziness, sedation, excitation (children), nervousness, seizure

Dermatologic: Urticaria, drug rash

Gastrointestinal: Dry mouth, anorexia, nausea, vomiting, diarrhea, constipation, GI upset

Genitourinary: Urinary frequency, urinary retention

(Continued)

Chlorpheniramine, Phenylephrine, and Phenyltoloxamine *(Continued)*

Hematologic: Agranulocytosis, leukopenia, thrombocytopenia

Ocular: Blurred vision

Respiratory: Dry nose/throat, thickening of bronchial secretions, wheezing, stuffy nose, tightness of chest

Drug Interactions

Cytochrome P450 Effect: Chlorpheniramine: **Substrate** of CYP2D6 (minor), 3A4 (major); **Inhibits** CYP2D6 (weak)

Increased Effect/Toxicity: See individual agents.

Decreased Effect: See individual agents.

Pregnancy Risk Factor C

Chlorpheniramine, Phenylephrine, Codeine, and Potassium Iodide

(klor fen IR a meen, fen il EF rin, KOE deen, & poe TASS ee um EYE oh dide)

Related Information

Chlorpheniramine *on page 338*

Codeine *on page 404*

Phenylephrine *on page 1293*

Potassium Iodide *on page 1330*

U.S. Brand Names Pediacof® [DSC]

Generic Available No

Index Terms Codeine, Chlorpheniramine, Phenylephrine, and Potassium Iodide; Phenylephrine, Chlorpheniramine, Codeine, and Potassium Iodide; Potassium Iodide, Chlorpheniramine, Phenylephrine, and Codeine

Pharmacologic Category Antihistamine/Decongestant/Antitussive/Expectorant

Use Symptomatic relief of rhinitis, nasal congestion and cough due to colds or allergy

Local Anesthetic/Vasoconstrictor Precautions Use with caution since phenylephrine is a sympathomimetic amine which could interact with epinephrine to cause a pressor response

Effects on Dental Treatment Key adverse event(s) related to dental treatment:

Chlorpheniramine: Prolonged use will cause significant xerostomia (normal salivary flow resumes upon discontinuation).

Phenylephrine: Up to 10% of patients could experience tachycardia, palpitations, and xerostomia (prolonged use worsens); use vasoconstrictor with caution.

Restrictions C-V

Drug Interactions

Cytochrome P450 Effect: Chlorpheniramine: **Substrate** of CYP2D6 (minor), 3A4 (major); **Inhibits** CYP2D6 (weak)

Increased Effect/Toxicity: See individual agents.

Decreased Effect: See individual agents.

Chlorpheniramine, Pseudoephedrine, and Acetaminophen *see* Acetaminophen, Chlorpheniramine, and Pseudoephedrine *on page 43*

Chlorpheniramine, Pseudoephedrine, and Codeine

(klor fen IR a meen, soo doe e FED rin, & KOE deen)

Related Information

Chlorpheniramine *on page 338*

Codeine *on page 404*

Pseudoephedrine *on page 1381*

U.S. Brand Names Dihistine® DH [DSC]

Generic Available No

Index Terms Codeine, Chlorpheniramine, and Pseudoephedrine; Pseudoephedrine, Chlorpheniramine, and Codeine

Pharmacologic Category Antihistamine/Decongestant/Antitussive

Use Temporary relief of cough associated with minor throat or bronchial irritation or nasal congestion due to common cold, allergic rhinitis, or sinusitis

Local Anesthetic/Vasoconstrictor Precautions Use with caution since pseudoephedrine is a sympathomimetic amine which could interact with epinephrine to cause a pressor response

Effects on Dental Treatment Key adverse event(s) related to dental treatment:

Chlorpheniramine: Significant xerostomia with prolonged use (normal salivary flow resumes upon discontinuation).

Pseudoephedrine: Xerostomia (normal salivary flow resumes upon discontinuation).

Common Adverse Effects See individual agents.

Restrictions C-V

Drug Interactions

Cytochrome P450 Effect: Chlorpheniramine: **Substrate** of CYP2D6 (minor), 3A4 (major); **Inhibits** CYP2D6 (weak)

Increased Effect/Toxicity: See individual agents.

Decreased Effect: See individual agents.

Pharmacodynamics/Kinetics See individual agents.

Pregnancy Risk Factor C

Chlorpheniramine, Pseudoephedrine, and Dihydrocodeine *see* Pseudoephedrine, Dihydrocodeine, and Chlorpheniramine *on page 1385*

Chlorpheniramine Tannate and Phenylephrine Tannate *see* Chlorpheniramine and Phenylephrine *on page 340*

Chlorpheniramine Tannate and Pseudoephedrine Tannate *see* Chlorpheniramine and Pseudoephedrine *on page 340*

ChlorproMAZINE (klor PROE ma zeen)

Canadian Brand Names Largactil®; Novo-Chlorpromazine

Mexican Brand Names Largactil

Generic Available Yes

Index Terms Chlorpromazine Hydrochloride; CPZ

Pharmacologic Category Antipsychotic Agent, Typical, Phenothiazine

Use Control of mania; treatment of schizophrenia; control of nausea and vomiting; relief of restlessness and apprehension before surgery; acute intermittent porphyria; adjunct in the treatment of tetanus; intractable hiccups; combativeness and/or explosive hyperexcitable behavior in children 1-12 years of age and in short-term treatment of hyperactive children

Unlabeled/Investigational Use Management of psychotic disorders; behavioral symptoms associated with dementia (elderly)

Local Anesthetic/Vasoconstrictor Precautions Most pharmacology textbooks state that in presence of phenothiazines, systemic doses of epinephrine paradoxically decrease the blood pressure. This is the so called "epinephrine reversal" phenomenon. This has never been observed when epinephrine is given by infiltration as part of the anesthesia procedure. Chlorpromazine is one of the drugs confirmed to prolong the QT interval and is accepted as having a risk of causing torsade de pointes. The risk of drug-induced torsade de pointes is extremely low when a single QT interval prolonging drug is prescribed. In terms of epinephrine, it is not known what effect vasoconstrictors in the local anesthetic regimen will have in patients with a known history of congenital prolonged QT interval or in patients taking any medication that prolongs the QT interval. Until more information is obtained, it is suggested that the clinician consult with the physician prior to the use of a vasoconstrictor in suspected patients, and that the vasoconstrictor (epinephrine, levonordefrin [Neo-Cobefrin®]) be used with caution.

Effects on Dental Treatment Key adverse event(s) related to dental treatment:

Xerostomia (normal salivary flow resumes upon discontinuation).

Significant hypotension may occur, especially when the drug is administered parenterally. Orthostatic hypotension is due to alpha-receptor blockade; elderly are at greater risk.

Tardive dyskinesia: Prevalence rate may be 40% in elderly; development of the syndrome and the irreversible nature are proportional to duration and total cumulative dose over time. Extrapyramidal reactions are more common in elderly with up to 50% developing these reactions after 60 years of age. Drug-induced Parkinson's syndrome occurs often; akathisia is the most common extrapyramidal reaction in elderly.

Increased confusion, memory loss, psychotic behavior, and agitation frequently occur as a consequence of anticholinergic effects. Antipsychotic-associated sedation in nonpsychotic patients is extremely unpleasant due to feelings of depersonalization, derealization, and dysphoria.

Common Adverse Effects Frequency not defined.

Cardiovascular: Postural hypotension, tachycardia, dizziness, nonspecific QT changes

(Continued)

ChlorproMAZINE *(Continued)*

Central nervous system: Drowsiness, dystonias, akathisia, pseudoparkinsonism, tardive dyskinesia, neuroleptic malignant syndrome, seizure

Dermatologic: Photosensitivity, dermatitis, skin pigmentation (slate gray)

Endocrine & metabolic: Lactation, breast engorgement, false-positive pregnancy test, amenorrhea, gynecomastia, hyper- or hypoglycemia

Gastrointestinal: Xerostomia, constipation, nausea

Genitourinary: Urinary retention, ejaculatory disorder, impotence

Hematologic: Agranulocytosis, eosinophilia, leukopenia, hemolytic anemia, aplastic anemia, thrombocytopenic purpura

Hepatic: Jaundice

Ocular: Blurred vision, corneal and lenticular changes, epithelial keratopathy, pigmentary retinopathy

Mechanism of Action Chlorpromazine is an aliphatic phenothiazine antipsychotic which blocks postsynaptic mesolimbic dopaminergic receptors in the brain; exhibits a strong alpha-adrenergic blocking effect and depresses the release of hypothalamic and hypophyseal hormones; believed to depress the reticular activating system, thus affecting basal metabolism, body temperature, wakefulness, vasomotor tone, and emesis

Drug Interactions

Cytochrome P450 Effect: Substrate of CYP1A2 (minor), 2D6 (major), 3A4 (minor); **Inhibits** CYP2D6 (strong), 2E1 (weak)

Increased Effect/Toxicity: The levels/effects of chlorpromazine may be increased by delavirdine, fluoxetine, miconazole, paroxetine, pergolide, quinidine, quinine, ritonavir, ropinirole, and other CYP2D6 inhibitors. Effects on CNS depression may be additive when chlorpromazine is combined with CNS depressants (opioid analgesics, ethanol, barbiturates, cyclic antidepressants, antihistamines, or sedative-hypnotics). Chlorpromazine may increase the levels/effects of amphetamines, selected beta-blockers, dextromethorphan, fluoxetine, lidocaine, mirtazapine, nefazodone, paroxetine, risperidone, ritonavir, thioridazine, tricyclic antidepressants, and venlafaxine and other CYP2D6 substrates. Chlorpromazine may increase the effects/toxicity of anticholinergics, antihypertensives, lithium (rare neurotoxicity), trazodone, or valproic acid. Concurrent use with TCA may produce increased toxicity or altered therapeutic response. Chloroquine and propranolol may increase chlorpromazine concentrations. Hypotension may occur when chlorpromazine is combined with epinephrine. May increase the risk of arrhythmia when combined with antiarrhythmics, cisapride, pimozide, sparfloxacin, or other drugs which prolong QT interval. Metoclopramide may increase risk of extrapyramidal symptoms (EPS). Acetylcholinesterase inhibitors (central) may increase the risk of antipsychotic-related EPS.

Decreased Effect: Chlorpromazine may decrease the levels/effects of CYP2D6 prodrug substrates; example prodrug substrates include codeine, hydrocodone, oxycodone, and tramadol. Phenothiazines inhibit the ability of bromocriptine to lower serum prolactin concentrations. Benztropine (and other anticholinergics) may inhibit the therapeutic response to chlorpromazine and excess anticholinergic effects may occur. Antihypertensive effects of guanethidine and guanadrel may be inhibited by chlorpromazine. Chlorpromazine may inhibit the antiparkinsonian effect of levodopa. Chlorpromazine and possibly other low potency antipsychotics may reverse the pressor effects of epinephrine.

Pharmacodynamics/Kinetics

Onset of action: I.M.: 15 minutes; Oral: 30-60 minutes

Absorption: Rapid

Distribution: V_d: 20 L/kg; crosses the placenta; enters breast milk

Protein binding: 92% to 97%

Metabolism: Extensively hepatic to active and inactive metabolites

Bioavailability: 20%

Half-life, biphasic: Initial: 2 hours; Terminal: 30 hours

Excretion: Urine (<1% as unchanged drug) within 24 hours

Pregnancy Risk Factor C

Chlorpromazine Hydrochloride *see* ChlorproMAZINE *on page 345*

ChlorproPAMIDE *(klor PROE pa mide)*

Related Information

Endocrine Disorders and Pregnancy *on page 1750*

U.S. Brand Names Diabinese®

Canadian Brand Names Apo-Chlorpropamide®; Novo-Propamide

Mexican Brand Names Diabenese; Insogen

Generic Available Yes

Pharmacologic Category Antidiabetic Agent, Sulfonylurea

Use Management of blood sugar in type 2 diabetes mellitus (noninsulin dependent, NIDDM)

Unlabeled/Investigational Use Neurogenic diabetes insipidus

Effects on Dental Treatment Chlorpropamide-dependent diabetics (noninsulin dependent, Type 2) should be appointed for dental treatment in morning in order to minimize chance of stress-induced hypoglycemia.

Common Adverse Effects Frequency not defined.

Central nervous system: Dizziness, headache

Dermatologic: Erythema multiforme, exfoliative dermatitis, maculopapular eruptions, photosensitivity, pruritus, urticaria

Endocrine & metabolic: Disulfiram-like reactions, hypoglycemia, SIADH

Gastrointestinal: Anorexia, diarrhea, hunger, nausea, proctocolitis, vomiting

Hematologic: Agranulocytosis, aplastic anemia, eosinophilia, hemolytic anemia, leukopenia, pancytopenia, porphyria cutanea tarda, thrombocytopenia

Hepatic: Cholestatic jaundice, hepatic porphyria

Mechanism of Action Stimulates insulin release from the pancreatic beta cells; reduces glucose output from the liver; insulin sensitivity is increased at peripheral target sites

Drug Interactions

Cytochrome P450 Effect: Substrate of CYP2C9 (minor)

Increased Effect/Toxicity: Allopurinol and fluconazole may increase the serum concentration of chlorpropamide. Cyclic antidepressants, fibric acid derivatives, pegvisomant, salicylates (high doses, not sporadic, low doses), and sulfonamide derivatives (except sulfacetamide) may enhance the hypoglycemic effect of chlorpropamide. Beta-blockers may enhance the hypoglycemic effect of chlorpropamide and mask tachycardia as an initial symptom of hypoglycemia. Chloramphenicol and cimetidine may decrease the metabolism of chlorpropamide. Chlorpropamide may increase the serum concentration of cyclosporine.

Decreased Effect: Rifampin may increase the metabolism, via CYP isoenzymes, of chlorpropamide.

Pharmacodynamics/Kinetics

Onset of action: 1 hour

Peak effect: 3-6 hours

Duration of action: 24 hours

Absorption: Rapid

Distribution: V_d: 0.13-0.23 L/kg

Protein binding: 90%

Metabolism: Extensively hepatic (~80%), primarily via CYP2C9; forms metabolites

Half-life elimination: ~36 hours; prolonged in elderly or with renal impairment

End-stage renal disease: 50-200 hours

Time to peak, serum: 2-4 hours

Excretion: Urine

Pregnancy Risk Factor C

Chlorthalidone (klor THAL i done)

Related Information

Cardiovascular Diseases *on page 1726*

U.S. Brand Names Thalitone®

Canadian Brand Names Apo-Chlorthalidone®

Mexican Brand Names Higroton

Generic Available Yes

Index Terms Hygroton

Pharmacologic Category Diuretic, Thiazide

Use Management of mild-to-moderate hypertension when used alone or in combination with other agents; treatment of edema associated with congestive heart failure or nephrotic syndrome. Recent studies have found chlorthalidone effective in the treatment of isolated systolic hypertension in the elderly.

Unlabeled/Investigational Use Pediatric hypertension

Effects on Dental Treatment No significant effects or complications reported

Common Adverse Effects 1% to 10%:

Dermatologic: Photosensitivity

Endocrine & metabolic: Hypokalemia

Gastrointestinal: Anorexia, epigastric distress

(Continued)

Chlorthalidone (Continued)

Mechanism of Action Sulfonamide-derived diuretic that inhibits sodium and chloride reabsorption in the cortical-diluting segment of the ascending loop of Henle

Drug Interactions

Increased Effect/Toxicity: Increased effect of chlorthalidone with furosemide and other loop diuretics. Increased hypotension and/or renal adverse effects of ACE inhibitors may result in aggressively diuresed patients. Beta-blockers increase hyperglycemic effects of thiazides in Type 2 diabetes mellitus. Cyclosporine and thiazides can increase the risk of gout or renal toxicity. Digoxin toxicity can be exacerbated if a thiazide induces hypokalemia or hypomagnesemia. Lithium toxicity can occur with thiazides due to reduced renal excretion of lithium. Thiazides may prolong the duration of action with neuromuscular blocking agents.

Decreased Effect: Effects of oral hypoglycemics may be decreased. Decreased absorption of chlorthalidone with cholestyramine and colestipol. NSAIDs can decrease the efficacy of chlorthalidone, reducing the diuretic and antihypertensive effects.

Pharmacodynamics/Kinetics

Onset of action: Peak effect: 2-6 hours

Duration: 24-72 hours

Absorption: 65%

Distribution: Crosses placenta; enters breast milk

Metabolism: Hepatic

Half-life elimination: 35-55 hours; may be prolonged with renal impairment; Anuria: 81 hours

Excretion: Urine (~50% to 65% as unchanged drug)

Pregnancy Risk Factor B (manufacturer); D (expert analysis)

Chlorthalidone and Atenolol *see* Atenolol and Chlorthalidone *on page 160*

Chlorthalidone and Clonidine *see* Clonidine and Chlorthalidone *on page 394*

Chlor-Trimeton® [OTC] *see* Chlorpheniramine *on page 338*

Chlor-Trimeton® Allergy D [OTC] [DSC] *see* Chlorpheniramine and Pseudoephedrine *on page 340*

Chlorzoxazone (klor ZOKS a zone)

Related Information

Temporomandibular Dysfunction (TMD) *on page 1822*

U.S. Brand Names Parafon Forte® DSC

Canadian Brand Names Parafon Forte®; Strifon Forte®

Generic Available Yes

Pharmacologic Category Skeletal Muscle Relaxant

Dental Use Treatment of muscle spasm and pain associated with acute temporomandibular joint pain (TMJ)

Use Symptomatic treatment of muscle spasm and pain associated with acute musculoskeletal conditions

Local Anesthetic/Vasoconstrictor Precautions No information available to require special precautions

Effects on Dental Treatment No significant effects or complications reported

Significant Adverse Effects Frequency not defined.

Central nervous system: Dizziness, drowsiness, lightheadedness, paradoxical stimulation, malaise

Dermatologic: Rash, petechiae, ecchymoses (rare), angioneurotic edema

Gastrointestinal: Nausea, vomiting, stomach cramps

Genitourinary: Urine discoloration

Hepatic: Liver dysfunction

Miscellaneous: Anaphylaxis (very rare)

Dental Usual Dosing Treatment of muscle spasm and pain associated with acute TMJ pain: Oral:

Children: 20 mg/kg/day or 600 mg/m^2/day in 3-4 divided doses

Adults: 250-500 mg 3-4 times/day up to 750 mg 3-4 times/day

Dosage Oral:

Children: 20 mg/kg/day or 600 mg/m^2/day in 3-4 divided doses

Adults: 250-500 mg 3-4 times/day up to 750 mg 3-4 times/day

Mechanism of Action Acts on the spinal cord and subcortical levels by depressing polysynaptic reflexes

Contraindications Hypersensitivity to chlorzoxazone or any component of the formulation; impaired liver function

Drug Interactions Substrate of CYP1A2 (minor), 2A6 (minor), 2D6 (minor), 2E1 (major), 3A4 (minor); **Inhibits** CYP2E1 (weak), 3A4 (weak)

CNS depressants: Effects may be increased by chlorzoxazone.

CYP2E1 inhibitors: May increase the levels/effects of chlorzoxazone. Example inhibitors include disulfiram, isoniazid, and miconazole.

Disulfiram: May increase chlorzoxazone concentration; monitor.

Isoniazid: May increase chlorzoxazone concentration; monitor.

Ethanol/Nutrition/Herb Interactions Ethanol: Avoid ethanol (may increase CNS depression).

Pharmacodynamics/Kinetics
Onset of action: ~1 hour
Duration: 6-12 hours
Absorption: Readily absorbed
Metabolism: Extensively hepatic via glucuronidation
Excretion: Urine (as conjugates)

Pregnancy Risk Factor C

Lactation Excretion in breast milk unknown/not recommended

Dosage Forms Excipient information presented when available (limited, particularly for generics); consult specific product labeling.
Caplet (Parafon Forte® DSC): 500 mg
Tablet: 250 mg, 500 mg

Cholecalciferol (kole e kal SI fer ole)

U.S. Brand Names Delta-D®
Canadian Brand Names D-Vi-Sol®
Generic Available Yes
Index Terms D_3
Pharmacologic Category Vitamin D Analog
Use Dietary supplement, treatment of vitamin D deficiency, or prophylaxis of deficiency
Local Anesthetic/Vasoconstrictor Precautions No information available to require special precautions
Effects on Dental Treatment Key adverse event(s) related to dental treatment: Metallic taste and xerostomia (normal salivary flow resumes upon discontinuation).
Common Adverse Effects Frequency not defined.
Cardiovascular: Arrhythmia, hyper-/hypotension, cardiac arrhythmia
Central nervous system: Irritability, headache, somnolence, overt psychosis (rare)
Dermatologic: Pruritus
Endocrine & metabolic: Polydipsia
Gastrointestinal: Nausea, vomiting, anorexia, pancreatitis, metallic taste, dry mouth, constipation, weight loss
Genitourinary: Albuminuria, polyuria
Hepatic: Increased liver function test
Neuromuscular & skeletal: Bone pain, myalgia, weakness, muscle pain
Ocular: Conjunctivitis, photophobia
Renal: Azotemia, nephrocalcinosis
Drug Interactions
Cytochrome P450 Effect: Inhibits CYP2C9 (weak), 2C19 (weak), 2D6 (weak)
Pharmacodynamics/Kinetics
Distribution: Primarily hepatic
Protein binding: Extensively to vitamin D-binding protein
Metabolism: Primary liver and kidney hydroxylation; glucuronidation (minimal)
Half-life elimination: 14 hours
Time to peak, plasma: 11 hours
Excretion: As metabolites, urine (2.4%) and feces (4.9%)
Pregnancy Risk Factor C

Cholecalciferol and Alendronate see Alendronate and Cholecalciferol on page 67

Cholestyramine Resin (koe LES teer a meen REZ in)

Related Information
Cardiovascular Diseases on page 1726
U.S. Brand Names Prevalite®; Questran®; Questran® Light
Canadian Brand Names Novo-Cholamine; Novo-Cholamine Light; PMS-Cholestyramine; Questran®; Questran® Light Sugar Free
Mexican Brand Names Questran
Generic Available Yes
(Continued)

Cholestyramine Resin *(Continued)*

Pharmacologic Category Antilipemic Agent, Bile Acid Sequestrant

Use Adjunct in the management of primary hypercholesterolemia; pruritus associated with elevated levels of bile acids; diarrhea associated with excess fecal bile acids; binding toxicologic agents; pseudomembraneous colitis

Local Anesthetic/Vasoconstrictor Precautions No information available to require special precautions

Effects on Dental Treatment No significant effects or complications reported

Common Adverse Effects

>10%: Gastrointestinal: Constipation, heartburn, nausea, vomiting, stomach pain

1% to 10%:

Central nervous system: Headache

Gastrointestinal: Belching, bloating, diarrhea

Mechanism of Action Forms a nonabsorbable complex with bile acids in the intestine, releasing chloride ions in the process; inhibits enterohepatic reuptake of intestinal bile salts and thereby increases the fecal loss of bile salt-bound low density lipoprotein cholesterol

Drug Interactions

Decreased Effect:

Cholestyramine can reduce the absorption of numerous medications when used concurrently. Give other medications 1 hour before or 4-6 hours after giving cholestyramine. Medications which may be affected include HMG-CoA reductase inhibitors, thiazide diuretics, propranolol (and potentially other beta-blockers), corticosteroids, thyroid hormones, digoxin, valproic acid, NSAIDs, loop diuretics, sulfonylureas, troglitazone (and potentially other agents in this class).

Warfarin and other oral anticoagulants: Hypoprothrombinemic effects may be reduced by cholestyramine. Separate administration times (as detailed above) and monitor INR closely when initiating or discontinuing.

Pharmacodynamics/Kinetics

Onset of action: Peak effect: 21 days

Absorption: None

Excretion: Feces (as insoluble complex with bile acids)

Pregnancy Risk Factor C

Choline Magnesium Trisalicylate

(KOE leen mag NEE zhum trye sa LIS i late)

Related Information

Rheumatoid Arthritis, Osteoarthritis, and Osteoporosis *on page 1759*

Temporomandibular Dysfunction (TMD) *on page 1822*

U.S. Brand Names Trilisate® [DSC]

Generic Available Yes

Index Terms Tricosal

Pharmacologic Category Salicylate

Use Management of osteoarthritis, rheumatoid arthritis, and other arthritis; acute painful shoulder

Local Anesthetic/Vasoconstrictor Precautions No information available to require special precautions

Effects on Dental Treatment NSAID formulations are known to reversibly decrease platelet aggregation via mechanisms different than observed with aspirin. The dentist should be aware of the potential of abnormal coagulation. Caution should also be exercised in the use of NSAIDs in patients already on anticoagulant therapy with drugs such as warfarin (Coumadin®).

Common Adverse Effects

<20%:

Gastrointestinal: Nausea, vomiting, diarrhea, heartburn, dyspepsia, epigastric pain, constipation

Otic: Tinnitus

<2%:

Central nervous system: Headache, lightheadedness, dizziness, drowsiness, lethargy

Otic: Hearing impairment

Dosage Oral (based on total salicylate content):

Children <37 kg: 50 mg/kg/day given in 2 divided doses; 2250 mg/day for heavier children

Adults: 500 mg to 1.5 g 2-3 times/day **or** 3 g at bedtime; usual maintenance dose: 1-4.5 g/day

Elderly: 750 mg 3 times/day

Dosing adjustment/comments in renal impairment: Avoid use in severe renal impairment

Mechanism of Action Inhibits prostaglandin synthesis; acts on the hypothalamus heat-regulating center to reduce fever; blocks the generation of pain impulses

Contraindications Hypersensitivity to salicylates, other nonacetylated salicylates, other NSAIDs, or any component of the formulation; bleeding disorders; pregnancy (3rd trimester)

Warnings/Precautions Salicylate salts may not inhibit platelet aggregation and, therefore, should not be substituted for aspirin in the prophylaxis of thrombosis. Use with caution in patients with impaired hepatic or renal function, dehydration, erosive gastritis, asthma, or peptic ulcer. Children and teenagers who have or are recovering from chickenpox or flu-like symptoms should not use this product. Changes in behavior (along with nausea and vomiting) may be an early sign of Reye's syndrome; patients should be instructed to contact their healthcare provider if these occur.

Elderly are a high-risk population for adverse effects from NSAIDs. As many as 60% of elderly can develop peptic ulceration and/or hemorrhage asymptomatically. Use lowest effective dose for shortest period possible. Tinnitus or impaired hearing may indicate toxicity. Tinnitus may be a difficult and unreliable indication of toxicity due to age-related hearing loss or eighth cranial nerve damage. CNS adverse effects may be observed in the elderly at lower doses than younger adults.

Drug Interactions

Increased Effect/Toxicity: Choline magnesium trisalicylate may increase the hypoprothrombinemic effect of warfarin.

Decreased Effect: Antacids may decrease choline magnesium trisalicylate absorption/salicylate concentrations.

Ethanol/Nutrition/Herb Interactions

Ethanol: Avoid ethanol (may enhance gastric mucosal irritation).

Food: May decrease the rate but not the extent of oral absorption.

Herb/Nutraceutical: Avoid cat's claw, dong quai, evening primrose, feverfew, garlic, ginger, ginkgo, red clover, horse chestnut, green tea, ginseng (all have additional antiplatelet activity). Limit curry powder, paprika, licorice, Benedictine liqueur, prunes, raisins, tea, and gherkins; may cause salicylate accumulation. These foods contain 6 mg salicylate/100 g.

Dietary Considerations Take with food or large volume of water or milk to minimize GI upset. Liquid may be mixed with fruit juice just before drinking. Hypermagnesemia resulting from magnesium salicylate; avoid or use with caution in renal insufficiency.

Pharmacodynamics/Kinetics

Onset of action: Peak effect: ~2 hours

Absorption: Stomach and small intestines

Distribution: Readily into most body fluids and tissues; crosses placenta; enters breast milk

Half-life elimination (dose dependent): Low dose: 2-3 hours; High dose: 30 hours

Time to peak, serum: ~2 hours

Pregnancy Risk Factor C/D (3rd trimester)

Dosage Forms

Liquid: 500 mg/5 mL

Tablet: 500 mg, 750 mg, 1000 mg

Cholografin® Meglumine *see* Iodipamide Meglumine *on page 901*

Chondroitin Sulfate and Sodium Hyaluronate
(kon DROY tin SUL fate & SOW de um hye al yoor ON ate)

Related Information

Chondroitin Sulfate *on page 1705*

U.S. Brand Names DisCoVisc™; Viscoat®

Generic Available No

Index Terms Sodium Chondroitin Sulfate and Sodium Hyaluronate; Sodium Hyaluronate and Chondroitin Sulfate

Pharmacologic Category Ophthalmic Agent, Viscoelastic

Use Ophthalmic surgical aid in the anterior segment during cataract extraction and intraocular lens implantation

Local Anesthetic/Vasoconstrictor Precautions No information available to require special precautions

Effects on Dental Treatment No significant effects or complications reported

Mechanism of Action Ophthalmic viscosurgical device which modulates the interactions between adjacent tissues by space creation, tissue stabilization, (Continued)

Chondroitin Sulfate and Sodium Hyaluronate
(Continued)

balancing pressure, and providing protection of the corneal endothelial cells during surgery.

Pregnancy Risk Factor C

Chooz® [OTC] *see* Calcium Carbonate *on page 260*

Choriogonadotropin Alfa *see* Chorionic Gonadotropin (Recombinant) *on page 352*

Chorionic Gonadotropin (Human)
(kor ee ON ik goe NAD oh troe pin, HYU man)

Related Information
Chorionic Gonadotropin (Recombinant) *on page 352*
U.S. Brand Names Novarel®; Pregnyl®
Canadian Brand Names Humegon®; Pregnyl®; Profasi® HP
Generic Available Yes
Index Terms CG; hCG
Pharmacologic Category Gonadotropin; Ovulation Stimulator
Use Induces ovulation and pregnancy in anovulatory, infertile females; treatment of hypogonadotropic hypogonadism, prepubertal cryptorchidism; spermatogenesis induction with follitropin alfa

Local Anesthetic/Vasoconstrictor Precautions No information available to require special precautions

Effects on Dental Treatment No significant effects or complications reported
Common Adverse Effects Frequency not defined.
Cardiovascular: Edema
Central nervous system: Depression, fatigue, headache, irritability, restlessness
Endocrine & metabolic: Gynecomastia, precocious puberty
Local: Injection site reaction
Miscellaneous: Hypersensitivity reaction (local or systemic)
Mechanism of Action Luteinizing hormone obtained from the urine of pregnant women. Stimulates production of gonadal steroid hormones by causing production of androgen by the testes; as a substitute for luteinizing hormone (LH) to stimulate ovulation

Drug Interactions
Increased Effect/Toxicity: No data reported
Decreased Effect: No data reported
Pharmacodynamics/Kinetics
Half-life elimination: Biphasic: Initial: 11 hours; Terminal: 23 hours
Excretion: Urine
Pregnancy Risk Factor X

Chorionic Gonadotropin (Recombinant)
(kor ee ON ik goe NAD oh troe pin ree KOM be nant)

Related Information
Chorionic Gonadotropin (Human) *on page 352*
U.S. Brand Names Ovidrel®
Canadian Brand Names Ovidrel®
Generic Available No
Index Terms Choriogonadotropin Alfa; r-hCG
Pharmacologic Category Gonadotropin; Ovulation Stimulator
Use As part of an assisted reproductive technology (ART) program, induces ovulation in infertile females who have been pretreated with follicle stimulating hormones (FSH); induces ovulation and pregnancy in infertile females when the cause of infertility is functional

Local Anesthetic/Vasoconstrictor Precautions No information available to require special precautions

Effects on Dental Treatment No significant effects or complications reported
Common Adverse Effects
2% to 10%:
Endocrine & metabolic: Ovarian cyst (3%), ovarian hyperstimulation (<2% to 3%)
Gastrointestinal: Abdominal pain (3% to 4%), nausea (3%), vomiting (3%)
Local: Injection site: Pain (8%), bruising (3% to 5%), reaction (<2% to 3%), inflammation (<2% to 2%)
Miscellaneous: Postoperative pain (5%)
<2%:
Cardiovascular: Cardiac arrhythmia, heart murmur

Central nervous system: Dizziness, emotional lability, fever, headache, insomnia, malaise

Dermatologic: Pruritus, rash

Endocrine & metabolic: Breast pain, hot flashes, hyperglycemia, intermenstrual bleeding, vaginal hemorrhage

Gastrointestinal: Abdominal enlargement, diarrhea, flatulence

Genitourinary: Cervical carcinoma, cervical lesion, dysuria, genital herpes, genital moniliasis, leukorrhea, urinary incontinence, urinary tract infection, vaginitis

Hematologic: Leukocytosis

Neuromuscular & skeletal: Back pain, paresthesia

Renal: Albuminuria

Respiratory: Cough, pharyngitis, upper respiratory tract infection

Miscellaneous: Ectopic pregnancy, hiccups

In addition, the following have been reported with menotropin therapy: Adnexal torsion, hemoperitoneum, mild-to-moderate ovarian enlargement, pulmonary and vascular complications. Ovarian neoplasms have also been reported (rare) with multiple drug regimens used for ovarian induction (relationship not established).

Mechanism of Action Luteinizing hormone analogue produced by recombinant DNA techniques; stimulates rupture of the ovarian follicle once follicular development has occurred.

Drug Interactions

Increased Effect/Toxicity: Specific drug interaction studies have not been conducted.

Decreased Effect: Specific drug interaction studies have not been conducted.

Pharmacodynamics/Kinetics

Distribution: V_d: 5.9 ± 1 L

Bioavailability: 40%

Half-life elimination: Initial: 4 hours; Terminal: 29 hours

Time to peak: 12-24 hours

Excretion: Urine (10% of dose)

Pregnancy Risk Factor X

Chromium see Trace Metals *on page 1595*

CI-1008 *see* Pregabalin *on page 1345*

Cialis® *see* Tadalafil *on page 1520*

Ciclesonide (sye KLES oh nide)

U.S. Brand Names Omnaris™

Canadian Brand Names Alvesco®

Generic Available No

Pharmacologic Category Corticosteroid, Nasal

Use Management of seasonal and perennial allergic rhinitis

Local Anesthetic/Vasoconstrictor Precautions No information available to require special precautions

Effects on Dental Treatment No significant effects or complications reported

Common Adverse Effects 1% to 10%:

Central nervous system: Headache (6%)

Otic: Ear pain (2%)

Respiratory: Epistaxis (5%), nasopharyngitis (4%), nasal discomfort

Dosage Intranasal: Children ≥12 years and Adults: Rhinitis: 2 sprays (50 mcg/spray) per nostril once daily; maximum: 200 mcg/day

Mechanism of Action Ciclesonide is a nonhalogenated, glucocorticoid prodrug that is hydrolyzed to the pharmacologically active metabolite des-ciclesonide following intranasal application. Des-ciclesonide has a high affinity for the glucocorticoid receptor and exhibits anti-inflammatory activity. The precise mechanism in allergic rhinitis is unknown; however, the mechanism of action for all topical corticosteroids is believed to be a combination of three important properties - anti-inflammatory activity, immunosuppressive properties, and antiproliferative actions.

Contraindications Hypersensitivity to ciclesonide or any component of the formulation

Warnings/Precautions May cause hypercorticism or suppression of hypothalamic-pituitary-adrenal (HPA) axis, particularly in younger children or in patients receiving high doses for prolonged periods. HPA axis suppression may lead to adrenal crisis. Withdrawal and discontinuation of a corticosteroid should be done slowly and carefully. Particular care is required when patients are transferred from systemic corticosteroids to inhaled products due to possible adrenal insufficiency or withdrawal from steroids, including an increase in allergic symptoms. Patients receiving >20 mg per day of prednisone (or equivalent) may be

(Continued)

Ciclesonide *(Continued)*

most susceptible. Fatalities have occurred due to adrenal insufficiency in asthmatic patients during and after transfer from systemic corticosteroids to aerosol steroids; aerosol steroids do **not** provide the systemic steroid needed to treat patients having trauma, surgery, or infections.

Bronchospasm may occur with wheezing after inhalation; if this occurs stop steroid and treat with a fast-acting bronchodilator. Supplemental steroids (oral or parenteral) may be needed during stress or severe asthma attacks. Not to be used in status asthmaticus or for the relief of acute bronchospasm. Corticosteroid use may cause psychiatric disturbances, including depression, euphoria, insomnia, mood swings, and personality changes. Pre-existing psychiatric conditions may be exacerbated by corticosteroid use. Prolonged use of corticosteroids may also increase the incidence of secondary infection, mask acute infection (including fungal infections), prolong or exacerbate viral infections, or limit response to vaccines. Exposure to chickenpox should be avoided; corticosteroids should not be used to treat ocular herpes simplex. Corticosteroids should not be used for cerebral malaria. Close observation is required in patients with latent tuberculosis and/or TB reactivity; restrict use in active TB (only in conjunction with antituberculosis treatment). Prolonged treatment with corticosteroids has been associated with the development of Kaposi's sarcoma (case reports); if noted, discontinuation of therapy should be considered.

Use with caution in patients with thyroid disease, hepatic impairment, renal impairment, cardiovascular disease, diabetes, glaucoma, cataracts, myasthenia gravis, patients at risk for osteoporosis, patients at risk for seizures, or GI diseases (diverticulitis, peptic ulcer, ulcerative colitis) due to perforation risk. Use caution following acute MI (corticosteroids have been associated with myocardial rupture). Because of the risk of adverse effects, systemic corticosteroids should be used cautiously in the elderly in the smallest possible effective dose for the shortest duration. Avoid nasal corticosteroid use in patients with recent nasal septal ulcers, nasal surgery or nasal trauma until healing has occurred.

Orally-inhaled and intranasal corticosteroids may cause a reduction in growth velocity in pediatric patients (~1 centimeter per year [range 0.3-1.8 cm per year] and related to dose and duration of exposure). To minimize the systemic effects of orally-inhaled and intranasal corticosteroids, each patient should be titrated to the lowest effective dose. Growth should be routinely monitored in pediatric patients. Safety and efficacy have not been established in children <12 years of age.

Drug Interactions

Cytochrome P450 Effect: Substrate (minor) of CYP3A4, 2D6

Increased Effect/Toxicity: Ciclesonide effects are increased by ketoconazole.

Pharmacodynamics/Kinetics

Onset of action: 24-48 hours; further improvement observed over 1-2 weeks in seasonal allergic rhinitis or 5 weeks in perennial allergic rhinitis

Absorption: Intranasal: Minimal systemic absorption

Protein binding: ≥99%

Metabolism: Ciclesonide hydrolyzed to active metabolite, des-ciclesonide via esterases in nasal mucosa; further metabolism via hepatic CYP3A4 and 2D6

Bioavailability: <1%

Excretion: Feces (~66%); urine (≤20%)

Pregnancy Risk Factor C

Dosage Forms

Suspension, intranasal [spray]:

Omnaris™: 50 mcg/inhalation (12.5 g)

Selected Readings

Nave R, Wingertzahn MA, Brookman S, et al, "Safety, Tolerability, and Exposure of Ciclesonide Nasal Spray in Healthy and Asymptomatic Subjects with Seasonal Allergic Rhinitis," *J Clin Pharmacol*, 2006, 46 (4):461-7.

Ciclopirox *(sye kloe PEER oks)*

U.S. Brand Names Loprox®; Penlac®

Canadian Brand Names Loprox®; Penlac®; Stieprox®

Mexican Brand Names Loprox; Loprox Laca; Stiprox

Generic Available Yes: Cream, topical suspension

Index Terms Ciclopirox Olamine
Pharmacologic Category Antifungal Agent, Topical
Use
 Cream/suspension: Treatment of tinea pedis (athlete's foot), tinea cruris (jock itch), tinea corporis (ringworm), cutaneous candidiasis, and tinea versicolor (pityriasis)
 Gel: Treatment of tinea pedis (athlete's foot), tinea corporis (ringworm); seborrheic dermatitis of the scalp
 Lacquer (solution): Topical treatment of mild-to-moderate onychomycosis of the fingernails and toenails due to *Trichophyton rubrum* (not involving the lunula) and the immediately-adjacent skin
 Shampoo: Treatment of seborrheic dermatitis of the scalp
Local Anesthetic/Vasoconstrictor Precautions No information available to require special precautions
Effects on Dental Treatment No significant effects or complications reported
Common Adverse Effects
 Central nervous system: Headache
 Dermatologic: Alopecia, dry skin, erythema, facial edema, hair discoloration (rare; shampoo formulation in light-haired individuals), nail disorder (shape or color change with lacquer), pruritus, rash
 Local: Burning sensation (gel: 34%; ≤1% with other forms), irritation, redness, or pain
Mechanism of Action Inhibiting transport of essential elements in the fungal cell disrupting the synthesis of DNA, RNA, and protein
Drug Interactions
 Increased Effect/Toxicity: No data reported
 Decreased Effect: No data reported
Pharmacodynamics/Kinetics
 Absorption: Cream, suspension: <2% through intact skin; increased with gel; <5% with lacquer
 Distribution: Scalp application: To epidermis, corium (dermis), including hair, hair follicles, and sebaceous glands
 Protein binding: 94% to 98%
 Half-life elimination: Biologic: 1.7 hours (suspension); elimination: 5.5 hours (gel)
 Excretion: Urine (gel: 3% to 10%); feces (small amounts)
Pregnancy Risk Factor B

Ciclopirox Olamine *see* Ciclopirox *on page 354*
Cidecin *see* Daptomycin *on page 443*

Cidofovir (si DOF o veer)

Related Information
 Systemic Viral Diseases *on page 1767*
U.S. Brand Names Vistide®
Generic Available No
Pharmacologic Category Antiviral Agent
Use Treatment of cytomegalovirus (CMV) retinitis in patients with acquired immunodeficiency syndrome (AIDS). **Note:** Should be administered with probenecid.
Local Anesthetic/Vasoconstrictor Precautions No information available to require special precautions
Effects on Dental Treatment Key adverse event(s) related to dental treatment: Stomatitis and abnormal taste.
Common Adverse Effects
 >10%:
  Central nervous system: Chills, fever, headache, pain
  Dermatologic: Alopecia, rash
  Gastrointestinal: Nausea, vomiting, diarrhea, anorexia
  Hematologic: Anemia, neutropenia
  Neuromuscular & skeletal: Weakness
  Ocular: Intraocular pressure decreased, iritis, ocular hypotony, uveitis
  Renal: Creatinine increased, proteinuria, renal toxicity
  Respiratory: Cough, dyspnea
  Miscellaneous: Infection, oral moniliasis, serum bicarbonate decreased
 1% to 10%:
  Renal: Fanconi syndrome
  Respiratory: Pneumonia
 Frequency not defined (limited to important or life-threatening reactions):
  Cardiovascular: Cardiomyopathy, cardiovascular disorder, CHF, edema, postural hypotension, shock, syncope, tachycardia
  Central nervous system: Agitation, amnesia, anxiety, confusion, convulsion, dizziness, hallucinations, insomnia, malaise, vertigo
 (Continued)

Cidofovir (Continued)

Dermatologic: Photosensitivity reaction, skin discoloration, urticaria

Endocrine & metabolic: Adrenal cortex insufficiency

Gastrointestinal: Abdominal pain, aphthous stomatitis, colitis, constipation, dysphagia, fecal incontinence, gastritis, GI hemorrhage, gingivitis, melena, proctitis, splenomegaly, stomatitis, tongue discoloration

Genitourinary: Urinary incontinence

Hematologic: Hypochromic anemia, leukocytosis, leukopenia, lymphadenopathy, lymphoma-like reaction, pancytopenia, thrombocytopenia, thrombocytopenic purpura

Hepatic: Hepatomegaly, hepatosplenomegaly, jaundice, liver function tests abnormal, liver damage, liver necrosis

Local: Injection site reaction

Neuromuscular & skeletal: Tremor

Ocular: Amblyopia, blindness, cataract, conjunctivitis, corneal lesion, diplopia, vision abnormal

Otic: Hearing loss

Miscellaneous: Allergic reaction, sepsis

Mechanism of Action Cidofovir is converted to cidofovir diphosphate which is the active intracellular metabolite; cidofovir diphosphate suppresses CMV replication by selective inhibition of viral DNA synthesis. Incorporation of cidofovir into growing viral DNA chain results in reductions in the rate of viral DNA synthesis.

Drug Interactions

Increased Effect/Toxicity: Drugs with nephrotoxic potential (eg, amphotericin B, aminoglycosides, foscarnet, and I.V. pentamidine) should not be used with or within 7 days of cidofovir therapy. Due to concomitant probenecid administration, temporarily discontinue or decrease zidovudine dose by 50% on the day of cidofovir administration only.

Pharmacodynamics/Kinetics The following pharmacokinetic data is based on a combination of cidofovir administered with probenecid:

Distribution: V_d: 0.54 L/kg; does not cross significantly into CSF

Protein binding: <6%

Metabolism: Minimal; phosphorylation occurs intracellularly

Half-life elimination, plasma: ~2.6 hours

Excretion: Urine

Pregnancy Risk Factor C

Cilazapril (sye LAY za pril)

Canadian Brand Names Apo-Cilazapril®; Inhibace®; Novo-Cilazapril

Index Terms Cilazapril Monohydrate

Pharmacologic Category Angiotensin-Converting Enzyme (ACE) Inhibitor

Use Management of hypertension; treatment of congestive heart failure

Local Anesthetic/Vasoconstrictor Precautions No information available to require special precautions

Effects on Dental Treatment Key adverse event(s) related to dental treatment: Orthostatic hypotension.

Common Adverse Effects 1% to 10%:

Cardiovascular: Palpitation (up to 1%), hypotension (symptomatic, up to 1% in CHF patients), orthostatic hypotension (2%)

Central nervous system: Headache (3% to 5%), dizziness (3% to 8%), fatigue (2% to 3%)

Gastrointestinal: Nausea (1% to 3%)

Neuromuscular & skeletal: Weakness (0.3% to 2%)

Renal: Serum creatinine increased

Respiratory: Cough (2% in hypertension, up to 7.5% in CHF patients)

Restrictions Not available in U.S.

Mechanism of Action Competitive inhibitor of angiotensin-converting enzyme (ACE); prevents conversion of angiotensin I to angiotensin II, a potent vasoconstrictor; results in lower levels of angiotensin II which causes an increase in plasma renin activity and a reduction in aldosterone secretion.

Drug Interactions

Increased Effect/Toxicity: Potassium supplements, sulfamethoxazole/trimethoprim (high dose), angiotensin II receptor antagonists (eg, candesartan, losartan, irbesartan), or potassium-sparing diuretics (amiloride, spironolactone, triamterene) may result in elevated serum potassium levels when combined with cilazapril. ACE inhibitor effects may be increased by phenothiazines or probenecid (increases levels of other ACE inhibitors). ACE inhibitors may increase serum concentrations/effects of lithium. ACE inhibitors may enhance the adverse/toxic effects (nitritoid reaction) of gold sodium thiomalate.

Diuretics have additive hypotensive effects with ACE inhibitors, and hypovolemia increases the potential for adverse renal effects of ACE inhibitors. In patients with compromised renal function, coadministration with nonsteroidal anti-inflammatory drugs may result in further deterioration of renal function. Allopurinol and ACE inhibitors may cause a higher risk of hypersensitivity reaction when taken concurrently.

Decreased Effect: Aspirin (high dose) may reduce the therapeutic effects of ACE inhibitors; at low dosages this does not appear to be significant. Rifampin may decrease the effect of ACE inhibitors. Antacids may decrease the bioavailability of ACE inhibitors (may be more likely to occur with captopril); separate administration times by 1-2 hours. NSAIDs, specifically indomethacin, may reduce the hypotensive effects of ACE inhibitors. More likely to occur in low renin or volume-dependent hypertensive patients.

Pharmacodynamics/Kinetics
Onset of action: Antihypertensive: ~1 hour
Duration: Therapeutic effect: 24 hours
Absorption: Rapid
Metabolism: To active form (cilazaprilat)
Bioavailability: 57%
Half-life elimination: Cilazaprilat: Terminal: 36-49 hours
Time to peak: 3-7 hours
Excretion: In urine (91%)

Pregnancy Risk Factor Not assigned; C/D (2nd and 3rd trimesters) based on other ACE inhibitors

Cilazapril Monohydrate see Cilazapril on page 356

Cilostazol (sil OH sta zol)

U.S. Brand Names Pletal®
Canadian Brand Names Pletal®
Generic Available Yes
Index Terms OPC-13013
Pharmacologic Category Antiplatelet Agent; Phosphodiesterase Enzyme Inhibitor
Use Symptomatic management of peripheral vascular disease, primarily intermittent claudication
Unlabeled/Investigational Use Treatment of acute coronary syndromes and for graft patency improvement in percutaneous coronary interventions with or without stenting
Local Anesthetic/Vasoconstrictor Precautions No information available to require special precautions
Effects on Dental Treatment No significant effects or complications reported
Common Adverse Effects
>10%:
Central nervous system: Headache (27% to 34%)
Gastrointestinal: Abnormal stools (12% to 15%), diarrhea (12% to 19%)
Respiratory: Rhinitis (7% to 12%)
Miscellaneous: Infection (10% to 14%)
2% to 10%:
Cardiovascular: Peripheral edema (7% to 9%), palpitation (5% to 10%), tachycardia (4%)
Central nervous system: Dizziness (9% to 10%), vertigo (up to 3%)
Gastrointestinal: Dyspepsia (6%), nausea (6% to 7%), abdominal pain (4% to 5%), flatulence (2% to 3%)
Neuromuscular & skeletal: Back pain (6% to 7%), myalgia (2% to 3%)
Respiratory: Pharyngitis (7% to 10%), cough (3% to 4%)
Mechanism of Action Cilostazol and its metabolites are inhibitors of phosphodiesterase III. As a result, cyclic AMP is increased leading to reversible inhibition of platelet aggregation and vasodilation. Other effects of phosphodiesterase III inhibition include increased cardiac contractility, accelerated AV nodal conduction, increased ventricular automaticity, heart rate, and coronary blood flow.
Drug Interactions
Cytochrome P450 Effect: Substrate of CYP1A2 (minor), 2C19 (minor), 2D6 (minor), 3A4 (major)
Increased Effect/Toxicity: Cilostazol serum concentrations may be increased by antifungal agents (midazole), macrolide antibiotics, and omeprazole. Increased concentrations of cilostazol may be anticipated during concurrent therapy with other inhibitors of CYP3A4 (eg, clarithromycin, diclofenac, doxycycline, erythromycin, imatinib, isoniazid, nefazodone, nicardipine, (Continued)

Cilostazol *(Continued)*

propofol, protease inhibitors, quinidine, telithromycin, and verapamil) or inhibitors of CYP2C19 (eg, delavirdine, fluconazole, fluvoxamine, gemfibrozil, isoniazid, omeprazole, and ticlopidine). Aspirin-induced inhibition of platelet aggregation is potentiated by concurrent cilostazol. Concurrent use of drotrecogin alfa, NSAIDs, or treprostinil may cause increased bleeding.

Pharmacodynamics/Kinetics
Onset of action: 2-4 weeks; may require up to 12 weeks
Protein binding: 97% to 98%
Metabolism: Hepatic via CYP3A4 (primarily), 1A2, 2C19, and 2D6; at least one metabolite has significant activity
Half-life elimination: 11-13 hours
Excretion: Urine (74%) and feces (20%) as metabolites

Pregnancy Risk Factor C

Ciloxan® *see* Ciprofloxacin *on page 359*

Cimetidine (sye MET i deen)

Related Information
Gastrointestinal Disorders *on page 1745*
U.S. Brand Names Tagamet® [DSC]; Tagamet® HB 200 [OTC]
Canadian Brand Names Apo-Cimetidine®; Gen-Cimetidine; Novo-Cimetidine; Nu-Cimet; PMS-Cimetidine; Tagamet® HB
Mexican Brand Names Cimetase; Tagamet
Generic Available Yes
Pharmacologic Category Histamine H_2 Antagonist
Use Short-term treatment of active duodenal ulcers and benign gastric ulcers; long-term prophylaxis of duodenal ulcer; gastric hypersecretory states; gastroesophageal reflux; prevention of upper GI bleeding in critically-ill patients; labeled for OTC use for prevention or relief of heartburn, acid indigestion, or sour stomach
Unlabeled/Investigational Use Part of a multidrug regimen for *H. pylori* eradication to reduce the risk of duodenal ulcer recurrence
Local Anesthetic/Vasoconstrictor Precautions No information available to require special precautions
Effects on Dental Treatment No significant effects or complications reported
Common Adverse Effects
1% to 10%:
Central nervous system: Headache (2% to 4%), dizziness (1%), somnolence (1%), agitation
Endocrine & metabolic: Gynecomastia (<1% to 4%)
Gastrointestinal: Diarrhea (1%)
Frequency not defined:
Cardiovascular: AV block, bradycardia, hypotension, tachycardia, vasculitis
Central nervous system: Confusion, fever
Dermatologic: Alopecia, erythema multiforme, exfoliative dermatitis, Stevens-Johnson syndrome, toxic epidermal necrolysis, rash
Endocrine & metabolic: Edema of the breasts, sexual ability decreased
Gastrointestinal: Nausea, pancreatitis, vomiting
Hematologic: Agranulocytosis, aplastic anemia, hemolytic anemia (immune-based), neutropenia, pancytopenia, thrombocytopenia
Hepatic: AST/ALT increased, hepatic fibrosis (case report)
Neuromuscular & skeletal: Arthralgia, myalgia, polymyositis
Renal: Creatinine increased, interstitial nephritis
Miscellaneous: Anaphylaxis, pneumonia (causal relationship not established)
Mechanism of Action Competitive inhibition of histamine at H_2 receptors of the gastric parietal cells resulting in reduced gastric acid secretion, gastric volume and hydrogen ion concentration reduced
Drug Interactions
Cytochrome P450 Effect: Inhibits CYP1A2 (moderate), 2C9 (weak), 2C19 (moderate), 2D6 (moderate), 2E1 (weak), 3A4 (moderate)
Increased Effect/Toxicity: Cimetidine may increase the levels/effects of aminophylline, amphetamines, selected beta-blockers, selected benzodiazepines, calcium channel blockers, cyclosporine, dextromethorphan, dofetilide, ergot derivatives, lidocaine, meperidine, metformin, methsuximide, metronidazole, mexiletine, mirtazapine, moricizine, nateglinide, nefazodone, paroxetine (and other SSRIs), phenytoin, procainamide, propafenone, propranolol, quinidine, quinolone antibiotics, risperidone, ritonavir, ropinirole, sildenafil (and other PDE-5 inhibitors), sulfonylureas, tacrine, tacrolimus, theophylline, thioridazine, triamterene, tricyclic antidepressants, trifluoperazine, venlafaxine, and other CYP1A2, 2C19, or 2D6 substrates.

Cimetidine increases warfarin's effect in a dose-related manner. Cimetidine increases carmustine's myelotoxicity; avoid concurrent use.

Decreased Effect: Cimetidine may decrease the levels/effects of CYP2D6 prodrug substrates (eg, codeine, hydrocodone, oxycodone, and tramadol). Ketoconazole, fluconazole, itraconazole (especially capsule) decrease serum concentration; avoid concurrent use with H_2 antagonists. Absorption of delavirdine and atazanavir may be decreased; avoid concurrent use of delavirdine with H_2 antagonists.

Pharmacodynamics/Kinetics
Onset of action: 1 hour
Duration: 4-8 hours
Absorption: Rapid
Distribution: Crosses placenta; enters breast milk
Protein binding: 20%
Metabolism: Partially hepatic, forms metabolites
Bioavailability: 60% to 70%
Half-life elimination: Neonates: 3.6 hours; Children: 1.4 hours; Adults: Normal renal function: 2 hours
Time to peak, serum: Oral: 1-2 hours
Excretion: Primarily urine (48% as unchanged drug); feces (some)

Pregnancy Risk Factor B

Cinacalcet (sin a KAL cet)

U.S. Brand Names Sensipar™
Generic Available No
Index Terms AMG 073; Cinacalcet Hydrochloride
Pharmacologic Category Calcimimetic
Use Treatment of secondary hyperparathyroidism in dialysis patients; treatment of hypercalcemia in patients with parathyroid carcinoma
Unlabeled/Investigational Use Primary hyperparathyroidism
Local Anesthetic/Vasoconstrictor Precautions No information available to require special precautions
Effects on Dental Treatment No significant effects or complications reported
Common Adverse Effects
>10%:
Endocrine & metabolic: Hypocalcemia
Gastrointestinal: Nausea (31%), vomiting (27%), diarrhea (21%)
Neuromuscular & skeletal: Myalgia (15%)
1% to 10%:
Cardiovascular: Hypertension (7%)
Central nervous system: Dizziness (10%), seizure (1%)
Endocrine & metabolic: Testosterone decreased
Gastrointestinal: Anorexia (6%)
Neuromuscular & skeletal: Weakness (7%), chest pain (6%)
Mechanism of Action Increases the sensitivity of the calcium-sensing receptor on the parathyroid gland.
Drug Interactions
Cytochrome P450 Effect: Substrate of CYP1A2, 2D6, 3A4; **Inhibits** CYP2D6
Increased Effect/Toxicity: Cinacalcet increases levels of amitriptyline and nortriptyline. Ketoconazole may increase cinacalcet levels.
Pharmacodynamics/Kinetics
Distribution: V_d: 1000 L
Protein binding: 93% to 97%
Metabolism: Hepatic via CYP3A4, 2D6, 1A2; forms inactive metabolites
Half-life elimination: Terminal: 30-40 hours
Time to peak, plasma: Nadir in iPTH levels: 2-6 hours postdose
Excretion: Urine 80% (as metabolites); feces 15%
Pregnancy Risk Factor C

Cinacalcet Hydrochloride *see* Cinacalcet *on page 359*
Cipro® *see* Ciprofloxacin *on page 359*
Ciprodex® *see* Ciprofloxacin and Dexamethasone *on page 364*

Ciprofloxacin (sip roe FLOKS a sin)

Related Information
Periodontal Diseases *on page 1801*
Sexually-Transmitted Diseases *on page 1766*
Tuberculosis Treatment *on page 1909*
(Continued)

Ciprofloxacin *(Continued)*

Related Sample Prescriptions

Bacterial Infections and Periodontal Diseases *on page 1837*

U.S. Brand Names Ciloxan®; Cipro®; Cipro® XR; Proquin® XR

Canadian Brand Names Apo-Ciprofllox®; Ciloxan®; Cipro®; Cipro® XL; CO Ciprofloxacin; Gen-Ciprofloxacin; Novo-Ciprofloxacin; PMS-Ciprofloxacin; RAN™-Ciprofloxacin; ratio-Ciprofloxacin; Rhoxal-ciprofloxacin; Sandoz-Ciprofloxacin; Taro-Ciprofloxacin

Mexican Brand Names Ciloxan; Cimogal; Ciprobac; Ciproflox; Ciproxina; Eni; Floxager; Floxantina; Kenzoflex; Mitroken; Sophixin Ofteno; Zipra

Generic Available Yes: Excludes infusion, suspension, ointment

Index Terms Ciprofloxacin Hydrochloride

Pharmacologic Category Antibiotic, Ophthalmic; Antibiotic, Quinolone

Dental Use Useful as a single agent or in combination with metronidazole in the treatment of periodontitis associated with the presence of *Actinobacillus actinomycetemcomitans* (AA), as well as enteric rods/pseudomonads

Use

Children: Complicated urinary tract infections and pyelonephritis due to *E. coli.* **Note:** Although effective, ciprofloxacin is not the drug of first choice in children.

Children and adults: To reduce incidence or progression of disease following exposure to aerolized *Bacillus anthracis.* Ophthalmologically, for superficial ocular infections (corneal ulcers, conjunctivitis) due to susceptible strains

Adults: Treatment of the following infections when caused by susceptible bacteria: Urinary tract infections; acute uncomplicated cystitis in females; chronic bacterial prostatitis; lower respiratory tract infections (including acute exacerbations of chronic bronchitis); acute sinusitis; skin and skin structure infections; bone and joint infections; complicated intra-abdominal infections (in combination with metronidazole); infectious diarrhea; typhoid fever due to *Salmonella typhi* (eradication of chronic typhoid carrier state has not been proven); uncomplicated cervical and urethra gonorrhea (due to *N. gonorrhoeae*); nosocomial pneumonia; empirical therapy for febrile neutropenic patients (in combination with piperacillin)

Note: As of April 2007, the CDC no longer recommends the use of fluoroquinolones for the treatment of gonococcal disease.

Unlabeled/Investigational Use Acute pulmonary exacerbations in cystic fibrosis (children); cutaneous/gastrointestinal/oropharyngeal anthrax (treatment, children and adults); disseminated gonococcal infection (adults); chancroid (adults); prophylaxis to *Neisseria meningitidis* following close contact with an infected person; empirical therapy (oral) for febrile neutropenia in low-risk cancer patients; infectious diarrhea (children)

Local Anesthetic/Vasoconstrictor Precautions No information available to require special precautions

Effects on Dental Treatment No significant effects or complications reported

Significant Adverse Effects

1% to 10%:

Central nervous system: Neurologic events (children 2%, includes dizziness, insomnia, nervousness, somnolence); fever (children 2%); headache (I.V. administration); restlessness (I.V. administration)

Dermatologic: Rash (children 2%, adults 1%)

Gastrointestinal: Nausea (children/adults 3%); diarrhea (children 5%, adults 2%); vomiting (children 5%, adults 1%); abdominal pain (children 3%, adults <1%); dyspepsia (children 3%)

Hepatic: ALT/AST increased (adults 1%)

Local: Injection site reactions (I.V. administration)

Respiratory: Rhinitis (children 3%)

<1% (Limited to important or life-threatening): Abnormal gait, acute renal failure, agitation, agranulocytosis, albuminuria, allergic reactions, anaphylactic shock, anaphylaxis, anemia, angina pectoris, angioedema, anorexia, anosmia, arthralgia, ataxia, atrial flutter, bone marrow depression (life-threatening), breast pain, bronchospasm, candidiasis, candiduria, cardiopulmonary arrest, cerebral thrombosis, chills, cholestatic jaundice, chromatopsia, confusion, constipation, crystalluria (particularly in alkaline urine), cylindruria, delirium, depersonalization, depression, dizziness, drowsiness, dyspepsia (adults), dysphagia, dyspnea, edema, eosinophilia, erythema multiforme, erythema nodosum, exfoliative dermatitis, fever (adults), fixed eruption, flatulence, gastrointestinal bleeding, hallucinations, headache (oral), hematuria, hemolytic anemia, hepatic failure, hepatic necrosis, hyperesthesia, hyperglycemia, hyperpigmentation, hyper-/hypotension, hypertonia, insomnia, interstitial nephritis, intestinal perforation, irritability, jaundice, joint pain, laryngeal

edema, lightheadedness, lymphadenopathy, malaise, manic reaction, methemoglobinemia, MI, migraine, moniliasis, myalgia, myasthenia gravis, myoclonus, nephritis, nightmares, nystagmus, orthostatic hypotension, palpitation, pancreatitis, pancytopenia (life-threatening or fatal), paranoia, paresthesia, peripheral neuropathy, petechia, photosensitivity, prolongation of PT/INR, pseudomembranous colitis, psychosis, pulmonary edema, renal calculi, seizure; serum cholesterol, glucose, triglycerides increased; serum sickness-like reactions, Stevens-Johnson syndrome, syncope, tachycardia, taste loss, tendon rupture, tendonitis, thrombophlebitis, tinnitus, torsade de pointes, toxic epidermal necrolysis (Lyell's syndrome), tremor, twitching, urethral bleeding, vaginal candidiasis, vaginitis, vasculitis, ventricular ectopy, visual disturbance, weakness

Dental Usual Dosing Treatment of periodontitis: Adults: Oral: 500 mg every 12 hours for 8-10 days

Dosage Note: Extended release tablets and immediate release formulations are not interchangeable. Unless otherwise specified, oral dosing reflects the use of immediate release formulations.

Usual dosage ranges:
Children (see Warnings/Precautions):
Oral: 20-30 mg/kg/day in 2 divided doses; maximum dose: 1.5 g/day
I.V.: 20-30 mg/kg/day divided every 12 hours; maximum dose: 800 mg/day
Adults:
Oral: 250-750 mg every 12 hours
I.V.: 200-400 mg every 12 hours

Indication-specific dosing:
Children:
Anthrax:
Inhalational (postexposure prophylaxis):
Oral: 15 mg/kg/dose every 12 hours for 60 days; maximum: 500 mg/dose
I.V.: 10 mg/kg/dose every 12 hours for 60 days; do **not** exceed 400 mg/dose (800 mg/day)
Cutaneous (treatment, CDC guidelines): Oral: 10-15 mg/kg every 12 hours for 60 days (maximum: 1 g/day); amoxicillin 80 mg/kg/day divided every 8 hours is an option for completion of treatment after clinical improvement. **Note:** In the presence of systemic involvement, extensive edema, lesions on head/neck, refer to I.V. dosing for treatment of inhalational/gastrointestinal/oropharyngeal anthrax.
Inhalational/gastrointestinal/oropharyngeal (treatment, CDC guidelines): I.V.: Initial: 10-15 mg/kg every 12 hours for 60 days (maximum: 500 mg/dose); switch to oral therapy when clinically appropriate; refer to adult dosing for notes on combined therapy and duration
Bacterial conjunctivitis: See adult dosing
Corneal ulcer: See adult dosing
Cystic fibrosis (unlabeled use):
Oral: 40 mg/kg/day divided every 12 hours administered following 1 week of I.V. therapy has been reported in a clinical trial; total duration of therapy: 10-21 days
I.V.: 30 mg/kg/day divided every 8 hours for 1 week, followed by oral therapy, has been reported in a clinical trial
Urinary tract infection (complicated) or pyelonephritis:
Oral: 20-30 mg/kg/day in 2 divided doses (every 12 hours) for 10-21 days; maximum: 1.5 g/day
I.V.: 6-10 mg/kg every 8 hours for 10-21 days (maximum: 400 mg/dose)
Adults:
Anthrax:
Inhalational (postexposure prophylaxis):
Oral: 500 mg every 12 hours for 60 days
I.V.: 400 mg every 12 hours for 60 days
Cutaneous (treatment, CDC guidelines): Oral: Immediate release formulation: 500 mg every 12 hours for 60 days. **Note:** In the presence of systemic involvement, extensive edema, lesions on head/neck, refer to I.V. dosing for treatment of inhalational/gastrointestinal/oropharyngeal anthrax
Inhalational/gastrointestinal/oropharyngeal (treatment, CDC guidelines): I.V.: 400 mg every 12 hours. **Note:** Initial treatment should include two or more agents predicted to be effective (per CDC recommendations). Continue combined therapy for 60 days.
Bacterial conjunctivitis:
Ophthalmic solution: Instill 1-2 drops in eye(s) every 2 hours while awake for 2 days and 1-2 drops every 4 hours while awake for the next 5 days
Ophthalmic ointment: Apply a ½" ribbon into the conjunctival sac 3 times/day for the first 2 days, followed by a ½" ribbon applied twice daily for the next 5 days

(Continued)

Ciprofloxacin *(Continued)*

Bone/joint infections:
Oral: 500-750 mg twice daily for 4-6 weeks
I.V.: Mild to moderate: 400 mg every 12 hours for 4-6 weeks; Severe/complicated: 400 mg every 8 hours for 4-6 weeks

Chancroid (CDC guidelines): Oral: 500 mg twice daily for 3 days

Corneal ulcer: Ophthalmic solution: Instill 2 drops into affected eye every 15 minutes for the first 6 hours, then 2 drops into the affected eye every 30 minutes for the remainder of the first day. On day 2, instill 2 drops into the affected eye hourly. On days 3-14, instill 2 drops into affected eye every 4 hours. Treatment may continue after day 14 if re-epithelialization has not occurred.

Febrile neutropenia*: I.V.: 400 mg every 8 hours for 7-14 days

Gonococcal infections:
Urethral/cervical gonococcal infections: Oral: 250-500 mg as a single dose (CDC recommends concomitant doxycycline or azithromycin due to possible co-infection with *Chlamydia*; **Note:** As of April 2007, the CDC no longer recommends the use of fluoroquinolones for the treatment of uncomplicated gonococcal disease.

Disseminated gonococcal infection (CDC guidelines): Oral: 500 mg twice daily to complete 7 days of therapy (initial treatment with ceftriaxone 1 g I.M./I.V. daily for 24-48 hours after improvement begins); **Note:** As of April 2007, the CDC no longer recommends the use of fluoroquinolones for the treatment of more serious gonococcal disease, unless no other options exist and susceptibility can be confirmed via culture.

Infectious diarrhea: Oral:
Salmonella: 500 mg twice daily for 5-7 days
Shigella: 500 mg twice daily for 3 days
Traveler's diarrhea: Mild: 750 mg for one dose; Severe: 500 mg twice daily for 3 days
Vibrio cholerae: 1 g for one dose

Intra-abdominal*:
Oral: 500 mg every 12 hours for 7-14 days
I.V.: 400 mg every 12 hours for 7-14 days

Lower respiratory tract, skin/skin structure infections:
Oral: 500-750 mg twice daily for 7-14 days
I.V.: Mild to moderate: 400 mg every 12 hours for 7-14 days; Severe/complicated: 400 mg every 8 hours for 7-14 days

Nosocomial pneumonia: I.V.: 400 mg every 8 hours for 10-14 days

Prostatitis (chronic, bacterial): Oral: 500 mg every 12 hours for 28 days

Sinusitis (acute): Oral: 500 mg every 12 hours for 10 days

Typhoid fever: Oral: 500 mg every 12 hours for 10 days

Urinary tract infection:
Acute uncomplicated, cystitis:
Oral:
Immediate release formulation: 250 mg every 12 hours for 3 days
Extended release formulation (Cipro® XR, Proquin® XR): 500 mg every 24 hours for 3 days
I.V.: 200 mg every 12 hours for 7-14 days
Complicated (including pyelonephritis):
Oral:
Immediate release formulation: 500 mg every 12 hours for 7-14 days
Extended release formulation (Cipro® XR): 1000 mg every 24 hours for 7-14 days
I.V.: 400 mg every 12 hours for 7-14 days

*Combination therapy generally recommended.

Elderly: No adjustment needed in patients with normal renal function

Dosing adjustment in renal impairment: Adults:
Cl_{cr} 30-50 mL/minute: Oral: 250-500 mg every 12 hours
Cl_{cr} <30 mL/minute: Acute uncomplicated pyelonephritis or complicated UTI:
Oral: Extended release formulation: 500 mg every 24 hours
Cl_{cr} 5-29 mL/minute:
Oral: 250-500 mg every 18 hours
I.V.: 200-400 mg every 18-24 hours
Dialysis: Only small amounts of ciprofloxacin are removed by hemo- or peritoneal dialysis (<10%); usual dose: Oral: 250-500 mg every 24 hours following dialysis
Continuous arteriovenous or venovenous hemodiafiltration effects: Administer 200-400 mg I.V. every 12 hours

Mechanism of Action Inhibits DNA-gyrase in susceptible organisms; inhibits relaxation of supercoiled DNA and promotes breakage of double-stranded DNA

Contraindications Hypersensitivity to ciprofloxacin, any component of the formulation, or other quinolones; concurrent administration of tizanidine

Warnings/Precautions CNS stimulation may occur (tremor, restlessness, confusion, and very rarely hallucinations or seizures). Use with caution in patients with known or suspected CNS disorder. Potential for seizures, although very rare, may be increased with concomitant NSAID therapy. Use with caution in individuals at risk of seizures. Fluoroquinolones may prolong QT_c interval; avoid use in patients with a history of QT_c prolongation, uncorrected hypokalemia, hypomagnesemia, or concurrent administration of other medications known to prolong the QT interval (including Class Ia and Class III antiarrhythmics, cisapride, erythromycin, antipsychotics, and tricyclic antidepressants). Prolonged use may result in fungal or bacterial superinfection, including *C. difficile*-associated diarrhea and pseudomembranous colitis. Tendon inflammation and/or rupture have been reported with ciprofloxacin and other quinolone antibiotics. Risk may be increased with concurrent corticosteroids, particularly in the elderly. Discontinue at first sign of tendon inflammation or pain. Adverse effects, including those related to joints and/or surrounding tissues, are increased in pediatric patients and therefore, ciprofloxacin should not be considered as drug of choice in children (exception is anthrax treatment). Rare cases of peripheral neuropathy may occur.

Severe hypersensitivity reactions, including anaphylaxis, have occurred with quinolone therapy. Quinolones may exacerbate myasthenia gravis, use with caution (rare, potentially life-threatening weakness of respiratory muscles may occur). Use caution in renal impairment. Avoid excessive sunlight; may cause moderate-to-severe phototoxicity reactions.

Ciprofloxacin is a potent inhibitor of CYP1A2. Coadministration of drugs which depend on this pathway may lead to substantial increases in serum concentrations and adverse effects.

Drug Interactions Inhibits CYP1A2 (strong), 3A4 (weak)

Caffeine: Ciprofloxacin may decrease the metabolism of caffeine.

Corticosteroids: Concurrent use may increase the risk of tendon rupture, particularly in elderly patients (overall incidence rare).

CYP1A2 substrates: Ciprofloxacin may increase the levels/effects of CYP1A2 substrates. Example substrates include aminophylline, fluvoxamine, mexiletine, mirtazapine, ropinirole, tizanidine, and trifluoperazine.

Foscarnet: Concomitant use with ciprofloxacin has been associated with an increased risk of seizures.

Glyburide: Quinolones may increase the effect of glyburide; monitor.

Metal cations (aluminum, calcium, iron, magnesium, and zinc) bind quinolones in the gastrointestinal tract and inhibit absorption. Concurrent administration of most antacids, oral electrolyte supplements, quinapril, sucralfate, some didanosine formulations (pediatric powder for oral suspension), and other highly-buffered oral drugs, should be avoided. Ciprofloxacin should be administered 2 hours before or 6 hours after these agents.

Methotrexate: Ciprofloxacin may decrease renal secretion of methotrexate; monitor.

NSAIDs: Risk of seizures may be increased with concomitant NSAID use. Risk is considered quite low and may only be a factor with high serum levels of either agent and/or in patients with additional predisposing factors (eg, renal dysfunction, history of seizure or other neurological disorder).

Pentoxifylline: Monitor for headache during concomitant therapy.

Phenytoin: Ciprofloxacin may decrease phenytoin levels; monitor.

Probenecid: May decrease renal secretion of quinolones.

Ropivacaine: Ciprofloxacin may decrease the metabolism of ropivacaine.

Sevelamer: May decrease absorption of oral ciprofloxacin.

Theophylline: Serum levels may be increased by ciprofloxacin; in addition, CNS stimulation/seizures may occur at lower theophylline serum levels due to additive CNS effects.

Tizanidine: Ciprofloxacin may increase serum levels of tizanidine. Concurrent administration is contraindicated.

Warfarin: The hypoprothrombinemic effect of warfarin may be enhanced by ciprofloxacin; monitor INR.

Ethanol/Nutrition/Herb Interactions

Food: Food decreases rate, but not extent, of absorption. Ciprofloxacin serum levels may be decreased if taken with dairy products or calcium-fortified juices. Ciprofloxacin may increase serum caffeine levels if taken with caffeine. Enteral feedings may decrease plasma concentrations of ciprofloxacin probably by >30% inhibition of absorption. Ciprofloxacin should not be administered with enteral feedings. The feeding would need to be discontinued for 1-2 hours prior to and after ciprofloxacin administration. Nasogastric administration produces a greater loss of ciprofloxacin bioavailability than does nasoduodenal administration.

Herb/Nutraceutical: Avoid dong quai, St John's wort (may also cause photosensitization).

(Continued)

Ciprofloxacin *(Continued)*

Dietary Considerations

Food: Drug may cause GI upset; take without regard to meals (manufacturer prefers that immediate release tablet is taken 2 hours after meals). Extended release tablet may be taken with meals that contain dairy products (calcium content <800 mg), but not with dairy products alone.

Dairy products, calcium-fortified juices, oral multivitamins, and mineral supplements: Absorption of ciprofloxacin is decreased by divalent and trivalent cations. The manufacturer states that the usual dietary intake of calcium (including meals which include dairy products) has not been shown to interfere with ciprofloxacin absorption. Immediate release ciprofloxacin and Cipro® XR may be taken 2 hours before or 6 hours after, and Proquin® XR may be taken 4 hours before or 6 hours after, any of these products.

Caffeine: Patients consuming regular large quantities of caffeinated beverages may need to restrict caffeine intake if excessive cardiac or CNS stimulation occurs.

Pharmacodynamics/Kinetics

Absorption: Oral: Immediate release tablet: Rapid (~50% to 85%)

Distribution: V_d: 2.1-2.7 L/kg; tissue concentrations often exceed serum concentrations especially in kidneys, gallbladder, liver, lungs, gynecological tissue, and prostatic tissue; CSF concentrations: 10% of serum concentrations (noninflamed meninges), 14% to 37% (inflamed meninges); crosses placenta; enters breast milk

Protein binding: 20% to 40%

Metabolism: Partially hepatic; forms 4 metabolites (limited activity)

Half-life elimination: Children: 2.5 hours; Adults: Normal renal function: 3-5 hours

Time to peak: Oral:
Immediate release tablet: 0.5-2 hours
Extended release tablet: Cipro® XR: 1-2.5 hours, Proquin® XR: 3.5-8.7 hours

Excretion: Urine (30% to 50% as unchanged drug); feces (15% to 43%)

Pregnancy Risk Factor C

Lactation Enters breast milk/not recommended (AAP rates "compatible")

Breast-Feeding Considerations Ciprofloxacin is excreted in breast milk; however, the exposure to the infant is considered small and one source suggests that the decision to breast-feed be independent of the need for the antibiotic in the mother. Another source recommends the mother wait 48 hours after the last dose of ciprofloxacin to continue nursing. The manufacturer recommends to discontinue nursing or to discontinue ciprofloxacin.

Dosage Forms Excipient information presented when available (limited, particularly for generics); consult specific product labeling.

Infusion [premixed in D_5W]:
Cipro®: 200 mg (100 mL); 400 mg (200 mL) [latex free]

Injection, solution: 10 mg/mL (20 mL, 40 mL)
Cipro®: 10 mg/mL (20 mL, 40 mL)

Microcapsules for suspension, oral:
Cipro®: 250 mg/5 mL (100 mL); 500 mg/5 mL (100 mL) [strawberry flavor]

Ointment, ophthalmic, as hydrochloride:
Ciloxan®: 3.33 mg/g [0.3% base] (3.5 g)

Solution, ophthalmic, as hydrochloride: 3.5 mg/mL (2.5 mL, 5mL, 10 mL) [0.3% base]
Ciloxin®: 3.5 mg/mL (2.5 mL, 5mL, 10 mL) [0.3% base; contains benzalkonium chloride]

Tablet: 250 mg, 500 mg, 750 mg
Cipro®: 250 mg, 500 mg, 750 mg

Tablet, extended release: 500 mg, 1000 mg
Cipro® XR: 500 mg [equivalent to ciprofloxacin hydrochloride 287.5 mg and ciprofloxacin base 212.6 mg]; 1000 mg [equivalent to ciprofloxacin hydrochloride 574.9 mg and ciprofloxacin base 425.2 mg]
Proquin® XR: 500 mg

Tablet, extended release [dose pack]:
Proquin® XR: 500 mg (3s)

Selected Readings

Rams TE and Slots J, "Antibiotics in Periodontal Therapy: An Update," *Compendium*, 1992, 13(12):1130, 1132, 1134.

Wynn RL, Bergman SA, Meiller TF, et al, "Antibiotics in Treating Oral-Facial Infections of Odontogenic Origin: An Update," *Gen Dent*, 2001, 49(3):238-40, 242, 244 passim.

Ciprofloxacin and Dexamethasone
(sip roe FLOKS a sin & deks a METH a sone)

Related Information

Ciprofloxacin *on page 359*

Dexamethasone *on page 464*
U.S. Brand Names Ciprodex®
Canadian Brand Names Ciprodex®
Generic Available No
Index Terms Ciprofloxacin Hydrochloride and Dexamethasone; Dexamethasone and Ciprofloxacin
Pharmacologic Category Antibiotic/Corticosteroid, Otic
Use Treatment of acute otitis media in pediatric patients with tympanostomy tubes or acute otitis externa in children and adults
Local Anesthetic/Vasoconstrictor Precautions No information available to require special precautions
Effects on Dental Treatment No significant effects or complications reported
Mechanism of Action Ciprofloxacin is a quinolone antibiotic; dexamethasone is a corticosteroid used to decrease inflammation accompanying bacterial infections
Pregnancy Risk Factor C

Ciprofloxacin and Hydrocortisone
(sip roe FLOKS a sin & hye droe KOR ti sone)

Related Information
Ciprofloxacin *on page 359*
Hydrocortisone *on page 836*
U.S. Brand Names Cipro® HC
Canadian Brand Names Cipro® HC
Generic Available No
Index Terms Ciprofloxacin Hydrochloride and Hydrocortisone; Hydrocortisone and Ciprofloxacin
Pharmacologic Category Antibiotic/Corticosteroid, Otic
Use Treatment of acute otitis externa, sometimes known as "swimmer's ear"
Local Anesthetic/Vasoconstrictor Precautions No information available to require special precautions
Effects on Dental Treatment No significant effects or complications reported

Ciprofloxacin Hydrochloride *see* Ciprofloxacin *on page 359*
Ciprofloxacin Hydrochloride and Dexamethasone *see* Ciprofloxacin and Dexamethasone *on page 364*
Ciprofloxacin Hydrochloride and Hydrocortisone *see* Ciprofloxacin and Hydrocortisone *on page 365*
Cipro® HC *see* Ciprofloxacin and Hydrocortisone *on page 365*
Cipro® XR *see* Ciprofloxacin *on page 359*

Cisapride (SIS a pride)

U.S. Brand Names Propulsid®
Mexican Brand Names Enteropride; Eriken; Kinestase; Prepulsid; Presiston; Unamol
Generic Available No
Pharmacologic Category Gastrointestinal Agent, Prokinetic
Use Treatment of nocturnal symptoms of gastroesophageal reflux disease (GERD); has demonstrated effectiveness for gastroparesis, refractory constipation, and nonulcer dyspepsia
Local Anesthetic/Vasoconstrictor Precautions Cisapride is one of the drugs confirmed to prolong the QT interval and is accepted as having a risk of causing torsade de pointes. The risk of drug-induced torsade de pointes is extremely low when a single QT interval prolonging drug is prescribed. In terms of epinephrine, it is not known what effect vasoconstrictors in the local anesthetic regimen will have in patients with a known history of congenital prolonged QT interval or in patients taking any medication that prolongs the QT interval. Until more information is obtained, it is suggested that the clinician consult with the physician prior to the use of a vasoconstrictor in suspected patients, and that the vasoconstrictor (epinephrine, levonordefrin [Neo-Cobefrin®]) be used with caution.
Effects on Dental Treatment Key adverse event(s) related to dental treatment: Xerostomia (normal salivary flow resumes upon discontinuation).
Common Adverse Effects
>5%:
  Central nervous system: Headache
  Dermatologic: Rash
  Gastrointestinal: Diarrhea, GI cramping, dyspepsia, flatulence, nausea, xerostomia
(Continued)

Cisapride *(Continued)*

Respiratory: Rhinitis

<5%:

Cardiovascular: Tachycardia

Central nervous system: Extrapyramidal effects, somnolence, fatigue, seizure, insomnia, anxiety

Hematologic: Thrombocytopenia, increased LFTs, pancytopenia, leukopenia, granulocytopenia, aplastic anemia

Respiratory: Sinusitis, cough, upper respiratory tract infection, increased incidence of viral infection

Restrictions In U.S., available via limited-access protocol only (1-800-JANSSEN).

Mechanism of Action Enhances the release of acetylcholine at the myenteric plexus. *In vitro* studies have shown cisapride to have serotonin-4 receptor agonistic properties which may increase gastrointestinal motility and cardiac rate; increases lower esophageal sphincter pressure and lower esophageal peristalsis; accelerates gastric emptying of both liquids and solids.

Drug Interactions

Cytochrome P450 Effect: Substrate of CYP1A2 (minor), 2A6 (minor), 2B6 (minor), 2C9 (minor), 2C19 (minor), 3A4 (major); **Inhibits** CYP2D6 (weak), 3A4 (weak)

Increased Effect/Toxicity: Cisapride may increase blood levels of warfarin, diazepam, cimetidine, ranitidine, and CNS depressants. The risk of cisapride-induced malignant arrhythmias may be increased by azole antifungals (fluconazole, itraconazole, ketoconazole, miconazole), antiarrhythmics (Class Ia; quinidine, procainamide, and Class III; amiodarone, sotalol), bepridil, cimetidine, maprotiline, macrolide antibiotics (erythromycin, clarithromycin, troleandomycin), molindone, nefazodone, protease inhibitors (amprenavir, atazanavir, indinavir, nelfinavir, ritonavir), phenothiazines (eg, prochlorperazine, promethazine), sertindole, tricyclic antidepressants (eg amitriptyline), and some quinolone antibiotics (sparfloxacin, gatifloxacin, moxifloxacin). Other strong inhibitors of CYP3A4 (including diclofenac, doxycycline, imatinib, isoniazid, nefazodone, nicardipine, propofol, telithromycin, and verapamil) should be avoided. Cardiovascular disease or electrolyte imbalances (potentially due to diuretic therapy) increase the risk of malignant arrhythmias.

Decreased Effect: Cisapride may decrease the effect of atropine and digoxin.

Pharmacodynamics/Kinetics

Onset of action: 0.5-1 hour

Protein binding: 97.5% to 98%

Metabolism: Extensively hepatic to norcisapride

Bioavailability: 35% to 40%

Half-life elimination: 6-12 hours

Excretion: Urine and feces (<10%)

Pregnancy Risk Factor C

Cisaplatin (SIS pla tin)

U.S. Brand Names Platinol®-AQ [DSC]

Mexican Brand Names Blastolem; Niyaplat; Tecnoplatin

Generic Available Yes

Index Terms CDDP

Pharmacologic Category Antineoplastic Agent, Alkylating Agent

Use Treatment of bladder, testicular, and ovarian cancer

Unlabeled/Investigational Use Treatment of head and neck, breast, gastric, lung, esophageal, cervical, prostate and small cell lung cancer; Hodgkin's and non-Hodgkin's lymphoma; neuroblastoma; sarcomas, myeloma, melanoma, mesothelioma, and osteosarcoma

Local Anesthetic/Vasoconstrictor Precautions No information available to require special precautions

Effects on Dental Treatment No significant effects or complications reported

Common Adverse Effects

>10%:

Central nervous system: Neurotoxicity: Peripheral neuropathy is dose- and duration-dependent.

Dermatologic: Mild alopecia

Gastrointestinal: Nausea and vomiting (76% to 100%)

Hematologic: Myelosuppression (25% to 30%; mild with moderate doses, mild to moderate with high-dose therapy)

WBC: Mild

Platelets: Mild

Onset: 10 days
Nadir: 14-23 days
Recovery: 21-39 days
Hepatic: Liver enzymes increased
Renal: Nephrotoxicity (acute renal failure and chronic renal insufficiency)
Otic: Ototoxicity (10% to 30%; manifested as high frequency hearing loss; ototoxicity is especially pronounced in children)
1% to 10%:
Gastrointestinal: Diarrhea
Local: Tissue irritation

Mechanism of Action Inhibits DNA synthesis by the formation of DNA cross-links; denatures the double helix; covalently binds to DNA bases and disrupts DNA function; may also bind to proteins; the *cis*-isomer is 14 times more cytotoxic than the *trans*-isomer; both forms cross-link DNA but cis-platinum is less easily recognized by cell enzymes and, therefore, not repaired. Cisplatin can also bind two adjacent guanines on the same strand of DNA producing intrastrand cross-linking and breakage.

Drug Interactions

Increased Effect/Toxicity: Cisplatin and ethacrynic acid have resulted in severe ototoxicity in animals. Delayed bleomycin elimination with decreased glomerular filtration rate. When administered as sequential infusions, observational studies indicate a potential for increased toxicity when platinum derivatives (carboplatin, cisplatin) are administered before taxane derivatives (docetaxel, paclitaxel).

Decreased Effect: Sodium thiosulfate and amifostine theoretically inactivate drug systemically; have been used clinically to reduce systemic toxicity with administration of cisplatin.

Pharmacodynamics/Kinetics
Distribution: I.V.: Rapidly into tissue; high concentrations in kidneys, liver, ovaries, uterus, and lungs
Protein binding: >90%
Metabolism: Nonenzymatic; inactivated (in both cell and bloodstream) by sulfhydryl groups; covalently binds to glutathione and thiosulfate
Half-life elimination: Initial: 20-30 minutes; Beta: 60 minutes; Terminal: ~24 hours; Secondary half-life: 44-73 hours
Excretion: Urine (>90%); feces (10%)

Pregnancy Risk Factor D

13-*cis*-Retinoic Acid *see* Isotretinoin *on page 918*

Citalopram (sye TAL oh pram)

Related Information
Escitalopram *on page 596*
U.S. Brand Names Celexa®
Canadian Brand Names Apo-Citalopram®; Celexa®; CO Citalopram; Dom-Citalopram; Gen-Citalopram; Novo-Citalopram; PHL-Citalopram; PMS-Citalopram; RAN™-Citalopram; ratio-Citalopram; Rhoxal-citalopram; Sandoz-Citalopram
Mexican Brand Names Seropram
Generic Available Yes
Index Terms Citalopram Hydrobromide; Nitalapram
Pharmacologic Category Antidepressant, Selective Serotonin Reuptake Inhibitor
Use Treatment of depression
Unlabeled/Investigational Use Treatment of dementia, smoking cessation, ethanol abuse, obsessive-compulsive disorder (OCD) in children, diabetic neuropathy
Local Anesthetic/Vasoconstrictor Precautions Although caution should be used in patients taking tricyclic antidepressants, no interactions have been reported with vasoconstrictors and citalopram, a nontricyclic antidepressant which acts to increase serotonin; no precautions appear to be needed
Effects on Dental Treatment Key adverse event(s) related to dental treatment: Xerostomia (normal salivary flow resumes upon discontinuation). Premarketing trials reported abnormal taste. See Dental Comment.

Common Adverse Effects
>10%:
Central nervous system: Somnolence, insomnia
Gastrointestinal: Nausea, xerostomia
Miscellaneous: Diaphoresis
<10%:
Central nervous system: Anxiety, anorexia, agitation, yawning
Dermatologic: Rash, pruritus
(Continued)

Citalopram *(Continued)*

Endocrine & metabolic: Sexual dysfunction

Gastrointestinal: Diarrhea, dyspepsia, vomiting, abdominal pain, weight gain

Neuromuscular & skeletal: Tremor, arthralgia, myalgia

Respiratory: Cough, rhinitis, sinusitis

Restrictions An FDA-approved medication guide concerning the use of antide-pressants in children, adolescents, and young adults must be distributed when dispensing an outpatient prescription (new or refill) where this medication is to be used without direct supervision of a healthcare provider. Medication guides are available at http://www.fda.gov/cder/Offices/ODS/medication_guides.htm. Dispense to parents or guardians of children and adolescents receiving this medication.

Dosage Oral:

Children and Adolescents: OCD (unlabeled use): 10-40 mg/day

Adults: Depression: Initial: 20 mg/day, generally with an increase to 40 mg/day; doses of more than 40 mg are not usually necessary. Should a dose increase be necessary, it should occur in 20 mg increments at intervals of no less than 1 week. Maximum dose: 60 mg/day; reduce dosage in elderly or those with hepatic impairment.

Mechanism of Action A bicyclic phthalane derivative, citalopram selectively inhibits serotonin reuptake in the presynaptic neurons

Contraindications Hypersensitivity to citalopram or any component of the formulation; hypersensitivity or other adverse sequelae during therapy with other SSRIs; concomitant use with MAO inhibitors or within 2 weeks of discontinuing MAO inhibitors

Warnings/Precautions [U.S. Boxed Warning]: Antidepressants increase the risk of suicidal thinking and behavior in children, adolescents, and young adults (18-24 years of age) with major depressive disorder (MDD) and other psychiatric disorders; consider risk prior to prescribing. Short-term studies did not show an increased risk in patients >24 years of age and showed a decreased risk in patients ≥65 years. Closely monitor patients for clinical worsening, suicidality, or unusual changes in behavior, particularly during the initial 1-2 months of therapy or during periods of dosage adjustments (increases or decreases); the patient's family or caregiver should be instructed to closely observe the patient and communicate condition with healthcare provider. A medication guide concerning the use of antidepressants should be dispensed with each prescription. **Citalopram is not FDA approved for use in children.**

The possibility of a suicide attempt is inherent in major depression and may persist until remission occurs. Use caution in high-risk patients. Worsening depression and severe abrupt suicidality that are not part of the presenting symptoms may require discontinuation or modification of drug therapy. The patient's family or caregiver should be alerted to monitor patients for the emergence of suicidality and associated behaviors (such as agitation, irritability, hostility, impulsivity, and hypomania) and call healthcare provider.

May worsen psychosis in some patients or precipitate a shift to mania or hypomania in patients with bipolar disorder. Patients presenting with depressive symptoms should be screened for bipolar disorder. Monotherapy in patients with bipolar disorder should be avoided. **Citalopram is not FDA approved for the treatment of bipolar depression.**

The potential for severe reaction exists when used with MAO inhibitors, SSRIs/SNRIs or triptans; serotonin syndrome (hyperthermia, muscular rigidity, mental status changes/agitation, autonomic instability) may occur. Concurrent use with MAO inhibitors is contraindicated. May increase the risks associated with electroconvulsive therapy. Has a low potential to impair cognitive or motor performance; caution operating hazardous machinery or driving.

Use with caution in patients with hepatic or renal dysfunction, in elderly patients, concomitant CNS depressants, and pregnancy (high doses of citalopram have been associated with teratogenicity in animals). Use caution with concomitant use of NSAIDs, ASA, or other drugs that affect coagulation; the risk of bleeding is potentiated. May cause hyponatremia/SIADH. May cause or exacerbate sexual dysfunction. Upon discontinuation of citalopram therapy, gradually taper dose. If intolerable symptoms occur following a decrease in dosage or upon discontinuation of therapy, then resuming the previous dose with a more gradual taper should be considered.

Drug Interactions

Cytochrome P450 Effect: Substrate of CYP2C19 (major), 2D6 (minor), 3A4 (major); **Inhibits** CYP1A2 (weak), 2B6 (weak), 2C19 (weak), 2D6 (weak)

Increased Effect/Toxicity: Citalopram should not be used with nonselective MAO inhibitors (phenelzine, isocarboxazid) or other drugs with MAO inhibition (linezolid); fatal reactions have been reported. Wait 2 weeks after stopping an MAO inhibitor before starting citalopram. Concurrent selegiline has been associated with mania, hypertension, or serotonin syndrome (risk may be reduced relative to nonselective MAO inhibitors).

CYP2C19 inhibitors may increase the levels/effects of citalopram; example inhibitors include delavirdine, fluconazole, fluvoxamine, gemfibrozil, isoniazid, omeprazole, and ticlopidine. CYP3A4 inhibitors may increase the levels/effects of citalopram; example inhibitors include azole antifungals, clarithromycin, diclofenac, doxycycline, erythromycin, imatinib, isoniazid, nefazodone, nicardipine, propofol, protease inhibitors, quinidine, telithromycin, and verapamil.

Combined use of SSRIs and amphetamines, buspirone, meperidine, nefazodone, serotonin agonists (such as sumatriptan), sibutramine, other SSRIs/SNRIs, sympathomimetics, ritonavir, tramadol, and venlafaxine may increase the risk of serotonin syndrome. Risk of hyponatremia may increase with concurrent use of loop diuretics (bumetanide, furosemide, torsemide). Citalopram may increase the hypoprothrombinemic response to warfarin. Concomitant use of citalopram and NSAIDs, aspirin, or other drugs affecting coagulation has been associated with an increased risk of bleeding; monitor.

Combined use of sumatriptan (and other serotonin agonists) may result in toxicity; weakness, hyper-reflexia, and incoordination have been observed with sumatriptan and SSRIs. In addition, concurrent use may theoretically increase the risk of serotonin syndrome; includes sumatriptan, naratriptan, rizatriptan, and zolmitriptan.

Decreased Effect: CYP2C19 inducers may decrease the levels/effects of citalopram; example inducers include aminoglutethimide, carbamazepine, phenytoin, and rifampin. Cyproheptadine may inhibit the effects of serotonin reuptake inhibitors. CYP3A4 inducers may decrease the levels/effects of citalopram; example inducers include aminoglutethimide, carbamazepine, nafcillin, nevirapine, phenobarbital, phenytoin, and rifamycins.

Ethanol/Nutrition/Herb Interactions

Ethanol: Avoid ethanol (may increase CNS depression).

Herb/Nutraceutical: Avoid valerian, St John's wort, SAMe, kava kava, and gotu kola (may increase CNS depression).

Dietary Considerations May be taken without regard to food.

Pharmacodynamics/Kinetics

Distribution: V_d: 12 L/kg

Protein binding, plasma: ~80%

Metabolism: Extensively hepatic, primarily via CYP3A4 and 2C19; forms metabolites, N-demethylcitalopram (DCT) and didemethylcitalopram (DDCT) which are ~ eight times less potent than citalopram

Bioavailability: 80%

Half-life elimination: 24-48 hours (average: 35 hours); doubled with hepatic impairment

Time to peak, serum: 1-6 hours, average within 4 hours

Excretion: Urine (Citalopram 10% and DCT 5%)

Note: Clearance was decreased, while AUC and half-life were significantly increased in elderly patients and in patients with hepatic impairment. Mild-to-moderate renal impairment may reduce clearance (17%) and prolong half-life of citalopram. No pharmacokinetic information is available concerning patients with severe renal impairment.

Pregnancy Risk Factor C

Dosage Forms

Solution, oral: 10 mg/5 mL

Celexa®: 10 mg/5 mL

Tablet: 10 mg, 20 mg, 40 mg

Celexa®: 10 mg, 20 mg, 40 mg

Dental Comment Problems with SSRI-induced bruxism have been reported and may preclude their use; clinicians attempting to evaluate any patient with bruxism or involuntary muscle movement, who is simultaneously being treated with an SSRI drug, should be aware of the potential association.

Citric Acid, Magnesium Carbonate, and Glucono-Delta-Lactone
(SI trik AS id, mag NEE see um KAR bo nate, and GLOO kon o DEL ta LAK tone)

U.S. Brand Names Renacidin®
Generic Available No
Index Terms Citric Acid and d-gluconic Acid Irrigant; Citric Acid Bladder Mixture; Citric Acid, Magnesium Hydroxycarbonate, D-Gluconic Acid, Magnesium Acid Citrate, and Calcium Carbonate; Hemiacidrin
Pharmacologic Category Genitourinary Irrigant; Urinary Tract Product
Use Prevention of formation of calcifications of indwelling urinary tract catheters; treatment of renal and bladder calculi of the apatite or struvite type
Local Anesthetic/Vasoconstrictor Precautions No information available to require special precautions
Effects on Dental Treatment No significant effects or complications reported
Common Adverse Effects
>10%:
   Central nervous system: Fever (20% to 40%)
   Genitourinary: Urothelial ulceration with or without edema (13%)
   Miscellaneous: Transient flank pain
1% to 10%:
   Endocrine & metabolic: Hypermagnesemia, hyperphosphatemia
   Genitourinary: Urinary tract infection, dysuria, hematuria, bladder irritability
   Neuromuscular & skeletal: Back pain
   Renal: Creatinine increased
Mechanism of Action Magnesium from the irrigating solution is exchanged for calcium in the stone matrix. The magnesium stones are soluble and are able to dissolve in the acidic pH of the solution.
Pregnancy Risk Factor C

Citric Acid, Magnesium Hydroxycarbonate, D-Gluconic Acid, Magnesium Acid Citrate, and Calcium Carbonate see Citric Acid, Magnesium Carbonate, and Glucono-Delta-Lactone on page 370

Citric Acid, Sodium Citrate, and Potassium Citrate
(SIT rik AS id, SOW dee um SIT rate, & poe TASS ee um SIT rate)

Related Information
   Potassium Citrate on page 1329
U.S. Brand Names Cytra-3; Polycitra®; Polycitra®-LC
Generic Available Yes
Index Terms Potassium Citrate, Citric Acid, and Sodium Citrate; Sodium Citrate, Citric Acid, and Potassium Citrate
Pharmacologic Category Alkalinizing Agent, Oral
Use Conditions where long-term maintenance of an alkaline urine is desirable as in control and dissolution of uric acid and cystine calculi of the urinary tract
Local Anesthetic/Vasoconstrictor Precautions No information available to require special precautions
Effects on Dental Treatment No significant effects or complications reported
Common Adverse Effects Frequency not defined.
   Cardiovascular: Cardiac abnormalities
   Endocrine & metabolic: Metabolic alkalosis, calcium levels, hyperkalemia, hypernatremia
   Gastrointestinal: Diarrhea
   Neuromuscular & skeletal: Tetany
Drug Interactions
   Increased Effect/Toxicity: Increased toxicity/levels of amphetamines, ephedrine, pseudoephedrine, flecainide, quinidine, and quinine due to urinary alkalinization.
   Decreased Effect: Decreased effect/levels of lithium, chlorpropamide, and salicylates due to urinary alkalinization.
Pregnancy Risk Factor Not established

Citroma® [OTC] see Magnesium Citrate on page 1013
Citrovorum Factor see Leucovorin on page 957
Citrucel® [OTC] see Methylcellulose on page 1077
Citrucel® Fiber Shake [OTC] see Methylcellulose on page 1077
Citrucel® Fiber Smoothie [OTC] see Methylcellulose on page 1077
CL-118,532 see Triptorelin on page 1625
Cl-719 see Gemfibrozil on page 772

CL-825 *see* Pentostatin *on page 1277*
CL-184116 *see* Porfimer *on page 1324*

Cladribine (KLA dri been)

U.S. Brand Names Leustatin®
Canadian Brand Names Leustatin®
Generic Available Yes
Index Terms 2-CdA; 2-Chlorodeoxyadenosine; NSC-105014
Pharmacologic Category Antineoplastic Agent, Antimetabolite; Antineoplastic Agent, Antimetabolite (Purine Antagonist)
Use Treatment of hairy cell leukemia
Unlabeled/Investigational Use Treatment of chronic lymphocytic leukemia (CLL), chronic myelogenous leukemia (CML), non-Hodgkin's lymphomas, progressive multiple sclerosis
Local Anesthetic/Vasoconstrictor Precautions No information available to require special precautions
Effects on Dental Treatment No significant effects or complications reported
Common Adverse Effects
>10%:
    Central nervous system: Fever (69%; ≥104°F: 11%), fatigue (11% to 45%), headache (7% to 22%)
    Dermatologic: Rash (10% to 27%)
    Gastrointestinal: Nausea (28%), appetite decreased (17%), vomiting (13%)
    Hematologic: Myelosuppression, common, dose limiting (nadir: 5-10 days, recovery: 4-8 weeks); neutropenia (70%); anemia (37%); thrombocytopenia (12%)
    Local: Injection site reactions (9% to 19%)
    Respiratory: Abnormal breath sounds (11%)
    Miscellaneous: Infection (28%)
1% to 10%:
    Cardiovascular: Edema (6%), tachycardia (6%), thrombosis (2%)
    Central nervous system: Dizziness (9%), chills (9%), insomnia (7%), malaise (5% to 7%), pain (6%)
    Dermatologic: Purpura (10%), petechiae (8%), pruritus (6%), erythema (6%)
    Gastrointestinal: Diarrhea (10%), constipation (9%), abdominal pain (6%)
    Local: Phlebitis (2%)
    Neuromuscular & skeletal: Weakness (9%), myalgia (7%), arthralgia (5%)
    Respiratory: Cough (7% to 10%), abnormal chest sounds (9%), dyspnea (7%), epistaxis (5%)
    Miscellaneous: Diaphoresis (9%)
Mechanism of Action A purine nucleoside analogue; prodrug which is activated via phosphorylation by deoxycytidine kinase to a 5'-triphosphate derivative. This active form incorporates into DNA to result in the breakage of DNA strand and shutdown of DNA synthesis. This also results in a depletion of nicotinamide adenine dinucleotide and adenosine triphosphate (ATP). Cladribine is cell-cycle nonspecific.
Pharmacodynamics/Kinetics
Absorption: Oral: 55%; SubQ: 100%; Rectal: 20%
Distribution: V_d: 4.52 ± 2.82 L/kg
Protein binding: 20%
Metabolism: Hepatic; 5'-triphosphate moiety-active
Half-life elimination: Biphasic: Alpha: 25 minutes; Beta: 6.7 hours; Terminal, mean: Normal renal function: 5.4 hours
Excretion: Urine (18% to 44%)
    Clearance: Estimated systemic: 640 mL/hour/kg
Pregnancy Risk Factor D

Claforan® *see* Cefotaxime *on page 303*
Claravis™ *see* Isotretinoin *on page 918*
Clarinex® *see* Desloratadine *on page 460*
Clarinex-D® 12 Hour *see* Desloratadine and Pseudoephedrine *on page 461*
Clarinex-D® 24 Hour *see* Desloratadine and Pseudoephedrine *on page 461*
Claripel™ *see* Hydroquinone *on page 841*

Clarithromycin (kla RITH roe mye sin)

Related Information
    Antibiotic Prophylaxis *on page 1772*
    Bacterial Infections *on page 1793*
    Gastrointestinal Disorders *on page 1745*
    Respiratory Diseases *on page 1747*
    (Continued)

Clarithromycin *(Continued)*

U.S. Brand Names Biaxin®; Biaxin® XL

Canadian Brand Names Biaxin®; Biaxin® XL; ratio-Clarithromycin

Mexican Brand Names Adel; Gervaken; Klaricid; Klaricid H.P.; Klaricid O.D.; Macrobiol; Macrobiol S.R.

Generic Available Yes: Tablet

Pharmacologic Category Antibiotic, Macrolide

Dental Use Alternate oral antibiotic for prevention of infective endocarditis in individuals allergic to penicillins or ampicillin, when amoxicillin cannot be used; alternate antibiotic in the treatment of common orofacial infections caused by aerobic gram-positive cocci and susceptible anaerobes

Use

Children:

Acute otitis media (*H. influenzae, M. catarrhalis,* or *S. pneumoniae*)

Community-acquired pneumonia due to susceptible *Mycoplasma pneumoniae, S. pneumoniae,* or *Chlamydia pneumoniae* (TWAR)

Pharyngitis/tonsillitis, acute maxillary sinusitis, uncomplicated skin/skin structure infections, and mycobacterial infections

Prevention of disseminated mycobacterial infections due to MAC disease in patients with advanced HIV infection

Adults:

Pharyngitis/tonsillitis due to susceptible *S. pyogenes*

Acute maxillary sinusitis and acute exacerbation of chronic bronchitis due to susceptible *H. influenzae, M. catarrhalis,* or *S. pneumoniae*

Community-acquired pneumonia due to susceptible *H. influenzae, H. parainfluenzae, Mycoplasma pneumoniae, S. pneumoniae,* or *Chlamydia pneumoniae* (TWAR)

Uncomplicated skin/skin structure infections due to susceptible *S. aureus, S. pyogenes*

Disseminated mycobacterial infections due to *M. avium* or *M. intracellulare*

Prevention of disseminated mycobacterial infections due to *M. avium* complex (MAC) disease (eg, patients with advanced HIV infection)

Duodenal ulcer disease due to *H. pylori* in regimens with other drugs including amoxicillin and lansoprazole or omeprazole, ranitidine bismuth citrate, bismuth subsalicylate, tetracycline, and/or an H_2 antagonist

Unlabeled/Investigational Use Pertussis (CDC guidelines); alternate antibiotic for prophylaxis of bacterial endocarditis in patients who are allergic to penicillin and undergoing surgical or dental procedures (ACC/AHA guidelines)

Local Anesthetic/Vasoconstrictor Precautions Clarithromycin is one of the drugs confirmed to prolong the QT interval and is accepted as having a risk of causing torsade de pointes. In terms of epinephrine, it is not known what effect vasoconstrictors in the local anesthetic regimen will have in patients with a known history of congenital prolonged QT interval or in patients taking any medication that prolongs the QT interval. Until more information is obtained, it is suggested that the clinician consult with the physician prior to the use of a vasoconstrictor in suspected patients, and that the vasoconstrictor (epinephrine, levonordefrin [Neo-Cobefrin®]) be used with caution. See Dental Comment.

Effects on Dental Treatment Key adverse event(s) related to dental treatment: Abnormal taste.

Significant Adverse Effects

1% to 10%:

Central nervous system: Headache (adults and children 2%)

Dermatologic: Rash (children 3%)

Gastrointestinal: Abnormal taste (adults 3% to 7%), diarrhea (adults 3% to 6%; children 6%), vomiting (children 6%), nausea (adults 3%), abdominal pain (adults 2%; children 3%), dyspepsia 2%

Hepatic: Prothrombin time increased (1%)

Renal: BUN increased (4%)

<1% (Limited to important or life-threatening): *Clostridium difficile* colitis, alkaline phosphatase increased, anaphylaxis, anorexia, anxiety, behavioral changes, bilirubin increased, confusion, disorientation, GGT increased, glossitis, hallucinations, hearing loss (reversible), hepatic dysfunction, hepatic failure, hepatitis, hypoglycemia, insomnia, interstitial nephritis, jaundice, leukopenia, manic behavior, neutropenia, oral moniliasis, pancreatitis, psychosis, QT prolongation, seizure, serum creatinine increased, Stevens-Johnson syndrome, stomatitis, tinnitus, tongue discoloration, tooth discoloration, torsade de pointes, toxic epidermal necrolysis, transaminases increased, tremor, urticaria, ventricular tachycardia, ventricular arrhythmia, vertigo

Dental Usual Dosing Infective endocarditis prophylaxis: Oral:

Children: 15 mg/kg 30-60 minutes before procedure

Adolescents ≥16 years and Adults: 500 mg 30-60 minutes prior to procedure

Dosage

Usual dosage range:

Children ≥6 months: Oral: 7.5 mg/kg every 12 hours (maximum: 500 mg/dose)

Adults: Oral: 250-500 mg every 12 hours **or** 1000 mg (two 500 mg extended release tablets) once daily for 7-14 days

Indication-specific dosing:

Children: Oral:

Community-acquired pneumonia, sinusitis, bronchitis, skin infections: 15 mg/kg/day divided every 12 hours for 10 days

Endocarditis, prophylaxis (unlabeled use): 15 mg/kg 1 hour before procedure (maximum: 500 mg)

Mycobacterial infection (prevention and treatment): 7.5 mg/kg (up to 500 mg) twice daily. **Note:** Safety of clarithromycin for MAC not studied in children <20 months.

Pertussis (unlabeled use; CDC guidelines):

Children 1-5 months: 15 mg/kg/day divided every 12 hours for 7 days

Children ≥6 months: 15 mg/kg/day divided every 12 hours for 7 days (maximum: 1 g/day)

Adults: Oral:

Acute exacerbation of chronic bronchitis:

M. catarrhalis and *S. pneumoniae*: 250 mg every 12 hours for 7-14 days **or** 1000 mg (two 500 mg extended release tablets) once daily for 7 days

H. influenzae: 500 mg every 12 hours for 7-14 days or 1000 mg (two 500 mg extended release tablets) once daily for 7 days

H. parainfluenzae: 500 mg every 12 hours for 7 days or 1000 mg (two 500 mg extended release tablets) once daily for 7 days

Acute maxillary sinusitis: 500 mg every 12 hours **or** 1000 mg (two 500 mg extended release tablets) once daily for 14 days

Endocarditis, prophylaxis (unlabeled use): 500 mg 1 hour prior to procedure

Mycobacterial infection (prevention and treatment): 500 mg twice daily (use with other antimycobacterial drugs, eg, ethambutol or rifampin)

Peptic ulcer disease: Eradication of *Helicobacter pylori*: Dual or triple combination regimens with bismuth subsalicylate, amoxicillin, an H_2-receptor antagonist, or proton-pump inhibitor: 500 mg every 8-12 hours for 10-14 days

Pertussis (unlabeled use; CDC guidelines): 500 mg twice daily for 7 days

Pharyngitis, tonsillitis: 250 mg every 12 hours for 10 days

Pneumonia:

C. pneumoniae, *M. pneumoniae*, and *S. pneumoniae*: 250 mg every 12 hours for 7-14 days **or** 1000 mg (two 500 mg extended release tablets) once daily for 7 days

H. influenzae: 250 mg every 12 hours for 7 days **or** 1000 mg (two 500 mg extended release tablets) once daily for 7 days

Skin and skin structure infection, uncomplicated: 250 mg every 12 hours for 7-14 days

Elderly: Pharmacokinetics are similar to those in younger adults; may have age-related reductions in renal function; monitor and adjust dose if necessary

Dosing adjustment in renal impairment:

Cl_{cr} <30 mL/minute: Half the normal dose or double the dosing interval

In combination with ritonavir:

Cl_{cr} 30-60 mL/minute: Decrease clarithromycin dose by 50%

Cl_{cr} <30 mL/minute: Decrease clarithromycin dose by 75%

Dosing adjustment in hepatic impairment: No dosing adjustment is needed as long as renal function is normal

Mechanism of Action Exerts its antibacterial action by binding to 50S ribosomal subunit resulting in inhibition of protein synthesis. The 14-OH metabolite of clarithromycin is twice as active as the parent compound against certain organisms.

Contraindications Hypersensitivity to clarithromycin, erythromycin, or any macrolide antibiotic; use with ergot derivatives, pimozide, cisapride

Warnings/Precautions Dosage adjustment required with severe renal impairment; decreased dosage or prolonged dosing interval may be appropriate. Prolonged use may result in fungal or bacterial superinfection, including *C. difficile*-associated diarrhea and pseudomembranous colitis. Macrolides (including clarithromycin) have been associated with rare QT prolongation and ventricular arrhythmias, including torsade de pointes. Use caution in patients with coronary artery disease. Avoid use of extended release tablets (Biaxin® XL) in patients with known stricture/narrowing of the GI tract. Safety and efficacy in children <6 months of age have not been established.

Drug Interactions Substrate of CYP3A4 (major); **Inhibits** CYP1A2 (weak), 3A4 (strong)

(Continued)

Clarithromycin *(Continued)*

Alfentanil (and possibly other opioid analgesics): Serum levels may be increased by clarithromycin; monitor for increased effect.

Azole antifungal agents: Serum levels/effects may be increased by clarithromycin; monitor.

Benzodiazepines (those metabolized by CYP3A4, including alprazolam, midazolam, triazolam): Serum levels may be increased by clarithromycin; somnolence and confusion have been reported.

Bromocriptine: Serum levels/toxicity (eg, ergotism) may be increased by clarithromycin; monitor for increased effect.

Buspirone: Serum levels may be increased by clarithromycin; monitor.

Calcium channel blockers (felodipine, verapamil, and potentially others metabolized by CYP3A4): Serum levels may be increased by clarithromycin; monitor.

Carbamazepine: Serum levels may be increased by clarithromycin; monitor.

Cilostazol: Serum levels may be increased by clarithromycin; monitor.

Cisapride: Serum levels may be increased by clarithromycin; serious arrhythmias have occurred; concurrent use contraindicated.

Clopidogrel: Therapeutic effect may be decreased by clarithromycin; monitor.

Clozapine: Serum levels may be increased by clarithromycin; monitor.

Colchicine: Serum levels/toxicity may be increased by clarithromycin; monitor. Avoid use, if possible.

CYP3A4 inducers: CYP3A4 inducers may decrease the levels/effects of clarithromycin. Example inducers include aminoglutethimide, carbamazepine, nafcillin, nevirapine, phenobarbital, phenytoin, and rifamycins.

CYP3A4 inhibitors: May increase the levels/effects of clarithromycin. Example inhibitors include azole antifungals, diclofenac, doxycycline, erythromycin, imatinib, isoniazid, nefazodone, nicardipine, propofol, protease inhibitors, quinidine, telithromycin, and verapamil.

CYP3A4 substrates: Clarithromycin may increase the levels/effects of CYP3A4 substrates. Example substrates include benzodiazepines, calcium channel blockers, mirtazapine, nateglinide, nefazodone, tacrolimus, and venlafaxine. Selected benzodiazepines (midazolam and triazolam), cisapride, ergot alkaloids, selected HMG-CoA reductase inhibitors (lovastatin and simvastatin), and pimozide are generally contraindicated with strong CYP3A4 inhibitors.

Delavirdine: Serum levels may be increased by clarithromycin; monitor.

Digoxin: Serum levels may be increased by clarithromycin; digoxin toxicity and potentially fatal arrhythmias have been reported; monitor digoxin levels.

Disopyramide: Serum levels may be increased by clarithromycin; in addition, QT_c prolongation and risk of malignant arrhythmia may be increased; avoid combination.

Eletriptan: Serum levels/effects may be increased by clarithromycin; monitor.

Eplerenone: Serum levels/effects may be increased by clarithromycin; monitor.

Ergot alkaloids: Concurrent use may lead to acute ergot toxicity (severe peripheral vasospasm and dysesthesia); concurrent use contraindicated.

HMG-CoA reductase inhibitors (atorvastatin, lovastatin, and simvastatin): Clarithromycin may increase serum levels of "statins" metabolized by CYP3A4, increasing the risk of myopathy/rhabdomyolysis (does not include fluvastatin, pravastatin, or rosuvastatin). Switch to pravastatin, fluvastatin, or rosuvastatin or suspend treatment during course of clarithromycin therapy.

Immunosuppressants (eg, cyclosporine, sirolimus, tacrolimus): Serum levels/effects may be increased by clarithromycin; monitor serum concentrations and for increased immune suppression.

Methylprednisolone: Serum levels may be increased by clarithromycin; monitor.

Phenytoin: Serum levels may be increased by clarithromycin; other evidence suggested phenytoin levels may be decreased in some patients; monitor.

Phosphodiesterase 5 inhibitors (eg, sildenafil, tadalafil, vardenafil): Sildenafil levels may be increased by clarithromycin. Do not exceed single sildenafil doses of 25 mg in 48 hours, a single tadalafil dose of 10 mg in 72 hours, or a single vardenafil dose of 5 mg in 24 hours.

Pimozide: Serum levels may be increased, leading to malignant arrhythmias; concomitant use is contraindicated.

Protease inhibitors (amprenavir, nelfinavir, and ritonavir): May increase serum levels of clarithromycin.

QT_c-prolonging agents: Concomitant use may increase the risk of malignant arrhythmias.

Quinidine: Serum levels may be increased by clarithromycin; in addition, the risk of QT_c prolongation and malignant arrhythmias may be increased during concurrent use.

Quinolone antibiotics (sparfloxacin, gatifloxacin, or moxifloxacin): Concurrent use may increase the risk of malignant arrhythmias.

Rifamycin derivatives (eg, rifabutin): Serum levels may be increased by clarithromycin; monitor.

Selective serotonin reuptake inhibitors (SSRIs): Serum levels/effects may be increased by clarithromycin; monitor.

Theophylline: Serum levels may be increased by clarithromycin; monitor.

Thioridazine: Risk of QT_c prolongation and malignant arrhythmias may be increased.

Valproic acid (and derivatives): Serum levels may be increased by clarithromycin; monitor.

Warfarin: Effects may be potentiated; monitor INR closely and adjust warfarin dose as needed or choose another antibiotic

Zopiclone: Serum levels may be increased by clarithromycin; monitor.

Ethanol/Nutrition/Herb Interactions

Food: Immediate release: Food delays rate, but not extent of absorption; Extended release: Food increases clarithromycin AUC by ~30% relative to fasting conditions.

Herb/Nutraceutical: St John's wort may decrease clarithromycin levels.

Dietary Considerations Clarithromycin immediate release tablets and oral solution may be given with or without meals. May be taken with milk. Biaxin® XL should be taken with food.

Pharmacodynamics/Kinetics

Absorption: Immediate release: Rapid; food delays rate, but not extent of absorption

Distribution: Widely into most body tissues except CNS

Protein binding: 42% to 50%

Metabolism: Partially hepatic via CYP3A4; converted to 14-OH clarithromycin (active metabolite)

Bioavailability: 50%

Half-life elimination: Immediate release: Clarithromycin: 3-7 hours; 14-OH-clarithromycin: 5-9 hours

Time to peak: Immediate release: 2-3 hours

Excretion: Primarily urine (20% to 40% as unchanged drug; additional 10% to 15% as metabolite)

Clearance: Approximates normal GFR

Pregnancy Risk Factor C

Lactation Excretion in breast milk unknown/use caution

Breast-Feeding Considerations It is not known if clarithromycin is excreted in breast milk, but other macrolides are excreted in human milk and clarithromycin is known to be excreted into animal milk. The manufacturer recommends that caution be exercised when administering clarithromycin to nursing women.

No adverse effects were noted in rats exposed via breast milk. No data is available on infants exposed via human milk. Other macrolides are considered compatible with breast-feeding and clarithromycin is used therapeutically in infants. Nondose-related effects could include modification of bowel flora.

Based on available data, clarithromycin is generally considered compatible (low risk to infant) while breast-feeding [animal data].

Dosage Forms Excipient information presented when available (limited, particularly for generics); consult specific product labeling.

Granules for oral suspension:

Biaxin®: 125 mg/5 mL (50 mL, 100 mL); 250 mg/5 mL (50 mL, 100 mL) [fruit punch flavor]

Tablet: 250 mg, 500 mg

Biaxin®: 250 mg, 500 mg

Tablet, extended release: 500 mg

Biaxin® XL: 500 mg

Dental Comment The FDA issued a special alert in December 2005 stating that short-term therapy with clarithromycin in patients with stable coronary artery disease may cause significantly higher cardiovascular mortality. The use of 500 mg clarithromycin daily for 14 days in patients with the above condition resulted in significantly higher all-cause mortality compared to patients taking placebo. This information is provided to the dental practitioner on the possible association between short-term use of clarithromycin for infections and increases in mortality in patients with a history of stable coronary artery disease.

Clarithromycin is known to prolong the QT interval. The QT interval is measured as the time and distance between the Q point of the QRS complex and the end of the T wave in the ECG tracing. After adjustment for heart rate, the QT interval is defined as prolonged if it is more than 450 msec in men and 460 msec in women. A long QT syndrome was first described in the 1950s and 60s as a congenital syndrome involving QT interval prolongation and syncope and sudden death. Some of the congenital long QT syndromes were characterized by a peculiar electrocardiographic appearance of the QRS complex involving a premature atria beat followed by a pause, then a subsequent sinus beat showing marked QT prolongation and deformity. This type of cardiac arrhythmia (Continued)

Clarithromycin *(Continued)*

was originally termed "torsade de pointes" (translated from the French as "twisting of the points").

Prolongation of the QT interval is thought to result from delayed ventricular repolarization. The repolarization process within the myocardial cell is due to the efflux of intracellular potassium. The channels associated with this current can be blocked by many drugs and predispose the electrical propagation cycle to torsade de pointes.

Clarithromycin is considered as having a risk of causing torsade de pointes. The risk of drug-induced torsade de pointes is extremely low when a single QT interval prolonging drug is prescribed. It is not known what effect vasoconstrictors in the local anesthetic regimen will have in patients with a known history of congenital prolonged QT interval or in patients taking any medication that prolongs the QT interval. Until more information is obtained, it is suggested that the clinician consult with the physician prior to the use of a vasoconstrictor in suspected patients, and that the vasoconstrictor (epinephrine, levonordefrin [Neo-Cobefrin®]) be used with caution.

Selected Readings

ADA Division of Legal Affairs, "A Legal Perspective on Antibiotic Prophylaxis," *J Am Dent Assoc*, 2003, 134(9):1260.

American Dental Association Council on Scientific Affairs, "Combating Antibiotic Resistance," *J Am Dent Assoc*, 2004, 135(4):484-7.

Amsden GW, "Erythromycin, Clarithromycin, and Azithromycin: Are the Differences Real?" *Clin Ther*, 1996, 18(1):56-72.

Dajani AS, Taubert KA, Wilson W, et al, "Prevention of Bacterial Endocarditis. Recommendations by the American Heart Association," *JAMA*, 1997, 277(22):1794-801.

Dajani AS, Taubert KA, Wilson W, et al, "Prevention of Bacterial Endocarditis: Recommendations by the American Heart Association," *J Am Dent Assoc*, 1997, 128(8):1142-51.

Moore PA, "Dental Therapeutic Indications for the Newer Long-Acting Macrolide Antibiotics," *J Am Dent Assoc*, 1999, 130(9):1341-3.

"Pimozide (Orap) Contraindicated With Clarithromycin (Biaxin®) and Other Macrolide Antibiotics," *FDA Medical Bulletin*, October 1996, 26 (3).

Wynn RL, "New Erythromycins," *Gen Dent*, 1996, 44(4):304-7.

Wynn RL, Bergman SA, Meiller TF, et al, "Antibiotics in Treating Oral-Facial Infections of Odontogenic Origin: An Update," *Gen Dent*, 2001, 49(3):238-40, 242, 244 passim.

Clemastine *(KLEM as teen)*

U.S. Brand Names Dayhist® Allergy [OTC]; Tavist® Allergy [OTC]
Generic Available Yes
Index Terms Clemastine Fumarate
Pharmacologic Category Antihistamine
Use Perennial and seasonal allergic rhinitis and other allergic symptoms including urticaria
Local Anesthetic/Vasoconstrictor Precautions No information available to require special precautions
Effects on Dental Treatment Key adverse event(s) related to dental treatment: Xerostomia (normal salivary flow resumes upon discontinuation).
Common Adverse Effects Frequency not defined.

Cardiovascular: Palpitation, hypotension, tachycardia

Central nervous system: Dyscoordination, sedation, somnolence slight to moderate, sleepiness, confusion, restlessness, nervousness, insomnia, irritability, fatigue, headache, dizziness increased

Dermatologic: Rash, photosensitivity

Gastrointestinal: Diarrhea, nausea, xerostomia, epigastric distress, vomiting, constipation

Genitourinary: Urinary frequency, difficult urination, urinary retention

Hematologic: Hemolytic anemia, thrombocytopenia, agranulocytosis

Ocular: Blurred vision
Otic: Tinnitus
Respiratory: Thickening of bronchial secretions
Miscellaneous: Anaphylaxis

Mechanism of Action Competes with histamine for H_1-receptor sites on effector cells in the gastrointestinal tract, blood vessels, and respiratory tract

Drug Interactions

Cytochrome P450 Effect: Inhibits CYP2D6 (weak), 3A4 (weak)

Increased Effect/Toxicity: CNS depressants may increase the degree of sedation and respiratory depression with antihistamines. May increase the absorption of digoxin. Central and/or peripheral anticholinergic syndrome can occur when administered with amantadine, rimantadine, narcotic analgesics, phenothiazines and other antipsychotics (especially with high anticholinergic activity), tricyclic antidepressants, quinidine, disopyramide, procainamide, and antihistamines.

Decreased Effect: May increase gastric degradation of levodopa and decrease the amount of levodopa absorbed by delaying gastric emptying. Therapeutic effects of cholinergic agents (tacrine, donepezil) and neuroleptics may be antagonized.

Pharmacodynamics/Kinetics
Onset of action: Peak effect: Therapeutic: 5-7 hours
Duration: 8-16 hours
Absorption: Almost complete
Metabolism: Hepatic
Excretion: Urine

Pregnancy Risk Factor B

Clidinium and Chlordiazepoxide
(kli DI nee um & klor dye az e POKS ide)

Related Information
Chlordiazepoxide *on page 331*
U.S. Brand Names Librax® *[original formulation]*
Canadian Brand Names Apo-Chlorax®; Librax®
Generic Available Yes
Index Terms Chlordiazepoxide and Clidinium
Pharmacologic Category Antispasmodic Agent, Gastrointestinal; Benzodiazepine
Use Adjunct treatment of peptic ulcer; treatment of irritable bowel syndrome
Local Anesthetic/Vasoconstrictor Precautions No information available to require special precautions
Effects on Dental Treatment Key adverse event(s) related to dental treatment: Xerostomia and changes in salivation (normal salivary flow resumes upon discontinuation).
Common Adverse Effects 1% to 10%:
Central nervous system: Drowsiness, ataxia, confusion, anticholinergic side effects
Gastrointestinal: Dry mouth, constipation, nausea
Drug Interactions
Cytochrome P450 Effect: Chlordiazepoxide: **Substrate** of CYP3A4 (major)
Increased Effect/Toxicity: Additive effects may result from concomitant benzodiazepine and/or anticholinergic therapy. CYP3A4 inhibitors may increase the levels/effects of chlordiazepoxide; example inhibitors include azole antifungals, clarithromycin, diclofenac, doxycycline, erythromycin, imatinib, isoniazid, nefazodone, nicardipine, propofol, protease inhibitors, quinidine, telithromycin, and verapamil.
Decreased Effect: CYP3A4 inducers may decrease the levels/effects of chlordiazepoxide. Example inducers include aminoglutethimide, carbamazepine, nafcillin, nevirapine, phenobarbital, phenytoin, and rifamycins.
Pregnancy Risk Factor D

ClindaMax™ *see Clindamycin on page 378*

Clindamycin (klin da MYE sin)

Related Information
Antibiotic Prophylaxis *on page 1772*
Bacterial Infections *on page 1793*
Periodontal Diseases *on page 1801*
Sexually-Transmitted Diseases *on page 1766*

Related Sample Prescriptions
Bacterial Infections and Periodontal Diseases *on page 1837*
Infective Endocarditis (Prevention) *on page 1832*
Prosthetic Joint Late Infections (Prevention) *on page 1833*

U.S. Brand Names Cleocin®; Cleocin HCl®; Cleocin Pediatric®; Cleocin Phosphate®; Cleocin T®; Cleocin® Vaginal Ovule; Clindagel®; ClindaMax™; Clindesse™; Clindets® [DSC]; Evoclin™

Canadian Brand Names Alti-Clindamycin; Apo-Clindamycin; Clindamycin Injection, USP; Clindoxyl®; Dalacin® C; Dalacin® T; Dalacin® Vaginal; Novo-Clindamycin; Riva-Clindamycin; Taro-Clindamycin

Mexican Brand Names Dalacin C; Lisiken; Trexen

Generic Available Yes: Excludes foam, granules, vaginal suppositories, vaginal cream

Index Terms Clindamycin Hydrochloride; Clindamycin Palmitate; Clindamycin Phosphate

Pharmacologic Category Antibiotic, Lincosamide; Topical Skin Product, Acne

Dental Use Alternate oral antibiotic for prevention of infective endocarditis in individuals allergic to penicillins or ampicillin, when amoxicillin cannot be used; alternate I.M. or I.V. antibiotic for prevention of infective endocarditis in patients allergic to penicillins or ampicillin and unable to take oral medication; alternate oral antibiotic for prophylaxis for dental patients with total joint replacement who are allergic to penicillin; alternate I.V. antibiotic for prophylaxis for dental patients with total joint replacement who are allergic to penicillin and unable to take oral medications; alternate antibiotic in the treatment of common orofacial infections caused by aerobic gram-positive cocci and susceptible anaerobes; treatment of periodontal disease

Use Treatment against aerobic and anaerobic streptococci (except enterococci), most staphylococci, *Bacteroides* sp and *Actinomyces*; bacterial vaginosis (vaginal cream, vaginal suppository); pelvic inflammatory disease (I.V.); topically in treatment of severe acne; vaginally for *Gardnerella vaginalis*

Unlabeled/Investigational Use May be useful in PCP; alternate treatment for toxoplasmosis

Local Anesthetic/Vasoconstrictor Precautions No information available to require special precautions

Effects on Dental Treatment No significant effects or complications reported (see Dental Comment)

Significant Adverse Effects
Systemic:
>10%: Gastrointestinal: Diarrhea, abdominal pain
1% to 10%:
Cardiovascular: Hypotension
Dermatologic: Urticaria, rash, Stevens-Johnson syndrome
Gastrointestinal: Pseudomembranous colitis, nausea, vomiting
Local: Thrombophlebitis, sterile abscess at I.M. injection site
Miscellaneous: Fungal overgrowth, hypersensitivity
<1% (Limited to important or life-threatening): Granulocytopenia, neutropenia, polyarthritis, renal dysfunction (rare), thrombocytopenia

Topical:
>10%: Dermatologic: Dryness, burning, itching, scaliness, erythema, or peeling of skin (lotion, solution); oiliness (gel, lotion)
1% to 10%: Central nervous system: Headache
<1% (Limited to important or life-threatening): Pseudomembranous colitis, nausea, vomiting, diarrhea (severe), abdominal pain, folliculitis, hypersensitivity reactions

Vaginal:
>10%: Genitourinary: Fungal vaginosis, vaginitis or vulvovaginal pruritus (from *Candida albicans*)
1% to 10%:
Central nervous system: Back pain, headache
Gastrointestinal: Constipation, diarrhea
Genitourinary: Urinary tract infection
Respiratory: Nasopharyngitis

Miscellaneous: Fungal infection

<1% (Limited to important or life-threatening): Atrophic vaginitis, bladder infection, bladder spasm, cervical dysplasia, diarrhea, dizziness, epistaxis, erythema, fever, hypersensitivity, hyperthyroidism, local edema, menstrual disorder, nausea, pain, palpable lymph node, pruritus, pyelonephritis, pyrexia, rash, sciatica, stomach cramps, upper respiratory urticaria, uterine cervical disorder, uterine spasm, vaginal burning, vertigo, vomiting, vulvar erythema, vulvar laceration, wheezing

Dental Usual Dosing

Orofacial infection: Adults: Oral: 150-450 mg/dose every 6-8 hours; maximum dose: 1.8 g/day

Treatment of periodontal disease: Oral: 300 mg every 8 hours for 8 days

Infective endocarditis prophylaxis: Oral, I.M., I.V.:

Children: 20 mg/kg 30-60 minutes before procedure

Adults: 600 mg 30-60 minutes before procedure

Note: Intramuscular injections should be avoided in patients who are receiving anticoagulant therapy. In these circumstances, orally administered regimens should be given whenever possible. Intravenously administered antibiotics should be used for patients who are unable to tolerate or absorb oral medications.

Prophylaxis in total joint replacement patients undergoing dental procedures which produce bacteremia: Adults: Oral: 600 mg 1 hour prior to procedure

Dosage

Usual dosage ranges:

Infants and Children:

Oral: 8-20 mg/kg/day as hydrochloride; 8-25 mg/kg/day as palmitate in 3-4 divided doses (minimum dose of palmitate: 37.5 mg 3 times/day)

I.M., I.V.:

<1 month: 15-20 mg/kg/day

>1 month: 20-40 mg/kg/day in 3-4 divided doses

Adults:

Oral: 150-450 mg/dose every 6-8 hours; maximum dose: 1.8 g/day

I.M., I.V.: 1.2-1.8 g/day in 2-4 divided doses; maximum dose: 4.8 g/day

Indication-specific dosing:

Children:

Anthrax: I.V.: 7.5 mg/kg every 6 hours

Babesiosis: Oral: 20-40 mg/kg/day divided every 8 hours for 7 days plus quinine

Orofacial infections: 8-25 mg/kg in 3-4 equally divided doses

Prevention of bacterial endocarditis (unlabeled use):

Oral: 20 mg/kg 1 hour before procedure with no follow-up dose needed

I.V.: 20 mg/kg within 30 minutes before procedure

Children ≥12 years and Adults:

Acne vulgaris: Topical:

Gel, pledget, lotion, solution: Apply a thin film twice daily

Foam (Evoclin™): Apply once daily

Adults:

Amnionitis: I.V.: 450-900 mg every 8 hours

Anthrax: I.V.: 900 mg every 8 hours with ciprofloxacin or doxycycline

Babesiosis:

Oral: 600 mg 3 times/day for 7 days with quinine

I.V.: 1.2 g twice daily

Bacterial vaginosis: Intravaginal:

Suppositories: Insert one ovule (100 mg clindamycin) daily into vagina at bedtime for 3 days

Cream:

Cleocin®: One full applicator inserted intravaginally once daily before bedtime for 3 or 7 consecutive days in nonpregnant patients or for 7 consecutive days in pregnant patients

Clindesse™: One full applicator inserted intravaginally as a single dose at anytime during the day in nonpregnant patients

Bite wounds (canine): Oral: 300 mg 4 times/day with a fluoroquinolone

Gangrenous myositis: I.V.: 900 mg every 8 hours with penicillin G

Group B streptococcus (neonatal prophylaxis): I.V.: 900 mg every 8 hours until delivery

Orofacial/parapharyngeal space infections:

Oral: 150-450 mg every 6 hours for 7 days, maximum 1.8 g/day

I.V.: 600-900 mg every 8 hours

Pelvic inflammatory disease: I.V.: 900 mg every 8 hours with gentamicin 2 mg/kg, then 1.5 mg/kg every 8 hours; continue after discharge with doxycycline 100 mg twice daily to complete 14 days of total therapy

***Pneumocystis jiroveci* pneumonia (unlabeled use):**

Oral: 300-450 mg 4 times/day with primaquine

(Continued)

Clindamycin *(Continued)*

I.M., I.V.: 1200-2400 mg/day with pyrimethamine or 600 mg 4 times/day with primaquine

Prevention of bacterial endocarditis (unlabeled use):
Oral: 600 mg 1 hour before procedure with no follow-up dose needed
I.V.: 600 mg within 30 minutes before procedure

Toxic shock syndrome: I.V.: 900 mg every 8 hours with penicillin G or ceftriaxone

Toxoplasmosis (unlabeled use): Oral, I.V.: 600 mg every 6 hours with pyrimethamine and folinic acid

Dosing adjustment in hepatic impairment: Adjustment recommended in patients with severe hepatic disease

Mechanism of Action Reversibly binds to 50S ribosomal subunits preventing peptide bond formation thus inhibiting bacterial protein synthesis; bacteriostatic or bactericidal depending on drug concentration, infection site, and organism

Contraindications Hypersensitivity to clindamycin or any component of the formulation; previous pseudomembranous colitis; regional enteritis, ulcerative colitis

Warnings/Precautions Dosage adjustment may be necessary in patients with severe hepatic dysfunction. **[U.S. Boxed Warning]: Can cause severe and possibly fatal colitis.** Discontinue drug if significant diarrhea, abdominal cramps, or passage of blood and mucus occurs. Vaginal products may weaken latex or rubber condoms, or contraceptive diaphragms. Barrier contraceptives are not recommended concurrently or for 3-5 days (depending on the product) following treatment. Some dosage forms contain benzyl alcohol or tartrazine. Use caution in atopic patients.

Drug Interactions Increased duration of neuromuscular blockade from tubocurarine, pancuronium

Ethanol/Nutrition/Herb Interactions
Food: Peak concentrations may be delayed with food.
Herb/Nutraceutical: St John's wort may decrease clindamycin levels.

Dietary Considerations May be taken with food.

Pharmacodynamics/Kinetics
Absorption: Topical: ~10%; Oral: Rapid (90%)
Distribution: High concentrations in bone and urine; no significant levels in CSF, even with inflamed meninges; crosses placenta; enters breast milk
Metabolism: Hepatic
Bioavailability: Topical: <1%
Half-life elimination: Neonates: Premature: 8.7 hours; Full-term: 3.6 hours; Adults: 1.6-5.3 hours (average: 2-3 hours)
Time to peak, serum: Oral: Within 60 minutes; I.M.: 1-3 hours
Excretion: Urine (10%) and feces (~4%) as active drug and metabolites

Pregnancy Risk Factor B

Lactation Enters breast milk/compatible

Dosage Forms Excipient information presented when available (limited, particularly for generics); consult specific product labeling. [DSC] = Discontinued product
Note: Strength is expressed as base
Capsule, as hydrochloride: 150 mg, 300 mg
Cleocin HCl®: 75 mg [contains tartrazine], 150 mg [contains tartrazine], 300 mg
Cream, vaginal, as phosphate:
Cleocin®: 2% (40 g) [contains benzyl alcohol and mineral oil; packaged with 7 disposable applicators]
Clindesse™: 2% (5 g) [contains mineral oil; prefilled single disposable applicator]
Foam, topical, as phosphate:
Evoclin™: 1% (50 g, 100 g) [contains ethanol 58%]
Gel, topical, as phosphate: 1% (30 g, 60 g)
Cleocin T®: 1% (30 g, 60 g)
Clindagel®: 1% (40 mL, 75 mL)
ClindaMax™: 1% (30 g, 60 g)
Granules for oral solution, as palmitate:
Cleocin Pediatric®: 75 mg/5 mL (100 mL) [cherry flavor]
Infusion, as phosphate [premixed in D₅W]:
Cleocin Phosphate®: 300 mg (50 mL); 600 mg (50 mL); 900 mg (50 mL)
Injection, solution, as phosphate: 150 mg/mL (2 mL, 4 mL, 6 mL, 60 mL)
Cleocin Phosphate®: 150 mg/mL (2 mL, 4 mL, 6 mL, 60 mL) [contains benzyl alcohol and disodium edetate 0.5 mg]
Lotion, as phosphate: 1% (60 mL)
Cleocin T®, ClindaMax™: 1% (60 mL)
Pledgets, topical: 1% (60s) [contains alcohol]

Cleocin T®: 1% (60s) [contains isopropyl alcohol 50%]

Clindets®: 1% (69s) [contains isopropyl alcohol 52%] [DSC]

Solution, topical, as phosphate: 1% (30 mL, 60 mL)

Cleocin T®: 1% (30 mL, 60 mL) [contains isopropyl alcohol 50%]

Suppository, vaginal, as phosphate:

Cleocin® Vaginal Ovule: 100 mg (3s) [contains oleaginous base; single reusable applicator]

Dental Comment Clindamycin has not been shown to interfere with oral contraceptive activity; however, it reduces GI microflora, thus, oral contraceptive users should be advised to use additional methods of birth control. About 1% of clindamycin users develop pseudomembranous colitis. Symptoms may occur 2-9 days after initiation of therapy; however, it has never occurred with the 1-dose regimen of clindamycin used to prevent bacterial endocarditis.

Selected Readings

ADA Division of Legal Affairs, "A Legal Perspective on Antibiotic Prophylaxis," *J Am Dent Assoc*, 2003, 134(9):1260.

"Advisory Statement. Antibiotic Prophylaxis for Dental Patients With Total Joint Replacements. American Dental Association; American Academy of Orthopedic Surgeons," *J Am Dent Assoc*, 1997, 128(7):1004-8.

American Dental Association; American Academy of Orthopedic Surgeons, "Antibiotic Prophylaxis for Dental Patients With Total Joint Replacements," *J Am Dent Assoc*, 2003, 134(7):895-9.

American Dental Association Council on Scientific Affairs, "Combating Antibiotic Resistance," *J Am Dent Assoc*, 2004, 135(4):484-7.

Dajani AS, Taubert KA, Wilson W, et al, "Prevention of Bacterial Endocarditis. Recommendations by the American Heart Association," *JAMA*, 1997, 277(22):1794-801.

Dajani AS, Taubert KA, Wilson W, et al, "Prevention of Bacterial Endocarditis: Recommendations by the American Heart Association," *J Am Dent Assoc*, 1997, 128(8):1142-51.

Sandor GK, Low DE, Judd PL, et al, "Antimicrobial Treatment Options in the Management of Odontogenic Infections," *J Can Dent Assoc*, 1998, 64(7):508-14.

Wynn RL, "Clindamycin: An Often Forgotten But Important Antibiotic," *AGD Impact*, 1994, 22:10.

Wynn RL and Bergman SA, "Antibiotics and Their Use in the Treatment of Orofacial Infections, Part I," *Gen Dent*, 1994, 42(5):398, 400, 402.

Wynn RL and Bergman SA, "Antibiotics and Their Use in the Treatment of Orofacial Infections, Part II," *Gen Dent*, 1994, 42(6):498-502.

Wynn RL, Bergman SA, Meiller TF, et al, "Antibiotics in Treating Oral-Facial Infections of Odontogenic Origin: An Update," *Gen Dent*, 2001, 49(3):238-40, 242, 244 passim.

Clindamycin and Benzoyl Peroxide
(klin da MYE sin & BEN zoe il peer OKS ide)

Related Information
Benzoyl Peroxide *on page 200*
Clindamycin *on page 378*
U.S. Brand Names BenzaClin®; Duac™
Canadian Brand Names BenzaClin®
Mexican Brand Names Benzaclin
Generic Available No
Index Terms Benzoyl Peroxide and Clindamycin; Clindamycin Phosphate and Benzoyl Peroxide
Pharmacologic Category Acne Products; Topical Skin Product; Topical Skin Product, Acne
Use Topical treatment of acne vulgaris
Local Anesthetic/Vasoconstrictor Precautions No information available to require special precautions
Effects on Dental Treatment No significant effects or complications reported
Common Adverse Effects
>10%: Dermatologic: Peeling (2% to 17%), dry skin (1% to 15%)
1% to 10%: Dermatologic: Pruritus (2%), erythema (1% to 5%), sunburn (1%), burning (<1% to 5%)
Mechanism of Action Clindamycin and benzoyl peroxide have activity against *Propionibacterium acnes in vitro*. This organism has been associated with acne vulgaris. Benzoyl peroxide releases free-radical oxygen which oxidizes bacterial proteins in the sebaceous follicles decreasing the number of anaerobic bacteria and decreasing irritating-type free fatty acids. Clindamycin reversibly binds to 50S ribosomal subunits preventing peptide bond formation thus inhibiting bacterial protein synthesis; bacteriostatic or bactericidal depending on drug concentration, infection site, and organism.
Drug Interactions
Increased Effect/Toxicity: Tretinoin may cause increased adverse events with concurrent use.
Decreased Effect: Erythromycin may antagonize clindamycin's effects.
Pharmacodynamics/Kinetics See individual agents.
Pregnancy Risk Factor C

Clindamycin and Tretinoin (klin da MYE sin & TRET i noyn)

U.S. Brand Names Ziana™
Generic Available No
Index Terms Clindamycin Phosphate and Tretinoin; Tretinoin and Clindamycin
Pharmacologic Category Acne Products; Retinoic Acid Derivative; Topical Skin Product; Topical Skin Product, Acne
Use Treatment of acne vulgaris
Local Anesthetic/Vasoconstrictor Precautions No information available to require special precautions
Effects on Dental Treatment No significant effects or complications reported
Common Adverse Effects
Dermatologic: Burning, dry skin, erythema, itching, scaling, stinging
Gastrointestinal: GI symptoms, unspecified
Respiratory: Nasopharyngitis
Mechanism of Action Clindamycin reversibly binds to 50S ribosomal subunits preventing peptide chain elongation thus inhibiting bacterial protein synthesis. Clindamycin exhibits *in vitro* activity against *Propionibacterium acnes*, an organism associated with acne vulgaris. Topical tretinoin is believed to decrease follicular epithelial cells cohesiveness and increase follicular epithelial cell turnover resulting in decreased microcomedo formation and increased expulsion of comedones.
Drug Interactions
Increased Effect/Toxicity: See individual agents.
Pharmacodynamics/Kinetics Absorption: Topical: Tretinoin: Minimal systemic absorption; Clindamycin: Low, but variable systemic absorption
Pregnancy Risk Factor C

Clobazam (KLOE ba zam)

Canadian Brand Names Alti-Clobazam; Apo-Clobazam®; Clobazam-10; Dom-Clobazam; Frisium®; Novo-Clobazam; PMS-Clobazam; ratio-Clobazam
Generic Available Yes
Pharmacologic Category Benzodiazepine
Use Adjunctive treatment of epilepsy
Unlabeled/Investigational Use Monotherapy for epilepsy or intermittent seizures
Local Anesthetic/Vasoconstrictor Precautions No information available to require special precautions
Effects on Dental Treatment Key adverse event(s) related to dental treatment: Xerostomia (normal salivary flow resumes upon discontinuation). Paradoxical reactions (including excitation, agitation, hallucinations, and psychosis) are known to occur with benzodiazepines.
Common Adverse Effects
Central nervous system: Drowsiness (17%), ataxia (4%), dizziness (2%), behavior disorder (1%), confusion, depression, lethargy, slurred speech, tremor, anterograde amnesia. In addition, paradoxical reactions (including excitation, agitation, hallucinations, and psychosis) are known to occur with benzodiazepines.
Dermatologic: Rash, pruritus, urticaria
Gastrointestinal: Weight gain (2%); dose related: Xerostomia, constipation, nausea
Hematologic: Decreased WBCs and other hematologic abnormalities have been rarely associated with benzodiazepines
Neuromuscular & skeletal: Muscle spasm
Ocular: Blurred vision (1%)
Restrictions Not available in U.S.
Mechanism of Action Clobazam is a 1,5 benzodiazepine which binds to stereospecific benzodiazepine receptors on the postsynaptic GABA neuron at several sites within the central nervous system, including the limbic system,

reticular formation. Enhancement of the inhibitory effect of GABA on neuronal excitability results by increased neuronal membrane permeability to chloride ions. This shift in chloride ions results in hyperpolarization (a less excitable state) and stabilization.

Drug Interactions

Cytochrome P450 Effect: Substrate (major) of CYP2C19 and 3A4

Increased Effect/Toxicity: Benzodiazepines potentiate the CNS depressant effects of opioid analgesics, barbiturates, phenothiazines, ethanol, antihistamines, MAO inhibitors, sedative-hypnotics, and cyclic antidepressants. CYP2C19 inhibitors may increase the levels/effects of clobazam; example inhibitors include delavirdine, fluconazole, fluvoxamine, gemfibrozil, isoniazid, omeprazole, and ticlopidine. CYP3A4 inhibitors may increase the levels/effects of clobazam; example inhibitors include azole antifungals, clarithromycin, diclofenac, doxycycline, erythromycin, imatinib, isoniazid, nefazodone, nicardipine, propofol, protease inhibitors, quinidine, telithromycin, and verapamil.

Decreased Effect: CYP3A4 inducers may decrease the levels/effects of clobazam; example inducers include aminoglutethimide, carbamazepine, nafcillin, nevirapine, phenobarbital, phenytoin, and rifamycins.

Pharmacodynamics/Kinetics

Absorption: Rapid

Protein binding: 85% to 91%

Metabolism: Hepatic via N-dealkylation (likely via CYP) to active metabolite (N-desmethyl), and glucuronidation

Bioavailability: 87%

Half-life elimination: 18 hours; N-desmethyl (active): 42 hours

Time to peak: 15 minutes to 4 hours

Excretion: Urine (90%), as metabolites

Pregnancy Risk Factor Not assigned; similar agents rated D. Contraindicated in 1st trimester (per manufacturer).

Clobetasol (kloe BAY ta sol)

Related Information
Ulcerative and Erosive Disorders *on page 1809*

Related Sample Prescriptions
Erosive Lichen Planus and Major Aphthae *on page 1845*
Recurrent Aphthous Stomatitis *on page 1844*

U.S. Brand Names Clobevate®; Clobex®; Cormax®; Olux®; Olux-E™; Temovate®; Temovate E®

Canadian Brand Names Clobex®; Dermovate®; Gen-Clobetasol; Novo-Clobetasol; Taro-Clobetasol

Mexican Brand Names Dermatovate; Lobevat

Generic Available Yes: Excludes foam, lotion, shampoo, spray

Index Terms Clobetasol Propionate

Pharmacologic Category Corticosteroid, Topical

Dental Use Short-term relief of oral mucosal inflammation

Use Short-term relief of inflammation of moderate-to-severe corticosteroid-responsive dermatoses (very high potency topical corticosteroid)

Local Anesthetic/Vasoconstrictor Precautions No information available to require special precautions

Effects on Dental Treatment No significant effects or complications reported

Significant Adverse Effects Frequency not defined; may depend upon formulation used, length of application, surface area covered, and the use of occlusive dressings.

Endocrine & metabolic: Adrenal suppression, Cushing's syndrome, hyperglycemia

Local: Application site: Burning, cracking/fissuring of the skin, dryness, erythema, folliculitis, irritation, numbness, pruritus, skin atrophy, stinging, telangiectasia

Renal: Glucosuria

Effects reported with other high-potency topical steroids: Acneiform eruptions, allergic contact dermatitis, hypertrichosis, hypopigmentation, maceration of the skin, miliaria, perioral dermatitis, secondary infection

Dental Usual Dosing Oral mucosal inflammation: Children ≥12 years and Adults: Cream: Apply twice daily for up to 2 weeks (maximum dose: 50 g/week); discontinue application when control is achieved; if no improvement is seen, reassessment of diagnosis may be necessary

Dosage Topical: Discontinue when control achieved; if improvement not seen within 2 weeks, reassessment of diagnosis may be necessary.

Children <12 years: Use is not recommended

(Continued)

Clobetasol (Continued)

Children ≥12 years and Adults:

Oral mucosal inflammation, dental (unlabeled use): Cream: Apply twice daily for up to 2 weeks (maximum dose: 50 g/week); discontinue application when control is achieved; if no improvement is seen, reassessment of diagnosis may be necessary

Steroid-responsive dermatoses:

Cream, emollient cream, gel, ointment: Apply twice daily for up to 2 weeks (maximum dose: 50 g/week)

Foam (Olux-E™): Apply to affected area twice daily for up to 2 weeks (maximum dose: 50 g/week); do not apply to face or intertriginous areas

Steroid-responsive dermatoses: Foam (Olux®), solution: Apply to affected scalp twice daily for up to 2 weeks (maximum dose: 50 g/week or 50 mL/week)

Mild-to-moderate plaque-type psoriasis of nonscalp areas: Foam (Olux®): Apply to affected area twice daily for up to 2 weeks (maximum dose: 50 g/week); do not apply to face or intertriginous areas

Children ≥16 years and Adults: Moderate-to-severe plaque-type psoriasis: Emollient cream, lotion: Apply twice daily for up to 2 weeks, has been used for up to 4 weeks when application is <10% of body surface area; use with caution (maximum dose: 50 g/week)

Children ≥18 years and Adults:

Moderate-to-severe plaque-type psoriasis: Spray: Apply by spraying directly onto affected area twice daily; should be gently rubbed into skin. Should be used for not longer than 4 weeks; treatment beyond 2 weeks should be limited to localized lesions which have not improved sufficiently. Total dose should not exceed 50 g/week or 59 mL/week.

Scalp psoriasis: Shampoo: Apply thin film to dry scalp once daily; leave in place for 15 minutes, then add water, lather; rinse thoroughly

Steroid-responsive dermatoses: Lotion: Apply twice daily for up to 2 weeks (maximum dose: 50 g/week)

Mechanism of Action Stimulates the synthesis of enzymes needed to decrease inflammation, suppress mitotic activity, and cause vasoconstriction

Contraindications Hypersensitivity to clobetasol or any component of the formulation; viral, fungal, or tubercular skin lesions

Warnings/Precautions Systemic absorption of topical corticosteroids may cause hypothalamic-pituitary-adrenal (HPA) axis suppression (reversible) particularly in younger children. HPA axis suppression may lead to adrenal crisis. Risk is increased when used over large surface areas, for prolonged periods, or with occlusive dressings. Allergic contact dermatitis can occur, it is usually diagnosed by failure to heal rather than clinical exacerbation. Prolonged treatment with corticosteroids has been associated with the development of Kaposi's sarcoma (case reports); if noted, discontinuation of therapy should be considered. Adverse systemic effects including hyperglycemia, glycosuria, fluid and electrolyte changes, and HPA suppression may occur when used on large surface areas, for prolonged periods, or with an occlusive dressing. Use in children <12 years of age is not recommended. Do not use on the face, axillae, or groin.

Drug Interactions No data reported

Pharmacodynamics/Kinetics

Absorption: Percutaneous absorption is variable and dependent upon many factors including vehicle used, integrity of epidermis, dose, and use of occlusive dressings

Metabolism: Hepatic

Excretion: Urine and feces

Pregnancy Risk Factor C

Lactation Excretion in breast milk unknown/use caution

Breast-Feeding Considerations It is not known if topical application will result in detectable quantities in breast milk.

Dosage Forms Excipient information presented when available (limited, particularly for generics); consult specific product labeling.

Cream, as propionate: 0.05% (15 g, 30 g, 45 g, 60 g)

Cormax®: 0.05% (30 g)

Temovate®: 0.05% (30 g, 60 g)

Cream, as propionate [in emollient base]: 0.05% (15 g, 30 g, 60 g)

Temovate E®: 0.05% (60 g)

Foam, topical, as propionate:

Olux®: 0.05% (50 g, 100 g) [contains ethanol 60%]

Olux-E™: 0.05% (50 g, 100 g)

Gel, as propionate: 0.05% (15 g, 30 g, 60 g)

Clobevate®: 0.05% (45 g)

Temovate®: 0.05% (60 g)

Lotion, as propionate:
Clobex®: 0.05% (30 mL, 59 mL)
Ointment, as propionate: 0.05% (15 g, 30 g, 45 g, 60 g)
Cormax®: 0.05% (15 g, 45 g)
Temovate®: 0.05% (15 g, 30 g)
Shampoo, as propionate:
Clobex®: 0.05% (120 mL) [contains alcohol]
Solution, topical, as propionate [for scalp application]: 0.05% (25 mL, 50 mL)
Cormax®: 0.05% (25 mL, 50 mL) [contains isopropyl alcohol 40%]
Temovate®: 0.05% (50 mL) [contains isopropyl alcohol 40%]
Solution, topical, as propionate [spray]:
Clobex®: 0.05% (60 mL, 125 mL) [contains alcohol]

Clobetasol Propionate *see* Clobetasol *on page 383*

Clobevate® *see* Clobetasol *on page 383*

Clobex® *see* Clobetasol *on page 383*

Clocortolone (kloe KOR toe lone)

U.S. Brand Names Cloderm®
Canadian Brand Names Cloderm®
Generic Available No
Index Terms Clocortolone Pivalate
Pharmacologic Category Corticosteroid, Topical
Use Inflammation of corticosteroid-responsive dermatoses (intermediate-potency topical corticosteroid)
Local Anesthetic/Vasoconstrictor Precautions No information available to require special precautions
Effects on Dental Treatment No significant effects or complications reported
Common Adverse Effects 1% to 10%:
Dermatologic: Itching, erythema
Local: Burning, dryness, irritation, papular rash
Mechanism of Action Stimulates the synthesis of enzymes needed to decrease inflammation, suppress mitotic activity, and cause vasoconstriction
Drug Interactions
Increased Effect/Toxicity: No data reported
Decreased Effect: No data reported
Pharmacodynamics/Kinetics
Absorption: Percutaneous absorption is variable and dependent upon many factors including vehicle used, integrity of epidermis, dose, and use of occlusive dressings; small amounts enter circulatory system via skin
Metabolism: Hepatic
Excretion: Urine and feces
Pregnancy Risk Factor C

Clocortolone Pivalate *see* Clocortolone *on page 385*

Cloderm® *see* Clocortolone *on page 385*

Clodronate (KLOE droh nate)

Related Information
Management of Patients Undergoing Cancer Therapy *on page 1826*
Canadian Brand Names Bonefos®; Clasteon®; Ostac®
Index Terms Clodronate Disodium
Pharmacologic Category Bisphosphonate Derivative
Use Management of hypercalcemia of malignancy
Local Anesthetic/Vasoconstrictor Precautions No information available to require special precautions
Effects on Dental Treatment Osteonecrosis of the jaw (ONJ), generally associated with local infection and/or tooth extraction and often with delayed healing, has been reported in patients taking bisphosphonates. Most reported cases of bisphosphonate-associated osteonecrosis have been in cancer patients treated with intravenous bisphosphonates. However, some have occurred in patients with postmenopausal osteoporosis taking oral bisphosphonates. Dental surgery may exacerbate ONJ. For patients requiring dental procedures, there are no data available to suggest whether discontinuation of bisphosphonate treatment reduces the risk of ONJ. See Dental Comment.
Common Adverse Effects 1% to 10%:
Endocrine & metabolic: Hypocalcemia (2%)
Gastrointestinal: Incidence highest with oral administration: Vomiting (4%), nausea (3%), diarrhea (2%), anorexia (1%)
Renal: Serum creatinine increased (1%), BUN increased
(Continued)

Clodronate *(Continued)*

Restrictions Not available in U.S.

Mechanism of Action A bisphosphonate which inhibits bone resorption via actions on osteoclasts or on osteoclast precursors.

Drug Interactions

Increased Effect/Toxicity: Aminoglycosides may lower serum calcium levels with prolonged administration; concomitant use may have an additive hypocalcemic effect. NSAIDs may enhance the gastrointestinal adverse/toxic effects (increased incidence of GI ulcers) of bisphosphonate derivatives. Bisphosphonate derivatives may enhance the hypocalcemic effect of phosphate supplements.

Decreased Effect: The following agents may decrease the absorption of oral bisphosphonate derivatives: Antacids (aluminum, calcium, magnesium), oral calcium salts, oral iron salts, and oral magnesium salts.

Pharmacodynamics/Kinetics

Onset of effect: 24-48 hours
  Peak effect: 5-7 days
Duration: 2-3 weeks
Distribution: V_d: 20 L
Bioavailability: Oral: 1% to 3%
Half-life (terminal): 13 hours (serum); prolonged in bone tissue
Elimination: Urine (as unchanged drug)

Pregnancy Risk Factor Not assigned; similar agents rated X

Dental Comment Novartis Pharmaceuticals Corporation has notified dental health professionals of the risk of **osteonecrosis of the jaw (ONJ)** and the use of the bisphosphonates, pamidronate (Zometa®) and zoledronic acid (Aredia®): *"Dear Dental Health Professional" Letter Issued for Intravenous Bisphosphonates, Pamidronate and Zoledronic Acid, Regarding the Risk of Osteonecrosis of the Jaw (ONJ) in Cancer Patients* - May 2005.

Often observed in patients receiving chemotherapy and corticosteroids, reports of ONJ (the majority being associated with dental procedures) have been documented in cancer patients. Dental exams and preventative dentistry should be performed prior to placing patients with risk factors (chemotherapy, corticosteroids, poor oral hygiene) on intravenous bisphosphonate therapy. Additionally, invasive dental procedures should be avoided during therapy; patients developing ONJ while on bisphosphonate therapy should not have invasive dental procedures because the condition may be exacerbated. It has not been determined whether the discontinuation of bisphosphonate therapy in patients requiring dental surgery decreases the risk of ONJ. The treating healthcare professional is encouraged to assess the benefits and risks.

Bisphosphonates are widely used in the management of metastatic bone disease to treat hypercalcemia associated with malignancies and to treat osteoporosis. It is suggested that because of the trend in the use of chronic bisphosphonate therapy, the observation of an associated risk of osteonecrosis of the jaw should alert practitioners to monitor for this previously unrecognized potential complication.

Additional information is available at http://www.fda.gov/medwatch/SAFETY/2005/safety05.htm#zometa2, or by contacting Novartis Oncology Medical Services at 1-888-669-6682.

Estimates of Percent Incidence of ONJ in Treated Cancer Patients

Two reports have attempted to assess the percent of cancer patients developing ONJ after bisphosphonate treatment. Maerevoet et al, reported that among 194 patients treated with Zometa® every 3-4 weeks, nine developed ONJ. Before receiving Zometa®, six had received Aredia® 90 mg every 3-4 weeks. The median duration of treatment with Aredia® was 39 months and for Zometa® 18 months. The incidence of ONJ in these patients was calculated to be 4.6%. Durie et al, described the results of a survey by the International Myeloma Foundation in 2004 to assess the risk factors of ONJ. Out of 1203 respondents, 904 had myeloma and 299 breast cancer. Of the myeloma patients, 62 developed ONJ and 54 had suspicious findings. Of the breast cancer patients, 13 had ONJ and 23 had suspicious findings. The total number of cases of either ONJ or suspicious findings was 152. ONJ developed in 10% of 211 patients receiving Zometa® compared to 4% of 413 receiving Aredia®. The mean time to onset of ONJ among patients taking Zometa® was 18 months; the mean time to onset after Aredia® was 6 years. It should be noted that an early report by authors from Novartis Pharmaceuticals Corporation (Tarassoff, 2003) stressed that Aredia® and Zometa® had been used in 2.5 million patients world wide and reports of ONJ during their extensive use had been rare. In addition, these authors stated that review of the reported cases revealed multiple risk factors for avascular necrosis. McMahon et al, followed up with a report that, along with other factors, bisphosphonates are additional stressors of bone health that can tip the balance to osteonecrosis. They suggested that the prevention of ONJ should be stressed such as the elimination of chronic dental infections prior to chemotherapy and bisphosphonate use in cancer patients.

Clodronate Disodium see Clodronate on page 385

Clofarabine (klo FARE a been)

U.S. Brand Names Clolar™
Generic Available No
Index Terms Clofarex; NSC606869
Pharmacologic Category Antineoplastic Agent, Antimetabolite (Purine Antagonist)
Use Treatment of relapsed or refractory acute lymphoblastic leukemia
Unlabeled/Investigational Use Adults: Relapsed and refractory acute myeloid leukemia (AML), chronic myeloid leukemia (CML) in blast phase, acute lymphocytic leukemia (ALL), myelodysplastic syndrome
Local Anesthetic/Vasoconstrictor Precautions No information available to require special precautions
Effects on Dental Treatment Key adverse event(s) related to dental treatment: Mucosal inflammation and gingival bleeding.
Common Adverse Effects
>10%:
Cardiovascular: Pericardial effusion (35%), tachycardia (34%), hypotension (29%), left ventricular systolic dysfunction (27%), edema (20%), flushing (18%), hypertension (11%)
Central nervous system: Headache (46%), pyrexia (41%), fatigue (36%) anxiety (22%), pain (19%), dizziness (16%), depression (11%), irritability (11%), lethargy (1%)
Dermatologic: Pruritus (47%), dermatitis (41%), petechiae (29%), erythema (18%), palmar-plantar erythrodysesthesia syndrome (13%), oral candidiasis (13%), cellulitis (11%)
Gastrointestinal: Vomiting (83%), nausea (75%), diarrhea (53%), abdominal pain (36%), anorexia (30%), constipation (21%), mucosal inflammation (18%), gingival bleeding (15%), sore throat (14%), appetite decreased (11%)
Genitourinary: Hematuria (17%)
Hematologic: Febrile neutropenia (57%)
Hepatic: ALT increased (44%), AST increased (38%), bilirubin increased (15%), hepatomegaly (15%), jaundice (15%)
Neuromuscular & skeletal: Rigors (38%), pain in limb (29%), myalgia (14%), back pain (13%), arthralgia (11%)
Respiratory: Epistaxis (31%), cough (19%), respiratory distress (14%), dyspnea (13%)
Miscellaneous: Infection (85%), injection site pain (14%), staphylococcal infection (13%), herpes simplex (11%)
1% to 10%:
Central nervous system: Somnolence (10%)
Gastrointestinal: Weight gain (10%)
Genitourinary: Creatinine increased (6%)
Neuromuscular & skeletal: Tremor (10%)
Respiratory: Pleural effusion (10%), pneumonia (10%), systemic inflammatory response syndrome (SIRS)/capillary leak syndrome
Miscellaneous: Transfusion reaction (10%), bacteremia (10%)
Mechanism of Action Clofarabine, a purine (deoxyadenosine) nucleoside analog, is metabolized to clofarabine 5'-triphosphate. Clofarabine 5'-triphosphate decreases cell replication and repair as well as causing cell death. To decrease cell replication and repair, clofarabine 5'-triphosphate competes with deoxyadenosine triphosphate for the enzymes ribonucleotide reductase and DNA polymerase. Cell replication is decreased when clofarabine 5'-triphosphate inhibits ribonucleotide reductase from reacting with deoxyadenosine triphosphate to produce deoxynucleotide triphosphate which is needed for DNA synthesis. Cell replication is also decreased when clofarabine 5'-triphosphate competes with DNA polymerase for incorporation into the DNA chain; when done during the repair process, cell repair is affected. To cause cell death, clofarabine 5'-triphosphate alters the mitochondrial membrane by releasing proteins, an inducing factor and cytochrome C.
Drug Interactions
Increased Effect/Toxicity: None known
Decreased Effect: None known
Pharmacodynamics/Kinetics
Distribution: V_d: 172 L/m^2
Protein binding: 47%
(Continued)

Clofarabine *(Continued)*

Metabolism: Intracellulary by deoxycytidine kinase and mono- and diphosphokinases to active metabolite clofarabine 5′-triphosphate

Half-life elimination: ~5.2 hours

Excretion: Urine (49% to 60% unchanged)

Pregnancy Risk Factor D

Clofarex *see Clofarabine on page 387*

Clolar™ *see Clofarabine on page 387*

Clomid® *see ClomiPHENE on page 388*

ClomiPHENE (KLOE mi feen)

U.S. Brand Names Clomid®; Serophene®

Canadian Brand Names Clomid®; Milophene®; Serophene®

Mexican Brand Names Omifin; Serofene

Generic Available Yes

Index Terms Clomiphene Citrate

Pharmacologic Category Ovulation Stimulator

Use Treatment of ovulatory failure in patients desiring pregnancy

Unlabeled/Investigational Use Male infertility

Local Anesthetic/Vasoconstrictor Precautions No information available to require special precautions

Effects on Dental Treatment No significant effects or complications reported

Common Adverse Effects

>10%: Endocrine & metabolic: Hot flashes, ovarian enlargement

1% to 10%:

Cardiovascular: Thromboembolism

Central nervous system: Mental depression, headache

Endocrine & metabolic: Breast enlargement (males), breast discomfort (females), abnormal menstrual flow

Gastrointestinal: Distention, bloating, nausea, vomiting

Hepatic: Hepatotoxicity

Ocular: Blurring of vision, diplopia, floaters, after-images, phosphenes, photophobia

Mechanism of Action Induces ovulation by stimulating the release of pituitary gonadotropins

Drug Interactions

Decreased Effect: Decreased response when used with danazol. Decreased estradiol response when used with clomiphene.

Pharmacodynamics/Kinetics

Metabolism: Undergoes enterohepatic recirculation

Half-life elimination: 5-7 days

Excretion: Primarily feces; urine (small amounts)

Pregnancy Risk Factor X

Clomiphene Citrate *see ClomiPHENE on page 388*

ClomiPRAMINE (kloe MI pra meen)

U.S. Brand Names Anafranil®

Canadian Brand Names Anafranil®; Apo-Clomipramine®; CO Clomipramine; Gen-Clomipramine

Mexican Brand Names Anafranil

Generic Available Yes

Index Terms Clomipramine Hydrochloride

Pharmacologic Category Antidepressant, Tricyclic (Tertiary Amine)

Use Treatment of obsessive-compulsive disorder (OCD)

Unlabeled/Investigational Use Depression, panic attacks, chronic pain

Local Anesthetic/Vasoconstrictor Precautions Use with caution; epinephrine and levonordefrin have been shown to have an increased pressor response in combination with TCAs. Clomipramine is one of the drugs confirmed to prolong the QT interval and is accepted as having a risk of causing torsade de pointes. The risk of drug-induced torsade de pointes is extremely low when a single QT interval prolonging drug is prescribed. In terms of epinephrine, it is not known what effect vasoconstrictors in the local anesthetic regimen will have in patients with a known history of congenital prolonged QT interval or in patients taking any medication that prolongs the QT interval. Until more information is obtained, it is suggested that the clinician consult with the physician prior to the use of a vasoconstrictor in suspected patients, and that the vasoconstrictor (epinephrine, levonordefrin [Neo-Cobefrin®]) be used with caution.

Effects on Dental Treatment Key adverse event(s) related to dental treatment: Xerostomia and changes in salivation (normal salivary flow resumes upon discontinuation). Long-term treatment with TCAs, such as clomipramine, increases the risk of caries by reducing salivation and salivary buffer capacity.

Common Adverse Effects

>10%:

Central nervous system: Dizziness, drowsiness, headache, insomnia, nervousness

Endocrine & metabolic: Libido changes

Gastrointestinal: Xerostomia, constipation, appetite increased, nausea, weight gain, dyspepsia, anorexia, abdominal pain

Neuromuscular & skeletal: Fatigue, tremor, myoclonus

Miscellaneous: Diaphoresis increased

1% to 10%:

Cardiovascular: Hypotension, palpitation, tachycardia

Central nervous system: Confusion, hypertonia, sleep disorder, yawning, speech disorder, abnormal dreaming, paresthesia, memory impairment, anxiety, twitching, coordination impaired, agitation, migraine, depersonalization, emotional lability, flushing, fever

Dermatologic: Rash, pruritus, dermatitis

Gastrointestinal: Diarrhea, vomiting

Genitourinary: Difficult urination

Ocular: Blurred vision, eye pain

Restrictions An FDA-approved medication guide concerning the use of antidepressants in children, adolescents, and young adults must be distributed when dispensing an outpatient prescription (new or refill) where this medication is to be used without direct supervision of a healthcare provider. Medication guides are available at http://www.fda.gov/cder/Offices/ODS/medication_guides.htm. Dispense to parents or guardians of children and adolescents receiving this medication.

Mechanism of Action Clomipramine appears to affect serotonin uptake while its active metabolite, desmethylclomipramine, affects norepinephrine uptake

Drug Interactions

Cytochrome P450 Effect: Substrate of CYP1A2 (major), 2C19 (major), 2D6 (major), 3A4 (minor); **Inhibits** CYP2D6 (moderate)

Increased Effect/Toxicity: The levels/effects of clomipramine may be increased by amiodarone, chlorpromazine, ciprofloxacin, delavirdine, fluconazole, fluoxetine, fluvoxamine, gemfibrozil, isoniazid, ketoconazole, miconazole, norfloxacin, ofloxacin, omeprazole, paroxetine, pergolide, quinidine, quinine, ritonavir, rofecoxib, ropinirole, ticlopidine, and other CYP1A2, 2C19, or 2D6 inhibitors. Clomipramine may increase the levels/effects of amphetamines, selected beta-blockers, dextromethorphan, fluoxetine, lidocaine, mirtazapine, nefazodone, paroxetine, risperidone, ritonavir, thioridazine, tricyclic antidepressants, venlafaxine, and other CYP2D6 substrates.

Clomipramine increases the effects of amphetamines, anticholinergics, lithium, other CNS depressants (sedatives, hypnotics, ethanol), chlorpropamide, tolazamide, phenothiazines, and warfarin. When used with MAO inhibitors or other serotonergic drugs, serotonin syndrome may occur. Serotonin syndrome has also been reported with ritonavir (rare). Pressor response to I.V. epinephrine, norepinephrine, and phenylephrine may be enhanced in patients receiving TCAs. (**Note:** Effect is unlikely with epinephrine or levonordefrin dosages typically administered as infiltration in combination with local anesthetics.) Combined use of beta-agonists or drugs which prolong QT_c (including quinidine, procainamide, disopyramide, cisapride, sparfloxacin, gatifloxacin, moxifloxacin) with TCAs may predispose patients to cardiac arrhythmias.

Decreased Effect: The levels/effects of clomipramine may be decreased by aminoglutethimide, carbamazepine, phenobarbital, phenytoin, rifampin, and other CYP1A2 or 2C19 inducers. Clomipramine may decrease the levels/effects of CYP2D6 prodrug substrates (eg, codeine, hydrocodone, oxycodone, tramadol). Clomipramine inhibits the antihypertensive response to bethanidine, clonidine, debrisoquin, guanadrel, guanethidine, guanabenz, and guanfacine. Cholestyramine and colestipol may decrease the absorption of clomipramine.

Pharmacodynamics/Kinetics

Absorption: Rapid

Metabolism: Hepatic to desmethylclomipramine (active); extensive first-pass effect

Half-life elimination: 20-30 hours

Pregnancy Risk Factor C

Clomipramine Hydrochloride see ClomiPRAMINE on page 388

Clonazepam (kloe NA ze pam)

U.S. Brand Names Klonopin®

Canadian Brand Names Alti-Clonazepam; Apo-Clonazepam®; Clonapam; CO Clonazepam; Gen-Clonazepam; Klonopin®; Novo-Clonazepam; Nu-Clonazepam; PMS-Clonazepam; Rho®-Clonazepam; Rivotril®; Sandoz-Clonazepam

Mexican Brand Names Kenoket; Kriadex; Rivotril

Generic Available Yes

Pharmacologic Category Benzodiazepine

Dental Use Burning mouth syndrome

Use Alone or as an adjunct in the treatment of petit mal variant (Lennox-Gastaut), akinetic, and myoclonic seizures; petit mal (absence) seizures unresponsive to succimides; panic disorder with or without agoraphobia

Unlabeled/Investigational Use Restless legs syndrome; neuralgia; multifocal tic disorder; parkinsonian dysarthria; bipolar disorder; adjunct therapy for schizophrenia

Local Anesthetic/Vasoconstrictor Precautions No information available to require special precautions

Effects on Dental Treatment Key adverse event(s) related to dental treatment: Xerostomia and changes in salivation (normal salivary flow resumes upon discontinuation), gum soreness, and coated tongue

Significant Adverse Effects Reactions reported in patients with seizure and/or panic disorder. Frequency not defined.

Cardiovascular: Edema (ankle or facial), palpitation

Central nervous system: Amnesia, ataxia (seizure disorder ~30%; panic disorder 5%), behavior problems (seizure disorder ~25%), coma, confusion, depression, dizziness, drowsiness (seizure disorder ~50%), emotional lability, fatigue, fever, hallucinations, headache, hypotonia, hysteria, insomnia, intellectual ability reduced, memory disturbance, nervousness; paradoxical reactions (including aggressive behavior, agitation, anxiety, excitability, hostility, irritability, nervousness, nightmares, sleep disturbance, vivid dreams); psychosis, slurred speech, somnolence (panic disorder 37%), suicidal attempt, vertigo

Dermatologic: Hair loss, hirsutism, skin rash

Endocrine & metabolic: Dysmenorrhea, libido increased/decreased

Gastrointestinal: Abdominal pain, anorexia, appetite increased/decreased, coated tongue, constipation, dehydration, diarrhea, gastritis, gum soreness, nausea, weight changes (loss/gain), xerostomia

Genitourinary: Colpitis, dysuria, ejaculation delayed, enuresis, impotence, micturition frequency, nocturia, urinary retention, urinary tract infection

Hematologic: Anemia, eosinophilia, leukopenia, thrombocytopenia

Hepatic: Alkaline phosphatase increased (transient), hepatomegaly, transaminases increased (transient)

Neuromuscular & skeletal: Choreiform movements, coordination abnormal, dysarthria, muscle pain, muscle weakness, myalgia, tremor

Ocular: Blurred vision, eye movements abnormal, diplopia, nystagmus

Respiratory: Chest congestion, cough, bronchitis, hypersecretions, pharyngitis, respiratory depression, respiratory tract infection, rhinitis, rhinorrhea, shortness of breath, sinusitis

Miscellaneous: Allergic reaction, aphonia, dysdiadochokinesis, encopresis, "glassy-eyed" appearance, hemiparesis, lymphadenopathy

Restrictions C-IV

Dental Usual Dosing Burning mouth syndrome: Adults: Oral: 0.25-3 mg/day in 2 divided doses, in morning and evening

Dosage Oral:

Children <10 years or 30 kg: Seizure disorders:

Initial daily dose: 0.01-0.03 mg/kg/day (maximum: 0.05 mg/kg/day) given in 2-3 divided doses; increase by no more than 0.5 mg every third day until seizures are controlled or adverse effects seen

Usual maintenance dose: 0.1-0.2 mg/kg/day divided 3 times/day, not to exceed 0.2 mg/kg/day

Adults:

Burning mouth syndrome (dental use): 0.25-3 mg/day in 2 divided doses, in morning and evening

Seizure disorders:

Initial daily dose not to exceed 1.5 mg given in 3 divided doses; may increase by 0.5-1 mg every third day until seizures are controlled or adverse effects seen (maximum: 20 mg/day)

Usual maintenance dose: 0.05-0.2 mg/kg; do not exceed 20 mg/day

Panic disorder: 0.25 mg twice daily; increase in increments of 0.125-0.25 mg twice daily every 3 days; target dose: 1 mg/day (maximum: 4 mg/day)

Discontinuation of treatment: To discontinue, treatment should be withdrawn gradually. Decrease dose by 0.125 mg twice daily every 3 days until medication is completely withdrawn.

Elderly: Initiate with low doses and observe closely

Hemodialysis: Supplemental dose is not necessary

Mechanism of Action The exact mechanism is unknown, but believed to be related to its ability to enhance the activity of GABA; suppresses the spike-and-wave discharge in absence seizures by depressing nerve transmission in the motor cortex

Contraindications Hypersensitivity to clonazepam or any component of the formulation (cross-sensitivity with other benzodiazepines may exist); significant liver disease; narrow-angle glaucoma; pregnancy

Warnings/Precautions Use with caution in elderly or debilitated patients, patients with hepatic disease (including alcoholics), or renal impairment. Use with caution in patients with respiratory disease or impaired gag reflex or ability to protect the airway from secretions (salivation may be increased). Worsening of seizures may occur when added to patients with multiple seizure types. Concurrent use with valproic acid may result in absence status. Monitoring of CBC and liver function tests has been recommended during prolonged therapy.

Causes CNS depression (dose related) resulting in sedation, dizziness, confusion, or ataxia which may impair physical and mental capabilities. Use with caution in patients receiving other CNS depressants or ethanol. Benzodiazepines have been associated with falls and traumatic injury and should be used with extreme caution in patients who are at risk of these events (especially the elderly).

Use caution in patients with depression, particularly if suicidal risk may be present. Use with caution in patients with a history of drug dependence. Benzodiazepines have been associated with dependence and acute withdrawal symptoms, including seizures, on discontinuation or reduction in dose.

Benzodiazepines have been associated with anterograde amnesia. Paradoxical reactions, including hyperactive or aggressive behavior, have been reported with benzodiazepines, particularly in adolescent/pediatric or psychiatric patients. Does not have analgesic, antidepressant, or antipsychotic properties.

Drug Interactions Substrate of CYP3A4 (major)

CNS depressants: Sedative effects and/or respiratory depression may be additive with CNS depressants; includes ethanol, barbiturates, opioid analgesics, and other sedative agents; monitor for increased effect.

CYP3A4 inducers: CYP3A4 inducers may decrease the levels/effects of clonazepam. Example inducers include aminoglutethimide, carbamazepine, nafcillin, nevirapine, phenobarbital, phenytoin, and rifamycins.

CYP3A4 inhibitors: May increase the levels/effects of clonazepam. Example inhibitors include azole antifungals, clarithromycin, diclofenac, doxycycline, erythromycin, imatinib, isoniazid, nefazodone, nicardipine, propofol, protease inhibitors, quinidine, telithromycin, and verapamil.

Disulfiram: Disulfiram may inhibit the metabolism of clonazepam; monitor for increased benzodiazepine effect.

Levodopa: Therapeutic effects may be diminished in some patients following the addition of a benzodiazepine; limited/inconsistent data.

Oral contraceptives: May decrease the clearance of some benzodiazepines (those which undergo oxidative metabolism); monitor for increased benzodiazepine effect.

Theophylline: May partially antagonize some of the effects of benzodiazepines; monitor for decreased response; may require higher doses for sedation.

Valproic acid: The combined use of clonazepam and valproic acid has been associated with absence seizures.

Ethanol/Nutrition/Herb Interactions

Ethanol: Avoid ethanol (may increase CNS depression).

Food: Clonazepam serum concentration is unlikely to be increased by grapefruit juice because of clonazepam's high oral bioavailability.

Herb/Nutraceutical: St John's wort may decrease clonazepam levels. Avoid valerian, St John's wort, kava kava, gotu kola (may increase CNS depression).

Pharmacodynamics/Kinetics

Onset of action: 20-60 minutes

Duration: Infants and young children: 6-8 hours; Adults: $\leq$12 hours

Absorption: Well absorbed

Distribution: Adults: V_d: 1.5-4.4 L/kg

Protein binding: 85%

Metabolism: Extensively hepatic via glucuronide and sulfate conjugation

Half-life elimination: Children: 22-33 hours; Adults: 19-50 hours

(Continued)

Clonazepam *(Continued)*

Time to peak, serum: 1-3 hours; Steady-state: 5-7 days

Excretion: Urine (<2% as unchanged drug); metabolites excreted as glucuronide or sulfate conjugates

Pregnancy Risk Factor D

Lactation Enters breast milk/not recommended

Breast-Feeding Considerations Clonazepam enters breast milk; clinical effects on the infant include CNS depression, respiratory depression reported (no recommendation from the AAP).

Dosage Forms Excipient information presented when available (limited, particularly for generics); consult specific product labeling.

Tablet: 0.5 mg, 1 mg, 2 mg

Tablet, orally disintegrating [wafer]: 0.125 mg, 0.25 mg, 0.5 mg, 1 mg, 2 mg

---

Clonidine (KLON i deen)

Related Information

Cardiovascular Diseases *on page 1726*

U.S. Brand Names Catapres®; Catapres-TTS®; Duraclon™

Canadian Brand Names Apo-Clonidine®; Carapres®; Dixarit®; Novo-Clonidine; Nu-Clonidine

Generic Available Yes: Tablet

Index Terms Clonidine Hydrochloride

Pharmacologic Category Alpha$_2$-Adrenergic Agonist

Use Management of mild-to-moderate hypertension; either used alone or in combination with other antihypertensives

Orphan drug: Duraclon™: For continuous epidural administration as adjunctive therapy with intraspinal opiates for treatment of cancer pain in patients tolerant to or unresponsive to intraspinal opiates

Unlabeled/Investigational Use Heroin or nicotine withdrawal; severe pain; dysmenorrhea; vasomotor symptoms associated with menopause; ethanol dependence; prophylaxis of migraines; glaucoma; diabetes-associated diarrhea; impulse control disorder, attention-deficit/hyperactivity disorder (ADHD), clozapine-induced sialorrhea

Local Anesthetic/Vasoconstrictor Precautions No information available to require special precautions

Effects on Dental Treatment Key adverse event(s) related to dental treatment: Significant xerostomia (normal salivary flow resumes upon discontinuation), orthostatic hypotension, and abnormal taste.

Common Adverse Effects Incidence of adverse events is not always reported.

>10%:

Central nervous system: Drowsiness (35% oral, 12% transdermal), dizziness (16% oral, 2% transdermal)

Dermatologic: Transient localized skin reactions characterized by pruritus, and erythema (15% to 50% transdermal)

Gastrointestinal: Dry mouth (40% oral, 25% transdermal)

1% to 10%:

Cardiovascular: Orthostatic hypotension (3% oral)

Central nervous system: Headache (1% oral, 5% transdermal), sedation (3% transdermal), fatigue (6% transdermal), lethargy (3% transdermal), insomnia (2% transdermal), nervousness (3% oral, 1% transdermal), mental depression (1% oral)

Dermatologic: Rash (1% oral), allergic contact sensitivity (5% transdermal), localized vesiculation (7%), hyperpigmentation (5% at application site), edema (3%), excoriation (3%), burning (3%), throbbing, blanching (1%), papules (1%), and generalized macular rash (1%) has occurred in patients receiving transdermal clonidine.

Endocrine & metabolic: Sodium and water retention, sexual dysfunction (3% oral, 2% transdermal), impotence (3% oral, 2% transdermal), weakness (10% transdermal)

Gastrointestinal: Nausea (5% oral, 1% transdermal), vomiting (5% oral), anorexia and malaise (1% oral), constipation (10% oral, 1% transdermal), dry throat (2% transdermal), taste disturbance (1% transdermal), weight gain (1% oral)

Genitourinary: Nocturia (1% oral)

Hepatic: Liver function test (mild abnormalities, 1% oral)

Miscellaneous: Withdrawal syndrome (1% oral)

Dosage

Children:

Oral:

Hypertension: Children ≥12 years: Initial: 0.2 mg/day in 2 divided doses; increase gradually at 5- to 7-day intervals; maximum: 2.4 mg/day

Clonidine tolerance test (test of growth hormone release from pituitary): 0.15 mg/m^2 or 4 mcg/kg as single dose

ADHD (unlabeled use): Initial: 0.05 mg/day; increase every 3-7 days by 0.05 mg/day to 3-5 mcg/kg/day given in divided doses 3-4 times/day (maximum dose: 0.3-0.4 mg/day)

Epidural infusion: Pain management: Reserved for patients with severe intractable pain, unresponsive to other analgesics or epidural or spinal opiates: Initial: 0.5 mcg/kg/hour; adjust with caution, based on clinical effect

Adults:

Oral:

Acute hypertension (urgency): Initial 0.1-0.2 mg; may be followed by additional doses of 0.1 mg every hour, if necessary, to a maximum total dose of 0.6 mg.

Unlabeled route of administration: Sublingual clonidine 0.1-0.2 mg twice daily may be effective in patients unable to take oral medication

Hypertension: Initial dose: 0.1 mg twice daily (maximum recommended dose: 2.4 mg/day); usual dose range (JNC 7): 0.1-0.8 mg/day in 2 divided doses

Nicotine withdrawal symptoms: 0.1 mg twice daily to maximum of 0.4 mg/day for 3-4 weeks

Transdermal: Hypertension: Apply once every 7 days; for initial therapy start with 0.1 mg and increase by 0.1 mg at 1- to 2-week intervals (dosages >0.6 mg do not improve efficacy); usual dose range (JNC 7): 0.1-0.3 mg once weekly

Note: If transitioning from oral to transdermal therapy, overlap oral regimen for 1-2 days; transdermal route takes 2-3 days to achieve therapeutic effects.

Conversion from oral to transdermal:

Day 1: Place Catapres-TTS® 1; administer 100% of oral dose.

Day 2: Administer 50% of oral dose.

Day 3: Administer 25% of oral dose.

Day 4: Patch remains, no further oral supplement necessary.

Epidural infusion: Pain management: Starting dose: 30 mcg/hour; titrate as required for relief of pain or presence of side effects; minimal experience with doses >40 mcg/hour; should be considered an adjunct to intraspinal opiate therapy

Elderly: Initial: 0.1 mg once daily at bedtime, increase gradually as needed

Dosing adjustment in renal impairment: Cl$_{cr}$ <10 mL/minute: Administer 50% to 75% of normal dose initially

Dialysis: Not dialyzable (0% to 5%) via hemo- or peritoneal dialysis; supplemental dose not necessary

Mechanism of Action Stimulates alpha$_2$-adrenoceptors in the brain stem, thus activating an inhibitory neuron, resulting in reduced sympathetic outflow from the CNS, producing a decrease in peripheral resistance, renal vascular resistance, heart rate, and blood pressure; epidural clonidine may produce pain relief at spinal presynaptic and postjunctional alpha$_2$-adrenoceptors by preventing pain signal transmission; pain relief occurs only for the body regions innervated by the spinal segments where analgesic concentrations of clonidine exist

Contraindications Hypersensitivity to clonidine hydrochloride or any component of the formulation

Warnings/Precautions Gradual withdrawal is needed (over 1 week for oral, 2-4 days with epidural) if drug needs to be stopped. Patients should be instructed about abrupt discontinuation (causes rapid increase in BP and symptoms of sympathetic overactivity). In patients on both a beta-blocker and clonidine where withdrawal of clonidine is necessary, withdraw the beta-blocker first and several days before clonidine. Then slowly decrease clonidine.

Use with caution in patients with severe coronary insufficiency; conduction disturbances; recent MI, CVA, or chronic renal insufficiency. Caution in sinus node dysfunction. Discontinue within 4 hours of surgery then restart as soon as possible after. Clonidine injection should be administered via a continuous epidural infusion device. **[U.S. Boxed Warning]: Epidural clonidine is not recommended for perioperative, obstetrical, or postpartum pain.** It is not recommended for use in patients with severe cardiovascular disease or hemodynamic instability. In all cases, the epidural may lead to cardiovascular instability (hypotension, bradycardia). Transdermal patch may contain conducting metal (eg, aluminum); remove patch prior to MRI. Due to the potential for altered electrical conductivity, remove transdermal patch before cardioversion or defibrillation. Clonidine cause significant CNS depression and xerostomia. (Continued)

Clonidine *(Continued)*

Caution in patients with pre-existing CNS disease or depression. Elderly may be at greater risk for CNS depressive effects, favoring other agents in this population.

Drug Interactions

Increased Effect/Toxicity: Concurrent use with antipsychotics (especially low potency), opioid analgesics, or nitroprusside may produce additive hypotensive effects. Clonidine may decrease the symptoms of hypoglycemia with oral hypoglycemic agents or insulin. Alcohol, barbiturates, and other CNS depressants may have additive CNS effects when combined with clonidine. Epidural clonidine may prolong the sensory and motor blockade of local anesthetics. Clonidine may increase cyclosporine (and perhaps tacrolimus) serum concentrations. Beta-blockers may potentiate bradycardia in patients receiving clonidine and may increase the rebound hypertension of withdrawal. Tricyclic antidepressants may also enhance the hypertensive response associated with abrupt clonidine withdrawal.

Decreased Effect: Tricyclic antidepressants (TCAs) antagonize the hypotensive effects of clonidine.

Ethanol/Nutrition/Herb Interactions

Ethanol: Avoid ethanol (may increase CNS depression).

Herb/Nutraceutical: Avoid dong quai if using for hypertension (has estrogenic activity). Avoid ephedra, yohimbe, ginseng (may worsen hypertension). Avoid valerian, St John's wort, kava kava, gotu kola (may increase CNS depression).

Dietary Considerations Hypertensive patients may need to decrease sodium and calories in diet.

Pharmacodynamics/Kinetics

Onset of action: Oral: 0.5-1 hour; Transdermal: Initial application: 2-3 days

Duration: 6-10 hours

Distribution: V_d: Adults: 2.1 L/kg; highly lipid soluble; distributes readily into extravascular sites

Protein binding: 20% to 40%

Metabolism: Extensively hepatic to inactive metabolites; undergoes enterohepatic recirculation

Bioavailability: 75% to 95%

Half-life elimination: Adults: Normal renal function: 6-20 hours; Renal impairment: 18-41 hours

Time to peak: 2-4 hours

Excretion: Urine (65%, 32% as unchanged drug); feces (22%)

Pregnancy Risk Factor C

Dosage Forms

Injection, epidural solution [preservative free]:

Duraclon™: 100 mcg/mL (10 mL); 500 mcg/mL (10 mL)

Patch, transdermal [once-weekly patch]:

Catapres-TTS®-1: 0.1 mg/24 hours (4s)

Catapres-TTS®-2: 0.2 mg/24 hours (4s)

Catapres-TTS®-3: 0.3 mg/24 hours (4s)

Tablet: 0.1 mg, 0.2 mg, 0.3 mg

Catapres®: 0.1 mg, 0.2 mg, 0.3 mg

Clonidine and Chlorthalidone *(KLON i deen & klor THAL i done)*

Related Information

Chlorthalidone *on page 347*
Clonidine *on page 392*

U.S. Brand Names Clorpres®; Combipres® [DSC]

Generic Available No

Index Terms Chlorthalidone and Clonidine

Pharmacologic Category Antihypertensive Agent, Combination

Use Management of mild-to-moderate hypertension

Local Anesthetic/Vasoconstrictor Precautions No information available to require special precautions

Effects on Dental Treatment Key adverse event(s) related to dental treatment: Clonidine: Significant xerostomia (normal salivary flow resumes upon discontinuation), orthostatic hypotension, and abnormal taste.

Common Adverse Effects See individual agents.

Drug Interactions

Increased Effect/Toxicity: See individual agents.

Decreased Effect: See individual agents.

Pharmacodynamics/Kinetics See individual agents.

Pregnancy Risk Factor C

Clonidine Hydrochloride *see* Clonidine *on page 392*

Clopidogrel (kloh PID oh grel)

Related Information
Cardiovascular Diseases *on page 1726*
U.S. Brand Names Plavix®
Canadian Brand Names Plavix®
Mexican Brand Names Plavix
Generic Available No
Index Terms Clopidogrel Bisulfate
Pharmacologic Category Antiplatelet Agent
Use Reduces rate of atherothrombotic events (myocardial infarction, stroke, vascular deaths) in patients with recent MI or stroke, or established peripheral arterial disease; reduces rate of atherothrombotic events in patients with unstable angina or non-ST-segment elevation acute coronary syndromes (unstable angina and non-ST-segment elevation MI) managed medically or through PCI (with or without stent) or CABG; reduces rate of death and athero-thrombotic events in patients with ST-segment elevation MI (STEMI) managed medically

Unlabeled/Investigational Use In aspirin-allergic patients, prevention of coronary artery bypass graft closure (saphenous vein)

Local Anesthetic/Vasoconstrictor Precautions No information available to require special precautions

Effects on Dental Treatment Aspirin and clopidogrel (Plavix®) in combination is the primary prevention strategy against stent thrombosis after placement of drug-eluting metal stents in coronary patients. Premature discontinuation of this combination antiplatelet therapy strongly increases the risk of a catastrophic event of stent thrombosis leading to myocardial infarction and/or death, so says a science advisory issued in January 2007 from the American Heart Association in collaboration with the American Dental Association and other professional healthcare organizations. The advisory stresses a 12-month therapy of aspirin and Plavix® combination after placement of a drug-eluting stent in order to prevent thrombosis at the stent site. Any elective surgery should be postponed for 1 year after stent implantation, and if surgery must be performed, consideration should be given to continuing the antiplatelet therapy during the perioperative period in high-risk patients with drug-eluting stents.

This advisory was issued from a science panel made up of representatives from the American Heart Association (AHA), the American College of Cardiology, the Society for Cardiovascular Angiography and Interventions, the American College of Surgeons, the American Dental Association (ADA), and the American College of Physicians (Grines, 2007).

Common Adverse Effects As with all drugs which may affect hemostasis, bleeding is associated with clopidogrel. Hemorrhage may occur at virtually any site. Risk is dependent on multiple variables, including the concurrent use of multiple agents which alter hemostasis and patient susceptibility.

>10%: Gastrointestinal: The overall incidence of gastrointestinal events (including abdominal pain, vomiting, dyspepsia, gastritis and constipation) has been documented to be 27% compared to 30% in patients receiving aspirin.
3% to 10%:
Cardiovascular: Chest pain (8%), edema (4%), hypertension (4%)
Central nervous system: Headache (3% to 8%), dizziness (2% to 6%), depression (4%), fatigue (3%), general pain (6%)
Dermatologic: Rash (4%), pruritus (3%)
Endocrine & metabolic: Hypercholesterolemia (4%)
Gastrointestinal: Abdominal pain (2% to 6%), dyspepsia (2% to 5%), diarrhea (2% to 5%), nausea (3%)
Genitourinary: Urinary tract infection (3%)
Hematologic: Bleeding (major 4%; minor 5%), purpura (5%), epistaxis (3%)
Hepatic: Liver function test abnormalities (<3%; discontinued in 0.11%)
Neuromuscular & skeletal: Arthralgia (6%), back pain (6%)
Respiratory: Dyspnea (5%), rhinitis (4%), bronchitis (4%), cough (3%), upper respiratory infection (9%)
Miscellaneous: Flu-like syndrome (8%)
1% to 3%:
Cardiovascular: Atrial fibrillation, cardiac failure, palpitation, syncope
Central nervous system: Fever, insomnia, vertigo, anxiety
Dermatologic: Eczema
Endocrine & metabolic: Gout, hyperuricemia
Gastrointestinal: Constipation, GI hemorrhage, vomiting
Genitourinary: Cystitis
Hematologic: Hematoma, anemia
(Continued)

Clopidogrel *(Continued)*

Neuromuscular & skeletal: Arthritis, leg cramps, neuralgia, paresthesia, weakness

Ocular: Cataract, conjunctivitis

Dosage Oral: Adults:

Recent MI, recent stroke, or established arterial disease: 75 mg once daily

Non-ST-segment elevation acute coronary syndrome: Initial: 300 mg loading dose, followed by 75 mg once daily (in combination with aspirin 75-325 mg once daily). **Note:** A loading dose of 600 mg has been used in some investigations; limited research exists comparing the two doses.

Note: Drug-eluting stents: Duration of clopidogrel (in combination with aspirin): Ideally 12 months following drug-eluting stent placement in patients not at high risk for bleeding; at a minimum, 1-, 3-, and 6 months for bare metal, sirolimus, and paclitaxel stents, respectively, for uninterrupted therapy.

ST-segment elevation MI: 75 mg once daily (in combination with aspirin 75-162 mg/day). CLARITY used a 300 mg loading dose of clopidogrel. The duration of therapy was <28 days (usually until hospital discharge).

Prevention of coronary artery bypass graft closure (saphenous vein): Aspirin-allergic patients (unlabeled use): Loading dose: 300 mg 6 hours following procedure; maintenance: 50-100 mg/day

Dosing adjustment in renal impairment and elderly: None necessary

Mechanism of Action Blocks the ADP receptors, which prevent fibrinogen binding at that site and thereby reduce the possibility of platelet adhesion and aggregation

Contraindications Hypersensitivity to clopidogrel or any component of the formulation; active pathological bleeding such as PUD or intracranial hemorrhage; coagulation disorders

Warnings/Precautions Use with caution in patients who may be at risk of increased bleeding, including patients with peptic ulcer disease, trauma, or surgery. Consider discontinuing 5 days before elective surgery (except in patients with cardiac stents that have not completed their full course of dual antiplatelet therapy; AHA/ACC/SCAI/ACS/ADA Science Advisory provides recommendations). Use caution in concurrent treatment with other antiplatelet drugs; bleeding risk is increased. Use with caution in patients with severe liver or renal disease (experience is limited). Cases of thrombotic thrombocytopenic purpura (usually occurring within the first 2 weeks of therapy) have been reported; urgent plasmapheresis is required. Safety and efficacy have not been established in pediatric patients.

Drug Interactions

Cytochrome P450 Effect: Substrate (minor) of CYP1A2, 3A4; **Inhibits** CYP2C9 (weak)

Increased Effect/Toxicity: Anticoagulants, antiplatelet agents, drotrecogin alfa, NSAIDs, salicylates, thrombolytics, and treprostinil may increase the risk of bleeding with concurrent use. Rifampin may increase the effects of clopidogrel (monitor).

Decreased Effect: Atorvastatin may attenuate the effects of clopidogrel; monitor. CYP3A4-inhibiting macrolide antibiotics may attenuate the effects of clopidogrel (including clarithromycin, erythromycin, and troleandomycin); monitor.

Ethanol/Nutrition/Herb Interactions Herb/Nutraceutical: Avoid cat's claw, dong quai, evening primrose, feverfew, garlic, ginger, ginkgo, red clover, horse chestnut, green tea, ginseng (all have additional antiplatelet activity).

Dietary Considerations May be taken without regard to meals.

Pharmacodynamics/Kinetics

Onset of action: Inhibition of platelet aggregation detected: 2 hours after 300 mg administered; after second day of treatment with 50-100 mg/day

Peak effect: 50-100 mg/day: Bleeding time: 5-6 days; Platelet function: 3-7 days

Absorption: Well absorbed

Protein binding: Parent drug: 98%; metabolite: 94%

Metabolism: Extensively hepatic via hydrolysis; biotransformation primarily to carboxyl acid derivative (inactive). The active metabolite that inhibits platelet aggregation has not been isolated.

Half-life elimination: ~8 hours

Time to peak, serum: ~1 hour

Excretion: Urine (50%); feces (46%)

Pregnancy Risk Factor B

Dosage Forms

Tablet:

Plavix®: 75 mg

Dental Comment There is no scientific evidence to warrant the discontinuance of clopidogrel prior to dental surgery. Patients taking one clopidogrel tablet daily as an antithrombotic and who require dental surgery should be given special consideration in consultation with physician.

Selected Readings

Daniel NG, Goulet J, Bergeron M, et al, "Antiplatelet Drugs: Is There a Surgical Risk?" *J Can Dent Assoc*, 2002, 68(11):683-7.

Grines CL, Bonow RO, Casey DE, et al, "AHA/ACC/SCAI/ACS/ADA Science Advisory, Prevention of Premature Discontinuation of Dual Antiplatelet Therapy in Patients With Coronary Artery Stents. A Science Advisory From the American Heart Association, American College of Cardiology, Society of Cardiovascular Angiography and Interventions, American College of Surgeons, and American Dental Association With Representation From The Amercian College Of Physicians," *Circulation*, 2007, 115(6):813-8. Available at http://www.acc.org/qualityandscience/clinical/pdfs/Final_Dual_Antiplatelet_Statement_010507.pdf.

Jeske AH, Suchko GD, ADA Council on Scientific Affairs and Division of Science, et al, "Lack of a Scientific Basis for Routine Discontinuation of Oral Anticoagulation Therapy Before Dental Treatment," *J Am Dent Assoc*, 2003, 134(11):1492-7.

Little JW, Miller CS, Henry RG, et al, "Antithrombotic Agents: Implications in Dentistry," *Oral Surg Oral Med Oral Pathol Oral Radiol Endod*, 2002, 93(5):544-51.

Scully C and Wolff A, "Oral Surgery in Patients on Anticoagulant Therapy," *Oral Surg Oral Med Oral Pathol Oral Radiol Endod*, 2002, 94(1):57-64.

Wynn RL, "Clopidogrel (Plavix): Dental Considerations of an Antiplatelet Drug," *Gen Dent*, 2001, 49(6):564-8.

Clopidogrel Bisulfate *see* Clopidogrel *on page 395*

Clorazepate (klor AZ e pate)

U.S. Brand Names Tranxene® SD™; Tranxene® SD™-Half Strength; Tranxene® T-Tab®

Canadian Brand Names Apo-Clorazepate®; Novo-Clopate

Mexican Brand Names Tranxene

Generic Available Yes

Index Terms Clorazepate Dipotassium; Tranxene T-Tab®

Pharmacologic Category Benzodiazepine

Use Treatment of generalized anxiety disorder; management of ethanol withdrawal; adjunct anticonvulsant in management of partial seizures

Local Anesthetic/Vasoconstrictor Precautions No information available to require special precautions

Effects on Dental Treatment Key adverse event(s) related to dental treatment: Xerostomia (normal salivary flow resumes upon discontinuation). Many patients will experience drowsiness; orthostatic hypotension is possible. It is suggested that narcotic analgesics not be given for pain control to patients taking clorazepate due to enhanced sedation.

Common Adverse Effects Frequency not defined.

Cardiovascular: Hypotension

Central nervous system: Drowsiness, fatigue, ataxia, lightheadedness, memory impairment, insomnia, anxiety, headache, depression, slurred speech, confusion, nervousness, dizziness, irritability

Dermatologic: Rash

Endocrine & metabolic: Libido decreased

Gastrointestinal: Xerostomia, constipation, diarrhea, nausea, salivation decreased, vomiting, appetite increased or decreased

Neuromuscular & skeletal: Dysarthria, tremor

Ocular: Blurred vision, diplopia

Restrictions C-IV

Mechanism of Action Binds to stereospecific benzodiazepine receptors on the postsynaptic GABA neuron at several sites within the central nervous system, including the limbic system, reticular formation. Enhancement of the inhibitory effect of GABA on neuronal excitability results by increased neuronal membrane permeability to chloride ions. This shift in chloride ions results in hyperpolarization (a less excitable state) and stabilization.

Drug Interactions

Cytochrome P450 Effect: Substrate of CYP3A4 (major)

Increased Effect/Toxicity: Clorazepate potentiates the CNS depressant effects of opioid analgesics, barbiturates, phenothiazines, ethanol, antihistamines, MAO inhibitors, sedative-hypnotics, and cyclic antidepressants. CYP3A4 inhibitors may increase the levels/effects of clorazepate; example inhibitors include azole antifungals, clarithromycin, diclofenac, doxycycline, erythromycin, imatinib, isoniazid, nefazodone, nicardipine, propofol, protease inhibitors, quinidine, telithromycin, and verapamil.

Decreased Effect: CYP3A4 inducers may decrease the levels/effects of clorazepate; example inducers include aminoglutethimide, carbamazepine, nafcillin, nevirapine, phenobarbital, phenytoin, and rifamycins.

Pharmacodynamics/Kinetics

Onset of action: 1-2 hours

(Continued)

Clorazepate (Continued)

Duration: Variable, 8-24 hours

Distribution: Crosses placenta; appears in urine

Metabolism: Rapidly decarboxylated to desmethyldiazepam (active) in acidic stomach prior to absorption; hepatically to oxazepam (active)

Half-life elimination: Adults: Desmethyldiazepam: 48-96 hours; Oxazepam: 6-8 hours

Time to peak, serum: ~1 hour

Excretion: Primarily urine

Pregnancy Risk Factor D

Clorazepate Dipotassium *see* Clorazepate *on page 397*

Clorpactin® WCS-90 [OTC] *see* Oxychlorosene *on page 1225*

Clorpres® *see* Clonidine and Chlorthalidone *on page 394*

Clotrimazole (kloe TRIM a zole)

Related Information

Fungal Infections *on page 1804*

Sexually-Transmitted Diseases *on page 1766*

Related Sample Prescriptions

Topical Fungal Infections *on page 1841*

U.S. Brand Names Cruex® Cream [OTC]; Gyne-Lotrimin® 3 [OTC]; Lotrimin® AF Athlete's Foot Cream [OTC]; Lotrimin® AF Athlete's Foot Solution [OTC]; Lotrimin® AF Jock Itch Cream [OTC]; Mycelex®; Mycelex®-7 [OTC]; Mycelex® Twin Pack [OTC]

Canadian Brand Names Canesten® Topical; Canesten® Vaginal; Clotrimaderm; Trivagizole-3®

Mexican Brand Names Candimon; Canesten; Dermasten

Generic Available Yes: Cream, solution, troche

Pharmacologic Category Antifungal Agent, Oral Nonabsorbed; Antifungal Agent, Topical; Antifungal Agent, Vaginal

Dental Use Treatment of susceptible fungal infections, including oropharyngeal candidiasis; limited data suggests that the use of clotrimazole troches may be effective for prophylaxis against oropharyngeal candidiasis in neutropenic patients

Use Treatment of susceptible fungal infections, including oropharyngeal candidiasis, dermatophytoses, superficial mycoses, and cutaneous candidiasis, as well as vulvovaginal candidiasis; limited data suggest that clotrimazole troches may be effective for prophylaxis against oropharyngeal candidiasis in neutropenic patients

Local Anesthetic/Vasoconstrictor Precautions No information available to require special precautions

Effects on Dental Treatment No significant effects or complications reported

Significant Adverse Effects

Oral:

>10%: Hepatic: Abnormal liver function tests

1% to 10%:

Gastrointestinal: Nausea and vomiting may occur in patients on clotrimazole troches

Local: Mild burning, irritation, stinging to skin or vaginal area

Vaginal:

1% to 10%: Genitourinary: Vulvar/vaginal burning

<1% (Limited to important or life-threatening): Burning or itching of penis of sexual partner; polyuria; vulvar itching, soreness, edema, or discharge

Dental Usual Dosing

Oropharyngeal candidiasis: Children >3 years and Adults: Oral:

Prophylaxis: 10 mg troche dissolved 3 times/day for the duration of chemotherapy or until steroids are reduced to maintenance levels

Treatment: 10 mg troche dissolved slowly 5 times/day for 14 consecutive days

Cutaneous candidiasis: Children >3 years and Adults: Topical (cream, solution): Apply twice daily; if no improvement occurs after 4 weeks of therapy, re-evaluate diagnosis.

Dosage

Children >3 years and Adults:

Oral:

Prophylaxis: 10 mg troche dissolved 3 times/day for the duration of chemotherapy or until steroids are reduced to maintenance levels

Treatment: 10 mg troche dissolved slowly 5 times/day for 14 consecutive days

Topical (cream, solution): Apply twice daily; if no improvement occurs after 4 weeks of therapy, re-evaluate diagnosis

Children >12 years and Adults:
Vaginal:
Cream:
1%: Insert 1 applicatorful vaginal cream daily (preferably at bedtime) for 7 consecutive days
2%: Insert 1 applicatorful vaginal cream daily (preferably at bedtime) for 3 consecutive days
Tablet: Insert 100 mg/day for 7 days or 500 mg single dose
Topical (cream, solution): Apply to affected area twice daily (morning and evening) for 7 consecutive days

Mechanism of Action Binds to phospholipids in the fungal cell membrane altering cell wall permeability resulting in loss of essential intracellular elements

Contraindications Hypersensitivity to clotrimazole or any component of the formulation

Warnings/Precautions Clotrimazole should not be used for treatment of ocular or systemic fungal infection. Use with caution with hepatic impairment. Safety and effectiveness of clotrimazole lozenges (troches) in children <3 years of age have not been established. When using topical formulation, avoid contact with eyes.

Drug Interactions Inhibits CYP1A2 (weak), 2A6 (weak), 2B6 (weak), 2C8 (weak), 2C9 (weak), 2C19 (weak), 2D6 (weak), 2E1 (weak), 3A4 (moderate)
CYP3A4 substrates: Clotrimazole may increase the levels/effects of CYP3A4 substrates. Example substrates include benzodiazepines, calcium channel blockers, cyclosporine, mirtazapine, nateglinide, nefazodone, sildenafil (and other PDE-5 inhibitors), tacrolimus, and venlafaxine. Selected benzodiazepines (midazolam and triazolam), cisapride, ergot alkaloids, selected HMG-CoA reductase inhibitors (lovastatin and simvastatin), and pimozide are generally contraindicated with strong CYP3A4 inhibitors.

Pharmacodynamics/Kinetics
Absorption: Topical: Negligible through intact skin
Time to peak, serum:
Oral topical (troche): Salivary levels occur within 3 hours following 30 minutes of dissolution time
Vaginal cream: High vaginal levels: 8-24 hours
Vaginal tablet: High vaginal levels: 1-2 days
Excretion: Feces (as metabolites)

Pregnancy Risk Factor B (topical); C (troches)

Lactation Excretion in breast milk unknown

Dosage Forms Excipient information presented when available (limited, particularly for generics); consult specific product labeling.
Combination pack (Mycelex®-7): Vaginal tablet 100 mg (7s) and vaginal cream 1% (7 g)
Cream, topical: 1% (15 g, 30 g, 45 g)
Cruex®: 1% (15 g)
Lotrimin® AF Athlete's Foot: 1% (12 g, 24 g)
Lotrimin® AF Jock Itch: 1% (12 g)
Cream, vaginal: 2% (21 g)
Mycelex®-7: 1% (45 g)
Solution, topical: 1% (10 mL, 30 mL)
Lotrimin® AF Athlete's Foot: 1% (10 mL)
Tablet, vaginal (Gyne-Lotrimin® 3): 200 mg (3s)
Troche (Mycelex®): 10 mg

Clotrimazole and Betamethasone *see* Betamethasone and Clotrimazole *on page 209*

Cloxacillin (kloks a SIL in)

Canadian Brand Names Apo-Cloxi®; Novo-Cloxin; Nu-Cloxi; Riva-Cloxacillin
Generic Available Yes
Index Terms Cloxacillin Sodium
Pharmacologic Category Antibiotic, Penicillin
Dental Use Treatment of susceptible orofacial infections (notably penicillinase-producing staphylococci)
Use Treatment of susceptible bacterial infections, notably penicillinase-producing staphylococci causing respiratory tract, skin and skin structure, bone and joint, urinary tract infections
Local Anesthetic/Vasoconstrictor Precautions No information available to require special precautions
Effects on Dental Treatment Key adverse event(s) related to dental treatment: Prolonged use of penicillins may lead to development of oral candidiasis.
Significant Adverse Effects
1% to 10%: Gastrointestinal: Nausea, diarrhea, abdominal pain, oral candidiasis
(Continued)

Cloxacillin (Continued)

<1% (Limited to important or life-threatening): Agranulocytosis, anemia, BUN increased, creatinine increased, eosinophilia, fever, hematuria, hemolytic anemia, hepatotoxicity, hypersensitivity, interstitial nephritis, leukopenia, neutropenia, PT prolonged, pseudomembranous colitis, rash (maculopapular to exfoliative), seizure with extremely high doses and/or renal failure, serum sickness-like reactions, thrombocytopenia, transient elevated LFTs, vaginitis, vomiting

Restrictions Not available in U.S.

Dental Usual Dosing Susceptible orofacial infections: Children >20 kg and Adults: Oral: 250-500 mg every 6 hours

Dosage

Usual dosage range:

Children >1 month and <20 kg: Oral: 50-100 mg/kg/day in divided doses every 6 hours; (maximum: 4 g/day)

Children >20 kg and Adults: Oral: 250-500 mg every 6 hours

Hemodialysis: Not dialyzable (0% to 5%)

Mechanism of Action Inhibits bacterial cell wall synthesis by binding to one or more of the penicillin-binding proteins (PBPs) which in turn inhibits the final transpeptidation step of peptidoglycan synthesis in bacterial cell walls, thus inhibiting cell wall biosynthesis. Bacteria eventually lyse due to ongoing activity of cell wall autolytic enzymes (autolysins and murein hydrolases) while cell wall assembly is arrested.

Contraindications Hypersensitivity to cloxacillin, any component of the formulation, or penicillins

Warnings/Precautions Monitor PT if patient is concurrently on warfarin. Elimination of drug is slow in renally impaired. Serious and occasionally severe or fatal hypersensitivity (anaphylactoid) reactions have been reported in patients on penicillin therapy, especially with a history of beta-lactam hypersensitivity, history of sensitivity to multiple allergens, or previous IgE-mediated reactions (eg, anaphylaxis, angioedema, urticaria). Use with caution in asthmatic patients. Prolonged use may result in fungal or bacterial superinfection, including *C. difficile*-associated diarrhea and pseudomembranous colitis.

Drug Interactions

Methotrexate: Penicillins may increase the exposure to methotrexate during concurrent therapy; monitor.

Oral contraceptives: Anecdotal reports suggesting decreased contraceptive efficacy with penicillins have been refuted by more rigorous scientific and clinical data.

Probenecid, disulfiram: May increase levels of penicillins (cloxacillin).

Warfarin: Effects of warfarin may be increased.

Dietary Considerations Should be taken 1 hour before or 2 hours after meals with water.

Sodium content of 250 mg capsule: 13.8 mg (0.6 mEq)

Sodium content of suspension 5 mL of 125 mg/5 mL: 11 mg (0.48 mEq)

Pharmacodynamics/Kinetics

Absorption: Oral: ~50%

Distribution: Widely to most body fluids and bone; penetration into cells, into eye, and across normal meninges is poor; crosses placenta; enters breast milk; inflammation increases amount that crosses blood-brain barrier

Protein binding: 90% to 98%

Metabolism: Extensively hepatic to active and inactive metabolites

Half-life elimination: 0.5-1.5 hours; prolonged with renal impairment and in neonates

Time to peak, serum: 0.5-2 hours

Excretion: Urine and feces

Pregnancy Risk Factor B

Lactation Excretion in breast milk unknown

Breast-Feeding Considerations No data reported; however, other penicillins may be taken while breast-feeding.

Dosage Forms Excipient information presented when available (limited, particularly for generics); consult specific product labeling.

Capsule, as sodium: 250 mg, 500 mg

Powder for oral suspension, as sodium: 125 mg/5 mL (100 mL, 200 mL)

Cloxacillin Sodium *see* Cloxacillin *on page 399*

Clozapine (KLOE za peen)

U.S. Brand Names Clozaril®; FazaClo®
Canadian Brand Names Apo-Clozapine®; Clozaril®; Gen-Clozapine
Mexican Brand Names Clopsine; Leponex
Generic Available Yes
Pharmacologic Category Antipsychotic Agent, Atypical
Use Treatment-refractory schizophrenia; to reduce risk of recurrent suicidal behavior in schizophrenia or schizoaffective disorder
Unlabeled/Investigational Use Schizoaffective disorder, bipolar disorder, childhood psychosis, severe obsessive-compulsive disorder
Local Anesthetic/Vasoconstrictor Precautions Most pharmacology textbooks state that in presence of phenothiazines, systemic doses of epinephrine paradoxically decrease the blood pressure. This is the so called "epinephrine reversal" phenomenon. This has never been observed when epinephrine is given by infiltration as part of the local anesthesia procedure.
Effects on Dental Treatment Key adverse event(s) related to dental treatment: Sialorrhea and xerostomia (normal salivary flow resumes upon discontinuation). Many patients may experience orthostatic hypotension with clozapine; precautions should be taken; do not use atropine-like drugs for xerostomia in patients taking clozapine due to significant potentiation.
Common Adverse Effects
>10%:
Cardiovascular: Tachycardia (25%)
Central nervous system: Drowsiness (39% to 46%), dizziness (19% to 27%), insomnia (2% to 20%)
Gastrointestinal: Constipation (14% to 25%), weight gain (4% to 31%), sialorrhea (31% to 48%), nausea/vomiting (3% to 17%)
1% to 10%:
Cardiovascular: Angina (1%), ECG changes (1%), hypertension (4%), hypotension (9%), syncope (6%)
Central nervous system: Akathisia (3%), seizure (3%), headache (7%), nightmares (4%), akinesia (4%), confusion (3%), myoclonic jerks (1%), restlessness (4%), agitation (4%), lethargy (1%), ataxia (1%), slurred speech (1%), depression (1%), anxiety (1%)
Dermatologic: Rash (2%)
Gastrointestinal: Abdominal discomfort/heartburn (4% to 14%), anorexia (1%), diarrhea (2%), xerostomia (6%), throat discomfort (1%)
Genitourinary: Urinary abnormalities (eg, abnormal ejaculation, retention, urgency, incontinence; 1% to 2%)
Hematologic: Eosinophilia (1%), leukopenia, leukocytosis, agranulocytosis (1%)
Hepatic: Liver function tests abnormal (1%)
Neuromuscular & skeletal: Tremor (6%), hypokinesia (4%), rigidity (3%), hyperkinesia (1%), weakness (1%), pain (1%), spasm (1%)
Ocular: Visual disturbances (5%)
Respiratory: Dyspnea (1%), nasal congestion (1%)
Miscellaneous: Diaphoresis increased, fever, tongue numbness (1%)
Restrictions Patient-specific registration is required to dispense clozapine. Monitoring systems for individual clozapine manufacturers are independent. If a patient is switched from one brand/manufacturer of clozapine to another, the patient must be entered into a new registry (must be completed by the prescriber and delivered to the dispensing pharmacy). Healthcare providers, including pharmacists dispensing clozapine, should verify the patient's hematological status and qualification to receive clozapine with all existing registries. The manufacturer of Clozaril® requests that healthcare providers submit all WBC/ANC values following discontinuation of therapy to the Clozaril National Registry for all nonrechallengable patients until WBC is $\geq 3500/mm^3$ and ANC is $\geq 2000/mm^3$.
Mechanism of Action Clozapine (dibenzodiazepine antipsychotic) exhibits weak antagonism of D_1, D_2, D_3, and D_5 dopamine receptor subtypes, but shows high affinity for D_4; in addition, it blocks the serotonin ($5HT_2$), alpha-adrenergic, histamine H_1, and cholinergic receptors
Drug Interactions
Cytochrome P450 Effect: Substrate of CYP1A2 (major), 2A6 (minor), 2C9 (minor), 2C19 (minor), 2D6 (minor), 3A4 (minor); **Inhibits** CYP1A2 (weak), 2C9 (weak), 2C19 (weak), 2D6 (moderate), 2E1 (weak), 3A4 (weak)
Increased Effect/Toxicity: May potentiate anticholinergic and hypotensive effects of other drugs. Benzodiazepines in combination with clozapine may produce respiratory depression and hypotension, especially during the first few weeks of therapy. May potentiate effect/toxicity of risperidone. Clozapine serum concentrations may be increased by inhibitors of CYP1A2; example
(Continued)

Clozapine *(Continued)*

inhibitors include ciprofloxacin, fluvoxamine, ketoconazole, norfloxacin, ofloxacin, and rofecoxib. Clozapine may increase the levels/effects of amphetamines, selected beta-blockers, substrates; example substrates include dextromethorphan, fluoxetine, lidocaine, mirtazapine, nefazodone, paroxetine, risperidone, ritonavir, thioridazine, tricyclic antidepressants, venlafaxine, and other CYP2D6 substrates. Sedative effects may be additive with other CNS depressants (eg, ethanol, barbiturates, benzodiazepines, opioid analgesics, and other sedatives). Metoclopramide may increase risk of extrapyramidal symptoms (EPS). Acetylcholinesterase inhibitors (central) may increase the risk of antipsychotic-related EPS. Citalopram may increase the levels/effects of clozapine. Omeprazole may alter the concentrations/effects of clozapine.

Decreased Effect: Clozapine may decrease the levels/effects of CYP2D6 prodrug substrates; example prodrug substrates include codeine, hydrocodone, oxycodone, and tramadol. The levels/effects of clozapine may be decreased by carbamazepine, phenobarbital, primidone, rifampin, and other CYP1A2 inducers. Clozapine may reverse the pressor effect of epinephrine (avoid in treatment of drug-induced hypotension). Omeprazole may alter the concentrations/effects of clozapine.

Pharmacodynamics/Kinetics

Protein binding: 97% to serum proteins
Metabolism: Extensively hepatic; forms metabolites with limited or no activity
Bioavailability: 12% to 81% (not affected by food)
Half-life elimination: Steady state: 12 hours (range: 4-66 hours)
Time to peak: 2.5 hours (range: 1-6 hours)
Excretion: Urine (~50%) and feces (30%) with trace amounts of unchanged drug

Pregnancy Risk Factor B

Clozaril® *see* Clozapine *on page 401*

CMA-676 *see* Gemtuzumab Ozogamicin *on page 774*

CNJ-016™ *see* Vaccinia Immune Globulin (Intravenous) *on page 1634*

Coagulant Complex Inhibitor *see* Anti-inhibitor Coagulant Complex *on page 133*

Coagulation Factor VIIa *see* Factor VIIa (Recombinant) *on page 666*

Coal Tar *(KOLE tar)*

U.S. Brand Names Balnetar® [OTC]; Betatar® Gel [OTC]; Cutar® [OTC]; Denorex® Original Therapeutic Strength [OTC]; DHS™ Tar [OTC]; DHS™ Targel [OTC]; Doak® Tar [OTC]; Exorex®; Fototar® [OTC]; Ionil T® [OTC]; Ionil T® Plus [OTC]; MG 217® [OTC]; MG 217® Medicated Tar [OTC]; Neutrogena® T/Gel [OTC]; Neutrogena® T/Gel Extra Strength [OTC]; Neutrogena® T/Gel Stubborn Itch Control [OTC]; Oxipor® VHC [OTC]; Polytar® [OTC]; PsoriGel® [OTC] [DSC]; Reme-T™ [OTC]; Tera-Gel™ [OTC]; Zetar® [OTC]

Canadian Brand Names Balnetar®; Estar®; Targel®

Generic Available No

Index Terms Crude Coal Tar; LCD; Pix Carbonis

Pharmacologic Category Topical Skin Product

Use Topically for controlling dandruff, seborrheic dermatitis, or psoriasis

Local Anesthetic/Vasoconstrictor Precautions No information available to require special precautions

Effects on Dental Treatment No significant effects or complications reported

Pregnancy Risk Factor C

Coal Tar and Salicylic Acid *(KOLE tar & sal i SIL ik AS id)*

Related Information

Coal Tar *on page 402*
Salicylic Acid *on page 1451*

U.S. Brand Names Tarsum® [OTC]; X-Seb T® Pearl [OTC]; X-Seb T® Plus [OTC]

Canadian Brand Names Sebcur/T®

Generic Available Yes

Index Terms Salicylic Acid and Coal Tar

Pharmacologic Category Topical Skin Product

Use Seborrheal dermatitis, dandruff, psoriasis

Local Anesthetic/Vasoconstrictor Precautions No information available to require special precautions

Effects on Dental Treatment No significant effects or complications reported

Pregnancy Risk Factor C

Cocaine (koe KANE)

Generic Available Yes
Index Terms Cocaine Hydrochloride
Pharmacologic Category Local Anesthetic
Use Topical anesthesia for mucous membranes
Local Anesthetic/Vasoconstrictor Precautions Although plain local anesthetic is not contraindicated, vasoconstrictor is absolutely contraindicated in any patient under the influence of or within 2 hours of cocaine use
Effects on Dental Treatment Key adverse event(s) related to dental treatment: Loss of taste perception. See Dental Comment.

Common Adverse Effects
>10%:
Central nervous system: CNS stimulation
Gastrointestinal: Loss of taste perception
Respiratory: Rhinitis, nasal congestion
Miscellaneous: Loss of smell
1% to 10%:
Cardiovascular: Heart rate (decreased) with low doses, tachycardia with moderate doses, hypertension, cardiomyopathy, cardiac arrhythmia, myocarditis, QRS prolongation, Raynaud's phenomenon, cerebral vasculitis, thrombosis, fibrillation (atrial), flutter (atrial), sinus bradycardia, CHF, pulmonary hypertension, sinus tachycardia, tachycardia (supraventricular), arrhythmia (ventricular), vasoconstriction
Central nervous system: Fever, nervousness, restlessness, euphoria, excitation, headache, psychosis, hallucinations, agitation, seizure, slurred speech, hyperthermia, dystonic reactions, cerebral vascular accident, vasculitis, clonic-tonic reactions, paranoia, sympathetic storm
Dermatologic: Skin infarction, pruritus, madarosis
Gastrointestinal: Nausea, anorexia, colonic ischemia, spontaneous bowel perforation
Genitourinary: Priapism, uterine rupture
Hematologic: Thrombocytopenia
Neuromuscular & skeletal: Chorea (extrapyramidal), paresthesia, tremor, fasciculations
Ocular: Mydriasis (peak effect at 45 minutes; may last up to 12 hours), sloughing of the corneal epithelium, ulceration of the cornea, iritis, mydriasis, chemosis
Renal: Myoglobinuria, necrotizing vasculitis
Respiratory: Tachypnea, nasal mucosa damage (when snorting), hyposmia, bronchiolitis obliterans organizing pneumonia
Miscellaneous: "Washed-out" syndrome

Restrictions C-II
Mechanism of Action Ester local anesthetic blocks both the initiation and conduction of nerve impulses by decreasing the neuronal membrane's permeability to sodium ions, which results in inhibition of depolarization with resultant blockade of conduction; interferes with the uptake of norepinephrine by adrenergic nerve terminals producing vasoconstriction

Drug Interactions
Cytochrome P450 Effect: Substrate of CYP3A4 (major); **Inhibits** CYP2D6 (strong), 3A4 (weak)
Increased Effect/Toxicity: Cocaine may increase the levels/effects of CYP2D6 substrates (eg, amphetamines, selected beta-blockers, dextromethorphan, fluoxetine, lidocaine, mirtazapine, nefazodone, paroxetine, risperidone, ritonavir, thioridazine, tricyclic antidepressants, venlafaxine). Increased toxicity with MAO inhibitors. Use with epinephrine may cause extreme hypertension and/or cardiac arrhythmias. CYP3A4 inhibitors may increase the levels/effects of cocaine (eg, azole antifungals, clarithromycin, diclofenac, doxycycline, erythromycin, imatinib, isoniazid, nefazodone, nicardipine, propofol, protease inhibitors, quinidine, telithromycin, verapamil).

Pharmacodynamics/Kinetics Following topical administration to mucosa:
Onset of action: ~1 minute
Peak effect: ~5 minutes
Duration (dose dependent): ≥30 minutes; cocaine metabolites may appear in urine of neonates up to 5 days after birth due to maternal cocaine use shortly before birth
Absorption: Well absorbed through mucous membranes; limited by drug-induced vasoconstriction; enhanced by inflammation
Distribution: Enters breast milk
(Continued)

Cocaine *(Continued)*

Metabolism: Hepatic; major metabolites are ecgonine methyl ester and benzoyl ecgonine

Half-life elimination: 75 minutes

Excretion: Primarily urine (<10% as unchanged drug and metabolites)

Pregnancy Risk Factor C/X (nonmedicinal use)

Dental Comment The cocaine user, regardless of how the cocaine was administered, presents a potential life-threatening situation in the dental operatory. A patient under the influence of cocaine could be compared to a car going 100 mph. Blood pressure is elevated, heart rate is likely increased, and the use of a local anesthetic with epinephrine may result in a medical emergency. Such patients can be identified by their jitteriness, irritability, talkativeness, tremors, and short, abrupt speech patterns. These same signs and symptoms may also be seen in a normal dental patient with preoperative dental anxiety; therefore, the dentist must be particularly alert in order to identify the potential cocaine abuser. If cocaine use is suspected, the patient should never be given a local anesthetic with vasoconstrictor, for fear of exacerbating the cocaine-induced sympathetic response. Life-threatening episodes of cardiac arrhythmias and hypertensive crises have been reported when local anesthetic with vasoconstrictor was administered to a patient under the influence of cocaine. No local anesthetic, used by any dentist, can interfere with, nor test positive by cocaine in any urine testing screen. Therefore, the dentist does not need to be concerned with any false drug-use accusations associated with dental anesthesia.

Cocaine Hydrochloride *see* Cocaine *on page 403*

Codeine (KOE deen)

Related Information
Oral Pain *on page 1788*

Canadian Brand Names Codeine Contin®

Generic Available Yes

Index Terms Codeine Phosphate; Codeine Sulfate; Methylmorphine

Pharmacologic Category Analgesic, Opioid; Antitussive

Dental Use Treatment of postoperative pain

Use Treatment of mild-to-moderate pain; antitussive in lower doses; dextromethorphan has equivalent antitussive activity but has much lower toxicity in accidental overdose

Local Anesthetic/Vasoconstrictor Precautions No information available to require special precautions

Effects on Dental Treatment No significant effects or complications reported (see Dental Comment)

Significant Adverse Effects

Frequency not defined: AST/ALT increased

>10%:
Central nervous system: Drowsiness
Gastrointestinal: Constipation

1% to 10%:
Cardiovascular: Tachycardia or bradycardia, hypotension
Central nervous system: Dizziness, lightheadedness, false feeling of well being, malaise, headache, restlessness, paradoxical CNS stimulation, confusion
Dermatologic: Rash, urticaria
Gastrointestinal: Dry mouth, anorexia, nausea, vomiting
Genitourinary: Urination decreased, ureteral spasm
Hepatic: LFTs increased
Local: Burning at injection site
Neuromuscular & skeletal: Weakness
Ocular: Blurred vision
Respiratory: Dyspnea
Miscellaneous: Histamine release

<1% (Limited to important or life-threatening): Convulsions, hallucinations, insomnia, mental depression, nightmares

Restrictions C-II

Dental Usual Dosing Postoperative pain: Adults: Oral: 30 mg every 4-6 hours as needed; patients with prior opiate exposure may require higher initial doses. Usual range: 15-120 mg every 4-6 hours as needed

Dosage Note: These are guidelines and do not represent the maximum doses that may be required in all patients. Doses should be titrated to pain relief/prevention. Doses >1.5 mg/kg body weight are not recommended.

Analgesic:
Children: Oral, I.M., SubQ: 0.5-1 mg/kg/dose every 4-6 hours as needed; maximum: 60 mg/dose
Adults:
Oral: 30 mg every 4-6 hours as needed; patients with prior opiate exposure may require higher initial doses. Usual range: 15-120 mg every 4-6 hours as needed
Oral, controlled release formulation (Codeine Contin®, not available in U.S.): 50-300 mg every 12 hours. **Note:** A patient's codeine requirement should be established using prompt release formulations; conversion to long acting products may be considered when chronic, continuous treatment is required. Higher dosages should be reserved for use only in opioid-tolerant patients.
I.M., SubQ: 30 mg every 4-6 hours as needed; patients with prior opiate exposure may require higher initial doses. Usual range: 15-120 mg every 4-6 hours as needed; more frequent dosing may be needed
Antitussive: Oral (for nonproductive cough):
Children: 1-1.5 mg/kg/day in divided doses every 4-6 hours as needed: Alternative dose according to age:
2-6 years: 2.5-5 mg every 4-6 hours as needed; maximum: 30 mg/day
6-12 years: 5-10 mg every 4-6 hours as needed; maximum: 60 mg/day
Adults: 10-20 mg/dose every 4-6 hours as needed; maximum: 120 mg/day
Dosing adjustment in renal impairment:
Cl_{cr} 10-50 mL/minute: Administer 75% of dose
Cl_{cr} <10 mL/minute: Administer 50% of dose
Dosing adjustment in hepatic impairment: Probably necessary in hepatic insufficiency
Mechanism of Action Binds to opiate receptors in the CNS, causing inhibition of ascending pain pathways, altering the perception of and response to pain; causes cough supression by direct central action in the medulla; produces generalized CNS depression
Contraindications Hypersensitivity to codeine or any component of the formulation; pregnancy (prolonged use or high doses at term)
Warnings/Precautions

Use with caution in patients with hypersensitivity reactions to other phenanthrene derivative opioid agonists (morphine, hydrocodone, hydromorphone, levorphanol, oxycodone, oxymorphone); respiratory diseases including asthma, emphysema, COPD, adrenal insufficiency, biliary tract impairment, CNS depression/coma, head trauma, morbid obesity, prostatic hyperplasia, urinary stricture, thyroid dysfunction, or severe liver or renal insufficiency; some preparations contain sulfites which may cause allergic reactions; tolerance or drug dependence may result from extended use. May obscure diagnosis or clinical course of patients with acute abdominal conditions. May cause CNS depression, which may impair physical or mental abilities; patients must be cautioned about performing tasks which require mental alertness (eg, operating machinery or driving). May cause hypotension; use with caution in patients with hypovolemia, cardiovascular disease (including acute MI), or drugs which may exaggerate hypotensive effects (including phenothiazines or general anesthetics).

Not recommended for use for cough control in patients with a productive cough; not recommended as an antitussive for children <2 years of age; the elderly and debilitated patients may be particularly susceptible to adverse effects of narcotics.

Not approved for I.V. administration (although this route has been used clinically). If given intravenously, must be given slowly and the patient should be lying down. Rapid intravenous administration of narcotics may increase the incidence of serious adverse effects, in part due to limited opportunity to assess response prior to administration of the full dose. Access to respiratory support should be immediately available.

Concurrent use of agonist/antagonist analgesics may precipitate withdrawal symptoms and/or reduced analgesic efficacy in patients following prolonged therapy with mu opioid agonists. Abrupt discontinuation following prolonged use may also lead to withdrawal symptoms.
Drug Interactions Substrate of CYP2D6 (major), 3A4 (minor); **Inhibits** CYP2D6 (weak)
CYP2D6 inhibitors: May decrease the effects of codeine. Example inhibitors include chlorpromazine, delavirdine, fluoxetine, miconazole, paroxetine, pergolide, quinidine, quinine, ritonavir, and ropinirole.
Decreased effect with cigarette smoking
Increased toxicity: CNS depressants, phenothiazines, TCAs, other opioid analgesics, guanabenz, MAO inhibitors, neuromuscular blockers
Ethanol/Nutrition/Herb Interactions
Ethanol: Avoid or limit ethanol (may increase CNS depression).
(Continued)

Codeine *(Continued)*

Herb/Nutraceutical: St John's wort may decrease codeine levels. Avoid valerian, St John's wort, kava kava, gotu kola (may increase CNS depression).

Pharmacodynamics/Kinetics

Onset of action: Oral: 0.5-1 hour; I.M.: 10-30 minutes
Peak effect: Oral: 1-1.5 hours; I.M.: 0.5-1 hour
Duration: 4-6 hours
Absorption: Oral: Adequate
Distribution: Crosses placenta; enters breast milk
Protein binding: 7%
Metabolism: Hepatic to morphine (active)
Half-life elimination: 2.5-3.5 hours
Excretion: Urine (3% to 16% as unchanged drug, norcodeine, and free and conjugated morphine)

Pregnancy Risk Factor C/D (prolonged use or high doses at term)

Lactation Enters breast milk/use caution (AAP rates "compatible")

Dosage Forms Excipient information presented when available (limited, particularly for generics); consult specific product labeling. [CAN] = Canadian brand name

Injection, as phosphate: 15 mg/mL (2 mL); 30 mg/mL (2 mL) [contains sodium metabisulfite]
Tablet, as phosphate: 30 mg, 60 mg
Tablet, as sulfate: 15 mg, 30 mg, 60 mg
Tablet, controlled release (Codeine Contin®) [CAN]: 50 mg, 100 mg, 150 mg, 200 mg [not available in U.S.]

Dental Comment It is recommended that codeine not be used as the sole entity for analgesia because of moderate efficacy along with relatively high incidence of nausea, sedation, and constipation. In addition, codeine has some narcotic addiction liability. Codeine in combination with acetaminophen or aspirin is recommended. Maximum effective analgesic dose of codeine is 60 mg (1 grain). Beyond 60 mg increases respiratory depression only. Sodium thiosulfate is an effective chemical antidote for codeine poisoning.

Selected Readings

Desjardins PJ, Cooper SA, Gallegos TL, et al, "The Relative Analgesic Efficacy of Propiram Fumarate, Codeine, Aspirin, and Placebo in Postimpaction Dental Pain," *J Clin Pharmacol*, 1984, 24(1):35-42.

Forbes JA, Keller CK, Smith JW, et al, "Analgesic Effect of Naproxen Sodium, Codeine, a Naproxen-Codeine Combination and Aspirin on the Postoperative Pain of Oral Surgery," *Pharmacotherapy*, 1986, 6(5):211-8.

Colchicine (KOL chi seen)

Mexican Brand Names Colchiquim
Generic Available Yes
Pharmacologic Category Colchicine
Use Treatment of acute gouty arthritis attacks and prevention of recurrences of such attacks
Unlabeled/Investigational Use Primary biliary cirrhosis; management of familial Mediterranean fever; pericarditis
Local Anesthetic/Vasoconstrictor Precautions No information available to require special precautions
Effects on Dental Treatment No significant effects or complications reported
Common Adverse Effects
>10%: Gastrointestinal: Nausea, vomiting, diarrhea, abdominal pain
1% to 10%:
Dermatologic: Alopecia
Gastrointestinal: Anorexia
Mechanism of Action Decreases leukocyte motility, decreases phagocytosis in joints and lactic acid production, thereby reducing the deposition of urate crystals that perpetuates the inflammatory response
Drug Interactions
Cytochrome P450 Effect: Substrate of CYP3A4 (major); **Induces** CYP2C8 (weak), 2C9 (weak), 2E1 (weak), 3A4 (weak)
Increased Effect/Toxicity: Concurrent use of cyclosporine with colchicine may increase toxicity of colchicine. CYP3A4 inhibitors may increase the levels/effects of colchicine (example inhibitors include azole antifungals, diclofenac, doxycycline, imatinib, isoniazid, nefazodone, nicardipine, propofol, protease inhibitors, quinidine, and verapamil. Macrolide antibiotics (clarithromycin, erythromycin, troleandomycin) and telithromycin may decrease the metabolism of colchicine resulting in severe colchicine toxicity; avoid, if possible. Verapamil may increase colchicine toxicity (especially nephrotoxicity).
Pharmacodynamics/Kinetics
Onset of action: Oral: Pain relief: ~12 hours if adequately dosed
Distribution: Concentrates in leukocytes, kidney, spleen, and liver; does not distribute in heart, skeletal muscle, and brain
Protein binding: 10% to 31%
Metabolism: Partially hepatic via deacetylation
Half-life elimination: 12-30 minutes; End-stage renal disease: 45 minutes
Time to peak, serum: Oral: 0.5-2 hours, declining for the next 2 hours before increasing again due to enterohepatic recycling
Excretion: Primarily feces; urine (10% to 20%)
Pregnancy Risk Factor C (oral); D (parenteral)

Colchicine and Probenecid (KOL chi seen & proe BEN e sid)

Related Information
Colchicine *on page 407*
Probenecid *on page 1354*
Generic Available Yes
Index Terms ColBenemid; Probenecid and Colchicine
Pharmacologic Category Anti-inflammatory Agent; Antigout Agent; Uricosuric Agent
Use Treatment of chronic gouty arthritis when complicated by frequent, recurrent acute attacks of gout
Local Anesthetic/Vasoconstrictor Precautions No information available to require special precautions
Effects on Dental Treatment No significant effects or complications reported
Common Adverse Effects 1% to 10%:
Cardiovascular: Flushing
Central nervous system: Headache, dizziness
Dermatologic: Rash, alopecia
Gastrointestinal: Anorexia, nausea, vomiting, diarrhea, abdominal pain
Hematologic: Anemia, leukopenia, aplastic anemia, agranulocytosis
Hepatic: Hepatic necrosis, hepatotoxicity
Neuromuscular & skeletal: Peripheral neuritis, myopathy
Renal: Nephrotic syndrome, uric acid stones, polyuria
(Continued)

Colchicine and Probenecid (Continued)

Miscellaneous: Hypersensitivity reactions

Drug Interactions

Cytochrome P450 Effect:

Colchicine: **Substrate** of CYP3A4 (major); **Induces** CYP2C8 (weak), 2C9 (weak), 2E1 (weak), 3A4 (weak)

Probenecid: **Inhibits** CYP2C19 (weak)

Pharmacodynamics/Kinetics See individual agents.

Pregnancy Risk Factor C

Coldcough *see* Pseudoephedrine, Dihydrocodeine, and Chlorpheniramine *on page 1385*

Coldcough PD *see* Dihydrocodeine, Chlorpheniramine, and Phenylephrine *on page 502*

Coldmist DM *see* Guaifenesin, Pseudoephedrine, and Dextromethorphan *on page 800*

Coldtuss DR [DSC] *see* Chlorpheniramine, Phenylephrine, and Dextromethorphan *on page 342*

Colesevelam (koh le SEV a lam)

Related Information

Cardiovascular Diseases *on page 1726*

U.S. Brand Names WelChol®

Canadian Brand Names WelChol®

Generic Available No

Pharmacologic Category Antilipemic Agent, Bile Acid Sequestrant

Use Adjunctive therapy to diet and exercise in the management of elevated LDL in primary hypercholesterolemia (Fredrickson type IIa) when used alone or in combination with an HMG-CoA reductase inhibitor

Local Anesthetic/Vasoconstrictor Precautions No information available to require special precautions

Effects on Dental Treatment No significant effects or complications reported

Common Adverse Effects

>10%: Gastrointestinal: Constipation (11%)

2% to 10%:

Gastrointestinal: Dyspepsia (8%)

Neuromuscular & skeletal: Weakness (4%), myalgia (2%)

Respiratory: Pharyngitis (3%)

Incidence less than or equal to placebo: Infection, headache, pain, back pain, abdominal pain, flu syndrome, flatulence, diarrhea, nausea, sinusitis, rhinitis, cough

Dosage Adult: Oral:

Monotherapy: 3 tablets twice daily with meals or 6 tablets once daily with a meal; maximum dose: 7 tablets/day

Combination therapy with an HMG-CoA reductase inhibitor: 4-6 tablets daily; maximum dose: 6 tablets/day

Dosage adjustment in renal impairment: No recommendations made

Dosage adjustment in hepatic impairment: No recommendations made

Elderly: No recommendations made

Mechanism of Action Colesevelam binds bile acids including glycocholic acid in the intestine, impeding their reabsorption. Increases the fecal loss of bile salt-bound LDL-C

Contraindications Hypersensitivity to colesevelam or any component of the formulation; bowel obstruction

Warnings/Precautions Use caution in treating patients with serum triglyceride levels >300 mg/dL (may cause increased levels). Use caution in dysphagia, swallowing disorders, severe GI motility disorders, major GI tract surgery, and in patients susceptible to fat-soluble vitamin deficiencies. Minimal effects are seen on HDL-C and triglyceride levels. Secondary causes of hypercholesterolemia should be excluded before initiation. Safety and efficacy have not been established in pediatric patients.

Drug Interactions

Decreased Effect: The absorption of thyroid supplements may be reduced by colesevelam (may be noted by elevation in TSH). Separate administration times by least 1 hour before or 4 hours after dose and monitor TSH levels during concurrent therapy. The absorption of corticosteroids, diuretics, ezetimibe, fibric acid derivatives, methotrexate, niacin, NSAIDs, raloxifene, tetracyclines, and thiazolidinediones may be reduced by concurrent colesevelam. Separate administration times by at least 1 hour before or 4 hours after dose. The absorption of amiodarone may also be reduced by concurrent colesevelam and close monitoring is recommended.

A number of medications, including digoxin, HMG-CoA reductase inhibitors (atorvastatin, lovastatin, simvastatin), metoprolol, quinidine, valproic acid, verapamil, or warfarin absorption have been specifically evaluated and were not found to be significantly affected with concurrent administration.

Dietary Considerations Should be taken with meal(s) and a liquid. Follow dietary guidelines.

Pharmacodynamics/Kinetics

Onset of action: Peak effect: Therapeutic: ~2 weeks

Absorption: Insignificant

Excretion: Urine (0.05%) after 1 month of chronic dosing

Pregnancy Risk Factor B

Dosage Forms

Tablet:

WelChol®: 625 mg

Selected Readings

Davidson MH, Dillon MA, Gordon B, et al, "Colesevelam Hydrochloride (Cholestagel): A New, Potent Bile Acid Sequestrant Associated With a Low Incidence of Gastrointestinal Side Effects," *Arch Intern Med*, 1999, 159(16):1893-900.

"Executive Summary of The Third Report of The National Cholesterol Education Program (NCEP) Expert Panel on Detection, Evaluation, And Treatment of High Blood Cholesterol In Adults (Adult Treatment Panel III)," *JAMA*, 2001, 285(19):2486-97.

Steinmetz KL, "Colesevelam Hydrochloride," *Am J Health Syst Pharm*, 2002, 59:932-9.

Colestid® *see* Colestipol *on page 409*

Colestipol (koe LES ti pole)

Related Information

Cardiovascular Diseases *on page 1726*

U.S. Brand Names Colestid®

Canadian Brand Names Colestid®

Generic Available No

Index Terms Colestipol Hydrochloride

Pharmacologic Category Antilipemic Agent, Bile Acid Sequestrant

Use Adjunct in management of primary hypercholesterolemia; regression of arteriosclerosis; relief of pruritus associated with elevated levels of bile acids; possibly used to decrease plasma half-life of digoxin in toxicity

Local Anesthetic/Vasoconstrictor Precautions No information available to require special precautions

Effects on Dental Treatment No significant effects or complications reported

Common Adverse Effects

>10%: Gastrointestinal: Constipation

1% to 10%:

Central nervous system: Headache, dizziness, anxiety, vertigo, drowsiness, fatigue

Gastrointestinal: Abdominal pain and distention, belching, flatulence, nausea, vomiting, diarrhea

Mechanism of Action Binds with bile acids to form an insoluble complex that is eliminated in feces; it thereby increases the fecal loss of bile acid-bound low density lipoprotein cholesterol

Drug Interactions

Decreased Effect: Colestipol can reduce the absorption of numerous medications when used concurrently. Give other medications 1 hour before or 4 hours after giving colestipol. Medications which may be affected include HMG-CoA reductase inhibitors, thiazide diuretics, propranolol (and potentially other beta-blockers), corticosteroids, thyroid hormones, digoxin, valproic acid, NSAIDs, loop diuretics, sulfonylureas, troglitazone (and potentially other agents in this class - pioglitazone and rosiglitazone).

Warfarin and other oral anticoagulants: Absorption is reduced by cholestyramine and may also be reduced by colestipol. Separate administration times (as detailed above).

Pharmacodynamics/Kinetics

Absorption: None

Excretion: Feces

Pregnancy Risk Factor C

Colestipol Hydrochloride *see* Colestipol *on page 409*

Colgate Total® *see* Triclosan and Fluoride *on page 1616*

Colistimethate (koe lis ti METH ate)

U.S. Brand Names Coly-Mycin® M
Canadian Brand Names Coly-Mycin® M
Generic Available Yes
Index Terms Colistimethate Sodium
Pharmacologic Category Antibiotic, Miscellaneous
Use Treatment of infections due to sensitive strains of certain gram-negative bacilli which are resistant to other antibacterials or in patients allergic to other antibacterials
Unlabeled/Investigational Use Used as inhalation in the prevention of *Pseudomonas aeruginosa* respiratory tract infections in immunocompromised patients, and used as inhalation adjunct agent for the treatment of *P. aeruginosa* infections in patients with cystic fibrosis and other seriously ill or chronically ill patients
Local Anesthetic/Vasoconstrictor Precautions No information available to require special precautions
Effects on Dental Treatment No significant effects or complications reported
Common Adverse Effects 1% to 10%:
Central nervous system: Vertigo, slurring of speech
Dermatologic: Urticaria
Gastrointestinal: GI upset
Respiratory: Respiratory arrest
Renal: Nephrotoxicity
Mechanism of Action Hydrolyzed to colistin, which acts as a cationic detergent which damages the bacterial cytoplasmic membrane causing leaking of intracellular substances and cell death
Drug Interactions
Increased Effect/Toxicity: Other nephrotoxic drugs, neuromuscular blocking agents.
Pharmacodynamics/Kinetics
Distribution: Widely, except for CNS, synovial, pleural, and pericardial fluids
Half-life elimination: 1.5-8 hours; Anuria: ≤2-3 days
Time to peak: ~2 hours
Excretion: Primarily urine (as unchanged drug)
Pregnancy Risk Factor C

Colistimethate Sodium *see* Colistimethate *on page 410*

CollaCote® *see* Collagen (Absorbable) *on page 410*

Collagen *see* Collagen Hemostat *on page 411*

Collagen (Absorbable) (KOL la jen, ab SORB able)

U.S. Brand Names CollaCote®; CollaPlug®; CollaTape®
Generic Available Yes
Pharmacologic Category Hemostatic Agent
Dental Use Control of bleeding created during dental surgery
Use Hemostatic
Local Anesthetic/Vasoconstrictor Precautions No information available to require special precautions
Effects on Dental Treatment No significant effects or complications reported
Significant Adverse Effects No data reported.
Dental Usual Dosing Control of bleeding: Children and Adults: Topical: A sufficiently large dressing should be selected so as to completely cover the oral wound
Dosage Children and Adults: A sufficiently large dressing should be selected so as to completely cover the oral wound
Mechanism of Action The highly porous sponge structure absorbs blood and wound exudate. The collagen component causes aggregation of platelets which bind to collagen fibrils. The aggregated platelets degranulate, releasing coagulation factors that promote the formation of fibrin.
Contraindications No data reported
Warnings/Precautions Should not be used on infected or contaminated wounds
Drug Interactions No data reported
Lactation Compatible
Dosage Forms Excipient information presented when available (limited, particularly for generics); consult specific product labeling.
Wound dressing:
³/₈" x ³/₄"
³/₄" x 1 ¹/₂"
1" x 3"

Collagen Absorbable Hemostat *see* Collagen Hemostat *on page 411*

Collagenase (KOL la je nase)

U.S. Brand Names Santyl®
Generic Available No
Pharmacologic Category Enzyme, Topical Debridement
Use Promotes debridement of necrotic tissue in dermal ulcers and severe burns
 Orphan drug: Injection: Treatment of Peyronie's disease; treatment of Dupytren's disease
Local Anesthetic/Vasoconstrictor Precautions No information available to require special precautions
Effects on Dental Treatment No significant effects or complications reported
Common Adverse Effects Frequency not defined.
 Local: Irritation, pain and burning may occur at site of application
Mechanism of Action Collagenase is an enzyme derived from the fermentation of *Clostridium histolyticum* and differs from other proteolytic enzymes in that its enzymatic action has a high specificity for native and denatured collagen. Collagenase will not attack collagen in healthy tissue or newly formed granulation tissue. In addition, it does not act on fat, fibrin, keratin, or muscle.
Drug Interactions
 Decreased Effect: Enzymatic activity is inhibited by detergents, benzalkonium chloride, hexachlorophene, nitrofurazone, tincture of iodine, and heavy metal ions (silver and mercury).
Pregnancy Risk Factor C

Collagen Hemostat (KOL la jen HEE moe stat)

U.S. Brand Names Avitene®; Avitene® Flour; Avitene® Ultrafoam; Avitene® UltraWrap™; EndoAvitene®; Helistat®; Helitene®; Instat™; Instat™ MCH; SyringeAvitene™
Generic Available No
Index Terms Collagen; Collagen Absorbable Hemostat; MCH; Microfibrillar Collagen Hemostat
Pharmacologic Category Hemostatic Agent
Dental Use Adjunct to hemostasis when control of bleeding by ligature is ineffective or impractical
Use Adjunct to hemostasis when control of bleeding by ligature is ineffective or impractical
Local Anesthetic/Vasoconstrictor Precautions No information available to require special precautions
Effects on Dental Treatment No significant effects or complications reported
Significant Adverse Effects Frequency not defined.
 Miscellaneous: Adhesion formation, allergic reaction, edema, foreign body reaction, hematoma, inflammation, potentiation of infection
 Postmarketing and/or case reports: Numbness, pain, paralysis, subgaleal seroma; alveolalgia and transient laryngospasm with dental use
Dental Usual Dosing Hemostasis: Adults: Topical: Apply dry directly to source of bleeding; remove excess material after ~10-15 minutes
Dosage Apply dry directly to source of bleeding; remove excess material after ~10-15 minutes
Mechanism of Action Collagen hemostat is an absorbable topical hemostatic agent prepared from purified bovine corium collagen and shredded into fibrils. Physically, microfibrillar collagen hemostat yields a large surface area. Chemically, it is collagen with hydrochloric acid noncovalently bound to some of the available amino groups in the collagen molecules. When in contact with a bleeding surface, collagen hemostat attracts platelets which adhere to its fibrils and undergo the release phenomenon. This triggers aggregation of the platelets into thrombi in the interstices of the fibrous mass, initiating the formation of a physiologic platelet plug.
Contraindications Hypersensitivity to any component of the formulation; products of bovine origin; closure of skin incisions, contaminated wounds; application to bone surfaces to which prosthetic materials are attached with methylmethacrylate adhesives
Warnings/Precautions Pain, numbness, or paralysis have been reported if used near a bony or neural space and left inside patient; use minimum amount necessary to achieve hemostasis. Remove as much of agent as possible after hemostasis is achieved. Do not leave in a contaminated or infected space. Fragments of MCH may pass through filters of blood scavenging systems; avoid reintroduction of blood from operative sites treated with MCH. Not intended to
(Continued)

411

Collagen Hemostat *(Continued)*

treat systemic coagulation disorders. Not for use when origin of bleeding is unknown.

Drug Interactions No data reported

Pharmacodynamics/Kinetics

Onset: Hemostasis: 2-5 minutes

Absorption: ≥8 weeks

Dosage Forms Excipient information presented when available (limited, particularly for generics); consult specific product labeling.

Pad (Instat™) [bovine derived]: 1 inch x 2 inch (24s); 3 inch x 4 inch (24s)

Powder:

Avitene® Flour [microfibrillar product, bovine derived]: 0.5 g, 1 g, 5 g

Helitene® [bovine derived]: 0.5 g, 1 g

Instat™ MCH [microfibrillar product, bovine derived]: 0.5 g, 1 g

SyringeAvitene™ [microfibrillar product, bovine derived, prefilled syringe]: 1 g

Sheet:

Avitene® [microfibrillar product, bovine derived, nonwoven web]: 35 mm x 35 mm (1s); 70 mm x 35 mm (6s, 12s); 70 mm x 70 mm (6s, 12s)

EndoAvitene® [microfibrillar product, bovine derived, preloaded applicator]: 5 mm diameter (6s); 10 mm diameter (6s)

Sponge:

Avitene® Ultrafoam [microfibrillar product, bovine derived]: 2 cm x 6.25 cm x 7 mm (12s); 8 cm x 6.25 cm x 1 cm (6s); 8 cm x 12.5 cm x 1 cm (6s); 8 cm x 12.5 cm x 3 mm (6s)

Avitene® UltraWrap™ [microfibrillar product, bovine derived]: 8 cm x 12.5 cm (6s)

Helistat® [bovine derived]: 0.5 inch x 1 inch x 7 mm (18s) [packaged as 3 strips of 6 sponges]; 3 inch x 4 inch x 5 inch (10s)

Conivaptan (koe NYE vap tan)

U.S. Brand Names Vaprisol®
Generic Available No
Index Terms Conivaptan Hydrochloride; YM087
Pharmacologic Category Vasopressin Antagonist
Use Treatment of euvolemic and hypervolemic hyponatremia in hospitalized patients
Local Anesthetic/Vasoconstrictor Precautions No information available to require special precautions
Effects on Dental Treatment Key adverse event(s) related to dental treatment: Dry mouth, oral candidiasis, orthostatic hypotension.
Common Adverse Effects
>10%:
  Cardiovascular: Orthostatic hypotension (6% to 14%)
  Central nervous system: Fever (5% to 11%)
  Endocrine & metabolic: Hypokalemia (10% to 22%)
  Local: Injection site reactions including pain, erythema, phlebitis, swelling (63% to 73%)
1% to 10%:
  Cardiovascular: Hypertension (6% to 8%), hypotension (5% to 8%), edema (3% to 8%), phlebitis (5%), atrial fibrillation (2% to 5%), ECG abnormality (up to 5%)
  Central nervous system: Headache (8% to 10%), insomnia (4% to 5%), confusion (up to 5%), pain (2%)
  Dermatologic: Pruritus (1% to 5%), erythema (3%)
  Endocrine & metabolic: Hyponatremia (3% to 8%), hypomagnesemia (2% to 5%), hyper-/hypoglycemia (3%)
  Gastrointestinal: Constipation (6% to 8%), vomiting (5% to 7%), diarrhea (up to 7%), nausea (5%), dry mouth (4%), dehydration (2%), oral candidiasis (2%)
  Genitourinary: Urinary tract infection (4% to 5%)
  Hematologic: Anemia (4%)
  Renal: Polyuria (5% to 6%), hematuria (2%)
  Respiratory: Pneumonia (2% to 5%)
  Miscellaneous: Thirst (3% to 6%)
Mechanism of Action Conivaptan is an arginine vasopressin (AVP) receptor antagonist with affinity for AVP receptor subtypes V_{1A} and V_2. The antidiuretic action of AVP is mediated through activation of the V_2 receptor, which functions to regulate water and electrolyte balance at the level of the collecting ducts in the kidney. Serum levels of AVP are commonly elevated in euvolemic or hypervolemic hyponatremia, which results in the dilution of serum sodium and the relative hyponatremic state. Antagonism of the V_2 receptor by conivaptan promotes the excretion of free water (without loss of serum electrolytes) resulting in net fluid loss, increased urine output, decreased urine osmolality, and subsequent restoration of normal serum sodium levels.
Drug Interactions
  Cytochrome P450 Effect: Substrate of CYP3A4 (major); **Inhibits** CYP3A4 (strong)
  Increased Effect/Toxicity: Conivaptan may increase the levels/effects of CYP3A4 substrates (eg, benzodiazepines, calcium channel blockers, clarithromycin, cyclosporine, erythromycin, estrogens, mirtazapine, nateglinide, nefazodone, nevirapine, protease inhibitors, tacrolimus, and venlafaxine), digoxin, and pimecrolimus. CYP3A4 inhibitors may increase the levels/effects of conivaptan; example inhibitors include ketoconazole, itraconazole, ritonavir, indinavir, and clarithromycin. Concurrent use of conivaptan and strong CYP3A4 inhibitors is contraindicated.
  Decreased Effect: CYP3A4 inducers may decrease the levels/effects of conivaptan; example inducers include aminoglutethimide, carbamazepine, nafcillin, nevirapine, phenobarbital, phenytoin, and rifamycins.
Pharmacodynamics/Kinetics
  Protein binding: 99%
  Metabolism: Hepatic via CYP3A4 to four minimally-active metabolites
  Half-life elimination: 6.7-8.6 hours
  Excretion: Feces (83%); urine (12%, primarily as metabolites)
Pregnancy Risk Factor C

Conray® 43 *see* Iothalamate Meglumine *on page 903*

Conray® 400 *see* Iothalamate Sodium *on page 903*

Constulose *see* Lactulose *on page 943*

Contac® Cold [OTC] [DSC] *see* Pseudoephedrine *on page 1381*

ControlRx® *see* Fluoride *on page 710*

Copaxone® *see* Glatiramer Acetate *on page 778*

Copegus® *see* Ribavirin *on page 1420*

Copolymer-1 *see* Glatiramer Acetate *on page 778*

Copper *see* Trace Metals *on page 1595*

Cordarone® *see* Amiodarone *on page 92*

Cordran® *see* Flurandrenolide *on page 720*

Cordran® SP *see* Flurandrenolide *on page 720*

Cordron-D NR [DSC] *see* Carbinoxamine and Pseudoephedrine *on page 282*

Cordron-DM NR [DSC] *see* Carbinoxamine, Pseudoephedrine, and Dextromethorphan *on page 282*

Coreg® *see* Carvedilol *on page 291*

Coreg CR™ *see* Carvedilol *on page 291*

Corfen DM *see* Chlorpheniramine, Phenylephrine, and Dextromethorphan *on page 342*

Corgard® *see* Nadolol *on page 1139*

Coricidin HBP® Chest Congestion and Cough [OTC] *see* Guaifenesin and Dextromethorphan *on page 796*

Coricidin HBP® Cold and Flu [OTC] *see* Chlorpheniramine and Acetaminophen *on page 339*

Corlopam® *see* Fenoldopam *on page 676*

Cormax® *see* Clobetasol *on page 383*

Correctol® Tablets [OTC] *see* Bisacodyl *on page 216*

Cortaid® Intensive Therapy [OTC] *see* Hydrocortisone *on page 836*

Cortaid® Maximum Strength [OTC] *see* Hydrocortisone *on page 836*

Cortaid® Sensitive Skin [OTC] *see* Hydrocortisone *on page 836*

Cortef® *see* Hydrocortisone *on page 836*

Corticool® [OTC] *see* Hydrocortisone *on page 836*

Corticorelin (kor ti koe REL in)

U.S. Brand Names Acthrel®

Generic Available No

Index Terms Corticorelin Ovine Triflutate; Human Corticotrophin-Releasing Hormone, Analogue; Ovine Corticotrophin-Releasing Hormone

Pharmacologic Category Diagnostic Agent, ACTH-Dependent Hypercortisolism

Use Diagnostic test used in adrenocorticotropic hormone (ACTH)-dependent Cushing's syndrome to differentiate between pituitary and ectopic production of ACTH

Local Anesthetic/Vasoconstrictor Precautions No information available to require special precautions

Effects on Dental Treatment No significant effects or complications reported

Common Adverse Effects

>10%: Cardiovascular: Flushing (face, neck and upper chest, 16%)

1% to 10%:

Gastrointestinal: Metallic taste (transient, 5%)

Respiratory: Dyspnea (urge to inspire, 6%)

Mechanism of Action Stimulates adrenocorticotropic hormone (ACTH) release from anterior pituitary. ACTH stimulates the adrenal cortex to produce cortisol.

Drug Interactions

Increased Effect/Toxicity: Corticorelin administration with heparin has been implicated in a case of severe hypotension (mechanism and confidence level unknown).

Decreased Effect: Corticorelin response may be decreased via a decreased plasma ACTH level. Other corticosteroids would theoretically exhibit this same blunting effect, secondary to suppression of the hypothalamic-pituitary-adrenal axis mechanism in normal patients.

Pharmacodynamics/Kinetics

Onset: I.V.: Plasma ACTH level increases 2 minutes after injection; plasma cortisol level increases within 10 minutes after injection

Duration: I.V.: Plasma ACTH and cortisol levels remain elevated for up to 2 hours

Time to peak, plasma: ACTH: 15-60 minutes; cortisol: 30-120 minutes; both levels show a dose-dependent, biphasic response with a second lower peak 2-3 hours after injection

Pregnancy Risk Factor C

Corticorelin Ovine Triflutate *see* Corticorelin *on page 414*

Corticotropin (kor ti koe TROE pin)

U.S. Brand Names H.P. Acthar® Gel
Generic Available No
Index Terms ACTH; Adrenocorticotropic Hormone; Corticotropin, Repository
Pharmacologic Category Corticosteroid, Systemic
Use Acute exacerbations of multiple sclerosis; diagnostic aid in adrenocortical insufficiency, severe muscle weakness in myasthenia gravis

Cosyntropin is preferred over corticotropin for diagnostic test of adrenocortical insufficiency (cosyntropin is less allergenic and test is shorter in duration)

Local Anesthetic/Vasoconstrictor Precautions No information available to require special precautions
Effects on Dental Treatment No significant effects or complications reported
Common Adverse Effects Frequency not defined.
Central nervous system: Insomnia, nervousness
Dermatologic: Hirsutism
Endocrine & metabolic: Diabetes mellitus
Gastrointestinal: Increased appetite, indigestion
Neuromuscular & skeletal: Arthralgia
Ocular: Cataracts
Respiratory: Epistaxis
Mechanism of Action Stimulates the adrenal cortex to secrete adrenal steroids (including hydrocortisone, cortisone), androgenic substances, and a small amount of aldosterone
Pregnancy Risk Factor C

Corticotropin, Repository *see* Corticotropin *on page 415*
Cortifoam® *see* Hydrocortisone *on page 836*
Cortisol *see* Hydrocortisone *on page 836*

Cortisone (KOR ti sone)

Related Information
Respiratory Diseases *on page 1747*
Triamcinolone *on page 1608*
Generic Available Yes
Index Terms Compound E; Cortisone Acetate
Pharmacologic Category Corticosteroid, Systemic
Use Management of adrenocortical insufficiency
Local Anesthetic/Vasoconstrictor Precautions No information available to require special precautions
Effects on Dental Treatment A compromised immune response may occur if patient has been taking systemic cortisone. The need for corticosteroid coverage in these patients should be considered before any dental treatment; consult with physician.
Common Adverse Effects
>10%:
Central nervous system: Insomnia, nervousness
Gastrointestinal: Increased appetite, indigestion
1% to 10%:
Dermatologic: Hirsutism
Endocrine & metabolic: Diabetes mellitus
Neuromuscular & skeletal: Arthralgia
Ocular: Cataracts, glaucoma
Respiratory: Epistaxis
Mechanism of Action Decreases inflammation by suppression of migration of polymorphonuclear leukocytes and reversal of increased capillary permeability
Drug Interactions
Increased Effect/Toxicity: Estrogens may increase cortisone effects. Cortisone may increase ulcerogenic potential of NSAIDs, and may increase potassium deletion due to diuretics.
Decreased Effect: Enzyme inducers (barbiturates, phenytoin, rifampin) may decrease cortisone effects. Effect of live virus vaccines may be decreased. Anticholinesterase agents may decrease effect of cortisone.
Cortisone may decrease effects of warfarin and salicylates.
(Continued)

Cortisone *(Continued)*

Pharmacodynamics/Kinetics

Onset of action: Peak effect: Oral: ~2 hours; I.M.: 20-48 hours

Duration: 30-36 hours

Absorption: Slow

Distribution: Muscles, liver, skin, intestines, and kidneys; crosses placenta; enters breast milk

Metabolism: Hepatic to inactive metabolites

Half-life elimination: 0.5-2 hours; End-stage renal disease: 3.5 hours

Excretion: Urine and feces

Pregnancy Risk Factor D

Cortisone Acetate *see* Cortisone *on page 415*

Cortisporin® Cream *see* Neomycin, Polymyxin B, and Hydrocortisone *on page 1162*

Cortisporin® Ointment *see* Bacitracin, Neomycin, Polymyxin B, and Hydrocortisone *on page 182*

Cortisporin® Ophthalmic *see* Neomycin, Polymyxin B, and Hydrocortisone *on page 1162*

Cortisporin® Otic *see* Neomycin, Polymyxin B, and Hydrocortisone *on page 1162*

Cortizone®-10 Maximum Strength [OTC] *see* Hydrocortisone *on page 836*

Cortizone®-10 Plus Maximum Strength [OTC] *see* Hydrocortisone *on page 836*

Cortizone®-10 Quick Shot [OTC] *see* Hydrocortisone *on page 836*

Cortrosyn® *see* Cosyntropin *on page 416*

Corvert® *see* Ibutilide *on page 858*

Corzide® *see* Nadolol and Bendroflumethiazide *on page 1140*

Cosmegen® *see* Dactinomycin *on page 437*

Cosopt® *see* Dorzolamide and Timolol *on page 528*

Cosyntropin *(koe sin TROE pin)*

U.S. Brand Names Cortrosyn®

Canadian Brand Names Cortrosyn®

Generic Available No

Index Terms Synacthen; Tetracosactide

Pharmacologic Category Diagnostic Agent

Use Diagnostic test to differentiate primary adrenal from secondary (pituitary) adrenocortical insufficiency

Local Anesthetic/Vasoconstrictor Precautions No information available to require special precautions

Effects on Dental Treatment No significant effects or complications reported

Common Adverse Effects Frequency not defined.

Cardiovascular: Bradycardia, hypertension, peripheral edema, tachycardia

Dermatologic: Rash

Local: Whealing with redness at the injection site

Miscellaneous: Anaphylaxis, hypersensitivity reaction

Mechanism of Action Stimulates the adrenal cortex to secrete adrenal steroids (including hydrocortisone, cortisone), androgenic substances, and a small amount of aldosterone

Pharmacodynamics/Kinetics Time to peak, serum: I.M., IVP: ~1 hour; plasma cortisol levels rise in healthy individuals within 5 minutes

Pregnancy Risk Factor C

Co-Trimoxazole *see* Sulfamethoxazole and Trimethoprim *on page 1504*

Coughcold HCM *see* Hydrocodone and Pseudoephedrine *on page 832*

Coumadin® *see* Warfarin *on page 1670*

Covera-HS® *see* Verapamil *on page 1654*

Co-Vidarabine *see* Pentostatin *on page 1277*

Coviracil *see* Emtricitabine *on page 562*

Cozaar® *see* Losartan *on page 1003*

CP358774 *see* Erlotinib *on page 587*

CPC *see* Cetylpyridinium *on page 324*

C-Phen *see* Chlorpheniramine and Phenylephrine *on page 340*

C-Phen DM *see* Chlorpheniramine, Phenylephrine, and Dextromethorphan *on page 342*

CPM *see* Cyclophosphamide *on page 423*

CPT-11 *see* Irinotecan *on page 909*

CPZ *see* ChlorproMAZINE *on page 345*

Crantex HC *see* Hydrocodone, Phenylephrine, and Guaifenesin *on page 834*

Cromolyn (KROE moe lin)

Related Information
Respiratory Diseases *on page 1747*
U.S. Brand Names Crolom®; Gastrocrom®; Intal®; NasalCrom® [OTC]; Opticrom®
Canadian Brand Names Apo-Cromolyn®; Intal®; Nalcrom®; Nu-Cromolyn; Opticrom®
Mexican Brand Names Intal; Opticrom; Rynacrom
Generic Available Yes: Excludes aerosol, oral solution
Index Terms Cromoglycic Acid; Cromolyn Sodium; Disodium Cromoglycate; DSCG
Pharmacologic Category Mast Cell Stabilizer
Use
Inhalation: May be used as an adjunct in the prophylaxis of allergic disorders, including asthma; prevention of exercise-induced bronchospasm
Nasal: Prevention and treatment of seasonal and perennial allergic rhinitis
Oral: Systemic mastocytosis
Ophthalmic: Treatment of vernal keratoconjunctivitis, vernal conjunctivitis, and vernal keratitis
Unlabeled/Investigational Use Oral: Food allergy, treatment of inflammatory bowel disease
Local Anesthetic/Vasoconstrictor Precautions No information available to require special precautions
Effects on Dental Treatment Key adverse event(s) related to dental treatment:
Inhalation: Unpleasant taste.
Systemic: Glossitis, stomatitis, and unpleasant taste.
Common Adverse Effects
Inhalation: >10%: Gastrointestinal: Unpleasant taste in mouth
Nasal:
>10%: Respiratory: Increase in sneezing, burning, stinging, or irritation inside of nose
1% to 10%:
Central nervous system: Headache
Gastrointestinal: Unpleasant taste
Respiratory: Hoarseness, cough, postnasal drip
<1% (Limited to important or life-threatening): Anaphylactic reactions, epistaxis
Ophthalmic: Frequency not defined:
Ocular: Conjunctival injection, dryness around the eye, edema, eye irritation, immediate hypersensitivity reactions, itchy eyes, puffy eyes, styes, rash, watery eyes
Respiratory: Dyspnea
Systemic: Frequency not defined:
Cardiovascular: Angioedema, chest pain, edema, flushing, palpitation, premature ventricular contractions, tachycardia
Central nervous system: Anxiety, behavior changes, convulsions, depression, dizziness, fatigue, hallucinations, headache, irritability, insomnia, lethargy, migraine, nervousness, hypoesthesia, postprandial lightheadedness, psychosis
Dermatologic: Erythema, photosensitivity, pruritus, purpura, rash, urticaria
Gastrointestinal: Abdominal pain, constipation, diarrhea, dyspepsia, dysphagia, esophagospasm, flatulence, glossitis, nausea, stomatitis, unpleasant taste, vomiting
Genitourinary: Dysuria, urinary frequency
Hematologic: Neutropenia, pancytopenia, polycythemia
Hepatic: Liver function test abnormal
Local: Burning
(Continued)

Cromolyn *(Continued)*

Neuromuscular & skeletal: Arthralgia, leg stiffness, leg weakness, myalgia, paresthesia

Otic: Tinnitus

Respiratory: Dyspnea, pharyngitis

Miscellaneous: Lupus erythematosus

Mechanism of Action Prevents the mast cell release of histamine, leukotrienes and slow-reacting substance of anaphylaxis by inhibiting degranulation after contact with antigens

Pharmacodynamics/Kinetics

Onset: Response to treatment:

Nasal spray: May occur at 1-2 weeks

Ophthalmic: May be seen within a few days; treatment for up to 6 weeks is often required

Oral: May occur within 2-6 weeks

Absorption:

Inhalation: ~8% reaches lungs upon inhalation; well absorbed

Oral: <1% of dose absorbed

Half-life elimination: 80-90 minutes

Time to peak, serum: Inhalation: ~15 minutes

Excretion: Urine and feces (equal amounts as unchanged drug); exhaled gases (small amounts)

Pregnancy Risk Factor B

Cromolyn Sodium *see Cromolyn on page 417*

Crosseal™ *see Fibrin Sealant Kit on page 690*

Crotamiton *(kroe TAM i tonn)*

U.S. Brand Names Eurax®

Mexican Brand Names Eurax

Generic Available No

Pharmacologic Category Scabicidal Agent

Use Treatment of scabies (*Sarcoptes scabiei*) and symptomatic treatment of pruritus

Local Anesthetic/Vasoconstrictor Precautions No information available to require special precautions

Effects on Dental Treatment No significant effects or complications reported

Common Adverse Effects Frequency not defined. Topical:

Dermatologic: Contact dermatitis, pruritus, rash

Local: Local irritation

Miscellaneous: Allergic sensitivity reactions, warm sensation

Mechanism of Action Crotamiton has scabicidal activity against *Sarcoptes scabiei*; mechanism of action unknown

Pregnancy Risk Factor C

Crude Coal Tar *see Coal Tar on page 402*

Cruex® Cream [OTC] *see Clotrimazole on page 398*

Cryselle™ *see Ethinyl Estradiol and Norgestrel on page 649*

Crystalline Penicillin *see Penicillin G (Parenteral/Aqueous) on page 1269*

Crystal Violet *see Gentian Violet on page 777*

CsA *see CycloSPORINE on page 426*

CSP *see Cellulose Sodium Phosphate on page 317*

CTLA-4Ig *see Abatacept on page 25*

CTM *see Chlorpheniramine on page 338*

CTX *see Cyclophosphamide on page 423*

Cubicin® *see Daptomycin on page 443*

Culturelle® [OTC] *see Lactobacillus on page 942*

Cuprimine® *see Penicillamine on page 1267*

Curasore® [OTC] *see Pramoxine on page 1334*

Curosurf® *see Poractant Alfa on page 1323*

Cutar® [OTC] *see Coal Tar on page 402*

Cutivate® *see Fluticasone on page 725*

CyA *see CycloSPORINE on page 426*

Cyanocobalamin *(sye an oh koe BAL a min)*

U.S. Brand Names Nascobal®; Twelve Resin-K

Generic Available Yes: Excludes nasal spray

Index Terms Vitamin B_{12}

Pharmacologic Category Vitamin, Water Soluble

Use Treatment of pernicious anemia; vitamin B_{12} deficiency due to dietary deficiencies or malabsorption diseases, inadequate secretion of intrinsic factor, and inadequate utilization of B_{12} (eg, during neoplastic treatment); increased B_{12} requirements due to pregnancy, thyrotoxicosis, hemorrhage, malignancy, liver or kidney disease

Local Anesthetic/Vasoconstrictor Precautions No information available to require special precautions

Effects on Dental Treatment No significant effects or complications reported

Significant Adverse Effects Frequency not defined.

Cardiovascular: CHF, peripheral vascular disorder, peripheral vascular thrombosis

Central nervous system: Anxiety, dizziness, headache, hypoesthesia, incoordination, pain, nervousness

Dermatologic: Itching, urticaria, exanthema (transient)

Gastrointestinal: Diarrhea, dyspepsia, glossitis, nausea, sore throat, vomiting

Hematologic: Polycythemia vera

Neuromuscular & skeletal: Abnormal gait, arthritis, back pain, myalgia, paresthesia, weakness

Respiratory: Dyspnea, pulmonary edema, rhinitis

Miscellaneous: Anaphylaxis (parenteral) and infection

Dosage

Adequate intake:

Children:

0-6 months: 0.4 mcg/day

7-12 months: 0.5 mcg/day

Recommended intake:

Children:

1-3 years: 0.9 mcg/day

4-8 years: 1.2 mcg/day

9-13 years: 1.8 mcg/day

Children >14 years and Adults: 2.4 mcg/day

Pregnancy: 2.6 mcg/day

Lactation: 2.8 mcg/day

Vitamin B_{12} deficiency:

I.M., deep SubQ:

Children (dosage not well established): 0.2 mcg/kg for 2 days, followed by 1000 mcg/day for 2-7 days, followed by 100 mcg/week for one month; for malabsorptive causes of B_{12} deficiency, monthly maintenance doses of 100 mcg have been recommended **or** as an alternative 100 mcg/day for 10-15 days, then once or twice weekly for several months

Adults: Initial: 30 mcg/day for 5-10 days; maintenance: 100-200 mcg/month

Intranasal: Adults: 500 mcg in one nostril once weekly

Oral: Adults: 250 mcg/day

Pernicious anemia: I.M., deep SubQ (administer concomitantly with folic acid if needed, 1 mg/day for 1 month):

Children: 30-50 mcg/day for 2 or more weeks (to a total dose of 1000-5000 mcg), then follow with 100 mcg/month as maintenance dosage

Adults: 100 mcg/day for 6-7 days; if improvement, administer same dose on alternate days for 7 doses, then every 3-4 days for 2-3 weeks; once hematologic values have returned to normal, maintenance dosage: 100 mcg/month. **Note:** Alternative dosing of 1000 mcg/day for 5 days (followed by 500-1000 mcg/month) has been used.

Hematologic remission (without evidence of nervous system involvement): Adults:

Intranasal: 500 mcg in one nostril once weekly

Oral: 1000-2000 mcg/day

I.M., SubQ: 100-1000 mcg/month

Schilling test: Adults: I.M.: 1000 mcg

Mechanism of Action Coenzyme for various metabolic functions, including fat and carbohydrate metabolism and protein synthesis, used in cell replication and hematopoiesis

Contraindications Hypersensitivity to cyanocobalamin, cobalt, or any component of the formulation

Warnings/Precautions I.M./SubQ routes are used to treat pernicious anemia; oral and intranasal administration are not indicated until hematologic remission and no signs of nervous system involvement. Treatment of severe vitamin B_{12} megaloblastic anemia may result in thrombocytosis and severe hypokalemia, sometimes fatal, due to intracellular potassium shift upon anemia resolution. Vitamin B_{12} deficiency masks signs of polycythemia vera; use caution in other conditions where folic acid or vitamin B_{12} administration alone might mask true diagnosis, despite hematologic response. Vitamin B_{12} deficiency for >3 months (Continued)

Cyanocobalamin *(Continued)*

results in irreversible degenerative CNS lesions; neurologic manifestations will not be prevented with folic acid unless vitamin B_{12} is also given. Spinal cord degeneration might also occur when folic acid used as a substitute for vitamin B_{12} in anemia prevention. Use caution in Leber's disease patients; B_{12} treatment may result in rapid optic atrophy. Some parenteral products contain aluminum; use caution in patients with impaired renal function and neonates. Some parenteral products contain benzyl alcohol; use caution in neonates. Avoid intravenous route; anaphylactic shock has occurred. Intradermal test dose of vitamin B_{12} is recommended for any patient suspected of cyanocobalamin sensitivity prior to intranasal or injectable administration.

Drug Interactions Chloramphenicol: Therapeutic effect of cyanocobalamin may be diminished with concurrent chloramphenicol.

Ethanol/Nutrition/Herb Interactions Ethanol: Heavy consumption >2 weeks may impair vitamin B_{12} absorption.

Dietary Considerations Strict vegetarian diets (eg, without eggs or dairy products) may result in vitamin B_{12} deficiency.

Pharmacodynamics/Kinetics

Absorption: Oral: Variable from the terminal ileum; requires the presence of calcium and gastric "intrinsic factor" to transfer the compound across the intestinal mucosa

Distribution: Principally stored in the liver and bone marrow, also stored in the kidneys and adrenals

Protein binding: Transcobalamins

Metabolism: Converted in tissues to active coenzymes, methylcobalamin and deoxyadenosylcobalamin; undergoes some enterohepatic recycling

Bioavailability: Intranasal solution: 6.1% (relative to I.M.)

Pregnancy Risk Factor A/C (dose exceeding RDA recommendation); C (intranasal)

Lactation Enters breast milk/compatible

Breast-Feeding Considerations Vegetarian diets which contain no animal products do not supply any vitamin B_{12}. Deficiency recognized in infants of vegetarian mothers who were breast-fed; consider supplementation during breast-feeding.

Dosage Forms Excipient information presented when available (limited, particularly for generics); consult specific product labeling.

Injection, solution: 1000 mcg/mL (1 mL, 10 mL, 30 mL) [may contain benzyl alcohol and/or aluminum]

Lozenge [OTC]: 100 mcg, 250 mcg, 500 mcg

Solution, intranasal [spray]:

Nascobal®: 500 mcg/0.1 mL actuation (2.3 mL) [contains benzalkonium chloride; delivers 8 doses]

Tablet [OTC]: 50 mcg, 100 mcg, 250 mcg, 500 mcg, 1000 mcg, 5000 mcg

Twelve Resin-K: 1000 mcg [may be used as oral, sublingual, or buccal]

Tablet, extended release [OTC]: 1000 mcg, 1500 mcg

Tablet, sublingual [OTC]: 2500 mcg

Cyanocobalamin, Folic Acid, and Pyridoxine *see* Folic Acid, Cyanocobalamin, and Pyridoxine *on page 738*

Cyanokit® *see* Hydroxocobalamin *on page 842*

Cyclessa® *see* Ethinyl Estradiol and Desogestrel *on page 621*

Cyclizine *(SYE kli zeen)*

U.S. Brand Names Marezine® [OTC]

Generic Available No

Index Terms Cyclizine Hydrochloride; Cyclizine Lactate

Pharmacologic Category Antihistamine

Use Prevention and treatment of nausea, vomiting, and vertigo associated with motion sickness; control of postoperative nausea and vomiting

Local Anesthetic/Vasoconstrictor Precautions No information available to require special precautions

Effects on Dental Treatment Key adverse event(s) related to dental treatment: Xerostomia (normal salivary flow resumes upon discontinuation).

Common Adverse Effects

>10%:

Central nervous system: Drowsiness

Gastrointestinal: Xerostomia

1% to 10%:

Central nervous system: Headache

Dermatologic: Dermatitis

Gastrointestinal: Nausea

Genitourinary: Urinary retention
Ocular: Diplopia
Renal: Polyuria

Mechanism of Action Cyclizine is a piperazine derivative with properties of histamines. The precise mechanism of action in inhibiting the symptoms of motion sickness is not known. It may have effects directly on the labyrinthine apparatus and central actions on the labyrinthine apparatus and on the chemoreceptor trigger zone. Cyclizine exerts a central anticholinergic action.

Drug Interactions
Increased Effect/Toxicity: Increased effect/toxicity with CNS depressants, alcohol.

Pregnancy Risk Factor B

Cyclizine Hydrochloride *see* Cyclizine *on page 420*
Cyclizine Lactate *see* Cyclizine *on page 420*

Cyclobenzaprine (sye kloe BEN za preen)

Related Information
Temporomandibular Dysfunction (TMD) *on page 1822*
U.S. Brand Names Flexeril®
Canadian Brand Names Apo-Cyclobenzaprine®; Flexeril®; Flexitec; Gen-Cyclobenzaprine; Novo-Cycloprine; Nu-Cyclobenzaprine
Generic Available Yes
Index Terms Cyclobenzaprine Hydrochloride
Pharmacologic Category Skeletal Muscle Relaxant
Dental Use Treatment of muscle spasm associated with acute temporomandibular joint pain (TMJ)
Use Treatment of muscle spasm associated with acute painful musculoskeletal conditions
Local Anesthetic/Vasoconstrictor Precautions No information available to require special precautions
Effects on Dental Treatment Key adverse event(s) related to dental treatment: Xerostomia and changes in salivation (normal salivary flow resumes upon discontinuation).
Significant Adverse Effects
>10%:
Central nervous system: Drowsiness (29% to 39%), dizziness (1% to 11%)
Gastrointestinal: Xerostomia (21% to 32%)
1% to 10%:
Central nervous system: Fatigue (1% to 6%), confusion (1% to 3%), headache (1% to 3%), irritability (1% to 3%), mental acuity decreased (1% to 3%), nervousness (1% to 3%)
Gastrointestinal: Abdominal pain (1% to 3%), constipation (1% to 3%), diarrhea (1% to 3%), dyspepsia (1% to 3%), nausea (1% to 3%)
Neuromuscular & skeletal: Muscle weakness (1% to 3%)
Ocular: Blurred vision (1% to 3%)
Respiratory: Pharyngitis (1% to 3%)
<1% (Limited to important or life-threatening): Ageusia, agitation, anaphylaxis, angioedema, anorexia, arrhythmia, cholestasis, diplopia, facial edema, gastritis, hallucinations, hepatitis (rare), hypertonia, hypotension, insomnia, jaundice, liver function tests abnormal, malaise, palpitation, paresthesia, pruritus, psychosis, rash, seizure, tachycardia, thinking abnormal, tinnitus, tongue edema, tremor, urinary frequency, urinary retention, urticaria, vertigo, vomiting
Dental Usual Dosing Treatment of muscle spasm associated with acute TMJ pain (**Note:** Do not use longer than 2-3 weeks): Oral:
Adults: Initial: 5 mg 3 times/day; may increase to 10 mg 3 times/day if needed
Elderly: 5 mg 3 times/day; plasma concentration and incidence of adverse effects are increased in the elderly; dose should be titrated slowly
Dosage Oral: **Note:** Do not use longer than 2-3 weeks
Adults: Initial: 5 mg 3 times/day; may increase to 10 mg 3 times/day if needed
Elderly: 5 mg 3 times/day; plasma concentration and incidence of adverse effects are increased in the elderly; dose should be titrated slowly
Dosage adjustment in hepatic impairment:
Mild: 5 mg 3 times/day; use with caution and titrate slowly
Moderate to severe: Use not recommended
Mechanism of Action Centrally-acting skeletal muscle relaxant pharmacologically related to tricyclic antidepressants; reduces tonic somatic motor activity influencing both alpha and gamma motor neurons
Contraindications Hypersensitivity to cyclobenzaprine or any component of the formulation; do not use concomitantly or within 14 days of MAO inhibitors; (Continued)

Cyclobenzaprine *(Continued)*

hyperthyroidism; congestive heart failure; arrhythmias; acute recovery phase of MI

Warnings/Precautions Cyclobenzaprine shares the toxic potentials of the tricyclic antidepressants and the usual precautions of tricyclic antidepressant therapy should be observed; use with caution in patients with urinary hesitancy, angle-closure glaucoma, hepatic impairment, or in the elderly. Do not use concomitantly or within 14 days after MAO inhibitors; combination may cause hypertensive crisis, severe convulsions. Effects may be potentiated when used with other sedative drugs or ethanol. Safety and efficacy have not been established in patients <15 years of age.

Drug Interactions Substrate of CYP1A2 (major), 2D6 (minor), 3A4 (minor)

Anticholinergics: Because of cyclobenzaprine's anticholinergic action, use with caution in patients receiving these agents.

CNS depressants: Effects may be enhanced by cyclobenzaprine.

CYP1A2 inhibitors: May increase the levels/effects of cyclobenzaprine. Example inhibitors include ciprofloxacin, fluvoxamine, ketoconazole, norfloxacin, ofloxacin, and rofecoxib.

Guanethidine: Antihypertensive effect of guanethidine may be decreased; effect seen with tricyclic antidepressants.

MAO inhibitors: Do not use concomitantly or within 14 days after MAO inhibitors.

Tramadol: May increase risk of seizure; effect seen with tricyclic antidepressants and tramadol.

Ethanol/Nutrition/Herb Interactions

Ethanol: Avoid ethanol (may increase CNS depression).

Herb/Nutraceutical: Avoid valerian, kava kava, gotu kola (may increase CNS depression).

Pharmacodynamics/Kinetics

Onset of action: ~1 hour

Duration: 12-24 hours

Absorption: Complete

Metabolism: Hepatic via CYP3A4, 1A2, and 2D6; may undergo enterohepatic recirculation

Bioavailability: 33% to 55%

Half-life elimination: 18 hours (range: 8-37 hours)

Time to peak, serum: 3-8 hours

Excretion: Urine (as inactive metabolites); feces (as unchanged drug)

Pregnancy Risk Factor B

Lactation Excretion in breast milk unknown/not recommended

Dosage Forms Excipient information presented when available (limited, particularly for generics); consult specific product labeling.

Tablet, as hydrochloride: 5 mg, 10 mg

Flexeril®: 5 mg, 10 mg

Cyclobenzaprine Hydrochloride *see* Cyclobenzaprine *on page 421*

Cyclocort® [DSC] *see* Amcinonide *on page 84*

Cyclogyl® *see* Cyclopentolate *on page 422*

Cyclomydril® *see* Cyclopentolate and Phenylephrine *on page 422*

Cyclopentolate *(sye kloe PEN toe late)*

U.S. Brand Names AK-Pentolate® [DSC]; Cyclogyl®; Cylate®

Canadian Brand Names Cyclogyl®; Diopentolate®

Generic Available Yes

Index Terms Cyclopentolate Hydrochloride

Pharmacologic Category Anticholinergic Agent, Ophthalmic

Use Diagnostic procedures requiring mydriasis and cycloplegia

Local Anesthetic/Vasoconstrictor Precautions No information available to require special precautions

Effects on Dental Treatment No significant effects or complications reported

Mechanism of Action Prevents the muscle of the ciliary body and the sphincter muscle of the iris from responding to cholinergic stimulation, causing mydriasis and cycloplegia

Pregnancy Risk Factor C

Cyclopentolate and Phenylephrine
(sye kloe PEN toe late & fen il EF rin)

Related Information

Cyclopentolate *on page 422*

Phenylephrine *on page 1293*
U.S. Brand Names Cyclomydril®
Generic Available No
Index Terms Phenylephrine and Cyclopentolate
Pharmacologic Category Ophthalmic Agent, Antiglaucoma
Use Induce mydriasis greater than that produced with cyclopentolate HCl alone
Local Anesthetic/Vasoconstrictor Precautions No information available to require special precautions
Effects on Dental Treatment No significant effects or complications reported
Pregnancy Risk Factor C

Cyclopentolate Hydrochloride *see* Cyclopentolate *on page 422*

Cyclophosphamide (sye kloe FOS fa mide)

U.S. Brand Names Cytoxan®
Canadian Brand Names Cytoxan®; Procytox®
Mexican Brand Names Ledoxina
Generic Available Yes: Tablet
Index Terms CPM; CTX; CYT; Neosar; NSC-26271
Pharmacologic Category Antineoplastic Agent, Alkylating Agent
Dental Use Treatment of Wegener's granulomatosis, systemic lupus erythematosus
Use

Oncologic: Treatment of Hodgkin's and non-Hodgkin's lymphoma, Burkitt's lymphoma, chronic lymphocytic leukemia (CLL), chronic myelocytic leukemia (CML), acute myelocytic leukemia (AML), acute lymphocytic leukemia (ALL), mycosis fungoides, multiple myeloma, neuroblastoma, retinoblastoma, rhabdomyosarcoma, Ewing's sarcoma; breast, testicular, endometrial, ovarian, and lung cancers; and in conditioning regimens for bone marrow transplantation

Nononcologic: Prophylaxis of rejection for kidney, heart, liver, and bone marrow transplants, severe rheumatoid disorders, nephrotic syndrome, Wegener's granulomatosis, idiopathic pulmonary hemosideroses, myasthenia gravis, multiple sclerosis, systemic lupus erythematosus, lupus nephritis, autoimmune hemolytic anemia, idiopathic thrombocytic purpura (ITP), macroglobulinemia, and antibody-induced pure red cell aplasia

Local Anesthetic/Vasoconstrictor Precautions No information available to require special precautions

Effects on Dental Treatment Key adverse event(s) related to dental treatment: Mucositis and stomatitis.

Significant Adverse Effects

>10%:

Dermatologic: Alopecia (40% to 60%) but hair will usually regrow although it may be a different color and/or texture. Hair loss usually begins 3-6 weeks after the start of therapy.

Endocrine & metabolic: Fertility: May cause sterility; interferes with oogenesis and spermatogenesis; may be irreversible in some patients; gonadal suppression (amenorrhea)

Gastrointestinal: Nausea and vomiting, usually beginning 6-10 hours after administration; anorexia, diarrhea, mucositis, and stomatitis are also seen

Genitourinary: Severe, potentially fatal acute hemorrhagic cystitis (7% to 40%)

Hematologic: Thrombocytopenia and anemia are less common than leukopenia

Onset: 7 days

Nadir: 10-14 days

Recovery: 21 days

1% to 10%:

Cardiovascular: Facial flushing

Central nervous system: Headache

Dermatologic: Skin rash

Renal: SIADH may occur, usually with doses >50 mg/kg (or 1 g/m^2); renal tubular necrosis, which usually resolves with discontinuation of the drug, is also reported

Respiratory: Nasal congestion occurs when I.V. doses are administered too rapidly; patients experience runny eyes, rhinorrhea, sinus congestion, and sneezing during or immediately after the infusion.

<1% (Limited to important or life-threatening): High-dose therapy may cause cardiac dysfunction manifested as CHF; cardiac necrosis or hemorrhagic myocarditis has occurred rarely, but may be fatal. Interstitial pneumonitis and pulmonary fibrosis are occasionally seen with high doses. Cyclophosphamide may also potentiate the cardiac toxicity of anthracyclines. Other adverse
(Continued)

Cyclophosphamide *(Continued)*

reactions include anaphylactic reactions, darkening of skin/fingernails, dizziness, hemorrhagic colitis, hemorrhagic ureteritis, hepatotoxicity, hyperuricemia, hypokalemia, jaundice, malaise, neutrophilic eccrine hidradenitis, radiation recall, renal tubular necrosis, secondary malignancy (eg, bladder carcinoma), SAIDH, Stevens-Johnson syndrome, toxic epidermal necrolysis, weakness.

BMT:

Cardiovascular: Heart failure, cardiac necrosis, pericardial tamponade

Endocrine & metabolic: Hyponatremia

Hematologic: Methemoglobinemia

Gastrointestinal: Severe nausea and vomiting

Miscellaneous: Hemorrhagic cystitis, secondary malignancy

Dosage Refer to individual protocols

Children:

SLE: I.V.: 500-750 mg/m^2 every month; maximum dose: 1 g/m^2

JRA/vasculitis: I.V.: 10 mg/kg every 2 weeks

Children and Adults:

Oral: 50-100 mg/m^2/day as continuous therapy or 400-1000 mg/m^2 in divided doses over 4-5 days as intermittent therapy

I.V.:

Single doses: 400-1800 mg/m^2 (30-50 mg/kg) per treatment course (1-5 days) which can be repeated at 2-4 week intervals

Continuous daily doses: 60-120 mg/m^2 (1-2.5 mg/kg) per day

Autologous BMT: IVPB: 50 mg/kg/dose x 4 days or 60 mg/kg/dose for 2 days; total dose is usually divided over 2-4 days

Nephrotic syndrome: Oral: 2-3 mg/kg/day every day for up to 12 weeks when corticosteroids are unsuccessful

Dosing adjustment in renal impairment: A large fraction of cyclophosphamide is eliminated by hepatic metabolism

Some authors recommend no dose adjustment unless severe renal insufficiency (Cl$_{cr}$ <20 mL/minute)

Cl$_{cr}$ >10 mL/minute: Administer 100% of normal dose

Cl$_{cr}$ <10 mL/minute: Administer 75% of normal dose

Hemodialysis: Moderately dialyzable (20% to 50%); administer dose posthemodialysis

CAPD effects: Unknown

CAVH effects: Unknown

Dosing adjustment in hepatic impairment: The pharmacokinetics of cyclophosphamide are not significantly altered in the presence of hepatic insufficiency. No dosage adjustments are recommended.

Mechanism of Action Cyclophosphamide is an alkylating agent that prevents cell division by cross-linking DNA strands and decreasing DNA synthesis. It is a cell cycle phase nonspecific agent. Cyclophosphamide also possesses potent immunosuppressive activity. Cyclophosphamide is a prodrug that must be metabolized to active metabolites in the liver.

Contraindications Hypersensitivity to cyclophosphamide or any component of the formulation; pregnancy

Warnings/Precautions Hazardous agent - use appropriate precautions for handling and disposal. Dosage adjustment may be needed for renal or hepatic failure. Hemorrhagic cystitis may occur; increased hydration and frequent voiding is recommended. Immunosuppression may occur; monitor for infections. May cause cardiotoxicity (CHF, usually with higher doses); may potentiate the cardiotoxicity of anthracyclines. May impair fertility; interferes with oogenesis and spermatogenesis. Secondary malignancies (usually delayed) have been reported

Drug Interactions Substrate of CYP2A6 (minor), 2B6 (major), 2C9 (minor), 2C19 (minor), 3A4 (major); **Inhibits** CYP3A4 (weak); **Induces** CYP2B6 (weak), 2C8 (weak), 2C9 (weak)

Allopurinol may cause increase in bone marrow depression and may result in significant elevations of cyclophosphamide cytotoxic metabolites.

Anesthetic agents: Cyclophosphamide reduces serum pseudocholinesterase concentrations and may prolong the neuromuscular blocking activity of succinylcholine; use with caution with halothane, nitrous oxide, and succinylcholine.

Cardiac glycosides: Cyclophosphamide may decrease the absorption of digoxin tablets.

CYP2B6 inducers: May increase the levels/effects of acrolein (the active metabolite of cyclophosphamide). Example inducers include carbamazepine, nevirapine, phenobarbital, phenytoin, and rifampin.

CYP2B6 inhibitors: May decrease the levels/effects of acrolein (the active metabolite of cyclophosphamide). Example inhibitors include desipramine, paroxetine, and sertraline.

CYP3A4 inducers: CYP3A4 inducers may increase the levels/effects of acrolein (the active metabolite of cyclophosphamide). Example inducers include aminoglutethimide, carbamazepine, nafcillin, nevirapine, phenobarbital, phenytoin, and rifamycins.

CYP3A4 inhibitors: May decrease the levels/effects of acrolein (the active metabolite of cyclophosphamide). Example inhibitors include azole antifungals, ciprofloxacin, clarithromycin, diclofenac, doxycycline, erythromycin, imatinib, isoniazid, nefazodone, nicardipine, propofol, protease inhibitors, quinidine, and verapamil.

Etanercept: May enhance the adverse/toxic effects of cyclophosphamide.

Mivacurium: Cyclophosphamide may increase the levels/effects of mivacurium.

Phenytoin: May decrease the levels/effects of cyclophosphamide; may increase the levels/effects of 4-hydroxycyclophosphamide.

Succinylcholine: Cyclophosphamide may increase the levels/effects of succinylcholine.

Ethanol/Nutrition/Herb Interactions Herb/Nutraceutical: Avoid black cohosh, dong quai in estrogen-dependent tumors.

Dietary Considerations Tablets should be administered during or after meals.

Pharmacodynamics/Kinetics
Absorption: Oral: Well absorbed
Distribution: V_d: 0.48-0.71 L/kg; crosses placenta; crosses into CSF (not in high enough concentrations to treat meningeal leukemia)
Protein binding: 10% to 60%
Metabolism: Hepatic to active metabolites acrolein, 4-aldophosphamide, 4-hydroperoxycyclophosphamide, and nor-nitrogen mustard
Bioavailability: >75%
Half-life elimination: 3-12 hours
Time to peak, serum: Oral: ~1 hour
Excretion: Urine (<30% as unchanged drug, 85% to 90% as metabolites)

Pregnancy Risk Factor D

Lactation Enters breast milk/contraindicated

Dosage Forms Excipient information presented when available (limited, particularly for generics); consult specific product labeling.
Injection, powder for reconstitution:
Cytoxan®: 500 mg, 1 g, 2 g [contains mannitol 75 mg per cyclophosphamide 100 mg
Tablet: 25 mg, 50 mg
Cytoxan®: 25 mg, 50 mg

CycloSERINE (sye kloe SER een)

Related Information
Tuberculosis on page 1765
U.S. Brand Names Seromycin®
Generic Available No
Pharmacologic Category Antibiotic, Miscellaneous; Antitubercular Agent
Use Adjunctive treatment in pulmonary or extrapulmonary tuberculosis
Unlabeled/Investigational Use Treatment of Gaucher's disease
Local Anesthetic/Vasoconstrictor Precautions No information available to require special precautions
Effects on Dental Treatment No significant effects or complications reported
Common Adverse Effects Frequency not defined.
Cardiovascular: Cardiac arrhythmia
Central nervous system: Drowsiness, headache, dizziness, vertigo, seizure, confusion, psychosis, paresis, coma
Dermatologic: Rash
Endocrine & metabolic: Vitamin B_{12} deficiency
Hematologic: Folate deficiency
Hepatic: Liver enzymes increased
Neuromuscular & skeletal: Tremor
Mechanism of Action Inhibits bacterial cell wall synthesis by competing with amino acid (D-alanine) for incorporation into the bacterial cell wall; bacteriostatic or bactericidal
Drug Interactions
Increased Effect/Toxicity: Alcohol, isoniazid, and ethionamide increase toxicity of cycloserine. Cycloserine inhibits the hepatic metabolism of phenytoin and may increase risk of epileptic seizures.
Pharmacodynamics/Kinetics
Absorption: ~70% to 90%
(Continued)

CycloSERINE (Continued)

Distribution: Widely to most body fluids and tissues including CSF, breast milk, bile, sputum, lymph tissue, lungs, and ascitic, pleural, and synovial fluids; crosses placenta

Half-life elimination: Normal renal function: 10 hours

Metabolism: Hepatic

Time to peak, serum: 3-4 hours

Excretion: Urine (60% to 70% as unchanged drug) within 72 hours; feces (small amounts); remainder metabolized

Pregnancy Risk Factor C

Cyclosporin A see CycloSPORINE on page 426

CycloSPORINE (SYE kloe spor een)

U.S. Brand Names Gengraf®; Neoral®; Restasis®; Sandimmune®

Canadian Brand Names Neoral®; Rhoxal-cyclosporine; Sandimmune® I.V.; Sandoz-Cyclosporine

Mexican Brand Names Sandimmun; Sandimmun Neoral

Generic Available Yes

Index Terms CsA; CyA; Cyclosporin A

Pharmacologic Category Immunosuppressant Agent

Dental Use Used as an immunosuppressive agent

Use Prophylaxis of organ rejection in kidney, liver, and heart transplants, has been used with azathioprine and/or corticosteroids; severe, active rheumatoid arthritis (RA) not responsive to methotrexate alone; severe, recalcitrant plaque psoriasis in nonimmunocompromised adults unresponsive to or unable to tolerate other systemic therapy

Ophthalmic emulsion (Restasis®): Increase tear production when suppressed tear production is presumed to be due to keratoconjunctivitis sicca-associated ocular inflammation (in patients not already using topical anti-inflammatory drugs or punctal plugs)

Unlabeled/Investigational Use Short-term, high-dose cyclosporine as a modulator of multidrug resistance in cancer treatment; allogenic bone marrow transplants for prevention and treatment of graft-versus-host disease; also used in some cases of severe autoimmune disease (eg, SLE, myasthenia gravis) that are resistant to corticosteroids and other therapy; focal segmental glomerulosclerosis

Local Anesthetic/Vasoconstrictor Precautions No information available to require special precautions

Effects on Dental Treatment Key adverse event(s) related to dental treatment: Mouth sores, swallowing difficulty, gingivitis, gum hyperplasia, xerostomia (normal salivary flow resumes upon discontinuation), abnormal taste, tongue disorder, tooth disorder, and gingival bleeding.

Significant Adverse Effects Adverse reactions reported with systemic use, including rheumatoid arthritis, psoriasis, and transplantation (kidney, liver, and heart). Percentages noted include the highest frequency regardless of indication/dosage. Frequencies may vary for specific conditions or formulation.

>10%:

Cardiovascular: Hypertension (8% to 53%), edema (5% to 14%)

Central nervous system: Headache (2% to 25%)

Dermatologic: Hirsutism (21% to 45%), hypertrichosis (5% to 19%)

Endocrine & metabolic: Triglycerides increased (15%), female reproductive disorder (9% to 11%)

Gastrointestinal: Nausea (23%), diarrhea (3% to 13%), gum hyperplasia (2% to 16%), abdominal discomfort (<1% to 15%), dyspepsia (2% to 12%)

Neuromuscular & skeletal: Tremor (7% to 55%), paresthesia (1% to 11%), leg cramps/muscle contractions (2% to 12%)

Renal: Renal dysfunction/nephropathy (10% to 38%), creatinine increased (16% to ≥50%)

Respiratory: Upper respiratory infection (1% to 14%)

Miscellaneous: Infection (3% to 25%)

1% to 10%:

Cardiovascular: Chest pain (4% to 6%), arrhythmia (2% to 5%), abnormal heart sounds, cardiac failure, flushes (<1% to 5%), MI, peripheral ischemia

Central nervous system: Dizziness (8%), pain (6%), convulsions (1% to 5%), insomnia (4%), psychiatric events (4% to 5%), pain (3% to 4%), depression (1% to 6%), migraine (2% to 3%), anxiety, confusion, fever, hypoesthesia, emotional lability, impaired concentration, lethargy, malaise, nervousness, paranoia, somnolence, vertigo

Dermatologic: Purpura (3% to 4%), acne (1% to 6%), brittle fingernails, hair breaking, abnormal pigmentation, angioedema, cellulitis, dermatitis, dry skin, eczema, folliculitis, keratosis, pruritus, rash, skin disorder, skin malignancies, urticaria

Endocrine & metabolic: Gynecomastia (<1% to 4%), menstrual disorder (1% to 3%), breast fibroadenosis, breast pain, hyper-/hypoglycemia, diabetes mellitus, goiter, hot flashes, hyperkalemia, hyperuricemia, libido increased/decreased

Gastrointestinal: Vomiting (2% to 10%), flatulence (5%), gingivitis (up to 4%), cramps (up to 4%), anorexia, constipation, dry mouth, dysphagia, enanthema, eructation, esophagitis, gastric ulcer, gastritis, gastroenteritis, gastrointestinal bleeding (upper), gingival bleeding, glossitis, mouth sores, peptic ulcer, pancreatitis, swallowing difficulty, salivary gland enlargement, taste perversion, tongue disorder, tooth disorder, weight loss/gain

Genitourinary: Leukorrhea (1%), abnormal urine, micturition increased, micturition urgency, nocturia, polyuria, pyelonephritis, urinary incontinence, uterine hemorrhage

Hematologic: Leukopenia (<1% to 6%), anemia, bleeding disorder, clotting disorder, platelet disorder, red blood cell disorder, thrombocytopenia

Hepatic: Hepatotoxicity (<1% to 7%), hyperbilirubinemia

Neuromuscular & skeletal: Arthralgia (1% to 6%), bone fracture, joint dislocation, joint pain, muscle pain, myalgia, neuropathy, stiffness, synovial cyst, tendon disorder, tingling, weakness

Ocular: Abnormal vision, cataract, conjunctivitis, eye pain, visual disturbance

Otic: Deafness, hearing loss, tinnitus, vestibular disorder

Renal: BUN increased, hematuria, renal abscess

Respiratory: Sinusitis (<1% to 7%), bronchospasm (up to 5%), cough (3% to 5%), pharyngitis (3% to 5%), dyspnea (1% to 5%), rhinitis (up to 5%), abnormal chest sounds, epistaxis, respiratory infection, pneumonia (up to 1%)

Miscellaneous: Flu-like syndrome (8% to 10%), lymphoma (<1% to 6% reported in transplant), abscess, allergic reactions, bacterial infection, carcinoma, diaphoresis increased, fungal infection, herpes simplex, herpes zoster, hiccups, lymphadenopathy, moniliasis, night sweats, tonsillitis, viral infection

Postmarketing and/or case reports (any indication): Anaphylaxis/anaphylactoid reaction (possibly associated with Cremophor® EL vehicle in injection formulation), benign intracranial hypertension, cholesterol increased, death (due to renal deterioration), encephalopathy, gout, hyperbilirubinemia, hyperkalemia, hypomagnesemia (mild), impaired consciousness, neurotoxicity, papilloedema, pulmonary edema (noncardiogenic), uric acid increased

Ophthalmic emulsion (Restasis®):

>10%: Ocular: Burning (17%)

1% to 10%: Ocular: Hyperemia (conjunctival 5%), eye pain, pruritus, stinging

Dental Usual Dosing Note: Neoral®/Genraf® and Sandimmune® are not bioequivalent and cannot be used interchangeably.

Autoimmune diseases: Adults: 1-3 mg/kg/day

Dosage Neoral®/Genraf® and Sandimmune® are not bioequivalent and cannot be used interchangeably.

Children: Transplant: Refer to adult dosing; children may require, and are able to tolerate, larger doses than adults.

Adults:

Newly-transplanted patients: Adjunct therapy with corticosteroids is recommended. Initial dose should be given 4-12 hours prior to transplant or may be given postoperatively; adjust initial dose to achieve desired plasma concentration

Oral: Dose is dependent upon type of transplant and formulation:

Cyclosporine (modified):

Renal: 9 ± 3 mg/kg/day, divided twice daily

Liver: 8 ± 4 mg/kg/day, divided twice daily

Heart: 7 ± 3 mg/kg/day, divided twice daily

Cyclosporine (non-modified): Initial dose: 15 mg/kg/day as a single dose (range 14-18 mg/kg); lower doses of 10-14 mg/kg/day have been used for renal transplants. Continue initial dose daily for 1-2 weeks; taper by 5% per week to a maintenance dose of 5-10 mg/kg/day; some renal transplant patients may be dosed as low as 3 mg/kg/day

Note: When using the non-modified formulation, cyclosporine levels may increase in liver transplant patients when the T-tube is closed; dose may need decreased

I.V.: Cyclosporine (non-modified): Manufacturer's labeling: Initial dose: 5-6 mg/kg/day as a single dose ($\frac{1}{3}$ the oral dose), infused over 2-6 hours; use should be limited to patients unable to take capsules or oral solution; patients should be switched to an oral dosage form as soon as possible

Note: Many transplant centers administer cyclosporine as "divided dose" infusions (in 2-3 doses/day) or as a continuous (24-hour) infusion;

(Continued)

CycloSPORINE *(Continued)*

dosages range from 3-7.5 mg/kg/day. Specific institutional protocols should be consulted.

Conversion to cyclosporine (modified) from cyclosporine (non-modified): Start with daily dose previously used and adjust to obtain preconversion cyclosporine trough concentration. Plasma concentrations should be monitored every 4-7 days and dose adjusted as necessary, until desired trough level is obtained. When transferring patients with previously poor absorption of cyclosporine (non-modified), monitor trough levels at least twice weekly (especially if initial dose exceeds 10 mg/kg/day); high plasma levels are likely to occur.

Rheumatoid arthritis: Oral: Cyclosporine (modified): Initial dose: 2.5 mg/kg/day, divided twice daily; salicylates, NSAIDs, and oral glucocorticoids may be continued (refer to Drug Interactions); dose may be increased by 0.5-0.75 mg/kg/day if insufficient response is seen after 8 weeks of treatment; additional dosage increases may be made again at 12 weeks (maximum dose: 4 mg/kg/day). Discontinue if no benefit is seen by 16 weeks of therapy.

Note: Increase the frequency of blood pressure monitoring after each alteration in dosage of cyclosporine. Cyclosporine dosage should be decreased by 25% to 50% in patients with no history of hypertension who develop sustained hypertension during therapy and, if hypertension persists, treatment with cyclosporine should be discontinued.

Psoriasis: Oral: Cyclosporine (modified): Initial dose: 2.5 mg/kg/day, divided twice daily; dose may be increased by 0.5 mg/kg/day if insufficient response is seen after 4 weeks of treatment. Additional dosage increases may be made every 2 weeks if needed (maximum dose: 4 mg/kg/day). Discontinue if no benefit is seen by 6 weeks of therapy. Once patients are adequately controlled, the dose should be decreased to the lowest effective dose. Doses lower than 2.5 mg/kg/day may be effective. Treatment longer than 1 year is not recommended.

Note: Increase the frequency of blood pressure monitoring after each alteration in dosage of cyclosporine. Cyclosporine dosage should be decreased by 25% to 50% in patients with no history of hypertension who develop sustained hypertension during therapy and, if hypertension persists, treatment with cyclosporine should be discontinued.

Focal segmental glomerulosclerosis (unlabeled use): Initial: 3 mg/kg/day divided every 12 hours

Autoimmune diseases (unlabeled use): 1-3 mg/kg/day

Keratoconjunctivitis sicca: Ophthalmic (Restasis®): Children ≥16 years and Adults: Instill 1 drop in each eye every 12 hours

Dosage adjustment in renal impairment: For severe psoriasis:

Serum creatinine levels ≥25% above pretreatment levels: Take another sample within 2 weeks; if the level remains ≥25% above pretreatment levels, decrease dosage of cyclosporine (modified) by 25% to 50%. If two dosage adjustments do not reverse the increase in serum creatinine levels, treatment should be discontinued.

Serum creatinine levels ≥50% above pretreatment levels: Decrease cyclosporine dosage by 25% to 50%. If two dosage adjustments do not reverse the increase in serum creatinine levels, treatment should be discontinued.

Hemodialysis: Supplemental dose is not necessary.

Peritoneal dialysis: Supplemental dose is not necessary.

Dosage adjustment in hepatic impairment: Probably necessary; monitor levels closely

Mechanism of Action Inhibition of production and release of interleukin II and inhibits interleukin II-induced activation of resting T-lymphocytes.

Contraindications Hypersensitivity to cyclosporine or any component of the formulation. Rheumatoid arthritis and psoriasis: Abnormal renal function, uncontrolled hypertension, malignancies. Concomitant treatment with PUVA or UVB therapy, methotrexate, other immunosuppressive agents, coal tar, or radiation therapy are also contraindications for use in patients with psoriasis. Ophthalmic emulsion is contraindicated in patients with active ocular infections.

Warnings/Precautions [U.S. Boxed Warning]: Renal impairment, including structural kidney damage has occurred (when used at high doses); monitor renal function closely. Use caution with other potentially nephrotoxic drugs (eg, acyclovir, aminoglycoside antibiotics, amphotericin B, ciprofloxacin). Increased risk of lymphomas and other malignancies. **[U.S. Boxed Warning]: Increased risk of infection. [U.S. Boxed Warning]: May cause hypertension.** Use caution when changing dosage forms. **[U.S. Boxed Warning]: Cyclosporine (modified) has increased bioavailability as compared to cyclosporine (non-modified) and cannot be used interchangeably without close monitoring.** Monitor cyclosporine concentrations closely following the addition, modification, or deletion of other medications; live, attenuated vaccines may be less effective; use should be avoided. Increased hepatic enzymes and bilirubin have occurred (when used at high doses); improvement usually seen with dosage reduction.

Transplant patients: To be used initially with corticosteroids. May cause significant hyperkalemia and hyperuricemia, seizures (particularly if used with high dose corticosteroids), and encephalopathy. Make dose adjustments based on cyclosporine blood concentrations. **[U.S. Boxed Warning]: Adjustment of dose should only be made under the direct supervision of an experienced physician.** Anaphylaxis has been reported with I.V. use; reserve for patients who cannot take oral form.

Psoriasis: Patients should avoid excessive sun exposure; safety and efficacy in children <18 years of age have not been established. **[U.S. Boxed Warning]: Risk of skin cancer may be increased with a history of PUVA and possibly methotrexate or other immunosuppressants, UVB, coal tar, or radiation.**

Rheumatoid arthritis: Safety and efficacy for use in juvenile rheumatoid arthritis have not been established. If receiving other immunosuppressive agents, radiation or UV therapy, concurrent use of cyclosporine is not recommended.

Ophthalmic emulsion: Safety and efficacy have not been established in patients <16 years of age.

Products may contain corn oil, castor oil, ethanol, or propylene glycol; injection also contains Cremophor® EL (polyoxyethylated castor oil), which has been associated with rare anaphylactic reactions.

Drug Interactions Substrate of CYP3A4 (major); **Inhibits** CYP2C9 (weak), 3A4 (moderate)

ACE inhibitors: May enhance nephrotoxic effects of cyclosporine.

Allopurinol: Increases cyclosporine concentrations by inhibiting cyclosporine metabolism.

Amiodarone: May increase cyclosporine concentrations by inhibiting cyclosporine metabolism.

Antibiotics: Concomitant use may potentiate renal dysfunction (seen with ciprofloxacin, gentamicin, tobramycin, vancomycin, trimethoprim and sulfamethoxazole); increased cyclosporine concentrations by inhibiting cyclosporine metabolism (seen with azithromycin, clarithromycin, erythromycin, and norfloxacin, quinupristin/dalfopristin); may decrease cyclosporine concentrations by inducing cyclosporine metabolism (seen with nafcillin, and rifampin); may decrease immunosuppressant effects (seen with ciprofloxacin); CNS disturbances, seizures (seen with imipenem).

Anticonvulsants: May decrease cyclosporine concentrations by inducing cyclosporine metabolism (seen with carbamazepine, phenobarbital, and phenytoin)

Antineoplastics: Concomitant use may potentiate renal dysfunction (seen with melphalan)

Antifungals: Concomitant use may potentiate renal dysfunction (seen with amphotericin B, ketoconazole); increase cyclosporine concentrations by inhibiting cyclosporine metabolism (seen with fluconazole, itraconazole, and ketoconazole)

Bosentan: Cyclosporine may increase the serum concentration of bosentan. Bosentan may decrease the serum concentration of cyclosporine. Concurrent use is contraindicated..

Bromocriptine: Increases cyclosporine concentrations by inhibiting cyclosporine metabolism

Calcium channel blockers (diltiazem, nicardipine, verapamil): Increase cyclosporine concentrations by inhibiting cyclosporine metabolism. Nifedipine has been reported to increase the risk of gingival hyperplasia.

Colchicine: May potentiate renal dysfunction; colchicine may increase cyclosporine concentrations by inhibiting metabolism. Cyclosporine may decrease the clearance of colchicine.

Corticosteroids: Systemic corticosteroids may increase the serum concentration of cyclosporine (reported with methylprednisolone). Cyclosporine may increase the serum concentration of systemic corticosteroids. Convulsions have been reported with high-dose methylprednisolone.

CYP3A4 inducers: CYP3A4 inducers may decrease the levels/effects of cyclosporine. Example inducers include aminoglutethimide, carbamazepine, nafcillin, nevirapine, phenobarbital, phenytoin, and rifamycins.

CYP3A4 inhibitors: May increase the levels/effects of cyclosporine. Example inhibitors include azole antifungals, clarithromycin, diclofenac, doxycycline, erythromycin, imatinib, isoniazid, nefazodone, nicardipine, propofol, protease inhibitors, quinidine, telithromycin, and verapamil.

CYP3A4 substrates: Cyclosporine may increase the levels/effects of CYP3A4 substrates. Example substrates include benzodiazepines, calcium channel blockers, cyclosporine, mirtazapine, nateglinide, nefazodone, sildenafil (and other PDE-5 inhibitors), tacrolimus, and venlafaxine. Selected benzodiazepines (midazolam and triazolam), cisapride, ergot alkaloids, selected
(Continued)

CycloSPORINE *(Continued)*

HMG-CoA reductase inhibitors (lovastatin and simvastatin), and pimozide are generally contraindicated with strong CYP3A4 inhibitors.

Danazol: Increases cyclosporine concentrations by inhibiting cyclosporine metabolism

Digoxin: Decreased clearance and decreased volume of distribution of digoxin; severe digitalis toxicity has been observed.

Fibric acid derivatives: May increase the risk of renal dysfunction and may alter cyclosporine concentrations; monitor

H_2 blockers: Concomitant use may potentiate renal dysfunction (seen with cimetidine, ranitidine).

HMG-CoA reductase inhibitors: Cyclosporine may increase levels/effects of HMG-CoA reductase inhibitors, resulting in myalgias, rhabdomyolysis, acute renal failure; dosage adjustments of HMG-CoA reductase inhibitors are recommended.

Imatinib: May increase cyclosporine serum concentrations by inhibiting cyclosporine metabolism.

Immunosuppressives: Concomitant use may potentiate renal dysfunction (seen with tacrolimus, muromonab-CD3).

Metoclopramide: Increases cyclosporine concentrations by inhibiting cyclosporine metabolism.

Methotrexate: Cyclosporine increases plasma levels of methotrexate and decreases plasma levels of its metabolite; monitor closely for signs of toxicity.

Minoxidil: Concomitant use may lead to severe hypertrichosis.

NSAIDs: Concomitant use may potentiate renal dysfunction, especially in dehydrated patients (seen with diclofenac, naproxen, sulindac). In addition, diclofenac plasma levels are doubled when given with cyclosporine; the lowest possible dose of diclofenac should be used. Monitor serum creatinine.

Octreotide: May decrease cyclosporine concentrations by inducing cyclosporine metabolism.

Oral contraceptives (hormonal): May increase serum levels of cyclosporine; monitor for signs of toxicity.

Orlistat: May decrease absorption of cyclosporine; avoid concomitant use.

Protease inhibitors: Formal interaction studies have not been done; protease inhibitors are known to induce CYP3A4; use caution when using cyclosporine with indinavir, nelfinavir, ritonavir, or saquinavir.

Rifabutin: Formal interaction studies have not been done; rifabutin is known to increase the metabolism of medications via CYP3A4.

Sirolimus: Cyclosporine may increase serum levels/effects; monitor. Concurrent therapy may increase the risk of HUS/TTP/TMA. Administer sirolimus 4 hours after cyclosporine to minimize the increase in sirolimus blood levels.

Sulfasalazine: May decrease cyclosporine levels.

Sulfinpyrazone: May decrease cyclosporine levels by inducing cyclosporine metabolism; monitor.

Ticlopidine: May decrease cyclosporine concentrations by inducing cyclosporine metabolism.

Vaccines: Vaccination may be less effective; avoid use of live vaccines during therapy.

Voriconazole: Cyclosporine serum concentrations may be increased; monitor serum concentrations and renal function. Decrease cyclosporine dosage by 50% when initiating voriconazole.

Ethanol/Nutrition/Herb Interactions

Food: Grapefruit juice increases absorption; unsupervised use should be avoided.

Herb/Nutraceutical: Avoid St John's wort; as an enzyme inducer, it may increase the metabolism of and decrease plasma levels of cyclosporine; organ rejection and graft loss have been reported. Avoid cat's claw, echinacea (have immunostimulant properties).

Dietary Considerations
Administer this medication consistently with relation to time of day and meals. Avoid grapefruit juice.

Pharmacodynamics/Kinetics

Absorption:

Ophthalmic emulsion: Serum concentrations not detectable.

Oral:

Cyclosporine (non-modified): Erratic and incomplete; dependent on presence of food, bile acids, and GI motility; larger oral doses are needed in pediatrics due to shorter bowel length and limited intestinal absorption

Cyclosporine (modified): Erratic and incomplete; increased absorption, up to 30% when compared to cyclosporine (non-modified); less dependent on food, bile acids, or GI motility when compared to cyclosporine (non-modified)

Distribution: Widely in tissues and body fluids including the liver, pancreas, and lungs; crosses placenta; enters breast milk

V_{dss}: 4-6 L/kg in renal, liver, and marrow transplant recipients (slightly lower values in cardiac transplant patients; children <10 years have higher values)

Protein binding: 90% to 98% to lipoproteins

Metabolism: Extensively hepatic via CYP3A4; forms at least 25 metabolites; extensive first-pass effect following oral administration

Bioavailability: Oral:

Cyclosporine (non-modified): Dependent on patient population and transplant type (<10% in adult liver transplant patients and as high as 89% in renal transplant patients); bioavailability of Sandimmune® capsules and oral solution are equivalent; bioavailability of oral solution is ~30% of the I.V. solution

Children: 28% (range: 17% to 42%); gut dysfunction common in BMT patients and oral bioavailability is further reduced

Cyclosporine (modified): Bioavailability of Neoral® capsules and oral solution are equivalent:

Children: 43% (range: 30% to 68%)

Adults: 23% greater than with cyclosporine (non-modified) in renal transplant patients; 50% greater in liver transplant patients

Half-life elimination: Oral: May be prolonged in patients with hepatic impairment and shorter in pediatric patients due to the higher metabolism rate

Cyclosporine (non-modified): Biphasic: Alpha: 1.4 hours; Terminal: 19 hours (range: 10-27 hours)

Cyclosporine (modified): Biphasic: Terminal: 8.4 hours (range: 5-18 hours)

Time to peak, serum: Oral:

Cyclosporine (non-modified): 2-6 hours; some patients have a second peak at 5-6 hours

Cyclosporine (modified): Renal transplant: 1.5-2 hours

Excretion: Primarily feces; urine (6%, 0.1% as unchanged drug and metabolites)

Pregnancy Risk Factor C

Lactation Enters breast milk/not recommended

Breast-Feeding Considerations The AAP does not recommend breast-feeding during therapy due to possible immune suppression in the infant as well as the unknown effects on growth or association with carcinogenesis.

Dosage Forms Excipient information presented when available (limited, particularly for generics); consult specific product labeling.

Capsule, soft gel, modified: 25 mg, 100 mg [contains castor oil, ethanol]

Gengraf®: 25 mg, 100 mg [contains ethanol, castor oil, propylene glycol]

Neoral®: 25 mg, 100 mg [contains dehydrated ethanol, corn oil, castor oil, propylene glycol]

Capsule, soft gel, non-modified (Sandimmune®): 25 mg, 100 mg [contains dehydrated ethanol, corn oil]

Emulsion, ophthalmic [preservative free, single-use vial] (Restasis®): 0.05% (0.4 mL) [contains glycerin, castor oil, polysorbate 80, carbomer 1342; 32 vials/box]

Injection, solution, non-modified (Sandimmune®): 50 mg/mL (5 mL) [contains Cremophor® EL (polyoxyethylated castor oil), ethanol]

Solution, oral, modified:

Gengraf®: 100 mg/mL (50 mL) [contains castor oil, propylene glycol]

Neoral®: 100 mg/mL (50 mL) [contains dehydrated ethanol, corn oil, castor oil, propylene glycol]

Solution, oral, non-modified (Sandimmune®): 100 mg/mL (50 mL) [contains olive oil, ethanol]

Selected Readings

Ferrari SL, Goffin E, Mourad M, et al, "The Interaction Between Clarithromycin and Cyclosporine in Kidney Transplant Recipients," *Transplantation*, 1994, 58(6):725-7.

Harnett JD, Parfrey PS, Paul MD, et al, "Erythromycin-Cyclosporine Interaction in Renal Transplant Recipients," *Transplantation*, 1987, 43(2):316-8.

Cyklokapron® *see* Tranexamic Acid *on page 1600*

Cylate® *see* Cyclopentolate *on page 422*

Cylex® [OTC] *see* Benzocaine *on page 195*

Cymbalta® *see* Duloxetine *on page 549*

Cyproheptadine (si proe HEP ta deen)

Generic Available Yes

Index Terms Cyproheptadine Hydrochloride; Periactin

Pharmacologic Category Antihistamine

Use Perennial and seasonal allergic rhinitis and other allergic symptoms including urticaria

Unlabeled/Investigational Use Appetite stimulation, blepharospasm, cluster headaches, migraine headaches, Nelson's syndrome, pruritus, schizophrenia, spinal cord damage associated spasticity, and tardive dyskinesia

(Continued)

Cyproheptadine *(Continued)*

Local Anesthetic/Vasoconstrictor Precautions No information available to require special precautions

Effects on Dental Treatment Key adverse event(s) related to dental treatment: Xerostomia (normal salivary flow resumes upon discontinuation)

Common Adverse Effects

>10%:

Central nervous system: Slight to moderate drowsiness

Respiratory: Thickening of bronchial secretions

1% to 10%:

Central nervous system: Dizziness, fatigue, headache, nervousness

Gastrointestinal: Abdominal pain, appetitie stimulation, diarrhea, nausea, xerostomia

Neuromuscular & skeletal: Arthralgia

Respiratory: Pharyngitis

Mechanism of Action A potent antihistamine and serotonin antagonist, competes with histamine for H_1-receptor sites on effector cells in the gastrointestinal tract, blood vessels, and respiratory tract

Drug Interactions

Increased Effect/Toxicity: Cyproheptadine may potentiate the effect of CNS depressants. MAO inhibitors may cause hallucinations when taken with cyproheptadine.

Pharmacodynamics/Kinetics

Absorption: Completely

Metabolism: Almost completely hepatic

Excretion: Urine (>50% primarily as metabolites); feces (~25%)

Pregnancy Risk Factor B

Cyproheptadine Hydrochloride *see* Cyproheptadine *on page 431*

Cystadane® *see* Betaine *on page 205*

Cystagon® *see* Cysteamine *on page 432*

Cysteamine (sis TEE a meen)

U.S. Brand Names Cystagon®

Generic Available No

Index Terms Cysteamine Bitartrate

Pharmacologic Category Anticystine Agent; Urinary Tract Product

Use Orphan drug: Treatment of nephropathic cystinosis

Local Anesthetic/Vasoconstrictor Precautions No information available to require special precautions

Effects on Dental Treatment No significant effects or complications reported

Mechanism of Action Reacts with cystine in the lysosome to convert it to cysteine and to a cysteine-cysteamine mixed disulfide, both of which can then exit the lysosome in patients with cystinosis, an inherited defect of lysosomal transport

Pregnancy Risk Factor C

Cysteamine Bitartrate *see* Cysteamine *on page 432*

Cysteine (SIS te een)

Generic Available Yes

Index Terms Cysteine Hydrochloride

Pharmacologic Category Nutritional Supplement

Use Supplement to crystalline amino acid solutions, in particular the specialized pediatric formulas (eg, Aminosyn® PF, TrophAmine®) to meet the intravenous amino acid nutritional requirements of infants receiving parenteral nutrition (PN)

Local Anesthetic/Vasoconstrictor Precautions No information available to require special precautions

Effects on Dental Treatment No significant effects or complications reported

Mechanism of Action Cysteine is a sulfur-containing amino acid synthesized from methionine via the transulfuration pathway. It is a precursor of the tripeptide glutathione and also of taurine. Newborn infants have a relative deficiency of the enzyme necessary to affect this conversion. Cysteine may be considered an essential amino acid in infants.

Cysteine Hydrochloride *see* Cysteine *on page 432*

Cysto-Conray® II *see* Iothalamate Meglumine *on page 903*

Cystografin® *see* Diatrizoate Meglumine *on page 479*

Cystografin® Dilute *see* Diatrizoate Meglumine *on page 479*

Cystospaz® *see* Hyoscyamine *on page 847*

Cystospaz-M® [DSC] *see* Hyoscyamine *on page 847*
CYT *see* Cyclophosphamide *on page 423*
Cytadren® *see* Aminoglutethimide *on page 89*

Cytarabine (sye TARE a been)

U.S. Brand Names Cytosar-U®
Canadian Brand Names Cytosar®
Mexican Brand Names Laracit
Generic Available Yes
Index Terms Arabinosylcytosine; Ara-C; Cytarabine Hydrochloride; Cytosine Arabinoside Hydrochloride; NSC-63878
Pharmacologic Category Antineoplastic Agent, Antimetabolite; Antineoplastic Agent, Antimetabolite (Purine Antagonist)
Use Treatment of acute myeloid leukemia (AML), acute lymphocytic leukemia (ALL), chronic myelocytic leukemia (CML; blast phase), and lymphomas; prophylaxis and treatment of meningeal leukemia
Local Anesthetic/Vasoconstrictor Precautions No information available to require special precautions
Effects on Dental Treatment Key adverse event(s) related to dental treatment: Mucositis
Common Adverse Effects Note: Frequencies not defined; CNS, gastrointestinal, ocular and pulmonary toxicities are more common with high-dose cytarabine regimens.

More frequent:
Central nervous system: Fever (>80%)
Dermatologic: Alopecia, rash
Gastrointestinal: Nausea, vomiting, diarrhea, mucositis, anal inflammation, anal ulceration, anorexia; GI effects may be more pronounced with divided I.V. bolus doses than with continuous infusion
Hematologic: Myelosuppression, neutropenia (onset: 1-7 days; nadir [biphasic]: 7-9 and at 15-24 days; recovery [biphasic]: 9-12 and at 24-34 days), thrombocytopenia (onset: 5 days; nadir: 12-15 days; recovery 15-25 days), anemia, leukopenia, megaloblastosis, reticulocytes decreased, bleeding
Hepatic: Hepatic dysfunction, transaminases increased (acute)
Local: Thrombophlebitis
Ocular: Tearing, ocular pain, foreign body sensation, photophobia, and blurred vision may occur with high-dose therapy; ophthalmic corticosteroids or 0.9% NaCl usually prevents or relieves the condition
Less frequent:
Cardiovascular: Chest pain, pericarditis
Central nervous system: Dizziness, headache, somnolence, confusion, malaise, neural toxicity, neuritis; a severe cerebellar toxicity occurs in about 8% of patients receiving a high dose (>36-48 g/m^2/cycle); it is irreversible or fatal in about 1%
Dermatologic: Skin freckling, itching, pruritus, ulceration, urticaria, pain, erythema, and skin sloughing of the palmar and plantar surfaces may occur with high-dose therapy. Prophylactic topical steroids and/or skin moisturizers may be useful.
Gastrointestinal: Abdominal pain, bowel necrosis, esophageal irritation, esophagitis, pancreatitis, sore throat
Genitourinary: Urinary retention
Hepatic: Jaundice
Local: Injection site cellulitis
Neuromuscular & skeletal: Myalgia, bone pain
Ocular: Conjunctivitis
Renal: Renal dysfunction
Respiratory: Syndrome of sudden respiratory distress, including tachypnea, hypoxemia, interstitial and alveolar infiltrates progressing to pulmonary edema, pneumonia, dyspnea
Miscellaneous: Allergic edema, anaphylaxis, sepsis
Adverse events associated with intrathecal cytarabine administration: Dysphagia, accessory nerve paralysis, diplopia, cough, hoarseness, aphonia, blindness (with concurrent systemic chemotherapy and cranial irradiation), fever, nausea, necrotizing leukoencephalopathy (with concurrent cranial irradiation, I.T. methotrexate, and I.T. hydrocortisone), neurotoxicity, paraplegia, vomiting

Mechanism of Action Inhibition of DNA synthesis. Cytosine gains entry into cells by a carrier process, and then must be converted to its active compound, aracytidine triphosphate. Cytosine is a purine analog and is incorporated into DNA; however, the primary action is inhibition of DNA polymerase resulting in (Continued)

433

Cytarabine *(Continued)*

decreased DNA synthesis and repair. The degree of cytotoxicity correlates linearly with incorporation into DNA; therefore, incorporation into the DNA is responsible for drug activity and toxicity. Cytarabine is specific for the S phase of the cell cycle.

Drug Interactions

Decreased Effect: Decreased effect of flucytosine; decreases digoxin oral tablet absorption.

Pharmacodynamics/Kinetics

Distribution: V_d: Total body water; widely and rapidly since it enters the cells readily; crosses blood-brain barrier with CSF levels of 40% to 50% of plasma level

Metabolism: Primarily hepatic; metabolized by deoxycytidine kinase and other nucleotide kinases to aracytidine triphosphate (active); about 86% to 96% of dose is metabolized to inactive uracil arabinoside

Half-life elimination: Initial: 7-20 minutes; Terminal: 0.5-2.6 hours

Excretion: Urine (~80% as metabolites) within 24-36 hours

Pregnancy Risk Factor D

Cytarabine Hydrochloride *see* Cytarabine *on page 433*

Cytarabine (Liposomal) *(sye TARE a been lip po SOE mal)*

U.S. Brand Names DepoCyt®
Canadian Brand Names DepoCyt®
Generic Available No
Pharmacologic Category Antineoplastic Agent, Antimetabolite
Use Treatment of neoplastic (lymphomatous) meningitis
Local Anesthetic/Vasoconstrictor Precautions No information available to require special precautions
Effects on Dental Treatment No significant effects or complications reported
Common Adverse Effects

>10%:

Central nervous system: Headache (28%), confusion (14%), somnolence (12%), fever (11%), pain (11%); chemical arachnoiditis is commonly observed, and may include neck pain, neck rigidity, headache, fever, nausea, vomiting, and back pain; may occur in up to 100% of cycles without dexamethasone prophylaxis; incidence is reduced to 33% when dexamethasone is used concurrently

Gastrointestinal: Vomiting (12%), nausea (11%)

Neuromuscular & skeletal: Weakness (19%)

1% to 10%:

Cardiovascular: Peripheral edema (7%)

Gastrointestinal: Constipation (7%)

Genitourinary: Incontinence (3%)

Hematologic: Neutropenia (9%), thrombocytopenia (8%), anemia (1%)

Neuromuscular & skeletal: Back pain (7%), abnormal gait (4%)

Mechanism of Action This is a sustained-release formulation of the active ingredient cytarabine, which acts through inhibition of DNA synthesis; cell cycle-specific for the S phase of cell division; cytosine gains entry into cells by a carrier process, and then must be converted to its active compound; cytosine acts as an analog and is incorporated into DNA; however, the primary action is inhibition of DNA polymerase resulting in decreased DNA synthesis and repair; degree of its cytotoxicity correlates linearly with its incorporation into DNA; therefore, incorporation into the DNA is responsible for drug activity and toxicity

Drug Interactions

Increased Effect/Toxicity: No formal studies of interactions with other medications have been conducted. The limited systemic exposure minimizes the potential for interaction between liposomal cytarabine and other medications.

Decreased Effect: No formal studies of interactions with other medications have been conducted. The limited systemic exposure minimizes the potential for interaction between liposomal cytarabine and other medications.

Pharmacodynamics/Kinetics

Absorption: Systemic exposure following intrathecal administration is negligible since transfer rate from CSF to plasma is slow

Metabolism: In plasma to ara-U (inactive)

Half-life elimination, CSF: 100-263 hours

Time to peak, CSF: Intrathecal: ~5 hours

Excretion: Primarily urine (as metabolites - ara-U)

Pregnancy Risk Factor D

Cytomel® *see* Liothyronine *on page 987*
Cytosar-U® *see* Cytarabine *on page 433*

Dacarbazine (da KAR ba zeen)

U.S. Brand Names DTIC-Dome®
Canadian Brand Names DTIC®
Mexican Brand Names Deticene; Detilem
Generic Available Yes
Index Terms DIC; Dimethyl Triazeno Imidazole Carboxamide; DTIC; Imidazole Carboxamide; Imidazole Carboxamide Dimethyltriazene; WR-139007
Pharmacologic Category Antineoplastic Agent, Alkylating Agent (Triazene)
Use Treatment of malignant melanoma, Hodgkin's disease, soft-tissue sarcomas, fibrosarcomas, rhabdomyosarcoma, islet cell carcinoma, medullary carcinoma of the thyroid, and neuroblastoma
Local Anesthetic/Vasoconstrictor Precautions No information available to require special precautions
Effects on Dental Treatment Key adverse event(s) related to dental treatment: Metallic taste
Common Adverse Effects
>10%:
  Gastrointestinal: Nausea and vomiting (>90%), can be severe and dose limiting; nausea and vomiting decrease on successive days when dacarbazine is given daily for 5 days; diarrhea
  Hematologic: Myelosuppression, leukopenia, thrombocytopenia - dose limiting
    Onset: 5-7 days
    Nadir: 7-10 days
    Recovery: 21-28 days
  Local: Pain on infusion, may be minimized by administration through a central line, or by administration as a short infusion (eg, 1-2 hours as opposed to bolus injection)
1% to 10%:
  Dermatologic: Alopecia, rash, photosensitivity
  Gastrointestinal: Anorexia, metallic taste
  Miscellaneous: Flu-like syndrome (fever, myalgia, malaise)
Mechanism of Action Alkylating agent which appears to form methyl-carbonium ions that attack nucleophilic groups in DNA; cross-links strands of DNA resulting in the inhibition of DNA, RNA, and protein synthesis, the exact mechanism of action is still unclear.
Drug Interactions
Cytochrome P450 Effect: Substrate (major) of CYP1A2, 2E1
Increased Effect/Toxicity: CYP1A2 inhibitors may increase the levels/effects of dacarbazine; example inhibitors include ciprofloxacin, fluvoxamine, ketoconazole, norfloxacin, ofloxacin, and rofecoxib. CYP2E1 inhibitors may increase the levels/effects of dacarbazine; example inhibitors include disulfiram, isoniazid, and miconazole.
Decreased Effect: CYP1A2 inducers may decrease the levels/effects of dacarbazine; example inducers include aminoglutethimide, carbamazepine, phenobarbital, and rifampin. Patients may experience impaired immune
(Continued)

Dacarbazine *(Continued)*

response to vaccines; possible infection after administration of live vaccines in patients receiving immunosuppressants.

Pharmacodynamics/Kinetics

Onset of action: I.V.: 18-24 days

Distribution: V_d: 0.6 L/kg, exceeding total body water; suggesting binding to some tissue (probably liver)

Protein binding: 5%

Metabolism: Extensively hepatic; hepatobiliary excretion is probably of some importance; metabolites may also have an antineoplastic effect

Half-life elimination: Biphasic: Initial: 20-40 minutes; Terminal: 5 hours

Excretion: Urine (~30% to 50% as unchanged drug)

Pregnancy Risk Factor C

Dacex-DM *see* Guaifenesin, Dextromethorphan, and Phenylephrine *on page 798*

Daclizumab *(dac KLYE zue mab)*

U.S. Brand Names Zenapax®
Canadian Brand Names Zenapax®
Mexican Brand Names Zenapax
Generic Available No
Pharmacologic Category Immunosuppressant Agent
Use Part of an immunosuppressive regimen (including cyclosporine and corticosteroids) for the prophylaxis of acute organ rejection in patients receiving renal transplant
Unlabeled/Investigational Use Graft-versus-host disease; prevention of organ rejection after heart transplant
Local Anesthetic/Vasoconstrictor Precautions No information available to require special precautions
Effects on Dental Treatment No significant effects or complications reported
Common Adverse Effects Although reported adverse events are frequent, when daclizumab is compared with placebo the incidence of adverse effects is similar between the two groups. Many of the adverse effects reported during clinical trial use of daclizumab may be related to the patient population, transplant procedure, and concurrent transplant medications. Diarrhea, fever, postoperative pain, pruritus, respiratory tract infection, urinary tract infection, and vomiting occurred more often in children than adults.

≥5%:

Cardiovascular: Chest pain, edema, hyper-/hypotension, tachycardia, thrombosis

Central nervous system: Dizziness, fatigue, fever, headache, insomnia, pain, post-traumatic pain, tremor

Dermatologic: Acne, cellulitis, wound healing impaired

Gastrointestinal: Abdominal distention, abdominal pain, constipation, diarrhea, dyspepsia, epigastric pain, nausea, pyrosis, vomiting

Genitourinary: Dysuria

Hematologic: Bleeding

Neuromuscular & skeletal: Back pain, musculoskeletal pain

Renal: Oliguria, renal tubular necrosis

Respiratory: Cough, dyspnea, pulmonary edema

Miscellaneous: Lymphocele, wound infection

≥2% to <5%:

Central nervous system: Anxiety, depression, shivering

Dermatologic: Hirsutism, pruritus, rash

Endocrine & metabolic: Dehydration, diabetes mellitus, fluid overload

Gastrointestinal: Flatulence, gastritis, hemorrhoids

Genitourinary: Urinary retention, urinary tract bleeding

Local: Application site reaction

Neuromuscular & skeletal: Arthralgia, leg cramps, myalgia, weakness

Ocular: Vision blurred

Renal: Hydronephrosis, renal damage, renal insufficiency

Respiratory: Atelectasis, congestion, hypoxia, pharyngitis, pleural effusion, rales, rhinitis

Miscellaneous: Night sweats, prickly sensation, diaphoresis

Mechanism of Action Daclizumab is a chimeric (90% human, 10% murine) monoclonal IgG antibody produced by recombinant DNA technology. Daclizumab inhibits immune reactions by binding and blocking the alpha-chain of the interleukin-2 receptor (CD25) located on the surface of activated lymphocytes.

Drug Interactions
  Increased Effect/Toxicity: The combined use of daclizumab, cyclosporine, mycophenolate mofetil, and corticosteroids has been associated with an increased mortality in a population of cardiac transplant recipients, particularly in patients who received antilymphocyte globulin and in patients with severe infections.
Pharmacodynamics/Kinetics
  Distribution: V_d:
    Adults: Central compartment: 0.031 L/kg; Peripheral compartment: 0.043 L/kg
    Children: Central compartment: 0.067 L/kg; Peripheral compartment: 0.047 L/kg
  Half-life elimination (estimated): Adults: Terminal: 20 days; Children: 13 days
Pregnancy Risk Factor C

Dacodyl™ [OTC] *see* Bisacodyl *on page 216*
Dacogen™ *see* Decitabine *on page 451*
DACT *see* Dactinomycin *on page 437*

Dactinomycin (dak ti noe MYE sin)

U.S. Brand Names Cosmegen®
Canadian Brand Names Cosmegen®
Mexican Brand Names Ac-De
Generic Available No
Index Terms ACT; Act-D; Actinomycin; Actinomycin Cl; Actinomycin D; DACT; NSC-3053
Pharmacologic Category Antineoplastic Agent, Antibiotic
Use Treatment of testicular tumors, melanoma, gestational trophoblastic neoplasm, Wilms' tumor, neuroblastoma, retinoblastoma, rhabdomyosarcoma, uterine sarcomas, Ewing's sarcoma, Kaposi's sarcoma, sarcoma botryoides, and soft tissue sarcoma
Local Anesthetic/Vasoconstrictor Precautions No information available to require special precautions
Effects on Dental Treatment Key adverse event(s) related to dental treatment: Stomatitis and mucositis
Common Adverse Effects Frequency not defined.
  Central nervous system: Fatigue, fever, lethargy, malaise
  Dermatologic: Acne, alopecia (reversible), cheilitis; increased pigmentation, sloughing, or erythema of previously irradiated skin; skin eruptions
  Endocrine & metabolic: Growth retardation, hypocalcemia
  Gastrointestinal: Abdominal pain, anorexia, diarrhea, dysphagia, esophagitis, GI ulceration, mucositis, nausea, pharyngitis, proctitis, stomatitis, vomiting
  Hematologic: Agranulocytosis, anemia, aplastic anemia, leukopenia, pancytopenia, reticulocytopenia, thrombocytopenia, myelosuppression (onset: 7 days, nadir: 14-21 days, recovery: 21-28 days)
  Hepatic: Ascites, hepatic failure, hepatitis, hepatomegaly, hepatotoxicity, liver function test abnormality, veno-occlusive disease
  Local: Erythema, edema, epidermolysis, pain, tissue necrosis, and ulceration (following extravasation)
  Neuromuscular & skeletal: Myalgia
  Renal: Renal function abnormality
  Respiratory: Pneumonitis
  Miscellaneous: Anaphylactoid reaction, infection
Mechanism of Action Binds to the guanine portion of DNA intercalating between guanine and cytosine base pairs inhibiting DNA and RNA synthesis and protein synthesis
Drug Interactions
  Increased Effect/Toxicity: Administration of live vaccines during treatment with dactinomycin should be avoided.
Pharmacodynamics/Kinetics
  Distribution: High concentrations found in bone marrow and tumor cells, submaxillary gland, liver, and kidney; crosses placenta; poor CSF penetration
  Metabolism: Hepatic, minimal
  Half-life elimination: ~36 hours
  Time to peak, serum: I.V.: 2-5 minutes
  Excretion: Bile (50%); feces (14%); urine (~10% as unchanged drug)
Pregnancy Risk Factor D

DAD *see* Mitoxantrone *on page 1113*
Dakin's Solution *see* Sodium Hypochlorite Solution *on page 1482*
Dallergy® *see* Chlorpheniramine, Phenylephrine, and Methscopolamine *on page 342*
Dallergy-JR® *see* Chlorpheniramine and Phenylephrine *on page 340*

Dalmane® *see* Flurazepam *on page 720*

d-Alpha-Gems™ [OTC] *see* Vitamin E *on page 1664*

d-Alpha Tocopherol *see* Vitamin E *on page 1664*

Dalteparin (dal TE pa rin)

Related Information
Cardiovascular Diseases *on page 1726*

U.S. Brand Names Fragmin®

Canadian Brand Names Fragmin®

Generic Available No

Index Terms Dalteparin Sodium; NSC-714371

Pharmacologic Category Low Molecular Weight Heparin

Use Prevention of deep vein thrombosis which may lead to pulmonary embolism, in patients requiring abdominal surgery who are at risk for thromboembolism complications (eg, patients >40 years of age, obesity, patients with malignancy, history of deep vein thrombosis or pulmonary embolism, and surgical procedures requiring general anesthesia and lasting >30 minutes); prevention of DVT in patients undergoing hip-replacement surgery; patients immobile during an acute illness; acute treatment of unstable angina or non-Q-wave myocardial infarction; prevention of ischemic complications in patients on concurrent aspirin therapy; in patients with cancer, extended treatment (6 months) of acute symptomatic venous thromboembolism (DVT and/or PE) to reduce the recurrence of venous thromboembolism

Unlabeled/Investigational Use Active treatment of deep vein thrombosis (noncancer patients)

Local Anesthetic/Vasoconstrictor Precautions No information available to require special precautions

Effects on Dental Treatment Key adverse event(s) related to dental treatment: As with all anticoagulants, bleeding is the major adverse effect of bivalirudin. Hemorrhage may occur at virtually any site. Risk is dependent on multiple variables, including the intensity of anticoagulation and patient susceptibility. Additional adverse effects are often related to idiosyncratic reactions, and the frequency is difficult to estimate. Adverse reactions reported were generally less than those seen with heparin.

Common Adverse Effects Note: As with all anticoagulants, bleeding is the major adverse effect of dalteparin. Hemorrhage may occur at virtually any site. Risk is dependent on multiple variables.

>10%:

Hematologic: Bleeding (3% to 14%)

1% to 10%:

Hematologic: Wound hematoma (up to 3%)

Hepatic: AST >3 times upper limit of normal (5% to 9%), ALT >3 times upper limit of normal (4% to 10%)

Local: Pain at injection site (up to 12%), injection site hematoma (up to 7%)

Mechanism of Action Low molecular weight heparin analog with a molecular weight of 4000-6000 daltons; the commercial product contains 3% to 15% heparin with a molecular weight <3000 daltons, 65% to 78% with a molecular weight of 3000-8000 daltons and 14% to 26% with a molecular weight >8000 daltons; while dalteparin has been shown to inhibit both factor Xa and factor IIa (thrombin), the antithrombotic effect of dalteparin is characterized by a higher ratio of antifactor Xa to antifactor IIa activity (ratio = 4)

Drug Interactions
Increased Effect/Toxicity: Anticoagulants, antiplatelet agents, dasatinib, NSAIDs, salicylates, and treprostinil may enhance the anticoagulant effect of dalteparin. Dalteparin, particularly at therapeutic doses, may enhance the bleeding complications of drotrecogin alfa.

Pharmacodynamics/Kinetics
Onset of action: 1-2 hours

Duration: >12 hours

Distribution: V_d: 40-60 mL/kg

Bioavailability: SubQ: 81% to 93%

Half-life elimination (route dependent): 2-5 hours

Time to peak, serum: 4 hours

Pregnancy Risk Factor B

Dalteparin Sodium *see* Dalteparin *on page 438*

Damason-P® *see* Hydrocodone and Aspirin *on page 825*

Danaparoid (da NAP a roid)

Canadian Brand Names Orgaran®
Generic Available No
Index Terms Danaparoid Sodium
Pharmacologic Category Anticoagulant
Use Prevention of postoperative deep vein thrombosis following elective hip replacement surgery
Unlabeled/Investigational Use Systemic anticoagulation for patients with heparin-induced thrombocytopenia: factor Xa inhibition is used to monitor degree of anticoagulation if necessary
Local Anesthetic/Vasoconstrictor Precautions No information available to require special precautions
Effects on Dental Treatment Key adverse event(s) related to dental treatment: As with all anticoagulants, bleeding is the major adverse effect of danaparoid. Hemorrhage may occur at virtually any site; risk is dependent on multiple variables.
Common Adverse Effects As with all anticoagulants, bleeding is the major adverse effect of danaparoid. Hemorrhage may occur at virtually any site. Risk is dependent on multiple variables.

>10%:
 Central nervous system: Fever (22%)
 Gastrointestinal: Nausea (4% to 14%), constipation (4% to 11%)
1% to 10%:
 Cardiovascular: Peripheral edema (3%), edema (3%)
 Central nervous system: Insomnia (3%), headache (3%), asthenia (2%), dizziness (2%), pain (9%)
 Dermatologic: Rash (2% to 5%), pruritus (4%)
 Gastrointestinal: Vomiting (3%)
 Genitourinary: Urinary tract infection (3% to 4%), urinary retention (2%)
 Hematologic: Anemia (2%)
 Local: Injection site pain (8% to 14%), injection site hematoma (5%)
 Neuromuscular & skeletal: Joint disorder (3%)
 Miscellaneous: Infection (2%)
Restrictions Not available in U.S.
Mechanism of Action Prevents fibrin formation in coagulation pathway via thrombin generation inhibition by anti-Xa and anti-IIa effects.
Drug Interactions
 Increased Effect/Toxicity: The risk of hemorrhage associated with danaparoid may be increased with thrombolytic agents, oral anticoagulants (warfarin) and drugs which affect platelet function (eg, aspirin, NSAIDs, dipyridamole, ticlopidine, clopidogrel).
Pharmacodynamics/Kinetics
 Onset of action: Peak effect: SubQ: Maximum antifactor Xa and antithrombin (antifactor IIa) activities occur in 2-5 hours
 Half-life elimination, plasma: Mean: Terminal: ~24 hours
 Excretion: Primarily urine
Pregnancy Risk Factor B

Danaparoid Sodium *see* Danaparoid *on page 439*

Danazol (DA na zole)

U.S. Brand Names Danocrine® [DSC]
Canadian Brand Names Cyclomen®; Danocrine®
Mexican Brand Names Ladogal
Generic Available Yes
Pharmacologic Category Androgen
Use Treatment of endometriosis, fibrocystic breast disease, and hereditary angioedema
Local Anesthetic/Vasoconstrictor Precautions No information available to require special precautions
Effects on Dental Treatment No significant effects or complications reported
Common Adverse Effects Frequency not defined.
 Cardiovascular: Benign intracranial hypertension (rare), edema, flushing, hypertension
 Central nervous system: Anxiety (rare), chills (rare), convulsions (rare), depression, dizziness, emotional lability, fainting, fever (rare), Guillain-Barré syndrome, headache, nervousness, sleep disorders, tremor
(Continued)

Danazol *(Continued)*

Dermatologic: Acne, hair loss, mild hirsutism, maculopapular rash, papular rash, petechial rash, pruritus, purpuric rash, seborrhea, Stevens-Johnson syndrome (rare), photosensitivity (rare), urticaria, vesicular rash

Endocrine & metabolic: Amenorrhea (which may continue post therapy), breast size reduction, clitoris hypertrophy, glucose intolerance, HDL decreased, LDL increased, libido changes, nipple discharge, menstrual disturbances (spotting, altered timing of cycle), semen abnormalities (changes in volume, viscosity, sperm count/motility), spermatogenesis reduction

Gastrointestinal: Appetite changes (rare), bleeding gums (rare), constipation, gastroenteritis, nausea, pancreatitis (rare), vomiting, weight gain

Genitourinary: Vaginal dryness, vaginal irritation, pelvic pain

Hematologic: Eosinophilia, erythrocytosis (reversible), leukocytosis, leukopenia, platelet count increased, polycythemia, RBC increased, thrombocytopenia

Hepatic: Cholestatic jaundice, hepatic adenoma, jaundice, liver enzymes (elevated), malignant tumors (after prolonged use), peliosis hepatis

Neuromuscular & skeletal: Back pain, carpal tunnel syndrome (rare), extremity pain, joint lockup, joint pain, joint swelling, muscle cramps, neck pain, paresthesia, spasms, weakness

Ocular: Cataracts (rare), visual disturbances

Renal: Hematuria

Respiratory: Nasal congestion (rare)

Miscellaneous: Voice change (hoarseness, sore throat, instability, deepening of pitch), diaphoresis

Mechanism of Action Suppresses pituitary output of follicle-stimulating hormone and luteinizing hormone that causes regression and atrophy of normal and ectopic endometrial tissue; decreases rate of growth of abnormal breast tissue; reduces attacks associated with hereditary angioedema by increasing levels of C4 component of complement

Drug Interactions

Cytochrome P450 Effect: Inhibits CYP3A4 (weak)

Increased Effect/Toxicity: Danazol may increase serum levels of carbamazepine, cyclosporine, tacrolimus, and warfarin leading to toxicity; dosage adjustment may be needed; monitor. Concomitant use of danazol and HMG-CoA reductase inhibitors may lead to severe myopathy or rhabdomyolysis. Danazol may enhance the glucose-lowering effect of hypoglycemic agents.

Decreased Effect: Danazol may decrease effectiveness of hormonal contraceptives. Nonhormonal birth control methods are recommended.

Pharmacodynamics/Kinetics

Onset of action: Therapeutic: ~4 weeks

Metabolism: Extensively hepatic, primarily to 2-hydroxymethylethisterone

Half-life elimination: 4.5 hours (variable)

Time to peak, serum: Within 2 hours

Excretion: Urine

Pregnancy Risk Factor X

Danocrine® [DSC] *see* Danazol *on page 439*

Dantrium® *see* Dantrolene *on page 440*

Dantrolene *(DAN troe leen)*

U.S. Brand Names Dantrium®

Canadian Brand Names Dantrium®

Generic Available Yes: Capsule

Index Terms Dantrolene Sodium

Pharmacologic Category Skeletal Muscle Relaxant

Use Treatment of spasticity associated with spinal cord injury, stroke, cerebral palsy, or multiple sclerosis; treatment of malignant hyperthermia

Unlabeled/Investigational Use Neuroleptic malignant syndrome (NMS)

Local Anesthetic/Vasoconstrictor Precautions No information available to require special precautions

Effects on Dental Treatment No significant effects or complications reported

Common Adverse Effects

>10%:

Central nervous system: Drowsiness, dizziness, lightheadedness, fatigue

Dermatologic: Rash

Gastrointestinal: Diarrhea (mild), nausea, vomiting

Neuromuscular & skeletal: Muscle weakness

1% to 10%:

Cardiovascular: Pleural effusion with pericarditis

Central nervous system: Chills, fever, headache, insomnia, nervousness, mental depression

Gastrointestinal: Diarrhea (severe), constipation, anorexia, stomach cramps

Ocular: Blurred vision

Respiratory: Respiratory depression

Mechanism of Action Acts directly on skeletal muscle by interfering with release of calcium ion from the sarcoplasmic reticulum; prevents or reduces the increase in myoplasmic calcium ion concentration that activates the acute catabolic processes associated with malignant hyperthermia

Drug Interactions

Cytochrome P450 Effect: Substrate of CYP3A4 (major)

Increased Effect/Toxicity: Increased toxicity with estrogens (hepatotoxicity), CNS depressants (sedation), MAO inhibitors, phenothiazines, clindamycin (increased neuromuscular blockade), verapamil (hyperkalemia and cardiac depression), warfarin, clofibrate, and tolbutamide. CYP3A4 inhibitors may increase the levels/effects of dantrolene; example inhibitors include azole antifungals, clarithromycin, diclofenac, doxycycline, erythromycin, imatinib, isoniazid, nefazodone, nicardipine, propofol, protease inhibitors, quinidine, telithromycin, and verapamil.

Decreased Effect: CYP3A4 inducers may decrease the levels/effects of dantrolene; example inducers include aminoglutethimide, carbamazepine, nafcillin, nevirapine, phenobarbital, phenytoin, and rifamycins.

Pharmacodynamics/Kinetics

Absorption: Oral: Slow and incomplete

Metabolism: Hepatic

Half-life elimination: 8.7 hours

Excretion: Feces (45% to 50%); urine (25% as unchanged drug and metabolites)

Pregnancy Risk Factor C

Dantrolene Sodium *see* Dantrolene *on page 440*

Dapcin *see* Daptomycin *on page 443*

Dapiprazole (DA pi pray zole)

U.S. Brand Names Rēv-Eyes™

Generic Available No

Index Terms Dapiprazole Hydrochloride

Pharmacologic Category Alpha₁ Blocker, Ophthalmic

Use Reverse dilation due to drugs (adrenergic or parasympathomimetic) after eye exams

Local Anesthetic/Vasoconstrictor Precautions No information available to require special precautions

Effects on Dental Treatment No significant effects or complications reported

Mechanism of Action Dapiprazole is a selective alpha-adrenergic blocking agent, exerting effects primarily on alpha₁-adrenoreceptors. It induces miosis via relaxation of the smooth dilator (radial) muscle of the iris, which causes pupillary constriction. It is devoid of cholinergic effects. Dapiprazole also partially reverses the cycloplegia induced with parasympatholytic agents such as tropicamide. Although the drug has no significant effect on the ciliary muscle *per se*, it may increase accommodative amplitude, therefore relieving the symptoms of paralysis of accommodation.

Pregnancy Risk Factor B

Dapiprazole Hydrochloride *see* Dapiprazole *on page 441*

Dapsone (DAP sone)

Related Information

HIV Infection and AIDS *on page 1753*

U.S. Brand Names Aczone™

Mexican Brand Names Dapsoderm-X; Novasulfon

Generic Available Yes: Tablet

Index Terms Diaminodiphenylsulfone

Pharmacologic Category Antibiotic, Miscellaneous; Topical Skin Product, Acne

Dental Use Used in lupus and in selected ulcerative conditions in consult with patient's physician

Use Treatment of leprosy and dermatitis herpetiformis (infections caused by *Mycobacterium leprae*); treatment of acne vulgaris

Unlabeled/Investigational Use Prophylaxis of toxoplasmosis in severely-immunocompromised patients; alternative agent for *Pneumocystis*

(Continued)

Dapsone (Continued)

carinii pneumonia prophylaxis (monotherapy) and treatment (in combination with trimethoprim)

Local Anesthetic/Vasoconstrictor Precautions No information available to require special precautions

Effects on Dental Treatment No significant effects or complications reported

Significant Adverse Effects

>10%: Hematologic: Hemolysis (dose related; seen in patients with and without G6PD deficiency), hemoglobin decrease (1-2 g/dL; almost all patients), reticulocyte increase (2% to 12%), methemoglobinemia, red cell life span shortened

Frequency not defined.

Cardiovascular: Tachycardia

Central nervous system: Fever, headache, insomnia, psychosis, tonic-clonic movement (topical), vertigo

Dermatologic: Bullous and exfoliative dermatitis, erythema nodosum, exfoliative dermatitis (oral), morbilliform and scarlatiniform reactions, phototoxicity (oral), Stevens-Johnson syndrome, toxic epidural necrolysis, urticaria

Endocrine & metabolic: Hypoalbuminemia (without proteinuria), male infertility

Gastrointestinal: Abdominal pain (oral, topical), nausea, pancreatitis (oral, topical), vomiting

Hematologic: Agranulocytosis, anemia, leukopenia, pure red cell aplasia (case report)

Hepatic: Cholestatic jaundice, hepatitis

Neuromuscular & skeletal: Drug-induced lupus erythematosus, lower motor neuron toxicity (prolonged therapy), peripheral neuropathy (rare, nonleprosy patients)

Ocular: Blurred vision

Otic: Tinnitus

Renal: Albuminuria, nephrotic syndrome, renal papillary necrosis

Respiratory: Interstitial pneumonitis, pharyngitis (topical), pulmonary eosinophilia

Miscellaneous: Infectious mononucleosis-like syndrome (rash, fever, lymphadenopathy, hepatic dysfunction)

Dosage Oral:

Leprosy:

Children: 1-2 mg/kg/24 hours, up to a maximum of 100 mg/day

Adults: 50-100 mg/day for 3-10 years

Dermatitis herpetiformis: Adults: Start at 50 mg/day, increase to 300 mg/day, or higher to achieve full control, reduce dosage to minimum level as soon as possible

Pneumocystis carinii pneumonia (unlabeled use):

Prophylaxis:

Children >1 month: 2 mg/kg/day once daily (maximum dose: 100 mg/day) or 4 mg/kg/dose once weekly (maximum dose: 200 mg)

Adults: 100 mg/day

Treatment: Adults: 100 mg/day in combination with trimethoprim (15-20 mg/kg/day) for 21 days

Topical: Acne vulgaris: Children ≥12 years and Adults: Apply pea-sized amount twice daily

Dosing in renal impairment: No specific guidelines are available

Mechanism of Action Competitive antagonist of para-aminobenzoic acid (PABA) and prevents normal bacterial utilization of PABA for the synthesis of folic acid

Contraindications Hypersensitivity to dapsone or any component of the formulation

Warnings/Precautions Use with caution in patients with severe anemia, G6PD deficiency, hypersensitivity to other sulfonamides, or restricted hepatic function. Safety and efficacy of topical dapsone has not been adequately evaluated in patient with G6PD deficiency or in patients <12 years of age.

Drug Interactions Substrate of CYP2C8 (minor), 2C9 (major), 2C19 (minor), 2E1 (minor), 3A4 (major)

CYP2C9 Inducers may decrease the levels/effects of dapsone. Example inducers include carbamazepine, phenobarbital, phenytoin, rifampin, rifapentine, and secobarbital.

CYP2C9 Inhibitors may increase the levels/effects of dapsone. Example inhibitors include delavirdine, fluconazole, gemfibrozil, ketoconazole, nicardipine, NSAIDs, sulfonamides and tolbutamide.

CYP3A4 inducers: May decrease the levels/effects of dapsone. Example inducers include aminoglutethimide, carbamazepine, efavirenz, fosphenytoin, nafcillin, nevirapine, oxcarbazine, phenobarbital, phenytoin, primidone, and rifamycins.

CYP3A4 inhibitors: May increase the levels/effects of dapsone. Example inhibitors include azole antifungals, clarithromycin, diclofenac, doxycycline, erythromycin, imatinib, isoniazid, nefazodone, nicardipine, propofol, protease inhibitors, quinidine, telithromycin, and verapamil.

Didanosine: May decrease absorption of dapsone. Didanosine enteric coated capsules should not affect dapsone. Avoid other forms of didanosine.

Folic acid antagonists: May increase the risk of hematologic reactions of dapsone.

Probenecid: Decreases dapsone excretion.

Rifamycin derivatives: Increase metabolism of dapsone.

Trimethoprim: May increase toxic effects of both drugs.

Ethanol/Nutrition/Herb Interactions Herb/Nutraceutical: St John's wort may decrease dapsone levels.

Dietary Considerations Do not administer with antacids, alkaline foods, or drugs.

Pharmacodynamics/Kinetics

Absorption:

Oral: Well absorbed

Topical: ~1% of the absorption of 100 mg tablet

Distribution: V_d: 1.5 L/kg; throughout total body water and present in all tissues, especially liver and kidney

Metabolism: Hepatic; forms metabolite

Half-life elimination: 30 hours (range: 10-50 hours)

Excretion: Urine (~85%)

Pregnancy Risk Factor C

Lactation Enters breast milk/not recommended (AAP rates "compatible")

Dosage Forms Excipient information presented when available (limited, particularly for generics); consult specific product labeling.

Gel, topical (Aczone™): 5% (30 g)

Tablet: 25 mg, 100 mg

Daptomycin (DAP toe mye sin)

U.S. Brand Names Cubicin®

Generic Available No

Index Terms Cidecin; Dapcin; LY146032

Pharmacologic Category Antibiotic, Cyclic Lipopeptide

Use Treatment of complicated skin and skin structure infections caused by susceptible aerobic Gram-positive organisms; *Staphylococcus aureus* bacteremia, including right-sided infective endocarditis caused by MSSA or MRSA

Unlabeled/Investigational Use Treatment of severe infections caused by MRSA or VRE

Local Anesthetic/Vasoconstrictor Precautions No information available to require special precautions

Effects on Dental Treatment No significant effects or complications reported

Common Adverse Effects

>10%:

Cardiovascular: Anemia (2% to 13%)

Gastrointestinal: Diarrhea (5% to 12%), vomiting (3% to 12%), constipation (6% to 11%)

1% to 10%:

Cardiovascular: Peripheral edema (7%), chest pain (7%), hypertension (1% to 6%), hypotension (2% to 5%)

Central nervous system: Insomnia (5% to 9%), headache (5% to 7%), fever (2% to 7%), dizziness (2% to 6%), anxiety (5%)

Dermatologic: Rash (4% to 7%), pruritus (3% to 6%), erythema (5%)

Endocrine & metabolic: Hypokalemia (9%), hyperkalemia (5%), hyperphosphatemia (3%)

Gastrointestinal: Nausea (6% to 10%), abdominal pain (6%), dyspepsia (1% to 4%), loose stool (4%), GI hemorrhage (2%)

Genitourinary: Urinary tract infection (2% to 7%)

Hematologic: INR increased (2%), eosinophilia (2%)

Hepatic: Transaminases increased (2% to 3%), alkaline phosphatase increased (2%)

Local: Injection site reaction (3% to 6%)

Neuromuscular & skeletal: CPK increased (3% to 9%), limb pain (2% to 9%), back pain (7%), weakness (5%), arthralgia (1% to 3%)

Renal: Renal failure (2% to 3%)

Respiratory: Pharyngolaryngeal pain (8%), pleural effusion (6%), cough (3%), pneumonia (3%), dyspnea (2% to 3%)

Miscellaneous: Osteomyelitis (6%), bacteremia (5%), diaphoresis (5%), sepsis (5%), infection (fungal, 2% to 3%)

(Continued)

Daptomycin *(Continued)*

Mechanism of Action Daptomycin binds to components of the cell membrane of susceptible organisms and causes rapid depolarization, inhibiting intracellular synthesis of DNA, RNA, and protein. Daptomycin is bactericidal in a concentration-dependent manner.

Drug Interactions
Increased Effect/Toxicity: No clinically-significant interactions have been identified.

Pharmacodynamics/Kinetics
Distribution: 0.1 L/kg
Protein binding: 90% to 93%; 84% to 88% in patients with Cl_{cr}<30 mL/minute
Half-life elimination: 8-9 hours (up to 28 hours in renal impairment)
Excretion: Urine (78%; primarily as unchanged drug); feces (6%)

Pregnancy Risk Factor B

Daranide® *see* Dichlorphenamide *on page 485*
Daraprim® *see* Pyrimethamine *on page 1390*

Darbepoetin Alfa *(dar be POE e tin AL fa)*

U.S. Brand Names Aranesp®
Canadian Brand Names Aranesp®
Generic Available No
Index Terms Erythropoiesis-Stimulating Agent (ESA); Erythropoiesis-Stimulating Protein; NSC-729969
Pharmacologic Category Colony Stimulating Factor; Growth Factor; Recombinant Human Erythropoietin
Use Treatment of anemia associated with chronic renal failure (CRF), including patients on dialysis (ESRD) and patients not on dialysis; anemia associated with concurrent chemotherapy for nonmyeloid malignancies
Local Anesthetic/Vasoconstrictor Precautions No information available to require special precautions
Effects on Dental Treatment No significant effects or complications reported
Common Adverse Effects
>10%:
Cardiovascular: Hypertension (4% to 23%), hypotension (22%), edema (21%), peripheral edema (11%)
Central nervous system: Fatigue (9% to 33%), fever (4% to 19%), headache (12% to 16%), dizziness (8% to 14%)
Gastrointestinal: Diarrhea (16% to 22%), constipation (5% to 18%), vomiting (2% to 15%), nausea (14%), abdominal pain (12%)
Neuromuscular & skeletal: Myalgia (8% to 21%), arthralgia (11% to 13%)
Respiratory: Upper respiratory infection (14%), dyspnea (2% to 12%)
Miscellaneous: Infection (27%)
1% to 10%:
Cardiovascular: Arrhythmia (10%), angina/chest pain (6% to 8%), fluid overload (6%), CHF (6%), thrombosis (6%), MI (2%)
Central nervous system: Seizure (≤1%), stroke (1%), TIA (1%)
Dermatologic: Pruritus (8%), rash (7%)
Endocrine & metabolic: Dehydration (3% to 5%)
Local: Vascular access thrombosis (8%), injection site pain (7%), vascular access hemorrhage (6%), vascular access infection (6%)
Neuromuscular & skeletal: Limb pain (10%), back pain (8%), weakness (5%)
Respiratory: Cough (10%), bronchitis (6%), pneumonia (3%), pulmonary embolism (1%)
Miscellaneous: Death (7% to 10 %; similar to placebo), flu-like syndrome (6%)
Postmarketing and/or case reports: Deep vein thrombosis, pure red cell aplasia, severe anemia (with or without other cytopenias), thromboembolism, thrombophlebitis
Mechanism of Action Induces erythropoiesis by stimulating the division and differentiation of committed erythroid progenitor cells; induces the release of reticulocytes from the bone marrow into the bloodstream, where they mature to erythrocytes. There is a dose response relationship with this effect. This results in an increase in reticulocyte counts followed by a rise in hematocrit and hemoglobin levels. When administered SubQ or I.V., darbepoetin's half-life is ~3 times that of epoetin alfa concentrations.
Pharmacodynamics/Kinetics
Onset of action: Increased hemoglobin levels not generally observed until 2-6 weeks after initiating treatment
Absorption: SubQ: Slow
Distribution: V_d: 0.06 L/kg

Bioavailability: CRF: SubQ: Adults: ~37% (range: 30% to 50%); Children: 54% (range: 32% to 70%)

Half-life elimination: CRF: Terminal: I.V.: 21 hours, SubQ: 49 hours; cancer: SubQ: 74 hours

Note: Half-life is approximately threefold longer than epoetin alfa following I.V. administration

Time to peak: SubQ: CRF: 34 hours (range: 24-72 hours); Cancer: 71-90 hours

Pregnancy Risk Factor C

Darifenacin (dar i FEN a sin)

U.S. Brand Names Enablex®
Canadian Brand Names Enablex®
Generic Available No
Index Terms Darifenacin Hydrobromide; UK-88,525
Pharmacologic Category Anticholinergic Agent
Use Management of symptoms of bladder overactivity (urge incontinence, urgency, and frequency)
Local Anesthetic/Vasoconstrictor Precautions No information available to require special precautions
Effects on Dental Treatment Key adverse event(s) related to dental treatment: Xerostomia (normal salivary flow resumes upon discontinuation). Prolonged xerostomia may contribute to discomfort and dental disease (eg, caries, periodontal disease, and oral candidiasis).
Common Adverse Effects
>10%: Gastrointestinal: Xerostomia (19% to 35%), constipation (15% to 21%)
1% to 10%:
  Cardiovascular: Hypertension, peripheral edema
  Central nervous system: Headache (7%), dizziness (1% to 2%)
  Dermatological: Dry skin, pruritis, rash
  Gastrointestinal: Dyspepsia (3% to 8%), abdominal pain (2% to 4%), nausea (2% to 4%), diarrhea (1% to 2%), vomiting, weight gain
  Genitourinary: Urinary tract infection (4% to 5%), urinary retention, urinary tract disorder, vaginitis
  Neuromuscular & skeletal: Weakness (2% to 3%), arthralgia, back pain
  Ocular: Dry eyes (2%), abnormal vision
  Respiratory: Bronchitis, pharyngitis, rhinitis, sinusitis
  Miscellaneous: Flu-like syndrome (<1% to 3%), accidental injury (<1% to 3%)
Mechanism of Action Selective antagonist of the M3 muscarinic (cholinergic) receptor subtype. Blockade of the receptor limits bladder contractions, reducing the symptoms of bladder irritability/overactivity (urge incontinence, urgency and frequency).
Drug Interactions
  Cytochrome P450 Effect: Substrate of CYP2D6 (minor), CYP3A4 (major); **Inhibits** CYP2D6 (moderate), 3A4 (weak)
  Increased Effect/Toxicity: Adverse anticholinergic effects may be additive with other anticholinergic agents (includes tricyclic antidepressants, antihistamines, and phenothiazines). Coadministration with pramlintide may result an additive reduction in gut motility. Darifenacin may increase the levels/effects of CYP2D6 substrates; example substrates include amphetamines, selected beta-blockers, dextromethorphan, fluoxetine, lidocaine, mirtazapine, nefazodone, paroxetine, risperidone, ritonavir, thioridazine, tricyclic antidepressants, and venlafaxine. CYP3A4 inhibitors may increase the levels/effects of darifenacin; example inhibitors include azole antifungals, clarithromycin, diclofenac, doxycycline, erythromycin, imatinib, isoniazid, nefazodone, nicardipine, propofol, protease inhibitors, quinidine, telithromycin, and verapamil.
  Decreased Effect: Darifenacin may decrease the levels/effects of CYP2D6 prodrug substrates; example prodrug substrates include codeine, hydrocodone, oxycodone, and tramadol. CYP3A4 inducers may decrease the levels/effects of darifenacin; example inducers include aminoglutethimide, carbamazepine, nafcillin, nevirapine, phenobarbital, phenytoin, and rifamycins. Concomitant use with acetylcholinesterase inhibitors may reduce the therapeutic efficacy of darifenacin.
Pharmacodynamics/Kinetics
  Distribution: V_{dss}: 163 L
  Protein binding: 98%
  Metabolism: Hepatic, via CYP3A4 (major) and CYP2D6 (minor)
  Bioavailability: 15% to 19%
  Half-life elimination: 13-19 hours
  Time to peak, plasma: 7 hours
  Excretion: As metabolites (inactive); urine (60%), feces (40%)
Pregnancy Risk Factor C

Darifenacin Hydrobromide *see* Darifenacin *on page 445*

Darunavir (dar OO na veer)

U.S. Brand Names Prezista™

Generic Available No

Index Terms Darunavir Ethanolate; TMC-114

Pharmacologic Category Antiretroviral Agent, Protease Inhibitor

Use Treatment of HIV-1 infections in combination with ritonavir and other antiretroviral agents; limited to highly treatment-experienced or multiprotease inhibitor-resistant patients

Local Anesthetic/Vasoconstrictor Precautions No information available to require special precautions

Effects on Dental Treatment No significant effects or complications reported

Common Adverse Effects As a class, protease inhibitors potentially cause dyslipidemias which includes elevated cholesterol and triglycerides and a redistribution of body fat centrally to cause increased abdominal girth, buffalo hump, facial atrophy, and breast enlargement. These agents also cause hyperglycemia. Frequency of adverse events is reported for darunavir/ritonavir where incidence was greater than in the comparator protease inhibitor group. See also Ritonavir monograph.

>10%:
Gastrointestinal: Nausea (18%), amylase increased (11% to 17%)
Hematologic: Neutropenia (7% to 12%)
Respiratory: Nasopharyngitis (14%)

2% to 10%:
Central nervous system: Headache (1% to 4%)
Dermatologic: Rash (7%)
Endocrine & metabolic: Hypercholesterolemia (≥240 mg/dL: 8% to 9%), hypoglycemia (2% to 4%), hypocalcemia (up to 4%), hyponatremia (1% to 3%), hypernatremia (up to 2%)
Gastrointestinal: Lipase increased (6% to 9%), diarrhea (2% to 3%), vomiting (2%), abdominal pain (1% to 2%), constipation (<1% to 2%)
Hematologic: Thromboplastin time increased (4% to 8%), hypoalbuminemia (3% to 4%), prothrombin time increased (1% to 4%), thrombocytopenia (3%)
Hepatic: Alkaline phosphatase increased (3% to 5%)

Mechanism of Action Darunavir binds to the HIV-1 protease activity site and inhibits the activity of the enzyme. HIV protease is required for the cleavage of viral Gag-Pol polyprotein precursors into individual functional proteins found in infectious HIV. Inhibition prevents cleavage of these polyproteins, resulting in the formation of immature, noninfectious viral particles.

Drug Interactions

Cytochrome P450 Effect: Substrate of CYP3A4 (major)

Increased Effect/Toxicity: Listed interactions include interactions resulting from coadministration with ritonavir. Refer to Ritonavir monograph for additional interaction concerns.

The serum concentrations of darunavir may be increased by ritonavir. This combination is recommended to enhance the effect ("boost") darunavir. Darunavir/ritonavir may increase the levels/effects of CYP3A4 substrates. Darunavir/ritonavir may increase the toxicity of benzodiazepines; concurrent use of midazolam and triazolam is specifically contraindicated. Darunavir may increase serum concentrations of cisapride, increasing the risk of malignant arrhythmias; use is contraindicated. Toxicity of pimozide is significantly increased by darunavir/ritonavir; concurrent use is contraindicated. Darunavir/ritonavir may increase serum concentrations/toxicity of several antiarrhythmic agents, including amiodarone, quinidine, and systemic lidocaine. Darunavir/ritonavir may also increase serum concentrations/effects of calcium channel blockers, immunosuppressants (cyclosporine, sirolimus, tacrolimus), inhaled corticosteroids, trazodone and warfarin; use reduced dose of trazodone, monitor INR with warfarin, and monitor for adrenal suppression with steroids.

Serum concentrations of HMG-CoA reductase inhibitors (atorvastatin, pravastatin, lovastatin, simvastatin) may be increased by darunavir/ritonavir, increasing the risk of myopathy/rhabdomyolysis. Lovastatin and simvastatin are not recommended. Use lowest possible dose of atorvastatin and pravastatin. Serum concentrations of rifabutin may be increased by darunavir/ritonavir; dosage adjustment of rifabutin is required. The toxicity of ergot alkaloids (dihydroergotamine, ergotamine, ergonovine, methylergonovine) is increased by darunavir; concurrent use is contraindicated. The serum concentrations of sildenafil, tadalafil, and vardenafil may be increased by darunavir/ritonavir; dose adjustment and limitations related to ritonavir coadministration must be recognized. Darunavir/ritonavir may increase serum concentrations of clarithromycin. Use with caution and adjust dose of clarithromycin during concurrent therapy in renally impaired patients. Ketoconazole may increase the serum levels of darunavir, while darunavir/ritonavir may increase the levels of ketoconazole; monitor.

Decreased Effect: CYP3A4 inducers may decrease the levels/effects of darunavir. Example inducers include aminoglutethimide, carbamazepine, nafcillin, nevirapine, phenobarbital, phenytoin, and rifamycins. Rifampin may decrease serum concentrations of darunavir; concurrent use of rifampin is not recommended. Darunavir/ritonavir may decrease the serum concentrations of ethinyl estradiol; nonhormonal contraception recommended. The effect of methadone may be reduced by darunavir (dosage increase of methadone may be required). Serum concentrations of darunavir may be decreased by lopinavir/ritonavir or saquinavir (hard gel cap); concurrent therapy not recommended. Darunavir may decrease the levels/effects of sertraline or paroxetine.

Pharmacodynamics/Kinetics All kinetic parameters derived in the presence of ritonavir coadministration.

Absorption: Increased 30% with food
Protein binding: 95%
Metabolism: Hepatic, via CYP3A4 to minimally-active metabolites
Bioavailability: 82% (with ritonavir)
Half-life elimination: 15 hours (with ritonavir)
Time to peak, plasma: 2.5-4 hours
Excretion: Feces (~80%, 41% as unchanged drug); urine (~14%, 8% as unchanged drug)

Pregnancy Risk Factor B

Dasatinib (da SA ti nib)

U.S. Brand Names Sprycel™
Canadian Brand Names Sprycel™
Generic Available No
Index Terms BMS-354825; NSC-732517
Pharmacologic Category Antineoplastic Agent, Tyrosine Kinase Inhibitor
Use Treatment of chronic myelogenous leukemia (CML); treatment of Philadelphia chromosome-positive (Ph+) acute lymphoblastic leukemia (ALL)
Local Anesthetic/Vasoconstrictor Precautions Dasatinib is one of the drugs confirmed to prolong the QT interval and is accepted as having a risk of causing torsade de pointes. The risk of drug-induced torsade de pointes is extremely low when a single QT interval prolonging drug is prescribed. In terms of epinephrine, it is not known what effect vasoconstrictors in the local anesthetic regimen will have in patients with a known history of congenital prolonged QT interval or in patients taking any medication that prolongs the QT interval. Until more information is obtained, it is suggested that the clinician consult with the physician prior to the use of a vasoconstrictor in suspected patients, and that the vasoconstrictor (epinephrine, levonordefrin [Neo-Cobefrin®]) be used with caution.
Effects on Dental Treatment Key adverse event(s) related to dental treatment: Mucositis/stomatitis, taste perversion.
Common Adverse Effects
≥10%:
  Cardiovascular: Fluid retention (14% to 50%), superficial edema (36%), chest pain (13%), arrhythmia (11%)
  Central nervous system: Headache (40%), fatigue (39%), fever (39%), pain (26%), dizziness (14%), chills (11%)
  Dermatologic: Rash (35%), pruritus (11%)
  Endocrine & metabolic: Hypophosphatemia (grades 3/4: 11% to 23%), hypocalcemia (grades 3/4 : 2% to 20%)
(Continued)

Dasatinib *(Continued)*

Gastrointestinal: Diarrhea (49%; grades 3/4: 5%), nausea (34%), abdominal pain (25%), vomiting (22%), anorexia (19%), mucositis/stomatitis (16%), gastrointestinal hemorrhage (14%; grades 3/4: 7%), constipation (14%), weight loss (14%), abdominal distention (11%), weight gain (11%)

Hematologic: Neutropenia (grades 3/4: 49% to 83%), thrombocytopenia (grades 3/4: 48% to 83%), anemia (grades 3/4: 18% to 70%), hemorrhage (40%; grades 3/4: 10%)

Hepatic: ALT increased (grades 3/4: 1% to 11%)

Neuromuscular & skeletal: Musculoskeletal pain (39%), arthralgia (19%), weakness (19%), neuropathy (including peripheral; 13%), myalgia (12%)

Respiratory: Dyspnea (32%; grades 3/4: 6%), cough (28%), upper respiratory tract infection/inflammation (26%), pleural effusion (22%; grades 3/4: 5%), pneumonia (11%)

Miscellaneous: Infection (34%; grades 3/4: 7%)

1% to <10%:

Cardiovascular: Generalized edema (5%), CHF/cardiac dysfunction (4%; grades 3/4: 2%), pericardial effusion (4%; grades 3/4: 1%), angina, cardiomegaly, flushing, hyper-/hypotension, MI, palpitation, syncope

Central nervous system: CNS bleeding (2%), affect lability, anxiety, confusion, depression, insomnia, malaise, seizure, somnolence, vertigo

Dermatologic: Acne, alopecia, dermatitis, dry skin, hyperhydrosis, nail disorder, photosensitivity, pigmentation disorder, urticaria

Endocrine & metabolic: Gynecomastia, hyperuricemia, libido decreased

Gastrointestinal: Anal fissure, colitis, dyspepsia, dysphagia, enterocolitis, gastritis, oral soft tissue disorder, taste perversion

Genitourinary: Polyuria, renal failure

Hematologic: Febrile neutropenia (9%; grades 3/4: 8%), contusion, pancytopenia

Hepatic: AST increased (grades 3/4: 1% to 8%), bilirubin increased (grades 3/4: <1% to 8%), ascites (1%; grades 3/4: 1%)

Neuromuscular & skeletal: Creatine phosphokinase increased, muscle inflammation, muscle weakness, musculoskeletal stiffness, tremor, troponin increased

Ocular: Conjunctivitis, periorbital edema, xerophthalmia

Otic: Tinnitus

Renal: Serum creatinine increased (grades 3/4: up to 2%)

Respiratory: Pulmonary edema (4%; grades 3/4: 1%), pulmonary hypertension (1%), asthma, lung infiltration, pneumonitis

Miscellaneous: Herpesvirus infection, sepsis, tumor lysis syndrome

Mechanism of Action BCR-ABL tyrosine kinase inhibitor; targets most imatinib-resistant BCR-ABL mutations (except the T315I and F317V mutants) by distinctly binding to ABL-kinase. Kinase inhibition halts proliferation of leukemia cells. Also inhibits SRC family (including SRC, LKC, YES, FYN); c-KIT, EPHA2 and platelet derived growth factor receptor (PDGFRβ)

Drug Interactions

Cytochrome P450 Effect: Substrate of CYP3A4 (major); **Inhibits** CYP3A4 (weak)

Increased Effect/Toxicity:

The levels/effects of dasatinib may be increased by azole antifungals, clarithromycin, diclofenac, doxycycline, erythromycin, imatinib, isoniazid, nefazodone, nicardipine, propofol, protease inhibitors, quinidine, telithromycin, verapamil, and other CYP3A4 inhibitors. Concurrent use of dasatinib with other drugs which may prolong QT_c interval may increase the risk of potentially-fatal arrhythmias. Anticoagulants and antiplatelet agents may increase the risk of bleeding.

Decreased Effect: The levels/effects of dasatinib may be decreased by aminoglutethimide, carbamazepine, nafcillin, nevirapine, phenobarbital, phenytoin, rifamycins, and other CYP3A4 inducers. Antacids, H_2 blockers and proton pump inhibitors may decrease the absorption of dasatinib.

Pharmacodynamics/Kinetics

Distribution: 2505 L

Protein binding: Dasatinib: 96%; metabolite: 93%

Metabolism: Hepatic; metabolized by CYP3A4 (primarily), flavin-containing mono-oxygenase-3 (FOM-3) and uridine diphosphate-glucuronosyltransferase (UGT) to an active metabolite and other inactive metabolites (the active metabolite plays only a minor role in the pharmacology of dasatinib)

Half-life elimination: Terminal: 3-5 hours

Time to peak, plasma: 0.5-6 hours

Excretion: Feces (85%, 19% as unchanged drug); urine (4%, 0.1% as unchanged drug)

Pregnancy Risk Factor D

Daunomycin *see* DAUNOrubicin Hydrochloride *on page 450*

DAUNOrubicin Citrate (Liposomal)
(daw noe ROO bi sin SI trate lip po SOE mal)

U.S. Brand Names DaunoXome®

Generic Available No

Index Terms DAUNOrubicin Liposomal; Liposomal DAUNOrubicin; NSC-697732

Pharmacologic Category Antineoplastic Agent, Anthracycline

Use First-line treatment of advanced HIV-associated Kaposi's sarcoma (KS)

Local Anesthetic/Vasoconstrictor Precautions No information available to require special precautions

Effects on Dental Treatment Key adverse event(s) related to dental treatment: Stomatitis.

Common Adverse Effects

>10%:

Cardiovascular: Edema (11%)

Central nervous system: Fatigue (49%), fever (47%), headache (25%), neutropenic fever (17%)

Gastrointestinal: Nausea (54%), diarrhea (38%), abdominal pain (23%), anorexia (23%), vomiting (23%)

Hematologic: Myelosuppression (onset: 7 days; nadir: 14 days; recovery 21 days), neutropenia (up to 55%; grade 4: 15%), anemia (up to 55%; grade 4: 2%), thrombocytopenia (up to 12%; grade 4: 1%)

Neuromuscular & skeletal: Rigors (19%), back pain (16%), neuropathy (13%)

Respiratory: Cough (28%), dyspnea (26%), rhinitis (12%)

Miscellaneous: Opportunistic infections (40%), allergic reactions (24%), diaphoresis (14%), infusion-related reactions (14%; includes back pain, flushing, chest tightness)

1% to 10%:

Cardiovascular: Chest pain (10%), hypertension (≤5%), palpitation (≤5%), syncope (≤5%), tachycardia (≤5%), LVEF decreased (3%), CHF/cardiomyopathy

Central nervous system: Depression (10%), malaise (10%), dizziness (8%), insomnia (6%), abnormal thinking (≤5%), amnesia (≤5%), anxiety (≤5%), ataxia (≤5%), confusion (≤5%), emotional lability (≤5%), hallucination (≤5%), meningitis (≤5%), seizure (≤5%), somnolence (≤5%)

Dermatologic: Alopecia (8%), pruritus (7%), dry skin (≤5%), folliculitis (≤5%), seborrhea (≤5%)

Endocrine & metabolic: Dehydration (≤5%), hot flashes (≤5%)

Gastrointestinal: Stomatitis (10%), constipation (7%), tenesmus (5%), appetite increased (≤5%), dental caries (≤5%), dysphagia (≤5%), gastrointestinal hemorrhage (≤5%), gastritis (≤5%), gingival bleeding (≤5%), hemorrhoids (≤5%), melena (≤5%), splenomegaly (≤5%), taste perversion (≤5%), xerostomia (≤5%)

Genitourinary: Dysuria (≤5%), nocturia (≤5%), polyuria (≤5%)

Hepatic: Hepatomegaly (≤5%)

Local: Injection site inflammation (≤5%)

Neuromuscular & skeletal: Arthralgia (7%), myalgia (7%), gait abnormal (≤5%), hyperkinesia (≤5%), hypertonia (≤5%), tremor (≤5%)

Ocular: Abnormal vision (5%) conjunctivitis (≤5%), eye pain (≤5%)

Otic: Deafness (≤5%), earache (≤5%), tinnitus (≤5%)

Respiratory: Sinusitis (8%), hemoptysis (≤5%), pulmonary infiltrate (≤5%), sputum increased (≤5%)

Miscellaneous: Flu-like syndrome (5%), hiccups (≤5%), lymphadenopathy (≤5%), thirst (≤5%)

Mechanism of Action Liposomes have been shown to penetrate solid tumors more effectively, possibly because of their small size and longer circulation time. Once in tissues, daunorubicin is released. Daunorubicin inhibits DNA and RNA synthesis by intercalation between DNA base pairs and by steric obstruction; and intercalates at points of local uncoiling of the double helix. Although the exact mechanism is unclear, it appears that direct binding to DNA (intercalation) and inhibition of DNA repair (topoisomerase II inhibition) result in blockade of DNA and RNA synthesis and fragmentation of DNA.

Drug Interactions

Increased Effect/Toxicity: Bevacizumab and trastuzumab may increase the cardiotoxic effects of anthracyclines. Daunorubicin citrate liposomal may increase the risk of vaccinal infection.

Decreased Effect: Daunorubicin citrate liposomal may decrease the effect of vaccines.

(Continued)

DAUNOrubicin Citrate (Liposomal) *(Continued)*

Pharmacodynamics/Kinetics
Distribution: V_d: 5-8 L
Metabolism: Similar to daunorubicin, but metabolite plasma levels are low
Half-life elimination: Distribution: 4.4 hours; Terminal: 3-5 hours
Excretion: Primarily feces; some urine
Clearance, plasma: 17.3 mL/minute
Pregnancy Risk Factor D

DAUNOrubicin Hydrochloride
(daw noe ROO bi sin hye droe KLOR ide)

U.S. Brand Names Cerubidine®
Canadian Brand Names Cerubidine®
Mexican Brand Names Rubilem; Trixilem RU
Generic Available Yes
Index Terms Daunomycin; DNR; NSC-82151; Rubidomycin Hydrochloride
Pharmacologic Category Antineoplastic Agent, Anthracycline
Use Treatment of acute lymphocytic (ALL) and nonlymphocytic (ANLL) leukemias
Local Anesthetic/Vasoconstrictor Precautions No information available to require special precautions
Effects on Dental Treatment Key adverse event(s) related to dental treatment: Stomatitis and discoloration of saliva.
Common Adverse Effects
>10%:
Cardiovascular: Transient ECG abnormalities (supraventricular tachycardia, S-T wave changes, atrial or ventricular extrasystoles); generally asymptomatic and self-limiting. CHF, dose related, may be delayed for 7-8 years after treatment.
Dermatologic: Alopecia, radiation recall
Gastrointestinal: Mild nausea or vomiting, stomatitis
Genitourinary: Discoloration of urine (red)
Hematologic: Myelosuppression, primarily leukopenia; thrombocytopenia and anemia
Onset: 7 days
Nadir: 10-14 days
Recovery: 21-28 days
1% to 10%:
Dermatologic: Skin "flare" at injection site; discoloration of saliva, sweat, or tears
Endocrine & metabolic: Hyperuricemia
Gastrointestinal: Abdominal pain, GI ulceration, diarrhea
Mechanism of Action Inhibition of DNA and RNA synthesis by intercalation between DNA base pairs and by steric obstruction. Daunomycin intercalates at points of local uncoiling of the double helix. Although the exact mechanism is unclear, it appears that direct binding to DNA (intercalation) and inhibition of DNA repair (topoisomerase II inhibition) result in blockade of DNA and RNA synthesis and fragmentation of DNA.
Drug Interactions
Decreased Effect: Patients may experience impaired immune response to vaccines; possible infection after administration of live vaccines in patients receiving immunosuppressants.
Pharmacodynamics/Kinetics
Distribution: Many body tissues, particularly the liver, kidneys, lung, spleen, and heart; not into CNS; crosses placenta; V_d: 40 L/kg
Metabolism: Primarily hepatic to daunorubicinol (active), then to inactive aglycones, conjugated sulfates, and glucuronides
Half-life elimination: Distribution: 2 minutes; Elimination: 14-20 hours; Terminal: 18.5 hours; Daunorubicinol plasma half-life: 24-48 hours
Excretion: Feces (40%); urine (~25% as unchanged drug and metabolites)
Pregnancy Risk Factor D

Decitabine (de SYE ta been)

U.S. Brand Names Dacogen™
Generic Available No
Index Terms 5-Aza-2'-deoxycytidine; 5-AzaC; NSC-127716
Pharmacologic Category Antineoplastic Agent, DNA Methylation Inhibitor
Use Treatment of myelodysplastic syndrome (MDS)
Unlabeled/Investigational Use Treatment of acute myelogenous leukemia (AML), chronic myelogenous leukemia (CML), sickle cell anemia
Local Anesthetic/Vasoconstrictor Precautions No information available to require special precautions
Effects on Dental Treatment Key adverse event(s) related to dental treatment: Oral mucosal petechiae, stomatitis, gingival bleeding, tongue ulceration, oral candidiasis, lip ulceration, mucosal inflammation, gingival pain have been reported.
Common Adverse Effects
>10%:
Cardiovascular: Peripheral edema (25%), pallor (23%), edema (18%), cardiac murmur (16%)
Central nervous system: Pyrexia (6% to 53%), headache (28%), insomnia (28%), dizziness (18%), pain (13%), confusion (12%), lethargy (12%), anxiety (11%), hypoesthesia (11%)
Dermatologic: Petechiae (39%), bruising (22%), rash (19%), erythema (14%), cellulitis (12%), lesions (11%), pruritus (11%)
Endocrine & metabolic: Hyperglycemia (33%), hypoalbuminemia (7% to 24%), hypomagnesemia (24%), hypokalemia (22%), hyperkalemia (13%), hyponatremia (13%)
Gastrointestinal: Nausea (42%), constipation (35%), diarrhea (34%), vomiting (25%), anorexia (16%), appetite decreased (16%), abdominal pain (5% to 14%), oral mucosal petechiae (13%), stomatitis (12%), dyspepsia (12%)
Hematologic: Neutropenia (90%; recovery 28-50 days), thrombocytopenia (89%), anemia (82%), febrile neutropenia (29%), leukopenia (28%), lymphadenopathy (12%)
Hepatic: Hyperbilirubinemia (14%), alkaline phosphatase increased (11%)
Local: Tenderness (11%)
Neuromuscular & skeletal: Rigors (22%), arthralgia (20%), limb pain (19%), back pain (17%)
Respiratory: Cough (40%), pneumonia (22%), pharyngitis (16%), lung crackles (14%)
5% to 10%:
Cardiovascular: Chest discomfort (7%), facial swelling (6%), hypotension (6%)
Central nervous system: Malaise (5%)
Dermatologic: Alopecia (8%), urticaria (6%)
Endocrine & metabolic: Hyperuricemia (10%), LDH increased (8%), bicarbonate increased (6%), dehydration (6%), hypochloremia (6%), bicarbonate decreased (5%), hypoproteinemia (5%)
Gastrointestinal: Gingival bleeding (8%), hemorrhoids (8%), loose stools (7%), tongue ulceration (7%), dysphagia (6%), oral candidiasis (6%), lip ulceration (5%), abdominal distension (5%), gastroesophageal reflux (5%), glossodynia (5%)
Genitourinary: Urinary tract infection (7%), dysuria (6%), polyuria (5%)
Hematologic: Hematoma (5%), thrombocythemia (5%), bacteremia (5%)
Hepatic: Ascites (10%), AST increased (10%), hypobilirubinemia (5%)
Local: Catheter infection (8%), catheter site erythema (5%), catheter site pain (5%), injection site swelling (5%)
(Continued)

Decitabine *(Continued)*

Neuromuscular & skeletal: Falling (8%), chest wall pain (7%), musculoskeletal discomfort (6%), crepitation (5%), myalgia (5%)

Ocular: Blurred vision (6%)

Respiratory: Breath sounds diminished (10%), hypoxia (10%), rales (8%), pulmonary edema (6%), postnasal drip (5%), sinusitis (5%)

Miscellaneous: Candidal infection (10%), staphylococcal infection (7%), transfusion reaction (7%)

Mechanism of Action After phosphorylation, decitabine is incorporated into DNA and inhibits DNA methyltransferase causing hypomethylation and subsequent cell death.

Pharmacodynamics/Kinetics
Protein binding: <1%
Half-life elimination: ~30 minutes

Pregnancy Risk Factor D

Declomycin® *see* Demeclocycline *on page 456*

Deconamine® *see* Chlorpheniramine and Pseudoephedrine *on page 340*

Deconamine® SR *see* Chlorpheniramine and Pseudoephedrine *on page 340*

Deconsal® II *see* Guaifenesin and Phenylephrine *on page 797*

Deep Sea [OTC] *see* Sodium Chloride *on page 1480*

Deferasirox *(de FER a sir ox)*

U.S. Brand Names Exjade®
Canadian Brand Names Exjade®
Generic Available No
Index Terms ICL670
Pharmacologic Category Antidote; Chelating Agent
Use Treatment of chronic iron overload due to blood transfusions
Local Anesthetic/Vasoconstrictor Precautions No information available to require special precautions
Effects on Dental Treatment No significant effects or complications reported
Common Adverse Effects
>10%:
Central nervous system: Fever (19%), headache (16%):
Gastrointestinal: Abdominal pain (8% to 14%), diarrhea (12%), nausea (11%)
Renal: Serum creatinine increased (2% to 38%), proteinuria (19%)
Respiratory: Cough (14%), nasopharyngitis (13%), pharyngolaryngeal pain (11%)
Miscellaneous: Influenza (11%)
1% to 10%:
Central nervous system: Fatigue (6%)
Dermatologic: Rash (8% to 11%), urticaria (4%)
Gastrointestinal: Vomiting (10%)
Hepatic: ALT increased (6% to 8%), transaminitis (4%)
Neuromuscular & skeletal: Arthralgia (7%), back pain (6%)
Otic: Ear infection (5%)
Respiratory: Respiratory tract infection (10%), bronchitis (9%), pharyngitis (8%), acute tonsillitis (6%), rhinitis (6%)

Mechanism of Action Selectively binds iron, forming a complex which is excreted primarily through the feces.

Drug Interactions
Decreased Effect: Aluminum-containing antacids may decrease absorption of deferasirox.

Pharmacodynamics/Kinetics
Distribution: Adults: 14 L
Protein binding: 99% to serum albumin
Metabolism: Hepatic via glucuronidation by UGT1A1 and UGT1A3; minor oxidation by CYP450; undergoes enterohepatic recirculation
Bioavailability: 70%
Half-life elimination: 8-16 hours
Time to peak, plasma: 1-4 hours
Excretion: Feces (84%), urine (6% to 8%)

Pregnancy Risk Factor B

Deferoxamine *(de fer OKS a meen)*

U.S. Brand Names Desferal®
Canadian Brand Names Desferal®; PMS-Deferoxamine
Generic Available Yes

Index Terms Deferoxamine Mesylate; Desferrioxamine; NSC-644468

Pharmacologic Category Antidote; Chelating Agent

Use Acute iron intoxication or when clinical signs of significant iron toxicity exist; chronic iron overload secondary to multiple transfusions

Unlabeled/Investigational Use Removal of corneal rust rings following surgical removal of foreign bodies; diagnosis or treatment of aluminum induced toxicity associated with chronic kidney disease (CKD)

Local Anesthetic/Vasoconstrictor Precautions No information available to require special precautions

Effects on Dental Treatment No significant effects or complications reported

Common Adverse Effects Frequency not defined.

Cardiovascular: Flushing, hypotension, tachycardia, shock, edema

Central nervous system: Fever, dizziness, neuropathy, seizure, exacerbation of aluminum-related encephalopathy (dialysis), headache

Dermatologic: Angioedema, rash, urticaria

Endocrine & metabolic: Growth retardation (children), hypocalcemia

Gastrointestinal: Abdominal discomfort, abdominal pain, diarrhea, nausea, vomiting

Genitourinary: Dysuria

Hematologic: Thrombocytopenia, leukopenia

Local: Injection site: Burning, crust, edema, erythema, eschar, induration, infiltration, irritation, pain, pruritus, swelling, vesicles, wheal formation

Neuromuscular & skeletal: Arthralgia, leg cramps, metaphyseal dysplasia (dose related), myalgia, paresthesia

Ocular: Acuity decreased, blurred vision, dichromatopsia, maculopathy, night vision impaired, peripheral vision impaired, visual loss, scotoma, visual field defects, optic neuritis, cataracts, retinal pigmentary abnormalities, night blindness

Otic: Hearing loss, tinnitus

Renal: Renal impairment, urine discoloration (vin-rose color)

Respiratory: Acute/adult respiratory distress syndrome, asthma

Miscellaneous: Anaphylaxis, hypersensitivity reaction, infections (*Yersinia*, mucormycosis)

Mechanism of Action Complexes with trivalent ions (ferric ions) to form ferrioxamine, which are removed by the kidneys

Drug Interactions

Increased Effect/Toxicity: May cause loss of consciousness or coma when administered with prochlorperazine. Vitamin C (>500 mg/day) may increase the adverse/toxic effects of deferoxamine; may cause left ventricular dysfunction; avoid concomitant use.

Pharmacodynamics/Kinetics

Absorption: I.M.: Erratic

Metabolism: Plasma enzymes; binds with iron to form ferrioxamine

Half-life elimination: Parent drug: 6.1 hours; Ferrioxamine: 5.8 hours

Excretion: Primarily urine (as unchanged drug and ferrioxamine); feces (via bile)

Pregnancy Risk Factor C

Delavirdine (de la VIR deen)

Related Information

HIV Infection and AIDS *on page 1753*

Tuberculosis Treatment *on page 1909*

U.S. Brand Names Rescriptor®

Canadian Brand Names Rescriptor®

Generic Available No

Index Terms U-90152S

Pharmacologic Category Antiretroviral Agent, Reverse Transcriptase Inhibitor (Non-nucleoside)

Use Treatment of HIV-1 infection in combination with at least two additional antiretroviral agents

Local Anesthetic/Vasoconstrictor Precautions No information available to require special precautions

Effects on Dental Treatment No significant effects or complications reported

(Continued)

Delavirdine *(Continued)*

Common Adverse Effects

Frequency of adverse reactions reported from occurrence in clinical trials with delavirdine when used as part of combination antiretroviral therapy.

>10%:

Central nervous system: Headache (19% to 20%), depressive symptoms (10% to 15%), fever (4% to 12%)

Dermatologic: Rash (16% to 32%)

Gastrointestinal: Nausea (20% to 25%), vomiting (3% to 11%)

1% to 10%:

Central nervous system: Anxiety (6% to 8%)

Endocrine & metabolic: Transaminases increased (2% to 5%), amylase increased (3%), bilirubin increased (2%)

Gastrointestinal: Diarrhea, vomiting, abdominal pain (4% to 6%)

Hematologic: Prothrombin time increased (2%), hemoglobin decreased (1% to 3%)

Respiratory: Bronchitis (6% to 8%)

Frequency not defined (limited to important or life threatening): Abscess, adenopathy, alkaline phosphatase increased, allergic reaction, angioedema, anorexia, arrhythmia, bloody stool, bone pain, bruising, cardiac insufficiency, cardiac rate abnormal, cardiomyopathy, chest congestion, cognitive impairment, colitis, confusion, conjunctivitis, dermal leukocytoclastic vasculitis, desquamation, diverticulitis, dyspnea, emotional lability, eosinophilia, erythema multiforme, fecal incontinence, fungal dermatitis, gamma glutamyl transpeptidase increased, gastroenteritis, gastrointestinal bleeding, granulocytosis, gum hemorrhage, hallucination, hematuria, hepatomegaly, hyperglycemia, hyperkalemia, hypertension, hypertriglyceridemia, hyperuricemia, hypocalcemia, hyponatremia, hypophosphatemia, infection, jaundice, kidney pain, leukopenia, lipase increased, menstrual irregularities, moniliasis (oral/vaginal), pancreatitis, pancytopenia, paralysis, peripheral vascular disorder, pneumonia, postural hypotension, purpura, redistribution of body fat, renal calculi, serum creatinine increased, spleen disorder, Stevens-Johnson syndrome, tetany, thrombocytopenia, urinary tract infection, vertigo

Mechanism of Action Delavirdine binds directly to reverse transcriptase, blocking RNA-dependent and DNA-dependent DNA polymerase activities

Drug Interactions

Cytochrome P450 Effect: Substrate of CYP2D6 (minor), 3A4 (major); **Inhibits** CYP1A2 (weak), 2C9 (strong), 2C19 (strong), 2D6 (strong), 3A4 (strong)

Increased Effect/Toxicity: Delavirdine has been reported to increase the serum concentrations of amprenavir, indinavir, nelfinavir, ritonavir, saquinavir, inhaled corticosteroids, and trazodone. Dose reduction of indinavir, saquinavir, and trazodone should be considered. Plasma concentrations of delavirdine may be increased by fluoxetine and ketoconazole. Clarithromycin, rifabutin, and methadone serum concentrations may be increased by delavirdine.

Delavirdine may increase the levels/effects of CYP2C9, 2C19, or 2D6 substrates. Example substrates include amiodarone, amphetamines, selected beta-blockers, bosentan, citalopram, dapsone, dextromethorphan, diazepam, fluoxetine, glimepiride, glipizide, lidocaine, methsuximide, nateglinide, nefazodone, paroxetine, phenytoin, pioglitazone, propranolol, risperidone, ritonavir, rosiglitazone, sertraline, thioridazine, tricyclic antidepressants, venlafaxine, and warfarin.

Delavirdine may increase the levels/effects of CYP3A4 substrates. Example substrates include benzodiazepines, calcium channel blockers, cisapride, cyclosporine, mirtazapine, nateglinide, nefazodone, sildenafil (and other PDE-5 inhibitors), tacrolimus, and venlafaxine. Concomitant use with alprazolam, cisapride, ergot alkaloids, midazolam, pimozide, or triazolam is contraindicated. Use with lovastatin or simvastatin is not recommended.

Decreased Effect: Antacids, histamine-2 receptor antagonists, or proton pump inhibitors (omeprazole, lansoprazole) may reduce the absorption of delavirdine. Separate administration of didanosine buffered tablets or antacids and delavirdine by 1 hour. Concomitant use with histamine-2 receptor antagonists, omeprazole, or lansoprazole is not recommended.

Decreased delavirdine concentrations may occur when used with amprenavir, nelfinavir, or rifamycin derivatives. Delavirdine decreases plasma concentrations of didanosine and didanosine may decrease plasma concentrations of delavirdine. Separate administration of didanosine buffered tablets and delavirdine by 1 hour. Concomitant use with rifampin is contraindicated.

Delavirdine may decrease the levels/effects of CYP2D6 prodrug substrates. Example prodrug substrates include codeine, hydrocodone, oxycodone, and tramadol. CYP3A4 inducers may decrease the levels/effects of delavirdine. Example inducers include aminoglutethimide, carbamazepine, nafcillin, nevirapine, phenobarbital, phenytoin, and rifamycins. Carbamazepine, phenobarbital, phenytoin and rifamycins should not be coadministered with delavirdine. Dexamethasone may decrease the plasma concentrations of delavirdine.

Pharmacodynamics/Kinetics

Absorption: Rapid

Distribution: Low concentration in saliva and semen; CSF 0.4% concurrent plasma concentration

Protein binding: ~98%, primarily albumin

Metabolism: Hepatic via CYP3A4 and 2D6 (**Note:** May reduce CYP3A activity and inhibit its own metabolism.)

Bioavailability: Tablet: 85% as tablet; ~100% as oral slurry

Half-life elimination: 5.8 hours (range: 2-11 hours)

Time to peak, plasma: 1 hour

Excretion: Urine (51%, <5% as unchanged drug); feces (44%); nonlinear kinetics exhibited

Pregnancy Risk Factor C

Delestrogen® *see* Estradiol *on page 602*

Delfen® [OTC] *see* Nonoxynol 9 *on page 1185*

Delmopinol (del MOE pi nol)

U.S. Brand Names Decapinol®

Generic Available No

Index Terms Delmopinol Hydrochloride

Pharmacologic Category Antibacterial, Oral Rinse

Dental Use Treatment of gingivitis; used to decrease the adhesion of oral plaque

Local Anesthetic/Vasoconstrictor Precautions No information available to require special precautions

Effects on Dental Treatment No significant effects or complications reported

Significant Adverse Effects

Local: Anesthetic effect (transient, local), taste alteration, dry mouth, dental calculus increased

Restrictions

Decapinol® is regulated as a medical device in both the U.S. and in Europe.

Preliminary monograph: At the time of publication, it is not possible to determine when this product will be available in the U.S. market.

Additional detail concerning FDA approval may be found at: www.fda.gov/bbs/topics/news/2005/NEW01174.html

Dental Usual Dosing Treatment of gingivitis; used to decrease the adhesion of oral plaque: Adults: Oral: Rinse mouth with 10 mL for 1 minute twice daily (after brushing and flossing)

Mechanism of Action Reduces adhesion of plaque-causing bacteria, reducing the formation of new plaque and promoting the removal of deposits with normal mechanical disruption (brushing and flossing). Ultimately causes a reduction in both plaque and gingivitis. Decapinol® is regulated as a medical device because the primary mode of action is to serve as a physical barrier without chemical activity.

Contraindications Hypersensitivity to delmopinol or any component of the formulation

Warnings/Precautions Not for ingestion, patients should be instructed not to swallow solution. May cause transient anesthetic effects, dry mouth, or changes in taste following use. Light staining may occur, which may be removed by brushing the teeth. Patients should be instructed to avoid eating or drinking for 30 minutes following use. Should be used as an adjunct to normal mechanical hygiene. Avoid use in pregnant women (lack of data). Not recommended for use in children <12 years of age.

Note: Preliminary monograph: A decision to market this product within the U.S. is pending. At the time of publication, it is not possible to determine when this product will be available in the U.S. market.

Drug Interactions

Delmopinol does not interact with toothpaste.

Pregnancy Risk Factor

The manufacturer does not recommend use in pregnant women.

Lactation Excretion unknown/not recommended

Dosage Forms Liquid, oral rinse: 0.2%

Selected Readings

Hase JC, Attstrom R, Edwardsson S, et al, "6-Month Use of 0.2% Delmopinol Hydrochloride in Comparison With 0.2% Chlorhexidine Digluconate and Placebo (I). Effect on Plaque Formation and Gingivitis," *J Clin Periodontol*, 1998, 25(9):746-53.

(Continued)

Delmopinol *(Continued)*

Klinge B, Matsson L, Attstrom R, et al, "Effect of Local Application of Delmopinol Hydrochloride on Developing and Early Established Supragingival Plaque in Humans," *J Clin Periodontol*, 1996, 23(6):543-7.

Lang NP, Hase JC, Grassi M, et al, "Plaque Formation and Gingivitis After Supervised Mouthrinsing With 0.2% Delmopinol Hydrochloride, 0.2% Chlorhexidine Digluconate and Placebo for 6 Months," *Oral Dis*, 1998, 4(2):105-13.

Demeclocycline *(dem e kloe SYE kleen)*

U.S. Brand Names Declomycin®

Canadian Brand Names Declomycin®

Generic Available Yes

Index Terms Demeclocycline Hydrochloride; Demethylchlortetracycline

Pharmacologic Category Antibiotic, Tetracycline Derivative

Use Treatment of susceptible bacterial infections (acne, gonorrhea, pertussis and urinary tract infections) caused by both gram-negative and gram-positive organisms

Unlabeled/Investigational Use Treatment of chronic syndrome of inappropriate secretion of antidiuretic hormone (SIADH)

Local Anesthetic/Vasoconstrictor Precautions No information available to require special precautions

Effects on Dental Treatment Tetracyclines are not recommended for use during pregnancy or in children ≤8 years of age since they have been reported to cause enamel hypoplasia and permanent teeth discoloration. Tetracyclines should only be used in these patients if other agents are contraindicated or alternative antimicrobials will not eradicate the organism. Long-term use associated with oral candidiasis.

Common Adverse Effects Frequency not defined.

Cardiovascular: Pericarditis

Central nervous system: Bulging fontanels (infants), dizziness, headache, pseudotumor cerebri (adults)

Dermatologic: Angioneurotic edema, erythema multiforme, erythematous rash, maculopapular rash, photosensitivity, pigmentation of skin, Stevens-Johnson syndrome (rare), urticaria

Endocrine & metabolic: Discoloration of thyroid gland (brown/black), nephrogenic diabetes insipidus

Gastrointestinal: Anorexia, diarrhea, dysphagia, enterocolitis, esophageal ulcerations, glossitis, nausea, pancreatitis, vomiting

Genitourinary: Balanitis

Hematologic: Eosinophilia, neutropenia, hemolytic anemia, thrombocytopenia

Hepatic: Hepatitis (rare), hepatotoxicity (rare), liver enzymes increased, liver failure (rare)

Neuromuscular & skeletal: Myasthenic syndrome, polyarthralgia, tooth discoloration (children <8 years, rarely in adults)

Ocular: Visual disturbances

Otic: Tinnitus

Renal: Acute renal failure

Respiratory: Pulmonary infiltrates

Miscellaneous: Anaphylaxis, anaphylactoid purpura, lupus-like syndrome, systemic lupus erythematosus exacerbation

Mechanism of Action Inhibits protein synthesis by binding with the 30S and possibly the 50S ribosomal subunit(s) of susceptible bacteria; may also cause alterations in the cytoplasmic membrane; inhibits the action of ADH in patients with chronic SIADH

Drug Interactions

Increased Effect/Toxicity: Methoxyflurane anesthesia may cause fatal nephrotoxicity; retinoic acid derivatives may increase adverse and toxic effects; warfarin may result in increased anticoagulation; methotrexate levels may be increased

Decreased Effect: Antacid preparations containing calcium, magnesium, aluminum bismuth, or sodium bicarbonate may decrease tetracycline absorption; bile acid sequestrants, quinapril (magnesium-containing formulation), iron, or zinc may also decrease absorption; penicillin decrease therapeutic effect of tetracyclines. Although anecdotal reports suggest oral contraceptive efficacy could be reduced by tetracyclines, this has been refuted by more rigorous scientific and clinical data.

Pharmacodynamics/Kinetics

Onset of action: SIADH: Several days

Absorption: ~50% to 80%; reduced by food and dairy products

Protein binding: 41% to 50%

Metabolism: Hepatic (small amounts) to inactive metabolites; undergoes enterohepatic recirculation

Half-life elimination: 10-17 hours

Time to peak, serum: 3-6 hours

Excretion: Urine (42% to 50% as unchanged drug)

Pregnancy Risk Factor D

Denileukin Diftitox (de ni LOO kin DIF ti toks)

U.S. Brand Names ONTAK®

Generic Available No

Index Terms DAB$_{389}$IL-2; NSC-714744

Pharmacologic Category Antineoplastic Agent, Miscellaneous

Use Treatment of persistent or recurrent cutaneous T-cell lymphoma whose malignant cells express the CD25 component of the IL-2 receptor

Local Anesthetic/Vasoconstrictor Precautions No information available to require special precautions

Effects on Dental Treatment No significant effects or complications reported

Common Adverse Effects

>10%:

Cardiovascular: Edema (47%; grade 3 and 4, 15%), hypotension (36%), chest pain (24%), vasodilation (22%), tachycardia (12%)

Central nervous system: Fever/chills (81%; grade 3 and 4, 22%), headache (26%), pain (48%; grade 3 and 4, 13%), dizziness (22%), nervousness (11%)

Dermatologic: Rash (34%; grade 3 and 4, 13%), pruritus (20%)

Endocrine & metabolic: Hypoalbuminemia (83%; grade 3 and 4, 14%), hypocalcemia (17%), weight loss (14%)

Gastrointestinal: Nausea/vomiting (64%; grade 3 and 4, 14%), anorexia (36%), diarrhea (29%)

Hematologic: Lymphocyte count decreased (34%), anemia (18%)

Hepatic: Transaminases increased (61%; grade 3 and 4, 15%)

Neuromuscular & skeletal: Weakness (66%; grade 3 and 4, 22%), myalgia (17%), paresthesia (13%)

Respiratory: Dyspnea (29%; grade 3 and 4, 14%), cough increased (26%), pharyngitis (17%), rhinitis (13%)

Miscellaneous: Flu-like syndrome (91%; beginning several hours to days following infusion), hypersensitivity (69%; reactions are variable, but may include hypotension, back pain, dyspnea, vasodilation, rash, chest pain, tachycardia, dysphagia, syncope, or anaphylaxis), infection (48%; grade 3 and 4, 24%), vascular leak syndrome (DIF; characterized by hypotension, edema, or hypoalbuminemia; the syndrome usually developed within the first 2 weeks of infusion; 6% of patients who developed this syndrome required hospitalization; the symptoms may persist or even worsen despite cessation of denileukin diftitox)

1% to 10%:

Cardiovascular: Thrombotic events (7%), hypertension (6%), arrhythmia (6%), MI (1%)

Central nervous system: Insomnia (9%), confusion (8%)

Endocrine & metabolic: Dehydration (9%), hypokalemia (6%), hyperthyroidism (<5%), hypothyroidism (<5%)

Gastrointestinal: Constipation (9%), dyspepsia (7%), dysphagia (6%), oral ulcer (<5%), pancreatitis (<5%)

(Continued)

Denileukin Diftitox *(Continued)*

Hematologic: Thrombocytopenia (8%), leukopenia (6%)

Local: Injection site reaction (8%), anaphylaxis (1%)

Neuromuscular & skeletal: Arthralgia (8%)

Renal: Hematuria (10%), albuminuria (10%), pyuria (10%), creatinine increased (7%), acute renal insufficiency (<5%)

Respiratory: Lung disorder (8%)

Miscellaneous: Anaphylaxis (1%), diaphoresis decreased (10%)

Mechanism of Action Denileukin diftitox is a fusion protein (a combination of amino acid sequences from diphtheria toxin and interleukin-2) which selectively delivers the cytotoxic activity of diphtheria toxin to targeted cells. It interacts with the high-affinity IL-2 receptor on the surface of malignant cells to inhibit intracellular protein synthesis, rapidly leading to cell death.

Pharmacodynamics/Kinetics

Distribution: V_d: 0.06-0.08 L/kg

Metabolism: Hepatic via proteolytic degradation (animal studies)

Half-life elimination: Distribution: 2-5 minutes; Terminal: 70-80 minutes

Pregnancy Risk Factor C

Desipramine (des IP ra meen)

U.S. Brand Names Norpramin®
Canadian Brand Names Alti-Desipramine; Apo-Desipramine®; Norpramin®; Nu-Desipramine; PMS-Desipramine
Mexican Brand Names Norpramin
Generic Available Yes
Index Terms Desipramine Hydrochloride; Desmethylimipramine Hydrochloride
Pharmacologic Category Antidepressant, Tricyclic (Secondary Amine)
Use Treatment of depression
Unlabeled/Investigational Use Analgesic adjunct in chronic pain; peripheral neuropathies; substance-related disorders (eg, cocaine withdrawal); attention-deficit/hyperactivity disorder (ADHD); depression in children ≤12 years of age
Local Anesthetic/Vasoconstrictor Precautions Use with caution; epinephrine and levonordefrin have been shown to have an increased pressor response in combination with TCAs. Desipramine is one of the drugs confirmed to prolong the QT interval and is accepted as having a risk of causing torsade de pointes. The risk of drug-induced torsade de pointes is extremely low when a single QT interval prolonging drug is prescribed. In terms of epinephrine, it is not known what effect vasoconstrictors in the local anesthetic regimen will have in patients with a known history of congenital prolonged QT interval or in patients taking any medication that prolongs the QT interval. Until more information is obtained, it is suggested that the clinician consult with the physician prior to the use of a vasoconstrictor in suspected patients, and that the vasoconstrictor (epinephrine, levonordefrin [Neo-Cobefrin®]) be used with caution.
Effects on Dental Treatment Key adverse event(s) related to dental treatment: Xerostomia and changes in salivation (normal salivary flow resumes upon discontinuation), unpleasant taste, stomatitis, and black tongue. Long-term treatment with TCAs increases the risk of caries by reducing salivation and salivary buffer capacity.
Common Adverse Effects Frequency not defined.

Cardiovascular: Arrhythmias, edema, flushing, heart block, hyper-/hypotension, MI, palpitation, stroke, tachycardia

Central nervous system: Agitation, anxiety, ataxia, confusion, delirium, disorientation, dizziness, drowsiness, drug fever, exacerbation of psychosis, extrapyramidal symptoms, fatigue, hallucinations, headache, hypomania, incoordination, insomnia, nervousness, parkinsonian syndrome, restlessness, seizure

Dermatologic: Alopecia, itching, petechiae, photosensitivity, skin rash, urticaria

Endocrine & metabolic: Breast enlargement, galactorrhea, hyper-/hypoglycemia, impotence, libido changes, SIADH

Gastrointestinal: Abdominal cramps, anorexia, black tongue, constipation, decreased lower esophageal sphincter tone may cause GE reflux, diarrhea, heartburn, nausea, paralytic ileus, stomatitis, unpleasant taste, vomiting, weight gain/loss, xerostomia

Genitourinary: Difficult urination, polyuria, sexual dysfunction, testicular edema, urinary retention

Hematologic: Agranulocytosis, eosinophilia, purpura, thrombocytopenia

Hepatic: Cholestatic jaundice, hepatitis, liver enzymes increased

Neuromuscular & skeletal: Fine muscle tremor, numbness, paresthesia of extremities, peripheral neuropathy, tingling, weakness

Ocular: Blurred vision, disturbances of accommodation, intraocular pressure increased, mydriasis

Otic: Tinnitus

Miscellaneous: Allergic reaction, diaphoresis (excessive)

Restrictions An FDA-approved medication guide concerning the use of antidepressants in children, adolescents, and young adults must be distributed when dispensing an outpatient prescription (new or refill) where this medication is to be used without direct supervision of a healthcare provider. Medication guides are available at http://www.fda.gov/cder/Offices/ODS/medication_guides.htm. Dispense to parents or guardians of children and adolescents receiving this medication.
Mechanism of Action Traditionally believed to increase the synaptic concentration of norepinephrine (and to a lesser extent, serotonin) in the central nervous system by inhibition of its reuptake by the presynaptic neuronal membrane. However, additional receptor effects have been found including desensitization of adenyl cyclase, down regulation of beta-adrenergic receptors, and down regulation of serotonin receptors.
(Continued)

Desipramine *(Continued)*

Drug Interactions

Cytochrome P450 Effect: Substrate of CYP1A2 (minor), 2D6 (major); **Inhibits** CYP2A6 (moderate), 2B6 (moderate), 2D6 (moderate), 2E1 (weak), 3A4 (moderate)

Increased Effect/Toxicity: Desipramine increases the effects of amphetamines, anticholinergics, other CNS depressants (sedatives, hypnotics, or ethanol), chlorpropamide, tolazamide, and warfarin. When used with MAO inhibitors, or other serotonin modulators (eg, SSRIs), enhanced serotonergic effects, including serotonin syndrome may occur. Concurrent use with sibutramine is contraindicated. Serotonin syndrome has also been reported with ritonavir (rare). The levels/effects of desipramine may be increased by chlorpromazine, delavirdine, fluoxetine, miconazole, paroxetine, pergolide, quinidine, quinine, ritonavir, ropinirole, and other CYP2D6 inhibitors.

Cimetidine, grapefruit juice, indinavir, methylphenidate, diltiazem, and verapamil may increase the serum concentration of TCAs. Use of lithium with a TCA may increase the risk for neurotoxicity. Phenothiazines may increase concentration of some TCAs and TCAs may increase concentration of phenothiazines. Pressor response to I.V. epinephrine, norepinephrine, and phenylephrine may be enhanced in patients receiving TCAs. (**Note:** Effect is unlikely with epinephrine or levonordefrin dosages typically administered as infiltration in combination with local anesthetics.) Combined use of beta-agonists or drugs which prolong QT$_c$ (including quinidine, procainamide, disopyramide, cisapride, sparfloxacin, gatifloxacin, moxifloxacin) with TCAs may predispose patients to cardiac arrhythmias.

Desipramine may increase the levels/effects of selected benzodiazepines, bupropion, calcium channel blockers, cisapride, dexmedetomidine, dextromethorphan, ergot derivatives, ifosfamide, fluoxetine, selected HMG-CoA reductase inhibitors, lidocaine, mesoridazine, mirtazapine, nateglinide, nefazodone, paroxetine, pimozide, promethazine, propofol, quinidine, risperidone, ritonavir, selegiline, sertraline, sildenafil (and other PDE-5 inhibitors), tacrolimus, thioridazine, tricyclic antidepressants, venlafaxine, and other CYP2A6, 2B6, 2D6, or 3A4 substrates.

Decreased Effect: Desipramine may decrease the levels/effects of CYP2D6 prodrug substrates (eg, codeine, hydrocodone, oxycodone, tramadol). Desipramine's serum levels/effect may be decreased by carbamazepine, cholestyramine, colestipol, phenobarbital, and rifampin. Desipramine may inhibit the antihypertensive effect of clonidine, guanadrel, or methyldopa.

Pharmacodynamics/Kinetics

Onset of action: 1-3 weeks; Maximum antidepressant effect: >2 weeks
Absorption: Well absorbed
Metabolism: Hepatic
Half-life elimination: Adults: 7-60 hours
Time to peak, plasma: 4-6 hours
Excretion: Urine (70%)

Pregnancy Risk Factor C

Desipramine Hydrochloride *see Desipramine on page 459*
Desitin® [OTC] *see Zinc Oxide on page 1683*
Desitin® Creamy [OTC] *see Zinc Oxide on page 1683*

Desloratadine *(des lor AT a deen)*

U.S. Brand Names Clarinex®
Canadian Brand Names Aerius®
Mexican Brand Names Aviant
Generic Available No
Pharmacologic Category Antihistamine, Nonsedating
Use Relief of nasal and non-nasal symptoms of seasonal allergic rhinitis (SAR) and perennial allergic rhinitis (PAR); treatment of chronic idiopathic urticaria (CIU)
Local Anesthetic/Vasoconstrictor Precautions No information available to require special precautions
Effects on Dental Treatment Key adverse event(s) related to dental treatment: Xerostomia (normal salivary flow resumes upon discontinuation)
Common Adverse Effects
>10%: Central nervous system: Headache (14%)
1% to 10%:
Central nervous system: Fatigue (2% to 5%), somnolence (2%), dizziness (4%)
Endocrine & metabolic: Dysmenorrhea (2%)

Gastrointestinal: Xerostomia (3%), nausea (5%), dyspepsia (3%)
Neuromuscular & skeletal: Myalgia (2% to 3%)
Respiratory: Pharyngitis (3% to 4%)

Dosage Oral:
Children:
6-11 months: 1 mg once daily
12 months to 5 years: 1.25 mg once daily
6-11 years: 2.5 mg once daily
Children ≥12 years and Adults: 5 mg once daily
Dosage adjustment in renal/hepatic impairment:
Children: Not established
Adults: 5 mg every other day

Mechanism of Action Desloratadine, a major metabolite of loratadine, is a long-acting tricyclic antihistamine with selective peripheral histamine H_1 receptor antagonistic activity and additional anti-inflammatory properties.

Contraindications Hypersensitivity to desloratadine, loratadine, or any component of the formulation

Warnings/Precautions Dose should be adjusted in patients with liver or renal impairment. Use with caution in patients known to be slow metabolizers of desloratadine (incidence of side effects may be increased). RediTabs® contain phenylalanine. Safety and efficacy have not been established for children <6 months of age.

Drug Interactions
Increased Effect/Toxicity: With concurrent use of desloratadine and erythromycin or ketoconazole, the C_{max} and AUC of desloratadine and its metabolite are increased; however, no clinically-significant changes in the safety profile of desloratadine were observed in clinical studies. CNS depressants may cause increased risk of sedation when combined with desloratadine; use caution.

Ethanol/Nutrition/Herb Interactions
Ethanol: Avoid ethanol (may increase risk of sedation).
Food: Does not affect bioavailability.

Dietary Considerations May be taken with or without food. Orally-disintegrating tablets contain phenylalanine.

Pharmacodynamics/Kinetics
Protein binding: Desloratadine: 82% to 87%; 3-hydroxydesloratadine: 85% to 89%
Metabolism: Hepatic to active metabolite, 3-hydroxydesloratadine (specific enzymes not identified); undergoes glucuronidation. Decreased in slow metabolizers of desloratadine. Not expected to affect or be affected by medications metabolized by CYP with normal doses.
Half-life elimination: 27 hours
Time to peak: 3 hours
Excretion: Urine and feces (as metabolites)

Pregnancy Risk Factor C

Dosage Forms
Syrup:
Clarinex®: 0.5 mg/mL
Tablet:
Clarinex®: 5 mg
Tablet, orally disintegrating:
Clarinex® RediTabs®: 2.5 mg, 5 mg

Desloratadine and Pseudoephedrine
(des lor AT a deen & soo doe e FED rin)

U.S. Brand Names Clarinex-D® 12 Hour; Clarinex-D® 24 Hour
Generic Available No
Index Terms Pseudoephedrine and Desloratadine
Pharmacologic Category Antihistamine/Decongestant Combination, Nonsedating
Use Relief of symptoms of seasonal allergic rhinitis, in children ≥12 years of age and adults
Local Anesthetic/Vasoconstrictor Precautions No information available to require special precautions
Effects on Dental Treatment Key adverse event(s) related to dental treatment: Pseudoephedrine: Xerostomia (normal salivary flow resumes upon discontinuation).
Common Adverse Effects See also individual agents. Percentages as reported with the combination products.
(Continued)

Desloratadine and Pseudoephedrine *(Continued)*

1% to 10%:

Central nervous system: Insomnia (5% to 10%), headache (6% to 8%), fatigue (3% to 4%), somnolence (3%), dizziness (2% to 3%), hyperactivity (2%), nervousness (2%)

Gastrointestinal: Xerostomia (8%), anorexia (2%), nausea (2%)

Respiratory: Pharyngitis (3%)

Miscellaneous: Infection (2%)

Mechanism of Action

Desloratadine, a major metabolite of loratadine, is a long-acting tricyclic antihistamine with selective peripheral histamine H_1 receptor antagonistic activity and additional anti-inflammatory properties.

Pseudoephedrine directly stimulates alpha-adrenergic receptors of respiratory mucosa causing vasoconstriction; directly stimulates beta-adrenergic receptors causing bronchial relaxation, increased heart rate and contractility.

Drug Interactions

Increased Effect/Toxicity: See individual agents.

Decreased Effect: See individual agents.

Pharmacodynamics/Kinetics Also see individual agents.

Onset: Antihistaminic activity: 1 hour

Time to peak, plasma: Desloratadine: 4-7 hours; pseudoephedrine: 6-9 hours

Pregnancy Risk Factor C

Desmethylimipramine Hydrochloride *see* Desipramine *on page 459*

Desmopressin *(des moe PRES in)*

U.S. Brand Names DDAVP®; Stimate™

Canadian Brand Names Apo-Desmopressin®; DDAVP®; Minirin®; Nove-Desmopressin®; Octostim®

Mexican Brand Names Minirin

Generic Available Yes

Index Terms 1-Deamino-8-D-Arginine Vasopressin; Desmopressin Acetate

Pharmacologic Category Antihemophilic Agent; Hemostatic Agent; Vasopressin Analog, Synthetic

Use

Injection: Treatment of diabetes insipidus; control of bleeding in hemophilia A, and mild-to-moderate classic von Willebrand disease (type I)

Tablet, nasal solution: Treatment of diabetes insipidus; primary nocturnal enuresis

Local Anesthetic/Vasoconstrictor Precautions No information available to require special precautions

Effects on Dental Treatment No significant effects or complications reported

Common Adverse Effects Frequency not defined (may be dose or route related).

Cardiovascular: Acute cerebrovascular thrombosis, acute MI, blood pressure increased/decreased, chest pain, edema, facial flushing, palpitation

Central nervous system: Agitation, chills, coma, dizziness, headache, insomnia, somnolence

Dermatologic: Rash

Endocrine & metabolic: Hyponatremia, water intoxication

Gastrointestinal: Abdominal cramps, dyspepsia, nausea, sore throat, vomiting

Genitourinary: Balanitis, vulval pain

Local: Injection: Burning pain, erythema, and swelling at the injection site

Ocular: Conjunctivitis, eye edema, lacrimation disorder

Respiratory: Cough, epistaxis, nasal congestion, rhinitis

Miscellaneous: Allergic reactions (rare), anaphylaxis (rare)

Mechanism of Action Enhances reabsorption of water in the kidneys by increasing cellular permeability of the collecting ducts; possibly causes smooth muscle constriction with resultant vasoconstriction; raises plasma levels of von Willebrand factor and factor VIII

Drug Interactions

Increased Effect/Toxicity: Chlorpropamide, fludrocortisone may increase ADH response.

Decreased Effect: Demeclocycline and lithium may decrease ADH response.

Pharmacodynamics/Kinetics

Intranasal administration:

Onset of increased factor VIII activity: 30 minutes (dose related)

Peak effect 1.5 hours

Bioavailability: 3.2%

I.V. infusion:
  Onset of increased factor VIII activity: 30 minutes (dose related)
    Peak effect: 1.5-2 hours
  Half-life elimination: Terminal: 3 hours (up to 9 hours in renal dysfunction)
  Excretion: Urine
Oral tablet:
  Onset of action: ADH: ~1 hour
    Peak effect: 4-7 hours
  Bioavailability: 5% compared to intranasal; 0.16% compared to I.V.
  Half-life elimination: 1.5-2.5 hours
Pregnancy Risk Factor B

Desmopressin Acetate *see* Desmopressin *on page 462*

Desogen® *see* Ethinyl Estradiol and Desogestrel *on page 621*

Desogestrel and Ethinyl Estradiol *see* Ethinyl Estradiol and Desogestrel *on page 621*

Desonate™ *see* Desonide *on page 463*

Desonide (DES oh nide)

U.S. Brand Names Desonate™; DesOwen®; LoKara™; Verdeso™
Canadian Brand Names Desocort®; PMS-Desonide
Mexican Brand Names Desowen
Generic Available Yes: Excludes aerosol, gel
Pharmacologic Category Corticosteroid, Topical
Use Adjunctive therapy for inflammation in acute and chronic corticosteroid responsive dermatosis (low potency corticosteroid); mild-to-moderate atopic dermatitis
Local Anesthetic/Vasoconstrictor Precautions No information available to require special precautions
Effects on Dental Treatment No significant effects or complications reported
Mechanism of Action Stimulates the synthesis of enzymes needed to decrease inflammation, suppress mitotic activity, and cause vasoconstriction
Pharmacodynamics/Kinetics
  Absorption: Extensive from scalp, face, axilla, and scrotum; adequate through epidermis on appendages; may be increased with inflammation or occlusion
  Metabolism: Hepatic
  Excretion: Primarily urine
Pregnancy Risk Factor C

DesOwen® *see* Desonide *on page 463*

Desoximetasone (des oks i MET a sone)

U.S. Brand Names Topicort®; Topicort®-LP
Canadian Brand Names Taro-Desoximetasone; Topicort®
Generic Available Yes
Pharmacologic Category Corticosteroid, Topical
Dental Use Short-term relief of inflammation of moderate to severe corticosteroid-responsive dermatosis (intermediate- to high-potency topical corticosteroid)
Use Relieves inflammation and pruritic symptoms of corticosteroid-responsive dermatosis (intermediate- to high-potency topical corticosteroid)
Local Anesthetic/Vasoconstrictor Precautions No information available to require special precautions
Effects on Dental Treatment No significant effects or complications reported
Significant Adverse Effects <1% (Limited to important or life-threatening): Acneiform eruptions, allergic contact dermatitis, burning, dry skin, erythema, folliculitis, folliculopustular lesions, hypertrichosis, hypopigmentation, itching; local burning, irritation, miliaria; perioral dermatitis, secondary infection, skin atrophy, skin maceration, striae, vesiculation
Dosage Desoximetasone is a potent fluorinated topical corticosteroid. Therapy should be discontinued when control is achieved; if no improvement is seen, reassessment of diagnosis may be necessary.

  Cream, gel: Children and Adults: Apply a thin film to affected area twice daily
  Ointment: Children ≥10 years and Adults: Apply a thin film to affected area twice daily
Mechanism of Action Stimulates the synthesis of enzymes needed to decrease inflammation, suppress mitotic activity, and cause vasoconstriction
Contraindications Hypersensitivity to desoximetasone or any component of the formulation; topical fungal infections; tuberculosis of skin herpes simplex
Warnings/Precautions Systemic absorption of topical corticosteroids may cause hypothalamic-pituitary-adrenal (HPA) axis suppression (reversible)
(Continued)

Desoximetasone *(Continued)*

particularly in younger children. HPA axis suppression may lead to adrenal crisis. Risk is increased when used over large surface areas, for prolonged periods, or with occlusive dressings. Prolonged treatment with corticosteroids has been associated with the development of Kaposi's sarcoma (case reports); if noted, discontinuation of therapy should be considered. Adverse systemic effects including hyperglycemia, glycosuria, fluid and electrolyte changes, and HPA suppression may occur when used on large surface areas, for prolonged periods, or with an occlusive dressing. Chronic use of corticosteroids in children may interfere with growth and development. Safety and efficacy of desoximetasone ointment have not been established in children <10 years of age.

Drug Interactions No data reported

Pharmacodynamics/Kinetics

Absorption: May be increased with occlusion, inflammation, or vary with site of application

Ointment: Systemic absorption with occlusion: 7%

Metabolism: Hepatic

Half-life elimination: Emollient cream: 15-17 hours

Excretion: Urine, feces

Pregnancy Risk Factor C

Lactation Excretion in breast milk unknown/use caution

Dosage Forms Excipient information presented when available (limited, particularly for generics); consult specific product labeling.

Cream, topical: 0.25% (15 g, 60 g); 0.05% (15 g, 60 g)

Topicort®: 0.25% (15 g, 60 g)

Topicort®-LP: 0.05% (15 g, 60 g)

Gel, topical (Topicort®): 0.05% (15 g, 60 g) [contains alcohol 20%]

Ointment, topical (Topicort®): 0.25% (15 g, 60 g)

Dexamethasone (deks a METH a sone)

Related Information

Respiratory Diseases *on page 1747*

Ulcerative and Erosive Disorders *on page 1809*

Related Sample Prescriptions

Erosive Lichen Planus and Major Aphthae *on page 1845*

Recurrent Aphthous Stomatitis *on page 1844*

U.S. Brand Names Dexamethasone Intensol™; DexPak® TaperPak®; Maxidex®

Canadian Brand Names Apo-Dexamethasone®; Dexasone®; Diodex®; Maxidex®; PMS-Dexamethasone

Mexican Brand Names Adrecort; Alin; Decadron; Decadronal; Dibasona

Generic Available Yes; Excludes ophthalmic suspension

Index Terms Dexamethasone Sodium Phosphate

Pharmacologic Category Anti-inflammatory Agent; Anti-inflammatory Agent, Ophthalmic; Antiemetic; Corticosteroid, Ophthalmic; Corticosteroid, Otic; Corticosteroid, Systemic

Dental Use Treatment of a variety of oral diseases of allergic, inflammatory or autoimmune origin

Use

Systemic: Primarily as an anti-inflammatory or immunosuppressant agent in the treatment of a variety of diseases including those of allergic, dermatologic, endocrine, hematologic, inflammatory, neoplastic, nervous system, renal, respiratory, rheumatic, and autoimmune origin; may be used in management of cerebral edema, septic shock, chronic swelling, as a diagnostic agent, diagnosis of Cushing's syndrome, antiemetic

Ophthalmic: Treatment of palpebral and bulbar conjunctivitis; corneal injury from chemical, radiation, thermal burns, or foreign body penetration

Otic: Treatment of inflammation of external auditory meatus; treatment of edema associated with infective otitis externa

Unlabeled/Investigational Use Dexamethasone suppression test: General indicator consistent with depression and/or suicide

Local Anesthetic/Vasoconstrictor Precautions No information available to require special precautions

Effects on Dental Treatment No significant effects or complications reported

Significant Adverse Effects Frequency not defined.

Cardiovascular: Arrhythmia, bradycardia, cardiac arrest, cardiomyopathy, CHF, circulatory collapse, edema, hypertension, myocardial rupture (post-MI), syncope, thromboembolism, vasculitis

Central nervous system: Depression, emotional instability, euphoria, headache, intracranial pressure increased, insomnia, malaise, mood swings, neuritis, personality changes, pseudotumor cerebri (usually following discontinuation), psychic disorders, seizure, vertigo

Dermatologic: Acne, allergic dermatitis, alopecia, angioedema, bruising, dry skin, erythema, fragile skin, hirsutism, hyper-/hypopigmentation, hypertrichosis, perianal pruritus (following I.V. injection), petechiae, rash, skin atrophy, skin test reaction impaired, striae, urticaria, wound healing impaired

Endocrine & metabolic: Adrenal suppression, carbohydrate tolerance decreased, Cushing's syndrome, diabetes mellitus, glucose intolerance decreased, growth suppression (children), hyperglycemia, hypokalemic alkalosis, menstrual irregularities, negative nitrogen balance, pituitary-adrenal axis suppression, protein catabolism, sodium retention

Gastrointestinal: Abdominal distention, appetite increased, gastrointestinal hemorrhage, gastrointestinal perforation, nausea, pancreatitis, peptic ulcer, ulcerative esophagitis, weight gain

Genitourinary: Altered (increased or decreased) spermatogenesis

Hepatic: Hepatomegaly, transaminases increased

Local: Postinjection flare (intra-articular use), thrombophlebitis

Neuromuscular & skeletal: Arthropathy, aseptic necrosis (femoral and humoral heads), fractures, muscle mass loss, myopathy (particularly in conjunction with neuromuscular disease or neuromuscular-blocking agents), neuropathy, osteoporosis, parasthesia, tendon rupture, vertebral compression fractures, weakness

Ocular: Cataracts, exophthalmos, glaucoma, intraocular pressure increased

Renal: Glucosuria

Respiratory: Pulmonary edema

Miscellaneous: Abnormal fat deposition, anaphylactoid reaction, anaphylaxis, avascular necrosis, diaphoresis, hiccups, hypersensitivity, impaired wound healing, infections, Kaposi's sarcoma, moon face, secondary malignancy

Dosage Refer to individual protocols.

Children:

Antiemetic (prior to chemotherapy): I.V.: 10 mg/m^2 (initial dose) followed by 5 mg/m^2 every 6 hours as needed **or** 5-20 mg given 15-30 minutes before treatment

Anti-inflammatory immunosuppressant: Oral, I.M., I.V.: 0.08-0.3 mg/kg/day **or** 2.5-10 mg/m^2/day in divided doses every 6-12 hours

Extubation or airway edema: Oral, I.M., I.V.: 0.5-2 mg/kg/day in divided doses every 6 hours beginning 24 hours prior to extubation and continuing for 4-6 doses afterwards

Cerebral edema: I.V.: Loading dose: 1-2 mg/kg/dose as a single dose; maintenance: 1-1.5 mg/kg/day (maximum: 16 mg/day) in divided doses every 4-6 hours, taper off over 1-6 weeks

Bacterial meningitis in infants and children >2 months: I.V.: 0.6 mg/kg/day in 4 divided doses every 6 hours for the first 4 days of antibiotic treatment; start dexamethasone at the time of the first dose of antibiotic

Physiologic replacement: Oral, I.M., I.V.: 0.03-0.15 mg/kg/day **or** 0.6-0.75 mg/m^2/day in divided doses every 6-12 hours

Adults:

Antiemetic:

Prophylaxis: Oral, I.V.: 10-20 mg 15-30 minutes before treatment on each treatment day

Continuous infusion regimen: Oral or I.V.: 10 mg every 12 hours on each treatment day

Mildly emetogenic therapy: Oral, I.M., I.V.: 4 mg every 4-6 hours

Delayed nausea/vomiting: Oral: 4-10 mg 1-2 times/day for 2-4 days **or**

8 mg every 12 hours for 2 days; then

4 mg every 12 hours for 2 days **or**

20 mg 1 hour before chemotherapy; then

10 mg 12 hours after chemotherapy; then

8 mg every 12 hours for 4 doses; then

4 mg every 12 hours for 4 doses

(Continued)

Dexamethasone *(Continued)*

Anti-inflammatory:

Oral, I.M., I.V. (injections should be given as sodium phosphate): 0.75-9 mg/day in divided doses every 6-12 hours

Intra-articular, intralesional, or soft tissue (as sodium phosphate): 0.4-6 mg/day

Ophthalmic:

Solution: Instill 1-2 drops into conjunctival sac every hour during the day and every other hour during the night; gradually reduce dose to every 3-4 hours, then to 3-4 times/day

Suspension: Instill 1-2 drops into conjunctival sac up to 4-6 times per day; may use hourly in severe disease; taper prior to discontinuation

Otic: Instill 3-4 drops 2-3 times a day; reduce dose gradually prior to discontinuation

Multiple myeloma: Oral, I.V.: 40 mg/day, days 1 to 4, 9 to 12, and 17 to 20, repeated every 4 weeks (alone or as part of a regimen)

Cerebral edema: I.V. 10 mg stat, 4 mg I.M./I.V. every 6 hours until response is maximized, then switch to oral regimen, then taper off if appropriate; dosage may be reduced after 24 days and gradually discontinued over 5-7 days

Extubation or airway edema: Oral, I.M., I.V. (injections should be given as sodium phosphate): 0.5-2 mg/kg/day in divided doses every 6 hours beginning 24 hours prior to extubation and continuing for 4-6 doses afterwards

Dexamethasone suppression test (depression/suicide indicator) (unlabeled use): Oral: 1 mg at 11 PM, draw blood at 8 AM the following day for plasma cortisol determination

Cushing's syndrome, diagnostic: Oral: 1 mg at 11 PM, draw blood at 8 AM; greater accuracy for Cushing's syndrome may be achieved by the following:

Dexamethasone 0.5 mg by mouth every 6 hours for 48 hours (with 24-hour urine collection for 17-hydroxycorticosteroid excretion)

Differentiation of Cushing's syndrome due to ACTH excess from Cushing's due to other causes: Oral: Dexamethasone 2 mg every 6 hours for 48 hours (with 24-hour urine collection for 17-hydroxycorticosteroid excretion)

Multiple sclerosis (acute exacerbation): 30 mg/day for 1 week, followed by 4-12 mg/day for 1 month

Physiological replacement: Oral, I.M., I.V. (should be given as sodium phosphate): 0.03-0.15 mg/kg/day **or** 0.6-0.75 mg/m^2/day in divided doses every 6-12 hours

Treatment of shock:

Addisonian crisis/shock (ie, adrenal insufficiency/responsive to steroid therapy): I.V. (given as sodium phosphate): 4-10 mg as a single dose, which may be repeated if necessary

Unresponsive shock (ie, unresponsive to steroid therapy): I.V. (given as sodium phosphate): 1-6 mg/kg as a single I.V. dose or up to 40 mg initially followed by repeat doses every 2-6 hours while shock persists

Hemodialysis: Supplemental dose is not necessary

Peritoneal dialysis: Supplemental dose is not necessary

Mechanism of Action Decreases inflammation by suppression of neutrophil migration, decreased production of inflammatory mediators, and reversal of increased capillary permeability; suppresses normal immune response. Dexamethasone's mechanism of antiemetic activity is unknown.

Contraindications Hypersensitivity to dexamethasone or any component of the formulation; systemic fungal infections; cerebral malaria; ophthalmic use in viral (active ocular herpes simplex), fungal, or tuberculosis diseases of the eye

Warnings/Precautions Use with caution in patients with thyroid disease, hepatic impairment, renal impairment, cardiovascular disease, diabetes, glaucoma, cataracts, myasthenia gravis, patients at risk for osteoporosis, patients at risk for seizures, or GI diseases (diverticulitis, peptic ulcer, ulcerative colitis) due to perforation risk. Use caution following acute MI (corticosteroids have been associated with myocardial rupture). Because of the risk of adverse effects, systemic corticosteroids should be used cautiously in the elderly in the smallest possible effective dose for the shortest duration. May affect growth velocity; growth should be routinely monitored in pediatric patients. Withdraw therapy with gradual tapering of dose.

May cause hypercorticism or suppression of hypothalamic-pituitary-adrenal (HPA) axis, particularly in younger children or in patients receiving high doses for prolonged periods. HPA axis suppression may lead to adrenal crisis. Withdrawal and discontinuation of a corticosteroid should be done slowly and carefully. Particular care is required when patients are transferred from systemic corticosteroids to inhaled products due to possible adrenal insufficiency or withdrawal from steroids, including an increase in allergic symptoms. Patients receiving >20 mg per day of prednisone (or equivalent) may be most susceptible. Fatalities have occurred due to adrenal insufficiency in asthmatic patients during and after transfer from systemic corticosteroids to aerosol steroids; aerosol steroids do not provide the systemic steroid needed to treat patients having trauma, surgery, or infections. Dexamethasone does not provide adequate mineralocorticoid activity in adrenal insufficiency (may be employed as a single dose while cortisol assays are performed). The lowest possible dose should be used during treatment; discontinuation and/or dose reductions should be gradual.

Acute myopathy has been reported with high dose corticosteroids, usually in patients with neuromuscular transmission disorders; may involve ocular and/or respiratory muscles; monitor creatine kinase; recovery may be delayed. Corticosteroid use may cause psychiatric disturbances, including depression, euphoria, insomnia, mood swings, and personality changes. Pre-existing psychiatric conditions may be exacerbated by corticosteroid use. Prolonged use of corticosteroids may also increase the incidence of secondary infection, mask acute infection (including fungal infections), prolong or exacerbate viral infections, or limit response to vaccines. Exposure to chickenpox should be avoided; corticosteroids should not be used to treat ocular herpes simplex. Corticosteroids should not be used for cerebral malaria. Close observation is required in patients with latent tuberculosis and/or TB reactivity; restrict use in active TB (only in conjunction with antituberculosis treatment). Prolonged treatment with corticosteroids has been associated with the development of Kaposi's sarcoma (case reports); if noted, discontinuation of therapy should be considered.

Drug Interactions **Substrate** of CYP3A4 (minor); **Induces** CYP2A6 (weak), 2B6 (weak), 2C8 (weak), 2C9 (weak), 3A4 (weak)

Aminoglutethimide: May reduce the serum levels/effects of dexamethasone; likely via induction of microsomal isoenzymes.

Antacids: May increase the absorption of corticosteroids; separate administration by 2 hours.

Anticholinesterases: Concurrent use may lead to severe weakness in patients with myasthenia gravis.

Aprepitant: May increase the serum levels of corticosteroids; monitor.

Azole antifungals: May increase the serum levels of corticosteroids; monitor.

Barbiturates: May decrease the levels/effects of dexamethasone (systemic).

Bile acid sequestrants: May reduce the absorption of corticosteroids; separate administration by 2 hours.

Calcium channel blockers (nondihydropyridine): May increase the serum levels of corticosteroids; monitor.

Cyclosporine: Corticosteroids may increase the serum levels of cyclosporine. In addition, cyclosporine may increase levels of corticosteroids.

Estrogens: May increase the serum levels of corticosteroids; monitor.

Fluoroquinolones: Concurrent use may increase the risk of tendon rupture, particularly in elderly patients (overall incidence rare).

Isoniazid: Serum concentrations may be decreased by corticosteroids.

Macrolide antibiotics: May increase the levels/effects of dexamethasone (systemic).

Neuromuscular-blocking agents: Concurrent use with corticosteroids may increase the risk of myopathy.

Nonsteroidal anti-inflammatory drugs (NSAIDs): Concurrent use with corticosteroids may lead to an increased incidence of gastrointestinal adverse effects; use caution. NSAID (ophthalmic) may enhance the adverse/toxic effect of dexamethasone (ophthalmic).

Primidone: May decrease the levels/effects of dexamethasone (systemic); monitor.

Rifamycins: May decrease the levels/effects of dexamethasone (systemic); monitor.

Salicylates: Salicylates may increase the gastrointestinal adverse effects of corticosteroids.

Thalidomide: Concurrent use with corticosteroids may increase the risk of selected adverse effects (toxic epidermal necrolysis and DVT); use caution.

Vaccine (dead organism): Dexamethasone may decrease the effect of vaccines (dead organisms). In patients receiving high doses of systemic corticosteroids for ≥14 days, wait at least 1 month between discontinuing steroid therapy and administering immunization.

Vaccine (live organism): Dexamethasone may increase the risk of vaccinal infection. The use of live vaccines is contraindicated in immunosuppressed patients.

Ethanol/Nutrition/Herb Interactions

Ethanol: Avoid ethanol (may enhance gastric mucosal irritation).

Food: Dexamethasone interferes with calcium absorption. Limit caffeine.

Herb/Nutraceutical: Avoid cat's claw, echinacea (have immunostimulant properties).

(Continued)

Dexamethasone *(Continued)*

Dietary Considerations May be taken with meals to decrease GI upset. May need diet with increased potassium, pyridoxine, vitamin C, vitamin D, folate, calcium, and phosphorus.

Pharmacodynamics/Kinetics
Onset of action: Acetate: Prompt
Duration of metabolic effect: 72 hours; acetate is a long-acting repository preparation
Metabolism: Hepatic
Half-life elimination: Normal renal function: 1.8-3.5 hours; Biological half-life: 36-54 hours
Time to peak, serum: Oral: 1-2 hours; I.M.: ~8 hours
Excretion: Urine and feces

Pregnancy Risk Factor C

Lactation Enters breast milk/use caution

Dosage Forms Excipient information presented when available (limited, particularly for generics); consult specific product labeling. [DSC] = Discontinued product
Elixir, as base: 0.5 mg/5 mL (240 mL)
Injection, solution, as sodium phosphate: 4 mg/mL (1 mL, 5 mL, 30 mL); 10 mg/mL (10 mL)
Injection, solution, as sodium phosphate [preservative free]: 10 mg/mL (1 mL)
Solution, ophthalmic, as sodium phosphate: 0.1% (5 mL)
Solution, oral: 0.5 mg/5 mL (500 mL)
Solution, oral concentrate:
Dexamethasone Intensol™: 1 mg/mL (30 mL) [contains alcohol 30%]
Suspension, ophthalmic:
Maxidex®: 0.1% (5 mL; 15 mL [DSC]) [contains benzalkonium chloride]
Tablet [scored]: 0.5 mg, 0.75 mg, 1 mg, 1.5 mg, 2 mg, 4 mg, 6 mg
DexPak® TaperPak®: 1.5 mg [51 tablets on taper dose card]

Dexamethasone and Ciprofloxacin *see* Ciprofloxacin and Dexamethasone *on page 364*

Dexamethasone and Tobramycin *see* Tobramycin and Dexamethasone *on page 1580*

Dexamethasone Intensol™ *see* Dexamethasone *on page 464*

Dexamethasone, Neomycin, and Polymyxin B *see* Neomycin, Polymyxin B, and Dexamethasone *on page 1161*

Dexamethasone Sodium Phosphate *see* Dexamethasone *on page 464*

Dexbrompheniramine and Pseudoephedrine
(deks brom fen EER a meen & soo doe e FED rin)

Related Information
Pseudoephedrine *on page 1381*
U.S. Brand Names Drixoral® Cold & Allergy [OTC]
Canadian Brand Names Drixoral®
Generic Available Yes
Index Terms Pseudoephedrine and Dexbrompheniramine
Pharmacologic Category Antihistamine/Decongestant Combination
Use Relief of symptoms of upper respiratory mucosal congestion in seasonal and perennial nasal allergies, acute rhinitis, rhinosinusitis and eustachian tube blockage
Local Anesthetic/Vasoconstrictor Precautions Use with caution since pseudoephedrine is a sympathomimetic amine which could interact with epinephrine to cause a pressor response
Effects on Dental Treatment Key adverse event(s) related to dental treatment: Pseudoephedrine: Xerostomia (normal salivary flow resumes upon discontinuation)
Pregnancy Risk Factor B

Dexchlorpheniramine (deks klor fen EER a meen)

Mexican Brand Names Polaramine
Generic Available Yes
Index Terms Dexchlorpheniramine Maleate
Pharmacologic Category Antihistamine
Use Perennial and seasonal allergic rhinitis and other allergic symptoms including urticaria
Local Anesthetic/Vasoconstrictor Precautions No information available to require special precautions

Effects on Dental Treatment Key adverse event(s) related to dental treatment: Significant xerostomia (normal salivary flow resumes upon discontinuation)

Common Adverse Effects

>10%:
Central nervous system: Slight to moderate drowsiness
Respiratory: Thickening of bronchial secretions

1% to 10%:
Central nervous system: Headache, fatigue, nervousness, dizziness
Gastrointestinal: Appetite increase, weight gain, nausea, diarrhea, abdominal pain, xerostomia
Neuromuscular & skeletal: Arthralgia
Respiratory: Pharyngitis

Mechanism of Action Competes with histamine for H_1-receptor sites on effector cells in the gastrointestinal tract, blood vessels, and respiratory tract. Dexchlorpheniramine is the predominant active isomer of chlorpheniramine and is approximately twice as active as the racemic compound.

Drug Interactions

Increased Effect/Toxicity: CNS depressants may increase the degree of sedation and respiratory depression with antihistamines. May increase the absorption of digoxin. Central and/or peripheral anticholinergic syndrome can occur when administered with amantadine, rimantadine, narcotic analgesics, phenothiazines and other antipsychotics (especially with high anticholinergic activity), tricyclic antidepressants, quinidine, disopyramide, procainamide, and antihistamines.

Decreased Effect: May increase gastric degradation of levodopa and decrease the amount of levodopa absorbed by delaying gastric emptying. Therapeutic effects of cholinergic agents (tacrine, donepezil) and neuroleptics may be antagonized.

Pharmacodynamics/Kinetics

Onset of action: ~1 hour
Duration: 3-6 hours
Absorption: Well absorbed
Metabolism: Hepatic

Pregnancy Risk Factor B

Dexchlorpheniramine and Pseudoephedrine
(deks klor fen EER a meen & soo doe e FED rin)

U.S. Brand Names Duotan PD; Tanafed DP™
Generic Available Yes
Index Terms Pseudoephedrine Tannate and Dexchlorpheniramine Tannate
Pharmacologic Category Alpha/Beta Agonist; Antihistamine
Use Relief of nasal congestion associated with the common cold, hay fever, and other allergies, sinusitis, and vasomotor and allergic rhinitis
Local Anesthetic/Vasoconstrictor Precautions No information available to require special precautions
Effects on Dental Treatment Key adverse event(s) related to dental treatment: Significant xerostomia (normal salivary flow resumes upon discontinuation)
Common Adverse Effects See individual agents.
Mechanism of Action
Chlorpheniramine competes with histamine for H_1-receptor sites on effector cells in the gastrointestinal tract, blood vessels, and respiratory tract. Dexchlorpheniramine is the predominant active isomer of chlorpheniramine and is approximately twice as active as the racemic compound.
Pseudoephedrine is a sympathomimetic amine and isomer of ephedrine; acts as a decongestant in respiratory tract mucous membranes with less vasoconstrictor action than ephedrine in normotensive individuals.

Drug Interactions
Cytochrome P450 Effect: See individual monographs for dexchlorpheniramine and pseudoephedrine.
Increased Effect/Toxicity: See individual monographs for dexchlorpheniramine and pseudoephedrine.
Decreased Effect: See individual monographs for chlorpheniramine and pseudoephedrine.

Pregnancy Risk Factor C

Dexedrine® *see* Dextroamphetamine *on page 473*
Dexferrum® *see* Iron Dextran Complex *on page 910*
DexFol™ *see* Vitamin B Complex Combinations *on page 1664*

Dexmedetomidine (deks MED e toe mi deen)

U.S. Brand Names Precedex™
Canadian Brand Names Precedex™
Mexican Brand Names Precedex
Generic Available No
Index Terms Dexmedetomidine Hydrochloride
Pharmacologic Category Alpha$_2$-Adrenergic Agonist; Sedative
Use Sedation of initially intubated and mechanically ventilated patients during treatment in an intensive care setting; duration of infusion should not exceed 24 hours
Unlabeled/Investigational Use Unlabeled uses include premedication prior to anesthesia induction with thiopental; relief of pain and reduction of opioid dose following laparoscopic tubal ligation; as an adjunct anesthetic in ophthalmic surgery; treatment of shivering; premedication to attenuate the cardiostimulatory and postanesthetic delirium of ketamine
Local Anesthetic/Vasoconstrictor Precautions No information available to require special precautions
Effects on Dental Treatment Key adverse event(s) related to dental treatment: Xerostomia and changes in salivation (normal salivary flow resumes upon discontinuation)
Common Adverse Effects
>10%:
   Cardiovascular: Hypotension (30%)
   Gastrointestinal: Nausea (11%)
1% to 10%:
   Cardiovascular: Bradycardia (8%), atrial fibrillation (7%)
   Central nervous system: Pain (3%)
   Gastrointestinal: Xerostomia
   Hematologic: Anemia (3%), leukocytosis (2%)
   Renal: Oliguria
   Respiratory: Hypoxia (6%), pulmonary edema (2%), pleural effusion (3%)
   Miscellaneous: Infection (2%), thirst (2%)
Mechanism of Action Selective alpha$_2$-adrenoceptor agonist with sedative properties; alpha$_1$ activity was observed at high doses or after rapid infusions
Drug Interactions
   Cytochrome P450 Effect: Substrate of CYP2A6 (major); **Inhibits** CYP1A2 (weak), 2C9 (weak), 2D6 (strong), 3A4 (weak)
   Increased Effect/Toxicity: The levels/effects of dexmedetomidine may be increased by isoniazid, methoxsalen, miconazole, and other CYP2A6 inhibitors. Dexmedetomidine may increase the levels/effects of amphetamines, selected beta-blockers, dextromethorphan, fluoxetine, lidocaine, mirtazapine, nefazodone, paroxetine, risperidone, ritonavir, thioridazine, tricyclic antidepressants, venlafaxine, and other CYP2D6 substrates. Hypotension and/or bradycardia may be increased by vasodilators and heart rate-lowering agents.
   Decreased Effect: Dexmedetomidine may decrease the levels/effects of CYP2D6 prodrug substrates; example prodrug substrates include codeine, hydrocodone, oxycodone, and tramadol.
Pharmacodynamics/Kinetics
   Onset of action: Rapid
   Distribution: V$_{ss}$: Approximately 118 L; rapid
   Protein binding: 94%
   Metabolism: Hepatic via glucuronidation and CYP2A6
   Half-life elimination: 6 minutes; Terminal: 2 hours
   Excretion: Urine (95%); feces (4%)
Pregnancy Risk Factor C

Dexmedetomidine Hydrochloride *see* Dexmedetomidine *on page 470*

Dexmethylphenidate (dex meth il FEN i date)

U.S. Brand Names Focalin®; Focalin® XR
Generic Available No
Index Terms Dexmethylphenidate Hydrochloride
Pharmacologic Category Central Nervous System Stimulant
Use Treatment of attention-deficit/hyperactivity disorder (ADHD)
Local Anesthetic/Vasoconstrictor Precautions No information available to require special precautions

Effects on Dental Treatment Key adverse event(s) related to dental treatment: Xerostomia (normal salivary flow resumes upon discontinuation).

Common Adverse Effects

>10%:

Central nervous system: Headache (25% to 26%), restlessness (12%)

Gastrointestinal: Appetite decreased (30%), abdominal pain (15%)

1% to 10%:

Cardiovascular: Tachycardia (3%)

Central nervous system: Dizziness (6%), anxiety (5% to 6%), fever (5%)

Gastrointestinal: Nausea (9%), dyspepsia (5% to 8%), xerostomia (7%), anorexia (6%), pharyngolaryngeal pain (4%)

Frequency not defined: Ocular: Accommodation difficulties, blurred vision

Also refer to Methylphenidate for adverse effects seen with other methylphenidate products.

Restrictions C-II

An FDA-approved medication guide must be distributed when dispensing an outpatient prescription (new or refill) where this medication is to be used without direct supervision of a healthcare provider. Medication guides are available at http://www.fda.gov/cder/drug/infopage/ADHD/default.htm.

Mechanism of Action Dexmethylphenidate is the more active, *d-threo*-enantiomer, of racemic methylphenidate. It is a CNS stimulant; blocks the reuptake of norepinephrine and dopamine, and increases their release into the extraneuronal space.

Drug Interactions

Increased Effect/Toxicity: Methylphenidate may cause hypertensive effects when used in combination with MAO inhibitors or drugs with MAO-inhibiting activity (linezolid). Risk may be less with selegiline (MAO type B selective at low doses); it is best to avoid this combination. NMS has been reported in a patient receiving methylphenidate and venlafaxine. Methylphenidate may increase levels of phenytoin and TCAs. Increased toxicity with clonidine, sibutramine, or other sympathomimetics.

Decreased Effect: Effectiveness of antihypertensive agents may be decreased. Carbamazepine may decrease the effect of methylphenidate.

Pharmacodynamics/Kinetics

Duration of action: Capsule: 12 hours

Absorption: Tablet: Rapid; Capsule: Bimodal

Distribution: V_d: 1.54-3.76 L/kg

Protein binding: 12% to 15%

Metabolism: Via de-esterification to inactive metabolite, d-α-phenyl-piperidine acetate (d-ritalinic acid)

Bioavailability: 22% to 25%

Half-life elimination: Immediate release: Adults: 2-4.5 hours; Children: 2-3 hours

Time to peak: Fasting:

Tablet: 1-1.5 hours

Capsule: First peak: 1.5 hours (range: 1-4 hours); Second peak: 6.5 hours (range: 4.5-7 hours)

Excretion: Urine (90%, primarily as inactive metabolite)

Pregnancy Risk Factor C

Dexmethylphenidate Hydrochloride see Dexmethylphenidate on page 470

DexPak® TaperPak® see Dexamethasone on page 464

Dexpanthenol (deks PAN the nole)

U.S. Brand Names Panthoderm® [OTC]

Generic Available Yes: Injection

Index Terms Pantothenyl Alcohol

Pharmacologic Category Gastrointestinal Agent, Stimulant; Topical Skin Product

Use Prophylactic use to minimize paralytic ileus; treatment of postoperative distention; topical to relieve itching and to aid healing of minor dermatoses

Local Anesthetic/Vasoconstrictor Precautions No information available to require special precautions

Effects on Dental Treatment No significant effects or complications reported

Common Adverse Effects Frequency not defined.

Cardiovascular: Slight drop in blood pressure

Central nervous system: Agitation

Dermatologic: Dermatitis, irritation, itching, urticaria

Gastrointestinal: Diarrhea, hyperperistalsis, vomiting

Neuromuscular & skeletal: Paresthesia

Respiratory: Dyspnea

Miscellaneous: Allergic reactions

(Continued)

Dexpanthenol *(Continued)*

Mechanism of Action A pantothenic acid B vitamin analog that is converted to coenzyme A internally; coenzyme A is essential to normal fatty acid synthesis, amino acid synthesis and acetylation of choline in the production of the neurotransmitter, acetylcholine

Drug Interactions
Increased Effect/Toxicity: Increased/prolonged effect when dexpanthenol injection is given with succinylcholine; do not give dexpanthenol within 1 hour of succinylcholine.

Pregnancy Risk Factor C

Dex PC *see* Chlorpheniramine, Phenylephrine, and Dextromethorphan *on page 342*

Dexrazoxane *(deks ray ZOKS ane)*

U.S. Brand Names Zinecard®
Canadian Brand Names Zinecard®
Mexican Brand Names Cardioxane
Generic Available No
Index Terms ICRF-187
Pharmacologic Category Cardioprotectant
Use Reduction of the incidence and severity of cardiomyopathy associated with doxorubicin administration in women with metastatic breast cancer who have received a cumulative doxorubicin dose of 300 mg/m^2 and who would benefit from continuing therapy with doxorubicin. It is not recommended for use with the initiation of doxorubicin therapy.

Local Anesthetic/Vasoconstrictor Precautions No information available to require special precautions
Effects on Dental Treatment No significant effects or complications reported
Common Adverse Effects Adverse reactions listed are those which were greater in the dexrazoxane arm in a trial comparison of dexrazoxane plus fluorouracil, doxorubicin, and cyclophosphamide (FAC) to FAC alone. (Most adverse reactions are thought to be attributed to FAC except for myelosuppression (increased) and pain at injection site).

Central nervous system: Fatigue/malaise, fever
Dermatologic: Alopecia, extravasation, streaking/erythema
Endocrine & metabolic: Serum amylase increased, serum calcium decreased, serum triglycerides increased
Hematologic: Hemorrhage, granulocytopenia, leukopenia, myelosuppression, thrombocytopenia
Hepatic: AST/ALT increased, bilirubin increased
Local: Pain at injection site, phlebitis
Neuromuscular & skeletal: Neurotoxicity
Miscellaneous: Infection, sepsis

Mechanism of Action Derivative of EDTA; potent intracellular chelating agent. The mechanism of cardioprotectant activity is not fully understood. Appears to be converted intracellularly to a ring-opened chelating agent that interferes with iron-mediated oxygen free radical generation thought to be responsible, in part, for anthracycline-induced cardiomyopathy.

Pharmacodynamics/Kinetics
Distribution: V_d: 22-22.4 L/m^2
Protein binding: None
Half-life elimination: 2.1-2.5 hours
Excretion: Urine (42%)
Clearance, renal: 3.35 L/hour/m^2; Plasma: 6.25-7.88 L/hour/m^2

Pregnancy Risk Factor C

Dextran *(DEKS tran)*

Related Information
Dextran 1 *on page 473*
U.S. Brand Names Gentran®; LMD®
Canadian Brand Names Gentran®
Generic Available Yes
Index Terms Dextran 40; Dextran 70; Dextran, High Molecular Weight; Dextran, Low Molecular Weight
Pharmacologic Category Plasma Volume Expander
Use Blood volume expander used in treatment of shock or impending shock when blood or blood products are not available; dextran 40 is also used as a

priming fluid in cardiopulmonary bypass and for prophylaxis of venous thrombosis and pulmonary embolism in surgical procedures associated with a high risk of thromboembolic complications

Local Anesthetic/Vasoconstrictor Precautions No information available to require special precautions

Effects on Dental Treatment No significant effects or complications reported

Mechanism of Action Produces plasma volume expansion by virtue of its highly colloidal starch structure, similar to albumin

Drug Interactions
Increased Effect/Toxicity: Dextran may enhance the anticoagulant effect of abciximab; avoid concurrent use.

Pharmacodynamics/Kinetics
Onset of action: Minutes to 1 hour (depending upon the molecular weight polysaccharide administered)
Excretion: Urine (~75%) within 24 hours

Pregnancy Risk Factor C

Dextran 40 *see* Dextran *on page 472*

Dextran 70 *see* Dextran *on page 472*

Dextran 1 (DEKS tran won)

Related Information
Dextran *on page 472*
U.S. Brand Names Promit® [DSC]
Generic Available No
Pharmacologic Category Plasma Volume Expander
Use Prophylaxis of serious anaphylactic reactions to I.V. infusion of dextran
Local Anesthetic/Vasoconstrictor Precautions No information available to require special precautions
Effects on Dental Treatment No significant effects or complications reported
Mechanism of Action Binds to dextran-reactive immunoglobulin without bridge formation and no formation of large immune complexes
Pregnancy Risk Factor C

Dextran, High Molecular Weight *see* Dextran *on page 472*

Dextran, Low Molecular Weight *see* Dextran *on page 472*

Dextroamphetamine (deks troe am FET a meen)

U.S. Brand Names Dexedrine®; Dextrostat®
Canadian Brand Names Dexedrine®
Generic Available Yes
Index Terms Dextroamphetamine Sulfate
Pharmacologic Category Stimulant
Use Narcolepsy; attention-deficit/hyperactivity disorder (ADHD)
Unlabeled/Investigational Use Exogenous obesity; depression; abnormal behavioral syndrome in children (minimal brain dysfunction)
Local Anesthetic/Vasoconstrictor Precautions Use vasoconstrictor with caution in patients taking dextroamphetamine. Amphetamines enhance the sympathomimetic response of epinephrine and norepinephrine leading to potential hypertension and cardiotoxicity.
Effects on Dental Treatment Key adverse event(s) related to dental treatment: Xerostomia (normal salivary flow resumes upon discontinuation). Up to 10% of patients taking dextroamphetamines may present with hypertension. Monitor blood pressure prior to using local anesthetic with vasoconstrictors.
Common Adverse Effects Frequency not defined.
Cardiovascular: Cardiomyopathy, hypertension, palpitation, tachycardia
Central nervous system: Aggression, dizziness, dyskinesia, dysphoria, euphoria, exacerbation of motor and phonic tics, headache, insomnia, mania, overstimulation, psychosis, restlessness, Tourette's syndrome
Dermatologic: Rash, urticaria
Endocrine & metabolic: Libido changes
Gastrointestinal: Anorexia, constipation, diarrhea, unpleasant taste, weight loss, xerostomia
Genitourinary: Impotence
Neuromuscular & skeletal: Tremor
Ocular: Accommodation abnormalities, blurred vision
Restrictions C-II

An FDA-approved medication guide must be distributed when dispensing an outpatient prescription (new or refill) where this medication is to be used without
(Continued)

Dextroamphetamine *(Continued)*

direct supervision of a healthcare provider. Medication guides are available at http://www.fda.gov/cder/drug/infopage/ADHD/default.htm.

Mechanism of Action Amphetamines are noncatecholamine, sympathomimetic amines. Blocks reuptake of dopamine and norepinephrine from the synapse, thus increases the amount of circulating dopamine and norepinephrine in cerebral cortex to reticular activating system; inhibits the action of monoamine oxidase and causes catecholamines to be released. Peripheral actions include elevated blood pressure, weak bronchodilator, and respiratory stimulant action.

Drug Interactions

Cytochrome P450 Effect: Substrate of CYP2D6 (major)

Increased Effect/Toxicity: CYP2D6 inhibitors may increase the levels/ effects of dextroamphetamine; example inhibitors include chlorpromazine, delavirdine, fluoxetine, miconazole, paroxetine, pergolide, quinidine, quinine, ritonavir, and ropinirole. Dextroamphetamine may precipitate hypertensive crisis or serotonin syndrome in patients receiving MAO inhibitors (selegiline >10 mg/day, isocarboxazid, phenelzine, tranylcypromine, furazolidone). Serotonin syndrome has also been associated with combinations of amphetamines and SSRIs; these combinations should be avoided. TCAs may enhance the effects of amphetamines. Large doses of antacids or urinary alkalinizers increase the half-life and duration of action of amphetamines. May precipitate arrhythmias in patients receiving general anesthetics.

Decreased Effect: Amphetamines inhibit the antihypertensive response to guanethidine, guanadrel, and other antihypertensives. Urinary acidifiers decrease the half-life and duration of action of amphetamines.

Pharmacodynamics/Kinetics

Onset of action: 1-1.5 hours

Distribution: V_d: Adults: 3.5-4.6 L/kg; distributes into CNS; mean CSF concentrations are 80% of plasma; enters breast milk

Metabolism: Hepatic via CYP monooxygenase and glucuronidation

Half-life elimination: Adults: 10-13 hours

Time to peak, serum: T_{max}: Immediate release: 3 hours; sustained release: 8 hours

Excretion: Urine (as unchanged drug and inactive metabolites)

Pregnancy Risk Factor C

Dextroamphetamine and Amphetamine

(deks troe am FET a meen & am FET a meen)

Related Information

Dextroamphetamine *on page 473*

U.S. Brand Names Adderall®; Adderall XR®

Canadian Brand Names Adderall XR®

Generic Available Yes: Tablet

Index Terms Amphetamine and Dextroamphetamine

Pharmacologic Category Stimulant

Use Attention-deficit/hyperactivity disorder (ADHD); narcolepsy

Local Anesthetic/Vasoconstrictor Precautions Use vasoconstrictor with caution in patients taking dextroamphetamine. Amphetamines enhance the sympathomimetic response of epinephrine and norepinephrine leading to potential hypertension and cardiotoxicity.

Effects on Dental Treatment Key adverse event(s) related to dental treatment: Tooth disorder; up to 10% of patients taking dextroamphetamines may present with hypertension. Monitor blood pressure prior to using local anesthetic with vasoconstrictors.

Common Adverse Effects

As reported with Adderall XR®:

>10%:

Central nervous system: Insomnia (12% to 27%), headache (up to 26% in adults)

Gastrointestinal: Appetite decreased (22% to 36%), abdominal pain (11% to 14%), dry mouth (2% to 35%), weight loss (4% to 11%)

1% to 10%:

Cardiovascular: Tachycardia (up to 6% in adults), palpitation (2% to 4%)

Central nervous system: Emotional lability (2% to 9%), agitation (up to 8% in adults), anxiety (8%), dizziness (2% to 7%), nervousness (6%), fever (5%), somnolence (2% to 4%)

Dermatologic: Photosensitization (2% to 4%)

Endocrine & metabolic: Dysmenorrhea (2% to 4%), impotence (2% to 4%), libido decreased (2% to 4%)

Gastrointestinal: Nausea (2% to 8%), vomiting (2% to 7%), diarrhea (2% to 6%), constipation (2% to 4%), dyspepsia (2% to 4%), tooth disorder (2% to 4%)

Genitourinary: Urinary tract infection (5%)

Neuromuscular & skeletal: Twitching (2% to 4%), weakness (2% to 6%)

Respiratory: Dyspnea (2% to 4%)

Miscellaneous: Diaphoresis (2% to 4%), infection (2% to 4%), speech disorder (2% to 4%)

Adverse reactions reported with other amphetamines include: Adverse reactions reported with other amphetamines include: Anaphylaxis, angioedema, anorexia, cardiomyopathy, depression, dyskinesia, dysphoria, euphoria, exacerbation of motor and phonic tics, exacerbation of Tourette's syndrome, hypertension, MI, overstimulation, psychosis, rash, restlessness, seizure, stroke, taste disturbance, tremor, urticaria

Restrictions C-II

An FDA-approved medication guide must be distributed when dispensing an outpatient prescription (new or refill) where this medication is to be used without direct supervision of a healthcare provider. Medication guides are available at http://www.fda.gov/cder/drug/infopage/ADHD/default.htm.

Dosage Oral: **Note:** Use lowest effective individualized dose; administer first dose as soon as awake

ADHD:

Children: <3 years: Not recommended

Children: 3-5 years (Adderall®): Initial 2.5 mg/day given every morning; increase daily dose in 2.5 mg increments at weekly intervals until optimal response is obtained (maximum dose: 40 mg/day given in 1-3 divided doses); use intervals of 4-6 hours between additional doses

Children: ≥6 years:

Adderall®: Initial: 5 mg 1-2 times/day; increase daily dose in 5 mg increments at weekly intervals until optimal response is obtained (usual maximum dose: 40 mg/day given in 1-3 divided doses); use intervals of 4-6 hours between additional doses

Adderall XR®: 5-10 mg once daily in the morning; if needed, may increase daily dose in 5-10 mg increments at weekly intervals (maximum dose: 30 mg/day)

Adolescents 13-17 years (Adderall XR®): 10 mg once daily in the morning; maybe increased to 20 mg/day after 1 week if symptoms are not controlled; higher doses (up to 60 mg/day) have been evaluated; however, there is not adequate evidence that higher doses afford additional benefit

Adults (Adderall XR®): Initial: 20 mg once daily in the morning; higher doses (up to 60 mg once daily) have been evaluated; however, there is not adequate evidence that higher doses afforded additional benefit

Narcolepsy (Adderall®):

Children: 6-12 years: Initial: 5 mg/day; increase daily dose in 5 mg at weekly intervals until optimal response is obtained (maximum dose: 60 mg/day given in 1-3 divided doses with intervals of 4-6 hours between doses)

Children >12 years and Adults: Initial: 10 mg/day; increase daily dose in 10 mg increments at weekly intervals until optimal response is obtained (maximum dose: 60 mg/day given in 1-3 divided doses with intervals of 4-6 hours between doses)

Mechanism of Action Blocks reuptake of dopamine and norepinephrine from the synapse, thus increases the amount of circulating dopamine and norepinephrine in cerebral cortex to reticular activating system; inhibits the action of monoamine oxidase and causes catecholamines to be released. Peripheral actions include elevation of blood pressure, weak bronchodilation, and respiratory stimulation.

Contraindications Hypersensitivity to dextroamphetamine, amphetamine, or any component of the formulation; advanced arteriosclerosis; symptomatic cardiovascular disease; moderate to severe hypertension; hyperthyroidism; hypersensitivity or idiosyncrasy to the sympathomimetic amines; glaucoma; agitated states; patients with a history of drug abuse; with or within 14 days following MAO inhibitor (hypertensive crisis)

Warnings/Precautions [U.S. Boxed Warning]: Use has been associated with serious cardiovascular events including sudden death in patients with pre-existing structural cardiac abnormalities or other serious heart problems (sudden death in children and adolescents; sudden death, stroke and MI in adults. These products should be avoided in the patients with known serious structural cardiac abnormalities, cardiomyopathy, serious heart rhythm abnormalities, or other serious cardiac problems that could increase the risk of sudden death that these conditions alone carry. Patients should be carefully evaluated for cardiac disease prior to initiation of therapy. Use with caution in patients with hypertension and other cardiovascular conditions that (Continued)

Dextroamphetamine and Amphetamine *(Continued)*

might be exacerbated by increases in blood pressure or heart rate. Amphetamines may impair the ability to engage in potentially hazardous activities. May cause visual disturbances.

Use with caution in patients with psychiatric or seizure disorders. May exacerbate symptoms of behavior and thought disorder in psychotic patients. Stimulants may unmask tics in individuals with coexisting Tourette's syndrome. **[U.S. Boxed Warning]: Potential for drug dependency exists; prolonged use may lead to drug dependency.** Use is contraindicated in patients with history of ethanol or drug abuse. Prescriptions should be written for the smallest quantity consistent with good patient care to minimize possibility of overdose. Abrupt discontinuation following high doses or for prolonged periods may result in symptoms for withdrawal. Safety and efficacy have not been established in children <3 years of age. Appetite suppression may occur; monitor weight during therapy, particularly in children. Use of stimulants has been associated with suppression of growth; monitor growth rate during treatment.

Drug Interactions
Cytochrome P450 Effect:
Dextroamphetamine: **Substrate** of CYP2D6 (major)

Amphetamine: **Substrate** of CYP2D6 (major); **Inhibits** CYP2D6 (weak)

Increased Effect/Toxicity: CYP2D6 inhibitors may increase the levels/effects of amphetamine and dextroamphetamine; example inhibitors include chlorpromazine, delavirdine, fluoxetine, miconazole, paroxetine, pergolide, quinidine, quinine, ritonavir, and ropinirole. Dextroamphetamine and amphetamine may precipitate hypertensive crisis or serotonin syndrome in patients receiving MAO inhibitors (selegiline >10 mg/day, isocarboxazid, phenelzine, tranylcypromine, furazolidone). Serotonin syndrome has also been associated with combinations of amphetamines and SSRIs; these combinations should be avoided. TCAs may enhance the effects of amphetamines, potentially leading to hypertensive crisis. Large doses of antacids or urinary alkalinizers increase the half-life and duration of action of amphetamines. May precipitate arrhythmias in patients receiving general anesthetics.

Decreased Effect: Urinary acidifiers decrease the half-life and duration of action of amphetamines. Efficacy of amphetamines may be decreased by antipsychotics.

Ethanol/Nutrition/Herb Interactions
Ethanol: Avoid ethanol (may increase CNS depression).

Food: Dextroamphetamine serum levels may be altered if taken with acidic food, juices, or vitamin C. Avoid caffeine.

Herb/Nutraceutical: Avoid ephedra (may cause hypertension or arrhythmias).

Pharmacodynamics/Kinetics
Onset: 30-60 minutes

Duration: 4-6 hours

Absorption: Well-absorbed

Distribution: V_d: Adults: 3.5-4.6 L/kg; concentrates in breast milk (avoid breast-feeding); distributes into CNS, mean CSF concentrations are 80% of plasma

Half-life elimination:

Children 6-12 years: d-amphetamine: 9 hours; l-amphetamine: 11 hours

Adolescents 13-17 years: d-amphetamine: 11 hours; l-amphetamine: 13-14 hours

Adults: d-amphetamine: 10 hours; l-amphetamine: 13 hours

Metabolism: Hepatic via cytochrome P450 monooxygenase and glucuronidation

Time to peak: T_{max}: Adderall®: 3 hours; Adderall XR®: 7 hours

Excretion: Urine (highly dependent on urinary pH); 70% of a single dose is eliminated within 24 hours; excreted as unchanged amphetamine (30%, may range from ~1% in alkaline urine to ~75% in acidic urine), benzoic acid, hydroxyamphetamine, hippuric acid, norephedrine, and *p*-hydroxynorephedrine

Pregnancy Risk Factor C
Dosage Forms
Capsule, extended release:
Adderall XR®:

5 mg [dextroamphetamine 1.25 mg, dextroamphetamine saccharate 1.25 mg, amphetamine aspartate monohydrate 1.25 mg, amphetamine sulfate 1.25 mg]

10 mg [dextroamphetamine sulfate 2.5 mg, dextroamphetamine saccharate 2.5 mg, amphetamine aspartate monohydrate 2.5 mg, amphetamine sulfate 2.5 mg]

15 mg [dextroamphetamine sulfate 3.75 mg, dextroamphetamine saccharate 3.75 mg, amphetamine aspartate monohydrate 3.75 mg, amphetamine sulfate 3.75 mg]

20 mg [dextroamphetamine sulfate 5 mg, dextroamphetamine saccharate 5 mg, amphetamine aspartate monohydrate 5 mg, amphetamine sulfate 5 mg]

25 mg [dextroamphetamine sulfate 6.25 mg, dextroamphetamine saccharate 6.25 mg, amphetamine aspartate monohydrate 6.25 mg, amphetamine sulfate 6.25 mg]

30 mg [dextroamphetamine sulfate 7.5 mg, dextroamphetamine saccharate 7.5 mg, amphetamine aspartate monohydrate 7.5 mg, amphetamine sulfate 7.5 mg]

Tablet: 5 mg, 7.5 mg, 10 mg, 12.5 mg, 15 mg, 20 mg, 30 mg

Adderall®:

5 mg [dextroamphetamine sulfate 1.25 mg, dextroamphetamine saccharate 1.25 mg, amphetamine aspartate 1.25 mg, amphetamine sulfate 1.25 mg]

7.5 mg [dextroamphetamine 1.875 mg, dextroamphetamine saccharate 1.875 mg, amphetamine aspartate 1.875 mg, amphetamine sulfate 1.875 mg]

10 mg [dextroamphetamine sulfate 2.5 mg, dextroamphetamine saccharate 2.5 mg, amphetamine aspartate 2.5 mg, amphetamine sulfate 2.5 mg]

12.5 mg [dextroamphetamine sulfate 3.125 mg, dextroamphetamine saccharate 3.125 mg, amphetamine aspartate 3.125 mg, amphetamine sulfate 3.125 mg]

15 mg [dextroamphetamine sulfate 3.75 mg, dextroamphetamine saccharate 3.75 mg, amphetamine aspartate 3.75 mg, amphetamine sulfate 3.75 mg]

20 mg [dextroamphetamine sulfate 5 mg, dextroamphetamine saccharate 5 mg, amphetamine aspartate 5 mg, amphetamine sulfate 5 mg]

30 mg [dextroamphetamine sulfate 7.5 mg, dextroamphetamine saccharate 7.5 mg, amphetamine aspartate 7.5 mg, amphetamine sulfate 7.5 mg]

Dextroamphetamine Sulfate *see* Dextroamphetamine *on page 473*

Dextromethorphan (deks troe meth OR fan)

U.S. Brand Names Babee® Cof Syrup [OTC]; Creomulsion® Cough [OTC]; Creomulsion® for Children [OTC]; Creo-Terpin® [OTC]; Delsym® [OTC]; Elix-Sure® Cough [OTC]; Hold® DM [OTC]; PediaCare® Children's Medicated Freezer Pops Long Acting Cough [OTC] [DSC]; PediaCare® Infants' Long-Acting Cough [OTC]; Robitussin® CoughGels™ [OTC]; Robitussin® Maximum Strength Cough [OTC]; Robitussin® Pediatric Cough [OTC]; Scot-Tussin DM® Cough Chasers [OTC]; Silphen DM® [OTC]; Simply Cough® [OTC] [DSC]; Triaminic® Thin Strips™ Long Acting Cough [OTC]; Vicks® 44® Cough Relief [OTC]

Generic Available Yes: Excludes strip, liquid freezer pop

Pharmacologic Category Antitussive

Use Symptomatic relief of coughs caused by minor viral upper respiratory tract infections or inhaled irritants; most effective for a chronic nonproductive cough

Unlabeled/Investigational Use *N*-methyl-D-aspartate (NMDA) antagonist in cerebral injury

Local Anesthetic/Vasoconstrictor Precautions No information available to require special precautions

Effects on Dental Treatment No significant effects or complications reported

Mechanism of Action Chemical relative of morphine lacking narcotic properties except in overdose; controls cough by depressing the medullary cough center

Drug Interactions

Cytochrome P450 Effect: Substrate of CYP2B6 (minor), 2C9 (minor), 2C19 (minor), 2D6 (major), 2E1 (minor), 3A4 (minor); **Inhibits** CYP2D6 (weak)

Increased Effect/Toxicity: CYP2D6 inhibitors may increase the levels/ effects of dextromethorphan; example inhibitors include chlorpromazine, delavirdine, fluoxetine, miconazole, paroxetine, pergolide, quinidine, quinine, ritonavir, and ropinirole. Dextromethorphan may increase effect/toxicity of MAO inhibitors.

Pharmacodynamics/Kinetics

Onset of action: Antitussive: 15-30 minutes

Duration: ≤6 hours

Pregnancy Risk Factor C

Dextromethorphan, Acetaminophen, and Pseudoephedrine *see* Acetaminophen, Dextromethorphan, and Pseudoephedrine *on page 44*

Dextromethorphan and Guaifenesin *see* Guaifenesin and Dextromethorphan *on page 796*

Dextromethorphan and Promethazine *see* Promethazine and Dextromethorphan *on page 1363*

DEXTROSE

Dextromethorphan and Pseudoephedrine *see* Pseudoephedrine and Dextromethorphan *on page 1383*

Dextromethorphan, Carbinoxamine, and Pseudoephedrine *see* Carbinoxamine, Pseudoephedrine, and Dextromethorphan *on page 282*

Dextromethorphan, Chlorpheniramine, and Phenylephrine *see* Chlorpheniramine, Phenylephrine, and Dextromethorphan *on page 342*

Dextromethorphan, Guaifenesin, and Pseudoephedrine *see* Guaifenesin, Pseudoephedrine, and Dextromethorphan *on page 800*

Dextromethorphan, Pseudoephedrine, and Carbinoxamine *see* Carbinoxamine, Pseudoephedrine, and Dextromethorphan *on page 282*

Dextropropoxyphene *see* Propoxyphene *on page 1368*

Dextrose (DEKS trose)

U.S. Brand Names B-D™ Glucose [OTC]; Dex4® Glucose [OTC]; Enfamil® Glucose; Glutol™ [OTC]; Glutose™ [OTC]; Insta-Glucose® [OTC]; Similac® Glucose

Generic Available Yes

Index Terms Anhydrous Glucose; Dextrose Monohydrate; D_5W; $D_{10}W$; $D_{25}W$; $D_{30}W$; $D_{40}W$; $D_{50}W$; $D_{60}W$; $D_{70}W$; Glucose; Glucose Monohydrate; Glycosum

Pharmacologic Category Antidote, Hypoglycemia; Intravenous Nutritional Therapy

Use
Oral: Treatment of hypoglycemia

5% and 10% solutions: Peripheral infusion to provide calories and fluid replacement

25% (hypertonic) solution: Treatment of acute symptomatic episodes of hypoglycemia in infants and children to restore depressed blood glucose levels; adjunctive treatment of hyperkalemia when combined with insulin

50% (hypertonic) solution: Treatment of insulin-induced hypoglycemia (hyperinsulinemia or insulin shock) and adjunctive treatment of hyperkalemia in adolescents and adults

≥10% solutions: Infusion after admixture with amino acids for nutritional support

Local Anesthetic/Vasoconstrictor Precautions No information available to require special precautions

Effects on Dental Treatment No significant effects or complications reported

Common Adverse Effects Frequency not defined. **Note:** Most adverse effects are associated with excessive dosage or rate of infusion.

Cardiovascular: Venous thrombosis, phlebitis, hypovolemia, hypervolemia, dehydration, edema

Central nervous system: Fever, mental confusion, unconsciousness, hyperosmolar syndrome

Endocrine & metabolic: Hyperglycemia, hypokalemia, acidosis, hypophosphatemia, hypomagnesemia

Genitourinary: Polyuria, glycosuria, ketonuria

Gastrointestinal: Polydipsia, nausea, diarrhea (oral)

Local: Pain, vein irritation, tissue necrosis

Respiratory: Tachypnea, pulmonary edema

Mechanism of Action Dextrose, a monosaccharide, is a source of calories and fluid for patients unable to obtain an adequate oral intake; may decrease body protein and nitrogen losses; promotes glycogen deposition in the liver. When used in the treatment of hyperkalemia (combined with insulin), dextrose stimulates the uptake of potassium by cells, especially in muscle tissue, lowering serum potassium.

Pharmacodynamics/Kinetics
Onset of action: Treatment of hypoglycemia: Oral: 10 minutes
Maximum effect: Treatment of hyperkalemia: I.V.: 30 minutes
Absorption: Rapidly from the small intestine by an active mechanism
Metabolism: Metabolized to carbon dioxide and water
Time to peak, serum: Oral: 40 minutes

Pregnancy Risk Factor C/A (oral)

Dextrose, Levulose, and Phosphoric Acid *see* Fructose, Dextrose, and Phosphoric Acid *on page 754*

Dextrose Monohydrate *see* Dextrose *on page 478*

Dextrostat® *see* Dextroamphetamine *on page 473*

DFMO *see* Eflornithine *on page 560*

DHAD *see* Mitoxantrone *on page 1113*

DHAQ *see* Mitoxantrone *on page 1113*

DHE *see* Dihydroergotamine *on page 504*

D.H.E. 45® *see* Dihydroergotamine *on page 504*

DHPG Sodium *see* Ganciclovir *on page 763*

DHS™ Sal [OTC] *see* Salicylic Acid *on page 1451*

DHS™ Tar [OTC] *see* Coal Tar *on page 402*

DHS™ Targel [OTC] *see* Coal Tar *on page 402*

DHS™ Zinc [OTC] *see* Pyrithione Zinc *on page 1391*

DHT™ [DSC] *see* Dihydrotachysterol *on page 504*

DHT™ Intensol™ [DSC] *see* Dihydrotachysterol *on page 504*

Diabeta *see* GlyBURIDE *on page 786*

DiabetAid™ Antifungal Foot Bath [OTC] *see* Miconazole *on page 1097*

DiabetAid Gingivitis Mouth Rinse [OTC] *see* Cetylpyridinium *on page 324*

Diabetic Tussin C® *see* Guaifenesin and Codeine *on page 795*

Diabetic Tussin® Allergy Relief [OTC] *see* Chlorpheniramine *on page 338*

Diabetic Tussin® DM [OTC] *see* Guaifenesin and Dextromethorphan *on page 796*

Diabetic Tussin® DM Maximum Strength [OTC] *see* Guaifenesin and Dextromethorphan *on page 796*

Diabetic Tussin® EX [OTC] *see* Guaifenesin *on page 795*

Diabinese® *see* ChlorproPAMIDE *on page 346*

Diaβeta® *see* GlyBURIDE *on page 786*

Diaminocyclohexane Oxalatoplatinum *see* Oxaliplatin *on page 1216*

Diaminodiphenylsulfone *see* Dapsone *on page 441*

Diamode [OTC] *see* Loperamide *on page 996*

Diamox® Sequels® *see* AcetaZOLAMIDE *on page 45*

Diasorb® [OTC] *see* Attapulgite *on page 170*

Diastat® *see* Diazepam *on page 480*

Diastat® AcuDial™ *see* Diazepam *on page 480*

Diatrizoate Meglumine (dye a tri ZOE ate MEG loo meen)

U.S. Brand Names Cystografin®; Cystografin® Dilute; Hypaque™ Meglumine; Reno-30®; Reno-60®; Reno-Dip®

Generic Available No

Pharmacologic Category Iodinated Contrast Media; Radiological/Contrast Media, Ionic

Use

Solution for instillation: Retrograde cystourethrography; retrograde or ascending pyelography

Solution for injection: Arthrography, cerebral angiography, direct cholangiography, discography, drip infusion pyelography, excretory urography, peripheral arteriography, splenoportography, venography; contrast enhancement of computed tomographic head imaging

Local Anesthetic/Vasoconstrictor Precautions No information available to require special precautions

Effects on Dental Treatment No significant effects or complications reported

Pregnancy Risk Factor C

Diatrizoate Meglumine and Diatrizoate Sodium
(dye a tri ZOE ate MEG loo meen & dye a tri ZOE ate SOW dee um)

U.S. Brand Names Gastrografin®; Hypaque™-76; MD-76®R; MD-Gastroview®; RenoCal-76®; Renografin®-60

Generic Available No

Index Terms Diatrizoate Sodium and Diatrizoate Meglumine

Pharmacologic Category Iodinated Contrast Media; Radiological/Contrast Media, Ionic

Use

Oral/rectal: Examination of GI tract; adjunct to contrast enhancement in computed tomography of the torso

Injection: Angiocardiography, aortography, central venography, cerebral angiography, cholangiography, digital arteriography, excretory urography, nephrotomography, peripheral angiography, peripheral arteriography, renal arteriography, renal venography, splenoportography, visceral arteriography; contrast enhancement of computed tomographic imaging

Local Anesthetic/Vasoconstrictor Precautions No information available to require special precautions

Effects on Dental Treatment No significant effects or complications reported

Pregnancy Risk Factor B/C (manufacturer dependent)

Diatrizoate Meglumine and Iodipamide Meglumine
(dye a tri ZOE ate MEG loo meen & eye oh DI pa mide MEG loo meen)

U.S. Brand Names Sinografin®
Generic Available No
Index Terms Iodipamide Meglumine and Diatrizoate Meglumine
Pharmacologic Category Iodinated Contrast Media; Radiological/Contrast Media, Ionic
Use Hysterosalpingography
Local Anesthetic/Vasoconstrictor Precautions No information available to require special precautions
Effects on Dental Treatment No significant effects or complications reported

Diatrizoate Sodium (dye a tri ZOE ate SOW dee um)

U.S. Brand Names Hypaque™ Sodium
Generic Available No
Pharmacologic Category Iodinated Contrast Media; Radiological/Contrast Media, Ionic
Use Radiographic examination of GI tract
Local Anesthetic/Vasoconstrictor Precautions No information available to require special precautions
Effects on Dental Treatment No significant effects or complications reported
Mechanism of Action When administered orally or given as an enema, the medium produces excellent opacification and delineation of the upper and lower gastrointestinal tract; however, because of dilution, contrast in the small bowel may be unsatisfactory.
Pregnancy Risk Factor C

Diatrizoate Sodium and Diatrizoate Meglumine *see* Diatrizoate Meglumine and Diatrizoate Sodium *on page 479*

Diatx™ *see* Vitamin B Complex Combinations *on page 1664*

Diazepam (dye AZ e pam)

Related Information
Sedation *on page 1825*
Temporomandibular Dysfunction (TMD) *on page 1822*
Related Sample Prescriptions
Sedation (Prior to Dental Treatment) *on page 1846*
U.S. Brand Names Diastat®; Diastat® AcuDial™; Diazepam Intensol®; Valium®
Canadian Brand Names Apo-Diazepam®; Diastat®; Diastat® Rectal Delivery System; Diazemuls®; Novo-Dipam; Valium®
Mexican Brand Names Alboral; Diapanil; Ortopsique; Valium
Generic Available Yes: Injection, tablet, solution only
Pharmacologic Category Benzodiazepine
Dental Use Oral medication for preoperative dental anxiety; sedative component in I.V. conscious sedation in oral surgery patients; skeletal muscle relaxant
Use Management of anxiety disorders, ethanol withdrawal symptoms; skeletal muscle relaxant; treatment of convulsive disorders
Rectal gel: Management of selected, refractory epilepsy patients on stable regimens of antiepileptic drugs (AEDs) requiring intermittent use of diazepam to control episodes of increased seizure activity
Unlabeled/Investigational Use Panic disorders; preoperative sedation, light anesthesia, amnesia
Local Anesthetic/Vasoconstrictor Precautions No information available to require special precautions
Effects on Dental Treatment Key adverse event(s) related to dental treatment: Xerostomia and changes in salivation (normal salivary flow resumes upon discontinuation).
Significant Adverse Effects Frequency not defined. Adverse reactions may vary by route of administration.

Cardiovascular: Hypotension, vasodilatation
Central nervous system: Agitation, amnesia, anxiety, ataxia, confusion, depression, dizziness, drowsiness, emotional lability, euphoria, fatigue, headache, incoordination, insomnia, memory impairment, paradoxical excitement or rage, seizure, slurred speech, somnolence, vertigo
Dermatologic: Rash
Endocrine & metabolic: Libido changes
Gastrointestinal: Constipation, diarrhea, nausea, salivation changes

Genitourinary: Incontinence, urinary retention
Hepatic: Jaundice
Local: Phlebitis, pain with injection
Neuromuscular & skeletal: Dysarthria, tremor, weakness
Ocular: Blurred vision, diplopia
Respiratory: Apnea, asthma, respiratory rate decreased

Restrictions C-IV

Dental Usual Dosing

Anxiety/sedation/skeletal muscle relaxant: Adults:
Oral: 2-10 mg 2-4 times/day
I.M., I.V.: 2-10 mg, may repeat in 3-4 hours if needed

Anxiety: Elderly: Oral: Initial: 1-2 mg 1-2 times/day; increase gradually as needed, rarely need to use >10 mg/day (watch for hypotension and excessive sedation)

Skeletal muscle relaxant: Elderly: Oral: Initial: 2-5 mg 2-4 times/day

Dosage Oral absorption is more reliable than I.M.

Children:
Conscious sedation for procedures: Oral: 0.2-0.3 mg/kg (maximum: 10 mg) 45-60 minutes prior to procedure

Sedation/muscle relaxant/anxiety:
Oral: 0.12-0.8 mg/kg/day in divided doses every 6-8 hours
I.M., I.V.: 0.04-0.3 mg/kg/dose every 2-4 hours to a maximum of 0.6 mg/kg within an 8-hour period if needed

Status epilepticus:
Infants 30 days to 5 years: I.V.: 0.05-0.3 mg/kg/dose given over 2-3 minutes, every 15-30 minutes to a maximum total dose of 5 mg; repeat in 2-4 hours as needed **or** 0.2-0.5 mg/dose every 2-5 minutes to a maximum total dose of 5 mg
>5 years: I.V.: 0.05-0.3 mg/kg/dose given over 2-3 minutes every 15-30 minutes to a maximum total dose of 10 mg; repeat in 2-4 hours as needed **or** 1 mg/dose given over 2-3 minutes, every 2-5 minutes to a maximum total dose of 10 mg

Rectal: 0.5 mg/kg, then 0.25 mg/kg in 10 minutes if needed (prepare dose using parenteral formulation)

Anticonvulsant (acute treatment): Rectal gel:
Children <2 years: Safety and efficacy have not been studied
Children 2-5 years: 0.5 mg/kg
Children 6-11 years: 0.3 mg/kg
Children ≥12 years: 0.2 mg/kg
Note: Dosage should be rounded upward to the next available dose, 2.5, 5, 7.5, 10, 12.5, 15, 17.5, and 20 mg/dose; dose may be repeated in 4-12 hours if needed; do not use for more than 5 episodes per month or more than one episode every 5 days

Adolescents: Conscious sedation for procedures:
Oral: 10 mg
I.V.: 5 mg, may repeat with ¹/₂ dose if needed

Adults:
Anticonvulsant (acute treatment): Rectal gel: 0.2 mg/kg
Note: Dosage should be rounded upward to the next available dose, 2.5, 5, 7.5, 10, 12.5, 15, 17.5, and 20 mg/dose; dose may be repeated in 4-12 hours if needed; do not use for more than 5 episodes per month or more than one episode every 5 days.

Anxiety/sedation/skeletal muscle relaxant:
Oral: 2-10 mg 2-4 times/day
I.M., I.V.: 2-10 mg, may repeat in 3-4 hours if needed

Sedation in the ICU patient: I.V.: 0.03-0.1 mg/kg every 30 minutes to 6 hours

Status epilepticus: I.V.: 5-10 mg every 10-20 minutes, up to 30 mg in an 8-hour period; may repeat in 2-4 hours if necessary

Rapid tranquilization of agitated patient (administer every 30-60 minutes): Oral: 5-10 mg; average total dose for tranquilization: 20-60 mg

Elderly:
Anticonvulsant: Rectal gel: Due to the increased half-life in elderly and debilitated patients, consider reducing dose.
Anxiety: Oral: Initial: 1-2 mg 1-2 times/day; increase gradually as needed, rarely need to use >10 mg/day (watch for hypotension and excessive sedation)
Skeletal muscle relaxant: Oral: Initial: 2-5 mg 2-4 times/day

Hemodialysis: Not dialyzable (0% to 5%); supplemental dose is not necessary

Dosing adjustment in hepatic impairment: Reduce dose by 50% in cirrhosis and avoid in severe/acute liver disease

Mechanism of Action Binds to stereospecific benzodiazepine receptors on the postsynaptic GABA neuron at several sites within the central nervous system, including the limbic system, reticular formation. Enhancement of the inhibitory
(Continued)

Diazepam (Continued)

effect of GABA on neuronal excitability results by increased neuronal membrane permeability to chloride ions. This shift in chloride ions results in hyperpolarization (a less excitable state) and stabilization.

Contraindications Hypersensitivity to diazepam or any component of the formulation (cross-sensitivity with other benzodiazepines may exist); narrow-angle glaucoma; not for use in children <6 months of age (oral); pregnancy

Warnings/Precautions Withdrawal has also been associated with an increase in the seizure frequency. Use with caution with drugs which may decrease diazepam metabolism. Use with caution in elderly or debilitated patients, obese patients, patients with hepatic disease (including alcoholics), respiratory disease, impaired gag reflex, or renal impairment. Active metabolites with extended half-lives may lead to delayed accumulation and adverse effects.

Acute hypotension, muscle weakness, apnea, and cardiac arrest have occurred with parenteral administration. Acute effects may be more prevalent in patients receiving concurrent barbiturates, narcotics, or ethanol. Appropriate resuscitative equipment and qualified personnel should be available during administration and monitoring. Avoid use of the injection in patients with shock, coma, or acute ethanol intoxication. Intra-arterial injection or extravasation of the parenteral formulation should be avoided. Parenteral formulation contains propylene glycol, which has been associated with toxicity when administered in high dosages. Administration of rectal gel should only be performed by individuals trained to recognize characteristic seizure activity and monitor response.

Causes CNS depression (dose-related) resulting in sedation, dizziness, confusion, or ataxia which may impair physical and mental capabilities. Use with caution in patients receiving other CNS depressants or psychoactive agents. Effects with other sedative drugs or ethanol may be potentiated. The dosage of narcotics should be reduced by approximately $\frac{1}{3}$ when diazepam is added. Benzodiazepines have been associated with falls and traumatic injury and should be used with extreme caution in patients who are at risk of these events (especially the elderly). Use with caution in patients taking strong CYP3A4 inhibitors, moderate or strong CYP3A4 and CYP2C19 inducers and major CYP3A4 substrates.

Use caution in patients with depression, particularly if suicidal risk may be present, or in patients with a history of drug dependence. Benzodiazepines have been associated with dependence and acute withdrawal symptoms on discontinuation or reduction in dose. Acute withdrawal, including seizures, may be precipitated in patients after administration of flumazenil to patients receiving long-term benzodiazepine therapy.

Diazepam has been associated with anterograde amnesia. Paradoxical reactions, including hyperactive or aggressive behavior, have been reported with benzodiazepines, particularly in adolescent/pediatric or psychiatric patients. Does not have analgesic, antidepressant, or antipsychotic properties.

Rectal gel: Safety and efficacy have not been established in children <2 years of age.

Oral: Safety and efficacy have not been established in children <6 months of age.

Injection: Safety and efficacy have not been established in children <30 days of age. Solution for injection may contain sodium benzoate, benzyl alcohol, or benzoic acid. Large amounts have been associated with "gasping syndrome" in neonates.

Drug Interactions Substrate of CYP1A2 (minor), 2B6 (minor), 2C9 (minor), 2C19 (major), 3A4 (major); **Inhibits** CYP2C19 (weak), 3A4 (weak)

Calcium channel blockers, nondihydropyridine (diltiazem, verapamil): May decrease the metabolism, via CYP isoenzymes, of diazepam.

Clozapine: Benzodiazepines may enhance the adverse/toxic effect of clozapine.

CNS depressants: Sedative effects and/or respiratory depression may be additive with CNS depressants; includes ethanol, barbiturates, opioid analgesics, and other sedative agents; monitor for increased effect.

CYP2C19 inducers: May decrease the levels/effects of diazepam. Example inducers include aminoglutethimide, carbamazepine, phenytoin, and rifampin.

CYP2C19 inhibitors: May increase the levels/effects of diazepam. Example inhibitors include delavirdine, fluconazole, fluvoxamine, gemfibrozil, isoniazid, omeprazole, and ticlopidine.

CYP3A4 inducers: CYP3A4 inducers may decrease the levels/effects of diazepam. Example inducers include aminoglutethimide, carbamazepine, nafcillin, nevirapine, phenobarbital, phenytoin, and rifamycins.

CYP3A4 inhibitors: May increase the levels/effects of diazepam. Example inhibitors include azole antifungals, clarithromycin, diclofenac, doxycycline, erythromycin, imatinib, isoniazid, nefazodone, nicardipine, propofol, protease inhibitors, quinidine, telithromycin, and verapamil.

Levodopa: Therapeutic effects may be diminished in some patients following the addition of a benzodiazepine; limited/inconsistent data.

Oral contraceptives: May decrease the clearance of some benzodiazepines (those which undergo oxidative metabolism); monitor for increased benzodiazepine effect.

Theophylline: May partially antagonize some of the effects of benzodiazepines; monitor for decreased response; may require higher doses for sedation.

Ethanol/Nutrition/Herb Interactions

Ethanol: Avoid ethanol (may increase CNS depression).

Food: Diazepam serum levels may be increased if taken with food. Diazepam effect/toxicity may be increased by grapefruit juice; avoid concurrent use.

Herb/Nutraceutical: St John's wort may decrease diazepam levels. Avoid valerian, St John's wort, kava kava, gotu kola (may increase CNS depression).

Pharmacodynamics/Kinetics

I.V.: Status epilepticus:
Onset of action: Almost immediate
Duration: 20-30 minutes

Absorption: Oral: 85% to 100%, more reliable than I.M.

Protein binding: 98%

Metabolism: Hepatic

Half-life elimination: Parent drug: Adults: 20-50 hours; increased half-life in neonates, elderly, and those with severe hepatic disorders; Active major metabolite (desmethyldiazepam): 50-100 hours; may be prolonged in neonates

Pregnancy Risk Factor D

Lactation Enters breast milk/contraindicated (AAP rates "of concern")

Breast-Feeding Considerations Clinical effects on the infant include sedation; AAP reports that USE MAY BE OF CONCERN.

Dosage Forms Excipient information presented when available (limited, particularly for generics); consult specific product labeling.

Gel, rectal:
Diastat® Pediatric rectal tip [4.4 cm]: 5 mg/mL (2.5 mg, 5 mg) [contains ethyl alcohol 10%, sodium benzoate, benzyl alcohol 1.5%; twin pack]
Diastat® AcuDial™ delivery system:
10 mg: Pediatric/adult rectal tip [4.4 cm]: 5 mg/mL (delivers set doses of 5 mg, 7.5 mg, and 10 mg) [contains ethyl alcohol 10%, sodium benzoate, benzyl alcohol 1.5%; twin pack]
20 mg: Adult rectal tip [6 cm]: 5 mg/mL (delivers set doses of 10 mg, 12.5 mg, 15 mg, 17.5 mg, and 20 mg) [contains ethyl alcohol 10%, sodium benzoate, benzyl alcohol 1.5%; twin pack]
Injection, solution: 5 mg/mL (2 mL, 10 mL) [may contain benzyl alcohol, sodium benzoate, benzoic acid]
Solution, oral: 5 mg/5 mL (5 mL, 500 mL) [wintergreen-spice flavor]
Solution, oral concentrate:
Diazepam Intensol®: 5 mg/mL (30 mL)
Tablet: 2 mg, 5 mg, 10 mg
Valium®: 2 mg, 5 mg, 10 mg

Diazepam Intensol® see Diazepam on page 480

Diazoxide (dye az OKS ide)

U.S. Brand Names Hyperstat® [DSC]; Proglycem®
Canadian Brand Names Proglycem®
Generic Available No
Pharmacologic Category Antihypertensive; Antihypoglycemic Agent
Use
Oral: Hypoglycemia related to islet cell adenoma, carcinoma, hyperplasia, or adenomatosis, nesidioblastosis, leucine sensitivity, or extrapancreatic malignancy
I.V.: Severe hypertension

Local Anesthetic/Vasoconstrictor Precautions No information available to require special precautions

Effects on Dental Treatment No significant effects or complications reported

Common Adverse Effects 1% to 10%:
Cardiovascular: Hypotension
Central nervous system: Dizziness
Gastrointestinal: Nausea, vomiting
Neuromuscular & skeletal: Weakness
(Continued)

Diazoxide *(Continued)*

Mechanism of Action Activates potassium channels. Inhibits insulin release from the pancreas; produces direct smooth muscle relaxation of the peripheral arterioles which results in decrease in blood pressure and reflex increase in heart rate and cardiac output

Drug Interactions

Increased Effect/Toxicity: Diuretics and hypotensive agents may potentiate diazoxide adverse effects. Diazoxide may decrease warfarin protein binding.

Decreased Effect: Diazoxide may increase phenytoin metabolism or free fraction.

Pharmacodynamics/Kinetics

Onset of action: Hyperglycemic: Oral: ~1 hour
  Peak effect: Hypotensive: I.V.: ~5 minutes
Duration: Hyperglycemic: Oral: Normal renal function: 8 hours; Hypotensive: I.V.: Usually 3-12 hours
Protein binding: 90%
Half-life elimination: Children: 9-24 hours; Adults: 20-36 hours; End-stage renal disease: >30 hours
Excretion: Urine (50% as unchanged drug)

Pregnancy Risk Factor C

Dibenzyline® *see* Phenoxybenzamine *on page 1290*

Dibucaine (DYE byoo kane)

U.S. Brand Names Nupercainal® [OTC]
Generic Available Yes
Pharmacologic Category Local Anesthetic
Dental Use Amide derivative local anesthetic for minor skin conditions
Use Fast, temporary relief of pain and itching due to hemorrhoids, minor burns
Local Anesthetic/Vasoconstrictor Precautions No information available to require special precautions
Effects on Dental Treatment No significant effects or complications reported
Significant Adverse Effects 1% to 10%:
  Dermatologic: Angioedema, contact dermatitis
  Local: Burning
Dental Usual Dosing Local pain (local anesthetic): Children and Adults: Topical: Apply gently to the affected areas; no more than 30 g for adults or 7.5 g for children should be used in any 24-hour period
Dosage Children and Adults: Topical: Apply gently to the affected areas; no more than 30 g for adults or 7.5 g for children should be used in any 24-hour period
Mechanism of Action Local anesthetics bind selectively to the intracellular surface of sodium channels to block influx of sodium into the axon. As a result, depolarization necessary for action potential propagation and subsequent nerve function is prevented. The block at the sodium channel is reversible. When drug diffuses away from the axon, sodium channel function is restored and nerve propagation returns.
Contraindications Hypersensitivity to amide-type anesthetics, ophthalmic use
Drug Interactions No data reported
Pharmacodynamics/Kinetics
  Onset of action: ~15 minutes
  Duration: 2-4 hours
  Absorption: Poor through intact skin; well absorbed through mucous membranes and excoriated skin
Pregnancy Risk Factor C
Breast-Feeding Considerations No data reported; however, topical administration is probably compatible.
Dosage Forms Excipient information presented when available (limited, particularly for generics); consult specific product labeling.
  Ointment: 1% (30 g, 454 g)
    Nupercainal®: 1% (30 g, 60g) [contains sodium bisulfite]

DIC *see* Dacarbazine *on page 435*

Dicel™ *see* Chlorpheniramine and Pseudoephedrine *on page 340*

Dichloralphenazone, Acetaminophen, and Isometheptene *see* Acetaminophen, Isometheptene, and Dichloralphenazone *on page 45*

Dichloralphenazone, Isometheptene, and Acetaminophen *see* Acetaminophen, Isometheptene, and Dichloralphenazone *on page 45*

6,7-Dichloro-1,5-Dihydroimidazo [2,1b] quinazolin-2(3H)-one Monohydrochloride *see* Anagrelide *on page 127*

Dichlorodifluoromethane and Trichloromonofluoromethane
(dye klor oh dye flor oh METH ane & tri klor oh mon oh flor oh METH ane)

Related Information
Temporomandibular Dysfunction (TMD) *on page 1822*
U.S. Brand Names Fluori-Methane®
Generic Available No
Index Terms Trichloromonofluoromethane and Dichlorodifluoromethane
Pharmacologic Category Analgesic, Topical
Dental Use Topical application in the management of myofascial pain, restricted motion, and muscle spasm
Use Management of pain associated with injections
Local Anesthetic/Vasoconstrictor Precautions No information available to require special precautions
Effects on Dental Treatment No significant effects or complications reported
Significant Adverse Effects No data reported.
Dosage Invert bottle over treatment area approximately 12" away from site of application; open dispenseal spring valve completely, allowing liquid to flow in a stream from the bottle. The rate of spraying is approximately 10 cm/second and should be continued until entire muscle has been covered.
Contraindications Hypersensitivity to dichlorofluoromethane and/or trichloromonofluoromethane, or any component of the formulation; patients having vascular impairment of the extremities
Warnings/Precautions For external use only; care should be taken to minimize inhalation of vapors, especially with application to head and neck; avoid contact with eyes; should not be applied to the point of frost formation
Drug Interactions No data reported
Pharmacodynamics/Kinetics No data reported
Dosage Forms Excipient information presented when available (limited, particularly for generics); consult specific product labeling.
Aerosol, topical: Dichlorodifluoromethane 15% and trichloromonofluoromethane 85% (103 mL) [contains chlorofluorocarbons]

Dichlorotetrafluoroethane and Ethyl Chloride *see* Ethyl Chloride and Dichlorotetrafluoroethane *on page 654*

Dichlorphenamide (dye klor FEN a mide)

U.S. Brand Names Daranide®
Canadian Brand Names Daranide®
Generic Available No
Index Terms Diclofenamide
Pharmacologic Category Carbonic Anhydrase Inhibitor; Diuretic, Carbonic Anhydrase Inhibitor; Ophthalmic Agent, Antiglaucoma
Use Adjunct in treatment of open-angle glaucoma and perioperative treatment for angle-closure glaucoma
Local Anesthetic/Vasoconstrictor Precautions No information available to require special precautions
Effects on Dental Treatment Key adverse event(s) related to dental treatment: Metallic taste.
Pregnancy Risk Factor C

Dichysterol *see* Dihydrotachysterol *on page 504*

Diclofenac (dye KLOE fen ak)

Related Information
Rheumatoid Arthritis, Osteoarthritis, and Osteoporosis *on page 1759*
Temporomandibular Dysfunction (TMD) *on page 1822*
U.S. Brand Names Cataflam®; Solaraze®; Voltaren®; Voltaren Ophthalmic®; Voltaren®-XR
Canadian Brand Names Apo-Diclo®; Apo-Diclo Rapide®; Apo-Diclo SR®; Cataflam®; Novo-Difenac; Novo-Difenac K; Novo-Difenac-SR; Nu-Diclo; Nu-Diclo-SR; Pennsaid®; PMS-Diclofenac; PMS-Diclofenac SR; Riva-Diclofenac; Riva-Diclofenac-K; Voltaren®; Voltaren Ophtha®; Voltaren Rapide®
Mexican Brand Names Artrenac; Cataflam; Clonodifen; Dioxaflex; Dolaren; Dolflam-Retard; Evadol; Lifenac; Voltaren; Voltaren Emulgel; Voltaren Ofta; Voltaren Retard
Generic Available Yes: Excludes gel, ophthalmic solution
(Continued)

Diclofenac *(Continued)*

Index Terms Diclofenac Potassium; Diclofenac Sodium

Pharmacologic Category Nonsteroidal Anti-inflammatory Drug (NSAID); Nonsteroidal Anti-inflammatory Drug (NSAID), Ophthalmic; Nonsteroidal Anti-inflammatory Drug (NSAID), Oral

Dental Use Immediate-release tablets: Acute treatment of mild to moderate pain

Use

Immediate release: Ankylosing spondylitis; primary dysmenorrhea; acute and chronic treatment of rheumatoid arthritis, osteoarthritis

Delayed-release tablets: Acute and chronic treatment of rheumatoid arthritis, osteoarthritis, ankylosing spondylitis

Extended-release tablets: Chronic treatment of osteoarthritis, rheumatoid arthritis

Ophthalmic solution: Postoperative inflammation following cataract extraction; temporary relief of pain and photophobia in patients undergoing corneal refractive surgery

Topical gel: Actinic keratosis (AK) in conjunction with sun avoidance

Unlabeled/Investigational Use Juvenile rheumatoid arthritis

Local Anesthetic/Vasoconstrictor Precautions No information available to require special precautions

Effects on Dental Treatment NSAID formulations are known to reversibly decrease platelet aggregation via mechanisms different than observed with aspirin. The dentist should be aware of the potential of abnormal coagulation. Caution should also be exercised in the use of NSAIDs in patients already on anticoagulant therapy with drugs such as warfarin (Coumadin®).

Significant Adverse Effects

>10%:
  Local: Application site reactions (gel): Pruritus (31% to 52%), rash (35% to 46%), contact dermatitis (19% to 33%), dry skin (25% to 27%), pain (15% to 26%), exfoliation (6% to 24%), paresthesia (8% to 20%)
  Ocular: Ophthalmic drops (incidence may be dependent upon indication): Lacrimation (30%), keratitis (28%), elevated IOP (15%), transient burning/stinging (15%)

1% to 10%:
  Central nervous system: Headache (7%), dizziness (3%)
  Dermatologic: Pruritus (1% to 3%), rash (1% to 3%)
  Endocrine & metabolic: Fluid retention (1% to 3%)
  Gastrointestinal: Abdominal cramps (3% to 9%), abdominal pain (3% to 9%), constipation (3% to 9%), diarrhea (3% to 9%), flatulence (3% to 9%), indigestion (3% to 9%), nausea (3% to 9%), abdominal distention (1% to 3%), peptic ulcer/GI bleed (0.6% to 2%)
  Hepatic: ALT/AST increased (2%)
  Local: Application site reactions (gel): Edema (4%)
  Ocular: Ophthalmic drops: Abnormal vision, acute elevated IOP, blurred vision, conjunctivitis, corneal deposits, corneal edema, corneal opacity, corneal lesions, discharge, eyelid swelling, injection, iritis, irritation, itching, lacrimation disorder, ocular allergy
  Otic: Tinnitus (1% to 3%)

<1% (Limited to important or life-threatening): Oral dosage forms: Acute renal failure, agranulocytosis, allergic purpura, alopecia, anaphylactoid reactions, anaphylaxis, angioedema, aplastic anemia, aseptic meningitis, asthma, bullous eruption, cirrhosis, CHF, eosinophilia, erythema multiforme major, GI hemorrhage, hearing loss, hemolytic anemia, hepatic necrosis, hepatitis, hepatorenal syndrome, interstitial nephritis, jaundice, laryngeal edema, leukopenia, nephrotic syndrome, pancreatitis, papillary necrosis, photosensitivity, purpura, Stevens-Johnson syndrome, swelling of lips and tongue, thrombocytopenia, urticaria, visual changes, vomiting

Restrictions An FDA-approved medication guide must be distributed when dispensing an oral outpatient prescription (new or refill) where this medication is to be used without direct supervision of a healthcare provider. Medication guides are available at http://www.fda.gov/cder/Offices/ODS/medication_guides.htm.

Dental Usual Dosing Pain: Adults: Oral: Starting dose: 50 mg 3 times/day; maximum dose: 150 mg/day

Dosage Adults:

Oral:

Analgesia/primary dysmenorrhea: Starting dose: 50 mg 3 times/day; maximum dose: 150 mg/day

Rheumatoid arthritis: 150-200 mg/day in 2-4 divided doses (100 mg/day of sustained release product)

Osteoarthritis: 100-150 mg/day in 2-3 divided doses (100-200 mg/day of sustained release product)

Ankylosing spondylitis: 100-125 mg/day in 4-5 divided doses

Ophthalmic:

Cataract surgery: Instill 1 drop into affected eye 4 times/day beginning 24 hours after cataract surgery and continuing for 2 weeks

Corneal refractive surgery: Instill 1-2 drops into affected eye within the hour prior to surgery, within 15 minutes following surgery, and then continue for 4 times/day, up to 3 days

Topical: Apply gel to lesion area twice daily for 60-90 days

Dosage adjustment in renal impairment: Not recommended in patients with advanced renal disease

Dosage adjustment in hepatic impairment: No specific dosing recommendations

Elderly: No specific dosing recommendations; elderly may demonstrate adverse effects at lower doses than younger adults, and >60% may develop asymptomatic peptic ulceration with or without hemorrhage; monitor renal function

Mechanism of Action Inhibits prostaglandin synthesis by decreasing the activity of the enzyme, cyclooxygenase, which results in decreased formation of prostaglandin precursors. Mechanism of action for the treatment of AK has not been established.

Contraindications Hypersensitivity to diclofenac, aspirin, other NSAIDs, or any component of the formulation; perioperative pain in the setting of coronary artery bypass surgery (CABG); pregnancy (3rd trimester)

Warnings/Precautions [U.S. Boxed Warning]: NSAIDs are associated with an increased risk of adverse cardiovascular events, including MI, stroke, and new onset or worsening of pre-existing hypertension. Risk may be increased with duration of use or pre-existing cardiovascular risk factors or disease. Carefully evaluate individual cardiovascular risk profiles prior to prescribing. Use caution with fluid retention, CHF, or hypertension. Concurrent administration of ibuprofen, and potentially other nonselective NSAIDs, may interfere with aspirin's cardioprotective effect.

Use of NSAIDs can compromise existing renal function. Renal toxicity can occur in patient with impaired renal function, dehydration, heart failure, liver dysfunction, those taking diuretics and ACEI, and the elderly. Rehydrate patient before starting therapy. Monitor renal function closely. Not recommended for use in patients with advanced renal disease.

[U.S. Boxed Warning]: NSAIDs may increase risk of gastrointestinal irritation, ulceration, bleeding, and perforation. These events may occur at any time during therapy and without warning. Use caution with a history of GI disease (bleeding or ulcers), concurrent therapy with aspirin, anticoagulants and/or corticosteroids, smoking, use of alcohol, the elderly or debilitated patients.

Use the lowest effective dose for the shortest duration of time, consistent with individual patient goals, to reduce risk of cardiovascular or GI adverse events. Alternate therapies should be considered for patients at high risk.

NSAIDs may cause serious skin adverse events including exfoliative dermatitis, Stevens-Johnson syndrome (SJS), and toxic epidermal necrolysis (TEN). Anaphylactoid reactions may occur, even without prior exposure; patients with "aspirin triad" (bronchial asthma, aspirin intolerance, rhinitis) may be at increased risk. Do not use in patients who experience bronchospasm, asthma, rhinitis, or urticaria with NSAID or aspirin therapy. Use caution in other forms of asthma.

Use with caution in patients with decreased hepatic function. Closely monitor patients with any abnormal LFT. Severe hepatic reactions (eg, fulminant hepatitis, liver failure) have occurred with NSAID use, rarely; discontinue if signs or symptoms of liver disease develop, or if systemic manifestations occur.

The elderly are at increased risk for adverse effects (especially peptic ulceration, CNS effects, renal toxicity) from NSAIDs even at low doses.

Withhold for at least 4-6 half-lives prior to surgical or dental procedures. Safety and efficacy have not been established in children.

Topical gel should not be applied to the eyes, open wounds, infected areas, or to exfoliative dermatitis. Monitor patients for 1 year following application of ophthalmic drops for corneal refractive procedures. Patients using ophthalmic drops should not wear soft contact lenses. Ophthalmic drops may slow/delay healing or prolong bleeding time following surgery.

Drug Interactions Substrate (minor) of CYP1A2, 2B6, 2C8, 2C9, 2C19, 2D6, 3A4; **Inhibits** CYP1A2 (moderate), 2C9 (weak), 2E1 (weak), 3A4 (strong)

ACE inhibitors: Antihypertensive effects may be decreased by concurrent therapy with NSAIDs; monitor blood pressure.

Angiotensin II antagonists: Antihypertensive effects may be decreased by concurrent therapy with NSAIDs; monitor blood pressure.

(Continued)

Diclofenac *(Continued)*

Anticoagulants (warfarin, heparin, LMWHs) in combination with NSAIDs can cause increased risk of bleeding.

Antiplatelet drugs (ticlopidine, clopidogrel, aspirin, abciximab, dipyridamole, eptifibatide, tirofiban) can cause an increased risk of bleeding.

Beta-blockers: NSAIDs may decrease the antihypertensive effect of beta-blockers; monitor.

Cholestyramine (and other bile acid sequestrants): May decrease the absorption of NSAIDs. Separate by at least 2 hours.

Corticosteroids may increase the risk of GI ulceration; avoid concurrent use.

Cyclosporine: NSAIDs may increase serum creatinine, potassium, blood pressure, and cyclosporine levels; monitor cyclosporine levels and renal function carefully.

CYP1A2 substrates: Diclofenac may increase the levels/effects of CYP1A2 substrates. Example substrates include aminophylline, fluvoxamine, mexiletine, mirtazapine, ropinirole, theophylline, and trifluoperazine.

CYP3A4 substrates: Diclofenac may increase the levels/effects of CYP3A4 substrates. Example substrates include benzodiazepines, calcium channel blockers, mirtazapine, nateglinide, nefazodone, tacrolimus, and venlafaxine. Selected benzodiazepines (midazolam and triazolam), cisapride, ergot alkaloids, selected HMG-CoA reductase inhibitors (lovastatin and simvastatin), and pimozide are generally contraindicated with strong CYP3A4 inhibitors.

Fluoroquinolone antibiotics: Risk of seizures may be increased with concomitant quinolone use. Risk is considered quite low and may only be a factor with high serum levels of either agent and/or in patients with additional predisposing factors (eg, renal dysfunction, history of seizure or other neurological disorder).

Gentamicin and amikacin serum concentrations are increased by indomethacin in premature infants. Results may apply to other aminoglycosides and NSAIDs.

Hydralazine's antihypertensive effect is decreased; avoid concurrent use.

Lithium levels can be increased; avoid concurrent use if possible or monitor lithium levels and adjust dose. Sulindac may have the least effect. When NSAID is stopped, lithium will need adjustment again.

Loop diuretics efficacy (diuretic and antihypertensive effect) is reduced. Indomethacin reduces this efficacy, however, it may be anticipated with any NSAID.

Methotrexate: Severe bone marrow suppression, aplastic anemia, and GI toxicity have been reported with concomitant NSAID therapy. Avoid use during moderate or high-dose methotrexate (increased and prolonged methotrexate levels). NSAID use during low-dose treatment of rheumatoid arthritis has not been fully evaluated; extreme caution is warranted.

Thiazides antihypertensive effects are decreased; avoid concurrent use.

Verapamil plasma concentration is decreased by diclofenac; avoid concurrent use.

Warfarin's INRs may be increased by piroxicam. Other NSAIDs may have the same effect depending on dose and duration. Monitor INR closely. Use the lowest dose of NSAIDs possible and for the briefest duration.

Ethanol/Nutrition/Herb Interactions

Ethanol: Avoid ethanol (may enhance gastric mucosal irritation).

Herb/Nutraceutical: Avoid alfalfa, anise, bilberry, bladderwrack, bromelain, cat's claw, celery, coleus, cordyceps, dong quai, evening primrose, feverfew, fenugreek, garlic, ginger, ginkgo biloba, red clover, horse chestnut, grapeseed, green tea, ginseng, guggul, horse chestnut seed, horseradish, licorice, prickly ash, red clover, reishi, SAMe, sweet clover, turmeric, white willow (all have additional antiplatelet activity).

Dietary Considerations
May be taken with food to decrease GI distress.

Diclofenac potassium = Cataflam®; potassium content: 5.8 mg (0.15 mEq) per 50 mg tablet

Pharmacodynamics/Kinetics

Onset of action: Cataflam® is more rapid than sodium salt (Voltaren®) because it dissolves in the stomach instead of the duodenum

Absorption: Topical gel: 10%

Protein binding: 99% to albumin

Metabolism: Hepatic to several metabolites

Half-life elimination: 2 hours

Time to peak, serum: Cataflam®: ~1 hour; Voltaren®: ~2 hours

Excretion: Urine (65%); feces (35%)

Pregnancy Risk Factor
B (topical); C (oral)/D (3rd trimester)

Lactation
Excretion in breast milk unknown/not recommended

Dosage Forms
Excipient information presented when available (limited, particularly for generics); consult specific product labeling. [DSC] = Discontinued product

Gel, as sodium:
  Solaraze®: 30 mg/g (50 g)
Solution, ophthalmic, as sodium:
  Voltaren Ophthalmic®: 0.1% (2.5 mL, 5 mL)
Tablet, as potassium: 50 mg
  Cataflam®: 50 mg
Tablet, delayed release, enteric coated, as sodium: 50 mg, 75 mg
  Voltaren®: 25 mg [DSC], 50 mg [DSC], 75 mg
Tablet, extended release, as sodium: 100 mg
  Voltaren®-XR: 100 mg

Selected Readings
  Kubitzek F, Ziegler G, Gold MS, et al, "Analgesic Efficacy of Low-Dose Diclofenac Versus Paracetamol and Placebo in Postoperative Dental Pain," *J Orofac Pain*, 2003, 17(3):237-44.

Diclofenac and Misoprostol
(dye KLOE fen ak & mye soe PROST ole)

Related Information
  Diclofenac *on page 485*
  Misoprostol *on page 1111*
  Rheumatoid Arthritis, Osteoarthritis, and Osteoporosis *on page 1759*
U.S. Brand Names Arthrotec®
Canadian Brand Names Arthrotec®
Mexican Brand Names Artrotec
Generic Available No
Index Terms Misoprostol and Diclofenac
Pharmacologic Category Nonsteroidal Anti-inflammatory Drug (NSAID), Oral; Prostaglandin
Use The diclofenac component is indicated for the treatment of osteoarthritis and rheumatoid arthritis; the misoprostol component is indicated for the prophylaxis of NSAID-induced gastric and duodenal ulceration
Local Anesthetic/Vasoconstrictor Precautions No information available to require special precautions
Effects on Dental Treatment No significant effects or complications reported
Common Adverse Effects Also see individual agents.
  >10%: Gastrointestinal: Abdominal pain (21%), diarrhea (19%), nausea (11%), dyspepsia (14%)
  1% to 10%:
    Endocrine & metabolic: Transaminases increased
    Gastrointestinal: Flatulence (9%)
    Hematologic: Anemia
    Miscellaneous: Anaphylactic reactions
Restrictions An FDA-approved medication guide must be distributed when dispensing an oral outpatient prescription (new or refill) where this medication is to be used without direct supervision of a healthcare provider. Medication guides are available at http://www.fda.gov/cder/Offices/ODS/medication_guides.htm.
Mechanism of Action See individual agents.
Drug Interactions
  Cytochrome P450 Effect: Diclofenac: **Substrate** (minor) of CYP1A2, 2B6, 2C8, 2C9, 2C19, 2D6, 3A4; **Inhibits** CYP1A2 (moderate), 2C9 (weak), 2E1 (weak), 3A4 (strong)
  Increased Effect/Toxicity: Aspirin (shared toxicity), digoxin (elevated digoxin levels), warfarin (synergistic bleeding potential), methotrexate (increased methotrexate levels), cyclosporine (increased nephrotoxicity), lithium (increased lithium levels). Diclofenac may increase the levels/effects of CYP3A4 substrates (eg, benzodiazepines, calcium channel blockers, mirtazapine, nateglinide, nefazodone, tacrolimus, and venlafaxine). Selected benzodiazepines (midazolam and triazolam), cisapride, ergot alkaloids, selected HMG-CoA reductase inhibitors (lovastatin and simvastatin), and pimozide are generally contraindicated with strong CYP3A4 inhibitors. Concomitant use with fluoroquinolones may rarely increase risk of seizure.
  Decreased Effect: Aspirin (displaces diclofenac from binding sites), antihypertensive agents (decreased blood pressure control), antacids (may decrease absorption). Antihypertensive effects of ACE inhibitors, angiotensin antagonists, beta blockers, hydralazine, and thiazides may be decreased by concurrent therapy with NSAIDs. Cholestyramine (and other bile acid sequestrants) may decrease the absorption of NSAIDs; separate by at least 2 hours.
Pharmacodynamics/Kinetics See individual agents.
Pregnancy Risk Factor X

Diclofenac Potassium *see* Diclofenac *on page 485*
Diclofenac Sodium *see* Diclofenac *on page 485*

Diclofenamide *see* Dichlorphenamide *on page 485*

Dicloxacillin (dye kloks a SIL in)

Related Information
Bacterial Infections *on page 1793*
Canadian Brand Names Dycill®; Pathocil®
Mexican Brand Names Brispen; Posipen
Generic Available Yes
Index Terms Dicloxacillin Sodium
Pharmacologic Category Antibiotic, Penicillin
Dental Use Treatment of susceptible orofacial infections (notably penicillinase-producing staphylococci)
Use Treatment of systemic infections such as pneumonia, skin and soft tissue infections, and osteomyelitis caused by penicillinase-producing staphylococci
Local Anesthetic/Vasoconstrictor Precautions No information available to require special precautions
Effects on Dental Treatment Key adverse event(s) related to dental treatment: Prolonged use of penicillins may lead to development of oral candidiasis.
Significant Adverse Effects
1% to 10%: Gastrointestinal: Nausea, diarrhea, abdominal pain
<1% (Limited to important or life-threatening): Agranulocytosis, eosinophilia, hemolytic anemia, hepatotoxicity, hypersensitivity, interstitial nephritis, leukopenia, neutropenia, prolonged PT, pseudomembranous colitis, rash (maculopapular to exfoliative), seizure with extremely high doses and/or renal failure, serum sickness-like reactions, thrombocytopenia, vaginitis, vomiting
Dental Usual Dosing Susceptible orofacial infections: Children >40 kg and Adults: 125-250 mg every 6 hours
Dosage
Usual dosage range:
Newborns: Use not recommended
Children <40 kg: Oral: 12.5-100 mg/kg/day divided every 6 hours
Children >40 kg: Oral: 125-250 mg every 6 hours
Adults: Oral: 125-1000 mg every 6 hours
Indication-specific dosing:
Children: Oral:
Furunculosis: 25-50 mg/kg/day divided every 6 hours
Osteomyelitis: 50-100 mg/kg/day in divided doses every 6 hours
Adults: Oral:
Erysipelas, furunculosis, mastitis, otitis externa, septic bursitis, skin abscess: 500 mg every 6 hours
Impetigo: 250 mg every 6 hours
Prosthetic joint (long-term suppression therapy): 250 mg twice daily
***Staphylococcus aureus*, methicillin susceptible infection if no I.V. access:** 500-1000 mg every 6-8 hours
Dosage adjustment in renal impairment: Not necessary
Hemodialysis: Not dialyzable (0% to 5%); supplemental dosage not necessary
Peritoneal dialysis: Supplemental dosage not necessary
Continuous arteriovenous or venovenous hemofiltration: Supplemental dosage not necessary
Mechanism of Action Inhibits bacterial cell wall synthesis by binding to one or more of the penicillin binding proteins (PBPs) which in turn inhibits the final transpeptidation step of peptidoglycan synthesis in bacterial cell walls, thus inhibiting cell wall biosynthesis. Bacteria eventually lyse due to ongoing activity of cell wall autolytic enzymes (autolysins and murein hydrolases) while cell wall assembly is arrested.
Contraindications Hypersensitivity to dicloxacillin, penicillin, or any component of the formulation
Warnings/Precautions Monitor PT if patient concurrently on warfarin. Serious and occasionally severe or fatal hypersensitivity (anaphylactoid) reactions have been reported in patients on penicillin therapy, especially with a history of beta-lactam hypersensitivity, history of sensitivity to multiple allergens, or previous IgE-mediated reactions (eg, anaphylaxis, angioedema, urticaria). Use with caution in asthmatic patients. Prolonged use may result in fungal or bacterial superinfection, including *C. difficile*-associated diarrhea and pseudomembranous colitis.
Drug Interactions Induces CYP3A4 (weak)
Methotrexate: Penicillins may increase the exposure to methotrexate during concurrent therapy; monitor.
Oral contraceptives: Anecdotal reports suggesting decreased contraceptive efficacy with penicillins have been refuted by more rigorous scientific and clinical data.

Probenecid, disulfiram: May increase levels of penicillins (dicloxacillin).
Warfarin: Concurrent use may decrease effect of warfarin.

Ethanol/Nutrition/Herb Interactions Food: Decreases drug absorption rate; decreases drug serum concentration.

Dietary Considerations Administer on an empty stomach 1 hour before or 2 hours after meals. Sodium content of 250 mg capsule: 13 mg (0.6 mEq).

Pharmacodynamics/Kinetics
Absorption: 35% to 76%; rate and extent reduced by food
Distribution: Throughout body with highest concentrations in kidney and liver; CSF penetration is low; crosses placenta; enters breast milk
Protein binding: 96%
Half-life elimination: 0.6-0.8 hour; slightly prolonged with renal impairment
Time to peak, serum: 0.5-2 hours
Excretion: Feces; urine (56% to 70% as unchanged drug); prolonged in neonates

Pregnancy Risk Factor B

Lactation Excretion in breast milk unknown (probably similar to penicillin G)

Breast-Feeding Considerations No data reported; however, other penicillins may be taken while breast-feeding.

Dosage Forms Excipient information presented when available (limited, particularly for generics); consult specific product labeling.
Capsule: 250 mg, 500 mg

Dicloxacillin Sodium *see* Dicloxacillin *on page 490*

Dicyclomine (dye SYE kloe meen)

U.S. Brand Names Bentyl®
Canadian Brand Names Bentylol®; Formulex®; Lomine; Riva-Dicyclomine
Mexican Brand Names Bentyl
Generic Available Yes: Excludes syrup
Index Terms Dicyclomine Hydrochloride; Dicyloverine Hydrochloride
Pharmacologic Category Anticholinergic Agent
Use Treatment of functional bowel/irritable bowel syndrome
Unlabeled/Investigational Use Urinary incontinence
Local Anesthetic/Vasoconstrictor Precautions No information available to require special precautions
Effects on Dental Treatment Key adverse event(s) related to dental treatment: Xerostomia and changes in salivation (normal salivary flow resumes upon discontinuation)
Common Adverse Effects Adverse reactions are included here that have been reported for pharmacologically similar drugs with anticholinergic/antispasmodic action.

Cardiovascular: Syncope, tachycardia, palpitation
Central nervous system: Dizziness (29%), lightheadedness (11%), drowsiness (9%), tingling, headache, nervousness (6%), numbness, mental confusion and/or excitement, dyskinesia, lethargy, speech disturbance, insomnia
Dermatologic: Rash, urticaria, itching, and other dermal manifestations
Endocrine & metabolic: Suppression of lactation
Gastrointestinal: Xerostomia (33%), nausea (14%), vomiting, constipation, bloated feeling, abdominal pain, taste loss, anorexia
Genitourinary: Urinary hesitancy, urinary retention, impotence
Local: Irritation (injection), focal coagulation necrosis (injection)
Neuromuscular & skeletal: Weakness (7%)
Ocular: Blurred vision (27%), diplopia, mydriasis, cycloplegia, increased ocular tension
Respiratory: Dyspnea, apnea, asphyxia, nasal stuffiness or congestion, sneezing, throat congestion
Miscellaneous: Anaphylaxis, diaphoresis decreased, severe allergic reaction

Mechanism of Action Blocks the action of acetylcholine at parasympathetic sites in smooth muscle, secretory glands and the CNS

Drug Interactions
Increased Effect/Toxicity: The anticholinergic effects of dicyclomine are additive with other anticholinergic agents, including antihistamines, amantadine, opioids, phenothiazines, and tricyclic antidepressants. Pramlintide may enhance the gastrointestinal anticholinergic effect of dicyclomine.
Decreased Effect: Effects of dicyclomine may be diminished by central acetylcholinesterase inhibitors; in addition the effects of acetylcholinesterase inhibitors may be diminished by drugs with anticholinergic effects such as dicyclomine.

Pharmacodynamics/Kinetics
Onset of action: 1-2 hours
(Continued)

Dicyclomine *(Continued)*

Duration: ≤4 hours
Absorption: Oral: Well absorbed
Metabolism: Extensive
Half-life elimination: Initial: 1.8 hours; Terminal: 9-10 hours
Excretion: Urine (small amounts as unchanged drug)
Pregnancy Risk Factor B

Dicyclomine Hydrochloride *see* Dicyclomine *on page 491*
Dicycloverine Hydrochloride *see* Dicyclomine *on page 491*
Di-Dak-Sol *see* Sodium Hypochlorite Solution *on page 1482*

Didanosine *(dye DAN oh seen)*

Related Information
HIV Infection and AIDS *on page 1753*
U.S. Brand Names Videx®; Videx® EC
Canadian Brand Names Videx®; Videx® EC
Mexican Brand Names Videx
Generic Available Yes: Delayed release capsule
Index Terms ddI; Dideoxyinosine
Pharmacologic Category Antiretroviral Agent, Reverse Transcriptase Inhibitor (Nucleoside)
Use Treatment of HIV infection; always to be used in combination with at least two other antiretroviral agents
Local Anesthetic/Vasoconstrictor Precautions No information available to require special precautions
Effects on Dental Treatment Key adverse event(s) related to dental treatment: Xerostomia (normal salivary flow resumes upon discontinuation).
Common Adverse Effects As reported in monotherapy studies; risk of toxicity may increase when combined with other agents.

>10%:
  Gastrointestinal: Diarrhea (19% to 28%), amylase increased (15% to 17%), abdominal pain (7% to 13%)
  Neuromuscular & skeletal: Peripheral neuropathy (17% to 20%)
1% to 10%:
  Dermatologic: Rash/pruritus (7% to 9%)
  Endocrine & metabolic: Uric acid increased (2% to 3%)
  Gastrointestinal: Pancreatitis (1% to 7% dose dependent); patients >65 years of age had a higher frequency of pancreatitis than younger patients
  Hepatic: AST/ALT increased (6% to 9%), alkaline phosphatase increased (1% to 4%)

Mechanism of Action Didanosine, a purine nucleoside (adenosine) analog and the deamination product of dideoxyadenosine (ddA), inhibits HIV replication *in vitro* in both T cells and monocytes. Didanosine is converted within the cell to the mono-, di-, and triphosphates of ddA. These ddA triphosphates act as substrate and inhibitor of HIV reverse transcriptase substrate and inhibitor of HIV reverse transcriptase thereby blocking viral DNA synthesis and suppressing HIV replication.
Drug Interactions
  Increased Effect/Toxicity: Concomitant administration of other drugs which have the potential to cause peripheral neuropathy or pancreatitis may increase the risk of these toxicities. Allopurinol may increase didanosine concentration; avoid concurrent use. Ganciclovir may increase didanosine concentration; monitor. Coadministration with ribavirin, tenofovir, hydroxyurea or stavudine may increase exposure to didanosine and/or its active metabolite increasing the risk of hepatic decompensation (or other signs of mitochondrial toxicity), including pancreatitis, lactic acidosis, and peripheral neuropathy; monitor closely and suspend therapy if signs or symptoms of toxicity are noted. Additionally, concomitant tenofovir administration has been associated with hyperglycemia, decreased CD4 cell counts, and reduced virologic response.
  Decreased Effect: Didanosine buffered tablets and pediatric oral solution may decrease absorption of dapsone, quinolones or tetracyclines (administer 2 hours prior to didanosine buffered formulations). Didanosine should be held during PCP treatment with pentamidine. Didanosine may decrease levels of indinavir and atazanavir. Drugs whose absorption depends on the level of acidity in the stomach such as ketoconazole, itraconazole, and dapsone should be administered at least 2 hours prior to the buffered formulations of didanosine (not affected by delayed release capsules). Methadone may decrease didanosine concentrations.

Pharmacodynamics/Kinetics

Absorption: Subject to degradation by acidic pH of stomach; some formulations are buffered to resist acidic pH; ≤50% reduction in peak plasma concentration is observed in presence of food. Delayed release capsules contain enteric-coated beadlets which dissolve in the small intestine.

Distribution: V_d: Children: 35.6 L/m^2; Adults: 1.08 L/kg

Protein binding: <5%

Metabolism: Has not been evaluated in humans; studies conducted in dogs show extensive metabolism with allantoin, hypoxanthine, xanthine, and uric acid being the major metabolites found in urine

Bioavailability: 42%

Half-life elimination:

Children and Adolescents: 0.8 hour

Adults: Normal renal function: 1.5 hours; active metabolite, ddATP, has an intracellular half-life >12 hours *in vitro*; Renal impairment: 2.5-5 hours

Time to peak: Delayed release capsules: 2 hours; Powder for suspension: 0.25-1.5 hours

Excretion: Urine (~55% as unchanged drug)

Clearance: Total body: Averages 800 mL/minute

Pregnancy Risk Factor B

Diethylene Triamine Penta-Acetic Acid
(dye ETH i leen TRYE a meen PEN ta a SEE tik AS id)

Generic Available No

Index Terms Ca-DTPA; Diethylenetriamine Pentaacetic Acid; DTPA; Pentetate Calcium Trisodium; Pentetate Zinc Trisodium; Trisodium Calcium Diethylene-triaminepentaacetate (Ca-DTPA); Zinc Diethylenetriaminepentaacetate (Zn-DTPA); Zn-DTPA

Pharmacologic Category Antidote

Use Treatment of known or suspected internal contamination with plutonium, americium, or curium

Local Anesthetic/Vasoconstrictor Precautions No information available to require special precautions

Effects on Dental Treatment Key adverse event(s) related to dental treatment: Metallic taste

Mechanism of Action Ca-DTPA and Zn-DTPA form chelates with metal ions. The radioactive chelates are then excreted in the urine. Treatment is most effective when radiocontaminants are in circulation or interstitial fluids. Radiocontaminants eventually sequester in liver and bone, therefore, effectiveness of treatment decreases with time after exposure.

Pregnancy Risk Factor C (Ca-DTPA)/B (Zn-DTPA)

Diethylpropion (dye eth il PROE pee on)

U.S. Brand Names Tenuate® [DSC]; Tenuate® Dospan® [DSC]

Canadian Brand Names Tenuate®; Tenuate® Dospan®

Generic Available Yes

Index Terms Amfepramone; Diethylpropion Hydrochloride

Pharmacologic Category Anorexiant; Sympathomimetic

Use Short-term (few weeks) adjunct in the management of exogenous obesity

Local Anesthetic/Vasoconstrictor Precautions Use vasoconstrictor with caution in patients taking diethylpropion. Amphetamine-like drugs such as diethylpropion enhance the sympathomimetic response of epinephrine and norepinephrine leading to potential hypertension and cardiotoxicity.

Effects on Dental Treatment Key adverse event(s) related to dental treatment: Xerostomia and changes in salivation (normal salivary flow resumes upon discontinuation), and metallic taste (the use of local anesthetic without vasoconstrictor is recommended in these patients).

Mechanism of Action Diethylpropion s a sympathomimetic amine with pharmacologic properties similar to the amphetamines. It is also structurally similar to bupropion. The mechanism of action in reducing appetite appears to be secondary to CNS effects, including stimulation of the hypothalamus to release norepinephrine

Pregnancy Risk Factor B

Diethylpropion Hydrochloride *see* Diethylpropion *on page 493*

Difenoxin and Atropine (dye fen OKS in & A troe peen)

Related Information
Atropine *on page 166*
U.S. Brand Names Motofen®
Generic Available No
Index Terms Atropine and Difenoxin
Pharmacologic Category Antidiarrheal
Use Treatment of diarrhea
Local Anesthetic/Vasoconstrictor Precautions No information available to require special precautions
Effects on Dental Treatment Key adverse event(s) related to dental treatment: Xerostomia (normal salivary flow resumes upon discontinuation)
Common Adverse Effects 1% to 10%:
Central nervous system: Dizziness, drowsiness, lightheadedness, headache
Gastrointestinal: Nausea, vomiting, xerostomia, epigastric distress
Restrictions C-IV
Drug Interactions
Increased Effect/Toxicity: Concurrent use with MAO inhibitors may precipitate hypertensive crisis. May potentiate action of barbiturates, tranquilizers, narcotics, and alcohol. Difenoxin has the potential to prolong biological half-life of drugs for which the rate of elimination is dependent on the microsomal drug metabolizing enzyme system.
Pharmacodynamics/Kinetics
Absorption: Rapid and well absorbed
Metabolism: To inactive hydroxylated metabolite
Time to peak, plasma: Within 40-60 minutes
Excretion: Urine and feces (primarily as conjugates)
Pregnancy Risk Factor C

Differin® *see* Adapalene *on page 54*

Diflorasone (dye FLOR a sone)

U.S. Brand Names ApexiCon™; ApexiCon™ E; Florone®; Psorcon® e™ [DSC]
Canadian Brand Names Florone®; Psorcon®
Generic Available Yes
Index Terms Diflorasone Diacetate
Pharmacologic Category Corticosteroid, Topical
Use Relieves inflammation and pruritic symptoms of corticosteroid-responsive dermatosis (high to very high potency topical corticosteroid)

Maxiflor®: High potency topical corticosteroid
Psorcon®: Very high potency topical corticosteroid
Local Anesthetic/Vasoconstrictor Precautions No information available to require special precautions
Effects on Dental Treatment No significant effects or complications reported
Mechanism of Action Decreases inflammation by suppression of migration of polymorphonuclear leukocytes and reversal of increased capillary permeability
Pharmacodynamics/Kinetics
Absorption: Negligible, around 1% reaches dermal layers or systemic circulation; occlusive dressings increase absorption percutaneously
Metabolism: Primarily hepatic
Pregnancy Risk Factor C

Diflorasone Diacetate *see* Diflorasone *on page 494*
Diflucan® *see* Fluconazole *on page 697*

Diflunisal (dye FLOO ni sal)

Related Information
Oral Pain *on page 1788*
Rheumatoid Arthritis, Osteoarthritis, and Osteoporosis *on page 1759*
Temporomandibular Dysfunction (TMD) *on page 1822*
Related Sample Prescriptions
Mild/Moderate Oral Pain *on page 1834*
U.S. Brand Names Dolobid® [DSC]
Canadian Brand Names Apo-Diflunisal®; Novo-Diflunisal; Nu-Diflunisal
Mexican Brand Names Dolobid
Generic Available Yes

Pharmacologic Category Nonsteroidal Anti-inflammatory Drug (NSAID), Oral

Dental Use Treatment of postoperative pain

Use Management of inflammatory disorders usually including rheumatoid arthritis and osteoarthritis; can be used as an analgesic for treatment of mild to moderate pain

Local Anesthetic/Vasoconstrictor Precautions No information available to require special precautions

Effects on Dental Treatment NSAID formulations are known to reversibly decrease platelet aggregation via mechanisms different than observed with aspirin. The dentist should be aware of the potential of abnormal coagulation. Caution should also be exercised in the use of NSAIDs in patients already on anticoagulant therapy with drugs such as warfarin (Coumadin®). See Dental Comment.

Significant Adverse Effects

1% to 10%:

Central nervous system: Headache (3% to 9%), dizziness (1% to 3%), insomnia (1% to 3%), somnolence (1% to 3%), fatigue (1% to 3%)

Dermatologic: Rash (3% to 9%)

Gastrointestinal: Nausea (3% to 9%), dyspepsia (3% to 9%), GI pain (3% to 9%), diarrhea (3% to 9%), constipation (1% to 3%), flatulence (1% to 3%), vomiting (1% to 3%), GI ulceration

Otic: Tinnitus (1% to 3%)

<1% (Limited to important or life-threatening): Acute anaphylactic reaction, agranulocytosis, allergic reactions, angioedema, anorexia, blurred vision, bronchospasm, confusion, chest pain, cholestasis, cystitis, depression, diaphoresis, disorientation, dry mucous membranes, dyspnea, dysuria, edema, eructation, erythema multiforme, esophagitis, exfoliative dermatitis, flushing, gastritis, GI bleeding, GI perforation, hallucinations, hearing decreased, hearing loss, hematuria, hemolytic anemia, hepatitis, hypersensitivity syndrome, hypersensitivity vasculitis, interstitial nephritis, itching, jaundice, mental depression, muscle cramps, necrotizing fasciitis, nephrotic syndrome, nervousness, palpitation, paresthesia, peptic ulcer, peripheral neuropathy, photosensitivity, proteinuria, pruritus, renal impairment, renal failure, seizure, Stevens-Johnson syndrome, stomatitis, syncope, tachycardia, thrombocytopenia, toxic epidermal necrolysis, trembling, urticaria, vasculitis, vertigo, weakness, wheezing

Restrictions An FDA-approved medication guide must be distributed when dispensing an oral outpatient prescription (new or refill) where this medication is to be used without direct supervision of a healthcare provider. Medication guides are available at http://www.fda.gov/cder/Offices/ODS/medication_guides.htm.

Dental Usual Dosing Mild-to-moderate pain: Adults: Oral: Initial: 500-1000 mg followed by 250-500 mg every 8-12 hours; maximum daily dose: 1.5 g

Dosage Adults: Oral:

Mild-to-moderate pain: Initial: 500-1000 mg followed by 250-500 mg every 8-12 hours; maximum daily dose: 1.5 g

Arthritis: 500-1000 mg/day in 2 divided doses; maximum daily dose: 1.5 g

Dosing adjustment in renal impairment: Use with caution; Cl_{cr} <50 mL/minute: Administer 50% of normal dose (Aronoff, 1998)

Hemodialysis: No supplement required

CAPD: No supplement require

CAVH: Dose for GFR 10-50

Mechanism of Action Inhibits prostaglandin synthesis by decreasing the activity of the enzyme, cyclooxygenase, which results in decreased formation of prostaglandin precursors

Contraindications Hypersensitivity to diflunisal, aspirin, other NSAIDs, or any component of the formulation; perioperative pain in the setting of coronary artery bypass surgery (CABG); pregnancy (3rd trimester)

Warnings/Precautions [U.S. Boxed Warning]: NSAIDs are associated with an increased risk of adverse cardiovascular events, including MI, stroke, and new onset or worsening of pre-existing hypertension. Risk may be increased with duration of use or pre-existing cardiovascular risk factors or disease. Carefully evaluate individual cardiovascular risk profiles prior to prescribing. Use caution with fluid retention, CHF, or hypertension. Concurrent administration of ibuprofen, and potentially other nonselective NSAIDs, may interfere with aspirin's cardioprotective effect.

[U.S. Boxed Warning]: NSAIDs may increase risk of gastrointestinal irritation, ulceration, bleeding, and perforation. These events may occur at any time during therapy and without warning. Use caution with a history of GI disease (bleeding or ulcers), concurrent therapy with aspirin, anticoagulants and/or corticosteroids, smoking, use of alcohol, the elderly or debilitated patients.

(Continued)

Diflunisal *(Continued)*

Use of NSAIDs can compromise existing renal function. Renal toxicity can occur in patient with impaired renal function, dehydration, heart failure, liver dysfunction, those taking diuretics and ACEI and the elderly. Rehydrate patient before starting therapy. Monitor renal function closely. Diflunisal is not recommended for patients with advanced renal disease.

Use the lowest effective dose for the shortest duration of time, consistent with individual patient goals, to reduce risk of cardiovascular or GI adverse events. Alternate therapies should be considered for patients at high risk.

NSAIDs may cause serious skin adverse events including exfoliative dermatitis, Stevens-Johnson syndrome (SJS), and toxic epidermal necrolysis (TEN). Anaphylactoid reactions may occur, even without prior exposure; patients with "aspirin triad" (bronchial asthma, aspirin intolerance, rhinitis) may be at increased risk. Do not use in patients who experience bronchospasm, asthma, rhinitis, or urticaria with NSAID or aspirin therapy. Use caution in other forms of asthma.

A hypersensitivity syndrome has been reported; monitor for constitutional symptoms and cutaneous findings; other organ dysfunction may be involved.

Use with caution in patients with decreased hepatic function. Closely monitor patients with any abnormal LFT. Severe hepatic reactions (eg, fulminant hepatitis, liver failure) have occurred with NSAID use, rarely; discontinue if signs or symptoms of liver disease develop, or if systemic manifestations occur.

Diflunisal is a derivative of acetylsalicylic acid and therefore may be associated with Reye's syndrome. Withhold for at least 4-6 half-lives prior to surgical or dental procedures. Safety and efficacy have not been established in children <12 years of age.

Drug Interactions

ACE inhibitors: Antihypertensive effects may be decreased by concurrent therapy with NSAIDs; monitor blood pressure.

Aminoglycosides: NSAIDs may decrease the excretion of aminoglycosides.

Angiotensin II antagonists: Antihypertensive effects may be decreased by concurrent therapy with NSAIDs; monitor blood pressure.

Anticoagulants (warfarin, heparin, LMWHs) in combination with NSAIDs can cause increased risk of bleeding.

Antiplatelet agents (ticlopidine, clopidogrel, aspirin, abciximab, dipyridamole, eptifibatide, tirofiban) can cause an increased risk of bleeding.

Beta-blockers: NSAIDs may diminish the antihypertensive effects of beta-blockers.

Bisphosphonates: NSAIDs may increase the risk of gastrointestinal ulceration.

Cholestyramine (and other bile acid sequestrants): May decrease the absorption of NSAIDs. Separate by at least 2 hours.

Corticosteroids may increase the risk of GI ulceration; avoid concurrent use.

Cyclosporine: NSAIDs may increase serum creatinine, potassium, blood pressure, and cyclosporine levels; monitor cyclosporine levels and renal function carefully.

Fluoroquinolone antibiotics: Risk of seizures may be increased with concomitant quinolone use. Risk is considered quite low and may only be a factor with high serum levels of either agent and/or in patients with additional predisposing factors (eg, renal dysfunction, history of seizure or other neurological disorder).

Hydralazine's antihypertensive effect is decreased; avoid concurrent use.

Lithium levels can be increased; avoid concurrent use if possible or monitor lithium levels and adjust dose.

Sulindac may have the least effect. When NSAID is stopped, lithium will need adjustment again.

Loop diuretics efficacy (diuretic and antihypertensive effect) is reduced. Indomethacin reduces this efficacy, however, it may be anticipated with any NSAID.

Methotrexate: Severe bone marrow suppression, aplastic anemia, and GI toxicity have been reported with concomitant NSAID therapy. Avoid use during moderate or high-dose methotrexate (increased and prolonged methotrexate levels). NSAID use during low-dose treatment of rheumatoid arthritis has not been fully evaluated; extreme caution is warranted.

Pemetrexed: NSAIDs may decrease the excretion of pemetrexed. Patients with Cl_{cr} 45-79 mL/minute should avoid long acting NSAIDs for 5 days before and 2 days after pemetrexed treatment.

Salicylates: NSAIDs (nonselective) may diminish the cardioprotective effect of acetylated salicylates. Avoid regular use of NSAIDs if possible; consider alternatives (eg, acetaminophen). Give salicylate before NSAID; for example ibuprofen should be given 30-120 minutes after aspirin (immediate release).

Thiazides antihypertensive effects are decreased; avoid concurrent use.

Treprostinil: May enhance the risk of bleeding with concurrent use.

Vancomycin: NSAID©s may decrease the excretion of vancomycin.

Ethanol/Nutrition/Herb Interactions

Ethanol: Avoid ethanol (may enhance gastric mucosal irritation).

Herb/Nutraceutical: Avoid alfalfa, anise, bilberry, bladderwrack, bromelain, cat's claw, celery, coleus, cordyceps, dong quai, evening primrose, feverfew, fenugreek, garlic, ginger, ginkgo biloba, red clover, horse chestnut, grapeseed, green tea, ginseng, guggul, horse chestnut seed, horseradish, licorice, prickly ash, red clover, reishi, SAMe, sweet clover, turmeric, white willow (all have additional antiplatelet activity).

Dietary Considerations Should be taken with food to decrease GI distress.

Pharmacodynamics/Kinetics

Onset of action: Analgesic: ~1 hour; maximal effect: 2-3 hours

Duration: 8-12 hours

Absorption: Well absorbed

Protein binding: >99%

Distribution: Enters breast milk

Metabolism: Extensively hepatic; metabolic pathways are saturable

Half-life elimination: 8-12 hours; prolonged with renal impairment

Time to peak, serum: 2-3 hours

Excretion: Urine (~3% as unchanged drug, 90% as glucuronide conjugates) within 72-96 hours

Pregnancy Risk Factor C (1st and 2nd trimesters)/D (3rd trimester)

Lactation Enters breast milk/not recommended

Dosage Forms Excipient information presented when available (limited, particularly for generics); consult specific product labeling. [DSC] = Discontinued product

Tablet: 500 mg

Dolobid®: 250 mg, 500 mg [DSC]

Dental Comment The advantage of diflunisal as a pain reliever is its 12-hour duration of effect. In many cases, this long effect will ensure a full night sleep during the postoperative pain period.

Selected Readings

Ahmad N, Grad HA, Haas DA, et al, "The Efficacy of Nonopioid Analgesics for Postoperative Dental Pain: A Meta-Analysis," *Anesth Prog*, 1997, 44(4):119-26.

Brooks PM and Day RO, "Nonsteroidal Anti-inflammatory Drugs - Differences and Similarities," *N Engl J Med*, 1991, 324(24):1716-25.

Dionne R, "Additive Analgesia Without Opioid Side Effects," *Compend Contin Educ Dent*, 2000, 21(7):572-4, 576-7.

Dionne RA, "New Approaches to Preventing and Treating Postoperative Pain," *J Am Dent Assoc*, 1992, 123(6):26-34.

Dionne RA and Berthold CW, "Therapeutic Uses of Nonsteroidal Anti-inflammatory Drugs in Dentistry," *Crit Rev Oral Biol Med*, 2001, 12(4):315-30.

Forbes JA, Calderazzo JP, Bowser MW, et al, "A 12-Hour Evaluation of the Analgesic Efficacy of Diflunisal, Aspirin, and Placebo in Postoperative Dental Pain," *J Clin Pharmacol*, 1982, 22(2-3):89-96.

Gobetti JP, "Controlling Dental Pain," *J Am Dent Assoc*, 1992, 123(6):47-52.

Nguyen AM, Graham DY, Gage T, et al, "Nonsteroidal Anti-inflammatory Drug Use in Dentistry: Gastrointestinal Implications," *Gen Dent*, 1999, 47(6):590-6.

Selcuk E, Gomel M, Bellibas SE, et al, "Comparison of the Analgesic Effects of Diflunisal and Paracetamol in the Treatment of Postoperative Dental Pain," *Int J Clin Pharmacol Res*, 1996, 16(2-3):57-65.

Digibind® *see* Digoxin Immune Fab *on page 500*

DigiFab™ *see* Digoxin Immune Fab *on page 500*

Digitek® *see* Digoxin *on page 497*

Digoxin (di JOKS in)

Related Information

Cardiovascular Diseases *on page 1726*

U.S. Brand Names Digitek®; Lanoxicaps®; Lanoxin®

Canadian Brand Names Apo-Digoxin®; Digoxin CSD; Lanoxicaps®; Lanoxin®; Novo-Digoxin; Pediatric Digoxin CSD

Mexican Brand Names Lanoxin; Mapluxin

Generic Available Yes: Excludes capsule

Pharmacologic Category Antiarrhythmic Agent, Class IV; Cardiac Glycoside

Use Treatment of congestive heart failure and to slow the ventricular rate in tachyarrhythmias such as atrial fibrillation, atrial flutter, and supraventricular tachycardia (paroxysmal atrial tachycardia); cardiogenic shock

Local Anesthetic/Vasoconstrictor Precautions Use vasoconstrictor with caution due to risk of cardiac arrhythmias with digoxin

Effects on Dental Treatment Sensitive gag reflex may cause difficulty in taking a dental impression.

Common Adverse Effects Incidence not always reported.

(Continued)

Digoxin *(Continued)*

Cardiovascular: Heart block; first-, second- (Wenckebach), or third-degree heart block; asystole; atrial tachycardia with block; AV dissociation; accelerated junctional rhythm; ventricular tachycardia or ventricular fibrillation; PR prolongation; ST segment depression

Central nervous system: Visual disturbances (blurred or yellow vision), headache (3%), dizziness (5%), apathy, confusion, mental disturbances (4%), anxiety, depression, delirium, hallucinations, fever

Dermatologic: Maculopapular rash (2%), erythematous, scarlatiniform, papular, vesicular or bullous rash, urticaria, pruritus, facial, angioneurotic or laryngeal edema, shedding of fingernails or toenails, alopecia

Gastrointestinal: Nausea (3%), vomiting (2%), diarrhea (3%), abdominal pain

Neuromuscular & skeletal: Weakness

Children are more likely to experience cardiac arrhythmia as a sign of excessive dosing. The most common are conduction disturbances or tachyarrhythmia (atrial tachycardia with or without block) and junctional tachycardia. Ventricular tachyarrhythmia are less common. In infants, sinus bradycardia may be a sign of digoxin toxicity. Any arrhythmia seen in a child on digoxin should be considered as digoxin toxicity. The gastrointestinal and central nervous system symptoms are not frequently seen in children.

Dosage When changing from oral (tablets or liquid) or I.M. to I.V. therapy, dosage should be reduced by 20% to 25%. Refer to the following: See table.

Dosage Recommendations for Digoxin

Age	Total Digitalizing Dose[2] (mcg/kg[1])		Daily Maintenance Dose[3] (mcg/kg[1])	
	P.O.	I.V. or I.M.	P.O.	I.V. or I.M.
Preterm infant[1]	20-30	15-25	5-7.5	4-6
Full-term infant[1]	25-35	20-30	6-10	5-8
1 mo - 2 y[1]	35-60	30-50	10-15	7.5-12
2-5 y[1]	30-40	25-35	7.5-10	6-9
5-10 y[1]	20-35	15-30	5-10	4-8
>10 y[1]	10-15	8-12	2.5-5	2-3
Adults	0.75-1.5 mg	0.5-1 mg	0.125-0.5 mg	0.1-0.4 mg

[1]Based on lean body weight and normal renal function for age. Decrease dose in patients with ↓ renal function; digitalizing dose often not recommended in infants and children.

[2]Give one-half of the total digitalizing dose (TDD) in the initial dose, then give one-quarter of the TDD in each of two subsequent doses at 8- to 12-hour intervals. Obtain ECG 6 hours after each dose to assess potential toxicity.

[3]Divided every 12 hours in infants and children <10 years of age. Given once daily to children >10 years of age and adults.

Dosing adjustment/interval in renal impairment:

Cl_{cr} 10-50 mL/minute: Administer 25% to 75% of dose or every 36 hours

Cl_{cr} <10 mL/minute: Administer 10% to 25% of dose or every 48 hours

Reduce loading dose by 50% in ESRD

Hemodialysis: Not dialyzable (0% to 5%)

Mechanism of Action

Congestive heart failure: Inhibition of the sodium/potassium ATPase pump which acts to increase the intracellular sodium-calcium exchange to increase intracellular calcium leading to increased contractility

Supraventricular arrhythmias: Direct suppression of the AV node conduction to increase effective refractory period and decrease conduction velocity - positive inotropic effect, enhanced vagal tone, and decreased ventricular rate to fast atrial arrhythmias. Atrial fibrillation may decrease sensitivity and increase tolerance to higher serum digoxin concentrations.

Contraindications Hypersensitivity to digoxin or any component of the formulation; hypersensitivity to cardiac glycosides (another may be tried); history of toxicity; ventricular tachycardia or fibrillation; idiopathic hypertrophic subaortic stenosis; constrictive pericarditis; amyloid disease; second- or third-degree heart block (except in patients with a functioning artificial pacemaker); Wolff-Parkinson-White syndrome and atrial fibrillation concurrently

Warnings/Precautions Watch for proarrhythmic effects (especially with digoxin toxicity); monitor and adjust dose to prevent QT_c prolongation. Use with caution in patients with hypoxia, myxedema, hypothyroidism, acute myocarditis; patients with incomplete AV block (Stokes-Adams attack) may progress to complete block with digitalis drug administration; use with caution in patients with acute myocardial infarction, severe pulmonary disease, advanced heart failure, idiopathic hypertrophic subaortic stenosis, Wolff-Parkinson-White syndrome, sick-sinus syndrome (bradyarrhythmias), amyloid heart disease, and constrictive cardiomyopathies; adjust dose with renal impairment and when verapamil, quinidine or amiodarone are added to a patient on digoxin; elderly and neonates may develop exaggerated serum/tissue concentrations due to age-related alterations in clearance and pharmacodynamic differences; exercise will reduce serum concentrations of digoxin due to increased skeletal muscle uptake; recent studies indicate photopsia, chromatopsia and decreased visual acuity may occur even with therapeutic serum drug levels; reduce or hold dose 1-2 days before elective electrical cardioversion. In the Cardiac Arrhythmia Suppression Trial (CAST), recent (>6 days but <2 years ago) myocardial infarction patients with asymptomatic, nonlife-threatening ventricular arrhythmias did not benefit and may have been harmed by attempts to suppress the arrhythmia with flecainide or encainide. An increased mortality or nonfatal cardiac arrest rate (7.7%) was seen in the active treatment group compared with patients in the placebo group (3%). The applicability of the CAST results to other populations is unknown. Antiarrhythmic agents should be reserved for patients with life-threatening ventricular arrhythmias.

Drug Interactions

Cytochrome P450 Effect: Substrate of CYP3A4 (minor)

Increased Effect/Toxicity: Beta-blocking agents (propranolol), verapamil, and diltiazem may have additive effects on heart rate. Carvedilol has additive effects on heart rate and inhibits the metabolism of digoxin. Digoxin levels may be increased by amiodarone (reduce digoxin dose 50%), bepridil, cyclosporine, diltiazem, indomethacin, itraconazole, some macrolides (erythromycin, clarithromycin), methimazole, propafenone, propylthiouracil, quinidine (reduce digoxin dose 33% to 50% on initiation), tetracyclines, and verapamil. Moricizine may increase the toxicity of digoxin (mechanism undefined). Spironolactone may interfere with some digoxin assays, but may also increase blood levels directly. Succinylcholine administration to patients on digoxin has been associated with an increased risk of arrhythmias. Rare cases of acute digoxin toxicity have been associated with parenteral calcium (bolus) administration. The following medications have been associated with increased digoxin blood levels which appear to be of limited clinical significance: Famciclovir, flecainide, ibuprofen, fluoxetine, nefazodone, cimetidine, famotidine, ranitidine, omeprazole, trimethoprim.

Decreased Effect: Amiloride and spironolactone may reduce the inotropic response to digoxin. Cholestyramine, colestipol, kaolin-pectin, and metoclopramide may reduce digoxin absorption. Levothyroxine (and other thyroid supplements) may decrease digoxin blood levels. Penicillamine has been associated with reductions in digoxin blood levels The following reported interactions appear to be of limited clinical significance: Aminoglutethimide, aminosalicylic acid, aluminum-containing antacids, sucralfate, sulfasalazine, neomycin, ticlopidine.

Ethanol/Nutrition/Herb Interactions

Food: Digoxin peak serum levels may be decreased if taken with food. Meals containing increased fiber (bran) or foods high in pectin may decrease oral absorption of digoxin.

Herb/Nutraceutical: Avoid ephedra (risk of cardiac stimulation). Avoid natural licorice (causes sodium and water retention and increases potassium loss).

Dietary Considerations Maintain adequate amounts of potassium in diet to decrease risk of hypokalemia (hypokalemia may increase risk of digoxin toxicity).

Pharmacodynamics/Kinetics

Onset of action: Oral: 1-2 hours; I.V.: 5-30 minutes

Peak effect: Oral: 2-8 hours; I.V.: 1-4 hours

Duration: Adults: 3-4 days both forms

Absorption: By passive nonsaturable diffusion in the upper small intestine; food may delay, but does not affect extent of absorption

Distribution:

Normal renal function: 6-7 L/kg

V_d: Extensive to peripheral tissues, with a distinct distribution phase which lasts 6-8 hours; concentrates in heart, liver, kidney, skeletal muscle, and intestines. Heart/serum concentration is 70:1. Pharmacologic effects are delayed and do not correlate well with serum concentrations during distribution phase.

Hyperthyroidism: Increased V_d

Hyperkalemia, hyponatremia: Decreased digoxin distribution to heart and muscle

Hypokalemia: Increased digoxin distribution to heart and muscles

Concomitant quinidine therapy: Decreased V_d

Chronic renal failure: 4-6 L/kg

Decreased sodium/potassium ATPase activity - decreased tissue binding

Neonates, full-term: 7.5-10 L/kg

Children: 16 L/kg

Adults: 7 L/kg, decreased with renal disease

(Continued)

Digoxin *(Continued)*

Protein binding: 30%; in uremic patients, digoxin is displaced from plasma protein binding sites

Metabolism: Via sequential sugar hydrolysis in the stomach or by reduction of lactone ring by intestinal bacteria (in ~10% of population, gut bacteria may metabolize up to 40% of digoxin dose); metabolites may contribute to therapeutic and toxic effects of digoxin; metabolism is reduced with CHF

Bioavailability: Oral (formulation dependent): Elixir: 75% to 85%; Tablet: 70% to 80%

Half-life elimination (age, renal and cardiac function dependent):
Neonates: Premature: 61-170 hours; Full-term: 35-45 hours
Infants: 18-25 hours
Children: 35 hours
Adults: 38-48 hours
Adults, anephric: 4-6 days

Half-life elimination: Parent drug: 38 hours; Metabolites: Digoxigenin: 4 hours; Monodigitoxoside: 3-12 hours

Time to peak, serum: Oral: ~1 hour

Excretion: Urine (50% to 70% as unchanged drug)

Pregnancy Risk Factor C

Dosage Forms

Capsule:
Lanoxicaps®: 100 mcg, 200 mcg

Injection: 250 mcg/mL (1 mL, 2 mL)
Lanoxin®: 250 mcg/mL (2 mL)

Injection, pediatric: 100 mcg/mL (1 mL)

Solution, oral: 50 mcg/mL (2.5 mL, 5 mL, 60 mL)

Tablet: 125 mcg, 250 mcg
Digitek®, Lanoxin®: 125 mcg, 250 mcg

Digoxin Immune Fab *(di JOKS in i MYUN fab)*

U.S. Brand Names Digibind®; DigiFab™
Canadian Brand Names Digibind®
Generic Available No
Index Terms Antidigoxin Fab Fragments, Ovine
Pharmacologic Category Antidote
Use Treatment of life-threatening or potentially life-threatening digoxin intoxication, including:
- acute digoxin ingestion (ie, >10 mg in adults or >4 mg in children)
- chronic ingestions leading to steady-state digoxin concentrations >6 ng/mL in adults or >4 ng/mL in children
- manifestations of digoxin toxicity due to overdose (life-threatening ventricular arrhythmias, progressive bradycardia, second- or third-degree heart block not responsive to atropine, serum potassium >5 mEq/L in adults or >6 mEq in children)

Local Anesthetic/Vasoconstrictor Precautions No information available to require special precautions
Effects on Dental Treatment No significant effects or complications reported
Common Adverse Effects Frequency not defined.
Cardiovascular: Effects (due to withdrawal of digitalis) include exacerbation of low cardiac output states and CHF, rapid ventricular response in patients with atrial fibrillation; postural hypotension
Endocrine & metabolic: Hypokalemia
Local: Phlebitis
Miscellaneous: Allergic reactions, serum sickness
Mechanism of Action Digoxin immune antigen-binding fragments (Fab) are specific antibodies for the treatment of digitalis intoxication in carefully selected patients; binds with molecules of digoxin or digitoxin and then is excreted by the kidneys and removed from the body
Drug Interactions
Increased Effect/Toxicity: Digoxin: Following administration of digoxin immune Fab, serum digoxin levels are markedly increased due to bound complexes (may be clinically misleading, since bound complex cannot interact with receptors).
Pharmacodynamics/Kinetics
Onset of action: I.V.: Improvement in 2-30 minutes for toxicity
Half-life elimination: 15-20 hours; prolonged with renal impairment
Excretion: Urine; undetectable amounts within 5-7 days
Pregnancy Risk Factor C

Dihematoporphyrin Ether *see* Porfimer *on page 1324*

Dihistine® DH [DSC] *see* Chlorpheniramine, Pseudoephedrine, and Codeine *on page 344*

Dihydrocodeine, Aspirin, and Caffeine
(dye hye droe KOE deen, AS pir in, & KAF een)

Related Information
Aspirin *on page 149*
Caffeine *on page 255*
Oral Pain *on page 1788*
U.S. Brand Names Synalgos®-DC
Generic Available No
Index Terms Dihydrocodeine Compound
Pharmacologic Category Analgesic, Opioid
Dental Use Management of postoperative pain
Use Management of mild to moderate pain that requires relaxation
Local Anesthetic/Vasoconstrictor Precautions No information available to require special precautions
Effects on Dental Treatment Key adverse event(s) related to dental treatment: Dihydrocodeine: nausea, followed by sedation and constipation. Elderly are a high-risk population for adverse effects from nonsteroidal anti-inflammatory agents. As many as 60% of elderly patients with GI complications from NSAIDs can develop peptic ulceration and/or hemorrhage asymptomatically. Concomitant disease and drug use contribute to the risk of GI adverse effects. Use lowest effective dose for shortest period possible. Consider renal function decline with age.
Aspirin: As with all drugs which may affect hemostasis, bleeding is associated with aspirin. Hemorrhage may occur at virtually any site; risk is dependent on multiple variables including dosage, concurrent use of multiple agents which alter hemostasis, and patient susceptibility. Many adverse effects of aspirin are dose related, and are rare at low dosages. Other serious reactions are idiosyncratic, related to allergy or individual sensitivity (see Dental Comment).

Significant Adverse Effects
>10%:
Central nervous system: Lightheadedness, dizziness, drowsiness, sedation
Dermatologic: Pruritus, skin reactions
Gastrointestinal: Nausea, vomiting, constipation
1% to 10%:
Cardiovascular: Hypotension, palpitation, bradycardia, peripheral vasodilation
Central nervous system: Increased intracranial pressure
Endocrine & metabolic: Antidiuretic hormone release
Gastrointestinal: Biliary tract spasm
Genitourinary: Urinary tract spasm
Ocular: Miosis
Respiratory: Respiratory depression
Miscellaneous: Histamine release, physical and psychological dependence with prolonged use

Restrictions C-III
Dental Usual Dosing Management of postoperative pain: Oral:
Adults: 1-2 capsules every 4-6 hours as needed for pain
Elderly: Initial dosing should be cautious (low end of adult dosing range)
Dosage
Adults: Oral: 1-2 capsules every 4-6 hours as needed for pain
Elderly: Initial dosing should be cautious (low end of adult dosing range)
Mechanism of Action Binds to opiate receptors in the CNS, causing inhibition of ascending pain pathways, altering the perception of and response to pain; causes cough suppression by direct central action in the medulla; produces generalized CNS depression
Contraindications Hypersensitivity to dihydrocodeine or any component of the formulation; pregnancy (prolonged use or high doses at term)
Warnings/Precautions Use with caution in patients with hypersensitivity reactions to other phenanthrene-derivative opioid agonists (morphine, hydrocodone, hydromorphone, levorphanol, oxycodone, oxymorphone); respiratory diseases including asthma, emphysema, COPD; or severe liver or renal insufficiency. Some preparations contain sulfites which may cause allergic reactions. May be habit-forming. Dextromethorphan has equivalent antitussive activity but has much lower toxicity in accidental overdose.
Drug Interactions Substrate of CYP2D6 (major) based on dihydrocodeine
CYP2D6 inhibitors: May decrease the effects of dihydrocodeine. Example inhibitors include chlorpromazine, delavirdine, fluoxetine, miconazole, paroxetine, pergolide, quinidine, quinine, ritonavir, and ropinirole.
MAO inhibitors may increase adverse symptoms
(Continued)

Dihydrocodeine, Aspirin, and Caffeine *(Continued)*

Ethanol/Nutrition/Herb Interactions Ethanol: Avoid ethanol (may increase CNS depression).

Pharmacodynamics/Kinetics

Onset of action: 10-30 minutes

Duration: 4-6 hours

Metabolism: Hepatic

Half-life elimination, serum: 3.8 hours

Time to peak, serum: 30-60 minutes

Pregnancy Risk Factor B/D (prolonged use or high doses at term)

Lactation Excretion in breast milk unknown/use caution

Breast-Feeding Considerations

Acetaminophen: May be taken while breast-feeding.

Aspirin: Use cautiously due to potential adverse effects in nursing infants.

Dihydrocodeine: No data reported.

Dosage Forms Excipient information presented when available (limited, particularly for generics); consult specific product labeling.

Capsule: Dihydrocodeine bitartrate 16 mg, aspirin 356.4 mg, and caffeine 30 mg

Dental Comment There is no scientific evidence to warrant discontinuance of aspirin prior to dental surgery. Patients taking one aspirin tablet daily as an antithrombotic and who require dental surgery should be given special consideration in consultation with the physician before removal of the aspirin relative to prevention of postoperative bleeding.

The Food and Drug Administration (FDA), has issued a letter updating information and considerations regarding the use of ibuprofen (400 mg doses) in patients who are taking low dose aspirin (81 mg, immediate release; not enteric coated) for cardioprotection and stroke prevention. Ibuprofen, at these doses, may interfere with aspirin's antiplatelet effect depending upon when it is administered. Patients initiated on aspirin first (for ~1 week) then ibuprofen (400 mg tid for 10 days) seem to maintain aspirin's platelet effect (Cryer B, 2005). Ibuprofen has the greatest impact on aspirin if administered less than 8 hours before aspirin (Catella-Lawson F, 2001).

Patients may require counseling about the appropriate timing of ibuprofen dosing in relationship to aspirin therapy. With occasional use of ibuprofen, a clinically-significant interaction with aspirin is unlikely. To avoid interference during chronic dosing, a single dose of ibuprofen should be taken 30-120 minutes after aspirin ingestion or at least 8 hours should elapse after ibuprofen dosing before giving aspirin (FDA, 2006; Catella-Lawson F, 2001).

The clinical implications of the interaction are unclear. There have not been any clinical endpoint studies conducted at this time. Avoidance of this interaction is potentially important because aspirin's vascular protection could be decreased or negated.

Other nonselective NSAIDs may have potential for a similar interaction with aspirin. Such has been described with naproxen (Capone ML, 2005). Acetaminophen does not appear to interfere with the antiplatelet effect of aspirin. Other clinical scenarios (use of smaller ibuprofen doses, other aspirin products, other doses of aspirin) have not been evaluated.

Additional information is available at: http://www.fda.gov/cder/drug/infopage/aspirin/default.htm.

Dihydrocodeine Bitartrate, Acetaminophen, and Caffeine *see* Acetaminophen, Caffeine, and Dihydrocodeine *on page 42*

Dihydrocodeine Bitartrate, Pseudoephedrine Hydrochloride, and Chlorpheniramine Maleate *see* Pseudoephedrine, Dihydrocodeine, and Chlorpheniramine *on page 1385*

Dihydrocodeine, Chlorpheniramine, and Phenylephrine

(dye hye droe KOE deen, klor fen IR a meen, & fen il EF rin)

Related Information

Chlorpheniramine *on page 338*

Codeine *on page 404*

Phenylephrine *on page 1293*

U.S. Brand Names Baltussin; Coldcough PD; Pancof®-PD

Generic Available Yes

Index Terms Chlorpheniramine Maleate, Dihydrocodeine Bitartrate, and Phenylephrine Hydrochloride; Phenylephrine, Chlorpheniramine, and Dihydrocodeine

Pharmacologic Category Antihistamine; Antihistamine/Decongestant/Antitussive; Antitussive; Decongestant

Use Symptomatic relief of cough and congestion associated with the upper respiratory tract

Local Anesthetic/Vasoconstrictor Precautions No information available to require special precautions

Effects on Dental Treatment Key adverse event(s) related to dental treatment:

Chlorpheniramine: Prolonged use will cause significant xerostomia (normal salivary flow resumes upon discontinuation).

Phenylephrine: Up to 10% of patients could experience tachycardia, palpitations, and xerostomia; use vasoconstrictor with caution.

Common Adverse Effects Refer to individual agents.

Restrictions C-III/C-V

Mechanism of Action

Dihydrocodeine: Binds to opiate receptors in the CNS; suppresses cough in medullary center; produces generalized CNS depression

Chlorpheniramine: Competes with histamine for H_1-receptor sites on effector cells in the gastrointestinal tract, blood vessels, and respiratory tract

Phenylephrine: Potent, direct-acting alpha-adrenergic stimulator with weak beta-adrenergic activity; causes vasoconstriction of the arterioles of the nasal mucosa and conjunctiva

Drug Interactions
Increased Effect/Toxicity: Refer to individual monographs for codeine, chlorpheniramine, and phenylephrine.

Pregnancy Risk Factor C

Dihydrocodeine Compound *see* Dihydrocodeine, Aspirin, and Caffeine *on page 501*

Dihydrocodeine, Pseudoephedrine, and Guaifenesin
(dye hye droe KOE deen, soo doe e FED rin, & gwye FEN e sin)

Related Information
Codeine *on page 404*
Guaifenesin *on page 795*
Pseudoephedrine *on page 1381*

U.S. Brand Names DiHydro-GP; Hydro-Tussin™ EXP; Pancof®-EXP

Generic Available Yes

Index Terms Guaifenesin, Dihydrocodeine, and Pseudoephedrine; Pseudoephedrine Hydrochloride, Guaifenesin, and Dihydrocodeine Bitartrate

Pharmacologic Category Antitussive/Decongestant/Expectorant

Use Temporary relief of cough and congestion associated with upper respiratory tract infections and allergies

Local Anesthetic/Vasoconstrictor Precautions Use with caution since pseudoephedrine is a sympathomimetic amine which could interact with epinephrine to cause a pressor response

Effects on Dental Treatment No significant effects or complications reported

Common Adverse Effects Refer to individual agents.

Mechanism of Action

Dihydrocodeine is an antitussive and analgesic chemically related to codeine. Codeine binds to opiate receptors in the CNS, causing inhibition of ascending pain pathways, altering the perception of and response to pain; causes cough supression by direct central action in the medulla; produces generalized CNS depression.

Pseudoephedrine directly stimulates alpha-adrenergic receptors of respiratory mucosa causing vasoconstriction; directly stimulates beta-adrenergic receptors causing bronchial relaxation, increased heart rate and contractility.

Guaifenesin is thought to act as an expectorant by irritating the gastric mucosa and stimulating respiratory tract secretions, thereby increasing respiratory fluid volumes and decreasing phlegm viscosity.

Drug Interactions
Increased Effect/Toxicity: Refer to individual monographs for Codeine, Pseudoephedrine, and Guaifenesin.

Pregnancy Risk Factor C

DiHydro-CP *see* Pseudoephedrine, Dihydrocodeine, and Chlorpheniramine *on page 1385*

Dihydroergotamine (dye hye droe er GOT a meen)

U.S. Brand Names D.H.E. 45®; Migranal®
Canadian Brand Names Migranal®
Mexican Brand Names Dihydergot
Generic Available Yes: Injection
Index Terms DHE; Dihydroergotamine Mesylate
Pharmacologic Category Antimigraine Agent; Ergot Derivative
Use Treatment of migraine headache with or without aura; injection also indicated for treatment of cluster headaches
Unlabeled/Investigational Use Adjunct for DVT prophylaxis for hip surgery, for orthostatic hypotension, xerostomia secondary to antidepressant use, and pelvic congestion with pain
Local Anesthetic/Vasoconstrictor Precautions No information available to require special precautions
Effects on Dental Treatment Key adverse event(s) related to dental treatment: Rhinitis and abnormal taste.
Common Adverse Effects
>10%: Nasal spray: Respiratory: Rhinitis (26%)
1% to 10%: Nasal spray:
Central nervous system: Dizziness (4%), somnolence (3%)
Endocrine & metabolic: Hot flashes (1%)
Gastrointestinal: Nausea (10%), taste disturbance (8%), vomiting (4%), diarrhea (2%)
Local: Application site reaction (6%)
Neuromuscular & skeletal: Weakness (1%), stiffness (1%)
Respiratory: Pharyngitis (3%)
Mechanism of Action Ergot alkaloid alpha-adrenergic blocker directly stimulates vascular smooth muscle to vasoconstrict peripheral and cerebral vessels; also has effects on serotonin receptors
Drug Interactions
Cytochrome P450 Effect: Substrate of CYP3A4 (major); **Inhibits** CYP3A4 (weak)
Increased Effect/Toxicity: CYP3A4 inhibitors may increase the levels/effects of dihydroergotamine; example inhibitors include azole antifungals, clarithromycin, diclofenac, doxycycline, erythromycin, imatinib, isoniazid, nefazodone, nicardipine, propofol, protease inhibitors, quinidine, telithromycin, and verapamil. Ergot alkaloids are contraindicated with potent CYP3A4 inhibitors. Dihydroergotamine may increase the effects of 5-HT$_1$ agonists (eg, sumatriptan), MAO inhibitors, sibutramine, and other serotonin agonists (serotonin syndrome). Severe vasoconstriction may occur when peripheral vasoconstrictors or beta-blockers are used in patients receiving ergot alkaloids; concurrent use is contraindicated.
Decreased Effect: Effects of dihydroergotamine may be diminished by antipsychotics, metoclopramide. Antianginal effects of nitrates may be reduced by ergot alkaloids.
Pharmacodynamics/Kinetics
Onset of action: 15-30 minutes
Duration: 3-4 hours
Distribution: V_d: 14.5 L/kg
Protein binding: 93%
Metabolism: Extensively hepatic
Half-life elimination: 1.3-3.9 hours
Time to peak, serum: I.M.: 15-30 minutes
Excretion: Primarily feces; urine (10% mostly as metabolites)
Pregnancy Risk Factor X

Dihydroergotamine Mesylate *see* Dihydroergotamine *on page 504*
Dihydroergotoxine *see* Ergoloid Mesylates *on page 584*
Dihydrogenated Ergot Alkaloids *see* Ergoloid Mesylates *on page 584*
DiHydro-GP *see* Dihydrocodeine, Pseudoephedrine, and Guaifenesin *on page 503*
Dihydrohydroxycodeinone *see* Oxycodone *on page 1225*
Dihydromorphinone *see* Hydromorphone *on page 840*

Dihydrotachysterol (dye hye droe tak ISS ter ole)

U.S. Brand Names DHT™ [DSC]; DHT™ Intensol™ [DSC]; Hytakerol® [DSC]
Canadian Brand Names Hytakerol®
Generic Available No

Index Terms Dichysterol

Pharmacologic Category Vitamin D Analog

Use Treatment of hypocalcemia associated with hypoparathyroidism; prophylaxis of hypocalcemic tetany following thyroid surgery

Local Anesthetic/Vasoconstrictor Precautions No information available to require special precautions

Effects on Dental Treatment No significant effects or complications reported

Common Adverse Effects >10%:

Endocrine & metabolic: Hypercalcemia

Renal: Serum creatinine increased, hypercalciuria

Mechanism of Action Synthetic analogue of vitamin D with a faster onset of action; stimulates calcium and phosphate absorption from the small intestine, promotes secretion of calcium from bone to blood; promotes renal tubule resorption of phosphate

Drug Interactions

Increased Effect/Toxicity: Thiazide diuretics may increase calcium levels.

Decreased Effect: Decreased effect/levels of vitamin D if taken with cholestyramine, colestipol, or mineral oil. Phenytoin and phenobarbital may inhibit activation leading to decreased effectiveness.

Pharmacodynamics/Kinetics

Onset of action: Peak effect: Calcium: 2-4 weeks

Duration: ≤9 weeks

Absorption: Well absorbed

Distribution: Stored in liver, fat, skin, muscle, and bone

Excretion: Feces

Pregnancy Risk Factor A/D (dose exceeding RDA recommendation)

Diltiazem (dil TYE a zem)

Related Information

Cardiovascular Diseases *on page 1726*

U.S. Brand Names Cardizem®; Cardizem® CD; Cardizem® LA; Cartia XT™; Dilacor® XR; Diltia XT®; Dilt-XR; Taztia XT™; Tiazac®

Canadian Brand Names Alti-Diltiazem CD; Apo-Diltiaz®; Apo-Diltiaz CD®; Apo-Diltiaz® Injectable; Apo-Diltiaz SR®; Apo-Diltiaz TZ®; Cardizem®; Cardizem® CD; Cardizem® SR; Diltiazem HCl ER®; Diltiazem Hydrochloride Injection; Gen-Diltiazem; Gen-Diltiazem CD; Med-Diltiazem; Novo-Diltiazem; Novo-Diltiazem-CD; Novo-Diltiazem HCl ER; Nu-Diltiaz; Nu-Diltiaz-CD; ratio-Diltiazem CD; Rhoxal-diltiazem CD; Rhoxal-diltiazem SR; Rhoxal-diltiazem T; Sandoz-Diltiazem CD; Sandoz-Diltiazem T; Syn-Diltiazem®; Tiazac®; Tiazac® XC

Mexican Brand Names Angiotrofin; Angiotrofin Retard; Presoken; Tilazem

Generic Available Yes: Excludes extended release tablet

Index Terms Diltiazem Hydrochloride

Pharmacologic Category Calcium Channel Blocker

Use

Oral: Essential hypertension; chronic stable angina or angina from coronary artery spasm

Injection: Atrial fibrillation or atrial flutter; paroxysmal supraventricular tachycardia (PSVT)

Unlabeled/Investigational Use Investigational: Therapy of Duchenne muscular dystrophy

Local Anesthetic/Vasoconstrictor Precautions No information available to require special precautions

Effects on Dental Treatment Key adverse event(s) related to dental treatment: Diltiazem has been reported to cause >10% incidence of gingival hyperplasia; usually disappears with discontinuation (consultation with physician is suggested).

(Continued)

Diltiazem (Continued)

Common Adverse Effects Note: Frequencies represent ranges for various dosage forms. Patients with impaired ventricular function and/or conduction abnormalities may have higher incidence of adverse reactions.

>10%:
Cardiovascular: Edema (2% to 15%)
Central nervous system: Headache (5% to 12%)
2% to 10%:
Cardiovascular: AV block (first degree 2% to 8%), edema (lower limb 2% to 8%), pain (6%), bradycardia (2% to 6%), hypotension (<2% to 4%), vasodilation (2% to 3%), extrasystoles (2%), flushing (1% to 2%), palpitation (1% to 2%)
Central nervous system: Dizziness (3% to 10%), nervousness (2%)
Dermatologic: Rash (1% to 4%)
Endocrine & metabolic: Gout (1% to 2%)
Gastrointestinal: Dyspepsia (1% to 6%), constipation (<2% to 4%), vomiting (2%), diarrhea (1% to 2%)
Local: Injection site reactions: Burning, itching (4%)
Neuromuscular & skeletal: Weakness (1% to 4%), myalgia (2%)
Respiratory: Rhinitis (<2% to 10%), pharyngitis (2% to 6%), dyspnea (1% to 6%), bronchitis (1% to 4%), sinus congestion (1% to 2%)

Dosage Adults:
Oral:
Angina:
Capsule, extended release (Cardizem® CD, Cartia XT™, Dilacor® XR, Diltia XT®, Tiazac®): Initial: 120-180 mg once daily (maximum dose: 480 mg/day)
Tablet, extended release (Cardizem® LA): 180 mg once daily; may increase at 7- to 14-day intervals (maximum recommended dose: 360 mg/day)
Tablet, immediate release (Cardizem®): Usual starting dose: 30 mg 4 times/day; usual range: 180-360 mg/day
Hypertension:
Capsule, extended release (Cardizem® CD, Cartia XT™, Dilacor® XR, Diltia XT®, Tiazac®): Initial: 180-240 mg once daily; dose adjustment may be made after 14 days; usual dose range (JNC 7): 180-420 mg/day; Tiazac®: usual dose range: 120-540 mg/day
Capsule, sustained release: Initial: 60-120 mg twice daily; dose adjustment may be made after 14 days; usual range: 240-360 mg/day
Tablet, extended release (Cardizem® LA): Initial: 180-240 mg once daily; dose adjustment may be made after 14 days; usual dose range (JNC 7): 120-540 mg/day
Note: Elderly: Patients ≥60 years may respond to a lower initial dose (ie, 120 mg once daily using extended release capsule)
I.V.: Atrial fibrillation, atrial flutter, PSVT:
Initial bolus dose: 0.25 mg/kg actual body weight over 2 minutes (average adult dose: 20 mg)
Repeat bolus dose (may be administered after 15 minutes if the response is inadequate.): 0.35 mg/kg actual body weight over 2 minutes (average adult dose: 25 mg)
Continuous infusion (requires an infusion pump; infusions >24 hours or infusion rates >15 mg/hour are not recommended.): Initial infusion rate of 10 mg/hour; rate may be increased in 5 mg/hour increments up to 15 mg/hour as needed; some patients may respond to an initial rate of 5 mg/hour.
If diltiazem injection is administered by continuous infusion for >24 hours, the possibility of decreased diltiazem clearance, prolonged elimination half-life, and increased diltiazem and/or diltiazem metabolite plasma concentrations should be considered.
Conversion from I.V. diltiazem to oral diltiazem: Start oral approximately 3 hours after bolus dose.
Oral dose (mg/day) is approximately equal to [rate (mg/hour) x 3 + 3] x 10.
3 mg/hour = 120 mg/day
5 mg/hour = 180 mg/day
7 mg/hour = 240 mg/day
11 mg/hour = 360 mg/day
Dosing comments in renal/hepatic impairment: Use with caution as extensively metabolized by the liver and excreted in the kidneys and bile.
Dialysis: Not removed by hemo- or peritoneal dialysis; supplemental dose is not necessary.

Mechanism of Action Inhibits calcium ion from entering the "slow channels" or select voltage-sensitive areas of vascular smooth muscle and myocardium during depolarization, producing a relaxation of coronary vascular smooth muscle and coronary vasodilation; increases myocardial oxygen delivery in patients with vasospastic angina

Contraindications Hypersensitivity to diltiazem or any component of the formulation; sick sinus syndrome; second- or third-degree AV block (except in patients with a functioning artificial pacemaker); hypotension (systolic <90 mm Hg); acute MI and pulmonary congestion

Warnings/Precautions Increased angina and/or MI has occurred with initiation or dosage titration of calcium channel blockers. Can cause first-degree AV block or sinus bradycardia; other conduction abnormalities are rare. The most common side effect is peripheral edema; occurs within 2-3 weeks of starting therapy. Symptomatic hypotension with or without syncope can rarely occur; blood pressure must be lowered at a rate appropriate for the patient's clinical condition. Concomitant use with beta-blockers or digoxin can result in conduction disturbances. Avoid concurrent I.V. use of diltiazem and a beta-blocker. Use caution in left ventricular dysfunction (can exacerbate condition). Use with caution with hypertrophic cardiomyopathy. Use with caution in hepatic or renal dysfunction.

Drug Interactions

Cytochrome P450 Effect: Substrate of CYP2C9 (minor), 2D6 (minor), 3A4 (major); **Inhibits** CYP2C9 (weak), 2D6 (weak), 3A4 (moderate)

Increased Effect/Toxicity: Diltiazem effects may be additive with amiodarone, beta-blockers, or digoxin, which may lead to bradycardia, other conduction delays, and decreased cardiac output. The levels/effects of diltiazem may be increased by azole antifungals, clarithromycin, diclofenac, doxycycline, erythromycin, imatinib, isoniazid, nefazodone, nicardipine, propofol, protease inhibitors, quinidine, telithromycin, verapamil, and other CYP3A4 inhibitors.

Diltiazem may increase the levels/effects of selected benzodiazepines, calcium channel blockers, cisapride, cyclosporine, ergot alkaloids, selected HMG-CoA reductase inhibitors, mesoridazine, mirtazapine, nateglinide, nefazodone, pimozide, quinidine, sildenafil (and other PDE-5 inhibitors), tacrolimus, thioridazine, venlafaxine, and other CYP3A4 substrates. Blood pressure-lowering effects may be additive with sildenafil, tadalafil, and vardenafil (use caution).

Decreased Effect: Levels/effects of diltiazem may be decreased by aminoglutethimide, carbamazepine, nafcillin, nevirapine, phenobarbital, phenytoin, rifamycins, and other CYP3A4 inducers.

Ethanol/Nutrition/Herb Interactions

Ethanol: Avoid ethanol (may increase risk of hypotension or vasodilation).

Food: Diltiazem serum levels may be elevated if taken with food. Serum concentrations were not altered by grapefruit juice in small clinical trials.

Herb/Nutraceutical: St John's wort may decrease diltiazem levels. Avoid dong quai if using for hypertension (has estrogenic activity). Avoid ephedra (may worsen arrhythmia or hypertension). Avoid yohimbe, ginseng (may worsen hypertension). Avoid garlic (may have increased antihypertensive effect).

Pharmacodynamics/Kinetics

Onset of action: Oral: Immediate release tablet: 30-60 minutes

Absorption: 70% to 80%

Distribution: V_d: 3-13 L/kg; enters breast milk

Protein binding: 70% to 80%

Metabolism: Hepatic; extensive first-pass effect; following single I.V. injection, plasma concentrations of N-monodesmethyldiltiazem and desacetyldiltiazem are typically undetectable; however, these metabolites accumulate to detectable concentrations following 24-hour constant rate infusion. N-monodesmethyldiltiazem appears to have 20% of the potency of diltiazem; desacetyldiltiazem is about 25% to 50% as potent as the parent compound.

Bioavailability: Oral: ~40%

Half-life elimination: Immediate release tablet: 3-4.5 hours, may be prolonged with renal impairment

Time to peak, serum: Immediate release tablet: 2-4 hours

Excretion: Urine and feces (primarily as metabolites)

Pregnancy Risk Factor C

Dosage Forms

Capsule, extended release [once-daily dosing]: 120 mg, 180 mg, 240 mg, 300 mg, 360 mg, 420 mg

Cardizem® CD, Taztia XT™: 120 mg, 180 mg, 240 mg, 300 mg, 360 mg

Cartia XT™: 120 mg, 180 mg, 240 mg, 300 mg

Dilacor® XR, Diltia XT®: 120 mg, 180 mg, 240 mg

Tiazac®: 120 mg, 180 mg, 240 mg, 300 mg, 360 mg, 420 mg

Capsule, sustained release [twice-daily dosing]: 60 mg, 90 mg, 120 mg

Injection, solution: 5 mg/mL (5 mL, 10 mL, 25 mL)

Injection, powder for reconstitution:

Cardizem®: 25 mg

(Continued)

Diltiazem *(Continued)*

Tablet: 30 mg, 60 mg, 90 mg, 120 mg
Cardizem®: 30 mg, 60 mg, 90 mg, 120 mg
Tablet, extended release:
Cardizem® LA: 120 mg, 180 mg, 240 mg, 300 mg, 360 mg, 420 mg

Diltiazem Hydrochloride *see* Diltiazem *on page 505*

Dilt-XR *see* Diltiazem *on page 505*

Dimaphen [OTC] *see* Brompheniramine and Pseudoephedrine *on page 231*

DimenhyDRINATE *(dye men HYE dri nate)*

U.S. Brand Names Dramamine® [OTC]; TripTone® [OTC] [DSC]
Canadian Brand Names Apo-Dimenhydrinate®; Children's Motion Sickness Liquid; Dinate®; Gravol®; Jamp® Travel Tablet; Nauseatol; Novo-Dimenate; SAB-Dimenhydrinate
Mexican Brand Names Vomisin
Generic Available Yes
Pharmacologic Category Antihistamine
Use Treatment and prevention of nausea, vertigo, and vomiting associated with motion sickness

Dosage forms available in Canada (not available in the U.S.), including parenteral formulations and suppositories, are also approved for the treatment of postoperative nausea and vomiting and treatment of radiation sickness.

Unlabeled/Investigational Use Treatment of Meniere's disease

Local Anesthetic/Vasoconstrictor Precautions No information available to require special precautions

Effects on Dental Treatment Key adverse event(s) related to dental treatment: Significant xerostomia (normal salivary flow resumes upon discontinuation).

Common Adverse Effects

>10%:
Central nervous system: Slight to moderate drowsiness
Respiratory: Thickening of bronchial secretions

1% to 10%:
Central nervous system: Headache, fatigue, nervousness, dizziness
Gastrointestinal: Abdominal pain, diarrhea, increased appetite, nausea, weight gain, xerostomia
Neuromuscular & skeletal: Arthralgia
Respiratory: Pharyngitis

Mechanism of Action Competes with histamine for H_1-receptor sites on effector cells in the gastrointestinal tract, blood vessels, and respiratory tract; blocks chemoreceptor trigger zone, diminishes vestibular stimulation, and depresses labyrinthine function through its central anticholinergic activity

Drug Interactions

Increased Effect/Toxicity: CNS depressants may increase the degree of sedation and respiratory depression with antihistamines. May increase the absorption of digoxin. Central and/or peripheral anticholinergic syndrome can occur when administered with amantadine, rimantadine, narcotic analgesics, phenothiazines and other antipsychotics (especially with high anticholinergic activity), tricyclic antidepressants, quinidine, disopyramide, procainamide, and antihistamines.

Decreased Effect: May increase gastric degradation of levodopa and decrease the amount of levodopa absorbed by delaying gastric emptying. Therapeutic effects of cholinergic agents (tacrine, donepezil) and neuroleptics may be antagonized.

Pharmacodynamics/Kinetics
Onset of action: Oral: ~15-30 minutes
Absorption: Oral: Well absorbed
Pregnancy Risk Factor B

Dimercaprol *(dye mer KAP role)*

U.S. Brand Names BAL in Oil®
Generic Available No
Index Terms BAL; British Anti-Lewisite; Dithioglycerol
Pharmacologic Category Antidote
Use Antidote to gold, arsenic (except arsine), and mercury poisoning (except nonalkyl mercury); adjunct to edetate calcium disodium in lead poisoning; possibly effective for antimony, bismuth, chromium, copper, nickel, tungsten, or zinc

Local Anesthetic/Vasoconstrictor Precautions No information available to require special precautions

Effects on Dental Treatment No significant effects or complications reported

Common Adverse Effects

>10%:
Cardiovascular: Hypertension, tachycardia (dose related)
Central nervous system: Headache
1% to 10%: Gastrointestinal: Nausea, vomiting

Mechanism of Action Sulfhydryl group combines with ions of various heavy metals to form relatively stable, nontoxic, soluble chelates which are excreted in urine

Drug Interactions

Increased Effect/Toxicity: Toxic complexes with iron, cadmium, selenium, or uranium.

Pharmacodynamics/Kinetics

Distribution: To all tissues including the brain
Metabolism: Rapidly hepatic to inactive metabolites
Time to peak, serum: 0.5-1 hour
Excretion: Urine

Pregnancy Risk Factor C

Dimetapp® 12-Hour Non-Drowsy Extentabs® [OTC] [DSC] *see* Pseudoephedrine on page 1381

Dimetapp® Decongestant Infant [OTC] [DSC] *see* Pseudoephedrine on page 1381

Dimetapp® Infant Decongestant Plus Cough [OTC] [DSC] *see* Pseudoephedrine and Dextromethorphan on page 1383

Dimetapp® Toddler's [OTC] *see* Phenylephrine on page 1293

β,β-Dimethylcysteine *see* Penicillamine on page 1267

Dimethyl Triazeno Imidazole Carboxamide *see* Dacarbazine on page 435

Dinoprostone (dye noe PROST one)

U.S. Brand Names Cervidil®; Prepidil®; Prostin E₂®
Canadian Brand Names Cervidil®; Prepidil®; Prostin E₂®
Generic Available No
Index Terms PGE₂; Prostaglandin E₂
Pharmacologic Category Abortifacient; Prostaglandin
Use

Gel: Promote cervical ripening in patients at or near term in whom there is a medical or obstetrical indication for the induction of labor

Suppositories: Terminate pregnancy from 12th through 20th week of gestation; evacuate uterus in cases of missed abortion or intrauterine fetal death up to 28 weeks of gestation; manage benign hydatidiform mole (nonmetastatic gestational trophoblastic disease)

Vaginal insert: Initiation and/or continuation of cervical ripening in patients at or near term in whom there is a medical or obstetrical indication for the induction of labor

Local Anesthetic/Vasoconstrictor Precautions No information available to require special precautions

Effects on Dental Treatment No significant effects or complications reported

Common Adverse Effects

Gel: 1% to 10%:
Central nervous system: Fever (1%)
Gastrointestinal: GI upset (6%)
Genitourinary: Abnormal uterine contractions (7%), warm feeling in vagina (2%)
Neuromuscular & skeletal: Back pain (3%)

Suppository: Frequency not defined:
Cardiovascular: Arrhythmia, chest pain, chest tightness, hypotension, syncope
Central nervous system: Chills, dizziness, fever, headache, shivering, tension
Dermatologic: Rash, skin discoloration
Endocrine & metabolic: Breast tenderness, endometritis, hot flashes
Gastrointestinal: Dehydration, diarrhea, nausea, vomiting
Genitourinary: uterine rupture, urinary retention, vaginal pain, vaginismus, vaginitis, vulvitis
Neuromuscular & skeletal: Arthralgia, backache, joint inflammation/pain (new or exacerbated), leg cramps (nocturnal), muscle cramp/pain, myalgia, paresthesia, stiff neck, tremor, weakness
Ocular: Blurred vision, eye pain
Otic: Hearing impairment
(Continued)

Dinoprostone *(Continued)*

Respiratory: Cough, dyspnea, laryngitis, pharyngitis, wheezing
Miscellaneous: Diaphoresis

Vaginal insert: 1% to 10%: Genitourinary: Uterine hyperstimulation *without* fetal distress (2% to 5%), uterine hyperstimulation *with* fetal distress (3%)

Mechanism of Action A synthetic prostaglandin E$_2$ abortifacient that stimulates uterine contractions similar to those seen during natural labor. Prostaglandin E$_2$ plays a role in cervical ripening, which allows the fetus to pass through the birth canal.

Drug Interactions

Increased Effect/Toxicity: Dinoprostone may increase the effect of oxytocin; wait 6-12 hours after dinoprostone gel administration or at least 30 minutes after removal of vaginal insert before initiating oxytocin.

Pharmacodynamics/Kinetics

Onset of action (uterine contractions): Vaginal suppository: Within 10 minutes
Duration: Vaginal insert: 0.3 mg/hour over 12 hours; Vaginal suppository: Up to 2-3 hours
Absorption: Vaginal suppository: Slow
Metabolism: In many tissues including lungs, liver, and kidney
Half-life elimination: 2.5-5 minutes
Time to peak, plasma: Gel: 30-45 minutes
Excretion: Primarily urine; feces (small amounts)

Pregnancy Risk Factor C

Diocto® [OTC] *see* Docusate *on page 522*

Dioctyl Calcium Sulfosuccinate *see* Docusate *on page 522*

Dioctyl Sodium Sulfosuccinate *see* Docusate *on page 522*

Diotame® [OTC] *see* Bismuth *on page 217*

Diovan® *see* Valsartan *on page 1643*

Diovan HCT® *see* Valsartan and Hydrochlorothiazide *on page 1644*

Dipentum® *see* Olsalazine *on page 1205*

Diphen® [OTC] *see* DiphenhydrAMINE *on page 510*

Diphen® AF [OTC] *see* DiphenhydrAMINE *on page 510*

Diphenhist [OTC] *see* DiphenhydrAMINE *on page 510*

DiphenhydrAMINE *(dye fen HYE dra meen)*

Related Information

Management of Patients Undergoing Cancer Therapy *on page 1826*
Ulcerative and Erosive Disorders *on page 1809*
Viral Infections *on page 1806*

Related Sample Prescriptions

Recurrent Aphthous Stomatitis *on page 1844*

U.S. Brand Names Aler-Cap [OTC]; Aler-Dryl [OTC]; Aler-Tab [OTC]; AllerMax® [OTC]; Altaryl [OTC]; Banophen® [OTC]; Banophen® Anti-Itch [OTC]; Benadryl® Allergy [OTC]; Benadryl® Children's Allergy [OTC]; Benadryl® Children's Allergy Fastmelt® [OTC]; Benadryl® Dye-Free Allergy [OTC]; Benadryl® Injection; Benadryl® Itch Stopping [OTC]; Benadryl® Itch Stopping Extra Strength [OTC]; Ben-Tann; Compoz® Nighttime Sleep Aid [OTC]; Dermamycin® [OTC]; Diphen® [OTC]; Diphen® AF [OTC]; Diphenhist [OTC]; Dytan™; Genahist® [OTC]; Hydramine® [OTC]; Nytol® Quick Caps [OTC]; Nytol® Quick Gels [OTC]; Siladryl® Allergy [OTC]; Silphen® [OTC]; Simply Sleep® [OTC]; Sleep-ettes D [OTC]; Sleepinal® [OTC]; Sominex® [OTC]; Sominex® Maximum Strength [OTC]; Triaminic® Thin Strips™ Cough and Runny Nose [OTC]; Twilite® [OTC]; Unisom® Maximum Strength SleepGels® [OTC]

Canadian Brand Names Allerdryl®; Allernix; Benadryl®; Nytol®; Nytol® Extra Strength; PMS-Diphenhydramine; Simply Sleep®

Mexican Brand Names Nytol Quickgels; Unisom

Generic Available Yes: Excludes chewable tablet, gel, orally-disintegrating tablet, stick, strip

Index Terms Diphenhydramine Citrate; Diphenhydramine Hydrochloride; Diphenhydramine Tannate

Pharmacologic Category Antihistamine

Dental Use Symptomatic relief of nasal mucosal congestion

Use Symptomatic relief of allergic symptoms caused by histamine release including nasal allergies and allergic dermatosis; adjunct to epinephrine in the treatment of anaphylaxis; nighttime sleep aid; prevention or treatment of motion sickness; antitussive; management of Parkinsonian syndrome including drug-induced extrapyramidal symptoms; topically for relief of pain and itching associated with insect bites, minor cuts and burns, or rashes due to poison ivy, poison oak, and poison sumac

Local Anesthetic/Vasoconstrictor Precautions No information available to require special precautions

Effects on Dental Treatment Key adverse event(s) related to dental treatment: Xerostomia (normal salivary flow resumes upon discontinuation) and dry mucous membranes. Chronic use of antihistamines will inhibit salivary flow, particularly in elderly patients; may contribute to periodontal disease and oral discomfort. See Dental Comment.

Significant Adverse Effects Frequency not defined.

Cardiovascular: Chest tightness, extrasystoles, hypotension, palpitation, tachycardia

Central nervous system: Chills, confusion, convulsion, disturbed coordination, dizziness, euphoria, excitation, fatigue, headache, insomnia, irritability, nervousness, paradoxical excitement, restlessness, sedation, sleepiness, vertigo

Dermatologic: Photosensitivity, rash, urticaria

Endocrine & metabolic: Menstrual irregularities (early menses)

Gastrointestinal: Anorexia, constipation, diarrhea, dry mucous membranes, epigastric distress, nausea, throat tightness, vomiting, xerostomia

Genitourinary: Difficult urination, urinary frequency, urinary retention

Hematologic: Agranulocytosis, hemolytic anemia, thrombocytopenia

Neuromuscular & skeletal: Neuritis, paresthesia, tremor

Ocular: Blurred vision, diplopia

Otic: Labyrinthitis (acute), tinnitus

Respiratory: Nasal stuffiness, thickening of bronchial secretions, wheezing

Miscellaneous: Anaphylactic shock, diaphoresis

Dental Usual Dosing Symptomatic relief of nasal mucosal congestion: Adults: Oral: 25-50 mg every 6-8 hours

Dosage Note: Dosages are expressed as the hydrochloride salt.

Children:

Allergic reactions or motion sickness: Oral, I.M., I.V.: 5 mg/kg/day or 150 mg/m^2/day in divided doses every 6-8 hours, not to exceed 300 mg/day

Alternate dosing by age: Oral:

2 to <6 years: 6.25 mg every 4-6 hours; maximum: 37.5 mg/day

6 to <12 years: 12.5-25 mg every 4-6 hours; maximum: 150 mg/day

≥12 years: 25-50 mg every 4-6 hours; maximum: 300 mg/day

Night-time sleep aid: Oral: Children ≥12 years: 50 mg at bedtime

Antitussive: Oral:

2 to <6 years: 6.25 mg every 4 hours; maximum 37.5 mg/day

6 to <12 years: 12.5 mg every 4 hours; maximum 75 mg/day

≥12 years: 25 mg every 4 hours; maximum 150 mg/day

Treatment of dystonic reactions: I.M., I.V.: 0.5-1 mg/kg/dose

Relief of pain and itching: Topical: Children ≥2 years: Apply 1% or 2% to affected area up to 3-4 times/day

Adults:

Allergic reactions or motion sickness: Oral: 25-50 mg every 6-8 hours

Antitussive: Oral: 25 mg every 4 hours; maximum 150 mg/24 hours

Nighttime sleep aid: Oral: 50 mg at bedtime

Allergic reactions or motion sickness: I.M., I.V.: 10-50 mg per dose; single doses up to 100 mg may be used if needed; not to exceed 400 mg/day

Dystonic reaction: I.M., I.V.: 50 mg in a single dose; may repeat in 20-30 minutes if necessary

Relief of pain and itching: Topical: Apply 1% or 2% to affected area up to 3-4 times/day

Elderly: Initial: 25 mg 2-3 times/day increasing as needed

Mechanism of Action Competes with histamine for H$_1$-receptor sites on effector cells in the gastrointestinal tract, blood vessels, and respiratory tract; anticholinergic and sedative effects are also seen

Contraindications Hypersensitivity to diphenhydramine or any component of the formulation; acute asthma; neonates or premature infants; breast-feeding; use as a local anesthetic (injection)

Warnings/Precautions Causes sedation, caution must be used in performing tasks which require alertness (eg, operating machinery or driving). Sedative effects of CNS depressants or ethanol are potentiated. Diphenhydramine has high sedative and anticholinergic properties, so it may not be considered the antihistamine of choice for prolonged use in the elderly. Use caution in children; may cause paradoxical excitation in pediatric patients, toxicity can result in hallucinations, coma, and death. Use with caution in patients with angle-closure glaucoma, pyloroduodenal obstruction (including stenotic peptic ulcer), urinary tract obstruction (including bladder neck obstruction and symptomatic prostatic hyperplasia), asthma, hyperthyroidism, increased intraocular pressure, and cardiovascular disease (including hypertension and tachycardia). Some preparations contain soy protein; avoid use in patients with soy protein or peanut allergies.

(Continued)

DiphenhydrAMINE *(Continued)*

Self-medication (OTC use): Do not use with other products containing diphenhydramine, even ones used on the skin. Oral products are not for OTC use in children <6 years of age. Topical products should not be used on large areas of the body, or on chicken pox or measles. Healthcare provider should be contacted if topical use is needed for >7 days. Topical products are not for OTC use in children <2 years of age.

Drug Interactions Inhibits CYP2D6 (moderate)

Acetylcholinesterase inhibitors (central): Acetylcholinesterase inhibitors, central (donepezil, galantamine, rivastigmine, tacrine) may diminish the therapeutic effect of anticholinergics. If the anticholinergic action is a side effect of the agent, the result may be beneficial. Anticholinergics may diminish the therapeutic effect of acetylcholinesterase inhibitors (central). Monitor for reduced therapeutic effects of either drug.

Anticholinergic agents: Diphenhydramine may enhance the adverse/toxic effect of other anticholinergics; monitor for additive effects.

Antipsychotic agents (phenothiazines): Antihistamines may enhance the arrhythmogenic effect of antipsychotic agents (phenothiazines).

Betahistine: Antihistamines may diminish the therapeutic effect of betahistine.

CNS depressants: Sedative effects may be additive with other CNS depressants; includes ethanol, benzodiazepines, barbiturates, opioid analgesics, and other sedative agents; monitor for increased effect

CYP2D6 substrates: Diphenhydramine may increase the levels/effects of CYP2D6 substrates. Example substrates include amphetamines, selected beta-blockers, dextromethorphan, fluoxetine, lidocaine, mirtazapine, nefazodone, paroxetine, risperidone, ritonavir, thioridazine, tricyclic antidepressants, and venlafaxine.

CYP2D6 prodrug substrates: Diphenhydramine may decrease the levels/effects of CYP2D6 prodrug substrates. Example prodrug substrates include codeine, hydrocodone, oxycodone, and tramadol.

Pramlintide: Pramlintide may enhance the anticholinergic GI effect of anticholinergics.

Ethanol/Nutrition/Herb Interactions

Ethanol: Avoid ethanol (may increase CNS depression).

Herb/Nutraceutical: Avoid valerian, St John's wort, kava kava, gotu kola (may increase CNS depression).

Dietary Considerations

Benadryl® Allergy strips contain sodium 4 mg per 25 mg strip.

Benadryl® Children's Allergy chewable tablets contain phenylalanine 4.2 mg, magnesium 15 mg, and sodium 2 mg per 12.5 mg tablet.

Benadryl® Children's Allergy Fastmelt® contains phenylalanine 4.5 mg/tablet and soy protein isolate (contraindicated in patients with soy protein allergies; use caution in peanut allergic individuals, ~10% are estimated to also have soy protein allergies).

Dytan™ chewable tablets contain phenylalanine.

Pharmacodynamics/Kinetics

Onset of action: Maximum sedative effect: 1-3 hours

Duration: 4-7 hours

Distribution: V_d: 3-22 L/kg

Protein binding: 78%

Metabolism: Extensively hepatic n-demethylation via CYP2D6; minor demethylation via CYP1A2, 2C9 and 2C19; smaller degrees in pulmonary and renal systems; significant first-pass effect

Bioavailability: Oral: ~40% to 70%

Half-life elimination: 2-10 hours; Elderly: 13.5 hours

Time to peak, serum: 2-4 hours

Excretion: Urine (as unchanged drug)

Pregnancy Risk Factor B

Lactation Enters breast milk/contraindicated

Breast-Feeding Considerations Infants may be more sensitive to the effects of antihistamines. Use while breastfeeding is contraindicated.

Dosage Forms Excipient information presented when available (limited, particularly for generics); consult specific product labeling.

Caplet, as hydrochloride: 25 mg, 50 mg

Aler-Dryl, AllerMax®, Compoz® Nighttime Sleep Aid, Sleep-ettes D, Sominex® Maximum Strength, Twilite®: 50 mg

Nytol® Quick Caps, Simply Sleep®: 25 mg

Capsule, as hydrochloride: 25 mg, 50 mg

Aler-Cap, Banophen®, Benadryl® Allergy, Diphen®, Diphenhist, Genahist®: 25 mg

Sleepinal®: 50 mg

Capsule, softgel, as hydrochloride: 50 mg

Benadryl® Dye-Free Allergy: 25 mg [dye-free]

Compoz® Nighttime Sleep Aid, Nytol® Quick Gels, Sleepinal®, Unisom® Maximum Strength SleepGels®: 50 mg

Captab, as hydrochloride:
Diphenhist®: 25 mg

Cream, as hydrochloride: 2% (30 g)
Banophen® Anti-Itch: 2% (30 g) [contains zinc acetate 0.1%]
Benadryl® Itch Stopping: 1% (30 g) [contains zinc acetate 0.1%]
Benadryl® Itch Stopping Extra Strength: 2% (30 g) [contains zinc acetate 0.1%]
Diphenhist®: 2% (30 g) [contains zinc acetate 0.1%]

Elixir, as hydrochloride:
Altaryl: 12.5 mg/5 mL (120 mL, 480 mL, 3840 mL) [cherry flavor]
Banophen®: 12.5 mg/5 mL (120 mL)
Diphen AF: 12.5 mg/5 mL (120 mL, 240 mL, 480 mL) [alcohol free; cherry flavor]

Gel, topical, as hydrochloride:
Benadryl® Itch Stopping Extra Strength: 2% (120 mL)

Injection, solution, as hydrochloride: 50 mg/mL (1 mL)
Benadryl®: 50 mg/mL (1 mL; 10 mL [DSC])

Liquid, as hydrochloride:
AllerMax®: 12.5 mg/5 mL (120 mL)
Benadryl® Allergy: 12.5 mg/5 mL (120 mL, 240 mL) [alcohol free; contains sodium benzoate; cherry flavor]
Benadryl® Dye-Free Allergy: 12.5 mg/5 mL (120 mL) [alcohol free, dye free, sugar free; contains sodium benzoate; bubble gum flavor]
Genahist®: 12.5 mg/5 mL (120 mL) [alcohol free, sugar free; contains sodium benzoate; cherry flavor]
Hydramine®: 12.5 mg/5 mL (120 mL, 480 mL) [alcohol free]
Siladryl® Allergy: 12.5 mg/5 mL (120 mL, 240 mL, 480 mL) [alcohol free, sugar free; black cherry flavor]

Liquid, topical, as hydrochloride [stick]:
Benadryl® Itch Stopping Extra Strength: 2% (14 mL) [contains zinc acetate 0.1% and alcohol]

Solution, oral, as hydrochloride:
Diphenhist: 12.5 mg/5 mL (120 mL, 480 mL) [alcohol free; contains sodium benzoate]

Solution, topical, as hydrochloride [spray]:
Benadryl® Itch Stopping Extra Strength: 2% (60 mL) [contains zinc acetate 0.1% and alcohol]
Dermamycin®: 2% (60 mL) [contains menthol 1%]

Strips, oral, as hydrochloride:
Benadryl® Allergy: 25 mg (10s) [contains sodium 4 mg/strip; vanilla mint flavor]
Benadryl® Children's Allergy: 12.5 mg (10s) [vanilla mint flavor]
Triaminic® Thin Strips™ Cough and Runny Nose: 12. 5 mg (16s) [grape flavor]

Suspension, as tannate:
Ben-Tann: 25 mg/5 mL (120 ml) [contains sodium benzoate; strawberry flavor]
Dytan™: 25 mg/5 mL (120 mL) [strawberry flavor]

Syrup, as hydrochloride:
Silphen® Cough: 12.5 mg/5 mL (120 mL, 240 mL, 480 mL) [contains alcohol; 5%; strawberry flavor]

Tablet, as hydrochloride: 25 mg, 50 mg
Aler-Tab, Benadryl® Allergy, Genahist®, Sominex®: 25 mg

Tablet, chewable, as hydrochloride:
Benadryl® Children's Allergy: 12.5 mg [contains phenylalanine 4.2 mg, magnesium 15 mg, and sodium 2 mg per tablet; grape flavor]

Tablet, chewable, as tannate:
Dytan™: 25 mg [contains phenylalanine; strawberry flavor]

Tablet, orally disintegrating, as citrate:
Benadryl® Children's Allergy Fastmelt®: 19 mg [equivalent to diphenhydramine hydrochloride 12.5 mg; contains phenylalanine 4.5 mg/tablet and soy protein isolate; cherry flavor]

Dental Comment 25-50 mg of diphenhydramine orally every 4-6 hours can be used to treat mild dermatologic manifestations of allergic reactions to penicillin and other antibiotics. Diphenhydramine is not recommended as local anesthetic for either infiltration route or nerve block since the vehicle has caused local necrosis upon injection. A 50:50 mixture of diphenhydramine liquid (12.5 mg/5 mL) in Kaopectate® or Maalox® is used as a local application for recurrent aphthous ulcers; swish 1 tablespoonful for 2 minutes 4 times/day.

Diphenhydramine and Acetaminophen see Acetaminophen and Diphenhydramine on page 38

Diphenhydramine and Pseudoephedrine
(dye fen HYE dra meen & soo doe e FED rin)

Related Information
DiphenhydrAMINE *on page 510*
Pseudoephedrine *on page 1381*

U.S. Brand Names Benadryl® Children's Allergy and Cold Fastmelt™ [OTC]; Benadryl-D™ Allergy and Sinus Fastmelt™ [OTC]; Benadryl-D™ Children's Allergy and Sinus [OTC]

Generic Available No

Index Terms Pseudoephedrine and Diphenhydramine

Pharmacologic Category Antihistamine/Decongestant Combination

Use Relief of symptoms of upper respiratory mucosal congestion in seasonal and perennial nasal allergies, acute rhinitis, rhinosinusitis, and eustachian tube blockage

Local Anesthetic/Vasoconstrictor Precautions Use with caution since pseudoephedrine is a sympathomimetic amine which could interact with epinephrine to cause a pressor response

Effects on Dental Treatment Key adverse event(s) related to dental treatment: Pseudoephedrine: Xerostomia (normal salivary flow resumes upon discontinuation). Chronic use of antihistamines will inhibit salivary flow, particularly in elderly patients; this may contribute to periodontal disease and oral discomfort.

Common Adverse Effects See individual agents.

Drug Interactions
Cytochrome P450 Effect: Diphenhydramine: **Inhibits** CYP2D6 (moderate)
Increased Effect/Toxicity: See individual agents.
Decreased Effect: See individual agents.

Diphenhydramine Citrate *see* DiphenhydrAMINE *on page 510*

Diphenhydramine Hydrochloride *see* DiphenhydrAMINE *on page 510*

Diphenhydramine, Hydrocodone, and Phenylephrine *see* Hydrocodone, Phenylephrine, and Diphenhydramine *on page 834*

Diphenhydramine Tannate *see* DiphenhydrAMINE *on page 510*

Diphenoxylate and Atropine (dye fen OKS i late & A troe peen)

Related Information
Atropine *on page 166*

U.S. Brand Names Lomotil®; Lonox®

Canadian Brand Names Lomotil®

Generic Available Yes

Index Terms Atropine and Diphenoxylate

Pharmacologic Category Antidiarrheal

Use Treatment of diarrhea

Local Anesthetic/Vasoconstrictor Precautions No information available to require special precautions

Effects on Dental Treatment Key adverse event(s) related to dental treatment: Significant xerostomia (normal salivary flow resumes upon discontinuation).

Common Adverse Effects Frequency not defined.
Cardiovascular: Tachycardia
Central nervous system: Confusion, depression, dizziness, drowsiness, euphoria, flushing, headache, hyperthermia, lethargy, malaise, restlessness, sedation
Dermatologic: Angioneurotic edema, dry skin, pruritus, urticaria
Gastrointestinal: Abdominal discomfort, anorexia, gum swelling, nausea, pancreatitis, paralytic ileus, toxic megacolon, vomiting, xerostomia
Genitourinary: Urinary retention
Neuromuscular & skeletal: Numbness
Miscellaneous: Anaphylaxis

Restrictions C-V

Mechanism of Action Diphenoxylate inhibits excessive GI motility and GI propulsion; commercial preparations contain a subtherapeutic amount of atropine to discourage abuse

Drug Interactions
Increased Effect/Toxicity: Pramlintide: Pramlintide may enhance the anticholinergic effect of anticholinergics; additive effects on reduced GI motility may occur.

Pharmacodynamics/Kinetics

Atropine: See Atropine monograph.

Diphenoxylate:

Onset of action: Antidiarrheal: 45-60 minutes

Duration: Antidiarrheal: 3-4 hours

Absorption: Well absorbed

Metabolism: Extensively hepatic via ester hydrolysis to diphenoxylic acid (active)

Half-life elimination: Diphenoxylate: 2.5 hours; Diphenoxylic acid: 12-14 hours

Time to peak, serum: 2 hours

Excretion: Primarily feces (49% as unchanged drug and metabolites); urine (~14%, <1% as unchanged drug)

Pregnancy Risk Factor C

Diphenylhydantoin *see* Phenytoin *on page 1295*

Diphtheria and Tetanus Toxoids and Acellular Pertussis Adsorbed, Hepatitis B (Recombinant) and Inactivated Poliovirus Vaccine Combined *see* Diphtheria, Tetanus Toxoids, Acellular Pertussis, Hepatitis B (Recombinant), and Poliovirus (Inactivated) Vaccine *on page 515*

Diphtheria CRM$_{197}$ Protein *see* Pneumococcal Conjugate Vaccine (7-Valent) *on page 1318*

Diphtheria CRM$_{197}$ Protein Conjugate *see Haemophilus* b Conjugate Vaccine *on page 802*

Diphtheria, Tetanus Toxoids, Acellular Pertussis, Hepatitis B (Recombinant), and Poliovirus (Inactivated) Vaccine

(dif THEER ee a, TET a nus TOKS oyds, ay CEL yoo lar per TUS sis, hep a TYE tis bee ree KOM be nant, & POE lee oh VYE rus, in ak ti VAY ted vak SEEN)

Related Information

Hepatitis B Vaccine *on page 811*

Immunizations (Vaccines) *on page 1886*

Poliovirus Vaccine (Inactivated) *on page 1544*

Tetanus Toxoid (Adsorbed) *on page 1544*

Tetanus Toxoid (Fluid) *on page 1545*

U.S. Brand Names Pediarix®

Canadian Brand Names Pediarix®

Generic Available No

Index Terms Diphtheria and Tetanus Toxoids and Acellular Pertussis Adsorbed, Hepatitis B (Recombinant) and Inactivated Poliovirus Vaccine Combined

Pharmacologic Category Vaccine

Use Combination vaccine for the active immunization against diphtheria, tetanus, pertussis, hepatitis B virus (all known subtypes), and poliomyelitis (caused by poliovirus types 1, 2, and 3)

Local Anesthetic/Vasoconstrictor Precautions No information available to require special precautions

Effects on Dental Treatment No significant effects or complications reported

Common Adverse Effects All serious adverse reactions must be reported to the U.S. Department of Health and Human Services (DHHS) Vaccine Adverse Event Reporting System (VAERS) 1-800-822-7967.

Adverse events reported within 4 days of vaccination at 2-, 4-, and 6 months of age in patients given Pediarix® concomitantly with Hib conjugate vaccine and PCV7 vaccine.

>10%:

Central nervous system: Central nervous system: Irritability/fussiness (61% to 65%; grade 3: 3% to 4%), drowsiness (41% to 57%), fever ≥100.4°F (28% to 39%)

Gastrointestinal: Loss of appetite (26% to 31%; grade 3: <1%)

Local: Injection site: Redness (25% to 40%; >20 mm: 2% to 3%), pain (31% to 36%; grade 3: 2% to 3%), swelling (17% to 29%; >20 mm: 2% to 3%)

1% to 10%: Central nervous system: Fever ≥103.1°F (≤1%)

Additional and postmarketing events: Anaphylactic/anaphylactoid reaction, angioedema, anorexia, apnea, arthus-type hypersensitivity reactions, brachial neuritis, bronchitis, bulging fontanelle, consciousness depressed, cranial mononeuropathy, crying, cyanosis, demyelinating disease, dermatitis, diarrhea, dyspnea, erythema, fatigue, febrile convulsion, Guillain-Barré syndrome, hypersensitivity reaction, hypotonia, hypotonic-hyporesposnive episode, injection site reactions (cellulitis, induration, itching, nodule, warmth), insomnia, lethargy, limb pain, limb swelling, liver function test abnormalities,

(Continued)

Diphtheria, Tetanus Toxoids, Acellular Pertussis, Hepatitis B (Recombinant), and Poliovirus (Inactivated) Vaccine *(Continued)*

nervousness, pallor, peripheral mononeruopathy, petechiae, pyrexia, rash, restlessness, screaming, seizure, SIDS, somnolence, upper respiratory tract infection, urticaria, vomiting

Mechanism of Action Promotes active immunity to diphtheria, tetanus, pertussis, hepatitis B and poliovirus (types 1, 2 and 3) by inducing production of specific antibodies and antitoxins.

Drug Interactions

Decreased Effect: Immunosuppressant medications or therapies (antimetabolites, alkylating agents, cytotoxic drugs, corticosteroids, irradiation) may decrease vaccine effectiveness, consider deferring vaccination for 3 months after immunosuppressant therapy is discontinued.

Pharmacodynamics/Kinetics Onset of action: Immune response observed to all components 1 month following the 3-dose series

Pregnancy Risk Factor C

Diphtheria Toxoid Conjugate *see* Haemophilus b Conjugate Vaccine *on page 802*

Dipivalyl Epinephrine *see* Dipivefrin *on page 516*

Dipivefrin *(dye PI ve frin)*

U.S. Brand Names Propine®
Canadian Brand Names Ophtho-Dipivefrin™; PMS-Dipivefrin; Propine®
Mexican Brand Names Diopine-C
Generic Available Yes
Index Terms Dipivalyl Epinephrine; Dipivefrin Hydrochloride; DPE
Pharmacologic Category Alpha/Beta Agonist; Ophthalmic Agent, Antiglaucoma; Ophthalmic Agent, Vasoconstrictor
Use Reduces elevated intraocular pressure in chronic open-angle glaucoma; also used to treat ocular hypertension, low tension, and secondary glaucomas
Local Anesthetic/Vasoconstrictor Precautions No information available to require special precautions
Effects on Dental Treatment No significant effects or complications reported
Mechanism of Action Dipivefrin is a prodrug of epinephrine which is the active agent that stimulates alpha- and/or beta-adrenergic receptors increasing aqueous humor outflow
Pregnancy Risk Factor B

Dipivefrin Hydrochloride *see* Dipivefrin *on page 516*
Diprivan® *see* Propofol *on page 1367*
Diprolene® *see* Betamethasone *on page 206*
Diprolene® AF *see* Betamethasone *on page 206*
Dipropylacetic Acid *see* Valproic Acid and Derivatives *on page 1638*

Dipyridamole *(dye peer ID a mole)*

U.S. Brand Names Persantine®
Canadian Brand Names Apo-Dipyridamole FC®; Persantine®
Mexican Brand Names Persantin
Generic Available Yes
Pharmacologic Category Antiplatelet Agent; Vasodilator
Use
Oral: Used with warfarin to decrease thrombosis in patients after artificial heart valve replacement
I.V.: Diagnostic agent in CAD
Local Anesthetic/Vasoconstrictor Precautions No information available to require special precautions
Effects on Dental Treatment No significant effects or complications reported
Common Adverse Effects
Oral:
>10%: Dizziness (14%)
1% to 10%:
Central nervous system: Headache (2%)
Dermatologic: Rash (2%)
Gastrointestinal: Abdominal distress (6%)
Frequency not defined: Diarrhea, vomiting, flushing, pruritus, angina pectoris, liver dysfunction

I.V.:
>10%:
Cardiovascular: Exacerbation of angina pectoris (20%)
Central nervous system: Dizziness (12%), headache (12%)
1% to 10%:
Cardiovascular: Hypotension (5%), hypertension (2%), blood pressure lability (2%), ECG abnormalities (ST-T changes, extrasystoles; 5% to 8%), pain (3%), tachycardia (3%)
Central nervous system: Flushing (3%), fatigue (1%)
Gastrointestinal: Nausea (5%)
Neuromuscular & skeletal: Paresthesia (1%)
Respiratory: Dyspnea (3%)
Mechanism of Action Inhibits the activity of adenosine deaminase and phosphodiesterase, which causes an accumulation of adenosine, adenine nucleotides, and cyclic AMP; these mediators then inhibit platelet aggregation and may cause vasodilation; may also stimulate release of prostacyclin or PGD_2; causes coronary vasodilation
Drug Interactions
Increased Effect/Toxicity: Adenosine blood levels and pharmacologic effects are increased with dipyridamole; consider reduced doses of adenosine.
Decreased Effect: Decreased vasodilation from I.V. dipyridamole when given to patients taking theophylline. Theophylline may reduce the pharmacologic effects of dipyridamole (hold theophylline preparations for 36-48 hours before dipyridamole facilitated stress test). Dipyridamole may counteract effect of cholinesterase inhibitor and may aggravate myasthenia gravis.
Pharmacodynamics/Kinetics
Absorption: Readily, but variable
Distribution: Adults: V_d: 2-3 L/kg
Protein binding: 91% to 99%
Metabolism: Hepatic
Half-life elimination: Terminal: 10-12 hours
Time to peak, serum: 2-2.5 hours
Excretion: Feces (as glucuronide conjugates and unchanged drug)
Pregnancy Risk Factor B

Dipyridamole and Aspirin *see* Aspirin and Dipyridamole *on page 154*

Dirithromycin (dye RITH roe mye sin)

U.S. Brand Names Dynabac® [DSC]
Generic Available No
Pharmacologic Category Antibiotic, Macrolide
Use Treatment of mild to moderate upper and lower respiratory tract infections due to *Moraxella catarrhalis, Streptococcus pneumoniae, Legionella pneumophila, H. influenzae,* or *S. pyogenes,* ie, acute exacerbation of chronic bronchitis, secondary bacterial infection of acute bronchitis, community-acquired pneumonia, pharyngitis/tonsillitis, and uncomplicated infections of the skin and skin structure due to *Staphylococcus aureus*
Local Anesthetic/Vasoconstrictor Precautions No information available to require special precautions
Effects on Dental Treatment No significant effects or complications reported
Common Adverse Effects 1% to 10%:
Central nervous system: Headache, dizziness, vertigo, insomnia
Dermatologic: Rash, pruritus, urticaria
Endocrine & metabolic: Hyperkalemia
Gastrointestinal: Abdominal pain, nausea, diarrhea, vomiting, dyspepsia, flatulence
Hematologic: Thrombocytosis, eosinophilia, segmented neutrophils
Neuromuscular & skeletal: Weakness, pain, increased CPK
Respiratory: Cough increased, dyspnea
Mechanism of Action After being converted during intestinal absorption to its active form, erythromycylamine, dirithromycin inhibits protein synthesis by binding to the 50S ribosomal subunits of susceptible microorganisms
Drug Interactions
Cytochrome P450 Effect: Substrate of CYP3A4 (minor)
Increased Effect/Toxicity: Absorption of dirithromycin is slightly enhanced with concomitant antacids and H_2 antagonists. Dirithromycin may, like erythromycin, increase the effect of alfentanil, anticoagulants, bromocriptine, carbamazepine, cyclosporine, digoxin, disopyramide, ergots, methylprednisolone, cisapride, and triazolam.
(Continued)

Dirithromycin *(Continued)*

Note: Interactions with nonsedating antihistamines (eg, astemizole) or theophylline are not known to occur; however, caution is advised with coadministration.

Pharmacodynamics/Kinetics

Absorption: Rapid

Distribution: V_d: 800 L; rapidly and widely (higher levels in tissues than plasma)

Protein binding: 14% to 30%

Metabolism: Hydrolyzed to erythromycylamine

Bioavailability: 10%

Half-life elimination: 8 hours (range: 2-36 hours)

Time to peak: 4 hours

Excretion: Feces (81% to 97%)

Pregnancy Risk Factor C

Disalicylic Acid *see* Salsalate *on page 1454*

DisCoVisc™ *see* Chondroitin Sulfate and Sodium Hyaluronate *on page 351*

Disodium Cromoglycate *see* Cromolyn *on page 417*

Disodium Thiosulfate Pentahydrate *see* Sodium Thiosulfate *on page 1484*

d-Isoephedrine Hydrochloride *see* Pseudoephedrine *on page 1381*

Disopyramide *(dye soe PEER a mide)*

Related Information

Cardiovascular Diseases *on page 1726*

U.S. Brand Names Norpace®; Norpace® CR

Canadian Brand Names Norpace®; Rythmodan®; Rythmodan®-LA

Mexican Brand Names Dismodan

Generic Available Yes

Index Terms Disopyramide Phosphate

Pharmacologic Category Antiarrhythmic Agent, Class Ia

Use Suppression and prevention of unifocal and multifocal atrial and premature, ventricular premature complexes, coupled ventricular tachycardia; effective in the conversion of atrial fibrillation, atrial flutter, and paroxysmal atrial tachycardia to normal sinus rhythm and prevention of the recurrence of these arrhythmias after conversion by other methods

Unlabeled/Investigational Use Hypertrophic obstructive cardiomyopathy (HOCM)

Local Anesthetic/Vasoconstrictor Precautions Disopyramide is one of the drugs confirmed to prolong the QT interval and is accepted as having a risk of causing torsade de pointes. The risk of drug-induced torsade de pointes is extremely low when a single QT interval prolonging drug is prescribed. In terms of epinephrine, it is not known what effect vasoconstrictors in the local anesthetic regimen will have in patients with a known history of congenital prolonged QT interval or in patients taking any medication that prolongs the QT interval. Until more information is obtained, it is suggested that the clinician consult with the physician prior to the use of a vasoconstrictor in suspected patients, and that the vasoconstrictor (epinephrine, levonordefrin [Neo-Cobefrin®]) be used with caution.

Effects on Dental Treatment Key adverse event(s) related to dental treatment: Xerostomia (normal salivary flow resumes upon discontinuation).

Common Adverse Effects The most common adverse effects are related to cholinergic blockade. The most serious adverse effects of disopyramide are hypotension and CHF.

>10%:

Gastrointestinal: Xerostomia (32%), constipation (11%)

Genitourinary: Urinary hesitancy (14% to 23%)

1% to 10%:

Cardiovascular: CHF, hypotension, cardiac conduction disturbance, edema, syncope, chest pain

Central nervous system: Fatigue, headache, malaise, dizziness, nervousness

Dermatologic: Rash, generalized dermatoses, pruritus

Endocrine & metabolic: Hypokalemia, elevated cholesterol, elevated triglycerides

Gastrointestinal: Dry throat, nausea, abdominal distension, flatulence, abdominal bloating, anorexia, diarrhea, vomiting, weight gain

Genitourinary: Urinary retention, urinary frequency, urinary urgency, impotence (1% to 3%)

Neuromuscular & skeletal: Muscle weakness, muscular pain

Ocular: Blurred vision, dry eyes

Respiratory: Dyspnea

Mechanism of Action Class Ia antiarrhythmic: Decreases myocardial excitability and conduction velocity; reduces disparity in refractory between normal and infarcted myocardium; possesses anticholinergic, peripheral vasoconstrictive, and negative inotropic effects

Drug Interactions
Cytochrome P450 Effect: Substrate of CYP3A4 (major)
Increased Effect/Toxicity: Disopyramide may increase the effects/toxicity of anticholinergics, beta-blockers, flecainide, procainamide, quinidine, or propafenone. Digoxin and quinidine serum concentrations may be increased by disopyramide.

CYP3A4 inhibitors may increase the levels/effects of disopyramide. Example inhibitors include azole antifungals, clarithromycin, diclofenac, doxycycline, erythromycin, imatinib, isoniazid, nefazodone, nicardipine, propofol, protease inhibitors, quinidine, telithromycin, and verapamil.

Disopyramide effect/toxicity may be additive with drugs which may prolong the QT interval - amiodarone, amitriptyline, bepridil, cisapride (use is contraindicated), disopyramide, erythromycin, haloperidol, imipramine, pimozide, quinidine, sotalol, and thioridazine. In addition concurrent use with sparfloxacin, gatifloxacin, and moxifloxacin may result in additional prolongation of the QT interval; concurrent use is contraindicated.

Decreased Effect: CYP3A4 inducers may decrease the levels/effects of disopyramide; example inducers include aminoglutethimide, carbamazepine, nafcillin, nevirapine, phenobarbital, phenytoin, and rifamycins.

Pharmacodynamics/Kinetics
Onset of action: 0.5-3.5 hours
Duration: 1.5-8.5 hours
Absorption: 60% to 83%
Protein binding (concentration dependent): 20% to 60%
Metabolism: Hepatic to inactive metabolites
Half-life elimination: Adults: 4-10 hours; prolonged with hepatic or renal impairment
Excretion: Urine (40% to 60% as unchanged drug); feces (10% to 15%)

Pregnancy Risk Factor C

Disopyramide Phosphate *see* Disopyramide *on page 518*

Disulfiram (dye SUL fi ram)

U.S. Brand Names Antabuse®
Mexican Brand Names Antabuse
Generic Available No
Pharmacologic Category Aldehyde Dehydrogenase Inhibitor
Use Management of chronic alcoholism
Local Anesthetic/Vasoconstrictor Precautions No information available to require special precautions
Effects on Dental Treatment No significant effects or complications reported
Common Adverse Effects Frequency not defined.
Central nervous system: Drowsiness, headache, fatigue, psychosis
Dermatologic: Rash, acneiform eruptions, allergic dermatitis
Gastrointestinal: Metallic or garlic-like aftertaste
Genitourinary: Impotence
Hepatic: Hepatitis (cholestatic and fulminant), hepatic failure (multiple case reports)
Neuromuscular & skeletal: Peripheral neuritis, polyneuritis, peripheral neuropathy
Ocular: Optic neuritis

Mechanism of Action Disulfiram is a thiuram derivative which interferes with aldehyde dehydrogenase. When taken concomitantly with alcohol, there is an increase in serum acetaldehyde levels. High acetaldehyde causes uncomfortable symptoms including flushing, nausea, thirst, palpitations, chest pain, vertigo, and hypotension. This reaction is the basis for disulfiram use in postwithdrawal long-term care of alcoholism.

Drug Interactions
Cytochrome P450 Effect: Substrate (minor) of CYP1A2, 2A6, 2B6, 2D6, 2E1, 3A4; **Inhibits** CYP1A2 (weak), 2A6 (weak), 2B6 (weak), 2C9 (weak), 2D6 (weak), 2E1 (strong), 3A4 (weak)
Increased Effect/Toxicity: Disulfiram results in severe ethanol intolerance (disulfiram reaction) secondary to disulfiram's ability to inhibit aldehyde dehydrogenase; this combination should be avoided. Combined use with isoniazid, metronidazole, or MAO inhibitors may result in adverse CNS effects; this combination should be avoided. Some pharmaceutic dosage forms include ethanol, including elixirs and intravenous trimethoprim-sulfamethoxazole
(Continued)

Disulfiram (Continued)

(contains 10% ethanol as a solubilizing agent); these may inadvertently provoke a disulfiram reaction. Disulfiram may increase the levels/effects of inhalational anesthetics, trimethadione, and other CYP2E1 substrates. Disulfiram may increase serum concentrations of benzodiazepines that undergo oxidative metabolism (all but oxazepam, lorazepam, temazepam). Disulfiram increases phenytoin and theophylline serum concentrations; toxicity may occur. Disulfiram inhibits the metabolism of warfarin resulting in an increased hypoprothrombinemic response.

Pharmacodynamics/Kinetics
Onset of action: Full effect: 12 hours
Duration: ~1-2 weeks after last dose
Absorption: Rapid
Metabolism: To diethylthiocarbamate
Excretion: Feces and exhaled gases (as metabolites)

Pregnancy Risk Factor C

Dithioglycerol see Dimercaprol on page 508

Dithranol see Anthralin on page 130

Ditropan® see Oxybutynin on page 1224

Ditropan® XL see Oxybutynin on page 1224

Diuril® see Chlorothiazide on page 337

Divalproex Sodium see Valproic Acid and Derivatives on page 1638

5071-1DL(6) see Megestrol on page 1030

dl-Alpha Tocopherol see Vitamin E on page 1664

4-DMDR see Idarubicin on page 860

DNA-Derived Humanized Monoclonal Antibody see Alemtuzumab on page 64

DNase see Dornase Alfa on page 527

DNR see DAUNOrubicin Hydrochloride on page 450

Doak® Tar [OTC] see Coal Tar on page 402

Doan's® Extra Strength [OTC] see Magnesium Salicylate on page 1016

DOBUTamine (doe BYOO ta meen)

Related Information
Cardiovascular Diseases on page 1726
Canadian Brand Names Dobutamine Injection, USP; Dobutrex®
Mexican Brand Names Cryobutol; Dobuject; Dobutrex; Oxiken
Generic Available Yes
Index Terms Dobutamine Hydrochloride
Pharmacologic Category Adrenergic Agonist Agent
Use Short-term management of patients with cardiac decompensation
Unlabeled/Investigational Use Positive inotropic agent for use in myocardial dysfunction of sepsis
Local Anesthetic/Vasoconstrictor Precautions No information available to require special precautions
Effects on Dental Treatment No significant effects or complications reported
Common Adverse Effects Incidence of adverse events is not always reported.

Cardiovascular: Increased heart rate, increased blood pressure, increased ventricular ectopic activity, hypotension, premature ventricular beats (5%, dose related), anginal pain (1% to 3%), nonspecific chest pain (1% to 3%), palpitation (1% to 3%)
Central nervous system: Fever (1% to 3%), headache (1% to 3%), paresthesia
Endocrine & metabolic: Slight decrease in serum potassium
Gastrointestinal: Nausea (1% to 3%)
Hematologic: Thrombocytopenia (isolated cases)
Local: Phlebitis, local inflammatory changes and pain from infiltration, cutaneous necrosis (isolated cases)
Neuromuscular & skeletal: Mild leg cramps
Respiratory: Dyspnea (1% to 3%)

Mechanism of Action Stimulates beta$_1$-adrenergic receptors, causing increased contractility and heart rate, with little effect on beta$_2$- or alpha-receptors

Drug Interactions
Increased Effect/Toxicity: General anesthetics (eg, halothane or cyclopropane) and usual doses of dobutamine have resulted in ventricular arrhythmias in animals. Bretylium and may potentiate dobutamine's effects. Beta-blockers (nonselective ones) may increase hypertensive effect; avoid concurrent use. Cocaine may cause malignant arrhythmias. Guanethidine, MAO inhibitors,

methyldopa, reserpine, and tricyclic antidepressants can increase the pressor response to sympathomimetics.

Decreased Effect: Beta-adrenergic blockers may decrease effect of dobutamine and increase risk of severe hypotension.

Pharmacodynamics/Kinetics

Onset of action: I.V.: 1-10 minutes

Peak effect: 10-20 minutes

Metabolism: In tissues and hepatically to inactive metabolites

Half-life elimination: 2 minutes

Excretion: Urine (as metabolites)

Pregnancy Risk Factor B

Dobutamine Hydrochloride *see* DOBUTamine *on page 520*

Docetaxel (doe se TAKS el)

U.S. Brand Names Taxotere®

Canadian Brand Names Taxotere®

Mexican Brand Names Taxotere

Generic Available No

Index Terms NSC-628503; RP-6976

Pharmacologic Category Antineoplastic Agent, Natural Source (Plant) Derivative

Use Treatment of breast cancer; locally-advanced or metastatic nonsmall cell lung cancer (NSCLC); hormone refractory, metastatic prostate cancer; advanced gastric adenocarcinoma; locally-advanced squamous cell head and neck cancer

Unlabeled/Investigational Use Investigational: Treatment of pancreatic cancer, ovarian cancer, soft tissue sarcoma, and melanoma

Local Anesthetic/Vasoconstrictor Precautions No information available to require special precautions

Effects on Dental Treatment Key adverse event(s) related to dental treatment: Mucositis, stomatitis, and taste perversion.

Common Adverse Effects Percentages reported for docetaxel monotherapy; frequency may vary depending on diagnosis, dose, liver function, prior treatment, and premedication. The incidence of adverse events was usually higher in patients with elevated liver function tests.

>10%:

Cardiovascular: Fluid retention (13% to 60%; dose dependent)

Central nervous system: Neurosensory events (20% to 58%; including neuropathy), fever (31% to 35%), neuromotor events (16%)

Dermatologic: Alopecia (56% to 76%), cutaneous events (20% to 48%), nail disorder (11% to 41%)

Gastrointestinal: Stomatitis (19% to 53%; severe 1% to 8%), diarrhea (23% to 43%; severe: 5% to 6%), nausea (34% to 42%), vomiting (22% to 23%)

Hematologic: Neutropenia (84% to 99%; grade 4: 75% to 86%; onset: 4-7 days, nadir: 5-9 days, recovery: 21 days; dose dependent), leukopenia (84% to 99%; grade 4: 32% to 44%), anemia (8% to 94%; dose dependent), thrombocytopenia (8% to 14%; grade 4: 1%; dose dependent), febrile neutropenia (6% to 12%; dose dependent)

Hepatic: Transaminases increased (4% to 19%)

Neuromuscular and skeletal: Weakness (53% to 66%; severe 13% to 18%), myalgia (3% to 23%)

Respiratory: Pulmonary events (41%)

Miscellaneous: Infection (1% to 34%; dose dependent), hypersensitivity (1% to 21%; with premedication 15%)

1% to 10%:

Cardiovascular: Hypotension (3%)

Dermatologic: Rash/erythema (2%)

Gastrointestinal: Taste perversion (6%)

Hepatic: Bilirubin increased (9%), alkaline phosphatase increased (4% to 7%)

Local: Infusion-site reactions (4%, including hyperpigmentation, inflammation, redness, dryness, phlebitis, extravasation, swelling of the vein)

Neuromuscular and skeletal: Arthralgia (3% to 9%)

Ocular: Epiphora associated with canalicular stenosis (up to 77% with weekly administration; up to 1% with every-3-week administration)

Mechanism of Action Docetaxel promotes the assembly of microtubules from tubulin dimers, and inhibits the depolymerization of tubulin which stabilizes microtubules in the cell. This results in inhibition of DNA, RNA, and protein synthesis. Most activity occurs during the M phase of the cell cycle.

(Continued)

Docetaxel *(Continued)*

Drug Interactions

Cytochrome P450 Effect: Substrate of CYP3A4 (major); **Inhibits** CYP3A4 (weak)

Increased Effect/Toxicity: CYP3A4 inhibitors may increase the levels/effects of docetaxel; example inhibitors include azole antifungals, clarithromycin, diclofenac, doxycycline, erythromycin, imatinib, isoniazid, nefazodone, nicardipine, propofol, protease inhibitors, quinidine, telithromycin, and verapamil. When administered as sequential infusions, observational studies indicate a potential for increased toxicity when platinum derivatives (carboplatin, cisplatin) are administered before taxane derivatives (docetaxel, paclitaxel).

Decreased Effect: CYP3A4 inducers may decrease the levels/effects of docetaxel; example inducers include aminoglutethimide, carbamazepine, nafcillin, nevirapine, phenobarbital, phenytoin, and rifamycins.

Pharmacodynamics/Kinetics Exhibits linear pharmacokinetics at the recommended dosage range

Distribution: Extensive extravascular distribution and/or tissue binding; V_d: 80-90 L/m^2, V_{dss}: 113 L (mean steady state)

Protein binding: >94%, primarily to alpha$_1$-acid glycoprotein, albumin, and lipoproteins

Metabolism: Hepatic; oxidation via CYP3A4 to metabolites

Half-life elimination: Terminal: 11 hours

Excretion: Feces (75%, <8% as unchanged drug); urine (6%); ~80% within 48 hours

Clearance: Total body: Mean: 21 $L/hour/m^2$

Pregnancy Risk Factor D

Docosanol *(doe KOE san ole)*

Related Sample Prescriptions

Herpes Simplex (Recurrent) *on page 1843*

U.S. Brand Names Abreva® [OTC]

Generic Available No

Index Terms Behenyl Alcohol; *n*-Docosanol

Pharmacologic Category Antiviral Agent, Topical

Dental Use Treatment of herpes simplex of the face or lips

Use Treatment of herpes simplex of the face or lips

Local Anesthetic/Vasoconstrictor Precautions No information available to require special precautions

Effects on Dental Treatment No significant effects or complications reported (see Dental Comment)

Significant Adverse Effects Limited information; headache reported (frequency similar to placebo)

Dental Usual Dosing Herpes simplex (face/lips): Children ≥12 years and Adults: Topical: Apply 5 times/day to affected area of face or lips. Start at first sign of cold sore or fever blister and continue until healed.

Dosage Children ≥12 years and Adults: Topical: Apply 5 times/day to affected area of face or lips. Start at first sign of cold sore or fever blister and continue until healed.

Mechanism of Action Prevents viral entry and replication at the cellular level

Contraindications Hypersensitivity to docosanol or any component of the formulation

Warnings/Precautions For external use only. Do not apply to inside of mouth or around eyes. Not for use in children <12 years of age.

Dosage Forms Excipient information presented when available (limited, particularly for generics); consult specific product labeling.

Cream: 10% (2 g)

Dental Comment Wash hands before and after applying cream. Begin treatment at first tingle of cold sore or fever blister. Rub into area gently, but completely. Do not apply directly to inside of mouth or around eyes. Contact healthcare provider if sore gets worse or does not heal within 10 days. Do not share this product with others, may spread infection. Notify healthcare professional if pregnant or breast-feeding.

Docusate *(DOK yoo sate)*

U.S. Brand Names Colace® [OTC]; Diocto® [OTC]; Docusoft-S™ [OTC]; DOK™ [OTC]; DOS® [OTC]; D-S-S® [OTC]; Dulcolax® Stool Softener [OTC]; Enemeez® [OTC]; Fleet® Sof-Lax® [OTC]; Genasoft® [OTC]; Phillips'® Stool Softener Laxative [OTC]; Silace [OTC]; Surfak® [OTC]

Canadian Brand Names Apo-Docusate-Sodium®; Colace®; Colax-C®; Novo-Docusate Calcium; Novo-Docusate Sodium; PMS-Docusate Calcium; PMS-Docusate Sodium; Regulex®; Selax®; Soflax™

Generic Available Yes: Excludes gelcap

Index Terms Dioctyl Calcium Sulfosuccinate; Dioctyl Sodium Sulfosuccinate; Docusate Calcium; Docusate Potassium; Docusate Sodium; DOSS; DSS

Pharmacologic Category Stool Softener

Use Stool softener in patients who should avoid straining during defecation and constipation associated with hard, dry stools; prophylaxis for straining (Valsalva) following myocardial infarction. A safe agent to be used in elderly; some evidence that doses <200 mg are ineffective; stool softeners are unnecessary if stool is well hydrated or "mushy" and soft; shown to be ineffective used long-term.

Unlabeled/Investigational Use Ceruminolytic

Local Anesthetic/Vasoconstrictor Precautions No information available to require special precautions

Effects on Dental Treatment Key adverse event(s) related to dental treatment: Throat irritation.

Common Adverse Effects 1% to 10%:
Gastrointestinal: Intestinal obstruction, diarrhea, abdominal cramping
Miscellaneous: Throat irritation

Mechanism of Action Reduces surface tension of the oil-water interface of the stool resulting in enhanced incorporation of water and fat allowing for stool softening

Pharmacodynamics/Kinetics
Onset of action: 12-72 hours
Excretion: Feces

Pregnancy Risk Factor C

Docusate Calcium *see* Docusate *on page 522*

Docusate Potassium *see* Docusate *on page 522*

Docusate Sodium *see* Docusate *on page 522*

Docusoft-S™ [OTC] *see* Docusate *on page 522*

Dofetilide (doe FET il ide)

Related Information
Cardiovascular Diseases *on page 1726*

U.S. Brand Names Tikosyn®

Canadian Brand Names Tikosyn®

Generic Available No

Pharmacologic Category Antiarrhythmic Agent, Class III

Use Maintenance of normal sinus rhythm in patients with chronic atrial fibrillation/atrial flutter of longer than 1-week duration who have been converted to normal sinus rhythm; conversion of atrial fibrillation and atrial flutter to normal sinus rhythm

Local Anesthetic/Vasoconstrictor Precautions Dofetilide is one of the drugs confirmed to prolong the QT interval and is accepted as having a risk of causing torsade de pointes. The risk of drug-induced torsade de pointes is extremely low when a single QT interval prolonging drug is prescribed. In terms of epinephrine, it is not known what effect vasoconstrictors in the local anesthetic regimen will have in patients with a known history of congenital prolonged QT interval or in patients taking any medication that prolongs the QT interval. Until more information is obtained, it is suggested that the clinician consult with the physician prior to the use of a vasoconstrictor in suspected patients, and that the vasoconstrictor (epinephrine, levonordefrin [Neo-Cobefrin®]) be used with caution.

Effects on Dental Treatment No significant effects or complications reported

Common Adverse Effects
Supraventricular arrhythmia patients (incidence > placebo)
>10%: Central nervous system: Headache (11%)
2% to 10%:
Central nervous system: Dizziness (8%), insomnia (4%)
Cardiovascular: Ventricular tachycardia (2.6% to 3.7%), chest pain (10%), torsade de pointes (3.3% in CHF patients and 0.9% in patients with a recent MI; up to 10.5% in patients receiving doses in excess of those recommended). Torsade de pointes occurs most frequently within the first 3 days of therapy.
Dermatologic: Rash (3%)
Gastrointestinal: Nausea (5%), diarrhea (3%), abdominal pain (3%)
Neuromuscular & skeletal: Back pain (3%)
Respiratory: Dyspnea (6%), respiratory tract infection (7%)
(Continued)

Dofetilide *(Continued)*

Miscellaneous: Flu syndrome (4%)

<2%:

Central nervous system: CVA, facial paralysis, flaccid paralysis, migraine, paralysis

Cardiovascular: AV block (0.4% to 1.5%), ventricular fibrillation (0% to 0.4%), bundle branch block, heart block, edema, heart arrest, myocardial infarct, sudden death, syncope

Dermatologic: Angioedema

Gastrointestinal: Liver damage

Neuromuscular & skeletal: Paresthesia

Respiratory: Cough

>2% (incidence ≤ placebo): Anxiety, pain, angina, atrial fibrillation, hypertension, palpitation, supraventricular tachycardia, peripheral edema, urinary tract infection, weakness, arthralgia, diaphoresis

Restrictions Tikosyn® is only available to prescribers and hospitals that have confirmed their participation in a designated Tikosyn® Education Program. The program provides comprehensive education about the importance of in-hospital treatment initiation and individualized dosing.

T.I.P.S. is the Tikosyn® In Pharmacy System designated to allow retail pharmacies to stock and dispense Tikosyn® once they have been enrolled. A participating pharmacy must confirm receipt of the T.I.P.S. program materials and educate its pharmacy staff about the procedures required to fill an outpatient prescription for Tikosyn®. The T.I.P.S. enrollment form is available at www.tikosyn.com. Tikosyn® is only available from a special mail order pharmacy, and enrolled retail pharmacies. Pharmacists must verify that the hospital/prescriber is a confirmed participant before Tikosyn® is provided. For participant verification, the pharmacist may call 1-800-788-7353 or use the web site located at www.tikosynlist.com. Further details and directions on the program are provided at www.tikosyn.com.

Dofetilide therapy must be initiated/adjusted in a hospital setting with proper monitoring under the guidance of experienced personnel.

Mechanism of Action Vaughan Williams Class III antiarrhythmic activity. Blockade of the cardiac ion channel carrying the rapid component of the delayed rectifier potassium current. Dofetilide has no effect on sodium channels, adrenergic alpha-receptors, or adrenergic beta-receptors. It increases the monophasic action potential duration due to delayed repolarization. The increase in the QT interval is a function of prolongation of both effective and functional refractory periods in the His-Purkinje system and the ventricles. Changes in cardiac conduction velocity and sinus node function have not been observed in patients with or without structural heart disease. PR and QRS width remain the same in patients with pre-existing heart block and or sick sinus syndrome.

Drug Interactions

Cytochrome P450 Effect: Substrate of CYP3A4 (minor)

Increased Effect/Toxicity: Dofetilide concentrations are increased by cimetidine, verapamil, hydrochlorothiazide, ketoconazole, and trimethoprim (concurrent use of these agents is contraindicated). Dofetilide levels may also be increased by renal cationic transport inhibitors (including triamterene, metformin, amiloride, and megestrol). Diuretics and other drugs which may deplete potassium and/or magnesium (aminoglycoside antibiotics, amphotericin, cyclosporine) may increase dofetilide's toxicity (torsade de pointes); concurrent use of hydrochlorothiazide is contraindicated. Use of QT_c-prolonging agents (including bepridil, cisapride, clarithromycin, erythromycin, tricyclic antidepressants, phenothiazines, sparfloxacin, gatifloxacin, moxifloxacin) is contraindicated. Itraconazole may decrease the metabolism of dofetilide (concurrent use is contraindicated).

Pharmacodynamics/Kinetics

Absorption: >90%

Distribution: V_d: 3 L/kg

Protein binding: 60% to 70%

Metabolism: Hepatic via CYP3A4, but low affinity for it; metabolites formed by N-dealkylation and N-oxidation

Bioavailability: >90%

Half-life elimination: 10 hours

Time to peak: Fasting: 2-3 hours

Excretion: Urine (80%, 80% as unchanged drug, 20% as inactive or minimally active metabolites); renal elimination consists of glomerular filtration and active tubular secretion via cationic transport system

Pregnancy Risk Factor C

Dofus [OTC] *see Lactobacillus on page 942*

DOK™ [OTC] *see* Docusate *on page 522*

Dolasetron (dol A se tron)

U.S. Brand Names Anzemet®
Canadian Brand Names Anzemet®
Mexican Brand Names Anzemet
Generic Available No
Index Terms Dolasetron Mesylate; MDL 73,147EF
Pharmacologic Category Antiemetic; Selective 5-HT₃ Receptor Antagonist
Use Prevention of nausea and vomiting associated with emetogenic cancer chemotherapy; prevention of postoperative nausea and vomiting; treatment of postoperative nausea and vomiting (injectable form only).

Note: In Canada, the use of dolasetron is contraindicated for all uses in children <18 years of age or in the treatment of postoperative nausea and vomiting in adults. These are not labeled contraindications in the U.S.

Local Anesthetic/Vasoconstrictor Precautions Dolasetron is one of the drugs confirmed to prolong the QT interval and is accepted as having a risk of causing torsade de pointes. The risk of drug-induced torsade de pointes is extremely low when a single QT interval prolonging drug is prescribed. In terms of epinephrine, it is not known what effect vasoconstrictors in the local anesthetic regimen will have in patients with a known history of congenital prolonged QT interval or in patients taking any medication that prolongs the QT interval. Until more information is obtained, it is suggested that the clinician consult with the physician prior to the use of a vasoconstrictor in suspected patients, and that the vasoconstrictor (epinephrine, levonordefrin [Neo-Cobefrin®]) be used with caution.

Effects on Dental Treatment Key adverse event(s) related to dental treatment: Taste alterations.

Common Adverse Effects Adverse events may vary according to indication
>10%:
  Central nervous system: Headache (7% to 24%)
  Gastrointestinal: Diarrhea (2% to 12%)
1% to 10%:
  Cardiovascular: Bradycardia (5%), hypotension (5%), hypertension (2% to 3%), tachycardia (2% to 3%)
  Central nervous system: Dizziness (1% to 6%), fatigue (3% to 6%), fever (3% to 5%), chills/shivering (1% to 2%), sedation (2%)
  Dermatological: Pruritus (3% to 4%)
  Gastrointestinal: Dyspepsia (2% to 3%), abdominal pain (3%)
  Hepatic: Abnormal hepatic function (4%)
  Neuromuscular & skeletal: Pain (3%)
  Renal: Oliguria (1% to 3%), urinary retention (2%)

Mechanism of Action Selective serotonin receptor (5-HT₃) antagonist, blocking serotonin both peripherally (primary site of action) and centrally at the chemoreceptor trigger zone

Drug Interactions
  Cytochrome P450 Effect: Substrate (minor) of CYP2C9, 3A4; **Inhibits** CYP2D6 (weak)
  Increased Effect/Toxicity: Due to reports of profound hypotension during concomitant therapy with ondansetron, the manufacturer of apomorphine contraindicates its use with all 5-HT₃ antagonists. Use caution with QT_c-prolonging agents (includes but may not be limited to amitriptyline, bepridil, disopyramide, erythromycin, haloperidol, imipramine, quinidine, pimozide, procainamide, sotalol, and thioridazine); effect/toxicity of dolasetron and other QT_c-prolonging agents may be increased
  Decreased Effect: Blood levels of active metabolite are decreased during coadministration of rifampin.

Pharmacodynamics/Kinetics
  Absorption: Rapid and complete
  Distribution: 5.8 L/kg
  Protein binding: Hydrodolasetron: 69% to 77% (50% bound to alpha₁-acid glycoprotein)
  Metabolism: Hepatic; reduction by carbonyl reductase to hydrodolasetron (active metabolite); further metabolized by CYP3A and flavin monooxygenase
  Bioavailability: 75%
  Half-life elimination: Dolasetron: 10 minutes; hydrodolasetron: Adults: 6-8 hours; Children: 4-6 hours
  Time to peak, plasma: I.V.: 0.6 hours; Oral: 1 hour
  Excretion: Urine ~67% (53% to 61% as active metabolite hydrodolasetron); feces ~33%

Pregnancy Risk Factor B

Dolasetron Mesylate *see* Dolasetron *on page 525*

Dolgic® LQ *see* Butalbital, Acetaminophen, and Caffeine *on page 247*

Dolgic® Plus *see* Butalbital, Acetaminophen, and Caffeine *on page 247*

Dolobid® [DSC] *see* Diflunisal *on page 494*

Dologesic® *see* Acetaminophen and Phenyltoloxamine *on page 38*

Dolophine® *see* Methadone *on page 1059*

Domeboro® [OTC] *see* Aluminum Sulfate and Calcium Acetate *on page 83*

Dome Paste Bandage *see* Zinc Gelatin *on page 1682*

Donatussin *see* Guaifenesin and Phenylephrine *on page 797*

Donatussin DC *see* Hydrocodone, Phenylephrine, and Guaifenesin *on page 834*

Donepezil (doh NEP e zil)

U.S. Brand Names Aricept®; Aricept® ODT
Canadian Brand Names Aricept®; Aricept® RDT
Mexican Brand Names Eranz
Generic Available No
Index Terms E2020
Pharmacologic Category Acetylcholinesterase Inhibitor (Central)
Use Treatment of mild, moderate, or severe dementia of the Alzheimer's type
Unlabeled/Investigational Use Attention-deficit/hyperactivity disorder (ADHD), behavioral syndromes in dementia
Local Anesthetic/Vasoconstrictor Precautions No information available to require special precautions
Effects on Dental Treatment No significant effects or complications reported
Common Adverse Effects
>10%:
    Central nervous system: Insomnia (5% to 14%)
    Gastrointestinal: Nausea (5% to 19%), diarrhea (8% to 15%)
    Miscellaneous: Accident (7% to 13%), infection (11%)
1% to 10%:
    Cardiovascular: Hypertension (3%), chest pain (2%), hemorrhage (2%), syncope (2%), hypotension, atrial fibrillation, bradycardia, ECG abnormal, edema, heart failure, hot flashes, peripheral edema, vasodilation
    Central nervous system: Headache (4% to 10%), pain (3% to 9%), fatigue (3% to 8%), dizziness (2% to 8%), abnormal dreams (3%), depression (2% to 3%), hostility (3%), nervousness (3%), hallucinations (3%), confusion (2%), emotional lability (2%), personality disorder (2%), fever (2%), somnolence (2%), abnormal crying, aggression, agitation, anxiety, aphasia, delusions, irritability, restlessness, seizure
    Dermatologic: Bruising (4% to 5%), eczema (3%), pruritus, rash, skin ulcer, urticaria
    Endocrine & metabolic: Dehydration (2%), hyperlipemia (2%), libido increased
    Gastrointestinal: Anorexia (3% to 8%), vomiting (3% to 8%), weight loss (3%), abdominal pain, constipation, dyspepsia, fecal incontinence, gastroenteritis, GI bleeding, bloating, epigastric pain, toothache
    Genitourinary: Urinary frequency (2%), urinary incontinence (2%), hematuria, glycosuria, nocturia, UTI
    Hematologic: Anemia
    Hepatic: Alkaline phosphatase increased
    Neuromuscular & skeletal: Muscle cramps (3% to 8%), back pain (3%), CPK increased (3%), arthritis (2%), ataxia, bone fracture, gait abnormal, lactate dehydrogenase increased, paresthesia, tremor, weakness
    Ocular: Blurred vision, cataract, eye irritation
    Respiratory: Cough increased, dyspnea, bronchitis, pharyngitis, pneumonia, sore throat
    Miscellaneous: Diaphoresis, fungal infection, flu symptoms, wandering
Mechanism of Action Alzheimer's disease is characterized by cholinergic deficiency in the cortex and basal forebrain, which contributes to cognitive deficits. Donepezil reversibly and noncompetitively inhibits centrally-active acetylcholinesterase, the enzyme responsible for hydrolysis of acetylcholine. This appears to result in increased concentrations of acetylcholine available for synaptic transmission in the central nervous system.
Drug Interactions
Cytochrome P450 Effect: Substrate (minor) of CYP2D6, 3A4
Increased Effect/Toxicity: A synergistic effect may be seen with concurrent administration of succinylcholine or cholinergic agonists (bethanechol).

Cholineresterase inhibitors may enhance the bradycardic effects of beta-blockers.

Decreased Effect: Anticholinergic agents (benztropine) may inhibit the effects of donepezil. Acetylcholinesterase inhibitors (central) may increase the risk of antipsychotic-related extrapyramidal symptoms. Acetylcholinesterase inhibitors may diminish the neuromuscular-blocking effects of nondepolarizing bllockers.

Pharmacodynamics/Kinetics

Absorption: Well absorbed

Protein binding: 96%, primarily to albumin (75%) and α_1-acid glycoprotein (21%)

Metabolism: Extensively to four major metabolites (two are active) via CYP2D6 and 3A4; undergoes glucuronidation

Bioavailability: 100%

Half-life elimination: 70 hours; time to steady-state: 15 days

Time to peak, plasma: 3-4 hours

Excretion: Urine 57% (17% as unchanged drug); feces 15%

Pregnancy Risk Factor C

Donnatal® see Hyoscyamine, Atropine, Scopolamine, and Phenobarbital on page 848

Donnatal Extentabs® see Hyoscyamine, Atropine, Scopolamine, and Phenobarbital on page 848

Dopram® see Doxapram on page 529

Doral® see Quazepam on page 1391

Dornase Alfa (DOOR nase AL fa)

U.S. Brand Names Pulmozyme®

Canadian Brand Names Pulmozyme™

Mexican Brand Names Pulmozyme

Generic Available No

Index Terms DNase; Recombinant Human Deoxyribonuclease

Pharmacologic Category Enzyme

Use Management of cystic fibrosis patients to reduce the frequency of respiratory infections that require parenteral antibiotics, and to improve pulmonary function

Unlabeled/Investigational Use Treatment of chronic bronchitis

Local Anesthetic/Vasoconstrictor Precautions No information available to require special precautions

Effects on Dental Treatment Key adverse event(s) related to dental treatment: Pharyngitis

Common Adverse Effects

>10%:

Respiratory: Pharyngitis

Miscellaneous: Voice alteration

1% to 10%:

Cardiovascular: Chest pain

Dermatologic: Rash

Ocular: Conjunctivitis

Respiratory: Laryngitis, cough, dyspnea, hemoptysis, rhinitis, hoarse throat, wheezing

Mechanism of Action The hallmark of cystic fibrosis lung disease is the presence of abundant, purulent airway secretions composed primarily of highly polymerized DNA. The principal source of this DNA is the nuclei of degenerating neutrophils, which is present in large concentrations in infected lung secretions. The presence of this DNA produces a viscous mucous that may contribute to the decreased mucociliary transport and persistent infections that are commonly seen in this population. Dornase alfa is a deoxyribonuclease (DNA) enzyme produced by recombinant gene technology. Dornase selectively cleaves DNA, thus reducing mucous viscosity and as a result, airflow in the lung is improved and the risk of bacterial infection may be decreased.

Pharmacodynamics/Kinetics

Onset of action: Nebulization: Enzyme levels are measured in sputum in ~15 minutes

Duration: Rapidly declines

Pregnancy Risk Factor B

Doryx® see Doxycycline (Systemic) on page 541

Dorzolamide (dor ZOLE a mide)

U.S. Brand Names Trusopt®
Canadian Brand Names Trusopt®
Mexican Brand Names Trusopt
Generic Available No
Index Terms Dorzolamide Hydrochloride
Pharmacologic Category Carbonic Anhydrase Inhibitor; Ophthalmic Agent, Antiglaucoma
Use Lowers intraocular pressure in patients with ocular hypertension or open-angle glaucoma
Local Anesthetic/Vasoconstrictor Precautions No information available to require special precautions
Effects on Dental Treatment No significant effects or complications reported
Mechanism of Action Reversible inhibition of the enzyme carbonic anhydrase resulting in reduction of hydrogen ion secretion at renal tubule and an increased renal excretion of sodium, potassium, bicarbonate, and water to decrease production of aqueous humor; also inhibits carbonic anhydrase in central nervous system to retard abnormal and excessive discharge from CNS neurons
Pregnancy Risk Factor C

Dorzolamide and Timolol (dor ZOLE a mide & TYE moe lole)

Related Information
Dorzolamide *on page 528*
Timolol *on page 1570*
U.S. Brand Names Cosopt®
Canadian Brand Names Cosopt®; Preservative-Free Cosopt®
Mexican Brand Names Cosopt
Generic Available No
Index Terms Timolol and Dorzolamide
Pharmacologic Category Beta-Adrenergic Blocker, Nonselective; Carbonic Anhydrase Inhibitor; Ophthalmic Agent, Antiglaucoma
Use Reduction of intraocular pressure in patients with ocular hypertension or open-angle glaucoma
Local Anesthetic/Vasoconstrictor Precautions No information available to require special precautions
Effects on Dental Treatment Key adverse event(s) related to dental treatment: Taste perversion.
Common Adverse Effects Percentages as reported with combination product. Also see individual agents.

>5%:
Gastrointestinal: Taste perversion (≤30%)
Ocular: Burning/stinging (≤30%), conjunctival hyperemia (5% to 15%), blurred vision (5% to 15%), superficial punctuate keratitis (5% to 15%), itching (5% to 15%)
1% to 5%:
Cardiovascular: Hypertension
Central nervous system: Dizziness, headache
Gastrointestinal: Abdominal pain, dyspepsia, nausea
Genitourinary: Urinary tract infection
Neuromuscular & skeletal: Back pain
Ocular: Blepharitis, cloudy vision, conjunctival discharge, conjunctival edema, conjunctival follicles, conjunctivitis, corneal erosion, corneal staining, cortical lens opacity, dryness, eye debris, eye/eyelid discharge, eye/eyelid pain, eyelid edema, eyelid erythema, eyelid exudate/scales, foreign body sensation, glaucomatous cupping, lens nucleus discoloration, lens opacity, post-capsular cataract, tearing, visual field defect, vitreous detachment
Respiratory: Bronchitis, cough, pharyngitis, sinusitis, upper respiratory infection
Miscellaneous: Flu
Drug Interactions
Cytochrome P450 Effect:
Dorzolamide: **Substrate** (minor) of CYP2C8/9, 3A4
Timolol: **Substrate** of CYP2D6 (major); **Inhibits** CYP2D6 (weak)
Increased Effect/Toxicity: See individual agents.
Decreased Effect: See individual agents.
Pharmacodynamics/Kinetics See individual agents.
Pregnancy Risk Factor C

Dorzolamide Hydrochloride *see* Dorzolamide *on page 528*

Doxapram (DOKS a pram)

U.S. Brand Names Dopram®
Generic Available Yes
Index Terms Doxapram Hydrochloride
Pharmacologic Category Respiratory Stimulant; Stimulant
Use Respiratory and CNS stimulant for respiratory depression secondary to anesthesia, drug-induced CNS depression; acute hypercapnia secondary to COPD
Local Anesthetic/Vasoconstrictor Precautions No information available to require special precautions
Effects on Dental Treatment No significant effects or complications reported
Common Adverse Effects Frequency not defined.
  Cardiovascular: Arrhythmia, blood pressure increased, chest pain, chest tightness, flushing, heart rate changes, T waves lowered, ventricular tachycardia, ventricular fibrillation
  Central nervous system: Apprehension, Babinski turns positive, disorientation, dizziness, hallucinations, headache, hyperactivity, pyrexia, seizure
  Dermatologic: Burning sensation, pruritus
  Gastrointestinal: Defecation urge, diarrhea, nausea, vomiting
  Genitourinary: Spontaneous voiding, urinary retention
  Hematologic: Hematocrit decreased, hemoglobin decreased, hemolysis, red blood cell count decreased
  Local: Phlebitis
  Neuromuscular & skeletal: Clonus, deep tendon reflexes increase, fasciculations, involuntary muscle movement, muscle spasm, paresthesia
  Ocular: Pupillary dilatation
  Renal: Albuminuria, BUN increased
  Respiratory: Bronchospasm, cough, dyspnea, hiccups, hyperventilation, laryngospasm, rebound hypoventilation, tachypnea
  Miscellaneous: Diaphoresis
Mechanism of Action Stimulates respiration through action on respiratory center in medulla or indirectly on peripheral carotid chemoreceptors
Drug Interactions
  Increased Effect/Toxicity: Increased blood pressure with sympathomimetics, MAO inhibitors. Halothane, cyclopropane, and enflurane may sensitize the myocardium to catecholamine and epinephrine which is released at the initiation of doxapram, hence, separate discontinuation of anesthetics and start of doxapram until the volatile agent has been excreted.
Pharmacodynamics/Kinetics
  Onset of action: Respiratory stimulation: I.V.: 20-40 seconds
    Peak effect: 1-2 minutes
  Duration: 5-12 minutes
  Half-life elimination, serum: Adults: Mean: 3.4 hours
Pregnancy Risk Factor B

Doxapram Hydrochloride *see* Doxapram *on page 529*

Doxazosin (doks AY zoe sin)

Related Information
  Cardiovascular Diseases *on page 1726*
U.S. Brand Names Cardura®; Cardura® XL
Canadian Brand Names Alti-Doxazosin; Apo-Doxazosin®; Cardura-1™; Cardura-2™; Cardura-4™; Gen-Doxazosin; Novo-Doxazosin
Mexican Brand Names Cardura
Generic Available Yes:Excludes extended release tablet
Index Terms Doxazosin Mesylate
Pharmacologic Category Alpha₁ Blocker
Use Treatment of hypertension alone or in conjunction with diuretics, ACE inhibitors, beta-blockers, or calcium antagonists; treatment of urinary outflow obstruction and/or obstructive and irritative symptoms associated with benign prostatic hyperplasia (BPH), particularly useful in patients with troublesome symptoms who are unable or unwilling to undergo invasive procedures, but who require rapid symptomatic relief; can be used in combination with finasteride
Unlabeled/Investigational Use Pediatric hypertension
  (Continued)

Doxazosin *(Continued)*

Local Anesthetic/Vasoconstrictor Precautions No information available to require special precautions

Effects on Dental Treatment Key adverse event(s) related to dental treatment: Xerostomia (normal salivary flow resumes upon discontinuation) and orthostatic hypotension

Common Adverse Effects Note: Type and frequency of adverse reactions reflect combined data from trials with immediate release and extended release products.

>10%: Central nervous system: Dizziness (5% to 19%), headache (5% to 14%)

1% to 10%:

Cardiovascular: Orthostatic hypotension (dose related; 0.3% up to 2%), edema (3% to 4%), hypotension (2%), palpitation (1% to 2%), chest pain (1% to 2%), arrhythmia (1%), syncope (2%), flushing (1%)

Central nervous system: Fatigue (8% to 12%), somnolence (1% to 5%), nervousness (2%), pain (2%), vertigo (2% to 4%), insomnia (1%), anxiety (1%), paresthesia (1%), movement disorder (1%), ataxia (1%), hypertonia (1%), depression (1%)

Dermatologic: Rash (1%), pruritus (1%)

Endocrine & metabolic: Sexual dysfunction (2%)

Gastrointestinal: Abdominal pain (2%), diarrhea (2%), dyspepsia (1% to 2%), nausea (1% to 3%), xerostomia (1% to 2%), constipation (1%), flatulence (1%)

Genitourinary: Urinary tract infection (1%), impotence (1%), polyuria (2%), incontinence (1%)

Neuromuscular & skeletal: Back pain (2% to 3%), weakness (1% to 7%), arthritis (1%), muscle weakness (1%), myalgia (≤1%), muscle cramps (1%)

Ocular: Abnormal vision (1% to 2%), conjunctivitis (1%)

Otic: Tinnitus (1%)

Respiratory: Respiratory tract infection (5%), rhinitis (3%), dyspnea (1% to 3%), respiratory disorder (1%), epistaxis (1%)

Miscellaneous: Diaphoresis increased (1%), flu-like syndrome (1%)

Dosage Oral:

Children (unlabeled use): Hypertension: Immediate release: Initial: 1 mg once daily; maximum: 4 mg/day

Adults:

Immediate release: 1 mg once daily in morning or evening; may be increased to 2 mg once daily. Thereafter titrate upwards, if needed, over several weeks, balancing therapeutic benefit with doxazosin-induced postural hypotension. In the elderly, initiate at 0.5 mg once daily

Hypertension: Maximum dose: 16 mg/day

BPH: Goal: 4-8 mg/day; maximum dose: 8 mg/day

Extended release: BPH: 4 mg once daily with breakfast; titrate based on response and tolerability every 3-4 weeks to maximum recommended dose of 8 mg/day

Reinitiation of therapy: If therapy is discontinued for several days, restart at 4 mg dose and titrate as before.

Conversion to extended release from immediate release: Initiate with 4 mg once daily; omit final evening dose of immediate release prior to starting morning dosing with extended release product.

Dosing adjustment in hepatic impairment: Use with caution in mild-to-moderate hepatic dysfunction. Do not use with severe impairment.

Mechanism of Action

Hypertension: Competitively inhibits postsynaptic alpha$_1$-adrenergic receptors which results in vasodilation of veins and arterioles and a decrease in total peripheral resistance and blood pressure; ~50% as potent on a weight by weight basis as prazosin.

BPH: Competitively inhibits postsynaptic alpha$_1$-adrenergic receptors in prostatic stromal and bladder neck tissues. This reduces the sympathetic tone-induced urethral stricture causing BPH symptoms.

Contraindications Hypersensitivity to quinazolines (prazosin, terazosin), doxazosin, or any component of the formulation

Warnings/Precautions Can cause significant orthostatic hypotension and syncope, especially with first dose; anticipate a similar effect if therapy is interrupted for a few days, if dosage is rapidly increased, or if another antihypertensive drug (particularly vasodilators) or a PDE5 inhibitor is introduced. Discontinue if symptoms of angina occur or worsen. Patients should be cautioned about performing hazardous tasks when starting new therapy or adjusting dosage upward. Prostate cancer should be ruled out before starting for BPH. Use with caution in mild to moderate hepatic impairment; not recommended in severe dysfunction. Intraoperative floppy iris syndrome has been observed in cataract surgery patients who were on or were previously treated with alpha$_1$-blockers. Causality has not been established and there appears to be no benefit in discontinuing alpha-blocker therapy prior to surgery. Safety and efficacy in children have not been established.

The extended release formulation consists of drug within a nondeformable matrix; following drug release/absorption, the matrix/shell is expelled in the stool. The use of nondeformable products in patients with known stricture/narrowing of the GI tract has been associated with symptoms of obstruction. Use caution in patients with increased GI retention (eg, chronic constipation) as doxazosin exposure may be increased. Extended release formulation is not approved for the treatment of hypertension.

Drug Interactions

Increased Effect/Toxicity: Increased hypotensive effect with beta-blockers, diuretics, ACE inhibitors, calcium channel blockers, other antihypertensive medications, sildenafil (use with extreme caution at a dose ≤25 mg), tadalafil, and vardenafil.

Ethanol/Nutrition/Herb Interactions Herb/Nutraceutical: Avoid dong quai if using for hypertension (has estrogenic activity). Avoid ephedra, yohimbe, ginseng (may worsen hypertension). Avoid saw palmetto when used for BPH (due to limited experience with this combination). Avoid garlic (may have increased antihypertensive effect).

Dietary Considerations Cardura® XL: Take with morning meal.

Pharmacodynamics/Kinetics Not significantly affected by increased age

Duration: >24 hours

Protein binding: Extended release: 98%

Metabolism: Extensively hepatic to active metabolites; primarily via CYP3A4; secondary pathways involve CYP2D6 and 2C19

Bioavailability: Extended release relative to immediate release: 54% to 59%

Half-life elimination: 15-22 hours

Time to peak, serum: Immediate release: 2-3 hours; extended release: 8-9 hours

Excretion: Feces (63% primarily as metabolites); urine (9%)

Pregnancy Risk Factor C

Dosage Forms

Tablet: 1 mg, 2 mg, 4 mg, 8 mg

Cardura®: 1 mg, 2 mg, 4 mg, 8 mg

Tablet, extended release:

Cardura® XL: 4 mg, 8 mg

Doxazosin Mesylate *see* Doxazosin *on page 529*

Doxepin (DOKS e pin)

Related Information

Sedation *on page 1825*

U.S. Brand Names Prudoxin™; Sinequan® [DSC]; Zonalon®

Canadian Brand Names Apo-Doxepin®; Novo-Doxepin; Sinequan®; Zonalon®

Generic Available Yes: Capsule, solution

Index Terms Doxepin Hydrochloride

Pharmacologic Category Antidepressant, Tricyclic (Tertiary Amine); Topical Skin Product

Dental Use Cream: Treatment of burning mouth syndrome and neuropathic pain

Use

Oral: Depression

Topical: Short-term (<8 days) management of moderate pruritus in adults with atopic dermatitis or lichen simplex chronicus

Unlabeled/Investigational Use Analgesic for certain chronic and neuropathic pain; anxiety

Local Anesthetic/Vasoconstrictor Precautions Doxepin is one of the drugs confirmed to prolong the QT interval and is accepted as having a risk of causing torsade de pointes. In terms of epinephrine, it is not known what effect vasoconstrictors in the local anesthetic regimen will have in patients with a known history of congenital prolonged QT interval or in patients taking any medication that prolongs the QT interval. Until more information is obtained, it is suggested that the clinician consult with the physician prior to the use of a vasoconstrictor in suspected patients, and that the vasoconstrictor (epinephrine, levonordefrin [Neo-Cobefrin®]) be used with caution. See Dental Comment.

Effects on Dental Treatment Key adverse event(s) related to dental treatment: Xerostomia and changes in salivation (normal salivary flow resumes upon discontinuation)

Oral: Aphthous stomatitis, unpleasant taste, trouble with gums

Topical: Taste alteration

(Continued)

Doxepin (Continued)

Long-term treatment with TCAs increases the risk of caries by reducing salivation and salivary buffer capacity.

Significant Adverse Effects

Oral: Frequency not defined.

Cardiovascular: Hyper-/hypotension, tachycardia

Central nervous system: Drowsiness, dizziness, headache, disorientation, ataxia, confusion, seizure

Dermatologic: Alopecia, photosensitivity, rash, pruritus

Endocrine & metabolic: Breast enlargement, galactorrhea, SIADH, blood sugar increased/decreased, libido increased/decreased

Gastrointestinal: Xerostomia, constipation, vomiting, indigestion, anorexia, aphthous stomatitis, nausea, unpleasant taste, weight gain, diarrhea, trouble with gums, lower esophageal sphincter tone decrease may cause GE reflux

Genitourinary: Urinary retention, testicular edema

Hematologic: Agranulocytosis, leukopenia, eosinophilia, thrombocytopenia, purpura

Neuromuscular & skeletal: Weakness, tremor, numbness, paresthesia, extrapyramidal symptoms, tardive dyskinesia

Ocular: Blurred vision

Otic: Tinnitus

Miscellaneous: Diaphoresis (excessive), allergic reactions

Topical:

>10%:

Central nervous system: Drowsiness (22%)

Dermatologic: Stinging/burning (23%)

1% to 10%:

Cardiovascular: Edema: (1%)

Central nervous system: Dizziness (2%), emotional changes (2%)

Gastrointestinal: Xerostomia (10%), taste alteration (2%)

<1% (Limited to important or life-threatening): Contact dermatitis, tongue numbness, anxiety

Restrictions An FDA-approved medication guide concerning the use of antidepressants in children, adolescents, and young adults must be distributed when dispensing an outpatient prescription (new or refill) where this medication is to be used without direct supervision of a healthcare provider. Medication guides are available at http://www.fda.gov/cder/Offices/ODS/medication_guides.htm. Dispense to parents or guardians of children and adolescents receiving this medication.

Dental Usual Dosing Treatment of burning mouth syndrome and neuropathic pain: Adults: Oral: Topical: Cream: Apply 3-4 times daily

Dosage

Oral: Topical: Burning mouth syndrome (dental use): Cream: Apply 3-4 times daily

Oral (entire daily dose may be given at bedtime):

Depression or anxiety:

Children (unlabeled use): 1-3 mg/kg/day in single or divided doses

Adolescents: Initial: 25-50 mg/day in single or divided doses; gradually increase to 100 mg/day

Adults: Initial: 25-150 mg/day at bedtime or in 2-3 divided doses; may gradually increase up to 300 mg/day; single dose should not exceed 150 mg; select patients may respond to 25-50 mg/day

Elderly: Use a lower dose and adjust gradually

Chronic urticaria, angioedema, nocturnal pruritus: Adults and Elderly: 10-30 mg/day

Dosing adjustment in hepatic impairment: Use a lower dose and adjust gradually

Topical: Pruritus: Adults and Elderly: Apply a thin film 4 times/day with at least 3- to 4-hour interval between applications; not recommended for use >8 days. **Note:** Low-dose (25-50 mg) oral administration has also been used to treat pruritus, but systemic effects are increased.

Mechanism of Action Increases the synaptic concentration of serotonin and norepinephrine in the central nervous system by inhibition of their reuptake by the presynaptic neuronal membrane

Contraindications Hypersensitivity to doxepin, drugs from similar chemical class, or any component of the formulation; narrow-angle glaucoma; urinary retention; use of MAO inhibitors within 14 days; use in a patient during acute recovery phase of MI

Warnings/Precautions [U.S. Boxed Warning]: Antidepressants increase the risk of suicidal thinking and behavior in children, adolescents, and young adults (18-24 years of age) with major depressive disorder (MDD) and other psychiatric disorders; consider risk prior to prescribing. Short-term studies did not show an increased risk in patients >24 years of age and showed a decreased risk in patients ≥65 years. Closely monitor for clinical worsening, suicidality, or unusual changes in behavior; the patient's family or caregiver should be instructed to closely observe the patient and communicate condition with healthcare provider. A medication guide should be dispensed with each prescription. **Doxepin is approved for treatment of depression in adolescents.**

The possibility of a suicide attempt is inherent in major depression and may persist until remission occurs. Monitor for worsening of depression or suicidality, especially during initiation of therapy (generally first 1-2 months) or with dose increases or decreases. Use caution in high-risk patients. Worsening depression and severe abrupt suicidality that are not part of the presenting symptoms may require discontinuation or modification of drug therapy. The patient's family or caregiver should be alerted to monitor patients for the emergence of suicidality and associated behaviors (such as agitation, irritability, hostility, impulsivity, and hypomania) and call healthcare provider.

May worsen psychosis in some patients or precipitate a shift to mania or hypomania in patients with bipolar disorder. Patients presenting with depressive symptoms should be screened for bipolar disorder. Monotherapy in patients with bipolar disorder should be avoided. **Doxepin is not FDA approved for the treatment of bipolar depression.**

The risks of sedative and anticholinergic effects are high relative to other antidepressant agents. Doxepin frequently causes sedation, which may result in impaired performance of tasks requiring alertness (eg, operating machinery or driving). Sedative effects may be additive with other CNS depressants and/or ethanol. Also use caution in patients with benign prostatic hyperplasia, xerostomia, visual problems, constipation, or history of bowel obstruction.

May cause orthostatic hypotension or conduction disturbances (risks are moderate relative to other antidepressants). Use with caution in patients with a history of cardiovascular disease (including previous MI, stroke, tachycardia, or conduction abnormalities). Consider discontinuation, when possible, prior to elective surgery. Therapy should not be abruptly discontinued in patients receiving high doses for prolonged periods.

Use caution in patients with a previous seizure disorder or condition predisposing to seizures such as brain damage, alcoholism, or concurrent therapy with other drugs which lower the seizure threshold. Use with caution in hyperthyroid patients or those receiving thyroid supplementation. Use with caution in patients with hepatic or renal dysfunction and in elderly patients.

Cream formulation is for external use only (not for ophthalmic, vaginal, or oral use). Do not use occlusive dressings. Use for >8 days may increase risk of contact sensitization. Doxepin is significantly absorbed following topical administration; plasma levels may be similar to those achieved with oral administration.

Drug Interactions Substrate (major) of CYP1A2, 2D6, 3A4

Altretamine: Concurrent use may cause orthostatic hypertension.

Amphetamines: TCAs may enhance the effect of amphetamines; monitor for adverse CV effects.

Anticholinergics: Combined use with TCAs may produce additive anticholinergic effects

Antihypertensives: TCAs may inhibit the antihypertensive response to bethanidine, clonidine, debrisoquin, guanadrel, guanethidine, guanabenz, guanfacine; monitor BP; consider alternate antihypertensive agent.

Beta-agonists (nonselective): When combined with TCAs may predispose patients to cardiac arrhythmias.

Bupropion: May increase the levels of tricyclic antidepressants; based on limited information; monitor response.

Carbamazepine: Tricyclic antidepressants may increase carbamazepine levels; monitor.

Cholestyramine and colestipol: May bind TCAs and reduce their absorption; monitor for altered response.

Clonidine: Abrupt discontinuation of clonidine may cause hypertensive crisis, amitriptyline may enhance the response.

CNS depressants: Sedative effects may be additive with TCAs; monitor for increased effect; includes benzodiazepines, barbiturates, antipsychotics, ethanol and other sedative medications.

CYP1A2 inducers: May decrease the levels/effects of doxepin. Example inducers include aminoglutethimide, carbamazepine, phenobarbital, and rifampin.

CYP1A2 inhibitors: May increase the levels/effects of doxepin. Example inhibitors include ciprofloxacin, fluvoxamine, ketoconazole, norfloxacin, ofloxacin, and rofecoxib.

(Continued)

Doxepin *(Continued)*

CYP2D6 inhibitors: May increase the levels/effects of doxepin. Example inhibitors include chlorpromazine, delavirdine, fluoxetine, miconazole, paroxetine, pergolide, quinidine, quinine, ritonavir, and ropinirole.

CYP3A4 inducers: CYP3A4 inducers may decrease the levels/effects of doxepin. Example inducers include aminoglutethimide, carbamazepine, nafcillin, nevirapine, phenobarbital, phenytoin, and rifamycins.

CYP3A4 inhibitors: May increase the levels/effects of doxepin. Example inhibitors include azole antifungals, clarithromycin, diclofenac, doxycycline, erythromycin, imatinib, isoniazid, nefazodone, nicardipine, propofol, protease inhibitors, quinidine, telithromycin, and verapamil.

Epinephrine (and other direct alpha-agonists): Pressor response to I.V. epinephrine, norepinephrine, and phenylephrine may be enhanced in patients receiving TCAs. (**Note:** Effect is unlikely with epinephrine or levonordefrin dosages typically administered as infiltration in combination with local anesthetics.)

Fenfluramine: May increase tricyclic antidepressant levels/effects.

Hypoglycemic agents (including insulin): TCAs may enhance the hypoglycemic effects of tolazamide, chlorpropamide, or insulin; monitor for changes in blood glucose levels; reported with chlorpropamide, tolazamide, and insulin.

Levodopa: Tricyclic antidepressants may decrease the absorption (bioavailability) of levodopa; rare hypertensive episodes have also been attributed to this combination.

Linezolid: Hyperpyrexia, hypertension, tachycardia, confusion, seizures, and **deaths have been reported** with agents which inhibit MAO (serotonin syndrome); this combination should be avoided.

Lithium: Concurrent use with a TCA may increase the risk for neurotoxicity.

MAO inhibitors: Hyperpyrexia, hypertension, tachycardia, confusion, seizures, and **deaths have been reported** (serotonin syndrome); this combination is contraindicated.

Methylphenidate: Metabolism of TCAs may be decreased.

Phenothiazines: Serum concentrations of some TCAs may be increased; in addition, TCAs may increase concentration of phenothiazines; monitor for altered clinical response.

QT_c-prolonging agents: Concurrent use of tricyclic agents with other drugs which may prolong QT_c interval may increase the risk of potentially fatal arrhythmias; includes type Ia and type III antiarrhythmics agents, selected quinolones (sparfloxacin, gatifloxacin, moxifloxacin, grepafloxacin), cisapride, and other agents.

Ritonavir: Combined use of high-dose tricyclic antidepressants with ritonavir may cause serotonin syndrome in HIV-positive patients; monitor.

Sucralfate: Absorption of tricyclic antidepressants may be reduced with coadministration.

Sympathomimetics, indirect-acting: Tricyclic antidepressants may result in a decreased sensitivity to indirect-acting sympathomimetics; includes dopamine and ephedrine; also see interaction with epinephrine (and direct-acting sympathomimetics).

Tramadol: Tramadol's risk of seizures may be increased with TCAs.

Valproic acid: May increase serum concentrations/adverse effects of some tricyclic antidepressants.

Warfarin (and other oral anticoagulants): TCAs may increase the anticoagulant effect in patients stabilized on warfarin; monitor INR.

Ethanol/Nutrition/Herb Interactions

Ethanol: Avoid ethanol (may increase CNS depression).

Food: Grapefruit juice may inhibit the metabolism of some TCAs and clinical toxicity may result.

Herb/Nutraceutical: Avoid valerian, St John's wort, SAMe, kava kava (may increase risk of serotonin syndrome and/or excessive sedation).

Pharmacodynamics/Kinetics

Onset of action: Peak effect: Antidepressant: Usually >2 weeks; Anxiolytic: may occur sooner

Absorption: Following topical application, plasma levels may be similar to those achieved with oral administration

Distribution: Crosses placenta; enters breast milk

Protein binding: 80% to 85%

Metabolism: Hepatic; metabolites include desmethyldoxepin (active)

Half-life elimination: Adults: 6-8 hours

Excretion: Urine

Pregnancy Risk Factor B (cream); C (all other forms)

Lactation Enters breast milk/not recommended (AAP rates "of concern")

Breast-Feeding Considerations Generally, it is not recommended to breast-feed if taking antidepressants because of the long half-life, active metabolites, and the potential for side effects in the infant.

Dosage Forms Excipient information presented when available (limited, particularly for generics); consult specific product labeling. [DSC] = Discontinued product

Capsule, as hydrochloride: 10 mg, 25 mg, 50 mg, 75 mg, 100 mg, 150 mg
   Sinequan®: 10 mg, 25 mg, 50 mg, 75 mg, 100 mg, 150 mg [DSC]
Cream, as hydrochloride:
   Prudoxin™: 5% (45 g) [contains benzyl alcohol]
   Zonalon®: 5% (30 g, 45 g) [contains benzyl alcohol]
Solution, oral concentrate, as hydrochloride: 10 mg/mL (120 mL)
   Sinequan®: 10 mg/mL (120 mL) [DSC]

Dental Comment Doxepin is known to prolong the QT interval. The QT interval is measured as the time and distance between the Q point of the QRS complex and the end of the T wave in the ECG tracing. After adjustment for heart rate, the QT interval is defined as prolonged if it is more than 450 msec in men and 460 msec in women. A long QT syndrome was first described in the 1950s and 60s as a congenital syndrome involving QT interval prolongation and syncope and sudden death. Some of the congenital long QT syndromes were characterized by a peculiar electrocardiographic appearance of the QRS complex involving a premature atria beat followed by a pause, then a subsequent sinus beat showing marked QT prolongation and deformity. This type of cardiac arrhythmia was originally termed "torsade de pointes" (translated from the French as "twisting of the points").

Prolongation of the QT interval is thought to result from delayed ventricular repolarization. The repolarization process within the myocardial cell is due to the efflux of intracellular potassium. The channels associated with this current can be blocked by many drugs and predispose the electrical propagation cycle to torsade de pointes.

Doxepin is considered as having a risk of causing torsade de pointes. The risk of drug-induced torsade de pointes is extremely low when a single QT interval prolonging drug is prescribed. It is not known what effect vasoconstrictors in the local anesthetic regimen will have in patients with a known history of congenital prolonged QT interval or in patients taking any medication that prolongs the QT interval. Until more information is obtained, it is suggested that the clinician consult with the physician prior to the use of a vasoconstrictor in suspected patients, and that the vasoconstrictor (epinephrine, levonordefrin [Neo-Cobefrin®]) be used with caution.

Selected Readings

Friedlander AH and Mahler ME, "Major Depressive Disorder. Psychopathology, Medical Management, and Dental Implications," *J Am Dent Assoc*, 2001, 132(5):629-38.

Ganzberg S, "Psychoactive Drugs," *ADA Guide to Dental Therapeutics*, 2nd ed, Chicago, IL: ADA Publishing, a Division of ADA Business Enterprises, Inc, 2000, 376-405.

Jastak JT and Yagiela JA, "Vasoconstrictors and Local Anesthesia: A Review and Rationale for Use," *J Am Dent Assoc*, 1983, 107(4):623-30.

Rundegren J, van Dijken J, Mörnstad H, et al, "Oral Conditions in Patients Receiving Long-Term Treatment With Cyclic Antidepressant Drugs," *Swed Dent J*, 1985, 9(2):55-64.

Yagiela JA, "Adverse Drug Interactions in Dental Practice: Interactions Associated With Vasoconstrictors. Part V of a Series," *J Am Dent Assoc*, 1999, 130(5):701-9.

Doxepin Hydrochloride *see* Doxepin *on page 531*

Doxercalciferol (doks er kal si fe FEER ole)

U.S. Brand Names Hectorol®
Canadian Brand Names Hectorol®
Generic Available No
Index Terms 1α-Hydroxyergocalciferol
Pharmacologic Category Vitamin D Analog
Use Treatment of secondary hyperparathyroidism in patients with chronic kidney disease

Local Anesthetic/Vasoconstrictor Precautions No information available to require special precautions
Effects on Dental Treatment No significant effects or complications reported
Common Adverse Effects
   Note: As reported in dialysis patients.
   >10%:
      Cardiovascular: Edema (34%)
      Central nervous system: Headache (28%), malaise (28%), dizziness (12%)
      Gastrointestinal: Nausea/vomiting (24%)
      Respiratory: Dyspnea (12%)
   1% to 10%:
      Cardiovascular: Bradycardia (7%)
      Central nervous system: Sleep disorder (3%)
      Dermatologic: Pruritus (8%)
(Continued)

Doxercalciferol *(Continued)*

Gastrointestinal: Anorexia (5%), constipation (3%), dyspepsia (5%), weight gain (5%)

Neuromuscular & skeletal: Arthralgia (5%)

Miscellaneous: Abscess (3%)

Mechanism of Action Doxercalciferol is metabolized to the active form of vitamin D. The active form of vitamin D controls the intestinal absorption of dietary calcium, the tubular reabsorption of calcium by the kidneys, and in conjunction with PTH, the mobilization of calcium from the skeleton.

Drug Interactions

Increased Effect/Toxicity: Doxercalciferol toxicity may be increased by concurrent use of other vitamin D supplements or magnesium-containing antacids and supplements.

Decreased Effect: Absorption of doxercalciferol is reduced with mineral oil and cholestyramine.

Pharmacodynamics/Kinetics

Metabolism: Hepatic via CYP27

Half-life elimination: Active metabolite: 32-37 hours; up to 96 hours

Pregnancy Risk Factor B

Doxidan® [OTC] *see* Bisacodyl *on page 216*

Doxil® *see* DOXOrubicin (Liposomal) *on page 537*

DOXOrubicin *(doks oh ROO bi sin)*

Related Information

DOXOrubicin (Liposomal) *on page 537*

U.S. Brand Names Adriamycin PFS®; Adriamycin RDF®; Rubex®

Canadian Brand Names Adriamycin®

Generic Available Yes

Index Terms ADR (error-prone abbreviation); Adria; Doxorubicin Hydrochloride; Hydroxydaunomycin Hydrochloride; Hydroxyldaunorubicin Hydrochloride; NSC-123127

Pharmacologic Category Antineoplastic Agent, Anthracycline

Use Treatment of leukemias, lymphomas, multiple myeloma, osseous and nonosseous sarcomas, mesotheliomas, germ cell tumors of the ovary or testis, and carcinomas of the head and neck, thyroid, lung, breast, stomach, pancreas, liver, ovary, bladder, prostate, uterus, neuroblastoma, and Wilms' tumor.

Local Anesthetic/Vasoconstrictor Precautions No information available to require special precautions

Effects on Dental Treatment Key adverse event(s) related to dental treatment: Stomatitis and mucositis.

Common Adverse Effects

>10%:

Dermatologic: Alopecia, radiation recall

Gastrointestinal: Nausea, vomiting, stomatitis, GI ulceration, anorexia, diarrhea

Genitourinary: Discoloration of urine, mild dysuria, urinary frequency, hematuria, bladder spasms, cystitis following bladder instillation

Hematologic: Myelosuppression, primarily leukopenia (75%); thrombocytopenia and anemia

Onset: 7 days

Nadir: 10-14 days

Recovery: 21-28 days

1% to 10%:

Cardiovascular: Transient ECG abnormalities (supraventricular tachycardia, S-T wave changes, atrial or ventricular extrasystoles); generally asymptomatic and self-limiting. CHF, dose related, may be delayed for 7-8 years after treatment. Cumulative dose, mediastinal/pericardial radiation therapy, cardiovascular disease, age, and use of cyclophosphamide (or other cardiotoxic agents) all increase the risk.

Recommended maximum cumulative doses:

No risk factors: 550 mg/m^2

Concurrent radiation: 450 mg/m^2

Note: Regardless of cumulative dose, if the left ventricular ejection fraction is <30% to 40%, the drug is usually not given.

Dermatologic: Skin "flare" at injection site; discoloration of saliva, sweat, or tears

Endocrine & metabolic: Hyperuricemia

Mechanism of Action Inhibition of DNA and RNA synthesis by intercalation between DNA base pairs by inhibition of topoisomerase II and by steric obstruction. Doxorubicin intercalates at points of local uncoiling of the double helix.

Although the exact mechanism is unclear, it appears that direct binding to DNA (intercalation) and inhibition of DNA repair (topoisomerase II inhibition) result in blockade of DNA and RNA synthesis and fragmentation of DNA. Doxorubicin is also a powerful iron chelator; the iron-doxorubicin complex can bind DNA and cell membranes and produce free radicals that immediately cleave the DNA and cell membranes.

Drug Interactions

Cytochrome P450 Effect: Substrate (major) of CYP2D6, 3A4; **Inhibits** CYP2B6 (moderate), 2D6 (weak), 3A4 (weak)

Increased Effect/Toxicity: Allopurinol may enhance the antitumor activity of doxorubicin (animal data only). Cyclosporine may increase doxorubicin levels, enhancing hematologic toxicity or may induce coma or seizures. Cyclophosphamide enhances the cardiac toxicity of doxorubicin by producing additional myocardial cell damage. Mercaptopurine increases doxorubicin toxicities. Streptozocin greatly enhances leukopenia and thrombocytopenia. Verapamil alters the cellular distribution of doxorubicin and may result in increased cell toxicity by inhibition of the P-glycoprotein pump. Paclitaxel reduces doxorubicin clearance and increases toxicity if administered prior to doxorubicin. High doses of progesterone enhance toxicity (neutropenia and thrombocytopenia).

Doxorubicin may increase the levels/effects of bupropion, promethazine, propofol, selegiline, sertraline, and other CYP2B6 substrates. The levels/effects of doxorubicin may be increased by azole antifungals, chlorpromazine, clarithromycin, delavirdine, diclofenac, doxycycline, erythromycin, fluoxetine, imatinib, isoniazid, miconazole, nefazodone, nicardipine, paroxetine, pergolide, propofol, protease inhibitors, quinidine, quinine, ritonavir, ropinirole, telithromycin, verapamil and other inhibitors of CYP2D6 or 3A4. Based on mouse studies, cardiotoxicity may be enhanced by verapamil. Concurrent therapy with actinomycin-D may result in recall pneumonitis following radiation.

Decreased Effect: The levels/effects of doxorubicin may be decreased by aminoglutethimide, carbamazepine, nafcillin, nevirapine, phenobarbital, phenytoin, rifamycins, and other CYP3A4 inducers. Doxorubicin may decrease plasma levels and effectiveness of digoxin. Doxorubicin may decrease the antiviral activity of zidovudine.

Pharmacodynamics/Kinetics

Absorption: Oral: Poor (<50%)

Distribution: V_d: 25 L/kg; to many body tissues, particularly liver, spleen, kidney, lung, heart; does not distribute into the CNS; crosses placenta

Protein binding, plasma: 70%

Metabolism: Primarily hepatic to doxorubicinol (active), then to inactive aglycones, conjugated sulfates, and glucuronides

Half-life elimination:

Distribution: 10 minutes

Elimination: Doxorubicin: 1-3 hours; Metabolites: 3-3.5 hours

Terminal: 17-30 hours

Male: 54 hours; Female: 35 hours

Excretion: Feces (~40% to 50% as unchanged drug); urine (~3% to 10% as metabolites, 1% doxorubicinol, <1% Adriamycin aglycones, and unchanged drug)

Clearance: Male: 113 L/hour; Female: 44 L/hour

Pregnancy Risk Factor D

Doxorubicin Hydrochloride *see* DOXOrubicin *on page 536*

DOXOrubicin Hydrochloride (Liposomal) *see* DOXOrubicin (Liposomal) *on page 537*

DOXOrubicin (Liposomal) (doks oh ROO bi sin lip pah SOW mal)

Related Information
DOXOrubicin *on page 536*
U.S. Brand Names Doxil®
Canadian Brand Names Caelyx®
Mexican Brand Names Caelyx; Doxolem
Generic Available No
Index Terms DOXOrubicin Hydrochloride (Liposomal); Liposomal DOXOrubicin
Pharmacologic Category Antineoplastic Agent, Anthracycline
Use Treatment of AIDS-related Kaposi's sarcoma, breast cancer, ovarian cancer, solid tumors
Local Anesthetic/Vasoconstrictor Precautions No information available to require special precautions
(Continued)

DOXOrubicin (Liposomal) *(Continued)*

Effects on Dental Treatment Key adverse event(s) related to dental treatment: Xerostomia (normal salivary flow resumes upon discontinuation), mucositis, gingivitis, glossitis, mouth ulceration, taste perversion, and stomatitis.

Common Adverse Effects

>10%:

Cardiovascular: Peripheral edema (up to 11%)

Central nervous system: Fever (8% to 12%), headache (up to 11%), pain (up to 21%)

Dermatologic: Alopecia (9% to 19%); palmar-plantar erythrodysesthesia/hand-foot syndrome (up to 51% in ovarian cancer, 4% in Kaposi's sarcoma), rash (up to 29% in ovarian cancer, up to 5% in Kaposi's sarcoma)

Gastrointestinal: Stomatitis (5% to 41%), vomiting (8% to 33%), nausea (18% to 46%), mucositis (up to 14%), constipation (up to 30%), anorexia (up to 20%), diarrhea (5% to 21%), dyspepsia (up to 12%), intestinal obstruction (up to 11%)

Hematologic: Myelosuppression, neutropenia (12% to 62%), leukopenia (36%), thrombocytopenia (13% to 65%), anemia (6% to 74%)

Onset: 7 days

Nadir: 10-14 days

Recovery: 21-28 days

Neuromuscular & skeletal: Weakness (7% to 40%), back pain (up to 12%)

Respiratory: Pharyngitis (up to 16%), dyspnea (up to 15%)

1% to 10%:

Cardiovascular: Cardiac arrest, chest pain, edema, hypotension, pallor, tachycardia, vasodilation

Central nervous system: Agitation, anxiety, chills, confusion, depression, dizziness, emotional lability, insomnia, somnolence, vertigo

Dermatologic: Acne, dry skin (6%), dermatitis, furunculosis, maculopapular rash, pruritus, rash, skin discoloration, vesiculobullous rash

Endocrine & metabolic: Dehydration, hyperbilirubinemia, hyperglycemia, hypocalcemia, hypokalemia, hyponatremia

Gastrointestinal: Abdomen enlarged, ascites, cachexia, dyspepsia, dysphagia, esophagitis, flatulence, gingivitis, glossitis, ileus, mouth ulceration, rectal bleeding, taste perversion, weight loss, xerostomia

Genitourinary: Cystitis, dysuria, leukorrhea, pelvic pain, polyuria, urinary incontinence, urinary tract infection, urinary urgency, vaginal bleeding

Hematologic: Ecchymosis, hemolysis, prothrombin time increased

Hepatic: ALT increased

Local: Thrombophlebitis

Neuromuscular & skeletal: Arthralgia, hypertonia, myalgia, neuralgia, neuritis (peripheral), neuropathy, paresthesia (up to 10%), pathological fracture,

Ocular: Conjunctivitis, dry eyes, retinitis

Otic: Ear pain

Renal: Albuminuria, hematuria

Respiratory: Apnea, cough increased (up to 10%), epistaxis, pleural effusion, pneumonia, rhinitis, sinusitis

Miscellaneous: Allergic reaction; infusion-related reactions (bronchospasm, chest tightness, chills, dyspnea, facial edema, flushing, headache, herpes simplex/zoster, hypotension, pruritus); moniliasis, diaphoresis

Mechanism of Action Doxorubicin inhibits DNA and RNA synthesis by intercalating between DNA base pairs causing steric obstruction and inhibits topoisomerase-II at the point of DNA cleavage. Doxorubicin is also a powerful iron chelator. The iron-doxorubicin complex can bind DNA and cell membranes, producing free hydroxyl (OH) radicals that cleave DNA and cell membranes. Active throughout entire cell cycle.

Drug Interactions

Cytochrome P450 Effect: Substrate (major) of CYP2D6, 3A4; **Inhibits** CYP2B6 (moderate), 2D6 (weak), 3A4 (weak)

Increased Effect/Toxicity: Allopurinol may enhance the antitumor activity of doxorubicin (animal data only). Cyclosporine may increase doxorubicin levels, enhancing hematologic toxicity or may induce coma or seizures. Cyclophosphamide enhances the cardiac toxicity of doxorubicin by producing additional myocardial cell damage. Mercaptopurine increases doxorubicin toxicities. Streptozocin greatly enhances leukopenia and thrombocytopenia. Verapamil alters the cellular distribution of doxorubicin and may result in increased cell toxicity by inhibition of the P-glycoprotein pump. Paclitaxel reduces doxorubicin clearance and increases toxicity if administered prior to doxorubicin. High doses of progesterone enhance toxicity (neutropenia and thrombocytopenia).

Doxorubicin may increase the levels/effects of bupropion, promethazine, propofol, selegiline, sertraline, and other CYP2B6 substrates. The levels/

effects of doxorubicin may be increased by azole antifungals, chlorpromazine, clarithromycin, delavirdine, diclofenac, doxycycline, erythromycin, fluoxetine, imatinib, isoniazid, miconazole, nefazodone, nicardipine, paroxetine, pergolide, propofol, protease inhibitors, quinidine, ritonavir, ropinirole, telithromycin, verapamil and other inhibitors of CYP2D6 or 3A4. Based on mouse studies, cardiotoxicity may be enhanced by verapamil. Concurrent therapy with actinomycin-D may result in recall pneumonitis following radiation.

Decreased Effect: The levels/effects of doxorubicin may be decreased by aminoglutethimide, carbamazepine, nafcillin, nevirapine, phenobarbital, phenytoin, rifamycins, and other CYP3A4 inducers. Doxorubicin may decrease plasma levels and effectiveness of digoxin. Doxorubicin may decrease the antiviral activity of zidovudine.

Pharmacodynamics/Kinetics

Distribution: V_{dss}: 2.8 L/m^2

Protein binding, plasma: Unknown; nonliposomal doxorubicin 70%

Half-life elimination: Terminal: Distribution: 4.7-5.2 hours, Elimination: 44-55 hours

Metabolism: Hepatic and in plasma to doxorubicinol and the sulfate and glucuronide conjugates of 4-demethyl,7-deoxyaglycones

Excretion: Urine (5% as doxorubicin or doxorubicinol)

Clearance: Mean: 0.041 L/hour/m^2

Pregnancy Risk Factor D

Doxy-100® *see* Doxycycline (Systemic) *on page 541*

Doxycycline Calcium *see* Doxycycline (Systemic) *on page 541*

Doxycycline Hyclate *see* Doxycycline (Systemic) *on page 541*

Doxycycline Hyclate (Periodontal)
(doks i SYE kleen HI klayt pair ee oh DON tol)

Related Information
Doxycycline (Systemic) *on page 541*
Periodontal Diseases *on page 1801*

U.S. Brand Names Atridox™

Canadian Brand Names Atridox™

Generic Available No

Pharmacologic Category Antibiotic, Tetracycline Derivative

Dental Use Treatment of chronic adult periodontitis for gain in clinical attachment, reduction in probing depth, and reduction in bleeding upon probing

Use Used exclusively in dental applications

Local Anesthetic/Vasoconstrictor Precautions No information available to require special precautions

Effects on Dental Treatment Key adverse event(s) related to dental treatment: Discoloration of teeth (in children), gum discomfort, toothache, periodontal abscess, tooth sensitivity, broken tooth, tooth mobility, endodontic abscess, and jaw pain

Mechanical oral hygiene procedures (ie, tooth brushing, flossing) should be avoided in any treated area for 7 days.

Effects reported in clinical trials were similar in incidence between doxycycline-containing product and vehicle alone; comparable to standard therapies including scaling and root planing or oral hygiene. Although there is no known relationship between doxycycline and hypertension, unspecified essential hypertension was noted in 1.6% of the doxycycline gel group, as compared to 0.2% in the vehicle group (allergic reactions to the vehicle were also reported in two patients).

Significant Adverse Effects Systemic: Gastrointestinal: Diarrhea (3%)

Dental Usual Dosing Oral, subgingival: Dose depends on size, shape and number of pockets treated. Application may be repeated four months after initial treatment. The delivery system consists of 2 separate syringes in a single pouch. Syringe A contains 450 mg of a bioabsorbable polymer gel; syringe B contains doxycycline hyclate 50 mg. To prepare for instillation, couple syringe A to syringe B. Inject contents of syringe A (purple stripe) into syringe B, then push contents back into syringe A. Repeat this mixing cycle at a rate of one cycle per second for 100 cycles. If syringes are stored prior to use (a maximum of 3 days), repeat mixing cycle 10 times before use. After appropriate mixing, contents should be in syringe A. Holding syringes vertically, with syringe A at the bottom, pull back on the syringe A plunger, allowing contents to flow down barrel for several seconds. Uncouple syringes and attach enclosed blunt cannula to syringe A. Local anesthesia is not required for placement. Cannula tip may be bent to resemble periodontal probe and used to explore pocket. (Continued)

Doxycycline Hyclate (Periodontal) *(Continued)*

Express product from syringe until pocket is filled. To separate tip from formulation, turn tip towards the tooth and press against tooth surface to achieve separation. An appropriate dental instrument may be used to pack gel into the pocket. Pockets may be covered with either Coe-pak™ or Octyldent™ dental adhesive.

Dosage Oral, subgingival: Dose depends on size, shape and number of pockets treated. Application may be repeated four months after initial treatment. The delivery system consists of 2 separate syringes in a single pouch. Syringe A contains 450 mg of a bioabsorbable polymer gel; syringe B contains doxycycline hyclate 50 mg. To prepare for instillation, couple syringe A to syringe B. Inject contents of syringe A (purple stripe) into syringe B, then push contents back into syringe A. Repeat this mixing cycle at a rate of one cycle per second for 100 cycles. If syringes are stored prior to use (a maximum of 3 days), repeat mixing cycle 10 times before use. After appropriate mixing, contents should be in syringe A. Holding syringes vertically, with syringe A at the bottom, pull back on the syringe A plunger, allowing contents to flow down barrel for several seconds. Uncouple syringes and attach enclosed blunt cannula to syringe A. Local anesthesia is not required for placement. Cannula tip may be bent to resemble periodontal probe and used to explore pocket. Express product from syringe until pocket is filled. To separate tip from formulation, turn tip towards the tooth and press against tooth surface to achieve separation. An appropriate dental instrument may be used to pack gel into the pocket. Pockets may be covered with either Coe-pak™ or Octyldent™ dental adhesive.

Mechanism of Action Inhibits protein synthesis by binding with the 30S and possibly the 50S ribosomal subunit(s) of susceptible bacteria; may also cause alterations in the cytoplasmic membrane

Doxycycline inhibits collagenase *in vitro* and has been shown to inhibit collagenase in the gingival crevicular fluid in adults with periodontitis

Contraindications Hypersensitivity to doxycycline, tetracycline or any component of the formulation; children <8 years of age; severe hepatic dysfunction; pregnancy

Warnings/Precautions Do not use during pregnancy; use of tetracyclines during tooth development may cause permanent discoloration of the teeth and enamel hypoplasia. Prolonged use may result in superinfection, including oral or vaginal candidiasis. Photosensitivity may occur; avoid prolonged exposure to sunlight or tanning equipment. Atridox™ has not been evaluated or tested in immunocompromised patients, those with oral candidiasis, or conditions characterized by severe periodontal defects with little remaining periodontium. May result in overgrowth of nonsusceptible organisms, including fungi. Effects of treatment >6 months have not been evaluated; has not been evaluated for use in regeneration of alveolar bone.

Drug Interactions Iron and bismuth subsalicylate may decrease doxycycline bioavailability; barbiturates, phenytoin, and carbamazepine decrease doxycycline's half-life; increased effect of warfarin. Concurrent use of tetracycline and Penthrane® has been reported to result in fatal renal toxicity.

Dietary Considerations May be taken with food, milk, or water.

Pharmacodynamics/Kinetics Systemic absorption from dental subgingival gel may occur, but is limited by the slow rate of dissolution from this formulation over 7 days.

Pregnancy Risk Factor D

Breast-Feeding Considerations Tetracyclines enter breast milk and breast-feeding is not recommended. Use of tetracyclines during tooth development may cause permanent discoloration of the teeth and enamel hypoplasia. Tetracyclines also form a complex in bone-forming tissue, leading to a decreased fibula growth rate when given to premature infants.

Dosage Forms Gel, subgingival (Atridox™): 50 mg in each 500 mg of blended formulation [2-syringe system includes doxycycline syringe (50 mg) and delivery system syringe (450 mg) with a blunt cannula]

Doxycycline Monohydrate *see* Doxycycline (Systemic) *on page 541*

Doxycycline (Subantimicrobial)
(doks i SYE kleen, sub an tee mye KROE bee ul)

Related Information
Doxycycline (Systemic) *on page 541*
U.S. Brand Names Periostat®
Generic Available No
Pharmacologic Category Antibiotic, Tetracycline Derivative
Dental Use Treatment of periodontitis associated with presence of *Actinobacillus actinomycetemcomitans* (AA). Periostat® is indicated for use as an adjunct to

scaling and root planing to promote attachment level gain and to reduce pocket depth in adult periodontitis (systemic levels are subinhibitory against bacteria)

Local Anesthetic/Vasoconstrictor Precautions No information available to require special precautions

Effects on Dental Treatment No significant effects or complications reported

Dental Usual Dosing Adjunctive treatment for periodontitis: Adults: Oral: 20 mg twice daily at least 1 hour before or 2 hours after morning and evening meals for up to 9 months

Dosage Adults: **Adjunctive treatment for periodontitis:** Oral: 20 mg twice daily at least 1 hour before or 2 hours after morning and evening meals for up to 9 months

Mechanism of Action Has been shown to inhibit collagenase activity *in vitro*; has been noted to reduce elevated collagenase activity in the gingival crevicular fluid of patients with periodontal disease; systemic levels do not reach inhibitory concentrations against bacteria

Contraindications Hypersensitivity to doxycycline, tetracycline or any component of the formulation; children <8 years of age; pregnancy

Warnings/Precautions Do not use during pregnancy; use of tetracyclines during tooth development may cause permanent discoloration of the teeth and enamel hypoplasia. Prolonged use may result in superinfection, including oral or vaginal candidiasis. Photosensitivity may occur; avoid prolonged exposure to sunlight or tanning equipment. Effectiveness has not been established in patients with coexisting oral candidiasis; use with caution in patients with a history or predisposition to oral candidiasis.

Breast-Feeding Considerations Tetracyclines enter breast milk and breast-feeding is not recommended. Use of tetracyclines during tooth development may cause permanent discoloration of the teeth and enamel hypoplasia. Tetracyclines also form a complex in bone-forming tissue, leading to a decreased fibula growth rate when given to premature infants.

Dosage Forms Tablet (Periostat®): 20 mg

Selected Readings

Lee HM, Ciancio SG, Tuter G, et al, "Subantimicrobial Dose Doxycycline Efficacy as a Matrix Metalloproteinase Inhibitor in Chronic Periodontitis Patients is Enhanced When Combined With a Non-Steroidal Anti-inflammatory Drug," *J Periodontol*, 2004, 75(3):453-63.

Doxycycline (Systemic) (doks i SYE kleen sis TEM ik)

Related Information
Periodontal Diseases *on page 1801*
Sexually-Transmitted Diseases *on page 1766*

Related Sample Prescriptions
Bacterial Infections and Periodontal Diseases *on page 1837*

U.S. Brand Names Adoxa™; Doryx®; Doxy-100®; Monodox®; Vibramycin®; Vibra-Tabs®

Canadian Brand Names Apo-Doxy®; Apo-Doxy Tabs®; Doxycin; Doxytec; Novo-Doxylin; Nu-Doxycycline; Vibra-Tabs®

Mexican Brand Names Vibramicina

Generic Available Yes: Excludes powder for oral solution, syrup

Index Terms Doxycycline Calcium; Doxycycline Hyclate; Doxycycline Monohydrate

Pharmacologic Category Antibiotic, Tetracycline Derivative

Dental Use See Dental Use in Doxycycline Hyclate (Periodontal) *on page 539* and Doxycycline (Subantimicrobial) *on page 540*.

Use Principally in the treatment of infections caused by susceptible *Rickettsia*, *Chlamydia*, and *Mycoplasma*; alternative to mefloquine for malaria prophylaxis; treatment for syphilis, uncomplicated *Neisseria gonorrhoeae*, *Listeria*, *Actinomyces israelii*, and *Clostridium* infections in penicillin-allergic patients; for community-acquired pneumonia and other common infections due to susceptible organisms; anthrax due to *Bacillus anthracis,* including inhalational anthrax (postexposure); treatment of infections caused by uncommon susceptible gram-negative and gram-positive organisms including *Borrelia recurrentis*, *Ureaplasma urealyticum*, *Haemophilus ducreyi*, *Yersinia pestis*, *Francisella tularensis*, *Vibrio cholerae*, *Campylobacter fetus*, *Brucella* spp, *Bartonella bacilliformis*, and *Calymmatobacterium granulomatis*

Unlabeled/Investigational Use Sclerosing agent for pleural effusion injection; treatment of vancomycin-resistant enterococci (VRE)

Local Anesthetic/Vasoconstrictor Precautions No information available to require special precautions

Effects on Dental Treatment Key adverse event(s) related to dental treatment: Glossitis and tooth discoloration (children). Opportunistic "superinfection" with *Candida albicans*; tetracyclines are not recommended for use during pregnancy or in children ≤8 years of age since they have been reported to cause (Continued)

Doxycycline (Systemic) *(Continued)*

enamel hypoplasia and permanent teeth discoloration. The use of tetracyclines should only be used in these patients if other agents are contraindicated or alternative antimicrobials will not eradicate the organism.

Significant Adverse Effects Frequency not defined:

Cardiovascular: Intracranial hypertension, pericarditis

Dermatologic: Angioneurotic edema, exfoliative dermatitis (rare), photosensitivity, rash, urticaria

Endocrine & metabolic: Brown/black discoloration of thyroid gland (no dysfunction reported)

Gastrointestinal: Anorexia, diarrhea, enterocolitis, inflammatory lesions in anogenital region

Hematologic: Eosinophilia, hemolytic anemia, neutropenia, thrombocytopenia

Renal: Increased BUN

Miscellaneous: Anaphylactoid purpura, bulging fontanels (infants), SLE exacerbation

Dental Usual Dosing

Adults: Oral: Treatment of periodontal disease: 100-200 mg once daily for 21 days. **Note:** A specific formulation (Periostat®) containing a subantimicrobial dosage is also available for use as an adjunct to scaling and root planing (see Doxycycline (Subantimicrobial) monograph). In addition, doxycycline gel (Atridox™) is available for subgingival application (see Doxycycline Hyclate (Periodontal)).

Dosage

Children:

Anthrax: Doxycycline should be used in children if antibiotic susceptibility testing, exhaustion of drug supplies, or allergic reaction preclude use of penicillin or ciprofloxacin. For treatment, the consensus recommendation does not include a loading dose for doxycycline.

Inhalational (postexposure prophylaxis) *(MMWR, 2001, 50:889-893)*: Oral, I.V. (use oral route when possible):

≤8 years: 2.2 mg/kg every 12 hours for 60 days

>8 years and ≤45 kg: 2.2 mg/kg every 12 hours for 60 days

>8 years and >45 kg: 100 mg every 12 hours for 60 days

Cutaneous (treatment): Oral: See dosing for "Inhalational (postexposure prophylaxis)"

Note: In the presence of systemic involvement, extensive edema, and/or lesions on head/neck, doxycycline should initially be administered I.V.

Inhalational/GI/oropharyngeal (treatment): I.V.: Refer to dosing for inhalational anthrax (postexposure prophylaxis). Switch to oral therapy when clinically appropriate; refer to "Note" on combined therapy and duration under Adult dosing.

Note: If liquid doxycycline is unavailable for the treatment of anthrax, emergency doses may be prepared for children using the tablets: Crush one 100 mg tablet and grind into a fine powder. Mix with 4 teaspoons of food or drink (lowfat milk, chocolate milk, chocolate pudding, or apple juice). Appropriate dose may be taken from this mixture. Mixture may be stored for up to 24 hours. Dairy mixtures should be refrigerated; apple juice may be stored at room temperature.

U.S. Food and Drug Administration, Center for Drug Evaluation and Research, "How to Prepare Emergency Dosages of Doxycycline at Home for Infants and Children," April 25, 2003, viewable at http://www.fda.gov/cder/drug/infopage/penG_doxy/doxycyclinePeds.htm, last accessed May 8, 2003.

Children ≥8 years (<45 kg): **Susceptible infections:** Oral, I.V.: 2-5 mg/kg/day in 1-2 divided doses, not to exceed 200 mg/day

Children >8 years (>45 kg) and Adults: **Susceptible infections:** Oral, I.V.: 100-200 mg/day in 1-2 divided doses

Acute gonococcal infection (PID) in combination with another antibiotic: 100 mg every 12 hours until improved, followed by 100 mg orally twice daily to complete 14 days

Community-acquired pneumonia: 100 mg twice daily

Lyme disease: Oral: 100 mg twice daily for 14-21 days

Early syphilis: 200 mg/day in divided doses for 14 days

Late syphilis: 200 mg/day in divided doses for 28 days

Uncomplicated chlamydial infections: 100 mg twice daily for ≥7 days

Endometritis, salpingitis, parametritis, or peritonitis: 100 mg I.V. twice daily with cefoxitin 2 g every 6 hours for 4 days and for ≥48 hours after patient improves; then continue with oral therapy 100 mg twice daily to complete a 10- to 14-day course of therapy

Sclerosing agent for pleural effusion injection (unlabeled use): 500 mg as a single dose in 30-50 mL of NS or SWI

Adults:

Anthrax:

Inhalational (postexposure prophylaxis): Oral, I.V. (use oral route when possible): 100 mg every 12 hours for 60 days (*MMWR*, 2001, 50:889-93); **Note:** Preliminary recommendation, FDA review and update is anticipated.

Cutaneous (treatment): Oral: 100 mg every 12 hours for 60 days. **Note:** In the presence of systemic involvement, extensive edema, lesions on head/neck, refer to I.V. dosing for treatment of inhalational/GI/oropharyngeal anthrax

Inhalational/GI/oropharyngeal (treatment): I.V.: Initial: 100 mg every 12 hours; switch to oral therapy when clinically appropriate; some recommend initial loading dose of 200 mg, followed by 100 mg every 8-12 hours (*JAMA*, 1997, 278:399-411). **Note:** Initial treatment should include two or more agents predicted to be effective (per CDC recommendations). Agents suggested for use in conjunction with doxycycline or ciprofloxacin include rifampin, vancomycin, imipenem, penicillin, ampicillin, chloramphenicol, clindamycin, and clarithromycin. May switch to oral antimicrobial therapy when clinically appropriate. Continue combined therapy for 60 days

Dialysis: Not dialyzable; 0% to 5% by hemo- and peritoneal methods or by continuous arteriovenous or venovenous hemofiltration. Supplemental dosage unnecessary.

Mechanism of Action Inhibits protein synthesis by binding with the 30S and possibly the 50S ribosomal subunit(s) of susceptible bacteria; may also cause alterations in the cytoplasmic membrane

Doxycycline inhibits collagenase *in vitro* and has been shown to inhibit collagenase in the gingival crevicular fluid in adults with periodontitis

Contraindications Hypersensitivity to doxycycline, tetracycline or any component of the formulation; children <8 years of age, except in treatment of anthrax (including inhalational anthrax postexposure prophylaxis); severe hepatic dysfunction; pregnancy

Warnings/Precautions Do not use during pregnancy - use of tetracyclines during tooth development may cause permanent discoloration of the teeth and enamel hypoplasia. Prolonged use may result in fungal or bacterial superinfection, including *C. difficile*-associated diarrhea and pseudomembranous colitis. Photosensitivity reaction may occur with this drug; avoid prolonged exposure to sunlight or tanning equipment. Antianabolic effects of tetracyclines can increase BUN (dose-related). Autoimmune syndromes have been reported. Hepatotoxicity rarely occurs: if symptomatic, conduct LFT and discontinue drug. Tetracyclines have been associated with pseudotumor cerebri. Avoid in children ≤8 years of age (except in treatment of anthrax exposure).

Additional specific warnings: Periostat®: Effectiveness has not been established in patients with coexistent oral candidiasis; use with caution in patients with a history or predisposition to oral candidiasis. Oracea™: Should not be used for the treatment or prophylaxis of bacterial infections, since the lower dose of drug per capsule may be subefficacious and promote resistance.

Drug Interactions Substrate of CYP3A4 (major); **Inhibits** CYP3A4 (strong)

Antacids (containing aluminum, calcium, or magnesium): Decreased absorption of tetracyclines

Anticoagulants: Tetracyclines may decrease plasma thrombin activity; monitor

Barbiturates: Decreased half-life of doxycycline

Carbamazepine: Decreased half-life of doxycycline

CYP3A4 inducers: CYP3A4 inducers may decrease the levels/effects of doxycycline. Example inducers include aminoglutethimide, carbamazepine, nafcillin, nevirapine, phenobarbital, phenytoin, and rifamycins.

CYP3A4 substrates: Doxycycline may increase the levels/effects of CYP3A4 substrates. Example substrates include benzodiazepines, calcium channel blockers, mirtazapine, nateglinide, nefazodone, tacrolimus, and venlafaxine. Selected benzodiazepines (midazolam and triazolam), cisapride, ergot alkaloids, selected HMG-CoA reductase inhibitors (lovastatin and simvastatin), and pimozide are generally contraindicated with strong CYP3A4 inhibitors.

Iron-containing products: Decreased absorption of tetracyclines

Methoxyflurane: Concomitant use may cause fatal renal toxicity.

Oral contraceptives: Anecdotal reports suggesting decreased contraceptive efficacy with tetracyclines have been refuted by more rigorous scientific and clinical data.

Phenytoin: Decreased half-life of doxycycline

Ethanol/Nutrition/Herb Interactions

Ethanol: Avoid or limit use (<3 drinks/day); chronic ingestion may decrease serum concentration.

Food: Administer with food or milk due to GI intolerance; may decrease absorption up to 20%. Of currently available tetracyclines, doxycycline has the least

(Continued)

Doxycycline (Systemic) *(Continued)*

affinity for calcium; may decrease absorption of amino acids, calcium, iron, magnesium, and zinc. Administration with calcium or iron may decrease doxycycline absorption. Boiled milk, buttermilk, or yogurt may reduce diarrhea.

Crushed tablets may be mixed with 4 teaspoons of food or drink (lowfat milk, chocolate milk, chocolate pudding, or apple juice) for emergency pediatric dosing if liquid unavailable for treatment of anthrax (see Dosage).

Herb/Nutraceutical: Avoid dong quai; may cause additional photosensitization. Avoid St John's wort; may decrease serum concentration and cause additional photosensitization.

Dietary Considerations

Tetracyclines (in general): Take with food if gastric irritation occurs. While administration with food may decrease GI absorption of doxycycline by up to 20%, administration on an empty stomach is not recommended due to GI intolerance. Of currently available tetracyclines, doxycycline has the least affinity for calcium.

Oracea™: Take on an empty stomach 1 hour before or 2 hours after meals.

Doryx® 75 mg and 100 mg tablets contain sodium 4.5 mg and 6 mg, respectively.

Pharmacodynamics/Kinetics

Absorption: Oral: Almost complete; reduced by food or milk by 20%

Distribution: Widely into body tissues and fluids including synovial, pleural, prostatic, seminal fluids, and bronchial secretions; saliva, aqueous humor, and CSF penetration is poor; readily crosses placenta; enters breast milk

Protein binding: 90%

Metabolism: Not hepatic; partially inactivated in GI tract by chelate formation

Half-life elimination: 12-15 hours (usually increases to 22-24 hours with multiple doses); End-stage renal disease: 18-25 hours

Time to peak, serum: 1.5-4 hours

Excretion: Feces (30%); urine (23%)

Pregnancy Risk Factor D

Lactation Enters breast milk/not recommended

Breast-Feeding Considerations Tetracyclines enter breast milk and breast-feeding is not recommended. Use of tetracyclines during tooth development may cause permanent discoloration of the teeth and enamel hypoplasia. Tetracyclines also form a complex in bone-forming tissue, leading to a decreased fibula growth rate when given to premature infants.

Dosage Forms

Capsule, as hyclate: 50 mg, 100 mg

Vibramycin®: 100 mg

Capsule, as monohydrate (Monodox®): 50 mg, 100 mg

Capsule, coated pellets, as hyclate (Doryx®): 75 mg, 100 mg

Injection, powder for reconstitution, as hyclate (Doxy-100®): 100 mg

Powder for oral suspension, as monohydrate (Vibramycin®): 25 mg/5 mL (60 mL) [raspberry flavor]

Syrup, as calcium (Vibramycin®): 50 mg/5 mL (480 mL) [contains sodium metabisulfite; raspberry-apple flavor]

Tablet, as hyclate: 100 mg

Vibra-Tabs®: 100 mg

Tablet, as monohydrate (Adoxa™): 50 mg, 75 mg, 100 mg

Doxylamine *(dox IL a meen)*

U.S. Brand Names Good Sense Sleep Aid [OTC]; Unisom® SleepTabs® [OTC]

Canadian Brand Names Unisom®-2

Generic Available Yes

Index Terms Doxylamine Succinate

Pharmacologic Category Antihistamine

Use Treatment of short-term insomnia

Local Anesthetic/Vasoconstrictor Precautions No information available to require special precautions

Effects on Dental Treatment Key adverse event(s) related to dental treatment: Dry mucous membranes and significant xerostomia (normal salivary flow resumes upon discontinuation)

Common Adverse Effects Frequency not defined.

Cardiovascular: Palpitation, tachycardia

Central nervous system: Dizziness, disorientation, drowsiness, headache, paradoxical CNS stimulation, vertigo

Gastrointestinal: Anorexia, dry mucous membranes, diarrhea, constipation, epigastric pain, xerostomia

Genitourinary: Dysuria, urinary retention

Ocular: Blurred vision, diplopia

Mechanism of Action Doxylamine competes with histamine for H₁-receptor sites on effector cells; blocks chemoreceptor trigger zone, diminishes vestibular stimulation, and depresses labyrinthine function through its central anticholinergic activity.

Drug Interactions

Increased Effect/Toxicity: Enhances sedative effects of other CNS depressants, may potentiate anticholinergic effects of opioid analgesics, phenothiazines (and other antipsychotics with high anticholinergic activity), tricyclic antidepressants, quinidine and some other antiarrhythmics, and antihistamines.

Decreased Effect: Theoretically, may decrease the effect of cholinergic agents (donepezil, rivastigmine, and tacrine).

Pharmacodynamics/Kinetics

Absorption: Well absorbed

Distribution: V_d: 2.5 L/kg

Metabolism: Via multiple metabolic pathways including N-demethylation, oxidation, hydroxylation, N-acetylation to metabolites including nordoxylamine, dinordoxylamine

Half-life elimination: 10-12 hours

Excretion: Urine (primarily as metabolites)

Pregnancy Risk Factor B

Dronabinol (droe NAB i nol)

U.S. Brand Names Marinol®

Canadian Brand Names Marinol®

Generic Available No

Index Terms Delta-9-tetrahydro-cannabinol; Delta-9 THC; Tetrahydrocannabinol; THC

Pharmacologic Category Antiemetic; Appetite Stimulant

Use Chemotherapy-associated nausea and vomiting refractory to other antiemetic(s); AIDS-related anorexia

Unlabeled/Investigational Use Cancer-related anorexia

Local Anesthetic/Vasoconstrictor Precautions No information available to require special precautions

Effects on Dental Treatment Key adverse event(s) related to dental treatment: Xerostomia (normal salivary flow resumes upon discontinuation) and orthostatic hypotension

Common Adverse Effects Frequency not always specified.

>1%:

Cardiovascular: Palpitations, tachycardia, vasodilation/facial flushing

Central nervous system: Euphoria (8% to 24%, dose related), abnormal thinking (3% to 10%), dizziness (3% to 10%), paranoia (3% to 10%), somnolence (3% to 10%), amnesia, anxiety, ataxia, confusion, depersonalization, hallucination

Gastrointestinal: Abdominal pain (3% to 10%), nausea (3% to 10%), vomiting (3% to 10%)

Neuromuscular & skeletal: Weakness

Restrictions C-III

Mechanism of Action Unknown, may inhibit endorphins in the brain's emetic center, suppress prostaglandin synthesis, and/or inhibit medullary activity through an unspecified cortical action. Some pharmacologic effects appear to involve sympathimometic activity; tachyphylaxis to some effect (eg, tachycardia) may occur, but appetite-stimulating effects do not appear to wane over time. (Continued)

545

Dronabinol *(Continued)*

Antiemetic activity may be due to effect on cannabinoid receptors (CB1) within the central nervous system.

Drug Interactions

Increased Effect/Toxicity: Sedative effects may be additive with CNS depressants (includes barbiturates, opioid analgesics, and other sedative agents). Use in combination with phenothiazines (prochlorperazine) may result in additive or synergistic effects (as antiemetics), but sedation must be monitored.

Pharmacodynamics/Kinetics

Onset of action: Within 1 hour
  Peak effect: 2-4 hours
Duration: 24 hours (appetite stimulation)
Absorption: Oral: 90% to 95%; 10% to 20% of dose gets into systemic circulation
Distribution: V_d: 10 L/kg; dronabinol is highly lipophilic and distributes to adipose tissue
Protein binding: 97% to 99%
Metabolism: Hepatic to at least 50 metabolites, some of which are active; 11-hydroxy-delta-9-tetrahydrocannabinol (11-OH-THC) is the major metabolite; extensive first-pass effect
Half-life elimination: Dronabinol: 25-36 hours (terminal); Dronabinol metabolites: 44-59 hours
Time to peak, serum: 0.5-4 hours
Excretion: Feces (50% as unconjugated metabolites, 5% as unchanged drug); urine (10% to 15% as acid metabolites and conjugates)

Pregnancy Risk Factor C

Droperidol *(droe PER i dole)*

U.S. Brand Names Inapsine®
Canadian Brand Names Droperidol Injection, USP
Generic Available Yes
Index Terms Dehydrobenzperidol
Pharmacologic Category Antiemetic; Antipsychotic Agent, Typical
Use Antiemetic in surgical and diagnostic procedures; preoperative medication in patients when other treatments are ineffective or inappropriate
Local Anesthetic/Vasoconstrictor Precautions Manufacturer's information states that droperidol may block vasopressor activity of epinephrine. This has not been observed during use of epinephrine as a vasoconstrictor in local anesthesia. Droperidol is one of the drugs confirmed to prolong the QT interval and is accepted as having a risk of causing torsade de pointes. The risk of drug-induced torsade de pointes is extremely low when a single QT interval prolonging drug is prescribed. In terms of epinephrine, it is not known what effect vasoconstrictors in the local anesthetic regimen will have in patients with a known history of congenital prolonged QT interval or in patients taking any medication that prolongs the QT interval. Until more information is obtained, it is suggested that the clinician consult with the physician prior to the use of a vasoconstrictor in suspected patients, and that the vasoconstrictor (epinephrine, levonordefrin [Neo-Cobefrin®]) be used with caution.
Effects on Dental Treatment Key adverse event(s) related to dental treatment: Orthostatic hypotension
Common Adverse Effects
>10%:
  Cardiovascular: QT_c prolongation (dose dependent)
  Central nervous system: Restlessness, anxiety, extrapyramidal symptoms, dystonic reactions, pseudoparkinsonian signs and symptoms, tardive dyskinesia, seizure, altered central temperature regulation, sedation, drowsiness
  Endocrine & metabolic: Swelling of breasts
  Gastrointestinal: Weight gain, constipation
1% to 10%:
  Cardiovascular: Hypotension (especially orthostatic), tachycardia, abnormal T waves with prolonged ventricular repolarization, hypertension
  Central nervous system: Hallucinations, persistent tardive dyskinesia, akathisia
  Gastrointestinal: Nausea, vomiting
  Genitourinary: Dysuria
Mechanism of Action Droperidol is a butyrophenone antipsychotic; antiemetic effect is a result of blockade of dopamine stimulation of the chemoreceptor trigger zone. Other effects include alpha-adrenergic blockade, peripheral vascular dilation, and reduction of the pressor effect of epinephrine resulting in

hypotension and decreased peripheral vascular resistance; may also reduce pulmonary artery pressure

Drug Interactions

Increased Effect/Toxicity: Droperidol in combination with certain forms of conduction anesthesia may produce peripheral vasodilitation and hypotension. Droperidol and CNS depressants will likely have additive CNS effects. Droperidol and cyclobenzaprine may have an additive effect on prolonging the QT interval. Use caution with other agents known to prolong QT interval (Class I or Class III antiarrhythmics, some quinolone antibiotics, cisapride, some phenothiazines, pimozide, tricyclic antidepressants). Potassium- or magnesium-depleting agents (diuretics, aminoglycosides, amphotericin B, cyclosporine) may increase risk of arrhythmias. Metoclopramide may increase risk of extrapyramidal symptoms (EPS). Acetylcholinesterase inhibitors (central) may increase the risk of antipsychotic-related EPS.

Pharmacodynamics/Kinetics

Onset of action: Peak effect: Parenteral: ~30 minutes

Duration: Parenteral: 2-4 hours, may extend to 12 hours

Absorption: I.M.: Rapid

Distribution: Crosses blood-brain barrier and placenta

V_d: Children: ~0.25-0.9 L/kg; Adults: ~2 L/kg

Protein binding: Extensive

Metabolism: Hepatic, to p-fluorophenylacetic acid, benzimidazolone, p-hydroxypiperidine

Half-life elimination: Adults: 2.3 hours

Excretion: Urine (75%, <1% as unchanged drug); feces (22%, 11% to 50% as unchanged drug)

Pregnancy Risk Factor C

Drospirenone and Estradiol (droh SPYE re none & es tra DYE ole)

U.S. Brand Names Angeliq®
Canadian Brand Names Angeliq®
Generic Available No
Index Terms E2 and DRSP; Estradiol and Drospirenone
Pharmacologic Category Estrogen and Progestin Combination
Use Treatment of moderate-to-severe vasomotor symptoms associated with menopause; treatment of vulvar and vaginal atrophy associated with menopause
Local Anesthetic/Vasoconstrictor Precautions No information available to require special precautions
Effects on Dental Treatment When prescribing antibiotics, patient must be warned to use additional methods of birth control if on oral contraceptives.

Common Adverse Effects

>10%:
Endocrine & metabolic: Breast pain (19%)
Gastrointestinal: Abdominal pain (11%)
Respiratory: Upper respiratory tract infection (19%)

1% to 10%:
Cardiovascular: Peripheral edema (2%)
Central nervous system: Headache (10%), pain (8%)
Gastrointestinal: Abdomen enlarged (7%)
Genitourinary: Vaginal hemorrhage (9%), endometrial disorder (2%), leukorrhea (1%)
Neuromuscular & skeletal: Back pain (7%)
Respiratory: Flu-like syndrome (7%), sinusitis (5%)

Additional adverse effects reported with estrogens and/or progestins: Abdominal cramps, acne, abnormal uterine bleeding, aggravation of porphyria, amenorrhea, anaphylactoid reactions, anaphylaxis, antifactor Xa decreased, antithrombin III decreased, appetite changes, bloating, breast enlargement, breast tenderness, cerebral embolism, cerebral thrombosis, chloasma, cholestatic jaundice, cholecystitis, cholelithiasis, chorea, contact lens intolerance, corneal curvature steepening, cystitis-like syndrome, decreased carbohydrate tolerance, depression, dementia, dizziness, dysmenorrhea; factors VII, VIII, IX, X, XII, VII-X complex, and II-VII-X complex increased; endometrial hyperplasia, erythema multiforme, erythema nodosum, galactorrhea, hemorrhagic eruption, fatigue, fibrinogen increased, impaired glucose tolerance, HDL-cholesterol increased, hirsutism, hypertension, gallbladder disease, insomnia, LDL-cholesterol decreased, libido changes, melasma, migraine, mood disturbances, nausea, nervousness, optic neuritis, pancreatitis, platelet aggregability and platelet count increased, premenstrual-like syndrome, PT and PTT accelerated, pulmonary embolism, pyrexia, retinal thrombosis, scalp hair loss, somnolence, stroke, thrombophlebitis, thyroid-binding globulin (Continued)

Drospirenone and Estradiol *(Continued)*

increased, total thyroid hormone (T₄) increased, triglycerides increased, urticaria, uterine leiomyomata size increased, vaginal candidiasis, vomiting, weight gain/loss

Mechanism of Action

Drospirenone is a synthetic progestin and spironolactone analog with antimineralocorticoid and antiandrogenic activity. Counteracts estrogen effects causing endometrial thinning.

Estrogens are responsible for the development and maintenance of the female reproductive system and secondary sexual characteristics. Estradiol is the principal intracellular human estrogen and is more potent than estrone and estriol at the receptor level; it is the primary estrogen secreted prior to menopause. Following menopause, estrone and estrone sulfate are more highly produced. Estrogens modulate the pituitary secretion of gonadotropins, luteinizing hormone, and follicle-stimulating hormone through a negative feedback system; estrogen replacement reduces elevated levels of these hormones in postmenopausal women.

Drug Interactions

Cytochrome P450 Effect:

Drospirenone: **Substrate** of CYP3A4 (minor); **Inhibits** CYP1A2 (weak), 2C9 (weak), 2C19 (weak), 3A4 (weak)

Estradiol: **Substrate** of CYP1A2 (major), 2A6 (minor), 2B6 (minor), 2C9 (minor), 2C19 (minor), 2D6 (minor), 2E1 (minor), 3A4 (major); **Inhibits** CYP1A2 (weak), 2C8 (weak); **Induces** CYP3A4 (weak)

Increased Effect/Toxicity: Potential for hyperkalemia with concomitant use of ACE inhibitors, aldosterone, angiotensin II receptor antagonists, heparin, NSAIDs (when taken daily, long term), and potassium-sparing diuretics; monitor serum potassium during first cycle. Potential for hyperkalemia with concomitant use of aldosterone antagonists; monitor serum potassium during first cycle. Aminoglutethimide may increase CYP metabolism of progestins. Oral contraceptives may increase or decrease the effects of coumarin derivatives.

Decreased Effect: Pregnancy has been reported following concomitant use of antibiotics (ampicillin, griseofulvin, tetracycline), however, pharmacokinetic studies have not shown consistent effects with these antibiotics on plasma concentrations of synthetic steroids. Oral contraceptives may increase or decrease the effects of coumarin derivatives. Anticonvulsants (carbamazepine, felbamate, phenobarbital, phenytoin, topiramate) increase the metabolism of ethinyl estradiol and/or some progestins, leading to possible decrease in contraceptive effectiveness. Phenylbutazones may decrease contraceptive effectiveness and increase menstrual irregularities.

Pharmacodynamics/Kinetics

Distribution: Drospirenone: 4.2 L/kg

Protein binding:

Drospirenone: 97%; does not bind to sex hormone binding globulin or corticosteroid binding globulin

Estradiol: 37% bound to sex hormone binding globulin; 61% bound to albumin

Metabolism: Hepatic

Drospirenone forms two metabolites (inactive)

Estradiol: Converted to estrone and estriol; also undergoes enterohepatic recirculation; estrone sulfite is the main metabolite in postmenopausal women

Bioavailability: Drospirenone: 76% to 85%

Time to peak, plasma: Drospirenone: 1 hour; Estradiol: 6-8 hours

Drospirenone and Ethinyl Estradiol *see* Ethinyl Estradiol and Drospirenone *on page 625*

Drotrecogin Alfa *(dro TRE coe jin AL fa)*

U.S. Brand Names Xigris®

Canadian Brand Names Xigris®

Generic Available No

Index Terms Activated Protein C, Human, Recombinant; Drotrecogin Alfa, Activated; Protein C (Activated), Human, Recombinant

Pharmacologic Category Protein C (Activated)

Use Reduction of mortality from severe sepsis (associated with organ dysfunction) in adults at high risk of death (eg, APACHE II score ≥25)

Unlabeled/Investigational Use Purpura fulminans

Local Anesthetic/Vasoconstrictor Precautions No information available to require special precautions

Effects on Dental Treatment Key adverse event(s) related to dental treatment: As with all drugs which may affect hemostasis, bleeding is the major adverse effect associated with drotrecogin alfa. Hemorrhage may occur at virtually any site; risk is dependent on multiple variables, including the dosage administered, concurrent use of multiple agents which alter hemostasis, and patient predisposition.

Common Adverse Effects As with all drugs which may affect hemostasis, bleeding is the major adverse effect associated with drotrecogin alfa. Hemorrhage may occur at virtually any site. Risk is dependent on multiple variables, including the dosage administered, concurrent use of multiple agents which alter hemostasis, and patient predisposition.

>10%:
   Dermatologic: Bruising
   Gastrointestinal: Gastrointestinal bleeding
   1% to 10%: Hematologic: Bleeding (serious 2.4% during infusion vs 3.5% during 28-day study period; individual events listed as <1%)

Mechanism of Action Inhibits factors Va and VIIIa, limiting thrombotic effects. Additional *in vitro* data suggest inhibition of plasminogen activator inhibitor-1 (PAF-1) resulting in profibrinolytic activity, inhibition of macrophage production of tumor necrosis factor, blocking of leukocyte adhesion, and limitation of thrombin-induced inflammatory responses. Relative contribution of effects on the reduction of mortality from sepsis is not completely understood.

Drug Interactions

   Increased Effect/Toxicity: Concurrent use of antiplatelet agents, including aspirin (>650 mg/day, recent use within 7 days), cilostazol, clopidogrel, dipyridamole, ticlopidine, NSAIDs, or glycoprotein IIb/IIIa antagonists (recent use within 7 days) may increase risk of bleeding. Concurrent use of low molecular weight heparins or heparin at therapeutic rates of infusion may increase the risk of bleeding. However, the use of low-dose prophylactic heparin does not appear to affect safety. Recent use of thrombolytic agents (within 3 days) may increase the risk of bleeding. Recent use of warfarin (within 7 days or elevation of INR ≥3) may increase the risk of bleeding. Other drugs which interfere with coagulation may increase risk of bleeding (including antithrombin III, danaparoid, direct thrombin inhibitors)

Pharmacodynamics/Kinetics
   Duration: Plasma nondetectable within 2 hours of discontinuation
   Metabolism: Inactivated by endogenous plasma protease inhibitors; mean clearance: 40 L/hour; increased with severe sepsis (~50%)
   Half-life elimination: 1.6 hours

Pregnancy Risk Factor C

Duloxetine (doo LOX e teen)

U.S. Brand Names Cymbalta®
Mexican Brand Names Cymbalta; Yentreve
Generic Available No
Index Terms Duloxetine Hydrochloride; LY248686; (+)-(*S*)-*N*-Methyl-γ-(1-naphthyloxy)-2-thiophenepropylamine Hydrochloride
Pharmacologic Category Antidepressant, Serotonin/Norepinephrine Reuptake Inhibitor
(Continued)

Duloxetine (Continued)

Use Treatment of major depressive disorder (MDD); management of pain associated with diabetic neuropathy; treatment of generalized anxiety disorder (GAD)

Unlabeled/Investigational Use Treatment of stress incontinence; management of chronic pain syndromes; management of fibromyalgia

Local Anesthetic/Vasoconstrictor Precautions Although duloxetine is not a tricyclic antidepressant, it does block norepinephrine reuptake within the CNS synapses as part of its mechanism. It has been suggested that vasoconstrictors be administered with caution and to monitor vital signs in dental patients taking antidepressants that affect norepinephrine in this way.

Effects on Dental Treatment Key adverse event(s) related to dental treatment: Xerostomia and changes in salivation (normal salivary flow resumes upon discontinuation).

Common Adverse Effects

>10%:

Central nervous system: Somnolence (7% to 15%), dizziness (1% to 14%), headache (13%), insomnia (8% to 11%)

Gastrointestinal: Nausea (4% to 22%), xerostomia (5% to 15%), diarrhea (8% to 13%), constipation (5% to 11%)

1% to 10%:

Cardiovascular: Palpitation (1%)

Central nervous system: Fatigue (2% to 10%), anxiety (3%), fever (1% to 2%), hypoesthesia (1%), irritability (1%), lethargy (1%), nervousness (1%), nightmares (1%), restlessness (1%), sleep disorder (1%), vertigo (1%), yawning (1%)

Dermatologic: Hyperhydrosis (6%), pruritus (1%), rash (1%)

Endocrine & metabolic: Libido decreased (3% to 6%), orgasm abnormality (3% to 4%), hot flushes (2%), anorgasmia (1%), hypoglycemia (1%)

Gastrointestinal: Appetite decreased (3% to 8%), vomiting (1% to 6%), dyspepsia (4%), loose stools (2% to 3%), weight loss (1% to 2%), gastritis (1%)

Genitourinary: Erectile dysfunction (1% to 4%), ejaculation delayed (3%), ejaculatory dysfunction (3%), pollakiuria (1% to 3%), dysuria (1%), urinary symptoms (hesitancy, obstructive symptoms; 1%)

Hepatic: Transaminases increased: Occasionally associated with hyperbilirubinemia and/or increased alkaline phosphatase (1%)

Neuromuscular & skeletal: Muscle cramp (4% to 5%), weakness (2% to 4%), myalgia (1% to 3%), tremor (1% to 3%), muscle tightness (1%), muscle twitching (1%), rigors (1%)

Ocular: Blurred vision (4%)

Respiratory: Nasopharyngitis (7% to 9%), cough (3% to 6%), pharyngolaryngeal pain (1% to 3%)

Miscellaneous: Diaphoresis increased (6%), night sweats (1%)

Restrictions An FDA-approved medication guide concerning the use of antidepressants in children, adolescents, and young adults must be distributed when dispensing an outpatient prescription (new or refill) where this medication is to be used without direct supervision of a healthcare provider. Medication guides are available at http://www.fda.gov/cder/Offices/ODS/medication_guides.htm. Dispense to parents or guardians of children and adolescents receiving this medication.

Mechanism of Action Duloxetine is a potent inhibitor of neuronal serotonin and norepinephrine reuptake and a weak inhibitor of dopamine reuptake. Duloxetine has no significant activity for muscarinic cholinergic, H_1-histaminergic, or alpha$_2$-adrenergic receptors. Duloxetine does not possess MAO-inhibitory activity.

Drug Interactions

Cytochrome P450 Effect: Substrate (major) of CYP1A2, 2D6; **inhibits** CYP2D6 (moderate)

Increased Effect/Toxicity: Hyperpyrexia, hypertension, tachycardia, confusion, seizures, and deaths have been reported with MAO inhibitors (serotonin syndrome); this combination is contraindicated. Avoid use of linezolid (due to MAO activity). Duloxetine may increase serum concentrations of thioridazine, which has been associated with the development of malignant ventricular arrhythmias. Serum levels/effects of tricyclic antidepressants may be increased by duloxetine.

Concurrent use of duloxetine with buspirone, meperidine, moclobemide, nefazodone, SSRIs/SNRIs, serotonin agonists (eg, triptans), sibutramine, tramadol and trazodone and venlafaxine may cause serotonin syndrome; avoid concurrent use. Concurrent use of selegiline with SSRIs has been reported to cause serotonin syndrome (less than with nonselective MAO inhibitors).

CYP1A2 and CYP2D6 inhibitors may increase the levels/effects of duloxetine. Example inhibitors include amiodarone, chlorpromazine, ciprofloxacin, delavirdine, fluvoxamine, fluoxetine, ketoconazole, miconazole, norfloxacin, ofloxacin, paroxetine, pergolide, quinidine, quinine, rofecoxib, ritonavir, and ropinirole.

Decreased Effect: CYP1A2 inducers may decrease the levels/effects of duloxetine. Example inducers include aminoglutethimide, carbamazepine, phenobarbital, and rifampin.

Pharmacodynamics/Kinetics
Absorption: Well absorbed, 2-hour delay in absorption after ingestion
Distribution: 1640 L
Protein binding: >90%
Metabolism: Hepatic, via CYP1A2 and CYP2D6; forms multiple metabolites (inactive)
Half-life elimination: 12 hours (range 8-17 hours)
Time to peak: 6 hours
Excretion: As metabolites; urine (70%), feces (20%)

Pregnancy Risk Factor C

Duloxetine Hydrochloride see Duloxetine on page 549

Duocaine™ see Lidocaine and Bupivacaine on page 976

DuoFilm® [OTC] see Salicylic Acid on page 1451

Duomax see Guaifenesin and Phenylephrine on page 797

DuoNeb™ see Ipratropium and Albuterol on page 905

DuoPlant® [DSC] [OTC] see Salicylic Acid on page 1451

Duotan PD see Dexchlorpheniramine and Pseudoephedrine on page 469

DuP 753 see Losartan on page 1003

Duraclon™ see Clonidine on page 392

Duradrin® see Acetaminophen, Isometheptene, and Dichloralphenazone on page 45

Duradryl® see Chlorpheniramine, Phenylephrine, and Methscopolamine on page 342

Duragesic® see Fentanyl on page 679

Durahist™ PE see Chlorpheniramine, Phenylephrine, and Methscopolamine on page 342

Duramist® Plus [OTC] see Oxymetazoline on page 1236

Duramorph® see Morphine Sulfate on page 1123

Duraphen™ II DM see Guaifenesin, Dextromethorphan, and Phenylephrine on page 798

Duraphen™ DM see Guaifenesin, Dextromethorphan, and Phenylephrine on page 798

Duraphen™ Forte see Guaifenesin, Dextromethorphan, and Phenylephrine on page 798

Duration® [OTC] see Oxymetazoline on page 1236

Duratuss® see Guaifenesin and Phenylephrine on page 797

Duratuss® DM see Guaifenesin and Dextromethorphan on page 796

Duratuss GP® see Guaifenesin and Phenylephrine on page 797

Duratuss® HD see Hydrocodone, Phenylephrine, and Guaifenesin on page 834

Duricef® see Cefadroxil on page 297

Dutasteride (doo TAS teer ide)

U.S. Brand Names Avodart™
Canadian Brand Names Avodart™
Mexican Brand Names Avodart
Generic Available No
Pharmacologic Category 5 Alpha-Reductase Inhibitor
Use Treatment of symptomatic benign prostatic hyperplasia (BPH)
Unlabeled/Investigational Use Treatment of male patterned baldness
Local Anesthetic/Vasoconstrictor Precautions No information available to require special precautions
Effects on Dental Treatment No significant effects or complications reported
Common Adverse Effects
>10%: Endocrine & metabolic: Serum testosterone increased, thyroid-stimulating hormone increased
1% to 10%: Endocrine & metabolic: Impotence (1% to 5%), libido decreased (1% to 3%), ejaculation disorders (1%), gynecomastia (including breast tenderness, breast enlargement) (1%)
Note: Frequency of adverse events (except gynecomastia) tends to decrease with continued use (>6 months).
(Continued)

Dutasteride *(Continued)*

Mechanism of Action Dutasteride is a 4-azo analog of testosterone and is a competitive, selective inhibitor of both reproductive tissues (type 2) and skin and hepatic (type 1) 5α-reductase. This results in inhibition of the conversion of testosterone to dihydrotestosterone and markedly suppresses serum dihydrotestosterone levels.

Drug Interactions

Cytochrome P450 Effect: Substrate of CYP3A4 (minor)

Increased Effect/Toxicity: Calcium channel blockers, nondihydropyridine (diltiazem, verapamil) increase dutasteride levels with concurrent use.

Pharmacodynamics/Kinetics

Absorption: Via skin when handling capsules

Distribution: ~12% of serum concentrations partitioned into semen

Protein binding: 99% to albumin; ~97% to α1-acid glycoprotein; >96% to semen protein

Metabolism: Hepatic via CYP3A4 isoenzyme; forms metabolites: 6-hydroxydutasteride has activity similar to parent compound, 4'-hydroxydutasteride and 1,2-dihydrodutasteride are much less potent than parent *in vitro*

Bioavailability: 60% (range: 40% to 94%)

Half-life elimination: Terminal: ~5 weeks

Time to peak: 2-3 hours

Excretion: Feces (40% as metabolites, 5% as unchanged drug); urine (<1% as unchanged drug); 55% of dose unaccounted for

Pregnancy Risk Factor X

Dyclonine *(DYE kloe neen)*

U.S. Brand Names Cēpacol® Dual Action Maximum Strength [OTC]; Sucrets® [OTC]

Generic Available No

Index Terms Dyclonine Hydrochloride

Pharmacologic Category Local Anesthetic, Oral

Use Temporary relief of pain associated with oral mucosa

Local Anesthetic/Vasoconstrictor Precautions No information available to require special precautions

Effects on Dental Treatment No significant effects or complications reported

Common Adverse Effects The following were reported with the previously available 0.5% and 1% topical solutions; effects are similar to other local anesthetic agents and are generally dose related; frequency not defined:

Cardiovascular: Bradycardia, hypotension

Central nervous system: Apprehension, confusion, convulsion, dizziness, drowsiness, euphoria, lightheadedness, nervousness

Gastrointestinal: Vomiting

Neuromuscular & skeletal: Numbness, tremor, twitching

Ocular: Blurred vision, double vision

Otic: Tinnitus

Respiratory: Respiratory depression

Miscellaneous: Allergic reactions, cold/heat sensation

Pharmacodynamics/Kinetics

Onset of action: Local anesthetic: 2-10 minutes

Duration: ~30 minutes

Absorption: Systemic absorption increased in presence of severely traumatized mucosa

Dyphylline (DYE fi lin)

U.S. Brand Names Dylix; Lufyllin®
Canadian Brand Names Dilor®; Lufyllin®
Generic Available Yes: Elixir
Index Terms Dihydroxypropyl Theophylline
Pharmacologic Category Theophylline Derivative
Use Bronchodilator in reversible airway obstruction due to asthma, chronic bronchitis, or emphysema
Local Anesthetic/Vasoconstrictor Precautions No information available to require special precautions
Effects on Dental Treatment Do not prescribe any erythromycin product to patients taking theophylline products. Erythromycin will delay the normal metabolic inactivation of theophyllines leading to increased blood levels; this has resulted in nausea, vomiting and CNS restlessness.
Mechanism of Action Causes bronchodilatation, through phosphodiesterase inhibition which increases concentrations of cyclic adenine monophosphate (cAMP) and produces relaxation of bronchial smooth muscle.
Pregnancy Risk Factor C

Dyrenium® see Triamterene on page 1613
Dytan™ see DiphenhydrAMINE on page 510
E2 and DRSP see Drospirenone and Estradiol on page 547
7E3 see Abciximab on page 26
E2020 see Donepezil on page 526
EarSol® HC see Hydrocortisone on page 836
Easprin® see Aspirin on page 149

Echothiophate Iodide (ek oh THYE oh fate EYE oh dide)

U.S. Brand Names Phospholine Iodide®
Generic Available No
Index Terms Ecostigmine Iodide
Pharmacologic Category Acetylcholinesterase Inhibitor; Ophthalmic Agent, Antiglaucoma; Ophthalmic Agent, Miotic
Use Used as miotic in treatment of chronic, open-angle glaucoma; may be useful in specific cases of angle-closure glaucoma (postiridectomy or where surgery refused/contraindicated); postcataract surgery-related glaucoma; accommodative esotropia
Local Anesthetic/Vasoconstrictor Precautions No information available to require special precautions
Effects on Dental Treatment No significant effects or complications reported
Mechanism of Action Long-acting inhibition of cholinesterase enhances activity of endogenous acetylcholine. Reduced degradation of acetylcholine leads to continuous stimulation of the ciliary muscle producing miosis; other effects include potentiation of accommodation and facilitation of aqueous humor outflow, with attendant reduction in intraocular pressure.
Pregnancy Risk Factor C

EC-Naprosyn® see Naproxen on page 1148
E. coli Asparaginase see Asparaginase on page 148

Econazole (e KONE a zole)

U.S. Brand Names Spectazole®
Canadian Brand Names Ecostatin®; Spectazole™
Mexican Brand Names Micostyl
Generic Available Yes
Index Terms Econazole Nitrate
Pharmacologic Category Antifungal Agent, Topical
Use Topical treatment of tinea pedis (athlete's foot), tinea cruris (jock itch), tinea corporis (ringworm), tinea versicolor, and cutaneous candidiasis
Local Anesthetic/Vasoconstrictor Precautions No information available to require special precautions
Effects on Dental Treatment No significant effects or complications reported
Common Adverse Effects 1% to 10%: Genitourinary: Vulvar/vaginal burning
Mechanism of Action Alters fungal cell wall membrane permeability; may interfere with RNA and protein synthesis, and lipid metabolism
(Continued)

Econazole *(Continued)*

Drug Interactions
Cytochrome P450 Effect: Inhibits CYP2E1 (weak)
Pharmacodynamics/Kinetics
Absorption: <10%
Metabolism: Hepatic to more than 20 metabolites
Excretion: Urine; feces (<1%)
Pregnancy Risk Factor C

Econazole Nitrate *see* Econazole *on page 553*

Econopred® Plus *see* PrednisoLONE *on page 1339*

Ecostigmine Iodide *see* Echothiophate Iodide *on page 553*

Ecotrin® [OTC] *see* Aspirin *on page 149*

Ecotrin® Low Strength [OTC] *see* Aspirin *on page 149*

Ecotrin® Maximum Strength [OTC] *see* Aspirin *on page 149*

Eculizumab *(e kue LIZ oo mab)*

U.S. Brand Names Soliris™
Generic Available No
Pharmacologic Category Monoclonal Antibody; Monoclonal Antibody, Complement Inhibitor
Use Treatment of paroxysmal nocturnal hemoglobinuria (PNH) to reduce hemolysis
Local Anesthetic/Vasoconstrictor Precautions No information available to require special precautions
Effects on Dental Treatment No significant effects or complications reported
Common Adverse Effects
>10%:
Central nervous system: Headache (2% to 44%), fatigue (12%)
Gastrointestinal: Nausea (16%)
Neuromuscular & skeletal: Back pain (19%)
Respiratory: Nasopharyngitis (23%), cough (12%)
1% to 10%:
Central nervous system: Fever (2%)
Gastrointestinal: Constipation (7%)
Hematologic: Anemia (2%)
Neuromuscular & skeletal: Limb pain (7%), myalgia (7%)
Respiratory: Respiratory tract infection (7%), sinusitis (7%)
Miscellaneous: Herpes infections (7%), flu-like syndrome (5%), viral infection (2%), meningococcal infection (1%)
Restrictions Patients and providers must enroll with Soliris™ OneSource™ (1-888-765-4747) prior to treatment initiation.

An FDA-approved medication guide is available; distribute to each patient to whom this medication is dispensed.
Mechanism of Action Eculizumab is a humanized monoclonal IgG antibody that binds to complement protein C5, preventing cleavage into C5a and C5b. Blocking the formation of C5b inhibits the subsequent formation of terminal complex C5b-9 or membrane attack complex (MAC). Terminal complement-mediated intravascular hemolysis is a key clinical feature of paroxysmal nocturnal hemoglobinuria. Blocking the formation of MAC results in stabilization of hemoglobin and a reduction in the need for RBC transfusions.
Pharmacodynamics/Kinetics
Onset of action: PNH: Reduced hemolysis: ≤1 week
Distribution: 7.7 L
Half-life elimination: ~11 days (range: ~8-15 days)
Pregnancy Risk Factor C

Ed A-Hist® *see* Chlorpheniramine and Phenylephrine *on page 340*

Edathamil Disodium *see* Edetate Disodium *on page 555*

Edecrin® *see* Ethacrynic Acid *on page 619*

Edetate Calcium Disodium
(ED e tate KAL see um dye SOW dee um)

U.S. Brand Names Calcium Disodium Versenate®
Generic Available No
Index Terms CaEDTA; Calcium Disodium Edetate; Calcium EDTA; EDTA (Calcium Disodium)

Pharmacologic Category Chelating Agent

Use Treatment of symptomatic acute and chronic lead poisoning or for symptomatic patients with high blood lead levels; used as an aid in the diagnosis of lead poisoning; possibly useful in poisoning by zinc, manganese, and certain heavy radioisotopes

Local Anesthetic/Vasoconstrictor Precautions No information available to require special precautions

Effects on Dental Treatment No significant effects or complications reported

Common Adverse Effects Frequency not defined.

Cardiovascular: Arrhythmias, ECG changes, hypotension

Central nervous system: Chills, fever, headache

Dermatologic: Cheilosis, skin lesions

Endocrine & metabolic: Hypercalcemia

Gastrointestinal: Anorexia, GI upset, nausea, vomiting

Hematologic: Anemia, bone marrow suppression (transient)

Hepatic: Liver function test increased (mild)

Local: Thrombophlebitis following I.V. infusion (when concentration >5 mg/mL), pain at injection site following I.M. injection

Neuromuscular & skeletal: Arthralgia, numbness, tremor, paresthesia

Ocular: Lacrimation

Renal: Renal tubular necrosis, microscopic hematuria, proteinuria

Respiratory: Nasal congestion, sneezing

Miscellaneous: Zinc deficiency

Mechanism of Action Calcium is displaced by divalent and trivalent heavy metals, forming a nonionizing soluble complex that is excreted in urine

Drug Interactions

Decreased Effect: Do not use simultaneously with zinc insulin preparations; do not mix in the same syringe with dimercaprol.

Pharmacodynamics/Kinetics

Onset of action: Chelation of lead: I.V.: 1 hour

Absorption: I.M., SubQ: Well absorbed

Distribution: Into extracellular fluid; minimal CSF penetration

Half-life elimination, plasma: I.M.: 1.5 hours; I.V.: 20 minutes

Excretion: Urine (as metal chelates or unchanged drug); decreased GFR decreases elimination

Pregnancy Risk Factor B

Edetate Disodium (ED e tate dye SOW dee um)

U.S. Brand Names Endrate®

Generic Available Yes

Index Terms Edathamil Disodium; EDTA (Disodium); Na2EDTA; Sodium Edetate

Pharmacologic Category Chelating Agent

Use Emergency treatment of hypercalcemia; control digitalis-induced cardiac dysrhythmias (ventricular arrhythmias)

Local Anesthetic/Vasoconstrictor Precautions No information available to require special precautions

Effects on Dental Treatment No significant effects or complications reported

Common Adverse Effects Rapid I.V. administration or excessive doses may cause a sudden drop in serum calcium concentration which may lead to hypocalcemic tetany, seizure, arrhythmia, and death from respiratory arrest. Do **not** exceed recommended dosage and rate of administration.

1% to 10%: Gastrointestinal: Nausea, vomiting, abdominal cramps, diarrhea

Mechanism of Action Chelates with divalent or trivalent metals to form a soluble complex that is then eliminated in urine

Drug Interactions

Increased Effect/Toxicity: Increased effect of insulin (edetate disodium may decrease blood glucose concentrations and reduce insulin requirements in diabetic patients treated with insulin).

Pharmacodynamics/Kinetics

Metabolism: None

Half-life elimination: 20-60 minutes

Time to peak: I.V.: 24-48 hours

Excretion: Following chelation: Urine (95%); chelates within 24-48 hours

Pregnancy Risk Factor C

Edex® *see* Alprostadil *on page 78*

Edrophonium (ed roe FOE nee um)

U.S. Brand Names Enlon®; Reversol®
Canadian Brand Names Enlon®; Tensilon®
Generic Available No
Index Terms Edrophonium Chloride
Pharmacologic Category Antidote; Cholinergic Agonist; Diagnostic Agent
Use Diagnosis of myasthenia gravis; differentiation of cholinergic crises from myasthenia crises; reversal of nondepolarizing neuromuscular blockers; adjunct treatment of respiratory depression caused by curare overdose
Local Anesthetic/Vasoconstrictor Precautions No information available to require special precautions
Effects on Dental Treatment No significant effects or complications reported
Common Adverse Effects Frequency not defined.
  Cardiovascular: Arrhythmias (especially bradycardia), AV block, cardiac arrest, decreased carbon monoxide, flushing, hypotension, nodal rhythm, nonspecific ECG changes, syncope, tachycardia
  Central nervous system: Convulsions, dizziness, drowsiness, dysarthria, dysphonia, headache, loss of consciousness
  Dermatologic: Skin rash, thrombophlebitis (I.V.), urticaria
  Gastrointestinal: Diarrhea, dysphagia, flatulence, hyperperistalsis, nausea, salivation, stomach cramps, vomiting
  Genitourinary: Urinary urgency
  Neuromuscular & skeletal: Arthralgias, fasciculations, muscle cramps, spasms, weakness
  Ocular: Lacrimation, small pupils
  Respiratory: Bronchiolar constriction, bronchospasm, dyspnea, bronchial secretions increased, laryngospasm, respiratory arrest, respiratory depression, respiratory muscle paralysis
  Miscellaneous: Allergic reactions, anaphylaxis, diaphoresis increased
Mechanism of Action Inhibits destruction of acetylcholine by acetylcholinesterase. This facilitates transmission of impulses across myoneural junction and results in increased cholinergic responses such as miosis, increased tonus of intestinal and skeletal muscles, bronchial and ureteral constriction, bradycardia, and increased salivary and sweat gland secretions.
Drug Interactions
  Increased Effect/Toxicity: Digoxin may enhance bradycardia potential of edrophonium. Effects of succinylcholine, decamethonium, nondepolarizing muscle relaxants (eg, pancuronium, vecuronium) are prolonged by edrophonium. I.V. acetazolamide, neostigmine, physostigmine, and acute muscle weakness may increase the effects of edrophonium.
  Decreased Effect: Atropine, nondepolarizing muscle relaxants, procainamide, and quinidine may antagonize the effects of edrophonium.
Pharmacodynamics/Kinetics
  Onset of action: I.M.: 2-10 minutes; I.V.: 30-60 seconds
  Duration: I.M.: 5-30 minutes; I.V.: 10 minutes
  Distribution: V_d: Adults: 1.1 L/kg
  Half-life elimination: Adults: 1.2-2.4 hours; Anephric patients: 2.4-4.4 hours
  Excretion: Adults: Primarily urine (67%)
Pregnancy Risk Factor C

Edrophonium and Atropine (ed roe FOE nee um & A troe peen)

Related Information
  Atropine on page 166
  Edrophonium on page 556
U.S. Brand Names Enlon-Plus™
Generic Available No
Index Terms Atropine Sulfate and Edrophonium Chloride; Edrophonium Chloride and Atropine Sulfate
Pharmacologic Category Anticholinergic Agent; Antidote; Cholinergic Agonist
Use Reversal of nondepolarizing neuromuscular blockers; adjunct treatment of respiratory depression caused by curare overdose
Local Anesthetic/Vasoconstrictor Precautions Bradyarrhythmias, tachycardia, and premature ventricular contractions have been reported; use vasoconstrictor with caution
Effects on Dental Treatment No significant effects or complications reported
Common Adverse Effects Also see individual agents.
  >10%: Cardiovascular: Bradycardia, junctional rhythm, tachycardia

1% to 10%: Cardiovascular: Atrial premature contractions (3% to 10%), first-degree AV block (3% to 10%), P-wave changes (3% to 10%), second-degree AV block (3% to 10%), third-degree AV block (1% to 3%), premature ventricular contractions (1% to 3%)

Mechanism of Action

Edrophonium: Inhibits destruction of acetylcholine by acetylcholinesterase. This facilitates transmission of impulses across myoneural junction and results in increased cholinergic response.

Atropine: Minimizes or prevents the muscarinic cholinergic effects caused by edrophonium (eg, bradycardia, bronchocontriction, and increased secretions).

Drug Interactions

Increased Effect/Toxicity: Concurrent use with opioid analgesics (without an inhaled anesthetic), beta blockers, or nondepolarizing-neuromuscular blockers without vagolytic activity may result in increased bradyarrhythmias. Concurrent use with other anticholinergics may increase incidence of anticholinergic adverse events.

Pharmacodynamics/Kinetics See individual agents.

Onset of action: Edrophonium: Antagonism of nondepolarizing muscle relaxants: 3 minutes; Atropine: Heart rate: Immediate

Duration: Edrophonium: Antagonism of nondepolarizing muscle relaxants: 70 minutes; Atropine: Heart rate: 170 minutes

Protein binding: Atropine: 14%

Half-life elimination: Edrophonium: Adults: 1.2-2.4 hours; Anephric patients: 2.4-4.4 hours

Time to peak, plasma: Edrophonium: Antagonism of nondepolarizing muscle relaxants: 1.2 minutes; Atropine: Heart rate: 2-16 minutes

Excretion: Edrophonium: Primarily urine (67%)

Pregnancy Risk Factor C

Efalizumab (e fa li ZOO mab)

U.S. Brand Names Raptiva®
Mexican Brand Names Raptiva
Generic Available No
Index Terms Anti-CD11a; hu1124
Pharmacologic Category Immunosuppressant Agent; Monoclonal Antibody
Use Treatment of chronic moderate-to-severe plaque psoriasis in patients who are candidates for systemic therapy or phototherapy
Local Anesthetic/Vasoconstrictor Precautions No information available to require special precautions
Effects on Dental Treatment No significant effects or complications reported
Common Adverse Effects

>10%:
Central nervous system: Headache (32%), chills (13%)
Gastrointestinal: Nausea (11%)
Hematologic: Lymphocytosis (40%), leukocytosis (26%)
Miscellaneous: First-dose reaction (29%, described as chills, fever, headache, myalgia, and nausea occurring within 2 days of the first injection; percent reported in patients receiving a 1 mg/kg dose; severity decreased with 0.7 mg/kg dose); infection (29%, serious infection <1%)

1% to 10%:
Cardiovascular: Peripheral edema (1% to 2%)
Central nervous system: Pain (10%), fever (7%)
Dermatologic: Acne (4%), psoriasis (1% to 2%), urticaria (1%)
Hepatic: Alkaline phosphatase elevated (4%)
Neuromuscular & skeletal: Myalgia (8%), back pain (4%), arthralgia (1% to 2%), weakness (1% to 2%)
Miscellaneous: Antibodies to efalizumab (6%); hypersensitivity reaction, including asthma, dyspnea, angioedema, urticaria, or maculopapular rash (8%); flu-like syndrome (7%)

Mechanism of Action Efalizumab is a recombinant monoclonal antibody which binds to CD11a, a subunit of leukocyte function antigen-1 (LFA-1) found on leukocytes. By binding to CD11a, efalizumab blocks multiple T-cell mediated responses involved in the pathogenesis of psoriatic plaques.
(Continued)

Efalizumab (Continued)

Drug Interactions

Increased Effect/Toxicity: Concurrent use of immunosuppressants may increase risk of infection.

Decreased Effect: Note: Formal drug interaction studies have not been conducted. Acellular, live, and live-attenuated vaccines should not be administered during therapy.

Pharmacodynamics/Kinetics

Onset: Reduction of CD11a expression and free CD11a-binding sites seen 1-2 days after the first dose; time to steady state serum concentration: 4 weeks
Response to therapy (75% reduction from baseline of PASI score): Observed after 12 weeks

Duration: CD11a expression was ~74% of baseline at 5-13 weeks after discontinuing dose; free CD11a binding sites were at ~86% of baseline at 8-13 weeks following discontinuation; response to therapy (75% reduction from baseline PASI score) continued 1-2 months after discontinuation

Bioavailability: SubQ: 50%

Excretion: Time to eliminate (at steady state): 25 days (range: 13-35 days)

Pregnancy Risk Factor C

Efavirenz (e FAV e renz)

Related Information
HIV Infection and AIDS *on page 1753*
Tuberculosis Treatment *on page 1909*

U.S. Brand Names Sustiva®

Canadian Brand Names Sustiva®

Mexican Brand Names Stocrin

Generic Available No

Pharmacologic Category Antiretroviral Agent, Reverse Transcriptase Inhibitor (Non-nucleoside)

Use Treatment of HIV-1 infections in combination with at least two other antiretroviral agents

Local Anesthetic/Vasoconstrictor Precautions No information available to require special precautions

Effects on Dental Treatment Key adverse event(s) related to dental treatment: Abnormal taste

Common Adverse Effects

Unless otherwise noted, frequency of adverse events is as reported in adults receiving combination antiretroviral therapy. Events marked with an asterisk (*), identify adverse effects reported in ≥10% of patients 3-16 years of age.

>10%:

Central nervous system: Dizziness* (2% to 28%), depression (up to 19%; severe: 1% to 2%), insomnia (up to 16%), anxiety (2% to 13%), pain* (1% to 13%)

Dermatologic: Rash (5% to 26%, grade 3/4: <1%; pediatric: up to 46%, grade 3/4: 2% to 4%)

Endocrine & metabolic: HDL increased (25% to 35%), total cholesterol increased (20% to 40%), triglycerides increased (≥751 mg/dL: 6% to 11%)

Gastrointestinal: Diarrhea (3% to 14%; children: up to 39%), nausea (2% to 12%)

1% to 10%:

Central nervous system: Impaired concentration (up to 8%), headache* (2% to 8%;), somnolence (up to 7%), fatigue (up to 8%), abnormal dreams (1% to 6%), nervousness (2% to 7%), hallucinations (1%)

Dermatologic: Pruritus (1% to 9%)

Endocrine & metabolic: Hyperglycemia (>250 mg/dL: 2% to 5%)

Gastrointestinal: Vomiting* (3% to 6%), dyspepsia (up to 4%), abdominal pain (2% to 3%), anorexia (up to 2%), amylase increased (grade 3/4: up to 6%)

Hepatic: Transaminases increased (grade 3/4: 2% to 8%, incidence higher with hepatitis B and/or C coinfection)

Miscellaneous: Diaphoresis increased (1% to 2%)

Mechanism of Action As a non-nucleoside reverse transcriptase inhibitor, efavirenz has activity against HIV-1 by binding to reverse transcriptase. It consequently blocks the RNA-dependent and DNA-dependent DNA polymerase activities including HIV-1 replication. It does not require intracellular phosphorylation for antiviral activity.

Drug Interactions

Cytochrome P450 Effect: Substrate (major) of CYP2B6, 3A4; **Inhibits** CYP2C9 (moderate), 2C19 (moderate), 3A4 (moderate); **Induces** CYP2B6 (weak), 3A4 (strong)

Increased Effect/Toxicity: Coadministration with medications metabolized by these enzymes may lead to increased concentration-related effects. Cisapride, midazolam, triazolam, and ergot alkaloids may result in life-threatening toxicities; concurrent use is contraindicated. May increase (or decrease) effect of warfarin. Efavirenz may increase the levels/effects of CYP2C9 substrates; example substrates include bosentan, dapsone, fluoxetine, glimepiride, glipizide, losartan, montelukast, nateglinide, paclitaxel, phenytoin, warfarin, and zafirlukast. CYP2C19 substrates: Efavirenz may increase the levels/effects of CYP2C19 substrates; example substrates include citalopram, diazepam, methsuximide, phenytoin, propranolol, and sertraline. Efavirenz may alter the levels/effects of CYP3A4 substrates; example substrates include benzodiazepines, calcium channel blockers, ergot derivatives, mirtazapine, nateglinide, nefazodone, tacrolimus, and venlafaxine.

Decreased Effect: CYP2B6 inducers may decrease the levels/effects of efavirenz; example inducers include carbamazepine, nevirapine, phenobarbital, phenytoin, and rifampin. St John's wort may decrease serum concentrations of efavirenz. Concentrations of atazanavir, indinavir, and/or lopinavir may be reduced; dosage adjustments required. Concentrations of saquinavir may be decreased (use as sole protease inhibitor is not recommended). Serum concentrations of methadone may be decreased; monitor for withdrawal. May decrease (or increase) effect of warfarin. Serum concentrations of sertraline may be decreased by efavirenz. CYP3A4 inducers may decrease the levels/effects of efavirenz; example inducers include aminoglutethimide, carbamazepine, nafcillin, nevirapine, phenobarbital, phenytoin, and rifamycins. Voriconazole serum levels may be reduced by efavirenz (concurrent use is contraindicated). Efavirenz may alter the levels/effects of CYP3A4 substrates; example substrates include benzodiazepines, calcium channel blockers, ergot derivatives, mirtazapine, nateglinide, nefazodone, tacrolimus, and venlafaxine.

Pharmacodynamics/Kinetics

Absorption: Increased by fatty meals

Distribution: CSF concentrations exceed free fraction in serum

Protein binding: >99%, primarily to albumin

Metabolism: Hepatic via CYP3A4 and 2B6 to inactive hydroxylated metabolites; may induce its own metabolism

Half-life elimination: Single dose: 52-76 hours; Multiple doses: 40-55 hours

Time to peak: 3-5 hours

Excretion: Feces (16% to 61% primarily as unchanged drug); urine (14% to 34% as metabolites)

Pregnancy Risk Factor D

Efavirenz, Emtricitabine, and Tenofovir
(e FAV e renz, em trye SYE ta been, & te NOE fo veer)

U.S. Brand Names Atripla™

Index Terms Emtricitabine, Efavirenz, and Tenofovir; Tenofovir Disoproxil Fumarate, Efavirenz, and Emtricitabine

Pharmacologic Category Antiretroviral Agent, Reverse Transcriptase Inhibitor (Non-nucleoside); Antiretroviral Agent, Reverse Transcriptase Inhibitor (Nucleoside); Antiretroviral Agent, Reverse Transcriptase Inhibitor (Nucleotide)

Use Treatment of HIV infection

Local Anesthetic/Vasoconstrictor Precautions No information available to require special precautions

Effects on Dental Treatment Key adverse event(s) related to dental treatment: Efavirenz alone has caused xerostomia (normal salivary flow resumes upon discontinuation) and abnormal taste (see individual monograph). No significant effects or complications reported with combination drug.

Common Adverse Effects The complete adverse reaction profile of combination therapy has not been established. See individual agents. The following adverse effects were noted in clinical trials with combination therapy:

>10%: Endocrine & metabolic: Bone mineral density decreased (28% vs 21% in comparator group had >5% loss of BMD in the spine and >7% loss in hip)

1% to 10%:

Central nervous system: Dizziness (8%), fatigue (7%), headache (5%), somnolence (4%), depression (4%), insomnia (4%), abnormal dreams (4%)

Dermatologic: Rash (5%)

Endocrine & metabolic: Triglycerides increased (4%)

Gastrointestinal: Nausea (8%), diarrhea (7%), serum amylase increased (7%), vomiting (1%)

Hepatic: AST increased (3%), alkaline phosphatase increased (1%)

Respiratory: Sinusitis (4%), upper respiratory infection (3%), nasopharyngitis (3%)

(Continued)

Efavirenz, Emtricitabine, and Tenofovir *(Continued)*

Additional severe effects associated with individual agents include: Severe rash, lactic acidosis, hepatomegaly with steatosis, psychiatric disturbances, hepatotoxicity, renal failure, nephrotoxicity, Fanconi syndrome, immune reconstitution syndrome.

Mechanism of Action See individual agents.

Drug Interactions

Cytochrome P450 Effect:

Efaviranz: **Substrate** (major) of CYP2B6, 3A4; **Inhibits** CYP2C9 (moderate), 2C19 (moderate), 3A4 (moderate); **Induces** CYP2B6 (weak), 3A4 (strong)

Tenofovir: **Inhibits** CYP1A2 (weak)

Increased Effect/Toxicity: See individual agents.

Decreased Effect: See individual agents.

Pharmacodynamics/Kinetics See individual agents.

Pregnancy Risk Factor D

Effer-K™ *see* Potassium Bicarbonate and Potassium Citrate *on page 1329*

Effexor® *see* Venlafaxine *on page 1651*

Effexor® XR *see* Venlafaxine *on page 1651*

Eflone® [DSC] *see* Fluorometholone *on page 712*

Eflornithine (ee FLOR ni theen)

U.S. Brand Names Vaniqa™

Canadian Brand Names Vaniqa™

Generic Available No

Index Terms DFMO; Eflornithine Hydrochloride

Pharmacologic Category Antiprotozoal; Topical Skin Product

Use Cream: Females ≥12 years: Reduce unwanted hair from face and adjacent areas under the chin

Orphan status: Injection: Treatment of meningoencephalitic stage of *Trypanosoma brucei gambiense* infection (sleeping sickness)

Local Anesthetic/Vasoconstrictor Precautions No information available to require special precautions

Effects on Dental Treatment No significant effects or complications reported

Common Adverse Effects

Injection:

>10%: Hematologic (reversible): Anemia (55%), leukopenia (37%), thrombocytopenia (14%)

1% to 10%:

Central nervous system: Seizures (may be due to the disease) (8%), dizziness

Dermatologic: Alopecia

Gastrointestinal: Vomiting, diarrhea

Hematologic: Eosinophilia

Otic: Hearing impairment

Topical:

>10%: Dermatologic: Acne (11% to 21%), pseudofolliculitis barbae (5% to 15%)

1% to 10%:

Central nervous system: Headache (4% to 5%), dizziness (1%), vertigo (0.3% to 1%)

Dermatologic: Pruritus (3% to 4%), burning skin (2% to 4%), tingling skin (1% to 4%), dry skin (2% to 3%), rash (1% to 3%), facial edema (0.3% to 3%), alopecia (1% to 2%), skin irritation (1% to 2%), erythema (0% to 2%), ingrown hair (0.3% to 2%), folliculitis (0% to 1%)

Gastrointestinal: Dyspepsia (2%), anorexia (0.7% to 2%)

Mechanism of Action Eflornithine exerts antitumor and antiprotozoal effects through specific, irreversible ("suicide") inhibition of the enzyme ornithine decarboxylase (ODC). ODC is the rate-limiting enzyme in the biosynthesis of putrescine, spermine, and spermidine, the major polyamines in nucleated cells. Polyamines are necessary for the synthesis of DNA, RNA, and proteins and are, therefore, necessary for cell growth and differentiation. Although many microorganisms and higher plants are able to produce polyamines from alternate biochemical pathways, all mammalian cells depend on ornithine decarboxylase to produce polyamines. Eflornithine inhibits ODC and rapidly depletes animal cells of putrescine and spermidine; the concentration of spermine remains the same or may even increase. Rapidly dividing cells appear to be most susceptible to the effects of eflornithine. Topically, the inhibition of ODC in the skin leads to a decreased rate of hair growth.

Drug Interactions

Increased Effect/Toxicity: Cream: Possible interactions with other topical products have not been studied.

Decreased Effect: Cream: Possible interactions with other topical products have not been studied.

Pharmacodynamics/Kinetics
Absorption: Topical: <1%
Half-life elimination: I.V.: 3-3.5 hours; Topical: 8 hours
Excretion: Primarily urine (as unchanged drug)

Pregnancy Risk Factor C

Eflornithine Hydrochloride *see* Eflornithine *on page 560*

Efudex® *see* Fluorouracil *on page 713*

E-Gems® [OTC] *see* Vitamin E *on page 1664*

E-Gems Elite® [OTC] *see* Vitamin E *on page 1664*

E-Gems Plus® [OTC] *see* Vitamin E *on page 1664*

EHDP *see* Etidronate Disodium *on page 654*

Elaprase™ *see* Idursulfase *on page 860*

Elavil *see* Amitriptyline *on page 94*

Eldepryl® *see* Selegiline *on page 1460*

Eldisine Lilly 99094 *see* Vindesine *on page 1660*

Eldopaque® [OTC] *see* Hydroquinone *on page 841*

Eldopaque Forte® *see* Hydroquinone *on page 841*

Eldoquin® [OTC] *see* Hydroquinone *on page 841*

Eldoquin Forte® *see* Hydroquinone *on page 841*

Electrolyte Lavage Solution *see* Polyethylene Glycol-Electrolyte Solution *on page 1321*

Elestat™ *see* Epinastine *on page 572*

Elestrin™ *see* Estradiol *on page 602*

Eletriptan (el e TRIP tan)

U.S. Brand Names Relpax®
Canadian Brand Names Relpax®
Mexican Brand Names Relpax
Generic Available No
Index Terms Eletriptan Hydrobromide
Pharmacologic Category Antimigraine Agent; Serotonin 5-HT$_{1B, 1D}$ Receptor Agonist
Use Acute treatment of migraine, with or without aura
Local Anesthetic/Vasoconstrictor Precautions No information available to require special precautions
Effects on Dental Treatment Key adverse event(s) related to dental treatment: Xerostomia (normal salivary flow resumes upon discontinuation)
Common Adverse Effects 1% to 10%:
Cardiovascular: Chest pain/tightness (1% to 4%; placebo 1%), palpitation
Central nervous system: Dizziness (3% to 7%; placebo 3%), somnolence (3% to 7%; placebo 4%), headache (3% to 4%; placebo 3%), chills, pain, vertigo
Gastrointestinal: Nausea (4% to 8%; placebo 5%), xerostomia (2% to 4%, placebo 2%), dysphagia (1% to 2%), abdominal pain/discomfort (1% to 2%; placebo 1%), dyspepsia (1% to 2%; placebo 1%)
Neuromuscular & skeletal: Weakness (4% to 10%), paresthesia (3% to 4%), back pain, hypertonia, hypoesthesia
Respiratory: Pharyngitis
Miscellaneous: Diaphoresis
Mechanism of Action Selective agonist for serotonin (5-HT$_{1B}$, 5-HT$_{1D}$, 5-HT$_{1F}$ receptors) in cranial arteries; causes vasoconstriction and reduce sterile inflammation associated with antidromic neuronal transmission correlating with relief of migraine
Drug Interactions
Cytochrome P450 Effect: Substrate of CYP3A4 (major)
Increased Effect/Toxicity: CYP3A4 inhibitors increase serum concentration and half-life of eletriptan; do not use eletriptan within 72 hours of potent CYP3A4 inhibitors (eg, azole antifungals, clarithromycin, diclofenac, doxycycline, erythromycin, imatinib, isoniazid, nefazodone, nicardipine, propofol, protease inhibitors, quinidine, telithromycin, verapamil). Ergot-containing drugs prolong vasospastic reactions; do not use within 24 hours of eletriptan. SSRIs/SNRIs or other serotonin agonists may increase symptoms of hyper-reflexia, weakness, and incoordination.
Pharmacodynamics/Kinetics
Absorption: Well absorbed
Distribution: V$_d$: 138 L
Protein binding: ~85%
Metabolism: Hepatic via CYP3A4; forms one metabolite (active)
(Continued)

Eletriptan *(Continued)*

Bioavailability: ~50%, increased with high-fat meal

Half-life elimination: 4 hours (Elderly: 4.4-5.7 hours); Metabolite: ~13 hours

Time to peak, plasma: 1.5-2 hours

Pregnancy Risk Factor C

Eletriptan Hydrobromide *see* Eletriptan *on page 561*

Elidel® *see* Pimecrolimus *on page 1303*

Eligard® *see* Leuprolide *on page 958*

Elimite® *see* Permethrin *on page 1284*

Elipten *see* Aminoglutethimide *on page 89*

Elitek™ *see* Rasburicase *on page 1413*

Elixophyllin® *see* Theophylline *on page 1554*

Elixophyllin-GG® *see* Theophylline and Guaifenesin *on page 1555*

ElixSure® Cough [OTC] *see* Dextromethorphan *on page 477*

ElixSure™ IB [OTC] *see* Ibuprofen *on page 853*

Ellence® *see* Epirubicin *on page 579*

Elmiron® *see* Pentosan Polysulfate Sodium *on page 1276*

Elocon® *see* Mometasone Furoate *on page 1118*

Eloxatin® *see* Oxaliplatin *on page 1216*

Elspar® *see* Asparaginase *on page 148*

Emadine® *see* Emedastine *on page 562*

Emcyt® *see* Estramustine *on page 605*

Emedastine (em e DAS teen)

U.S. Brand Names Emadine®

Index Terms Emedastine Difumarate

Pharmacologic Category Antihistamine, H$_1$ Blocker, Ophthalmic

Use Treatment of allergic conjunctivitis

Local Anesthetic/Vasoconstrictor Precautions No information available to require special precautions

Effects on Dental Treatment No significant effects or complications reported

Mechanism of Action Selective histamine H$_1$-receptor antagonist for topical ophthalmic use

Pregnancy Risk Factor B

Emedastine Difumarate *see* Emedastine *on page 562*

Emend® *see* Aprepitant *on page 137*

Emetrol® [OTC] *see* Fructose, Dextrose, and Phosphoric Acid *on page 754*

Emko® [OTC] [DSC] *see* Nonoxynol 9 *on page 1185*

EMLA® *see* Lidocaine and Prilocaine *on page 981*

Emsam® *see* Selegiline *on page 1460*

Emtricitabine (em trye SYE ta been)

U.S. Brand Names Emtriva®

Canadian Brand Names Emtriva®

Mexican Brand Names Emtriva

Generic Available No

Index Terms BW524W91; Coviracil; FTC

Pharmacologic Category Antiretroviral Agent, Reverse Transcriptase Inhibitor (Nucleoside)

Use Treatment of HIV infection in combination with at least two other antiretroviral agents

Unlabeled/Investigational Use Hepatitis B (with HIV coinfection)

Local Anesthetic/Vasoconstrictor Precautions No information available to require special precautions

Effects on Dental Treatment No significant effects or complications reported

Common Adverse Effects Clinical trials were conducted in patients receiving other antiretroviral agents, and it is not possible to correlate frequency of adverse events with emtricitabine alone. The range of frequencies of adverse events is generally comparable to comparator groups, with the exception of hyperpigmentation, which occurred more frequently in patients receiving emtricitabine. Unless otherwise noted, percentages are as reported in adults.

>10%:

Central nervous system: Dizziness (4% to 25%), headache (13% to 22%), fever (children 18%), insomnia (7% to 16%), abnormal dreams (2% to 11%)

Dermatologic: Hyperpigmentation (adults 2% to 4%; children 32%; primarily of palms and/or soles but may include tongue, arms, lip and nails; generally mild and nonprogressive without associated local reactions such as pruritus or rash); rash (17% to 30%; includes pruritus, maculopapular rash, vesiculobullous rash, pustular rash, and allergic reaction)

Gastrointestinal: Diarrhea (adults 23%; children 20%), vomiting (adults 9%; children 23%), nausea (13% to 18%), abdominal pain (8% to 14%), gastroenteritis (children 11%)

Neuromuscular & skeletal: Weakness (12% to 16%), CPK increased (grades 3/4: 11% to 12%)

Otic: Otitis media (children 23%)

Respiratory: Cough (adults 14%; children 28%), rhinitis (adults 12% to 18%; children 20%), pneumonia (children 15%)

Miscellaneous: Infection (children 44%)

1% to 10%:

Central nervous system: Depression (6% to 9%), neuropathy/neuritis (4%)

Endocrine & metabolic: Serum triglycerides increased (grades 3/4: 9% to 10%), disordered glucose homeostasis (grades 3/4: 2% to 3%), serum amylase increased (grades 3/4: adults 2% to 5%; children 9%), serum lipase increased (grades 3/4: ≤1%)

Gastrointestinal: Dyspepsia (4% to 8%)

Hematologic: Anemia (children: 7%), neutropenia (grades 3/4: adults 5%, children 2%)

Hepatic: Transaminases increased (grades 3/4: 2% to 6%), bilirubin increased (grades 3/4: 1%)

Neuromuscular & skeletal: Myalgia (4% to 6%), paresthesia (5% to 6%), arthralgia (3% to 5%)

Mechanism of Action Nucleoside reverse transcriptase inhibitor; emtricitabine is a cytosine analogue which is phosphorylated intracellularly to emtricitabine 5'-triphosphate which interferes with HIV viral RNA dependent DNA polymerase resulting in inhibition of viral replication.

Drug Interactions

Increased Effect/Toxicity: Concomitant use of ribavirin with or without interferon alfa and nucleoside analogues may increase the risk of developing hepatic decompensation or other signs of mitochondrial toxicity, including pancreatitis or lactic acidosis. Ganciclovir and valganciclovir may enhance hematologic toxicity of emtricitabine; avoid concurrent use.

Pharmacodynamics/Kinetics

Absorption: Rapid, extensive

Protein binding: <4%

Metabolism: Limited, via oxidation and conjugation (not via CYP isoenzymes)

Bioavailability: Capsule: 93%; solution: 75%

Half-life elimination: Normal renal function: Adults: 10 hours; children: 5-18 hours

Time to peak, plasma: 1-2 hours

Excretion: Urine (86% primarily as unchanged drug, 13% as metabolites); feces (14%)

Pregnancy Risk Factor B

Emtricitabine and Tenofovir
(em trye SYE ta been & te NOE fo veer)

Related Information

Emtricitabine *on page 562*

Tenofovir *on page 1537*

U.S. Brand Names Truvada®

Canadian Brand Names Truvada®

Mexican Brand Names Truvada

Generic Available No

Index Terms Tenofovir and Emtricitabine

Pharmacologic Category Antiretroviral Agent, Reverse Transcriptase Inhibitor (Nucleoside); Antiretroviral Agent, Reverse Transcriptase Inhibitor (Nucleotide)

Use Treatment of HIV infection in combination with other antiretroviral agents

Local Anesthetic/Vasoconstrictor Precautions No information available to require special precautions

Effects on Dental Treatment No significant effects or complications reported

Common Adverse Effects The adverse reaction profile of combination therapy has not been established. See individual agents.

Mechanism of Action Nucleoside and nucleotide reverse transcriptase inhibitor combination; emtricitabine is a cytosine analogue while tenofovir disoproxil
(Continued)

Emtricitabine and Tenofovir *(Continued)*

fumarate (TDF) is an analog of adenosine 5'-monophosphate. Each drug interferes with HIV viral RNA dependent DNA polymerase resulting in inhibition of viral replication.

Drug Interactions
Increased Effect/Toxicity: Refer to individual agents.
Pharmacodynamics/Kinetics Refer to individual monographs.
Pregnancy Risk Factor B

Enalapril *(e NAL a pril)*

Related Information
Cardiovascular Diseases *on page 1726*
U.S. Brand Names Vasotec®
Canadian Brand Names Vasotec®
Mexican Brand Names Enaladil; Glioten; Renitec
Generic Available Yes
Index Terms Enalaprilat; Enalapril Maleate
Pharmacologic Category Angiotensin-Converting Enzyme (ACE) Inhibitor
Use Management of mild to severe hypertension; treatment of congestive heart failure, left ventricular dysfunction after myocardial infarction
Unlabeled/Investigational Use
Unlabeled: Hypertensive crisis, diabetic nephropathy, rheumatoid arthritis, diagnosis of anatomic renal artery stenosis, hypertension secondary to scleroderma renal crisis, diagnosis of aldosteronism, idiopathic edema, Bartter's syndrome, postmyocardial infarction for prevention of ventricular failure
Investigational: Severe congestive heart failure in infants, neonatal hypertension, acute pulmonary edema
Local Anesthetic/Vasoconstrictor Precautions No information available to require special precautions
Effects on Dental Treatment Key adverse event(s) related to dental treatment: Abnormal taste and orthostatic hypotension
Common Adverse Effects Note: Frequency ranges include data from hypertension and heart failure trials. Higher rates of adverse reactions have generally been noted in patients with CHF. However, the frequency of adverse effects associated with placebo is also increased in this population.

1% to 10%:
Cardiovascular: Hypotension (0.9% to 7%), chest pain (2%), syncope (0.5% to 2%), orthostasis (2%), orthostatic hypotension (2%)
Central nervous system: Headache (2% to 5%), dizziness (4% to 8%), fatigue (2% to 3%)
Dermatologic: Rash (2%)
Gastrointestinal: Abnormal taste, abdominal pain, vomiting, nausea, diarrhea, anorexia, constipation
Neuromuscular & skeletal: Weakness
Renal: Serum creatinine increased (0.2% to 20%), worsening of renal function (in patients with bilateral renal artery stenosis or hypovolemia)
Respiratory (1% to 2%): Bronchitis, cough, dyspnea

Dosage Use lower listed initial dose in patients with hyponatremia, hypovolemia, severe congestive heart failure, decreased renal function, or in those receiving diuretics.

Oral: **Enalapril**: Children 1 month to 17 years: Hypertension: Initial: 0.08 mg/kg/d (up to 5 mg) in 1-2 divided doses; adjust dosage based on patient response; doses >0.58 mg/kg (40 mg) have not been evaluated in pediatric patients
Investigational: Congestive heart failure: Initial oral doses of **enalapril**: 0.1 mg/kg/day increasing as needed over 2 weeks to 0.5 mg/kg/day have been used in infants
Investigational: Neonatal hypertension: I.V. doses of **enalaprilat**: 5-10 mcg/kg/dose administered every 8-24 hours have been used; monitor patients carefully; select patients may require higher doses
Adults:
Oral: **Enalapril**:
Hypertension: 2.5-5 mg/day then increase as required, usually at 1- to 2-week intervals; usual dose range (JNC 7): 2.5-40 mg/day in 1-2 divided

doses. **Note:** Initiate with 2.5 mg if patient is taking a diuretic which cannot be discontinued. May add a diuretic if blood pressure cannot be controlled with enalapril alone.

Heart failure: Initial: 2.5 mg once or twice daily (usual range: 5-40 mg/day in 2 divided doses). Titrate slowly at 1- to 2-week intervals. Target dose: 10-20 mg twice daily (ACC/AHA 2005 Heart Failure Guidelines)

Asymptomatic left ventricular dysfunction: 2.5 mg twice daily, titrated as tolerated to 20 mg/day

I.V.: **Enalaprilat:**

Hypertension: 1.25 mg/dose, given over 5 minutes every 6 hours; doses as high as 5 mg/dose every 6 hours have been tolerated for up to 36 hours. **Note:** If patients are concomitantly receiving diuretic therapy, begin with 0.625 mg I.V. over 5 minutes; if the effect is not adequate after 1 hour, repeat the dose and administer 1.25 mg at 6-hour intervals thereafter; if adequate, administer 0.625 mg I.V. every 6 hours.

Heart failure: Avoid I.V. administration in patients with unstable heart failure or those suffering acute myocardial infarction.

Conversion from I.V. to oral therapy if not concurrently on diuretics: 5 mg once daily; subsequent titration as needed; if concurrently receiving diuretics and responding to 0.625 mg I.V. every 6 hours, initiate with 2.5 mg/day.

Dosing adjustment in renal impairment:

Oral: Enalapril:

Cl_{cr} 30-80 mL/minute: Administer 5 mg/day titrated upwards to maximum of 40 mg.

Cl_{cr} <30 mL/minute: Administer 2.5 mg day; titrated upward until blood pressure is controlled.

For heart failure patients with sodium <130 mEq/L or serum creatinine >1.6 mg/dL, initiate dosage with 2.5 mg/day, increasing to twice daily as needed. Increase further in increments of 2.5 mg/dose at >4-day intervals to a maximum daily dose of 40 mg.

I.V.: Enalaprilat:

Cl_{cr} >30 mL/minute: Initiate with 1.25 mg every 6 hours and increase dose based on response.

Cl_{cr} <30 mL/minute: Initiate with 0.625 mg every 6 hours and increase dose based on response.

Hemodialysis: Moderately dialyzable (20% to 50%); administer dose postdialysis (eg, 0.625 mg I.V. every 6 hours) or administer 20% to 25% supplemental dose following dialysis; Clearance: 62 mL/minute.

Peritoneal dialysis: Supplemental dose is not necessary, although some removal of drug occurs.

Dosing adjustment in hepatic impairment: Hydrolysis of enalapril to enalaprilat may be delayed and/or impaired in patients with severe hepatic impairment, but the pharmacodynamic effects of the drug do not appear to be significantly altered; no dosage adjustment.

Mechanism of Action Competitive inhibitor of angiotensin-converting enzyme (ACE); prevents conversion of angiotensin I to angiotensin II, a potent vasoconstrictor; results in lower levels of angiotensin II which causes an increase in plasma renin activity and a reduction in aldosterone secretion

Contraindications Hypersensitivity to enalapril or enalaprilat; angioedema related to previous treatment with an ACE inhibitor; patients with idiopathic or hereditary angioedema; bilateral renal artery stenosis; pregnancy (2nd and 3rd trimesters)

Warnings/Precautions Anaphylactic reactions can occur. Angioedema can occur at any time during treatment (especially following first dose). It may involve head and neck (potentially affecting the airway) or the intestine (presenting with abdominal pain). Prolonged monitoring may be required especially if tongue, glottis, or larynx are involved as they are associated with airway obstruction. Those with a history of airway surgery in this situation have a higher risk. Careful blood pressure monitoring with first dose (hypotension can occur especially in volume-depleted patients). **[U.S. Boxed Warning]: Based on human data, ACEIs can cause injury and death to the developing fetus when used in the second and third trimesters. ACEIs should be discontinued as soon as possible once pregnancy is detected.** Dosage adjustment needed in renal impairment. Use with caution in hypovolemia; collagen vascular diseases; valvular stenosis (particularly aortic stenosis); hyperkalemia; or before, during, or immediately after anesthesia. Avoid rapid dosage escalation which may lead to renal insufficiency.

Rare toxicities associated with ACE inhibitors include cholestatic jaundice (which may progress to hepatic necrosis) and neutropenia/agranulocytosis with myeloid hyperplasia. Hyperkalemia may rarely occur. May be associated with deterioration of renal function and/or increases in serum creatinine, particularly in patients dependent on renin-angiotensin-aldosterone system. Use with (Continued)

Enalapril *(Continued)*

caution in unilateral renal artery stenosis and pre-existing renal insufficiency; if patient has renal impairment then a baseline WBC with differential and serum creatinine should be evaluated and monitored closely during the first 3 months of therapy. Hypersensitivity reactions may be seen during hemodialysis with high-flux dialysis membranes (eg, AN69).

Drug Interactions

Cytochrome P450 Effect: Substrate of CYP3A4 (major)

Increased Effect/Toxicity: Potassium supplements, co-trimoxazole (high dose), angiotensin II receptor antagonists (eg, candesartan, losartan, irbesartan), or potassium-sparing diuretics (amiloride, spironolactone, triam-terene) may result in elevated serum potassium levels when combined with enalapril. ACE inhibitor effects may be increased by phenothiazines or probenecid (increases levels of captopril). ACE inhibitors may increase serum concentrations/effects of lithium.

Diuretics have additive hypotensive effects with ACE inhibitors, and hypovo-lemia increases the potential for adverse renal effects of ACE inhibitors. In patients with compromised renal function, coadministration with NSAIDs may result in further deterioration of renal function. Allopurinol and ACE inhibitors may cause a higher risk of hypersensitivity reaction when taken concurrently.

Decreased Effect: Aspirin (high dose) may reduce the therapeutic effects of ACE inhibitors; at low dosages this does not appear to be significant. Antacids may decrease the bioavailability of ACE inhibitors (may be more likely to occur with captopril); separate administration times by 1-2 hours. NSAIDs may reduce the hypotensive effects of ACE inhibitors. More likely to occur in low renin or volume-dependent hypertensive patients. CYP3A4 inducers may decrease the levels/effects of enalapril; example inducers include aminoglu-tethimide, carbamazepine, nafcillin, nevirapine, phenobarbital, phenytoin, and rifamycins.

Ethanol/Nutrition/Herb Interactions Herb/Nutraceutical: St John's wort may decrease enalapril levels. Avoid dong quai if using for hypertension (has estro-genic activity). Avoid ephedra, yohimbe, ginseng (may worsen hypertension). Avoid natural licorice (causes sodium and water retention and increases potas-sium loss). Avoid garlic (may have increased antihypertensive effect).

Dietary Considerations Limit salt substitutes or potassium-rich diet.

Pharmacodynamics/Kinetics

Onset of action: Oral: ~1 hour

Duration: Oral: 12-24 hours

Absorption: Oral: 55% to 75%

Protein binding: 50% to 60%

Metabolism: Prodrug, undergoes hepatic biotransformation to enalaprilat

Half-life elimination:

Enalapril: Adults: Healthy: 2 hours; Congestive heart failure: 3.4-5.8 hours

Enalaprilat: Infants 6 weeks to 8 months old: 6-10 hours; Adults: 35-38 hours

Time to peak, serum: Oral: Enalapril: 0.5-1.5 hours; Enalaprilat (active): 3-4.5 hours

Excretion: Urine (60% to 80%); some feces

Pregnancy Risk Factor C (1st trimester)/D (2nd and 3rd trimesters)

Dosage Forms

Injection, solution: 1.25 mg/mL (1 mL, 2 mL)

Tablet: 2.5 mg, 5 mg, 10 mg, 20 mg

Vasotec®: 2.5 mg, 5 mg, 10 mg, 20 mg

Enalapril and Felodipine *(e NAL a pril & fe LOE di peen)*

Related Information

Enalapril *on page 564*

Felodipine *on page 673*

U.S. Brand Names Lexxel®

Canadian Brand Names Lexxel®

Generic Available No

Index Terms Felodipine and Enalapril

Pharmacologic Category Antihypertensive Agent, Combination

Use Treatment of hypertension, however, not indicated for initial treatment of hypertension; replacement therapy in patients receiving separate dosage forms (for patient convenience); when monotherapy with one component fails to achieve desired antihypertensive effect, or when dose-limiting adverse effects limit upward titration of monotherapy

Local Anesthetic/Vasoconstrictor Precautions No information available to require special precautions

Effects on Dental Treatment Key adverse event(s) related to dental treatment: Gingival hyperplasia (fewer reports with felodipine than with other CCBs); resolves upon discontinuation (consultation with physician is suggested).
Common Adverse Effects See individual agents.
Mechanism of Action See individual agents.
Drug Interactions
  Cytochrome P450 Effect:
    Enalapril: **Substrate** of CYP3A4 (major)
    Felodipine: **Substrate** of CYP3A4 (major); **Inhibits** CYP2C8 (moderate), 2C9 (weak), 2D6 (weak), 3A4 (weak)
  Increased Effect/Toxicity: See individual agents.
  Decreased Effect: See individual agents.
Pharmacodynamics/Kinetics See individual agents.
Pregnancy Risk Factor C/D (2nd and 3rd trimesters)

Enalapril and Hydrochlorothiazide
(e NAL a pril & hye droe klor oh THYE a zide)

Related Information
  Cardiovascular Diseases *on page 1726*
  Enalapril *on page 564*
  Hydrochlorothiazide *on page 819*
U.S. Brand Names Vaseretic®
Canadian Brand Names Vaseretic®
Mexican Brand Names Co-Renitec
Generic Available Yes
Index Terms Hydrochlorothiazide and Enalapril
Pharmacologic Category Antihypertensive Agent, Combination
Use Treatment of hypertension
Local Anesthetic/Vasoconstrictor Precautions No information available to require special precautions
Effects on Dental Treatment No significant effects or complications reported
Common Adverse Effects See individual agents.
Drug Interactions
  Cytochrome P450 Effect: Enalapril: **Substrate** of CYP3A4 (major)
Pharmacodynamics/Kinetics See individual agents.
Pregnancy Risk Factor C/D (2nd and 3rd trimesters)

Enalaprilat *see* Enalapril *on page 564*
Enalapril Maleate *see* Enalapril *on page 564*
Enbrel® *see* Etanercept *on page 617*
Encare® [OTC] *see* Nonoxynol 9 *on page 1185*
Encort™ *see* Hydrocortisone *on page 836*
EndaCof *see* Hydrocodone and Guaifenesin *on page 828*
EndaCof-XP *see* Hydrocodone and Guaifenesin *on page 828*
EndoAvitene® *see* Collagen Hemostat *on page 411*
Endocet® *see* Oxycodone and Acetaminophen *on page 1228*
Endodan® *see* Oxycodone and Aspirin *on page 1231*
Endrate® *see* Edetate Disodium *on page 555*
Enduron® [DSC] *see* Methyclothiazide *on page 1077*
Enemeez® [OTC] *see* Docusate *on page 522*
Enerjets [OTC] *see* Caffeine *on page 255*
Enfamil® Glucose *see* Dextrose *on page 478*

Enfuvirtide (en FYOO vir tide)

U.S. Brand Names Fuzeon®
Canadian Brand Names Fuzeon®
Mexican Brand Names Fuzeon
Generic Available No
Index Terms T-20
Pharmacologic Category Antiretroviral Agent, Fusion Protein Inhibitor
Use Treatment of HIV-1 infection in combination with other antiretroviral agents in treatment-experienced patients with evidence of HIV-1 replication despite ongoing antiretroviral therapy
Local Anesthetic/Vasoconstrictor Precautions No information available to require special precautions
Effects on Dental Treatment Key adverse event(s) related to dental treatment: Xerostomia (normal salivary flow resumes upon discontinuation) and taste disturbance
(Continued)

Enfuvirtide *(Continued)*

Common Adverse Effects

>10%:

Gastrointestinal: Diarrhea (32%), nausea (23%)

Local: Injection site reactions (98%; may include pain, erythema, induration, pruritus, ecchymosis, nodule or cyst formation)

1% to 10%:

Dermatologic: Folliculitis (2%)

Gastrointestinal: Weight loss (7%), abdominal pain (4%), appetite decreased (3%), pancreatitis (3%), anorexia (2%), xerostomia (2%)

Hematologic: Eosinophilia (2% to 9%)

Hepatic: Transaminases increased (4%, grade 4: 1%)

Local: Injection site infection (2%)

Neuromuscular & skeletal: CPK increased (3% to 7%), limb pain (3%), myalgia (3%)

Ocular: Conjunctivitis (2%)

Respiratory: Sinusitis (6%), cough (4%), pneumonia (3%)

Miscellaneous: Infections (4% to 6%), herpes simplex (4%), flu-like syndrome (2%)

Mechanism of Action Binds to the first heptad-repeat (HR1) in the gp41 subunit of the viral envelope glycoprotein. Inhibits the fusion of HIV-1 virus with CD4 cells by blocking the conformational change in gp41 required for membrane fusion and entry into CD4 cells

Drug Interactions

Increased Effect/Toxicity: No significant interactions identified.

Decreased Effect: No significant interactions identified.

Pharmacodynamics/Kinetics

Distribution: V_d: 5.5 L

Protein binding: 92%

Metabolism: Proteolytic hydrolysis (CYP isoenzymes do not appear to contribute to metabolism)

Clearance: Adults: 24.8 mL/hour/kg

Bioavailability: 84% ± 16%

Half-life elimination: 3.8 hours

Time to peak: 4-8 hours

Pregnancy Risk Factor B

Enoxaparin *(ee noks a PA rin)*

Related Information

Cardiovascular Diseases *on page 1726*

U.S. Brand Names Lovenox®

Canadian Brand Names Enoxaparin Injection; Lovenox®; Lovenox® HP

Mexican Brand Names Clexane

Generic Available No

Index Terms Enoxaparin Sodium

Pharmacologic Category Low Molecular Weight Heparin

Use

DVT treatment (acute): Inpatient treatment (patients with and without pulmonary embolism) and outpatient treatment (patients without pulmonary embolism)

DVT prophylaxis: Following hip or knee replacement surgery, abdominal surgery, or in medical patients with severely-restricted mobility during acute illness in patients at risk of thromboembolic complications

Note: High-risk patients include those with one or more of the following risk factors: >40 years of age, obesity, general anesthesia lasting >30 minutes, malignancy, history of deep vein thrombosis or pulmonary embolism

Unstable angina and non-Q-wave myocardial infarction (to prevent ischemic complications)

Unlabeled/Investigational Use Prophylaxis and treatment of thromboembolism in children

Local Anesthetic/Vasoconstrictor Precautions No information available to require special precautions

Effects on Dental Treatment Key adverse event(s) related to dental treatment: As with all anticoagulants, bleeding is the major adverse effect of enoxaparin. Hemorrhage may occur at virtually any site; risk is dependent on multiple variables. At the recommended doses, single injections of enoxaparin do not significantly influence platelet aggregation or affect global clotting time (ie, PT or aPTT)

Common Adverse Effects As with all anticoagulants, bleeding is the major adverse effect of enoxaparin. Hemorrhage may occur at virtually any site. Risk is dependent on multiple variables. At the recommended doses, single injections of enoxaparin do not significantly influence platelet aggregation or affect global clotting time (ie, PT or aPTT).

1% to 10%:
> Central nervous system: Fever (5% to 8%), confusion, pain
> Dermatologic: Erythema, bruising
> Gastrointestinal: Nausea (3%), diarrhea
> Hematologic: Hemorrhage (5% to 13%), thrombocytopenia (2%), hypochromic anemia (2%)
> Hepatic: ALT/AST increased
> Local: Injection site hematoma (9%), local reactions (irritation, pain, ecchymosis, erythema)

Thrombocytopenia with thrombosis: Cases of heparin-induced thrombocytopenia (some complicated by organ infarction, limb ischemia, or death) have been reported.

Mechanism of Action Standard heparin consists of components with molecular weights ranging from 4000-30,000 daltons with a mean of 16,000 daltons. Heparin acts as an anticoagulant by enhancing the inhibition rate of clotting proteases by antithrombin III impairing normal hemostasis and inhibition of factor Xa. Low molecular weight heparins have a small effect on the activated partial thromboplastin time and strongly inhibit factor Xa. Enoxaparin is derived from porcine heparin that undergoes benzylation followed by alkaline depolymerization. The average molecular weight of enoxaparin is 4500 daltons which is distributed as ($\leq$20%) 2000 daltons ($\geq$68%) 2000-8000 daltons, and ($\leq$15%) >8000 daltons. Enoxaparin has a higher ratio of antifactor Xa to antifactor IIa activity than unfractionated heparin.

Drug Interactions

Increased Effect/Toxicity: Risk of bleeding with enoxaparin may be increased with thrombolytic agents, oral anticoagulants (warfarin), drugs which affect platelet function (eg, aspirin, NSAIDs, dipyridamole, ticlopidine, clopidogrel, and IIb/IIIa antagonists). Although the risk of bleeding may be increased during concurrent therapy with warfarin, enoxaparin is commonly continued during the initiation of warfarin therapy to assure anticoagulation and to protect against possible transient hypercoagulability. Some cephalosporins and penicillins may block platelet aggregation, theoretically increasing the risk of bleeding.

Pharmacodynamics/Kinetics

Onset of action: Peak effect: SubQ: Antifactor Xa and antithrombin (antifactor IIa): 3-5 hours

Duration: 40 mg dose: Antifactor Xa activity: ~12 hours

Metabolism: Hepatic, to lower molecular weight fragments (little activity)

Protein binding: Does not bind to heparin binding proteins

Half-life elimination, plasma: 2-4 times longer than standard heparin, independent of dose; based on anti-Xa activity: 4.5-7 hours

Excretion: Urine (40% of dose; 10% as active fragments)

Pregnancy Risk Factor B

Enoxaparin Sodium *see* Enoxaparin *on page 568*

Enpresse™ *see* Ethinyl Estradiol and Levonorgestrel *on page 633*

Entacapone (en TA ka pone)

U.S. Brand Names Comtan®
Canadian Brand Names Comtan®
Mexican Brand Names Comtan
Generic Available No
Pharmacologic Category Anti-Parkinson's Agent, COMT Inhibitor
Use Adjunct to levodopa/carbidopa therapy in patients with idiopathic Parkinson's disease who experience "wearing-off" symptoms at the end of a dosing interval

Local Anesthetic/Vasoconstrictor Precautions No information available to require special precautions
(Continued)

Entacapone *(Continued)*

Effects on Dental Treatment Key adverse event(s) related to dental treatment: Orthostatic hypotension and abnormal taste. Dopaminergic therapy in Parkinson's disease (ie, treatment with levodopa) is associated with orthostatic hypotension. Entacapone enhances levodopa bioavailability and may increase the occurrence of hypotension/syncope in the dental patient. The patient should be carefully assisted from the chair and observed for signs of orthostatic hypotension.

Common Adverse Effects
>10%:
Gastrointestinal: Nausea (14%)
Neuromuscular & skeletal: Dyskinesia (25%), placebo (15%)
1% to 10%:
Cardiovascular: Orthostatic hypotension (4%), syncope (1%)
Central nervous system: Dizziness (8%), fatigue (6%), hallucinations (4%), anxiety (2%), somnolence (2%), agitation (1%)
Dermatologic: Purpura (2%)
Gastrointestinal: Diarrhea (10%), abdominal pain (8%), constipation (6%), vomiting (4%), dry mouth (3%), dyspepsia (2%), flatulence (2%), gastritis (1%), taste perversion (1%)
Genitourinary: Brown-orange urine discoloration (10%)
Neuromuscular & skeletal: Hyperkinesia (10%), hypokinesia (9%), back pain (4%), weakness (2%)
Respiratory: Dyspnea (3%)
Miscellaneous: Diaphoresis increased (2%), bacterial infection (1%)

Mechanism of Action Entacapone is a reversible and selective inhibitor of catechol-O-methyltransferase (COMT). When entacapone is taken with levodopa, the pharmacokinetics are altered, resulting in more sustained levodopa serum levels compared to levodopa taken alone. The resulting levels of levodopa provide for increased concentrations available for absorption across the blood-brain barrier, thereby providing for increased CNS levels of dopamine, the active metabolite of levodopa.

Drug Interactions
Cytochrome P450 Effect: Inhibits CYP1A2 (weak), 2A6 (weak), 2C9 (weak), 2C19 (weak), 2D6 (weak), 2E1 (weak), 3A4 (weak)
Increased Effect/Toxicity: Entacapone may decrease the metabolism and increase the side effects of COMT substrates (eg, apomorphine, bitolterol, dobutamine, dopamine, epinephrine, norepinephrine, isoproterenol, isoetharine, and methyldopa). Effects on mental status may be additive with other CNS depressants; includes barbiturates, benzodiazepines, TCAs, antipsychotics, ethanol, opioid analgesics, and other sedative-hypnotics. Concurrent use of nonselective MAO inhibitors with entacapone may increase the risk of cardiovascular side effects; selective MAO inhibitors (eg, selegiline) appear to pose limited risk.

Pharmacodynamics/Kinetics
Onset of action: Rapid
Peak effect: 1 hour
Absorption: Rapid
Distribution: I.V.: V_{dss}: 20 L
Protein binding: 98%, primarily to albumin
Metabolism: Isomerization to the *cis*-isomer, followed by direct glucuronidation of the parent and *cis*-isomer
Bioavailability: 35%
Half-life elimination: B phase: 0.4-0.7 hours; Y phase: 2.4 hours
Time to peak, serum: 1 hour
Excretion: Feces (90%); urine (10%)

Pregnancy Risk Factor C

Entacapone, Carbidopa, and Levodopa *see* Levodopa, Carbidopa, and Entacapone *on page 965*

Entecavir *(en TE ka veer)*

U.S. Brand Names Baraclude™
Canadian Brand Names Baraclude™
Generic Available No
Pharmacologic Category Antiretroviral Agent, Reverse Transcriptase Inhibitor (Nucleoside)
Use Treatment of chronic hepatitis B infection in adults with evidence of active viral replication and either evidence of persistent transaminase elevations or histologically-active disease

Local Anesthetic/Vasoconstrictor Precautions No information available to require special precautions

Effects on Dental Treatment No significant effects or complications reported

Common Adverse Effects

>10%: Hepatic: ALT increased (>5 x ULN: 11% to 12%; >10 x ULN and >2 x baseline [post-treatment flare in lamivudine refractory]: 12%)

1% to 10%:

Central nervous system: Headache (2% to 4%), fatigue (1% to 3%)

Endocrine & metabolic: Hyperglycemia (2% to 3%)

Gastrointestinal: Lipase increased (7% to 8%), amylase increased (2% to 3%), diarrhea (≤1%), dyspepsia (≤1%)

Hepatic: AST increased (>5 x ULN: 5%), bilirubin increased (2% to 3%), ALT increased (>10 x ULN and >2 x baseline, including post-treatment flare in nucleoside naive: 2%)

Renal: Hematuria (9%), glycosuria (4%), creatinine increased (1% to 2%)

Mechanism of Action Entecavir is intracellularly phosphorylated to guanosine triphosphate which competes with natural substrates to effectively inhibit hepatitis B viral polymerase; enzyme inhibition blocks reverse transcriptase activity thereby reducing viral DNA synthesis.

Drug Interactions

Increased Effect/Toxicity:

Concomitant use of ribavirin with or without interferon alfa and nucleoside analogues may increase the risk of developing hepatic decompensation or other signs of mitochondrial toxicity, including pancreatitis or lactic acidosis. Ganciclovir/valganciclovir may increase the adverse effects/toxicity (eg, hematologic) of nucleoside reverse transcriptase inhibitors.

Pharmacodynamics/Kinetics

Distribution: Extensive (V_d in excess of body water)

Protein binding: 13%

Metabolism: Minor hepatic glucuronide/sulfate conjugation

Half-life elimination: Terminal: 5-6 days; accumulation: 24 hours

Time to peak, plasma: 0.5-1.5 hours

Excretion: Urine (60% to 70% as unchanged drug)

Pregnancy Risk Factor C

Ephedrine (e FED rin)

U.S. Brand Names Pretz-D® [OTC]

Generic Available Yes

Index Terms Ephedrine Sulfate

Pharmacologic Category Alpha/Beta Agonist

Use Treatment of bronchial asthma, nasal congestion, acute bronchospasm, idiopathic orthostatic hypotension, hypotension induced by spinal anesthesia

Local Anesthetic/Vasoconstrictor Precautions Use vasoconstrictor with caution since ephedrine may enhance cardiostimulation and vasopressor effects of sympathomimetics such as epinephrine

Effects on Dental Treatment Key adverse event(s) related to dental treatment: Xerostomia (normal salivary flow resumes upon discontinuation)

Common Adverse Effects Frequency not defined.

Cardiovascular: Arrhythmias, chest pain, elevation or depression of blood pressure, hypertension, palpitation, tachycardia, unusual pallor

Central nervous system: Agitation, anxiety, apprehension, CNS stimulating effects, dizziness, excitation, fear, headache hyperactivity, insomnia, irritability, nervousness, restlessness, tension

Gastrointestinal: Anorexia, GI upset, nausea, vomiting, xerostomia

Genitourinary: Painful urination

(Continued)

Ephedrine *(Continued)*

Neuromuscular & skeletal: Trembling, tremor (more common in the elderly), weakness

Respiratory: Dyspnea

Miscellaneous: Diaphoresis increased

Mechanism of Action Releases tissue stores of epinephrine and thereby produces an alpha- and beta-adrenergic stimulation; longer-acting and less potent than epinephrine

Drug Interactions

Increased Effect/Toxicity: Increased (toxic) cardiac stimulation with other sympathomimetic agents, theophylline, cardiac glycosides, or general anesthetics. Increased blood pressure with atropine or MAO inhibitors.

Decreased Effect: Alpha- and beta-adrenergic blocking agents decrease ephedrine vasopressor effects.

Pharmacodynamics/Kinetics

Onset of action: Oral: Bronchodilation: 0.25-1 hour

Duration: Oral: 3-6 hours

Distribution: Crosses placenta; enters breast milk

Metabolism: Minimally hepatic

Half-life elimination: 2.5-3.6 hours

Excretion: Urine (60% to 77% as unchanged drug) within 24 hours

Pregnancy Risk Factor C

Ephedrine, Chlorpheniramine, Phenylephrine, and Carbetapentane *see* Chlorpheniramine, Ephedrine, Phenylephrine, and Carbetapentane *on page 341*

Ephedrine Sulfate *see* Ephedrine *on page 571*

Epidermal Thymocyte Activating Factor *see* Aldesleukin *on page 62*

Epifoam® *see* Pramoxine and Hydrocortisone *on page 1335*

Epinastine *(ep i NAS teen)*

U.S. Brand Names Elestat™

Generic Available No

Index Terms Epinastine Hydrochloride

Pharmacologic Category Antihistamine, H₁ Blocker, Ophthalmic

Use Treatment of allergic conjunctivitis

Local Anesthetic/Vasoconstrictor Precautions No information available to require special precautions

Effects on Dental Treatment No significant effects or complications reported

Mechanism of Action Selective H₁-receptor antagonist; inhibits release of histamine from the mast cell

Pregnancy Risk Factor C

Epinastine Hydrochloride *see* Epinastine *on page 572*

Epinephrine *(ep i NEF rin)*

Related Information

Respiratory Diseases *on page 1747*

U.S. Brand Names Adrenalin®; EpiPen®; EpiPen® Jr; Primatene® Mist [OTC]; Raphon [OTC]; S2® [OTC]; Twinject™

Canadian Brand Names Adrenalin®; EpiPen®; EpiPen® Jr; Twinject™

Generic Available Yes: Solution for injection

Index Terms Adrenaline; Epinephrine Bitartrate; Epinephrine Hydrochloride; Racepinephrine

Pharmacologic Category Alpha/Beta Agonist; Antidote

Dental Use Emergency drug for treatment of anaphylactic reactions; used as vasoconstrictor to prolong local anesthesia

Use Treatment of bronchospasms, bronchial asthma, nasal congestion, viral croup, anaphylactic reactions, cardiac arrest; added to local anesthetics to decrease systemic absorption of local anesthetics and increase duration of action; decrease superficial hemorrhage

Unlabeled/Investigational Use ACLS guidelines: Ventricular fibrillation (VF) or pulseless ventricular tachycardia (VT) unresponsive to initial defibrillatory shocks; pulseless electrical activity, asystole, hypotension unresponsive to volume resuscitation; symptomatic bradycardia or hypotension unresponsive to atropine or pacing; inotropic support

Local Anesthetic/Vasoconstrictor Precautions No information available to require special precautions

Effects on Dental Treatment Key adverse event(s) related to dental treatment: Xerostomia (normal salivary flow resumes upon discontinuation) and dry throat.

Significant Adverse Effects Frequency not defined.

Cardiovascular: Angina, cardiac arrhythmia, chest pain, flushing, hypertension, increased myocardial oxygen consumption, pallor, palpitation, sudden death, tachycardia (parenteral), vasoconstriction, ventricular ectopy

Central nervous system: Anxiety, dizziness, headache, insomnia, lightheadedness, nervousness, restlessness

Gastrointestinal: Dry throat, nausea, vomiting, xerostomia

Genitourinary: Acute urinary retention in patients with bladder outflow obstruction

Neuromuscular & skeletal: Trembling, weakness

Ocular: Allergic lid reaction, burning, eye pain, ocular irritation, precipitation of or exacerbation of narrow-angle glaucoma, transient stinging

Renal: Decreased renal and splanchnic blood flow

Respiratory: Dyspnea, wheezing

Miscellaneous: Diaphoresis increased

Dental Usual Dosing Hypersensitivity reaction:

Infants and Children:

SubQ, I.V.: 0.01 mg/kg every 20 minutes; larger doses or continuous infusion may be needed for some anaphylactic reactions

SubQ, I.M.:

15-30 kg: Twinject™: 0.15 mg (for self-administration following severe allergic reactions to insect stings, food, etc)

>30 kg: Refer to adult dosing

I.M.:

<30 kg: Epipen® Jr: 0.15 mg (for self-administration following severe allergic reactions to insect stings, food, etc)

>30 kg: Refer to adult dosing

Adults:

I.M., SubQ: 0.3-0.5 mg (1:1000) every 15-20 minutes if condition requires (I.M route is preferred)

>30 kg: Twinject™: 0.3 mg (for self-administration following severe allergic reactions to insect stings, food, etc)

I.M.: >30 kg: Epipen®: 0.3 mg (for self-administration following severe allergic reactions to insect stings, food, etc)

I.V.: 0.1 mg (1:10,000) over 5 minutes. May infuse at 1-4 mcg/minute to prevent the need to repeat injections frequently.

Dosage

Neonates: Cardiac arrest: I.V.: 0.01-0.03 mg/kg (0.1-0.3 mL/kg of **1:10,000** solution) every 3-5 minutes as needed. Although I.V. route is preferred, may consider administration of doses up to 0.1 mg/kg through the endotracheal tube until I.V. access established; dilute intratracheal doses to 1-2 mL with normal saline.

Infants and Children:

Asystole/pulseless arrest, bradycardia, VT/VF (after failed defibrillations):

I.V., I.O.: 0.01 mg/kg (0.1 mL/kg of **1:10,000** solution) every 3-5 minutes as needed (maximum: 1 mg)

Intratracheal: 0.1 mg/kg (0.1 mL/kg of **1:1000** solution) every 3-5 minutes (maximum: 10 mg)

Continuous I.V. infusion: 0.1-1 mcg/kg/minute; doses <0.3 mcg/kg/minute generally produce β-adrenergic effects and higher doses generally produce α-adrenergic vasoconstriction; titrate dosage to desired effect

Bronchodilator: SubQ: 0.01 mg/kg (0.01 mL/kg of **1:1000**) (single doses not to exceed 0.5 mg) every 20 minutes for 3 doses

Nebulization: 1-3 inhalations up to every 3 hours using solution prepared with 10 drops of 1:100

Children <4 years: S2® (racepinephrine, OTC labeling): Croup: 0.05 mL/kg (max 0.5 mL/dose); dilute in NS 3 mL. Administer over ~15 minutes; do not administer more frequently than every 2 hours.

Inhalation: Children ≥4 years: Primatene® Mist: Refer to adult dosing.

Decongestant: Children ≥6 years: Refer to adult dosing

Hypersensitivity reaction:

SubQ, I.V.: 0.01 mg/kg every 20 minutes; larger doses or continuous infusion may be needed for some anaphylactic reactions

Self-administration following severe allergic reactions (eg, insect stings, food): **Note:** World Health Organization (WHO) and Anaphylaxis Canada recommend the availability of 1 dose for every 10-20 minutes of travel time to a medical emergency facility:

Twinject™: SubQ, I.M.:

Children 15-30 kg: 0.15 mg

Children >30 kg: 0.3 mg

(Continued)

Epinephrine *(Continued)*

Epipen® Jr: I.M.: Children <30 kg: 0.15 mg
Epipen®: I.M.: Children ≥30 kg: 0.3 mg

Adults:

Asystole/pulseless arrest, bradycardia, VT/VF:

I.V., I.O.: 1 mg every 3-5 minutes; if this approach fails, higher doses of epinephrine (up to 0.2 mg/kg) may be indicated for treatment of specific problems (eg, beta-blocker or calcium channel blocker overdose)

Intratracheal: Administer 2-2.5 mg for VF or pulseless VT if I.V./I.O. access is delayed or cannot be established; dilute in 5-10 mL NS or distilled water. **Note:** Absorption is greater with distilled water, but causes more adverse effects on PaO_2.

Bradycardia (symptomatic) or hypotension (not responsive to atropine or pacing): I.V. infusion: 2-10 mcg/minute; titrate to desired effect

Bronchodilator:

SubQ: 0.3-0.5 mg **(1:1000)** every 20 minutes for 3 doses

Nebulization: 1-3 inhalations up to every 3 hours using solution prepared with 10 drops of the **1:100** product

S2® (racepinephrine, OTC labeling): 0.5 mL (~10 drops). Dose may be repeated not more frequently than very 3-4 hours if needed. Solution should be diluted if using jet nebulizer.

Inhalation: Primatene® Mist (OTC labeling): One inhalation, wait at least 1 minute; if relieved, may use once more. Do not use again for at least 3 hours.

Decongestant: Intranasal: Apply 1:1000 locally as drops or spray or with sterile swab

Hypersensitivity reaction:

SubQ, I.M.: 0.3-0.5 mg (1:1000) every 15-20 minutes if condition requires (I.M route is preferred)

I.V.: 0.1 mg (1:10,000) over 5 minutes. May infuse at 1-4 mcg/minute to prevent the need to repeat injections frequently.

Self-administration following severe allergic reactions (eg, insect stings, food): **Note:** The World Health Organization (WHO) and Anaphylaxis Canada recommend the availability of one dose for every 10 to 20 minutes of travel time to a medical emergency facility. More than 2 doses should only be administered under direct medical supervision.

Twinject™: SubQ, I.M.: 0.3 mg

Epipen®: I.M.: 0.3 mg

Mechanism of Action Stimulates alpha-, $beta_1$-, and $beta_2$-adrenergic receptors resulting in relaxation of smooth muscle of the bronchial tree, cardiac stimulation, and dilation of skeletal muscle vasculature; small doses can cause vasodilation via $beta_2$-vascular receptors; large doses may produce constriction of skeletal and vascular smooth muscle

Contraindications Hypersensitivity to epinephrine or any component of the formulation; cardiac arrhythmias; angle-closure glaucoma

Warnings/Precautions Use with caution in elderly patients, patients with diabetes mellitus, cardiovascular diseases (angina, tachycardia, prostatic hyperplasia, history of seizures, renal dysfunction, myocardial infarction), thyroid disease, cerebrovascular disease, Parkinson's or taking MAO inhibitors. Some products contain sulfites as preservatives. Rapid I.V. infusion may cause death from cerebrovascular hemorrhage or cardiac arrhythmias. Oral inhalation of epinephrine is **not** the preferred route of administration. Avoid topical application where reduced perfusion could lead to ischemic tissue damage (eg, penis, ears, digits).

Drug Interactions Increased toxicity: Increased cardiac irritability if administered concurrently with halogenated inhalational anesthetics, beta-blocking agents, alpha-blocking agents

Ethanol/Nutrition/Herb Interactions Herb/Nutraceutical: Avoid ephedra, yohimbe (may cause CNS stimulation).

Pharmacodynamics/Kinetics

Onset of action: Bronchodilation: SubQ: ~5-10 minutes; Inhalation: ~1 minute

Distribution: Crosses placenta

Metabolism: Taken up into the adrenergic neuron and metabolized by monoamine oxidase and catechol-o-methyltransferase; circulating drug hepatically metabolized

Excretion: Urine (as inactive metabolites, metanephrine, and sulfate and hydroxy derivatives of mandelic acid, small amounts as unchanged drug)

Pregnancy Risk Factor C

Lactation Excretion in breast milk unknown

Dosage Forms Excipient information presented when available (limited, particularly for generics); consult specific product labeling.

Aerosol for oral inhalation:
  Primatene® Mist: 0.22 mg/inhalation (15 mL, 22.5 mL) [contains CFCs]
Injection, solution [prefilled auto injector]:
  EpiPen®: 0.3 mg/0.3 mL [1:1000] (2 mL) [contains sodium metabisulfite; available as single unit or in double-unit pack with training unit]
  EpiPen® Jr: 0.15 mg/0.3 mL [1:2000] (2 mL) [contains sodium metabisulfite; available as single unit or in double-unit pack with training unit]
  Twinject™: 0.15 mg/0.15 mL [1:1000] (1.1 mL) [contains sodium bisulfite; two 0.15 mg doses per injector]; 0.3 mg/0.3 mL [1:1000] (1.1 mL) [contains sodium bisulfite; two 0.3 mg doses per injector]
Injection, solution, as hydrochloride: 0.1 mg/mL [1:10,000] (10 mL); 1 mg/mL [1:1000] (1 mL) [products may contain sodium metabisulfite]
  Adrenalin®: 1 mg/mL [1:1000] (1 mL, 30 mL) [contains sodium bisulfite]
Solution for oral inhalation, as hydrochloride:
  Adrenalin®: 1% [10 mg/mL, 1:100] (7.5 mL) [contains sodium bisulfite]
Solution for oral inhalation [racepinephrine]:
  S2®: 2.25% (0.5 mL, 15 mL) [as d-epinephrine 1.125% and l-epinephrine 1.125%; contains metabisulfites]
Solution, topical [racepinephrine]:
  Raphon: 2.25% (15 mL) [as d-epinephrine 1.125% and l-epinephrine 1.125%; contains metabisulfites]

Selected Readings

"2005 American Heart Association Guidelines for Cardiopulmonary Resuscitation and Emergency Cardiovascular Care," *Circulation*, 2005, 112(24 Suppl): 1-211.

Cydulka R, Davison R, Grammer L, et al, "The Use of Epinephrine in the Treatment of Older Adult Asthmatics," *Ann Emerg Med*, 1988, 17(4):322-6.

Davis C and Wax P, "Subcutaneous Epinephrine O.D. in a Child Resulting in Dysrhythmias and Myocardial Ischemia," *Vet Hum Toxicol*, 1994, 36:367.

Illi A, Sundberg S, Ojala-Karlsson P, et al, "The Effect of Entacapone on the Disposition and Hemodynamic Effects of Intravenous Isoproterenol and Epinephrine," *Clin Pharmacol Ther*, 1995, 58(2):221-7.

Klein JS, Rich MR, and Yunginger JW, "Myocardial Ischemia Without Coronary Artery Disease After Epinephrine Overdose for Insect Sting Reaction," *J Allergy Clin Immunol*, 1995, 95(2):371.

Kuracheck SC and Rockoff MA, "Inadvertent Intravenous Administration of Racemic Epinephrine," *JAMA*, 1984, 253(10):1441-2.

Murphy FT, Manown TJ, Knutson SW, et al, "Epinephrine-Induced Lactic Acidosis in the Setting of Status Asthmaticus," *South Med J*, 1995, 88(5):577-9.

National Asthma Education and Prevention Program, "Expert Panel Report 2: Guidelines for the Diagnosis and Management of Asthma," Bethesda, MD, National Institutes of Health, 1997. NIH publication 97-4051.

Nicholson KE and Rogers JE, "Cocaine and Adrenaline Paste: A Fatal Combination?" *BMJ*, 1995, 311(6999):250-1.

Riou B, Barriot P, Rimailho A, et al, "Treatment of Severe Chloroquine Poisoning," *N Engl J Med*, 1988, 318(1):1-6.

Scalzo A, Keith G, and Thompson M, "Fatal Outcome After Massive Epinephrine Overdose by Intravenous Injection of an OTC Asthma Inhaler," *Clin Toxicol*, 1995, 33(5):501-2.

Stiell IG, Hebert PC, Wells GA, et al, "Vasopressin Versus Epinephrine for Inhospital Cardiac Arrest: A Randomised Controlled Trial," *Lancet*, 2001, 358(9276):105-9.

Waisman Y, Klein BL, Boenning DA, et al, "Prospective Randomized Double-Blind Study Comparing L-Epinephrine and Racemic Epinephrine Aerosols in the Treatment of Laryngotracheitis (Croup)," *Pediatrics*, 1992, 89(2):302-6.

Wenzel V, Krismer AC, Arntz HR, et al, "A Comparison of Vasopressin and Epinephrine for Out-of-Hospital Cardiopulmonary Resuscitation. European Resuscitation Council Vasopressor during Cardiopulmonary Resuscitation Study Group," *N Engl J Med*, 2004, 350(2):105-13.

Epinephrine and Articaine Hydrochloride *see* Articaine and Epinephrine *on page 143*

Epinephrine and Chlorpheniramine
(ep i NEF rin & klor fen IR a meen)

Related Information
Chlorpheniramine *on page 338*
Epinephrine *on page 572*

U.S. Brand Names Ana-Kit®

Generic Available No

Index Terms Insect Sting Kit

Pharmacologic Category Antidote

Use Anaphylaxis emergency treatment of insect bites or stings by the sensitive patient that may occur within minutes of insect sting or exposure to an allergic substance

Local Anesthetic/Vasoconstrictor Precautions No information available to require special precautions

Effects on Dental Treatment No significant effects or complications reported

Drug Interactions
Cytochrome P450 Effect: Chlorpheniramine: **Substrate** of CYP2D6 (minor), 3A4 (major); **Inhibits** CYP2D6 (weak)

Epinephrine and Lidocaine *see* Lidocaine and Epinephrine *on page 977*

Epinephrine and Prilocaine (Dental) *see* Prilocaine and Epinephrine *on page 1350*

Epinephrine Bitartrate *see* Epinephrine *on page 572*

Epinephrine Bitartrate and Bupivacaine Hydrochloride *see* Bupivacaine and Epinephrine *on page 237*

Epinephrine Hydrochloride *see* Epinephrine *on page 572*

Epinephrine (Racemic) (ep i NEF rin, ra SEE mik)

U.S. Brand Names AsthmaNefrin®; microNefrin®; S-2®

Generic Available Yes

Pharmacologic Category Alpha/Beta Agonist; Vasoconstrictor

Dental Use Emergency drug for treatment of bronchoconstriction

Use Emergency drug for treatment of bronchoconstriction

Local Anesthetic/Vasoconstrictor Precautions No information available to require special precautions

Effects on Dental Treatment No significant effects or complications reported

Significant Adverse Effects Refer to Epinephrine monograph.

Dental Usual Dosing Bronchoconstriction: Oral Inhalation: 1-3 inhalations (via nebulization); use minimum number of inhalations necessary to achieve response

Dosage Bronchoconstriction: Oral Inhalation: 1-3 inhalations (via nebulization); use minimum number of inhalations necessary to achieve response

Contraindications Hypersensitivity to epinephrine or any component of the formulation; cardiac arrhythmias; angle-closure glaucoma

Warnings/Precautions Use with caution in elderly patients, patients with diabetes mellitus, cardiovascular diseases (angina, tachycardia, myocardial infarction), thyroid disease, cerebrovascular disease, or Parkinson's.

Drug Interactions Refer to Epinephrine monograph.

Pharmacodynamics/Kinetics Onset of action: Bronchodilation: Inhalation: ~1 minute

Dosage Forms Excipient information presented when available (limited, particularly for generics); consult specific product labeling.

Solution for oral inhalation (AsthmaNefrin®, microNefrin®, S-2®): Racepinephrine 2.25% [epinephrine base 1.125%] (7.5 mL, 15 mL, 30 mL)

Epinephrine (Racemic) and Aluminum Potassium Sulfate

(ep i NEF rin, ra SEE mik a LOO mi num poe TASS ee um SUL fate)

Related Information

Epinephrine *on page 572*

U.S. Brand Names Van R Gingibraid®

Generic Available No

Index Terms Aluminum Potassium Sulfate and Epinephrine (Racemic) (Dental)

Pharmacologic Category Adrenergic Agonist Agent; Alpha/Beta Agonist; Astringent; Vasoconstrictor

Dental Use Gingival retraction

Local Anesthetic/Vasoconstrictor Precautions No information available to require special precautions

Effects on Dental Treatment Key adverse event(s) related to dental treatment: Tissue retraction around base of the tooth (therapeutic effect)..

Significant Adverse Effects No data reported.

Dental Usual Dosing Gingival retraction: Adults: Pass the impregnated yarn around the neck of the tooth and place into gingival sulcus; normal tissue moisture, water, or gingival retraction solutions activate impregnated yarn. Limit use to one quadrant of the mouth at a time; recommended use is for 3-8 minutes in the mouth.

Mechanism of Action Epinephrine stimulates alpha$_1$ adrenergic receptors to cause vasoconstriction in blood vessels in gingiva; aluminum potassium sulfate, precipitates tissue and blood proteins

Contraindications Hypersensitivity to epinephrine or any component of the formulation; cardiovascular disease, hyperthyroidism, or diabetes; do not apply to areas of heavy or deep bleeding or over exposed bone

Warnings/Precautions Caution should be exercised whenever using gingival retraction cords with epinephrine since it delivers vasoconstrictor doses of racemic epinephrine to patients; the general medical history should be thoroughly evaluated before using in any patient

Drug Interactions No data reported.

Pharmacodynamics/Kinetics No data reported.

Dosage Forms Excipient information presented when available (limited, particularly for generics); consult specific product labeling.

Yarn, saturated in solution of 8% racemic epinephrine and 7% aluminum potassium sulfate:

Type "0e": 0.20 ± 0.10 mg epinephrine/inch

Type "1e": 0.40 ± 0.20 mg epinephrine/inch

Type "2e": 0.60 ± 0.20 mg epinephrine/inch

EpiPen® *see* Epinephrine *on page 572*

EpiPen® Jr *see* Epinephrine *on page 572*

Epipodophyllotoxin *see* Etoposide *on page 660*

EpiQuin™ Micro *see* Hydroquinone *on page 841*

Epirubicin (ep i ROO bi sin)

U.S. Brand Names Ellence®

Canadian Brand Names Ellence®; Pharmorubicin®

Mexican Brand Names Binarin; Epilem; Farmorubicin; Farmorubicin RD

Generic Available Yes

Index Terms Epirubicin Hydrochloride; NSC-256942; Pidorubicin; Pidorubicin Hydrochloride

Pharmacologic Category Antineoplastic Agent, Anthracycline

Use Adjuvant therapy for primary breast cancer

Local Anesthetic/Vasoconstrictor Precautions No information available to require special precautions

Effects on Dental Treatment Key adverse event(s) related to dental treatment: Mucositis

Common Adverse Effects Percentages reported as part of combination chemotherapy regimens.

>10%:

Central nervous system: Lethargy (1% to 46%)

Dermatologic: Alopecia (69% to 96%)

Endocrine & metabolic: Amenorrhea (69% to 72%), hot flashes (5% to 39%)

Gastrointestinal: Nausea/vomiting (83% to 92%), mucositis (9% to 59%), diarrhea (7% to 25%)

Hematologic: Leukopenia (50% to 80%; grades 3/4: 2% to 59%), neutropenia (54% to 80%; grades 3/4: 11% to 67%; nadir: 10-14 days; recovery: 21 days), anemia (13% to 72%; grades 3/4: 6%), thrombocytopenia (5% to 49%; grades 3/4: 5%)

Local: Injection site reactions (3% to 20%)

Ocular: Conjunctivitis (1% to 15%)

Miscellaneous: Infection (15% to 21%)

1% to 10%:

Cardiovascular: CHF (0.4% to 1.5%), decreased LVEF (asymptomatic) (1% to 2%); recommended maximum cumulative dose: 900 mg/m^2

Central nervous system: Fever (1% to 5%)

Dermatologic: Rash (1% to 9%), skin changes (1% to 5%)

Gastrointestinal: Anorexia (2% to 3%)

Hematologic: Neutropenic fever (grades 3/4: 6%)

Mechanism of Action Epirubicin is an anthracycline antibiotic; known to inhibit DNA and RNA synthesis by steric obstruction after intercalating between DNA base pairs; active throughout entire cell cycle. Intercalation triggers DNA cleavage by topoisomerase II, resulting in cytocidal activity. Also inhibits DNA helicase, and generates cytotoxic free radicals.

Drug Interactions

Increased Effect/Toxicity: Cimetidine may increase the levels/effects of epirubicin. Bevacizumab and trastuzumab may enhance the cardiotoxic effects of epirubicin.

Pharmacodynamics/Kinetics

Distribution: V_{ss} 21-27 L/kg

Protein binding: 77% to albumin

Metabolism: Extensively via hepatic and extrahepatic (including RBCs) routes

Half-life elimination: Triphasic; Mean terminal: 33 hours

Excretion: Feces (34% to 35%); urine (20% to 27%)

Pregnancy Risk Factor D

Epirubicin Hydrochloride *see* Epirubicin *on page 577*

Epitol® *see* Carbamazepine *on page 272*

Epivir® *see* Lamivudine *on page 944*

Epivir-HBV® *see* Lamivudine *on page 944*

Eplerenone (e PLER en one)

U.S. Brand Names Inspra™
Mexican Brand Names Inspra IC
Generic Available No
Pharmacologic Category Diuretic, Potassium-Sparing; Selective Aldosterone Blocker
Use Treatment of hypertension (may be used alone or in combination with other antihypertensive agents); treatment of CHF following acute MI
Local Anesthetic/Vasoconstrictor Precautions No information available to require special precautions
Effects on Dental Treatment No significant effects or complications reported
Common Adverse Effects
>10%: Endocrine & metabolic: Hypertriglyceridemia (1% to 15%, dose related)
1% to 10%:
Central nervous system: Dizziness (3%), fatigue (2%)
Endocrine & metabolic: Breast pain (males <1% to 1%), serum creatinine increased (6% in CHF), gynecomastia (males <1% to 1%), hyponatremia (2%, dose related), hypercholesterolemia (<1% to 1%); hyperkalemia (mild-to-moderate hypertension <1%; left ventricular dysfunction ~6% had serum potassium ≥6 mEq/L)
Gastrointestinal: Diarrhea (2%), abdominal pain (1%)
Genitourinary: Abnormal vaginal bleeding (<1% to 2%)
Renal: Albuminuria (1%)
Respiratory: Cough (2%)
Miscellaneous: Flu-like syndrome (2%)
Mechanism of Action Aldosterone increases blood pressure primarily by inducing sodium reabsorption. Eplerenone reduces blood pressure by blocking aldosterone binding at mineralocorticoid receptors found in the kidney, heart, blood vessels and brain.
Drug Interactions
Cytochrome P450 Effect: Substrate of CYP3A4 (major)
Increased Effect/Toxicity: ACE inhibitors, angiotensin II receptor antagonists, NSAIDs, potassium supplements, and potassium-sparing diuretics increase the risk of hyperkalemia; concomitant use with potassium supplements and potassium-sparing diuretics is contraindicated; monitor potassium levels with ACE inhibitors and angiotensin II receptor antagonists. Potent CYP3A4 inhibitors (eg, itraconazole, ketoconazole) lead to fivefold increase in eplerenone; concurrent use is contraindicated. Less potent CYP3A4 inhibitors (eg, erythromycin, fluconazole, saquinavir, verapamil) lead to approximately twofold increase in eplerenone; starting dose should be decreased to 25 mg/day. Although interaction studies have not been conducted, monitoring of lithium levels is recommended.
Decreased Effect: NSAIDs may decrease the antihypertensive effects of eplerenone. CYP3A4 inducers may decrease the levels/effects of eplerenone; example inducers include aminoglutethimide, carbamazepine, nafcillin, nevirapine, phenobarbital, phenytoin, and rifamycins.
Pharmacodynamics/Kinetics
Distribution: V_d: 43-90 L
Protein binding: ~50%; primarily to alpha$_1$-acid glycoproteins
Metabolism: Primarily hepatic via CYP3A4; metabolites inactive
Half-life elimination: 4-6 hours
Time to peak, plasma: 1.5 hours; may take up to 4 weeks for full therapeutic effect
Excretion: Urine (67%; <5% as unchanged drug), feces (32%)
Pregnancy Risk Factor B

EPO see Epoetin Alfa on page 578

Epoetin Alfa (e POE e tin AL fa)

U.S. Brand Names Epogen®; Procrit®
Canadian Brand Names Eprex®
Mexican Brand Names Eprex
Generic Available No
Index Terms EPO; Erythropoiesis-Stimulating Agent (ESA); Erythropoietin; NSC-724223; rHuEPO-α
Pharmacologic Category Colony Stimulating Factor
Use Treatment of anemia related to HIV (zidovudine) therapy, chronic renal failure, antineoplastic therapy (for nonmyeloid malignancies); reduction of allogeneic blood transfusion for elective, noncardiac, nonvascular surgery

Unlabeled/Investigational Use Anemia associated with rheumatic disease; hypogenerative anemia of Rh hemolytic disease; sickle cell anemia; acute renal failure; Gaucher's disease; Castleman's disease; paroxysmal nocturnal hemoglobinuria; anemia of critical illness (limited documentation); anemia of prematurity

Local Anesthetic/Vasoconstrictor Precautions No information available to require special precautions

Effects on Dental Treatment No significant effects or complications reported

Common Adverse Effects
>10%:
  Cardiovascular: Hypertension (5% to 24%), thrombotic/vascular events (coronary artery bypass graft surgery: 23%), edema (6% to 17%), deep vein thrombosis (3% to 11%)
  Central nervous system: Fever (29% to 51%), dizziness (<7% to 21%), insomnia (13% to 21%), headache (10% to 19%)
  Dermatologic: Pruritus (14% to 22%), skin pain (4% to 18%), rash (≤16%)
  Gastrointestinal: Nausea (11% to 58%), constipation (42% to 53%), vomiting (8% to 29%), diarrhea (9% to 21%), dyspepsia (7% to 11%)
  Genitourinary: Urinary tract infection (3% to 12%)
  Local: Injection site reaction (<10% to 29%)
  Neuromuscular & skeletal: Arthralgia (11%), paresthesia (11%)
  Respiratory: Cough (18%), congestion (15%), dyspnea (13% to 14%), upper respiratory infection (11%)
1% to 10%:
  Central nervous system: Seizure (1% to 3%)
  Local: Clotted vascular access (7%)

Mechanism of Action Induces erythropoiesis by stimulating the division and differentiation of committed erythroid progenitor cells; induces the release of reticulocytes from the bone marrow into the bloodstream, where they mature to erythrocytes. There is a dose response relationship with this effect. This results in an increase in reticulocyte counts followed by a rise in hematocrit and hemoglobin levels.

Pharmacodynamics/Kinetics
Onset of action: Several days
Peak effect: 2-3 weeks
Distribution: V_d: 9 L; rapid in the plasma compartment; concentrated in liver, kidneys, and bone marrow
Metabolism: Some degradation does occur
Bioavailability: SubQ: ~21% to 31%; intraperitoneal epoetin: 3% (a few patients)
Half-life elimination: Cancer: SubQ: 16-67 hours; Chronic renal failure: 4-13 hours
Time to peak, serum: Chronic renal failure: 5-24 hours
Excretion: Feces (majority); urine (small amounts, 10% unchanged in normal volunteers)

Pregnancy Risk Factor C

Epogen® *see* Epoetin Alfa *on page 578*

Epoprostenol (e poe PROST en ole)

U.S. Brand Names Flolan®
Canadian Brand Names Flolan®
Generic Available No
Index Terms Epoprostenol Sodium; PGI_2; PGX; Prostacyclin
Pharmacologic Category Prostaglandin
Use Treatment of idiopathic pulmonary arterial hypertension [IPAH]; pulmonary hypertension associated with the scleroderma spectrum of disease [SSD] in NYHA Class III and Class IV patients who do not respond adequately to conventional therapy

Local Anesthetic/Vasoconstrictor Precautions No information available to require special precautions

Effects on Dental Treatment No significant effects or complications reported

Common Adverse Effects
Note: Adverse events reported during dose initiation and escalation include flushing (58%), headache (49%), nausea/vomiting (32%), hypotension (16%), anxiety/nervousness/agitation (11%), chest pain (11%); abdominal pain, back pain, bradycardia, diaphoresis, dizziness, dyspepsia, dyspnea, hypoesthesia/paresthesia, musculoskeletal pain, and tachycardia are also reported. The following adverse events have been reported during chronic administration for IPAH. Although some may be related to the underlying disease state, anxiety, diarrhea, flu-like syndrome, flushing, headache, jaw pain, nausea, nervousness, and vomiting are clearly contributed to epoprostenol.
(Continued)

Epoprostenol *(Continued)*

>10%:
    Cardiovascular: Chest pain (67%), palpitation (63%), flushing (42%), tachycardia (35%), arrhythmia (27%), hemorrhage (19%), bradycardia (15%)

    Central nervous system: Dizziness (83%), headache (83%), chills/fever/sepsis/flu-like syndrome (25%), anxiety/nervousness/tremor (21%)

    Gastrointestinal: Nausea/vomiting (67%), diarrhea (37%)

    Genitourinary: Weight loss (27%)

    Local: Injection site reactions: Infection (21%), pain (13%)

    Neuromuscular & skeletal: Weakness (87%), jaw pain (54%), myalgia (44%), musculoskeletal pain (35%; predominantly involving legs and feet), hypoesthesia/hyperparesthesia/paresthesia (12%)

    Respiratory: Dyspnea (90%)

1% to 10%:
    Cardiovascular: Supraventricular tachycardia (8%), cerebrovascular accident (4%)

    Central nervous system: Convulsion (4%)

    Dermatologic: Rash (10%; conventional therapy 13%), pruritus (4%)

    Endocrine & metabolic: Hypokalemia (6%)

    Gastrointestinal: Constipation (6%), weight gain (6%)

    Neuromuscular & skeletal: Arthralgia (6%)

    Ocular: Amblyopia (8%), vision abnormality (4%)

    Respiratory: Epistaxis (4%), pleural effusion (4%)

Restrictions Orders for epoprostenol are distributed by two sources in the United States. Information on orders or reimbursement assistance may be obtained from either Accredo Health, Inc (1-800-935-6526) or TheraCom, Inc (1-877-356-5264).

Mechanism of Action Epoprostenol is also known as prostacyclin and PGI_2. It is a strong vasodilator of all vascular beds. In addition, it is a potent endogenous inhibitor of platelet aggregation. The reduction in platelet aggregation results from epoprostenol's activation of intracellular adenylate cyclase and the resultant increase in cyclic adenosine monophosphate concentrations within the platelets. Additionally, it is capable of decreasing thrombogenesis and platelet clumping in the lungs by inhibiting platelet aggregation.

Drug Interactions
    Increased Effect/Toxicity: The hypotensive effects of epoprostenol may be exacerbated by other vasodilators, diuretics, or by using acetate in dialysis fluids. Patients treated with anticoagulants (heparins, warfarin, thrombin inhibitors) or antiplatelet agents (ticlopidine, clopidogrel, IIb/IIIa antagonists, aspirin) and epoprostenol should be monitored for increased bleeding risk.

Pharmacodynamics/Kinetics
    Metabolism: Rapidly hydrolyzed; subject to some enzymatic degradation; forms one active metabolite and 13 inactive metabolites

    Half-life elimination: 6 minutes

    Excretion: Urine (84%); feces (4%)

Pregnancy Risk Factor B

Epoprostenol Sodium *see* Epoprostenol *on page 579*

Eprosartan *(ep roe SAR tan)*

Related Information
    Cardiovascular Diseases *on page 1726*

U.S. Brand Names Teveten®

Canadian Brand Names Teveten®

Generic Available No

Pharmacologic Category Angiotensin II Receptor Blocker

Use Treatment of hypertension; may be used alone or in combination with other antihypertensives

Local Anesthetic/Vasoconstrictor Precautions No information available to require special precautions

Effects on Dental Treatment No significant effects or complications reported

Common Adverse Effects 1% to 10%:
    Central nervous system: Fatigue (2%), depression (1%)

    Endocrine & metabolic: Hypertriglyceridemia (1%)

    Gastrointestinal: Abdominal pain (2%)

    Genitourinary: Urinary tract infection (1%)

    Respiratory: Upper respiratory tract infection (8%), rhinitis (4%), pharyngitis (4%), cough (4%)

    Miscellaneous: Viral infection (2%), injury (2%)

Dosage Adults: Oral: Dosage must be individualized; can administer once or twice daily with total daily doses of 400-800 mg. Usual starting dose is 600 mg once daily as monotherapy in patients who are euvolemic. Limited clinical experience with doses >800 mg.

Dosage adjustment in renal impairment: No starting dosage adjustment is necessary; however, carefully monitor the patient

Dosage adjustment in hepatic impairment: No starting dosage adjustment is necessary; however, carefully monitor the patient

Elderly: No starting dosage adjustment is necessary; however, carefully monitor the patient

Mechanism of Action Angiotensin II is formed from angiotensin I in a reaction catalyzed by angiotensin-converting enzyme (ACE, kininase II). Angiotensin II is the principal pressor agent of the renin-angiotensin system, with effects that include vasoconstriction, stimulation of synthesis and release of aldosterone, cardiac stimulation, and renal reabsorption of sodium. Eprosartan blocks the vasoconstrictor and aldosterone-secreting effects of angiotensin II by selectively blocking the binding of angiotensin II to the AT1 receptor in many tissues, such as vascular smooth muscle and the adrenal gland. Its action is therefore independent of the pathways for angiotensin II synthesis. Blockade of the renin-angiotensin system with ACE inhibitors, which inhibit the biosynthesis of angiotensin II from angiotensin I, is widely used in the treatment of hypertension. ACE inhibitors also inhibit the degradation of bradykinin, a reaction also catalyzed by ACE. Because eprosartan does not inhibit ACE (kininase II), it does not affect the response to bradykinin. Whether this difference has clinical relevance is not yet known. Eprosartan does not bind to or block other hormone receptors or ion channels known to be important in cardiovascular regulation.

Contraindications Hypersensitivity to eprosartan or any component of the formulation; sensitivity to other A-II receptor antagonists; bilateral renal artery stenosis; pregnancy

Warnings/Precautions [U.S. Boxed Warning]: Based on human data, drugs that act on the angiotensin system can cause injury and death to the developing fetus when used in the second and third trimesters. Angiotensin receptor blockers should be discontinued as soon as possible once pregnancy is detected. May cause hyperkalemia; avoid potassium supplementation unless specifically required by healthcare provider. Avoid use or use a smaller dose in patients who are volume depleted; correct depletion first. May be associated with deterioration of renal function and/or increases in serum creatinine, particularly in patients dependent on renin-angiotensin-aldosterone system. Use with caution in unilateral renal artery stenosis and pre-existing renal insufficiency; significant aortic/mitral stenosis. Safety and efficacy not established in pediatric patients.

Drug Interactions

Cytochrome P450 Effect: Inhibits CYP2C9 (weak)

Increased Effect/Toxicity: Eprosartan may increase risk of lithium toxicity. May increase risk of hyperkalemia with potassium-sparing diuretics (eg, amiloride, potassium, spironolactone, triamterene), potassium supplements, or high doses of trimethoprim.

Ethanol/Nutrition/Herb Interactions Herb/Nutraceutical: Avoid dong quai if using for hypertension (has estrogenic activity). Avoid ephedra, yohimbe, ginseng (may worsen hypertension). Avoid garlic (may have increased antihypertensive effect).

Pharmacodynamics/Kinetics

Protein binding: 98%

Metabolism: Minimally hepatic

Bioavailability: 300 mg dose: 13%

Half-life elimination: Terminal: 5-9 hours

Time to peak, serum: Fasting: 1-2 hours

Excretion: Feces (90%); urine (7%, mostly as unchanged drug)

Clearance: 7.9 L/hour

Pregnancy Risk Factor C (1st trimester); D (2nd and 3rd trimesters)

Dosage Forms

Tablet:

Teveten®: 400 mg, 600 mg

Eprosartan and Hydrochlorothiazide
(ep roe SAR tan & hye droe klor oh THYE a zide)

Related Information

Eprosartan *on page 580*
Hydrochlorothiazide *on page 819*

U.S. Brand Names Teveten® HCT

Canadian Brand Names Teveten® HCT; Teveten® Plus

Generic Available No

(Continued)

Eprosartan and Hydrochlorothiazide *(Continued)*

Index Terms Eprosartan Mesylate and Hydrochlorothiazide; Hydrochlorothiazide and Eprosartan

Pharmacologic Category Angiotensin II Receptor Blocker Combination; Antihypertensive Agent, Combination; Diuretic, Thiazide

Use Treatment of hypertension (not indicated for initial treatment)

Local Anesthetic/Vasoconstrictor Precautions No information available to require special precautions

Effects on Dental Treatment No significant effects or complications reported

Common Adverse Effects Percentages reported with combination product; other reactions have been reported (see individual agents for additional information).

1% to 10%:
Central nervous system: Dizziness (4%), headache (3%), fatigue (2%)
Hematologic: Neutrophil count decreased (1%)
Neuromuscular & skeletal: Back pain (3%)
Renal: BUN increased (1%)

Mechanism of Action Hydrochlorothiazide inhibits sodium reabsorption in the distal tubules causing increased excretion of sodium and water as well as potassium and hydrogen ions. **Eprosartan** blocks the vasoconstrictor and aldosterone-secreting effects of angiotensin II by selectively blocking the binding of angiotensin II to the AT1 receptor in many tissues, such as vascular smooth muscle and the adrenal gland.

Drug Interactions
Increased Effect/Toxicity: See individual agents.
Decreased Effect: See individual agents.
Pharmacodynamics/Kinetics See individual agents.
Pregnancy Risk Factor C/D (2nd and 3rd trimesters)

Eptifibatide *(ep TIF i ba tide)*

Related Information
Cardiovascular Diseases *on page 1726*
U.S. Brand Names Integrilin®
Canadian Brand Names Integrilin®
Generic Available No
Index Terms Intrifiban
Pharmacologic Category Antiplatelet Agent, Glycoprotein IIb/IIIa Inhibitor

Use Treatment of patients with acute coronary syndrome (unstable angina/non-Q wave myocardial infarction [UA/NQMI]), including patients who are to be managed medically and those undergoing percutaneous coronary intervention (PCI including angioplasty, intracoronary stenting)

Local Anesthetic/Vasoconstrictor Precautions No information available to require special precautions

Effects on Dental Treatment Key adverse event(s) related to dental treatment: Bleeding; patients weighing <70 kg may have an increased risk of major bleeding.

Common Adverse Effects Bleeding is the major drug-related adverse effect. Access site is often primary source of bleeding complications. Incidence of bleeding is also related to heparin intensity. Patients weighing <70 kg may have an increased risk of major bleeding.

>10%: Hematologic: Bleeding (major: 1% to 11%; minor: 3% to 14%; transfusion required: 2% to 13%)
1% to 10%:
Cardiovascular: Hypotension (up to 7%)
Hematologic: Thrombocytopenia (1% to 3%)
Local: Injection site reaction

Mechanism of Action Eptifibatide is a cyclic heptapeptide which blocks the platelet glycoprotein IIb/IIIa receptor, the binding site for fibrinogen, von Willebrand factor, and other ligands. Inhibition of binding at this final common receptor reversibly blocks platelet aggregation and prevents thrombosis.

Drug Interactions

Increased Effect/Toxicity: Eptifibatide effect may be increased by other drugs which affect hemostasis include thrombolytics, oral anticoagulants, NSAIDs, dipyridamole, heparin, low molecular weight heparins, ticlopidine, and clopidogrel. Avoid concomitant use of other IIb/IIIa inhibitors. Cephalosporins which contain the MTT side chain may theoretically increase the risk of hemorrhage. Use with aspirin and heparin may increase bleeding over aspirin and heparin alone. However, aspirin and heparin were used concurrently in the majority of patients in the major clinical studies of eptifibatide. Antiplatelet agents (eg, eptifibatide) may enhance the adverse/toxic effect of drotrecogin alfa; bleeding may occur.

Pharmacodynamics/Kinetics

Onset of action: Within 1 hour

Duration: Platelet function restored ~4 hours following discontinuation

Protein binding: ~25%

Half-life elimination: 2.5 hours

Excretion: Primarily urine (as eptifibatide and metabolites); significant renal impairment may alter disposition of this compound

Clearance: Total body: 55-58 mL/kg/hour; Renal: ~50% of total in healthy subjects

Pregnancy Risk Factor B

Epzicom™ see Abacavir and Lamivudine on page 23

Equagesic® see Meprobamate and Aspirin on page 1049

Equalactin® [OTC] see Polycarbophil on page 1320

Equalizer Gas Relief [OTC] see Simethicone on page 1472

Equanil see Meprobamate on page 1048

Equetro™ see Carbamazepine on page 272

Eraxis™ see Anidulafungin on page 130

Erbitux® see Cetuximab on page 323

Ergocalciferol (er goe kal SIF e role)

U.S. Brand Names Calciferol™; Drisdol®

Canadian Brand Names Drisdol®; Ostoforte®

Generic Available Yes: Capsule

Index Terms Activated Ergosterol; Viosterol; Vitamin D_2

Pharmacologic Category Vitamin D Analog

Use Treatment of refractory rickets, hypophosphatemia, hypoparathyroidism; dietary supplement

Local Anesthetic/Vasoconstrictor Precautions No information available to require special precautions

Effects on Dental Treatment Key adverse event(s) related to dental treatment: Metallic taste and xerostomia (normal salivary flow resumes upon discontinuation).

Common Adverse Effects Generally well tolerated

Frequency not defined: Cardiac arrhythmia, hypertension (late), irritability, headache, psychosis (rare), somnolence, hyperthermia (late), pruritus, libido decreased (late), hypercholesterolemia, mild acidosis (late), polydipsia (late), nausea, vomiting, anorexia, pancreatitis, metallic taste, weight loss (rare), xerostomia, constipation, polyuria (late), BUN increased (late), LFTs increased (late), bone pain, myalgia, weakness, conjunctivitis, photophobia (late), vascular/nephrocalcinosis (rare)

Mechanism of Action Stimulates calcium and phosphate absorption from the small intestine, promotes secretion of calcium from bone to blood; promotes renal tubule phosphate resorption

Drug Interactions

Increased Effect/Toxicity: Thiazide diuretics may increase vitamin D effects. Cardiac glycosides may increase toxicity.

Decreased Effect: Cholestyramine, colestipol, mineral oil may decrease oral absorption.

Pharmacodynamics/Kinetics

Onset of action: Peak effect: ~1 month following daily doses

Absorption: Readily; requires bile

Metabolism: Inactive until hydroxylated hepatically and renally to calcifediol and then to calcitriol (most active form)

Pregnancy Risk Factor A/C (dose exceeding RDA recommendation)

Ergoloid Mesylates (ER goe loid MES i lates)

Canadian Brand Names Hydergine®
Mexican Brand Names Hydergina
Generic Available Yes
Index Terms Dihydroergotoxine; Dihydrogenated Ergot Alkaloids; Hydergine [DSC]
Pharmacologic Category Ergot Derivative
Use Treatment of cerebrovascular insufficiency in primary progressive dementia, Alzheimer's dementia, and senile onset

Local Anesthetic/Vasoconstrictor Precautions No information available to require special precautions

Effects on Dental Treatment Key adverse event(s) related to dental treatment: Orthostatic hypotension.

Common Adverse Effects Adverse effects are minimal; most common include transient nausea, gastrointestinal disturbances and sublingual irritation with SL tablets; other common side effects include:

Cardiovascular: Orthostatic hypotension, bradycardia
Dermatologic: Skin rash, flushing
Ocular: Blurred vision
Respiratory: Nasal congestion

Mechanism of Action Ergoloid mesylates do not have the vasoconstrictor effects of the natural ergot alkaloids; exact mechanism in dementia is unknown; originally classed as peripheral and cerebral vasodilator, now considered a "metabolic enhancer"; there is no specific evidence which clearly establishes the mechanism by which ergoloid mesylate preparations produce mental effects, nor is there conclusive evidence that the drug particularly affects cerebral arteriosclerosis or cerebrovascular insufficiency

Drug Interactions
Cytochrome P450 Effect: Substrate of CYP3A4 (major)
Increased Effect/Toxicity: CYP3A4 inhibitors may increase the levels/effects of ergoloid mesylates; example inhibitors include azole antifungals, clarithromycin, diclofenac, doxycycline, erythromycin, imatinib, isoniazid, nefazodone, nicardipine, propofol, protease inhibitors, quinidine, telithromycin, and verapamil. Ergot alkaloids are contraindicated with potent CYP3A4 inhibitors. Ergoloid mesylates may increase the effects of 5-HT$_1$ agonists (eg, sumatriptan), MAO inhibitors, sibutramine, and other serotonin agonists (serotonin syndrome). Severe vasoconstriction may occur when peripheral vasoconstrictors or beta-blockers are used in patients receiving ergot alkaloids; concurrent use is contraindicated.
Decreased Effect: Effects of ergoloid mesylates may be diminished by antipsychotics, metoclopramide. Antianginal effects of nitrates may be reduced by ergot alkaloids.

Pharmacodynamics/Kinetics
Absorption: Rapid yet incomplete
Half-life elimination, serum: 3.5 hours
Time to peak, serum: ~1 hour

Pregnancy Risk Factor C

Ergomar® *see* Ergotamine *on page 585*
Ergometrine Maleate *see* Ergonovine *on page 584*

Ergonovine (er goe NOE veen)

U.S. Brand Names Ergotrate®
Mexican Brand Names Ergotrate
Generic Available No
Index Terms Ergometrine Maleate; Ergonovine Maleate
Pharmacologic Category Ergot Derivative
Use Prevention and treatment of postpartum and postabortion hemorrhage caused by uterine atony or subinvolution

Unlabeled/Investigational Use Diagnostically to identify Prinzmetal's angina

Local Anesthetic/Vasoconstrictor Precautions No information available to require special precautions

Effects on Dental Treatment No significant effects or complications reported
Common Adverse Effects Frequency not defined.
Cardiovascular: Hypertension, MI, shock
Gastrointestinal: Nausea, vomiting
Miscellaneous: Allergic reactions, ergotism

Mechanism of Action Similar smooth muscle actions as seen with ergotamine; however, it affects primarily uterine smooth muscles producing sustained contractions and thereby shortens the third stage of labor.

Drug Interactions

Cytochrome P450 Effect: Substrate of CYP3A4 (major)

Increased Effect/Toxicity: CYP3A4 inhibitors may increase the levels/ effects of ergonovine; example inhibitors include azole antifungals, clarithromycin, diclofenac, doxycycline, erythromycin, imatinib, isoniazid, nefazodone, nicardipine, propofol, protease inhibitors, quinidine, telithromycin, troleandomycin, and verapamil. Ergot alkaloids are contraindicated with potent CYP3A4 inhibitors. Ergonovine may increase the effects of MAO inhibitors, sibutramine, and other serotonin modulators (eg, 5-HT$_{1D}$ receptor agonists, buspirone, SSRIs, TCAs, nefazodone, and trazodone). Severe vasoconstriction may occur when peripheral vasoconstrictors or beta-blockers are used in patients receiving ergot alkaloids; concurrent use is contraindicated.

Decreased Effect: Effects of ergonovine may be diminished by antipsychotics, metoclopramide. Antianginal effects of nitrates may be reduced by ergot alkaloids.

Pharmacodynamics/Kinetics
Onset of action: I.M.: ~2-5 minutes; Oral: 6-15 minutes
Duration: I.M.: Uterine effect: 3 hours; I.V.: ~45 minutes; Oral: 3 hours
Absorption: Oral: Rapid
Metabolism: Hepatic
Half-life elimination: I.V.: 120 minutes
Excretion: Primarily feces; urine

Ergonovine Maleate see Ergonovine on page 584

Ergotamine (er GOT a meen)

U.S. Brand Names Ergomar®
Generic Available No
Index Terms Ergotamine Tartrate
Pharmacologic Category Antimigraine Agent; Ergot Derivative
Use Abort or prevent vascular headaches, such as migraine, migraine variants, or so-called "histaminic cephalalgia"
Local Anesthetic/Vasoconstrictor Precautions No information available to require special precautions
Effects on Dental Treatment No significant effects or complications reported
Common Adverse Effects Frequency not defined.
Cardiovascular: Absence of pulse, bradycardia, cardiac valvular fibrosis, cyanosis, edema, ECG changes, gangrene, hypertension, ischemia, precordial distress and pain, tachycardia, vasospasm
Central nervous system: Vertigo
Dermatologic: Itching
Gastrointestinal: Nausea, vomiting
Genitourinary: Retroperitoneal fibrosis
Neuromuscular & skeletal: Muscle pain, numbness, paresthesia, weakness
Respiratory: Pleuropulmonary fibrosis
Miscellaneous: Cold extremities

Mechanism of Action Has partial agonist and/or antagonist activity against tryptaminergic, dopaminergic and alpha-adrenergic receptors depending upon their site; is a highly active uterine stimulant; it causes constriction of peripheral and cranial blood vessels and produces depression of central vasomotor centers

Drug Interactions

Cytochrome P450 Effect: Substrate of CYP3A4 (major); Inhibits CYP3A4 (weak)

Increased Effect/Toxicity: CYP3A4 inhibitors may increase the levels/ effects of ergotamine; example inhibitors include azole antifungals, clarithromycin, diclofenac, doxycycline, erythromycin, imatinib, isoniazid, nefazodone, nicardipine, propofol, protease inhibitors, quinidine, telithromycin, troleandomycin, and verapamil. Ergot alkaloids are contraindicated with strong CYP3A4 inhibitors. Ergotamine may increase the effects of 5-HT$_1$ agonists (eg, sumatriptan), MAO inhibitors, sibutramine, and other serotonin agonists (serotonin syndrome). Severe vasoconstriction may occur when peripheral vasoconstrictors or beta-blockers are used in patients receiving ergot alkaloids; concurrent use is contraindicated.

Decreased Effect: Effects of ergotamine may be diminished by antipsychotics, metoclopramide. Antianginal effects of nitrates may be reduced by ergot alkaloids.

Pharmacodynamics/Kinetics
Absorption: Oral: Erratic; enhanced by caffeine coadministration
(Continued)

Ergotamine *(Continued)*

Metabolism: Extensively hepatic
Time to peak, serum: 0.5-3 hours
Half-life elimination: 2 hours
Excretion: Feces (90% as metabolites)
Pregnancy Risk Factor X

Ergotamine and Caffeine *(er GOT a meen & KAF een)*

Related Information
Caffeine *on page 255*
Ergotamine *on page 585*
U.S. Brand Names Cafergot®; Migergot
Canadian Brand Names Cafergor®
Mexican Brand Names Cafergot; Ergocaf; Trinergot
Generic Available Yes
Index Terms Caffeine and Ergotamine; Ergotamine Tartrate and Caffeine
Pharmacologic Category Antimigraine Agent; Ergot Derivative; Stimulant
Use Abort or prevent vascular headaches, such as migraine, migraine variants, or so-called "histaminic cephalalgia"
Local Anesthetic/Vasoconstrictor Precautions No information available to require special precautions
Effects on Dental Treatment No significant effects or complications reported
Common Adverse Effects Frequency not defined.
Cardiovascular: Absence of pulse, bradycardia, cardiac valvular fibrosis, cyanosis, edema, ECG changes, gangrene, hypertension, ischemia, precordial distress and pain, tachycardia, vasospasm
Central nervous system: Vertigo
Dermatologic: Itching
Gastrointestinal: Anal or rectal ulcer (with overuse of suppository), nausea, vomiting
Genitourinary: Retroperitoneal fibrosis
Neuromuscular & skeletal: Muscle pain, numbness, paresthesia, weakness
Respiratory: Pleuropulmonary fibrosis
Miscellaneous: Cold extremities
Mechanism of Action Has partial agonist and/or antagonist activity against tryptaminergic, dopaminergic and alpha-adrenergic receptors depending upon their site; is a highly active uterine stimulant; it causes constriction of peripheral and cranial blood vessels and produces depression of central vasomotor centers
Drug Interactions
Cytochrome P450 Effect:
Ergotamine: **Substrate** of CYP3A4 (major); **Inhibits** CYP3A4 (weak)
Caffeine: **Substrate** of CYP1A2 (major), 2C9 (minor), 2D6 (minor), 2E1 (minor), 3A4 (minor); **Inhibits** CYP1A2 (weak), 3A4 (moderate)
Increased Effect/Toxicity: See Ergotamine monograph for related interactions. CYP1A2 inhibitors may increase the levels/effects of caffeine; example inhibitors include amiodarone, fluvoxamine, ketoconazole, and rofecoxib. CYP3A4 inhibitors may increase the levels/effects of ergotamine; example inhibitors include azole antifungals, ciprofloxacin, clarithromycin, diclofenac, doxycycline, erythromycin, imatinib, isoniazid, nefazodone, nicardipine, propofol, protease inhibitors, quinidine, and verapamil. Caffeine may increase the levels/effects of CYP3A4 substrates; example substrates include benzodiazepines, calcium channel blockers, ergot derivatives, mirtazapine, nateglinide, nefazodone, tacrolimus, and venlafaxine. Caffeine levels may be increased by selected quinolone antibiotics (ciprofloxacin, norfloxacin, ofloxacin).
Decreased Effect: See Ergotamine monograph for related interactions.
Pharmacodynamics/Kinetics
Absorption: Ergotamine: Oral, rectal: Erratic; enhanced by caffeine coadministration
Metabolism: Extensively hepatic
Time to peak, serum: Ergotamine: 0.5-3 hours
Half-life elimination: 2 hours
Excretion: Feces (90% as metabolites)
Pregnancy Risk Factor X

Erlotinib (er LOE tye nib)

U.S. Brand Names Tarceva®
Canadian Brand Names Tarceva®
Generic Available No
Index Terms CP358774; Erlotinib Hydrochloride; NSC-718781; OSI-774; R 14-15
Pharmacologic Category Antineoplastic Agent, Tyrosine Kinase Inhibitor; Epidermal Growth Factor Receptor (EGFR) Inhibitor
Use Treatment of refractory advanced or metastatic nonsmall cell lung cancer (NSCLC); pancreatic cancer (first-line therapy in combination with gemcitabine)
Unlabeled/Investigational Use Treatment of advanced or metastatic breast cancer, colorectal cancer, head and neck tumors, ovarian cancer, and renal cell cancer
Local Anesthetic/Vasoconstrictor Precautions No information available to require special precautions
Effects on Dental Treatment Key adverse event(s) related to dental treatment: Xerostomia (normal salivary flow resumes upon discontinuation), mucositis, abnormal taste, and stomatitis.
Common Adverse Effects Percentages as reported with monotherapy; frequency of adverse event with combination chemotherapy (gemcitabine) noted where applicable

>10%:
  Cardiovascular: Edema (37% combination)
  Central nervous system: Fatigue (14% to 55%; 73% combination), pyrexia (36% combination), anxiety (21%), headache (17%), depression (16%; 19% combination), dizziness (15% combination), insomnia (12%; 15% combination)
  Dermatologic: Acneiform rash (50% to 88%; grade 3/4: 9%), pruritus (13% to 55%), dry skin (12% to 35%), erythema (18%), alopecia (14% combination)
  Gastrointestinal: Diarrhea (30% to 56%; grade 3/4: 6%), anorexia (23% to 52%), nausea (11% to 33%; 60% combination), vomiting (23%; 42% combination), mucositis (17% to 18%), glossodynia (18%), stomatitis (17%; 22% combination), xerostomia (17%), pain (14%), flatulence (13% combination); constipation (12%; 31% combination), dyspepsia (12%; 17% combination), dysphagia (12%), weight loss (12%; 39% combination), abnormal taste (11%), abdominal pain (11%; 46% combination)
  Hepatic: ALT increased (4%; combination grade 2: 31%, grade 3: 13%, grade 4: <1%), AST increased (combination grade 2: 24%, grade 3: 10%, grade 4 <1%), hyperbilirubinemia (20%; combination grade 2: 17%, grade 3: 10%, grade 4: <1%)
  Neuromuscular & skeletal: Bone pain (25% combination), myalgia (21% combination), arthralgia (14%), neuropathy (13% combination), rigors (12% combination), paresthesia (11%)
  Ocular: Conjunctivitis (12%; <1% combination), keratoconjunctivitis sicca (12%)
  Respiratory: Dyspnea (21% to 41%), cough (16% to 33%)
  Miscellaneous: Infection (24%; 39% combination)
1% to 10%:
  Cardiovascular (reported with combination chemotherapy): Deep venous thrombosis (4%), arrhythmia, cerebrovascular accidents (including cerebral hemorrhage), MI, myocardial ischemia, syncope
  Gastrointestinal (reported with combination chemotherapy): Ileus, pancreatitis
  Hematologic (reported with combination chemotherapy): Hemolytic anemia, microangiopathic hemolytic anemia with thrombocytopenia
  Ocular: Keratitis (6%; <1% combination)
  Renal (reported with combination chemotherapy): Renal insufficiency
  Respiratory: Pneumonitis (6%)
Mechanism of Action The mechanism of erlotinib's antitumor action is not fully characterized. The drug is known to inhibit overall epidermal growth factor receptor (HER1/EGFR)- tyrosine kinase. Active competitive inhibition of adenosine triphosphate inhibits downstream signal transduction of ligand dependent HER1/EGFR activation.
Drug Interactions
  Cytochrome P450 Effect: Substrate of CYP1A2 (minor), 3A4 (major)
  Increased Effect/Toxicity: Ketoconazole and CYP3A4 inhibitors may increase erlotinib levels/effects; example inhibitors include azole antifungals, clarithromycin, diclofenac, doxycycline, erythromycin, imatinib, isoniazid, nefazodone, nicardipine, propofol, protease inhibitors, quinidine, telithromycin, and verapamil.
  (Continued)

Erlotinib *(Continued)*

Decreased Effect: Rifamycins and CYP3A4 inducers may decrease erlotinib levels/effects; example inducers include aminoglutethimide, carbamazepine, nafcillin, nevirapine, phenobarbital, and phenytoin. Erlotinib may decrease the absorption of digoxin tablets.

Pharmacodynamics/Kinetics

Absorption: Oral: 60% on an empty stomach; ~100% on a full stomach

Distribution: 94-232 L

Protein binding: 92% to 95%, albumin and α_1-acid glycoprotein

Metabolism: Hepatic, CYP3A4 (major), CYP1A1 (minor), CYP1A2 (minor), and CYP1C (minor)

Bioavailability: 100% when given with food; 60% without food

Half-life elimination: 24-36 hours

Time to peak, plasma: 1-7 hours

Excretion: Primarily as metabolites: Feces (83%); urine (8%)

Pregnancy Risk Factor D

Erlotinib Hydrochloride *see* Erlotinib *on page 587*

Errin™ *see* Norethindrone *on page 1186*

Ertaczo™ *see* Sertaconazole *on page 1463*

Ertapenem *(er ta PEN em)*

U.S. Brand Names Invanz®

Canadian Brand Names Invanz®

Mexican Brand Names Invanz

Generic Available No

Index Terms Ertapenem Sodium; L-749,345; MK0826

Pharmacologic Category Antibiotic, Carbapenem

Use Treatment of the following moderate-severe infections: Complicated intra-abdominal infections, complicated skin and skin structure infections (including diabetic foot infections without osteomyelitis), complicated UTI (including pyelonephritis), acute pelvic infections, and community-acquired pneumonia. Prophylaxis of surgical site infection following elective colorectal surgery. Antibacterial coverage includes aerobic gram-positive organisms, aerobic gram-negative organisms, anaerobic organisms.

Note: Methicillin-resistant *Staphylococcus*, *Enterococcus* spp, penicillin-resistant strains of *Streptococcus pneumoniae*, beta-lactamase-positive strains of *Haemophilus influenzae* are **resistant** to ertapenem, as are most *Pseudomonas aeruginosa*.

Local Anesthetic/Vasoconstrictor Precautions No information available to require special precautions

Effects on Dental Treatment Key adverse event(s) related to dental treatment: Oral candidiasis

Common Adverse Effects Note: Percentages reported in adults.

1% to 10%:

Cardiovascular: Swelling/edema (3%), chest pain (1% to 2%), hypertension (1% to 2%), hypotension (1% to 2%), tachycardia (1% to 2%)

Central nervous system: Headache (6% to 7%), altered mental status (ie, agitation, confusion, disorientation, decreased mental acuity, changed mental status, somnolence, stupor) (3% to 5%), fever (2% to 5%), insomnia (3%), dizziness (2%), fatigue (1%), anxiety (1%)

Dermatologic: Rash (2% to 3%), pruritus (1% to 2%), erythema (1% to 2%), wound complication (3%)

Gastrointestinal: Diarrhea (9% to 10%), nausea (6% to 9%), abdominal pain (4%), vomiting (4%), constipation (3% to 4%), acid regurgitation (1% to 2%), dyspepsia (1%), oral candidiasis (≤1%)

Genitourinary: Vaginitis (1% to 3%), dysuria (1%), proteinuria

Hematologic: Platelet count increased (3% to 7%), leukopenia (1% to 2%), neutrophils decreased (1% to 2%), prothrombin time increased (1% to 2%)

Hepatic: Hepatic enzyme increased (5% to 9%), alkaline phosphatase increase (3% to 7%)

Local: Infused vein complications (5% to 7%), phlebitis/thrombophlebitis (2%), extravasation (1% to 2%)

Neuromuscular & skeletal: Leg pain (≤1%), weakness (1%)

Respiratory: Atelectasis (3%), dyspnea (1% to 3%), cough (1% to 2%), pharyngitis (1%), rales/rhonchi (1%), respiratory distress (≤1%)

Mechanism of Action Inhibits bacterial cell wall synthesis by binding to one or more of the penicillin binding proteins; which in turn inhibits the final transpeptidation step of peptidoglycan synthesis in bacterial cell walls, thus inhibiting cell wall biosynthesis. Bacteria eventually lyse due to ongoing activity of cell wall autolytic enzymes (autolysins and murein hydrolases) while cell wall assembly is arrested.

Drug Interactions

Increased Effect/Toxicity: Probenecid may increase serum concentrations of ertapenem; use caution.

Decreased Effect: Ertapenem may decrease valproic acid serum concentrations to subtherapeutic levels; monitor. Antibiotics may decrease effectiveness of the Ty21a live, attenuated typhoid vaccine; delay vaccination for >24 hours after administration of antibiotic

Pharmacodynamics/Kinetics

Absorption: I.M.: Almost complete

Distribution: V_{dss}:

Children 3 months to 12 years: 0.2 L/kg

Children 13-17 years: 0.16 L/kg

Adults: 0.12 L/kg

Protein binding (concentration dependent): 85% at 300 mcg/mL, 95% at <100 mcg/mL

Metabolism: Non-CYP-mediated hydrolysis to inactive metabolite

Bioavailability: I.M.: ~90%

Half-life elimination:

Children 3 months to 12 years: 2.5 hours

Children ≥13 years and Adults: 4 hours

Time to peak: I.M.: ~2.3 hours

Excretion: Urine (80% as unchanged drug and metabolite); feces (10%)

Pregnancy Risk Factor B

Ertapenem Sodium *see Ertapenem on page 588*

***Erwinia* Asparaginase** *see Asparaginase on page 148*

Eryc® [DSC] *see Erythromycin on page 589*

Eryderm® *see Erythromycin on page 589*

Erygel® *see Erythromycin on page 589*

EryPed® *see Erythromycin on page 589*

Ery-Tab® *see Erythromycin on page 589*

Erythrocin® *see Erythromycin on page 589*

Erythromycin (er ith roe MYE sin)

Related Information

Bacterial Infections *on page 1793*

Cardiovascular Diseases *on page 1726*

Respiratory Diseases *on page 1747*

Treatment of Sexually-Transmitted Infections *on page 1920*

Related Sample Prescriptions

Bacterial Infections and Periodontal Diseases *on page 1837*

U.S. Brand Names Akne-Mycin®; E.E.S.®; Eryc® [DSC]; Eryderm®; Erygel®; EryPed®; Ery-Tab®; Erythrocin®; PCE®; Romycin®

Canadian Brand Names Apo-Erythro Base®; Apo-Erythro E-C®; Apo-Erythro-ES®; Apo-Erythro-S®; Diomycin®; EES®; Erybid™; Eryc®; Novo-Rythro Estolate; Novo-Rythro Ethylsuccinate; Nu-Erythromycin-S; PCE®; PMS-Erythromycin; Sans Acne®

Mexican Brand Names Bestocin; Eritrowel; Ilosone; Lauritran; Lederpax; Pantomicina; Sans-acne

Generic Available Yes: Capsule, gel, ophthalmic ointment, topical solution, suspension (as ethylsuccinate), swab, tablet (as base, ethylsuccinate, and stearate)

Index Terms Erythromycin Base; Erythromycin Ethylsuccinate; Erythromycin Lactobionate; Erythromycin Stearate

Pharmacologic Category Acne Products; Antibiotic, Macrolide; Antibiotic, Ophthalmic; Antibiotic, Topical; Topical Skin Product; Topical Skin Product, Acne

Dental Use Systemic: Alternative to penicillin VK for treatment of orofacial infections

Use

Systemic: Treatment of susceptible bacterial infections including *S. pyogenes*, some *S. pneumoniae*, some *S. aureus*, *M. pneumoniae*, *Legionella pneumophila*, diphtheria, pertussis, *Chlamydia*, erythrasma, *N. gonorrhoeae*, *E. histolytica*, syphilis and nongonococcal urethritis, and *Campylobacter* gastroenteritis; used in conjunction with neomycin for decontaminating the bowel

Ophthalmic: Treatment of superficial eye infections involving the conjunctiva or cornea; neonatal ophthalmia

Topical: Treatment of acne vulgaris

(Continued)

Erythromycin *(Continued)*

Unlabeled/Investigational Use Systemic: Treatment of gastroparesis, chancroid; preoperative gut sterilization

Local Anesthetic/Vasoconstrictor Precautions Erythromycin is one of the drugs confirmed to prolong the QT interval and is accepted as having a risk of causing torsade de pointes. In terms of epinephrine, it is not known what effect vasoconstrictors in the local anesthetic regimen will have in patients with a known history of congenital prolonged QT interval or in patients taking any medication that prolongs the QT interval. Until more information is obtained, it is suggested that the clinician consult with the physician prior to the use of a vasoconstrictor in suspected patients, and that the vasoconstrictor (epinephrine, levonordefrin [Neo-Cobefrin®]) be used with caution. See Dental Comment.

Effects on Dental Treatment Key adverse event(s) related to dental treatment: Oral candidiasis.

Significant Adverse Effects Frequency not defined. Incidence may vary with formulation.

Systemic:

Cardiovascular: QT_c prolongation, torsade de pointes, ventricular arrhythmia, ventricular tachycardia

Central nervous system: Seizure

Dermatitis: Pruritus, rash

Gastrointestinal: Abdominal pain, anorexia, diarrhea, infantile hypertrophic pyloric stenosis, nausea, oral candidiasis, pancreatitis, pseudomembranous colitis, vomiting

Hepatic: Cholestatic jaundice (most common with estolate), hepatitis, liver function tests abnormal

Local: Phlebitis at the injection site, thrombophlebitis

Neuromuscular & skeletal: Weakness

Otic: Hearing loss

Miscellaneous: Allergic reactions, anaphylaxis, hypersensitivity reactions, urticaria

Topical: 1% to 10%: Dermatologic: Erythema, desquamation, dryness, pruritus

Dental Usual Dosing Treatment of orofacial infections: Adults: Oral:

Base: 250-500 mg every 6-12 hours

Ethylsuccinate: 400-800 mg every 6-12 hours

Dosage Note: Due to differences in absorption, 400 mg erythromycin ethylsuccinate produces the same serum levels as 250 mg erythromycin base or stearate.

Usual dosage range:

Neonates: Ophthalmic: Prophylaxis of neonatal gonococcal or chlamydial conjunctivitis: 0.5-1 cm ribbon of ointment should be instilled into each conjunctival sac

Infants and Children:

Oral:

Base: 30-50 mg/kg/day in 2-4 divided doses; maximum: 2 g/day

Ethylsuccinate: 30-50 mg/kg/day in 2-4 divided doses; maximum: 3.2 g/day

Stearate: 30-50 mg/kg/day in 2-4 divided doses; maximum: 2 g/day

I.V.: Lactobionate: 15-50 mg/kg/day divided every 6 hours, not to exceed 4 g/day

Children and Adults:

Ophthalmic: Instill ½" (1.25 cm) 2-6 times/day depending on the severity of the infection

Topical: Acne: Apply over the affected area twice daily after the skin has been thoroughly washed and patted dry

Adults:

Oral:

Base: 250-500 mg every 6-12 hours; maximum 4 g/day

Ethylsuccinate: 400-800 mg every 6-12 hours; maximum 4 g/day

I.V.: Lactobionate: 15-20 mg/kg/day divided every 6 hours or 500 mg to 1 g every 6 hours, or given as a continuous infusion over 24 hours; maximum: 4 g/24 hours

Indication-specific dosing:

Children:

***Bartonella* sp infections (bacillary angiomatosis [BA], peliosis hepatis [PH]) (unlabeled use):** Oral: 40 mg/kg/day (ethylsuccinate) in 4 divided doses (maximum: 2 g/day) for 3 months (BA) or 4 months (PH)

Conjunctivitis, neonatal *(C. trachomatis)*: Oral: 50 mg/kg/day (base or ethylsuccinate) in 4 divided doses for 14 days

Mild/moderate infection: Oral: 30-50 mg/kg/day in divided doses every 6-12 hours

Pertussis: Oral: 40-50 mg/kg/day in 4 divided doses for 14 days; maximum 2 g/day (not preferred agent for infants <1 month due to IHPS)

Pharyngitis, tonsillitis (streptococcal): Oral: 20 mg (base)/kg/day or 40 mg (ethylsuccinate)/kg/day in 2 divided doses for 10 days. **Note:** No longer preferred therapy due to increased organism resistance.

Pneumonia *(C. trachomatis):* Oral: 50 mg/kg/day (base or ethylsuccinate) in 4 divided doses for 14-21 days

Preop bowel preparation: Oral: 20 mg (base)/kg at 1, 2, and 11 PM on the day before surgery combined with mechanical cleansing of the large intestine and oral neomycin

Severe infection: I.V.: 15-50 mg/kg/day; maximum: 4 g/day

Adults:

Bartonella sp infections (bacillary angiomatosis [BA], peliosis hepatis [PH]) (unlabeled use): Oral: 500 mg (base) 4 times/day for 3 months (BA) or 4 months (PH)

Chancroid (unlabeled use): Oral: 500 mg (base) 3 times/day for 7 days; Note: Not a preferred agent; isolates with intermediate resistance have been documented

Gastrointestinal prokinetic (unlabeled use): I.V.: 200 mg initially followed by 250 mg (base) orally 3 times/day 30 minutes before meals. Lower dosages have been used in some trials.

Granuloma inguinale (*K. granulomatis*) (unlabeled use): Oral: 500 mg (base) 4 times/day for 21 days

Legionnaires' disease: Oral: 1.6-4 g (ethylsuccinate)/day or 1-4 g (base)/day in divided doses for 21 days. **Note:** No longer preferred therapy and only used in nonhospitalized patients.

Lymphogranuloma venereum: Oral: 500 mg (base) 4 times/day for 21 days

Nongonococcal urethritis (including coinfection with *C. trachomatis*): Oral: 500 mg (base) 4 times/day for 7 days or 800 mg (ethylsuccinate) 4 times/day for 7 days. **Note:** May use 250 mg (base) or 400 mg (ethylsuccinate) 4 times/day for 14 days if gastrointestinal intolerance.

Pelvic inflammatory disease: I.V.: 500 mg every 6 hours for 3 days, followed by 1000 mg (base)/day orally in 2-4 divided doses for 7 days. **Note:** Not recommended therapy per current treatment guidelines.

Pertussis: Oral: 500 mg (base) every 6 hours for 14 days

Preop bowel preparation (unlabeled use): Oral: 1 g erythromycin base at 1, 2, and 11 PM on the day before surgery combined with mechanical cleansing of the large intestine and oral neomycin

Syphilis, primary: Oral: 48-64 g (ethylsuccinate) or 30-40 g (base) in divided doses over 10-15 days. **Note:** Not recommended therapy per current treatment guidelines.

Dosage adjustment in renal impairment: Dialysis: Slightly dialyzable (5% to 20%); no supplemental dosage necessary in hemo- or peritoneal dialysis or in continuous arteriovenous or venovenous hemofiltration

Mechanism of Action Inhibits RNA-dependent protein synthesis at the chain elongation step; binds to the 50S ribosomal subunit resulting in blockage of transpeptidation

Contraindications Hypersensitivity to erythromycin or any component of the formulation

Systemic: Concomitant use with pimozide or cisapride

Warnings/Precautions Systemic: Use caution with hepatic impairment with or without jaundice has occurred, it may be accompanied by malaise, nausea, vomiting, abdominal colic, and fever; discontinue use if these occur. Use caution with other medication relying on CYP3A4 metabolism; high potential for drug interactions exists. Prolonged use may result in fungal or bacterial superinfection, including *C. difficile*-associated diarrhea and pseudomembranous colitis. Use in infants has been associated with infantile hypertrophic pyloric stenosis (IHPS). Macrolides have been associated with rare QT_c prolongation and ventricular arrhythmias, including torsade de pointes. Use caution in elderly patients, as risk of adverse events may be increased. Use caution in myasthenia gravis patients; erythromycin may aggravate muscular weakness.

Drug Interactions Substrate of CYP2B6 (minor), 3A4 (major); **Inhibits** CYP1A2 (weak), 3A4 (moderate)

Alfentanil (and possibly other opioid analgesics): Serum levels may be increased by erythromycin; monitor for increased effect.

Antifungal agents (imidazole): Reciprocal inhibition of metabolism may lead to increased levels/effects of both azole antifungal and erythromycin; monitor.

Antipsychotic agents (particularly mesoridazine and thioridazine): Risk of QT_c prolongation and malignant arrhythmias may be increased.

Benzodiazepines (those metabolized by CYP3A4, including alprazolam and triazolam): Serum levels may be increased by erythromycin; somnolence and confusion have been reported.

Bromocriptine: Serum levels may be increased by erythromycin; monitor for increased effect (eg, ergotism).

(Continued)

Erythromycin *(Continued)*

Buspirone: Serum levels may be increased by erythromycin; monitor.

Calcium channel blockers (felodipine, verapamil, and potentially others metabolized by CYP3A4): Serum levels may be increased by erythromycin; monitor.

Carbamazepine: Serum levels may be increased by erythromycin; monitor.

Cilostazol: Serum levels may be increased by erythromycin; monitor.

Cisapride: Serum levels may be increased by erythromycin; serious arrhythmias have occurred; concurrent use contraindicated.

Clindamycin (and lincomycin): Use with erythromycin may result in pharmacologic antagonism; manufacturer recommends avoiding this combination.

Clopidogrel: Erythromycin may decrease the anticoagulant effects of clopidogrel; monitor.

Clozapine: Serum levels may be increased by erythromycin; monitor.

Colchicine: serum levels/toxicity may be increased by erythromycin; monitor. Avoid use, if possible.

Corticosteroids: Erythromycin may increase the levels/effects of systemic steroids; monitor for increased effects.

Cyclosporine: Serum levels may be increased by erythromycin; monitor serum levels.

CYP3A4 inducers: CYP3A4 inducers may decrease the levels/effects of erythromycin. Example inducers include aminoglutethimide, carbamazepine, nafcillin, nevirapine, phenobarbital, phenytoin, and rifamycins.

CYP3A4 inhibitors: May increase the levels/effects of erythromycin. Example inhibitors include azole antifungals, clarithromycin, diclofenac, doxycycline, imatinib, isoniazid, nefazodone, nicardipine, propofol, protease inhibitors, quinidine, telithromycin, and verapamil.

CYP3A4 substrates: Erythromycin may increase the levels/effects of CYP3A4 substrates. Example substrates include benzodiazepines, calcium channel blockers, cyclosporine, mirtazapine, nateglinide, nefazodone, sildenafil (and other PDE-5 inhibitors), tacrolimus, and venlafaxine. Selected benzodiazepines (midazolam and triazolam), cisapride, ergot alkaloids, selected HMG-CoA reductase inhibitors (lovastatin and simvastatin), and pimozide are generally contraindicated with strong CYP3A4 inhibitors.

Delavirdine: Serum levels of erythromycin may be increased; also, serum levels of delavirdine may increased by erythromycin (low risk); monitor.

Digoxin: Serum levels may be increased by erythromycin; monitor digoxin levels.

Disopyramide: Serum levels may be increased by erythromycin; in addition, QT_c prolongation and risk of malignant arrhythmia may be increased; avoid combination.

Eletriptan: Serum levels/effects may be increased by erythromycin; monitor.

Eplerenone: Serum levels/effects may be increased by erythromycin; monitor.

Ergot alkaloids: Concurrent use may lead to acute ergot toxicity (severe peripheral vasospasm and dysesthesia).

HMG-CoA reductase inhibitors (atorvastatin, lovastatin, and simvastatin): Erythromycin may increase serum levels of "statins" metabolized by CYP3A4, increasing the risk of myopathy/rhabdomyolysis (does not include fluvastatin, pravastatin, and rosuvastatin). Switch to pravastatin/fluvastatin/rosuvastatin or suspend treatment during course of erythromycin therapy.

Immunosuppressants (eg, cyclosporine, tacrolimus, sirolimus): Serum levels/effects may be increased by erythromycin; monitor.

Phenytoin: Serum levels may be increased by erythromycin; other evidence suggested phenytoin levels may be decreased in some patients; monitor.

Phosphodiesterase-5 inhibitors (eg, sildenafil, tadalafil, vardenafil): Serum concentration may be substantially increased by erythromycin. Do not exceed single sildenafil doses of 25 mg in 48 hours, a single tadalafil dose of 10 mg in 72 hours, or a single vardenafil dose of 2.5 mg in 24 hours.

Pimozide: Serum levels may be increased, leading to malignant arrhythmias; concomitant use is contraindicated.

QT_c-prolonging agents: Concomitant use may increase the risk of malignant arrhythmias.

Quinidine: Serum levels may be increased by erythromycin; in addition, the risk of QT_c prolongation and malignant arrhythmias may be increased during concurrent use.

Repaglinide: Serum levels/effects may be increased by erythromycin; monitor.

Rifamycin derivatives (eg, rifabutin, rifampin): Serum levels may be increased by erythromycin; monitor.

SSRIs: Macrolides may increase the levels/effects; monitor.

Theophylline: Serum levels may be increased by erythromycin; monitor.

Thioridazine: Risk of QT_c prolongation may be increased; concomitant use not recommended.

Valproic acid (and derivatives): Serum levels may be increased by erythromycin; monitor.

Vinblastine (and vincristine): Serum levels may be increased by erythromycin.
Warfarin: Effects may be potentiated; monitor INR closely and adjust warfarin dose as needed or choose another antibiotic.
Zafirlukast: Serum levels may be decreased by erythromycin; monitor.
Zopiclone: Serum levels may be increased by erythromycin; monitor.

Ethanol/Nutrition/Herb Interactions
Ethanol: Avoid ethanol (may decrease absorption of erythromycin or enhance ethanol effects).
Food: Erythromycin serum levels may be altered if taken with food (formulation"dependent).
Herb/Nutraceutical: St John's wort may decrease erythromycin levels.

Dietary Considerations
Systemic: Drug may cause GI upset; may take with food.
E.E.S.® granules for oral suspension contain sodium 25.9 mg (1.1 mEq)/5 mL
EryPed® powder for oral suspension contains sodium 117.5 mg (5.1 mEq)/5 mL; powder for oral suspension (drops) contains sodium 58.8 mg (2.6 mEq)/dropperful dose

Pharmacodynamics/Kinetics
Absorption: Oral: Variable but better with salt forms than with base form; 18% to 45%; ethylsuccinate may be better absorbed with food
Distribution:
Relative diffusion from blood into CSF: Minimal even with inflammation
CSF:blood level ratio: Normal meninges: 2% to 13%; Inflamed meninges: 7% to 25%
Protein binding: Base: 73% to 81%
Metabolism: Demethylation primarily via hepatic CYP3A4
Half-life elimination: Peak: 1.5-2 hours; End-stage renal disease: 5-6 hours
Time to peak, serum: Base: 4 hours; Ethylsuccinate: 0.5-2.5 hours; delayed with food due to differences in absorption
Excretion: Primarily feces; urine (2% to 15% as unchanged drug)

Pregnancy Risk Factor B
Lactation Enters breast milk/use caution (AAP considers "compatible")
Breast-Feeding Considerations Erythromycin is excreted in breast milk. The manufacturer recommends that caution be exercised when administering erythromycin to nursing women. The American Academy of Pediatrics considers erythromycin to be "usually compatible with breast-feeding."

Due to the low concentrations in human milk, minimal toxicity would be expected in the nursing infant. One case report and a cohort study raise the possibility for a connection with pyloric stenosis in neonates exposed to erythromycin via breast milk and an alternative antibiotic may be preferred for breast-feeding mothers of infants in this age group. Nondose-related effects could include modification of bowel flora.

Based on available data, for neonates, erythromycin should be used with caution (high risk to neonates) while breast-feeding [human data]. For older infants, erythromycin is generally considered compatible (low risk to infant) while breast-feeding [human data].

Dosage Forms Excipient information presented when available (limited, particularly for generics); consult specific product labeling. [DSC] = Discontinued product; [CAN] = Canadian brand name
Note: Strength expressed as base
Capsule, delayed release, enteric-coated pellets, as base: 250 mg
Eryc®: 250 mg [DSC]
Gel, topical: 2% (30 g, 60 g)
Erygel®: 2% (30 g, 60 g) [contains alcohol 92%]
Granules for oral suspension, as ethylsuccinate:
E.E.S.®: 200 mg/5 mL (100 mL, 200 mL) [contains sodium 25.9 mg (1.1 mEq)/5 mL; cherry flavor]
Injection, powder for reconstitution, as lactobionate:
Erythrocin®: 500 mg, 1 g
Ointment, ophthalmic: 0.5% [5 mg/g] (1 g, 3.5 g)
Romycin®: 0.5% [5 mg/g] (3.5 g)
Ointment, topical:
Akne-Mycin®: 2% (25 g)
Powder for oral suspension, as ethylsuccinate:
EryPed®: 200 mg/5 mL (100 mL, 200 mL) [contains sodium 117.5 mg (5.1 mEq)/5 mL; fruit flavor]; 400 mg/5 mL (100 mL, 200 mL) [contains sodium 117.5 mg (5.1 mEq)/5 mL; banana flavor]
Powder for oral suspension, as ethylsuccinate [drops]:
EryPed®: 100 mg/2.5 mL (50 mL) [contains sodium 58.8 mg (2.6 mEq)/dropperful; fruit flavor]
Solution, topical: 2% (60 mL)
Eryderm®: 2% (60 mL) [contain alcohol]
(Continued)

Erythromycin *(Continued)*

Sans acne [CAN]: 2% (60 mL) [contains ethyl alcohol 44%; not available in U.S.]

Suspension, oral, as ethylsuccinate: 200 mg/5 mL (480 mL); 400 mg/5 mL (480 mL)

E.E.S.®: 200 mg/5 mL (100 mL, 480 mL) [fruit flavor]; 400 mg/5 mL (100 mL, 480 mL) [orange flavor]

Tablet, as base: 250 mg, 500 mg

Tablet, as base [polymer-coated particles]:

PCE®: 333 mg, 500 mg

Tablet, as ethylsuccinate: 400 mg

E.E.S.®: 400 mg

Tablet, as stearate: 250 mg, 500 mg

Erythrocin®: 250 mg, 500 mg

Tablet, delayed release, enteric coated, as base:

Ery-Tab®: 250 mg, 333 mg, 500 mg

Dental Comment Erythromycin is known to prolong the QT interval. The QT interval is measured as the time and distance between the Q point of the QRS complex and the end of the T wave in the ECG tracing. After adjustment for heart rate, the QT interval is defined as prolonged if it is more than 450 msec in men and 460 msec in women. A long QT syndrome was first described in the 1950s and 60s as a congenital syndrome involving QT interval prolongation and syncope and sudden death. Some of the congenital long QT syndromes were characterized by a peculiar electrocardiographic appearance of the QRS complex involving a premature atria beat followed by a pause, then a subsequent sinus beat showing marked QT prolongation and deformity. This type of cardiac arrhythmia was originally termed "torsade de pointes" (translated from the French as "twisting of the points").

Prolongation of the QT interval is thought to result from delayed ventricular repolarization. The repolarization process within the myocardial cell is due to the efflux of intracellular potassium. The channels associated with this current can be blocked by many drugs and predispose the electrical propagation cycle to torsade de pointes.

Erythromycin is considered as having a risk of causing torsade de pointes. The risk of drug-induced torsade de pointes is extremely low when a single QT interval prolonging drug is prescribed. It is not known what effect vasoconstrictors in the local anesthetic regimen may have in patients with a known history of congenital prolonged QT interval or in patients taking any medication that prolongs the QT interval. Until more information is obtained, it is suggested that the clinician consult with the physician prior to the use of a vasoconstrictor in suspected patients, and that the vasoconstrictor (epinephrine, levonordefrin [Neo-Cobefrin®]) be used with caution.

Many patients cannot tolerate erythromycin because of abdominal pain and nausea; the mechanism of this adverse effect appears to be the motilin agonistic properties of erythromycin in the GI tract. For these patients, clindamycin is indicated as the alternative antibiotic for treatment of orofacial infections.

HMG-CoA reductase inhibitors, also known as the statins, effectively decrease the hepatic cholesterol biosynthesis resulting in the reduction of blood LDL-cholesterol concentrations. The AUC of atorvastatin (Lipitor®) was increased 33% by erythromycin administration. Combination of erythromycin and lovastatin (Mevacor®) has been associated with rhabdomyolysis (Ayanian, et al). The mechanism of erythromycin is inhibiting the CYP3A4 metabolism of atorvastatin, lovastatin, and cerivastatin. Simvastatin (Zocor®) would likely be affected in a similar manner by the coadministration of erythromycin. Clarithromycin (Biaxin®) may exert a similar effect as erythromycin on atorvastatin, lovastatin, cerivastatin, and simvastatin. Erythromycin 3 times/day had no effect on pravastatin (Pravachol®) plasma concentrations (Bottorff, et al).

Selected Readings

American Dental Association Council on Scientific Affairs, "Combating Antibiotic Resistance," *J Am Dent Assoc*, 2004, 135(4):484-7.

Ayanian JZ, Fuchs CS, and Stone RM, "Lovastatin and Rhabdomyolysis," *Ann Intern Med*, 1988, 109(8):682-3.

"Pimozide (Orap) Contraindicated With Clarithromycin (Biaxin®) and Other Macrolide Antibiotics," *FDA Medical Bulletin*, October 1996, 26(3).

Wynn RL and Bergman SA, "Antibiotics and Their Use in the Treatment of Orofacial Infections, Part I," *Gen Dent*, 1994, 42(5):398, 400, 402.

Wynn RL and Bergman SA, "Antibiotics and Their Use in the Treatment of Orofacial Infections, Part II," *Gen Dent*, 1994, 42(6):498-502.

Wynn RL, "Current Concepts of the Erythromycins," *Gen Dent*, 1991, 39(6):408,10-1.

Erythromycin and Benzoyl Peroxide
(er ith roe MYE sin & BEN zoe il per OKS ide)

Related Information
Benzoyl Peroxide *on page 200*
Erythromycin *on page 589*
U.S. Brand Names Benzamycin®; Benzamycin® Pak
Mexican Brand Names Benzamycin
Generic Available Yes
Index Terms Benzoyl Peroxide and Erythromycin
Pharmacologic Category Acne Products; Topical Skin Product, Acne
Use Topical control of acne vulgaris
Local Anesthetic/Vasoconstrictor Precautions No information available to require special precautions
Effects on Dental Treatment No significant effects or complications reported
Drug Interactions
Cytochrome P450 Effect: Erythromycin: **Substrate** of CYP2B6 (minor), 3A4 (major); **Inhibits** CYP1A2 (weak), 3A4 (moderate)
Pharmacodynamics/Kinetics See individual agents.
Pregnancy Risk Factor C

Erythromycin and Sulfisoxazole
(er ith roe MYE sin & sul fi SOKS a zole)

Related Information
Erythromycin *on page 589*
SulfiSOXAZOLE *on page 1508*
U.S. Brand Names Pediazole® [DSC]
Canadian Brand Names Pediazole®
Generic Available Yes
Index Terms Sulfisoxazole and Erythromycin
Pharmacologic Category Antibiotic, Macrolide; Antibiotic, Macrolide Combination; Antibiotic, Sulfonamide Derivative
Use Treatment of susceptible bacterial infections of the upper and lower respiratory tract, otitis media in children caused by susceptible strains of *Haemophilus influenzae*, and many other infections in patients allergic to penicillin
Local Anesthetic/Vasoconstrictor Precautions No information available to require special precautions
Effects on Dental Treatment Key adverse event(s) related to dental treatment: Oral candidiasis.
Common Adverse Effects Frequency not defined.
Cardiovascular: Ventricular arrhythmia,
Central nervous system: Headache, fever
Dermatologic: Rash, Stevens-Johnson syndrome, toxic epidermal necrolysis
Gastrointestinal: Abdominal pain, cramping, nausea, vomiting, oral candidiasis, hypertrophic pyloric stenosis, diarrhea, pseudomembranous colitis
Hematologic: Agranulocytosis, aplastic anemia, eosinophilia
Hepatic: Hepatic necrosis, cholestatic jaundice
Local: Phlebitis at the injection site, thrombophlebitis
Renal: Toxic nephrosis, crystalluria
Miscellaneous: Hypersensitivity reactions
Mechanism of Action Erythromycin inhibits bacterial protein synthesis; sulfisoxazole competitively inhibits bacterial synthesis of folic acid from para-aminobenzoic acid
Drug Interactions
Cytochrome P450 Effect:
Erythromycin: **Substrate** of CYP2B6 (minor), 3A4 (major); **Inhibits** CYP1A2 (weak), 3A4 (moderate)
Sulfisoxazole: **Substrate** of CYP2C8/9 (major); **Inhibits** CYP2C8/9 (strong)
Increased Effect/Toxicity: See individual agents.
Decreased Effect: See individual agents.
Pharmacodynamics/Kinetics See individual agents.
Pregnancy Risk Factor C

Erythropoiesis-Stimulating Protein *see Darbepoetin Alfa on page 444*
Erythropoietin *see Epoetin Alfa on page 578*

Escitalopram (es sye TAL oh pram)

Related Information
Citalopram *on page 367*

U.S. Brand Names Lexapro®

Canadian Brand Names Cipralex®

Generic Available No

Index Terms Escitalopram Oxalate; Lu-26-054; S-Citalopram

Pharmacologic Category Antidepressant, Selective Serotonin Reuptake Inhibitor

Use Treatment of major depressive disorder; generalized anxiety disorders (GAD)

Local Anesthetic/Vasoconstrictor Precautions Although caution should be used in patients taking tricyclic antidepressants, no interactions have been reported with vasoconstrictors and escitalopram, a nontricyclic antidepressant which acts to increase serotonin; no precautions appear to be needed

Effects on Dental Treatment Key adverse event(s) related to dental treatment: Xerostomia (normal salivary flow resumes upon discontinuation) and toothache

Common Adverse Effects

>10%:
  Central nervous system: Headache (24%), somnolence (6% to 13%), insomnia (9% to 12%)
  Gastrointestinal: Nausea (15%)
  Genitourinary: Ejaculation disorder (9% to 14%)

1% to 10%:
  Cardiovascular: Chest pain, hypertension, palpitation
  Central nervous system: Dizziness (5%), fatigue (5% to 8%), dreaming abnormal, concentration impaired, fever, irritability, lethargy, lightheadedness, migraine, vertigo, yawning
  Dermatologic: Rash
  Endocrine & metabolic: Libido decreased (3% to 7%), anorgasmia (2% to 6%), hot flashes, menstrual cramps, menstrual disorder
  Gastrointestinal: Diarrhea (8%), xerostomia (6% to 9%), appetite decreased (3%), constipation (3% to 5%), indigestion (3%), abdominal pain (2%), abdominal cramps, appetite increased, flatulence, gastroenteritis, gastroesophageal reflux, heartburn, toothache, vomiting, weight gain/loss
  Genitourinary: Impotence (3%), urinary tract infection, urinary frequency
  Neuromuscular & skeletal: Arthralgia, limb pain, muscle cramp, myalgia, neck/shoulder pain, paresthesia, tremor
  Ocular: Blurred vision
  Otic: Earache, tinnitus
  Respiratory: Rhinitis (5%), sinusitis (3%), bronchitis, cough, nasal or sinus congestion, sinus headache
  Miscellaneous: Diaphoresis (4% to 5%), flu-like syndrome (5%), allergy

Restrictions An FDA-approved medication guide concerning the use of antidepressants in children, adolescents, and young adults must be distributed when dispensing an outpatient prescription (new or refill) where this medication is to be used without direct supervision of a healthcare provider. Medication guides are available at http://www.fda.gov/cder/Offices/ODS/medication_guides.htm. Dispense to parents or guardians of children and adolescents receiving this medication.

Dosage Oral:
  Adults: Depression, GAD: Initial: 10 mg/day; dose may be increased to 20 mg/day after at least 1 week
  Elderly: 10 mg/day; bioavailability and half-life are increased by 50% in the elderly
  Dosage adjustment in renal impairment:
    Mild-to-moderate impairment: No dosage adjustment needed
    Severe impairment: Cl$_{cr}$ <20 mL/minute: Use caution
  Dosage adjustment in hepatic impairment: 10 mg/day

Mechanism of Action Escitalopram is the S-enantiomer of the racemic derivative citalopram, which selectively inhibits the reuptake of serotonin with little to no effect on norepinephrine or dopamine reuptake. It has no or very low affinity for 5-HT$_{1-7}$, alpha- and beta-adrenergic, D$_{1-5}$, H$_{1-3}$, M$_{1-5}$, and benzodiazepine receptors. Escitalopram does not bind or has low affinity for Na$^+$, K$^+$, Cl$^-$, and Ca^{++} ion channels.

Contraindications Hypersensitivity to escitalopram, citalopram, or any component of the formulation; concomitant use or within 2 weeks of MAO inhibitors

Warnings/Precautions [U.S. Boxed Warning]: **Antidepressants increase the risk of suicidal thinking and behavior in children, adolescents, and young adults (18-24 years of age) with major depressive disorder (MDD) and other psychiatric disorders;** consider risk prior to prescribing. Short-term studies did not show an increased risk in patients >24 years of age and showed a decreased risk in patients ≥65 years. Closely monitor patients for clinical worsening, suicidality, or unusual changes in behavior, particularly during the initial 1-2 months of therapy or during periods of dosage adjustments (increases or decreases); the patient's family or caregiver should be instructed to closely observe the patient and communicate condition with healthcare provider. A medication guide concerning the use of antidepressants should be dispensed with each prescription. **Escitalopram is not FDA approved for use in children.**

The possibility of a suicide attempt is inherent in major depression and may persist until remission occurs. Use caution in high-risk patients. Worsening depression and severe abrupt suicidality that are not part of the presenting symptoms may require discontinuation or modification of drug therapy. The patient's family or caregiver should be alerted to monitor patients for the emergence of suicidality and associated behaviors (such as agitation, irritability, hostility, impulsivity, and hypomania) and call healthcare provider.

May worsen psychosis in some patients or precipitate a shift to mania or hypomania in patients with bipolar disorder. Patients presenting with depressive symptoms should be screened for bipolar disorder. Monotherapy in patients with bipolar disorder should be avoided. Escitalopram is not FDA approved for the treatment of bipolar depression.

The potential for a severe reaction exists when used with MAO inhibitors, SSRIs/SNRIs or triptans; serotonin syndrome (hyperthermia, muscular rigidity, mental status changes/agitation, autonomic instability) may occur. Concurrent use with MAO inhibitors is contraindicated. May increase the risks associated with electroconvulsive therapy. Has a low potential to impair cognitive or motor performance; caution operating hazardous machinery or driving.

Use caution with a previous seizure disorder or condition predisposing to seizures such as brain damage, alcoholism, or concurrent therapy with other drugs which lower the seizure threshold. May cause hyponatremia/SIADH. May cause or exacerbate sexual dysfunction. Use caution with renal or liver impairment; concomitant CNS depressants; pregnancy (high doses of citalopram has been associated with teratogenicity in animals). Use caution with concomitant use of NSAIDs, ASA, or other drugs that affect coagulation; the risk of bleeding is potentiated.

Upon discontinuation of escitalopram therapy, gradually taper dose. If intolerable symptoms occur following a decrease in dosage or upon discontinuation of therapy, then resuming the previous dose with a more gradual taper should be considered.

Drug Interactions

Cytochrome P450 Effect: Substrate (major) of CYP2C19, 3A4; **Inhibits** CYP2D6 (weak)

Increased Effect/Toxicity: Escitalopram should not be used with nonselective MAO inhibitors (phenelzine, isocarboxazid) or other drugs with MAO inhibition (linezolid); fatal reactions have been reported. Wait 2 weeks after stopping an MAO inhibitor before starting escitalopram. Concurrent selegiline has been associated with mania, hypertension, or serotonin syndrome (risk may be reduced relative to nonselective MAO inhibitors).

CYP2C19 inhibitors may increase the levels/effects of imipramine; example inhibitors include delavirdine, fluconazole, fluvoxamine, gemfibrozil, isoniazid, omeprazole, and ticlopidine. CYP3A4 inhibitors may increase the levels/effects of escitalopram; example inhibitors include azole antifungals, clarithromycin, diclofenac, doxycycline, erythromycin, imatinib, isoniazid, nefazodone, nicardipine, propofol, protease inhibitors, quinidine, telithromycin, and verapamil.

Combined use of SSRIs and buspirone, meperidine, moclobemide, nefazodone, other SSRIs/SNRIs, tramadol, trazodone, triptans and venlafaxine may increase the risk of serotonin syndrome. Escitalopram increases serum levels/effects of CYP2D6 substrates (tricyclic antidepressants). Escitalopram may increase desipramine levels.

Combined use of sumatriptan (and other serotonin agonists) may result in toxicity; weakness, hyper-reflexia, and incoordination have been observed with sumatriptan and SSRIs. In addition, concurrent use may theoretically increase the risk of serotonin syndrome; includes sumatriptan, naratriptan, rizatriptan, and zolmitriptan.

(Continued)

Escitalopram *(Continued)*

Concomitant use of escitalopram and NSAIDs, aspirin, or other drugs affecting coagulation has been associated with an increased risk of bleeding; monitor.

Decreased Effect: CYP2C19 inducers may decrease the levels/effects of imipramine; example inducers include aminoglutethimide, carbamazepine, phenytoin, and rifampin. CYP3A4 inducers may decrease the levels/effects of escitalopram; example inducers include aminoglutethimide, carbamazepine, nafcillin, nevirapine, phenobarbital, phenytoin, and rifamycins.

Ethanol/Nutrition/Herb Interactions

Ethanol: Avoid ethanol (may increase CNS depression).

Herb/Nutraceutical: Avoid valerian, St John's wort, SAMe, kava kava, and gotu kola (may increase CNS depression).

Dietary Considerations May be taken with or without food.

Pharmacodynamics/Kinetics

Protein binding: 56% to plasma proteins

Metabolism: Hepatic via CYP2C19 and 3A4 to an active metabolite, S-desmethylcitalopram (S-DCT; 1/7 the activity); S-DCT is metabolized to S-didesmethylcitalopram (S-DDCT; active; 1/27 the activity) via CYP2D6

Half-life elimination: Escitalopram: 27-32 hours; S-desmethylcitalopram: 59 hours

Time to peak: Escitalopram: 5 ± 1.5 hours; S-desmethylcitalopram: 14 hours

Excretion: Urine (Escitalopram: 8%; S-DCT: 10%)

Clearance: Total body: 37-40 L/hour; Renal: Escitalopram: 2.7 L/hour; S-desmethylcitalopram: 6.9 L/hour

Pregnancy Risk Factor C

Dosage Forms

Solution, oral:

Lexapro®: 1 mg/mL

Tablet:

Lexapro®: 5 mg, 10 mg, 20 mg

Note: Cipralex® [CAN] is available only in 10 mg and 20 mg strengths.

Esmolol *(ES moe lol)*

U.S. Brand Names Brevibloc®

Canadian Brand Names Brevibloc®

Mexican Brand Names Brevibloc

Generic Available Yes: Excludes infusion

Index Terms Esmolol Hydrochloride

Pharmacologic Category Antiarrhythmic Agent, Class II; Beta Blocker, Beta₁ Selective

Use Treatment of supraventricular tachycardia (SVT) and atrial fibrillation/flutter (control ventricular rate); treatment of tachycardia and/or hypertension (especially intraoperative or postoperative); treatment of noncompensatory sinus tachycardia

Unlabeled/Investigational Use In children, for SVT and postoperative hypertension

Local Anesthetic/Vasoconstrictor Precautions No information available to require special precautions

Effects on Dental Treatment Esmolol is a cardioselective beta-blocker. Local anesthetic with vasoconstrictor can be safely used in patients medicated with esmolol. Nonselective beta-blockers (ie, propranolol, nadolol) enhance the pressor response to epinephrine, resulting in hypertension and bradycardia; this has not been reported for esmolol. Many nonsteroidal anti-inflammatory drugs, such as ibuprofen and indomethacin, can reduce the hypotensive effect of beta-blockers after 3 or more weeks of therapy with the NSAID. Short-term NSAID use (ie, 3 days) requires no special precautions in patients taking beta-blockers.

Common Adverse Effects

>10%:

Cardiovascular: Asymptomatic hypotension (dose related: 25% to 38%), symptomatic hypotension (dose related: 12%)

Miscellaneous: Diaphoresis (10%)
1% to 10%:
Cardiovascular: Peripheral ischemia (1%)
Central nervous system: Dizziness (3%), somnolence (3%), confusion (2%), headache (2%), agitation (2%), fatigue (1%)
Gastrointestinal: Nausea (7%), vomiting (1%)
Local: Pain on injection (8%), infusion site reaction

Mechanism of Action Class II antiarrhythmic: Competitively blocks response to beta$_1$-adrenergic stimulation with little or no effect of beta$_2$-receptors except at high doses, no intrinsic sympathomimetic activity, no membrane stabilizing activity

Drug Interactions
Increased Effect/Toxicity: Anticholinesterase inhibitors, amiodarone, cardia glycosides dipyridamole (I.V.) increase bradycardia; beta-blockers increase alpha$_1$ blockers orthostasis, alpha-/beta-agonists (direct acting) vasopressor effects, alpha$_2$-agonists rebound hypertension when withdrawn. Beta-blockers may enhance the hypoglycemia and mask most symptoms of hypoglycemia in patients on insulin or sulfonylureas. Calcium channel blockers increase hypotension

Decreased Effect: Alpha$_2$-agonists decrease the effectiveness of beta-blockers (beta$_1$ selective). NSAIDs may diminish the antihypertensive effects of beta-blockers.

Pharmacodynamics/Kinetics
Onset of action: Beta-blockade: I.V.: 2-10 minutes (quickest when loading doses are administered)
Duration of hemodynamic effects: 10-30 minutes; prolonged following higher cumulative doses, extended duration of use
Protein binding: 55%
Metabolism: In blood by red blood cell esterases
Half-life elimination: Adults: 9 minutes; elimination of metabolite decreases with end stage renal disease
Excretion: Urine (~69% as metabolites, 2% unchanged drug)

Pregnancy Risk Factor C (manufacturer); D (2nd and 3rd trimesters - expert analysis)

Esmolol Hydrochloride *see* Esmolol *on page 598*

Esomeprazole (es oh ME pray zol)

Related Information
Omeprazole *on page 1206*
U.S. Brand Names Nexium®
Canadian Brand Names Nexium®
Mexican Brand Names Nexium; Nexium-MUPS
Generic Available No
Index Terms Esomeprazole Magnesium; Esomeprazole Sodium
Pharmacologic Category Proton Pump Inhibitor; Substituted Benzimidazole
Use
Oral: Short-term (4-8 weeks) treatment of erosive esophagitis; maintaining symptom resolution and healing of erosive esophagitis; treatment of symptomatic gastroesophageal reflux disease (GERD); as part of a multidrug regimen for *Helicobacter pylori* eradication in patients with duodenal ulcer disease (active or history of within the past 5 years); prevention of gastric ulcers in patients at risk (age ≥60 years and/or history of gastric ulcer) associated with continuous NSAID therapy; long-term treatment of pathological hypersecretory conditions including Zollinger-Ellison syndrome
I.V.: Short-term (≤10 days) treatment of gastroesophageal reflux disease (GERD) when oral therapy is not possible or appropriate

Local Anesthetic/Vasoconstrictor Precautions No information available to require special precautions

Effects on Dental Treatment Key adverse event(s) related to dental treatment: Xerostomia (normal salivary flow resumes upon discontinuation)

Common Adverse Effects Unless otherwise specified, percentages represent adverse reactions identified in clinical trials evaluating the intravenous formulation.

>10%: Central nervous system: Headache (I.V. 11%; oral 4% to 8%)
1% to 10%:
Central nervous system: Dizziness (3%)
Dermatologic: Pruritus (≤1%)
Gastrointestinal: Flatulence (10%), nausea (I.V. 6%; oral 2%), abdominal pain (6%; oral 3% to 4%), diarrhea (4%), xerostomia (I.V. 4%; oral ≥1%), dyspepsia (<1% to 6%), constipation (3%)
(Continued)

Esomeprazole *(Continued)*

Local: Injection site reaction (2%)
Respiratory: Sinusitis (I.V. 2%; oral <1%), respiratory infection (1%)

Dosage

Adolescents 12-17 years: Oral: GERD: 20-40 mg once daily for up to 8 weeks
Adults:
Oral:
Erosive esophagitis (healing): Initial: 20-40 mg once daily for 4-8 weeks; if incomplete healing, may continue for an additional 4-8 weeks; maintenance: 20 mg once daily

Symptomatic GERD: 20 mg once daily for 4 weeks; may continue an additional 4 weeks if symptoms persist

Helicobacter pylori eradication: 40 mg once daily for 10 days; requires combination therapy

Prevention of NSAID-induced gastric ulcers: 20-40 mg once daily for up to 6 months

Pathological hypersecretory conditions (Zollinger-Ellison syndrome): 40 mg twice daily; adjust regimen to individual patient needs; doses up to 240 mg/day have been administered

I.V.: GERD: 20 mg or 40 mg once daily for ≤10 days; change to oral therapy as soon as appropriate

Elderly: No dosage adjustment needed.

Dosage adjustment in renal impairment: No dosage adjustment needed

Dosage adjustment in hepatic impairment:
Mild-to-moderate hepatic impairment (Child-Pugh Class A or B): No dosage adjustment needed
Severe hepatic impairment (Child-Pugh Class C): Dose should not exceed 20 mg/day

Mechanism of Action Proton pump inhibitor suppresses gastric acid secretion by inhibition of the H$^+$/K$^+$-ATPase in the gastric parietal cell

Contraindications Hypersensitivity to esomeprazole, substituted benzimidazoles (ie, lansoprazole, omeprazole, pantoprazole, rabeprazole), or any component of the formulation

Warnings/Precautions Relief of symptoms does not preclude the presence of a gastric malignancy. Atrophic gastritis (by biopsy) has been noted with long-term omeprazole therapy; this may also occur with esomeprazole. No reports of enterochromaffin-like (ECL) cell carcinoids, dysplasia, or neoplasia have occurred. Severe liver dysfunction may require dosage reductions. Safety and efficacy in children <12 years of age have not been established.

Drug Interactions

Cytochrome P450 Effect: Substrate of CYP2C19 (major), 3A4 (minor); **Inhibits** CYP2C19 (moderate)

Increased Effect/Toxicity: Esomeprazole and omeprazole may increase the levels of carbamazepine, HMG-CoA reductase inhibitors, methotrexate, and CYP2C19 substrates, including benzodiazepines metabolized by oxidation (eg, diazepam, midazolam, triazolam)

Decreased Effect: CYP2C19 inducers may decrease the levels/effects of esomeprazole; example inducers include aminoglutethimide, carbamazepine, phenytoin, and rifampin. Proton pump inhibitors may decrease the absorption of atazanavir, indinavir, iron salts, itraconazole, and ketoconazole.

Ethanol/Nutrition/Herb Interactions Food: Absorption is decreased by 43% to 53% when taken with food.

Dietary Considerations Take at least 1 hour before meals; best if taken before breakfast. The contents of the capsule may be mixed in applesauce or water; pellets also remain intact when exposed to orange juice, apple juice, and yogurt.

Pharmacodynamics/Kinetics

Distribution: V_{dss}: 16 L
Protein binding: 97%
Metabolism: Hepatic via CYP2C19 and 3A4 enzymes to hydroxy, desmethyl, and sulfone metabolites (all inactive)
Bioavailability: 90% with repeat dosing
Half-life elimination: 1-1.5 hours
Time to peak: 1.5 hours
Excretion: Urine (80%, primarily as inactive metabolites); feces (20%)

Pregnancy Risk Factor B

Dosage Forms Note: Strength expressed as base
Capsule, delayed release:
Nexium®: 20 mg, 40 mg
Granules, for oral suspension, delayed release, as magnesium:
Nexium®: 20 mg, 40 mg
Injection, powder for reconstitution:
Nexium®: 20 mg, 40 mg

Esomeprazole Magnesium *see* Esomeprazole *on page 599*
Esomeprazole Sodium *see* Esomeprazole *on page 599*
Esopho-Cat® *see* Barium *on page 185*
Esoterica® Regular [OTC] *see* Hydroquinone *on page 841*
Especol® [OTC] *see* Fructose, Dextrose, and Phosphoric Acid *on page 754*

Estazolam (es TA zoe lam)

U.S. Brand Names ProSom®
Mexican Brand Names Tasedan
Generic Available Yes
Pharmacologic Category Benzodiazepine
Use Short-term management of insomnia

Local Anesthetic/Vasoconstrictor Precautions No information available to require special precautions

Effects on Dental Treatment Key adverse event(s) related to dental treatment: Significant xerostomia (normal salivary flow resumes upon discontinuation)

Common Adverse Effects
>10%:
Central nervous system: Somnolence
Neuromuscular & skeletal: Weakness
1% to 10%:
Cardiovascular: Flushing, palpitation
Central nervous system: Anxiety, confusion, dizziness, hypokinesia, abnormal coordination, hangover effect, agitation, amnesia, apathy, emotional lability, euphoria, hostility, seizure, sleep disorder, stupor, twitch
Dermatologic: Dermatitis, pruritus, rash, urticaria
Gastrointestinal: Xerostomia, constipation, appetite increased/decreased, flatulence, gastritis, perverse taste
Genitourinary: Frequent urination, menstrual cramps, urinary hesitancy, urinary frequency, vaginal discharge/itching
Neuromuscular & skeletal: Paresthesia
Ocular: Photophobia, eye pain, eye swelling
Respiratory: Cough, dyspnea, asthma, rhinitis, sinusitis
Miscellaneous: Diaphoresis

Restrictions C-IV

Mechanism of Action Binds to stereospecific benzodiazepine receptors on the postsynaptic GABA neuron at several sites within the central nervous system, including the limbic system, reticular formation. Enhancement of the inhibitory effect of GABA on neuronal excitability results by increased neuronal membrane permeability to chloride ions. This shift in chloride ions results in hyperpolarization (a less excitable state) and stabilization.

Drug Interactions
Cytochrome P450 Effect: Substrate of CYP3A4 (minor)
Increased Effect/Toxicity: Sedative effects and/or respiratory depression may be additive with CNS depressants; includes ethanol, barbiturates, opioid analgesics, and other sedative agents; monitor for increased effect. Levodopa therapeutic effects may be diminished in some patients following the addition of a benzodiazepine; limited/inconsistent data. Oral contraceptives may decrease the clearance of some benzodiazepines (those which undergo oxidative metabolism); monitor for increased benzodiazepine effect. Theophylline may partially antagonize some of the effects of benzodiazepines; monitor for decreased response; may require higher doses for sedation. Concurrent use with itraconazole or ketoconazole is contraindicated (per manufacturer); however, estazolam is a minor CYP3A4 substrate and an effect has not been documented in clinical studies.

Pharmacodynamics/Kinetics
Onset of action: ~1 hour
Duration: Variable
Metabolism: Extensively hepatic
Half-life elimination: 10-24 hours (no significant changes in elderly)
Time to peak, serum: 0.5-1.6 hours
Excretion: Urine (<5% as unchanged drug)

Pregnancy Risk Factor X

Ester-E™ [OTC] *see* Vitamin E *on page 1664*
Esterified Estrogen and Methyltestosterone *see* Estrogens (Esterified) and Methyltestosterone *on page 614*
Esterified Estrogens *see* Estrogens (Esterified) *on page 613*
Estrace® *see* Estradiol *on page 602*
Estraderm® *see* Estradiol *on page 602*

Estradiol (es tra DYE ole)

Related Information
Endocrine Disorders and Pregnancy *on page 1750*
Rheumatoid Arthritis, Osteoarthritis, and Osteoporosis *on page 1759*

U.S. Brand Names Alora®; Climara®; Delestrogen®; Depo®-Estradiol; Elestrin™; Esclim®; Estrace®; Estraderm®; Estrasorb™; Estring®; EstroGel®; Femring®; Femtrace®; Gynodiol®; Menostar™; Vagifem®; Vivelle®; Vivelle-Dot®

Canadian Brand Names Climara®; Depo®-Estradiol; Estrace®; Estraderm®; Estradot®; Estring®; EstroGel®; Menostar™; Oesclim®; Sandoz-Estradiol Derm 50; Sandoz-Estradiol Derm 75; Sandoz-Estradiol Derm 100; Vagifem®

Mexican Brand Names Climaderm; Evorel; Ginedisc; Oestrogel; Sandrena; Systen

Generic Available Yes: Oral tablet, patch

Index Terms Estradiol Acetate; Estradiol Cypionate; Estradiol Hemihydrate; Estradiol Transdermal; Estradiol Valerate

Pharmacologic Category Estrogen Derivative

Use Treatment of moderate-to-severe vasomotor symptoms associated with menopause; treatment of vulvar and vaginal atrophy; hypoestrogenism (due to hypogonadism, castration, or primary ovarian failure); prostatic cancer (palliation), breast cancer (palliation), osteoporosis (prophylaxis); abnormal uterine bleeding due to hormonal imbalance; postmenopausal urogenital symptoms of the lower urinary tract (urinary urgency, dysuria)

Local Anesthetic/Vasoconstrictor Precautions No information available to require special precautions

Effects on Dental Treatment No significant effects or complications reported

Common Adverse Effects Frequency not defined. Some adverse reactions observed with estrogen and/or progestin combination therapy.

Cardiovascular: DVT, edema, hypertension, MI, stroke, venous thromboembolism

Central nervous system: Anxiety, dementia, dizziness, epilepsy exacerbation, headache, irritability, mental depression, migraine, mood disturbances, nervousness

Dermatologic: Angioedema, chloasma, erythema multiforme, erythema nodosum, hemorrhagic eruption, hirsutism, loss of scalp hair, melasma, rash, pruritus, urticaria

Endocrine & metabolic: Breast cancer, breast enlargement, breast pain, breast tenderness, fibrocystic breast changes, HDL-cholesterol increased, galactorrhea, glucose intolerance, hypocalcemia, LDL-cholesterol decreased, libido changes, nipple pain, serum triglycerides/phospholipids increased, thyroid-binding globulin increased, total thyroid hormone (T_4) increased, vaginal discharge, vaginitis

Gastrointestinal: Abdominal cramps, abdominal distension, abdominal pain, bloating, cholecystitis, cholelithiasis, diarrhea, flatulence, gallbladder disease, nausea, pancreatitis, vomiting, weight gain/loss

Genitourinary: Alterations in frequency and flow of menses, cervical secretion changes, endometrial cancer, endometrial hyperplasia, ovarian cancer, Pap smear suspicious, urinary tract infection, uterine leiomyomata size increased, uterine pain, vaginal candidiasis

Vaginal: Trauma from applicator insertion may occur in women with severely atrophic vaginal mucosa

Hematologic: Aggravation of porphyria, antithrombin III and antifactor Xa decreased, fibrinogen levels increased, platelet aggregability increased, platelet count increased, prothrombin increased; factors VII, VIII, IX, X increased

Hepatic: Cholestatic jaundice, hepatic hemangioma enlargement

Local: Thrombophlebitis
Transdermal patches: Burning, erythema, irritation

Neuromuscular & skeletal: Arthralgia, back pain, chorea, leg cramps

Ocular: Contact lens intolerance, corneal curvature steepening, retinal vascular thrombosis

Respiratory: Asthma exacerbation, pulmonary thromboembolism

Miscellaneous: Anaphylactoid/anaphylactic reactions

Mechanism of Action Estrogens are responsible for the development and maintenance of the female reproductive system and secondary sexual characteristics. Estradiol is the principle intracellular human estrogen and is more potent than estrone and estriol at the receptor level; it is the primary estrogen secreted prior to menopause. Following menopause, estrone and estrone sulfate are more highly produced. Estrogens modulate the pituitary secretion of gonadotropins, luteinizing hormone, and follicle-stimulating hormone through a negative feedback system; estrogen replacement reduces elevated levels of these hormones in postmenopausal women.

Drug Interactions

Cytochrome P450 Effect: Substrate of CYP1A2 (major), 2A6 (minor), 2B6 (minor), 2C9 (minor), 2C19 (minor), 2D6 (minor), 2E1 (minor), 3A4 (major); **Inhibits** CYP1A2 (weak), 2C8 (weak); **Induces** CYP3A4 (weak)

Increased Effect/Toxicity: Estradiol with hydrocortisone increases corticosteroid toxic potential. Anticoagulants and estradiol increase the potential for thromboembolic events. Estrogen derivatives may enhance the hepatotoxic effect of cyclosporine. Estrogen derivatives may increase the serum concentration of cyclosporine.

Decreased Effect: CYP1A2 inducers may decrease the levels/effects of estradiol; example inducers include aminoglutethimide, carbamazepine, phenobarbital, and rifampin. CYP3A4 inducers may decrease the levels/effects of estradiol; example inducers include aminoglutethimide, carbamazepine, nafcillin, nevirapine, phenobarbital, phenytoin, and rifamycins. Estrogen derivatives may diminish the therapeutic effect of thyroid products.

Pharmacodynamics/Kinetics

Absorption: Oral, topical: Well absorbed

Protein binding: 37% to sex hormone-binding globulin; 61% to albumin

Metabolism: Hepatic via oxidation and conjugation in GI tract; hydroxylated via CYP3A4 to metabolites; first-pass effect; enterohepatic recirculation; reversibly converted to estrone and estriol

Excretion: Primarily urine (as metabolites estrone and estriol); feces (small amounts)

Pregnancy Risk Factor X

Estradiol Acetate *see* Estradiol *on page 602*

Estradiol and Drospirenone *see* Drospirenone and Estradiol *on page 547*

Estradiol and NGM *see* Estradiol and Norgestimate *on page 604*

Estradiol and Norethindrone (es tra DYE ole & nor eth IN drone)

Related Information

Estradiol *on page 602*

Norethindrone *on page 1186*

U.S. Brand Names Activella®; CombiPatch®

Canadian Brand Names Estalis®; Estalis-Sequi®

Generic Available No

Index Terms Norethindrone and Estradiol

Pharmacologic Category Estrogen and Progestin Combination

Use Women with an intact uterus:

Tablet: Treatment of moderate-to-severe vasomotor symptoms associated with menopause; treatment of vulvar and vaginal atrophy; prophylaxis for postmenopausal osteoporosis

Transdermal patch: Treatment of moderate-to-severe vasomotor symptoms associated with menopause; treatment of vulvar and vaginal atrophy; treatment of hypoestrogenism due to hypogonadism, castration, or primary ovarian failure

Local Anesthetic/Vasoconstrictor Precautions No information available to require special precautions

Effects on Dental Treatment No significant effects or complications reported

Common Adverse Effects Frequency not defined.

Cardiovascular: Altered blood pressure, cardiovascular accident, edema, MI, stroke, venous thromboembolism, thrombophlebitis

Central nervous system: Dementia, dizziness, emotional lability, fatigue, headache, insomnia, irritability, mental depression, migraine, mood changes, nervousness, seizures

Dermatologic: Chloasma, erythema multiforme, erythema nodosum, hemorrhagic eruption, hirsutism, itching, loss of scalp hair, melasma, pruritus, seborrhea, skin rash

Endocrine & metabolic: Breast cancer, breast enlargement, breast tenderness, breast pain, fibrocystic breast changes, galactorrhea, hypocalcemia, libido changes, nipple discharge, triglycerides increased

Gastrointestinal: Abdominal pain, bloating, changes in appetite, cramps, flatulence, gallbladder disease, gastroenteritis, nausea, pancreatitis, vomiting, weight gain/loss

Genitourinary: Alterations in frequency and flow of menses, changes in cervical secretions, cystitis-like syndrome, endometrial cancer, endometrial hyperplasia, endometrial thickening, endometriosis exacerbation, genital moniliasis, ovarian cancer, ovarian cyst, postmenopausal bleeding, premenstrual-like syndrome, size of uterine leiomyomata increased, uterine fibroid, vaginal candidiasis, vaginal hemorrhage, vaginitis

Hematologic: Aggravation of porphyria

Hepatic: Cholestatic jaundice

(Continued)

Estradiol and Norethindrone *(Continued)*

Local: Application site reaction (transdermal patch)

Neuromuscular & skeletal: Arthralgia, back pain, chorea, extremity pain, leg cramps, myalgia, weakness

Ocular: Contact lens intolerance, corneal curvature steepening, retinal vascular thrombosis

Respiratory: Asthma exacerbation, nasopharyngitis, pharyngitis, pulmonary thromboembolism, rhinitis, sinusitis, upper respiratory tract infection

Miscellaneous: Allergic reactions, carbohydrate intolerance, flu-like syndrome, viral infection

Drug Interactions

Cytochrome P450 Effect:

Estradiol: **Substrate** of CYP1A2 (major), 2A6 (minor), 2B6 (minor), 2C9 (minor), 2C19 (minor), 2D6 (minor), 2E1 (minor), 3A4 (major); **Inhibits** CYP1A2 (weak), 2C8 (weak); **Induces** CYP3A4 (weak)

Norethindrone: **Substrate** of CYP3A4 (major); **Induces** CYP2C19 (weak)

Pharmacodynamics/Kinetics

Activella®:

Bioavailability: Estradiol: 50%; Norethindrone: 100%

Half-life elimination: Estradiol: 12-14 hours; Norethindrone: 8-11 hours

Time to peak: Estradiol: 5-8 hours

See individual agents.

Estradiol and Norgestimate *(es tra DYE ole & nor JES ti mate)*

Related Information

Estradiol *on page 602*

U.S. Brand Names Prefest™

Generic Available No

Index Terms Estradiol and NGM; Norgestimate and Estradiol; Ortho Prefest

Pharmacologic Category Estrogen and Progestin Combination

Use Women with an intact uterus: Treatment of moderate to severe vasomotor symptoms associated with menopause; treatment of atrophic vaginitis; prevention of osteoporosis

Local Anesthetic/Vasoconstrictor Precautions No information available to require special precautions

Effects on Dental Treatment No significant effects or complications reported

Common Adverse Effects

>10%:

Central nervous system: Headache (23%)

Endocrine & metabolic: Breast pain (16%)

Gastrointestinal: Abdominal pain (12%)

Neuromuscular & skeletal: Back pain (12%)

Respiratory: Upper respiratory tract infection (21%)

Miscellaneous: Flu-like syndrome (11%)

1% to 10%:

Central nervous system: Fatigue (6%), pain (6%), depression (5%), dizziness (5%)

Endocrine & metabolic: Vaginal bleeding (9%), dysmenorrhea (8%), vaginitis (7%)

Gastrointestinal: Nausea (6%), flatulence (5%)

Neuromuscular & skeletal: Arthralgia (9%), myalgia (5%)

Respiratory: Sinusitis (8%), pharyngitis (7%), cough (5%)

Miscellaneous: Viral infection (6%)

Additional adverse effects associated with **estrogens and progestins**; frequency not defined:

Cardiovascular: Edema, hypertension, MI, stroke, venous thrombosis

Central nervous system: Anxiety, epilepsy exacerbation, insomnia, irritability, migraine, mood disturbances, nervousness, pyrexia, somnolence

Dermatologic: Acne, chloasma, erythema multiforme, erythema nodosum, hemorrhagic eruptions, hirsutism, itching, melasma, pruritus, rash, scalp hair loss, urticaria

Endocrine & metabolic: Amenorrhea, breast cancer, breast discharge, breast enlargement, Breast tenderness, carbohydrate tolerance decreased, endometrial cancer, endometrial hyperplasia, fibrocystic breast changes, galactorrhea, hypocalcemia, libido changes, ovarian cancer, triglycerides increased

Gastrointestinal: Abdominal cramps, appetite changes, bloating, gallbladder disease, pancreatitis, vomiting, weight gain/loss

Genitourinary: Abnormal withdrawal bleeding/flow, breakthrough bleeding, cervical secretion changes, cystitis syndrome, uterine leiomyomata size increased, vaginal candidiasis, vaginal bleeding/spotting

Hematologic: Anemia, porphyria

Hepatic: Cholestatic jaundice

Local: Thrombophlebitis

Neuromuscular & skeletal: Chorea

Ocular: Contact lens intolerance, corneal curvature steepening, neuro-ocular lesions

Respiratory: Asthma exacerbation, pulmonary embolism

Miscellaneous: Anaphylaxis

Mechanism of Action Estrogens are responsible for the development and maintenance of the female reproductive system and secondary sexual characteristics. Estradiol is the principle intracellular human estrogen and is more potent than estrone and estriol at the receptor level; it is the primary estrogen secreted prior to menopause. Following menopause, estrone and estrone sulfate are more highly produced. Estrogens modulate the pituitary secretion of gonadotropins, luteinizing hormone, and follicle-stimulating hormone through a negative feedback system; estrogen replacement reduces elevated levels of these hormones in postmenopausal women.

Progestins inhibit gonadotropin production which then prevents follicular maturation and ovulation. In women with adequate estrogen, progestins transform a proliferative endometrium into a secretory endometrium; when administered with estradiol, reduces the incidence of endometrial hyperplasia and risk of adenocarcinoma.

Drug Interactions

Cytochrome P450 Effect:

Estradiol: **Substrate** of CYP1A2 (major), 2A6 (minor), 2B6 (minor), 2C9 (minor), 2C19 (minor), 2D6 (minor), 2E1 (minor), 3A4 (major); **Inhibits** CYP1A2 (weak), 2C8 (weak); **Induces** CYP3A4 (weak)

Increased Effect/Toxicity: Acetaminophen and ascorbic acid may increase plasma levels of estrogen component. Atorvastatin and indinavir increase plasma levels of estrogen/progestin combinations. Estrogen/progestin combinations increase the plasma levels of alprazolam, chlordiazepoxide, cyclosporine, diazepam, prednisolone, selegiline, theophylline, tricyclic antidepressants. Estrogen/progestin combinations may increase (or decrease) the effects of coumarin derivatives.

Decreased Effect: Estrogen/progestin combinations may decrease plasma levels of acetaminophen, clofibric acid, lorazepam, morphine, oxazepam, salicylic acid, temazepam. Estrogen/progestin levels decreased by aminoglutethimide, amprenavir, anticonvulsants, griseofulvin, lopinavir, nelfinavir, nevirapine, rifampin, and ritonavir. Estrogen/progestin combinations may decrease (or increase) the effects of coumarin derivatives.

Pharmacodynamics/Kinetics

Estradiol: See Estradiol monograph.

Norgestimate:

Protein binding: 17-deacetylnorgestimate: 99%

Metabolism: Forms 17-deacetylnorgestimate (major active metabolite) and other metabolites; first-pass effect

Half-life elimination: 17-deacetylnorgestimate: 37 hours

Excretion: Norgestimate metabolites: Urine and feces

Pregnancy Risk Factor X

Estradiol Cypionate *see* Estradiol *on page 602*

Estradiol Hemihydrate *see* Estradiol *on page 602*

Estradiol Transdermal *see* Estradiol *on page 602*

Estradiol Valerate *see* Estradiol *on page 602*

Estramustine (es tra MUS teen)

U.S. Brand Names Emcyt®

Canadian Brand Names Emcyt®

Mexican Brand Names Emcyt

Generic Available No

Index Terms Estramustine Phosphate; Estramustine Phosphate Sodium; NSC-89199

Pharmacologic Category Antineoplastic Agent, Alkylating Agent; Antineoplastic Agent, Hormone; Antineoplastic Agent, Hormone (Estrogen/Nitrogen Mustard)

Use Palliative treatment of prostatic carcinoma (progressive or metastatic)

Local Anesthetic/Vasoconstrictor Precautions No information available to require special precautions

Effects on Dental Treatment No significant effects or complications reported

(Continued)

Estramustine *(Continued)*

Common Adverse Effects

>10%:

Cardiovascular: Edema (20%)

Endocrine & metabolic: Gynecomastia (75%), breast tenderness (71%), libido decreased

Gastrointestinal: Nausea (16%), diarrhea (13%), gastrointestinal upset (12%)

Hepatic: LDH increased (2% to 33%), AST increased (2% to 33%)

Respiratory: Dyspnea (12%)

1% to 10%:

Cardiovascular: CHF (3%), MI (3%), cerebrovascular accident (2%), chest pain (1%), flushing (1%)

Central nervous system: Lethargy (4%), insomnia (3%), emotional lability (2%), anxiety (1%), headache (1%)

Dermatologic: Bruising (3%), pruritus (2%), dry skin (1%), hair thinning (1%), rash (1%), skin peeling (1%)

Gastrointestinal: Anorexia (4%), flatulence (2%), burning throat (1%), gastrointestinal bleeding (1%), thirst (1%), vomiting (1%)

Hematologic: Leukopenia (4%), thrombocytopenia (1%)

Hepatic: Bilirubin increased (1% to 2%)

Local: Thrombophlebitis (3%)

Neuromuscular & skeletal: Leg cramps (9%)

Ocular: Tearing (1%)

Respiratory: Pulmonary embolism (2%), upper respiratory discharge (1%), hoarseness (1%)

Mechanism of Action Combines the effects of estradiol and nitrogen mustard. It appears to bind to microtubule proteins, preventing normal tubulin function. The antitumor effect may be due solely to an estrogenic effect. Estramustine causes a marked decrease in plasma testosterone and an increase in estrogen levels.

Drug Interactions

Decreased Effect: Antacids containing calcium and calcium salts may decrease the absorption of estramustine.

Pharmacodynamics/Kinetics

Absorption: Oral: 75%

Metabolism:

GI tract: Initial dephosphorylation

Hepatic: Oxidation and hydrolysis; metabolites include estramustine, estrone analog, estrone, and estradiol

Half-life elimination: Terminal: 20-24 hours

Time to peak, serum: 2-3 hours

Excretion: Feces (2.9% to 4.8% as unchanged drug)

Estramustine Phosphate *see* Estramustine *on page 605*

Estramustine Phosphate Sodium *see* Estramustine *on page 605*

Estrasorb™ *see* Estradiol *on page 602*

Estratest® *see* Estrogens (Esterified) and Methyltestosterone *on page 614*

Estratest® H.S. *see* Estrogens (Esterified) and Methyltestosterone *on page 614*

Estring® *see* Estradiol *on page 602*

EstroGel® *see* Estradiol *on page 602*

Estrogenic Substances, Conjugated *see* Estrogens (Conjugated/Equine) *on page 609*

Estrogens (Conjugated A/Synthetic)

(ES troe jenz, KON joo gate ed, aye, sin THET ik)

Related Information

Endocrine Disorders and Pregnancy *on page 1750*

U.S. Brand Names Cenestin®

Canadian Brand Names Cenestin

Generic Available No

Pharmacologic Category Estrogen Derivative

Use Treatment of moderate-to-severe vasomotor symptoms of menopause; treatment of vulvar and vaginal atrophy

Local Anesthetic/Vasoconstrictor Precautions No information available to require special precautions

Effects on Dental Treatment No significant effects or complications reported

Common Adverse Effects

>10%:

Central nervous system: Headache (11% to 68%), dizziness (11%), pain (11%)

Endocrine & metabolic: Breast pain (29%), endometrial thickening (19%), metrorrhagia (14%)
Gastrointestinal: Abdominal pain (9% to 28%), nausea (9% to 18%)
Neuromuscular & skeletal: Paresthesia (8% to 33%), back pain (14%)
Respiratory: Upper respiratory tract infection (13%)
Miscellaneous: Infection (2% to 14%)

1% to 10%:
Central nervous system: Anxiety (6%), fever (1%)
Gastrointestinal: Dyspepsia (10%), vomiting (7%), constipation (6%), diarrhea (6%), weight gain (6%)
Genitourinary: Vaginitis (8%)
Neuromuscular & skeletal: Leg cramps (10%), hypertonia (6%)
Respiratory: Rhinitis (6% to 8%), cough (6%)

In addition, the following have been reported with estrogen and/or progestin therapy:
Cardiovascular: Edema, hypertension, MI, stroke, venous thromboembolism
Central nervous system: Epilepsy exacerbation, irritability, mental depression, migraine, mood disturbances, nervousness
Dermatologic: Angioedema, chloasma, erythema multiforme, erythema nodosum, hemorrhagic eruption, hirsutism, melasma, pruritus, rash, scalp hair loss, urticaria
Endocrine & metabolic: Breast cancer, breast enlargement, breast tenderness, glucose tolerance impaired, HDL-cholesterol increased, hyper-/hypocalcemia, LDL-cholesterol decreased, libido changes, serum triglycerides/phospholipids increased, thyroid-binding globulin increased, total thyroid hormone (T_4) increased
Gastrointestinal: Abdominal cramps, bloating, cholecystitis, cholelithiasis, gallbladder disease, pancreatitis, weight gain/loss
Genitourinary: Alterations in frequency and flow of menses, cervical secretion changes, endometrial cancer, endometrial hyperplasia, uterine leiomyomata size increased, vaginal candidiasis
Hematologic: Aggravation of porphyria, antithrombin III and antifactor Xa decreased, fibrinogen levels increased, platelet aggregability and platelet count increased; prothrombin and factors VII, VIII, IX, X increased
Hepatic: Cholestatic jaundice, hepatic hemangiomas enlarged
Neuromuscular & skeletal: Arthralgias, chorea, leg cramps
Local: Thrombophlebitis
Ocular: Contact lens intolerance, retinal vascular thrombosis, corneal curvature steepening
Respiratory: Asthma exacerbation, pulmonary thromboembolism
Miscellaneous: Anaphylactoid/anaphylactic reactions, carbohydrate intolerance

Mechanism of Action Conjugated A/synthetic estrogens contain a mixture of 9 synthetic estrogen substances, including sodium estrone sulfate, sodium equilin sulfate, sodium 17 alpha-dihydroequilin, sodium 17 alpha-estradiol and sodium 17 beta-dihydroequilin. Estrogens are responsible for the development and maintenance of the female reproductive system and secondary sexual characteristics. Estradiol is the principle intracellular human estrogen and is more potent than estrone and estriol at the receptor level; it is the primary estrogen secreted prior to menopause. Following menopause, estrone and estrone sulfate are more highly produced. Estrogens modulate the pituitary secretion of gonadotropins, luteinizing hormone, and follicle-stimulating hormone through a negative feedback system; estrogen replacement reduces elevated levels of these hormones in postmenopausal women.

Drug Interactions
Cytochrome P450 Effect: Based on estradiol and estrone: **Substrate** of CYP1A2 (major), 2A6 (minor), 2B6 (minor), 2C9 (minor), 2C19 (minor), 2D6 (minor), 2E1 (minor), 3A4 (major); **Inhibits** CYP1A2 (weak); **Induces** CYP3A4 (weak)

Increased Effect/Toxicity: Anticoagulants increase the potential for thromboembolic events. Estrogens may enhance the effects of hydrocortisone and prednisone. Estrogen derivatives may enhance the hepatotoxic effect of cyclosporine. Estrogen derivatives may increase the serum concentration of cyclosporine.

Decreased Effect: CYP1A2 inducers may decrease the levels/effects of estrogens; example inducers include aminoglutethimide, carbamazepine, phenobarbital, and rifampin. CYP3A4 inducers may decrease the levels/effects of estrogen; example inducers include aminoglutethimide, carbamazepine, nafcillin, nevirapine, phenobarbital, phenytoin, and rifamycins. Estrogen derivatives may diminish the therapeutic effect of thyroid products.

Pharmacodynamics/Kinetics
Absorption: Well absorbed over a period of several hours
Protein-binding: Sex hormone-binding globulin (SHBG) and albumin
(Continued)

Estrogens (Conjugated A/Synthetic) *(Continued)*

Metabolism: Hepatic via CYP3A4; estradiol is converted to estrone and estriol; also undergoes enterohepatic recirculation; estrone sulfate is the main metabolite in postmenopausal women

Excretion: Urine (primarily estriol, also as estradiol, estrone, and conjugates)

Estrogens (Conjugated B/Synthetic)
(ES troe jenz, KON joo gate ed, bee, sin THET ik)

U.S. Brand Names Enjuvia™

Generic Available No

Pharmacologic Category Estrogen Derivative

Use Treatment of moderate-to-severe vasomotor symptoms of menopause

Local Anesthetic/Vasoconstrictor Precautions No information available to require special precautions

Effects on Dental Treatment No significant effects or complications reported

Common Adverse Effects

>10%:
  Central nervous system: Headache (15% to 25%), pain (10% to 19%)
  Endocrine & metabolic: Breast pain (up to 14%)
  Gastrointestinal: Abdominal pain (4% to 15%), nausea (7% to 12%)

1% to 10%:
  Central nervous system: Dizziness (1% to 7%)
  Endocrine & metabolic: Dysmenorrhea (1% to 8%)
  Gastrointestinal: Flatulence (4% to 7%)
  Genitourinary: Vaginitis (2% to 7%)
  Neuromuscular & skeletal: Paresthesia (up to 6%)
  Respiratory: Bronchitis (up to 7%), rhinitis (4% to 7%), sinusitis (3% to 7%)
  Miscellaneous: Flu-like syndrome (4% to 7%)

In addition, the following have been reported with estrogen and/or progestin therapy:

Cardiovascular: Edema, hypertension, MI, stroke, venous thromboembolism

Central nervous system: Epilepsy exacerbation, irritability, mental depression, migraine, mood disturbances, nervousness

Dermatologic: Angioedema, chloasma, erythema multiforme, erythema nodosum, hemorrhagic eruption, hirsutism, loss of scalp hair, melasma, pruritus, rash, urticaria

Endocrine & metabolic: Breast cancer, breast enlargement, breast tenderness, HDL-cholesterol increased, hyper-/hypocalcemia, impaired glucose tolerance, LDL-cholesterol decreased, libido (changes in), serum triglycerides/phospholipids increased, thyroid-binding globulin increased, total thyroid hormone (T_4) increased

Gastrointestinal: Abdominal cramps, bloating, cholecystitis, cholelithiasis, gallbladder disease, pancreatitis, weight gain/loss

Genitourinary: Alterations in frequency and flow of menses, changes in cervical secretions, endometrial cancer, endometrial hyperplasia, increased size of uterine leiomyomata, vaginal candidiasis

Hematologic: Aggravation of porphyria; antithrombin III and antifactor Xa decreased; fibrinogen levels increased; platelet aggregability and platelet count increased; prothrombin and factors VII, VIII, IX, X increased

Hepatic: Cholestatic jaundice, hepatic hemangiomas enlarged

Local: Thrombophlebitis

Neuromuscular & skeletal: Arthralgias, chorea, leg cramps

Ocular: Contact lens intolerance, corneal curvature steepening, retinal vascular thrombosis

Respiratory: Asthma exacerbation, pulmonary thromboembolism

Miscellaneous: Anaphylactoid/anaphylactic reactions, carbohydrate intolerance

Mechanism of Action Conjugated B/synthetic estrogens contain a mixture of 10 synthetic estrogen substances, including sodium estrone sulfate, sodium equilin sulfate, sodium 17-alpha-dihydroequilin, sodium 17-alpha-estradiol, and sodium 17-beta-dihydroequilin. Estrogens are responsible for the development and maintenance of the female reproductive system and secondary sexual characteristics. Estradiol is the principle intracellular human estrogen and is more potent than estrone and estriol at the receptor level; it is the primary estrogen secreted prior to menopause. Following menopause, estrone and estrone sulfate are more highly produced. Estrogens modulate the pituitary secretion of gonadotropins, luteinizing hormone, and follicle-stimulating hormone through a negative feedback system; estrogen replacement reduces elevated levels of these hormones in postmenopausal women.

Drug Interactions

Cytochrome P450 Effect: Based on estradiol and estrone: **Substrate** of CYP1A2 (major), 2A6 (minor), 2B6 (minor), 2C9 (minor), 2C19 (minor), 2D6 (minor), 2E1 (minor), 3A4 (major); **Inhibits** CYP1A2 (weak); **Induces** CYP3A4 (weak)

Increased Effect/Toxicity: Anticoagulants increase the potential for thromboembolic events. Estrogens may enhance the effects of hydrocortisone and prednisone. Estrogen derivatives may enhance the hepatotoxic effect of cyclosporine. Estrogen derivatives may increase the serum concentration of cyclosporine.

Decreased Effect: CYP1A2 inducers may decrease the levels/effects of estrogens; example inducers include aminoglutethimide, carbamazepine, phenobarbital, and rifampin. CYP3A4 inducers may decrease the levels/effects of estrogen; example inducers include aminoglutethimide, carbamazepine, nafcillin, nevirapine, phenobarbital, phenytoin, and rifamycins. Estrogen derivatives may diminish the therapeutic effect of thyroid products.

Pharmacodynamics/Kinetics

Absorption: Well absorbed over a period of several hours

Protein-binding: Sex hormone-binding globulin (SHBG) and albumin

Metabolism: Hepatic via CYP3A4; estradiol is converted to estrone and estriol; also undergoes enterohepatic recirculation; estrone sulfate is the main metabolite in postmenopausal women

Excretion: Urine (primarily estriol, also as estradiol, estrone, and conjugates)

Estrogens (Conjugated/Equine)
(ES troe jenz KON joo gate ed, EE kwine)

Related Information

Endocrine Disorders and Pregnancy *on page 1750*

U.S. Brand Names Premarin®

Canadian Brand Names C.E.S.®; Premarin®

Generic Available No

Index Terms CEE; C.E.S.; Estrogenic Substances, Conjugated

Pharmacologic Category Estrogen Derivative

Use Treatment of moderate-to-severe vasomotor symptoms associated with menopause; treatment of vulvar and vaginal atrophy; hypoestrogenism (due to hypogonadism, castration, or primary ovarian failure); prostatic cancer (palliation); breast cancer (palliation); osteoporosis (prophylaxis, postmenopausal women at significant risk only); abnormal uterine bleeding

Unlabeled/Investigational Use Uremic bleeding

Local Anesthetic/Vasoconstrictor Precautions No information available to require special precautions

Effects on Dental Treatment No significant effects or complications reported

Common Adverse Effects

Note: Percentages reported in postmenopausal women.

>10%:

Central nervous system: Headache (26% to 32%; placebo 28%)

Endocrine & metabolic: Breast pain (7% to 12%; placebo 9%)

Gastrointestinal: Abdominal pain (15% to 17%)

Genitourinary: Vaginal hemorrhage (2% to 14%)

Neuromuscular & skeletal: Back pain (13% to 14%)

1% to 10%:

Central nervous system: Nervousness (2% to 5%)

Endocrine & metabolic: Leukorrhea (4% to 7%)

Gastrointestinal: Flatulence (6% to 7%)

Genitourinary: Vaginitis (5% to 7%), vaginal moniliasis (5% to 6%)

Neuromuscular & skeletal: Weakness (7% to 8%), leg cramps (3% to 7%)

In addition, the following have been reported with estrogen and/or progestin therapy:

Cardiovascular: Edema, hypertension, MI, stroke, venous thromboembolism

Central nervous system: Dizziness, epilepsy exacerbation, headache, irritability, mental depression, migraine, mood disturbances, nervousness

Dermatologic: Angioedema, chloasma, erythema multiforme, erythema nodosum, hemorrhagic eruption, hirsutism, loss of scalp hair, melasma, pruritus, rash, urticaria

Endocrine & metabolic: Breast cancer, breast enlargement, breast tenderness, libido (changes in), increased thyroid-binding globulin, increased total thyroid hormone (T_4), increased serum triglycerides/phospholipids, increased HDL-cholesterol, decreased LDL-cholesterol, impaired glucose tolerance, hypercalcemia, hypocalcemia

Gastrointestinal: Abdominal cramps, bloating, cholecystitis, cholelithiasis, gallbladder disease, nausea, pancreatitis, vomiting, weight gain/loss

(Continued)

Estrogens (Conjugated/Equine) *(Continued)*

Genitourinary: Alterations in frequency and flow of menses, changes in cervical secretions, endometrial cancer, endometrial hyperplasia, increased size of uterine leiomyomata, vaginal candidiasis

Hematologic: Aggravation of porphyria, decreased antithrombin III and antifactor Xa, increased levels of fibrinogen, increased platelet aggregability and platelet count; increased prothrombin and factors VII, VIII, IX, X

Hepatic: Cholestatic jaundice, hepatic hemangiomas enlarged

Neuromuscular & skeletal: Arthralgias, chorea, leg cramps

Local: Thrombophlebitis

Ocular: Contact lens intolerance, corneal curvature steepening, retinal vascular thrombosis

Respiratory: Asthma exacerbation, pulmonary thromboembolism

Miscellaneous: Anaphylactoid/anaphylactic reactions, carbohydrate intolerance

Dosage Adults:

Male: Androgen-dependent prostate cancer palliation: Oral: 1.25-2.5 mg 3 times/day

Female:

Prevention of postmenopausal osteoporosis: Oral: Initial: 0.3 mg/day cyclically* or daily, depending on medical assessment of patient. Dose may be adjusted based on bone mineral density and clinical response. The lowest effective dose should be used.

Moderate to severe vasomotor symptoms associated with menopause: Oral: Initial: 0.3 mg/day, cyclically* or daily, depending on medical assessment of patient. The lowest dose that will control symptoms should be used. Medication should be discontinued as soon as possible.

Vulvar and vaginal atrophy:

Oral: Initial: 0.3 mg/day; the lowest dose that will control symptoms should be used. May be given cyclically* or daily, depending on medical assessment of patient. Medication should be discontinued as soon as possible.

Vaginal cream: Intravaginal: $1/2$ to 2 g/day given cyclically*

Abnormal uterine bleeding:

Acute/heavy bleeding:

Oral (unlabeled route): 1.25 mg, may repeat every 4 hours for 24 hours, followed by 1.25 mg once daily for 7-10 days

I.M., I.V.: 25 mg, may repeat in 6-12 hours if needed

Note: Treatment should be followed by a low-dose oral contraceptive; medroxyprogesterone acetate along with or following estrogen therapy can also be given

Nonacute/lesser bleeding: Oral (unlabeled route): 1.25 mg once daily for 7-10 days

Female hypogonadism: Oral: 0.3-0.625 mg/day given cyclically*; dose may be titrated in 6- to 12-month intervals; progestin treatment should be added to maintain bone mineral density once skeletal maturity is achieved.

Female castration, primary ovarian failure: Oral: 1.25 mg/day given cyclically*; adjust according to severity of symptoms and patient response. For maintenance, adjust to the lowest effective dose.

*Cyclic administration: Either 3 weeks on, 1 week off **or** 25 days on, 5 days off

Male and Female:

Breast cancer palliation, metastatic disease in selected patients: Oral: 10 mg 3 times/day for at least 3 months

Uremic bleeding (unlabeled use): I.V.: 0.6 mg/kg/day for 5 days

Elderly: Refer to adult dosing; a higher incidence of stroke and invasive breast cancer was observed in women >75 years in a WHI substudy.

Mechanism of Action Conjugated estrogens contain a mixture of estrone sulfate, equilin sulfate, 17 alpha-dihydroequilin, 17 alpha-estradiol and 17 beta-dihydroequilin. Estrogens are responsible for the development and maintenance of the female reproductive system and secondary sexual characteristics. Estradiol is the principle intracellular human estrogen and is more potent than estrone and estriol at the receptor level; it is the primary estrogen secreted prior to menopause. Following menopause, estrone and estrone sulfate are more highly produced. Estrogens modulate the pituitary secretion of gonadotropins, luteinizing hormone, and follicle-stimulating hormone through a negative feedback system; estrogen replacement reduces elevated levels of these hormones in postmenopausal women.

Contraindications Hypersensitivity to estrogens or any component of the formulation; undiagnosed abnormal vaginal bleeding; history of or current thrombophlebitis or venous thromboembolic disorders (including DVT, PE); active or recent (within 1 year) arterial thromboembolic disease (eg, stroke, MI); carcinoma of the breast (except in appropriately selected patients being treated for metastatic disease); estrogen-dependent tumor; hepatic dysfunction or disease; pregnancy

Warnings/Precautions

Cardiovascular-related considerations: **[U.S. Boxed Warning]: Estrogens with or without progestin should not be used to prevent coronary heart disease.** Use caution with cardiovascular disease or dysfunction. May increase the risks of hypertension, myocardial infarction (MI), stroke, pulmonary emboli (PE), and deep vein thrombosis; incidence of these effects was shown to be significantly increased in postmenopausal women using conjugated equine estrogens (CEE) in combination with medroxyprogesterone acetate (MPA). Nonfatal MI, PE, and thrombophlebitis have also been reported in males taking high doses of CEE (eg, for prostate cancer). Estrogen compounds are generally associated with lipid effects such as increased HDL-cholesterol and decreased LDL-cholesterol. Triglycerides may also be increased; use with caution in patients with familial defects of lipoprotein metabolism. Whenever possible, estrogens should be discontinued at least 4 weeks prior to and for 2 weeks following elective surgery associated with an increased risk of thromboembolism or during periods of prolonged immobilization.

Neurological considerations: **[U.S. Boxed Warning]: The risk of dementia may be increased in postmenopausal women;** increased incidence was observed in women ≥65 years of age taking CEE alone or in combination with MPA.

Cancer-related considerations: **[U.S. Boxed Warning]: Unopposed estrogens may increase the risk of endometrial carcinoma in postmenopausal women.** Estrogens may exacerbate endometriosis. Malignant transformation of residual endometrial implants has been reported posthysterectomy with estrogen only therapy. Consider adding a progestin in women with residual endometriosis posthysterectomy. Estrogens may increase the risk of breast cancer. An increased risk of invasive breast cancer was observed in postmenopausal women using CEE in combination with MPA; a smaller increase in risk was seen with estrogen therapy alone in observational studies. An increase in abnormal mammograms has also been reported with estrogen and progestin therapy. Estrogen use may lead to severe hypercalcemia in patients with breast cancer and bone metastases; discontinue estrogen if hypercalcemia occurs.

Estrogens may cause retinal vascular thrombosis; discontinue permanently if papilledema or retinal vascular lesions are observed on examination. Use with caution in patients with diseases which may be exacerbated by fluid retention, including asthma, epilepsy, migraine, diabetes or renal dysfunction. Use with caution in patients with a history of severe hypocalcemia, SLE, hepatic hemangiomas, porphyria, endometriosis, and gallbladder disease. Use caution with history of cholestatic jaundice associated with past estrogen use or pregnancy. Safety and efficacy in pediatric patients have not been established. Prior to puberty, estrogens may cause premature closure of the epiphyses, premature breast development in girls or gynecomastia in boys. Vaginal bleeding and vaginal cornification may also be induced in girls.

Before prescribing estrogen therapy to postmenopausal women, the risks and benefits must be weighed for each patient. Women should be informed of these risks and benefits, as well as possible effects of progestin when added to estrogen therapy. Estrogens with or without progestin should be used for shortest duration possible consistent with treatment goals. Conduct periodic risk:benefit assessments.

When used solely for prevention of osteoporosis in women at significant risk, nonestrogen treatment options should be considered. When used solely for the treatment of vulvar and vaginal atrophy, topical vaginal products should be considered. Use caution applying topical products to severely atrophic vaginal mucosa.

Drug Interactions
Cytochrome P450 Effect:

Based on estradiol and estrone: **Substrate** of CYP1A2 (major), 2A6 (minor), 2B6 (minor), 2C9 (minor), 2C19 (minor), 2D6 (minor), 2E1 (minor), 3A4 (major); Inhibits CYP1A2 (weak), 2C8 (weak); Induces CYP3A4 (weak)

Increased Effect/Toxicity: Hydrocortisone taken with estrogen may cause corticosteroid-induced toxicity. Increased potential for thromboembolic events with anticoagulants. Estrogen derivatives may enhance the hepatotoxic effect of cyclosporine. Estrogen derivatives may increase the serum concentration of cyclosporine.

Decreased Effect: CYP1A2 inducers may decrease the levels/effects of estrogens; example inducers include aminoglutethimide, carbamazepine, phenobarbital, and rifampin. CYP3A4 inducers may decrease the levels/ (Continued)

Estrogens (Conjugated/Equine) *(Continued)*

effects of estrogens; example inducers include aminoglutethimide, carbamazepine, nafcillin, nevirapine, phenobarbital, phenytoin, and rifamycins. Estrogen derivatives may diminish the therapeutic effect of thyroid products.

Ethanol/Nutrition/Herb Interactions

Ethanol: Avoid ethanol (routine use increases estrogen level and risk of breast cancer). Ethanol may also increase the risk of osteoporosis.

Food: Folic acid absorption may be decreased.

Herb/Nutraceutical: St John's wort may decrease levels. Herbs with estrogenic properties may enhance the adverse/toxic effect of estrogen derivatives; examples include alfalfa, black cohosh, bloodroot, hops, kudzu, licorice, red clover, saw palmetto, soybean, thyme, wild yam, yucca.

Dietary Considerations Ensure adequate calcium and vitamin D intake when used for the prevention of osteoporosis. Powder for reconstitution for injection (25 mg) contains lactose 200 mg.

Pharmacodynamics/Kinetics

Absorption: Well absorbed

Metabolism: Hepatic via CYP3A4; estradiol is converted to estrone and estriol; also undergoes enterohepatic recirculation; estrone sulfite is the main metabolite in postmenopausal women

Excretion: Urine (primarily estriol, also as estradiol, estrone, and conjugates

Dosage Forms

Cream, vaginal:

Premarin®: 0.625 mg/g (42.5 g)

Injection, powder for reconstitution:

Premarin®: 25 mg

Tablet:

Premarin®: 0.3 mg, 0.45 mg, 0.625 mg, 0.9 mg, 1.25 mg

Estrogens (Conjugated/Equine) and Medroxyprogesterone

(ES troe jenz KON joo gate ed/EE kwine & me DROKS ee proe JES te rone)

Related Information

Endocrine Disorders and Pregnancy *on page 1750*
Estrogens (Conjugated/Equine) *on page 609*
MedroxyPROGESTERone *on page 1026*

U.S. Brand Names Premphase®; Prempro™

Canadian Brand Names Premphase®; Premplus®; Prempro™

Mexican Brand Names Premelle

Generic Available No

Index Terms Medroxyprogesterone and Estrogens (Conjugated); MPA and Estrogens (Conjugated)

Pharmacologic Category Estrogen and Progestin Combination

Use Women with an intact uterus: Treatment of moderate-to-severe vasomotor symptoms associated with menopause; treatment of atrophic vaginitis; osteoporosis (prophylaxis)

Local Anesthetic/Vasoconstrictor Precautions No information available to require special precautions

Effects on Dental Treatment No significant effects or complications reported

Common Adverse Effects

>10%:

Central nervous system: Headache (28% to 37%), pain (11% to 13%), depression (6% to 11%)

Endocrine & metabolic: Breast pain (32% to 38%), dysmenorrhea (8% to 13%)

Gastrointestinal: Abdominal pain (16% to 23%), nausea (9% to 11%)

Neuromuscular & skeletal: Back pain (13% to 16%)

Respiratory: Pharyngitis (11% to 13%)

Miscellaneous: Infection (16% to 18%), flu-like syndrome (10% to 13%)

1% to 10%:

Cardiovascular: Peripheral edema (3% to 4%)

Central nervous system: Dizziness (3% to 5%)

Dermatologic: Pruritus (5% to 10%), rash (4% to 6%)

Endocrine & metabolic: Leukorrhea (5% to 9%)

Gastrointestinal: Flatulence (8% to 9%), diarrhea (5% to 6%), dyspepsia (5% to 6%)

Genitourinary: Vaginitis (5% to 7%), cervical changes (4% to 5%), vaginal hemorrhage (1% to 3%)

Neuromuscular & skeletal: Weakness (6% to 10%), arthralgia (7% to 9%), leg cramps (3% to 5%), hypertonia (3% to 4%)

Respiratory: Sinusitis (7% to 8%), rhinitis (6% to 8%)

Additional adverse effects reported with conjugated estrogens and/or progestins: Abdominal cramps, acne, abnormal uterine bleeding, aggravation of porphyria, amenorrhea, anaphylactoid reactions, anaphylaxis, antifactor Xa decreased, antithrombin III decreased, appetite changes, bloating, breast enlargement, breast tenderness, cerebral embolism, cerebral thrombosis, chloasma, cholestatic jaundice, cholecystitis, cholelithiasis, chorea, contact lens intolerance, cystitis-like syndrome, decreased carbohydrate tolerance, dizziness; factors VII, VIII, IX, X, XII, VII-X complex, and II-VII-X complex increased; endometrial hyperplasia, erythema multiforme, erythema nodosum, galactorrhea, hemorrhagic eruption, fatigue, fibrinogen increased, impaired glucose tolerance, HDL-cholesterol increased, hirsutism, hypertension, increase in size of uterine leiomyomata, gallbladder disease, insomnia, LDL-cholesterol decreased, libido changes, loss of scalp hair, melasma, migraine, nervousness, optic neuritis, pancreatitis, platelet aggregability and platelet count increased, premenstrual like syndrome, PT and PTT accelerated, pulmonary embolism, pyrexia, retinal thrombosis, somnolence, steepening of corneal curvature, thrombophlebitis, thyroid-binding globulin increased, total thyroid hormone (T_4) increased, triglycerides increased, urticaria, vaginal candidiasis, vomiting, weight gain/loss

Mechanism of Action

Conjugated estrogens contain a mixture of estrone sulfate, equilin sulfate, 17 alpha-dihydroequilin, 17 alpha-estradiol, and 17 beta-dihydroequilin. Estrogens are responsible for the development and maintenance of the female reproductive system and secondary sexual characteristics. Estradiol is the principle intracellular human estrogen and is more potent than estrone and estriol at the receptor level; it is the primary estrogen secreted prior to menopause. Following menopause, estrone and estrone sulfate are more highly produced. Estrogens modulate the pituitary secretion of gonadotropins, luteinizing hormone, and follicle-stimulating hormone through a negative feedback system; estrogen replacement reduces elevated levels of these hormones in postmenopausal women.

MPA inhibits gonadotropin production which then prevents follicular maturation and ovulation. In women with adequate estrogen, MPA transforms a proliferative endometrium into a secretory endometrium; when administered with conjugated estrogens, reduces the incidence of endometrial hyperplasia and risk of adenocarcinoma.

Drug Interactions

Cytochrome P450 Effect:

Based on estradiol and estrone: **Substrate** of CYP1A2 (major), 2A6 (minor), 2B6 (minor), 2C9 (minor), 2C19 (minor), 2D6 (minor), 2E1 (minor), 3A4 (major); **Inhibits** CYP1A2 (weak), 2C8 (weak); **Induces** CYP3A4 (weak)

Medroxyprogesterone: **Substrate** of CYP3A4 (major); **Induces** CYP3A4 (weak)

Increased Effect/Toxicity: Hydrocortisone taken with estrogen may cause corticosteroid-induced toxicity. Increased potential for thromboembolic events with anticoagulants.

Decreased Effect:

Conjugated estrogens:

Anticonvulsants which are enzyme inducers (barbiturates, carbamazepine, phenobarbital, phenytoin, primidone) may potentially decrease estrogen levels.

Rifampin, nelfinavir, and ritonavir decrease estradiol serum concentrations

MPA: Aminoglutethimide: May decrease effects by increasing hepatic metabolism

Pharmacodynamics/Kinetics See individual agents.

Estrogens (Esterified) (ES troe jenz, es TER i fied)

Related Information

Endocrine Disorders and Pregnancy *on page 1750*

U.S. Brand Names Menest®

Canadian Brand Names Estratab®; Menest®

Generic Available No

Index Terms Esterified Estrogens

Pharmacologic Category Estrogen Derivative

Use Treatment of moderate to severe vasomotor symptoms associated with menopause; treatment of vulvar and vaginal atrophy; hypoestrogenism (due to hypogonadism, castration, or primary ovarian failure); prostatic cancer (palliation); breast cancer (palliation); osteoporosis (prophylaxis, in women at significant risk only)

(Continued)

613

Estrogens (Esterified) *(Continued)*

Local Anesthetic/Vasoconstrictor Precautions No information available to require special precautions

Effects on Dental Treatment No significant effects or complications reported

Common Adverse Effects Frequency not defined.

Cardiovascular: Edema, hypertension, venous thromboembolism

Central nervous system: Dizziness, headache, mental depression, migraine

Dermatologic: Chloasma, erythema multiforme, erythema nodosum, hemorrhagic eruption, hirsutism, loss of scalp hair, melasma

Endocrine & metabolic: Breast enlargement, breast tenderness, libido (changes in), increased thyroid-binding globulin, increased total thyroid hormone (T_4), increased serum triglycerides/phospholipids, increased HDL-cholesterol, decreased LDL-cholesterol, impaired glucose tolerance, hypercalcemia

Gastrointestinal: Abdominal cramps, bloating, cholecystitis, cholelithiasis, gallbladder disease, nausea, pancreatitis, vomiting, weight gain/loss

Genitourinary: Alterations in frequency and flow of menses, changes in cervical secretions, endometrial cancer, increased size of uterine leiomyomata, vaginal candidiasis

Hematologic: Aggravation of porphyria, decreased antithrombin III and antifactor Xa, increased levels of fibrinogen, increased platelet aggregability and platelet count; increased prothrombin and factors VII, VIII, IX, X

Hepatic: Cholestatic jaundice

Neuromuscular & skeletal: Chorea

Ocular: Ocular: Contact lens intolerance, corneal curvature steepening

Respiratory: Pulmonary thromboembolism

Miscellaneous: Carbohydrate intolerance

Mechanism of Action Esterified estrogens contain a mixture of estrogenic substances; the principle component is estrone. Preparations contain 75% to 85% sodium estrone sulfate and 6% to 15% sodium equilin sulfate such that the total is not <90%. Estrogens are responsible for the development and maintenance of the female reproductive system and secondary sexual characteristics. Estradiol is the principle intracellular human estrogen and is more potent than estrone and estriol at the receptor level; it is the primary estrogen secreted prior to menopause. In males and following menopause in females, estrone and estrone sulfate are more highly produced. Estrogens modulate the pituitary secretion of gonadotropins, luteinizing hormone, and follicle-stimulating hormone through a negative feedback system; estrogen replacement reduces elevated levels of these hormones.

Drug Interactions

Cytochrome P450 Effect: Based on estrone: **Substrate** of CYP1A2 (major), 2B6 (minor), 2C9 (minor), 2E1 (minor), 3A4 (major)

Increased Effect/Toxicity: Hydrocortisone taken with estrogen may cause corticosteroid-induced toxicity. Increased potential for thromboembolic events with anticoagulants. Estrogen derivatives may enhance the hepatotoxic effect of cyclosporine. Estrogen derivatives may increase the serum concentration of cyclosporine.

Decreased Effect: CYP1A2 inducers may decrease the levels/effects of estrogens; example inducers include aminoglutethimide, carbamazepine, phenobarbital, and rifampin. CYP3A4 inducers may decrease the levels/effects of estrogens; example inducers include aminoglutethimide, carbamazepine, nafcillin, nevirapine, phenobarbital, phenytoin, and rifamycins. Estrogen derivatives may diminish the therapeutic effect of thyroid products.

Pharmacodynamics/Kinetics

Absorption: Readily

Metabolism: Rapidly hepatic to estrone sulfate, conjugated and unconjugated metabolites; first-pass effect

Excretion: Urine (as unchanged drug and as glucuronide and sulfate conjugates)

Pregnancy Risk Factor X

Estrogens (Esterified) and Methyltestosterone

(ES troe jenz es TER i fied & meth il tes TOS te rone)

Related Information

Endocrine Disorders and Pregnancy *on page 1750*

Estrogens (Esterified) *on page 613*

MethylTESTOSTERone *on page 1085*

U.S. Brand Names Estratest®; Estratest® H.S.; Syntest D.S.; Syntest H.S.

Canadian Brand Names Estratest®

Generic Available Yes

Index Terms Conjugated Estrogen and Methyltestosterone; Esterified Estrogen and Methyltestosterone

Pharmacologic Category Estrogen and Progestin Combination
Use Vasomotor symptoms of menopause
Local Anesthetic/Vasoconstrictor Precautions No information available to require special precautions
Effects on Dental Treatment No significant effects or complications reported
Common Adverse Effects 1% to 10%:
    Cardiovascular: Increase in blood pressure, edema, thromboembolic disorder
    Central nervous system: Depression, headache
    Dermatologic: Chloasma, melasma
    Endocrine & metabolic: Breast tenderness, change in menstrual flow, hypercalcemia
    Gastrointestinal: Nausea, vomiting
    Hepatic: Cholestatic jaundice
Mechanism of Action
    Conjugated estrogens: Activate estrogen receptors (DNA protein complex) located in estrogen-responsive tissues. Once activated, regulate transcription of certain genes leading to observed effects.
    Testosterone: Increases synthesis of DNA, RNA, and various proteins in target tissues
Drug Interactions
    Cytochrome P450 Effect: Based on estrone: **Substrate** of CYP1A2 (major), 2B6 (minor), 2C9 (minor), 2E1 (minor), 3A4 (major)
Pharmacodynamics/Kinetics See individual agents.
Pregnancy Risk Factor X

Estropipate (ES troe pih pate)

Related Information
    Endocrine Disorders and Pregnancy *on page 1750*
U.S. Brand Names Ogen®; Ortho-Est®
Canadian Brand Names Ogen®
Generic Available Yes
Index Terms Ortho Est; Piperazine Estrone Sulfate
Pharmacologic Category Estrogen Derivative
Use Treatment of moderate to severe vasomotor symptoms associated with menopause; treatment of vulvar and vaginal atrophy; hypoestrogenism (due to hypogonadism, castration, or primary ovarian failure); osteoporosis (prophylaxis, in women at significant risk only)
Local Anesthetic/Vasoconstrictor Precautions No information available to require special precautions
Effects on Dental Treatment No significant effects or complications reported
Common Adverse Effects Frequency not defined.
    Cardiovascular: Edema, hypertension, venous thromboembolism
    Central nervous system: Dizziness, headache, mental depression, migraine
    Dermatologic: Chloasma, erythema multiforme, erythema nodosum, hemorrhagic eruption, hirsutism, loss of scalp hair, melasma
    Endocrine & metabolic: Breast enlargement, breast tenderness, libido (changes in), increased thyroid-binding globulin, increased total thyroid hormone (T_4), increased serum triglycerides/phospholipids, increased HDL-cholesterol, decreased LDL-cholesterol, impaired glucose tolerance, hypercalcemia
    Gastrointestinal: Abdominal cramps, bloating, cholecystitis, cholelithiasis, gallbladder disease, nausea, pancreatitis, vomiting, weight gain/loss
    Genitourinary: Alterations in frequency and flow of menses, changes in cervical secretions, endometrial cancer, increased size of uterine leiomyomata, vaginal candidiasis
    Hematologic: Aggravation of porphyria, decreased antithrombin III and antifactor Xa, increased levels of fibrinogen, increased platelet aggregability and platelet count; increased prothrombin and factors VII, VIII, IX, X
    Hepatic: Cholestatic jaundice
    Neuromuscular & skeletal: Chorea
    Ocular: Ocular: Contact lens intolerance, corneal curvature steepening
    Respiratory: Pulmonary thromboembolism
    Miscellaneous: Carbohydrate intolerance
Mechanism of Action Estrogens are responsible for the development and maintenance of the female reproductive system and secondary sexual characteristics. Estradiol is the principle intracellular human estrogen and is more potent than estrone and estriol at the receptor level; it is the primary estrogen secreted prior to menopause. In males and following menopause in females, estrone and estrone sulfate are more highly produced. Estrogens modulate the pituitary secretion of gonadotropins, luteinizing hormone, and follicle-stimulating hormone through a negative feedback system; estrogen replacement reduces
(Continued)

Estropipate (Continued)

elevated levels of these hormones. Estropipate is prepared from purified crystal-line estrone that has been solubilized as the sulfate and stabilized with pipera-zine.

Drug Interactions

Cytochrome P450 Effect: Based on estrone: **Substrate** of CYP1A2 (major), 2B6 (minor), 2C9 (minor), 2E1 (minor), 3A4 (major)

Increased Effect/Toxicity: Hydrocortisone taken with estrogen may cause corticosteroid-induced toxicity. Increased potential for thromboembolic events with anticoagulants. Estrogen derivatives may enhance the hepatotoxic effect of cyclosporine. Estrogen derivatives may increase the serum concentration of cyclosporine.

Decreased Effect: CYP1A2 inducers may decrease the levels/effects of estrogens; example inducers include aminoglutethimide, carbamazepine, phenobarbital, and rifampin. CYP3A4 inducers may decrease the levels/ effects of estrogens; example inducers include aminoglutethimide, carbamaz-epine, nafcillin, nevirapine, phenobarbital, phenytoin, and rifamycins. Estrogen derivatives may diminish the therapeutic effect of thyroid products.

Pharmacodynamics/Kinetics

Absorption: Well absorbed

Metabolism: Hepatic and in target tissues; first-pass effect

Pregnancy Risk Factor X

Estrostep® Fe *see* Ethinyl Estradiol and Norethindrone *on page 640*

Eszopiclone (es zoe PIK lone)

U.S. Brand Names Lunesta™

Generic Available No

Pharmacologic Category Hypnotic, Nonbenzodiazepine

Dental Use Not established at this time

Use Treatment of insomnia

Local Anesthetic/Vasoconstrictor Precautions No information available to require special precautions

Effects on Dental Treatment Key adverse event(s) related to dental treat-ment: Unpleasant taste and xerostomia (normal salivary flow resumes upon discontinuation).

Common Adverse Effects

>10%:

Central nervous system: Headache (15% to 21%)

Gastrointestinal: Unpleasant taste (8% to 34%)

1% to 10%:

Cardiovascular: Chest pain, peripheral edema

Central nervous system: Somnolence (8% to 10%), dizziness (5% to 7%), hallucinations (1% to 3%), anxiety (1% to 3%), nervousness (up to 5%), confusion (up to 3%), depression (1% to 4%), abnormal dreams (1% to 3%), migraine

Dermatologic: Rash (3% to 4%), pruritus (1% to 4%)

Endocrine & metabolic: Libido decreased (up to 3%), dysmenorrhea (up to 3%), gynecomastia (males up to 3%)

Gastrointestinal: Xerostomia (3% to 7%), dyspepsia (5% to 6%), nausea (5%), diarrhea (2% to 4%), vomiting (up to 3%)

Genitourinary: Urinary tract infection (up to 3%)

Neuromuscular & skeletal: Neuralgia (up to 3%)

Miscellaneous: Infection (5% to 10%), viral infection (3%)

Restrictions C-IV

Dosage Oral:

Adults: Insomnia: Initial: 2 mg before bedtime (maximum dose: 3 mg)

Concurrent use with strong CYP3A4 inhibitor: 1 mg before bedtime; if needed, dose may be increased to 2 mg

Elderly:

Difficulty **falling** asleep: Initial: 1 mg before bedtime; maximum dose: 2 mg

Difficulty **staying** asleep: 2 mg before bedtime

Dosage adjustment in renal impairment: None required

Dosage adjustment in hepatic impairment:

Mild-to-moderate: Use with caution; dosage adjustment unnecessary

Severe: Maximum dose: 2 mg

Mechanism of Action May interact with GABA-receptor complexes at binding domains located close to or allosterically coupled to benzodiazepine receptors.

Contraindications Hypersensitivity to eszopiclone or any component of the formulation

Warnings/Precautions Symptomatic treatment of insomnia should be initiated only after careful evaluation of potential causes of sleep disturbance. Tolerance did not develop over 6 months of use. Use with caution in patients with depression or a history of drug dependence. Abrupt discontinuance may lead to withdrawal symptoms. Use with caution in patients receiving other CNS depressants or psychoactive medications. Hypnotics/sedatives have been associated with abnormal thinking and behavior changes including decreased inhibition, aggression, bizarre behavior, agitation, hallucinations, and depersonalization. These changes may occur unpredictably and may indicate previously unrecognized psychiatric disorders; evaluate appropriately. Amnesia may occur. May impair physical and mental capabilities. Postmarketing studies have indicated that the use of hypnotic/sedative agents for sleep has been associated with hypersensitivity reactions including anaphylaxis as well as angioedema. An increased risk for hazardous sleep-related activities such as sleep-driving; cooking and eating food, and making phone calls while asleep have also been noted. Use caution in patients with respiratory compromise, hepatic dysfunction, elderly or those taking strong CYP3A4 inhibitors. Because of the rapid onset of action, administer immediately prior to bedtime or after the patient has gone to bed and is having difficulty falling asleep. Safety and efficacy in children have not been established.

Drug Interactions

Cytochrome P450 Effect: Substrate of CYP2E1 (minor), 3A4 (major)

Increased Effect/Toxicity: CYP3A4 inhibitors may increase the levels/effects of eszopiclone; example inhibitors include azole antifungals, clarithromycin, diclofenac, doxycycline, erythromycin, imatinib, isoniazid, nefazodone, nicardipine, propofol, protease inhibitors, quinidine, telithromycin, and verapamil. Concurrent use with olanzapine may lead to decreased psychomotor function.

Decreased Effect: CYP3A4 inducers may decrease the levels/effects of eszopiclone; example inducers include aminoglutethimide, carbamazepine, nafcillin, nevirapine, phenobarbital, phenytoin, and rifamycins.

Ethanol/Nutrition/Herb Interactions

Ethanol: Use caution with concurrent use. Effects are additive and may decrease psychomotor function.

Food: Onset of action may be reduced if taken with or immediately after a heavy meal.

Herb/Nutraceutical: Avoid valerian, St John's wort, kava kava, gotu kola (may increase CNS depression).

Dietary Considerations Avoid taking after a heavy meal; may delay onset.

Pharmacodynamics/Kinetics

Absorption: Rapid; high-fat/heavy meal may delay absorption

Protein binding: 52% to 59%

Metabolism: Hepatic via oxidation and demethylation (CYP2E1, 3A4); 2 primary metabolites; one with activity less than parent.

Half-life elimination: 6 hours; Elderly (≥65 years): ~9 hours

Time to peak, plasma: 1 hour

Excretion: Urine (75%, primarily as metabolites; <10% as parent drug)

Pregnancy Risk Factor C

Dosage Forms

Tablet:

Lunesta™: 1 mg, 2 mg, 3 mg

Selected Readings

Krystal AD, Walsh JK, Laska E, et al, "Sustained Efficacy of Eszopiclone Over 6 Months of Nightly Treatment: Results of a Randomized, Double-Blind, Placebo-Controlled Study in Adults With Chronic Insomnia," *Sleep*, 2003, 26(7):793-9.

ETAF *see* Aldesleukin *on page 62*

Etanercept (et a NER sept)

Related Information

Rheumatoid Arthritis, Osteoarthritis, and Osteoporosis *on page 1759*

U.S. Brand Names Enbrel®

Canadian Brand Names Enbrel®

Mexican Brand Names Enbrel

Generic Available No

Pharmacologic Category Antirheumatic, Disease Modifying; Tumor Necrosis Factor (TNF) Blocking Agent

Use Treatment of moderately- to severely-active rheumatoid arthritis (RA); moderately- to severely-active polyarticular juvenile rheumatoid arthritis (JRA) in patients with inadequate response to at least one disease-modifying antirheumatic drug; psoriatic arthritis; active ankylosing spondylitis (AS); moderate-to-severe chronic plaque psoriasis

(Continued)

Etanercept *(Continued)*

Local Anesthetic/Vasoconstrictor Precautions No information available to require special precautions

Effects on Dental Treatment No significant effects or complications reported

Common Adverse Effects

>10%:

Central nervous system: Headache (17%)

Local: Injection site reaction (14% to 37%; erythema, itching, pain or swelling)

Respiratory: Respiratory tract infection (upper, 20% to 29%), rhinitis (12%)

Miscellaneous: Infection (35%), positive ANA (11%), positive antidouble-stranded DNA antibodies (15% by RIA, 3% by *Crithidia luciliae* assay)

≥3% to 10%:

Central nervous system: Dizziness (7%)

Dermatologic: Rash (5%)

Gastrointestinal: Abdominal pain (5%), dyspepsia (4%), nausea (9%), vomiting (3%)

Neuromuscular & skeletal: Weakness (5%)

Respiratory: Pharyngitis (7%), respiratory disorder (5%), sinusitis (3%), cough (6%)

Pediatric patients (JRA): The percentages of patients reporting abdominal pain (17%) and vomiting (13%) were higher than in adult RA. Two patients developed varicella infection associated with aseptic meningitis which resolved without complications (see Warnings/Precautions). Other severe reactions included gastroenteritis, depression, cutaneous ulcer, esophagitis/gastritis, group A streptococcal septic shock, and wound infections.

Dosage SubQ

Children 4-17 years: Juvenile rheumatoid arthritis:

Once-weekly dosing (patients weighing <31 kg or ≥63 kg): 0.8 mg/kg (maximum: 50 mg/dose) once weekly

Twice-weekly dosing (patients weighing 31-62 kg): 0.4 mg/kg (maximum: 25 mg/dose) twice weekly (individual doses should be separated by 72-96 hours)

Adults:

Rheumatoid arthritis, psoriatic arthritis, ankylosing spondylitis:

Once-weekly dosing: 50 mg once weekly

Twice weekly dosing: 25 mg given twice weekly (individual doses should be separated by 72-96 hours)

Plaque psoriasis:

Initial: 50 mg twice weekly, 3-4 days apart (starting doses of 25 or 50 mg once weekly have also been used successfully); maintain initial dose for 3 months

Maintenance dose: 50 mg weekly

Elderly: Refer to adult dosing. Although greater sensitivity of some elderly patients cannot be ruled out, no overall differences in safety or effectiveness were observed.

Mechanism of Action Etanercept is a recombinant DNA-derived protein composed of tumor necrosis factor receptor (TNFR) linked to the Fc portion of human IgG1. Etanercept binds tumor necrosis factor (TNF) and blocks its interaction with cell surface receptors. TNF plays an important role in the inflammatory processes and the resulting joint pathology of rheumatoid arthritis (RA), polyarticular-course juvenile arthritis (JRA), ankylosing spondylitis (AS), and plaque psoriasis.

Contraindications Hypersensitivity to etanercept or any component of the formulation; patients with sepsis (mortality may be increased); active infections (including chronic or local infection)

Warnings/Precautions Serious and potentially fatal rare infections, including reactivation of hepatitis or cases of tuberculosis have been reported. Discontinue administration if patient develops a serious infection. Caution should be exercised when considering the use in patients with chronic infection, history of recurrent infection, or predisposition to infection (such as poorly-controlled diabetes). Do not give to patients with an active chronic or localized infection. Patients who develop a new infection while undergoing treatment should be monitored closely. If a patient develops a serious infection, therapy should be discontinued. Patients should be brought up to date with all immunizations before initiating therapy. Live vaccines should not be given concurrently. Patients with a significant exposure to varicella virus should temporarily discontinue etanercept. Treatment with varicella zoster immune globulin should be considered.

Impact on the development and course of malignancies is not fully defined. As compared to the general population, an increased risk of lymphoma has been noted in clinical trials; however, rheumatoid arthritis has been previously associated with an increased rate of lymphoma. Etanercept is not recommended for use in patients with Wegener's granulomatosis who are receiving immunosuppressive therapy. Treatment may result in the formation of autoimmune antibodies; cases of autoimmune disease have not been described. Non-neutralizing antibodies to etanercept may also be formed. Rarely, a reversible lupus-like syndrome has occurred. Safety and efficacy have not been established in children <4 years of age.

Use caution in patients with pre-existing or recent-onset demyelinating CNS disorders; cases of optic neuritis, demyelinating disease and/or seizures have been reported. Use caution in patients with CHF; has been associated with worsening and new-onset CHF. Use caution in patients with a history of significant hematologic abnormalities; has been associated with pancytopenia and aplastic anemia (rare). Discontinue if significant hematologic abnormalities are confirmed.

Should not be used in combination with anakinra, unless no satisfactory alternatives exist, and then only with extreme caution. Some dosage forms may contain dry natural rubber (latex).

Drug Interactions
Increased Effect/Toxicity: Abatacept and anakinra may increase the risk of infection. Cyclophosphamide may increase the risk of noncutaneous solid malignancy. Etanercept may increase the risk of vaccinal infection (live organism vaccine).
Decreased Effect: Etanercept may decrease the effect of killed organism or component vaccines.
Ethanol/Nutrition/Herb Interactions Herb/Nutraceutical: Echinacea may decrease the therapeutic effects of etanercept (avoid concurrent use).
Pharmacodynamics/Kinetics
Onset of action: ~2-3 weeks; RA: 1-2 weeks
Half-life elimination: RA: SubQ: 72-132 hours
Time to peak: RA: SubQ: 35-103 hours
Excretion: Clearance: Children: 45.9 mL/hour/m^2; Adults: 89 mL/hour (52 mL/hour/m^2)
Pregnancy Risk Factor B
Dosage Forms
Injection, powder for reconstitution:
Enbrel®: 25 mg
Injection, solution:
Enbrel®: 50 mg/mL (0.98 mL)

Ethacrynate Sodium *see* Ethacrynic Acid *on page 619*

Ethacrynic Acid (eth a KRIN ik AS id)

Related Information
Cardiovascular Diseases *on page 1726*
U.S. Brand Names Edecrin®
Canadian Brand Names Edecrin®
Generic Available No
Index Terms Ethacrynate Sodium
Pharmacologic Category Diuretic, Loop
Use Management of edema associated with congestive heart failure; hepatic cirrhosis or renal disease; short-term management of ascites due to malignancy, idiopathic edema, and lymphedema
Local Anesthetic/Vasoconstrictor Precautions No information available to require special precautions
Effects on Dental Treatment No significant effects or complications reported
Common Adverse Effects Frequency not defined.
Central nervous system: Headache, fatigue, apprehension, confusion, fever, chills, encephalopathy (patients with pre-existing liver disease); vertigo
Dermatologic: Skin rash, Henoch-Schönlein purpura (in patient with rheumatic heart disease)
Endocrine & metabolic: Hyponatremia, hyperglycemia, variations in phosphorus, CO_2 content, bicarbonate, and calcium; reversible hyperuricemia, gout, hyperglycemia, hypoglycemia (occurred in two uremic patients who received doses above those recommended)
Gastrointestinal: Anorexia, malaise, abdominal discomfort or pain, dysphagia, nausea, vomiting, diarrhea, gastrointestinal bleeding, acute pancreatitis (rare)
Genitourinary: Hematuria
Hepatic: Jaundice, abnormal liver function tests
Hematology: Agranulocytosis, severe neutropenia, thrombocytopenia
Local: Thrombophlebitis (with intravenous use), local irritation and pain
(Continued)

Ethacrynic Acid *(Continued)*

Ocular: Blurred vision
Otic: Tinnitus, temporary or permanent deafness
Renal: Serum creatinine increased

Mechanism of Action Inhibits reabsorption of sodium and chloride in the ascending loop of Henle and distal renal tubule, interfering with the chloride-binding cotransport system, thus causing increased excretion of water, sodium, chloride, magnesium, and calcium

Drug Interactions

Increased Effect/Toxicity: Ethacrynic acid-induced hypokalemia may predispose to digoxin toxicity and may increase the risk of arrhythmia with drugs which may prolong QT interval, including type Ia and type III antiarrhythmic agents, cisapride, and some quinolones (sparfloxacin, gatifloxacin, and moxifloxacin). The risk of toxicity from lithium and salicylates (high dose) may be increased by loop diuretics. Hypotensive effects and/or adverse renal effects of ACE inhibitors and NSAIDs are potentiated by ethacrynic acid-induced hypovolemia. The effects of peripheral adrenergic-blocking drugs or ganglionic blockers may be increased by ethacrynic acid.

Ethacrynic acid may increase the risk of ototoxicity with other ototoxic agents (aminoglycosides, cis-platinum), especially in patients with renal dysfunction. Synergistic diuretic effects occur with thiazide-type diuretics. Diuretics tend to be synergistic with other antihypertensive agents, and hypotension may occur. Nephrotoxicity has been associated with concomitant use of cephaloridine or cephalexin.

Decreased Effect: Probenecid decreases diuretic effects of ethacrynic acid. Glucose tolerance may be decreased by loop diuretics, requiring adjustment of hypoglycemic agents. Cholestyramine or colestipol may reduce bioavailability of ethacrynic acid. Indomethacin (and other NSAIDs) may reduce natriuretic and hypotensive effects of diuretics.

Pharmacodynamics/Kinetics

Onset of action: Diuresis: Oral: ~30 minutes; I.V.: 5 minutes
Peak effect: Oral: 2 hours; I.V.: 30 minutes
Duration: Oral: 12 hours; I.V.: 2 hours
Absorption: Oral: Rapid
Protein binding: >90%
Metabolism: Hepatic (35% to 40%) to active cysteine conjugate
Half-life elimination: Normal renal function: 2-4 hours
Excretion: Feces and urine (30% to 60% as unchanged drug)

Pregnancy Risk Factor B

Ethambutol *(e THAM byoo tole)*

Related Information
Tuberculosis *on page 1765*
U.S. Brand Names Myambutol®
Canadian Brand Names Etibi®
Mexican Brand Names Myambutol
Generic Available Yes
Index Terms Ethambutol Hydrochloride
Pharmacologic Category Antitubercular Agent
Use Treatment of tuberculosis and other mycobacterial diseases in conjunction with other antituberculosis agents
Local Anesthetic/Vasoconstrictor Precautions No information available to require special precautions
Effects on Dental Treatment No significant effects or complications reported
Common Adverse Effects Frequency not defined.
Cardiovascular: Myocarditis, pericarditis
Central nervous system: Headache, confusion, disorientation, malaise, mental confusion, fever, dizziness, hallucinations
Dermatologic: Rash, pruritus, dermatitis, exfoliative dermatitis
Endocrine & metabolic: Acute gout or hyperuricemia
Gastrointestinal: Abdominal pain, anorexia, nausea, vomiting
Hematologic: Leukopenia, thrombocytopenia, eosinophilia, neutropenia, lymphadenopathy
Hepatic: Abnormal LFTs, hepatotoxicity (possibly related to concurrent therapy), hepatitis
Neuromuscular & skeletal: Peripheral neuritis, arthralgia
Ocular: Optic neuritis; symptoms may include decreased acuity, scotoma, color blindness, or visual defects (usually reversible with discontinuation, irreversible blindness has been described)
Renal: Nephritis

Respiratory: Infiltrates (with or without eosinophilia), pneumonitis
Miscellaneous: Anaphylaxis, anaphylactoid reaction; hypersensitivity syndrome (rash, eosinophilia, and organ-specific inflammation)
Mechanism of Action Suppresses mycobacteria multiplication by interfering with RNA synthesis
Drug Interactions
Decreased Effect: Decreased absorption with aluminum hydroxide. Avoid concurrent administration of aluminum-containing antacids for at least 4 hours following ethambutol.
Pharmacodynamics/Kinetics
Absorption: ~80%
Distribution: Widely throughout body; concentrated in kidneys, lungs, saliva, and red blood cells
Relative diffusion from blood into CSF: Adequate with or without inflammation (exceeds usual MICs)
CSF:blood level ratio: Normal meninges: 0%; Inflamed meninges: 25%
Protein binding: 20% to 30%
Metabolism: Hepatic (20%) to inactive metabolite
Half-life elimination: 2.5-3.6 hours; End-stage renal disease: 7-15 hours
Time to peak, serum: 2-4 hours
Excretion: Urine (~50%) and feces (20%) as unchanged drug
Pregnancy Risk Factor C

Ethambutol Hydrochloride *see* Ethambutol *on page 620*
Ethamolin® *see* Ethanolamine Oleate *on page 621*

Ethanolamine Oleate (ETH a nol a meen OH lee ate)

U.S. Brand Names Ethamolin®
Generic Available No
Index Terms Monoethanolamine
Pharmacologic Category Sclerosing Agent
Use Orphan drug: Sclerosing agent used for bleeding esophageal varices
Local Anesthetic/Vasoconstrictor Precautions No information available to require special precautions
Effects on Dental Treatment No significant effects or complications reported
Common Adverse Effects 1% to 10%:
Central nervous system: Pyrexia (1.8%)
Gastrointestinal: Esophageal ulcer (2%), esophageal stricture (1.3%)
Respiratory: Pleural effusion (2%), pneumonia (1.2%)
Miscellaneous: Retrosternal pain (1.6%)
Mechanism of Action Derived from oleic acid and similar in physical properties to sodium morrhuate; however, the exact mechanism of the hemostatic effect used in endoscopic injection sclerotherapy is not known. Intravenously injected ethanolamine oleate produces a sterile inflammatory response resulting in fibrosis and occlusion of the vein; a dose-related extravascular inflammatory reaction occurs when the drug diffuses through the venous wall. Autopsy results indicate that variceal obliteration occurs secondary to mural necrosis and fibrosis. Thrombosis appears to be a transient reaction.
Pregnancy Risk Factor C

EtheDent™ *see* Fluoride *on page 710*
Ethezyme™ *see* Papain and Urea *on page 1251*
Ethezyme™ 830 *see* Papain and Urea *on page 1251*

Ethinyl Estradiol and Desogestrel (ETH in il es tra DYE ole & des oh JES trel)

U.S. Brand Names Apri®; Cesia™; Cyclessa®; Desogen®; Kariva™; Mircette®; Ortho-Cept®; Reclipsen™; Solia™; Velivet™
Canadian Brand Names Cyclessa®; Linessa®; Marvelon®; Ortho-Cept®
Mexican Brand Names Marvelon
Generic Available Yes
Index Terms Desogestrel and Ethinyl Estradiol; Ortho Cept
Pharmacologic Category Contraceptive; Estrogen and Progestin Combination
Use Prevention of pregnancy
Unlabeled/Investigational Use Treatment of hypermenorrhea (menorrhagia); pain associated with endometriosis; dysmenorrhea; dysfunctional uterine bleeding
Local Anesthetic/Vasoconstrictor Precautions No information available to require special precautions
(Continued)

Ethinyl Estradiol and Desogestrel *(Continued)*

Effects on Dental Treatment When prescribing antibiotics, patient must be warned to use additional methods of birth control if on oral contraceptives.

Common Adverse Effects Frequency not defined.

Cardiovascular: Arterial thromboembolism, cerebral hemorrhage, cerebral thrombosis, edema, hypertension, mesenteric thrombosis, MI

Central nervous system: Depression, dizziness, headache, migraine, nervousness, premenstrual syndrome, stroke

Dermatologic: Acne, erythema multiforme, erythema nodosum, hirsutism, loss of scalp hair, melasma (may persist), rash (allergic)

Endocrine & metabolic: Amenorrhea, breakthrough bleeding, breast enlargement, breast secretion, breast tenderness, carbohydrate intolerance, lactation decreased (postpartum), glucose tolerance decreased, libido changes, menstrual flow changes, sex hormone-binding globulins (SHBG) increased, spotting, temporary infertility (following discontinuation), thyroid-binding globulin increased, triglycerides increased

Gastrointestinal: Abdominal cramps, appetite changes, bloating, cholestasis, colitis, gallbladder disease, jaundice, nausea, vomiting, weight gain/loss

Genitourinary: Cervical erosion changes, cervical secretion changes, cystitis-like syndrome, vaginal candidiasis, vaginitis

Hematologic: Antithrombin III decreased, folate levels decreased, hemolytic uremic syndrome, norepinephrine induced platelet aggregability increased, porphyria, prothrombin increased; factors VII, VIII, IX, and X

Hepatic: Benign liver tumors, Budd-Chiari syndrome, cholestatic jaundice, hepatic adenomas

Local: Thrombophlebitis

Ocular: Cataracts, change in corneal curvature (steepening), contact lens intolerance, optic neuritis, retinal thrombosis

Renal: Impaired renal function

Respiratory: Pulmonary thromboembolism

Miscellaneous: Hemorrhagic eruption

Dosage Oral: Adults: Female: Contraception:

Schedule 1 (Sunday starter): Dose begins on first Sunday after onset of menstruation; if the menstrual period starts on Sunday, take first tablet that very same day. **With a Sunday start, an additional method of contraception should be used until after the first 7 days of consecutive administration.**

For 21-tablet package: Dosage is 1 tablet daily for 21 consecutive days, followed by 7 days off of the medication; a new course begins on the 8th day after the last tablet is taken.

For 28-tablet package: Dosage is 1 tablet daily without interruption.

Schedule 2 (Day 1 starter): Dose starts on first day of menstrual cycle taking 1 tablet daily.

For 21-tablet package: Dosage is 1 tablet daily for 21 consecutive days, followed by 7 days off of the medication; a new course begins on the 8th day after the last tablet is taken.

For 28-tablet package: Dosage is 1 tablet daily without interruption.

If all doses have been taken on schedule and one menstrual period is missed, continue dosing cycle. If two consecutive menstrual periods are missed, pregnancy test is required before new dosing cycle is started.

Missed doses **monophasic formulations** (refer to package insert for complete information):

One dose missed: Take as soon as remembered or take 2 tablets next day

Two consecutive doses missed in the first 2 weeks: Take 2 tablets as soon as remembered or 2 tablets next 2 days. **An additional method of contraception should be used for 7 days after missed dose.**

Two consecutive doses missed in week 3 or three consecutive doses missed at any time:

Schedule 1 (Sunday starter): Continue to take 1 tablet daily until Sunday, then discard the rest of the pack, and a new pack is started that same day.

Schedule 2 (Day 1 starter): Current pack should be discarded, and a new pack started that same day. **An additional method of contraception should be used for 7 days after missed dose.**

Missed doses **biphasic/triphasic formulations** (refer to package insert for complete information):

One dose missed: Take as soon as remembered or take 2 tablets next day.

Two consecutive doses missed in week 1 or week 2 of the pack: Take 2 tablets as soon as remembered and 2 tablets the next day. Resume taking 1 tablet daily until the pack is empty. **An additional method of contraception should be used for 7 days after a missed dose.**

Two consecutive doses missed in week 3 of the pack; **an additional method of contraception must be used for 7 days after a missed dose**:

Schedule 1 (Sunday starter): Take 1 tablet every day until Sunday. Discard the remaining pack and start a new pack of pills on the same day.

Schedule 2 (Day 1 starter): Discard the remaining pack and start a new pack the same day.

Three or more consecutive doses missed; **an additional method of contraception must be used for 7 days after a missed dose**:

Schedule 1 (Sunday starter): Take 1 tablet every day until Sunday; on Sunday, discard the pack and start a new pack.

Schedule 2 (Day 1 starter): Discard the remaining pack and begin new pack of tablets starting on the same day.

Dosage adjustment in renal impairment: Specific guidelines not available; use with caution and monitor blood pressure closely. Consider other forms of contraception.

Dosage adjustment in hepatic impairment: Contraindicated in patients with hepatic impairment

Mechanism of Action Combination hormonal contraceptives inhibit ovulation via a negative feedback mechanism on the hypothalamus, which alters the normal pattern of gonadotropin secretion of a follicle-stimulating hormone (FSH) and luteinizing hormone by the anterior pituitary. The follicular phase FSH and midcycle surge of gonadotropins are inhibited. In addition, combination hormonal contraceptives produce alterations in the genital tract, including changes in the cervical mucus, rendering it unfavorable for sperm penetration even if ovulation occurs. Changes in the endometrium may also occur, producing an unfavorable environment for nidation. Combination hormonal contraceptive drugs may alter the tubal transport of the ova through the fallopian tubes. Progestational agents may also alter sperm fertility.

Contraindications Hypersensitivity to ethinyl estradiol, etonogestrel, desogestrel, or any component of the formulation; history of or current thrombophlebitis or venous thromboembolic disorders (including DVT, PE); active or recent (within 1 year) arterial thromboembolic disease (eg, stroke, MI); cerebral vascular disease, coronary artery disease, valvular heart disease with complications, severe hypertension; diabetes mellitus with vascular involvement; severe headache with focal neurological symptoms; known or suspected breast carcinoma, endometrial cancer, estrogen-dependent neoplasms, undiagnosed abnormal genital bleeding; hepatic dysfunction or tumor, cholestatic jaundice of pregnancy, jaundice with prior combination hormonal contraceptive use; major surgery with prolonged immobilization; heavy smoking (≥15 cigarettes/day) in patients >35 years of age; pregnancy

Warnings/Precautions Combination hormonal contraceptives do not protect against HIV infection or other sexually-transmitted diseases. **[U.S. Boxed Warning]: The risk of cardiovascular side effects increases in women who smoke cigarettes, especially those who are >35 years of age; women who use combination hormonal contraceptives should be strongly advised not to smoke.** Combination hormonal contraceptives may lead to increased risk of myocardial infarction, use with caution in patients with risk factors for coronary artery disease. May increase the risk of thromboembolism. Whenever possible, combination hormonal contraceptives should be discontinued at least 4 weeks prior to and for 2 weeks following elective surgery associated with an increased risk of thromboembolism or during periods of prolonged immobilization. Combination hormonal contraceptives may have a dose-related risk of vascular disease, hypertension, and gallbladder disease. Women with hypertension or renal disease should be encouraged to use another form of contraception. The use of combination hormonal contraceptives has been associated with a slight increase in frequency of breast cancer, however, studies are not consistent. Combination hormonal contraceptives may cause glucose intolerance or effect serum triglyceride and lipoprotein levels. Retinal thrombosis has been reported (rarely). Use caution in conditions that may be aggravated by fluid retention, depression, or history of migraine. Not for use prior to menarche.

The minimum dosage combination of estrogen/progestin that will effectively treat the individual patient should be used. New patients should be started on products containing ≤0.035 mg of estrogen per tablet.

Drug Interactions

Cytochrome P450 Effect:

Ethinyl estradiol: **Substrate** of CYP2C9 (minor), 3A4 (major), 3A5-7 (minor); **Inhibits** CYP1A2 (weak), 2B6 (weak), 2C8 (weak), 2C19 (weak), 3A4 (weak)

Desogestrel: **Substrate** of CYP2C19 (major)

Increased Effect/Toxicity: Acetaminophen, ascorbic acid, and repaglinide may increase plasma levels of estrogen component. Atorvastatin and indinavir increase plasma levels of combination hormonal contraceptives. (Continued)

Ethinyl Estradiol and Desogestrel *(Continued)*

Combination hormonal contraceptives increase the plasma levels of alprazolam, chlordiazepoxide, cyclosporine, diazepam, prednisolone, selegiline, theophylline, tricyclic antidepressants. Combination hormonal contraceptives may increase (or decrease) the effects of coumarin derivatives.

Decreased Effect: CYP2C19 inducers may decrease the levels/effects of desogestrel; example inducers include aminoglutethimide, carbamazepine, phenytoin, and rifampin. CYP3A4 inducers may decrease the levels/effects of ethinyl estradiol; example inducers include aminoglutethimide, carbamazepine, nafcillin, phenobarbital, phenytoin, and rifamycins. Combination hormonal contraceptives may decrease plasma levels of acetaminophen, clofibric acid, lorazepam, morphine, oxazepam, salicylic acid, temazepam. Contraceptive effect decreased by acitretin, amprenavir, griseofulvin, lopinavir, nelfinavir, nevirapine, penicillins (effect not consistent), ritonavir, tetracyclines (effect not consistent), troglitazone. Combination hormonal contraceptives may decrease (or increase) the effects of coumarin derivatives. Aprepitant, modafinil, and topiramate may decrease the serum concentration of oral contraceptive (estrogens). Oral contraceptive (estrogens) may decrease the serum concentration of lamotrigine.

Ethanol/Nutrition/Herb Interactions

Food: CNS effects of caffeine may be enhanced if combination hormonal contraceptives are used concurrently with caffeine. Grapefruit juice increases ethinyl estradiol concentrations and would be expected to increase progesterone serum levels as well; clinical implications are unclear.

Herb/Nutraceutical: St John's wort may decrease levels. Herbs with estrogenic properties may enhance the adverse/toxic effect of estrogen derivatives; examples include alfalfa, black cohosh, bloodroot, hops, kudzu, licorice, red clover, saw palmetto, soybean, thyme, wild yam, yucca. Herbs with progestogenic properties may enhance the adverse/toxic effect of progestins; examples include bloodroot, chasteberry, damiana, oregano, yucca.

Dietary Considerations Should be taken at same time each day.

Pharmacodynamics/Kinetics

Desogestrel:

Absorption: Rapid and complete

Protein binding: Etonogestrel (active metabolite): 98%, primarily to sex hormone-binding globulin

Metabolism: Hepatic via CYP2C9 to active metabolite etonogestrel (3-keto-desogestrel); etonogestrel metabolized via CYP3A4

Half-life elimination: 37.1 hours

Excretion: Urine and feces (as metabolites)

Pregnancy Risk Factor X

Dosage Forms

Tablet, low-dose formulations:

Kariva™:

Day 1-21: Ethinyl estradiol 0.02 mg and desogestrel 0.15 mg [21 white tablets]

Day 22-23: 2 inactive light green tablets

Day 24-28: Ethinyl estradiol 0.01 mg [5 light blue tablets] (28s)

Mircette®:

Day 1-21: Ethinyl estradiol 0.02 mg and desogestrel 0.15 mg [21 white tablets]

Day 22-23: 2 inactive green tablets

Day 24-28: Ethinyl estradiol 0.01 mg [5 yellow tablets] (28s)

Tablet, monophasic formulations:

Apri® 28: Ethinyl estradiol 0.03 mg and desogestrel 0.15 mg [21 rose tablets and 7 white inactive tablets] (28s)

Desogen®, Reclipsen™, Solia™: Ethinyl estradiol 0.03 mg and desogestrel 0.15 mg [21 white tablets and 7 green inactive tablets] (28s)

Ortho-Cept® 28: Ethinyl estradiol 0.03 mg and desogestrel 0.15 mg [21 orange tablets and 7 green inactive tablets] (28s)

Tablet, triphasic formulations:

Cesia™, Cyclessa®:

Day 1-7:Ethinyl estradiol 0.025 mg and desogestrel 0.1 mg [7 light yellow tablets]

Day 8-14: Ethinyl estradiol 0.025 mg and desogestrel 0.125 mg [7 orange tablets]

Day 14-21: Ethinyl estradiol 0.025 mg and desogestrel 0.15 mg [7 red tablets]

Day 21-28: 7 green inactive tablets (28s)

Velivet™:

Day 1-7: Ethinyl estradiol 0.025 mg and desogestrel 0.1 mg [7 beige tablets]

Day 8-14: Ethinyl estradiol 0.025 mg and desogestrel 0.125 mg [7 orange tablets]

Day 14-21: Ethinyl estradiol 0.025 mg and desogestrel 0.15 mg [7 pink tablets]

Day 21-28: 7 white inactive tablets (28s)

Ethinyl Estradiol and Drospirenone
(ETH in il es tra DYE ole & droh SPYE re none)

U.S. Brand Names Yasmin®; Yaz

Canadian Brand Names Yasmin®

Mexican Brand Names Yasmin

Generic Available No

Index Terms Drospirenone and Ethinyl Estradiol

Pharmacologic Category Contraceptive; Estrogen and Progestin Combination

Use Females: Prevention of pregnancy; treatment of premenstrual dysphoric disorder (PMDD); treatment of acne

Unlabeled/Investigational Use Treatment of hypermenorrhea (menorrhagia); pain associated with endometriosis; dysmenorrhea; dysfunctional uterine bleeding

Local Anesthetic/Vasoconstrictor Precautions No information available to require special precautions

Effects on Dental Treatment When prescribing antibiotics, patient must be warned to use additional methods of birth control if on oral contraceptives.

Common Adverse Effects

>1%:
Central nervous system: Depression, dizziness, emotional lability, fever, headache, migraine, nervousness, pain

Dermatologic: Acne, pruritus, rash

Endocrine & metabolic: Amenorrhea, breast pain, dysmenorrhea, hyperlipidemia, intermenstrual bleeding, libido decreased, menstrual irregularities

Gastrointestinal: Abdomen enlarged, abdominal pain, diarrhea, dyspepsia, gastroenteritis, nausea, tooth disorder, vomiting, weight gain

Genitourinary: Cystitis, leukorrhea, papanicolaou smear suspicious, pelvic pain, UTI, vaginal moniliasis, vaginitis

Neuromuscular & skeletal: Back pain, extremity pain, weakness

Respiratory: Bronchitis, cough, pharyngitis, rhinitis, sinusitis, upper respiratory infection

Miscellaneous: Allergic reaction, flu-like syndrome, infection

Adverse reactions reported with other oral contraceptives: Appetite changes, antithrombin III decreased, arterial thromboembolism, benign liver tumors, breast changes, Budd-Chiari syndrome, carbohydrate intolerance, cataracts, cerebral hemorrhage, cerebral thrombosis, cervical changes, change in corneal curvature (steepening), cholestatic jaundice, colitis, contact lens intolerance, decreased lactation (postpartum), deep vein thrombosis, diplopia, edema, erythema multiforme, erythema nodosum; factors VII, VIII, IX, X increased; folate serum concentrations decreased, gallbladder disease, glucose intolerance, hemolytic uremic syndrome, hemorrhagic eruption, hepatic adenomas, hirsutism, hypercalcemia, hyperglycemia, hypertension, melasma, mesenteric thrombosis, MI, papilledema, platelet aggregability increased, porphyria, premenstrual syndrome, proptosis, prothrombin increased, pulmonary thromboembolism, renal function impairment, retinal thrombosis, sex hormone-binding globulin increased, thrombophlebitis, thyroid-binding globulin increased, total thyroid hormone (T_4) increased, triglycerides/phospholipids increased, vaginal candidiasis

Dosage Oral:
Children ≥14 years and Adults: Female: Acne (Yaz): Refer to dosing for contraception

Adults: Female: Contraception (Yasmin®, Yaz), PMDD (Yaz): Dosage is 1 tablet daily for 28 consecutive days. Dose should be taken at the same time each day, either after the evening meal or at bedtime. Dosing may be started on the first day of menstrual period (Day 1 starter) or on the first Sunday after the onset of the menstrual period (Sunday starter).

Day 1 starter: Dose starts on first day of menstrual cycle taking 1 tablet daily.

Sunday starter: Dose begins on first Sunday after onset of menstruation; if the menstrual period starts on Sunday, take first tablet that very same day. **With a Sunday start, an additional method of contraception should be used until after the first 7 days of consecutive administration.**

If all doses have been taken on schedule and one menstrual period is missed, continue dosing cycle. If two consecutive menstrual periods are missed, pregnancy test is required before new dosing cycle is started.

(Continued)

Ethinyl Estradiol and Drospirenone *(Continued)*

If doses have been missed during the first 3 weeks and the menstrual period is missed, pregnancy should be ruled out prior to continuing treatment.

Missed doses (monophasic formulations) (refer to package insert for complete information):

One dose missed: Take as soon as remembered or take 2 tablets next day

Two consecutive doses missed in the first 2 weeks: Take 2 tablets as soon as remembered or 2 tablets next 2 days. **An additional method of contraception should be used for 7 days after missed dose.**

Two consecutive doses missed in week 3 or three consecutive doses missed at any time: **An additional method of contraception must be used for 7 days after a missed dose.**

Day 1 starter: Current pack should be discarded, and a new pack should be started that same day.

Sunday starter: Continue dose of 1 tablet daily until Sunday, then discard the rest of the pack, and a new pack should be started that same day.

Any number of doses missed in week 4: Continue taking one pill each day until pack is empty; no back-up method of contraception is needed

Dosage adjustment in renal impairment: Contraindicated in patients with renal dysfunction (Cl_{cr} ≤50 mL/minute)

Dosage adjustment in hepatic impairment: Contraindicated in patients with hepatic dysfunction

Mechanism of Action Combination oral contraceptives inhibit ovulation via a negative feedback mechanism on the hypothalamus, which alters the normal pattern of gonadotropin secretion of a follicle-stimulating hormone (FSH) and luteinizing hormone by the anterior pituitary. The follicular phase FSH and midcycle surge of gonadotropins are inhibited. In addition, oral contraceptives produce alterations in the genital tract, including changes in the cervical mucus, rendering it unfavorable for sperm penetration even if ovulation occurs. Changes in the endometrium may also occur, producing an unfavorable environment for nidation. Oral contraceptive drugs may alter the tubal transport of the ova through the fallopian tubes. Progestational agents may also alter sperm fertility. Drospirenone is a spironolactone analogue with antimineralocorticoid and antiandrogenic activity.

Contraindications Hypersensitivity to ethinyl estradiol, drospirenone, or to any component of the formulation; history of or current thrombophlebitis or venous thromboembolic disorders (including DVT, PE); active or recent (within 1 year) arterial thromboembolic disease (eg, stroke, MI); cerebral vascular disease, coronary artery disease, severe hypertension, valvular heart disease with thrombogenic complications; diabetes with vascular involvement; headache with focal neurological symptoms; known or suspected breast carcinoma, endometrial cancer, estrogen-dependent neoplasms, undiagnosed abnormal genital bleeding; renal insufficiency, hepatic dysfunction or tumor, adrenal insufficiency, cholestatic jaundice of pregnancy, jaundice with prior oral contraceptive use; major surgery with prolonged immobilization; heavy smoking (≥15 cigarettes/day) in patients >35 years of age; pregnancy

Warnings/Precautions Oral contraceptives do not protect against HIV infection or other sexually-transmitted diseases. **[U.S. Boxed Warning]: The risk of cardiovascular side effects increases in women who smoke cigarettes, especially those who are >35 years of age; women who use oral contraceptives should be strongly advised not to smoke.** Oral contraceptives may lead to increased risk of myocardial infarction, use with caution in patients with risk factors for coronary artery disease. May increase the risk of thromboembolism. Whenever possible, combination hormonal contraceptives should be discontinued at least 4 weeks prior to and for 2 weeks following elective surgery associated with an increased risk of thromboembolism or during periods of prolonged immobilization. Oral contraceptives may have a dose-related risk of vascular disease, hypertension, and gallbladder disease. Women with hypertension should be encouraged to use another form of contraception. The use of combination hormonal contraceptives has been associated with a slight increase in frequency of breast cancer, however, studies are not consistent. Combination hormonal contraceptives may cause glucose intolerance or effect serum triglyceride and lipoprotein levels. Retinal thrombosis has been reported (rarely) with oral contraceptive use. Use with caution in patients with conditions that may be aggravated by fluid retention, depression, or patients with history of migraine. Not for use prior to menarche.

The minimum dosage combination of estrogen/progestin that will effectively treat the individual patient should be used.

Acne use: For use only in females ≥14 years who have reached menarche, who also desire combination hormonal contraceptive therapy, are unresponsive to topical treatments, and have no contraindications to combination hormonal contraceptive use.

PMDD use: For use only in females who desire combination hormonal contraceptive therapy; use for more than 3 menstrual cycles has not been evaluated. Has not been evaluated for the treatment of premenstrual syndrome

Drospirenone has antimineralocorticoid activity that may lead to hyperkalemia in patients with renal insufficiency, hepatic dysfunction, or adrenal insufficiency. Use caution with medications that may increase serum potassium.

Drug Interactions

Cytochrome P450 Effect:

Ethinyl estradiol: **Substrate** of CYP2C9 (minor), 3A4 (major), 3A5-7 (minor); **Inhibits** CYP1A2 (weak), 2B6 (weak), 2C8 (weak), 2C19 (weak), 3A4 (weak)

Drospirenone: **Substrate** of CYP3A4 (minor); **Inhibits** CYP1A2 (weak), 2C9 (weak), 2C19 (weak), 3A4 (weak)

Increased Effect/Toxicity: ACE inhibitors, aldosterone antagonists, angiotensin II receptor antagonists, heparin, NSAIDs (when taken daily, long term), and potassium salts increase risk of hyperkalemia with concomitant use. Estrogen derivatives may increase the serum concentration of systemic corticosteroids. Ethinyl estradiol may increase plasma concentrations of cyclosporine, prednisolone, and selegiline. Oral contraceptives may increase (or decrease) the effects of coumarin derivatives. Oral contraceptive (estrogens) may increase the serum concentration of tizanidine. Oral contraceptive (estrogens and progestins) may increase the serum concentration of voriconazole. Drospirenone may of the risk of systemic acidosis when used with ammonium chloride. Drospirenone may enhance the hyperkalemic effect of potassium-sparing diuretics. Estrogens may reduce the clearance of benzodiazepines that undergo oxidative metabolism; monitor for toxic effects of benzodiazepines which undergo oxidation (eg, diazepam, triazolam). Voriconazole may decrease the metabolism, via CYP isoenzymes, of oral contraceptive (estrogens and progestins).

Decreased Effect: Acitretin may diminish the therapeutic effect of progestins; contraceptive failure is possible. Oral contraceptives may decrease the plasma concentration of lamotrigine and morphine. Aminoglutethimide, anticonvulsants (carbamazepine, felbamate, oxcarbazepine, phenobarbital, phenytoin, topiramate), aprepitant, rifampin, and protease inhibitors (except atazanavir, tipranavir) may increase metabolism leading to decreased effect of oral contraceptives. Griseofulvin may diminish the therapeutic effect of contraceptive (progestins). Oral contraceptives may decrease (or increase) the effects of coumarin derivatives. Modafinil and topiramate may decrease the serum concentration of oral contraceptive (estrogens). Barbiturates and protease inhibitors (except atazanavir, tipranavir) may diminish the therapeutic effect of estrogen and progestin contraceptives.

Ethanol/Nutrition/Herb Interactions

Food: CNS effects of caffeine may be enhanced if oral contraceptives are used concurrently with caffeine. Grapefruit juice increases ethinyl estradiol concentrations; clinical implications are unclear.

Herb/Nutraceutical: St John's wort may decrease levels. Herbs with estrogenic properties may enhance the adverse/toxic effect of estrogen derivatives; examples include alfalfa, black cohosh, bloodroot, hops, kudzu, licorice, red clover, saw palmetto, soybean, thyme, wild yam, yucca. Herbs with progestogenic properties may enhance the adverse/toxic effect of progestins; examples include bloodroot, chasteberry, damiana, oregano, yucca.

Pharmacodynamics/Kinetics

Distribution: Drospirenone: 4 L/kg; Ethinyl estradiol: 4-5 L/kg

Protein binding: Drospirenone: Serum proteins (excluding sex hormone-binding globulin and corticosteroid-binding globulin): 97%; Ethinyl estradiol: ~98%

Metabolism: Drospirenone: To inactive metabolites, minor metabolism hepatically via CYP3A4; Ethinyl estradiol: Hepatic via CYP3A4; forms metabolites; undergoes enterohepatic circulation

Bioavailability: Drospirenone: 76%; Ethinyl estradiol: 40%

Half-life elimination: Drospirenone: 30 hours; Ethinyl estradiol: ~24 hours

Time to peak: 1-3 hours

Excretion: Drospirenone, ethinyl estradiol: Urine and feces

Pregnancy Risk Factor X

Dosage Forms

Tablet:

Yasmin®: Ethinyl estradiol 0.03 mg and drospirenone 3 mg [21 yellow active tablets and 7 white inactive tablets] (28s)

Yaz: Ethinyl estradiol 0.02 mg and drospirenone 3 mg [24 light pink tablets and 4 white inactive tablets] (28s)

Ethinyl Estradiol and Ethynodiol Diacetate
(ETH in il es tra DYE ole & e thye noe DYE ole dye AS e tate)

U.S. Brand Names Demulen® [DSC]; Kelnor™; Zovia™

Canadian Brand Names Demulen® 30

Generic Available Yes

Index Terms Ethynodiol Diacetate and Ethinyl Estradiol

Pharmacologic Category Contraceptive; Estrogen and Progestin Combination

Use Prevention of pregnancy

Unlabeled/Investigational Use Treatment of hypermenorrhea (menorrhagia); pain associated with endometriosis; dysmenorrhea; dysfunctional uterine bleeding

Local Anesthetic/Vasoconstrictor Precautions No information available to require special precautions

Effects on Dental Treatment When prescribing antibiotics, patient must be warned to use additional methods of birth control if on oral contraceptives.

Common Adverse Effects Frequency not defined.

Cardiovascular: Arterial thromboembolism, cerebral hemorrhage, cerebral thrombosis, edema, hypertension, mesenteric thrombosis, MI

Central nervous system: Depression, dizziness, headache, migraine, nervousness, premenstrual syndrome, stroke

Dermatologic: Acne, erythema multiforme, erythema nodosum, hirsutism, loss of scalp hair, melasma (may persist), rash (allergic)

Endocrine & metabolic: Amenorrhea, breakthrough bleeding, breast enlargement, breast secretion, breast tenderness, carbohydrate intolerance, lactation decreased (postpartum), glucose tolerance decreased, libido changes, menstrual flow changes, sex hormone-binding globulins (SHBG) increased, spotting, temporary infertility (following discontinuation), thyroid-binding globulin increased, triglycerides increased

Gastrointestinal: Abdominal cramps, appetite changes, bloating, cholestasis, colitis, gallbladder disease, jaundice, nausea, vomiting, weight gain/loss

Genitourinary: Cervical erosion changes, cervical secretion changes, cystitis-like syndrome, vaginal candidiasis, vaginitis

Hematologic: Antithrombin III decreased, folate levels decreased, hemolytic uremic syndrome, norepinephrine induced platelet aggregability increased, porphyria, prothrombin increased; factors VII, VIII, IX, and X increased

Hepatic: Benign liver tumors, Budd-Chiari syndrome, cholestatic jaundice, hepatic adenomas

Local: Thrombophlebitis

Ocular: Cataracts, change in corneal curvature (steepening), contact lens intolerance, optic neuritis, retinal thrombosis

Renal: Impaired renal function

Respiratory: Pulmonary thromboembolism

Miscellaneous: Hemorrhagic eruption

Dosage Oral: Adults: Female: Contraception:

Schedule 1 (Sunday starter): Dose begins on first Sunday after onset of menstruation; if the menstrual period starts on Sunday, take first tablet that very same day. **With a Sunday start, an additional method of contraception should be used until after the first 7 days of consecutive administration.**

For 21-tablet package: 1 tablet/day for 21 consecutive days, followed by 7 days off of the medication; a new course begins on the 8th day after the last tablet is taken.

For 28-tablet package: 1 tablet/day without interruption.

Schedule 2 (Day 1 starter): Dose starts on first day of menstrual cycle taking 1 tablet daily.

For 21-tablet package: 1 tablet/day for 21 consecutive days, followed by 7 days off of the medication; a new course begins on the 8th day after the last tablet is taken.

For 28-tablet package: 1 tablet/day without interruption.

If all doses have been taken on schedule and one menstrual period is missed, continue dosing cycle. If two consecutive menstrual periods are missed, pregnancy test is required before new dosing cycle is started.

Missed doses **monophasic formulations** (refer to package insert for complete information):

One dose missed: Take as soon as remembered or take 2 tablets next day

Two consecutive doses missed in the first 2 weeks: Take 2 tablets as soon as remembered or 2 tablets next 2 days. **An additional method of contraception should be used for 7 days after missed dose.**

Two consecutive doses missed in week 3 or three consecutive doses missed at any time: **An additional method of contraception should be used for 7 days after missed dose:**

Schedule 1 (Sunday starter): Continue dose of 1 tablet daily until Sunday, then discard the rest of the pack, and a new pack should be started that same day.

Schedule 2 (Day 1 starter): Current package should be discarded, and a new pack should be started that same day.

Dosage adjustment in renal impairment: Specific guidelines not available; use with caution and monitor blood pressure closely. Consider other forms of contraception.

Dosage adjustment in hepatic impairment: Contraindicated in patients with hepatic impairment

Mechanism of Action Combination hormonal contraceptives inhibit ovulation via a negative feedback mechanism on the hypothalamus, which alters the normal pattern of gonadotropin secretion of a follicle-stimulating hormone (FSH) and luteinizing hormone by the anterior pituitary. The follicular phase FSH and midcycle surge of gonadotropins are inhibited. In addition, combination hormonal contraceptives produce alterations in the genital tract, including changes in the cervical mucus, rendering it unfavorable for sperm penetration even if ovulation occurs. Changes in the endometrium may also occur, producing an unfavorable environment for nidation. Combination hormonal contraceptive drugs may alter the tubal transport of the ova through the fallopian tubes. Progestational agents may also alter sperm fertility.

Contraindications Hypersensitivity to ethinyl estradiol, ethynodiol diacetate, or any component of the formulation; history of or current thrombophlebitis or venous thromboembolic disorders (including DVT, PE); active or recent (within 1 year) arterial thromboembolic disease (eg, stroke, MI); cerebral vascular disease, coronary artery disease, valvular heart disease with complications, severe hypertension; diabetes mellitus with vascular involvement; severe headache with focal neurologic symptoms; known or suspected breast carcinoma, endometrial cancer, estrogen-dependent neoplasms, undiagnosed abnormal genital bleeding; hepatic dysfunction or tumor, cholestatic jaundice of pregnancy, jaundice with prior combination hormonal contraceptive use; major surgery with prolonged immobilization; heavy smoking (≥15 cigarettes/day) in patients >35 years of age; pregnancy

Warnings/Precautions Combination hormonal contraceptives do not protect against HIV infection or other sexually-transmitted diseases. **[U.S. Boxed Warning]: The risk of cardiovascular side effects increases in women who smoke cigarettes, especially those who are >35 years of age; women who use combination hormonal contraceptives should be strongly advised not to smoke.** Combination hormonal contraceptives may lead to increased risk of myocardial infarction, use with caution in patients with risk factors for coronary artery disease. May increase the risk of thromboembolism. Whenever possible, combination hormonal contraceptives should be discontinued at least 4 weeks prior to and for 2 weeks following elective surgery associated with an increased risk of thromboembolism or during periods of prolonged immobilization. Combination hormonal contraceptives may have a dose-related risk of vascular disease, hypertension, and gallbladder disease. Women with hypertension or renal disease should be encouraged to use a nonhormonal form of contraception. The use of combination hormonal contraceptives has been associated with a slight increase in frequency of breast cancer, however, studies are not consistent. Combination hormonal contraceptives may cause glucose intolerance or effect serum triglyceride and lipoprotein levels. Retinal thrombosis has been reported (rarely). Use caution with conditions that may be aggravated by fluid retention, depression, or history of migraine. Not for use prior to menarche.

The minimum dosage combination of estrogen/progestin that will effectively treat the individual patient should be used. New patients should be started on products containing ≤0.035 mg of estrogen per tablet.

Drug Interactions

Cytochrome P450 Effect: Ethinyl estradiol: **Substrate** of CYP2C9 (minor), 3A4 (major), 3A5-7 (minor); **Inhibits** CYP1A2 (weak), 2B6 (weak), 2C8 (weak), 2C19 (weak), 3A4 (weak)

Increased Effect/Toxicity: Acetaminophen and ascorbic acid may increase plasma levels of estrogen component. Atorvastatin and indinavir increase plasma levels of combination hormonal contraceptives. Combination hormonal contraceptives increase the plasma levels of alprazolam, chlordiazepoxide, cyclosporine, diazepam, prednisolone, selegiline, theophylline, tricyclic antidepressants. Combination hormonal contraceptives may increase (or decrease) the effects of coumarin derivatives.

(Continued)

Ethinyl Estradiol and Ethynodiol Diacetate *(Continued)*

Decreased Effect: CYP3A4 inducers may decrease the levels/effects of ethinyl estradiol; example inducers include aminoglutethimide, carbamazepine, nafcillin, nevirapine, phenobarbital, phenytoin, and rifamycins. Combination hormonal contraceptives may decrease plasma levels of acetaminophen, clofibric acid, lorazepam, morphine, oxazepam, salicylic acid, temazepam. Contraceptive effect decreased by acitretin, aminoglutethimide, amprenavir, anticonvulsants, griseofulvin, lopinavir, nelfinavir, penicillins (effect not consistent), rifampin, ritonavir, tetracyclines (effect not consistent). Combination hormonal contraceptives may decrease (or increase) the effects of coumarin derivatives. Aprepitant, modafinil, and topiramate may decrease the serum concentration of oral contraceptive (estrogens). Oral contraceptive (estrogens) may decrease the serum concentration of lamotrigine.

Ethanol/Nutrition/Herb Interactions

Food: CNS effects of caffeine may be enhanced if combination hormonal contraceptives are used concurrently with caffeine. Grapefruit juice increases ethinyl estradiol concentrations and would be expected to increase progesterone serum levels as well; clinical implications are unclear.

Herb/Nutraceutical: St John's wort may decrease levels. Herbs with estrogenic properties may enhance the adverse/toxic effect of estrogen derivatives; examples include alfalfa, black cohosh, bloodroot, hops, kudzu, licorice, red clover, saw palmetto, soybean, thyme, wild yam, yucca. Herbs with progestogenic properties may enhance the adverse/toxic effect of progestins; examples include bloodroot, chasteberry, damiana, oregano, yucca.

Dietary Considerations Should be taken with food at same time each day.

Pharmacodynamics/Kinetics

Ethynodiol diacetate (converted to norethindrone)

Metabolism: Hepatic conjugation

Half-life elimination: Terminal: 5-14 hours

See Norethindrone monograph.

Pregnancy Risk Factor X

Dosage Forms

Tablet, monophasic formulations:

Kelnor™ 1/35: Ethinyl estradiol 0.035 mg and ethynodiol diacetate 1 mg [21 light yellow tablets and 7 white inactive tablets] (28s)

Zovia™ 1/35-28: Ethinyl estradiol 0.035 mg and ethynodiol diacetate 1 mg [21 light pink tablets and 7 white inactive tablets] (28s)

Zovia™ 1/50-28: Ethinyl estradiol 0.05 mg and ethynodiol diacetate 1 mg [21 pink tablets and 7 white inactive tablets] (28s)

Ethinyl Estradiol and Etonogestrel

(ETH in il es tra DYE ole & et oh noe JES trel)

U.S. Brand Names NuvaRing®

Canadian Brand Names NuvaRing®

Mexican Brand Names NuvaRing

Generic Available No

Index Terms Etonogestrel and Ethinyl Estradiol

Pharmacologic Category Contraceptive; Estrogen and Progestin Combination

Use Prevention of pregnancy

Unlabeled/Investigational Use Treatment of hypermenorrhea (menorrhagia); pain associated with endometriosis; dysmenorrhea; dysfunctional uterine bleeding

Local Anesthetic/Vasoconstrictor Precautions No information available to require special precautions

Effects on Dental Treatment When prescribing antibiotics, patient must be warned to use additional methods of birth control if on oral contraceptives.

Common Adverse Effects Adverse reactions associated with oral combination hormonal contraceptive agents are also likely to appear with vaginally-administered products (frequency difficult to anticipate). Refer to oral contraceptive monographs for additional information.

5% to 14%:

Central nervous system: Headache

Gastrointestinal: Nausea, weight gain

Genitourinary: Leukorrhea, vaginitis

Respiratory: Sinusitis, upper respiratory tract infection

Frequency not defined:

Central nervous system: Emotional lability

Genitourinary: Bleeding irregularities, coital problems, device expulsion, foreign body sensation, toxic shock syndrome (in some cases associated with tampon use), vaginal discomfort

Dosage Vaginal: Adults: Female: Contraception: One ring, inserted vaginally and left in place for 3 consecutive weeks, then removed for 1 week. A new ring is inserted 7 days after the last was removed (even if bleeding is not complete) and should be inserted at approximately the same time of day the ring was removed the previous week.

Initial treatment should begin as follows (pregnancy should always be ruled out first):

No hormonal contraceptive use in the past month: Using the first day of menstruation as "Day 1," insert the ring on or prior to "Day 5," even if bleeding is not complete. **An additional form of contraception should be used for the following 7 days.***

Switching from combination oral contraceptive: Ring can be inserted on any day within 7 days after the last **active** tablet in the cycle was taken and no later than the first day a new cycle of tablets would begin. Additional forms of contraception are not needed.

Switching from progestin-only contraceptive: **An additional form of contraception should be used for the following 7 days with any of the following.***

If previously using a progestin-only mini-pill, insert the ring on any day of the month; do not skip days between the last pill and insertion of the ring.

If previously using an implant, insert the ring on the same day of implant removal.

If previously using a progestin-containing IUD, insert the ring on day of IUD removal.

If previously using a progestin injection, insert the ring on the day the next injection would be given.

Following complete 1st trimester abortion: Insert ring within the first five days of abortion. If not inserted within five days, follow instructions for "No hormonal contraceptive use within the past month" and instruct patient to use a nonhormonal contraceptive in the interim.

Following delivery or 2nd trimester abortion: Insert ring 4 weeks postpartum (in women who are not breast-feeding) or following 2nd trimester abortion. **An additional form of contraception should be used for the following 7 days.***

If the ring is accidentally removed from the vagina at anytime during the 3-week period of use, it may be rinsed with cool or lukewarm water (not hot) and reinserted as soon as possible. If the ring is not reinserted within three hours, contraceptive effectiveness will be decreased. **An additional form of contraception should be used until the ring has been in place for 7 consecutive days.***

If the ring has been removed for longer than 1 week, pregnancy must be ruled out prior to restarting therapy. **An additional form of contraception should be used for the following 7 days.***

If the ring has been left in place for >3 weeks, a new ring should be inserted following a 1-week (ring-free) interval. Pregnancy must be ruled out prior to insertion and **an additional form of contraception should be used for the following 7 days.***

Disconnected ring: In the event the ring disconnects at the weld joint, discard and replace with a new ring.

***Note:** Diaphragms may interfere with proper ring placement, and therefore, are not recommended for use as an additional form of contraception.

Dosage adjustment in renal impairment: Specific guidelines not available; use with caution and monitor blood pressure closely. Consider other forms of contraception.

Dosage adjustment in hepatic impairment: Contraindicated in patients with hepatic impairment

Mechanism of Action Combination hormonal contraceptives inhibit ovulation via a negative feedback mechanism on the hypothalamus, which alters the normal pattern of gonadotropin secretion of a follicle-stimulating hormone (FSH) and luteinizing hormone by the anterior pituitary. The follicular phase FSH and midcycle surge of gonadotropins are inhibited. In addition, combination hormonal contraceptives produce alterations in the genital tract, including changes in the cervical mucus, rendering it unfavorable for sperm penetration even if ovulation occurs. Changes in the endometrium may also occur, producing an unfavorable environment for nidation. Combination hormonal contraceptive drugs may alter the tubal transport of the ova through the fallopian tubes. Progestational agents may also alter sperm fertility.

Contraindications Hypersensitivity to ethinyl estradiol, etonogestrel, or any component of the formulation; history of or current thrombophlebitis or venous thromboembolic disorders (including DVT, PE); active or recent (within 1 year) arterial thromboembolic disease (eg, stroke, MI); major surgery with prolonged immobilization, cerebral vascular disease, coronary artery disease, valvular heart disease with complications, severe hypertension; diabetes mellitus with (Continued)

Ethinyl Estradiol and Etonogestrel *(Continued)*

vascular involvement; severe headache with focal neurological symptoms; known or suspected breast carcinoma, endometrial cancer, estrogen-dependent neoplasms, undiagnosed abnormal genital bleeding; hepatic dysfunction or tumor, cholestatic jaundice of pregnancy, jaundice with prior combination hormonal contraceptive use; heavy smoking (≥15 cigarettes/day) in patients >35 years of age; conditions which make the vagina susceptible to irritation or ulceration; pregnancy

Warnings/Precautions Combination hormonal contraceptive agents do not protect against HIV infection or other sexually-transmitted diseases. **[U.S. Boxed Warning]: The risk of cardiovascular side effects increases in women who smoke cigarettes, especially those who are >35 years of age; women who use combination hormonal contraceptives should be strongly advised not to smoke.** May lead to increased risk of myocardial infarction, use with caution in patients with risk factors for coronary artery disease. May increase the risk of thromboembolism. Whenever possible, combination hormonal contraceptives should be discontinued at least 4 weeks prior to and for 2 weeks following elective surgery associated with an increased risk of thromboembolism or during periods of prolonged immobilization. May have a dose-related risk of vascular disease, hypertension, and gallbladder disease. Women with hypertension or renal disease should be encouraged to use another form of contraception. The use of combination hormonal contraceptives has been associated with a slight increase in frequency of breast cancer, however, studies are not consistent. Combination hormonal contraceptives may cause glucose intolerance or effect serum triglyceride and lipoprotein levels. Retinal thrombosis has been reported (rarely). Use caution with conditions that may be aggravated by fluid retention, depression, or history of migraine. Not for use prior to menarche.

Vaginally-administered combination hormonal contraceptive agents may have a similar adverse effects associated with oral contraceptive products. In order to reduce some of the possible risks, the minimum dosage combination of estrogen/progestin that will effectively treat the individual patient should be used.

Drug Interactions

Cytochrome P450 Effect:

Ethinyl estradiol: **Substrate** of CYP2C9 (minor), 3A4 (major), 3A5-7 (minor); **Inhibits** CYP1A2 (weak), 2B6 (weak), 2C8 (weak), 2C19 (weak), 3A4 (weak)

Etonogestrel: **Substrate** of CYP3A4 (minor)

Increased Effect/Toxicity: Acetaminophen and ascorbic acid may increase plasma levels of estrogen component. Atorvastatin and indinavir increase plasma levels of combination hormonal contraceptives. Combination hormonal contraceptives increase the plasma levels of alprazolam, chlordiazepoxide, cyclosporine, diazepam, prednisolone, selegiline, theophylline, tricyclic antidepressants. Combination hormonal contraceptives may increase (or decrease) the effects of coumarin derivatives.

Decreased Effect: Combination hormonal contraceptives may decrease plasma levels of acetaminophen, clofibric acid, lorazepam, morphine, oxazepam, salicylic acid, temazepam. Contraceptive effect decreased by acitretin, aminoglutethimide, amprenavir, anticonvulsants, griseofulvin, lopinavir, nelfinavir, nevirapine, penicillins (effect not consistent), rifampin, ritonavir, tetracyclines (effect not consistent). Combination hormonal contraceptives may decrease (or increase) the effects of coumarin derivatives. Aprepitant, modafinil, and topiramate may decrease the serum concentration of oral contraceptive (estrogens). Oral contraceptive (estrogens) may decrease the serum concentration of lamotrigine.

Ethanol/Nutrition/Herb Interactions

Food: CNS effects of caffeine may be enhanced if combination hormonal contraceptives are used concurrently with caffeine. Grapefruit juice increases ethinyl estradiol concentrations and would be expected to increase progesterone serum levels as well; clinical implications are unclear.

Herb/Nutraceutical: St John's wort may decrease levels. Herbs with estrogenic properties may enhance the adverse/toxic effect of estrogen derivatives; examples include alfalfa, black cohosh, bloodroot, hops, kudzu, licorice, red clover, saw palmetto, soybean, thyme, wild yam, yucca. Herbs with progestogenic properties may enhance the adverse/toxic effect of progestins; examples include bloodroot, chasteberry, damiana, oregano, yucca.

Pharmacodynamics/Kinetics

Duration: Serum levels (contraceptive effectiveness) decrease after 3 weeks of continuous use

Absorption: Ethinyl estradiol and etonogestrel: Rapid
Tampons do not interfere with absorption.

Protein binding:
Ethinyl estradiol: 98%, primarily to albumin
Etonogestrel: 32% to sex hormone-binding globulin (SHBG) and 66% to albumin; SHBG capacity is affected by plasma ethinyl estradiol levels
Metabolism:
Ethinyl estradiol: Hepatic via CYP3A4; forms metabolites (weak estrogenic activity)
Etonogestrel: Hepatic via CYP3A4; forms metabolites (activity not known)
Bioavailability: Ethinyl estradiol: ~56% Etonogestrel: 100%
Half-life elimination: Ethinyl estradiol: 45 hours; Etonogestrel: 29 hours
Excretion: Ethinyl estradiol and etonogestrel: Urine, bile, and feces

Pregnancy Risk Factor X

Dosage Forms
Ring, vaginal:
NuvaRing®: Ethinyl estradiol 0.015 mg/day and etonogestrel 0.12 mg/day (1s) [3-week duration]

Ethinyl Estradiol and Levonorgestrel

(ETH in il es tra DYE ole & LEE voe nor jes trel)

Related Information
Levonorgestrel on page 968

U.S. Brand Names Alesse®; Aviane™; Enpresse™; Jolessa™; Lessina™; Levlen®; Levlite™; Levora®; Lutera™; Nordette®; Portia™; Quasense™; Seasonale®; Seasonique™; Sronyx™; Tri-Levlen®; Triphasil®; Trivora®

Canadian Brand Names Alesse®; Min-Ovral®; Triphasil®; Triquilar®

Mexican Brand Names Microgynon; Microgynon CD; Nordet; Trinordiol; Triquilar

Generic Available Yes

Index Terms Levonorgestrel and Ethinyl Estradiol

Pharmacologic Category Contraceptive; Estrogen and Progestin Combination

Use Prevention of pregnancy; postcoital contraception

Unlabeled/Investigational Use Treatment of hypermenorrhea (menorrhagia); pain associated with endometriosis; dysmenorrhea; dysfunctional uterine bleeding

Local Anesthetic/Vasoconstrictor Precautions No information available to require special precautions

Effects on Dental Treatment When prescribing antibiotics, patient must be warned to use additional methods of birth control if on oral contraceptives.

Common Adverse Effects Frequency not defined.
Cardiovascular: Arterial thromboembolism, cerebral hemorrhage, cerebral thrombosis, edema, hypertension, mesenteric thrombosis, MI
Central nervous system: Depression, dizziness, headache, migraine, nervousness, premenstrual syndrome, stroke
Dermatologic: Acne, erythema multiforme, erythema nodosum, hirsutism, loss of scalp hair, melasma (may persist), rash (allergic)
Endocrine & metabolic: Amenorrhea, breakthrough bleeding, breast enlargement, breast secretion, breast tenderness, carbohydrate intolerance, lactation decreased (postpartum), glucose tolerance decreased, libido changes, menstrual flow changes, sex hormone-binding globulins (SHBG) increased, spotting, temporary infertility (following discontinuation), thyroid-binding globulin increased, triglycerides increased
Gastrointestinal: Abdominal cramps, appetite changes, bloating, cholestasis, colitis, gallbladder disease, jaundice, nausea, vomiting, weight gain/loss
Genitourinary: Cervical erosion changes, cervical secretion changes, cystitis-like syndrome, vaginal candidiasis, vaginitis
Hematologic: Antithrombin III decreased, folate levels decreased, hemolytic uremic syndrome, norepinephrine induced platelet aggregability increased, porphyria, prothrombin increased; factors VII, VIII, IX, and X increased
Hepatic: Benign liver tumors, Budd-Chiari syndrome, cholestatic jaundice, hepatic adenomas
Local: Thrombophlebitis
Ocular: Cataracts, change in corneal curvature (steepening), contact lens intolerance, optic neuritis, retinal thrombosis
Renal: Impaired renal function
Respiratory: Pulmonary thromboembolism
Miscellaneous: Hemorrhagic eruption

Dosage Oral: Adults: Female:
Contraception, 28-day cycle:
Schedule 1 (Sunday starter): Dose begins on first Sunday after onset of menstruation; if the menstrual period starts on Sunday, take first tablet that
(Continued)

Ethinyl Estradiol and Levonorgestrel *(Continued)*

very same day. With a Sunday start, an additional method of contraception should be used until after the first 7 days of consecutive administration:

For 21-tablet package: 1 tablet/day for 21 consecutive days, followed by 7 days off of the medication; a new course begins on the 8th day after the last tablet is taken

For 28-tablet package: 1 tablet/day without interruption

Schedule 2 (Day 1 starter): Dose starts on first day of menstrual cycle taking 1 tablet/day:

For 21-tablet package: 1 tablet/day for 21 consecutive days, followed by 7 days off of the medication; a new course begins on the 8th day after the last tablet is taken

For 28-tablet package: 1 tablet/day without interruption

If all doses have been taken on schedule and one menstrual period is missed, continue dosing cycle. If two consecutive menstrual periods are missed, pregnancy test is required before new dosing cycle is started.

Missed doses **monophasic formulations** (refer to package insert for complete information):

One dose missed: Take as soon as remembered or take 2 tablets next day

Two consecutive doses missed in the first 2 weeks: Take 2 tablets as soon as remembered or 2 tablets next 2 days. An additional method of contraception should be used for 7 days after missed dose.

Two consecutive doses missed in week 3 or three consecutive doses missed at any time: An additional method of contraception must be used for 7 days after a missed dose:

Schedule 1 (Sunday starter): Continue dose of 1 tablet daily until Sunday, then discard the rest of the pack, and a new pack should be started that same day.

Schedule 2 (Day 1 starter): Current pack should be discarded, and a new pack should be started that same day.

Missed doses **biphasic/triphasic formulations** (refer to package insert for complete information):

One dose missed: Take as soon as remembered or take 2 tablets next day.

Two consecutive doses missed in week 1 or week 2 of the pack: Take 2 tablets as soon as remembered and 2 tablets the next day. Resume taking 1 tablet daily until the pack is empty. An additional method of contraception should be used for 7 days after a missed dose.

Two consecutive doses missed in week 3 of the pack: An additional method of contraception must be used for 7 days after a missed dose.

Schedule 1 (Sunday starter): Take 1 tablet every day until Sunday. Discard the remaining pack and start a new pack of pills on the same day.

Schedule 2 (Day 1 starter): Discard the remaining pack and start a new pack the same day.

Three or more consecutive doses missed: An additional method of contraception must be used for 7 days after a missed dose.

Schedule 1 (Sunday starter): Take 1 tablet every day until Sunday; on Sunday, discard the pack and start a new pack.

Schedule 2 (Day 1 starter): Discard the remaining pack and begin new pack of tablets starting on the same day.

Contraception, 91-day cycle (extended cycle regimen): Dose begins on first Sunday after onset of menstruation; if the menstrual period starts on Sunday, take first tablet that very same day. An additional method of contraception should be used until after the first 7 days of consecutive administration:

Seasonale®: One active tablet/day for 84 consecutive days, followed by 1 inactive tablet/day for 7 days; if all doses have been taken on schedule and one menstrual period is missed, pregnancy should be ruled out prior to continuing therapy.

Seasonique™: One active tablet/day for 84 consecutive days, followed by 1 low dose estrogen tablet/day for 7 days; if all doses have been taken on schedule and one menstrual period is missed, pregnancy should be ruled out prior to continuing therapy.

Missed doses:

One dose missed: Take as soon as remembered or take 2 tablets the next day

Two consecutive doses missed: Take 2 tablets as soon as remembered or 2 tablets the next 2 days. An additional nonhormonal method of contraception should be used for 7 consecutive days after the missed dose.

Three or more consecutive doses missed: Do not take the missed doses; continue taking 1 tablet/day until pack is complete. Bleeding may occur during the following week. An additional nonhormonal method of contraception should be used for 7 consecutive days after the missed dose.

Any number of pills during week 13: Throw away the missed pills and keep taking scheduled pills until the pack is finished. A back-up method of contraception is not needed

Dosage adjustment in renal impairment: Specific guidelines not available; use with caution and monitor blood pressure closely. Consider other forms of contraception.

Dosage adjustment in hepatic impairment: Contraindicated in patients with hepatic impairment

Mechanism of Action Combination hormonal contraceptives inhibit ovulation via a negative feedback mechanism on the hypothalamus, which alters the normal pattern of gonadotropin secretion of a follicle-stimulating hormone (FSH) and luteinizing hormone by the anterior pituitary. The follicular phase FSH and midcycle surge of gonadotropins are inhibited. In addition, combination hormonal contraceptives produce alterations in the genital tract, including changes in the cervical mucus, rendering it unfavorable for sperm penetration even if ovulation occurs. Changes in the endometrium may also occur, producing an unfavorable environment for nidation. Combination hormonal contraceptive drugs may alter the tubal transport of the ova through the fallopian tubes. Progestational agents may also alter sperm fertility.

Contraindications Hypersensitivity to ethinyl estradiol, levonorgestrel, or any component of the formulation; history of or current thrombophlebitis or venous thromboembolic disorders (including DVT, PE); active or recent (within 1 year) arterial thromboembolic disease (eg, stroke, MI); cerebral vascular disease, coronary artery disease, valvular heart disease with complications, severe hypertension; diabetes mellitus with vascular involvement; severe headache with focal neurological symptoms; known or suspected breast carcinoma, endometrial cancer, estrogen-dependent neoplasms, undiagnosed abnormal genital bleeding; hepatic dysfunction or tumor, cholestatic jaundice of pregnancy, jaundice with prior combination hormonal contraceptive use; major surgery with prolonged immobilization; heavy smoking (≥15 cigarettes/day) in patients >35 years of age; pregnancy

Warnings/Precautions Combination hormonal contraceptives do not protect against HIV infection or other sexually-transmitted diseases. **[U.S. Boxed Warning]: The risk of cardiovascular side effects increases in women who smoke cigarettes, especially those who are >35 years of age; women who use combination hormonal contraceptives should be strongly advised not to smoke.** Combination hormonal contraceptives may lead to increased risk of myocardial infarction, use with caution in patients with risk factors for coronary artery disease. May increase the risk of thromboembolism. Whenever possible, combination hormonal contraceptives should be discontinued at least 4 weeks prior to and for 2 weeks following elective surgery associated with an increased risk of thromboembolism or during periods of prolonged immobilization. Combination hormonal contraceptives may have a dose-related risk of vascular disease, hypertension, and gallbladder disease. Women with hypertension or renal disease should be encouraged to use another form of contraception. The use of combination hormonal contraceptives has been associated with a slight increase in frequency of breast cancer, however, studies are not consistent. Combination hormonal contraceptives may cause glucose intolerance or effect serum triglyceride and lipoprotein levels. Retinal thrombosis has been reported (rarely). Use caution with conditions that may be aggravated by fluid retention, depression, or history of migraine. Not for use prior to menarche.

The minimum dosage combination of estrogen/progestin that will effectively treat the individual patient should be used. New patients should be started on products containing ≤0.035 mg of estrogen per tablet. Extended cycle regimen contraceptives provide more hormonal exposure per year than conventional monthly contraceptives.

Drug Interactions
  Cytochrome P450 Effect:
    Ethinyl estradiol: **Substrate** of CYP2C9 (minor), 3A4 (major), 3A5-7 (minor); **Inhibits** CYP1A2 (weak), 2B6 (weak), 2C8 (weak), 2C19 (weak), 3A4 (weak)
    Levonorgestrel: **Substrate** of CYP3A4 (major)
  Increased Effect/Toxicity: Acetaminophen and ascorbic acid may increase plasma levels of estrogen component. Atorvastatin and indinavir increase plasma levels of combination hormonal contraceptives. Combination hormonal contraceptives increase the plasma levels of alprazolam, chlordiazepoxide, cyclosporine, diazepam, prednisolone, selegiline, theophylline, tricyclic antidepressants. Combination hormonal contraceptives may increase (or decrease) the effects of coumarin derivatives.
  Decreased Effect: CYP3A4 inducers may decrease the levels/effects of ethinyl estradiol and/or levonorgestrel; example inducers include aminoglutethimide, carbamazepine, nafcillin, nevirapine, phenobarbital, phenytoin, and
(Continued)

Ethinyl Estradiol and Levonorgestrel *(Continued)*

rifamycins. Combination hormonal contraceptives may decrease plasma levels of acetaminophen, clofibric acid, lorazepam, morphine, oxazepam, salicylic acid, temazepam. Contraceptive effect decreased by acitretin, aminoglutethimide, amprenavir, anticonvulsants, griseofulvin, lopinavir, nelfinavir, penicillins (effect not consistent), rifampin, ritonavir, tetracyclines (effect not consistent). Combination hormonal contraceptives may decrease (or increase) the effects of coumarin derivatives. Aprepitant, modafinil, and topiramate may decrease the serum concentration of oral contraceptive (estrogens). Oral contraceptive (estrogens) may decrease the serum concentration of lamotrigine.

Ethanol/Nutrition/Herb Interactions

Food: CNS effects of caffeine may be enhanced if combination hormonal contraceptives are used concurrently with caffeine. Grapefruit juice increases ethinyl estradiol concentrations and would be expected to increase progesterone serum levels as well; clinical implications are unclear.

Herb/Nutraceutical: St John's wort may decrease levels. Herbs with estrogenic properties may enhance the adverse/toxic effect of estrogen derivatives; examples include alfalfa, black cohosh, bloodroot, hops, kudzu, licorice, red clover, saw palmetto, soybean, thyme, wild yam, yucca. Herbs with progestogenic properties may enhance the adverse/toxic effect of progestins; examples include bloodroot, chasteberry, damiana, oregano, yucca.

Dietary Considerations Should be taken at the same time each day.

Pharmacodynamics/Kinetics

Absorption: Rapid

Distribution: Ethinyl estradiol: 4.3 L/kg; Levonorgestrel: 1.8 L/kg

Protein binding:

Ethinyl estradiol: 95% to 97% to albumin

Levonorgestrel: 97% to 99% primarily to sex hormone binding globulin (SHBG), lesser amounts to albumin

Metabolism:

Ethinyl estradiol: Hepatic via CYP3A4; undergoes first-pass metabolism; forms metabolites

Levonorgestrel: Forms conjugated in unconjugated metabolites

Bioavailability: Ethinyl estradiol: 38% to 48%; Levonorgestrel: 100%

Half-life elimination: Ethinyl estradiol: 13-22 hours; Levonorgestrel: 23-49 hours

Excretion:

Ethinyl estradiol: Urine and feces

Levonorgestrel: Urine (40% to 68%, parent drug and metabolites); feces (16% to 48% as metabolites)

Pregnancy Risk Factor X

Dosage Forms

Tablet, low-dose formulations:

Alesse® 28: Ethinyl estradiol 0.02 mg and levonorgestrel 0.1 mg [21 pink tablets and 7 light green inactive tablets] (28s)

Aviane™ 28: Ethinyl estradiol 0.02 mg and levonorgestrel 0.1 mg [21 orange tablets and 7 light green inactive tablets] (28s)

Lessina™ 28, Levlite™ 28: Ethinyl estradiol 0.02 mg and levonorgestrel 0.1 mg [21 pink tablets and 7 white inactive tablets] (28s)

Lutera™, Sronyx™: Ethinyl estradiol 0.02 mg and levonorgestrel 0.1 mg [21 white tablets and 7 peach inactive tablets] (28s)

Tablet, monophasic formulations:

Levlen® 28: Ethinyl estradiol 0.03 mg and levonorgestrel 0.15 mg [21 light orange tablets and 7 pink inactive tablets] (28s)

Levora® 28: Ethinyl estradiol 0.03 mg and levonorgestrel 0.15 mg [21 white tablets and 7 peach inactive tablets] (28s)

Nordette® 28: Ethinyl estradiol 0.03 mg and levonorgestrel 0.15 mg [21 light orange tablets and 7 pink inactive tablets] (28s)

Portia™ 28: Ethinyl estradiol 0.03 mg and levonorgestrel 0.15 mg [21 pink tablets and 7 white inactive tablets] (28s)

Tablet, monophasic formulations [extended cycle regimen]:

Jolessa™, Seasonale®: Ethinyl estradiol 0.03 mg and levonorgestrel 0.15 mg [84 pink tablets and 7 white inactive tablets] (91s)

Quasense™: Ethinyl estradiol 0.03 mg and levonorgestrel 0.15 mg [84 white tablets and 7 peach inactive tablets] (91s)

Seasonique™: Ethinyl estradiol 0.03 mg and levonorgestrel 0.15 mg [84 light blue-green tablets] and ethinyl estradiol 0.01 mg [7 yellow tablets] (91s)

Tablet, triphasic formulations:

Enpresse™:

Day 1-6: Ethinyl estradiol 0.03 mg and levonorgestrel 0.05 mg [6 pink tablets]

  Day 7-11: Ethinyl estradiol 0.04 mg and levonorgestrel 0.075 mg [5 white tablets]

  Day 12-21: Ethinyl estradiol 0.03 mg and levonorgestrel 0.125 mg [10 orange tablets]

  Day 22-28: 7 light green inactive tablets (28s)

 Tri-Levlen® 28, Triphasil® 28:

  Day 1-6: Ethinyl estradiol 0.03 mg and levonorgestrel 0.05 mg [6 brown tablets]

  Day 7-11: Ethinyl estradiol 0.04 mg and levonorgestrel 0.075 mg [5 white tablets]

  Day 12-21: Ethinyl estradiol 0.03 mg and levonorgestrel 0.125 mg [10 light yellow tablets]

  Day 22-28: 7 light green inactive tablets (28s)

 Trivora® 28:

  Day 1-6: Ethinyl estradiol 0.03 mg and levonorgestrel 0.05 mg [6 blue tablets]

  Day 7-11: Ethinyl estradiol 0.04 mg and levonorgestrel 0.075 mg [5 white tablets]

  Day 12-21: Ethinyl estradiol 0.03 mg and levonorgestrel 0.125 mg [10 pink tablets]

  Day 22-28: 7 peach inactive tablets (28s)

Ethinyl Estradiol and NGM *see* Ethinyl Estradiol and Norgestimate *on page 645*

Ethinyl Estradiol and Norelgestromin
(ETH in il es tra DYE ole & nor el JES troe min)

U.S. Brand Names Ortho Evra®

Canadian Brand Names Evra®

Index Terms Norelgestromin and Ethinyl Estradiol; Ortho-Evra

Pharmacologic Category Contraceptive; Estrogen and Progestin Combination

Use Prevention of pregnancy

Local Anesthetic/Vasoconstrictor Precautions No information available to require special precautions

Effects on Dental Treatment When prescribing antibiotics, patient must be warned to use additional methods of birth control if on oral contraceptives.

Common Adverse Effects The following reactions have been reported with the contraceptive patch. Adverse reactions associated with oral combination hormonal contraceptive agents are also likely to appear with the topical contraceptive patch (frequency difficult to anticipate). Refer to individual **oral** contraceptive monographs for additional information.

9% to 22%: Abdominal pain, application site reaction, breast symptoms, headache, menstrual cramps, nausea, upper respiratory infection

Dosage Topical: Adults: Female:

 Contraception: Apply one patch each week for 3 weeks (21 total days); followed by one week that is patch-free. Each patch should be applied on the same day each week ("patch change day") and only one patch should be worn at a time. No more than 7 days should pass during the patch-free interval.

  Schedule 1 (Sunday starter): Dose begins on first Sunday after onset of menstruation; if the menstrual period starts on Sunday, apply one patch that very same day. **With a Sunday start, an additional method of contraception (nonhormonal) should be used until after the first 7 days of consecutive administration.** Each patch change will then occur on Sunday.

  Schedule 2 (Day 1 starter): Dose starts on first day of menstrual cycle, applying one patch during the first 24 hours of menstrual cycle. No back-up method of contraception is needed as long as the patch is applied on the first day of cycle. Each patch change will then occur on that same day of the week.

 Additional dosing considerations:

 No bleeding during patch-free week/missed menstrual period: If patch has been applied as directed, continue treatment on usual "patch change day". If used correctly, no bleeding during patch-free week does not necessarily indicate pregnancy. However, if no withdrawal bleeding occurs for 2 consecutive cycles, pregnancy should be ruled out. If patch has not been applied as directed, and one menstrual period is missed, pregnancy should be ruled out prior to continuing treatment.

 If a patch becomes partially or completely detached for <24 hours: Try to reapply to same place, or replace with a new patch immediately. Do not reapply if patch is no longer sticky, if it is sticking to itself or another surface, or if it has material sticking to it.

(Continued)

Ethinyl Estradiol and Norelgestromin *(Continued)*

If a patch becomes partially or completely detached for >24 hours (or time period is unknown): Apply a new patch and use this day of the week as the new "patch change day" from this point on. **An additional method of contraception (nonhormonal) should be used until after the first 7 days of consecutive administration.**

Switching from oral contraceptives: Apply first patch on the first day of withdrawal bleeding. If there is no bleeding within 5 days of taking the last active tablet, pregnancy must first be ruled out. If patch is applied later than the first day of bleeding, **an additional method of contraception (nonhormonal) should be used until after the first 7 days of consecutive administration**

Use after childbirth: Therapy should not be started <4 weeks after childbirth. Pregnancy should be ruled out prior to treatment if menstrual periods have not restarted. **An additional method of contraception (nonhormonal) should be used until after the first 7 days of consecutive administration.**

Use after abortion or miscarriage: Therapy may be started immediately if abortion/miscarriage occur within the first trimester. If therapy is not started within 5 days, follow instructions for first time use. If abortion/miscarriage occur during the second trimester, therapy should not be started for at least 4 weeks. Follow directions for use after childbirth.

Dosage adjustment in renal impairment: Specific guidelines not available; use with caution and monitor blood pressure closely. Consider other forms of contraception.

Dosage adjustment in hepatic impairment: Contraindicated in patients with hepatic impairment

Mechanism of Action Combination hormonal contraceptives inhibit ovulation via a negative feedback mechanism on the hypothalamus, which alters the normal pattern of gonadotropin secretion of a follicle-stimulating hormone (FSH) and luteinizing hormone by the anterior pituitary. The follicular phase FSH and midcycle surge of gonadotropins are inhibited. In addition, combination hormonal contraceptives produce alterations in the genital tract, including changes in the cervical mucus, rendering it unfavorable for sperm penetration even if ovulation occurs. Changes in the endometrium may also occur, producing an unfavorable environment for nidation. Combination hormonal contraceptive drugs may alter the tubal transport of the ova through the fallopian tubes. Progestational agents may also alter sperm fertility.

Contraindications Hypersensitivity to ethinyl estradiol, norelgestromin, or any component of the formulation; history of or current thrombophlebitis or venous thromboembolic disorders (including DVT, PE); active or recent (within 1 year) arterial thromboembolic disease (eg, stroke, MI); cerebral vascular disease, coronary artery disease, valvular heart disease with complications, severe hypertension; diabetes mellitus with vascular involvement; severe headache with focal neurological symptoms; known or suspected breast carcinoma, endometrial cancer, estrogen-dependent neoplasms, undiagnosed abnormal genital bleeding; hepatic dysfunction or tumor, cholestatic jaundice of pregnancy, jaundice with prior combination hormonal contraceptive use; major surgery with prolonged immobilization; heavy smoking (≥15 cigarettes/day) in patients >35 years of age; pregnancy

Warnings/Precautions

The amount of ethinyl estradiol absorbed from the transdermal patch results in higher but more variable exposure than achieved if administered orally. The increased estrogen exposure may increase the risk of adverse events, including venous thromboembolism. The combination hormonal contraceptive patch may have adverse effects similar to those associated with oral contraceptive products. Risk of complications increases with other risk factors such as hypertension, hyperlipidemias, obesity and diabetes. The topical patch may be less effective in patients weighing ≥90 kg (198 lb) and an increased incidence of pregnancy has been reported in this population; consider another form of contraception. Transdermal patch may contain conducting metal (eg, aluminum); remove patch prior to MRI.

Combination hormonal contraceptives do not protect against HIV infection or other sexually-transmitted diseases. **[U.S. Boxed Warning]: The risk of cardiovascular side effects increases in women who smoke cigarettes, especially those who are >35 years of age; women who use combination hormonal contraceptives should be strongly advised not to smoke.** Combination hormonal contraceptives may lead to increased risk of myocardial infarction, use with caution in patients with risk factors for coronary artery disease. May increase the risk of thromboembolism. Whenever possible, combination hormonal contraceptives should be discontinued at least 4 weeks prior to and for 2 weeks following elective surgery associated with an increased risk of thromboembolism or during periods of prolonged immobilization. Combination hormonal contraceptives may have a dose-related risk of vascular disease, hypertension, and gallbladder disease. Women with hypertension or renal disease should be encouraged to use a nonhormonal form of contraception. The use of combination hormonal contraceptives has been associated with a slight increase in frequency of breast cancer, however, studies are not consistent. Combination hormonal contraceptives may cause glucose intolerance or effect serum triglyceride and lipoprotein levels. Retinal thrombosis has been reported (rarely). Use caution with conditions that may be aggravated by fluid retention, depression, or history of migraine. The minimum dosage combination of estrogen/progestin that will effectively treat the individual patient should be used. Not for use prior to menarche.

Drug Interactions

Cytochrome P450 Effect:

Ethinyl estradiol: **Substrate** of CYP2C9 (minor), 3A4 (major), 3A5-7 (minor); **Inhibits** CYP1A2 (weak), 2B6 (weak), 2C8 (weak), 2C19 (weak), 3A4 (weak)

Norelgestromin: **Substrate** of CYP3A4 (minor)

Increased Effect/Toxicity: Acetaminophen and ascorbic acid may increase plasma levels of estrogen component. Atorvastatin and indinavir increase plasma levels of combination hormonal contraceptives. Combination hormonal contraceptives increase the plasma levels of alprazolam, chlordiazepoxide, cyclosporine, diazepam, prednisolone, selegiline, theophylline, tricyclic antidepressants. Combination hormonal contraceptives may increase (or decrease) the effects of coumarin derivatives.

Decreased Effect: CYP3A4 inducers may decrease the levels/effects of ethinyl estradiol; example inducers include aminoglutethimide, carbamazepine, nafcillin, nevirapine, phenobarbital, phenytoin, and rifamycins. Combination hormonal contraceptives may decrease plasma levels of acetaminophen, clofibric acid, lorazepam, morphine, oxazepam, salicylic acid, temazepam. Contraceptive effect decreased by acitretin, aminoglutethimide, amprenavir, anticonvulsants, griseofulvin, lopinavir, nelfinavir, penicillins (effect not consistent), rifampin, ritonavir, tetracyclines (effect not consistent), troglitazone. Combination hormonal contraceptives may decrease (or increase) the effects of coumarin derivatives. Aprepitant, modafinil, and topiramate may decrease the serum concentration of oral contraceptive (estrogens). Oral contraceptive (estrogens) may decrease the serum concentration of lamotrigine.

Ethanol/Nutrition/Herb Interactions

Food: CNS effects of caffeine may be enhanced if combination hormonal contraceptives are used concurrently with caffeine. Grapefruit juice increases ethinyl estradiol concentrations and would be expected to increase progesterone serum levels as well; clinical implications are unclear.

Herb/Nutraceutical: St John's wort may decrease levels. Herbs with estrogenic properties may enhance the adverse/toxic effect of estrogen derivatives; examples include alfalfa, black cohosh, bloodroot, hops, kudzu, licorice, red clover, saw palmetto, soybean, thyme, wild yam, yucca. Herbs with progestogenic properties may enhance the adverse/toxic effect of progestins; examples include bloodroot, chasteberry, damiana, oregano, yucca.

Pharmacodynamics/Kinetics

Ortho Evra®:

Absorption: Topical: Equivalent when applied to abdomen, buttock, upper outer arm, and upper torso

Ethinyl estradiol and norelgestromin: Rapid; reaches plateau by ~48 hours. Absorption of ethinyl estradiol may be increased with heat exposure due to sauna, whirlpool, or treadmill.

The amount of ethinyl estradiol absorbed is 20 mcg/day and results in greater exposure than produced by oral ethinyl estradiol 20 mcg. In contrast, peak levels of ethinyl estradiol are higher in women taking oral tablets.

Protein binding: Norelgestromin: >97% to albumin

Metabolism: Topical:

Ethinyl estradiol: First-pass effect avoided; forms metabolites

Norelgestromin: Hepatic to norgestrel and others; first-pass effect avoided

Bioavailability: Ethinyl estradiol: ~60% greater using the topical patch when compared to oral tablets.

Half-life elimination: Topical:

Ethinyl estradiol: 17 hours

Norelgestromin: 28 hours

Excretion: Ethinyl estradiol and norelgestromin: Urine and feces

Pregnancy Risk Factor X

Dosage Forms The Canadian formulation differs from the U.S. product in both composition and manufacturing process (although delivery rates appear similar). [CAN] = Canadian brand name.

(Continued)

Ethinyl Estradiol and Norelgestromin *(Continued)*

Patch, transdermal:
Evra® [CAN]: Ethinyl estradiol 0.6 mg and norelgestromin 6 mg [releases ethinyl estradiol 20 mcg and norelgestromin 150 mcg per day] (1s, 3s) [not available in the U.S.]
Ortho Evra®: Ethinyl estradiol 0.75 mg and norelgestromin 6 mg [releases ethinyl estradiol 20 mcg and norelgestromin 150 mcg per day] (1s, 3s)

Ethinyl Estradiol and Norethindrone
(ETH in il es tra DYE ole & nor eth IN drone)

Related Information
Norethindrone *on page 1186*

U.S. Brand Names Aranelle™; Brevicon®; Estrostep® Fe; Femcon™ Fe; femhrt®; Junel™; Junel™ Fe; Leena™; Loestrin®; Loestrin® 24 Fe; Loestrin® Fe; Microgestin™; Microgestin™ Fe; Modicon®; Necon® 0.5/35; Necon® 1/35; Necon® 7/7/7; Necon® 10/11; Norinyl® 1+35; Nortrel™; Nortrel™ 7/7/7; Ortho-Novum®; Ovcon®; Tri-Norinyl®; Zenchent™

Canadian Brand Names Brevicon® 0.5/35; Brevicon® 1/35; FemHRT®; Loestrin™ 1.5/30; Minestrin™ 1/20; Ortho® 0.5/35; Ortho® 1/35; Ortho® 7/7/7; Select™ 1/35; Synphasic®

Mexican Brand Names Evorelconti; Ortho-Novum 1 35; Trinovum

Generic Available Yes

Index Terms Norethindrone Acetate and Ethinyl Estradiol; Ortho Novum

Pharmacologic Category Contraceptive; Estrogen and Progestin Combination

Use Prevention of pregnancy; treatment of acne; moderate to severe vasomotor symptoms associated with menopause; prevention of osteoporosis (in women at significant risk only)

Unlabeled/Investigational Use Treatment of hypermenorrhea (menorrhagia); pain associated with endometriosis, dysmenorrhea; dysfunctional uterine bleeding

Local Anesthetic/Vasoconstrictor Precautions No information available to require special precautions

Effects on Dental Treatment When prescribing antibiotics, patient must be warned to use additional methods of birth control if on oral contraceptives.

Common Adverse Effects As reported with oral contraceptive agents. Frequency not defined.
Cardiovascular: Arterial thromboembolism, cerebral hemorrhage, cerebral thrombosis, edema, hypertension, mesenteric thrombosis, MI
Central nervous system: Depression, dizziness, headache, migraine, nervousness, premenstrual syndrome, stroke
Dermatologic: Acne, erythema multiforme, erythema nodosum, hirsutism, loss of scalp hair, melasma (may persist), rash (allergic)
Endocrine & metabolic: Amenorrhea, breakthrough bleeding, breast enlargement, breast secretion, breast tenderness, carbohydrate intolerance, lactation decreased (postpartum), glucose tolerance decreased, libido changes, menstrual flow changes, sex hormone-binding globulins (SHBG) increased, spotting, temporary infertility (following discontinuation), thyroid-binding globulin increased, triglycerides increased
Gastrointestinal: Abdominal cramps, appetite changes, bloating, cholestasis, colitis, gallbladder disease, jaundice, nausea, vomiting, weight gain/loss
Genitourinary: Cervical erosion changes, cervical secretion changes, cystitis-like syndrome, vaginal candidiasis, vaginitis
Hematologic: Antithrombin III decreased, folate levels decreased, hemolytic uremic syndrome, norepinephrine induced platelet aggregability increased, porphyria, prothrombin increased; factors VII, VIII, IX, and X
Hepatic: Benign liver tumors, Budd-Chiari syndrome, cholestatic jaundice, hepatic adenomas
Local: Thrombophlebitis
Ocular: Cataracts, change in corneal curvature (steepening), contact lens intolerance, optic neuritis, retinal thrombosis
Renal: Impaired renal function
Respiratory: Pulmonary thromboembolism
Miscellaneous: Hemorrhagic eruption

Dosage Oral:
Adolescents ≥15 years and Adults: Female: Acne: Estrostep®: Refer to dosing for contraception

Adults: Female:
Moderate-to-severe vasomotor symptoms associated with menopause: Initial: femhrt® 0.5/2.5: 1 tablet daily; patient should be re-evaluated at 3- to 6-month

intervals to determine if treatment is still necessary; patient should be maintained at the lowest effective dose

Prevention of osteoporosis: Initial: femhrt® 0.5/2.5: 1 tablet daily; patient should be maintained on the lowest effective dose

Contraception:

Schedule 1 (Sunday starter): Dose begins on first Sunday after onset of menstruation; if the menstrual period starts on Sunday, take first tablet that very same day. With a Sunday start, an additional method of contraception should be used until after the first 7 days of consecutive administration.

For 21-tablet package: Dosage is 1 tablet daily for 21 consecutive days, followed by 7 days off of the medication; a new course begins on the 8th day after the last tablet is taken.

For 28-tablet package: Dosage is 1 tablet daily without interruption.

Schedule 2 (Day 1 starter): Dose starts on first day of menstrual cycle taking 1 tablet daily.

For 21-tablet package: Dosage is 1 tablet daily for 21 consecutive days, followed by 7 days off of the medication; a new course begins on the 8th day after the last tablet is taken.

For 28-tablet package: Dosage is 1 tablet daily without interruption.

If all doses have been taken on schedule and one menstrual period is missed, continue dosing cycle. If two consecutive menstrual periods are missed, pregnancy test is required before new dosing cycle is started.

Missed doses **monophasic formulations** (refer to package insert for complete information):

One dose missed: Take as soon as remembered or take 2 tablets next day

Two consecutive doses missed in the first 2 weeks: Take 2 tablets as soon as remembered or 2 tablets next 2 days. An additional method of contraception should be used for 7 days after missed dose.

Two consecutive doses missed in week 3 or three consecutive doses missed at any time: An additional method of contraception must be used for 7 days after a missed dose.

Schedule 1 (Sunday starter): Continue dose of 1 tablet daily until Sunday, then discard the rest of the pack, and a new pack should be started that same day.

Schedule 2 (Day 1 starter): Current pack should be discarded, and a new pack should be started that same day.

Missed doses **biphasic/triphasic formulations** (refer to package insert for complete information):

One dose missed: Take as soon as remembered or take 2 tablets next day.

Two consecutive doses missed in week 1 or week 2 of the pack: Take 2 tablets as soon as remembered and 2 tablets the next day. Resume taking 1 tablet daily until the pack is empty. An additional method of contraception should be used for 7 days after a missed dose.

Two consecutive doses missed in week 3 of the pack: An additional method of contraception must be used for 7 days after a missed dose.

Schedule 1 (Sunday Starter): Take 1 tablet every day until Sunday. Discard the remaining pack and start a new pack of pills on the same day.

Schedule 2 (Day 1 starter): Discard the remaining pack and start a new pack the same day.

Three or more consecutive doses missed: An additional method of contraception must be used for 7 days after a missed dose.

Schedule 1 (Sunday Starter): Take 1 tablet every day until Sunday; on Sunday, discard the pack and start a new pack.

Schedule 2 (Day 1 Starter): Discard the remaining pack and begin new pack of tablets starting on the same day.

Dosage adjustment in renal impairment: Specific guidelines not available; use with caution and monitor blood pressure closely. Consider other forms of contraception.

Dosage adjustment in hepatic impairment: Contraindicated in patients with hepatic impairment.

Mechanism of Action Combination oral contraceptives inhibit ovulation via a negative feedback mechanism on the hypothalamus, which alters the normal pattern of gonadotropin secretion of a follicle-stimulating hormone (FSH) and luteinizing hormone by the anterior pituitary. The follicular phase FSH and midcycle surge of gonadotropins are inhibited. In addition, combination hormonal contraceptives produce alterations in the genital tract, including changes in the cervical mucus, rendering it unfavorable for sperm penetration even if ovulation occurs. Changes in the endometrium may also occur, producing an unfavorable environment for nidation. Combination hormonal contraceptive drugs may alter the tubal transport of the ova through the fallopian tubes. Progestational agents may also alter sperm fertility.

(Continued)

Ethinyl Estradiol and Norethindrone *(Continued)*

In postmenopausal women, exogenous estrogen is used to replace decreased endogenous production. The addition of progestin reduces the incidence of endometrial hyperplasia and risk of endometrial cancer in women with an intact uterus.

Contraindications Hypersensitivity to ethinyl estradiol, norethindrone, norethindrone acetate, or any component of the formulation; history of or current thrombophlebitis or venous thromboembolic disorders (including DVT, PE); active or recent (within 1 year) arterial thromboembolic disease (eg, stroke, MI); cerebral vascular disease, coronary artery disease, severe hypertension; diabetes mellitus with vascular involvement; severe headache with focal neurological symptoms; known or suspected breast carcinoma, endometrial cancer, estrogen-dependent neoplasms, undiagnosed abnormal genital bleeding; hepatic dysfunction or tumor, cholestatic jaundice of pregnancy, jaundice with prior combination hormonal contraceptive use; major surgery with prolonged immobilization; heavy smoking (≥15 cigarettes/day) in patients >35 years of age; pregnancy

Warnings/Precautions

Cardiovascular-related considerations: Use caution with cardiovascular disease or dysfunction. Combination estrogen/progestin therapy has been associated with an increased risk of cardiovascular disease, which may be dose related. May increase the risks of hypertension, myocardial infarction (MI), stroke, pulmonary emboli (PE), and deep vein thrombosis; incidence of these effects was shown to be significantly increased in postmenopausal women using conjugated equine estrogens (CEE) in combination with medroxyprogesterone acetate (MPA). Nonfatal MI, PE, and thrombophlebitis have also been reported in males taking high doses of CEE (eg, for prostate cancer). An increased risk of MI has been noted with use of combination hormonal contraceptives, primarily in women with underlying risk factors. The risk of cardiovascular events increases in women who smoke cigarettes, especially those who are >35 years of age; women who use combination hormonal contraceptives should be strongly advised not to smoke. Women with hypertension or renal disease should be encouraged to use another form of contraception. Estrogen compounds are generally associated with lipid effects such as increased HDL-cholesterol and decreased LDL-cholesterol. Triglycerides may also be increased; use with caution in patients with familial defects of lipoprotein metabolism. Estrogens with or without progestin should not be used to prevent coronary heart disease in postmenopausal women. Whenever possible, combination hormonal contraceptives should be discontinued at least 4 weeks prior to and for 2 weeks following elective surgery associated with an increased risk of thromboembolism or during periods of prolonged immobilization.

Cancer-related considerations: Estrogens may increase the risk of breast cancer. The use of combination hormonal contraceptives has been associated with a slight increase in frequency of breast cancer, however studies are not consistent. An increased risk of invasive breast cancer was observed in postmenopausal women using CEE in combination with MPA; a smaller increase in risk was seen with estrogen therapy alone in observational studies. An increase in abnormal mammograms has also been reported with estrogen and progestin therapy in postmenopausal women. Unopposed estrogens may increase the risk of endometrial carcinoma in postmenopausal women. Estrogens may exacerbate endometriosis. Malignant transformation of residual endometrial implants has been reported post-hysterectomy with estrogen only therapy. Consider adding a progestin in women with residual endometriosis post-hysterectomy. Estrogen use may lead to severe hypercalcemia in postmenopausal patients with breast cancer and bone metastases; discontinue estrogen if hypercalcemia occurs.

Use with caution in patients with diseases which may be exacerbated by fluid retention, including asthma, epilepsy, migraine, or diabetes. Use with caution in patients with a history of severe hypocalcemia, SLE, hepatic hemangiomas, porphyria, endometriosis, and gallbladder disease. Use caution with history of cholestatic jaundice associated with past estrogen use or pregnancy.

Estrogens may cause retinal vascular thrombosis. Discontinue pending examination in cases of sudden partial or complete vision loss, sudden onset of proptosis, diplopia, or migraine; discontinue permanently if papilledema or retinal vascular lesions are observed on examination.

Combination hormonal contraceptives do not protect against HIV infection or other sexually-transmitted diseases. The minimum dosage combination of estrogen/progestin that will effectively treat the individual patient should be used. New patients should be started on products containing ≤0.035 mg of estrogen per tablet. When used for acne, use only in females ≥15 years, who also desire combination hormonal contraceptive therapy, are unresponsive to topical treatments, and have no contraindications to combination hormonal contraceptive use. Not for use prior to menarche.

The risk of dementia may be increased in postmenopausal women; increased incidence was observed in women ≥65 years of age taking CEE alone or in combination with MPA. Before prescribing estrogen therapy to postmenopausal women, the risks and benefits must be weighed for each patient. Women should be informed of these risks and benefits, as well as possible effects of progestin when added to estrogen therapy. Estrogens with or without progestin should be used for shortest duration possible consistent with treatment goals. Conduct periodic risk:benefit assessments. When used solely for prevention of osteoporosis in women at significant risk, nonestrogen treatment options should be considered.

Drug Interactions
Cytochrome P450 Effect:
Ethinyl estradiol: **Substrate** of CYP2C9 (minor), 3A4 (major), 3A5-7 (minor); **Inhibits** CYP1A2 (weak), 2B6 (weak), 2C8 (weak), 2C19 (weak), 3A4 (weak)

Norethindrone: **Substrate** of CYP3A4 (major); Induces CYP2C19 (weak)

Increased Effect/Toxicity: Acetaminophen and ascorbic acid may increase plasma levels of estrogen component. Atorvastatin and indinavir increase plasma levels of combination hormonal contraceptives. Combination hormonal contraceptives increase the plasma levels of alprazolam, chlordiazepoxide, cyclosporine, diazepam, prednisolone, selegiline, theophylline, tricyclic antidepressants. Combination hormonal contraceptives may increase (or decrease) the effects of coumarin derivatives.

Decreased Effect: CYP3A4 inducers may decrease the levels/effects of ethinyl estradiol and norethindrone; example inducers include aminoglutethimide, carbamazepine, nafcillin, nevirapine, phenobarbital, phenytoin, and rifamycins. Combination hormonal contraceptives may decrease plasma levels of acetaminophen, clofibric acid, lorazepam, morphine, oxazepam, salicylic acid, temazepam. Contraceptive effect decreased by acitretin, aminoglutethimide, amprenavir, anticonvulsants, griseofulvin, lopinavir, nelfinavir, penicillins (effect not consistent), rifampin, ritonavir, tetracyclines (effect not consistent), troglitazone. Oral contraceptives may decrease (or increase) the effects of coumarin derivatives. Aprepitant, modafinil, and topiramate may decrease the serum concentration of oral contraceptive (estrogens). Oral contraceptive (estrogens) may decrease the serum concentration of lamotrigine.

Ethanol/Nutrition/Herb Interactions
Ethanol: Routine use increases estrogen level and risk of breast cancer; avoid ethanol. Ethanol may also increase the risk of osteoporosis.

Food: CNS effects of caffeine may be enhanced if combination hormonal contraceptives are used concurrently with caffeine. Grapefruit juice increases ethinyl estradiol concentrations and would be expected to increase progesterone serum levels as well; clinical implications are unclear. Norethindrone absorption is increased by 27% following administration with food.

Herb/Nutraceutical: St John's wort may decrease levels. Herbs with estrogenic properties may enhance the adverse/toxic effect of estrogen derivatives; examples include alfalfa, black cohosh, bloodroot, hops, kudzu, licorice, red clover, saw palmetto, soybean, thyme, wild yam, yucca. Herbs with progestogenic properties may enhance the adverse/toxic effect of progestins; examples include bloodroot, chasteberry, damiana, oregano, yucca.

Dietary Considerations Should be taken at same time each day. May be taken with or without food. Ensure adequate calcium and vitamin D intake when used for the prevention of osteoporosis.

Pharmacodynamics/Kinetics
Norethindrone: See individual monograph.

Ethinyl estradiol:

Absorption: Rapid

Bioavailability: 43% to 55%

Distribution: V_d: 2-4 L/kg

Protein binding: >95% to albumin

Metabolism: Hepatic via oxidation and conjugation in GI tract; hydroxylated via CYP3A4 to metabolites; first-pass effect; enterohepatic recirculation; reversibly converted to estrone and estriol

Half-life elimination: 19-24 hours

Excretion: Urine (as estradiol, estrone, and estriol); feces

Pregnancy Risk Factor X
Dosage Forms
Tablet:
femhrt®: 1/5: Ethinyl estradiol 5 mcg and norethindrone 1 mg [white tablets]; 0.5/2.5: Ethinyl estradiol 2.5 mcg and norethindrone 0.5 mg [white tablets]
(Continued)

Ethinyl Estradiol and Norethindrone *(Continued)*

Tablet, monophasic formulations:

Brevicon®: Ethinyl estradiol 0.035 mg and norethindrone 0.5 mg [21 blue tablets and 7 orange inactive tablets] (28s)

Junel™ 21 1/20: Ethinyl estradiol 0.02 mg and norethindrone 1 mg [yellow tablets] (21s)

Junel™ 21 1.5/30: Ethinyl estradiol 0.03 mg and norethindrone 1.5 mg [pink tablets] (21s)

Junel™ Fe 1/20: Ethinyl estradiol 0.02 mg and norethindrone 1 mg [21 yellow tablets] and ferrous fumarate 75 mg [7 brown tablets] (28s)

Junel™ Fe 1.5/30: Ethinyl estradiol 0.03 mg and norethindrone 1.5 mg [21 pink tablets] and ferrous fumarate 75 mg [7 brown tablets] (28s)

Loestrin® 21 1/20, Microgestin™ 1/20: Ethinyl estradiol 0.02 mg and norethindrone 1 mg [white tablets] (21s)

Loestrin® 21 1.5/30, Microgestin™ 1.5/30: Ethinyl estradiol 0.03 mg and norethindrone 1.5 mg [green tablets] (21s)

Loestrin® 24 Fe: 1/20: Ethinyl estradiol 0.02 mg and norethindrone acetate 1 mg [24 white tablets] and ferrous fumarate 75 mg [4 brown tablets] (28s)

Loestrin® Fe 1/20, Microgestin™ Fe 1/20: Ethinyl estradiol 0.02 mg and norethindrone 1 mg [21 white tablets] and ferrous fumarate 75 mg [7 brown tablets] (28s)

Loestrin® Fe 1.5/30, Microgestin™ Fe 1.5/30: Ethinyl estradiol 0.03 mg and norethindrone 1.5 mg [21 green tablets] and ferrous fumarate 75 mg [7 brown tablets] (28s)

Modicon® 28: Ethinyl estradiol 0.035 mg and norethindrone 0.5 mg [21 white tablets and 7 green inactive tablets] (28s)

Necon® 0.5/35-28: Ethinyl estradiol 0.035 mg and norethindrone 0.5 mg [21 light yellow tablets and 7 white inactive tablets] (28s)

Necon® 1/35-28: Ethinyl estradiol 0.035 mg and norethindrone 1 mg [21 dark yellow tablets and 7 white inactive tablets] (28s)

Norinyl® 1+35: Ethinyl estradiol 0.035 mg and norethindrone 1 mg [21 yellow-green tablets and 7 orange inactive tablets] (28s)

Nortrel™ 0.5/35 mg:

Ethinyl estradiol 0.035 mg and norethindrone 0.5 mg [light yellow tablets] (21s)

Ethinyl estradiol 0.035 mg and norethindrone 0.5 mg [21 light yellow tablets and 7 white inactive tablets] (28s)

Nortrel™ 1/35 mg:

Ethinyl estradiol 0.035 mg and norethindrone 1 mg [yellow tablets] (21s)

Ethinyl estradiol 0.035 mg and norethindrone 1 mg [21 yellow tablets and 7 white inactive tablets] (28s)

Ortho-Novum® 1/35 28: Ethinyl estradiol 0.035 mg and norethindrone 1 mg [21 peach tablets and 7 green inactive tablets] (28s)

Ovcon® 35 21-day: Ethinyl estradiol 0.035 mg and norethindrone 0.4 mg [peach tablets] (21s)

Ovcon® 35 28-day: Ethinyl estradiol 0.035 mg and norethindrone 0.4 mg [21 peach tablets and 7 green inactive tablets] (28s)

Ovcon® 50: Ethinyl estradiol 0.05 mg and norethindrone 1 mg [21 yellow tablets and 7 green inactive tablets] (28s)

Zenchent™: Ethinyl estradiol 0.035 mg and norethindrone 0.4 mg [21 light peach tablets and 7 white inactive tablets] (28s)

Tablet, chewable, monophasic formulations:

Femcon™ Fe: Ethinyl estradiol 0.035 mg and norethindrone 0.4 mg [21 white tablets and 7 brown inactive tablets] (28s) [spearmint flavor]

Tablet, biphasic formulations:

Necon® 10/11-28:

Day 1-10: Ethinyl estradiol 0.035 mg and norethindrone 0.5 mg [10 light yellow tablets]

Day 11-21: Ethinyl estradiol 0.035 mg and norethindrone 1 mg [11 dark yellow tablets]

Day 22-28: 7 white inactive tablets (28s)

Ortho-Novum® 10/11-28:

Day 1-10: Ethinyl estradiol 0.035 mg and norethindrone 0.5 mg [10 white tablets]

Day 11-21: Ethinyl estradiol 0.035 mg and norethindrone 1 mg [11 peach tablets]

Day 22-28: 7 green inactive tablets (28s)

Tablet, triphasic formulations:

Aranelle™:

Day 1-7: Ethinyl estradiol 0.035 mg and norethindrone 0.5 mg [7 light yellow tablets]

Day 8-16: Ethinyl estradiol 0.035 mg and norethindrone 1 mg [9 white tablets]

Day 17-21: Ethinyl estradiol 0.035 mg and norethindrone 0.5 mg [5 light yellow tablets]

Day 22-28: 7 peach inactive tablets (28s)

Estrostep® Fe:

Day 1-5: Ethinyl estradiol 0.02 mg and norethindrone 1 mg [5 white triangular tablets]

Day 6-12: Ethinyl estradiol 0.03 mg and norethindrone 1 mg [7 white square tablets]

Day 13-21: Ethinyl estradiol 0.035 mg and norethindrone 1 mg [9 white round tablets]

Day 22-28: Ferrous fumarate 75 mg [7 brown tablets] (28s)

Leena™:

Day 1-7: Ethinyl estradiol 0.035 mg and norethindrone 0.5 mg [7 light blue tablets]

Day 8-16: Ethinyl estradiol 0.035 mg and norethindrone 1 mg [9 light yellow-green tablets]

Day 17-21: Ethinyl estradiol 0.035 mg and norethindrone 0.5 mg [5 light blue tablets]

Day 22-28: 7 orange inactive tablets (28s)

Necon® 7/7/7, Ortho-Novum® 7/7/7 28:

Day 1-7: Ethinyl estradiol 0.035 mg and norethindrone 0.5 mg [7 white tablets]

Day 8-14: Ethinyl estradiol 0.035 mg and norethindrone 0.75 mg [7 light peach tablets]

Day 15-21: Ethinyl estradiol 0.035 mg and norethindrone 1 mg [7 peach tablets]

Day 22-28: 7 green inactive tablets (28s)

Nortrel™ 7/7/7 28:

Day 1-7: Ethinyl estradiol 0.035 mg and norethindrone 0.5 mg [7 light yellow tablets]

Day 8-14: Ethinyl estradiol 0.035 mg and norethindrone 0.75 mg [7 blue tablets]

Day 15-21: Ethinyl estradiol 0.035 mg and norethindrone 1 mg [7 peach tablets]

Day 22-28: 7 white inactive tablets (28s)

Ortho-Novum® 7/7/7 28:

Day 1-7: Ethinyl estradiol 0.035 mg and norethindrone 0.5 mg [7 white tablets]

Day 8-14: Ethinyl estradiol 0.035 mg and norethindrone 0.75 mg [7 light peach tablets]

Day 15-21: Ethinyl estradiol 0.035 mg and norethindrone 1 mg [7 peach tablets]

Day 22-28: 7 green inactive tablets (28s)

Tri-Norinyl® 28:

Day 1-7: Ethinyl estradiol 0.035 mg and norethindrone 0.5 mg [7 blue tablets]

Day 8-16: Ethinyl estradiol 0.035 mg and norethindrone 1 mg [9 yellow-green tablets]

Day 17-21: Ethinyl estradiol 0.035 mg and norethindrone 0.5 mg [5 blue tablets]

Day 22-28: 7 orange inactive tablets (28s)

Ethinyl Estradiol and Norgestimate
(ETH in il es tra DYE ole & nor JES ti mate)

U.S. Brand Names MonoNessa™; Ortho-Cyclen®; Ortho Tri-Cyclen®; Ortho Tri-Cyclen® Lo; Previfem™; Sprintec™; TriNessa™; Tri-Previfem™; Tri-Sprintec™

Canadian Brand Names Cyclen®; Tri-Cyclen®; Tri-Cyclen® Lo

Mexican Brand Names Cilest

Generic Available Yes

Index Terms Ethinyl Estradiol and NGM; Norgestimate and Ethinyl Estradiol; Ortho Cyclen; Ortho Tri Cyclen

Pharmacologic Category Contraceptive; Estrogen and Progestin Combination

Use Prevention of pregnancy; treatment of acne

Unlabeled/Investigational Use Treatment of hypermenorrhea (menorrhagia); pain associated with endometriosis; dysmenorrhea; dysfunctional uterine bleeding

Local Anesthetic/Vasoconstrictor Precautions No information available to require special precautions

(Continued)

Ethinyl Estradiol and Norgestimate *(Continued)*

Effects on Dental Treatment When prescribing antibiotics, patient must be warned to use additional methods of birth control if on oral contraceptives.

Common Adverse Effects Frequency not defined.

Cardiovascular: Arterial thromboembolism, cerebral hemorrhage, cerebral thrombosis, edema, hypertension, mesenteric thrombosis, MI

Central nervous system: Depression, dizziness, headache, migraine, nervousness, premenstrual syndrome, stroke

Dermatologic: Acne, erythema multiforme, erythema nodosum, hirsutism, loss of scalp hair, melasma (may persist), rash (allergic)

Endocrine & metabolic: Amenorrhea, breakthrough bleeding, breast enlargement, breast secretion, breast tenderness, carbohydrate intolerance, lactation decreased (postpartum), glucose tolerance decreased, libido changes, menstrual flow changes, sex hormone-binding globulins (SHBG) increased, spotting, temporary infertility (following discontinuation), thyroid-binding globulin increased, triglycerides increased

Gastrointestinal: Abdominal cramps, appetite changes, bloating, cholestasis, colitis, gallbladder disease, jaundice, nausea, vomiting, weight gain/loss

Genitourinary: Cervical erosion changes, cervical secretion changes, cystitis-like syndrome, vaginal candidiasis, vaginitis

Hematologic: Antithrombin III decreased, folate levels decreased, hemolytic uremic syndrome, norepinephrine induced platelet aggregability increased, porphyria, prothrombin increased; factors VII, VIII, IX, and X increased

Hepatic: Benign liver tumors, Budd-Chiari syndrome, cholestatic jaundice, hepatic adenomas

Local: Thrombophlebitis

Ocular: Cataracts, change in corneal curvature (steepening), contact lens intolerance, optic neuritis, retinal thrombosis

Renal: Impaired renal function

Respiratory: Pulmonary thromboembolism

Miscellaneous: Hemorrhagic eruption

Dosage Oral:

Children ≥15 years and Adults: Female: Acne (Ortho Tri-Cyclen®): Refer to dosing for contraception

Adults: Female:

Contraception:

Schedule 1 (Sunday starter): Dose begins on first Sunday after onset of menstruation; if the menstrual period starts on Sunday, take first tablet that very same day. **With a Sunday start, an additional method of contraception should be used until after the first 7 days of consecutive administration.**

For 21-tablet package: Dosage is 1 tablet daily for 21 consecutive days, followed by 7 days off of the medication; a new course begins on the 8th day after the last tablet is taken.

For 28-tablet package: Dosage is 1 tablet daily without interruption.

Schedule 2 (Day 1 starter): Dose starts on first day of menstrual cycle taking 1 tablet daily.

For 21-tablet package: Dosage is 1 tablet daily for 21 consecutive days, followed by 7 days off of the medication; a new course begins on the 8th day after the last tablet is taken.

For 28-tablet package: Dosage is 1 tablet daily without interruption.

If all doses have been taken on schedule and one menstrual period is missed, continue dosing cycle. If two consecutive menstrual periods are missed, pregnancy test is required before new dosing cycle is started.

Missed doses **monophasic formulations** (refer to package insert for complete information):

One dose missed: Take as soon as remembered or take 2 tablets next day

Two consecutive doses missed in the first 2 weeks: Take 2 tablets as soon as remembered or 2 tablets next 2 days. **An additional method of contraception should be used for 7 days after missed dose.**

Two consecutive doses missed in week 3 or three consecutive doses missed at any time: **An additional method of contraception must be used for 7 days after a missed dose:**

Schedule 1 (Sunday starter): Continue dose of 1 tablet daily until Sunday, then discard the rest of the pack, and a new pack should be started that same day.

Schedule 2 (Day 1 starter): Current pack should be discarded, and a new pack should be started that same day.

Missed doses **biphasic/triphasic formulations** (refer to package insert for complete information):

One dose missed: Take as soon as remembered or take 2 tablets next day.

Two consecutive doses missed in week 1 or week 2 of the pack: Take 2 tablets as soon as remembered and 2 tablets the next day. Resume taking 1 tablet daily until the pack is empty. **An additional method of contraception must be used for 7 days after a missed dose.**

Two consecutive doses missed in week 3 of the pack. **An additional method of contraception must be used for 7 days after a missed dose.**

Schedule 1 (Sunday starter): Take 1 tablet every day until Sunday. Discard the remaining pack and start a new pack of pills on the same day.

Schedule 2 (Day 1 starter): Discard the remaining pack and start a new pack the same day.

Three or more consecutive doses missed. **An additional method of contraception must be used for 7 days after a missed dose.**

Schedule 1 (Sunday starter): Take 1 tablet every day until Sunday; on Sunday, discard the pack and start a new pack.

Schedule 2 (Day 1 starter): Discard the remaining pack and begin new pack of tablets starting on the same day.

Dosage adjustment in renal impairment: Specific guidelines not available; use with caution and monitor blood pressure closely. Consider other forms of contraception.

Dosage adjustment in hepatic impairment: Contraindicated in patients with hepatic impairment.

Mechanism of Action Combination hormonal contraceptives inhibit ovulation via a negative feedback mechanism on the hypothalamus, which alters the normal pattern of gonadotropin secretion of a follicle-stimulating hormone (FSH) and luteinizing hormone by the anterior pituitary. The follicular phase FSH and midcycle surge of gonadotropins are inhibited. In addition, combination hormonal contraceptives produce alterations in the genital tract, including changes in the cervical mucus, rendering it unfavorable for sperm penetration even if ovulation occurs. Changes in the endometrium may also occur, producing an unfavorable environment for nidation. Combination hormonal contraceptive drugs may alter the tubal transport of the ova through the fallopian tubes. Progestational agents may also alter sperm fertility.

Contraindications Hypersensitivity to ethinyl estradiol, norgestimate, or any component of the formulation; history of or current thrombophlebitis or venous thromboembolic disorders (including DVT, PE); active or recent (within 1 year) arterial thromboembolic disease (eg, stroke, MI); cerebral vascular disease, coronary artery disease, valvular heart disease with complications, severe hypertension; severe headache with focal neurological symptoms; known or suspected breast carcinoma, endometrial cancer, estrogen-dependent neoplasms, undiagnosed abnormal genital bleeding; hepatic dysfunction or tumor, cholestatic jaundice of pregnancy, jaundice with prior combination hormonal contraceptive use; heavy smoking (≥15 cigarettes/day) in patients >35 years of age; pregnancy

Warnings/Precautions Combination hormonal contraceptives do not protect against HIV infection or other sexually-transmitted diseases. **[U.S. Boxed Warning]: The risk of cardiovascular side effects increases in women who smoke cigarettes, especially those who are >35 years of age; women who use combination hormonal contraceptives should be strongly advised not to smoke.** Combination hormonal contraceptives may lead to increased risk of myocardial infarction, use with caution in patients with risk factors for coronary artery disease. May increase the risk of thromboembolism. Whenever possible, combination hormonal contraceptives should be discontinued at least 4 weeks prior to and for 2 weeks following elective surgery associated with an increased risk of thromboembolism or during periods of prolonged immobilization. Combination hormonal contraceptives may have a dose-related risk of vascular disease, hypertension, and gallbladder disease. Women with hypertension or renal disease should be encouraged to use a nonhormonal form of contraception. The use of combination hormonal contraceptives has been associated with a slight increase in frequency of breast cancer, however, studies are not consistent. Combination hormonal contraceptives may cause glucose intolerance or effect serum triglyceride and lipoprotein levels. Retinal thrombosis has been reported (rarely). Use caution with conditions that may be aggravated by fluid retention, depression, or history of migraine. Not for use prior to menarche.

The minimum dosage combination of estrogen/progestin that will effectively treat the individual patient should be used. New patients should be started on products containing ≤0.035 mg of estrogen per tablet.

Acne: For use only in females ≥15 years, who also desire combination hormonal contraceptive therapy, are unresponsive to topical treatments, and have no contraindications to combination hormonal contraceptive use. (Continued)

Ethinyl Estradiol and Norgestimate *(Continued)*

Drug Interactions

Cytochrome P450 Effect: Ethinyl estradiol: **Substrate** of CYP2C9 (minor), 3A4 (major), 3A5-7 (minor); **Inhibits** CYP1A2 (weak), 2B6 (weak), 2C8 (weak), 2C19 (weak), 3A4 (weak)

Increased Effect/Toxicity: Acetaminophen and ascorbic acid may increase plasma levels of estrogen component. Atorvastatin and indinavir increase plasma levels of combination hormonal contraceptives. Combination hormonal contraceptives increase the plasma levels of alprazolam, chlordiazepoxide, cyclosporine, diazepam, prednisolone, selegiline, theophylline, tricyclic antidepressants. Combination hormonal contraceptives may increase (or decrease) the effects of coumarin derivatives.

Decreased Effect: CYP3A4 inducers may decrease the levels/effects of ethinyl estradiol; example inducers include aminoglutethimide, carbamazepine, nafcillin, nevirapine, phenobarbital, phenytoin, and rifamycins. Combination hormonal contraceptives may decrease plasma levels of acetaminophen, clofibric acid, lorazepam, morphine, oxazepam, salicylic acid, temazepam. Contraceptive effect decreased by acitretin, aminoglutethimide, amprenavir, anticonvulsants, griseofulvin, lopinavir, nelfinavir, nevirapine, penicillins (effect not consistent), rifampin, ritonavir, tetracyclines (effect not consistent). Combination hormonal contraceptives may decrease (or increase) the effects of coumarin derivatives. Aprepitant, modafinil, and topiramate may decrease the serum concentration of oral contraceptive (estrogens). Oral contraceptive (estrogens) may decrease the serum concentration of lamotrigine.

Ethanol/Nutrition/Herb Interactions

Food: CNS effects of caffeine may be enhanced if combination hormonal contraceptives are used concurrently with caffeine. Grapefruit juice increases ethinyl estradiol concentrations and would be expected to increase progesterone serum levels as well; clinical implications are unclear.

Herb/Nutraceutical: St John's wort may decrease levels. Herbs with estrogenic properties may enhance the adverse/toxic effect of estrogen derivatives; examples include alfalfa, black cohosh, bloodroot, hops, kudzu, licorice, red clover, saw palmetto, soybean, thyme, wild yam, yucca. Herbs with progestogenic properties may enhance the adverse/toxic effect of progestins; examples include bloodroot, chasteberry, damiana, oregano, yucca.

Dietary Considerations Should be taken at same time each day.

Pharmacodynamics/Kinetics

Norgestimate:

Absorption: Well absorbed

Protein binding: To albumin and sex hormone-binding globulin (SHBG); SHBG capacity is affected by plasma ethinyl estradiol levels

Metabolism: Hepatic; forms 17-deacetylnorgestimate (major active metabolite) and other metabolites

Half-life elimination: 17-deacetylnorgestimate: 12-30 hours

Excretion: Urine and feces

Pregnancy Risk Factor X

Dosage Forms

Tablet, monophasic formulations:

MonoNessa™, Ortho-Cyclen®: Ethinyl estradiol 0.035 mg and norgestimate 0.25 mg [21 blue tablets and 7 green inactive tablets] (28s)

Previfem™: Ethinyl estradiol 0.035 mg and norgestimate 0.25 mg [21 blue tablets and 7 teal inactive tablets] (28s)

Sprintec™: Ethinyl estradiol 0.035 mg and norgestimate 0.25 mg [21 blue tablets and 7 white inactive tablets] (28s)

Tablet, triphasic formulations:

Ortho Tri-Cyclen®, TriNessa™:

Day 1-7: Ethinyl estradiol 0.035 mg and norgestimate 0.18 mg [7 white tablets]

Day 8-14: Ethinyl estradiol 0.035 mg and norgestimate 0.215 mg [7 light blue tablets]

Day 15-21: Ethinyl estradiol 0.035 mg and norgestimate 0.25 mg [7 blue tablets]

Day 22-28: 7 green inactive tablets (28s)

Tri-Previfem™:

Day 1-7: Ethinyl estradiol 0.035 mg and norgestimate 0.18 mg [7 white tablets]

Day 8-14: Ethinyl estradiol 0.035 mg and norgestimate 0.215 mg [7 light blue tablets]

Day 15-21: Ethinyl estradiol 0.035 mg and norgestimate 0.25 mg [7 blue tablets]

Day 22-28: 7 teal inactive tablets (28s)

Tri-Sprintec™:
Day 1-7: Ethinyl estradiol 0.035 mg and norgestimate 0.18 mg [7 gray tablets]
Day 8-14: Ethinyl estradiol 0.035 mg and norgestimate 0.215 mg [7 light blue tablets]
Day 15-21: Ethinyl estradiol 0.035 mg and norgestimate 0.25 mg [7 blue tablets]
Day 22-28: 7 white inactive tablets (28s)

Ortho Tri-Cyclen® Lo:
Day 1-7: Ethinyl estradiol 0.025 mg and norgestimate 0.18 mg [7 white tablets]
Day 8-14: Ethinyl estradiol 0.025 mg and norgestimate 0.215 mg [7 light blue tablets]
Day 15-21: Ethinyl estradiol 0.025 mg and norgestimate 0.25 mg [7 dark blue tablets]
Day 22-28: 7 green inactive tablets (28s)

Ethinyl Estradiol and Norgestrel
(ETH in il es tra DYE ole & nor JES trel)

U.S. Brand Names Cryselle™; Lo/Ovral®; Low-Ogestrel®; Ogestrel®
Canadian Brand Names Ovral®
Mexican Brand Names Ovral
Generic Available Yes
Index Terms Morning After Pill; Norgestrel and Ethinyl Estradiol
Pharmacologic Category Contraceptive; Estrogen and Progestin Combination
Use Prevention of pregnancy; postcoital contraceptive or "morning after" pill
Unlabeled/Investigational Use Treatment of hypermenorrhea (menorrhagia); pain associated with endometriosis; dysmenorrhea; dysfunctional uterine bleeding
Local Anesthetic/Vasoconstrictor Precautions No information available to require special precautions
Effects on Dental Treatment When prescribing antibiotics, patient must be warned to use additional methods of birth control if on oral contraceptives.
Common Adverse Effects Frequency not defined.
Cardiovascular: Arterial thromboembolism, cerebral hemorrhage, cerebral thrombosis, edema, hypertension, mesenteric thrombosis, MI
Central nervous system: Depression, dizziness, headache, migraine, nervousness, premenstrual syndrome, stroke
Dermatologic: Acne, erythema multiforme, erythema nodosum, hirsutism, loss of scalp hair, melasma (may persist), rash (allergic)
Endocrine & metabolic: Amenorrhea, breakthrough bleeding, breast enlargement, breast secretion, breast tenderness, carbohydrate intolerance, lactation decreased (postpartum), glucose tolerance decreased, libido changes, menstrual flow changes, sex hormone-binding globulins (SHBG) increased, spotting, temporary infertility (following discontinuation), thyroid-binding globulin increased, triglycerides increased
Gastrointestinal: Abdominal cramps, appetite changes, bloating, cholestasis, colitis, gallbladder disease, jaundice, nausea, vomiting, weight gain/loss
Genitourinary: Cervical erosion changes, cervical secretion changes, cystitis-like syndrome, vaginal candidiasis, vaginitis
Hematologic: Antithrombin III decreased, folate levels decreased, hemolytic uremic syndrome, norepinephrine induced platelet aggregability increased, porphyria, prothrombin increased; factors VII, VIII, IX, and X
Hepatic: Benign liver tumors, Budd-Chiari syndrome, cholestatic jaundice, hepatic adenomas
Local: Thrombophlebitis
Ocular: Cataracts, change in corneal curvature (steepening), contact lens intolerance, optic neuritis, retinal thrombosis
Renal: Impaired renal function
Respiratory: Pulmonary thromboembolism
Miscellaneous: Hemorrhagic eruption
Dosage Oral: Adults: Female:
Contraception:
Schedule 1 (Sunday starter): Dose begins on first Sunday after onset of menstruation; if the menstrual period starts on Sunday, take first tablet that very same day. **With a Sunday start, an additional method of contraception should be used until after the first 7 days of consecutive administration.**
(Continued)

Ethinyl Estradiol and Norgestrel *(Continued)*

For 21-tablet package: Dosage is 1 tablet daily for 21 consecutive days, followed by 7 days off of the medication; a new course begins on the 8th day after the last tablet is taken.

For 28-tablet package: Dosage is 1 tablet daily without interruption.

Schedule 2 (Day 1 starter): Dose starts on first day of menstrual cycle taking 1 tablet daily.

For 21-tablet package: Dosage is 1 tablet daily for 21 consecutive days, followed by 7 days off of the medication; a new course begins on the 8th day after the last tablet is taken.

For 28-tablet package: Dosage is 1 tablet daily without interruption.

If all doses have been taken on schedule and one menstrual period is missed, continue dosing cycle. If two consecutive menstrual periods are missed, pregnancy test is required before new dosing cycle is started.

Missed doses **monophasic formulations** (refer to package insert for complete information):

One dose missed: Take as soon as remembered or take 2 tablets next day

Two consecutive doses missed in the first 2 weeks: Take 2 tablets as soon as remembered or 2 tablets next 2 days. **An additional method of contraception should be used for 7 days after missed dose.**

Two consecutive doses missed in week 3 or three consecutive doses missed at any time:

Schedule 1 (Sunday starter): Continue to take 1 tablet daily until Sunday, then discard the rest of the pack, and a new pack is started that same day.

Schedule 2 (Day 1 starter): Current pack should be discarded, and a new pack started that same day. **An additional method of contraception should be used for 7 days after missed dose.**

Postcoital contraception:

Ethinyl estradiol 0.03 mg and norgestrel 0.3 mg formulation: 4 tablets within 72 hours of unprotected intercourse and 4 tablets 12 hours after first dose

Ethinyl estradiol 0.05 mg and norgestrel 0.5 mg formulation: 2 tablets within 72 hours of unprotected intercourse and 2 tablets 12 hours after first dose

Dosage adjustment in renal impairment: Specific guidelines not available; use with caution and monitor blood pressure closely. Consider other forms of contraception.

Dosage adjustment in hepatic impairment: Contraindicated in patients with hepatic impairment.

Mechanism of Action Combination hormonal contraceptives inhibit ovulation via a negative feedback mechanism on the hypothalamus, which alters the normal pattern of gonadotropin secretion of a follicle-stimulating hormone (FSH) and luteinizing hormone by the anterior pituitary. The follicular phase FSH and midcycle surge of gonadotropins are inhibited. In addition, combination hormonal contraceptives produce alterations in the genital tract, including changes in the cervical mucus, rendering it unfavorable for sperm penetration even if ovulation occurs. Changes in the endometrium may also occur, producing an unfavorable environment for nidation. Combination hormonal contraceptive drugs may alter the tubal transport of the ova through the fallopian tubes. Progestational agents may also alter sperm fertility.

Contraindications Hypersensitivity to ethinyl estradiol, norgestrel, or any component of the formulation; history of or current thrombophlebitis or venous thromboembolic disorders (including DVT, PE); active or recent (within 1 year) arterial thromboembolic disease (eg, stroke, MI); cerebral vascular disease, coronary artery disease, valvular heart disease with complications, severe hypertension; diabetes mellitus with vascular involvement; severe headache with focal neurological symptoms; known or suspected breast carcinoma, endometrial cancer, estrogen-dependent neoplasms, undiagnosed abnormal genital bleeding; hepatic dysfunction or tumor, cholestatic jaundice of pregnancy, jaundice with prior combination hormonal contraceptive use; major surgery with prolonged immobilization; heavy smoking ($\geq$15 cigarettes/day) in patients >35 years of age; pregnancy

Warnings/Precautions Combination hormonal contraceptives do not protect against HIV infection or other sexually-transmitted diseases. **[U.S. Boxed Warning]: The risk of cardiovascular side effects increases in women who smoke cigarettes, especially those who are >35 years of age; women who use combination hormonal contraceptives should be strongly advised not to smoke.** Combination hormonal contraceptives may lead to increased risk of myocardial infarction, use with caution in patients with risk factors for coronary artery disease. May increase the risk of thromboembolism. Whenever possible, combination hormonal contraceptives should be discontinued at least 4 weeks prior to and for 2 weeks following elective surgery associated with an increased risk of thromboembolism or during periods of prolonged immobilization. Combination hormonal contraceptives may have a dose-related risk of vascular disease, hypertension, and gallbladder disease. Women with hypertension or renal disease should be encouraged to use another form of contraception. The use of combination hormonal contraceptives has been associated with a slight increase in frequency of breast cancer, however, studies are not consistent. Combination hormonal contraceptives may cause glucose intolerance or effect serum triglyceride and lipoprotein levels. Retinal thrombosis has been reported (rarely). Use caution with conditions that may be aggravated by fluid retention, depression, or history of migraine. Not for use prior to menarche.

The minimum dosage combination of estrogen/progestin that will effectively treat the individual patient should be used. New patients should be started on products containing ≤0.035 mg of estrogen per tablet.

Drug Interactions

Cytochrome P450 Effect:

Ethinyl estradiol: **Substrate** of CYP2C9 (minor), 3A4 (major), 3A5-7 (minor); **Inhibits** CYP1A2 (weak), 2B6 (weak), 2C8 (weak), 2C19 (weak), 3A4 (weak)

Norgestrel: **Substrate** of CYP3A4 (major)

Increased Effect/Toxicity: Acetaminophen and ascorbic acid may increase plasma levels of estrogen component. Atorvastatin and indinavir increase plasma levels of combination hormonal contraceptives. Combination hormonal contraceptives increase the plasma levels of alprazolam, chlordiaz-epoxide, cyclosporine, diazepam, prednisolone, selegiline, theophylline, tricyclic antidepressants. Combination hormonal contraceptives may increase (or decrease) the effects of coumarin derivatives.

Decreased Effect: CYP3A4 inducers may decrease the levels/effects of norgestrel; example inducers include aminoglutethimide, carbamazepine, nafcillin, nevirapine, phenobarbital, phenytoin, and rifamycins. Combination hormonal contraceptives may decrease plasma levels of acetaminophen, clofibric acid, lorazepam, morphine, oxazepam, salicylic acid, temazepam. Contraceptive effect decreased by acitretin, aminoglutethimide, amprenavir, anticonvulsants, griseofulvin, lopinavir, nelfinavir, nevirapine, penicillins (effect not consistent), rifampin, ritonavir, tetracyclines (effect not consistent). Combination hormonal contraceptives may decrease (or increase) the effects of coumarin derivatives. Aprepitant, modafinil, and topiramate may decrease the serum concentration of oral contraceptive (estrogens). Oral contraceptive (estrogens) may decrease the serum concentration of lamotrigine.

Ethanol/Nutrition/Herb Interactions

Food: CNS effects of caffeine may be enhanced if combination hormonal contraceptives are used concurrently with caffeine. Grapefruit juice increases ethinyl estradiol concentrations and would be expected to increase progesterone serum levels as well; clinical implications are unclear.

Herb/Nutraceutical: St John's wort may decrease levels. Herbs with estrogenic properties may enhance the adverse/toxic effect of estrogen derivatives; examples include alfalfa, black cohosh, bloodroot, hops, kudzu, licorice, red clover, saw palmetto, soybean, thyme, wild yam, yucca. Herbs with progestogenic properties may enhance the adverse/toxic effect of progestins; examples include bloodroot, chasteberry, damiana, oregano, yucca.

Dietary Considerations Should be taken at same time each day.

Pregnancy Risk Factor X

Dosage Forms

Tablet, monophasic formulations:

Cryselle™: Ethinyl estradiol 0.03 mg and norgestrel 0.3 mg [21 white tablets and 7 light green inactive tablets] (28s)

Low-Ogestrel® 28: Ethinyl estradiol 0.03 mg and norgestrel 0.3 mg [21 white tablets and 7 peach inactive tablets] (28s)

Lo/Ovral® 28: Ethinyl estradiol 0.03 mg and norgestrel 0.3 mg [21 white tablets and 7 pink inactive tablets] (28s)

Ogestrel® 28: Ethinyl estradiol 0.05 mg and norgestrel 0.5 mg [21 white tablets and 7 peach inactive tablets] (28s)

Ethiofos *see* Amifostine *on page 85*

Ethionamide (e thye on AM ide)

Related Information

Tuberculosis *on page 1765*

U.S. Brand Names Trecator®

Canadian Brand Names Trecator®

Generic Available No

Pharmacologic Category Antitubercular Agent

Use Treatment of tuberculosis and other mycobacterial diseases, in conjunction with other antituberculosis agents, when first-line agents have failed or resistance has been demonstrated

(Continued)

Ethionamide (Continued)

Local Anesthetic/Vasoconstrictor Precautions No information available to require special precautions

Effects on Dental Treatment Key adverse event(s) related to dental treatment: Postural hypotension, metallic taste, and stomatitis.

Common Adverse Effects Frequency not defined.

Cardiovascular: Postural hypotension

Central nervous system: Depression, dizziness, drowsiness, headache, psychiatric disturbances, restlessness, seizure

Dermatologic: Acne, alopecia, photosensitivity, purpura, rash

Endocrine & metabolic: Gynecomastia, hypoglycemia, hypothyroidism or goiter, pellagra-like syndrome

Gastrointestinal: Abdominal pain, anorexia, diarrhea, excessive salivation, metallic taste, nausea, stomatitis, vomiting, weight loss

Genitourinary: Impotence

Hematologic: Thrombocytopenia

Hepatic: Hepatitis, jaundice, liver function tests increased

Neuromuscular & skeletal: Peripheral neuritis, weakness (common)

Ocular: Blurred vision, diplopia, optic neuritis

Respiratory: Olfactory disturbances

Miscellaneous: Hypersensitivity reaction

Mechanism of Action Inhibits peptide synthesis

Pharmacodynamics/Kinetics

Absorption: Rapid, complete

Distribution: Crosses placenta; V_d: 93.5 L

Protein binding: ~30%

Metabolism: Extensively hepatic to active and inactive metabolites

Bioavailability: 80%

Half-life elimination: 2-3 hours

Time to peak, serum: 1 hour

Excretion: Urine (<1% as unchanged drug; as active and inactive metabolites)

Pregnancy Risk Factor C

Ethmozine® *see* Moricizine *on page 1123*

Ethosuximide (eth oh SUKS i mide)

U.S. Brand Names Zarontin®

Canadian Brand Names Zarontin®

Generic Available Yes

Pharmacologic Category Anticonvulsant, Succinimide

Use Management of absence (petit mal) seizures

Local Anesthetic/Vasoconstrictor Precautions No information available to require special precautions

Effects on Dental Treatment No significant effects or complications reported

Common Adverse Effects Frequency not defined.

Central nervous system: Aggressiveness, ataxia, disturbance in sleep, dizziness, drowsiness, euphoria, fatigue, headache, hyperactivity, inability to concentrate, irritability, lethargy, mental depression (with cases of overt suicidal intentions), night terrors, paranoid psychosis

Dermatologic: Hirsutism, pruritus, rash, Stevens-Johnson syndrome, urticaria

Endocrine & metabolic: Libido increased

Gastrointestinal: Abdominal pain, anorexia, cramps, diarrhea, epigastric pain, gastric upset, gum hypertrophy, nausea, tongue swelling, vomiting, weight loss

Genitourinary: Hematuria (microscopic), vaginal bleeding

Hematologic: Agranulocytosis, eosinophilia, leukopenia, pancytopenia

Ocular: Myopia

Miscellaneous: Hiccups, systemic lupus erythematosus

Mechanism of Action Increases the seizure threshold and suppresses paroxysmal spike-and-wave pattern in absence seizures; depresses nerve transmission in the motor cortex

Drug Interactions

Cytochrome P450 Effect: Substrate of CYP3A4 (major)

Increased Effect/Toxicity: Sedative effects may be additive with other CNS depressants. CYP3A4 inhibitors may increase the levels/effects of ethosuximide; example inhibitors include azole antifungals, clarithromycin, diclofenac, doxycycline, erythromycin, imatinib, isoniazid, nefazodone, nicardipine, propofol, protease inhibitors, quinidine, telithromycin, and verapamil.

Decreased Effect: CYP3A4 inducers may decrease the levels/effects of ethosuximide; example inducers include aminoglutethimide, carbamazepine, nafcillin, nevirapine, phenobarbital, phenytoin, and rifamycins.

Pharmacodynamics/Kinetics
Distribution: Adults: V_d: 0.62-0.72 L/kg
Metabolism: Hepatic (~80% to 3 inactive metabolites)
Half-life elimination, serum: Children: 30 hours; Adults: 50-60 hours
Time to peak, serum: Capsule: ~2-4 hours; Syrup: <2-4 hours
Excretion: Urine, slowly (50% as metabolites, 10% to 20% as unchanged drug);
feces (small amounts)

Ethotoin (ETH oh toyn)

U.S. Brand Names Peganone®
Canadian Brand Names Peganone®
Generic Available No
Index Terms Ethylphenylhydantoin
Pharmacologic Category Anticonvulsant, Hydantoin
Use Generalized tonic-clonic or complex-partial seizures
Local Anesthetic/Vasoconstrictor Precautions No information available to require special precautions
Effects on Dental Treatment No significant effects or complications reported
Common Adverse Effects Frequency not defined.
Cardiovascular: Chest pain
Central nervous system: Ataxia, dizziness, fatigue, fever, headache, insomnia
Dermatologic: Skin rash, Stevens-Johnson syndrome
Gastrointestinal: Diarrhea, gingival hyperplasia, nausea, vomiting
Hematologic: Blood dyscrasias
Neuromuscular & skeletal: Numbness
Ocular: Diplopia, nystagmus
Miscellaneous: Lymphadenopathy, SLE-like syndrome
Mechanism of Action Stabilizes the seizure threshold and prevents the spread of seizure activity
Drug Interactions
Cytochrome P450 Effect: Inhibits CYP2C19 (weak)
Increased Effect/Toxicity: Carbonic anhydrase inhibitors may enhance the adverse/toxic effect hydantoin anticonvulsants; monitor for evidence of osteomalacia and rickets if these 2 agents are used concomitantly. Monitor for additive CNS-depressant effects if 2 or more CNS depressants are concomitantly used.
Decreased Effect: Hydantoin anticonvulsants may increase the metabolism of acetaminophen; monitor for decreased effects of acetaminophen and hepatotoxicity. Chloramphenicol may decrease the metabolism, via CYP isoenzymes, of hydantoin anticonvulsants. Hydantoin anticonvulsants may decrease the serum concentration of chloramphenicol; monitor for toxic effects. Antacids may decrease the serum concentration of hydantoin anticonvulsants.
Pharmacodynamics/Kinetics
Absorption: Rapid
Metabolism: Hepatic; forms metabolites
Half-life elimination: 3-9 hours
Excretion: Urine, feces, saliva (minimal)
Pregnancy Risk Factor D

ETH-Oxydose™ see Oxycodone on page 1225
Ethoxynaphthamido Penicillin Sodium see Nafcillin on page 1141
Ethyl Aminobenzoate see Benzocaine on page 195

Ethyl Chloride (ETH il KLOR ide)

U.S. Brand Names Gebauer's Ethyl Chloride®
Generic Available No
Index Terms Chloroethane
Pharmacologic Category Local Anesthetic
Use Local anesthetic in minor operative procedures and to relieve pain caused by insect stings and burns, and irritation caused by myofascial and visceral pain syndromes
Local Anesthetic/Vasoconstrictor Precautions No information available to require special precautions
Effects on Dental Treatment Key adverse event(s) related to dental treatment: Mucous membrane irritation. See Dental Comment.
Common Adverse Effects 1% to 10%: Mucous membrane irritation, freezing may alter skin pigment
Pregnancy Risk Factor C
(Continued)

Ethyl Chloride *(Continued)*

Dental Comment Spray for a few seconds to the point of frost formation when the tissue becomes white; avoid prolonged spraying of skin beyond this point

Ethyl Chloride and Dichlorotetrafluoroethane

(ETH il KLOR ide & dye klor oh te tra floo or oh ETH ane)

Related Information
Ethyl Chloride *on page 653*

U.S. Brand Names Fluro-Ethyl®

Generic Available No

Index Terms Dichlorotetrafluoroethane and Ethyl Chloride

Pharmacologic Category Local Anesthetic

Use Topical refrigerant anesthetic to control pain associated with minor surgical procedures, dermabrasion, injections, contusions, and minor strains

Local Anesthetic/Vasoconstrictor Precautions No information available to require special precautions

Effects on Dental Treatment No significant effects or complications reported

Pregnancy Risk Factor C

Ethylphenylhydantoin *see* Ethotoin *on page 653*

Ethynodiol Diacetate and Ethinyl Estradiol *see* Ethinyl Estradiol and Ethynodiol Diacetate *on page 628*

Ethyol® *see* Amifostine *on page 85*

Etidronate and Calcium (e ti DROE nate & KAL see um)

Related Information
Calcium Carbonate *on page 260*
Etidronate Disodium *on page 654*

Canadian Brand Names Didrocal™

Index Terms Calcium Carbonate and Etidronate Disodium

Pharmacologic Category Bisphosphonate Derivative; Calcium Salt

Use Treatment and prevention of postmenopausal osteoporosis; prevention of corticosteroid-induced osteoporosis

Local Anesthetic/Vasoconstrictor Precautions No information available to require special precautions

Effects on Dental Treatment Osteonecrosis of the jaw (ONJ), generally associated with local infection and/or tooth extraction and often with delayed healing, has been reported in patients taking bisphosphonates. Symptoms included nonhealing extraction socket or an exposed jawbone. Most reported cases of bisphosphonate-associated osteonecrosis have been in cancer patients treated with intravenous bisphosphonates. However, some have occurred in patients with postmenopausal osteoporosis taking oral bisphosphonates. Dental surgery may exacerbate ONJ. For patients requiring dental procedures, there are no data available to suggest whether discontinuation of bisphosphonate treatment reduces the risk of ONJ. Patients who develop ONJ while on bisphosphonate therapy should receive care by an oral surgeon. See Dental Comment in Etidronate Disodium monograph.

Common Adverse Effects >10%:
Central nervous system: Dizziness (16%), headache (13%)
Gastrointestinal: Diarrhea (37%), nausea (18%), flatulence (17%), constipation (13%), dyspepsia (12%), vomiting (11%)

Restrictions Not available in U.S.

Mechanism of Action See individual agents.

Drug Interactions
Decreased Effect: See individual agents. **Note:** Since etidronate and calcium carbonate are administered sequentially, there is no interaction between the two components. Concurrent administration may result in reduced absorption of etidronate.

Pharmacodynamics/Kinetics See individual agents.

Pregnancy Risk Factor C (based on U.S. labeling)

Dental Comment See Etidronate Disodium monograph.

Etidronate Disodium (e ti DROE nate dye SOW dee um)

Related Information
Rheumatoid Arthritis, Osteoarthritis, and Osteoporosis *on page 1759*

U.S. Brand Names Didronel®

Canadian Brand Names Didronel®; Gen-Etidronate

Generic Available No

Index Terms EHDP; Sodium Etidronate

Pharmacologic Category Bisphosphonate Derivative

Use Symptomatic treatment of Paget's disease; prevention and treatment of heterotopic ossification due to spinal cord injury or after total hip replacement

Unlabeled/Investigational Use Postmenopausal osteoporosis

Local Anesthetic/Vasoconstrictor Precautions No information available to require special precautions

Effects on Dental Treatment Key adverse event(s) related to dental treatment: Abnormal taste.

Osteonecrosis of the jaw (ONJ), generally associated with local infection and/or tooth extraction and often with delayed healing, has been reported in patients taking bisphosphonates. Symptoms included nonhealing extraction socket or an exposed jawbone. Most reported cases of bisphosphonate-associated osteonecrosis have been in cancer patients treated with intravenous bisphosphonates. However, some have occurred in patients with postmenopausal osteoporosis taking oral bisphosphonates. Dental surgery may exacerbate ONJ. For patients requiring dental procedures, there are no data available to suggest whether discontinuation of bisphosphonate treatment reduces the risk of ONJ. Patients who develop ONJ while on bisphosphonate therapy should receive care by an oral surgeon. See Dental Comment.

Common Adverse Effects Frequency not defined.

Gastrointestinal: Diarrhea, nausea

Neuromuscular & skeletal: Bone pain

Mechanism of Action Decreases bone resorption by inhibiting osteocystic osteolysis; decreases mineral release and matrix or collagen breakdown in bone

Drug Interactions

Increased Effect/Toxicity: Aminoglycosides may lower serum calcium levels with prolonged administration; concomitant use may have an additive hypocalcemic effect. NSAIDs may enhance the gastrointestinal adverse/toxic effects (increased incidence of GI ulcers) of bisphosphonate derivatives. Bisphosphonate derivatives may enhance the hypocalcemic effect of phosphate supplements.

Decreased Effect: The following agents may decrease the absorption of oral bisphosphonate derivatives: Antacids (aluminum, calcium, magnesium), oral calcium salts, oral iron salts, and oral magnesium salts

Pharmacodynamics/Kinetics

Onset of action: 1-3 months

Duration: Can persist for 12 months without continuous therapy

Absorption: ~3%

Metabolism: None

Half-life elimination: 1-6 hours

Excretion: Primarily urine (as unchanged drug); feces (as unabsorbed drug)

Pregnancy Risk Factor C

Dental Comment There is no data on the incidence of ONJ associated with use of etidronate disodium. A report by the Council of Scientific Affairs of the American Dental Association (accessed at: http://www.ada.org/prof/resources/topics/osteonecrosis.asp) as of July 2006 gave an estimated incidence of 0.7 cases for every 100,000 person-years of exposure to alendronate (Fosamax®). This translates to one case for every 142,857 person-years exposure. This figure from the ADA report was based on information received from Merck & Co citing 170 worldwide cases for alendronate (Fosamax®). In addition, Procter & Gamble Pharmaceuticals has cited 20 cases for risedronate (Actonel®) and Roche Laboratories has cited one case for ibandronate (Boniva®).

Consumer Reports On Health stated that the risk of jaw bone osteonecrosis due to alendronate (Fosamax®), risedronate (Actonel®), or ibandronate (Boniva®) taken to prevent osteoporosis is very low and is estimated to be one out of every 20,000 users. That report mentioned that tooth extraction or implants increase the risk of developing osteonecrosis in patients taking any of these drugs for osteoporosis. The report also recommended that patients should stop taking any of these oral drugs 1-2 months before and after such dental treatment. No evidence was presented to support this statement.

In terms of length of exposure to oral bisphosphonates prior to onset of ONJ, data from large population studies or controlled studies is lacking. A report by Marx et al, observed that of three cases of ONJ associated with Fosamax® exposure, one patient had been taking 10 mg/day by mouth for 6 years and the other two patients 10 mg/day by mouth for 3 and 2 years respectively. In contrast, they observed that in cancer patients receiving intravenous bisphosphonates, the time period between the first doses of the bisphosphonate *(Continued)*

Etidronate Disodium *(Continued)*

to first recognition of exposed bone either by the patients or by the clinician, was 9.4 months for zoledronate (Zometa®), 14.3 months for pamidronate (Aredia®), and 12.1 months for pamidronate then to zoledronate.

Etodolac *(ee toe DOE lak)*

Related Information
Oral Pain *on page 1788*
Rheumatoid Arthritis, Osteoarthritis, and Osteoporosis *on page 1759*
Temporomandibular Dysfunction (TMD) *on page 1822*
U.S. Brand Names Lodine® [DSC]; Lodine® XL [DSC]
Canadian Brand Names Apo-Etodolac®; Lodine®; Utradol™
Mexican Brand Names Lodine; Lodine Retard
Generic Available Yes
Index Terms Etodolic Acid
Pharmacologic Category Nonsteroidal Anti-inflammatory Drug (NSAID), Oral
Dental Use Management of postoperative pain
Use Acute and long-term use in the management of signs and symptoms of osteoarthritis; rheumatoid arthritis and juvenile rheumatoid arthritis; management of acute pain
Local Anesthetic/Vasoconstrictor Precautions No information available to require special precautions
Effects on Dental Treatment NSAID formulations are known to reversibly decrease platelet aggregation via mechanisms different than observed with aspirin. The dentist should be aware of the potential of abnormal coagulation. Caution should also be exercised in the use of NSAIDs in patients already on anticoagulant therapy with drugs such as warfarin (Coumadin®).
Significant Adverse Effects
1% to 10%:
  Central nervous system: Dizziness (3% to 9 %), chills/fever (1% to 3%), depression (1% to 3%), nervousness (1% to 3%)
  Dermatologic: Rash (1% to 3%), pruritus (1% to 3%)
  Gastrointestinal: Abdominal cramps (3% to 9%), nausea (3% to 9%), vomiting (1% to 3%), dyspepsia (10%), diarrhea (3% to 9%), constipation (1% to 3%), flatulence (3% to 9%), melena (1% to 3%), gastritis (1% to 3%)
  Genitourinary: Dysuria (1% to 3%)
  Neuromuscular & skeletal: Weakness (3% to 9%)
  Ocular: Blurred vision (1% to 3%)
  Otic: Tinnitus (1% to 3%)
  Renal: Polyuria (1% to 3%)
<1% (Limited to important or life-threatening): Agranulocytosis, allergic reaction, allergic/necrotizing vasculitis, alopecia, anaphylactic/anaphylactoid reactions, anemia, angioedema, anorexia, arrhythmia, aseptic meningitis, asthma, bleeding time increased, CHF, confusion, conjunctivitis, CVA, cystitis, duodenitis, dyspnea, ecchymosis, edema, erythema multiforme, esophagitis (+/- stricture or cardiospasm), exfoliative dermatitis, GI ulceration, hallucinations, headache, hearing decreased, hematemesis, hematuria, hepatic failure, hepatitis, hyperglycemia (in controlled diabetics), hyperpigmentation, hypertension, infection, insomnia, interstitial nephritis, irregular uterine bleeding, jaundice, LFTs increased, leukopenia, MI, Palpitation, pancreatitis, pancytopenia, paresthesia, peptic ulcer (+/- bleeding/perforation), peripheral neuropathy, photophobia, photosensitivity, pulmonary infiltration (eosinophilia), rectal bleeding, renal calculus, renal failure, renal insufficiency, shock, Stevens-Johnson syndrome, syncope, thrombocytopenia, toxic epidermal necrolysis, ulcerative stomatitis, urticaria, vesiculobullous rash, renal papillary necrosis, visual disturbances
Restrictions An FDA-approved medication guide must be distributed when dispensing an oral outpatient prescription (new or refill) where this medication is to be used without direct supervision of a healthcare provider. Medication guides are available at http://www.fda.gov/cder/Offices/ODS/medication_guides.htm.
Dental Usual Dosing Acute pain: Adults: Oral: 200-400 mg every 6-8 hours, as needed, not to exceed total daily doses of 1000 mg
Dosage Note: For chronic conditions, response is usually observed within 2 weeks.
  Children 6-16 years: Oral: Juvenile rheumatoid arthritis (Lodine® XL):
    20-30 kg: 400 mg once daily
    31-45 kg: 600 mg once daily
    46-60 kg: 800 mg once daily
    >60 kg: 1000 mg once daily

Adults: Oral:

Acute pain: 200-400 mg every 6-8 hours, as needed, not to exceed total daily doses of 1000 mg

Rheumatoid arthritis, osteoarthritis: 400 mg 2 times/day **or** 300 mg 2-3 times/day **or** 500 mg 2 times/day (doses >1000 mg/day have not been evaluated)

Lodine® XL: 400-1000 mg once daily

Elderly: Refer to adult dosing; in patients ≥65 years, no dosage adjustment required based on pharmacokinetics. The elderly are more sensitive to antiprostaglandin effects and may need dosage adjustments.

Dosage adjustment in renal impairment:
Mild to moderate: No adjustment required
Severe: Use not recommended; use with caution
Hemodialysis: Not removed

Dosage adjustment in hepatic impairment: No adjustment required.

Mechanism of Action Inhibits prostaglandin synthesis by decreasing the activity of the enzyme, cyclooxygenase, which results in decreased formation of prostaglandin precursors

Contraindications Hypersensitivity to etodolac, aspirin, other NSAIDs, or any component of the formulation; perioperative pain in the setting of coronary artery bypass surgery (CABG); pregnancy

Warnings/Precautions [U.S. Boxed Warning]: NSAIDs are associated with an increased risk of adverse cardiovascular events, including MI, stroke, and new onset or worsening of pre-existing hypertension. Risk may be increased with duration of use or pre-existing cardiovascular risk factors or disease. Carefully evaluate individual cardiovascular risk profiles prior to prescribing. Use caution with fluid retention, CHF, or hypertension. Concurrent administration of ibuprofen, and potentially other nonselective NSAIDs, may interfere with aspirin's cardioprotective effect.

[U.S. Boxed Warning]: NSAIDs may increase risk of gastrointestinal irritation, ulceration, bleeding, and perforation. These events may occur at any time during therapy and without warning. Use caution with a history of GI disease (bleeding or ulcers), concurrent therapy with aspirin, anticoagulants and/or corticosteroids, smoking, use of alcohol, the elderly or debilitated patients.

Use of NSAIDs can compromise existing renal function. Renal toxicity can occur in patient with impaired renal function, dehydration, heart failure, liver dysfunction, those taking diuretics and ACE inhibitors and the elderly. Rehydrate patient before starting therapy. Monitor renal function closely. Etodolac is not recommended for patients with advanced renal disease.

Use the lowest effective dose for the shortest duration of time, consistent with individual patient goals, to reduce risk of cardiovascular or GI adverse events. Alternate therapies should be considered for patients at high risk.

NSAIDs may cause serious skin adverse events including exfoliative dermatitis, Stevens-Johnson syndrome (SJS), and toxic epidermal necrolysis (TEN). Anaphylactoid reactions may occur, even without prior exposure; patients with "aspirin triad" (bronchial asthma, aspirin intolerance, rhinitis) may be at increased risk. Do not use in patients who experience bronchospasm, asthma, rhinitis, or urticaria with NSAID or aspirin therapy. Use caution in other forms of asthma.

Use with caution in patients with decreased hepatic function. Closely monitor patients with any abnormal LFT. Severe hepatic reactions (eg, fulminant hepatitis, liver failure) have occurred with NSAID use, rarely; discontinue if signs or symptoms of liver disease develop, or if systemic manifestations occur. The elderly are at increased risk for adverse effects (especially peptic ulceration, CNS effects, renal toxicity) from NSAIDs even at low doses.

Withhold for at least 4-6 half-lives prior to surgical or dental procedures. Safety and efficacy have not been established in children.

Use of extended release product consisting of a nondeformable matrix should be avoided in patients with stricture/narrowing of the GI tract; symptoms of obstruction have been associated with nondeformable products.

Drug Interactions

ACE inhibitors: Antihypertensive effects may be decreased by concurrent therapy with NSAIDs; monitor blood pressure.

Aminoglycosides: NSAIDs may decrease the excretion of aminoglycosides.

Angiotensin II antagonists: Antihypertensive effects may be decreased by concurrent therapy with NSAIDs; monitor blood pressure.

Anticoagulants (warfarin, heparin, LMWHs) in combination with NSAIDs can cause increased risk of bleeding.

Antiplatelet agents (ticlopidine, clopidogrel, aspirin, abciximab, dipyridamole, eptifibatide, tirofiban) can cause an increased risk of bleeding.

(Continued)

Etodolac *(Continued)*

Beta-blockers: NSAIDs may diminish the antihypertensive effects of beta-blockers.

Bisphosphonates: NSAIDs may increase the risk of gastrointestinal ulceration.

Cholestyramine and colestipol reduce the bioavailability of some NSAIDs; separate administration times.

Corticosteroids may increase the risk of GI ulceration; avoid concurrent use.

Cyclosporine: NSAIDs may increase serum creatinine, potassium, blood pressure, and cyclosporine levels; monitor cyclosporine levels and renal function carefully.

Fluoroquinolone antibiotics: Risk of seizures may be increased with concomitant quinolone use. Risk is considered quite low and may only be a factor with high serum levels of either agent and/or in patients with additional predisposing factors (eg, renal dysfunction, history of seizure or other neurological disorder).

Hydralazine's antihypertensive effect is decreased; avoid concurrent use.

Lithium levels can be increased; avoid concurrent use if possible or monitor lithium levels and adjust dose. Sulindac may have the least effect. When NSAID is stopped, lithium will need adjustment again.

Loop diuretics efficacy (diuretic and antihypertensive effect) is reduced. Indomethacin reduces this efficacy, however, it may be anticipated with any NSAID.

Methotrexate: Severe bone marrow suppression, aplastic anemia, and GI toxicity have been reported with concomitant NSAID therapy. Avoid use during moderate or high-dose methotrexate (increased and prolonged methotrexate levels). NSAID use during low-dose treatment of rheumatoid arthritis has not been fully evaluated; extreme caution is warranted.

Pemetrexed: NSAIDs may decrease the excretion of pemetrexed. Patients with Cl_{cr} 45-79 mL/minute should avoid short acting NSAIDs for 2 days before and 2 days after pemetrexed treatment.

Salicylates: NSAIDs (nonselective) may diminish the cardioprotective effect of acetylated salicylates. Avoid regular use of NSAIDs if possible; consider alternatives (eg, acetaminophen). Give salicylate before NSAID; for example ibuprofen should be given 30-120 minutes after aspirin (immediate release).

Thiazides antihypertensive effects are decreased; avoid concurrent use.

Treprostinil: May enhance the risk of bleeding with concurrent use.

Vancomycin: NSAIDs may decrease the excretion of vancomycin. Avoid concurrent use.

Verapamil plasma concentration is decreased by some NSAIDs; avoid concurrent use.

Ethanol/Nutrition/Herb Interactions

Ethanol: Avoid ethanol (may enhance gastric mucosal irritation).

Food: Etodolac peak serum levels may be decreased if taken with food.

Herb/Nutraceutical: Avoid alfalfa, anise, bilberry, bladderwrack, bromelain, cat's claw, celery, coleus, cordyceps, dong quai, evening primrose, feverfew, fenugreek, garlic, ginger, ginkgo biloba, red clover, horse chestnut, grapeseed, green tea, ginseng, guggul, horse chestnut seed, horseradish, licorice, prickly ash, red clover, reishi, SAMe, sweet clover, turmeric, white willow (all have additional antiplatelet activity)

Dietary Considerations May be taken with food to decrease GI distress.

Pharmacodynamics/Kinetics

Onset of action: Analgesic: 2-4 hours; Maximum anti-inflammatory effect: A few days

Absorption: ≥80%

Distribution: V_d:

Immediate release: Adults:0.4 L/kg

Extended release: Adults: 0.57 L/kg; Children (6-16 years): 0 .08 L/kg

Protein binding: ≥99%, primarily albumin

Metabolism: Hepatic

Half-life elimination: Terminal: Adults: 5-8 hours

Extended release: Children (6-16 years): 12 hours

Time to peak, serum:

Immediate release: Adults: 1-2 hours

Extended release: Extended release: 5-7 hours, increased 1.4-3.8 hours with food

Excretion: Urine 73% (1% unchanged); feces 16%

Pregnancy Risk Factor C/D (3rd trimester)

Lactation Excretion in breast milk unknown/not recommended

Dosage Forms Excipient information presented when available (limited, particularly for generics); consult specific product labeling. [DSC] = Discontinued product

Capsule: 200 mg, 300 mg

Lodine®: 200 mg, 300 mg [DSC]

Tablet: 400 mg, 500 mg

Tablet, extended release (Lodine® XL): 400 mg, 500 mg [DSC]

Selected Readings

Brooks PM and Day RO, "Nonsteroidal Anti-inflammatory Drugs - Differences and Similarities," *N Engl J Med*, 1991, 324(24):1716-25.

Tucker PW, Smith JR, and Adams DF, "A Comparison of 2 Analgesic Regimens for the Control of Postoperative Periodontal Discomfort," *J Periodontol*, 1996, 67(2):125-9.

Etodolic Acid *see* Etodolac *on page 656*

Etomidate (e TOM i date)

U.S. Brand Names Amidate®

Canadian Brand Names Amidate®

Mexican Brand Names Hypnomidate

Generic Available Yes

Pharmacologic Category General Anesthetic

Use Induction and maintenance of general anesthesia

Unlabeled/Investigational Use Sedation for diagnosis of seizure foci

Local Anesthetic/Vasoconstrictor Precautions No information available to require special precautions

Effects on Dental Treatment Key adverse event(s) related to dental treatment: Hiccups.

Common Adverse Effects

>10%:

Endocrine & metabolic: Adrenal suppression

Gastrointestinal: Nausea, vomiting on emergence from anesthesia

Local: Pain at injection site (30% to 80%)

Neuromuscular & skeletal: Myoclonus (33%), transient skeletal movements, uncontrolled eye movements

1% to 10%: Hiccups

Mechanism of Action Ultrashort-acting nonbarbiturate hypnotic (benzylimidazole) used for the induction of anesthesia; chemically, it is a carboxylated imidazole which produces a rapid induction of anesthesia with minimal cardiovascular effects; produces EEG burst suppression at high doses

Drug Interactions

Increased Effect/Toxicity: Fentanyl decreases etomidate elimination. Verapamil may increase the anesthetic and respiratory depressant effects of etomidate.

Pharmacodynamics/Kinetics

Onset of action: 30-60 seconds

Peak effect: 1 minute

Duration: 3-5 minutes; terminated by redistribution

Distribution: V_d: 2-4.5 L/kg

Protein binding: 76%;

Metabolism: Hepatic and plasma esterases

Half-life elimination: Terminal: 2.6 hours

Pregnancy Risk Factor C

Etonogestrel (e toe noe JES trel)

U.S. Brand Names Implanon™

Generic Available No

Index Terms ENG; 3-Keto-desogestrel

Pharmacologic Category Contraceptive; Progestin

Use Prevention of pregnancy; for use in women who request long-acting (up to 3 years) contraception

Local Anesthetic/Vasoconstrictor Precautions No information available to require special precautions

Effects on Dental Treatment Key adverse event(s) related to dental treatment: Until more is known about the mechanism of interaction, use caution in prescribing antibiotics to female patients taking progestin-only contraceptives.

Common Adverse Effects

>10%:

Central nervous system: Headache (25%)

Dermatologic: Acne (14%)

Endocrine & metabolic: Infrequent menstrual bleeding (<3 episodes/90 days: 34%), amenorrhea (no bleeding in 90 days: 22%), prolonged menstrual bleeding (lasting >14 days: 18%), breast pain (13%), menstrual bleeding irregularities requiring discontinuation (11%)

Gastrointestinal: Weight gain (14%), abdominal pain (11%)

Genitourinary: Vaginitis (15%)

Respiratory: Upper respiratory tract infection (13%), pharyngitis (11%)

(Continued)

Etonogestrel *(Continued)*

5% to 10%:
  Central nervous system: Dizziness (7%), emotional lability (7%), depression (6%), nervousness (6%), pain (6%)
  Endocrine & metabolic: Dysmenorrhea (7%), frequent menstrual bleeding (>5 episodes/90 days: 7%)
  Gastrointestinal: Nausea (6%)
  Genitourinary: Leukorrhea (10%)
  Local: Insertion site pain (5%)
  Neuromuscular & skeletal: Back pain (7%)
  Respiratory: Sinusitis (6%)
  Miscellaneous: Flu-like syndrome (8%)

Restrictions Only healthcare providers who have undergone training in the insertion and removal procedures will be able to order Implanon™.

Mechanism of Action Etonogestrel is the active metabolite of desogestrel. It prevents pregnancy by suppressing ovulation, increasing the viscosity of cervical mucous, and inhibiting endometrial proliferation.

Drug Interactions

  Cytochrome P450 Effect: Substrate of CYP3A4 (minor)

  Increased Effect/Toxicity: Progestins may enhance the hepatotoxic effect of cyclosporine. Progestins may increase the serum concentration of cyclosporine. Progestin contraceptives may increase the serum concentration of selegiline. Progestin contraceptives may diminish the anticoagulant effect of coumarin derivatives. In contrast, enhanced anticoagulant effects have also been noted with some products.

  Decreased Effect: Specific drug interaction studies have not been conducted with strong CYP3A4 inducers; however, strong CYP3A4 inducers may increase the metabolism of etonogestrel. Chronic use of these agents is not recommended with the etonogestrel implant. Felbamate, griseofulvin, retinoic acid, and retinoids may decrease the serum concentration of progestin contraceptives. Progestin contraceptives may diminish the anticoagulant effect of coumarin derivatives. In contrast, enhanced anticoagulant effects have also been noted with some products.

Pharmacodynamics/Kinetics

  Onset of action: Serum levels sufficient to inhibit ovulation: ≤8 hours of implant
  Duration: Implant: Each rod maintains etonogestrel levels sufficient to inhibit ovulation for 3 years
  Distribution: V_d: 201 L
  Protein binding: Albumin (66%) and sex hormone binding globulin (32%)
  Metabolism: Hepatic via CYP3A4; forms metabolites (activity not known)
  Bioavailability: Implant: 100%
  Half-life, elimination: 25 hours
  Excretion: Urine (primarily); feces

Etonogestrel and Ethinyl Estradiol *see* Ethinyl Estradiol and Etonogestrel *on page 630*

Etopophos® *see* Etoposide Phosphate *on page 661*

Etoposide *(e toe POE side)*

U.S. Brand Names Toposar®; VePesid®
Canadian Brand Names VePesid®
Mexican Brand Names Etopos; Kenazol; Lastet; VP-TEC
Generic Available Yes
Index Terms Epipodophyllotoxin; VP-16; VP-16-213
Pharmacologic Category Antineoplastic Agent, Podophyllotoxin Derivative
Use Treatment of refractory testicular tumors; treatment of small cell lung cancer
Unlabeled/Investigational Use Treatment of lymphomas, acute nonlymphocytic leukemia (ANLL); lung, bladder, and prostate carcinoma; hepatoma, rhabdomyosarcoma, uterine carcinoma, neuroblastoma, mycosis fungoides, Kaposi's sarcoma, histiocytosis, gestational trophoblastic disease, Ewing's sarcoma, Wilms' tumor, brain tumors
Local Anesthetic/Vasoconstrictor Precautions No information available to require special precautions
Effects on Dental Treatment Key adverse event(s) related to dental treatment: Mucositis (especially at high doses) and stomatitis.
Common Adverse Effects
  >10%:
    Dermatologic: Alopecia (8% to 66%)
    Endocrine & metabolic: Ovarian failure (38%), amenorrhea
    Gastrointestinal: Nausea/vomiting (31% to 43%), anorexia (10% to 13%), diarrhea (1% to 13%), mucositis/esophagitis (with high doses)

Hematologic: Leukopenia (60% to 91%; grade 4: 3% to 17%; onset: 5-7 days; nadir: 7-14 days; recovery: 21-28 days), thrombocytopenia (22% to 41%; grades 3/4: 1% to 20%; nadir 9-16 days), anemia (up to 33%)

1% to 10%:

Cardiovascular: Hypotension (1% to 2%; due to rapid infusion)

Gastrointestinal: Stomatitis (1% to 6%), abdominal pain (up to 2%)

Hepatic: Hepatic toxicity (up to 3%)

Neuromuscular & skeletal: Peripheral neuropathy (1% to 2%)

Miscellaneous: Anaphylactic-like reaction (I.V. infusion: 1% to 2%; including chills, fever, tachycardia, bronchospasm, dyspnea)

Mechanism of Action Etoposide has been shown to delay transit of cells through the S phase and arrest cells in late S or early G_2 phase. The drug may inhibit mitochondrial transport at the NADH dehydrogenase level or inhibit uptake of nucleosides into HeLa cells. It is a topoisomerase II inhibitor and appears to cause DNA strand breaks. Etoposide does not inhibit microtubular assembly.

Drug Interactions

Cytochrome P450 Effect: Substrate of CYP1A2 (minor), 2E1 (minor), 3A4 (major); **Inhibits** CYP2C9 (weak), 3A4 (weak)

Increased Effect/Toxicity: Cyclosporine may increase the levels of etoposide; consider reducing the dose of etoposide by 50%. Etoposide may increase the effects/toxicity of warfarin. CYP3A4 inhibitors may increase the levels/effects of etoposide; example inhibitors include azole antifungals, clarithromycin, diclofenac, doxycycline, erythromycin, imatinib, isoniazid, nefazodone, nicardipine, propofol, protease inhibitors, quinidine, telithromycin, and verapamil.

Decreased Effect: Barbiturates and phenytoin may decrease the levels/effects of etoposide; monitor. CYP3A4 inducers may decrease the levels/effects of etoposide; example inducers include aminoglutethimide, carbamazepine, nafcillin, nevirapine, phenobarbital, phenytoin, and rifamycins.

Pharmacodynamics/Kinetics

Absorption: Oral: 25% to 75%; significant inter- and intrapatient variation

Distribution: Average V_d: 7-17 L/m²; poor penetration across the blood-brain barrier; CSF concentrations <10% of plasma concentrations

Protein binding: 94% to 97%

Metabolism: Hepatic to hydroxy acid and cislactone metabolites

Bioavailability: Oral: ~50% (range 25% to 75%)

Half-life elimination: Terminal: 4-11 hours; Children: Normal renal/hepatic function: 6-8 hours

Time to peak, serum: Oral: 1-1.5 hours

Excretion:

Children: Urine (≤55% as unchanged drug)

Adults: Urine (42% to 67%; 8% to 35% as unchanged drug) within 24 hours; feces (up to 44%)

Pregnancy Risk Factor D

Etoposide Phosphate (e toe POE side FOS fate)

Related Information

Etoposide *on page 660*

U.S. Brand Names Etopophos®

Mexican Brand Names Etopos

Generic Available No

Pharmacologic Category Antineoplastic Agent, Podophyllotoxin Derivative

Use Treatment of refractory testicular tumors; treatment of small cell lung cancer

Local Anesthetic/Vasoconstrictor Precautions No information available to require special precautions

Effects on Dental Treatment Key adverse event(s) related to dental treatment: Mucositis (especially at high doses), stomatitis, and taste perversion.

Common Adverse Effects Note: Also see adverse reactions for **etoposide**. Since etoposide phosphate is converted to etoposide, adverse reactions experienced with etoposide would also be expected with etoposide phosphate.

>10%:

Central nervous system: Chills/fever (24%)

Dermatologic: Alopecia (33% to 44%)

Gastrointestinal: Nausea/vomiting (37%), anorexia (16%), mucositis (11%)

Hematologic: Leukopenia (91%; grade 4: 17%), neutropenia (88%; grade 4: 37%), anemia (72%; grades 3/4: 19%), thrombocytopenia (23%; grade 4: 9%)

Neuromuscular and skeletal: Weakness/malaise (39%)

1% to 10%:

Cardiovascular: Hypotension (5%), hypertension (3%), facial flushing (2%)

(Continued)

Etoposide Phosphate (Continued)

Central nervous system: Dizziness (5%)

Dermatologic: Skin rash (3%)

Gastrointestinal: Constipation (8%), abdominal pain (7%), diarrhea (6%), taste perversion (6%)

Local: Extravasation/phlebitis (5%)

Miscellaneous: Anaphylactic-type reactions (3%; including chills, diaphoresis, fever, rigor, tachycardia, bronchospasm, dyspnea, pruritus)

Mechanism of Action Etoposide phosphate is converted *in vivo* to the active moiety, etoposide, by dephosphorylation. Etoposide inhibits mitotic activity; inhibits cells from entering prophase; inhibits DNA synthesis. Initially thought to be mitotic inhibitors similar to podophyllotoxin, but actually have no effect on microtubule assembly. However, later shown to induce DNA strand breakage and inhibition of topoisomerase II (an enzyme which breaks and repairs DNA); etoposide acts in late S or early G2 phases.

Drug Interactions

Cytochrome P450 Effect: Substrate of CYP1A2 (minor), 2E1 (minor), 3A4 (major); **Inhibits** CYP2C9 (weak), 3A4 (weak)

Increased Effect/Toxicity: Cyclosporine may increase the levels of etoposide; consider reducing the dose of etoposide by 50%. Etoposide may increase the effects/toxicity of warfarin. CYP3A4 inhibitors may increase the levels/effects of etoposide; example inhibitors include azole antifungals, clarithromycin, diclofenac, doxycycline, erythromycin, imatinib, isoniazid, nefazodone, nicardipine, propofol, protease inhibitors, quinidine, telithromycin, and verapamil.

Decreased Effect: Barbiturates and phenytoin may decrease the levels/effects of etoposide; monitor. CYP3A4 inducers may decrease the levels/effects of etoposide; example inducers include aminoglutethimide, carbamazepine, nafcillin, nevirapine, phenobarbital, phenytoin, and rifamycins.

Pharmacodynamics/Kinetics

Distribution: Average V_d: 7-17 L/m²; poor penetration across blood-brain barrier; concentrations in CSF being <10% that of plasma

Protein binding: 94% to 97%

Metabolism:

Etoposide phosphate: Rapidly and completely converted to etoposide in plasma

Etoposide: Hepatic to hydroxy acid and cislactone metabolites

Half-life elimination: Terminal: 4-11 hours; Children: Normal renal/hepatic function: 6-8 hours

Excretion: Urine (as unchanged drug and metabolites); feces (2% to 16%)

Children: I.V.: Urine (≤55% as unchanged drug)

Pregnancy Risk Factor D

Exemestane (ex e MES tane)

U.S. Brand Names Aromasin®

Canadian Brand Names Aromasin®

Generic Available No

Pharmacologic Category Antineoplastic Agent, Aromatase Inactivator

Use Treatment of advanced breast cancer in postmenopausal women whose disease has progressed following tamoxifen therapy; adjuvant treatment of postmenopausal estrogen receptor-positive early breast cancer following 2-3 years of tamoxifen (for a total of 5 years of adjuvant therapy)

Local Anesthetic/Vasoconstrictor Precautions No information available to require special precautions

Effects on Dental Treatment No significant effects or complications reported

Common Adverse Effects
>10%:
Cardiovascular: Hypertension (5% to 15%)
Central nervous system: Fatigue (8% to 22%), insomnia (11% to 14%), pain (13%), headache (7% to 13%), depression (6% to 13%)
Dermatological: Hyperhidrosis (4% to 18%), alopecia (15%)
Endocrine & metabolic: Hot flashes (13% to 21%)
Gastrointestinal: Nausea (9% to 18%), abdominal pain (6% to 11%)
Hepatic: Alkaline phosphatase increased (14% to 15%)
Neuromuscular & skeletal: Arthralgia (15% to 29%)
1% to 10%:
Cardiovascular: Edema (6% to 7%); cardiac ischemic events (2%: MI, angina, myocardial ischemia); chest pain
Central nervous system: Dizziness (8% to 10%), anxiety (4% to 10%), fever (5%), confusion, hypoesthesia
Dermatologic: Dermatitis (8%), itching, rash
Endocrine & metabolic: Weight gain (8%)
Gastrointestinal: Diarrhea (4% to 10%), vomiting (7%), anorexia (6%), constipation (5%), appetite increased (3%), dyspepsia
Genitourinary: Urinary tract infection
Hepatic: Bilirubin increased (5% to 7%)
Neuromuscular & skeletal: Back pain (9%), limb pain (9%), osteoarthritis (6%), weakness (6%), osteoporosis (5%), pathological fracture (4%), paresthesia (3%), carpal tunnel syndrome (2%), cramps (2%)
Ocular: Visual disturbances (5%)
Renal: Creatinine increased (6%)
Respiratory: Dyspnea (10%), cough (6%), bronchitis, pharyngitis, rhinitis, sinusitis, upper respiratory infection
Miscellaneous: Influenza-like symptoms (6%), diaphoresis (6%), lymphedema, infection

A dose-dependent decrease in sex hormone-binding globulin has been observed with daily doses of 25 mg or more. Serum luteinizing hormone and follicle-stimulating hormone levels have increased with this medicine.

Mechanism of Action Exemestane is an irreversible, steroidal aromatase inactivator. It prevents conversion of androgens to estrogens by tying up the enzyme aromatase. In breast cancers where growth is estrogen-dependent, this medicine will lower circulating estrogens.

Drug Interactions
Cytochrome P450 Effect: Substrate of CYP3A4 (major)
Decreased Effect: CYP3A4 inducers may decrease the levels/effects of exemestane; example inducers include aminoglutethimide, carbamazepine, efavirenz, fosphenytoin, nafcillin, nevirapine, oxcarbazepine, pentobarbital, phenobarbital, phenytoin, primidone, rifabutin, rifampin, and rifapentine; adjustment required with potent inducers.

Pharmacodynamics/Kinetics
Absorption: Rapid and moderate (~42%) following oral administration; absorption increases ~40% following high-fat meal
Distribution: Extensive
Protein binding: 90%, primarily to albumin and α_1-acid glycoprotein
Metabolism: Extensively hepatic; oxidation (CYP3A4) of methylene group, reduction of 17-keto group with formation of many secondary metabolites; metabolites are inactive
Half-life elimination: 24 hours
Time to peak: Women with breast cancer: 1.2 hours
Excretion: Urine (<1% as unchanged drug, 39% to 45% as metabolites); feces (36% to 48%)

Pregnancy Risk Factor D

Exenatide (ex EN a tide)

U.S. Brand Names Byetta™
Generic Available No
(Continued)

Exenatide *(Continued)*

Index Terms AC002993; Exendin-4; LY2148568

Pharmacologic Category Antidiabetic Agent, Incretin Mimetic

Use Management (adjunctive) of type 2 diabetes mellitus (noninsulin dependent, NIDDM) in patients receiving a sulfonylurea, thiazolidinedione, or metformin (or a combination of these agents)

Local Anesthetic/Vasoconstrictor Precautions No information available to require special precautions

Effects on Dental Treatment No significant effects or complications reported

Common Adverse Effects

>10%:

Endocrine & metabolic: Hypoglycemia (with concurrent sulfonylurea therapy 14% to 36%; frequency similar to placebo with metformin therapy)

Gastrointestinal: Nausea (44%), vomiting (13%), diarrhea (13%)

Miscellaneous: Anti-exenatide antibodies (low titers 38%, high titers 6%)

1% to 10%:

Central nervous system: Dizziness (9%), headache (9%)

Endocrine & metabolic: Appetite decreased (<5%)

Gastrointestinal: Dyspepsia (6%), GERD (<5%)

Neuromuscular & skeletal: Weakness (<5%)

Miscellaneous: Feeling jittery (9%), diaphoresis increased (<5%)

Mechanism of Action Exenatide is an analog of the hormone incretin (glucagon-like peptide 1 or GLP-1) which increases insulin secretion, increases B-cell growth/replication, slows gastric emptying, and may decrease food intake. When added to sulfonylureas, thiazolidinediones, and/or metformin, it results in additional lowering of hemoglobin A_{1c} by approximately 0.5% to 1%.

Drug Interactions

Decreased Effect: Note: Due to its effects on gastric emptying, exenatide may reduce the rate and extent of absorption of orally-administered drugs. Should be used with caution in patients receiving medications which require rapid absorption from the gastrointestinal tract. Administration of medications 1 hour prior to the use of exenatide has been recommended by the manufacturer when optimal drug absorption and peak levels are important to the overall therapeutic effect (such as with antibiotics and/or oral contraceptives).

Pharmacodynamics/Kinetics

Distribution: V_d: 28.3 L

Metabolism: Minimal systemic metabolism; proteolytic degradation may occur following glomerular filtration

Half-life elimination: 2.4 hours

Time to peak, plasma: SubQ: 2.1 hours

Excretion: Urine (majority of dose)

Pregnancy Risk Factor C

Ezetimibe (ez ET i mibe)

U.S. Brand Names Zetia™
Canadian Brand Names Ezetrol®
Mexican Brand Names Ezetrol
Generic Available No
Pharmacologic Category Antilipemic Agent, 2-Azetidinone
Use Use in combination with dietary therapy for the treatment of primary hyper-cholesterolemia (as monotherapy or in combination with HMG-CoA reductase inhibitors); homozygous sitosterolemia; homozygous familial hypercholesterol-emia (in combination with atorvastatin or simvastatin); mixed hyperlipidemia (in combination with fenofibrate)
Local Anesthetic/Vasoconstrictor Precautions No information available to require special precautions
Effects on Dental Treatment No significant effects or complications reported
Common Adverse Effects 1% to 10%:
  Cardiovascular: Chest pain (3%), dizziness (3%), fatigue (2%)
  Central nervous system: Headache (8%)
  Gastrointestinal: Diarrhea (3% to 4%), abdominal pain (3%)
  Neuromuscular & skeletal: Arthralgia (4%)
  Respiratory: Sinusitis (4% to 5%), pharyngitis (2% to 3%, placebo 2%)
Dosage Oral:
  Hyperlipidemias: Children ≥10 years and Adults: 10 mg/day
  Sitosterolemia: Adults: 10 mg/day
  Elderly: Refer to adult dosing
  Dosage adjustment in renal impairment: Bioavailability increased with severe impairment; no dosing adjustment recommended
  Dosage adjustment in hepatic impairment: Bioavailability increased with hepatic impairment
    Mild impairment (Child-Pugh score 5-6): No dosing adjustment necessary
    Moderate to severe impairment (Child-Pugh score 7-15): Use of ezetimibe not recommended
Mechanism of Action Inhibits absorption of cholesterol at the brush border of the small intestine via the sterol transporter, Niemann-Pick C1-Like 1 (NPC1L1). This leads to a decreased delivery of cholesterol to the liver, reduction of hepatic cholesterol stores and an increased clearance of cholesterol from the blood; decreases total C, LDL-cholesterol (LDL-C), ApoB, and triglycerides (TG) while increasing HDL-cholesterol (HDL-C).
Contraindications Hypersensitivity to ezetimibe or any component of the formulation
Warnings/Precautions Secondary causes of hyperlipidemia should be ruled out prior to therapy. Use caution with renal or mild hepatic impairment; not recommended for use with moderate or severe hepatic impairment. Use of ezetimibe and fenofibrate (160 mg daily) may increase rate of cholecystectomy. Safety and efficacy have not been established in patients <10 years of age.
Drug Interactions
  Increased Effect/Toxicity: Cyclosporine may increase plasma levels of ezetimibe. Fibric acid derivatives may increase serum concentrations of ezetimibe. Ezetimibe may increase serum levels of cyclosporine.
  Decreased Effect: Bile acid sequestrants may decrease ezetimibe bioavaila-bility; administer ezetimibe ≥2 hours before or ≥4 hours after bile acid seques-trants.
Dietary Considerations May be taken without regard to meals. Before initia-tion of therapy, patients should be placed on a standard cholesterol-lowering diet for 6 weeks and the diet should be continued during drug therapy.
Pharmacodynamics/Kinetics
  Protein binding: >90% to plasma proteins
  Metabolism: Undergoes conjugation in the small intestine and liver; forms metabolite (active); may undergo enterohepatic recycling
  Bioavailability: Variable
  Half-life elimination: 22 hours (ezetimibe and metabolite)
  Time to peak, plasma: 4-12 hours
  Excretion: Feces (78%, 69% as ezetimibe); urine (11%, 9% as metabolite)
Pregnancy Risk Factor C
Dosage Forms
  Tablet:
    Zetia™: 10 mg

Ezetimibe and Simvastatin (ez ET i mibe & SIM va stat in)

Related Information
Ezetimibe *on page 665*
Simvastatin *on page 1472*
U.S. Brand Names Vytorin®
Mexican Brand Names Zintrepid
Generic Available No
Pharmacologic Category Antilipemic Agent, 2-Azetidinone; Antilipemic Agent, HMG-CoA Reductase Inhibitor
Use Used in combination with dietary modification for the treatment of primary hypercholesterolemia and homozygous familial hypercholesterolemia
Local Anesthetic/Vasoconstrictor Precautions No information available to require special precautions
Effects on Dental Treatment No significant effects or complications reported
Common Adverse Effects Percentages below refer to combination Vytorin®. Also see individual agents.

1% to 10%:
Central nervous system: Headache (7%)
Neuromuscular & skeletal: Myalgia (4%), pain in extremity (2%)
Respiratory: Upper respiratory infection (4%)
Miscellaneous: Influenza (3%)

Mechanism of Action
Ezetimibe: Inhibits absorption of cholesterol at the brush border of the small intestine, leading to a decreased delivery of cholesterol to the liver.
Simvastatin: A methylated derivative of lovastatin that acts by competitively inhibiting 3-hydroxy-3-methylglutaryl-coenzyme A (HMG-CoA) reductase, the enzyme that catalyzes the rate-limiting step in cholesterol biosynthesis.

Drug Interactions
Cytochrome P450 Effect: Simvastatin: **Substrate** of CYP3A4 (major); **Inhibits** CYP2C8 (weak), 2C9 (weak), 2D6 (weak)
Increased Effect/Toxicity: Risk of myopathy/rhabdomyolysis may be increased by concurrent use of strong CYP3A4 inhibitors. CYP3A4 inhibitors may increase the levels/effects of simvastatin; example inhibitors include azole antifungals, clarithromycin, diclofenac, diltiazem, doxycycline, erythromycin, imatinib, isoniazid, nefazodone, nicardipine, propofol, protease inhibitors, quinidine, telithromycin, and verapamil. Manufacturer recommends avoiding concurrent use with clarithromycin, erythromycin, fibric acid derivatives, itraconazole, ketoconazole, nefazodone, protease inhibitors, telithromycin. Manufacturer recommends limiting simvastatin dose to 20 mg/day when used with amiodarone or verapamil, and 10 mg/day when used with cyclosporine or danazol. The anticoagulant effect of warfarin may be increased by simvastatin. Diclofenac, imatinib, proton pump inhibitors, ranolazine, and sildenafil may increase levels/effects of simvastatin.
Decreased Effect: Bile acid sequestrants may decrease the absorption of ezetimibe; administer Vytorin® at least 2 hours before or 4 hours after the bile acid sequestrant. Bosentan, phenytoin, and rifamycin derivatives may decrease levels/effects of HMG-CoA reductase inhibitors.
Pharmacodynamics/Kinetics See individual agents.
Bioavailability: Vytorin® is equivalent to coadministered ezetimibe and simvastatin.

Pregnancy Risk Factor X

E•R•O [OTC] *see Carbamide Peroxide on page 276*
F₃T *see Trifluridine on page 1618*
Fabrazyme® *see Agalsidase Beta on page 56*
Factive® *see Gemifloxacin on page 773*

Factor VIIa (Recombinant) (FAK ter SEV en aye ree KOM be nant)

U.S. Brand Names NovoSeven®
Canadian Brand Names Niastase®
Generic Available No
Index Terms Coagulation Factor VIIa; Eptacog Alfa (Activated); rFVIIa
Pharmacologic Category Antihemophilic Agent; Blood Product Derivative
Use Treatment of bleeding episodes and prevention of bleeding in surgical interventions in patients with hemophilia A or B with inhibitors to factor VIII or factor IX and in patients with congenital factor VII deficiency
Local Anesthetic/Vasoconstrictor Precautions No information available to require special precautions
Effects on Dental Treatment No significant effects or complications reported

Common Adverse Effects 1% to 10%:
Cardiovascular: Hypertension
Central nervous system: Fever
Hematologic: Hemorrhage, plasma fibrinogen decreased
Neuromuscular & skeletal: Hemarthrosis

Mechanism of Action Recombinant factor VIIa, a vitamin K-dependent glycoprotein, promotes hemostasis by activating the extrinsic pathway of the coagulation cascade. It replaces deficient activated coagulation factor VII, which
complexes with tissue factor and may activate coagulation factor X to Xa and
factor IX to IXa. When complexed with other factors, coagulation factor Xa
converts prothrombin to thrombin, a key step in the formation of a fibrin-platelet
hemostatic plug.

Pharmacodynamics/Kinetics
Distribution: V_d: 103 mL/kg (78-139)
Half-life elimination: 2.3 hours (1.7-2.7)
Excretion: Clearance: 33 mL/kg/hour (27-49)

Pregnancy Risk Factor C

Factor VIII (Human) *see* Antihemophilic Factor (Human) *on page 131*

Factor VIII (Human) *see* Antihemophilic Factor/von Willebrand Factor Complex
(Human) *on page 132*

Factor VIII (Recombinant) *see* Antihemophilic Factor (Recombinant) *on
page 132*

Factor IX (FAK ter nyne)

U.S. Brand Names AlphaNine® SD; BeneFix®; Mononine®
Canadian Brand Names BeneFix®; Immunine® VH; Mononine®
Generic Available No
Pharmacologic Category Antihemophilic Agent; Blood Product Derivative
Use Control bleeding in patients with factor IX deficiency (hemophilia B or
Christmas disease)
Local Anesthetic/Vasoconstrictor Precautions No information available to
require special precautions
Effects on Dental Treatment No significant effects or complications reported
Common Adverse Effects Frequency not defined.
Cardiovascular: Angioedema, cyanosis, flushing, hypotension, tightness in
chest, tightness in neck, (thrombosis following high dosages because of pres-
ence of activated clotting factors)
Central nervous system: Fever, headache, chills, somnolence, dizziness,
drowsiness, lightheadedness
Dermatologic: Urticaria, rash
Gastrointestinal: Nausea, vomiting, abnormal taste
Hematologic: Disseminated intravascular coagulation (DIC)
Local: Injection site discomfort
Neuromuscular & skeletal: Tingling
Respiratory: Dyspnea, laryngeal edema, allergic rhinitis
Miscellaneous: Transient fever (following rapid administration), anaphylaxis,
burning sensation in jaw/skull

Mechanism of Action Replaces deficient clotting factor IX; concentrate of
factor IX; hemophilia B, or Christmas disease, is an X-linked inherited disorder
of blood coagulation characterized by insufficient or abnormal synthesis of the
clotting protein factor IX. Factor IX is a vitamin K-dependent coagulation factor
which is synthesized in the liver. Factor IX is activated by factor XIa in the
intrinsic coagulation pathway. Activated factor IX (IXa), in combination with
factor VII:C activates factor X to Xa, resulting ultimately in the conversion of
prothrombin to thrombin and the formation of a fibrin clot. The infusion of
exogenous factor IX to replace the deficiency present in hemophilia B temporarily restores hemostasis.

Drug Interactions
Increased Effect/Toxicity: Do not coadminister with aminocaproic acid; may
increase risk for thrombosis.
Pharmacodynamics/Kinetics Half-life elimination: IX component: 23-31 hours
Pregnancy Risk Factor C

Factor IX Complex (Human) (FAK ter nyne KOM pleks HYU man)

U.S. Brand Names Bebulin® VH; Profilnine® SD; Proplex® T [DSC]
Generic Available No
(Continued)

Factor IX Complex (Human) *(Continued)*

Index Terms Prothrombin Complex Concentrate

Pharmacologic Category Antihemophilic Agent; Blood Product Derivative

Use

Control bleeding in patients with factor IX deficiency (hemophilia B or Christmas disease) **Note:** Factor IX concentrate containing **only** factor IX is also available and preferable for this indication.

Prevention/control of bleeding in hemophilia A patients with inhibitors to factor VIII.

Prevention/control of bleeding in patients with factor VII deficiency.

Emergency correction of the coagulopathy of warfarin excess in critical situations.

Local Anesthetic/Vasoconstrictor Precautions No information available to require special precautions

Effects on Dental Treatment No significant effects or complications reported

Common Adverse Effects 1% to 10%:

Central nervous system: Fever, headache, chills

Neuromuscular & skeletal: Tingling

Miscellaneous: Following rapid administration: Transient fever

Mechanism of Action Replaces deficient clotting factor including factor X; hemophilia B, or Christmas disease, is an X-linked recessively inherited disorder of blood coagulation characterized by insufficient or abnormal synthesis of the clotting protein factor IX. Factor IX is a vitamin K-dependent coagulation factor which is synthesized in the liver. Factor IX is activated by factor XIa in the intrinsic coagulation pathway. Activated factor IX (IXa), in combination with factor VII:C, activates factor X to Xa, resulting ultimately in the conversion of prothrombin to thrombin and the formation of a fibrin clot. The infusion of exogenous factor IX to replace the deficiency present in hemophilia B temporarily restores hemostasis.

Drug Interactions

Increased Effect/Toxicity: Do not coadminister with aminocaproic acid; may increase risk for thrombosis.

Pharmacodynamics/Kinetics

Half-life elimination:

VII component: Initial: 4-6 hours; Terminal: 22.5 hours

IX component: 24 hours

Pregnancy Risk Factor C

Factrel® *see* Gonadorelin *on page 792*

Famciclovir *(fam SYE kloe veer)*

Related Information

Systemic Viral Diseases *on page 1767*

Treatment of Sexually-Transmitted Infections *on page 1920*

Viral Infections *on page 1806*

Related Sample Prescriptions

Herpes Simplex (Recurrent) *on page 1843*

Shingles (Varicella-Zoster Virus) *on page 1843*

U.S. Brand Names Famvir®

Canadian Brand Names Apo-Famciclovir; Famvir®; PMS-Famciclovir

Generic Available No

Pharmacologic Category Antiviral Agent

Dental Use Management of acute herpes zoster (shingles); treatment of recurrent herpes labialis in immunocompetent patients

Use Treatment of acute herpes zoster (shingles); treatment and suppression of recurrent episodes of genital herpes in immunocompetent patients; treatment of herpes labialis (cold sores) in immunocompetent patients; treatment of recurrent mucocutaneous/genital herpes simplex in HIV-infected patients

Local Anesthetic/Vasoconstrictor Precautions No information available to require special precautions

Effects on Dental Treatment No significant effects or complications reported

Significant Adverse Effects

Note: Frequencies vary with dose and duration. Single-dose treatment (herpes labialis) was associated only with headache (10%), diarrhea (2%), fatigue (1%), and dysmenorrhea (1%).

>10%:

Central nervous system: Headache (17% to 39%)

Gastrointestinal: Nausea (7% to 13%)

1% to 10%:

Central nervous system: Fatigue (4% to 6%), migraine (1% to 3%)

Dermatologic: Pruritus (1% to 4%), rash (<1% to 3%)
Endocrine and metabolic: Dysmenorrhea (up to 8%)
Gastrointestinal: Diarrhea (5% to 9%), flatulence (2% to 5%), vomiting (1% to 5%), abdominal pain (1% to 8%)
Hematologic: Neutropenia (3%), leukopenia (1%)
Hepatic: Transaminases increased (2% to 3%), bilirubin increased (2%)
Neuromuscular & skeletal: Paresthesia (1% to 3%)
Postmarketing and/or case reports: Confusion, delirium, disorientation, dizziness, erythema multiforme, hallucinations, jaundice, somnolence, thrombocytopenia, urticaria

Dosage Adults: Oral:

Acute herpes zoster: 500 mg every 8 hours for 7 days (**Note:** Initiate therapy within 72 hours of rash onset.)

Recurrent genital herpes simplex in immunocompetent patients:
Initial: 1000 mg twice daily for 1 day (**Note:** Initiate therapy within 6 hours of symptoms/lesions.)
Suppressive therapy: 250 mg twice daily for up to 1 year

Recurrent herpes labialis (cold sores): 1500 mg as a single dose; initiate therapy at first sign or symptom such as tingling, burning, or itching (initiated within 1 hour in clinical studies)

Recurrent mucocutaneous/genital herpes simplex in HIV patients: 500 mg twice daily for 7 days

Dosing interval in renal impairment:

Herpes zoster:
Cl_{cr} 40-59 mL/minute: Administer 500 mg every 12 hours
Cl_{cr} 20-39 mL/minute: Administer 500 mg every 24 hours
Cl_{cr} <20 mL/minute: Administer 250 mg every 24 hours
Hemodialysis: Administer 250 mg after each dialysis session.

Recurrent genital herpes: Treatment (single day regimen):
Cl_{cr} 40-59 mL/minute: Administer 500 mg every 12 hours for 1 day
Cl_{cr} 20-39 mL/minute: Administer 500 mg as a single dose
Cl_{cr} <20 mL/minute: Administer 250 mg as a single dose
Hemodialysis: Administer 250 mg as a single dose after dialysis session.

Recurrent genital herpes: Suppression:
Cl_{cr} 20-39 mL/minute: Administer 125 mg every 12 hours
Cl_{cr} <20 mL/minute: Administer 125 mg every 24 hours
Hemodialysis: Administer 125 mg after each dialysis session.

Recurrent herpes labialis: Treatment (single dose regimen):
Cl_{cr} 40-59 mL/minute: Administer 750 mg as a single dose
Cl_{cr} 20-39 mL/minute: Administer 500 mg as a single dose
Cl_{cr} <20 mL/minute: Administer 250 mg as a single dose
Hemodialysis: Administer 250 mg as a single dose after dialysis session.

Recurrent orolabial or genital herpes in HIV-infected patients:
Cl_{cr} 20-39 mL/minute: Administer 500 mg every 12 hours
Cl_{cr} <20 mL/minute: Administer 250 mg every 24 hours
Hemodialysis: Administer 250 mg after each dialysis session.

Mechanism of Action Famciclovir undergoes rapid biotransformation to the active compound, penciclovir, which is phosphorylated by viral thymidine kinase in HSV-1, HSV-2, and VZV-infected cells to a monophosphate form; this is then converted to penciclovir triphosphate and competes with deoxyguanosine triphosphate to inhibit HSV-2 polymerase (eg, herpes viral DNA synthesis/replication is selectively inhibited)

Contraindications Hypersensitivity to famciclovir, penciclovir, or any component of the formulation

Warnings/Precautions Has not been studied in immunocompromised patients or patients with ophthalmic, disseminated zoster, or with initial episode of genital herpes. Dosage adjustment is required in patients with renal insufficiency. Tablets contain lactose; do not use with galactose intolerance, severe lactase deficiency, or glucose-galactose malabsorption syndromes. Safety and efficacy have not been established in children <18 years of age

Ethanol/Nutrition/Herb Interactions Food: Rate of absorption and/or conversion to penciclovir and peak concentration are reduced with food, but bioavailability is not affected.

Dietary Considerations May be taken with food or on an empty stomach.

Pharmacodynamics/Kinetics

Absorption: Food decreases maximum peak concentration and delays time to peak; AUC remains the same

Distribution: V_{dss}: 0.91-1.25 L/kg

Protein binding: ≤20%

Metabolism: Rapidly deacetylated and oxidized to penciclovir; not via CYP

Bioavailability: 69% to 85%

Half-life elimination: Penciclovir: 2-3 hours (10, 20, and 7 hours in HSV-1, HSV-2, and VZV-infected cells, respectively); prolonged with renal impairment

(Continued)

Famciclovir (Continued)

Time to peak: 0.9 hours; C_{max} and T_{max} are decreased and prolonged with noncompensated hepatic impairment

Excretion: Urine (73% primarily as penciclovir); feces (27%)

Pregnancy Risk Factor B

Lactation Excretion in breast milk unknown/use caution

Breast-Feeding Considerations There is no specific data describing the excretion of famciclovir in breast milk. If herpes lesions are on breast, breast feeding should be avoided in order to avoid transmission to infant.

Dosage Forms Excipient information presented when available (limited, particularly for generics); consult specific product labeling.

Tablet: 125 mg, 250 mg, 500 mg [contains lactose]

Famotidine (fa MOE ti deen)

Related Information

Gastrointestinal Disorders *on page 1745*

U.S. Brand Names Pepcid®; Pepcid® AC [OTC]

Canadian Brand Names Apo-Famotidine®; Apo-Famotidine® Injectable; Famotidine Omega; Gen-Famotidine; Novo-Famotidine; Nu-Famotidine; Pepcid®; Pepcid® AC; Pepcid® I.V.; ratio-Famotidine; Riva-Famotidine; Ulcidine

Mexican Brand Names Durater; Famoxal; Pepcidine

Generic Available Yes: Injection, tablet

Pharmacologic Category Histamine H_2 Antagonist

Use Therapy and treatment of duodenal ulcer, gastric ulcer; control gastric pH in critically-ill patients; symptomatic relief in gastritis, gastroesophageal reflux, active benign ulcer, and pathological hypersecretory conditions

OTC labeling: Relief of heartburn, acid indigestion, and sour stomach

Unlabeled/Investigational Use Part of a multidrug regimen for *H. pylori* eradication to reduce the risk of duodenal ulcer recurrence

Local Anesthetic/Vasoconstrictor Precautions No information available to require special precautions

Effects on Dental Treatment No significant effects or complications reported

Common Adverse Effects

Note: Agitation and vomiting have been reported in up to 14% of pediatric patients <1 year of age.

1% to 10%:

Central nervous system: Dizziness (1%), headache (5%)

Gastrointestinal: Constipation (1%), diarrhea (2%)

Dosage

Children: Treatment duration and dose should be individualized

Peptic ulcer: 1-16 years:

Oral: 0.5 mg/kg/day at bedtime or divided twice daily (maximum dose: 40 mg/day); doses of up to 1 mg/kg/day have been used in clinical studies

I.V.: 0.25 mg/kg every 12 hours (maximum dose: 40 mg/day); doses of up to 0.5 mg/kg have been used in clinical studies

GERD: Oral:

<3 months: 0.5 mg/kg once daily

3-12 months: 0.5 mg/kg twice daily

1-16 years: 1 mg/kg/day divided twice daily (maximum dose: 40 mg twice daily); doses of up to 2 mg/kg/day have been used in clinical studies

Children ≥12 years and Adults: Heartburn, indigestion, sour stomach: OTC labeling: Oral: 10-20 mg every 12 hours; dose may be taken 15-60 minutes before eating foods known to cause heartburn

Adults:

Duodenal ulcer: Oral: Acute therapy: 40 mg/day at bedtime for 4-8 weeks; maintenance therapy: 20 mg/day at bedtime

Helicobacter pylori eradication (unlabeled use): 40 mg once daily; requires combination therapy with antibiotics

Gastric ulcer: Oral: Acute therapy: 40 mg/day at bedtime

Hypersecretory conditions: Oral: Initial: 20 mg every 6 hours, may increase in increments up to 160 mg every 6 hours

GERD: Oral: 20 mg twice daily for 6 weeks

Esophagitis and accompanying symptoms due to GERD: Oral: 20 mg or 40 mg twice daily for up to 12 weeks

Patients unable to take oral medication: I.V.: 20 mg every 12 hours

Dosing adjustment in renal impairment: Cl_{cr} <50 mL/minute: Manufacturer recommendation: Administer 50% of dose **or** increase the dosing interval to every 36-48 hours (to limit potential CNS adverse effects).

Mechanism of Action Competitive inhibition of histamine at H_2 receptors of the gastric parietal cells, which inhibits gastric acid secretion

Contraindications Hypersensitivity to famotidine, other H_2 antagonists, or any component of the formulation

Warnings/Precautions Modify dose in patients with renal impairment. Chewable tablets contain phenylalanine; multidose vials contain benzyl alcohol.

OTC labeling: When used for self-medication, patients should be instructed not to use if they have difficulty swallowing, have vomiting with blood, or bloody or black stools. Not for use with other acid reducers.

Drug Interactions

Increased Effect/Toxicity:

H_2 antagonists may increase levels/effects of cyclosporine; monitor.

Decreased Effect: Histamine H_2 antagonists may decrease the serum levels of azole antifungals (eg, itraconazole, ketoconazole), delviradine (avoid concurrent use), cefpodoxime, cefuroxime; separate oral dose of cephalosporin and H_2 antagonist by at least 2 hours.

Ethanol/Nutrition/Herb Interactions

Ethanol: Avoid ethanol (may cause gastric mucosal irritation).

Food: Famotidine bioavailability may be increased if taken with food.

Dietary Considerations Phenylalanine content: Pepcid® AC chewable: Each 10 mg tablet contains phenylalanine 1.4 mg

Pharmacodynamics/Kinetics

Onset of action: GI: Oral: Within 1-3 hour

Duration: 10-12 hours

Protein binding: 15% to 20%

Bioavailability: Oral: 40% to 50%

Half-life elimination: Injection, oral suspension, tablet: 2.5-3.5 hours; prolonged with renal impairment; Oliguria: 20 hours

Time to peak, serum: Oral: ~1-3 hours

Excretion: Urine (as unchanged drug)

Pregnancy Risk Factor B

Dosage Forms

Infusion [premixed in NS]:

Pepcid®: 20 mg (50 mL)

Injection, solution: 10 mg/mL (4 mL, 20 mL, 50 mL)

Pepcid®: 10 mg/mL (20 mL)

Injection, solution [preservative free]: 10 mg/mL (2 mL)

Pepcid®: 10 mg/mL (2 mL)

Powder for oral suspension:

Pepcid®: 40 mg/5 mL

Tablet: 10 mg [OTC], 20 mg, 40 mg

Pepcid®: 20 mg, 40 mg

Pepcid® AC [OTC]: 10 mg, 20 mg

Tablet, chewable:

Pepcid® AC [OTC]: 10 mg

Famotidine, Calcium Carbonate, and Magnesium Hydroxide

(fa MOE ti deen, KAL see um KAR bun ate, & mag NEE zhum hye DROKS ide)

Related Information

Calcium Carbonate *on page 260*

Famotidine *on page 670*

Magnesium Hydroxide *on page 1014*

U.S. Brand Names Pepcid® Complete [OTC]

Canadian Brand Names Pepcid® Complete [OTC]

Generic Available No

Index Terms Calcium Carbonate, Magnesium Hydroxide, and Famotidine; Magnesium Hydroxide, Famotidine, and Calcium Carbonate

Pharmacologic Category Antacid; Histamine H_2 Antagonist

Use Relief of heartburn due to acid indigestion

Local Anesthetic/Vasoconstrictor Precautions No information available to require special precautions

Effects on Dental Treatment No significant effects or complications reported

Common Adverse Effects See individual agents.

Mechanism of Action

Famotidine: H_2 antagonist

Calcium carbonate: Antacid

Magnesium hydroxide: Antacid

(Continued)

Famotidine, Calcium Carbonate, and Magnesium Hydroxide *(Continued)*

Drug Interactions
Increased Effect/Toxicity: See individual agents.
Decreased Effect: See individual agents.
Pharmacodynamics/Kinetics See individual agents.

Famvir® *see* Famciclovir *on page 668*
Fansidar® *see* Sulfadoxine and Pyrimethamine *on page 1503*
Fareston® *see* Toremifene *on page 1593*
Faslodex® *see* Fulvestrant *on page 755*

Fat Emulsion *(fat e MUL shun)*

U.S. Brand Names Intralipid®; Liposyn® III
Canadian Brand Names Intralipid®; Liposyn® II
Mexican Brand Names Liposyn II
Generic Available No
Index Terms Intravenous Fat Emulsion
Pharmacologic Category Caloric Agent
Use Source of calories and essential fatty acids for patients requiring parenteral nutrition of extended duration
Local Anesthetic/Vasoconstrictor Precautions No information available to require special precautions
Effects on Dental Treatment No significant effects or complications reported
Common Adverse Effects Frequency not defined.
Cardiovascular: Chest pain, cyanosis, flushing
Central nervous system: Dizziness, headache
Endocrine & metabolic: Hyperlipemia, hypertriglyceridemia
Gastrointestinal: Diarrhea, nausea, vomiting
Hematologic: Hypercoagulability, thrombocytopenia in neonates (rare)
Hepatic: Hepatomegaly, pancreatitis
Local: Thrombophlebitis
Respiratory: Dyspnea
Miscellaneous: Brown pigment deposition in the reticuloendothelial system (significance unknown), diaphoresis, sepsis
Mechanism of Action Essential for normal structure and function of cell membranes
Pharmacodynamics/Kinetics
Metabolism: Undergoes lipolysis to free fatty acids which are utilized by reticuloendothelial cells
Half-life elimination: 0.5-1 hour
Pregnancy Risk Factor C

FazaClo® *see* Clozapine *on page 401*
5-FC *see* Flucytosine *on page 699*
FC1157a *see* Toremifene *on page 1593*
Feiba VH *see* Anti-inhibitor Coagulant Complex *on page 133*

Felbamate *(FEL ba mate)*

U.S. Brand Names Felbatol®
Generic Available No
Pharmacologic Category Anticonvulsant, Miscellaneous
Use Not as a first-line antiepileptic treatment; only in those patients who respond inadequately to alternative treatments and whose epilepsy is so severe that a substantial risk of aplastic anemia and/or liver failure is deemed acceptable in light of the benefits conferred by its use. Patient must be fully advised of risk and provide signed written informed consent. Felbamate can be used as either monotherapy or adjunctive therapy in the treatment of partial seizures (with and without generalization) and in adults with epilepsy.
Orphan drug: Adjunctive therapy in the treatment of partial and generalized seizures associated with Lennox-Gastaut syndrome in children
Local Anesthetic/Vasoconstrictor Precautions No information available to require special precautions
Effects on Dental Treatment Key adverse event(s) related to dental treatment: Xerostomia (normal salivary flow resumes upon discontinuation) and abnormal taste.
Common Adverse Effects
>10%:
Central nervous system: Somnolence, headache, fatigue, dizziness

Gastrointestinal: Nausea, anorexia, vomiting, constipation

1% to 10%:

Cardiovascular: Chest pain, palpitation, tachycardia

Central nervous system: Depression or behavior changes, nervousness, anxiety, ataxia, stupor, malaise, agitation, psychological disturbances, aggressive reaction

Dermatologic: Skin rash, acne, pruritus

Gastrointestinal: Xerostomia, diarrhea, abdominal pain, weight gain, taste perversion

Neuromuscular & skeletal: Tremor, abnormal gait, paresthesia, myalgia

Ocular: Diplopia, abnormal vision

Respiratory: Sinusitis, pharyngitis

Miscellaneous: ALT increased

Restrictions A patient "informed consent" form should be completed and signed by the patient and physician. Copies are available from Wallace Pharmaceuticals by calling 609-655-6147.

Mechanism of Action Mechanism of action is unknown but has properties in common with other marketed anticonvulsants; has weak inhibitory effects on GABA-receptor binding, benzodiazepine receptor binding, and is devoid of activity at the MK-801 receptor binding site of the NMDA receptor-ionophore complex.

Drug Interactions

Cytochrome P450 Effect: Substrate of CYP2E1 (minor), 3A4 (major); **Inhibits** CYP2C19 (weak); **Induces** CYP3A4 (weak)

Increased Effect/Toxicity: Felbamate increases serum phenytoin, phenobarbital, and valproic acid concentrations which may result in toxicity; consider decreasing phenytoin or phenobarbital dosage by 25%. A decrease in valproic acid dosage may also be necessary. CYP3A4 inhibitors may increase the levels/effects of felbamate; example inhibitors include azole antifungals, clarithromycin, diclofenac, doxycycline, erythromycin, imatinib, isoniazid, nefazodone, nicardipine, propofol, protease inhibitors, quinidine, telithromycin, and verapamil.

Decreased Effect: Felbamate may decrease carbamazepine levels and increase levels of the active metabolite of carbamazepine (10,11-epoxide) resulting in carbamazepine toxicity; monitor for signs of carbamazepine toxicity (dizziness, ataxia, nystagmus, drowsiness). CYP3A4 inducers may decrease the levels/effects of felbamate; example inducers include aminoglutethimide, carbamazepine, nafcillin, nevirapine, phenobarbital, phenytoin, and rifamycins.

Pharmacodynamics/Kinetics

Absorption: Rapid and almost complete; food has no effect upon the tablet's absorption

Distribution: V_d: 0.7-1 L/kg

Protein binding: 22% to 25%, primarily to albumin

Half-life elimination: 20-23 hours (average); prolonged in renal dysfunction

Time to peak, serum: ~3 hours

Excretion: Urine (40% to 50% as unchanged drug, 40% as inactive metabolites)

Pregnancy Risk Factor C

Felbatol® see Felbamate on page 672

Feldene® see Piroxicam on page 1315

Felodipine (fe LOE di peen)

Related Information

Cardiovascular Diseases on page 1726

U.S. Brand Names Plendil®

Canadian Brand Names Plendil®; Renedil®

Mexican Brand Names Munobal; Plendil

Generic Available No

Pharmacologic Category Calcium Channel Blocker

Use Treatment of hypertension

Unlabeled/Investigational Use Pediatric hypertension

Local Anesthetic/Vasoconstrictor Precautions No information available to require special precautions

Effects on Dental Treatment Key adverse event(s) related to dental treatment: Gingival hyperplasia (fewer reports than other CCBs, resolves upon discontinuation, consultation with physician is suggested).

Common Adverse Effects

>10%: Central nervous system: Headache (11% to 15%)

2% to 10%: Cardiovascular: Peripheral edema (2% to 17%), tachycardia (0.4% to 2.5%), flushing (4% to 7%)

(Continued)

Felodipine *(Continued)*

Mechanism of Action Inhibits calcium ions from entering the "slow channels" or select voltage-sensitive areas of vascular smooth muscle and myocardium during depolarization, producing a relaxation of coronary vascular smooth muscle and coronary vasodilation; increases myocardial oxygen delivery in patients with vasospastic angina

Drug Interactions

Cytochrome P450 Effect: Substrate of CYP3A4 (major); **Inhibits** CYP2C8 (moderate), 2C9 (weak), 2D6 (weak), 3A4 (weak)

Increased Effect/Toxicity: Felodipine may increase the levels/effects of CYP2C8 substrates; example substrates include amiodarone, paclitaxel, pioglitazone, repaglinide, and rosiglitazone. CYP3A4 inhibitors may increase the levels/effects of felodipine; example inhibitors include azole antifungals, clarithromycin, diclofenac, doxycycline, erythromycin, imatinib, isoniazid, nefazodone, nicardipine, propofol, protease inhibitors, quinidine, telithromycin, and verapamil. Beta-blockers may have increased pharmacokinetic or pharmacodynamic interactions with felodipine. Cyclosporine increases felodipine's serum concentration. Blood pressure-lowering effects may be additive with sildenafil, tadalafil, and vardenafil (use caution). Felodipine may increase tacrolimus serum levels (monitor).

Decreased Effect: Felodipine may decrease pharmacologic actions of theophylline. Calcium may reduce the calcium channel blocker's effects, particularly hypotension. Felodipine may decrease pharmacologic actions of theophylline. CYP3A4 inducers may decrease the levels/effects of felodipine; example inducers include aminoglutethimide, carbamazepine, nafcillin, nevirapine, phenobarbital, phenytoin, and rifamycins.

Pharmacodynamics/Kinetics

Onset of action: Antihypertensive: 2-5 hours

Duration of antihypertensive effect: 24 hours

Absorption: 100%; Absolute: 20% due to first-pass effect

Protein binding: >99%

Metabolism: Hepatic; CYP3A4 substrate (major); extensive first-pass effect

Half-life elimination: Immediate release: 11-16 hours

Excretion: Urine (70% as metabolites); feces 10%

Pregnancy Risk Factor C

Fenofibrate *(fen oh FYE brate)*

Related Information

Cardiovascular Diseases on page 1726

U.S. Brand Names Antara™; Lipofen™; Lofibra™; TriCor®; Triglide™

Canadian Brand Names Apo-Fenofibrate®; Apo-Feno-Micro®; Dom-Fenofibrate Supra; Gen-Fenofibrate Micro; Lipidil EZ®; Lipidil Micro®; Lipidil Supra®; Novo-Fenofibrate; Novo-Fenofibrate-S; Nu-Fenofibrate; PHL-Fenofibrate Supra; PMS-Fenofibrate Micro; PMS-Fenofibrate Supra; ratio-Fenofibrate MC; Sandoz Fenofibrate S; TriCor®

Mexican Brand Names Controlip

Generic Available Yes: Micronized capsule and tablet

Index Terms Procetofene; Proctofene

Pharmacologic Category Antilipemic Agent, Fibric Acid

Use Adjunct to dietary therapy for the treatment of adults with elevations of serum triglyceride levels (types IV and V hyperlipidemia); adjunct to dietary therapy for the reduction of low density lipoprotein cholesterol (LDL-C), total cholesterol (total-C), triglycerides, and apolipoprotein B (apo B) in adult patients with primary hypercholesterolemia or mixed dyslipidemia (Fredrickson types IIa and IIb)

Local Anesthetic/Vasoconstrictor Precautions No information available to require special precautions

Effects on Dental Treatment Key adverse event(s) related to dental treatment: Dry mouth and tooth disorder.

Common Adverse Effects
>10%: Hepatic: ALT/AST increased (3% to 13%)
1% to 10%:
Gastrointestinal: Abdominal pain (5%), constipation (2%)
Neuromuscular & skeletal: Back pain (3%)
Respiratory: Respiratory disorder (6%), rhinitis (2%)

Frequency not defined:
Cardiovascular: Angina pectoris, arrhythmia, atrial fibrillation, cardiovascular disorder, chest pain, coronary artery disorder, edema, electrocardiogram abnormality, extrasystoles, hyper-/hypotension, MI, palpitation, peripheral edema, peripheral vascular disorder, phlebitis, tachycardia, varicose veins, vasodilatation
Central nervous system: Anxiety, depression, dizziness, fever, headache, insomnia, malaise, nervousness, neuralgia, pain, somnolence, vertigo
Dermatologic: Acne, alopecia, bruising, contact dermatitis, eczema, fungal dermatitis, maculopapular rash, nail disorder, photosensitivity reaction, pruritus, skin ulcer, Stevens-Johnson syndrome, toxic epidermal necrolysis, urticaria
Endocrine & metabolic: Diabetes mellitus, gout, gynecomastia, hypoglycemia, hyperuricemia, libido decreased
Gastrointestinal: Anorexia, appetite increased, colitis, diarrhea, dry mouth, duodenal ulcer, dyspepsia, eructation, esophagitis, flatulence, gastroenteritis, gastritis, gastrointestinal disorder, nausea, peptic ulcer, rectal disorder, rectal hemorrhage, tooth disorder, vomiting, weight gain/loss
Genitourinary: Cystitis, dysuria, prostatic disorder, libido decreased, pregnancy (unintended), urinary frequency, urolithiasis, vaginal moniliasis
Hematologic: Agranulocytosis, anemia, eosinophilia, leukopenia, lymphadenopathy, thrombocytopenia
Hepatic: Cholelithiasis, cholecystitis, creatine phosphokinase increased, fatty liver deposits, liver function tests abnormal
Neuromuscular & skeletal: Arthralgia, arthritis, arthrosis, bursitis, hypertonia, joint disorder, leg cramps, muscle pain, myalgia, myasthenia, myopathy, myositis, paresthesia, rhabdomyolysis, tenderness, tenosynovitis, weakness
Ocular: Abnormal vision, amblyopia, cataract, conjunctivitis, eye disorder, refraction disorder
Otic: Ear pain, otitis media
Renal: Creatinine increased, kidney function abnormality
Respiratory: Asthma, bronchitis, cough increased, dyspnea, laryngitis, pharyngitis, pneumonia, sinusitis
Miscellaneous: Allergic reaction, cyst, diaphoresis, hernia, herpes simplex, herpes zoster, hypersensitivity reaction, infection

Dosage Oral:
Adults:
Hypertriglyceridemia: Initial:
Antara™: 43-130 mg/day
Lipofen™: 50-150 mg/day; maximum dose: 150 mg/day
Lofibra™: 67 mg/day with meals, up to 200 mg/day
TriCor®: 48 mg/day, up to 145 mg/day
Triglide™: 50-160 mg/day
Hypercholesterolemia or mixed hyperlipidemia:
Antara™: 130 mg/day
Lipofen™: 150 mg/day
Lofibra™: 200 mg/day with meals
TriCor®: 145 mg/day
Triglide™: 160 mg/day
Elderly: Initial:
Antara™: 43 mg/day
Lipofen™: 50 mg/day
Lofibra™: 67 mg/day
TriCor®: 48 mg/day
Triglide™: 50 mg/day
Dosage adjustment/interval in renal impairment: Monitor renal function and lipid panel before adjusting. Decrease dose or increase dosing interval for patients with renal failure: Initial:
Antara™: 43 mg/day
Lipofen™: 50 mg/day
Lofibra™: 67 mg/day
TriCor®: 48 mg/day
Triglide™: 50 mg/day
Mechanism of Action Fenofibric acid is believed to increase VLDL catabolism by enhancing the synthesis of lipoprotein lipase; as a result of a decrease in
(Continued)

Fenofibrate *(Continued)*

VLDL levels, total plasma triglycerides are reduced by 30% to 60%; modest increase in HDL occurs in some hypertriglyceridemic patients

Contraindications Hypersensitivity to fenofibrate or any component of the formulation; hepatic dysfunction including primary biliary cirrhosis and unexplained persistent liver function abnormalities; severe renal dysfunction; pre-existing gallbladder disease

Warnings/Precautions Hepatic transaminases can become significantly elevated (dose-related); hepatocellular, chronic active, and cholestatic hepatitis have been reported. Regular monitoring of liver function tests is required. May cause cholelithiasis. Use caution with warfarin; adjustments in warfarin therapy may be required. Use caution with HMG-CoA reductase inhibitors (may lead to myopathy, rhabdomyolysis). Therapy should be withdrawn if an adequate response is not obtained after 2 months of therapy at the maximal daily dose. May cause mild to moderate decreases in hemoglobin, hematocrit and WBC upon initiation of therapy which usually stabilizes with long-term therapy. Rare hypersensitivity reactions may occur. Dose adjustment is required for renal impairment and elderly patients. Safety and efficacy in children have not been established.

Drug Interactions

Cytochrome P450 Effect: Substrate of CYP3A4 (minor); **Inhibits** CYP2A6 (weak), 2C8 (moderate), 2C9 (moderate), 2C19 weak

Increased Effect/Toxicity: Fenofibrate may increase the effects of sulfonylureas and warfarin. Concurrent use of fenofibrate with HMG-CoA reductase inhibitors may increase the risk of myopathy and rhabdomyolysis. Ezetimibe's serum concentration may be increased with concurrent use. Fenofibrate may increase the levels/effects of CYP2C8 substrates (example substrates include amiodarone, paclitaxel, pioglitazone, repaglinide, and rosiglitazone). Fenofibrate may increase the levels/effects of CYP2C9 substrates (example substrates include bosentan, dapsone, fluoxetine, glimepiride, glipizide, losartan, montelukast, nateglinide, paclitaxel, phenytoin, warfarin, and zafirlukast).

Decreased Effect: Bile acid sequestrants may decrease absorption of fenofibrate (separate administration).

Dietary Considerations

Lofibra™: Take with meals.

Antara™, Lipofen™, TriCor®, Triglide™: May be taken with or without food.

Pharmacodynamics/Kinetics

Absorption: Increased when taken with meals

Distribution: Widely to most tissues

Protein binding: >99%

Metabolism: Tissue and plasma via esterases to active form, fenofibric acid; undergoes inactivation by glucuronidation hepatically or renally

Half-life elimination: Fenofibric acid: Mean: 20 hours (range: 10-35 hours)

Time to peak: 3-8 hours

Excretion: Urine (60% as metabolites); feces (25%); hemodialysis has no effect on removal of fenofibric acid from plasma

Pregnancy Risk Factor C

Dosage Forms

Capsule:

Lipofen™: 50 mg, 100 mg, 150 mg

Capsule [micronized]: 67 mg, 134 mg, 200 mg

Antara™: 43 mg, 130 mg

Lofibra™: 67 mg, 134 mg, 200 mg

Tablet: 54 mg, 160 mg

TriCor®: 48 mg, 145 mg

Triglide™: 50 mg, 160 mg

Fenoldopam *(fe NOL doe pam)*

U.S. Brand Names Corlopam®

Canadian Brand Names Corlopam®

Generic Available Yes

Index Terms Fenoldopam Mesylate

Pharmacologic Category Dopamine Agonist

Use Treatment of severe hypertension (up to 48 hours in adults), including in patients with renal compromise; short-term (up to 4 hours) blood pressure reduction in pediatric patients

Local Anesthetic/Vasoconstrictor Precautions No information available to require special precautions

Effects on Dental Treatment Key adverse event(s) related to dental treatment: Xerostomia and changes in salivation (normal salivary flow resumes upon discontinuation).

Common Adverse Effects Frequency not always defined.

Cardiovascular: Angina, asymptomatic T wave flattening on ECG, chest pain, edema, facial flushing (>5%), fibrillation (atrial), flutter (atrial), hypotension (>5%), tachycardia

Central nervous system: Dizziness, headache (>5%)

Endocrine & metabolic: Hypokalemia

Gastrointestinal: Abdominal pain/fullness, diarrhea, nausea (>5%), vomiting, xerostomia

Local: Injection site reactions

Ocular: Intraocular pressure (increased), blurred vision

Hepatic: Increases in portal pressure in cirrhotic patients

Mechanism of Action A selective postsynaptic dopamine agonist (D_1-receptors) which exerts hypotensive effects by decreasing peripheral vasculature resistance with increased renal blood flow, diuresis, and natriuresis; 6 times as potent as dopamine in producing renal vasodilitation; has minimal adrenergic effects

Drug Interactions

Increased Effect/Toxicity: Concurrent acetaminophen may increase fenoldopam levels (30% to 70%). Beta-blockers increase the risk of hypotension; avoid concurrent use. If used concurrently with beta-blockers, close monitoring is recommended.

Pharmacodynamics/Kinetics

Onset of action: I.V.: 10 minutes

Duration: I.V.: 1 hour

Distribution: V_d: 0.6 L/kg

Half-life elimination: I.V.: Children: 3-5 minutes; Adults: ~5 minutes

Metabolism: Hepatic via methylation, glucuronidation, and sulfation; the 8-sulfate metabolite may have some activity; extensive first-pass effect

Excretion: Urine (90%); feces (10%)

Pregnancy Risk Factor B

Fenoldopam Mesylate *see* Fenoldopam *on page 676*

Fenoprofen (fen oh PROE fen)

Related Information

Rheumatoid Arthritis, Osteoarthritis, and Osteoporosis *on page 1759*

Temporomandibular Dysfunction (TMD) *on page 1822*

U.S. Brand Names Nalfon®

Canadian Brand Names Nalfon®

Mexican Brand Names Nalfon

Generic Available Yes: Tablet

Index Terms Fenoprofen Calcium

Pharmacologic Category Nonsteroidal Anti-inflammatory Drug (NSAID), Oral

Use Symptomatic treatment of acute and chronic rheumatoid arthritis and osteoarthritis; relief of mild to moderate pain

Local Anesthetic/Vasoconstrictor Precautions No information available to require special precautions

Effects on Dental Treatment NSAID formulations are known to reversibly decrease platelet aggregation via mechanisms different than observed with aspirin. The dentist should be aware of the potential of abnormal coagulation. Caution should also be exercised in the use of NSAIDs in patients already on anticoagulant therapy with drugs such as warfarin (Coumadin®).

Common Adverse Effects

>10%:

Central nervous system: Dizziness (7% to 15%), somnolence (9% to 15%)

Gastrointestinal: Abdominal cramps (2% to 4%), heartburn, indigestion, nausea (8% to 14%), dyspepsia (10% to 14%), flatulence (14%), anorexia (14%), constipation (7% to 14%), occult blood in stool (14%), vomiting (3% to 14%), diarrhea (2% to 14%)

1% to 10%:

Central nervous system: Headache (9%)

Dermatologic: Itching

Endocrine & metabolic: Fluid retention

Restrictions An FDA-approved medication guide must be distributed when dispensing an oral outpatient prescription (new or refill) where this medication is to be used without direct supervision of a healthcare provider. Medication guides are available at http://www.fda.gov/cder/Offices/ODS/medication_guides.htm.

(Continued)

Fenoprofen (Continued)

Dosage Adults: Oral:

Rheumatoid arthritis: 300-600 mg 3-4 times/day up to 3.2 g/day

Mild to moderate pain: 200 mg every 4-6 hours as needed

Dosage adjustment in renal impairment: Not recommended in patients with advanced renal disease

Mechanism of Action Inhibits prostaglandin synthesis by decreasing the activity of the enzyme, cyclooxygenase, which results in decreased formation of prostaglandin precursors

Contraindications Hypersensitivity to fenoprofen, aspirin, or other NSAIDs, or any component of the formulation; perioperative pain in the setting of coronary artery bypass surgery (CABG); significant renal dysfunction; pregnancy (3rd trimester)

Warnings/Precautions [U.S. Boxed Warning]: NSAIDs are associated with an increased risk of adverse cardiovascular events, including MI, stroke, and new onset or worsening of pre-existing hypertension. Risk may be increased with duration of use or pre-existing cardiovascular risk factors or disease. Carefully evaluate individual cardiovascular risk profiles prior to prescribing. Use caution with fluid retention, CHF, or hypertension. Concurrent administration of ibuprofen, and potentially other nonselective NSAIDs, may interfere with aspirin's cardioprotective effect.

Use of NSAIDs can compromise existing renal function. Renal toxicity can occur in patient with impaired renal function, dehydration, heart failure, liver dysfunction, those taking diuretics and ACEI, and the elderly. Rehydrate patient before starting therapy. Monitor renal function closely. Not recommended for use in patients with advanced renal disease.

[U.S. Boxed Warning]: NSAIDs may increase risk of gastrointestinal irritation, ulceration, bleeding, and perforation. These events may occur at any time during therapy and without warning. Use caution with a history of GI disease (bleeding or ulcers), concurrent therapy with aspirin, anticoagulants and/or corticosteroids, smoking, use of alcohol, the elderly or debilitated patients.

Use the lowest effective dose for the shortest duration of time, consistent with individual patient goals, to reduce risk of cardiovascular or GI adverse events. Alternate therapies should be considered for patients at high risk.

NSAIDs may cause serious skin adverse events including exfoliative dermatitis, Stevens-Johnson syndrome (SJS), and toxic epidermal necrolysis (TEN). Anaphylactoid reactions may occur, even without prior exposure; patients with "aspirin triad" (bronchial asthma, aspirin intolerance, rhinitis) may be at increased risk. Do not use in patients who experience bronchospasm, asthma, rhinitis, or urticaria with NSAID or aspirin therapy. Use caution in other forms of asthma.

Use with caution in patients with decreased hepatic function. Closely monitor patients with any abnormal LFT. Severe hepatic reactions (eg, fulminant hepatitis, liver failure) have occurred with NSAID use, rarely; discontinue if signs or symptoms of liver disease develop, or if systemic manifestations occur.

The elderly are at increased risk for adverse effects (especially peptic ulceration, CNS effects, renal toxicity) from NSAIDs even at low doses.

Withhold for at least 4-6 half-lives prior to surgical or dental procedures. Safety and efficacy have not been established in children.

Drug Interactions

Increased Effect/Toxicity: Increased effect/toxicity of phenytoin, sulfonamides, sulfonylureas, salicylates, and oral anticoagulants. Serum concentration/toxicity of methotrexate may be increased. Concomitant use with fluoroquinolones may rarely increase risk of seizure.

Decreased Effect: Decreased effect with phenobarbital. Thiazide efficacy (diuretic and antihypertensive effect) may be reduced (indomethacin may reduce this efficacy and it may be anticipated with any NSAID). NSAIDs may decrease the antihypertensive effect of ACE inhibitors, angiotensin antagonists, beta-blockers, or hydralazine. Cholestyramine (and other bile acid sequestrants) may decrease the absorption of NSAIDs; separate by at least 2 hours. Salicylates' antiplatelet effect may be reduced.

Ethanol/Nutrition/Herb Interactions

Ethanol: Avoid ethanol (may enhance gastric mucosal irritation).

Food: Fenoprofen peak serum levels may be decreased if taken with food.

Herb/Nutraceutical: Avoid alfalfa, anise, bilberry, bladderwrack, bromelain, cat's claw, celery, coleus, cordyceps, dong quai, evening primrose, feverfew, fenugreek, garlic, ginger, ginkgo biloba, red clover, horse chestnut, grapeseed, green tea, ginseng, guggul, horse chestnut seed, horseradish, licorice, prickly ash, red clover, reishi, SAMe, sweet clover, turmeric, white willow (all have additional antiplatelet activity).

Dietary Considerations May be taken with food to decrease GI distress.
Pharmacodynamics/Kinetics
Onset of action: A few days
Absorption: Rapid, 80%
Distribution: Does not cross the placenta
Protein binding: 99%
Metabolism: Extensively hepatic
Half-life elimination: 2.5-3 hours
Time to peak, serum: ~2 hours
Excretion: Urine (2% to 5% as unchanged drug); feces (small amounts)
Pregnancy Risk Factor C/D (3rd trimester)
Dosage Forms
Capsule:
Nalfon®: 200 mg, 300 mg
Tablet: 600 mg

Fenoprofen Calcium *see* Fenoprofen *on page 677*

Fenoterol (fen oh TER ole)

Canadian Brand Names Berotec®
Index Terms Fenoterol Hydrobromide
Pharmacologic Category Beta₂-Adrenergic Agonist
Use Treatment and prevention of symptoms of reversible obstructive pulmonary disease (including asthma and acute bronchospasm), chronic bronchitis, emphysema
Local Anesthetic/Vasoconstrictor Precautions No information available to require special precautions
Effects on Dental Treatment No significant effects or complications reported
Common Adverse Effects Note: Frequency of most effects may be dose related, approximate frequencies noted below. In the treatment of acute bronchospasm (high-dose nebulization), symptoms of headache (up to 12%), tremor (32%), and tachycardia (up to 21%) are frequently noted.

>10%: Endocrine & metabolic: Serum glucose increased, serum potassium decreased
1% to 10%:
Cardiovascular: Palpitation, tachycardia
Central nervous system: Headache, dizziness, nervousness
Neuromuscular & skeletal: Tremor, muscle cramps
Respiratory: Pharyngeal irritation, cough
Restrictions Not available in U.S.
Mechanism of Action Relaxes bronchial smooth muscle by action on beta₂-receptors with little effect on heart rate.
Drug Interactions
Increased Effect/Toxicity: When used with inhaled ipratropium, an increased duration of bronchodilation may occur. Cardiovascular effects are potentiated in patients also receiving MAO inhibitors, tricyclic antidepressants, and sympathomimetic agents (eg, amphetamine, dopamine, dobutamine). Fenoterol may increase the risk of malignant arrhythmias with inhaled anesthetics (eg, enflurane, halothane). Concurrent use with diuretics may increase the risk of hypokalemia.
Decreased Effect: When used with nonselective beta-adrenergic blockers (eg, propranolol), the effect of fenoterol is decreased.
Pharmacodynamics/Kinetics
Onset of action: 5 minutes
Peak effect: 30-60 minutes
Duration: 3-4 hours (up to 6-8 hours)
Pregnancy Risk Factor Not available; similar agents rated C

Fenoterol Hydrobromide *see* Fenoterol *on page 679*

Fentanyl (FEN ta nil)

U.S. Brand Names Actiq®; Duragesic®; Fentora™; Ionsys™; Sublimaze®
Canadian Brand Names Actiq®; Duragesic®; Fentanyl Citrate Injection, USP
Mexican Brand Names Fentanest
Generic Available Yes: Excludes buccal tablet and iontophoretic transdermal system
Index Terms Fentanyl Citrate; Fentanyl Hydrochloride; OTFC (Oral Transmucosal Fentanyl Citrate)
(Continued)

Fentanyl *(Continued)*

Pharmacologic Category Analgesic, Opioid; General Anesthetic

Dental Use Adjunct in preoperative intravenous conscious sedation in patients undergoing dental surgery

Use

Injection: Sedation, relief of pain, preoperative medication, adjunct to general or regional anesthesia

Iontophoretic transdermal system (Ionsys™): Short-term in-hospital management of acute postoperative pain

Transdermal patch (eg, Duragesic®): Management of moderate-to-severe chronic pain

Transmucosal lozenge (eg, Actiq®), buccal tablet (Fentora™): Management of breakthrough cancer pain

Local Anesthetic/Vasoconstrictor Precautions No information available to require special precautions

Effects on Dental Treatment Key adverse event(s) related to dental treatment: Xerostomia, changes in salivation (normal salivary flow resumes upon discontinuation), and orthostatic hypotension. Actiq® may contribute to dental carries due to sugar content of oral lozenge; advise patients to maintain good oral hygiene. See Dental Comment.

Significant Adverse Effects

>10%:

Cardiovascular: Hypotension, bradycardia

Central nervous system: CNS depression, confusion, drowsiness, sedation

Gastrointestinal: Nausea, vomiting, constipation, xerostomia

Local: Application-site reaction (iontophoretic system 14%)

Neuromuscular & skeletal: Chest wall rigidity (high dose I.V.), weakness

Ocular: Miosis

Respiratory: Respiratory depression

Miscellaneous: Diaphoresis

1% to 10%:

Cardiovascular: Cardiac arrhythmia, edema, orthostatic hypotension, hypertension, syncope, tachycardia

Central nervous system: Abnormal dreams, abnormal thinking, agitation, amnesia, anxiety, dizziness, euphoria, fatigue, fever, hallucinations, headache, insomnia, nervousness, paranoid reaction

Dermatologic: Erythema, papules, pruritus (iontophoretic system 6%), rash

Gastrointestinal: Abdominal pain, anorexia, biliary tract spasm, diarrhea, dyspepsia, flatulence, ileus

Genitourinary: Urinary retention (iontophoretic transdermal system 3%)

Hematologic: Anemia

Local: Application site reactions (buccal tablet)

Neuromuscular & skeletal: Abnormal coordination, abnormal gait, back pain, paresthesia, rigors, tremor

Respiratory: Apnea, bronchitis, dyspnea, hemoptysis, hypoxia, pharyngitis, rhinitis, sinusitis, upper respiratory infection

Miscellaneous: Hiccups, flu-like syndrome, speech disorder

<1% (Limited to important or life-threatening): Amblyopia, anorgasmia, aphasia, bradycardia, bronchospasm, circulatory depression, CNS excitation or delirium, convulsions, dental caries (Actiq®), depersonalization, dysesthesia, ejaculatory difficulty, exfoliative dermatitis, gum line erosion (Actiq®), hyper-/hypotonia, laryngospasm, paradoxical dizziness, physical and psychological dependence with prolonged use, stertorous breathing, stupor, tachycardia, tooth loss (Actiq®), urinary tract spasm, urticaria, vertigo

Restrictions C-II

An FDA-approved medication guide for buccal tablet (Fentora™) and transmucosal lozenge (eg, Actiq®) must be distributed when dispensing an outpatient prescription (new or refill) where this medication is to be used without direct supervision of a healthcare provider. Medication guides are available at http://www.fda.gov/cder/Offices/ODS/medication_guides.htm.

Dental Usual Dosing Surgery: Adults:

Premedication: I.M., slow I.V.: 25-100 mcg/dose 30-60 minutes prior to surgery

Adjunct to regional anesthesia: Slow I.V.: 25-100 mcg/dose over 1-2 minutes.

Note: An I.V. should be in place with regional anesthesia so the I.M. route is rarely used but still maintained as an option in the package labeling.

Dosage Note: These are guidelines and do not represent the maximum doses that may be required in all patients. Doses should be titrated to pain relief/prevention. Monitor vital signs routinely. Single I.M. doses have a duration of 1-2 hours, single I.V. doses last 0.5-1 hour.

Sedation for minor procedures/analgesia:

Children 1-12 years:

Sedation for minor procedures/analgesia: I.M., I.V.: 1-2 mcg/kg/dose; may repeat at 30- to 60-minute intervals. **Note:** Children 18-36 months of age may require 2-3 mcg/kg/dose

Continuous sedation/analgesia: Initial I.V. bolus: 1-2 mcg/kg; then 1-3 mcg/kg/hour to a maximum dose of 5 mcg/kg/hour

Children >12 years and Adults: I.V.: 25-50 mcg; may repeat every 3-5 minutes to desired effect or adverse event; maximum dose of 500 mcg/4 hours; higher doses are used for major procedures

Surgery: Adults:

Premedication: I.M., slow I.V.: 25-100 mcg/dose 30-60 minutes prior to surgery

Adjunct to regional anesthesia: Slow I.V.: 25-100 mcg/dose over 1-2 minutes. **Note:** An I.V. should be in place with regional anesthesia so the I.M. route is rarely used but still maintained as an option in the package labeling.

Adjunct to general anesthesia: Slow I.V.:

Low dose: 0.5-2 mcg/kg/dose depending on the indication. For example, 0.5 mcg/kg will provide analgesia or reduce the amount of propofol needed for laryngeal mask airway insertion with minimal respiratory depression. However, to blunt the hemodynamic response to intubation 2 mcg/kg is often necessary.

Moderate dose: Initial: 2-15 mcg/kg/dose; Maintenance (bolus or infusion): 1-2 mcg/kg/hour. Discontinuing fentanyl infusion 30-60 minutes prior to the end of surgery will usually allow adequate ventilation upon emergence from anesthesia. For "fast-tracking" and early extubation following major surgery, total fentanyl doses are limited to 10-15 mcg/kg.

High dose: **Note:** High-dose (20-50 mcg/kg/dose) fentanyl is rarely used, but is still maintained in the package labeling.

Acute pain management: Adults:

Severe: I.M, I.V.: 50-100 mcg/dose every 1-2 hours as needed; patients with prior opiate exposure may tolerate higher initial doses

Patient-controlled analgesia (PCA): I.V.: Usual concentration: 10 mcg/mL

Demand dose: Usual: 10 mcg; range: 10-50 mcg

Lockout interval: 5-8 minutes

Mechanically-ventilated patients (based on 70 kg patient): Slow I.V.: 0.35-1.5 mcg/kg every 30-60 minutes as needed; infusion: 0.7-10 mcg/kg/hour

Iontophoretic transdermal system: 40 mcg per activation on-demand (maximum: 6 doses/hour). **Note:** Patient's pain should be controlled prior to initiating system. Instruct patient how to operate system. Only the patient should initiate system. Each system operates for 24 hours or until 80 doses have been administered, whichever comes first.

Breakthrough cancer pain: For patients who are tolerant to and currently receiving opioid therapy for persistent cancer pain; dosing should be individually titrated to provide adequate analgesia with minimal side effects. Dose titration should be done if patient requires more than 1 dose/breakthrough pain episode for several consecutive episodes. Patients experiencing >4 breakthrough pain episodes/day should have the dose of their long-term opioid re-evaluated.

Children ≥16 years and Adults: Lozenge: Initial dose: 200 mcg; the second dose may be started 15 minutes after completion of the first dose. Consumption should be limited to ≤4 units/day.

Adults: Buccal tablet (Fentora™): Initial dose: 100 mcg; a second 100 mcg dose, if needed, may be started 30 minutes after the start of the first dose. Dose titration, if required, should be done using multiples of the 100 mcg tablets. Patient can take two 100 mcg tablets (one on each side of mouth). If that dose is not successful, can use four 100 mcg tablets (two on each side of mouth). If titration requires >400 mcg, then use 200 mcg tablets.

Conversion from lozenge to buccal tablet (Fentora™):

Lozenge dose 200-400 mcg, then buccal tablet 100 mcg

Lozenge dose 600-800 mcg, then buccal tablet 200 mcg

Lozenge dose 1200 mcg, then buccal tablet 400 mcg

Note: Four 100 mcg buccal tablets deliver approximately 12% and 13% higher values of C_{max} and AUC, respectively, compared to one 400 mcg buccal tablet. To prevent confusion, patient should only have one strength available at a time. Using more than four buccal tablets at a time has not been studied.

Elderly >65 years: Transmucosal lozenge (eg, Actiq®): Dose should be reduced to 2.5-5 mcg/kg

(Continued)

Fentanyl *(Continued)*

Chronic pain management: Children ≥2 years and Adults (opioid-tolerant patients): Transdermal patch (eg, Duragesic®):

Initial: To convert patients from oral or parenteral opioids to transdermal patch, a 24-hour analgesic requirement should be calculated (based on prior opiate use). Using the tables, the appropriate initial dose can be determined. The initial fentanyl dosage may be approximated from the 24-hour morphine dosage and titrated to minimize adverse effects and provide analgesia. With the initial application, the absorption of transdermal fentanyl requires several hours to reach plateau; therefore transdermal fentanyl is inappropriate for management of acute pain. Change patch every 72 hours.

Conversion from continuous infusion of fentanyl: In patients who have adequate pain relief with a fentanyl infusion, fentanyl may be converted to transdermal dosing at a rate equivalent to the intravenous rate. A two-step taper of the infusion to be completed over 12 hours has been recommended (Kornick, 2001) after the patch is applied. The infusion is decreased to 50% of the original rate six hours after the application of the first patch, and subsequently discontinued twelve hours after application.

Titration: Short-acting agents may be required until analgesic efficacy is established and/or as supplements for "breakthrough" pain. The amount of supplemental doses should be closely monitored. Appropriate dosage increases may be based on daily supplemental dosage using the ratio of 45 mg/24 hours of oral morphine to a 12.5 mcg/hour increase in fentanyl dosage.

Frequency of adjustment: The dosage should not be titrated more frequently than every 3 days after the initial dose or every 6 days thereafter. Patients should wear a consistent fentanyl dosage through two applications (6 days) before dosage increase based on supplemental opiate dosages can be estimated.

Frequency of application: The majority of patients may be controlled on every 72-hour administration; however, a small number of patients require every 48-hour administration.

Dose conversion guidelines for transdermal fentanyl[1] (see tables below and on next page).

Dosing adjustment in hepatic impairment: Actiq®: Although fentanyl kinetics may be altered in hepatic disease, Actiq® can be used successfully in the management of breakthrough cancer pain. Doses should be titrated to reach clinical effect with careful monitoring of patients with severe hepatic disease.

Dosing Conversion Guidelines[1,2]

Current Analgesic	Daily Dosage (mg/day)			
Morphine (I.M./I.V.)	10-22	23-37	38-52	53-67
Oxycodone (oral)	30-67	67.5-112	112.5-157	157.5-202
Oxycodone (I.M./I.V.)	15-33	33.1-56	56.1-78	78.1-101
Codeine (oral)	150-447	448-747	748-1047	1048-1347
Hydromorphone (oral)	8-17	17.1-28	28.1-39	39.1-51
Hydromorphone (I.V.)	1.5-3.4	3.5-5.6	5.7-7.9	8-10
Meperidine (I.M.)	75-165	166-278	279-390	391-503
Methadone (oral)	20-44	45-74	75-104	105-134
Methadone (I.M.)	10-22	23-37	38-52	53-67
Fentanyl transdermal recommended dose (mcg/h)	25 mcg/h	50 mcg/h	75 mcg/h	100 mcg/h

[1] The table should NOT be used to convert from transdermal fentanyl (eg, Duragesic®) to other opioid analgesics. Rather, following removal of the patch, titrate the dose of the new opioid until adequate analgesia is achieved.

[2] Duragesic® product insert, Janssen Pharmaceutica, Feb 2005.

Recommended Initial Duragesic® Dose Based Upon Daily Oral Morphine Dose[1]

Oral 24-Hour Morphine (mg/d)	Duragesic® Dose (mcg/h)
60-134[2]	25
135-224	50
225-314	75
315-404	100
405-494	125
495-584	150
585-674	175
675-764	200
765-854	225
855-944	250
945-1034	275
1035-1124	300

[1]The table should NOT be used to convert from transdermal fentanyl (eg, Duragesic®) to other opioid analgesics. Rather, following removal of the patch, titrate the dose of the new opioid until adequate analgesia is achieved.

[2]Pediatric patients initiating therapy on a 25 mcg/hour Duragesic® system should be opioid-tolerant and receiving at least 60 mg oral morphine equivalents per day.

Opioid Analgesics Initial Oral Dosing Commonly Used for Severe Pain

Drug	Equianalgesic Dose (mg)		Initial Oral Dose	
	Oral[1]	Parenteral[2]	Children (mg/kg)	Adults (mg)
Buprenorphine	—	0.4	—	—
Butorphanol	—	2	—	—
Hydromorphone	7.5	1.5	0.06	4-8
Levorphanol	4 (acute) 1 (chronic)	2 (acute) 1 (chronic)	0.04	2-4
Meperidine	300	75	Not Recommended	
Methadone	10	5	0.2	0.2
Morphine	30	10	0.3	15-30
Nalbuphine	—	10	—	—
Pentazocine	50	30	—	—
Oxycodone	20	—	0.3	10-20
Oxymorphone	1	—	—	—

From "Principles of Analgesic Use in the Treatment of Acute Pain and Cancer Pain," *Am Pain Soc*, Fifth Ed.

[1]Elderly: Starting dose should be lower for this population group

[2]Standard parenteral doses for acute pain in adults; can be used to doses for I.V. infusions and repeated small I.V. boluses. Single I.V. boluses, use half the I.M. dose. Children >6 months: I.V. dose = parenteral equianalgesic dose x weight (kg)/100

Mechanism of Action Binds with stereospecific receptors at many sites within the CNS, increases pain threshold, alters pain reception, inhibits ascending pain pathways

Contraindications Hypersensitivity to fentanyl or any component of the formulation; increased intracranial pressure; severe respiratory disease or depression including acute asthma (unless patient is mechanically ventilated); paralytic ileus; severe liver or renal insufficiency; pregnancy (prolonged use or high doses near term)

Iontophoretic transdermal system (Ionsys™): Hypersensitivity to fentanyl, cetylpyridinium chloride (eg, Cepacol®) or any component of Ionsys™ system

Transmucosal buccal tablets (Fentora™), lozenges (eg, Actiq®), and/or transdermal patches (eg, Duragesic®) are recommended for use only in patients who are opioid-tolerant. Patients are considered opioid-tolerant if they are taking at least 60 mg morphine/day, 30 mg oral oxycodone/day, 8 mg oral hydromorphone/day, 25 mcg transdermal fentanyl/hour, or an equivalent dose of another opioid for ≥1 week. Transmucosal buccal tablets (Fentora™), lozenges (eg, Actiq®), and transdermal patches (eg, Duragesic®) are not for use in acute pain, mild pain, intermittent pain, or postoperative pain management. (Continued)

Fentanyl *(Continued)*

Warnings/Precautions An opioid-containing analgesic regimen should be tailored to each patient's needs and based upon the type of pain being treated (acute versus chronic), the route of administration, degree of tolerance for opioids (naive versus chronic user), age, weight, and medical condition. The optimal analgesic dose varies widely among patients. Doses should be titrated to pain relief/prevention. When using with other CNS depressants, reduce dose of one or both agents. Fentanyl shares the toxic potentials of opiate agonists, and precautions of opiate agonist therapy should be observed; use with caution in patients with bradycardia; rapid I.V. infusion may result in skeletal muscle and chest wall rigidity leading to respiratory distress and/or apnea, bronchoconstriction, laryngospasm; inject slowly over 3-5 minutes. Tolerance or drug dependence may result from extended use. Use caution in patients with a history of drug dependence or abuse. The elderly may be particularly susceptible to the CNS depressant and constipating effects of narcotics. Use extreme caution in patients with COPD or other chronic respiratory conditions. Use caution with head injuries, morbid obesity, or hepatic dysfunction. **[U.S. Boxed Warning]: Use with strong or moderate CYP3A4 inhibitors may result in increased effects and potential respiratory depression.** Concurrent use of agonist/antagonist analgesics may precipitate withdrawal symptoms and/or reduced analgesic efficacy in patients following prolonged therapy with mu opioid agonists. Abrupt discontinuation following prolonged use may also lead to withdrawal symptoms. Opioid-nontolerant patients should not receive some formulations/strengths of fentanyl, including buccal tablets (Fentora™), lozenges (Actiq®), or transdermal patches.

Transmucosal: Lozenge (eg, Actiq®), buccal tablet (Fentora™): **[U.S. Boxed Warning]: Do not substitute Fentora™ on a mcg-per-mcg basis when converting from transmucosal lozenge to buccal tablet. Buccal tablet has higher bioavailability. [U.S. Boxed Warning]: Should be used only for the care of opioid-tolerant cancer patients.** Not approved for use in management of acute or postoperative pain. **[U.S. Boxed Warning]: Buccal tablet and lozenge contain an amount of medication that can be fatal to children.** Keep all units out of the reach of children and discard any open units properly. Safety and efficacy have not been established in children <16 years of age for the lozenge and <18 years of age for the buccal tablet.

Transdermal patches (eg, Duragesic®): **[U.S. Boxed Warning]: Serious or life-threatening hypoventilation may occur, even in opioid-tolerant patients.** Serum fentanyl concentrations may increase approximately one-third for patients with a body temperature of 40°C secondary to a temperature-dependent increase in fentanyl release from the patch and increased skin permeability. Avoid exposure of application site to direct external heat sources. Patients who experience adverse reactions should be monitored for at least 24 hours after removal of the patch. Transdermal patch does not contain any metal-based compounds; the printed ink used to indicate strength on the outer surface of the patch does contain titanium dioxide but the amount is minimal; adverse events have not been reported while wearing during an MRI. **[U.S. Boxed Warning]: Safety and efficacy of transdermal patch have been limited to children ≥2 years of age who are opioid tolerant.**

Iontophoretic transdermal system (Ionsys™): **[U.S. Boxed Warning]: Should only be used for the treatment of hospitalized patients. To avoid overdose, the patient should be the only one to activate the system. Unintended exposure to fentanyl hydrogel could lead to absorption of fatal dose; hydrogel should not come in contact with fingers or mouth.** Should be used only in patients who are able to understand and follow instructions to operate the system. The error detection circuit uses a series of audible signals to alert the patient when a dose is not being delivered; use caution in patients who have high frequency hearing impairment. Remove prior to MRI procedure, cardioversion, or defibrillation. May interfere with radiographic image or CAT scan. Patients on chronic opioids or with a history of opioid abuse may require higher analgesic doses than Ionsys™ is able to provide. Prior to patient's hospital discharge, the system must be removed and disposed of in accordance with State and Federal regulations for a C-II substance. **[U.S. Boxed Warning]: Even if all 80 doses are used, a significant amount of fentanyl remains in the iontophoretic transdermal system and requires proper removal and disposal to avoid misuse, abuse, or diversion.** Safety and efficacy of iontophoretic transdermal system have not been established in children <18 years of age.

Drug Interactions Substrate of CYP3A4 (major); **Inhibits** CYP3A4 (weak)

Ammonium chloride: May increase the excretion of analgesics (opioid).

Antipsychotic agents (phenothiazines): May enhance the hypotensive effect of analgesics (opioid).

CNS depressants: Increased sedation with fentanyl; monitor closely.

CYP3A4 inhibitors: May increase the levels/effects of fentanyl. Potentially fatal respiratory depression may occur when a potent inhibitor is used in a patient receiving chronic fentanyl (eg, transdermal patch). Example inhibitors include azole antifungals, clarithromycin, diclofenac, doxycycline, erythromycin, imatinib, isoniazid, nefazodone, nicardipine, propofol, protease inhibitors, quinidine, telithromycin, and verapamil.

MAO inhibitors: Not recommended to use Actiq® within 14 days. Severe and unpredictable potentiation by MAO inhibitors has been reported with opioid analgesics.

Pegvisomant: Analgesics (opioid) may diminish the therapeutic effect of pegvisomant.

Protease inhibitors: May decrease the metabolism, via CYP isoenzymes, of fentanyl.

Rifamycin derivatives: May decrease the serum concentration of fentanyl.

Selective serotonin reuptake inhibitors (SSRIs): Analgesics (opioid) may enhance the serotonergic effect of SSRIs. This may cause serotonin syndrome.

Sibutramine: Fentanyl may enhance the serotonergic effect of sibutramine.

Ethanol/Nutrition/Herb Interactions

Ethanol: Avoid ethanol (may increase CNS depression).

Food: Glucose may cause hyperglycemia.

Herb/Nutraceutical: St John's wort may decrease fentanyl levels. Avoid valerian, St John's wort, kava kava, gotu kola (may increase CNS depression).

Dietary Considerations Transmucosal lozenge contains 2 g sugar per unit.

Pharmacodynamics/Kinetics

Onset of action: Analgesic: I.M.: 7-15 minutes; I.V.: Almost immediate; Transmucosal: 5-15 minutes

Peak effect: Transmucosal: Analgesic: 15-30 minutes

Duration: I.M.: 1-2 hours; I.V.: 0.5-1 hour; Transmucosal: Related to blood level; respiratory depressant effect may last longer than analgesic effect

Absorption:

Transmucosal, buccal tablet: Rapid, ~50% from the buccal mucosa; remaining 50% swallowed with saliva and slowly absorbed from GI tract

Transmucosal, lozenge: Rapid, ~25% from the buccal mucosa; 75% swallowed with saliva and slowly absorbed from GI tract

Iontophoretic transdermal system (Ionsys™): Fentanyl levels continue to rise for 5 minutes after the completion of each 10-minute dose

Distribution: Highly lipophilic, redistributes into muscle and fat

Protein binding: 80% to 85%

Metabolism: Hepatic, primarily via CYP3A4

Bioavailability: Total (transmucosal and GI absorption): Buccal: 65% (range: 45% to 85%); Lozenge: 47% (range: 37% to 57%)

Half-life elimination:

I.V.: 2-4 hours

Iontophoretic transdermal system (Ionsys™): 11 hours

Transdermal patch: 17 hours (half-life is influenced by absorption rate)

Transmucosal: Lozenge: 7 hours; Buccal tablet: 100-200 mcg: 3-4 hours, 400-800 mcg: 11-12 hours

Time to peak: Buccal tablet: 46 minutes; Lozenge: ~91 minutes; Transdermal patch: 24-72 hours

Excretion: Urine (primarily as metabolites, <7% to 10% as unchanged drug)

Pregnancy Risk Factor C/D (prolonged use or high doses at term)

Lactation Enters breast milk/not recommended (AAP rates "compatible")

Breast-Feeding Considerations Fentanyl is excreted in low concentrations into breast milk. Breast-feeding is considered acceptable following single doses to the mother; however, no information is available when used long-term. **Note:** Iontophoretic transdermal system (Ionsys™), transdermal patch, transmucosal lozenge, and buccal tablet (Fentora™) are not recommended in nursing women due to potential for sedation and/or respiratory depression.

Dosage Forms Excipient information presented when available (limited, particularly for generics); consult specific product labeling.

Note: Strengths expressed as base.

Infusion, as citrate [premixed in NS]: 0.05 mg (10 mL); 1 mg (100 mL); 1.25 mg (250 mL); 2 mg (100 mL); 2.5 mg (250 mL)

Injection, solution, as citrate [preservative free]: 0.05 mg/mL (2 mL, 5 mL, 10 mL, 20 mL, 30 mL, 50 mL)

Sublimaze®: 0.05 mg/mL (2 mL, 5 mL, 10 mL, 20 mL)

Lozenge, oral, as citrate [transmucosal]: 200 mcg, 400 mcg, 600 mcg, 800 mcg, 1200 mcg, 1600 mcg

Actiq®: 200 mcg, 400 mcg, 600 mcg, 800 mcg, 1200 mcg, 1600 mcg [mounted on a plastic radiopaque handle; contains sugar 2 g/unit; raspberry flavor]

Tablet, for buccal application, as citrate:

Fentora™: 100 mcg, 200 mcg, 300 mcg, 400 mcg, 600 mcg, 800 mcg

(Continued)

Fentanyl *(Continued)*

Transdermal system, topical, as base: 25 mcg/hour [6.25 cm²] (5s); 50 mcg/hour [12.5 cm²] (5s); 75 mcg/hour [18.75 cm²]; 100 mcg/hour [25 cm²] (5s)

Duragesic®: 12 [delivers 12.5 mcg/hour; 5 cm²; contains alcohol 0.1 mL/10 cm²] (5s); 25 [delivers 25 mcg/hour; 10 cm²; contains alcohol 0.1 mL/10 cm²] (5s); 50 [delivers 50 mcg/hour; 20 cm²; contains alcohol 0.1 mL/10 cm²] (5s); 75 [delivers 75 mcg/hour; 30 cm²; contains alcohol 0.1 mL/10 cm²]; 100 [delivers 100 mcg/hour; 40 cm²; contains alcohol 0.1 mL/10 cm²] (5s)

Transdermal iontophoretic system, topical, as hydrochloride:

Ionsys™: Fentanyl 40 mcg/dose [80 doses/patch; contains 3-volt lithium battery]

Dental Comment Transdermal fentanyl should not be used as a pain reliever in dentistry due to danger of hypoventilation

Selected Readings

Dionne RA, Yagiela JA, Moore PA, et al, "Comparing Efficacy and Safety of Four Intravenous Sedation Regimens in Dental Outpatients," *Am Dent Assoc*, 2001, 132(6):740-51.

Fentanyl Citrate *see* Fentanyl *on page 679*

Fentanyl Hydrochloride *see* Fentanyl *on page 679*

Fentora™ *see* Fentanyl *on page 679*

Feosol® [OTC] *see* Ferrous Sulfate *on page 688*

Feostat® [OTC] [DSC] *see* Ferrous Fumarate *on page 687*

Feratab® [OTC] *see* Ferrous Sulfate *on page 688*

Fer-Gen-Sol [OTC] *see* Ferrous Sulfate *on page 688*

Fergon® [OTC] *see* Ferrous Gluconate *on page 687*

Feridex I.V.® *see* Ferumoxides *on page 688*

Fer-In-Sol® [OTC] *see* Ferrous Sulfate *on page 688*

Fer-Iron® [OTC] *see* Ferrous Sulfate *on page 688*

Fero-Grad 500® [OTC] *see* Ferrous Sulfate and Ascorbic Acid *on page 688*

Ferretts [OTC] *see* Ferrous Fumarate *on page 687*

Ferrex 150 [OTC] *see* Polysaccharide-Iron Complex *on page 1323*

Ferric (III) Hexacyanoferrate (II) *see* Ferric Hexacyanoferrate *on page 687*

Ferric Gluconate *(FER ik GLOO koe nate)*

U.S. Brand Names Ferrlecit®
Canadian Brand Names Ferrlecit®
Generic Available No
Index Terms Sodium Ferric Gluconate
Pharmacologic Category Iron Salt
Use Repletion of total body iron content in patients with iron-deficiency anemia who are undergoing hemodialysis in conjunction with erythropoietin therapy
Local Anesthetic/Vasoconstrictor Precautions No information available to require special precautions
Effects on Dental Treatment Key adverse event(s) related to dental treatment: Xerostomia (normal salivary flow resumes upon discontinuation). Do not prescribe tetracyclines simultaneously with iron since GI tract absorption of both tetracycline and iron may be inhibited.
Common Adverse Effects

Cardiovascular: Angina, bradycardia, chest pain, edema, hyper-/hypotension, hypervolemia, MI, pulmonary edema, syncope, tachycardia, thrombosis, vasodilation

Central nervous system: Agitation, chills, dizziness, fatigue, fever, headache, insomnia, malaise, pain, somnolence

Dermatologic: Pruritus, rash

Endocrine & metabolic: Hyper-/hypokalemia, hypoglycemia

Gastrointestinal: Abdominal pain, anorexia, diarrhea, dyspepsia, epigastric pain, eructation, flatulence, melena, nausea, vomiting

Genitourinary: Urinary tract infection

Hematologic: Abnormal erythrocytes, leukocytosis, lymphadenopathy

Local: Injection site reactions, injection site pain

Neuromuscular & skeletal: Arthralgia, back pain, cramps, groin pain, leg cramps, myalgia, paresthesia, rigors, weakness

Ocular: Blurred vision, conjunctivitis

Respiratory: Cough, dyspnea, pneumonia, rhinitis, upper respiratory infection

Miscellaneous: Carcinoma, diaphoresis increased, flu-like syndrome, hypersensitivity reactions, infection, sepsis

Mechanism of Action Supplies a source to elemental iron necessary to the function of hemoglobin, myoglobin and specific enzyme systems; allows transport of oxygen via hemoglobin

Drug Interactions
Decreased Effect: Ferric gluconate injection may decrease the absorption of oral iron.
Pharmacodynamics/Kinetics Half-life elimination: Bound: 1 hour
Pregnancy Risk Factor B

Ferric Hexacyanoferrate (FER ik hex a SYE an oh fer ate)

U.S. Brand Names Radiogardase™
Generic Available No
Index Terms Ferric (III) Hexacyanoferrate (II); Insoluble Prussian Blue; Prussian Blue
Pharmacologic Category Antidote
Use Treatment of known or suspected internal contamination with radioactive cesium and/or radioactive or nonradioactive thallium
Local Anesthetic/Vasoconstrictor Precautions No information available to require special precautions
Effects on Dental Treatment No significant effects or complications reported
Common Adverse Effects
>10%: Gastrointestinal: Constipation (24%)
1% to 10%: Endocrine & metabolic: Hypokalemia (7%)
Frequency not defined: Gastrointestinal: Gastric distress, fecal discoloration (blue)
Mechanism of Action Binds to cesium and thallium isotopes in the gastrointestinal tract following their ingestion or excretion in the bile; reduces their gastrointestinal reabsorption (enterohepatic circulation)
Pharmacodynamics/Kinetics
Absorption: Ferric hexacyanoferrate: Oral: None
Half-life elimination:
Cesium-137: Effective: Adults: 80 days, decreased by 69% with ferric hexacyanoferrate; adolescents: 62 days, decreased by 46% with ferric hexacyanoferrate; children: 42 days, decreased by 43% with ferric hexacyanoferrate
Nonradioactive thallium: Biological: 8-10 days; with ferric hexacyanoferrate: 3 days
Excretion:
Cesium-137: Without ferric hexacyanoferrate: Urine (~80%); feces (~20%)
Thallium: Without ferric hexacyanoferrate: Fecal to urine excretion ration: 2:1
Ferric hexacyanoferrate: Feces (99%, unchanged)
Pregnancy Risk Factor C

Ferrlecit® see Ferric Gluconate on page 686
Ferro-Sequels® [OTC] see Ferrous Fumarate on page 687

Ferrous Fumarate (FER us FYOO ma rate)

U.S. Brand Names Femiron® [OTC]; Feostat® [OTC] [DSC]; Ferretts [OTC]; Ferro-Sequels® [OTC]; Hemocyte® [OTC]; Ircon® [OTC]; Nephro-Fer® [OTC]
Canadian Brand Names Palafer®
Generic Available Yes: Tablet
Index Terms Iron Fumarate
Pharmacologic Category Iron Salt
Use Prevention and treatment of iron-deficiency anemias
Local Anesthetic/Vasoconstrictor Precautions No information available to require special precautions
Effects on Dental Treatment Key adverse event(s) related to dental treatment: Staining of teeth. Do not prescribe tetracyclines simultaneously with iron since GI tract absorption of both tetracycline and iron may be inhibited.
Mechanism of Action Replaces iron found in hemoglobin, myoglobin, and enzymes; allows the transportation of oxygen via hemoglobin
Pregnancy Risk Factor A

Ferrous Gluconate (FER us GLOO koe nate)

U.S. Brand Names Fergon® [OTC]
Canadian Brand Names Apo-Ferrous Gluconate®; Novo-Ferrogluc
Generic Available Yes
Index Terms Iron Gluconate
Pharmacologic Category Iron Salt
Use Prevention and treatment of iron-deficiency anemias
Local Anesthetic/Vasoconstrictor Precautions No information available to require special precautions
(Continued)

Ferrous Gluconate *(Continued)*

Effects on Dental Treatment Key adverse event(s) related to dental treatment: Staining of teeth. Do not prescribe tetracyclines simultaneously with iron since GI tract absorption of both tetracycline and iron may be inhibited.

Mechanism of Action Replaces iron found in hemoglobin, myoglobin, and enzymes; allows the transportation of oxygen via hemoglobin

Pregnancy Risk Factor A

Ferrous Sulfate *(FER us SUL fate)*

U.S. Brand Names Feosol® [OTC]; Feratab® [OTC]; Fer-Gen-Sol [OTC]; Fer-In-Sol® [OTC]; Fer-Iron® [OTC]; Slow FE® [OTC]

Canadian Brand Names Apo-Ferrous Sulfate®; Fer-In-Sol®; Ferodan™

Mexican Brand Names Hemobion

Generic Available Yes

Index Terms FeSO₄; Iron Sulfate

Pharmacologic Category Iron Salt

Use Prevention and treatment of iron-deficiency anemias

Local Anesthetic/Vasoconstrictor Precautions No information available to require special precautions

Effects on Dental Treatment Do not prescribe tetracyclines simultaneously with iron since GI tract absorption of both tetracycline and iron may be inhibited. Liquid preparations may temporarily stain the teeth.

Mechanism of Action Replaces iron, found in hemoglobin, myoglobin, and other enzymes; allows the transportation of oxygen via hemoglobin

Pregnancy Risk Factor A

Ferrous Sulfate and Ascorbic Acid
(FER us SUL fate & a SKOR bik AS id)

Related Information
Ascorbic Acid *on page 148*
Ferrous Sulfate *on page 688*

U.S. Brand Names Fero-Grad 500® [OTC]; Vitelle™ Irospan® [OTC] [DSC]

Generic Available No

Index Terms Ascorbic Acid and Ferrous Sulfate; Iron Sulfate and Vitamin C

Pharmacologic Category Iron Salt; Vitamin

Use Treatment of iron deficiency in nonpregnant adults; treatment and prevention of iron deficiency in pregnant adults

Local Anesthetic/Vasoconstrictor Precautions No information available to require special precautions

Effects on Dental Treatment Do not prescribe tetracyclines simultaneously with iron since GI tract absorption of both tetracycline and iron may be inhibited. Liquid preparations may temporarily stain the teeth.

Common Adverse Effects Based on **ferrous sulfate** component:
>10%: Gastrointestinal: GI irritation, epigastric pain, nausea, dark stools, vomiting, stomach cramping, constipation
1% to 10%:
Gastrointestinal: Heartburn, diarrhea
Genitourinary: Discoloration of urine
Miscellaneous: Liquid preparations may temporarily stain the teeth

Drug Interactions
Increased Effect/Toxicity: Concurrent administration of ≥200 mg vitamin C per 30 mg elemental iron increases absorption of oral iron.
Decreased Effect: Absorption of oral preparation of iron and tetracyclines are decreased when both of these drugs are given together. Absorption of quinolones may be decreased due to formation of a ferric ion-quinolone complex when given concurrently. Concurrent administration of antacids and H₂ blockers (cimetidine) may decrease iron absorption. Iron may decrease absorption of levodopa, methyldopa, penicillamine when given at the same time. Response to iron therapy may be delayed by chloramphenicol.

Pharmacodynamics/Kinetics See individual agents.

Ferumoxides *(fer yoo MOX ides)*

U.S. Brand Names Feridex I.V.®

Generic Available No

Pharmacologic Category Radiological/Contrast Media, Nonionic

Use For I.V. administration as an adjunct to MRI (in adult patients) to enhance the T2 weighted images used in the detection and evaluation of lesions of the liver

Local Anesthetic/Vasoconstrictor Precautions No information available to require special precautions

Effects on Dental Treatment No significant effects or complications reported

Pregnancy Risk Factor C

FeSO$_4$ *see Ferrous Sulfate on page 688*

FeverALL® [OTC] *see Acetaminophen on page 31*

Fexofenadine (feks oh FEN a deen)

U.S. Brand Names Allegra®

Canadian Brand Names Allegra®

Mexican Brand Names Allegra

Generic Available Yes: Excludes suspension

Index Terms Fexofenadine Hydrochloride

Pharmacologic Category Antihistamine, Nonsedating

Use Relief of symptoms associated with seasonal allergic rhinitis; treatment of chronic idiopathic urticaria

Local Anesthetic/Vasoconstrictor Precautions No information available to require special precautions

Effects on Dental Treatment No significant effects or complications reported

Common Adverse Effects

>10%:

Central nervous system: Headache (5% to 11%)

Gastrointestinal: Vomiting (children 6 months to 5 years): 4% to 12%

1% to 10%:

Central nervous system: Somnolence (1% to 3%), dizziness (2%), drowsiness (2%), pain (2%), fatigue (1%)

Endocrine & metabolic: Dysmenorrhea (2%)

Gastrointestinal: Dyspepsia (1% to 5%), diarrhea (3% to 4%), nausea (2%)

Neuromuscular & skeletal: Myalgia (3%), back pain (2% to 3%)

Otic: Otitis media (2%)

Respiratory: Upper respiratory tract infection (4%), cough (2% to 4%), nasopharyngitis (2%)

Miscellaneous: Viral infection (3%)

Dosage Oral:

Chronic idiopathic urticaria: Children 6 months to <2 years: 15 mg twice daily

Chronic idiopathic urticaria, seasonal allergic rhinitis:

Children 2-11 years: 30 mg twice daily

Children ≥12 years and Adults: 60 mg twice daily **or** 180 mg once daily

Elderly: Starting dose: 60 mg once daily; adjust for renal impairment

Dosing adjustment in renal impairment: Cl$_{cr}$ <80 mL/minute:

Children 6 months to <2 years: Initial: 15 mg once daily

Children 2-11 years: Initial: 30 mg once daily

Children ≥12 years and Adults: Initial: 60 mg once daily

Mechanism of Action Fexofenadine is an active metabolite of terfenadine and like terfenadine it competes with histamine for H$_1$-receptor sites on effector cells in the gastrointestinal tract, blood vessels and respiratory tract; it appears that fexofenadine does not cross the blood brain barrier to any appreciable degree, resulting in a reduced potential for sedation

Contraindications Hypersensitivity to fexofenadine or any component of the formulation

Warnings/Precautions Safety and efficacy in children <6 months of age have not been established.

Drug Interactions

Cytochrome P450 Effect: Substrate of CYP3A4 (minor); **Inhibits** CYP2D6 (weak)

Increased Effect/Toxicity: Anticholinergics, CNS depressants may have increased adverse/toxic effects. Verapamil increases levels/effects of fexofenadine.

Decreased Effect: Acetylcholinesterase inhibitors (central) may decrease the adverse effects of fexofenadine. Acetylcholinesterase inhibitor, betahistine may be less effective. Pramlintide may increase the adverse GI effects of fexofenadine. Rifampin decreases levels/effects of fexofenadine.

Ethanol/Nutrition/Herb Interactions

Ethanol: Avoid ethanol (although limited with fexofenadine, may increase risk of sedation).

Food: Fruit juice (apple, grapefruit, orange) may decrease bioavailability of fexofenadine by ~36%.

Herb/Nutraceutical: St John's wort may decrease fexofenadine levels.

Pharmacodynamics/Kinetics

Onset of action: 60 minutes

(Continued)

Fexofenadine *(Continued)*

Duration: Antihistaminic effect: ≥12 hours
Protein binding: 60% to 70%, primarily albumin and alpha₁-acid glycoprotein
Metabolism: Minimal (~5%)
Half-life elimination: 14.4 hours
Time to peak, serum: ~2.6 hours
Excretion: Feces (~80%) and urine (~11%) as unchanged drug

Pregnancy Risk Factor C

Dosage Forms

Suspension:
Allegra®: 6 mg/mL
Tablet: 30 mg, 60 mg, 180 mg
Allegra®: 30 mg, 60 mg, 180 mg

Fexofenadine and Pseudoephedrine
(feks oh FEN a deen & soo doe e FED rin)

Related Information
Fexofenadine *on page 689*
Pseudoephedrine *on page 1381*

U.S. Brand Names Allegra-D® 12 Hour; Allegra-D® 24 Hour

Canadian Brand Names Allegra-D®

Mexican Brand Names Allegra-D

Generic Available No

Index Terms Pseudoephedrine and Fexofenadine

Pharmacologic Category Antihistamine/Decongestant Combination

Use Relief of symptoms associated with seasonal allergic rhinitis in adults and children ≥12 years of age

Local Anesthetic/Vasoconstrictor Precautions Use with caution since pseudoephedrine is a sympathomimetic amine which could interact with epinephrine to cause a pressor response

Effects on Dental Treatment Key adverse event(s) related to dental treatment: Pseudoephedrine: Xerostomia (normal salivary flow resumes upon discontinuation).

Common Adverse Effects See individual agents.

Drug Interactions
Cytochrome P450 Effect: Fexofenadine: **Substrate** of CYP3A4 (minor); **Inhibits** CYP2D6 (weak)

Pharmacodynamics/Kinetics See individual agents.

Pregnancy Risk Factor C

Fexofenadine Hydrochloride *see* Fexofenadine *on page 689*

Fiberall® *see* Psyllium *on page 1386*

FiberCon® [OTC] *see* Polycarbophil *on page 1320*

Fiber-Lax® [OTC] *see* Polycarbophil *on page 1320*

Fiber-Tabs™ [OTC] *see* Polycarbophil *on page 1320*

Fibrin Sealant Kit (FI brin SEEL ent kit)

U.S. Brand Names Crosseal™; Tisseel® VH

Canadian Brand Names Tisseel® VH

Generic Available No

Index Terms FS

Pharmacologic Category Hemostatic Agent

Use
Crosseal™: Adjunct to hemostasis in liver surgery
Tisseel® VH: Adjunct to hemostasis in cardiopulmonary bypass surgery and splenic injury (due to blunt or penetrating trauma to the abdomen) when the control of bleeding by conventional surgical techniques is ineffective or impractical; adjunctive sealant for closure of colostomies; hemostatic agent in heparinized patients undergoing cardiopulmonary bypass

Local Anesthetic/Vasoconstrictor Precautions No information available to require special precautions

Effects on Dental Treatment No significant effects or complications reported

Mechanism of Action Formation of a biodegradable adhesive is done by duplicating the last step of the coagulation cascade, the formation of fibrin from fibrinogen. Fibrinogen is the main component of the sealant solution. The solution also contains thrombin, which transforms fibrinogen from the sealer protein solution into fibrin, and fibrinolysis inhibitor (aprotinin), which prevents the premature degradation of fibrin. When mixed as directed, a viscous solution forms that sets into an elastic coagulum.

Drug Interactions
  Decreased Effect: Decreased effect (Tisseel® VH): Local concentrations/ applications of alcohol, heavy-metal ions, iodine; oxycellulose preparations
Pharmacodynamics/Kinetics Onset of action:
  Crosseal™: Time to hemostasis: 5.3 minutes
  Tisseel® VH: Time to hemostasis: 5 minutes (65% of patients); Final prepared sealant: 70% strength: ~10 minutes; Full strength: ~2 hours
Pregnancy Risk Factor C

Fibro-XL [OTC] *see* Psyllium *on page 1386*
Fibro-Lax [OTC] *see* Psyllium *on page 1386*

Filgrastim (fil GRA stim)

U.S. Brand Names Neupogen®
Canadian Brand Names Neupogen®
Mexican Brand Names Neupogen
Generic Available No
Index Terms G-CSF; Granulocyte Colony Stimulating Factor; NSC-614629
Pharmacologic Category Colony Stimulating Factor
Use Stimulation of granulocyte production in chemotherapy-induced neutropenia (nonmyeloid malignancies, acute myeloid leukemia, and bone marrow transplantation; severe chronic neutropenia (SCN); patients undergoing peripheral blood progenitor cell (PBPC) collection
Unlabeled/Investigational Use Treatment of anemia in myelodysplastic syndrome; treatment of drug-induced (nonchemotherapy) agranulocytosis in the elderly
Local Anesthetic/Vasoconstrictor Precautions No information available to require special precautions
Effects on Dental Treatment No significant effects or complications reported
Common Adverse Effects
  >10%:
    Central nervous system: Fever (12%)
    Dermatologic: Petechiae (17%), rash (12%)
    Gastrointestinal: Splenomegaly (severe chronic neutropenia: 30%; rare in other patients)
    Hepatic: Alkaline phosphatase increased (21%)
    Neuromuscular & skeletal: Bone pain (22% to 33%), commonly in the lower back, posterior iliac crest, and sternum
    Respiratory: Epistaxis (9% to 15%)
  1% to 10%:
    Cardiovascular: Hyper-/hypotension (4%), S-T segment depression (3%), myocardial infarction/arrhythmias (3%)
    Central nervous system: Headache (7%)
    Gastrointestinal: Nausea (10%), vomiting (7%), peritonitis (2%)
    Hematologic: Leukocytosis (2%)
    Miscellaneous: Transfusion reaction (10%)
Mechanism of Action Stimulates the production, maturation, and activation of neutrophils; filgrastim activates neutrophils to increase both their migration and cytotoxicity.
Pharmacodynamics/Kinetics
  Onset of action: ~24 hours; plateaus in 3-5 days
  Duration: ANC decreases by 50% within 2 days after discontinuing filgrastim; white counts return to the normal range in 4-7 days; peak plasma levels can be maintained for up to 12 hours
  Absorption: SubQ: 100%
  Distribution: V_d: 150 mL/kg; no evidence of drug accumulation over a 11- to 20-day period
  Metabolism: Systemically degraded
  Half-life elimination: 1.8-3.5 hours
  Time to peak, serum: SubQ: 2-8 hours
Pregnancy Risk Factor C

Finacea® *see* Azelaic Acid *on page 174*

Finasteride (fi NAS teer ide)

U.S. Brand Names Propecia®; Proscar®
Canadian Brand Names Propecia®; Proscar®
Mexican Brand Names Propeshia; Proscar
Generic Available Yes
(Continued)

Finasteride *(Continued)*

Pharmacologic Category 5 Alpha-Reductase Inhibitor

Use

Propecia®: Treatment of male pattern hair loss in **men only**. Safety and efficacy were demonstrated in men between 18-41 years of age.

Proscar®: Treatment of symptomatic benign prostatic hyperplasia (BPH); can be used in combination with an alpha-blocker, doxazosin

Unlabeled/Investigational Use Adjuvant monotherapy after radical prostatectomy in the treatment of prostatic cancer; female hirsutism

Local Anesthetic/Vasoconstrictor Precautions No information available to require special precautions

Effects on Dental Treatment No significant effects or complications reported

Common Adverse Effects Note: "Combination therapy" refers to finasteride and doxazosin.

>10%:

Endocrine & metabolic: Impotence (19%; combination therapy 23%), libido decreased (10%; combination therapy 12%)

Genitourinary: Neuromuscular & skeletal: Weakness (5%; combination therapy 17%)

1% to 10%:

Cardiovascular: Postural hypotension (9%; combination therapy 18%), edema (1%, combination therapy 3%)

Central nervous system: Dizziness (7%; combination therapy 23%), somnolence (2%; combination therapy 3%)

Genitourinary: Ejaculation disturbances (7%; combination therapy 14%), decreased volume of ejaculate

Endocrine & metabolic: Gynecomastia (2%)

Respiratory: Dyspnea (1%; combination therapy 2%), rhinitis (1%; combination therapy 2%)

Mechanism of Action Finasteride is a competitive inhibitor of both tissue and hepatic 5-alpha reductase. This results in inhibition of the conversion of testosterone to dihydrotestosterone and markedly suppresses serum dihydrotestosterone levels

Drug Interactions

Cytochrome P450 Effect: Substrate of CYP3A4 (minor)

Pharmacodynamics/Kinetics

Onset of action: 3-6 months of ongoing therapy

Duration:

After a single oral dose as small as 0.5 mg: 65% depression of plasma dihydrotestosterone levels persists 5-7 days

After 6 months of treatment with 5 mg/day: Circulating dihydrotestosterone levels are reduced to castrate levels without significant effects on circulating testosterone; levels return to normal within 14 days of discontinuation of treatment

Distribution: V_{dss}: 76 L

Protein binding: 90%

Metabolism: Hepatic via CYP3A4; two active metabolites (<20% activity of finasteride)

Bioavailability: Mean: 63%

Half-life elimination, serum: Elderly: 8 hours; Adults: 6 hours (3-16)

Time to peak, serum: 2-6 hours

Excretion: Feces (57%) and urine (39%) as metabolites

Pregnancy Risk Factor X

Flavocoxid (fla vo KOKS id)

U.S. Brand Names Limbrel™
Index Terms Flavan; Flavonoid
Pharmacologic Category Anti-inflammatory Agent
Use Clinical dietary management of osteoarthritis, including associated inflammation
Local Anesthetic/Vasoconstrictor Precautions No information available to require special precautions
Effects on Dental Treatment No significant effects or complications reported
Common Adverse Effects
≥2%:
  Cardiovascular: Hypertension, varicose veins
  Dermatologic: Psoriasis
  Gastrointestinal: Occult stools (statistically similar to placebo)
  Neuromuscular & skeletal: Fluid on the knee
Mechanism of Action Exerts anti-inflammatory properties through nonspecific inhibition of cyclooxygenase (COX) and lipoxygenase (5-LOX) pathways; may also possess general analgesic and antioxidant/anticytokine properties
Drug Interactions
  Cytochrome P450 Effect: Inhibits CYP1A2 (weak), 2C9 (weak), 2C19 (weak), 2D6 (weak), 3A4 (weak)
  Increased Effect/Toxicity:
    Concomitant use with NSAIDs may increase the risk of gastrointestinal bleeding.
Pharmacodynamics/Kinetics
  Onset of action: 1-2 hours
  Metabolism: Primarily via glucuronidation and sulfation

Flavonoid see Flavocoxid on page 693

Flavoxate (fla VOKS ate)

U.S. Brand Names Urispas®
Canadian Brand Names Apo-Flavoxate®; Urispas®
Generic Available Yes
Index Terms Flavoxate Hydrochloride
Pharmacologic Category Antispasmodic Agent, Urinary
Use Antispasmodic to provide symptomatic relief of dysuria, nocturia, suprapubic pain, urgency, and incontinence due to detrusor instability and hyper-reflexia in elderly with cystitis, urethritis, urethrocystitis, urethrotrigonitis, and prostatitis
Local Anesthetic/Vasoconstrictor Precautions No information available to require special precautions
Effects on Dental Treatment Key adverse event(s) related to dental treatment: Xerostomia and changes in salivation (normal salivary flow resumes upon discontinuation), and dry throat.
Common Adverse Effects Frequency not defined.
  Cardiovascular: Tachycardia, palpitation
  Central nervous system: Drowsiness, confusion (especially in the elderly), nervousness, fatigue, vertigo, headache, hyperpyrexia
  Dermatologic: Rash, urticaria
  Gastrointestinal: Constipation, nausea, vomiting, xerostomia, dry throat
  Genitourinary: Dysuria
  Hematologic: Leukopenia
  Ocular: Increased intraocular pressure, blurred vision
Mechanism of Action Synthetic antispasmotic with similar actions to that of propantheline; it exerts a direct relaxant effect on smooth muscles via phosphodiesterase inhibition, providing relief to a variety of smooth muscle spasms; it is especially useful for the treatment of bladder spasticity, whereby it produces an increase in urinary capacity
Pharmacodynamics/Kinetics
  Onset of action: 55-60 minutes
  Metabolism: To methyl; flavone carboxylic acid active
  Excretion: Urine (10% to 30%) within 6 hours
Pregnancy Risk Factor B

Flavoxate Hydrochloride see Flavoxate on page 693
Flebogamma® see Immune Globulin (Intravenous) on page 870

Flecainide (fle KAY nide)

Related Information
Cardiovascular Diseases *on page 1726*

U.S. Brand Names Tambocor™

Canadian Brand Names Apo-Flecainide®; Tambocor™

Mexican Brand Names Tambocor

Generic Available Yes

Index Terms Flecainide Acetate

Pharmacologic Category Antiarrhythmic Agent, Class Ic

Use Prevention and suppression of documented life-threatening ventricular arrhythmias (eg, sustained ventricular tachycardia); controlling symptomatic, disabling supraventricular tachycardias in patients without structural heart disease in whom other agents fail

Local Anesthetic/Vasoconstrictor Precautions Flecainide is one of the drugs confirmed to prolong the QT interval and is accepted as having a risk of causing torsade de pointes. The risk of drug-induced torsade de pointes is extremely low when a single QT interval prolonging drug is prescribed. In terms of epinephrine, it is not known what effect vasoconstrictors in the local anesthetic regimen will have in patients with a known history of congenital prolonged QT interval or in patients taking any medication that prolongs the QT interval. Until more information is obtained, it is suggested that the clinician consult with the physician prior to the use of a vasoconstrictor in suspected patients, and that the vasoconstrictor (epinephrine, levonordefrin [Neo-Cobefrin®]) be used with caution.

Effects on Dental Treatment No significant effects or complications reported

Common Adverse Effects
>10%:
 Central nervous system: Dizziness (19% to 30%)
 Ocular: Visual disturbances (16%)
 Respiratory: Dyspnea (~10%)

1% to 10%:
 Cardiovascular: Palpitation (6%), chest pain (5%), edema (3.5%), tachycardia (1% to 3%), proarrhythmic (4% to 12%), sinus node dysfunction (1.2%)
 Central nervous system: Headache (4% to 10%), fatigue (8%), nervousness (5%) additional symptoms occurring at a frequency between 1% and 3%: fever, malaise, hypoesthesia, paresis, ataxia, vertigo, syncope, somnolence, tinnitus, anxiety, insomnia, depression
 Dermatologic: Rash (1% to 3%)
 Gastrointestinal: Nausea (9%), constipation (1%), abdominal pain (3%), anorexia (1% to 3%), diarrhea (0.7% to 3%)
 Neuromuscular & skeletal: Tremor (5%), weakness (5%), paresthesia (1%)
 Ocular: Diplopia (1% to 3%), blurred vision

Mechanism of Action Class Ic antiarrhythmic; slows conduction in cardiac tissue by altering transport of ions across cell membranes; causes slight prolongation of refractory periods; decreases the rate of rise of the action potential without affecting its duration; increases electrical stimulation threshold of ventricle, His-Purkinje system; possesses local anesthetic and moderate negative inotropic effects

Drug Interactions
Cytochrome P450 Effect: Substrate of CYP1A2 (minor), 2D6 (major); Inhibits CYP2D6 (weak)

Increased Effect/Toxicity: CYP2D6 inhibitors may increase the levels/effects of flecainide; example inhibitors include chlorpromazine, delavirdine, fluoxetine, miconazole, paroxetine, pergolide, quinidine, quinine, ritonavir, and ropinirole. Flecainide concentrations may be increased by amiodarone (reduce flecainide 25% to 33%), and propranolol. Beta-adrenergic blockers, disopyramide, verapamil may enhance flecainide's negative inotropic effects. Alkalinizing agents (ie, high-dose antacids, cimetidine, carbonic anhydrase inhibitors, sodium bicarbonate) may decrease flecainide clearance, potentially increasing toxicity. Propranolol blood levels are increased by flecainide.

Decreased Effect: Smoking and acid urine increase flecainide clearance.

Pharmacodynamics/Kinetics
Absorption: Oral: Rapid
Distribution: Adults: V$_d$: 5-13.4 L/kg
Protein binding: Alpha$_1$ glycoprotein: 40% to 50%
Metabolism: Hepatic
Bioavailability: 85% to 90%
Half-life elimination: Infants: 11-12 hours; Children: 8 hours; Adults: 7-22 hours, increased with congestive heart failure or renal dysfunction; End-stage renal disease: 19-26 hours
Time to peak, serum: ~1.5-3 hours

Excretion: Urine (80% to 90%, 10% to 50% as unchanged drug and metabolites)

Pregnancy Risk Factor C

Floctafenine (flok ta FEN een)

Canadian Brand Names Apo-Floctafenine®; Idarac®
Generic Available Yes
Index Terms Floctafenina; Floctafeninum
Pharmacologic Category Nonsteroidal Anti-inflammatory Drug (NSAID), Oral
Use Short-term management of acute, mild-to-moderate pain
Local Anesthetic/Vasoconstrictor Precautions No information available to require special precautions
Effects on Dental Treatment Key adverse event(s) related to dental treatment: Xerostomia and changes in salivation (normal salivary flow resumes upon discontinuation), bitter taste.
Common Adverse Effects Frequency not defined.
Cardiovascular: Edema, flushing, tachycardia
Central nervous system: Depression, dizziness, drowsiness, fatigue, headache, insomnia, irritability, malaise, nervousness, vertigo
Dermatologic: Angioedema, pruritus, rash, urticaria
Endocrine & metabolic: Fluid retention, hyperkalemia
Gastrointestinal: Abdominal pain, bitter taste, constipation, diarrhea, dyspepsia, flatulence, gastrointestinal bleeding, gastrointestinal ulcer, gross bleeding with perforation, heartburn, nausea, vomiting, xerostomia
Hematologic: Agranulocytosis, aplastic anemia, bleeding, leukopenia, neutropenia, thrombocytopenia
Hepatic: Hepatotoxicity, liver enzymes increased
Ocular: Blurred and/or diminished vision
Otic: Tinnitus
Renal: Burning micturition, cystitis, dysuria, hematuria, interstitial nephritis, polyuria, reversible acute renal insufficiency with or without oliguria/anuria, strong smelling urine, urethritis
Respiratory: Asthmatic-type dyspnea
Miscellaneous: Anaphylaxis, diaphoresis, thirst
Restrictions Not available in U.S.
Mechanism of Action Inhibits prostaglandin synthesis by decreasing the activity of the enzyme, cyclooxygenase, which results in decreased formation of prostaglandin precursors
Drug Interactions
Increased Effect/Toxicity: Floctafenine may increase effect/toxicity of anticoagulants (bleeding), antiplatelet agents (bleeding), corticosteroids (GI irritation), cyclosporine (nephrotoxicity), lithium, methotrexate, phenytoin, sulfonylureas, hypoglycemic agents, and sulfonamides. The renal adverse effects of ACE inhibitors may be potentiated by NSAIDS.
Decreased Effect: Floctafenine may decrease the antihypertensive effects of ACE-inhibitors, Angiotensin II antagonists, beta-blockers, and diuretics.
Pharmacodynamics/Kinetics
Duration: 6-8 hours
Absorption: Rapid, well absorbed
Metabolism: Hepatic
(Continued)

Floctafenine *(Continued)*

Half-life elimination: Initial phase (distribution): 1 hour; second phase (elimination): 8 hours

Time to peak, plasma: 1-2 hours

Excretion: Feces and bile (60%); urine (40%)

Pregnancy Risk Factor Risk factor not assigned. Floctafenic acid (active metabolite) crosses the placenta; therefore, the benefits of use must be weighed against risk to mother and fetus.

Floxuridine *(floks YOOR i deen)*

U.S. Brand Names FUDR®

Canadian Brand Names FUDR®

Generic Available Yes

Index Terms Fluorodeoxyuridine; FUDR; 5-FUDR; NSC-27640

Pharmacologic Category Antineoplastic Agent, Antimetabolite (Pyrimidine Antagonist)

Use Management of hepatic metastases of colorectal and gastric cancers

Local Anesthetic/Vasoconstrictor Precautions No information available to require special precautions

Effects on Dental Treatment Key adverse event(s) related to dental treatment: Stomatitis.

Common Adverse Effects

>10%:

Gastrointestinal: Stomatitis, diarrhea; may be dose-limiting

Hematologic: Myelosuppression, may be dose-limiting; leukopenia, thrombocytopenia, anemia

Onset: 4-7 days

Nadir: 5-9 days

Recovery: 21 days

1% to 10%:

Dermatologic: Alopecia, photosensitivity, hyperpigmentation of the skin, localized erythema, dermatitis

Gastrointestinal: Anorexia

Hepatic: Biliary sclerosis, cholecystitis, jaundice

Mechanism of Action Mechanism of action and pharmacokinetics are very similar to fluorouracil; floxuridine is the deoxyribonucleotide of fluorouracil. Floxuridine is a fluorinated pyrimidine antagonist which inhibits DNA and RNA synthesis and methylation of deoxyuridylic acid to thymidylic acid.

Drug Interactions

Increased Effect/Toxicity: Any form of therapy which adds to the stress of the patient, interferes with nutrition, or depresses bone marrow function will increase the toxicity of floxuridine.

Decreased Effect: Patients may experience impaired immune response to vaccines; possible infection after administration of live vaccines in patients receiving immunosuppressants.

Pharmacodynamics/Kinetics

Metabolism: Hepatic; Active metabolites: Floxuridine monophosphate (FUDR-MP) and fluorouracil; Inactive metabolites: Urea, CO_2, α-fluoro-β-alanine, α-fluoro-β-guanidopropionic acid, α-fluoro-β-ureidopropionic acid, and dihydrofluorouracil

Excretion: Urine: Fluorouracil, urea, α-fluoro-β-alanine, α-fluoro-β-guanidopropionic acid, α-fluoro-β-ureidopropionic acid, and dihydrofluorouracil; exhaled gases (CO_2)

Pregnancy Risk Factor D

Flubenisolone *see* Betamethasone *on page 206*
Flucaine® *see* Proparacaine and Fluorescein *on page 1367*

Fluconazole (floo KOE na zole)

Related Information
Fungal Infections *on page 1804*
Treatment of Sexually-Transmitted Infections *on page 1920*
Related Sample Prescriptions
Systemic Fungal Infections *on page 1841*
U.S. Brand Names Diflucan®
Canadian Brand Names Apo-Fluconazole®; Diflucan®; Fluconazole Injection; Fluconazole Omega; Gen-Fluconazole; GMD-Fluconazole; Novo-Fluconazole; Riva-Fluconazole
Mexican Brand Names Diflucan; Flukazol; Oxifungol; Zoldicam
Generic Available Yes
Pharmacologic Category Antifungal Agent, Oral; Antifungal Agent, Parenteral
Dental Use Treatment of susceptible fungal infections in the oral cavity including candidiasis, oral thrush, and chronic mucocutaneous candidiasis treatment of esophageal and oropharyngeal candidiasis caused by *Candida* species; treatment of severe, chronic mucocutaneous candidiasis caused by *Candida* species
Use Treatment of candidiasis (vaginal, oropharyngeal, esophageal, urinary tract infections, peritonitis, pneumonia, and systemic infections); cryptococcal meningitis; antifungal prophylaxis in allogeneic bone marrow transplant recipients
Local Anesthetic/Vasoconstrictor Precautions No information available to require special precautions
Effects on Dental Treatment Key adverse event(s) related to dental treatment: Abnormal taste.
Significant Adverse Effects Frequency not always defined.
Cardiovascular: Angioedema, pallor, QT prolongation (rare, case reports), torsade de pointes(rare, case reports)
Central nervous system: Headache (2% to 13%), seizure, dizziness
Dermatologic: Rash (2%), alopecia, toxic epidermal necrolysis, Stevens-Johnson syndrome
Endocrine & metabolic: Hypercholesterolemia, hypertriglyceridemia, hypokalemia
Gastrointestinal: Nausea (4% to 7%), vomiting (2%), abdominal pain (2% to 6%), diarrhea (2% to 3%), taste perversion, dyspepsia
Hematologic: Agranulocytosis, leukopenia, neutropenia, thrombocytopenia
Hepatic: Hepatic failure (rare), hepatitis, cholestasis, jaundice, increased ALT/AST, increased alkaline phosphatase
Respiratory: Dyspnea
Miscellaneous: Anaphylactic reactions (rare)
Dental Usual Dosing Candidiasis: Adults:
Usual dosage range: 200-400 mg/day; duration and dosage depends on severity of infection
Oropharyngeal (long-term suppression): 200 mg/day; chronic therapy is recommended in immunocompromised patients with history of oropharyngeal candidiasis (OPC)
Dosage The daily dose of fluconazole is the same for oral and I.V. administration
Usual dosage ranges:
Neonates: First 2 weeks of life, especially premature neonates: Same dose as older children every 72 hours
Children: Loading dose: 6-12 mg/kg; maintenance: 3-12 mg/kg/day; duration and dosage depends on severity of infection
Adults: 200-400 mg/day; duration and dosage depends on severity of infection

Indication-specific dosing:
Children:
Candidiasis:
Oropharyngeal: Loading dose: 6 mg/kg; maintenance: 3 mg/kg/day for 2 weeks
Esophageal: Loading dose: 6 mg/kg; maintenance: 3-12 mg/kg/day for 21 days and at least 2 weeks following resolution of symptoms
Systemic infection: 6 mg/kg every 12 hours for 28 days
Meningitis, cryptococcal: Loading dose: 12 mg/kg; maintenance: 6-12 mg/kg/day for 10-12 weeks following negative CSF culture; relapse suppression: 6 mg/kg/day
(Continued)

Fluconazole *(Continued)*

Adults:

Candidiasis:

Candidemia, primary therapy, non-neutropenic: 400-800 mg/day for 14 days after last positive blood culture and resolution of signs/symptoms

Alternate therapy: 800 mg/day with amphotericin B for 4-7 days followed by 800 mg/day for 14 days after last positive blood culture and resolution of signs/symptoms

Candidemia, secondary, neutropenic: 6-12 mg/kg/day for 14 days after last positive blood culture and resolution of signs/symptoms

Chronic, disseminated: 6 mg/kg/day for 3-6 months

Oropharyngeal (long-term suppression): 200 mg/day; chronic therapy is recommended in immunocompromised patients with history of oropharyngeal candidiasis (OPC)

Osteomyelitis: 6 mg/kg/day for 6-12 months

Esophageal: 200 mg on day 1, then 100-200 mg/day for 2-3 weeks after clinical improvement

Prophylaxis in bone marrow transplant: 400 mg/day; begin 3 days before onset of neutropenia and continue for 7 days after neutrophils >1000 cells/mm^3

Urinary: 200 mg/day for 1-2 weeks

Vaginal: 150 mg as a single dose

Coccidiomycosis: 400 mg/day; doses of 800-1000 mg/day have been used for meningeal disease; usual duration of therapy ranges from 3-6 months for primary uncomplicated infections and up to 1 year for pulmonary (chronic and diffuse) infection

Endocarditis, prosthetic valve, early: 6-12 mg/kg/day for 6 weeks after valve replacement

Endophthalmitis: 6-12 mg/kg/day or 400-800 mg/day for 6-12 weeks after surgical intervention. **Note:** *C. krusei* and *C. galbrata* infection acquired exogenously should be treated with voriconazole.

Meningitis, cryptococcal: 400-800 mg/day for 10-12 weeks or with flucytosine 100-150 mg/day for 6 weeks; maintenance: 200-400 mg/day

Pneumonia, cryptococcal (mild-to-moderate): 200-400 mg/day for 6-12 months (life-long in HIV-positive patients)

Dosing adjustment/interval in renal impairment:

No adjustment for vaginal candidiasis single-dose therapy

For multiple dosing, administer usual load then adjust daily doses

Cl$_{cr}$ ≤50 mL/minute (no dialysis): Administer 50% of recommended dose or administer every 48 hours.

Hemodialysis: 50% is removed by hemodialysis; administer 100% of daily dose (according to indication) after each dialysis treatment.

Continuous arteriovenous or venovenous hemofiltration: Dose as for Cl$_{cr}$ 10-50 mL/minute.

Mechanism of Action Interferes with cytochrome P450 activity, decreasing ergosterol synthesis (principal sterol in fungal cell membrane) and inhibiting cell membrane formation

Contraindications Hypersensitivity to fluconazole, other azoles, or any component of the formulation; concomitant administration with cisapride

Warnings/Precautions Should be used with caution in patients with renal and hepatic dysfunction or previous hepatotoxicity from other azole derivatives. Patients who develop abnormal liver function tests during fluconazole therapy should be monitored closely and discontinued if symptoms consistent with liver disease develop. Rare exfoliative skin disorders have been observed; monitor closely if rash develops. the manufacturer reports rare cases of QT$_c$ prolongation and TdP associated with fluconazole use and advises caution in patients with concomitant medications or conditions which are arrhythmogenic. However, given the limited number of cases and the presence of multiple confounding variables, the likelihood that fluconazole causes conduction abnormalities appears remote.

Drug Interactions Inhibits CYP1A2 (weak), 2C9 (strong), 2C19 (strong), 3A4 (moderate)

Benzodiazepines (metabolized by oxidation, eg, alprazolam, triazolam, midazolam, diazepam) serum concentrations are increased by fluconazole which may cause increased CNS sedation. Consider a benzodiazepine not metabolized by CYP3A4 or another antifungal.

Caffeine's metabolism is decreased; monitor for tachycardia, nervousness, and anxiety.

Calcium channel blockers may have increased serum concentrations; consider another agent instead of a calcium channel blocker, another antifungal, or reduce the dose of the calcium channel blocker. Monitor blood pressure.

Cisapride's serum concentration is increased which may lead to malignant arrhythmias; concurrent use is contraindicated.

Cyclosporine's serum concentration is increased; monitor cyclosporine's serum concentration and renal function.

CYP2C9 Substrates: Fluconazole may increase the levels/effects of CYP2C9 substrates. Example substrates include bosentan, dapsone, fluoxetine, glimepiride, glipizide, losartan, montelukast, nateglinide, paclitaxel, phenytoin, warfarin, and zafirlukast.

CYP2C19 substrates: Fluconazole may increase the levels/effects of CYP2C19 substrates. Example substrates include citalopram, diazepam, methsuximide, phenytoin, propranolol, and sertraline.

CYP3A4 substrates: Fluconazole may increase the levels/effects of CYP3A4 substrates. Example substrates include benzodiazepines, calcium channel blockers, cyclosporine, mirtazapine, nateglinide, nefazodone, sildenafil (and other PDE-5 inhibitors), tacrolimus, and venlafaxine. Selected benzodiazepines (midazolam and triazolam), cisapride, ergot alkaloids, selected HMG-CoA reductase inhibitors (lovastatin and simvastatin), and pimozide are generally contraindicated with strong CYP3A4 inhibitors.

HMG-CoA reductase inhibitors (except pravastatin and fluvastatin) have increased serum concentrations; switch to pravastatin/fluvastatin or monitor for development of myopathy.

Losartan's active metabolite is reduced in concentration; consider another antihypertensive agent unaffected by the azole antifungals, another antifungal, or monitor blood pressure closely.

Phenytoin's serum concentration is increased; monitor phenytoin levels and adjust dose as needed.

Rifampin decreases fluconazole's serum concentration; monitor infection status.

Tacrolimus's serum concentration is increased; monitor tacrolimus's serum concentration and renal function.

Warfarin's effects are increased; monitor INR and adjust warfarin's dose as needed.

Dietary Considerations Take with or without regard to food.

Pharmacodynamics/Kinetics

Distribution: Widely throughout body with good penetration into CSF, eye, peritoneal fluid, sputum, skin, and urine

Relative diffusion blood into CSF: Adequate with or without inflammation (exceeds usual MICs)

CSF:blood level ratio: Normal meninges: 70% to 80%; Inflamed meninges: >70% to 80%

Protein binding, plasma: 11% to 12%

Bioavailability: Oral: >90%

Half-life elimination: Normal renal function: ~30 hours

Time to peak, serum: Oral: 1-2 hours

Excretion: Urine (80% as unchanged drug)

Pregnancy Risk Factor C

Lactation Enters breast/not recommended (AAP rates "compatible")

Breast-Feeding Considerations Fluconazole is found in breast milk at concentration similar to plasma.

Dosage Forms Excipient information presented when available (limited, particularly for generics); consult specific product labeling.

Infusion [premixed in sodium chloride or dextrose]: 200 mg (100 mL); 400 mg (200 mL)

Diflucan® [premixed in sodium chloride or dextrose]: 200 mg (100 mL); 400 mg (200 mL)

Powder for oral suspension: 10 mg/mL (35 mL); 40 mg/mL (35 mL)

Diflucan®: 10 mg/mL (35 mL); 40 mg/mL (35 mL) [contains sodium benzoate; orange flavor]

Tablet: 50 mg, 100 mg, 150 mg, 200 mg

Diflucan®: 50 mg, 100 mg, 150 mg, 200 mg

Flucytosine (floo SYE toe seen)

U.S. Brand Names Ancobon®
Canadian Brand Names Ancobon®
Generic Available No
Index Terms 5-FC; 5-Fluorocytosine; 5-Flurocytosine
Pharmacologic Category Antifungal Agent, Oral
Use Adjunctive treatment of systemic fungal infections (eg, septicemia, endocarditis, UTI, meningitis, or pulmonary) caused by susceptible strains of *Candida* or *Cryptococcus*
(Continued)

Flucytosine *(Continued)*

Local Anesthetic/Vasoconstrictor Precautions No information available to require special precautions

Effects on Dental Treatment No significant effects or complications reported

Common Adverse Effects Frequency not defined.

Cardiovascular: Cardiac arrest, myocardial toxicity, ventricular dysfunction, chest pain

Central nervous system: Ataxia, confusion, dizziness, drowsiness, fatigue, hallucinations, headache, parkinsonism, psychosis, pyrexia, sedation, seizure, vertigo

Dermatologic: Rash, photosensitivity, pruritus, toxic epidermal necrolysis, urticaria

Endocrine & metabolic: Hypoglycemia, hypokalemia

Gastrointestinal: Abdominal pain, diarrhea, dry mouth, duodenal ulcer, hemorrhage, loss of appetite, nausea, ulcerative colitis, vomiting

Hematologic: Agranulocytosis, anemia, aplastic anemia, eosinophilia, leukopenia, pancytopenia, thrombocytopenia

Hepatic: Acute hepatic injury, bilirubin increased, hepatic dysfunction, jaundice, liver enzymes increased

Neuromuscular & skeletal: Paresthesia, peripheral neuropathy, weakness

Otic: Hearing loss

Renal: Azotemia, BUN increased, crystalluria, renal failure, serum creatinine increased

Respiratory: Dyspnea, respiratory arrest

Miscellaneous: Allergic reaction

Mechanism of Action Penetrates fungal cells and is converted to fluorouracil which competes with uracil interfering with fungal RNA and protein synthesis

Drug Interactions

Decreased Effect: Cytarabine may decrease levels/effects of flucytosine.

Pharmacodynamics/Kinetics

Absorption: 76% to 89%

Distribution: Into CSF, aqueous humor, joints, peritoneal fluid, and bronchial secretions; V_d: 0.6 L/kg

Protein binding: 3% to 4%

Metabolism: Minimally hepatic; deaminated, possibly via gut bacteria, to 5-fluorouracil

Half-life elimination:

Normal renal function: 2-5 hours

Anuria: 85 hours (range: 30-250)

End stage renal disease: 75-200 hours

Time to peak, serum: ~1-2 hours

Excretion: Urine (>90% as unchanged drug)

Pregnancy Risk Factor C

Fludara® *see Fludarabine on page 700*

Fludarabine *(floo DARE a been)*

U.S. Brand Names Fludara®

Canadian Brand Names Beneflur®; Fludara®

Mexican Brand Names Fludara

Generic Available Yes

Index Terms Fludarabine Phosphate; NSC-312887

Pharmacologic Category Antineoplastic Agent, Antimetabolite (Purine Antagonist)

Use

I.V.: Treatment of chronic lymphocytic leukemia (CLL) (including refractory CLL); non-Hodgkin's lymphoma in adults

Oral (formulation not available in U.S.): Approved in Canada for treatment of CLL

Unlabeled/Investigational Use Treatment of non-Hodgkin's lymphoma and acute leukemias in pediatric patients; reduced-intensity conditioning regimens prior to allogeneic hematopoietic stem cell transplantation (generally administered in combination with busulfan and antithymocyte globulin or lymphocyte immune globulin, or in combination with melphalan and alemtuzumab)

Local Anesthetic/Vasoconstrictor Precautions No information available to require special precautions

Effects on Dental Treatment Key adverse event(s) related to dental treatment: Stomatitis.

Common Adverse Effects

>10%:

Cardiovascular: Edema (8% to 19%)

Central nervous system: Fever (60% to 69%), fatigue (10% to 38%), pain (20% to 22%), chills (11% to 19%)

Dermatologic: Rash (15%)

Gastrointestinal: Nausea/vomiting (mild: 31% to 36%), anorexia (7% to 34%), diarrhea (13% to 15%), gastrointestinal bleeding (3% to 13%)

Genitourinary: Urinary tract infection (2% to 15%)

Hematologic: Myelosuppression (nadir: 10-14 days; recovery: 5-7 weeks; dose-limiting toxicity), anemia (60%), neutropenia (grade 4: 59%; nadir: ~13 days), thrombocytopenia (50% to 55%; nadir: ~16 days)

Neuromuscular & skeletal: Weakness (9% to 65%), myalgia (4% to 16%), paresthesia (4% to 12%)

Ocular: Visual disturbance (3% to 15%)

Respiratory: Cough (10% to 44%), pneumonia (16% to 22%), dyspnea (9% to 22%), upper respiratory infection (2% to 16%)

Miscellaneous: Infection (33% to 44%), diaphoresis (1% to 13%)

1% to 10%:

Cardiovascular: Angina (≤6%), CHF (≤3%), arrhythmia (≤3%), cerebrovascular accident (≤3%), MI (≤3%), supraventricular tachycardia (≤3%), deep vein thrombosis (1% to 3%), phlebitis (1% to 3%), aneurysm (≤1%), transient ischemic attack (≤1%)

Central nervous system: Malaise (6% to 8%), headache (≤3%), sleep disorder (1% to 3%), cerebellar syndrome (≤1%), depression (≤1%), mentation impaired (≤1%)

Dermatologic: Alopecia (≤3%), pruritus (1% to 3%), seborrhea (≤1%)

Endocrine & metabolic: Hyperglycemia (1% to 6%), dehydration (≤1%)

Gastrointestinal: Stomatitis (≤9%), esophagitis (≤3%), constipation (1% to 3%), mucositis (≤2%), dysphagia (≤1%)

Genitourinary: Dysuria (3% to 4%), hesitancy (≤3%)

Hematologic: Hemorrhage (≤1%)

Hepatic: Cholelithiasis (≤3%), liver function tests abnormal (1% to 3%), liver failure (≤1%)

Neuromuscular & skeletal: Osteoporosis (≤2%), arthralgia (≤1%)

Otic: Hearing loss (2% to 6%)

Renal: Hematuria (2% to 3%), renal failure (≤1%), renal function test abnormal (≤1%), proteinuria (≤1%)

Respiratory: Pharyngitis (≤9%), allergic pneumonitis (≤6%), hemoptysis (1% to 6%), sinusitis (≤5%), bronchitis (≤1%), epistaxis (≤1%), hypoxia (≤1%)

Miscellaneous: Anaphylaxis (≤1%), tumor lysis syndrome (1%)

Mechanism of Action Fludarabine inhibits DNA synthesis by inhibition of DNA polymerase, ribonucleotide reductase and DNA primase.

Drug Interactions

Increased Effect/Toxicity: Combined use with pentostatin may lead to severe, even fatal, pulmonary toxicity.

Pharmacodynamics/Kinetics

Distribution: V_d: 38-96 L/m^2; widely with extensive tissue binding

Metabolism: I.V.: Fludarabine phosphate is rapidly dephosphorylated to 2-fluoro-vidarabine, which subsequently enters tumor cells and is phosphorylated by deoxycytidine kinase to the active triphosphate derivative; rapidly dephosphorylated in the serum

Bioavailability: 75%

Half-life elimination: 2-fluoro-vidarabine: 9 hours

Excretion: Urine (60%, 23% as 2-fluoro-vidarabine) within 24 hours

Pregnancy Risk Factor D

Fludarabine Phosphate see Fludarabine on page 700

Fludrocortisone (floo droe KOR ti sone)

U.S. Brand Names Florinef®

Canadian Brand Names Florinef®

Generic Available Yes

Index Terms 9α-Fluorohydrocortisone Acetate; Fludrocortisone Acetate; Fluohydrisone Acetate; Fluohydrocortisone Acetate

Pharmacologic Category Corticosteroid, Systemic

Use Partial replacement therapy for primary and secondary adrenocortical insufficiency in Addison's disease; treatment of salt-losing adrenogenital syndrome

Local Anesthetic/Vasoconstrictor Precautions No information available to require special precautions

Effects on Dental Treatment No significant effects or complications reported

Significant Adverse Effects Frequency not defined.

Cardiovascular: Hypertension, edema, CHF

Central nervous system: Convulsions, headache, dizziness

Dermatologic: Acne, rash, bruising

(Continued)

Fludrocortisone *(Continued)*

Endocrine & metabolic: Hypokalemic alkalosis, suppression of growth, hyperglycemia, HPA suppression

Gastrointestinal: Peptic ulcer

Neuromuscular & skeletal: Muscle weakness

Ocular: Cataracts

Miscellaneous: Diaphoresis, anaphylaxis (generalized)

Dosage Oral:

Infants and Children: 0.05-0.1 mg/day

Adults: 0.1-0.2 mg/day with ranges of 0.1 mg 3 times/week to 0.2 mg/day

Addison's disease: Initial: 0.1 mg/day; if transient hypertension develops, reduce the dose to 0.05 mg/day. Preferred administration with cortisone (10-37.5 mg/day) or hydrocortisone (10-30 mg/day).

Salt-losing adrenogenital syndrome: 0.1-0.2 mg/day

Mechanism of Action Promotes increased reabsorption of sodium and loss of potassium from renal distal tubules

Contraindications Hypersensitivity to fludrocortisone or any component of the formulation; systemic fungal infections

Warnings/Precautions May cause hypercorticism or suppression of hypothalamic-pituitary-adrenal (HPA) axis, particularly in younger children or in patients receiving high doses for prolonged periods. HPA axis suppression may lead to adrenal crisis. Withdrawal and discontinuation of a corticosteroid should be done slowly and carefully. Fludrocortisone is primarily a mineralocorticoid agonist, but may also inhibit the HPA axis. May increase risk of infection and/or limit response to vaccinations; close observation is required in patients with latent tuberculosis and/or TB reactivity. Restrict use in active TB (only in conjunction with antituberculosis treatment). Use with caution in patients with sodium retention and potassium loss, hepatic impairment, myocardial infarction, osteoporosis, and/or renal impairment. Use with caution in the elderly. Withdraw therapy with gradual tapering of dose. Safety and efficacy have not been established in children.

Drug Interactions Decreased effect:

Anticholinesterases effects are antagonized

Decreased corticosteroid effects by rifampin, barbiturates, and hydantoins

Decreased salicylate levels

Dietary Considerations Systemic use of mineralocorticoids/corticosteroids may require a diet with increased potassium, vitamins A, B_6, C, D, folate, calcium, zinc, and phosphorus, and decreased sodium. With fludrocortisone, a decrease in dietary sodium is often not required as the increased retention of sodium is usually the desired therapeutic effect.

Pharmacodynamics/Kinetics

Absorption: Rapid and complete

Protein binding: 42%

Metabolism: Hepatic

Half-life elimination, plasma: 30-35 minutes; Biological: 18-36 hours

Time to peak, serum: ~1.7 hours

Pregnancy Risk Factor C

Lactation Excretion in breast milk unknown

Dosage Forms Excipient information presented when available (limited, particularly for generics); consult specific product labeling.

Tablet, as acetate: 0.1 mg

Fludrocortisone Acetate *see* Fludrocortisone *on page 701*

FluLaval™ *see* Influenza Virus Vaccine *on page 880*

Flumadine® *see* Rimantadine *on page 1427*

Flumazenil *(FLOO may ze nil)*

U.S. Brand Names Romazicon®

Canadian Brand Names Anexate®; Flumazenil Injection; Flumazenil Injection, USP; Romazicon®

Mexican Brand Names Lanexat

Generic Available Yes

Pharmacologic Category Antidote

Use Benzodiazepine antagonist; reverses sedative effects of benzodiazepines used in conscious sedation and general anesthesia; treatment of benzodiazepine overdose

Local Anesthetic/Vasoconstrictor Precautions No information available to require special precautions

Effects on Dental Treatment Key adverse event(s) related to dental treatment: Xerostomia (normal salivary flow resumes upon discontinuation).

Common Adverse Effects

>10%: Gastrointestinal: Vomiting, nausea

1% to 10%:

Cardiovascular: Palpitation

Central nervous system: Headache, anxiety, nervousness, insomnia, abnormal crying, euphoria, depression, agitation, dizziness, emotional lability, ataxia, depersonalization, increased tears, dysphoria, paranoia, fatigue, vertigo

Endocrine & metabolic: Hot flashes

Gastrointestinal: Xerostomia

Local: Pain at injection site

Neuromuscular & skeletal: Tremor, weakness, paresthesia

Ocular: Abnormal vision, blurred vision

Respiratory: Dyspnea, hyperventilation

Miscellaneous: Diaphoresis

Dosage

Children and Adults: I.V.: See table.

Flumazenil

Pediatric Dosage (further studies needed)	
Pediatric dosage for **reversal of conscious sedation and general anesthesia:**	
Initial dose	0.01 mg/kg over 15 seconds (maximum: 0.2 mg)
Repeat doses (maximum: 4 doses)	0.005-0.01 mg/kg (maximum: 0.2 mg) repeated at 1-minute intervals
Maximum total cumulative dose	1 mg or 0.05 mg/kg (whichever is lower)
Adult Dosage	
Adult dosage for **reversal of conscious sedation and general anesthesia:**	
Initial dose	0.2 mg intravenously over 15 seconds
Repeat doses	If desired level of consciousness is not obtained, 0.2 mg may be repeated at 1-minute intervals.
Maximum total cumulative dose	1 mg (usual dose: 0.6-1 mg) **In the event of resedation:** Repeat doses may be given at 20-minute intervals with maximum of 1 mg/dose and 3 mg/hour.
Adult dosage for **suspected benzodiazepine overdose:**	
Initial dose	0.2 mg intravenously over 30 seconds; if the desired level of consciousness is not obtained, 0.3 mg can be given over 30 seconds
Repeat doses	0.5 mg over 30 seconds repeated at 1-minute intervals
Maximum total cumulative dose	3 mg (usual dose 1-3 mg) Patients with a partial response at 3 mg may require additional titration up to a total dose of 5 mg. If a patient has not responded 5 minutes after cumulative dose of 5 mg, the major cause of sedation is not likely due to benzodiazepines. **In the event of resedation:** May repeat doses at 20-minute intervals with maximum of 1 mg/dose and 3 mg/hour.

Resedation: Repeated doses may be given at 20-minute intervals as needed; repeat treatment doses of 1 mg (at a rate of 0.5 mg/minute) should be given at any time and no more than 3 mg should be given in any hour. After intoxication with high doses of benzodiazepines, the duration of a single dose of flumazenil is not expected to exceed 1 hour; if desired, the period of wakefulness may be prolonged with repeated low intravenous doses of flumazenil, or by an infusion of 0.1-0.4 mg/hour. Most patients with benzodiazepine overdose will respond to a cumulative dose of 1-3 mg and doses >3 mg do not reliably produce additional effects. Rarely, patients with a partial response at 3 mg may require additional titration up to a total dose of 5 mg. **If a patient has not responded 5 minutes after receiving a cumulative dose of 5 mg, the major cause of sedation is not likely to be due to benzodiazepines.**

Elderly: No differences in safety or efficacy have been reported. However, increased sensitivity may occur in some elderly patients.

Dosing in renal impairment: Not significantly affected by renal failure (Cl_{cr} <10 mL/minute) or hemodialysis beginning 1 hour after drug administration

Dosing in hepatic impairment: Initial dose of flumazenil used for initial reversal of benzodiazepine effects is not changed; however, subsequent doses in liver disease patients should be reduced in size or frequency

Mechanism of Action Competitively inhibits the activity at the benzodiazepine recognition site on the GABA/benzodiazepine receptor complex. Flumazenil does not antagonize the CNS effect of drugs affecting GABA-ergic neurons by means other than the benzodiazepine receptor (ethanol, barbiturates, general anesthetics) and does not reverse the effects of opioids

(Continued)

Flumazenil (Continued)

Contraindications Hypersensitivity to flumazenil, benzodiazepines, or any component of the formulation; patients given benzodiazepines for control of potentially life-threatening conditions (eg, control of intracranial pressure or status epilepticus); patients who are showing signs of serious cyclic-antidepressant overdosage

Warnings/Precautions **[U.S. Boxed Warning]: Benzodiazepine reversal may result in seizures in some patients.** Patients who may develop seizures include patients on benzodiazepines for long-term sedation, tricyclic antidepressant overdose patients, concurrent major sedative-hypnotic drug withdrawal, recent therapy with repeated doses of parenteral benzodiazepines, myoclonic jerking or seizure activity prior to flumazenil administration. Flumazenil does not reverse respiratory depression/hypoventilation or cardiac depression. Resedation occurs more frequently in patients where a large single dose or cumulative dose of a benzodiazepine is administered along with a neuromuscular blocking agent and multiple anesthetic agents. Flumazenil should be used with caution in the intensive care unit because of increased risk of unrecognized benzodiazepine dependence in such settings. Should not be used to diagnose benzodiazepine-induced sedation. Reverse neuromuscular blockade before considering use. Flumazenil does not antagonize the CNS effects of other GABA agonists (such as ethanol, barbiturates, or general anesthetics); nor does it reverse narcotics. Use with caution in patients with a history of panic disorder; may provoke panic attacks. Use caution in drug and ethanol-dependent patients; these patients may also be dependent on benzodiazepines. Not recommended for treatment of benzodiazepine dependence. Use with caution in head injury patients. Use caution in patients with mixed drug overdoses; toxic effects of other drugs taken may emerge once benzodiazepine effects are reversed. Flumazenil does not consistently reverse amnesia; patient may not recall verbal instructions after procedure. Use caution in severe hepatic dysfunction and in patients relying on a benzodiazepine for seizure control. Safety and efficacy have not been established in children <1 year of age.

Drug Interactions

Increased Effect/Toxicity: Flumazenil reverses the effects of these nonbenzodiazepine hypnotics (zaleplon, zolpidem, zopiclone).

Pharmacodynamics/Kinetics

Onset of action: 1-3 minutes; 80% response within 3 minutes
Peak effect: 6-10 minutes
Duration: Resedation: ~1 hour; duration related to dose given and benzodiazepine plasma concentrations; reversal effects of flumazenil may wear off before effects of benzodiazepine
Distribution: Initial V_d: 0.5 L/kg; V_{dss} 0.77-1.6 L/kg
Protein binding: 40% to 50%
Metabolism: Hepatic; dependent upon hepatic blood flow
Half-life elimination: Adults: Alpha: 7-15 minutes; Terminal: 41-79 minutes
Excretion: Feces; urine (0.2% as unchanged drug)

Pregnancy Risk Factor C

Dosage Forms

Injection, solution: 0.1 mg/mL (5 mL, 10 mL)
Romazicon®: 0.1 mg/mL (5 mL, 10 mL)

fluMist® *see* Influenza Virus Vaccine *on page 880*

Flunarizine (floo NAR i zeen)

Canadian Brand Names Apo-Flunarizine®; Novo-Flunarizine; Sibelium®
Generic Available Yes
Index Terms Flunarizine Hydrochloride
Pharmacologic Category Calcium Channel Antagonist
Use Prophylaxis of classic (with aura) or common (without aura) migraine; symptomatic treatment of vestibular vertigo (due to a diagnosed functional disorder of the vestibular system)
Local Anesthetic/Vasoconstrictor Precautions No information available to require special precautions
Effects on Dental Treatment Key adverse event(s) related to dental treatment: Xerostomia and changes in salivation (normal salivary flow resumes upon discontinuation).
Common Adverse Effects Frequency not defined.
Central nervous system: Anxiety, dizziness, drowsiness, fatigue, insomnia, vertigo
Dermatologic: Rash
Endocrine & metabolic: Galactorrhea, prolactin levels increased

Gastrointestinal: Appetite increased, epigastric pain, heartburn, nausea, vomiting, weight gain, xerostomia

Neuromuscular & skeletal: Asthenia/weakness, muscle ache

Restrictions Not available in U.S.

Mechanism of Action Flunarizine is a selective calcium channel antagonist that prevents cellular calcium overload by reducing transmembrane calcium influx; also has antihistamine properties.

Drug Interactions

Cytochrome P450 Effect: Substrate of CYP2D6

Increased Effect/Toxicity: Sedative effects and/or respiratory depression may be additive with CNS depressants; includes ethanol, barbiturates, narcotic analgesics, and other sedative agents; monitor for increased effect. CYP2D6 inhibitors may increase the levels/effects of flunarizine (example inhibitors include delavirdine, fluoxetine, miconazole, paroxetine, pergolide, quinidine, quinine, ritonavir, and ropinirole). Concurrent use with oral contraceptives has been reported to cause galactorrhea (case reports). Blood pressure-lowering effects of PDE-5 inhibitors (sildenafil, tadalafil, vardenafil) may be additive; use caution. Effect of antihypertensive agents may be potentiated by flunarizine.

Decreased Effect: Hepatic enzyme inducing drugs may increase metabolism/decrease serum concentrations of flunarizine. Flunarizine may decrease mephenytoin levels.

Pharmacodynamics/Kinetics

Absorption: Well absorbed

Distribution: V_d: Mean: 43.2 L/kg

Protein binding: 99%

Metabolism: Hepatic: N-oxidation, aromatic hydroxylation

Half-life elimination: ~19 days

Time to peak, plasma: 2-4 hours

Excretion: Urine (minimal)

Flunarizine Hydrochloride see Flunarizine on page 704

Flunisolide (floo NISS oh lide)

Related Information

Respiratory Diseases on page 1747

U.S. Brand Names AeroBid®; AeroBid®-M; Aerospan™; Nasarel®

Canadian Brand Names Alti-Flunisolide; Apo-Flunisolide®; Nasalide®; PMS-Flunisolide; Rhinalar®

Generic Available Yes: Nasal spray

Pharmacologic Category Corticosteroid, Inhalant (Oral); Corticosteroid, Nasal

Use Steroid-dependent asthma; nasal solution is used for seasonal or perennial rhinitis

Local Anesthetic/Vasoconstrictor Precautions No information available to require special precautions

Effects on Dental Treatment Key adverse event(s) related to dental treatment: *Candida* infections of the nose or pharynx, atrophic rhinitis, sore throat, bitter taste, palpitations, dizziness, headache, nervousness, GI irritation, sneezing, coughing, upper respiratory tract infection, bronchitis, nasal congestion, nasal dryness and burning, increased susceptibility to infections, xerostomia (normal salivary flow resumes upon discontinuation), dry throat, loss of taste, epistaxis, and diaphoresis.

Common Adverse Effects

>10%:

Central nervous system: Headache (intranasal <5%; oral 9% to 25%)

Gastrointestinal: Aftertaste (10% to 17%)

Respiratory: Nasal burning (intranasal 45%), pharyngitis (14% to 20%), rhinitis (<15%), nasal irritation (>1% to 13%)

1% to 10%:

Cardiovascular: Chest pain (1% to 3%), edema (1% to 3%), chest tightness, hypertension, palpitation, tachycardia

Central nervous system: Fever (1% to 9%), dizziness (1% to 3%), insomnia (1% to 3%), migraine (1% to 3%), chills, malaise, irritability, shakiness, anxiety, depression, faintness, fatigue, moodiness, vertigo

Dermatologic: Erythema multiform (1% to 3%), acne, eczema, pruritus, urticaria

Endocrine & metabolic: Dysmenorrhea (1% to 3%)

Gastrointestinal: Dyspepsia (2% to 4%), abdominal pain (1% to 3%), diarrhea (1% to 10%), gastroenteritis (1% to 3%), nausea (Aerospan™: 1% to 3%), (Continued)

Flunisolide (Continued)

oral candidiasis (1% to 3%), taste perversion (1% to 3%), abdominal full-ness, constipation, gas, heartburn, sore throat, dry throat, mouth discomfort, throat irritation

Genitourinary: Vaginitis (1% to 3%), urinary tract infection (1% to 4%)

Neuromuscular & skeletal: Myalgia (1% to 3%), neck pain (1% to 3%), numb-ness, weakness

Ocular: Conjunctivitis (1% to 3%), blurred vision

Renal: Laryngitis (1% to 3%)

Respiratory: Sinusitis (<9%), epistaxia (<3%), bronchospasm, cough increased, dyspnea, hoarseness, nasal ulcer, sneezing, wheezing

Miscellaneous: Allergy (4% to 5%), infection (3% to 9%), loss of smell, voice alteration (1% to 3%), flu-like syndrome, diaphoresis

<1%: Adrenal suppression

Mechanism of Action Decreases inflammation by suppression of migration of polymorphonuclear leukocytes and reversal of increased capillary permeability; does not depress hypothalamus

Drug Interactions

Cytochrome P450 Effect:

Substrate of CYP3A4 (major)

Increased Effect/Toxicity: Expected interactions similar to other corticoste-roids. CYP3A4 inhibitors may increase the levels/effects of flunisolide; monitor for HPA axis suppression. Salmeterol has been demonstrated to improve response to inhaled corticosteroids (as compared to increasing steroid dosage).

Pharmacodynamics/Kinetics

Absorption: Nasal inhalation: ~50%

Metabolism: Rapidly hepatic to active metabolites

Bioavailability: 40% to 50%

Half-life elimination: 1.8 hours

Excretion: Urine and feces (equal amounts)

Pregnancy Risk Factor C

Fluocinolone (floo oh SIN oh lone)

U.S. Brand Names Capex™; Derma-Smoothe/FS®; Retisert™; Synalar®

Canadian Brand Names Capex™; Derma-Smoothe/FS®; Synalar®

Mexican Brand Names Cortilona; Fusalar; Synalar Simple

Generic Available Yes: Excludes ocular implant, oil, shampoo

Index Terms Fluocinolone Acetonide

Pharmacologic Category Corticosteroid, Ophthalmic; Corticosteroid, Topical

Dental Use Relief of inflammatory and pruritic manifestations (low, medium, high potency topical corticosteroid)

Use Relief of susceptible inflammatory dermatosis [low, medium, high potency topical corticosteroid]; psoriasis of the scalp; atopic dermatitis in children ≥2 years of age

Ocular implant (Retisert™): Treatment of chronic, noninfectious uveitis affecting the posterior segment of the eye.

Local Anesthetic/Vasoconstrictor Precautions No information available to require special precautions

Effects on Dental Treatment No significant effects or complications reported

Significant Adverse Effects Topical: Frequency not defined.

Dermatologic: Acneiform eruptions, allergic contact dermatitis, burning, dryness, folliculitis, irritation, itching, hypertrichosis, hypopigmentation, mili-aria, perioral dermatitis, skin atrophy, striae

Endocrine & metabolic: Cushing's syndrome, HPA axis suppression

Miscellaneous: Secondary infection

Ocular implant:

>50%: Ocular: Cataract, intraocular pressure increased, eye pain; procedural complications (eg, cataract fragments, implant migration, wound complica-tions)

10% to 35%:

Central nervous system: Dizziness (5% to 15%), headache (31%), pain (5% to 15%), pyrexia (5% to 15%)

Dermatologic: Rash (5% to 15%)

Gastrointestinal (5% to 15%): Nausea, vomiting

Neuromuscular & skeletal (5% to 15%): Arthralgia, back pain, limb pain

Ocular: Blurred vision, conjunctival hemorrhage, conjunctival hyperemia, dry eye, eye irritation/inflammation, eyelid edema, glaucoma, hypotony, maculopathy, pruritus, ptosis, tearing, visual acuity decrease, vitreous floaters, vitreous hemorrhage

Respiratory (5% to 15%): Cough, influenza, nasopharyngitis, sinusitis, upper respiratory infection

5% to 9%: Ocular: Blepharitis, choroidal detachment, conjunctival edema/chemosis, corneal edema, eye discharge, eye swelling, macular edema, photophobia, photopsia, retinal hemorrhage, visual disturbance, vitreous opacitites

Frequency not specified: Miscellaneous: Secondary infection (bacterial, viral, or fungal)

Dental Usual Dosing Inflammatory and pruritic manifestations: Adults: Topical: Apply to oral lesion 4 times/day, after meals and at bedtime

Dosage

Children ≥2 years: Topical: Atopic dermatitis (Derma-Smoothe/FS®): Moisten skin; apply to affected area twice daily; do not use for longer than 4 weeks

Children and Adults: Topical: Corticosteroid-responsive dermatoses: Cream, ointment, solution: Apply a thin layer to affected area 2-4 times/day; may use occlusive dressings to manage psoriasis or recalcitrant conditions

Adults:

Topical:

Atopic dermatitis (Derma-Smoothe/FS®): Apply thin film to affected area 3 times/day

Inflammatory and pruritic manifestations (dental use): Apply to oral lesion 4 times/day , after meals and at bedtime

Scalp psoriasis (Derma-Smoothe/FS®): Massage thoroughly into wet or dampened hair/scalp; cover with shower cap. Leave on overnight (or for at least 4 hours). Remove by washing hair with shampoo and rinsing thoroughly.

Seborrheic dermatitis of the scalp (Capex™): Apply no more than 1 ounce to scalp once daily; work into lather and allow to remain on scalp for ~5 minutes. Remove from hair and scalp by rinsing thoroughly with water.

Ocular implant: Chronic uveitis: One silicone-encased tablet (0.59 mg) surgically implanted into the posterior segment of the eye is designed to release 0.6 mcg/day, decreasing over 30 days to a steady-state release rate of 0.3-0.4 mcg/day for 30 months. Recurrence of uveitis denotes depletion of tablet, requiring reimplantation.

Mechanism of Action A synthetic corticosteroid which differs structurally from triamcinolone acetonide in the presence of an additional fluorine atom in the 6-alpha position on the steroid nucleus. The mechanism of action for all topical corticosteroids is not well defined, however, is believed to be a combination of anti-inflammatory, antipruritic, and vasoconstrictive properties.

Contraindications Hypersensitivity to fluocinolone or any component of the formulation; TB of skin; herpes (including varicella)

Ocular implant: Additional contraindications include ocular infections of viral or fungal origin

Warnings/Precautions Adverse systemic effects may occur when used on large areas of the body, denuded areas, for prolonged periods of time, with an occlusive dressing, and/or in infants or small children. Infants and small children may be more susceptible to adrenal axis suppression from topical corticosteroid therapy. Derma-Smoothe/FS® contains peanut oil; use caution in peanut-sensitive children.

Ocular implant: May cause transient decrease in visual acuity of 1-4 weeks duration; caution with use in glaucoma patients; routine monitoring of IOP recommended. May require IOP-lowering treatments within 2 years postimplantation. Prolonged use of ocular corticosteroids may increase risk of secondary infection, cataract formation, optic nerve damage, and/or glaucoma. Recommend unilateral implantation only to minimize risk of postoperative infections developing in both eyes. Safety and efficacy have not been established in children <12 years of age.

Drug Interactions No data reported

Pharmacodynamics/Kinetics

Absorption:

Topical: Dependent on strength of preparation, amount applied, nature of skin at application site, vehicle, and use of occlusive dressing; increased in areas of skin damage, inflammation, or occlusion

Ocular implant: Systemic absorption is negligible

Duration: Ocular implant: Releases fluocinolone acetonide at a rate of 0.6 mcg/day, decreasing over 30 days to a steady-state release rate of 0.3-0.4 mcg/day for 30 months

Distribution:

Topical: Throughout local skin; absorbed drug is distributed rapidly into muscle, liver, skin, intestines, and kidneys

Ocular implant: Aqueous and vitreous humor

Metabolism: Primarily in skin; small amount absorbed into systemic circulation is primarily hepatic to inactive compounds

(Continued)

Fluocinolone *(Continued)*

Excretion: Urine (primarily as glucuronide and sulfate, also as unconjugated products); feces (small amounts)

Pregnancy Risk Factor C

Lactation Excretion in breast milk unknown/use caution

Breast-Feeding Considerations Systemic corticosteroids are excreted in human milk. It is not known if sufficient quantities of fluocinolone are absorbed following topical or ocular administration to produce detectable amounts in breast milk. Hypertension in the nursing infant has been reported following corticosteroid ointment applied to the nipples. Use with caution.

Dosage Forms Excipient information presented when available (limited, particularly for generics); consult specific product labeling.

Cream, as acetonide: 0.01% (15 g, 60 g); 0.025% (15 g, 60 g)
Synalar®: 0.025% (15 g, 60 g)

Oil, as acetonide:
Derma-Smoothe/FS® [eczema oil]: 0.01% (120 mL) [contains peanut oil]
Derma-Smoothe/FS® [scalp oil]: 0.01% (120 mL) [contains peanut oil; packaged with shower caps]

Ointment, as acetonide (Synalar®): 0.025% (15 g, 60 g)

Shampoo, as acetonide (Capex™): 0.01% (120 mL)

Solution, as acetonide: 0.01% (60 mL)
Synalar®: 0.01% (20 mL, 60 mL)

Tablet, ocular implant, as acetonide (Retisert™): 0.59 mg [enclosed in silicone elastomer]

Fluocinolone Acetonide *see* Fluocinolone *on page 706*

Fluocinolone, Hydroquinone, and Tretinoin
(floo oh SIN oh lone, HYE droe kwin one, & TRET i noyn)

Related Information
Fluocinolone *on page 706*
Hydroquinone *on page 841*

U.S. Brand Names Tri-Luma™

Generic Available No

Index Terms Hydroquinone, Fluocinolone Acetonide, and Tretinoin; Tretinoin, Fluocinolone Acetonide, and Hydroquinone

Pharmacologic Category Corticosteroid, Topical; Depigmenting Agent; Retinoic Acid Derivative

Use Short-term treatment of moderate to severe melasma of the face

Local Anesthetic/Vasoconstrictor Precautions No information available to require special precautions

Effects on Dental Treatment Key adverse event(s) related to dental treatment: Xerostomia (normal salivary flow resumes upon discontinuation).

Common Adverse Effects
>10%:
Dermatologic: Erythema (41%), desquamation (38%), burning (18%), dry skin (14%), pruritus (11%)

1% to 10%:
Cardiovascular: Telangiectasia (3%)
Central nervous system: Paresthesia (3%), hyperesthesia (2%)
Dermatologic: Acne (5%), pigmentation change (2%), irritation (2%), papules (1%), rash (1%), rosacea (1%), vesicles (1%)
Gastrointestinal: Xerostomia (1%)

Mechanism of Action Not clearly defined. Hydroquinone may interrupt melanin synthesis (tyrosine-tyrosinase pathway); reduces hyperpigmentation.

Drug Interactions
Cytochrome P450 Effect: Tretinoin: **Substrate** (minor) of CYP2A6, 2B6, 2C8/9; **Inhibits** CYP2C8/9 (weak); **Induces** CYP2E1 (weak)

Increased Effect/Toxicity: Avoid soaps/cosmetic preparations which are medicated, abrasive, irritating, or any product with strong drying effects (including alcohol, astringent, benzoyl peroxide, resorcinol, salicylic acid, sulfur). Drugs with photosensitizing effects should also be avoided (includes tetracyclines, thiazides, fluoroquinolones, phenothiazines, sulfonamides).

Pharmacodynamics/Kinetics
Absorption: Minimal
Metabolism: Hepatic for the small amount absorbed
Excretion: Urine and feces

Pregnancy Risk Factor C

Fluocinonide (floo oh SIN oh nide)

Related Information
Ulcerative and Erosive Disorders *on page 1809*

Related Sample Prescriptions
Mild Lichen Planus *on page 1845*
Recurrent Aphthous Stomatitis *on page 1844*

U.S. Brand Names Lidex®; Lidex-E®; Vanos™

Canadian Brand Names Lidemol®; Lidex®; Lyderm®; Tiamol®; Topsyn®

Generic Available Yes

Pharmacologic Category Corticosteroid, Topical

Dental Use Relief of inflammatory and pruritic manifestations (high potency topical corticosteroid)

Use Anti-inflammatory, antipruritic; treatment of plaque-type psoriasis (up to 10% of body surface area) [high-potency topical corticosteroid]

Local Anesthetic/Vasoconstrictor Precautions No information available to require special precautions

Effects on Dental Treatment No significant effects or complications reported

Significant Adverse Effects Frequency not defined.
Cardiovascular: Intracranial hypertension
Dermatologic: Acne, allergic dermatitis, contact dermatitis, dry skin, folliculitis, hypertrichosis, hypopigmentation, maceration of the skin, miliaria, perioral dermatitis, pruritus, skin atrophy, striae, telangiectasia
Endocrine & metabolic: Cushing's syndrome, growth retardation, HPA suppression, hyperglycemia
Local: Burning, irritation
Renal: Glycosuria
Miscellaneous: Secondary infection

Dental Usual Dosing Pruritus and inflammation: Children and Adults: Topical (0.5% cream): Apply thin layer to affected area 2-4 times/day depending on the severity of the condition. Therapy should be discontinued when control is achieved; if no improvement is seen, reassessment of diagnosis may be necessary.

Dosage
Children and Adults: Pruritus and inflammation: Topical (0.5% cream): Apply thin layer to affected area 2-4 times/day depending on the severity of the condition. Therapy should be discontinued when control is achieved; if no improvement is seen, reassessment of diagnosis may be necessary.
Children ≥12 years and Adults: Plaque-type psoriasis (Vanos™): Topical (0.1% cream): Apply a thin layer once or twice daily to affected areas (limited to <10% of body surface area). **Note:** Not recommended for use >2 consecutive weeks or >60 g/week total exposure. Discontinue when control is achieved.

Mechanism of Action Fluorinated topical corticosteroid considered to be of high potency. The mechanism of action for all topical corticosteroids is not well defined, however, is felt to be a combination of three important properties: anti-inflammatory activity, immunosuppressive properties, and antiproliferative actions.

Contraindications Hypersensitivity to fluocinonide or any component of the formulation; viral, fungal, or tubercular skin lesions, herpes simplex

Warnings/Precautions Systemic absorption of topical corticosteroids may cause hypothalamic-pituitary-adrenal (HPA) axis suppression (reversible) particularly in younger children. HPA axis suppression may lead to adrenal crisis. Risk is increased when used over large surface areas, for prolonged periods, or with occlusive dressings. Allergic contact dermatitis can occur, it is usually diagnosed by failure to heal rather than clinical exacerbation. Prolonged treatment with corticosteroids has been associated with the development of Kaposi's sarcoma (case reports); if noted, discontinuation of therapy should be considered. Adverse systemic effects including hyperglycemia, glycosuria, fluid and electrolyte changes, and HPA suppression may occur when used on large surface areas, for prolonged periods, or with an occlusive dressing. Lower-strength cream (0.05%) may be used cautiously on face or opposing skin surfaces that may rub or touch (eg, skin folds of the groin, axilla, and breasts); higher-strength (0.1%) should not be used on the face, groin, or axillae. Use of the 0.1% cream for >2 weeks or in patients <12 years of age is not recommended. Chronic use of corticosteroids in children may interfere with growth and development.

Drug Interactions No data reported. Concomitant use with other corticosteroids (by any route) may increase the risk of HPA axis suppression.

Pharmacodynamics/Kinetics
Absorption: Dependent on strength of product, amount applied, and nature of skin at application site; ranges from ~1% in areas of thick stratum corneum
(Continued)

Fluocinonide *(Continued)*

(palms, soles, elbows, etc) to 36% in areas of thin stratum corneum (face, eyelids, etc); increased in areas of skin damage, inflammation, or occlusion

Distribution: Throughout local skin; absorbed drug into muscle, liver, skin, intestines, and kidneys

Metabolism: Primarily in skin; small amount absorbed into systemic circulation is primarily hepatic to inactive compounds

Excretion: Urine (primarily as glucuronide and sulfate, also as unconjugated products); feces (small amounts as metabolites)

Pregnancy Risk Factor C

Dosage Forms Excipient information presented when available (limited, particularly for generics); consult specific product labeling.

Cream, anhydrous, emollient (Lidex®): 0.05% (15 g, 30 g, 60 g)

Cream, aqueous, emollient (Lidex-E®): 0.05% (15 g, 30 g, 60 g)

Cream (Vanos™): 0.1% (30 g, 60 g)

Gel (Lidex®): 0.05% (15 g, 30 g, 60 g)

Ointment (Lidex®): 0.05% (15 g, 30 g, 60 g)

Solution (Lidex®): 0.05% (60 mL) [contains alcohol 35%]

Fluohydrisone Acetate *see* Fludrocortisone *on page 701*

Fluohydrocortisone Acetate *see* Fludrocortisone *on page 701*

Fluoracaine® *see* Proparacaine and Fluorescein *on page 1367*

Fluor-A-Day *see* Fluoride *on page 710*

Fluorescein and Proparacaine *see* Proparacaine and Fluorescein *on page 1367*

Fluoride *(FLOR ide)*

Related Information

Dentin Hypersensitivity, High Caries Index, and Xerostomia *on page 1812*

Management of Patients Undergoing Cancer Therapy *on page 1826*

U.S. Brand Names ACT® [OTC]; ACT® Plus [OTC]; ACT® x2™ [OTC]; CaviRinse™; ControlRx®; Denta 5000 Plus; DentaGel; EtheDent™; Fluor-A-Day; Fluorigard® [OTC]; Fluorinse®; Flura-Drops®; Gel-Kam® [OTC]; Gel-Kam® Rinse; Just for Kids™ [OTC]; Lozi-Flur™; Luride®; Luride® Lozi-Tab®; Neutra-Care®; NeutraGard® [OTC]; NeutraGard® Advanced; NeutraGard® Plus; Omnii Gel™ [OTC]; Pediaflor® [DSC]; PerioMed™; Pharmaflur®; Pharmaflur® 1.1; Phos-Flur®; Phos-Flur® Rinse [OTC]; PreviDent®; PreviDent® 5000 Plus™; StanGard®; StanGard® Perio; Stop®; Thera-Flur-N®

Canadian Brand Names Fluor-A-Day; Fluotic®

Generic Available Yes: Excludes lozenge, gel drops

Index Terms Acidulated Phosphate Fluoride; Sodium Fluoride; Stannous Fluoride

Pharmacologic Category Nutritional Supplement

Dental Use Prevention of dental caries

Use Prevention of dental caries

Local Anesthetic/Vasoconstrictor Precautions No information available to require special precautions

Effects on Dental Treatment Key adverse event(s) related to dental treatment: Products containing stannous fluoride may stain teeth. See Dental Comment.

Fluoride Ion

Fluoride Content of Drinking Water	Daily Dose, Oral (mg)
<0.3 ppm	
Birth - 6 mo	None
6 mo - 3 y	0.25
3-6 y	0.5
6-16 y	1
0.3-0.6 ppm	
Birth - 6 mo	None
6 mo - 3 y	None
3-6 y	0.25
6-16 y	0.5

Adapted from Recommended Dosage Schedule of The American Dental Association, The American Academy of Pediatric Dentistry, and The American Academy of Pediatrics.

Significant Adverse Effects <1% (Limited to important or life-threatening): Discoloration of teeth, rash, nausea, vomiting

Dosage Oral:

The recommended daily dose of oral fluoride supplement (mg), based on fluoride ion content (ppm) in drinking water (2.2 mg of sodium fluoride is equivalent to 1 mg of fluoride ion): See table on previous page.

Cream: Children ≥6 years and Adults: Brush teeth with cream once daily regardless of fluoride content of drinking water

Dental rinse or gel:

Children 6-12 years: 5-10 mL rinse or apply to teeth and spit daily after brushing

Adults: 10 mL rinse or apply to teeth and spit daily after brushing

PreviDent® rinse: Children >6 years and Adults: Once weekly, rinse 10 mL vigorously around and between teeth for 1 minute, then spit; this should be done preferably at bedtime, after thoroughly brushing teeth; for maximum benefit, do not eat, drink, or rinse mouth for at least 30 minutes after treatment; do not swallow

Fluorinse®: Children >6 years and Adults: Once weekly, vigorously swish 5-10 mL in mouth for 1 minute, then spit

Lozenge (Lozi-Flur™): Adults: One lozenge daily regardless of fluoride content of drinking water

Mechanism of Action Promotes remineralization of decalcified enamel; inhibits the cariogenic microbial process in dental plaque; increases tooth resistance to acid dissolution

Contraindications Hypersensitivity to fluoride, tartrazine, or any component of the formulation; when fluoride content of drinking water exceeds 0.7 ppm; low sodium or sodium-free diets; do not use 1 mg tablets in children <3 years of age or when drinking water fluoride content is ≥0.3 ppm; do not use 1 mg/5 mL rinse (as supplement) in children <6 years of age

Warnings/Precautions Prolonged ingestion with excessive doses may result in dental fluorosis and osseous changes; do **not** exceed recommended dosage. Some products contain tartrazine.

Drug Interactions Decreased effect/absorption with magnesium-, aluminum-, and calcium-containing products.

Dietary Considerations Do not administer with milk; do **not** allow eating or drinking for 30 minutes after use.

Pharmacodynamics/Kinetics

Absorption: Oral: Rapid and complete; sodium fluoride; other soluble fluoride salts; calcium, iron, or magnesium may delay absorption

Distribution: 50% of fluoride is deposited in teeth and bone after ingestion; topical application works superficially on enamel and plaque; crosses placenta; enters breast milk

Excretion: Urine and feces

Pregnancy Risk Factor C

Dosage Forms Excipient information presented when available (limited, particularly for generics); consult specific product labeling. [DSC] = Discontinued product

Cream, oral, as sodium [toothpaste]: 1.1% (51 g) [fluoride 2.5 mg/dose]

Denta 5000 Plus: 1.1% (51g) [fluoride 2.5 mg/dose; spearmint flavor]

EtheDent™: 1.1% (51g) [fluoride 2.5 mg/dose]

Gel-drops, as sodium fluoride (Thera-Flur-N®): 1.1% (24 mL) [fluoride 0.5%; neutral pH; no artificial color or flavor]

Gel, topical, as acidulated phosphate fluoride (Phos-Flur®): 1.1% (60 g) [fluoride 0.5%; cherry and mint flavors]

Gel, topical, as sodium fluoride: 1.1% (56 g) [fluoride 2 mg/dose]

DentaGel, EtheDent™: 1.1% (56 g) [fluoride 2 mg/dose; fresh mint flavor]

NeutraCare®: 1.1% (60 g) [neutral pH; grape and mint flavors]

NeutraGard® Advanced: 1.1% (60 g) [cinnamon and mint flavors]

PreviDent®: 1.1% (60 g) [fluoride 2 mg/dose; berry, cherry, and mint flavors]

Gel, topical, as stannous fluoride:

Gel-Kam®: 0.4% (129 g) [bubble gum, cinnamon, fruit/berry, and mint flavors]

Just for Kids™: 0.4% (122 g) [bubble gum, fruit punch, and grapey grape flavors]

Omnii Gel™: 0.4% (122 g) [cinnamon, grape, natural, mint, and raspberry flavors]

StanGard®: 0.4% (122 g) [bubble gum, cherry, mint, and raspberry flavors]

Stop®: 0.4% (120 g) [bubble gum, cinnamon, grape, and mint flavors]

Lozenge, as sodium (Lozi-Flur™): 2.21 mg [fluoride 1 mg; cherry flavor]

Paste, oral, as sodium [toothpaste] (ControlRx®): 1.1% (56 g) [vanilla mint flavor]

Solution, oral drops, as sodium: 1.1 mg/mL (50 mL) [fluoride 0.5 mg/mL]

Flura-Drops®: 0.55 mg/drop (24 mL) [fluoride 0.25 mg/drop; dye free, sugar free]

(Continued)

Fluoride *(Continued)*

Luride®: 1.1 mg/mL (50 mL) [fluoride 0.5 mg/mL; sugar free]
Pediaflor®: 1.1 mg/mL (50 mL) [fluoride 0.5 mg/mL; contains alcohol <0.5%; sugar free; cherry flavor] [DSC]
Solution, oral rinse, as sodium:
ACT®: 0.05% (530 mL) [fluoride 0.02%; bubble gum, cinnamon (contains tartrazine), and mint flavors]
ACT® Plus: 0.05% (530 mL) [fluoride 0.02%; alcohol free; icy cool mint flavor]
ACT® x2™: 0.5% (530 mL) [fluoride 0.02%; contains alcohol 11%; icy cool mint and spearmint flavors]
CaviRinse™: 0.2% (240 mL) [mint flavor]
Fluorigard®: 0.05% (480 mL) [alcohol free, sugar free; contains sodium benzoate and tartrazine; mint flavor]
Fluorinse®: 0.2% (480 mL) [alcohol free; cinnamon and mint flavors]
NeutraGard®: 0.05% (480 mL) [neutral pH; mint and tropical blast flavors]
NeutraGard® Plus: 0.2% (480 mL) [neutral pH; mint and tropical blast flavors]
Phos-Flur®: 0.44% (500 mL) [bubble gum, cherry, grape, and mint flavors]
PreviDent®: 0.2% (250 mL) [contains alcohol; mint flavor]
Solution, oral rinse concentrate, as stannous fluoride:
Gel-Kam®: 0.63% (300 mL) [fluoride 0.1%/dose; cinnamon and mint flavors]
PerioMed™: 0.63% (284 mL) [fluoride 7 mg/30 mL; alcohol free; cinnamon, mint and tropical fruit flavors]
StanGard® Perio: 0.63% (284 mL) [mint flavor]
Tablet, chewable, as sodium: 0.5 mg [fluoride 0.25 mg]; 1.1 mg [fluoride 0.5 mg]; 2.2 mg [fluoride 1 mg]
EtheDent™:
0.55 mg [fluoride 0.25 mg; sugar free; contains aspartame; vanilla flavor]
1.1 mg [fluoride 0.5 mg; sugar free; contains aspartame; grape flavor]
2.2 mg [fluoride 1 mg; sugar free; contains aspartame; cherry flavor]
Fluor-A-Day:
0.56 mg [fluoride 0.25 mg; raspberry flavor]
1.1 mg [fluoride 0.5 mg; raspberry flavor]
2.21 mg [fluoride 1 mg; raspberry flavor]
Luride® Lozi-Tab®:
0.55 mg [fluoride 0.25 mg; sugar free; vanilla flavor]
1.1 mg [fluoride 0.5 mg; sugar free; grape flavor]
2.2 mg [fluoride 1 mg; sugar free; cherry flavor]
Pharmaflur®: 2.2 mg [fluoride 1 mg; dye free, sugar free; cherry flavor]
Pharmaflur® 1.1: 1.1 mg [fluoride 0.5 mg; dye free, sugar free; grape flavor]
Dental Comment Neutral pH fluoride preparations are preferred in patients with oral mucositis to reduce tissue irritation; long-term use of acidulated fluorides has been associated with enamel demineralization and damage to porcelain crowns

Selected Readings
Wynn RC, "Fluoride: After 50 Years, a Clearer Picture of Its Mechanism," *Gen Dent*, 2002, 50(2):118-22, 124, 126.

Fluoride and Triclosan (Dental) *see* Triclosan and Fluoride *on page 1616*
Fluorigard® [OTC] *see* Fluoride *on page 710*
Fluori-Methane® *see* Dichlorodifluoromethane and Trichloromonofluoromethane *on page 485*
Fluorinse® *see* Fluoride *on page 710*
5-Fluorocytosine *see* Flucytosine *on page 699*
Fluorodeoxyuridine *see* Floxuridine *on page 696*
9α-Fluorohydrocortisone Acetate *see* Fludrocortisone *on page 701*

Fluorometholone *(flure oh METH oh lone)*

U.S. Brand Names Eflone® [DSC]; Flarex®; Fluor-Op® [DSC]; FML®; FML® Forte
Canadian Brand Names Flarex®; FML®; FML Forte®; PMS-Fluorometholone
Mexican Brand Names Fluforte Liquifilm (MX, MX); Flumetol NF (MX, MX); Flumetol Ofteno
Generic Available Yes: Suspension (as base)
Pharmacologic Category Corticosteroid, Ophthalmic
Use Treatment of steroid-responsive inflammatory conditions of the eye
Local Anesthetic/Vasoconstrictor Precautions No information available to require special precautions
Effects on Dental Treatment No significant effects or complications reported
Mechanism of Action Decreases inflammation by suppression of migration of polymorphonuclear leukocytes and reversal of increased capillary permeability
Pregnancy Risk Factor C

Fluorometholone and Sulfacetamide *see* Sulfacetamide and Fluorometholone *on page 1502*

Fluor-Op® [DSC] *see* Fluorometholone *on page 712*

Fluoroplex® *see* Fluorouracil *on page 713*

Fluorouracil (flure oh YOOR a sil)

Related Information
Capecitabine *on page 267*

U.S. Brand Names Adrucil®; Carac™; Efudex®; Fluoroplex®

Canadian Brand Names Efudex®

Mexican Brand Names Efudix; Ifacil

Generic Available Yes: Injection, topical solution

Index Terms 5-Fluorouracil; FU; 5-FU

Pharmacologic Category Antineoplastic Agent, Antimetabolite (Pyrimidine Antagonist)

Use Treatment of carcinoma of the breast, colon, head and neck, pancreas, rectum, or stomach; topically for the management of actinic or solar keratoses and superficial basal cell carcinomas

Local Anesthetic/Vasoconstrictor Precautions No information available to require special precautions

Effects on Dental Treatment Key adverse event(s) related to dental treatment: Stomatitis.

Common Adverse Effects Toxicity depends on route and duration of treatment

I.V.:

Cardiovascular: Angina, myocardial ischemia, nail changes

Central nervous system: Acute cerebellar syndrome, confusion, disorientation, euphoria, headache, nystagmus

Dermatologic: Alopecia, dermatitis, dry skin, fissuring, palmar-plantar erythrodysesthesia syndrome, pruritic maculopapular rash, photosensitivity, vein pigmentations

Gastrointestinal: Anorexia, bleeding, diarrhea, esophagopharyngitis, nausea, sloughing, stomatitis, ulceration, vomiting

Hematologic: Agranulocytosis, anemia, leukopenia, pancytopenia, thrombocytopenia

Myelosuppression:
Onset: 7-10 days
Nadir: 9-14 days
Recovery: 21-28 days

Local: Thrombophlebitis

Ocular: Lacrimation, lacrimal duct stenosis, photophobia, visual changes

Respiratory: Epistaxis

Miscellaneous: Anaphylaxis, generalized allergic reactions, nail loss

Topical: Note: Systemic toxicity normally associated with parenteral administration (including neutropenia, neurotoxicity, and gastrointestinal toxicity) has been associated with topical use particularly in patients with a genetic deficiency of dihydropyrimidine dehydrogenase (DPD).

Central nervous system: Headache, insomnia, irritability

Dermatologic: Alopecia, photosensitivity, pruritus, rash, scarring, telangiectasia

Gastrointestinal: Medicinal taste, stomatitis

Hematologic: Leukocytosis, thrombocytopenia

Local: Application site reactions: Allergic contact dermatitis, burning, crusting, dryness, edema, erosion, erythema, hyperpigmentation, irritation, pain, soreness, ulceration

Ocular: Eye irritation (burning, watering, sensitivity, stinging, itching)

Miscellaneous: Birth defects, herpes simplex, miscarriage

Mechanism of Action A pyrimidine antimetabolite that interferes with DNA synthesis by blocking the methylation of deoxyuridylic acid; fluorouracil inhibits thymidylate synthetase (TS), or is incorporated into RNA. The reduced folate cofactor is required for tight binding to occur between the 5-FdUMP and TS.

Drug Interactions
Increased Effect/Toxicity: Fluorouracil may increase effects of warfarin.

Pharmacodynamics/Kinetics
Duration: ~3 weeks

Distribution: V_d: ~22% of total body water; penetrates extracellular fluid, CSF, and third space fluids (eg, pleural effusions and ascitic fluid)

Metabolism: Hepatic (90%); via a dehydrogenase enzyme; FU must be metabolized to be active

Bioavailability: <75%, erratic and undependable

(Continued)

Fluorouracil *(Continued)*

Half-life elimination: Biphasic: Initial: 6-20 minutes; two metabolites, FdUMP and FUTP, have prolonged half-lives depending on the type of tissue

Excretion: Lung (large amounts as CO_2); urine (5% as unchanged drug) in 6 hours

Pregnancy Risk Factor D (injection); X (topical)

5-Fluorouracil *see* Fluorouracil *on page 713*

Fluoxetine *(floo OKS e teen)*

Related Information
Sedation *on page 1825*

U.S. Brand Names Prozac®; Prozac® Weekly™; Sarafem®

Canadian Brand Names Alti-Fluoxetine; Apo-Fluoxetine®; BCI-Fluoxetine; CO Fluoxetine; FXT; Gen-Fluoxetine; Novo-Fluoxetine; Nu-Fluoxetine; PMS-Fluoxetine; Prozac®; Rhoxal-fluoxetine; Sandoz-Fluoxetine

Mexican Brand Names Auroken; Fluoxac; Prozac 20

Generic Available Yes: Excludes delayed release capsule

Index Terms Fluoxetine Hydrochloride

Pharmacologic Category Antidepressant, Selective Serotonin Reuptake Inhibitor

Use Treatment of major depressive disorder (MDD); treatment of binge-eating and vomiting in patients with moderate-to-severe bulimia nervosa; obsessive-compulsive disorder (OCD); premenstrual dysphoric disorder (PMDD); panic disorder with or without agoraphobia

Unlabeled/Investigational Use Selective mutism

Local Anesthetic/Vasoconstrictor Precautions Although caution should be used in patients taking tricyclic antidepressants, no interactions have been reported with vasoconstrictors and fluoxetine, a nontricyclic antidepressant which acts to increase serotonin; no precautions appear to be needed. Fluoxetine is one of the drugs confirmed to prolong the QT interval and is accepted as having a risk of causing torsade de pointes. The risk of drug-induced torsade de pointes is extremely low when a single QT interval prolonging drug is prescribed. In terms of epinephrine, it is not known what effect vasoconstrictors in the local anesthetic regimen will have in patients with a known history of congenital prolonged QT interval or in patients taking any medication that prolongs the QT interval. Until more information is obtained, it is suggested that the clinician consult with the physician prior to the use of a vasoconstrictor in suspected patients, and that the vasoconstrictor (epinephrine, levonordefrin [Neo-Cobefrin®]) be used with caution.

Effects on Dental Treatment Key adverse event(s) related to dental treatment: Xerostomia (normal salivary flow resumes upon discontinuation) and taste perversion. Problems with SSRI-induced bruxism have been reported and may preclude their use. Clinicians attempting to evaluate any patient with bruxism or involuntary muscle movement, who is simultaneously being treated with an SSRI drug, should be aware of this potential association.

Common Adverse Effects Percentages listed for adverse effects as reported in placebo-controlled trials and were generally similar in adults and children; actual frequency may be dependent upon diagnosis and in some cases the range presented may be lower than or equal to placebo for a particular disorder.

>10%:

Central nervous system: Insomnia (10% to 33%), headache (21%), anxiety (6% to 15%), nervousness (8% to 14%), somnolence (5% to 17%)

Endocrine & metabolic: Libido decreased (1% to 11%)

Gastrointestinal: Nausea (12% to 29%), diarrhea (8% to 18%), anorexia (4% to 11%), xerostomia (4% to 12%)

Neuromuscular & skeletal: Weakness (7% to 21%), tremor (3% to 13%)

Respiratory: Pharyngitis (3% to 11%), yawn (<1% to 11%)

1% to 10%:

Cardiovascular: Vasodilation (1% to 5%), fever (2%), chest pain, hemorrhage, hypertension, palpitation

Central nervous system: Dizziness (9%), dream abnormality (1% to 5%), thinking abnormality (2%), agitation, amnesia, chills, confusion, emotional lability, sleep disorder

Dermatologic: Rash (2% to 6%), pruritus (4%)

Endocrine & metabolic: Ejaculation abnormal (<1% to 7%), impotence (<1% to 7%)

Gastrointestinal: Dyspepsia (6% to 10%), constipation (5%), flatulence (3%), vomiting (3%), weight loss (2%), appetite increased, taste perversion, weight gain

Genitourinary: Urinary frequency

Ocular: Vision abnormal (2%)

Otic: Ear pain, tinnitus

Respiratory: Sinusitis (1% to 6%)

Miscellaneous: Flu-like syndrome (3% to 10%), diaphoresis (2% to 8%)

Restrictions An FDA-approved medication guide concerning the use of antidepressants in children, adolescents, and young adults must be distributed when dispensing an outpatient prescription (new or refill) where this medication is to be used without direct supervision of a healthcare provider. Medication guides are available at http://www.fda.gov/cder/Offices/ODS/medication_guides.htm. Dispense to parents or guardians of children and adolescents receiving this medication.

Dosage Oral: **Note:** Upon discontinuation of fluoxetine therapy, gradually taper dose. If intolerable symptoms occur following a dose reduction, consider resuming the previously prescribed dose and/or decrease dose at a more gradual rate.

Children:

Depression: 8-18 years: 10-20 mg/day; lower-weight children can be started at 10 mg/day, may increase to 20 mg/day after 1 week if needed

OCD: 7-18 years: Initial: 10 mg/day; in adolescents and higher-weight children, dose may be increased to 20 mg/day after 2 weeks. Range: 10-60 mg/day.

Selective mutism (unlabeled use):

<5 years: No dosing information available

5-18 years: Initial: 5-10 mg/day; titrate upwards as needed (usual maximum dose: 60 mg/day)

Adults: 20 mg/day in the morning; may increase after several weeks by 20 mg/day increments; maximum: 80 mg/day; doses >20 mg may be given once daily or divided twice daily. **Note:** Lower doses of 5-10 mg/day have been used for initial treatment.

Usual dosage range:

Bulimia nervosa: 60-80 mg/day

Depression: 20-40 mg/day; patients maintained on Prozac® 20 mg/day may be changed to Prozac® Weekly™ 90 mg/week, starting dose 7 days after the last 20 mg/day dose

OCD: 40-80 mg/day

Panic disorder: Initial: 10 mg/day; after 1 week, increase to 20 mg/day; may increase after several weeks; doses >60 mg/day have not been evaluated

PMDD (Sarafem™): 20 mg/day continuously, **or** 20 mg/day starting 14 days prior to menstruation and through first full day of menses (repeat with each cycle)

Elderly: Depression: Some patients may require an initial dose of 10 mg/day with dosage increases of 10 and 20 mg every several weeks as tolerated; should not be taken at night unless patient experiences sedation

Dosing adjustment in renal impairment:

Single dose studies: Pharmacokinetics of fluoxetine and norfluoxetine were similar among subjects with all levels of impaired renal function, including anephric patients on chronic hemodialysis

Chronic administration: Additional accumulation of fluoxetine or norfluoxetine may occur in patients with severely impaired renal function

Hemodialysis: Not removed by hemodialysis; use of lower dose or less frequent dosing is not usually necessary.

Dosing adjustment in hepatic impairment: Elimination half-life of fluoxetine is prolonged in patients with hepatic impairment; a lower or less frequent dose of fluoxetine should be used in these patients

Cirrhosis patients: Administer a lower dose or less frequent dosing interval

Compensated cirrhosis without ascites: Administer 50% of normal dose

Mechanism of Action Inhibits CNS neuron serotonin reuptake; minimal or no effect on reuptake of norepinephrine or dopamine; does not significantly bind to alpha-adrenergic, histamine, or cholinergic receptors

Contraindications Hypersensitivity to fluoxetine or any component of the formulation; patients currently receiving MAO inhibitors, pimozide, or thioridazine

Note: MAO inhibitor therapy must be stopped for 14 days before fluoxetine is initiated. Treatment with MAO inhibitors, thioridazine, or mesoridazine should not be initiated until 5 weeks after the discontinuation of fluoxetine.

Warnings/Precautions [U.S. Boxed Warning]: Antidepressants increase the risk of suicidal thinking and behavior in children, adolescents, and young adults (18-24 years of age) with major depressive disorder (MDD) and other psychiatric disorders; consider risk prior to prescribing. Short-term studies did not show an increased risk in patients >24 years of age and showed a decreased risk in patients ≥65 years. Closely monitor patients for clinical worsening, suicidality, or unusual changes in behavior, particularly during the initial 1-2 months of therapy or during periods of dosage adjustments (increases

(Continued)

Fluoxetine *(Continued)*

or decreases); the patient's family or caregiver should be instructed to closely observe the patient and communicate condition with healthcare provider. A medication guide concerning the use of antidepressants should be dispensed with each prescription. **Fluoxetine is FDA approved for the treatment of OCD in children ≥7 years of age and MDD in children ≥8 years of age.**

The possibility of a suicide attempt is inherent in major depression and may persist until remission occurs. Use caution in high-risk patients. Worsening depression and severe abrupt suicidality that are not part of the presenting symptoms may require discontinuation or modification of drug therapy. The patient's family or caregiver should be alerted to monitor patients for the emergence of suicidality and associated behaviors (such as agitation, irritability, hostility, impulsivity, and hypomania) and call healthcare provider.

May worsen psychosis in some patients or precipitate a shift to mania or hypomania in patients with bipolar disorder. Patients presenting with depressive symptoms should be screened for bipolar disorder. Monotherapy in patients with bipolar disorder should be avoided. **Fluoxetine is not FDA approved for the treatment of bipolar depression.** May cause insomnia, anxiety, nervousness, or anorexia. Use with caution in patients where weight loss is undesirable. May impair cognitive or motor performance; caution operating hazardous machinery or driving.

The potential for severe reactions exists when used with MAO inhibitors, SSRIs/SNRIs or triptans; serotonin syndrome (hyperthermia, muscular rigidity, mental status changes/agitation, autonomic instability) may occur. Concurrent use with MAO inhibitors is contraindicated. Fluoxetine may elevate plasma levels of thioridazine and increase the risk of QT_c interval prolongation. This may lead to serious ventricular arrhythmias, such as torsade de pointes-type arrhythmias, and sudden death. Fluoxetine use has been associated with occurrences of significant rash and allergic events, including vasculitis, lupus-like syndrome, laryngospasm, anaphylactoid reactions, and pulmonary inflammatory disease. Discontinue if underlying cause of rash cannot be identified.

Use caution in patients with a previous seizure disorder or condition predisposing to seizures such as brain damage, alcoholism, or concurrent therapy with other drugs which lower the seizure threshold. Use with caution in patients with hepatic or renal dysfunction and in elderly patients. May cause hyponatremia/SIADH. May increase the risks associated with electroconvulsive treatment. Use with caution in patients at risk of bleeding or receiving concurrent anticoagulant therapy - may cause impairment in platelet function. Use caution with history of MI or unstable heart disease; use in these patients is limited. May alter glycemic control in patients with diabetes. Due to the long half-life of fluoxetine and its metabolites, the effects and interactions noted may persist for prolonged periods following discontinuation. May cause or exacerbate sexual dysfunction. Discontinuation symptoms (eg, dysphoric mood, irritability, agitation, confusion, anxiety, insomnia, hypomania) may occur upon abrupt discontinuation. Taper dose when discontinuing therapy.

Drug Interactions

Cytochrome P450 Effect: Substrate of CYP1A2 (minor), 2B6 (minor), 2C9 (major), 2C19 (minor), 2D6 (major), 2E1 (minor), 3A4 (minor); **Inhibits** CYP1A2 (moderate), 2B6 (weak), 2C9 (weak), 2C19 (moderate), 2D6 (strong), 3A4 (weak)

Increased Effect/Toxicity: Fluoxetine should not be used with nonselective MAO inhibitors (phenelzine, isocarboxazid) or other drugs with MAO inhibition (linezolid); fatal reactions have been reported. Wait 5 weeks after stopping fluoxetine before starting a nonselective MAO inhibitor and 2 weeks after stopping an MAO inhibitor before starting fluoxetine. Concurrent selegiline has been associated with mania, hypertension, or serotonin syndrome (risk may be reduced relative to nonselective MAO inhibitors).

Due to potential QT_c interval prolongation, concomitant use of pimozide is contraindicated. Fluoxetine may inhibit the metabolism of thioridazine, resulting in increased plasma levels and increasing the risk of QT_c interval prolongation. This may lead to serious ventricular arrhythmias, such as torsade de pointes-type arrhythmias, and sudden death. Do not use together. Wait at least 5 weeks after discontinuing fluoxetine prior to starting thioridazine.

Fluoxetine may increase the levels/effects of aminophylline, amphetamines, selected beta-blockers, citalopram, dextromethorphan, diazepam, fluvoxamine, lidocaine, mexiletine, methsuximide, mirtazapine, nefazodone, paroxetine, phenytoin, propranolol, risperidone, ritonavir, ropinirole, sertraline, theophylline, thioridazine, tricyclic antidepressants, trifluoperazine, venlafaxine, and other substrates of CYP1A2, 2C19, or 2D6.

Combined use of SSRIs and amphetamines, buspirone, meperidine, nefazodone, serotonin agonists (such as sumatriptan), sibutramine, other SSRIs/SNRIs, sympathomimetics, ritonavir, tramadol, and venlafaxine may increase the risk of serotonin syndrome. Combined use of sumatriptan (and other serotonin agonists) may result in toxicity; weakness, hyper-reflexia, and incoordination have been observed with sumatriptan and SSRIs. In addition, concurrent use may theoretically increase the risk of serotonin syndrome.

Concurrent lithium may increase risk of neurotoxicity, and lithium levels may be increased. Risk of hyponatremia may increase with concurrent use of loop diuretics (bumetanide, furosemide, torsemide). Fluoxetine may increase the hypoprothrombinemic response to warfarin. Concomitant use of fluoxetine and NSAIDs, aspirin, or other drugs affecting coagulation has been associated with an increased risk of bleeding; monitor.

The levels/effects of fluoxetine may be increased by chlorpromazine, delavirdine, fluconazole, gemfibrozil, ketoconazole, miconazole, nicardipine, NSAIDs, paroxetine, pergolide, quinidine, quinine, ritonavir, sulfonamides, ropinirole, tolbutamide, and other CYP2C9 or 2D6 inhibitors.

Decreased Effect: The levels/effects of fluoxetine may be decreased by carbamazepine, phenobarbital, phenytoin, rifampin, rifapentine, secobarbital, and other CYP2C9 inducers. Fluoxetine may decrease the levels/effects of CYP2D6 prodrug substrates (eg, codeine, hydrocodone, oxycodone, tramadol). Cyproheptadine may inhibit the effects of serotonin reuptake inhibitors. Lithium levels may be decreased by fluoxetine (in addition to reports of increased lithium levels).

Ethanol/Nutrition/Herb Interactions

Ethanol: Avoid ethanol (may increase CNS depression). Depressed patients should avoid/limit intake.

Herb/Nutraceutical: Avoid valerian, St John's wort, kava kava, gotu kola (may increase CNS depression).

Dietary Considerations May be taken with or without food.

Pharmacodynamics/Kinetics

Onset of action: Depression: ≥4 weeks; OCD: ≥5 weeks

Absorption: Well absorbed; delayed 1-2 hours with weekly formulation

Distribution: V_d: 12-43 L/kg

Protein binding: 95% to albumin and alpha$_1$ glycoprotein

Metabolism: Hepatic, via CYP2C19 and 2D6, to norfluoxetine (activity equal to fluoxetine)

Half-life elimination: Adults:

Parent drug: 1-3 days (acute), 4-6 days (chronic), 7.6 days (cirrhosis)

Metabolite (norfluoxetine): 9.3 days (range: 4-16 days), 12 days (cirrhosis)

Time to peak, serum: 6-8 hours

Excretion: Urine (10% as norfluoxetine, 2.5% to 5% as fluoxetine)

Note: Weekly formulation results in greater fluctuations between peak and trough concentrations of fluoxetine and norfluoxetine compared to once-daily dosing (24% daily/164% weekly; 17% daily/43% weekly, respectively). Trough concentrations are 76% lower for fluoxetine and 47% lower for norfluoxetine than the concentrations maintained by 20 mg once-daily dosing. Steady-state fluoxetine concentrations are ~50% lower following the once-weekly regimen compared to 20 mg once daily. Average steady-state concentrations of once-daily dosing were highest in children ages 6 to <13 (fluoxetine 171 ng/mL; norfluoxetine 195 ng/mL), followed by adolescents ages 13 to <18 (fluoxetine 86 ng/mL; norfluoxetine 113 ng/mL); concentrations were considered to be within the ranges reported in adults (fluoxetine 91-302 ng/mL; norfluoxetine 72-258 ng/mL).

Pregnancy Risk Factor C

Dosage Forms

Capsule: 10 mg, 20 mg, 40 mg

Prozac®: 10 mg, 20 mg, 40 mg

Sarafem®: 10 mg, 20 mg

Capsule, delayed release:

Prozac® Weekly™: 90 mg

Solution, oral: 20 mg/5 mL

Prozac®: 20 mg/5 mL

Tablet: 10 mg, 20 mg

Selected Readings

Friedlander AH and Mahler ME, "Major Depressive Disorder. Psychopathology, Medical Management, and Dental Implications," *J Am Dent Assoc*, 2001, 132(5):629-38.

Gerber PE and Lynd LD, "Selective Serotonin Reuptake Inhibitor-induced Movement Disorders," *Ann Pharmacother*, 1998, 32(6):692-8.

Wynn RL, "New Antidepressant Medications," *Gen Dent*, 1997, 45(1):24-8.

Fluoxetine and Olanzapine *see* Olanzapine and Fluoxetine *on page 1202*

Fluoxetine Hydrochloride *see* Fluoxetine *on page 714*

Fluoxymesterone (floo oks i MES te rone)

U.S. Brand Names Halotestin®
Mexican Brand Names Stenox
Generic Available Yes
Pharmacologic Category Androgen
Use Replacement of endogenous testicular hormone; in females, palliative treatment of breast cancer
Unlabeled/Investigational Use Stimulation of erythropoiesis, angioneurotic edema
Local Anesthetic/Vasoconstrictor Precautions No information available to require special precautions
Effects on Dental Treatment No significant effects or complications reported
Common Adverse Effects
>10%:
  Male: Priapism
  Female: Menstrual problems (amenorrhea), virilism, breast soreness
  Cardiovascular: Edema
  Dermatologic: Acne
1% to 10%:
  Male: Prostatic carcinoma, hirsutism (increase in pubic hair growth), impotence, testicular atrophy
  Cardiovascular: Edema
  Gastrointestinal: GI irritation, nausea, vomiting
  Genitourinary: Prostatic hyperplasia
  Hepatic: Hepatic dysfunction
Restrictions C-III
Mechanism of Action Synthetic androgenic anabolic hormone responsible for the normal growth and development of male sex hormones and development of male sex organs and maintenance of secondary sex characteristics; synthetic testosterone derivative with significant androgen activity; stimulates RNA polymerase activity resulting in an increase in protein production; increases bone development; halogenated derivative of testosterone with up to 5 times the activity of methyltestosterone
Drug Interactions
  Increased Effect/Toxicity: Fluoxymesterone may suppress clotting factors II, V, VII, and X; therefore, bleeding may occur in patients on anticoagulant therapy May elevate cyclosporine serum levels. May enhance hypoglycemic effect of insulin therapy; may decrease blood glucose concentrations and insulin requirements in patients with diabetes. Lithium may potentiate EPS and other CNS effect. May potentiate the effects of narcotics including respiratory depression
  Decreased Effect: May decrease barbiturate levels and fluphenazine effectiveness.
Pharmacodynamics/Kinetics
  Absorption: Rapid
  Protein binding: 98%
  Metabolism: Hepatic; enterohepatic recirculation
  Half-life elimination: 10-100 minutes
  Excretion: Urine (90%)
Pregnancy Risk Factor X

Fluphenazine (floo FEN a zeen)

U.S. Brand Names Prolixin® [DSC]; Prolixin Decanoate®
Canadian Brand Names Apo-Fluphenazine®; Apo-Fluphenazine Decanoate®; Modecate®; Modecate® Concentrate; PMS-Fluphenazine Decanoate
Generic Available Yes: Injection, tablet
Index Terms Fluphenazine Decanoate
Pharmacologic Category Antipsychotic Agent, Typical, Phenothiazine
Use Management of manifestations of psychotic disorders and schizophrenia; depot formulation may offer improved outcome in individuals with psychosis who are nonadherent with oral antipsychotics
Unlabeled/Investigational Use Pervasive developmental disorder; nonpsychotic patient, dementia behavior in the elderly
Local Anesthetic/Vasoconstrictor Precautions Most pharmacology textbooks state that in presence of phenothiazines, systemic doses of epinephrine paradoxically decrease the blood pressure. This is the so called "epinephrine reversal" phenomenon. This has never been observed when epinephrine is given by infiltration as part of the anesthesia procedure.

Effects on Dental Treatment Key adverse event(s) related to dental treatment: Xerostomia and increased salivation (normal salivary flow resumes upon discontinuation). Orthostatic hypotension and nasal congestion are possible and since the drug is a dopamine antagonist, extrapyramidal symptoms of the TMJ are a possibility.

Common Adverse Effects Frequency not defined.

Cardiovascular: Hyper-/hypotension, tachycardia, fluctuations in blood pressure, arrhythmia, edema

Central nervous system: Parkinsonian symptoms, akathisia, dystonias, tardive dyskinesia, dizziness, hyper-reflexia, headache, cerebral edema, drowsiness, lethargy, restlessness, excitement, bizarre dreams, EEG changes, depression, seizure, NMS, altered central temperature regulation

Dermatologic: Dermatitis, eczema, erythema, itching, photosensitivity, rash, seborrhea, skin pigmentation, urticaria

Endocrine & metabolic: Menstrual cycle changes, breast pain, amenorrhea, galactorrhea, gynecomastia, libido changes, prolactin increased, SIADH

Gastrointestinal: Weight gain, appetite loss, salivation, xerostomia, constipation, paralytic ileus, laryngeal edema

Genitourinary: Ejaculatory disturbances, impotence, polyuria, bladder paralysis, enuresis

Hematologic: Agranulocytosis, leukopenia, thrombocytopenia, nonthrombocytopenic purpura, eosinophilia, pancytopenia

Hepatic: Cholestatic jaundice, hepatotoxicity

Neuromuscular & skeletal: Trembling of fingers, SLE, facial hemispasm

Ocular: Pigmentary retinopathy, cornea and lens changes, blurred vision, glaucoma

Respiratory: Nasal congestion, asthma

Mechanism of Action Fluphenazine is a piperazine phenothiazine antipsychotic which blocks postsynaptic mesolimbic dopaminergic D_1 and D_2 receptors in the brain; depresses the release of hypothalamic and hypophyseal hormones; believed to depress the reticular activating system, thus affecting basal metabolism, body temperature, wakefulness, vasomotor tone, and emesis

Drug Interactions

Cytochrome P450 Effect: **Substrate** of CYP2D6 (major); **Inhibits** CYP1A2 (weak), 2C9 (weak), 2D6 (weak), 2E1 (weak)

Increased Effect/Toxicity: CYP2D6 inhibitors may increase the levels/effects of fluphenazine; example inhibitors include chlorpromazine, delavirdine, fluoxetine, miconazole, paroxetine, pergolide, quinidine, quinine, ritonavir, and ropinirole. Effects on CNS depression may be additive when fluphenazine is combined with CNS depressants (opioid analgesics, ethanol, barbiturates, cyclic antidepressants, antihistamines, sedative-hypnotics). Fluphenazine may increase the effects/toxicity of anticholinergics, antihypertensives, lithium (rare neurotoxicity), trazodone, or valproic acid. Concurrent use with TCA may produce increased toxicity or altered therapeutic response. Chloroquine and propranolol may increase chlorpromazine concentrations. Hypotension may occur when fluphenazine is combined with epinephrine. May increase the risk of arrhythmia when combined with antiarrhythmics, cisapride, pimozide, sparfloxacin, or other drugs which prolong QT interval. Metoclopramide may increase risk of extrapyramidal symptoms (EPS). Acetylcholinesterase inhibitors (central) may increase the risk of antipsychotic-related EPS.

Decreased Effect: Phenothiazines inhibit the activity of guanethidine, guanadrel, levodopa, and bromocriptine. Barbiturates and cigarette smoking may enhance the hepatic metabolism of fluphenazine. Fluphenazine and possibly other low potency antipsychotics may reverse the pressor effects of epinephrine.

Pharmacodynamics/Kinetics

Onset of action: I.M., SubQ (derivative dependent): Hydrochloride salt: ~1 hour
Peak effect: Neuroleptic: Decanoate: 48-96 hours

Duration: Hydrochloride salt: 6-8 hours; Decanoate: 24-72 hours

Absorption: Oral: Erratic and variable

Distribution: Crosses placenta; enters breast milk

Protein binding: 91% and 99%

Metabolism: Hepatic

Half-life elimination (derivative dependent): Hydrochloride: 33 hours; Decanoate: 163-232 hours

Excretion: Urine (as metabolites)

Pregnancy Risk Factor C

Fluphenazine Decanoate see Fluphenazine on page 718
Flura-Drops® see Fluoride on page 710

Flurandrenolide (flure an DREN oh lide)

U.S. Brand Names Cordran®; Cordran® SP
Canadian Brand Names Cordran®
Generic Available No
Index Terms Flurandrenolone
Pharmacologic Category Corticosteroid, Topical
Use Inflammation of corticosteroid-responsive dermatoses [medium potency topical corticosteroid]
Local Anesthetic/Vasoconstrictor Precautions No information available to require special precautions
Effects on Dental Treatment No significant effects or complications reported
Common Adverse Effects Frequency not defined.
  Cardiovascular: Intracranial hypertension
  Dermatologic: Acne, acneiform eruptions, allergic contact dermatitis, dry skin, folliculitis, hyperpigmentation, hypertrichosis, itching, maceration of the skin, miliaria, perioral dermatitis, skin atrophy, striae
  Endocrine & metabolic: Cushing's syndrome, growth retardation, HPA suppression
  Local: Burning, irritation
  Miscellaneous: Secondary infection
Mechanism of Action Decreases inflammation by suppression of migration of polymorphonuclear leukocytes and reversal of increased capillary permeability
Pharmacodynamics/Kinetics
  Absorption: Adequate with intact skin; repeated applications lead to depot effects on skin, potentially resulting in enhanced percutaneous absorption
  Metabolism: Hepatic
  Excretion: Urine; feces (small amounts)
Pregnancy Risk Factor C

Flurandrenolone see Flurandrenolide on page 720

Flurazepam (flure AZ e pam)

U.S. Brand Names Dalmane®
Canadian Brand Names Apo-Flurazepam®; Dalmane®; Som Pam
Generic Available Yes
Index Terms Flurazepam Hydrochloride
Pharmacologic Category Hypnotic, Benzodiazepine
Use Short-term treatment of insomnia
Local Anesthetic/Vasoconstrictor Precautions No information available to require special precautions
Effects on Dental Treatment Key adverse event(s) related to dental treatment: Xerostomia and changes in salivation (normal salivary flow resumes upon discontinuation), and bitter taste.
Common Adverse Effects Frequency not defined.
  Cardiovascular: Chest pain, flushing, hypotension, palpitation
  Central nervous system: Apprehension, ataxia, confusion, depression, dizziness, drowsiness, euphoria, faintness, falling, hallucinations, hangover effect, headache, irritability, lightheadedness, memory impairment, nervousness, paradoxical reactions, restlessness, slurred speech, staggering, talkativeness
  Dermatologic: Pruritus, rash
  Gastrointestinal: Appetite increased/decreased, bitter taste, constipation, diarrhea, GI pain, heartburn, nausea, salivation increased/excessive, upset stomach, vomiting, weight gain/loss, xerostomia
  Hematologic: Granulocytopenia, leukopenia
  Hepatic: Alkaline phosphatase increased, ALT/AST increased, cholestatic jaundice, total bilirubin increased
  Neuromuscular & skeletal: Body/joint pain, dysarthria, reflex slowing, weakness
  Ocular: Blurred vision, burning eyes, difficulty focusing
  Respiratory: Apnea, dyspnea
  Miscellaneous: Diaphoresis, drug dependence
  Postmarketing and/or case reports: Anaphylaxis, angioedema, complex sleep-related behavior (sleep-driving, cooking or eating food, making phone calls)
Restrictions C-IV
Dosage Oral:
  Children: Insomnia:
    <15 years: Dose not established
    ≥15 years: 15 mg at bedtime
  Adults: Insomnia: 15-30 mg at bedtime

Elderly: Insomnia: Oral: 15 mg at bedtime; avoid use if possible

Mechanism of Action Binds to stereospecific benzodiazepine receptors on the postsynaptic GABA neuron at several sites within the central nervous system, including the limbic system, reticular formation. Enhancement of the inhibitory effect of GABA on neuronal excitability results by increased neuronal membrane permeability to chloride ions. This shift in chloride ions results in hyperpolarization (a less excitable state) and stabilization.

Contraindications Hypersensitivity to flurazepam or any component of the formulation (cross-sensitivity with other benzodiazepines may exist); narrow-angle glaucoma; pregnancy

Warnings/Precautions Use with caution in elderly or debilitated patients, patients with hepatic disease (including alcoholics), or renal impairment. Use with caution in patients with respiratory disease or impaired gag reflex. Avoid use in patients with sleep apnea.

Causes CNS depression (dose related); patients must be cautioned about performing tasks which require mental alertness (eg, operating machinery or driving). Use with caution in patients receiving other CNS depressants or psychoactive agents. Benzodiazepines have been associated with falls and traumatic injury and should be used with extreme caution in patients who are at risk of these events (especially the elderly).

Use caution in patients with depression, particularly if suicidal risk may be present. Use with caution in patients with a history of drug dependence. Benzodiazepines have been associated with dependence and acute withdrawal symptoms on discontinuation or reduction in dose (may occur after as little as 10 days of use).

As a hypnotic, should be used only after evaluation of potential causes of sleep disturbance. Failure of sleep disturbance to resolve after 7-10 days may indicate psychiatric or medical illness. A worsening of insomnia or the emergence of new abnormalities of thought or behavior may represent unrecognized psychiatric or medical illness and requires immediate and careful evaluation. Postmarketing studies have indicated that the use of hypnotic/sedative agents for sleep has been associated with hypersensitivity reactions including anaphylaxis as well as angioedema. An increased risk for hazardous sleep-related activities such as sleep-driving; cooking and eating food, and making phone calls while asleep have also been noted.

Benzodiazepines have been associated with anterograde amnesia. Paradoxical reactions have been reported, particularly in adolescent/pediatric or psychiatric patients. Does not have analgesic, antidepressant, or antipsychotic properties.

Safety and efficacy have not been established in children <15 years of age.

Drug Interactions

Cytochrome P450 Effect: Substrate of CYP3A4 (major); **Inhibits** CYP2E1 (weak)

Increased Effect/Toxicity: CYP3A4 inhibitors may increase the levels/effects of flurazepam; example inhibitors include azole antifungals, clarithromycin, diclofenac, doxycycline, erythromycin, imatinib, isoniazid, nefazodone, nicardipine, propofol, protease inhibitors, quinidine, telithromycin, and verapamil. Serum levels and response to flurazepam may be increased by cimetidine, clozapine, CNS depressants, diltiazem, disulfiram, digoxin, ethanol, fluconazole, fluoxetine, fluvoxamine, grapefruit juice, labetalol, levodopa, loxapine, metoprolol, metronidazole, nelfinavir, omeprazole, and valproic acid.

Decreased Effect: CYP3A4 inducers may decrease the levels/effects of flurazepam; example inducers include aminoglutethimide, carbamazepine, nafcillin, nevirapine, phenobarbital, phenytoin, and rifamycins.

Ethanol/Nutrition/Herb Interactions

Ethanol: Avoid ethanol (may increase CNS depression).

Food: Serum levels and response to flurazepam may be increased by grapefruit juice, but unlikely because of flurazepam's high oral bioavailability.

Herb/Nutraceutical: Avoid valerian, St John's wort, kava kava, gotu kola (may increase CNS depression).

Pharmacodynamics/Kinetics

Onset of action: Hypnotic: 15-20 minutes

Peak effect: 3-6 hours

Duration: 7-8 hours

Metabolism: Hepatic to N-desalkylflurazepam (active) and N-hydroxyethylflurazepam

Half-life elimination:

Flurazepam: 2.3 hours

N-desalkylflurazepam:

Adults: Single dose: 74-90 hours; Multiple doses: 111-113 hours

Elderly (61-85 years): Single dose: 120-160 hours; Multiple doses: 126-158 hours

(Continued)

Flurazepam *(Continued)*

Excretion: Urine: N-hydroxyethylflurazepam (22% to 55%); N-desalkyl-flurazepam (<1%)

Pregnancy Risk Factor X

Dosage Forms

Capsule: 15 mg, 30 mg
Dalmane®: 15 mg, 30 mg

Flurazepam Hydrochloride *see* Flurazepam *on page 720*

Flurbiprofen *(flure BI proe fen)*

Related Information

Rheumatoid Arthritis, Osteoarthritis, and Osteoporosis *on page 1759*
Temporomandibular Dysfunction (TMD) *on page 1822*

U.S. Brand Names Ansaid® [DSC]; Ocufen®

Canadian Brand Names Alti-Flurbiprofen; Ansaid®; Apo-Flurbiprofen®; Froben®; Froben-SR®; Novo-Flurprofen; Nu-Flurprofen; Ocufen®

Mexican Brand Names Ansaid; Ocufen

Generic Available Yes

Index Terms Flurbiprofen Sodium

Pharmacologic Category Nonsteroidal Anti-inflammatory Drug (NSAID), Ophthalmic; Nonsteroidal Anti-inflammatory Drug (NSAID), Oral

Dental Use Oral: Management of postoperative pain

Use

Oral: Treatment of rheumatoid arthritis and osteoarthritis
Ophthalmic: Inhibition of intraoperative miosis

Local Anesthetic/Vasoconstrictor Precautions No information available to require special precautions

Effects on Dental Treatment NSAID formulations are known to reversibly decrease platelet aggregation via mechanisms different than observed with aspirin. The dentist should be aware of the potential of abnormal coagulation. Caution should also be exercised in the use of NSAIDs in patients already on anticoagulant therapy with drugs such as warfarin (Coumadin®).

Significant Adverse Effects

Ophthalmic: Frequency not defined: Ocular: Slowing of corneal wound healing, mild ocular stinging, itching and burning, ocular irritation, fibrosis, miosis, mydriasis, bleeding tendency increased

Oral:

>1%:

Cardiovascular: Edema

Central nervous system: Amnesia, anxiety, depression, dizziness, headache, insomnia, malaise, nervousness, somnolence, vertigo

Dermatologic: Rash

Gastrointestinal: Abdominal pain, constipation, diarrhea, dyspepsia, flatulence, GI bleeding, nausea, vomiting, weight changes

Hepatic: Liver enzymes increased

Neuromuscular & skeletal: Reflexes increased, tremor, weakness

Ocular: Vision changes

Otic: Tinnitus

Respiratory: Rhinitis

<1% (Limited to important or life-threatening): Anaphylactic reaction, anemia, angioedema, asthma, bruising, cerebrovascular ischemia, CHF, confusion, eczema, eosinophilia, epistaxis, exfoliative dermatitis, fever, gastric/peptic ulcer, hematocrit decreased, hematuria, hemoglobin decreased, hepatitis, hypertension, hyperuricemia, interstitial nephritis, jaundice, leukopenia, paresthesia, parosmia, photosensitivity, pruritus, purpura, renal failure, stomatitis, thrombocytopenia, toxic epidermal necrolysis, urticaria, vasodilation

Restrictions An FDA-approved medication guide must be distributed when dispensing an oral outpatient prescription (new or refill) where this medication is to be used without direct supervision of a healthcare provider. Medication guides are available at http://www.fda.gov/cder/Offices/ODS/medication_guides.htm.

Dental Usual Dosing Management of postoperative pain: Adults: Oral: 100 mg every 12 hours

Dosage

Oral:

Rheumatoid arthritis and osteoarthritis: 200-300 mg/day in 2-, 3-, or 4 divided doses; do not administer more than 100 mg for any single dose; maximum: 300 mg/day

Dental: Management of postoperative pain: 100 mg every 12 hours

Ophthalmic: Instill 1 drop every 30 minutes, beginning 2 hours prior to surgery (total of 4 drops in each affected eye)

Dosage adjustment in renal impairment: Not recommended in patients with advanced renal disease

Mechanism of Action Inhibits prostaglandin synthesis by decreasing the activity of the enzyme, cyclooxygenase, which results in decreased formation of prostaglandin precursors

Contraindications Hypersensitivity to flurbiprofen, aspirin, other NSAIDs, or any component of the formulation; perioperative pain in the setting of coronary artery bypass surgery (CABG); dendritic keratitis; pregnancy (3rd trimester)

Warnings/Precautions [U.S. Boxed Warning]: NSAIDs are associated with an increased risk of adverse cardiovascular events, including MI, stroke, and new onset or worsening of pre-existing hypertension. Risk may be increased with duration of use or pre-existing cardiovascular risk factors or disease. Carefully evaluate individual cardiovascular risk profiles prior to prescribing. Use caution with fluid retention, CHF, or hypertension. Concurrent administration of ibuprofen, and potentially other nonselective NSAIDs, may interfere with aspirin's cardioprotective effect.

Use of NSAIDs can compromise existing renal function. Renal toxicity can occur in patient with impaired renal function, dehydration, heart failure, liver dysfunction, those taking diuretics and ACEIs, and the elderly. Rehydrate patient before starting therapy. Monitor renal function closely. Not recommended for use in patients with advanced renal disease.

[U.S. Boxed Warning]: NSAIDs may increase risk of gastrointestinal irritation, ulceration, bleeding, and perforation. These events may occur at any time during therapy and without warning. Use caution with a history of GI disease (bleeding or ulcers), concurrent therapy with aspirin, anticoagulants and/or corticosteroids, smoking, use of alcohol, the elderly, or debilitated patients.

Use the lowest effective dose for the shortest duration of time, consistent with individual patient goals, to reduce risk of cardiovascular or GI adverse events. Alternate therapies should be considered for patients at high risk.

NSAIDs may cause serious skin adverse events including exfoliative dermatitis, Stevens-Johnson syndrome (SJS), and toxic epidermal necrolysis (TEN). Anaphylactoid reactions may occur, even without prior exposure; patients with "aspirin triad" (bronchial asthma, aspirin intolerance, rhinitis) may be at increased risk. Do not use in patients who experience bronchospasm, asthma, rhinitis, or urticaria with NSAID or aspirin therapy. Use caution in other forms of asthma.

Use with caution in patients with decreased hepatic function. Closely monitor patients with any abnormal LFT. Severe hepatic reactions (eg, fulminant hepatitis, liver failure) have occurred with NSAID use, rarely; discontinue if signs or symptoms of liver disease develop, or if systemic manifestations occur.

The elderly are at increased risk for adverse effects (especially peptic ulceration, CNS effects, renal toxicity) from NSAIDs even at low doses.

Withhold for at least 4-6 half-lives prior to surgical or dental procedures. Safety and efficacy have not been established in children.

Drug Interactions Substrate of CYP2C9 (minor); **Inhibits** CYP2C9 (strong)

ACE inhibitors: Antihypertensive effects may be decreased by concurrent therapy with NSAIDs; monitor blood pressure.

Angiotensin II antagonists: Antihypertensive effects may be decreased by concurrent therapy with NSAIDs; monitor blood pressure.

Anticoagulants (warfarin, heparin, LMWHs) in combination with NSAIDs can cause increased risk of bleeding.

Antiplatelet drugs (ticlopidine, clopidogrel, aspirin, abciximab, dipyridamole, eptifibatide, tirofiban) can cause an increased risk of bleeding.

Beta-blockers: NSAIDs may decrease the antihypertensive effect of beta-blockers. Monitor.

Cholestyramine (and other bile acid sequestrants): May decrease the absorption of NSAIDs. Separate by at least 2 hours.

Corticosteroids may increase the risk of GI ulceration; avoid concurrent use.

Cyclosporine: NSAIDs may increase serum creatinine, potassium, blood pressure, and cyclosporine levels; monitor cyclosporine levels and renal function carefully.

CYP2C9 Substrates: Flurbiprofen may increase the levels/effects of CYP2C9 substrates. Example substrates include bosentan, dapsone, fluoxetine, glimepiride, glipizide, losartan, montelukast, nateglinide, paclitaxel, phenytoin, warfarin, and zafirlukast.

Gentamicin and amikacin serum concentrations are increased by indomethacin in premature infants. Results may apply to other aminoglycosides and NSAIDs.

(Continued)

Flurbiprofen *(Continued)*

Hydralazine's antihypertensive effect is decreased; avoid concurrent use.

Lithium levels can be increased; avoid concurrent use if possible or monitor lithium levels and adjust dose. Sulindac may have the least effect. When NSAID is stopped, lithium will need adjustment again.

Loop diuretics efficacy (diuretic and antihypertensive effect) is reduced. Indomethacin reduces this efficacy, however, it may be anticipated with any NSAID.

Methotrexate: Severe bone marrow suppression, aplastic anemia, and GI toxicity have been reported with concomitant NSAID therapy. Avoid use during moderate or high-dose methotrexate (increased and prolonged methotrexate levels). NSAID use during low-dose treatment of rheumatoid arthritis has not been fully evaluated; extreme caution is warranted.

Salicylates: NSAIDs (nonselective) may diminish the cardioprotective effect of acetylated salicylates. Avoid regular use of NSAIDs if possible; consider alternatives (eg, acetaminophen). Give salicylate before NSAID; for example ibuprofen should be given 30-120 minutes after aspirin (immediate release).

Thiazides antihypertensive effects are decreased; avoid concurrent use.

Warfarin's INRs may be increased by piroxicam. Other NSAIDs may have the same effect depending on dose and duration. Monitor INR closely. Use the lowest dose of NSAIDs possible and for the briefest duration.

Verapamil plasma concentration is decreased by some NSAIDs; avoid concurrent use.

Ethanol/Nutrition/Herb Interactions

Ethanol: Avoid ethanol (may enhance gastric mucosal irritation).

Food: Food may decrease the rate but not the extent of absorption.

Herb/Nutraceutical: Avoid alfalfa, anise, bilberry, bladderwrack, bromelain, cat's claw, celery, coleus, cordyceps, dong quai, evening primrose, feverfew, fenugreek, garlic, ginger, ginkgo biloba, red clover, horse chestnut, horse chestnut seed, horseradish, licorice, prickly ash, red clover, reishi, SAMe, sweet clover, turmeric, white willow (all have additional antiplatelet activity).

Dietary Considerations
Tablet may be taken with food, milk, or antacid to decrease GI effects.

Pharmacodynamics/Kinetics

Onset of action: ~1-2 hours

Distribution: V_d: 0.12 L/kg

Protein binding: 99%, primarily albumin

Metabolism: Hepatic via CYP2C9; forms metabolites such as 4-hydroxy-flurbiprofen (inactive)

Half-life elimination: 5.7 hours

Time to peak: 1.5 hours

Excretion: Urine (primarily as metabolites)

Pregnancy Risk Factor
C/D (3rd trimester)

Lactation
Enters breast milk/not recommended

Dosage Forms
Excipient information presented when available (limited, particularly for generics); consult specific product labeling. [DSC] = Discontinued product

Solution, ophthalmic, as sodium (Ocufen®): 0.03% (2.5 mL) [contains thimerosal]

Tablet: 50 mg, 100 mg

Ansaid®: 50 mg, 100 mg [DSC]

Selected Readings

Ahmad N, Grad HA, Haas DA, et al, "The Efficacy of Nonopioid Analgesics for Postoperative Dental Pain: A Meta-Analysis," *Anesth Prog*, 1997, 44(4):119-26.

Bragger U, Muhle T, Fourmousis I, et al, "Effect of the NSAID Flurbiprofen on Remodeling After Periodontal Surgery," *J Periodontal Res*, 1997, 32(7):575-82.

Cooper SA and Kupperman A, "The Analgesic Efficacy of Flurbiprofen Compared to Acetaminophen With Codeine," *J Clin Dent*, 1991, 2(3):70-4.

Dionne R, "Additive Analgesia Without Opioid Side Effects," *Compend Contin Educ Dent*, 2000, 21(7):572-4, 576-7.

Dionne RA, "Suppression of Dental Pain by the Preoperative Administration of Flurbiprofen," *Am J Med*, 1986, 80(3A):41-9.

Dionne RA and Berthold CW, "Therapeutic Uses of Nonsteroidal Anti-inflammatory Drugs in Dentistry," *Crit Rev Oral Biol Med*, 2001, 12(4):315-30.

Dionne RA, Snyder J, and Hargreaves KM, "Analgesic Efficacy of Flurbiprofen in Comparison With Acetaminophen, Acetaminophen Plus Codeine, and Placebo After Impacted Third Molar Removal," *J Oral Maxillofac Surg*, 1994, 52(9):919-24.

Doroschak AM, Bowles WR, and Hargreaves KM, "Evaluation of the Combination of Flurbiprofen and Tramadol for Management of Endodontic Pain," *J Endod*, 1999, 25(10):660-3.

Forbes JA, Yorio CC, Selinger LR, et al, "An Evaluation of Flurbiprofen, Aspirin, and Placebo in Postoperative Oral Surgery Pain," *Pharmacotherapy*, 1989, 9(2):66-73.

Gallardo F and Rossi E, "Analgesic Efficacy of Flurbiprofen as Compared to Acetaminophen and Placebo After Periodontal Surgery," *J Periodontol*, 1990, 11(2):224-7.

Jeffcoat MK, Reddy MS, Haigh S, et al, "A Comparison of Topical Ketorolac, Systemic Flurbiprofen, and Placebo for the Inhibition of Bone Loss in Adult Periodontitis," *J Periodontol*, 1995, 66(5):329-38.

Jeffcoat MK, Reddy MS, Wang IC, et al, "The Effect of Systemic Flurbiprofen on Bone Supporting Dental Implants," *J Am Dent Assoc*, 1995, 126(3):305-11.

Malmberg AB and Yaksh TL, "Antinociception Produced by Spinal Delivery of the S and R Enantiomers of Flurbiprofen in the Formalin Test," *Eur J Pharmacol*, 1994, 256(2):205-9.

Nguyen AM, Graham DY, Gage T, et al, "Nonsteroidal Anti-inflammatory Drug Use in Dentistry: Gastrointestinal Implications," *Gen Dent*, 1999, 47(6):590-6.

Flurbiprofen Sodium *see* Flurbiprofen *on page 722*

5-Flurocytosine *see* Flucytosine *on page 699*

Fluro-Ethyl® *see* Ethyl Chloride and Dichlorotetrafluoroethane *on page 654*

Flutamide (FLOO ta mide)

U.S. Brand Names Eulexin®

Canadian Brand Names Apo-Flutamide®; Euflex®; Eulexin®; Novo-Flutamide

Mexican Brand Names Eulexin; Fluken; Flulem; Tafenil

Generic Available Yes

Index Terms Niftolid; NSC-147834; 4'-Nitro-3'-Trifluoromethylisobutyrantide; SCH 13521

Pharmacologic Category Antineoplastic Agent, Antiandrogen

Use Treatment of metastatic prostatic carcinoma in combination therapy with LHRH agonist analogues

Unlabeled/Investigational Use Female hirsutism

Local Anesthetic/Vasoconstrictor Precautions No information available to require special precautions

Effects on Dental Treatment No significant effects or complications reported

Common Adverse Effects

>10%:

Endocrine & metabolic: Gynecomastia, hot flashes, breast tenderness, galactorrhea (9% to 42%), impotence, libido decreased, tumor flare

Gastrointestinal: Nausea, vomiting (11% to 12%)

Hepatic: AST and LDH levels increased, transient, mild

1% to 10%:

Cardiovascular: Hypertension (1%), edema

Central nervous system: Drowsiness, confusion, depression, anxiety, nervousness, headache, dizziness, insomnia

Dermatologic: Pruritus, ecchymosis, photosensitivity

Gastrointestinal: Anorexia, appetite increased, constipation, indigestion, upset stomach (4% to 6%); diarrhea

Hematologic: Anemia (6%), leukopenia (3%), thrombocytopenia (1%)

Neuromuscular & skeletal: Weakness (1%)

Miscellaneous: Herpes zoster

Mechanism of Action Nonsteroidal antiandrogen that inhibits androgen uptake or inhibits binding of androgen in target tissues

Drug Interactions

Cytochrome P450 Effect: Substrate (major) of CYP1A2, 3A4; **Inhibits** CYP1A2 (weak)

Increased Effect/Toxicity: CYP1A2 inhibitors may increase the levels/effects of flutamide; example inhibitors include ciprofloxacin, fluvoxamine, ketoconazole, lomefloxacin, ofloxacin, and rofecoxib. CYP3A4 inhibitors may increase the levels/effects of flutamide; example inhibitors include azole antifungals, clarithromycin, diclofenac, doxycycline, erythromycin, imatinib, isoniazid, nefazodone, nicardipine, propofol, protease inhibitors, quinidine, telithromycin, and verapamil. Warfarin effects may be increased.

Decreased Effect: CYP1A2 inducers may decrease the levels/effects of flutamide; example inducers include aminoglutethimide, carbamazepine, phenobarbital, and rifampin. CYP3A4 inducers may decrease the levels/effects of flutamide; example inducers include aminoglutethimide, carbamazepine, nafcillin, nevirapine, phenobarbital, phenytoin, and rifamycins.

Pharmacodynamics/Kinetics

Absorption: Oral: Rapid and complete

Protein binding: Parent drug: 94% to 96%; 2-hydroxyflutamide: 92% to 94%

Metabolism: Extensively hepatic to more than 10 metabolites, primarily 2-hydroxyflutamide (active)

Half-life elimination: 5-6 hours (2-hydroxyflutamide)

Excretion: Primarily urine (as metabolites)

Pregnancy Risk Factor D

Fluticasone (floo TIK a sone)

Related Information

Respiratory Diseases *on page 1747*

(Continued)

Fluticasone (Continued)

U.S. Brand Names Cutivate®; Flonase®; Flovent® HFA

Canadian Brand Names Cutivate™; Flonase®; Flovent® Diskus®; Flovent® HFA

Mexican Brand Names Cutivate; Flixonase; Flixotide

Generic Available Yes: Cream, nasal spray, ointment

Index Terms Fluticasone Propionate

Pharmacologic Category Corticosteroid, Inhalant (Oral); Corticosteroid, Nasal; Corticosteroid, Topical; Corticosteroid, Topical (Medium Potency)

Use

Inhalation: Maintenance treatment of asthma as prophylactic therapy; also indicated for patients requiring oral corticosteroid therapy for asthma to assist in total discontinuation or reduction of total oral dose

Intranasal: Management of seasonal and perennial allergic rhinitis and nonallergic rhinitis

Topical: Relief of inflammation and pruritus associated with corticosteroid-responsive dermatoses; atopic dermatitis

Local Anesthetic/Vasoconstrictor Precautions No information available to require special precautions

Effects on Dental Treatment Localized infections with *Candida albicans* or *Aspergillus niger* have occurred frequently in the mouth and pharynx with repetitive use of oral inhaler of corticosteroids. These infections may require treatment with appropriate antifungal therapy or discontinuance of treatment with corticosteroid inhaler.

Common Adverse Effects

Oral inhalation:

>10%:

Central nervous system: Headache (5% to 11%)

Respiratory: Upper respiratory tract infection (16% to 18%)

3% to 10%:

Respiratory: Throat irritation (8% to 10%), sinusitis/sinus infection (4% to 7%), cough (4% to 6%), bronchitis (2% to 6%), hoarseness/dysphonia (2% to 6%), upper respiratory tract inflammation (2% to 5%)

Miscellaneous: Candidiasis (2% to 5%)

1% to 3%:

Cardiovascular: Chest symptoms

Central nervous system: Dizziness, fever, migraine, pain

Gastrointestinal: Diarrhea, dyspepsia, gastrointestinal infection (viral), gastrointestinal discomfort/pain, hyposalivation

Genitourinary: Urinary tract infection

Neuromuscular & skeletal: Musculoskeletal pain, muscle pain, muscle stiffness/tightness/rigidity

Respiratory: Rhinitis, pharyngitis/throat infection, rhinorrhea/postnasal drip, nasal sinus disorder, laryngitis

Miscellaneous: Viral infection, injuries (including muscle, soft tissue)

Nasal inhalation:

>10%: Central nervous system: Headache (7% to 16%)

1% to 10%:

Central nervous system: Dizziness (1% to 3%), fever (1% to 3%)

Gastrointestinal: Nausea/vomiting (3% to 5%), abdominal pain (1% to 3%), diarrhea (1% to 3%)

Respiratory: Pharyngitis (6% to 8%), epistaxis (6% to 7%), asthma symptoms (3% to 7%), cough (4%), blood in nasal mucous (1% to 3%), runny nose (1% to 3%), bronchitis (1% to 3%)

Miscellaneous: Aches and pains (1% to 3%), flu-like syndrome (1% to 3%)

Topical: 1% to 10%:

Dermatologic: Dry skin (7%), skin burning/stinging (2% to 5%), pruritus (3%), skin irritation (3%), viral skin infection (1% to 3%), exacerbation of eczema (2%)

Neuromuscular & skeletal: Numbness of fingers (1%)

Reported with other topical corticosteroids (in decreasing order of occurrence): Irritation, folliculitis, acneiform eruptions, hypopigmentation, perioral dermatitis, allergic contact dermatitis, secondary infection, skin atrophy, striae, miliaria, pustular psoriasis from chronic plaque psoriasis

Dosage

Children:

Asthma: Inhalation, oral:

Flovent® HFA:

Children 4-11 years: 88 mcg twice daily

Children ≥12 years: Refer to adult dosing.

Note: NIH Asthma Guidelines (administer in divided doses twice daily):
"Low" dose: 88-176 mcg/day
"Medium" dose: 176-440 mcg/day
"High" dose: >440 mcg/day
Flovent® Diskus® [CAN]:
Children 4-16 years: Usual starting dose: 50-100 mcg twice daily; may increase to 200 mcg twice daily in patients not adequately controlled; titrate to the lowest effective dose once asthma stability is achieved
Children ≥16 years: Refer to adult dosing

Corticosteroid-responsive dermatoses: Topical: Children ≥3 months: Cream: Apply sparingly to affected area twice daily. If no improvement is seen within 2 weeks, reassessment of diagnosis may be necessary. **Note:** Safety and efficacy of treatment >4 weeks duration have not been established.

Atopic dermatitis: Topical:
Children ≥3 months: Cream: Apply sparingly to affected area 1-2 times/day. If no improvement is seen within 2 weeks, reassessment of diagnosis may be necessary.
Children ≥1 year: Lotion: Apply sparingly to affected area once daily
Note: Safety and efficacy of treatment >4 weeks duration have not been established.

Rhinitis: Intranasal: Children ≥4 years and Adolescents: Initial: 1 spray (50 mcg/spray) per nostril once daily; patients not adequately responding or patients with more severe symptoms may use 2 sprays (100 mcg) per nostril. Depending on response, dosage may be reduced to 100 mcg daily. Total daily dosage should not exceed 2 sprays in each nostril (200 mcg)/day. Dosing should be at regular intervals.

Adults:

Asthma: Inhalation, oral: **Note:** Titrate to the lowest effective dose once asthma stability is achieved
Flovent® HFA: Manufacturers labeling: Dosing based on previous therapy
Bronchodilator alone: Recommended starting dose: 88 mcg twice daily; highest recommended dose: 440 mcg twice daily
Inhaled corticosteroids: Recommended starting dose: 88-220 mcg twice daily; highest recommended dose: 440 mcg twice daily; a higher starting dose may be considered in patients previously requiring higher doses of inhaled corticosteroids
Oral corticosteroids: Recommended starting dose:
Flovent® HFA: 440 mcg twice daily
Highest recommended dose: 880 mcg twice daily; starting dose is patient dependent. In patients on chronic oral corticosteroids therapy, reduce prednisone dose no faster than 2.5-5 mg/day on a weekly basis; begin taper after 1 week of fluticasone therapy.
NIH Asthma Guidelines (administer in divided doses twice daily).
"Low" dose: 88-264 mcg/day
"Medium" dose: 264-660 mcg/day
"High" dose: >660 mcg/day
Flovent® Diskus® [CAN]:
Mild asthma: 100-250 mcg twice daily
Moderate asthma: 250-500 mcg twice daily
Severe asthma: 500 mcg twice daily; may increase to 1000 mcg twice daily in very severe patients requiring high doses of corticosteroids

Corticosteroid-responsive dermatoses: Topical: Cream, lotion, ointment: Apply sparingly to affected area twice daily. If no improvement is seen within 2 weeks, reassessment of diagnosis may be necessary.

Atopic dermatitis: Topical: Cream, lotion: Apply sparingly to affected area once or twice daily. If no improvement is seen within 2 weeks, reassessment of diagnosis may be necessary.

Rhinitis: Intranasal: Initial: 2 sprays (50 mcg/spray) per nostril once daily; may also be divided into 100 mcg twice a day. After the first few days, dosage may be reduced to 1 spray per nostril once daily for maintenance therapy. Dosing should be at regular intervals.

Elderly: No differences in safety have been observed in the elderly when compared to younger patients. Based on current data, no dosage adjustment is needed based on age.

Dosage adjustment in hepatic impairment: Fluticasone is primarily cleared in the liver. Fluticasone plasma levels may be increased in patients with hepatic impairment, use with caution; monitor.

Mechanism of Action Fluticasone belongs to a new group of corticosteroids which utilizes a fluorocarbothioate ester linkage at the 17 carbon position; extremely potent vasoconstrictive and anti-inflammatory activity; has a weak HPA inhibitory potency when applied topically, which gives the drug a high therapeutic index. The effectiveness of inhaled fluticasone is due to its direct
(Continued)

Fluticasone *(Continued)*

local effect. The mechanism of action for all topical corticosteroids is believed to be a combination of three important properties: anti-inflammatory activity, immunosuppressive properties, and antiproliferative actions.

Contraindications Hypersensitivity to fluticasone or any component of the formulation; primary treatment of status asthmaticus or acute bronchospasm

Topical: Do not use if infection is present at treatment site, in the presence of skin atrophy, or for the treatment of rosacea or perioral dermatitis

Warnings/Precautions May cause hypercorticism or suppression of hypothalamic-pituitary-adrenal (HPA) axis, particularly in younger children or in patients receiving high doses for prolonged periods. HPA axis suppression may lead to adrenal crisis. Withdrawal and discontinuation of a corticosteroid should be done slowly and carefully. Particular care is required when patients are transferred from systemic corticosteroids to inhaled products due to possible adrenal insufficiency or withdrawal from steroids, including an increase in allergic symptoms. Patients receiving >20 mg per day of prednisone (or equivalent) may be most susceptible. Concurrent use of ritonavir (and potentially other strong inhibitors of CYP3A4) may increase fluticasone levels and effects on HPA suppression. Fatalities have occurred due to adrenal insufficiency in asthmatic patients during and after transfer from systemic corticosteroids to aerosol steroids; aerosol steroids do **not** provide the systemic steroid needed to treat patients having trauma, surgery, or infections.

Bronchospasm may occur with wheezing after inhalation; if this occurs, stop steroid and treat with a fast-acting bronchodilator. Supplemental steroids (oral or parenteral) may be needed during stress or severe asthma attacks. Corticosteroid use may cause psychiatric disturbances, including depression, euphoria, insomnia, mood swings, and personality changes. Pre-existing psychiatric conditions may be exacerbated by corticosteroid use. Prolonged use of corticosteroids may also increase the incidence of secondary infection, mask acute infection (including fungal infections), prolong or exacerbate viral infections, or limit response to vaccines. Exposure to chickenpox should be avoided; corticosteroids should not be used to treat ocular herpes simplex. Corticosteroids should not be used for cerebral malaria. Close observation is required in patients with latent tuberculosis and/or TB reactivity; restrict use in active TB (only in conjunction with antituberculosis treatment). Rare cases of vasculitis (Churg-Strauss syndrome) or other eosinophilic conditions can occur. Prolonged treatment with corticosteroids has been associated with the development of Kaposi's sarcoma (case reports); if noted, discontinuation of therapy should be considered.

Use with caution in patients with thyroid disease, hepatic impairment, renal impairment, cardiovascular disease, diabetes, glaucoma, cataracts, myasthenia gravis, patients at risk for osteoporosis, patients at risk for seizures, or GI diseases (diverticulitis, peptic ulcer, ulcerative colitis) due to perforation risk. Use caution following acute MI (corticosteroids have been associated with myocardial rupture). Because of the risk of adverse effects, systemic corticosteroids should be used cautiously in the elderly in the smallest possible effective dose for the shortest duration. Avoid nasal corticosteroid use in patients with recent nasal septal ulcers, nasal surgery, or nasal trauma until healing has occurred.

Orally-inhaled and intranasal corticosteroids may cause a reduction in growth velocity in pediatric patients (~1 centimeter per year [range 0.3-1.8 cm per year] and related to dose and duration of exposure). To minimize the systemic effects of orally-inhaled and intranasal corticosteroids, each patient should be titrated to the lowest effective dose. Growth should be routinely monitored in pediatric patients.

Inhalation: Not to be used in status asthmaticus or for the relief of acute bronchospasm. Flovent® Diskus® [CAN] contains lactose; very rare anaphylactic reactions have been reported in patients with severe milk protein allergy. There have been reports of systemic corticosteroid withdrawal symptoms (eg, joint/muscle pain, lassitude, depression) when withdrawing oral inhalation therapy.

Topical: May also cause suppression of HPA axis, especially when used on large areas of the body, denuded areas, for prolonged periods of time, or with an occlusive dressing. Pediatric patients may be more susceptible to systemic toxicity.

Drug Interactions

Cytochrome P450 Effect: Substrate of CYP3A4 (major)

Increased Effect/Toxicity: CYP3A4 inhibitors: May increase the levels/effects of fluticasone; example inhibitors include azole antifungals, clarithromycin, diclofenac, doxycycline, erythromycin, imatinib, isoniazid, nefazodone, nicardipine, propofol, protease inhibitors, quinidine, telithromycin, and verapamil. Ritonavir may increase serum levels (due to CYP3A4 inhibition) and the potential for steroid-related adverse effects (eg, Cushing syndrome, adrenal suppression).

The addition of salmeterol has been demonstrated to improve response to inhaled corticosteroids (as compared to increasing steroid dosage).

Ethanol/Nutrition/Herb Interactions Herb/Nutraceutical: In theory, St John's wort may decrease serum levels of fluticasone by inducing CYP3A4 isoenzymes.

Dietary Considerations Flovent® Diskus® [CAN] contains lactose; very rare anaphylactic reactions have been reported with Flovent® Rotadisk® in patients with severe milk protein allergy.

Pharmacodynamics/Kinetics
Onset of action: Flovent® HFA: Maximal benefit may take 1-2 weeks or longer
Absorption:
Topical cream: 5% (increased with inflammation)
Oral inhalation: Absorbed systemically (DISKUS®: ~18%) primarily via lungs, minimal GI absorption (<1%) due to presystemic metabolism
Distribution: 4.2 L/kg
Protein binding: 91%
Metabolism: Hepatic via CYP3A4 to 17β-carboxylic acid (negligible activity)
Bioavailability: Nasal: ≤2%; Oral inhalation: (~18% to 21%)
Excretion: Feces (as parent drug and metabolites); urine (<5% as metabolites)

Pregnancy Risk Factor C
Dosage Forms [CAN] = Canadian brand name
Aerosol for oral inhalation [CFC free]:
Flovent® HFA: 44 mcg/inhalation (10.6 g); 110 mcg/inhalation (12 g); 220 mcg/inhalation (12 g)
Cream: 0.05% (15 g, 30 g, 60 g)
Cutivate®: 0.05% (15 g, 30 g, 60 g)
Lotion:
Cutivate®: 0.05% (60 mL)
Ointment: 0.005% (15 g, 30 g, 60 g)
Cutivate®: 0.005% (15 g, 30 g, 60 g)
Powder for oral inhalation [prefilled blister pack]:
Flovent® Diskus® [CAN]: 50 mcg (28s, 60s); 100 mcg (28s, 60s); 250 mcg (28s, 60s); 500 mcg (28s, 60s) [not available in the U.S.]
Suspension, intranasal spray: 50 mcg/inhalation (16 g)
Flonase®: 50 mcg/inhalation (16 g)

Fluticasone and Salmeterol (floo TIK a sone & sal ME te role)

Related Information
Fluticasone *on page 725*
Salmeterol *on page 1453*
U.S. Brand Names Advair Diskus®; Advair® HFA
Canadian Brand Names Advair Diskus®
Mexican Brand Names Seretide Accuhaler
Generic Available No
Index Terms Fluticasone Propionate and Salmeterol Xinafoate; Salmeterol and Fluticasone
Pharmacologic Category Beta₂-Adrenergic Agonist; Corticosteroid, Inhalant (Oral)
Use Maintenance treatment of asthma; maintenance treatment of COPD associated with chronic bronchitis
Local Anesthetic/Vasoconstrictor Precautions No information available to require special precautions
Effects on Dental Treatment Localized infections with *Candida albicans* or *Aspergillus niger* have occurred frequently in the mouth and pharynx with repetitive use of oral inhaler of corticosteroids. These infections may require treatment with appropriate antifungal therapy or discontinuance of treatment with corticosteroid inhaler.
Common Adverse Effects Percentages reported in patients with asthma; also see individual agents:
>10%:
Central nervous system: Headache (12% to 21%)
Respiratory: Upper respiratory tract infection (16% to 27%), pharyngitis (9% to 13%)
>3% to 10%:
Central nervous system: Dizziness (1% to 4%)
Gastrointestinal: Nausea/vomiting (4% to 6%), diarrhea (2% to 4%), pain/discomfort (1% to 4%), oral candidiasis (1% to 4%)
(Continued)

Fluticasone and Salmeterol *(Continued)*

Neuromuscular & skeletal: Musculoskeletal pain (2% to 7%)

Respiratory: Bronchitis (2% to 8%), upper respiratory tract inflammation (4% to 7%), cough (3% to 6%), sinusitis (4% to 5%), hoarseness/dysphonia (1% to 5%), viral respiratory tract infection (4%), epistaxis (1% to 4%)

1% to 3%:

Cardiovascular: Arrhythmia, chest symptoms, fluid retention, MI, palpitation, syncope, tachycardia

Central nervous system: Compressed nerve syndromes, hypnagogic effects, migraine, pain, sleep disorders, tremor

Dermatologic: Dermatitis, dermatosis, eczema, hives, skin flakiness, urticaria, viral skin infection

Endocrine & metabolic: Hypothyroidism

Gastrointestinal: Appendicitis, constipation, dental discomfort/pain, gastrointestinal infection, gastrointestinal signs and symptoms (nonspecified), hemorrhoids, oral discomfort/pain, oral erythema/rash, oral ulcerations, unusual taste, viral GI infection (0% to 3%), weight gain

Genitourinary: Urinary tract infection

Hematologic: Contusions/hematomas, lymphatic signs and symptoms (nonspecified)

Hepatic: Abnormal liver function tests

Neuromuscular & skeletal: Arthralgia, articular rheumatism, bone/cartilage disorders, bone pain, cramps, fractures, muscle injuries, muscle spasm, muscle stiffness, tightness/rigidity

Ocular: Conjunctivitis, edema, eye redness, keratitis, xerophthalmia

Otic: Ear signs and symptoms (nonspecified)

Respiratory: Blood in nasal mucosa, congestion, ear/nose/throat infection, laryngitis, lower respiratory tract infection, lower respiratory signs and symptoms (nonspecified), nasal irritation, nasal signs and symptoms (nonspecified), nasal sinus disorders, pneumonia, rhinitis, rhinorrhea/postnasal drip, sneezing, wheezing

Miscellaneous: Allergies/allergic reactions, bacterial infection, burns, candidiasis (0% to 3%), diaphoresis, sweat/sebum disorders, viral infection, wounds and lacerations

Restrictions An FDA-approved medication guide must be distributed when dispensing an outpatient prescription (new or refill) where this medication is to be used without direct supervision of a healthcare provider. Medication guides are available at http://www.fda.gov/cder/Offices/ODS/medication_guides.htm.

Dosage Oral inhalation: **Note:** Do not use to transfer patients from systemic corticosteroid therapy.

COPD: Adults: Advair Diskus®: Fluticasone 250 mcg/salmeterol 50 mcg twice daily, 12 hours apart. **Note:** This is the maximum dose.

Asthma:

Children 4-11 years: Advair Diskus®: Fluticasone 100 mcg/salmeterol 50 mcg twice daily, 12 hours apart. **Note:** This is the maximum dose.

Children ≥12 and Adults:

Advair Diskus®: One inhalation twice daily, morning and evening, 12 hours apart

Maximum dose: Fluticasone 500 mcg/salmeterol 50 mcg per inhalation

Advair® HFA: Two inhalations twice daily, morning and evening, 12 hours apart

Maximum dose: Fluticasone 230 mcg/salmeterol 21 mcg per inhalation

Note: Initial dose prescribed should be based upon previous dose of inhaled-steroid asthma therapy. Dose should be increased after 2 weeks if adequate response is not achieved. Patients should be titrated to lowest effective dose once stable. Each suggestion below specifies the product strength to use; remember to **use 1 inhalation for Diskus® and 2 inhalations for HFA.**

Patients not currently on inhaled corticosteroids:

Advair Diskus®: Fluticasone 100 mcg/salmeterol 50 mcg **or** fluticasone 250 mcg/salmeterol 50 mcg

Advair® HFA: Fluticasone 45 mcg/salmeterol 21 mcg **or** fluticasone 115 mcg/salmeterol 21 mcg

Patients currently using inhaled beclomethasone dipropionate:

≤160 mcg/day: Advair Diskus®: Fluticasone 100 mcg/salmeterol 50 mcg **or** Advair® HFA: Fluticasone 45 mcg/salmeterol 21 mcg

320 mcg/day: Advair Diskus®:Fluticasone 250 mcg/salmeterol 50 mcg **or** Advair® HFA: Fluticasone 115 mcg/salmeterol 21 mcg

640 mcg/day: Advair Diskus®: Fluticasone 500 mcg/salmeterol 50 mcg **or** Advair® HFA: Fluticasone 230 mcg/salmeterol 21 mcg

Patients currently using inhaled budesonide:
≤400 mcg/day: Advair Diskus®: Fluticasone 100 mcg/salmeterol 50 mcg **or** Advair® HFA: Fluticasone 45 mcg/salmeterol 21 mcg

800-1200 mcg/day: Advair Diskus®: Fluticasone 250 mcg/salmeterol 50 mcg **or** Advair® HFA: Fluticasone 115 mcg/salmeterol 21mcg

1600 mcg/day: Advair Diskus®: Fluticasone 500 mcg/salmeterol 50 mcg **or** Advair® HFA: Fluticasone 230 mcg/salmeterol 21 mcg

Patients currently using inhaled flunisolide CFC aerosol:
≤1000 mcg/day: Advair Diskus®: Fluticasone 100 mcg/salmeterol 50 mcg **or** Advair® HFA: Fluticasone 45 mcg/salmeterol 21 mcg

1250-2000 mcg/day: Advair Diskus®: Fluticasone 250 mcg/salmeterol 50 mcg **or** Advair® HFA: Fluticasone 115 mcg/salmeterol 21 mcg

Patients currently using inhaled fluticasone HFA aerosol:
≤176 mcg/day: Advair Diskus®: Fluticasone 100 mcg/salmeterol 50 mcg **or** Advair® HFA: Fluticasone 45 mcg/salmeterol 21 mcg

440 mcg/day: Advair Diskus®: Fluticasone 250 mcg/salmeterol 50 mcg **or** Advair® HFA: Fluticasone 115 mcg/salmeterol 21 mcg

660-880 mcg/day: Advair Diskus®: Fluticasone 500 mcg/salmeterol 50 mcg **or** Advair® HFA: Fluticasone 230 mcg/salmeterol 21 mcg

Patients currently using inhaled fluticasone propionate powder:
≤200 mcg/day: Advair Diskus®: Fluticasone 100 mcg/salmeterol 50 mcg **or** Advair® HFA: Fluticasone 45 mcg/salmeterol 21 mcg

500 mcg/day: Advair Diskus®: Fluticasone 250 mcg/salmeterol 50 mcg **or** Advair® HFA: Fluticasone 115 mcg/salmeterol 21 mcg

1000 mcg/day: Advair Diskus®: Fluticasone 500 mcg/salmeterol 50 mcg **or** Advair® HFA: Fluticasone 230 mcg/salmeterol 21 mcg

Patients currently using inhaled mometasone furoate powder:
220 mcg/day: Advair Diskus®: Fluticasone 100 mcg/salmeterol 50 mcg **or** Advair® HFA: Fluticasone 45 mcg/salmeterol 21 mcg

440 mcg/day: Advair Diskus®: Fluticasone 250 mcg/salmeterol 50 mcg **or** Advair® HFA: Fluticasone 115 mcg/salmeterol 21 mcg

880 mcg/day: Advair Diskus®: Fluticasone 500 mcg/salmeterol 50 mcg **or** Advair® HFA: Fluticasone 230 mcg/salmeterol 21 mcg

Patients currently using inhaled triamcinolone acetonide:
≤1000 mcg/day: Advair Diskus®: Fluticasone 100 mcg/salmeterol 50 mcg **or** Advair® HFA: Fluticasone 45 mcg/salmeterol 21 mcg

1100-1600 mcg/day: Advair Diskus®: Fluticasone 250 mcg/salmeterol 50 mcg **or** Advair® HFA: Fluticasone 115 mcg/salmeterol 21 mcg

Elderly: No differences in safety or effectiveness have been seen in studies of patients ≥65 years of age. However, increased sensitivity may be seen in the elderly. Use with caution in patients with concomitant cardiovascular disease.

Dosage adjustment in renal impairment: Specific guidelines are not available
Dosage adjustment in hepatic impairment: Systemic absorption is poor from inhalation therapy; therefore, no dosage adjustment recommended. Manufacturer suggests close monitoring of patients with hepatic impairment.

Mechanism of Action Combination of fluticasone (corticosteroid) and salmeterol (long-acting beta$_2$-agonist) designed to improve pulmonary function and control over what is produced by either agent when used alone. Because fluticasone and salmeterol act locally in the lung, plasma levels do not predict therapeutic effect.

Fluticasone: The mechanism of action for all topical corticosteroids is believed to be a combination of three important properties: Anti-inflammatory activity, immunosuppressive properties, and antiproliferative actions. Fluticasone has extremely potent vasoconstrictive and anti-inflammatory activity.

Salmeterol: Relaxes bronchial smooth muscle by selective action on beta$_2$-receptors with little effect on heart rate

Contraindications Hypersensitivity to fluticasone, salmeterol, or any component of the formulation; status asthmaticus; acute episodes of asthma or COPD

Warnings/Precautions
Asthma treatment: Long-acting beta$_2$ agonists may increase the risk of asthma-related deaths. In a large, randomized clinical trial (SMART, 2006), salmeterol was associated with an increase in asthma-related deaths (when added to usual asthma therapy); risk may be greater in African-American patients versus Caucasians. Should only be used as adjuvant therapy in patients not adequately controlled on inhaled corticosteroids or whose disease requires two maintenance therapies. Salmeterol is not meant to relieve acute asthmatic symptoms, should not be initiated in patients with significantly worsening or acutely deteriorating asthma, and is not a substitute for inhaled or oral corticosteroids. Short-acting beta$_2$ agonist should be used for acute symptoms and symptoms occurring between treatments. Corticosteroids should not be stopped or reduced when salmeterol is initiated. During the initiation of salmeterol watch for signs of worsening asthma. Patients must be instructed to seek medical attention in cases where acute symptoms are not relieved or a previous (Continued)

Fluticasone and Salmeterol *(Continued)*

level of response is diminished. The need to increase frequency of use may indicate deterioration of asthma, and treatment must not be delayed.

Concurrent diseases: Use caution in patients with cardiovascular disease (eg, arrhythmia, hypertension, or CHF), seizure disorders, diabetes, ocular disease, thyroid disease, osteoporosis, gastrointestinal disease, hepatic impairment, renal impairment, myasthenia gravis, osteoporosis, or hypokalemia. Beta-agonists may cause elevation in blood pressure, heart rate, CNS stimulation/excitation, increase risk of arrhythmia, increase serum glucose, decrease serum potassium.

Adverse events: Salmeterol should not be used more than twice daily; do not exceed recommended dose. Do not use with other long-acting beta₂ agonists; serious adverse events, have been associated with excessive use of inhaled sympathomimetics. There have been reports of laryngeal spasm, irritation, and swelling (stridor, choking) with use. Rarely, paradoxical bronchospasm may occur with use of inhaled bronchodilating agents; this should be distinguished from inadequate response. Powder for oral inhalation contains lactose; very rare anaphylactic reactions have been reported in patients with severe milk protein allergy. Immediate hypersensitivity reactions (urticaria, angioedema, rash, bronchospasm) have been reported. Rare cases of vasculitis (Churg-Strauss syndrome) have been reported with fluticasone use. Glaucoma, increased intraocular pressure, and cataracts have occurred with fluticasone inhalation; consider routine eye exams in chronic users. Local yeast infections (eg, oral pharyngeal candidiasis) may occur. Corticosteroid use may cause psychiatric manifestations, including depression, euphoria, insomnia, mood swings, and personality changes. Pre-existing psychiatric conditions may be exacerbated by corticosteroid use.

Adrenal suppression: Fluticasone may cause hypercorticism or suppression of hypothalamic-pituitary-adrenal (HPA) axis, particularly in younger children or in patients receiving high doses for prolonged periods. Withdrawal and discontinuation of a corticosteroid should be done slowly and carefully. Particular care is required when patients are transferred from systemic corticosteroids to inhaled products. Patients receiving >20 mg per day of prednisone (or equivalent) may be most susceptible. Concurrent use of ritonavir (and potentially other strong inhibitors of CYP3A4) may increase fluticasone levels and effects on HPA suppression. Fatalities have occurred due to adrenal insufficiency in asthmatic patients during and after transfer from systemic corticosteroids to aerosol steroids; aerosol steroids do not provide the systemic steroid needed to treat patients having trauma, surgery, or infections. Do not use this product to transfer patients from oral corticosteroid therapy.

Immune system: Prolonged use of corticosteroids may also increase the incidence of secondary infection, mask acute infection (including fungal infections), prolong or exacerbate viral infections, or limit response to vaccines. Exposure to chickenpox should be avoided; corticosteroids should not be used to treat ocular herpes simplex. Corticosteroids should not be used for cerebral malaria. Close observation is required in patients with latent tuberculosis and/or TB reactivity; restrict use in active TB (only in conjunction with antituberculosis treatment).

Growth: Orally-inhaled and intranasal corticosteroids may cause a reduction in growth velocity in pediatric patients (~1 centimeter per year [range 0.3-1.8 cm per year] and related to dose and duration of exposure). To minimize the systemic effects of orally-inhaled and intranasal corticosteroids, each patient should be titrated to the lowest effective dose. Growth should be routinely monitored in pediatric patients.

There have been reports of systemic corticosteroid withdrawal symptoms (eg, joint/muscle pain, lassitude, depression) when withdrawing oral inhalation therapy. Advair Diskus®: Safety and efficacy have not been established in children <4 years of age. Advair® HFA: Safety and efficacy have not been established in children <12 years of age.

Drug Interactions

Cytochrome P450 Effect: Fluticasone: **Substrate** of CYP3A4 (major); Salmeterol: **Substrate** of CYP3A4 (major)

Increased Effect/Toxicity: Atomoxetine may enhance the tachycardia effect of beta₂-agonists. Protease inhibitors may decrease the metabolism, via CYP isoenzymes, of corticosteroids (orally inhaled); examples include amprenavir, atazanavir, fosamprenavir, indinavir, lopinavir, nelfinavir, ritonavir, and saquinavir; **exception** is tipranavir. Sympathomimetics may enhance the adverse/toxic effect of salmeterol. Antifungal agents (imidazole) may decrease the metabolism, via CYP isoenzymes, of corticosteroids (orally inhaled).

Decreased Effect: Beta₂-agonists may diminish the bradycardia effect of beta-blockers (beta₁ selective). Beta-blockers (nonselective) may diminish the bronchodilator effect of beta₂-agonists.

Dietary Considerations Advair Diskus® powder for oral inhalation contains lactose; very rare anaphylactic reactions have been reported in patients with severe milk protein allergy.

Pharmacodynamics/Kinetics See individual agents.
Duration: 12 hours

Pregnancy Risk Factor C

Dosage Forms

Aerosol, for oral inhalation:
Advair® HFA:
45/21: Fluticasone 45 mcg and salmeterol 30.45 mcg (12 g)
115/21: Fluticasone 115 mcg and salmeterol 30.45 mcg (12 g)
230/21: Fluticasone 230 mcg and salmeterol 30.45 mcg (12 g)

Powder for oral inhalation:
Advair Diskus®:
100/50: Fluticasone 100 mcg and salmeterol 50 mcg (28s, 60s)
250/50: Fluticasone 250 mcg and salmeterol 50 mcg (28s, 60s)
500/50: Fluticasone 500 mcg and salmeterol 50 mcg (28s, 60s)

Fluticasone Propionate see Fluticasone on page 725

Fluticasone Propionate and Salmeterol Xinafoate see Fluticasone and Salmeterol on page 729

Fluvastatin (FLOO va sta tin)

Related Information
Cardiovascular Diseases on page 1726

U.S. Brand Names Lescol®; Lescol® XL

Canadian Brand Names Lescol®; Lescol® XL

Mexican Brand Names Lescol; Lescol XL

Generic Available No

Pharmacologic Category Antilipemic Agent, HMG-CoA Reductase Inhibitor

Use To be used as a component of multiple risk factor intervention in patients at risk for atherosclerosis vascular disease due to hypercholesterolemia

Adjunct to dietary therapy to reduce elevated total cholesterol (total-C), LDL-C, triglyceride, and apolipoprotein B (apo-B) levels and to increase HDL-C in primary hypercholesterolemia and mixed dyslipidemia (Fredrickson types IIa and IIb); to slow the progression of coronary atherosclerosis in patients with coronary heart disease; reduce risk of coronary revascularization procedures in patients with coronary heart disease

Local Anesthetic/Vasoconstrictor Precautions No information available to require special precautions

Effects on Dental Treatment No significant effects or complications reported

Common Adverse Effects As reported with fluvastatin capsules; in general, adverse reactions reported with fluvastatin extended release tablet were similar, but the incidence was less.

1% to 10%:
Central nervous system: Headache (9%), fatigue (3%), insomnia (3%)
Gastrointestinal: Dyspepsia (8%), diarrhea (5%), abdominal pain (5%), nausea (3%)
Genitourinary: Urinary tract infection (2%)
Neuromuscular & skeletal: Myalgia (5%)
Respiratory: Sinusitis (3%), bronchitis (2%)

Mechanism of Action Acts by competitively inhibiting 3-hydroxyl-3-methylglutaryl-coenzyme A (HMG-CoA) reductase, the enzyme that catalyzes the reduction of HMG-CoA to mevalonate; this is an early rate-limiting step in cholesterol biosynthesis. HDL is increased while total, LDL, and VLDL cholesterols; apolipoprotein B; and plasma triglycerides are decreased.

Drug Interactions

Cytochrome P450 Effect: Substrate of CYP2C9 (major), 2C8 (minor), 2D6 (minor), 3A4 (minor); **Inhibits** CYP1A2 (weak), 2C8 (weak), 2C9 (moderate), 2D6 (weak), 3A4 (weak)

Increased Effect/Toxicity: Fibric acid derivatives may increase the risk of myopathy and rhabdomyolysis. Fluvastatin levels/effects may be increased by omeprazole, phenytoin, fluconazole, NSAIDs, sulfonamides, or other CYP2C9 inhibitors. The anticoagulant effect of warfarin may be increased by fluvastatin. Cholestyramine effect may be additive with fluvastatin if administration times are separated. Fluvastatin may increase the levels/effects of fluoxetine, glimepiride, glipizide, and other CYP2C9 substrates.

(Continued)

Fluvastatin (Continued)

Decreased Effect: Administration of cholestyramine at the same time with fluvastatin reduces absorption and clinical effect of fluvastatin. Separate administration times by at least 4 hours. Rifampin and rifabutin may decrease fluvastatin blood levels.

Pharmacodynamics/Kinetics

Onset of action: Peak effect: Maximal LDL-C reductions achieved within 4 weeks

Distribution: V_d: 0.35 L/kg

Protein binding: >98%

Metabolism: To inactive and active metabolites (oxidative metabolism via CYP2C9 [75%], 2C8 [~5%], and 3A4 [~20%] isoenzymes); active forms do not circulate systemically; extensive (saturable) first-pass hepatic extraction

Bioavailability: Absolute: Capsule: 24%; Extended release tablet: 29%

Half-life elimination: Capsule: <3 hours; Extended release tablet: 9 hours

Time to peak: Capsule: 1 hour; Extended release tablet: 3 hours

Excretion: Feces (90%): urine (5%)

Pregnancy Risk Factor X

Fluvirin® see Influenza Virus Vaccine on page 880

Fluvoxamine (floo VOKS a meen)

Related Information

Sedation on page 1825

Canadian Brand Names Alti-Fluvoxamine; Apo-Fluvoxamine®; Luvox®; Novo-Fluvoxamine; Nu-Fluvoxamine; PMS-Fluvoxamine; Rhoxal-fluvoxamine; Sandoz-Fluvoxamine

Generic Available Yes

Index Terms Luvox

Pharmacologic Category Antidepressant, Selective Serotonin Reuptake Inhibitor

Use Treatment of obsessive-compulsive disorder (OCD) in children ≥8 years of age and adults

Unlabeled/Investigational Use Treatment of major depression; panic disorder; anxiety disorders in children

Local Anesthetic/Vasoconstrictor Precautions Although caution should be used in patients taking tricyclic antidepressants, no interactions have been reported with vasoconstrictors and fluvoxamine, a nontricyclic antidepressant which acts to increase serotonin; no precautions appear to be needed

Effects on Dental Treatment Key adverse event(s) related to dental treatment: Xerostomia (normal salivary flow resumes upon discontinuation) and abnormal taste. Problems with SSRI-induced bruxism have been reported and may preclude their use; clinicians attempting to evaluate any patient with bruxism or involuntary muscle movement, who is simultaneously being treated with an SSRI drug, should be aware of the potential association. See Dental Comment.

Common Adverse Effects

>10%:

Central nervous system: Headache (22%), somnolence (22%), insomnia (21%), nervousness (12%), dizziness (11%)

Gastrointestinal: Nausea (40%), diarrhea (11%), xerostomia (14%)

Neuromuscular & skeletal: Weakness (14%)

1% to 10%:

Cardiovascular: Palpitation

Central nervous system: Somnolence, mania, hypomania, vertigo, abnormal thinking, agitation, anxiety, malaise, amnesia, yawning, hypertonia, CNS stimulation, depression

Endocrine & metabolic: Libido decreased

Gastrointestinal: Abdominal pain, vomiting, dyspepsia, constipation, abnormal taste, anorexia, flatulence, weight gain

Genitourinary: Ejaculation delayed, impotence, anorgasmia, urinary frequency, urinary retention

Neuromuscular & skeletal: Tremors

Ocular: Blurred vision

Respiratory: Dyspnea

Miscellaneous: Diaphoresis

Restrictions An FDA-approved medication guide concerning the use of antidepressants in children, adolescents, and young adults must be distributed when dispensing an outpatient prescription (new or refill) where this medication is to be used without direct supervision of a healthcare provider. Medication guides are available at http://www.fda.gov/cder/Offices/ODS/medication_guides.htm.

Dispense to parents or guardians of children and adolescents receiving this medication.

Dosage Oral: **Note:** When total daily dose exceeds 50 mg, the dose should be given in 2 divided doses:

Children 8-17 years: Initial: 25 mg at bedtime; adjust in 25 mg increments at 4- to 7-day intervals, as tolerated, to maximum therapeutic benefit: Range: 50-200 mg/day

Maximum: Children: 8-11 years: 200 mg/day, adolescents: 300 mg/day; lower doses may be effective in female versus male patients

Adults: Initial: 50 mg at bedtime; adjust in 50 mg increments at 4- to 7-day intervals; usual dose range: 100-300 mg/day; divide total daily dose into 2 doses; administer larger portion at bedtime

Elderly: Reduce dose, titrate slowly

Dosage adjustment in hepatic impairment: Reduce dose, titrate slowly

Mechanism of Action Inhibits CNS neuron serotonin uptake; minimal or no effect on reuptake of norepinephrine or dopamine; does not significantly bind to alpha-adrenergic, histamine or cholinergic receptors

Contraindications Hypersensitivity to fluvoxamine or any component of the formulation; concurrent use with alosetron, pimozide, thioridazine, tizanidine, mesoridazine, or cisapride; use of MAO inhibitors within 14 days

Warnings/Precautions [U.S. Boxed Warning]: Antidepressants increase the risk of suicidal thinking and behavior in children, adolescents, and young adults (18-24 years of age) with major depressive disorder (MDD) and other psychiatric disorders; consider risk prior to prescribing. Short-term studies did not show an increased risk in patients >24 years of age and showed a decreased risk in patients ≥65 years. Closely monitor patients for clinical worsening, suicidality, or unusual changes in behavior, particularly during the initial 1-2 months of therapy or during periods of dosage adjustments (increases or decreases); the patient's family or caregiver should be instructed to closely observe the patient and communicate condition with healthcare provider. A medication guide concerning the use of antidepressants should be dispensed with each prescription. **Fluvoxamine is FDA approved for the treatment of OCD in children ≥8 years of age.**

The possibility of a suicide attempt is inherent in major depression and may persist until remission occurs. Use caution in high-risk patients. Worsening depression and severe abrupt suicidality that are not part of the presenting symptoms may require discontinuation or modification of drug therapy. The patient's family or caregiver should be alerted to monitor patients for the emergence of suicidality and associated behaviors (such as agitation, irritability, hostility, impulsivity, and hypomania) and call healthcare provider.

May worsen psychosis in some patients or precipitate a shift to mania or hypomania in patients with bipolar disorder. Patients presenting with depressive symptoms should be screened for bipolar disorder. Monotherapy in patients with bipolar disorder should be avoided. **Fluvoxamine is not FDA approved for the treatment of bipolar depression.**

The potential for severe reaction exits when used with MAO inhibitors, SSRIs/SNRIs, or triptans; serotonin syndrome (hyperthermia, muscular rigidity, mental status changes/agitation, autonomic instability) may occur. Concurrent use with MAO inhibitors is contraindicated. Fluvoxamine has a low potential to impair cognitive or motor performance; caution operating hazardous machinery or driving. Use caution in patients with a previous seizure disorder or condition predisposing to seizures such as brain damage, alcoholism, or concurrent therapy with other drugs which lower the seizure threshold.

May increase the risks associated with electroconvulsive therapy. Use with caution in patients with hepatic or renal dysfunction and in elderly patients. May cause hyponatremia/SIADH. Use with caution in patients with renal insufficiency or other concurrent illness (cardiovascular disease). Use with caution in patients at risk of bleeding or receiving concurrent anticoagulant therapy, although not consistently noted, fluvoxamine may cause impairment in platelet function. May cause or exacerbate sexual dysfunction.

Drug Interactions

Cytochrome P450 Effect: Substrate (major) of CYP1A2, 2D6; **Inhibits** CYP1A2 (strong), 2B6 (weak), 2C9 (weak), 2C19 (strong), 2D6 (weak), 3A4 (weak)

Increased Effect/Toxicity: Fluvoxamine should not be used with nonselective MAO inhibitors (phenelzine, isocarboxazid) and drugs with MAO inhibitor properties (linezolid); fatal reactions have been reported. Wait 2 weeks after stopping an MAO inhibitor before starting fluvoxamine. Concurrent selegiline has been associated with mania, hypertension, or serotonin syndrome (risk may be reduced relative to nonselective MAO inhibitors).

(Continued)

Fluvoxamine *(Continued)*

Fluvoxamine may inhibit the metabolism of thioridazine or mesoridazine, resulting in increased plasma levels and increasing the risk of QT$_c$ interval prolongation. This may lead to serious ventricular arrhythmias, such as torsade de pointes-type arrhythmias, and sudden death. Do not use together. Wait at least 5 weeks after discontinuing fluvoxamine prior to starting thioridazine. Fluvoxamine may increase the levels/effects of aminophylline, citalopram, diazepam, mexiletine, mirtazapine, methsuximide, phenytoin, propranolol, ropinirole, sertraline, theophylline, trifluoperazine, and other substrates of CYP1A2 or 2C19. Fluvoxamine may increase the concentrations of alosetron and tizanidine; concurrent use is not recommended.

The levels/effects of fluvoxamine may be increased by amphetamines, selected beta-blockers, chlorpromazine, ciprofloxacin, delavirdine, fluoxetine, ketoconazole, miconazole, norfloxacin, ofloxacin, paroxetine, pergolide, quinidine, quinine, ritonavir, rofecoxib, ropinirole, and other CYP1A2 or 2D6 inhibitors.

Combined use of SSRIs and amphetamines, buspirone, meperidine, nefazodone, serotonin agonists (such as sumatriptan), sibutramine, other SSRIs/SNRIs, sympathomimetics, ritonavir, tramadol, and venlafaxine may increase the risk of serotonin syndrome. Combined use of sumatriptan (and other serotonin agonists) may result in toxicity; weakness, hyper-reflexia, and incoordination have been observed with sumatriptan and SSRIs. In addition, concurrent use may theoretically increase the risk of serotonin syndrome; includes sumatriptan, naratriptan, rizatriptan, and zolmitriptan.

Concurrent lithium may increase risk of nephrotoxicity. Risk of hyponatremia may increase with concurrent use of loop diuretics (bumetanide, furosemide, torsemide). Fluvoxamine may increase the hypoprothrombinemic response to warfarin. Concomitant use of fluvoxamine and NSAIDs, aspirin, or other drugs affecting coagulation has been associated with an increased risk of bleeding; monitor.

Decreased Effect: The levels/effects of fluvoxamine may be decreased by aminoglutethimide, carbamazepine, phenobarbital, rifampin, and other CYP1A2 inducers. Cyproheptadine, a serotonin antagonist, may inhibit the effects of serotonin reuptake inhibitors (fluvoxamine); monitor for altered antidepressant response.

Ethanol/Nutrition/Herb Interactions

Ethanol: Avoid ethanol. Depressed patients should avoid/limit intake.

Food: The bioavailability of melatonin has been reported to be increased by fluvoxamine.

Herb/Nutraceutical: Avoid valerian, St John's wort, SAMe, kava kava (may increase risk of serotonin syndrome and/or excessive sedation).

Pharmacodynamics/Kinetics

Absorption: Steady-state plasma concentrations have been noted to be 2-3 times higher in children than those in adolescents; female children demonstrated a significantly higher AUC than males

Distribution: V$_d$: ~25 L/kg

Protein binding: ~80%, primarily to albumin

Metabolism: Hepatic

Bioavailability: 53%; not significantly affected by food

Half-life elimination: 15 hours

Time to peak, plasma: 3-8 hours

Excretion: Urine

Pregnancy Risk Factor C

Dosage Forms

Tablet: 25 mg, 50 mg, 100 mg

Dental Comment Problems with SSRI-induced bruxism have been reported and may preclude their use. Clinicians attempting to evaluate any patient with bruxism or involuntary muscle movement, who is simultaneously being treated with an SSRI drug, should be aware of the potential association.

Selected Readings

Friedlander AH and Mahler ME, "Major Depressive Disorder. Psychopathology, Medical Management, and Dental Implications," *J Am Dent Assoc*, 2001, 132(5):629-38.

Gerber PE and Lynd LD, "Selective Serotonin Reuptake Inhibitor-induced Movement Disorders," *Ann Pharmacother*, 1998, 32(6):692-8.

Wynn RL, "New Antidepressant Medications," *Gen Dent*, 1997, 45(1):24-8.

Fluzone® *see* Influenza Virus Vaccine *on page 880*

FML® *see* Fluorometholone *on page 712*

FML® Forte *see* Fluorometholone *on page 712*

FML-S® *see* Sulfacetamide and Fluorometholone *on page 1502*

Focalin® *see* Dexmethylphenidate *on page 470*

Focalin® XR *see* Dexmethylphenidate *on page 470*

Folic Acid (FOE lik AS id)

Canadian Brand Names Apo-Folic®
Generic Available Yes
Index Terms Folacin; Folate; Pteroylglutamic Acid
Pharmacologic Category Vitamin, Water Soluble
Use Treatment of megaloblastic and macrocytic anemias due to folate deficiency; dietary supplement to prevent neural tube defects
Local Anesthetic/Vasoconstrictor Precautions No information available to require special precautions
Effects on Dental Treatment No significant effects or complications reported
Significant Adverse Effects Frequency not defined.
  Allergic reaction, bronchospasm, flushing (slight), malaise (general), pruritus, rash
Dosage
  Oral, I.M., I.V., SubQ: Anemia:
    Infants: 0.1 mg/day
    Children <4 years: Up to 0.3 mg/day
    Children >4 years and Adults: 0.4 mg/day
    Pregnant and lactating women: 0.8 mg/day
  Oral:
    RDA: Expressed as dietary folate equivalents:
      Children:
        1-3 years: 150 mcg/day
        4-8 years: 200 mcg/day
        9-13 years: 300 mcg/day
      Children ≥14 years and Adults: 400 mcg/day
      Elderly: Vitamin B$_{12}$ deficiency must be ruled out before initiating folate therapy due to frequency of combined nutritional deficiencies: RDA requirements (1999): 400 mcg/day (0.4 mg) minimum
    Prevention of neural tube defects:
      Females of childbearing potential: 400 mcg/day
      Females at high risk or with family history of neural tube defects: 4 mg/day
Mechanism of Action Folic acid is necessary for formation of a number of coenzymes in many metabolic systems, particularly for purine and pyrimidine synthesis; required for nucleoprotein synthesis and maintenance in erythropoiesis; stimulates WBC and platelet production in folate deficiency anemia
Contraindications Hypersensitivity to folic acid or any component of the formulation
Warnings/Precautions Not appropriate for monotherapy with pernicious, aplastic, or normocytic anemias when anemia is present with vitamin B$_{12}$ deficiency. Doses >0.1 mg/day may obscure pernicious anemia with continuing irreversible nerve damage progression. Resistance to treatment may occur with depressed hematopoiesis, alcoholism, and deficiencies of other vitamins. Injection contains benzyl alcohol (1.5%) as preservative (use care in administration to neonates).
Drug Interactions
  Phenytoin: Folic acid may decrease phenytoin concentrations.
  Raltitrexed: Folic acid may diminish the therapeutic effect of raltitrexed.
Dietary Considerations As of January 1998, the FDA has required manufacturers of enriched flour, bread, corn meal, pasta, rice, and other grain products to add folic acid to their products. The intent is to help decrease the risk of neural tube defects by increasing folic acid intake. Other foods which contain folic acid include dark green leafy vegetables, citrus fruits and juices, and lentils.
Pharmacodynamics/Kinetics
  Onset of action: Peak effect: Oral: 0.5-1 hour
  Absorption: Proximal part of small intestine
Pregnancy Risk Factor A
Lactation Enters breast milk/compatible
Dosage Forms Excipient information presented when available (limited, particularly for generics); consult specific product labeling.
  (Continued)

Folic Acid *(Continued)*

Injection, solution, as sodium folate: 5 mg/mL (10 mL) [contains benzyl alcohol]
Tablet: 0.4 mg, 0.8 mg, 1 mg

Folic Acid, Cyanocobalamin, and Pyridoxine
(FOE lik AS id, sye an oh koe BAL a min, & peer i DOKS een)

Related Information
Cyanocobalamin *on page 418*
Folic Acid *on page 737*
Pyridoxine *on page 1389*
U.S. Brand Names AllanFol RX; Folbee; Folgard® [OTC]; Folgard RX 2.2®
[DSC]; Foltx®; Tricardio B
Generic Available Yes
Index Terms Cyanocobalamin, Folic Acid, and Pyridoxine; Folacin, Vitamin B₁₂,
and Vitamin B₆; Pyridoxine, Folic Acid, and Cyanocobalamin
Pharmacologic Category Vitamin
Use Nutritional supplement in end-stage renal failure, dialysis, hyperhomocys-
teinemia, homocystinuria, malabsorption syndromes, dietary deficiencies
Local Anesthetic/Vasoconstrictor Precautions No information available to
require special precautions
Effects on Dental Treatment No significant effects or complications reported
Common Adverse Effects See individual agents.

Folinic Acid *see Leucovorin on page 957*

Follicle-Stimulating Hormone, Human *see Urofollitropin on page 1633*

Follicle Stimulating Hormone, Recombinant *see Follitropin Alfa on page 738*

Follicle Stimulating Hormone, Recombinant *see Follitropin Beta on
page 739*

Follistim® AQ *see Follitropin Beta on page 739*

Follistim® AQ Cartridge *see Follitropin Beta on page 739*

Follitropin Alfa *(foe li TRO pin AL fa)*

U.S. Brand Names Gonal-f®; Gonal-f® RFF
Canadian Brand Names Gonal-f®; Gonal-f® Pen
Mexican Brand Names Gonal-F
Generic Available No
Index Terms Follicle Stimulating Hormone, Recombinant; FSH; rFSH-alpha;
rhFSH-alpha
Pharmacologic Category Gonadotropin; Ovulation Stimulator
Use
Gonal-f®: Ovulation induction in patients in whom the cause of infertility is
functional and not caused by primary ovarian failure; development of multiple
follicles with Assisted Reproductive Technology (ART); spermatogenesis
induction
Gonal-f® RFF: Ovulation induction in patients in whom the cause of infertility is
functional and not caused by primary ovarian failure; development of multiple
follicles with ART
Local Anesthetic/Vasoconstrictor Precautions No information available to
require special precautions
Effects on Dental Treatment Key adverse event(s) related to dental treat-
ment: Stomatitis and toothache.
Common Adverse Effects Percentage may vary by indication, product formu-
lation
>10%:
Central nervous system: Headache
Endocrine & metabolic: Ovarian cyst
Gastrointestinal: Abdomen enlarged, abdominal pain, nausea
Miscellaneous: Upper respiratory infection
1% to 10%:
Central nervous system: Dizziness, emotional lability, fever, malaise,
migraine, pain
Dermatologic: Acne
Endocrine & metabolic: Breast pain, cervix lesion, hot flashes, intermenstrual
bleeding, menstrual disorder, ovarian disorder, ovarian hyperstimulation
Gastrointestinal: Constipation, diarrhea, dyspepsia, flatulence, pelvic pain,
stomatitis (ulcerative), toothache, vomiting, weight gain
Genitourinary: Cystitis, leukorrhea, micturition frequency, urinary tract infec-
tion, uterine hemorrhage, vaginal hemorrhage
Local: Injection site bruising, edema, inflammation, pain, reaction

Neuromuscular & skeletal: Back pain
Respiratory: Cough, flu-like symptoms, pharyngitis, rhinitis, sinusitis
Miscellaneous: Infection, moniliasis
Mechanism of Action Follitropin alfa is a human FSH preparation of recombinant DNA origin. Follitropins stimulate ovarian follicular growth in women who do not have primary ovarian failure, and stimulate spermatogenesis in men with hypogonadotrophic hypogonadism. FSH is required for normal follicular growth, maturation, gonadal steroid production, and spermatogenesis.
Pharmacodynamics/Kinetics
Onset of action: Peak effect:
Spermatogenesis, median: 6.8-12.4 months (range 2.7-15.7 months)
Follicle development: Within cycle
Absorption: I.M., SubQ: Absorption rate is slower than the elimination rate
Distribution: Mean V_d: 10 L with *in vitro* fertilization/embryo transfer patients
Bioavailability: ~66% to 76% in healthy female volunteers
Half-life elimination:
I.M.: 50 hours in healthy female volunteers
SubQ: 24 hours in healthy female volunteers; 32 hours with *in vitro* fertilization/embryo transfer patients; 32-41 hours in healthy male volunteers
Time to peak: In healthy volunteers:
Females: SubQ: 8-16 hours; I.M.: 25 hours
Males: SubQ: 11-20 hours
Excretion: Clearance: I.V.: 0.6 L/hour in healthy female volunteers
Pregnancy Risk Factor X

Follitropin Beta (foe li TRO pin BAY ta)

U.S. Brand Names Follistim® AQ; Follistim® AQ Cartridge
Canadian Brand Names Puregon®
Mexican Brand Names Puregon
Generic Available No
Index Terms Follicle Stimulating Hormone, Recombinant; FSH; rFSH-beta; rhFSH-beta
Pharmacologic Category Gonadotropin; Ovulation Stimulator
Use Ovulation induction in patients in whom the cause of infertility is functional and not caused by primary ovarian failure; development of multiple follicles with Assisted Reproductive Technology (ART)
Local Anesthetic/Vasoconstrictor Precautions No information available to require special precautions
Effects on Dental Treatment No significant effects or complications reported
Common Adverse Effects Percentage may vary by indication, product formulation
>10%:
Endocrine & metabolic: Breast pain
Gastrointestinal: Abdominal pain, flatulence, nausea
Miscellaneous: Miscarriage
1% to 10%:
Central nervous system: Headache
Endocrine & metabolic: Ovarian hyperstimulation syndrome, ovarian pain
Gastrointestinal: Abdomen enlarged, constipation
Local: Injection site reaction
Neuromuscular & skeletal: Back pain
Respiratory: Sinusitis, upper respiratory tract infection
Mechanism of Action Follitropin beta is a human FSH preparation of recombinant DNA origin. Follitropins stimulate ovarian follicular growth in women who do not have primary ovarian failure. FSH is required for normal follicular growth, maturation, gonadal steroid production, and spermatogenesis.
Pharmacodynamics/Kinetics
Onset of action: Peak effect: Follicle development: Within cycle
Absorption: I.M.: 76%; SubQ: 78%
Distribution: 8 L
Half-life elimination: I.M.: 44 hours (single dose), 27-30 hours (multiple doses); SubQ: 33 hours (single dose)
Time to peak: SubQ: 13 hours
Pregnancy Risk Factor X

Foltx® see Folic Acid, Cyanocobalamin, and Pyridoxine on page 738

Fomepizole (foe ME pi zole)

U.S. Brand Names Antizol®
Generic Available No
(Continued)

Fomepizole *(Continued)*

Index Terms 4-Methylpyrazole; 4-MP

Pharmacologic Category Antidote

Use Orphan drug: Treatment of methanol or ethylene glycol poisoning alone or in combination with hemodialysis

Unlabeled/Investigational Use Known or suspected propylene glycol toxicity

Local Anesthetic/Vasoconstrictor Precautions No information available to require special precautions

Effects on Dental Treatment Key adverse event(s) related to dental treatment: Bad/metallic taste.

Common Adverse Effects

>10%:

Central nervous system: Headache (14%)

Gastrointestinal: Nausea (11%)

1% to 10% (≤3% unless otherwise noted):

Cardiovascular: Bradycardia, facial flush, hypotension, phlebosclerosis, shock, tachycardia

Central nervous system: Dizziness (6%), drowsiness increased (6%), agitation, anxiety, lightheadedness, seizure, vertigo

Dermatologic: Rash

Gastrointestinal: Bad/metallic taste (6%), abdominal pain, appetite decreased, diarrhea, heartburn, vomiting

Hematologic: Anemia, disseminated intravascular coagulation (DIC), eosinophilia, lymphangitis

Hepatic: Liver function tests increased

Local: Application site reaction, injection site inflammation, pain during injection, phlebitis

Neuromuscular & skeletal: Backache

Ocular: Nystagmus, transient blurred vision, visual disturbances

Renal: Anuria

Respiratory: Abnormal smell, hiccups, pharyngitis

Miscellaneous: Multiorgan failure, speech disturbances

Mechanism of Action Fomepizole competitively inhibits alcohol dehydrogenase, an enzyme which catalyzes the metabolism of ethanol, ethylene glycol, and methanol to their toxic metabolites. Ethylene glycol is metabolized to glycoaldehyde, then oxidized to glycolate, glyoxylate, and oxalate. Glycolate and oxalate are responsible for metabolic acidosis and renal damage. Methanol is metabolized to formaldehyde, then oxidized to formic acid. Formic acid is responsible for metabolic acidosis and visual disturbances.

Pharmacodynamics/Kinetics

Onset of effect: Peak effect: Maximum: 1.5-2 hours

Absorption: Oral: Readily absorbed

Distribution: V_d: 0.6-1.02 L/kg; rapidly into total body water

Protein binding: Negligible

Metabolism: Hepatic to 4-carboxypyrazole (80% to 85% of dose), 4-hydroxymethylpyrazole, and their N-glucuronide conjugates; following multiple doses, induces its own metabolism via CYP oxidases after 30-40 hours

Half-life elimination: Has not been calculated; varies with dose

Excretion: Urine (1% to 3.5% as unchanged drug and metabolites)

Pregnancy Risk Factor C

Fomivirsen *(foe MI vir sen)*

Related Information

Systemic Viral Diseases *on page 1767*

U.S. Brand Names Vitravene™ [DSC]

Canadian Brand Names Vitravene™

Generic Available No

Index Terms Fomivirsen Sodium

Pharmacologic Category Antiviral Agent, Ophthalmic

Use Local treatment of cytomegalovirus (CMV) retinitis in patients with acquired immunodeficiency syndrome who are intolerant or insufficiently responsive to other treatments for CMV retinitis or when other treatments for CMV retinitis are contraindicated

Local Anesthetic/Vasoconstrictor Precautions No information available to require special precautions

Effects on Dental Treatment No significant effects or complications reported

Mechanism of Action Inhibits synthesis of viral protein by binding to mRNA which blocks replication of cytomegalovirus through an antisense mechanism

Fomivirsen Sodium *see* Fomivirsen *on page 740*

Fondaparinux (fon da PARE i nuks)

U.S. Brand Names Arixtra®

Canadian Brand Names Arixtra®

Mexican Brand Names Arixtra

Generic Available No

Index Terms Fondaparinux Sodium

Pharmacologic Category Factor Xa Inhibitor

Use Prophylaxis of deep vein thrombosis (DVT) in patients undergoing surgery for hip replacement, knee replacement, hip fracture (including extended prophylaxis following hip fracture surgery), or abdominal surgery (in patients at risk for thromboembolic complications); treatment of acute pulmonary embolism (PE); treatment of acute DVT without PE

Unlabeled/Investigational Use Prophylaxis of DVT in patients with a history of heparin-induced thrombocytopenia (HIT)

Local Anesthetic/Vasoconstrictor Precautions No information available to require special precautions

Effects on Dental Treatment Key adverse event(s) related to dental treatment: Hemorrhage may occur at any site; risk increased in renal dysfunction, patients >75 years and/or <50 kg; major bleeding increased as high as 5% in patients receiving initial dose <6 hours postsurgery.

Common Adverse Effects As with all anticoagulants, bleeding is the major adverse effect. Hemorrhage may occur at any site. Risk appears increased by a number of factors including renal dysfunction, age (>75 years), and weight (<50 kg).

>10%:

Central nervous system: Fever (4% to 14%)

Gastrointestinal: Nausea (11%)

Hematologic: Anemia (20%)

1% to 10%:

Cardiovascular: Edema (9%), hypotension (4%), confusion (3%)

Central nervous system: Insomnia (5%), dizziness (4%), headache (2% to 5%), pain (2%)

Dermatologic: Rash (8%), purpura (4%), bullous eruption (3%)

Endocrine & metabolic: Hypokalemia (1% to 4%)

Gastrointestinal: Constipation (5% to 9%), nausea (3%), vomiting (6%), diarrhea (3%), dyspepsia (2%)

Genitourinary: Urinary tract infection (4%), urinary retention (3%)

Hematologic: Moderate thrombocytopenia (50,000-100,000/mm^3: 3%), major bleeding (1% to 3%), minor bleeding (2% to 4%), hematoma (3%); risk of major bleeding increased as high as 5% in patients receiving initial dose <6 hours following surgery

Hepatic: AST increased (2%), ALT increased (3%)

Local: Injection site reaction (bleeding, rash, pruritus)

Miscellaneous: Wound drainage increased (5%)

Mechanism of Action Fondaparinux is a synthetic pentasaccharide that causes an antithrombin III-mediated selective inhibition of factor Xa. Neutralization of factor Xa interrupts the blood coagulation cascade and inhibits thrombin formation and thrombus development.

Drug Interactions

Increased Effect/Toxicity: Anticoagulants, antiplatelet agents, drotrecogin alfa, NSAIDs, salicylates, and thrombolytic agents may enhance the anticoagulant effect and/or increase the risk of bleeding.

Pharmacodynamics/Kinetics

Absorption: Rapid and complete

Distribution: V$_d$: 7-11 L; mainly in blood

Protein binding: ≥94% to antithrombin III

Bioavailability: 100%

Half-life elimination: 17-21 hours; prolonged with worsening renal impairment

Time to peak: 2-3 hours

Excretion: Urine (as unchanged drug); decreased clearance in patients <50 kg

Pregnancy Risk Factor B

Fondaparinux Sodium *see* Fondaparinux *on page 741*

Foradil® Aerolizer™ *see* Formoterol *on page 742*

Formoterol (for MOH te rol)

U.S. Brand Names Foradil® Aerolizer™
Canadian Brand Names Foradil®; Oxeze® Turbuhaler®
Mexican Brand Names Foradil
Generic Available No
Index Terms Formoterol Fumarate
Pharmacologic Category Beta₂-Adrenergic Agonist
Use Maintenance treatment of asthma and prevention of bronchospasm in patients ≥5 years of age with reversible obstructive airway disease, including patients with symptoms of nocturnal asthma, who require regular treatment with inhaled, short-acting beta₂-agonists; maintenance treatment of bronchoconstriction in patients with COPD; prevention of exercise-induced bronchospasm in patients ≥5 years of age

Note: Oxeze® is also approved in Canada for acute relief of symptoms ("on demand" treatment) in patients ≥6 years of age.

Local Anesthetic/Vasoconstrictor Precautions No information available to require special precautions
Effects on Dental Treatment Key adverse event(s) related to dental treatment: Xerostomia (normal salivary flow resumes upon discontinuation).
Common Adverse Effects
>10%: Miscellaneous: Viral infection (17%)
1% to 10%:
  Cardiovascular: Chest pain (2%)
  Central nervous system: Anxiety (2%), dizziness (2%), fever (2%), insomnia (2%), dysphonia (1%)
  Dermatologic: Rash (1%)
  Gastrointestinal: Abdominal pain, dyspepsia, gastroenteritis, nausea, xerostomia (1%)
  Respiratory: Asthma exacerbation (age 5-12 years: 5% to 6%; age >12 years: <4%), bronchitis (5%), infection (3% to 7%), pharyngitis (4%), sinusitis (3%), dyspnea (2%), tonsillitis (1%)
Restrictions An FDA-approved medication guide must be distributed when dispensing an outpatient prescription (new or refill) where this medication is to be used without direct supervision of a healthcare provider. Medication guides are available at http://www.fda.gov/cder/Offices/ODS/medication_guides.htm.
Mechanism of Action Relaxes bronchial smooth muscle by selective action on beta₂ receptors with little effect on heart rate. Formoterol has a long-acting effect.
Drug Interactions
Cytochrome P450 Effect: Substrate (minor) of CYP2A6, 2C9, 2C19, 2D6
Increased Effect/Toxicity: Sympathomimetics may enhance the adverse/toxic effects of formoterol. Atomoxetine may increase the tachycardia of formoterol.
Decreased Effect: Formoterol may decrease the bradycardic effect of beta-blockers (beta₁ selective). Beta-blockers (nonselective) may decrease the bronchodilatory effect of beta₂-agonists.
Pharmacodynamics/Kinetics
Onset: Within 3 minutes
  Peak effect: 80% of peak effect within 15 minutes
Duration: Improvement in FEV_1 observed for 12 hours in most patients
Absorption: Rapidly into plasma
Protein binding: 61% to 64% *in vitro* at higher concentrations than achieved with usual dosing
Metabolism: Hepatic via direct glucuronidation and O-demethylation; CYP2D6, CYP2C8/9, CYP2C19, CYP2A6 involved in O-demethylation
Half-life elimination: ~10-14 hours
Time to peak: Maximum improvement in FEV_1 in 1-3 hours
Excretion:
  Children 5-12 years: Urine (7% to 9% as direct glucuronide metabolites, 6% as unchanged drug)
  Adults: Urine (15% to 18% as direct glucuronide metabolites, 10% as unchanged drug)
Pregnancy Risk Factor C

Formoterol Fumarate *see* Formoterol *on page 742*
Formula EM [OTC] *see* Fructose, Dextrose, and Phosphoric Acid *on page 754*
Formulation R™ [OTC] *see* Phenylephrine *on page 1293*
5-Formyl Tetrahydrofolate *see* Leucovorin *on page 957*
Fortamet® *see* Metformin *on page 1056*
Fortaz® *see* Ceftazidime *on page 307*

Fosamprenavir (FOS am pren a veer)

Related Information
  HIV Infection and AIDS *on page 1753*
U.S. Brand Names Lexiva®
Canadian Brand Names Telzir®
Mexican Brand Names Telzir
Generic Available No
Index Terms Fosamprenavir Calcium; GW433908G
Pharmacologic Category Antiretroviral Agent, Protease Inhibitor
Use Treatment of HIV infections in combination with at least two other antiretroviral agents
Local Anesthetic/Vasoconstrictor Precautions No information available to require special precautions
Effects on Dental Treatment No significant effects or complications reported
Common Adverse Effects Incidence data is compiled from use of fosamprenavir with and without concurrent ritonavir in combination with other antiretrovirals.
>10%:
  Central nervous system: Headache (19% to 27%), fatigue (9% to 18%), depression (8% to 11%)
  Dermatologic: Rash (9% to 35%; moderate-to-severe reactions 3% to 8%; onset ~11 days; duration ~13 days)
  Endocrine & metabolic: Hypertriglyceridemia (>750 mg/dL: up to 11%)
  Gastrointestinal: Diarrhea (34% to 52%), nausea (20% to 39%), vomiting (10% to 20%), abdominal pain (5% to 11%)
1% to 10%:
  Dermatologic: Pruritus (7% to 8%)
  Endocrine & metabolic: Hyperglycemia (>251 mg/dL: <1% to 2%)
  Gastrointestinal: Serum lipase increased (5% to 8%)
  Hematologic: Neutropenia (3%)
  Hepatic: Transaminases increased (4% to 8%)
  Neuromuscular & skeletal: Oral paresthesia (<1% to 10%)
Mechanism of Action Fosamprenavir is rapidly and almost completely converted to amprenavir by cellular phosphatases *in vivo*. Amprenavir binds to the active site of HIV protease activity and inhibits cleavage of viral polyprotein precursors (eg, Gag and Gag-Pol) into individual functional proteins found in infectious HIV. Inhibition prevents cleavage of these polyproteins, resulting in the formation of immature, noninfectious viral particles.

Drug Interactions
  Cytochrome P450 Effect: As amprenavir: **Substrate** of CYP2C9 (minor), 3A4 (major); **Inhibits** CYP2C19 (weak), 3A4 (strong)
  Increased Effect/Toxicity: Concurrent use of cisapride, midazolam, pimozide, quinidine, or triazolam is contraindicated. Concurrent use of ergot alkaloids (dihydroergotamine, ergotamine, ergonovine, methylergonovine) with amprenavir is also contraindicated (may cause vasospasm and peripheral ischemia). Concurrent use of oral suspension (Telzir® [CAN]) with disulfiram or metronidazole is contraindicated, due to the risk of propylene glycol toxicity.

  Serum concentrations of orally-inhaled corticosteroids, trazodone, and some antiarrhythmics (eg, amiodarone, lidocaine, and quinidine) may be increased, potentially leading to toxicity; when amprenavir is coadministered with ritonavir, flecainide, and propafenone are contraindicated. HMG-CoA reductase inhibitors serum concentrations may be increased by amprenavir, increasing the risk of myopathy/rhabdomyolysis; lovastatin and simvastatin are not recommended.

  Amprenavir may increase the levels/effects of selected benzodiazepines (midazolam and triazolam are contraindicated), calcium channel blockers, cyclosporine, eplerenone, fentanyl, mirtazapine, nateglinide, nefazodone, sildenafil (and other PDE-5 inhibitors), tacrolimus, venlafaxine, and other CYP3A4 substrates. When used with strong CYP3A4 inhibitors, dosage adjustment/limits are recommended for sildenafil and other PDE-5 inhibitors; refer to individual monographs.

  Concurrent therapy with ritonavir may result in increased serum concentrations: dosage adjustment is recommended. Indinavir, nelfinavir may increase serum concentrations of amprenavir.
(Continued)

Fosamprenavir *(Continued)*

Decreased Effect: CYP3A4 inducers may decrease the levels/effects of amprenavir; example inducers include aminoglutethimide, carbamazepine, nafcillin, nevirapine, phenobarbital, phenytoin, and rifamycins. Serum concentrations of estrogen (oral contraceptives) may be decreased, use alternative (nonhormonal) forms of contraception. Serum concentrations of delavirdine may be decreased by amprenavir; may lead to loss of virologic response and possible resistance; concomitant use of amprenavir with delavirdine is not recommended. Efavirenz and nevirapine may decrease serum concentrations of amprenavir (dosing for combinations not established). Avoid St John's wort (may lead to subtherapeutic concentrations of amprenavir). Effect of amprenavir may be diminished when administered with methadone (consider alternative antiretroviral); in addition, effect of methadone may be reduced (dosage increase may be required). Antacids and H_2-blockers may impair absorption of fosamprenavir, leading to reduced serum levels of amprenavir; separate doses.

Pharmacodynamics/Kinetics

Absorption: 63%

Bioavailability: Not established; food does not have a significant effect on absorption

Protein-binding: 90%

Half-life elimination: 7.7 hours (amprenavir)

Time to peak, plasma: 1.5-4 hours (median: 2.5 hours)

Metabolism: Fosamprenavir is rapidly and almost completely converted to amprenavir by cellular phosphatases in gut epithelium; amprenavir is hepatically metabolized via CYP isoenzymes (primarily CYP3A4)

Excretion: Feces (75% as metabolites, <1% as unchanged drug); urine (14% as metabolites, <1% as unchanged drug)

Pregnancy Risk Factor C

Fosamprenavir Calcium *see* Fosamprenavir *on page 743*

Foscarnet *(fos KAR net)*

Related Information

Systemic Viral Diseases *on page 1767*

U.S. Brand Names Foscavir®

Canadian Brand Names Foscavir®

Generic Available Yes

Index Terms PFA; Phosphonoformate; Phosphonoformic Acid

Pharmacologic Category Antiviral Agent

Dental Use Treatment of mucotaneous herpesvirus infections suspected to be caused by acyclovir (HSV, VZV) or ganciclovir (CMV) resistant strains (this occurs almost exclusively in persons with advanced AIDS who have received prolonged treatment for herpes infection)

Use

Treatment of mucotaneous herpesvirus infections suspected to be caused by acyclovir-resistant (HSV, VZV) or ganciclovir-resistant (CMV) strains; this occurs almost exclusively in immunocompromised persons (eg, with advanced AIDS) who have received prolonged treatment for a herpesvirus infection

Treatment of CMV retinitis in persons with AIDS

Unlabeled/Investigational Use Other CMV infections (eg, colitis, esophagitis, neurological disease)

Local Anesthetic/Vasoconstrictor Precautions Foscarnet is one of the drugs confirmed to prolong the QT interval and is accepted as having a risk of causing torsade de pointes. In terms of epinephrine, it is not known what effect vasoconstrictors in the local anesthetic regimen will have in patients with a known history of congenital prolonged QT interval or in patients taking any medication that prolongs the QT interval. Until more information is obtained, it is suggested that the clinician consult with the physician prior to the use of a vasoconstrictor in suspected patients, and that the vasoconstrictor (epinephrine, levonordefrin [Neo-Cobefrin®]) be used with caution. See Dental Comment.

Effects on Dental Treatment Key adverse event(s) related to dental treatment: Xerostomia (normal salivary flow resumes upon discontinuation), taste perversion, and ulcerative stomatitis.

Significant Adverse Effects

>10%:

Central nervous system: Fever (65%), headache (26%)

Endocrine & metabolic: Hypokalemia (16% to 48%), hypocalcemia (15% to 30%), hypomagnesemia (15% to 30%), hypophosphatemia (8% to 26%)

Gastrointestinal: Nausea (47%), diarrhea (30%), vomiting (26%)

Hematologic: Anemia (33%), granulocytopenia (17%)

Renal: Abnormal renal function/decreased creatinine clearance (27%)

1% to 10%:

Cardiovascular: Chest pain (1% to 5%), edema (1% to 5%), facial edema (1% to 5%), flushing (1% to 5%), hyper-/hypotension (1% to 5%), palpitation (1% to 5%), sinus tachycardia, first degree AV block, nonspecific ST-T segment changes

Central nervous system: Seizure (10%), fatigue (>5%), malaise (>5%), dizziness (>5%), hypoesthesia (>5%), depression (>5%), confusion (>5%), anxiety (≥5%), aphasia (1% to 5%), ataxia (1% to 5%), dementia (1% to 5%), meningitis (1% to 5%), stupor (1% to 5%), insomnia (1% to 5%), somnolence (1% to 5%), nervousness (1% to 5%), amnesia (1% to 5%), agitation (1% to 5%), aggressiveness (1% to 5%), hallucination (1% to 5%)

Dermatologic: Rash (>5%), pruritus (1% to 5%), skin ulceration (1% to 5%), seborrhea (1% to 5%), erythematous rash, maculopapular rash, skin discoloration

Endocrine & metabolic: Hyperphosphatemia (6%), acidosis (1% to 5%), hyponatremia (1% to 5%)

Gastrointestinal: Anorexia (>5%), abdominal pain (>5%), constipation (1% to 5%), dysphasia (1% to 5%), dyspepsia (1% to 5%), flatulence (1% to 5%), melena (1% to 5%), pancreatitis (1% to 5%), rectal hemorrhage (1% to 5%), taste perversion (1% to 5%), ulcerative stomatitis (1% to 5%), weight loss (1% to 5%), xerostomia (1% to 5%)

Genitourinary: Urinary retention (1% to 5%), dysuria (1% to 5%), nocturia (1% to 5%)

Hematologic: Leukopenia (≥5%), thrombocytopenia (1% to 5%), thrombosis (1% to 5%), lymphadenopathy (1% to 5%)

Local: Injection site pain

Neuromuscular & skeletal: Paresthesia (>5%), involuntary muscle contractions (>5%), rigors (>5%), neuropathy (peripheral; >5%), weakness (>5%), arthralgia (1% to 5%), back pain (1% to 5%), leg cramps (1% to 5%), myalgia (1% to 5%), tremor (1% to 5%)

Ocular: Vision abnormalities (>5%), conjunctivitis (1% to 5%), eye pain (1% to 5%)

Renal: Acute renal failure (1% to 5%), albuminuria (1% to 5%), BUN increased (1% to 5%), polyuria (1% to 5%), urinary tract infection (1% to 5%)

Respiratory: Cough (>5%), dyspnea (≥5%), bronchospasm (1% to 5%), hemoptysis (1% to 5%), pharyngitis (1% to 5%), pneumonia (1% to 5%), pneumothorax (1% to 5%), rhinitis (1% to 5%), sinusitis (1% to 5%), stridor (1% to 5%)

Miscellaneous: Sepsis (>5%), diaphoresis (increased), flu-like syndrome (1% to 5%), infection (1% to 5%), thirst (1% to 5%)

<1% (Limited to important or life-threatening): Amylase increased, cardiac arrest, coma, creatinine phosphokinase increased, dehydration, diabetes insipidus (usually nephrogenic), erythema multiforme, hematuria, hypoproteinemia, muscle weakness, myopathy, myositis, neutropenia, pancytopenia, QT_c prolongation, renal calculus, rhabdomyolysis, Stevens-Johnson syndrome, syndrome of inappropriate antidiuretic hormone (SIADH), toxic epidermal necrolysis, ventricular arrhythmia, vesiculobullous eruptions

Induction Dosing of Foscarnet in Patients With Abnormal Renal Function

Cl_{cr} (mL/min/kg)	HSV Equivalent to 40 mg/kg q12h	HSV Equivalent to 40 mg/kg q8h	CMV Equivalent to 60 mg/kg q8h	CMV Equivalent to 90 mg/kg q12h
<0.4	Not recommended	Not recommended	Not recommended	Not recommended
≥0.4-0.5	20 mg/kg every 24 hours	35 mg/kg every 24 hours	50 mg/kg every 24 hours	50 mg/kg every 24 hours
>0.5-0.6	25 mg/kg every 24 hours	40 mg/kg every 24 hours	60 mg/kg every 24 hours	60 mg/kg every 24 hours
>0.6-0.8	35 mg/kg every 24 hours	25 mg/kg every 12 hours	40 mg/kg every 12 hours	80 mg/kg every 24 hours
>0.8-1.0	20 mg/kg every 12 hours	35 mg/kg every 12 hours	50 mg/kg every 12 hours	50 mg/kg every 12 hours
>1.0-1.4	30 mg/kg every 12 hours	30 mg/kg every 8 hours	45 mg/kg every 8 hours	70 mg/kg every 12 hours
>1.4	40 mg/kg every 12 hours	40 mg/kg every 8 hours	60 mg/kg every 8 hours	90 mg/kg every 12 hours

Dental Usual Dosing Herpes simplex infections (acyclovir-resistant): Induction: I.V.: 40 mg/kg/dose every 8-12 hours for 14-21 days

(Continued)

Foscarnet (Continued)

Dosage

CMV retinitis: I.V.:

Induction treatment: 60 mg/kg/dose every 8 hours **or** 90 mg/kg every 12 hours for 14-21 days

Maintenance therapy: 90-120 mg/kg/day as a single infusion

Herpes simplex infections (acyclovir-resistant): Induction: I.V.: 40 mg/kg/dose every 8-12 hours for 14-21 days

Dosage adjustment in renal impairment:

Induction and maintenance dosing schedules based on creatinine clearance (mL/minute/kg): See tables below and on previous page.

Maintenance Dosing of Foscarnet in Patients With Abnormal Renal Function

Cl_{cr} (mL/min/kg)	CMV Equivalent to 90 mg/kg q24h	CMV Equivalent to 120 mg/kg q24h
<0.4	Not recommended	Not recommended
≥0.4-0.5	50 mg/kg every 48 hours	65 mg/kg every 48 hours
>0.5-0.6	60 mg/kg every 48 hours	80 mg/kg every 48 hours
>0.6-0.8	80 mg/kg every 48 hours	105 mg/kg every 48 hours
>0.8-1.0	50 mg/kg every 24 hours	65 mg/kg every 24 hours
>1.0-1.4	70 mg/kg every 24 hours	90 mg/kg every 24 hours
>1.4	90 mg/kg every 24 hours	120 mg/kg every 24 hours

Hemodialysis:

Foscarnet is highly removed by hemodialysis (30% in 4 hours HD)

Doses of 50 mg/kg/dose posthemodialysis have been found to produce similar serum concentrations as doses of 90 mg/kg twice daily in patients with normal renal function

Doses of 60-90 mg/kg/dose loading dose (posthemodialysis) followed by 45 mg/kg/dose posthemodialysis (3 times/week) with the monitoring of weekly plasma concentrations to maintain peak plasma concentrations in the range of 400-800 µMolar have been recommended by some clinicians

Continuous arteriovenous or venovenous hemodiafiltration effects: Dose as for Cl_{cr} 10-50 mL/minute

Mechanism of Action Pyrophosphate analogue which acts as a noncompetitive inhibitor of many viral RNA and DNA polymerases as well as HIV reverse transcriptase. Similar to ganciclovir, foscarnet is a virostatic agent. Foscarnet does not require activation by thymidine kinase.

Contraindications Hypersensitivity to foscarnet or any component of the formulation; Cl_{cr} <0.4 mL/minute/kg during therapy

Warnings/Precautions Hazardous agent - use appropriate precautions for handling and disposal. **[U.S. Boxed Warning]: Indicated only for immuno-compromised patients with CMV retinitis and mucocutaneous acyclovir-resistant HSV infection. [U.S. Boxed Warning]: Renal impairment occurs to some degree in the majority of patients treated with foscarnet;** renal impairment may occur at any time and is usually reversible within 1 week following dose adjustment or discontinuation of therapy, however, several patients have died with renal failure within 4 weeks of stopping foscarnet; therefore, renal function should be closely monitored. To reduce the risk of nephrotoxicity and the potential to administer a relative overdose, always calculate the Cl_{cr} even if serum creatinine is within the normal range. Adequate hydration may reduce the risk of nephrotoxicity; the manufacturer makes specific recommendations regarding this.

Imbalance of serum electrolytes or minerals occurs in at least 15% of patients (hypocalcemia, low ionized calcium, hypophosphatemia, hypomagnesemia, or hypokalemia). Patients with low ionized calcium may experience perioral tingling, numbness, paresthesias, tetany, and seizures. Correct electrolytes before initiating therapy. Use caution when administering other medications that cause electrolyte imbalances. Patients who experience signs or symptoms of an electrolyte imbalance should be assessed immediately. **[U.S. Boxed Warning]: Seizures related to plasma electrolyte/mineral imbalance may occur;** incidence has been reported in up to 10% of AIDS patients. Risk factors for seizures include impaired baseline renal function and low total serum calcium. May cause anemia and granulocytopenia. Safety and efficacy in children have not been established.

Drug Interactions

Ciprofloxacin: May enhance the neuroexcitatory and/or seizure-potentiating effect of foscarnet.

Nephrotoxic drugs (amphotericin B, I.V. pentamidine, aminoglycosides, etc): Should be avoided, if possible, to minimize additive renal risk with foscarnet.

QT_c-prolonging agents: May enhance the adverse/toxic effect of other QT_c-prolonging agents such as foscarnet. Any electrolyte abnormalities caused by foscarnet may exacerbate the situation.

Pentamidine: Increases risk of severe hypocalcemia.

Ritonavir, saquinavir: Increased risk of renal impairment has been associated with concurrent use with foscarnet.

Thioridazine: Foscarnet may enhance the QT_c-prolonging effect of thioridazine.

Zalcitabine: Foscarnet may enhance the neurotoxic (peripheral) effect of zalcitabine.

Pharmacodynamics/Kinetics

Distribution: Up to 28% of cumulative I.V. dose may be deposited in bone

Metabolism: Biotransformation does not occur

Half-life elimination: ~3 hours

Excretion: Urine (≤28% as unchanged drug)

Pregnancy Risk Factor C

Lactation Excretion in breast milk unknown/contraindicated

Breast-Feeding Considerations The CDC recommends **not** to breast-feed if diagnosed with HIV to avoid postnatal transmission of the virus.

Dosage Forms Excipient information presented when available (limited, particularly for generics); consult specific product labeling.

Injection, solution: 24 mg/mL (250 mL, 500 mL)

Foscavir®: 24 mg/mL (500 mL)

Dental Comment Foscarnet is known to prolong the QT interval. The QT interval is measured as the time and distance between the Q point of the QRS complex and the end of the T wave in the ECG tracing. After adjustment for heart rate, the QT interval is defined as prolonged if it is more than 450 msec in men and 460 msec in women. A long QT syndrome was first described in the 1950s and 60s as a congenital syndrome involving QT interval prolongation and syncope and sudden death. Some of the congenital long QT syndromes were characterized by a peculiar electrocardiographic appearance of the QRS complex involving a premature atria beat followed by a pause, then a subsequent sinus beat showing marked QT prolongation and deformity. This type of cardiac arrhythmia was originally termed "torsade de pointes" (translated from the French as "twisting of the points").

Prolongation of the QT interval is thought to result from delayed ventricular repolarization. The repolarization process within the myocardial cell is due to the efflux of intracellular potassium. The channels associated with this current can be blocked by many drugs and predispose the electrical propagation cycle to torsade de pointes.

Foscarnet is considered as having a risk of causing torsade de pointes. The risk of drug-induced torsade de pointes is extremely low when a single QT interval prolonging drug is prescribed. It is not known what effect vasoconstrictors in the local anesthetic regimen will have in patients with a known history of congenital prolonged QT interval or in patients taking any medication that prolongs the QT interval. Until more information is obtained, it is suggested that the clinician consult with the physician prior to the use of a vasoconstrictor in suspected patients, and that the vasoconstrictor (epinephrine, levonordefrin [Neo-Cobefrin®]) be used with caution.

Selected Readings

Chilukuri S and Rosen T, "Management of Acyclovir-Resistant Herpes Simplex Virus," *Dermatol Clin*, 2003, 21(2):311-20.

Foscavir® *see Foscarnet on page 744*

Fosfomycin (fos foe MYE sin)

U.S. Brand Names Monurol™

Canadian Brand Names Monurol™

Mexican Brand Names Monurol

Generic Available No

Index Terms Fosfomycin Tromethamine

Pharmacologic Category Antibiotic, Miscellaneous

Use Single oral dose in the treatment of uncomplicated urinary tract infections in women due to susceptible strains of *E. coli* and *Enterococcus*; may have an advantage over other agents since it maintains high concentration in the urine for up to 48 hours

Unlabeled/Investigational Use Multiple doses have been investigated for complicated urinary tract infections in men

Local Anesthetic/Vasoconstrictor Precautions No information available to require special precautions

(Continued)

Fosfomycin *(Continued)*

Effects on Dental Treatment No significant effects or complications reported

Common Adverse Effects
1% to 10%:
    Central nervous system: Headache (47%), dizziness (1%)
    Dermatologic: Rash (1%)
    Gastrointestinal: Diarrhea (2% to 10%), nausea (4%), epigastric discomfort (1%), abdominal pain
    Genitourinary: Vaginitis
    Neuromuscular & skeletal: Weakness (1%)

Mechanism of Action As a phosphoric acid derivative, fosfomycin inhibits bacterial wall synthesis (bactericidal) by inactivating the enzyme, pyruvyl transferase, which is critical in the synthesis of cell walls by bacteria; the tromethamine salt is preferable to the calcium salt due to its superior absorption

Drug Interactions
Decreased Effect: Antacids or calcium salts may cause precipitate formation and decrease fosfomycin absorption. Increased gastrointestinal motility due to metoclopramide may lower fosfomycin tromethamine serum concentrations and urinary excretion. This drug interaction possibly could be extrapolated to other medications which increase gastrointestinal motility.

Pharmacodynamics/Kinetics
Absorption: Well absorbed
Distribution: V_d: 2 L/kg; high concentrations in urine; well into other tissues; crosses maximally into CSF with inflamed meninges
Protein binding: <3%
Bioavailability: 34% to 58%
Half-life elimination: 4-8 hours; Cl_{cr} <10 mL/minute: 50 hours
Time to peak, serum: 2 hours
Excretion: Urine (as unchanged drug); high urinary levels (100 mcg/mL) persist for >48 hours

Pregnancy Risk Factor B

Fosfomycin Tromethamine *see* Fosfomycin *on page 747*

Fosinopril *(foe SIN oh pril)*

Related Information
    Cardiovascular Diseases *on page 1726*
U.S. Brand Names Monopril®
Canadian Brand Names Apo-Fosinopril®; Monopril®; Novo-Fosinopril; ratio-Fosinopril; Riva-Fosinopril
Mexican Brand Names Monopril
Generic Available Yes
Index Terms Fosinopril Sodium
Pharmacologic Category Angiotensin-Converting Enzyme (ACE) Inhibitor
Use Treatment of hypertension, either alone or in combination with other antihypertensive agents; treatment of congestive heart failure, left ventricular dysfunction after myocardial infarction
Local Anesthetic/Vasoconstrictor Precautions No information available to require special precautions
Effects on Dental Treatment Key adverse event(s) related to dental treatment: Orthostatic hypotension.
Common Adverse Effects Note: Frequency ranges include data from hypertension and heart failure trials. Higher rates of adverse reactions have generally been noted in patients with CHF. However, the frequency of adverse effects associated with placebo is also increased in this population.

>10%: Central nervous system: Dizziness (2% to 12%)
1% to 10%:
    Cardiovascular: Orthostatic hypotension (1% to 2%), palpitation (1%)
    Central nervous system: Dizziness (1% to 2%; up to 12% in CHF patients), headache (3%), fatigue (1% to 2%)
    Endocrine & metabolic: Hyperkalemia (2.6%)
    Gastrointestinal: Diarrhea (2%), nausea/vomiting (1.2% to 2.2%)
    Hepatic: Transaminases increased
    Neuromuscular & skeletal: Musculoskeletal pain (<1% to 3%), noncardiac chest pain (<1% to 2%), weakness (1%)
    Renal: Serum creatinine increased, renal function worsening (in patients with bilateral renal artery stenosis or hypovolemia)
    Respiratory: Cough (2% to 10%)
    Miscellaneous: Upper respiratory infection (2%)
>1% but ≤ frequency in patients receiving placebo: Sexual dysfunction, fever, flu-like syndrome, dyspnea, rash, headache, insomnia

Other events reported with ACE inhibitors: Neutropenia, agranulocytosis, eosinophilic pneumonitis, cardiac arrest, pancytopenia, hemolytic anemia, anemia, aplastic anemia, thrombocytopenia, acute renal failure, hepatic failure, jaundice, symptomatic hyponatremia, bullous pemphigus, exfoliative dermatitis, Stevens-Johnson syndrome. In addition, a syndrome which may include fever, myalgia, arthralgia, interstitial nephritis, vasculitis, rash, eosinophilia and positive ANA, and elevated ESR has been reported for other ACE inhibitors.

Dosage Oral:

Children ≥6 years and >50 kg: Hypertension: Initial: 5-10 mg once daily (maximum: 40 mg/day)

Adults:

Hypertension: Initial: 10 mg/day; most patients are maintained on 20-40 mg/day. May need to divide the dose into two if trough effect is inadequate; discontinue the diuretic, if possible 2-3 days before initiation of therapy; resume diuretic therapy carefully, if needed.

Heart failure: Initial: 10 mg/day (5 mg if renal dysfunction present) and increase, as needed, to a maximum of 40 mg once daily over several weeks; usual dose: 20-40 mg/day. If hypotension, orthostasis, or azotemia occur during titration, consider decreasing concomitant diuretic dose, if any.

Dosing adjustment/comments in renal impairment: None needed since hepatobiliary elimination compensates adequately diminished renal elimination.

Hemodialysis: Moderately dialyzable (20% to 50%)

Mechanism of Action Competitive inhibitor of angiotensin-converting enzyme (ACE); prevents conversion of angiotensin I to angiotensin II, a potent vasoconstrictor; results in lower levels of angiotensin II which causes an increase in plasma renin activity and a reduction in aldosterone secretion; a CNS mechanism may also be involved in hypotensive effect as angiotensin II increases adrenergic outflow from CNS; vasoactive kallikreins may be decreased in conversion to active hormones by ACE inhibitors, thus reducing blood pressure

Contraindications Hypersensitivity to fosinopril or any component of the formulation; angioedema related to previous treatment with an ACE inhibitor; idiopathic or hereditary angioedema; bilateral renal artery stenosis; pregnancy (2nd and 3rd trimesters)

Warnings/Precautions Anaphylactic reactions can occur. Angioedema can occur at any time during treatment (especially following first dose). It may involve head and neck (potentially affecting the airway) or the intestine (presenting with abdominal pain). Prolonged monitoring may be required, especially if tongue, glottis, or larynx are involved as they are associated with airway obstruction. Those with a history of airway surgery in this situation have a higher risk. Careful blood pressure monitoring (hypotension can occur especially in volume-depleted patients). **[U.S. Boxed Warning]: Based on human data, ACEIs can cause injury and death to the developing fetus when used in the second and third trimesters. ACEIs should be discontinued as soon as possible once pregnancy is detected.** Dosage adjustment needed in severe renal impairment (Cl_{cr} <10 mL/minute). Use with caution in hypovolemia; collagen vascular diseases; valvular stenosis (particularly aortic stenosis); hyperkalemia; or before, during, or immediately after anesthesia. Avoid rapid dosage escalation which may lead to renal insufficiency. Rare toxicities associated with ACE inhibitors include cholestatic jaundice (which may progress to hepatic necrosis) and neutropenia/agranulocytosis with myeloid hyperplasia. Hyperkalemia may rarely occur. May be associated with deterioration of renal function and/or increases in serum creatinine, particularly in patients dependent on renin-angiotensin-aldosterone system. Use with caution in unilateral renal artery stenosis and pre-existing renal insufficiency; if patient has renal impairment, then a baseline WBC with differential and serum creatinine should be evaluated and monitored closely during the first 3 months of therapy. Hypersensitivity reactions may be seen during hemodialysis with high-flux dialysis membranes (eg, AN69). Safety and efficacy have not been established in children <6 years of age.

Drug Interactions

Increased Effect/Toxicity: Potassium supplements, co-trimoxazole (high dose), angiotensin II receptor antagonists (eg, candesartan, losartan, irbesartan), or potassium-sparing diuretics (amiloride, spironolactone, triamterene) may result in elevated serum potassium levels when combined with fosinopril. ACE inhibitor effects may be increased by phenothiazines or probenecid (increases levels of captopril). ACE inhibitors may increase serum concentrations/effects of lithium. ACE inhibitors may enhance the adverse/toxic effects (nitritoid reaction) of gold sodium thiomalate.

Diuretics have additive hypotensive effects with ACE inhibitors, and hypovolemia increases the potential for adverse renal effects of ACE inhibitors. In patients with compromised renal function, coadministration with NSAIDs may (Continued)

Fosinopril *(Continued)*

result in further deterioration of renal function. Allopurinol and ACE inhibitors may cause a higher risk of hypersensitivity reaction when taken concurrently.

Decreased Effect: Aspirin (high dose) may reduce the therapeutic effects of ACE inhibitors; at low dosages this does not appear to be significant. Rifampin may decrease the effect of ACE inhibitors. Antacids may decrease the bioavailability of ACE inhibitors (may be more likely to occur with captopril); separate administration times by 1-2 hours. NSAIDs, specifically indomethacin, may reduce the hypotensive effects of ACE inhibitors. More likely to occur in low renin or volume-dependent hypertensive patients.

Ethanol/Nutrition/Herb Interactions Herb/Nutraceutical: Avoid dong quai if using for hypertension (has estrogenic activity). Avoid ephedra, garlic, yohimbe, ginseng (may worsen hypertension).

Dietary Considerations Should not take a potassium salt supplement without the advice of healthcare provider.

Pharmacodynamics/Kinetics

Onset of action: 1 hour

Duration: 24 hours

Absorption: 36%

Protein binding: 95%

Metabolism: Prodrug, hydrolyzed to its active metabolite fosinoprilat by intestinal wall and hepatic esterases

Bioavailability: 36%

Half-life elimination, serum (fosinoprilat): 12 hours

Time to peak, serum: ~3 hours

Excretion: Urine and feces (as fosinoprilat and other metabolites in roughly equal proportions, 45% to 50%)

Pregnancy Risk Factor C (1st trimester)/D (2nd and 3rd trimesters)

Dosage Forms

Tablet: 10 mg, 20 mg, 40 mg

Monopril®: 10 mg, 20 mg, 40 mg

Fosinopril and Hydrochlorothiazide

(foe SIN oh pril & hye droe klor oh THYE a zide)

Related Information

Fosinopril *on page 748*
Hydrochlorothiazide *on page 819*

U.S. Brand Names Monopril-HCT®

Canadian Brand Names Monopril-HCT®

Generic Available Yes

Index Terms Hydrochlorothiazide and Fosinopril

Pharmacologic Category Antihypertensive Agent, Combination

Use Treatment of hypertension; not indicated for first-line treatment

Local Anesthetic/Vasoconstrictor Precautions No information available to require special precautions

Effects on Dental Treatment No significant effects or complications reported

Common Adverse Effects

2% to 10%:

Central nervous system: Headache (7%, less than placebo), fatigue (4%), dizziness (3%), orthostatic hypotension (2%)

Neuromuscular & skeletal: Musculoskeletal pain (2%)

Respiratory: Cough (6%), upper respiratory infection (2%, less than placebo)

<2%: Abdominal pain, angioedema, breast mass, BUN elevation (similar to placebo), chest pain, creatinine elevation (similar to placebo), depression, diarrhea, dyspepsia, dysuria, edema, eosinophilia, esophagitis, fever, flushing, gastritis, gout, heartburn, hepatic necrosis, leukopenia, libido change, liver function test elevations (transaminases, LDH, alkaline phosphatase, serum bilirubin), muscle cramps, myalgia, nausea, neutropenia, numbness, paresthesia, pharyngitis, pruritus, rash, rhinitis, sexual dysfunction, sinus congestion, somnolence, syncope, tinnitus, urinary frequency, urinary tract infection, viral infection, vomiting, weakness

Other adverse events reported with **ACE inhibitors**: Aplastic anemia, bullous pemphigus, cardiac arrest, cholestatic jaundice, exfoliative dermatitis, hemolytic anemia, hyperkalemia, pancreatitis, pancytopenia, photosensitivity; syndrome that may include one or more of arthralgia/arthritis, vasculitis, serositis, myalgia, fever, rash or other dermopathy, positive ANA titer, leukocytosis, eosinophilia, and elevated ESR; thrombocytopenia

Other adverse events reported with **hydrochlorothiazide**: Agranulocytosis, anaphylactic reactions, anorexia, blurred vision (transient), constipation, cramping, glucosuria, hemolytic anemia, hypercalcemia, hyperglycemia, hyperuricemia, hypokalemia, jaundice (intrahepatic cholestatic), lightheadedness, muscle spasm, necrotizing angiitis, pancreatitis, photosensitivity, pneumonitis, pulmonary edema, purpura, respiratory distress, restlessness, sialadenitis, SLE, Stevens-Johnson syndrome, urticaria, vertigo, xanthopsia

Mechanism of Action Fosinopril is a competitive inhibitor of angiotensin-converting enzyme (ACE); prevents conversion of angiotensin I to angiotensin II, a potent vasoconstrictor; results in lower levels of angiotensin II which causes an increase in plasma renin activity and a reduction in aldosterone secretion; a CNS mechanism may also be involved in hypotensive effect as angiotensin II increases adrenergic outflow from CNS; vasoactive kallikreins may be decreased in conversion to active hormones by ACE inhibitors, thus reducing blood pressure. Hydrochlorothiazide inhibits sodium reabsorption in the distal tubules causing increased excretion of sodium and water as well as potassium and hydrogen ions.

Drug Interactions

Increased Effect/Toxicity: Alpha$_1$-blockers, diuretics increase hypotension. Beta-blockers may increase hyperglycemic effect. Cyclosporine may increase risk of gout or renal toxicity. Risk of lithium toxicity may be increased. Mercaptopurine may increase risk of neutropenia. Digoxin and neuromuscular-blocking agents: Effects may be increased with hypokalemia. Potassium-sparing diuretics, potassium supplements, trimethoprim may increase risk of hyperkalemia. ACE inhibitors may enhance the adverse/toxic effects (nitritoid reaction) of gold sodium thiomalate.

Decreased Effect: Aspirin, NSAIDs may decrease antihypertensive effect. Antacids, cholestyramine, colestipol may decrease absorption.

Pharmacodynamics/Kinetics See individual agents.

Pregnancy Risk Factor C (1st trimester); D (2nd and 3rd trimester)

Fosinopril Sodium *see Fosinopril on page 748*

Fosphenytoin (FOS fen i toyn)

Related Information
Phenytoin *on page 1295*

U.S. Brand Names Cerebyx®

Canadian Brand Names Cerebyx®

Generic Available No

Index Terms Fosphenytoin Sodium

Pharmacologic Category Anticonvulsant, Hydantoin

Use Used for the control of generalized convulsive status epilepticus and prevention and treatment of seizures occurring during neurosurgery; indicated for short-term parenteral administration when other means of phenytoin administration are unavailable, inappropriate, or deemed less advantageous (the safety and effectiveness of fosphenytoin in this use has not been systematically evaluated for more than 5 days)

Local Anesthetic/Vasoconstrictor Precautions No information available to require special precautions

Effects on Dental Treatment Key adverse event(s) related to dental treatment: Tongue disorder and dry mouth.

Common Adverse Effects The more important adverse clinical events caused by the I.V. use of fosphenytoin or phenytoin are cardiovascular collapse and/or central nervous system depression. Hypotension can occur when either drug is administered rapidly by the I.V. route. Do not exceed a rate of 150 mg phenytoin equivalent/minute when administering fosphenytoin.

The adverse clinical events most commonly observed with the use of fosphenytoin in clinical trials were nystagmus, dizziness, pruritus, paresthesia, headache, somnolence, and ataxia. Paresthesia and pruritus were seen more often following fosphenytoin (versus phenytoin) administration and occurred more often with I.V. fosphenytoin than with I.M. administration. These events were dose and rate related (doses ≥15 mg/kg at a rate of 150 mg/minute). These sensations, generally described as itching, burning, or tingling are usually not at the infusion site. The location of the discomfort varied with the groin mentioned most frequently. The paresthesia and pruritus were transient events that occurred within several minutes of the start of infusion and generally resolved within 10 minutes after completion of infusion.

Transient pruritus, tinnitus, nystagmus, somnolence, and ataxia occurred 2-3 times more often at doses ≥15 mg/kg and rates ≥150 mg/minute.

I.V. administration (maximum dose/rate):

>10%:
Central nervous system: Nystagmus, dizziness, somnolence, ataxia
Dermatologic: Pruritus

(Continued)

Fosphenytoin (Continued)

1% to 10%:

    Cardiovascular: Hypotension, vasodilation, tachycardia

    Central nervous system: Stupor, incoordination, paresthesia, extrapyramidal syndrome, tremor, agitation, hypoesthesia, dysarthria, vertigo, brain edema, headache

    Gastrointestinal: Nausea, tongue disorder, dry mouth, vomiting

    Neuromuscular & skeletal: Pelvic pain, muscle weakness, back pain

    Ocular: Diplopia, amblyopia

    Otic: Tinnitus, deafness

    Miscellaneous: Taste perversion

I.M. administration (substitute for oral phenytoin):

1% to 10%:

    Central nervous system: Nystagmus, tremor, ataxia, headache, incoordination, somnolence, dizziness, paresthesia, reflexes decreased

    Dermatologic: Pruritus

    Gastrointestinal: Nausea, vomiting

    Hematologic/lymphatic: Ecchymosis

    Neuromuscular & skeletal: Muscle weakness

Mechanism of Action Diphosphate ester salt of phenytoin which acts as a water soluble prodrug of phenytoin; after administration, plasma esterases convert fosphenytoin to phosphate, formaldehyde, and phenytoin as the active moiety; phenytoin works by stabilizing neuronal membranes and decreasing seizure activity by increasing efflux or decreasing influx of sodium ions across cell membranes in the motor cortex during generation of nerve impulses

Drug Interactions

Cytochrome P450 Effect: As phenytoin: **Substrate** of CYP2C9 (major), 2C19 (major), 3A4 (minor); **Induces** CYP2B6 (strong), 2C8 (strong), 2C9 (strong), 2C19 (strong), 3A4 (strong)

Increased Effect/Toxicity: The sedative effects of phenytoin may be additive with other CNS depressants including ethanol, barbiturates, sedatives, antidepressants, opioid analgesics, and benzodiazepines. Selected anticonvulsants (felbamate, gabapentin, and topiramate) have been reported to increase phenytoin levels/effects. In addition, serum phenytoin concentrations may be increased by allopurinol, amiodarone, calcium channel blockers (including diltiazem and nifedipine), cimetidine, disulfiram, methylphenidate, metronidazole, omeprazole, selective serotonin reuptake inhibitors (SSRIs), ticlopidine, tricyclic antidepressants, trazodone, and trimethoprim. Case reports indicate ciprofloxacin may increase or decrease serum phenytoin concentrations.

The levels/effects of phenytoin may be increased by delavirdine, fluconazole, fluvoxamine, gemfibrozil, isoniazid, ketoconazole, nicardipine, NSAIDs, omeprazole, pioglitazone, sulfonamides, ticlopidine, and other CYP2C9 or 2C19 inhibitors.

Phenytoin enhances the conversion of primidone to phenobarbital resulting in elevated phenobarbital serum concentrations. Concurrent use of acetazolamide with phenytoin may result in an increased risk of osteomalacia. Concurrent use of phenytoin and lithium has resulted in lithium intoxication. Valproic acid (and sulfisoxazole) may displace phenytoin from binding sites; valproic acid may increase, decrease, or have no effect on phenytoin serum concentrations. Phenytoin transiently increased the response to warfarin initially; this is followed by an inhibition of the hypoprothrombinemic response. Phenytoin may enhance the hepatotoxic potential of acetaminophen overdoses. Concurrent use of dopamine and intravenous phenytoin may lead to an increased risk of hypotension.

Decreased Effect: Phenytoin may enhance the metabolism of estrogen and/or oral contraceptives, decreasing their clinical effect; an alternative method of contraception should be considered. Phenytoin may increase the metabolism of anticonvulsants including barbiturates, carbamazepine, ethosuximide, felbamate, lamotrigine, tiagabine, topiramate, and zonisamide. Valproic acid may increase, decrease, or have no effect on phenytoin serum concentrations. Phenytoin may also decrease the serum concentrations/effects of some antiarrhythmics (disopyramide, propafenone, quinidine, quetiapine) and tricyclic antidepressants may be reduced by phenytoin. Phenytoin may enhance the metabolism of doxycycline, decreasing its clinical effect; higher dosages may be required. Phenytoin may increase the metabolism of chloramphenicol or itraconazole.

Phenytoin may decrease the levels/effects of amiodarone, benzodiazepines, bupropion, calcium channel blockers, carbamazepine, citalopram, clarithromycin, cyclosporine, efavirenz, erythromycin, estrogens, fluoxetine, glimepiride, glipizide, losartan, methsuximide, mirtazapine, nateglinide, nefazodone, nevirapine, phenytoin, pioglitazone, promethazine, propranolol, protease inhibitors, proton pump inhibitors, rosiglitazone, selegiline, sertraline, sulfona-mides, tacrolimus, venlafaxine. voriconazole, warfarin, zafirlukast, and other CYP2B6, 2C8, 2C9, 2C19, or 3A4 substrates.

The levels/effects of phenytoin may be decreased by aminoglutethimide, carbamazepine, phenobarbital, rifampin, rifapentine, secobarbital, and other CYP2C8/9 or 2C19 inducers. Clozapine and vigabatrin may reduce phenytoin serum concentrations. Case reports indicate ciprofloxacin may increase or decrease serum phenytoin concentrations. Dexamethasone may decrease serum phenytoin concentrations. Replacement of folic acid has been reported to increase the metabolism of phenytoin, decreasing its serum concentrations and/or increasing seizures.

Initially, phenytoin increases the response to warfarin; this is followed by a decrease in response to warfarin. Phenytoin may inhibit the anti-Parkinson effect of levodopa. The duration of neuromuscular blockade from neuromus-cular-blocking agents may be decreased by phenytoin. Phenytoin may enhance the metabolism of methadone resulting in methadone withdrawal. Phenytoin may decrease serum levels/effects of digitalis glycosides, theophyl-line, and thyroid hormones.

Several chemotherapeutic agents have been associated with a decrease in serum phenytoin levels; includes cisplatin, bleomycin, carmustine, metho-trexate, and vinblastine. Enzyme-inducing anticonvulsant therapy may reduce the effectiveness of some chemotherapy regimens (specifically in ALL). Teni-poside and methotrexate may be cleared more rapidly in these patients.

Pharmacodynamics/Kinetics Also refer to Phenytoin monograph for addi-tional information.
Protein binding: Fosphenytoin: 95% to 99% to albumin; can displace phenytoin and increase free fraction (up to 30% unbound) during the period required for conversion of fosphenytoin to phenytoin
Metabolism: Fosphenytoin is rapidly converted via hydrolysis to phenytoin; phenytoin is metabolized in the liver and forms metabolites
Bioavailability: I.M.: Fosphenytoin: 100%
Half-life elimination:
Fosphenytoin: 15 minutes
Phenytoin: Variable (mean: 12-29 hours); kinetics of phenytoin are saturable
Time to peak: Conversion to phenytoin: Following I.V. administration (maximum rate of administration): 15 minutes; following I.M. administration, peak phen-ytoin levels are reached in 3 hours
Excretion: Phenytoin: Urine (as inactive metabolites)
Pregnancy Risk Factor D

Frovatriptan (froe va TRIP tan)

Related Information
Temporomandibular Dysfunction (TMD) *on page 1822*
U.S. Brand Names Frova®
Generic Available No
Index Terms Frovatriptan Succinate
Pharmacologic Category Antimigraine Agent; Serotonin 5-HT$_{1B, 1D}$ Receptor Agonist
Use Acute treatment of migraine with or without aura in adults
Local Anesthetic/Vasoconstrictor Precautions No information available to require special precautions
Effects on Dental Treatment No significant effects or complications reported
Common Adverse Effects 1% to 10%:
Cardiovascular: Chest pain (2%), flushing (4%), palpitation (1%)
Central nervous system: Dizziness (8%), fatigue (5%), headache (4%), hot or cold sensation (3%), anxiety (1%), dysesthesia (1%), hypoesthesia (1%), insomnia (1%), pain (1%)
Gastrointestinal: Hyposalivation (3%), dyspepsia (2%), abdominal pain (1%), diarrhea (1%), vomiting (1%)
Neuromuscular & skeletal: Paresthesia (4%), skeletal pain (3%)
Ocular: Visual abnormalities (1%)
Otic: Tinnitus (1%)
(Continued)

Frovatriptan *(Continued)*

Respiratory: Rhinitis (1%), sinusitis (1%)

Miscellaneous: Diaphoresis (1%)

Dosage Oral: Adults: Migraine: 2.5 mg; if headache recurs, a second dose may be given if first dose provided some relief and at least 2 hours have elapsed since the first dose (maximum daily dose: 7.5 mg)

Dosage adjustment in renal impairment: No adjustment necessary

Dosage adjustment in hepatic impairment: No adjustment necessary in mild-to-moderate hepatic impairment; use with caution in severe impairment

Mechanism of Action Selective agonist for serotonin (5-HT$_{1B}$ and 5-HT$_{1D}$ receptor) in cranial arteries to cause vasoconstriction and reduces sterile inflammation associated with antidromic neuronal transmission correlating with relief of migraine.

Contraindications Hypersensitivity to frovatriptan or any component of the formulation; patients with ischemic heart disease or signs or symptoms of ischemic heart disease (including Prinzmetal's angina, angina pectoris, myocardial infarction, silent myocardial ischemia); cerebrovascular syndromes (including strokes, transient ischemic attacks); peripheral vascular syndromes (including ischemic bowel disease); uncontrolled hypertension; use within 24 hours of ergotamine derivatives; use within 24 hours of another 5-HT$_1$ agonist; management of hemiplegic or basilar migraine; prophylactic treatment of migraine; severe hepatic impairment

Warnings/Precautions Not intended for migraine prophylaxis, or treatment of cluster headaches, hemiplegic or basilar migraines. Cardiac events (coronary artery vasospasm, transient ischemia, MI, ventricular tachycardia/fibrillation, cardiac arrest, and death), cerebral/subarachnoid hemorrhage, stroke, peripheral vascular ischemia, and colonic ischemia have been reported with 5-HT$_1$ agonist administration. May cause vasospastic reactions resulting in colonic, peripheral, or coronary ischemia. Do not give to patients with risk factors for CAD until a cardiovascular evaluation has been performed; if evaluation is satisfactory, the healthcare provider should administer the first dose and cardiovascular status should be periodically evaluated. Significant elevation in blood pressure, including hypertensive crisis, has also been reported on rare occasions in patients using other 5-HT$_{1D}$ agonists with and without a history of hypertension. Symptoms of agitation, confusion, hallucinations, hyper-reflexia, myoclonus, shivering, and tachycardia (serotonin syndrome) may occur with concomitant proserotonergic drugs (ie, SSRIs/SNRIs or triptans) or agents which reduce frovatriptan's metabolism. Safety and efficacy in pediatric patients have not been established.

Drug Interactions

Cytochrome P450 Effect: Substrate of CYP1A2 (minor)

Increased Effect/Toxicity: The effects of frovatriptan may be increased by estrogen derivatives and propranolol. Ergot derivatives may increase the effects of frovatriptan (do not use within 24 hours of each other). SSRIs/SNRIs may exhibit additive toxicity with frovatriptan or other serotonin agonists (eg, antidepressants, dextromethorphan, tramadol) leading to serotonin syndrome.

Ethanol/Nutrition/Herb Interactions Food: Food does not affect frovatriptan bioavailability.

Pharmacodynamics/Kinetics

Distribution: Male: 4.2 L/kg; Female: 3.0 L/kg

Protein binding: 15%

Metabolism: Primarily hepatic via CYP1A2

Bioavailability: 20% to 30%

Half-life elimination: 26 hours

Time to peak: 2-4 hours

Excretion: Feces (62%); urine (32%)

Pregnancy Risk Factor C

Dosage Forms

Tablet:

Frova®: 2.5 mg

Frovatriptan Succinate *see* Frovatriptan *on page 753*

Fructose, Dextrose, and Phosphoric Acid

(FRUK tose, DEKS trose, & foss FOR ik AS id)

U.S. Brand Names Emetrol® [OTC]; Especol® [OTC]; Formula EM [OTC]; Kalmz [OTC]; Nausea Relief [OTC]; Nausetrol® [OTC]

Generic Available Yes

Index Terms Dextrose, Levulose, and Phosphoric Acid; Levulose, Dextrose, and Phosphoric Acid; Phosphorated Carbohydrate Solution; Phosphoric Acid, Levulose, and Dextrose

Pharmacologic Category Antiemetic

Use Relief of nausea associated with upset stomach that occurs with intestinal or stomach flu, and food indiscretions

Local Anesthetic/Vasoconstrictor Precautions No information available to require special precautions

Effects on Dental Treatment No significant effects or complications reported

Fulvestrant (fool VES trant)

U.S. Brand Names Faslodex®

Generic Available No

Index Terms ICI-182,780; Zeneca 182,780; ZM-182,780

Pharmacologic Category Antineoplastic Agent, Estrogen Receptor Antagonist

Use Treatment of hormone receptor positive metastatic breast cancer in postmenopausal women with disease progression following antiestrogen therapy

Unlabeled/Investigational Use Endometriosis; uterine bleeding

Local Anesthetic/Vasoconstrictor Precautions No information available to require special precautions

Effects on Dental Treatment No significant effects or complications reported

Common Adverse Effects

>10%:
  Cardiovascular: Vasodilation (18%)
  Central nervous system: Pain (19%), headache (15%)
  Endocrine & metabolic: Hot flushes (19% to 24%)
  Gastrointestinal: Nausea (26%), vomiting (13%), constipation (13%), diarrhea (12%), abdominal pain (12%)
  Local: Injection site reaction (11%)
  Neuromuscular & skeletal: Weakness (23%), bone pain (16%), back pain (14%)
  Respiratory: Pharyngitis (16%), dyspnea (15%)

1% to 10%:
  Cardiovascular: Edema (9%), chest pain (7%)
  Central nervous system: Dizziness (7%), insomnia (7%), paresthesia (6%), fever (6%), depression (6%), anxiety (5%)
  Dermatologic: Rash (7%)
  Gastrointestinal: Anorexia (9%), weight gain (1% to 2%)
  Genitourinary: Pelvic pain (10%), urinary tract infection (6%), vaginitis (2% to 3%)
  Hematologic: Anemia (5%)
  Neuromuscular and skeletal: Arthritis (3%)
  Respiratory: Cough (10%)
  Miscellaneous: Diaphoresis increased (5%)

Mechanism of Action Steroidal compound which competitively binds to estrogen receptors on tumors and other tissue targets, producing a nuclear complex that decreases DNA synthesis and inhibits estrogen effects. Fulvestrant has no estrogen-receptor agonist activity. Causes down-regulation of estrogen receptors and inhibits tumor growth.

Drug Interactions
  Cytochrome P450 Effect: Substrate of CYP3A4 (minor)

Pharmacodynamics/Kinetics
  Duration: I.M.: Plasma levels maintained for at least 1 month
  Distribution: V_d: 3-5 L/kg
  Protein binding: 99%
  Metabolism: Hepatic via multiple pathways (CYP3A4 substrate, relative contribution to metabolism unknown)
  (Continued)

Fulvestrant *(Continued)*

Bioavailability: Oral: Poor
Half-life elimination: ~40 days
Time to peak, plasma: I.M.: 7-9 days
Excretion: Feces (>90%); urine (<1%)
Pregnancy Risk Factor D

Fungi-Guard [OTC] *see* Tolnaftate *on page 1587*

Fungi-Nail® [OTC] *see* Undecylenic Acid and Derivatives *on page 1631*

Fung-O® [OTC] *see* Salicylic Acid *on page 1451*

Fungoid® Tincture [OTC] *see* Miconazole *on page 1097*

Furadantin® *see* Nitrofurantoin *on page 1180*

Furazolidone *(fyoor a ZOE li done)*

Canadian Brand Names Furoxone®
Mexican Brand Names Furoxona
Generic Available No
Index Terms Furoxone
Pharmacologic Category Antiprotozoal
Use Treatment of bacterial or protozoal diarrhea and enteritis caused by suscep-
tible organisms *Giardia lamblia* and *Vibrio cholerae*
Local Anesthetic/Vasoconstrictor Precautions No information available to
require special precautions
Effects on Dental Treatment No significant effects or complications reported
Common Adverse Effects
>10%: Genitourinary: Discoloration of urine (dark yellow to brown)
1% to 10%:
Central nervous system: Headache
Gastrointestinal: Abdominal pain, diarrhea, nausea, vomiting
Restrictions Not available in U.S.
Mechanism of Action Inhibits several vital enzymatic reactions causing anti-
bacterial and antiprotozoal action
Drug Interactions
Increased Effect/Toxicity: Increased effect with sympathomimetic amines,
tricyclic antidepressants, tyramine-containing foods, MAO inhibitors, meperi-
dine, anorexiants, dextromethorphan, fluoxetine, paroxetine, sertraline, and
trazodone. Increased effect/toxicity of levodopa. Disulfiram-like reaction with
alcohol.
Pharmacodynamics/Kinetics
Absorption: Poor
Excretion: Urine (33% as active drug and metabolites)
Pregnancy Risk Factor C

Furazosin *see* Prazosin *on page 1337*

Furosemide *(fyoor OH se mide)*

Related Information
Cardiovascular Diseases *on page 1726*
U.S. Brand Names Lasix®
Canadian Brand Names Apo-Furosemide®; Furosemide Injection, USP; Furo-
semide Special; Lasix®; Lasix® Special; Novo-Semide
Mexican Brand Names Edenol; Lasix; Zafurida
Generic Available Yes
Index Terms Frusemide
Pharmacologic Category Diuretic, Loop
Use Management of edema associated with congestive heart failure and hepatic
or renal disease; alone or in combination with antihypertensives in treatment of
hypertension
Local Anesthetic/Vasoconstrictor Precautions No information available to
require special precautions
Effects on Dental Treatment No significant effects or complications reported
Common Adverse Effects Frequency not defined.
Cardiovascular: Acute hypotension, chronic aortitis, necrotizing angiitis, ortho-
static hypotension, thrombophlebitis, sudden death from cardiac arrest (with
I.V. or I.M. administration)
Central nervous system: Blurred vision, dizziness, fever, headache, lighthead-
edness, restlessness, vertigo, xanthopsia
Dermatologic: Cutaneous vasculitis, erythema multiforme, exfoliative dermatitis,
photosensitivity, pruritus, purpura, rash, urticaria

Endocrine & metabolic: Gout, hyperglycemia, hyperuricemia, hypocalcemia, hypochloremia, hypokalemia, hypomagnesemia, hyponatremia, metabolic alkalosis

Gastrointestinal: Anorexia, constipation, cramping, diarrhea, intrahepatic cholestatic jaundice, ischemia hepatitis, nausea, oral and gastric irritation, pancreatitis, vomiting

Genitourinary: Urinary bladder spasm, urinary frequency

Hematological: Agranulocytosis (rare), anemia, aplastic anemia (rare), hemolytic anemia, leukopenia, purpura, thrombocytopenia

Neuromuscular & skeletal: Muscle spasm, paresthesia, weakness

Otic: Hearing impairment (reversible or permanent with rapid I.V. or I.M. administration), reversible deafness (with rapid I.V. or I.M. administration), tinnitus

Renal: Allergic interstitial nephritis, fall in glomerular filtration rate and renal blood flow (due to overdiuresis), glycosuria, transient rise in BUN, vasculitis

Miscellaneous: Anaphylaxis (rare), exacerbate or activate systemic lupus erythematosus

Dosage

Infants and Children:

Oral: 0.5-2 mg/kg/dose increased in increments of 1 mg/kg/dose with each succeeding dose until a satisfactory effect is achieved to a maximum of 6 mg/kg/dose no more frequently than 6 hours.

I.M., I.V.: 1 mg/kg/dose, increasing by each succeeding dose at 1 mg/kg/dose at intervals of 6-12 hours until a satisfactory response up to 6 mg/kg/dose.

Adults:

Oral: 20-80 mg/dose initially increased in increments of 20-40 mg/dose at intervals of 6-8 hours; usual maintenance dose interval is twice daily or every day; may be titrated up to 600 mg/day with severe edematous states. Hypertension (JNC 7): 20-80 mg/day in 2 divided doses

I.M., I.V.: 20-40 mg/dose, may be repeated in 1-2 hours as needed and increased by 20 mg/dose until the desired effect has been obtained. Usual dosing interval: 6-12 hours; for acute pulmonary edema, the usual dose is 40 mg I.V. over 1-2 minutes. If not adequate, may increase dose to 80 mg. **Note:** ACC/AHA 2005 guidelines for chronic congestive heart failure recommend a maximum single dose of 160-200 mg.

Continuous I.V. infusion: Initial I.V. bolus dose 20-40 mg, followed by continuous I.V. infusion doses of 10-40 mg/hour. If urine output is <1 mL/kg/hour, double as necessary to a maximum of 80-160 mg/hour. The risk associated with higher infusion rates (80-160 mg/hour) must be weighed against alternative strategies. **Note:** ACC/AHA 2005 guidelines for chronic congestive heart failure recommend 40 mg I.V. load, then 10-40 mg/hour infusion.

Refractory heart failure: Oral, I.V.: Doses up to 8 g/day have been used.

Elderly: Oral, I.M., I.V.: Initial: 20 mg/day; increase slowly to desired response.

Dosing adjustment/comments in renal impairment: Acute renal failure: High doses (up to 1-3 g/day - oral/I.V.) have been used to initiate desired response; avoid use in oliguric states.

Dialysis: Not removed by hemo- or peritoneal dialysis; supplemental dose is not necessary.

Dosing adjustment/comments in hepatic disease: Diminished natriuretic effect with increased sensitivity to hypokalemia and volume depletion in cirrhosis; monitor effects, particularly with high doses.

Mechanism of Action Inhibits reabsorption of sodium and chloride in the ascending loop of Henle and distal renal tubule, interfering with the chloride-binding cotransport system, thus causing increased excretion of water, sodium, chloride, magnesium, and calcium

Contraindications Hypersensitivity to furosemide, any component, or sulfonylureas; anuria; patients with hepatic coma or in states of severe electrolyte depletion until the condition improves or is corrected

Warnings/Precautions Loop diuretics are potent diuretics; excess amounts can lead to profound diuresis with fluid and electrolyte loss; close medical supervision and dose evaluation are required. Watch for and correct electrolyte disturbances; adjust dose to avoid dehydration. In cirrhosis, avoid electrolyte and acid/base imbalances that might lead to hepatic encephalopathy. Coadministration of antihypertensives may increase the risk of hypotension.

Monitor fluid status and renal function in an attempt to prevent oliguria, azotemia, and reversible increases in BUN and creatinine; close medical supervision of aggressive diuresis is required. Rapid I.V. administration, renal impairment, excessive doses, and concurrent use of other ototoxins is associated with ototoxicity. Asymptomatic hyperuricemia has been reported with use.

Chemical similarities are present among sulfonamides, sulfonylureas, carbonic anhydrase inhibitors, thiazides, and loop diuretics (except ethacrynic acid). Use in patients with sulfonylurea allergy is specifically contraindicated in product labeling, however, a risk of cross-reaction exists in patients with allergy to any of (Continued)

Furosemide (Continued)

these compounds; avoid use when previous reaction has been severe. Discontinue if signs of hypersensitivity are noted.

Drug Interactions

Increased Effect/Toxicity: Furosemide-induced hypokalemia may predispose to digoxin toxicity and may increase the risk of arrhythmia with drugs which may prolong QT interval, including type Ia and type III antiarrhythmic agents, cisapride, and some quinolones (sparfloxacin, gatifloxacin, and moxifloxacin). The risk of toxicity from lithium and salicylates (high dose) may be increased by loop diuretics. Hypotensive effects and/or adverse renal effects of ACE inhibitors and NSAIDs are potentiated by furosemide-induced hypovolemia. The effects of peripheral adrenergic-blocking drugs or ganglionic blockers may be increased by furosemide.

Furosemide may increase the risk of ototoxicity with other ototoxic agents (aminoglycosides, cis-platinum), especially in patients with renal dysfunction. Synergistic diuretic effects occur with thiazide-type diuretics. Diuretics tend to be synergistic with other antihypertensive agents, and hypotension may occur.

Decreased Effect: Indomethacin, aspirin, phenobarbital, phenytoin, and NSAIDs may reduce natriuretic and hypotensive effects of furosemide. Colestipol, cholestyramine, and sucralfate may reduce the effect of furosemide; separate administration by 2 hours. Furosemide may antagonize the effect of skeletal muscle relaxants (tubocurarine). Glucose tolerance may be decreased by furosemide, requiring an adjustment in the dose of hypoglycemic agents. Metformin may decrease furosemide concentrations.

Ethanol/Nutrition/Herb Interactions

Food: Furosemide serum levels may be decreased if taken with food.

Herb/Nutraceutical: Avoid dong quai if using for hypertension (has estrogenic activity). Avoid ephedra, yohimbe, and ginseng (may worsen hypertension). Limit intake of natural licorice. Avoid garlic (may have increased antihypertensive effect).

Dietary Considerations May cause a potassium loss; potassium supplement or dietary changes may be required. Administer on an empty stomach. May be administered with food or milk if GI distress occurs. Do not mix with acidic solutions.

Pharmacodynamics/Kinetics

Onset of action: Diuresis: Oral: 30-60 minutes; I.M.: 30 minutes; I.V.: ~5 minutes

Peak effect: Oral: 1-2 hours

Duration: Oral: 6-8 hours; I.V.: 2 hours

Absorption: Oral: 60% to 67%

Protein binding: >98%

Metabolism: Minimally hepatic

Half-life elimination: Normal renal function: 0.5-1.1 hours; End-stage renal disease: 9 hours

Excretion: Urine (Oral: 50%, I.V.: 80%) within 24 hours; feces (as unchanged drug); nonrenal clearance prolonged in renal impairment

Pregnancy Risk Factor C

Dosage Forms

Injection, solution: 10 mg/mL (2 mL, 4 mL, 8 mL, 10 mL)

Solution, oral: 10 mg/mL, 40 mg/5 mL

Tablet: 20 mg, 40 mg, 80 mg

Lasix®: 20 mg, 40 mg, 80 mg

Furoxone see Furazolidone on page 756

Fuzeon® see Enfuvirtide on page 567

FVIII/vWF see Antihemophilic Factor/von Willebrand Factor Complex (Human) on page 132

Gabapentin (GA ba pen tin)

Related Information

Temporomandibular Dysfunction (TMD) on page 1822

U.S. Brand Names Neurontin®

Canadian Brand Names Apo-Gabapentin®; BCI-Gabapentin; Gen-Gabapentin; Neurontin®; Novo-Gabapentin; Nu-Gabapentin; PMS-Gabapentin

Mexican Brand Names Neurontin

Generic Available Yes: Capsule, tablet

Pharmacologic Category Anticonvulsant, Miscellaneous

Dental Use Neuropathic pain (consult with physician)

Use Adjunct for treatment of partial seizures with and without secondary generalized seizures in patients >12 years of age with epilepsy; adjunct for treatment of partial seizures in pediatric patients 3-12 years of age; management of postherpetic neuralgia (PHN) in adults

Unlabeled/Investigational Use Social phobia; chronic pain

Local Anesthetic/Vasoconstrictor Precautions No information available to require special precautions

Effects on Dental Treatment Key adverse event(s) related to dental treatment: Xerostomia (normal salivary flow resumes upon discontinuation), dry throat, and dental abnormalities.

Significant Adverse Effects As reported in patients >12 years of age, unless otherwise noted in children (3-12 years)

>10%:

Central nervous system: Somnolence (20%; children 8%), dizziness (17% to 28%; children 3%), ataxia (13%), fatigue (11%)

Miscellaneous: Viral infection (children 11%)

1% to 10%:

Cardiovascular: Peripheral edema (2% to 8%), vasodilatation (1%)

Central nervous system: Fever (children 10%), hostility (children 8%), emotional lability (children 4%), fatigue (children 3%), headache (3%), ataxia (3%), abnormal thinking (2% to 3%; children 2%), amnesia (2%), depression (2%), dysarthria (2%), nervousness (2%), abnormal coordination (1% to 2%), twitching (1%), hyperesthesia (1%)

Dermatologic: Pruritus (1%), rash (1%)

Endocrine & metabolic: Hyperglycemia (1%)

Gastrointestinal: Diarrhea (6%), nausea/vomiting (3% to 4%; children 8%), abdominal pain (3%), weight gain (adults and children 2% to 3%), dyspepsia (2%), flatulence (2%), dry throat (2%), xerostomia (2% to 5%), constipation (2% to 4%), dental abnormalities (2%), appetite stimulation (1%)

Genitourinary: Impotence (2%)

Hematologic: Leukopenia (1%), decreased WBC (1%)

Neuromuscular & skeletal: Tremor (7%), weakness (6%), hyperkinesia (children 3%), abnormal gait (2%), back pain (2%), myalgia (2%), fracture (1%)

Ocular: Nystagmus (8%), diplopia (1% to 6%), blurred vision (3% to 4%), conjunctivitis (1%)

Otic: Otitis media (1%)

Respiratory: Rhinitis (4%), bronchitis (children 3%), respiratory infection (children 3%), pharyngitis (1% to 3%), cough (2%)

Miscellaneous: Infection (5%)

Postmarketing and additional clinical reports (limited to important or life-threatening): Acute renal failure, anemia, angina, angioedema, aphasia, arrhythmias (various), aspiration pneumonia, blindness, bradycardia, bronchospasm, cerebrovascular accident, CNS tumors, coagulation defect, colitis, Cushingoid appearance, dyspnea, encephalopathy, facial paralysis, fecal incontinence, glaucoma, glycosuria, heart block, hearing loss, hematemesis, hematuria, hemiplegia, hemorrhage, hepatitis, hepatomegaly, hyper-/hypotension, hyperlipidemia, hyper-/hypothyroidism, hyper-/hypoventilation, gastroenteritis, heart failure, leukocytosis, liver function tests increased, local myoclonus, lymphadenopathy, lymphocytosis, meningismus, MI, migraine, nephrosis, nerve palsy, non-Hodgkin's lymphoma, ovarian failure, pulmonary thrombosis, pericardial rub, pulmonary embolus, pericardial effusion, pericarditis, pancreatitis, peptic ulcer, purpura, paresthesia, palpitation, peripheral vascular disorder, pneumonia, psychosis, renal stone, retinopathy, skin necrosis, status epilepticus, subdural hematoma, syncope, tachycardia, thrombocytopenia, thrombophlebitis

Dental Usual Dosing

Pain (unlabeled use): Children >12 years and Adults: Oral: 300-1800 mg/day given in 3 divided doses has been the most common dosage range

Postherpetic neuralgia or neuropathic pain: Adults: Oral: Day 1: 300 mg, Day 2: 300 mg twice daily, Day 3: 300 mg 3 times/day; dose may be titrated as needed for pain relief (range: 1800-3600 mg/day, daily doses >1800 mg do not generally show greater benefit)

Dosage Oral:

Children: Anticonvulsant:

3-12 years: Initial: 10-15 mg/kg/day in 3 divided doses; titrate to effective dose over ~3 days; dosages of up to 50 mg/kg/day have been tolerated in clinical studies

3-4 years: Effective dose: 40 mg/kg/day in 3 divided doses

≥5-12 years: Effective dose: 25-35 mg/kg/day in 3 divided doses

See "Note" in adult dosing.

Children >12 years and Adults:

Anticonvulsant: Initial: 300 mg 3 times/day; if necessary the dose may be increased up to 1800 mg/day. Doses of up to 2400 mg/day have been

(Continued)

Gabapentin *(Continued)*

tolerated in long-term clinical studies; up to 3600 mg/day has been tolerated in short-term studies.

Note: If gabapentin is discontinued or if another anticonvulsant is added to therapy, it should be done slowly over a minimum of 1 week

Pain (unlabeled use): 300-1800 mg/day given in 3 divided doses has been the most common dosage range

Adults: Postherpetic neuralgia or neuropathic pain: Day 1: 300 mg, Day 2: 300 mg twice daily, Day 3: 300 mg 3 times/day; dose may be titrated as needed for pain relief (range: 1800-3600 mg/day, daily doses >1800 mg do not generally show greater benefit)

Elderly: Studies in elderly patients have shown a decrease in clearance as age increases. This is most likely due to age-related decreases in renal function; dose reductions may be needed.

Dosing adjustment in renal impairment: Children ≥12 years and Adults: See table.

Hemodialysis: Dialyzable

Gabapentin Dosing Adjustments in Renal Impairment

Creatinine Clearance (mL/min)	Daily Dose Range
≥60	300-1200 mg tid
>30-59	200-700 mg bid
>15-29	200-700 mg daily
15[1]	100-300 mg daily
Hemodialysis[2]	125-350 mg

[1]Cl_{cr}<15 mL/minute: Reduce daily dose in proportion to creatinine clearance.
[2]Single supplemental dose administered after each 4 hours of hemodialysis

Mechanism of Action Gabapentin is structurally related to GABA. However, it does not bind to $GABA_A$ or $GABA_B$ receptors, and it does not appear to influence synthesis or uptake of GABA. High affinity gabapentin binding sites have been located throughout the brain; these sites correspond to the presence of voltage-gated calcium channels specifically possessing the alpha-2-delta-1 subunit. This channel appears to be located presynaptically, and may modulate the release of excitatory neurotransmitters which participate in epileptogenesis and nociception.

Contraindications Hypersensitivity to gabapentin or any component of the formulation

Warnings/Precautions Avoid abrupt withdrawal, may precipitate seizures; use cautiously in patients with severe renal dysfunction; male rat studies demonstrated an association with pancreatic adenocarcinoma (clinical implication unknown). May cause CNS depression, which may impair physical or mental abilities. Patients must be cautioned about performing tasks which require mental alertness (eg, operating machinery or driving). Effects with other sedative drugs or ethanol may be potentiated. Pediatric patients (3-12 years of age) have shown increased incidence of CNS-related adverse effects, including emotional lability, hostility, thought disorder, and hyperkinesia. Safety and efficacy in children <3 years of age have not been established.

Drug Interactions CNS depressants: Sedative effects may be additive with CNS depressants; includes ethanol, barbiturates, opioid analgesics, and other sedative agents. Monitor for increased effect.

Ethanol/Nutrition/Herb Interactions

Ethanol: Avoid ethanol (may increase CNS depression).

Food: Does not change rate or extent of absorption.

Herb/Nutraceutical: Avoid evening primrose (seizure threshold decreased). Avoid valerian, St John's wort, kava kava, gotu kola (may increase CNS depression).

Dietary Considerations May be taken without regard to meals.

Pharmacodynamics/Kinetics

Absorption: 50% to 60% from proximal small bowel by L-amino transport system

Distribution: V_d: 0.6-0.8 L/kg

Protein binding: <3%

Bioavailability: Inversely proportional to dose due to saturable absorption:
900 mg/day: 60%
1200 mg/day: 47%
2400 mg/day: 34%
3600 mg/day: 33%
4800 mg/day: 27%

Half-life elimination: 5-7 hours; anuria 132 hours; during dialysis 3.8 hours

Excretion: Proportional to renal function; urine (as unchanged drug)

Pregnancy Risk Factor C

Lactation Enters breast milk/use caution

Breast-Feeding Considerations Gabapentin is excreted in human breast milk. A nursed infant could be exposed to ~1 mg/kg/day of gabapentin; the effect on the child is not known. Use in breast-feeding women only if the benefits to the mother outweigh the potential risk to the infant.

Dosage Forms Excipient information presented when available (limited, particularly for generics); consult specific product labeling.

Capsule: 100 mg, 300 mg, 400 mg

   Neurontin®: 100 mg, 300 mg, 400 mg

Solution, oral:

   Neurontin®: 250 mg/5 mL (480 mL) [cool strawberry anise flavor]

Tablet: 100 mg, 300 mg, 400 mg, 600 mg, 800 mg

   Neurontin®: 600 mg, 800 mg

Selected Readings

Laird MA and Gidal BE, "Use of Gabapentin in the Treatment of Neuropathic Pain," *Ann Pharmacother*, 2000, 34(6):802-7.

Rose MA and Kam PCA, "Gabapentin: Pharmacology and Its Use in Pain Management," *Anaesthesia*, 2002, 57:451-62.

Rosenberg JM, Harrell C, Ristic H, et al, "The Effect of Gabapentin on Neuropathic Pain," *Clin J Pain*, 1997, 13(3):251-5.

Rowbotham M, Harden N, Stacey B, et al, "Gabapentin for the Treatment of Postherpetic Neuralgia: A Randomized Controlled Trial," *JAMA*, 1998, 280(21):1837-42.

Gabitril® *see* Tiagabine *on page 1564*

Gadolinium-DTPA *see* Gadopentetate Dimeglumine *on page 761*

Gadolinium-HP-DO3A *see* Gadoteridol *on page 761*

Gadopentetate Dimeglumine (gad oh PEN te tate dye MEG loo meen)

U.S. Brand Names Magnevist®

Canadian Brand Names Magnevist®

Generic Available No

Index Terms Gadolinium-DTPA; Gd-DTPA

Pharmacologic Category Radiological/Contrast Media, Paramagnetic Agent

Use Contrast medium for magnetic resonance imaging (MRI) to visualize lesions with abnormal vascularity in the brain, spine and associated tissues, head and neck, and body (excluding the heart)

Local Anesthetic/Vasoconstrictor Precautions No information available to require special precautions

Effects on Dental Treatment No significant effects or complications reported

Mechanism of Action Exposure to an external magnetic field induces a large local magnetic field in gadopentetate exposed tissues. This local magnetism disrupts water protons in the vicinity, resulting in a change in proton density and spin characteristics, which can be detected by the imaging device.

Pregnancy Risk Factor C

Gadoteridol (gad oh TER i dol)

U.S. Brand Names ProHance®

Generic Available No

Index Terms Gadolinium-HP-DO3A; Gd-HP-DO3A

Pharmacologic Category Radiological/Contrast Media, Nonionic

Use Contrast medium for magnetic resonance imaging (MRI) to visualize CNS lesions with abnormal vascularity in the brain, spine, and associated tissues and to visualize extracranial/extraspinal tissues in the head and neck

Local Anesthetic/Vasoconstrictor Precautions No information available to require special precautions

Effects on Dental Treatment No significant effects or complications reported

Mechanism of Action Gadoteridol is a gadolinium-containing paramagnetic agent. Exposure to an external magnetic field induces a large local magnetic field in exposed tissues. This local magnetism disrupts water protons in the vicinity, resulting in a change in proton density and spin characteristics, which can be detected by the imaging device.

Pregnancy Risk Factor C

Galantamine (ga LAN ta meen)

U.S. Brand Names Razadyne™; Razadyne™ ER; Reminyl® [DSC]
Canadian Brand Names Reminyl®; Reminyl® ER
Mexican Brand Names Reminyl
Generic Available No
Index Terms Galantamine Hydrobromide
Pharmacologic Category Acetylcholinesterase Inhibitor (Central)
Use Treatment of mild-to-moderate dementia of Alzheimer's disease
Local Anesthetic/Vasoconstrictor Precautions No information available to require special precautions
Effects on Dental Treatment No significant effects or complications reported
Common Adverse Effects
>10%: Gastrointestinal: Nausea (6% to 24%), vomiting (4% to 13%), diarrhea (6% to 12%)
1% to 10%:
Cardiovascular: Bradycardia (2% to 3%), syncope (0.4% to 2.2%: dose related), chest pain (≥1%)
Central nervous system: Dizziness (9%), headache (8%), depression (7%), fatigue (5%), insomnia (5%), somnolence (4%)
Gastrointestinal: Anorexia (7% to 9%), weight loss (5% to 7%), abdominal pain (5%), dyspepsia (5%), flatulence (≥1%)
Genitourinary: Urinary tract infection (8%), hematuria (<1% to 3%), incontinence (≥1%)
Hematologic: Anemia (3%)
Neuromuscular & skeletal: Tremor (3%)
Respiratory: Rhinitis (4%)
Mechanism of Action Centrally-acting cholinesterase inhibitor (competitive and reversible). It elevates acetylcholine in cerebral cortex by slowing the degradation of acetylcholine. Modulates nicotinic acetylcholine receptor to increase acetylcholine from surviving presynaptic nerve terminals. May increase glutamate and serotonin levels.
Drug Interactions
Cytochrome P450 Effect: Substrate (minor) of CYP2D6, 3A4
Increased Effect/Toxicity: Succinylcholine: increased neuromuscular blockade. Amiodarone, beta-blockers without ISA activity, diltiazem, verapamil may increase bradycardia. NSAIDs increase risk of peptic ulcer. Other CYP3A4 inhibitors and other CYP2D6 inhibitors increase levels of galantamine. Concurrent cholinergic agents may have synergistic effects. Digoxin may lead to AV block. Acetylcholinesterase inhibitors (central) may increase the risk of antipsychotic-related extrapyramidal symptoms.
Decreased Effect: Anticholinergic agents are antagonized by galantamine. CYP inducers may decrease galantamine levels.
Pharmacodynamics/Kinetics
Duration: 3 hours; maximum inhibition of erythrocyte acetylcholinesterase ~40% at 1 hour post 8 mg oral dose; levels return to baseline at 30 hours
Absorption: Rapid and complete
Distribution: 175 L; levels in the brain are 2-3 times higher than in plasma
Protein binding: 18%
Metabolism: Hepatic; linear, CYP2D6 and 3A4; metabolized to epigalanthaminone and galanthaminone both of which have acetylcholinesterase inhibitory activity 130 times less than galantamine
Bioavailability: ~90%
Half-life elimination: 7 hours
Time to peak: Immediate release: 1 hour (2.5 hours with food); extended release: 4.5-5 hours
Excretion: Urine (25%)
Pregnancy Risk Factor B

Galantamine Hydrobromide *see* Galantamine *on page 762*

Gallium Nitrate (GAL ee um NYE trate)

U.S. Brand Names Ganite™
Generic Available No
Index Terms NSC-15200
Pharmacologic Category Calcium-Lowering Agent
Use Treatment of hypercalcemia
Local Anesthetic/Vasoconstrictor Precautions No information available to require special precautions
Effects on Dental Treatment No significant effects or complications reported

Mechanism of Action Inhibits bone resorption by inhibiting osteoclast function
Pregnancy Risk Factor C

Galsulfase (gal SUL fase)

U.S. Brand Names Naglazyme™
Generic Available No
Index Terms Recombinant N-Acetylgalactosamine 4-Sulfatase; rhASB
Pharmacologic Category Enzyme
Use Replacement therapy in mucopolysaccharidosis VI (MPS VI; Maroteaux-Lamy Syndrome) for improvement of walking and stair-climbing capacity
Local Anesthetic/Vasoconstrictor Precautions No information available to require special precautions
Effects on Dental Treatment No significant effects or complications reported
Common Adverse Effects
Note: Percentages reported are from a placebo-controlled study (39 patients, 19 on galsulfase); also included are adverse effects noted during other clinical studies.
Cardiovascular: Chest pain (16%), facial edema (11%), hypertension (11%)
Central nervous system: Pain (26%), malaise (11%), fever, headache
Gastrointestinal: Abdominal pain (53%), gastroenteritis (11%), diarrhea, vomiting
Neuromuscular & skeletal: Rigors (21%), areflexia (11%), arthralgia
Ocular: Conjunctivitis (21%), corneal opacification increased (11%)
Otic: Ear pain (42%), otitis media
Respiratory: Dyspnea (21%), pharyngitis (16%), nasal congestion (11%), cough, upper respiratory tract infections
Miscellaneous: Antigalsulfase antibodies (98%), umbilical hernia (11%)
Infusion-related reactions: Angioedema, apnea, bronchospasm, chills, facial and neck urticaria, hypotension, rash, respiratory distress
Mechanism of Action Galsulfase is a recombinant form of N-acetyl-galactosamine 4-sulfatase, produced in Chinese hamster cells. A deficiency of this enzyme leads to accumulation of the glycosaminoglycan dermatan sulfate in various tissues, causing progressive disease which includes decreased growth, skeletal deformities, upper airway obstruction, clouding of the cornea, heart disease, and coarse facial features. Replacement of this enzyme has been shown to improve mobility and physical function (measured by walking and stair-climbing).
Pharmacodynamics/Kinetics
Half-life elimination: Week 1: Median 9 hours (range: 6-21 hours); Week 24: Median 26 hours (range: 8-40 hours)
Pregnancy Risk Factor B

Gamma Benzene Hexachloride see Lindane on page 985
Gamma E-Gems® [OTC] see Vitamin E on page 1664
Gamma-E Plus [OTC] see Vitamin E on page 1664
Gammagard® Liquid see Immune Globulin (Intravenous) on page 870
Gammagard® S/D see Immune Globulin (Intravenous) on page 870
Gamma Globulin see Immune Globulin (Intramuscular) on page 869
Gamma Hydroxybutyric Acid see Sodium Oxybate on page 1482
Gammaphos see Amifostine on page 85
Gammar®-P I.V. see Immune Globulin (Intravenous) on page 870
GammaSTAN™ S/D see Immune Globulin (Intramuscular) on page 869
Gamunex® see Immune Globulin (Intravenous) on page 870

Ganciclovir (gan SYE kloe veer)

Related Information
Systemic Viral Diseases on page 1767
Valganciclovir on page 1637
U.S. Brand Names Cytovene®; Vitrasert®
Canadian Brand Names Cytovene®; Vitrasert®
Mexican Brand Names Cymevene
Generic Available Yes: Capsule
(Continued)

Ganciclovir *(Continued)*

Index Terms DHPG Sodium; GCV Sodium; Nordeoxyguanosine

Pharmacologic Category Antiviral Agent

Use

Parenteral: Treatment of CMV retinitis in immunocompromised individuals, including patients with acquired immunodeficiency syndrome; prophylaxis of CMV infection in transplant patients

Oral: Alternative to the I.V. formulation for maintenance treatment of CMV retinitis in immunocompromised patients, including patients with AIDS, in whom retinitis is stable following appropriate induction therapy and for whom the risk of more rapid progression is balanced by the benefit associated with avoiding daily I.V. infusions.

Implant: Treatment of CMV retinitis

Unlabeled/Investigational Use May be given in combination with foscarnet in patients who relapse after monotherapy with either drug

Local Anesthetic/Vasoconstrictor Precautions No information available to require special precautions

Effects on Dental Treatment No significant effects or complications reported

Common Adverse Effects

\>10%:

Central nervous system: Fever (38% to 48%)

Dermatologic: Rash (15% oral, 10% I.V.)

Gastrointestinal: Abdominal pain (17% to 19%), diarrhea (40%), nausea (25%), anorexia (15%), vomiting (13%)

Hematologic: Anemia (20% to 25%), leukopenia (30% to 40%)

1% to 10%:

Central nervous system: Confusion, neuropathy (8% to 9%), headache (4%)

Dermatologic: Pruritus (5%)

Hematologic: Thrombocytopenia (6%), neutropenia with ANC <500/mm^3 (5% oral, 14% I.V.)

Neuromuscular & skeletal: Paresthesia (6% to 10%), weakness (6%)

Ocular: Retinal detachment (8% oral, 11% I.V.; relationship to ganciclovir not established)

Miscellaneous: Sepsis (4% oral, 15% I.V.)

Dosage

CMV retinitis: Slow I.V. infusion (dosing is based on total body weight):

Children >3 months and Adults:

Induction therapy: 5 mg/kg/dose every 12 hours for 14-21 days followed by maintenance therapy

Maintenance therapy: 5 mg/kg/day as a single daily dose for 7 days/week or 6 mg/kg/day for 5 days/week

CMV retinitis: Oral: 1000 mg 3 times/day with food **or** 500 mg 6 times/day with food

Prevention of CMV disease in patients with advanced HIV infection and normal renal function: Oral: 1000 mg 3 times/day with food

Prevention of CMV disease in transplant patients: Same initial and maintenance dose as CMV retinitis except duration of initial course is 7-14 days, duration of maintenance therapy is dependent on clinical condition and degree of immunosuppression

Intravitreal implant: One implant for 5- to 8-month period; following depletion of ganciclovir, as evidenced by progression of retinitis, implant may be removed and replaced

Elderly: Refer to adult dosing; in general, dose selection should be cautious, reflecting greater frequency of organ impairment

Dosing adjustment in renal impairment:

I.V. (Induction):

Cl$_{cr}$ 50-69 mL/minute: Administer 2.5 mg/kg/dose every 12 hours

Cl$_{cr}$ 25-49 mL/minute: Administer 2.5 mg/kg/dose every 24 hours

Cl$_{cr}$ 10-24 mL/minute: Administer 1.25 mg/kg/dose every 24 hours

Cl$_{cr}$ <10 mL/minute: Administer 1.25 mg/kg/dose 3 times/week following hemodialysis

I.V. (Maintenance):

Cl$_{cr}$ 50-69 mL/minute: Administer 2.5 mg/kg/dose every 24 hours

Cl$_{cr}$ 25-49 mL/minute: Administer 1.25 mg/kg/dose every 24 hours

Cl$_{cr}$ 10-24 mL/minute: Administer 0.625 mg/kg/dose every 24 hours

Cl$_{cr}$ <10 mL/minute: Administer 0.625 mg/kg/dose 3 times/week following hemodialysis

Oral:

Cl$_{cr}$ 50-69 mL/minute: Administer 1500 mg/day or 500 mg 3 times/day

Cl$_{cr}$ 25-49 mL/minute: Administer 1000 mg/day or 500 mg twice daily

Cl$_{cr}$ 10-24 mL/minute: Administer 500 mg/day

Cl$_{cr}$ <10 mL/minute: Administer 500 mg 3 times/week following hemodialysis

Hemodialysis effects: Dialyzable (50%) following hemodialysis; administer dose postdialysis. During peritoneal dialysis, dose as for Cl_{cr} <10 mL/minute. During continuous arteriovenous or venovenous hemofiltration, administer 2.5 mg/kg/dose every 24 hours.

Mechanism of Action Ganciclovir is phosphorylated to a substrate which competitively inhibits the binding of deoxyguanosine triphosphate to DNA polymerase resulting in inhibition of viral DNA synthesis

Contraindications Hypersensitivity to ganciclovir, acyclovir, or any component of the formulation; absolute neutrophil count <500/mm³; platelet count <25,000/mm³

Warnings/Precautions Hazardous agent - use appropriate precautions for handling and disposal. **[U.S. Boxed Warning]: Granulocytopenia, anemia, and thrombocytopenia may occur.** Dosage adjustment or interruption of ganciclovir therapy may be necessary in patients with neutropenia and/or thrombocytopenia and patients with impaired renal function. Use with extreme caution in children since long-term safety has not been determined and **[U.S. Boxed Warning]: Animal studies have demonstrated carcinogenic and teratogenic effects, and inhibition of spermatogenesis;** contraceptive precautions for female and male patients need to be followed during and for at least 90 days after therapy with the drug; take care to administer only into veins with good blood flow. **[U.S. Boxed Warning]: Indicated only for treatment of CMV retinitis in the immunocompromised patient and CMV prevention in transplant patients at risk.**

Drug Interactions
Increased Effect/Toxicity: Immunosuppressive agents may increase hematologic toxicity of ganciclovir. Imipenem/cilastatin may increase seizure potential. Oral ganciclovir increases blood levels of zidovudine, although zidovudine decreases steady-state levels of ganciclovir. Since both drugs have the potential to cause neutropenia and anemia, some patients may not tolerate concomitant therapy with these drugs at full dosage. Didanosine levels are increased with concurrent ganciclovir. Other nephrotoxic drugs (eg, amphotericin and cyclosporine) may have additive nephrotoxicity with ganciclovir.

Decreased Effect: A decrease in blood levels of ganciclovir AUC may occur when used with didanosine.

Dietary Considerations Sodium content of 500 mg vial: 46 mg

Pharmacodynamics/Kinetics
Distribution: V_d: 15.26 L/1.73 m²; widely to all tissues including CSF and ocular tissue

Protein binding: 1% to 2%

Bioavailability: Oral: Fasting: 5%; Following food: 6% to 9%; Following fatty meal: 28% to 31%

Half-life elimination: 1.7-5.8 hours; prolonged with renal impairment; End-stage renal disease: 5-28 hours

Excretion: Urine (80% to 99% as unchanged drug)

Pregnancy Risk Factor C

Dosage Forms
Capsule: 250 mg, 500 mg
Implant, intravitreal:
Vitrasert®: 4.5 mg [released gradually over 5-8 months]
Injection, powder for reconstitution:
Cytovene®: 500 mg

Ganidin NR *see* Guaifenesin *on page 795*

Ganirelix (ga ni REL ix)

Canadian Brand Names Orgalutran®
Mexican Brand Names Orgalutran
Generic Available No
Index Terms Ganirelix Acetate
Pharmacologic Category Gonadotropin Releasing Hormone Antagonist
Use Inhibits premature luteinizing hormone (LH) surges in women undergoing controlled ovarian hyperstimulation in fertility clinics.
Local Anesthetic/Vasoconstrictor Precautions No information available to require special precautions
Effects on Dental Treatment No significant effects or complications reported
Common Adverse Effects 1% to 10%:
Central nervous system: Headache (3%)
Endocrine & metabolic: Ovarian hyperstimulation syndrome (2%)
Gastrointestinal: Abdominal pain (5%), nausea (1%)
Genitourinary: Vaginal bleeding (2%)
Local: Injection site reaction (1%)
(Continued)

Ganirelix (Continued)

Mechanism of Action Competitively blocks the gonadotropin-release hormone receptors on the pituitary gonadotroph and transduction pathway. This suppresses gonadotropin secretion and luteinizing hormone secretion preventing ovulation until the follicles are of adequate size.

Drug Interactions

Increased Effect/Toxicity: No formal studies have been performed.

Decreased Effect: No formal studies have been performed.

Pharmacodynamics/Kinetics

Absorption: SubQ: Rapid

Distribution: Mean V_d: 43.7 L

Protein binding: 81.9%

Metabolism: Hepatic to two primary metabolites (1-4 and 1-6 peptide)

Bioavailability: 91.1%

Half-life elimination: 16.2 hours

Time to peak: 1.1 hours

Excretion: Feces (75%) within 288 hours; urine (22%) within 24 hours

Pregnancy Risk Factor X

Ganirelix Acetate *see* Ganirelix *on page 765*

Ganite™ *see* Gallium Nitrate *on page 762*

Gani-Tuss DM NR *see* Guaifenesin and Dextromethorphan *on page 796*

Gani-Tuss® NR *see* Guaifenesin and Codeine *on page 795*

Gantrisin® *see* SulfiSOXAZOLE *on page 1508*

GAR-936 *see* Tigecycline *on page 1567*

Gardasil® *see* Papillomavirus (Types 6, 11, 16, 18) Recombinant Vaccine *on page 1252*

Gas-X® [OTC] *see* Simethicone *on page 1472*

Gas-X® Extra Strength [OTC] *see* Simethicone *on page 1472*

Gas-X® Maximum Strength [OTC] *see* Simethicone *on page 1472*

GasAid [OTC] *see* Simethicone *on page 1472*

Gas Ban™ [OTC] *see* Calcium Carbonate and Simethicone *on page 261*

Gastrocrom® *see* Cromolyn *on page 417*

Gastrografin® *see* Diatrizoate Meglumine and Diatrizoate Sodium *on page 479*

Gatifloxacin (gat i FLOKS a sin)

Related Information

Bacterial Infections *on page 1793*

Respiratory Diseases *on page 1747*

U.S. Brand Names Tequin® [DSC]; Zymar™

Canadian Brand Names Tequin®; Zymar™

Mexican Brand Names Tequin

Generic Available No

Pharmacologic Category Antibiotic, Ophthalmic; Antibiotic, Quinolone

Use

Oral, I.V.: Treatment of the following infections when caused by susceptible bacteria: Acute bacterial exacerbation of chronic bronchitis; acute sinusitis; community-acquired pneumonia including pneumonia caused by multi-drug-resistant *S. pneumoniae* (MDRSP); uncomplicated skin and skin structure infection; uncomplicated urinary tract infections (cystitis); complicated urinary tract infections; pyelonephritis; uncomplicated urethral and cervical gonorrhea; acute, uncomplicated rectal infections in women caused by gonorrhea

Ophthalmic: Bacterial conjunctivitis

Local Anesthetic/Vasoconstrictor Precautions Gatifloxacin is one of the drugs confirmed to prolong the QT interval and is accepted as having a risk of causing torsade de pointes. The risk of drug-induced torsade de pointes is extremely low when a single QT interval prolonging drug is prescribed. In terms of epinephrine, it is not known what effect vasoconstrictors in the local anesthetic regimen will have in patients with a known history of congenital prolonged QT interval or in patients taking any medication that prolongs the QT interval. Until more information is obtained, it is suggested that the clinician consult with the physician prior to the use of a vasoconstrictor in suspected patients, and that the vasoconstrictor (epinephrine, levonordefrin [Neo-Cobefrin®]) be used with caution.

Effects on Dental Treatment Key adverse event(s) related to dental treatment: Taste disturbance.

Common Adverse Effects
Systemic therapy:
3% to 10%:
Central nervous system: Headache (3%), dizziness (3%)
Gastrointestinal: Nausea (8%), diarrhea (4%)
Genitourinary: Vaginitis (6%)
Local: Injection site reactions (5%)
0.1% to ≤3%: Abdominal pain, abnormal dreams, abnormal vision, agitation, alkaline phosphatase increased, allergic reaction, anorexia, anxiety, arthralgia, back pain, chest pain, chills, confusion, constipation, diaphoresis, dry skin, dyspepsia, dyspnea, dysuria, electrolyte abnormalities, facial edema, fever, flatulence, gastritis, glossitis, hematuria, hyperglycemia, hypertension, insomnia, leg cramps, mouth ulceration, nervousness, neutropenia, oral candidiasis, palpitation, paresthesia, peripheral edema, pharyngitis, pruritus, rash, serum amylase increased, serum bilirubin increased, serum transaminases increased, somnolence, stomatitis, taste perversion, thirst, tinnitus, tremor, weakness, vasodilation, vertigo, vomiting

Ophthalmic therapy:
5% to 10%: Ocular: Conjunctival irritation, keratitis, lacrimation increased, papillary conjunctivitis
1% to 4%:
Central nervous system: Headache
Gastrointestinal: Taste disturbance
Ocular: Chemosis, conjunctival hemorrhage, discharge, dry eye, edema, irritation, pain, visual acuity decreased

Dosage
Usual dosage range:
Adults: Oral, I.V.: 400 mg once daily
Indication-specific dosing:
Children ≥1 year and Adults:
Bacterial conjunctivitis: Ophthalmic:
Days 1 and 2: Instill 1 drop into affected eye(s) every 2 hours while awake (maximum: 8 times/day)
Days 3-7: Instill 1 drop into affected eye(s) up to 4 times/day while awake
Adults: Oral, I.V.:
Acute bacterial exacerbation of chronic bronchitis: 400 mg every 24 hours for 5 days
Acute sinusitis: 400 mg every 24 hours for 10 days
Community-acquired pneumonia (including atypical organisms): 400 mg every 24 hours for 7-14 days
Pyelonephritis (acute): 400 mg every 24 hours for 7-10 days
Skin/skin structure infections (uncomplicated): 400 mg every 24 hours for 7-10 days
Traveler's diarrhea (unlabeled use): 400 mg once daily for 3 days
Urinary tract infections:
Complicated: 400 mg every 24 hours for 7-10 days
Uncomplicated, cystitis: 400 mg single dose or 200 mg every 24 hours for 3 days
Urethral gonorrhea in men (uncomplicated), cervical or rectal gonorrhea in women and pharyngitis (gonococcal): 400 mg single dose
Elderly: No dosage adjustment is required based on age, however, assessment of renal function is particularly important in this population.

Dosage adjustment in renal impairment: Creatinine clearance <40 mL/minute (or patients on hemodialysis/CAPD) should receive an initial dose of 400 mg, followed by a subsequent dose of 200 mg every 24 hours. Patients receiving single-dose or 3-day therapy for appropriate indications do not require dosage adjustment. Administer after hemodialysis.
Dosage adjustment in hepatic impairment: No dosage adjustment is required in mild-moderate hepatic disease. No data are available in severe hepatic impairment (Child-Pugh Class C).
Mechanism of Action Gatifloxacin is a DNA gyrase inhibitor, and also inhibits topoisomerase IV. DNA gyrase (topoisomerase II) is an essential bacterial enzyme that maintains the superhelical structure of DNA. DNA gyrase is required for DNA replication and transcription, DNA repair, recombination, and transposition; inhibition is bactericidal.
Contraindications Hypersensitivity to gatifloxacin, other quinolone antibiotics, or any component of the formulation; diabetes mellitus
Warnings/Precautions Use with caution in patients with significant bradycardia or acute myocardial ischemia. May prolong QT interval (concentration related). Use caution in patients with known prolongation of QT interval, uncorrected hypokalemia, or concurrent administration of other medications known to prolong the QT interval (including Class Ia and Class III antiarrhythmics, cisapride, erythromycin, antipsychotics, and tricyclic antidepressants). May
(Continued)

Gatifloxacin *(Continued)*

cause increased CNS stimulation, increased intracranial pressure, convulsions, or psychosis. Use with caution in individuals at risk of seizures. Potential for seizures, although very rare, may be increased with concomitant NSAID therapy. Discontinue in patients who experience significant CNS adverse effects. Use caution in renal dysfunction (dosage adjustment required) and in severe hepatic insufficiency (no data available). Serious disruptions in glucose regulation (including hyperglycemia and severe hypoglycemia) may occur, usually (but not always) in patients with diabetes. Other risk factors for glucose dysregulation include advanced age, renal insufficiency, and use of concurrent medications which alter glucose utilization. Hypoglycemia may be more prevalent in the initial 3 days of therapy while a greater risk of hyperglycemia may be present after the initial 3 days (particularly days 4-10). Monitor closely and discontinue if hyper- or hypoglycemia occur. Tendon inflammation and/or rupture has been reported with this and other quinolone antibiotics. Discontinue at first signs or symptoms of tendon or pain. Quinolones may exacerbate myasthenia gravis. May cause peripheral neuropathy (rare); discontinue if symptoms of sensory or sensorimotor neuropathy occur.

Severe hypersensitivity reactions, including anaphylaxis, have occurred with quinolone therapy. Prolonged use may result in fungal or bacterial superinfection, including *C. difficile*-associated diarrhea and pseudomembranous colitis. Avoid excessive sunlight; other quinolones have been associated with moderate-to-severe phototoxicity reactions. Do not inject ophthalmic solution subconjunctivally or introduce directly into the anterior chamber of the eye.

Safety and efficacy for ophthalmic use have not been established in children <1 year of age. Safety and efficacy for systemic use have not been established in patients <18 years of age.

Drug Interactions
Increased Effect/Toxicity: Gatifloxacin may increase the effects/toxicity of hypoglycemic agents and warfarin. Concomitant use with corticosteroids may increase the risk of tendon rupture. Concomitant use with other QT_c-prolonging agents (eg, Class Ia and Class III antiarrhythmics, erythromycin, cisapride, antipsychotics, and cyclic antidepressants) may result in arrhythmias, such as torsade de pointes. Probenecid may increase gatifloxacin levels. Atypical antipsychotics and protease inhibitors may cause hyperglycemia; use with caution and monitor. Concomitant use with NSAIDs may rarely increase risk of seizure.

Decreased Effect: Concurrent administration of metal cations, including most antacids (not calcium carbonate), oral electrolyte supplements, quinapril, sucralfate, some didanosine formulations (pediatric powder for oral suspension), and other highly-buffered oral drugs, may decrease quinolone levels; separate doses.

Ethanol/Nutrition/Herb Interactions
Ethanol: Caution with ethanol (may cause hypoglycemia).

Herb/Nutraceutical: Avoid dong quai, St John's wort (may also cause photosensitization); caution with chromium, garlic, gymnema (may cause hypoglycemia).

Dietary Considerations
May take tablets with or without food, milk, or calcium supplements. Gatifloxacin should be taken 4 hours before supplements (including multivitamins) containing iron, zinc, or magnesium.

Pharmacodynamics/Kinetics
Absorption: Oral: Well absorbed; Ophthalmic: Not measurable

Distribution: V_d: 1.5-2.0 L/kg; concentrates in alveolar macrophages and lung parenchyma

Protein binding: 20%

Metabolism: Only 1%; no interaction with CYP

Bioavailability: 96%

Half-life elimination: 7.1-13.9 hours; ESRD/CAPD: 30-40 hours

Time to peak: Oral: 1 hour

Excretion: Urine (70% as unchanged drug, <1% as metabolites); feces (5%)

Pregnancy Risk Factor C
Dosage Forms
Solution, ophthalmic:

Zymar™: 0.3% (2.5 mL, 5 mL)

Gaviscon® Extra Strength [OTC] *see* Aluminum Hydroxide and Magnesium Carbonate *on page 81*

Gaviscon® Liquid [OTC] *see* Aluminum Hydroxide and Magnesium Carbonate *on page 81*

Gaviscon® Tablet [OTC] *see* Aluminum Hydroxide and Magnesium Trisilicate *on page 82*

G-CSF *see* Filgrastim *on page 691*

Gefitinib (ge FI tye nib)

U.S. Brand Names IRESSA®
Generic Available No
Index Terms NSC-715055; ZD1839
Pharmacologic Category Antineoplastic Agent, Tyrosine Kinase Inhibitor
Use
  U.S. labeling: Treatment of locally advanced or metastatic nonsmall cell lung cancer after failure of platinum-based and docetaxel therapies. Treatment is limited to patients who are benefiting or have benefited from treatment with gefitinib.
  Note: Due to the lack of improved survival data from clinical trials of gefitinib, and in response to positive survival data with another EGFR inhibitor, physicians are advised to use other treatment options in advanced nonsmall cell lung cancer patients following one or two prior chemotherapy regimens when they are refractory/intolerant to their most recent regimen.
  Canada labeling: Approved indication is limited to NSCLC patients with epidermal growth factor receptor (EGFR) expression status positive or unknown.
Local Anesthetic/Vasoconstrictor Precautions No information available to require special precautions
Effects on Dental Treatment Key adverse event(s) related to dental treatment: Mouth ulceration.
Common Adverse Effects
  >10%:
    Dermatologic: Rash (43% to 54%), acne (25% to 33%), dry skin (13% to 26%)
    Gastrointestinal: Diarrhea (48% to 76%), nausea (13% to 18%), vomiting (9% to 12%)
  1% to 10%:
    Cardiovascular: Peripheral edema (2%)
    Dermatologic: Pruritus (8% to 9%)
    Gastrointestinal: Anorexia (7% to 10%), weight loss (3% to 5%), mouth ulceration (1%)
    Neuromuscular & skeletal: Weakness (4% to 6%)
    Ocular: Amblyopia (2%), conjunctivitis (1%)
    Respiratory: Dyspnea (2%), interstitial lung disease (1% to 2%)
Restrictions As of September 15, 2005, distribution will be limited to patients enrolled in the Iressa Access Program. Under this program, access to gefitinib will be limited to the following groups:
    Patients who are currently receiving and benefitting from gefitinib (IRESSA®)
    Patients who have previously received and benefited from gefitinib (IRESSA®)
    Previously-enrolled patients or new patients in non-Investigational New Drug (IND) clinical trials involving gefitinib (IRESSA®) if these protocols were approved by an IRB prior to June 17, 2005
    New patients may also receive Iressa if the manufacturer (AstraZeneca) decides to make it available under IND, and the patients meet the criteria for enrollment under the IND
  Additional information on the IRESSA® Access Program, including enrollment forms, may be obtained by calling AstraZeneca at 1-800-601-8933 or via the web at www.Iressa-access.com
Mechanism of Action The mechanism of antineoplastic action is not fully understood. Gefitinib inhibits tyrosine kinases (TK) associated with transmembrane cell surface receptors found on both normal and cancer cells. One such receptor is epidermal growth factor receptor. TK activity appears to be vitally important to cell proliferation and survival.
Drug Interactions
  Cytochrome P450 Effect: Substrate of CYP3A4 (major); **Inhibits** CYP2C19 (weak), 2D6 (weak)
  (Continued)

Gefitinib *(Continued)*

Increased Effect/Toxicity: Gefitinib may increase the effects of warfarin. CYP3A4 inhibitors may increase the levels/effects of gefitinib; example inhibitors include azole antifungals, clarithromycin, diclofenac, doxycycline, erythromycin, imatinib, isoniazid, nefazodone, nicardipine, propofol, protease inhibitors, quinidine, telithromycin, and verapamil.

Decreased Effect: Gefitinib effects may be decreased by H_2-receptor blockers and sodium bicarbonate. CYP3A4 inducers may decrease the levels/effects of gefitinib; example inducers include aminoglutethimide, carbamazepine, nafcillin, nevirapine, phenobarbital, phenytoin, and rifamycins.

Pharmacodynamics/Kinetics

Absorption: Oral: slow

Distribution: I.V.: 1400 L

Protein binding: 90%, albumin and alpha$_1$-acid glycoprotein

Metabolism: Hepatic, primarily via CYP3A4; forms metabolites

Bioavailability: 60%

Half-life elimination: I.V.: 48 hours

Time to peak, plasma: Oral: 3-7 hours

Excretion: Feces (86%); urine (<4%)

Pregnancy Risk Factor D

Gelatin (Absorbable) *(JEL a tin, ab SORB a ble)*

U.S. Brand Names Gelfilm®; Gelfoam®

Generic Available No

Index Terms Absorbable Gelatin Sponge

Pharmacologic Category Hemostatic Agent

Dental Use Adjunct to provide hemostasis in oral and dental surgery

Use Adjunct to provide hemostasis in surgery; open prostatic surgery

Local Anesthetic/Vasoconstrictor Precautions No information available to require special precautions

Effects on Dental Treatment Key adverse event(s) related to dental treatment: Local infection and abscess formation.

Significant Adverse Effects 1% to 10%: Local: Infection and abscess formation

Dosage Hemostasis: Apply packs or sponges dry or saturated with sodium chloride. When applied dry, hold in place with moderate pressure. When applied wet, squeeze to remove air bubbles. The powder is applied as a paste prepared by adding approximately 4 mL of sterile saline solution to the powder.

Contraindications Should not be used in closure of skin incisions since they may interfere with the healing of skin edges

Warnings/Precautions Do not sterilize by heat; do not use in the presence of infection

Drug Interactions No data reported

Pregnancy Risk Factor No data reported

Dosage Forms Excipient information presented when available (limited, particularly for generics); consult specific product labeling.

Film, ophthalmic (Gelfilm®): 25 mm x 50 mm (6s)

Film, topical (Gelfilm®): 100 mm x 125 mm (1s)

Powder, topical (Gelfoam®): 1 g

Sponge, dental (Gelfoam®): Size 4 (12s)

Sponge, topical (Gelfoam®):

Size 50 (4s)

Size 100 (6s)

Size 200 (6s)

Size 2 cm (1s)

Size 6 cm (6s)

Size 12-7 mm (12s)

Gelclair® *see* Maltodextrin *on page 1017*

Gelfilm® *see* Gelatin (Absorbable) *on page 770*

Gelfoam® *see* Gelatin (Absorbable) *on page 770*

Gel-Kam® [OTC] *see* Fluoride *on page 710*

Gel-Kam® Rinse *see* Fluoride *on page 710*

Gelucast® *see* Zinc Gelatin *on page 1682*

Gelusil® [OTC] *see* Aluminum Hydroxide, Magnesium Hydroxide, and Simethicone *on page 82*

Gemcitabine (jem SITE a been)

U.S. Brand Names Gemzar®

Canadian Brand Names Gemzar®

Mexican Brand Names Gemzar

Generic Available No

Index Terms Gemcitabine Hydrochloride; NSC-613327

Pharmacologic Category Antineoplastic Agent, Antimetabolite (Pyrimidine Antagonist)

Use Treatment of metastatic breast cancer; locally-advanced or metastatic nonsmall cell lung cancer (NSCLC) or pancreatic cancer; advanced, relapsed ovarian cancer

Unlabeled/Investigational Use Treatment of bladder cancer, acute leukemia

Local Anesthetic/Vasoconstrictor Precautions No information available to require special precautions

Effects on Dental Treatment Key adverse event(s) related to dental treatment: Stomatitis.

Common Adverse Effects

>10%:

Cardiovascular: Peripheral edema (20%), edema (13%)

Central nervous system: Pain (10% to 48%), fever (30% to 41%), somnolence (5% to 11%)

Dermatologic: Rash (24% to 30%), alopecia (15% to 18%), pruritus (13%)

Gastrointestinal: Nausea/vomiting (64% to 71%; grades 3/4: 1% to 13%), constipation (10% to 31%), diarrhea (19% to 30%), stomatitis (10% to 14%)

Hematologic: Anemia (65% to 73%; grade 4: 1% to 3%), leukopenia (62% to 71%; grade 4: ≤1%), neutropenia (61% to 63%; grade 4: 6% to 7%), thrombocytopenia (24% to 47%; grade 4: ≤1%), hemorrhage (4% to 17%; grades 3/4: <1% to 2%); myelosuppression is the dose-limiting toxicity

Hepatic: Transaminases increased (67% to 78%; grades 3/4: 1% to 12%), alkaline phosphatase increased (55% to 77%; grades 3/4: 2% to 16%), bilirubin increased (13% to 26%; grades 3/4: <1% to 6%)

Renal: Proteinuria (10% to 45%; grades 3/4: <1%), hematuria (13% to 35%; grades 3/4: <1%), BUN increased (8% to 16%; grades 3/4: 0%)

Respiratory: Dyspnea (6% to 23%)

Miscellaneous: Flu-like syndrome (19%), infection (8% to 16%; grades 3/4: <1% to 2%)

1% to 10%:

Local: Injection site reactions (4%)

Neuromuscular & skeletal: Paresthesia (2% to 10%)

Renal: Creatinine increased (2% to 8%)

Respiratory: Bronchospasm (<2%)

Mechanism of Action A pyrimidine antimetabolite that inhibits DNA synthesis by inhibition of DNA polymerase and ribonucleotide reductase, specific for the S-phase of the cycle. Gemcitabine is phosphorylated intracellularly by deoxycytidine kinase to gemcitabine monophosphate, which is further phosphorylated to active metabolites gemcitabine diphosphate and gemcitabine triphosphate. Gemcitabine diphosphate inhibits DNA synthesis by inhibiting ribonucleotide reductase; gemcitabine triphosphate incorporates into DNA and inhibits DNA polymerase.

Drug Interactions

Increased Effect/Toxicity: Gemcitabine may increase the levels/effects of fluorouracil. Gemcitabine may enhance the adverse pulmonary effects of bleomycin.

Pharmacodynamics/Kinetics

Distribution: Infusions <70 minutes: 50 L/m²; Long infusion times: 370 L/m²

Protein binding: Low

Metabolism: Metabolized intracellularly by nucleoside kinases to the active diphosphate (dFdCDP) and triphosphate (dFdCTP) nucleoside metabolites

Half-life elimination:

Gemcitabine: Infusion time ≤1 hour: 42-94 minutes; infusion time 3-4 hours: 4-10.5 hours

Metabolite (gemcitabine triphosphate), terminal phase: 1.7-19.4 hours

Time to peak, plasma: 30 minutes after completion of infusion

Excretion: Urine (92% to 98%; primarily as inactive uracil metabolite); feces (<1%)

Pregnancy Risk Factor D

Gemcitabine Hydrochloride see Gemcitabine on page 771

Gemfibrozil (jem FI broe zil)

Related Information
  Cardiovascular Diseases *on page 1726*
U.S. Brand Names Lopid®
Canadian Brand Names Apo-Gemfibrozil®; Gen-Gemfibrozil; GMD-Gemfibrozil; Lopid®; Novo-Gemfibrozil; Nu-Gemfibrozil; PMS-Gemfibrozil
Mexican Brand Names Lopid
Generic Available Yes
Index Terms CI-719
Pharmacologic Category Antilipemic Agent, Fibric Acid
Use Treatment of hypertriglyceridemia in types IV and V hyperlipidemia for patients who are at greater risk for pancreatitis and who have not responded to dietary intervention
Local Anesthetic/Vasoconstrictor Precautions No information available to require special precautions
Effects on Dental Treatment No significant effects or complications reported
Common Adverse Effects
  >10%: Gastrointestinal: Dyspepsia (20%)
  1% to 10%:
    Central nervous system: Fatigue (4%), vertigo (2%), headache (1%)
    Dermatologic: Eczema (2%), rash (2%)
    Gastrointestinal: Abdominal pain (10%), diarrhea (7%), nausea/vomiting (3%), constipation (1%)

  Reports where causal relationship has not been established: Weight loss, extrasystoles, pancreatitis, hepatoma, colitis, confusion, seizure, syncope, retinal edema, decreased fertility (male), renal dysfunction, positive ANA, drug-induced lupus-like syndrome, thrombocytopenia, anaphylaxis, vasculitis, alopecia, photosensitivity
Dosage Adults: Oral: 1200 mg/day in 2 divided doses, 30 minutes before breakfast and dinner
  Hemodialysis: Not removed by hemodialysis; supplemental dose is not necessary
Mechanism of Action The exact mechanism of action of gemfibrozil is unknown, however, several theories exist regarding the VLDL effect; it can inhibit lipolysis and decrease subsequent hepatic fatty acid uptake as well as inhibit hepatic secretion of VLDL; together these actions decrease serum VLDL levels; increases HDL-cholesterol; the mechanism behind HDL elevation is currently unknown
Contraindications Hypersensitivity to gemfibrozil or any component of the formulation; significant hepatic or renal dysfunction; primary biliary cirrhosis; pre-existing gallbladder disease
Warnings/Precautions Abnormal elevation of AST, ALT, LDH, bilirubin, and alkaline phosphatase has occurred; if no appreciable triglyceride or cholesterol lowering effect occurs after 3 months, the drug should be discontinued; not useful for type I hyperlipidemia; myositis may be more common in patients with poor renal function
Drug Interactions
  Cytochrome P450 Effect: Substrate of CYP3A4 (minor); **Inhibits** CYP1A2 (moderate), 2C8 (strong), 2C9 (strong), 2C19 (strong)
  Increased Effect/Toxicity: Gemfibrozil may potentiate the effects of bexarotene (avoid concurrent use), sulfonylureas (including glyburide, chlorpropamide), and warfarin. HMG-CoA reductase inhibitors (atorvastatin, fluvastatin, lovastatin, pravastatin, simvastatin) may increase the risk of myopathy and rhabdomyolysis. The manufacturer warns against the concurrent use of lovastatin (if unavoidable, limit lovastatin to <20 mg/day). Combination therapy with statins has been used in some patients with resistant hyperlipidemias (with great caution). Gemfibrozil may increase the serum concentration of repaglinide (resulting in severe, prolonged hypoglycemia); the addition of itraconazole may augment the effects of gemfibrozil on repaglinide (consider alternative therapy). Gemfibrozil may increase the levels/effects of aminophylline, amiodarone, bosentan, citalopram, dapsone, diazepam, fluoxetine, fluvoxamine, glimepiride, glipizide, losartan, methsuximide, mexiletine, mirtazapine, montelukast, nateglinide, paclitaxel, phenytoin, pioglitazone, propranolol, repaglinide, ropinirole, rosiglitazone, sertraline, theophylline, trifluoperazine, warfarin, zafirlukast, and other substrates of CYP1A2, 2C8, 2C9, or 2C19.
  Decreased Effect: Cyclosporine's blood levels may be reduced during concurrent therapy. Rifampin may decrease gemfibrozil blood levels.
Ethanol/Nutrition/Herb Interactions Ethanol: Avoid ethanol to decrease triglycerides.

Dietary Considerations Before initiation of therapy, patients should be placed on a standard cholesterol-lowering diet for 3-6 months and the diet should be continued during drug therapy.

Pharmacodynamics/Kinetics

Onset of action: May require several days

Absorption: Well absorbed

Protein binding: 99%

Metabolism: Hepatic via oxidation to two inactive metabolites; undergoes enterohepatic recycling

Half-life elimination: 1.4 hours

Time to peak, serum: 1-2 hours

Excretion: Urine (70% primarily as conjugated drug); feces (6%)

Pregnancy Risk Factor C

Dosage Forms

Tablet: 600 mg

Lopid®: 600 mg

Gemifloxacin (je mi FLOKS a sin)

Related Information

Bacterial Infections *on page 1793*

U.S. Brand Names Factive®

Canadian Brand Names Factive®

Generic Available No

Index Terms DW286; Gemifloxacin Mesylate; LA 20304a; SB-265805

Pharmacologic Category Antibiotic, Quinolone

Use Treatment of acute exacerbation of chronic bronchitis; treatment of community-acquired pneumonia (CAP), including pneumonia caused by multidrug-resistant strains of *S. pneumoniae* (MDRSP)

Unlabeled/Investigational Use Acute sinusitis

Local Anesthetic/Vasoconstrictor Precautions No information available to require special precautions

Effects on Dental Treatment No significant effects or complications reported

Common Adverse Effects

1% to 10%:

Central nervous system: Headache (1%), dizziness (1%)

Dermatologic: Rash (3%)

Gastrointestinal: Diarrhea (4%), nausea (3%), abdominal pain (1%), vomiting (1%)

Hepatic: Transaminases increased (1% to 2%)

Important adverse effects reported with other agents in this drug class include (not reported for gemifloxacin): Allergic reactions, CNS stimulation, hepatitis, jaundice, peripheral neuropathy, pneumonitis (eosinophilic), seizure; sensorimotor-axonal neuropathy (paresthesia, hypoesthesias, dysesthesias, weakness); severe dermatologic reactions (toxic epidermal necrolysis, Stevens-Johnson syndrome); tendon rupture, torsade de pointes, vasculitis

Dosage

Usual dosage range:

Adults: Oral: 320 mg once daily

Indication-specific dosing:

Adults: Oral:

Acute exacerbations of chronic bronchitis: 320 mg once daily for 5 days

Community-acquired pneumonia (mild to moderate): 320 mg once daily for 5 or 7 days (decision to use 5- or 7-day regimen should be guided by initial sputum culture; 7 days are recommended for MDRSP, *Klebsiella*, or *M. catarrhalis* infection)

Sinusitis (unlabeled use): 320 mg once daily for 10 days

Elderly: Refer to adult dosing.

Dosage adjustment in renal impairment: Cl_{cr} ≤40 mL/minute (or patients on hemodialysis/CAPD): 160 mg once daily (administer dose following hemodialysis)

Dosage adjustment in hepatic impairment: No adjustment required.

Mechanism of Action Gemifloxacin is a DNA gyrase inhibitor and also inhibits topoisomerase IV. DNA gyrase (topoisomerase IV) is an essential bacterial enzyme that maintains the superhelical structure of DNA. DNA gyrase is required for DNA replication and transcription, DNA repair, recombination, and transposition; bactericidal

Contraindications Hypersensitivity to gemifloxacin, other fluoroquinolones, or any component of the formulation

Warnings/Precautions Fluoroquinolones may prolong QT_c interval; avoid use of gemifloxacin in patients with a history of QT_c prolongation, uncorrected hypokalemia, hypomagnesemia, or concurrent administration of other medications (Continued)

Gemifloxacin *(Continued)*

known to prolong the QT interval (including Class Ia and Class III antiarrhythmics, cisapride, erythromycin, antipsychotics, and tricyclic antidepressants). Use with caution in patients with significant bradycardia or acute myocardial ischemia. Use with caution in individuals at risk of seizures (CNS disorders or concurrent therapy with medications which may lower seizure threshold). Potential for seizures, although very rare, may be increased with concomitant NSAID therapy. Discontinue in patients who experience significant CNS adverse effects (dizziness, hallucinations, suicidal ideation or actions). Use caution in renal dysfunction; dosage adjustment required for Cl_{cr} ≤40 mL/minute.

Severe hypersensitivity reactions, including anaphylaxis, have occurred with quinolone therapy. If an allergic reaction occurs (itching, urticaria, dyspnea or facial edema, loss of consciousness, tingling, cardiovascular collapse), discontinue drug immediately. May cause mild-to-moderate maculopapular rash, usually 8-10 days after treatment initiation; risk factors may include age <40 years, female gender (including postmenopausal women on HRT), and treatment duration >7 days; discontinue therapy if rash develops. Avoid excessive sunlight; may rarely cause moderate-to-severe phototoxicity reactions similar to ciprofloxacin. Prolonged use may result in fungal or bacterial superinfection, including *C. difficile*-associated diarrhea and pseudomembranous colitis. Tendon inflammation and/or rupture has been reported with other quinolone antibiotics; risk may increase with concurrent corticosteroids, particularly in the elderly. Discontinue at first sign of tendon inflammation or pain. Peripheral neuropathy has been linked to the use of quinolones; these cases were rare. Safety and effectiveness in pediatric patients (<18 years of age) have not been established.

Drug Interactions

Increased Effect/Toxicity: Gemifloxacin may increase the effects/toxicity of glyburide and warfarin. Concomitant use with corticosteroids may increase the risk of tendon rupture. Concomitant use with other QT_c-prolonging agents (eg, Class Ia and Class III antiarrhythmics, erythromycin, cisapride, antipsychotics, and cyclic antidepressants) may result in arrhythmias, such as torsade de pointes. Probenecid may increase gemifloxacin levels. Concomitant use with NSAIDs may rarely increase risk of seizure.

Decreased Effect: Concurrent administration of metal cations, including most antacids, oral electrolyte supplements, quinapril, sucralfate, some didanosine formulations (pediatric powder for oral suspension), and other highly-buffered oral drugs, may decrease quinolone levels; separate doses. Gemifloxacin may diminish the therapeutic effect of the live, attenuated Ty21a strain of typhoid vaccine.

Ethanol/Nutrition/Herb Interactions Herb/Nutraceutical: Avoid dong quai, St John's wort (may also cause photosensitization).

Dietary Considerations May take tablets with or without food, milk, or calcium supplements. Gemifloxacin should be taken 3 hours before or 2 hours after supplements (including multivitamins) containing iron, zinc, or magnesium.

Pharmacodynamics/Kinetics

Absorption: Well absorbed from the GI tract

Distribution: V_{dss}: 4.2 L/kg

Bioavailability: 71%

Metabolism: Hepatic (minor); forms metabolites (CYP isoenzymes are not involved)

Time to peak, plasma: 0.5-2 hours

Protein binding: 60% to 70%

Half-life elimination: 7 hours (range 4-12 hours)

Excretion: Feces (61%); urine (36%)

Pregnancy Risk Factor C

Dosage Forms

Tablet:

Factive®: 320 mg

Gemifloxacin Mesylate *see* Gemifloxacin *on page 773*

Gemtuzumab Ozogamicin *(gem TOO zoo mab oh zog a MY sin)*

U.S. Brand Names Mylotarg®

Canadian Brand Names Mylotarg®

Generic Available No

Index Terms CMA-676; NSC-720568

Pharmacologic Category Antineoplastic Agent, Monoclonal Antibody

Use Treatment of relapsed CD33 positive acute myeloid leukemia (AML) in patients ≥60 years of age who are not candidates for cytotoxic chemotherapy

Unlabeled/Investigational Use Salvage therapy for acute promyelocytic leukemia (APL), relapsed/ refractory CD33 positive acute myeloid leukemia in children and adults <60 years

Local Anesthetic/Vasoconstrictor Precautions No information available to require special precautions

Effects on Dental Treatment Key adverse event(s) related to dental treatment: Stomatitis, gingival hemorrhage, and mucositis.

Common Adverse Effects Percentages established in adults ≥60 years of age. **Note:** A postinfusion symptom complex (fever, chills, less commonly hypertension, and/or dyspnea) may occur within 24 hours of administration; the incidence of infusion-related events decreases with repeat administration.

>10%:
   Cardiovascular: Peripheral edema (19%), hypotension (18%), hypertension (17%), tachycardia (11%)
   Central nervous system: Fever (78%), chills (64%), headache (27%), pain (18%), insomnia (11%)
   Dermatologic: Petechiae (19%), rash (18%), bruising (11%)
   Endocrine & metabolic: Hypokalemia (24%), hyperglycemia (11%)
   Gastrointestinal: Nausea (63%), vomiting (53%), diarrhea (30%), anorexia (27%), abdominal pain (26%), constipation (23%), stomatitis/mucositis (22%)
   Hematologic: Neutropenia (grades 3/4: 98%; median recovery 40.5 days), lymphopenia (grades 3/4: 93%), thrombocytopenia (49%; grades 3/4: 48%; median recovery 39 days), hemoglobin decreased (grades 3/4: 50%), leukopenia (grades 3/4: 43%), anemia (22%, grades 3/4: 12%)
   Hepatic: Abnormal liver function tests (20%; grade 3/4: 7%), LDH increased (18%), hyperbilirubinemia (11%)
   Local: Local reaction (17%)
   Neuromuscular & skeletal: Weakness (36%), back pain (12%)
   Respiratory: Dyspnea (26%), epistaxis (24%; grade 3/4: 3%), cough (18%), pneumonia (13%)
   Miscellaneous: Sepsis (25%), neutropenic fever (19%), cutaneous herpes simplex (18%),
1% to 10%:
   Central nervous system: Anxiety (10%), depression (10%), dizziness (10%), cerebral hemorrhage (2%), intracranial hemorrhage (1%)
   Dermatologic: Pruritus (4%)
   Endocrine & metabolic: Hypocalcemia (10%), hypophosphatemia (6%) hypomagnesemia (3%)
   Gastrointestinal: Dyspepsia (8%), gingival hemorrhage (5%)
   Genitourinary: Vaginal hemorrhage (5%), vaginal bleeding 2%, hematuria (grade 3/4: 1%)
   Hematologic: Hemorrhage (9%), disseminated intravascular coagulation (DIC) (1%)
   Hepatic: Alkaline phosphatase increased (10%), PT/PTT increased, veno-occlusive disease (5% to 10%; up to 20% in relapsed patients; higher frequency in patients with prior history of subsequent hematopoietic stem cell transplant)
   Neuromuscular & skeletal: Arthralgia (10%), myalgia (3%)
   Respiratory: Pharyngitis (10%), rhinitis (7%), hypoxia (5%)
   Miscellaneous: Infection (10%)

Mechanism of Action Antibody to CD33 antigen. Binding results in internalization of the antibody-antigen complex. Following internalization, the calicheamicin derivative is released inside the myeloid cell. The calicheamicin derivative binds to DNA resulting in double strand breaks and cell death. Pluripotent stem cells and nonhematopoietic cells are not affected.

Drug Interactions
   Increased Effect/Toxicity: Monoclonal antibodies may increase the risk for allergic reactions to gemtuzumab due to the presence of HACA antibodies

Pharmacodynamics/Kinetics
   Distribution: V_{ss}: Adults: Initial dose: 21 L; Repeat dose: 10 L
   Half-life elimination: Total calicheamicin: Initial: 41-45 hours, Repeat dose: 60-64 hours; Unconjugated: 100-143 hours (no change noted in repeat dosing)
   Time to peak, plasma: Immediate; higher concentrations observed after repeat dose

Pregnancy Risk Factor D

Genapap™ [OTC] *see* Acetaminophen *on page 31*

Genapap™ Children [OTC] *see* Acetaminophen *on page 31*

Genapap™ Extra Strength [OTC] *see* Acetaminophen *on page 31*

Genapap™ Infant [OTC] *see* Acetaminophen *on page 31*

Genapap™ Sinus Maximum Strength [OTC] *see* Acetaminophen and Pseudoephedrine *on page 38*

Genaphed® [OTC] *see* Pseudoephedrine *on page 1381*

Genasal [OTC] *see* Oxymetazoline *on page 1236*

Genasec™ [OTC] *see* Acetaminophen and Phenyltoloxamine *on page 38*

Genasoft® [OTC] *see* Docusate *on page 522*

Genasyme® [OTC] *see* Simethicone *on page 1472*

Genaton™ [OTC] *see* Aluminum Hydroxide and Magnesium Carbonate *on page 81*

Genaton Tablet [OTC] *see* Aluminum Hydroxide and Magnesium Trisilicate *on page 82*

Genatuss DM® [OTC] *see* Guaifenesin and Dextromethorphan *on page 796*

Genebs [OTC] *see* Acetaminophen *on page 31*

Genebs Extra Strength [OTC] *see* Acetaminophen *on page 31*

Generlac *see* Lactulose *on page 943*

Geneye® [OTC] *see* Tetrahydrozoline *on page 1551*

Genfiber® [OTC] *see* Psyllium *on page 1386*

Gengraf® *see* CycloSPORINE *on page 426*

Genoptic® [DSC] *see* Gentamicin *on page 776*

Genotropin® *see* Somatropin *on page 1486*

Genotropin Miniquick® *see* Somatropin *on page 1486*

Genpril® [OTC] *see* Ibuprofen *on page 853*

Gentak® *see* Gentamicin *on page 776*

Gentamicin (jen ta MYE sin)

Related Information
Treatment of Sexually-Transmitted Infections *on page 1920*

U.S. Brand Names Genoptic® [DSC]; Gentak®

Canadian Brand Names Alcomicin®; Diogent®; Garamycin®; Gentamicin Injection, USP; SAB-Gentamicin

Mexican Brand Names Garamicina; Garamicina Crema; Garamicina Oftalmica; Genrex; Genta Grin; Yectamicina

Generic Available Yes

Index Terms Gentamicin Sulfate

Pharmacologic Category Antibiotic, Aminoglycoside; Antibiotic, Ophthalmic; Antibiotic, Topical

Dental Use Prevention of bacterial endocarditis prior to dental or surgical procedures

Use Treatment of susceptible bacterial infections, normally gram-negative organisms including *Pseudomonas*, *Proteus*, *Serratia*, and gram-positive *Staphylococcus*; treatment of bone infections, respiratory tract infections, skin and soft tissue infections, as well as abdominal and urinary tract infections, endocarditis, and septicemia; used topically to treat superficial infections of the skin or ophthalmic infections caused by susceptible bacteria; prevention of bacterial endocarditis prior to dental or surgical procedures

Local Anesthetic/Vasoconstrictor Precautions No information available to require special precautions

Effects on Dental Treatment No significant effects or complications reported

Common Adverse Effects
>10%:
Central nervous system: Neurotoxicity (vertigo, ataxia)
Neuromuscular & skeletal: Gait instability
Otic: Ototoxicity (auditory), ototoxicity (vestibular)
Renal: Nephrotoxicity, decreased creatinine clearance
1% to 10%:
Cardiovascular: Edema
Dermatologic: Skin itching, reddening of skin, rash

Mechanism of Action Interferes with bacterial protein synthesis by binding to 30S and 50S ribosomal subunits resulting in a defective bacterial cell membrane

Drug Interactions
Increased Effect/Toxicity: Penicillins, cephalosporins, amphotericin B, loop diuretics may increase nephrotoxic potential. Aminoglycosides may potentiate the effects of neuromuscular blocking agents.

Pharmacodynamics/Kinetics
Absorption:
Intramuscular: Rapid and complete
Oral: None
Distribution: Primarily into extracellular fluid (highly hydrophilic); high concentration in the renal cortex; minimal penetration to ocular tissues via I.V. route
V_d: Increased by edema, ascites, fluid overload; decreased with dehydration
Neonates: 0.4-0.6 L/kg
Children: 0.3-0.35 L/kg
Adults: 0.2-0.3 L/kg
Relative diffusion from blood into CSF: Minimal even with inflammation
CSF:blood level ratio: Normal meninges: Nil; Inflamed meninges: 10% to 30%
Protein binding: <30%
Half-life elimination:
Infants: <1 week: 3-11.5 hours; 1 week to 6 months: 3-3.5 hours
Adults: 1.5-3 hours; End-stage renal disease: 36-70 hours
Time to peak, serum: I.M.: 30-90 minutes; I.V.: 30 minutes after 30-minute infusion
Excretion: Urine (as unchanged drug)
Clearance: Directly related to renal function
Pregnancy Risk Factor C (ophthalmic, topical); C/D (injection; varies per manufacturer)

Gentamicin and Prednisolone *see* Prednisolone and Gentamicin *on page 1342*
Gentamicin Sulfate *see* Gentamicin *on page 776*
GenTeal® [OTC] *see* Hydroxypropyl Methylcellulose *on page 844*
GenTeal® Mild [OTC] *see* Hydroxypropyl Methylcellulose *on page 844*
Gentex HC *see* Hydrocodone, Phenylephrine, and Guaifenesin *on page 834*
Gentex LA *see* Guaifenesin and Phenylephrine *on page 797*
Gentex LQ *see* Carbetapentane, Guaifenesin, and Phenylephrine *on page 279*

Gentian Violet (JEN shun VYE oh let)

Generic Available Yes
Index Terms Crystal Violet; Methylrosaniline Chloride
Pharmacologic Category Antibiotic, Topical; Antifungal Agent, Topical
Use Treatment of cutaneous or mucocutaneous infections caused by *Candida albicans* and other superficial skin infections
Local Anesthetic/Vasoconstrictor Precautions No information available to require special precautions
Effects on Dental Treatment Key adverse event(s) related to dental treatment: Ulceration of mucous membranes.
Common Adverse Effects Frequency not defined.
Dermatologic: Vesicle formation
Gastrointestinal: Esophagitis, ulceration of mucous membranes
Local: Burning, irritation
Respiratory: Laryngitis, laryngeal obstruction, tracheitis
Miscellaneous: Sensitivity reactions
Mechanism of Action Topical antiseptic/germicide effective against some vegetative gram-positive bacteria, particularly *Staphylococcus* sp, and some yeast; it is much less effective against gram-negative bacteria and is ineffective against acid-fast bacteria
Pregnancy Risk Factor C

Gentran® *see* Dextran *on page 472*
Gentuss-HC *see* Hydrocodone, Phenylephrine, and Diphenhydramine *on page 834*
Geocillin® *see* Carbenicillin *on page 278*
Geodon® *see* Ziprasidone *on page 1683*
Geref® Diagnostic *see* Sermorelin Acetate *on page 1462*
Geriation [OTC] *see* Vitamins (Multiple/Oral) *on page 1665*
Geri-Hydrolac™ [OTC] *see* Lactic Acid and Ammonium Hydroxide *on page 941*
Geri-Hydrolac™-12 [OTC] *see* Lactic Acid and Ammonium Hydroxide *on page 941*
Geritol Complete® [OTC] *see* Vitamins (Multiple/Oral) *on page 1665*
Geritol Extend® [OTC] *see* Vitamins (Multiple/Oral) *on page 1665*
Geritol® Tonic [OTC] *see* Vitamins (Multiple/Oral) *on page 1665*
German Measles Vaccine *see* Rubella Virus Vaccine (Live) *on page 1450*
Gevrabon® [OTC] *see* Vitamin B Complex Combinations *on page 1664*
GF196960 *see* Tadalafil *on page 1520*
GG *see* Guaifenesin *on page 795*

Glatiramer Acetate (gla TIR a mer AS e tate)

U.S. Brand Names Copaxone®
Canadian Brand Names Copaxone®
Generic Available No
Index Terms Copolymer-1
Pharmacologic Category Biological, Miscellaneous
Use Treatment of relapsing-remitting type multiple sclerosis; studies indicate that it reduces the frequency of attacks and the severity of disability; appears to be most effective for patients with minimal disability

Local Anesthetic/Vasoconstrictor Precautions No information available to require special precautions

Effects on Dental Treatment Key adverse event(s) related to dental treatment: Ulcerative stomatitis, salivary gland enlargement, and oral moniliasis.

Common Adverse Effects Reported in >2% of patients in placebo-controlled trials:

>10%:
  Cardiovascular: Chest pain (21%), vasodilation (27%), palpitation (17%)
  Central nervous system: Pain (28%), anxiety (23%)
  Dermatologic: Pruritus (18%), rash (18%), diaphoresis (15%)
  Gastrointestinal: Nausea (22%), diarrhea (12%)
  Local: Injection site reactions: Pain (73%), erythema (66%), inflammation (49%), pruritus (40%), mass (27%), induration (13%), welt (11%)
  Neuromuscular & skeletal: Weakness (41%), arthralgia (24%), hypertonia (22%), back pain (16%)
  Respiratory: Dyspnea (19%), rhinitis (14%)
  Miscellaneous: Infection (50%), flu-like syndrome (19%), lymphadenopathy (12%)
1% to 10%:
  Cardiovascular: Peripheral edema (7%), facial edema (6%), edema (3%), tachycardia (5%)
  Central nervous system: Fever (8%), vertigo (6%), migraine (5%), syncope (5%), agitation (4%), chills (4%), confusion (2%), nervousness (2%), speech disorder (2%)
  Dermatologic: Bruising (8%), erythema (4%), urticaria (4%), skin nodule (2%)
  Endocrine & metabolic: Dysmenorrhea (6%)
  Gastrointestinal: Anorexia (8%), vomiting (6%), gastrointestinal disorder (5%), gastroenteritis (3%), weight gain (3%)
  Genitourinary: Urinary urgency (10%), vaginal moniliasis (8%)
  Local: Injection site reactions: Hemorrhage (5%), urticaria (5%)
  Neuromuscular & skeletal: Tremor (7%), foot drop (3%)
  Ocular: Eye disorder (4%), nystagmus (2%)
  Otic: Ear pain (7%)
  Respiratory: Bronchitis (9%), laryngismus (5%)
  Miscellaneous: Neck pain (8%), bacterial infection (5%), herpes simplex (4%), cyst (2%), herpes zoster

Mechanism of Action Glatiramer is a mixture of random polymers of four amino acids; L-alanine, L-glutamic acid, L-lysine and L-tyrosine, the resulting mixture is antigenically similar to myelin basic protein, which is an important component of the myelin sheath of nerves; glatiramer is thought to suppress T-lymphocytes specific for a myelin antigen, it is also proposed that glatiramer interferes with the antigen-presenting function of certain immune cells opposing pathogenic T-cell function

Pharmacodynamics/Kinetics
  Distribution: Small amounts of intact and partial hydrolyzed drug enter lymphatic circulation
  Metabolism: SubQ: Large percentage hydrolyzed locally
Pregnancy Risk Factor B

Gleevec® see Imatinib on page 863

Gliadel® *see* Carmustine *on page 288*
Glibenclamide *see* GlyBURIDE *on page 786*

Gliclazide (GLYE kla zide)

Canadian Brand Names Apo-Gliclazide®; Diamicron®; Diamicron® MR; Novo-Gliclazide; Rhoxal-gliclazide; Sandoz-Gliclazide

Generic Available Yes: 80 mg tablet

Pharmacologic Category Antidiabetic Agent, Sulfonylurea

Use Management of type 2 diabetes mellitus (noninsulin dependent, NIDDM)

Local Anesthetic/Vasoconstrictor Precautions No information available to require special precautions

Effects on Dental Treatment Gliclazide-dependent diabetics (noninsulin dependent, type 2) should be appointed for dental treatment in morning in order to minimize chance of stress-induced hypoglycemia.

Common Adverse Effects Frequency not defined.

Central nervous system: Headache, nervousness, dizziness

Dermatologic: Rash, erythema, pruritus, urticaria. Sulfonylureas have also been associated with rare photosensitivity and porphyria cutanea tarda

Endocrine & metabolic: Hypoglycemia (dose dependent), hyponatremia (rare)

Gastrointestinal: Nausea, vomiting, diarrhea, epigastric fullness, gastritis

Hematologic: Agranulocytosis, leukopenia, thrombocytopenia, anemia

Hepatic: Jaundice, LDH increased, transaminases increased

Miscellaneous: Disulfiram reaction (very low potential)

Restrictions Not available in U.S.

Dosage Oral: Adults:

Immediate release tablet: Initial: 80-160 mg/day; typical dose range 80-320 mg/day; dosage of ≥160 mg should be divided into 2 equal parts for twice-daily administration; maximum dose: 320 mg/day; should be taken with meals

Sustained release tablet: 30-120 mg once daily

Note: There is no fixed dosage regimen for the management of diabetes mellitus with gliclazide or any other hypoglycemic agent. Dose must be individualized based on frequent determinations of blood glucose during dose titration and throughout maintenance.

Dosage adjustment in renal/hepatic impairment: Contraindicated in severe impairment

Mechanism of Action Stimulates insulin release from the pancreatic beta cells; reduces glucose output from the liver; lowers plasma glucose concentrations. Gliclazide has also been shown to decrease platelet aggregation at therapeutic doses.

Contraindications Hypersensitivity to gliclazide, sulfonylureas, or any component of the formulation; type 1 diabetes mellitus (insulin dependent, IDDM), diabetic ketoacidosis with or without coma; renal or hepatic impairment; pregnancy (per manufacturer); breast-feeding

Warnings/Precautions All sulfonylurea drugs are capable of producing severe hypoglycemia. Hypoglycemia is more likely to occur when caloric intake is deficient, after severe or prolonged exercise, when ethanol is ingested, or when more than one glucose-lowering drug is used. Hypoglycemia is also more likely in elderly patients, malnourished patients or in impaired renal or hepatic function.

Chemical similarities are present among sulfonamides, sulfonylureas, carbonic anhydrase inhibitors, thiazides, and loop diuretics (except ethacrynic acid). Use in patients with sulfonamide allergy is specifically contraindicated in product labeling, however, a risk of cross-reaction exists in patients with allergy to any of these compounds; avoid use when previous reaction has been severe.

Product labeling of sulfonylureas (in U.S.) states oral hypoglycemic drugs may be associated with an increased cardiovascular mortality as compared to treatment with diet alone or diet plus insulin. Data to support this association are limited, and several studies, including a large prospective trial (UKPDS), have not supported an association.

It may be necessary to discontinue therapy and administer insulin if the patient is exposed to stress (fever, trauma, infection, surgery). Safety and efficacy have not been established in children.

Drug Interactions

Increased Effect/Toxicity: Anabolic steroids, ACE inhibitors, H₂ antagonists, antacids, oral sodium bicarbonate, salicylates, and sulfonamides may increase the hypoglycemic effect of gliclazide. A possible interaction between sulfonylureas and fluoroquinolone antibiotics has been reported resulting in a potentiation of hypoglycemic action of sulfonylureas. Warfarin's anticoagulant effects may be increased by sulfonylureas. Rare disulfiram reactions may (Continued)

Gliclazide *(Continued)*

occur with ethanol. Gliclazide may increase serum concentrations of cyclosporine.

Decreased Effect: Beta-blockers may decrease gliclazide's hypoglycemic effect, mask most hypoglycemic symptoms, and decrease glycogenolysis; avoid use in patients with diabetes with frequent hypoglycemic episodes (particularly nonselective beta-blockers). Corticosteroids and thiazide diuretics may cause hyperglycemia; adjustment of hypoglycemic agent may be necessary. Ethanol (large amounts) and/or rifampin may decrease gliclazide's hypoglycemic effect; avoid concurrent use.

Ethanol/Nutrition/Herb Interactions

Ethanol: Avoid ethanol (may cause hypoglycemia and/or rare disulfiram reactions).

Herb/Nutraceutical: Avoid chromium, garlic, gymnema (may cause hypoglycemia).

Dietary Considerations Should be taken with meals. Dietary modification based on ADA recommendations is a part of therapy. Decreases blood glucose concentration. Hypoglycemia may occur. Must be able to recognize symptoms of hypoglycemia (palpitations, sweaty palms, lightheadedness).

Pharmacodynamics/Kinetics

Absorption: Rapid

Protein binding: 94%

Metabolism: Hepatic, to inactive metabolites

Half-life elimination: 10 hours

Time to peak: 4-6 hours

Excretion: Urine (60% to 70%) and feces (10% to 20%) as metabolites

Pregnancy Risk Factor Not available (similar agents rated C); manufacturer contraindicates use

Dosage Forms

[CAN] = Canadian brand name

Tablet: 80 mg [not available in the U.S.]

Diamicron® [CAN]: 80 mg [not available in the U.S.]

Tablet, sustained release:

Diamicron® MR [CAN]: 30 mg [not available in the U.S.]

Glimepiride *(GLYE me pye ride)*

Related Information

Endocrine Disorders and Pregnancy *on page 1750*

U.S. Brand Names Amaryl®

Canadian Brand Names Amaryl®; CO Glimepiride; Novo-Glimepiride; ratio-Glimepiride; Rhoxal-glimepiride; Sandoz-Glimepiride

Mexican Brand Names Amaryl

Generic Available Yes

Pharmacologic Category Antidiabetic Agent, Sulfonylurea

Use Management of type 2 diabetes mellitus (noninsulin dependent, NIDDM) as an adjunct to diet and exercise to lower blood glucose; may be used in combination with metformin or insulin in patients whose hyperglycemia cannot be controlled by diet and exercise in conjunction with a single oral hypoglycemic agent

Local Anesthetic/Vasoconstrictor Precautions No information available to require special precautions

Effects on Dental Treatment Glimepiride-dependent diabetics (noninsulin dependent, type 2) should be appointed for dental treatment in morning in order to minimize chance of stress-induced hypoglycemia.

Common Adverse Effects

1% to 10%:

Central nervous system: Dizziness (2%), headache (2%)

Endocrine & metabolic: Hypoglycemia (1% to 2%)

Gastrointestinal: Nausea (1%)

Neuromuscular & skeletal: Weakness (2%)

Dosage Oral:

Children 10-18 years (unlabeled use): Initial: 1 mg once daily; maintenance: 1-4 mg once daily

Adults: Initial: 1-2 mg once daily, administered with breakfast or the first main meal; usual maintenance dose: 1-4 mg once daily; after a dose of 2 mg once daily, increase in increments of 2 mg at 1- to 2-week intervals based upon the patient's blood glucose response to a maximum of 8 mg once daily. If inadequate response to maximal dose, combination therapy with metformin may be considered.

Combination with insulin therapy (fasting glucose level for instituting combination therapy is in the range of >150 mg/dL in plasma or serum depending on the patient): initial recommended dose: 8 mg once daily with the first main meal

After starting with low-dose insulin, upward adjustments of insulin can be done approximately weekly as guided by frequent measurements of fasting blood glucose. Once stable, combination-therapy patients should monitor their capillary blood glucose on an ongoing basis, preferably daily.

Conversion from therapy with long half-life agents: Observe patient carefully for 1-2 weeks when converting from a longer half-life agent (eg, chlorpropamide) to glimepiride due to overlapping hypoglycemic effects.

Dosing adjustment/comments in renal impairment: Cl_{cr} <22 mL/minute: Initial starting dose should be 1 mg and dosage increments should be based on fasting blood glucose levels

Dosing adjustment in hepatic impairment: No data available

Elderly: Initial: 1 mg/day; dose titration and maintenance dosing should be conservative to avoid hypoglycemia

Mechanism of Action Stimulates insulin release from the pancreatic beta cells; reduces glucose output from the liver; insulin sensitivity is increased at peripheral target sites

Contraindications Hypersensitivity to glimepiride, any component of the formulation, or sulfonamides; diabetic ketoacidosis (with or without coma)

Warnings/Precautions All sulfonylurea drugs are capable of producing severe hypoglycemia. Hypoglycemia is more likely to occur when caloric intake is deficient, after severe or prolonged exercise, when ethanol is ingested, or when more than one glucose-lowering drug is used. It is also more likely in elderly patients, malnourished patients and in patients with impaired renal or hepatic function; use with caution.

Chemical similarities are present among sulfonamides, sulfonylureas, carbonic anhydrase inhibitors, thiazides, and loop diuretics (except ethacrynic acid). Use in patients with sulfonamide allergy is specifically contraindicated in product labeling, however, a risk of cross-reaction exists in patients with allergy to any of these compounds; avoid use when previous reaction has been severe.

Product labeling states oral hypoglycemic drugs may be associated with an increased cardiovascular mortality as compared to treatment with diet alone or diet plus insulin. Data to support this association are limited, and several studies, including a large prospective trial (UKPDS) have not supported an association.

It may be necessary to discontinue therapy and administer insulin if the patient is exposed to stress (fever, trauma, infection, surgery). Safety and efficacy have not been established in children.

Drug Interactions

Cytochrome P450 Effect: Substrate of CYP2C9 (major)

Increased Effect/Toxicity: CYP2C9 inhibitors may increase the levels/effects of glimepiride; example inhibitors include delavirdine, ketoconazole, nicardipine, NSAIDs, sulfonamides, and tolbutamide. Beta-blockers, chloramphenicol, cimetidine, fibric acid derivatives, fluconazole, pegvisomant, salicylates, sulfonamides, and tricyclic antidepressants may increase the hypoglycemic effects of glimepiride. Glimepiride may increase effects of cyclosporine. Sulfonylureas may induce a disulfiram-like reaction with ethanol.

Decreased Effect: CYP2C9 inducers may decrease the levels/effects of glimepiride; example inducers include carbamazepine, phenobarbital, phenytoin, rifampin, rifapentine, and secobarbital. There may be a decreased effect of glimepiride with corticosteroids, estrogens, oral contraceptives, thiazide and other diuretics, phenothiazines, NSAIDs, thyroid products, nicotinic acid, isoniazid, sympathomimetics, urinary alkalinizers, and charcoal. **Note:** However, pooled data did **not** demonstrate drug interactions with calcium channel blockers, estrogens, NSAIDs, HMG-CoA reductase inhibitors, sulfonamides, or thyroid hormone.

Ethanol/Nutrition/Herb Interactions

Ethanol: Caution with ethanol (may cause hypoglycemia).

Herb/Nutraceutical: Caution with chromium, garlic, gymnema (may cause hypoglycemia).

Dietary Considerations Administer with breakfast or the first main meal of the day. Dietary modification based on ADA recommendations is a part of therapy. Decreases blood glucose concentration. Hypoglycemia may occur. Must be able to recognize symptoms of hypoglycemia (palpitations, sweaty palms, lightheadedness).

Pharmacodynamics/Kinetics

Onset of action: Peak effect: Blood glucose reductions: 2-3 hours

Duration: 24 hours

(Continued)

Glimepiride *(Continued)*

Absorption: 100%; delayed when given with food

Distribution: V$_d$: 8.8 L

Protein binding: >99.5%

Metabolism: Hepatic oxidation via CYP2C9 to M1 metabolite (~33% activity of parent compound); further oxidative metabolism to inactive M2 metabolite

Half-life elimination: 5-9 hours

Time to peak, plasma: 2-3 hours

Excretion: Urine (60%, 80% to 90% M1 and M2); feces (40%, 70% M1 and M2)

Pregnancy Risk Factor C

Dosage Forms

Tablet: 1 mg, 2 mg, 4 mg

Amaryl®: 1 mg, 2 mg, 4 mg

Glimepiride and Pioglitazone *see* Pioglitazone and Glimepiride *on page 1309*

Glimepiride and Pioglitazone Hydrochloride *see* Pioglitazone and Glimepiride *on page 1309*

Glimepiride and Rosiglitazone Maleate *see* Rosiglitazone and Glimepiride *on page 1446*

GlipiZIDE (GLIP i zide)

Related Information

Endocrine Disorders and Pregnancy *on page 1750*

U.S. Brand Names Glucotrol®; Glucotrol® XL

Mexican Brand Names Glupitel; Minodiab

Generic Available Yes

Index Terms Glydiazinamide

Pharmacologic Category Antidiabetic Agent, Sulfonylurea

Use Management of type 2 diabetes mellitus (noninsulin dependent, NIDDM)

Local Anesthetic/Vasoconstrictor Precautions No information available to require special precautions

Effects on Dental Treatment Glipizide-dependent diabetics (noninsulin dependent, type 2) should be appointed for dental treatment in morning in order to minimize chance of stress-induced hypoglycemia.

Common Adverse Effects Frequency not defined.

Cardiovascular: Edema, syncope

Central nervous system: Anxiety, depression, dizziness, drowsiness, headache, hypoesthesia, insomnia, nervousness, pain

Dermatologic: Eczema, erythema, maculopapular eruptions, morbilliform eruptions, photosensitivity, pruritus, rash, urticaria

Endocrine & metabolic: Disulfiram-like reaction, hypoglycemia, hyponatremia, SIADH (rare)

Gastrointestinal: Anorexia, constipation, diarrhea, epigatsric fullness, flatulence, gastralgia, hearburn, nausea, vomiting

Hematologic: Agranulocytopenia, aplastic anemia, blood dyscrasias, hemolytic anemia, leukopenia, pancytopenia, porphyria cutanea tarda, thrombocytopenia

Hepatic: Cholestatic jaundice, hepatic porphyria

Neuromuscular & skeletal: Arthralgia, leg cramps, myalgia, paresthesia, tremor

Ocular: Blurred vision

Renal: Diuretic effect (minor)

Respiratory: Rhinitis

Miscellaneous: Diaphoresis

Dosage Oral (allow several days between dose titrations): Adults: Initial: 5 mg/day; adjust dosage at 2.5-5 mg daily increments as determined by blood glucose response at intervals of several days.

Immediate release tablet: Maximum recommended once-daily dose: 15 mg; maximum recommended total daily dose: 40 mg. Doses >15 mg/day should be administered in divided doses.

Extended release tablet (Glucotrol® XL): Maximum recommended dose: 20 mg

When transferring from insulin to glipizide:

Current insulin requirement ≤20 units: Discontinue insulin and initiate glipizide at usual dose

Current insulin requirement >20 units: Decrease insulin by 50% and initiate glipizide at usual dose; gradually decrease insulin dose based on patient response. Several days should elapse between dosage changes.

Elderly: Initial: 2.5 mg/day; increase by 2.5-5 mg/day at 1- to 2-week intervals

Dosing adjustment/comments in renal impairment: Cl$_{cr}$ <10 mL/minute: Some investigators recommend not using

Dosing adjustment in hepatic impairment: Initial dosage should be 2.5 mg/day

Mechanism of Action Stimulates insulin release from the pancreatic beta cells; reduces glucose output from the liver; insulin sensitivity is increased at peripheral target sites

Contraindications Hypersensitivity to glipizide or any component of the formulation, other sulfonamides; type 1 diabetes mellitus (insulin dependent, IDDM); diabetic ketoacidosis

Warnings/Precautions All sulfonylurea drugs are capable of producing severe hypoglycemia. Hypoglycemia is more likely to occur when caloric intake is deficient, after severe or prolonged exercise, when ethanol is ingested, or when more than one glucose-lowering drug is used. It is also more likely in elderly patients, malnourished patients and in patients with impaired renal or hepatic function; use with caution.

Chemical similarities are present among sulfonamides, sulfonylureas, carbonic anhydrase inhibitors, thiazides, and loop diuretics (except ethacrynic acid). Use in patients with sulfonamide allergy is specifically contraindicated in product labeling, however, a risk of cross-reaction exists in patients with allergy to any of these compounds; avoid use when previous reaction has been severe.

Product labeling states oral hypoglycemic drugs may be associated with an increased cardiovascular mortality as compared to treatment with diet alone or diet plus insulin. Data to support this association are limited, and several studies, including a large prospective trial (UKPDS) have not supported an association.

Use with caution in patients with severe hepatic disease. It may be necessary to discontinue therapy and administer insulin if the patient is exposed to stress (fever, trauma, infection, surgery). Safety and efficacy have not been established in children.

Avoid use of extended release tablets (Glucotrol® XL) in patients with known stricture/narrowing of the GI tract.

Drug Interactions
Cytochrome P450 Effect: Substrate of 2C9 (major)
Increased Effect/Toxicity: Beta-blockers decrease hypoglycemic effect and mask most hypoglycemic symptoms. Cyclic antidepressants, fibric acid derivatives, pegvisomant, salicylates (higher doses, not sporadic, low doses) and sulfonamide derivatives (except sulfacetamide) may enhance the hypoglycemic effect of glipizide. Cyclosporine serum concentration is increased; monitor cyclosporine levels and renal function. CYP2C9 inhibitor may increase the levels/effects of glipizide; example inhibitors include delavirdine, fluconazole, gemfibrozil, ketoconazole, nicardipine, NSAIDs, pioglitazone, and sulfonamides). Chloramphenicol and cimetidine may decrease the metabolism of glipizide.
Decreased Effect: CYP2C9 inducers may decrease the levels/effects of glipizide; example inducers include carbamazepine, phenobarbital, phenytoin, rifampin, rifapentine, and secobarbital.

Ethanol/Nutrition/Herb Interactions
Ethanol: Caution with ethanol (may cause hypoglycemia or rare disulfiram reaction).
Food: A delayed release of insulin may occur if glipizide is taken with food. Immediate release tablets should be administered 30 minutes before meals to avoid erratic absorption.
Herb/Nutraceutical: Herbs with hypoglycemic properties may enhance the hypoglycemic effect of glipizide. This includes alfalfa, aloe, bilberry, bitter melon, burdock, celery, damiana, fenugreek, garcinia, garlic, ginger, ginseng (American), gymnema, marshmallow, stinging nettle

Dietary Considerations Take immediate release tablets 30 minutes before meals; extended release tablets should be taken with breakfast. Dietary modification based on ADA recommendations is a part of therapy. Decreases blood glucose concentration. Hypoglycemia may occur. Must be able to recognize symptoms of hypoglycemia (palpitations, sweaty palms, lightheadedness).

Pharmacodynamics/Kinetics
Duration: 12-24 hours
Absorption: Rapid and complete; delayed with food
Distribution: 10-11 L
Protein binding: 98% to 99%; primarily to albumin
Bioavailability: 90% to 100%
Metabolism: Hepatic via CYP2C9; forms metabolites (inactive)
Half-life elimination: 2-5 hours
Time to peak: 1-3 hours; extended release tablets: 6-12 hours
Excretion: Urine (60% to 80%, 91% to 97% as metabolites); feces (11%)

Pregnancy Risk Factor C

(Continued)

GlipiZIDE *(Continued)*

Dosage Forms
    Tablet: 5 mg, 10 mg
      Glucotrol®: 5 mg, 10 mg
    Tablet, extended release:2.5 mg, 5 mg, 10 mg
      Glucotrol® XL: 2.5 mg, 5 mg, 10 mg

Glipizide and Metformin *(GLIP i zide & met FOR min)*

Related Information
    GlipiZIDE *on page 782*
    Metformin *on page 1056*
U.S. Brand Names Metaglip™
Generic Available Yes
Index Terms Glipizide and Metformin Hydrochloride; Metformin and Glipizide
Pharmacologic Category Antidiabetic Agent, Biguanide; Antidiabetic Agent, Sulfonylurea
Use Initial therapy for management of type 2 diabetes mellitus (noninsulin dependent, NIDDM) when hyperglycemia cannot be managed with diet and exercise alone. Second-line therapy for management of type 2 diabetes (NIDDM) when hyperglycemia cannot be managed with a sulfonylurea or metformin along with diet and exercise.
Local Anesthetic/Vasoconstrictor Precautions No information available to require special precautions
Effects on Dental Treatment Key adverse event(s) related to dental treatment: Upper respiratory tract infection (8% to 10%). Dependent diabetics (noninsulin dependent, type 2) should be appointed for dental treatment in the morning in order to minimize chance of stress-induced hypoglycemia.
Common Adverse Effects Also see individual agents.
    >10%:
      Central nervous system: Headache (12%)
      Endocrine & metabolic: Hypoglycemia (8% to 13%)
      Gastrointestinal: Diarrhea (2% to 18%)
    1% to 10%:
      Cardiovascular: Hypertension (3%)
      Central nervous system: Dizziness (2% to 5%)
      Gastrointestinal: Nausea/vomiting (<1% to 8%), abdominal pain (6%)
      Neuromuscular & skeletal: Musculoskeletal pain (8%)
      Renal: Urinary tract infection (1%)
      Respiratory: Upper respiratory tract infection (8% to 10%)
Mechanism of Action The combination of glipizide and metformin is used to improve glycemic control in patients with type 2 diabetes mellitus (noninsulin dependent, NIDDM) by using two different, but complementary, mechanisms of action:
    Glipizide: Stimulates insulin release from the pancreatic beta cells; reduces glucose output from the liver; insulin sensitivity is increased at peripheral target sites
    Metformin: Decreases hepatic glucose production, decreasing intestinal absorption of glucose and improves insulin sensitivity (increases peripheral glucose uptake and utilization)
Drug Interactions
    Cytochrome P450 Effect: Glipizide: **Substrate** of 2C8/9 (major)
    Increased Effect/Toxicity: See individual agents.
    Decreased Effect: See individual agents.
Pharmacodynamics/Kinetics See individual agents.
Pregnancy Risk Factor C

Glipizide and Metformin Hydrochloride *see* Glipizide and Metformin *on page 784*

Glivec *see* Imatinib *on page 863*

Gln *see* Glutamine *on page 786*

GlucaGen® *see* Glucagon *on page 784*

GlucaGen® Diagnostic Kit *see* Glucagon *on page 784*

GlucaGen® HypoKit™ *see* Glucagon *on page 784*

Glucagon *(GLOO ka gon)*

U.S. Brand Names GlucaGen®; GlucaGen® Diagnostic Kit; GlucaGen® HypoKit™; Glucagon Diagnostic Kit [DSC]; Glucagon Emergency Kit
Generic Available No

Index Terms Glucagon Hydrochloride

Pharmacologic Category Antidote; Diagnostic Agent

Use Management of hypoglycemia; diagnostic aid in radiologic examinations to temporarily inhibit GI tract movement

Unlabeled/Investigational Use Used with some success as a cardiac stimulant in management of severe cases of beta-adrenergic blocking agent overdosage; treatment of myocardial depression due to calcium channel blocker overdose

Local Anesthetic/Vasoconstrictor Precautions No information available to require special precautions

Effects on Dental Treatment No significant effects or complications reported

Common Adverse Effects Frequency not defined.

Cardiovascular: Hypotension (up to 2 hours after GI procedures), hypertension, tachycardia

Gastrointestinal: Nausea, vomiting (high incidence with rapid administration of high doses)

Miscellaneous: Hypersensitivity reactions, anaphylaxis

Mechanism of Action Stimulates adenylate cyclase to produce increased cyclic AMP, which promotes hepatic glycogenolysis and gluconeogenesis, causing a raise in blood glucose levels

Drug Interactions

Increased Effect/Toxicity: Oral anticoagulant: Hypoprothrombinemic effects may be increased possibly with bleeding; effect seen with glucagon doses of 50 mg administered over 1-2 days

Pharmacodynamics/Kinetics

Onset of action: Peak effect: Blood glucose levels: Parenteral:

I.V.: 5-20 minutes

I.M.: 30 minutes

SubQ: 30-45 minutes

Duration: Hyperglycemia: 60-90 minutes

Metabolism: Primarily hepatic; some inactivation occurring renally and in plasma

Half-life elimination, plasma: 3-10 minutes

Pregnancy Risk Factor B

Glucagon Diagnostic Kit [DSC] *see* Glucagon *on page 784*

Glucagon Emergency Kit *see* Glucagon *on page 784*

Glucagon Hydrochloride *see* Glucagon *on page 784*

Glucocerebrosidase *see* Alglucerase *on page 69*

Glucophage® *see* Metformin *on page 1056*

Glucophage® XR *see* Metformin *on page 1056*

Glucose *see* Dextrose *on page 478*

Glucose Monohydrate *see* Dextrose *on page 478*

Glucose Polymers (GLOO kose POL i merz)

U.S. Brand Names Moducal® [OTC]; Polycose® [OTC]

Generic Available No

Pharmacologic Category Nutritional Supplement

Use Supplies calories for those persons not able to meet the caloric requirement with usual food intake

Local Anesthetic/Vasoconstrictor Precautions No information available to require special precautions

Effects on Dental Treatment No significant effects or complications reported

Glucotrol® *see* GlipiZIDE *on page 782*

Glucotrol® XL *see* GlipiZIDE *on page 782*

Glucovance® *see* Glyburide and Metformin *on page 787*

Glu-K® [OTC] *see* Potassium Gluconate *on page 1330*

Glulisine Insulin *see* Insulin Glulisine *on page 885*

Glumetza™ *see* Metformin *on page 1056*

Glutamic Acid (gloo TAM ik AS id)

Generic Available Yes

Index Terms Glutamic Acid Hydrochloride

Pharmacologic Category Gastrointestinal Agent, Miscellaneous

Use Treatment of hypochlorhydria and achlorhydria

Local Anesthetic/Vasoconstrictor Precautions No information available to require special precautions

Effects on Dental Treatment No significant effects or complications reported

Pregnancy Risk Factor C

Glutamic Acid Hydrochloride *see* Glutamic Acid *on page 785*

Glutamine (GLOO ta meen)

U.S. Brand Names Enterex® Glutapak-10® [OTC]; NutreStore™; Resource® GlutaSolve® [OTC]; Sympt-X [OTC]; Sympt-X G.I. [OTC]
Index Terms Gln; L-Glutamine
Pharmacologic Category Amino Acid
Use Treatment of short bowel syndrome when used in combination with nutritional support and growth hormone therapy; a medical food used to promote GI tract healing and nutritional supplementation with GI disorders, HIV/AIDS, cancer, and other critical illnesses
Local Anesthetic/Vasoconstrictor Precautions No information available to require special precautions
Effects on Dental Treatment No significant effects or complications reported
Common Adverse Effects Frequency not defined.
Cardiovascular: Facial edema, peripheral edema
Central nervous system: Dizziness, fever, headache, pain
Dermatologic: Pruritus, rash
Gastrointestinal: Abdominal pain, flatulence, nausea, pancreatitis, tenesmus, vomiting
Neuromuscular & skeletal: Arthralgia, back pain, hypoesthesia
Otic: Ear or hearing symptoms
Respiratory: Rhinitis
Miscellaneous: Flu-like syndrome, infection, sepsis
Mechanism of Action Glutamine regulates gastrointestinal cell growth, function, and regeneration. Considered a "conditionally essential" amino acid during metabolic stress and injury.
Pharmacodynamics/Kinetics As reported in healthy adults; parameters may vary following oral administration in patients with short bowel syndrome.
Distribution: I.V.: V_d: 200 mL/kg
Metabolism: Via splanchnic tissue, lymphocytes, kidney, and liver to glutamate and ammonia
Half-life elimination: I.V.: 1 hour
Pregnancy Risk Factor C

Glutofac®-MX *see* Vitamins (Multiple/Oral) *on page 1665*

Glutofac®-ZX *see* Vitamins (Multiple/Oral) *on page 1665*

Glutol™ [OTC] *see* Dextrose *on page 478*

Glutose™ [OTC] *see* Dextrose *on page 478*

Glybenclamide *see* GlyBURIDE *on page 786*

Glybenzcyclamide *see* GlyBURIDE *on page 786*

GlyBURIDE (GLYE byoor ide)

Related Information
Endocrine Disorders and Pregnancy *on page 1750*
U.S. Brand Names Diaβeta®; Glynase® PresTab®; Micronase®
Canadian Brand Names Albert® Glyburide; Apo-Glyburide®; Diaβeta®; Euglucon®; Gen-Glybe; Novo-Glyburide; Nu-Glyburide; PMS-Glyburide; ratio-Glyburide; Sandoz-Glyburide
Mexican Brand Names Daonil; Euglucon; Glucal; Norboral
Generic Available Yes
Index Terms Diabeta; Glibenclamide; Glybenclamide; Glybenzcyclamide
Pharmacologic Category Antidiabetic Agent, Sulfonylurea
Use Management of type 2 diabetes mellitus (noninsulin dependent, NIDDM)
Unlabeled/Investigational Use Alternative to insulin in women for the treatment of gestational diabetes (11-33 weeks gestation)
Local Anesthetic/Vasoconstrictor Precautions No information available to require special precautions
Effects on Dental Treatment Glyburide-dependent diabetics (noninsulin dependent, type 2) should be appointed for dental treatment in morning in order to minimize chance of stress-induced hypoglycemia.
Common Adverse Effects Frequency not defined.
Cardiovascular: Vasculitis
Central nervous system: Headache, dizziness
Dermatologic: Erythema, maculopapular eruptions, morbilliform eruptions, pruritus, purpura, rash, urticaria, photosensitivity reaction

Endocrine & metabolic: Disulfiram-like reaction, hypoglycemia, hyponatremia (SIADH reported with other sulfonylureas)

Gastrointestinal: Nausea, epigastric fullness, heartburn, constipation, diarrhea, anorexia

Genitourinary: Nocturia

Hematologic: Leukopenia, thrombocytopenia, hemolytic anemia, agranulocytosis, aplastic anemia, pancytopenia, porphyria cutanea tarda

Hepatic: Cholestatic jaundice, hepatitis, transaminase increased

Neuromuscular & skeletal: Arthralgia, myalgia, paresthesia

Ocular: Blurred vision

Renal: Diuretic effect (minor)

Miscellaneous: Allergic reaction

Mechanism of Action Stimulates insulin release from the pancreatic beta cells; reduces glucose output from the liver; insulin sensitivity is increased at peripheral target sites

Drug Interactions

Cytochrome P450 Effect: Inhibits CYP2C8 (weak), 3A4 (weak)

Increased Effect/Toxicity: Cyclic antidepressants, fibric acid derivatives, pegvisomant, quinolone antibiotics, salicylates (regular, higher doses, not sporadic, low doses), and sulfonamide derivatives (except sulfacetamide) may enhance the hypoglycemic effect of glyburide. Beta-blockers may enhance the hypoglycemic effect of glyburide and mask tachycardia as an initial symptom of hypoglycemia. Chloramphenicol and cimetidine may decrease the metabolism of glyburide. Fluconazole may increase the serum concentration of glyburide.

Glyburide may enhance the hepatotoxic effect and increase the metabolism of bosentan; concomitant use is contraindicated. Glyburide may increase the serum concentration of cyclosporine.

Decreased Effect: Bosentan may increase the metabolism of glyburide; concomitant use is contraindicated. Rifampin may increase the metabolism, of glyburide.

Pharmacodynamics/Kinetics

Onset of action: Serum insulin levels begin to increase 15-60 minutes after a single dose

Duration: ≤24 hours

Absorption: Significant within 1 hour

Distribution: 9-10 L

Protein binding, plasma: >99% primarily to albumin

Metabolism: Hepatic; forms metabolites (weakly active)

Half-life elimination: Diabeta®, Micronase®: 10 hours; Glynase® PresTab®: ~4 hours; may be prolonged with renal or hepatic impairment

Time to peak, serum: Adults: 2-4 hours

Excretion: Feces (50%) and urine (50%) as metabolites

Pregnancy Risk Factor B/C (manufacturer dependent)

Glyburide and Metformin (GLYE byoor ide & met FOR min)

Related Information

Endocrine Disorders and Pregnancy on page 1750
GlyBURIDE on page 786
Metformin on page 1056

U.S. Brand Names Glucovance®

Mexican Brand Names Bi-Euglucon M "5"

Generic Available Yes

Index Terms Glyburide and Metformin Hydrochloride; Metformin and Glyburide

Pharmacologic Category Antidiabetic Agent, Biguanide; Antidiabetic Agent, Sulfonylurea

Use Initial therapy for management of type 2 diabetes mellitus (noninsulin dependent, NIDDM). Second-line therapy for management of type 2 diabetes (NIDDM) when hyperglycemia cannot be managed with a sulfonylurea or metformin; combination therapy with a thiazolidinedione may be required to achieve additional control.

Local Anesthetic/Vasoconstrictor Precautions No information available to require special precautions

Effects on Dental Treatment Glyburide-dependent diabetics (noninsulin dependent, type 2) should be appointed for dental treatment in morning in order to minimize chance of stress-induced hypoglycemia. Metformin-dependent diabetics (noninsulin dependent, type 2) should be appointed for dental treatment in morning in order to minimize chance of stress-induced hypoglycemia. (Continued)

Glyburide and Metformin *(Continued)*

Common Adverse Effects (Also refer to individual agents)

>10%:

Endocrine & metabolic: Hypoglycemia (11% to 38%, effects higher when increased doses were used as initial therapy)

Gastrointestinal: Diarrhea (17%)

Respiratory: Upper respiratory infection (17%)

1% to 10%:

Central nervous system: Headache (9%), dizziness (6%)

Gastrointestinal: Nausea (8%), vomiting (8%), abdominal pain (7%) (combined GI effects increased to 38% in patients taking high doses as initial therapy)

Dosage Note: Dose must be individualized. Dosages expressed as glyburide/metformin components.

Adults: Oral:

Initial therapy (no prior treatment with sulfonylurea or metformin): 1.25 mg/250 mg once daily with a meal; patients with Hb A_{1c} >9% or fasting plasma glucose (FPG) >200 mg/dL may start with 1.25 mg/250 mg twice daily

Dosage may be increased in increments of 1.25 mg/250 mg, at intervals of not less than 2 weeks; maximum daily dose: 10 mg/2000 mg (limited experience with higher doses)

Previously treated with a sulfonylurea or metformin alone: Initial: 2.5 mg/500 mg or 5 mg/500 mg twice daily; increase in increments no greater than 5 mg/500 mg; maximum daily dose: 20 mg/2000 mg

When switching patients previously on a sulfonylurea and metformin together, do not exceed the daily dose of glyburide (or glyburide equivalent) or metformin.

Note: May combine with a thiazolidinedione in patients with an inadequate response to glyburide/metformin therapy (risk of hypoglycemia may be increased).

Elderly: Oral: Conservative doses are recommended in the elderly due to potentially decreased renal function; **do not titrate to maximum dose**; should not be used in patients ≥80 years of age unless renal function is verified as normal

Dosage adjustment in renal impairment: Risk of lactic acidosis increases with degree of renal impairment; contraindicated in renal disease or renal dysfunction (see Contraindications)

Dosage adjustment in hepatic impairment: Use conservative initial and maintenance doses and avoid use in severe hepatic disease

Mechanism of Action The combination of glyburide and metformin is used to improve glycemic control in patients with type 2 diabetes mellitus by using two different, but complementary, mechanisms of action:

Glyburide: Stimulates insulin release from the pancreatic beta cells; reduces glucose output from the liver; insulin sensitivity is increased at peripheral target sites

Metformin: Decreases hepatic glucose production, decreasing intestinal absorption of glucose and improves insulin sensitivity (increases peripheral glucose uptake and utilization)

Contraindications Hypersensitivity to glyburide or other sulfonamides, metformin, or any component of the formulation; renal disease or renal dysfunction (serum creatinine ≥1.5 mg/dL in males or ≥1.4 mg/dL in females, or abnormal creatinine clearance which may also result from conditions such as cardiovascular collapse, acute myocardial infarction, and septicemia); acute or chronic metabolic acidosis with or without coma (including diabetic ketoacidosis); congestive heart failure requiring pharmacologic treatment

Note: Temporarily discontinue in patients undergoing radiologic studies in which intravascular iodinated contrast materials are utilized.

Warnings/Precautions Age, hepatic and renal impairment are independent risk factors for hypoglycemia. Use with caution in patients with hepatic impairment, malnourished or debilitated conditions, or adrenal or pituitary insufficiency. Use caution in patients with renal impairment.

[U.S. Boxed Warning]: Lactic acidosis is a rare, but potentially severe consequence of therapy with metformin. Withhold therapy in hypoxemia, dehydration, or sepsis. The risk of lactic acidosis is increased in any patient with CHF requiring pharmacologic management. This risk is particularly high during acute or unstable CHF because of the risk of hypoperfusion and hypoxemia. Metformin is substantially excreted by the kidney. The risk of accumulation and lactic acidosis increases with the degree of impairment of renal function. Patients with renal function below the limit of normal for their age should not receive metformin. In elderly patients, renal function should be monitored regularly; should not be used in any patient ≥80 years of age unless measurement of creatinine clearance verifies normal renal function. Use of concomitant medications that may affect renal function (ie, affect tubular secretion) may also affect metformin disposition. Metformin should be suspended in patients with dehydration and/or prerenal azotemia. Therapy should be suspended for any surgical procedures (resume only after normal intake resumed and normal renal function is verified).Intravascular iodinated contrast materials used for radiologic studies are associated with alteration of renal function and may increase risk of lactic acidosis. Discontinue Glucovance® at the time of or prior to the procedure and withhold for 48 hours subsequent to the procedure; reinstitute only after renal function function has been re-evaluated and found to be normal.

Chemical similarities are present among sulfonamides, sulfonylureas, carbonic anhydrase inhibitors, thiazides, and loop diuretics (except ethacrynic acid). Use in patients with sulfonamide allergy is specifically contraindicated in product labeling, however a risk of cross-reaction exists in patients with allergy to any of these compounds; avoid use when previous reaction has been severe.

Product labeling states oral hypoglycemic drugs may be associated with an increased cardiovascular mortality as compared to treatment with diet alone or diet plus insulin. Data to support this association are limited, and several studies, including a large prospective trial (UKPDS), have not supported an association.

Drug Interactions
  Increased Effect/Toxicity: See individual agents.
  Decreased Effect: See individual agents.
Ethanol/Nutrition/Herb Interactions
  Ethanol: May cause hypoglycemia; incidence of lactic acidosis may be increased; a disulfiram-like reaction characterized by flushing, headache, nausea, vomiting, sweating, or tachycardia has been reported with sulfonylureas; avoid or limit use.
  Food: Metformin decreases absorption of vitamin B_{12}. Metformin decreases absorption of folic acid.
Dietary Considerations May cause GI upset; take with food to decrease GI upset. Dietary modification based on ADA recommendations is a part of therapy. Decreases blood glucose concentration. Hypoglycemia may occur. Must be able to recognize symptoms of hypoglycemia (palpitations, sweaty palms, lightheadedness). Monitor for signs and symptoms of vitamin B_{12} deficiency. Monitor for signs and symptoms of folic acid deficiency.
Pharmacodynamics/Kinetics
  Glucovance®:
    Bioavailability: 18% with 2.5 mg glyburide/500 mg metformin dose; 7% with 5 mg glyburide/500 mg metformin dose; bioavailability is greater than that of Micronase® brand of glyburide and therefore not bioequivalent
    Time to peak: 2.75 hours when taken with food
  Glyburide: See Glyburide monograph.
  Metformin: This component of Glucovance® is bioequivalent to metformin coadministration with glyburide.
Pregnancy Risk Factor B (manufacturer); C (expert analysis)
Dosage Forms
  Tablet: Glyburide 1.25 mg and metformin 250 mg; glyburide 2.5 mg and metformin 500 mg; glyburide 5 mg and metformin 500 mg
    Glucovance®: 1.25 mg/250 mg: Glyburide 1.25 mg and metformin 250 mg; 2.5 mg/500 mg: Glyburide 2.5 mg and metformin 500 mg; 5 mg/500 mg: Glyburide 5 mg and metformin 500 mg

Glyburide and Metformin Hydrochloride see Glyburide and Metformin on page 787

Glycerin (GLIS er in)

U.S. Brand Names Bausch & Lomb® Computer Eye Drops [OTC]; Colace® Adult/Children Suppositories [OTC]; Colace® Infant/Children Suppositories [OTC]; Fleet® Babylax® [OTC]; Fleet® Glycerin Suppositories [OTC]; Fleet® Glycerin Suppositories Maximum Strength [OTC]; Fleet® Liquid Glycerin Suppositories [OTC]; Osmoglyn® [DSC]; Sani-Supp® [OTC]
Generic Available Yes: Suppositories
Index Terms Glycerol
Pharmacologic Category Laxative, Osmotic; Ophthalmic Agent, Miscellaneous
Use Constipation; reduction of intraocular pressure; reduction of corneal edema; glycerin has been administered orally to reduce intracranial pressure
Local Anesthetic/Vasoconstrictor Precautions No information available to require special precautions
Effects on Dental Treatment No significant effects or complications reported
(Continued)

Glycerin (Continued)

Common Adverse Effects Frequency not defined.
Cardiovascular: Arrhythmias
Central nervous system: Headache, confusion, dizziness, hyperosmolar nonketotic coma
Endocrine: Polydipsia, hyperglycemia, dehydration
Gastrointestinal: Nausea, vomiting, tenesmus, rectal irritation, cramping pain, diarrhea, dry mouth

Mechanism of Action Osmotic dehydrating agent which increases osmotic pressure; draws fluid into colon and thus stimulates evacuation

Pharmacodynamics/Kinetics
Onset of action:
Decrease in intraocular pressure: Oral: 10-30 minutes
Reduction of intracranial pressure: Oral: 10-60 minutes
Constipation: Suppository: 15-30 minutes
Peak effect:
Decrease in intraocular pressure: Oral: 60-90 minutes
Reduction of intracranial pressure: Oral: 60-90 minutes
Duration:
Decrease in intraocular pressure: Oral: 4-8 hours
Reduction of intracranial pressure: Oral: ~2-3 hours
Absorption: Oral: Well absorbed; Rectal: Poorly absorbed
Half-life elimination, serum: 30-45 minutes

Pregnancy Risk Factor C

Glycerol see Glycerin on page 789
Glycerol Guaiacolate see Guaifenesin on page 795
Glycerol Triacetate see Triacetin on page 1608
Glyceryl Trinitrate see Nitroglycerin on page 1181
GlycoLax® see Polyethylene Glycol 3350 on page 1321

Glycopyrrolate (glye koe PYE roe late)

U.S. Brand Names Robinul®; Robinul® Forte
Canadian Brand Names Glycopyrrolate Injection, USP
Generic Available Yes
Index Terms Glycopyrronium Bromide
Pharmacologic Category Anticholinergic Agent
Use Inhibit salivation and excessive secretions of the respiratory tract preoperatively; reversal of neuromuscular blockade; control of upper airway secretions; adjunct in treatment of peptic ulcer
Local Anesthetic/Vasoconstrictor Precautions No information available to require special precautions
Effects on Dental Treatment Key adverse event(s) related to dental treatment: Significant xerostomia (normal salivary flow resumes upon discontinuation).
Common Adverse Effects Frequency not defined. **Note:** Includes adverse effects which may occur as an extension of the pharmacologic action of anticholinergics (including glycopyrrolate) and adverse effects reported postmarketing with glycopyrrolate.
Cardiovascular: Arrhythmias, cardiac arrest, heart block, hyper-/hypotension, malignant hyperthermia, palpitation, QT_c interval prolongation, tachycardia
Central nervous system: Confusion, dizziness, drowsiness, excitement, headache, insomnia, nervousness, seizures
Dermatologic: Dry skin, pruritus, sensitivity to light increased
Endocrine & metabolic: Lactation suppression
Gastrointestinal: Bloated feeling, constipation, loss of taste, nausea, vomiting, xerostomia
Genitourinary: Impotence, urinary hesitancy, urinary retention
Local: Irritation at injection site
Neuromuscular & skeletal: Weakness
Ocular: Blurred vision, cycloplegia, mydriasis, ocular tension increased, photophobia, sensitivity to light increased
Respiratory: Respiratory depression
Miscellaneous: Anaphylactoid reactions, diaphoresis decreased, hypersensitivity reactions

Mechanism of Action Blocks the action of acetylcholine at parasympathetic sites in smooth muscle, secretory glands, and the CNS

Drug Interactions
Increased Effect/Toxicity: Effects of other anticholinergic agents or medications with anticholinergic activity may be increased by glycopyrrolate. Severity of potassium chloride-induced gastrointestinal lesions (when potassium is

given in a wax matrix formulation, eg, Klor-Con®) may be increased by glycopyrrolate. Pramlinitide may enhance the anticholinergic effects of
anticholinergics (effects are specific to the GI tract).

Pharmacodynamics/Kinetics

Onset of action: Oral: 50 minutes; I.M.: 15-30 minutes; I.V.: ~1 minute

Peak effect: Oral: ~1 hour; I.M.: 30-45 minutes

Duration: Vagal effect: 2-3 hours; Inhibition of salivation: Up to 7 hours; Anticholinergic: Oral: 8-12 hours

Absorption: Oral: Poor and erratic

Distribution: V_d: 0.2-0.62 L/kg

Metabolism: Hepatic (minimal)

Bioavailability: ~10%

Half-life elimination: Infants: 22-130 minutes; Children 19-99 minutes; Adults: ~30-75 minutes

Excretion: Urine (as unchanged drug, I.M.: 80%, I.V.: 85%); bile (as unchanged drug)

Pregnancy Risk Factor B

Glycopyrronium Bromide see Glycopyrrolate on page 790

Glycosum see Dextrose on page 478

Glydiazinamide see GlipiZIDE on page 782

Glynase® PresTab® see GlyBURIDE on page 786

Gly-Oxide® [OTC] see Carbamide Peroxide on page 276

Glyquin® see Hydroquinone on page 841

Glyquin-XM™ see Hydroquinone on page 841

Glyset® see Miglitol on page 1104

GM-CSF see Sargramostim on page 1456

GnRH see Gonadorelin on page 792

GnRH Agonist see Histrelin on page 814

Gold Bond® Antifungal [OTC] [DSC] see Tolnaftate on page 1587

Gold Sodium Thiomalate (gold SOW dee um thye oh MAL ate)

Related Information

Rheumatoid Arthritis, Osteoarthritis, and Osteoporosis on page 1759

U.S. Brand Names Aurolate®

Canadian Brand Names Myochrysine®

Generic Available No

Pharmacologic Category Gold Compound

Use Treatment of progressive rheumatoid arthritis

Local Anesthetic/Vasoconstrictor Precautions No information available to require special precautions

Effects on Dental Treatment Key adverse event(s) related to dental treatment: Stomatitis, gingivitis, and glossitis.

Common Adverse Effects

>10%:

Dermatologic: Itching, rash

Gastrointestinal: Stomatitis, gingivitis, glossitis

Ocular: Conjunctivitis

1% to 10%:

Dermatologic: Urticaria, alopecia

Hematologic: Eosinophilia, leukopenia, thrombocytopenia

Renal: Proteinuria, hematuria

Mechanism of Action Unknown, may decrease prostaglandin synthesis or may alter cellular mechanisms by inhibiting sulfhydryl systems

Drug Interactions

Increased Effect/Toxicity: ACE inhibitors may enhance the adverse/toxic effects (nitritoid reaction) of gold sodium thiomalate.

Decreased Effect: Penicillamine and acetylcysteine may decrease effect of gold sodium thiomalate.

Pharmacodynamics/Kinetics

Onset of action: Delayed; may require up to 3 months

Half-life elimination: 5 days; may be prolonged with multiple doses

Time to peak, serum: 4-6 hours

Excretion: Urine (60% to 90%); feces (10% to 40%)

Pregnancy Risk Factor C

GoLYTELY® see Polyethylene Glycol-Electrolyte Solution on page 1321

Gonadorelin (goe nad oh RELL in)

U.S. Brand Names Factrel®
Canadian Brand Names Lutrepulse™
Generic Available No
Index Terms GnRH; Gonadorelin Acetate; Gonadorelin Hydrochloride; Gonadotropin Releasing Hormone; LHRH; LRH; Luteinizing Hormone Releasing Hormone
Pharmacologic Category Diagnostic Agent; Gonadotropin
Use Evaluation of functional capacity and response of gonadotrophic hormones; evaluate abnormal gonadotropin regulation as in precocious puberty and delayed puberty.
    Orphan drug: Lutrepulse®: Induction of ovulation in females with hypothalamic amenorrhea
Local Anesthetic/Vasoconstrictor Precautions No information available to require special precautions
Effects on Dental Treatment No significant effects or complications reported
Common Adverse Effects 1% to 10%: Local: Pain at injection site
Mechanism of Action Stimulates the release of luteinizing hormone (LH) from the anterior pituitary gland
Drug Interactions
    Increased Effect/Toxicity: Increased levels/effect with androgens, estrogens, progestins, glucocorticoids, spironolactone, and levodopa.
    Decreased Effect: Decreased levels/effect with oral contraceptives, digoxin, phenothiazines, and dopamine antagonists.
Pharmacodynamics/Kinetics
    Onset of action: Peak effect: Maximal LH release: ~20 minutes
    Duration: 3-5 hours
    Half-life elimination: 4 minutes
Pregnancy Risk Factor B

Gonadorelin Acetate *see* Gonadorelin *on page 792*

Gonadorelin Hydrochloride *see* Gonadorelin *on page 792*

Gonadotropin Releasing Hormone *see* Gonadorelin *on page 792*

Gonak™ [OTC] *see* Hydroxypropyl Methylcellulose *on page 844*

Gonal-f® *see* Follitropin Alfa *on page 738*

Gonal-f® RFF *see* Follitropin Alfa *on page 738*

Gonioscopic Ophthalmic Solution *see* Hydroxypropyl Methylcellulose *on page 844*

Goniosoft™ *see* Hydroxypropyl Methylcellulose *on page 844*

Goniosol® [OTC] [DSC] *see* Hydroxypropyl Methylcellulose *on page 844*

Good Sense Sleep Aid [OTC] *see* Doxylamine *on page 544*

Goody's® Extra Strength Headache Powder [OTC] *see* Acetaminophen, Aspirin, and Caffeine *on page 41*

Goody's® Extra Strength Pain Relief [OTC] *see* Acetaminophen, Aspirin, and Caffeine *on page 41*

Goody's PM® [OTC] *see* Acetaminophen and Diphenhydramine *on page 38*

Gordofilm® [OTC] *see* Salicylic Acid *on page 1451*

Gordon Boro-Packs [OTC] *see* Aluminum Sulfate and Calcium Acetate *on page 83*

Gormel® [OTC] *see* Urea *on page 1632*

Goserelin (GOE se rel in)

U.S. Brand Names Zoladex®
Canadian Brand Names Zoladex®; Zoladex® LA
Generic Available No
Index Terms D-Ser(Bu^t)^6,Azgly^{10}-LHRH; Goserelin Acetate; ICI-118630; NSC-606864
Pharmacologic Category Gonadotropin Releasing Hormone Agonist
Use Palliative treatment of advanced breast cancer and carcinoma of the prostate; treatment of endometriosis, including pain relief and reduction of endometriotic lesions; endometrial thinning agent as part of treatment for dysfunctional uterine bleeding
Local Anesthetic/Vasoconstrictor Precautions No information available to require special precautions
Effects on Dental Treatment Key adverse event(s) related to dental treatment: Xerostomia (normal salivary flow resumes upon discontinuation) and taste disturbances.

Common Adverse Effects Percentages reported in males with prostatic carcinoma and females with endometriosis using the 1-month implant:

>10%:

Central nervous system: Headache (female 75%, male 1% to 5%), emotional lability (female 60%), depression (female 54%, male 1% to 5%), pain (female 17%, male 8%), insomnia (female 11%, male 5%)

Endocrine & metabolic: Hot flashes (female 96%, male 62%), sexual dysfunction (21%), erections decreased (18%), libido decreased (female 61%), breast enlargement (female 18%)

Genitourinary: Lower urinary symptoms (male 13%), vaginitis (75%), dyspareunia (female 14%)

Miscellaneous: Diaphoresis (female 45%, male 6%); infection (female 13%)

1% to 10%:

Cardiovascular: CHF (male 5%), arrhythmia, cerebrovascular accident, hypertension, MI, peripheral vascular disorder, chest pain, palpitation, tachycardia, edema

Central nervous system: Lethargy (male 8%), dizziness (female 6%, male 5%), abnormal thinking, anxiety, chills, fever, malaise, migraine, somnolence

Dermatologic: Rash (female >1%, male 6%), alopecia, bruising, dry skin, skin discoloration

Endocrine & metabolic: Breast pain (female 7%), breast swelling/tenderness (male 1% to 5%), dysmenorrhea, gout, hyperglycemia

Gastrointestinal: Anorexia (female >1%, male 5%), nausea (male 5%), constipation, diarrhea, flatulence, dyspepsia, ulcer, vomiting, weight increased, xerostomia

Genitourinary: Renal insufficiency, urinary frequency, urinary obstruction, urinary tract infection, vaginal hemorrhage

Hematologic: Anemia, hemorrhage

Neuromuscular & skeletal: Arthralgia, bone mineral density decreased (female; ~4% decrease in 6 months), joint disorder, paresthesia

Ocular: Amblyopia, dry eyes

Respiratory: Upper respiratory tract infection (male 7%), COPD (male 5%), pharyngitis (female 5%), bronchitis, cough, epistaxis, rhinitis, sinusitis

Miscellaneous: Allergic reaction

Mechanism of Action Goserelin is a synthetic analog of luteinizing-hormone-releasing hormone (LHRH). Following an initial increase in luteinizing hormone (LH) and follicle stimulating hormone (FSH), chronic administration of goserelin results in a sustained suppression of pituitary gonadotropins. Serum testosterone falls to levels comparable to surgical castration. The exact mechanism of this effect is unknown, but may be related to changes in the control of LH or down-regulation of LH receptors.

Pharmacodynamics/Kinetics Note: Data reported using the 1-month implant.

Absorption: SubQ: Rapid and can be detected in serum in 10 minutes

Distribution: V_d: Male: 44.1 L; Female: 20.3 L

Time to peak, serum: SubQ: Male: 12-15 days, Female: 8-22 days

Half-life elimination: SubQ: Male: ~4 hours, Female: ~2 hours; Renal impairment: Male: 12 hours

Excretion: Urine (90%)

Pregnancy Risk Factor X (endometriosis, endometrial thinning); D (advanced breast cancer)

Goserelin Acetate *see* Goserelin *on page 792*

GP 47680 *see* Oxcarbazepine *on page 1221*

GR38032R *see* Ondansetron *on page 1209*

Gramicidin, Neomycin, and Polymyxin B *see* Neomycin, Polymyxin B, and Gramicidin *on page 1161*

Granisetron (gra NI se tron)

U.S. Brand Names Kytril®
Canadian Brand Names Kytril®
Mexican Brand Names Kytril
Generic Available No
Index Terms BRL 43694
Pharmacologic Category Antiemetic; Selective 5-HT$_3$ Receptor Antagonist
Use Prophylaxis of nausea and vomiting associated with emetogenic chemotherapy and radiation therapy, (including total body irradiation and fractionated abdominal radiation); prophylaxis and treatment of postoperative nausea and vomiting (PONV)

Generally **not** recommended for treatment of existing chemotherapy-induced emesis (CIE) or for prophylaxis of nausea from agents with a low emetogenic potential.

(Continued)

Granisetron *(Continued)*

Local Anesthetic/Vasoconstrictor Precautions No information available to require special precautions

Effects on Dental Treatment No significant effects or complications reported

Common Adverse Effects
>10%:
Central nervous system: Headache (9% to 21%)
Gastrointestinal: Constipation (3% to 18%)
Neuromuscular & skeletal: Weakness (5% to 18%)
1% to 10%:
Cardiovascular: Hypertension (1% to 2%)
Central nervous system: Pain (10%), fever (3% to 9%), dizziness (4% to 5%), insomnia (<2% to 5%), somnolence (1% to 4%), anxiety (2%), agitation (<2%), CNS stimulation (<2%)
Dermatologic: Rash (1%)
Gastrointestinal: Diarrhea (3% to 9%), abdominal pain (4% to 6%), dyspepsia (3% to 6%), taste perversion (2%)
Hepatic: Liver enzymes increased (5% to 6%)
Renal: Oliguria (2%)
Respiratory: Cough (2%)
Miscellaneous: Infection (3%)

Mechanism of Action Selective 5-HT$_3$-receptor antagonist, blocking serotonin, both peripherally on vagal nerve terminals and centrally in the chemoreceptor trigger zone

Drug Interactions
Cytochrome P450 Effect: Substrate of CYP3A4 (minor)
Increased Effect/Toxicity: Granisetron may enhance the hypotensive effect of apomorphine.

Pharmacodynamics/Kinetics
Duration: Generally up to 24 hours
Absorption: Tablets and oral solution are bioequivalent
Distribution: V$_d$: 2-4 L/kg; widely throughout body
Protein binding: 65%
Metabolism: Hepatic via N-demethylation, oxidation, and conjugation; some metabolites may have 5-HT$_3$ antagonist activity
Half-life elimination: Terminal: 5-9 hours
Excretion: Urine (12% as unchanged drug, 48% to 49% as metabolites); feces (34% to 38% as metabolites)

Pregnancy Risk Factor B

Granulex® *see* Trypsin, Balsam Peru, and Castor Oil *on page 1628*

Granulocyte Colony Stimulating Factor *see* Filgrastim *on page 691*

Granulocyte Colony Stimulating Factor (PEG Conjugate) *see* Pegfilgrastim *on page 1261*

Granulocyte-Macrophage Colony Stimulating Factor *see* Sargramostim *on page 1456*

Grifulvin® V *see* Griseofulvin *on page 794*

Griseofulvin *(gri see oh FUL vin)*

U.S. Brand Names Grifulvin® V; Gris-PEG®
Mexican Brand Names Fulvina P G; Grisovin
Generic Available Yes: Suspension, ultramicrosized product
Index Terms Griseofulvin Microsize; Griseofulvin Ultramicrosize
Pharmacologic Category Antifungal Agent, Oral
Use Treatment of susceptible tinea infections of the skin, hair, and nails
Local Anesthetic/Vasoconstrictor Precautions No information available to require special precautions
Effects on Dental Treatment Key adverse event(s) related to dental treatment: May cause soreness or irritation of mouth or tongue. May cause oral thrush.

Common Adverse Effects Frequency not defined.
Central nervous system: Dizziness, fatigue, headache, insomnia, mental confusion
Dermatologic: Angioneurotic edema (rare), erythema multiforme-like drug reaction, photosensitivity, rash (most common), urticaria (most common),
Gastrointestinal: Nausea, vomiting, epigastric distress, diarrhea, GI bleeding
Genitourinary: Menstrual irregularities (rare)
Hematologic: Granulocytopenia, leukopenia
Hepatic: Hepatotoxicity
Neuromuscular & skeletal: Paresthesia (rare)
Renal: Nephrosis, proteinuria

Miscellaneous: Drug-induced lupus-like syndrome (rare), oral thrush

Mechanism of Action Inhibits fungal cell mitosis at metaphase; binds to human keratin making it resistant to fungal invasion

Drug Interactions

Cytochrome P450 Effect: Induces CYP1A2 (weak), 2C8 (weak), 2C9 (weak), 3A4 (weak)

Decreased Effect: Barbiturates may decrease levels/effects of griseofulvin. Griseofulvin may decrease the levels/effects of cyclosporine and warfarin. The effectiveness of estrogen and hormonal contraceptives may be decreased by griseofulvin.

Pharmacodynamics/Kinetics

Absorption: Ultramicrosize griseofulvin absorption is almost complete; absorption of microsize griseofulvin is variable (25% to 70% of an oral dose); enhanced by ingestion of a fatty meal (GI absorption of ultramicrosize is ~1.5 times that of microsize)

Distribution: Crosses placenta

Metabolism: Extensively hepatic

Half-life elimination: 9-22 hours

Excretion: Urine (<1% as unchanged drug); feces; perspiration

Pregnancy Risk Factor C

Griseofulvin Microsize see Griseofulvin on page 794

Griseofulvin Ultramicrosize see Griseofulvin on page 794

Gris-PEG® see Griseofulvin on page 794

Guaicon DM [OTC] see Guaifenesin and Dextromethorphan on page 796

Guaicon DMS [OTC] see Guaifenesin and Dextromethorphan on page 796

Guaifed® see Guaifenesin and Phenylephrine on page 797

Guaifed-PD® see Guaifenesin and Phenylephrine on page 797

Guaifen™ DM see Guaifenesin, Dextromethorphan, and Phenylephrine on page 798

Guaifenesin (gwye FEN e sin)

U.S. Brand Names Allfen Jr; Diabetic Tussin® EX [OTC]; Ganidin NR; Guiatuss™ [OTC]; Mucinex® [OTC]; Mucinex®, Children's [OTC]; Mucinex®, Children's Mini-Melts™ [OTC]; Mucinex®, Junior Mini-Melts™ [OTC]; Organidin® NR; Phanasin® [OTC]; Phanasin® Diabetic Choice [OTC]; Robitussin® [OTC]; Scot-Tussin® Expectorant [OTC]; Siltussin DAS [OTC]; Siltussin SA [OTC]; Vicks® Casero™ Chest Congestion Relief [OTC]; XPECT™ [OTC]

Canadian Brand Names Balminil Expectorant; Benylin® E Extra Strength; Koffex Expectorant; Robitussin®

Mexican Brand Names 44 Exp; Robitussin

Generic Available Yes: Excludes extended release and granules

Index Terms GG; Glycerol Guaiacolate

Pharmacologic Category Expectorant

Use Help loosen phlegm and thin bronchial secretions to make coughs more productive

Local Anesthetic/Vasoconstrictor Precautions No information available to require special precautions

Effects on Dental Treatment No significant effects or complications reported

Common Adverse Effects Frequency not defined.

Central nervous system: Dizziness, drowsiness, headache

Dermatologic: Rash

Endocrine & metabolic: Uric acid levels decreased

Gastrointestinal: Nausea, vomiting, stomach pain

Postmarketing and/or case reports: Kidney stone formation (with consumption of large quantities)

Mechanism of Action Thought to act as an expectorant by irritating the gastric mucosa and stimulating respiratory tract secretions, thereby increasing respiratory fluid volumes and decreasing mucous viscosity

Pharmacodynamics/Kinetics

Absorption: Well absorbed

Half-life elimination: ~1 hour

Excretion: Urine (as unchanged drug and metabolites)

Pregnancy Risk Factor C

Guaifenesin AC see Guaifenesin and Codeine on page 795

Guaifenesin and Codeine (gwye FEN e sin & KOE deen)

Related Information

Codeine on page 404

(Continued)

Guaifenesin and Codeine *(Continued)*

Guaifenesin *on page 795*

U.S. Brand Names Brontex®; Cheracol®; Diabetic Tussin C®; Gani-Tuss® NR; Guaifenesin AC; Guaituss AC; Kolephrin® #1; Mytussin® AC; Robafen® AC; Romilar® AC; Tussi-Organidin® NR; Tussi-Organidin® S-NR

Generic Available Yes

Index Terms Codeine and Guaifenesin

Pharmacologic Category Antitussive; Cough Preparation; Expectorant

Use Temporary control of cough due to minor throat and bronchial irritation

Local Anesthetic/Vasoconstrictor Precautions No information available to require special precautions

Effects on Dental Treatment Key adverse event(s) related to dental treatment: Xerostomia (normal salivary flow resumes upon discontinuation).

Common Adverse Effects Frequency not defined; also see individual agents.

Cardiovascular: Bradycardia, circulatory depression, flushing, orthostatic hypotension, palpitation, syncope, tachycardia

Central nervous system: Convulsions, CNS depression, disorientation, dizziness, dysphoria, euphoria, faintness, hallucinations (transient), headache, lightheadedness, sedation

Dermatologic: Angioneurotic edema, pruritus, urticaria

Gastrointestinal: Biliary tract spasm, colonic motility increase (with chronic ulcerative colitis), constipation, nausea, stomach pain, toxic dilation (with acute ulcerative colitis), vomiting

Genitourinary: Oliguria, urinary retention

Neuromuscular & skeletal: Weakness

Ocular: Visual disturbances

Respiratory: Laryngeal edema, respiratory depression

Miscellaneous: Anaphylaxis, diaphoresis

Restrictions C-V

Mechanism of Action

Guaifenesin may act as an expectorant by irritating the gastric mucosa and stimulating respiratory tract secretions, thereby increasing respiratory fluid volumes and decreasing phlegm viscosity

Codeine is an antitussive that controls cough by depressing the medullary cough center

Drug Interactions

Increased Effect/Toxicity: See individual agents.

Decreased Effect: See individual agents.

Pharmacodynamics/Kinetics See individual agents.

Pregnancy Risk Factor C

Guaifenesin and Dextromethorphan

(gwye FEN e sin & deks troe meth OR fan)

Related Information

Dextromethorphan *on page 477*

Guaifenesin *on page 795*

U.S. Brand Names Allfen-DM; Altarussin DM [OTC]; Amibid DM [DSC]; Cheracol® D [OTC]; Cheracol® Plus [OTC]; Coricidin HBP® Chest Congestion and Cough [OTC]; Diabetic Tussin® DM [OTC]; Diabetic Tussin® DM Maximum Strength [OTC]; Duratuss® DM; Gani-Tuss DM NR; Genatuss DM® [OTC]; Guaicon DM [OTC]; Guaicon DMS [OTC]; Guaifenex® DM; Guia-D; Guiatuss-DM® [OTC]; Hydro-Tussin™ DM; Kolephrin® GG/DM [OTC]; Mintab DM; Mucinex® Children's Cough [OTC]; Mucinex® DM [OTC]; Phanatuss® DM [OTC]; Phlemex; Respa-DM®; Robafen DM [OTC]; Robafen DM Clear [OTC]; Robitussin® Cough and Congestion [OTC]; Robitussin® DM [OTC]; Robitussin® DM Infant [OTC]; Robitussin® Sugar Free Cough [OTC]; Safe Tussin® [OTC]; Scot-Tussin® Senior [OTC]; Silexin [OTC]; Siltussin DM [OTC]; Siltussin DM DAS [OTC]; Simuc-DM; Su-Tuss DM; Touro® DM; Tussi-Organidin® DM NR; Tussi-Organidin® DM-S NR; Vicks® 44E [OTC]; Vicks® Pediatric Formula 44E [OTC]; Z-Cof LA™

Canadian Brand Names Balminil DM E; Benylin® DM-E; Koffex DM-Expectorant; Robitussin® DM

Generic Available Yes

Index Terms Dextromethorphan and Guaifenesin

Pharmacologic Category Antitussive; Cough Preparation; Expectorant

Use Temporary control of cough due to minor throat and bronchial irritation

Local Anesthetic/Vasoconstrictor Precautions No information available to require special precautions

Effects on Dental Treatment No significant effects or complications reported

Common Adverse Effects See individual agents.

Mechanism of Action
Guaifenesin is thought to act as an expectorant by irritating the gastric mucosa and stimulating respiratory tract secretions, thereby increasing respiratory fluid volumes and decreasing phlegm viscosity

Dextromethorphan is a chemical relative of morphine lacking narcotic properties except in overdose; controls cough by depressing the medullary cough center

Drug Interactions
Cytochrome P450 Effect: Dextromethorphan: **Substrate** of CYP2B6 (minor), 2C9 (minor), 2C19 (minor), 2D6 (major), 2E1 (minor), 3A4 (minor); **Inhibits** CYP2D6 (weak)

Increased Effect/Toxicity: See individual agents.

Decreased Effect: See individual agents.

Pharmacodynamics/Kinetics See individual agents.

Pregnancy Risk Factor C

Guaifenesin and Hydrocodone *see* Hydrocodone and Guaifenesin *on page 828*

Guaifenesin and Phenylephrine (gwye FEN e sin & fen il EF rin)

Related Information
Guaifenesin *on page 795*
Phenylephrine *on page 1293*

U.S. Brand Names Aldex™; Amidal [DSC]; Ami-Tex LA [DSC]; Crantex LA; Deconsal® II; Donatussin; Duomax; Duratuss®; Duratuss GP®; Entex® [DSC]; Entex® ER [DSC]; Entex® LA [DSC]; ExeFen-PD; ExeTuss; ExeTuss-GP; Gentex LA; Gilphex TR®; Guaifed®; Guaifed-PD®; Guaiphen-D; Guaiphen-D 1200; Guaiphen-PD; Liquibid-D®; Liquibid-D® 1200; Liquibid®-PD [DSC]; Nasex-G; Nexphen PD; norel® EX; Pendex; PhenaVent™; PhenaVent™ D; PhenaVent™ LA; PhenaVent™ Ped; Prolex®-D; Prolex®-PD; Rescon GG; Sil-Tex; Simuc; Sina-12X; SINUvent® PE; XPECT-PE™

Generic Available Yes: Excludes suspension

Index Terms Guaifenesin and Phenylephrine Tannate; Phenylephrine Hydrochloride and Guaifenesin

Pharmacologic Category Decongestant; Expectorant

Use Temporary relief of nasal congestion, sinusitis, rhinitis and hay fever; temporary relief of cough associated with upper respiratory tract conditions, especially when associated with dry, nonproductive cough

Local Anesthetic/Vasoconstrictor Precautions Use with caution since phenylephrine is a sympathomimetic amine which could interact with epinephrine to cause a pressor response

Effects on Dental Treatment Key adverse event(s) related to dental treatment:

Guaifenesin: No significant effects or complications reported

Phenylephrine: Up to 10% of patients could experience tachycardia, palpitations, and xerostomia (normal salivary flow resumes upon discontinuation); use vasoconstrictor with caution

Common Adverse Effects See individual agents.

Mechanism of Action See individual agents.

Drug Interactions
Increased Effect/Toxicity: See individual agents.

Decreased Effect: See individual agents.

Pharmacodynamics/Kinetics See individual agents.

Pregnancy Risk Factor C

Guaifenesin and Phenylephrine Tannate *see* Guaifenesin and Phenylephrine *on page 797*

Guaifenesin and Potassium Guaiacolsulfonate
(gwye FEN e sin & poe TASS ee um gwye a kole SUL foe nate)

Related Information
Guaifenesin *on page 795*

U.S. Brand Names Allfen *(reformulation)*; Humibid® LA *(reformulation)*

Generic Available No

Index Terms Potassium Guaiacolsulfonate and Guaifenesin

Pharmacologic Category Expectorant

Use Temporary control of cough associated with respiratory tract infections and related conditions which are complicated by tenacious mucus and/or mucous plugs and congestion

Local Anesthetic/Vasoconstrictor Precautions No information available to require special precautions

(Continued)

Guaifenesin and Potassium Guaiacolsulfonate
(Continued)

Effects on Dental Treatment No significant effects or complications reported

Mechanism of Action Guaifenesin and potassium guaiacolsulfonate are both expectorants. Guaifenesin is thought to act as an expectorant by irritating the gastric mucosa and stimulating respiratory tract secretions, thereby increasing respiratory fluid volumes and decreasing mucous viscosity.

Pregnancy Risk Factor C

Guaifenesin and Pseudoephedrine
(gwye FEN e sin & soo doe e FED rin)

Related Information
Guaifenesin *on page 795*
Pseudoephedrine *on page 1381*

U.S. Brand Names Ambifed-G; Congestac® [OTC]; Dynex; Entex® PSE; Eudal®-SR; Guaifenex® GP; Guaifenex® PSE; Guaimax-D®; Levall G; Maxifed®; Maxifed-G®; Mucinex®-D [OTC]; Nasatab® LA; Pseudo GG TR; Pseudo Max; Pseudovent™; Pseudovent™ 400; Pseudovent™-Ped; Refenesen Plus [OTC]; Respaire®-60 SR; Respaire®-120 SR; Robitussin-PE® [OTC] [DSC]; Robitussin® Severe Congestion [OTC] [DSC]; Sinutab® Non-Drying [OTC]; Sudafed® Non-Drying Sinus [OTC] [DSC]; Touro LA®; Zephrex LA® [DSC]

Canadian Brand Names Contac® Cold-Chest Congestion, Non Drowsy, Regular Strength; Entex® LA; Novahistex® Expectorant with Decongestant

Generic Available Yes

Index Terms Pseudoephedrine and Guaifenesin

Pharmacologic Category Alpha/Beta Agonist; Expectorant

Use Temporary relief of nasal congestion and to help loosen phlegm and thin bronchial secretions in the treatment of cough

Local Anesthetic/Vasoconstrictor Precautions Use with caution since pseudoephedrine is a sympathomimetic amine which could interact with epinephrine to cause a pressor response

Effects on Dental Treatment Key adverse event(s) related to dental treatment:
Guaifenesin: No significant effects or complications reported
Pseudoephedrine: Xerostomia (normal salivary flow resumes upon discontinuation).

Common Adverse Effects See individual agents.

Drug Interactions
Increased Effect/Toxicity: See individual agents.
Decreased Effect: See individual agents.

Pharmacodynamics/Kinetics See individual agents.

Pregnancy Risk Factor C

Guaifenesin and Theophylline *see* Theophylline and Guaifenesin *on page 1555*

Guaifenesin, Carbetapentane Citrate, and Phenylephrine Hydrochloride *see* Carbetapentane, Guaifenesin, and Phenylephrine *on page 279*

Guaifenesin, Dextromethorphan, and Phenylephrine
(gwye FEN e sin, deks troe meth OR fan, & fen il EF rin)

Related Information
Dextromethorphan *on page 477*
Guaifenesin *on page 795*
Phenylephrine *on page 1293*

U.S. Brand Names Anextuss; Certuss-D®; Dacex-DM; Dexcon-DM [DSC]; Dexcon-PE; Duraphen™ DM; Duraphen™ Forte; Duraphen™ II DM; Dynatuss-EX; Giltuss®; Giltuss Pediatric®; Giltuss TR®; Guaifen™ DM; Maxiphen DM; SINUtuss® DM; TriTuss®; TriTuss® ER

Generic Available Yes

Index Terms Guaifenesin, Dextromethorphan Hydrobromide, and Phenylephrine Hydrochloride; Phenylephrine Hydrochloride, Guaifenesin, and Dextromethorphan Hydrobromide

Pharmacologic Category Antitussive; Decongestant

Use Symptomatic relief of dry nonproductive coughs and upper respiratory symptoms associated with hay fever, colds, or the flu

Local Anesthetic/Vasoconstrictor Precautions Use with caution since phenylephrine is a sympathomimetic amine which could interact with epinephrine to cause a pressor response

Effects on Dental Treatment Key adverse event(s) related to dental treatment:

Dextromethorphan: No significant effects or complications reported

Guaifenesin: No significant effects or complications reported

Phenylephrine: Up to 10% of patients could experience tachycardia, palpitations, and xerostomia (normal salivary flow resumes upon discontinuation); use vasoconstrictor with caution

Common Adverse Effects Reactions which follow have been reported with the combination product; see individual drug monographs for additional adverse reactions that may be expected from each agent.

Cardiovascular: Cardiovascular collapse, palpitation, tachycardia

Central nervous system: Anxiety, CNS depression, convulsions, dizziness, drowsiness, excitability increased, fear, hallucinations, headache, insomnia, irritability increased, lightheadedness, nervousness

Gastrointestinal: Nausea, vomiting

Neuromuscular & skeletal: Tremor, weakness

Respiratory: Respiratory difficulties

Mechanism of Action See individual agents.

Drug Interactions

Cytochrome P450 Effect: Dextromethorphan: **Substrate** of CYP2B6 (minor), 2C9 (minor), 2C19 (minor), 2D6 (major), 2E1 (minor), 3A4 (minor); **Inhibits** CYP2D6 (weak)

Pharmacodynamics/Kinetics See individual agents.

Pregnancy Risk Factor C

Guaifenesin, Dextromethorphan Hydrobromide, and Phenylephrine Hydrochloride see Guaifenesin, Dextromethorphan, and Phenylephrine on page 798

Guaifenesin, Dihydrocodeine, and Pseudoephedrine see Dihydrocodeine, Pseudoephedrine, and Guaifenesin on page 503

Guaifenesin, Hydrocodone, and Pseudoephedrine see Hydrocodone, Pseudoephedrine, and Guaifenesin on page 835

Guaifenesin, Hydrocodone Bitartrate, and Phenylephrine Hydrochloride see Hydrocodone, Phenylephrine, and Guaifenesin on page 834

Guaifenesin, Pseudoephedrine, and Codeine
(gwye FEN e sin, soo doe e FED rin, & KOE deen)

Related Information
Codeine on page 404
Guaifenesin on page 795
Pseudoephedrine on page 1381

U.S. Brand Names Guiatuss DAC; Mytussin® DAC; Nucofed® Expectorant [DSC]; Nucofed® Pediatric Expectorant [DSC]

Canadian Brand Names Benylin® 3.3 mg-D-E; Calmylin with Codeine

Generic Available Yes

Index Terms Codeine, Guaifenesin, and Pseudoephedrine; Pseudoephedrine, Guaifenesin, and Codeine

Pharmacologic Category Antitussive/Decongestant/Expectorant

Use Temporarily relieves nasal congestion and controls cough associated with upper respiratory infections and related conditions (common cold, sinusitis, bronchitis, influenza)

Local Anesthetic/Vasoconstrictor Precautions Use with caution since pseudoephedrine is a sympathomimetic amine which could interact with epinephrine to cause a pressor response

Effects on Dental Treatment Key adverse event(s) related to dental treatment:

Codeine: Xerostomia (normal salivary flow resumes upon discontinuation).

Guaifenesin: No significant effects or complications reported

Pseudoephedrine: Xerostomia (normal salivary flow resumes upon discontinuation).

Common Adverse Effects See individual agents.

Restrictions C-III; C-V

Drug Interactions
Increased Effect/Toxicity: See individual agents.

Decreased Effect: See individual agents.

Pharmacodynamics/Kinetics See individual agents.

Pregnancy Risk Factor C

Guaifenesin, Pseudoephedrine, and Dextromethorphan
(gwye FEN e sin, soo doe e FED rin, & deks troe meth OR fan)

Related Information
Dextromethorphan *on page 477*
Guaifenesin *on page 795*
Pseudoephedrine *on page 1381*

U.S. Brand Names Ambifed-G DM; Coldmist DM; Maxifed DM; Maxifed DMX; Medent-DM; Profen Forte™ DM; Profen II DM®; Pseudo Max DMX; Pseudovent™ DM; Relacon-DM NR; Robitussin® Cough and Cold [OTC]; Robitussin® Cough and Cold CF [OTC]; Robitussin® Cough and Cold Infant CF [OTC]; Ru-Tuss DM; Touro® CC; Touro® CC-LD; Tri-Vent™ DM; Tusnel Pediatric®; Z-Cof™ DM

Canadian Brand Names Balminil DM + Decongestant + Expectorant; Benylin® DM-D-E; Koffex DM + Decongestant + Expectorant; Novahistex® DM Decongestant Expectorant; Novahistine® DM Decongestant Expectorant; Robitussin® Cough & Cold®

Generic Available Yes

Index Terms Dextromethorphan, Guaifenesin, and Pseudoephedrine; Pseudoephedrine, Dextromethorphan, and Guaifenesin

Pharmacologic Category Antitussive/Decongestant/Expectorant

Use Temporarily relieves nasal congestion and controls cough due to minor throat and bronchial irritation; helps loosen phlegm and thin bronchial secretions to make coughs more productive

Local Anesthetic/Vasoconstrictor Precautions Use with caution since pseudoephedrine is a sympathomimetic amine which could interact with epinephrine to cause a pressor response

Effects on Dental Treatment Key adverse event(s) related to dental treatment:
Dextromethorphan: No significant effects or complications reported
Guaifenesin: No significant effects or complications reported
Pseudoephedrine: Xerostomia (normal salivary flow resumes upon discontinuation).

Common Adverse Effects See individual agents.

Mechanism of Action See individual agents.

Drug Interactions
Cytochrome P450 Effect: Dextromethorphan: **Substrate** of CYP2B6 (minor), 2C9 (minor), 2C19 (minor), 2D6 (major), 2E1 (minor), 3A4 (minor); **Inhibits** CYP2D6 (weak)
Increased Effect/Toxicity: See individual agents.
Decreased Effect: See individual agents.

Pharmacodynamics/Kinetics See individual agents.

Pregnancy Risk Factor C

Guaifenex® DM *see* Guaifenesin and Dextromethorphan *on page 796*

Guaifenex® GP *see* Guaifenesin and Pseudoephedrine *on page 798*

Guaifenex® PSE *see* Guaifenesin and Pseudoephedrine *on page 798*

Guaimax-D® *see* Guaifenesin and Pseudoephedrine *on page 798*

Guaiphen-D *see* Guaifenesin and Phenylephrine *on page 797*

Guaiphen-D 1200 *see* Guaifenesin and Phenylephrine *on page 797*

Guaiphen-PD *see* Guaifenesin and Phenylephrine *on page 797*

Guaituss AC *see* Guaifenesin and Codeine *on page 795*

Guanabenz (GWAHN a benz)

Related Information
Cardiovascular Diseases *on page 1726*
Canadian Brand Names Wytensin®
Generic Available Yes
Index Terms Guanabenz Acetate
Pharmacologic Category Alpha₂-Adrenergic Agonist
Use Management of hypertension
Local Anesthetic/Vasoconstrictor Precautions No information available to require special precautions
Effects on Dental Treatment Key adverse event(s) related to dental treatment: Taste disorder, nasal congestion, dyspnea, significant xerostomia (normal salivary flow resumes upon discontinuation).
Common Adverse Effects Higher rates with larger doses

>5% (at doses of 16 mg/day):
Cardiovascular: Orthostasis
Central nervous system: Drowsiness or sedation (39%), dizziness (12% to 17%), headache (5%)
Gastrointestinal: Xerostomia (28% to 38%)
Neuromuscular & skeletal: Weakness (~10%)
≤3% (may be similar to placebo):
Cardiovascular: Arrhythmias, chest pain, edema, palpitation
Central nervous system: Anxiety, ataxia, depression, sleep disturbances
Dermatologic: Pruritus, rash
Endocrine & metabolic: Disturbances of sexual function, gynecomastia, decreased sexual function
Gastrointestinal: Constipation, diarrhea, nausea, vomiting
Genitourinary: Polyuria
Neuromuscular & skeletal: Myalgia
Ocular: Blurring of vision
Respiratory: Dyspnea, nasal congestion
Miscellaneous: Taste disorders

Mechanism of Action Stimulates alpha$_2$-adrenoreceptors in the brain stem, thus activating an inhibitory neuron, resulting in reduced sympathetic outflow, producing a decrease in vasomotor tone and heart rate

Drug Interactions
Cytochrome P450 Effect: Substrate of CYP1A2 (major)
Increased Effect/Toxicity: CYP1A2 inhibitors may increase the levels/effects of guanabenz; example inhibitors include ciprofloxacin, fluvoxamine, ketoconazole, norfloxacin, ofloxacin, and rofecoxib. Nitroprusside and guanabenz have additive hypotensive effects. Noncardioselective beta-blockers (nadolol, propranolol, timolol) may exacerbate rebound hypertension when guanabenz is withdrawn. The beta-blocker should be withdrawn first. The gradual withdrawal of guanabenz or a cardioselective beta-blocker could be substituted.

Hypoglycemic agents: Hypoglycemic symptoms may be reduced. Educate patient about decreased signs and symptoms of hypoglycemia or avoid use in patients with frequent episodes of hypoglycemia.
Decreased Effect: CYP1A2 inducers may decrease the levels/effects of guanabenz; example inducers include aminoglutethimide, carbamazepine, phenobarbital, and rifampin. TCAs decrease the hypotensive effect of guanabenz.

Pharmacodynamics/Kinetics
Onset of action: Antihypertensive: ~1 hour
Absorption: ~75%
Half-life elimination, serum: 7-10 hours

Pregnancy Risk Factor C

Guanabenz Acetate *see* Guanabenz *on page 800*

Guanfacine (GWAHN fa seen)

Related Information
Cardiovascular Diseases *on page 1726*
U.S. Brand Names Tenex®
Canadian Brand Names Tenex®
Generic Available Yes
Index Terms Guanfacine Hydrochloride
Pharmacologic Category Alpha$_2$-Adrenergic Agonist
Use Management of hypertension
Unlabeled/Investigational Use ADHD, tic disorder, aggression
Local Anesthetic/Vasoconstrictor Precautions No information available to require special precautions
Effects on Dental Treatment Key adverse event(s) related to dental treatment: Xerostomia and changes in salivation (normal salivary flow resumes upon discontinuation).

Common Adverse Effects
>10%:
Central nervous system: Somnolence (5% to 40%), headache (3% to 13%), dizziness (2% to 15%)
Gastrointestinal: Xerostomia (10% to 54%), constipation (2% to 15%)
1% to 10%:
Central nervous system: Fatigue (2% to 10%)
Endocrine & metabolic: Impotence (up to 7%)
(Continued)

Guanfacine (Continued)

Mechanism of Action Stimulates alpha$_2$-adrenoreceptors in the brain stem, thus activating an inhibitory neuron, resulting in reduced sympathetic outflow, producing a decrease in vasomotor tone and heart rate

Drug Interactions

Increased Effect/Toxicity: Nitroprusside and guanfacine have additive hypotensive effects. Noncardioselective beta-blockers (nadolol, propranolol, timolol) may exacerbate rebound hypertension when guanfacine is withdrawn. The beta-blocker should be withdrawn first. The gradual withdrawal of guanfacine or a cardioselective beta-blocker could be substituted.

Decreased Effect: TCAs decrease the hypotensive effect of guanfacine.

Pharmacodynamics/Kinetics

Onset of action: Peak effect: 8-11 hours

Duration: 24 hours following single dose

Half-life elimination, serum: 17 hours

Time to peak, serum: 1-4 hours

Pregnancy Risk Factor B

Guanfacine Hydrochloride see Guanfacine on page 801

Guanidine (GWAHN i deen)

Generic Available No

Index Terms Guanidine Hydrochloride

Pharmacologic Category Cholinergic Agonist

Use Reduction of the symptoms of muscle weakness associated with the myasthenic syndrome of Eaton-Lambert, not for myasthenia gravis

Local Anesthetic/Vasoconstrictor Precautions No information available to require special precautions

Effects on Dental Treatment No significant effects or complications reported

Guanidine Hydrochloride see Guanidine on page 802

Guia-D see Guaifenesin and Dextromethorphan on page 796

Guiaplex™ HC see Hydrocodone, Phenylephrine, and Guaifenesin on page 834

Guiatuss™ [OTC] see Guaifenesin on page 795

Guiatuss DAC see Guaifenesin, Pseudoephedrine, and Codeine on page 799

Guiatuss-DM® [OTC] see Guaifenesin and Dextromethorphan on page 796

Gum Benjamin see Benzoin on page 200

GW506U78 see Nelarabine on page 1157

GW-1000-02 see Tetrahydrocannabinol and Cannabidiol on page 1550

GW433908G see Fosamprenavir on page 743

GW572016 see Lapatinib on page 950

Gynazole-1® see Butoconazole on page 253

Gyne-Lotrimin® 3 [OTC] see Clotrimazole on page 398

Gynodiol® see Estradiol on page 602

Gynol II® [OTC] see Nonoxynol 9 on page 1185

Gynovite® Plus [OTC] see Vitamins (Multiple/Oral) on page 1665

H5N1 Influenza Vaccine see Influenza Virus Vaccine (H5N1) on page 882

Habitrol see Nicotine on page 1169

Haemophilus b Conjugate Vaccine
(he MOF fi lus bee KON joo gate vak SEEN)

Related Information

Immunizations (Vaccines) on page 1886

U.S. Brand Names ActHIB®; HibTITER®; PedvaxHIB®

Canadian Brand Names ActHIB®; PedvaxHIB®

Generic Available No

Index Terms Diphtheria CRM$_{197}$ Protein Conjugate; Diphtheria Toxoid Conjugate; Haemophilus b Oligosaccharide Conjugate Vaccine; Haemophilus b Polysaccharide Vaccine; HbCV; HbOC; Hib Conjugate Vaccine; Hib Polysaccharide Conjugate; PRP-OMP; PRP-T

Pharmacologic Category Vaccine

Use Routine immunization of children 2 months to 5 years of age against invasive disease caused by H. influenzae type b

Unimmunized children ≥5 years of age with a chronic illness known to be associated with increased risk of Haemophilus influenzae type b disease, specifically, persons with anatomic or functional asplenia or sickle cell anemia or those who have undergone splenectomy, should receive Haemophilus influenzae type b (Hib) vaccine.

Haemophilus b conjugate vaccines are not indicated for prevention of bronchitis or other infections due to *H. influenzae* in adults; adults with specific dysfunction or certain complement deficiencies who are at especially high risk of *H. influenzae* type b infection (HIV-infected adults); patients with Hodgkin's disease (vaccinated at least 2 weeks before the initiation of chemotherapy or 3 months after the end of chemotherapy)

Local Anesthetic/Vasoconstrictor Precautions No information available to require special precautions

Effects on Dental Treatment No significant effects or complications reported

Common Adverse Effects All serious adverse reactions must be reported to the U.S. Department of Health and Human Services (DHHS) Vaccine Adverse Event Reporting System (VAERS) 1-800-822-7967. Frequency not defined:

Central nervous system: Crying (unusual, high pitched, prolonged), fever, irritability, pain, sleepiness

Dermatologic: Rash

Gastrointestinal: Anorexia, diarrhea, vomiting

Local: Injection site: Erythema, induration, pain, soreness, swelling, warmth

Otic: Otitis media

Respiratory: Upper respiratory tract infection

Mechanism of Action Stimulates production of anticapsular antibodies and provides active immunity to *Haemophilus influenzae* type b

Drug Interactions

Decreased Effect: The effect of the vaccine may be decreased with immunosuppressive agents; consider deferring vaccination for 3 months after immunosuppressant therapy is discontinued.

Pharmacodynamics/Kinetics Seroconversion following one dose of Hib vaccine for children 18 months or 24 months of age or older is 75% to 90%, respectively.

Onset of action: Serum antibody response: 1-2 weeks

Duration: Immunity: 1.5 years

Pregnancy Risk Factor C

Haemophilus b Oligosaccharide Conjugate Vaccine *see Haemophilus* b Conjugate Vaccine *on page 802*

Haemophilus b Polysaccharide Vaccine *see Haemophilus* b Conjugate Vaccine *on page 802*

Halcinonide (hal SIN oh nide)

U.S. Brand Names Halog®

Canadian Brand Names Halog®

Generic Available No

Pharmacologic Category Corticosteroid, Topical

Use Inflammation of corticosteroid-responsive dermatoses [high potency topical corticosteroid]

Local Anesthetic/Vasoconstrictor Precautions No information available to require special precautions

Effects on Dental Treatment No significant effects or complications reported

Common Adverse Effects Frequency not defined: Itching; dry skin; folliculitis; hypertrichosis; acneiform eruptions; hypopigmentation; perioral dermatitis; allergic contact dermatitis; skin maceration; skin atrophy; striae; local burning, irritation, miliaria; secondary infection

Mechanism of Action Decreases inflammation by suppression of migration of polymorphonuclear leukocytes and reversal of increased capillary permeability

Pharmacodynamics/Kinetics

Absorption: Percutaneous absorption varies by location of topical application and use of occlusive dressings

Metabolism: Primarily hepatic

Excretion: Urine

Pregnancy Risk Factor C

Halcion® [DSC] *see* Triazolam *on page 1613*

Haldol® *see* Haloperidol *on page 805*

Haldol® Decanoate *see* Haloperidol *on page 805*

Haley's M-O *see* Magnesium Hydroxide and Mineral Oil *on page 1014*

Halfprin® [OTC] *see* Aspirin *on page 149*

Halobetasol (hal oh BAY ta sol)

U.S. Brand Names Ultravate®
Canadian Brand Names Ultravate®
Generic Available Yes
Index Terms Halobetasol Propionate
Pharmacologic Category Corticosteroid, Topical
Dental Use Relief of inflammatory and pruritic manifestations (super high potency topical corticosteroid)
Use Relief of inflammatory and pruritic manifestations of corticosteroid-response dermatoses [super high potency topical corticosteroid]
Local Anesthetic/Vasoconstrictor Precautions No information available to require special precautions
Effects on Dental Treatment No significant effects or complications reported
Significant Adverse Effects
1% to 4%: Dermatologic: Burning, itching, stinging
<1% (Limited to important or life-threatening): Acneiform eruptions, allergic contact dermatitis, dry skin, erythema, HPA axis suppression, hypopigmentation, leukoderma, miliaria, perioral dermatitis, pustulation, rash, secondary infection, skin atrophy, striae, vesicles
Dental Usual Dosing Inflammatory and pruritic manifestations: Children ≥12 years and Adults: Topical: Cream: Apply sparingly to lesion twice daily. Treatment should not exceed 2 consecutive weeks and total dosage should not exceed 50 g/week. Therapy should be discontinued when control is achieved; if no improvement is seen, reassessment of diagnosis may be necessary.
Dosage Children ≥12 years and Adults: Topical:
Inflammatory and pruritic manifestations (dental use): Cream: Apply sparingly to lesion twice daily. Treatment should not exceed 2 consecutive weeks and total dosage should not exceed 50 g/week. Therapy should be discontinued when control is achieved; if no improvement is seen, reassessment of diagnosis may be necessary.
Steroid-responsive dermatoses: Apply sparingly to skin twice daily, rub in gently and completely; treatment should not exceed 2 consecutive weeks and total dosage should not exceed 50 g/week. Therapy should be discontinued when control is achieved; if no improvement is seen, reassessment of diagnosis may be necessary.
Mechanism of Action Corticosteroids inhibit the initial manifestations of the inflammatory process (ie, capillary dilation and edema, fibrin deposition, and migration and diapedesis of leukocytes into the inflamed site) as well as later sequelae (angiogenesis, fibroblast proliferation)
Contraindications Hypersensitivity to halobetasol or any component of the formulation; viral, fungal, or tubercular skin lesions
Warnings/Precautions Systemic absorption of topical corticosteroids may cause hypothalamic-pituitary-adrenal (HPA) axis suppression (reversible) particularly in younger children. HPA axis suppression may lead to adrenal crisis. Risk is increased when used over large surface areas, for prolonged periods, or with occlusive dressings. Allergic contact dermatitis can occur, it is usually diagnosed by failure to heal rather than clinical exacerbation. Prolonged treatment with corticosteroids has been associated with the development of Kaposi's sarcoma (case reports); if noted, discontinuation of therapy should be considered. Adverse systemic effects including hyperglycemia, glycosuria, fluid and electrolyte changes, and HPA suppression may occur when used on large surface areas, for prolonged periods, or with an occlusive dressing. Not for ophthalmic use. Topical halobetasol should not be used for the treatment of rosacea or perioral dermatitis. Not recommended for application to the face, groin, or axillae. Safety and efficacy have not been established in pediatric patients; use in children <12 years of age is not recommended.
Drug Interactions No data reported
Pharmacodynamics/Kinetics
Absorption: Percutaneous absorption varies by location of topical application; ~6% of a topically applied dose of ointment enters circulation within 96 hours
Metabolism: Primarily hepatic
Excretion: Urine
Pregnancy Risk Factor C
Lactation Excretion in breast milk unknown/use caution
Breast-Feeding Considerations Systemically administered corticosteroids appear in human milk and may cause adverse effects in a nursing infant. It is not known if the systemic absorption of topical halobetasol results in detectable quantities in human milk.
Dosage Forms Excipient information presented when available (limited, particularly for generics); consult specific product labeling.

Cream, as propionate: 0.05% (15 g, 50 g)
Ointment, as propionate: 0.05% (15 g, 50 g)

Halobetasol Propionate *see* Halobetasol *on page 804*
Halog® *see* Halcinonide *on page 803*

Haloperidol (ha loe PER i dole)

U.S. Brand Names Haldol®; Haldol® Decanoate
Canadian Brand Names Apo-Haloperidol®; Apo-Haloperidol LA®; Haloperidol Injection, USP; Haloperidol-LA; Haloperidol-LA Omega; Haloperidol Long Acting; Novo-Peridol; Peridol; PMS-Haloperidol LA
Mexican Brand Names Haldol; Haldol Decanoas
Generic Available Yes
Index Terms Haloperidol Decanoate; Haloperidol Lactate
Pharmacologic Category Antipsychotic Agent, Typical
Use Management of schizophrenia; control of tics and vocal utterances of Tourette's disorder in children and adults; severe behavioral problems in children
Unlabeled/Investigational Use Treatment of psychosis; may be used for the emergency sedation of severely-agitated or delirious patients; adjunctive treatment of ethanol dependence; antiemetic
Local Anesthetic/Vasoconstrictor Precautions Manufacturer's information states that haloperidol may block vasopressor activity of epinephrine. This has not been observed during use of epinephrine as a vasoconstrictor in local anesthesia. Haloperidol is one of the drugs confirmed to prolong the QT interval and is accepted as having a risk of causing torsade de pointes. The risk of drug-induced torsade de pointes is extremely low when a single QT interval prolonging drug is prescribed. In terms of epinephrine, it is not known what effect vasoconstrictors in the local anesthetic regimen will have in patients with a known history of congenital prolonged QT interval or in patients taking any medication that prolongs the QT interval. Until more information is obtained, it is suggested that the clinician consult with the physician prior to the use of a vasoconstrictor in suspected patients, and that the vasoconstrictor (epinephrine, levonordefrin [Neo-Cobefrin®]) be used with caution.
Effects on Dental Treatment Key adverse event(s) related to dental treatment: Xerostomia (normal salivary flow resumes upon discontinuation). Orthostatic hypotension, and nasal congestion are possible; since the drug is a dopamine antagonist, extrapyramidal symptoms of the TMJ are a possibility.
Common Adverse Effects Frequency not defined.
Cardiovascular: Hyper-/hypotension, tachycardia, arrhythmia, abnormal T waves with prolonged ventricular repolarization, torsade de pointes (case-control study ~4%)
Central nervous system: Restlessness, anxiety, extrapyramidal symptoms, dystonic reactions, pseudoparkinsonian signs and symptoms, tardive dyskinesia, neuroleptic malignant syndrome (NMS), altered central temperature regulation, akathisia, tardive dystonia, insomnia, euphoria, agitation, drowsiness, depression, lethargy, headache, confusion, vertigo, seizure
Dermatologic: Hyperpigmentation, pruritus, rash, contact dermatitis, alopecia, photosensitivity (rare)
Endocrine & metabolic: Amenorrhea, galactorrhea, gynecomastia, sexual dysfunction, lactation, breast engorgement, mastalgia, menstrual irregularities, hyperglycemia, hypoglycemia, hyponatremia
Gastrointestinal: Nausea, vomiting, anorexia, constipation, diarrhea, hypersalivation, dyspepsia, xerostomia
Genitourinary: Urinary retention, priapism
Hematologic: Cholestatic jaundice, obstructive jaundice
Ocular: Blurred vision
Respiratory: Laryngospasm, bronchospasm
Miscellaneous: Heat stroke, diaphoresis
Mechanism of Action Haloperidol is a butyrophenone antipsychotic which blocks postsynaptic mesolimbic dopaminergic D_1 and D_2 receptors in the brain; depresses the release of hypothalamic and hypophyseal hormones; believed to depress the reticular activating system thus affecting basal metabolism, body temperature, wakefulness, vasomotor tone, and emesis
Drug Interactions
Cytochrome P450 Effect: Substrate of CYP1A2 (minor), 2D6 (major), 3A4 (major); **Inhibits** CYP2D6 (moderate), 3A4 (moderate)
Increased Effect/Toxicity: Haloperidol concentrations/effects may be increased by chloroquine, propranolol, and sulfadoxine-pyridoxine. The levels/effects of haloperidol may be increased by azole antifungals, chlorpromazine, clarithromycin, delavirdine, diclofenac, doxycycline, erythromycin, (Continued)

Haloperidol *(Continued)*

fluoxetine, imatinib, isoniazid, miconazole, nefazodone, nicardipine, paroxetine, pergolide, propofol, protease inhibitors, quinidine, quinine, ritonavir, ropinirole, telithromycin, verapamil, and other CYP2D6 or 3A4 inhibitors.

Haloperidol may increase the levels/effects of amphetamines, selected beta-blockers, selected benzodiazepines, calcium channel blockers, cisapride, cyclosporine, dextromethorphan, ergot alkaloids, fluoxetine, selected HMG-CoA reductase inhibitors, lidocaine, mesoridazine, mirtazapine, nateglinide, nefazodone, paroxetine, risperidone, ritonavir, sildenafil (and other PDE-5 inhibitors), tacrolimus, thioridazine, tricyclic antidepressants, venlafaxine, and other substrates of CYP2D6 or 3A4.

Haloperidol may increase the effects of antihypertensives, CNS depressants (ethanol, opioid analgesics, sedative-hypnotics), lithium, trazodone, and TCAs. Haloperidol in combination with indomethacin may result in drowsiness, tiredness, and confusion. Metoclopramide may increase risk of extrapyramidal symptoms (EPS). Acetylcholinesterase inhibitors (central) may increase the risk of antipsychotic-related EPS.

Decreased Effect: Haloperidol may inhibit the ability of bromocriptine to lower serum prolactin concentrations. Benztropine (and other anticholinergics) may inhibit the therapeutic response to haloperidol and excess anticholinergic effects may occur. Barbiturates, carbamazepine, and cigarette smoking may enhance the hepatic metabolism of haloperidol. Haloperidol may inhibit the antiparkinsonian effect of levodopa; avoid this combination. The levels/effects of haloperidol may be decreased by aminoglutethimide, carbamazepine, nafcillin, nevirapine, phenobarbital, phenytoin, rifamycins, and other CYP3A4 inducers. Haloperidol may decrease the levels/effects of CYP2D6 prodrug substrates (eg, codeine, hydrocodone, oxycodone, tramadol).

Pharmacodynamics/Kinetics

Onset of action: Sedation: I.V.: ~1 hour
Duration: Decanoate: ~3 weeks
Distribution: Crosses placenta; enters breast milk
Protein binding: 90%
Metabolism: Hepatic to inactive compounds
Bioavailability: Oral: 60%
Half-life elimination: 20 hours
Time to peak, serum: 20 minutes
Excretion: Urine (33% to 40% as metabolites) within 5 days; feces (15%)

Pregnancy Risk Factor C

Hemin (HEE min)

U.S. Brand Names Panhematin®
Generic Available No
Index Terms Hematin
Pharmacologic Category Blood Modifiers
Use Treatment of recurrent attacks of acute intermittent porphyria (AIP)
Local Anesthetic/Vasoconstrictor Precautions No information available to require special precautions
Effects on Dental Treatment No significant effects or complications reported
Common Adverse Effects Frequency not defined.
   Central nervous system: Pyrexia
   Hematologic: Leukocytosis
   Local: Phlebitis
Mechanism of Action Inhibits the hepatic and/or marrow synthesis of ALA synthase, the enzyme that regulates the porphyrin/heme pathway
Pregnancy Risk Factor C

Heparin (HEP a rin)

U.S. Brand Names HepFlush®-10; Hep-Lock®; Hep-Lock U/P
Canadian Brand Names Hepalean®; Hepalean® Leo; Hepalean®-LOK
Generic Available Yes
Index Terms Heparin Calcium; Heparin Lock Flush; Heparin Sodium
Pharmacologic Category Anticoagulant
Use Prophylaxis and treatment of thromboembolic disorders
   Note: Heparin lock flush solution is intended only to maintain patency of I.V. devices and is **not** to be used for anticoagulant therapy.
Unlabeled/Investigational Use Acute MI - combination regimen of heparin (unlabeled dose), tenecteplase (half dose), and abciximab (full dose)
Local Anesthetic/Vasoconstrictor Precautions No information available to require special precautions
Effects on Dental Treatment Key adverse event(s) related to dental treatment: Bleeding from the gums.
Common Adverse Effects
   Cardiovascular: Chest pain, hemorrhagic shock, thrombosis, vasospasm (possibly related to thrombosis)
   Central nervous system: Fever, headache, chills
   Dermatologic: Unexplained bruising, urticaria, alopecia, dysesthesia pedis, purpura, eczema, cutaneous necrosis (following deep SubQ injection), erythematous plaques (case reports)
   Endocrine & metabolic: Hyperkalemia (supression of aldosterone), rebound hyperlipidemia on discontinuation
   Gastrointestinal: Nausea, vomiting, constipation, hematemesis
   Genitourinary: Frequent or persistent erection
   Hematologic: Hemorrhage, blood in urine, bleeding from gums, epistaxis, adrenal hemorrhage, ovarian hemorrhage, retroperitoneal hemorrhage, thrombocytopenia (see note)
   Hepatic: Elevated liver enzymes (AST/ALT)
   Local: Irritation, ulceration, cutaneous necrosis have been rarely reported with deep SubQ injections, I.M. injection (not recommended) is associated with a high incidence of these effects
   (Continued)

Heparin *(Continued)*

Neuromuscular & skeletal: Peripheral neuropathy, osteoporosis (chronic therapy effect)

Ocular: Conjunctivitis (allergic reaction)

Respiratory: Hemoptysis, pulmonary hemorrhage, asthma, rhinitis, bronchospasm (case reports)

Miscellaneous: Allergic reactions, anaphylactoid reactions

Note: Thrombocytopenia has been reported to occur at an incidence between 0% and 30%. It is often of no clinical significance. However, immunologically mediated heparin-induced thrombocytopenia has been estimated to occur in 1% to 2% of patients, and is marked by a progressive fall in platelet counts and, in some cases, thromboembolic complications (skin necrosis, pulmonary embolism, gangrene of the extremities, stroke or MI). For recommendations regarding platelet monitoring during heparin therapy, consult "Seventh ACCP Consensus Conference on Antithrombotic and Thrombolytic Therapy."

Mechanism of Action Potentiates the action of antithrombin III and thereby inactivates thrombin (as well as activated coagulation factors IX, X, XI, XII, and plasmin) and prevents the conversion of fibrinogen to fibrin; heparin also stimulates release of lipoprotein lipase (lipoprotein lipase hydrolyzes triglycerides to glycerol and free fatty acids)

Drug Interactions

Increased Effect/Toxicity: The risk of hemorrhage associated with heparin may be increased by oral anticoagulants (warfarin), thrombolytics, dextran, and drugs which affect platelet function (eg, aspirin, NSAIDs, dipyridamole, ticlopidine, clopidogrel, IIb/IIIa antagonists). However, heparin is often used in conjunction with thrombolytic therapy or during the initiation of warfarin therapy to assure anticoagulation and to protect against possible transient hypercoagulability. Cephalosporins which contain the MTT side chain and parenteral penicillins (may inhibit platelet aggregation) may increase the risk of hemorrhage. Other drugs reported to increase heparin's anticoagulant effect include antihistamines, tetracycline, quinine, nicotine, and cardiac glycosides (digoxin).

Decreased Effect: Nitroglycerin (I.V.) may decrease heparin's anticoagulant effect. This interaction has not been validated in some studies, and may only occur at high nitroglycerin dosages.

Pharmacodynamics/Kinetics

Onset of action: Anticoagulation: I.V.: Immediate; SubQ: ~20-30 minutes

Absorption: Oral, rectal, I.M.: Erratic at best from all these routes of administration; SubQ absorption is also erratic, but considered acceptable for prophylactic use

Distribution: Does not cross placenta; does not enter breast milk

Metabolism: Hepatic; may be partially metabolized in the reticuloendothelial system

Half-life elimination: Mean: 1.5 hours; Range: 1-2 hours; affected by obesity, renal function, hepatic function, malignancy, presence of pulmonary embolism, and infections

Excretion: Urine (small amounts as unchanged drug)

Pregnancy Risk Factor C

Heparin Calcium *see* Heparin *on page 807*

Heparin Cofactor I *see* Antithrombin III *on page 134*

Heparin Lock Flush *see* Heparin *on page 807*

Heparin Sodium *see* Heparin *on page 807*

Hepatitis A Inactivated and Hepatitis B (Recombinant) Vaccine

(hep a TYE tis aye in ak ti VAY ted & hep a TYE tis bee ree KOM be nant vak SEEN)

Related Information

Immunizations (Vaccines) *on page 1886*

Systemic Viral Diseases *on page 1767*

U.S. Brand Names Twinrix®

Canadian Brand Names Twinrix®

Mexican Brand Names Twinrix

Generic Available No

Index Terms Engerix-B® and Havrix®; Havrix® and Engerix-B®; Hepatitis B (Recombinant) and Hepatitis A Inactivated Vaccine

Pharmacologic Category Vaccine

Use Active immunization against disease caused by hepatitis A virus and hepatitis B virus (all known subtypes) in populations desiring protection against or at high risk of exposure to these viruses.

Populations include travelers to areas of intermediate/high endemicity for **both** HAV and HBV; those at increased risk of HBV infection due to behavioral or occupational factors; patients with chronic liver disease; laboratory workers who handle live HAV and HBV; healthcare workers, police, and other personnel who render first-aid or medical assistance; workers who come in contact with sewage; employees of day care centers and correctional facilities; patients/staff of hemodialysis units; male homosexuals; patients frequently receiving blood products; military personnel; users of injectable illicit drugs; close household contacts of patients with hepatitis A and hepatitis B infection; residents of drug and alcohol treatment centers

Local Anesthetic/Vasoconstrictor Precautions No information available to require special precautions

Effects on Dental Treatment Key adverse event(s) related to dental treatment: Flu-like syndrome and upper respiratory tract infection.

Common Adverse Effects All serious adverse reactions must be reported to the U.S. Department of Health and Human Services (DHHS) Vaccine Adverse Event Reporting System (VAERS) 1-800-822-7967.

Incidence of adverse effects of the combination product were similar to those occurring after administration of hepatitis A vaccine and hepatitis B vaccine alone. (Incidence reported is not versus placebo.)

>10%:

Central nervous system: Headache (13% to 22%), fatigue (11% to 14%)

Local: Injection site reaction: Soreness (37% to 41%), redness (8% to 11%)

1% to 10%:

Central nervous system: Fever (2% to 4%)

Gastrointestinal: Diarrhea (4% to 6%), nausea (2% to 4%), vomiting (≤1%)

Local: Injection site reaction: Swelling (4% to 6%), induration

Respiratory: Upper respiratory tract infection

Mechanism of Action

Hepatitis A vaccine, an inactivated virus vaccine, offers active immunization against hepatitis A virus infection at an effective immune response rate in up to 99% of subjects.

Recombinant hepatitis B vaccine is a noninfectious subunit viral vaccine. The vaccine is derived from hepatitis B surface antigen (HB_sAg) produced through recombinant DNA techniques from yeast cells. The portion of the hepatitis B gene which codes for HB_sAg is cloned into yeast which is then cultured to produce hepatitis B vaccine.

In immunocompetent people, Twinrix® provides active immunization against hepatitis A virus infection (at an effective immune response rate >99% of subjects) and against hepatitis B virus infection (at an effective immune response rate of 93% to 97%) 30 days after completion of the 3-dose series. This is comparable to using hepatitis A vaccine and hepatitis B vaccine concomitantly.

Drug Interactions

Decreased Effect: Immunosuppressant agents: May decrease immune response to vaccine

Pharmacodynamics/Kinetics

Onset of action: Seroconversion for antibodies against HAV and HBV were detected 1 month after completion of the 3-dose series.

Duration: Patients remained seropositive for at least 4 years during clinical studies.

Pregnancy Risk Factor C

Hepatitis A Vaccine (hep a TYE tis aye vak SEEN)

Related Information

Immunizations (Vaccines) *on page 1886*
Systemic Viral Diseases *on page 1767*

U.S. Brand Names Havrix®; VAQTA®

Canadian Brand Names Avaxim®; Avaxim®-Pediatric; Havrix®; VAQTA®

Mexican Brand Names Havrix 1440; Havrix Junior; Vaqta

Generic Available No

Pharmacologic Category Vaccine

Use

Active immunization against disease caused by hepatitis A virus in populations desiring protection against or at high risk of exposure

(Continued)

Hepatitis A Vaccine *(Continued)*

Populations at high risk of exposure to hepatitis A virus may include children and adolescents in selected states and regions, travelers to developing countries, household and sexual contacts of persons infected with hepatitis A, child day care employees, patients with chronic liver disease, illicit drug users, male homosexuals, institutional workers (eg, institutions for the mentally and physically handicapped persons, prisons), and healthcare workers who may be exposed to hepatitis A virus (eg, laboratory employees)

Local Anesthetic/Vasoconstrictor Precautions No information available to require special precautions

Effects on Dental Treatment No significant effects or complications reported

Common Adverse Effects All serious adverse reactions must be reported to the U.S. Department of Health and Human Services (DHHS) Vaccine Adverse Event Reporting System (VAERS) 1-800-822-7967.

Frequency dependent upon age, product used, and concomitant vaccine administration. In general, injection site reactions were less common in younger children.

>10%:

Central nervous system: Irritability (11% to 36%), drowsiness (15% to 17%), headache (≤1% to 16%), fever ≥100.4°F (9% to 11%)

Gastrointestinal: Anorexia (1% to 19%)

Local: Injection site: Pain, soreness, tenderness (3% to 56%), erythema (1% to 22%), warmth (<1% to 17%), swelling (1% to 14%)

1% to 10%:

Central nervous system: Fever ≥102°F (3% to 4%)

Dermatologic: Rash (≤1% to 5%)

Endocrine & metabolic: Menstrual disorder (1%)

Gastrointestinal: Diarrhea (<1% to 6%), vomiting (<1% to 4%), nausea (2%), abdominal pain (<1% to 2%), anorexia (1%)

Local: Injection site bruising (1% to 2%)

Neuromuscular & skeletal: Weakness/fatigue (4%), myalgia (<1% to 2%), arm pain (1%), back pain (1%), stiffness (1%)

Ocular: Conjunctivitis (1%)

Otic: Otitis media (8%), otitis (2%)

Respiratory: Upper respiratory tract infection (<1% to 10%), rhinorrhea (6%), cough (1% to 5%), pharyngitis (<1% to 3%), respiratory congestion (2%), nasal congestion (1%), laryngotracheobronchitis (1%)

Miscellaneous: Crying (2%), viral exanthema (1%)

Mechanism of Action As an inactivated virus vaccine, hepatitis A vaccine offers active immunization against hepatitis A virus infection at an effective immune response rate in up to 99% of subjects

Pharmacodynamics/Kinetics

Onset of action (protection): 4 weeks after a single dose

Duration: Neutralizing antibodies have persisted for up to 8 years; based on kinetic models, antibodies may be present >20 years

Pregnancy Risk Factor C

Hepatitis B Immune Globulin

(hep a TYE tis bee i MYUN GLOB yoo lin)

Related Information

Immunizations (Vaccines) *on page 1886*

Occupational Exposure to Bloodborne Pathogens (Standard / Universal Precautions) *on page 1871*

Systemic Viral Diseases *on page 1767*

U.S. Brand Names HepaGam B™; HyperHEP B™ S/D; Nabi-HB®

Canadian Brand Names HepaGam B™; HyperHep B®

Generic Available No

Index Terms HBIG

Pharmacologic Category Immune Globulin

Use

Passive prophylactic immunity to hepatitis B following: Acute exposure to blood containing hepatitis B surface antigen (HBsAg); perinatal exposure of infants born to HBsAg-positive mothers; sexual exposure to HBsAg-positive persons; household exposure to persons with acute HBV infection

Prevention of hepatitis B virus recurrence after liver transplantation in HBsAg-positive transplant patients

Note: Hepatitis B immune globulin is not indicated for treatment of active hepatitis B infection and is ineffective in the treatment of chronic active hepatitis B infection.

Local Anesthetic/Vasoconstrictor Precautions No information available to require special precautions

Effects on Dental Treatment No significant effects or complications reported

Common Adverse Effects Reported with postexposure prophylaxis; frequency not defined. Adverse events reported in liver transplant patients included tremor and hypotension, were associated with a single infusion during the first week of treatment, and did not recur with additional infusions.

Central nervous system: Fainting, headache, lightheadedness, malaise

Dermatologic: Angioedema, bruising, urticaria

Gastrointestinal: Nausea, vomiting

Hematologic: WBC decreased

Hepatic: Alkaline phosphatase increased, AST increased

Local: Ache, erythema, pain, and/or tenderness at injection site

Neuromuscular & skeletal: Arthralgia, joint stiffness, myalgia

Renal: Creatinine increased

Respiratory: Cold symptoms

Miscellaneous: Anaphylaxis, flu-like syndrome

Mechanism of Action Hepatitis B immune globulin (HBIG) is a nonpyrogenic sterile solution containing immunoglobulin G (IgG) specific to hepatitis B surface antigen (HB_sAg). HBIG differs from immune globulin in the amount of anti-HB_s. Immune globulin is prepared from plasma that is not preselected for anti-HB_s content. HBIG is prepared from plasma preselected for high titer anti-HB_s. In the U.S., HBIG has an anti-HB_s high titer >1:100,000 by IRA.

Drug Interactions

Decreased Effect:

Interferes with immune response of live virus vaccines; defer live virus vaccine for about 3 months after immune globulin

Note: HBIG may be administered at the same time (but at a different site) or up to 1 month preceding hepatitis B vaccination without impairing the active immune response

Pharmacodynamics/Kinetics

Duration of action: Postexposure prophylaxis: 3-6 months

Absorption: I.M.: Slow

Half-life: 17-25 days

Distribution: V_d: 7-15 L

Time to peak, serum: I.M.: 2-10 days

Pregnancy Risk Factor C

Hepatitis B Inactivated Virus Vaccine (recombinant DNA) *see* Hepatitis B Vaccine *on page 811*

Hepatitis B (Recombinant) and Hepatitis A Inactivated Vaccine *see* Hepatitis A Inactivated and Hepatitis B (Recombinant) Vaccine *on page 808*

Hepatitis B Vaccine (hep a TYE tis bee vak SEEN)

Related Information

Immunizations (Vaccines) *on page 1886*

Systemic Viral Diseases *on page 1767*

U.S. Brand Names Engerix-B®; Recombivax HB®

Canadian Brand Names Engerix-B®; Recombivax HB®

Mexican Brand Names Engerix-B

Generic Available No

Index Terms Hepatitis B Inactivated Virus Vaccine (recombinant DNA)

Pharmacologic Category Vaccine

Dental Use Immunization is recommended for dentists, oral surgeons, dental hygienists, dental nurses, and dental students

Use Immunization against infection caused by all known subtypes of hepatitis B virus (HBV), in individuals seeking protection from HBV infection and/or in the following individuals considered at high risk of potential exposure to hepatitis B virus or HB_sAg-positive materials:

Workplace Exposure:

- Healthcare workers[1] (including students, custodial staff, lab personnel, etc)
- Police and fire personnel
- Military personnel
- Morticians and embalmers
- Clients/staff of institutions for the developmentally disabled

Lifestyle Factors:

- Homosexual men
- Heterosexually-active persons with multiple partners in a 6-month period or those with recently acquired sexually-transmitted disease
- Intravenous drug users

(Continued)

Hepatitis B Vaccine (Continued)

Specific Patient Groups:
- Those on hemodialysis[2], receiving transfusions[3], or in hematology/oncology units
- Adolescents
- Infants born of HBsAG-positive mothers
- Individuals with chronic liver disease
- Individual with HIV infection

Others:
- Prison inmates and staff of correctional facilities
- Household and sexual contacts of HBV carriers
- Residents, immigrants, adoptees, and refugees from areas with endemic HBV infection (eg, Alaskan Eskimos, Pacific Islanders, Indochinese, and Haitian descent)
- International travelers to areas of endemic HBV
- Children born after 11/21/1991

[1]The risk of hepatitis B virus (HBV) infection for healthcare workers varies both between hospitals and within hospitals. Hepatitis B vaccination is recommended for all healthcare workers with blood exposure.

[2]Hemodialysis patients often respond poorly to hepatitis B vaccination; higher vaccine doses or increased number of doses are required. A special formulation of one vaccine is now available for such persons (Recombivax HB®, 40 mcg/mL). The anti-HB$_s$(antibody to hepatitis B surface antigen) response of such persons should be tested after they are vaccinated, and those who have not responded should be revaccinated with 1-3 additional doses. Patients with chronic renal disease should be vaccinated as early as possible, ideally before they require hemodialysis. In addition, their anti-HB$_s$ levels should be monitored at 6- to 12-month intervals to assess the need for revaccination.

[3]Patients with hemophilia should be immunized subcutaneously, not intramuscularly.

Local Anesthetic/Vasoconstrictor Precautions No information available to require special precautions

Effects on Dental Treatment No significant effects or complications reported

Common Adverse Effects All serious adverse reactions must be reported to the U.S. Department of Health and Human Services (DHHS) Vaccine Adverse Event Reporting System (VAERS) 1-800-822-7967.

Frequency not defined. The most common adverse effects reported with both products included injection site reactions (>10%).

Cardiovascular: Flushing, hypotension

Central nervous system: Agitation, chills, dizziness, fatigue, fever (≥37.5°C / 100°F), headache, insomnia, irritability, lightheadedness, malaise, somnolence, vertigo

Dermatologic: Angioedema, petechiae, pruritus, rash, urticaria

Gastrointestinal: Abdominal pain, appetite decreased, constipation, cramps, diarrhea, dyspepsia, nausea, vomiting

Genitourinary: Dysuria

Local: Injection site reactions: Ecchymosis, erythema, induration, pain, nodule formation, soreness, swelling, tenderness, warmth

Neuromuscular & skeletal: Achiness, arthralgia, back pain, myalgia, neck pain, neck stiffness, paresthesia, shoulder pain, tingling, weakness

Otic: Earache

Respiratory: Cough, pharyngitis, rhinitis, upper respiratory tract infection

Miscellaneous: Diaphoresis, lymphadenopathy, flu-like syndrome

Mechanism of Action Recombinant hepatitis B vaccine is a noninfectious subunit viral vaccine, which confers active immunity via formation of antihepatitis B antibodies. The vaccine is derived from hepatitis B surface antigen (HB$_s$Ag) produced through recombinant DNA techniques from yeast cells. The portion of the hepatitis B gene which codes for HB$_s$Ag is cloned into yeast which is then cultured to produce hepatitis B vaccine.

Drug Interactions

Decreased Effect: Concomitant immunosuppressive agents may decrease efficacy of vaccine; consider deferring vaccination for at least 3 months after immunosuppressant therapy is discontinued.

Pharmacodynamics/Kinetics Duration of action: Following a 3-dose series in children, up to 50% of patients will have low or undetectable anti-HB antibody 5-15 years postvaccination. However, anamnestic increases in anti-HB have been shown up to 23 years later suggesting a lifelong immune memory response.

Pregnancy Risk Factor C

HepFlush®-10 see Heparin on page 807
Hep-Lock® see Heparin on page 807

Hetastarch (HET a starch)

U.S. Brand Names Hespan®; Hextend®
Canadian Brand Names Hextend®; Voluven®
Generic Available Yes: Sodium chloride infusion
Index Terms HES; Hydroxyethyl Starch
Pharmacologic Category Plasma Volume Expander, Colloid
Use Blood volume expander used in treatment of hypovolemia
    Hespan®: Adjunct in leukapheresis to improve harvesting and increasing the
    yield of granulocytes by centrifugal means
Unlabeled/Investigational Use Hextend®: Priming fluid in pump oxygenators
    during cardiopulmonary bypass, and as a plasma volume expander during
    cardiopulmonary bypass
Local Anesthetic/Vasoconstrictor Precautions No information available to
    require special precautions
Effects on Dental Treatment No significant effects or complications reported
Common Adverse Effects Frequency not defined.
    Cardiovascular: Circulatory overload, heart failure, peripheral edema
    Central nervous system: Chills, fever, headache, intracranial bleeding
    Dermatologic: Itching, pruritus, rash
    Endocrine & metabolic: Amylase levels increased, parotid gland enlargement,
        indirect bilirubin increased, metabolic acidosis
    Gastrointestinal: Vomiting
    Hematologic: Bleeding, factor VIII:C plasma levels decreased, decreased
        plasma aggregation decreased, von Willebrand factor decreased, dilutional
        coagulopathy; prolongation of PT, PTT, clotting time, and bleeding time;
        thrombocytopenia, anemia, disseminated intravascular coagulopathy (rare),
        hemolysis (rare)
    Neuromuscular & skeletal: Myalgia
    Miscellaneous: Anaphylactoid reactions, hypersensitivity, flu-like syndrome
        (mild)
Mechanism of Action Produces plasma volume expansion by virtue of its
    highly colloidal starch structure, similar to albumin
Pharmacodynamics/Kinetics
    Onset of action: Volume expansion: I.V.: ~30 minutes
    Duration: 24-36 hours
    Metabolism: Molecules >50,000 daltons require enzymatic degradation by the
        reticuloendothelial system or amylases in the blood
    Excretion: Urine (~40%) within 24 hours; smaller molecular weight molecules
        readily excreted
Pregnancy Risk Factor C

Hexachlorophene (heks a KLOR oh feen)

U.S. Brand Names pHisoHex®
Canadian Brand Names pHisoHex®
Generic Available No
Pharmacologic Category Antibiotic, Topical
Use Surgical scrub and as a bacteriostatic skin cleanser; control an outbreak of
    gram-positive infection when other procedures have been unsuccessful
Local Anesthetic/Vasoconstrictor Precautions No information available to
    require special precautions
Effects on Dental Treatment No significant effects or complications reported
Mechanism of Action Bacteriostatic polychlorinated biphenyl which inhibits
    membrane-bound enzymes and disrupts the cell membrane
Pharmacodynamics/Kinetics
    Absorption: Percutaneously through inflamed, excoriated, and intact skin
    Distribution: Crosses placenta
    Half-life elimination: Infants: 6.1-44.2 hours
Pregnancy Risk Factor C

Hexamethylmelamine *see* Altretamine *on page 79*
HEXM *see* Altretamine *on page 79*
Hextend® *see* Hetastarch *on page 813*

Hexylresorcinol (heks il re ZOR si nole)

U.S. Brand Names S.T. 37® [OTC]; Sucrets® Original [OTC]
Generic Available No
Pharmacologic Category Antiseptic, Topical; Local Anesthetic
Use Minor antiseptic and local anesthetic for sore throat; topical antiseptic for minor cuts or abrasions
Local Anesthetic/Vasoconstrictor Precautions No information available to require special precautions
Effects on Dental Treatment No significant effects or complications reported

hFSH *see* Urofollitropin *on page 1633*
hGH *see* Somatropin *on page 1486*
Hib Conjugate Vaccine *see* Haemophilus b Conjugate Vaccine *on page 802*
Hibiclens® [OTC] *see* Chlorhexidine Gluconate *on page 332*
Hibistat® [OTC] *see* Chlorhexidine Gluconate *on page 332*
Hib Polysaccharide Conjugate *see* Haemophilus b Conjugate Vaccine *on page 802*
HibTITER® *see* Haemophilus b Conjugate Vaccine *on page 802*
High Gamma Vitamin E Complete™ [OTC] *see* Vitamin E *on page 1664*
Hi-Kovite [OTC *see* Vitamins (Multiple/Oral) *on page 1665*
Hiprex® *see* Methenamine *on page 1063*
Hirulog *see* Bivalirudin *on page 220*
Histade™ *see* Chlorpheniramine and Pseudoephedrine *on page 340*
Hista-Vent® DA *see* Chlorpheniramine, Phenylephrine, and Methscopolamine *on page 342*
Histex™ *see* Chlorpheniramine and Pseudoephedrine *on page 340*
Histex™ HC *see* Hydrocodone, Carbinoxamine, and Pseudoephedrine *on page 832*
Histex™ SR *see* Brompheniramine and Pseudoephedrine *on page 231*

Histrelin (his TREL in)

U.S. Brand Names Vantas™
Canadian Brand Names Vantas™
Generic Available No
Index Terms GnRH Agonist; Histrelin Acetate; LH-RH Agonist
Pharmacologic Category Gonadotropin Releasing Hormone Agonist
Use Palliative treatment of advanced prostate cancer
Local Anesthetic/Vasoconstrictor Precautions No information available to require special precautions
Effects on Dental Treatment No significant effects or complications reported
Common Adverse Effects
>10%: Endocrine & metabolic: Expected pharmacological consequence of testosterone suppression: Hot flashes (66%)
2% to 10%:
Central nervous system: Fatigue (10%), headache (3%), insomnia (3%)
Endocrine & metabolic: Expected pharmacological consequences of testosterone suppression: Gynecomastia (4%), sexual dysfunction (4%), libido decreased (2%)
Gastrointestinal: Constipation (4%), weight gain (2%)
Genitourinary: Expected pharmacological consequence of testosterone suppression: Testicular atrophy (5%)
Local: Implant site reaction (6%)
Renal: Renal impairment (5%)
Mechanism of Action Potent inhibitor of gonadotropin secretion; continuous administration results in, after an initiation phase, the suppression of luteinizing hormone (LH), follicle-stimulating hormone (FSH), and a subsequent decrease in testosterone.
Drug Interactions
Increased Effect/Toxicity: Not studied
Pharmacodynamics/Kinetics
Onset: Chemical castration: 14 days
Duration: 1 year
Distribution: V_d: ~58 L
Protein binding: 70% ± 9%

Metabolism: Hepatic via C-terminal dealkylation and hydrolysis
Bioavailability: 92%
Half-life elimination: Terminal: ~4 hours
Time to peak, serum: 12 hours
Pregnancy Risk Factor X

Histrelin Acetate *see* Histrelin *on page 814*

Histussin D® [DSC] *see* Hydrocodone and Pseudoephedrine *on page 832*

Hi-Vegi-Lip [OTC] *see* Pancreatin *on page 1247*

Hivid® [DSC] *see* Zalcitabine *on page 1675*

hMG *see* Menotropins *on page 1037*

HMM *see* Altretamine *on page 79*

HMR 3647 *see* Telithromycin *on page 1528*

HMS Liquifilm® [DSC] *see* Medrysone *on page 1027*

Hold® DM [OTC] *see* Dextromethorphan *on page 477*

Homatropine (hoe MA troe peen)

U.S. Brand Names Isopto® Homatropine
Generic Available No
Index Terms Homatropine Hydrobromide
Pharmacologic Category Anticholinergic Agent, Ophthalmic; Ophthalmic Agent, Mydriatic
Use Producing cycloplegia and mydriasis for refraction; treatment of acute inflammatory conditions of the uveal tract
Local Anesthetic/Vasoconstrictor Precautions No information available to require special precautions
Effects on Dental Treatment Key adverse event(s) related to dental treatment: Nasal congestion.
Mechanism of Action Blocks response of iris sphincter muscle and the accommodative muscle of the ciliary body to cholinergic stimulation resulting in dilation and loss of accommodation
Pregnancy Risk Factor C

Homatropine and Hydrocodone *see* Hydrocodone and Homatropine *on page 829*

Homatropine Hydrobromide *see* Homatropine *on page 815*

Horse Antihuman Thymocyte Gamma Globulin *see* Antithymocyte Globulin (Equine) *on page 134*

H.P. Acthar® Gel *see* Corticotropin *on page 415*

HPV Vaccine *see* Papillomavirus (Types 6, 11, 16, 18) Recombinant Vaccine *on page 1252*

HTF919 *see* Tegaserod *on page 1527*

hu1124 *see* Efalizumab *on page 557*

Humalog® *see* Insulin Lispro *on page 887*

Humalog® Mix 50/50™ *see* Insulin Lispro Protamine and Insulin Lispro *on page 887*

Humalog® Mix 75/25™ *see* Insulin Lispro Protamine and Insulin Lispro *on page 887*

Human Antitumor Necrosis Factor Alpha *see* Adalimumab *on page 53*

Human Corticotrophin-Releasing Hormone, Analogue *see* Corticorelin *on page 414*

Human Diploid Cell Cultures Rabies Vaccine *see* Rabies Virus Vaccine *on page 1403*

Human Growth Hormone *see* Somatropin *on page 1486*

Humanized IgG1 Anti-CD52 Monoclonal Antibody *see* Alemtuzumab *on page 64*

Human LFA-3/IgG(1) Fusion Protein *see* Alefacept *on page 63*

Human Menopausal Gonadotropin *see* Menotropins *on page 1037*

Human Papillomavirus Vaccine *see* Papillomavirus (Types 6, 11, 16, 18) Recombinant Vaccine *on page 1252*

Human Thyroid Stimulating Hormone *see* Thyrotropin Alpha *on page 1563*

Humate-P® *see* Antihemophilic Factor/von Willebrand Factor Complex (Human) *on page 132*

Humatin® *see* Paromomycin *on page 1254*

Humatrope® *see* Somatropin *on page 1486*

Humibid® LA *(reformulation) see* Guaifenesin and Potassium Guaiacolsulfonate *on page 797*

Humira® *see* Adalimumab *on page 53*

Humulin® 50/50 *see* Insulin NPH and Insulin Regular *on page 888*

Humulin® 70/30 *see* Insulin NPH and Insulin Regular *on page 888*

Humulin® N *see* Insulin NPH *on page 888*

Humulin® R *see* Insulin Regular *on page 889*

Humulin® R (Concentrated) U-500 *see* Insulin Regular *on page 889*

Hurricaine® [OTC] *see* Benzocaine *on page 195*

HXM *see* Altretamine *on page 79*

Hyalgan® *see* Hyaluronate and Derivatives *on page 816*

Hyaluronan *see* Hyaluronate and Derivatives *on page 816*

Hyaluronate and Derivatives
(hye al yoor ON ate & dah RIV ah tives)

U.S. Brand Names Biolon™ [DSC]; Euflexxa™; Healon®; Healon®5; Healon GV®; Hyalgan®; Hylaform®; Hylaform® Plus; IPM Wound Gel™ [OTC]; Juvederm™ 24HV; Juvederm™ 30; Juvederm™ 30HV; Orthovisc®; Provisc®; Restylane®; Supartz™; Synvisc®; Vitrax®

Canadian Brand Names Cystistat®; Durolane®; Eyestil; Healon®; Healon GV®; OrthoVisc®; Suplasyn®

Mexican Brand Names Synvisc

Generic Available No

Index Terms Hyaluronan; Hyaluronic Acid; Hylan Polymers; Sodium Hyaluronate

Pharmacologic Category Antirheumatic Miscellaneous; Ophthalmic Agent, Viscoelastic; Skin and Mucous Membrane Agent, Miscellaneous

Use

Intra-articular injection: Treatment of pain in osteoarthritis in knee in patients who have failed nonpharmacologic treatment and simple analgesics

Intradermal: Correction of moderate-to-severe facial wrinkles or folds

Ophthalmic: Surgical aid in cataract extraction, intraocular implantation, corneal transplant, glaucoma filtration, and retinal attachment surgery

Topical: Management of skin ulcers and wounds

Local Anesthetic/Vasoconstrictor Precautions No information available to require special precautions

Effects on Dental Treatment No significant effects or complications reported

Common Adverse Effects Frequencies and/or type of local reaction may vary by formulation and site of application/injection.

>10%:

Local: Injection site (intradermal): Bruising (52% to 61%), erythema (85% to 93%), lumps/bumps (79% to 83%), pain (57% to 90%), swelling (86% to 89%); pruritus (28% to 36%), skin discoloration (31% to 34%)

Respiratory: Infection (12%)

1% to 10%:

Cardiovascular: Blood pressure increased (2% to 4%)

Central nervous system: Fatigue (1%)

Gastrointestinal: Nausea (≤2%)

Local: Dry skin (intradermal >1%), peeling (intradermal >1%)

Neuromuscular & skeletal: Back pain (<1% to 6%), tendonitis (2%), paresthesia (1%)

Respiratory: Rhinitis (3%)

Frequency not defined:

Cardiovascular: Edema, flushing, hypotension, tachycardia

Central nervous system: Dizziness, headache

Dermatologic: Rash

Local: Injection site: Arthralgia, nodule

Neuromuscular & skeletal: Hypokinesia (knee)

Ocular (with ophthalmic formulation): Postoperative inflammatory reactions (iritis, hypopyon), corneal edema, corneal decompensation, transient postoperative increase in IOP

Miscellaneous: Abscess formation, allergic reactions, anaphylaxis, respiratory difficulties

Mechanism of Action Sodium hyaluronate is a polysaccharide which is distributed widely in the extracellular matrix of connective tissue in man (vitreous and aqueous humor of the eye, synovial fluid, skin, and umbilical cord). Sodium hyaluronate and its derivatives form a viscoelastic solution in water (at physiological pH and ionic strength) which makes it suitable for aqueous and vitreous humor in ophthalmic surgery, and functions as a tissue and/or joint lubricant which plays an important role in modulating the interactions between adjacent tissues. Intradermal injection may decrease the depth of facial wrinkles.

Drug Interactions

Increased Effect/Toxicity: Anticoagulants or antiplatelet agents may increase the risk of injection site bleeding or hematoma.

Pharmacodynamics/Kinetics

Distribution: Intravitreous injection: Diffusion occurs slowly

Excretion: Ophthalmic: Via Canal of Schlemm
Pregnancy Risk Factor C

Hyaluronic Acid *see* Hyaluronate and Derivatives *on page 816*

Hyaluronidase (hye al yoor ON i dase)

U.S. Brand Names Amphadase™; Hydase™; Hylenex™; Vitrase®
Generic Available No
Pharmacologic Category Enzyme
Use Increase the dispersion and absorption of other drugs; increase rate of absorption of parenteral fluids given by hypodermoclysis; adjunct in subcutaneous urography for improving resorption of radiopaque agents
Unlabeled/Investigational Use Management of drug extravasations
Local Anesthetic/Vasoconstrictor Precautions No information available to require special precautions
Effects on Dental Treatment No significant effects or complications reported
Common Adverse Effects
Frequency not defined:
Cardiovascular: Edema
Local: Injection site reactions
Mechanism of Action Modifies the permeability of connective tissue through hydrolysis of hyaluronic acid, one of the chief components of tissue cement which offers resistance to diffusion of liquids through tissues; hyaluronidase increases both the distribution and absorption of locally injected substances.
Drug Interactions
Increased Effect/Toxicity: Absorption and toxicity of local anesthetics may be increased.
Pharmacodynamics/Kinetics
Onset of action: SubQ: Immediate
Duration: 24-48 hours
Pregnancy Risk Factor C

Hycamptamine *see* Topotecan *on page 1592*

Hycamtin® *see* Topotecan *on page 1592*

hycet™ *see* Hydrocodone and Acetaminophen *on page 822*

Hycodan® *see* Hydrocodone and Homatropine *on page 829*

Hycomine® Compound *see* Hydrocodone, Chlorpheniramine, Phenylephrine, Acetaminophen, and Caffeine *on page 833*

Hycotuss® *see* Hydrocodone and Guaifenesin *on page 828*

Hydase™ *see* Hyaluronidase *on page 817*

Hydergine [DSC] *see* Ergoloid Mesylates *on page 584*

HydrALAZINE (hye DRAL a zeen)

Related Information
Cardiovascular Diseases *on page 1726*
Canadian Brand Names Apo-Hydralazine®; Apresoline®; Novo-Hylazin; Nu-Hydral
Mexican Brand Names Apresolina
Generic Available Yes
Index Terms Apresoline [DSC]; Hydralazine Hydrochloride
Pharmacologic Category Vasodilator
Use Management of moderate to severe hypertension, congestive heart failure, hypertension secondary to pre-eclampsia/eclampsia; treatment of primary pulmonary hypertension
Local Anesthetic/Vasoconstrictor Precautions No information available to require special precautions
Effects on Dental Treatment No significant effects or complications reported
Common Adverse Effects Frequency not defined.
Cardiovascular: Tachycardia, angina pectoris, orthostatic hypotension (rare), dizziness (rare), paradoxical hypertension, peripheral edema, vascular collapse (rare), flushing
Central nervous system: Increased intracranial pressure (I.V., in patient with pre-existing increased intracranial pressure), fever (rare), chills (rare), anxiety*, disorientation*, depression*, coma*
Dermatologic: Rash (rare), urticaria (rare), pruritus (rare)
Gastrointestinal: Anorexia, nausea, vomiting, diarrhea, constipation, adynamic ileus
Genitourinary: Difficulty in micturition, impotence
(Continued)

HydrALAZINE *(Continued)*

Hematologic: Hemolytic anemia (rare), eosinophilia (rare), decreased hemoglobin concentration (rare), reduced erythrocyte count (rare), leukopenia (rare), agranulocytosis (rare), thrombocytopenia (rare)

Neuromuscular & skeletal: Rheumatoid arthritis, muscle cramps, weakness, tremor, peripheral neuritis (rare)

Ocular: Lacrimation, conjunctivitis

Respiratory: Nasal congestion, dyspnea

Miscellaneous: Drug-induced lupus-like syndrome (dose related; fever, arthralgia, splenomegaly, lymphadenopathy, asthenia, myalgia, malaise, pleuritic chest pain, edema, positive ANA, positive LE cells, maculopapular facial rash, positive direct Coombs' test, pericarditis, pericardial tamponade), diaphoresis

*Seen in uremic patients and severe hypertension where rapidly escalating doses may have caused hypotension leading to these effects.

Mechanism of Action Direct vasodilation of arterioles (with little effect on veins) with decreased systemic resistance

Drug Interactions

Cytochrome P450 Effect: Inhibits CYP3A4 (weak)

Increased Effect/Toxicity: Hydralazine may increase levels of beta-blockers (metoprolol, propranolol). Some beta-blockers (acebutolol, atenolol, and nadolol) are unlikely to be affected due to limited hepatic metabolism. Concurrent use of hydralazine with MAO inhibitors may cause a significant decrease in blood pressure. Propranolol may increase hydralazine serum concentrations.

Decreased Effect: NSAIDs (eg, indomethacin) may decrease the hemodynamic effects of hydralazine.

Pharmacodynamics/Kinetics

Onset of action: Oral: 20-30 minutes; I.V.: 5-20 minutes

Duration: Oral: Up to 8 hours; I.V.: 1-4 hours; **Note:** May vary depending on acetylator status of patient

Distribution: Crosses placenta; enters breast milk

Protein binding: 85% to 90%

Metabolism: Hepatically acetylated; extensive first-pass effect (oral)

Bioavailability: 30% to 50%; increased with food

Half-life elimination: Normal renal function: 2-8 hours; End-stage renal disease: 7-16 hours

Excretion: Urine (14% as unchanged drug)

Pregnancy Risk Factor C

Hydralazine and Hydrochlorothiazide

(hye DRAL a zeen & hye droe klor oh THYE a zide)

Related Information

HydrALAZINE *on page 817*

Hydrochlorothiazide *on page 819*

Generic Available Yes

Index Terms Apresazide [DSC]; Hydrochlorothiazide and Hydralazine

Pharmacologic Category Antihypertensive Agent, Combination

Use Management of moderate to severe hypertension and treatment of congestive heart failure

Local Anesthetic/Vasoconstrictor Precautions No information available to require special precautions

Effects on Dental Treatment No significant effects or complications reported

Common Adverse Effects See individual agents.

Drug Interactions

Cytochrome P450 Effect: Hydralazine: **Inhibits** CYP3A4 (weak)

Increased Effect/Toxicity: See individual agents.

Pharmacodynamics/Kinetics See individual agents.

Pregnancy Risk Factor C

Hydralazine and Isosorbide Dinitrate *see* Isosorbide Dinitrate and Hydralazine *on page 915*

Hydralazine Hydrochloride *see* HydrALAZINE *on page 817*

Hydramine® [OTC] *see* DiphenhydrAMINE *on page 510*

Hydrated Chloral *see* Chloral Hydrate *on page 327*

Hydrea® *see* Hydroxyurea *on page 845*

Hydrisalic™ [OTC] *see* Salicylic Acid *on page 1451*

Hydrochlorothiazide (hye droe klor oh THYE a zide)

Related Information
Cardiovascular Diseases *on page 1726*
U.S. Brand Names Microzide™
Canadian Brand Names Apo-Hydro®; Novo-Hydrazide; PMS-Hydrochlorothiazide
Generic Available Yes
Index Terms HCTZ (error-prone abbreviation)
Pharmacologic Category Diuretic, Thiazide
Use Management of mild to moderate hypertension; treatment of edema in congestive heart failure and nephrotic syndrome
Unlabeled/Investigational Use Treatment of lithium-induced diabetes insipidus
Local Anesthetic/Vasoconstrictor Precautions No information available to require special precautions
Effects on Dental Treatment Key adverse event(s) related to dental treatment: Orthostatic hypotension and hypotension.
Common Adverse Effects
1% to 10%:
Cardiovascular: Orthostatic hypotension, hypotension
Dermatologic: Photosensitivity
Endocrine & metabolic: Hypokalemia
Gastrointestinal: Anorexia, epigastric distress
Dosage Oral (effect of drug may be decreased when used every day):
Children (in pediatric patients, chlorothiazide may be preferred over hydrochlorothiazide as there are more dosage formulations [eg, suspension] available):
Edema, hypertension:
<6 months: 1-3 mg/kg/day in 2 divided doses
>6 months to 2 years: 1-3 mg/kg/day in 2 divided doses; maximum: 37.5 mg/day
>2-17 years: Initial: 1 mg/kg/day; maximum: 3 mg/kg/day (50 mg/day)
Adults:
Edema: 25-100 mg/day in 1-2 doses; maximum: 200 mg/day
Hypertension: 12.5-50 mg/day; minimal increase in response and more electrolyte disturbances are seen with doses >50 mg/day
Elderly: 12.5-25 mg once daily

Dosing adjustment/comments in renal impairment: Cl_{cr} <10 mL/minute: Avoid use. Usually ineffective with GFR <30 mL/minute. Effective at lower GFR in combination with a loop diuretic.
Mechanism of Action Inhibits sodium reabsorption in the distal tubules causing increased excretion of sodium and water as well as potassium and hydrogen ions
Contraindications Hypersensitivity to hydrochlorothiazide or any component of the formulation, thiazides, or sulfonamide-derived drugs; anuria; renal decompensation; pregnancy
Warnings/Precautions Avoid in severe renal disease (ineffective). Electrolyte disturbances (hypokalemia, hypochloremic alkalosis, hyponatremia) can occur. Use with caution in severe hepatic dysfunction; hepatic encephalopathy can be caused by electrolyte disturbances. Gout can be precipitate in certain patients with a history of gout, a familial predisposition to gout, or chronic renal failure. Cautious use in prediabetics and diabetics; may see a change in glucose control. Can cause SLE exacerbation or activation. Use with caution in patients with moderate or high cholesterol concentrations. Photosensitization may occur. Correct hypokalemia before initiating therapy.

Chemical similarities are present among sulfonamides, sulfonylureas, carbonic anhydrase inhibitors, thiazides, and loop diuretics (except ethacrynic acid). Use in patients with sulfonamide allergy is specifically contraindicated in product labeling, however, a risk of cross-reaction exists in patients with allergy to any of these compounds; avoid use when previous reaction has been severe. Discontinue if signs of hypersensitivity are noted.
Drug Interactions
Increased Effect/Toxicity: Increased effect of hydrochlorothiazide with furosemide and other loop diuretics. Increased hypotension and/or renal adverse effects of ACE inhibitors may result in aggressively diuresed patients. Beta-blockers increase hyperglycemic effects of thiazides in type 2 diabetes mellitus. Cyclosporine and thiazides can increase the risk of gout or renal toxicity. Digoxin toxicity can be exacerbated if a thiazide induces hypokalemia or hypomagnesemia. Lithium toxicity can occur with thiazides due to reduced renal excretion of lithium. Thiazides may prolong the duration of action with neuromuscular blocking agents.
(Continued)

Hydrochlorothiazide *(Continued)*

Decreased Effect: Effects of oral hypoglycemics may be decreased. Decreased absorption of hydrochlorothiazide with cholestyramine and colestipol. NSAIDs can decrease the efficacy of thiazides, reducing the diuretic and antihypertensive effects.

Ethanol/Nutrition/Herb Interactions

Food: Hydrochlorothiazide peak serum levels may be decreased if taken with food. This product may deplete potassium, sodium, and magnesium.

Herb/Nutraceutical: Avoid dong quai if using for hypertension (has estrogenic activity). Dong quai may also cause photosensitization. Avoid ephedra, ginseng, yohimbe (may worsen hypertension). Avoid garlic (may have increased antihypertensive effect).

Pharmacodynamics/Kinetics

Onset of action: Diuresis: ~2 hours

Peak effect: 4-6 hours

Duration: 6-12 hours

Absorption: ~50% to 80%

Distribution: 3.6-7.8 L/kg

Protein binding: 68%

Metabolism: Not metabolized

Bioavailability: 50% to 80%

Half-life elimination: 5.6-14.8 hours

Time to peak: 1-2.5 hours

Excretion: Urine (as unchanged drug)

Pregnancy Risk Factor B (manufacturer); D (expert analysis)

Dosage Forms

Capsule: 12.5 mg

Microzide™: 12.5 mg

Tablet: 25 mg, 50 mg

Hydrochlorothiazide and Spironolactone

(hye droe klor oh THYE a zide & speer on oh LAK tone)

Related Information

Cardiovascular Diseases *on page 1726*

Hydrochlorothiazide *on page 819*

Spironolactone *on page 1492*
U.S. Brand Names Aldactazide®
Canadian Brand Names Aldactazide 25®; Aldactazide 50®; Novo-Spirozine
Generic Available Yes
Index Terms Spironolactone and Hydrochlorothiazide
Pharmacologic Category Antihypertensive Agent, Combination
Use Management of mild- to-moderate hypertension; treatment of edema in congestive heart failure and nephrotic syndrome, and cirrhosis of the liver accompanied by edema and/or ascites
Local Anesthetic/Vasoconstrictor Precautions No information available to require special precautions
Effects on Dental Treatment No significant effects or complications reported
Common Adverse Effects See individual agents.
Drug Interactions
  Increased Effect/Toxicity: See individual agents.
Pharmacodynamics/Kinetics See individual agents.
Pregnancy Risk Factor C

Hydrochlorothiazide and Telmisartan *see* Telmisartan and Hydrochlorothiazide *on page 1532*

Hydrochlorothiazide and Triamterene
(hye droe klor oh THYE a zide & trye AM ter een)

Related Information
Cardiovascular Diseases *on page 1726*
Hydrochlorothiazide *on page 819*
Triamterene *on page 1613*
U.S. Brand Names Dyazide®; Maxzide®; Maxzide®-25
Canadian Brand Names Apo-Triazide®; Novo-Triamzide; Nu-Triazide; Penta-Triamterene HCTZ; Riva-Zide
Mexican Brand Names Dyazide
Generic Available Yes
Index Terms Triamterene and Hydrochlorothiazide
Pharmacologic Category Antihypertensive Agent, Combination; Diuretic, Potassium-Sparing; Diuretic, Thiazide
Use Management of mild to moderate hypertension; treatment of edema in congestive heart failure and nephrotic syndrome
Local Anesthetic/Vasoconstrictor Precautions No information available to require special precautions
Effects on Dental Treatment No significant effects or complications reported
Common Adverse Effects Also see individual agents. Frequency not defined.
  Central nervous system: Dizziness, fatigue
  Dermatologic: Purpura, cracked corners of mouth
  Endocrine & metabolic: Electrolyte disturbances
  Gastrointestinal: Bright orange tongue, burning of tongue, loss of appetite, nausea, vomiting, stomach cramps, diarrhea, upset stomach
  Hematologic: Aplastic anemia, agranulocytosis, hemolytic anemia, leukopenia, thrombocytopenia, megaloblastic anemia
  Neuromuscular & skeletal: Muscle cramps
  Ocular: Xanthopsia, transient blurred vision
  Respiratory: Allergic pneumonitis, pulmonary edema, respiratory distress
Dosage Adults: Oral:
  Hydrochlorothiazide 25 mg and triamterene 37.5 mg: 1-2 tablets/capsules once daily
  Hydrochlorothiazide 50 mg and triamterene 75 mg: $^1/_2$-1 tablet daily
Mechanism of Action
  Based on **triamterene** component: Interferes with potassium/sodium exchange (active transport) in the distal tubule, cortical collecting tubule and collecting duct by inhibiting sodium, potassium-ATPase; decreases calcium excretion; increases magnesium loss
  Based on **hydrochlorothiazide** component: Inhibits sodium reabsorption in the distal tubules causing increased excretion of sodium and water as well as potassium and hydrogen ions
Contraindications
  Based on **hydrochlorothiazide** component: Hypersensitivity to hydrochlorothiazide or any component of the formulation, thiazides, or sulfonamide-derived drugs; anuria; renal decompensation; pregnancy
  Based on **triamterene** component: Hypersensitivity to triamterene or any component of the formulation; patients receiving other potassium-sparing diuretics; anuria; severe hepatic disease; hyperkalemia or history of hyperkalemia; severe or progressive renal disease
(Continued)

Hydrochlorothiazide and Triamterene *(Continued)*

Warnings/Precautions See individual agents.

Drug Interactions
Increased Effect/Toxicity: See individual agents.

Ethanol/Nutrition/Herb Interactions Food: Avoid food with high potassium content and potassium-containing salt substitutes.

Dietary Considerations Should be taken after meals.

Pharmacodynamics/Kinetics See individual agents.

Pregnancy Risk Factor C (per manufacturer)

Dosage Forms
Capsule: Hydrochlorothiazide 25 mg and triamterene 37.5 mg
Dyazide®: Hydrochlorothiazide 25 mg and triamterene 37.5 mg
Tablet: Hydrochlorothiazide 50 mg and triamterene 75 mg; hydrochlorothiazide 25 mg and triamterene 37.5 mg
Maxzide®: Hydrochlorothiazide 50 mg and triamterene 75 mg
Maxzide®-25: Hydrochlorothiazide 25 mg and triamterene 37.5 mg

Hydrochlorothiazide and Valsartan *see* Valsartan and Hydrochlorothiazide *on page 1644*

Hydrocil® Instant [OTC] *see* Psyllium *on page 1386*

Hydrocodone and Acetaminophen
(hye droe KOE done & a seet a MIN oh fen)

Related Information
Acetaminophen *on page 31*
Oral Pain *on page 1788*

Related Sample Prescriptions
Moderate/Moderately Severe Oral Pain *on page 1834*

U.S. Brand Names Anexsia®; Ceta-Plus®; Co-Gesic®; hycet™; Lorcet® 10/650; Lorcet® Plus; Lortab®; Margesic® H; Maxidone™; Norco®; Stagesic®; Vicodin®; Vicodin® ES; Vicodin® HP; Xodol®; Xodol® 5/300; Zydone®

Generic Available Yes

Index Terms Acetaminophen and Hydrocodone

Pharmacologic Category Analgesic Combination (Opioid)

Dental Use Treatment of postoperative pain

Use Relief of moderate to severe pain

Local Anesthetic/Vasoconstrictor Precautions No information available to require special precautions

Effects on Dental Treatment Key adverse event(s) related to dental treatment: Xerostomia (normal salivary flow resumes upon discontinuation). See Dental Comment.

Significant Adverse Effects Frequency not defined.
Cardiovascular: Bradycardia, cardiac arrest, circulatory collapse, coma, hypotension
Central nervous system: Anxiety, dizziness, drowsiness, dysphoria, euphoria, fear, lethargy, lightheadedness, malaise, mental clouding, mental impairment, mood changes, physiological dependence, sedation, somnolence, stupor
Dermatologic: Pruritus, rash
Endocrine & metabolic: Hypoglycemic coma
Gastrointestinal: Abdominal pain, constipation, gastric distress, heartburn, nausea, peptic ulcer, vomiting, xerostomia
Genitourinary: Ureteral spasm, urinary retention, vesical sphincter spasm
Hematologic: Agranulocytosis, bleeding time prolonged, hemolytic anemia, iron deficiency anemia, occult blood loss, thrombocytopenia
Hepatic: Hepatic necrosis, hepatitis
Neuromuscular & skeletal: Skeletal muscle rigidity
Otic: Hearing impairment or loss (chronic overdose)
Renal: Renal toxicity, renal tubular necrosis
Respiratory: Acute airway obstruction, apnea, dyspnea, respiratory depression (dose related)
Miscellaneous: Allergic reactions, clamminess, diaphoresis

Restrictions C-III

Dental Usual Dosing Postoperative pain: Oral:
Children and Adults ≥50 kg: Average starting dose in opioid naive patients: Hydrocodone 5-10 mg 4 times/day; the dosage of acetaminophen should be limited to ≤4 g/day (and possibly less in patients with hepatic impairment or ethanol use).
Dosage ranges (based on specific product labeling): Hydrocodone 2.5-10 mg every 4-6 hours; maximum: 60 mg hydrocodone/day (maximum dose of hydrocodone may be limited by the acetaminophen content of specific product)

Elderly: Doses should be titrated to appropriate analgesic effect; 2.5-5 mg of the hydrocodone component every 4-6 hours. Do not exceed 4 g/day of acetaminophen.

Dosage Oral (doses should be titrated to appropriate analgesic effect): Analgesic:

Children 2-13 years or <50 kg: Hydrocodone 0.135 mg/kg/dose every 4-6 hours; do not exceed 6 doses/day or the maximum recommended dose of acetaminophen

Children and Adults ≥50 kg: Average starting dose in opioid naive patients: Hydrocodone 5-10 mg 4 times/day; the dosage of acetaminophen should be limited to ≤4 g/day (and possibly less in patients with hepatic impairment or ethanol use).

Dosage ranges (based on specific product labeling): Hydrocodone 2.5-10 mg every 4-6 hours; maximum: 60 mg hydrocodone/day (maximum dose of hydrocodone may be limited by the acetaminophen content of specific product)

Elderly: Doses should be titrated to appropriate analgesic effect; 2.5-5 mg of the hydrocodone component every 4-6 hours. Do not exceed 4 g/day of acetaminophen.

Dosage adjustment in hepatic impairment: Use with caution. Limited, low-dose therapy usually well tolerated in hepatic disease/cirrhosis; however, cases of hepatotoxicity at daily acetaminophen dosages <4 g/day have been reported. Avoid chronic use in hepatic impairment.

Mechanism of Action Hydrocodone, as with other narcotic (opiate) analgesics, blocks pain perception in the cerebral cortex by binding to specific receptor molecules (opiate receptors) within the neuronal membranes of synapses. This binding results in a decreased synaptic chemical transmission throughout the CNS thus inhibiting the flow of pain sensations into the higher centers. Mu and kappa are the two subtypes of the opiate receptor which hydrocodone binds to cause analgesia.

Acetaminophen inhibits the synthesis of prostaglandins in the CNS and peripherally blocks pain impulse generation; produces antipyresis from inhibition of hypothalamic heat-regulating center.

Contraindications Hypersensitivity to hydrocodone, acetaminophen, or any component of the formulation; CNS depression; severe respiratory depression

Warnings/Precautions Use with caution in patients with hypersensitivity reactions to other phenanthrene derivative opioid agonists (morphine, hydromorphone, levorphanol, oxycodone, oxymorphone); tolerance or drug dependence may result from extended use.

Respiratory depressant effects may be increased with head injuries. Use caution with acute abdominal conditions; clinical course may be obscured. Use caution with thyroid dysfunction, prostatic hyperplasia, hepatic or renal disease, and in the elderly. Causes sedation; caution must be used in performing tasks which require alertness (eg, operating machinery or driving).

Limit acetaminophen to <4 g/day. May cause severe hepatic toxicity in acute overdose; in addition, chronic daily dosing in adults has resulted in liver damage in some patients. Use with caution in patients with alcoholic liver disease; consuming ≥3 alcoholic drinks/day may increase the risk of liver damage. Use caution in patients with known G6PD deficiency.

Drug Interactions

Hydrocodone: **Substrate** of CYP2D6 (major)

Acetaminophen: **Substrate** (minor) of CYP1A2, 2A6, 2C9, 2D6, 2E1, 3A4; **Inhibits** CYP3A4 (weak)

Acetaminophen component: Refer to Acetaminophen monograph.

Hydrocodone component:

CYP2D6 inhibitors may decrease the effects of hydrocodone. Example inhibitors include chlorpromazine, delavirdine, fluoxetine, miconazole, paroxetine, pergolide, quinidine, quinine, ritonavir, and ropinirole.

CNS depressants (including antianxiety agents, antihistamines, antipsychotics, narcotics): CNS depression is additive; dose adjustment may be needed

MAO inhibitors: May see increased effects of MAO inhibitor and hydrocodone.

Tricyclic antidepressants (TCAs): May see increased effects of TCA and hydrocodone.

Ethanol/Nutrition/Herb Interactions

Ethanol: Avoid ethanol (may increase CNS depression); consuming ≥3 alcoholic drinks/day may increase the risk of liver damage

Herb/Nutraceutical: Avoid valerian, St John's wort, SAMe, kava kava (may increase risk of excessive sedation).

Pharmacodynamics/Kinetics

Acetaminophen: See Acetaminophen monograph.

(Continued)

Hydrocodone and Acetaminophen *(Continued)*

Hydrocodone:

Onset of action: Narcotic analgesic: 10-20 minutes

Duration: 4-8 hours

Distribution: Crosses placenta

Metabolism: Hepatic; O-demethylation; N-demethylation and 6-ketosteroid reduction

Half-life elimination: 3.3-4.4 hours

Excretion: Urine

Pregnancy Risk Factor C/D (prolonged use or high doses near term)

Lactation Excretion in breast milk unknown/contraindicated

Breast-Feeding Considerations Acetaminophen is excreted in breast milk. The AAP considers it to be "compatible" with breast-feeding. Information is not available for hydrocodone; codeine and other opioids are excreted in breast milk and the AAP considers codeine to be "compatible" with breast-feeding. The manufacturers recommend discontinuing the medication or to discontinue nursing during therapy.

Dosage Forms Excipient information presented when available (limited, particularly for generics); consult specific product labeling. [DSC] = Discontinued product

Capsule:

Ceta-Plus®, Margesic® H, Stagesic®: Hydrocodone bitartrate 5 mg and acetaminophen 500 mg

Elixir: Hydrocodone bitartrate 7.5 mg and acetaminophen 500 mg per 15 mL (480 mL)

Lortab®: Hydrocodone bitartrate 7.5 mg and acetaminophen 500 mg per 15 mL (480 mL) [contains alcohol 7%; tropical fruit punch flavor]

Solution, oral:

hycet™: Hydrocodone bitartrate 7.5 mg and acetaminophen 325 mg per 15 mL (480 mL) [contains alcohol 7%; tropical fruit punch flavor]

Tablet:

Hydrocodone bitartrate 2.5 mg and acetaminophen 500 mg

Hydrocodone bitartrate 5 mg and acetaminophen 325 mg

Hydrocodone bitartrate 5 mg and acetaminophen 500 mg

Hydrocodone bitartrate 7.5 mg and acetaminophen 325 mg

Hydrocodone bitartrate 7.5 mg and acetaminophen 500 mg

Hydrocodone bitartrate 7.5 mg and acetaminophen 650 mg

Hydrocodone bitartrate 7.5 mg and acetaminophen 750 mg

Hydrocodone bitartrate 10 mg and acetaminophen 325 mg

Hydrocodone bitartrate 10 mg and acetaminophen 500 mg

Hydrocodone bitartrate 10 mg and acetaminophen 650 mg

Hydrocodone bitartrate 10 mg and acetaminophen 660 mg

Hydrocodone bitartrate 10 mg and acetaminophen 750 mg

Anexsia®:

5/325: Hydrocodone bitartrate 5 mg and acetaminophen 325 mg

5/500: Hydrocodone bitartrate 5 mg and acetaminophen 500 mg [DSC]

7.5/325: Hydrocodone bitartrate 7.5 mg and acetaminophen 325 mg

7.5/650: Hydrocodone bitartrate 7.5 mg and acetaminophen 650 mg [DSC]

Co-Gesic® 5/500: Hydrocodone bitartrate 5 mg and acetaminophen 500 mg

Lorcet® 10/650: Hydrocodone bitartrate 10 mg and acetaminophen 650 mg

Lorcet® Plus: Hydrocodone bitartrate 7.5 mg and acetaminophen 650 mg

Lortab®:

5/500: Hydrocodone bitartrate 5 mg and acetaminophen 500 mg

7.5/500: Hydrocodone bitartrate 7.5 mg and acetaminophen 500 mg

10/500: Hydrocodone bitartrate 10 mg and acetaminophen 500 mg

Maxidone™: Hydrocodone bitartrate 10 mg and acetaminophen 750 mg

Norco®:

Hydrocodone bitartrate 5 mg and acetaminophen 325 mg

Hydrocodone bitartrate 7.5 mg and acetaminophen 325 mg

Hydrocodone bitartrate 10 mg and acetaminophen 325 mg

Vicodin®: Hydrocodone bitartrate 5 mg and acetaminophen 500 mg

Vicodin® ES: Hydrocodone bitartrate 7.5 mg and acetaminophen 750 mg

Vicodin® HP: Hydrocodone bitartrate 10 mg and acetaminophen 660 mg

Xodol®: Hydrocodone bitartrate 10 mg and acetaminophen 300 mg

Xodol® 5/300: Hydrocodone bitartrate 5 mg and acetaminophen 300 mg

Zydone®:

Hydrocodone bitartrate 5 mg and acetaminophen 400 mg

Hydrocodone bitartrate 7.5 mg and acetaminophen 400 mg

Hydrocodone bitartrate 10 mg and acetaminophen 400 mg

Dental Comment Neither hydrocodone nor acetaminophen elicit anti-inflammatory effects. Because of addiction liability of opiate analgesics, the use of hydrocodone should be limited to 2-3 days postoperatively for treatment of dental pain. Nausea is the most common adverse effect seen after use in dental patients; sedation and constipation are second. Nausea elicited by narcotic analgesics is centrally mediated and the presence or absence of food will not affect the degree nor incidence of nausea.

Acetaminophen:

A study by Hylek, et al, suggested that the combination of acetaminophen with warfarin (Coumadin®) may cause enhanced anticoagulation. The following recommendations have been made by Hylek, et al, and supported by an editorial in *JAMA* by Bell.

Dose and duration of acetaminophen should be as low as possible, individualized and monitored

The study by Hylek reported the following:

For patients who reported taking the equivalent of at least 4 regular strength (325 mg) tablets for longer than a week, the odds of having an INR >6.0 were increased 10-fold above those not taking acetaminophen. Risk decreased with lower intakes of acetaminophen reaching a background level of risk at a dose of 6 or fewer 325 mg tablets per week.

Selected Readings

Bell WR, "Acetaminophen and Warfarin: Undesirable Synergy," *JAMA*, 1998, 279(9):702-3.

Botting RM, "Mechanism of Action of Acetaminophen: Is There a Cyclooxygenase 3?" *Clin Infect Dis*, 2000, Suppl 5:S202-10.

Dart RC, Kuffner EK, and Rumack BH, "Treatment of Pain or Fever With Paracetamol (Acetaminophen) in the Alcoholic Patient: A Systematic Review," *Am J Ther*, 2000, 7(2):123-34.

Dionne RA, "New Approaches to Preventing and Treating Postoperative Pain," *J Am Dent Assoc*, 1992, 123(6):26-34.

Gobetti JP, "Controlling Dental Pain," *J Am Dent Assoc*, 1992, 123(6):47-52.

Grant JA and Weiler JM, "A Report of a Rare Immediate Reaction After Ingestion of Acetaminophen," *Ann Allergy Asthma Immunol*, 2001, 87(3):227-9.

Hylek EM, Heiman H, Skates SJ, et al, "Acetaminophen and Other Risk factors for excessive warfarin anticoagulation," *JAMA*, 1998, 279(9):657-62.

Kwan D, Bartle WR, and Walker SE, "The Effects of Acetaminophen on Pharmacokinetics and Pharmacodynamics of Warfarin," *J Clin Pharmacol*, 1999, 39(1):68-75.

McClain CJ, Price S, Barve S, et al, "Acetaminophen Hepatotoxicity: An Update," *Curr Gastroenterol Rep*, 1999, 1(1):42-9.

Shek KL, Chan LN, and Nutescu E, "Warfarin-Acetaminophen Drug Interaction Revisited," *Pharmacotherapy*, 1999, 19(10):1153-8.

Tanaka E, Yamazaki K, and Misawa S, "Update: The Clinical Importance of Acetaminophen Hepatotoxicity in Nonalcoholic and Alcoholic Subjects," *J Clin Pharm Ther*, 2000, 25(5):325-32.

Wynn RL, "Narcotic Analgesics for Dental Pain: Available Products, Strengths, and Formulations," *Gen Dent*, 2001, 49(2):126-8, 130, 132 passim.

Hydrocodone and Aspirin (hye droe KOE done & AS pir in)

Related Information
Aspirin *on page 149*

U.S. Brand Names Damason-P®

Generic Available No

Index Terms Aspirin and Hydrocodone

Pharmacologic Category Analgesic Combination (Opioid)

Dental Use Treatment of postoperative pain

Use Relief of moderate to moderately severe pain

Local Anesthetic/Vasoconstrictor Precautions No information available to require special precautions

Effects on Dental Treatment Key adverse event(s) related to dental treatment: Nausea is the most common adverse effect seen after use in dental patients. Sedation and constipation are second.

Aspirin: As with all drugs which may affect hemostasis, bleeding is associated with aspirin. Hemorrhage may occur at virtually any site; risk is dependent on multiple variables including dosage, concurrent use of multiple agents which alter hemostasis, and patient susceptibility. Many adverse effects of aspirin are dose related, and are rare at low dosages. Other serious reactions are idiosyncratic, related to allergy or individual sensitivity (see Dental Comment).

Significant Adverse Effects

>10%:

Cardiovascular: Hypotension

Central nervous system: Lightheadedness, dizziness, sedation, drowsiness, fatigue

Gastrointestinal: Nausea, heartburn, stomach pain, heartburn, epigastric discomfort

Neuromuscular & skeletal: Weakness

1% to 10%:

Cardiovascular: Bradycardia

Central nervous system: Confusion

Dermatologic: Rash

Gastrointestinal: Vomiting, gastrointestinal ulceration

Genitourinary: Decreased urination

Hematologic: Hemolytic anemia

(Continued)

Hydrocodone and Aspirin *(Continued)*

Respiratory: Dyspnea

Miscellaneous: Anaphylactic shock

<1% (Limited to important or life-threatening): Biliary tract spasm, broncho-spasm, hallucinations, hepatotoxicity, histamine release, leukopenia, occult bleeding, physical and psychological dependence with prolonged use, prolon-gated bleeding time, thrombocytopenia, urinary tract spasm

Restrictions C-III

Dental Usual Dosing Postoperative pain: Adults: Oral: 1-2 tablets every 4-6 hours as needed for pain

Dosage Adults: Oral: 1-2 tablets every 4-6 hours as needed for pain

Mechanism of Action

Based on **hydrocodone** component: Binds to opiate receptors in the CNS, altering the perception of and response to pain; suppresses cough in medul-lary center; produces generalized CNS depression

Based on **aspirin** component: Inhibits prostaglandin synthesis, acts on the hypothalamus heat-regulating center to reduce fever, blocks prostaglandin synthetase action which prevents formation of the platelet-aggregating substance thromboxane A_2

Contraindications

Based on **hydrocodone** component: Hypersensitivity to hydrocodone or any component of the formulation

Based on **aspirin** component: Hypersensitivity to salicylates, other NSAIDs, or any component of the formulation; asthma; rhinitis; nasal polyps; inherited or acquired bleeding disorders (including factor VII and factor IX deficiency); pregnancy (in 3rd trimester especially); do not use in children (<16 years) for viral infections (chickenpox or flu symptoms), with or without fever, due to a potential association with Reye's syndrome

Warnings/Precautions Use with caution in patients with impaired renal func-tion, erosive gastritis, or peptic ulcer disease. Children and teenagers should not use for chickenpox or flu symptoms before a physician is consulted about Reye's syndrome.

Drug Interactions

Based on **hydrocodone** component: **Substrate** of CYP2D6 (major)

CNS depressants, MAO inhibitors, general anesthetics, and tricyclic antide-pressants: May potentiate the effects of opiate agonists; dextroampheta-mine may enhance the analgesic effect of opiate agonists.

CYP2D6 inhibitors: May decrease the effects of hydrocodone. Example inhibi-tors include chlorpromazine, delavirdine, fluoxetine, miconazole, paroxetine, pergolide, quinidine, quinine, ritonavir, and ropinirole.

Based on **aspirin** component: **Substrate** of CYP2C9 (minor)

ACE inhibitors: The effects of ACE inhibitors may be blunted by aspirin admin-istration, particularly at higher dosages.

Buspirone increases aspirin's free % *in vitro*.

Carbonic anhydrase inhibitors and corticosteroids have been associated with alteration in salicylate serum concentrations.

Heparin and low molecular weight heparins: Concurrent use may increase the risk of bleeding

Methotrexate serum levels may be increased; consider discontinuing aspirin 2-3 days before high-dose methotrexate treatment or avoid concurrent use.

NSAIDs may increase the risk of gastrointestinal adverse effects and bleeding. Serum concentrations of some NSAIDs may be decreased by aspirin.

Platelet inhibitors (IIb/IIIa antagonists): Risk of bleeding may be increased.

Probenecid effects may be antagonized by aspirin.

Sulfonylureas: The effects of older sulfonylurea agents (tolazamide, tolbuta-mide) may be potentiated due to displacement from plasma proteins. This effect does not appear to be clinically significant for newer sulfonylurea agents (glyburide, glipizide, glimepiride).

Valproic acid may be displaced from its binding sites which can result in toxicity.

Verapamil may potentiate the prolongation of bleeding time associated with aspirin.

Warfarin and oral anticoagulants may increase the risk of bleeding.

Ethanol/Nutrition/Herb Interactions

Based on **hydrocodone** component: Ethanol: Avoid or limit ethanol (may increase CNS depression). Watch for sedation.

Based on **aspirin** component:

Ethanol: Avoid ethanol (may enhance gastric mucosal damage).

Food: Food may decrease the rate but not the extent of oral absorption. Take with food or large volume of water or milk to minimize GI upset.

Herb/Nutraceutical: Avoid cat's claw, dong quai, evening primrose, feverfew, garlic, ginger, ginkgo, red clover, horse chestnut, green tea, ginseng (all have additional antiplatelet activity).

Pharmacodynamics/Kinetics

Aspirin: See Aspirin monograph.

Hydrocodone:

Onset of action: Narcotic analgesic: 10-20 minutes

Duration: 4-8 hours

Distribution: Crosses placenta

Metabolism: Hepatic; O-demethylation; N-demethylation and 6-ketosteroid reduction

Half-life elimination: 3.3-4.4 hours

Excretion: Urine

Pregnancy Risk Factor D

Lactation Enters breast milk/contraindicated

Breast-Feeding Considerations

Hydrocodone: No data reported.

Aspirin: Cautious use due to potential adverse effects in nursing infants.

Dosage Forms Excipient information presented when available (limited, particularly for generics); consult specific product labeling.

Tablet: Hydrocodone bitartrate 5 mg and aspirin 500 mg

Dental Comment Because of addiction liability of opiate analgesics, the use of hydrocodone should be limited to 2-3 days postoperatively for treatment of dental pain; nausea is the most common adverse effect seen after use in dental patients; sedation and constipation are second; aspirin component affects bleeding times and could influence time of wound healing

There is no scientific evidence to warrant discontinuance of aspirin prior to dental surgery. Patients taking one aspirin tablet daily as an antithrombotic and who require dental surgery should be given special consideration in consultation with the physician before removal of the aspirin relative to prevention of postoperative bleeding.

The Food and Drug Administration (FDA), has issued a letter updating information and considerations regarding the use of ibuprofen (400 mg doses) in patients who are taking low dose aspirin (81 mg, immediate release; not enteric coated) for cardioprotection and stroke prevention. Ibuprofen, at these doses, may interfere with aspirin's antiplatelet effect depending upon when it is administered. Patients initiated on aspirin first (for ~1 week) then ibuprofen (400 mg tid for 10 days) seem to maintain aspirin's platelet effect (Cryer B, 2005). Ibuprofen has the greatest impact on aspirin if administered less than 8 hours before aspirin (Catella-Lawson F, 2001).

Patients may require counseling about the appropriate timing of ibuprofen dosing in relationship to aspirin therapy. With occasional use of ibuprofen, a clinically-significant interaction with aspirin in unlikely. To avoid interference during chronic dosing, a single dose of ibuprofen should be taken 30-120 minutes after aspirin ingestion or at least 8 hours should elapse after ibuprofen dosing before giving aspirin (FDA, 2006; Catella-Lawson F, 2001).

The clinical implications of the interaction are unclear. There have not been any clinical endpoint studies conducted at this time. Avoidance of this interaction is potentially important because aspirin's vascular protection could be decreased or negated.

Other nonselective NSAIDs may have potential for a similar interaction with aspirin. Such has been described with naproxen (Capone ML, 2005). Acetaminophen does not appear to interfere with the antiplatelet effect of aspirin. Other clinical scenarios (use of smaller ibuprofen doses, other aspirin products, other doses of aspirin) have not been evaluated.

Additional information is available at: http://www.fda.gov/cder/drug/infopage/aspirin/default.htm.

Selected Readings

Dionne RA, "New Approaches to Preventing and Treating Postoperative Pain," *J Am Dent Assoc*, 1992, 123(6):26-34.

Gobetti JP, "Controlling Dental Pain," *J Am Dent Assoc*, 1992, 123(6):47-52.

Wynn RL, "Narcotic Analgesics for Dental Pain: Available Products, Strengths, and Formulations," *Gen Dent*, 2001, 49(2):126-8, 130, 132 passim.

Hydrocodone and Chlorpheniramine
(hye droe KOE done & klor fen IR a meen)

Related Information

Chlorpheniramine on page 338

U.S. Brand Names HyTan™ [DSC]; Tussionex®

Generic Available No

(Continued)

Hydrocodone and Chlorpheniramine *(Continued)*

Index Terms Chlorpheniramine Maleate and Hydrocodone Bitartrate; Hydrocodone Tannate and Chlorpheniramine Tannate

Pharmacologic Category Antihistamine/Antitussive

Use Symptomatic relief of cough and upper respiratory symptoms associated with cold and allergy

Local Anesthetic/Vasoconstrictor Precautions No information available to require special precautions

Effects on Dental Treatment Key adverse event(s) related to dental treatment: Prolonged use will cause significant xerostomia (normal salivary flow resumes upon discontinuation).

Common Adverse Effects Frequency not defined.

Central nervous system: Anxiety, dizziness, drowsiness, dysphoria, euphoria, fear, lethargy, mental impairment, mood changes, sedation

Dermatologic: Pruritus, rash

Gastrointestinal: Constipation, nausea, vomiting

Genitourinary: Ureteral spasm, urinary retention, vesicle sphincter spasm

Respiratory: Dryness of pharynx, respiratory depression

Restrictions C-III

Mechanism of Action

Hydrocodone binds to opiate receptors in the CNS, altering the perception of and response to pain; suppresses cough in medullary center; produces generalized CNS depression

Chlorpheniramine competes with histamine for H_1-receptor sites on effector cells in the gastrointestinal tract, blood vessels, and respiratory tract

Drug Interactions

Cytochrome P450 Effect:

Hydrocodone: **Substrate** of CYP2D6 (major)

Chlorpheniramine: **Substrate** of CYP2D6 (minor), 3A4 (major); **Inhibits** CYP2D6 (weak)

Increased Effect/Toxicity: Anticholinergics may enhance the adverse/toxic effect of chlorpheniramine; CNS depressants may enhance the adverse/toxic effects of hydrocodone and chlorpheniramine

Pharmacodynamics/Kinetics

Chlorpheniramine: See Chlorpheniramine monograph.

Hydrocodone:

Onset of action: Narcotic analgesic: 10-20 minutes

Duration: 4-8 hours

Distribution: Crosses placenta

Metabolism: Hepatic; O-demethylation; N-demethylation and 6-ketosteroid reduction

Half-life elimination: 3.3-4.4 hours

Excretion: Urine

Pregnancy Risk Factor C

Hydrocodone and Guaifenesin

(hye droe KOE done & gwye FEN e sin)

Related Information

Guaifenesin *on page 795*

U.S. Brand Names Atuss® HX; Codiclear® DH; EndaCof; EndaCof-XP; ExeClear; ExeCof-XP; Extendryl® HC; Hycotuss®; Hydro-Tussin™ HG; Kwelcof®; Maxi-Tuss HCG; Pancof-XP; Phanatuss® HC; Pneumotussin®; Touro® HC; Tusso-DF®; Vitussin; Xpect-HC™; Ztuss™ ZT

Generic Available Yes: Liquid, syrup

Index Terms Guaifenesin and Hydrocodone

Pharmacologic Category Antitussive/Expectorant

Use Symptomatic relief of nonproductive coughs associated with upper and lower respiratory tract congestion

Local Anesthetic/Vasoconstrictor Precautions No information available to require special precautions

Effects on Dental Treatment Key adverse event(s) related to dental treatment: Xerostomia (normal salivary flow resumes upon discontinuation).

Common Adverse Effects Frequency not defined.

Cardiovascular: Hypertension, postural hypotension, palpitation

Central nervous system: Drowsiness, sedation, mental clouding, mental and physical impairment, anxiety, fear, dysphoria, dizziness, psychotic dependence, mood changes

Gastrointestinal: Nausea, vomiting, constipation with prolonged use, xerostomia

Genitourinary: Ureteral spasm, urinary retention

Ocular: Blurred vision

Respiratory: Respiratory depression (dose related)

Restrictions C-III

Mechanism of Action

Hydrocodone binds to opiate receptors in the CNS, altering the perception of and response to pain; suppresses cough in medullary center; produces generalized CNS depression

Guaifenesin is thought to act as an expectorant by irritating the gastric mucosa and stimulating respiratory tract secretions, thereby increasing respiratory fluid volumes and decreasing phlegm viscosity

Drug Interactions

Cytochrome P450 Effect: Hydrocodone: **Substrate** of CYP2D6 (major)

Increased Effect/Toxicity:

Based on **hydrocodone** component: CNS depressants, MAO inhibitors, general anesthetics, and tricyclic antidepressants may potentiate the effects of opiate agonists; dextroamphetamine may enhance the analgesic effect of opiate agonists

Also refer to individual monograph for Guaifenesin.

Pharmacodynamics/Kinetics

Guaifenesin: See Guaifenesin monograph.

Hydrocodone:

Onset of action: Narcotic analgesic: 10-20 minutes

Duration: 4-8 hours

Distribution: Crosses placenta

Metabolism: Hepatic; O-demethylation; N-demethylation and 6-ketosteroid reduction

Half-life elimination: 3.3-4.4 hours

Excretion: Urine

Pregnancy Risk Factor C

Hydrocodone and Homatropine
(hye droe KOE done & hoe MA troe peen)

Related Information

Homatropine *on page 815*

U.S. Brand Names Hycodan®; Hydromet®; Tussigon®

Mexican Brand Names Hydromet

Generic Available Yes

Index Terms Homatropine and Hydrocodone

Pharmacologic Category Antitussive

Use Symptomatic relief of cough

Local Anesthetic/Vasoconstrictor Precautions No information available to require special precautions

Effects on Dental Treatment Key adverse event(s) related to dental treatment: Xerostomia (normal salivary flow resumes upon discontinuation).

Common Adverse Effects Frequency not defined.

Central nervous system: Anxiety, dizziness, drowsiness, dysphoria, fear, lethargy, mental clouding, mental impairment, mood changes, sedation

Dermatologic: Pruritus, rash

Gastrointestinal: Constipation, nausea, vomiting

Genitourinary: Urinary retention, urinary tract spasm

Respiratory: Respiratory depression

Miscellaneous: Physical and psychological dependence with prolonged use

Restrictions C-III

Mechanism of Action

Hydrocodone binds to opiate receptors in the CNS, altering the perception of and response to pain; suppresses cough in medullary center; produces generalized CNS depression.

Homatropine is an anticholinergic agent, present in a subtherapeutic amount to discourage deliberate overdose.

Drug Interactions

Cytochrome P450 Effect: Hydrocodone: **Substrate** of CYP2D6 (major)

Increased Effect/Toxicity: CNS depressants may enhance the adverse/toxic effect of hydrocodone. Hydrocodone may enhance the serotonergic effect of SSRIs.

Decreased Effect: Ammonium chloride may increase the excretion of hydrocodone. CYP2D6 inhibitors and quinidine may decrease the effects of hydrocodone. Hydrocodone may diminish the therapeutic effect of pegvisomant.

Pregnancy Risk Factor C

Hydrocodone and Ibuprofen
(hye droe KOE done & eye byoo PROE fen)

Related Information
Ibuprofen *on page 853*
Oral Pain *on page 1788*

Related Sample Prescriptions
Moderate/Moderately Severe Oral Pain *on page 1834*

U.S. Brand Names Reprexain™; Vicoprofen®

Canadian Brand Names Vicoprofen®

Generic Available Yes

Index Terms Ibuprofen and Hydrocodone

Pharmacologic Category Analgesic, Opioid; Nonsteroidal Anti-inflammatory Drug (NSAID), Oral

Dental Use Short-term management (generally <10 days) of moderate-to-severe acute postoperative dental pain where an anti-inflammatory effect is desired

Use Short-term (generally <10 days) management of moderate to severe acute pain; is not indicated for treatment of such conditions as osteoarthritis or rheumatoid arthritis

Local Anesthetic/Vasoconstrictor Precautions No information available to require special precautions

Effects on Dental Treatment Key adverse event(s) related to dental treatment: Xerostomia (normal salivary flow resumes upon discontinuation).

Significant Adverse Effects
>10%:
　　Central nervous system: Headache (27%), somnolence (22%), dizziness (14%)
　　Gastrointestinal: Constipation (22%), nausea (21%), dyspepsia (12%)
1% to 10%:
　　Cardiovascular: Edema (3% to 9%), palpitation (<3%), vasodilation (<3%)
　　Central nervous system: Anxiety (3% to 9%), insomnia (3% to 9%), nervousness (3% to 9%), confusion (<3%), fever (<3%), thought abnormalities (<3%)
　　Dermatologic: Itching (3% to 9%)
　　Gastrointestinal: Abdominal pain (3% to 9%), diarrhea (3% to 9%), flatulence (3% to 9%), vomiting (3% to 9%), xerostomia (3% to 9%), gastritis (<3%), melena (<3%), mouth ulcers (<3%)
　　Genitourinary: Polyuria (<3%)
　　Neuromuscular & skeletal: Hypertonia (<3%), paresthesia (<3%)
　　Otic: Tinnitus (<3%)
　　Respiratory: Dyspnea (<3%), pharyngitis (<3%), rhinitis (<3%)
　　Miscellaneous: Diaphoresis (3% to 9%), infection (3% to 9%), flu-like syndrome (<3%), hiccups (<3%)
<1% (Limited to important or life-threatening): Abnormal dreams, agitation, allergic reactions, arthralgia, bronchitis, cough increased, dependence with prolonged use, depression, dry eyes, esophageal spasm, esophagitis, euphoria, gastroenteritis, glossitis, glycosuria, hoarseness, hypotension, impotence, libido decreased, liver enzymes increased, mood changes, myalgia, neuralgia, pneumonia, psychological dependence with prolonged use, pulmonary edema, respiratory depression, sinusitis, slurred speech, tachycardia, taste (unpleasant), tremor, urinary incontinence, urinary retention, urticaria, vertigo, vision change, weight loss

Restrictions C-III; An FDA-approved medication guide for NSAIDs must be distributed when dispensing an oral outpatient prescription (new or refill) where this medication is to be used without direct supervision of a healthcare provider. Medication guides are available at http://www.fda.gov/cder/Offices/ODS/medication_guides.htm.

Dental Usual Dosing Moderate-to-severe acute postoperative dental pain: Adults: Oral: 1-2 tablets every 4-6 hours as needed for pain; maximum: 5 tablets/day

Dosage Adults: Oral: 1 tablet every 4-6 hours as needed for pain; maximum: 5 tablets/day

Mechanism of Action
　　Based on **hydrocodone** component: Binds to opiate receptors in the CNS, altering the perception of and response to pain; suppresses cough in medullary center; produces generalized CNS depression
　　Based on **ibuprofen** component: Inhibits prostaglandin synthesis by decreasing the activity of the enzyme, cyclooxygenase, which results in decreased formation of prostaglandin precursors

Contraindications Hypersensitivity to hydrocodone, ibuprofen, aspirin, other NSAIDs, or any component of the formulation; perioperative pain in the setting of coronary artery bypass surgery (CABG); pregnancy (3rd trimester)

Warnings/Precautions [U.S. Boxed Warning]: NSAIDs are associated with an increased risk of adverse cardiovascular events, including MI, stroke, and new onset or worsening of pre-existing hypertension. Risk may be increased with duration of use or pre-existing cardiovascular risk factors or disease. Use caution with fluid retention, CHF, or hypertension. Use of NSAIDs can compromise existing renal function. Rehydrate patient before starting therapy. Monitor renal function closely. Ibuprofen is not recommended for patients with advanced renal disease. **[U.S. Boxed Warning]: NSAIDs may increase risk of gastrointestinal irritation, ulceration, bleeding, and perforation.** NSAIDs may cause serious skin adverse events. Anaphylactoid reactions may occur, even without prior exposure. Do not use in patients who experience bronchospasm, asthma, rhinitis, or urticaria with NSAID or aspirin therapy. Use caution in other forms of asthma. The elderly are at increased risk for adverse effects (especially peptic ulceration, CNS effects, renal toxicity) from NSAIDs even at low doses.

Hydrocodone: May cause CNS depression. Use with caution in patients with pre-existing respiratory compromise, and kyphoscoliosis or other skeletal disorder which may alter respiratory function. Use with caution in patients with hypersensitivity reactions to other phenanthrene derivative opioid agonists (codeine, hydrocodone, hydromorphone, levorphanol, oxycodone, oxymorphone). Use with extreme caution in patients with head injury, intracranial lesions, or elevated intracranial pressure. May obscure diagnosis or clinical course of patients with acute abdominal conditions. Use with caution in patients with severe hepatic dysfunction. Use with caution in patients with biliary tract dysfunction; acute pancreatitis may cause constriction of sphincter of Oddi. Use with caution in patients with prostatic hyperplasia and/or urinary stricture, severe hepatic dysfunction, or a history of drug abuse or acute alcoholism. Tolerance, psychological and physical dependence may occur with prolonged use.

Safety and efficacy in children <16 years have not been established.

Drug Interactions
Hydrocodone: **Substrate** of CYP2D6 (major)

Ibuprofen: **Substrate** (minor) of CYP2C9, 2C19; **Inhibits** CYP2C9 (strong)

Also see individual agents.

Ethanol/Nutrition/Herb Interactions
Based on **hydrocodone** component: Ethanol: Avoid or limit ethanol (may increase CNS depression). Watch for sedation.

Based on **ibuprofen** component:

Ethanol: Avoid ethanol (may enhance gastric mucosal irritation).

Food: Ibuprofen peak serum levels may be decreased if taken with food.

Herb/Nutraceutical: Avoid alfalfa, anise, bilberry, bladderwrack, bromelain, cat's claw, celery, coleus, cordyceps, dong quai, evening primrose, feverfew, fenugreek, garlic, ginger, ginkgo biloba, red clover, horse chestnut, grapeseed, green tea, ginseng, guggul, horse chestnut seed, horseradish, licorice, prickly ash, red clover, reishi, SAMe, sweet clover, turmeric, white willow (all have additional antiplatelet activity).

Pharmacodynamics/Kinetics
Ibuprofen: See Ibuprofen monograph.

Hydrocodone:

Onset of action: Narcotic analgesic: 10-20 minutes

Duration: 4-8 hours

Distribution: Crosses placenta

Protein binding: 19% to 45%

Metabolism: Hepatic; O-demethylation; N-demethylation and 6-ketosteroid reduction

Half-life elimination: 3.3-4.4 hours

Time to peak: 1.7 hours

Excretion: Urine

Pregnancy Risk Factor C/D (3rd trimester)

Lactation Excretion in breast milk unknown/contraindicated

Dosage Forms Excipient information presented when available (limited, particularly for generics); consult specific product labeling.

Tablet: Hydrocodone bitartrate 5 mg and ibuprofen 200 mg; hydrocodone bitartrate 7.5 mg and ibuprofen 200 mg

Reprexain™: Hydrocodone bitartrate 5 mg and ibuprofen 200 mg

Vicoprofen®: Hydrocodone bitartrate 7.5 mg and ibuprofen 200 mg

Selected Readings
Dionne R, "To Tame the Pain?" *Compend Contin Educ Dent*, 1998, 19(4):426-8, 430-1.

Hargreaves KM, "Management of Pain in Endodontic Patients," *Tex Dent J*, 1997, 114(10):27-31.

Sunshine A, Olson NZ, O'Neill E, et al, "Analgesic Efficacy of a Hydrocodone With Ibuprofen Combination Compared With Ibuprofen Alone for the Treatment of Acute Postoperative Pain," *J Clin Pharmacol*, 1997, 37(10):908-15.

Wynn RL, "Narcotic Analgesics for Dental Pain: Available Products, Strengths, and Formulations," *Gen Dent*, 2001, 49(2):126-8, 130, 132 passim.

Hydrocodone and Pseudoephedrine
(hye droe KOE done & soo doe e FED rin)

Related Information
Pseudoephedrine *on page 1381*
U.S. Brand Names Coughcold HCM; Histussin D® [DSC]; Pancof-HC; P-V Tussin Tablet
Generic Available Yes: Syrup
Index Terms Pseudoephedrine and Hydrocodone
Pharmacologic Category Antitussive/Decongestant
Use Symptomatic relief of cough due to colds, nasal congestion, and cough
Local Anesthetic/Vasoconstrictor Precautions Use with caution since pseudoephedrine is a sympathomimetic amine which could interact with epinephrine to cause a pressor response
Effects on Dental Treatment Key adverse event(s) related to dental treatment: Pseudoephedrine: Xerostomia (normal salivary flow resumes upon discontinuation).
Common Adverse Effects See individual agents.
Restrictions C-III
Mechanism of Action
Based on **hydrocodone** component: Binds to opiate receptors in the CNS, altering the perception of and response to pain; suppresses cough in medullary center; produces generalized CNS depression
Based on **pseudoephedrine** component: Directly stimulates alpha-adrenergic receptors of respiratory mucosa causing vasoconstriction; directly stimulates beta-adrenergic receptors causing bronchial relaxation, increased heart rate and contractility
Drug Interactions
Cytochrome P450 Effect: Hydrocodone: **Substrate** of CYP2D6 (major)
Increased Effect/Toxicity:
Based on **hydrocodone** component: Increased toxicity: CNS depressants, MAO inhibitors, general anesthetics, and tricyclic antidepressants may potentiate the effects of opiate agonists; dextroamphetamine may enhance the analgesic effect of opiate agonists
Based on **pseudoephedrine** component: Increased toxicity: MAO inhibitors may increase blood pressure effects of pseudoephedrine; propranolol, sympathomimetic agents may increase toxicity
Decreased Effect: Based on **pseudoephedrine** component: Decreased effect of methyldopa, reserpine
Pharmacodynamics/Kinetics
Pseudoephedrine: See Pseudoephedrine monograph.
Hydrocodone:
Onset of action: Narcotic analgesic: 10-20 minutes
Duration: 4-8 hours
Distribution: Crosses placenta
Metabolism: Hepatic; O-demethylation; N-demethylation and 6-ketosteroid reduction
Half-life elimination: 3.3-4.4 hours
Excretion: Urine

Hydrocodone Bitartrate, Carbinoxamine Maleate, and Pseudoephedrine Hydrochloride *see* Hydrocodone, Carbinoxamine, and Pseudoephedrine *on page 832*

Hydrocodone Bitartrate, Phenylephrine Hydrochloride, and Diphenhydramine Hydrochloride *see* Hydrocodone, Phenylephrine, and Diphenhydramine *on page 834*

Hydrocodone, Carbinoxamine, and Pseudoephedrine
(hye droe KOE done, kar bi NOKS a meen, & soo doe e FED rin)

Related Information
Carbinoxamine *on page 281*
Pseudoephedrine *on page 1381*
U.S. Brand Names Histex™ HC; Tri-Vent™ HC
Generic Available No
Index Terms Carbinoxamine, Pseudoephedrine, and Hydrocodone; Hydrocodone Bitartrate, Carbinoxamine Maleate, and Pseudoephedrine Hydrochloride; Pseudoephedrine, Hydrocodone, and Carbinoxamine

Pharmacologic Category Antihistamine/Decongestant/Antitussive

Use Symptomatic relief of cough, congestion, and rhinorrhea associated with the common cold, influenza, bronchitis, or sinusitis

Local Anesthetic/Vasoconstrictor Precautions Use with caution since pseudoephedrine is a sympathomimetic amine which could interact with epinephrine to cause a pressor response

Effects on Dental Treatment Key adverse event(s) related to dental treatment: Pseudoephedrine: Xerostomia (normal salivary flow resumes upon discontinuation).

Common Adverse Effects See individual agents.

Restrictions C-III

Mechanism of Action

Hydrocodone binds to opiate receptors in the CNS, altering the perception of and response to pain; suppresses cough in medullary center; produces generalized CNS depression.

Carbinoxamine competes with histamine for H_1-receptor sites on effector cells in the gastrointestinal tract, blood vessels, and respiratory tract.

Pseudoephedrine is a sympathomimetic amine and isomer of ephedrine; acts as a decongestant in respiratory tract mucous membranes with less vasoconstrictor action than ephedrine in normotensive individuals.

Pharmacodynamics/Kinetics See individual agents.

Pregnancy Risk Factor C

Hydrocodone, Chlorpheniramine, Phenylephrine, Acetaminophen, and Caffeine

(hye droe KOE done, klor fen IR a meen, fen il EF rin, a seet a MIN oh fen, & KAF een)

Related Information

Acetaminophen *on page 31*
Caffeine *on page 255*
Chlorpheniramine *on page 338*
Phenylephrine *on page 1293*

U.S. Brand Names Hycomine® Compound

Generic Available No

Index Terms Acetaminophen, Caffeine, Hydrocodone, Chlorpheniramine, and Phenylephrine; Caffeine, Hydrocodone, Chlorpheniramine, Phenylephrine, and Acetaminophen; Chlorpheniramine, Hydrocodone, Phenylephrine, Acetaminophen, and Caffeine; Phenylephrine, Hydrocodone, Chlorpheniramine, Acetaminophen, and Caffeine

Pharmacologic Category Antitussive/Decongestant

Use Symptomatic relief of cough and symptoms of upper respiratory infection

Local Anesthetic/Vasoconstrictor Precautions Use with caution since phenylephrine is a sympathomimetic amine which could interact with epinephrine to cause a pressor response

Effects on Dental Treatment Key adverse event(s) related to dental treatment:

Acetaminophen: No significant effects or complications reported.

Chlorpheniramine: Prolonged use will cause significant xerostomia (normal salivary flow resumes upon discontinuation).

Phenylephrine: Up to 10% of patients could experience tachycardia, palpitations, and xerostomia; use vasoconstrictor with caution.

Common Adverse Effects Frequency not defined.

Cardiovascular: Hypertension, postural hypotension, tachycardia, palpitation

Central nervous system: Sedation, drowsiness, mental clouding, lethargy, impairment of mental and physical performance, anxiety, fear, dysphoria, dizziness, psychic dependence, mood changes

Dermatologic: Rash, pruritus

Gastrointestinal: Nausea, vomiting, constipation with prolonged use

Genitourinary: Ureteral spasms, spasm of vesical sphincters and urinary retention

Ocular: Blurred vision

Respiratory: Respiratory depression

Restrictions C-III

Drug Interactions

Cytochrome P450 Effect:

Hydrocodone: **Substrate** of CYP2D6 (major)

Chlorpheniramine: **Substrate** of CYP2D6 (minor), 3A4 (major); **Inhibits** CYP2D6 (weak)

Acetaminophen: **Substrate** (minor) of CYP1A2, 2A6, 2C9, 2D6, 2E1, 3A4; (Continued)

Hydrocodone, Chlorpheniramine, Phenylephrine, Acetaminophen, and Caffeine *(Continued)*

Caffeine: **Substrate** of CYP1A2 (major), 2C9 (minor), 2D6 (minor), 2E1 (minor), 3A4 (minor); **Inhibits** CYP1A2 (weak), 3A4 (moderate)

Increased Effect/Toxicity: See individual agents.

Pharmacodynamics/Kinetics

See Chlorpheniramine, Phenylephrine, and Acetaminophen monographs.

Hydrocodone:

Onset of action: Narcotic analgesic: 10-20 minutes

Duration: 4-8 hours

Distribution: Crosses placenta

Metabolism: Hepatic; O-demethylation; N-demethylation and 6-ketosteroid reduction

Half-life elimination: 3.3-4.4 hours

Excretion: Urine

Pregnancy Risk Factor C

Hydrocodone, Phenylephrine, and Diphenhydramine

(hye droe KOE done, fen il EF rin, & dye fen HYE dra meen)

Related Information

DiphenhydrAMINE *on page 510*

Phenylephrine *on page 1293*

U.S. Brand Names D-Tann HC; Gentuss-HC; Hydro DP; Rindal HPD; TussiNate™

Generic Available Yes: Syrup

Index Terms Diphenhydramine, Hydrocodone, and Phenylephrine; Hydrocodone Bitartrate, Phenylephrine Hydrochloride, and Diphenhydramine Hydrochloride; Hydrocodone Tannate, Phenylephrine Tannate, and Diphenhydramine Tannate; Phenylephrine, Diphenhydramine, and Hydrocodone

Pharmacologic Category Antihistamine/Decongestant/Antitussive; Antitussive; Decongestant; Histamine H₁ Antagonist

Use Symptomatic relief of cough and congestion associated with the common cold, sinusitis, or acute upper respiratory tract infections

Local Anesthetic/Vasoconstrictor Precautions Use with caution since phenylephrine is a sympathomimetic amine which could interact with epinephrine to cause a pressor response

Effects on Dental Treatment Key adverse event(s) related to dental treatment: Xerostomia (normal salivary flow resumes upon discontinuation).

Common Adverse Effects See individual agents.

Restrictions C-III

Mechanism of Action

Hydrocodone binds to opiate receptors in the CNS; suppresses cough in medullary center.

Phenylephrine is a potent, direct-acting alpha-adrenergic stimulator.

Diphenhydramine is an H₁-receptor antagonist.

Pharmacodynamics/Kinetics See individual agents.

Pregnancy Risk Factor C

Hydrocodone, Phenylephrine, and Guaifenesin

(hye droe KOE done, fen il EF rin, & gwye FEN e sin)

Related Information

Guaifenesin *on page 795*

Phenylephrine *on page 1293*

U.S. Brand Names Crantex HC; De-Chlor G; Donatussin DC; Duratuss® HD; Gentex HC; Giltuss HC®; Guiaplex™ HC; HydroFed; Hydro-GP; Levall 5.0; Mintuss G; Tussafed® HC; Tussafed® HCG

Generic Available Yes

Index Terms Guaifenesin, Hydrocodone Bitartrate, and Phenylephrine Hydrochloride; Phenylephrine, Guaifenesin, and Hydrocodone

Pharmacologic Category Antitussive/Decongestant/Expectorant

Use Temporary relief of cough, congestion, and other symptoms associated with colds or allergies

Local Anesthetic/Vasoconstrictor Precautions Use with caution since pseudoephedrine is a sympathomimetic amine which could interact with epinephrine to cause a pressor response

Effects on Dental Treatment Key adverse event(s) related to dental treatment: Tachycardia, palpitations, and xerostomia (normal salivary flow resumes upon discontinuation).

Common Adverse Effects Frequency not defined.
Central nervous system: Drowsiness, giddiness, lassitude
Gastrointestinal: Constipation, GI upset, nausea

Restrictions C-III

Mechanism of Action
Hydrocodone binds to opiate receptors in the CNS, altering the perception of and response to pain; suppresses cough in medullary center; produces generalized CNS depression.

Phenylephrine is a direct-acting alpha-adrenergic stimulator with weak beta-adrenergic activity; causes vasoconstriction of the arterioles of the nasal mucosa and conjunctiva; activates the dilator muscle of the pupil to cause contraction; produces vasoconstriction of arterioles in the body; produces systemic arterial vasoconstriction.

Guaifenesin is thought to act as an expectorant by irritating the gastric mucosa and stimulating respiratory tract secretions, thereby increasing respiratory fluid volumes and decreasing phlegm viscosity.

Drug Interactions
Cytochrome P450 Effect: Hydrocodone: **Substrate** of CYP2D6 (major)

Increased Effect/Toxicity: CNS depressants, MAO inhibitors, general anesthetics, and tricyclic antidepressants may potentiate the effects of opiate agonists. Dextroamphetamine may enhance the analgesic effect of opiate agonists.

Also refer to individual monographs for Phenylephrine and Guaifenesin.

Decreased Effect: CYP2D6 inhibitors may decrease the effects of hydrocodone (example inhibitors include chlorpromazine, delavirdine, fluoxetine, miconazole, paroxetine, pergolide, quinidine, quinine, ritonavir, and ropinirole).

Also refer to individual monographs for Phenylephrine and Guaifenesin.

Pregnancy Risk Factor C

Hydrocodone, Pseudoephedrine, and Guaifenesin
(hye droe KOE done, soo doe e FED rin & gwye FEN e sin)

Related Information
Guaifenesin *on page 795*
Pseudoephedrine *on page 1381*

Guaifenesin *on page 795*
Pseudoephedrine *on page 1381*

U.S. Brand Names Hydro-Tussin™ HD; Hydro-Tussin™ XP; Su-Tuss®-HD; Tussend® Expectorant [DSC]; Ztuss™ Tablet

Generic Available Yes: Excludes tablet

Index Terms Guaifenesin, Hydrocodone, and Pseudoephedrine; Pseudoephedrine, Hydrocodone, and Guaifenesin

Pharmacologic Category Antitussive/Decongestant/Expectorant

Use Symptomatic relief of irritating, nonproductive cough associated with upper respiratory conditions and allergies

Local Anesthetic/Vasoconstrictor Precautions Use with caution since pseudoephedrine is a sympathomimetic amine which could interact with epinephrine to cause a pressor response

Effects on Dental Treatment Key adverse event(s) related to dental treatment:
Guaifenesin: No significant effects or complications reported
Pseudoephedrine: Xerostomia (normal salivary flow resumes upon discontinuation).

Common Adverse Effects Frequency not defined.
Cardiovascular: Arrhythmias, tachycardia, hypertension
Central nervous system: Drowsiness, fear, anxiety, tenseness, restlessness, pallor, insomnia, hallucinations, CNS depression
Gastrointestinal: GI upset, nausea, constipation with prolonged use
Genitourinary: Dysuria
Hepatic: Transaminases increased (slight)
Neuromuscular & skeletal: Weakness, tremor
Respiratory: Respiratory difficulty
Patients hyper-reactive to pseudoephedrine may display ephedrine-like reactions such as tachycardia, palpitation, headache, dizziness, or nausea; patient idiosyncrasy to adrenergic agents may be manifested by insomnia, dizziness, weakness, tremor, or arrhythmia.

Restrictions C-III

Mechanism of Action
Hydrocodone binds to opiate receptors in the CNS, altering the perception of and response to pain; suppresses cough in medullary center; produces generalized CNS depression.
(Continued)

Hydrocodone, Pseudoephedrine, and Guaifenesin
(Continued)

Pseudoephedrine directly stimulates alpha-adrenergic receptors of respiratory mucosa causing vasoconstriction; directly stimulates beta-adrenergic receptors causing bronchial relaxation, increased heart rate and contractility.

Guaifenesin is thought to act as an expectorant by irritating the gastric mucosa and stimulating respiratory tract secretions, thereby increasing respiratory fluid volumes and decreasing phlegm viscosity.

Drug Interactions

Cytochrome P450 Effect: Hydrocodone: **Substrate** of CYP2D6 (major)

Increased Effect/Toxicity: CNS depressants, MAO inhibitors, general anesthetics, and tricyclic antidepressants may potentiate the effects of opiate agonists. Dextroamphetamine may enhance the analgesic effect of opiate agonists.

Also refer to individual monographs for Pseudoephedrine and Guaifenesin.

Decreased Effect: CYP2D6 inhibitors may decrease the effects of hydrocodone (example inhibitors include chlorpromazine, delavirdine, fluoxetine, miconazole, paroxetine, pergolide, quinidine, quinine, ritonavir, and ropinirole).

Also refer to individual monographs for Pseudoephedrine and Guaifenesin.

Pharmacodynamics/Kinetics

See Guaifenesin and Pseudoephedrine monographs.

Hydrocodone:

Onset of action: Narcotic analgesic: 10-20 minutes

Duration: 4-8 hours

Distribution: Crosses placenta

Metabolism: Hepatic; O-demethylation; N-demethylation and 6-ketosteroid reduction

Half-life elimination: 3.3-4.4 hours

Excretion: Urine

Pregnancy Risk Factor C

Hydrocodone Tannate and Chlorpheniramine Tannate *see* Hydrocodone and Chlorpheniramine *on page 827*

Hydrocodone Tannate, Phenylephrine Tannate, and Diphenhydramine Tannate *see* Hydrocodone, Phenylephrine, and Diphenhydramine *on page 834*

Hydrocortisone (hye droe KOR ti sone)

U.S. Brand Names Anucort-HC®; Anusol-HC®; Anusol® HC-1 [OTC]; Aquanil™ HC [OTC]; Beta-HC®; Caldecort® [OTC]; Cetacort®; Colocort®; Cortaid® Intensive Therapy [OTC]; Cortaid® Maximum Strength [OTC]; Cortaid® Sensitive Skin [OTC]; Cortef®; Corticool® [OTC]; Cortifoam®; Cortizone®-10 Maximum Strength [OTC]; Cortizone®-10 Plus Maximum Strength [OTC]; Cortizone®-10 Quick Shot [OTC]; Dermarest Dricort® [OTC]; Dermtex® HC [OTC]; EarSol® HC; Encort™; Hemril®-30; HydroZone Plus [OTC]; Hytone®; IvySoothe® [OTC]; Locoid®; Locoid Lipocream®; Nupercainal® Hydrocortisone Cream [OTC]; Nutracort®; Pandel®; Post Peel Healing Balm [OTC]; Preparation H® Hydrocortisone [OTC]; Proctocort®; ProctoCream® HC; Procto-Kit™; Procto-Pak™; Proctosert; Proctosol-HC®; Proctozone-HC™; Sarnol®-HC [OTC]; Solu-Cortef®; Summer's Eve® SpecialCare™ Medicated Anti-Itch Cream [OTC]; Texacort®; Tucks® Anti-Itch [OTC]; Westcort®

Canadian Brand Names Aquacort®; Cortamed®; Cortef®; Cortenema®; Cortifoam™; Emo-Cort®; Hycort™; Hyderm; HydroVal®; Locoid®; Prevex® HC; Sarna® HC; Solu-Cortef®; Westcort®

Mexican Brand Names Aquanil HC; Flebocortid; Lacticare HC; Locoid; Nositrol

Generic Available Yes: Excludes acetate foam, butyrate cream and ointment, gel as base, otic drops as base, probutate cream, sodium succinate injection

Index Terms A-hydroCort; Compound F; Cortisol; Hemorrhoidal HC; Hydrocortisone Acetate; Hydrocortisone Butyrate; Hydrocortisone Probutate; Hydrocortisone Sodium Succinate; Hydrocortisone Valerate

Pharmacologic Category Corticosteroid, Rectal; Corticosteroid, Systemic; Corticosteroid, Topical

Dental Use Treatment of a variety of oral diseases of allergic, inflammatory, or autoimmune origin

Use Management of adrenocortical insufficiency; relief of inflammation of corticosteroid-responsive dermatoses (low and medium potency topical corticosteroid); adjunctive treatment of ulcerative colitis

Local Anesthetic/Vasoconstrictor Precautions No information available to require special precautions

Effects on Dental Treatment No significant effects or complications reported

Significant Adverse Effects
Systemic:
>10%:
  Central nervous system: Insomnia, nervousness
  Gastrointestinal: Increased appetite, indigestion
1% to 10%:
  Dermatologic: Hirsutism
  Endocrine & metabolic: Diabetes mellitus
  Neuromuscular & skeletal: Arthralgia
  Ocular: Cataracts
  Respiratory: Epistaxis
<1% (Limited to important or life-threatening): Hypertension, edema, euphoria, headache, delirium, hallucinations, seizure, mood swings, acne, dermatitis, skin atrophy, bruising, hyperpigmentation, hypokalemia, hyperglycemia, Cushing's syndrome, sodium and water retention, bone growth suppression, amenorrhea, peptic ulcer, abdominal distention, ulcerative esophagitis, pancreatitis, muscle wasting, hypersensitivity reactions, immunosuppression

Topical:
>10%: Dermatologic: Eczema (12.5%)
1% to 10%: Dermatologic: Pruritus (6%), stinging (2%), dry skin (2%)
<1% (Limited to important or life-threatening): Allergic contact dermatitis, burning, dermal atrophy, folliculitis, HPA axis suppression, hypopigmentation; metabolic effects (hyperglycemia, hypokalemia); striae

Dental Usual Dosing
Treatment of a variety of oral diseases of allergic, inflammatory, or autoimmune origin: Children >2 years and Adults: Topical: Apply to affected area 2-4 times/day (Buteprate: Apply once or twice daily). Therapy should be discontinued when control is achieved; if no improvement is seen, reassessment of diagnosis may be necessary.

Dosage
Dose should be based on severity of disease and patient response
Acute adrenal insufficiency: I.M., I.V.:
  Infants and young Children: Succinate: 1-2 mg/kg/dose bolus, then 25-150 mg/day in divided doses every 6-8 hours
  Older Children: Succinate: 1-2 mg/kg bolus then 150-250 mg/day in divided doses every 6-8 hours
  Adults: Succinate: 100 mg I.V. bolus, then 300 mg/day in divided doses every 8 hours or as a continuous infusion for 48 hours; once patient is stable change to oral, 50 mg every 8 hours for 6 doses, then taper to 30-50 mg/day in divided doses
Chronic adrenal corticoid insufficiency: Adults: Oral: 20-30 mg/day
Anti-inflammatory or immunosuppressive:
  Infants and Children:
    Oral: 2.5-10 mg/kg/day **or** 75-300 mg/m^2/day every 6-8 hours
    I.M., I.V.: Succinate: 1-5 mg/kg/day **or** 30-150 mg/m^2/day divided every 12-24 hours
  Adolescents and Adults: Oral, I.M., I.V.: Succinate: 15-240 mg every 12 hours
Congenital adrenal hyperplasia: Oral: Initial: 10-20 mg/m^2/day in 3 divided doses; a variety of dosing schedules have been used. **Note:** Inconsistencies have occurred with liquid formulations; tablets may provide more reliable levels. Doses must be individualized by monitoring growth, bone age, and hormonal levels. Mineralocorticoid and sodium supplementation may be required based upon electrolyte regulation and plasma renin activity.
Physiologic replacement: Children:
  Oral: 0.5-0.75 mg/kg/day **or** 20-25 mg/m^2/day every 8 hours
  I.M.: Succinate: 0.25-0.35 mg/kg/day **or** 12-15 mg/m^2/day once daily
Shock: I.M., I.V.: Succinate:
  Children: Initial: 50 mg/kg, then repeated in 4 hours and/or every 24 hours as needed
  Adolescents and Adults: 500 mg to 2 g every 2-6 hours
Status asthmaticus: Children and Adults: I.V.: Succinate: 1-2 mg/kg/dose every 6 hours for 24 hours, then maintenance of 0.5-1 mg/kg every 6 hours
Adults:
  Rheumatic diseases:
    Intralesional, intra-articular, soft tissue injection: Acetate:
      Large joints: 25 mg (up to 37.5 mg)
      Small joints: 10-25 mg
    Tendon sheaths: 5-12.5 mg
    Soft tissue infiltration: 25-50 mg (up to 75 mg)
    Bursae: 25-37.5 mg
    Ganglia: 12.5-25 mg
  Stress dosing (surgery) in patients known to be adrenally-suppressed or on chronic systemic steroids: I.V.:
    Minor stress (ie, inguinal herniorrhaphy): 25 mg/day for 1 day
(Continued)

Hydrocortisone *(Continued)*

Moderate stress (ie, joint replacement, cholecystectomy): 50-75 mg/day (25 mg every 8-12 hours) for 1-2 days

Major stress (pancreatoduodenectomy, esophagogastrectomy, cardiac surgery): 100-150 mg/day (50 mg every 8-12 hours) for 2-3 days

Dermatosis: Children >2 years and Adults: Topical: Apply to affected area 2-4 times/day (Buteprate: Apply once or twice daily). Therapy should be discontinued when control is achieved; if no improvement is seen, reassessment of diagnosis may be necessary.

Ulcerative colitis: Adults: Rectal: 10-100 mg 1-2 times/day for 2-3 weeks

Mechanism of Action Decreases inflammation by suppression of migration of polymorphonuclear leukocytes and reversal of increased capillary permeability

Contraindications Hypersensitivity to hydrocortisone or any component of the formulation; serious infections, except septic shock or tuberculous meningitis; viral, fungal, or tubercular skin lesions

Warnings/Precautions Use with caution in patients with thyroid disease, hepatic impairment, renal impairment, cardiovascular disease, diabetes, glaucoma, cataracts, myasthenia gravis, patients at risk for osteoporosis, patients at risk for seizures, or GI diseases (diverticulitis, peptic ulcer, ulcerative colitis) due to perforation risk. Use caution following acute MI (corticosteroids have been associated with myocardial rupture). Because of the risk of adverse effects, systemic corticosteroids should be used cautiously in the elderly in the smallest possible effective dose for the shortest duration. May affect growth velocity; growth should be routinely monitored in pediatric patients. Withdraw therapy with gradual tapering of dose.

May cause hypercorticism or suppression of hypothalamic-pituitary-adrenal (HPA) axis, particularly in younger children or in patients receiving high doses for prolonged periods. HPA axis suppression may lead to adrenal crisis. Withdrawal and discontinuation of a corticosteroid should be done slowly and carefully. Particular care is required when patients are transferred from systemic corticosteroids to inhaled products due to possible adrenal insufficiency or withdrawal from steroids, including an increase in allergic symptoms. Patients receiving >20 mg per day of prednisone (or equivalent) may be most susceptible. Fatalities have occurred due to adrenal insufficiency in asthmatic patients during and after transfer from systemic corticosteroids to aerosol steroids; aerosol steroids do not provide the systemic steroid needed to treat patients having trauma, surgery, or infections. Avoid use of topical preparations with occlusive dressings or on weeping or exudative lesions.

Acute myopathy has been reported with high dose corticosteroids, usually in patients with neuromuscular transmission disorders; may involve ocular and/or respiratory muscles; monitor creatine kinase; recovery may be delayed. Corticosteroid use may cause psychiatric disturbances, including depression, euphoria, insomnia, mood swings, and personality changes. Pre-existing psychiatric conditions may be exacerbated by corticosteroid use. Prolonged use of corticosteroids may also increase the incidence of secondary infection, mask acute infection (including fungal infections), prolong or exacerbate viral infections, or limit response to vaccines. Exposure to chickenpox should be avoided; corticosteroids should not be used to treat ocular herpes simplex. Corticosteroids should not be used for cerebral malaria. Close observation is required in patients with latent tuberculosis and/or TB reactivity; restrict use in active TB (only in conjunction with antituberculosis treatment). Prolonged treatment with corticosteroids has been associated with the development of Kaposi's sarcoma (case reports); if noted, discontinuation of therapy should be considered.

Drug Interactions **Substrate** of CYP3A4 (minor); **Induces** CYP3A4 (weak)

Decreased effect:

Insulin decreases hypoglycemic effect

Phenytoin, phenobarbital, ephedrine, and rifampin increase metabolism of hydrocortisone and decrease steroid blood level

Increased toxicity:

Oral anticoagulants change prothrombin time

Potassium-depleting diuretics increase risk of hypokalemia

Cardiac glucosides increase risk of arrhythmias or digitalis toxicity secondary to hypokalemia

Ethanol/Nutrition/Herb Interactions

Ethanol: Avoid ethanol (may enhance gastric mucosal irritation).

Food: Hydrocortisone interferes with calcium absorption.

Herb/Nutraceutical: St John's wort may decrease hydrocortisone levels. Avoid cat's claw, echinacea (have immunostimulant properties).

Dietary Considerations Systemic use of corticosteroids may require a diet with increased potassium, vitamins A, B_6, C, D, folate, calcium, zinc, phosphorus, and decreased sodium. Sodium content of 1 g (sodium succinate injection): 47.5 mg (2.07 mEq)

Pharmacodynamics/Kinetics
Onset of action:
Hydrocortisone acetate: Slow
Hydrocortisone sodium succinate (water soluble): Rapid
Duration: Hydrocortisone acetate: Long
Absorption: Rapid by all routes, except rectally
Metabolism: Hepatic
Half-life elimination: Biologic: 8-12 hours
Excretion: Urine (primarily as 17-hydroxysteroids and 17-ketosteroids)

Pregnancy Risk Factor C

Lactation Excretion in breast milk unknown/use caution

Breast-Feeding Considerations It is not known if hydrocortisone is excreted in breast milk, however, other corticosteroids are excreted. Prednisone and prednisolone are excreted in breast milk; the AAP considers them to be "usually compatible" with breast-feeding. Hypertension was reported in a nursing infant when a topical corticosteroid was applied to the nipples of the mother.

Dosage Forms Excipient information presented when available (limited, particularly for generics); consult specific product labeling. [DSC] = Discontinued product
Aerosol, rectal, as acetate (Cortifoam®): 10% (15 g) [90 mg/applicator]
Cream, rectal, as acetate (Nupercainal® Hydrocortisone Cream): 1% (30 g) [strength expressed as base]
Cream, rectal, as base:
Cortizone®-10: 1% (30 g) [contains aloe]
Preparation H® Hydrocortisone: 1% (27 g)
Cream, topical, as acetate: 0.5% (9 g, 30 g, 60 g) [available with aloe]; 1% (30 g, 454 g) [available with aloe]
Cream, topical, as base: 0.5% (30 g); 1% (1.5 g, 30 g, 114 g, 454 g); 2.5% (20 g, 30 g, 454 g)
Anusol-HC®: 2.5% (30 g) [contains benzyl alcohol]
Caldecort®: 1% (30 g) [contains aloe vera gel]
Cortaid® Intensive Therapy: 1% (60 g)
Cortaid® Maximum Strength: 1% (15 g, 30 g, 40 g, 60 g) [contains aloe vera gel and benzyl alcohol]
Cortaid® Sensitive Skin: 0.5% (15 g) [contains aloe vera gel]
Cortizone®-10 Maximum Strength: 1% (15 g, 30 g, 60 g) [contains aloe]
Cortizone®-10 Plus Maximum Strength: 1% (30 g, 60 g) [contains vitamins A, D, E and aloe]
Dermarest® Dricort®: 1% (15 g, 30 g)
HydroZone Plus, Proctocort®, Procto-Pak™: 1% (30 g)
Hytone®: 2.5% (30 g, 60 g)
IvySoothe®: 1% (30 g) [contains aloe]
Post Peel Healing Balm: 1% (23 g)
ProctoCream® HC: 2.5% (30 g) [contains benzyl alcohol]
Procto-Kit™: 1% (30 g) [packaged with applicator tips and finger cots]; 2.5% (30 g) [packaged with applicator tips and finger cots]
Proctosol-HC®, Proctozone-HC™: 2.5% (30 g)
Summer's Eve® SpecialCare™ Medicated Anti-Itch Cream: 1% (30 g)
Cream, topical, as butyrate (Locoid®, Locoid Lipocream®): 0.1% (15 g, 45 g)
Cream, topical, as probutate (Pandel®): 0.1% (15 g, 45 g, 80 g)
Cream, topical, as valerate (Westcort®): 0.2% (15 g, 45 g, 60 g)
Gel, topical, as base (Corticool®): 1% (45 g)
Injection, powder for reconstitution, as sodium succinate (Solu-Cortef®): 100 mg, 250 mg, 500 mg, 1 g [diluent contains benzyl alcohol; strength expressed as base]
Lotion, topical, as base: 1% (120 mL); 2.5% (60 mL)
Aquanil™ HC: 1% (120 mL)
Beta-HC®, Cetacort®, Sarnol®-HC: 1% (60 mL)
HydroZone Plus: 1% (120 mL)
Hytone®: 2.5% (60 mL)
Nutracort®: 1% (60 mL, 120 mL); 2.5% (60 mL, 120 mL)
Ointment, topical, as acetate: 1% (30 g) [strength expressed as base; available with aloe]
Anusol® HC-1: 1% (21 g) [strength expressed as base]
Cortaid® Maximum Strength: 1% (15 g, 30 g) [strength expressed as base]
Ointment, topical, as base: 0.5% (30 g); 1% (30 g, 454 g); 2.5% (20 g, 30 g, 454 g)
Cortizone®-10 Maximum Strength: 1% (30 g, 60 g)
Hytone®: 2.5% (30 g) [DSC]
Ointment, topical, as butyrate (Locoid®): 0.1% (15 g, 45 g)
Ointment, topical, as valerate (Westcort®): 0.2% (15 g, 45 g, 60 g)
Solution, otic, as base (EarSol® HC): 1% (30 mL) [contains alcohol 44%, benzyl benzoate, yerba santa]
(Continued)

Hydrocortisone *(Continued)*

Solution, topical, as base (Texacort®): 2.5% (30 mL) [contains alcohol]
Solution, topical, as butyrate (Locoid®): 0.1% (20 mL, 60 mL) [contains alcohol 50%]
Solution, topical spray, as base:
Cortaid® Intensive Therapy: 1% (60 mL) [contains alcohol]
Cortizone®-10 Quick Shot: 1% (44 mL) [contains benzyl alcohol]
Dermtex® HC: 1% (52 mL) [contains menthol 1%]
Suppository, rectal, as acetate: 25 mg (12s, 24s, 100s)
Anucort-HC®, Tucks® Anti-Itch: 25 mg (12s, 24s, 100s) [strength expressed as base; Anucort-HC® *renamed* Tucks® Anti-Itch]
Anusol-HC®, Proctosol-HC®: 25 mg (12s, 24s)
Encort™: 30 mg (12s)
Hemril®-30, Proctocort®, Proctosert: 30 mg (12s, 24s)
Suspension, rectal, as base: 100 mg/60 mL (7s)
Colocort®: 100 mg/60 mL (1s, 7s)
Tablet, as base: 20 mg
Cortef®: 5 mg, 10 mg, 20 mg

Hydrocortisone Acetate *see* Hydrocortisone *on page 836*

Hydrocortisone, Acetic Acid, and Propylene Glycol Diacetate *see* Acetic Acid, Propylene Glycol Diacetate, and Hydrocortisone *on page 45*

Hydrocortisone and Benzoyl Peroxide *see* Benzoyl Peroxide and Hydrocortisone *on page 201*

Hydrocortisone and Ciprofloxacin *see* Ciprofloxacin and Hydrocortisone *on page 365*

Hydrocortisone and Iodoquinol *see* Iodoquinol and Hydrocortisone *on page 902*

Hydrocortisone and Lidocaine *see* Lidocaine and Hydrocortisone *on page 980*

Hydrocortisone and Pramoxine *see* Pramoxine and Hydrocortisone *on page 1335*

Hydrocortisone and Urea *see* Urea and Hydrocortisone *on page 1633*

Hydrocortisone, Bacitracin, Neomycin, and Polymyxin B *see* Bacitracin, Neomycin, Polymyxin B, and Hydrocortisone *on page 182*

Hydrocortisone Butyrate *see* Hydrocortisone *on page 836*

Hydrocortisone, Neomycin, and Polymyxin B *see* Neomycin, Polymyxin B, and Hydrocortisone *on page 1162*

Hydrocortisone Probutate *see* Hydrocortisone *on page 836*

Hydrocortisone Sodium Succinate *see* Hydrocortisone *on page 836*

Hydrocortisone Valerate *see* Hydrocortisone *on page 836*

Hydro DP *see* Hydrocodone, Phenylephrine, and Diphenhydramine *on page 834*

HydroFed *see* Hydrocodone, Phenylephrine, and Guaifenesin *on page 834*

Hydro-GP *see* Hydrocodone, Phenylephrine, and Guaifenesin *on page 834*

Hydromet® *see* Hydrocodone and Homatropine *on page 829*

Hydromorphone *(hye droe MOR fone)*

Related Information
Oral Pain *on page 1788*
Oxymorphone *on page 1237*
U.S. Brand Names Dilaudid®; Dilaudid-HP®
Canadian Brand Names Dilaudid®; Dilaudid-HP®; Dilaudid-HP-Plus®; Dilaudid® Sterile Powder; Dilaudid-XP®; Hydromorph Contin®; Hydromorph-IR®; Hydromorphone HP; Hydromorphone HP® 10; Hydromorphone HP® 20; Hydromorphone HP® 50; Hydromorphone HP® Forte; Hydromorphone Hydrochloride Injection, USP; PMS-Hydromorphone
Generic Available Yes: Excludes capsule, liquid, powder for injection
Index Terms Dihydromorphinone; Hydromorphone Hydrochloride
Pharmacologic Category Analgesic, Opioid
Dental Use Management of moderate-to-severe pain
Use Management of moderate-to-severe pain
Unlabeled/Investigational Use Antitussive
Local Anesthetic/Vasoconstrictor Precautions No information available to require special precautions
Effects on Dental Treatment Key adverse event(s) related to dental treatment: Xerostomia (normal salivary flow resumes upon discontinuation).
Common Adverse Effects Frequency not defined.
Cardiovascular: Bradycardia, flushing of face, hyper-/hypotension, palpitation, peripheral vasodilation, syncope, tachycardia

Central nervous system: Agitation, chills, CNS depression, dizziness, drowsiness, dysphoria, euphoria, fatigue, hallucinations, headache, increased intracranial pressure, insomnia, lightheadedness, mental depression, nervousness, restlessness, sedation, seizure

Dermatologic: Pruritus, rash, urticaria

Endocrine & metabolic: Antidiuretic hormone release

Gastrointestinal: Anorexia, biliary tract spasm, constipation, diarrhea, nausea, paralytic ileus, stomach cramps, taste perversion, vomiting, xerostomia

Genitourinary: Ureteral spasm, urinary retention, urinary tract spasm, urination decreased

Hepatic: AST/ALT increased, LFTs increased

Local: Pain at injection site (I.M.), wheal/flare over vein (I.V.)

Neuromuscular & skeletal: Myoclonus, paresthesia, trembling, tremor, weakness

Ocular: Blurred vision, diplopia, miosis, nystagmus

Respiratory: Apnea, bronchospasm, dyspnea, laryngospasm, respiratory depression

Miscellaneous: Diaphoresis, histamine release, physical and psychological dependence

Restrictions C-II

Mechanism of Action Binds to opiate receptors in the CNS, causing inhibition of ascending pain pathways, altering the perception of and response to pain; causes cough supression by direct central action in the medulla; produces generalized CNS depression

Drug Interactions

Increased Effect/Toxicity: Effects may be additive with CNS depressants; hypotensive effects may be increased with phenothiazines or general anesthetics; serotonergic effects may be additive with SSRIs

Decreased Effect: Hydromorphone may diminish the effects of pegvisomant. Ammonium chloride may decrease the levels/effects of hydromorphone.

Pharmacodynamics/Kinetics

Onset of action: Analgesic: Immediate release formulations:
Oral: 15-30 minutes
Peak effect: Oral: 30-60 minutes
Duration: Immediate release formulations: 4-5 hours
Absorption: I.M.: Variable and delayed
Distribution: V_d: 4 L/kg
Protein binding: ~8% to 19%
Metabolism: Hepatic via glucuronidation; to inactive metabolites
Bioavailability: 62%
Half-life elimination: Immediate release formulations: 1-3 hours
Excretion: Urine (primarily as glucuronide conjugates)

Pregnancy Risk Factor C/D (prolonged use or high doses at term)

Hydromorphone Hydrochloride *see* Hydromorphone *on page 840*

Hydroquinol *see* Hydroquinone *on page 841*

Hydroquinone (HYE droe kwin one)

U.S. Brand Names Alphaquin HP®; Claripel™; Dermarest® Skin Correction Cream Plus [OTC]; Eldopaque® [OTC]; Eldopaque Forte®; Eldoquin® [OTC]; Eldoquin Forte®; EpiQuin™ Micro; Esoterica® Regular [OTC]; Glyquin®; Glyquin-XM™; Lustra®; Lustra-AF™; Melanex®; Melpaque HP®; Melquin-3®; Melquin HP®; NeoStrata® AHA [OTC]; Nuquin HP®; Palmer's® Skin Success Eventone® Fade Cream [OTC]; Solaquin® [OTC]; Solaquin Forte®

Canadian Brand Names Eldopaque®; Eldoquin®; Glyquin® XM; Lustra®; NeoStrata® HQ; Solaquin®; Solaquin Forte®; Ultraquin™

Mexican Brand Names Crema Blanca Bustillos; Eldoquin

Generic Available Yes

Index Terms Hydroquinol; Quinol

Pharmacologic Category Depigmenting Agent

Use Gradual bleaching of hyperpigmented skin conditions

Local Anesthetic/Vasoconstrictor Precautions No information available to require special precautions

Effects on Dental Treatment No significant effects or complications reported

Common Adverse Effects Frequency not defined.

Dermatologic: Dermatitis, dryness, erythema, stinging, inflammatory reaction, sensitization

Local: Irritation

Mechanism of Action Produces reversible depigmentation of the skin by suppression of melanocyte metabolic processes, in particular the inhibition of the enzymatic oxidation of tyrosine to DOPA (3,4-dihydroxyphenylalanine); sun exposure reverses this effect and will cause repigmentation.

(Continued)

Hydroquinone *(Continued)*

Pharmacodynamics/Kinetics Onset and duration of depigmentation produced by hydroquinone varies among individuals

Pregnancy Risk Factor C

Hydroquinone, Fluocinolone Acetonide, and Tretinoin *see* Fluocinolone, Hydroquinone, and Tretinoin *on page 708*

Hydro-Tussin™-CBX *see* Carbinoxamine and Pseudoephedrine *on page 282*

Hydro-Tussin™ DHC *see* Pseudoephedrine, Dihydrocodeine, and Chlorpheniramine *on page 1385*

Hydro-Tussin™ DM *see* Guaifenesin and Dextromethorphan *on page 796*

Hydro-Tussin™ EXP *see* Dihydrocodeine, Pseudoephedrine, and Guaifenesin *on page 503*

Hydro-Tussin™ HD *see* Hydrocodone, Pseudoephedrine, and Guaifenesin *on page 835*

Hydro-Tussin™ HG *see* Hydrocodone and Guaifenesin *on page 828*

Hydro-Tussin™ XP *see* Hydrocodone, Pseudoephedrine, and Guaifenesin *on page 835*

Hydroxocobalamin *(hye droks oh koe BAL a min)*

U.S. Brand Names Cyanokit®
Mexican Brand Names Axofor
Generic Available Yes: Excludes powder for injection
Index Terms Vitamin B_{12a}
Pharmacologic Category Antidote; Vitamin, Water Soluble
Use Treatment of pernicious anemia, vitamin B_{12} deficiency due to dietary deficiencies or malabsorption diseases, inadequate secretion of intrinsic factor, and inadequate utilization of B_{12} (eg, during neoplastic treatment); diagnostic agent for Schilling test

Cyanokit®: Treatment of cyanide poisoning (known or suspected)
Unlabeled/Investigational Use Neuropathies
Local Anesthetic/Vasoconstrictor Precautions No information available to require special precautions
Effects on Dental Treatment No significant effects or complications reported
Common Adverse Effects
I.M. injection: Frequency not defined:
Dermatologic: Exanthema (transient), itching
Gastrointestinal: Diarrhea (mild, transient)
Local: Injection site pain
Miscellaneous: Anaphylaxis

I.V. infusion (Cyanokit®):
>10%:
Cardiovascular: Blood pressure increased (18% to 28%; systolic ≥180 mm Hg or diastolic ≥110 mm Hg)
Central nervous system: Headache (6% to 33%)
Dermatologic: Erythema (94% to 100%; may last up to 2 weeks), rash (predominantly acneiform; 20% to 44%; can appear 7-28 days after administration and usually resolves within a few weeks)
Gastrointestinal: Nausea (6% to 11%)
Genitourinary: Chromaturia (100%; may last up to 5 weeks after administration)
Hematologic: Lymphocytes decreased (8% to 17%)
Local: Infusion site reaction (6% to 39%)
Frequency not defined:
Cardiovascular: Chest discomfort, heart rate increased/decreased, hot flashes, peripheral edema
Central nervous system: Dizziness, memory impairment, restlessness
Dermatologic: Pruritus, urticaria
Gastrointestinal: Abdominal discomfort, diarrhea, dyspepsia, dysphagia, hematochezia, vomiting
Ocular: Irritation, redness, swelling
Respiratory: Dry throat, dyspnea, throat tightness
Miscellaneous: Allergic reaction (including anaphylaxis)
Mechanism of Action Hydroxocobalamin (vitamin B_{12a}) is a precursor to cyanocobalamin (vitamin B_{12}). Cyanocobalamin acts as a coenzyme for various metabolic functions, including fat and carbohydrate metabolism and protein synthesis, used in cell replication and hematopoiesis. In the presence of cyanide, each hydroxocobalamin molecule can bind one cyanide ion by displacing it for the hydroxo ligand linked to the trivalent cobalt ion, forming cyanocobalamin.

Pharmacodynamics/Kinetics Following I.V. administration of Cyanokit®:
Protein binding: Significant; forms various cobalamin-(III) complexes
Half-life elimination: 26-31 hours
Excretion: Urine (50% to 60% within initial 72 hours)
Pregnancy Risk Factor C

Hydroxyamphetamine and Tropicamide
(hye droks ee am FET a meen & troe PIK a mide)

Related Information
Tropicamide *on page 1627*
U.S. Brand Names Paremyd®
Generic Available No
Index Terms Hydroxyamphetamine Hydrobromide and Tropicamide; Tropicamide and Hydroxyamphetamine
Pharmacologic Category Adrenergic Agonist Agent, Ophthalmic
Use Short-term pupil dilation for diagnostic procedures and exams
Local Anesthetic/Vasoconstrictor Precautions No information available to require special precautions
Effects on Dental Treatment No significant effects or complications reported
Mechanism of Action Hydroxyamphetamine hydrobromide is an indirect acting sympathomimetic agent which causes the release of norepinephrine from adrenergic nerve terminals, resulting in mydriasis. Tropicamide is a parasympatholytic agent which produces mydriasis and paralysis by blocking the sphincter muscle in the iris and the ciliary muscle.
Pregnancy Risk Factor C

Hydroxyamphetamine Hydrobromide and Tropicamide *see* Hydroxyamphetamine and Tropicamide *on page 843*

4-Hydroxybutyrate *see* Sodium Oxybate *on page 1482*

Hydroxycarbamide *see* Hydroxyurea *on page 845*

Hydroxychloroquine (hye droks ee KLOR oh kwin)

Related Information
Rheumatoid Arthritis, Osteoarthritis, and Osteoporosis *on page 1759*
U.S. Brand Names Plaquenil®
Canadian Brand Names Apo-Hydroxyquine®; Gen-Hydroxychloroquine; Plaquenil®
Mexican Brand Names Plaquenil Sulfate
Generic Available Yes
Index Terms Hydroxychloroquine Sulfate
Pharmacologic Category Aminoquinoline (Antimalarial)
Use Suppression and treatment of acute attacks of malaria; treatment of systemic lupus erythematosus and rheumatoid arthritis
Unlabeled/Investigational Use Porphyria cutanea tarda, polymorphous light eruptions
Local Anesthetic/Vasoconstrictor Precautions No information available to require special precautions
Effects on Dental Treatment No significant effects or complications reported
Common Adverse Effects Frequency not defined.
Cardiovascular: Cardiomyopathy (rare, relationship to hydroxychloroquine unclear)
Central nervous system: Irritability, nervousness, emotional changes, nightmares, psychosis, headache, dizziness, vertigo, seizure, ataxia, lassitude
Dermatologic: Bleaching of hair, alopecia, pigmentation changes (skin and mucosal; black-blue color), rash (urticarial, morbilliform, lichenoid, maculopapular, purpuric, erythema annulare centrifugum, Stevens-Johnson syndrome, acute generalized exanthematous pustulosis, and exfoliative dermatitis)
Endocrine & metabolic: Weight loss
Gastrointestinal: Anorexia, nausea, vomiting, diarrhea, abdominal cramping
Hematologic: Aplastic anemia, agranulocytosis, leukopenia, thrombocytopenia, hemolysis (in patients with glucose-6-phosphate deficiency)
Hepatic: Abnormal liver function/hepatic failure (isolated cases)
Neuromuscular & skeletal: Myopathy, palsy, or neuromyopathy leading to progressive weakness and atrophy of proximal muscle groups (may be associated with mild sensory changes, loss of deep tendon reflexes, and abnormal nerve conduction)
Ocular: Disturbance in accommodation, keratopathy, corneal changes/deposits (visual disturbances, blurred vision, photophobia - reversible on discontinuation), macular edema, atrophy, abnormal pigmentation, retinopathy (early
(Continued)

Hydroxychloroquine *(Continued)*

changes reversible - may progress despite discontinuation if advanced), optic disc pallor/atrophy, attenuation of retinal arterioles, pigmentary retinopathy, scotoma, decreased visual acuity, nystagmus

Otic: Tinnitus, deafness

Miscellaneous: Exacerbation of porphyria and nonlight sensitive psoriasis

Mechanism of Action Interferes with digestive vacuole function within sensitive malarial parasites by increasing the pH and interfering with lysosomal degradation of hemoglobin; inhibits locomotion of neutrophils and chemotaxis of eosinophils; impairs complement-dependent antigen-antibody reactions

Drug Interactions

Increased Effect/Toxicity: Cimetidine increases levels of chloroquine and probably other 4-aminoquinolones.

Decreased Effect: Chloroquine and other 4-aminoquinolones absorption may be decreased due to GI binding with kaolin or magnesium trisilicate.

Pharmacodynamics/Kinetics

Onset of action: Rheumatic disease: May require 4-6 weeks to respond

Absorption: Complete

Protein binding: 55%

Metabolism: Hepatic

Half-life elimination: 32-50 days

Time to peak: Rheumatic disease: Several months

Excretion: Urine (as metabolites and unchanged drug); may be enhanced by urinary acidification

Pregnancy Risk Factor C

Hydroxychloroquine Sulfate *see* Hydroxychloroquine *on page 843*

Hydroxydaunomycin Hydrochloride *see* DOXOrubicin *on page 536*

1α-Hydroxyergocalciferol *see* Doxercalciferol *on page 535*

Hydroxyethylcellulose *see* Artificial Tears *on page 147*

Hydroxyethyl Starch *see* Hetastarch *on page 813*

Hydroxyldaunorubicin Hydrochloride *see* DOXOrubicin *on page 536*

Hydroxypropyl Cellulose (hye droks ee PROE pil SEL yoo lose)

Related Information

Hydroxypropyl Methylcellulose *on page 844*

U.S. Brand Names Lacrisert®

Canadian Brand Names Lacrisert®

Generic Available No

Pharmacologic Category Ophthalmic Agent, Miscellaneous

Use Dry eyes (moderate to severe)

Local Anesthetic/Vasoconstrictor Precautions No information available to require special precautions

Effects on Dental Treatment No significant effects or complications reported

---

Hydroxypropyl Methylcellulose (hye droks ee PROE pil meth il SEL yoo lose)

Related Information

Hydroxypropyl Cellulose *on page 844*

U.S. Brand Names Cellugel®; GenTeal® [OTC]; GenTeal® Mild [OTC]; Gonak™ [OTC]; Goniosoft™; Goniosol® [OTC] [DSC]; Isopto® Tears [OTC]; Tearisol® [OTC]; Tears Again® MC [OTC]

Canadian Brand Names Genteal®; Isopto® Tears

Mexican Brand Names Celulose Grin; Naturalag

Generic Available Yes: Solution

Index Terms Gonioscopic Ophthalmic Solution; Hypromellose

Pharmacologic Category Diagnostic Agent, Ophthalmic; Lubricant, Ocular

Use Relief of burning and minor irritation due to dry eyes; diagnostic agent in gonioscopic examination

Local Anesthetic/Vasoconstrictor Precautions No information available to require special precautions

Effects on Dental Treatment No significant effects or complications reported

Pregnancy Risk Factor C

9-hydroxy-risperidone *see* Paliperidone *on page 1243*

Hydroxyurea (hye droks ee yoor EE a)

U.S. Brand Names Droxia®; Hydrea®; Mylocel™
Canadian Brand Names Apo-Hydroxyurea®; Gen-Hydroxyurea; Hydrea®
Mexican Brand Names Hydrea
Generic Available Yes: Capsule
Index Terms Hydroxycarbamide
Pharmacologic Category Antineoplastic Agent, Antimetabolite
Use Treatment of melanoma, refractory chronic myelocytic leukemia (CML), relapsed and refractory metastatic ovarian cancer; radiosensitizing agent in the treatment of squamous cell head and neck cancer (excluding lip cancer); adjunct in the management of sickle cell patients who have had at least three painful crises in the previous 12 months (to reduce frequency of these crises and the need for blood transfusions)
Unlabeled/Investigational Use Treatment of HIV; treatment of psoriasis, treatment of hematologic conditions such as essential thrombocythemia, polycythemia vera, hypereosinophilia, and hyperleukocytosis due to acute leukemia; treatment of uterine, cervix and nonsmall cell lung cancers; radiosensitizing agent in the treatment of primary brain tumors; has shown activity against renal cell cancer and prostate cancer
Local Anesthetic/Vasoconstrictor Precautions No information available to require special precautions
Effects on Dental Treatment No significant effects or complications reported
Common Adverse Effects Frequency not defined.

Cardiovascular: Edema

Central nervous system: Chills, disorientation, dizziness, drowsiness (dose-related), fever, hallucinations, headache, malaise, seizure

Dermatologic: Alopecia (rare), cutaneous vasculitic toxicities, dermatomyositis-like skin changes, dry skin, facial erythema, gangrene, hyperpigmentation, maculopapular rash, nail atrophy, nail pigmentation, peripheral erythema, scaling, skin atrophy, skin cancer, skin ulcer, vasculitis ulcerations, violet papules

Endocrine & metabolic: Hyperuricemia

Gastrointestinal: Anorexia, constipation, diarrhea, gastrointestinal irritation and mucositis, (potentiated with radiation therapy), nausea, pancreatitis, stomatitis, vomiting

Genitourinary: Dysuria (rare)

Hematologic: Myelosuppression (primarily leukopenia; onset: 24-48 hours; nadir: 10 days; recovery: 7 days after stopping drug; reversal of WBC count occurs rapidly but the platelet count may take 7-10 days to recover); thrombocytopenia and anemia, megaloblastic erythropoiesis, macrocytosis, hemolysis, serum iron decreased, persistent cytopenias, secondary leukemias (long-term use)

Hepatic: Hepatic enzymes increased, hepatotoxicity

Neuromuscular & skeletal: Peripheral neuropathy, weakness

Renal: BUN increased, creatinine increased

Respiratory: Acute diffuse pulmonary infiltrates (rare), dyspnea, pulmonary fibrosis (rare)

Mechanism of Action Thought to interfere (unsubstantiated hypothesis) with synthesis of DNA, during the S phase of cell division, without interfering with RNA synthesis; inhibits ribonucleoside diphosphate reductase, preventing conversion of ribonucleotides to deoxyribonucleotides; cell-cycle specific for the S phase and may hold other cells in the G_1 phase of the cell cycle. In sickle cell anemia, hydroxyurea increases red blood cell (RBC) hemoglobin F levels, RBC water content, deformability of sickled cells, and alters adhesion of RBCs to endothelium.

Drug Interactions
Increased Effect/Toxicity: Hydroxyurea may increase the toxicity of didanosine.

Pharmacodynamics/Kinetics
Absorption: Readily ($\geq 80\%$)
Distribution: Readily crosses blood-brain barrier; distributes into intestine, brain, lung, kidney tissues, effusions and ascites
Metabolism: 60% via hepatic and GI tract
Half-life elimination: 3-4 hours
Time to peak: 1-4 hours
Excretion: Urine (80%, 50% as unchanged drug, 30% as urea); exhaled gases (as CO_2)
Pregnancy Risk Factor D

HydrOXYzine (hye DROKS i zeen)

Related Information
Sedation *on page 1825*

Related Sample Prescriptions
Sedation (Prior to Dental Treatment) *on page 1846*

U.S. Brand Names Vistaril®

Canadian Brand Names Apo-Hydroxyzine®; Atarax®; Hydroxyzine Hydrochloride Injection, USP; Novo-Hydroxyzin; PMS-Hydroxyzine; Vistaril®

Mexican Brand Names Atarax

Generic Available Yes

Index Terms Hydroxyzine Hydrochloride; Hydroxyzine Pamoate

Pharmacologic Category Antiemetic; Antihistamine

Dental Use Treatment of anxiety, as a preoperative sedative in pediatric dentistry

Use Treatment of anxiety; preoperative sedative; antipruritic

Unlabeled/Investigational Use Antiemetic; ethanol withdrawal symptoms

Local Anesthetic/Vasoconstrictor Precautions No information available to require special precautions

Effects on Dental Treatment Key adverse event(s) related to dental treatment: Xerostomia (normal salivary flow resumes upon discontinuation).

Significant Adverse Effects Frequency not defined.
Central nervous system: Dizziness, drowsiness, fatigue, hallucination, headache, nervousness, seizure
Dermatologic: Pruritus, rash, urticaria
Gastrointestinal: Xerostomia
Neuromuscular & skeletal: Involuntary movements, paresthesia, tremor
Ocular: Blurred vision
Respiratory: Thickening of bronchial secretions
Miscellaneous: Allergic reaction

Dental Usual Dosing
Anxiety: Adults: Oral: 50-100 mg 4 times/day
Preoperative sedation:
Children:
Oral: 0.6 mg/kg/dose
I.M.: 0.5-1 mg/kg/dose
Adults:
Oral: 50-100 mg
I.M.: 25-100 mg

Dosage
Children:
Preoperative sedation:
Oral: 0.6 mg/kg/dose
I.M.: 0.5-1 mg/kg/dose
Pruritus, anxiety: Oral:
<6 years: 50 mg daily in divided doses
≥6 years: 50-100 mg daily in divided doses
Adults:
Antiemetic (unlabeled use): I.M.: 25-100 mg/dose every 4-6 hours as needed
Anxiety: Oral, I.M.: 50-100 mg 4 times/day
Preoperative sedation:
Oral: 50-100 mg
I.M.: 25-100 mg
Pruritus: Oral, I.M.: 25 mg 3-4 times/day

Dosing interval in hepatic impairment: Change dosing interval to every 24 hours in patients with primary biliary cirrhosis

Mechanism of Action Competes with histamine for H_1-receptor sites on effector cells in the gastrointestinal tract, blood vessels, and respiratory tract. Possesses skeletal muscle relaxing, bronchodilator, antihistamine, antiemetic, and analgesic properties.

Contraindications Hypersensitivity to hydroxyzine or any component of the formulation; early pregnancy; SubQ, intra-arterial, or I.V. administration of injection

Warnings/Precautions Causes sedation, caution must be used in performing tasks which require alertness (eg, operating machinery or driving). Sedative effects of CNS depressants or ethanol are potentiated. SubQ, I.V., and intra-arterial administration are contraindicated since tissue damage, intravascular hemolysis, thrombosis, and digital gangrene can occur. Use with caution with narrow-angle glaucoma, prostatic hyperplasia, bladder neck obstruction, asthma, or COPD. Not recommended for use as a sedative or anxiolytic in the elderly.

Drug Interactions Inhibits CYP2D6 (weak)

Acetylcholinesterase Inhibitors (Central): May diminish the anticholinergic of hydroxyzine. If the anticholinergic effect is a side effect of the agent, as is the case with hydroxyzine, the result may be beneficial.

Anticholinergic agents: Central and/or peripheral anticholinergic syndrome can occur when administered with opioid analgesics, phenothiazines and other antipsychotics (especially with high anticholinergic activity), tricyclic antidepressants, quinidine and some other antiarrhythmics, and antihistamines

CNS depressants: Sedative effects of hydroxyzine may be additive with CNS depressants; includes ethanol, benzodiazepines, barbiturates, opioid analgesics, and other sedative agents; monitor for increased effect

Pramlintide: May enhance the GI-related anticholinergic effect of hydroxyzine.

Ethanol/Nutrition/Herb Interactions

Ethanol: Avoid ethanol (may increase CNS depression).

Herb/Nutraceutical: Avoid valerian, St John's wort, kava kava, gotu kola (may increase CNS depression).

Pharmacodynamics/Kinetics

Onset of action: Oral: 15-30 minutes

Duration: 4-6 hours

Absorption: Oral: Rapid

Metabolism: Forms metabolites

Half-life elimination: 3-7 hours

Time to peak: ~2 hours

Excretion: Urine

Pregnancy Risk Factor C

Lactation Excretion in breast milk unknown/not recommended

Dosage Forms Excipient information presented when available (limited, particularly for generics); consult specific product labeling.

Capsule, as pamoate: 25 mg, 50 mg, 100 mg

Vistaril®: 25 mg, 50 mg

Injection, solution, as hydrochloride: 25 mg/mL (1 mL); 50 mg/mL (1 mL, 2 mL, 10 mL)

Suspension, oral, as pamoate:

Vistaril®: 25 mg/5 mL (120 mL, 480 mL) [lemon flavor]

Syrup, as hydrochloride: 10 mg/5 mL (120 mL, 480 mL)

Tablet, as hydrochloride: 10 mg, 25 mg, 50 mg

Hyoscyamine (hye oh SYE a meen)

U.S. Brand Names Anaspaz®; Cystospaz®; Cystospaz-M® [DSC]; Hyosine; Levbid®; Levsin®; Levsinex®; Levsin/SL®; NuLev™; Spacol [DSC]; Spacol T/S [DSC]; Symax SL; Symax SR

Canadian Brand Names Cystospaz®; Levsin®

Generic Available Yes

Index Terms Hyoscyamine Sulfate; *l*-Hyoscyamine Sulfate

Pharmacologic Category Anticholinergic Agent

Use

Oral: Adjunctive therapy for peptic ulcers, irritable bowel, neurogenic bladder/bowel; treatment of infant colic, GI tract disorders caused by spasm; to reduce rigidity, tremors, sialorrhea, and hyperhidrosis associated with parkinsonism; as a drying agent in acute rhinitis

Injection: Preoperative antimuscarinic to reduce secretions and block cardiac vagal inhibitory reflexes; to improve radiologic visibility of the kidneys; symptomatic relief of biliary and renal colic; reduce GI motility to facilitate diagnostic procedures (ie, endoscopy, hypotonic duodenography); reduce pain and hypersecretion in pancreatitis, certain cases of partial heart block associated with vagal activity; reversal of neuromuscular blockade

Local Anesthetic/Vasoconstrictor Precautions No information available to require special precautions

(Continued)

Hyoscyamine *(Continued)*

Effects on Dental Treatment Key adverse event(s) related to dental treatment: Xerostomia (normal salivary flow resumes upon discontinuation).

Mechanism of Action Blocks the action of acetylcholine at parasympathetic sites in smooth muscle, secretory glands and the CNS; increases cardiac output, dries secretions, antagonizes histamine and serotonin

Pregnancy Risk Factor C

Hyoscyamine, Atropine, Scopolamine, and Phenobarbital

(hye oh SYE a meen, A troe peen, skoe POL a meen, & fee noe BAR bi tal)

Related Information

Atropine *on page 166*
Hyoscyamine *on page 847*
Phenobarbital *on page 1288*
Scopolamine *on page 1457*

U.S. Brand Names Donnatal®; Donnatal Extentabs®

Generic Available Yes: Elixir, tablet

Index Terms Atropine, Hyoscyamine, Scopolamine, and Phenobarbital; Belladonna Alkaloids With Phenobarbital; Phenobarbital, Hyoscyamine, Atropine, and Scopolamine; Scopolamine, Hyoscyamine, Atropine, and Phenobarbital

Pharmacologic Category Anticholinergic Agent; Antispasmodic Agent, Gastrointestinal

Use Adjunct in treatment of irritable bowel syndrome, acute enterocolitis, duodenal ulcer

Local Anesthetic/Vasoconstrictor Precautions No information available to require special precautions

Effects on Dental Treatment Key adverse event(s) related to dental treatment: Xerostomia (normal salivary flow resumes upon discontinuation).

Common Adverse Effects Frequency not defined.

Cardiovascular: Palpitation, tachycardia

Central nervous system: Dizziness, drowsiness, headache, insomnia, nervousness

Dermatologic: Urticaria

Gastrointestinal: Bloating, constipation, nausea, taste loss, vomiting, xerostomia

Genitourinary: Impotence, urinary hesitancy, urinary retention

Neuromuscular & skeletal: Musculoskeletal pain, weakness

Ocular: Blurred vision, cycloplegia, mydriasis, ocular tension increased

Miscellaneous: Allergic reaction (may be severe), anaphylaxis, lactation suppressed, diaphoresis decreased

Mechanism of Action A fixed combination of belladonna alkaloids and phenobarbital which provides anticholinergic/antispasmodic action and mild sedation.

Drug Interactions

Cytochrome P450 Effect: Phenobarbital: **Substrate** (minor) of CYP2C8/9, 2C19, 2E1; **Induces** CYP1A2 (strong), 2A6 (strong), 2B6 (strong), 2C8/9 (strong), 3A4 (strong)

Increased Effect/Toxicity: Anticholinergic effects may be additive with other anticholinergic agents, or drugs with significant anticholinergic activity (antihistamine, tricyclic antidepressants, phenothiazines). When combined with other CNS depressants, ethanol, narcotic analgesics, antidepressants, or benzodiazepines, additive respiratory and CNS depression may occur. Barbiturates may enhance the hepatotoxic potential of acetaminophen overdoses. Chloramphenicol, MAO inhibitors, valproic acid, and felbamate may inhibit barbiturate metabolism. Barbiturates may impair the absorption of griseofulvin, and may enhance the nephrotoxic effects of methoxyflurane. Concurrent use of phenobarbital with meperidine may result in increased CNS depression. Concurrent use of phenobarbital with primidone may result in elevated phenobarbital serum concentrations. The levels/effects of phenobarbital may be increased by delavirdine, fluconazole, fluvoxamine, gemfibrozil, isoniazid, omeprazole, ticlopidine, and other CYP2C19 inhibitors.

Decreased Effect: Barbiturates may increase the metabolism of estrogens and reduce the efficacy of oral contraceptives; an alternative method of contraception should be considered. Barbiturates inhibit the hypoprothrombinemic effects of oral anticoagulants via increased metabolism. Barbiturates may enhance the metabolism of methadone resulting in methadone withdrawal. The levels/effects of phenobarbital may be decreased by aminoglutethimide, carbamazepine, phenytoin, rifampin, and other CYP2C19 inducers.

Phenobarbital may decrease the levels/effects of aminophylline, amiodarone, benzodiazepines, bupropion, calcium channel blockers, carbamazepine, citalopram, clarithromycin, cyclosporine diazepam, efavirenz, erythromycin, estrogens, fluoxetine, fluvoxamine, glimepiride, glipizide, ifosfamide, losartan, methsuximide, mirtazapine, nateglinide, nefazodone, nevirapine, phenytoin, pioglitazone, promethazine, propranolol, protease inhibitors, proton pump inhibitors, rifampin, ropinirole, rosiglitazone, selegiline, sertraline, sulfonamides, tacrolimus, theophylline, venlafaxine. voriconazole warfarin, zafirlukast, and other CYP1A2, 2A6, 2B6, 2C8/9, or 3A4 substrates.

Pregnancy Risk Factor C

Ibandronate (eye BAN droh nate)

Related Information
Rheumatoid Arthritis, Osteoarthritis, and Osteoporosis *on page 1759*

U.S. Brand Names Boniva®

Canadian Brand Names Bondronat®

Generic Available No

Index Terms Ibandronate Sodium; Ibandronic Acid; NSC-722623

Pharmacologic Category Bisphosphonate Derivative

Use Treatment and prevention of osteoporosis in postmenopausal females

Unlabeled/Investigational Use Hypercalcemia of malignancy; corticosteroid-induced osteoporosis; Paget's disease; reduce bone pain and skeletal complications from metastatic bone disease

Local Anesthetic/Vasoconstrictor Precautions No information available to require special precautions

Effects on Dental Treatment Key adverse event(s) related to dental treatment: Tooth disorder.

Osteonecrosis of the jaw (ONJ), generally associated with local infection and/or tooth extraction and often with delayed healing, has been reported in patients taking bisphosphonates. Symptoms included nonhealing extraction socket or an exposed jawbone. Most reported cases of bisphosphonate-associated osteonecrosis have been in cancer patients treated with intravenous bisphosphonates. However, some have occurred in patients with postmenopausal osteoporosis taking oral bisphosphonates. Dental surgery may exacerbate ONJ. For patients requiring dental procedures, there are no data available to suggest whether discontinuation of bisphosphonate treatment reduces the risk of ONJ. Patients who develop ONJ while on bisphosphonate therapy should receive care by an oral surgeon. See Dental Comment.

Common Adverse Effects Percentages vary based on frequency of administration (daily vs monthly). Unless specified, percentages are reported with oral use.

>10%:
Gastrointestinal: Dyspepsia (6% to 12%)
Neuromuscular & skeletal: Back pain (4% to 14%)

1% to 10%:
Central nervous system: Headache (3% to 7%), dizziness (1% to 4%), insomnia (1% to 2%)
Dermatologic: Rash (1% to 2%)
Endocrine & metabolic: Hypercholesterolemia (5%)

(Continued)

Ibandronate *(Continued)*

Gastrointestinal: Abdominal pain (5% to 8%), diarrhea (4% to 7%), nausea (5%), tooth disorder (4%), vomiting (3%), constipation (3% to 4%)

Genitourinary: Urinary tract infection (2% to 6%)

Hepatic: Alkaline phosphatase decreased (frequency not defined)

Local: Injection site reaction (<2%)

Neuromuscular & skeletal: Pain in extremity (8%), myalgia (1% to 6%), joint disorder (4%), weakness (4%), muscle cramp (2%)

Respiratory: Bronchitis (3% to 10%), pneumonia (6%), pharyngitis/nasopharyngitis (3% to 4%), upper respiratory infection (2%)

Miscellaneous: Acute phase reaction (I.V. 10%; oral 4%), allergic reaction (3%), flu-like syndrome (1% to 3%)

Dosage

Oral:

Treatment of postmenopausal osteoporosis: 2.5 mg/day or 150 mg once a month

Prevention of postmenopausal osteoporosis: 2.5 mg/day; 150 mg once a month may be considered

Metastatic bone disease (unlabeled use): 50 mg once daily

I.V.:

Treatment of postmenopausal osteoporosis: 3 mg every 3 months

Hypercalcemia of malignancy (unlabeled use): 2-4 mg over 2 hours

Metastatic bone disease (unlabeled use): 6 mg over 1 hour every 3-4 weeks

Dosage adjustment in renal impairment:

Mild or moderate impairment: Dosing adjustment not needed

Severe impairment (Cl$_{cr}$ <30 mL/minute): Use not recommended

Dose adjustment in renal impairment for oncologic uses (unlabeled): Severe impairment (Cl$_{cr}$ <30 mL/minute):

Oral: 50 mg once weekly

I.V.: 2 mg over 1 hour every 3-4 weeks

Dosage adjustment in hepatic impairment: Dosing adjustment not needed

Mechanism of Action A bisphosphonate which inhibits bone resorption via actions on osteoclasts or on osteoclast precursors; decreases the rate of bone resorption, leading to an indirect increase in bone mineral density.

Contraindications Hypersensitivity to ibandronate, other bisphosphonates, or any component of the formulation; hypocalcemia; oral tablets are also contraindicated in patients unable to stand or sit upright for at least 60 minutes

Warnings/Precautions Hypocalcemia must be corrected before therapy initiation. Ensure adequate calcium and vitamin D intake. Bisphosphonate therapy has been associated with osteonecrosis, primarily of the jaw; this has been observed mostly in cancer patients, but also in patients with postmenopausal osteoporosis and other diagnoses. Dental exams and preventative dentistry should be performed prior to placing patients with risk factors on chronic bisphosphonate therapy. Invasive dental procedures should be avoided during treatment.

Infrequently, severe (and occasionally debilitating) bone, joint, and/or muscle pain have been reported during bisphosphonate treatment. The onset of pain ranged from a single day to several months. Symptoms usually resolve upon discontinuation. Some patients experienced recurrence when rechallenged with same drug or another bisphosphonate; avoid use in patients with a history of these symptoms in association with bisphosphonate therapy.

Oral bisphosphonates may cause dysphagia, esophagitis, esophageal or gastric ulcer; risk may increase in patients unable to comply with dosing instructions. Intravenous bisphosphonates may cause transient decreases in serum calcium and have also been associated with renal toxicity.

Use not recommended with severe renal impairment (Cl$_{cr}$ <30 mL/minute or serum creatinine >2.3 mg/dL). Safety and efficacy have not been established in patients <18 years of age.

Drug Interactions

Increased Effect/Toxicity: Aminoglycosides may lower serum calcium levels with prolonged administration; concomitant use may have an additive hypocalcemic effect. Nonsteroidal anti-inflammatory drugs may enhance the gastrointestinal adverse/toxic effects (increased incidence of GI ulcers) of bisphosphonate derivatives. Bisphosphonate derivatives may enhance the hypocalcemic effect of phosphate supplements.

Decreased Effect: The following agents may decrease the absorption of oral bisphosphonate derivatives: Antacids (aluminum, calcium, magnesium), oral calcium salts, oral iron salts, and oral magnesium salts

Ethanol/Nutrition/Herb Interactions

Ethanol: Avoid ethanol (may increase risk of osteoporosis).

Food: May reduce absorption; mean oral bioavailability is decreased up to 90% when given with food.

Dietary Considerations Supplemental calcium or vitamin D may be required if dietary intake is not adequate. Tablet should be taken with a full glass (6-8 oz) of plain water, at least 60 minutes prior to any food, beverages, or medications. Mineral water with a high calcium content should be avoided.

Pharmacodynamics/Kinetics

Distribution: Terminal V_d: 90 L; 40% to 50% of circulating ibandronate binds to bone

Protein binding: 85% to 99%

Bioavailability: Oral: Reduced by 90% following standard breakfast

Half-life elimination:

Oral: 150 mg dose: Terminal: 37-157 hours

I.V.: Terminal: ~5-25 hours

Time to peak, plasma: Oral: 0.5-2 hours

Excretion: Urine (50% to 60% of absorbed dose, excreted as unchanged drug); feces (unabsorbed drug)

Pregnancy Risk Factor C

Dosage Forms

Injection, solution:

Boniva®: 1 mg/mL (3 mL)

Tablet:

Boniva®: 2.5 mg [once-daily formulation]; 150 mg [once-monthly formulation]

Dental Comment Cases of oral bisphosphonate-associated ONJ have been reported. A report by the Council of Scientific Affairs of the American Dental Association (accessed at: http://www.ada.org/prof/resources/topics/osteone-crosis.asp) as of July 2006 gave an estimated incidence of 0.7 cases for every 100,000 person-years of exposure to alendronate (Fosamax®). This translates to one case for every 142,857 person-years exposure. This figure from the ADA report was based on information received from Merck & Co citing 170 worldwide cases for alendronate (Fosamax®). In addition, Procter & Gamble Pharmaceuticals has cited 20 cases for risedronate (Actonel®) and Roche Laboratories has cited one case for ibandronate (Boniva®).

Consumer Reports On Health stated that the risk of jaw bone osteoporosis due to alendronate (Fosamax®), risedronate (Actonel®), or ibandronate (Boniva®) taken to prevent osteoporosis is very low and is estimated to be one out of every 20,000 users. That report mentioned that tooth extraction or implants increase the risk of developing osteonecrosis in patients taking any of these drugs for osteoporosis. The report also recommended that patients should stop taking any of these oral drugs 1-2 months before and after such dental treatment. No evidence was presented to support this statement.

In terms of length of exposure to oral bisphosphonates prior to onset of ONJ, data from large population studies or controlled studies is lacking. A report by Marx et al, observed that of three cases of ONJ associated with Fosamax® exposure, one patient had been taking 10 mg/day by mouth for 6 years and the other two patients 10 mg/day by mouth for 3 and 2 years respectively. In contrast, they observed that in cancer patients receiving intravenous bisphosphonates, the time period between the first doses of the bisphosphonate to first recognition of exposed bone either by the patients or by the clinician, was 9.4 months for zoledronate (Zometa®), 14.3 months for pamidronate (Aredia®), and 12.1 months for pamidronate then to zoledronate.

Selected Readings

Author Unknown, "Safety Update: Bone-Building Drugs: Risks Explained," *Consumer Reports on Health*, 2006, 18(5):3.

Barrett J, Worth E, Bauss F, et al, "Ibandronate: A Clinical Pharmacological and Pharmacokinetic Update," *J Clin Pharmacol*, 2004, 44(9):951-65.

French AE, Kaplan N, Lishner M, et al, "Taking Bisphosphonates During Pregnancy," *Can Fam Physician*, 2003, 49:1281-2.

Marx RE, Sawatari Y, Fortin M, et al, "Bisphosphonate-Induced Exposed Bone (Osteonecrosis/ Osteopetrosis) of the Jaws: Risk Factors, Recognition, Prevention, and Treatment," *J Oral Maxillofac Surg*, 2005, 63(11):1567-75.

Ibritumomab (ib ri TYOO mo mab)

U.S. Brand Names Zevalin®

Canadian Brand Names Zevalin®

Generic Available No

(Continued)

Ibritumomab *(Continued)*

Index Terms Ibritumomab Tiuxetan; IDEC-Y2B8; In-111 Ibritumomab; In-111 Zevalin; Y-90 Ibritumomab; Y-90 Zevalin

Pharmacologic Category Antineoplastic Agent, Monoclonal Antibody; Radiopharmaceutical

Use Treatment of relapsed or refractory low-grade, follicular, or transformed B-cell non-Hodgkin's lymphoma

Local Anesthetic/Vasoconstrictor Precautions No information available to require special precautions

Effects on Dental Treatment Key adverse event(s) related to dental treatment: Hypotension, cough, throat irritation, rhinitis.

Common Adverse Effects Severe, potentially life-threatening allergic reactions have occurred in association with infusions. Also refer to Rituximab monograph.

>10%:

Central nervous system: Chills (24%), fever (17%), pain (13%), headache (12%)

Gastrointestinal: Nausea (31%), abdominal pain (16%), vomiting (12%)

Hematologic: Thrombocytopenia (95%; grades 3/4: 63%; nadir: 53 days), neutropenia (77%; grades 3/4: 60%; nadir: 62 days), anemia (61%; grades 3/4: 17%; nadir: 68 days), myelosuppression (nadir: 7-9 weeks; duration: 22-35 days)

Neuromuscular & skeletal: Weakness (43%)

Respiratory: Dyspnea (14%)

Miscellaneous: Infection (29%)

1% to 10%:

Cardiovascular: Peripheral edema (8%), hypotension (6%), flushing (6%)

Central nervous system: Dizziness (10%), insomnia (5%), anxiety (4%)

Dermatologic: Pruritus (9%), rash (8%), bruising (7%), angioedema (5%; severe: <1%), urticaria (4%), petechia (3%)

Gastrointestinal: Diarrhea (9%), anorexia (8%), abdominal distension (5%), constipation (5%), dyspepsia (4%), melena (2%; life threatening in 1%), gastrointestinal hemorrhage (1%)

Hematologic: Pancytopenia (2%), secondary malignancies (2% to 6%; includes acute myelogenous leukemia and myelodysplastic syndrome)

Neuromuscular & skeletal: Back pain (8%), arthralgia (7%), myalgia (7%)

Respiratory: Cough (10%), throat irritation (10%), rhinitis (6%), bronchospasm (5%), epistaxis (3%), apnea (1%)

Miscellaneous: Diaphoresis (4%), allergic reaction (2%; life-threatening in 1%)

Mechanism of Action Ibritumomab is a monoclonal antibody directed against the CD20 antigen found on B lymphocytes (normal and malignant). Ibritumomab binding induces apoptosis in B lymphocytes *in vitro*. It is combined with the chelator tiuxetan, which acts as a specific chelation site for either Indium-111 (In-111) or Yttrium-90 (Y-90). The monoclonal antibody acts as a delivery system to direct the radioactive isotope to the targeted cells, however, binding has been observed in lymphoid cells throughout the body and in lymphoid nodules in organs such as the large and small intestines. Indium-111 is a gamma-emitter used to assess biodistribution of ibritumomab, while Y-90 emits beta particles. Beta-emission induces cellular damage through the formation of free radicals (in both target cells and surrounding cells).

Drug Interactions

Increased Effect/Toxicity: Due to the high incidence of thrombocytopenia associated with ibritumomab, the use of agents which decrease platelet function may be associated with a higher risk of bleeding (includes aspirin, NSAIDs, glycoprotein IIb/IIIa antagonists, clopidogrel and ticlopidine). In addition, the risk of bleeding may be increased with anticoagulant agents, including heparin, low molecular weight heparins, thrombolytics, and warfarin. The safety of live viral vaccines has not been established.

Decreased Effect: Response to vaccination may be impaired.

Pharmacodynamics/Kinetics

Duration: Beta cell recovery begins in ~12 weeks; generally in normal range within 9 months

Distribution: To lymphoid cells throughout the body and in lymphoid nodules in organs such as the large and small intestines, spleen, testes, and liver

Metabolism: Has not been characterized; the product of yttrium-90 radioactive decay is zirconium-90 (nonradioactive); Indium-111 decays to cadmium-111 (nonradioactive)

Half-life elimination: Y-90 ibritumomab: 30 hours; Indium-111 decays with a physical half-life of 67 hours; Yttrium-90 decays with a physical half-life of 64 hours

Excretion: A median of 7.2% of the radiolabeled activity was excreted in urine over 7 days

Pregnancy Risk Factor D

Ibritumomab Tiuxetan *see* Ibritumomab *on page 851*

Ibu-200 [OTC] *see* Ibuprofen *on page 853*

Ibuprofen (eye byoo PROE fen)

Related Information
Oral Pain *on page 1788*
Rheumatoid Arthritis, Osteoarthritis, and Osteoporosis *on page 1759*
Temporomandibular Dysfunction (TMD) *on page 1822*

Related Sample Prescriptions
Mild/Moderate Oral Pain *on page 1834*
Moderate/Moderately Severe Oral Pain *on page 1834*

U.S. Brand Names Advil® [OTC]; Advil® Children's [OTC]; Advil® Infants' [OTC]; Advil® Junior [OTC]; Advil® Migraine [OTC]; ElixSure™ IB [OTC]; Genpril® [OTC]; Ibu-200 [OTC]; I-Prin [OTC]; Midol® Cramp and Body Aches [OTC]; Motrin®; Motrin® Children's [OTC]; Motrin® IB [OTC]; Motrin® Infants' [OTC]; Motrin® Junior Strength [OTC]; NeoProfen®; Proprinal [OTC]; Ultraprin [OTC]

Canadian Brand Names Advil®; Apo-Ibuprofen®; Motrin® (Children's); Motrin® IB; Novo-Profen; Nu-Ibuprofen

Mexican Brand Names Advil; Advil Infantil; Bestafen; Dolval; Febratic; Ibuflam; Motrin; Proartinal; Quadrax; Tabalon 400

Generic Available Yes: Caplet, suspension, tablet

Index Terms Ibuprofen Lysine; *p*-Isobutylhydratropic Acid

Pharmacologic Category Nonsteroidal Anti-inflammatory Drug (NSAID), Oral; Nonsteroidal Anti-inflammatory Drug (NSAID), Parenteral

Dental Use Management of pain and swelling

Use
Oral: Inflammatory diseases and rheumatoid disorders including juvenile rheumatoid arthritis, mild-to-moderate pain, fever, dysmenorrhea

Injection: Ibuprofen lysine is for use in premature infants weighing between 500-1500 g and who are ≤32 weeks gestational age (GA) to induce closure of a clinically-significant patent ductus arteriosus (PDA) when usual treatments are ineffective

Unlabeled/Investigational Use Cystic fibrosis, gout, ankylosing spondylitis, acute migraine headache

Local Anesthetic/Vasoconstrictor Precautions No information available to require special precautions

Effects on Dental Treatment In a statement released on September 8, 2006, the FDA notified consumers and healthcare professionals that the administration of ibuprofen for pain relief to patients taking aspirin for cardioprotection may interfere with aspirin's cardiovascular benefits. The FDA states that ibuprofen can interfere with the antiplatelet effect of low-dose aspirin (81 mg/day). This could result in diminished effectiveness of aspirin as used for cardioprotection and stroke prevention. The FDA adds that although ibuprofen and aspirin can be taken together, it is recommended that consumers talk with their healthcare providers for additional information. For more information, including how to advise aspirin patients requiring ibuprofen for pain relief, see Dental Comment.

Significant Adverse Effects
Oral:
1% to 10%:
Cardiovascular: Edema (1% to 3%)
Central nervous system: Dizziness (3% to 9%), headache (1% to 3%), nervousness (1% to 3%)
Dermatologic: Itching (1% to 3%), rash (3% to 9%)
Endocrine & metabolic: Fluid retention (1% to 3%)
Gastrointestinal: Dyspepsia (1% to 3%), vomiting (1% to 3%), abdominal pain/cramps/distress (1% to 3%), heartburn (3% to 9%), nausea (3% to 9%), diarrhea (1% to 3%), constipation (1% to 3%), flatulence (1% to 3%), epigastric pain (3% to 9%), appetite decreased (1% to 3%)
Otic: Tinnitus (3% to 9%)

<1% (Limited to important or life-threatening): Acute renal failure, agranulocytosis, anaphylaxis, aplastic anemia, azotemia, blurred vision, bone marrow suppression, confusion, creatinine clearance decreased, duodenal ulcer, edema, eosinophilia, epistaxis, erythema multiforme, gastric ulcer, GI bleed, GI hemorrhage, GI ulceration, hallucinations, hearing decreased, hematuria, hematocrit decreased, hemoglobin decreased, hemolytic anemia, hepatitis, hypertension, inhibition of platelet aggregation, jaundice, liver function tests abnormal, leukopenia, melena, neutropenia, pancreatitis, photosensitivity, Stevens-Johnson syndrome, thrombocytopenia, toxic amblyopia, toxic epidermal necrolysis, urticaria, vesiculobullous eruptions, vision changes
(Continued)

Ibuprofen (Continued)

Injection:

>10%:

Cardiovascular: Intraventricular hemorrhage (29%; grade 3/4: 15%)

Dermatologic: Skin irritation (16%)

Endocrine & metabolic: Hypocalcemia (12%), hypoglycemia (12%)

Gastrointestinal: GI disorders, non NEC (22%)

Hematologic: Anemia (32%)

Respiratory: Apnea (28%), respiratory infection (19%)

Miscellaneous: Sepsis (43%)

1% to 10%:

Cardiovascular: Edema (4%)

Endocrine & metabolic: Adrenal insufficiency (7%), hypernatremia (7%)

Genitourinary: Urinary tract infection (9%)

Renal: Urea increased (7%), renal impairment (6%), creatinine increased (3%), urine output decreased (3%; small decrease reported on days 2-6 with compensatory increase in output on day 9)

Respiratory: Respiratory failure (10%), atelectasis (4%)

Frequency not defined: Abdominal distension, cardiac failure, cholestasis, convulsions, feeding problems, gastritis, GI reflux, hyperglycemia, hypotension, ileus, infection, inguinal hernia, injection site reaction, jaundice, neutropenia, tachycardia, thrombocytopenia

Restrictions An FDA-approved medication guide must be distributed when dispensing an oral outpatient prescription (new or refill) where this medication is to be used without direct supervision of a healthcare provider. Medication guides are available at http://www.fda.gov/cder/Offices/ODS/medication_guides.htm.

Dental Usual Dosing

Analgesic/pain/fever: Oral:

Children: 4-10 mg/kg/dose every 6-8 hours

Adults: 200-400 mg/dose every 4-6 hours (maximum daily dose: 1.2 g, unless directed by physician)

OTC labeling (analgesic, antipyretic): Oral:

Children 6 months to 11 years: See table; use of weight to select dose is preferred; doses may be repeated every 6-8 hours (maximum: 4 doses/day)

Children ≥12 years and Adults: 200 mg every 4-6 hours as needed (maximum: 1200 mg/24 hours)

Ibuprofen Dosing

Weight (lb)	Age	Dosage (mg)
12-17	6-11 mo	50
18-23	12-23 mo	75
24-35	2-3 y	100
35-47	4-5 y	150
48-59	6-8 y	200
60-71	9-10 y	250
72-95	11 y	300

Dosage

I.V.: Infants between 500-1500 g and ≤32 weeks GA: Patent ductus arteriosus: Initial dose: Ibuprofen 10 mg/kg, followed by two doses of 5 mg/kg at 24 and 48 hours. Dose should be based on birth weight.

Oral:

Children:

Antipyretic: 6 months to 12 years: Temperature <102.5°F (39°C): 5 mg/kg/dose; temperature >102.5°F: 10 mg/kg/dose given every 6-8 hours (maximum daily dose: 40 mg/kg/day)

Juvenile rheumatoid arthritis: 30-50 mg/kg/24 hours divided every 8 hours; start at lower end of dosing range and titrate upward (maximum: 2.4 g/day)

Analgesic: 4-10 mg/kg/dose every 6-8 hours

Cystic fibrosis (unlabeled use): Chronic (>4 years) twice daily dosing adjusted to maintain serum levels of 50-100 mcg/mL has been associated with slowing of disease progression in younger patients with mild lung disease

OTC labeling (analgesic, antipyretic):

Children 6 months to 11 years: See table. Use of weight to select dose is preferred; doses may be repeated every 6-8 hours (maximum: 4 doses/day)

Children ≥12 years: 200 mg every 4-6 hours as needed (maximum: 1200 mg/24 hours)

Adults:

Inflammatory disease: 400-800 mg/dose 3-4 times/day (maximum dose: 3.2 g/day)

Analgesia/pain/fever/dysmenorrhea: 200-400 mg/dose every 4-6 hours (maximum daily dose: 1.2 g, unless directed by physician)

OTC labeling (analgesic, antipyretic): 200 mg every 4-6 hours as needed (maximum: 1200 mg/24 hours)

Dosing adjustment/comments in severe hepatic impairment: Avoid use

Mechanism of Action Inhibits prostaglandin synthesis by decreasing the activity of the enzyme, cyclooxygenase, which results in decreased formation of prostaglandin precursors

Contraindications Hypersensitivity to ibuprofen, aspirin, other NSAIDs, or any component of the formulation; perioperative pain in the setting of coronary artery bypass surgery (CABG); pregnancy (3rd trimester)

Ibuprofen lysine is contraindicated in preterm infants with untreated proven or suspected infection; congenital heart disease where patency of the PDA is necessary for pulmonary or systemic blood flow; bleeding (especially with active intracranial hemorrhage or GI bleed); thrombocytopenia; coagulation defects; proven or suspected necrotizing enterocolitis (NEC); significant renal dysfunction

Warnings/Precautions [U.S. Boxed Warning]: NSAIDs are associated with an increased risk of adverse cardiovascular events, including MI, stroke, and new onset or worsening of pre-existing hypertension. Risk may be increased with duration of use or pre-existing cardiovascular risk factors or disease. Carefully evaluate individual cardiovascular risk profiles prior to prescribing. Use caution with fluid retention, CHF or hypertension. Concurrent administration of ibuprofen, and potentially other nonselective NSAIDs, may interfere with aspirin's cardioprotective effect.

Use of NSAIDs can compromise existing renal function. Renal toxicity can occur in patient with impaired renal function, dehydration, heart failure, liver dysfunction, those taking diuretics and ACEI and the elderly. Rehydrate patient before starting therapy. Monitor renal function closely. Ibuprofen is not recommended for patients with advanced renal disease.

NSAIDs may increase risk of gastrointestinal irritation, ulceration, bleeding, and perforation. These events may occur at any time during therapy and without warning. Use caution with a history of GI disease (bleeding or ulcers), concurrent therapy with aspirin, anticoagulants and/or corticosteroids, smoking, use of alcohol, the elderly or debilitated patients.

Use the lowest effective dose for the shortest duration of time, consistent with individual patient goals, to reduce risk of cardiovascular or GI adverse events. Alternate therapies should be considered for patients at high risk.

NSAIDs may cause serious skin adverse events including exfoliative dermatitis, Stevens-Johnson syndrome (SJS) and toxic epidermal necrolysis (TEN). Anaphylactoid reactions may occur, even without prior exposure; patients with "aspirin triad" (bronchial asthma, aspirin intolerance, rhinitis) may be at increased risk. Do not use in patients who experience bronchospasm, asthma, rhinitis, or urticaria with NSAID or aspirin therapy. Use caution in other forms of asthma.

Use with caution in patients with decreased hepatic function. Closely monitor patients with any abnormal LFT. Severe hepatic reactions (eg, fulminant hepatitis, liver failure) have occurred with NSAID use, rarely; discontinue if signs or symptoms of liver disease develop, or if systemic manifestations occur.

The elderly are at increased risk for adverse effects (especially peptic ulceration, CNS effects, renal toxicity) from NSAIDs even at low doses.

Withhold for at least 4-6 half-lives prior to surgical or dental procedures.

Injection: Hold second or third doses if urinary output is <0.6 mL/kg/hour. May alter signs of infection. May inhibit platelet aggregation; monitor for signs of bleeding. May displace bilirubin; use caution when total bilirubin is elevated. Long-term evaluations of neurodevelopment, growth, or diseases associated with prematurity following treatment have not been conducted. A second course of treatment, alternative pharmacologic therapy or surgery may be needed if the ductus arteriosus fails to close or reopens following the initial course of therapy.

OTC labeling: Prior to self-medication, patients should contact healthcare provider if they have had recurring stomach pain or upset, ulcers, bleeding problems, high blood pressure, heart or kidney disease, other serious medical problems, are currently taking a diuretic, or are ≥60 years of age. Recommended dosages should not be exceeded, due to an increased risk of GI bleeding. Consuming ≥3 alcoholic beverages/day or taking longer than recommended may increase the risk of GI bleeding.

(Continued)

Ibuprofen *(Continued)*

Drug Interactions **Substrate** (minor) of CYP2C9, 2C19; **Inhibits** CYP2C9 (strong)

ACE inhibitors: Antihypertensive effects may be decreased by concurrent therapy with NSAIDs; monitor blood pressure.

Aminoglycosides: NSAIDs may decrease the excretion of aminoglycosides; this is of particular concern in preterm infants.

Angiotensin II antagonists: Antihypertensive effects may be decreased by concurrent therapy with NSAIDs; monitor blood pressure.

Anticoagulants (warfarin, heparin, LMWHs) in combination with NSAIDs can cause increased risk of bleeding.

Antiplatelet drugs (ticlopidine, clopidogrel, aspirin, abciximab, dipyridamole, eptifibatide, tirofiban) can cause an increased risk of bleeding.

Aspirin: Ibuprofen and other COX-1 inhibitors may reduce the cardioprotective effects of aspirin. Avoid giving prior to aspirin therapy or on a regular basis in patients with CAD.

Beta-blockers: NSAIDs may decrease the antihypertensive effect of beta-blockers. Monitor.

Bisphosphonate derivatives: NSAIDs may enhance the adverse/toxic effect of bisphosphonate derivatives. An increased incidence of gastrointestinal ulceration is of concern.

Cholestyramine (and other bile acid sequestrants): May decrease the absorption of NSAIDs. Separate by at least 2 hours.

Corticosteroids: May increase the risk of GI ulceration; avoid concurrent use

Cyclosporine: NSAIDs may increase serum creatinine, potassium, blood pressure, and cyclosporine levels; monitor cyclosporine levels and renal function carefully.

CYP2C9 Substrates: Ibuprofen may increase the levels/effects of CYP2C9 substrates. Example substrates include bosentan, dapsone, fluoxetine, glimepiride, glipizide, losartan, montelukast, nateglinide, paclitaxel, phenytoin, warfarin, and zafirlukast.

Fluoroquinolone antibiotics: Risk of seizures may be increased with concomitant quinolone use. Risk is considered quite low and may only be a factor with high serum levels of either agent and/or in patients with additional predisposing factors (eg, renal dysfunction, history of seizure or other neurological disorder).

Hydralazine's antihypertensive effect is decreased; avoid concurrent use

Lithium levels can be increased; avoid concurrent use if possible or monitor lithium levels and adjust dose. Sulindac may have the least effect. When NSAID is stopped, lithium will need adjustment again.

Loop diuretics efficacy (diuretic and antihypertensive effect) is reduced. Indomethacin reduces this efficacy, however, it may be anticipated with any NSAID.

Methotrexate: Severe bone marrow suppression, aplastic anemia, and GI toxicity have been reported with concomitant NSAID therapy. Avoid use during moderate or high-dose methotrexate (increased and prolonged methotrexate levels). NSAID use during low-dose treatment of rheumatoid arthritis has not been fully evaluated; extreme caution is warranted.

Pemetrexed: NSAIDs may decrease the excretion of pemetrexed.

Probenecid: Probenecid may increase the serum concentration of NSAIDs.

Salicylates: NSAIDs (nonselective) may diminish the cardioprotective effect of acetylated salicylates. Avoid regular use of NSAIDs if possible; consider alternatives (eg, acetaminophen). If ibuprofen is used occasionally, give ½® hour to 2 hours after aspirin (immediate release; not enteric coated) ingestion.

Vancomycin: NSAIDs may decrease the excretion of vancomycin; this is of particular concern in preterm infants.

Warfarin's INRs may be increased by piroxicam. Other NSAIDs may have the same effect depending on dose and duration. Monitor INR closely. Use the lowest dose of NSAIDs possible and for the briefest duration. May alter the anticoagulant effects of warfarin; concurrent use with other antiplatelet agents or anticoagulants may increase risk of bleeding.

Ethanol/Nutrition/Herb Interactions

Ethanol: Avoid ethanol (may enhance gastric mucosal irritation).

Food: Ibuprofen peak serum levels may be decreased if taken with food.

Herb/Nutraceutical: Avoid alfalfa, anise, bilberry, bladderwrack, bromelain, cat's claw, celery, coleus, cordyceps, dong quai, evening primrose, feverfew, fenugreek, garlic, ginger, ginkgo biloba, red clover, horse chestnut, grapeseed, green tea, ginseng, guggul, horse chestnut seed, horseradish, licorice, prickly ash, red clover, reishi, SAMe, sweet clover, turmeric, white willow (all have additional antiplatelet activity).

Dietary Considerations Should be taken with food. Chewable tablets may contain phenylalanine; amount varies by product, consult manufacturers labeling.

Pharmacodynamics/Kinetics

Onset of action: Analgesic: 30-60 minutes; Anti-inflammatory: ≤7 days
  Peak effect: 1-2 weeks
Duration: 4-6 hours
Absorption: Oral: Rapid (85%)
Distribution: Premature infants with ductal closure (highly variable between studies):
  Day 3: 145-349 mL/kg
  Day 5: 72-222 mL/kg
Protein binding: 90% to 99%
Metabolism: Hepatic via oxidation
Half-life elimination:
  Premature infants (highly variable between studies):
    Day 3: 35-51 hours
    Day 5: 20-33 hours
  Children 3 months to 10 years: 1.6 ± 0.7 hours
  Adults: 2-4 hours; End-stage renal disease: Unchanged
Time to peak: ~1-2 hours
Excretion: Urine (1% as free drug); some feces

Pregnancy Risk Factor C/D (3rd trimester)

Lactation Enters breast milk/use caution (AAP rates "compatible")

Breast-Feeding Considerations Limited data suggests minimal excretion in breast milk.

Dosage Forms Excipient information presented when available (limited, particularly for generics); consult specific product labeling. [DSC] = Discontinued product

Caplet: 200 mg [OTC]
  Advil®: 200 mg [contains sodium benzoate]
  Ibu-200, Motrin® IB: 200 mg
  Motrin® Junior Strength: 100 mg
Capsule, liqui-gel:
  Advil®: 200 mg
  Advil® Migraine: 200 mg [solubilized ibuprofen; contains potassium 20 mg]
Gelcap:
  Advil®: 200 mg [contains coconut oil]
Injection, solution, as lysine [preservative free]:
  NeoProfen®: 17.1 mg/mL (2 mL) [equivalent to ibuprofen 10 mg/mL]
Suspension, oral: 100 mg/5 mL (5 mL, 120 mL, 480 mL)
  Advil® Children's: 100 mg/5 mL (60 mL, 120 mL) [contains sodium benzoate; blue raspberry, fruit, and grape flavors]
  ElixSure™ IB: 100 mg/5 mL (120 mL) [berry flavor]
  Motrin® Children's: 100 mg/5 mL (60 mL, 120 mL) [contains sodium benzoate; berry, dye free berry, bubble gum, and grape flavors]
Suspension, oral drops: 40 mg/mL (15 mL)
  Advil® Infants': 40 mg/mL (15 mL) [contains sodium benzoate; fruit and grape flavors]
  Motrin® Infants': 40 mg/mL (15 mL, 30 mL) [contains sodium benzoate; berry and dye-free berry flavors]
Tablet: 200 mg [OTC], 400 mg, 600 mg, 800 mg
  Advil®: 200 mg [contains sodium benzoate]
  Advil® Junior: 100 mg [contains sodium benzoate; coated tablets]
  Genpril®, I-Prin, Midol® Cramp and Body Aches, Motrin® IB, Proprinal, Ultraprin: 200 mg
  Motrin®: 400 mg [DSC], 600 mg, 800 mg
Tablet, chewable:
  Advil® Children's: 50 mg [contains phenylalanine 2.1 mg; grape flavors]
  Advil® Junior: 100 mg [contains phenylalanine 4.2 mg; grape flavors]
  Motrin® Children's: 50 mg [contains phenylalanine 1.4 mg; grape and orange flavor]
  Motrin® Junior Strength: 100 mg [contains phenylalanine 2.1 mg; grape and orange flavors]

Dental Comment Preoperative use of ibuprofen at a dose of 400-600 mg every 6 hours 24 hours before the appointment decreases postoperative edema and hastens healing time.

New information from the FDA states that ibuprofen can interfere with the antiplatelet effect of low-dose aspirin (81 mg/day), potentially rendering aspirin less effective when used for cardioprotection and stroke protection. In situations where these drugs could be used concomitantly, the FDA has provided the following information.

Patients who use immediate release aspirin (not enteric-coated aspirin) and take a single dose or chronic doses of ibuprofen 400 mg, should dose the ibuprofen at least **30 minutes or longer after aspirin ingestion or more than 8 hours before aspirin ingestion** to avoid attenuation of aspirin's effect.
(Continued)

Ibuprofen (Continued)

At this time, recommendations about the timing of ibuprofen 400 mg in patients taking enteric-coated low-dose aspirin cannot be made based on available data. One study however, showed that the antiplatelet effect of enteric-coated low-dose aspirin was attenuated when ibuprofen 400 mg was dosed 2, 7, and 12 hours after aspirin (Catella-Lawson, 2001).

With occasional use of ibuprofen, there is likely to be minimal risk from any attenuation of the antiplatelet effect of low-dose aspirin, because of a long-lasting effect of aspirin on platelets.

Other over-the-counter (OTC) NSAIDs (ie, naproxen sodium and ketoprofen) should be viewed as having the potential to interfere with the antiplatelet effect of low-dose aspirin until proven otherwise. However, the FDA is unaware of any studies that have looked at the same type of interference by ketoprofen with low-dose aspirin. One study of naproxen and low-dose aspirin has suggested that naproxen may interfere with aspirin's antiplatelet activity when they are coadministered (Steinhubl, 2005). However, naproxen 500 mg administered 2 hours before or after aspirin 100 mg, did not interfere with aspirin's antiplatelet effect. The FDA stated that there is no data looking at doses of naproxen <500 mg. Naproxen OTC strength is 220 mg tablets.

Selected Readings

Ahmad N, Grad HA, Haas DA, et al, "The Efficacy of Nonopioid Analgesics for Postoperative Dental Pain: A Meta-Analysis," *Anesth Prog*, 1997, 44(4):119-26.

Beaver WT, "Review of the Analgesic Efficacy of Ibuprofen," *Int J Clin Pract*, 2003, (Suppl 135):13-7.

Dionne R, "Additive Analgesia Without Opioid Side Effects," *Compend Contin Educ Dent*, 2000, 21(7):572-4, 576-7.

Dionne R, "Relative Efficacy of Selective COX-2 Inhibitors Compared With Over-The-Counter Ibuprofen," *Int J Clin Pract Suppl*, 2003, (135):18-22.

Dionne RA and Berthold CW, "Therapeutic Uses of Nonsteroidal Anti-inflammatory Drugs in Dentistry," *Crit Rev Oral Biol Med*, 2001, 12(4):315-30.

Doyle G, Jayawardena S, Ashraf E, et al, "Efficacy and Tolerability of Nonprescription Ibuprofen Versus Celecoxib for Dental Pain," *J Clin Pharmacol*, 2002, 42(8):912-9.

Gobetti JP, "Controlling Dental Pain," *J Am Dent Assoc*, 1992, 123(6):47-52.

Hersh EV, Levin LM, Cooper SA, et al, "Ibuprofen Liquigel for Oral Surgery Pain," *Clin Ther*, 2000, 22(11):1306-18.

Olson NZ, Otero AM, Marrero I, et al, "Onset of Analgesia for Liquigel Ibuprofen 400 mg, Acetaminophen 1000 mg, Ketoprofen 25 mg, and Placebo in the Treatment of Postoperative Dental Pain," *J Clin Pharmacol*, 2001, 41(11):1238-47.

Pearlman B, Boyatzis S, Daly C, et al, "The Analgesic Efficacy of Ibuprofen in Periodontal Surgery: A Multicentre Study," *Aust Dent J*, 1997, 42(5):328-34.

Nguyen AM, Graham DY, Gage T, et al, "Nonsteroidal Anti-inflammatory Drug Use in Dentistry: Gastrointestinal Implications," *Gen Dent*, 1999, 47(6):590-6.

Steinhubl SR, "The Use of Anti-Inflammatory Analgesics in the Patient With Cardiovascular Disease: What a Pain," *J Am Coll Cardiol*, 2005, 45(8):1302-3.

Wynn RL, "Update on Nonprescription Pain Relievers for Dental Pain," *Gen Dent*, 2004, 52(2):94-8.

Ibuprofen and Hydrocodone *see* Hydrocodone and Ibuprofen *on page 830*

Ibuprofen and Oxycodone *see* Oxycodone and Ibuprofen *on page 1233*

Ibuprofen and Pseudoephedrine *see* Pseudoephedrine and Ibuprofen *on page 1384*

Ibuprofen Lysine *see* Ibuprofen *on page 853*

Ibutilide (i BYOO ti lide)

Related Information
Cardiovascular Diseases *on page 1726*

U.S. Brand Names Corvert®

Generic Available No

Index Terms Ibutilide Fumarate

Pharmacologic Category Antiarrhythmic Agent, Class III

Use Acute termination of atrial fibrillation or flutter of recent onset; the effectiveness of ibutilide has not been determined in patients with arrhythmias >90 days in duration

Local Anesthetic/Vasoconstrictor Precautions Ibutilide is one of the drugs confirmed to prolong the QT interval and is accepted as having a risk of causing torsade de pointes. The risk of drug-induced torsade de pointes is extremely low when a single QT interval prolonging drug is prescribed. In terms of epinephrine, it is not known what effect vasoconstrictors in the local anesthetic regimen will have in patients with a known history of congenital prolonged QT interval or in patients taking any medication that prolongs the QT interval. Until more information is obtained, it is suggested that the clinician consult with the physician prior to the use of a vasoconstrictor in suspected patients, and that the vasoconstrictor (epinephrine, levonordefrin [Neo-Cobefrin®]) be used with caution.

Effects on Dental Treatment No significant effects or complications reported

Common Adverse Effects 1% to 10%:

Cardiovascular: Ventricular extrasystoles (5.1%), nonsustained monomorphic ventricular tachycardia (4.9%), nonsustained polymorphic ventricular tachycardia (2.7%), tachycardia/supraventricular tachycardia (2.7%), hypotension (2%), bundle branch block (1.9%), sustained polymorphic ventricular tachycardia (eg, torsade de pointes) (1.7%, often requiring cardioversion), AV block (1.5%), bradycardia (1.2%), QT segment prolongation, hypertension (1.2%), palpitation (1%)

Central nervous system: Headache (3.6%)

Gastrointestinal: Nausea (>1%)

Mechanism of Action Exact mechanism of action is unknown; prolongs the action potential in cardiac tissue

Drug Interactions

Increased Effect/Toxicity: Class Ia antiarrhythmic drugs (disopyramide, quinidine, and procainamide) and other class III drugs such as amiodarone and sotalol should not be given concomitantly with ibutilide due to their potential to prolong refractoriness. Signs of digoxin toxicity may be masked when coadministered with ibutilide. Toxicity of ibutilide is potentiated by concurrent administration of other drugs which may prolong QT interval: phenothiazines, tricyclic and tetracyclic antidepressants, cisapride, sparfloxacin, gatifloxacin, moxifloxacin, and erythromycin.

Pharmacodynamics/Kinetics

Onset of action: ~90 minutes after start of infusion ($\frac{1}{2}$ of conversions to sinus rhythm occur during infusion)

Distribution: V_d: 11 L/kg

Protein binding: 40%

Metabolism: Extensively hepatic; oxidation

Half-life elimination: 2-12 hours (average: 6 hours)

Excretion: Urine (82%, 7% as unchanged drug and metabolites); feces (19%)

Pregnancy Risk Factor C

Ibutilide Fumarate see Ibutilide on page 858

IC-Green™ see Indocyanine Green on page 876

ICI-182,780 see Fulvestrant on page 755

ICI-204,219 see Zafirlukast on page 1675

ICI-46474 see Tamoxifen on page 1522

ICI-118630 see Goserelin on page 792

ICI-176334 see Bicalutamide on page 214

ICI-D1033 see Anastrozole on page 128

ICL670 see Deferasirox on page 452

Icodextrin (eye KOE dex trin)

U.S. Brand Names Adept®; Extraneal®

Generic Available No

Pharmacologic Category Adhesiolytic; Peritoneal Dialysate, Osmotic

Use

Adept®: Reduction of postsurgical adhesions in gynecologic laparoscopic procedures

Extraneal®: Daily exchange for the long dwell (8- to 16-hour) during continuous ambulatory peritoneal dialysis (CAPD) or automated peritoneal dialysis (APD) for the management of end-stage renal disease (ESRD); improvement of long-dwell ultrafiltration and clearance of creatinine and urea nitrogen (compared to 4.25% dextrose) in patients with high/average or greater transport characteristics as measured by peritoneal equilibration test (PET)

Local Anesthetic/Vasoconstrictor Precautions No information available to require special precautions

Effects on Dental Treatment No significant effects or complications reported

Mechanism of Action When used for dialysis, icodextrin exerts osmotic pressure across small intercellular pores resulting in transcapillary ultrafiltration throughout the dwell while providing electrolytes and lactate for the maintenance of both the electrolyte and acid-base balance. When used for laparoscopic surgery, the colloidal osmotic action allows the fluid to be retained in the peritoneal cavity for 3-4 days, physically providing a temporary separation of peritoneal surfaces and minimizing adhesion formation.

Pregnancy Risk Factor C

ICRF-187 see Dexrazoxane on page 472

Idamycin PFS® see Idarubicin on page 860

Idarubicin (eye da ROO bi sin)

U.S. Brand Names Idamycin PFS®
Canadian Brand Names Idamycin®
Mexican Brand Names Idamycin; Idaralem
Generic Available Yes
Index Terms 4-Demethoxydaunorubicin; 4-DMDR; Idarubicin Hydrochloride; IDR; IMI 30; NSC-256439; SC 33428
Pharmacologic Category Antineoplastic Agent, Anthracycline; Antineoplastic Agent, Antibiotic
Use Treatment of acute leukemias (AML, ANLL, ALL), accelerated phase or blast crisis of chronic myelogenous leukemia (CML), breast cancer
Unlabeled/Investigational Use Autologous hematopoietic stem cell transplantation
Local Anesthetic/Vasoconstrictor Precautions No information available to require special precautions
Effects on Dental Treatment Key adverse event(s) related to dental treatment: Stomatitis.
Common Adverse Effects
>10%:
  Cardiovascular: Transient ECG abnormalities (supraventricular tachycardia, S-T wave changes, atrial or ventricular extrasystoles); generally asymptomatic and self-limiting. CHF, dose related. The relative cardiotoxicity of idarubicin compared to doxorubicin is unclear. Some investigators report no increase in cardiac toxicity at cumulative oral idarubicin doses up to 540 mg/m^2; other reports suggest a maximum cumulative intravenous dose of 150 mg/m^2.
  Central nervous system: Headache
  Dermatologic: Alopecia (25% to 30%), radiation recall, skin rash (11%), urticaria
  Gastrointestinal: Nausea, vomiting (30% to 60%); diarrhea (9% to 22%); stomatitis (11%); GI hemorrhage (30%)
  Genitourinary: Discoloration of urine (darker yellow)
  Hematologic: Myelosuppression, primarily leukopenia; thrombocytopenia and anemia. Effects are generally less severe with oral dosing.
    Nadir: 10-15 days
    Recovery: 21-28 days
  Hepatic: Bilirubin and transaminases increased (44%)
1% to 10%:
  Central nervous system: Seizure
  Neuromuscular & skeletal: Peripheral neuropathy
Mechanism of Action Similar to doxorubicin and daunorubicin; inhibition of DNA and RNA synthesis by intercalation between DNA base pairs
Drug Interactions
Decreased Effect: Patients may experience impaired immune response to vaccines; possible infection after administration of live vaccines in patients receiving immunosuppressants.
Pharmacodynamics/Kinetics
Absorption: Oral: Variable (4% to 77%; mean: ~30%)
Distribution: V$_d$: 64 L/kg (some reports indicate 2250 L); extensive tissue binding; CSF
Protein binding: 94% to 97%
Metabolism: Hepatic to idarubicinol (pharmacologically active)
Half-life elimination: Oral: 14-35 hours; I.V.: 12-27 hours
Time to peak, serum: 1-5 hours
Excretion:
  Oral: Urine (~5% of dose; 0.5% to 0.7% as unchanged drug, 4% as idarubicinol); hepatic (8%)
  I.V.: Urine (13% as idarubicinol, 3% as unchanged drug); hepatic (17%)
Pregnancy Risk Factor D

Idursulfase (eye dur SUL fase)

U.S. Brand Names Elaprase™
Generic Available No

Pharmacologic Category Enzyme

Use Replacement therapy in mucopolysaccharidosis II (MPS II, Hunter syndrome) for improvement of walking capacity

Local Anesthetic/Vasoconstrictor Precautions No information available to require special precautions

Effects on Dental Treatment No significant effects or complications reported

Common Adverse Effects

>10%:

Cardiovascular: Hypertension (25%), atrial abnormality (13%)

Central nervous system: Pyrexia (63%), headache (59%), malaise (22%), anxiety (13%), irritability (13%)

Dermatologic: Pruritus (28%), urticaria (16%), pruritic rash (13%), skin disorder (13%)

Gastrointestinal: Dyspepsia (13%)

Local: Abscess (16%), infusion-site edema (13%)

Neuromuscular & skeletal: Arthralgia (31%), limb pain (28%), chest wall musculoskeletal pain (16%), musculoskeletal dysfunction (16%)

Ocular: visual disturbance (22%)

Respiratory: Wheezing (19%)

Miscellaneous: Antibody development (51%), superficial injury (13%)

<1: Angioedema, cardiac arrhythmia, cyanosis, hypotension, infection, pulmonary embolism, respiratory distress, respiratory failure, seizure

Mechanism of Action Idursulfase is a recombinant form of iduronate-2-sulfatase, an enzyme needed to hydrolyze the mucopolysaccharides dermatan sulfate and heparan sulfate in various cells. Accumulation of these polysaccharides can lead to various manifestations of disease, including physical changes, CNS involvement, cardiac, respiratory and, mobility dysfunction. Replacement of this enzyme has been shown to improve walking capacity in patients with a deficiency.

Pharmacodynamics/Kinetics Half-life elimination: 44-48 minutes

Pregnancy Risk Factor C

Ifex® *see* Ifosfamide *on page 861*
IFLrA *see* Interferon Alfa-2a *on page 890*

Ifosfamide (eye FOSS fa mide)

U.S. Brand Names Ifex®

Canadian Brand Names Ifex®

Mexican Brand Names Ifolem

Generic Available Yes

Index Terms Isophosphamide; NSC-109724; Z4942

Pharmacologic Category Antineoplastic Agent, Alkylating Agent; Antineoplastic Agent, Alkylating Agent (Nitrogen Mustard)

Use Treatment of lung cancer, Hodgkin's and non-Hodgkin's lymphoma, breast cancer, acute and chronic lymphocytic leukemias, ovarian cancer, sarcomas, pancreatic and gastric carcinomas

Orphan drug: Treatment of testicular cancer

Local Anesthetic/Vasoconstrictor Precautions No information available to require special precautions

Effects on Dental Treatment No significant effects or complications reported

Common Adverse Effects

>10%:

Central nervous system: Somnolence, confusion, hallucinations (12%)

Dermatologic: Alopecia (75% to 100%)

Endocrine & metabolic: Metabolic acidosis (31%)

Gastrointestinal: Nausea and vomiting (58%), may be more common with higher doses or bolus infusions; constipation

Genitourinary: Hemorrhagic cystitis (40% to 50%), patients should be vigorously hydrated (at least 2 L/day) and receive mesna

Hematologic: Myelosuppression, leukopenia (65% to 100%), thrombocytopenia (10%) - dose related

Onset: 7-14 days

Nadir: 21-28 days

Recovery: 21-28 days

Renal: Hematuria (6% to 92%)

1% to 10%:

Central nervous system: Hallucinations, depressive psychoses, polyneuropathy

Dermatologic: Dermatitis, nail banding/ridging, hyperpigmentation

Endocrine & metabolic: SIADH, sterility

Hematologic: Anemia

Hepatic: Transaminases increased (3%)

(Continued)

Ifosfamide (Continued)

Local: Phlebitis
Renal: BUN/creatinine increased (6%)
Respiratory: Nasal stuffiness

Mechanism of Action Causes cross-linking of strands of DNA by binding with nucleic acids and other intracellular structures; inhibits protein synthesis and DNA synthesis

Drug Interactions

Cytochrome P450 Effect: Substrate of CYP2A6 (minor), 2B6 (minor), 2C8 (minor), 2C9 (minor), 2C19 (minor), 3A4 (major); **Inhibits** CYP3A4 (weak); **Induces** CYP2C8 (weak), 2C9 (weak)

Increased Effect/Toxicity: CYP3A4 inducers may increase the levels/effects of acrolein (the active metabolite of ifosfamide); example inducers include aminoglutethimide, carbamazepine, nafcillin, nevirapine, phenobarbital, phenytoin, and rifamycins.

Decreased Effect: CYP3A4 inhibitors may decrease the levels/effects of acrolein (the active metabolite of ifosfamide); example inhibitors include azole antifungals, clarithromycin, diclofenac, doxycycline, erythromycin, imatinib, isoniazid, nefazodone, nicardipine, propofol, protease inhibitors, quinidine, telithromycin, and verapamil.

Pharmacodynamics/Kinetics Pharmacokinetics are dose dependent

Distribution: V_d: 5.7-49 L; does penetrate CNS, but not in therapeutic levels

Protein binding: Negligible

Metabolism: Hepatic to active metabolites phosphoramide mustard, acrolein, and inactive dichloroethylated and carboxy metabolites; acrolein is the agent implicated in development of hemorrhagic cystitis

Bioavailability: Estimated at 100%

Half-life elimination: Beta: High dose: 11-15 hours (3800-5000 mg/m²); Lower dose: 4-7 hours (1800 mg/m²)

Time to peak, plasma: Oral: Within 1 hour

Excretion: Urine (15% to 50% as unchanged drug, 41% as metabolites)

Pregnancy Risk Factor D

Iloprost (EYE loe prost)

U.S. Brand Names Ventavis™

Generic Available No

Index Terms Iloprost Tromethamine; Prostacyclin PGI₂

Pharmacologic Category Prostaglandin

Use Treatment of idiopathic pulmonary arterial hypertension in patients with NYHA Class III or IV symptoms

Local Anesthetic/Vasoconstrictor Precautions No information available to require special precautions

Effects on Dental Treatment Key adverse event(s) related to dental treatment: Jaw pain (reported in >10% of patients).

Common Adverse Effects

>10%:

Cardiovascular: Flushing (27%), hypotension (11%)

Central nervous system: Headache (30%)

Gastrointestinal: Nausea (13%)

Neuromuscular & skeletal: Trismus (12%)

Respiratory: Cough increased (39%)

Miscellaneous: Flu-like syndrome (14%), jaw pain (12%)

1% to 10%:

Cardiovascular: Syncope (8%), palpitation (7%)

Central nervous system: Insomnia (8%)

Gastrointestinal: Vomiting (7%)

Hepatic: Alkaline phosphatase increased (6%), GGT increased (6%)

Neuromuscular & skeletal: Back pain (7%), muscle cramps (6%)

Respiratory: Hemoptysis (5%), pneumonia (4%)

Mechanism of Action Acutely, iloprost dilates systemic and pulmonary arterial vascular beds. In longer-term use, alters pulmonary vascular resistance and suppresses vascular smooth muscle proliferation. In addition, it is a potent endogenous inhibitor of platelet aggregation.

Drug Interactions

Increased Effect/Toxicity: Vasodilators and antihypertensives may increase the hypotensive effects; anticoagulants and antiplatelet medications may increase the risk of bleeding.

Pharmacodynamics/Kinetics

Duration: 30-90 minutes

Protein binding: ~60%, primarily to albumin

Metabolism: Hepatic via beta oxidation of the carboxyl side chain; main metabolite, tetranor-iloprost (inactive in animal studies)

Half-life elimination: 20-30 minutes

Pregnancy Risk Factor C

Iloprost Tromethamine *see* Iloprost *on page 862*

Imatinib (eye MAT eh nib)

U.S. Brand Names Gleevec®

Canadian Brand Names Gleevec®

Mexican Brand Names Glivec

Generic Available No

Index Terms CGP-57148B; Glivec; Imatinib Mesylate; NSC-716051; STI571

Pharmacologic Category Antineoplastic Agent, Tyrosine Kinase Inhibitor

Use Treatment of:

Aggressive systemic mastocytosis (ASM) without D816V c-kit mutation (or c-Kit mutation status unknown)

Dermatofibrosarcoma protuberans (DFSP) (unresectable, recurrent and metastatic)

Gastrointestinal stromal tumors (GIST) kit-positive (CD117) unresectable and/or (metastatic) malignant

Hypereosinophilic syndrome (HES) and/or chronic eosinophilic leukemia (CEL)

Myelodysplastic/myeloproliferative disease (MDS/MPD) associated with platelet-derived growth factor receptor (PDGFR) gene rearrangements

Philadelphia chromosome-positive (Ph+) chronic myeloid leukemia (CML) in chronic phase (newly-diagnosed)

Ph+ acute lymphoblastic leukemia (ALL) (relapsed or refractory)

Ph+ CML in blast crisis, accelerated phase, or chronic phase after failure of interferon therapy

Ph+ CML in chronic phase in pediatric patients recurring following stem cell transplant or who are resistant to interferon-alpha therapy

Local Anesthetic/Vasoconstrictor Precautions No information available to require special precautions

Effects on Dental Treatment Key adverse event(s) related to dental treatment: Mouth ulceration and taste disturbance.

Common Adverse Effects

>10%:

Cardiovascular: Chest pain (7% to 11%)

Central nervous system: Fatigue (30% to 53%), pyrexia (15% to 41%), headache (27% to 39%), insomnia (10% to 19%), dizziness (11% to 16%), depression (13%), anxiety (7% to 12%)

Dermatologic: Rash (36% to 53%), pruritus (8% to 14%)

Endocrine & metabolic: Fluid retention (7% to 81% includes aggravated edema, anasarca, ascites, pericardial effusion, pleural effusion, pulmonary edema); hypokalemia (6% to 13%)

Gastrointestinal: Nausea (47% to 74%), diarrhea (39% to 70%), vomiting (21% to 58%), abdominal pain (30% to 40%), flatulence (30% to 34%), weight gain (5% to 32%), dyspepsia (12% to 27%), anorexia (7% to 17%), constipation (9% to 16%), sore throat (10% to 15%), taste disturbance (3% to 15%), loose stools (10% to 12%)

Hematologic: Hemorrhage (24% to 53%; grades 3/4: 1% to 19%), neutropenia (grade 4: 3% to 48%), anemia (grade 4: <1% to 11%), thrombocytopenia (grade 4: <1% to 33%)

Hepatic: Ascites or pleural effusion (GIST: 12% to 15%), hepatotoxicity (6% to 12%)

Neuromuscular & skeletal: Muscle cramps (28% to 62%), musculoskeletal pain (30% to 49%), arthralgia (25% to 40%), joint pain (11 to 30%), myalgia (9% to 27%), back pain (23% to 26%), weakness (15% to 21%), rigors (10% to 12%)

Ocular: Lacrimation increased (16% to 18%)

Respiratory: Cough (14% to 27%), nasopharyngitis (10% to 27%), dyspnea (12% to 21%), upper respiratory tract infection (3% to 19%), pharyngolaryngeal pain (7% to 17%), pneumonia (4% to 13%), sinusitis (4% to 11%)

Miscellaneous: Superficial edema (58% to 81%), night sweats (13% to 17%), influenza (1% to 11%)

(Continued)

Imatinib *(Continued)*

1% to 10%:

Central nervous system: CNS hemorrhage (<1% to 9%)

Dermatologic: Alopecia, dry skin

Gastrointestinal: Gastrointestinal hemorrhage (1% to 8%), abdominal distension, gastroesophageal reflux, mouth ulceration

Hepatic: Alkaline phosphatase increased (grade 3: <1% to 6%), ALT increased (grades 3/4: <1% to 7%), bilirubin increased (grades 3/4: <1% to 3%), AST increased (grades 3/4: <1% to 4%)

Neuromuscular & skeletal: Joint swelling, paresthesia

Ocular: Blurred vision, conjunctivitis

Renal: Albumin decreased (grade 3: 3% to 4%), creatinine increased (grades 3/4: <1% to 3%)

Miscellaneous: Flu-like syndrome (<1% to 10%)

Mechanism of Action Inhibits Bcr-Abl tyrosine kinase, the constitutive abnormal gene product of the Philadelphia chromosome in chronic myeloid leukemia (CML). Inhibition of this enzyme blocks proliferation and induces apoptosis in Bcr-Abl positive cell lines as well as in fresh leukemic cells in Philadelphia chromosome positive CML. Also inhibits tyrosine kinase for platelet-derived growth factor (PDGF), stem cell factor (SCF), c-kit, and cellular events mediated by PDGF and SCF.

Drug Interactions

Cytochrome P450 Effect: Substrate of CYP1A2 (minor), 2D6 (minor), 2C9 (minor), 2C19 (minor), 3A4 (major), **Inhibits** CYP2C9 (weak), 2D6 (moderate), 3A4 (strong)

Increased Effect/Toxicity: Imatinib may increase the levels/effects of amphetamines, selected beta-blockers, dextromethorphan, fluoxetine, lidocaine, mirtazapine, nefazodone, paroxetine, risperidone, ritonavir, thioridazine, tricyclic antidepressants, venlafaxine and other CYP2D6 substrates. Imatinib may increase the risk of myopathy/rhabdomyolysis with HMG-CoA reductase inhibitors (except pravastatin/fluvastatin). Imatinib may increase the toxicity of pimecrolimus (in patients with widespread and/or erythrodermic disease). Imatinib may increase the levels/effects of benzodiazepines, calcium channel blockers, clarithromycin, cyclosporine, erythromycin, estrogens, mirtazapine, nateglinide, nefazodone, nevirapine, protease inhibitors, tacrolimus, venlafaxine and other CYP3A4 substrates. (Selected benzodiazepines [midazolam and triazolam], cisapride, ergot alkaloids, selected HMG-CoA reductase inhibitors [lovastatin and simvastatin], and pimozide are generally contraindicated with strong CYP3A4 inhibitors.)

The levels/effects of imatinib may be increased by azole antifungals, clarithromycin, diclofenac, doxycycline, erythromycin, isoniazid, nefazodone, nicardipine, propofol, protease inhibitors, quinidine, telithromycin, verapamil, and other CYP3A4 inhibitors. Lansoprazole may enhance the dermatologic adverse effects of Imatinib.

Decreased Effect: The levels/effects of imatinib may be decreased by aminoglutethimide, carbamazepine, nafcillin, nevirapine, phenobarbital, phenytoin, rifamycins, and other CYP3A4 inducers. Dosage of imatinib should be increased by at least 50% (with careful monitoring) when used concurrently with a strong inducer.

Imatinib may decrease the levels/effects of codeine, hydrocodone, oxycodone, tramadol, and other CYP2D6 prodrug substrates. Imatinib may decrease the absorption of digoxin (tablet formulation).

Pharmacodynamics/Kinetics

Protein binding: 95% to albumin and alpha$_1$-acid glycoprotein

Metabolism: Hepatic via CYP3A4 (minor metabolism via CYP1A2, CYP2D6, CYP2C9, CYP2C19); primary metabolite (active): N-demethylated piperazine derivative (CGP74588); severe hepatic impairment (bilirubin >3-10 times ULN) increases AUC by 45% to 55% for imatinib and its active metabolite, respectively

Bioavailability: 98%

Half-life elimination: Parent drug: 18 hours; N-desmethyl metabolite: 40 hours

Time to peak: 2-4 hours

Excretion: Feces (68% primarily as metabolites, 20% as unchanged drug); urine (13% primarily as metabolites, 5% as unchanged drug)

Clearance: Highly variable; Mean: 8-14 L/hour (for 50 kg and 100 kg male, respectively)

Pregnancy Risk Factor D

Imiglucerase (i mi GLOO ser ace)

U.S. Brand Names Cerezyme®
Canadian Brand Names Cerezyme®
Generic Available No
Pharmacologic Category Enzyme
Use Long-term enzyme replacement therapy for patients with Type 1 Gaucher's disease

Local Anesthetic/Vasoconstrictor Precautions No information available to require special precautions

Effects on Dental Treatment No significant effects or complications reported
Common Adverse Effects
  1% to 10%: Miscellaneous: Hypersensitivity reaction (7%; symptoms may include pruritus, flushing, urticaria, angioedema, bronchospasm)
  Individual frequency not defined, but <1.5%:
    Cardiovascular: Tachycardia
    Central nervous system: Headache, dizziness, fatigue, fever
    Dermatologic: Rash, pruritus
    Gastrointestinal: Nausea, abdominal discomfort, vomiting, diarrhea
  Local: Injection site burning, swelling, or sterile abscess (<1%)
    Neuromuscular & skeletal: Backache
    Miscellaneous: Anaphylactoid reactions (<1%)
Mechanism of Action Imiglucerase is an analogue of glucocerebrosidase; it is produced by recombinant DNA technology using mammalian cell culture. Glucocerebrosidase is an enzyme deficient in Gaucher's disease. It is needed to catalyze the hydrolysis of glucocerebroside to glucose and ceramide.
Pharmacodynamics/Kinetics
  Distribution: V_d: 0.09-0.15 L/kg
  Half-life elimination: 3.6-10.4 minutes
Pregnancy Risk Factor C

Imipenem and Cilastatin (i mi PEN em & sye la STAT in)

U.S. Brand Names Primaxin®
Canadian Brand Names Primaxin®; Primaxin® I.V.
Mexican Brand Names Tienam
Generic Available No
Index Terms Imipemide
Pharmacologic Category Antibiotic, Carbapenem
Use Treatment of lower respiratory tract, urinary tract, intra-abdominal, gynecologic, bone and joint, skin and skin structure, and polymicrobic infections as well as bacterial septicemia and endocarditis. Antibacterial activity includes resistant gram-negative bacilli (*Pseudomonas aeruginosa* and *Enterobacter* sp), gram-positive bacteria (methicillin-sensitive *Staphylococcus aureus* and *Streptococcus* sp) and anaerobes.
Unlabeled/Investigational Use Hepatic abscess; neutropenic fever; melioidosis

Local Anesthetic/Vasoconstrictor Precautions No information available to require special precautions

Effects on Dental Treatment No significant effects or complications reported
Common Adverse Effects Adverse reactions reported with use for both I.V. and I.M. formulations in adults, except where noted.
  1% to 10%:
    Cardiovascular: Tachycardia (infants 2%; adults <1%)
    Central nervous system: Seizure (infants 6%; adults <1%)
    Dermatologic: Rash (≤1%, children 2%)
    Gastrointestinal: Nausea (1% to 2%), diarrhea (children 3% to 4%; adults 1% to 2%), vomiting (≤2%)
    Genitourinary: Oliguria/anuria (infants 2%; adults <1%)
    Local: Phlebitis/thrombophlebitis (3%), pain at I.M. injection site (1.2%)
Mechanism of Action Inhibits bacterial cell wall synthesis by binding to one or more of the penicillin binding proteins (PBPs); which in turn inhibits the final transpeptidation step of peptidoglycan synthesis in bacterial cell walls, thus inhibiting cell wall biosynthesis. Bacteria eventually lyse due to ongoing activity of cell wall autolytic enzymes (autolysins and murein hydrolases) while cell wall assembly is arrested. Cilastatin prevents renal metabolism of imipenem by
(Continued)

Imipenem and Cilastatin (Continued)

competitive inhibition of dehydropeptidase along the brush border of the renal tubules.

Drug Interactions

Increased Effect/Toxicity: Ganciclovir may increase the risk of seizures; concomitant use not recommended. Uricosuric agents (eg, probenecid) may increase the levels/effects of imipenem; monitor. Concurrent cyclosporine may increase the neurotoxic effects of imipenem and cyclosporine levels may also be increased; monitor.

Decreased Effect: Imipenem may decrease valproic acid concentrations to subtherapeutic levels; monitor. Antibiotics may decrease therapeutic effects of Ty21a typhoid vaccine.

Pharmacodynamics/Kinetics

Absorption: I.M.: Imipenem: 60% to 75%; cilastatin: 95% to 100%

Distribution: Rapidly and widely to most tissues and fluids including sputum, pleural fluid, peritoneal fluid, interstitial fluid, bile, aqueous humor, and bone; highest concentrations in pleural fluid, interstitial fluid, and peritoneal fluid; low concentrations in CSF

Protein binding: Imipenem: 20%; cilastatin: 40%

Metabolism: Imipenem is metabolized in the kidney by dehydropeptidase I; cilastatin prevents imipenem metabolism by this enzyme; cilastatin is partially metabolized renally

Half-life elimination: I.V.: Both drugs: 60 minutes; prolonged with renal impairment; I.M.: Imipenem: 2-3 hours

Time to peak: I.M.: 3.5 hours

Excretion: Both drugs: Urine (~70% as unchanged drug)

Pregnancy Risk Factor C

Imipramine (im IP ra meen)

U.S. Brand Names Tofranil®; Tofranil-PM®

Canadian Brand Names Apo-Imipramine®; Novo-Pramine; Tofranil®

Mexican Brand Names Talpramin; Tofranil; Tofranil-PM

Generic Available Yes

Index Terms Imipramine Hydrochloride; Imipramine Pamoate

Pharmacologic Category Antidepressant, Tricyclic (Tertiary Amine)

Use Treatment of depression; treatment of nocturnal enuresis in children

Unlabeled/Investigational Use Analgesic for certain chronic and neuropathic pain; panic disorder; attention-deficit/hyperactivity disorder (ADHD)

Local Anesthetic/Vasoconstrictor Precautions Use with caution; epinephrine and levonordefrin have been shown to have an increased pressor response in combination with TCAs. Imipramine is one of the drugs confirmed to prolong the QT interval and is accepted as having a risk of causing torsade de pointes. The risk of drug-induced torsade de pointes is extremely low when a single QT interval prolonging drug is prescribed. In terms of epinephrine, it is not known what effect vasoconstrictors in the local anesthetic regimen will have in patients with a known history of congenital prolonged QT interval or in patients taking any medication that prolongs the QT interval. Until more information is obtained, it is suggested that the clinician consult with the physician prior to the use of a vasoconstrictor in suspected patients, and that the vasoconstrictor (epinephrine, levonordefrin [Neo-Cobefrin®]) be used with caution.

Effects on Dental Treatment Key adverse event(s) related to dental treatment: Xerostomia and changes in salivation (normal salivary flow resumes upon discontinuation). Long-term treatment with TCAs, such as imipramine, increases the risk of caries by reducing salivation and salivary buffer capacity. In a study by Rundergren, et al, pathological alterations were observed in the oral mucosa of 72% of 58 patients; 55% had new carious lesions after taking TCAs for a median of 5½ years. Current research is investigating the use of the salivary stimulant pilocarpine to overcome the xerostomia from imipramine.

Common Adverse Effects Frequency not defined.

Cardiovascular: Orthostatic hypotension, arrhythmia, tachycardia, hypertension, palpitation, MI, heart block, ECG changes, CHF, stroke

Central nervous system: Dizziness, drowsiness, headache, agitation, insomnia, nightmares, hypomania, psychosis, fatigue, confusion, hallucinations, disorientation, delusions, anxiety, restlessness, seizure

Endocrine & metabolic: Gynecomastia, breast enlargement, galactorrhea, increase or decrease in libido, increase or decrease in blood sugar, SIADH

Gastrointestinal: Nausea, unpleasant taste, weight gain, xerostomia, constipation, ileus, stomatitis, abdominal cramps, vomiting, anorexia, epigastric disorders, diarrhea, black tongue, weight loss

Genitourinary: Urinary retention, impotence

Neuromuscular & skeletal: Weakness, numbness, tingling, paresthesia, incoordination, ataxia, tremor, peripheral neuropathy, extrapyramidal symptoms

Ocular: Blurred vision, disturbances of accommodation, mydriasis

Otic: Tinnitus

Miscellaneous: Diaphoresis

Restrictions An FDA-approved medication guide concerning the use of antidepressants in children, adolescents, and young adults must be distributed when dispensing an outpatient prescription (new or refill) where this medication is to be used without direct supervision of a healthcare provider. Medication guides are available at http://www.fda.gov/cder/Offices/ODS/medication_guides.htm. Dispense to parents or guardians of children and adolescents receiving this medication.

Mechanism of Action Traditionally believed to increase the synaptic concentration of serotonin and/or norepinephrine in the central nervous system by inhibition of their reuptake by the presynaptic neuronal membrane. However, additional receptor effects have been found including desensitization of adenyl cyclase, down regulation of beta-adrenergic receptors, and down regulation of serotonin receptors.

Drug Interactions

Cytochrome P450 Effect: Substrate of CYP1A2 (minor), 2B6 (minor), 2C19 (major), 2D6 (major), 3A4 (minor); **Inhibits** CYP1A2 (weak), 2C19 (weak), 2D6 (moderate), 2E1 (weak)

Increased Effect/Toxicity: When used with MAO inhibitors, hyperpyrexia, hypertension, tachycardia, confusion, seizures, and **deaths have been reported** (serotonin syndrome). Serotonin syndrome has also been reported with ritonavir (rare). Use of lithium with a TCA may increase the risk for neurotoxicity.

CYP2C19 inhibitors may increase the levels/effects of imipramine; example inhibitors include delavirdine, fluconazole, fluvoxamine, gemfibrozil, isoniazid, omeprazole, and ticlopidine. Imipramine increases the effects of amphetamines, anticholinergics, other CNS depressants (sedatives, hypnotics, or ethanol), chlorpropamide, tolazamide, and warfarin. CYP2D6 inhibitors may increase the levels/effects of imipramine; example inhibitors include chlorpromazine, delavirdine, fluoxetine, miconazole, paroxetine, pergolide, quinidine, quinine, ritonavir, and ropinirole.

Phenothiazines may increase concentration of some TCAs and TCAs may increase concentration of phenothiazines. Pressor response to I.V. epinephrine, norepinephrine, and phenylephrine may be enhanced in patients receiving TCAs (**Note:** Effect is unlikely with epinephrine or levonordefrin dosages typically administered as infiltration in combination with local anesthetics).

Combined use of beta-agonists or drugs which prolong QT_c (including quinidine, procainamide, disopyramide, cisapride, sparfloxacin, gatifloxacin, moxifloxacin) with TCAs may predispose patients to cardiac arrhythmias.

Decreased Effect: CYP2C19 inducers may decrease the levels/effects of imipramine; example inducers include aminoglutethimide, carbamazepine, phenytoin, and rifampin. Imipramine inhibits the antihypertensive response to bethanidine, clonidine, debrisoquin, guanadrel, guanethidine, guanabenz, and guanfacine. Cholestyramine and colestipol may bind TCAs and reduce their absorption; monitor for altered response.

Pharmacodynamics/Kinetics

Onset of action: Peak antidepressant effect: Usually after ≥2 weeks

Absorption: Well absorbed

Distribution: Crosses placenta

Metabolism: Hepatic via CYP to desipramine (active) and other metabolites; significant first-pass effect

Half-life elimination: 6-18 hours

Excretion: Urine (as metabolites)

Pregnancy Risk Factor D

Imipramine Hydrochloride *see* Imipramine *on page 866*

Imipramine Pamoate *see* Imipramine *on page 866*

Imiquimod (i mi KWI mod)

Related Information

Systemic Viral Diseases *on page 1767*

Viral Infections *on page 1806*

U.S. Brand Names Aldara™

Canadian Brand Names Aldara™

Mexican Brand Names Aldara

Generic Available No

(Continued)

Imiquimod *(Continued)*

Pharmacologic Category Skin and Mucous Membrane Agent; Topical Skin Product

Dental Use Treatment of oral warts

Use Treatment of external genital and perianal warts/condyloma acuminata; nonhyperkeratotic, nonhypertrophic actinic keratosis on face or scalp; superficial basal cell carcinoma (sBCC) with a maximum tumor diameter of 2 cm located on the trunk, neck, or extremities (excluding hands or feet)

Unlabeled/Investigational Use Treatment of common warts

Local Anesthetic/Vasoconstrictor Precautions No information available to require special precautions

Effects on Dental Treatment No significant effects or complications reported

Significant Adverse Effects

>10%:

Local: Application site reactions are common. Frequency of reactions vary, and are related to the degree of inflammation associated with the treated disease, number of weekly applications, and individual sensitivity.

Edema, erosion/ulceration, erythema, excoriation, flaking, induration, itching, scabbing/crusting, scaling/dryness, vesicles, weeping/exudate

Respiratory: Upper respiratory infection (3% to 15%)

1% to 10%:

Cardiovascular: Chest pain (1%)

Central nervous system: Headache (4% to 8%), fatigue (2%), fever (1% to 2%), anxiety (1%), dizziness (1%)

Dermatologic: Eczema (2%), alopecia (1%)

Gastrointestinal: Diarrhea (3%), dyspepsia (2% to 3%), nausea (1%), vomiting (1%)

Genitourinary: Urinary tract infection (1%)

Local: Bleeding, burning, hypopigmentation, infection, irritation, pain, papule, rash, sensitivity, soreness, stinging, tenderness

Neuromuscular & skeletal: Myalgia (1%), back pain (4%), rigors (1%)

Respiratory: Sinusitis (2% to 7%), rhinitis (3%), pharyngitis (1%), coughing (2%)

Miscellaneous: Squamous cell carcinoma (4%), influenza-like syndrome (1% to 3%), lymphadenopathy (3%)

Postmarketing and/or case reports (limited to important and/or life-threatening): Agitation, anemia, angioedema, arrhythmias, capillary leak syndrome, cardiac failure, cardiomyopathy, cerebrovascular accident, depression, dyspnea, erythema multiforme, exfoliative dermatitis, Henoch-Schönlein purpura syndrome, idiopathic thrombocytopenia purpura, insomnia, ischemia, leukopenia, liver function abnormal, lymphoma, MI, multiple sclerosis aggravated, paresis, proteinuria, pulmonary edema, seizure, syncope, thrombocytopenia, thyroiditis

Dental Usual Dosing Common oral warts: Adults: Topical: Apply once daily prior to bedtime

Dosage Topical: **Note:** A rest period of several days may be taken if required by the patient's discomfort or severity of the local skin reaction. Treatment may resume once the reaction subsides.

Children ≥12 years and Adults: Perianal warts/condyloma acuminata: Apply a thin layer 3 times/week prior to bedtime and leave on skin for 6-10 hours. Remove with mild soap and water. Examples of 3 times/week application schedules are: Monday, Wednesday, Friday; or Tuesday, Thursday, Saturday. Continue imiquimod treatment until there is total clearance of the genital/perianal warts for ≤16 weeks.

Adults:

Actinic keratosis: Apply twice weekly for 16 weeks to a treatment area on face or scalp (but not both concurrently); apply prior to bedtime and leave on skin for 8 hours. Remove with mild soap and water.

Common oral warts (dental use): Apply once daily prior to bedtime

Common warts (unlabeled use): Apply once daily prior to bedtime

Superficial basal cell carcinoma: Apply once daily prior to bedtime, 5 days/week for 6 weeks. Treatment area should include a 1 cm margin of skin around the tumor. Leave on skin for 8 hours. Remove with mild soap and water.

Mechanism of Action Mechanism of action is unknown; however, induces cytokines, including interferon-alpha and others

Contraindications Hypersensitivity to imiquimod or any component of the formulation

Warnings/Precautions Imiquimod is not intended for oral, intravaginal, or ophthalmic use. Topical imiquimod administration is not recommended until tissue is healed from any previous drug or surgical treatment. Imiquimod has the potential to exacerbate inflammatory conditions of the skin. Intense inflammatory reactions may occur, and may be accompanied by systemic symptoms (fever, malaise, myalgia); interruption of therapy should be considered. May increase sunburn susceptibility; patients should protect themselves from the sun and artificial forms of sunlight. Safety and efficacy in immunosuppressed patients or in patients <12 years of age have not been established. Safety and efficacy have not been established for basal cell nevus syndrome or xeroderma pigmentosum; efficacy was not established for molluscum contagiosum in children 2-12 years of age.

Basal cell carcinoma: Use in basal cell carcinoma should be limited to superficial carcinomas with a maximum diameter of 2 cm. Safety and efficacy in treatment of sBCC lesions of the face, head, and anogenital area, or other subtypes of basal cell carcinoma (including nodular and morpheaform), have not been established.

Actinic keratosis: Treatment should be limited to areas ≤25 cm². Safety and efficacy of repeated use in the same 25 cm² area has not been established.

External genital warts: Imiquimod has not been evaluated for the treatment of urethral, intravaginal, cervical, rectal, or intra-anal human papilloma viral disease and is not recommended for these conditions.

Drug Interactions Substrate (minor) of CYP1A2, 3A4

Pharmacodynamics/Kinetics
Absorption: Minimal; systemic absorption more dependant upon surface area of application as opposed to dose
Excretion: Urine (≤2% of applied dose as imiquimod and metabolites)

Pregnancy Risk Factor C

Lactation Excretion in breast milk unknown/use caution

Dosage Forms Excipient information presented when available (limited, particularly for generics); consult specific product labeling.
Cream:
Aldara™: 5% (12s) [contains benzyl alcohol; single-dose packets]

Imitrex® see Sumatriptan on page 1511

Immune Globulin (Intramuscular)
(i MYUN GLOB yoo lin, IN tra MUS kyoo ler)

Related Information
Immunizations (Vaccines) on page 1886
Systemic Viral Diseases on page 1767
U.S. Brand Names BayGam® [DSC]; GammaSTAN™ S/D
Canadian Brand Names BayGam®
Generic Available No
Index Terms Gamma Globulin; IG; IGIM; Immune Serum Globulin; ISG
Pharmacologic Category Immune Globulin
Use To provide passive immunity in susceptible individuals under the following circumstances:
Hepatitis A: Within 14 days of exposure and prior to manifestation of disease
Measles: For use within 6 days of exposure in an unvaccinated person, who has not previously had measles
Varicella: When Varicella Zoster Immune Globulin is not available
Rubella: Post exposure prophylaxis (within 72 hours) to reduce the risk of infection in exposed pregnant women who will not consider therapeutic abortion
Immunoglobulin deficiency: To help prevent serious infections
Local Anesthetic/Vasoconstrictor Precautions No information available to require special precautions
Effects on Dental Treatment No significant effects or complications reported
Common Adverse Effects Frequency not defined.
Cardiovascular: Flushing, angioedema
Central nervous system: Chills, lethargy, fever
Dermatologic: Urticaria, erythema
Gastrointestinal: Nausea, vomiting
Local: Pain, tenderness, muscle stiffness at I.M. site
Neuromuscular & skeletal: Myalgia
Miscellaneous: Hypersensitivity reactions
Dosage I.M.: Children and Adults:
Hepatitis A:
Pre-exposure prophylaxis upon travel into endemic areas (hepatitis A vaccine preferred):
0.02 mL/kg for anticipated risk of exposure <3 months
0.06 mL/kg for anticipated risk of exposure ≥3 months
Repeat approximate dose every 5 months if exposure continues
(Continued)

Immune Globulin (Intramuscular) *(Continued)*

Postexposure prophylaxis: 0.02 mL/kg given within 14 days of exposure. IG is not needed if at least 1 dose of hepatitis A vaccine was given at ≥1 month before exposure

Measles:

Prophylaxis, immunocompetent: 0.25 mL/kg/dose (maximum dose: 15 mL) given within 6 days of exposure followed by live attenuated measles vaccine in 5-6 months when indicated

Prophylaxis, immunocompromised: 0.5 mL/kg (maximum dose: 15 mL) immediately following exposure

Rubella: Prophylaxis during pregnancy: 0.55 mL/kg/dose within 72 hours of exposure

Varicella: Prophylaxis: 0.6-1.2 mL/kg (varicella zoster immune globulin preferred) within 72 hours of exposure

IgG deficiency: 0.66 mL/kg/dose every 3-4 weeks. A double dose may be given at onset of therapy; some patients may require more frequent injections.

Mechanism of Action Provides passive immunity by increasing the antibody titer and antigen-antibody reaction potential

Contraindications Hypersensitivity to immune globulin or any component of the formulation; IgA deficiency; severe thrombocytopenia or coagulation disorders where I.M. injections are contraindicated

Warnings/Precautions Hypersensitivity and anaphylactic reactions can occur; immediate treatment (including epinephrine 1:1000) should be available. Product of human plasma; may potentially contain infectious agents which could transmit disease. Screening of donors, as well as testing and/or inactivation or removal of certain viruses, reduces the risk. Infections thought to be transmitted by this product should be reported to the manufacturer. Skin testing should not be performed as local irritation can occur and be misinterpreted as a positive reaction. Not for I.V. administration.

Drug Interactions

Decreased Effect:

Do not administer MMR within 3 months after administration of IGIM; do not administer varicella vaccine within 5 months. If IG is given <2 weeks after MMR vaccine or <3 weeks after varicella vaccine, revaccination is required.

Pharmacodynamics/Kinetics

Duration: Immune effect: Usually 3-4 weeks

Half-life elimination: 23 days

Time to peak, serum: I.M.: ~48 hours

Pregnancy Risk Factor C

Dosage Forms

Injection, solution [preservative free]:

GammaSTAN™ S/D: 15% to 18% (2 mL, 10 mL)

Selected Readings

ASHP Commission on Therapeutics, "ASHP Therapeutic Guidelines for Intravenous Immune Globulin," *Clin Pharm*, 1992, 11(2):117-36.

Berkman SA, Lee ML, and Gale RP, "Clinical Uses of Intravenous Immunoglobulins," *Ann Intern Med*, 1990, 112(4):278-92.

Immune Globulin (Intravenous)
(i MYUN GLOB yoo lin, IN tra VEE nus)

Related Information

Systemic Viral Diseases *on page 1767*

U.S. Brand Names Carimune™ NF; Flebogamma®; Gammagard® Liquid; Gammagard® S/D; Gammar®-P I.V.; Gamunex®; Iveegam EN; Octagam®; Panglobulin® NF; Polygam® S/D

Canadian Brand Names Gamimune® N; Gammagard® Liquid; Gammagard® S/D; Gamunex®; Iveegam Immuno®

Generic Available No

Index Terms IVIG

Pharmacologic Category Immune Globulin

Use

Treatment of primary immunodeficiency syndromes (congenital agammaglobulinemia, severe combined immunodeficiency syndromes [SCIDS], common variable immunodeficiency, X-linked immunodeficiency, Wiskott-Aldrich syndrome); idiopathic thrombocytopenic purpura (ITP); Kawasaki disease (in combination with aspirin)

Prevention of bacterial infection in B-cell chronic lymphocytic leukemia (CLL); pediatric HIV infection; bone marrow transplant (BMT)

Unlabeled/Investigational Use Autoimmune diseases (myasthenia gravis, SLE, bullous pemphigoid, severe rheumatoid arthritis), Guillain-Barré syndrome; used in conjunction with appropriate anti-infective therapy to prevent or modify acute bacterial or viral infections in patients with iatrogenically-induced or disease-associated immunodepression; autoimmune hemolytic anemia or neutropenia, refractory dermatomyositis/polymyositis

Local Anesthetic/Vasoconstrictor Precautions No information available to require special precautions

Effects on Dental Treatment No significant effects or complications reported

Common Adverse Effects Frequency not defined.

Cardiovascular: Flushing of the face, tachycardia, hyper-/hypotension, chest tightness, angioedema, lightheadedness, chest pain, MI, CHF, pulmonary embolism

Central nervous system: Anxiety, chills, dizziness, drowsiness, fatigue, fever, headache, irritability, lethargy, malaise, aseptic meningitis syndrome

Dermatologic: Pruritus, rash, urticaria

Gastrointestinal: Abdominal cramps, diarrhea, nausea, sore throat, vomiting

Hematologic: Autoimmune hemolytic anemia, hematocrit decreased, leukopenia, mild hemolysis

Hepatic: Liver function test increased

Local: Pain or irritation at the infusion site

Neuromuscular & skeletal: Arthralgia, back or hip pain, myalgia, nuchal rigidity

Ocular: Photophobia, painful eye movements

Renal: Acute renal failure, acute tubular necrosis, anuria, BUN increased, creatinine increased, nephrotic syndrome, oliguria, proximal tubular nephropathy, osmotic nephrosis

Respiratory: Cough, dyspnea, wheezing, nasal congestion, pharyngeal pain, rhinorrhea, sinusitis

Miscellaneous: Diaphoresis, hypersensitivity reactions, anaphylaxis

Dosage Approved doses and regimens may vary between brands; check manufacturer guidelines. **Note:** Some clinicians dose IVIG on ideal body weight or an adjusted ideal body weight in morbidly obese patients.

Infants and Children: Prevention of gastroenteritis (unlabeled use): Oral: 50 mg/kg/day divided every 6 hours

Children: I.V.:

Pediatric HIV: 400 mg/kg every 28 days

Severe systemic viral and bacterial infections (unlabeled use): 500-1000 mg/kg/week

Children and Adults: I.V.:

Primary immunodeficiency disorders: 200-400 mg/kg every 4 weeks or as per monitored serum IgG concentrations

Flebogamma®, Gammagard® Liquid, Gamunex®, Octagam®: 300-600 mg/kg every 3-4 weeks; adjusted based on dosage and interval in conjunction with monitored serum IgG concentrations.

B-cell chronic lymphocytic leukemia (CLL): 400 mg/kg/dose every 3 weeks

Idiopathic thrombocytopenic purpura (ITP):

Acute: 400 mg/kg/day for 5 days or 1000 mg/kg/day for 1-2 days

Chronic: 400 mg/kg as needed to maintain platelet count >30,000/mm^3; may increase dose to 800 mg/kg (1000 mg/kg if needed)

Kawasaki disease: Initiate therapy within 10 days of disease onset: 2 g/kg as a single dose administered over 10 hours, or 400 mg/kg/day for 4 days. **Note:** Must be used in combination with aspirin: 80-100 mg/kg/day in 4 divided doses for 14 days; when fever subsides, dose aspirin at 3-5 mg/kg once daily for ≥6-8 weeks

Acquired immunodeficiency syndrome (patients must be symptomatic) (unlabeled use): Various regimens have been used, including:

200-250 mg/kg/dose every 2 weeks

or

400-500 mg/kg/dose every month or every 4 weeks

Autoimmune hemolytic anemia and neutropenia (unlabeled use): 1000 mg/kg/dose for 2-3 days

Autoimmune diseases (unlabeled use): 400 mg/kg/day for 4 days

Bone marrow transplant: 500 mg/kg beginning on days 7 and 2 pretransplant, then 500 mg/kg/week for 90 days post-transplant

Adjuvant to severe cytomegalovirus infections (unlabeled use): 500 mg/kg/dose every other day for 7 doses

Guillain-Barré syndrome (unlabeled use): Various regimens have been used, including:

400 mg/kg/day for 4 days

or

1000 mg/kg/day for 2 days

or

2000 mg/kg/day for one day

Refractory dermatomyositis (unlabeled use): 2 g/kg/dose every month x 3-4 doses

(Continued)

Immune Globulin (Intravenous) *(Continued)*

Refractory polymyositis (unlabeled use): 1 g/kg/day x 2 days every month x 4 doses

Chronic inflammatory demyelinating polyneuropathy (unlabeled use): Various regimens have been used, including:

400 mg/kg/day for 5 doses once each month

or

800 mg/kg/day for 3 doses once each month

or

1000 mg/kg/day for 2 days once each month

Dosing adjustment/comments in renal impairment: Cl_{cr} <10 mL/minute: Avoid use; in patients at risk of renal dysfunction, consider infusion at a rate less than maximum.

Mechanism of Action Replacement therapy for primary and secondary immunodeficiencies; interference with F_c receptors on the cells of the reticuloendothelial system for autoimmune cytopenias and ITP; possible role of contained antiviral-type antibodies

Contraindications Hypersensitivity to immune globulin or any component of the formulation; selective IgA deficiency

Warnings/Precautions [U.S. Boxed Warning]: Acute renal dysfunction (increased serum creatinine, oliguria, acute renal failure) can rarely occur; usually within 7 days of use (more likely with products stabilized with sucrose). Use with caution in the elderly, patients with renal disease, diabetes mellitus, volume depletion, sepsis, paraproteinemia, and nephrotoxic medications due to risk of renal dysfunction. In patients at risk of renal dysfunction, the rate of infusion and concentration of solution should be minimized. discontinue if renal function deteriorates. Hypersensitivity and anaphylactic reactions can occur; immediate treatment (including epinephrine 1:1000) should be available; product of human plasma; may potentially contain infectious agents which could transmit disease. Screening of donors, as well as testing and/or inactivation or removal of certain viruses, reduces the risk. Infections thought to be transmitted by this product should be reported to the manufacturer; aseptic meningitis may occur with high doses (≥2 g/kg). Intravenous immune globulin has been associated with antiglobulin hemolysis; monitor for signs of hemolytic anemia. Patients should be adequately hydrated prior to therapy. Use caution in patients with a history of thrombotic events or cardiovascular disease; there is clinical evidence of a possible association between thrombotic events and administration of intravenous immune globulin. For intravenous administration only. Patients should be monitored for adverse events during and after the infusion. Stop administration with signs of infusion reaction (fever, chills, nausea, vomiting, and rarely shock). Risk may be increased with initial treatment, when switching brands of immune globulin, and with treatment interruptions of >8 weeks. Monitor for transfusion-related acute lung injury (TRALI); noncardiogenic pulmonary edema has been reported with intravenous immune globulin use. Some products may contain maltose, which may result in falsely-elevated blood glucose readings. Product may contain sucrose.

Drug Interactions

Decreased Effect: Decreased effect of live virus vaccines (eg, measles, mumps, rubella); separate administration by at least 3 months

Dietary Considerations Octagam® contains sodium 30 mmol/L

Pharmacodynamics/Kinetics

Onset of action: I.V.: Provides immediate antibody levels

Duration: Immune effect: 3-4 weeks (variable)

Distribution: V_d: 0.09-0.13 L/kg

Intravascular portion (primarily): Healthy subjects: 41% to 57%; Patients with congenital humoral immunodeficiencies: ~70%

Half-life elimination: IgG (variable among patients): Healthy subjects: 14-24 days; Patients with congenital humoral immunodeficiencies: 26-40 days; hypermetabolism associated with fever and infection have coincided with a shortened half-life

Pregnancy Risk Factor C

Dosage Forms

Injection, powder for reconstitution [preservative free]:

Gammar®-P I.V.: 5 g, 10 g

Iveegam EN: 5 g

Injection, powder for reconstitution [preservative free, nanofiltered]:

Carimune™ NF: 3 g, 6 g, 12 g

Panglobulin® NF: 6 g, 12 g

Injection, powder for reconstitution [preservative free, solvent detergent-treated]:

Gammagard® S/D: 2.5 g, 5 g, 10 g

Polygam® S/D: 5 g, 10 g

Injection, solution [preservative free; solvent detergent-treated]:
    Gammagard® Liquid: 10% (10 mL, 25 mL, 50 mL, 100 mL, 200 mL)
    Octagam®: 5% (20 mL, 50 mL, 100 mL, 200 mL)
Injection, solution [preservative free]:
    Flebogamma®: 5% (10 mL, 50 mL, 100 mL, 200 mL)
    Gamunex®: 10% (10 mL, 25 mL, 50 mL, 100 mL, 200 mL)

Selected Readings

ASHP Commission on Therapeutics, "ASHP Therapeutic Guidelines for Intravenous Immune Globulin," *Am J Hosp Pharm*, 1992, 49(3):652-4.

Blanchette VS, Luke B, Andrew M, et al, "A Prospective Randomized Trial of High-Dose Intravenous Immune Globulin G Therapy, Oral Prednisone Therapy, and No Therapy in Childhood Acute Immune Thrombocytopenic Purpura," *J Pediatr*, 1993, 123(6):989-95.

Grillo JA, Gorson, KC, Ropper AH, et al, "Rapid Infusion of Intravenous Immune Globulin in Patients With Neuromuscular Disorders," *Neurology*, 2001; 57:1699-1701.

Morrell A, "Pharmacokinetics of Intravenous Immunoglobulin Preparations," *Intravenous Immunoglobulins in Clinical Practice*, Lee ML and Strand V eds, New York, NY: Marcel Dekker, Inc, 1997, 1-18.

NIH Consensus Conference, "Intravenous Immunoglobulin, Prevention and Treatment of Disease," *JAMA*, 1990, 264(24):3189-93.

Skvaril F and Gardi A, "Differences Among Available Immunoglobulin Preparations for Intravenous Use," *Pediatr Infect Dis J*, 1988, 7:543-48.

"University Hospital Consortium Expert Panel for Off-Label Use of Polyvalent Intravenously Administered Immunoglobulin Preparations Consensus Statement," *JAMA*, 1995, 273(23):1865-70.

Immune Globulin (Subcutaneous)
(i MYUN GLOB yoo lin sub kyoo TAY nee us)

U.S. Brand Names Vivaglobin®
Generic Available No
Index Terms Immune Globulin Subcutaneous (Human); SCIG
Pharmacologic Category Immune Globulin
Use Treatment of primary immune deficiency (PID)
Local Anesthetic/Vasoconstrictor Precautions No information available to require special precautions
Effects on Dental Treatment No significant effects or complications reported
Common Adverse Effects Adverse reactions can be expected to be similar to those experienced with other immune globulin products; percentages are reported as adverse events per patient; injection site reactions decreased with subsequent infusions
  >10%:
    Central nervous system: Headache (32% to 48%), fever (3% to 25%)
    Dermatologic: Rash (6% to 17%)
    Gastrointestinal: Gastrointestinal disorder (5% to 37%), nausea (11% to 18%), sore throat (17%)
    Local: Injection site reactions (swelling, redness, itching; 92%)
    Miscellaneous: Allergic reaction (11%)
  1% to 10%:
    Cardiovascular: Tachycardia (3%)
    Central nervous system: Pain (10%)
    Dermatologic: Skin disorder (3%)
    Gastrointestinal: Diarrhea (10%)
    Genitourinary: Urine abnormality (3%)
    Neuromuscular & skeletal: Weakness (5%)
    Respiratory: Cough (10%)
Mechanism of Action Immune globulin replacement therapy of IgG antibodies against bacteria and viral agents.
Drug Interactions
  Decreased Effect: Immune globulin may decrease the efficacy of immune response to live vaccines.
Pharmacodynamics/Kinetics
  Bioavailability: 73% (compared to I.V.)
  Time to peak, plasma: 2.5 days
Pregnancy Risk Factor C

Immune Globulin Subcutaneous (Human) *see* Immune Globulin (Subcutaneous) *on page 873*

Immune Serum Globulin *see* Immune Globulin (Intramuscular) *on page 869*

Imodium® A-D [OTC] *see* Loperamide *on page 996*

Imodium® Advanced *see* Loperamide and Simethicone *on page 996*

Imogam® Rabies-HT *see* Rabies Immune Globulin (Human) *on page 1402*

Imovax® Rabies *see* Rabies Virus Vaccine *on page 1403*

Implanon™ *see* Etonogestrel *on page 659*

Imuran® *see* Azathioprine *on page 172*

In-111 Ibritumomab *see* Ibritumomab *on page 851*

In-111 Zevalin *see* Ibritumomab *on page 851*

Inamrinone (eye NAM ri none)

Related Information
Cardiovascular Diseases *on page 1726*

Generic Available Yes

Index Terms Amrinone Lactate

Pharmacologic Category Phosphodiesterase Enzyme Inhibitor

Use Infrequently used as a last resort, short-term therapy in patients with intractable heart failure

Local Anesthetic/Vasoconstrictor Precautions No information available to require special precautions

Effects on Dental Treatment No significant effects or complications reported

Common Adverse Effects
1% to 10%:
Cardiovascular: Arrhythmias (3%, especially in high-risk patients), hypotension (1% to 2%), (may be infusion rate-related)
Gastrointestinal: Nausea (1% to 2%)
Hematologic: Thrombocytopenia (may be dose related)

Mechanism of Action Inhibits myocardial cyclic adenosine monophosphate (cAMP) phosphodiesterase activity and increases cellular levels of cAMP resulting in a positive inotropic effect and increased cardiac output; also possesses systemic and pulmonary vasodilator effects resulting in pre- and afterload reduction; slightly increases atrioventricular conduction

Drug Interactions
Increased Effect/Toxicity: Diuretics may cause significant hypovolemia and decrease filling pressure. Inotropic effects with digitalis are additive.

Pharmacodynamics/Kinetics
Onset of action: I.V.: 2-5 minutes
Peak effect: ~10 minutes
Duration (dose dependent): Low dose: ~30 minutes; Higher doses: ~2 hours
Half-life elimination, serum: Adults: Healthy volunteers: 3.6 hours, Congestive heart failure: 5.8 hours

Pregnancy Risk Factor C

Inapsine® *see* Droperidol *on page 546*
Increlex™ *see* Mecasermin *on page 1023*

Indapamide (in DAP a mide)

Related Information
Cardiovascular Diseases *on page 1726*

U.S. Brand Names Lozol® [DSC]

Canadian Brand Names Apo-Indapamide®; Gen-Indapamide; Lozide®; Lozol®; Novo-Indapamide; Nu-Indapamide; PMS-Indapamide

Generic Available Yes

Pharmacologic Category Diuretic, Thiazide-Related

Use Management of mild to moderate hypertension; treatment of edema in congestive heart failure and nephrotic syndrome

Local Anesthetic/Vasoconstrictor Precautions Indapamide is one of the drugs confirmed to prolong the QT interval and is accepted as having a risk of causing torsade de pointes. The risk of drug-induced torsade de pointes is extremely low when a single QT interval prolonging drug is prescribed. In terms of epinephrine, it is not known what effect vasoconstrictors in the local anesthetic regimen will have in patients with a known history of congenital prolonged QT interval or in patients taking any medication that prolongs the QT interval. Until more information is obtained, it is suggested that the clinician consult with the physician prior to the use of a vasoconstrictor in suspected patients, and that the vasoconstrictor (epinephrine, levonordefrin [Neo-Cobefrin®]) be used with caution.

Effects on Dental Treatment Key adverse event(s) related to dental treatment: Orthostatic hypotension, palpitations, flushing, xerostomia (normal salivary flow resumes upon discontinuation), and rhinorrhea.

Common Adverse Effects 1% to 10%:
Cardiovascular: Orthostatic hypotension, palpitation (<5%), flushing
Central nervous system: Dizziness (<5%), lightheadedness (<5%), vertigo (<5%), headache (≥5%), restlessness (<5%), drowsiness (<5%), fatigue, lethargy, malaise, lassitude, anxiety, agitation, depression, nervousness (≥5%)
Dermatologic: Rash (<5%), pruritus (<5%), hives (<5%)
Endocrine & metabolic: Hyperglycemia (<5%), hyperuricemia (<5%)
Gastrointestinal: Anorexia, gastric irritation, nausea, vomiting, abdominal pain, cramping, bloating, diarrhea, constipation, dry mouth, weight loss

Genitourinary: Nocturia, frequent urination, polyuria, impotence (<5%), reduced libido (<5%), glycosuria (<5%)

Neuromuscular & skeletal: Muscle cramps, spasm, weakness (≥5%)

Ocular: Blurred vision (<5%)

Renal: Necrotizing angiitis, vasculitis, cutaneous vasculitis (<5%)

Respiratory: Rhinorrhea (<5%)

Mechanism of Action Diuretic effect is localized at the proximal segment of the distal tubule of the nephron; it does not appear to have significant effect on glomerular filtration rate nor renal blood flow; like other diuretics, it enhances sodium, chloride, and water excretion by interfering with the transport of sodium ions across the renal tubular epithelium

Drug Interactions

Increased Effect/Toxicity: The diuretic effect of indapamide is synergistic with furosemide and other loop diuretics. Increased hypotension and/or renal adverse effects of ACE inhibitors may result in aggressively diuresed patients. Cyclosporine and thiazide-type diuretics can increase the risk of gout or renal toxicity. Digoxin toxicity can be exacerbated if a diuretic induces hypokalemia or hypomagnesemia. Lithium toxicity can occur with thiazide-type diuretics due to reduced renal excretion of lithium. Thiazide-type diuretics may prolong the duration of action of neuromuscular blocking agents.

Decreased Effect: Effects of oral hypoglycemics may be decreased. Decreased absorption of indapamide with cholestyramine and colestipol. NSAIDs can decrease the efficacy of thiazide-type diuretics, reducing the diuretic and antihypertensive effects.

Pharmacodynamics/Kinetics

Onset of action: 1-2 hours

Duration: ≤36 hours

Absorption: Complete

Protein binding, plasma: 71% to 79%

Metabolism: Extensively hepatic

Half-life elimination: 14-18 hours

Time to peak: 2-2.5 hours

Excretion: Urine (~60%) within 48 hours; feces (~16% to 23%)

Pregnancy Risk Factor B (manufacturer); D (expert analysis)

Inderal® see Propranolol on page 1373

Inderal® LA see Propranolol on page 1373

Inderide® see Propranolol and Hydrochlorothiazide on page 1376

Indinavir (in DIN a veer)

Related Information

HIV Infection and AIDS on page 1753

Tuberculosis on page 1765

U.S. Brand Names Crixivan®

Canadian Brand Names Crixivan®

Mexican Brand Names Crixivan

Generic Available No

Index Terms Indinavir Sulfate

Pharmacologic Category Antiretroviral Agent, Protease Inhibitor

Use Treatment of HIV infection; should always be used as part of a multidrug regimen (at least three antiretroviral agents)

Local Anesthetic/Vasoconstrictor Precautions No information available to require special precautions

Effects on Dental Treatment Key adverse event(s) related to dental treatment: Abnormal taste.

Common Adverse Effects

>10%:

Gastrointestinal: Abdominal pain (17%), nausea (12%)

Hepatic: Hyperbilirubinemia (14%; dose dependent)

Renal: Nephrolithiasis/urolithiasis, including flank pain with/without hematuria (29%, pediatric patients; 12% adult patients; dose dependent)

1% to 10%:

Central nervous system: Headache (5%), dizziness (3%), somnolence (2%), fever (2%), malaise (2%), fatigue (2%)

Dermatologic: Pruritus (4%), rash (1%)

Gastrointestinal: Vomiting (8%), diarrhea (3%), taste perversion (3%), acid reflux (3%), anorexia (3%), appetite increased (2%), dyspepsia (2%), serum amylase increased (2%)

Hematologic: Neutropenia (2%)

Hepatic: Transaminases increased (4% to 5%), jaundice (2%)

Neuromuscular & skeletal: Back pain (8%), weakness (2%)

Renal: Dysuria (2%)

(Continued)

Indinavir (Continued)

Respiratory: Cough (2%)

Mechanism of Action Indinavir is a human immunodeficiency virus protease inhibitor, binding to the protease activity site and inhibiting the activity of this enzyme. HIV protease is an enzyme required for the cleavage of viral polyprotein precursors into individual functional proteins found in infectious HIV. Inhibition prevents cleavage of these polyproteins resulting in the formation of immature noninfectious viral particles.

Drug Interactions

Cytochrome P450 Effect: Substrate of CYP2D6 (minor), 3A4 (major); **Inhibits** CYP2C9 (weak), 2C19 (weak), 2D6 (weak), 3A4 (strong)

Increased Effect/Toxicity: Indinavir may increase the levels/effects of selected benzodiazepines, calcium channel blockers, cyclosporine, fentanyl, mirtazapine, nateglinide, nefazodone, quinidine, sildenafil (and other PDE-5 inhibitors), tacrolimus, trazodone, and other CYP3A4 substrates. Indinavir may also increase the levels of orally inhaled corticosteroids (eg, fluticasone); concomitant use not recommended. Selected benzodiazepines (alprazolam, midazolam, triazolam), cisapride, ergot alkaloids, selected HMG-CoA reductase inhibitors (lovastatin and simvastatin), mesoridazine, pimozide, and thioridazine are generally contraindicated with strong CYP3A4 inhibitors. When used with strong CYP3A4 inhibitors, dosage adjustment/limits are recommended for sildenafil and other PDE-5 inhibitors; refer to individual monographs.

Itraconazole or ketoconazole may increase the serum concentrations of indinavir; dosage adjustment is recommended. The levels/effects of indinavir may be increased by azole antifungals, clarithromycin, diclofenac, doxycycline, erythromycin, imatinib, isoniazid, nefazodone, nicardipine, propofol, protease inhibitors, quinidine, telithromycin, verapamil, and other CYP3A4 inhibitors.

When used with delavirdine, serum levels of indinavir are increased; dosage adjustment of indinavir may be required for this combination. Serum levels of both nelfinavir and indinavir are increased with concurrent use. Serum concentrations of indinavir may be increased by ritonavir; serum levels of ritonavir and saquinavir may be increased; dosage adjustments of indinavir are required during concurrent therapy. Rifabutin serum concentrations has been increased when coadministered with indinavir; dosage adjustments of both agents required. Concurrent use or atazanavir with indinavir may increase the risk of hyperbilirubinemia. Serum concentrations of lidocaine (systemic) may be increased; monitor serum concentrations.

Decreased Effect: The levels/effects of indinavir may be decreased by aminoglutethimide, antacids carbamazepine, nafcillin, nevirapine, phenobarbital, phenytoin, rifamycins, and other CYP3A4 inducers; dosage adjustment may be recommended (see individual agents). Rifampin and/or St John's wort (*Hypericum perforatum*); should not be used with indinavir. Venlafaxine and proton pump inhibitors may decrease indinavir levels/effects.

Pharmacodynamics/Kinetics

Absorption: Administration with a high fat, high calorie diet resulted in a reduction in AUC and in maximum serum concentration (77% and 84% respectively); lighter meal resulted in little or no change in these parameters.

Protein binding, plasma: 60%

Metabolism: Hepatic via CYP3A4; seven metabolites of indinavir identified

Bioavailability: Good

Half-life elimination: 1.8 ± 0.4 hour

Time to peak: 0.8 ± 0.3 hour

Excretion: Feces (83%, 19% as unchanged drug); urine (19%, 9% as unchanged drug)

Pregnancy Risk Factor C

Indinavir Sulfate *see* Indinavir *on page 875*

Indocin® *see* Indomethacin *on page 877*

Indocin® I.V. *see* Indomethacin *on page 877*

Indocyanine Green *(in doe SYE a neen green)*

U.S. Brand Names IC-Green™

Generic Available No

Pharmacologic Category Diagnostic Agent

Use Determining hepatic function, cardiac output, and liver blood flow; ophthalmic angiography

Local Anesthetic/Vasoconstrictor Precautions No information available to require special precautions

Effects on Dental Treatment No significant effects or complications reported

Common Adverse Effects Frequency not defined.

Central nervous system: Headache

Dermatologic: Pruritus, urticaria

Gastrointestinal: Feces discoloration (green)

Miscellaneous: Diaphoresis, anaphylactoid reactions

Pharmacodynamics/Kinetics

Protein binding: 95% to albumin

Half-life elimination: 2.5-3 minutes

Excretion: Bile

Pregnancy Risk Factor C

Indometacin *see* Indomethacin *on page 877*

Indomethacin (in doe METH a sin)

Related Information

Rheumatoid Arthritis, Osteoarthritis, and Osteoporosis *on page 1759*

Temporomandibular Dysfunction (TMD) *on page 1822*

U.S. Brand Names Indocin®; Indocin® I.V.

Canadian Brand Names Apo-Indomethacin®; Indocid® P.D.A.; Indocin®; Indo-Lemmon; Indotec; Novo-Methacin; Nu-Indo; Rhodacine®

Mexican Brand Names Antalgin Dialicels; Indocid; Malival; Malival AP

Generic Available Yes: Capsule

Index Terms Indometacin; Indomethacin Sodium Trihydrate

Pharmacologic Category Nonsteroidal Anti-inflammatory Drug (NSAID), Oral; Nonsteroidal Anti-inflammatory Drug (NSAID), Parenteral

Use Acute gouty arthritis, acute bursitis/tendonitis, moderate to severe osteoarthritis, rheumatoid arthritis, ankylosing spondylitis; I.V. form used as alternative to surgery for closure of patent ductus arteriosus in neonates

Local Anesthetic/Vasoconstrictor Precautions No information available to require special precautions

Effects on Dental Treatment NSAID formulations are known to reversibly decrease platelet aggregation via mechanisms different than observed with aspirin. The dentist should be aware of the potential of abnormal coagulation. Caution should also be exercised in the use of NSAIDs in patients already on anticoagulant therapy with drugs such as warfarin (Coumadin®).

Common Adverse Effects

>10%: Central nervous system: Headache (12%)

1% to 10%:

Central nervous system: Dizziness (3% to 9%), fatigue (<3%), vertigo (<3%), depression (<3%), malaise (<3%), somnolence (<3%)

Gastrointestinal: Nausea (3% to 9%), epigastric pain (3% to 9%), abdominal pain/cramps/distress (<3%), heartburn (3% to 9%), indigestion (3% to 9%), constipation (<3%), diarrhea (<3%), dyspepsia (3% to 9%), vomiting

Otic: Tinnitus (<3%)

Restrictions An FDA-approved medication guide must be distributed when dispensing an oral outpatient prescription (new or refill) where this medication is to be used without direct supervision of a healthcare provider. Medication guides are available at http://www.fda.gov/cder/Offices/ODS/medication_guides.htm.

Dosage

Patent ductus arteriosus:

Neonates: I.V.: Initial: 0.2 mg/kg, followed by 2 doses depending on postnatal age (PNA):

PNA **at time of first dose** <48 hours: 0.1 mg/kg at 12- to 24-hour intervals

PNA **at time of first dose** 2-7 days: 0.2 mg/kg at 12- to 24-hour intervals

PNA **at time of first dose** >7 days: 0.25 mg/kg at 12- to 24-hour intervals

In general, may use 12-hour dosing interval if urine output >1 mL/kg/hour after prior dose; use 24-hour dosing interval if urine output is <1 mL/kg/hour but >0.6 mL/kg/hour; doses should be withheld if patient has oliguria (urine output <0.6 mL/kg/hour) or anuria

Inflammatory/rheumatoid disorders: Oral: Use lowest effective dose.

Children ≥2 years: 1-2 mg/kg/day in 2-4 divided doses; maximum dose: 4 mg/kg/day; not to exceed 150-200 mg/day

Adults: 25-50 mg/dose 2-3 times/day; maximum dose: 200 mg/day. In patients with arthritis and persistent night pain and/or morning stiffness may give the larger portion (up to 100 mg) of the total daily dose at bedtime.

Bursitis/tendonitis: Oral: Adults: Initial dose: 75-150 mg/day in 3-4 divided doses; usual treatment is 7-14 days

Acute gouty arthritis: Oral: Adults: 50 mg 3 times daily until pain is tolerable then reduce dose; usual treatment <3-5 days

(Continued)

Indomethacin *(Continued)*

Elderly: Refer to adult dosing; best to start older adults on 25 mg dose given 2-3 times/day

Dosage adjustment in renal impairement: Not recommended in patients with advanced renal disease

Mechanism of Action Inhibits prostaglandin synthesis by decreasing the activity of the enzyme, cyclooxygenase, which results in decreased formation of prostaglandin precursors

Contraindications Hypersensitivity to indomethacin, aspirin, other NSAIDs, or any component of the formulation; perioperative pain in the setting of coronary artery bypass surgery (CABG); pregnancy (3rd trimester)

Neonates: Necrotizing enterocolitis, impaired renal function, active bleeding, thrombocytopenia, coagulation defects, untreated infection

Warnings/Precautions [U.S. Boxed Warning]: NSAIDs are associated with an increased risk of adverse cardiovascular events, including MI, stroke, and new onset or worsening of pre-existing hypertension. Risk may be increased with duration of use or pre-existing cardiovascular risk factors or disease. Use caution with fluid retention, CHF or hypertension. Concurrent administration of ibuprofen, and potentially other nonselective NSAIDs, may interfere with aspirin's cardioprotective effect.

Use of NSAIDs can compromise existing renal function. Indomethacin is not recommended for patients with advanced renal disease. Use with caution in patients with decreased hepatic function.

[U.S. Boxed Warning]: NSAIDs may increase risk of gastrointestinal irritation, ulceration, bleeding, and perforation. Use caution with a history of GI disease (bleeding or ulcers), concurrent therapy with aspirin, anticoagulants and/or corticosteroids, smoking, use of alcohol, the elderly or debilitated patients.

Use the lowest effective dose for the shortest duration of time, consistent with individual patient goals, to reduce risk of cardiovascular or GI adverse events.

NSAIDs may cause serious skin adverse events including exfoliative dermatitis, Stevens-Johnson syndrome (SJS) and toxic epidermal necrolysis (TEN). Do not use in patients who experience bronchospasm, asthma, rhinitis, or urticaria with NSAID or aspirin therapy. Use caution in other forms of asthma.

The elderly are at increased risk for adverse effects (especially peptic ulceration, CNS effects, renal toxicity) from NSAIDs even at low doses. Prolonged use may cause corneal deposits and retinal disturbances; discontinue if visual changes are observed. Use caution with depression, epilepsy or Parkinson's disease.

Withhold for at least 4-6 half-lives prior to surgical or dental procedures.

Oral: Safety and efficacy have not been established in children <14 years of age. Hepatotoxicity has been reported in younger children treated for JRA. Closely monitor if use is needed in children ≥2 years of age.

Drug Interactions

Cytochrome P450 Effect: Substrate (minor) of CYP2C9, 2C19; **Inhibits** CYP2C9 (strong), 2C19 (weak)

Increased Effect/Toxicity: Indomethacin may increase effect/toxicity of anticoagulants (bleeding), antiplatelet agents (bleeding), aminoglycosides, biphosphonates (GI irritation), cyclosporine (nephrotoxicity), lithium, methotrexate, pemetrexed, treprostinil (bleeding), vancomycin. Tilundronate serum concentrations may be increased. Indomethacin may increase the levels/effects of bosentan, dapsone, fluoxetine, glimepiride, glipizide, losartan, montelukast, nateglinide, paclitaxel, phenytoin, warfarin, zafirlukast, and other CYP2C9 substrates. Concomitant use with fluoroquinolones may rarely increase risk of seizure. Indomethacin may enhance the nephrotoxic effect of triamterene. Probenecid may increase the serum concentration of NSAIDs.

Decreased Effect: May reduce effect of some diuretics and antihypertensive effect of beta-blockers, ACE inhibitors, hydralazine Cholestyramine and colestipol may reduce absorption of indomethacin. Salicylates' antiplatelet effect may be reduced.

Ethanol/Nutrition/Herb Interactions

Ethanol: Avoid ethanol (may enhance gastric mucosal irritation).

Food: Food may decrease the rate but not the extent of absorption. Indomethacin peak serum levels may be delayed if taken with food.

Herb/Nutraceutical: Avoid alfalfa, anise, bilberry, bladderwrack, bromelain, cat's claw, celery, coleus, cordyceps, dong quai, evening primrose, feverfew, fenugreek, garlic, ginger, ginkgo biloba, ginseng, grapeseed, green tea, guggul, horse chestnut seed, horseradish, licorice, prickly ash, red clover, reishi, SAMe, sweet clover, turmeric, white willow (all have additional antiplatelet activity).

Dietary Considerations May cause GI upset; take with food or milk to minimize

Pharmacodynamics/Kinetics
Onset of action: ~30 minutes
Duration: 4-6 hours
Absorption: Prompt and extensive
Distribution: V_d: 0.34-1.57 L/kg; crosses blood brain barrier and placenta; enters breast milk
Protein binding: 99%
Metabolism: Hepatic; significant enterohepatic recirculation
Bioavailability: 100%
Half-life elimination: 4.5 hours; prolonged in neonates
Time to peak: Oral: 2 hours
Excretion: Urine (60%, primarily as glucuronide conjugates); feces (33%, primarily as metabolites)

Pregnancy Risk Factor C/D (3rd trimester)

Dosage Forms
Capsule: 25 mg, 50 mg
Injection, powder for reconstitution:
Indocin® I.V.: 1 mg
Suspension, oral: 25 mg/5 mL
Indocin®: 25 mg/5 mL

Infliximab (in FLIKS e mab)

U.S. Brand Names Remicade®
Canadian Brand Names Remicade®
Mexican Brand Names Remicade
Generic Available No
Index Terms Infliximab, Recombinant; NSC-728729
Pharmacologic Category Antirheumatic, Disease Modifying; Gastrointestinal Agent, Miscellaneous; Monoclonal Antibody; Tumor Necrosis Factor (TNF) Blocking Agent
Use Treatment of rheumatoid arthritis (moderate-to-severe, with methotrexate); treatment of Crohn's disease (moderate-to-severe with inadequate response to conventional therapy) for induction and maintenance of remission, and/or to reduce the number of draining enterocutaneous and rectovaginal fistulas, and to maintain fistula closure; treatment of psoriatic arthritis; treatment of plaque psoriasis (chronic severe); treatment of ankylosing spondylitis; treatment of and maintenance of healing of ulcerative colitis (moderately- to severely-active with inadequate response to conventional therapy)

Note: In Canada, infliximab is not approved for use in children.

Unlabeled/Investigational Use Acute graft-versus-host disease (GVHD)
Local Anesthetic/Vasoconstrictor Precautions No information available to require special precautions
Effects on Dental Treatment No significant effects or complications reported
Common Adverse Effects Although profile is similar, frequency of adverse effects may vary with disease state. Except where noted, percentages reported in adults with rheumatoid arthritis:

>10%:
Central nervous system: Headache (18%)
Gastrointestinal: Nausea (21%), diarrhea (12%), abdominal pain (12%, Crohn's 26%)
Hepatic: ALT increased (risk increased with concomitant methotrexate)
Local: Infusion reactions (20%; severe: <1%)
Respiratory: Upper respiratory tract infection (32%), sinusitis (14%), cough (12%), pharyngitis (12%)
Miscellaneous: Development of antinuclear antibodies (~50%), infection (36%), development of antibodies to double-stranded DNA (17%); Crohn's patients with fistulizing disease: Development of new abscess (15%)
5% to 10%:
Cardiovascular: Hypertension (7%)
(Continued)

Infliximab (Continued)

Central nervous system: Fatigue (9%), pain (8%), fever (7%)
Dermatologic: Rash (1% to 10%), pruritus (7%)
Gastrointestinal: Dyspepsia (10%)
Genitourinary: Urinary tract infection (8%)
Neuromuscular & skeletal: Arthralgia (1% to 8%), back pain (8%)
Respiratory: Bronchitis (10%), rhinitis (8%), dyspnea (6%)
Miscellaneous: Moniliasis (5%)

The following adverse events were reported in children with Crohn's disease and were found more frequently in children than adults:
>10%:
Hepatic: Liver enzymes increased (18%; ≥5 times ULN: 1%)
Hematologic: Anemia (11%)
Miscellaneous: Infections (56%; more common with every 8-week versus every 12-week infusions)
1% to 10%:
Central nervous system: Flushing (9%)
Gastrointestinal: Blood in stool (10%)
Hematologic: Leukopenia (9%), neutropenia (7%)
Neuromuscular & skeletal: Bone fracture (7%)
Respiratory: Respiratory tract allergic reaction (6%)
Miscellaneous: Viral infection (8%), bacterial infection (6%), antibodies to infliximab (3%)

Restrictions An FDA-approved medication guide is available at www.fda.gov/cder/Offices/ODS/labeling.htm; distribute to each patient to whom this medication is dispensed.

Mechanism of Action Infliximab is a chimeric monoclonal antibody that binds to human tumor necrosis factor alpha (TNFα), thereby interfering with endogenous TNFα activity. Biological activities of TNFα include the induction of proinflammatory cytokines (interleukins), enhancement of leukocyte migration, activation of neutrophils and eosinophils, and the induction of acute phase reactants and tissue degrading enzymes. Animal models have shown TNFα expression causes polyarthritis, and infliximab can prevent disease as well as allow diseased joints to heal.

Drug Interactions
Increased Effect/Toxicity: Specific drug interaction studies have not been conducted. Anti-TNF agents may be associated with increased risk of serious infection when used in combination with anakinra. Abciximab may increase potential for hypersensitivity reaction to infliximab, and may increase risk of thrombocytopenia and/or reduced therapeutic efficacy of infliximab. Infliximab may enhance the adverse/toxic effects of abatacept and live vaccines.

Decreased Effect: Infliximab may decrease the effect of vaccines (dead organisms).

Pharmacodynamics/Kinetics
Onset of action: Crohn's disease: ~2 weeks
Half-life elimination: 8-9.5 days

Pregnancy Risk Factor B

Infliximab, Recombinant see Infliximab on page 879

Influenza Virus Vaccine (in floo EN za VYE rus vak SEEN)

Related Information
Immunizations (Vaccines) on page 1886
U.S. Brand Names Fluarix®; FluLaval™; fluMist®; Fluvirin®; Fluzone®
Canadian Brand Names Fluviral S/F®; Vaxigrip®
Mexican Brand Names Fluarix
Generic Available No
Index Terms Influenza Virus Vaccine (Purified Surface Antigen); Influenza Virus Vaccine (Split-Virus); Influenza Virus Vaccine (Trivalent, Live); Live Attenuated Influenza Vaccine (LAIV); Trivalent Inactivated Influenza Vaccine (TIV)
Pharmacologic Category Vaccine
Use Provide active immunity to influenza virus strains contained in the vaccine

Groups at Increased Risk for Influenza-Related Complications: Advisory Committee on Immunization Practices (ACIP) recommendations for vaccination:
• Persons ≥50 years of age
• Residents of nursing homes and other chronic-care facilities that house persons of any age with chronic medical conditions
• Adults and children with chronic disorders of the pulmonary or cardiovascular systems, including asthma

- Adults and children who have required regular medical follow-up or hospitalization during the preceding year because of chronic metabolic diseases (including diabetes mellitus), renal dysfunction, hemoglobinopathies, or immunosuppression (including immunosuppression caused by medications or HIV)
- Adults and children with conditions which may compromise respiratory function, the handling of respiratory secretions, or that can increase the risk of aspiration (eg, cognitive dysfunction, spinal; cord injuries, seizure disorders, other neuromuscular disorders)
- Children and adolescents (6 months to 18 years of age) who are receiving long-term aspirin therapy and therefore, may be at risk for developing Reye's syndrome after influenza
- Women who will be pregnant during the influenza season
- Children 6-59 months of age

Vaccination is also recommended for close contacts of children 0-59 months of age, healthy persons who may transmit influenza to those at risk, and all healthcare workers.

Local Anesthetic/Vasoconstrictor Precautions No information available to require special precautions

Effects on Dental Treatment No significant effects or complications reported

Common Adverse Effects All serious adverse reactions must be reported to the U.S. Department of Health and Human Services (DHHS) Vaccine Adverse Event Reporting System (VAERS) 1-800-822-7967.

Injection:

Frequency not defined.

Central nervous system: Chills; fever and malaise (may start within 6-12 hours and last 1-2 days; incidence equal to placebo in adults; occurs more frequently than placebo in children); Guillain-Barré syndrome (GBS)

Dermatologic: Angioedema, rash, urticaria

Local: Tenderness, redness, or induration at the site of injection (10% to 64%; may last up to 2 days); injection site pain

Neuromuscular & skeletal: Myalgia (may start within 6-12 hours and last 1-2 days; incidence equal to placebo in adults; occurs more frequently than placebo in children)

Miscellaneous: Allergic or anaphylactoid reactions (most likely to residual egg protein; includes allergic asthma, angioedema, hives, systemic anaphylaxis)

Postmarketing and/or case reports: Seizure (rare; majority associated with fever)

Nasal spray: Frequency of events reported within 10 days

>10%:

Central nervous system: Headache (children 18% after first dose, < placebo after second dose; adults 40%) irritability (children 10% to 18%)

Neuromuscular & skeletal: Tiredness/weakness (adults 26%), muscle aches (children 5% to 6%; adults 17%)

Respiratory: Cough (children 26% to 38%; adults 14%), nasal congestion/runny nose (children 46% to 48%; adults 9% to 45%), sore throat (children < placebo; adults 28%)

Miscellaneous: Activity decreased (children 14% after first dose, < placebo after second dose)

1% to 10%:

Central nervous system: Chills

Gastrointestinal: Abdominal pain, diarrhea, vomiting

Otic: Otitis media

Respiratory: Rhinitis, sinusitis

Mechanism of Action Promotes immunity to influenza virus by inducing specific antibody production. Each year the formulation is standardized according to the U.S. Public Health Service. Preparations from previous seasons must not be used.

Drug Interactions

Increased Effect/Toxicity: Concomitant use of aspirin and the nasal spray formulation may increase the risk of Reye syndrome in patients 5-17 years; concomitant use in this age group is contraindicated.

Decreased Effect: Decreased effect with immunosuppressive agents; some manufacturers and clinicians recommend that the flu vaccine not be administered concomitantly with DTP due to the potential for increased febrile reactions (specifically whole-cell pertussis) and that one should wait at least 3 days. However, ACIP recommends that children at high risk for influenza may get the vaccine concomitantly with DTP. Safety and efficacy of nasal spray with other vaccines have not been established; do not give within 1 month of other live virus vaccines or within 2 weeks of inactivated or subunit vaccines. Live virus vaccines may diminish the diagnostic effect of tuberculin tests. Efficacy of influenza (live) vaccines may be diminished (live virus vaccinations should be withheld for as long as 6 months).

(Continued)

Influenza Virus Vaccine *(Continued)*

Pharmacodynamics/Kinetics
Onset: Protective antibody titers achieved ~2 weeks after vaccination
Duration: Protective antibody titers persist approximately ≥6 months. Elderly: Protective antibody titers may fall ≤4 months after vaccination.

Pregnancy Risk Factor C

Influenza Virus Vaccine (H5N1)
(in floo EN za VYE rus vak SEEN H5N1)

Generic Available No

Index Terms Avian Influenza Virus Vaccine; Bird Flu Vaccine; H5N1 Influenza Vaccine; Influenza Virus Vaccine (Monovalent)

Pharmacologic Category Vaccine

Use Active immunization of adults at increased risk of exposure to the H5N1 viral subtype of influenza

Local Anesthetic/Vasoconstrictor Precautions No information available to require special precautions

Effects on Dental Treatment No significant effects or complications reported

Common Adverse Effects All serious adverse reactions must be reported to the U.S. Department of Health and Human Services (DHHS) Vaccine Adverse Event Reporting System (VAERS) 1-800-822-7967.

>10%:
Central nervous system: Headache (3% to 36%), malaise (22%)
Local: Pain (74%), tenderness (70%), erythema/redness (20%), induration/swelling (15%)
Neuromuscular & skeletal: Myalgia (16%)

1% to 10%:
Central nervous system: Fever (up to 7%)
Gastrointestinal: Nausea (10%), diarrhea (6%)
Respiratory: Nasopharyngitis (2%), upper respiratory infection (2%), nasal congestion (1%)

Additional reactions observed with other influenza vaccine formulations: Allergic reaction, anaphylaxis, angioedema, asthma, encephalopathy, facial paralysis, hives, GBS, neuropathy, optic neuritis, vasculitis

Restrictions Commercial distribution is not planned. The vaccine will be included as part of the U.S. Strategic National Stockpile. It will be distributed by public health officials if needed.

Mechanism of Action A monovalent, split virus (inactivated) preparation of the H5N1 avian strain of influenza virus (A/Vietnam/1203/2004) which promotes active immunity to avian influenza.

Drug Interactions
Decreased Effect: Decreased protective effect of vaccine with immunosuppressive agents.

Pharmacodynamics/Kinetics Onset of action: Four-fold increase in antibody titers occurred in up to 58% of patients 28 days after second dose.

Pregnancy Risk Factor C

Insulin Aspart (IN soo lin AS part)

Related Information
Insulin Regular *on page 889*
U.S. Brand Names NovoLog®
Canadian Brand Names NovoRapid®
Generic Available No
Index Terms Aspart Insulin
Pharmacologic Category Antidiabetic Agent, Insulin
Use Treatment of type 1 diabetes mellitus (insulin dependent, IDDM); type 2 diabetes mellitus (noninsulin dependent, NIDDM) to control hyperglycemia
Local Anesthetic/Vasoconstrictor Precautions No information available to require special precautions
Effects on Dental Treatment Type 1 diabetics (insulin dependent) should be appointed for dental treatment in the morning in order to minimize chance of stress-induced hypoglycemia.
Mechanism of Action Refer to Insulin Regular *on page 889*. Insulin aspart is a rapid-acting insulin analog.
Drug Interactions
Increased Effect/Toxicity: Refer to Insulin Regular *on page 889*.
Pharmacodynamics/Kinetics
Onset of action: 0.2-0.5 hours
Duration: 3-5 hours
Protein binding: 0% to 9%
Half-life elimination: 81 minutes
Time to peak: 1-3 hours
Excretion: Urine
Pregnancy Risk Factor B

Insulin Aspart and Insulin Aspart Protamine *see* Insulin Aspart Protamine and Insulin Aspart *on page 883*

Insulin Aspart Protamine and Insulin Aspart
(IN soo lin AS part PROE ta meen & IN soo lin AS part)

Related Information
Insulin Regular *on page 889*
U.S. Brand Names NovoLog® Mix 70/30
Canadian Brand Names NovoMix® 30
Generic Available No
Index Terms Insulin Aspart and Insulin Aspart Protamine
Pharmacologic Category Antidiabetic Agent, Insulin
Use Treatment of type 1 diabetes mellitus (insulin dependent, IDDM); type 2 diabetes mellitus (noninsulin dependent, NIDDM) to control hyperglycemia
Local Anesthetic/Vasoconstrictor Precautions No information available to require special precautions
Effects on Dental Treatment Type 1 diabetics (insulin dependent) should be appointed for dental treatment in the morning in order to minimize chance of stress-induced hypoglycemia.
Common Adverse Effects Refer to Insulin Regular *on page 889*.
Mechanism of Action Refer to Insulin Regular *on page 889*. Insulin aspart protamine and insulin aspart is a combination insulin product with intermediate-acting characteristics. Normally administered twice daily.
Pharmacodynamics/Kinetics
Onset of action: 0.2 hours
Duration: 18-24 hours
Half-life: 8-9 hours
Time to peak: 1-4 hours
Excretion: Urine
Pregnancy Risk Factor C

Insulin Detemir (IN soo lin DE te mir)

Related Information
Insulin Regular *on page 889*
U.S. Brand Names Levemir®
Canadian Brand Names Levemir®
Generic Available No
(Continued)

Insulin Detemir *(Continued)*

Index Terms Detemir Insulin

Pharmacologic Category Antidiabetic Agent, Insulin

Use Treatment of type 1 diabetes mellitus (insulin dependent, IDDM); type 2 diabetes mellitus (noninsulin dependent, NIDDM) to control hyperglycemia

Local Anesthetic/Vasoconstrictor Precautions No information available to require special precautions

Effects on Dental Treatment Type 1 diabetics (insulin dependent) should be appointed for dental treatment in the morning in order to minimize chance of stress-induced hypoglycemia.

Common Adverse Effects Refer to Insulin Regular *on page 889*.

Mechanism of Action Refer to Insulin Regular *on page 889*. Insulin detemir differs from human insulin by a single amino acid omission (threonine at B30) and the addition of a 14-carbon fatty acid chain attached at the B29 position. On injection, the fatty acid chain facilitates self-association between the molecules as well as binding to albumin. The delayed release of insulin from the injection site and albumin binding sites result in more prolonged action and limits variability in the amount of free insulin at steady-state. Insulin detemir has a duration of action which is dose-dependent. The FDA-approved product labeling identifies this product as a long-acting insulin analog; however, at lower dosages (<0.6 units/kg) published data regarding its duration of action is consistent with an intermediate insulin form (12-20 hours). In clinical trials it has been compared primarily with NPH insulin and dosed in a similar manner. In some patients, or at higher dosages, it may have a duration of action up to 24 hours, which is consistent with a long-acting insulin.

Drug Interactions

Cytochrome P450 Effect: Refer to Insulin Regular *on page 889*.

Increased Effect/Toxicity: Refer to Insulin Regular *on page 889*.

Pharmacodynamics/Kinetics

Onset of action: 3-4 hours

Duration: Dose dependent: 6-23 hours

Note: Duration is dose-dependent. At lower dosages (0.1-0.2 units/kg), mean duration is variable (5.7-12.1 hours). At 0.6 units/kg, the mean duration was 19.9 hours. At high dosages (>0.6 units/kg) the duration is longer and less variable (mean of 22-23 hours).

Bioavailability: 60%

Half-life: 5-7 hours (dose dependent)

Protein binding: >98% (albumin)

Distribution: V_d: 0.1 L/kg

Time to peak: 6-8 hours

Excretion: Urine

Pregnancy Risk Factor C

Insulin Glargine *(IN soo lin GLAR jeen)*

Related Information

Insulin Regular *on page 889*

U.S. Brand Names Lantus®

Canadian Brand Names Lantus®; Lantus® OptiSet®

Mexican Brand Names Lantus

Generic Available No

Index Terms Glargine Insulin

Pharmacologic Category Antidiabetic Agent, Insulin

Use Treatment of type 1 diabetes mellitus (insulin dependent, IDDM); type 2 diabetes mellitus (noninsulin dependent, NIDDM) requiring basal (long-acting) insulin to control hyperglycemia

Local Anesthetic/Vasoconstrictor Precautions No information available to require special precautions

Effects on Dental Treatment Type 1 diabetics (insulin dependent) should be appointed for dental treatment in the morning in order to minimize chance of stress-induced hypoglycemia.

Common Adverse Effects Refer to Insulin Regular *on page 889*.

Mechanism of Action Refer to Insulin Regular *on page 889*. Insulin glargine is a long-acting insulin analog.

Drug Interactions

Cytochrome P450 Effect: Refer to Insulin Regular *on page 889*.

Increased Effect/Toxicity: Refer to Insulin Regular *on page 889*.

Pharmacodynamics/Kinetics

Onset of action: 3-4 hours

Duration: 24 hours

Absorption: Slow; forms microprecipitates which allow small amounts to release over time

Metabolism: Partially metabolized in the skin to form teo active metabolites

Time to peak: No pronounced peak

Excretion: Urine

Pregnancy Risk Factor C

Insulin Glulisine (IN soo lin gloo LIS een)

Related Information
Insulin Regular on page 889

U.S. Brand Names Apidra®

Canadian Brand Names Apidra®

Generic Available No

Index Terms Glulisine Insulin

Pharmacologic Category Antidiabetic Agent, Insulin

Use Treatment of type 1 diabetes mellitus (insulin dependent, IDDM); type 2 diabetes mellitus (noninsulin dependent, NIDDM) to control hyperglycemia

Local Anesthetic/Vasoconstrictor Precautions No information available to require special precautions

Effects on Dental Treatment Type 1 diabetics (insulin dependent) should be appointed for dental treatment in the morning in order to minimize chance of stress-induced hypoglycemia.

Common Adverse Effects Refer to Insulin Regular on page 889.

Mechanism of Action Refer to Insulin Regular on page 889. Insulin glulisine is a rapid-acting insulin analog. Insulin glulisine differs from human insulin by the replacement of two amino acids on the B-chain (positions B3 and B29).

Drug Interactions
Increased Effect/Toxicity: Refer to Insulin Regular on page 889.

Pharmacodynamics/Kinetics
Onset of action: 0.2-0.5 hours
Duration: 3-4 hours
Time to Peak: 30-90 minutes
Excretion: Urine

Pregnancy Risk Factor C

Insulin Inhalation (IN soo lin in ha LAY shun)

Related Information
Insulin Regular on page 889

U.S. Brand Names Exubera®

Canadian Brand Names Exubera®

Index Terms Inhaled Insulin

Pharmacologic Category Antidiabetic Agent, Insulin

Use Treatment of type 1 diabetes mellitus (insulin dependent, IDDM); type 2 diabetes mellitus (noninsulin dependent, NIDDM)

Local Anesthetic/Vasoconstrictor Precautions No information available to require special precautions

Effects on Dental Treatment Key adverse event(s) related to dental treatment: Xerostomia and changes in salivation (normal salivary flow resumes upon discontinuation). Type 1 diabetics (insulin dependent) should be appointed for dental treatment in the morning in order to minimize chance of stress-induced hypoglycemia.

Common Adverse Effects Also refer to Insulin Regular on page 889.

Cardiovascular: Chest pain (5%; usually mild to moderate)

Dermatologic: Rash (rare)

Endocrine & metabolic: Hypoglycemia

Gastrointestinal: Xerostomia (2%)

Otic: Otitis media (pediatric patients 7%), ear pain (4%), ear disorder (1%)

Respiratory: Respiratory infection (30% to 43%), cough increased (22% to 30%), pharyngitis (10% to 18%), rhinitis (9% to 15%), sinusitis (5% to 10%), dyspnea (3% to 4%), sputum increased (3% to 4%), bronchitis (3% to 5%), epistaxis (1%), laryngitis (1%), voice alteration (1%), bronchospasm (rare)

    Note: Decreases in pulmonary function (reduced FEV1, DLco) have been associated with use, usually noted in the initial weeks of therapy; declines from baseline of 20% in, respectively, FEV1 and DLco, were reported in 1.5% and 5.1% of patients as compared to 1.3% and 3.6% in comparator-treated patients.

Miscellaneous: Allergic reactions, anaphylaxis (including tachycardia and hypotension), diaphoresis increased

(Continued)

Insulin Inhalation *(Continued)*

Restrictions An FDA-approved medication guide must be distributed when dispensing an outpatient prescription (new or refill) where this medication is to be used without direct supervision of a healthcare provider. Medication guides are available at http://www.fda.gov/cder/Offices/ODS/medication_guides.htm.

Dosage Inhalation: Children ≥6 years and Adults:

Initial: 0.05 mg/kg (rounded down to nearest whole milligram) 3 times/daily administered within 10 minutes of a meal

Adjustment: Dosage may be increased or decreased based on serum glucose monitoring, meal size, nutrient composition, time of day, and exercise patterns.

Note: A 1 mg blister is approximately equivalent to 3 units of regular insulin, while a 3 mg blister is approximately equivalent to 8 units of regular insulin administered subcutaneously. Patients should combine 1 mg and 3 mg blisters so that the fewest blisters are required to achieve the prescribed dose. Consecutive inhalation of three 1 mg blisters results in significantly higher insulin levels as compared to inhalation of a single 3 mg blister (do not substitute). In a patient stabilized on a dosage which uses 3 mg blisters, if 3 mg blister is temporarily unavailable, inhalation of two 1 mg blisters may be substituted.

Dosing adjustment in renal impairment: Insulin requirements are reduced due to changes in insulin clearance or metabolism.

Mechanism of Action Refer to Insulin Regular *on page 889*. Insulin inhalation is a rapid-acting form of human insulin.

Contraindications Hypersensitivity to any component of the formulation; smokers or patients who have discontinued smoking for <6 months; poorly-controlled or unstable lung disease

Warnings/Precautions Also refer to Insulin Regular *on page 889*.

Due to increased systemic absorption, the risk of hypoglycemia is greatly increased in patients who smoke or who have stopped smoking for less than 6 months. The effect of passive exposure to smoke has not been fully evaluated but may result in alteration in absorption and/or hypoglycemia. Insulin inhalation should be immediately discontinued in any patient who resumes smoking.

Decreases in pulmonary function have been associated with use. Due the potential impact on pulmonary function, testing should be performed prior to the initiation of inhaled insulin therapy. Not recommended for use in patients with lung disease (asthma, COPD). Monitor closely during periods of intercurrent respiratory illness.

In type 1 diabetes mellitus (insulin dependent, IDDM), rapid-acting insulins including insulin inhalation should be used in combination with a long-acting insulin. However, in type 2 diabetes mellitus (noninsulin dependent, NIDDM), rapid-acting agents may be used without a long-acting insulin when used as monotherapy or combined with an oral antidiabetic agent.

Use caution in renal and/or hepatic impairment.

Drug Interactions

Cytochrome P450 Effect: Refer to Insulin Regular *on page 889*.

Increased Effect/Toxicity: Refer to Insulin Regular *on page 889*.

Decreased Effect: Refer to Insulin Regular *on page 889*.

Ethanol/Nutrition/Herb Interactions Refer to Insulin Regular *on page 889*.

Dietary Considerations Dietary modification based on ADA recommendations is a key component of therapy.

Pharmacodynamics/Kinetics

Onset of action: 0.2-0.4 hours

Duration: 6-8 hours

Absorption: Rapid

Bioavailability: Absolute bioavailability not defined (depends on inspiratory flow characteristics); systemic exposure may be up to 2-5 times higher in smokers

Time to peak, plasma: 30-90 minutes

Excretion: Urine

Pregnancy Risk Factor C

Dosage Forms

Combination package:

Exubera® Kit [packaged with inhaler, chamber and release unit]:

Powder for oral inhalation: 1 mg/blister (180s) and 3 mg/blister (90s)

Exubera® Combination Pack 15 [packaged with 2 release units]:

Powder for oral inhalation: 1 mg/blister (180s) and 3 mg/blister (90s)

Exubera® Combination Pack 12 [packaged with 2 release units:]

Powder for oral inhalation 1 mg/blister (90s) and 3 mg/blister (90s)

Selected Readings
Skyler JS, Weinstock RS, and Raskin P, "Use of Inhaled Insulin in a Basal/Bolus Insulin Regimen in Type 1 Diabetic Subjects: A 6-Month, Randomized, Comparative Trial," *Diabetes Care*, 2005, 28(7):1630-5.

Insulin Lispro (IN soo lin LYE sproe)

Related Information
Insulin Regular *on page 889*
U.S. Brand Names Humalog®
Canadian Brand Names Humalog®
Mexican Brand Names Humalog Lispro
Generic Available No
Index Terms Lispro Insulin
Pharmacologic Category Antidiabetic Agent, Insulin
Use Treatment of type 1 diabetes mellitus (insulin dependent, IDDM); type 2 diabetes mellitus (noninsulin dependent, NIDDM) to control hyperglycemia
  Note: In type 1 diabetes mellitus (insulin dependent, IDDM), insulin lispro (Humalog®) should be used in combination with a long-acting insulin. However, in type 2 diabetes mellitus (noninsulin dependent, NIDDM), insulin lispro (Humalog®) may be used without a long-acting insulin when used in combination with a sulfonylurea.
Local Anesthetic/Vasoconstrictor Precautions No information available to require special precautions
Effects on Dental Treatment Type 1 diabetics (insulin dependent) should be appointed for dental treatment in the morning in order to minimize chance of stress-induced hypoglycemia.
Common Adverse Effects Refer to Insulin Regular *on page 889*.
Mechanism of Action Refer to Insulin Regular *on page 889*. Insulin lispro is a rapid-acting form of insulin.
Drug Interactions
  Cytochrome P450 Effect: Refer to Insulin Regular *on page 889*.
  Increased Effect/Toxicity: Refer to Insulin Regular *on page 889*.
Pharmacodynamics/Kinetics
  Onset of action: 0.2-0.5 hours
  Duration: 3-4 hours
  Distribution: 0.26-0.36 L/kg
  Bioavailability: 55% to 77%
  Time to peak: 30-90 minutes
  Excretion: Urine
Pregnancy Risk Factor B

Insulin Lispro and Insulin Lispro Protamine *see* Insulin Lispro Protamine and Insulin Lispro *on page 887*

Insulin Lispro Protamine and Insulin Lispro
(IN soo lin LYE sproe PROE ta meen & IN soo lin LYE sproe)

Related Information
Insulin Regular *on page 889*
U.S. Brand Names Humalog® Mix 50/50™; Humalog® Mix 75/25™
Canadian Brand Names Humalog® Mix 25
Mexican Brand Names Humalog Mix 25
Generic Available No
Index Terms Insulin Lispro and Insulin Lispro Protamine
Pharmacologic Category Antidiabetic Agent, Insulin
Use Treatment of type 1 diabetes mellitus (insulin dependent, IDDM); type 2 diabetes mellitus (noninsulin dependent, NIDDM) to control hyperglycemia
Local Anesthetic/Vasoconstrictor Precautions No information available to require special precautions
Effects on Dental Treatment Type 1 diabetics (insulin-dependent) should be appointed for dental treatment in the morning in order to minimize chance of stress-induced hypoglycemia.
Common Adverse Effects Refer to Insulin Regular *on page 889*.
Mechanism of Action Refer to Insulin Regular *on page 889*. Insulin lispro protamine and insulin lispro is a combination product with a rapid onset, and a duration of action which is similar to intermediate-acting insulin products.
Drug Interactions
  Increased Effect/Toxicity: Refer to Insulin Regular *on page 889*.
Pharmacodynamics/Kinetics
  Onset of action: 0.2-0.5 hours
  Duration: 18-24 hours
  (Continued)

Insulin Lispro Protamine and Insulin Lispro
(Continued)
Time to peak: 2-12 hours
Excretion: Urine
Pregnancy Risk Factor B

Insulin NPH (IN soo lin N P H)

Related Information
Insulin Regular *on page 889*
U.S. Brand Names Humulin® N; Novolin® N
Canadian Brand Names Humulin® N; Novolin® ge NPH
Mexican Brand Names Humulin N; Novolin N
Generic Available No
Index Terms Isophane Insulin; NPH Insulin
Pharmacologic Category Antidiabetic Agent, Insulin
Use Treatment of type 1 diabetes mellitus (insulin dependent, IDDM); type 2 diabetes mellitus (noninsulin dependent, NIDDM) to control hyperglycemia
Local Anesthetic/Vasoconstrictor Precautions No information available to require special precautions
Effects on Dental Treatment Type 1 diabetics (insulin dependent) should be appointed for dental treatment in the morning in order to minimize chance of stress-induced hypoglycemia.
Common Adverse Effects Refer to Insulin Regular *on page 889*.
Mechanism of Action Refer to Insulin Regular *on page 889*. Insulin NPH is an intermediate-acting form of insulin.
Drug Interactions
Cytochrome P450 Effect: Refer to Insulin Regular *on page 889*.
Increased Effect/Toxicity: Refer to Insulin Regular *on page 889*.
Pharmacodynamics/Kinetics
Onset of action: 1-2 hours
Duration: 18-24 hours
Time to peak: 6-12 hours
Excretion: Urine
Pregnancy Risk Factor B

Insulin NPH and Insulin Regular
(IN soo lin N P H & IN soo lin REG yoo ler)

Related Information
Insulin Regular *on page 889*
U.S. Brand Names Humulin® 50/50; Humulin® 70/30; Novolin® 70/30
Canadian Brand Names Humulin® 20/80; Humulin® 70/30; Novolin® ge 10/90; Novolin® ge 20/80; Novolin® ge 30/70; Novolin® ge 40/60; Novolin® ge 50/50
Mexican Brand Names Humulin 30 70; Novolin 70/30
Generic Available No
Index Terms Insulin Regular and Insulin NPH; Isophane Insulin and Regular Insulin; NPH Insulin and Regular Insulin
Pharmacologic Category Antidiabetic Agent, Insulin
Use Treatment of type 1 diabetes mellitus (insulin dependent, IDDM); type 2 diabetes mellitus (noninsulin dependent, NIDDM) to control hyperglycemia
Local Anesthetic/Vasoconstrictor Precautions No information available to require special precautions
Effects on Dental Treatment Type 1 diabetics (insulin dependent) should be appointed for dental treatment in the morning in order to minimize chance of stress-induced hypoglycemia.
Mechanism of Action Refer to Insulin Regular *on page 889*. Insulin NPH and insulin regular is a combination insulin product with intermediate-acting characteristics. It may be administered once or twice daily.
Pharmacodynamics/Kinetics
Onset of action: 0.5 hours
Duration: 18-24 hours
Time to peak: 2-12 hours
Excretion: Urine
Pregnancy Risk Factor C

Insulin Regular (IN soo lin REG yoo ler)

Related Information
Insulin Aspart *on page 883*
Insulin Aspart Protamine and Insulin Aspart *on page 883*
Insulin Detemir *on page 883*
Insulin Glargine *on page 884*
Insulin Glulisine *on page 885*
Insulin Lispro *on page 887*
Insulin Lispro Protamine and Insulin Lispro *on page 887*
Insulin NPH *on page 888*
Insulin NPH and Insulin Regular *on page 888*

U.S. Brand Names Humulin® R; Humulin® R (Concentrated) U-500; Novolin® R

Canadian Brand Names Humulin® R; Novolin® ge Toronto

Generic Available No

Index Terms Regular Insulin

Pharmacologic Category Antidiabetic Agent, Insulin; Antidote

Use Treatment of type 1 diabetes mellitus (insulin dependent, IDDM); type 2 diabetes mellitus (noninsulin dependent, NIDDM) unresponsive to treatment with diet and/or oral hypoglycemics, to control hyperglycemia; adjunct to parenteral nutrition; diabetic ketoacidosis (DKA)

Unlabeled/Investigational Use Hyperkalemia (regular insulin only; use with glucose to shift potassium into cells to lower serum potassium levels)

Local Anesthetic/Vasoconstrictor Precautions No information available to require special precautions

Effects on Dental Treatment Type 1 diabetics (insulin dependent) should be appointed for dental treatment in the morning in order to minimize chance of stress-induced hypoglycemia.

Common Adverse Effects Frequency not defined.
Cardiovascular: Palpitation, pallor, tachycardia
Central nervous system: Fatigue, headache, hypothermia, loss of consciousness, mental confusion
Dermatologic: Urticaria, redness
Endocrine & metabolic: Hypoglycemia
Gastrointestinal: Hunger, nausea, numbness of mouth
Local: Atrophy or hypertrophy of SubQ fat tissue; edema, itching, pain or warmth at injection site; stinging
Neuromuscular & skeletal: Muscle weakness, paresthesia, tremor
Ocular: Transient presbyopia or blurred vision
Miscellaneous: Anaphylaxis, diaphoresis, local allergy, systemic allergic symptoms

Mechanism of Action Insulin acts via specific membrane-bound receptors on target tissues to regulate metabolism of carbohydrate, protein, and fats. Insulin facilitates entry of glucose into muscle, adipose, and other tissues via hexose transporters, including GLUT4. Insulin stimulates the cellular uptake of amino acids and increases cellular permeability to several ions, including potassium, magnesium, and phosphate. By activating sodium-potassium ATPases, insulin promotes the intracellular movement of potassium.

Target organs for insulin include the liver, skeletal muscle, and adipose tissue. Within the liver, insulin stimulates hepatic glycogen synthesis through the activation of the enzymes hexokinase, phosphofructokinase, and glycogen synthase as well as the inhibition of glucose-6 phosphatase. Insulin promotes hepatic synthesis of fatty acids, which are released into the circulation as lipoproteins. Skeletal muscle effects of insulin include increased protein synthesis and increased glycogen synthesis. Within adipose tissue, insulin stimulates the processing of circulating lipoproteins to provide free fatty acids, facilitating triglyceride synthesis and storage by adipocytes. Insulin also directly inhibits the hydrolysis of triglycerides.

Normally secreted by the pancreas, insulin products are manufactured for pharmacologic use through recombinant DNA technology using either *E. coli* or *Saccharomyces cerevisiae*. Insulins are categorized based on promptness and duration of effect, including rapid-, short-, intermediate-, and long-acting insulins.

Drug Interactions
Cytochrome P450 Effect: Induces CYP1A2 (weak)

Increased Effect/Toxicity: Increased hypoglycemic effect of insulin with alcohol, alpha-blockers, anabolic steroids, beta-blockers (nonselective beta-blockers may delay recovery from hypoglycemic episodes and mask signs/symptoms of hypoglycemia; cardioselective beta-blocker agents may be alternatives), clofibrate, guanethidine, MAO inhibitors, pentamidine, phenylbutazone, salicylates, sulfinpyrazone, and tetracyclines.
(Continued)

Insulin Regular (Continued)

Insulin increases the risk of hypoglycemia associated with oral hypoglycemic agents (including sulfonylureas, metformin, pioglitazone, rosiglitazone, and troglitazone).

Decreased Effect: Decreased hypoglycemic effect of insulin with corticosteroids, dextrothyroxine, diltiazem, dobutamine, epinephrine, niacin, oral contraceptives, thiazide diuretics, thyroid hormone, and smoking.

Pharmacodynamics/Kinetics
Onset of action: 0.5 hours
Duration: 6-8 hours (may increase with dose)
Time to peak: 2-4 hours
Excretion: Urine

Pregnancy Risk Factor B

Insulin Regular and Insulin NPH see Insulin NPH and Insulin Regular on page 888

Intal® see Cromolyn on page 417

Integrilin® see Eptifibatide on page 582

α-2-interferon see Interferon Alfa-2b on page 891

Interferon Alfa-2a (PEG Conjugate) see Peginterferon Alfa-2a on page 1262

Interferon Alfa-2b and Ribavirin Combination Pack see Interferon Alfa-2b and Ribavirin on page 895

Interferon Alfa-2b (PEG Conjugate) see Peginterferon Alfa-2b on page 1263

Interferon Alfa-2a (in ter FEER on AL fa too aye)

Related Information
Systemic Viral Diseases on page 1767
U.S. Brand Names Roferon®-A
Canadian Brand Names Roferon®-A
Mexican Brand Names Roferon-A; Roquiferon
Generic Available No
Index Terms IFLrA; Interferon Alpha-2a; NSC-367982; rIFN-A
Pharmacologic Category Interferon
Use

Patients >18 years of age: Treatment of hairy cell leukemia, chronic hepatitis C
Children and Adults: Treatment of Philadelphia chromosome-positive (Ph+) chronic myelogenous leukemia (CML) in chronic phase, within 1 year of diagnosis (limited experience in children)

Unlabeled/Investigational Use Adjuvant therapy for malignant melanoma; treatment of AIDS-related Kaposi's sarcoma, carcinoid tumors; bladder, cervical, and ovarian cancers; hemangioma; chronic hepatitis D; low-grade non-Hodgkin's lymphoma; multiple myeloma; renal cell carcinoma; basal and squamous cell skin cancer; cutaneous T-cell lymphoma

Local Anesthetic/Vasoconstrictor Precautions No information available to require special precautions

Effects on Dental Treatment Key adverse event(s) related to dental treatment: Significant xerostomia (normal salivary flow resumes upon discontinuation), metallic taste, taste change, loss of taste, cough, irritation of oropharynx, dry throat, and stomatitis.

Common Adverse Effects Note: A flu-like syndrome (fever, chills, tachycardia, malaise, myalgia, arthralgia, headache) occurs within 1-2 hours of administration; may last up to 24 hours and may be dose-limiting.

>10%:
Cardiovascular: Chest pain (<4% to 11%), edema (1% to 11%), hypertension (11%)
Central nervous system: Fever (28% to 92%), fatigue (58% with 88%), headache (44% to 64%), chills (23% to 64%), depression (16% to 28%), pain (24%), dizziness (11% to 21%), mental status decreased (10% to 16%), irritability (15%), insomnia (14%), sleep disturbances (10% to 11%)
Dermatologic: Rash (8% to 44%), alopecia (17% to 19%), pruritus (7% to 13%), dry skin (7% to 17%)
Endocrine & metabolic: Hypocalcemia (28%), hypophosphatemia (22%)
Gastrointestinal: Anorexia (14% to 48%), nausea (33% to 39%), vomiting (33% to 39%), diarrhea (20% to 37%), weight loss (33%), throat irritation (21%), abdominal pain (12%)
Hematologic (often due to underlying disease): Myelosuppression (onset: 7-10 days; nadir 14 days [may be delayed 20-40 days in hairy cell leukemia], recovery: 21 days), neutropenia (≤68%; dose dependant); thrombocytopenia (5% to 62%), leukopenia (2% to 45%), anemia (≤31%)

Hepatic: Alkaline phosphatase increased (≤50%), transaminases increased (≤50%)

Local: Injection site reaction (29%)

Neuromuscular & skeletal: Weakness (6% to 88%) myalgia (51% to 71%), arthralgia (47% to 51%), bone pain (25% to 47%), joint pain (25%), back pain (16%), numbness (12%), paresthesia (7% to 12%)

Respiratory: Cough (1% to 19%), rhinorrhea/rhinitis (3% to 12%), dyspnea (1% to 12%), pneumonia (11%), sinusitis (11%)

Miscellaneous: Flu-like syndrome (16% to 33%), diaphoresis (1% to 22%)

1% to 10%:

Cardiovascular: Dysrhythmia (7%), hypotension (<5%), syncope (<5%), murmur (<5%), thrombophlebitis (<5%), palpitations (<3%), vasculitis (<3%), arrhythmia (1%)

Central nervous system: Confusion (<4% to 7%), anxiety (5% to 6%), lethargy (1% to 6%), nervousness (<5%), vertigo (<5%), concentration impaired (4%), memory loss (<4%), seizure (<4%), behavior disturbances (3%), malaise (1%)

Dermatologic: Bruising (<4%), skin lesions (1% to 3%)

Endocrine & metabolic: Hyperphosphatemia (9%), diabetes (<5%), hyper-/hypothyroidism (<5%), hypertriglyceridemia (<4%), libido changes (<4%), sexual dysfunction (1% to 3%), menstrual irregularity (2%)

Gastrointestinal: Colitis (<5%), gastrointestinal hemorrhage (<5%), pancreatitis (<5%), flatulence (3%), taste change (3% to <4%), stomatitis (1% to <5%), constipation (<3%), digestion impaired (2%), gingival bleeding (≤2%)

Genitourinary: Impotence (<4%), urinary tract infection (1% to 3%)

Hematologic: Coagulopathy (<4%), hemolytic anemia (<3%), hematoma (1%)

Hepatic: Liver pain (3%)

Neuromuscular & skeletal: Involuntary movements (7%), arthritis (≤5%), polyarthritis (5%), gait disturbance (<5%), leg cramps (3%), muscle cramps (1% to 3%)

Ocular: Visual disturbance (6%), conjunctivitis (4%), eye pain (1% to 3%)

Otic: Hearing alteration (<4%)

Renal: Proteinuria (≤10%)

Respiratory: Oropharynx dryness/inflammation (6%), pneumonitis (<5%), epistaxis (≤4%), bronchospasm (<4%), chest congestion (<3%)

Miscellaneous: Herpes virus reactivation (1% to 3%), lupus erythematosus syndrome (<3%)

Restrictions An FDA-approved medication guide must be distributed when dispensing an outpatient prescription (new or refill) where this medication is to be used without direct supervision of a healthcare provider. Medication guides are available at http://www.fda.gov/cder/Offices/ODS/medication_guides.htm.

Mechanism of Action Following activation, multiple effects can be detected including induction of gene transcription. Inhibits cellular growth, alters the state of cellular differentiation, interferes with oncogene expression, alters cell surface antigen expression, increases phagocytic activity of macrophages, and augments cytotoxicity of lymphocytes for target cells

Drug Interactions

Cytochrome P450 Effect: Inhibits CYP1A2 (weak)

Increased Effect/Toxicity: Concurrent therapy with ribavirin may increase the risk of hemolytic anemia. Interferon alfa may increase the levels/effects of theophylline derivatives. Interferons may decrease the metabolism of zidovudine; the neutropenic effects of zidovudine and interferon may be synergistic.

Pharmacodynamics/Kinetics

Distribution: V_d: 0.223-0.748 L/kg

Metabolism: Primarily renal; filtered through glomeruli and undergoes rapid proteolytic degradation during tubular reabsorption

Bioavailability: I.M.: 83%; SubQ: 90%

Half-life elimination: I.V.: 3.7-8.5 hours (mean ~5 hours)

Time to peak, serum: I.M., SubQ: ~4-7 hours

Pregnancy Risk Factor C

Interferon Alfa-2b (in ter FEER on AL fa too bee)

Related Information

Systemic Viral Diseases *on page 1767*

U.S. Brand Names Intron® A

Canadian Brand Names Intron® A

Mexican Brand Names Intron-A

Generic Available No

Index Terms α-2-interferon; INF-alpha 2; Interferon Alpha-2b; NSC-377523; rLFN-α2

(Continued)

Interferon Alfa-2b *(Continued)*

Pharmacologic Category Interferon

Use

Patients ≥1 year of age: Chronic hepatitis B

Patients ≥3 years of age: Chronic hepatitis C (in combination with ribavirin)

Patients ≥18 years of age: Condyloma acuminata, chronic hepatitis B, chronic hepatitis C, hairy cell leukemia, malignant melanoma, AIDS-related Kaposi's sarcoma, follicular non-Hodgkin's lymphoma

Unlabeled/Investigational Use AIDS-related thrombocytopenia, cutaneous ulcerations of Behçet's disease, carcinoid syndrome, cervical cancer, cutaneous T-Cell lymphoma, lymphomatoid granulomatosis, genital herpes, hepatitis D, chronic myelogenous leukemia (CML), non-Hodgkin's lymphomas (other than follicular lymphoma, see approved use), polycythemia vera, medullary thyroid carcinoma, multiple myeloma, renal cell carcinoma, basal and squamous cell skin cancers, essential thrombocytopenia, thrombocytopenic purpura, West Nile virus

Local Anesthetic/Vasoconstrictor Precautions No information available to require special precautions

Effects on Dental Treatment Key adverse event(s) related to dental treatment: Xerostomia (normal salivary flow resumes upon discontinuation), metallic taste, taste alteration, and gingivitis.

Common Adverse Effects Note: In a majority of patients, a flu-like syndrome (fever, chills, tachycardia, malaise, myalgia, headache), occurs within 1-2 hours of administration; may last up to 24 hours and may be dose-limiting.

>10%:

Cardiovascular: Chest pain (≤28%)

Central nervous system: Fatigue (8% to 96%), fever (34% to 94%), headache (21% to 62%), chills (≤54%), depression (3% to 40%; grades 3/4: 2%), somnolence (≤33%), dizziness (≤24%), irritability (≤22%), pain (≤18%), amnesia (≤14%), concentration impaired (≤14%), malaise (≤14%), confusion (≤12%), insomnia (≤12%)

Dermatologic: Alopecia (≤38%), rash (≤25%), pruritus (≤11%)

Endocrine & metabolic: Amenorrhea (≤12%)

Gastrointestinal: Anorexia (1% to 69%), nausea, (17% to 66%), diarrhea (2% to 45%), vomiting (2% to 32%), xerostomia (≤28%), taste alteration (≤24%), abdominal pain (1% to 23%), constipation (≤14%), gingivitis (≤14%), weight loss (<1% to 13%)

Hematologic: Neutropenia (≤92%; grade 4: 1% to 4%), leukopenia (≤68%), anemia (≤32%), thrombocytopenia (≤15%)

Hepatic: AST increased (≤63%; grades 3/4: 14%), ALT increased (≤15%), pain (upper right quadrant: up to 15%); alkaline phosphatase increased (≤13%)

Local: Injection site reaction (≤20%)

Neuromuscular & skeletal: Myalgia (28% to 75%), weakness (≤63%), rigors (≤42%), paresthesia (1% to 21%), skeletal pain (≤21%), arthralgia (≤19%), back pain (≤19%)

Renal: BUN increased (≤12%)

Respiratory: Dyspnea (≤34%), cough (≤31%), pharyngitis (≤31%), sinusitis (≤21%)

Miscellaneous: Flu-like syndrome (≤79%), diaphoresis (1% to 21%), moniliasis (≤17%)

5% to 10%:

Cardiovascular: Edema (≤10%), hypertension (≤9%)

Central nervous system: Hypoesthesia (≤10%), anxiety (≤9%), vertigo (≤8%), agitation (≤7%)

Dermatologic: Dry skin (≤10%), dermatitis (≤8%), purpura (≤5%)

Endocrine & metabolic: Libido decreased (≤5%)

Gastrointestinal: Loose stools (≤10%), dyspepsia (≤8%)

Genitourinary: Urinary tract infection (≤5%)

Renal: Polyuria (≤10%), serum creatinine increased (≤6%)

Respiratory: Bronchitis (≤10%), nasal congestion (≤10%), epistaxis (≤7%)

Miscellaneous: Herpesvirus infections (≤5%), infection (≤7%)

Restrictions An FDA-approved medication guide is available at http://www.fda.gov/cder/Offices/ODS/labeling.htm; distribute to each patient to whom this medication is dispensed.

Dosage Refer to individual protocols. **Note:** Withhold treatment for ANC <500/mm³ or platelets <25,000/mm³. Consider premedication with acetaminophen prior to administration to reduce the incidence of some adverse reactions. Not all dosage forms and strengths are appropriate for all indications; refer to product labeling for details.

Children 1-17 years: Chronic hepatitis B: SubQ: 3 million units/m^2 3 times/week for 1 week; then 6 million units/m^2 3 times/week; maximum: 10 million units 3 times/week; total duration of therapy 16-24 weeks

Children ≥3 years: Chronic hepatitis C: In combination with ribavirin (refer to Interferon Alfa-2b/Ribavirin combination pack monograph)

Adults:

Hairy cell leukemia: I.M., SubQ: 2 million units/m^2 3 times/week for up to 6 months (may continue treatment with continued treatment response)

Lymphoma (follicular): SubQ: 5 million units 3 times/week for up to 18 months

Malignant melanoma: Induction: 20 million units/m^2 I.V. for 5 consecutive days per week for 4 weeks, followed by maintenance dosing of 10 million units/m^2 SubQ 3 times/week for 48 weeks

AIDS-related Kaposi's sarcoma: I.M., SubQ: 30 million units/m^2 3 times/week

Chronic hepatitis B: I.M., SubQ: 5 million units/day or 10 million units 3 times/week for 16 weeks

Chronic hepatitis C: I.M., SubQ: 3 million units 3 times/week for 16 weeks. In patients with normalization of ALT at 16 weeks, continue treatment for 18-24 months; consider discontinuation if normalization does not occur at 16 weeks. **Note:** May be used in combination therapy with ribavirin in previously untreated patients or in patients who relapse following alpha interferon therapy.

Condyloma acuminata: Intralesionally: 1 million units/lesion (maximum: 5 lesions/treatment) 3 times/week (on alternate days) for 3 weeks; may administer a second course at 12-16 weeks

Dosage adjustment in renal impairment: Combination therapy with ribavirin (hepatitis C) should not be used in patients with reduced renal function (Cl$_{cr}$ <50 mL/minute).

Not removed by peritoneal or hemodialysis

Dosage adjustment for toxicity: Manufacturer-recommended adjustments, listed according to indication:

Lymphoma (follicular):

Neutrophils >1000/mm^3 to <1500/mm^3: Reduce dose by 50%; may re-escalate to starting dose when neutrophils return to >1500/mm^3

Severe toxicity (neutrophils <1000/mm^3 or platelets <50,000/mm^3): Temporarily withhold

AST >5 times ULN or serum creatinine >2 mg/dL: Permanently discontinue

Hairy cell leukemia, chronic hepatitis C: Severe toxicity: Reduce dose by 50% or temporarily withhold and resume with 50% dose reduction; permanently discontinue if persistent or recurrent severe toxicity is noted

Chronic hepatitis B:

WBC <1500/mm^3, granulocytes <750/mm^3, or platelet count <50,000/mm, or other laboratory abnormality or severe adverse reaction: Reduce dose by 50%; may re-escalate to starting dose upon resolution of hematologic toxicity. Discontinue for persistent intolerance.

WBC <1000/mm^3, granulocytes <500/mm^3, or platelet count <25,000/mm^3: Permanently discontinue

Kaposi sarcoma: Severe toxicity: Reduce dose by 50% or temporarily withhold; may resume at reduced dose with toxicity resolution; permanently discontinue for persistent/recurrent toxicities

Malignant melanoma:

Severe toxicity (neutrophils >250/mm^3 to <500/mm^3 or AST/ALT >5-10 times ULN): Temporarily withhold; resume with a 50% dose reduction when adverse reaction abates

Neutrophils <250/mm^3, AST/ALT >10 times ULN, or severe/persistent adverse reactions: Permanently discontinue

Mechanism of Action Following activation, multiple effects can be detected including induction of gene transcription. Inhibits cellular growth, alters the state of cellular differentiation, interferes with oncogene expression, alters cell surface antigen expression, increases phagocytic activity of macrophages, and augments cytotoxicity of lymphocytes for target cells

Contraindications Hypersensitivity to interferon alfa or any component of the formulation; decompensated liver disease; autoimmune hepatitis; pre-existing autoimmune disease; immunosuppressed transplant patients

Warnings/Precautions Hazardous agent - use appropriate precautions for handling and disposal.

[U.S. Boxed Warning]: May cause or aggravate fatal or life-threatening autoimmune disorders, neuropsychiatric symptoms (including depression and/or suicidal thoughts/behaviors), ischemic, and/or infectious disorders; discontinue treatment for persistent severe or worsening symptoms.

Neuropsychiatric disorders: May cause severe psychiatric adverse events (eg, depression, psychosis, mania, suicidal behavior/ideation) in patients with and

(Continued)

Interferon Alfa-2b *(Continued)*

without previous psychiatric symptoms, avoid use in severe psychiatric disorders or in patients with a history of severe depression; careful neuropsychiatric monitoring is required. Suicidal ideation or attempts may occur more frequently in pediatric patients when compared to adults. Discontinue in patients developing severe depression or psychiatric disorders. Higher doses in elderly patients, or diseases other than hairy cell leukemia, may result in increased CNS toxicity.

Hepatic disease: May cause hepatotoxicity; monitor closely if abnormal liver function tests develop. A transient increase in ALT (≥2 times baseline) may occur in patients treated with interferon alfa-2b for chronic hepatitis B. Therapy generally may continue; monitor. Worsening and potentially fatal liver disease, including jaundice, hepatic encephalopathy, and hepatic failure have been reported in patients receiving interferon alfa for chronic hepatitis B and C with decompensated liver disease, autoimmune hepatitis, history of autoimmune disease, and immunosuppressed transplant recipients; avoid use in these patients. Discontinue treatment in any patient developing signs or symptoms of liver failure.

Bone marrow suppression: Causes bone marrow suppression, including potentially severe cytopenias, and very rarely, aplastic anemia. Hemolytic anemia (hemoglobin <10 g/dL) was observed when combined with ribavirin; anemia occurred within 1-2 weeks of initiation of therapy. Use caution in patients with pre-existing myelosuppression and in patients with concomitant medications which cause myelosuppression.

Autoimmune disorders: Avoid use in patients with history of autoimmune disorders; development of autoimmune disorders (thrombocytopenia, vasculitis, Raynaud's disease, rheumatoid arthritis, lupus erythematosus and rhabdomyolysis) has been associated with use. Monitor closely; consider discontinuing. Worsening of psoriasis and sarcoidosis (and the development of new sarcoidosis) have been reported; use caution.

Cardiovascular disease/coagulation disorders: Use caution and monitor closely in patients with cardiovascular disease (ischemic or thromboembolic), arrhythmias, hypertension, and in patients with a history of MI or prior therapy with cardiotoxic drugs. Patients with pre-existing cardiac disease and/or advanced cancer should have baseline and periodic ECGs. May cause hypotension (during administration or delayed), arrhythmia, tachycardia, cardiomyopathy (~2% in AIDS-related Kaposi's Sarcoma patients) and/or MI. Use caution in patients with coagulopathy.

Endocrine disorders: Thyroid disorders (possibly reversible) have been reported; use caution in patients with pre-existing thyroid disease. Discontinue use in patients who cannot maintain normal ranges with thyroid medication. Diabetes mellitus has been reported; discontinue if cannot effectively manage with medication. Use caution in patients with a history of diabetes mellitus, particularly if prone to DKA. Hypertriglyceridemia has been reported; discontinue if severe, and/or combined with symptoms of pancreatitis.

Pulmonary disease: Pulmonary infiltrates, pneumonitis and pneumonia have been reported with interferon alfa therapy; occurs more frequently in patients being treated for chronic hepatitis C. Patients with fever, cough, dyspnea or other respiratory symptoms should be evaluated with a chest x-ray; monitor closely and consider discontinuing treatment with evidence of impaired pulmonary function. Use caution in patients with a history of pulmonary disease.

Ophthalmic disorders: Decreased/loss of vision, retinal hemorrhages, cotton wool spots, papilledema, and retinal artery or vein obstruction have occurred in patients receiving alpha interferons. Use caution in patients with pre-existing eye disorders; monitor closely; discontinue with new or worsening ophthalmic disorders.

Commonly associated with fever and flu-like symptoms; use with caution in patients with debilitating conditions. Acute hypersensitivity reactions have been reported. Do not treat patients with visceral AIDS-related Kaposi's sarcoma associated with rapidly-progressing or life-threatening disease. Some formulations contain albumin, which may carry a remote risk of viral transmission. Due to differences in dosage, patients should not change brands of interferons without the concurrence of their healthcare provider. Safety and efficacy in children <1 year of age have not been established.

Drug Interactions

Cytochrome P450 Effect: Inhibits CYP1A2 (weak)

Increased Effect/Toxicity: Interferons may increase serum levels and neutropenic effects of zidovudine. Concurrent therapy with ribavirin may increase the risk of hemolytic anemia. Interferon alfa may increase the levels/effects of theophylline.

Pharmacodynamics/Kinetics

Distribution: V_d: 31 L; but has been noted to be much greater (370-720 L) in leukemia patients receiving continuous infusion IFN; IFN does not penetrate the CSF

Metabolism: Primarily renal

Bioavailability: I.M.: 83%; SubQ: 90%

Half-life elimination: I.V.: 2 hours; I.M., SubQ: 2-3 hours

Time to peak, serum: I.M., SubQ: ~3-12 hours

Pregnancy Risk Factor C

Dosage Forms

Injection, powder for reconstitution:

Intron® A: 10 million units; 18 million units; 50 million units

Injection, solution [multidose prefilled pen]:

Intron® A:

Delivers 3 million units/0.2 mL (1.5 mL)

Delivers 5 million units/0.2 mL (1.5 mL)

Delivers 10 million units/0.2 mL (1.5 mL)

Injection, solution [multidose vial]:

Intron® A: 6 million units/mL (3 mL); 10 million units/mL (2.5 mL)

Injection, solution [single-dose vial]:

Intron® A: 10 million units/ mL (1 mL)

Interferon Alfa-2b and Ribavirin

(in ter FEER on AL fa too bee & rye ba VYE rin)

Related Information

Interferon Alfa-2b *on page 891*

Ribavirin *on page 1420*

Systemic Viral Diseases *on page 1767*

U.S. Brand Names Rebetron®

Mexican Brand Names Hepatron C

Generic Available No

Index Terms Interferon Alfa-2b and Ribavirin Combination Pack; Ribavirin and Interferon Alfa-2b Combination Pack

Pharmacologic Category Antiviral Agent; Interferon

Use Combination therapy for the treatment of chronic hepatitis C in patients with compensated liver disease previously untreated with alpha interferon or who have relapsed after alpha interferon therapy

Local Anesthetic/Vasoconstrictor Precautions No information available to require special precautions

Effects on Dental Treatment Key adverse event(s) related to dental treatment: Xerostomia (normal salivary flow resumes upon discontinuation), metallic taste, and taste perversion.

Common Adverse Effects Note: Adverse reactions listed are specific to combination regimen in previously untreated hepatitis patients. See individual agents for additional adverse reactions reported with each agent during therapy for other diseases.

>10%:

Central nervous system: Fatigue (children 61%; adults 68%), headache (63%), insomnia (children 14%; adults 39%), fever (children 61%; adults 37%), depression (children 13%; adults 32% to 36%), irritability (children 10%; adults 23% to 32%), dizziness (17% to 23%), emotional lability (children 16%; adults 7% to 11%), impaired concentration (5% to 14%)

Dermatologic: Alopecia (23% to 32%), pruritus (children 12%; adults 19% to 21%), rash (17% to 28%)

Gastrointestinal: Nausea (33% to 46%), anorexia (children 51%; adults 25% to 27%), dyspepsia (children <1%; adults 14% to 16%), vomiting (children 42%; adults 9% to 11%)

Hematologic: Leukopenia, neutropenia (usually recovers within 4 weeks of treatment discontinuation), anemia

Hepatic: Hyperbilirubinemia (27%; only 0.9% to 2% >3.0-6 mg/dL)

Local: Injection site inflammation (13%)

Neuromuscular & skeletal: Myalgia (children 32%; adults 61% to 64%), rigors (40%), arthralgia (children 15%; adults 30% to 33%), musculoskeletal pain (20% to 28%)

Respiratory: Dyspnea (children 5%; adults 18% to 19%)

Miscellaneous: Flu-like syndrome (children 31%; adults 14% to 18%)

1% to 10%:

Cardiovascular: Chest pain (5% to 9%)

Central nervous system: Nervousness (3% to 4%)

Endocrine & metabolic: Thyroid abnormalities (hyper- or hypothyroidism), serum uric acid increased, hyperglycemia

(Continued)

Interferon Alfa-2b and Ribavirin *(Continued)*

Gastrointestinal: Taste perversion (children <1%; adults 7% to 8%)

Hematologic: Hemolytic anemia (10%), thrombocytopenia, anemia

Local: Injection site reaction (7%)

Neuromuscular & skeletal: Weakness (5% to 9%)

Respiratory: Sinusitis (children <1%; adults 9% to 10%)

Restrictions An FDA-approved medication guide must be distributed when dispensing an outpatient prescription (new or refill) for treatment of hepatitis C where this medication is to be used without direct supervision of a healthcare provider. Medication guides are available at http://www.fda.gov/cder/Offices/ODS/medication_guides.htm.

Mechanism of Action

Interferon Alfa-2b: Alpha interferons are a family of proteins, produced by nucleated cells, that have antiviral, antiproliferative, and immune-regulating activity. There are 16 known subtypes of alpha interferons. Interferons interact with cells through high affinity cell surface receptors. Following activation, multiple effects can be detected including induction of gene transcription. Inhibits cellular growth, alters the state of cellular differentiation, interferes with oncogene expression, alters cell surface antigen expression, increases phagocytic activity of macrophages, and augments cytotoxicity of lymphocytes for target cells

Ribavirin: Inhibits replication of RNA and DNA viruses; inhibits influenza virus RNA polymerase activity and inhibits the initiation and elongation of RNA fragments resulting in inhibition of viral protein synthesis

Drug Interactions

Cytochrome P450 Effect: Interferon Alfa-2b: **Inhibits** CYP1A2 (weak)

Increased Effect/Toxicity: Interferon alpha: Cimetidine may augment the antitumor effects of interferon in melanoma. Theophylline clearance has been reported to be decreased in hepatitis patients receiving interferon. Vinblastine enhances interferon toxicity in several patients; increased incidence of paresthesia has also been noted. Interferons may increase the adverse/toxic effects of ACE inhibitors, specifically the development of granulocytopenia. Agranulocytosis has been reported with concurrent use of clozapine (case report). Interferons may increase the anticoagulant effects of warfarin, and interferons may increase serum levels of zidovudine. Concurrent therapy with ribavirin may increase the risk of hemolytic anemia. Concomitant use of ribavirin and nucleoside analogues may increase the risk of developing lactic acidosis. Concomitant therapy of interferon (alfa) and ribavirin may increase the risk of hemolytic anemia.

Decreased Effect:

Interferon alpha: Prednisone may decrease the therapeutic effects of interferon alpha. A decreased response to erythropoietin has been reported (case reports) in patients receiving interferons. Interferon alpha may decrease the serum concentrations of melphalan (may or may not decrease toxicity of melphalan). Thyroid dysfunction has been reported during treatment; monitor response to thyroid hormones.

Ribavirin: Decreased effect of stavudine and zidovudine.

Pharmacodynamics/Kinetics See individual agents.

Pregnancy Risk Factor X

Interferon Alfa-n3 (in ter FEER on AL fa en three)

Related Information

Systemic Viral Diseases *on page 1767*

U.S. Brand Names Alferon® N

Canadian Brand Names Alferon® N

Generic Available No

Pharmacologic Category Interferon

Use Patients ≥18 years of age: Intralesional treatment of refractory or recurring genital or venereal warts (condylomata acuminata)

Local Anesthetic/Vasoconstrictor Precautions No information available to require special precautions

Effects on Dental Treatment Key adverse event(s) related to dental treatment: Xerostomia (normal salivary flow resumes upon discontinuation), metallic taste, tongue hyperesthesia, abnormal taste, thirst, rhinitis, pharyngitis, nosebleed, increased diaphoresis, taste disturbance, and gingivitis.

Common Adverse Effects Note: Adverse reaction incidence noted below is specific to intralesional administration in patients with condylomata acuminata. Flu-like reactions, consisting of headache, fever, and/or myalgia, was reported in 30% of patients, and abated with repeated dosing.

>10%:
  Central nervous system: Fever (40%), headache (31%), chills (14%), fatigue (14%)
  Hematologic: Decreased WBC (11%)
  Neuromuscular & skeletal: Myalgia (45%)
  Miscellaneous: Flu-like syndrome (30%)
1% to 10%:
  Central nervous system: Malaise (9%), dizziness (9%), depression (2%), insomnia (2%), thirst (1%)
  Dermatologic: Pruritus (2%)
  Gastrointestinal: Nausea (45), vomiting (3%), dyspepsia (3%), diarrhea (2%), tongue hyperesthesia (1%), taste disturbance (1%)
  Genitourinary: Groin lymph node swelling (1%)
  Neuromuscular & skeletal: Arthralgia (5%), back pain (4%), cramps (1%), paresthesia (1%)
  Ocular: Visual disturbance (1%)
  Respiratory: Rhinitis (2%), pharyngitis (1%), nosebleed (1%)
  Miscellaneous: Diaphoresis increased (2%), vasovagal reaction (2%)

Mechanism of Action Interferons interact with cells through high affinity cell surface receptors. Following activation, multiple effects can be detected including induction of gene transcription. Inhibits cellular growth, alters the state of cellular differentiation, interferes with oncogene expression, alters cell surface antigen expression, increases phagocytic activity of macrophages, and augments cytotoxicity of lymphocytes for target cells

Drug Interactions
  Increased Effect/Toxicity: Interferons may increase the adverse/toxic effects of ACE inhibitors, specifically the development of granulocytopenia. Risk: Monitor A case report of agranulocytosis has been reported with concurrent use of clozapine. Case reports of decreased hematopoietic effect with erythropoietin. Interferon alpha may decrease the P450 isoenzyme metabolism of theophylline. Interferons may increase the anticoagulant effects of warfarin. Interferons may decrease the metabolism of zidovudine.
  Decreased Effect: Interferon alpha may decrease the serum concentrations of melphalan; this may or may not decrease the potential toxicity of melphalan. Prednisone may decrease the therapeutic effects of Interferon alpha.

Pregnancy Risk Factor C

Interferon Alpha-2a *see* Interferon Alfa-2a *on page 890*
Interferon Alpha-2b *see* Interferon Alfa-2b *on page 891*

Interferon Beta-1a (in ter FEER on BAY ta won aye)

U.S. Brand Names Avonex®: Rebif®
Canadian Brand Names Avonex®; Rebif®
Mexican Brand Names Rebif
Generic Available No
Index Terms rIFN beta-1a
Pharmacologic Category Interferon
Use Treatment of relapsing forms of multiple sclerosis (MS)
Local Anesthetic/Vasoconstrictor Precautions No information available to require special precautions
Effects on Dental Treatment Key adverse event(s) related to dental treatment: Xerostomia and changes in salivation (normal salivary flow resumes upon discontinuation), and toothache.
Common Adverse Effects
>10%:
  Central nervous system: Headache (Avonex® 58%; Rebif® 65% to 70%), fatigue (Rebif® 33% to 41%), fever (Avonex® 20%; Rebif® 25% to 28%), pain (Avonex® 23%), chills (Avonex® 19%), depression (Avonex® 18%), dizziness (Avonex® 14%)
  Gastrointestinal: Nausea (Avonex® 23%), abdominal pain (Avonex® 8%; Rebif® 20% to 22%)
  Genitourinary: Urinary tract infection (Avonex® 17%)
  Hematologic: Leukopenia (Rebif® 28% to 36%)
  Hepatic: ALT increased (Rebif® 20% to 27%), AST increased (Rebif® 10% to 17%)
  Local: Injection site reaction (Avonex® 3%; Rebif® 89% to 92%)
  Neuromuscular & skeletal: Myalgia (Avonex® 29%; Rebif® 25%), back pain (Rebif® 23% to 25%), weakness (Avonex® 24%), skeletal pain (Rebif® 10% to 15%), rigors (Rebif® 6% to 13%)
  Ocular: Vision abnormal (Rebif® 7% to 13%)
(Continued)

Interferon Beta-1a *(Continued)*

Respiratory: Sinusitis (Avonex® 14%), upper respiratory tract infection (Avonex® 14%)

Miscellaneous: Flu-like syndrome (Avonex® 49%; Rebif® 56% to 59%), neutralizing antibodies (significance not known; Avonex® 5%; Rebif® 24%), lymphadenopathy (Rebif® 11% to 12%)

1% to 10% (reported with one or both products):

Cardiovascular: Chest pain, vasodilation

Central nervous system: Convulsions, malaise, migraine, somnolence

Dermatologic: Alopecia, erythematous rash, maculopapular rash, urticaria

Endocrine & metabolic: Thyroid disorder

Gastrointestinal: Toothache, xerostomia

Genitourinary: Micturition frequency, urinary incontinence

Hematologic: Anemia, thrombocytopenia

Hepatic: Bilirubinemia, hepatic function abnormal

Local: Injection site bruising, injection site inflammation, injection site necrosis, injection site pain

Neuromuscular & skeletal: Arthralgia, coordination abnormal, hypertonia

Ocular: Eye disorder, xerophthalmia

Respiratory: Bronchitis

Miscellaneous: Infection

Restrictions An FDA-approved medication guide must be distributed when dispensing an outpatient prescription (new or refill) where this medication is to be used without direct supervision of a healthcare provider. Medication guides are available at http://www.fda.gov/cder/Offices/ODS/medication_guides.htm.

Mechanism of Action Interferon beta differs from naturally occurring human protein by a single amino acid substitution and the lack of carbohydrate side chains; alters the expression and response to surface antigens and can enhance immune cell activities. Properties of interferon beta that modify biologic responses are mediated by cell surface receptor interactions; mechanism in the treatment of MS is unknown.

Drug Interactions

Increased Effect/Toxicity: Interferons may increase the adverse/toxic effects of ACE inhibitors, specifically the development of granulocytopenia. Agranulocytosis has been reported with concurrent use of clozapine (case report). Interferons may increase the anticoagulant effects of warfarin, and interferons may increase serum levels of zidovudine. Concurrent use of hepatotoxic drugs may increase the risk of hepatic injury in patients receiving interferon beta-1a.

Pharmacodynamics/Kinetics Limited data due to small doses used

Half-life elimination: Avonex®: 10 hours; Rebif®: 69 hours

Time to peak, serum: Avonex® (I.M.): 3-15 hours; Rebif® (SubQ): 16 hours

Pregnancy Risk Factor C

Interferon Beta-1b *(in ter FEER on BAY ta won bee)*

U.S. Brand Names Betaseron®

Canadian Brand Names Betaseron®

Mexican Brand Names Betaferon

Generic Available No

Index Terms rIFN beta-1b

Pharmacologic Category Interferon

Use Treatment of relapsing forms of multiple sclerosis (MS); treatment of first clinical episode with MRI features consistent with MS

Local Anesthetic/Vasoconstrictor Precautions No information available to require special precautions

Effects on Dental Treatment No significant effects or complications reported

Common Adverse Effects Note: Flu-like syndrome (including at least two of the following - headache, fever, chills, malaise, diaphoresis, and myalgia) are reported in the majority of patients (60%) and decrease over time (average duration ~1 week).

>10%:

Cardiovascular: Peripheral edema (15%), chest pain (11%)

Central nervous system: Headache (57%), fever (36%), pain (51%), chills (25%), dizziness (24%), insomnia (24%)

Dermatologic: Rash (24%), skin disorder (12%)

Endocrine & metabolic: Metrorrhagia (11%)

Gastrointestinal: Nausea (27%), diarrhea (19%), abdominal pain (19%), constipation (20%), dyspepsia (14%)

Genitourinary: Urinary urgency (13%)

Hematologic: Lymphopenia (88%), neutropenia (14%), leukopenia (14%)

Local: Injection site reaction (85%), inflammation (53%), pain (18%)
Neuromuscular & skeletal: Weakness (61%), myalgia (27%), hypertonia (50%), myasthenia (46%), arthralgia (31%), incoordination (21%)
Miscellaneous: Flu-like syndrome (decreases over treatment course; 60%)
1% to 10%:
Cardiovascular: Palpitation (4%), vasodilation (8%), hypertension (7%), tachycardia (4%), peripheral vascular disorder (6%)
Central nervous system: Anxiety (10%), malaise (8%), nervousness (7%)
Dermatologic: Alopecia (4%)
Endocrine & metabolic: Menorrhagia (8%), dysmenorrhea (7%)
Gastrointestinal: Weight gain (7%)
Genitourinary: Impotence (9%), pelvic pain (6%), cystitis (8%), urinary frequency (7%), prostatic disorder (3%)
Hematologic: Lymphadenopathy (8%)
Hepatic: ALT increased >5x baseline (10%), AST increased >5x baseline (3%)
Local: Injection site necrosis (4% to 5%), edema (3%), mass (2%)
Neuromuscular & skeletal: Leg cramps (4%)
Respiratory: Dyspnea (7%)
Miscellaneous: Diaphoresis (8%), hypersensitivity (3%)

Restrictions An FDA-approved medication guide must be distributed when dispensing an outpatient prescription (new or refill) where this medication is to be used without direct supervision of a healthcare provider. Medication guide is available at http://www.berlex.com/html/products/pi/Betaseron_Medication_Guide.pdf.

Mechanism of Action Interferon beta-1b differs from naturally occurring human protein by a single amino acid substitution and the lack of carbohydrate side chains; mechanism in the treatment of MS is unknown; however, immunomodulatory effects attributed to interferon beta-1b include enhancement of suppressor T cell activity, reduction of proinflammatory cytokines, down-regulation of antigen presentation, and reduced trafficking of lymphocytes into the central nervous system. Improves MRI lesions, decreases relapse rate, and disease severity in patients with secondary progressive MS.

Drug Interactions
Increased Effect/Toxicity: Interferons may decrease the metabolism of theophylline derivatives.
Pharmacodynamics/Kinetics Limited data due to small doses used
Half-life elimination: 8 minutes to 4.3 hours
Time to peak, serum: 1-8 hours
Pregnancy Risk Factor C

Interferon Gamma-1b (in ter FEER on GAM ah won bee)

U.S. Brand Names Actimmune®
Canadian Brand Names Actimmune®
Generic Available No
Pharmacologic Category Interferon
Use Reduce frequency and severity of serious infections associated with chronic granulomatous disease; delay time to disease progression in patients with severe, malignant osteopetrosis
Local Anesthetic/Vasoconstrictor Precautions No information available to require special precautions
Effects on Dental Treatment No significant effects or complications reported
Common Adverse Effects Based on 50 mcg/m² dose administered 3 times weekly for chronic granulomatous disease
>10%:
Central nervous system: Fever (52%), headache (33%), chills (14%), fatigue (14%)
Dermatologic: Rash (17%)
Gastrointestinal: Diarrhea (14%), vomiting (13%)
Local: Injection site erythema or tenderness (14%)
1% to 10%:
Central nervous system: Depression (3%)
Gastrointestinal: Nausea (10%), abdominal pain (8%)
Neuromuscular & skeletal: Myalgia (6%), arthralgia (2%), back pain (2%)

Additional adverse reactions noted at doses >100 mcg/m² administered 3 times weekly: ALT increased, AST increased, autoantibodies increased, bronchospasm, chest discomfort, confusion, dermatomyositis exacerbation, disorientation, DVT, gait disturbance, GI bleeding, hallucinations, heart block, heart failure, hepatic insufficiency, hyperglycemia, hypertriglyceridemia, hyponatremia, hypotension, interstitial pneumonitis, lupus-like syndrome, MI, neutropenia, pancreatitis (may be fatal), Parkinsonian symptoms, PE, proteinuria, (Continued)

Interferon Gamma-1b (Continued)

renal insufficiency (reversible), seizure, syncope, tachyarrhythmia, tachypnea, thrombocytopenia, TIA

Mechanism of Action Interferon gamma participates in immunoregulation by enhancing the oxidative metabolism of macrophages; it also enhances antibody dependent cellular cytotoxicity, activates natural killer cells and has a role in the expression of Fc receptors and histocompatibility antigens. The exact mechanism of action for the treatment of chronic granulomatous disease or osteopetrosis has not been defined.

Drug Interactions

Cytochrome P450 Effect: Inhibits CYP1A2 (weak), 2E1 (weak)

Increased Effect/Toxicity: Interferons may decrease the metabolism of theophylline derivatives.

Pharmacodynamics/Kinetics

Absorption: I.M., SubQ: >89%

Half-life elimination: I.V.: 38 minutes; I.M.: ~3 hours, SubQ: ~6 hours

Time to peak, plasma: I.M.: 4 hours (1.5 ng/mL); SubQ: 7 hours (0.6 ng/mL)

Pregnancy Risk Factor C

Interleukin-1 Receptor Antagonist see Anakinra on page 128

Interleukin-2 see Aldesleukin on page 62

Interleukin-11 see Oprelvekin on page 1210

Intralipid® see Fat Emulsion on page 672

Intravenous Fat Emulsion see Fat Emulsion on page 672

Intrifiban see Eptifibatide on page 582

Intron® A see Interferon Alfa-2b on page 891

Intropaste see Barium on page 185

Invanz® see Ertapenem on page 588

Invega™ see Paliperidone on page 1243

Inversine® see Mecamylamine on page 1022

Invirase® see Saquinavir on page 1455

Iodex [OTC] see Iodine on page 900

Iodine (EYE oh dyne)

Related Information

Trace Metals on page 1595

U.S. Brand Names Iodex [OTC]; Iodoflex™; Iodosorb®

Generic Available Yes: Tincture

Pharmacologic Category Antiseptic, Topical

Use Used topically as an antiseptic in the management of minor, superficial skin wounds and has been used to disinfect the skin preoperatively

Local Anesthetic/Vasoconstrictor Precautions No information available to require special precautions

Effects on Dental Treatment No significant effects or complications reported

Common Adverse Effects Reactions reported following topical application: Frequency not defined:

Endocrine & metabolic: TSH increased

Local: Eczema, edema, irritation, pain, redness

Miscellaneous: Allergic reaction

Reactions reported more likely observed following large doses or chronic iodine intoxication; Frequency not defined:

Central nervous system: Fever, headache

Dermatologic: Skin rash, angioedema, urticaria, acne

Endocrine & metabolic: Hypothyroidism

Gastrointestinal: Metallic taste, diarrhea

Hematologic: Eosinophilia, hemorrhage (mucosal)

Neuromuscular & skeletal: Arthralgia

Ocular: Swelling of eyelids

Respiratory: Pulmonary edema

Miscellaneous: Ioderma, lymph node enlargement

Mechanism of Action Iodine is required for thyroid hormone synthesis. Iodine is also known to be a powerful broad spectrum germicidal agent effective against a wide range of bacteria, viruses, fungi, protozoa, and spores. Iodosorb® and Iodoflex™ contain iodine in hydrophilic beads of cadexomer which allows a slow release of iodine into the wound and absorption of fluid, bacteria, and other substances from the wound

Pharmacodynamics/Kinetics

Absorption: Topical: Amount absorbed systemically depends upon concentration and characteristics of skin

Distribution: Primarily trapped by the thyroid
Bioavailability: Oral: >90%
Excretion: Urine (>90%)

Iodine *see* Trace Metals *on page 1595*

Iodipamide Meglumine (eye oh DI pa mide MEG loo meen)

U.S. Brand Names Cholografin® Meglumine
Generic Available No
Pharmacologic Category Iodinated Contrast Media; Radiological/Contrast Media, Ionic
Use Contrast medium for intravenous cholangiography and cholecystography
Local Anesthetic/Vasoconstrictor Precautions No information available to require special precautions
Effects on Dental Treatment No significant effects or complications reported

Iodipamide Meglumine and Diatrizoate Meglumine *see* Diatrizoate Meglumine and Iodipamide Meglumine *on page 480*

Iodixanol (EYE oh dix an ole)

U.S. Brand Names Visipaque™
Generic Available No
Pharmacologic Category Iodinated Contrast Media; Radiological/Contrast Media, Nonionic
Use
Intra-arterial: Digital subtraction angiography, angiocardiography, peripheral arteriography, visceral arteriography, cerebral arteriography
Intravenous: Contrast enhanced computed tomography imaging, excretory urography, and peripheral venography
Local Anesthetic/Vasoconstrictor Precautions No information available to require special precautions
Effects on Dental Treatment Key adverse event(s) related to dental treatment: Taste perversion.
Mechanism of Action Opacifies vessels in the path of flow permitting radiographic imaging of internal structures.
Pregnancy Risk Factor B

Iodoflex™ *see* Iodine *on page 900*
Iodopen® *see* Trace Metals *on page 1595*

Iodoquinol (eye oh doe KWIN ole)

U.S. Brand Names Yodoxin®
Canadian Brand Names Diodoquin®
Mexican Brand Names Depofin
Generic Available No
Index Terms Diiodohydroxyquin
Pharmacologic Category Amebicide
Use Treatment of acute and chronic intestinal amebiasis; asymptomatic cyst passers; *Blastocystis hominis* infections; ineffective for amebic hepatitis or hepatic abscess
Local Anesthetic/Vasoconstrictor Precautions No information available to require special precautions
Effects on Dental Treatment No significant effects or complications reported
Common Adverse Effects Frequency not defined.
Central nervous system: Fever, chills, agitation, retrograde amnesia, headache
Dermatologic: Rash, urticaria, pruritus
Endocrine & metabolic: Thyroid gland enlargement
Gastrointestinal: Diarrhea, nausea, vomiting, stomach pain, abdominal cramps
Neuromuscular & skeletal: Peripheral neuropathy, weakness
Ocular: Optic neuritis, optic atrophy, visual impairment
Miscellaneous: Itching of rectal area
Mechanism of Action Contact amebicide that works in the lumen of the intestine by an unknown mechanism
Pharmacodynamics/Kinetics
Absorption: Poor and erratic
Metabolism: Hepatic
Excretion: Feces (high percentage)
Pregnancy Risk Factor C

Iodoquinol and Hydrocortisone
(eye oh doe KWIN ole & hye droe KOR ti sone)

Related Information
Hydrocortisone *on page 836*
Iodoquinol *on page 901*

Related Sample Prescriptions
Angular Cheilitis *on page 1842*

U.S. Brand Names Dermazene®; Vytone®

Generic Available Yes

Index Terms Hydrocortisone and Iodoquinol

Pharmacologic Category Antifungal Agent, Topical; Corticosteroid, Topical

Dental Use Reported to be useful in the treatment of angular cheilitis

Use Treatment of eczema; infectious dermatitis; chronic eczematoid otitis externa; mycotic dermatoses

Local Anesthetic/Vasoconstrictor Precautions No information available to require special precautions

Effects on Dental Treatment No significant effects or complications reported

Significant Adverse Effects See individual agents.

Dental Usual Dosing Angular cheilitis: Adults: Topical: Apply 3-4 times/day

Dosage Apply 3-4 times/day

Contraindications
Based on **iodoquinol** component: Hypersensitivity to iodine or iodoquinol or any component of the formulation; hepatic damage; pre-existing optic neuropathy

Based on **hydrocortisone** component: Hypersensitivity to hydrocortisone or any component of the formulation; serious infections, except septic shock or tuberculous meningitis; viral, fungal, or tubercular skin lesions

Warnings/Precautions
Based on **iodoquinol** component: Optic neuritis, optic atrophy, and peripheral neuropathy have occurred following prolonged use; avoid long-term therapy

Based on **hydrocortisone** component:
Use with caution in patients with hyperthyroidism, cirrhosis, nonspecific ulcerative colitis, hypertension, osteoporosis, thromboembolic tendencies, CHF, convulsive disorders, myasthenia gravis, thrombophlebitis, peptic ulcer, diabetes

Acute adrenal insufficiency may occur with abrupt withdrawal (depending on degree of systemic absorption) after long-term therapy or with stress; young pediatric patients may be more susceptible to adrenal axis suppression from topical therapy

Drug Interactions Hydrocortisone: **Substrate** of CYP3A4 (minor); **Induces** CYP3A4 (weak)
Also see individual agents.

Pharmacodynamics/Kinetics See individual agents.

Pregnancy Risk Factor C

Lactation Excretion in breast milk unknown

Dosage Forms Excipient information presented when available (limited, particularly for generics); consult specific product labeling.
Cream: Iodoquinol 1% and hydrocortisone acetate 1% (30 g)
Dermazene®: Iodoquinol 1% and hydrocortisone acetate 1% (30 g, 45 g)
Vytone®: Iodoquinol 1% and hydrocortisone acetate 1% (30 g)

Iodosorb® *see* Iodine *on page 900*

Iohexol (eye oh HEX ole)

U.S. Brand Names Omnipaque™

Generic Available No

Pharmacologic Category Polypeptide Hormone; Radiological/Contrast Media, Nonionic

Use
Intrathecal: Myelography; contrast enhancement for computerized tomography
Intravascular: Angiocardiography, aortography, digital subtraction angiography, peripheral arteriography, excretory urography; contrast enhancement for computed tomographic imaging
Oral/body cavity: Arthrography, GI tract examination, hysterosalpingography, pancreatography, cholangiopancreatography, herniography, cystourethrography; enhanced computed tomography of the abdomen

Local Anesthetic/Vasoconstrictor Precautions No information available to require special precautions

Effects on Dental Treatment No significant effects or complications reported

Pregnancy Risk Factor B

Ionamin® *see* Phentermine *on page 1291*

Ionil® [OTC] *see* Salicylic Acid *on page 1451*

Ionil® Plus [OTC] *see* Salicylic Acid *on page 1451*

Ionil T® [OTC] *see* Coal Tar *on page 402*

Ionil T® Plus [OTC] *see* Coal Tar *on page 402*

Ionsys™ *see* Fentanyl *on page 679*

Iopamidol (eye oh PA mi dole)

U.S. Brand Names Isovue®; Isovue-M®; Isovue Multipack®
Generic Available No
Pharmacologic Category Iodinated Contrast Media; Radiological/Contrast Media, Nonionic
Use
Intrathecal (Isovue-M®): Neuroradiology; contrast enhancement of computed tomographic cisternography and ventriculography; thoraco-lumbar myelography

Intravascular (Isovue®, Isovue Multipack®): Angiography, excretory urography; contrast enhancement of computed tomographic imaging; evaluation of certain malignancies; image enhancement of non-neoplastic lesions

Local Anesthetic/Vasoconstrictor Precautions No information available to require special precautions
Effects on Dental Treatment No significant effects or complications reported
Pregnancy Risk Factor B

Iopidine® *see* Apraclonidine *on page 136*

Iopromide (eye oh PROE mide)

U.S. Brand Names Ultravist®
Generic Available No
Pharmacologic Category Radiological/Contrast Media, Nonionic
Use Enhance imaging in cerebral arteriography and peripheral arteriography; coronary arteriography and left ventriculography, visceral angiography and aortography; contrast-enhanced computed tomographic imaging of the head and body, excretory urography, intra-arterial digital subtraction angiography, peripheral venography
Local Anesthetic/Vasoconstrictor Precautions No information available to require special precautions
Effects on Dental Treatment Key adverse event(s) related to dental treatment: Abnormal taste.
Mechanism of Action Iopromide opacifies vessels in its path of flow, permitting radiographic visualization of internal structures.
Pregnancy Risk Factor B

Iosat™ [OTC] *see* Potassium Iodide *on page 1330*

Iothalamate Meglumine (eye oh thal A mate MEG loo meen)

U.S. Brand Names Conray®; Conray® 30; Conray® 43; Cysto-Conray® II
Generic Available No
Pharmacologic Category Iodinated Contrast Media; Radiological/Contrast Media, Ionic
Use
Solution for injection: Arthrography, cerebral angiography, cranial computerized angiotomography, digital subtraction angiography, direct cholangiography, endoscopic retrograde cholangiopancreatography, excretory urography, peripheral arteriography, urography, venography; contrast enhancement of computed tomographic images
Solution for instillation: Retrograde cystography and cystourethrography

Local Anesthetic/Vasoconstrictor Precautions No information available to require special precautions
Effects on Dental Treatment No significant effects or complications reported
Pregnancy Risk Factor B/C (product dependent)

Iothalamate Sodium (eye oh thal A mate SOW dee um)

U.S. Brand Names Conray® 400
Generic Available No
(Continued)

Iothalamate Sodium *(Continued)*

Pharmacologic Category Iodinated Contrast Media; Radiological/Contrast Media, Ionic

Use Excretory urography, angiocardiography, aortography; contrast enhancement of computed tomographic brain images

Local Anesthetic/Vasoconstrictor Precautions No information available to require special precautions

Effects on Dental Treatment No significant effects or complications reported

Pregnancy Risk Factor B

Ioversol *(EYE oh ver sole)*

U.S. Brand Names Optiray®
Generic Available No
Pharmacologic Category Iodinated Contrast Media; Radiological/Contrast Media, Nonionic

Use Arteriography, angiography, angiocardiography, ventriculography, excretory urography, and venography procedures; contrast enhanced tomographic imaging

Local Anesthetic/Vasoconstrictor Precautions No information available to require special precautions

Effects on Dental Treatment No significant effects or complications reported

Pregnancy Risk Factor B

Ioxaglate Meglumine and Ioxaglate Sodium
(eye ox AG late MEG loo meen & eye ox AG late SOW dee um)

U.S. Brand Names Hexabrix™
Generic Available No
Index Terms Ioxaglate Sodium and Ioxaglate Meglumine
Pharmacologic Category Iodinated Contrast Media; Radiological/Contrast Media, Ionic

Use Angiocardiography, arteriography, aortography, arthrography, angiography, hysterosalpingography, venography, and urography procedures; contrast enhancement of computed tomographic imaging

Local Anesthetic/Vasoconstrictor Precautions No information available to require special precautions

Effects on Dental Treatment No significant effects or complications reported

Pregnancy Risk Factor B

Ioxaglate Sodium and Ioxaglate Meglumine *see* Ioxaglate Meglumine and Ioxaglate Sodium *on page 904*

Ipecac Syrup *(IP e kak SIR up)*

Generic Available Yes
Index Terms Syrup of Ipecac
Pharmacologic Category Antidote
Use Treatment of acute oral drug overdosage and in certain poisonings

Local Anesthetic/Vasoconstrictor Precautions No information available to require special precautions

Effects on Dental Treatment No significant effects or complications reported

Common Adverse Effects Frequency not defined.
  Cardiovascular: Cardiotoxicity
  Central nervous system: Lethargy
  Gastrointestinal: Protracted vomiting, diarrhea
  Neuromuscular & skeletal: Myopathy

Mechanism of Action Irritates the gastric mucosa and stimulates the medullary chemoreceptor trigger zone to induce vomiting

Drug Interactions
  Increased Effect/Toxicity: Phenothiazines (chlorpromazine has been associated with serious dystonic reactions).
  Decreased Effect: Activated charcoal, milk, carbonated beverages decrease the effect of ipecac syrup.

Pharmacodynamics/Kinetics
  Onset of action: 15-30 minutes
  Duration: 20-25 minutes; 60 minutes in some cases
  Absorption: Significant amounts, mainly when it does not produce emesis
  Excretion: Urine; emetine (alkaloid component) may be detected in urine 60 days after excess dose or chronic use

Pregnancy Risk Factor C

Iplex™ *see* Mecasermin *on page 1023*

IPM Wound Gel™ [OTC] *see* Hyaluronate and Derivatives *on page 816*

IPOL® *see* Poliovirus Vaccine (Inactivated) *on page 1320*

Ipratropium (i pra TROE pee um)

Related Information
Respiratory Diseases *on page 1747*
U.S. Brand Names Atrovent®; Atrovent® HFA
Canadian Brand Names Alti-Ipratropium; Apo-Ipravent®; Atrovent®; Atrovent® HFA; Gen-Ipratropium; Novo-Ipramide; Nu-Ipratropium; PMS-Ipratropium
Mexican Brand Names Atrovent
Generic Available Yes: Excludes solution for oral inhalation, aerosol for oral inhalation
Index Terms Ipratropium Bromide
Pharmacologic Category Anticholinergic Agent
Use Anticholinergic bronchodilator used in bronchospasm associated with COPD, bronchitis, and emphysema; symptomatic relief of rhinorrhea associated with the common cold and allergic and nonallergic rhinitis
Local Anesthetic/Vasoconstrictor Precautions No information available to require special precautions
Effects on Dental Treatment Key adverse event(s) related to dental treatment: Xerostomia and changes in salivation (normal salivary flow resumes upon discontinuation), and dry mucous membranes.
Common Adverse Effects
Inhalation aerosol and inhalation solution:
>10%: Bronchitis (10% to 23%), upper respiratory tract infection (13%)
1% to 10%:
Cardiovascular: Palpitation
Central nervous system: Dizziness (2% to 3%)
Dermatologic: Rash (1%)
Gastrointestinal: Nausea, xerostomia, stomach upset, dry mucous membranes
Renal: Urinary tract infection
Respiratory: Nasal congestion, dyspnea (10%), sputum increased (1%), bronchospasm (2%), pharyngitis (3%), rhinitis (2%), sinusitis (5%)
Miscellaneous: Flu-like syndrome

Nasal spray: Respiratory: Epistaxis (8%), nasal dryness (5%), nausea (2%)
Mechanism of Action Blocks the action of acetylcholine at parasympathetic sites in bronchial smooth muscle causing bronchodilation
Drug Interactions
Increased Effect/Toxicity: Increased toxicity with anticholinergics or drugs with anticholinergic properties.
Pharmacodynamics/Kinetics
Onset of action: Bronchodilation: 1-3 minutes
Peak effect: 1.5-2 hours
Duration: ≤4 hours
Absorption: Negligible
Distribution: Inhalation: 15% of dose reaches lower airways
Pregnancy Risk Factor B

Ipratropium and Albuterol (i pra TROE pee um & al BYOO ter ole)

Related Information
Albuterol *on page 58*
Ipratropium *on page 905*
U.S. Brand Names Combivent®; DuoNeb™
Canadian Brand Names CO Ipra-Sal; Combivent®; Gen-Combo Sterinebs
Mexican Brand Names Combivent
Generic Available No
Index Terms Albuterol and Ipratropium; Salbutamol and Ipratropium
Pharmacologic Category Bronchodilator
Use Treatment of COPD in those patients who are currently on a regular bronchodilator who continue to have bronchospasms and require a second bronchodilator
Local Anesthetic/Vasoconstrictor Precautions No information available to require special precautions
(Continued)

Ipratropium and Albuterol *(Continued)*

Effects on Dental Treatment Key adverse event(s) related to dental treatment: Xerostomia (normal salivary flow resumes upon discontinuation), dry mucous membrane, and unusual taste.

Common Adverse Effects

Based on **ipratropium** component: **Note:** Ipratropium is poorly absorbed from the lung, so systemic effects are rare.

Inhalation aerosol and inhalation solution:

<10%: Respiratory: Upper respiratory infection (13%), bronchitis (15%)

1% to 10%:

Cardiovascular: Palpitation (2%)

Central nervous system: Nervousness (3%), dizziness (2%), fatigue, headache (6%), pain (4%)

Dermatologic: Rash (1%)

Gastrointestinal: Nausea, xerostomia, stomach upset, dry mucous membranes

Respiratory: Nasal congestion, dyspnea (10%), increased sputum (1%), bronchospasm (2%), pharyngitis (3%), rhinitis (2%), sinusitis (5%)

Miscellaneous: Influenza-like symptoms

Based on **albuterol** component:

>10%:

Cardiovascular: Tachycardia, palpitation, pounding heartbeat

Gastrointestinal: GI upset, nausea

1% to 10%:

Cardiovascular: Flushing of face, hypertension or hypotension

Central nervous system: Nervousness, CNS stimulation, hyperactivity, insomnia, dizziness, lightheadedness, drowsiness, headache

Gastrointestinal: Xerostomia, heartburn, vomiting, unusual taste

Genitourinary: Dysuria

Neuromuscular & skeletal: Muscle cramping, tremor, weakness

Respiratory: Coughing

Miscellaneous: Diaphoresis (increased)

Dosage Adults:

Inhalation: 2 inhalations 4 times/day (maximum: 12 inhalations/24 hours)

Inhalation via nebulization: Initial: 3 mL every 6 hours (maximum: 3 mL every 4 hours)

Mechanism of Action See individual agents.

Contraindications

Based on **ipratropium** component: Hypersensitivity to atropine, its derivatives, or any component of the formulation

In addition, Combivent® inhalation aerosol is contraindicated in patients with hypersensitivity to soya lecithin or related food products (eg, soybean and peanut). **Note:** Other formulations may include these components; refer to product-specific labeling.

Based on **albuterol** component: Hypersensitivity to albuterol, adrenergic amines, or any component of the formulation

Drug Interactions

Cytochrome P450 Effect: Albuterol: **Substrate** of CYP3A4 (major)

Increased Effect/Toxicity: See individual agents.

Decreased Effect: See individual agents.

Dietary Considerations Some dosage forms may contain soya lecithin. Do not use in patients allergic to soya lecithin or related food products such as soybean and peanut.

Pharmacodynamics/Kinetics See individual agents.

Pregnancy Risk Factor C

Dosage Forms

Aerosol for oral inhalation:

Combivent®: Ipratropium 18 mcg and albuterol 103 mcg per actuation [200 doses] (14.7 g)

Solution for nebulization:

DuoNeb™: Ipratropium 0.5 mg [0.017%] and albuterol 2.5 mg [0.083%] per 3 mL vial (30s, 60s)

Ipratropium Bromide *see* Ipratropium *on page 905*

I-Prin [OTC] *see* Ibuprofen *on page 853*

Iproveratril Hydrochloride *see* Verapamil *on page 1654*

IPV *see* Poliovirus Vaccine (Inactivated) *on page 1320*

Iquix® *see* Levofloxacin *on page 965*

Irbesartan (ir be SAR tan)

Related Information
Cardiovascular Diseases *on page 1726*

U.S. Brand Names Avapro®

Canadian Brand Names Avapro®

Mexican Brand Names Aprovel; Avapro

Generic Available No

Pharmacologic Category Angiotensin II Receptor Blocker

Use Treatment of hypertension alone or in combination with other antihypertensives; treatment of diabetic nephropathy in patients with type 2 diabetes mellitus (noninsulin dependent, NIDDM) and hypertension

Local Anesthetic/Vasoconstrictor Precautions No information available to require special precautions

Effects on Dental Treatment Key adverse event(s) related to dental treatment: Orthostatic hypotension.

Common Adverse Effects Unless otherwise indicated, percentage of incidence is reported for patients with hypertension.

>10%: Endocrine & metabolic: Hyperkalemia (19%, diabetic nephropathy; rarely seen in HTN)

1% to 10%:

Cardiovascular: Orthostatic hypotension (5%, diabetic nephropathy)

Central nervous system: Fatigue (4%), dizziness (10%, diabetic nephropathy)

Gastrointestinal: Diarrhea (3%), dyspepsia (2%)

Respiratory: Upper respiratory infection (9%), cough (2.8% versus 2.7% in placebo)

>1% but frequency ≤ placebo: Abdominal pain, anxiety, chest pain, edema, headache, influenza, musculoskeletal pain, nausea, nervousness, pharyngitis, rash, rhinitis, sinus abnormality, syncope, tachycardia, urinary tract infection, vertigo, vomiting

Dosage Oral:

Hypertension:

Children:

<6 years: Safety and efficacy have not been established.

≥6-12 years: Initial: 75 mg once daily; may be titrated to a maximum of 150 mg once daily

Children ≥13 years and Adults: 150 mg once daily; patients may be titrated to 300 mg once daily

Note: Starting dose in volume-depleted patients should be 75 mg

Nephropathy in patients with type 2 diabetes and hypertension: Adults: Target dose: 300 mg once daily

Dosage adjustment in renal impairment: No dosage adjustment necessary with mild to severe impairment unless the patient is also volume depleted.

Mechanism of Action Irbesartan is an angiotensin receptor antagonist. Angiotensin II acts as a vasoconstrictor. In addition to causing direct vasoconstriction, angiotensin II also stimulates the release of aldosterone. Once aldosterone is released, sodium as well as water are reabsorbed. The end result is an elevation in blood pressure. Irbesartan binds to the AT1 angiotensin II receptor. This binding prevents angiotensin II from binding to the receptor thereby blocking the vasoconstriction and the aldosterone secreting effects of angiotensin II.

Contraindications Hypersensitivity to irbesartan or any component of the formulation; hypersensitivity to other A-II receptor antagonists; bilateral renal artery stenosis; pregnancy

Warnings/Precautions [U.S. Boxed Warning]: Based on human data, drugs that act on the angiotensin system can cause injury and death to the developing fetus when used in the second and third trimesters. Angiotensin receptor blockers should be discontinued as soon as possible once pregnancy is detected. May cause hyperkalemia; avoid potassium supplementation unless specifically required by healthcare provider. May be associated with deterioration of renal function and/or increases in serum creatinine, particularly in patients dependent on renin-angiotensin-aldosterone system. Avoid use or use a much smaller dose in patients who are intravascularly volume-depleted; use caution in patients with unilateral or bilateral renal artery stenosis to avoid a decrease in renal function; AUCs of irbesartan (not the active metabolite) are about 50% greater in patients with Cl_{cr} <30 mL/minute and are doubled in hemodialysis patients. Safety and efficacy have not been established in pediatric patients <6 years of age.

Drug Interactions

Cytochrome P450 Effect: Substrate of CYP2C9 (minor); **Inhibits** CYP2C8 (moderate), 2C9 (moderate), 2D6 (weak), 3A4 (weak)

(Continued)

Irbesartan *(Continued)*

Increased Effect/Toxicity: Potassium salts/supplements, co-trimoxazole (high dose), ACE inhibitors, and potassium-sparing diuretics (amiloride, spironolactone, triamterene) may increase the risk of hyperkalemia. Irbesartan may increase the levels/effects of amiodarone, bosentan, dapsone, fluoxetine, glimepiride, glipizide, losartan, montelukast, nateglinide, paclitaxel, phenytoin, pioglitazone, repaglinide, rosiglitazone, warfarin, zafirlukast, and other CYP2C8 and 2C9 substrates.

Ethanol/Nutrition/Herb Interactions Herb/Nutraceutical: Avoid dong quai if using for hypertension (has estrogenic activity). Avoid ephedra, yohimbe, ginseng (may worsen hypertension). Avoid garlic (may have increased antihypertensive effect).

Dietary Considerations May be taken with or without food.

Pharmacodynamics/Kinetics

Onset of action: Peak effect: 1-2 hours

Duration: >24 hours

Distribution: V_d: 53-93 L

Protein binding, plasma: 90%

Metabolism: Hepatic, primarily CYP2C9

Bioavailability: 60% to 80%

Half-life elimination: Terminal: 11-15 hours

Time to peak, serum: 1.5-2 hours

Excretion: Feces (80%); urine (20%)

Pregnancy Risk Factor C/D (2nd and 3rd trimesters)

Dosage Forms

Tablet:

Avapro®: 75 mg, 150 mg, 300 mg

Irbesartan and Hydrochlorothiazide

(ir be SAR tan & hye droe klor oh THYE a zide)

Related Information

Cardiovascular Diseases *on page 1726*
Hydrochlorothiazide *on page 819*
Irbesartan *on page 907*

U.S. Brand Names Avalide®

Canadian Brand Names Avalide®

Mexican Brand Names Co-Aprovel

Generic Available No

Index Terms Avapro® HCT; Hydrochlorothiazide and Irbesartan

Pharmacologic Category Angiotensin II Receptor Blocker Combination; Antihypertensive Agent, Combination; Diuretic, Thiazide

Use Combination therapy for the management of hypertension

Local Anesthetic/Vasoconstrictor Precautions No information available to require special precautions

Effects on Dental Treatment No significant effects or complications reported

Common Adverse Effects See individual agents.

Mechanism of Action

Irbesartan: Irbesartan is an angiotensin receptor antagonist. Angiotensin II acts as a vasoconstrictor. In addition to causing direct vasoconstriction, angiotensin II also stimulates the release of aldosterone. Once aldosterone is released, sodium as well as water are reabsorbed. The end result is an elevation in blood pressure. Irbesartan binds to the AT1 angiotensin II receptor. This binding prevents angiotensin II from binding to the receptor thereby blocking the vasoconstriction and the aldosterone secreting effects of angiotensin II.

Hydrochlorothiazide: Inhibits sodium reabsorption in the distal tubules causing increased excretion of sodium and water as well as potassium and hydrogen ions

Drug Interactions

Cytochrome P450 Effect: Irbesartan: **Substrate** of CYP2C9 (minor); **Inhibits** CYP2C8 (moderate), 2C9 (moderate), 2D6 (weak), 3A4 (weak)

Increased Effect/Toxicity: See individual agents.

Decreased Effect: See individual agents.

Pregnancy Risk Factor C/D (2nd and 3rd trimesters)

Ircon® [OTC] *see* Ferrous Fumarate *on page 687*
IRESSA® *see* Gefitinib *on page 769*

Irinotecan (eye rye no TEE kan)

U.S. Brand Names Camptosar®
Canadian Brand Names Camptosar®; Irinotecan Hydrochloride Trihydrate
Mexican Brand Names Camptosar
Generic Available No
Index Terms Camptothecin-11; CPT-11; NSC-616348
Pharmacologic Category Antineoplastic Agent, Natural Source (Plant) Derivative
Use Treatment of metastatic carcinoma of the colon or rectum
Unlabeled/Investigational Use Lung cancer (small cell and nonsmall cell), cervical cancer, gastric cancer, pancreatic cancer, leukemia, lymphoma, breast cancer
Local Anesthetic/Vasoconstrictor Precautions No information available to require special precautions
Effects on Dental Treatment Key adverse event(s) related to dental treatment: Increased salivation, mucositis, and stomatitis.
Common Adverse Effects Frequency of adverse reactions reported for single-agent use of irinotecan only.
>10%:
Cardiovascular: Vasodilation (9% to 11%)
Central nervous system: Cholinergic toxicity (47% - includes rhinitis, increased salivation, miosis, lacrimation, diaphoresis, flushing and intestinal hyperperistalsis); fever (44% to 45%), pain (23% to 24%), dizziness (15% to 21%), insomnia (19%), headache (17%), chills (14%)
Dermatologic: Alopecia (46% to 72%), rash (13% to 14%)
Endocrine & metabolic: Dehydration (15%)
Gastrointestinal: Diarrhea, late (83% to 88%; grade 3/4: 5% to 31%), diarrhea, early (43% to 51%; grade 3/4: 6% to 22%), nausea (70% to 86%), abdominal pain (57% to 68%), vomiting (62% to 67%), cramps (57%), anorexia (44% to 55%), constipation (30% to 32%), mucositis (30%), weight loss (30%), flatulence (12%), stomatitis (12%)
Hematologic: Anemia (60% to 97%; grades 3/4: 5% to 22%), leukopenia (63% to 96%, grades 3/4: 14% to 28%), thrombocytopenia (96%, grades 3/4: 1% to 4%), neutropenia (30% to 96%; grades 3/4: 14% to 31%)
Hepatic: Bilirubin increased (84%), alkaline phosphatase increased (13%)
Neuromuscular & skeletal: Weakness (69% to 76%), back pain (14%)
Respiratory: Dyspnea (22%), cough (17% to 20%), rhinitis (16%)
Miscellaneous: Diaphoresis (16%), infection (14%)
1% to 10%:
Cardiovascular: Edema (10%), hypotension (6%), thromboembolic events (5%)
Central nervous system: Somnolence (9%), confusion (3%)
Gastrointestinal: Abdominal fullness (10%), dyspepsia (10%)
Hematologic: Neutropenic fever (grades 3/4: 2% to 6%), hemorrhage (grades 3/4: 1% to 5%), neutropenic infection (grades 3/4: 1% to 2%)
Hepatic: AST increased (10%), ascites and/or jaundice (grades 3/4: 9%)
Respiratory: Pneumonia (4%)
Note: In limited pediatric experience, dehydration (often associated with severe hypokalemia and hyponatremia) was among the most significant grade 3/4 adverse events, with a frequency up to 29%. In addition, grade 3/4 infection was reported in 24%.
Mechanism of Action Irinotecan and its active metabolite (SN-38) bind reversibly to topoisomerase I-DNA complex preventing religation of the cleaved DNA strand. This results in the accumulation of cleavable complexes and double-strand DNA breaks. As mammalian cells cannot efficiently repair these breaks, cell death consistent with S-phase cell cycle specificity occurs, leading to termination of cellular replication.
Drug Interactions
Cytochrome P450 Effect: Substrate (major) of CYP2B6, 3A4
Increased Effect/Toxicity: CYP2B6 inhibitors may increase the levels/effects of irinotecan; example inhibitors include desipramine, paroxetine, and sertraline. CYP3A4 inhibitors may increase the levels/effects of irinotecan; example inhibitors include azole antifungals, clarithromycin, diclofenac, doxycycline, erythromycin, imatinib, isoniazid, nefazodone, nicardipine, propofol, protease inhibitors, quinidine, telithromycin, and verapamil. Atazanavir may increase the levels/effects of irinotecan (SN-38) by CYP3A4 and UGT1A1 inhibition. Bevacizumab may increase the adverse effects of irinotecan (eg, diarrhea, neutropenia). Ketoconazole increases the levels/effects of irinotecan and active metabolite; discontinue ketoconazole 1 week prior to irinotecan therapy; **concurrent use is contraindicated.**
(Continued)

Irinotecan *(Continued)*

Decreased Effect: CYP2B6 inducers may decrease the levels/effects of irinotecan; example inducers include carbamazepine, nevirapine, phenobarbital, phenytoin, and rifampin. CYP3A4 inducers may decrease the levels/effects of irinotecan; example inducers include aminoglutethimide, carbamazepine, nafcillin, nevirapine, phenobarbital, phenytoin, and rifamycins. St John's wort decreases therapeutic effect of irinotecan; discontinue ≥2 weeks prior to irinotecan therapy; **concurrent use is contraindicated.**

Pharmacodynamics/Kinetics

Distribution: V_d: 33-150 L/m^2

Protein binding, plasma: Predominantly albumin; Parent drug: 30% to 68%, SN-38 (active drug): ~95%

Metabolism: Primarily hepatic to SN-38 (active metabolite) by carboxylesterase enzymes; SN-38 undergoes conjugation by UDP- glucuronosyl transferase 1A1 (UGT1A1) to form a glucuronide metabolite. SN-38 is increased by UGT1A1*28 polymorphism (10% of North Americans are homozygous for UGT1A1*28 allele). The lactones of both irinotecan and SN-38 undergo hydrolysis to inactive hydroxy acid forms.

Half-life elimination: SN-38: Mean terminal: 10-20 hours

Time to peak: SN-38: Following 90-minute infusion: ~1 hour

Excretion: Within 24 hours: Urine: Irinotecan (11% to 20%), metabolites (SN-38 <1%, SN-38 glucuronide, 3%)

Pregnancy Risk Factor D

Iron Dextran Complex *(EYE ern DEKS tran KOM pleks)*

U.S. Brand Names Dexferrum®; INFeD®

Canadian Brand Names Dexiron™; Infufer®

Mexican Brand Names Driken

Generic Available No

Pharmacologic Category Iron Salt

Use Treatment of microcytic hypochromic anemia resulting from iron deficiency in patients in whom oral administration is infeasible or ineffective

Local Anesthetic/Vasoconstrictor Precautions No information available to require special precautions

Effects on Dental Treatment Key adverse event(s) related to dental treatment: Metallic taste.

Common Adverse Effects

>10%:

Cardiovascular: Flushing

Central nervous system: Dizziness, fever, headache, pain

Gastrointestinal: Nausea, vomiting, metallic taste

Local: Staining of skin at the site of I.M. injection

Miscellaneous: Diaphoresis

1% to 10%:

Cardiovascular: Hypotension (1% to 2%)

Dermatologic: Urticaria (1% to 2%), phlebitis (1% to 2%)

Gastrointestinal: Diarrhea

Genitourinary: Discoloration of urine

Note: Diaphoresis, urticaria, arthralgia, fever, chills, dizziness, headache, and nausea may be delayed 24-48 hours after I.V. administration or 3-4 days after I.M. administration.

Anaphylactoid reactions: Respiratory difficulties and cardiovascular collapse have been reported and occur most frequently within the first several minutes of administration.

Mechanism of Action The released iron, from the plasma, eventually replenishes the depleted iron stores in the bone marrow where it is incorporated into hemoglobin

Drug Interactions

Decreased Effect: Decreased effect with chloramphenicol.

Pharmacodynamics/Kinetics

Absorption:

I.M.: 50% to 90% is promptly absorbed, balance is slowly absorbed over month

I.V.: Uptake of iron by the reticuloendothelial system appears to be constant at about 10-20 mg/hour

Excretion: Urine and feces via reticuloendothelial system

Pregnancy Risk Factor C

Iron Fumarate *see* Ferrous Fumarate *on page 687*

Iron Gluconate *see* Ferrous Gluconate *on page 687*

Iron-Polysaccharide Complex *see* Polysaccharide-Iron Complex *on page 1323*

Iron Sucrose (EYE ern SOO krose)

U.S. Brand Names Venofer®
Canadian Brand Names Venofer®
Generic Available No
Pharmacologic Category Iron Salt
Use Treatment of iron-deficiency anemia in chronic renal failure, including nondialysis-dependent patients (with or without erythropoietin therapy) and dialysis-dependent patients receiving erythropoietin therapy
Local Anesthetic/Vasoconstrictor Precautions No information available to require special precautions
Effects on Dental Treatment Key adverse event(s) related to dental treatment: Taste perversion.
Common Adverse Effects
>10%:
Cardiovascular: Hypotension (1% to 7%; 39% in hemodialysis patients; may be related to total dose or rate of administration), peripheral edema (2% to 13%)
Central nervous system: Headache (3% to 13%)
Gastrointestinal: Nausea (1% to 15%)
Neuromuscular & skeletal: Muscle cramps (1% to 3%; 29% in hemodialysis patients)
1% to 10%:
Cardiovascular: Hypertension (6% to 8%), edema (1% to 7%), chest pain (1% to 6%), murmur (<1% to 3%), CHF
Central nervous system: Dizziness (1% to 10%), fatigue (2% to 5%), fever (1% to 3%), anxiety
Dermatologic: Pruritus (1% to 7%), rash (<1% to 2%)
Endocrine & metabolic: Gout (2% to 7%), hypoglycemia (<1% to 4%), hyperglycemia (3% to 4%), fluid overload (1% to 3%)
Gastrointestinal: Diarrhea (1% to 10%), vomiting (5% to 9%), taste perversion (1% to 9%), peritoneal infection (8%), constipation (1% to 7%), abdominal pain (1% to 4%), positive fecal occult blood (1% to 3%)
Genitourinary: Urinary tract infection (≤1%)
Local: Injection site reaction (2% to 4%), catheter site infection (4%)
Neuromuscular & skeletal: Muscle pain (1% to 7%), extremity pain (3% to 6%), arthralgia (1% to 4%), weakness (1% to 3%), back pain (1% to 3%)
Ocular: Conjunctivitis (<1% to 3%)
Otic: Ear pain (1% to 7%)
Respiratory: Dyspnea (1% to 10%), pharyngitis (<1% to 7%), cough (1% to 7%), sinusitis (1% to 4%), rhinitis (1% to 3%), upper respiratory infection (1% to 3%), nasal congestion (1%)
Miscellaneous: Graft complication (1% to 10%), hypersensitivity, sepsis
Mechanism of Action Iron sucrose is dissociated by the reticuloendothelial system into iron and sucrose. The released iron increases serum iron concentrations and is incorporated into hemoglobin.
Drug Interactions
Increased Effect/Toxicity: Iron sucrose injection may reduce the absorption of oral iron preparations.
Pharmacodynamics/Kinetics
Distribution: V_{dss}: Healthy adults: 7.9 L
Metabolism: Dissociated into iron and sucrose by the reticuloendothelial system
Half-life elimination: Healthy adults: 6 hours
Excretion: Healthy adults: Urine (5%) within 24 hours
Pregnancy Risk Factor B

Isocarboxazid (eye soe kar BOKS a zid)

U.S. Brand Names Marplan®
Generic Available No
(Continued)

Isocarboxazid *(Continued)*

Pharmacologic Category Antidepressant, Monoamine Oxidase Inhibitor
Use Treatment of depression

Local Anesthetic/Vasoconstrictor Precautions Attempts should be made to avoid use of vasoconstrictor due to possibility of hypertensive episodes with monoamine oxidase inhibitors

Effects on Dental Treatment Key adverse event(s) related to dental treatment: Orthostatic hypotension, xerostomia (normal salivary flow resumes upon discontinuation).

Common Adverse Effects
>10%:
Cardiovascular: Orthostatic hypotension
Central nervous system: Drowsiness
Endocrine & metabolic: Decreased sexual ability
Neuromuscular & skeletal: Weakness, trembling
Ocular: Blurred vision
1% to 10%:
Cardiovascular: Tachycardia, peripheral edema
Central nervous system: Nervousness, chills
Dermatologic: Xerostomia
Gastrointestinal: Diarrhea, anorexia, constipation, xerostomia

Restrictions An FDA-approved medication guide concerning the use of antidepressants in children, adolescents, and young adults must be distributed when dispensing an outpatient prescription (new or refill) where this medication is to be used without direct supervision of a healthcare provider. Medication guides are available at http://www.fda.gov/cder/Offices/ODS/medication_guides.htm. Dispense to parents or guardians of children and adolescents receiving this medication.

Mechanism of Action Thought to act by increasing endogenous concentrations of epinephrine, norepinephrine, dopamine, and serotonin through inhibition of the enzyme (monoamine oxidase) responsible for the breakdown of these neurotransmitters

Drug Interactions
Increased Effect/Toxicity: In general, the combined use with TCAs, venlafaxine, trazodone, dexfenfluramine, sibutramine, lithium, meperidine, fenfluramine, dextromethorphan, and SSRIs should be avoided due to the potential for severe adverse reactions (serotonin syndrome, death). MAO inhibitors (including isocarboxazid) may inhibit the metabolism of barbiturates and prolong their effect. Isocarboxazid in combination with amphetamines, other stimulants (methylphenidate), levodopa, metaraminol, reserpine, and decongestants (pseudoephedrine) may result in severe hypertensive reactions. Isocarboxazid may increase the pressor response of norepinephrine and may prolong neuromuscular blockade produced by succinylcholine. Tramadol may increase the risk of seizures and serotonin syndrome in patients receiving an MAO inhibitor. Isocarboxazid may produce additive hypoglycemic effect in patients receiving hypoglycemic agents and may produce delirium in patients receiving disulfiram.
Decreased Effect: MAO inhibitors may inhibit the antihypertensive response to guanadrel or guanethidine.

Pregnancy Risk Factor C

Isochron™ *see* Isosorbide Dinitrate *on page 914*

Isometheptene, Acetaminophen, and Dichloralphenazone *see* Acetaminophen, Isometheptene, and Dichloralphenazone *on page 45*

Isometheptene, Dichloralphenazone, and Acetaminophen *see* Acetaminophen, Isometheptene, and Dichloralphenazone *on page 45*

IsonaRif™ *see* Rifampin and Isoniazid *on page 1424*

Isoniazid *(eye soe NYE a zid)*

Related Information
Tuberculosis *on page 1765*
U.S. Brand Names Nydrazid® [DSC]
Canadian Brand Names Isotamine®; PMS-Isoniazid
Mexican Brand Names Valifol
Generic Available Yes
Index Terms INH; Isonicotinic Acid Hydrazide
Pharmacologic Category Antitubercular Agent
Use Treatment of susceptible tuberculosis infections; treatment of latent tuberculosis infection (LTBI)
Local Anesthetic/Vasoconstrictor Precautions No information available to require special precautions

Effects on Dental Treatment Key adverse event(s) related to dental treatment: Xerostomia (normal salivary flow resumes upon discontinuation).

Common Adverse Effects Frequency not defined.

Cardiovascular: Hypertension, palpitation, tachycardia, vasculitis

Central nervous system: Dizziness, encephalopathy, memory impairment, slurred speech, lethargy, fever, depression, psychosis, seizure

Dermatologic: Rash (morbilliform, maculopapular, pruritic, or exfoliative), flushing

Endocrine & metabolic: Hyperglycemia, metabolic acidosis, gynecomastia, pellagra, pyridoxine deficiency

Gastrointestinal: Anorexia, nausea, vomiting, stomach pain

Hematologic: Agranulocytosis, anemia (sideroblastic, hemolytic, or aplastic), thrombocytopenia, eosinophilia, lymphadenopathy

Hepatic: LFTs mildly increased (10% to 20%); hyperbilirubinemia, jaundice, hepatitis (may involve progressive liver damage; risk increases with age; 2.3% in patients >50 years)

Neuromuscular & skeletal: Weakness, peripheral neuropathy (dose-related incidence, 10% to 20% incidence with 10 mg/kg/day), hyper-reflexia, arthralgia, lupus-like syndrome

Ocular: Blurred vision, loss of vision, optic neuritis and atrophy

Mechanism of Action Unknown, but may include the inhibition of myocolic acid synthesis resulting in disruption of the bacterial cell wall

Drug Interactions

Cytochrome P450 Effect: Substrate of CYP2E1 (major); **Inhibits** CYP1A2 (weak), 2A6 (moderate), 2C9 (weak), 2C19 (strong), 2D6 (moderate), 2E1 (moderate), 3A4 (strong); **Induces** CYP2E1 (after discontinuation) (weak)

Increased Effect/Toxicity: Concurrent use of disulfiram may result in acute intolerance reactions. Isoniazid may increase the levels/effects of amphetamines, benzodiazepines, beta-blockers, calcium channel blockers, citalopram, dexmedetomidine, dextromethorphan, diazepam, fluoxetine, ifosfamide, inhalational anesthetics, lidocaine, methsuximide, mirtazapine, nateglinide, nefazodone, phenytoin, propranolol, risperidone, ritonavir, sertraline, tacrolimus, theophylline, thioridazine, tricyclic antidepressants, trimethadione, venlafaxine, and other substrates of CYP2A6, 2C19, 2D6, 2E1, or 3A4. Selected benzodiazepines (midazolam and triazolam), cisapride, ergot alkaloids, selected HMG-CoA reductase inhibitors (lovastatin and simvastatin), and pimozide are generally contraindicated with strong CYP3A4 inhibitors. Mesoridazine and thioridazine are generally contraindicated with strong CYP2D6 inhibitors. When used with strong CYP3A4 inhibitors, dosage adjustment/limits are recommended for sildenafil and other PDE-5 inhibitors; consult individual monographs.

Decreased Effect: Decreased effect/levels of isoniazid with aluminum salts or antacids. Isoniazid may decrease the levels/effects of CYP2D6 prodrug substrates (eg, codeine, hydrocodone, oxycodone, tramadol).

Pharmacodynamics/Kinetics

Absorption: Rapid and complete; rate can be slowed with food

Distribution: All body tissues and fluids including CSF; crosses placenta; enters breast milk

Protein binding: 10% to 15%

Metabolism: Hepatic with decay rate determined genetically by acetylation phenotype

Half-life elimination: Fast acetylators: 30-100 minutes; Slow acetylators: 2-5 hours; may be prolonged with hepatic or severe renal impairment

Time to peak, serum: 1-2 hours

Excretion: Urine (75% to 95%); feces; saliva

Pregnancy Risk Factor C

Isoproterenol (eye soe proe TER e nole)

U.S. Brand Names Isuprel®
Generic Available Yes
(Continued)

Isoproterenol *(Continued)*

Index Terms Isoproterenol Hydrochloride

Pharmacologic Category Beta$_1$- & Beta$_2$-Adrenergic Agonist Agent

Use Ventricular arrhythmias due to AV nodal block; hemodynamically compromised bradyarrhythmias or atropine- and dopamine-resistant bradyarrhythmias (when transcutaneous/venous pacing is not available); temporary use in third-degree AV block until pacemaker insertion

Unlabeled/Investigational Use Pharmacologic overdrive pacing for torsade de pointes; diagnostic aid (vasovagal syncope)

Local Anesthetic/Vasoconstrictor Precautions Isoproterenol is selective for beta-adrenergic receptors and not alpha-receptors; therefore, there is no precaution in the use of vasoconstrictor such as epinephrine

Effects on Dental Treatment Key adverse event(s) related to dental treatment: Xerostomia and changes in salivation (normal salivary flow resumes upon discontinuation).

Common Adverse Effects Frequency not defined.

Cardiovascular: Premature ventricular beats, bradycardia, hyper-/hypotension, chest pain, palpitation, tachycardia, ventricular arrhythmia, MI size increased

Central nervous system: Headache, nervousness or restlessness

Endocrine & metabolic: Serum glucose increased, serum potassium decreased, hypokalemia

Gastrointestinal: Nausea, vomiting

Respiratory: Dyspnea

Mechanism of Action Stimulates beta$_1$- and beta$_2$-receptors resulting in relaxation of bronchial, GI, and uterine smooth muscle, increased heart rate and contractility, vasodilation of peripheral vasculature

Drug Interactions

Increased Effect/Toxicity: Sympathomimetic agents may cause headaches and elevate blood pressure. General anesthetics may cause arrhythmias.

Pharmacodynamics/Kinetics

Onset of action: Bronchodilation: I.V.: Immediate

Duration: I.V.: 10-15 minutes

Metabolism: Via conjugation in many tissues including hepatic and pulmonary

Half-life elimination: 2.5-5 minutes

Excretion: Urine (primarily as sulfate conjugates)

Pregnancy Risk Factor C

Isoproterenol Hydrochloride *see* Isoproterenol *on page 913*

Isoptin® SR *see* Verapamil *on page 1654*

Isopto® Atropine *see* Atropine *on page 166*

Isopto® Carbachol *see* Carbachol *on page 272*

Isopto® Carpine *see* Pilocarpine (Ophthalmic) *on page 1300*

Isopto® Homatropine *see* Homatropine *on page 815*

Isopto® Hyoscine *see* Scopolamine *on page 1457*

Isopto® Tears [OTC] *see* Hydroxypropyl Methylcellulose *on page 844*

Isordil® *see* Isosorbide Dinitrate *on page 914*

Isosorbide Dinitrate *(eye soe SOR bide dye NYE trate)*

Related Information

Cardiovascular Diseases *on page 1726*

Isosorbide Mononitrate *on page 916*

U.S. Brand Names Dilatrate®-SR; Isochron™; Isordil®

Canadian Brand Names Apo-ISDN®; Cedocard®-SR; Coronex®; Novo-Sorbide; PMS-Isosorbide

Mexican Brand Names Isorbid

Generic Available Yes: Tablet, sublingual tablet

Index Terms ISD; ISDN

Pharmacologic Category Vasodilator

Use Prevention and treatment of angina pectoris; for congestive heart failure; to relieve pain, dysphagia, and spasm in esophageal spasm with GE reflux

Unlabeled/Investigational Use Esophageal spastic disorders

Local Anesthetic/Vasoconstrictor Precautions No information available to require special precautions

Effects on Dental Treatment Key adverse event(s) related to dental treatment: Xerostomia and changes in salivation (normal salivary flow resumes upon discontinuation).

Common Adverse Effects Frequency not defined.

Cardiovascular: Hypotension (infrequent), postural hypotension, crescendo angina (uncommon), rebound hypertension (uncommon), pallor, cardiovascular collapse, tachycardia, shock, flushing, peripheral edema

Central nervous system: Headache (most common), lightheadedness (related to blood pressure changes), syncope (uncommon), dizziness, restlessness
Gastrointestinal: Nausea, vomiting, bowel incontinence, xerostomia
Genitourinary: Urinary incontinence
Hematologic: Methemoglobinemia (rare, overdose)
Neuromuscular & skeletal: Weakness
Ocular: Blurred vision
Miscellaneous: Cold sweat

The incidence of hypotension and adverse cardiovascular events may be increased when used in combination with sildenafil (Viagra®).

Mechanism of Action Stimulation of intracellular cyclic-GMP results in vascular smooth muscle relaxation of both arterial and venous vasculature. Increased venous pooling decreases left ventricular pressure (preload) and arterial dilatation decreases arterial resistance (afterload). Therefore, this reduces cardiac oxygen demand by decreasing left ventricular pressure and systemic vascular resistance by dilating arteries. Additionally, coronary artery dilation improves collateral flow to ischemic regions; esophageal smooth muscle is relaxed via the same mechanism.

Drug Interactions

Cytochrome P450 Effect: Substrate of CYP3A4 (major)

Increased Effect/Toxicity: CYP3A4 inhibitors may increase the levels/ effects of isosorbide dinitrate; example inhibitors include azole antifungals, clarithromycin, diclofenac, doxycycline, erythromycin, imatinib, isoniazid, nefazodone, nicardipine, propofol, protease inhibitors, quinidine, telithromycin, and verapamil. Significant reduction of systolic and diastolic blood pressure with concurrent use of sildenafil, tadalafil, or vardenafil (contraindicated). Do not administer sildenafil, tadalafil, or vardenafil within 24 hours of a nitrate preparation.

Decreased Effect: CYP3A4 inducers may decrease the levels/effects of isosorbide dinitrate; example inducers include aminoglutethimide, carbamazepine, nafcillin, nevirapine, phenobarbital, phenytoin, and rifamycins.

Pharmacodynamics/Kinetics

Onset of action: Sublingual tablet: 2-10 minutes; Chewable tablet: 3 minutes; Oral tablet: 45-60 minutes

Duration: Sublingual tablet: 1-2 hours; Chewable tablet: 0.5-2 hours; Oral tablet: 4-6 hours

Metabolism: Extensively hepatic to conjugated metabolites, including isosorbide 5-mononitrate (active) and 2-mononitrate (active)

Half-life elimination: Parent drug: 1-4 hours; Metabolite (5-mononitrate): 4 hours

Excretion: Urine and feces

Pregnancy Risk Factor C

Isosorbide Dinitrate and Hydralazine
(eye soe SOR bide dye NYE trate & hye DRAL a zeen)

U.S. Brand Names BiDil®
Generic Available No
Index Terms Hydralazine and Isosorbide Dinitrate
Pharmacologic Category Vasodilator
Use Treatment of heart failure, adjunct to standard therapy, in self-identified African-Americans

Local Anesthetic/Vasoconstrictor Precautions No information available to require special precautions

Effects on Dental Treatment No significant effects or complications reported

Common Adverse Effects The following events were reported in the A-HeFT Study using the combination isosorbide dinitrate/hydralazine product. See individual drug monographs for additional information.

>10%:
Cardiovascular: Chest pain (16%)
Central nervous system: Headache (50%), dizziness (32%)
Neuromuscular & skeletal: Weakness (14%)

1% to 10%:
Cardiovascular: Hypotension (8%), ventricular tachycardia (4%), palpitation (4%), tachycardia (2%)
Dermatologic: Alopecia (1%), angioedema (1%)
Endocrine & metabolic: Hyperglycemia (4%), hyperlipidemia (3%), hypercholesterolemia (1%)
Gastrointestinal: Nausea (10%), vomiting (4%)
Hepatic: Cholecystitis (1%)
Neuromuscular & skeletal: Paresthesia (4%), arthralgia (1%), myalgia (1%), tendon disorder (1%)
Respiratory: Bronchitis (8%), sinusitis (4%), rhinitis (4%)

(Continued)

Isosorbide Dinitrate and Hydralazine *(Continued)*

Miscellaneous: Allergic reaction (1%), diaphoresis (1%)

Dosage Oral: Adults: Initial: 1 tablet 3 times/day; titrate to a maximum dose of 2 tablets 3 times/day

Dosage adjustment for toxicity: If patient experiences persistent headache, adjust dosing to twice daily.

Mechanism of Action

Hydralazine: Direct vasodilation of arterioles (with little effect on veins) resulting in decreased systemic resistance

Isosorbide Dinitrate: Nitric oxide release causes stimulation of intracellular guanylyl cyclase leading to increased cyclic GMP. This results in vascular smooth muscle relaxation of both arterial and venous vasculature. Increased venous pooling decreases left ventricular pressure (preload) and arterial dilatation decreases arterial resistance (afterload). Therefore, this reduces cardiac oxygen demand by decreasing left ventricular pressure and systemic vascular resistance by dilating arteries. Additionally, coronary artery dilation improves collateral flow to ischemic regions.

Contraindications Hypersensitivity to isosorbide dinitrate, hydralazine, or any component of the formulation; hypersensitivity to organic nitrates; concurrent use with phosphodiesterase-5 inhibitors (sildenafil, tadalafil, or vardenafil); angle-closure glaucoma (intraocular pressure may be increased); head trauma or cerebral hemorrhage (increase intracranial pressure); severe anemia; mitral valve rheumatic heart disease

Warnings/Precautions May cause a drug-induced lupus-like syndrome (more likely on larger doses, longer duration). Adjust dose in severe renal dysfunction. Use with caution in CAD (increase in tachycardia may increase myocardial oxygen demand). Use with caution in pulmonary hypertension; severe hypotension can occur. Use with caution in volume depletion, hypotension, and right ventricular infarctions. Hydralazine-induced fluid and sodium retention may require addition or increased dosage of a diuretics. Paradoxical bradycardia and increased angina pectoris can accompany hypotension. Postural hypotension can also occur. Nitrates may aggravate angina caused by hypertrophic cardiomyopathy. Tolerance may develop to nitrates and appropriate dosing is needed to minimize this. Avoid concurrent use with PDE-5 inhibitors. Safety and efficacy have not been established in pediatric patients.

Drug Interactions

Cytochrome P450 Effect: Hydralazine: **Inhibits** CYP3A4 (weak); Isosorbide dinitrate: **Substrate** of CYP3A4 (major)

Increased Effect/Toxicity: See individual agents.

Pharmacodynamics/Kinetics The following values are from administration of isosorbide dinitrate 40 mg and hydralazine 75 mg in healthy adults. Also see individual drug monographs.

Half-life elimination: Hydralazine: 4 hours; Isosorbide dinitrate: 2 hours

Time to peak, plasma: 1 hour (both agents)

Pregnancy Risk Factor C

Dosage Forms

Tablet:

BiDil®: Isosorbide 20 mg and hydralazine 37.5 mg

Selected Readings

Cohn JN, Archibald DG, Francis GS, et al, "Effect of Vasodilator Therapy on Mortality in Chronic Congestive Heart Failure: Results of a Veterans Administration Cooperative Study," *N Engl J Med*, 1986, 314 (24):1547-52.

Cohn JN, Johnson G, Ziesche S, et al, "A Comparison of Enalapril With Hydralazine " Isosorbide Dinitrate in the Treatment of Chronic Congestive Heart Failure," *N Engl J Med*, 1991, 325(5):303-10.

Hunt SA, Abraham WT, Chin MH, et al, "ACC/AHA 2005 Guideline Update for the Diagnosis and Management of Chronic Heart Failure in the Adult-Summary Article A Report of the American College of Cardiology/American Heart Association Task Force on Practice Guidelines (Writing Committee to Update the 2001 Guidelines for the Evaluation and Management of Heart Failure)," *J Am Coll Cardiol*, 2005, 46(6):1116-43.

Taylor AL, Ziesche S, Yancy C, et al, "Combination of Isosorbide Dinitrate and Hydralazine in Blacks With Heart Failure," *N Engl J Med*, 2004, 351(20):2049-57.

Isosorbide Mononitrate *(eye soe SOR bide mon oh NYE trate)*

Related Information

Cardiovascular Diseases *on page 1726*
Isosorbide Dinitrate *on page 914*

U.S. Brand Names Imdur®; Ismo®; Monoket®

Canadian Brand Names Apo-ISMN; Imdur®

Mexican Brand Names Elantan; Imdur 60; Mono Mack

Generic Available Yes

Index Terms ISMN

Pharmacologic Category Vasodilator

Use Long-acting metabolite of the vasodilator isosorbide dinitrate used for the prophylactic treatment of angina pectoris

Local Anesthetic/Vasoconstrictor Precautions No information available to require special precautions

Effects on Dental Treatment No significant effects or complications reported

Common Adverse Effects

>10%: Central nervous system: Headache (19% to 38%)

1% to 10%:

Central nervous system: Dizziness (3% to 5%)

Gastrointestinal: Nausea/vomiting (2% to 4%)

The incidence of hypotension and adverse cardiovascular events may be increased when used in combination with sildenafil (Viagra®).

Dosage Adults and Geriatrics (start with lowest recommended dose): Oral:

Regular tablet: 5-20 mg twice daily with the two doses given 7 hours apart (eg, 8 AM and 3 PM) to decrease tolerance development; then titrate to 10 mg twice daily in first 2-3 days.

Extended release tablet: Initial: 30-60 mg given in morning as a single dose; titrate upward as needed, giving at least 3 days between increases; maximum daily single dose: 240 mg

Dosing adjustment in renal impairment: Not necessary for elderly or patients with altered renal or hepatic function.

Tolerance to nitrate effects develops with chronic exposure. Dose escalation does not overcome this effect. Tolerance can only be overcome by short periods of nitrate absence from the body. Short periods (10-12 hours) of nitrate withdrawal help minimize tolerance. Recommended dosage regimens incorporate this interval. General recommendations are to take the last dose of short-acting agents no later than 7 PM; administer 2 times/day rather than 4 times/day. Administer sustained release tablet once daily in the morning.

Mechanism of Action Prevailing mechanism of action for nitroglycerin (and other nitrates) is systemic venodilation, decreasing preload as measured by pulmonary capillary wedge pressure and left ventricular end diastolic volume and pressure; the average reduction in left ventricular end diastolic volume is 25% at rest, with a corresponding increase in ejection fractions of 50% to 60%. This effect improves congestive symptoms in heart failure and improves the myocardial perfusion gradient in patients with coronary artery disease.

Contraindications Hypersensitivity to isosorbide or any component of the formulation; hypersensitivity to organic nitrates; concurrent use with phosphodiesterase-5 (PDE-5) inhibitors (sildenafil, tadalafil, or vardenafil); angle-closure glaucoma (intraocular pressure may be increased); head trauma or cerebral hemorrhage (increase intracranial pressure); severe anemia

Warnings/Precautions Postural hypotension, transient episodes of weakness, dizziness, or syncope may occur even with small doses; ethanol accentuates these effects; tolerance and cross-tolerance to nitrate antianginal and hemodynamic effects may occur during prolonged isosorbide mononitrate therapy; (minimized by using the smallest effective dose, by alternating coronary vasodilators or offering drug-free intervals of as little as 12 hours). Excessive doses may result in severe headache, blurred vision, or xerostomia; increased anginal symptoms may be a result of dosage increases. Nitrates may aggravate angina caused by hypertrophic cardiomyopathy. Avoid concurrent use with PDE-5 inhibitors (eg, sildenafil, tadalafil, vardenafil). Safety and efficacy have not been established in children.

Drug Interactions

Cytochrome P450 Effect: Substrate of CYP3A4 (major)

Increased Effect/Toxicity: CYP3A4 inhibitors may increase the levels/effects of isosorbide dinitrate; example inhibitors include azole antifungals, clarithromycin, diclofenac, doxycycline, erythromycin, imatinib, isoniazid, nefazodone, nicardipine, propofol, protease inhibitors, quinidine, telithromycin, and verapamil. Significant reduction of systolic and diastolic blood pressure with concurrent use of sildenafil, tadalafil, or vardenafil (contraindicated). Do not administer sildenafil, tadalafil, or vardenafil within 24 hours of a nitrate preparation.

Ethanol/Nutrition/Herb Interactions Ethanol: Caution with ethanol (may increase risk of hypotension).

Pharmacodynamics/Kinetics

Onset of action: 30-60 minutes

Absorption: Nearly complete and low intersubject variability in its pharmacokinetic parameters and plasma concentrations

Metabolism: Hepatic

Half-life elimination: Mononitrate: ~4 hours

Excretion: Urine and feces

(Continued)

Isosorbide Mononitrate *(Continued)*

Pregnancy Risk Factor C
Dosage Forms
Tablet: 10 mg, 20 mg
Ismo®: 20 mg
Monoket®: 10 mg, 20 mg
Tablet, extended release: 30 mg, 60 mg, 120 mg
Imdur®: 30 mg, 60 mg, 120 mg

Isotretinoin *(eye soe TRET i noyn)*

U.S. Brand Names Accutane®; Amnesteem™; Claravis™; Sotret®
Canadian Brand Names Accutane®; Clarus™; Isotrex®
Mexican Brand Names Isotrex Gel; Roaccutan
Generic Available Yes
Index Terms 13-*cis*-Retinoic Acid
Pharmacologic Category Acne Products; Retinoic Acid Derivative
Use Treatment of severe recalcitrant nodular acne unresponsive to conventional therapy
Unlabeled/Investigational Use Investigational: Treatment of children with metastatic neuroblastoma or leukemia that does not respond to conventional therapy
Local Anesthetic/Vasoconstrictor Precautions No information available to require special precautions
Effects on Dental Treatment Key adverse event(s) related to dental treatment: Xerostomia and changes in salivation (normal salivary flow resumes upon discontinuation).
Common Adverse Effects Frequency not defined.
Cardiovascular: Palpitation, tachycardia, vascular thrombotic disease, stroke, chest pain, syncope, flushing
Central nervous system: Edema, fatigue, pseudotumor cerebri, dizziness, drowsiness, headache, insomnia, lethargy, malaise, nervousness, paresthesia, seizure, stroke, suicidal ideation, suicide attempts, suicide, depression, psychosis, aggressive or violent behavior, emotional instability
Dermatologic: Cutaneous allergic reactions, purpura, acne fulminans, alopecia, bruising, cheilitis, dry mouth, dry nose, dry skin, epistaxis, eruptive xanthomas, fragility of skin, hair abnormalities, hirsutism, hyperpigmentation, hypopigmentation, peeling of palms, peeling of soles, photoallergic reactions, photosensitizing reactions, pruritus, rash, dystrophy, paronychia, facial erythema, seborrhea, eczema, increased sunburn susceptibility, diaphoresis, urticaria, abnormal wound healing
Endocrine & metabolic: Triglycerides increased (25%), abnormal menses, blood glucose increased, cholesterol increased, HDL decreased
Gastrointestinal: Weight loss, inflammatory bowel disease, regional ileitis, pancreatitis, bleeding and inflammation of the gums, colitis, nausea, nonspecific gastrointestinal symptoms
Genitourinary: Nonspecific urogenital findings
Hematologic: Anemia, thrombocytopenia, neutropenia, agranulocytosis, pyogenic granuloma
Hepatic: Hepatitis
Neuromuscular & skeletal: Skeletal hyperostosis, calcification of tendons and ligaments, premature epiphyseal closure, arthralgia, CPK elevations, arthritis, tendonitis, bone abnormalities, weakness, back pain (29% in pediatric patients), rhabdomyolysis (rare), bone mineral density decreased
Ocular: Corneal opacities, decreased night vision, cataracts, color vision disorder, conjunctivitis, dry eyes, eyelid inflammation, keratitis, optic neuritis, photophobia, visual disturbances
Otic: Hearing impairment, tinnitus
Renal: Vasculitis, glomerulonephritis,
Respiratory: Bronchospasms, respiratory infection, voice alteration, Wegener's granulomatosis
Miscellaneous: Allergic reactions, anaphylactic reactions, lymphadenopathy, infection, disseminated herpes simplex, diaphoresis
Restrictions All patients (male and female), prescribers, wholesalers, and dispensing pharmacists must register and be active in the iPLEDGE™ risk management program, designed to eliminate fetal exposures to isotretinoin. This program covers all isotretinoin products (brand and generic). The iPLEDGE™ program requires that all patients meet qualification criteria and monthly program requirements. Registration, activation, and additional information are provided at www.ipledgeprogram.com or by calling 866-495-0654.

An FDA-approved medication guide must be distributed when dispensing an outpatient prescription (new or refill) where this medication is to be used without direct supervision of a healthcare provider. Medication guides are available at http://www.fda.gov/cder/Offices/ODS/medication_guides.htm.

Mechanism of Action Reduces sebaceous gland size and reduces sebum production; regulates cell proliferation and differentiation

Drug Interactions

Increased Effect/Toxicity: Cases of pseudotumor cerebri have been reported in concurrent use with tetracycline; avoid combination.

Decreased Effect: Isotretinoin may increase clearance of carbamazepine resulting in reduced carbamazepine levels. Retinoic acid derivatives may diminish the therapeutic effect of oral contraceptives (two forms of contraception are recommended in females of childbearing potential during retinoic acid therapy).

Pharmacodynamics/Kinetics

Distribution: Crosses placenta

Protein binding: 99% to 100%; primarily albumin

Metabolism: Hepatic via CYP2B6, 2C8, 2C9, 2D6, 3A4; forms metabolites; major metabolite: 4-oxo-isotretinoin (active)

Half-life elimination: Terminal: Parent drug: 21 hours; Metabolite: 21-24 hours

Time to peak, serum: 3-5 hours

Excretion: Urine and feces (equal amounts)

Pregnancy Risk Factor X

Isovue® *see* Iopamidol *on page 903*

Isovue-M® *see* Iopamidol *on page 903*

Isovue Multipack® *see* Iopamidol *on page 903*

Isoxsuprine (eye SOKS syoo preen)

U.S. Brand Names Vasodilan® [DSC]

Generic Available Yes

Index Terms Isoxsuprine Hydrochloride

Pharmacologic Category Vasodilator

Use Treatment of peripheral vascular diseases, such as arteriosclerosis obliterans and Raynaud's disease

Local Anesthetic/Vasoconstrictor Precautions No information available to require special precautions

Effects on Dental Treatment May enhance effects of other vasodilators.

Common Adverse Effects Frequency not defined.

Cardiovascular: Hypotension, chest pain, tachycardia

Central nervous system: Dizziness

Dermatologic: Rash

Gastrointestinal: Nausea, vomiting

Neuromuscular & skeletal: Weakness

Mechanism of Action In studies on normal human subjects, isoxsuprine increases muscle blood flow, but skin blood flow is usually unaffected. Rather than increasing muscle blood flow by beta-receptor stimulation, isoxsuprine probably has a direct action on vascular smooth muscle. The generally accepted mechanism of action of isoxsuprine on the uterus is beta-adrenergic stimulation. Isoxsuprine was shown to inhibit prostaglandin synthetase at high serum concentrations, with low concentrations there was an increase in the P-G synthesis.

Drug Interactions

Increased Effect/Toxicity: May enhance effects of other vasodilators/hypotensive agents.

Pharmacodynamics/Kinetics

Absorption: Nearly complete

Half-life elimination, serum: Mean: 1.25 hours

Time to peak, serum: ~1 hour

Pregnancy Risk Factor C

Isoxsuprine Hydrochloride *see* Isoxsuprine *on page 919*

Isradipine (iz RA di peen)

Related Information

Cardiovascular Diseases *on page 1726*

U.S. Brand Names DynaCirc® [DSC]; DynaCirc® CR

Canadian Brand Names DynaCirc®

Mexican Brand Names Dynacirc; Dynacirc SRO

Generic Available Yes: Capsule

(Continued)

Isradipine (Continued)

Pharmacologic Category Calcium Channel Blocker

Use Treatment of hypertension

Unlabeled/Investigational Use Pediatric hypertension

Local Anesthetic/Vasoconstrictor Precautions Isradipine is one of the drugs confirmed to prolong the QT interval and is accepted as having a risk of causing torsade de pointes. The risk of drug-induced torsade de pointes is extremely low when a single QT interval prolonging drug is prescribed. In terms of epinephrine, it is not known what effect vasoconstrictors in the local anesthetic regimen will have in patients with a known history of congenital prolonged QT interval or in patients taking any medication that prolongs the QT interval. Until more information is obtained, it is suggested that the clinician consult with the physician prior to the use of a vasoconstrictor in suspected patients, and that the vasoconstrictor (epinephrine, levonordefrin [Neo-Cobefrin®]) be used with caution.

Effects on Dental Treatment No significant effects or complications reported

Common Adverse Effects Percentages reported with capsule formulation.

>10%: Central nervous system: Headache (dose related 2% to 22%)

1% to 10%:

Cardiovascular: Edema (dose related 1% to 9%), palpitation (dose related 1% to 5%), flushing (dose related 1% to 5%), tachycardia (1% to 3%), chest pain (2% to 3%)

Central nervous system: Dizziness (2% to 8%), fatigue (dose related 1% to 9%)

Dermatologic: Rash (2%)

Gastrointestinal: Nausea (1% to 5%), abdominal discomfort (≤3%), vomiting (≤1%), diarrhea (≤3%)

Neuromuscular & skeletal: Weakness (≤1%)

Renal: Urinary frequency (1% to 3%)

Respiratory: Dyspnea (1% to 3%)

Mechanism of Action Inhibits calcium ion from entering the "slow channels" or select voltage-sensitive areas of vascular smooth muscle and myocardium during depolarization, producing a relaxation of coronary vascular smooth muscle and coronary vasodilation; increases myocardial oxygen delivery in patients with vasospastic angina

Drug Interactions

Cytochrome P450 Effect: Substrate of CYP3A4 (major); **Inhibits** CYP3A4 (weak)

Increased Effect/Toxicity: Isradipine may increase cardiovascular adverse effects of beta-blockers. Alpha$_1$-blockers may enhance the hypotensive effect of isradipine. Calcium channel blockers may enhance the adverse/toxic effect of magnesium salts. Isradipine may minimally increase cyclosporine levels. CYP3A4 inhibitors may increase the levels/effects of isradipine; example inhibitors include azole antifungals, clarithromycin, diclofenac, doxycycline, erythromycin, imatinib, isoniazid, nefazodone, nicardipine, propofol, protease inhibitors, quinidine, telithromycin, and verapamil. Blood pressure-lowering effects may be additive with sildenafil, tadalafil, and vardenafil (use caution). Cimetidine and cyclosporine may decrease the metabolism, via CYP isoenzymes, of israpidine. Isradipine may enhance the adverse/toxic effect of other QT$_c$-prolonging agents. Isradipine may enhance the QT$_c$-prolonging effect of thioridazine.

Decreased Effect: NSAIDs (diclofenac) may decrease the antihypertensive response of isradipine. Isradipine may cause a decrease in lovastatin effect. CYP3A4 inducers may decrease the levels/effects of isradipine; example inducers include aminoglutethimide, carbamazepine, nafcillin, nevirapine, phenobarbital, phenytoin, and rifamycins.

Pharmacodynamics/Kinetics

Onset of action: Immediate release: 2-3 hours

Duration: Immediate release: >12 hours

Absorption: 90% to 95%

Distribution: V$_d$: 3 L/kg

Protein binding: 95%

Metabolism: Hepatic; CYP3A4 substrate (major); extensive first-pass effect; forms metabolites (inactive)

Bioavailability: 15% to 24%

Half-life elimination: Terminal: 8 hours

Time to peak, serum: 1-1.5 hours

Excretion: Urine (60% to 65% as metabolites); feces (25% to 30%)

Pregnancy Risk Factor C

Itraconazole (i tra KOE na zole)

Related Information
Fungal Infections *on page 1804*

U.S. Brand Names Sporanox®

Canadian Brand Names Sporanox®

Mexican Brand Names Isox; Itranax; Sinozol; Sporanox 15 D

Generic Available No

Pharmacologic Category Antifungal Agent, Oral

Dental Use Treatment of susceptible fungal infections in immunocompromised and immunocompetent patients including blastomycosis and histoplasmosis; has activity against *Aspergillus, Candida, Coccidioides, Cryptococcus, Sporothrix,* and chromomycosis. Useful in superficial mycoses including dermatophytoses (eg, tinea capitis), pityriasis versicolor, sebopsoriasis, vaginal and chronic mucocutaneous candidiases; systemic mycoses including candidiasis, meningeal and disseminated cryptococcal infections, paracoccidioidomycosis, coccidioidomycoses; miscellaneous mycoses such as sporotrichosis, chromomycosis, leishmaniasis, fungal keratitis, alternariosis, zygomycosis.

Use Treatment of susceptible fungal infections in immunocompromised and immunocompetent patients including blastomycosis and histoplasmosis; indicated for aspergillosis, and onychomycosis of the toenail; treatment of onychomycosis of the fingernail without concomitant toenail infection via a pulse-type dosing regimen; has activity against *Aspergillus, Candida, Coccidioides, Cryptococcus, Sporothrix,* tinea unguium

Oral: Useful in superficial mycoses including dermatophytoses (eg, tinea capitis), pityriasis versicolor, sebopsoriasis, vaginal and chronic mucocutaneous candidiases; systemic mycoses including candidiasis, meningeal and disseminated cryptococcal infections, paracoccidioidomycoses, coccidioidomycoses; miscellaneous mycoses such as sporotrichosis, chromomycosis, leishmaniasis, fungal keratitis, alternariosis, zygomycosis

Oral solution: Treatment of oral and esophageal candidiasis

Intravenous solution: Indicated in the treatment of blastomycosis, histoplasmosis (nonmeningeal), and aspergillosis (in patients intolerant or refractory to amphotericin B therapy); empiric therapy of febrile neutropenic fever

Local Anesthetic/Vasoconstrictor Precautions No information available to require special precautions

Effects on Dental Treatment No significant effects or complications reported

Significant Adverse Effects Listed incidences are for higher doses appropriate for systemic fungal infection.

>10%: Gastrointestinal: Nausea (11%)

1% to 10%:

Cardiovascular: Edema (4%), hypertension (3%)

Central nervous system: Headache (4%), fatigue (2% to 3%), malaise (1%), fever (3%), dizziness (2%)

Dermatologic: Rash (9%), pruritus (3%)

Endocrine & metabolic: Decreased libido (1%), hypertriglyceridemia, hypokalemia (2%)

Gastrointestinal: Abdominal pain (2%), anorexia (1%), vomiting (5%), diarrhea (3%)

Hepatic: Abnormal LFTs (3%), hepatitis

Renal: Albuminuria (1%)

<1% (Limited to important or life-threatening): Adrenal suppression; allergic reactions (urticaria, angioedema); alopecia, anaphylactoid reactions, anaphylaxis, arrhythmia, CHF, constipation, gastritis, gynecomastia, hepatic failure, impotence, neutropenia, peripheral neuropathy, photosensitivity, pulmonary edema, somnolence, Stevens-Johnson syndrome, tinnitus

Dental Usual Dosing Oropharyngeal candidiasis: Adults: Oral solution: 200 mg once daily for 1-2 weeks; in patients unresponsive or refractory to fluconazole: 100 mg twice daily (clinical response expected in 1-2 weeks)

Dosage

Usual dosage ranges:

Children: Efficacy and safety have not been established; a small number of patients 3-16 years of age have been treated with 100 mg/day for systemic fungal infections with no serious adverse effects reported. A dose of 5 mg/kg once daily was used in a pharmacokinetic study using the oral solution in patients 6 months to 12 years; duration of study was 2 weeks.

Adults: Oral, I.V.: 100-400 mg/day; doses >200 mg/day are given in 2 divided doses; length of therapy varies from 1 day to >6 months depending on the condition and mycological response

(Continued)

Itraconazole *(Continued)*

Indication-specific dosing:

Adults:

Aspergillosis:
Oral: 200-400 mg/day
I.V.: 200 mg twice daily for 4 doses, followed by 200 mg daily

Blastomycosis/histoplasmosis:
Oral: 200 mg once daily, if no obvious improvement or there is evidence of progressive fungal disease, increase the dose in 100 mg increments to a maximum of 400 mg/day; doses >200 mg/day are given in 2 divided doses; length of therapy varies from 1 day to >6 months depending on the condition and mycological response
I.V.: 200 mg twice daily for 4 doses, followed by 200 mg/day

Brain abscess: Cerebral phaeohyphomycosis (dematiaceous): Oral: 200 mg twice daily for at least 6 months with amphotericin

Candidiasis:
Oropharyngeal: Oral solution: 200 mg once daily for 1-2 weeks; in patients unresponsive or refractory to fluconazole: 100 mg twice daily (clinical response expected in 1-2 weeks)
Esophageal: Oral solution: 100-200 mg once daily for a minimum of 3 weeks; continue dosing for 2 weeks after resolution of symptoms
Coccidioides: Oral: 200 mg twice daily

Infections, life-threatening:
Oral: 200 mg 3 times/day (600 mg/day) should be given for the first 3 days of therapy
I.V.: 200 mg twice daily for 4 doses, followed by 200 mg/day

Meningitis:
Coccidioides: Oral: 400-800 mg/day
Cryptococcal: HIV positive (unlabeled use): Induction: Oral: 400 mg/day for 10-12 weeks; maintenance: 200 mg twice daily lifelong

Onychomycosis: Oral: 200 mg once daily for 12 consecutive weeks

Pneumonia:
Coccidioides: Mild to moderate: Oral, I.V.: 200 mg twice daily
Cryptococcal: Mild to moderate (unlabeled use): 200-400 mg/day for 6-12 months (lifelong for HIV positive)

Prototechal infection: 200 mg once daily for 2 months

Sporotrichosis: Oral:
Lymphocutaneous: 100-200 mg/day for 3-6 months
Osteoarticular and pulmonary: 200 mg twice daily for 1-2 years (may use amphotericin B initially for stabilization)

Dosing adjustment in renal impairment: Not necessary; itraconazole injection is not recommended in patients with Cl$_{cr}$ <30 mL/minute; hydroxypropyl-β-cyclodextrin (the excipient) is eliminated primarily by the kidneys. Hemodialysis: Not dialyzable

Dosing adjustment in hepatic impairment: May be necessary, but specific guidelines are not available. Risk-to-benefit evaluation should be undertaken in patients who develop liver function abnormalities during treatment.

Mechanism of Action Interferes with cytochrome P450 activity, decreasing ergosterol synthesis (principal sterol in fungal cell membrane) and inhibiting cell membrane formation

Contraindications Hypersensitivity to itraconazole, any component of the formulation, or to other azoles; concurrent administration with cisapride, dofetilide, ergot derivatives, levomethadyl, lovastatin, midazolam, pimozide, quinidine, simvastatin, or triazolam; treatment of onychomycosis in patients with evidence of left ventricular dysfunction, CHF, or a history of CHF

Warnings/Precautions Discontinue if signs or symptoms of CHF or neuropathy occur during treatment. **[U.S. Boxed Warning]: Rare cases of serious cardiovascular adverse events (including death), ventricular tachycardia, and torsade de pointes have been observed due to increased cisapride, pimozide, quinidine, dofetilide or levomethadyl concentrations induced by itraconazole; concurrent use is contraindicated. Use with caution in patients with left ventricular dysfunction or a history of CHF; not recommended for treatment of onychomycosis in these patients.** Not recommended for use in patients with active liver disease, elevated liver enzymes, or prior hepatotoxic reactions to other drugs. Itraconazole has been associated with rare cases of serious hepatotoxicity (including fatal cases and cases within the first week of treatment); treatment should be discontinued in patients who develop clinical symptoms of liver dysfunction or abnormal liver function tests during itraconazole therapy except in cases where expected benefit exceeds risk. Large differences in itraconazole pharmacokinetic parameters have been observed in cystic fibrosis patients receiving the solution; if a patient with cystic fibrosis does not respond to therapy, alternate therapies should be considered.

Due to differences in bioavailability, oral capsules and oral solution **cannot be used interchangeably.** Intravenous formulation should be used with caution in renal impairment; consider conversion to oral therapy if renal dysfunction/toxicity is noted. Initiation of treatment with oral solution is not recommended in patients at immediate risk for systemic candidiasis (eg, patients with severe neutropenia).

Drug Interactions Substrate of CYP3A4 (major); **Inhibits** CYP3A4 (strong)

Antacids: May decrease serum concentration of itraconazole. Administer antacids 1 hour before or 2 hours after itraconazole capsules.

Alfentanil: Serum concentrations may be increased; monitor.

Anticonvulsants: Itraconazole may increase the serum concentration of carbamazepine; carbamazepine, phenobarbital, and phenytoin may decrease the serum concentration of itraconazole.

Benzodiazepines: Alprazolam, diazepam, temazepam, triazolam, and midazolam serum concentrations may be increased; consider a benzodiazepine not metabolized by CYP3A4 (such as lorazepam) or another antifungal that is metabolized by CYP3A4

Buspirone: Serum concentrations may be increased; monitor for sedation

Busulfan: Serum concentrations may be increased; avoid concurrent use

Calcium channel blockers: Serum concentrations may be increased (applies to those agents metabolized by CYP3A4, including felodipine, nifedipine, and verapamil); consider another agent instead of a calcium channel blocker, another antifungal, or reduce the dose of the calcium channel blocker; monitor blood pressure

Cisapride; Serum concentration is increased which may lead to malignant arrhythmias; concurrent use is contraindicated

Corticosteroids: Serum levels/effects of the corticosteroid may be increased; use caution.

CYP3A4 inducers: CYP3A4 inducers may decrease the levels/effects of itraconazole. Example inducers include aminoglutethimide, carbamazepine, nafcillin, nevirapine, phenobarbital, phenytoin, and rifamycins.

CYP3A4 substrates: Itraconazole may increase the levels/effects of CYP3A4 substrates. Example substrates include benzodiazepines, calcium channel blockers, mirtazapine, nateglinide, nefazodone, tacrolimus, and venlafaxine. Selected benzodiazepines (midazolam and triazolam), cisapride, ergot alkaloids, selected HMG-CoA reductase inhibitors (lovastatin and simvastatin), and pimozide are generally contraindicated with strong CYP3A4 inhibitors.

Didanosine: May decrease absorption of itraconazole (due to buffering capacity of oral solution); applies only to oral solution formulation of didanosine

Digoxin: Serum concentrations may be increased; monitor.

Disopyramide: Serum levels/effects (including QT_c prolongation) may be increased; use caution.

Docetaxel: Serum concentrations may be increased; avoid concurrent use

Dofetilide: Serum levels/toxicity may be increased; concurrent use is contraindicated.

Eletriptan: Serum level/toxicity of eletriptan may be increased; use caution.

Ergot alkaloids: Toxicity (vasospasm, ischemia) may be significantly increased by itraconazole; concurrent use is contraindicated.

Erythromycin (and clarithromycin): May increase serum concentrations of itraconazole.

H_2 blockers: May decrease itraconazole absorption. Itraconazole depends on gastric acidity for absorption. Avoid concurrent use.

HMG-CoA reductase inhibitors (except pravastatin and fluvastatin): Serum concentrations may be increased. The risk of myopathy/rhabdomyolysis may be increased. Switch to pravastatin/fluvastatin or suspend treatment during course of itraconazole therapy.

Hypoglycemic agents, oral: Serum concentrations may be increased; monitor.

Immunosuppressants: Cyclosporine, sirolimus, and tacrolimus: Serum concentrations may be increased; monitor serum concentrations and renal function.

Levomethadyl: Serum levels/effects may be increased by itraconazole, potentially resulting in malignant arrhythmia; concurrent use is contraindicated.

Nevirapine: May decrease serum concentrations of itraconazole; monitor

Oral contraceptives: Efficacy may be reduced by itraconazole (limited data); use barrier birth control method during concurrent use

Pimozide: Serum levels/toxicity may be increased; concurrent use is contraindicated.

Protease inhibitors: May increase serum concentrations of itraconazole. Includes amprenavir, indinavir, nelfinavir, ritonavir, and saquinavir; monitor. Serum concentrations of indinavir, ritonavir, or saquinavir may be increased by itraconazole.

Proton pump inhibitors: May decrease itraconazole absorption. Itraconazole depends on gastric acidity for absorption. Avoid concurrent use (includes omeprazole, lansoprazole).

Quinidine: Serum levels may be increased. Concurrent use is contraindicated. (Continued)

Itraconazole *(Continued)*

Rifabutin: Serum concentrations may be increased; monitor.

Sildenafil: Serum concentrations may be increased by itraconazole; consider dosage reduction. A maximum sildenafil dose of 25 mg in 48 hours is recommended with other strong CYP3A4 inhibitors.

Tadalafil: Serum concentrations may be increased by itraconazole. A maximum tadalafil dose of 10 mg in 72 hours is recommended with strong CYP3A4 inhibitors.

Trimetrexate: Serum concentrations may be increased; monitor

Vardenafil: Serum concentrations may be increased by itraconazole. If itraconazole dose is 200 mg/day, limit vardenafil dose to a maximum of 5 mg/24 hours. If itraconazole dose is 400 mg/day, limit vardenafil dose to a maximum of 2.5 mg/24 hours.

Warfarin: Anticoagulant effects may be increased; monitor INR and adjust warfarin's dose as needed

Vinca alkaloids: Serum concentrations may be increased.

Zolpidem: Serum levels may be increased; monitor

Ethanol/Nutrition/Herb Interactions

Food:
Capsules: Enhanced by food and possibly by gastric acidity. cola drinks have been shown to increase the absorption of the capsules in patients with achlorhydria or those taking H_2-receptor antagonists or other gastric acid suppressors. Avoid grapefruit juice.
Solution: Decreased by food, time to peak concentration prolonged by food.
Herb/Nutraceutical: St John's wort may decrease itraconazole levels.

Dietary Considerations

Capsule: Administer with food.
Solution: Take without food, if possible.

Pharmacodynamics/Kinetics

Absorption: Requires gastric acidity; capsule better absorbed with food, solution better absorbed on empty stomach

Distribution: V_d (average): 796 ± 185 L or 10 L/kg; highly lipophilic and tissue concentrations are higher than plasma concentrations. The highest concentrations: adipose, omentum, endometrium, cervical and vaginal mucus, and skin/nails. Aqueous fluids (eg, CSF and urine) contain negligible amounts.

Protein binding, plasma: 99.9%; metabolite hydroxy-itraconazole: 99.5%

Metabolism: Extensively hepatic via CYP3A4 into >30 metabolites including hydroxy-itraconazole (major metabolite); appears to have *in vitro* antifungal activity. Main metabolic pathway is oxidation; may undergo saturation metabolism with multiple dosing.

Bioavailability: Variable, ~55% (oral solution) in 1 small study; **Note:** Oral solution has a higher degree of bioavailability (149% ± 68%) relative to oral capsules; should not be interchanged

Half-life elimination: Oral: After single 200 mg dose: 21 ± 5 hours; 64 hours at steady-state; I.V.: steady-state: 35 hours; steady-state concentrations are achieved in 13 days with multiple administration of itraconazole 100-400 mg/day.

Excretion: Feces (~3% to 18%); urine (~0.03% as parent drug, 40% as metabolites)

Pregnancy Risk Factor C

Lactation Enters breast milk/not recommended

Dosage Forms Excipient information presented when available (limited, particularly for generics); consult specific product labeling.

Capsule: 100 mg

Injection, solution: 10 mg/mL (25 mL) [packaged in a kit containing sodium chloride 0.9% (50 mL); filtered infusion set (1)]

Solution, oral: 100 mg/10 mL (150 mL) [cherry flavor]

Iveegam EN *see* Immune Globulin (Intravenous) *on page 870*

Ivermectin *(eye ver MEK tin)*

U.S. Brand Names Stromectol®
Mexican Brand Names Ivexterm
Generic Available No
Pharmacologic Category Anthelmintic
Use Treatment of the following infections: Strongyloidiasis of the intestinal tract due to the nematode parasite *Strongyloides stercoralis*. Onchocerciasis due to the nematode parasite *Onchocerca volvulus*. Ivermectin is only active against the immature form of *Onchocerca volvulus*, and the intestinal forms of *Strongyloides stercoralis*.

Unlabeled/Investigational Use Has been used for other parasitic infections including *Ascaris lumbricoides*, Bancroftian filariasis, *Brugia malayi*, scabies, *Enterobius vermicularis*, *Mansonella ozzardi*, *Trichuris trichiura*.

Local Anesthetic/Vasoconstrictor Precautions No information available to require special precautions

Effects on Dental Treatment No significant effects or complications reported

Common Adverse Effects Frequency not defined.

Cardiovascular: Hypotension, mild ECG changes, orthostasis, peripheral and facial edema, transient tachycardia

Central nervous system: Dizziness, encephalopathy (rare; associated with loiasis), headache, hyperthermia, insomnia, seizure, somnolence, vertigo

Dermatologic: Pruritus, rash, Stevens-Johnson syndrome, toxic epidermal necrolysis, urticaria

Gastrointestinal: Abdominal pain, anorexia, constipation, diarrhea, nausea, vomiting

Hematologic: Anemia, eosinophilia, leukopenia

Hepatic: ALT/AST increased, bilirubin increased

Neuromuscular & skeletal: Limbitis, myalgia, tremor, weakness

Ocular: Blurred vision, mild conjunctivitis, punctate opacity

Respiratory: Asthma exacerbation

Miscellaneous: Mazzotti reaction (with onchocerciasis): Arthralgia, edema, fever, lymphadenopathy, ocular damage, pruritus, rash, synovitis

Mechanism of Action Ivermectin is a semisynthetic antihelminthic agent; it binds selectively and with strong affinity to glutamate-gated chloride ion channels which occur in invertebrate nerve and muscle cells. This leads to increased permeability of cell membranes to chloride ions then hyperpolarization of the nerve or muscle cell, and death of the parasite.

Drug Interactions

Cytochrome P450 Effect: Substrate of CYP3A4 (minor)

Pharmacodynamics/Kinetics

Onset of action: Peak effect: 3-6 months

Absorption: Well absorbed

Distribution: Does not cross blood-brain barrier

Half-life elimination: 16-35 hours

Metabolism: Hepatic (>97%)

Excretion: Urine (<1%); feces

Pregnancy Risk Factor C

IVIG see Immune Globulin (Intravenous) on page 870

IvyBlock® [OTC] see Bentoquatam on page 193

Ivy-Rid® [OTC] see Benzocaine on page 195

IvySoothe® [OTC] see Hydrocortisone on page 836

Jantoven™ see Warfarin on page 1670

Janumet™ see Sitagliptin and Metformin on page 1479

Januvia™ see Sitagliptin on page 1478

Japanese Encephalitis Virus Vaccine (Inactivated)

(jap a NEESE en sef a LYE tis VYE rus vak SEEN, in ak ti VAY ted)

Related Information

Immunizations (Vaccines) on page 1886

U.S. Brand Names JE-VAX®

Canadian Brand Names JE-VAX®

Generic Available No

Pharmacologic Category Vaccine

Use Active immunization against Japanese encephalitis

Local Anesthetic/Vasoconstrictor Precautions No information available to require special precautions

Effects on Dental Treatment No significant effects or complications reported

Common Adverse Effects Report allergic or unusual adverse reactions to the Vaccine Adverse Event Reporting System (VAERS) 1-800-822-7967. Percentage of adverse reactions may depend upon timing of vaccination. In general, adverse reactions occur more frequently following the first dose or when doses are administered closer together (abbreviated dosing schedule). However, reactions have been reported when previous doses were tolerated uneventfully.

>10%:

Central nervous system: Headache (<5% to 15%)

Local: Injection site reaction (<1% to 31%)

1% to 10%:

Central nervous system: Chills (~10%), dizziness (~10%), malaise (~10%), fever (<5% to 10%)

(Continued)

Japanese Encephalitis Virus Vaccine (Inactivated)
(Continued)

Dermatologic: Rash (≤10%)
Gastrointestinal: Abdominal pain (~10%), nausea (~10%), vomiting (~10%)
Neuromuscular & skeletal: Myalgia (~10%)
Miscellaneous: Flu-like syndrome (<5%)

Drug Interactions
Increased Effect/Toxicity: Hypersensitivity reactions may be increased when given within 7 day of other vaccines. When possible, administer concomitantly with other vaccines.

Pregnancy Risk Factor C

Kanamycin (kan a MYE sin)

Related Information
Tuberculosis *on page 1765*
U.S. Brand Names Kantrex®
Canadian Brand Names Kantrex®
Mexican Brand Names Kantrex
Generic Available No
Index Terms Kanamycin Sulfate
Pharmacologic Category Antibiotic, Aminoglycoside
Use Treatment of serious infections caused by susceptible strains of *E. coli*, *Proteus* species, *Enterobacter aerogenes*, *Klebsiella pneumoniae*, *Serratia marcescens*, and *Acinetobacter* species; second-line treatment of *Mycobacterium tuberculosis*

Local Anesthetic/Vasoconstrictor Precautions No information available to require special precautions
Effects on Dental Treatment Key adverse event(s) related to dental treatment: Salivation increased.
Common Adverse Effects Frequency not defined.
Cardiovascular: Edema
Central nervous system: Neurotoxicity, drowsiness, headache, pseudomotor cerebri
Dermatologic: Skin itching, redness, rash, photosensitivity, erythema
Gastrointestinal: Nausea, vomiting, diarrhea, malabsorption syndrome (with prolonged and high-dose therapy of hepatic coma), anorexia, weight loss, salivation increased, enterocolitis
Hematologic: Granulocytopenia, agranulocytosis, thrombocytopenia
Local: Burning, stinging
Neuromuscular & skeletal: Weakness, tremor, muscle cramps
Otic: Ototoxicity (auditory), ototoxicity (vestibular)
Renal: Nephrotoxicity
Respiratory: Dyspnea
Mechanism of Action Interferes with protein synthesis in bacterial cell by binding to ribosomal subunit
Drug Interactions
Increased Effect/Toxicity: Increased toxicity may occur with amphotericin B, cisplatin, loop diuretics, neuromuscular-blocking agents. Use with bisphosphonate derivatives may lead to hypocalcemia.
Pharmacodynamics/Kinetics
Absorption:
I.M.: Rapid
Oral: Minimal

Distribution:

Relative diffusion from blood into CSF: Good only with inflammation (exceeds usual MICs)

CSF:blood level ratio: Normal meninges: Nil; Inflamed meninges: 43%

Protein binding: 0%

Half-life elimination: 2-4 hours; Anuria: 80 hours; End-stage renal disease: 40-96 hours

Time to peak, serum: I.M.: 1-2 hours (decreased in burn patients)

Excretion: Urine (as unchanged drug)

Pregnancy Risk Factor D

Ketamine (KEET a meen)

U.S. Brand Names Ketalar®

Canadian Brand Names Ketalar®; Ketamine Hydrochloride Injection, USP

Mexican Brand Names Ketalin

Generic Available Yes

Index Terms Ketamine Hydrochloride

Pharmacologic Category General Anesthetic

Use Induction and maintenance of general anesthesia, especially when cardiovascular depression must be avoided (ie, hypotension, hypovolemia, cardiomyopathy, constrictive pericarditis); sedation; analgesia

Local Anesthetic/Vasoconstrictor Precautions No information available to require special precautions

Effects on Dental Treatment Key adverse event(s) related to dental treatment: Increased salivation.

Common Adverse Effects

>10%:

Cardiovascular: Cardiac output increased, hypertension, paradoxical direct myocardial depression, tachycardia

Central nervous system: Intracranial pressure increased, visual hallucinations, vivid dreams

Neuromuscular & skeletal: Tonic-clonic movements, tremor

Miscellaneous: Emergence reactions, vocalization

(Continued)

Ketamine *(Continued)*

1% to 10%:
Cardiovascular: Bradycardia, hypotension
Dermatologic: Pain at injection site, skin rash
Gastrointestinal: Anorexia, nausea, vomiting
Ocular: Diplopia, nystagmus
Respiratory: Respiratory depression

Restrictions C-III

Mechanism of Action Produces a cataleptic-like state in which the patient is dissociated from the surrounding environment by direct action on the cortex and limbic system. Releases endogenous catecholamines (epinephrine, norepinephrine) which maintain blood pressure and heart rate. Reduces polysynaptic spinal reflexes.

Drug Interactions

Cytochrome P450 Effect: Substrate (major) of CYP2B6, 2C9, 3A4

Increased Effect/Toxicity: CYP2B6 inhibitors may increase the levels/effects of ketamine; example inhibitors include desipramine, paroxetine, and sertraline. CYP2C9 inhibitors may increase the levels/effects of ketamine. Example inhibitors include delavirdine, fluconazole, gemfibrozil, ketoconazole, nicardipine, NSAIDs, sulfonamides, and tolbutamide. CYP3A4 inhibitors may increase the levels/effects of ketamine; example inhibitors include azole antifungals, clarithromycin, diclofenac, doxycycline, erythromycin, imatinib, isoniazid, nefazodone, nicardipine, propofol, protease inhibitors, quinidine, telithromycin, and verapamil. Barbiturates, narcotics, hydroxyzine increase prolonged recovery; nondepolarizing neuromuscular blockers may increase effects. Muscle relaxants, thyroid hormones may increase blood pressure and heart rate. Halothane may decrease BP.

Pharmacodynamics/Kinetics

Onset of action:
I.V.: General anesthesia: 1-2 minutes; Sedation: 1-2 minutes
I.M.: General anesthesia: 3-8 minutes

Duration: I.V.: 5-15 minutes; I.M.: 12-25 minutes

Metabolism: Hepatic via hydroxylation and N-demethylation; the metabolite norketamine is 25% as potent as parent compound

Half-life elimination: 11-17 minutes; Elimination: 2.5-3.1 hours

Excretion: Clearance: 18 mL/kg/minute

Pregnancy Risk Factor D

Ketamine Hydrochloride *see* Ketamine *on page 927*

Ketek® *see* Telithromycin *on page 1528*

Ketoconazole *(kee toe KOE na zole)*

Related Information
Fungal Infections *on page 1804*
Respiratory Diseases *on page 1747*

Related Sample Prescriptions
Systemic Fungal Infections *on page 1841*
Topical Fungal Infections *on page 1841*

U.S. Brand Names Kuric™; Nizoral®; Nizoral® A-D [OTC]; Xolegel™

Canadian Brand Names Apo-Ketoconazole®; Ketoderm®; Novo-Ketoconazole®; Xolegel™

Mexican Brand Names Akorazol; Conazol; Fungoral; Konaturil; Nastil; Nizoral Cream and Tablets; Termizol

Generic Available Yes: Cream, shampoo, tablet

Pharmacologic Category Antifungal Agent, Oral; Antifungal Agent, Topical

Dental Use Treatment of susceptible fungal infections in the oral cavity including candidiasis, oral thrush, and chronic mucocutaneous candidiasis

Use

Systemic: Treatment of susceptible fungal infections, including candidiasis, oral thrush, blastomycosis, histoplasmosis, paracoccidioidomycosis, coccidioidomycosis, chromomycosis, candiduria, chronic mucocutaneous candidiasis, as well as certain recalcitrant cutaneous dermatophytoses

Topical: Treatment of tinea corporis, tinea cruris, tinea versicolor, cutaneous candidiasis, seborrheic dermatitis

Unlabeled/Investigational Use Treatment of prostate cancer (androgen synthesis inhibitor)

Local Anesthetic/Vasoconstrictor Precautions No information available to require special precautions

Effects on Dental Treatment No significant effects or complications reported

Significant Adverse Effects

Oral:

1% to 10%:

Dermatologic: Pruritus (2%)

Gastrointestinal: Nausea/vomiting (3% to 10%), abdominal pain (1%)

<1% (Limited to important or life-threatening): Bulging fontanelles, chills, depression, diarrhea, dizziness, fever, gynecomastia, headache, hemolytic anemia, hepatotoxicity, impotence, leukopenia, photophobia, somnolence, thrombocytopenia

Topical cream/gel: Allergic reaction, contact dermatitis (possibly related to sulfites or propylene glycol), facial swelling, headache, impetigo, local burning, ocular irritation, paresthesia, pruritus, severe irritation, stinging (~5%)

Shampoo: Abnormal hair texture, hair loss increase, irritation (<1%), itching, mild dryness of skin, oiliness/dryness of hair, scalp pustules

Dental Usual Dosing Oral fungal infections: Oral:

Children ≥2 years: 3.3-6.6 mg/kg/day as a single dose for 1-2 weeks for candidiasis, for at least 4 weeks in recalcitrant dermatophyte infections, and for up to 6 months for other systemic mycoses

Adults: 200-400 mg/day as a single daily dose for durations as stated above

Dosage

Fungal infections:

Oral:

Children ≥2 years: 3.3-6.6 mg/kg/day as a single dose for 1-2 weeks for candidiasis, for at least 4 weeks in recalcitrant dermatophyte infections, and for up to 6 months for other systemic mycoses

Adults: 200-400 mg/day as a single daily dose for durations as stated above

Shampoo: Children >12 years and Adults: Apply twice weekly for 4 weeks with at least 3 days between each shampoo

Topical: Adults:

Tinea infections: Cream: Rub gently into the affected area once daily. Duration of treatment: Tinea corporis, cruris: 2 weeks; tinea pedis: 6 weeks

Seborrheic dermatitis:

Cream: Rub gently into the affected area twice daily for 4 weeks or until clinical response is noted

Gel: Rub gently into the affected area once daily for 2 weeks

Prostate cancer (unlabeled use): Oral: Adults: 400 mg 3 times/day

Dosing adjustment in hepatic impairment: Dose reductions should be considered in patients with severe liver disease

Hemodialysis: Not dialyzable (0% to 5%)

Mechanism of Action Alters the permeability of the cell wall by blocking fungal cytochrome P450; inhibits biosynthesis of triglycerides and phospholipids by fungi; inhibits several fungal enzymes that results in a build-up of toxic concentrations of hydrogen peroxide; also inhibits androgen synthesis

Contraindications Hypersensitivity to ketoconazole or any component of the formulation; CNS fungal infections (due to poor CNS penetration); coadministration with ergot derivatives or cisapride is contraindicated due to risk of potentially fatal cardiac arrhythmias

Warnings/Precautions [U.S. Boxed Warning]: Ketoconazole has been associated with hepatotoxicity, including some fatalities; use with caution in patients with impaired hepatic function and perform periodic liver function tests. **[U.S. Boxed Warning]: Concomitant use with cisapride is contraindicated due to the occurrence of ventricular arrhythmias.** High doses of ketoconazole may depress adrenocortical function.

Topical: Formulations may contain sulfites. Avoid exposure of gel to open flames during or immediately after application.

Drug Interactions Substrate of CYP3A4 (major); **Inhibits** CYP1A2 (strong), 2A6 (moderate), 2B6 (weak), 2C8 (weak), 2C9 (strong), 2C19 (moderate), 2D6 (moderate), 3A4 (strong)

Benzodiazepines: Alprazolam, diazepam, temazepam, triazolam, and midazolam serum concentrations may be increased; consider a benzodiazepine not metabolized by CYP3A4 (such as lorazepam) or another antifungal that is metabolized by CYP3A4. Concurrent use is contraindicated.

Buspirone: Serum concentrations may be increased; monitor for sedation.

Busulfan: Serum concentrations may be increased; avoid concurrent use.

Calcium channel blockers: Serum concentrations may be increased (applies to those agents metabolized by CYP3A4, including felodipine, nifedipine, and verapamil); consider another agent instead of a calcium channel blocker, another antifungal, or reduce the dose of the calcium channel blocker. Monitor blood pressure.

Cisapride: Serum concentration is increased which may lead to malignant arrhythmias; concurrent use is contraindicated.

(Continued)

Ketoconazole *(Continued)*

CYP1A2 substrates: Ketoconazole may increase the levels/effects of CYP1A2 substrates. Example substrates include aminophylline, fluvoxamine, mexiletine, mirtazapine, ropinirole, theophylline, and trifluoperazine.

CYP2A6 substrates: Ketoconazole may increase the levels/effects of CYP2A6 substrates. Example substrates include dexmedetomidine and ifosfamide.

CYP2C9 substrates: Ketoconazole may increase the levels/effects of CYP2C9 substrates. Example substrates include bosentan, dapsone, fluoxetine, glimepiride, glipizide, losartan, montelukast, nateglinide, paclitaxel, phenytoin, warfarin, and zafirlukast.

CYP2C19 substrates: Ketoconazole may increase the levels/effects of CYP2C19 substrates. Example substrates include citalopram, diazepam, methsuximide, phenytoin, propranolol, and sertraline.

CYP2D6 substrates: Ketoconazole may increase the levels/effects of CYP2D6 substrates. Example substrates include amphetamines, selected beta-blockers, dextromethorphan, fluoxetine, lidocaine, mirtazapine, nefazodone, paroxetine, risperidone, ritonavir, thioridazine, tricyclic antidepressants, and venlafaxine.

CYP2D6 prodrug substrates: Ketoconazole may decrease the levels/effects of CYP2D6 prodrug substrates. Example prodrug substrates include codeine, hydrocodone, oxycodone, and tramadol.

CYP3A4 inducers: CYP3A4 inducers may decrease the levels/effects of ketoconazole. Example inducers include aminoglutethimide, carbamazepine, nafcillin, nevirapine, phenobarbital, phenytoin, and rifamycins.

CYP3A4 substrates: Ketoconazole may increase the levels/effects of CYP3A4 substrates. Example substrates include benzodiazepines, calcium channel blockers, mirtazapine, nateglinide, nefazodone, tacrolimus, and venlafaxine. Selected benzodiazepines (midazolam and triazolam), cisapride, ergot alkaloids, selected HMG-CoA reductase inhibitors (lovastatin and simvastatin), and pimozide are generally contraindicated with strong CYP3A4 inhibitors.

Didanosine: May decrease absorption of ketoconazole (due to buffering capacity of oral solution); applies only to oral solution formulation of didanosine.

Docetaxel: Serum concentrations may be increased; avoid concurrent use.

Erythromycin (and clarithromycin): May increase serum concentrations of ketoconazole.

H$_2$ blockers: May decrease ketoconazole absorption. Ketoconazole depends on gastric acidity for absorption. Avoid concurrent use.

HMG-CoA reductase inhibitors (except pravastatin and fluvastatin): Serum concentrations may be increased. The risk of myopathy/rhabdomyolysis may be increased. Switch to pravastatin/fluvastatin or suspend treatment during course of ketoconazole therapy.

Immunosuppressants: Cyclosporine, sirolimus, and tacrolimus: Serum concentrations may be increased; monitor serum concentrations and renal function.

Methylprednisolone: Serum concentrations may be increased; monitor.

Nevirapine: May decrease serum concentrations of ketoconazole; monitor.

Oral contraceptives: Efficacy may be reduced by ketoconazole (limited data); use barrier birth control method during concurrent use.

Phenytoin: Serum concentrations may be increased; monitor phenytoin levels and adjust dose as needed.

Protease inhibitors: May increase serum concentrations of ketoconazole. Includes amprenavir, indinavir, nelfinavir, ritonavir, and saquinavir; monitor.

Proton pump inhibitors: May decrease ketoconazole absorption. Ketoconazole depends on gastric acidity for absorption. Avoid concurrent use (includes omeprazole, lansoprazole).

Quinidine: Serum levels may be increased; monitor.

Rifampin: Rifampin decreases ketoconazole's serum concentration to levels which are no longer effective; avoid concurrent use.

Sildenafil: Serum concentrations may be increased by ketoconazole; consider dosage reduction. A maximum sildenafil dose of 25 mg in 48 hours is recommended with other strong CYP3A4 inhibitors.

Tadalafil: Serum concentrations may be increased by ketoconazole. A maximum tadalafil dose of 10 mg in 72 hours is recommended with strong CYP3A4 inhibitors.

Trimetrexate: Serum concentrations may be increased; monitor.

Vardenafil: Serum concentrations may be increased by ketoconazole. If ketoconazole dose is 200 mg/day, limit vardenafil to a maximum of 5 mg/24 hours. If ketoconazole dose is 400 mg/day, limit vardenafil dose to a maximum of 2.5 mg/24 hours.

Warfarin: Anticoagulant effects may be increased; monitor INR and adjust warfarin's dose as needed.

Vinca alkaloids: Serum concentrations may be increased.

Zolpidem: Serum levels may be increased; monitor.

Ethanol/Nutrition/Herb Interactions
Food: Ketoconazole peak serum levels may be prolonged if taken with food.
Herb/Nutraceutical: St John's wort may decrease ketoconazole levels.

Dietary Considerations May be taken with food or milk to decrease GI adverse effects.

Pharmacodynamics/Kinetics
Absorption: Oral: Rapid (~75%); Shampoo: None; Gel: Minimal
Distribution: Well into inflamed joint fluid, saliva, bile, urine, breast milk, sebum, cerumen, feces, tendons, skin and soft tissue, and testes; crosses blood-brain barrier poorly; only negligible amounts reach CSF
Protein binding: 93% to 96%
Metabolism: Partially hepatic via CYP3A4 to inactive compounds
Bioavailability: Decreases as gastric pH increases
Half-life elimination: Biphasic: Initial: 2 hours; Terminal: 8 hours
Time to peak, serum: 1-2 hours
Excretion: Feces (57%); urine (13%)

Pregnancy Risk Factor C

Lactation Enters breast milk/not recommended

Dosage Forms Excipient information presented when available (limited, particularly for generics); consult specific product labeling.
Cream, topical: 2% (15 g, 30 g, 60 g)
Kuric™: 2%: (25 g, 75 g)
Gel, topical:
Xolegel™: 2% (15 g) [contains dehydrated alcohol 34%]
Shampoo, topical: 1% (120 mL), 2% (120 mL)
Nizoral® : 2% (120 mL)
Nizoral® A-D: 1% (120 mL, 210 mL)
Tablet: 200 mg
Nizoral®: 200 mg

3-Keto-desogestrel *see* Etonogestrel *on page 659*

Ketoprofen (kee toe PROE fen)

Related Information
Oral Pain *on page 1788*
Rheumatoid Arthritis, Osteoarthritis, and Osteoporosis *on page 1759*
Temporomandibular Dysfunction (TMD) *on page 1822*

U.S. Brand Names Orudis® KT [OTC] [DSC]

Canadian Brand Names Apo-Keto®; Apo-Keto-E®; Apo-Keto SR®; Novo-Keto; Novo-Keto-EC; Nu-Ketoprofen; Nu-Ketoprofen-E; Oruvail®; Rhodis™; Rhodis-EC™; Rhodis SR™

Mexican Brand Names Efiken; Keduril; Profenid

Generic Available Yes: Capsule

Pharmacologic Category Nonsteroidal Anti-inflammatory Drug (NSAID), Oral

Dental Use Management of pain and swelling

Use Acute and long-term treatment of rheumatoid arthritis and osteoarthritis; primary dysmenorrhea; mild-to-moderate pain

Local Anesthetic/Vasoconstrictor Precautions No information available to require special precautions

Effects on Dental Treatment Key adverse event(s) related to dental treatment: Stomatitis.
According to the FDA, the over-the-counter NSAID ketoprofen should be viewed as having the potential to interfere with the antiplatelet effect of low-dose aspirin until proven otherwise. This statement was provided in the same warning from the FDA that ibuprofen can interfere with the antiplatelet effect of low-dose aspirin (81 mg/day), potentially rendering aspirin less effective when used for cardioprotection and stroke protection. In situations where these drugs could be used concomitantly, the FDA has provided the following information: Patients who use immediate release aspirin (not enteric-coated aspirin) and take single doses of ibuprofen 400 mg, should dose the ibuprofen at least 30 minutes or longer after aspirin ingestion or more than 8 hours before aspirin ingestion to avoid attenuation of aspirin's effect. Similar recommendations may hold for concomitant ketoprofen and aspirin use.
At this time, recommendations about the timing of ibuprofen 400 mg or other NSAIDs (such as ketoprofen) in patients taking enteric-coated low-dose aspirin cannot be made based on available data.

Significant Adverse Effects
>10%: Gastrointestinal: Dyspepsia (11%)
1% to 10%:
Central nervous system: Headache (3% to 9%), depression, dizziness (>1%), dreams, insomnia, malaise, nervousness, somnolence
Dermatologic: Rash
(Continued)

Ketoprofen *(Continued)*

Gastrointestinal: Abdominal pain (3% to 9%), constipation (3% to 9%), diarrhea (3% to 9%), flatulence (3% to 9%), nausea (3% to 9%), anorexia (>1%), stomatitis (>1%), vomiting (>1%)

Genitourinary: Urinary tract infection (>1%)

Ocular: Visual disturbances

Otic: Tinnitus

Renal: Renal dysfunction (3% to 9%)

<1% (Limited to important or life-threatening): Agranulocytosis, allergic reaction, allergic rhinitis, alopecia, anaphylaxis, anemia, angioedema, arrhythmia, aseptic meningitis, blurred vision, bone marrow suppression, buccal necrosis, bullous rash, cholestatic hepatitis, confusion, CHF, conjunctivitis, cystitis, diabetes mellitus (aggravated), drowsiness, dry eyes, dysphoria, dyspnea, eczema, epistaxis, erythema multiforme, exfoliative dermatitis, gastritis, gastrointestinal perforation, GI ulceration, gynecomastia, hallucinations, hearing decreased, hemolytic anemia, hepatic dysfunction, hepatitis, hot flashes, hypertension, hyponatremia, impotence, interstitial nephritis, intestinal ulceration, jaundice, leukopenia, microvesicular steatosis, migraine, myocardial infarction, nephrotic syndrome, nightmares, onycholysis, pancreatitis, peptic ulcer, peripheral neuropathy, peripheral vascular disease, photosensitivity, polydipsia, polyuria, purpura, renal failure, retinal hemorrhage, Stevens-Johnson syndrome, tachycardia, taste perversion, thrombocytopenia, toxic amblyopia, toxic epidermal necrolysis, tubulopathy, ulcerative colitis, urticaria

Restrictions An FDA-approved medication guide must be distributed when dispensing an oral outpatient prescription (new or refill) where this medication is to be used without direct supervision of a healthcare provider. Medication guides are available at http://www.fda.gov/cder/Offices/ODS/medication_guides.htm.

Dental Usual Dosing Mild-to-moderate pain: Children ≥16 years and Adults:

Oral: Capsule: 25-50 mg every 6-8 hours up to a maximum of 300 mg/day

OTC labeling: 12.5 mg every 4-6 hours, up to a maximum of 6 tablets/24 hours

Dosage Oral:

Children ≥16 years and Adults:

Rheumatoid arthritis or osteoarthritis (lower doses may be used in small patients or in the elderly, or debilitated):

Capsule: 50-75 mg 3-4 times/day up to a maximum of 300 mg/day

Capsule, extended release: 200 mg once daily

Mild-to-moderate pain: Capsule: 25-50 mg every 6-8 hours up to a maximum of 300 mg/day

OTC labeling: 12.5 mg every 4-6 hours, up to a maximum of 6 tablets/24 hours

Elderly: Initial dose should be decreased in patients >75 years; use caution when dosage changes are made

Dosage adjustment in renal impairment: In general, NSAIDs are not recommended for use in patients with advanced renal disease, but the manufacturer of ketoprofen does provide some guidelines for adjustment in renal dysfunction:

Mild impairment: Maximum dose: 150 mg/day

Severe impairment: Cl_{cr} <25 mL/minute: Maximum dose: 100 mg/day

Dosage adjustment in hepatic impairment and serum albumin <3.5 g/dL: Maximum dose: 100 mg/day

Mechanism of Action Inhibits prostaglandin synthesis by decreasing the activity of the enzyme, cyclooxygenase, which results in decreased formation of prostaglandin precursors

Contraindications Hypersensitivity to ketoprofen, aspirin, other NSAIDs, or any component of the formulation; perioperative pain in the setting of coronary artery bypass surgery (CABG); pregnancy (3rd trimester)

Warnings/Precautions [U.S. Boxed Warning]: NSAIDs are associated with an increased risk of adverse cardiovascular events, including MI, stroke, and new onset or worsening of pre-existing hypertension. Risk may be increased with duration of use or pre-existing cardiovascular risk factors or disease. Carefully evaluate individual cardiovascular risk profiles prior to prescribing. Use caution with fluid retention, CHF or hypertension. Concurrent administration of ibuprofen, and potentially other nonselective NSAIDs, may interfere with aspirin's cardioprotective effect.

Use of NSAIDs can compromise existing renal function. Renal toxicity can occur in patient with impaired renal function, dehydration, heart failure, liver dysfunction, those taking diuretics and ACEI and the elderly. Rehydrate patient before starting therapy. Monitor renal function closely. Ketoprofen is not recommended for patients with advanced renal disease.

[U.S. Boxed Warning]: NSAIDs may increase risk of gastrointestinal irritation, ulceration, bleeding, and perforation. These events may occur at any time during therapy and without warning. Use caution with a history of GI disease (bleeding or ulcers), concurrent therapy with aspirin, anticoagulants and/or corticosteroids, smoking, use of alcohol, the elderly or debilitated patients.

Use the lowest effective dose for the shortest duration of time, consistent with individual patient goals, to reduce risk of cardiovascular or GI adverse events. Alternate therapies should be considered for patients at high risk.

NSAIDs may cause serious skin adverse events including exfoliative dermatitis, Stevens-Johnson syndrome (SJS), and toxic epidermal necrolysis (TEN). Anaphylactoid reactions may occur, even without prior exposure; patients with "aspirin triad" (bronchial asthma, aspirin intolerance, rhinitis) may be at increased risk. Do not use in patients who experience bronchospasm, asthma, rhinitis, or urticaria with NSAID or aspirin therapy. Use caution in other forms of asthma.

Use with caution in patients with decreased hepatic function. Closely monitor patients with any abnormal LFT. Severe hepatic reactions (eg, fulminant hepatitis, liver failure) have occurred with NSAID use, rarely; discontinue if signs or symptoms of liver disease develop, or if systemic manifestations occur.

The elderly are at increased risk for adverse effects (especially peptic ulceration, CNS effects, renal toxicity) from NSAIDs, even at low doses.

Withhold for at least 4-6 half-lives prior to surgical or dental procedures. Safety and efficacy have not been established in pediatric patients.

Drug Interactions Inhibits CYP2C9 (weak)

ACE inhibitors: Antihypertensive effects may be decreased by concurrent therapy with NSAIDs; monitor blood pressure.

Aminoglycosides: NSAIDs may decrease the excretion of aminoglycosides.

Angiotensin II antagonists: Antihypertensive effects may be decreased by concurrent therapy with NSAIDs; monitor blood pressure.

Anticoagulants (warfarin, heparin, LMWHs): In combination with NSAIDs can cause increased risk of bleeding.

Antiplatelet agents (ticlopidine, clopidogrel, aspirin, abciximab, dipyridamole, eptifibatide, tirofiban): In combination with NSAIDs can cause an increased risk of bleeding.

Beta-blockers: NSAIDs may decrease the antihypertensive effect of beta-blockers; monitor.

Bisphosphonates: NSAIDs may increase the risk of gastrointestinal ulceration.

Cholestyramine (and other bile acid sequestrants): May decrease the absorption of NSAIDs; separate by at least 2 hours.

Corticosteroids: May increase the risk of GI ulceration; avoid concurrent use.

Cyclosporine: NSAIDs may increase serum creatinine, potassium, blood pressure, and cyclosporine levels; monitor cyclosporine levels and renal function carefully.

Fluoroquinolone antibiotics: Risk of seizures may be increased with concomitant quinolone use. Risk is considered quite low and may only be a factor with high serum levels of either agent and/or in patients with additional predisposing factors (eg, renal dysfunction, history of seizure, or other neurological disorder).

Hydralazine: Antihypertensive effect is decreased; avoid concurrent use.

Lithium: Lithium levels can be increased; avoid concurrent use if possible or monitor lithium levels and adjust dose. Sulindac may have the least effect. When NSAID is stopped, lithium will need adjustment again.

Loop diuretics: Antihypertensive and diuretic effects may be diminished. Indomethacin reduces this efficacy, however, it may be anticipated with any NSAID.

Methotrexate: Severe bone marrow suppression, aplastic anemia, and GI toxicity have been reported with concomitant NSAID therapy. Avoid use during moderate or high-dose methotrexate (increased and prolonged methotrexate levels). NSAID use during low-dose treatment of rheumatoid arthritis has not been fully evaluated; extreme caution is warranted.

Pemetrexed: NSAIDs may decrease the excretion of pemetrexed. Patients with Cl$_{cr}$ 45-79 mL/minute should avoid long-acting NSAIDs for 5 days before and 2 days after pemetrexed treatment.

Probenecid: May increase the serum concentration of ketoprofen.

Salicylates: NSAIDs (nonselective) may diminish the cardioprotective effect of acetylated salicylates. Avoid regular use of NSAIDs if possible; consider alternatives (eg, acetaminophen). Give salicylate before NSAID; for example ibuprofen should be given 30-120 minutes after aspirin (immediate release).

Thiazides: Antihypertensive effects may be decreased; avoid concurrent use.

Treprostinil: May enhance the risk of bleeding with concurrent use.

Vancomycin: NSAIDs may decrease the excretion of vancomycin.

(Continued)

Ketoprofen *(Continued)*

Ethanol/Nutrition/Herb Interactions

Ethanol: Avoid ethanol (due to GI irritation).

Food: Food slows rate of absorption resulting in delayed and reduced peak serum concentrations.

Herb/Nutraceutical: Avoid alfalfa, anise, bilberry, bladderwrack, bromelain, cat's claw, celery, coleus, cordyceps, dong quai, evening primrose, feverfew, fenugreek, garlic, ginger, ginkgo biloba, red clover, horse chestnut, grapeseed, green tea, ginseng, guggul, horse chestnut seed, horseradish, licorice, prickly ash, red clover, reishi, SAMe, sweet clover, turmeric, and white willow (all have additional antiplatelet activity).

Dietary Considerations
In order to minimize gastrointestinal effects, ketoprofen can be prescribed to be taken with food or milk.

Pharmacodynamics/Kinetics

Absorption: Almost complete

Protein binding: >99%, primarily albumin

Metabolism: Hepatic via glucuronidation; metabolite can be converted back to parent compound; may have enterohepatic recirculation

Half-life elimination:
Capsule: 2-4 hours; moderate-to-severe renal impairment: 5-9 hours
Capsule, extended release: ~3-7.5 hours

Time to peak, serum:
Capsule: 0.5-2 hours
Capsule, extended release: 6-7 hours

Excretion: Urine (~80%, primarily as glucuronide conjugates)

Pregnancy Risk Factor C/D (3rd trimester)

Lactation
Excretion in breast milk unknown/not recommended

Dosage Forms
Excipient information presented when available (limited, particularly for generics); consult specific product labeling. [DSC] = Discontinued product

Capsule: 50 mg, 75 mg

Capsule, extended release: 200 mg

Tablet (Orudis® KT): 12.5 mg [contains tartrazine and sodium benzoate] [DSC]

Selected Readings

Brooks PM and Day RO, "Nonsteroidal Anti-inflammatory Drugs - Differences and Similarities," *N Engl J Med*, 1991, 324(24):1716-25.

Cooper SA, "Ketoprofen in Oral Surgery Pain: A Review," *J Clin Pharmacol*, 1988, 28(12 Suppl):S40-6.

Hersh EV, "The Efficacy and Safety of Ketoprofen in Postsurgical Dental Pain," *Compendium*, 1991, 12(4):234.

Ketorolac *(KEE toe role ak)*

Related Information

Oral Pain *on page 1788*
Rheumatoid Arthritis, Osteoarthritis, and Osteoporosis *on page 1759*
Temporomandibular Dysfunction (TMD) *on page 1822*

U.S. Brand Names Acular®; Acular LS™; Acular® PF; Toradol®

Canadian Brand Names Acular®; Acular LS™; Apo-Ketorolac®; Apo-Ketorolac Injectable®; Ketorolac Tromethamine Injection, USP; Novo-Ketorolac; ratio-Ketorolac; Toradol®; Toradol® IM

Mexican Brand Names Alidol; Dolac; Estopein; Supradol; Toloran; Toral; Tromedal

Generic Available Yes: Injection, tablet

Index Terms Ketorolac Tromethamine

Pharmacologic Category Nonsteroidal Anti-inflammatory Drug (NSAID), Ophthalmic; Nonsteroidal Anti-inflammatory Drug (NSAID), Oral; Nonsteroidal Anti-inflammatory Drug (NSAID), Parenteral

Dental Use Oral, injection: Short-term (≤5 days) management of moderate-to-severe acute pain requiring analgesia at the opioid level

Use

Oral, injection: Short-term (≤5 days) management of moderate-to-severe acute pain requiring analgesia at the opioid level

Ophthalmic: Temporary relief of ocular itching due to seasonal allergic conjunctivitis; postoperative inflammation following cataract extraction; reduction of ocular pain and photophobia following incisional refractive surgery; reduction of ocular pain, burning, and stinging following corneal refractive surgery

Local Anesthetic/Vasoconstrictor Precautions No information available to require special precautions

Effects on Dental Treatment Key adverse event(s) related to dental treatment: Xerostomia (normal salivary flow resumes upon discontinuation) and stomatitis.

NSAID formulations are known to reversibly decrease platelet aggregation via mechanisms different than observed with aspirin. The dentist should be aware of the potential of abnormal coagulation. Caution should also be exercised in the use of NSAIDs in patients already on anticoagulant therapy with drugs such as warfarin (Coumadin®). See Dental Comment.

Significant Adverse Effects
Systemic (frequencies noted for parenteral administration):
>10%:

Central nervous system: Headache (17%)

Gastrointestinal: Gastrointestinal pain (13%), dyspepsia (12%), nausea (12%)

>1% to 10%:

Cardiovascular: Edema (4%), hypertension

Central nervous system: Dizziness (7%), drowsiness (6%)

Dermatologic: Pruritus, purpura, rash

Gastrointestinal: Diarrhea (7%), constipation, flatulence, gastrointestinal fullness, vomiting, stomatitis

Local: Injection site pain (2%)

Miscellaneous: Diaphoresis

≤1% (Limited to important or life-threatening): Abnormal vision, acute renal failure, anaphylactoid reaction, anaphylaxis, asthma, azotemia, bronchospasm, cholestatic jaundice, convulsions, eosinophilia, epistaxis, esophagitis, extrapyramidal symptoms, GI hemorrhage, GI perforation, hallucinations, hearing loss, hematemesis, hematuria, hepatitis, hypersensitivity reactions, liver failure, Lyell's syndrome, maculopapular rash, nephritis, peptic ulceration, photosensitivity, Stevens-Johnson syndrome, tinnitus, toxic epidermal necrolysis, urticaria, vertigo, wound hemorrhage (postoperative)

Ophthalmic solution:
>10%: Ocular: Transient burning/stinging (Acular®: 40%; Acular® PF: 20%)

>1% to 10%:

Central nervous system: Headache

Ocular: Conjunctival hyperemia, corneal infiltrates, iritis, ocular edema, ocular inflammation, ocular irritation, ocular pain, superficial keratitis, superficial ocular infection

Miscellaneous: Allergic reactions

≤1% (Limited to important or life-threatening): Blurred vision, corneal ulcer, corneal erosion, corneal perforation, corneal thinning, dry eyes, epithelial breakdown

Restrictions An FDA-approved medication guide must be distributed when dispensing an oral outpatient prescription (new or refill) where this medication is to be used without direct supervision of a healthcare provider. Medication guides are available at http://www.fda.gov/cder/Offices/ODS/medication_guides.htm.

Dental Usual Dosing
Short-term (≤5 days) management of moderate-to-severe acute pain requiring analgesia at the opioid level (**Note:** The maximum combined duration of treatment (for parenteral and oral) is 5 days; do not increase dose or frequency; supplement with low-dose opioids if needed for breakthrough pain). For patients <50 kg and/or ≥65 years, see Elderly dosing.

Adults:

I.M.: 60 mg as a single dose or 30 mg every 6 hours (maximum daily dose: 120 mg)

I.V.: 30 mg as a single dose or 30 mg every 6 hours (maximum daily dose: 120 mg)

Oral: 20 mg, followed by 10 mg every 4-6 hours; do not exceed 40 mg/day; oral dosing is intended to be a continuation of I.M. or I.V. therapy only

Dosage adjustments in elderly (>65 years), renal insufficiency, or low body weight (<50 kg): Note: These groups have an increased incidence of GI bleeding, ulceration, and perforation. The maximum combined duration of treatment (for parenteral and oral) is 5 days.

I.M.: 30 mg as a single dose or 15 mg every 6 hours (maximum daily dose: 60 mg)

I.V.: 15 mg as a single dose or 15 mg every 6 hours (maximum daily dose: 60 mg)

Oral: 10 mg, followed by 10 mg every 4-6 hours; do not exceed 40 mg/day; oral dosing is intended to be a continuation of I.M. or I.V. therapy only

Dosage
Children 2-16 years: **Do not exceed adult doses:**

Single-dose treatment:

I.M.: 1 mg/kg (maximum: 30 mg)

I.V.: 0.5 mg/kg (maximum: 15 mg)

Oral (unlabeled): 1 mg/kg as a single dose reported in one study

Multiple-dose treatment (unlabeled): Limited pediatric studies. The maximum combined duration of treatment (for parenteral and oral) is 5 days.

(Continued)

Ketorolac *(Continued)*

I.V.: Initial dose: 0.5 mg/kg, followed by 0.25-1 mg/kg every 6 hours for up to 48 hours (maximum daily dose: 90 mg)

Oral: 0.25 mg/kg every 6 hours

Children ≥16 years and Adults (pain relief usually begins within 10 minutes with parenteral forms): **Note:** The maximum combined duration of treatment (for parenteral and oral) is 5 days; do not increase dose or frequency; supplement with low-dose opioids if needed for breakthrough pain. For patients <50 kg and/or ≥65 years, see Elderly dosing.

I.M.: 60 mg as a single dose or 30 mg every 6 hours (maximum daily dose: 120 mg)

I.V.: 30 mg as a single dose or 30 mg every 6 hours (maximum daily dose: 120 mg)

Oral: 20 mg, followed by 10 mg every 4-6 hours; do not exceed 40 mg/day; oral dosing is intended to be a continuation of I.M. or I.V. therapy only

Ophthalmic: Children ≥3 years and Adults:

Allergic conjunctivitis (relief of ocular itching) (Acular®): Instill 1 drop (0.25 mg) 4 times/day for seasonal allergic conjunctivitis

Inflammation following cataract extraction (Acular®): Instill 1 drop (0.25 mg) to affected eye(s) 4 times/day beginning 24 hours after surgery; continue for 2 weeks

Pain and photophobia following incisional refractive surgery (Acular® PF): Instill 1 drop (0.25 mg) 4 times/day to affected eye for up to 3 days

Pain following corneal refractive surgery (Acular LS™): Instill 1 drop 4 times/day as needed to affected eye for up to 4 days

Dosage adjustments in elderly (>65 years), renal insufficiency, or low body weight (<50 kg): Note: These groups have an increased incidence of GI bleeding, ulceration, and perforation. The maximum combined duration of treatment (for parenteral and oral) is 5 days.

I.M.: 30 mg as a single dose or 15 mg every 6 hours (maximum daily dose: 60 mg)

I.V.: 15 mg as a single dose or 15 mg every 6 hours (maximum daily dose: 60 mg)

Oral: 10 mg, followed by 10 mg every 4-6 hours; do not exceed 40 mg/day; oral dosing is intended to be a continuation of I.M. or I.V. therapy only

Dosage adjustment in renal impairment: Contraindicated in patients with advanced renal impairment. Patients with moderately-elevated serum creatinine should use half the recommended dose, not to exceed 60 mg/day I.M./I.V.

Dosage adjustment in hepatic impairment: Use with caution, may cause elevation of liver enzymes

Mechanism of Action Inhibits prostaglandin synthesis by decreasing the activity of the enzyme, cyclooxygenase, which results in decreased formation of prostaglandin precursors

Contraindications Hypersensitivity to ketorolac, aspirin, other NSAIDs, or any component of the formulation; active or history of peptic ulcer disease; recent or history of GI bleeding or perforation; patients with advanced renal disease or risk of renal failure; labor and delivery; nursing mothers; prophylaxis before major surgery; suspected or confirmed cerebrovascular bleeding; hemorrhagic diathesis or high risk of bleeding; concurrent ASA or other NSAIDs; concomitant probenecid or pentoxifylline; epidural or intrathecal administration; perioperative pain in the setting of coronary artery bypass surgery (CABG); pregnancy (3rd trimester)

Warnings/Precautions

Systemic: Treatment should be started with I.V./I.M. administration then changed to oral only as a continuation of treatment. Total therapy is not to exceed 5 days. Should not be used for minor or chronic pain.

May prolong bleeding time; do not use when hemostasis is critical. Patients should be euvolemic prior to treatment. Low doses of narcotics may be needed for breakthrough pain.

[U.S. Boxed Warning]: NSAIDs are associated with an increased risk of adverse cardiovascular events, including MI, stroke, and new onset or worsening of pre-existing hypertension. Risk may be increased with duration of use or pre-existing cardiovascular risk factors or disease. Carefully evaluate individual cardiovascular risk profiles prior to prescribing. Use caution with fluid retention, CHF or hypertension. Concurrent administration of ibuprofen, and potentially other nonselective NSAIDs, may interfere with aspirin's cardioprotective effect.

Use of NSAIDs can compromise existing renal function. Renal toxicity can occur in patient with impaired renal function, dehydration, heart failure, liver dysfunction, those taking diuretics and ACEI, and the elderly. Rehydrate patient before starting therapy. Monitor renal function closely. Ketorolac is not recommended for patients with advanced renal disease.

[U.S. Boxed Warning]: NSAIDs may increase risk of gastrointestinal irritation, ulceration, bleeding, and perforation. These events may occur at any time during therapy and without warning. Use caution with a history of GI disease (bleeding or ulcers), concurrent therapy with aspirin, anticoagulants and/or corticosteroids, smoking, use of alcohol, the elderly, or debilitated patients.

Use the lowest effective dose for the shortest duration of time, consistent with individual patient goals, to reduce risk of cardiovascular or GI adverse events. Alternate therapies should be considered for patients at high risk.

NSAIDs may cause serious skin adverse events including exfoliative dermatitis, Stevens-Johnson syndrome (SJS) and toxic epidermal necrolysis (TEN). Anaphylactoid reactions may occur, even without prior exposure; patients with "aspirin triad" (bronchial asthma, aspirin intolerance, rhinitis) may be at increased risk. Do not use in patients who experience bronchospasm, asthma, rhinitis, or urticaria with NSAID or aspirin therapy. Use caution in other forms of asthma.

Use with caution in patients with decreased hepatic function. Closely monitor patients with any abnormal LFT. Severe hepatic reactions (eg, fulminant hepatitis, liver failure) have occurred with NSAID use, rarely; discontinue if signs or symptoms of liver disease develop, or if systemic manifestations occur.

The elderly are at increased risk for adverse effects (especially peptic ulceration, CNS effects, renal toxicity) from NSAIDs, even at low doses. Patients with low body weight (<50 kg) or moderate elevation of serum creatinine require adjusted doses to limit risk of bleeding.

Withhold for at least 4-6 half-lives prior to surgical or dental procedures. Safety and efficacy for systemic preparations has not been established in children <2 years of age; a single-dose injection may be used in children 2-16 years of age.

Ophthalmic: May increase bleeding time associated with ocular surgery. Use with caution in patients with known bleeding tendencies or those receiving anticoagulants. Healing time may be slowed or delayed. Corneal thinning, erosion, or ulceration have been reported with topical NSAIDs; discontinue if corneal epithelial breakdown occurs. Use caution with complicated ocular surgery, corneal denervation, corneal epithelial defects, diabetes, rheumatoid arthritis, ocular surface disease, or ocular surgeries repeated within short periods of time; risk of corneal epithelial breakdown may be increased. Use for >24 hours prior to or for >14 days following surgery also increases risk of corneal adverse effects. Do not administer while wearing soft contact lenses. Safety and efficacy in pediatric patients <3 years of age have not been established.

Drug Interactions

ACE inhibitors: Antihypertensive effects may be decreased by concurrent therapy with NSAIDs; monitor blood pressure.

Angiotensin II antagonists: Antihypertensive effects may be decreased by concurrent therapy with NSAIDs; monitor blood pressure.

Anticoagulants: Increased risk of bleeding complications with concomitant use; monitor closely.

Antiepileptic drugs (carbamazepine, phenytoin): Sporadic cases of seizures have been reported with concomitant use.

Beta-blockers: NSAIDs may decrease the antihypertensive effect of beta-blockers; monitor.

Cholestyramine (and other bile acid sequestrants): May decrease the absorption of NSAIDs; separate by at least 2 hours.

Diuretics: May see decreased effect of diuretics.

Fluoroquinolone antibiotics: Risk of seizures may be increased with concomitant quinolone use. Risk is considered quite low and may only be a factor with high serum levels of either agent and/or in patients with additional predisposing factors (eg, renal dysfunction, history of seizure or other neurological disorder).

Hydralazine's antihypertensive effect may be reduced; monitor.

Lithium: May increase lithium levels; monitor.

Methotrexate: Severe bone marrow suppression, aplastic anemia, and GI toxicity have been reported with concomitant NSAID therapy. Avoid use during moderate or high-dose methotrexate (increased and prolonged methotrexate levels). NSAID use during low-dose treatment of rheumatoid arthritis has not been fully evaluated; extreme caution is warranted.

Nondepolarizing muscle relaxants: Concomitant use has resulted in apnea.

(Continued)

Ketorolac *(Continued)*

NSAIDs, salicylates: Concomitant use increases NSAID-induced adverse effects; contraindicated.

Pentoxifylline: Concomitant use may increase risk of bleeding; contraindicated.

Probenecid: Probenecid significantly decreases ketorolac clearance, increases ketorolac plasma levels, and doubles the half-life of ketorolac; concomitant use is contraindicated.

Psychoactive drugs (alprazolam, fluoxetine, thiothixene): Hallucinations have been reported with concomitant use.

Salicylates: NSAIDs (nonselective) may diminish the cardioprotective effect of acetylated salicylates. Avoid regular use of NSAIDs, if possible; consider alternatives (eg, acetaminophen). Give salicylate before NSAID; for example, ibuprofen should be given 30-120 minutes after aspirin (immediate release).

Ethanol/Nutrition/Herb Interactions

Ethanol: Avoid ethanol (may enhance gastric mucosal irritation).

Food: Oral: High-fat meals may delay time to peak (by ~1 hour) and decrease peak concentrations.

Herb/Nutraceuticals: Avoid alfalfa, anise, bilberry, bladderwrack, bromelain, cat's claw, celery, coleus, cordyceps, dong quai, evening primrose, feverfew, fenugreek, garlic, ginger, ginkgo biloba, red clover, horse chestnut, grapeseed, green tea, ginseng, guggul, horse chestnut seed, horseradish, licorice, prickly ash, red clover, reishi, SAMe, sweet clover, turmeric, and white willow (all have additional antiplatelet activity).

Dietary Considerations Administer tablet with food or milk to decrease gastro-intestinal distress.

Pharmacodynamics/Kinetics

Onset of action: Analgesic: I.M.: ~10 minutes
  Peak effect: Analgesic: 2-3 hours

Duration: Analgesic: 6-8 hours

Absorption: Oral: Well absorbed (100%)

Distribution: Poor penetration into CSF; crosses placenta; enters breast milk

Protein binding: 99%

Metabolism: Hepatic

Half-life elimination: 2-6 hours; prolonged 30% to 50% in elderly; up to 19 hours in renal impairment

Time to peak, serum: I.M.: 30-60 minutes

Excretion: Urine (92%, 61% as unchanged drug)

Pregnancy Risk Factor C/D (3rd trimester)

Lactation Enters breast milk/contraindicated

Dosage Forms Excipient information presented when available (limited, particularly for generics); consult specific product labeling. [DSC] = Discontinued product

Injection, solution, as tromethamine: 15 mg/mL (1 mL); 30 mg/mL (1 mL, 2 mL, 10 mL) [contains alcohol]

Solution, ophthalmic, as tromethamine:
  Acular®: 0.5% (3 mL, 5 mL, 10 mL) [contains benzalkonium chloride]
  Acular LS™: 0.4% (5 mL) [contains benzalkonium chloride]
  Acular® P.F. [preservative free]: 0.5% (0.4 mL)

Tablet, as tromethamine: 10 mg
  Toradol®: 10 mg [DSC]

Dental Comment According to the manufacturer, ketorolac has been used inappropriately by physicians in the past. The drug had been prescribed to NSAID-sensitive patients, patients with GI bleeding, and for long-term use; a warning has been issued regarding increased incidence and severity of GI complications with increasing doses and duration of use. Labeling now includes the statement that ketorolac inhibits platelet function and is indicated for up to 5 days use only.

Selected Readings

Ahmad N, Grad HA, Haas DA, et al, "The Efficacy of Nonopioid Analgesics for Postoperative Dental Pain: A Meta-Analysis," *Anesth Prog*, 1997, 44(4):119-26.

Balevi B, "Ketorolac Versus Ibuprofen: A Simple Cost-Efficacy Comparison for Dental Use," *J Can Dent Assoc*, 1994, 60(1):31-2.

Forbes JA, Butterworth GA, Burchfield WH, et al, "Evaluation of Ketorolac, Aspirin, and an Acetaminophen-Codeine Combination in Postoperative Oral Surgery Pain," *Pharmacotherapy*, 1990, 10(6 Pt 2): 77S-93S.

Forbes JA, Kehm CJ, Grodin CD, et al, "Evaluation of Ketorolac, Ibuprofen, Acetaminophen, and an Acetaminophen-Codeine Combination in Postoperative Oral Surgery Pain," *Pharmacotherapy*, 1990, 10(6 Pt 2):94S-105S.

Fricke JR Jr, Angelocci D, Fox K, et al, "Comparison of the Efficacy and Safety of Ketorolac and Meperidine in the Relief of Dental Pain," *J Clin Pharmacol*, 1992, 32(4):376-84.

Fricke J, Halladay SC, Bynum L, et al, "Pain Relief After Dental Impaction Surgery Using Ketorolac, Hydrocodone Plus Acetaminophen, or Placebo," *Clin Ther*, 1993, 15(3):500-9.

Pendeville PE, Van Boven MJ, Contreras V, et al, "Ketorolac Tromethamine for Postoperative Analgesia in Oral Surgery," *Acta Anaesthesiol Belg*, 1995, 46(1):25-30.

Swift JQ, Roszkowski MT, Alton T, "Effect of Intra-articular Versus Systemic Anti-inflammatory Drugs in a Rabbit Model of Temporomandibular Joint Inflammation," *J Oral Maxillofac Surg*, 1998, 56(11):1288-95; discussion 1295-6.

Walton GM, Rood JP, Snowdon AT, et al, "Ketorolac and Diclofenac for Postoperative Pain Relief Following Oral Surgery," *Br J Oral Maxillofac Surg*, 1993, 31(3):158-60.

Wynn RL, "Ketorolac (Toradol®) for Dental Pain," *Gen Dent*, 1992, 40(6):476-9.

Ketorolac Tromethamine *see* Ketorolac *on page 934*

Ketotifen (kee toe TYE fen)

U.S. Brand Names Alaway™ [OTC]; Zaditor® [OTC]
Canadian Brand Names Apo-Ketotifen®; Novo-Ketotifen; Zaditen®; Zaditor®
Mexican Brand Names Kasmal; Zaditen; Zaditen SRO
Generic Available Yes
Index Terms Ketotifen Fumarate
Pharmacologic Category Antihistamine, H$_1$ Blocker, Ophthalmic
Use Temporary prevention of eye itching due to allergic conjunctivitis
Local Anesthetic/Vasoconstrictor Precautions No information available to require special precautions
Effects on Dental Treatment Key adverse event(s) related to dental treatment: Pharyngitis.
Mechanism of Action Relatively selective, noncompetitive H$_1$-receptor antagonist and mast cell stabilizer, inhibiting the release of mediators from cells involved in hypersensitivity reactions
Pregnancy Risk Factor C

Ketotifen Fumarate *see* Ketotifen *on page 939*

Key-E® [OTC] *see* Vitamin E *on page 1664*

Key-E® Kaps [OTC] *see* Vitamin E *on page 1664*

Keygesic [OTC] *see* Magnesium Salicylate *on page 1016*

KI *see* Potassium Iodide *on page 1330*

Kidkare Decongestant [OTC] *see* Pseudoephedrine *on page 1381*

Kineret® *see* Anakinra *on page 128*

Kinevac® *see* Sincalide *on page 1475*

Klaron® *see* Sulfacetamide *on page 1502*

Klonopin® *see* Clonazepam *on page 390*

K-Lor® *see* Potassium Chloride *on page 1329*

Klor-Con® *see* Potassium Chloride *on page 1329*

Klor-Con® 8 *see* Potassium Chloride *on page 1329*

Klor-Con® 10 *see* Potassium Chloride *on page 1329*

Klor-Con®/25 *see* Potassium Chloride *on page 1329*

Klor-Con® M *see* Potassium Chloride *on page 1329*

Klor-Con®/EF *see* Potassium Bicarbonate and Potassium Citrate *on page 1329*

K-Lyte® *see* Potassium Bicarbonate and Potassium Citrate *on page 1329*

K-Lyte/Cl® *see* Potassium Bicarbonate and Potassium Chloride *on page 1328*

K-Lyte® DS *see* Potassium Bicarbonate and Potassium Citrate *on page 1329*

Kobee [OTC] *see* Vitamin B Complex Combinations *on page 1664*

Kodet SE [OTC] *see* Pseudoephedrine *on page 1381*

Kogenate® FS *see* Antihemophilic Factor (Recombinant) *on page 132*

Kolephrin® [OTC] *see* Acetaminophen, Chlorpheniramine, and Pseudoephedrine *on page 43*

Kolephrin® #1 *see* Guaifenesin and Codeine *on page 795*

Kolephrin® GG/DM [OTC] *see* Guaifenesin and Dextromethorphan *on page 796*

Konsyl® [OTC] *see* Psyllium *on page 1386*

Konsyl-D® [OTC] *see* Psyllium *on page 1386*

Konsyl® Easy Mix [OTC] *see* Psyllium *on page 1386*

Konsyl® Fiber Caplets [OTC] *see* Polycarbophil *on page 1320*

Konsyl® Orange [OTC] *see* Psyllium *on page 1386*

Kovia® *see* Papain and Urea *on page 1251*

Koāte®-DVI *see* Antihemophilic Factor (Human) *on page 131*

K-Pek II [OTC] *see* Loperamide *on page 996*

K-Phos® MF *see* Potassium Phosphate and Sodium Phosphate *on page 1332*

K-Phos® Neutral *see* Potassium Phosphate and Sodium Phosphate *on page 1332*

K-Phos® No. 2 *see* Potassium Phosphate and Sodium Phosphate *on page 1332*

K-Phos® Original *see* Potassium Acid Phosphate *on page 1328*

K+ Potassium *see* Potassium Chloride *on page 1329*

Kristalose® *see* Lactulose *on page 943*

Kronofed-A® *see* Chlorpheniramine and Pseudoephedrine *on page 340*

Kronofed-A®-Jr *see* Chlorpheniramine and Pseudoephedrine *on page 340*

Labetalol (la BET a lole)

Related Information
Cardiovascular Diseases *on page 1726*

U.S. Brand Names Trandate®

Canadian Brand Names Apo-Labetalol®; Labetalol Hydrochloride Injection, USP; Normodyne®; Trandate®

Generic Available Yes

Index Terms Ibidomide Hydrochloride; Labetalol Hydrochloride

Pharmacologic Category Beta Blocker With Alpha-Blocking Activity

Use Treatment of mild to severe hypertension; I.V. for hypertensive emergencies

Unlabeled/Investigational Use Pediatric hypertension

Local Anesthetic/Vasoconstrictor Precautions Use with caution; epinephrine has interacted with nonselective beta-blockers to result in initial hypertensive episode followed by bradycardia

Effects on Dental Treatment Key adverse event(s) related to dental treatment: Taste disorder.

Many nonsteroidal anti-inflammatory drugs, such as ibuprofen and indomethacin, can reduce the hypotensive effect of beta-blockers after 3 or more weeks of therapy with the NSAID. Short-term NSAID use (ie, 3 days) requires no special precautions in patients taking beta-blockers.

Common Adverse Effects
>10%:
  Central nervous system: Dizziness (1% to 16%)
  Gastrointestinal: Nausea (0% to 19%)
1% to 10%:
  Cardiovascular: Edema (0% to 2%), hypotension (1% to 5%); with I.V. use, hypotension may occur in up to 58%
  Central nervous system: Fatigue (1% to 10%), headache (2%), vertigo (2%)
  Dermatologic: Rash (1%), scalp tingling (1% to 5%)
  Gastrointestinal: Vomiting (<1% to 3%), dyspepsia (1% to 4%)
  Genitourinary: Ejaculatory failure (0% to 5%), impotence (1% to 4%)
  Hepatic: Transaminases increased (4%)
  Neuromuscular & skeletal: Paresthesia (1% to 5%), weakness (1%)
  Respiratory: Nasal congestion (1% to 6%), dyspnea (2%)
  Miscellaneous: Taste disorder (1%), abnormal vision (1%)
Other adverse reactions noted with beta-adrenergic blocking agents include mental depression, catatonia, disorientation, short-term memory loss, emotional lability, clouded sensorium, intensification of pre-existing AV block, laryngospasm, respiratory distress, agranulocytosis, thrombocytopenic purpura, nonthrombocytopenic purpura, mesenteric artery thrombosis, and ischemic colitis.

Mechanism of Action Blocks alpha-, beta$_1$-, and beta$_2$-adrenergic receptor sites; elevated renins are reduced

Drug Interactions

Cytochrome P450 Effect: Substrate of CYP2D6 (major); **Inhibits** CYP2D6 (weak)

Increased Effect/Toxicity: CYP2D6 inhibitors may increase the levels/effects of labetalol; example inhibitors include chlorpromazine, delavirdine, fluoxetine, miconazole, paroxetine, pergolide, quinidine, quinine, ritonavir, and ropinirole. Cimetidine increases the bioavailability of labetalol. Labetalol has additive hypotensive effects with other antihypertensive agents. Concurrent use with alpha-blockers (prazosin, terazosin) and beta-blockers increases the risk of orthostasis. Concurrent use with diltiazem, verapamil, or digoxin may increase the risk of bradycardia with beta-blocking agents. Halothane, enflurane, isoflurane, and potentially other inhalation anesthetics may cause synergistic hypotension. Beta-blockers may affect the action or levels of ethanol, disopyramide, nondepolarizing muscle relaxants, and theophylline although the effects are difficult to predict.

Decreased Effect: Decreased effect of beta-blockers with aluminum salts, barbiturates, calcium salts, cholestyramine, colestipol, NSAIDs, penicillins (ampicillin), rifampin, salicylates, and sulfinpyrazone due to decreased bioavailability and plasma levels. Beta-blockers may decrease the effect of sulfonylureas.

Pharmacodynamics/Kinetics
Onset of action: Oral: 20 minutes to 2 hours; I.V.: 2-5 minutes
Peak effect: Oral: 1-4 hours; I.V.: 5-15 minutes
Duration: Oral: 8-24 hours (dose dependent); I.V.: 2-4 hours
Distribution: V_d: Adults: 3-16 L/kg; mean: <9.4 L/kg; moderately lipid soluble, therefore, can enter CNS; crosses placenta; small amounts enter breast milk
Protein binding: 50%
Metabolism: Hepatic, primarily via glucuronide conjugation; extensive first-pass effect
Bioavailability: Oral: 25%; increased with liver disease, elderly, and concurrent cimetidine
Half-life elimination: Normal renal function: 2.5-8 hours
Excretion: Urine (<5% as unchanged drug)
Clearance: Possibly decreased in neonates/infants
Pregnancy Risk Factor C (manufacturer); D (2nd and 3rd trimesters - expert analysis)

Labetalol Hydrochloride see Labetalol on page 940

Lac-Hydrin® see Lactic Acid and Ammonium Hydroxide on page 941

Lac-Hydrin® Five [OTC] see Lactic Acid and Ammonium Hydroxide on page 941

LAClotion™ see Lactic Acid and Ammonium Hydroxide on page 941

Lacrisert® see Hydroxypropyl Cellulose on page 844

Lactaid® Extra Strength [OTC] [DSC] see Lactase on page 941

Lactaid® Fast Act [OTC] see Lactase on page 941

Lactaid® Original [OTC] see Lactase on page 941

Lactaid® Ultra [OTC] [DSC] see Lactase on page 941

Lactase (LAK tase)

U.S. Brand Names Lactaid® Extra Strength [OTC] [DSC]; Lactaid® Fast Act [OTC]; Lactaid® Original [OTC]; Lactaid® Ultra [OTC] [DSC]; Lactrase® [OTC]
Canadian Brand Names Dairyaid®
Generic Available No
Pharmacologic Category Enzyme
Use Help digest lactose in milk for patients with lactose intolerance
Local Anesthetic/Vasoconstrictor Precautions No information available to require special precautions
Effects on Dental Treatment No significant effects or complications reported

Lactic Acid (LAK tik AS id)

U.S. Brand Names LactiCare® [OTC]; Lactinol®; Lactinol-E®
Generic Available Yes
Index Terms Sodium-PCA and Lactic Acid
Pharmacologic Category Topical Skin Product
Use Lubricate and moisturize the skin counteracting dryness and itching
Local Anesthetic/Vasoconstrictor Precautions No information available to require special precautions
Effects on Dental Treatment No significant effects or complications reported
Common Adverse Effects Frequency not defined.
Dermatologic: Burning, mild stinging, peeling

Lactic Acid and Ammonium Hydroxide
(LAK tik AS id & a MOE nee um hye DROKS ide)

U.S. Brand Names AmLactin® [OTC]; Geri-Hydrolac™ [OTC]; Geri-Hydrolac™-12 [OTC]; Lac-Hydrin®; Lac-Hydrin® Five [OTC]; LAClotion™
Mexican Brand Names Lactrex
Generic Available Yes
Index Terms Ammonium Lactate
Pharmacologic Category Topical Skin Product
Use Treatment of moderate to severe xerosis and ichthyosis vulgaris
(Continued)

Lactic Acid and Ammonium Hydroxide *(Continued)*

Local Anesthetic/Vasoconstrictor Precautions No information available to require special precautions

Effects on Dental Treatment No significant effects or complications reported

Common Adverse Effects
>10%: Dermatologic: Rash, including erythema and irritation (2% to 15%); burning/stinging (2% to 15%)
1% to 10%: Dermatologic: Itching (5%), dry skin (2%)

Mechanism of Action Exact mechanism of action unknown; lactic acid is a normal component in blood and tissues. When applied topically to the skin, acts as a humectant.

Pharmacodynamics/Kinetics Absorption: 6%

Pregnancy Risk Factor B

LactiCare® [OTC] *see Lactic Acid on page 941*

Lactinex™ [OTC] *see Lactobacillus on page 942*

Lactinol® *see Lactic Acid on page 941*

Lactinol-E® *see Lactic Acid on page 941*

Lactobacillus (lak toe ba SIL us)

Related Information
Bifidobacterium bifidum / Lactobacillus acidophilus on page 1702
Ulcerative and Erosive Disorders on page 1809

U.S. Brand Names Bacid® [OTC]; Culturelle® [OTC]; Dofus [OTC]; Flora-Q™ [OTC]; Kala® [OTC]; Lactinex™ [OTC]; Lacto-Bifidus [OTC]; Lacto-Key [OTC]; Lacto-Pectin [OTC]; Lacto-TriBlend [OTC]; Megadophilus® [OTC]; MoreDophilus® [OTC]; Superdophilus® [OTC]

Canadian Brand Names Bacid®; Fermalac

Generic Available Yes

Index Terms *Lactobacillus acidophilus*; *Lactobacillus bifidus*; *Lactobacillus bulgaricus*; *Lactobacillus casei*; *Lactobacillus paracasei*; *Lactobacillus reuteri*; *Lactobacillus rhamnosus* GG

Pharmacologic Category Dietary Supplement; Probiotic

Dental Use Treatment of uncomplicated diarrhea, particularly that caused by antibiotic therapy; re-establish normal physiologic and bacterial flora of the intestinal tract

Use Promote normal bacterial flora of the intestinal tract

Local Anesthetic/Vasoconstrictor Precautions No information available to require special precautions

Effects on Dental Treatment No significant effects or complications reported

Significant Adverse Effects Gastrointestinal: Flatulence

Dosage Dietary supplement: Oral: Dosing varies by manufacturer; consult product labeling

Children (Culturelle®): 1 capsule daily
Adults:
Bacid®: 2 caplets/day
Culturelle®: 1 capsule daily; may increase to twice daily
Flora-Q™: 1 capsule/day
Lacto-Key 100 or 600: 1-2 capsules/day
Lactinex™: 1 packet or 4 tablets 3-4 times/day

Mechanism of Action Helps re-establish normal intestinal flora; suppresses the growth of potentially pathogenic microorganisms by producing lactic acid which favors the establishment of an aciduric flora.

Contraindications Hypersensitivity to any component of the formulation

Warnings/Precautions *Lactobacillus* species have been studied for various gastrointestinal disorders including diarrhea, inflammatory bowel disease, gastrointestinal infection. Effectiveness may be dependent upon actual species used; studies are ongoing. Currently, there are no FDA-approved disease-prevention or therapeutic indications for these products.

Drug Interactions No data reported

Dietary Considerations Products may contain whey, evaporated milk, soy peptone casein and/or beef extract; consult individual product labeling. Lactinex™ contains sodium 5.6 mg/4 tablets

Pharmacodynamics/Kinetics
Absorption: Oral: None
Distribution: Local, primarily colon
Excretion: Feces

Dosage Forms Excipient information presented when available (limited, particularly for generics); consult specific product labeling.

Capsule:
  Culturelle®: *L. rhamnosus* GG 10 billion colony-forming units [contains casein and whey]
  Dofus: *L. acidophilus* and *L. bifidus* 10:1 ratio [beet root powder base]
  Flora-Q™: *L. acidophilus* and *L. paracasei* ≥8 billion colony-forming units [also contains *Bifidobacterium* and *S. thermophilus*]
  Lacto-Key:
    100: *L. acidophilus* 1 billion colony-forming units [milk, soy, and yeast free; rice derived]
    600: *L. acidophilus* 6 billion colony-forming units [milk, soy, and yeast free; rice derived]
  Lacto-Bifidus:
    100: *L. bifidus* 1 billion colony-forming units [milk, soy, and yeast free; rice derived]
    600: *L. bifidus* 6 billion colony-forming units [milk, soy, and yeast free; rice derived]
  Lacto-Pectin: *L. acidophilus* and *L. casei* ≥5 billion colony-forming units [also contains *Bifidobacterium lactis* and citrus pectin cellulose complex]
  Lacto-TriBlend:
    100: *L. acidophilus*, *L. bifidus*, and *L. bulgaricus* 1 billion colony-forming units [milk, soy and yeast free; rice derived]
    600: *L. acidophilus*, *L. bifidus,* and *L. bulgaricus* 6 billion colony-forming units [milk, soy and yeast free; rice derived]
  Megadophilus®, Superdophilus®: *L. acidophilus* 2 billion units [available in dairy based or dairy free formulations]
Capsule, softgel: *L. acidophilus* 100 active units
Caplet (Bacid®): *L. acidophilus 80%* and *L. bulgaricus* 10% [also contains *Bifidobacterium biffidum* 5% and *S. thermophilus* 5%]

Granules (Lactinex™): *L. acidophilus* and *L. bulgaricus* 100 million live cells per 1 g packet (12s) [contains whey, evaporated milk, soy peptone, lactose, and beef extract]
Powder:
  Lacto-TriBlend: *L. acidophilus, L. bifidus,* and *L. bulgaricus* 10 billion colony-forming units per ¼ teaspoon (60 g) [milk, soy, and yeast free; rice derived]
  Megadophilus®, Superdophilus®: *L. acidophilus* 2 billion units per half-teaspoon (49 g, 70 g, 84 g, 126 g) [available in dairy based or dairy free (garbanzo bean) formulations]
  MoreDophilus®: *L. acidophilus* 12.4 billion units per teaspoon (30 g, 120 g) [dairy free, yeast free; soy and carrot derived]
Tablet:
  Kala®: *L. acidophilus* 200 million units [dairy free, yeast free; soy based]
  Lactinex™: *L. acidophilus* and *L. bulgaricus* 1 million live cells [contains whey, evaporated milk, soy peptone, lactose, and beef extract; contains sodium 5.6 mg/4 tablets]
Tablet, chewable: *L. reuteri* 100 million organisms
Wafer: *L. acidophilus* 90 mg and *L. bifidus* 25 mg (100s) [provides 1 billion organisms/wafer at time of manufacture; milk free]

Lactobacillus acidophilus see Lactobacillus on page 942
Lactobacillus bifidus see Lactobacillus on page 942
Lactobacillus bulgaricus see Lactobacillus on page 942
Lactobacillus casei see Lactobacillus on page 942
Lactobacillus paracasei see Lactobacillus on page 942
Lactobacillus reuteri see Lactobacillus on page 942
Lactobacillus rhamnosus GG see Lactobacillus on page 942
Lacto-Bifidus [OTC] see Lactobacillus on page 942
Lactoflavin see Riboflavin on page 1422
Lacto-Key [OTC] see Lactobacillus on page 942
Lacto-Pectin [OTC] see Lactobacillus on page 942
Lacto-TriBlend [OTC] see Lactobacillus on page 942
Lactrase® [OTC] see Lactase on page 941

Lactulose (LAK tyoo lose)

U.S. Brand Names Constulose; Enulose; Generlac; Kristalose®
Canadian Brand Names Acilac; Apo-Lactulose®; Laxilose; PMS-Lactulose
Mexican Brand Names Lactulax; Regulact
Generic Available Yes
Pharmacologic Category Ammonium Detoxicant; Laxative, Osmotic
Use Adjunct in the prevention and treatment of portal-systemic encephalopathy; treatment of chronic constipation
(Continued)

Lactulose (Continued)

Local Anesthetic/Vasoconstrictor Precautions No information available to require special precautions

Effects on Dental Treatment No significant effects or complications reported

Common Adverse Effects Frequency not defined: Gastrointestinal: Flatulence, diarrhea (excessive dose), abdominal discomfort, nausea, vomiting, cramping

Mechanism of Action The bacterial degradation of lactulose resulting in an acidic pH inhibits the diffusion of NH_3 into the blood by causing the conversion of NH_3 to NH_4+; also enhances the diffusion of NH_3 from the blood into the gut where conversion to NH_4+ occurs; produces an osmotic effect in the colon with resultant distention promoting peristalsis

Drug Interactions

Decreased Effect: Oral neomycin, laxatives, antacids

Pharmacodynamics/Kinetics

Absorption: Not appreciable

Metabolism: Via colonic flora to lactic acid and acetic acid; requires colonic flora for drug activation

Excretion: Primarily feces and urine (~3%)

Pregnancy Risk Factor B

Ladakamycin *see* Azacitidine *on page 171*

Lagesic™ *see* Acetaminophen and Phenyltoloxamine *on page 38*

L-All 12 *see* Carbetapentane and Phenylephrine *on page 279*

L-AmB *see* Amphotericin B (Liposomal) *on page 118*

Lamictal® *see* Lamotrigine *on page 945*

Lamisil® *see* Terbinafine *on page 1539*

Lamisil® AT™ [OTC] *see* Terbinafine *on page 1539*

Lamivudine (la MI vyoo deen)

Related Information

HIV Infection and AIDS *on page 1753*

U.S. Brand Names Epivir®; Epivir-HBV®

Canadian Brand Names Heptovir®; 3TC®

Mexican Brand Names 3TC

Generic Available No

Index Terms 3TC

Pharmacologic Category Antiretroviral Agent, Reverse Transcriptase Inhibitor (Nucleoside)

Use

Epivir®: Treatment of HIV infection when antiretroviral therapy is warranted; should always be used as part of a multidrug regimen (at least three antiretroviral agents)

Epivir-HBV®: Treatment of chronic hepatitis B associated with evidence of hepatitis B viral replication and active liver inflammation

Unlabeled/Investigational Use Prevention of HIV following needlesticks (with or without protease inhibitor)

Local Anesthetic/Vasoconstrictor Precautions No information available to require special precautions

Effects on Dental Treatment No significant effects or complications reported

Common Adverse Effects Reported for treatment of HIV or HBV in adults. Incidence data includes patients on combination therapy with other antiretroviral agents.

>10%:

Central nervous system: Headache (21% to 35%), fatigue (24% to 27%), insomnia (11%)

Gastrointestinal: Nausea (15% to 33%), diarrhea (14% to 18%), pancreatitis (range: 0.3% to 18%; higher percentage in pediatric patients), abdominal pain (9% to 16%), vomiting (13% to 15%)

Hematologic: Neutropenia (7% to 15%)

Hepatic: Transaminases increased (2% to 11%)

Neuromuscular & skeletal: Myalgia (8% to 14%), neuropathy (12%), musculoskeletal pain (12%)

Respiratory: Nasal signs and symptoms (20%), cough (18%), sore throat (13%)

Miscellaneous: Infections (25%; includes ear, nose, and throat)

1% to 10%:

Central nervous system: Dizziness (10%), depression (9%), fever (7% to 10%), chills (7% to 10%)

Dermatologic: Rash (5% to 9%)

Gastrointestinal: Anorexia (10%), lipase increased (10%), abdominal cramps (6%), dyspepsia (5%), amylase increased (<1% to 4%), heartburn
Hematologic: Thrombocytopenia (1% to 4%), hemoglobinemia (2% to 3%)
Neuromuscular & skeletal: Creatine phosphokinase increased (9%), arthralgia (5% to 7%)

Mechanism of Action Lamivudine is a cytosine analog. After lamivudine is triphosphorylated, the principle mode of action is inhibition of HIV reverse transcription via viral DNA chain termination; inhibits RNA- and DNA-dependent DNA polymerase activities of reverse transcriptase. The monophosphate form of lamivudine is incorporated into the viral DNA by hepatitis B virus polymerase, resulting in DNA chain termination.

Drug Interactions
Increased Effect/Toxicity: Sulfamethoxazole/trimethoprim increases lamivudine's blood levels. Concomitant use of ribavirin with or without interferon alfa and nucleoside analogues may increase the risk of developing hepatic decompensation or other signs of mitochondrial toxicity, including pancreatitis or lactic acidosis. Ganciclovir/valganciclovir may increase the adverse effects/toxicity (eg, hematologic) of nucleoside reverse transcriptase inhibitors. Trimethoprim (and other drugs excreted by organic cation transport) may increase serum levels/effects of lamivudine.
Decreased Effect: Zalcitabine and lamivudine may inhibit the intracellular phosphorylation of each other; concomitant use should be avoided.

Pharmacodynamics/Kinetics
Absorption: Rapid
Distribution: V_d: 1.3 L/kg
Protein binding, plasma: <36%
Metabolism: 5.2% to trans-sulfoxide metabolite
Bioavailability: Absolute; Cp_{max} decreased with food although AUC not significantly affected
 Children: 66%
 Adults: 86% to 87%
Half-life elimination: Children: 2 hours; Adults: 5-7 hours
Time to peak, plasma: Fed: 3.2 hours; Fasted: 0.9 hours
Excretion: Primarily urine (as unchanged drug)
Pregnancy Risk Factor C

Lamivudine, Abacavir, and Zidovudine see Abacavir, Lamivudine, and Zidovudine on page 23

Lamivudine and Abacavir see Abacavir and Lamivudine on page 23

Lamivudine and Zidovudine see Zidovudine and Lamivudine on page 1681

Lamotrigine (la MOE tri jeen)

U.S. Brand Names Lamictal®
Canadian Brand Names Apo-Lamotrigine®; Gen-Lamotrigine; Lamictal®; Novo-Lamotrigine; PMS-Lamotrigine; ratio-Lamotrigine
Mexican Brand Names Lamictal
Generic Available Yes: Chewable tablet
Index Terms BW-430C; LTG
Pharmacologic Category Anticonvulsant, Miscellaneous
Use Adjunctive therapy in the treatment of generalized seizures of Lennox-Gastaut syndrome, primary generalized tonic-clonic seizures, and partial seizures in adults and children ≥2 years of age; conversion to monotherapy in adults with partial seizures who are receiving treatment with valproic acid or a single enzyme-inducing antiepileptic drug (specifically carbamazepine, phenytoin, phenobarbital or primidone); maintenance treatment of bipolar I disorder
Local Anesthetic/Vasoconstrictor Precautions No information available to require special precautions
Effects on Dental Treatment Key adverse event(s) related to dental treatment: Xerostomia (normal salivary flow resumes upon discontinuation).
Common Adverse Effects Percentages reported in adults on monotherapy for epilepsy or bipolar disorder.
>10%: Gastrointestinal: Nausea (7% to 14%)
1% to 10%:
 Cardiovascular: Chest pain (5%), peripheral edema (2% to 5%), edema (1% to 5%)
 Central nervous system: Somnolence (9%), fatigue (8%), dizziness (7%), anxiety (5%), insomnia (5% to 10%), pain (5%), ataxia (2% to 5%), irritability (2% to 5%), suicidal ideation (2% to 5%), agitation (1% to 5%), amnesia (1% to 5%), depression (1% to 5%), dream abnormality (1% to 5%), emotional lability (1% to 5%), fever (1% to 5%), hypoesthesia (1% to 5%), migraine (1% to 5%), thought abnormality (1% to 5%), confusion (1%)
(Continued)

Lamotrigine *(Continued)*

Dermatologic: Rash (nonserious: 7%), dermatitis (2% to 5%), dry skin (2% to 5%)

Endocrine & metabolic: Dysmenorrhea (5%), libido increased (2% to 5%)

Gastrointestinal: Vomiting (5% to 9%), dyspepsia (7%), abdominal pain (6%), xerostomia (2% to 6%), constipation (5%), weight loss (5%), anorexia (2% to 5%), peptic ulcer (2% to 5%), rectal hemorrhage (2% to 5%), flatulence (1% to 5%), weight gain (1% to 5%)

Genitourinary: Urinary frequency (1% to 5%)

Neuromuscular & skeletal: Back pain (8%), coordination abnormal (7%), weakness (2% to 5%), arthralgia (1% to 5%), myalgia (1% to 5%), neck pain (1% to 5%), paresthesia (1%)

Ocular: Nystagmus (2% to 5%), vision abnormal (2% to 5%), amblyopia (1%)

Respiratory: Rhinitis (7%), cough (5%), pharyngitis (5%), bronchitis (2% to 5%), dyspnea (2% to 5%), epistaxis (2% to 5%), sinusitis (1% to 5%)

Miscellaneous: Infection (5%), diaphoresis (2% to 5%), reflexes increased/decreased (2% to 5%), dyspraxia (1% to 5%)

Mechanism of Action A triazine derivative which inhibits release of glutamate (an excitatory amino acid) and inhibits voltage-sensitive sodium channels, which stabilizes neuronal membranes. Lamotrigine has weak inhibitory effect on the 5-HT$_3$ receptor; *in vitro* inhibits dihydrofolate reductase.

Drug Interactions

Increased Effect/Toxicity: Lamotrigine may increase the epoxide metabolite of carbamazepine resulting in toxicity. Valproic acid increases blood levels of lamotrigine. Valproic acid inhibits the clearance of lamotrigine, dosage adjustment required when adding or withdrawing valproic acid; inhibition appears maximal at valproic acid 250-500 mg/day; the incidence of serious rash may be increased by valproic acid. Lamotrigine may enhance the adverse/toxic effect of other CNS depressants.

Decreased Effect: Carbamazepine, oral contraceptives (estrogens), phenytoin, phenobarbital, primidone may decrease concentrations of lamotrigine; dosage adjustments may be needed when adding or withdrawing agent; monitor. Rifampin may reduce serum concentrations and effects of lamotrigine.

Pharmacodynamics/Kinetics

Absorption: Rapid and complete

Distribution: V$_d$: ~1 L/kg

Protein binding: 55%

Metabolism: Hepatic and renal; metabolized by glucuronic acid conjugation to inactive metabolites

Bioavailability: 98%

Half-life elimination: Adults: 25-33 hours

Concomitant valproic acid therapy: 59-70 hours

Concomitant phenytoin or carbamazepine therapy: 13-14 hours

Chronic renal failure: 43 hours

Hemodialysis: 13 hours during dialysis; 57 hours between dialysis

Hepatic impairment: 26-148 hours

Time to peak, plasma: 1-5 hours

Excretion: Urine (94%, ~90% as glucuronide conjugates and ~10% unchanged); feces (2%)

Pregnancy Risk Factor C

Lanacane® [OTC] *see* Benzocaine *on page 195*

Lanacane® Maximum Strength [OTC] *see* Benzocaine *on page 195*

Lanaphilic® [OTC] *see* Urea *on page 1632*

Lanolin, Cetyl Alcohol, Glycerin, Petrolatum, and Mineral Oil

(LAN oh lin, SEE til AL koe hol, GLIS er in, pe troe LAY tum, & MIN er al oyl)

Related Information

Glycerin *on page 789*

U.S. Brand Names Lubriderm® [OTC]; Lubriderm® Fragrance Free [OTC]

Generic Available Yes

Index Terms Mineral Oil, Petrolatum, Lanolin, Cetyl Alcohol, and Glycerin

Pharmacologic Category Topical Skin Product

Use Treatment of dry skin

Local Anesthetic/Vasoconstrictor Precautions No information available to require special precautions

Effects on Dental Treatment No significant effects or complications reported

Common Adverse Effects 1% to 10%: Local irritation

Pregnancy Risk Factor C

Lanoxicaps® *see* Digoxin *on page 497*

Lanoxin® *see* Digoxin *on page 497*

Lansoprazole (lan SOE pra zole)

Related Information
Gastrointestinal Disorders *on page 1745*
Oral Pain *on page 1788*
U.S. Brand Names Prevacid®; Prevacid® SoluTab™
Canadian Brand Names Prevacid®
Mexican Brand Names Ilsatec; Keval; Ogastro; Ulpax
Generic Available No
Pharmacologic Category Proton Pump Inhibitor; Substituted Benzimidazole
Use
Oral: Short-term treatment of active duodenal ulcers; maintenance treatment of healed duodenal ulcers; as part of a multidrug regimen for *H. pylori* eradication to reduce the risk of duodenal ulcer recurrence; short-term treatment of active benign gastric ulcer; treatment of NSAID-associated gastric ulcer; to reduce the risk of NSAID-associated gastric ulcer in patients with a history of gastric ulcer who require an NSAID; short-term treatment of symptomatic GERD; short-term treatment for all grades of erosive esophagitis; to maintain healing of erosive esophagitis; long-term treatment of pathological hypersecretory conditions, including Zollinger-Ellison syndrome

I.V.: Short-term treatment (≤7 days) of erosive esophagitis in adults unable to take oral medications
Unlabeled/Investigational Use Active ulcer bleeding (parenteral formulation)
Local Anesthetic/Vasoconstrictor Precautions No information available to require special precautions
Effects on Dental Treatment No significant effects or complications reported
Common Adverse Effects 1% to 10%:
Central nervous system: Headache (children 1-11 years 3%, 12-17 years 7%)
Gastrointestinal: Abdominal pain (children 12-17 years 5%; adults 2%), constipation (children 1-11 years 5%; adults 1%), diarrhea (60 mg/day 7%), nausea (children 12-17 years 3%; adults 1%)
Local: Injection site reaction (1%)
Dosage
Children 1-11 years: GERD, erosive esophagitis: Oral:
≤30 kg: 15 mg once daily
>30 kg: 30 mg once daily
Note: Doses were increased in some pediatric patients if still symptomatic after 2 or more weeks of treatment (maximum dose: 30 mg twice daily)
Children 12-17 years: Oral:
Nonerosive GERD: 15 mg once daily for up to 8 weeks
Erosive esophagitis: 30 mg once daily for up to 8 weeks
Adults:
Duodenal ulcer: Oral: Short-term treatment: 15 mg once daily for 4 weeks; maintenance therapy: 15 mg once daily
Gastric ulcer: Oral: Short-term treatment: 30 mg once daily for up to 8 weeks
NSAID-associated gastric ulcer (healing): Oral: 30 mg once daily for 8 weeks; controlled studies did not extend past 8 weeks of therapy
NSAID-associated gastric ulcer (to reduce risk): Oral: 15 mg once daily for up to 12 weeks; controlled studies did not extend past 12 weeks of therapy
Symptomatic GERD: Oral: Short-term treatment: 15 mg once daily for up to 8 weeks
Erosive esophagitis:
Oral: Short-term treatment: 30 mg once daily for up to 8 weeks; continued treatment for an additional 8 weeks may be considered for recurrence or for patients who do not heal after the first 8 weeks of therapy; maintenance therapy: 15 mg once daily
I.V.: 30 mg once daily for up to 7 days; patients should be switched to an oral formulation as soon as they can take oral medications
Hypersecretory conditions: Oral: Initial: 60 mg once daily; adjust dose based upon patient response and to reduce acid secretion to <10 mEq/hour (5 mEq/hour in patients with prior gastric surgery); doses of 90 mg twice daily have been used; administer doses >120 mg/day in divided doses
Helicobacter pylori eradication: Oral: Currently accepted recommendations (may differ from product labeling): Dose varies with regimen: 30 mg once daily or 60 mg/day in 2 divided doses; requires combination therapy with antibiotics
Prevention of rebleeding in peptic ulcer bleed (unlabeled use): I.V.: 60 mg, followed by 6 mg/hour infusion for 72 hours
(Continued)

Lansoprazole (Continued)

Elderly: No dosage adjustment is needed in elderly patients with normal hepatic function

Dosage adjustment in renal impairment: No dosage adjustment is needed

Dosing adjustment in hepatic impairment: Dose reduction is necessary for severe hepatic impairment

Mechanism of Action Decreases acid secretion in gastric parietal cells through inhibition of (H+, K+)-ATPase enzyme system, blocking the final step in gastric acid production

Contraindications Hypersensitivity to lansoprazole, substituted benzimidazoles (ie, esomeprazole, omeprazole, pantoprazole, rabeprazole), or any component of the formulation

Warnings/Precautions Relief of symptoms does not preclude the presence of a gastric malignancy. Atrophic gastritis (by biopsy) has been noted with long-term omeprazole therapy; this may also occur with lansoprazole. No reports of enterochromaffin-like (ECL) cell carcinoids, dysplasia, or neoplasia have occurred. Severe liver dysfunction may require dosage reductions. Oral: Safety and efficacy have not been established in children <1 year of age; I.V.: Safety and efficacy have not been established in children.

Drug Interactions

Cytochrome P450 Effect: Substrate of CYP2C9 (minor), 2C19 (major), 3A4 (major); **Inhibits** CYP2C9 (weak), 2C19 (moderate), 2D6 (weak), 3A4 (weak); **Induces** CYP1A2 (weak)

Increased Effect/Toxicity: Lansoprazole may increase the levels/effects of citalopram, diazepam, HMG-CoA reductase inhibitors, methotrexate, methsuximide, phenytoin, propranolol, sertraline, and other CYP2C19 substrates. May enhance the dermatologic adverse effect of imatinib.

Decreased Effect: Proton pump inhibitors may decrease the absorption of atazanavir, indinavir, oral iron salts, itraconazole, and ketoconazole. The levels/effects of lansoprazole may be decreased by aminoglutethimide, carbamazepine, fosphenytoin, nafcillin, nevirapine, phenobarbital, phenytoin, rifamycins, and other CYP2C19 or 3A4 inducers.

Ethanol/Nutrition/Herb Interactions

Ethanol: Avoid ethanol (may cause gastric mucosal irritation).

Food: Lansoprazole serum concentrations may be decreased if taken with food.

Herb/Nutraceutical: Avoid St John's wort (may decrease the levels/effect of lansoprazole).

Dietary Considerations Should be taken before eating; best if taken before breakfast. Prevacid® SoluTab™ contains phenylalanine 2.5 mg per 15 mg tablet; phenylalanine 5.1 mg per 30 mg tablet.

Pharmacodynamics/Kinetics

Duration: >1 day

Absorption: Rapid

Distribution: V_d: 14-18 L

Protein binding: 97%

Metabolism: Hepatic via CYP2C19 and 3A4, and in parietal cells to two active metabolites that are not present in systemic circulation

Bioavailability: 80%; decreased 50% to 70% if given 30 minutes after food

Half-life elimination: 1-2 hours; Elderly: 2-3 hours; Hepatic impairment: ≤7 hours

Time to peak, plasma: 1.7 hours

Excretion: Feces (67%); urine (33%)

Pregnancy Risk Factor B

Dosage Forms

Capsule, delayed release:

Prevacid®: 15 mg, 30 mg

Granules, for oral suspension, delayed release:

Prevacid®: 15 mg/packet (30s), 30 mg/packet (30s)

Injection, powder for reconstitution:

Prevacid®: 30 mg

Tablet, orally disintegrating:

Prevacid® SoluTab™: 15 mg, 30 mg

Lansoprazole, Amoxicillin, and Clarithromycin

(lan SOE pra zole, a moks i SIL in, & kla RITH roe mye sin)

Related Information

Amoxicillin *on page 108*

Clarithromycin *on page 371*

Gastrointestinal Disorders *on page 1745*

Lansoprazole *on page 947*

U.S. Brand Names Prevpac®

Canadian Brand Names Hp-PAC®; Prevpac®

Generic Available No

Index Terms Amoxicillin, Lansoprazole, and Clarithromycin; Clarithromycin, Lansoprazole, and Amoxicillin

Pharmacologic Category Antibiotic, Macrolide Combination; Antibiotic, Penicillin; Gastrointestinal Agent, Miscellaneous

Use Eradication of *H. pylori* to reduce the risk of recurrent duodenal ulcer

Local Anesthetic/Vasoconstrictor Precautions No information available to require special precautions

Effects on Dental Treatment Key adverse event(s) related to dental treatment: Taste perversion.

Common Adverse Effects Note: Frequencies noted refer to experience with combination therapy. Also see individual agents.

3% to 10%:

Central nervous system: Headache (6%)

Gastrointestinal: Diarrhea (7%), taste perversion (5%)

Drug Interactions

Cytochrome P450 Effect:

Lansoprazole: **Substrate** of CYP2C9 (minor), 2C19 (major), 3A4 (major); **Inhibits** CYP2C9 (weak), 2C19 (moderate), 2D6 (weak), 3A4 (weak); **Induces** CYP1A2 (weak)

Clarithromycin: **Substrate** of CYP3A4 (major); **Inhibits** CYP1A2 (weak), 3A4 (strong)

Increased Effect/Toxicity: See individual agents.

Decreased Effect: See individual agents.

Pharmacodynamics/Kinetics See individual agents.

Pregnancy Risk Factor C (clarithromycin)

Lansoprazole and Naproxen (lan SOE pra zole & na PROKS en)

Related Information

Gastrointestinal Disorders *on page 1745*

Lansoprazole *on page 947*

Naproxen *on page 1148*

Oral Pain *on page 1788*

U.S. Brand Names Prevacid® NapraPAC™

Generic Available No

Index Terms NapraPAC™; Naproxen and Lansoprazole

Pharmacologic Category Nonsteroidal Anti-inflammatory Drug (NSAID), Oral; Proton Pump Inhibitor

Use Reduction of the risk of NSAID-associated gastric ulcers in patients with history of gastric ulcer who require an NSAID for the treatment of rheumatoid arthritis, osteoarthritis, and ankylosing spondylitis

Local Anesthetic/Vasoconstrictor Precautions No information available to require special precautions

Effects on Dental Treatment No significant effects or complications reported

Common Adverse Effects See individual agents.

Restrictions An FDA-approved medication guide must be distributed when dispensing an oral outpatient prescription (new or refill) where this medication is to be used without direct supervision of a healthcare provider. Medication guides are available at http://www.fda.gov/cder/Offices/ODS/medication_guides.htm.

Mechanism of Action Lansoprazole is a proton pump inhibitor which decreases acid secretion in gastric parietal cells; naproxen inhibits prostaglandin synthesis by decreasing the activity of the enzyme (cyclooxygenase) which results in decreased formation of prostaglandin precursors.

Drug Interactions

Cytochrome P450 Effect:

Lansoprazole: **Substrate** of CYP2C9 (minor), 2C19 (major), 3A4 (major); **Inhibits** CYP2C9 (weak), 2C19 (moderate), 2D6 (weak), 3A4 (weak); **Induces** CYP1A2 (weak)

Naproxen: **Substrate** (minor) of CYP1A2, 2C9

Increased Effect/Toxicity: See individual agents.

Decreased Effect: See individual agents.

Pharmacodynamics/Kinetics See individual agents.

Pregnancy Risk Factor C (naproxen: D/third trimester)

Lanthanum (LAN tha num)

U.S. Brand Names Fosrenol™
Generic Available No
Index Terms Lanthanum Carbonate
Pharmacologic Category Phosphate Binder
Use Reduction of serum phosphate in patients with stage 5 chronic kidney disease (kidney failure: GFR <15 mL/minute/1.73 m^2 or dialysis)
Local Anesthetic/Vasoconstrictor Precautions No information available to require special precautions
Effects on Dental Treatment No significant effects or complications reported
Common Adverse Effects Reported in short-term (4-6 weeks) trials at frequency > placebo:
>10%:
  Gastrointestinal: Nausea (11%), vomiting (9%), diarrhea (13%), abdominal pain (5%)
  Miscellaneous: Dialysis graft occlusion (8%)
1% to 10%: Endocrine & metabolic: Hypercalcemia was reported in longer-term trials at frequencies ≤4% (less frequently than with alternate therapy)

Note: Additional adverse effects noted in longer-term trials at rates higher than alternate therapy included headache, dialysis graft occlusion, and vomiting.
Mechanism of Action Disassociates in the upper gastrointestinal tract to lanthanum ions (La^{3+}) which bind to dietary phosphate resulting in insoluble lanthanum phosphate complexes and a net decrease in serum phosphate and calcium levels.
Drug Interactions
  Decreased Effect: Lanthanum may bind to some drugs in the gastrointestinal tract and decrease their absorption. It is recommended that compounds known to interact with antacids, especially those with significant clinical consequences (eg, antiarrhythmic and antiseizure medications), not be administered within 2 hours of the administration of lanthanum.
Pharmacodynamics/Kinetics
  Absorption: <0.002%
  Protein binding: 99%
  Metabolism: Not metabolized
  Half-life elimination: Plasma: 53 hours; Bone: 2-3.6 years
  Excretion: Feces primarily; urine <2%
Pregnancy Risk Factor C

Lanthanum Carbonate *see* Lanthanum *on page 950*
Lantus® *see* Insulin Glargine *on page 884*
Lapase *see* Pancreatin *on page 1247*

Lapatinib (la PA ti nib)

U.S. Brand Names Tykerb®
Generic Available No
Index Terms GW572016; Lapatinib Ditosylate; NSC-727989
Pharmacologic Category Antineoplastic Agent, Tyrosine Kinase Inhibitor; Epidermal Growth Factor Receptor (EGFR) Inhibitor
Use Treatment (in combination with capecitabine) of HER-2/neu overexpressing advanced or metastatic breast cancer, in patients who have received prior therapy (with an anthracycline, a taxane, and trastuzumab)
Unlabeled/Investigational Use Treatment of head and neck cancers
Local Anesthetic/Vasoconstrictor Precautions Lapatinib is one of the drugs confirmed to prolong the QT interval and is accepted as having a risk of causing torsade de pointes. The risk of drug-induced torsade de pointes is extremely low when a single QT interval prolonging drug is prescribed. In terms of epinephrine, it is not known what effect vasoconstrictors in the local anesthetic regimen will have in patients with a known history of congenital prolonged QT interval or in patients taking any medication that prolongs the QT interval. Until more information is obtained, it is suggested that the clinician consult with the physician prior to the use of a vasoconstrictor in suspected patients, and that the vasoconstrictor (epinephrine, levonordefrin [Neo-Cobefrin®]) be used with caution.
Effects on Dental Treatment Key adverse event(s) related to dental treatment: Stomatitis.
Common Adverse Effects Percentages reported for combination chemotherapy.
>10%:
  Central nervous system: Fatigue (10% to 18%)

Dermatologic: Palmar-plantar erythrodysesthesia (hand-and-foot syndrome) (53%; grade 3: 12%), rash (28%)

Gastrointestinal: Diarrhea (65%; grade 3: 13%; grade 4: 1%), nausea (44%), vomiting (26%), abdominal pain (15%), mucosal inflammation (15%), stomatitis (14%), dyspepsia (11%)

Hematologic: Anemia (56%; grade 3: <1%), neutropenia (22%; grade 3: 3%; grade 4: <1%), thrombocytopenia (18%; grade 3: <1%)

Hepatic:AST increased (49%; grade 3: 2%; grade 4: <1%), total bilirubin increased (45%; grade 3: 4%), ALT increased (37%; grade 3: 2%)

Neuromuscular and skeletal: Limb pain (12%), back pain (11%)

Respiratory: Dyspnea (12%)

1% to 10%:

Cardiovascular: LVEF decreased (grade 2: 2%; grade 3: <1%)

Central nervous system: Insomnia (10%)

Dermatologic: Dry skin (10%)

Restrictions Lapatinib is available at specialty pharmacies through a restricted-access program, Tykerb® CARES. Information is available at www.tykerbcares.com or 1-866-489-5372.

Mechanism of Action Tyrosine kinase (dual kinase) inhibitor; inhibitor of EGFR (ErbB1) and HER2 (ErbB2) by reversibly binding to tyrosine kinase, blocking phosphorylation and activation of downstream second messengers (Erk1/2 and Akt), regulating cellular proliferation and survival in ErbB- and ErbB2-expressing tumors.;

Drug Interactions

Cytochrome P450 Effect: Substrate of CYP2C8 (minor), 3A4 (major), **Inhibits** CYP2C8, 3A4

Increased Effect/Toxicity: CYP3A4 inhibitors may increase the levels/ effects of lapatinib; example inhibitors include azole antifungals, clarithromycin, diclofenac, doxycycline, erythromycin, imatinib, isoniazid, nefazodone, nicardipine, propofol, protease inhibitors, quinidine, telithromycin, and verapamil. Concurrent use of lapatinib with other drugs which may prolong QT_c interval may increase the risk of potentially-fatal arrhythmias; includes type Ia and type III antiarrhythmic agents, selected quinolones (eg, moxifloxacin), cisapride, dolasetron, palonosetron, thioridazine, and other agents.

Lapatinib may increase levels/effects of CYP2C8 substrates; example substrates include amiodarone, paclitaxel, pioglitazone, repaglinide and rosiglitazone. Lapatinib may increase the levels/effects of CYP3A4 substrates; example substrates include benzodiazepines, calcium channel blockers, cyclosporine, mirtazapine, nateglinide, nefazodone, sildenafil (and other PDE-5 inhibitors), tacrolimus, and venlafaxine. Selected benzodiazepines (midazolam, triazolam), cisapride, ergot alkaloids, selected HMG-CoA reductase inhibitors (lovastatin and simvastatin), and pimozide are generally contraindicated with strong CYP3A4 inhibitors.

Decreased Effect: CYP3A4 inducers may decrease the levels/effects of lapatinib; example inducers include aminoglutethimide, carbamazepine, dexamethasone, nafcillin, nevirapine, phenobarbital, phenytoin, and rifamycins.

Pharmacodynamics/Kinetics

Absorption: Incomplete and variable

Protein binding: >99% to albumin and alpha$_1$-acid glycoprotein

Metabolism: Hepatic; extensive via CYP3A4 and 3A5, and to a lesser extent via CYP2C19 and 2C8 to oxidized metabolites

Half-life elimination: ~24 hours

Time to peak, plasma: ~4 hours

Excretion: Feces (27% as unchanged drug; range 3% to 67%); urine (<2%)

Pregnancy Risk Factor D

Lapatinib Ditosylate *see* Lapatinib *on page 950*

Lariam® *see* Mefloquine *on page 1029*

Laronidase (lair OH ni days)

U.S. Brand Names Aldurazyme®
Canadian Brand Names Aldurazyme®
Generic Available No
Index Terms Recombinant α-L-Iduronidase (Glycosaminoglycan α-L-Iduronohydrolase)
Pharmacologic Category Enzyme
Use Treatment of Hurler and Hurler-Scheie forms of mucopolysaccharidosis I (MPS I); treatment of Scheie form of MPS I in patients with moderate to severe symptoms
Local Anesthetic/Vasoconstrictor Precautions No information available to require special precautions
(Continued)

Laronidase *(Continued)*

Effects on Dental Treatment No significant effects or complications reported

Common Adverse Effects

>10%:

Cardiovascular: Vein disorder (14%)

Dermatologic: Rash (36%)

Local: Infusion reactions [31%; may be severe; includes flushing (23%), fever, and headache; frequency decreased over time during open-label extension period], injection site reaction (18%)

Neuromuscular & skeletal: Hyper-reflexia (14%), paresthesia (14%)

Respiratory: Upper respiratory tract infection (32%)

Miscellaneous: Antibody development to laronidase (91%; significance unknown)

1% to 10%:

Cardiovascular: Chest pain (9%), edema (9%), facial edema (9%), hypotension (9%)

Hematologic: Thrombocytopenia (9%)

Hepatic: Bilirubinemia

Local: Abscess (9%), injection site pain (9%)

Ocular: Corneal opacity (9%)

Mechanism of Action Laronidase is a recombinant (replacement) form of α-L-iduronidase derived from Chinese hamster cells. α-L-iduronidase is an enzyme needed to break down endogenous glycosaminoglycans (GAGs) within lysosomes. A deficiency of α-L-iduronidase leads to an accumulation of GAGs, causing cellular, tissue, and organ dysfunction as seen in MPS I. Improved pulmonary function and walking capacity have been demonstrated with the administration of laronidase to patients with Hurler, Hurler-Scheie, or Scheie (with moderate to severe symptoms) forms of MPS.

Pharmacodynamics/Kinetics

Distribution: V_d: 0.24-0.6 L/kg

Half-life elimination: 1.5-3.6 hours

Excretion: Clearance: 1.7 to 2.7 mL/minute/kg; during the first 12 weeks of therapy the clearance of laronidase increases proportionally to the amount of antibodies a given patient develops against the enzyme. However, with long-term use (≥26 weeks) antibody titers have no effect on laronidase clearance.

Pregnancy Risk Factor B

Lasix® *see Furosemide on page 756*

L-asparaginase *see Asparaginase on page 148*

Lassar's Zinc Paste *see Zinc Oxide on page 1683*

Latanoprost *(la TA noe prost)*

U.S. Brand Names Xalatan®

Canadian Brand Names Xalatan®

Mexican Brand Names Xalatan

Generic Available No

Pharmacologic Category Ophthalmic Agent, Antiglaucoma; Prostaglandin, Ophthalmic

Use Reduction of elevated intraocular pressure in patients with open-angle glaucoma or ocular hypertension

Local Anesthetic/Vasoconstrictor Precautions No information available to require special precautions

Effects on Dental Treatment No significant effects or complications reported

Common Adverse Effects

>10%: Ocular: Blurred vision, burning and stinging, conjunctival hyperemia, foreign body sensation, itching, increased pigmentation of the iris, and punctate epithelial keratopathy

1% to 10%:

Cardiovascular: Chest pain, angina pectoris

Dermatologic: Rash, allergic skin reaction

Neuromuscular & skeletal: Myalgia, arthralgia, back pain

Ocular: Dry eye, excessive tearing, eye pain, lid crusting, lid edema, lid erythema, lid discomfort/pain, photophobia

Respiratory: Upper respiratory tract infection, cold, flu

Dosage Adults: Ophthalmic: 1 drop (1.5 mcg) in the affected eye(s) once daily in the evening; do not exceed the once daily dosage because it has been shown that more frequent administration may decrease the IOP lowering effect

Note: A medication delivery device (Xal-Ease™) is available for use with Xalatan®.

Mechanism of Action Latanoprost is a prostaglandin F_2-alpha analog believed to reduce intraocular pressure by increasing the outflow of the aqueous humor

Contraindications Hypersensitivity to latanoprost or any component of the formulation

Warnings/Precautions Latanoprost may gradually change eye color, increasing the amount of brown pigment in the iris by increasing the number of melanosome in melanocytes. The long-term effects on the melanocytes and the consequences of potential injury to the melanocytes or deposition of pigment granules to other areas of the eye is currently unknown. Patients should be examined regularly, and depending on the clinical situation, treatment may be stopped if increased pigmentation ensues.

There have been reports of bacterial keratitis associated with the use of multiple-dose containers of topical ophthalmic products. Do not administer while wearing contact lenses.

Drug Interactions

Increased Effect/Toxicity:

Combination therapy with bimatoprost may result in higher IOP than either agent alone.

Decreased Effect: Precipitation occurs when eye drops containing thimerosal are mixed with latanoprost. If such drugs are used, administer with an interval of at least 5 minutes between applications. May be used concomitantly with other topical ophthalmic drugs if administration is separated by at least 5 minutes.

Pharmacodynamics/Kinetics

Onset of action: 3-4 hours

Peak effect: Maximum: 8-12 hours

Absorption: Through the cornea where the isopropyl ester prodrug is hydrolyzed by esterases to the biologically active acid. Peak concentration is reached in 2 hours after topical administration in the aqueous humor.

Distribution: V_d: 0.16 L/kg

Metabolism: Primarily hepatic via fatty acid beta-oxidation

Half-life elimination: 17 minutes

Excretion: Urine (as metabolites)

Pregnancy Risk Factor C

Dosage Forms

Solution, ophthalmic:

Xalatan®: 0.005% (2.5 mL)

Leflunomide (le FLOO noh mide)

Related Information

Rheumatoid Arthritis, Osteoarthritis, and Osteoporosis *on page 1759*

U.S. Brand Names Arava®

Canadian Brand Names Apo-Leflunomide®; Arava®; Novo-Leflunomide

Mexican Brand Names Arava

Generic Available Yes

Pharmacologic Category Antirheumatic, Disease Modifying

Use Treatment of active rheumatoid arthritis; indicated to reduce signs and symptoms, and to retard structural damage and improve physical function

Orphan drug: Prevention of acute and chronic rejection in recipients of solid organ transplants

Unlabeled/Investigational Use Treatment of cytomegalovirus (CMV) disease

Local Anesthetic/Vasoconstrictor Precautions No information available to require special precautions

Effects on Dental Treatment Key adverse event(s) related to dental treatment: Xerostomia (normal salivary flow resumes upon discontinuation), stomatitis, oral candidiasis, abnormal taste, tooth disorder, enlarged salivary gland, esophagitis, and gingivitis.

Common Adverse Effects

>10%:

Gastrointestinal: Diarrhea (17%)

Respiratory: Respiratory tract infection (15%)

(Continued)

Leflunomide (Continued)

1% to 10%:

Cardiovascular: Hypertension (10%), chest pain (2%), palpitation, tachycardia, vasculitis, vasodilation, varicose vein, edema (peripheral)

Central nervous system: Headache (7%), dizziness (4%), pain (2%), fever, malaise, migraine, anxiety, depression, insomnia, sleep disorder

Dermatologic: Alopecia (10%), rash (10%), pruritus (4%), dry skin (2%), eczema (2%), acne, dermatitis, hair discoloration, hematoma, nail disorder, subcutaneous nodule, skin disorder/discoloration, skin ulcer, bruising

Endocrine & metabolic: Hypokalemia (1%), diabetes mellitus, hyperglycemia, hyperlipidemia, hyperthyroidism, menstrual disorder

Gastrointestinal: Nausea (9%), abdominal pain (5%), dyspepsia (5%), weight loss (4%), anorexia (3%), gastroenteritis (3%), stomatitis (3%), vomiting (3%), cholelithiasis, colitis, constipation, esophagitis, flatulence, gastritis, gingivitis, melena, candidiasis (oral), enlarged salivary gland, tooth disorder, xerostomia, taste disturbance

Genitourinary: Urinary tract infection (5%), albuminuria, cystitis, dysuria, hematuria, vaginal candidiasis, prostate disorder, urinary frequency

Hematologic: Anemia

Hepatic: Abnormal LFTs (5%)

Neuromuscular & skeletal: Back pain (5%), joint disorder (4%), weakness (3%), tenosynovitis (3%), synovitis (2%), arthralgia (1%), paresthesia (2%), muscle cramps (1%), neck pain, pelvic pain, increased CPK, arthrosis, bursitis, myalgia, bone necrosis, bone pain, tendon rupture, neuralgia, neuritis

Ocular: Blurred vision, cataract, conjunctivitis, eye disorder

Respiratory: Bronchitis (7%), cough (3%), pharyngitis (3%), pneumonia (2%), rhinitis (2%), sinusitis (2%), asthma, dyspnea, epistaxis

Miscellaneous: Infection (4%), accidental injury (5%), allergic reactions (2%), diaphoresis, herpes infection

Mechanism of Action Inhibits pyrimidine synthesis, resulting in antiproliferative and anti-inflammatory effects. For CMV, may interfere with virion assembly.

Drug Interactions

Cytochrome P450 Effect: Inhibits CYP2C9 (weak)

Increased Effect/Toxicity: Leflunomide may increase the risk of hepatotoxicity when combined with drugs which may cause hepatic injury. Concomitant treatment of methotrexate with leflunomide may increase the risk of hepatotoxicity or hematologic toxicity. Rifampin may increase the serum concentration of leflunomide's active metabolite. Leflunomide may increase the effects of warfarin.

Decreased Effect: Bile acid sequestrants (cholestyramine) may interfere with enterohepatic recycling of leflunomide; this is used emergently to remove drug from the circulation, but may decrease levels inadvertently if used concomitantly.

Pharmacodynamics/Kinetics

Distribution: V_d: 0.13 L/kg

Metabolism: Hepatic to A77 1726 (MI) which accounts for nearly all pharmacologic activity; further metabolism to multiple inactive metabolites; undergoes enterohepatic recirculation

Bioavailability: 80%

Half-life elimination: Mean: 14-15 days; enterohepatic recycling appears to contribute to the long half-life of this agent, since activated charcoal and cholestyramine substantially reduce plasma half-life

Time to peak: 6-12 hours

Excretion: Feces (48%); urine (43%)

Pregnancy Risk Factor X

Legatrin PM® [OTC] see Acetaminophen and Diphenhydramine on page 38

Lenalidomide (le na LID oh mide)

U.S. Brand Names Revlimid®

Generic Available No

Index Terms CC-5013; IMiD-3; NSC-703813

Pharmacologic Category Angiogenesis Inhibitor; Antineoplastic Agent; Immunosuppressant Agent; Tumor Necrosis Factor (TNF) Blocking Agent

Use Treatment of myelodysplastic syndrome (MDS) in patients with deletion 5q (del 5q) cytogenetic abnormality; treatment of multiple myeloma

Unlabeled/Investigational Use Treatment of metastatic malignant melanoma; treatment of myelofibrosis

Local Anesthetic/Vasoconstrictor Precautions No information available to require special precautions

Effects on Dental Treatment Key adverse event(s) related to dental treatment: Xerostomia (normal salivary flow resumes upon discontinuation), taste perversion.

Common Adverse Effects

>10%:

Cardiovascular: Peripheral edema (8% to 21%)

Central nervous system: Fatigue (31% to 38%), pyrexia (21% to 23%), dizziness (20% to 21%), headache (20%)

Dermatologic: Pruritus (42%), rash (16% to 36%), dry skin (14%)

Endocrine & metabolic: Hyperglycemia (15%), hypokalemia (11%)

Gastrointestinal: Diarrhea (29% to 49%), constipation (24% to 39%), nausea (22% to 24%), weight loss (18%), dyspepsia (14%), anorexia (10% to 14%), taste perversion (6% to 13%), abdominal pain (8% to 12%)

Genitourinary: Urinary tract infection (11%)

Hematologic: Thrombocytopenia (17% to 62%; grades 3/4: 10% to 50%), neutropenia (28% to 59%; grades 3/4: 21% to 53%), anemia (12% to 24%; grades 3/4: 6% to 9%); myelosuppression is dose-dependent and reversible with treatment interruption and/or dose reduction

Neuromuscular & skeletal: Muscle cramp (18% to 30%), arthralgia (10% to 22%), back pain (15% to 21%), tremor (20%), weakness (15%), paresthesia (12%), limb pain (11%)

Ocular: Blurred vision (15%)

Respiratory: Nasopharyngitis (23%), cough (20%), dyspnea (7% to 20%), pharyngitis (16%), epistaxis (15%), upper respiratory infection (14% to 15%), pneumonia (11% to 12%)

1% to 10%:

Cardiovascular: Edema (10%), deep vein thrombosis (≤8%; grades 3/4: 7%), hypertension (6%), chest pain (5%), palpitation (5%), atrial fibrillation (grades 3/4: 3%), syncope (grade 3: 2%)

Central nervous system: Insomnia (10%), hypoesthesia (7%), pain (7%), depression (5%)

Dermatologic: Bruising (5% to 8%), cellulitis (5%), erythema (5%)

Endocrine & metabolic: Hypothyroidism (7%), hypomagnesemia (6%), hypocalcemia (grades 3/4: 4%)

Gastrointestinal: Vomiting (10%), xerostomia (7%), loose stools (6%)

Genitourinary: Dysuria (7%)

Hematologic: Leukopenia (8%; grade 3: 4%), febrile neutropenia (5%), lymphopenia (grade 3: 2%)

Hepatic: ALT increased (8%)

Neuromuscular & skeletal: Myalgia (9%), rigors (6%), neuropathy (peripheral 5%)

Respiratory: Sinusitis (8%), rhinitis (7%), bronchitis (6%), pulmonary embolism (≤3%; grades 3/4: 3%)

Miscellaneous: Night sweats (8%), diaphoresis increased (7%)

Restrictions Lenalidomide is approved for marketing only under a Food and Drug Administration (FDA) approved, restricted distribution program called RevAssist[SM] (www.REVLIMID.com or 1-888-423-5436). Physicians, pharmacies, and patients must be registered; a maximum 28-day supply may be dispensed; a new prescription is required each time it is filled; pregnancy testing is required for females of childbearing potential.

An FDA-approved medication guide must be distributed when dispensing an outpatient prescription (new or refill) where this medication is to be used without direct supervision of a healthcare provider. Medication guides are available at http://www.fda.gov/cder/Offices/ODS/medication_guides.htm.

Mechanism of Action Immunomodulatory and antiangiogenic characteristics via multiple mechanisms. Selectively inhibits secretion of proinflammatory cytokines (potent inhibitor of tumor necrosis factor-alpha secretion); enhances cell-mediated immunity by stimulating proliferation of anti-CD3 stimulated T cells (resulting in increased IL-2 and interferon gamma secretion); inhibits trophic signals to angiogenic factors in cells. Inhibits the growth of myeloma cells by inducing cell cycle arrest and cell death.

Drug Interactions

Increased Effect/Toxicity: Abatacept and anakinra may increase the risk of serious infection when used in combination with lenalidomide. Lenalidomide may increase the risk of infections associated with vaccines (live organism).

Decreased Effect: Lenalidomide may decrease the effect of vaccines (dead organisms).

Pharmacodynamics/Kinetics

Absorption: Rapid

Protein binding: ~30%

Half-life elimination: ~3 hours

Time to peak, plasma: Healthy volunteers: 0.6-1.5 hours; Myeloma patients: 0.5-4 hours

(Continued)

Lenalidomide *(Continued)*
Excretion: Urine (~67% as unchanged drug)
Pregnancy Risk Factor X

Lepirudin *(leh puh ROO din)*

Related Information
Cardiovascular Diseases *on page 1726*
U.S. Brand Names Refludan®
Canadian Brand Names Refludan®
Generic Available No
Index Terms Lepirudin (rDNA); Recombinant Hirudin
Pharmacologic Category Anticoagulant, Thrombin Inhibitor
Use Indicated for anticoagulation in patients with heparin-induced thrombocytopenia (HIT) and associated thromboembolic disease in order to prevent further thromboembolic complications
Unlabeled/Investigational Use Investigational: Prevention or reduction of ischemic complications associated with unstable angina
Local Anesthetic/Vasoconstrictor Precautions No information available to require special precautions
Effects on Dental Treatment No significant effects or complications reported
Common Adverse Effects As with all anticoagulants, bleeding is the most common adverse event associated with lepirudin. Hemorrhage may occur at virtually any site. Risk is dependent on multiple variables.
HIT patients:
>10%: Hematologic: Anemia (12%), bleeding from puncture sites (11%), hematoma (11%)
1% to 10%:
Cardiovascular: Heart failure (3%), pericardial effusion (1%), ventricular fibrillation (1%)
Central nervous system: Fever (7%)
Dermatologic: Eczema (3%), maculopapular rash (4%)
Gastrointestinal: GI bleeding/rectal bleeding (5%)
Genitourinary: Vaginal bleeding (2%)
Hepatic: Transaminases increased (6%)
Renal: Hematuria (4%)
Respiratory: Epistaxis (4%)
Non-HIT populations (including those receiving thrombolytics and/or contrast media):
1% to 10%: Respiratory: Bronchospasm/stridor/dyspnea/cough
Mechanism of Action Lepirudin is a highly specific direct inhibitor of thrombin; lepirudin is a recombinant hirudin derived from yeast cells
Drug Interactions
Increased Effect/Toxicity: Thrombolytics may enhance anticoagulant properties of lepirudin on aPTT and can increase the risk of bleeding complications. Bleeding risk may also be increased by oral anticoagulants (warfarin) and platelet function inhibitors (NSAIDs, dipyridamole, ticlopidine, clopidogrel, IIb/IIIa antagonists, and aspirin).
Pharmacodynamics/Kinetics
Distribution: Two-compartment model; confined to extracellular fluids.
Metabolism: Via release of amino acids via catabolic hydrolysis of parent drug
Half-life elimination: Initial: ~10 minutes: Terminal: Healthy volunteers: 1.3 hours; Marked renal impairment (Cl_{cr} <15 mL/minute and on hemodialysis): ≤2 days
Excretion: Urine (~48%, 35% as unchanged drug and unchanged drug fragments of parent drug); systemic clearance is proportional to glomerular filtration rate or creatinine clearance
Pregnancy Risk Factor B

Letrozole *(LET roe zole)*

U.S. Brand Names Femara®
Canadian Brand Names Femara®
Mexican Brand Names Femara
Generic Available No

Index Terms CGS-20267; NSC-719345

Pharmacologic Category Antineoplastic Agent, Aromatase Inhibitor

Use Adjuvant treatment of postmenopausal hormone receptor positive early breast cancer; treatment of postmenopausal hormone receptor positive or hormone receptor unknown, locally-advanced, or metastatic breast cancer

Local Anesthetic/Vasoconstrictor Precautions No information available to require special precautions

Effects on Dental Treatment No significant effects or complications reported

Common Adverse Effects

>10%:

Cardiovascular: Edema (7% to 18%)

Central nervous system: Headache (4% to 20%), dizziness (2% to 14%), fatigue (6% to 13%)

Endocrine & metabolic: Hot flashes (5% to 50%), hypercholesterolemia (3% to 16%)

Gastrointestinal: Nausea (9% to 17%), constipation (2% to 11%), weight gain (2% to 11%),

Neuromuscular & skeletal: Weakness (4% to 34%), bone pain (22%), arthralgia (8% to 22%), arthritis (7% to 21%), back pain (5% to 18%)

Respiratory: Dyspnea (6% to 18%), cough (5% to 13%)

Miscellaneous: Diaphoresis (<5% to 24%), night sweats (14%)

2% to 10%:

Cardiovascular: Chest pain (3% to 8%), hypertension (5% to 8%), peripheral edema (5%)

Central nervous system: Insomnia (6% to 7%), pain (5%), somnolence (2% to 3%), depression (<5%), anxiety (<5%), vertigo (<5%)

Dermatologic: Rash (4% to 5%), alopecia (<5%), pruritus (1% to 2%)

Endocrine & metabolic: Breast pain (7%), hypercalcemia (<5%)

Gastrointestinal: Diarrhea (5% to 8%), vomiting (3% to 7%), weight loss (7%), abdominal pain (5% to 6%), anorexia (3% to 5%), dyspepsia (3% to 4%)

Genitourinary: Urinary tract infection (6%), vaginal bleeding (5%), vaginal dryness (5%), vaginal hemorrhage (5%), vaginal irritation (4%)

Hepatic: Transaminases increased (<1% to 3%)

Neuromuscular & skeletal: Limb pain (10%), myalgia (6% to 7%), bone fractures (<5% to 6%), bone mineral density decreased/osteoporosis (2% to 7%)

Renal: Renal disorder (5%)

Respiratory: Pleural effusion (<5%)

Miscellaneous: Infection (7%), flu (6%), viral infection (5% to 6%)

Mechanism of Action Nonsteroidal competitive inhibitor of the aromatase enzyme system which binds to the heme group of aromatase, a cytochrome P450 enzyme which catalyzes conversion of androgens to estrogens (specifically, androstenedione to estrone and testosterone to estradiol). This leads to inhibition of the enzyme and a significant reduction in plasma estrogen levels. Does not affect synthesis of adrenal or thyroid hormones, aldosterone, or androgens.

Drug Interactions

Cytochrome P450 Effect: Substrate (minor) of CYP2A6, 3A4; **Inhibits** CYP2A6 (strong), 2C19 (weak)

Increased Effect/Toxicity: Letrozole may increase the levels/effects of CYP2A6 substrates; example substrates include dexmedetomidine and ifosfamide.

Decreased Effect: Tamoxifen may decrease serum concentrations of letrozole.

Pharmacodynamics/Kinetics

Absorption: Rapid and well absorbed; not affected by food

Distribution: V_d: ~1.9 L/kg

Protein binding, plasma: Weak

Metabolism: Hepatic via CYP3A4 and 2A6 to an inactive carbinol metabolite

Half-life elimination: Terminal: ~2 days

Time to steady state, plasma: 2-6 weeks

Excretion: Urine (90%; 6% as unchanged drug, 75% as glucuronide carbinol metabolite, 9% as unidentified metabolites)

Pregnancy Risk Factor D

Leucovorin (loo koe VOR in)

Generic Available Yes

Index Terms Calcium Leucovorin; Citrovorum Factor; Folinic Acid; 5-Formyl Tetrahydrofolate; Leucovorin Calcium

(Continued)

Leucovorin (Continued)

Pharmacologic Category Antidote; Vitamin, Water Soluble

Use Antidote for folic acid antagonists (methotrexate, trimethoprim, pyrimethamine); treatment of megaloblastic anemias when folate is deficient as in infancy, sprue, pregnancy, and nutritional deficiency when oral folate therapy is not possible; in combination with fluorouracil in the treatment of colon cancer

Local Anesthetic/Vasoconstrictor Precautions No information available to require special precautions

Effects on Dental Treatment No significant effects or complications reported

Common Adverse Effects Frequency not defined.
Dermatologic: Rash, pruritus, erythema, urticaria
Hematologic: Thrombocytosis
Respiratory: Wheezing
Miscellaneous: Anaphylactoid reactions

Mechanism of Action A reduced form of folic acid, leucovorin supplies the necessary cofactor blocked by methotrexate, enters the cells via the same active transport system as methotrexate. Stabilizes the binding of 5-dUMP and thymidylate synthetase, enhancing the activity of fluorouracil.

Drug Interactions
Decreased Effect: May decrease efficacy of co-trimoxazole against *Pneumocystis carinii* pneumonitis

Pharmacodynamics/Kinetics
Onset of action: Oral: ~30 minutes; I.V.: ~5 minutes
Absorption: Oral, I.M.: Rapid and well absorbed
Metabolism: Intestinal mucosa and hepatically to 5-methyl-tetrahydrofolate (5MTHF; active)
Bioavailability: 31% following 200 mg dose; 98% following doses ≤25 mg
Half-life elimination: Leucovorin: 15 minutes; 5MTHF: 33-35 minutes
Excretion: Urine (80% to 90%); feces (5% to 8%)

Pregnancy Risk Factor C

Leucovorin Calcium *see* Leucovorin *on page 957*

Leukeran® *see* Chlorambucil *on page 329*

Leukine® *see* Sargramostim *on page 1456*

Leuprolide (loo PROE lide)

U.S. Brand Names Eligard®; Lupron®; Lupron Depot®; Lupron Depot-Ped®; Viadur®

Canadian Brand Names Eligard®; Lupron®; Lupron® Depot®; Viadur®

Mexican Brand Names Lucrin; Lucrin Depot

Generic Available Yes: Injection (solution)

Index Terms Abbott-43818; Leuprolide Acetate; Leuprorelin Acetate; NSC-377526; TAP-144

Pharmacologic Category Gonadotropin Releasing Hormone Agonist

Use Palliative treatment of advanced prostate carcinoma; management of endometriosis; treatment of anemia caused by uterine leiomyomata (fibroids); central precocious puberty

Unlabeled/Investigational Use Treatment of breast, ovarian, and endometrial cancer; infertility; prostatic hyperplasia

Local Anesthetic/Vasoconstrictor Precautions No information available to require special precautions

Effects on Dental Treatment Key adverse event(s) related to dental treatment: Gum hemorrhage, gingivitis, dry mucous membranes, and dysphagia

Common Adverse Effects
Children: 2% to 10%:
Central nervous system: Pain (2%)
Dermatologic: Acne (2%), rash (2% including erythema multiforme), seborrhea (2%)
Genitourinary: Vaginitis (2%), vaginal bleeding (2%), vaginal discharge (2%)
Local: Injection site reaction (5%)

Adults (frequency dependent upon formulation and indication):
Cardiovascular: Angina, atrial fibrillation, CHF, deep vein thrombosis, edema, hot flashes, hypertension, MI, peripheral edema, syncope, tachycardia
Central nervous system: Abnormal thinking, agitation, amnesia, anxiety, chills, confusion, convulsion, dementia, depression, dizziness, fatigue, fever, headache, insomnia, malaise, pain, vertigo
Dermatologic: Alopecia, bruising, burning, cellulitis, pruritus
Endocrine & metabolic: Bone density decreased, breast enlargement, breast tenderness, dehydration, hirsutism, hyperglycemia, hyperlipidemia, hyperphosphatemia, libido decreased, menstrual disorders, potassium decreased

Gastrointestinal: Anorexia, appetite increased, constipation, diarrhea, dry mucous membranes, dysphagia, eructation, GI hemorrhage, gingivitis, gum hemorrhage, intestinal obstruction, nausea, peptic ulcer, vomiting, weight gain/loss

Genitourinary: Balanitis, impotence, nocturia, penile shrinkage, testicular atrophy; urinary disorder (eg, urgency, incontinence, retention); UTI, vaginitis

Hematologic: Anemia, platelets decreased, PT prolonged, WBC increased

Hepatic: Hepatomegaly, liver function tests abnormal

Local: Abscess, injection site reaction

Neuromuscular & skeletal: Arthritis, bone pain, leg cramps, myalgia, paresthesia, tremor, weakness

Renal: BUN increased

Respiratory: Allergic reaction, dyspnea, emphysema, hemoptysis, hypoxia, lung edema, pulmonary embolism

Miscellaneous: Body odor, diaphoresis, flu-like syndrome, neoplasm, night sweats, voice alteration

Mechanism of Action Potent inhibitor of gonadotropin secretion; continuous daily administration results in suppression of ovarian and testicular steroidogenesis due to decreased levels of LH and FSH with subsequent decrease in testosterone (male) and estrogen (female) levels. Leuprolide may also have a direct inhibitory effect on the testes, and act by a different mechanism not directly related to reduction in serum testosterone.

Pharmacodynamics/Kinetics

Onset of action: Following transient increase, testosterone suppression occurs in ~2-4 weeks of continued therapy

Distribution: Males: V_d: 27 L

Protein binding: 43% to 49%

Metabolism: Major metabolite, pentapeptide (M-1)

Bioavailability: Oral: None; SubQ: 94%

Half-life elimination: I.V.: 3 hours

Excretion: Urine (<5% as parent and major metabolite)

Pregnancy Risk Factor X

Leuprolide Acetate *see* Leuprolide *on page 958*

Leuprorelin Acetate *see* Leuprolide *on page 958*

Leurocristine Sulfate *see* VinCRIStine *on page 1659*

Leustatin® *see* Cladribine *on page 371*

Levalbuterol (leve al BYOO ter ole)

U.S. Brand Names Xopenex®; Xopenex HFA™

Canadian Brand Names Xopenex®

Generic Available No

Index Terms Levalbuterol Hydrochloride; Levalbuterol Tartrate; R-albuterol

Pharmacologic Category Beta$_2$-Adrenergic Agonist

Use Treatment or prevention of bronchospasm in children and adults with reversible obstructive airway disease

Local Anesthetic/Vasoconstrictor Precautions No information available to require special precautions

Effects on Dental Treatment No significant effects or complications reported

Common Adverse Effects

>10%:

Endocrine & metabolic: Serum glucose increased, serum potassium decreased

Respiratory: Viral infection (7% to 12%), rhinitis (3% to 11%)

>2% to 10%:

Central nervous system: Nervousness (3% to 10%), tremor (≤7%), anxiety (≤3%), dizziness (1% to 3%), migraine (≤3%), pain (1% to 3%)

Cardiovascular: Tachycardia (~3%)

Gastrointestinal: Dyspepsia (1% to 3%)

Neuromuscular & skeletal: Leg cramps (≤3%)

Respiratory: Asthma (9%), pharyngitis (8%), cough (1% to 4%), nasal edema (1% to 3%), sinusitis (1% to 4%)

Miscellaneous: Flu-like syndrome (1% to 4%), accidental injury (≤3%)

Mechanism of Action Relaxes bronchial smooth muscle by action on beta$_2$-receptors with little effect on heart rate

Drug Interactions

Increased Effect/Toxicity: May add to effects of medications which deplete potassium (eg, loop or thiazide diuretics). Cardiac effects of levalbuterol may be potentiated in patients receiving MAO inhibitors, tricyclic antidepressants, sympathomimetics (eg, amphetamine, dobutamine), or inhaled anesthetics (eg, enflurane).

(Continued)

Levalbuterol *(Continued)*

Decreased Effect: Beta-blockers (particularly nonselective agents) block the effect of levalbuterol. Digoxin levels may be decreased.

Pharmacodynamics/Kinetics

Onset of action:

Aerosol: 5.5-10.2 minutes

Peak effect: ~77 minutes

Nebulization: 10-17 minutes (measured as a 15% increase in FEV_1)

Peak effect: 1.5 hours

Duration:

Aerosol: 3-4 hours (up to 6 hours in some patients)

Nebulization: 5-6 hours (up to 8 hours in some patients)

Absorption: A portion of inhaled dose is absorbed to systemic circulation

Half-life elimination: 3.3-4 hours

Time to peak, serum:

Aerosol: 0.5 hours

Nebulization: 0.2 hours

Pregnancy Risk Factor C

Levetiracetam *(lee va tye RA se tam)*

U.S. Brand Names Keppra®

Canadian Brand Names CO Levetiracetam; Keppra®

Mexican Brand Names Keppra

Generic Available No

Pharmacologic Category Anticonvulsant, Miscellaneous

Use Adjunctive therapy in the treatment of partial onset, myoclonic, and/or primary generalized tonic-clonic seizures

Unlabeled/Investigational Use Bipolar disorder

Local Anesthetic/Vasoconstrictor Precautions No information available to require special precautions

Effects on Dental Treatment No significant effects or complications reported

Common Adverse Effects

>10%:

Central nervous system: Behavioral symptoms (agitation, aggression, anger, anxiety, apathy, depersonalization, depression, emotional lability, hostility, hyperkinesias, irritability, nervousness, neurosis and personality disorder: adults 5% to 13%; children 5% to 38%), somnolence (12% to 23%), headache (14%), hostility (2% to 12%)

Gastrointestinal: Vomiting (15%), anorexia (3% to 13%)

Neuromuscular & skeletal: Weakness (9% to 15%)

Respiratory: Pharyngitis (6% to 14%), rhinitis (4% to 13%), cough (2% to 11%)

Miscellaneous: Accidental injury (17%), infection (2% to 13%)

1% to 10%:

Cardiovascular: Facial edema (2%)

Central nervous system: Fatigue (10%), nervousness (4% to 10%), dizziness (7% to 9%), personality disorder (8%), pain (6% to 7%), agitation (6%), irritability (6%), emotional lability (2% to 6%), mood swings (5%), depression (3% to 5%), vertigo (3% to 5%), ataxia (3%), amnesia (2%), anxiety (2%), confusion (2%)

Dermatologic: Bruising (4%), pruritus (2%), rash (2%), skin discoloration (2%)

Endocrine & metabolic: Dehydration (2%)

Gastrointestinal: Diarrhea (8%), gastroenteritis (4%), constipation (3%)

Genitourinary: Urine abnormality (2%)

Hematologic: Leukocytes decreased (2% to 3%)

Neuromuscular & skeletal: Neck pain (2% to 8%), paresthesia (2%), reflexes increased (2%)

Ocular: Conjunctivitis (3%), diplopia (2%), amblyopia (2%)

Otic: Ear pain (2%)

Renal: Albuminuria (4%)
Respiratory: Influenza (5%), asthma (2%), sinusitis (2%)
Miscellaneous: Flu-like syndrome (3%), viral infection (2%)

Mechanism of Action The precise mechanism by which levetiracetam exerts its antiepileptic effect is unknown. However, several studies have suggested the mechanism may involve one or more of the following central pharmacologic effects: inhibition of voltage-dependent N-type calcium channels; facilitation of GABA-ergic inhibitory transmission through displacement of negative modulators; reduction of delayed rectifier potassium current; and/or binding to synaptic proteins which modulate neurotransmitter release.

Drug Interactions
Increased Effect/Toxicity: CNS depressants may enhance the adverse/ toxic effect of levetiracetam.

Pharmacodynamics/Kinetics
Absorption: Oral: Rapid and complete
Distribution: V_d: Similar to total body water
Protein binding: <10%
Metabolism: Not extensive; primarily by enzymatic hydrolysis; forms metabolites (inactive)
Bioavailability: 100%
Half-life elimination: 6-8 hours
Time to peak, plasma: Oral: 1 hour
Excretion: Urine (66% as unchanged drug)

Pregnancy Risk Factor C

Levitra® *see* Vardenafil *on page 1647*

Levlen® *see* Ethinyl Estradiol and Levonorgestrel *on page 633*

Levlite™ *see* Ethinyl Estradiol and Levonorgestrel *on page 633*

Levobunolol (lee voe BYOO noe lole)

U.S. Brand Names Betagan®
Canadian Brand Names Apo-Levobunolol®; Betagan®; Novo-Levobunolol; Optho-Bunolol®; PMS-Levobunolol; Sandoz-Levobunolol
Mexican Brand Names Betagan
Generic Available Yes
Index Terms *l*-Bunolol Hydrochloride; Levobunolol Hydrochloride
Pharmacologic Category Beta-Adrenergic Blocker, Nonselective; Ophthalmic Agent, Antiglaucoma
Use To lower intraocular pressure in chronic open-angle glaucoma or ocular hypertension
Local Anesthetic/Vasoconstrictor Precautions No information available to require special precautions
Effects on Dental Treatment Key adverse event(s) related to dental treatment: Levobunolol is a nonselective beta-blocker and may enhance the pressor response to epinephrine, resulting in hypertension and bradycardia. Many nonsteroidal anti-inflammatory drugs, such as ibuprofen and indomethacin, can reduce the hypotensive effect of beta-blockers after 3 or more weeks of therapy with the NSAID. Short-term NSAID use (ie, 3 days) requires no special precautions in patients taking beta-blockers.
Mechanism of Action A nonselective beta-adrenergic blocking agent that lowers intraocular pressure by reducing aqueous humor production and possibly increases the outflow of aqueous humor
Pregnancy Risk Factor C

Levobunolol Hydrochloride *see* Levobunolol *on page 961*

Levobupivacaine (LEE voe byoo PIV a kane)

Related Information
Oral Pain *on page 1788*
U.S. Brand Names Chirocaine® [DSC]
Canadian Brand Names Chirocaine®
Mexican Brand Names Quirocaine
Generic Available No
Pharmacologic Category Local Anesthetic
Use Production of local or regional anesthesia for surgery and obstetrics, and for postoperative pain management
Local Anesthetic/Vasoconstrictor Precautions No information available to require special precautions
Effects on Dental Treatment No significant effects or complications reported
(Continued)

Levobupivacaine *(Continued)*

Common Adverse Effects

>10%:

Cardiovascular: Hypotension (20% to 31%)

Central nervous system: Pain (postoperative) (7% to 18%), fever (7% to 17%)

Gastrointestinal: Nausea (12% to 21%), vomiting (8% to 14%)

Hematologic: Anemia (10% to 12%)

1% to 10%:

Cardiovascular: Abnormal ECG (3%), bradycardia (2%), tachycardia (2%), hypertension (1%)

Central nervous system: Pain (4% to 8%), headache (5% to 7%), dizziness (5% to 6%), hypoesthesia (3%), somnolence (1%), anxiety (1%), hypothermia (2%)

Dermatologic: Pruritus (4% to 9%), purpura (1%)

Endocrine & metabolic: Breast pain - female (1%)

Gastrointestinal: Constipation (3% to 7%), enlarged abdomen (3%), flatulence (2%), abdominal pain (2%), dyspepsia (2%), diarrhea (1%)

Genitourinary: Urinary incontinence (1%), urine flow decreased (1%), urinary tract infection (1%)

Hematologic: Leukocytosis (1%)

Local: Anesthesia (1%)

Neuromuscular & skeletal: Back pain (6%), rigors (3%), paresthesia (2%)

Ocular: Diplopia (3%)

Renal: Albuminuria (3%), hematuria (2%)

Respiratory: Cough (1%)

Miscellaneous: Fetal distress (5% to 10%), delayed delivery (6%), hemorrhage in pregnancy (2%), uterine abnormality (2%), increased wound drainage (1%)

Mechanism of Action Levobupivacaine is the S-enantiomer of bupivacaine. It blocks both the initiation and transmission of nerve impulses by decreasing the neuronal membrane's permeability to sodium ions, which results in inhibition of depolarization with resultant blockade of conduction. Local anesthetics reversibly prevent generation and conduction of electrical impulses in neurons by decreasing the transient increase in permeability to sodium. The differential sensitivity generally depends on the size of the fiber; small fibers are more sensitive than larger fibers and require a longer period for recovery. Sensory pain fibers are usually blocked first, followed by fibers that transmit sensations of temperature, touch, and deep pressure. High concentrations block sympathetic somatic sensory and somatic motor fibers. The spread of anesthesia depends upon the distribution of the solution. This is primarily dependent on the site of administration and volume of drug injected.

Drug Interactions

Cytochrome P450 Effect: Substrate (minor) of CYP1A2, 3A4

Pharmacodynamics/Kinetics

Onset of action: Epidural: 10-14 minutes

Duration (dose dependent): 1-8 hours

Absorption: Dependent on route of administration and dose

Distribution: 67 L

Protein binding, plasma: >97%

Metabolism: Extensively hepatic via CYP3A4 and CYP1A2

Half-life elimination: 1.3 hours

Time to peak: Epidural: 30 minutes

Excretion: Urine (71%) and feces (24%) as metabolites

Pregnancy Risk Factor B

Levocabastine *(LEE voe kab as teen)*

U.S. Brand Names Livostin® [DSC]

Canadian Brand Names Livostin®

Mexican Brand Names Livostin

Generic Available No

Index Terms Levocabastine Hydrochloride

Pharmacologic Category Antihistamine, H₁ Blocker, Ophthalmic

Use Treatment of allergic conjunctivitis

Local Anesthetic/Vasoconstrictor Precautions No information available to require special precautions

Effects on Dental Treatment Key adverse event(s) related to dental treatment: Xerostomia (normal salivary flow resumes upon discontinuation).

Mechanism of Action Potent, selective histamine H₁-receptor antagonist for topical ophthalmic use

Pregnancy Risk Factor C

Levocabastine Hydrochloride *see* Levocabastine *on page 962*

Levocarnitine (lee voe KAR ni teen)

U.S. Brand Names Carnitor®; Carnitor® SF
Canadian Brand Names Carnitor®
Mexican Brand Names Cardispan
Generic Available Yes
Index Terms L-Carnitine
Pharmacologic Category Dietary Supplement
Use

Oral: Primary systemic carnitine deficiency; acute and chronic treatment of patients with an inborn error of metabolism which results in secondary carnitine deficiency

I.V.: Acute and chronic treatment of patients with an inborn error of metabolism which results in secondary carnitine deficiency; prevention and treatment of carnitine deficiency in patients with end-stage renal disease (ESRD) who are undergoing hemodialysis.

Local Anesthetic/Vasoconstrictor Precautions No information available to require special precautions

Effects on Dental Treatment Key adverse event(s) related to dental treatment: Taste perversion.

Common Adverse Effects Frequencies noted with I.V. therapy (hemodialysis patients).

>10%:

Cardiovascular: Hypertension (18% to 21%), chest pain (6% to 15%)

Central nervous system: Headache (3% to 37%), dizziness (10% to 18%), fever (5% to 12%)

Endocrine & metabolic: Hypercalcemia (6% to 15%)

Gastrointestinal: Diarrhea (9% to 35%), vomiting (9% to 21%), abdominal pain (5% to 21%), nausea (9% to 12%)

Hematologic: Anemia (3% to 12%)

Neuromuscular & skeletal: Weakness (8% to 12%), paresthesia (3% to 12%)

Respiratory: Cough (10% to 18%), rhinitis (6% to 11%)

Miscellaneous: Infection (10% to 24%)

1% to 10%:

Cardiovascular: Tachycardia (5% to 9%), hemorrhage (2% to 9%), palpitation (3% to 8%), peripheral edema (3% to 6%), atrial fibrillation (2% to 6%), ECG abnormality (2% to 6%), vascular disorder (2% to 6%)

Central nervous system: Depression (5% to 6%), vertigo (2% to 6%)

Dermatologic: Rash (3% to 5%)

Endocrine & metabolic: Parathyroid disorder (2% to 6%)

Gastrointestinal: Taste perversion (2% to 9%), weight loss (3% to 8%), anorexia (3% to 6%), gastrointestinal disorder (2% to 6%), melena (2% to 6%), weight gain (2% to 6%)

Ocular: Amblyopia (3% to 6%), eye disorder (3% to 6%)

Respiratory: Bronchitis (3% to 5%)

Miscellaneous: Allergic reaction (2% to 6%)

Frequency not defined: Body odor, gastritis, seizure

Mechanism of Action Carnitine is a naturally occurring metabolic compound which functions as a carrier molecule for long-chain fatty acids within the mitochondria, facilitating energy production. Carnitine deficiency is associated with accumulation of excess acyl CoA esters and disruption of intermediary metabolism. Carnitine supplementation increases carnitine plasma concentrations. The effects on specific metabolic alterations have not been evaluated. ESRD patients on maintenance HD may have low plasma carnitine levels because of reduced intake of meat and dairy products, reduced renal synthesis, and dialytic losses. Certain clinical conditions (malaise, muscle weakness, cardiomyopathy and arrhythmias) in HD patients may be related to carnitine deficiency.

Pharmacodynamics/Kinetics

Metabolism: Hepatic (limited with moderate renal impairment), to trimethylamine (TMA) and trimethylamine N-oxide (TMAO)

Bioavailability: Oral: ~10% to 20%

Half-life elimination: 17.4 hours

Time to peak: Oral: 3.3 hours

Excretion: Urine (76%, 4% to 9% as unchanged drug); feces (<1%)

Pregnancy Risk Factor B

Levodopa and Carbidopa (lee voe DOE pa & kar bi DOE pa)

Related Information
Carbidopa *on page 280*

U.S. Brand Names Parcopa™; Sinemet®; Sinemet® CR

Canadian Brand Names Apo-Levocarb®; Apo-Levocarb® CR; Endo®-Levodopa/Carbidopa; Novo-Levocarbidopa; Nu-Levocarb; Sinemet®; Sinemet® CR

Mexican Brand Names Racovel; Sinemet

Generic Available Yes: Excludes orally-disintegrating tablet

Index Terms Carbidopa and Levodopa

Pharmacologic Category Anti-Parkinson's Agent, Dopamine Agonist

Use Idiopathic Parkinson's disease; postencephalitic parkinsonism; symptomatic parkinsonism

Unlabeled/Investigational Use Restless leg syndrome

Local Anesthetic/Vasoconstrictor Precautions No information available to require special precautions

Effects on Dental Treatment Key adverse event(s) related to dental treatment: Xerostomia (normal salivary flow resumes upon discontinuation) and taste alterations. Dopaminergic therapy in Parkinson's disease (ie, treatment with levodopa and carbidopa combination) is associated with orthostatic hypotension. Patients medicated with this drug combination should be carefully assisted from the chair and observed for signs of orthostatic hypotension.

Common Adverse Effects Frequency not defined.

Cardiovascular: Orthostatic hypotension, arrhythmia, chest pain, hypertension, syncope, palpitation, phlebitis

Central nervous system: Dizziness, anxiety, confusion, nightmares, headache, hallucinations, on-off phenomenon, decreased mental acuity, memory impairment, disorientation, delusions, euphoria, agitation, somnolence, insomnia, gait abnormalities, nervousness, ataxia, EPS, falling, psychosis, peripheral neuropathy, seizure (causal relationship not established)

Dermatologic: Rash, alopecia, malignant melanoma, hypersensitivity (angioedema, urticaria, pruritus, bullous lesions, Henoch-Schönlein purpura)

Endocrine & metabolic: Increased libido

Gastrointestinal: Anorexia, nausea, vomiting, constipation, GI bleeding, duodenal ulcer, diarrhea, dyspepsia, taste alterations, sialorrhea, heartburn

Genitourinary: Discoloration of urine, urinary frequency

Hematologic: Hemolytic anemia, agranulocytosis, thrombocytopenia, leukopenia; decreased hemoglobin and hematocrit; abnormalities in AST and ALT, LDH, bilirubin, BUN, Coombs' test

Neuromuscular & skeletal: Choreiform and involuntary movements, paresthesia, bone pain, shoulder pain, muscle cramps, weakness

Ocular: Blepharospasm, oculogyric crises (may be associated with acute dystonic reactions)

Renal: Difficult urination

Respiratory: Dyspnea, cough

Miscellaneous: Hiccups, discoloration of sweat, diaphoresis (increased)

Mechanism of Action Parkinson's symptoms are due to a lack of striatal dopamine; levodopa circulates in the plasma to the blood-brain-barrier (BBB), where it crosses, to be converted by striatal enzymes to dopamine; carbidopa inhibits the peripheral plasma breakdown of levodopa by inhibiting its decarboxylation, and thereby increases available levodopa at the BBB

Drug Interactions

Increased Effect/Toxicity: Concurrent use of levodopa with nonselective MAO inhibitors may result in hypertensive reactions via an increased storage and release of dopamine, norepinephrine, or both. Use with carbidopa to minimize reactions if combination is necessary; otherwise avoid combination.

Decreased Effect: Antipsychotics, benzodiazepines, L-methionine, phenytoin, pyridoxine, spiramycin, and tacrine may inhibit the antiparkinsonian effects of levodopa; monitor for reduced effect. Antipsychotics may inhibit the antiparkinsonian effects of levodopa via dopamine receptor blockade. Use antipsychotics with low dopamine blockade (clozapine, olanzapine, quetiapine). High-protein diets may inhibit levodopa's efficacy; avoid high protein foods. Iron binds levodopa and reduces its bioavailability; separate doses of iron and levodopa.

Pharmacodynamics/Kinetics

Duration: Variable, 6-12 hours; longer with sustained release forms
See individual agents.

Pregnancy Risk Factor C

Levodopa, Carbidopa, and Entacapone
(lee voe DOE pa, kar bi DOE pa, & en TA ka pone)

Related Information
Carbidopa *on page 280*
Entacapone *on page 569*
U.S. Brand Names Stalevo™
Generic Available No
Index Terms Carbidopa, Levodopa, and Entacapone; Entacapone, Carbidopa, and Levodopa
Pharmacologic Category Anti-Parkinson's Agent, COMT Inhibitor; Anti-Parkinson's Agent, Dopamine Agonist
Use Treatment of idiopathic Parkinson's disease
Local Anesthetic/Vasoconstrictor Precautions No information available to require special precautions
Effects on Dental Treatment No significant effects or complications reported
Common Adverse Effects See individual agents.
Mechanism of Action
Levodopa: The metabolic precursor of dopamine, a chemical depleted in Parkinson's disease. Levodopa is able to circulate in the plasma and cross the blood-brain-barrier (BBB), where it is converted by striatal enzymes to dopamine.
Carbidopa: Inhibits the peripheral plasma breakdown of levodopa by inhibiting its decarboxylation; increases available levodopa at the BBB
Entacapone: A reversible and selective inhibitor of catechol-O-methyltransferase (COMT). Alters the pharmacokinetics of levodopa, resulting in more sustained levodopa serum levels and increased concentrations available for absorption across the BBB.
Pharmacodynamics/Kinetics See individual agents.
Pregnancy Risk Factor C

Levo-Dromoran® *see* Levorphanol *on page 969*

Levofloxacin (lee voe FLOKS a sin)

Related Information
Sexually-Transmitted Diseases *on page 1766*
Tuberculosis Treatment *on page 1909*
Related Sample Prescriptions
Bacterial Infections and Periodontal Diseases *on page 1837*
U.S. Brand Names Iquix®; Levaquin®; Quixin™
Canadian Brand Names Levaquin®; Novo-Levofloxacin
Mexican Brand Names Elequine; Tavanic
Generic Available No
Pharmacologic Category Antibiotic, Quinolone
Use
Systemic: Treatment of mild, moderate, or severe infections caused by susceptible organisms. Includes the treatment of community-acquired pneumonia, including multidrug resistant strains of *S. pneumoniae* (MDRSP); nosocomial pneumonia; chronic bronchitis (acute bacterial exacerbation); acute bacterial sinusitis; urinary tract infection (uncomplicated or complicated), including acute pyelonephritis caused by *E. coli*; prostatitis (chronic bacterial); skin or skin structure infections (uncomplicated or complicated); reduce incidence or disease progression of inhalational anthrax (postexposure)
Ophthalmic: Treatment of bacterial conjunctivitis caused by susceptible organisms (Quixin™ 0.5% ophthalmic solution); treatment of corneal ulcer caused by susceptible organisms (Iquix® 1.5% ophthalmic solution)
Unlabeled/Investigational Use Diverticulitis, enterocolitis (*Shigella* spp.), epididymitis (non-gonococcal), gonococcal infections, Legionnaires' disease, peritonitis, PID
Note: As of April 2007, the CDC no longer recommends the use of fluoroquinolones for the treatment of gonococcal disease.
Local Anesthetic/Vasoconstrictor Precautions Levofloxacin is one of the drugs confirmed to prolong the QT interval and is accepted as having a risk of causing torsade de pointes. The risk of drug-induced torsade de pointes is extremely low when a single QT interval prolonging drug is prescribed. In terms of epinephrine, it is not known what effect vasoconstrictors in the local anesthetic regimen will have in patients with a known history of congenital prolonged QT interval or in patients taking any medication that prolongs the QT interval. Until more information is obtained, it is suggested that the clinician consult with the physician prior to the use of a vasoconstrictor in suspected patients, and
(Continued)

Levofloxacin *(Continued)*

that the vasoconstrictor (epinephrine, levonordefrin [Neo-Cobefrin®]) be used with caution.

Effects on Dental Treatment No significant effects or complications reported

Common Adverse Effects 1% to 10%:

Cardiovascular: Chest pain (1%)

Central nervous system: Headache (6%), insomnia (5%), dizziness (2%), fatigue (1%), pain (1%), fever

Dermatologic: Pruritus (1%), rash (1%)

Gastrointestinal: Nausea (7%), diarrhea (5%), abdominal pain (3%), constipation (3%), dyspepsia (2%), vomiting (2%), flatulence (1%)

Genitourinary: Vaginitis (1%)

Hematologic: Lymphopenia (2%)

Ocular (with ophthalmic solution use): Decreased vision (transient), foreign body sensation, transient ocular burning, ocular pain or discomfort, photophobia

Respiratory: Pharyngitis (4%), dyspnea (1%), rhinitis (1%), sinusitis (1%)

Dosage Note: Sequential therapy (intravenous to oral) may be instituted based on prescriber's discretion.

Usual dosage range:

Children ≥1 year: Ophthalmic: 1-2 drops every 2-6 hours

Adults:

Ophthalmic: 1-2 drops every 2-6 hours

Oral, I.V.: 250-500 mg every 24 hours; severe or complicated infections: 750 mg every 24 hours

Indication-specific dosing:

Children ≥1 year and Adults: Ophthalmic:

Conjunctivitis (0.5% ophthalmic solution):

Treatment day 1 and day 2: Instill 1-2 drops into affected eye(s) every 2 hours while awake, up to 8 times/day

Treatment day 3 through day 7: Instill 1-2 drops into affected eye(s) every 4 hours while awake, up to 4 times/day

Children ≥6 years and Adults: Ophthalmic:

Corneal ulceration (1.5% ophthalmic solution): Treatment day 1 through day 3: Instill 1-2 drops into affected eye(s) every 30 minutes to 2 hours while awake and 4-6 hours after retiring.

Adults: Oral, I.V.:

Anthrax (inhalational): 500 mg every 24 hours for 60 days, beginning as soon as possible after exposure

Chronic bronchitis (acute bacterial exacerbation): 500 mg every 24 hours for at least 7 days

Diverticulitis, peritonitis (unlabeled use): 750 mg every 24 hours for 7-10 days; use adjunctive metronidazole therapy

Dysenteric enterocolitis, *Shigella* spp. (unlabeled use): 500 mg every 24 hours for 3-5 days

Epididymitis, nongonococcal (unlabeled use): 500 mg once daily for 10 days

Gonococcal infection (unlabeled use):

Cervicitis, urethritis: 250 mg for one dose with azithromycin or doxycycline; **Note:** As of April 2007, the CDC no longer recommends the use of fluoroquinolones for the treatment of uncomplicated gonococcal disease.

Disseminated infection: 250 mg I.V. once daily; 24 hours after symptoms improve may change to 500 mg orally every 24 hours to complete total therapy of 7 days; **Note:** As of April 2007, the CDC no longer recommends the use of fluoroquinolones for the treatment of more serious gonococcal disease, unless no other options exist and susceptibility can be confirmed via culture.

Pelvic inflammatory disease (unlabeled use): 500 mg once daily for 14 days with or without adjunctive metronidazole; **Note:** The CDC recommends use only if standard cephalosporin therapy is not feasible and community prevalence of quinolone-resistant gonococcal organisms is low. Culture sensitivity must be confirmed.

Pneumonia:

Community-acquired: 500 mg every 24 hours for 7-14 days or 750 mg every 24 hours for 5 days (efficacy of 5-day regimen for MDRSP not established)

Nosocomial: 750 mg every 24 hours for 7-14 days

Prostatitis (chronic bacterial): 500 mg every 24 hours for 28 days

Sinusitis (acute bacterial): 500 mg every 24 hours for 10-14 days or 750 mg every 24 hours for 5 days

Skin and skin structure infections:

Uncomplicated: 500 mg every 24 hours for 7-10 days

Complicated: 750 mg every 24 hours for 7-14 days
Traveler's diarrhea (unlabeled use): 500 mg for one dose
Urinary tract infections:
Uncomplicated: 250 mg once daily for 3 days
Complicated, including pyelonephritis: 250 mg once daily for 10 days

Dosing adjustment in renal impairment:
Chronic bronchitis, acute bacterial sinusitis, uncomplicated skin infection, community-acquired pneumonia, chronic bacterial prostatitis, or inhalational anthrax: Initial: 500 mg, then as follows:
Cl_{cr} 20-49 mL/minute: 250 mg every 24 hours
Cl_{cr} 10-19 mL/minute: 250 mg every 48 hours
Hemodialysis/CAPD: 250 mg every 48 hours
Uncomplicated UTI: No dosage adjustment required
Complicated UTI, acute pyelonephritis: Cl_{cr} 10-19 mL/minute: 250 mg every 48 hours
Complicated skin infection, acute bacterial sinusitis, community-acquired pneumonia, or nosocomial pneumonia: Initial: 750 mg, then as follows:
Cl_{cr} 20-49 mL/minute: 750 mg every 48 hours
Cl_{cr} 10-19 mL/minute: 500 mg every 48 hours
Hemodialysis/CAPD: 500 mg every 48 hours

Mechanism of Action As the S (-) enantiomer of the fluoroquinolone, ofloxacin, levofloxacin, inhibits DNA-gyrase in susceptible organisms thereby inhibits relaxation of supercoiled DNA and promotes breakage of DNA strands. DNA gyrase (topoisomerase II), is an essential bacterial enzyme that maintains the superhelical structure of DNA and is required for DNA replication and transcription, DNA repair, recombination, and transposition.

Contraindications Hypersensitivity to levofloxacin, any component of the formulation, or other quinolones

Warnings/Precautions
Systemic: Not recommended in children <18 years of age; CNS stimulation may occur (tremor, restlessness, confusion, and very rarely hallucinations or seizures). Potential for seizures, although very rare, may be increased with concomitant NSAID therapy. Use with caution in individuals at risk of seizures, with known or suspected CNS disorders or renal dysfunction; use caution to avoid possible photosensitivity reactions during and for several days following fluoroquinolone therapy
Rare cases of torsade de pointes have been reported in patients receiving levofloxacin. Use caution in patients with known prolongation of QT interval, bradycardia, hypokalemia, hypomagnesemia, or in those receiving concurrent therapy with Class Ia or Class III antiarrhythmics.
Severe hypersensitivity reactions, including anaphylaxis, have occurred with quinolone therapy. If an allergic reaction occurs (itching, urticaria, dyspnea or facial edema, loss of consciousness, tingling, cardiovascular collapse), discontinue drug immediately. Prolonged use may result in fungal or bacterial superinfection, including *C. difficile*-associated diarrhea and pseudomembranous colitis. Tendon inflammation and/or rupture has been reported; risk may be increased with concurrent corticosteroids, particularly in the elderly. Discontinue at first sign of tendon inflammation or pain. Peripheral neuropathies have been linked to levofloxacin use; discontinue if numbness, tingling, or weakness develops. Quinolones may exacerbate myasthenia gravis.
Ophthalmic solution: For topical use only. Do not inject subconjunctivally or introduce into anterior chamber of the eye. Contact lenses should not be worn during treatment for bacterial conjunctivitis. Safety and efficacy in children <1 year of age (Quixin™) or <6 years of age (Iquix®) have not been established. **Note:** Indications for ophthalmic solutions are product concentration-specific and should not be used interchangeably.

Drug Interactions
Increased Effect/Toxicity: Levofloxacin may increase the effects/toxicity of glyburide and warfarin. Concomitant use with corticosteroids may increase the risk of tendon rupture. Concomitant use with other QT_c-prolonging agents (eg, Class Ia and Class III antiarrhythmics, erythromycin, cisapride, antipsychotics, and cyclic antidepressants) may result in arrhythmias, such as torsade de pointes. Probenecid may increase levofloxacin levels. Concomitant use with NSAIDs may rarely increase risk of seizure.
Decreased Effect: Concurrent administration of metal cations, including most antacids, oral electrolyte supplements, quinapril, sucralfate, some didanosine formulations (pediatric powder for oral suspension), and other highly-buffered oral drugs, may decrease quinolone levels; separate doses.

Dietary Considerations Tablets may be taken without regard to meals. Oral solution should be administered on an empty stomach (1 hour before or 2 hours after a meal).

Pharmacodynamics/Kinetics
Absorption: Rapid and complete
(Continued)

Levofloxacin *(Continued)*

Distribution: V_d: 1.25 L/kg; CSF concentrations ~15% of serum levels; high concentrations are achieved in prostate, lung, and gynecological tissues, sinus, saliva

Protein binding: 50%

Metabolism: Minimally hepatic

Bioavailability: 99%

Half-life elimination: 6-8 hours

Time to peak, serum: 1-2 hours

Excretion: Primarily urine (as unchanged drug)

Pregnancy Risk Factor C

Dosage Forms

Infusion [premixed in D_5W]:
Levaquin®: 250 mg (50 mL); 500 mg (100 mL); 750 mg (150 mL)

Injection, solution [preservative free]:
Levaquin®: 25 mg/mL (20 mL, 30 mL)

Solution, ophthalmic:
Iquix®: 1.5% (5 mL)
Quixin™: 0.5% (5 mL)

Solution, oral:
Levaquin®: 25 mg/mL

Tablet:
Levaquin®: 250 mg, 500 mg, 750 mg
Levaquin® Leva-Pak: 750 mg (5s)

Levomepromazine *see* Methotrimeprazine *on page 1073*

Levonordefrin and Mepivacaine Hydrochloride *see* Mepivacaine and Levonordefrin *on page 1045*

Levonorgestrel *(LEE voe nor jes trel)*

Related Information
Endocrine Disorders and Pregnancy *on page 1750*

U.S. Brand Names Mirena®; Plan B® [RX/OTC]

Canadian Brand Names Mirena®; Norplant® Implant; Plan B™

Mexican Brand Names Postinor-2

Generic Available No

Index Terms LNg 20

Pharmacologic Category Contraceptive; Progestin

Use Prevention of pregnancy

Local Anesthetic/Vasoconstrictor Precautions No information available to require special precautions

Effects on Dental Treatment No significant effects or complications reported

Common Adverse Effects

Intrauterine system:

>5%:

Cardiovascular: Hypertension

Central nervous system: Headache, depression, nervousness

Dermatologic: Acne, skin disorder

Endocrine & metabolic: Breast pain, dysmenorrhea, decreased libido, abnormal Pap smear, amenorrhea (20% at 1 year), enlarged follicles (12%)

Gastrointestinal: Abdominal pain, nausea, weight gain

Genitourinary: Leukorrhea, vaginitis

Neuromuscular & skeletal: Back pain

Respiratory: Upper respiratory tract infection, sinusitis

<3% and postmarketing reports: Alopecia, anemia, cervicitis, dyspareunia, eczema, failed insertion, migraine, sepsis, vomiting

Oral tablets:

>10%:

Central nervous system: Fatigue (17%), headache (17%), dizziness (11%)

Endocrine & metabolic: Heavier menstrual bleeding (14%), lighter menstrual bleeding (12%), breast tenderness (11%)

Gastrointestinal: Nausea (23%), abdominal pain (18%)

1% to 10%: Gastrointestinal: Vomiting (6%), diarrhea (5%)

Restrictions Plan B® is approved for OTC use by women ≥18 years of age and available by prescription only for women ≤17 years of age. Sales of Plan B® will be limited to pharmacies or healthcare clinics with a valid license to distribute prescription products. Because there will be one package for both OTC and prescription use, pharmacies are required to keep the product behind the counter.

Mechanism of Action Pregnancy may be prevented through several mechanisms: Thickening of cervical mucus, which inhibits sperm passage through the uterus and sperm survival; inhibition of ovulation, from a negative feedback mechanism on the hypothalamus, leading to reduced secretion of follicle stimulating hormone (FSH) and luteinizing hormone (LH); inhibition of implantation. Levonorgestrel is not effective once the implantation process has begun.

Drug Interactions

Cytochrome P450 Effect: Substrate of CYP3A4 (major)

Decreased Effect: CYP3A4 inducers may decrease the levels/effects of levonorgestrel; example inducers include aminoglutethimide, carbamazepine, nafcillin, nevirapine, phenobarbital, phenytoin, and rifamycins.

Pharmacodynamics/Kinetics

Duration: Intrauterine system: Up to 5 years

Absorption: Oral: Rapid and complete

Protein binding: Highly bound to albumin (~50%) and sex hormone-binding globulin (~47%)

Metabolism: To inactive metabolites

Half-life elimination: Oral: ~24 hours

Excretion: Primarily urine

Pregnancy Risk Factor X

Levonorgestrel and Ethinyl Estradiol *see* Ethinyl Estradiol and Levonorgestrel *on page 633*

Levophed® *see* Norepinephrine *on page 1186*

Levora® *see* Ethinyl Estradiol and Levonorgestrel *on page 633*

Levorphanol (lee VOR fa nole)

U.S. Brand Names Levo-Dromoran®

Generic Available Yes: Tablet

Index Terms Levorphanol Tartrate; Levorphan Tartrate

Pharmacologic Category Analgesic, Opioid

Use Relief of moderate to severe pain; also used parenterally for preoperative sedation and an adjunct to nitrous oxide/oxygen anesthesia

Local Anesthetic/Vasoconstrictor Precautions No information available to require special precautions

Effects on Dental Treatment Key adverse event(s) related to dental treatment: Xerostomia (normal salivary flow resumes upon discontinuation).

Common Adverse Effects Frequency not defined.

Cardiovascular: Palpitation, hypotension, bradycardia, peripheral vasodilation, cardiac arrest, shock, tachycardia

Central nervous system: CNS depression, fatigue, drowsiness, dizziness, nervousness, headache, restlessness, anorexia, malaise, confusion, coma, convulsion, insomnia, amnesia, mental depression, hallucinations, paradoxical CNS stimulation, intracranial pressure (increased)

Dermatologic: Pruritus, urticaria, rash

Endocrine & metabolic: Antidiuretic hormone release

Gastrointestinal: Nausea, vomiting, dyspepsia, stomach cramps, xerostomia, constipation, abdominal pain, dry mouth, biliary tract spasm, paralytic ileus

Genitourinary: Decreased urination, urinary tract spasm, urinary retention

Local: Pain at injection site

Neuromuscular & skeletal: Weakness

Ocular: Miosis, diplopia

Respiratory: Respiratory depression, apnea, hypoventilation, cyanosis

Miscellaneous: Histamine release, physical and psychological dependence

Restrictions C-II

Mechanism of Action Levorphanol tartrate is a synthetic opioid agonist that is classified as a morphinan derivative. Opioids interact with stereospecific opioid receptors in various parts of the central nervous system and other tissues. Analgesic potency parallels the affinity for these binding sites. These drugs do not alter the threshold or responsiveness to pain, but the perception of pain.

Drug Interactions

Increased Effect/Toxicity: CNS depression is enhanced with coadministration of other CNS depressants.

Pharmacodynamics/Kinetics

Onset of action: Oral: 10-60 minutes

Duration: 4-8 hours

Metabolism: Hepatic

Half-life elimination: 11-16 hours

Excretion: Urine (as inactive metabolite)

Pregnancy Risk Factor B/D (prolonged use or high doses at term)

Levorphanol Tartrate *see* Levorphanol *on page 969*

Levorphan Tartrate *see* Levorphanol *on page 969*

Levothroid® *see* Levothyroxine *on page 970*

Levothyroxine (lee voe thye ROKS een)

Related Information
Endocrine Disorders and Pregnancy *on page 1750*

U.S. Brand Names Levothroid®; Levoxyl®; Synthroid®; Unithroid®

Canadian Brand Names Eltroxin®; Gen-Levothyroxine; Levothyroxine Sodium; Synthroid®

Mexican Brand Names Eutirox; Tiroidine

Generic Available Yes

Index Terms Levothyroxine Sodium; *L*-Thyroxine Sodium; T_4

Pharmacologic Category Thyroid Product

Use Replacement or supplemental therapy in hypothyroidism; pituitary TSH suppression

Local Anesthetic/Vasoconstrictor Precautions No precautions with vasoconstrictor are necessary if patient is well controlled with levothyroxine

Effects on Dental Treatment No significant effects or complications reported

Common Adverse Effects Frequency not defined.

Cardiovascular: Angina, arrhythmia, blood pressure increased, cardiac arrest, flushing, heart failure, MI, palpitation, pulse increased, tachycardia

Central nervous system: Anxiety, emotional lability, fatigue, fever, headache, hyperactivity, insomnia, irritability, nervousness, pseudotumor cerebri (children), seizure (rare)

Dermatologic: Alopecia

Endocrine & metabolic: Fertility impaired, menstrual irregularities

Gastrointestinal: Abdominal cramps, appetite increased, diarrhea, vomiting, weight loss

Hepatic: Liver function tests increased

Neuromuscular & skeletal: Bone mineral density decreased, muscle weakness, tremor, slipped capital femoral epiphysis (children)

Respiratory: Dyspnea

Miscellaneous: Diaphoresis, heat intolerance, hypersensitivity (to inactive ingredients, symptoms include urticaria, pruritus, rash, flushing, angioedema, GI symptoms, fever, arthralgia, serum sickness, wheezing)

Levoxyl®: Choking, dysphagia, gagging

Dosage Doses should be adjusted based on clinical response and laboratory parameters.

Oral:

Children: Hypothyroidism:

Newborns: Initial: 10-15 mcg/kg/day. Lower doses of 25 mcg/day should be considered in newborns at risk for cardiac failure. Newborns with T_4 levels <5 mcg/dL should be started at 50 mcg/day. Adjust dose at 4- to 6-week intervals.

Infants and Children: Dose based on body weight and age as listed below. Children with severe or chronic hypothyroidism should be started at 25 mcg/day; adjust dose by 25 mcg every 2-4 weeks. In older children, hyperactivity may be decreased by starting with ¼ of the recommended dose and increasing by ¼ dose each week until the full replacement dose is reached. Refer to adult dosing once growth and puberty are complete.

0-3 months: 10-15 mcg/kg/day

3-6 months: 8-10 mcg/kg/day

6-12 months: 6-8 mcg/kg/day

1-5 years: 5-6 mcg/kg/day

6-12 years: 4-5 mcg/kg/day

>12 years: 2-3 mcg/kg/day

Adults:

Hypothyroidism: 1.7 mcg/kg/day in otherwise healthy adults <50 years old, children in whom growth and puberty are complete, and older adults who have been recently treated for hyperthyroidism or who have been hypothyroid for only a few months. Titrate dose every 6 weeks. Average starting dose ~100 mcg; usual doses are ≤200 mcg/day; doses ≥300 mcg/day are rare (consider poor compliance, malabsorption, and/or drug interactions). **Note:** For patients >50 years or patients with cardiac disease, refer to Elderly dosing.

Severe hypothyroidism: Initial: 12.5-25 mcg/day; adjust dose by 25 mcg/day every 2-4 weeks as appropriate; **Note:** Oral agents are not recommended for myxedema (see I.V. dosing).

Subclinical hypothyroidism (if treated): 1 mcg/kg/day

TSH suppression:

Well-differentiated thyroid cancer: Highly individualized; Doses >2 mcg/kg/day may be needed to suppress TSH to <0.1 mU/L.

Benign nodules and nontoxic multinodular goiter: Goal TSH suppression: 0.1-0.3 mU/L

Elderly: Hypothyroidism:
> >50 years without cardiac disease **or** <50 years with cardiac disease: Initial: 25-50 mcg/day; adjust dose at 6- to 8-week intervals as needed
> >50 years with cardiac disease: Initial: 12.5-25 mcg/day; adjust dose by 12.5-25 mcg increments at 4- to 6-week intervals. (**Note:** Many clinicians prefer to adjust at 6- to 8-week intervals.)

Note: Elderly patients may require <1 mcg/kg/day

I.M., I.V.: Children, Adults, Elderly: Hypothyroidism: 50% of the oral dose
I.V.:
> Adults: Myxedema coma or stupor: 200-500 mcg, then 100-300 mcg the next day if necessary; smaller doses should be considered in patients with cardiovascular disease
>
> Elderly: Myxedema coma: Refer to adult dosing; lower doses may be needed

Mechanism of Action Exact mechanism of action is unknown; however, it is believed the thyroid hormone exerts its many metabolic effects through control of DNA transcription and protein synthesis; involved in normal metabolism, growth, and development; promotes gluconeogenesis, increases utilization and mobilization of glycogen stores, and stimulates protein synthesis, increases basal metabolic rate

Contraindications Hypersensitivity to levothyroxine sodium or any component of the formulation; recent MI or thyrotoxicosis; uncorrected adrenal insufficiency

Warnings/Precautions [U.S. Boxed Warning]: Ineffective and potentially toxic for weight reduction. High doses may produce serious or even life-threatening toxic effects particularly when used with some anorectic drugs. Use with caution and reduce dosage in patients with angina pectoris or other cardiovascular disease; use cautiously in elderly since they may be more likely to have compromised cardiovascular functions. Patients with adrenal insufficiency, myxedema, diabetes mellitus and insipidus may have symptoms exaggerated or aggravated. Chronic hypothyroidism predisposes patients to coronary artery disease. Levoxyl® may rapidly swell and disintegrate causing choking or gagging (should be administered with a full glass of water); use caution in patients with dysphagia or other swallowing disorders.

Drug Interactions
  Increased Effect/Toxicity: Levothyroxine may potentiate the hypoprothrombinemic effect of warfarin (and other oral anticoagulants). Tricyclic antidepressants (TCAs) coadministered with levothyroxine may increase potential for toxicity of both drugs. Coadministration with ketamine may lead to hypertension and tachycardia.

  Decreased Effect: Some medications may decrease absorption of levothyroxine: Cholestyramine, colestipol (separate administration by at least 2 hours); aluminum- and magnesium-containing antacids, iron preparations, sucralfate, Kayexalate® (separate administration by at least 4 hours). Enzyme inducers (phenytoin, phenobarbital, carbamazepine, and rifampin/rifabutin) may decrease levothyroxine levels. Levothyroxine may decrease effect of oral sulfonylureas. Serum levels of digoxin and theophylline may be altered by thyroid function. Estrogens may decrease serum free-thyroxine concentrations. Imatinib may decrease the effects of thyroid replacement therapy.

Ethanol/Nutrition/Herb Interactions Food: Taking levothyroxine with enteral nutrition may cause reduced bioavailability and may lower serum thyroxine levels leading to signs or symptoms of hypothyroidism. Soybean flour (infant formula), cottonseed meal, walnuts, and dietary fiber may decrease absorption of levothyroxine from the GI tract.

Dietary Considerations Should be taken on an empty stomach, at least 30 minutes before food.

Pharmacodynamics/Kinetics
Onset of action: Therapeutic: Oral: 3-5 days; I.V. 6-8 hours
  Peak effect: I.V.: ~24 hours
Absorption: Oral: Erratic (40% to 80%); decreases with age
Protein binding: >99%
Metabolism: Hepatic to triiodothyronine (active)
Time to peak, serum: 2-4 hours
Half-life elimination: Euthyroid: 6-7 days; Hypothyroid: 9-10 days; Hyperthyroid: 3-4 days
Excretion: Urine and feces; decreases with age

Pregnancy Risk Factor A

Dosage Forms
  Injection, powder for reconstitution: 0.2 mg, 0.5 mg
  Tablet: 25 mcg, 50 mcg, 75 mcg, 88 mcg, 100 mcg, 112 mcg, 125 mcg, 150 mcg, 175 mcg, 200 mcg, 300 mcg
    Levothroid®: 25 mcg, 50 mcg, 75 mcg, 88 mcg, 100 mcg, 112 mcg, 125 mcg, 150 mcg, 175 mcg, 200 mcg, 300 mcg
    Levoxyl®: 25 mcg, 50 mcg, 75 mcg, 88 mcg, 100 mcg, 112 mcg, 125 mcg, 137 mcg, 150 mcg, 175 mcg, 200 mcg
(Continued)

Levothyroxine (Continued)

Synthroid®: 25 mcg, 50 mcg, 75 mcg, 88 mcg, 100 mcg, 112 mcg, 125 mcg, 137 mcg, 150 mcg, 175 mcg, 200 mcg, 300 mcg

Unithroid®: 25 mcg, 50 mcg, 75 mcg, 88 mcg, 100 mcg, 112 mcg, 125 mcg, 150 mcg, 175 mcg, 200 mcg, 300 mcg

---

Lidocaine (LYE doe kane)

Related Information
Cardiovascular Diseases *on page 1726*
Management of Patients Undergoing Cancer Therapy *on page 1826*
Oral Pain *on page 1788*
Viral Infections *on page 1806*

U.S. Brand Names Anestacon®; Band-Aid® Hurt-Free™ Antiseptic Wash [OTC]; Burnamycin [OTC]; Burn Jel [OTC]; Burn-O-Jel [OTC]; LidaMantle®; Lidoderm®; L-M-X™ 4 [OTC]; L-M-X™ 5 [OTC]; LTA® 360; Premjact® [OTC]; Solarcaine® Aloe Extra Burn Relief [OTC]; Topicaine® [OTC]; Xylocaine®; Xylocaine® MPF; Xylocaine® Viscous; Zilactin-L® [OTC]

Canadian Brand Names Betacaine®; Lidodan™; Lidoderm®; Xylocaine®; Xylocard®; Zilactin®

Mexican Brand Names Xylocaina Ointment; Xylocaina Spray

Generic Available Yes: Cream, infusion, injection, jelly, lotion, ointment, solution

Index Terms Lidocaine Hydrochloride; Lignocaine Hydrochloride

Pharmacologic Category Analgesic, Topical; Antiarrhythmic Agent, Class Ib; Local Anesthetic

Dental Use Amide-type injectable local anesthetic and topical local anesthetic; Patch: Production of mild topical anesthesia of accessible mucous membranes of the mouth prior to superficial dental procedures

Use Local anesthetic and acute treatment of ventricular arrhythmias from myocardial infarction, or cardiac manipulation
Rectal: Temporary relief of pain and itching due to anorectal disorders
Topical: Local anesthetic for use in laser, cosmetic, and outpatient surgeries; minor burns, cuts, and abrasions of the skin
Lidoderm® Patch: Relief of allodynia (painful hypersensitivity) and chronic pain in postherpetic neuralgia

Unlabeled/Investigational Use ACLS guidelines (not considered drug of choice): Stable monomorphic VT (preserved ventricular function), polymorphic VT (preserved ventricular function), drug-induced monomorphic VT

Local Anesthetic/Vasoconstrictor Precautions No information available to require special precautions

Effects on Dental Treatment Key adverse event(s) related to dental treatment: Metallic taste.

Significant Adverse Effects Effects vary with route of administration. Many effects are dose related.

Frequency not defined.

Cardiovascular: Arrhythmia, bradycardia, arterial spasms, cardiovascular collapse, defibrillator threshold increased, edema, flushing, heart block, hypotension, sinus node supression, vascular insufficiency (periarticular injections)

Central nervous system: Agitation, anxiety, apprehension, coma, confusion, disorientation, dizziness, drowsiness, euphoria, hallucinations, headache, hyperesthesia, hypoesthesia, lethargy, lightheadedness, nervousness, psychosis, seizure, slurred speech, somnolence, unconsciousness

Dermatologic: Angioedema, bruising (transdermal system), contact dermatitis, depigmentation (transdermal system), edema of the skin, itching, petechia (transdermal system), pruritus, rash, urticaria

Gastrointestinal: Metallic taste, nausea, vomiting

Local: Irritation (transdermal system), thrombophlebitis

Neuromuscular & skeletal: Pain exacerbation (transdermal system), paresthesia, transient radicular pain (subarachnoid administration; up to 1.9%), tremor, twitching, weakness

Ocular: Diplopia, visual changes

Otic: Tinnitus

Respiratory: Bronchospasm, dyspnea, respiratory depression or arrest

Miscellaneous: Allergic reactions, anaphylactoid reaction, sensitivity to temperature extremes

Following spinal anesthesia positional headache (3%), shivering (2%) nausea, peripheral nerve symptoms, respiratory inadequacy and double vision (<1%), hypotension, cauda equina syndrome

Postmarketing and/or case reports: ARDS (inhalation), asystole, disorientation, methemoglobinemia, skin reaction

Dental Usual Dosing Anesthesia, topical:

Cold sores and fever blisters: Children ≥5 years and Adults: Liquid: Apply to affected area every 6 hours as needed

Postherpetic neuralgia: Adults: Patch: Apply patch to most painful area. Up to 3 patches may be applied in a single application. Patch may remain in place for up to 12 hours in any 24-hour period.

Dosage

Antiarrhythmic:

Children:

I.V., I.O.: **Note:** For use in pulseless VT or VF, give after defibrillation, CPR, and epinephrine:

Loading dose: 1 mg/kg (maximum 100 mg); follow with continuous infusion; may administer second bolus of 0.5-1 mg/kg if delay between bolus and start of infusion is >15 minutes

Continuous infusion: 20-50 mcg/kg/minute. Use 20 mcg/kg/minute in patients with shock, hepatic disease, cardiac arrest, mild CHF; moderate-to-severe CHF may require $1/2$ loading dose and lower infusion rates to avoid toxicity.

E.T. (loading dose only): 2-10 times the I.V. bolus dose; dilute with NS to a volume of 3-5 mL and follow with several positive-pressure ventilations

Adults:

Ventricular fibrillation or pulseless ventricular tachycardia (after defibrillation, CPR, and vasopressor administration): I.V.: Initial: 1-1.5 mg/kg. Refractory ventricular tachycardia or ventricular fibrillation, a repeat 0.5-0.75 mg/kg bolus may be given every 5-10 minutes after initial dose for a maximum of 3 doses. Total dose should not exceed 3 mg/kg. Follow with continuous infusion (1-4 mg/minute) after return of perfusion. Reappearance of arrhythmia during constant infusion: 0.5 mg/kg bolus and reassessment of infusion.

E.T. (loading dose only): 2-2.5 times the recommended I.V. dose; dilute in 10 mL NS or distilled water. **Note:** Absorption is greater with distilled water, but causes more adverse effects on PaO_2.

Hemodynamically stable VT: 0.5-0.75 mg/kg followed by synchronized cardioversion

Note: Decrease dose in patients with CHF, shock, or hepatic disease.

Anesthesia, topical:

Cream:

LidaMantle®: Skin irritation: Children and Adults: Apply to affected area 2-3 times/day as needed

L-M-X™ 4: Children ≥2 years and Adults: Apply $1/4$ inch thick layer to intact skin. Leave on until adequate anesthetic effect is obtained. Remove cream and cleanse area before beginning procedure.

(Continued)

Lidocaine *(Continued)*

L-M-X™ 5: Relief of anorectal pain and itching: Children ≥12 years and Adults: Rectal: Apply topically to clean, dry area **or** using applicator, insert rectally, up to 6 times/day

Gel, ointment, solution: Adults: Apply to affected area ≤3 times/day as needed (maximum dose: 4.5 mg/kg, not to exceed 300 mg)

Jelly:

Children ≥10 years: Dose varies with age and weight (maximum dose: 4.5 mg/kg)

Adults (maximum dose: 30 mL [600 mg] in any 12-hour period):

Anesthesia of male urethra: 5-30 mL

Anesthesia of female urethra: 3-5 mL

Lubrication of endotracheal tube: Apply a moderate amount to external surface only

Liquid: Cold sores and fever blisters: Children ≥5 years and Adults: Apply to affected area every 6 hours as needed

Patch: Postherpetic neuralgia: Adults: Apply patch to most painful area. Up to 3 patches may be applied in a single application. Patch may remain in place for up to 12 hours in any 24-hour period.

Anesthetic, local injectable: Children and Adults: Varies with procedure, degree of anesthesia needed, vascularity of tissue, duration of anesthesia required, and physical condition of patient; maximum: 4.5 mg/kg/dose; do not repeat within 2 hours.

Dosage adjustment in renal impairment: Not dialyzable (0% to 5%) by hemo- or peritoneal dialysis; supplemental dose is not necessary.

Dosage adjustment in hepatic impairment: Reduce dose in acute hepatitis and decompensated cirrhosis by 50%.

Mechanism of Action Class Ib antiarrhythmic; suppresses automaticity of conduction tissue, by increasing electrical stimulation threshold of ventricle, His-Purkinje system, and spontaneous depolarization of the ventricles during diastole by a direct action on the tissues; blocks both the initiation and conduction of nerve impulses by decreasing the neuronal membrane's permeability to sodium ions, which results in inhibition of depolarization with resultant blockade of conduction

Contraindications Hypersensitivity to lidocaine or any component of the formulation; hypersensitivity to another local anesthetic of the amide type; Adam-Stokes syndrome; severe degrees of SA, AV, or intraventricular heart block (except in patients with a functioning artificial pacemaker); premixed injection may contain corn-derived dextrose and its use is contraindicated in patients with allergy to corn-related products

Warnings/Precautions

Intravenous: Constant ECG monitoring is necessary during I.V. administration. Use cautiously in hepatic impairment, any degree of heart block, Wolff-Parkinson-White syndrome, CHF, marked hypoxia, severe respiratory depression, hypovolemia, history of malignant hyperthermia, or shock. Increased ventricular rate may be seen when administered to a patient with atrial fibrillation. Correct electrolyte disturbances, especially hypokalemia or hypomagnesemia, prior to use and throughout therapy. Correct any underlying causes of ventricular arrhythmias. Monitor closely for signs and symptoms of CNS toxicity. The elderly may be prone to increased CNS and cardiovascular side effects. Reduce dose in hepatic dysfunction and CHF.

Injectable anesthetic: Follow appropriate administration techniques so as not to administer any intravascularly. Solutions containing antimicrobial preservatives should not be used for epidural or spinal anesthesia. Some solutions contain a bisulfite; avoid in patients who are allergic to bisulfite. Resuscitative equipment, medicine and oxygen should be available in case of emergency. Use products containing epinephrine cautiously in patients with significant vascular disease, compromised blood flow, or during or following general anesthesia (increased risk of arrhythmias). Adjust the dose for the elderly, pediatric, acutely ill, and debilitated patients.

Topical: Do not leave on large body areas for >2 hours. Potentially life threatening side effects (eg, irregular heart beat, seizures, coma, respiratory depression, death) have occurred when used prior to cosmetic procedures. Observe young children closely to prevent accidental ingestion. Not for use ophthalmic use or for use on mucous membranes.

Transdermal patch: Safety and efficacy have not been established in children.

Drug Interactions Substrate of CYP1A2 (minor), 2A6 (minor), 2B6 (minor), 2C9 (minor), 2D6 (major), 3A4 (major); **Inhibits** CYP1A2 (strong), 2D6 (moderate), 3A4 (moderate)

Cimetidine increases lidocaine blood levels; monitor levels or use an alternative H₂ antagonist.

CYP1A2 substrates: Lidocaine may increase the levels/effects of CYP1A2 substrates. Example substrates include aminophylline, fluvoxamine, mexiletine, mirtazapine, ropinirole, theophylline, and trifluoperazine.

CYP2D6 inhibitors: May increase the levels/effects of lidocaine. Example inhibitors include chlorpromazine, delavirdine, fluoxetine, miconazole, paroxetine, pergolide, quinidine, quinine, ritonavir, and ropinirole.

CYP2D6 substrates: Lidocaine may increase the levels/effects of CYP2D6 substrates. Example substrates include amphetamines, selected beta-blockers, dextromethorphan, fluoxetine, mirtazapine, nefazodone, paroxetine, risperidone, ritonavir, thioridazine, tricyclic antidepressants, and venlafaxine.

CYP2D6 prodrug substrates: Lidocaine may decrease the levels/effects of CYP2D6 prodrug substrates. Example prodrug substrates include codeine, hydrocodone, oxycodone, and tramadol.

CYP3A4 inducers: CYP3A4 inducers may decrease the levels/effects of lidocaine. Example inducers include aminoglutethimide, carbamazepine, nafcillin, nevirapine, phenobarbital, phenytoin, and rifamycins.

CYP3A4 inhibitors: May increase the levels/effects of lidocaine. Example inhibitors include amiodarone (doses >400 mg/day), azole antifungals, clarithromycin, diclofenac, doxycycline, erythromycin, imatinib, isoniazid, nefazodone, nicardipine, propofol, protease inhibitors, quinidine, telithromycin, and verapamil.

CYP3A4 substrates: Lidocaine may increase the levels/effects of CYP3A4 substrates. Example substrates include benzodiazepines, calcium channel blockers, cyclosporine, mirtazapine, nateglinide, nefazodone, sildenafil (and other PDE-5 inhibitors), tacrolimus, and venlafaxine. Selected benzodiazepines (midazolam and triazolam), cisapride, ergot alkaloids, selected HMG-CoA reductase inhibitors (lovastatin and simvastatin), and pimozide are generally contraindicated with strong CYP3A4 inhibitors.

Propranolol: Increases lidocaine blood levels.

Protease inhibitors (eg, amprenavir, ritonavir): May increase lidocaine blood levels.

Ethanol/Nutrition/Herb Interactions Herb/Nutraceutical: St John's wort may decrease lidocaine levels; avoid concurrent use.

Dietary Considerations Premixed injection may contain corn-derived dextrose and its use is contraindicated in patients with allergy to corn-related products.

Pharmacodynamics/Kinetics

Onset of action: Single bolus dose: 45-90 seconds

Duration: 10-20 minutes

Distribution: V_d: 1.1-2.1 L/kg; alterable by many patient factors; decreased in CHF and liver disease; crosses blood-brain barrier

Protein binding: 60% to 80% to alpha$_1$ acid glycoprotein

Metabolism: 90% hepatic; active metabolites monoethylglycinexylidide (MEGX) and glycinexylidide (GX) can accumulate and may cause CNS toxicity

Half-life elimination: Biphasic: Prolonged with congestive heart failure, liver disease, shock, severe renal disease; Initial: 7-30 minutes; Terminal: Infants, premature: 3.2 hours, Adults: 1.5-2 hours

Pregnancy Risk Factor B

Lactation Enters breast milk (small amounts)/use caution (AAP rates "compatible")

Dosage Forms Excipient information presented when available (limited, particularly for generics); consult specific product labeling. [DSC] = Discontinued product

Cream, rectal (L-M-X™ 5): 5% (15 g) [contains benzyl alcohol; packaged with applicator]; (30 g) [contains benzyl alcohol]

Cream, topical (L-M-X™ 4): 4% (5 g) [contains benzyl alcohol; packaged with Tegaderm™ dressing]; (15 g, 30 g) [contains benzyl alcohol]

Cream, topical, as hydrochloride: 3% (30 g)

LidaMantle®: 3% (30 g, 85 g)

Gel, topical:

Burn-O-Jel: 0.5% (90 g)

Topicaine®: 4% (10 g, 30 g, 113 g) [contains alcohol 35%, benzyl alcohol, aloe vera, and jojoba]

Gel, topical, as hydrochloride:

Burn Jel: 2% (3.5 g, 120 g)

Solarcaine® Aloe Extra Burn Relief: 0.5% (113 g, 226 g) [contains aloe vera gel and tartrazine]

Infusion, as hydrochloride [premixed in D_5W]: 0.4% [4 mg/mL] (250 mL, 500 mL); 0.8% [8 mg/mL] (250 mL, 500 mL)

Injection, solution, as hydrochloride: 0.5% [5 mg/mL] (50 mL); 1% [10 mg/mL] (2 mL, 10 mL, 20 mL, 30 mL, 50 mL); 2% [20 mg/mL] (2 mL, 5 mL, 20 mL, 50 mL)

(Continued)

Lidocaine *(Continued)*

Xylocaine®: 0.5% [5 mg/mL] (50 mL); 1% [10 mg/mL] (10 mL, 20 mL, 50 mL); 2% [20 mg/mL] (1.8 mL, 10 mL, 20 mL, 50 mL)

Injection, solution, as hydrochloride [preservative free]: 0.5% [5 mg/mL] (50 mL); 1% [10 mg/mL] (2 mL, 5 mL, 30 mL); 1.5% [15 mg/mL] (20 mL); 2% [20 mg/mL] (2 mL, 5 mL, 10 mL); 4% [40 mg/mL] (5 mL)

Xylocaine®: 10% [100 mg/mL] (5 mL) [for ventricular arrhythmias]

Xylocaine® MPF: 0.5% [5 mg/mL] (50 mL); 1% [10 mg/mL] (2 mL, 5 mL, 10 mL, 30 mL); 1.5% [15 mg/mL] (10 mL, 20 mL); 2% [20 mg/mL] (2 mL, 5 mL, 10 mL); 4% [40 mg/mL] (5 mL)

Injection, solution, as hydrochloride [premixed in $D_{7.5}W$, preservative free]: 5% (2 mL)

Xylocaine® MPF: 1.5% (2 mL) [DSC]

Jelly, topical, as hydrochloride: 2% (5 mL, 30 mL)

Anestacon®: 2% (15 mL) [contains benzalkonium chloride]

Xylocaine®: 2% (5 mL, 30 mL)

Liquid, topical (Zilactin®-L): 2.5% (7.5 mL)

Lotion, topical, as hydrochloride (LidaMantle®): 3% (177 mL)

Ointment, topical: 5% (37 g, 50 g)

Solution, topical, as hydrochloride: 4% [40 mg/mL] (50 mL)

Band-Aid® Hurt-Free™ Antiseptic Wash: 2% (180 mL)

LTA® 360: 4% [40 mg/mL] (4 mL) [packaged with cannula for laryngotracheal administration]

Xylocaine®: 4% [40 mg/mL] (50 mL)

Solution, viscous, as hydrochloride: 2% [20 mg/mL] (20 mL, 100 mL)

Xylocaine® Viscous: 2% [20 mg/mL] (100 mL, 450 mL)

Spray, topical:

Burnamycin: 0.5% (60 mL) [contains aloe vera gel and menthol]

Premjact®: 9.6% (13 mL)

Solarcaine® Aloe Extra Burn Relief: 0.5% (127 g) [contains aloe vera]

Transdermal system, topical (Lidoderm®): 5% (30s)

Lidocaine and Bupivacaine *(LYE doe kane & byoo PIV a kane)*

Related Information

Bupivacaine *on page 236*
Lidocaine *on page 972*

U.S. Brand Names Duocaine™

Generic Available No

Index Terms Bupivacaine and Lidocaine; Lidocaine Hydrochloride and Bupivacaine Hydrochloride

Pharmacologic Category Local Anesthetic

Use Local or regional anesthesia in ophthalmologic surgery by peripheral nerve block techniques such as peribulbar, retrobulbar, and facial blocks; may be used with or without epinephrine

Local Anesthetic/Vasoconstrictor Precautions No information available to require special precautions

Effects on Dental Treatment No significant effects or complications reported

Common Adverse Effects Frequency not defined; reactions may be dose related or due to unintentional intravascular injection.

Cardiovascular: Bradycardia, cardiac arrest, cardiac output decreased, heart block, hypotension, myocardium depression, ventricular arrhythmia

Central nervous system: Anxiety, chills, convulsions, depression, dizziness, drowsiness, excitation, restlessness

Gastrointestinal: Nausea, vomiting

Neuromuscular & skeletal: Tremors

Ocular: Blurred vision, pupil constriction, permanent injury to extraocular muscle

Otic: Tinnitus

Respiratory: Respiratory arrest

Miscellaneous: Allergic reaction

Following unintentional subarachnoid injection: Backache, cranial nerve palsies, headache, incontinence (fecal or urinary), meningismus, paralysis, paresthesia, perineal sensation loss, persistent anesthesia, septic meningitis, sexual function loss, spinal block, urinary retention, weakness

Mechanism of Action Blocks both the initiation and conduction of nerve impulses by decreasing the neuronal membrane's permeability to sodium ions, which results in inhibition of depolarization with resultant blockade of conduction.

Drug Interactions

Cytochrome P450 Effect: Lidocaine: **Substrate** of CYP1A2 (minor), 2A6 (minor), 2B6 (minor), 2C9 (minor), 2D6 (major), 3A4 (major); **Inhibits** CYP1A2 (strong), 2D6 (moderate), 3A4 (moderate)

Decreased Effect: Epinephrine may be used to decrease systemic absorption of lidocaine/bupivacaine; if used, see Epinephrine monograph for Drug Interactions.

Pharmacodynamics/Kinetics Also see individual agents.

Protein binding: Lidocaine: Fraction bound decreases with increased concentration; also dependent upon plasma concentration of alpha$_1$-acid glycoprotein

Metabolism: Lidocaine: Hepatic, forms metabolites; Bupivacaine: hepatic, forms metabolites

Half-life elimination: Lidocaine: I.V.: 1.5-2 hours; Bupivacaine: I.V.: 2.7 hours

Time to peak, plasma: Following peribulbar block: Lidocaine: 20 minutes; Bupivacaine: 21 minutes

Excretion: Urine

Pregnancy Risk Factor C

Lidocaine and Epinephrine (LYE doe kane & ep i NEF rin)

Related Information

Epinephrine on page 572
Lidocaine on page 972
Oral Pain on page 1788

U.S. Brand Names LidoSite™; Xylocaine® MPF With Epinephrine; Xylocaine® With Epinephrine

Canadian Brand Names Xylocaine® With Epinephrine

Generic Available Yes: Excludes transdermal system

Index Terms Epinephrine and Lidocaine

Pharmacologic Category Local Anesthetic

Dental Use Amide-type anesthetic used for local infiltration anesthesia injection near nerve trunks to produce nerve block

Use Local infiltration anesthesia; AVS for nerve block; topical local analgesia for superficial dermatologic procedures

Local Anesthetic/Vasoconstrictor Precautions No information available to require special precautions

Effects on Dental Treatment It is common to misinterpret psychogenic responses to local anesthetic injection as an allergic reaction. Intraoral injections are perceived by many patients as a stressful procedure in dentistry. Common symptoms to this stress are diaphoresis, palpitations, hyperventilation. Patients may exhibit hypersensitivity to bisulfites contained in local anesthetic solution to prevent oxidation of epinephrine. In general, patients reacting to bisulfites have a history of asthma and their airways are hyper-reactive to asthmatic syndrome.

Degree of adverse effects in the CNS and cardiovascular system is directly related to the blood levels of lidocaine: Bradycardia, hypersensitivity reactions (rare; may be manifest as dermatologic reactions and edema at injection site), asthmatic syndromes

High blood levels: Anxiety, restlessness, disorientation, confusion, dizziness, tremors, seizures, CNS depression (resulting in somnolence, unconsciousness and possible respiratory arrest), nausea, and vomiting.

Significant Adverse Effects Degree of adverse effects in the central nervous system and cardiovascular system are directly related to the blood levels of lidocaine. The effects below are more likely to occur after systemic administration rather than infiltration.

Cardiovascular: Myocardial effects include a decrease in contraction force as well as a decrease in electrical excitability and myocardial conduction rate resulting in bradycardia and reduction in cardiac output.

Central nervous system: High blood levels result in anxiety, restlessness, disorientation, confusion, dizziness, tremor, and seizure. This is followed by depression of CNS resulting in somnolence, unconsciousness and possible respiratory arrest. In some cases, symptoms of CNS stimulation may be absent and the primary CNS effects are somnolence and unconsciousness.

Gastrointestinal: Nausea and vomiting may occur

Hypersensitivity reactions: Extremely rare, but may be manifest as dermatologic reactions and edema at injection site. Asthmatic syndromes have occurred. Patients may exhibit hypersensitivity to bisulfites contained in local anesthetic solution to prevent oxidation of epinephrine. In general, patients reacting to bisulfites have a history of asthma and their airways are hyper-reactive to asthmatic syndrome.

(Continued)

Lidocaine and Epinephrine *(Continued)*

Psychogenic reactions: It is common to misinterpret psychogenic responses to local anesthetic injection as an allergic reaction. Intraoral injections are perceived by many patients as a stressful procedure in dentistry. Common symptoms to this stress are diaphoresis, palpitation, hyperventilation, generalized pallor and a fainting feeling

Topical formulation:

>10%: Dermatologic: Papules (up to 12%)

1% to 10%: Dermatologic: Burns (up to 8%), rash (5%), skin irritation, burning sensation, blanching

<1% (Limited to important or life-threatening): Erythema, hematoma, urticaria

Dental Usual Dosing Dosage varies with the anesthetic procedure, degree of anesthesia needed, vascularity of tissue, duration of anesthesia required, and physical condition of patient.

Dental anesthesia, infiltration, or conduction block:

Children <10 years: 20-30 mg (1-1.5 mL) of lidocaine hydrochloride as a 2% solution with epinephrine 1:100,000; maximum: 4-5 mg of lidocaine hydrochloride/kg of body weight or 100-150 mg as a single dose

Children >10 years and Adults: Do not exceed 6.6 mg/kg body weight or 300 mg of lidocaine hydrochloride and 3 mcg (0.003 mg) of epinephrine/kg of body weight or 0.2 mg epinephrine per dental appointment. The effective anesthetic dose varies with procedure, intensity of anesthesia needed, duration of anesthesia required, and physical condition of the patient. Always use the lowest effective dose along with careful aspiration.

The following numbers of dental carpules (1.8 mL) provide the indicated amounts of lidocaine hydrochloride 2% and epinephrine 1:100,000 (see table):

# of Cartridges (1.8 mL)	Lidocaine HCl (2%) (mg)	Epinephrine 1:100,000 (mg)
1	36	0.018
2	72	0.036
3	108	0.054
4	144	0.072
5	180	0.090
6	216	0.108
7	252	0.126
8	288	0.144
9	324	0.162
10	360	0.180

For most routine dental procedures, lidocaine hydrochloride 2% with epinephrine 1:100,000 is preferred. When a more pronounced hemostasis is required, a 1:50,000 epinephrine concentration should be used. The following numbers of dental carpules (1.8 mL) provide the indicated amounts of lidocaine hydrochloride 2% and epinephrine 1:50,000 (see table):

# of Cartridges (1.8 mL)	Lidocaine HCl (2%) (mg)	Epinephrine 1:50,000 (mg)
1	36	0.036
2	72	0.072
3	108	0.108
4	144	0.144
5	180	0.180
6	216	0.216

Dermatologic procedure: Children ≥5 and Adults: Topical: Place 1 transdermal patch over area requiring analgesia; attach patch to iontophoretic controller and leave on for 10 minutes. Remove patch and perform procedure within 10-20 minutes of patch removal. Do not use another patch for 30 minutes.

Dosage Dosage varies with the anesthetic procedure, degree of anesthesia needed, vascularity of tissue, duration of anesthesia required, and physical condition of patient.

Dental anesthesia, infiltration, or conduction block:

Children <10 years: 20-30 mg (1-1.5 mL) of lidocaine hydrochloride as a 2% solution with epinephrine 1:100,000; maximum: 4-5 mg of lidocaine hydrochloride/kg of body weight or 100-150 mg as a single dose

Children >10 years and Adults: Do not exceed 6.6 mg/kg body weight or 300 mg of lidocaine hydrochloride and 3 mcg (0.003 mg) of epinephrine/kg of body weight or 0.2 mg epinephrine per dental appointment. The effective anesthetic dose varies with procedure, intensity of anesthesia needed, duration of anesthesia required, and physical condition of the patient. Always use the lowest effective dose along with careful aspiration.

For most routine dental procedures, lidocaine hydrochloride 2% with epinephrine 1:100,000 is preferred. When a more pronounced hemostasis is required, a 1:50,000 epinephrine concentration should be used.

Dermatologic procedure: Children ≥5 and Adults: Topical: Place 1 transdermal patch over area requiring analgesia; attach patch to iontophoretic controller and leave on for 10 minutes. Remove patch and perform procedure within 10-20 minutes of patch removal. Do not use another patch for 30 minutes.

Mechanism of Action Lidocaine blocks both the initiation and conduction of nerve impulses via decreased permeability of sodium ions; epinephrine increases the duration of action of lidocaine by causing vasoconstriction (via alpha effects) which slows the vascular absorption of lidocaine

Contraindications Hypersensitivity to lidocaine, epinephrine, or any component of the formulation; hypersensitivity to other local anesthetics of the amide type; myasthenia gravis; shock; cardiac conduction disease; angle-closure glaucoma

LidoSite™: Hypersensitivity to lidocaine, epinephrine, other local anesthetics of the amide type, or any component of the formulation; patients with electrically-sensitive devices (eg, pacemakers, implantable defibrillators)

Warnings/Precautions Aspirate the syringe (injection solution for infiltration formulation) after tissue penetration and before injection to minimize chance of direct vascular injection. Use caution in endocrine, hepatic, or thyroid disease. Avoid use in presence of flammable anesthetics. Avoid in patients with uncontrolled hyperthyroidism. Use minimal amounts in patients with significant cardiovascular problems (because of epinephrine component). May contain sodium metabisulfite; use caution in patients with a sulfite allergy. Avoid application of topical formulation to distal portions of body (eg, digits, nose, ears, penis). Transdermal patch may contain conducting metal (eg, aluminum); remove patch prior to MRI.

LidoSite™: Do not use near flammable anesthetics. Use with caution in patients with peripheral vascular disease; may have exaggerated vasoconstriction. Use with caution in patients with severe coronary artery disease, hypertension, cardiac dysrhythmias, or patients taking MAO inhibitors or tricyclic antidepressants. Use caution in patients with skin susceptible to injury.

Drug Interactions Lidocaine: **Substrate** of CYP1A2 (minor), 2A6 (minor), 2B6 (minor), 2C9 (minor), 2D6 (major), 3A4 (major); **Inhibits** CYP1A2 (strong), 2D6 (strong), 3A4 (moderate)

Also see individual agents. **Note:** Significance of interaction may depend on route of drug delivery and systemic exposure.

Beta-blockers, nonselective: Combination treatment may increase blood pressure.

Epinephrine (and other direct alpha-agonists): Pressor response to I.V. epinephrine, norepinephrine, and phenylephrine may be enhanced in patients receiving TCAs (**Note:** Effect is unlikely with epinephrine or levonordefrin dosages typically administered as infiltration in combination with local anesthetics)

General Anesthetics: May increase sensitivity of myocardium to dysrhythmic effects of epinephrine.

Tricyclic Antidepressants: Combination treatment may increase blood pressure.

Pharmacodynamics/Kinetics

Onset of action: Peak effect: ~5 minutes

Duration: ~2 hours; dose and anesthetic procedure dependent

Absorption: Topical: Lidocaine: Minimal; Epinephrine: Minimal

See individual agents.

Pregnancy Risk Factor B

Lactation Enters breast milk/compatible

Breast-Feeding Considerations Usual infiltration doses of lidocaine with epinephrine given to nursing mothers has not been shown to affect the health of the nursing infant.

Dosage Forms Excipient information presented when available (limited, particularly for generics); consult specific product labeling.

Injection, solution:

0.5% / 1:200,000: Lidocaine hydrochloride 0.5% and epinephrine 1:200,000 (50 mL)

1% / 1:100,000: Lidocaine hydrochloride 1% and epinephrine 1:100,000 (20 mL, 30 mL, 50 mL)

(Continued)

Lidocaine and Epinephrine *(Continued)*

1% / 1:200,000: Lidocaine hydrochloride 1% and epinephrine 1:200,000 (30 mL)

1.5% / 1:200,000: Lidocaine hydrochloride 1.5% and epinephrine 1:200,000 (30 mL)

2% / 1:50,000: Lidocaine hydrochloride 2% and epinephrine 1:50,000 (1.8 mL)

2% / 1:100,000: Lidocaine hydrochloride 2% and epinephrine 1:100,000 (1.8 mL, 30 mL, 50 mL)

2% / 1:200,000: Lidocaine hydrochloride 2% and epinephrine 1:200,000 (20 mL)

Xylocaine® with Epinephrine:

0.5% / 1:200,000: Lidocaine hydrochloride 0.5% and epinephrine 1:200,000 (50 mL) [contains methylparaben]

1% / 1:100,000: Lidocaine hydrochloride 1% and epinephrine 1:100,000 (10 mL, 20 mL, 50 mL) [contains methylparaben]

2% / 1:50,000: Lidocaine hydrochloride 2% and epinephrine 1:50,000 (1.8 mL) [contains sodium metabisulfite]

2% / 1:100,000: Lidocaine hydrochloride 2% and epinephrine 1:100,000 (1.8 mL) [contains sodium metabisulfite]; (10 mL, 20 mL, 50 mL) [contains methylparaben]

Xylocaine®-MPF with Epinephrine:

1% / 1:200,000: Lidocaine hydrochloride 1% and epinephrine 1:200,000 (5 mL, 10 mL, 30 mL) [contains sodium metabisulfite]

1.5% / 1:200,000: Lidocaine hydrochloride 1.5% and epinephrine 1:200,000 (5 mL, 10 mL, 30 mL) [contains sodium metabisulfite]

2% / 1:200,000: Lidocaine hydrochloride 2% and epinephrine 1:200,000 (5 mL, 10 mL, 20 mL) [contains sodium metabisulfite]

Transdermal system (LidoSite™): Lidocaine hydrochloride 10% and epinephrine 0.1% (25s) [contains sodium metabisulfite; for use only with LidoSite™ controller]

Selected Readings

Ayoub ST and Coleman AE, "A Review of Local Anesthetics," *Gen Dent*, 1992, 40(4):285-7, 289-90.

Budenz AW, "Local Anesthetics in Dentistry: Then and Now," *J Calif Dent Assoc*, 2003, 31(5):388-96.

Dower JS Jr, "A Review of Paresthesia in Association With Administration of Local Anesthesia," *Dent Today*, 2003, 22(2):64-9.

Finder RL and Moore PA, "Adverse Drug Reactions to Local Anesthesia," *Dent Clin North Am*, 2002, 46(4):747-57, x.

Haas DA, "An Update on Local Anesthetics in Dentistry," *J Can Dent Assoc*, 2002, 68(9):546-51.

Hawkins JM and Moore PA, "Local Anesthesia: Advances in Agents and Techniques," *Dent Clin North Am*, 2002, 46(4):719-32, ix.

"Injectable Local Anesthetics," *J Am Dent Assoc*, 2003, 134(5):628-9.

Jastak JT and Yagiela JA, "Vasoconstrictors and Local Anesthesia: A Review and Rationale for Use," *J Am Dent Assoc*, 1983, 107(4):623-30.

MacKenzie TA and Young ER, "Local Anesthetic Update," *Anesth Prog*, 1993, 40(2):29-34.

Malamed SF, "Allergy and Toxic Reactions to Local Anesthetics," *Dent Today*, 2003, 22(4):114-6, 118-21.

Nusstein J, Reader A, and Beck FM, "Anesthetic Efficacy of Different Volumes of Lidocaine With Epinephrine for Inferior Alveolar Nerve Blocks," *Gen Dent*, 2002, 50(4):372-5.

Wynn RL, "Epinephrine Interactions With Beta-Blockers," *Gen Dent*, 1994, 42(1):16, 18.

Wynn RL, "Recent Research on Mechanisms of Local Anesthetics," *Gen Dent*, 1995, 43(4):316-8.

Yagiela JA, "Local Anesthetics," *Anesth Prog*, 1991, 38(4-5):128-41.

Lidocaine and Hydrocortisone

(LYE doe kane & hye droe KOR ti sone)

Related Information

Hydrocortisone *on page 836*
Lidocaine *on page 972*

U.S. Brand Names AnaMantle® HC; Lida-Mantle® HC

Generic Available Yes: Topical cream

Index Terms Hydrocortisone and Lidocaine

Pharmacologic Category Anesthetic/Corticosteroid

Use Topical anti-inflammatory and anesthetic for skin disorders; rectal for the treatment of hemorrhoids, anal fissures, pruritus ani, or similar conditions

Local Anesthetic/Vasoconstrictor Precautions No information available to require special precautions

Effects on Dental Treatment No significant effects or complications reported

Drug Interactions

Cytochrome P450 Effect:

Lidocaine: **Substrate** of CYP1A2 (minor), 2A6 (minor), 2B6 (minor), 2C9 (minor), 2D6 (major), 3A4 (major); **Inhibits** CYP1A2 (strong), 2D6 (strong), 3A4 (moderate)

Hydrocortisone: **Substrate** of CYP3A4 (minor); **Induces** CYP3A4 (weak)

Increased Effect/Toxicity: See individual agents.
Decreased Effect: See individual agents.
Pharmacodynamics/Kinetics See individual agents.
Pregnancy Risk Factor B

Lidocaine and Prilocaine (LYE doe kane & PRIL oh kane)

Related Information
Lidocaine *on page 972*
Prilocaine *on page 1348*
U.S. Brand Names EMLA®; Oraqix®
Canadian Brand Names EMLA®
Generic Available Yes: Cream
Index Terms Prilocaine and Lidocaine
Pharmacologic Category Local Anesthetic
Dental Use

Periodontal gel (Oraqix®): Use in adults who require localized anesthesia in periodontal pockets during scaling and/or root planning.

Topical: Amide-type topical anesthetic for use on normal intact skin to provide local analgesia for minor procedures such as I.V. cannulation or venipuncture

Use Topical anesthetic for use on normal intact skin to provide local analgesia for minor procedures such as I.V. cannulation or venipuncture; has also been used for painful procedures such as lumbar puncture and skin graft harvesting; for superficial minor surgery of genital mucous membranes and as an adjunct for local infiltration anesthesia in genital mucous membranes.

Local Anesthetic/Vasoconstrictor Precautions No information available to require special precautions

Effects on Dental Treatment Key adverse event(s) related to dental treatment: Application site reactions in the oral cavity in 52/391 patients (13%) included pain, soreness, irritation, numbness, ulcerations, vesicles, edema, abscess and/or redness in the treated area. The 13% represented adverse effects occurring in more than one patient. Each patient was counted only once per adverse event. Taste perversion also reported (2%) including complaints of bad or bitter taste for up to 4 hours after administration.

Significant Adverse Effects Frequency not defined.

Cardiovascular: Hypotension, angioedema
Central nervous system: Shock
Dermatologic: Hyperpigmentation, erythema, itching, rash, burning, urticaria
Genitourinary: Blistering of foreskin (rare)
Local: Burning, stinging, edema
Respiratory: Bronchospasm
Miscellaneous: Alteration in temperature sensation, hypersensitivity reactions

Dental Usual Dosing Oraqix®: Gel: Apply on gingival margin around selected teeth using the blunt-tipped applicator included in package. Wait 30 seconds, then fill the periodontal pockets using the blunt-tipped applicator until gel becomes visible at the gingival margin. Wait another 30 seconds before starting treatment. Maximum recommended dose: One treatment session: 5 cartridges (8.5 g)

Dosage Although the incidence of systemic adverse effects with EMLA® is very low, caution should be exercised, particularly when applying over large areas and leaving on for >2 hours

Children (intact skin): EMLA® should **not** be used in neonates with a gestation age <37 weeks nor in infants <12 months of age who are receiving treatment with methemoglobin-inducing agents

Dosing is based on child's age and weight:

Age 0-3 months or <5 kg: Apply a maximum of 1 g over no more than 10 cm² of skin; leave on for no longer than 1 hour

Age 3 months to 12 months and >5 kg: Apply no more than a maximum 2 g total over no more than 20 cm² of skin; leave on for no longer than 4 hours

Age 1-6 years and >10 kg: Apply no more than a maximum of 10 g total over no more than 100 cm² of skin; leave on for no longer than 4 hours.

Age 7-12 years and >20 kg: Apply no more than a maximum 20 g total over no more than 200 cm² of skin; leave on for no longer than 4 hours.

Note: If a patient greater than 3 months old does not meet the minimum weight requirement, the maximum total dose should be restricted to the corresponding maximum based on patient weight.

Adults (intact skin):

EMLA® cream and EMLA® anesthetic disc: A thick layer of EMLA® cream is applied to intact skin and covered with an occlusive dressing, or alternatively, an EMLA® anesthetic disc is applied to intact skin

Minor dermal procedures (eg, I.V. cannulation or venipuncture): Apply 2.5 g of cream (1/2 of the 5 g tube) over 20-25 cm of skin surface area, or 1

(Continued)

Lidocaine and Prilocaine *(Continued)*

anesthetic disc (1 g over 10 cm²) for at least 1 hour. **Note:** In clinical trials, 2 sites were usually prepared in case there was a technical problem with cannulation or venipuncture at the first site.

Major dermal procedures (eg, more painful dermatological procedures involving a larger skin area such as split thickness skin graft harvesting): Apply 2 g of cream per 10 cm² of skin and allow to remain in contact with the skin for at least 2 hours.

Adult male genital skin (eg, pretreatment prior to local anesthetic infiltration): Apply a thick layer of cream (1 g/10 cm²) to the skin surface for 15 minutes. Local anesthetic infiltration should be performed immediately after removal of EMLA® cream.

Note: Dermal analgesia can be expected to increase for up to 3 hours under occlusive dressing and persist for 1-2 hours after removal of the cream

Adult females: Genital mucous membranes: Minor procedures (eg, removal of condylomata acuminata, pretreatment for local anesthetic infiltration): Apply 5-10 g (thick layer) of cream for 5-10 minutes

Periodontal gel (Oraqix®): Adults: Apply on gingival margin around selected teeth using the blunt-tipped applicator included in package. Wait 30 seconds, then fill the periodontal pockets using the blunt-tipped applicator until gel becomes visible at the gingival margin. Wait another 30 seconds before starting treatment. Maximum recommended dose: One treatment session: 5 cartridges (8.5 g)

Mechanism of Action Local anesthetic action occurs by stabilization of neuronal membranes and inhibiting the ionic fluxes required for the initiation and conduction of impulses

Contraindications Hypersensitivity to amide-type anesthetic agents (eg, lidocaine, prilocaine, dibucaine, mepivacaine, bupivacaine, etidocaine); hypersensitivity to any component of the formulation selected; application on mucous membranes or broken or inflamed skin; infants <1 month of age if gestational age is <37 weeks; infants <12 months of age receiving therapy with methemoglobin-inducing agents; children with congenital or idiopathic methemoglobinemia, or in children who are receiving medications associated with drug-induced methemoglobinemia (eg, acetaminophen [overdosage], benzocaine, chloroquine, dapsone, nitrofurantoin, nitroglycerin, nitroprusside, phenazopyridine, phenelzine, phenobarbital, phenytoin, quinine, sulfonamides)

Warnings/Precautions Use with caution in patients receiving class I and III antiarrhythmic drugs, since systemic absorption occurs and synergistic toxicity is possible. Although the incidence of systemic adverse reactions with EMLA® is very low, caution should be exercised, particularly when applying over large areas and leaving on for longer than 2 hours. Avoid use on open wounds or near the eyes.

Drug Interactions Lidocaine: **Substrate** of CYP1A2 (minor), 2A6 (minor), 2B6 (minor), 2C9 (minor), 2D6 (major), 3A4 (major); **Inhibits** CYP1A2 (strong), 2D6 (strong), 3A4 (moderate)

Also see individual agents.

Increased toxicity:

Class I antiarrhythmic drugs (eg, mexiletine): Effects are additive and potentially synergistic

Class III antiarrhythmic drugs (eg, amiodarone, sotalol, dofetilide): Cardiac ffects may be additive. Consider ECG monitoring.

Drugs known to induce methemoglobinemia

Pharmacodynamics/Kinetics

EMLA®:

Onset of action: 1 hour

Peak effect: 2-3 hours

Duration: 1-2 hours after removal

Absorption: Related to duration of application and area where applied

3-hour application: 3.6% lidocaine and 6.1% prilocaine

24-hour application: 16.2% lidocaine and 33.5% prilocaine

See individual agents.

Pregnancy Risk Factor B

Lactation Enters breast milk/compatible

Breast-Feeding Considerations Usual infiltration doses of lidocaine and prilocaine given to nursing mothers has not been shown to affect the health of the nursing infant.

Dosage Forms Excipient information presented when available (limited, particularly for generics); consult specific product labeling.

Cream, topical: Lidocaine 2.5% and prilocaine 2.5% (5 g, 30 g)

EMLA®: Lidocaine 2.5% and prilocaine 2.5% (5 g, 30 g) [each packaged with Tegaderm® dressings]

Disc, topical: Lidocaine 2.5% and prilocaine 2.5% per disc (2s, 10s) [each 1 g disc is 10 cm²]

Gel, periodontal: Lidocaine 2.5% and prilocaine 2.5% (1.7 g) [cartridge]

Selected Readings

Broadman LM, Soliman IE, Hannallah RS, et al, "Analgesic Efficacy of Eutectic Mixture of Local Anesthetics (EMLA®) vs Intradermal Infiltration Prior to Venous Cannulation in Children," *Am J Anaesth*, 1987, 34:S56.

Friskopp J and Huledal G, "Plasma Levels of Lidocaine and Prilocaine After Application of Oraqix, a New Intrapocket Anesthetic, in Patients With Advanced Periodontitis," *J Clin Periodontol*, 2001, 28(5):425-9.

Friskopp J, Nilsson M, and Isacsson G, "The Anesthetic Onset and Duration of a New Lidocaine/ Prilocaine Gel Intra-Pocket Anesthetic (Oraqix) for Periodontal Scaling/Root Planing," *J Clin Periodontol*, 2001, 28(5):453-8.

Halperin DL, Koren G, Attias D, et al, "Topical Skin Anesthesia for Venous Subcutaneous Drug Reservoir and Lumbar Puncture in Children," *Pediatrics*, 1989, 84(2):281-4.

Robieux I, Kumar R, Radhakrishnan S, et al, "Assessing Pain and Analgesia With a Lido-caine-Prilocaine Emulsion in Infants and Toddlers During Venipuncture," *J Pediatr*, 1991, 118(6):971-3.

Taddio A, Shennan AT, Stevens B, et al, "Safety of Lidocaine-Prilocaine Cream in the Treatment of Preterm Neonates," *J Pediatr*, 1995, 127(6):1002-5.

Vickers ER, Mazbani N, Gerzina TM, et al, "Pharmacokinetics of EMLA Cream 5% Application to Oral Mucosa," *Anesth Prog*, 1997, 44:32-7.

Lidocaine and Tetracaine (LYE doe kane & TET ra kane)

U.S. Brand Names Synera™
Generic Available No
Index Terms Tetracaine and Lidocaine
Pharmacologic Category Analgesic, Topical; Local Anesthetic
Use Topical anesthetic for use on normal intact skin for minor procedures (eg, I.V. cannulation or venipuncture) and superficial dermatologic procedures
Local Anesthetic/Vasoconstrictor Precautions No information available to require special precautions
Effects on Dental Treatment No significant effects or complications reported
Common Adverse Effects
>10%: Dermatologic: Erythema (71%), blanching (12%), edema (12%)
1% to 10%: Dermatologic: Application site reactions (contact dermatitis, rash, skin discoloration 4%)
Dosage Transdermal patch: Children ≥3 years and Adults:
Venipuncture or intravenous cannulation: Prior to procedure, apply to intact skin for 20-30 minutes
Superficial dermatological procedures: Prior to procedure, apply to intact skin for 30 minutes
Note: Adults can use another patch at a new location to facilitate venous access after a failed attempt; remove previous patch.

Dosage adjustment in hepatic impairment: Use caution in patients with severe hepatic dysfunction.
Mechanism of Action
Local anesthetic action occurs by stabilization of neuronal membranes and inhibiting the ionic fluxes required for the initiation and conduction of impulses. A heating mechanism within the patch enhances drug delivery.
Contraindications Hypersensitivity to amide or ester type anesthetic agents, para-aminobenzoid acid (PABA), or any other component of the formulation
Warnings/Precautions Use with caution in patients receiving class I antiar-rhythmic drugs, since systemic absorption occurs and synergistic toxicity is possible. Although the incidence of systemic adverse reactions is very low, caution should be exercised when applying simultaneous or sequential applica-tion of multiple patches to adults; this practice is not recommended with chil-dren. Use with caution in patients who may be sensitive to systemic effects (eg, acutely ill, debilitated). If being used with other products containing local anes-thetic, consider potential for additive effects. Avoid contact with eye; loss of protective reflexes may predispose to corneal irritation and/or abrasion. Applica-tion to broken or inflamed skin or mucous membranes may lead to increased systemic absorption. Use caution in patients with severe hepatic disease or pseudocholinesterase deficiency. Remove patch prior to MRI. Not for use at home.
Drug Interactions
Cytochrome P450 Effect: Lidocaine: **Substrate** of CYP1A2 (minor), 2A6 (minor), 2B6 (minor), 2C9 (minor), 2D6 (major), 3A4 (major); **Inhibits** CYP1A2 (strong), 2D6 (strong), 3A4 (moderate)
Increased Effect/Toxicity: See individual agents. With administration with class I antiarrhythmic agents (eg, mexiletine), effects are additive and poten-tially synergistic.
Pharmacodynamics/Kinetics
Also see individual agents.
(Continued)

Lidocaine and Tetracaine *(Continued)*

Absorption: Related to duration of application and area where applied.

Pregnancy Risk Factor B

Dosage Forms

Transdermal system:

Synera™: Lidocaine 70 mg and tetracaine 70 mg (10s)

Lidocaine (Transoral) *(LYE doe kane trans OR al)*

Related Information

Lidocaine *on page 972*

Oral Pain *on page 1788*

U.S. Brand Names DentiPatch®

Generic Available No

Pharmacologic Category Local Anesthetic, Transoral

Dental Use

Local anesthesia of the oral mucosa prior to oral injections and soft-tissue dental procedures

Use Local anesthesia of the oral mucosa prior to oral injections and soft-tissue dental procedures

Local Anesthetic/Vasoconstrictor Precautions No information available to require special precautions

Effects on Dental Treatment No significant effects or complications reported (see Dental Comment)

Significant Adverse Effects No data reported

Dental Usual Dosing Local anesthesia of the oral mucosa (prior to oral injections): Adults: Topical: One patch on selected area of oral mucosa

Dosage One patch on selected area of oral mucosa

Mechanism of Action Blocks both the initiation and conduction of nerve impulses by decreasing the neuronal membrane's permeability to sodium ions, which results in inhibition of depolarization with resultant blockade of conduction

Contraindications Hypersensitivity to lidocaine or any of component of the formulation

Dietary Considerations Oral patch with lidocaine 46.1 mg/2 cm^2 contains phenylalanine 0.62 mg.

Pharmacodynamics/Kinetics

Onset of action: 2 minutes

Duration: Anesthesia: 40 minutes after 15-minute wear period

Dosage Forms Excipient information presented when available (limited, particularly for generics); consult specific product labeling.

Patch, oral: 46.1 mg/2 cm^2 (50s, 100s) [contains phenylalanine 0.62 mg/patch; spearmint flavor]

Dental Comment Peak plasma levels were 10% of those seen following local infiltration anesthesia with 1.8 mL lidocaine and 1:100,000 epinephrine.

The manufacturer claims DentiPatch® is safe, with "negligible systemic absorption" of lidocaine. The agent is "clinically proven to prevent injection pain from 25-gauge needles that are inserted to the level of the bone." Data from controlled studies (235 patients) have shown no serious adverse effects with the application of lidocaine patch to the oral mucosa for 15 minutes.

Selected Readings

Hersh EV, Houpt MI, Cooper SA, et al, "Analgesic Efficacy and Safety of an Intraoral Lidocaine Patch," *J Am Dent Assoc*, 1996, 127(11):1626-34.

Houpt MI, Heins P, Lamster I, et al, "An Evaluation of Intraoral Lidocaine Patches in Reducing Needle-Insertion Pain," *Compend Contin Educ Dent*, 1997, 18(4):309-10, 312-4, 316.

"The Lidocaine Patch: A New Delivery System," *Biolog Ther Dent*, 1997, 13:17-22.

Lincomycin (lin koe MYE sin)

U.S. Brand Names Lincocin®
Canadian Brand Names Lincocin®
Mexican Brand Names Libiocid; Lincocin; Princol
Generic Available No
Index Terms Lincomycin Hydrochloride
Pharmacologic Category Antibiotic, Lincosamide
Use Treatment of serious susceptible bacterial infections, mainly those caused by streptococci and staphylococci resistant to other agents
Local Anesthetic/Vasoconstrictor Precautions No information available to require special precautions
Effects on Dental Treatment Key adverse event(s) related to dental treatment: Glossitis and stomatitis.
Common Adverse Effects Frequency not defined.
Cardiovascular: Cardiopulmonary arrest and hypotension (I.V. infusion, rate related)
Central nervous system: Vertigo
Dermatologic: Dermatitis (exfoliative, vesiculobullous); erythema multiforme, rash, urticaria
Gastrointestinal: Colitis, diarrhea, glossitis, nausea, pruritus ani, stomatitis, vomiting
Genitourinary: Vaginitis
Hematologic: Agranulocytosis, aplastic anemia, leukopenia, neutropenia, pancytopenia, thrombocytopenic purpura
Hepatic: Jaundice, liver function test abnormalities
Otic: Tinnitus
Renal: Azotemia, proteinuria, oliguria
Miscellaneous: Hypersensitivity reactions (anaphylaxis, angioneurotic edema, serum sickness)
Mechanism of Action Lincosamide antibiotic which was isolated from a strain of *Streptomyces lincolnensis*; lincomycin, like clindamycin, inhibits bacterial protein synthesis by specifically binding on the 50S subunit and affecting the process of peptide chain initiation. Other macrolide antibiotics (erythromycin) also bind to the 50S subunit. Since only one molecule of antibiotic can bind to a single ribosome, the concomitant use of erythromycin and lincomycin is not recommended.
Drug Interactions
Increased Effect/Toxicity: Lincomycin may enhance the neuromuscular-blocking effect; use with caution.
Decreased Effect: Lincomycin may diminish the therapeutic effect of erythromycin; concomitant use is not recommended.
Pharmacodynamics/Kinetics
Metabolism: Hepatic
Half-life elimination, serum: ~5 hours; prolonged with renal or hepatic impairment
Time to peak, serum: I.M.: 1 hour
Excretion: Urine (2% to 30%); bile
Pregnancy Risk Factor C

Lincomycin Hydrochloride *see* Lincomycin *on page 985*

Lindane (LIN dane)

Canadian Brand Names Hexit™; PMS-Lindane
Mexican Brand Names Scabisan
Generic Available Yes
Index Terms Benzene Hexachloride; Gamma Benzene Hexachloride; Hexachlorocyclohexane
Pharmacologic Category Antiparasitic Agent, Topical; Pediculocide; Scabicidal Agent
Use Treatment of *Sarcoptes scabiei* (scabies), *Pediculus capitis* (head lice), and *Phthirus pubis* (crab lice); FDA recommends reserving lindane as a second-line agent or with inadequate response to other therapies
Local Anesthetic/Vasoconstrictor Precautions No information available to require special precautions
Effects on Dental Treatment No significant effects or complications reported
Common Adverse Effects Frequency not defined (includes postmarketing and/or case reports).
Cardiovascular: Cardiac arrhythmia
(Continued)

Lindane *(Continued)*

Central nervous system: Ataxia, dizziness, headache, restlessness, seizure, pain

Dermatologic: Alopecia, contact dermatitis, skin and adipose tissue may act as repositories, eczematous eruptions, pruritus, urticaria

Gastrointestinal: Nausea, vomiting

Hematologic: Aplastic anemia

Hepatic: Hepatitis

Local: Burning and stinging

Neuromuscular & skeletal: Paresthesia

Renal: Hematuria

Respiratory: Pulmonary edema

Restrictions An FDA-approved medication guide must be distributed when dispensing an outpatient prescription (new or refill) where this medication is to be used without direct supervision of a healthcare provider. Medication guides are available at http://www.fda.gov/cder/Offices/ODS/medication_guides.htm.

Mechanism of Action Directly absorbed by parasites and ova through the exoskeleton; stimulates the nervous system resulting in seizures and death of parasitic arthropods

Drug Interactions

Increased Effect/Toxicity: Increased toxicity: Drugs which lower seizure threshold

Pharmacodynamics/Kinetics

Absorption: ≤13% systemically

Distribution: Stored in body fat; accumulates in brain; skin and adipose tissue may act as repositories

Metabolism: Hepatic

Half-life elimination: Children: 17-22 hours

Time to peak, serum: Children: 6 hours

Excretion: Urine and feces

Pregnancy Risk Factor C

Linezolid *(li NE zoh lid)*

U.S. Brand Names Zyvox®
Canadian Brand Names Zyvoxam®
Mexican Brand Names Zyvoxam
Generic Available No
Pharmacologic Category Antibiotic, Oxazolidinone

Use Treatment of vancomycin-resistant *Enterococcus faecium* (VRE) infections, nosocomial pneumonia caused by *Staphylococcus aureus* including MRSA or *Streptococcus pneumoniae* (including multidrug-resistant strains [MDRSP]), complicated and uncomplicated skin and skin structure infections (including diabetic foot infections without concomitant osteomyelitis), and community-acquired pneumonia caused by susceptible gram-positive organisms

Local Anesthetic/Vasoconstrictor Precautions Linezolid has mild monoamine oxidase inhibitor properties. The clinician is reminded that vasoconstrictors have the potential to interact with MAOIs to result in elevation of blood pressure. Caution is suggested.

Effects on Dental Treatment Key adverse event(s) related to dental treatment: Oral moniliasis, taste alteration, and tongue discoloration.

Common Adverse Effects Percentages as reported in adults; frequency similar in pediatric patients

>10%:

Central nervous system: Headache (<1% to 11%)

Gastrointestinal: Diarrhea (3% to 11%)

1% to 10%:

Central nervous system: Insomnia (3%), dizziness (0.4% to 2%), fever (2%)

Dermatologic: Rash (2%)

Gastrointestinal: Nausea (3% to 10%), vomiting (1% to 4%), pancreatic enzymes increased (<1% to 4%), constipation (2%), taste alteration (1% to 2%), tongue discoloration (0.2% to 1%), oral moniliasis (0.4% to 1%), pancreatitis

Genitourinary: Vaginal moniliasis (1% to 2%)

Hematologic: Thrombocytopenia (0.3% to 10%), hemoglobin decreased (0.9% to 7%), anemia, leukopenia, neutropenia; **Note:** Myelosuppression (including anemia, leukopenia, pancytopenia, and thrombocytopenia; may be more common in patients receiving linezolid for >2 weeks)

Hepatic: Abnormal LFTs (0.4% to 1%)

Renal: BUN increased (<1% to 2%)

Miscellaneous: Fungal infection (0.1% to 2%), lactate dehydrogenase increased (<1% to 2%)

Mechanism of Action Inhibits bacterial protein synthesis by binding to bacterial 23S ribosomal RNA of the 50S subunit. This prevents the formation of a functional 70S initiation complex that is essential for the bacterial translation process. Linezolid is bacteriostatic against enterococci and staphylococci and bactericidal against most strains of streptococci.

Drug Interactions

Increased Effect/Toxicity: Linezolid is a reversible, nonselective inhibitor of MAO. Serotonergic agents (eg, TCAs, venlafaxine, trazodone, sibutramine, meperidine, dextromethorphan, and SSRIs) may cause a serotonin syndrome (eg, hyperpyrexia, cognitive dysfunction) when used concomitantly. Adrenergic agents (eg, phenylpropanolamine, pseudoephedrine, sympathomimetic agents, vasopressor or dopaminergic agents) may cause hypertension. Tramadol may increase the risk of seizures when used concurrently with linezolid. Myelosuppressive medications may increase risk of myelosuppression when used concurrently with linezolid.

Pharmacodynamics/Kinetics

Absorption: Rapid and extensive

Distribution: V_{dss}: Adults: 40-50 L

Protein binding: Adults: 31%

Metabolism: Hepatic via oxidation of the morpholine ring, resulting in two inactive metabolites (aminoethoxyacetic acid, hydroxyethyl glycine); does not involve CYP

Bioavailability: 100%

Half-life elimination: Children ≥1 week (full-term) to 11 years: 1.5-3 hours; Adults: 4-5 hours

Time to peak: Adults: Oral: 1-2 hours

Excretion: Urine (30% as parent drug, 50% as metabolites); feces (9% as metabolites)

Nonrenal clearance: 65%; increased in children ≥1 week to 11 years

Pregnancy Risk Factor C

Lioresal® *see* Baclofen *on page 183*

Liothyronine (lye oh THYE roe neen)

Related Information

Endocrine Disorders and Pregnancy *on page 1750*

U.S. Brand Names Cytomel®; Triostat®

Canadian Brand Names Cytomel®

Mexican Brand Names Cynomel

Generic Available No

Index Terms Liothyronine Sodium; Sodium *L*-Triiodothyronine; T_3 Sodium (error-prone abbreviation)

Pharmacologic Category Thyroid Product

Use

Oral: Replacement or supplemental therapy in hypothyroidism; management of nontoxic goiter; a diagnostic aid

I.V.: Treatment of myxedema coma/precoma

Local Anesthetic/Vasoconstrictor Precautions No precautions with vasoconstrictor are necessary if patient is well controlled with liothyronine

Effects on Dental Treatment No significant effects or complications reported

Common Adverse Effects 1% to 10%: Cardiovascular: Arrhythmia (6%), tachycardia (3%), cardiopulmonary arrest (2%), hypotension (2%), MI (2%)

Mechanism of Action Exact mechanism of action is unknown; however, it is believed the thyroid hormone exerts its many metabolic effects through control of DNA transcription and protein synthesis; involved in normal metabolism, growth, and development; promotes gluconeogenesis, increases utilization and mobilization of glycogen stores, and stimulates protein synthesis, increases basal metabolic rate

Drug Interactions

Increased Effect/Toxicity: Thyroid products may potentiate the hypoprothrombinemic effect of warfarin (and other oral anticoagulants). Tricyclic antidepressants (TCAs) may increase potential for toxicity of both drugs. Coadministration with ketamine may lead to hypertension and tachycardia.

Decreased Effect: Some medications may decrease absorption of liothyronine: Cholestyramine, colestipol (separate administration by at least 2 hours); aluminum- and magnesium-containing antacids, iron preparations, sucralfate, Kayexalate® (separate administration by at least 4 hours). Enzyme inducers (phenytoin, phenobarbital, carbamazepine, and rifampin/rifabutin) may decrease thyroid hormone levels. Thyroid hormone may decrease effect of oral sulfonylureas. Serum levels of digoxin and theophylline may be altered by thyroid function. Estrogens may decrease serum free-thyroxine concentrations.

(Continued)

Liothyronine *(Continued)*

Pharmacodynamics/Kinetics
Onset of action: 2-4 hours
  Peak response: 2-3 days
Absorption: Oral: Well absorbed (95% in 4 hours)
Half-life elimination: 2.5 days
Excretion: Urine

Pregnancy Risk Factor A

Liothyronine Sodium *see* Liothyronine *on page 987*

Liotrix *(LYE oh triks)*

Related Information
Endocrine Disorders and Pregnancy *on page 1750*

U.S. Brand Names Thyrolar®

Canadian Brand Names Thyrolar®

Generic Available No

Index Terms T_3/T_4 Liotrix

Pharmacologic Category Thyroid Product

Use Replacement or supplemental therapy in hypothyroidism (uniform mixture of $T_4:T_3$ in 4:1 ratio by weight); little advantage to this product exists and cost is not justified

Local Anesthetic/Vasoconstrictor Precautions No precautions with vasoconstrictor are necessary if patient is well controlled with liotrix

Effects on Dental Treatment No significant effects or complications reported

Common Adverse Effects Frequency not defined.
Cardiovascular: Cardiac arrhythmia, chest pain, palpitation, tachycardia
Central nervous system: Ataxia, fever, headache, insomnia, nervousness
Dermatologic: Alopecia
Endocrine & metabolic: Changes in menstrual cycle, increased appetite, weight loss
Gastrointestinal: Abdominal cramps, constipation, diarrhea, vomiting
Neuromuscular & skeletal: Hand tremor, myalgia, tremor
Respiratory: Dyspnea
Miscellaneous: Allergic skin reactions (rare), diaphoresis

Mechanism of Action The primary active compound is T_3 (triiodothyronine), which may be converted from T_4 (thyroxine) and then circulates throughout the body to influence growth and maturation of various tissues. Liotrix is uniform mixture of synthetic T_4 and T_3 in 4:1 ratio; exact mechanism of action is unknown; however, it is believed the thyroid hormone exerts its many metabolic effects through control of DNA transcription and protein synthesis; involved in normal metabolism, growth, and development; promotes gluconeogenesis, increases utilization and mobilization of glycogen stores and stimulates protein synthesis, increases basal metabolic rate

Drug Interactions
Increased Effect/Toxicity: Thyroid products may potentiate the hypoprothrombinemic effect of warfarin (and other oral anticoagulants). Effect of warfarin may be dramatically increased when thyroid is added. However, the addition of warfarin in a patient previously receiving a stable dose of thyroid hormone does not require a significantly different dosing strategy. Tricyclic antidepressants (TCAs) may increase potential for toxicity of both drugs. Excessive thyroid replacement in patients receiving growth hormone may lead to accelerated epiphyseal closure; inadequate replacement interferes with growth response. Coadministration with ketamine may lead to hypertension and tachycardia.

Decreased Effect: Aluminum- and magnesium-containing antacids, iron preparations, sucralfate, cholestyramine, colestipol, and Kayexalate® may decrease absorption (separate administration by 8 hours). Thyroid hormone may decrease effect of oral sulfonylureas. Dosage of thyroid hormone may need to be increased when SSRIs are added. Serum levels of digoxin and theophylline may be altered by thyroid function.

Pharmacodynamics/Kinetics
Absorption: 50% to 95%
Metabolism: Partially hepatic, renal, and in intestines
Half-life elimination: 6-7 days
Time to peak, serum: 12-48 hours
Excretion: Partially feces (as conjugated metabolites)

Pregnancy Risk Factor A

Lipancreatin *see* Pancrelipase *on page 1248*
Lipitor® *see* Atorvastatin *on page 162*

Lipofen™ *see* Fenofibrate *on page 674*

Liposomal DAUNOrubicin *see* DAUNOrubicin Citrate (Liposomal) *on page 449*

Liposomal DOXOrubicin *see* DOXOrubicin (Liposomal) *on page 537*

Liposyn® III *see* Fat Emulsion *on page 672*

Lipram 4500 *see* Pancrelipase *on page 1248*

Lipram-CR *see* Pancrelipase *on page 1248*

Lipram-PN *see* Pancrelipase *on page 1248*

Lipram-UL *see* Pancrelipase *on page 1248*

Liqua-Cal [OTC] *see* Calcium and Vitamin D *on page 259*

Liquibid-D® *see* Guaifenesin and Phenylephrine *on page 797*

Liquibid-D® 1200 *see* Guaifenesin and Phenylephrine *on page 797*

Liquibid®-PD [DSC] *see* Guaifenesin and Phenylephrine *on page 797*

Liqui-Coat HD® *see* Barium *on page 185*

Liquid Antidote *see* Charcoal, Activated *on page 327*

Liquid Barosperse® *see* Barium *on page 185*

Liquifilm® Tears [OTC] *see* Artificial Tears *on page 147*

Lisdexamfetamine (lis dex am FET a meen)

U.S. Brand Names Vyvanse™

Generic Available No

Index Terms Lisdexamfetamine Dimesylate; NRP104

Pharmacologic Category Stimulant

Use Treatment of attention-deficit/hyperactivity disorder (ADHD)

Local Anesthetic/Vasoconstrictor Precautions Use vasoconstrictor with caution in patients taking lisdexamfetamine. Amphetamines enhance the sympathomimetic response of epinephrine and levonordefrin leading to potential hypertension and cardiotoxicity.

Effects on Dental Treatment Key adverse event(s) related to dental treatment: Xerostomia (normal salivary flow resumes upon discontinuation).

Lisdexamfetamine is a prodrug that is converted to the active component dextroamphetamine (a noncatecholamine, sympathomimetic amine); dextroamphetamine is known to increase blood pressure. Monitor blood pressure prior to using local anesthetic with vasoconstrictors.

Common Adverse Effects

>10%

Central nervous system: Insomnia (4% to 19%), headache (12%)

Gastrointestinal: Abdominal pain (12%)

Endocrine & metabolic: Appetite decreased (39%)

1% to 10%:

Central nervous system: Irritability (10%), dizziness (5%), affect lability (3%), fever (2%), somnolence (2%), tic (2%)

Gastrointestinal: Vomiting (9%), weight loss (9%), nausea (6%), xerostomia (5%)

Dermatologic: Rash (3%)

Additional adverse reaction; frequency not defined. **Note:** Some reactions reported with related compounds.

Cardiovascular: Cardiomyopathy, hypertension, MI, palpitation, sudden death, tachycardia

Central nervous system: Depression, dizziness, dyskinesia, dysphoria, euphoria, exacerbation of motor and phonic tics, Tourette's syndrome, overstimulation, psychotic episodes, restlessness, seizure, stroke

Dermatologic: Angioedema, Stevens-Johnson syndrome, toxic epidermal necrolysis, urticaria

Endocrine & metabolic: Libido changes

Gastrointestinal: Abnormal taste, constipation, diarrhea

Genitourinary: Impotence

Miscellaneous: Anaphylaxis

Restrictions C-II

An FDA-approved medication guide must be distributed when dispensing an outpatient prescription (new or refill) where this medication is to be used without direct supervision of a healthcare provider. Medication guides are available at http://www.fda.gov/cder/drug/infopage/ADHD/default.htm.

Mechanism of Action Lisdexamfetamine dimesylate is a prodrug that is converted to the active component dextroamphetamine (a noncatecholamine, sympathomimetic amine); CNS stimulant effects are thought to result from the interference of norepinephrine and dopamine reuptake into presynaptic neurons as well as increasing their release from nerve terminals; inhibits the actions of monoamine oxidase; peripheral actions include increase in systolic and (Continued)

Lisdexamfetamine *(Continued)*

diastolic blood pressure as well as weak bronchodilator and respiratory stimulant action.

Drug Interactions

Cytochrome P450 Effect: Dextroamphetamine: **Substrate** of CYP2D6 (major)

Increased Effect/Toxicity: CYP2D6 inhibitors may increase the levels/ effects of dextroamphetamine; example inhibitors include chlorpromazine, delavirdine, fluoxetine, miconazole, paroxetine, pergolide, quinidine, quinine, ritonavir, ropinirole, and terbinafine. Dextroamphetamine may precipitate hypertensive crisis or serotonin syndrome in patients receiving MAO inhibitors. Serotonin syndrome has also been associated with combinations of amphetamines and SSRIs; these combinations should be avoided. TCAs may enhance the effects of amphetamines, potentially leading to hypertensive crisis. Use with carbonic anhydrase inhibitors may increase effects/toxicity of amphetamines. Large doses of antacids may increase the half-life and duration of action of amphetamines. Concurrent use with phenobarbital or phenytoin may produce synergistic anticonvulsant effect. May increase adverse/ toxic effects of other sympathomimetics and propoxyphene. Amphetamines may enhance analgesic effect of meperidine.

Decreased Effect: Methenamine and acidifying agents (urinary) decrease the half-life and duration of action of amphetamines. Concurrent use with amphetamines may result in a decrease in the therapeutic effects of antihypertensive agents, antipsychotics, ethosuximide, and sedating antihistamines. Lithium may inhibit stimulatory and anorectic effects of amphetamines.

Pharmacodynamics/Kinetics

Absorption: Rapid

Distribution: Dextroamphetamine: V_d: Adults: 3.5-4.6 L/kg; distributes into CNS; mean CSF concentrations are 80% of plasma; enters breast milk

Metabolism: Non-cyp-mediated hepatic metabolism

Half-life elimination: Lisdexamfetamine: <1 hour; Dextroamphetamine: 10-13 hours

Time to peak, serum: T_{max}: Lisdexamfetamine: 1 hour; Dextroamphetamine: 3.5 hours

Excretion: Urine (42% amphetamine, 2% lisdexamfetamine, 25% hippuric acid); feces (minimal)

Pregnancy Risk Factor C

Lisdexamfetamine Dimesylate *see* Lisdexamfetamine *on page 989*

Lisinopril *(lyse IN oh pril)*

Related Information

Cardiovascular Diseases *on page 1726*

U.S. Brand Names Prinivil®; Zestril®

Canadian Brand Names Apo-Lisinopril®; Prinivil®; Zestril®

Mexican Brand Names Alfaken; Prinivil; Zestril

Generic Available Yes

Pharmacologic Category Angiotensin-Converting Enzyme (ACE) Inhibitor

Use Treatment of hypertension, either alone or in combination with other antihypertensive agents; adjunctive therapy in treatment of CHF (afterload reduction); treatment of acute myocardial infarction within 24 hours in hemodynamically-stable patients to improve survival; treatment of left ventricular dysfunction after myocardial infarction

Local Anesthetic/Vasoconstrictor Precautions No information available to require special precautions

Effects on Dental Treatment Key adverse event(s) related to dental treatment: Orthostatic effects.

Common Adverse Effects Note: Frequency ranges include data from hypertension and heart failure trials. Higher rates of adverse reactions have generally been noted in patients with CHF. However, the frequency of adverse effects associated with placebo is also increased in this population.

1% to 10%:

Cardiovascular: Orthostatic effects (1%), hypotension (1% to 4%)

Central nervous system: Headache (4% to 6%), dizziness (5% to 12%), fatigue (3%)

Dermatologic: Rash (1% to 2%)

Endocrine & metabolic: Hyperkalemia (2% to 5%)

Gastrointestinal: Diarrhea (3% to 4%), nausea (2%), vomiting (1%), abdominal pain (2%)

Genitourinary: Impotence (1%)

Hematologic: Decreased hemoglobin (small)

Neuromuscular & skeletal: Chest pain (3%), weakness (1%)

Renal: BUN increased (2%); deterioration in renal function (in patients with bilateral renal artery stenosis or hypovolemia); serum creatinine increased (often transient)

Respiratory: Cough (4% to 9%), upper respiratory infection (1% to 2%)

Dosage Oral:

Hypertension:

Children ≥6 years: Initial: 0.07 mg/kg once daily (up to 5 mg); increase dose at 1- to 2-week intervals; doses >0.61 mg/kg or >40 mg have not been evaluated.

Adults: Usual dosage range (JNC 7): 10-40 mg/day

Not maintained on diuretic: Initial: 10 mg/day

Maintained on diuretic: Initial: 5 mg/day

Note: Antihypertensive effect may diminish toward the end of the dosing interval especially with doses of 10 mg/day. An increased dose may aid in extending the duration of antihypertensive effect. Doses up to 80 mg/day have been used, but do not appear to give greater effect (Zestoril® Product Information, 12/04).

Elderly: Initial: 2.5-5 mg/day; increase doses 2.5-5 mg/day at 1- to 2-week intervals; maximum daily dose: 40 mg

Patients taking diuretics should have them discontinued 2-3 days prior to initiating lisinopril if possible. Restart diuretic after blood pressure is stable if needed. If diuretic cannot be discontinued prior to therapy, begin with 5 mg with close supervision until stable blood pressure. In patients with hyponatremia (<130 mEq/L), start dose at 2.5 mg/day

Congestive heart failure: Adults: Initial: 2.5-5 mg once daily; then increase by no more than 10 mg increments at intervals no less than 2 weeks to a maximum daily dose of 40 mg. Usual maintenance: 5-40 mg/day as a single dose. Target dose: 20-40 mg once daily (ACC/AHA 2005 Heart Failure Guidelines)

Note: If patient has hyponatremia (serum sodium <130 meq/L) or renal impairment (Cl_{cr} <30 mL/minute or creatinine >3 mg/dL), then initial dose should be 2.5 mg/day

Acute myocardial infarction (within 24 hours in hemodynamically stable patients): Oral: 5 mg immediately, then 5 mg at 24 hours, 10 mg at 48 hours, and 10 mg every day thereafter for 6 weeks. Patients should continue to receive standard treatments such as thrombolytics, aspirin, and beta-blockers.

Dosing adjustment in renal impairment:

Hypertension:

Adults: Initial doses should be modified and upward titration should be cautious, based on response (maximum: 40 mg/day)

Cl_{cr} >30 mL/minute: Initial: 10 mg/day

Cl_{cr} 10-30 mL/minute: Initial: 5 mg/day

Hemodialysis: Initial: 2.5 mg/day; dialyzable (50%)

Children: Use in not recommended in pediatric patients with GFR <30 mL/minute/1.73 m^2

Congestive heart failure: Adults: Cl_{cr} <30 mL/minute or creatinine >3 mg/dL): Initial: 2.5 mg/day

Mechanism of Action Competitive inhibitor of angiotensin-converting enzyme (ACE); prevents conversion of angiotensin I to angiotensin II, a potent vasoconstrictor; results in lower levels of angiotensin II which causes an increase in plasma renin activity and a reduction in aldosterone secretion; a CNS mechanism may also be involved in hypotensive effect as angiotensin II increases adrenergic outflow from CNS; vasoactive kallikreins may be decreased in conversion to active hormones by ACE inhibitors, thus reducing blood pressure

Contraindications Hypersensitivity to lisinopril or any component of the formulation; angioedema related to previous treatment with an ACE inhibitor; bilateral renal artery stenosis; pregnancy (2nd and 3rd trimesters)

Warnings/Precautions Anaphylactic reactions can occur. Angioedema can occur at any time during treatment (especially following first dose). It may involve head and neck (potentially affecting the airway) or the intestine (presenting with abdominal pain). Prolonged monitoring may be required especially if tongue, glottis, or larynx are involved as they are associated with airway obstruction. Those with a history of airway surgery in this situation have a higher risk. Careful blood pressure monitoring with first dose (hypotension can occur especially in volume-depleted patients). **[U.S. Boxed Warning]: Based on human data, ACEIs can cause injury and death to the developing fetus when used in the second and third trimesters. ACEIs should be discontinued as soon as possible once pregnancy is detected.**

Dosage adjustment needed in renal impairment. Use with caution in hypovolemia; collagen vascular diseases; valvular stenosis (particularly aortic stenosis); or before, during, or immediately after anesthesia. Hyperkalemia may occur; risk factors include renal dysfunction, diabetes mellitus, concomitant use (Continued)

Lisinopril *(Continued)*

of potassium-sparing diuretics, potassium supplements and/or potassium containing salts. Use cautiously, if at all, with these agents and monitor potassium closely. Avoid rapid dosage escalation, which may lead to renal insufficiency. Rare toxicities associated with ACE inhibitors include cholestatic jaundice (which may progress to hepatic necrosis) and neutropenia/agranulocytosis with myeloid hyperplasia. May be associated with deterioration of renal function and/or increases in serum creatinine, particularly in patients dependent on renin-angiotensin-aldosterone system. Use with caution in unilateral renal artery stenosis and pre-existing renal insufficiency; if patient has renal impairment then a baseline WBC with differential and serum creatinine should be evaluated and monitored closely during the first 3 months of therapy. Hypersensitivity reactions may be seen during hemodialysis with high-flux dialysis membranes (eg, AN69). Safety and efficacy have not been established in children <6 years of age.

Drug Interactions

Increased Effect/Toxicity: Allopurinol may cause a higher risk of hypersensitivity reaction when taken concurrently. Neutropenia from azathioprine may be enhanced by concurrent use. Adverse events/toxicity of azathioprine (neutropenia), cyclosporine (nephrotoxicity), ferric gluconate, insulin (hypoglycemia), lithium, mercaptopurine (neutropenia), NSAIDs (nephrotoxicity). Concurrent use of eplerenone, potassium-sparing diuretics, or trimethoprim with ACE inhibitor may increase risk of hyperkalemia. Loop and thiazide diuretics may increase risk of hypovolemia, increasing the risk of nephrotoxicity when used with ACE inhibitors. ACE inhibitors may enhance the adverse/toxic effects (nitritoid reaction) of gold sodium thiomalate.

Decreased Effect: Antacids may decrease serum concentrations of ACE inhibitors. Aprotinin may decrease the antihypertensive effect of ACE inhibitors during infusion. NSAIDs and salicylates may attenuate hypertensive efficacy of ACE inhibitors.

Ethanol/Nutrition/Herb Interactions

Food: Potassium-containing salt substitutes may increase risk of hyperkalemia. Herb/Nutraceutical: Avoid dong quai if using for hypertension (has estrogenic activity). Avoid ephedra, yohimbe, ginseng (may worsen hypertension). Avoid garlic (may have increased antihypertensive effect).

Dietary Considerations Use potassium-containing salt substitutes cautiously in diabetic patients, patients with renal dysfunction, or those maintained on potassium supplements or potassium-sparing diuretics.

Pharmacodynamics/Kinetics

Onset of action: 1 hour
  Peak effect: Hypotensive: Oral: ~6 hours
Duration: 24 hours
Absorption: Well absorbed; unaffected by food
Protein binding: 25%
Half-life elimination: 11-12 hours
Excretion: Primarily urine (as unchanged drug)

Pregnancy Risk Factor C (1st trimester)/D (2nd and 3rd trimesters)

Dosage Forms

Tablet: 2.5 mg, 5 mg, 10 mg, 20 mg, 30 mg, 40 mg
  Prinivil®: 5 mg, 10 mg, 20 mg, 30 mg
  Zestril®: 2.5 mg, 5 mg, 10 mg, 20 mg, 30 mg, 40 mg

Lisinopril and Hydrochlorothiazide
(lyse IN oh pril & hye droe klor oh THYE a zide)

Related Information

Cardiovascular Diseases *on page 1726*
Hydrochlorothiazide *on page 819*
Lisinopril *on page 990*

U.S. Brand Names Prinzide®; Zestoretic®
Canadian Brand Names Prinzide®; Zestoretic®
Mexican Brand Names Prinzide; Zestoretic
Generic Available Yes
Index Terms Hydrochlorothiazide and Lisinopril
Pharmacologic Category Antihypertensive Agent, Combination
Use Treatment of hypertension
Local Anesthetic/Vasoconstrictor Precautions No information available to require special precautions
Effects on Dental Treatment No significant effects or complications reported
Common Adverse Effects See individual agents.

Drug Interactions
Increased Effect/Toxicity: See individual agents.
Decreased Effect: See individual agents.
Pharmacodynamics/Kinetics See individual agents.
Pregnancy Risk Factor C/D (2nd and 3rd trimesters)

Lispro Insulin see Insulin Lispro on page 887

Lithium (LITH ee um)

U.S. Brand Names Eskalith® [DSC]; Eskalith CR® [DSC]; Lithobid®
Canadian Brand Names Apo-Lithium® Carbonate; Apo-Lithium® Carbonate SR; Carbolith™; Duralith®; Lithane™; PMS-Lithium Carbonate; PMS-Lithium Citrate
Mexican Brand Names Litheum 300
Generic Available Yes
Index Terms Lithium Carbonate; Lithium Citrate
Pharmacologic Category Lithium
Use Management of bipolar disorders; treatment of mania in individuals with bipolar disorder (maintenance treatment prevents or diminishes intensity of subsequent episodes)
Unlabeled/Investigational Use Potential augmenting agent for antidepressants; aggression, post-traumatic stress disorder, conduct disorder in children
Local Anesthetic/Vasoconstrictor Precautions No information available to require special precautions
Effects on Dental Treatment Key adverse event(s) related to dental treatment: Xerostomia and changes in salivation (normal salivary flow resumes upon discontinuation), salivary gland swelling, and metallic taste. Avoid NSAIDs if analgesics are required since lithium toxicity has been reported with concomitant administration; acetaminophen products (ie, singly or with narcotics) are recommended.
Common Adverse Effects Frequency not defined.
Cardiovascular: Cardiac arrhythmia, hypotension, sinus node dysfunction, flattened or inverted T waves (reversible), edema, bradycardia, syncope
Central nervous system: Dizziness, vertigo, slurred speech, blackout spells, seizure, sedation, restlessness, confusion, psychomotor retardation, stupor, coma, dystonia, fatigue, lethargy, headache, pseudotumor cerebri, slowed intellectual functioning, tics
Dermatologic: Dry or thinning of hair, folliculitis, alopecia, exacerbation of psoriasis, rash
Endocrine & metabolic: Euthyroid goiter and/or hypothyroidism, hyperthyroidism, hyperglycemia, diabetes insipidus
Gastrointestinal: Polydipsia, anorexia, nausea, vomiting, diarrhea, xerostomia, metallic taste, weight gain, salivary gland swelling, excessive salivation
Genitourinary: Incontinence, polyuria, glycosuria, oliguria, albuminuria
Hematologic: Leukocytosis
Neuromuscular & skeletal: Tremor, muscle hyperirritability, ataxia, choreoathetoid movements, hyperactive deep tendon reflexes, myasthenia gravis (rare)
Ocular: Nystagmus, blurred vision, transient scotoma
Miscellaneous: Coldness and painful discoloration of fingers and toes
Mechanism of Action Alters cation transport across cell membrane in nerve and muscle cells and influences reuptake of serotonin and/or norepinephrine; second messenger systems involving the phosphatidylinositol cycle are inhibited; postsynaptic D2 receptor supersensitivity is inhibited
Drug Interactions
Increased Effect/Toxicity: Concurrent use of lithium with carbamazepine, diltiazem, SSRIs (fluoxetine, fluvoxamine), haloperidol, methyldopa, metronidazole (rare), phenothiazines, phenytoin, TCAs, and verapamil may increase the risk for neurotoxicity. A rare encephalopathic syndrome has been reported in association with haloperidol (causal relationship not established). Lithium concentrations/toxicity may be increased by diuretics, NSAIDs (sulindac and aspirin may be exceptions), ACE inhibitors, angiotensin receptor antagonists (losartan), tetracyclines, or COX-2 inhibitors (celecoxib).

Lithium and MAO inhibitors should generally be avoided due to use reports of fatal malignant hyperpyrexia; risk with selective MAO type B inhibitors (selegiline) appears to be lower. Potassium iodide may enhance the hypothyroid effects of lithium. Combined use of lithium with tricyclic antidepressants or sibutramine may increase the risk of serotonin syndrome; this combination is best avoided. Lithium may potentiate effect of neuromuscular blockers.
Decreased Effect: Combined use of lithium and chlorpromazine may lower serum concentrations of both drugs. Lithium may blunt the pressor response
(Continued)

Lithium (Continued)

to sympathomimetics (epinephrine, norepinephrine). Caffeine (xanthine derivatives) may lower lithium serum concentrations by increasing urinary lithium excretion (monitor).

Pharmacodynamics/Kinetics

Absorption: Rapid and complete

Distribution: V_d: Initial: 0.3-0.4 L/kg; V_{dss}: 0.7-1 L/kg; crosses placenta; enters breast milk at 35% to 50% the concentrations in serum; distribution is complete in 6-10 hours

CSF, liver concentrations: $1/3$ to $1/2$ of serum concentration

Erythrocyte concentration: $\sim 1/2$ of serum concentration

Heart, lung, kidney, muscle concentrations: Equivalent to serum concentration

Saliva concentration: 2-3 times serum concentration

Thyroid, bone, brain tissue concentrations: Increase 50% over serum concentrations

Protein binding: Not protein bound

Metabolism: Not metabolized

Bioavailability: Not affected by food; Capsule, immediate release tablet: 95% to 100%; Extended release tablet: 60% to 90%; Syrup: 100%

Half-life elimination: 18-24 hours; can increase to more than 36 hours in elderly or with renal impairment

Time to peak, serum: Nonsustained release: ~0.5-2 hours; slow release: 4-12 hours; syrup: 15-60 minutes

Excretion: Urine (90% to 98% as unchanged drug); sweat (4% to 5%); feces (1%)

Clearance: 80% of filtered lithium is reabsorbed in the proximal convoluted tubules; therefore, clearance approximates 20% of GFR or 20-40 mL/minute

Pregnancy Risk Factor D

Lodoxamide (loe DOKS a mide)

U.S. Brand Names Alomide®
Canadian Brand Names Alomide®
Generic Available No
Index Terms Lodoxamide Tromethamine
Pharmacologic Category Mast Cell Stabilizer
Use Treatment of vernal keratoconjunctivitis, vernal conjunctivitis, and vernal keratitis
Local Anesthetic/Vasoconstrictor Precautions No information available to require special precautions
Effects on Dental Treatment No significant effects or complications reported
Common Adverse Effects

>10%: Local: Transient burning, stinging, discomfort

1% to 10%:

Central nervous system: Headache

Ocular: Blurred vision, corneal erosion/ulcer, eye pain, corneal abrasion, blepharitis

Mechanism of Action Mast cell stabilizer that inhibits the in vivo type I immediate hypersensitivity reaction to increase cutaneous vascular permeability associated with IgE and antigen-mediated reactions

Pharmacodynamics/Kinetics Absorption: Topical: Negligible

Pregnancy Risk Factor B

Lomustine (loe MUS teen)

U.S. Brand Names CeeNU®
Canadian Brand Names CeeNU®
Mexican Brand Names CEENU
Generic Available No
Index Terms CCNU; NSC-79037
Pharmacologic Category Antineoplastic Agent, Alkylating Agent
Use Treatment of brain tumors and Hodgkin's disease
Unlabeled/Investigational Use Non-Hodgkin's lymphoma, melanoma, renal carcinoma, lung cancer, colon cancer
Local Anesthetic/Vasoconstrictor Precautions No information available to require special precautions
Effects on Dental Treatment No significant effects or complications reported
Common Adverse Effects
>10%:
   Gastrointestinal: Nausea and vomiting, usually within 3-6 hours after oral administration. Administration of the dose at bedtime, with an antiemetic, significantly reduces both the incidence and severity of nausea.
   Hematologic: Myelosuppression, common, dose-limiting, may be cumulative and irreversible; leukopenia (65%; nadir: 5-6 weeks; recovery 6-8 weeks); thrombocytopenia (nadir: 4 weeks; recovery 5-6 weeks)
Frequency not defined: Acute leukemia, alkaline phosphatase increased, alopecia, anemia, ataxia, azotemia (progressive), bilirubin increased, blindness, bone marrow dysplasia, disorientation, dysarthria, kidney size decreased, lethargy, optic atrophy, pulmonary fibrosis, pulmonary infiltrates, renal failure, stomatitis, transaminases increased, visual disturbances
Mechanism of Action Inhibits DNA and RNA synthesis via carbamylation of DNA polymerase, alkylation of DNA, and alteration of RNA, proteins, and enzymes
Drug Interactions
   Cytochrome P450 Effect: Substrate of CYP2D6 (major); **Inhibits** CYP2D6 (weak), 3A4 (weak)
   Increased Effect/Toxicity: CYP2D6 inhibitors may increase the levels/effects of lomustine; example inhibitors include chlorpromazine, delavirdine, fluoxetine, miconazole, paroxetine, pergolide, quinidine, quinine, ritonavir, and ropinirole.
Pharmacodynamics/Kinetics
   Duration: Marrow recovery: ~5-8 weeks
   Absorption: Complete
   Distribution: Crosses blood-brain barrier to a greater degree than BCNU; CNS concentrations are ≥50% of plasma concentrations
   Metabolism: Rapidly hepatic via hydroxylation producing at least two active metabolites; enterohepatically recycled
   Half-life elimination: Parent drug: 16-72 hours; Active metabolite: 16-48 hours
   Time to peak, serum: Active metabolite: ~3 hours
   Excretion: Urine (~50%); feces (<5%); expired air (<10%)
Pregnancy Risk Factor D

Lo/Ovral® *see* Ethinyl Estradiol and Norgestrel *on page 649*

Loperamide (loe PER a mide)

U.S. Brand Names Diamode [OTC]; Imodium® A-D [OTC]; Kao-Paverin® [OTC]; K-Pek II [OTC]

Canadian Brand Names Apo-Loperamide®; Diarr-Eze; Imodium®; Loperacap; Novo-Loperamide; PMS-Loperamine; Rho®-Loperamine; Riva-Loperamine

Mexican Brand Names Acanol; Pramidal; Top-Dal

Generic Available Yes

Index Terms Loperamide Hydrochloride

Pharmacologic Category Antidiarrheal

Use Treatment of chronic diarrhea associated with inflammatory bowel disease; acute nonspecific diarrhea; increased volume of ileostomy discharge

OTC labeling: Control of symptoms of diarrhea, including Traveler's diarrhea

Unlabeled/Investigational Use Cancer treatment-induced diarrhea (eg, irinotecan induced); chronic diarrhea caused by bowel resection

Local Anesthetic/Vasoconstrictor Precautions No information available to require special precautions

Effects on Dental Treatment No significant effects or complications reported

Common Adverse Effects 1% to 10%:

Central nervous system: Dizziness (1%)

Gastrointestinal: Constipation (2% to 5%), abdominal cramping (<1% to 3%), nausea (<1% to 3%)

Postmarketing and/or case reports: Abdominal distention, abdominal pain, allergic reactions, anaphylactic shock, anaphylactoid reactions, angioedema, bullous eruption (rare), drowsiness, dry mouth, dyspepsia, erythema multiforme (rare), fatigue, flatulence, paralytic ileus, megacolon, pruritus, rash, Stevens-Johnson syndrome, toxic epidermal necrolysis, toxic megacolon, urinary retention, urticaria, vomiting

Mechanism of Action Acts directly on circular and longitudinal intestinal muscles, through the opioid receptor, to inhibit peristalsis and prolong transit time; reduces fecal volume, increases viscosity, and diminishes fluid and electrolyte loss; demonstrates antisecretory activity. Loperamide increases tone on the anal sphincter

Drug Interactions

Cytochrome P450 Effect: Substrate (minor) of CYP2B6

Increased Effect/Toxicity: P-glycoprotein Inhibitors may increase CNS depressant effects.

Decreased Effect: Loperamide may decrease levels/effects of saquinavir.

Pharmacodynamics/Kinetics

Absorption: Poor

Distribution: Poor penetration into brain; low amounts enter breast milk

Metabolism: Hepatic via oxidative N-demethylation

Half-life elimination: 7-14 hours

Time to peak, plasma: Liquid: 2.5 hours; Capsule: 5 hours

Excretion: Urine and feces (1% as metabolites, 30% to 40% as unchanged drug)

Pregnancy Risk Factor C

Loperamide and Simethicone
(loe PER a mide & sye METH i kone)

U.S. Brand Names Imodium® Advanced

Generic Available No

Index Terms Simethicone and Loperamide Hydrochloride

Pharmacologic Category Antidiarrheal; Antiflatulent

Use Control of symptoms of diarrhea and gas (bloating, pressure, and cramps)

Local Anesthetic/Vasoconstrictor Precautions No information available to require special precautions

Effects on Dental Treatment No significant effects or complications reported

Common Adverse Effects See individual agents.

Mechanism of Action

Loperamide acts by slowing intestinal motility and by affecting water and electrolyte movement through the bowel.

Simethicone acts in the stomach and intestines by altering the surface tension of gas bubbles enabling them to coalesce thereby freeing and eliminating the gas more easily by belching or passing flatus.

Drug Interactions

Increased Effect/Toxicity: CNS depressants, phenothiazines, tricyclic antidepressants may potentiate adverse effects. Also see individual agents.

Pharmacodynamics/Kinetics See individual agents.

Loperamide Hydrochloride *see* Loperamide *on page 996*

Lopid® *see* Gemfibrozil *on page 772*

Lopinavir and Ritonavir (loe PIN a veer & rit ON uh veer)

Related Information
 HIV Infection and AIDS *on page 1753*
 Ritonavir *on page 1436*
U.S. Brand Names Kaletra®
Canadian Brand Names Kaletra®
Mexican Brand Names Kaletra
Generic Available No
Index Terms Ritonavir and Lopinavir
Pharmacologic Category Antiretroviral Agent, Protease Inhibitor
Use Treatment of HIV infection in combination with other antiretroviral agents
Local Anesthetic/Vasoconstrictor Precautions No information available to require special precautions
Effects on Dental Treatment Key adverse event(s) related to dental treatment: Dysphagia.
Common Adverse Effects Protease inhibitors cause dyslipidemia which includes elevated cholesterol and triglycerides and a redistribution of body fat centrally to cause increased abdominal girth, buffalo hump, facial atrophy, and breast enlargement. These agents also cause hyperglycemia.

>10%:
 Endocrine & metabolic: Hypercholesterolemia (3% to 39%), triglycerides increased (4% to 36%)
 Gastrointestinal: Diarrhea (5% to 27%), nausea (5% to 16%)
 Hepatic: GGT increased (6% to 29%)
2% to 10%:
 Cardiovascular: Hypertension (up to 2%), vein distension (up to 2%)
 Central nervous system: Headache (2% to 7%), chills (up to 2%), depression (up to 2%), fever (2%), insomnia (up to 2%)
 Dermatologic: Rash (up to 4%)
 Endocrine & metabolic: Amylase increased (3% to 8%), amenorrhea (up to 5%), hyperglycemia (1% to 5%), hyperuricemia (up to 3%), sodium decreased or increased (3% children), hypogonadism (up to 2%), inorganic phosphorus decreased (up to 2%), libido decreased (up to 2%)
 Gastrointestinal: Abdominal pain (2% to 10%), abnormal stools (up to 6%), vomiting (2% to 6%), dyspepsia (up to 5%), flatulence (1% to 4%), weight loss (up to 3%), dysphagia (up to 2%), anorexia (1% to 2%)
 Hematologic: Platelets decreased (4% children), neutrophils decreased (1% to 5%)
 Hepatic: ALT increased (3% to 10%), AST increased (2% to 9%), bilirubin increased (children 3%)
 Neuromuscular & skeletal: Weakness (up to 9%), myalgia (up to 2%), paresthesia (up to 2%)
 Respiratory: Bronchitis (up to 2%)
Mechanism of Action A coformulation of lopinavir and ritonavir. The lopinavir component is the active inhibitor of HIV protease. Lopinavir inhibits HIV protease and renders the enzyme incapable of processing polyprotein precursor which leads to production of noninfectious immature HIV particles. The ritonavir component inhibits the CYP3A metabolism of lopinavir, allowing increased plasma levels of lopinavir.
Drug Interactions
 Cytochrome P450 Effect:
  Lopinavir: **Substrate** of 3A4 (minor)
  Ritonavir: **Substrate** of CYP1A2 (minor), 2B6 (minor), 2D6 (major), 3A4 (major); **Inhibits** CYP2C8 (strong), 2C9 (weak), 2C19 (weak), 2D6 (strong), 2E1 (weak), 3A4 (strong); **Induces** CYP1A2 (weak), 2C8 (weak), 2C9 (weak), 3A4 (weak)
 Increased Effect/Toxicity: Concurrent use of cisapride, ergot alkaloids, (dihydroergotamine, ergonovine, methylergonovine), lovastatin, midazolam, pimozide, simvastatin, and triazolam is contraindicated. Alfuzosin serum level may be increased by ritonavir; concurrent use is contraindicated (by the manufacturer of ritonavir). Antiarrhythmic agents (including amiodarone, bepridil, flecainide, propafenone, lidocaine (systemic), and quinidine) should be used with caution; life-threatening arrhythmias may result from concurrent use.

 Ritonavir may increase the levels/effects of amiodarone, amphetamines, selected beta-blockers, selected benzodiazepines (midazolam and triazolam
(Continued)

Lopinavir and Ritonavir (Continued)

contraindicated), calcium channel blockers, dextromethorphan, fluoxetine, lidocaine, HMG-CoA reductase inhibitors (lovastatin and simvastatin are not recommended), mesoridazine, mirtazapine, nateglinide, nefazodone, paclitaxel, paroxetine, pioglitazone, repaglinide, risperidone, rosiglitazone, sildenafil (and other PDE-5 inhibitors), thioridazine, tricyclic antidepressants, venlafaxine, and other substrates of CYP2D6 or 3A4. Mesoridazine and thioridazine are generally contraindicated with strong CYP2D6 inhibitors. When used with strong CYP3A4 inhibitors, dosage adjustment/limits are recommended for sildenafil and other PDE-5 inhibitors; refer to individual monographs. Warfarin levels/effects may also be increased. High dosages of itraconazole or ketoconazole (>200 mg/day) are not recommended.

Serum levels of protease inhibitors may be altered during concurrent therapy. Ritonavir may increase serum concentrations of amprenavir, indinavir, or saquinavir. Delavirdine increases levels of lopinavir; dosing recommendations are not yet established. Serum concentrations of corticosteroids (eg, budesonide, dexamethasone, fluticasone, prednisone) may be increased by lopinavir/ritonavir, resulting in decreased serum cortisol, HPA axis suppression; concurrent use is not recommended.

Lopinavir/ritonavir solution contains alcohol, concurrent use with disulfiram or metronidazole should be avoided. May cause disulfiram-like reaction. Serum concentrations of meperidine's neuroexcitatory metabolite (normeperidine) are increased by ritonavir, which may increase the risk of CNS toxicity/seizures. Rifabutin and rifabutin metabolite serum concentrations may be increased by ritonavir; reduce rifabutin dose to 150 mg every other day. Tenofovir serum concentration/effects may be increased by lopinavir/ritonavir. Trazodone serum concentration/effects may be increased by lopinavir/ritonavir; use caution and reduce trazodone dose.

Decreased Effect: The levels/effects of ritonavir may be decreased by aminoglutethimide, carbamazepine, nafcillin, nevirapine, phenobarbital, phenytoin, rifamycins, and other CYP3A4 inducers. Concurrent use of rifampin is not recommended. Ritonavir may decrease the levels/effects of CYP2D6 prodrug substrates (eg, codeine, hydrocodone, oxycodone, tramadol). Non-nucleoside reverse transcriptase inhibitors (efavirenz, nevirapine) may decrease levels of lopinavir. To avoid incompatibility with didanosine, administer didanosine 1 hour before or 2 hours after lopinavir/ritonavir. Decreased levels of ethinyl estradiol may result from concurrent use (alternative contraception is recommended). Lopinavir/ritonavir may decrease levels of abacavir, atovaquone, or zidovudine. Voriconazole serum levels are reduced by ritonavir. Lopinavir/ritonavir may decrease the concentration and effect of amprenavir when administered as fosamprenavir.

Pharmacodynamics/Kinetics
Ritonavir: See Ritonavir monograph.
Lopinavir:
Protein binding: 98% to 99%; decreased with mild-to-moderate hepatic dysfunction
Metabolism: Hepatic via CYP3A; 13 metabolites identified
Half-life elimination: 5-6 hours
Time to peak, plasma: ~4 hours
Excretion: Feces (83%, 20% as unchanged drug); urine (2%)

Pregnancy Risk Factor C

Lopremone *see* Protirelin *on page 1379*

Lopressor® *see* Metoprolol *on page 1088*

Lopressor HCT® *see* Metoprolol and Hydrochlorothiazide *on page 1090*

Loprox® *see* Ciclopirox *on page 354*

Lorabid® [DSC] *see* Loracarbef *on page 998*

Loracarbef (lor a KAR bef)

U.S. Brand Names Lorabid® [DSC]
Canadian Brand Names Lorabid®
Mexican Brand Names Carbac; Lorabid
Generic Available No
Pharmacologic Category Antibiotic, Carbacephem
Use Treatment of infections caused by susceptible organisms involving the upper and lower respiratory tract, uncomplicated skin and skin structure, and urinary tract (including uncomplicated pyelonephritis)
Local Anesthetic/Vasoconstrictor Precautions No information available to require special precautions
Effects on Dental Treatment No significant effects or complications reported

Common Adverse Effects

1% to 10%:

Central nervous system: Headache (1% to 3%), somnolence (<1% to 2%)

Dermatologic: Rash (1% to 3%)

Gastrointestinal: Diarrhea (4% to 6%), nausea (2% to 3%), vomiting (1% to 3%), anorexia (<1% to 2%), abdominal pain (1%)

Genitourinary: Vaginitis (1%), vaginal moniliasis (1%)

Respiratory: Rhinitis (2% to 6%)

Miscellaneous: Hypersensitivity reactions (1%; eg, urticaria, pruritus, erythema multiforme)

Other adverse reactions observed with beta-lactam antibiotics: Agranulocytosis, allergic reactions, aplastic anemia, hemolytic anemia, hemorrhage, interstitial nephritis, LDH increased, neutropenia, pancytopenia, positive direct Coombs' test, pseudomembranous colitis, seizure (with high doses and renal dysfunction), toxic epidermal necrolysis

Mechanism of Action Inhibits bacterial cell wall synthesis by binding to one or more of the penicillin binding proteins (PBPs); inhibits the final transpeptidation step of peptidoglycan synthesis in bacterial cell walls, thus inhibiting cell wall biosynthesis. It is thought that beta-lactam antibiotics inactivate transpeptidase via acylation of the enzyme with cleavage of the CO-N bond of the beta-lactam ring. Upon exposure to beta-lactam antibiotics, bacteria eventually lyse due to ongoing activity of cell wall autolytic enzymes (autolysins and murein hydrolases) while cell wall assembly is arrested.

Drug Interactions

Increased Effect/Toxicity: Loracarbef serum levels are increased with coadministered probenecid.

Pharmacodynamics/Kinetics

Absorption: Rapid

Protein binding: ~25%

Bioavailability: ~90%; decreased by food

Half-life elimination: ~1 hour

Time to peak, serum: ~1 hour

Excretion: Clearance: Plasma: ~200-300 mL/minute

Pregnancy Risk Factor B

Loratadine (lor AT a deen)

U.S. Brand Names Alavert® [OTC]; Claritin® 24 Hour Allergy [OTC]; Claritin® Hives Relief [OTC]; Tavist® ND [OTC]; Triaminic® Allerchews™ [OTC]

Canadian Brand Names Apo-Loratadine®; Claritin®; Claritin® Kids

Mexican Brand Names Analergal; Clarityne; Curyken; Lertamine; Lowadina; Sensibit

Generic Available Yes

Pharmacologic Category Antihistamine, Nonsedating

Use Relief of nasal and non-nasal symptoms of seasonal allergic rhinitis; treatment of chronic idiopathic urticaria

Local Anesthetic/Vasoconstrictor Precautions No information available to require special precautions

Effects on Dental Treatment Key adverse event(s) related to dental treatment: Xerostomia (normal salivary flow resumes upon discontinuation) and stomatitis in children (2-5 years).

Common Adverse Effects

Adults:

Central nervous system: Headache (12%), somnolence (8%), fatigue (4%)

Gastrointestinal: Xerostomia (3%)

Children:

Central nervous system: Nervousness (4% ages 6-12 years), fatigue (3% ages 6-12 years, 2% to 3% ages 2-5 years), malaise (2% ages 6-12 years)

Dermatologic: Rash (2% to 3% ages 2-5 years)

Gastrointestinal: Abdominal pain (2% ages 6-12 years), stomatitis (2% to 3% ages 2-5 years)

Neuromuscular & skeletal: Hyperkinesia (3% ages 6-12 years)

Ocular: Conjunctivitis (2% ages 6-12 years)

Respiratory: Wheezing (4% ages 6-12 years), dysphonia (2% ages 6-12 years), upper respiratory infection (2% ages 6-12 years), epistaxis (2% to 3% ages 2-5 years), pharyngitis (2% to 3% ages 2-5 years)

Miscellaneous: Flu-like syndrome (2% to 3% ages 2-5 years), viral infection (2% to 3% ages 2-5 years)

Mechanism of Action Long-acting tricyclic antihistamine with selective peripheral histamine H_1-receptor antagonistic properties

(Continued)

Loratadine *(Continued)*

Drug Interactions
Cytochrome P450 Effect: Substrate (minor) of CYP2D6, 3A4; **Inhibits** CYP2C8 (weak), 2C19 (moderate), 2D6 (weak)

Increased Effect/Toxicity: Increased toxicity with procarbazine, other anti-histamines. Protease inhibitors (amprenavir, ritonavir, nelfinavir) may increase the serum levels of loratadine. Loratadine may increase the levels/effects of citalopram, diazepam, methsuximide, phenytoin, propranolol, sertraline, and other CYP2C19 substrates.

Pharmacodynamics/Kinetics
Onset of action: 1-3 hours
Peak effect: 8-12 hours
Duration: >24 hours
Absorption: Rapid
Distribution: Significant amounts enter breast milk
Metabolism: Extensively hepatic via CYP2D6 and 3A4 to active metabolite
Half-life elimination: 12-15 hours
Excretion: Urine (40%) and feces (40%) as metabolites

Pregnancy Risk Factor B

Loratadine and Pseudoephedrine
(lor AT a deen & soo doe e FED rin)

Related Information
Bacterial Infections *on page 1793*
Loratadine *on page 999*
Pseudoephedrine *on page 1381*

U.S. Brand Names Alavert™ Allergy and Sinus [OTC]; Claritin-D® 12-Hour [OTC]; Claritin-D® 24-Hour [OTC]

Canadian Brand Names Chlor-Tripolon ND®; Claritin® Extra; Claritin® Liberator

Mexican Brand Names Clarityne D 24H; Clarityne D Pediatrico; Clarityne D Repetabs; Lertamine - D

Generic Available Yes

Index Terms Pseudoephedrine and Loratadine

Pharmacologic Category Antihistamine/Decongestant Combination

Use Temporary relief of symptoms of seasonal allergic rhinitis, other upper respiratory allergies, or the common cold

Local Anesthetic/Vasoconstrictor Precautions Use with caution since pseudoephedrine is a sympathomimetic amine which could interact with epinephrine to cause a pressor response

Effects on Dental Treatment Key adverse event(s) related to dental treatment: Pseudoephedrine: Xerostomia (normal salivary flow resumes upon discontinuation).

Common Adverse Effects See individual agents.

Dosage Children ≥12 years and Adults: Oral:
Claritin-D® 12-Hour: 1 tablet every 12 hours
Alavert™ Allergy and Sinus, Claritin-D® 24-Hour: 1 tablet daily

Dosage adjustment in renal impairment: Cl$_{cr}$ ≤30 mL/minute:
Claritin-D® 12-Hour: 1 tablet daily
Claritin-D® 24-Hour: 1 tablet every other day

Dosage adjustment in hepatic impairment: Should be avoided

Contraindications Hypersensitivity to loratadine, pseudoephedrine, or any component of the formulation; use with or within 14 days of MAO inhibitors

Warnings/Precautions Patients with renal impairment (Cl$_{cr}$ <30 mL/minute) should start with a lower dose since their ability to clear the drug will be reduced. Avoid use in hepatic dysfunction. Use with caution in lactation. Safety and efficacy in children <12 years of age have not been established. Use with caution in hypertension, diabetes mellitus, ischemic heart disease, increased intraocular pressure, hyperthyroidism, and prostatic hyperplasia. Do not take with MAO inhibitors and for 2 weeks after stopping MAO inhibitors. Patients with swallowing difficulties (eg, upper GI narrowing or abnormal esophageal peristalsis) should not use Claritin-D® 24-Hour.

Drug Interactions
Cytochrome P450 Effect: Loratadine: **Substrate** (minor) of CYP2D6, 3A4; **Inhibits** CYP2C8 (weak), 2C19 (moderate), 2D6 (weak)

Increased Effect/Toxicity: See individual agents.

Pharmacodynamics/Kinetics See individual agents.

Pregnancy Risk Factor B

Dosage Forms
Tablet, extended release: Loratadine 10 mg and pseudoephedrine 240 mg

Alavert™ Allergy and Sinus [OTC], Claritin-D® 12-hour [OTC]: Loratadine 5 mg and pseudoephedrine 120 mg

Claritin-D® 24-hour [OTC]: Loratadine 10 mg and pseudoephedrine 240 mg

Lorazepam (lor A ze pam)

Related Information
Sedation *on page 1825*
Temporomandibular Dysfunction (TMD) *on page 1822*
Related Sample Prescriptions
Sedation (Prior to Dental Treatment) *on page 1846*
U.S. Brand Names Ativan®; Lorazepam Intensol®
Canadian Brand Names Apo-Lorazepam®; Ativan®; Lorazepam Injection, USP; Novo-Lorazepam; Nu-Loraz; PMS-Lorazepam; Riva-Lorazepam
Mexican Brand Names Ativan
Generic Available Yes
Pharmacologic Category Benzodiazepine
Dental Use Short-term relief of anxiety prior to dental appointment
Use
Oral: Management of anxiety disorders or short-term relief of the symptoms of anxiety or anxiety associated with depressive symptoms
I.V.: Status epilepticus, preanesthesia for desired amnesia
Unlabeled/Investigational Use Ethanol detoxification; insomnia; psychogenic catatonia; partial complex seizures; agitation (I.V.); antiemetic adjunct
Local Anesthetic/Vasoconstrictor Precautions No information available to require special precautions
Effects on Dental Treatment Key adverse event(s) related to dental treatment: Xerostomia (normal salivary flow resumes upon discontinuation).
Significant Adverse Effects
>10%:
Central nervous system: Sedation
Respiratory: Respiratory depression
1% to 10%:
Cardiovascular: Hypotension
Central nervous system: Confusion, dizziness, akathisia, unsteadiness, headache, depression, disorientation, amnesia
Dermatologic: Dermatitis, rash
Gastrointestinal: Weight gain/loss, nausea, changes in appetite
Neuromuscular & skeletal: Weakness
Respiratory: Nasal congestion, hyperventilation, apnea
<1% (Limited to important or life-threatening): Menstrual irregularities, increased salivation, blood dyscrasias, reflex slowing, physical and psychological dependence with prolonged use, polyethylene glycol or propylene glycol poisoning (prolonged I.V. infusion)
Restrictions C-IV
Dental Usual Dosing
Anxiety and sedation: Adults: Oral: 1-10 mg/day in 2-3 divided doses; usual dose: 2-6 mg/day in divided doses
Preoperative: Adults:
I.M.: 0.05 mg/kg administered 2 hours before surgery (maximum: 4 mg/dose)
I.V.: 0.044 mg/kg 15-20 minutes before surgery (usual maximum: 2 mg/dose)
Preprocedural anxiety: Adults: Oral: 1-2 mg 1 hour before procedure
Dosage
Antiemetic (unlabeled use):
Children 2-15 years: I.V.: 0.05 mg/kg (up to 2 mg/dose) prior to chemotherapy
Adults: Oral, I.V. (**Note:** May be administered sublingually; not a labeled route): 0.5-2 mg every 4-6 hours as needed
Anxiety and sedation:
Infants and Children: Oral, I.M., I.V.: Usual: 0.05 mg/kg/dose (range: 0.02-0.09 mg/kg) every 4-8 hours
I.V.: May use smaller doses (eg, 0.01-0.03 mg/kg) and repeat every 20 minutes, as needed to titrate to effect
Adults: Oral: 1-10 mg/day in 2-3 divided doses; usual dose: 2-6 mg/day in divided doses
Elderly: 0.5-4 mg/day; initial dose not to exceed 2 mg
Insomnia: Adults: Oral: 2-4 mg at bedtime
Preoperative: Adults:
I.M.: 0.05 mg/kg administered 2 hours before surgery (maximum: 4 mg/dose)
I.V.: 0.044 mg/kg 15-20 minutes before surgery (usual maximum: 2 mg/dose)
Preprocedural anxiety (dental use): Adults: Oral: 1-2 mg 1 hour before procedure
Operative amnesia: Adults: I.V.: Up to 0.05 mg/kg (maximum: 4 mg/dose)
(Continued)

Lorazepam *(Continued)*

Sedation (preprocedure): Infants and Children:
Oral, I.M., I.V.: Usual: 0.05 mg/kg (range: 0.02-0.09 mg/kg)
  I.V.: May use smaller doses (eg, 0.01-0.03 mg/kg) and repeat every 20 minutes, as needed to titrate to effect

Status epilepticus: I.V.:
Infants and Children: 0.1 mg/kg slow I.V. over 2-5 minutes; do not exceed 4 mg/single dose; may repeat second dose of 0.05 mg/kg slow I.V. in 10-15 minutes if needed
Adolescents: 0.07 mg/kg slow I.V. over 2-5 minutes; maximum: 4 mg/dose; may repeat in 10-15 minutes
Adults: 4 mg/dose slow I.V. over 2-5 minutes; may repeat in 10-15 minutes; usual maximum dose: 8 mg

Rapid tranquilization of agitated patient (administer every 30-60 minutes):
Oral: 1-2 mg
I.M.: 0.5-1 mg
Average total dose for tranquilization: Oral, I.M.: 4-8 mg

Agitation in the ICU patient (unlabeled):
I.V.: 0.02-0.06 mg/kg every 2-6 hours
I.V. infusion: 0.01-0.1 mg/kg/hour
Concurrent use of probenecid or valproic acid: Reduce lorazepam dose by 50%

Dosage adjustment in renal impairment: I.V.: Risk of propylene glycol toxicity. Monitor closely if using for prolonged periods of time or at high doses.
Dosage adjustment in hepatic impairment: Use cautiously.

Mechanism of Action Binds to stereospecific benzodiazepine receptors on the postsynaptic GABA neuron at several sites within the central nervous system, including the limbic system, reticular formation. Enhancement of the inhibitory effect of GABA on neuronal excitability results by increased neuronal membrane permeability to chloride ions. This shift in chloride ions results in hyperpolarization (a less excitable state) and stabilization.

Contraindications Hypersensitivity to lorazepam or any component of the formulation (cross-sensitivity with other benzodiazepines may exist); acute narrow-angle glaucoma; sleep apnea (parenteral); intra-arterial injection of parenteral formulation; severe respiratory insufficiency (except during mechanical ventilation); pregnancy

Warnings/Precautions Causes CNS depression (dose-related) which may impair physical and mental capabilities. Use with caution in patients receiving other CNS depressants or psychoactive agents. Benzodiazepines have been associated with falls and traumatic injury and should be used with extreme caution in patients who are at risk of these events (especially the elderly). Use with caution in patients with a history of drug dependence.

Use with caution in elderly or debilitated patients, patients with hepatic disease (including alcoholics), renal impairment, respiratory disease, or impaired gag reflex. Use is not recommended in patients with depressive disorders or psychoses. Avoid use in patients with sleep apnea.

The parenteral formulation of lorazepam contains polyethylene glycol and propylene glycol. Also contains benzyl alcohol; avoid in neonates.

Benzodiazepines have been associated with anterograde amnesia. Paradoxical reactions, including hyperactive or aggressive behavior, have been reported with benzodiazepines, particularly in adolescent/pediatric or psychiatric patients. Does not have analgesic, antidepressant, or antipsychotic properties.

Drug Interactions
Clozapine: Benzodiazepines may enhance the adverse/toxic effect of Clozapine.
CNS depressants: Sedative effects and/or respiratory depression may be additive with CNS depressants; includes ethanol, barbiturates, opioid analgesics, and other sedative agents; monitor for increased effect
Loxapine: There are rare reports of significant respiratory depression, stupor, and/or hypotension with concomitant use of loxapine and lorazepam; use caution if concomitant administration of loxapine and CNS drugs is required
Theophylline: May partially antagonize some of the effects of benzodiazepines; monitor for decreased response; may require higher doses for sedation

Ethanol/Nutrition/Herb Interactions
Ethanol: Avoid or limit ethanol (may increase CNS depression).
Herb/Nutraceutical: Avoid valerian, St John's wort, kava kava, gotu kola (may increase CNS depression).

Pharmacodynamics/Kinetics
Onset of action:
Hypnosis: I.M.: 20-30 minutes
Sedation: I.V.: 5-20 minutes

Anticonvulsant: I.V.: 5 minutes, oral: 30-60 minutes
Duration: 6-8 hours
Absorption: Oral, I.M.: Prompt
Distribution:

V$_d$: Neonates: 0.76 L/kg, Adults: 1.3 L/kg; crosses placenta; enters breast milk
Protein binding: 85%; free fraction may be significantly higher in elderly
Metabolism: Hepatic to inactive compounds
Half-life elimination: Neonates: 40.2 hours; Older children: 10.5 hours; Adults: 12.9 hours; Elderly: 15.9 hours; End-stage renal disease: 32-70 hours
Excretion: Urine; feces (minimal)

Pregnancy Risk Factor D

Lactation Enters breast milk/contraindicated (AAP rates "of concern")

Breast-Feeding Considerations Crosses into breast milk and no data on clinical effects on the infant. AAP states MAY BE OF CONCERN.

Dosage Forms Excipient information presented when available (limited, particularly for generics); consult specific product labeling.
Injection, solution: 2 mg/mL (1 mL, 10 mL); 4 mg/mL (1 mL, 10 mL)
Ativan®: 2 mg/mL (1 mL, 10 mL); 4 mg/mL (1 mL, 10 mL) [contains benzyl alcohol and propylene glycol]
Solution, oral concentrate:
Lorazepam Intensol®: 2 mg/mL (30 mL) [alcohol free, dye free]
Tablet: 0.5 mg, 1 mg, 2 mg
Ativan®: 0.5 mg, 1 mg, 2 mg

Losartan (loe SAR tan)

Related Information
Cardiovascular Diseases on page 1726
U.S. Brand Names Cozaar®
Canadian Brand Names Cozaar®
Mexican Brand Names Cozaar
Generic Available No
Index Terms DuP 753; Losartan Potassium; MK594
Pharmacologic Category Angiotensin II Receptor Blocker
Use Treatment of hypertension (HTN); treatment of diabetic nephropathy in patients with type 2 diabetes mellitus (noninsulin dependent, NIDDM) and a history of hypertension; stroke risk reduction in patients with HTN and left ventricular hypertrophy (LVH)
Local Anesthetic/Vasoconstrictor Precautions No information available to require special precautions
Effects on Dental Treatment Key adverse event(s) related to dental treatment: Orthostatic hypotension.
Common Adverse Effects
>10%:
Cardiovascular: Chest pain (12% diabetic nephropathy)
Central nervous system: Fatigue (14% diabetic nephropathy)
Endocrine: Hypoglycemia (14% diabetic nephropathy)
Gastrointestinal: Diarrhea (2% hypertension to 15% diabetic nephropathy)
Genitourinary: Urinary tract infection (13% diabetic nephropathy)
Hematologic: Anemia (14% diabetic nephropathy)
Neuromuscular & skeletal: Weakness (14% diabetic nephropathy), back pain (2% hypertension to 12% diabetic nephropathy)
Respiratory: Cough (≤3% to 11%; similar to placebo; incidence higher in patients with previous cough related to ACE inhibitor therapy)
1% to 10%:
Cardiovascular: Hypotension (7% diabetic nephropathy), orthostatic hypotension (4% hypertension to 4% diabetic nephropathy), first-dose hypotension (dose related: <1% with 50 mg, 2% with 100 mg)
Central nervous system: Dizziness (4%), hypoesthesia (5% diabetic nephropathy), fever (4% diabetic nephropathy), insomnia (1%)
Dermatology: Cellulitis (7% diabetic nephropathy)
Endocrine: Hyperkalemia (<1% hypertension to 7% diabetic nephropathy)
Gastrointestinal: Gastritis (5% diabetic nephropathy), weight gain (4% diabetic nephropathy), dyspepsia (1% to 4%), abdominal pain (2%), nausea (2%)
(Continued)

Losartan *(Continued)*

Neuromuscular & skeletal: Muscular weakness (7% diabetic nephropathy), knee pain (5% diabetic nephropathy), leg pain (1% to 5%), muscle cramps (1%), myalgia (1%)

Respiratory: Bronchitis (10% diabetic nephropathy), upper respiratory infection (8%), nasal congestion (2%), sinusitis (1% hypertension to 6% diabetic nephropathy)

Miscellaneous: Infection (5% diabetic nephropathy), flu-like syndrome (10% diabetic nephropathy)

Dosage Oral:

Hypertension:

Children 6-16 years: 0.7 mg/kg once daily (maximum: 50 mg/day); adjust dose based on response; doses >1.4 mg/kg (maximum: 100 mg) have not been studied

Adults: Usual starting dose: 50 mg once daily; can be administered once or twice daily with total daily doses ranging from 25-100 mg

Patients receiving diuretics or with intravascular volume depletion: Usual initial dose: 25 mg

Nephropathy in patients with type 2 diabetes and hypertension: Adults: Initial: 50 mg once daily; can be increased to 100 mg once daily based on blood pressure response

Stroke reduction (HTN with LVH): Adults: 50 mg once daily (maximum daily dose: 100 mg); may be used in combination with a thiazide diuretic

Dosing adjustment in renal impairment:

Children: Use is not recommended if Cl$_{cr}$ <30 mL/minute.

Adults: No adjustment necessary.

Dosing adjustment in hepatic impairment: Reduce the initial dose to 25 mg/day; divide dosage intervals into two.

Mechanism of Action As a selective and competitive, nonpeptide angiotensin II receptor antagonist, losartan blocks the vasoconstrictor and aldosterone-secreting effects of angiotensin II; losartan interacts reversibly at the AT1 and AT2 receptors of many tissues and has slow dissociation kinetics; its affinity for the AT1 receptor is 1000 times greater than the AT2 receptor. Angiotensin II receptor antagonists may induce a more complete inhibition of the renin-angiotensin system than ACE inhibitors, they do not affect the response to bradykinin, and are less likely to be associated with nonrenin-angiotensin effects (eg, cough and angioedema). Losartan increases urinary flow rate and in addition to being natriuretic and kaliuretic, increases excretion of chloride, magnesium, uric acid, calcium, and phosphate.

Contraindications Hypersensitivity to losartan or any component of the formulation; hypersensitivity to other A-II receptor antagonists; bilateral renal artery stenosis; pregnancy

Warnings/Precautions [U.S. Boxed Warning]: **Based on human data, drugs that act on the angiotensin system can cause injury and death to the developing fetus when used in the second and third trimesters. Angiotensin receptor blockers should be discontinued as soon as possible once pregnancy is detected.** Avoid use or use a much smaller dose in patients who are volume-depleted; correct depletion first. Use with caution in patients with pre-existing renal insufficiency or significant aortic/mitral stenosis. May cause hyperkalemia; avoid potassium supplementation unless specifically required by healthcare provider. May be associated with deterioration of renal function and/or increases in serum creatinine, particularly in patients dependent on renin-angiotensin-aldosterone system. Use caution in patients with unilateral or bilateral renal artery stenosis to avoid a decrease in renal function. AUCs of losartan (not the active metabolite) are about 50% greater in patients with Cl$_{cr}$ <30 mL/minute and are doubled in hemodialysis patients. When used to reduce the risk of stroke in patients with HTN and LVH, may not be effective in African-American population. Use caution with hepatic dysfunction, dose adjustment may be needed. Safety and efficacy have not been established in children <6 years of age.

Drug Interactions

Cytochrome P450 Effect: Substrate (major) of CYP2C9, 3A4; **Inhibits** CYP1A2 (weak), 2C8 (moderate), 2C9 (moderate), 2C19 (weak), 3A4 (weak)

Increased Effect/Toxicity: Cimetidine may increase the absorption of losartan by 18% (clinical effect is unknown). Potassium salts/supplements, co-trimoxazole (high dose), ACE inhibitors, and potassium-sparing diuretics (amiloride, spironolactone, triamterene) may increase the risk of hyperkalemia. Risk of lithium toxicity may be increased by losartan. Losartan may increase the levels/effects of amiodarone, bosentan, dapsone, fluoxetine, glimepiride, glipizide, montelukast, nateglinide, paclitaxel, phenytoin, pioglitazone, repaglinide, rosiglitazone, warfarin, zafirlukast, and other CYP2C8 or 2C9 substrates. Fluconazole may increase the levels/effects of losartan.

Decreased Effect: The levels/effects of losartan may be decreased by amino-glutethimide, carbamazepine, nafcillin, nevirapine, phenobarbital, phenytoin, rifampin, rifapentine, secobarbital, and other CYP2C9 or 3A4 inducers. NSAIDs may decrease the efficacy of losartan.

Ethanol/Nutrition/Herb Interactions Herb/Nutraceutical: St John's wort may decrease levels. Avoid dong quai if using for hypertension (has estrogenic activity). Avoid ephedra, yohimbe, ginseng (may worsen hypertension). Avoid garlic (may have increased antihypertensive effect).

Dietary Considerations May be taken with or without food.

Pharmacodynamics/Kinetics

Onset of action: 6 hours

Distribution: V_d: Losartan: 34 L; E-3174: 12 L; does not cross blood brain barrier

Protein binding, plasma: High

Metabolism: Hepatic (14%) via CYP2C9 and 3A4 to active metabolite, E-3174 (40 times more potent than losartan); extensive first-pass effect

Bioavailability: 25% to 33%; AUC of E-3174 is four times greater than that of losartan

Half-life elimination: Losartan: 1.5-2 hours; E-3174: 6-9 hours

Time to peak, serum: Losartan: 1 hour; E-3174: 3-4 hours

Excretion: Urine (4% as unchanged drug, 6% as active metabolite)

Clearance: Plasma: Losartan: 600 mL/minute; Active metabolite: 50 mL/minute

Pregnancy Risk Factor C/D (2nd and 3rd trimesters)

Dosage Forms

Tablet:

Cozaar®: 25 mg, 50 mg, 100 mg

Losartan and Hydrochlorothiazide

(loe SAR tan & hye droe klor oh THYE a zide)

Related Information

Hydrochlorothiazide on page 819

Losartan on page 1003

U.S. Brand Names Hyzaar®

Canadian Brand Names Hyzaar®; Hyzaar® DS

Mexican Brand Names Hyzaar

Generic Available No

Index Terms Hydrochlorothiazide and Losartan

Pharmacologic Category Angiotensin II Receptor Blocker Combination; Antihypertensive Agent, Combination; Diuretic, Thiazide

Use Treatment of hypertension; stroke risk reduction in patients with HTN and left ventricular hypertrophy (LVH)

Local Anesthetic/Vasoconstrictor Precautions No information available to require special precautions

Effects on Dental Treatment No significant effects or complications reported

Common Adverse Effects Based on clinical trials of the combination product in patients with essential hypertension. Also see individual agents.

1% to 10%:

Cardiovascular: Edema (1%), palpitation (1%)

Central nervous system: Dizziness (6%)

Dermatologic: Skin rash (1%)

Gastrointestinal: Abdominal pain (1%)

Neuromuscular & skeletal: Back pain (2%)

Respiratory: Upper respiratory infection (6%), cough (3%), sinusitis (1%)

Dosage

Oral: Adults: Dose is individualized (combination substituted for individual components); dose may be titrated after 2-4 weeks of therapy

Hypertension/stroke reduction in hypertension (with LVH): Usual recommended starting dose of losartan: 50 mg once daily when used as monotherapy in patients who are not volume depleted

Dosage adjustment in renal impairment: Cl_{cr} ≤30 mL/minute: Use of combination formulation not recommended

Dosage adjustment in hepatic impairment: Use is not recommended

Contraindications

Hypersensitivity to hydrochlorothiazide, thiazides, sulfonamide-derived drugs, losartan, or any component of the formulation; hypersensitivity to other A-II receptor antagonists; bilateral renal artery stenosis, anuria, renal decompensation; pregnancy

Warnings/Precautions See individual agents.

(Continued)

Losartan and Hydrochlorothiazide *(Continued)*

Drug Interactions

Cytochrome P450 Effect: Losartan: **Substrate** (major) of CYP2C9, 3A4; **Inhibits** CYP1A2 (weak), 2C8 (moderate), 2C9 (moderate), 2C19 (weak), 3A4 (weak)

Increased Effect/Toxicity: See individual agents.

Pharmacodynamics/Kinetics See individual agents.

Pregnancy Risk Factor C/D (2nd and 3rd trimesters)

Dosage Forms

Tablet:

Hyzaar®: 50-12.5: Losartan 50 mg and hydrochlorothiazide 12.5 mg; 100-12.5: Losartan 100 mg and hydrochlorothiazide 12.5 mg; 100-25: Losartan 100 mg and hydrochlorothiazide 25 mg

Losartan Potassium *see* Losartan *on page 1003*

Lotemax® *see* Loteprednol *on page 1006*

Lotensin® *see* Benazepril *on page 191*

Lotensin® HCT *see* Benazepril and Hydrochlorothiazide *on page 193*

Loteprednol (loe te PRED nol)

U.S. Brand Names Alrex®; Lotemax®

Canadian Brand Names Alrex®; Lotemax®

Mexican Brand Names Loterex

Generic Available No

Index Terms Loteprednol Etabonate

Pharmacologic Category Corticosteroid, Ophthalmic

Use

Suspension, 0.2% (Alrex®): Temporary relief of signs and symptoms of seasonal allergic conjunctivitis

Suspension, 0.5% (Lotemax®): Inflammatory conditions (treatment of steroid-responsive inflammatory conditions of the palpebral and bulbar conjunctiva, cornea, and anterior segment of the globe such as allergic conjunctivitis, acne rosacea, superficial punctate keratitis, herpes zoster keratitis, iritis, cyclitis, selected infective conjunctivitis, when the inherent hazard of steroid use is accepted to obtain an advisable diminution in edema and inflammation) and treatment of postoperative inflammation following ocular surgery

Local Anesthetic/Vasoconstrictor Precautions No information available to require special precautions

Effects on Dental Treatment No significant effects or complications reported

Mechanism of Action Corticosteroids inhibit the inflammatory response including edema, capillary dilation, leukocyte migration, and scar formation. Loteprednol is highly lipid soluble and penetrates cells readily to induce the production of lipocortins. These proteins modulate the activity of prostaglandins and leukotrienes.

Pregnancy Risk Factor C

Loteprednol and Tobramycin (loe te PRED nol & toe bra MYE sin)

U.S. Brand Names Zylet™

Generic Available No

Index Terms Loteprednol Etabonate and Tobramycin; Tobramycin and Loteprednol Etabonate

Pharmacologic Category Antibiotic/Corticosteroid, Ophthalmic

Use Treatment of steroid-responsive ocular inflammatory conditions where either a superficial bacterial ocular infection or the risk of a superficial bacterial ocular infection exists

Local Anesthetic/Vasoconstrictor Precautions No information available to require special precautions

Effects on Dental Treatment No significant effects or complications reported

Mechanism of Action See individual agents.

Pregnancy Risk Factor C

Loteprednol Etabonate *see* Loteprednol *on page 1006*

Loteprednol Etabonate and Tobramycin *see* Loteprednol and Tobramycin *on page 1006*

Lotrel® *see* Amlodipine and Benazepril *on page 104*

Lotrimin® AF Athlete's Foot Cream [OTC] *see* Clotrimazole *on page 398*

Lotrimin® AF Athlete's Foot Solution [OTC] *see* Clotrimazole *on page 398*

Lotrimin® AF Jock Itch Cream [OTC] *see* Clotrimazole *on page 398*

Lovastatin (LOE va sta tin)

Related Information
Cardiovascular Diseases *on page 1726*

U.S. Brand Names Altoprev®; Mevacor®

Canadian Brand Names Apo-Lovastatin®; CO Lovastatin; Gen-Lovastatin; Mevacor®; Novo-Lovastatin; Nu-Lovastatin; PMS-Lovastatin; RAN™-Lovastatin; ratio-Lovastatin; Riva-Lovastatin; Sandoz-Lovastatin

Mexican Brand Names Mevacor

Generic Available Yes: Immediate release tablet

Index Terms Mevinolin; Monacolin K

Pharmacologic Category Antilipemic Agent, HMG-CoA Reductase Inhibitor

Use

Adjunct to dietary therapy to decrease elevated serum total and LDL-cholesterol concentrations in primary hypercholesterolemia

Primary prevention of coronary artery disease (patients without symptomatic disease with average to moderately elevated total and LDL-cholesterol and below average HDL-cholesterol); slow progression of coronary atherosclerosis in patients with coronary heart disease

Adjunct to dietary therapy in adolescent patients (10-17 years of age, females >1 year postmenarche) with heterozygous familial hypercholesterolemia having LDL >189 mg/dL, **or** LDL >160 mg/dL with positive family history of premature cardiovascular disease (CVD), **or** LDL >160 mg/dL with the presence of at least two other CVD risk factors

Local Anesthetic/Vasoconstrictor Precautions No information available to require special precautions

Effects on Dental Treatment No significant effects or complications reported

Common Adverse Effects Percentages as reported with immediate release tablets; similar adverse reactions seen with extended release tablets.

>10%: Neuromuscular & skeletal: Increased CPK (>2x normal) (11%)

1% to 10%:

Central nervous system: Headache (2% to 3%), dizziness (0.5% to 1%)

Dermatologic: Rash (0.8% to 1%)

Gastrointestinal: Abdominal pain (2% to 3%), constipation (2% to 4%), diarrhea (2% to 3%), dyspepsia (1% to 2%), flatulence (4% to 5%), nausea (2% to 3%)

Neuromuscular & skeletal: Myalgia (2% to 3%), weakness (1% to 2%), muscle cramps (0.6% to 1%)

Ocular: Blurred vision (0.8% to 1%)

Dosage Oral:

Adolescents 10-17 years: Immediate release tablet:

LDL reduction <20%: Initial: 10 mg/day with evening meal

LDL reduction ≥20%: Initial: 20 mg/day with evening meal

Usual range: 10-40 mg with evening meal, then adjust dose at 4-week intervals

Adults: Initial: 20 mg with evening meal, then adjust at 4-week intervals; maximum dose: 80 mg/day immediate release tablet **or** 60 mg/day extended release tablet

Dosage modification/limits based on concurrent therapy:

Cyclosporine and other immunosuppressant drugs: Initial dose: 10 mg/day with a maximum recommended dose of 20 mg/day

Concurrent therapy with fibrates, danazol, and/or lipid-lowering doses of niacin (>1 g/day): Maximum recommended dose: 20 mg/day. Concurrent use with fibrates should be avoided unless risk to benefit favors use.

Concurrent therapy with amiodarone or verapamil: Maximum recommended dose: 40 mg/day of regular release or 20 mg/day with extended release.

Dosage adjustment in renal impairment: Cl_{cr} <30 mL/minute: Use doses >20 mg/day with caution.

Mechanism of Action Lovastatin acts by competitively inhibiting 3-hydroxyl-3-methylglutaryl-coenzyme A (HMG-CoA) reductase, the enzyme that catalyzes the rate-limiting step in cholesterol biosynthesis

Contraindications Hypersensitivity to lovastatin or any component of the formulation; active liver disease; unexplained persistent elevations of serum transaminases; pregnancy; breast-feeding

Warnings/Precautions Secondary causes of hyperlipidemia should be ruled out prior to therapy. Liver function must be monitored by periodic laboratory (Continued)

Lovastatin *(Continued)*

assessment. Rhabdomyolysis with or without acute renal failure has occurred. Risk is dose-related and is increased with concurrent use of lipid-lowering agents which may cause rhabdomyolysis (gemfibrozil, fibric acid derivatives, or niacin at doses ≥1 g/day) or during concurrent use with potent CYP3A4 inhibitors. Avoid concurrent use of azole antifungals, macrolide antibiotics, and protease inhibitors. Use caution/limit dose with amiodarone, cyclosporine, danazol, gemfibrozil (or other fibrates), lipid-lowering doses of niacin, or verapamil. Patients should be instructed to report unexplained muscle pain or weakness; lovastatin should be discontinued if myopathy is suspected/confirmed. Temporarily discontinue in any patient experiencing an acute or serious condition predisposing to renal failure secondary to rhabdomyolysis. Use with caution in patients with advanced age, these patients are predisposed to myopathy. Use with caution in patients who consume large amounts of ethanol or have a history of liver disease. Safety and efficacy of the immediate release tablet have not been evaluated in prepubertal patients, patients <10 years of age, or doses >40 mg/day in appropriately-selected adolescents; extended release tablets have not been studied in patients <20 years of age.

Drug Interactions

Cytochrome P450 Effect: Substrate of CYP3A4 (major); **Inhibits** CYP2C9 (weak), 2D6 (weak), 3A4 (weak)

Increased Effect/Toxicity: CYP3A4 inhibitors may increase the levels/effects of lovastatin; example inhibitors include azole antifungals, clarithromycin, diclofenac, doxycycline, erythromycin, imatinib, isoniazid, nefazodone, nicardipine, propofol, protease inhibitors, quinidine, telithromycin, and verapamil. Suspend lovastatin therapy during concurrent clarithromycin, erythromycin, itraconazole, or ketoconazole therapy. Concurrent use of danazol may increase risk of myopathy (limit dose of lovastatin). Cyclosporine, clofibrate, diltiazem, fenofibrate, gemfibrozil, and niacin also may increase the risk of myopathy and rhabdomyolysis. The effect/toxicity of warfarin (elevated PT) and levothyroxine may be increased by lovastatin. Digoxin, norethindrone, and ethinyl estradiol levels may be increased. Effects are additive with other lipid-lowering therapies.

Decreased Effect: Cholestyramine taken with lovastatin reduces lovastatin absorption and effect.

Ethanol/Nutrition/Herb Interactions

Ethanol: Avoid excessive ethanol consumption (due to potential hepatic effects).

Food: Food **decreases** the bioavailability of lovastatin extended release tablets and **increases** the bioavailability of lovastatin immediate release tablets. Lovastatin serum concentrations may be increased if taken with grapefruit juice; avoid concurrent intake of large quantities (>1 quart/day). Red yeast rice contains an estimated 2.4 mg lovastatin per 600 mg rice.

Herb/Nutraceutical: St John's wort may decrease lovastatin levels.

Dietary Considerations Before initiation of therapy, patients should be placed on a standard cholesterol-lowering diet for 6 weeks and the diet should be continued during drug therapy. Avoid intake of large quantities of grapefruit juice (≥1 quart/day); may increase toxicity. Red yeast rice contains an estimated 2.4 mg lovastatin per 600 mg rice.

Pharmacodynamics/Kinetics

Onset of action: LDL-cholesterol reductions: 3 days

Absorption: 30%; increased with extended release tablets when taken in the fasting state

Protein binding: 95%

Metabolism: Hepatic; extensive first-pass effect; hydrolyzed to B-hydroxy acid (active)

Bioavailability: Increased with extended release tablets

Half-life elimination: 1.1-1.7 hours

Time to peak, serum: 2-4 hours

Excretion: Feces (~80% to 85%); urine (10%)

Pregnancy Risk Factor X

Dosage Forms

Tablet: 10 mg, 20 mg, 40 mg

Mevacor®: 20 mg, 40 mg

Tablet, extended release:

Altoprev®: 20 mg, 40 mg, 60 mg

Lovastatin and Niacin *see* Niacin and Lovastatin *on page 1167*

Lovenox® *see* Enoxaparin *on page 568*

Low-Ogestrel® *see* Ethinyl Estradiol and Norgestrel *on page 649*

Loxapine (LOKS a peen)

U.S. Brand Names Loxitane®
Canadian Brand Names Apo-Loxapine®; Loxapac® IM; Nu-Loxapine; PMS-Loxapine
Generic Available Yes
Index Terms Loxapine Succinate; Oxilapine Succinate
Pharmacologic Category Antipsychotic Agent, Typical
Use Management of psychotic disorders

Local Anesthetic/Vasoconstrictor Precautions Most pharmacology textbooks state that in presence of phenothiazines, systemic doses of epinephrine paradoxically decrease the taking blood pressure. This is the so called "epinephrine reversal" phenomenon. This has never been observed when epinephrine is given by infiltration as part of the anesthesia procedure. Loxapine is one of the drugs confirmed to prolong the QT interval and is accepted as having a risk of causing torsade de pointes. The risk of drug-induced torsade de pointes is extremely low when a single QT interval prolonging drug is prescribed. In terms of epinephrine, it is not known what effect vasoconstrictors in the local anesthetic regimen will have in patients with a known history of congenital prolonged QT interval or in patients taking any medication that prolongs the QT interval. Until more information is obtained, it is suggested that the clinician consult with the physician prior to the use of a vasoconstrictor in suspected patients, and that the vasoconstrictor (epinephrine, levonordefrin [Neo-Cobefrin®]) be used with caution.

Effects on Dental Treatment Key adverse event(s) related to dental treatment:

Xerostomia and changes in salivation (normal salivary flow resumes upon discontinuation).

Significant hypotension may occur, especially when the drug is administered parenterally; orthostatic hypotension is due to alpha-receptor blockade, the elderly are at greater risk for orthostatic hypotension.

Tardive dyskinesia: Prevalence rate may be 40% in elderly; development of the syndrome and the irreversible nature are proportional to duration and total cumulative dose over time. Extrapyramidal reactions are more common in elderly with up to 50% developing these reactions after 60 years of age. Drug-induced Parkinson's syndrome occurs often; akathisia is the most common extrapyramidal reaction in elderly.

Increased confusion, memory loss, psychotic behavior, and agitation frequently occur as a consequence of anticholinergic effects. Antipsychotic associated sedation in nonpsychotic patients is extremely unpleasant due to feelings of depersonalization, derealization, and dysphoria.

Common Adverse Effects Frequency not defined.

Cardiovascular: Abnormal T waves with prolonged ventricular repolarization, arrhythmia, hyper-/hypotension, orthostatic hypotension, tachycardia, syncope

Central nervous system: Agitation, altered central temperature regulation, ataxia, confusion, dizziness, drowsiness, extrapyramidal reactions (akathisia, akinesia, dystonia, pseudoparkinsonism, tardive dyskinesia), faintness, headache, insomnia, lightheadedness, neuroleptic malignant syndrome (NMS), seizure, slurred speech, tension

Dermatologic: Alopecia, dermatitis, photosensitivity, pruritus, rash, seborrhea

Endocrine & metabolic: Amenorrhea, enlargement of breasts, galactorrhea, gynecomastia, menstrual irregularity

Gastrointestinal: Adynamic ileus, constipation, nausea, polydipsia, vomiting, weight gain/loss, xerostomia

Genitourinary: Sexual dysfunction, urinary retention

Hematologic: Agranulocytosis, leukopenia, thrombocytopenia

Neuromuscular & skeletal: Weakness

Ocular: Blurred vision

Respiratory: Nasal congestion

Mechanism of Action Loxapine is a dibenzoxazepine antipsychotic which blocks postsynaptic mesolimbic D_1 and D_2 receptors in the brain, and also possesses serotonin 5-HT$_2$ blocking activity

Drug Interactions

Increased Effect/Toxicity: Loxapine concentrations may be increased by chloroquine, propranolol, sulfadoxine-pyrimethamine. Loxapine may increased the effect and/or toxicity of antihypertensives, lithium, TCAs, CNS depressants (ethanol, narcotics), and trazodone. There are rare reports of significant respiratory depression, stupor, and/or hypotension with the concomitant use of loxapine and lorazepam. Use caution if the concomitant administration of loxapine and CNS drugs is required. Metoclopramide may
(Continued)

Loxapine *(Continued)*

increase risk of extrapyramidal symptoms (EPS). Acetylcholinesterase inhibitors (central) may increase the risk of antipsychotic-related EPS. Effects on QT_c interval may be additive with antipsychotics, increasing the risk of malignant arrhythmias; other QT_c-prolonging agents include type Ia antiarrhythmics, TCAs, and some quinolone antibiotics (sparfloxacin, moxifloxacin and gatifloxacin). Concomitant use with thioridazine is contraindicated.

Decreased Effect: Antipsychotics inhibit the activity of bromocriptine and levodopa. Benztropine (and other anticholinergics) may inhibit the therapeutic response to loxapine and excess anticholinergic effects may occur. Loxapine and possibly other low potency antpsychotic may reverse the pressor effects of epinephrine.

Pharmacodynamics/Kinetics
Onset of action: Neuroleptic: Oral: 20-30 minutes
  Peak effect: 1.5-3 hours
Duration: ~12 hours
Metabolism: Hepatic to glucuronide conjugates
Half-life elimination: Biphasic: Initial: 5 hours; Terminal: 12-19 hours
Excretion: Urine; feces (small amounts)

Pregnancy Risk Factor C

Loxapine Succinate *see* Loxapine *on page 1009*

Loxitane® *see* Loxapine *on page 1009*

Lozi-Flur™ *see* Fluoride *on page 710*

Lozol® [DSC] *see* Indapamide *on page 874*

L-PAM *see* Melphalan *on page 1034*

LRH *see* Gonadorelin *on page 792*

L-Sarcolysin *see* Melphalan *on page 1034*

LTA® 360 *see* Lidocaine *on page 972*

LTG *see* Lamotrigine *on page 945*

Lu-26-054 *see* Escitalopram *on page 596*

Lubiprostone *(loo bi PROS tone)*

U.S. Brand Names Amitiza™
Generic Available No
Index Terms RU 0211; SPI 0211
Pharmacologic Category Gastrointestinal Agent, Miscellaneous
Use Treatment of chronic idiopathic constipation
Local Anesthetic/Vasoconstrictor Precautions No information available to require special precautions
Effects on Dental Treatment Key adverse event(s) related to dental treatment: Xerostomia (normal salivary flow resumes upon discontinuation).
Common Adverse Effects
>10%:
  Central nervous system: Headache (13%)
  Gastrointestinal: Nausea (31%; dose related), diarrhea (13%; severe 3%)
1% to 10%:
  Cardiovascular: Peripheral edema (4%), chest discomfort (2%), chest pain (1%), hypertension (1%)
  Central nervous system: Dizziness (4%), fatigue (2%), fever (1%), depression (1%), anxiety (1%), insomnia (1%)
  Gastrointestinal: Abdominal distention (7%), abdominal pain (7%), flatulence (6%), vomiting (5%), loose stools (3%), dyspepsia (3%), gastroesophageal reflux disease (2%), xerostomia (2%), weight gain (1%)
  Neuromuscular & skeletal: Arthralgia (3%), back pain (2%), muscle cramp (1%)
  Renal: Urinary tract infection (4%)
  Respiratory: Sinusitis (5%), upper respiratory tract infection (4%), nasopharyngitis (3%), bronchitis (2%), dyspnea (2%), cough (2%)
  Miscellaneous: Influenza (2%)
Mechanism of Action Bicyclic fatty acid that acts locally at the apical portion of the intestine as a chloride channel activator, increasing intestinal water secretion.
Pharmacodynamics/Kinetics
Absorption: Systemic: Parent drug: Poor (below levels of detection); Active metabolite (M3): Low
Distribution: Gastrointestinal tissue
Metabolism: Within stomach and jejunum by carbonyl reductase to M3 (active metabolite) and others
Bioavailability: Minimal

Half-life elimination: M3: 0.9-1.4 hours
Excretion: M3: Feces (trace amounts)
Pregnancy Risk Factor C

Lubriderm® [OTC] *see* Lanolin, Cetyl Alcohol, Glycerin, Petrolatum, and Mineral Oil *on page 946*

Lubriderm® Fragrance Free [OTC] *see* Lanolin, Cetyl Alcohol, Glycerin, Petrolatum, and Mineral Oil *on page 946*

Lucentis® *see* Ranibizumab *on page 1408*

Ludiomil *see* Maprotiline *on page 1018*

Lufyllin® *see* Dyphylline *on page 553*

Lugol's Solution *see* Potassium Iodide and Iodine *on page 1331*

Lumigan® *see* Bimatoprost *on page 215*

Luminal® Sodium *see* Phenobarbital *on page 1288*

Lumitene™ *see* Beta-Carotene *on page 205*

Lunesta™ *see* Eszopiclone *on page 616*

LupiCare™ II Psoriasis [OTC] *see* Salicylic Acid *on page 1451*

LupiCare™ Dandruff [OTC] *see* Salicylic Acid *on page 1451*

LupiCare™ Psoriasis [OTC] *see* Salicylic Acid *on page 1451*

Lupron® *see* Leuprolide *on page 958*

Lupron Depot® *see* Leuprolide *on page 958*

Lupron Depot-Ped® *see* Leuprolide *on page 958*

Luride® *see* Fluoride *on page 710*

Luride® Lozi-Tab® *see* Fluoride *on page 710*

LuSonal™ *see* Phenylephrine *on page 1293*

Lustra® *see* Hydroquinone *on page 841*

Lustra-AF™ *see* Hydroquinone *on page 841*

Luteinizing Hormone Releasing Hormone *see* Gonadorelin *on page 792*

Lutera™ *see* Ethinyl Estradiol and Levonorgestrel *on page 633*

Lutropin Alfa (LOO troe pin AL fa)

U.S. Brand Names Luveris®
Mexican Brand Names Luver-I.S.
Generic Available No
Index Terms Recombinant Human Luteinizing Hormone; r-hLH
Pharmacologic Category Gonadotropin; Ovulation Stimulator
Use Stimulation of follicular development in infertile hypogonadotropic hypogonadal (HH) women with profound luteinizing hormone (LH) deficiency; to be used in combination with follitropin alfa
Local Anesthetic/Vasoconstrictor Precautions No information available to require special precautions
Effects on Dental Treatment No significant effects or complications reported
Common Adverse Effects
1% to 10%:
Central nervous system: Headache (10%), fatigue (2% to 3%)
Endocrine & metabolic: Ovarian hyperstimulation (6%)
Gastrointestinal: Nausea (7%), constipation (2% to 3%), diarrhea (2% to 3%)
Adverse events reported with gonadotropin or menotropin therapy: Adnexal torsion, arterial thromboembolism, congenital abnormalities, ectopic pregnancy, hemoperitoneum, ovarian enlargement (mild-to-moderate), ovarian neoplasms (infrequent), postpartum fever, premature labor, pulmonary complications, spontaneous abortion, vascular complications
Mechanism of Action Lutropin alfa is a recombinant luteinizing hormone prepared using Chinese hamster cell ovaries. Administration leads to increased follicular estradiol secretion needed for follicle stimulating hormone induced follicular development.
Pharmacodynamics/Kinetics
Distribution: V_d: 10
Bioavailability: 56% ± 23%
Half-life elimination: Terminal: ~18 hours
Time to peak, serum: 4-16 hours
Excretion: Urine (<5% unchanged)
Pregnancy Risk Factor X

Luveris® *see* Lutropin Alfa *on page 1011*

Luvox *see* Fluvoxamine *on page 734*

Luxiq® *see* Betamethasone *on page 206*

LY139603 *see* Atomoxetine *on page 160*

LY146032 *see* Daptomycin *on page 443*

L-Lysine (el LYE seen)

U.S. Brand Names Lysinyl [OTC]
Generic Available Yes
Index Terms L-Lysine Hydrochloride
Pharmacologic Category Nutritional Supplement
Dental Use Prevention of recurrent herpes simplex infection
Use Improves utilization of vegetable proteins
Local Anesthetic/Vasoconstrictor Precautions No information available to require special precautions
Effects on Dental Treatment No significant effects or complications reported
Dental Usual Dosing Recurrent herpes simplex infection: Adults: Oral: 2000 mg every 4 hours until symptoms subside. Begin treatment during early stage of recurrence.
Dosage
Oral:
Adults: 334-1500 mg/day

Recurrent herpes simplex infection (dental use): 2000 mg every 4 hours until symptoms subside. Begin treatment during early stage of recurrence.
Pregnancy Risk Factor C
Dosage Forms Excipient information presented when available (limited, particularly for generics); consult specific product labeling.
Capsule (Lysinyl): 500 mg
Tablet: 500 mg, 1000 mg

Mafenide (MA fe nide)

U.S. Brand Names Sulfamylon®
Generic Available No
Index Terms Mafenide Acetate
Pharmacologic Category Antibiotic, Topical
Use Cream: Adjunctive antibacterial agent in the treatment of second- and third-degree burns
Solution: Adjunctive antibacterial agent for use under moist dressings over meshed autografts on excised burn wounds
Local Anesthetic/Vasoconstrictor Precautions No information available to require special precautions
Effects on Dental Treatment No significant effects or complications reported
Mechanism of Action As a sulfonamide, mafenide interferes with bacterial folic acid synthesis through competitive inhibition of para-aminobenzoic acid. Spectrum of activity encompasses both gram positive and negative organisms, including *Pseudomonas* and some anaerobes.
Pregnancy Risk Factor C

Magaldrate and Simethicone (MAG al drate & sye METH i kone)

Related Information
Simethicone *on page 1472*

U.S. Brand Names Riopan Plus® [OTC] [DSC]; Riopan Plus® Double Strength [OTC] [DSC]

Generic Available Yes

Index Terms Simethicone and Magaldrate

Pharmacologic Category Antacid; Antiflatulent

Use Relief of hyperacidity associated with peptic ulcer, gastritis, peptic esophagitis and hiatal hernia which are accompanied by symptoms of gas

Local Anesthetic/Vasoconstrictor Precautions No information available to require special precautions

Effects on Dental Treatment Key adverse event(s) related to dental treatment: Chalky taste.

Common Adverse Effects Frequency not defined.
Based on **magaldrate** component:
Central nervous system: Encephalopathy
Gastrointestinal: Constipation, chalky taste, stomach cramps, fecal impaction, diarrhea, nausea, vomiting, discoloration of feces (white speckles), rebound hyperacidity
Endocrine & metabolic: Hypophosphatemia, hypermagnesemia, milk-alkali syndrome
Neuromuscular & metabolic: Osteomalacia
Miscellaneous: Aluminum intoxication
Based on **simethicone** component: No data reported

Drug Interactions
Increased Effect/Toxicity: See individual agents.

Pregnancy Risk Factor C

Mag-Caps [OTC] *see* Magnesium Oxide *on page 1015*

Mag Delay® [OTC] *see* Magnesium Chloride *on page 1013*

Mag G® [OTC] *see* Magnesium Gluconate *on page 1014*

MagGel™ [OTC] *see* Magnesium Oxide *on page 1015*

Maginex™ [OTC] *see* Magnesium L-aspartate Hydrochloride *on page 1015*

Maginex™ DS [OTC] *see* Magnesium L-aspartate Hydrochloride *on page 1015*

Magnesia Magma *see* Magnesium Hydroxide *on page 1014*

Magnesium Carbonate and Aluminum Hydroxide *see* Aluminum Hydroxide and Magnesium Carbonate *on page 81*

Magnesium Chloride (mag NEE zhum KLOR ide)

U.S. Brand Names Chloromag®; Mag 64™ [OTC]; Mag Delay® [OTC]; Slow-Mag® [OTC]

Generic Available Yes

Pharmacologic Category Electrolyte Supplement, Oral; Electrolyte Supplement, Parenteral; Magnesium Salt

Use Correction or prevention of hypomagnesemia; dietary supplement

Local Anesthetic/Vasoconstrictor Precautions No information available to require special precautions

Effects on Dental Treatment Key adverse event(s) related to dental treatment: Magnesium products may prevent GI absorption of tetracyclines by forming a large ionized chelated molecule with the tetracyclines in the stomach. Tetracyclines should be given at least 1 hour before magnesium.

Mechanism of Action Magnesium is important as a cofactor in many enzymatic reactions in the body involving protein synthesis and carbohydrate metabolism (at least 300 enzymatic reactions require magnesium). Actions on lipoprotein lipase have been found to be important in reducing serum cholesterol and on sodium/potassium ATPase in promoting polarization (eg, neuromuscular functioning).

Pregnancy Risk Factor C

Magnesium Citrate (mag NEE zhum SIT rate)

U.S. Brand Names Citroma® [OTC]
Canadian Brand Names Citro-Mag®
Generic Available Yes
(Continued)

Magnesium Citrate *(Continued)*

Index Terms Citrate of Magnesia

Pharmacologic Category Laxative, Saline; Magnesium Salt

Use Evacuation of bowel prior to certain surgical and diagnostic procedures or overdose situations

Local Anesthetic/Vasoconstrictor Precautions No information available to require special precautions

Effects on Dental Treatment Key adverse event(s) related to dental treatment: Magnesium products may prevent GI absorption of tetracyclines by forming a large ionized chelated molecule with the tetracyclines in the stomach. Tetracyclines should be given at least 1 hour before magnesium.

Mechanism of Action Promotes bowel evacuation by causing osmotic retention of fluid which distends the colon with increased peristaltic activity

Pregnancy Risk Factor B

Magnesium Gluconate *(mag NEE zhum GLOO koe nate)*

U.S. Brand Names Almora® [OTC]; Mag G® [OTC]; Magonate® [OTC]; Magtrate® [OTC]

Generic Available Yes: Tablet

Pharmacologic Category Electrolyte Supplement, Oral; Magnesium Salt

Use Dietary supplement

Local Anesthetic/Vasoconstrictor Precautions No information available to require special precautions

Effects on Dental Treatment Key adverse event(s) related to dental treatment: Magnesium products may prevent GI absorption of tetracyclines by forming a large ionized chelated molecule with the tetracyclines in the stomach. Tetracyclines should be given at least 1 hour before magnesium.

Mechanism of Action Magnesium is important as a cofactor in many enzymatic reactions in the body involving protein synthesis and carbohydrate metabolism (at least 300 enzymatic reactions require magnesium). Actions on lipoprotein lipase have been found to be important in reducing serum cholesterol and on sodium/potassium ATPase in promoting polarization (eg, neuromuscular functioning).

Magnesium Hydroxide *(mag NEE zhum hye DROKS ide)*

U.S. Brand Names Phillips'® Chews [OTC]; Phillips'® Milk of Magnesia [OTC]

Generic Available Yes: Liquid

Index Terms Magnesia Magma; Milk of Magnesia; MOM

Pharmacologic Category Antacid; Laxative; Magnesium Salt

Use Short-term treatment of occasional constipation and symptoms of hyperacidity, laxative; dietary supplement

Local Anesthetic/Vasoconstrictor Precautions No information available to require special precautions

Effects on Dental Treatment Key adverse event(s) related to dental treatment: Magnesium products may prevent GI absorption of tetracyclines by forming a large ionized chelated molecule with the tetracyclines in the stomach. Tetracyclines should be given at least 1 hour before magnesium.

Mechanism of Action Promotes bowel evacuation by causing osmotic retention of fluid which distends the colon with increased peristaltic activity; reacts with hydrochloric acid in stomach to form magnesium chloride

Magnesium Hydroxide, Aluminum Hydroxide, and Simethicone *see* Aluminum Hydroxide, Magnesium Hydroxide, and Simethicone *on page 82*

Magnesium Hydroxide and Aluminum Hydroxide *see* Aluminum Hydroxide and Magnesium Hydroxide *on page 81*

Magnesium Hydroxide and Calcium Carbonate *see* Calcium Carbonate and Magnesium Hydroxide *on page 261*

Magnesium Hydroxide and Mineral Oil
(mag NEE zhum hye DROKS ide & MIN er al oyl)

Related Information
Magnesium Hydroxide *on page 1014*

U.S. Brand Names Phillips'® M-O [OTC]

Generic Available No

Index Terms Haley's M-O; MOM/Mineral Oil Emulsion

Pharmacologic Category Laxative

Use Short-term treatment of occasional constipation

Local Anesthetic/Vasoconstrictor Precautions No information available to require special precautions

Effects on Dental Treatment Key adverse event(s) related to dental treatment: Magnesium products may prevent GI absorption of tetracyclines by forming a large ionized chelated molecule with the tetracyclines in the stomach. Tetracyclines should be given at least 1 hour before magnesium.

Magnesium Hydroxide, Famotidine, and Calcium Carbonate *see* Famotidine, Calcium Carbonate, and Magnesium Hydroxide *on page 671*

Magnesium L-aspartate Hydrochloride
(mag NEE zhum el as PAR tate hye droe KLOR ide)

U.S. Brand Names Maginex™ [OTC]; Maginex™ DS [OTC]
Generic Available No
Index Terms MAH
Pharmacologic Category Electrolyte Supplement, Oral; Magnesium Salt
Use Dietary supplement
Local Anesthetic/Vasoconstrictor Precautions No information available to require special precautions
Effects on Dental Treatment Key adverse event(s) related to dental treatment: Magnesium ions prevent GI absorption of tetracycline by forming a large, ionized, chelated molecule with the magnesium ion and tetracyclines in the stomach. Magnesium supplement should not be taken within 2-4 hours of oral tetracycline or other members of the tetracycline family.
Common Adverse Effects Frequency not defined: Gastrointestinal: Diarrhea (excessive oral doses)
Mechanism of Action Magnesium is important as a cofactor in many enzymatic reactions in the body involving protein synthesis and carbohydrate metabolism (at least 300 enzymatic reactions require magnesium). Actions on lipoprotein lipase have been found to be important in reducing serum cholesterol and on sodium/potassium ATPase in promoting polarization (eg, neuromuscular functioning).
Drug Interactions
  Increased Effect/Toxicity: Calcium channel blockers may enhance the adverse/toxic effect of magnesium salts. Magnesium salts may enhance the hypotensive effect of calcium channel blockers. Magnesium salts may enhance the neuromuscular-blocking effect of neuromuscular-blocking agents; only of concern in patients with increased serum magnesium concentrations.
  Decreased Effect: Oral magnesium salts may decrease the absorption of bisphosphonate derivatives, mycophenolate, and phosphate supplements. Magnesium salts may decrease the absorption of quinolone and tetracycline antibiotics; of concern only with oral administration of both agents.
Pharmacodynamics/Kinetics
  Absorption: Oral: Inversely proportional to amount ingested; 40% to 60% under controlled dietary conditions; 15% to 36% at higher doses. Absorption of the Maginex™ formulation may be increased compared to other magnesium salts.
  Distribution: Bone (50% to 60%); extracellular fluid (1% to 2%)
  Protein binding: 30%, to albumin
  Excretion: Urine (as magnesium)

Magnesium Oxide (mag NEE zhum OKS ide)

U.S. Brand Names Mag-Caps [OTC]; MagGel™ [OTC]; Mag-Ox® 400 [OTC]; Uro-Mag® [OTC]
Generic Available Yes
Pharmacologic Category Electrolyte Supplement, Oral; Magnesium Salt
Use Electrolyte replacement
Local Anesthetic/Vasoconstrictor Precautions No information available to require special precautions
Effects on Dental Treatment Key adverse event(s) related to dental treatment: Magnesium products may prevent GI absorption of tetracyclines by forming a large ionized chelated molecule with the tetracyclines in the stomach. Tetracyclines should be given at least 1 hour before magnesium.
Mechanism of Action Magnesium is important as a cofactor in many enzymatic reactions in the body involving protein synthesis and carbohydrate metabolism (at least 300 enzymatic reactions require magnesium). Actions on lipoprotein lipase have been found to be important in reducing serum cholesterol and on sodium/potassium ATPase in promoting polarization (eg, neuromuscular functioning).

Magnesium Salicylate (mag NEE zhum sa LIS i late)

Related Information
Rheumatoid Arthritis, Osteoarthritis, and Osteoporosis *on page 1759*
Temporomandibular Dysfunction (TMD) *on page 1822*

U.S. Brand Names Doan's® Extra Strength [OTC]; Keygesic [OTC]; Momentum® [OTC]; Novasal™

Generic Available Yes

Pharmacologic Category Salicylate

Use Mild-to-moderate pain, fever, various inflammatory conditions; relief of pain and inflammation of rheumatoid arthritis and osteoarthritis

Local Anesthetic/Vasoconstrictor Precautions No information available to require special precautions

Effects on Dental Treatment NSAID formulations are known to reversibly decrease platelet aggregation via mechanisms different than observed with aspirin. The dentist should be aware of the potential of abnormal coagulation. Caution should also be exercised in the use of NSAIDs in patients already on anticoagulant therapy with drugs such as warfarin (Coumadin®).

Common Adverse Effects Refer to Aspirin monograph.

Dosage Oral:
Children ≥12 years and Adults: Relief of mild-to-moderate pain:
Doan's® Extra Strength, Momentum®: Two caplets every 6 hours as needed (maximum: 8 caplets/24 hours)
Keygesic: One tablet every 4 hours as needed (maximum 4 tablets/24 hours)
Adults: Treatment of arthritis (Novasal™): Initial: 1 tablet 3-4 times/day. Maximum: 8 tablets/day
Elderly: Treatment of arthritis (Novasal™): Reduce adult dose to lowest effective dose; monitor for signs of toxicity

Contraindications Hypersensitivity to magnesium salicylate, salicylates, other NSAIDs, or any component of the formulation; advanced chronic renal dysfunction; concomitant use with uricosuric agents

In patients ≥65 years of age: Also contraindicated with a history of chronic salicylate use, carditis, chronic liver dysfunction

Warnings/Precautions [U.S. Boxed Warnings]: Use caution with hepatic dysfunction, hypoprothrombinemia, vitamin K deficiency, and prior to surgery. Surgical patients should avoid salicylates if possible, for 1-2 weeks prior to surgery, to reduce the risk of excessive bleeding. Use with caution in bleeding disorders, renal dysfunction, dehydration, gastritis, or peptic ulcer disease. Heavy ethanol use (>3 drinks/day) can increase bleeding risks. Avoid use in renal or hepatic failure. Discontinue use if tinnitus or impaired hearing occurs. Patients with sensitivity to tartrazine dyes, nasal polyps, and asthma may have an increased risk of salicylate sensitivity. Children and teenagers who have or are recovering from chickenpox or flu-like symptoms should not use this product. Changes in behavior (along with nausea and vomiting) may be an early sign of Reye's syndrome; patients should be instructed to contact their healthcare provider if these occur. The lowest effective dose should be used in patients ≥65 years of age. Safety and efficacy have not been established in children <12 years.

Ethanol/Nutrition/Herb Interactions Refer to Aspirin monograph.

Pharmacodynamics/Kinetics
Absorption: Rapid from stomach and upper intestine
Distribution: Readily into most body fluids and tissues; crosses the placenta, enters breast milk
Protein binding: 50% to 90%; primarily albumin
Metabolism: Released into the plasma as salicylic acid which is enzymatically converted to salicyluric acid and salicylphenolic glucuronide
Half-life elimination: 2 hours; increased with repeated dosing
Time to peak: 1.5 hours
Excretion: Urine

Pregnancy Risk Factor C

Dosage Forms
Caplet: 467 mg
Doan's® Extra Strength [OTC]: 467 mg
Momentum® [OTC]: 467 mg
Tablet, chelated:
Keygesic [OTC]: 650 mg
Tablet, as tetrahydrate [scored]:
Novasal™: 600 mg

Magnesium Sulfate (mag NEE zhum SUL fate)

Generic Available Yes
Index Terms Epsom Salts; MgSO₄ (error-prone abbreviation)
Pharmacologic Category Anticonvulsant, Miscellaneous; Electrolyte Supplement, Parenteral; Laxative, Saline; Magnesium Salt
Use Treatment and prevention of hypomagnesemia; prevention and treatment of seizures in severe pre-eclampsia or eclampsia, pediatric acute nephritis; torsade de pointes; treatment of cardiac arrhythmias (VT/VF) caused by hypomagnesemia; short-term treatment of constipation; soaking aid
Local Anesthetic/Vasoconstrictor Precautions No information available to require special precautions
Effects on Dental Treatment Key adverse event(s) related to dental treatment: Magnesium products may prevent GI absorption of tetracyclines by forming a large ionized chelated molecule with the tetracyclines in the stomach. Tetracyclines should be given at least 1 hour before magnesium.
Mechanism of Action When taken orally, magnesium promotes bowel evacuation by causing osmotic retention of fluid which distends the colon with increased peristaltic activity; parenterally, magnesium decreases acetylcholine in motor nerve terminals and acts on myocardium by slowing rate of S-A node impulse formation and prolonging conduction time. Magnesium is necessary for the movement of calcium, sodium, and potassium in and out of cells, as well as stabilizing excitable membranes.
Pregnancy Risk Factor A/C (manufacturer dependent)

Magnesium Trisilicate and Aluminum Hydroxide see Aluminum Hydroxide and Magnesium Trisilicate on page 82

Magnevist® see Gadopentetate Dimeglumine on page 761

Magonate® [OTC] see Magnesium Gluconate on page 1014

Mag-Ox® 400 [OTC] see Magnesium Oxide on page 1015

Magtrate® [OTC] see Magnesium Gluconate on page 1014

MAH see Magnesium L-aspartate Hydrochloride on page 1015

Malarone® see Atovaquone and Proguanil on page 165

Maldemar™ see Scopolamine on page 1457

Maltodextrin (mal toe DEK strin)

U.S. Brand Names Gelclair®; Multidex® [OTC]; OraRinse™ [OTC]
Generic Available No
Pharmacologic Category Anti-inflammatory, Locally Applied
Dental Use Oral: Management and relief of pain due to oral lesions (including mucositis/stomatitis), oral ulcers, or irritation; treatment of aphthous ulcers
Use Topical: Treatment of infected or noninfected wounds
Local Anesthetic/Vasoconstrictor Precautions No information available to require special precautions
Effects on Dental Treatment No significant effects or complications reported (see Dental Comment)
Dental Usual Dosing
Management of pain due to oral lesions: Adults: Oral:
Gelclair®: Using contents of 1 reconstituted packet, rinse around mouth for ~1 minute, 3 times/day or more if needed; gargle and expectorate. May be used undiluted or with less dilution if adequate pain relief is not achieved.
OraRinse™: 1 tablespoonful, swish or gargle for ~1 minute, 4 times/day or more if needed
Dosage Adults:
Oral: Management of pain due to oral lesions:
Gelclair®: Using contents of 1 reconstituted packet, rinse around mouth for ~1 minute, 3 times/day or more if needed; gargle and expectorate. May be used undiluted or with less dilution if adequate pain relief is not achieved.
OraRinse™: 1 tablespoonful, swish or gargle for ~1 minute, 4 times/day or more if needed
Topical: Wound dressing: Multidex®: After debridement and irrigation of wound, apply and cover with a nonadherent, nonocclusive dressing. May be applied to moist or dry, infected or noninfected wounds.
Mechanism of Action Forms a protective barrier over wound providing an environment which promotes tissue growth.
Contraindications Hypersensitivity to maltodextrin or any component of the formulation
Warnings/Precautions Oral: Avoid eating or drinking for 1 hour; products are not harmful if accidentally swallowed; notify healthcare provider if improvement is not seen within 7 days
(Continued)

Maltodextrin *(Continued)*

Dosage Forms Excipient information presented when available (limited, particularly for generics); consult specific product labeling.

Gel, oral [concentrate] (Gelclair®): 15 mL/packet (21s) [contains benzalkonium chloride and sodium benzoate]

Gel, topical dressing (Multidex®): (4 mL, 7 mL, 14 mL, 85 mL)

Powder, for oral suspension (OraRinse™): (19 g) [contains phenylalanine; also contains aloe vera, fructose, and sodium benzoate; vanilla flavor]

Powder, topical dressing (Multidex®): (6 g, 12 g, 25 g, 45 g)

Dental Comment

Gelclair®: Store at room temperature away from direct sunlight. Do not refrigerate. Gel may become darker or thicker over time; efficacy and safety are not affected if used prior to labeled expiration date. Mix contents of one packet with 40 mL of water. Stir and use at once. Product may be used undiluted if water is unavailable.

OraRinse™: Fill bottle with water to first arrow; shake vigorously until suspended; continue to fill to second arrow; shake well

m-AMSA *see* Amsacrine *on page 126*

Mandelamine® *see* Methenamine *on page 1063*

Mandrake *see* Podophyllum Resin *on page 1319*

Manganese *see* Trace Metals *on page 1595*

Mantoux *see* Tuberculin Tests *on page 1628*

Mapap [OTC] *see* Acetaminophen *on page 31*

Mapap Children's [OTC] *see* Acetaminophen *on page 31*

Mapap Extra Strength [OTC] *see* Acetaminophen *on page 31*

Mapap Infants [OTC] *see* Acetaminophen *on page 31*

Mapap Sinus Maximum Strength [OTC] *see* Acetaminophen and Pseudoephedrine *on page 38*

Maprotiline *(ma PROE ti leen)*

Canadian Brand Names Novo-Maprotiline

Mexican Brand Names Ludiomil

Generic Available Yes

Index Terms Ludiomil; Maprotiline Hydrochloride

Pharmacologic Category Antidepressant, Tetracyclic

Use Treatment of depression and anxiety associated with depression

Unlabeled/Investigational Use Bulimia; duodenal ulcers; enuresis; urinary symptoms of multiple sclerosis; pain; panic attacks; tension headache; cocaine withdrawal

Local Anesthetic/Vasoconstrictor Precautions Although maprotiline is not a tricyclic antidepressant, it does block norepinephrine reuptake within CNS synapses as part of its mechanisms. It has been suggested that vasoconstrictor be administered with caution and to monitor vital signs in dental patients taking antidepressants that affect norepinephrine in this way, including maprotiline. Epinephrine and levonordefrin have been shown to have an increased pressor response in combination with TCAs. Maprotiline is one of the drugs confirmed to prolong the QT interval and is accepted as having a risk of causing torsade de pointes. The risk of drug-induced torsade de pointes is extremely low when a single QT interval prolonging drug is prescribed. In terms of epinephrine, it is not known what effect vasoconstrictors in the local anesthetic regimen will have in patients with a known history of congenital prolonged QT interval or in patients taking any medication that prolongs the QT interval. Until more information is obtained, it is suggested that the clinician consult with the physician prior to the use of a vasoconstrictor in suspected patients, and that the vasoconstrictor (epinephrine, levonordefrin [Neo-Cobefrin®]) be used with caution.

Effects on Dental Treatment Key adverse event(s) related to dental treatment: Xerostomia and changes in salivation (normal salivary flow resumes upon discontinuation).

Common Adverse Effects

>10%:

Central nervous system: Drowsiness

Gastrointestinal: Xerostomia

1% to 10%:

Central nervous system: Insomnia, nervousness, anxiety, agitation, dizziness, fatigue, headache

Gastrointestinal: Constipation, nausea

Neuromuscular & skeletal: Tremor, weakness

Ocular: Blurred vision

Restrictions An FDA-approved medication guide concerning the use of antidepressants in children, adolescents, and young adults must be distributed when dispensing an outpatient prescription (new or refill) where this medication is to be used without direct supervision of a healthcare provider. Medication guides are available at http://www.fda.gov/cder/Offices/ODS/medication_guides.htm. Dispense to parents or guardians of children and adolescents receiving this medication.

Mechanism of Action Traditionally believed to increase the synaptic concentration of norepinephrine in the central nervous system by inhibition of their reuptake by the presynaptic neuronal membrane. However, additional receptor effects have been found including desensitization of adenyl cyclase, down regulation of beta-adrenergic receptors, and down regulation of serotonin receptors.

Drug Interactions

Cytochrome P450 Effect: Substrate of CYP2D6 (major)

Increased Effect/Toxicity: Maprotiline may increase the effects of amphetamines, anticholinergics, other CNS depressants (sedatives, hypnotics, or ethanol), carbamazepine, tolazamide, chlorpropamide, and warfarin. When used with MAO inhibitors, hyperpyrexia, hypertension, tachycardia, confusion, seizures, and **deaths have been reported** (serotonin syndrome). CYP2D6 inhibitors may increase the levels/effects of maprotiline; example inhibitors include chlorpromazine, delavirdine, fluoxetine, miconazole, paroxetine, pergolide, quinidine, quinine, ritonavir, and ropinirole. Cimetidine, fenfluramine, grapefruit juice, indinavir, methylphenidate, diltiazem, valproate, and verapamil may increase the serum concentrations of cyclic antidepressants. Use of lithium with a cyclic antidepressant may increase the risk for neurotoxicity. Phenothiazines may increase concentration of some cyclic antidepressants and cyclic antidepressants may increase the concentration of phenothiazines. Pressor response to I.V. epinephrine, norepinephrine, and phenylephrine may be enhanced in patients receiving cyclic antidepressants (**Note:** Effect is unlikely with epinephrine or levonordefrin dosages typically administered as infiltration in combination with local anesthetics). Combined use of beta-agonists or drugs which prolong QT_c (including quinidine, procainamide, disopyramide, cisapride, sparfloxacin, gatifloxacin, moxifloxacin) with cyclic antidepressants may predispose patients to cardiac arrhythmias.

Decreased Effect: Maprotiline inhibits the antihypertensive response to bethanidine, clonidine, debrisoquin, guanadrel, guanethidine, guanabenz, or guanfacine. Cholestyramine and colestipol may bind cyclic antidepressants and reduce their absorption.

Pharmacodynamics/Kinetics

Absorption: Slow
Protein binding: 88%
Metabolism: Hepatic to active and inactive compounds
Half-life elimination, serum: 27-58 hours (mean: 43 hours)
Time to peak, serum: Within 12 hours
Excretion: Urine (70%); feces (30%)

Pregnancy Risk Factor B

Maxitrol® *see* Neomycin, Polymyxin B, and Dexamethasone *on page 1161*

Maxi-Tuss HCG *see* Hydrocodone and Guaifenesin *on page 828*

Maxzide® *see* Hydrochlorothiazide and Triamterene *on page 821*

Maxzide®-25 *see* Hydrochlorothiazide and Triamterene *on page 821*

May Apple *see* Podophyllum Resin *on page 1319*

3M™ Cavilon™ Skin Cleanser [OTC] [DSC] *see* Benzalkonium Chloride *on page 194*

MCH *see* Collagen Hemostat *on page 411*

m-Cresyl Acetate (em-KREE sil AS e tate)

U.S. Brand Names Cresylate®
Generic Available No
Pharmacologic Category Otic Agent, Anti-infective
Use Provides an acid medium; for external otitis infections caused by susceptible bacteria or fungus
Local Anesthetic/Vasoconstrictor Precautions No information available to require special precautions
Effects on Dental Treatment No significant effects or complications reported

MCT *see* Medium Chain Triglycerides *on page 1026*

MCT Oil® [OTC] *see* Medium Chain Triglycerides *on page 1026*

MCV4 *see* Meningococcal Polysaccharide (Groups A / C / Y and W-135) Diphtheria Toxoid Conjugate Vaccine *on page 1035*

MD-76®R *see* Diatrizoate Meglumine and Diatrizoate Sodium *on page 479*

MD-Gastroview® *see* Diatrizoate Meglumine and Diatrizoate Sodium *on page 479*

MDL 73,147EF *see* Dolasetron *on page 525*

Measles, Mumps, and Rubella Vaccines (Combined) (MEE zels, mumpz & roo BEL a vak SEENS, kom BINED)

Related Information
Immunizations (Vaccines) *on page 1886*
U.S. Brand Names M-M-R® II
Canadian Brand Names M-M-R® II; Priorix™
Mexican Brand Names Morupar
Generic Available No
Index Terms MMR; Mumps, Measles and Rubella Vaccines, Combined; Rubella, Measles and Mumps Vaccines, Combined
Pharmacologic Category Vaccine, Live Virus
Use Measles, mumps, and rubella prophylaxis
Local Anesthetic/Vasoconstrictor Precautions No information available to require special precautions
Effects on Dental Treatment No significant effects or complications reported
Common Adverse Effects All serious adverse reactions must be reported to the U.S. Department of Health and Human Services (DHHS) Vaccine Adverse Event Reporting System (VAERS) 1-800-822-7967.
Frequency not defined:
  Cardiovascular: Syncope, vasculitis
  Central nervous system: Ataxia, dizziness, febrile convulsions, fever, encephalitis, encephalopathy, Guillain-Barré syndrome, headache, irritability, malaise, measles inclusion body encephalitis, polyneuritis, polyneuropathy, seizure, subacute sclerosing panencephalitis
  Dermatologic: Angioneurotic edema, erythema multiforme, purpura, rash, Stevens-Johnson syndrome, urticaria
  Endocrine & metabolic: Diabetes mellitus, parotitis
  Gastrointestinal: Diarrhea, nausea, pancreatitis, sore throat, vomiting
  Genitourinary: Orchitis
  Hematologic: Leukocytosis, thrombocytopenia
  Local: Injection site reactions which include burning, induration, redness, stinging, swelling, tenderness, wheal and flare, vesiculation
  Neuromuscular & skeletal: Arthralgia/arthritis (variable; highest rates in women, 12% to 26% versus children, up to 3%), myalgia, paresthesia
  Ocular: Ocular palsies
  Otic: Otitis media
  Renal: Conjunctivitis, retinitis, optic neuritis, papillitis, retrobulbar neuritis
  Respiratory: Bronchospasm, cough, pneumonitis, rhinitis
  Miscellaneous: Anaphylactoid reactions, anaphylaxis, atypical measles, panniculitis, regional lymphadenopathy

Mechanism of Action As a live, attenuated vaccine, MMR vaccine offers active immunity to disease caused by the measles, mumps, and rubella viruses.

Drug Interactions

Decreased Effect: The effect of the vaccine may be decreased in individuals who are receiving immunosuppressant drugs (including high dose systemic corticosteroids). Effect of vaccine may be decreased when given with immune globulin. Live virus vaccination should be withheld for ~3-11 months following immune globulin administration; length of time depends on dose of IgG given.

Pregnancy Risk Factor C

Measles, Mumps, Rubella, and Varicella Virus Vaccine
(MEE zels, mumpz, roo BEL a, & var i SEL a VYE rus vak SEEN)

U.S. Brand Names ProQuad®

Generic Available No

Index Terms MMRV; Mumps, Rubella, Varicella, and Measles Vaccine; Rubella, Varicella, Measles, and Mumps Vaccine; Varicella, Measles, Mumps, and Rubella Vaccine

Pharmacologic Category Vaccine, Live Virus

Use To provide simultaneous active immunization against measles, mumps, rubella, and varicella

Local Anesthetic/Vasoconstrictor Precautions No information available to require special precautions

Effects on Dental Treatment No significant effects or complications reported

Common Adverse Effects All serious adverse reactions must be reported to the U.S. Department of Health and Human Services (DHHS) Vaccine Adverse Event Reporting System (VAERS) 1-800-822-7967.

With the exception of fever and measles-like rash, incidence of adverse events was generally lower in patients receiving ProQuad® compared to those receiving M-M-R® II and Varivax®. Also refer to M-M-R® II and Varivax® monographs for additional adverse reactions reported with those agents.

>10%:

Central nervous system: Fever ≥38.9°C (≥102°F) (22%)

Local: Injection site reaction including pain, tenderness, soreness (22%); erythema (14%)

1% to 10%:

Central nervous system: Irritability (7%)

Dermatologic: Measles-like rash (3%), varicella-like rash (2%), rash (2%), viral exanthema (1%)

Gastrointestinal: Diarrhea (1%)

Local: Injection site reaction: Swelling (8%), bruising (2%)

Respiratory: Upper respiratory tract infection (1%)

Mechanism of Action A live, attenuated virus; offers active immunity to disease caused by the measles, mumps, rubella, and varicella-zoster virus.

Drug Interactions

Increased Effect/Toxicity: Salicylates may increase the risk of Reye's syndrome following varicella vaccination; avoid use of salicylates for 6 weeks following vaccination.

Decreased Effect: In patients receiving high doses of systemic corticosteroids for ≥14 days, wait at least 1 month between discontinuing steroid therapy and administering vaccine. Do not administer with immune globulin (including varicella zoster immune globulin); vaccination should be deferred for at least 5 months following immune globulin administration; immune globulins should not be given for at least 2 months following vaccination (unless benefits of use outweigh benefits of vaccination). The effect of the vaccine may be decreased and the risk of varicella disease in individuals who are receiving immunosuppressant drugs may be increased.

Pregnancy Risk Factor C

Measles Virus Vaccine (Live) (MEE zels VYE rus vak SEEN, live)

Related Information

Immunizations (Vaccines) *on page 1886*

U.S. Brand Names Attenuvax®

Generic Available No

Index Terms More Attenuated Enders Strain; Rubeola Vaccine

Pharmacologic Category Vaccine, Live Virus

Use Active immunization against measles (rubeola)

Note: Trivalent measles - mumps - rubella (MMR) is the vaccine of choice if recipients are likely to be susceptible to rubella and/or mumps as well as to measles.

(Continued)

Measles Virus Vaccine (Live) *(Continued)*

Local Anesthetic/Vasoconstrictor Precautions No information available to require special precautions

Effects on Dental Treatment No significant effects or complications reported

Common Adverse Effects All serious adverse reactions must be reported to the U.S. Department of Health and Human Services (DHHS) Vaccine Adverse Event Reporting System (VAERS) 1-800-822-7967.

Frequency not defined.

Cardiovascular: Peripheral edema, syncope, vasculitis

Central nervous system: Ataxia, dizziness, encephalitis, encephalopathy, febrile seizure, fever, Guillain-Barré syndrome, headache, irritability, malaise, seizure

Dermatologic: Angioneurotic edema, erythema multiforme, panniculitis, purpura, rash, Stevens-Johnson syndrome, urticaria

Gastrointestinal: Diarrhea, nausea, vomiting

Hematologic: Leukocytosis, thrombocytopenia

Local: Injection site reactions: Burning, redness, stinging, swelling, vesiculation, wheal and flare

Neuromuscular & skeletal: Arthralgia, myalgia

Ocular: Conjunctivitis, ocular palsies, optic neuritis, papillitis, retinitis, retrobulbar neuritis

Otic: Nerve deafness, otitis media

Respiratory: Bronchial spasm, cough, pneumonitis, rhinitis

Miscellaneous: Anaphylaxis/anaphylactoid reactions, atypical measles, facial edema, lymphadenopathy, measles inclusion body encephalitis, subacute sclerosing pancephalitis

Mechanism of Action Promotes active immunity to measles virus by inducing specific measles IgG and IgM antibodies. Measles antibodies develop in ~95% of children vaccinated at 12 months of age and in 98% of children vaccinated at 15 months of age. Life-long immunity is induced in most persons completing vaccination schedule.

Drug Interactions

Decreased Effect: In patients receiving high doses of systemic corticosteroids for ≥14 days, wait at least 1 month between discontinuing steroid therapy and administering immunization. Do not administer immune globulin, whole blood, plasma together with this vaccine; immune response may be compromised (defer vaccine administration for ≥3 months). Immunosuppressants may enhance the adverse/toxic effect of live vaccines; vaccinial infections may develop.

Pregnancy Risk Factor C

Mebaral® *see* Mephobarbital *on page 1041*

Mebendazole *(me BEN da zole)*

U.S. Brand Names Vermox® [DSC]

Canadian Brand Names Vermox®

Mexican Brand Names Bestelar; Revapol; Soltric; Vermox

Generic Available Yes

Pharmacologic Category Anthelmintic

Use Treatment of pinworms (*Enterobius vermicularis*), whipworms (*Trichuris trichiura*), roundworms (*Ascaris lumbricoides*), and hookworms (*Ancylostoma duodenale*)

Local Anesthetic/Vasoconstrictor Precautions No information available to require special precautions

Effects on Dental Treatment No significant effects or complications reported

Mechanism of Action Selectively and irreversibly blocks glucose uptake and other nutrients in susceptible adult intestine-dwelling helminths

Pregnancy Risk Factor C

Mecamylamine *(mek a MIL a meen)*

U.S. Brand Names Inversine®

Canadian Brand Names Inversine®

Generic Available No

Index Terms Mecamylamine Hydrochloride

Pharmacologic Category Ganglionic Blocking Agent

Use Treatment of moderately severe to severe hypertension and in uncomplicated malignant hypertension

Unlabeled/Investigational Use Tourette's syndrome

Local Anesthetic/Vasoconstrictor Precautions No information available to require special precautions

Effects on Dental Treatment Key adverse event(s) related to dental treatment: Xerostomia (normal salivary flow resumes upon discontinuation).

Mechanism of Action Mecamylamine is a ganglionic blocker. This agent inhibits acetylcholine at the autonomic ganglia, causing a decrease in blood pressure. Mecamylamine also blocks central nicotinic cholinergic receptors, which inhibits the effects of nicotine and may suppress the desire to smoke.

Pregnancy Risk Factor C

Mecamylamine Hydrochloride *see Mecamylamine on page 1022*

Mecasermin (mek a SER min)

U.S. Brand Names Increlex™; Iplex™

Generic Available No

Index Terms Mecasermin (rDNA Origin); Mecasermin Rinfabate; Recombinant Human Insulin-Like Growth Factor-1; rhIGF-1; rhIGF-1/rhIGFBP-3

Pharmacologic Category Growth Hormone

Use Treatment of growth failure in children with severe primary insulin-like growth factor-1 deficiency (IGF-1 deficiency; primary IGFD), or with growth hormone (GH) gene deletions who have developed neutralizing antibodies to GH

Local Anesthetic/Vasoconstrictor Precautions No information available to require special precautions

Effects on Dental Treatment No significant effects or complications reported

Common Adverse Effects

≥5%:

Cardiovascular: Cardiac murmur

Central nervous system: Convulsion, dizziness, headache (Iplex™: 22%)

Endocrine & metabolic: Hyper-/hypoglycemia (Increlex™: 42%; Iplex™ 31%), iron-deficiency anemia, ovarian cysts, thymus hypertrophy, thyromegaly

Gastrointestinal: Vomiting

Hepatic: Liver enzymes increased

Local: Injection site reactions: Erythema, bruising, hair growth, lipohypertrophy

Neuromuscular & skeletal: Arthralgia, bone pain, extremity pain, muscular atrophy

Ocular: Papilledema

Otic: Ear pain, hypoacusis, middle ear fluid, otitis media, serous otitis media, tympanometry abnormal

Renal: Hematuria

Respiratory: Snoring, tonsillar hypertrophy (Increlex™: 15%; Iplex™ 19%)

Miscellanous: Lymphadenopathy

<5% or frequency not defined: Hypoglycemic seizure, intracranial hypertension, loss of consciousness secondary to hypoglycemia, thickening of soft facial tissue

Mechanism of Action Mecasermin is an insulin-like growth factor (IGF-1) produced using recombinant DNA technology to replace endogenous IGF-1. Endogenous IGF-1 circulates predominately bound to insulin-like growth factor-binding protein-3 (IGFBP-3) and a growth hormone-dependent acid-labile subunit (ALS). Acting at receptors in the liver and other tissues, endogenous growth hormone (GH) stimulates the synthesis and secretion of IGF-1. In patients with primary severe IGF-1 deficiency, growth hormone receptors in the liver are unresponsive to GH, leading to reduced endogenous IGF-I concentrations and decreased growth (skeletal, cell, and organ). Endogenous IGF-1 also suppresses liver glucose production, stimulates peripheral glucose utilization and has an inhibitory effect on insulin secretion.

Mecasermin rinfabate is a complex of IGF-1 and IGFBP-3, both produced by recombinant DNA technology.

Pharmacodynamics/Kinetics

Distribution: V_d: Severe primary IGFD: 0.184-0.33 L/kg

Protein binding: >80% bound to IGFBP-3 and an acid-labile subunit (IGFBP-3 reduced with severe primary IGFD)

Metabolism: Hepatic and renal

Half-life elimination: Severe primary IGFD: Mecasermin: 5.8 hours; Mecasermin rinfabate: >12 hours

Pregnancy Risk Factor C

Mecasermin (rDNA Origin) *see Mecasermin on page 1023*
Mecasermin Rinfabate *see Mecasermin on page 1023*

Meclizine (MEK li zeen)

U.S. Brand Names Antivert®; Bonine® [OTC]; Dramamine® Less Drowsy Formula [OTC]

Canadian Brand Names Bonamine™; Bonine®

Generic Available Yes

Index Terms Meclizine Hydrochloride; Meclozine Hydrochloride

Pharmacologic Category Antiemetic; Antihistamine

Use Prevention and treatment of symptoms of motion sickness; management of vertigo with diseases affecting the vestibular system

Local Anesthetic/Vasoconstrictor Precautions No information available to require special precautions

Effects on Dental Treatment Key adverse event(s) related to dental treatment: Slight to moderate drowsiness, thickening of bronchial secretions, significant xerostomia (normal salivary flow resumes upon discontinuation).

Common Adverse Effects

>10%:

Central nervous system: Slight to moderate drowsiness

Respiratory: Thickening of bronchial secretions

1% to 10%:

Central nervous system: Headache, fatigue, nervousness, dizziness

Gastrointestinal: Appetite increase, weight gain, nausea, diarrhea, abdominal pain, xerostomia

Respiratory: Pharyngitis

Mechanism of Action Has central anticholinergic action by blocking chemoreceptor trigger zone; decreases excitability of the middle ear labyrinth and blocks conduction in the middle ear vestibular-cerebellar pathways

Drug Interactions

Increased Effect/Toxicity: Increased toxicity with CNS depressants, neuroleptics, and anticholinergics.

Pharmacodynamics/Kinetics

Onset of action: ~1 hour

Duration: 8-24 hours

Metabolism: Hepatic

Half-life elimination: 6 hours

Excretion: Urine (as metabolites); feces (as unchanged drug)

Pregnancy Risk Factor B

Meclizine Hydrochloride *see* Meclizine *on page 1024*

Meclofenamate (me kloe fen AM ate)

Related Information

Rheumatoid Arthritis, Osteoarthritis, and Osteoporosis *on page 1759*

Temporomandibular Dysfunction (TMD) *on page 1822*

Canadian Brand Names Meclomen®

Generic Available Yes

Index Terms Meclofenamate Sodium

Pharmacologic Category Nonsteroidal Anti-inflammatory Drug (NSAID), Oral

Use Treatment of inflammatory disorders, arthritis, mild to moderate pain, dysmenorrhea

Local Anesthetic/Vasoconstrictor Precautions No information available to require special precautions

Effects on Dental Treatment NSAID formulations are known to reversibly decrease platelet aggregation via mechanisms different than observed with aspirin. The dentist should be aware of the potential of abnormal coagulation. Caution should also be exercised in the use of NSAIDs in patients already on anticoagulant therapy with drugs such as warfarin (Coumadin®). Recovery of platelet function usually occurs 1-2 days after discontinuation of NSAIDs.

Common Adverse Effects

>10%:

Central nervous system: Dizziness

Dermatologic: Rash

Gastrointestinal: Abdominal cramps, heartburn, indigestion, nausea

1% to 10%:

Central nervous system: Headache, nervousness

Dermatologic: Itching

Endocrine & metabolic: Fluid retention

Gastrointestinal: Vomiting

Otic: Tinnitus

Restrictions An FDA-approved medication guide must be distributed when dispensing an oral outpatient prescription (new or refill) where this medication is to be used without direct supervision of a healthcare provider. Medication guides are available at http://www.fda.gov/cder/Offices/ODS/medication_guides.htm.

Dosage Children >14 years and Adults: Oral:

Mild to moderate pain: 50 mg every 4-6 hours; increases to 100 mg may be required; maximum dose: 400 mg

Rheumatoid arthritis and osteoarthritis: 50 mg every 4-6 hours; increase, over weeks, to 200-400 mg/day in 3-4 divided doses; do not exceed 400 mg/day; maximal benefit for any dose may not be seen for 2-3 weeks

Mechanism of Action Inhibits prostaglandin synthesis by decreasing the activity of the enzyme, cyclooxygenase, which results in decreased formation of prostaglandin precursors

Contraindications Hypersensitivity to meclofenamate, aspirin, other NSAIDs, or any component of the formulation; perioperative pain in the setting of coronary artery bypass surgery (CABG); active GI bleeding, ulcer disease; pregnancy (3rd trimester)

Warnings/Precautions [U.S. Boxed Warning]: NSAIDs are associated with an increased risk of adverse cardiovascular events, including MI, stroke, and new onset or worsening of pre-existing hypertension. Risk may be increased with duration of use or pre-existing cardiovascular risk factors or disease. Carefully evaluate individual cardiovascular risk profiles prior to prescribing. Use caution with fluid retention, CHF or hypertension. Concurrent administration of ibuprofen, and potentially other nonselective NSAIDs, may interfere with aspirin's cardioprotective effect.

Use of NSAIDs can compromise existing renal function. Renal toxicity can occur in patient with impaired renal function, dehydration, heart failure, liver dysfunction, those taking diuretics and ACEI and the elderly. Rehydrate patient before starting therapy. Monitor renal function closely. Use caution in patients with advanced renal disease.

[U.S. Boxed Warning]: NSAIDs may increase risk of gastrointestinal irritation, ulceration, bleeding, and perforation. These events may occur at any time during therapy and without warning. Use caution with a history of GI disease (bleeding or ulcers), concurrent therapy with aspirin, anticoagulants and/or corticosteroids, smoking, use of alcohol, the elderly or debilitated patients.

Use the lowest effective dose for the shortest duration of time, consistent with individual patient goals, to reduce risk of cardiovascular or GI adverse events. Alternate therapies should be considered for patients at high risk.

NSAIDs may cause serious skin adverse events including exfoliative dermatitis, Stevens-Johnson syndrome (SJS) and toxic epidermal necrolysis (TEN). Anaphylactoid reactions may occur, even without prior exposure; patients with "aspirin triad" (bronchial asthma, aspirin intolerance, rhinitis) may be at increased risk. Do not use in patients who experience bronchospasm, asthma, rhinitis, or urticaria with NSAID or aspirin therapy. Use caution in other forms of asthma.

Use with caution in patients with decreased hepatic function. Closely monitor patients with any abnormal LFT. Severe hepatic reactions (eg, fulminant hepatitis, liver failure) have occurred with NSAID use, rarely; discontinue if signs or symptoms of liver disease develop, or if systemic manifestations occur.

The elderly are at increased risk for adverse effects (especially peptic ulceration, CNS effects, renal toxicity) from NSAIDs even at low doses

Withhold for at least 4-6 half-lives prior to surgical or dental procedures. Safety and efficacy have not been established in children <14 years of age.

Drug Interactions

Increased Effect/Toxicity: Anticoagulants (warfarin, heparin, LMWHs) in combination with NSAIDs can cause increased risk of bleeding. Other antiplatelet drugs (ticlopidine, clopidogrel, aspirin, abciximab, dipyridamole, eptifibatide, tirofiban) can cause an increased risk of bleeding. NSAIDs may increase serum creatinine, potassium, blood pressure, and cyclosporine levels during concurrent therapy; monitor cyclosporine levels and renal function carefully. Lithium levels can be increased; avoid concurrent use if possible or monitor lithium levels and adjust dose. Sulindac may have the least effect. When NSAID is stopped, lithium will need adjustment again. Corticosteroids may increase the risk of GI ulceration; avoid concurrent use. Serum concentration/toxicity of methotrexate may be increased. Concomitant use with fluoroquinolones may rarely increase risk of seizure.

Decreased Effect: Antihypertensive effects of ACE inhibitors, angiotensin antagonists, beta-blockers, diuretics, and hydralazine may be decreased by concurrent therapy with NSAIDs; monitor blood pressure. Cholestyramine

(Continued)

Meclofenamate *(Continued)*

(and other bile acid sequestrants) may decrease the absorption of NSAIDs; separate by at least 2 hours. Salicylates' antiplatelet effect may be reduced.

Ethanol/Nutrition/Herb Interactions

Ethanol: Avoid ethanol (may enhance gastric mucosal irritation).

Herb/Nutraceutical: Avoid alfalfa, anise, bilberry, bladderwrack, bromelain, cat's claw, celery, coleus, cordyceps, dong quai, evening primrose, feverfew, fenugreek, garlic, ginger, ginkgo biloba, red clover, horse chestnut, grapeseed, green tea, ginseng, guggul, horse chestnut seed, horseradish, licorice, prickly ash, red clover, reishi, SAMe, sweet clover, turmeric, white willow (all have additional antiplatelet activity).

Dietary Considerations May be taken with food, milk, or antacids.

Pharmacodynamics/Kinetics

Duration: 2-4 hours

Distribution: Crosses placenta

Protein binding: 99%

Half-life elimination: 2-3.3 hours

Time to peak, serum: 0.5-1.5 hours

Excretion: Primarily urine and feces (as metabolites)

Pregnancy Risk Factor C/D (3rd trimester)

Dosage Forms

Capsule: 50 mg, 100 mg

Meclofenamate Sodium *see* Meclofenamate *on page 1024*

Meclozine Hydrochloride *see* Meclizine *on page 1024*

Medebar® Plus *see* Barium *on page 185*

Medent-DM *see* Guaifenesin, Pseudoephedrine, and Dextromethorphan *on page 800*

Medicinal Carbon *see* Charcoal, Activated *on page 327*

Medicinal Charcoal *see* Charcoal, Activated *on page 327*

Medicone® Suppositories [OTC] *see* Phenylephrine *on page 1293*

Medigesic® *see* Butalbital, Acetaminophen, and Caffeine *on page 247*

Medi-Phenyl [OTC] *see* Phenylephrine *on page 1293*

Mediplast® [OTC] *see* Salicylic Acid *on page 1451*

Medi-Synal [OTC] *see* Acetaminophen and Pseudoephedrine *on page 38*

Medium Chain Triglycerides

(mee DEE um chane trye GLIS er ides)

U.S. Brand Names MCT Oil® [OTC]

Canadian Brand Names MCT Oil®

Generic Available No

Index Terms MCT; Triglycerides, Medium Chain

Pharmacologic Category Nutritional Supplement

Use Dietary supplement for those who cannot digest long chain fats; malabsorption associated with disorders such as pancreatic insufficiency, bile salt deficiency, short bowel syndrome, and bacterial overgrowth of the small bowel; induce ketosis as a prevention for seizures

Local Anesthetic/Vasoconstrictor Precautions No information available to require special precautions

Effects on Dental Treatment No significant effects or complications reported

Common Adverse Effects Frequency not defined.

Endocrine & metabolic: HDL serum levels decreased and triglycerides serum levels increased (>6 months daily use)

Gastrointestinal: Abdominal pain, bloating, cramping, diarrhea, nausea

Mechanism of Action MCTs are saturated fatty acids in chains of 6-12 carbon atoms. They are water soluble and can pass directly through intestinal cell membranes and blood stream. Once taken up by the liver, they are used for metabolic energy before being stored.

Medrol® *see* MethylPREDNISolone *on page 1083*

MedroxyPROGESTERone (me DROKS ee proe JES te rone)

Related Information

Endocrine Disorders and Pregnancy *on page 1750*

U.S. Brand Names Depo-Provera®; Depo-Provera® Contraceptive; depo-subQ provera 104™; Provera®

Canadian Brand Names Alti-MPA; Apo-Medroxy®; Depo-Prevera®; Depo-Provera®; Gen-Medroxy; Novo-Medrone; Provera®; Provera-Pak

Mexican Brand Names Cycrin
Generic Available Yes
Index Terms Acetoxymethylprogesterone; Medroxyprogesterone Acetate; Methylacetoxyprogesterone; MPA
Pharmacologic Category Contraceptive; Progestin
Use Endometrial carcinoma or renal carcinoma; secondary amenorrhea or abnormal uterine bleeding due to hormonal imbalance; reduction of endometrial hyperplasia in nonhysterectomized postmenopausal women receiving conjugated estrogens; prevention of pregnancy; management of endometriosis-associated pain
Local Anesthetic/Vasoconstrictor Precautions No information available to require special precautions
Effects on Dental Treatment Progestins may predispose the patient to gingival bleeding.
Common Adverse Effects Adverse effects as reported with any dosage form; percent ranges presented are noted with the MPA contraceptive injection:
>5%:
Central nervous system: Dizziness, headache, nervousness
Endocrine & metabolic: Libido decreased, menstrual irregularities (includes bleeding, amenorrhea, or both)
Gastrointestinal: Abdominal pain/discomfort, weight changes (average 3-5 pounds after 1 year, 8 pounds after 2 years)
Neuromuscular & skeletal: Weakness
1% to 5%:
Cardiovascular: Edema
Central nervous system: Depression, fatigue, insomnia, irritability, pain
Dermatologic: Acne, alopecia, rash
Endocrine & metabolic: Anorgasmia, breast pain, hot flashes
Gastrointestinal: Bloating, nausea
Genitourinary: Cervical smear abnormal, leukorrhea, menometrorrhagia, menorrhagia, pelvic pain, urinary tract infection, vaginitis, vaginal infection, vaginal hemorrhage
Local: Injection site atrophy, injection site reaction, injection site pain
Neuromuscular & skeletal: Arthralgia, backache, leg cramp
Respiratory: Respiratory tract infections
Mechanism of Action Inhibits secretion of pituitary gonadotropins, which prevents follicular maturation and ovulation; causes endometrial thinning
Drug Interactions
Cytochrome P450 Effect: Substrate of CYP3A4 (major); **Induces** CYP3A4 (weak)
Decreased Effect: Acitretin, and griseofulvin may diminish the therapeutic effect of progestin contraceptives (contraceptive failure is possible). CYP3A4 inducers may decrease the levels/effects of medroxyprogesterone; example inducers include aminoglutethimide, carbamazepine, nafcillin, nevirapine, phenobarbital, phenytoin, and rifamycins. Progestins may diminish the anticoagulant effect of coumarin derivatives; and in contrast, enhanced anticoagulant effects have also been noted with some products.
Pharmacodynamics/Kinetics
Absorption: Oral: Well absorbed; I.M.: Slow
Protein binding: 86% to 90% primarily to albumin; does not bind to sex hormone-binding globulin
Metabolism: Extensively hepatic via hydroxylation and conjugation; forms metabolites
Time to peak: Oral: 2-4 hours
Half-life elimination: Oral: 12-17 hours; I.M. (Depo-Provera® Contraceptive): 50 days; SubQ: ~40 days
Excretion: Urine
Pregnancy Risk Factor X

Medroxyprogesterone Acetate *see* MedroxyPROGESTERone *on page 1026*

Medroxyprogesterone and Estrogens (Conjugated) *see* Estrogens (Conjugated/Equine) and Medroxyprogesterone *on page 612*

Medrysone (ME dri sone)

U.S. Brand Names HMS Liquifilm® [DSC]
Mexican Brand Names Medrixon
Generic Available No
Pharmacologic Category Corticosteroid, Ophthalmic
Use Treatment of allergic conjunctivitis, vernal conjunctivitis, episcleritis, ophthalmic epinephrine sensitivity reaction
Local Anesthetic/Vasoconstrictor Precautions No information available to require special precautions
(Continued)

Medrysone *(Continued)*

Effects on Dental Treatment No significant effects or complications reported

Mechanism of Action Decreases inflammation by suppression of migration of polymorphonuclear leukocytes and reversal of increased capillary permeability

Pregnancy Risk Factor C

Mefenamic Acid *(me fe NAM ik AS id)*

Related Information

Rheumatoid Arthritis, Osteoarthritis, and Osteoporosis *on page 1759*

Temporomandibular Dysfunction (TMD) *on page 1822*

U.S. Brand Names Ponstel®

Canadian Brand Names Apo-Mefenamic®; Dom-Mefenamic Acid; Mefe-namic-250; Nu-Mefenamic; PMS-Mefenamic Acid; Ponstan®

Mexican Brand Names Ponstan-500

Generic Available Yes

Pharmacologic Category Nonsteroidal Anti-inflammatory Drug (NSAID), Oral

Use Short-term relief of mild to moderate pain including primary dysmenorrhea

Local Anesthetic/Vasoconstrictor Precautions No information available to require special precautions

Effects on Dental Treatment NSAID formulations are known to reversibly decrease platelet aggregation via mechanisms different than observed with aspirin. The dentist should be aware of the potential of abnormal coagulation. Caution should also be exercised in the use of NSAIDs in patients already on anticoagulant therapy with drugs such as warfarin (Coumadin®). Recovery of platelet function usually occurs 1-2 days after discontinuation of NSAIDs.

Common Adverse Effects 1% to 10%:

Central nervous system: Headache, nervousness, dizziness (3% to 9%)

Dermatologic: Itching, rash

Endocrine & metabolic: Fluid retention

Gastrointestinal: Abdominal cramps, heartburn, indigestion, nausea (1% to 10%), vomiting (1% to 10%), diarrhea (1% to 10%), constipation (1% to 10%), abdominal distress/cramping/pain (1% to 10%), dyspepsia (1% to 10%), flatulence (1% to 10%), gastric or duodenal ulcer with bleeding or perforation (1% to 10%), gastritis (1% to 10%)

Hematologic: Bleeding (1% to 10%)

Hepatic: Elevated LFTs (1% to 10%)

Otic: Tinnitus (1% to 10%)

Restrictions An FDA-approved medication guide must be distributed when dispensing an oral outpatient prescription (new or refill) where this medication is to be used without direct supervision of a healthcare provider. Medication guides are available at http://www.fda.gov/cder/Offices/ODS/medication_guides.htm.

Dosage Children >14 years and Adults: Oral: 500 mg to start then 250 mg every 4 hours as needed; maximum therapy: 1 week

Dosing adjustment/comments in renal impairment: Not recommended for use

Mechanism of Action Inhibits prostaglandin synthesis by decreasing the activity of the enzyme, cyclooxygenase, which results in decreased formation of prostaglandin precursors

Contraindications Hypersensitivity to mefenamic acid, aspirin, other NSAIDs, or any component of the formulation; perioperative pain in the setting of coronary artery bypass surgery (CABG); active ulceration or chronic inflammation of the GI tract; renal disease; pregnancy (3rd trimester)

Warnings/Precautions [U.S. Boxed Warning]: NSAIDs are associated with an increased risk of adverse cardiovascular events, including MI, stroke, and new onset or worsening of pre-existing hypertension. Risk may be increased with duration of use or pre-existing cardiovascular risk factors or disease. Carefully evaluate individual cardiovascular risk profiles prior to prescribing. Use caution with fluid retention, CHF or hypertension. Concurrent administration of ibuprofen, and potentially other nonselective NSAIDs, may interfere with aspirin's cardioprotective effect.

Use of NSAIDs can compromise existing renal function. Renal toxicity can occur in patient with impaired renal function, dehydration, heart failure, liver dysfunction, those taking diuretics and ACEI and the elderly. Rehydrate patient before starting therapy. Monitor renal function closely. Mefenamic acid is not recommended for patients with advanced renal disease.

[U.S. Boxed Warning]: NSAIDs may increase risk of gastrointestinal irritation, ulceration, bleeding, and perforation. These events may occur at any time during therapy and without warning. Use caution with a history of GI disease (bleeding or ulcers), concurrent therapy with aspirin, anticoagulants and/or corticosteroids, smoking, use of alcohol, the elderly or debilitated patients.

Use the lowest effective dose for the shortest duration of time, consistent with individual patient goals, to reduce risk of cardiovascular or GI adverse events. Alternate therapies should be considered for patients at high risk.

NSAIDs may cause serious skin adverse events including exfoliative dermatitis, Stevens-Johnson syndrome (SJS) and toxic epidermal necrolysis (TEN). Anaphylactoid reactions may occur, even without prior exposure; patients with "aspirin triad" (bronchial asthma, aspirin intolerance, rhinitis) may be at increased risk. Do not use in patients who experience bronchospasm, asthma, rhinitis, or urticaria with NSAID or aspirin therapy.

Use with caution in patients with decreased hepatic function. Closely monitor patients with any abnormal LFT. Severe hepatic reactions (eg, fulminant hepatitis, liver failure) have occurred with NSAID use, rarely; discontinue if signs or symptoms of liver disease develop, or if systemic manifestations occur.

The elderly are at increased risk for adverse effects (especially peptic ulceration, CNS effects, renal toxicity) from NSAIDs even at low doses.

Withhold for at least 4-6 half-lives prior to surgical or dental procedures. Safety and efficacy have not been established in children <14 years of age.

Drug Interactions
Cytochrome P450 Effect: Substrate of CYP2C9 (minor); **Inhibits** CYP2C9 (strong)

Increased Effect/Toxicity: Anticoagulants (warfarin, heparin, LMWHs) in combination with NSAIDs can cause increased risk of bleeding. Other antiplatelet drugs (ticlopidine, clopidogrel, aspirin, abciximab, dipyridamole, eptifibatide, tirofiban) can cause an increased risk of bleeding. Mefenamic acid may increase the levels/effects of CYP2C9 substrates. Example substrates include bosentan, dapsone, fluoxetine, glimepiride, glipizide, losartan, montelukast, nateglinide, paclitaxel, phenytoin, warfarin, and zafirlukast. NSAIDs may increase serum creatinine, potassium, blood pressure, and cyclosporine levels during concurrent therapy; monitor cyclosporine levels and renal function carefully. Lithium levels can be increased; avoid concurrent use if possible or monitor lithium levels and adjust dose. Sulindac may have the least effect. When NSAID is stopped, lithium will need adjustment again. Corticosteroids may increase the risk of GI ulceration; avoid concurrent use. Serum concentration/toxicity of methotrexate may be increased. Concomitant use with fluoroquinolones may rarely increase risk of seizure.

Decreased Effect: Antihypertensive effects of ACE inhibitors, angiotensin antagonists, beta-blockers, diuretics, and hydralazine may be decreased by concurrent therapy with NSAIDs; monitor blood pressure. Salicylates' antiplatelet effect may be reduced. Cholestyramine (and other bile acid sequestrants) may decrease the absorption of NSAIDs; separate by at least 2 hours.

Ethanol/Nutrition/Herb Interactions
Ethanol: Avoid ethanol (may enhance gastric mucosal irritation).

Herb/Nutraceutical: Avoid alfalfa, anise, bilberry, bladderwrack, bromelain, cat's claw, celery, coleus, cordyceps, dong quai, evening primrose, feverfew, fenugreek, garlic, ginger, ginkgo biloba, red clover, horse chestnut, grapeseed, green tea, ginseng, guggul, horse chestnut seed, horseradish, licorice, prickly ash, red clover, reishi, SAMe, sweet clover, turmeric, white willow (all have additional antiplatelet activity).

Pharmacodynamics/Kinetics
Onset of action: Peak effect: 2-4 hours
Duration: ≤6 hours
Protein binding: High
Metabolism: Conjugated hepatically
Half-life elimination: 3.5 hours
Excretion: Urine (50%) and feces as unchanged drug and metabolites

Pregnancy Risk Factor C/D (3rd trimester)

Dosage Forms
Capsule: 250 mg
Ponstel®: 250 mg

Mefloquine (ME floe kwin)

U.S. Brand Names Lariam®
Canadian Brand Names Apo-Mefloquine®; Lariam®
Generic Available Yes
(Continued)

Mefloquine (Continued)

Index Terms Mefloquine Hydrochloride

Pharmacologic Category Antimalarial Agent

Use Treatment of acute malarial infections and prevention of malaria

Local Anesthetic/Vasoconstrictor Precautions No information available to require special precautions

Effects on Dental Treatment No significant effects or complications reported

Common Adverse Effects

Frequency not defined: Neuropsychiatric events

1% to 10%:

Central nervous system: Headache, fever, chills, fatigue

Dermatologic: Rash

Gastrointestinal: Vomiting (3%), diarrhea, stomach pain, nausea, appetite decreased

Neuromuscular & skeletal: Myalgia

Otic: Tinnitus

Restrictions An FDA-approved medication guide and wallet card must be distributed when dispensing an outpatient prescription (new or refill) to prevent malaria where this medication is to be used without direct supervision of a healthcare provider. Medication guides are available at http://www.fda.gov/cder/Offices/ODS/medication_guides.htm.

Mechanism of Action Mefloquine is a quinoline-methanol compound structurally similar to quinine; mefloquine's effectiveness in the treatment and prophylaxis of malaria is due to the destruction of the asexual blood forms of the malarial pathogens that affect humans, *Plasmodium falciparum*, *P. vivax*, *P. malariae*, *P. ovale*

Drug Interactions

Cytochrome P450 Effect: Substrate of CYP3A4 (major); **Inhibits** CYP2D6 (weak), 3A4 (weak)

Increased Effect/Toxicity: Use caution with drugs that alter cardiac conduction; increased toxicity with chloroquine, quinine, and quinidine (hold treatment until at least 12 hours after these later drugs). CYP3A4 inhibitors may increase the levels/effects of mefloquine; example inhibitors include azole antifungals, clarithromycin, diclofenac, doxycycline, erythromycin, imatinib, isoniazid, nefazodone, nicardipine, propofol, protease inhibitors, quinidine, telithromycin, and verapamil.

Decreased Effect: Mefloquine may decrease the effect of valproic acid, carbamazepine, phenobarbital, and phenytoin. CYP3A4 inducers may decrease the levels/effects of mefloquine; example inducers include aminoglutethimide, carbamazepine, nafcillin, nevirapine, phenobarbital, phenytoin, and rifamycins. Vaccination with oral live attenuated Ty21a vaccine should be delayed for at least 24 hours after the administration of mefloquine.

Pharmacodynamics/Kinetics

Absorption: Well absorbed

Distribution: V_d: 19 L/kg; blood, urine, CSF, tissues; enters breast milk

Protein binding: 98%

Metabolism: Extensively hepatic; main metabolite is inactive

Bioavailability: Increased by food

Half-life elimination: 21-22 days

Time to peak, plasma: 6-24 hours (median: ~17 hours)

Excretion: Primarily bile and feces; urine (9% as unchanged drug, 4% as primary metabolite)

Pregnancy Risk Factor C

Megestrol (me JES trole)

U.S. Brand Names Megace®; Megace® ES

Canadian Brand Names Apo-Megestrol®; Megace®; Megace® OS; Nu-Megestrol

Mexican Brand Names Mestrel

Generic Available Yes

Index Terms 5071-1DL(6); Megestrol Acetate; NSC-71423

Pharmacologic Category Antineoplastic Agent, Hormone; Appetite Stimulant; Progestin

Use Palliative treatment of breast and endometrial carcinoma; treatment of anorexia, cachexia, or unexplained significant weight loss in patients with AIDS

Local Anesthetic/Vasoconstrictor Precautions No information available to require special precautions

Effects on Dental Treatment No significant effects or complications reported

Common Adverse Effects

Frequency not always defined.

Cardiovascular: Hypertension (≤8%), cardiomyopathy (1% to 3%), chest pain (1% to 3%), edema (1% to 3%), palpitation (1% to 3%), peripheral edema (1% to 3%), heart failure

Central nervous system: Headache (≤10%), insomnia (≤6%), fever (1% to 6%), pain (≤6%, similar to placebo), abnormal thinking (1% to 3%), confusion (1% to 3%), seizure (1% to 3%), depression (1% to 3%), hypoesthesia (1% to 3%), mood changes, malaise, lethargy

Dermatologic: Rash (2% to 12%), alopecia (1% to 3%), pruritus (1% to 3%), vesiculobullous rash (1% to 3%)

Endocrine & metabolic: Breakthrough bleeding and amenorrhea, spotting, changes in menstrual flow, changes in cervical erosion and secretions, increased breast tenderness, changes in vaginal bleeding pattern, hyperglycemia (≤6%), gynecomastia (1% to 3%), diabetes, HPA axis suppression, adrenal insufficiency, Cushing's syndrome, hypercalcemia, hot flashes

Gastrointestinal: Weight gain (not attributed to edema or fluid retention), diarrhea (6% to 15%, similar to placebo), flatulence (≤10%), vomiting (≤6%), nausea (≤5%), dyspepsia (≤4%), abdominal pain (1% to 3%), constipation (1% to 3%), salivation increased (1% to 3%), xerostomia (1% to 3%)

Genitourinary: Impotence (4% to 14%), decreased libido (≤5%), urinary incontinence (1% to 3%), urinary tract infection (1% to 3%), urinary frequency (≤2%)

Hematologic: Anemia (≤5%), leukopenia (1% to 3%)

Hepatic: Hepatomegaly (1% to 3%), LDH increased (1% to 3%), cholestatic jaundice, hepatotoxicity

Neuromuscular & skeletal: Carpal tunnel syndrome, weakness (2% to 8%), neuropathy (1% to 3%), paresthesia (1% to 3%)

Ocular: Amblyopia (1% to 3%)

Renal: Albuminuria (1% to 3%)

Respiratory: Dyspnea (1% to 3%), cough (1% to 3%), pharyngitis (1% to 3%), pneumonia (≤2%), hyperpnea

Miscellaneous: Diaphoresis (1% to 3%), herpes infection (1% to 3%), infection (1% to 3%), tumor flare

Mechanism of Action A synthetic progestin with antiestrogenic properties which disrupt the estrogen receptor cycle. Megestrol interferes with the normal estrogen cycle and results in a lower LH titer. May also have a direct effect on the endometrium. Megestrol is an antineoplastic progestin thought to act through an antileutenizing effect mediated via the pituitary. May stimulate appetite by antagonizing the metabolic effects of catabolic cytokines.

Drug Interactions

Increased Effect/Toxicity: Megestrol may enhance the hepatotoxic effect of cyclosporine; megestrol may increase the serum concentration of cyclosporine.

Decreased Effect: Aminoglutethimide may decrease the levels/effects of megestrol.

Pharmacodynamics/Kinetics

Absorption: Well absorbed orally

Metabolism: Hepatic (to free steroids and glucuronide conjugates)

Half-life elimination: 13-105 hours

Time to peak, serum: 1-3 hours

Excretion: Urine (57% to 78%; 5% to 8% as metabolites); feces (8% to 30%)

Pregnancy Risk Factor X

Megestrol Acetate see Megestrol on page 1030

Melanex® see Hydroquinone on page 841

Melfiat® [DSC] see Phendimetrazine on page 1286

Meloxicam (mel OKS i kam)

U.S. Brand Names Mobic®

Canadian Brand Names Apo-Meloxicam®; CO Meloxicam; Gen-Meloxicam; Mobic®; Mobicox®; Novo-Meloxicam; PMS-Meloxicam

Mexican Brand Names Aflamid; Exel; Loxibest; Melosteral; Mobicox

Generic Available Yes

Pharmacologic Category Nonsteroidal Anti-inflammatory Drug (NSAID), Oral

Use Relief of signs and symptoms of osteoarthritis, rheumatoid arthritis, and juvenile rheumatoid arthritis (JRA)

(Continued)

Meloxicam *(Continued)*

Local Anesthetic/Vasoconstrictor Precautions No information available to require special precautions

Effects on Dental Treatment Key adverse event(s) related to dental treatment: Taste perversion, ulcerative stomatitis, and xerostomia (normal salivary flow resumes upon discontinuation).

Common Adverse Effects Percentages reported in adult patients; abdominal pain, diarrhea, headache, pyrexia, and vomiting were reported more commonly in pediatric patients

2% to 10%:

Cardiovascular: Edema (<1% to 4%)

Central nervous system: Headache (2% to 8%), dizziness (<1% to 4%), insomnia (<1% to 4%)

Dermatologic: Pruritus (<1% to 2%), rash (<1% to 3%)

Gastrointestinal: Diarrhea (3% to 8%), dyspepsia (4% to 9%), abdominal pain (2% to 5%), nausea (2% to 7%), constipation (<1% to 3%), flatulence (<1% to 3%), vomiting (<1% to 3%)

Hematologic: Anemia (<1% to 4%)

Neuromuscular & skeletal: Arthralgia (<1% to 5%), back pain (<1% to 3%)

Respiratory: Cough (<1% to 2%), pharyngitis (<1% to 3%), upper respiratory infection (2% to 8%)

Miscellaneous: Flu-like syndrome (2% to 6%), falls (3%)

Restrictions An FDA-approved medication guide must be distributed when dispensing an oral outpatient prescription (new or refill) where this medication is to be used without direct supervision of a healthcare provider. Medication guides are available at http://www.fda.gov/cder/Offices/ODS/medication_guides.htm.

Dosage Oral:

Children ≥2 years: JRA: 0.125 mg/kg/day; maximum dose: 7.5 mg/day

Adults: Osteoarthritis, rheumatoid arthritis: Initial: 7.5 mg once daily; some patients may receive additional benefit from an increased dose of 15 mg once daily; maximum dose: 15 mg/day

Elderly: Increased concentrations may occur in elderly patients (particularly in females); however, no specific dosage adjustment is recommended

Dosage adjustment in renal impairment:

Mild-to-moderate impairment: No specific dosage recommendations

Significant impairment (Cl$_{cr}$ ≤15 mL/minute): Avoid use

Hemodialysis: Supplemental dose after dialysis not necessary.

Dosage adjustment in hepatic impairment:

Mild (Child-Pugh class A) to moderate (Child-Pugh class B) hepatic dysfunction: No dosage adjustment is necessary

Severe hepatic impairment: Patients with severe hepatic impairment have not been adequately studied

Mechanism of Action Inhibits prostaglandin synthesis by decreasing the activity of the enzyme, cyclooxygenase, which results in decreased formation of prostaglandin precursors

Contraindications Hypersensitivity to meloxicam, aspirin, other NSAIDs, or any component of the formulation; perioperative pain in the setting of coronary artery bypass surgery (CABG); pregnancy (3rd trimester)

Warnings/Precautions [U.S. Boxed Warning]: NSAIDs are associated with an increased risk of adverse cardiovascular events, including MI, stroke, and new onset or worsening of pre-existing hypertension. Risk may be increased with duration of use or pre-existing cardiovascular risk factors or disease. Carefully evaluate individual cardiovascular risk profiles prior to prescribing. Use caution with fluid retention, CHF or hypertension. Concurrent administration of ibuprofen, and potentially other nonselective NSAIDs, may interfere with aspirin's cardioprotective effect.

Use of NSAIDs can compromise existing renal function. Renal toxicity can occur in patient with impaired renal function, dehydration, heart failure, liver dysfunction, those taking diuretics, angiotensin antagonists, ACEIs, and the elderly. Rehydrate patient before starting therapy. Monitor renal function closely. Meloxicam is not recommended for patients with advanced renal disease

[U.S. Boxed Warning]: NSAIDs may increase risk of gastrointestinal irritation, ulceration, bleeding, and perforation. These events may occur at any time during therapy and without warning. Use caution with a history of GI disease (bleeding or ulcers), concurrent therapy with aspirin, anticoagulants and/or corticosteroids, smoking, use of alcohol, the elderly or debilitated patients.

Use the lowest effective dose for the shortest duration of time, consistent with individual patient goals, to reduce risk of cardiovascular or GI adverse events. Alternate therapies should be considered for patients at high risk.

NSAIDs may cause serious skin adverse events including exfoliative dermatitis, Stevens-Johnson syndrome (SJS) and toxic epidermal necrolysis (TEN). Anaphylactoid reactions may occur, even without prior exposure; patients with "aspirin triad" (bronchial asthma, aspirin intolerance, rhinitis) may be at increased risk. Do not use in patients who experience bronchospasm, asthma, rhinitis, or urticaria with NSAID or aspirin therapy. Use caution in other forms of asthma.

Use with caution in patients with decreased hepatic function. Closely monitor patients with any abnormal LFT. Severe hepatic reactions (eg, fulminant hepatitis, liver failure) have occurred with NSAID use, rarely; discontinue if signs or symptoms of liver disease develop, or if systemic manifestations occur.

The elderly are at increased risk for adverse effects (especially peptic ulceration, CNS effects, renal toxicity) from NSAIDs even at low doses.

Withhold for at least 4-6 half-lives prior to surgical or dental procedures. Safety and efficacy have not been established in pediatric patients <2 years of age.

Drug Interactions
Cytochrome P450 Effect: Substrate (minor) of CYP2C9, 3A4; **Inhibits** CYP2C9 (weak)

Increased Effect/Toxicity: Renal adverse effects of NSAIDs may be increased with ACE inhibitors and angiotensin antagonists. Anticoagulants (warfarin, heparin, LMWHs) in combination with NSAIDs can cause increased risk of bleeding. Antiplatelet drugs (ticlopidine, clopidogrel, aspirin, abciximab, dipyridamole, eptifibatide, tirofiban) can cause an increased risk of bleeding. Aspirin increases serum concentrations (AUC) of meloxicam (in addition to potential for additive adverse effects); concurrent use is not recommended. Corticosteroids may increase the risk of GI ulceration; avoid concurrent use. NSAIDs may increase serum creatinine, potassium, blood pressure, and cyclosporine levels; monitor cyclosporine levels and renal function carefully. Lithium levels can be increased; avoid concurrent use if possible or monitor lithium levels and adjust dose. When NSAID is stopped, lithium will need adjustment again. Serum concentration/toxicity of methotrexate may be increased. Warfarin INRs may be increased by meloxicam. Monitor INR closely, particularly during initiation or change in dose. May increase risk of bleeding. Use lowest possible dose for shortest duration possible. Concomitant use with fluoroquinolones may rarely increase risk of seizure.

Decreased Effect: Cholestyramine (and possibly colestipol) increases the clearance of meloxicam. Hydralazine's antihypertensive effect is decreased; avoid concurrent use. Loop diuretic efficacy (diuretic and antihypertensive effect) may be reduced by NSAIDs. Antihypertensive effects of thiazide diuretics are decreased; avoid concurrent use. Salicylates' antiplatelet effect may be reduced. NSAIDs may decrease the antihypertensive effect of beta-blockers, ACE inhibitors, and angiotensin antagonists. Cholestyramine (and other bile acid sequestrants) may decrease the absorption of NSAIDs; separate by at least 2 hours.

Ethanol/Nutrition/Herb Interactions
Ethanol: Avoid ethanol (may enhance gastric mucosal irritation).

Herb/Nutraceutical: Avoid alfalfa, anise, bilberry, bladderwrack, bromelain, cat's claw, celery, coleus, cordyceps, dong quai, evening primrose, feverfew, fenugreek, garlic, ginger, ginkgo biloba, red clover, horse chestnut, grapeseed, green tea, ginseng, guggul, horse chestnut seed, horseradish, licorice, prickly ash, red clover, reishi, SAMe, sweet clover, turmeric, white willow (all have additional antiplatelet activity).

Dietary Considerations Should be taken with food or milk to minimize gastrointestinal irritation.

Pharmacodynamics/Kinetics
Distribution: 10 L

Protein binding: 99.4%

Metabolism: Hepatic via CYP2C9 and CYP3A4 (minor); forms 4 metabolites (inactive)

Bioavailability: 89%

Half-life elimination: Adults: 15-20 hours

Time to peak: Initial: 5-10 hours; Secondary: 12-14 hours

Excretion: Urine and feces (as inactive metabolites)

Pregnancy Risk Factor C/D (3rd trimester)

Dosage Forms
Suspension: 7.5 mg/5 mL (100 mL)
Mobic®: 7.5 mg/5 mL
Tablet: 7.5 mg, 15 mg
Mobic®: 7.5 mg, 15 mg

Melpaque HP® *see Hydroquinone on page 841*

Melphalan (MEL fa lan)

U.S. Brand Names Alkeran®
Canadian Brand Names Alkeran®
Mexican Brand Names Alkeran
Generic Available No
Index Terms L-PAM; L-Sarcolysin; NSC-8806; Phenylalanine Mustard
Pharmacologic Category Antineoplastic Agent, Alkylating Agent
Use Palliative treatment of multiple myeloma and nonresectable epithelial ovarian carcinoma
Unlabeled/Investigational Use Treatment of neuroblastoma, rhabdomyosarcoma, breast cancer; part of an induction regimen for marrow and stem cell transplantation
Local Anesthetic/Vasoconstrictor Precautions No information available to require special precautions
Effects on Dental Treatment Key adverse event(s) related to dental treatment: Stomatitis.
Common Adverse Effects
>10%:
  Gastrointestinal: Vomiting (oral low-dose: <10%; I.V.: 30% to 90%)
  Hematologic: Myelosuppression, leukopenia (onset 7 days; nadir 14-35 days; recovery 28-56 days), thrombocytopenia (onset 7 days; nadir 14-35 days; recovery 28-56 days)
  Miscellaneous: Secondary malignancy (<2% to 20%; cumulative dose and duration dependent)
1% to 10%: Miscellaneous: Hypersensitivity (I.V.: 2%)
Mechanism of Action Alkylating agent which is a derivative of mechlorethamine that inhibits DNA and RNA synthesis via formation of carbonium ions; cross-links strands of DNA; acts on both resting and rapidly dividing tumor cells.
Drug Interactions
  Increased Effect/Toxicity: Risk of nephrotoxicity of cyclosporine is increased by melphalan. Concomitant use of I.V. melphalan may cause serious GI toxicity. Cisplatin may increase the levels/effects of melphalan (I.V.). Melphalan may increase risk of vaccinal infection.
  Decreased Effect: Melphalan may decrease the levels/effects of digoxin.
Pharmacodynamics/Kinetics
  Absorption: Oral: Variable and incomplete
  Distribution: V_d: 0.5-0.6 L/kg throughout total body water
  Protein binding: 60% to 90%; primarily to albumin, 20% to α_1-acid glycoprotein
  Metabolism: Hepatic; chemical hydrolysis to monohydroxymelphalan and dihydroxymelphalan
  Bioavailability: Unpredictable; 61% ± 26%, decreasing with repeated doses
  Half-life elimination: Terminal: I.V.: 1.5 hours; oral: 1-1.25 hours
  Time to peak, serum: ~1-2 hours
  Excretion: Oral: Feces (20% to 50%); urine (10% to 30% as unchanged drug)
Pregnancy Risk Factor D

Melquin-3® *see* Hydroquinone *on page 841*
Melquin HP® *see* Hydroquinone *on page 841*

Memantine (me MAN teen)

U.S. Brand Names Namenda™
Canadian Brand Names Ebixa®
Mexican Brand Names Ebixa
Generic Available No
Index Terms Memantine Hydrochloride
Pharmacologic Category N-Methyl-D-Aspartate Receptor Antagonist
Use Treatment of moderate-to-severe dementia of the Alzheimer's type
Unlabeled/Investigational Use Treatment of mild-to-moderate vascular dementia
Local Anesthetic/Vasoconstrictor Precautions No information available to require special precautions
Effects on Dental Treatment No significant effects or complications reported
Common Adverse Effects
1% to 10%:
  Cardiovascular: Hypertension (4%), cardiac failure, syncope, cerebrovascular accident, transient ischemic attack
  Central nervous system: Dizziness (7%), confusion (6%), headache (6%), hallucinations (3%), pain (3%), somnolence (3%), fatigue (2%), aggressive reaction, ataxia, vertigo

Dermatologic: Rash
Gastrointestinal: Constipation (5%), vomiting (3%), weight loss
Genitourinary: Micturition
Hematologic: Anemia
Hepatic: Alkaline phosphatase increased
Neuromuscular & skeletal: Back pain (3%), hypokinesia
Ocular: Cataract, conjunctivitis
Respiratory: Cough (4%), dyspnea (2%), pneumonia

Mechanism of Action Glutamate, the primary excitatory amino acid in the CNS, may contribute to the pathogenesis of Alzheimer's disease (AD) by over-stimulating various glutamate receptors leading to excitotoxicity and neuronal cell death. Memantine is an uncompetitive antagonist of the N-methyl-D-aspartate (NMDA) type of glutamate receptors, located ubiquitously throughout the brain. Under normal physiologic conditions, the (unstimulated) NMDA receptor ion channel is blocked by magnesium ions, which are displaced after agonist-induced depolarization. Pathologic or excessive receptor activation, as postulated to occur during AD, prevents magnesium from reentering and blocking the channel pore resulting in a chronically open state and excessive calcium influx. Memantine binds to the intra-pore magnesium site, but with longer dwell time, and thus functions as an effective receptor blocker only under conditions of excessive stimulation; memantine does not affect normal neurotransmission.

Drug Interactions
Increased Effect/Toxicity: Clearance of memantine is decreased 80% at urinary pH 8; use caution with medications (carbonic anhydrase inhibitors, sodium bicarbonate) which may increase urinary pH.

Pharmacodynamics/Kinetics
Distribution: 9-11 L/kg
Protein binding: 45%
Metabolism: Forms 3 metabolites (minimal activity)
Half-life elimination: Terminal: 60-80 hours; severe renal impairment (Cl$_{cr}$ 5-29 mL/minute): 117-156 hours
Time to peak, serum: 3-7 hours
Excretion: Urine (57% to 82% unchanged); excretion reduced by alkaline urine pH

Pregnancy Risk Factor B

Memantine Hydrochloride *see* Memantine *on page 1034*

Menactra® *see* Meningococcal Polysaccharide (Groups A / C / Y and W-135) Diphtheria Toxoid Conjugate Vaccine *on page 1035*

Menest® *see* Estrogens (Esterified) *on page 613*

Meningococcal Polysaccharide (Groups A / C / Y and W-135) Diphtheria Toxoid Conjugate Vaccine
(me NIN joe kok al pol i SAK a ride groops aye, see, why & dubl yoo won thur tee fyve dif THEER ee a TOKS oyds KON joo gate vak SEEN)

Related Information
Immunizations (Vaccines) *on page 1886*
U.S. Brand Names Menactra®
Generic Available No
Index Terms MCV4; Quadrivalent Meningococcal Conjugate Vaccine
Pharmacologic Category Vaccine
Use Provide active immunization of adolescents and adults (11-55 years of age) against invasive meningococcal disease caused by *N. meningitidis* serogroups A, C, Y and W-135

The ACIP recommends routine vaccination of all adolescents at age 11-12 years. For adolescents not previously vaccinated, vaccine should be administered prior to high school entry (~15 years of age).
The ACIP also recommends routine vaccination for persons at increased risk for meningococcal disease. (MCV4 is preferred for persons aged 11-55 years; MPSV4 may be used if MCV4 is not available). Persons at increased risk include:
College freshmen living in dormitories
Microbiologists routinely exposed to isolates of *N. meningitides*
Military recruits
Persons traveling to or who reside in countries where *N. meningitides* is hyperendemic or epidemic, particularly if contact with local population will be prolonged
Persons with terminal complement component deficiencies
Persons with anatomic or functional asplenia
(Continued)

Meningococcal Polysaccharide (Groups A / C / Y and W-135) Diphtheria Toxoid Conjugate Vaccine
(Continued)

Use is also recommended during meningococcal outbreaks caused by vaccine preventable serogroups.

Local Anesthetic/Vasoconstrictor Precautions No information available to require special precautions

Effects on Dental Treatment No significant effects or complications reported

Common Adverse Effects All serious adverse reactions must be reported to the U.S. Department of Health and Human Services Vaccine Adverse Event Reporting System (VAERS) 1-800-822-7967 or www.vaers.org.

>10%:
Central nervous system: Pain (54% to 59%), headache (36% to 41%), fatigue (30% to 35%), malaise (22% to 24%)
Gastrointestinal: Diarrhea (12% to 16%), anorexia (11% to 12%)
Local: Redness (11% to 14%), swelling (11% to 13%), induration (16% to 17%)
Neuromuscular & skeletal: Arthralgia (17% to 20%)
1% to 10%:
Central nervous system: Chills (7% to 10%), fever (2% to 5%)
Gastrointestinal: Vomiting (2%)
Local: Rash (1% to 2%)
Postmarketing and/or case reports: Guillain-Barré syndrome, transverse myelitis

Mechanism of Action Induces immunity against meningococcal disease via the formation of bactericidal antibodies directed toward the polysaccharide capsular components of *Neisseria meningitidis* serogroups A, C, Y and W-135.

Pregnancy Risk Factor C

Meningococcal Polysaccharide Vaccine (Groups A, C, Y, and W-135)
(me NIN joe kok al pol i SAK a ride vak SEEN groops aye, see, why & dubl yoo won thur tee fyve)

U.S. Brand Names Menomune®-A/C/Y/W-135
Generic Available No
Index Terms MPSV4; Quadrivalent Meningococcal Conjugate Vaccine
Pharmacologic Category Vaccine
Use Provide active immunity to meningococcal serogroups contained in the vaccine

The ACIP recommends routine vaccination for persons at increased risk for meningococcal disease. (Use of MPSV4 is recommended in children 2-10 years and adults > 55 years. MCV4 is preferred for persons aged 11-55 years; MPSV4 may be used if MCV4 is not available). Persons at increased risk include:
College freshmen living in dormitories
Microbiologists routinely exposed to isolates of *N. meningitides*
Military recruits
Persons traveling to or who reside in countries where *N. meningitides* is hyperendemic or epidemic, particularly if contact with local population will be prolonged
Persons with terminal complement component deficiencies
Persons with anatomic or functional asplenia
Use is also recommended during meningococcal outbreaks caused by vaccine preventable serogroups.

Local Anesthetic/Vasoconstrictor Precautions No information available to require special precautions

Effects on Dental Treatment No significant effects or complications reported

Common Adverse Effects All serious adverse reactions must be reported to the U.S. Department of Health and Human Services (DHHS) Vaccine Adverse Event Reporting System (VAERS) 1-800-822-7967. Percentages reported in adults; incidence of erythema, swelling, or tenderness may be higher in children
>10%: Local: Tenderness (9% to 36%)
1% to 10%:
Central nervous system: Headache (2% to 5%), malaise (2%), fever (100°F to 106°F: 3%), chills (2%)
Local: Pain at injection site (2% to 3%), erythema (1% to 4%), induration (1% to 4%)

Mechanism of Action Induces the formation of bactericidal antibodies to meningococcal antigens; the presence of these antibodies is strongly correlated with immunity to meningococcal disease caused by *Neisseria meningitidis* groups A, C, Y and W-135.

Drug Interactions
Increased Effect/Toxicity: Should not be administered with whole-cell pertussis or whole-cell typhoid vaccines due to combined endotoxin content.
Decreased Effect: Decreased effect with administration of immunoglobulin within 1 month.

Pharmacodynamics/Kinetics
Onset of action: Antibody levels: 7-10 days
Duration: Antibodies against group A and C polysaccharides decline markedly (to prevaccination levels) over the first 3 years following a single dose of vaccine, especially in children <4 years of age

Pregnancy Risk Factor C

Menomune®-A/C/Y/W-135 *see* Meningococcal Polysaccharide Vaccine (Groups A, C, Y, and W-135) *on page 1036*

Menopur® *see* Menotropins *on page 1037*

Menostar™ *see* Estradiol *on page 602*

Menotropins (men oh TROE pins)

U.S. Brand Names Menopur®; Repronex®
Canadian Brand Names Repronex®
Generic Available No
Index Terms hMG; Human Menopausal Gonadotropin
Pharmacologic Category Gonadotropin; Ovulation Stimulator
Use Female:
In conjunction with hCG to induce ovulation and pregnancy in infertile females experiencing oligoanovulation or anovulation when the cause of anovulation is functional and not caused by primary ovarian failure (Repronex®)
Stimulation of multiple follicle development in ovulatory patients as part of an assisted reproductive technology (ART) (Menopur®, Repronex®)
Unlabeled/Investigational Use Male: Stimulation of spermatogenesis in primary or secondary hypogonadotropic hypogonadism
Local Anesthetic/Vasoconstrictor Precautions No information available to require special precautions
Effects on Dental Treatment No significant effects or complications reported
Common Adverse Effects Adverse effects may vary according to specific product, route, and/or dosage.
>10%:
Central nervous system: Headache (up to 34%)
Gastrointestinal: Abdominal pain (up to 18%), nausea (up to 12%)
Genitourinary: OHSS (up to 13%, dose related)
Local: Injection site reaction (4% to 12%)
1% to 10%:
Cardiovascular: Flushing
Central nervous system: Dizziness, malaise, migraine
Endocrine & metabolic: Breast tenderness, hot flashes, menstrual irregularities
Gastrointestinal: Abdominal cramping, abdominal fullness, constipation, diarrhea, enlarged abdomen, vomiting
Genitourinary: Ectopic pregnancy, ovarian disease, vaginal hemorrhage
Local: Injection site edema/pain
Neuromuscular & skeletal: Back pain
Respiratory: Cough increased, respiratory disorder
Miscellaneous: Infection, flu-like syndrome

Frequency not defined:
Cardiovascular: Stroke, tachycardia, thrombosis (venous or arterial)
Central nervous system: Dizziness
Dermatologic: Angioedema, rash, urticaria
Genitourinary: Adnexal torsion, hemoperitoneum, ovarian enlargement
Neuromuscular & skeletal: Limb necrosis
Respiratory: Acute respiratory distress syndrome, atelectasis, dyspnea, embolism, laryngeal edema pulmonary infarction tachypnea
Miscellaneous: Allergic reaction, anaphylaxis

Mechanism of Action Actions occur as a result of both follicle stimulating hormone (FSH) effects and luteinizing hormone (LH) effects; menotropins stimulate the development and maturation of the ovarian follicle (FSH), cause ovulation (LH), and stimulate the development of the corpus luteum (LH); in males it stimulates spermatogenesis (LH)
(Continued)

Menotropins (Continued)

Pharmacodynamics/Kinetics Excretion: Urine (~10% as unchanged drug)
Pregnancy Risk Factor X

Mentax® *see Butenafine on page 253*

Mepenzolate (me PEN zoe late)

U.S. Brand Names Cantil® [DSC]
Canadian Brand Names Cantil®
Generic Available No
Index Terms Mepenzolate Bromide
Pharmacologic Category Anticholinergic Agent; Antispasmodic Agent, Gastrointestinal
Use Adjunctive treatment of peptic ulcer disease
Local Anesthetic/Vasoconstrictor Precautions No information available to require special precautions
Effects on Dental Treatment Key adverse event(s) related to dental treatment: Xerostomia (normal salivary flow resumes upon discontinuation), dry throat, dysphagia, and loss of taste.
Common Adverse Effects Frequency not defined.
Cardiovascular: Palpitation, tachycardia
Central nervous system: Headache, nervousness, drowsiness, dizziness, CNS stimulation may be produced with large doses, confusion, insomnia
Dermatologic: Dry skin, urticaria
Gastrointestinal: Constipation, xerostomia, dysphagia, nausea, vomiting, delayed gastric emptying, loss of taste
Genitourinary: Impotence, urinary hesitation, urinary retention
Neuromuscular & skeletal: Weakness
Ophthalmic: Cycloplegia, blurred vision, ocular tension increased, pupil dilation
Miscellaneous: Diaphoresis decreased, hypersensitivity reactions, anaphylaxis, lactation suppressed
Mechanism of Action Mepenzolate is a postganglionic parasympathetic inhibitor. It decreases gastric acid and pepsin secretion and suppresses spontaneous contractions of the colon.
Pharmacodynamics/Kinetics
Absorption: Oral: Low
Excretion: Urine (3% to 33%); feces
Pregnancy Risk Factor B

Mepenzolate Bromide *see Mepenzolate on page 1038*
Mepergan *see Meperidine and Promethazine on page 1041*

Meperidine (me PER i deen)

Related Information
Oral Pain *on page 1788*
Related Sample Prescriptions
Severe Oral Pain *on page 1835*
U.S. Brand Names Demerol®; Meperitab®
Canadian Brand Names Demerol®
Mexican Brand Names Demerol HCl
Generic Available Yes
Index Terms Isonipecaine Hydrochloride; Meperidine Hydrochloride; Pethidine Hydrochloride
Pharmacologic Category Analgesic, Opioid
Dental Use Adjunct in preoperative intravenous conscious sedation in patients undergoing dental surgery; alternate oral narcotic in patients allergic to codeine to treat moderate to moderate-severe pain
Use Management of moderate to severe pain; adjunct to anesthesia and preoperative sedation
Unlabeled/Investigational Use
Reduce postoperative shivering; reduce rigors from amphotericin
Local Anesthetic/Vasoconstrictor Precautions No information available to require special precautions
Effects on Dental Treatment Key adverse event(s) related to dental treatment: Xerostomia (normal salivary flow resumes upon discontinuation). See Dental Comment.
Significant Adverse Effects Frequency not defined.
Cardiovascular: Hypotension

Central nervous system: Fatigue, drowsiness, dizziness, nervousness, head-ache, restlessness, malaise, confusion, mental depression, hallucinations, paradoxical CNS stimulation, increased intracranial pressure, seizure (associated with metabolite accumulation), serotonin syndrome

Dermatologic: Rash, urticaria

Gastrointestinal: Nausea, vomiting, constipation, anorexia, stomach cramps, xerostomia, biliary spasm, paralytic ileus, sphincter of Oddi spasm

Genitourinary: Ureteral spasms, decreased urination

Local: Pain at injection site

Neuromuscular & skeletal: Weakness

Respiratory: Dyspnea

Miscellaneous: Histamine release, physical and psychological dependence

Restrictions C-II

Dental Usual Dosing Pain (analgesic): Adults: Oral: Initial: Opiate-naive: 50 mg every 3-4 hours as needed; usual dosage range: 50-150 mg every 2-4 hours as needed (manufacturers recommendation; oral route is not recommended for acute pain)

Dosage Note: Doses should be titrated to necessary analgesic effect. When changing route of administration, note that oral doses are about half as effective as parenteral dose. Not recommended for chronic pain. These are guidelines and do not represent the maximum doses that may be required in all patients. In patients with normal renal function, doses of ≤600 mg/24 hours and use for ≤48 hours are recommended (American Pain Society, 1999).

Children: Pain: Oral, I.M., I.V., SubQ: 1-1.5 mg/kg/dose every 3-4 hours as needed; 1-2 mg/kg as a single dose preoperative medication; maximum 100 mg/dose (Note: Oral route is not recommended for acute pain.)

Adults: Pain:

Oral: Initial: Opiate-naive: 50 mg every 3-4 hours as needed; usual dosage range: 50-150 mg every 2-4 hours as needed (manufacturers recommendation; oral route is not recommended for acute pain)

I.M., SubQ: Initial: Opiate-naive: 50-75 mg every 3-4 hours as needed; patients with prior opiate exposure may require higher initial doses

Preoperatively: 50-100 mg given 30-90 minutes before the beginning of anesthesia

Slow I.V.: Initial: 5-10 mg every 5 minutes as needed

Patient-controlled analgesia (PCA): Usual concentration: 10 mg/mL

Initial dose: 10 mg

Demand dose: 1-5 mg (manufacturer recommendations); range 5-25 mg (American Pain Society, 1999).

Lockout interval: 5-10 minutes

Elderly:

Oral: 50 mg every 4 hours

I.M.: 25 mg every 4 hours

Dosing adjustment in renal impairment: Avoid repeated administration of meperidine in renal dysfunction:

Cl$_{cr}$ 10-50 mL/minute: Administer at 75% of normal dose

Cl$_{cr}$ <10 mL/minute: Administer at 50% of normal dose

Dosing adjustment/comments in hepatic disease: Increased narcotic effect in cirrhosis; reduction in dose more important for oral than I.V. route

Mechanism of Action Binds to opiate receptors in the CNS, causing inhibition of ascending pain pathways, altering the perception of and response to pain; produces generalized CNS depression

Contraindications Hypersensitivity to meperidine or any component of the formulation; use with or within 14 days of MAO inhibitors; pregnancy (prolonged use or high doses near term)

Warnings/Precautions Meperidine is not recommended for the management of chronic pain. When used for acute pain (in patients without renal or CNS disease), treatment should be limited to 48 hours and doses should not exceed 600 mg/24 hours. Oral meperidine is not recommended for acute pain management. Normeperidine (an active metabolite and CNS stimulant) may accumulate and precipitate anxiety, tremors, or seizures; risk increases with renal dysfunction and cumulative dose. Effects may be potentiated when used with other sedative drugs or ethanol.

May cause CNS depression, which may impair physical or mental abilities; patients must be cautioned about performing tasks which require mental alertness (eg, operating machinery or driving). Use only with extreme caution (if at all) in patients with head injury or increased intracranial pressure (ICP); potential to elevate ICP may be greatly exaggerated in these patients. Use caution with pulmonary, hepatic, or renal disorders; supraventricular tachycardias, acute abdominal conditions, hypothyroidism, toxic psychosis, kyphoscoliosis, morbid obesity, Addison's disease, BPH, or urethral stricture. Use with caution in patients with biliary tract dysfunction; acute pancreatitis may cause constriction of sphincter of Oddi. May cause hypotension; use with caution in patients (Continued)

Meperidine *(Continued)*

with depleted blood volume or drugs which may exaggerate hypotensive effects (including phenothiazines or general anesthetics).

An opioid-containing analgesic regimen should be tailored to each patient's needs and based upon the type of pain being treated (acute versus chronic), the route of administration, degree of tolerance for opioids (naive versus chronic user), age, weight, and medical condition. The optimal analgesic dose varies widely among patients. Doses should be titrated to pain relief/prevention.

Some preparations contain sulfites which may cause allergic reaction. Tolerance or drug dependence may result from extended use. Healthcare provider should be alert to problems of abuse, misuse, and diversion. Concurrent use of agonist/antagonist analgesics may precipitate withdrawal symptoms and/or reduced analgesic efficacy in patients following prolonged therapy with mu opioid agonists. Abrupt discontinuation following prolonged use may also lead to withdrawal symptoms. Use with caution in the elderly and debilitated patients; may be more sensitive to adverse effects.

Drug Interactions

Substrate (minor) of CYP2B6, 2C19, 3A4

Acyclovir: May increase meperidine metabolite concentrations. Use caution.

Barbiturates: May decrease analgesic efficacy and increase sedative and/or respiratory depressive effects of meperidine.

Cimetidine: May increase meperidine metabolite concentrations; use caution.

CNS depressants (including benzodiazepines): May potentiate the sedative and/or respiratory depressive effects of meperidine.

MAO inhibitors: May enhance the serotonergic effect of meperidine, which may cause serotonin syndrome. Concurrent use with or within 14 days of an MAO inhibitor is contraindicated.

Phenothiazines: May potentiate the sedative and/or respiratory depressive effects of meperidine; may increase the incidence of hypotension.

Phenytoin: May decrease the analgesic effects of meperidine

Ritonavir: May increase meperidine metabolite concentrations; use caution.

Serotonin agonists: Serotonin agonists and meperidine may enhance serotonin levels in the brain. Serotonin syndrome may occur.

Serotonin reuptake inhibitors: May potentiate the effects of meperidine, increasing serotonin levels in the brain. Serotonin syndrome may occur.

Sibutramine: May enhance the serotonergic effect of meperidine. Serotonin syndrome may occur.

Tricyclic antidepressants: May potentiate the sedative and/or respiratory depressive effects of meperidine. In addition, potentially may increase the risk of serotonin syndrome.

Ethanol/Nutrition/Herb Interactions

Ethanol: Avoid or limit ethanol (may increase CNS depression). Watch for sedation.

Herb/Nutraceutical: Avoid valerian, St John's wort, kava kava, gotu kola (may increase CNS depression).

Pharmacodynamics/Kinetics

Onset of action: Analgesic: Oral, SubQ: 10-15 minutes; I.V.: ~5 minutes

  Peak effect: SubQ.: ~1 hour; Oral: 2 hours

Duration: Oral, SubQ.: 2-4 hours

Absorption: I.M.: Erratic and highly variable

Distribution: Crosses placenta; enters breast milk

Protein binding: 65% to 75%

Metabolism: Hepatic; hydrolyzed to meperidinic acid (inactive) or undergoes N-demethylation to normeperidine (active; has $\frac{1}{2}$ the analgesic effect and 2-3 times the CNS effects of meperidine)

Bioavailability: ~50% to 60%; increased with liver disease

Half-life elimination:

  Parent drug: Terminal phase: Adults: 2.5-4 hours, Liver disease: 7-11 hours

  Normeperidine (active metabolite): 15-30 hours; can accumulate with high doses or with decreased renal function

Excretion: Urine (as metabolites)

Pregnancy Risk Factor C/D (prolonged use or high doses at term)

Lactation Enters breast milk/contraindicated (AAP rates "compatible")

Breast-Feeding Considerations Meperidine is excreted in breast milk and may cause CNS and/or respiratory depression in the nursing infant.

Dosage Forms Excipient information presented when available (limited, particularly for generics); consult specific product labeling.

Injection, solution, as hydrochloride [ampul]: 25 mg/0.5 mL (0.5 mL); 25 mg/mL (1 mL); 50 mg/mL (1 mL, 1.5 mL, 2 mL); 75 mg/mL (1 mL); 100 mg/mL (1 mL)

Injection, solution, as hydrochloride [prefilled syringe]: 25 mg/mL (1 mL); 50 mg/mL (1 mL); 75 mg/mL (1 mL); 100 mg/mL (1 mL)

Injection, solution, as hydrochloride [for PCA pump]: 10 mg/mL (30 mL, 50 mL, 60 mL)

Injection, solution, as hydrochloride [vial]: 25 mg/mL (1 mL); 50 mg/mL (1 mL, 30 mL); 75 mg/mL (1 mL); 100 mg/mL (1 mL, 20 mL) [may contain sodium metabisulfite]

Solution, oral, as hydrochloride: 50 mg/5 mL (500 mL)

Syrup, as hydrochloride:
Demerol®: 50 mg/5 mL (480 mL) [contains benzoic acid; banana flavor]

Tablet, as hydrochloride: 50 mg, 100 mg
Demerol®, Meperitab®: 50 mg, 100 mg

Dental Comment Meperidine is not to be used as the narcotic drug of first choice. It is recommended only to be used in codeine-allergic patients when a narcotic analgesic is indicated. Meperidine is not an anti-inflammatory agent. Meperidine, as with other narcotic analgesics, is recommended only for limited acute dosing (ie, 3 days or less); common adverse effects in the dental patient are nausea, sedation, and constipation. Meperidine has a significant addiction liability, especially when given long-term.

Meperidine and Promethazine
(me PER i deen & proe METH a zeen)

Related Information
Meperidine *on page 1038*
Promethazine *on page 1361*

Generic Available Yes

Index Terms Mepergan; Promethazine and Meperidine

Pharmacologic Category Analgesic Combination (Opioid)

Use Management of moderate pain

Local Anesthetic/Vasoconstrictor Precautions No information available to require special precautions

Effects on Dental Treatment Key adverse event(s) related to dental treatment: Xerostomia (normal salivary flow resumes upon discontinuation).

Common Adverse Effects See individual agents.

Restrictions C-II

Drug Interactions
Cytochrome P450 Effect: Promethazine: **Substrate** (major) of CYP2B6, 2D6; **Inhibits** CYP2D6 (weak)

Pharmacodynamics/Kinetics See individual agents.

Meperidine Hydrochloride *see* Meperidine *on page 1038*

Meperitab® *see* Meperidine *on page 1038*

Mephobarbital (me foe BAR bi tal)

U.S. Brand Names Mebaral®

Canadian Brand Names Mebaral®

Generic Available No

Index Terms Methylphenobarbital

Pharmacologic Category Barbiturate

Use Sedative; treatment of grand mal and petit mal epilepsy

Local Anesthetic/Vasoconstrictor Precautions No information available to require special precautions

Effects on Dental Treatment No significant effects or complications reported

Common Adverse Effects
>10%: Central nervous system: Dizziness, lightheadedness, drowsiness, "hangover" effect
1% to 10%:
Central nervous system: Confusion, mental depression, unusual excitement, nervousness, faint feeling, headache, insomnia, nightmares
Gastrointestinal: Constipation, nausea, vomiting

Restrictions C-IV

Mechanism of Action Increases seizure threshold in the motor cortex; depresses monosynaptic and polysynaptic transmission in the CNS

Drug Interactions
Cytochrome P450 Effect: **Substrate** of CYP2B6 (minor), 2C9 (minor), 2C19 (major); **Inhibits** CYP2C19 (weak); **Induces** CYP2A6 (weak)

Increased Effect/Toxicity: When combined with other CNS depressants, ethanol, opioid analgesics, antidepressants, or benzodiazepines, additive respiratory and CNS depression may occur. Barbiturates may enhance the hepatotoxic potential of acetaminophen overdoses. Chloramphenicol, MAO inhibitors, valproic acid, and felbamate may inhibit barbiturate metabolism. Barbiturates may impair the absorption of griseofulvin, and may enhance the
(Continued)

Mephobarbital *(Continued)*

nephrotoxic effects of methoxyflurane. Concurrent use of phenobarbital with meperidine may result in increased CNS depression. CYP2C19 inhibitors may increase the levels/effects of mephobarbital; example inhibitors include delavirdine, fluconazole, fluvoxamine, gemfibrozil, isoniazid, omeprazole, and ticlopidine.

Decreased Effect: Barbiturates are hepatic enzyme inducers, and may increase the metabolism of antipsychotics, some beta-blockers (unlikely with atenolol and nadolol), calcium channel blockers, chloramphenicol, cimetidine, corticosteroids, cyclosporine, disopyramide, doxycycline, ethosuximide, felbamate, furosemide, griseofulvin, lamotrigine, phenytoin, propafenone, quinidine, tacrolimus, TCAs, and theophylline. Barbiturates may increase the metabolism of estrogens and reduce the efficacy of oral contraceptives; an alternative method of contraception should be considered. Barbiturates inhibit the hypoprothrombinemic effects of oral anticoagulants via increased metabolism. Barbiturates may enhance the metabolism of methadone resulting in methadone withdrawal. CYP2C19 inducers may decrease the levels/effects of mephobarbital; example inducers include aminoglutethimide, carbamazepine, phenytoin, and rifampin.

Pharmacodynamics/Kinetics
Onset of action: 20-60 minutes
Duration: 6-8 hours
Absorption: ~50%
Half-life elimination, serum: 34 hours
Pregnancy Risk Factor D

Mephyton® *see* Phytonadione *on page 1299*

Mepivacaine *(me PIV a kane)*

U.S. Brand Names Carbocaine®; Polocaine®; Polocaine® Dental; Polocaine® MPF

Canadian Brand Names Carbocaine®; Polocaine®

Generic Available No

Index Terms Mepivacaine Hydrochloride

Pharmacologic Category Local Anesthetic

Dental Use Local anesthesia by nerve block, infiltration in dental procedures

Use Local or regional analgesia; anesthesia by local infiltration, peripheral and central neural techniques including epidural and caudal blocks; **not** for use in spinal anesthesia

Local Anesthetic/Vasoconstrictor Precautions No information available to require special precautions

Effects on Dental Treatment Key adverse event(s) related to dental treatment: Degree of adverse effects in the CNS and cardiovascular system is directly related to blood levels of mepivacaine (frequency not defined; more likely to occur after systemic administration rather than infiltration): Bradycardia, cardiovascular collapse, hypotension, myocardial depression, ventricular arrhythmias, nausea, vomiting, respiratory arrest, anaphylactoid reactions, blurred vision, heart block, transient stinging or burning at injection site

High blood levels: Anxiety, restlessness, disorientation, confusion, dizziness, and seizures, followed by CNS depression resulting in somnolence, unconsciousness, and possible respiratory arrest.

In some cases, symptoms of CNS stimulation may be absent and the primary CNS effects are somnolence and unconsciousness.

Significant Adverse Effects Degree of adverse effects in the CNS and cardiovascular system is directly related to the blood levels of mepivacaine, route of administration, and physical status of the patient. The effects below are more likely to occur after systemic administration rather than infiltration.

Cardiovascular: Bradycardia, cardiac arrest, cardiac output decreased, heart block, hyper-/hypotension, myocardial depression, syncope, tachycardia, ventricular arrhythmias
Central nervous system: Anxiety, chills, convulsions, depression, dizziness, excitation, restlessness, tremors
Dermatologic: Angioneurotic edema, diaphoresis, erythema, pruritus, urticaria
Gastrointestinal: Fecal incontinence, nausea, vomiting
Genitourinary: Incontinence, urinary retention
Neuromuscular & skeletal: Paralysis
Ocular: Blurred vision, pupil constriction
Otic: Tinnitus
Respiratory: Apnea, hypoventilation, sneezing
Miscellaneous: Allergic reaction, anaphylactoid reaction

Dental Usual Dosing

Injectable local anesthetic: Children and Adults: Dose varies with procedure, degree of anesthesia needed, vascularity of tissue, duration of anesthesia required, and physical condition of patient. The smallest dose and concentration required to produce the desired effect should be used.

Children: Maximum dose: 5-6 mg/kg; only concentrations <2% should be used in children <3 years or <14 kg (30 lbs)

Adults: Dental anesthesia:

Single site in upper or lower jaw: 54 mg (1.8 mL) as a 3% solution

Infiltration and nerve block of entire oral cavity: 270 mg (9 mL) as a 3% solution. Manufacturer's maximum recommended dose is not more than 400 mg to normal healthy adults.

Dosage

Injectable local anesthetic: Dose varies with procedure, degree of anesthesia needed, vascularity of tissue, duration of anesthesia required, and physical condition of patient. The smallest dose and concentration required to produce the desired effect should be used.

Children: Maximum dose: 5-6 mg/kg; only concentrations <2% should be used in children <3 years or <14 kg (30 lbs)

Adults: Maximum dose: 400 mg; do not exceed 1000 mg/24 hours

Cervical, brachial, intercostal, pudenal nerve block: 5-40 mL of a 1% solution (maximum: 400 mg) **or** 5-20 mL of a 2% solution (maximum: 400 mg). For pudenal block, inject $^1/_2$ the total dose each side.

Transvaginal block (paracervical plus pudenal): Up to 30 mL (both sides) of a 1% solution (maximum: 300 mg). Inject $^1/_2$ the total dose each side.

Paracervical block: Up to 20 mL (both sides) of a 1% solution (maximum: 200 mg). Inject $^1/_2$ the total dose to each side. This is the maximum recommended dose per 90-minute procedure; inject slowly with 5 minutes between sides.

Caudal and epidural block (preservative free solutions only): 15-30 mL of a 1% solution (maximum: 300 mg) **or** 10-25 mL of a 1.5% solution (maximum: 375 mg) **or** 10-20 mL of a 2% solution (maximum: 400 mg)

Infiltration: Up to 40 mL of a 1% solution (maximum: 400 mg)

Therapeutic block (pain management): 1-5 mL of a 1% solution (maximum: 50 mg) **or** 1-5 mL of a 2% solution (maximum: 100 mg)

Dental anesthesia: Adults:

Single site in upper or lower jaw: 54 mg (1.8 mL) as a 3% solution

Infiltration and nerve block of entire oral cavity: 270 mg (9 mL) as a 3% solution. Manufacturer's maximum recommended dose is not more than 400 mg to normal healthy adults.

Mechanism of Action Mepivacaine is an amide local anesthetic similar to lidocaine; like all local anesthetics, mepivacaine acts by preventing the generation and conduction of nerve impulses

Contraindications Hypersensitivity to mepivacaine, other amide-type local anesthetics, or any component of the formulation

Warnings/Precautions Use with caution in patients with cardiac disease, hepatic or renal disease, or hyperthyroidism. Local anesthetics have been associated with rare occurrences of sudden respiratory arrest; convulsions due to systemic toxicity leading to cardiac arrest have been reported presumably due to intravascular injection. A test dose is recommended prior to epidural administration and all reinforcing doses with continuous catheter technique. Do not use solutions containing preservatives for caudal or epidural block. Use caution in debilitated, elderly, or acutely-ill patients; dose reduction may be required.

Pharmacodynamics/Kinetics

Onset of action (route and dose dependent): Range: 3-20 minutes

Duration (route and dose dependent): 2-2.5 hours

Protein binding: ~75%

Metabolism: Primarily hepatic via N-demethylation, hydroxylation, and glucuronidation

Half-life elimination: Neonates: 8.7-9 hours; Adults: 1.9-3 hours

Excretion: Urine (95% as metabolites)

Pregnancy Risk Factor C

Lactation Excretion in breast milk unknown/use caution

Dosage Forms Excipient information presented when available (limited, particularly for generics); consult specific product labeling.

Injection, solution, as hydrochloride [contains methylparabens]:

Carbocaine®: 1% (50 mL); 2% (50 mL)

Polocaine®: 1% (50 mL); 2% (50 mL)

Injection, solution, as hydrochloride [preservative free]:

Carbocaine®: 1% (30 mL); 1.5% (30 mL); 2% (20 mL); 3% (1.8 mL) [dental cartridge]

Polocaine® Dental: 3% (1.8 mL) [dental cartridge]

Polocaine® MPF: 1% (30 mL); 1.5% (30 mL); 2% (20 mL)

Mepivacaine (Dental Anesthetic) (me PIV a kane, DEN tl)

Related Information
Mepivacaine *on page 1042*
Oral Pain *on page 1788*

U.S. Brand Names Carbocaine®; Polocaine®

Canadian Brand Names Polocaine®

Generic Available No

Pharmacologic Category Local Anesthetic

Dental Use Amide-type anesthetic used for local infiltration anesthesia; injection near nerve trunks to produce nerve block

Local Anesthetic/Vasoconstrictor Precautions No information available to require special precautions

Effects on Dental Treatment It is common to misinterpret psychogenic responses to local anesthetic injection as an allergic reaction. Intraoral injections are perceived by many patients as a stressful procedure in dentistry. Common symptoms to this stress are diaphoresis, palpitations, hyperventilation, generalized pallor, and a fainting feeling.

Degree of adverse effects in the CNS and cardiovascular system is directly related to the blood levels of mepivacaine.

Frequency not defined: Bradycardia and reduction in cardiac output, nausea, vomiting, tremors, asthmatic syndromes, hypersensitivity reactions (may manifest as dermatologic reactions and edema at injection site)

High blood levels: Anxiety, restlessness, disorientation, confusion, dizziness, tremors and seizures, followed by CNS depression resulting in somnolence, unconsciousness and possible respiratory arrest. In some cases, symptoms of CNS stimulation may be absent and the primary CNS effects are somnolence and unconsciousness.

Significant Adverse Effects Degree of adverse effects in the CNS and cardiovascular system is directly related to the blood levels of local anesthetic.

Cardiovascular: Myocardial effects include a decrease in contraction force as well as a decrease in electrical excitability and myocardial conduction rate resulting in bradycardia and reduction in cardiac output

Central nervous system: High blood levels result in anxiety, restlessness, disorientation, confusion, dizziness, and seizure. This is followed by depression of CNS resulting in somnolence, unconsciousness and possible respiratory arrest. In some cases, symptoms of CNS stimulation may be absent and the primary CNS effects are somnolence and unconsciousness.

Gastrointestinal: Nausea and vomiting may occur

Hypersensitivity reactions: May manifest as dermatologic reactions and edema at injection site. Asthmatic syndromes have occurred.

Neuromuscular & skeletal: Tremors

Psychogenic reactions: It is common to misinterpret psychogenic responses to local anesthetic injection as an allergic reaction. Intraoral injection is perceived by many patients as a stressful procedure in dentistry. Common symptoms to this stress are diaphoresis, palpitation, hyperventilation, generalized pallor and a fainting feeling.

# of Cartridges (1.8 mL)	mg Mepivacaine (3%)
1	54
2	108
3	162
4	216
5	270
6	324
7	378
8	432

Dental Usual Dosing
Children <10 years: Up to 5-6 mg/kg of body weight; maximum pediatric dosage must be carefully calculated on the basis of patient's weight but must not exceed 270 mg (9 mL) of the 3% solution

Children >10 years and Adults:
Dental anesthesia, single site in upper or lower jaw: 54 mg (1.8 mL) as a 3% solution
Infiltration and nerve block of entire oral cavity: 270 mg (9 mL) as a 3% solution; up to a maximum of 6.6 mg/kg of body weight but not to exceed 300 mg per appointment. Manufacturer's maximum recommended dose is

not more than 400 mg to normal healthy adults. The effective anesthetic dose varies with procedure, intensity of anesthesia needed, duration of anesthesia required, and physical condition of the patient. Always use the lowest effective dose along with careful aspiration.

The following number of dental carpules (1.8 mL) provide the indicated amounts of mepivacaine dental anesthetic 3%. See table on previous page.

Note: Adult and children doses of mepivacaine dental anesthetic cited from USP Dispensing Information (USP DI), 17th ed, The United States Pharmacopeial Convention, Inc, Rockville, MD, 1997, 138-9.

Dosage

Children <10 years: Up to 5-6 mg/kg of body weight; maximum pediatric dosage must be carefully calculated on the basis of patient's weight but must not exceed 270 mg (9 mL) of the 3% solution

Children >10 years and Adults:
Dental anesthesia, single site in upper or lower jaw: 54 mg (1.8 mL) as a 3% solution

Infiltration and nerve block of entire oral cavity: 270 mg (9 mL) as a 3% solution; up to a maximum of 6.6 mg/kg of body weight but not to exceed 300 mg per appointment. Manufacturer's maximum recommended dose is not more than 400 mg to normal healthy adults. The effective anesthetic dose varies with procedure, intensity of anesthesia needed, duration of anesthesia required, and physical condition of the patient. Always use the lowest effective dose along with careful aspiration.

Note: Adult and children doses of mepivacaine dental anesthetic cited from USP Dispensing Information (USP DI), 17th ed, The United States Pharmacopeial Convention, Inc, Rockville, MD, 1997, 138-9.

Mechanism of Action Local anesthetics bind selectively to the intracellular surface of sodium channels to block influx of sodium into the axon. As a result, depolarization necessary for action potential propagation and subsequent nerve function is prevented. The block at the sodium channel is reversible. When drug diffuses away from the axon, sodium channel function is restored and nerve propagation returns.

Contraindications Hypersensitivity to local anesthetics of the amide type or any component of the formulation

Warnings/Precautions Aspirate the syringe after tissue penetration and before injection to minimize chance of direct vascular injection

Drug Interactions No data reported

Pharmacodynamics/Kinetics

Onset of action: Upper jaw: 30-120 seconds; Lower jaw: 1-4 minutes
Duration: Upper jaw: 20 minutes; Lower jaw: 40 minutes
Half-life elimination, serum: 1.9 hours

Pregnancy Risk Factor C

Breast-Feeding Considerations Usual infiltration doses of mepivacaine dental anesthetic given to nursing mothers has not been shown to affect the health of the nursing infant.

Dosage Forms Excipient information presented when available (limited, particularly for generics); consult specific product labeling.

Injection, solution, as hydrochloride: 3% (1.8 mL) [dental cartridges]

Selected Readings

Ayoub ST and Coleman AE, "A Review of Local Anesthetics," *Gen Dent*, 1992, 40(4):285-7, 289-90.
Budenz AW, "Local Anesthetics in Dentistry: Then and Now," *J Calif Dent Assoc*, 2003, 31(5):388-96.
Dower JS Jr, "A Review of Paresthesia in Association With Administration of Local Anesthesia," *Dent Today*, 2003, 22(2):64-9.
Finder RL and Moore PA, "Adverse Drug Reactions to Local Anesthesia," *Dent Clin North Am*, 2002, 46(4):747-57, x.
Haas DA, "An Update on Local Anesthetics in Dentistry," *J Can Dent Assoc*, 2002, 68(9):546-51.
Hawkins JM and Moore PA, "Local Anesthesia: Advances in Agents and Techniques," *Dent Clin North Am*, 2002, 46(4):719-32, ix.
"Injectable Local Anesthetics," *J Am Dent Assoc*, 2003, 134(5):628-9.
Malamed SF, "Allergy and Toxic Reactions to Local Anesthetics," *Dent Today*, 2003, 22(4):114-6, 118-21.
Wynn RL, "Recent Research on Mechanisms of Local Anesthetics," *Gen Dent*, 1995, 43(4):316-8.

Mepivacaine and Levonordefrin
(me PIV a kane & lee voe nor DEF rin)

Related Information
Mepivacaine *on page 1042*
Oral Pain *on page 1788*

U.S. Brand Names Carbocaine® 2% with Neo-Cobefrin®

Canadian Brand Names Polocaine® 2% and Levonordefrin 1:20,000

Generic Available No

(Continued)

Mepivacaine and Levonordefrin *(Continued)*

Index Terms Levonordefrin and Mepivacaine Hydrochloride

Pharmacologic Category Local Anesthetic

Dental Use Amide-type anesthetic used for local infiltration anesthesia; injection near nerve trunks to produce nerve block

Local Anesthetic/Vasoconstrictor Precautions No information available to require special precautions

Effects on Dental Treatment It is common to misinterpret psychogenic responses to local anesthetic injection as an allergic reaction. Intraoral injections are perceived by many patients as a stressful procedure in dentistry. Common symptoms to this stress are diaphoresis, palpitations, hyperventilation, generalized pallor and a fainting feeling. Patients may exhibit hypersensitivity to bisulfites contained in local anesthetic solution to prevent oxidation of levonordefrin. In general, patients reacting to bisulfites have a history of asthma and their airways are hyper-reactive to asthmatic syndrome.

Degree of adverse effects in the CNS and cardiovascular system is directly related to the blood levels of mepivacaine (frequency not defined; more likely to occur after systemic administration rather than infiltration): Bradycardia and reduction in cardiac output, nausea, vomiting, tremors, hypersensitivity reactions (extremely rare; may be manifest as dermatologic reactions and edema at injection site), asthmatic syndromes

High blood levels: Anxiety, restlessness, disorientation, confusion, dizziness, and seizures, followed by CNS depression resulting in somnolence, unconsciousness and possible respiratory arrest.

In some cases, symptoms of CNS stimulation may be absent and the primary CNS effects are somnolence and unconsciousness.

Significant Adverse Effects Degree of adverse effects in the CNS and cardiovascular system is directly related to the blood levels of mepivacaine. The effects below are more likely to occur after systemic administration rather than infiltration.

Cardiovascular: Myocardial effects include a decrease in contraction force as well as a decrease in electrical excitability and myocardial conduction rate resulting in bradycardia and reduction in cardiac output.

Central nervous system: High blood levels result in anxiety, restlessness, disorientation, confusion, dizziness, and seizure. This is followed by depression of CNS resulting in somnolence, unconsciousness and possible respiratory arrest. In some cases, symptoms of CNS stimulation may be absent and the primary CNS effects are somnolence and unconsciousness.

Gastrointestinal: Nausea and vomiting may occur

Hypersensitivity reactions: Extremely rare, but may be manifest as dermatologic reactions and edema at injection site. Asthmatic syndromes have occurred. Patients may exhibit hypersensitivity to bisulfites contained in local anesthetic solution to prevent oxidation of levonordefrin. In general, patients reacting to bisulfites have a history of asthma and their airways are hyper-reactive to asthmatic syndrome.

Neuromuscular & skeletal: Tremors

Psychogenic reactions: It is common to misinterpret psychogenic responses to local anesthetic injection as an allergic reaction. Intraoral injections are perceived by many patients as a stressful procedure in dentistry. Common symptoms to this stress are diaphoresis, palpitation, hyperventilation, generalized pallor and a fainting feeling.

Dental Usual Dosing

Children <10 years: Maximum pediatric dosage must be carefully calculated on the basis of patient's weight but should not exceed 6.6 mg/kg of body weight or 180 mg of mepivacaine hydrochloride as a 2% solution with levonordefrin 1:20,000

# of Cartridges (1.8 mL)	mg Mepivacaine (2%)	mg Vasoconstrictor (Levonordefrin 1:20,000)
1	36	0.090
2	72	0.180
3	108	0.270
4	144	0.360
5	180	0.450
6	216	0.540
7	252	0.630
8	288	0.720
9	324	0.810
10	360	0.900

Children >10 years and Adults:

Dental infiltration and nerve block, single site: 36 mg (1.8 mL) of mepivacaine hydrochloride as a 2% solution with levonordefrin 1:20,000

Entire oral cavity: 180 mg (9 mL) of mepivacaine hydrochloride as a 2% solution with levonordefrin 1:20,000; up to a maximum of 6.6 mg/kg of body weight but not to exceed 400 mg of mepivacaine hydrochloride per appointment. The effective anesthetic dose varies with procedure, intensity of anesthesia needed, duration of anesthesia required, and physical condition of the patient. Always use the lowest effective dose along with careful aspiration.

The following numbers of dental carpules (1.8 mL) provide the indicated amounts of mepivacaine hydrochloride 2% and levonordefrin 1:20,000. See table on previous page.

Note: Adult and children doses of mepivacaine hydrochloride with levonordefrin cited from USP Dispensing Information (USP DI), 17th ed, The United States Pharmacopeial Convention, Inc, Rockville, MD, 1997, 139.

Dosage

Children <10 years: Maximum pediatric dosage must be carefully calculated on the basis of patient's weight but should not exceed 6.6 mg/kg of body weight or 180 mg of mepivacaine hydrochloride as a 2% solution with levonordefrin 1:20,000

Children >10 years and Adults:

Dental infiltration and nerve block, single site: 36 mg (1.8 mL) of mepivacaine hydrochloride as a 2% solution with levonordefrin 1:20,000

Entire oral cavity: 180 mg (9 mL) of mepivacaine hydrochloride as a 2% solution with levonordefrin 1:20,000; up to a maximum of 6.6 mg/kg of body weight but not to exceed 400 mg of mepivacaine hydrochloride per appointment. The effective anesthetic dose varies with procedure, intensity of anesthesia needed, duration of anesthesia required, and physical condition of the patient. Always use the lowest effective dose along with careful aspiration.

Note: Adult and children doses of mepivacaine hydrochloride with levonordefrin cited from USP Dispensing Information (USP DI), 17th ed, The United States Pharmacopeial Convention, Inc, Rockville, MD, 1997, 139.

Mechanism of Action Local anesthetics bind selectively to the intracellular surface of sodium channels to block influx of sodium into the axon. As a result, depolarization necessary for action potential propagation and subsequent nerve function is prevented. The block at the sodium channel is reversible. When drug diffuses away from the axon, sodium channel function is restored and nerve propagation returns.

Levonordefrin prolongs the duration of the anesthetic actions of mepivacaine by causing vasoconstriction (alpha-adrenergic receptor agonist) of the vasculature surrounding the nerve axons. This prevents the diffusion of mepivacaine away from the nerves resulting in a longer retention in the axon.

Contraindications Hypersensitivity to local anesthetics of the amide-type or any component of the formulation

Warnings/Precautions Should be avoided in patients with uncontrolled hyperthyroidism. Should be used in minimal amounts in patients with significant cardiovascular problems (because of levonordefrin component). Aspirate the syringe after tissue penetration and before injection to minimize chance of direct vascular injection. Contains sodium bisulfite which may cause allergic reactions in some individuals.

Drug Interactions Due to levonordefrin component, use with tricyclic antidepressants or MAO inhibitors could result in increased pressor response; use with nonselective beta-blockers (ie, propranolol) could result in serious hypertension and reflex bradycardia

Pharmacodynamics/Kinetics

Duration: Upper jaw: 1-2.5 hours; Lower jaw: 2.5-5.5 hours

Infiltration: 50 minutes

Inferior alveolar block: 60-75 minutes

Pregnancy Risk Factor C

Breast-Feeding Considerations Usual infiltration doses of mepivacaine with levonordefrin given to nursing mothers has not been shown to affect the health of the nursing infant.

Dosage Forms Excipient information presented when available (limited, particularly for generics); consult specific product labeling.

Injection, solution: Mepivacaine hydrochloride 2% and levonordefrin 1:20,000 (1.8 mL) [dental cartridges; contains sodium bisulfite]

(Continued)

Mepivacaine and Levonordefrin (Continued)

Selected Readings

Ayoub ST and Coleman AE, "A Review of Local Anesthetics," Gen Dent, 1992, 40(4):285-7, 289-90.

Jastak JT and Yagiela JA, "Vasoconstrictors and Local Anesthesia: A Review and Rationale for Use," J Am Dent Assoc, 1983, 107(4):623-30.

MacKenzie TA and Young ER, "Local Anesthetic Update," Anesth Prog, 1993, 40(2):29-34.

Wynn RL, "Epinephrine Interactions With Beta-Blockers," Gen Dent, 1994, 42(1):16, 18.

Wynn RL, "Recent Research on Mechanisms of Local Anesthetics," Gen Dent, 1995, 43(4):316-8.

Yagiela JA, "Local Anesthetics," Anesth Prog, 1991, 38(4-5):128-41.

Mepivacaine Hydrochloride see Mepivacaine on page 1042

Meprobamate (me proe BA mate)

U.S. Brand Names Miltown® [DSC]

Canadian Brand Names Novo-Mepro

Generic Available Yes

Index Terms Equanil

Pharmacologic Category Antianxiety Agent, Miscellaneous

Dental Use Treatment of muscle spasm associated with acute temporomandibular joint (TMJ) pain; management of dental anxiety disorders

Use Management of anxiety disorders

Unlabeled/Investigational Use Demonstrated value for muscle contraction, headache, premenstrual tension, external sphincter spasticity, muscle rigidity, opisthotonos-associated with tetanus

Local Anesthetic/Vasoconstrictor Precautions No information available to require special precautions

Effects on Dental Treatment No significant effects or complications reported

Significant Adverse Effects Frequency not defined.

Cardiovascular: Syncope, peripheral edema, palpitation, tachycardia, arrhythmia

Central nervous system: Drowsiness, ataxia, dizziness, paradoxical excitement, confusion, slurred speech, headache, euphoria, chills, vertigo, paresthesia, overstimulation

Dermatologic: Rashes, purpura, dermatitis, Stevens-Johnson syndrome, petechiae, ecchymosis

Gastrointestinal: Diarrhea, vomiting, nausea

Hematologic: Leukopenia, eosinophilia, agranulocytosis, aplastic anemia

Neuromuscular & skeletal: Weakness

Ocular: Blurred vision, impairment of accommodation

Renal: Renal failure

Respiratory: Wheezing, dyspnea, bronchospasm, angioneurotic edema

Restrictions C-IV

Dental Usual Dosing Muscle spasm (TMJ) pain or anxiety: Adults: Oral: 400 mg 3-4 times/day, up to 2400 mg/day

Dosage Oral:

Children 6-12 years: Anxiety: 100-200 mg 2-3 times/day

Adults: Anxiety: 400 mg 3-4 times/day, up to 2400 mg/day

Dosing interval in renal impairment:

Cl_{cr} 10-50 mL/minute: Administer every 9-12 hours

Cl_{cr} <10 mL/minute: Administer every 12-18 hours

Hemodialysis: Moderately dialyzable (20% to 50%)

Dosing adjustment in hepatic impairment: Probably necessary in patients with liver disease

Mechanism of Action Affects the thalamus and limbic system; also appears to inhibit multineuronal spinal reflexes

Contraindications Hypersensitivity to meprobamate, related compounds (including carisoprodol), or any component of the formulation; acute intermittent porphyria; pre-existing CNS depression; narrow-angle glaucoma; severe uncontrolled pain; pregnancy

Warnings/Precautions Physical and psychological dependence and abuse may occur; abrupt cessation may precipitate withdrawal. Use with caution in patients with depression or suicidal tendencies, or in patients with a history of drug abuse. May cause CNS depression, which may impair physical or mental abilities. Patients must be cautioned about performing tasks which require mental alertness (eg, operating machinery or driving). Effects with other sedative drugs or ethanol may be potentiated. Not recommended in children <6 years of age; allergic reaction may occur in patients with history of dermatological condition (usually by fourth dose). Use with caution in patients with renal or hepatic impairment, or with a history of seizures. Use caution in the elderly as it may cause confusion, cognitive impairment, or excessive sedation.

Drug Interactions CNS depressants: Sedative effects may be additive with other CNS depressants; monitor for increased effect; includes barbiturates, benzodiazepines, opioid analgesics, ethanol, and other sedative agents

Ethanol/Nutrition/Herb Interactions
Ethanol: Avoid ethanol (may increase CNS depression).
Herb/Nutraceutical: Avoid valerian, St John's wort, kava kava, gotu kola (may increase CNS depression).

Pharmacodynamics/Kinetics
Onset of action: Sedation: ~1 hour
Distribution: Crosses placenta; enters breast milk
Metabolism: Hepatic
Half-life elimination: 10 hours
Excretion: Urine (8% to 20% as unchanged drug); feces (10% as metabolites)

Pregnancy Risk Factor D
Lactation Enters breast milk/not recommended
Breast-Feeding Considerations Breast milk concentrations are higher than plasma; effects are unknown.
Dosage Forms Excipient information presented when available (limited, particularly for generics); consult specific product labeling. [DSC] = Discontinued product
Tablet: 200 mg, 400 mg
Miltown®: 200 mg, 400 mg [DSC]

Meprobamate and Aspirin (me proe BA mate & AS pir in)

Related Information
Aspirin on page 149
Meprobamate on page 1048
U.S. Brand Names Equagesic®
Canadian Brand Names 292 MEP®
Generic Available No
Index Terms Aspirin and Meprobamate
Pharmacologic Category Antianxiety Agent, Miscellaneous; Salicylate
Use Adjunct to the short-term treatment of pain in patients with skeletal-muscular disease exhibiting tension and/or anxiety
Local Anesthetic/Vasoconstrictor Precautions No information available to require special precautions
Effects on Dental Treatment Key adverse event(s) related to dental treatment: Elderly are a high-risk population for adverse effects from nonsteroidal anti-inflammatory agents. As many as 60% of elderly patients with GI complications from NSAIDs can develop peptic ulceration and/or hemorrhage asymptomatically. Concomitant disease and drug use contribute to the risk of GI adverse effects. Use lowest effective dose for shortest period possible. Consider renal function decline with age.
Aspirin: As with all drugs which may affect hemostasis, bleeding is associated with aspirin. Hemorrhage may occur at virtually any site; risk is dependent on multiple variables including dosage, concurrent use of multiple agents which alter hemostasis, and patient susceptibility. Many adverse effects of aspirin are dose related, and are rare at low dosages. Other serious reactions are idiosyncratic, related to allergy or individual sensitivity (see Dental Comment).
Common Adverse Effects See individual agents.
Restrictions C-IV
Drug Interactions
Cytochrome P450 Effect: Aspirin: **Substrate** of CYP2C9 (minor)
Increased Effect/Toxicity: See individual agents.
Decreased Effect: See individual agents.
Pharmacodynamics/Kinetics See individual agents.
Pregnancy Risk Factor X
Dental Comment There is no scientific evidence to warrant discontinuance of aspirin prior to dental surgery. Patients taking one aspirin tablet daily as an antithrombotic and who require dental surgery should be given special consideration in consultation with the physician before removal of the aspirin relative to prevention of postoperative bleeding.

The Food and Drug Administration (FDA), has issued a letter updating information and considerations regarding the use of ibuprofen (400 mg doses) in patients who are taking low dose aspirin (81 mg, immediate release; not enteric coated) for cardioprotection and stroke prevention. Ibuprofen, at these doses, may interfere with aspirin's antiplatelet effect depending upon when it is administered. Patients initiated on aspirin first (for ~1 week) then ibuprofen (400 mg tid for 10 days) seem to maintain aspirin's platelet effect (Cryer B, 2005). Ibuprofen (Continued)

Meprobamate and Aspirin *(Continued)*

has the greatest impact on aspirin if administered less than 8 hours before aspirin (Catella-Lawson F, 2001).

Patients may require counseling about the appropriate timing of ibuprofen dosing in relationship to aspirin therapy. With occasional use of ibuprofen, a clinically-significant interaction with aspirin in unlikely. To avoid interference during chronic dosing, a single dose of ibuprofen should be taken 30-120 minutes after aspirin ingestion or at least 8 hours should elapse after ibuprofen dosing before giving aspirin (FDA, 2006; Catella-Lawson F, 2001).

The clinical implications of the interaction are unclear. There have not been any clinical endpoint studies conducted at this time. Avoidance of this interaction is potentially important because aspirin's vascular protection could be decreased or negated.

Other nonselective NSAIDs may have potential for a similar interaction with aspirin. Such has been described with naproxen (Capone ML, 2005). Acetaminophen does not appear to interfere with the antiplatelet effect of aspirin. Other clinical scenarios (use of smaller ibuprofen doses, other aspirin products, other doses of aspirin) have not been evaluated.

Additional information is available at: http://www.fda.gov/cder/drug/infopage/aspirin/default.htm.

Mepron® *see* Atovaquone *on page 164*

Mequinol and Tretinoin (ME kwi nole & TRET i noyn)

U.S. Brand Names Solagé™

Canadian Brand Names Solagé™

Generic Available No

Index Terms Tretinoin and Mequinol

Pharmacologic Category Retinoic Acid Derivative; Vitamin A Derivative; Vitamin, Topical

Use Treatment of solar lentigines; the efficacy of using Solagé™ daily for >24 weeks has not been established. The local cutaneous safety of Solagé™ in non-Caucasians has not been adequately established.

Local Anesthetic/Vasoconstrictor Precautions No information available to require special precautions

Effects on Dental Treatment No significant effects or complications reported

Common Adverse Effects

>10%: Dermatologic: Erythema (49%), burning, stinging or tingling (26%), desquamation (14%), pruritus (12%)

1% to 10%: Dermatologic: Skin irritation (5%), hypopigmentation (5%), halo hypopigmentation (7%), rash (3%), dry skin (3%), crusting (3%), vesicular bullae rash (2%), contact allergic reaction (1%)

Mechanism of Action Solar lentigines are localized, pigmented, macular lesions of the skin on areas of the body chronically exposed to the sun. Mequinol is a substrate for the enzyme tyrosinase and acts as a competitive inhibitor of the formation of melanin precursors. The mechanisms of depigmentation for both drugs is unknown.

Drug Interactions

Cytochrome P450 Effect: Tretinoin: **Substrate** (minor) of CYP2A6, 2B6, 2C8/9; **Inhibits** CYP2C8/9 (weak); **Induces** CYP2E1 (weak)

Increased Effect/Toxicity:

Topical products with skin drying effects (eg, those containing alcohol, astringents, spices, or lime; medicated soaps or shampoos; permanent wave solutions; hair depilatories or waxes; and others) may increase skin irritation. Avoid concurrent use.

Photosensitizing drugs (eg, thiazides, tetracyclines, fluoroquinolones, phenothiazines, sulfonamides) can further increase sun sensitivity. Avoid concurrent use.

Pharmacodynamics/Kinetics

Absorption: Percutaneous absorption was 4.4% of tretinoin when applied as 0.8 mL of Solagé™ to a 400 cm^2 area of the back

Time to peak: Mequinol: 2 hours

Pregnancy Risk Factor X

Mercaptopurine (mer kap toe PYOOR een)

U.S. Brand Names Purinethol®
Canadian Brand Names Purinethol®
Mexican Brand Names Purinethol
Generic Available Yes
Index Terms 6-Mercaptopurine (error-prone abbreviation); 6-MP (error-prone abbreviation); NSC-755
Pharmacologic Category Antineoplastic Agent, Antimetabolite; Immunosuppressant Agent
Use Treatment (maintenance and induction) of acute lymphoblastic leukemia (ALL)
Unlabeled/Investigational Use Steroid-sparing agent for corticosteroid-dependent Crohn's disease (CD) and ulcerative colitis (UC); maintenance of remission in CD; fistulizing Crohn's disease
Local Anesthetic/Vasoconstrictor Precautions No information available to require special precautions
Effects on Dental Treatment Key adverse event(s) related to dental treatment: Stomatitis and mucositis.
Common Adverse Effects
>10%:
  Hematologic: Myelosuppression; leukopenia, thrombocytopenia, anemia
    Onset: 7-10 days
    Nadir: 14-16 days
    Recovery: 21-28 days
  Hepatic: Intrahepatic cholestasis and focal centralobular necrosis (40%), characterized by hyperbilirubinemia, increased alkaline phosphatase and AST, jaundice, ascites, encephalopathy; more common at doses >2.5 mg/kg/day. Usually occurs within 2 months of therapy but may occur within 1 week, or be delayed up to 8 years.
1% to 10%:
  Central nervous system: Drug fever
  Dermatologic: Hyperpigmentation, rash
  Endocrine & metabolic: Hyperuricemia
  Gastrointestinal: Nausea, vomiting, diarrhea, stomatitis, anorexia, stomach pain, mucositis
  Renal: Renal toxicity
Mechanism of Action Purine antagonist which inhibits DNA and RNA synthesis; acts as false metabolite and is incorporated into DNA and RNA, eventually inhibiting their synthesis; specific for the S phase of the cell cycle
Drug Interactions
  Increased Effect/Toxicity: Allopurinol can cause increased levels of mercaptopurine by inhibition of xanthine oxidase. Decrease dose of mercaptopurine by 75% when both drugs are used concomitantly. May potentiate effect of bone marrow suppression (reduce mercaptopurine to 25% of dose). Synergistic liver toxicity between doxorubicin and mercaptopurine has been reported. Any agent which could potentially alter the metabolic function of the liver could produce higher drug levels and greater toxicities from either mercaptopurine or thioguanine (6-TG). Aminosalicylates (eg, olsalazine, mesalamine, sulfasalazine) may inhibit TPMT, increasing toxicity/myelosuppression of mercaptopurine. Azathioprine is metabolized to mercaptopurine; concomitant use may result in profound myelosuppression and should be avoided
  Decreased Effect: Mercaptopurine inhibits the anticoagulation effect of warfarin by an unknown mechanism.
Pharmacodynamics/Kinetics
  Absorption: Variable and incomplete (16% to 50%)
  Distribution: V_d = total body water; CNS penetration is poor
  Protein binding: 19%
  Metabolism: Hepatic and in GI mucosa; hepatically via xanthine oxidase and methylation via TPMT to sulfate conjugates, 6-thiouric acid, and other inactive compounds; first-pass effect
  Half-life elimination (age dependent): Children: 21 minutes; Adults: 47 minutes
  Time to peak, serum: ~2 hours
  Excretion: Urine (46% as mercaptopurine and metabolites)
Pregnancy Risk Factor D

Meropenem (mer oh PEN em)

U.S. Brand Names Merrem® I.V.
Canadian Brand Names Merrem®
Mexican Brand Names Merrem
Generic Available No
Pharmacologic Category Antibiotic, Carbapenem
Use Treatment of intra-abdominal infections (complicated appendicitis and peritonitis); treatment of bacterial meningitis in pediatric patients ≥3 months of age caused by *S. pneumoniae*, *H. influenzae*, and *N. meningitidis*; treatment of complicated skin and skin structure infections caused by susceptible organisms
Unlabeled/Investigational Use Febrile neutropenia, urinary tract infections
Local Anesthetic/Vasoconstrictor Precautions No information available to require special precautions
Effects on Dental Treatment Key adverse event(s) related to dental treatment: Oral moniliasis (pediatric patients) and glossitis.
Common Adverse Effects
1% to 10%:
Cardiovascular: Peripheral vascular disorder (<1%)
Central nervous system: Headache (2% to 8%), pain (5%)
Dermatologic: Rash (2% to 3%, includes diaper-area moniliasis in pediatrics), pruritus (1%)
Gastrointestinal: Diarrhea (4% to 5%), nausea/vomiting (1% to 8%), constipation (1% to 7%), oral moniliasis (up to 2% in pediatric patients), glossitis
Hematologic: Anemia (up to 6%)
Local: Inflammation at the injection site (2%), phlebitis/thrombophlebitis (1%), injection site reaction (1%)
Respiratory: Apnea (1%)
Miscellaneous: Sepsis (2%), septic shock (1%)
Mechanism of Action Inhibits bacterial cell wall synthesis by binding to several of the penicillin-binding proteins, which in turn inhibit the final transpeptidation step of peptidoglycan synthesis in bacterial cell walls, thus inhibiting cell wall biosynthesis; bacteria eventually lyse due to ongoing activity of cell wall autolytic enzymes (autolysins and murein hydrolases) while cell wall assembly is arrested
Drug Interactions
Increased Effect/Toxicity: Probenecid may increase meropenem serum concentrations.
Decreased Effect: Meropenem may decrease valproic acid serum concentrations to subtherapeutic levels.
Pharmacodynamics/Kinetics
Distribution: V_d: Adults: ~0.3 L/kg, Children: 0.4-0.5 L/kg; penetrates well into most body fluids and tissues; CSF concentrations approximate those of the plasma
Protein binding: 2%
Metabolism: Hepatic; metabolized to open beta-lactam form (inactive)
Half-life elimination:
Normal renal function: 1-1.5 hours
Cl_{cr} 30-80 mL/minute: 1.9-3.3 hours
Cl_{cr} 2-30 mL/minute: 3.82-5.7 hours
Time to peak, tissue: 1 hour following infusion
Excretion: Urine (~25% as inactive metabolites)
Pregnancy Risk Factor B

Merrem® I.V. *see* Meropenem *on page 1052*
Meruvax® II *see* Rubella Virus Vaccine (Live) *on page 1450*

Mesalamine (me SAL a meen)

U.S. Brand Names Asacol®; Canasa™; Lialda™; Pentasa®; Rowasa®
Canadian Brand Names Asacol®; Asacol® 800; Mesasal®; Novo-5 ASA; Pendo-5 ASA; Pentasa®; Quintasa®; Rowasa®; Salofalk®
Mexican Brand Names Asacol
Generic Available Yes: Rectal suspension
Index Terms 5-Aminosalicylic Acid; 5-ASA; Fisalamine; Mesalazine
Pharmacologic Category 5-Aminosalicylic Acid Derivative
Use
Oral: Treatment and maintenance of remission of mildly to moderately active ulcerative colitis
Rectal: Treatment of active mild to moderate distal ulcerative colitis, proctosigmoiditis, or proctitis

Local Anesthetic/Vasoconstrictor Precautions No information available to require special precautions

Effects on Dental Treatment Key adverse event(s) related to dental treatment: Pharyngitis.

Common Adverse Effects Adverse effects vary depending upon dosage form. Effects as reported with tablets, unless otherwise noted:

>10%:

Central nervous system: Headache (4% to 35% [capsule 2%; enema 7%; suppository 14%]), pain (14%)

Gastrointestinal: Abdominal pain (3% to 18% [capsule 1%; enema 8%; suppository 5%]), eructation (16%), nausea (13% [capsule 3%; enema 6%; suppository 3%])

Respiratory: Pharyngitis (11%)

1% to 10%:

Cardiovascular: Chest pain (3%), peripheral edema (3%)

Central nervous system: Chills (3%), dizziness (8% [enema 2%; suppository 3%]), fever (6% [capsule 1%; enema 3%; suppository 1%]), insomnia (2%), malaise (2% [enema 3%])

Dermatologic: Rash (6% [capsule 1%; enema 3%; suppository 1%]), pruritus (1% to 3%), acne (2% [suppository 1%]), alopecia (1%)

Gastrointestinal: Colitis exacerbation (3% [suppository 1%]), constipation (5%), diarrhea (7% [capsule 4%; enema 2%; suppository 3%]), dyspepsia (6%), flatulence (3% [enema 6%; suppository 5%]), hemorrhoids (enema 1%), rectal pain (enema 1%; suppository 2%), vomiting (5% [capsule 1%])

Hepatic: ALT increased (1%)

Local: Pain on insertion of enema tip (enema 1%)

Neuromuscular & skeletal: Back pain (7% [enema 1%]), arthralgia (5%), hypertonia (5%), myalgia (3%), arthritis (2%), leg/joint pain (enema 2%)

Ocular: Conjunctivitis (2%)

Respiratory: Flu-like syndrome (3% [enema 5%]), cough increased (2%)

Miscellaneous: Diaphoresis (3%), intolerance syndrome (3%)

Mechanism of Action Mesalamine (5-aminosalicylic acid) is the active component of sulfasalazine; the specific mechanism of action of mesalamine is unknown; however, it is thought that it modulates local chemical mediators of the inflammatory response, especially leukotrienes, and is also postulated to be a free radical scavenger or an inhibitor of tumor necrosis factor (TNF); action appears topical rather than systemic

Drug Interactions

Increased Effect/Toxicity: Mesalamine may increase the risk of myelosuppression from azathioprine, mercaptopurine, and thioguanine.

Decreased Effect: Decreased digoxin bioavailability.

Pharmacodynamics/Kinetics

Absorption: Rectal: Variable and dependent upon retention time, underlying GI disease, and colonic pH; Oral: Tablet: ~21% to 28%, Capsule: ~20% to 30%

Protein binding: 43%

Metabolism: Hepatic and via GI tract to acetyl-5-aminosalicylic acid

Half-life elimination: 5-ASA: 0.5-1.5 hours; acetyl-5-ASA: 5-12 hours

Time to peak, serum:

Capsule: Pentasa®: 3 hours

Rectal: 4-7 hours

Tablet: Asacol®: 4-12 hours; Lialda™: 9-12 hours

Excretion: Urine (primarily as metabolites, <8% as unchanged drug); feces (<2%)

Pregnancy Risk Factor B

Mesalazine see Mesalamine *on page 1052*

Mestinon® see Pyridostigmine *on page 1389*

Mestinon® Timespan® see Pyridostigmine *on page 1389*

Mestranol and Norethindrone (MES tra nole & nor eth IN drone)

Related Information

Endocrine Disorders and Pregnancy *on page 1750*

Norethindrone *on page 1186*

U.S. Brand Names Necon® 1/50; Norinyl® 1+50; Ortho-Novum® 1/50

Canadian Brand Names Ortho-Novum® 1/50

Mexican Brand Names Norace

Generic Available Yes

Index Terms Norethindrone and Mestranol; Ortho Novum 1/50

Pharmacologic Category Contraceptive; Estrogen and Progestin Combination

Use Prevention of pregnancy

(Continued)

Mestranol and Norethindrone *(Continued)*

Unlabeled/Investigational Use Treatment of hypermenorrhea (menorrhagia); pain associated with endometriosis; dysmenorrhea; dysfunctional uterine bleeding

Local Anesthetic/Vasoconstrictor Precautions No information available to require special precautions

Effects on Dental Treatment When prescribing antibiotics, patient must be advised to use additional methods of birth control if on hormonal contraceptives.

Common Adverse Effects Frequency not defined.

Cardiovascular: Arterial thromboembolism, cerebral hemorrhage, cerebral thrombosis, edema, hypertension, mesenteric thrombosis, MI

Central nervous system: Depression, dizziness, headache, migraine, nervousness, premenstrual syndrome, stroke

Dermatologic: Acne, erythema multiforme, erythema nodosum, hirsutism, loss of scalp hair, melasma (may persist), rash (allergic)

Endocrine & metabolic: Amenorrhea, breakthrough bleeding, breast enlargement, breast secretion, breast tenderness, carbohydrate intolerance, lactation decreased (postpartum), glucose tolerance decreased, libido changes, menstrual flow changes, sex hormone-binding globulins (SHBG) increased, spotting, temporary infertility (following discontinuation), thyroid-binding globulin increased, triglycerides increased

Gastrointestinal: Abdominal cramps, appetite changes, bloating, cholestasis, colitis, gallbladder disease, jaundice, nausea, vomiting, weight gain/loss

Genitourinary: Cervical erosion changes, cervical secretion changes, cystitis-like syndrome, vaginal candidiasis, vaginitis

Hematologic: Antithrombin III decreased, folate levels decreased, hemolytic uremic syndrome, norepinephrine induced platelet aggregability increased, porphyria, prothrombin increased; factors VII, VIII, IX, and X increased

Hepatic: Benign liver tumors, Budd-Chiari syndrome, cholestatic jaundice, hepatic adenomas

Local: Thrombophlebitis

Ocular: Cataracts, change in corneal curvature (steepening), contact lens intolerance, optic neuritis, retinal thrombosis

Renal: Impaired renal function

Respiratory: Pulmonary thromboembolism

Miscellaneous: Hemorrhagic eruption

Mechanism of Action Combination oral contraceptives inhibit ovulation via a negative feedback mechanism on the hypothalamus, which alters the normal pattern of gonadotropin secretion of a follicle-stimulating hormone (FSH) and luteinizing hormone by the anterior pituitary. The follicular phase FSH and midcycle surge of gonadotropins are inhibited. In addition, combination hormonal contraceptives produce alterations in the genital tract, including changes in the cervical mucus, rendering it unfavorable for sperm penetration even if ovulation occurs. Changes in the endometrium may also occur, producing an unfavorable environment for nidation. Combination hormonal contraceptive drugs may alter the tubal transport of the ova through the fallopian tubes. Progestational agents may also alter sperm fertility.

Drug Interactions

Cytochrome P450 Effect:

Mestranol: **Substrate** of CYP2C9 (major); Based on active metabolite ethinyl estradiol: **Substrate** of CYP3A4 (major), 3A5-7 (minor); **Inhibits** CYP1A2 (weak), 2B6 (weak), 2C19 (weak), 3A4 (weak)

Norethindrone: **Substrate** of CYP3A4 (major); **Induces** CYP2C19 (weak)

Increased Effect/Toxicity: Acetaminophen and ascorbic acid may increase plasma levels of estrogen component. Atorvastatin and indinavir increase plasma levels of combination hormonal contraceptives. Combination hormonal contraceptives increase the plasma levels of alprazolam, chlordiazepoxide, cyclosporine, diazepam, prednisolone, selegiline, theophylline, tricyclic antidepressants. Combination hormonal contraceptives may increase (or decrease) the effects of coumarin derivatives.

Decreased Effect: CYP2C9 Inhibitors may increase the levels/effects of (drugname). Example inhibitors include delavirdine, fluconazole, gemfibrozil, ketoconazole, nicardipine, NSAIDs, sulfonamides and tolbutamide. CYP3A4 inducers may decrease the levels of ethinyl estradiol (active metabolite of mestranol); example inducers include aminoglutethimide, carbamazepine, nafcillin, nevirapine, phenobarbital, phenytoin, and rifamycins. Combination hormonal contraceptives may decrease plasma levels of acetaminophen, clofibric acid, lorazepam, morphine, oxazepam, salicylic acid, temazepam. Contraceptive effect decreased by acitretin, aminoglutethimide, amprenavir, griseofulvin, lopinavir, nelfinavir, nevirapine, penicillins (effect not consistent), ritonavir, tetracyclines (effect not consistent) troglitazone. Combination hormonal contraceptives may decrease (or increase) the effects of coumarin derivatives.

Pharmacodynamics/Kinetics
Mestranol: Metabolism: Hepatic via demethylation to ethinyl estradiol
Norethindrone: See Norethindrone monograph for additional information.
Pregnancy Risk Factor X

Metacortandralone *see* PrednisoLONE *on page 1339*

Metadate® CD *see* Methylphenidate *on page 1079*

Metadate® ER *see* Methylphenidate *on page 1079*

Metaglip™ *see* Glipizide and Metformin *on page 784*

Metamucil® [OTC] *see* Psyllium *on page 1386*

Metamucil® Plus Calcium [OTC] *see* Psyllium *on page 1386*

Metamucil® Smooth Texture [OTC] *see* Psyllium *on page 1386*

Metaproterenol (met a proe TER e nol)

Related Information
Respiratory Diseases *on page 1747*
U.S. Brand Names Alupent®
Canadian Brand Names Apo-Orciprenaline®; Ratio-Orciprenaline®; Tanta-Orciprenaline®
Generic Available Yes: Excludes inhaler
Index Terms Metaproterenol Sulfate; Orciprenaline Sulfate
Pharmacologic Category Beta$_2$-Adrenergic Agonist
Use Bronchodilator in reversible airway obstruction due to asthma or COPD; because of its delayed onset of action (1 hour) and prolonged effect (4 or more hours), this may not be the drug of choice for assessing response to a bronchodilator
Local Anesthetic/Vasoconstrictor Precautions No information available to require special precautions
Effects on Dental Treatment Key adverse event(s) related to dental treatment: Bad taste and xerostomia (normal salivary flow resumes upon discontinuation).
Common Adverse Effects
>10%:
  Cardiovascular: Tachycardia (<17%)
  Central nervous system: Nervousness (3% to 14%)
  Endocrine & metabolic: Serum glucose increased, serum potassium decreased
  Neuromuscular & skeletal: Tremor (1% to 33%)
1% to 10%:
  Cardiovascular: Palpitation (<4%)
  Central nervous system: Headache (<4%), dizziness (1% to 4%), insomnia (2%)
  Gastrointestinal: Nausea, vomiting, bad taste, heartburn (≥4%), xerostomia
  Neuromuscular & skeletal: Trembling, muscle cramps, weakness (1%)
  Respiratory: Coughing, pharyngitis (≤4%)
  Miscellaneous: Diaphoresis (increased) (≤4%)
Mechanism of Action Relaxes bronchial smooth muscle by action on beta$_2$-receptors with very little effect on heart rate
Drug Interactions
Increased Effect/Toxicity: Sympathomimetics, TCAs, MAO inhibitors taken with metaproterenol may result in toxicity. Inhaled ipratropium may increase duration of bronchodilation. Halothane may increase risk of malignant arrhythmias; avoid concurrent use.
Decreased Effect: Decreased effect of beta-blockers.
Pharmacodynamics/Kinetics
Onset of action: Bronchodilation: Oral: ~15 minutes; Inhalation: ~60 seconds
  Peak effect: Oral: ~1 hour
Duration: ~1-5 hours
Pregnancy Risk Factor C

Metaproterenol Sulfate *see* Metaproterenol *on page 1055*

Metaxalone (me TAKS a lone)

U.S. Brand Names Skelaxin®
Canadian Brand Names Skelaxin®
Generic Available No
Pharmacologic Category Skeletal Muscle Relaxant
Use Relief of discomfort associated with acute, painful musculoskeletal conditions
(Continued)

Metaxalone (Continued)

Local Anesthetic/Vasoconstrictor Precautions No information available to require special precautions

Effects on Dental Treatment No significant effects or complications reported

Common Adverse Effects Frequency not defined.

Central nervous system: Dizziness, drowsiness, headache, irritability, paradoxical stimulation

Dermatologic: Rash (with or without pruritus)

Gastrointestinal: Gastrointestinal upset, nausea, vomiting

Hematologic: Hemolytic anemia, leukopenia

Hepatic: Jaundice

Miscellaneous: Hypersensitivity (including anaphylactoid reactions)

Dosage Children >12 years and Adults: Oral: 800 mg 3-4 times/day

Mechanism of Action Precise mechanism has not been established; however, efficacy appears to result from disruption of the spasm-pain-spasm cycle, probably by a general CNS depressant effect. Does not have a direct effect on skeletal muscle.

Contraindications Hypersensitivity to metaxalone or any component of the formulation; impaired hepatic or renal function, history of drug-induced hemolytic anemias or other anemias

Warnings/Precautions May cause CNS depression. CNS depressant effects may be augmented when used in conjunction with other depressants (eg, barbiturates, ethanol), when taken with food, or in the elderly. May impair mental and/or physical ability to perform hazardous tasks such as operating machinery or driving a motor vehicle. Use with caution in patients with impaired renal or hepatic function; routine monitoring of transaminases is recommended. An increase in bioavailability and half-life have been observed in female patients.

Drug Interactions

Increased Effect/Toxicity: Metaxalone may increase effects/toxicity of other CNS depressants such as anticonvulsants, antihistamines, antipsychotics, barbiturates, benzodiazepines, opiates, phenothiazines, selective serotonin reuptake inhibitors, and tricyclic antidepressants.

Ethanol/Nutrition/Herb Interactions

Ethanol: Avoid ethanol (may increase CNS depression).

Food: Bioavailability may be increased (may increase CNS depression).

Herb/Nutraceutical: Avoid valerian, St John's wort, kava kava, gotu kola (may increase CNS depression).

Dietary Considerations Administration with food may increase serum concentrations.

Pharmacodynamics/Kinetics

Onset of action: ~1 hour

Duration: ~4-6 hours

Metabolism: Hepatic

Bioavailability: Not established; food may increase

Half-life elimination: 9 hours

Time to peak: T_{max}: 3 hours

Excretion: Urine (as metabolites)

Pregnancy Risk Factor C

Dosage Forms

Tablet:

Skelaxin®: 800 mg

Metformin (met FOR min)

Related Information

Endocrine Disorders and Pregnancy *on page 1750*

U.S. Brand Names Fortamet®; Glucophage®; Glucophage® XR; Glumetza™; Riomet™

Canadian Brand Names Alti-Metformin; Apo-Metformin®; BCI-Metformin; Gen-Metformin; Glucophage®; Glumetza®; Glycon; Novo-Metformin; Nu-Metformin; PMS-Metformin; RAN™-Metformin; ratio-Metformin; Rho®-Metformin; Sandoz-Metformin FC

Mexican Brand Names Dabex; Dimefor; Glucophage Forte

Generic Available Yes: Excludes solution

Index Terms Metformin Hydrochloride

Pharmacologic Category Antidiabetic Agent, Biguanide

Use Management of type 2 diabetes mellitus (noninsulin dependent, NIDDM) as monotherapy when hyperglycemia cannot be managed on diet alone. May be used concomitantly with a sulfonylurea or insulin to improve glycemic control.

Unlabeled/Investigational Use Treatment of HIV lipodystrophy syndrome, gestational diabetes mellitus (GDM), polycystic ovary syndrome (PCOS)

Local Anesthetic/Vasoconstrictor Precautions No information available to require special precautions

Effects on Dental Treatment Key adverse event(s) related to dental treatment: Taste disorder.

Metformin-dependent diabetics (noninsulin dependent, Type 2) should be appointed for dental treatment in morning in order to minimize chance of stress-induced hypoglycemia.

Common Adverse Effects
>10%:
Gastrointestinal: Nausea/vomiting (6% to 25%), diarrhea (10% to 53%), flatulence (12%)

Neuromuscular & skeletal: Weakness (9%)

1% to 10%:
Cardiovascular: Chest discomfort, flushing, palpitation

Central nervous system: Headache (6%), chills, dizziness, lightheadedness

Dermatologic: Rash

Endocrine & metabolic: Hypoglycemia

Gastrointestinal: Indigestion (7%), abdominal discomfort (6%), abdominal distention, abnormal stools, constipation, dyspepsia/ heartburn, taste disorder

Neuromuscular & skeletal: Myalgia

Respiratory: Dyspnea, upper respiratory tract infection

Miscellaneous: Decreased vitamin B_{12} levels (7%), increased diaphoresis, flu-like syndrome, nail disorder

Dosage Note: Allow 1-2 weeks between dose titrations: Generally, clinically significant responses are not seen at doses <1500 mg daily; however, a lower recommended starting dose and gradual increased dosage is recommended to minimize gastrointestinal symptoms

Children 10-16 years: Management of type 2 diabetes mellitus: Oral (immediate release tablet or oral solution): Initial: 500 mg twice daily (given with the morning and evening meals); increases in daily dosage should be made in increments of 500 mg at weekly intervals, given in divided doses, up to a maximum of 2000 mg/day

Adults ≥17 years: Management of type 2 diabetes mellitus: Oral:
Immediate release tablet or oral solution: Initial: 500 mg twice daily (give with the morning and evening meals) **or** 850 mg once daily; increase dosage incrementally.

Incremental dosing recommendations based on dosage form:
500 mg tablet: One tablet/day at weekly intervals
850 mg tablet: One tablet/day every other week
Oral solution: 500 mg twice daily every other week

Doses of up to 2000 mg/day may be given twice daily. If a dose >2000 mg/day is required, it may be better tolerated in three divided doses. Maximum recommended dose 2550 mg/day.

Extended release tablet: Initial: 500 mg once daily (with the evening meal); dosage may be increased by 500 mg weekly; maximum dose: 2000 mg once daily. If glycemic control is not achieved at maximum dose, may divide dose to 1000 mg twice daily. If doses >2000 mg/day are needed, switch to regular release tablets and titrate to maximum dose of 2550 mg/day.

Elderly: The initial and maintenance dosing should be conservative, due to the potential for decreased renal function. Generally, elderly patients should not be titrated to the maximum dose of metformin. Do not use in patients ≥80 years of age unless normal renal function has been established.

Transfer from other antidiabetic agents: No transition period is generally necessary except when transferring from chlorpropamide. When transferring from chlorpropamide, care should be exercised during the first 2 weeks because of the prolonged retention of chlorpropamide in the body, leading to overlapping drug effects and possible hypoglycemia.

Concomitant metformin and oral sulfonylurea therapy: If patients have not responded to 4 weeks of the maximum dose of metformin monotherapy, consider a gradual addition of an oral sulfonylurea, even if prior primary or secondary failure to a sulfonylurea has occurred. Continue metformin at the maximum dose.

Failed sulfonylurea therapy: Patients with prior failure on glyburide may be treated by gradual addition of metformin. Initiate with glyburide 20 mg and metformin 500 mg daily. Metformin dosage may be increased by 500 mg/day at weekly intervals, up to a maximum of 2500 mg/day (dosage of glyburide maintained at 20 mg/day).

Concomitant metformin and insulin therapy: Initial: 500 mg metformin once daily, continue current insulin dose; increase by 500 mg metformin weekly until adequate glycemic control is achieved

Maximum dose: 2500 mg metformin; 2000 mg metformin extended release

(Continued)

Metformin *(Continued)*

Decrease insulin dose 10% to 25% when FPG <120 mg/dL; monitor and make further adjustments as needed

Dosing adjustment/comments in renal impairment: The plasma and blood half-life of metformin is prolonged and the renal clearance is decreased in proportion to the decrease in creatinine clearance. Per the manufacturer, metformin is contraindicated in the presence of renal dysfunction defined as a serum creatinine >1.5 mg/dL in males, or >1.4 mg/dL in females and in patients with abnormal clearance. Clinically, it has been recommended that metformin be avoided in patients with Cl_{cr} <60-70 mL/minute (DeFronzo, 1999).

Dosing adjustment in hepatic impairment: Avoid metformin; liver disease is a risk factor for the development of lactic acidosis during metformin therapy.

Mechanism of Action Decreases hepatic glucose production, decreasing intestinal absorption of glucose and improves insulin sensitivity (increases peripheral glucose uptake and utilization)

Contraindications Hypersensitivity to metformin or any component of the formulation; renal disease or renal dysfunction (serum creatinine ≥1.5 mg/dL in males or ≥1.4 mg/dL in females or abnormal creatinine clearance from any cause, including shock, acute myocardial infarction, or septicemia); acute or chronic metabolic acidosis with or without coma (including diabetic ketoacidosis)

Note: Temporarily discontinue in patients undergoing radiologic studies in which intravascular iodinated contrast materials are utilized.

Warnings/Precautions [U.S. Boxed Warning]: Lactic acidosis is a rare, but potentially severe consequence of therapy with metformin. Lactic acidosis should be suspected in any diabetic patient receiving metformin who has evidence of acidosis when evidence of ketoacidosis is lacking. Discontinue metformin in clinical situations predisposing to hypoxemia, including conditions such as cardiovascular collapse, respiratory failure, acute myocardial infarction, acute congestive heart failure, and septicemia. Use caution in patients with congestive heart failure requiring pharmacologic management, particularly in patients with unstable or acute CHF; risk of lactic acidosis may be increased secondary to hypoperfusion.

Metformin is substantially excreted by the kidney. The risk of accumulation and lactic acidosis increases with the degree of impairment of renal function. Patients with renal function below the limit of normal for their age should not receive metformin. In elderly patients, renal function should be monitored regularly; should not be used in any patient ≥80 years of age unless measurement of creatinine clearance verifies normal renal function. Use of concomitant medications that may affect renal function (ie, affect tubular secretion) may also affect metformin disposition. Metformin should be suspended in patients with dehydration and/or prerenal azotemia. Therapy should be suspended for any surgical procedures (resume only after normal intake resumed and normal renal function is verified). Metformin should also be temporarily discontinued for 48 hours in patients undergoing radiologic studies involving the intravascular administration of iodinated contrast materials (potential for acute alteration in renal function). It may be necessary to discontinue metformin and administer insulin if the patient is exposed to stress (fever, trauma, infection, surgery).

Avoid use in patients with impaired liver function. Patient must be instructed to avoid excessive acute or chronic ethanol use. Administration of oral antidiabetic drugs has been reported to be associated with increased cardiovascular mortality; metformin does not appear to share this risk. Safety and efficacy of metformin have been established for use in children ≥10 years of age; the extended release preparation is for use in patients ≥17 years of age.

Drug Interactions

Increased Effect/Toxicity: Furosemide and cimetidine may increase metformin blood levels. Cationic drugs (eg, amiloride, digoxin, morphine, procainamide, quinidine, quinine, ranitidine, triamterene, trimethoprim, and vancomycin) which are eliminated by renal tubular secretion have the potential to increase metformin levels by competing for common renal tubular transport systems. Contrast agents may increase the risk of metformin-induced lactic acidosis; discontinue metformin prior to exposure and withhold for 48 hours.

Decreased Effect: Drugs which tend to produce hyperglycemia (eg, diuretics, corticosteroids, phenothiazines, thyroid products, estrogens, oral contraceptives, phenytoin, nicotinic acid, sympathomimetics, calcium channel blocking drugs, isoniazid) may lead to a loss of glucose control.

Ethanol/Nutrition/Herb Interactions

Ethanol: Avoid or limit ethanol (incidence of lactic acidosis may be increased; may cause hypoglycemia).

Food: Food decreases the extent and slightly delays the absorption. May decrease absorption of vitamin B_{12} and/or folic acid.

Herb/Nutraceutical: Caution with chromium, garlic, gymnema (may cause hypoglycemia).

Dietary Considerations Drug may cause GI upset; take with food (to decrease GI upset). Take at the same time each day. Dietary modification based on ADA recommendations is a part of therapy. Monitor for signs and symptoms of vitamin B_{12} and/or folic acid deficiency; supplementation may be required.

Pharmacodynamics/Kinetics

Onset of action: Within days; maximum effects up to 2 weeks

Distribution: V_d: 654 ± 358 L; partitions into erythrocytes

Protein binding: Negligible

Metabolism: Not metabolized by the liver

Bioavailability: Absolute: Fasting: 50% to 60%

Half-life elimination:

Plasma: 6.2 hours

Blood: 17.6 hours

Time to peak, serum: Extended release: 7 hours (range: 4-8 hours)

Excretion: Urine (90% as unchanged drug)

Pregnancy Risk Factor B

Dosage Forms

Solution, oral:

Riomet™: 100 mg/mL

Tablet: 500 mg, 850 mg, 1000 mg

Glucophage®: 500 mg, 850 mg, 1000 mg

Tablet, extended release: 500 mg, 750 mg

Fortamet®: 500 mg, 1000 mg

Glucophage® XR: 500 mg, 750 mg

Glumetza™: 500 mg

Methadone (METH a done)

U.S. Brand Names Dolophine®; Methadone Diskets®; Methadone Intensol™; Methadose®

Canadian Brand Names Metadol™

Generic Available Yes

Index Terms Methadone Hydrochloride

Pharmacologic Category Analgesic, Opioid

Use Management of moderate-to-severe pain; detoxification and maintenance treatment of opioid addiction (if used for detoxification and maintenance treatment of narcotic addiction, it must be part of an FDA-approved program)

Local Anesthetic/Vasoconstrictor Precautions No information available to require special precautions

Effects on Dental Treatment Key adverse event(s) related to dental treatment: Significant xerostomia (normal salivary flow resumes upon discontinuation) and glossitis.

Common Adverse Effects Frequency not defined. During prolonged administration, adverse effects may decrease over several weeks; however, constipation and sweating may persist.

Cardiovascular: Bradycardia, peripheral vasodilation, cardiac arrest, syncope, faintness, shock, hypotension, edema, arrhythmia, bigeminal rhythms, extrasystoles, tachycardia, torsade de pointes, ventricular fibrillation, ventricular tachycardia, ECG changes, QT interval prolonged, T-wave inversion, cardiomyopathy, flushing, heart failure, palpitation, phlebitis, orthostatic hypotension

Central nervous system: Euphoria, dysphoria, hallucination, headache, insomnia, agitation, disorientation, drowsiness, dizziness, lightheadedness, sedation, confusion, seizure

Dermatologic: Pruritus, urticaria, rash, hemorrhagic urticaria

Endocrine & metabolic: Libido decreased, hypokalemia, hypomagnesemia, antidiuretic effect, amenorrhea

Gastrointestinal: Nausea, vomiting, constipation, anorexia, stomach cramps, xerostomia, biliary tract spasm, abdominal pain, glossitis, weight gain

(Continued)

Methadone (Continued)

Genitourinary: Urinary retention or hesitancy, impotence

Hematologic: Thrombocytopenia (reversible, reported in patients with chronic hepatitis)

Neuromuscular & skeletal: Weakness

Local: I.M./SubQ injection: Pain, erythema, swelling; I.V. injection: pruritus, urticaria, rash, hemorrhagic urticaria (rare)

Ocular: Miosis, visual disturbances

Respiratory: Respiratory depression, respiratory arrest, pulmonary edema

Miscellaneous: Physical and psychological dependence, death, diaphoresis

Restrictions C-II

When used for treatment of opioid addiction: May only be dispensed in accordance to guidelines established by the Substance Abuse and Mental Health Services Administration's (SAMHSA) Center for Substance Abuse Treatment (CSAT). Regulations regarding methadone use may vary by state and/or country. Obtain advice from appropriate regulatory agencies and/or consult with pain management/palliative care specialists.

Note: Regulatory Exceptions to the General Requirement to Provide Opioid Agonist Treatment (per manufacturer's labeling):

1. During inpatient care, when the patient was admitted for any condition other than concurrent opioid addiction, to facilitate the treatment of the primary admitting diagnosis.

2. During an emergency period of no longer than 3 days while definitive care for the addiction is being sought in an appropriately licensed facility.

Mechanism of Action Binds to opiate receptors in the CNS, causing inhibition of ascending pain pathways, altering the perception of and response to pain; produces generalized CNS depression

Drug Interactions

Cytochrome P450 Effect: Substrate of CYP2C9 (minor), 2C19 (minor), 2D6 (minor), 3A4 (major); **Inhibits** CYP2D6 (moderate), 3A4 (weak)

Increased Effect/Toxicity: CYP3A4 inhibitors may increase the levels/effects of methadone (eg, azole antifungals, clarithromycin, diclofenac, doxycycline, erythromycin, imatinib, isoniazid, nefazodone, nicardipine, propofol, protease inhibitors, quinidine, telithromycin, verapamil). Methadone may increase the levels/effects of CYP2D6 substrates (eg, amphetamines, selected beta-blockers, dextromethorphan, fluoxetine, lidocaine, mirtazapine, nefazodone, paroxetine, risperidone, ritonavir, thioridazine, tricyclic antidepressants, venlafaxine). Methadone may increase bioavailability and toxic effects of zidovudine. CNS depressants (including but not limited to opioid analgesics, general anesthetics, sedatives, hypnotics, ethanol) may cause respiratory depression, hypotension, profound sedation, or coma. Levels of desipramine may be increased by methadone. Effects/toxicity of QT_c interval-prolonging agents may be increased; use with caution (including but may not be limited to amitriptyline, astemizole, bepridil, disopyramide, erythromycin, haloperidol, imipramine, quinidine, pimozide, procainamide, sotalol, thioridazine). Ritonavir may increase levels/effects of methadone shortly after initiation. SSRIs may increase the levels/effects of methadone; the serotonergic effects of SSRIs or selegiline may be increased by methadone.

Decreased Effect: Agonist/antagonist analgesics (buprenorphine, butorphanol, nalbuphine, pentazocine) may decrease analgesic effect of methadone and precipitate withdrawal symptoms; use is not recommended. Efavirenz and nevirapine may decrease levels of methadone (opioid withdrawal syndrome has been reported). Methadone may decrease bioavailability of didanosine and stavudine. Ritonavir (and combinations) may decrease levels of methadone during prolonged therapy; withdrawal symptoms have inconsistently been observed, monitor. CYP3A4 inducers may decrease the levels/effects of methadone (eg, aminoglutethimide, carbamazepine, nafcillin, nevirapine, phenobarbital, phenytoin, rifamycins). Monitor for methadone withdrawal. Larger doses of methadone may be required. Methadone may decrease the levels/effects of CYP2D6 prodrug substrates (eg, codeine, hydrocodone, oxycodone, tramadol). Methadone may decrease the effects of pegvisomant.

Pharmacodynamics/Kinetics

Onset of action: Oral: Analgesic: 0.5-1 hour; Parenteral: 10-20 minutes

Peak effect: Parenteral: 1-2 hours; Oral: continuous dosing: 3-5 days

Duration of analgesia: Oral: 4-8 hours, increases to 22-48 hours with repeated doses

Distribution: V_{dss}: 1-8 L/kg

Protein binding: 85% to 90%

Metabolism: Hepatic; N-demethylation primarily via CYP3A4, CYP2B6, and CYP2C19 to inactive metabolites

Bioavailability: Oral: 36% to 100%

Half-life elimination: 8-59 hours; may be prolonged with alkaline pH, decreased during pregnancy

Time to peak, plasma: 1-7.5 hours

Excretion: Urine (<10% as unchanged drug); increased with urine pH <6

Pregnancy Risk Factor C/D (prolonged use or high doses at term)

Dental Comment This drug is known to prolong the QT interval. The QT interval is measured as the time and distance between the Q point of the QRS complex and the end of the T wave in the ECG tracing. After adjustment for heart rate, the QT interval is defined as prolonged if it is more than 450 msec in men and 460 msec in women. A long QT syndrome was first described in the 1950s and 60s as a congenital syndrome involving QT interval prolongation and syncope and sudden death. Some of the congenital long QT syndromes were character- ized by a peculiar electrocardiographic appearance of the QRS complex involving a premature atria beat followed by a pause, then a subsequent sinus beat showing marked QT prolongation and deformity. This type of cardiac arrhythmia was originally termed "torsade de pointes" (translated from the French as "twisting of the points").

Prolongation of the QT interval is thought to result from delayed ventricular repolarization. The repolarization process within the myocardial cell is due to the efflux of intracellular potassium. The channels associated with this current can be blocked by many drugs and predispose the electrical propagation cycle to torsade de pointes.

Methadone is one of the drugs confirmed to prolong the QT interval and is accepted as having a risk of causing torsade de pointes. The risk of drug-induced torsade de pointes is extremely low when a single QT interval prolonging drug is prescribed. In terms of epinephrine, it is not known what effect vasoconstrictors in the local anesthetic regimen will have in patients with a known history of congenital prolonged QT interval or in patients taking any medication that prolongs the QT interval. Until more information is obtained, it is suggested that the clinician consult with the physician prior to the use of a vasoconstrictor in suspected patients, and that the vasoconstrictor (epinephrine, levonordefrin [Neo-Cobefrin®]) be used with caution.

Methadone Diskets® *see* Methadone *on page 1059*

Methadone Hydrochloride *see* Methadone *on page 1059*

Methadone Intensol™ *see* Methadone *on page 1059*

Methadose® *see* Methadone *on page 1059*

Methaminodiazepoxide Hydrochloride *see* Chlordiazepoxide *on page 331*

Methamphetamine (meth am FET a meen)

U.S. Brand Names Desoxyn®

Canadian Brand Names Desoxyn®

Generic Available Yes

Index Terms Desoxyephedrine Hydrochloride; Methamphetamine Hydrochlo- ride

Pharmacologic Category Anorexiant; Stimulant; Sympathomimetic

Use Treatment of attention-deficit/hyperactivity disorder (ADHD); exogenous obesity (short-term adjunct)

Unlabeled/Investigational Use Narcolepsy

Local Anesthetic/Vasoconstrictor Precautions Use vasoconstrictor with caution in patients taking methamphetamine. Amphetamines enhance the sympathomimetic response of epinephrine and norepinephrine leading to potential hypertension and cardiotoxicity.

Effects on Dental Treatment Key adverse event(s) related to dental treat- ment: Xerostomia (normal salivary flow resumes upon discontinuation) and unpleasant taste. Up to 10% of patients taking methamphetamine may present with hypertension. Monitor blood pressure prior to using local anesthetic with vasoconstrictors.

Common Adverse Effects Frequency not defined.

Cardiovascular: Hypertension, tachycardia, palpitation

Central nervous system: Restlessness, headache, exacerbation of motor and phonic tics and Tourette's syndrome, dizziness, psychosis, dysphoria, overstimulation, euphoria, insomnia

Dermatologic: Rash, urticaria

Endocrine & metabolic: Change in libido

Gastrointestinal: Diarrhea, nausea, vomiting, stomach cramps, constipation, anorexia, weight loss, xerostomia, unpleasant taste

Genitourinary: Impotence

Neuromuscular & skeletal: Tremor

Miscellaneous: Suppression of growth in children, tolerance and withdrawal with prolonged use

(Continued)

Methamphetamine *(Continued)*

Restrictions C-II

An FDA-approved medication guide must be distributed when dispensing an outpatient prescription (new or refill) where this medication is to be used without direct supervision of a healthcare provider. Medication guides are available at http://www.fda.gov/cder/drug/infopage/ADHD/default.htm.

Pharmacotherapy for weight loss is recommended only for obese patients with a body mass index ≥30 kg/m², or ≥27 kg/m² in the presence of other risk factors such as hypertension, diabetes, and/or dyslipidemia or a high waist circumference; therapy should be used in conjunction with a comprehensive weight management program. Rule out organic causes of obesity (eg, untreated hypothyroidism) prior to use.

Note: Methamphetamine is not approved for long-term use. The limited usefulness of medications in this class should be weighed against possible risks associated with their use. Consult weight loss guidelines for current pharmacotherapy recommendations.

Mechanism of Action A sympathomimetic amine related to ephedrine and amphetamine with CNS stimulant activity; peripheral actions include elevation of systolic and diastolic blood pressure and weak bronchodilator and respiratory stimulant action

Drug Interactions

Cytochrome P450 Effect: Substrate of CYP2D6 (major)

Increased Effect/Toxicity: Amphetamines may precipitate hypertensive crisis or serotonin syndrome in patients receiving MAO inhibitors (selegiline >10 mg/day, isocarboxazid, phenelzine, tranylcypromine, furazolidone). Serotonin syndrome has also been associated with combinations of amphetamines and SSRIs; these combinations should be avoided. TCAs may enhance the effects of amphetamines, potentially leading to hypertensive crisis. CYP2D6 inhibitors may increase the levels/effects of methamphetamine; example inhibitors include chlorpromazine, delavirdine, fluoxetine, miconazole, paroxetine, pergolide, quinidine, quinine, ritonavir, and ropinirole. Large doses of antacids or urinary alkalinizers increase the half-life and duration of action of amphetamines. May precipitate arrhythmias in patients receiving general anesthetics. Inhibitors of CYP2D6 may increase the effects of amphetamines (includes amiodarone, cimetidine, delavirdine, fluoxetine, paroxetine, propafenone, quinidine, and ritonavir).

Decreased Effect: Amphetamines inhibit the antihypertensive response to guanethidine, methyldopa, and guanadrel. Enzyme inducers (barbiturates, carbamazepine, phenytoin, and rifampin) may decrease serum concentrations of amphetamines.

Pharmacodynamics/Kinetics

Absorption: Rapid from GI tract

Metabolism: Hepatic; forms metabolite

Half-life elimination: 4-5 hours

Excretion: Urine primarily (dependent on urine pH)

Pregnancy Risk Factor C

Methamphetamine Hydrochloride *see* Methamphetamine *on page 1061*

Methazolamide *(meth a ZOE la mide)*

Canadian Brand Names Apo-Methazolamide®

Generic Available Yes

Pharmacologic Category Carbonic Anhydrase Inhibitor; Diuretic, Carbonic Anhydrase Inhibitor; Ophthalmic Agent, Antiglaucoma

Use Adjunctive treatment of open-angle or secondary glaucoma; short-term therapy of narrow-angle glaucoma when delay of surgery is desired

Local Anesthetic/Vasoconstrictor Precautions No information available to require special precautions

Effects on Dental Treatment Key adverse event(s) related to dental treatment: Xerostomia (normal salivary flow resumes upon discontinuation) and metallic taste.

Common Adverse Effects Frequency not defined.

Central nervous system: Malaise, fever, mental depression, drowsiness, dizziness, nervousness, headache, confusion, seizure, fatigue, trembling, unsteadiness

Dermatologic: Urticaria, pruritus, photosensitivity, rash, Stevens-Johnson syndrome

Endocrine & metabolic: Hyperchloremic metabolic acidosis, hypokalemia, hyperglycemia

Gastrointestinal: Metallic taste, anorexia, nausea, vomiting, diarrhea, constipation, weight loss, GI irritation, xerostomia, black tarry stools

Genitourinary: Polyuria, crystalluria, hematuria, polyuria, renal calculi, impotence

Hematologic: Bone marrow depression, thrombocytopenia, thrombocytopenic purpura, hemolytic anemia, leukopenia, pancytopenia, agranulocytosis

Hepatic: Hepatic insufficiency

Neuromuscular & skeletal: Weakness, ataxia, paresthesia

Miscellaneous: Hypersensitivity

Mechanism of Action Noncompetitive inhibition of the enzyme carbonic anhydrase; thought that carbonic anhydrase is located at the luminal border of cells of the proximal tubule. When the enzyme is inhibited, there is an increase in urine volume and a change to an alkaline pH with a subsequent decrease in the excretion of titratable acid and ammonia.

Drug Interactions

Increased Effect/Toxicity: Methazolamide may induce hypokalemia which would sensitize a patient to digitalis toxicity. Hypokalemia may be compounded with concurrent diuretic use or steroids. Methazolamide may increase the potential for salicylate toxicity. Primidone absorption may be delayed.

Decreased Effect: Increased lithium excretion and altered excretion of other drugs by alkalinization of the urine, such as amphetamines, quinidine, procainamide, methenamine, phenobarbital, and salicylates.

Pharmacodynamics/Kinetics

Onset of action: Slow in comparison with acetazolamide (2-4 hours)

Peak effect: 6-8 hours

Duration: 10-18 hours

Absorption: Slow

Distribution: Well into tissue

Protein binding: ~55%

Metabolism: Slowly from GI tract

Half-life elimination: ~14 hours

Excretion: Urine (~25% as unchanged drug)

Pregnancy Risk Factor C

Methenamine (meth EN a meen)

U.S. Brand Names Hiprex®; Mandelamine®; Urex®

Canadian Brand Names Dehydral®; Hiprex®; Mandelamine®; Urasal®; Urex®

Mexican Brand Names Mandepiril-S

Generic Available Yes

Index Terms Hexamethylenetetramine; Methenamine Hippurate; Methenamine Mandelate

Pharmacologic Category Antibiotic, Miscellaneous

Use Prophylaxis or suppression of recurrent urinary tract infections; urinary tract discomfort secondary to hypermotility

Local Anesthetic/Vasoconstrictor Precautions No information available to require special precautions

Effects on Dental Treatment No significant effects or complications reported

Common Adverse Effects 1% to 10%:

Dermatologic: Rash (<4%)

Gastrointestinal: Nausea, dyspepsia (<4%)

Genitourinary: Dysuria (<4%)

Mechanism of Action Methenamine is hydrolyzed to formaldehyde and ammonia in acidic urine; formaldehyde has nonspecific bactericidal action

Drug Interactions

Increased Effect/Toxicity: Sulfonamides may precipitate in the urine; concurrent use is contraindicated.

Decreased Effect: Sodium bicarbonate and acetazolamide will decrease effect secondary to alkalinization of urine.

Pharmacodynamics/Kinetics

Absorption: Readily

Metabolism: Gastric juices: Hydrolyze 10% to 30% unless protected via enteric coating; Hepatic: ~10% to 25%

Half-life elimination: 3-6 hours

Excretion: Urine (~70% to 90% as unchanged drug) within 24 hours

Pregnancy Risk Factor C

Methenamine, Sodium Biphosphate, Phenyl Salicylate, Methylene Blue, and Hyoscyamine
(meth EN a meen, SOW dee um bye FOS fate, fen nil sa LIS i late, METH i leen bloo, & hye oh SYE a meen)

Related Information
Hyoscyamine *on page 847*
Methenamine *on page 1063*

U.S. Brand Names Urelle®; Urimar-T

Generic Available No

Index Terms Hyoscyamine, Methenamine, Sodium Biphosphate, Phenyl Salicylate, and Methylene Blue; Methylene Blue, Methenamine, Sodium Biphosphate, Phenyl Salicylate, and Hyoscyamine; Phenyl Salicylate, Methenamine, Methylene Blue, Sodium Biphosphate, and Hyoscyamine; Sodium Biphosphate, Methenamine, Methylene Blue, Phenyl Salicylate, and Hyoscyamine

Pharmacologic Category Antibiotic, Miscellaneous

Use Treatment of symptoms of irritative voiding; relief of local symptoms associated with urinary tract infections; relief of urinary tract symptoms caused by diagnostic procedures

Local Anesthetic/Vasoconstrictor Precautions No information available to require special precautions

Effects on Dental Treatment Key adverse event(s) related to dental treatment: Xerostomia (normal salivary flow resumes upon discontinuation).

Common Adverse Effects Frequency not defined.
Cardiovascular: Tachycardia, flushing
Central nervous system: Dizziness
Gastrointestinal: Xerostomia, nausea, vomiting
Genitourinary: Urinary retention (acute), micturition difficulty, discoloration of urine (blue)
Ocular: Blurred vision
Respiratory: Dyspnea, shortness of breath

Drug Interactions
Increased Effect/Toxicity: Refer to individual monographs for Hyoscyamine and Methenamine.
Decreased Effect: Refer to individual monographs for Hyoscyamine and Methenamine.

Pregnancy Risk Factor C

Methergine® *see* Methylergonovine *on page 1079*

Methimazole (meth IM a zole)

Related Information
Endocrine Disorders and Pregnancy *on page 1750*

U.S. Brand Names Tapazole®

Canadian Brand Names Dom-Methimazole; PHL-Methimazole; Tapazole®

Generic Available Yes

Index Terms Thiamazole

Pharmacologic Category Antithyroid Agent

Use Palliative treatment of hyperthyroidism, return the hyperthyroid patient to a normal metabolic state prior to thyroidectomy, and to control thyrotoxic crisis that may accompany thyroidectomy. The use of antithyroid thioamides is as effective in elderly as they are in younger adults; however, the expense, potential adverse effects, and inconvenience (compliance, monitoring) make them undesirable. The use of radioiodine due to ease of administration and less concern for long-term side effects and reproduction problems (some older males) makes it a more appropriate therapy.

Local Anesthetic/Vasoconstrictor Precautions No information available to require special precautions

Effects on Dental Treatment Key adverse event(s) related to dental treatment: Abnormal taste and salivary gland swelling.

Common Adverse Effects Frequency not defined.
Cardiovascular: Edema
Central nervous system: Headache, vertigo, drowsiness, CNS stimulation, depression
Dermatologic: Skin rash, urticaria, pruritus, erythema nodosum, skin pigmentation, exfoliative dermatitis, alopecia
Endocrine & metabolic: Goiter
Gastrointestinal: Nausea, vomiting, stomach pain, abnormal taste, constipation, weight gain, salivary gland swelling

Hematologic: Leukopenia, agranulocytosis, granulocytopenia, thrombocyto-penia, aplastic anemia, hypoprothrombinemia

Hepatic: Cholestatic jaundice, jaundice, hepatitis

Neuromuscular & skeletal: Arthralgia, paresthesia

Renal: Nephrotic syndrome

Miscellaneous: SLE-like syndrome

Mechanism of Action Inhibits the synthesis of thyroid hormones by blocking the oxidation of iodine in the thyroid gland, blocking iodine's ability to combine with tyrosine to form thyroxine and triiodothyronine (T_3), does not inactivate circulating T_4 and T_3

Drug Interactions

Cytochrome P450 Effect: Inhibits CYP1A2 (weak), 2A6 (weak), 2B6 (weak), 2C9 (weak), 2C19 (weak), 2D6 (moderate), 2E1 (weak), 3A4 (weak)

Increased Effect/Toxicity: Dosage of some drugs (including beta-blockers, digoxin, and theophylline) require adjustment during treatment of hyperthyroidism. Methimazole may increase the levels/effects of CYP2D6 substrates (eg, amphetamines, selected beta-blockers, dextromethorphan, fluoxetine, lidocaine, mirtazapine, nefazodone, paroxetine, risperidone, ritonavir, thioridazine, tricyclic antidepressants, venlafaxine).

Decreased Effect: Anticoagulant effect of warfarin may be decreased. Methimazole may decrease the levels/effects of CYP2D6 prodrug substrates (eg, codeine, hydrocodone, oxycodone, tramadol).

Pharmacodynamics/Kinetics

Onset of action: Antithyroid: Oral: 12-18 hours

Duration: 36-72 hours

Distribution: Concentrated in thyroid gland; crosses placenta; enters breast milk (1:1)

Protein binding, plasma: None

Metabolism: Hepatic

Bioavailability: 80% to 95%

Half-life elimination: 4-13 hours

Excretion: Urine (80%)

Pregnancy Risk Factor D

Methitest™ see MethylTESTOSTERone on page 1085

Methocarbamol (meth oh KAR ba mole)

Related Information

Temporomandibular Dysfunction (TMD) on page 1822

U.S. Brand Names Robaxin®

Canadian Brand Names Robaxin®

Generic Available Yes: Tablet

Pharmacologic Category Skeletal Muscle Relaxant

Dental Use Treatment of muscle spasm associated with acute temporomandibular joint pain (TMJ)

Use Treatment of muscle spasm associated with acute painful musculoskeletal conditions; supportive therapy in tetanus

Local Anesthetic/Vasoconstrictor Precautions No information available to require special precautions

Effects on Dental Treatment Key adverse event(s) related to dental treatment: Metallic taste.

Significant Adverse Effects Frequency not defined.

Cardiovascular: Flushing of face, bradycardia, hypotension, syncope

Central nervous system: Drowsiness, dizziness, lightheadedness, convulsion, vertigo, headache, fever, amnesia, confusion, insomnia, sedation, coordination impaired (mild)

Dermatologic: Allergic dermatitis, urticaria, pruritus, rash, angioneurotic edema

Gastrointestinal: Nausea, vomiting, metallic taste, dyspepsia

Hematologic: Leukopenia

Hepatic: Jaundice

Local: Pain at injection site, thrombophlebitis

Ocular: Nystagmus, blurred vision, diplopia, conjunctivitis

Renal: Renal impairment

Respiratory: Nasal congestion

Miscellaneous: Allergic manifestations, anaphylactic reaction

Dental Usual Dosing

Muscle spasm associated with acute TMJ pain: Children ≥16 years and Adults: Oral: 1.5 g 4 times/day for 2-3 days (up to 8 g/day may be given in severe conditions), then decrease to 4-4.5 g/day in 3-6 divided doses

(Continued)

Methocarbamol *(Continued)*

Dosage

Tetanus: I.V.:

Children: Recommended **only** for use in tetanus: 15 mg/kg/dose or 500 mg/m²/dose, may repeat every 6 hours if needed; maximum dose: 1.8 g/m²/day for 3 days only

Adults: Initial dose: 1-3 g; may repeat dose every 6 hours until oral dosing is possible; injection should not be used for more than 3 consecutive days

Muscle spasm: Children ≥16 years and Adults:

Oral: 1.5 g 4 times/day for 2-3 days (up to 8 g/day may be given in severe conditions), then decrease to 4-4.5 g/day in 3-6 divided doses

I.M., I.V.: 1 g every 8 hours if oral not possible; injection should not be used for more than 3 consecutive days. If condition persists, may repeat course of therapy after a drug-free interval of 48 hours.

Elderly: Muscle spasm: Oral: Initial: 500 mg 4 times/day; titrate to response

Dosing adjustment/comments in renal impairment: Do not administer parenteral formulation to patients with renal dysfunction.

Dosing adjustment in hepatic impairment: Specific dosing guidelines are not available; plasma protein binding and clearance are decreased; half-life is increased

Mechanism of Action Causes skeletal muscle relaxation by general CNS depression

Contraindications Hypersensitivity to methocarbamol or any component of the formulation; renal impairment (injection formulation)

Warnings/Precautions

May cause CNS depression, which may impair physical or mental abilities; patients must be cautioned about performing tasks which require mental alertness (eg, operating machinery or driving). Effects may be potentiated when used with other sedative drugs or ethanol.

Oral: Use caution with renal or hepatic impairment.

Injection: Rate of injection should not exceed 3 mL/minute; solution is hypertonic; avoid extravasation. Use with caution in patients with a history of seizures. Use caution with hepatic impairment. Vial stopper contains latex.

Safety and efficacy have not been established in children <12 years or age.

Drug Interactions Increased effect/toxicity with CNS depressants; pyridostigmine (a single case of worsening myasthenia has been reported following methocarbamol administration)

Ethanol/Nutrition/Herb Interactions

Ethanol: Avoid ethanol (may increase CNS depression).

Herb/Nutraceutical: Avoid valerian, St John's wort, kava kava, gotu kola (may increase CNS depression).

Pharmacodynamics/Kinetics

Onset of action: Muscle relaxation: Oral: ~30 minutes

Protein binding: 46% to 50%

Metabolism: Hepatic via dealkylation and hydroxylation

Half-life elimination: 1-2 hours

Time to peak, serum: ~2 hours

Excretion: Urine (as metabolites)

Pregnancy Risk Factor C

Lactation Excretion in breast milk unknown/use caution

Dosage Forms Excipient information presented when available (limited, particularly for generics); consult specific product labeling.

Injection, solution: 100 mg/mL (10 mL) [in polyethylene glycol; vial stopper contains latex]

Tablet: 500 mg, 750 mg

Methohexital *(meth oh HEKS i tal)*

U.S. Brand Names Brevital® Sodium

Canadian Brand Names Brevital®

Generic Available No

Index Terms Methohexital Sodium

Pharmacologic Category Barbiturate

Dental Use Induction and maintenance of general anesthesia for short procedures

Use Induction and maintenance of general anesthesia for short procedures

Can be used in pediatric patients ≥1 month of age as follows: For rectal or intramuscular induction of anesthesia prior to the use of other general anesthetic agents, as an adjunct to subpotent inhalational anesthetic agents for short surgical procedures, or for short surgical, diagnostic, or therapeutic procedures associated with minimal painful stimuli

Unlabeled/Investigational Use Wada test

Local Anesthetic/Vasoconstrictor Precautions No information available to require special precautions

Effects on Dental Treatment No significant effects or complications reported

Significant Adverse Effects Frequency not defined.

Cardiovascular: Hypotension, peripheral vascular collapse

Central nervous system: Seizure, headache

Gastrointestinal: Cramping, diarrhea, rectal bleeding, nausea, vomiting, abdominal pain

Hematologic: Hemolytic anemia, thrombophlebitis

Hepatic: Transaminases increased

Local: Pain on I.M. injection

Neuromuscular & skeletal: Tremor, twitching, rigidity, involuntary muscle movement, radial nerve palsy

Respiratory: Apnea, respiratory depression, laryngospasm, cough, hiccups

Restrictions C-IV

Dental Usual Dosing Induction and maintenance of general anesthesia for short procedures: Doses must be titrated to effect: Adults: I.V.: Induction: 50-120 mg to start; 20-40 mg every 4-7 minutes

Dosage Doses must be titrated to effect

Manufacturer's recommendations:

Infants <1 month: Safety and efficacy not established

Infants ≥1 month and Children:

I.M.: Induction: 6.6-10 mg/kg of a 5% solution

Rectal: Induction: Usual: 25 mg/kg of a 1% solution

Alternative pediatric dosing:

Children 3-12 years:

I.M.: Preoperative: 5-10 mg/kg/dose

I.V.: Induction: 1-2 mg/kg/dose

Rectal: Preoperative/induction: 20-35 mg/kg/dose; usual: 25 mg/kg/dose; maximum dose: 500 mg/dose; give as 10% aqueous solution

Adults: I.V.:

Induction: 50-120 mg to start; 20-40 mg every 4-7 minutes

Wada test (unlabeled): 3-4 mg over 3 second; following signs of recovery, administer a second dose of 2 mg over 2 seconds

Dosing adjustment/comments in hepatic impairment: Lower dosage and monitor closely

Mechanism of Action Ultra short-acting I.V. barbiturate anesthetic

Contraindications Hypersensitivity to methohexital or any component of the formulation; porphyria

Warnings/Precautions Use with extreme caution in patients with liver impairment, asthma, cardiovascular instability. **[U.S. Boxed Warning]: Should only be administered in hospitals or ambulatory care settings.**

Drug Interactions

Acetaminophen: Barbiturates may enhance the hepatotoxic potential of acetaminophen overdoses

Antiarrhythmics: Barbiturates may increase the metabolism of antiarrhythmics, decreasing their clinical effect; includes disopyramide, propafenone, and quinidine

Anticonvulsants: Barbiturates may increase the metabolism of anticonvulsants; includes ethosuximide, felbamate (possibly), lamotrigine, phenytoin, tiagabine, topiramate, and zonisamide; does not appear to affect gabapentin or levetiracetam

Antineoplastics: Limited evidence suggests that enzyme-inducing anticonvulsant therapy may reduce the effectiveness of some chemotherapy regimens (specifically in ALL); teniposide and methotrexate may be cleared more rapidly in these patients

Antipsychotics: Barbiturates may enhance the metabolism (decrease the efficacy) of antipsychotics; monitor for altered response; dose adjustment may be needed

Beta-blockers: Metabolism of beta-blockers may be increased and clinical effect decreased; atenolol and nadolol are unlikely to interact given their renal elimination

Calcium channel blockers: Barbiturates may enhance the metabolism of calcium channel blockers, decreasing their clinical effect

Chloramphenicol: Barbiturates may increase the metabolism of chloramphenicol and chloramphenicol may inhibit barbiturate metabolism; monitor for altered response

Cimetidine: Barbiturates may enhance the metabolism of cimetidine, decreasing its clinical effect

CNS depressants: Sedative effects and/or respiratory depression with barbiturates may be additive with other CNS depressants; monitor for increased

(Continued)

Methohexital (Continued)

effect; includes ethanol, sedatives, antidepressants, opioid analgesics, and benzodiazepines

Corticosteroids: Barbiturates may enhance the metabolism of corticosteroids, decreasing their clinical effect

Cyclosporine: Levels may be decreased by barbiturates; monitor

Doxycycline: Barbiturates may enhance the metabolism of doxycycline, decreasing its clinical effect; higher dosages may be required

Estrogens: Barbiturates may increase the metabolism of estrogens and reduce their efficacy

Felbamate may inhibit the metabolism of barbiturates and barbiturates may increase the metabolism of felbamate

Griseofulvin: Barbiturates may impair the absorption of griseofulvin, and griseofulvin metabolism may be increased by barbiturates, decreasing clinical effect

Guanfacine: Effect may be decreased by barbiturates

Immunosuppressants: Barbiturates may enhance the metabolism of immunosuppressants, decreasing its clinical effect; includes both cyclosporine and tacrolimus

Loop diuretics: Metabolism may be increased and clinical effects decreased; established for furosemide, effect with other loop diuretics not established

MAO inhibitors: Metabolism of barbiturates may be inhibited, increasing clinical effect or toxicity of the barbiturates

Methadone: Barbiturates may enhance the metabolism of methadone resulting in methadone withdrawal

Methoxyflurane: Barbiturates may enhance the nephrotoxic effects of methoxyflurane

Oral contraceptives: Barbiturates may enhance the metabolism of oral contraceptives, decreasing their clinical effect; an alternative method of contraception should be considered

Theophylline: Barbiturates may increase metabolism of theophylline derivatives and decrease their clinical effect

Tricyclic antidepressants: Barbiturates may increase metabolism of tricyclic antidepressants and decrease their clinical effect; sedative effects may be additive

Valproic acid: Metabolism of barbiturates may be inhibited by valproic acid; monitor for excessive sedation; a dose reduction may be needed

Warfarin: Barbiturates inhibit the hypoprothrombinemic effects of oral anticoagulants via increased metabolism; this combination should generally be avoided

Dietary Considerations Should not be given to patients with food in stomach because of danger of vomiting during anesthesia.

Pharmacodynamics/Kinetics
Onset of action: I.V.: Immediately
Duration: Single dose: 10-20 minutes

Pregnancy Risk Factor C

Dosage Forms Excipient information presented when available (limited, particularly for generics); consult specific product labeling.

Injection, powder for reconstitution, as sodium: 500 mg, 2.5 g, 5 g

Selected Readings
Buchtel HA, Passaro EA, Selwa LM, et al, "Sodium Methohexital (Brevital) as an Anesthetic in the Wada Test," *Epilepsia*, 2002, 43(9):1056-61.
Cote' CJ, "Sedation for the Pediatric Patient," *Pediatr Clin North Am*, 1994, 41(1):31-58.
Dionne RA, Yagiela JA, Moore PA, et al, "Comparing Efficacy and Safety of Four Intravenous Sedation Regimens in Dental Outpatients," *Am Dent Assoc*, 2001, 132(6):740-51.

Methohexital Sodium *see* Methohexital *on page 1066*

Methotrexate (meth oh TREKS ate)

Related Information
Rheumatoid Arthritis, Osteoarthritis, and Osteoporosis *on page 1759*

U.S. Brand Names Rheumatrex®; Trexall™

Canadian Brand Names Apo-Methotrexate®; ratio-Methotrexate

Mexican Brand Names Ifamet; Ledertrexate; Texate; Texate-T; Trixilem

Generic Available Yes

Index Terms Amethopterin; Methotrexate Sodium; MTX (error-prone abbreviation); NSC-740

Pharmacologic Category Antineoplastic Agent, Antimetabolite (Antifolate); Antirheumatic, Disease Modifying

Use Treatment of trophoblastic neoplasms; leukemias; psoriasis; rheumatoid arthritis (RA), including polyarticular-course juvenile rheumatoid arthritis (JRA); breast, head and neck, and lung carcinomas; osteosarcoma; soft-tissue sarcomas; carcinoma of gastrointestinal tract, esophagus, testes; lymphomas

Unlabeled/Investigational Use Treatment and maintenance of remission in Crohn's disease; ectopic pregnancy

Local Anesthetic/Vasoconstrictor Precautions No information available to require special precautions

Effects on Dental Treatment Key adverse event(s) related to dental treatment: Ulcerative stomatitis, gingivitis, glossitis, and mucositis (dose dependent; appears 3-7 days post-therapy and resolves within 2 weeks).

Common Adverse Effects Note: Adverse reactions vary by route and dosage. Hematologic and/or gastrointestinal toxicities may be common at dosages used in chemotherapy; these reactions are much less frequent when used at typical dosages for rheumatic diseases.

>10%:
Central nervous system (with I.T. administration or very high-dose therapy):
Arachnoiditis: Acute reaction manifested as severe headache, nuchal rigidity, vomiting, and fever; may be alleviated by reducing the dose
Subacute toxicity: 10% of patients treated with 12-15 mg/m^2 of I.T. methotrexate may develop this in the second or third week of therapy; consists of motor paralysis of extremities, cranial nerve palsy, seizure, or coma. This has also been seen in pediatric cases receiving very high-dose I.V. methotrexate.
Demyelinating encephalopathy: Seen months or years after receiving methotrexate; usually in association with cranial irradiation or other systemic chemotherapy
Dermatologic: Reddening of skin
Endocrine & metabolic: Hyperuricemia, defective oogenesis or spermatogenesis
Gastrointestinal: Ulcerative stomatitis, glossitis, gingivitis, nausea, vomiting, diarrhea, anorexia, intestinal perforation, mucositis (dose dependent; appears in 3-7 days after therapy, resolving within 2 weeks)
Hematologic: Leukopenia, thrombocytopenia
Renal: Renal failure, azotemia, nephropathy
Respiratory: Pharyngitis

1% to 10%:
Cardiovascular: Vasculitis
Central nervous system: Dizziness, malaise, encephalopathy, seizure, fever, chills
Dermatologic: Alopecia, rash, photosensitivity, depigmentation or hyperpigmentation of skin
Endocrine & metabolic: Diabetes
Genitourinary: Cystitis
Hematologic: Hemorrhage
Myelosuppressive: This is the primary dose-limiting factor (along with mucositis) of methotrexate; occurs about 5-7 days after methotrexate therapy, and should resolve within 2 weeks
WBC: Mild
Platelets: Moderate
Onset: 7 days
Nadir: 10 days
Recovery: 21 days
Hepatic: Cirrhosis and portal fibrosis have been associated with chronic methotrexate therapy; acute elevation of liver enzymes are common after high-dose methotrexate, and usually resolve within 10 days.
Neuromuscular & skeletal: Arthralgia
Ocular: Blurred vision
Renal: Renal dysfunction: Manifested by an abrupt rise in serum creatinine and BUN and a fall in urine output; more common with high-dose methotrexate, and may be due to precipitation of the drug.
Respiratory: Pneumonitis: Associated with fever, cough, and interstitial pulmonary infiltrates; treatment is to withhold methotrexate during the acute reaction; interstitial pneumonitis has been reported to occur with an incidence of 1% in patients with RA (dose 7.5-15 mg/week)

Dosage Refer to individual protocols.
Note: Doses between 100-500 mg/m^2 **may require** leucovorin rescue. Doses >500 mg/m^2 **require** leucovorin rescue: Oral, I.M., I.V.: Leucovorin 10-15 mg/m^2 every 6 hours for 8 or 10 doses, starting 24 hours after the start of methotrexate infusion. Continue until the methotrexate level is ≤0.1 micromolar (10^{-7}M). Some clinicians continue leucovorin until the methotrexate level is <0.05 micromolar (5 x 10^{-8}M) or 0.01 micromolar (10^{-8}M).
If the 48-hour methotrexate level is >1 micromolar (10^{-7}M) or the 72-hour methotrexate level is >0.2 micromolar (2 x 10^{-7}M): I.V., I.M, Oral: Leucovorin 100 mg/m^2 every 6 hours until the methotrexate level is ≤0.1 micromolar (10^{-7}M). Some clinicians continue leucovorin until the methotrexate level is <0.05 micromolar (5 x 10^{-8}M) or 0.01 micromolar (10^{-8}M).
(Continued)

Methotrexate *(Continued)*

Children:

Dermatomyositis: Oral: 15-20 mg/m^2/week as a single dose once weekly **or** 0.3-1 mg/kg/dose once weekly

Juvenile rheumatoid arthritis: Oral, I.M.: 10 mg/m^2 once weekly, then 5-15 mg/m^2/week as a single dose **or** as 3 divided doses given 12 hours apart

Antineoplastic dosage range:

Oral, I.M.: 7.5-30 mg/m^2/week **or** every 2 weeks

I.V.: 10-18,000 mg/m^2 bolus dosing **or** continuous infusion over 6-42 hours

Pediatric solid tumors (high-dose): I.V.:

<12 years: 12-25 g/m^2

≥12 years: 8 g/m^2

Acute lymphocytic leukemia (intermediate-dose): I.V.: Loading: 100 mg/m^2 bolus dose, followed by 900 mg/m^2/day infusion over 23-41 hours.

Meningeal leukemia: I.T.: 10-15 mg/m^2 (maximum dose: 15 mg) **or** an age-based dosing regimen; one possible system is:

≤3 months: 3 mg/dose

4-11 months: 6 mg/dose

1 year: 8 mg/dose

2 years: 10 mg/dose

≥3 years: 12 mg/dose

Adults: I.V.: Range is wide from 30-40 mg/m^2/week to 100-12,000 mg/m^2 with leucovorin rescue

Trophoblastic neoplasms:

Oral, I.M.: 15-30 mg/day for 5 days; repeat in 7 days for 3-5 courses

I.V.: 11 mg/m^2 days 1 through 5 every 3 weeks

Head and neck cancer: Oral, I.M., I.V.: 25-50 mg/m^2 once weekly

Mycosis fungoides (cutaneous T-cell lymphoma): Oral, I.M.: Initial (early stages):

5-50 mg once weekly **or**

15-37.5 mg twice weekly

Bladder cancer: I.V.:

30 mg/m^2 day 1 and 8 every 3 weeks **or**

30 mg/m^2 day 1, 15, and 22 every 4 weeks

Breast cancer: I.V.: 30-60 mg/m^2 days 1 and 8 every 3-4 weeks

Gastric cancer: I.V.: 1500 mg/m^2 every 4 weeks

Lymphoma, non-Hodgkin's: I.V.:

30 mg/m^2 days 3 and 10 every 3 weeks **or**

120 mg/m^2 day 8 and 15 every 3-4 weeks **or**

200 mg/m^2 day 8 and 15 every 3 weeks **or**

400 mg/m^2 every 4 weeks for 3 cycles **or**

1 g/m^2 every 3 weeks **or**

1.5 g/m^2 every 4 weeks

Sarcoma: I.V.: 8-12 g/m^2 weekly for 2-4 weeks

Rheumatoid arthritis: Oral: 7.5 mg once weekly **or** 2.5 mg every 12 hours for 3 doses/week, not to exceed 20 mg/week

Psoriasis:

Oral: 2.5-5 mg/dose every 12 hours for 3 doses given weekly **or**

Oral, I.M.: 10-25 mg/dose given once weekly

Ectopic pregnancy (unlabeled use): I.M.: 50 mg/m^2 as a single dose

Active Crohn's disease (unlabeled use): Induction of remission: I.M., SubQ: 15-25 mg once weekly; remission maintenance: 15 mg once weekly

Note: Oral dosing has been reported as effective but oral absorption is highly variable. If patient relapses after a switch to oral, may consider returning to injectable.

Elderly: Rheumatoid arthritis/psoriasis: Oral: Initial: 5-7.5 mg/week, not to exceed 20 mg/week

Dosing adjustment in renal impairment:

Cl$_{cr}$ 61-80 mL/minute: Reduce dose to 75% of usual dose

Cl$_{cr}$ 51-60 mL/minute: Reduce dose to 70% of usual dose

Cl$_{cr}$ 10-50 mL/minute: Reduce dose to 30% to 50% of usual dose

Cl$_{cr}$ <10 mL/minute: Avoid use

Hemodialysis: Not dialyzable (0% to 5%); supplemental dose is not necessary

Peritoneal dialysis: Supplemental dose is not necessary

Dosage adjustment in hepatic impairment:

Bilirubin 3.1-5 mg/dL **or** AST >180 units: Administer 75% of usual dose

Bilirubin >5 mg/dL: Do not use

Mechanism of Action Methotrexate is a folate antimetabolite that inhibits DNA synthesis. Methotrexate irreversibly binds to dihydrofolate reductase, inhibiting the formation of reduced folates, and thymidylate synthetase, resulting in inhibition of purine and thymidylic acid synthesis. Methotrexate is cell cycle specific for the S phase of the cycle.

The MOA in the treatment of rheumatoid arthritis is unknown, but may affect immune function. In psoriasis, methotrexate is thought to target rapidly proliferating epithelial cells in the skin.

In Crohn's disease, it may have immune modulator and anti-inflammatory activity

Contraindications Hypersensitivity to methotrexate or any component of the formulation; severe renal or hepatic impairment; pre-existing profound bone marrow suppression in patients with psoriasis or rheumatoid arthritis, alcoholic liver disease, AIDS, pre-existing blood dyscrasias; pregnancy (in patients with psoriasis or rheumatoid arthritis); breast-feeding

Warnings/Precautions Hazardous agent - use appropriate precautions for handling and disposal.

[U.S. Boxed Warning]: Methotrexate has been associated with acute (elevated transaminases) and potentially fatal chronic (fibrosis, cirrhosis) hepatotoxicity. Risk is related to cumulative dose and prolonged exposure. Monitor closely (with liver function tests, including serum albumin) for liver toxicities. Liver enzyme elevations may be noted, but may not be predictive of hepatic disease in long term treatment for psoriasis (but generally is predictive in rheumatoid arthritis [RA] treatment). With long-term use, liver biopsy may show histologic changes, fibrosis or cirrhosis; periodic liver biopsy is recommended with long-term use for psoriasis and for persistent abnormal liver function tests with RA; discontinue methotrexate with moderate-to-severe change in liver biopsy. Ethanol abuse, obesity, advanced age, and diabetes may increase the risk of hepatotoxic reactions. Use caution with preexisting liver impairment; may require dosage reduction. Use caution when used with other hepatotoxic agents (azathioprine, retinoids, sulfasalazine). **[U.S. Boxed Warning]: Methotrexate elimination is reduced in patients with ascites;** may require dose reduction or discontinuation. Monitor closely for toxicity.

[U.S. Boxed Warning]: May cause renal damage leading to acute renal failure, especially with high-dose methotrexate; monitor renal function and methotrexate levels closely, maintain adequate hydration and urinary alkalinization. Use caution in osteosarcoma patients treated with high-dose methotrexate in combination with nephrotoxic chemotherapy (eg, cisplatin). **[U.S. Boxed Warning]: Methotrexate elimination is reduced in patients with renal impairment;** may require dose reduction or discontinuation; monitor closely for toxicity. **[U.S. Boxed Warning]: Tumor lysis syndrome may occur in patients with high tumor burden;** use appropriate prevention and treatment.

[U.S. Boxed Warning]: May cause potentially life-threatening pneumonitis (may occur at any time during therapy and at any dosage); monitor closely for pulmonary symptoms, particularly dry, nonproductive cough. Other potential symptoms include fever, dyspnea, hypoxemia, or pulmonary infiltrate. **[U.S. Boxed Warning]: Methotrexate elimination is reduced in patients with pleural effusions;** may require dose reduction or discontinuation. Monitor closely for toxicity.

[U.S. Boxed Warning]: Bone marrow suppression may occur, resulting in anemia, aplastic anemia, pancytopenia, leukopenia, neutropenia, and/or thrombocytopenia. Use caution in patients with pre-existing bone marrow suppression. Discontinue therapy in RA or psoriasis if a significant decrease in hematologic components is noted. **[U.S. Boxed Warning]: Use of low dose methotrexate has been associated with the development of malignant lymphomas;** may regress upon discontinuation of therapy; treat lymphoma appropriately if regression is not induced by cessation of methotrexate.

[U.S. Boxed Warning]: Diarrhea and ulcerative stomatitis may require interruption of therapy; death from hemorrhagic enteritis or intestinal perforation has been reported. Use with caution in patients with peptic ulcer disease, ulcerative colitis.

May cause neurotoxicity including seizures (usually in pediatric ALL patients), leukoencephalopathy (usually with concurrent cranial irradiation) and stroke-like encephalopathy (usually with high-dose regimens). Chemical arachnoiditis (headache, back pain, nuchal rigidity, fever), myelopathy and chronic leukoencephalopathy may result from intrathecal administration.

[U.S. Boxed Warning]: Any dose level or route of administration may cause severe and potentially fatal dermatologic reactions, including toxic epidermal necrolysis, Stevens-Johnson syndrome, exfoliative dermatitis, skin necrosis, and erythema multiforme. Radiation dermatitis and sunburn may be precipitated by methotrexate administration. Psoriatic lesions may be worsened by concomitant exposure to ultraviolet radiation.

[U.S. Boxed Warning]: Concomitant administration with NSAIDs may cause severe bone marrow suppression, aplastic anemia, and GI toxicity. Do not administer NSAIDs prior to or during high dose methotrexate therapy; (Continued)

Methotrexate *(Continued)*

may increase and prolong serum methotrexate levels. Doses used for psoriasis may still lead to unexpected toxicities; use caution when administering NSAIDs or salicylates with lower doses of methotrexate for RA. Methotrexate may increase the levels and effects of mercaptopurine; may require dosage adjustments. Vitamins containing folate may decrease response to systemic methotrexate; folate deficiency may increase methotrexate toxicity. **[U.S. Boxed Warning]: Concomitant methotrexate administration with radiotherapy may increase the risk of soft tissue necrosis and osteonecrosis.**

[U.S. Boxed Warnings]: Should be administered under the supervision of a physician experienced in the use of antimetabolite therapy; serious and fatal toxicities have occurred at all dose levels. Immune suppression may lead to potentially fatal opportunistic infections. For rheumatoid arthritis and psoriasis, immunosuppressive therapy should only be used when disease is active and less toxic, traditional therapy is ineffective. Methotrexate formulations and/or diluents containing preservatives should not be used for intrathecal or high-dose therapy. May cause fetal death or congenital abnormalities; do not use for psoriasis or RA treatment in pregnant women. May cause impairment of fertility, oligospermia, and menstrual dysfunction. Toxicity from methotrexate or any immunosuppressive is increased in the elderly. Methotrexate injection may contain benzyl alcohol and should not be used in neonates.

Drug Interactions

Increased Effect/Toxicity: Concurrent therapy with NSAIDs has resulted in severe bone marrow suppression, aplastic anemia, and GI toxicity. NSAIDs should not be used during moderate or high-dose methotrexate due to increased and prolonged methotrexate levels (may increase toxicity); NSAID use during treatment of rheumatoid arthritis has not been fully explored, but continuation of prior regimen has been allowed in some circumstances, with cautious monitoring. Salicylates may increase methotrexate levels, however salicylate doses used for prophylaxis of cardiovascular events are not likely to be of concern.

Penicillins, probenecid, sulfonamides, tetracyclines may increase methotrexate concentrations due to a reduction in renal tubular secretion; primarily a concern with high doses of methotrexate. Hepatotoxic agents (acitretin, azathioprine, retinoids, sulfasalazine) may increase the risk of hepatotoxic reactions with methotrexate.

Concomitant administration of cyclosporine with methotrexate may increase levels and toxicity of each. Methotrexate may increase mercaptopurine or theophylline levels. Methotrexate, when administered prior to cytarabine, may enhance the efficacy and toxicity of cytarabine; some combination treatment regimens (eg, hyper-CVAD) have been designed to take advantage of this interaction.

Concurrent use of live virus vaccines may result in infections.

Decreased Effect: Cholestyramine may decrease levels of methotrexate. Corticosteroids may decrease uptake of methotrexate into leukemia cells. Administration of these drugs should be separated by 12 hours. Dexamethasone has been reported to not affect methotrexate influx into cells.

Ethanol/Nutrition/Herb Interactions

Ethanol: Avoid ethanol (may be associated with increased liver injury).

Food: Methotrexate peak serum levels may be decreased if taken with food. Milk-rich foods may decrease methotrexate absorption. Folate may decrease drug response.

Herb/Nutraceutical: Avoid echinacea (has immunostimulant properties).

Dietary Considerations

Sodium content of 100 mg injection: 20 mg (0.86 mEq)

Sodium content of 100 mg (low sodium) injection: 15 mg (0.65 mEq)

Pharmacodynamics/Kinetics

Onset of action: Antirheumatic: 3-6 weeks; additional improvement may continue longer than 12 weeks

Absorption: Oral: Rapid; well absorbed at low doses (<30 mg/m^2), incomplete after large doses; I.M.: Complete

Distribution: Penetrates slowly into 3rd space fluids (eg, pleural effusions, ascites), exits slowly from these compartments (slower than from plasma); crosses placenta; small amounts enter breast milk; sustained concentrations retained in kidney and liver

Protein binding: 50%

Metabolism: <10%; degraded by intestinal flora to DAMPA by carboxypeptidase; hepatic aldehyde oxidase converts methotrexate to 7-OH methotrexate;

polyglutamates are produced intracellularly and are just as potent as methotrexate; their production is dose- and duration-dependent and they are slowly eliminated by the cell once formed

Half-life elimination: Low dose: 3-10 hours; High dose: 8-12 hours

Time to peak, serum: Oral: 1-2 hours; I.M.: 30-60 minutes

Excretion: Urine (44% to 100%); feces (small amounts)

Pregnancy Risk Factor X (psoriasis, rheumatoid arthritis)

Dosage Forms

Injection, powder for reconstitution [preservative free]: 20 mg, 1 g

Injection, solution: 25 mg/mL (2 mL, 10 mL)

Injection, solution [preservative free]: 25 mg/mL (2 mL, 4 mL, 8 mL, 10 mL)

Tablet: 2.5 mg

Trexall™: 5 mg, 7.5 mg, 10 mg, 15 mg

Tablet [dose pack]: 2.5 mg (4 cards with 2, 3, 4, 5, or 6 tablets each)

Rheumatrex® Dose Pack: 2.5 mg (4 cards with 2, 3, 4, 5, or 6 tablets each)

Methotrexate Sodium *see* Methotrexate *on page 1068*

Methotrimeprazine (meth oh trye MEP ra zeen)

Canadian Brand Names Apo-Methoprazine®; Nozinan®

Mexican Brand Names Sinogan

Generic Available No

Index Terms Levomepromazine; Methotrimeprazine Hydrochloride

Pharmacologic Category Analgesic, Nonopioid

Use Treatment of schizophrenia or psychosis; management of pain, including pain caused by neuralgia or cancer; adjunct to general anesthesia; management of nausea and vomiting; sedation

Unlabeled/Investigational Use Bipolar disorder, agitation

Local Anesthetic/Vasoconstrictor Precautions No information available to require special precautions (see Dental Comment)

Effects on Dental Treatment Key adverse event(s) related to dental treatment: Anticholinergic side effects can cause a reduction of saliva production or secretion, contributing to discomfort and dental disease (ie, caries, oral candidiasis, and periodontal disease). Phenothiazines can cause extrapyramidal reactions which may appear as muscle twitching or increased motor activity of the face, neck, or head.

Common Adverse Effects Note: Frequencies not defined; some reactions listed are based on reports for other agents in this same pharmacologic class, and may not be specifically reported for methotrimeprazine.

Cardiovascular: Hypotension, orthostatic hypotension, tachycardia, QT_c prolongation (rare)

Central nervous system: Extrapyramidal symptoms (pseudoparkinsonism, akathisia, dystonias, tardive dyskinesia), dizziness, seizure, headache, drowsiness, neuroleptic malignant syndrome (NMS), impairment of temperature regulation

Dermatologic: Photosensitivity (rare), rash

Endocrine & metabolic: Gynecomastia, weight gain, menstrual irregularity, libido (changes in)

Gastrointestinal: Constipation, vomiting, nausea, xerostomia, ileus

Genitourinary: Difficulty in urination, ejaculatory disturbances, incontinence, polyuria, ejaculating dysfunction, priapism

Hematologic: Agranulocytosis (rare), leukopenia, eosinophilia, hemolytic anemia, thrombocytopenic purpura, pancytopenia

Hepatic: Cholestatic jaundice, hepatotoxicity

Miscellaneous: Diaphoresis

Restrictions Not available in U.S.

Mechanism of Action Dopamine antagonist; also binds alpha-1, alpha-2, and serotonin receptors

Drug Interactions

Cytochrome P450 Effect: Inhibits CYP2D6

Increased Effect/Toxicity: Concurrent use of MAO inhibitors may result in toxicity; these combinations are best avoided. Methotrimeprazine may produce additive CNS depressant effects with CNS depressants (ethanol, narcotics). If a patient is receiving methotrimeprazine, the dose of a barbiturate or narcotic should be reduced by 50%. Chloroquine, propranolol, and sulfadoxine-pyrimethamine may increase methotrimeprazine concentrations. Concurrent use with TCA may produce increased toxicity or altered therapeutic response. A phenothiazine plus lithium may rarely produce neurotoxicity. Metoclopramide may increase risk of extrapyramidal symptoms (EPS). Acetylcholinesterase inhibitors (central) may increase the risk of antipsychotic-related EPS.

(Continued)

Methotrimeprazine *(Continued)*

Methotrimeprazine may increase the levels/effects of amphetamines, selected beta blockers, dextromethorphan, fluoxetine, lidocaine, mesoridazine, mirtazapine, nefazodone, paroxetine, risperidone, ritonavir, thioridazine, tricyclic antidepressants, venlafaxine, and other CYP2D6 substrates.

Decreased Effect: Benztropine (and other anticholinergics) may inhibit the therapeutic response to phenothiazines. Antipsychotics such as methotrimeprazine inhibit the ability of bromocriptine to lower serum prolactin concentrations. The antihypertensive effects of guanethidine and guanadrel may be inhibited by phenothiazines. Methotrimeprazine may inhibit the antiparkinsonian effect of levodopa. Low potency antipsychotics may reverse the pressor effects of epinephrine. Methotrimeprazine may decrease the levels/effects of CYP2D6 prodrug substrates (eg, codeine, hydrocodone, oxycodone, tramadol).

Pharmacodynamics/Kinetics
Onset of action: Injection: 1 hour
Duration of action: 2-4 hours
Bioavailability: 50%
Time to peak, serum: I.M.: 0.5-1.5 hours; Oral: 1-3 hours
Half-life elimination: 30 hours

Pregnancy Risk Factor C

Dental Comment This drug is known to prolong the QT interval. The QT interval is measured as the time and distance between the Q point of the QRS complex and the end of the T wave in the ECG tracing. After adjustment for heart rate, the QT interval is defined as prolonged if it is more than 450 msec in men and 460 msec in women. A long QT syndrome was first described in the 1950s and 60s as a congenital syndrome involving QT interval prolongation and syncope and sudden death. Some of the congenital long QT syndromes were characterized by a peculiar electrocardiographic appearance of the QRS complex involving a premature atria beat followed by a pause, then a subsequent sinus beat showing marked QT prolongation and deformity. This type of cardiac arrhythmia was originally termed "torsade de pointes" (translated from the French as "twisting of the points").

Prolongation of the QT interval is thought to result from delayed ventricular repolarization. The repolarization process within the myocardial cell is due to the efflux of intracellular potassium. The channels associated with this current can be blocked by many drugs and predispose the electrical propagation cycle to torsade de pointes.

Methotrimeprazine is one of the drugs confirmed to prolong the QT interval and is accepted as having a risk of causing torsade de pointes. The risk of drug-induced torsade de pointes is extremely low when a single QT interval prolonging drug is prescribed. In terms of epinephrine, it is not known what effect vasoconstrictors in the local anesthetic regimen will have in patients with a known history of congenital prolonged QT interval or in patients taking any medication that prolongs the QT interval. Until more information is obtained, it is suggested that the clinician consult with the physician prior to the use of a vasoconstrictor in suspected patients, and that the vasoconstrictor (epinephrine, levonordefrin [Neo-Cobefrin®]) be used with caution.

Methotrimeprazine Hydrochloride *see* Methotrimeprazine *on page 1073*

Methoxsalen *(meth OKS a len)*

U.S. Brand Names 8-MOP®; Oxsoralen®; Oxsoralen-Ultra®; Uvadex®
Canadian Brand Names 8-MOP®; Oxsoralen®; Oxsoralen-Ultra®; Ultramop™; Uvadex®
Mexican Brand Names Meladinina
Generic Available No
Index Terms Methoxypsoralen; 8-Methoxypsoralen; 8-MOP
Pharmacologic Category Psoralen
Use
Oral: Symptomatic control of severe, recalcitrant disabling psoriasis; repigmentation of idiopathic vitiligo; palliative treatment of skin manifestations of cutaneous T-cell lymphoma (CTCL)
Topical: Repigmentation of idiopathic vitiligo
Extracorporeal: Palliative treatment of skin manifestations of CTCL
Local Anesthetic/Vasoconstrictor Precautions No information available to require special precautions
Effects on Dental Treatment No significant effects or complications reported
Common Adverse Effects Frequency not always defined.
Cardiovascular: Severe edema, hypotension

Central nervous system: Nervousness, vertigo, depression, dizziness, headache, malaise

Dermatologic: Painful blistering, burning, and peeling of skin; pruritus (10%), freckling, hypopigmentation, rash, cheilitis, erythema, itching, urticaria

Gastrointestinal: Nausea (10%)

Neuromuscular & skeletal: Loss of muscle coordination, leg cramps

Miscellaneous: Miliaria

Mechanism of Action Bonds covalently to pyrimidine bases in DNA, inhibits the synthesis of DNA, and suppresses cell division. The augmented sunburn reaction involves excitation of the methoxsalen molecule by radiation in the long-wave ultraviolet light (UVA), resulting in transference of energy to the methoxsalen molecule producing an excited state ("triplet electronic state"). The molecule, in this "triplet state", then reacts with cutaneous DNA.

Drug Interactions

Cytochrome P450 Effect: Substrate of CYP2A6 (minor); **Inhibits** CYP1A2 (strong), 2A6 (strong), 2C9 (weak), 2C19 (weak), 2D6 (weak), 2E1 (weak), 3A4 (weak)

Increased Effect/Toxicity: Methoxsalen may increase the levels/effects of CYP1A2 substrates (eg, aminophylline, fluvoxamine, mexiletine, mirtazapine, ropinirole, theophylline, trifluoperazine) and CYP2A6 substrates (eg, dexmedetomidine, ifosfamide).

Pharmacodynamics/Kinetics

Protein binding: Reversibly bound to albumin

Metabolism: Hepatic; forms metabolites

Bioavailability: Bioavailability increased with soft-gelatin capsules compared to hard-gelatin capsules; exposure using UVAR® system is ~200 times less than with oral administration

Time to peak, serum:

Hard-gelatin capsules: 1.5-6 hours (peak photosensitivity: ~4 hours)

Soft-gelatin capsules: 0.5-4 hours (peak photosensitivity: 1.5-2 hours)

Half-life elimination: ~2 hours

Excretion: Urine (~95% as metabolites)

Pregnancy Risk Factor C/D (Uvadex®)

Methoxypsoralen see Methoxsalen on page 1074

8-Methoxypsoralen see Methoxsalen on page 1074

Methscopolamine (meth skoe POL a meen)

U.S. Brand Names Pamine®; Pamine® Forte

Canadian Brand Names Pamine®

Generic Available No

Index Terms Methscopolamine Bromide

Pharmacologic Category Anticholinergic Agent

Use Adjunctive therapy in the treatment of peptic ulcer

Local Anesthetic/Vasoconstrictor Precautions No information available to require special precautions

Effects on Dental Treatment Key adverse event(s) related to dental treatment: Xerostomia and changes in salivation (normal salivary flow resumes upon discontinuation), and dry throat and nose. Anticholinergic side effects can cause a reduction of saliva production or secretion, contributing to discomfort and dental disease (ie, caries, oral candidiasis and periodontal disease).

Common Adverse Effects Frequency not defined.

Cardiovascular: Palpitation, tachycardia

Central nervous system: Headache, insomnia, flushing, nervousness, drowsiness, dizziness, confusion, fever, CNS stimulation may be produced with large doses

Dermatologic: Dry skin, urticaria

Endocrine & metabolic: Lactation suppressed

Gastrointestinal: Constipation, xerostomia, dry throat, dysphagia, nausea, vomiting, loss of taste

Genitourinary: Impotence, urinary hesitancy, urinary retention

Neuromuscular & skeletal: Weakness

Ocular: Blurred vision, cycloplegia, ocular tension increased, pupil dilation

Respiratory: Dry nose

Miscellaneous: Allergic reaction, diaphoresis decreased, hypersensitivity reactions, anaphylaxis

Mechanism of Action Methscopolamine is a peripheral anticholinergic agent with limited ability to cross the blood-brain barrier and provides a peripheral blockade of muscarinic receptors. This agent reduces the volume and the total acid content of gastric secretions, inhibits salivation, and reduces gastrointestinal motility.

(Continued)

Methscopolamine *(Continued)*

Drug Interactions

Increased Effect/Toxicity: Antipsychotic agents and TCAs may produce additive anticholinergic effects.

Decreased Effect: Antacids may decrease the absorption of methscopolamine.

Pharmacodynamics/Kinetics

Onset: 1 hour

Duration: 4-6 hours

Excretion: Bile, urine

Pregnancy Risk Factor C

Methscopolamine and Pseudoephedrine *see* Pseudoephedrine and Methscopolamine *on page 1384*

Methscopolamine Bromide *see* Methscopolamine *on page 1075*

Methscopolamine Nitrate and Chlordiazepoxide Hydrochloride *see* Chlordiazepoxide and Methscopolamine *on page 332*

Methscopolamine Nitrate, Chlorpheniramine Maleate, and Phenylephrine Hydrochloride *see* Chlorpheniramine, Phenylephrine, and Methscopolamine *on page 342*

Methsuximide *(meth SUKS i mide)*

U.S. Brand Names Celontin®

Canadian Brand Names Celontin®

Generic Available No

Pharmacologic Category Anticonvulsant, Succinimide

Use Control of absence (petit mal) seizures that are refractory to other drugs

Unlabeled/Investigational Use Partial complex (psychomotor) seizures

Local Anesthetic/Vasoconstrictor Precautions No information available to require special precautions

Effects on Dental Treatment No significant effects or complications reported

Common Adverse Effects Frequency not defined.

Cardiovascular: Hyperemia

Central nervous system: Ataxia, dizziness, drowsiness, headache, aggressiveness, mental depression, irritability, nervousness, insomnia, confusion, psychosis, suicidal behavior, auditory hallucinations

Dermatologic: Stevens-Johnson syndrome, rash, urticaria, pruritus

Gastrointestinal: Anorexia, nausea, vomiting, weight loss, diarrhea, epigastric and abdominal pain, constipation

Genitourinary: Proteinuria, hematuria (microscopic); cases of blood dyscrasias have been reported with succinimides

Hematologic: Leukopenia, pancytopenia, eosinophilia, monocytosis

Neuromuscular & skeletal: Cases of systemic lupus erythematosus have been reported

Ocular: Blurred vision, photophobia, peripheral edema

Mechanism of Action Increases the seizure threshold and suppresses paroxysmal spike-and-wave pattern in absence seizures; depresses nerve transmission in the motor cortex

Drug Interactions

Cytochrome P450 Effect: Substrate of CYP2C19 (major); **Inhibits** CYP2C19 (weak)

Increased Effect/Toxicity: CYP2C19 inhibitors may increase the levels/effects of methsuximide; example inhibitors include delavirdine, fluconazole, fluvoxamine, gemfibrozil, isoniazid, omeprazole, and ticlopidine. Sedative effects and/or respiratory depression may be additive with CNS depressants; includes ethanol, benzodiazepines, barbiturates, opioid analgesics, and other sedative agents. Methsuximide may increase phenobarbital and/or phenytoin concentration.

Decreased Effect: CYP2C19 inducers may decrease the levels/effects of methsuximide; example inducers include aminoglutethimide, carbamazepine, phenytoin, and rifampin.

Pharmacodynamics/Kinetics

Metabolism: Hepatic; rapidly demethylated to N-desmethylmethsuximide (active metabolite)

Half-life elimination: 2-4 hours

Time to peak, serum: Within 1-3 hours

Excretion: Urine (<1% as unchanged drug)

Pregnancy Risk Factor C

Methyclothiazide (meth i kloe THYE a zide)

Related Information
Cardiovascular Diseases *on page 1726*
U.S. Brand Names Enduron® [DSC]
Canadian Brand Names Aquatensen®; Enduron®
Generic Available Yes
Pharmacologic Category Diuretic, Thiazide
Use Management of mild to moderate hypertension; treatment of edema in congestive heart failure and nephrotic syndrome
Local Anesthetic/Vasoconstrictor Precautions No information available to require special precautions
Effects on Dental Treatment Key adverse event(s) related to dental treatment: Orthostatic hypotension.
Common Adverse Effects 1% to 10%:
Cardiovascular: Orthostatic hypotension
Dermatologic: Photosensitivity
Endocrine & metabolic: Hypokalemia
Gastrointestinal: Anorexia, epigastric distress
Mechanism of Action Inhibits sodium reabsorption in the distal tubules causing increased excretion of sodium and water, as well as, potassium and hydrogen ions
Drug Interactions
Increased Effect/Toxicity: Increased effect of methyclothiazide with furosemide and other loop diuretics. Increased hypotension and/or renal adverse effects of ACE inhibitors may result in aggressively diuresed patients. Beta-blockers increase hyperglycemic effects of thiazides in Type 2 diabetes mellitus. Cyclosporine and thiazides can increase the risk of gout or renal toxicity. Digoxin toxicity can be exacerbated if a thiazide induces hypokalemia or hypomagnesemia. Lithium toxicity can occur with thiazides due to reduced renal excretion of lithium. Thiazides may prolong the duration of action with neuromuscular blocking agents.
Decreased Effect: Effects of oral hypoglycemics may be decreased. Decreased absorption of thiazides with cholestyramine and colestipol. NSAIDs can decrease the efficacy of thiazides, reducing the diuretic and antihypertensive effects.
Pharmacodynamics/Kinetics
Onset of action: Diuresis: 2 hours
Peak effect: 6 hours
Duration: ~1 day
Distribution: Crosses placenta; enters breast milk
Excretion: Urine (as unchanged drug)
Pregnancy Risk Factor B

Methylacetoxyprogesterone *see* MedroxyPROGESTERone *on page 1026*

Methylcellulose (meth il SEL yoo lose)

U.S. Brand Names Citrucel® [OTC]; Citrucel® Fiber Shake [OTC]; Citrucel® Fiber Smoothie [OTC]
Generic Available Yes: Powder
Pharmacologic Category Laxative
Use Adjunct in treatment of constipation
Local Anesthetic/Vasoconstrictor Precautions No information available to require special precautions
Effects on Dental Treatment No significant effects or complications reported
Pregnancy Risk Factor C

Methyldopa (meth il DOE pa)

Related Information
Cardiovascular Diseases *on page 1726*
Canadian Brand Names Apo-Methyldopa®; Nu-Medopa
Mexican Brand Names Aldomet
Generic Available Yes
Index Terms Aldomet; Methyldopate Hydrochloride
Pharmacologic Category Alpha-Adrenergic Inhibitor; Alpha₂-Adrenergic Agonist
Use Management of moderate to severe hypertension
Local Anesthetic/Vasoconstrictor Precautions No information available to require special precautions
(Continued)

Methyldopa *(Continued)*

Effects on Dental Treatment Key adverse event(s) related to dental treatment: Xerostomia (normal salivary flow resumes upon discontinuation). Anticholinergic side effects can cause a reduction of saliva production or secretion, contributing to discomfort and dental disease (ie, caries, oral candidiasis, and periodontal disease).

Common Adverse Effects

>10%: Cardiovascular: Peripheral edema

1% to 10%:

Central nervous system: Drug fever, mental depression, anxiety, nightmares, drowsiness, headache

Gastrointestinal: Dry mouth

Mechanism of Action Stimulation of central alpha-adrenergic receptors by a false transmitter that results in a decreased sympathetic outflow to the heart, kidneys, and peripheral vasculature

Drug Interactions

Increased Effect/Toxicity: Beta-blockers, MAO inhibitors, phenothiazines, and sympathomimetics (including epinephrine) may result in hypertension (sometimes severe) when combined with methyldopa. Methyldopa may increase lithium serum levels resulting in lithium toxicity. Levodopa may cause enhanced blood pressure lowering; methyldopa may also potentiate the effect of levodopa. Tolbutamide, haloperidol, and anesthetics effects/toxicity are increased with methyldopa.

Decreased Effect: Iron supplements can interact and cause a significant **increase** in blood pressure. Ferrous sulfate and ferrous gluconate decrease bioavailability. Barbiturates and TCAs may reduce response to methyldopa.

Pharmacodynamics/Kinetics

Onset of action: Peak effect: Hypotensive: Oral/parenteral: 3-6 hours

Duration: 12-24 hours

Distribution: Crosses placenta; enters breast milk

Protein binding: <15%

Metabolism: Intestinal and hepatic

Half-life elimination: 75-80 minutes; End-stage renal disease: 6-16 hours

Excretion: Urine (85% as metabolites) within 24 hours

Pregnancy Risk Factor B

Methyldopa and Hydrochlorothiazide
(meth il DOE pa & hye droe klor oh THYE a zide)

Related Information

Hydrochlorothiazide *on page 819*

Methyldopa *on page 1077*

U.S. Brand Names Aldoril®

Canadian Brand Names Apo-Methazide®

Generic Available Yes

Index Terms Hydrochlorothiazide and Methyldopa

Pharmacologic Category Antihypertensive Agent, Combination

Use Management of moderate to severe hypertension

Local Anesthetic/Vasoconstrictor Precautions No information available to require special precautions

Effects on Dental Treatment Key adverse event(s) related to dental treatment: Anticholinergic side effects can cause a reduction of saliva production or secretion, contributing to discomfort and dental disease (ie, caries, oral candidiasis, and periodontal disease).

Common Adverse Effects See individual agents.

Drug Interactions

Increased Effect/Toxicity: See individual agents.

Decreased Effect: See individual agents.

Pharmacodynamics/Kinetics See individual agents.

Pregnancy Risk Factor C

Methyldopate Hydrochloride *see* Methyldopa *on page 1077*

Methylene Blue, Methenamine, Sodium Biphosphate, Phenyl Salicylate, and Hyoscyamine *see* Methenamine, Sodium Biphosphate, Phenyl Salicylate, Methylene Blue, and Hyoscyamine *on page 1064*

Methylergometrine Maleate *see* Methylergonovine *on page 1079*

Methylergonovine (meth il er goe NOE veen)

U.S. Brand Names Methergine®
Canadian Brand Names Methergine®
Mexican Brand Names Methergin
Generic Available No
Index Terms Methylergometrine Maleate; Methylergonovine Maleate
Pharmacologic Category Ergot Derivative
Use Prevention and treatment of postpartum and postabortion hemorrhage caused by uterine atony or subinvolution
Local Anesthetic/Vasoconstrictor Precautions No information available to require special precautions
Effects on Dental Treatment No significant effects or complications reported
Common Adverse Effects Frequency not defined.
Cardiovascular: Acute MI, arterial spasm, bradycardia, hyper-/hypotension, palpitation, tachycardia, temporary chest pain
Central nervous system: Dizziness, hallucinations, headache, seizure
Dermatologic: Rash
Endocrine & metabolic: Water intoxication
Gastrointestinal: Diarrhea, foul taste, nausea, vomiting
Local: Thrombophlebitis
Neuromuscular & skeletal: Leg cramps
Otic: Tinnitus
Renal: Hematuria
Respiratory: Dyspnea, nasal congestion
Miscellaneous: Anaphylaxis, diaphoresis
Mechanism of Action Similar smooth muscle actions as seen with ergotamine; however, it affects primarily uterine smooth muscles producing sustained contractions and thereby shortens the third stage of labor and reduces blood loss.

Drug Interactions
Cytochrome P450 Effect: Substrate of CYP3A4 (major)
Increased Effect/Toxicity: CYP3A4 inhibitors may increase the levels/effects of methylergonovine; example inhibitors include azole antifungals, clarithromycin, diclofenac, doxycycline, erythromycin, imatinib, isoniazid, nefazodone, nicardipine, propofol, protease inhibitors, quinidine, telithromycin, and verapamil. Ergot alkaloids are contraindicated with potent CYP3A4 inhibitors. Methylergonovine may increase the effects of 5-HT$_1$ agonists (eg, sumatriptan), MAO inhibitors, sibutramine, and other serotonin agonists (serotonin syndrome). Severe vasoconstriction may occur when peripheral vasoconstrictors are used in patients receiving ergot alkaloids; concurrent use is contraindicated. Ergot alkaloids may enhance the vasoconstricting effect of dopamine.
Decreased Effect: Ergot alkaloids may diminish the vasodilatory effect of nitroglycerin.

Pharmacodynamics/Kinetics
Onset of action: Oxytocic: Oral: 5-10 minutes; I.M.: 2-5 minutes; I.V.: Immediately
Duration: Oral: ~3 hours; I.M.: ~3 hours; I.V.: 45 minutes
Absorption: Rapid
Distribution: V$_d$: 39-73 L
Rapid; primarily to plasma and extracellular fluid following I.V. administration; tissues
Metabolism: Hepatic
Bioavailability: Oral: 60%; I.M.: 78%
Half-life elimination: Biphasic: Initial: 1-5 minutes; Terminal: 0.5-2 hours
Time to peak, serum: Oral: 0.3-2 hours; I.M.: 0.2-0.6 hours
Excretion: Urine and feces
Pregnancy Risk Factor C

Methylphenidate (meth il FEN i date)

U.S. Brand Names Concerta®; Daytrana™; Metadate® CD; Metadate® ER; Methylin®; Methylin® ER; Ritalin®; Ritalin® LA; Ritalin-SR®
(Continued)

Methylphenidate *(Continued)*

Canadian Brand Names Apo-Methylphenidate®; Apo-Methylphenidate® SR; Biphentin®; Concerta®; PMS-Methylphenidate; Riphenidate; Ritalin®; Ritalin® SR

Mexican Brand Names Ritalin

Generic Available Yes: Immediate release tablet, extended release 20 mg tablet

Index Terms Methylphenidate Hydrochloride

Pharmacologic Category Central Nervous System Stimulant

Use Treatment of attention-deficit/hyperactivity disorder (ADHD); symptomatic management of narcolepsy

Unlabeled/Investigational Use Depression (especially elderly or medically ill)

Local Anesthetic/Vasoconstrictor Precautions No information available to require special precautions

Effects on Dental Treatment Key adverse event(s) related to dental treatment: Up to 10% of patients taking amphetamine-like drugs may present with hypertension. Monitor blood pressure prior to using local anesthetic with vasoconstrictors.

Common Adverse Effects

Transdermal system: Frequency of adverse events as reported in trials of 7-week duration. Incidence of some events reportedly higher with extended use.

>10%:
Central nervous system: Insomnia (13%)
Endocrine & metabolic: Appetite decreased (26%)
Gastrointestinal: Nausea (12%)

1% to 10%:
Central nervous system: Tic (7%), emotional instability (6%)
Gastrointestinal: Vomiting (10%), anorexia (5%)
Respiratory: Nasal congestion (6%), nasopharyngitis (5%)
Endocrine & metabolic: Weight loss (9%)

All dosage forms: Frequency not defined:

Cardiovascular: Angina, cardiac arrhythmia, cerebral arteritis, cerebral occlusion, hyper-/hypotension, MI, necrotizing vasculitis, palpitation, pulse increase/decrease, tachycardia

Central nervous system: Depression, dizziness, drowsiness, fever, headache, insomnia, nervousness, neuroleptic malignant syndrome (NMS), Tourette's syndrome, toxic psychosis

Dermatologic: Erythema multiforme, exfoliative dermatitis, hair loss, rash, urticaria

Endocrine & metabolic: Growth retardation

Gastrointestinal: Abdominal pain, anorexia, diarrhea, nausea, vomiting, weight loss

Hematologic: Anemia, leukopenia, thrombocytopenic purpura, thrombocytopenia

Hepatic: Liver function tests abnormal, hepatic coma, transaminases increased

Neuromuscular & skeletal: Arthralgia, dyskinesia

Ocular: Blurred vision, visual accommodation disturbance

Renal: Necrotizing vasculitis

Respiratory: Cough increased, pharyngitis, sinusitis, upper respiratory tract infection

Miscellaneous: Accidental injury, hypersensitivity reactions

Restrictions C-II

An FDA-approved medication guide must be distributed when dispensing an outpatient prescription (new or refill) where this medication is to be used without direct supervision of a healthcare provider. Medication guides are available at http://www.fda.gov/cder/drug/infopage/ADHD/default.htm.

Dosage

ADHD:

Oral:

Immediate release products Children ≥6 years and Adults: Initial: 5 mg/dose (~0.3 mg/kg/dose) given twice daily before breakfast and lunch; increase by 5-10 mg/day (0.2 mg/kg/day) at weekly intervals; maximum dose: 60 mg/day (2 mg/kg/day). **Note:** Discontinue periodically to re-evaluate or if no improvement occurs within 1 month.

Extended release products:

Children ≥6 years and Adults:

Metadate® ER, Methylin® ER, Ritalin® SR: May be given in place of immediate release products, once the daily dose is titrated and the titrated 8-hour dosage corresponds to sustained or extended release tablet size; maximum: 60 mg/day

Metadate® CD, Ritalin® LA: Initial: 20 mg once daily; may be adjusted in 10-20 mg increments at weekly intervals; maximum: 60 mg/day

Children 6-12 years and Adolescents 13-17 years: *Concerta®:*

Patients not currently taking methylphenidate: Initial dose: 18 mg once daily in the morning

Patients currently taking methylphenidate: **Note:** Initial dose: Dosing based on current regimen and clinical judgment; suggested dosing listed below:

— Patients taking methylphenidate 5 mg 2-3 times/day **or** 20 mg/day sustained release formulation: 18 mg once every morning

— Patients taking methylphenidate 10 mg 2-3 times/day **or** 40 mg/day sustained release formulation: 36 mg once every morning

— Patients taking methylphenidate 15 mg 2-3 times/day **or** 60 mg/day sustained release formulation: 54 mg once every morning

Dose adjustment: May increase dose in increments of 18 mg; dose may be adjusted at weekly intervals. A dosage strength of 27 mg is available for situations in which a dosage between 18-36 mg is desired. Maximum dose should not exceed 2 mg/kg/day **or** 54 mg/day in children 6-12 years or 72 mg/day in children 13-17 years.

Transdermal (Daytrana™): Children 6-12 years: Initial: 10 mg patch once daily; remove up to 9 hours after application. Titrate based on response and tolerability; may increase to next transdermal dose no more frequently than every week. **Note:** Application should occur 2 hours prior to desired effect. Drug absorption may continue for a period of time after patch removal.

Narcolepsy: Oral: Adults: 10 mg 2-3 times/day, up to 60 mg/day

Depression (unlabeled use): Oral: Adults: Initial: 2.5 mg every morning before 9 AM; dosage may be increased by 2.5-5 mg every 2-3 days as tolerated to a maximum of 20 mg/day; may be divided (ie, 7 AM and 12 noon), but should not be given after noon; do not use sustained release product

Mechanism of Action Mild CNS stimulant; blocks the reuptake of norepinephrine and dopamine into presynaptic neurons; appears to stimulate the cerebral cortex and subcortical structures similar to amphetamines

Contraindications Hypersensitivity to methylphenidate, any component of the formulation, or idiosyncratic reactions to sympathomimetic amines; marked anxiety, tension, and agitation; glaucoma; use during or within 14 days following MAO inhibitor therapy; Tourette's syndrome or tics

Metadate CD™ is contraindicated in patients with severe hypertension, heart failure, arrhythmia, hyperthyroidism, recent MI or angina.

Warnings/Precautions CNS stimulant use has been associated with serious cardiovascular events including sudden death in patients with pre-existing structural cardiac abnormalities or other serious heart problems (sudden death in children and adolescents; sudden death, stroke, and MI in adults). These products should be avoided in patients with known serious structural cardiac abnormalities, cardiomyopathy, serious heart rhythm abnormalities, or other serious cardiac problems that could increase the risk of sudden death that these conditions alone carry. Patients should be carefully evaluated for cardiac disease prior to initiation of therapy. Some products are contraindicated in patients with heart failure, arrhythmias or recent MI. Use of stimulants can cause an increase in blood pressure (average 2-4 mm Hg) and increases in heart rate (average 3-6 bpm), although some patients may have larger than average increases. Use caution with hypertension, hyperthyroidism, or other cardiovascular conditions that might be exacerbated by increases in blood pressure or heart rate. Some products are contraindicated in patients with severe hypertension, hyperthyroidism or angina.

Has demonstrated value as part of a comprehensive treatment program for ADHD. Use with caution in patients with bipolar disorder (may induce mixed/manic episode). May exacerbate symptoms of behavior and thought disorder in psychotic patients; new onset psychosis or mania may occur with stimulant use; observe for symptoms of aggression and/or hostility. Use caution with seizure disorders (may reduce seizure threshold). Use caution in patients with history of ethanol or drug abuse. May exacerbate symptoms of behavior and thought disorder in psychotic patients. **[U.S. Boxed Warning]: Potential for drug dependency exists - avoid abrupt discontinuation in patients who have received for prolonged periods.** Visual disturbances have been reported (rare). Stimulant use has been associated with growth suppression. Growth should be monitored during treatment. Concerta® should not be used in patients with esophageal motility disorders or pre-existing severe gastrointestinal narrowing (small bowel disease, short gut syndrome, history of peritonitis, cystic fibrosis, chronic intestinal pseudo-obstruction, Meckel's diverticulum). Safety and efficacy in children <6 years of age have not been established. Transdermal system may cause allergic contact sensitization, characterized by (Continued)

Methylphenidate (Continued)

intense local reactions (edema, papules); sensitization may subsequently manifest systemically with other routes of methylphenidate administration; monitor closely. Avoid exposure of application site to any direct external heat sources (eg, heating pads, electric blankets). Efficacy of transdermal methylphenidate therapy for >7 weeks has not been established.

Drug Interactions

Cytochrome P450 Effect: Substrate of CYP2D6 (major); **Inhibits** CYP2D6 (weak)

Increased Effect/Toxicity: Methylphenidate may cause hypertensive effects when used in combination with MAO inhibitors or drugs with MAO-inhibiting activity (linezolid). Risk may be less with selegiline (MAO type B selective at low doses); it is best to avoid this combination. CYP2D6 inhibitors may increase the levels/effects of methylphenidate; example inhibitors include chlorpromazine, delavirdine, fluoxetine, miconazole, paroxetine, pergolide, quinidine, quinine, ritonavir, and ropinirole. Methylphenidate may increase levels of phenytoin, phenobarbital, and TCAs. Increased toxicity with clonidine and sibutramine.

Decreased Effect: Effectiveness of antihypertensive agents may be decreased. Carbamazepine may decrease the effect of methylphenidate.

Ethanol/Nutrition/Herb Interactions

Ethanol: Avoid ethanol (may cause CNS depression).

Food: Food may increase oral absorption; Concerta® formulation is not affected. Food delays early peak and high-fat meals increase C_{max} and AUC of Metadate® CD formulation.

Herb/Nutraceutical: Avoid ephedra (may cause hypertension or arrhythmias) and yohimbe (also has CNS stimulatory activity).

Dietary Considerations
Should be taken 30-45 minutes before meals. Concerta® is not affected by food and should be taken with water, milk, or juice. Metadate® CD should be taken before breakfast. Metadate® ER should be taken before breakfast and lunch. Methylin® chewable tablets contain phenylalanine 0.42 mg/methylphenidate 2.5 mg.

Pharmacodynamics/Kinetics

Onset of action: Peak effect:

Immediate release tablet: Cerebral stimulation: ~2 hours

Extended release capsule (Metadate® CD): Biphasic; initial peak similar to immediate release product, followed by second rising portion (corresponding to extended release portion)

Sustained release tablet: 4-7 hours

Osmotic release tablet (Concerta®): Initial: 1-2 hours

Transdermal: ~2 hours

Duration: Immediate release tablet: 3-6 hours; Sustained release tablet: 8 hours; Extended release tablet: Methylin® ER, Metadate® ER: 8 hours, Concerta®: 12 hours

Absorption:

Oral: Readily absorbed

Transdermal: Absorption increased when applied to inflamed skin or exposed to heat. Absorption is continuous for 9 hours after application.

Metabolism: Hepatic via de-esterification to minimally active metabolite

Half-life elimination: d-methylphenidate: 3-4 hours; l-methylphenidate: 1-3 hours

Time to peak: Concerta®: C_{max}: 6-8 hours; Daytrana™: 7.5-10.5 hours

Excretion: Urine (90% as metabolites and unchanged drug)

Pregnancy Risk Factor C

Dosage Forms

Capsule, extended release:

Metadate® CD: 10 mg, 20 mg, 30 mg, 40 mg, 50 mg, 60 mg

Ritalin® LA: 10 mg, 20 mg, 30 mg, 40 mg

Solution, oral:

Methylin®: 5 mg/5 mL, 10 mg/5 mL

Tablet: 5 mg, 10 mg, 20 mg

Methylin®, Ritalin®: 5 mg, 10 mg, 20 mg

Tablet, chewable:

Methylin®: 2.5 mg, 5 mg, 10 mg

Tablet, extended release: 20 mg

Concerta®: 18 mg, 27 mg, 36 mg, 54 mg

Metadate® ER, Methylin® ER: 10 mg, 20 mg

Tablet, sustained release:

Ritalin-SR®: 20 mg

Transdermal system [once-daily patch]:

Daytrana™: 10 mg/9 hours (10s, 30s); 15 mg/9 hours (10s, 30s); 20 mg/9 hours (10s, 30s); 30 mg/9 hours (10s, 30s)

Methylphenidate Hydrochloride *see* Methylphenidate *on page 1079*

MethylPREDNISolone (meth il pred NIS oh lone)

Related Information
Respiratory Diseases *on page 1747*
Related Sample Prescriptions
Erosive Lichen Planus and Major Aphthae *on page 1845*
U.S. Brand Names Depo-Medrol®; Medrol®; Solu-Medrol®
Canadian Brand Names Depo-Medrol®; Medrol®; Methylprednisolone Acetate; Solu-Medrol®
Mexican Brand Names Cryosolona; Solu Medrol
Generic Available Yes: Sodium succinate injection, tablet
Index Terms 6-α-Methylprednisolone; A-Methapred; Methylprednisolone Acetate; Methylprednisolone Sodium Succinate
Pharmacologic Category Corticosteroid, Systemic
Dental Use Treatment of a variety of oral diseases of allergic, inflammatory, or autoimmune origin
Use Primarily as an anti-inflammatory or immunosuppressant agent in the treatment of a variety of diseases including those of hematologic, allergic, inflammatory, neoplastic, and autoimmune origin. Prevention and treatment of graft-versus-host disease following allogeneic bone marrow transplantation.
Local Anesthetic/Vasoconstrictor Precautions No information available to require special precautions
Effects on Dental Treatment Key adverse event(s) related to dental treatment: Ulcerative esophagitis.
Significant Adverse Effects Frequency not defined.
Cardiovascular: Edema, hypertension, arrhythmia
Central nervous system: Insomnia, nervousness, vertigo, seizure, psychoses, pseudotumor cerebri, headache, mood swings, delirium, hallucinations, euphoria
Dermatologic: Hirsutism, acne, skin atrophy, bruising, hyperpigmentation
Endocrine & metabolic: Diabetes mellitus, adrenal suppression, hyperlipidemia, Cushing's syndrome, pituitary-adrenal axis suppression, growth suppression, glucose intolerance, hypokalemia, alkalosis, amenorrhea, sodium and water retention, hyperglycemia
Gastrointestinal: Increased appetite, indigestion, peptic ulcer, nausea, vomiting, abdominal distention, ulcerative esophagitis, pancreatitis
Hematologic: Transient leukocytosis
Neuromuscular & skeletal: Arthralgia, muscle weakness, osteoporosis, fractures
Ocular: Cataracts, glaucoma
Miscellaneous: Infections, hypersensitivity reactions, avascular necrosis, secondary malignancy, intractable hiccups
Dental Usual Dosing Anti-inflammatory or immunosuppressive: Adults: Oral: 2-60 mg/day in 1-4 divided doses to start, followed by gradual reduction in dosage to the lowest possible level consistent with maintaining an adequate clinical response.
Dosage Dosing should be based on the lesser of ideal body weight or actual body weight
Only sodium succinate may be given I.V.; methylprednisolone sodium succinate is highly soluble and has a rapid effect by I.M. and I.V. routes. Methylprednisolone acetate has a low solubility and has a sustained I.M. effect.
Children:
Anti-inflammatory or immunosuppressive: Oral, I.M., I.V. (sodium succinate): 0.5-1.7 mg/kg/day **or** 5-25 mg/m²/day in divided doses every 6-12 hours; "Pulse" therapy: 15-30 mg/kg/dose over ≥30 minutes given once daily for 3 days
Status asthmaticus: I.V. (sodium succinate): Loading dose: 2 mg/kg/dose, then 0.5-1 mg/kg/dose every 6 hours for up to 5 days
Acute spinal cord injury: I.V. (sodium succinate): 30 mg/kg over 15 minutes, followed in 45 minutes by a continuous infusion of 5.4 mg/kg/hour for 23 hours
Lupus nephritis: I.V. (sodium succinate): 30 mg/kg over ≥30 minutes every other day for 6 doses
Adults: **Only sodium succinate may be given I.V.;** methylprednisolone sodium succinate is highly soluble and has a rapid effect by I.M. and I.V. routes. Methylprednisolone acetate has a low solubility and has a sustained I.M. effect.
(Continued)

MethylPREDNISolone *(Continued)*

Acute spinal cord injury: I.V. (sodium succinate): 30 mg/kg over 15 minutes, followed in 45 minutes by a continuous infusion of 5.4 mg/kg/hour for 23 hours

Anti-inflammatory or immunosuppressive:

Oral: 2-60 mg/day in 1-4 divided doses to start, followed by gradual reduction in dosage to the lowest possible level consistent with maintaining an adequate clinical response.

I.M. (sodium succinate): 10-80 mg/day once daily

I.M. (acetate): 10-80 mg every 1-2 weeks

I.V. (sodium succinate): 10-40 mg over a period of several minutes and repeated I.V. or I.M. at intervals depending on clinical response; when high dosages are needed, give 30 mg/kg over a period ≥30 minutes and may be repeated every 4-6 hours for 48 hours.

Status asthmaticus: I.V. (sodium succinate): Loading dose: 2 mg/kg/dose, then 0.5-1 mg/kg/dose every 6 hours for up to 5 days

Lupus nephritis: High-dose "pulse" therapy: I.V. (sodium succinate): 1 g/day for 3 days

Aplastic anemia: I.V. (sodium succinate): 1 mg/kg/day or 40 mg/day (whichever dose is higher), for 4 days. After 4 days, change to oral and continue until day 10 or until symptoms of serum sickness resolve, then rapidly reduce over approximately 2 weeks.

Pneumocystis pneumonia in AIDs patients: I.V.: 40-60 mg every 6 hours for 7-10 days

Intra-articular (acetate): Administer every 1-5 weeks.

Large joints: 20-80 mg

Small joints: 4-10 mg

Intralesional (acetate): 20-60 mg every 1-5 weeks

Mechanism of Action In a tissue-specific manner, corticosteroids regulate gene expression subsequent to binding specific intracellular receptors and translocation into the nucleus. Corticosteroids exert a wide array of physiologic effects including modulation of carbohydrate, protein, and lipid metabolism and maintenance of fluid and electrolyte homeostasis. Moreover cardiovascular, immunologic, musculoskeletal, endocrine, and neurologic physiology are influenced by corticosteroids. Decreases inflammation by suppression of migration of polymorphonuclear leukocytes and reversal of increased capillary permeability.

Contraindications Hypersensitivity to methylprednisolone or any component of the formulation; viral, fungal, or tubercular skin lesions; administration of live virus vaccines; serious infections, except septic shock or tuberculous meningitis. Methylprednisolone formulations containing benzyl alcohol preservative are contraindicated in infants.

Warnings/Precautions Use with caution in patients with thyroid disease, hepatic impairment, renal impairment, cardiovascular disease, diabetes, glaucoma, cataracts, myasthenia gravis, patients at risk for osteoporosis, patients at risk for seizures, or GI diseases (diverticulitis, peptic ulcer, ulcerative colitis) due to perforation risk. Use caution following acute MI (corticosteroids have been associated with myocardial rupture). Because of the risk of adverse effects, systemic corticosteroids should be used cautiously in the elderly in the smallest possible effective dose for the shortest duration. May affect growth velocity; growth should be routinely monitored in pediatric patients. Withdraw therapy with gradual tapering of dose.

May cause hypercorticism or suppression of hypothalamic-pituitary-adrenal (HPA) axis, particularly in younger children or in patients receiving high doses for prolonged periods. HPA axis suppression may lead to adrenal crisis. Withdrawal and discontinuation of a corticosteroid should be done slowly and carefully. Particular care is required when patients are transferred from systemic corticosteroids to inhaled products due to possible adrenal insufficiency or withdrawal from steroids, including an increase in allergic symptoms. Patients receiving >20 mg per day of prednisone (or equivalent) may be most susceptible. Fatalities have occurred due to adrenal insufficiency in asthmatic patients during and after transfer from systemic corticosteroids to aerosol steroids; aerosol steroids do not provide the systemic steroid needed to treat patients having trauma, surgery, or infections.

Acute myopathy has been reported with high dose corticosteroids, usually in patients with neuromuscular transmission disorders; may involve ocular and/or respiratory muscles; monitor creatine kinase; recovery may be delayed. Corticosteroid use may cause psychiatric disturbances, including depression, euphoria, insomnia, mood swings, and personality changes. Pre-existing psychiatric conditions may be exacerbated by corticosteroid use. Prolonged use of corticosteroids may also increase the incidence of secondary infection, mask acute infection (including fungal infections), prolong or exacerbate viral infections, or limit response to vaccines. Exposure to chickenpox should be avoided; cortico-steroids should not be used to treat ocular herpes simplex. Corticosteroids should not be used for cerebral malaria. Close observation is required in patients with latent tuberculosis and/or TB reactivity; restrict use in active TB (only in conjunction with antituberculosis treatment). Prolonged treatment with corticosteroids has been associated with the development of Kaposi's sarcoma (case reports); if noted, discontinuation of therapy should be considered.

Drug Interactions Substrate of CYP3A4 (minor); **Inhibits** CYP2C8 (weak), 3A4 (weak)

Decreased effect:

Phenytoin, phenobarbital, rifampin increase clearance of methylprednisolone
Potassium depleting diuretics enhance potassium depletion

Increased toxicity:

Skin test antigens, immunizations decrease response and increase potential infections

Methylprednisolone may increase circulating glucose levels and may need adjustments of insulin or oral hypoglycemics

Ethanol/Nutrition/Herb Interactions

Ethanol: Avoid ethanol (may increase gastric mucosal irritation).

Food: Methylprednisolone interferes with calcium absorption. Limit caffeine.

Herb/Nutraceutical: St John's wort may decrease methylprednisolone levels. Avoid cat's claw, echinacea (have immunostimulant properties).

Dietary Considerations Should be taken after meals or with food or milk; need diet rich in pyridoxine, vitamin C, vitamin D, folate, calcium, phosphorus, and protein.

Sodium content of 1 g sodium succinate injection: 2.01 mEq; 53 mg of sodium succinate salt is equivalent to 40 mg of methylprednisolone base

Methylprednisolone acetate: Depo-Medrol®

Methylprednisolone sodium succinate: Solu-Medrol®

Pharmacodynamics/Kinetics

Onset of action: Peak effect (route dependent): Oral: 1-2 hours; I.M.: 4-8 days; Intra-articular: 1 week; methylprednisolone sodium succinate is highly soluble and has a rapid effect by I.M. and I.V. routes

Duration (route dependent): Oral: 30-36 hours; I.M.: 1-4 weeks; Intra-articular: 1-5 weeks; methylprednisolone acetate has a low solubility and has a sustained I.M. effect

Distribution: V_d: 0.7-1.5 L/kg

Half-life elimination: 3-3.5 hours; reduced in obese

Excretion: Clearance: Reduced in obese

Pregnancy Risk Factor C

Lactation Excretion in breast milk unknown

Dosage Forms Excipient information presented when available (limited, particularly for generics); consult specific product labeling.

Injection, powder for reconstitution, as sodium succinate: 125 mg [strength expressed as base]

Solu-Medrol®: 40 mg, 125 mg, 500 mg, 1 g, 2 g [packaged with diluent; diluent contains benzyl alcohol; strength expressed as base]

Solu-Medrol®: 500 mg, 1 g

Injection, suspension, as acetate (Depo-Medrol®): 20 mg/mL (5 mL); 40 mg/mL (5 mL); 80 mg/mL (5 mL) [contains benzyl alcohol; strength expressed as base]

Injection, suspension, as acetate [single-dose vial] (Depo-Medrol®): 40 mg/mL (1 mL, 10 mL); 80 mg/mL (1 mL)

Tablet: 4 mg

Medrol®: 2 mg, 4 mg, 8 mg, 16 mg, 32 mg

Tablet, dose-pack: 4 mg (21s)

Medrol® Dosepack™: 4 mg (21s)

6-α-**Methylprednisolone** see MethylPREDNISolone on page 1083

Methylprednisolone Acetate see MethylPREDNISolone on page 1083

Methylprednisolone Sodium Succinate see MethylPREDNISolone on page 1083

4-**Methylpyrazole** see Fomepizole on page 739

Methylrosaniline Chloride see Gentian Violet on page 777

MethylTESTOSTERone (meth il tes TOS te rone)

U.S. Brand Names Android®; Methitest™; Testred®; Virilon®

Generic Available No

Pharmacologic Category Androgen

Use

Male: Hypogonadism; delayed puberty; impotence and climacteric symptoms

Female: Palliative treatment of metastatic breast cancer

(Continued)

MethylTESTOSTERone *(Continued)*

Local Anesthetic/Vasoconstrictor Precautions No information available to require special precautions

Effects on Dental Treatment No significant effects or complications reported

Common Adverse Effects Frequency not defined.

Male: Virilism, priapism, prostatic hyperplasia, prostatic carcinoma, impotence, testicular atrophy, gynecomastia

Female: Virilism, menstrual problems (amenorrhea), breast soreness, hirsutism (increase in pubic hair growth) atrophy

Cardiovascular: Edema

Central nervous system: Headache, anxiety, depression

Dermatologic: Acne, "male pattern" baldness, seborrhea

Endocrine & metabolic: Hypercalcemia, hypercholesterolemia

Gastrointestinal: GI irritation, nausea, vomiting

Hematologic: Leukopenia, polycythemia

Hepatic: Hepatic dysfunction, hepatic necrosis, cholestatic hepatitis

Miscellaneous: Hypersensitivity reactions

Restrictions C-III

Mechanism of Action Stimulates receptors in organs and tissues to promote growth and development of male sex organs and maintains secondary sex characteristics in androgen-deficient males

Drug Interactions

Increased Effect/Toxicity: Effects of oral anticoagulants and hypoglycemic agents may be increased. Toxicity may occur with cyclosporine; avoid concurrent use.

Decreased Effect: Decreased oral anticoagulant effect

Pharmacodynamics/Kinetics

Metabolism: Hepatic

Excretion: Urine

Pregnancy Risk Factor X

Metipranolol *(met i PRAN oh lol)*

U.S. Brand Names OptiPranolol®

Canadian Brand Names OptiPranolol®

Generic Available Yes

Index Terms Metipranolol Hydrochloride

Pharmacologic Category Beta-Adrenergic Blocker, Nonselective; Ophthalmic Agent, Antiglaucoma

Use Agent for lowering intraocular pressure in patients with chronic open-angle glaucoma

Local Anesthetic/Vasoconstrictor Precautions No information available to require special precautions

Effects on Dental Treatment Metipranolol is a nonselective beta-blocker and may enhance the pressor response to epinephrine, resulting in hypertension and bradycardia. Many nonsteroidal anti-inflammatory drugs, such as ibuprofen and indomethacin, can reduce the hypotensive effect of beta-blockers after 3 or more weeks of therapy with the NSAID. Short-term NSAID use (ie, 3 days) requires no special precautions in patients taking beta-blockers.

Mechanism of Action Beta-adrenoceptor-blocking agent; lacks intrinsic sympathomimetic activity and membrane-stabilizing effects and possesses only slight local anesthetic activity; mechanism of action of metipranolol in reducing intraocular pressure appears to be via reduced production of aqueous humor. This effect may be related to a reduction in blood flow to the iris root-ciliary body. It remains unclear if the reduction in intraocular pressure observed with beta-blockers is actually secondary to beta-adrenoceptor blockade.

Pregnancy Risk Factor C

Metipranolol Hydrochloride *see* Metipranolol *on page 1086*

Metoclopramide *(met oh KLOE pra mide)*

Related Information

Endocrine Disorders and Pregnancy *on page 1750*

U.S. Brand Names Reglan®

Canadian Brand Names Apo-Metoclop®; Metoclopramide Hydrochloride Injection; Nu-Metoclopramide

Mexican Brand Names Carnotprim; Meclomid; Plasil; Primperan

Generic Available Yes

Pharmacologic Category Antiemetic; Gastrointestinal Agent, Prokinetic

Use

Oral: Symptomatic treatment of diabetic gastric stasis; gastroesophageal reflux

I.V., I.M.: Symptomatic treatment of diabetic gastric stasis; postpyloric placement of enteral feeding tubes; prevention and/or treatment of nausea and vomiting associated with chemotherapy, or postsurgery; to stimulate gastric emptying and intestinal transit of barium during radiological examination

Local Anesthetic/Vasoconstrictor Precautions No information available to require special precautions

Effects on Dental Treatment Key adverse event(s) related to dental treatment: Xerostomia (normal salivary flow resumes upon discontinuation).

Common Adverse Effects Frequency not always defined.

Cardiovascular: AV block, bradycardia, CHF, fluid retention, flushing (following high I.V. doses), hyper-/hypotension, supraventricular tachycardia

Central nervous system: Drowsiness (~10% to 70%; dose related), fatigue (~10%), restlessness (~10%), acute dystonic reactions (<1% to 25%; dose and age related), akathisia, confusion, depression, dizziness, hallucinations (rare), headache, insomnia, neuroleptic malignant syndrome (rare), Parkinsonian-like symptoms, suicidal ideation, seizure, tardive dyskinesia

Dermatologic: Angioneurotic edema (rare), rash, urticaria

Endocrine & metabolic: Amenorrhea, galactorrhea, gynecomastia, impotence

Gastrointestinal: Diarrhea, nausea

Genitourinary: Incontinence, urinary frequency

Hematologic: Agranulocytosis, leukopenia, neutropenia, porphyria

Hepatic: Hepatotoxicity (rare)

Ocular: Visual disturbance

Respiratory: Bronchospasm, laryngeal edema (rare)

Miscellaneous: Allergic reactions, methemoglobinemia, sulfhemoglobinemia

Mechanism of Action Blocks dopamine receptors and (when given in higher doses) also blocks serotonin receptors in chemoreceptor trigger zone of the CNS; enhances the response to acetylcholine of tissue in upper GI tract causing enhanced motility and accelerated gastric emptying without stimulating gastric, biliary, or pancreatic secretions; increases lower esophageal sphincter tone

Drug Interactions

Cytochrome P450 Effect: Substrate (minor) of CYP1A2, 2D6; **Inhibits** CYP2D6 (weak)

Increased Effect/Toxicity: Opiate analgesics may increase CNS depression. Metoclopramide may increase extrapyramidal symptoms (EPS) or risk when used concurrently with antipsychotic agents. Metoclopramide may increase cyclosporine levels.

Decreased Effect: Anticholinergic agents antagonize metoclopramide's actions.

Pharmacodynamics/Kinetics

Onset of action: Oral: 0.5-1 hour; I.V.: 1-3 minutes; I.M.: 10-15 minutes

Duration: Therapeutic: 1-2 hours, regardless of route

Distribution: V_d: 2-4 L/kg

Protein binding: 30%

Bioavailability: Oral: 65% to 95%

Half-life elimination: Normal renal function: 4-6 hours (may be dose dependent)

Time to peak, serum: Oral: 1-2 hours

Excretion: Urine (~85%)

Pregnancy Risk Factor B

Metolazone (me TOLE a zone)

Related Information

Cardiovascular Diseases on page 1726

U.S. Brand Names Zaroxolyn®

Canadian Brand Names Zaroxolyn®

Generic Available Yes

Pharmacologic Category Diuretic, Thiazide-Related

Use Management of mild to moderate hypertension; treatment of edema in congestive heart failure and nephrotic syndrome, impaired renal function

Local Anesthetic/Vasoconstrictor Precautions No information available to require special precautions

Effects on Dental Treatment Key adverse event(s) related to dental treatment: Xerostomia (normal salivary flow resumes upon discontinuation) and orthostatic hypotension.

Mechanism of Action Inhibits sodium reabsorption in the distal tubules causing increased excretion of sodium and water, as well as, potassium and hydrogen ions

Pregnancy Risk Factor B (manufacturer); D (expert analysis)

Metoprolol (me toe PROE lole)

Related Information
Cardiovascular Diseases *on page 1726*

U.S. Brand Names Lopressor®; Toprol-XL®

Canadian Brand Names Apo-Metoprolol®; Betaloc®; Betaloc® Durules®; Lopressor®; Metoprolol Tartrate Injection, USP; Novo-Metoprolol; Nu-Metop; PMS-Metoprolol; Sandoz-Metoprolol; Toprol-XL®

Mexican Brand Names Lopresor; Prolaken; Seloken-Zok

Generic Available Yes

Index Terms Metoprolol Succinate; Metoprolol Tartrate

Pharmacologic Category Beta Blocker, Beta$_1$ Selective

Use Treatment of hypertension and angina pectoris; prevention of myocardial infarction, atrial fibrillation, flutter, symptomatic treatment of hypertrophic subaortic stenosis

Extended release: To reduce mortality/hospitalization in patients with congestive heart failure (stable NYHA Class II or III) in patients already receiving ACE inhibitors, diuretics, and/or digoxin

Unlabeled/Investigational Use Treatment of ventricular arrhythmias, atrial ectopy, migraine prophylaxis, essential tremor, aggressive behavior

Local Anesthetic/Vasoconstrictor Precautions No information available to require special precautions

Effects on Dental Treatment Metoprolol is a cardioselective beta-blocker. Local anesthetic with vasoconstrictor can be safely used in patients medicated with metoprolol. Nonselective beta-blockers (ie, propranolol, nadolol) enhance the pressor response to epinephrine, resulting in hypertension and bradycardia; this has not been reported for metoprolol. Many nonsteroidal anti-inflammatory drugs, such as ibuprofen and indomethacin, can reduce the hypotensive effect of beta-blockers after 3 or more weeks of therapy with the NSAID. Short-term NSAID use (ie, 3 days) requires no special precautions in patients taking beta-blockers.

Common Adverse Effects Frequency may not be defined.

Cardiovascular: Bradycardia (2% to 16%), hypotension (1% to 2%), arterial insufficiency (usually Raynaud type; 1%), chest pain (1%), CHF (1%), edema (peripheral; 1%), palpitation (1%), syncope (1%), gangrene (rare)

Central nervous system: Dizziness (2% to 10%), fatigue (10%), depression (5%), confusion, headache, insomnia, memory loss (short-term), nightmares, somnolence

Dermatology: Pruritus (5%), rash (5%), psoriasis increased, alopecia (reversible; rare)

Endocrine & metabolic: Libido decreased, Peyronie's disease (<1%)

Gastrointestinal: Diarrhea (5%), constipation (1%), flatulence (1%), gastrointestinal pain (1%), heartburn (1%), nausea (1%), xerostomia (1%)

Hematologic: Agranulocytosis (rare)

Neuromuscular & skeletal: Musculoskeletal pain

Ocular: Blurred vision, dry eyes (rare), oculomucocutaneous syndrome

Otic: Tinnitus

Respiratory: Dyspnea (1% to 3%), bronchospasm (1%), wheezing (1%), rhinitis

Miscellaneous: Cold extremities (1%)

Other events reported with beta-blockers: AV block increased, catatonia, emotional lability, fever, hypersensitivity reactions, laryngospasm, nonthrombocytopenic purpura, respiratory distress, thrombocytopenic purpura

Dosage

Children 1-17 years: Hypertension (unlabeled use): Oral: Initial: 1-2 mg/kg/day; maximum 6 mg/kg/day (≤200 mg/day); administer in 2 divided doses

Adults:

Hypertension: Oral: 100-450 mg/day in 2-3 divided doses, begin with 50 mg twice daily and increase doses at weekly intervals to desired effect; usual dosage range (JNC 7): 50-100 mg/day

Extended release: Initial: 25-100 mg/day (maximum 400 mg/day)

Angina, SVT, MI prophylaxis: Oral: 100-450 mg/day in 2-3 divided doses, begin with 50 mg twice daily and increase doses at weekly intervals to desired effect

Extended release: Initial: 100 mg/day (maximum 400 mg/day)

Hypertension/ventricular rate control: I.V. (in patients having nonfunctioning GI tract): Initial: 1.25-5 mg every 6-12 hours; titrate initial dose to response. Initially, low doses may be appropriate to establish response; however, up to 15 mg every 3-6 hours has been employed.

Congestive heart failure: Oral (extended release): Initial: 25 mg once daily (reduce to 12.5 mg once daily in NYHA class higher than class II); may double dosage every 2 weeks as tolerated, up to 200 mg/day

Myocardial infarction (acute): I.V.: 5 mg every 2 minutes for 3 doses in early treatment of myocardial infarction; thereafter give 50 mg orally every 6 hours 15 minutes after last I.V. dose and continue for 48 hours; then administer a maintenance dose of 100 mg twice daily.

Note: When switching from immediate release metoprolol to extended release, the same total daily dose of metoprolol should be used.

Elderly: Oral: Initial: 25 mg/day; usual range: 25-300 mg/day

Extended release: 25-50 mg/day initially as a single dose; increase at 1- to 2-week intervals.

Hemodialysis: Administer dose posthemodialysis or administer 50 mg supplemental dose; supplemental dose is not necessary following peritoneal dialysis

Dosing adjustment/comments in hepatic disease: Reduced dose probably necessary

Mechanism of Action Selective inhibitor of beta$_1$-adrenergic receptors; competitively blocks beta$_1$-receptors, with little or no effect on beta$_2$-receptors at doses <100 mg; does not exhibit any membrane stabilizing or intrinsic sympathomimetic activity

Contraindications Hypersensitivity to metoprolol or any component of the formulation; sick sinus syndrome; sinus bradycardia; heart block greater than first degree (except in patients with a functioning artificial pacemaker); cardiogenic shock; uncompensated cardiac failure; severe peripheral arterial disease; pheochromocytoma (without alpha blockade); pregnancy (2nd and 3rd trimesters)

Warnings/Precautions [U.S. Boxed Warning]: Beta-blocker therapy should not be withdrawn abruptly (particularly in patients with CAD), but gradually tapered to avoid acute tachycardia, hypertension, and/or ischemia. Consider pre-existing conditions such as sick sinus syndrome before initiating. Use caution in patients with PVD (can aggravate arterial insufficiency). Use caution with concurrent use of beta-blockers and either verapamil or diltiazem; bradycardia or heart block can occur; avoid concurrent I.V. use of both agents. In general, beta-blockers should be avoided in patients with bronchospastic disease. Metoprolol, with B$_1$ selectivity, should be used cautiously in bronchospastic disease with close monitoring. Use cautiously in diabetics because it can mask prominent hypoglycemic symptoms. Use caution with hepatic dysfunction. Use with caution in patients with myasthenia gravis or psychiatric disease (may cause CNS depression). Use care with anesthetic agents which decrease myocardial function. Use of beta-blockers may unmask cardiac failure in patients without a history of dysfunction. Adequate alpha-blockade is required prior to use of any beta-blocker for patients with untreated pheochromocytoma. Safety and efficacy have not been established in children.

Extended release: Use care in compensated heart failure and monitor closely for a worsening of the condition.

Drug Interactions

Cytochrome P450 Effect: Substrate of CYP2C19 (minor), 2D6 (major); **Inhibits** CYP2D6 (weak)

Increased Effect/Toxicity: CYP2D6 inhibitors may increase the levels/ effects of metoprolol; example inhibitors include chlorpromazine, delavirdine, fluoxetine, miconazole, paroxetine, pergolide, quinidine, quinine, ritonavir, and ropinirole. Aminoquinolones (antimalarial), propafenone, and propoxyphene increase levels of metoprolol. Concomitant therapy with bupropion may result in bradycardia. Metoprolol may increase the effects of other drugs which slow AV conduction (digoxin, verapamil, diltiazem), dipyridamole, disopyramide, acetylcholinesterase inhibitors, amiodarone, alpha$_1$-blockers (prazosin, terazosin), and alpha-/beta-agonists (direct acting). Metoprolol may mask the tachycardia from hypoglycemia caused by insulin and sulfonylureas. In patients receiving concurrent therapy, the risk of hypertensive crisis is increased with clonidine (alpha$_2$-agonist). May increase the levels of antipsychotic agents (phenothiazines) and lidocaine.

Decreased Effect: Decreased effect of beta-blockers with barbiturates, NSAIDs, and rifampin, salicylates; beta-blockers may decrease the effect of theophylline derivatives.

Ethanol/Nutrition/Herb Interactions

Food: Food increases absorption. Metoprolol serum levels may be increased if taken with food.

Herb/Nutraceutical: Avoid dong quai if using for hypertension (has estrogenic activity). Avoid bayberry, blue cohosh, cayenne, ephedra, ginger, ginseng (american), gotu kola, licorice, yohimbe (may worsen hypertension). Avoid black cohosh, california poppy, coleus, garlic, golden seal, hawthorn, mistletoe, periwinkle, quinine, shepherd's purse (have antihypertensive activity, may cause hypotension).

Dietary Considerations Regular tablets should be taken with food. Extended release tablets may be taken without regard to meals.

(Continued)

Metoprolol *(Continued)*

Pharmacodynamics/Kinetics
Onset of action: Peak effect: Antihypertensive: Oral: 1.5-4 hours
Duration: 10-20 hours
Absorption: 95%
Protein binding: 12%
Metabolism: Extensively hepatic via CYP2D6; significant first-pass effect
Bioavailability: Oral: 40% to 50%
Half-life elimination: 3-8 hours
Excretion: Urine (3% to 10% as unchanged drug)

Pregnancy Risk Factor C (manufacturer); D (2nd and 3rd trimesters - expert analysis)

Dosage Forms
Injection, solution: 1 mg/mL (5 mL)
Lopressor®: 1 mg/mL (5 mL)
Tablet: 25 mg, 50 mg, 100 mg
Lopressor®: 50 mg, 100 mg
Tablet, extended release: 25 mg, 50 mg, 100 mg, 200 mg
Toprol-XL®: 25 mg, 50 mg, 100 mg, 200 mg

Selected Readings
Foster CA and Aston SJ, "Propranolol-Epinephrine Interaction: A Potential Disaster," *Plast Reconstr Surg*, 1983, 72(1):74-8.
Wong DG, Spence JD, Lamki L, et al, "Effect of Nonsteroidal Anti-inflammatory Drugs on Control of Hypertension of Beta-Blockers and Diuretics," *Lancet*, 1986, 1(8488):997-1001.
Wynn RL, "Dental Nonsteroidal Anti-inflammatory Drugs and Prostaglandin-Based Drug Interactions, Part Two," *Gen Dent*, 1992, 40(2):104, 106, 108.
Wynn RL, "Epinephrine Interactions With Beta-Blockers," *Gen Dent*, 1994, 42(1):16, 18.

Metoprolol and Hydrochlorothiazide
(me toe PROE lole & hye droe klor oh THYE a zide)

U.S. Brand Names Lopressor HCT®
Generic Available Yes
Index Terms Hydrochlorothiazide and Metoprolol; Hydrochlorothiazide and Metoprolol Tartrate; Metoprolol Tartrate and Hydrochlorothiazide
Pharmacologic Category Beta Blocker, Beta$_1$ Selective; Diuretic, Thiazide
Use Treatment of hypertension

Local Anesthetic/Vasoconstrictor Precautions No information available to require special precautions

Effects on Dental Treatment
Metoprolol: Treatment of oral soft tissue infections due to anaerobic bacteria including all anaerobic cocci, anaerobic gram-negative bacilli (*Bacteroides*), and gram-positive spore-forming bacilli (*Clostridium*). Useful as single agent or in combination with amoxicillin, Augmentin®, or ciprofloxacin in the treatment of periodontitis associated with the presence of *Actinobacillus actinomycetemcomitans* (AA).

Hydrochlorothiazide: Key adverse event(s) related to dental treatment: Orthostatic hypotension and hypotension.

Common Adverse Effects Reactions noted here have been reported with the combination product; see individual drug monographs for additional adverse reactions that may be expected from each agent.
1% to 10%:
Cardiovascular: Bradycardia (6%), edema (1%)
Central nervous system: Fatigue (10%), dizziness (10%), drowsiness (10%), headache (10%), vertigo (10%), abnormal dreams (1%)
Dermatologic: Purpura (1%)
Endocrine & metabolic: Hypokalemia, gout (1%)
Gastrointestinal: Anorexia (1%), constipation (1%), diarrhea (1%), nausea (1%), vomiting (1%), xerostomia (1%)
Genitourinary: Impotence (1%)
Neuromuscular & skeletal: Myalgia
Ocular: Blurred vision (1%)
Otic: Earache (1%), tinnitus (1%)
Respiratory: Dyspnea (1%)
Miscellaneous: Flu-like syndrome (10%), diaphoresis (1%), exercise tolerance decreased (1%)

Mechanism of Action See individual agents.

Drug Interactions
Cytochrome P450 Effect: Metoprolol: **Substrate** of CYP2C19 (minor), 2D6 (major); Inhibits CYP2D6 (weak)
Pharmacodynamics/Kinetics See individual agents.
Pregnancy Risk Factor C/D (expert analysis)

Metronidazole (met roe NYE da zole)

Related Information
Bacterial Infections *on page 1793*
Gastrointestinal Disorders *on page 1745*
Periodontal Diseases *on page 1801*
Sexually-Transmitted Diseases *on page 1766*
Ulcerative and Erosive Disorders *on page 1809*

Related Sample Prescriptions
Bacterial Infections and Periodontal Diseases *on page 1837*

U.S. Brand Names Flagyl®; Flagyl ER®; MetroCream®; MetroGel®; MetroGel-Vaginal®; MetroLotion®; Noritate®; Vandazole™

Canadian Brand Names Apo-Metronidazole®; Flagyl®; Florazole® ER; MetroCream®; Metrogel®; Nidagel™; Noritate®; Trikacide

Mexican Brand Names Epaq; Flagenase; Flagyl; MetroCream; MetroGel

Generic Available Yes: Capsule, cream, gel, infusion, lotion, tablet

Index Terms Metronidazole Hydrochloride

Pharmacologic Category Amebicide; Antibiotic, Miscellaneous; Antibiotic, Topical; Antiprotozoal, Nitroimidazole

Dental Use Treatment of oral soft tissue infections due to anaerobic bacteria including all anaerobic cocci, anaerobic gram-negative bacilli (*Bacteroides*), and gram-positive spore-forming bacilli (*Clostridium*). Useful as single agent or in combination with amoxicillin, Augmentin®, or ciprofloxacin in the treatment of periodontitis associated with the presence of *Actinobacillus actinomycetemcomitans* (AA).

Use Treatment of susceptible anaerobic bacterial and protozoal infections in the following conditions: Amebiasis, symptomatic and asymptomatic trichomoniasis; skin and skin structure infections; CNS infections; intra-abdominal infections (as part of combination regimen); systemic anaerobic infections; treatment of antibiotic-associated pseudomembranous colitis (AAPC), bacterial vaginosis; as part of a multidrug regimen for *H. pylori* eradication to reduce the risk of duodenal ulcer recurrence

Topical: Treatment of inflammatory lesions and erythema of rosacea

Unlabeled/Investigational Use Crohn's disease

Local Anesthetic/Vasoconstrictor Precautions No information available to require special precautions

Effects on Dental Treatment Key adverse event(s) related to dental treatment: Unusual/metallic taste, glossitis, stomatitis, xerostomia (normal salivary flow resumes upon discontinuation), and furry tongue.

Significant Adverse Effects

Systemic: Frequency not defined:

Cardiovascular: Flattening of the T-wave, flushing

Central nervous system: Ataxia, confusion, coordination impaired, dizziness, fever, headache, insomnia, irritability, seizure, vertigo

Dermatologic: Erythematous rash, urticaria

Endocrine & metabolic: Disulfiram-like reaction, dysmenorrhea, libido decreased

Gastrointestinal: Nausea (~12%), anorexia, abdominal cramping, constipation, diarrhea, furry tongue, glossitis, proctitis, stomatitis, unusual/metallic taste, vomiting, xerostomia

Genitourinary: Cystitis, darkened urine (rare), dysuria, incontinence, polyuria, vaginitis

Hematologic: Neutropenia (reversible), thrombocytopenia (reversible, rare)

Neuromuscular & skeletal: Peripheral neuropathy, weakness

Respiratory: Nasal congestion, rhinitis, sinusitis, pharyngitis

Miscellaneous: Flu-like syndrome, moniliasis

Topical: Frequency not defined:

Central nervous system: Headache

Dermatologic: Burning, contact dermatitis, dryness, erythema, irritation, pruritus, rash

Gastrointestinal: Unusual/metallic taste, nausea, constipation

Local: Local allergic reaction

(Continued)

Metronidazole *(Continued)*

Neuromuscular & skeletal: Tingling/numbness of extremities

Ocular: Eye irritation

Vaginal:

>10%: Genitourinary: Vaginal discharge (12%)

1% to 10%:

Central nervous system: Headache (5%), dizziness (2%)

Gastrointestinal: Gastrointestinal discomfort (7%), nausea and/or vomiting (4%), unusual/metallic taste (2%), diarrhea (1%)

Genitourinary: Vaginitis (10%), vulva/vaginal irritation (9%), pelvic discomfort (3%)

Hematologic: WBC increased (2%)

<1%: Abdominal bloating, abdominal gas, darkened urine, depression, fatigue, itching, rash, thirst, xerostomia

Dental Usual Dosing

Anaerobic infections/abscess: Adults: Oral, I.V.: 500 mg every 6-8 hours, not to exceed 4 g/day

Treatment of periodontitis (monotherapy or combination) associated with the presence of *Actinobacillus actinomycetemcomitans* (AA): Adults: Oral: 500 mg every 8 hours for 8 days.

Dosage

Infants and Children:

Amebiasis: Oral: 35-50 mg/kg/day in divided doses every 8 hours for 10 days

Trichomoniasis: Oral: 15-30 mg/kg/day in divided doses every 8 hours for 7 days

Anaerobic infections:

Oral: 15-35 mg/kg/day in divided doses every 8 hours

I.V.: 30 mg/kg/day in divided doses every 6 hours

Clostridium difficile (antibiotic-associated colitis): Oral: 20 mg/kg/day divided every 6 hours

Maximum dose: 2 g/day

Adults:

Anaerobic infections (diverticulitis, intra-abdominal, peritonitis, cholangitis, or abscess): Oral, I.V.: 500 mg every 6-8 hours, not to exceed 4 g/day

Acne rosacea: Topical:

0.75%: Apply and rub a thin film twice daily, morning and evening, to entire affected areas after washing. Significant therapeutic results should be noticed within 3 weeks. Clinical studies have demonstrated continuing improvement through 9 weeks of therapy.

1%: Apply thin film to affected area once daily

Amebiasis: Oral: 500-750 mg every 8 hours for 5-10 days

Antibiotic-associated pseudomembranous colitis: Oral: 250-500 mg 3-4 times/day for 10-14 days

Note: Due to the emergence of a new strain of *C. difficile*, some clinicians recommend converting to oral vancomycin therapy if the patient does not show a clear clinical response after 2 days of metronidazole therapy.

Giardiasis: 500 mg twice daily for 5-7 days

Helicobacter pylori eradication: Oral: 250-500 mg with meals and at bedtime for 14 days; requires combination therapy with at least one other antibiotic and an acid-suppressing agent (proton pump inhibitor or H_2 blocker)

Bacterial vaginosis or vaginitis due to *Gardnerella, Mobiluncus*:

Oral: 500 mg twice daily (regular release) or 750 mg once daily (extended release tablet) for 7 days

Vaginal: 1 applicatorful (~37.5 mg metronidazole) intravaginally once or twice daily for 5 days; apply once in morning and evening if using twice daily, if daily, use at bedtime

Trichomoniasis: Oral: 250 mg every 8 hours for 7 days **or** 375 mg twice daily for 7 days **or** 2 g as a single dose

Elderly: Use lower end of dosing recommendations for adults, do not administer as a single dose

Dosing adjustment in renal impairment: Cl_{cr} <10 mL/minute, but not on dialysis: Recommendations vary: To reduce possible accumulation in patients receiving multiple doses, consider reduction to 50% of dose or every 12 hours; **Note:** Dosage reduction is unnecessary in short courses of therapy. Clinical recommendations and practice vary. Some references do not recommend reduction at any level of renal impairment (Lamp, 1999).

Hemodialysis: Extensively removed by hemodialysis and peritoneal dialysis (50% to 100%); dosage reduction not recommended; administer full dose posthemodialysis

Peritoneal dialysis: Dose as for Cl_{cr} <10 mL/minute

Continuous arteriovenous or venovenous hemofiltration: Administer usual dose

Dosing adjustment/comments in hepatic disease: Unchanged in mild liver disease; reduce dosage in severe liver disease

Mechanism of Action After diffusing into the organism, interacts with DNA to cause a loss of helical DNA structure and strand breakage resulting in inhibition of protein synthesis and cell death in susceptible organisms

Contraindications Hypersensitivity to metronidazole, nitroimidazole derivatives, or any component of the formulation; pregnancy (1st trimester - found to be carcinogenic in rats)

Warnings/Precautions Use with caution in patients with liver impairment due to potential accumulation, blood dyscrasias; history of seizures, CHF, or other sodium retaining states; reduce dosage in patients with severe liver impairment, CNS disease, and consider dosage reduction in longer-term therapy with severe renal failure (Cl_{cr} <10 mL/minute); if *H. pylori* is not eradicated in patients being treated with metronidazole in a regimen, it should be assumed that metronidazole-resistance has occurred and it should not again be used; seizures and neuropathies have been reported especially with increased doses and chronic treatment; if this occurs, discontinue therapy. **[U.S. Boxed Warning]: Possibly carcinogenic based on animal data.**

Drug Interactions Inhibits CYP2C9 (weak), 3A4 (moderate)

Cimetidine may increase metronidazole levels.

Cisapride: May inhibit metabolism of cisapride, causing potential arrhythmias; avoid concurrent use

CYP3A4 substrates: Metronidazole may increase the levels/effects of CYP3A4 substrates. Example substrates include benzodiazepines, calcium channel blockers, cyclosporine, mirtazapine, nateglinide, nefazodone, sildenafil (and other PDE-5 inhibitors), tacrolimus, and venlafaxine. Selected benzodiazepines (midazolam and triazolam), cisapride, ergot alkaloids, selected HMG-CoA reductase inhibitors (lovastatin and simvastatin), and pimozide are generally contraindicated with strong CYP3A4 inhibitors.

Ethanol: Ethanol results in disulfiram-like reactions.

Lithium: Metronidazole may increase lithium levels/toxicity; monitor lithium levels.

Phenytoin, phenobarbital may increase metabolism of metronidazole, potentially decreasing its effect.

Warfarin: Metronidazole increases P-T prolongation with warfarin.

Ethanol/Nutrition/Herb Interactions

Ethanol: The manufacturer recommends to avoid all ethanol or any ethanol-containing drugs (may cause disulfiram-like reaction characterized by flushing, headache, nausea, vomiting, sweating or tachycardia).

Food: Peak antibiotic serum concentration lowered and delayed, but total drug absorbed not affected.

Dietary Considerations Take on an empty stomach. Drug may cause GI upset; if GI upset occurs, take with food. Extended release tablets should be taken on an empty stomach (1 hour before or 2 hours after meals). Sodium content of 500 mg (I.V.): 322 mg (14 mEq). The manufacturer recommends that ethanol be avoided during treatment and for 3 days after therapy is complete.

Pharmacodynamics/Kinetics

Absorption: Oral: Well absorbed; Topical: Concentrations achieved systemically after application of 1 g topically are 10 times less than those obtained after a 250 mg oral dose

Distribution: To saliva, bile, seminal fluid, breast milk, bone, liver, and liver abscesses, lung and vaginal secretions; crosses placenta and blood-brain barrier

CSF:blood level ratio: Normal meninges: 16% to 43%; Inflamed meninges: 100%

Protein binding: <20%

Metabolism: Hepatic (30% to 60%)

Half-life elimination: Neonates: 25-75 hours; Others: 6-8 hours, prolonged with hepatic impairment; End-stage renal disease: 21 hours

Time to peak, serum: Oral: Immediate release: 1-2 hours

Excretion: Urine (20% to 40% as unchanged drug); feces (6% to 15%)

Pregnancy Risk Factor B (may be contraindicated in 1st trimester)

Lactation Enters breast milk/not recommended (AAP rates "of concern")

Breast-Feeding Considerations It is suggested to stop breast-feeding for 12-24 hours following single dose therapy to allow excretion of dose.

Dosage Forms Excipient information presented when available (limited, particularly for generics); consult specific product labeling.

Capsule: 375 mg

Flagyl®: 375 mg

Cream, topical: 0.75% (45 g)

MetroCream®: 0.75% (45 g) [contains benzyl alcohol]

Noritate®: 1% (60 g)

Gel, topical: 0.75% (45 g)

(Continued)

Metronidazole *(Continued)*

MetroGel®: 1% (46 g, 60 g) [60 g tube also packaged in a kit with Cetaphil® skin cleanser]

Gel, vaginal: 0.75% (70 g)

MetroGel-Vaginal®, Vandazole™: 0.75% (70 g)

Infusion [premixed iso-osmotic sodium chloride solution]: 500 mg (100 mL)

Lotion, topical: 0.75% (60 mL)

MetroLotion®: 0.75% (60 mL) [contains benzyl alcohol]

Tablet: 250 mg, 500 mg

Flagyl®: 250 mg, 500 mg

Tablet, extended release:

Flagyl® ER: 750 mg

Selected Readings

Eisenberg L, Suchow R, Coles RS, et al, "The Effects of Metronidazole Administration on Clinical and Microbiologic Parameters of Periodontal Disease," *Clin Prev Dent,* 1991, 13(1):28-34.

Herrera D, Sanz M, Jepsen S, et al, "A Systematic Review on the Effect of Systemic Antimicrobials as an Adjunct to Scaling and Root Planing in Periodontitis Patients," *J Clin Periodontol,* 2002, 29(Suppl 3):136-59, discussion 160-2.

Jansson H, Bratthall G, and Soderholm G, "Clinical Outcome Observed in Subjects With Recurrent Periodontal Disease Following Local Treatment With 25% Metronidazole Gel," *J Periodontol,* 2003, 74(3):372-7.

Jenkins WM, MacFarlane TW, Gilmour WH, et al, "Systemic Metronidazole in the Treatment of Periodontitis," *J Clin Periodontol,* 1989, 16(7):433-50.

Loesche WJ, Giordano JR, Hujoel P, et al, "Metronidazole in Periodontitis: Reduced Need for Surgery," *J Clin Periodontol,* 1992, 19(2):103-12.

Loesche WJ, Schmidt E, Smith BA, et al, "Effects of Metronidazole on Periodontal Treatment Needs," *J Periodontol,* 1991, 62(4):247-57.

Noiri Y, Okami Y, Narimatsu M, et al, "Effects of Chlorhexidine, Minocycline, and Metronidazole on Porphyromonas Gingivalis Strain 381 in Biofilms," *J Periodontol,* 2003, 74(11):1647-51.

Soder PO, Frithiof L, Wikner S, et al, "The Effect of Systemic Metronidazole After Nonsurgical Treatment in Moderate and Advanced Periodontitis in Young Adults," *J Periodontol,* 1990, 61(5):281-8.

Wynn RL, Bergman SA, Meiller TF, et al, "Antibiotics in Treating Oral-Facial Infections of Odontogenic Origin: An Update," *Gen Dent,* 2001, 49(3):238-40, 242, 244 passim.

Metronidazole and Nystatin (met roe NYE da zole & nye STAT in)

Related Information

Metronidazole *on page 1091*

Nystatin *on page 1194*

Canadian Brand Names Flagystatin®

Pharmacologic Category Antifungal Agent, Vaginal; Antiprotozoal, Nitroimidazole

Use Treatment of mixed vaginal infection due to *T. vaginalis* and *C. albicans*

Local Anesthetic/Vasoconstrictor Precautions No information available to require special precautions

Effects on Dental Treatment Key adverse event(s) related to dental treatment: Taste disturbances (bitter) and coated tongue.

Common Adverse Effects Note: Adverse effects are infrequent and generally minor.

Central nervous system: Headache

Dermatologic: Pruritus, spots on skin (around knees), welts on body

Gastrointestinal: Coated tongue, nausea, taste disturbance (bitter), vomiting

Genitourinary: Vaginal: Burning, granular sensation

Neuromuscular & skeletal: Fatigue, swelling/aching or wrists

Restrictions Not available in U.S.

Mechanism of Action See individual agents.

Drug Interactions

Increased Effect/Toxicity: See individual agents. Due to low systemic absorption, the risk for interaction with other drugs is considered very low.

Metronidazole, Bismuth Subsalicylate, and Tetracycline *see* Bismuth Subsalicylate, Metronidazole, and Tetracycline *on page 218*

Metronidazole Hydrochloride *see* Metronidazole *on page 1091*

Metyrosine (me TYE roe seen)

U.S. Brand Names Demser®

Canadian Brand Names Demser®

Generic Available No

Index Terms AMPT; OGMT

Pharmacologic Category Tyrosine Hydroxylase Inhibitor

Use Short-term management of pheochromocytoma before surgery, long-term management when surgery is contraindicated or when chronic malignant pheochromocytoma exists

Local Anesthetic/Vasoconstrictor Precautions No information available to require special precautions

Effects on Dental Treatment Key adverse event(s) related to dental treatment: Xerostomia (normal salivary flow resumes upon discontinuation).

Common Adverse Effects

>10%:
Central nervous system: Drowsiness, extrapyramidal symptoms
Gastrointestinal: Diarrhea

1% to 10%:
Endocrine & metabolic: Galactorrhea, edema of the breasts
Gastrointestinal: Nausea, vomiting, xerostomia
Genitourinary: Impotence
Respiratory: Nasal congestion

Mechanism of Action Blocks the rate-limiting step in the biosynthetic pathway of catecholamines. It is a tyrosine hydroxylase inhibitor, blocking the conversion of tyrosine to dihydroxyphenylalanine. This inhibition results in decreased levels of endogenous catecholamines. Catecholamine biosynthesis is reduced by 35% to 80% in patients treated with metyrosine 1-4 g/day.

Drug Interactions
Increased Effect/Toxicity: Phenothiazines, haloperidol may potentiate EPS

Pharmacodynamics/Kinetics
Half-life elimination: 7.2 hours
Excretion: Primarily urine (as unchanged drug)

Pregnancy Risk Factor C

Mevacor® see Lovastatin on page 1007
Mevinolin see Lovastatin on page 1007
Mexar™ Wash see Sulfacetamide on page 1502

Mexiletine (meks IL e teen)

U.S. Brand Names Mexitil® [DSC]
Canadian Brand Names Novo-Mexiletine
Generic Available Yes
Pharmacologic Category Antiarrhythmic Agent, Class Ib
Use Management of serious ventricular arrhythmias; suppression of PVCs
Unlabeled/Investigational Use Diabetic neuropathy

Local Anesthetic/Vasoconstrictor Precautions No information available to require special precautions

Effects on Dental Treatment Key adverse event(s) related to dental treatment: Xerostomia (normal salivary flow resumes upon discontinuation).

Common Adverse Effects

>10%:
Central nervous system: Lightheadedness (11% to 25%), dizziness (20% to 25%), nervousness (5% to 10%), incoordination (10%)
Gastrointestinal: GI distress (41%), nausea/vomiting (40%)
Neuromuscular & skeletal: Trembling, unsteady gait, tremor (13%), ataxia (10% to 20%)

1% to 10%:
Cardiovascular: Chest pain (3% to 8%), premature ventricular contractions (1% to 2%), palpitation (4% to 8%), angina (2%), proarrhythmia (10% to 15% in patients with malignant arrhythmia)
Central nervous system: Confusion, headache, insomnia (5% to 7%), depression (2%)
Dermatologic: Rash (4%)
Gastrointestinal: Constipation or diarrhea (4% to 5%), xerostomia (3%), abdominal pain (1%)
Neuromuscular & skeletal: Weakness (5%), numbness of fingers or toes (2% to 4%), paresthesia (2%), arthralgia (1%)
Ocular: Blurred vision (5% to 7%), nystagmus (6%)
Otic: Tinnitus (2% to 3%)
Respiratory: Dyspnea (3%)

Mechanism of Action Class IB antiarrhythmic, structurally related to lidocaine, which inhibits inward sodium current, decreases rate of rise of phase 0, increases effective refractory period/action potential duration ratio

Drug Interactions
Cytochrome P450 Effect: Substrate (major) of CYP1A2, 2D6; Inhibits CYP1A2 (strong)
Increased Effect/Toxicity: Mexiletine may increase the levels/effects of aminophylline, fluvoxamine, mirtazapine, ropinirole, trifluoperazine, or other CYP1A2 substrates. The levels/effects of mexiletine may be increased by inhibitors of CYP1A2 or 2D6; example inhibitors include chlorpromazine, (Continued)

Mexiletine *(Continued)*

ciprofloxacin, delavirdine, fluoxetine, fluvoxamine, ketoconazole, miconazole, norfloxacin, ofloxacin, paroxetine, pergolide, quinidine, quinine, ritonavir, rofecoxib, ropinirole, and other CYP1A2 or 2D6 inhibitors. Mexiletine may increase levels of theophylline and caffeine. Quinidine and urinary alkalinizers (antacids, sodium bicarbonate, acetazolamide) may increase mexiletine blood levels.

Decreased Effect: The levels/effects of mexiletine may be decreased by aminoglutethimide, carbamazepine, phenobarbital, rifampin, and other CYP1A2 inducers. Urinary acidifying agents may decrease mexiletine levels.

Pharmacodynamics/Kinetics

Absorption: Elderly have a slightly slower rate, but extent of absorption is the same as young adults

Distribution: V_d: 5-7 L/kg

Protein binding: 50% to 70%

Metabolism: Hepatic; low first-pass effect

Half-life elimination: Adults: 10-14 hours (average: elderly: 14.4 hours, younger adults: 12 hours); prolonged with hepatic impairment or heart failure

Time to peak: 2-3 hours

Excretion: Urine (10% to 15% as unchanged drug); urinary acidification increases excretion, alkalinization decreases excretion

Pregnancy Risk Factor C

Micafungin *(mi ka FUN gin)*

U.S. Brand Names Mycamine®

Generic Available No

Index Terms Micafungin Sodium

Pharmacologic Category Antifungal Agent, Parenteral; Echinocandin

Use Esophageal candidiasis; *Candida* prophylaxis in patients undergoing hematopoietic stem cell transplant

Unlabeled/Investigational Use Treatment of infections due to *Aspergillus* spp; prophylaxis of HIV-related esophageal candidiasis

Local Anesthetic/Vasoconstrictor Precautions No information available to require special precautions

Effects on Dental Treatment No significant effects or complications reported

Common Adverse Effects 1% to 10%:

Cardiovascular: Phlebitis (2%), hypertension (1%), flushing (1%)

Central nervous system: Headache (2%), pyrexia (2%), delirium (1%), dizziness (1%), somnolence (1%)

Dermatologic: Rash (2%), pruritus (1%), febrile neutropenia (1%)

Endocrine & metabolic: Hypokalemia (1%), hypocalcemia (1%), hypomagnesemia (1%), hypophosphatemia (1%)

Gastrointestinal: Nausea (3%), diarrhea (2%), vomiting (2%), abdominal pain (1%), appetite decreased (1%), dysgeusia (1%), dyspepsia (1%)

Hematologic: Leukopenia (2%), neutropenia (1%), thrombocytopenia (1%), anemia (1%), lymphopenia (1%), eosinophilia (1%)

Hepatic: Transaminase increased (2% to 3%), serum alkaline phosphatase increased (2%), hyperbilirubinemia (1%)

Local: Infusion site inflammation (1%)

Neuromuscular & skeletal: Rigors (1%), lactate dehydrogenase increased (1%)

Renal: Serum creatinine increased (1%), serum urea increased (1%)

Mechanism of Action Concentration-dependent inhibition of 1,3-beta-D-glucan synthase resulting in reduced formation of 1,3-beta-D-glucan, an essential polysaccharide comprising 30% to 60% of *Candida* cell walls (absent in mammalian cells); decreased glucan content leads to osmotic instability and cellular lysis

Drug Interactions
  Cytochrome P450 Effect: Substrate of CYP3A4 (minor); **Inhibits** CYP3A4 (weak)
  Increased Effect/Toxicity: No clinically-significant interactions have been identified.
  Decreased Effect: No clinically-signficant interactions have been identified.
Pharmacodynamics/Kinetics
  Distribution: 0.28-0.5 L/kg
  Protein binding: >99%
  Metabolism: Hepatic; forms M-1 (catechol) and M-2 (methoxy) metabolites (activity unknown)
  Half-life elimination: 11-21 hours
  Excretion: Primarily feces (71%), urine (<15%, unchanged drug)
Pregnancy Risk Factor C

Micafungin Sodium *see Micafungin on page 1096*

Micardis® *see Telmisartan on page 1531*

Micardis® HCT *see Telmisartan and Hydrochlorothiazide on page 1532*

Micatin® Athlete's Foot [OTC] *see Miconazole on page 1097*

Micatin® Jock Itch [OTC] *see Miconazole on page 1097*

Miconazole (mi KON a zole)

Related Information
  Treatment of Sexually-Transmitted Infections *on page 1920*
U.S. Brand Names Aloe Vesta® 2-n-1 Antifungal [OTC]; Baza® Antifungal [OTC]; Carrington Antifungal [OTC]; DermaFungal [OTC]; Dermagran® AF [OTC]; DiabetAid™ Antifungal Foot Bath [OTC]; Fungoid® Tincture [OTC]; Lotrimin® AF Jock Itch Powder Spray [OTC]; Lotrimin® AF Powder/Spray [OTC]; Micaderm® [OTC]; Micatin® Athlete's Foot [OTC]; Micatin® Jock Itch [OTC]; Micro-Guard® [OTC]; Mitrazol™ [OTC]; Monistat® 1 Combination Pack [OTC]; Monistat® 3 [OTC]; Monistat® 3 Combination Pack [OTC]; Monistat® 7 [OTC]; Monistat-Derm® [DSC]; Neosporin® AF [OTC]; Podactin Cream [OTC]; Secura® Antifungal [OTC]; Zeasorb®-AF [OTC]
Canadian Brand Names Dermazole; Micatin®; Micozole; Monistat®; Monistat® 3
Mexican Brand Names Aloid; Daktarin; Neomicol
Generic Available Yes
Index Terms Miconazole Nitrate
Pharmacologic Category Antifungal Agent, Topical; Antifungal Agent, Vaginal
Use Treatment of vulvovaginal candidiasis and a variety of skin and mucous membrane fungal infections
Local Anesthetic/Vasoconstrictor Precautions No information available to require special precautions
Effects on Dental Treatment No significant effects or complications reported
Common Adverse Effects Frequency not defined.
  Topical: Allergic contact dermatitis, burning, maceration
  Vaginal: Abdominal cramps, burning, irritation, itching
Mechanism of Action Inhibits biosynthesis of ergosterol, damaging the fungal cell wall membrane, which increases permeability causing leaking of nutrients
Drug Interactions
  Cytochrome P450 Effect: Substrate of CYP3A4 (major); **Inhibits** CYP1A2 (moderate), 2A6 (strong), 2B6 (weak), 2C9 (strong), 2C19 (strong), 2D6 (strong), 2E1 (moderate), 3A4 (strong)
  Increased Effect/Toxicity: Note: The majority of reported drug interactions were observed following intravenous miconazole administration. Although systemic absorption following topical and/or vaginal administration is low, potential interactions due to CYP isoenzyme inhibition may occur (rarely). This may be particularly true in situations where topical absorption may be increased (ie, inflamed tissue).

  Miconazole coadministered with warfarin has increased the anticoagulant effect of warfarin (including reports associated with vaginal miconazole therapy of as little as 3 days). Concurrent administration of cisapride is contra-indicated due to an increased risk of cardiotoxicity. Miconazole may increase the serum levels/effects of amiodarone, amphetamines, benzodiazepines, beta-blockers, buspirone, busulfan, calcium channel blockers, citalopram, dexmedetomidine, dextromethorphan, diazepam, digoxin, docetaxel, fluoxe-tine, fluvoxamine, glimepiride, glipizide, ifosfamide, inhalational anesthetics, lidocaine, mesoridazine, methsuximide, mexiletine, mirtazapine, nateglinide, nefazodone, paroxetine, phenytoin, pioglitazone, propranolol, risperidone,
(Continued)

Miconazole (Continued)

ritonavir, ropinirole, rosiglitazone, sertraline, sirolimus, tacrolimus, theophylline, thioridazine, tricyclic antidepressants, trifluoperazine, trimetrexate, venlafaxine, vincristine, vinblastine, warfarin, zolpidem, and other substrates of CYP1A2, 2A6, 2C9, 2C19, 2D6, or 3A4. Selected benzodiazepines (midazolam and triazolam), cisapride, ergot alkaloids, selected HMG-CoA reductase inhibitors (lovastatin and simvastatin), and pimozide are generally contraindicated with strong CYP3A4 inhibitors. Mesoridazine and thioridazine are generally contraindicated with strong CYP2D6 inhibitors. When used with strong CYP3A4 inhibitors, dosage adjustment/limits are recommended for sildenafil and other PDE-5 inhibitors; consult individual monographs.

Decreased Effect: Amphotericin B may decrease antifungal effect of both agents. The levels/effects of miconazole may be decreased by aminoglutethimide, carbamazepine, nafcillin, nevirapine, phenobarbital, phenytoin, rifamycins or other CYP3A4 inducers. Miconazole may decrease the levels/effects of CYP2D6 prodrug substrates (eg, codeine, hydrocodone, oxycodone, tramadol).

Pharmacodynamics/Kinetics

Absorption: Topical: Negligible

Distribution: Widely to body tissues; penetrates well into inflamed joints, vitreous humor of eye, and peritoneal cavity, but poorly into saliva and sputum; crosses blood-brain barrier but only to a small extent

Protein binding: 91% to 93%

Metabolism: Hepatic

Half-life elimination: Multiphasic: Initial: 40 minutes; Secondary: 126 minutes; Terminal: 24 hours

Excretion: Feces (~50%); urine (<1% as unchanged drug)

Pregnancy Risk Factor C

Miconazole and Zinc Oxide (mi KON a zole & zink OKS ide)

U.S. Brand Names Vusion™

Generic Available No

Index Terms Zinc Oxide and Miconazole Nitrate

Pharmacologic Category Antifungal Agent, Topical

Use Adjunctive treatment of diaper dermatitis complicated by *Candida albicans* infection

Local Anesthetic/Vasoconstrictor Precautions No information available to require special precautions

Effects on Dental Treatment No significant effects or complications reported

Mechanism of Action

Miconazole inhibits the biosynthesis of ergosterol, damaging the fungal cell wall membrane.

Zinc oxide is a mild astringent with weak antiseptic properties.

Pharmacodynamics/Kinetics Absorption: Topical: Miconazole: Undetectable to 3.8 ng/mL in infants with dermatitis

Pregnancy Risk Factor C

Midazolam (MID aye zoe lam)

Canadian Brand Names Apo-Midazolam®; Midazolam Injection

Mexican Brand Names Dormicum; Hypnovel

Generic Available Yes

Index Terms Midazolam Hydrochloride; Versed

Pharmacologic Category Benzodiazepine

Dental Use Sedation component in I.V. conscious sedation in oral surgery patients; syrup formulation is used for children to help alleviate anxiety before a dental procedure

Use Preoperative sedation and provides conscious sedation prior to diagnostic or radiographic procedures; ICU sedation (continuous infusion); intravenous anesthesia (induction); intravenous anesthesia (maintenance)

Unlabeled/Investigational Use Anxiety, status epilepticus

Local Anesthetic/Vasoconstrictor Precautions No information available to require special precautions

Effects on Dental Treatment No significant effects or complications reported

Significant Adverse Effects As reported in adults unless otherwise noted:

>10%: Respiratory: Decreased tidal volume and/or respiratory rate decrease, apnea (3% children)

1% to 10%:

Cardiovascular: Hypotension (3% children)

Central nervous system: Drowsiness (1%), oversedation, headache (1%), seizure-like activity (1% children)

Gastrointestinal: Nausea (3%), vomiting (3%)

Local: Pain and local reactions at injection site (4% I.M., 5% I.V.; severity less than diazepam)

Ocular: Nystagmus (1% children)

Respiratory: Cough (1%)

Miscellaneous: Physical and psychological dependence with prolonged use, hiccups (4%, 1% children), paradoxical reaction (2% children)

<1% (Limited to important or life-threatening): Agitation, amnesia, bigeminy, bronchospasm, emergence delirium, euphoria, hallucinations, laryngospasm, rash

Restrictions C-IV

Dental Usual Dosing Adults:

Preoperative sedation:

I.M.: 0.07-0.08 mg/kg 30-60 minutes prior to surgery/procedure; usual dose: 5 mg; **Note:** Reduce dose in patients with COPD, high-risk patients, patients ≥60 years of age, and patients receiving other narcotics or CNS depressants

I.V.: 0.02-0.04 mg/kg; repeat every 5 minutes as needed to desired effect or up to 0.1-0.2 mg/kg

Intranasal (not an approved route): 0.2 mg/kg (up to 0.4 mg/kg in some studies); administer 30-45 minutes prior to surgery/procedure

Conscious sedation: I.V.: Initial: 0.5-2 mg slow I.V. over at least 2 minutes; slowly titrate to effect by repeating doses every 2-3 minutes if needed; usual total dose: 2.5-5 mg; use decreased doses in elderly.

Healthy Adults <60 years: Initial: Some patients respond to doses as low as 1 mg; no more than 2.5 mg should be administered over a period of 2 minutes. Additional doses of midazolam may be administered after a 2-minute waiting period and evaluation of sedation after each dose increment. A total dose >5 mg is generally not needed. If narcotics or other CNS depressants are administered concomitantly, the midazolam dose should be reduced by 30%.

Dosage The dose of midazolam needs to be individualized based on the patient's age, underlying diseases, and concurrent medications. Decrease dose (by ~30%) if narcotics or other CNS depressants are administered concomitantly. **Personnel and equipment needed for standard respiratory resuscitation should be immediately available during midazolam administration.**

Children <6 years may require higher doses and closer monitoring than older children; calculate dose on ideal body weight

Conscious sedation for procedures or preoperative sedation:

Oral: 0.25-0.5 mg/kg as a single dose preprocedure, up to a maximum of 20 mg; administer 30-45 minutes prior to procedure. Children <6 years or less cooperative patients may require as much as 1 mg/kg as a single dose; 0.25 mg/kg may suffice for children 6-16 years of age.

Intranasal (not an approved route): 0.2 mg/kg (up to 0.4 mg/kg in some studies), to a maximum of 15 mg; may be administered 30-45 minutes prior to procedure

I.M.: 0.1-0.15 mg/kg 30-60 minutes before surgery or procedure; range 0.05-0.15 mg/kg; doses up to 0.5 mg/kg have been used in more anxious patients; maximum total dose: 10 mg

I.V.:

Infants <6 months: Limited information is available in nonintubated infants; dosing recommendations not clear; infants <6 months are at higher risk for airway obstruction and hypoventilation; titrate dose in small increments to desired effect; monitor carefully

(Continued)

Midazolam *(Continued)*

Infants 6 months to Children 5 years: Initial: 0.05-0.1 mg/kg; titrate dose carefully; total dose of 0.6 mg/kg may be required; usual maximum total dose: 6 mg

Children 6-12 years: Initial: 0.025-0.05 mg/kg; titrate dose carefully; total doses of 0.4 mg/kg may be required; usual maximum total dose: 10 mg

Children 12-16 years: Dose as adults; usual maximum total dose: 10 mg

Conscious sedation during mechanical ventilation: Children: Loading dose: 0.05-0.2 mg/kg, followed by initial continuous infusion: 0.06-0.12 mg/kg/hour (1-2 mcg/kg/minute); titrate to the desired effect; usual range: 0.4-6 mcg/kg/minute

Status epilepticus refractory to standard therapy (unlabeled use): Infants >2 months and Children: Loading dose: 0.15 mg/kg followed by a continuous infusion of 1 mcg/kg/minute; titrate dose upward every 5 minutes until clinical seizure activity is controlled; mean infusion rate required in 24 children was 2.3 mcg/kg/minute with a range of 1-18 mcg/kg/minute

Adults:

Preoperative sedation:

I.M.: 0.07-0.08 mg/kg 30-60 minutes prior to surgery/procedure; usual dose: 5 mg; **Note:** Reduce dose in patients with COPD, high-risk patients, patients ≥60 years of age, and patients receiving other narcotics or CNS depressants

I.V.: 0.02-0.04 mg/kg; repeat every 5 minutes as needed to desired effect or up to 0.1-0.2 mg/kg

Intranasal (not an approved route): 0.2 mg/kg (up to 0.4 mg/kg in some studies); administer 30-45 minutes prior to surgery/procedure

Conscious sedation: I.V.: Initial: 0.5-2 mg slow I.V. over at least 2 minutes; slowly titrate to effect by repeating doses every 2-3 minutes if needed; usual total dose: 2.5-5 mg; use decreased doses in elderly

Healthy Adults <60 years: Some patients respond to doses as low as 1 mg; no more than 2.5 mg should be administered over a period of 2 minutes. Additional doses of midazolam may be administered after a 2-minute waiting period and evaluation of sedation after each dose increment. A total dose >5 mg is generally not needed. If narcotics or other CNS depressants are administered concomitantly, the midazolam dose should be reduced by 30%.

Anesthesia: I.V.:

Induction:

Unpremedicated patients: 0.3-0.35 mg/kg (up to 0.6 mg/kg in resistant cases)

Premedicated patients: 0.15-0.35 mg/kg

Maintenance: 0.05-0.3 mg/kg as needed, or continuous infusion 0.25-1.5 mcg/kg/minute

Sedation in mechanically-ventilated patients: I.V. continuous infusion: 100 mg in 250 mL D_5W or NS (if patient is fluid-restricted, may concentrate up to a maximum of 0.5 mg/mL); initial dose: 0.02-0.08 mg/kg (~1 mg to 5 mg in 70 kg adult) initially and either repeated at 5-15 minute intervals until adequate sedation is achieved or continuous infusion rates of 0.04-0.2 mg/kg/hour and titrate to reach desired level of sedation

Elderly: I.V.: Conscious sedation: Initial: 0.5 mg slow I.V.; give no more than 1.5 mg in a 2-minute period; if additional titration is needed, give no more than 1 mg over 2 minutes, waiting another 2 or more minutes to evaluate sedative effect; a total dose of >3.5 mg is rarely necessary

Dosage adjustment in renal impairment:

Hemodialysis: Supplemental dose is not necessary

Peritoneal dialysis: Significant drug removal is unlikely based on physiochemical characteristics

Mechanism of Action Binds to stereospecific benzodiazepine receptors on the postsynaptic GABA neuron at several sites within the central nervous system, including the limbic system, reticular formation. Enhancement of the inhibitory effect of GABA on neuronal excitability results by increased neuronal membrane permeability to chloride ions. This shift in chloride ions results in hyperpolarization (a less excitable state) and stabilization.

Contraindications Hypersensitivity to midazolam or any component of the formulation, including benzyl alcohol (cross-sensitivity with other benzodiazepines may exist); parenteral form is not for intrathecal or epidural injection; narrow-angle glaucoma; concurrent use of potent inhibitors of CYP3A4 (amprenavir, atazanavir, or ritonavir); pregnancy

Warnings/Precautions [U.S. Boxed Warning]: May cause severe respiratory depression, respiratory arrest, or apnea. Use with extreme caution, particularly in noncritical care settings. Appropriate resuscitative equipment and qualified personnel must be available for administration and monitoring.

Initial dosing must be cautiously titrated and individualized, particularly in elderly or debilitated patients, patients with hepatic impairment (including alcoholics), or in renal impairment, particularly if other CNS depressants (including opiates) are used concurrently. **[U.S. Boxed Warning]: Initial doses in elderly or debilitated patients should be conservative; as little as 1 mg, but not to exceed 2.5 mg.** Use with caution in patients with respiratory disease or impaired gag reflex. Use during upper airway procedures may increase risk of hypoventilation. Prolonged responses have been noted following extended administration by continuous infusion (possibly due to metabolite accumulation) or in the presence of drugs which inhibit midazolam metabolism.

Causes CNS depression (dose-related) resulting in sedation, dizziness, confusion, or ataxia which may impair physical and mental capabilities. Patients must be cautioned about performing tasks which require mental alertness (eg, operating machinery or driving). A minimum of 1 day should elapse after midazolam administration before attempting these tasks. Use with caution in patients receiving other CNS depressants or psychoactive agents. Effects with other sedative drugs or ethanol may be potentiated. Benzodiazepines have been associated with falls and traumatic injury and should be used with extreme caution in patients who are at risk of these events (especially the elderly).

May cause hypotension - hemodynamic events are more common in pediatric patients or patients with hemodynamic instability. Hypotension and/or respiratory depression may occur more frequently in patients who have received opioid analgesics. Use with caution in obese patients, chronic renal failure, and HF. Does not protect against increases in heart rate or blood pressure during intubation. Should not be used in shock, coma, or acute alcohol intoxication. **[U.S. Boxed Warning]: Parenteral form contains benzyl alcohol; avoid rapid injection in neonates or prolonged infusions.** Avoid intra-arterial administration or extravasation of parenteral formulation.

Midazolam causes anterograde amnesia. Paradoxical reactions, including hyperactive or aggressive behavior have been reported with benzodiazepines, particularly in adolescent/pediatric or psychiatric patients. Does not have analgesic, antidepressant, or antipsychotic properties.

Benzodiazepines have been associated with dependence and acute withdrawal symptoms on discontinuation or reduction in dose. Acute withdrawal, including seizures, may be precipitated after administration of flumazenil to patients receiving long-term benzodiazepine therapy.

Drug Interactions Substrate of CYP2B6 (minor), 3A4 (major); **Inhibits** CYP2C8 (weak), 2C9 (weak), 3A4 (weak)

CNS depressants: Sedative effects and/or respiratory depression may be additive with CNS depressants; includes ethanol, barbiturates, opioid analgesics, and other sedative agents; monitor for increased effect. **If narcotics or other CNS depressants are administered concomitantly, the midazolam dose should be reduced by 30% if <65 years of age, or by at least 50% if >65 years of age.**

CYP3A4 inducers: CYP3A4 inducers may decrease the levels/effects of midazolam. Example inducers include aminoglutethimide, carbamazepine, nafcillin, nevirapine, phenobarbital, phenytoin, and rifamycins.

CYP3A4 inhibitors: May increase the levels/effects of midazolam. Example inhibitors include azole antifungals, clarithromycin, diclofenac, doxycycline, erythromycin, imatinib, isoniazid, nefazodone, nicardipine, propofol, protease inhibitors, quinidine, telithromycin, and verapamil.

Levodopa: Therapeutic effects may be diminished in some patients following the addition of a benzodiazepine; limited/inconsistent data

Oral contraceptives: May decrease the clearance of some benzodiazepines (those which undergo oxidative metabolism); monitor for increased benzodiazepine effect

Saquinavir: A 56% reduction in clearance and a doubling of midazolam's half-life were seen with concurrent administration with saquinavir.

Theophylline: May partially antagonize some of the effects of benzodiazepines; monitor for decreased response; may require higher doses for sedation

Ethanol/Nutrition/Herb Interactions

Ethanol: Avoid ethanol (may increase CNS depression).

Food: Grapefruit juice may increase serum concentrations of midazolam; avoid concurrent use with oral form.

Herb/Nutraceutical: Avoid concurrent use with St John's wort (may decrease midazolam levels, may increase CNS depression). Avoid concurrent use with valerian, kava kava, gotu kola (may increase CNS depression).

Dietary Considerations Injection: Sodium content of 1 mL: 0.14 mEq

Pharmacodynamics/Kinetics

Onset of action: I.M.: Sedation: ~15 minutes; I.V.: 1-5 minutes

Peak effect: I.M.: 0.5-1 hour

Duration: I.M.: Up to 6 hours; Mean: 2 hours

(Continued)

Midazolam (Continued)

Absorption: Oral: Rapid

Distribution: V_d: 0.8-2.5 L/kg; increased with congestive heart failure (CHF) and chronic renal failure

Protein binding: 95%

Metabolism: Extensively hepatic via CYP3A4

Bioavailability: Mean: 45%

Half-life elimination: 1-4 hours; prolonged with cirrhosis, congestive heart failure, obesity, and elderly

Excretion: Urine (as glucuronide conjugated metabolites); feces (~2% to 10%)

Pregnancy Risk Factor D

Lactation Enters breast milk/not recommended (AAP rates "of concern")

Dosage Forms Excipient information presented when available (limited, particularly for generics); consult specific product labeling.

Injection, solution: 1 mg/mL (2 mL, 5 mL, 10 mL); 5 mg/mL (1 mL, 2 mL, 5 mL, 10 mL) [contains benzyl alcohol 1%]

Injection, solution [preservative free]: 1 mg/mL (2 mL, 5 mL); 5 mg/mL (1 mL, 2 mL)

Syrup: 2 mg/mL (118 mL) [contains sodium benzoate; cherry flavor]

Selected Readings

Dionne RA, Yagiela JA, Moore PA, et al, "Comparing Efficacy and Safety of Four Intravenous Sedation Regimens in Dental Outpatients," *Am Dent Assoc*, 2001, 132(6):740-51.

Midazolam Hydrochloride *see* Midazolam *on page 1098*

Midodrine (MI doe dreen)

U.S. Brand Names Orvaten™; ProAmatine®

Canadian Brand Names Amatine®; Apo-Midodrine®

Generic Available Yes

Index Terms Midodrine Hydrochloride

Pharmacologic Category Alpha₁ Agonist

Use Orphan drug: Treatment of symptomatic orthostatic hypotension

Unlabeled/Investigational Use Investigational: Management of urinary incontinence

Local Anesthetic/Vasoconstrictor Precautions No information available to require special precautions

Effects on Dental Treatment Key adverse event(s) related to dental treatment: Xerostomia (normal salivary flow resumes upon discontinuation).

Causes of Orthostatic Hypotension

Primary Autonomic Causes
Pure autonomic failure (Bradbury-Eggleston syndrome, idiopathic orthostatic hypotension)
Autonomic failure with multiple system atrophy (Shy-Drager syndrome)
Familial dysautonomia (Riley-Day syndrome)
Dopamine beta-hydroxylase deficiency
Secondary Autonomic Causes
Chronic alcoholism
Parkinson's disease
Diabetes mellitus
Porphyria
Amyloidosis
Various carcinomas
Vitamin B₁ or B₁₂ deficiency
Nonautonomic Causes
Hypovolemia (such as associated with hemorrhage, burns, or hemodialysis) and dehydration
Diminished homeostatic regulation (such as associated with aging, pregnancy, fever, or prolonged bedrest)
Medications (eg, antihypertensives, insulin, tricyclic antidepressants)

Common Adverse Effects

>10%:

Cardiovascular: Supine hypertension (7% to 13%)

Dermatologic: Piloerection (13%), pruritus (12%)

Genitourinary: Urinary urgency, retention, or polyuria, dysuria (up to 13%)

Neuromuscular & skeletal: Paresthesia (18%)

1% to 10%:
Central nervous system: Chills (5%), pain (5%)
Dermatologic: Rash (2%)
Gastrointestinal: Abdominal pain

Mechanism of Action Midodrine forms an active metabolite, desglymidodrine, that is an alpha$_1$-agonist. This agent increases arteriolar and venous tone resulting in a rise in standing, sitting, and supine systolic and diastolic blood pressure in patients with orthostatic hypotension. See table on previous page.

Drug Interactions

Increased Effect/Toxicity: Concomitant fludrocortisone results in hypernatremia or an increase in intraocular pressure and glaucoma. Bradycardia may be accentuated with concomitant administration of cardiac glycosides, psychotherapeutics, and beta-blockers. Alpha agonists may increase the pressure effects and alpha antagonists may negate the effects of midodrine.

Pharmacodynamics/Kinetics

Onset of action: ~1 hour

Duration: 2-3 hours

Absorption: Rapid

Distribution: V_d (desglymidodrine): <1.6 L/kg; poorly across membrane (eg, blood brain barrier)

Protein binding: Minimal

Metabolism: Hepatic; midodrine is a prodrug which undergoes rapid deglycination to desglymidodrine (active metabolite); metabolism occurs in many tissues and plasma

Bioavailability: Desglymidodrine: 93%

Half-life elimination: Desglymidodrine: ~3-4 hours; Midodrine: 25 minutes

Time to peak, serum: Desglymidodrine: 1-2 hours; Midodrine: 30 minutes

Excretion: Urine (2% to 4%)

Clearance: Desglymidodrine: 385 mL/minute (predominantly by renal secretion)

Pregnancy Risk Factor C

Midodrine Hydrochloride *see* Midodrine *on page 1102*

Midol® Cramp and Body Aches [OTC] *see* Ibuprofen *on page 853*

Midol® Extended Relief *see* Naproxen *on page 1148*

Midrin® *see* Acetaminophen, Isometheptene, and Dichloralphenazone *on page 45*

Mifeprex® *see* Mifepristone *on page 1103*

Mifepristone (mi FE pris tone)

Related Information
Endocrine Disorders and Pregnancy *on page 1750*

U.S. Brand Names Mifeprex®

Generic Available No

Index Terms RU-486; RU-38486

Pharmacologic Category Abortifacient; Antineoplastic Agent, Hormone Antagonist; Antiprogestin

Use Medical termination of intrauterine pregnancy, through day 49 of pregnancy. Patients may need treatment with misoprostol and possibly surgery to complete therapy

Unlabeled/Investigational Use Treatment of unresectable meningioma; has been studied in the treatment of breast cancer, ovarian cancer, and adrenal cortical carcinoma

Local Anesthetic/Vasoconstrictor Precautions No information available to require special precautions

Effects on Dental Treatment No significant effects or complications reported

Common Adverse Effects Vaginal bleeding and uterine cramping are expected to occur when this medication is used to terminate a pregnancy; 90% of women using this medication for this purpose also report adverse reactions. Bleeding or spotting occurs in most women for a period of 9-16 days. Up to 8% of women will experience some degree of bleeding or spotting for 30 days or more. In some cases, bleeding may be prolonged and heavy, potentially leading to hypovolemic shock.

>10%:
Central nervous system: Headache (2% to 31%), dizziness (1% to 12%)
Gastrointestinal: Abdominal pain (cramping) (96%), nausea (43% to 61%), vomiting (18% to 26%), diarrhea (12% to 20%)
Genitourinary: Uterine cramping (83%)

1% to 10%:
Cardiovascular: Syncope (1%)

(Continued)

Mifepristone *(Continued)*

Central nervous system: Fatigue (10%), fever (4%), insomnia (3%), anxiety (2%), fainting (2%)

Gastrointestinal: Dyspepsia (3%)

Genitourinary: Uterine hemorrhage (5%), vaginitis (3%), pelvic pain (2%), endometriosis/salpingitis/pelvic inflammatory disease (1%)

Hematologic: Decreased hemoglobin >2 g/dL (6%), anemia (2%), leukorrhea (2%)

Neuromuscular & skeletal: Back pain (9%), rigors (3%), leg pain (2%), weakness (2%)

Respiratory: Sinusitis (2%)

Miscellaneous: Viral infection (4%)

Restrictions Investigators wishing to obtain the agent for use in oncology patients must apply for a patient-specific IND from the FDA. Mifepristone will be supplied only to licensed physicians who sign and return a "Prescriber's Agreement." Distribution of mifepristone will be subject to specific requirements imposed by the distributor. Mifepristone will **not** be available to the public through licensed pharmacies. An FDA-approved medication guide must be distributed when dispensing an outpatient prescription (new or refill) where this medication is to be used without direct supervision of a healthcare provider. Medication guides are available at http://www.fda.gov/cder/Offices/ODS/medication_guides.htm.

Not available in Canada

Mechanism of Action Mifepristone, a synthetic steroid, competitively binds to the intracellular progesterone receptor, blocking the effects of progesterone. When used for the termination of pregnancy, this leads to contraction-inducing activity in the myometrium. In the absence of progesterone, mifepristone acts as a partial progesterone agonist. Mifepristone also has weak antiglucocorticoid and antiandrogenic properties; it blocks the feedback effect of cortisol on corticotropin secretion.

Drug Interactions

Cytochrome P450 Effect: Substrate of CYP3A4 (minor); **Inhibits** CYP2D6 (weak), 3A4 (weak)

Increased Effect/Toxicity: There are no reported interactions. It might be anticipated that the concurrent administration of mifepristone and a progestin would result in an attenuation of the effects of one or both agents.

Pharmacodynamics/Kinetics

Absorption: Oral: rapid

Protein binding: 98% to albumin and α_1-acid glycoprotein

Metabolism: Hepatic via CYP3A4 to three metabolites (may possess some antiprogestin and antiglucocorticoid activity)

Bioavailability: Oral: 69%

Half-life elimination: Terminal: 18 hours following a slower phase where 50% eliminated between 12-72 hours

Time to peak: Oral: 90 minutes

Excretion: Feces (83%); urine (9%)

Pregnancy Risk Factor X

Migergot *see* Ergotamine and Caffeine *on page 586*

Miglitol *(MIG li tol)*

Related Information

Endocrine Disorders and Pregnancy *on page 1750*

U.S. Brand Names Glyset®

Canadian Brand Names Glyset®

Mexican Brand Names Diastabol

Generic Available No

Pharmacologic Category Antidiabetic Agent, Alpha-Glucosidase Inhibitor

Use Type 2 diabetes mellitus (noninsulin-dependent, NIDDM):

Monotherapy adjunct to diet to improve glycemic control in patients with type 2 diabetes mellitus (noninsulin-dependent, NIDDM) whose hyperglycemia cannot be managed with diet alone

Combination therapy with a sulfonylurea when diet plus either miglitol or a sulfonylurea alone do not result in adequate glycemic control. The effect of miglitol to enhance glycemic control is additive to that of sulfonylureas when used in combination.

Local Anesthetic/Vasoconstrictor Precautions No information available to require special precautions

Effects on Dental Treatment No significant effects or complications reported

Common Adverse Effects

>10%: Gastrointestinal: Flatulence (42%), diarrhea (29%), abdominal pain (12%)

1% to 10%: Dermatologic: Rash

Mechanism of Action In contrast to sulfonylureas, miglitol does not enhance insulin secretion; the antihyperglycemic action of miglitol results from a reversible inhibition of membrane-bound intestinal alpha-glucosidases which hydrolyze oligosaccharides and disaccharides to glucose and other monosaccharides in the brush border of the small intestine; in diabetic patients, this enzyme inhibition results in delayed glucose absorption and lowering of postprandial hyperglycemia

Drug Interactions

Decreased Effect: Miglitol may decrease the absorption and bioavailability of digoxin, propranolol, and ranitidine. Digestive enzymes (amylase, pancreatin, charcoal) may reduce the effect of miglitol and should **not** be taken concomitantly.

Pharmacodynamics/Kinetics

Absorption: Saturable at high doses: 25 mg dose: Completely absorbed; 100 mg dose: 50% to 70% absorbed

Distribution: V_d: 0.18 L/kg

Protein binding: <4%

Metabolism: None

Half-life elimination: ~2 hours

Time to peak: 2-3 hours

Excretion: Urine (as unchanged drug)

Pregnancy Risk Factor B

Miglustat (MIG loo stat)

U.S. Brand Names Zavesca®

Canadian Brand Names Zavesca®

Generic Available No

Index Terms OGT-918

Pharmacologic Category Enzyme Inhibitor

Use Treatment of mild-to-moderate type 1 Gaucher disease when enzyme replacement therapy is not a therapeutic option

Local Anesthetic/Vasoconstrictor Precautions No information available to require special precautions

Effects on Dental Treatment No significant effects or complications reported

Common Adverse Effects Percentages reported from open-label, uncontrolled monotherapy trials.

>10%:

Central nervous system: Headache (21% to 22%), dizziness (up to 11%)

Gastrointestinal: Diarrhea (89%; up to 100% in other studies), weight loss (39% to 67%), abdominal pain (18% to 50%), flatulence (29% to 44%), nausea (14% to 22%), vomiting (4% to 11%), cramps (up to 11%)

Neuromuscular & skeletal: Tremor (11%; up to 30% in other studies), leg cramps (4% to 11%)

Ocular: visual disturbances (up to 17%)

1% to 10%:

Central nervous system: headache (up to 6%)

Endocrine & metabolic: Menstrual disorder (up to 6%)

Gastrointestinal: Anorexia (up to 7%), dyspepsia (up to 7%), epigastric pain (up to 6%)

Hematologic: Thrombocytopenia (6% to 7%)

Neuromuscular & skeletal: Paresthesia (up to 7%)

Mechanism of Action Miglustat inhibits the enzyme needed to produce glycosphingolipids and decreases the rate of glycosphingolipid glucosylceramide formation. Glucosylceramide accumulates in type 1 Gaucher disease, causing complications specific to this disease.

Drug Interactions

Decreased Effect: Miglustat increases the clearance of imiglucerase; combination therapy is not indicated.

Pharmacodynamics/Kinetics

Distribution: V_d: 83-105 L

Protein binding: No binding to plasma proteins

Bioavailability: 97%

Half-life elimination: 6-7 hours

Time to peak, plasma: 2-2.5 hours

Excretion: Urine (as unchanged drug)

Pregnancy Risk Factor X

Milrinone (MIL ri none)

Related Information
Cardiovascular Diseases *on page 1726*

U.S. Brand Names Primacor®

Canadian Brand Names Milrinone Lactate Injection; Primacor®

Generic Available Yes

Index Terms Milrinone Lactate

Pharmacologic Category Phosphodiesterase Enzyme Inhibitor

Use Short-term I.V. therapy of congestive heart failure; calcium antagonist intoxication

Local Anesthetic/Vasoconstrictor Precautions No information available to require special precautions

Effects on Dental Treatment No significant effects or complications reported

Common Adverse Effects
>10%: Cardiovascular: Ventricular arrhythmia (ectopy 9%, NSVT 3%, sustained ventricular tachycardia 1%, ventricular fibrillation <1%); life-threatening arrhythmia are infrequent, often associated with underlying factors (eg, pre-existing arrhythmia, electrolyte disturbances, catheter insertion)

1% to 10%:
Cardiovascular: Supraventricular arrhythmia (4%), hypotension
Central nervous system: Headache

Mechanism of Action Phosphodiesterase inhibitor resulting in vasodilation

Pharmacodynamics/Kinetics
Onset of action: I.V.: 5-15 minutes

Serum level: Following a 125 mcg/kg dose, peak plasma concentrations ~1000 ng/mL were observed at 2 minutes postinjection, decreasing to <100 ng/mL in 2 hours

Drug concentration levels:
Therapeutic:
Serum levels of 166 ng/mL, achieved during I.V. infusions of 0.25-1 mcg/kg/minute, were associated with sustained hemodynamic benefit in severe congestive heart failure patients over a 24-hour period
Maximum beneficial effects on cardiac output and pulmonary capillary wedge pressure following I.V. infusion have been associated with plasma milrinone concentrations of 150-250 ng/mL

Toxic: Serum concentrations >250-300 ng/mL have been associated with marked reductions in mean arterial pressure and tachycardia; however, more studies are required to determine the toxic serum levels for milrinone

Distribution: V_{dss}: 0.32 L/kg; Severe congestive heart failure (CHF): V_d: 0.33-0.47 L/kg; not significantly bound to tissues; excretion in breast milk unknown

Protein binding, plasma: ~70%

Metabolism: Hepatic (12%)

Half-life elimination: I.V.: 136 minutes in patients with CHF; patients with severe CHF have a more prolonged half-life, with values ranging from 1.7-2.7 hours. Patients with CHF have a reduction in the systemic clearance of milrinone, resulting in a prolonged elimination half-life. Alternatively, one study reported that 1 month of therapy with milrinone did not change the pharmacokinetic parameters for patients with CHF despite improvement in cardiac function.

Excretion: I.V.: Urine (85% as unchanged drug) within 24 hours; active tubular secretion is a major elimination pathway for milrinone

Clearance: I.V. bolus: 25.9 ± 5.7 L/hour (0.37 L/hour/kg); Severe congestive heart failure: 0.11-0.13 L/hour/kg. The reduction in clearance may be a result of reduced renal function. Creatinine clearance values were 1/2 those reported for healthy adults in patients with severe congestive heart failure (52 vs 119 mL/minute).

Pregnancy Risk Factor C

Mineral Oil, Petrolatum, Lanolin, Cetyl Alcohol, and Glycerin see Lanolin, Cetyl Alcohol, Glycerin, Petrolatum, and Mineral Oil on page 946

Minidyne® [OTC] see Povidone-Iodine on page 1332

Minipress® see Prazosin on page 1337

Minitran™ see Nitroglycerin on page 1181

Minizide® [DSC] see Prazosin and Polythiazide on page 1338

Minocin® PAC see Minocycline on page 1107

Minocycline (mi noe SYE kleen)

Related Sample Prescriptions
Bacterial Infections and Periodontal Diseases on page 1837

U.S. Brand Names Dynacin®; Minocin® PAC; myrac™; Solodyn™

Canadian Brand Names Alti-Minocycline; Apo-Minocycline®; Gen-Minocycline; Minocin®; Novo-Minocycline; PMS-Minocycline; Rhoxal-minocycline; Sandoz-Minocycline

Mexican Brand Names Micromycin; Minocin

Generic Available Yes: Excludes extended release tablet

Index Terms Minocycline Hydrochloride

Pharmacologic Category Antibiotic, Tetracycline Derivative

Use Treatment of susceptible bacterial infections of both gram-negative and gram-positive organisms; treatment of anthrax (inhalational, cutaneous, and gastrointestinal); acne; meningococcal (asymptomatic) carrier state; Rickettsial diseases (including Rocky Mountain spotted fever, Q fever); nongonococcal urethritis, gonorrhea; acute intestinal amebiasis

Local Anesthetic/Vasoconstrictor Precautions No information available to require special precautions

Effects on Dental Treatment Key adverse event(s) related to dental treatment: Discoloration of teeth (children). Opportunistic "superinfection" with *Candida albicans*; tetracyclines are not recommended for use during pregnancy or in children ≤8 years of age since they have been reported to cause enamel hypoplasia and permanent teeth discoloration. The use of tetracycline's should only be used in these patients if other agents are contraindicated or alternative antimicrobials will not eradicate the organism. Long-term use associated with oral candidiasis.

Common Adverse Effects Frequency not defined.

Cardiovascular: Myocarditis, pericarditis, vasculitis

Central nervous system: Bulging fontanels, dizziness, fatigue, fever, headache, hypoesthesia, malaise, mood changes, paresthesia, pseudotumor cerebri, sedation, seizure, somnolence, vertigo

Dermatologic: Alopecia, angioedema, erythema multiforme, erythema nodosum, erythematous rash, exfoliative dermatitis, hyperpigmentation of nails, maculopapular rash, photosensitivity, pigmentation of the skin and mucous membranes, pruritus, Stevens-Johnson syndrome, toxic epidermal necrolysis, urticaria

Endocrine & metabolic: Thyroid discoloration, thyroid dysfunction

Gastrointestinal: Anorexia, diarrhea, dyspepsia, dysphagia, enamel hypoplasia, enterocolitis, esophageal ulcerations, esophagitis, glossitis, inflammatory lesions (oral/anogenital), moniliasis, nausea, oral cavity discoloration, pancreatitis, pseudomembranous colitis, stomatitis, tooth discoloration, vomiting, xerostomia

Genitourinary: Balanitis, vulvovaginitis

Hematologic: Agranulocytosis, eosinophilia, hemolytic anemia, leukopenia, neutropenia, pancytopenia, thrombocytopenia

Hepatic: Hepatic cholestasis, hepatic failure, hepatitis, hyperbilirubinemia, jaundice, liver enzyme increases

Neuromuscular & skeletal: Arthralgia, arthritis, bone discoloration, joint stiffness, joint swelling, myalgia

Otic: Hearing loss, tinnitus

Renal: Acute renal failure, BUN increased, interstitial nephritis

Respiratory: Asthma, bronchospasm, cough, dyspnea, pneumonitis, pulmonary infiltrate (with eosinophilia)

Miscellaneous: Anaphylaxis, hypersensitivity, lupus erythematosus, lupus-like syndrome, serum sickness

Mechanism of Action Inhibits bacterial protein synthesis by binding with the 30S and possibly the 50S ribosomal subunit(s) of susceptible bacteria; cell wall synthesis is not affected

Drug Interactions

Increased Effect/Toxicity: Minocycline may increase the effect of warfarin. Retinoic acid derivatives may increase risk of pseudotumor cerebri.

(Continued)

Minocycline *(Continued)*

Decreased Effect: Calcium-, magnesium-, or aluminum-containing antacids, bile acid sequestrants, bismuth, oral contraceptives, iron, zinc, sodium bicarbonate, penicillins, cimetidine, quinapril may decrease absorption of tetracyclines. Methoxyflurane anesthesia (when concurrent with tetracyclines) may cause fatal nephrotoxicity. Tetracyclines may reduce bactericidal efficacy of penicillins and cephalosporins. Tetracycline may reduce the efficacy of the live, attenuated typhoid vaccine (Ty21a).

Pharmacodynamics/Kinetics

Absorption: Well absorbed

Protein binding: 70% to 75%

Metabolism: Hepatic to inactive metabolites

Half-life elimination: 16 hours (range: 11-23 hours)

Time to peak: Capsule, pellet filled: 1-4 hours; Extended release tablet: 3.5-4 hours

Excretion: Urine, feces

Pregnancy Risk Factor D

Minocycline Hydrochloride *see* Minocycline *on page 1107*

Minocycline Hydrochloride (Periodontal)

(mi noe SYE kleen hye droe KLOR ide pair ee oh DON tol)

Related Information

Minocycline *on page 1107*
Periodontal Diseases *on page 1801*

U.S. Brand Names Arestin™

Generic Available No

Pharmacologic Category Antibiotic, Tetracycline Derivative

Dental Use Adjunct to scaling and root planing procedures for reduction of pocket depth in patients with adult periodontitis. May be used as part of a periodontal maintenance program which includes good oral hygiene, scaling, and root planing.

Local Anesthetic/Vasoconstrictor Precautions No information available to require special precautions

Effects on Dental Treatment Key adverse event(s) related to dental treatment: Patients should avoid the following postadministration: Eating hard, crunchy, or sticky foods for 1 week; brushing for a 12-hour period; touching treated areas; use of interproximal cleaning devices for 10 days.

Significant Adverse Effects Frequency not defined.

Central nervous system: Headache, pain

Gastrointestinal: Periodontitis, tooth disorder, dental caries, dental pain, gingivitis, stomatitis, mouth ulceration, dyspepsia, dental infection, mucous membrane disorder

Respiratory: Pharyngitis

Miscellaneous: Infection, flu syndrome

Dental Usual Dosing Arestin™ is a variable-dose product; dependent upon the size, shape, and number of pockets being treated.

Administration of Arestin™ does not require local anesthesia. Professional subgingival administration is accomplished by inserting the unit-dose cartridge to the base of the periodontal pocket and then pressing the thumb ring in the handle mechanism to expel the powder while gradually withdrawing the tip from the base of the pocket. The handle mechanism should be sterilized between patients. Arestin™ does not have to be removed (it is bioresorbable) nor is an adhesive dressing required.

Dosage Variable-dose product; dependent upon the size, shape, and number of pockets being treated

Mechanism of Action Minocycline, a member of the tetracycline class of antibiotics, has a broad spectrum of activity. It is bacteriostatic and exerts its antimicrobial activity by inhibiting protein synthesis.

Contraindications Known hypersensitivity to minocycline, tetracyclines, or any component of the formulation; pregnancy

Warnings/Precautions The use of the tetracycline class during tooth development (last half of pregnancy, infancy, and childhood to 8 years of age) may cause permanent discoloration of the teeth (yellow-gray brown). This adverse reaction is more common during long-term use of the drugs, but has been observed following repeated short-term courses. Enamel hypoplasia has also been reported. Tetracycline drugs, therefore, should not be used in this age group, or in pregnant or nursing women, unless the potential benefits are considered to outweigh the potential risks. Results of animal studies indicate that tetracyclines cross the placenta, are found in fetal tissues, and can have toxic effects on the developing fetus (often related to retardation of skeletal development). Evidence of embryotoxicity has also been noted in animals treated early in pregnancy. If any tetracyclines are used during pregnancy, or if the patient becomes pregnant while taking this drug, the patient should be apprised of the potential hazard to the fetus. Photosensitivity manifested by an exaggerated sunburn reaction has been observed in some individuals taking tetracyclines. Patients apt to be exposed to direct sunlight or ultraviolet light should be advised that this reaction can occur with tetracycline drugs, and treatment should be discontinued at the first evidence of skin erythema.

The use of Arestin™ in an acutely abscessed periodontal pocket has not been studied and is not recommended. While not observed in clinical trials, prolonged use may result in fungal or bacterial superinfection, including *C. diffi-cile*-associated diarrhea and pseudomembranous colitis. The effects of treatment for >6 months have not been studied. Arestin™ should be used with caution in patients having a history of predisposition to oral candidiasis. The safety and effectiveness of Arestin™ have not been established for the treatment of periodontitis in patients with coexistent oral candidiasis. Arestin™ has not been clinically tested in immunocompromised patients (such as those immunocompromised by diabetes, chemotherapy, radiation therapy, or infection with HIV). Arestin™ has not been clinically tested for use in the regeneration of alveolar bone, either in preparation for or in conjunction with the placement of endosseous (dental) implants or in the treatment of failing implants.

Pregnancy Risk Factor D

Dosage Forms Excipient information presented when available (limited, particularly for generics); consult specific product labeling.

Injection, powder, sustained release [microspheres for subgingival application]: 1 mg (12s) [each unit-dose cartridge delivers minocycline hydrochloride equivalent to minocycline free base 1 mg]

Minoxidil (mi NOKS i dil)

Related Information
Cardiovascular Diseases *on page 1726*

U.S. Brand Names Rogaine® Extra Strength for Men [OTC]; Rogaine® for Men [OTC]; Rogaine® for Women [OTC]

Canadian Brand Names Apo-Gain®; Minox; Rogaine®

Generic Available Yes

Pharmacologic Category Topical Skin Product; Vasodilator

Use Management of severe hypertension (usually in combination with a diuretic and beta-blocker); treatment (topical formulation) of alopecia androgenetica in males and females

Local Anesthetic/Vasoconstrictor Precautions No information available to require special precautions

Effects on Dental Treatment No significant effects or complications reported

Common Adverse Effects

Oral: Incidence of reactions not always reported.

Cardiovascular: Peripheral edema (7%), sodium and water retention, CHF, tachycardia, angina pectoris, pericardial effusion with or without tamponade, pericarditis, ECG changes (T-wave changes, 60%), rebound hypertension (in children after a gradual withdrawal)

Central nervous system: Headache (rare), fatigue

Dermatologic: Hypertrichosis (common, 80%), transient pruritus, changes in pigmentation (rare), serosanguineous bullae (rare), rash (rare), Stevens-Johnson syndrome

Hepatic: Increased alkaline phosphatase

Renal: Transient increase in serum BUN and creatinine

Respiratory: Pulmonary edema

Topical: Incidence of adverse events is not always reported.

Cardiovascular: Increased left ventricular end-diastolic volume, increased cardiac output, increased left ventricular mass, dizziness, tachycardia, edema, transient chest pain, palpitation, increase or decrease in blood pressure, increase or decrease in pulse rate (1.5%, placebo 1.6%)

Central nervous system: Headache, dizziness, taste alterations, faintness, lightheadedness (3.4%, placebo 3.5%), vertigo (1.2%, placebo 1.2%), anxiety (rare), mental depression (rare), fatigue (rare 0.4%, placebo 1%)

Dermatologic: Local irritation, dryness, erythema, allergic contact dermatitis (7.4%, placebo 5.4%), pruritus, scaling/flaking, eczema, seborrhea, papular rash, folliculitis, local erythema, flushing, exacerbation of hair loss, alopecia, hypertrichosis, increased hair growth outside the area of application (face, beard, eyebrows, ear, arm)

Gastrointestinal: Diarrhea, nausea, vomiting (4.3%, placebo 6.6%), weight gain (1.2%, placebo 1.3%)

(Continued)

Minoxidil *(Continued)*

Neuromuscular & skeletal: Fractures, back pain, retrosternal chest pain of muscular origin, tendonitis (2.6%, placebo 2.2%), weakness

Ocular: Conjunctivitis, visual disturbances, decreased visual acuity

Respiratory: Bronchitis, upper respiratory infection, sinusitis (7.2%, placebo 8.6%)

Mechanism of Action Produces vasodilation by directly relaxing arteriolar smooth muscle, with little effect on veins; effects may be mediated by cyclic AMP; stimulation of hair growth is secondary to vasodilation, increased cutaneous blood flow and stimulation of resting hair follicles

Drug Interactions

Increased Effect/Toxicity: Concurrent use of guanethidine can cause severe orthostasis; avoid concurrent use - discontinue 1-3 weeks prior to initiating minoxidil. Effects of other antihypertensives may be additive with minoxidil.

Pharmacodynamics/Kinetics

Onset of action: Hypotensive: Oral: ~30 minutes

Peak effect: 2-8 hours

Duration: 2-5 days

Protein binding: None

Metabolism: 88%, primarily via glucuronidation

Bioavailability: Oral: 90%

Half-life elimination: Adults: 3.5-4.2 hours

Excretion: Urine (12% as unchanged drug)

Pregnancy Risk Factor C

Mintab DM *see* Guaifenesin and Dextromethorphan *on page 796*

Mintezol® *see* Thiabendazole *on page 1556*

Mintox Extra Strength [OTC] *see* Aluminum Hydroxide, Magnesium Hydroxide, and Simethicone *on page 82*

Mintox Plus [OTC] *see* Aluminum Hydroxide, Magnesium Hydroxide, and Simethicone *on page 82*

Mintuss G *see* Hydrocodone, Phenylephrine, and Guaifenesin *on page 834*

Miochol®-E *see* Acetylcholine *on page 46*

Miostat® *see* Carbachol *on page 272*

MiraLax® [OTC] *see* Polyethylene Glycol 3350 *on page 1321*

Mirapex® *see* Pramipexole *on page 1333*

Mircette® *see* Ethinyl Estradiol and Desogestrel *on page 621*

Mirena® *see* Levonorgestrel *on page 968*

Mirtazapine *(mir TAZ a peen)*

U.S. Brand Names Remeron®; Remeron SolTab®

Canadian Brand Names CO Mirtazapine; Gen-Mirtazapine; Novo-Mirtazapine; PMS-Mirtazapine; ratio-Mirtazapine; Remeron®; Remeron® RD; Rhoxal-mirtazapine; Rhoxal-mirtazapine FC; Riva-Mirtazapine; Sandoz-Mirtazapine; Sandoz-Mirtazapine FC

Mexican Brand Names Remeron

Generic Available Yes

Pharmacologic Category Antidepressant, Alpha-2 Antagonist

Use Treatment of depression

Local Anesthetic/Vasoconstrictor Precautions Although mirtazapine is not a tricyclic antidepressant, it does block norepinephrine reuptake within CNS synapses as part of its mechanisms. It has been suggested that vasoconstrictor be administered with caution and to monitor vital signs in dental patients taking antidepressants that affect norepinephrine in this way, including mirtazapine.

Effects on Dental Treatment Key adverse event(s) related to dental treatment: Significant xerostomia (normal salivary flow resumes upon discontinuation).

Common Adverse Effects

>10%:

Central nervous system: Somnolence (54%)

Endocrine & metabolic: Increased cholesterol

Gastrointestinal: Constipation (13%), xerostomia (25%), increased appetite (17%), weight gain (12%; weight gain of >7% reported in 8% of adults, ≤49% of pediatric patients)

1% to 10%:

Cardiovascular: Hypertension, vasodilatation, peripheral edema (2%), edema (1%)

Central nervous system: Dizziness (7%), abnormal dreams (4%), abnormal thoughts (3%), confusion (2%), malaise

Endocrine & metabolic: Increased triglycerides

Gastrointestinal: Vomiting, anorexia, abdominal pain

Genitourinary: Urinary frequency (2%)

Neuromuscular & skeletal: Myalgia (2%), back pain (2%), arthralgia, tremor (2%), weakness (8%)

Respiratory: Dyspnea (1%)

Miscellaneous: Flu-like syndrome (5%), thirst

Restrictions An FDA-approved medication guide concerning the use of antidepressants in children, adolescents, and young adults must be distributed when dispensing an outpatient prescription (new or refill) where this medication is to be used without direct supervision of a healthcare provider. Medication guides are available at http://www.fda.gov/cder/Offices/ODS/medication_guides.htm. Dispense to parents or guardians of children and adolescents receiving this medication.

Mechanism of Action Mirtazapine is a tetracyclic antidepressant that works by its central presynaptic alpha$_2$-adrenergic antagonist effects, which results in increased release of norepinephrine and serotonin. It is also a potent antagonist of 5-HT$_2$ and 5-HT$_3$ serotonin receptors and H1 histamine receptors and a moderate peripheral alpha$_1$-adrenergic and muscarinic antagonist; it does not inhibit the reuptake of norepinephrine or serotonin.

Drug Interactions

Cytochrome P450 Effect: Substrate of CYP1A2 (major), 2C9 (minor), 2D6 (major), 3A4 (major); **Inhibits** CYP1A2 (weak), 3A4 (weak)

Increased Effect/Toxicity: Contraindicated with drugs which inhibit MAO (including linezolid, selegiline, sibutramine, and MAOIs); severe/fatal reactions may occur. CYP1A2 inhibitors may increase the levels/effects of mirtazapine; example inhibitors include ciprofloxacin, fluvoxamine, ketoconazole, norfloxacin, ofloxacin, and rofecoxib. CYP2D6 inhibitors may increase the levels/effects of mirtazapine; example inhibitors include chlorpromazine, delavirdine, fluoxetine, miconazole, paroxetine, pergolide, quinidine, quinine, ritonavir, and ropinirole. CYP3A4 inhibitors may increase the levels/effects of mirtazapine; example inhibitors include azole antifungals, clarithromycin, diclofenac, doxycycline, erythromycin, imatinib, isoniazid, nefazodone, nicardipine, propofol, protease inhibitors, quinidine, telithromycin, and verapamil. Increased sedative effect seen with CNS depressants.

Decreased Effect: CYP1A2 inducers may decrease the levels/effects of mirtazapine; example inducers include aminoglutethimide, carbamazepine, phenobarbital, and rifampin. Decreased effect seen with clonidine. CYP3A4 inducers may decrease the levels/effects of mirtazapine; example inducers include aminoglutethimide, carbamazepine, nafcillin, nevirapine, phenobarbital, phenytoin, and rifamycins.

Pharmacodynamics/Kinetics

Protein binding: 85%

Metabolism: Extensively hepatic via CYP1A2, 2C9, 2D6, 3A4 and via demethylation and hydroxylation

Bioavailability: 50%

Half-life elimination: 20-40 hours; hampered with renal or hepatic impairment

Time to peak, serum: 2 hours

Excretion: Urine (75%) and feces (15%) as metabolites

Pregnancy Risk Factor C

Misoprostol (mye soe PROST ole)

U.S. Brand Names Cytotec®

Canadian Brand Names Apo-Misoprostol®; Novo-Misoprostol

Mexican Brand Names Cytotec

Generic Available Yes

Pharmacologic Category Prostaglandin

Use Prevention of NSAID-induced gastric ulcers; medical termination of pregnancy of ≤49 days (in conjunction with mifepristone)

Unlabeled/Investigational Use Cervical ripening and labor induction; NSAID-induced nephropathy; fat malabsorption in cystic fibrosis

Local Anesthetic/Vasoconstrictor Precautions No information available to require special precautions

Effects on Dental Treatment No significant effects or complications reported

Common Adverse Effects

>10%: Gastrointestinal: Diarrhea, abdominal pain

1% to 10%:

Central nervous system: Headache

Gastrointestinal: Constipation, flatulence, nausea, dyspepsia, vomiting

(Continued)

Misoprostol *(Continued)*

Mechanism of Action Misoprostol is a synthetic prostaglandin E$_1$ analog that replaces the protective prostaglandins consumed with prostaglandin-inhibiting therapies (eg, NSAIDs); has been shown to induce uterine contractions

Drug Interactions

Increased Effect/Toxicity: Misoprostol may increase the effect of oxytocin; wait 6-12 hours after misoprostol administration before initiating oxytocin.

Pharmacodynamics/Kinetics

Absorption: Rapid

Metabolism: Hepatic; rapidly de-esterified to misoprostol acid (active)

Half-life elimination: Metabolite: 20-40 minutes

Time to peak, serum: Active metabolite: Fasting: 15-30 minutes

Excretion: Urine (64% to 73%) and feces (15%) within 24 hours

Pregnancy Risk Factor X

Misoprostol and Diclofenac *see* Diclofenac and Misoprostol *on page 489*

Mitomycin *(mye toe MYE sin)*

U.S. Brand Names Mutamycin®

Canadian Brand Names Mutamycin®

Mexican Brand Names Mixandex

Generic Available Yes

Index Terms Mitomycin-C; Mitomycin-X; MTC; NSC-26980

Pharmacologic Category Antineoplastic Agent, Antibiotic

Use Treatment of adenocarcinoma of stomach or pancreas, bladder cancer, breast cancer, or colorectal cancer

Unlabeled/Investigational Use Prevention of excess scarring in glaucoma filtration procedures in patients at high risk of bleb failure

Local Anesthetic/Vasoconstrictor Precautions No information available to require special precautions

Effects on Dental Treatment Key adverse event(s) related to dental treatment: Stomatitis.

Common Adverse Effects

>10%:

Cardiovascular: CHF (3% to 15%) (doses >30 mg/m^2)

Central nervous system: Fever (14%)

Dermatologic: Alopecia, nail banding/discoloration

Gastrointestinal: Nausea, vomiting and anorexia (14%)

Hematologic: Anemia (19% to 24%); myelosuppression, common, dose-limiting, delayed

Onset: 3 weeks

Nadir: 4-6 weeks

Recovery: 6-8 weeks

1% to 10%:

Dermatologic: Rash

Gastrointestinal: Stomatitis

Neuromuscular: Paresthesia

Renal: Creatinine increase (2%)

Respiratory: Interstitial pneumonitis, infiltrates, dyspnea, cough (7%)

Mechanism of Action Acts like an alkylating agent and produces DNA cross-linking (primarily with guanine and cytosine pairs); cell-cycle nonspecific; inhibits DNA and RNA synthesis; degrades preformed DNA, causes nuclear lysis and formation of giant cells. While not phase-specific *per se*, mitomycin has its maximum effect against cells in late G and early S phases.

Drug Interactions

Increased Effect/Toxicity: *Vinca* alkaloids or doxorubicin may enhance cardiac toxicity when coadministered with mitomycin.

Pharmacodynamics/Kinetics

Distribution: V$_d$: 22 L/m^2; high drug concentrations found in kidney, tongue, muscle, heart, and lung tissue; probably not distributed into the CNS

Metabolism: Hepatic

Half-life elimination: 23-78 minutes; Terminal: 50 minutes

Excretion: Urine (<10% as unchanged drug), with elevated serum concentrations

Pregnancy Risk Factor D

Mitomycin-X *see* Mitomycin *on page 1112*
Mitomycin-C *see* Mitomycin *on page 1112*

Mitotane (MYE toe tane)

U.S. Brand Names Lysodren®
Canadian Brand Names Lysodren®
Generic Available No
Index Terms NSC-38721; o,p′-DDD
Pharmacologic Category Antineoplastic Agent, Miscellaneous
Use Treatment of adrenocortical carcinoma
Unlabeled/Investigational Use Treatment of Cushing's syndrome
Local Anesthetic/Vasoconstrictor Precautions No information available to require special precautions
Effects on Dental Treatment No significant effects or complications reported
Common Adverse Effects
>10%:
    Central nervous system: CNS depression (32%), somnolence (25%), dizziness/vertigo (15%)
    Dermatologic: Skin rash (15%)
    Gastrointestinal: Anorexia (24%), nausea (39%), vomiting (37%), diarrhea (13%)
    Neuromuscular & skeletal: Weakness (12%)
1% to 10%:
    Central nervous system: Headache (5%), confusion (3%)
    Neuromuscular & skeletal: Muscle tremor (3%)
Mechanism of Action Causes adrenal cortical atrophy; drug affects mitochondria in adrenal cortical cells and decreases production of cortisol; also alters the peripheral metabolism of steroids
Drug Interactions
Decreased Effect: Potassium-sparing diuretics (spironolactone) may decrease the effect of mitotane. Mitotane may decrease the effects of warfarin.
Pharmacodynamics/Kinetics
Absorption: Oral: ~35% to 40%
Distribution: Stored mainly in fat tissue but is found in all body tissues
Metabolism: Hepatic and other tissues
Half-life elimination: 18-159 days
Time to peak, serum: 3-5 hours
Excretion: Urine (10% as metabolites) and feces (1% to 17% as metabolites)
Pregnancy Risk Factor C

Mitoxantrone (mye toe ZAN trone)

U.S. Brand Names Novantrone®
Canadian Brand Names Mitoxantrone Injection®; Novantrone®
Mexican Brand Names Mitroxone
Generic Available Yes
Index Terms DAD; DHAD; DHAQ; Dihydroxyanthracenedione Dihydrochloride; Mitoxantrone Hydrochloride CL-232315; Mitozantrone; NSC-301739
Pharmacologic Category Antineoplastic Agent, Anthracenedione
Use Treatment of acute leukemias, lymphoma, breast cancer, pediatric sarcoma, secondary progressive or relapsing-remitting multiple sclerosis, prostate cancer
Local Anesthetic/Vasoconstrictor Precautions No information available to require special precautions
Effects on Dental Treatment Key adverse event(s) related to dental treatment: Mucositis and stomatitis.
Common Adverse Effects Includes events reported with any indication; incidence varies based on treatment/dose
>10%:
    Cardiovascular: Arrhythmia (3% to 18%), edema (10% to 31%), ECG changes (11%)
    Central nervous system: Pain (8% to 41%), fatigue (up to 39%), fever (6% to 78%), headache (6% to 13%)
    Dermatologic: Alopecia (20% to 61%), nail bed changes (11%)
    Endocrine & metabolic: Amenorrhea (28% to 53%), menstrual disorder (26% to 61%), hyperglycemia (10% to 31%)
    Gastrointestinal: Abdominal pain (9% to 15%), anorexia (22% to 25%), nausea (26% to 76%), constipation (10% to 16%), diarrhea (14% to 47%), GI bleeding (2% to 16%), mucositis (10% to 29%), stomatitis (8% to 29%), dyspepsia (5% to 14%), vomiting (6% to 11%), weight gain/loss (13% to 17%)
    Genitourinary: Abnormal urine (6% to 11%), urinary tract infection (7% to 32%)
(Continued)

Mitoxantrone (Continued)

Hematologic: Neutropenia (79% to 100%), leukopenia (9% to 100%), lympho-penia (72% to 95%), anemia (5% to 75%), hemoglobin decreased (43%), thrombocytopenia (33% to 39%), petechiae/bruising (6% to 11%); myelo-suppression (WBC: mild; platelets: mild; onset: 7-10 days; nadir: 14 days; recovery: 21 days)

Hepatic: Alkaline phosphatase increased (37%), transaminases increased (5% to 20%), GGT increased (3% to 15%)

Neuromuscular & skeletal: Weakness (24%)

Renal: BUN increased (22%), creatinine increased (13%), hematuria (11%)

Respiratory: Cough (5% to 13%), dyspnea (6% to 18%), upper respiratory tract infection (7% to 53%)

Miscellaneous: Fungal infection (9% to 15%), infection (4% to 18%), sepsis (ANLL 31% to 34%)

1% to 10%:

Cardiovascular: Ischemia (5%), LVEF decreased (≤5%), hypertension (4%), CHF (2% to 5%, risk is much lower with anthracyclines, some reports suggest cumulative doses >160 mg/mL cause CHF in ~10% of patients)

Central nervous system: Chills (5%), anxiety (5%), depression (5%), seizure (2% to 4%)

Dermatologic: Skin infection

Endocrine & metabolic: Hypocalcemia (10%), hypokalemia (7% to 10%), hyponatremia (9%), menorrhagia (7%)

Gastrointestinal: Aphthosis (10%)

Genitourinary: Impotence (7%), sterility (5%)

Hematologic: Granulocytopenia (6%), hemorrhage (6%)

Hepatic: Jaundice (3% to 7%)

Neuromuscular & skeletal: Back pain (8%), myalgia (5%), arthralgia (5%)

Ocular: Conjunctivitis (5%), blurred vision (3%)

Renal: Renal failure (8%), proteinuria (6%)

Respiratory: Rhinitis (10%), pneumonia (9%), sinusitis (6%)

Miscellaneous: Systemic infection, diaphoresis (9%), development of secon-dary leukemia (~1% to 2%)

Mechanism of Action Analogue of the anthracyclines, mitoxantrone interca-lates DNA; binds to nucleic acids and inhibits DNA and RNA synthesis by template disordering and steric obstruction; replication is decreased by binding to DNA topoisomerase II and seems to inhibit the incorporation of uridine into RNA and thymidine into DNA; active throughout entire cell cycle

Drug Interactions

Cytochrome P450 Effect: Inhibits CYP3A4 (weak)

Decreased Effect: Patients may experience impaired immune response to vaccines; possible infection after administration of live vaccines in patients receiving immunosuppressants.

Pharmacodynamics/Kinetics

Absorption: Oral: Poor

Distribution: V_d: 14 L/kg; distributes into pleural fluid, kidney, thyroid, liver, heart, and red blood cells

Protein binding: >95%, 76% to albumin

Metabolism: Hepatic; pathway not determined

Half-life elimination: Terminal: 23-215 hours; may be prolonged with hepatic impairment

Excretion: Urine (6% to 11%; 65% as unchanged drug); feces (25%; 65% as unchanged drug)

Pregnancy Risk Factor D

Mobic® *see* Meloxicam *on page 1031*
Mobisyl® [OTC] *see* Triethanolamine Salicylate *on page 1617*

Modafinil (moe DAF i nil)

U.S. Brand Names Provigil®
Canadian Brand Names Alertec®; Provigil®
Mexican Brand Names Modiodal
Generic Available No
Pharmacologic Category Stimulant
Use Improve wakefulness in patients with excessive daytime sleepiness associated with narcolepsy and shift work sleep disorder (SWSD); adjunctive therapy for obstructive sleep apnea/hypopnea syndrome (OSAHS)
Unlabeled/Investigational Use Attention-deficit/hyperactivity disorder (ADHD); treatment of fatigue in MS and other disorders
Local Anesthetic/Vasoconstrictor Precautions No information available to require special precautions
Effects on Dental Treatment Key adverse event(s) related to dental treatment: Xerostomia (normal salivary flow resumes upon discontinuation), oral ulceration, gingivitis, and taste perversion.

Common Adverse Effects
>10%:
  Central nervous system: Headache (34%, dose related)
  Gastrointestinal: Nausea (11%)
1% to 10%:
  Cardiovascular: Chest pain (3%), hypertension (3%), palpitation (2%), tachycardia (2%), vasodilation (2%), edema (1%)
  Central nervous system: Nervousness (7%), dizziness (5%), depression (2%), anxiety (5%; dose related), insomnia (5%), somnolence (2%), chills (1%), agitation (1%), confusion (1%), emotional lability (1%), vertigo (1%)
  Gastrointestinal: Diarrhea (6%), dyspepsia (5%), xerostomia (4%), anorexia (4%), constipation (2%), flatulence (1%), mouth ulceration (1%), taste perversion (1%)
  Genitourinary: Abnormal urine (1%), hematuria (1%), pyuria (1%)
  Hematologic: Eosinophilia (1%)
  Hepatic: LFTs abnormal (2%)
  Neuromuscular & skeletal: Back pain (6%), paresthesia (2%), dyskinesia (1%), hyperkinesia (1%), hypertonia (1%), neck rigidity (1%), tremor (1%)
  Ocular: Amblyopia (1%), eye pain (1%), vision abnormal (1%)
  Respiratory: Pharyngitis (4%), rhinitis (7%), lung disorder (2%), asthma (1%), epistaxis (1%)
  Miscellaneous: Diaphoresis

Restrictions C-IV
Mechanism of Action The exact mechanism of action is unclear, it does not appear to alter the release of dopamine or norepinephrine, it may exert its stimulant effects by decreasing GABA-mediated neurotransmission, although this theory has not yet been fully evaluated; several studies also suggest that an intact central alpha-adrenergic system is required for modafinil's activity; the drug increases high-frequency alpha waves while decreasing both delta and theta wave activity, and these effects are consistent with generalized increases in mental alertness

Drug Interactions
Cytochrome P450 Effect: Substrate of CYP3A4 (major); **Inhibits** CYP1A2 (weak), 2A6 (weak), 2C9 (weak), 2C19 (strong), 2E1 (weak), 3A4 (weak); **Induces** CYP1A2 (weak), 2B6 (weak), 3A4 (weak)
Increased Effect/Toxicity: Modafinil may increase the levels/effects of citalopram, diazepam, methsuximide, phenytoin, propranolol, sertraline, or other CYP2C19 substrates. Modafinil may increase levels of warfarin. In populations deficient in the CYP2D6 isoenzyme, where CYP2C19 acts as a secondary metabolic pathway, concentrations of tricyclic antidepressants and selective serotonin reuptake inhibitors may be increased during coadministration. The levels/effects of modafinil may be increased by azole antifungals, clarithromycin, diclofenac, doxycycline, erythromycin, imatinib, isoniazid, nefazodone, nicardipine, propofol, protease inhibitors, quinidine, telithromycin, verapamil, or other CYP3A4 inhibitors.
Decreased Effect: Modafinil may decrease serum concentrations of oral contraceptives, cyclosporine, and to a lesser degree, theophylline. The levels/effects of modafinil may be decreased by aminoglutethimide, carbamazepine, nafcillin, nevirapine, phenobarbital, phenytoin, rifamycins, and other CYP3A4 inducers. There is also evidence to suggest that modafinil may induce its own metabolism.
(Continued)

Modafinil *(Continued)*

Pharmacodynamics/Kinetics Modafinil is a racemic compound (10% *d*-isomer and 90% *l*-isomer at steady state) whose enantiomers have different pharmacokinetics

Distribution: V_d: 0.9 L/kg
Protein binding: 60%, primarily to albumin
Metabolism: Hepatic; multiple pathways including CYP3A4
Half-life elimination: Effective half-life: 15 hours; Steady-state: 2-4 days
Time to peak, serum: 2-4 hours
Excretion: Urine (as metabolites, <10% as unchanged drug)
Pregnancy Risk Factor C

Modane® Bulk [OTC] *see* Psyllium *on page 1386*

Modicon® *see* Ethinyl Estradiol and Norethindrone *on page 640*

Modified Dakin's Solution *see* Sodium Hypochlorite Solution *on page 1482*

Modified Shohl's Solution *see* Sodium Citrate and Citric Acid *on page 1481*

Moducal® [OTC] *see* Glucose Polymers *on page 785*

Moexipril *(mo EKS i pril)*

Related Information
Cardiovascular Diseases *on page 1726*

U.S. Brand Names Univasc®
Generic Available Yes
Index Terms Moexipril Hydrochloride
Pharmacologic Category Angiotensin-Converting Enzyme (ACE) Inhibitor
Use Treatment of hypertension, alone or in combination with thiazide diuretics; treatment of left ventricular dysfunction after myocardial infarction
Local Anesthetic/Vasoconstrictor Precautions No information available to require special precautions
Effects on Dental Treatment No significant effects or complications reported
Common Adverse Effects 1% to 10%:
Cardiovascular: Hypotension, peripheral edema
Central nervous system: Headache, dizziness, fatigue
Dermatologic: Rash, alopecia, flushing, rash
Endocrine & metabolic: Hyperkalemia, hyponatremia
Gastrointestinal: Diarrhea, nausea, heartburn
Genitourinary: Polyuria
Neuromuscular & skeletal: Myalgia
Renal: Reversible increases in creatinine or BUN
Respiratory: Cough, pharyngitis, upper respiratory infection, sinusitis
Mechanism of Action Competitive inhibitor of angiotensin-converting enzyme (ACE); prevents conversion of angiotensin I to angiotensin II, a potent vasoconstrictor; results in lower levels of angiotensin II which causes an increase in plasma renin activity and a reduction in aldosterone secretion
Drug Interactions
Increased Effect/Toxicity: Potassium supplements, co-trimoxazole (high dose), angiotensin II receptor antagonists (eg, candesartan, losartan, irbesartan), or potassium-sparing diuretics (amiloride, spironolactone, triamterene) may result in elevated serum potassium levels when combined with moexipril. ACE inhibitor effects may be increased by probenecid (increases levels of captopril). ACE inhibitors may increase serum concentrations/effects of lithium. ACE inhibitors may enhance the adverse/toxic effects (nitritoid reaction) of gold sodium thiomalate.

Diuretics have additive hypotensive effects with ACE inhibitors, and hypovolemia increases the potential for adverse renal effects of ACE inhibitors. In patients with compromised renal function, coadministration with NSAIDs may result in further deterioration of renal function. Allopurinol and ACE inhibitors may cause a higher risk of hypersensitivity reaction when taken concurrently.

Decreased Effect: Aspirin (high dose) may reduce the therapeutic effects of ACE inhibitors; at low dosages this does not appear to be significant. Rifampin may decrease the effect of ACE inhibitors. Antacids may decrease the bioavailability of ACE inhibitors (may be more likely to occur with captopril); separate administration times by 1-2 hours. NSAIDs, specifically indomethacin, may reduce the hypotensive effects of ACE inhibitors. More likely to occur in low renin or volume dependent hypertensive patients.
Pharmacodynamics/Kinetics
Onset of action: Peak effect: 1-2 hours
Duration: >24 hours
Distribution: V_d (moexiprilat): 180 L
Protein binding, plasma: Moexipril: 90%; Moexiprilat: 50% to 70%

Metabolism: Parent drug: Hepatic and via GI tract to moexiprilat, 1000 times more potent than parent

Bioavailability: Moexiprilat: 13%; reduced with food (AUC decreased by ~40%)

Half-life elimination: Moexipril: 1 hour; Moexiprilat: 2-9 hours

Time to peak: 1.5 hours

Excretion: Feces (50%)

Pregnancy Risk Factor C (1st trimester)/D (2nd and 3rd trimesters)

Moexipril and Hydrochlorothiazide
(mo EKS i pril & hye droe klor oh THYE a zide)

Related Information
Hydrochlorothiazide *on page 819*
Moexipril *on page 1116*

U.S. Brand Names Uniretic®

Canadian Brand Names Uniretic®

Generic Available No

Index Terms Hydrochlorothiazide and Moexipril

Pharmacologic Category Antihypertensive Agent, Combination

Use Combination therapy for hypertension, however, not indicated for initial treatment of hypertension; replacement therapy in patients receiving separate dosage forms (for patient convenience); when monotherapy with one component fails to achieve desired antihypertensive effect, or when dose-limiting adverse effects limit upward titration of monotherapy

Local Anesthetic/Vasoconstrictor Precautions No information available to require special precautions

Effects on Dental Treatment No significant effects or complications reported

Common Adverse Effects See individual agents.

Mechanism of Action See individual agents.

Drug Interactions
Increased Effect/Toxicity: See individual agents.
Decreased Effect: See individual agents.

Pharmacodynamics/Kinetics See individual agents.

Pregnancy Risk Factor C/D (2nd and 3rd trimesters)

Moexipril Hydrochloride *see Moexipril on page 1116*

Moi-Stir® [OTC] *see Saliva Substitute on page 1452*

Moisture® Eyes [OTC] *see Artificial Tears on page 147*

Moisture® Eyes PM [OTC] *see Artificial Tears on page 147*

Molindone (moe LIN done)

U.S. Brand Names Moban®

Canadian Brand Names Moban®

Generic Available No

Index Terms Molindone Hydrochloride

Pharmacologic Category Antipsychotic Agent, Typical

Use Management of schizophrenia

Unlabeled/Investigational Use Management of psychotic disorders; behavioral symptoms associated with dementia (elderly)

Local Anesthetic/Vasoconstrictor Precautions No information available to require special precautions

Effects on Dental Treatment Key adverse event(s) related to dental treatment: Xerostomia and changes in salivation (normal salivary flow resumes upon discontinuation) and orthostatic hypotension. Anticholinergic side effects can cause a reduction of saliva production or secretion, contributing to discomfort and dental disease (ie, caries, oral candidiasis, and periodontal disease). Molindone can cause extrapyramidal reactions which may appear as muscle twitching or increased motor activity of the face, neck, or head.

Common Adverse Effects Frequency not defined.

Cardiovascular: Orthostatic hypotension, tachycardia, arrhythmia

Central nervous system: Extrapyramidal reactions (akathisia, pseudoparkinsonism, dystonia, tardive dyskinesia), mental depression, altered central temperature regulation, sedation, drowsiness, restlessness, anxiety, hyperactivity, euphoria, seizure, neuroleptic malignant syndrome (NMS)

Dermatologic: Pruritus, rash, photosensitivity

Endocrine & metabolic: Change in menstrual periods, edema of breasts, amenorrhea, galactorrhea, gynecomastia

Gastrointestinal: Constipation, xerostomia, nausea, salivation, weight gain (minimal compared to other antipsychotics), weight loss

Genitourinary: Urinary retention, priapism

(Continued)

Molindone *(Continued)*

Hematologic: Leukopenia, leukocytosis
Ocular: Blurred vision, retinal pigmentation
Miscellaneous: Diaphoresis (decreased)

Mechanism of Action Molindone is a dihydroindoline antipsychotic whose mechanism of action mimics that of chlorpromazine; however, it produces more extrapyramidal symptoms and less sedation than chlorpromazine

Drug Interactions

Increased Effect/Toxicity: Molindone concentrations may be increased by chloroquine, propranolol, sulfadoxine-pyrimethamine. Molindone may increase the effect and/or toxicity of antihypertensives, lithium, TCAs, CNS depressants (ethanol, opioid analgesics), and trazodone. Metoclopramide may increase risk of extrapyramidal symptoms (EPS). Acetylcholinesterase inhibitors (central) may increase the risk of antipsychotic-related EPS.

Decreased Effect: Antipsychotics inhibit the activity of bromocriptine and levodopa. Benztropine (and other anticholinergics) may inhibit the therapeutic response to molindone and excess anticholinergic effects may occur. Barbiturates and cigarette smoking may enhance the hepatic metabolism of molindone. Molindone and possibly other low potency antipsychotic may reverse the pressor effects of epinephrine.

Pharmacodynamics/Kinetics

Metabolism: Hepatic
Half-life elimination: 1.5 hours
Time to peak, serum: ~1.5 hours
Excretion: Urine and feces (90%) within 24 hours

Pregnancy Risk Factor C

Molindone Hydrochloride *see* Molindone *on page 1117*

Molybdenum *see* Trace Metals *on page 1595*

Molypen® *see* Trace Metals *on page 1595*

MOM *see* Magnesium Hydroxide *on page 1014*

Momentum® [OTC] *see* Magnesium Salicylate *on page 1016*

Mometasone Furoate *(moe MET a sone FYOOR oh ate)*

Related Information
Respiratory Diseases *on page 1747*

U.S. Brand Names Asmanex® Twisthaler®; Elocon®; Nasonex®

Canadian Brand Names Elocom®; Nasonex®; PMS-Mometasone; ratio-Mometasone; Taro-Mometasone

Mexican Brand Names Elica; Elomet; Rinelon; Uniclar

Generic Available Yes: Ointment

Pharmacologic Category Corticosteroid, Inhalant (Oral); Corticosteroid, Nasal; Corticosteroid, Topical

Use Relief of the inflammatory and pruritic manifestations of corticosteroid-responsive dermatoses (medium potency topical corticosteroid); treatment of nasal symptoms of seasonal and perennial allergic rhinitis; prevention of nasal symptoms associated with seasonal allergic rhinitis; treatment of nasal polyps in adults; maintenance treatment of asthma as prophylactic therapy or as a supplement in asthma patients requiring oral corticosteroids for the purpose of decreasing or eliminating the oral corticosteroid requirement

Local Anesthetic/Vasoconstrictor Precautions No information available to require special precautions

Effects on Dental Treatment No significant effects or complications reported

Common Adverse Effects

Nasal/oral inhalation:
>10%:
Central nervous system: Headache (17% to 22%), fatigue (oral inhalation 1% to 13%), depression (oral inhalation 11%)
Neuromuscular & skeletal: Musculoskeletal pain (1% to 22%), arthralgia (oral inhalation 13%)
Respiratory: Sinusitis (oral inhalation 22%), rhinitis (2% to 20%), upper respiratory infection (8% to 15%), pharyngitis (8% to 13%), cough (nasal inhalation 7% to 13%), epistaxis (1% to 11%)
Miscellaneous: Viral infection (nasal inhalation 8% to 14%), oral candidiasis (oral inhalation 4% to 22%)
1% to 10%:
Cardiovascular: Chest pain
Gastrointestinal: Abdominal pain, dry throat (oral inhalation), vomiting (1% to 5%), diarrhea, dyspepsia, flatulence, gastroenteritis, nausea, vomiting
Genitourinary: Dysmenorrhea
Neuromuscular & skeletal: Back pain, myalgia

Ocular: Conjunctivitis

Otic: Earache, otitis media

Respiratory: Asthma, bronchitis, dysphonia, epistaxis, nasal irritation, rhinitis, wheezing

Miscellaneous: Accidental injury, flu-like syndrome

Topical:

1% to 10%: Dermatologic: Bacterial skin infection, burning, furunculosis, pruritus, skin atrophy, tingling/stinging

Cataract formation, reduction in growth velocity, and HPA axis suppression have been reported with other corticosteroids

Dosage

Oral inhalation: Children ≥12 years and Adults: Previous therapy:

Bronchodilators or inhaled corticosteroids: Initial: 1 inhalation (220 mcg) daily (maximum 2 inhalations or 440 mcg/day); may be given in the evening or in divided doses twice daily

Oral corticosteroids: Initial: 440 mcg twice daily (maximum 880 mcg/day); prednisone should be reduced no faster than 2.5 mg/day on a weekly basis, beginning after at least 1 week of mometasone furoate use

Note: Maximum effects may not be evident for 1-2 weeks or longer; dose should be titrated to effect, using the lowest possible dose

Nasal spray:

Allergic rhinitis:

Children 2-11 years: 1 spray (50 mcg) in each nostril daily

Children ≥12 years and Adults: 2 sprays (100 mcg) in each nostril daily; when used for the prevention of allergic rhinitis, treatment should begin 2-4 weeks prior to pollen season

Nasal polyps: Adults: 2 sprays (100 mcg) in each nostril twice daily; 2 sprays (100 mcg) once daily may be effective in some patients

Topical: Apply sparingly, do not use occlusive dressings. Therapy should be discontinued when control is achieved; if no improvement is seen in 2 weeks, reassessment of diagnosis may be necessary.

Cream, ointment: Children ≥2 years and Adults: Apply a thin film to affected area once daily; do not use in pediatric patients for longer than 3 weeks

Lotion: Children ≥12 years and Adults: Apply a few drops to affected area once daily

Mechanism of Action May depress the formation, release, and activity of endogenous chemical mediators of inflammation (kinins, histamine, liposomal enzymes, prostaglandins). Leukocytes and macrophages may have to be present for the initiation of responses mediated by the above substances. Inhibits the margination and subsequent cell migration to the area of injury, and also reverses the dilatation and increased vessel permeability in the area resulting in decreased access of cells to the sites of injury.

Contraindications Hypersensitivity to mometasone or any component of the formulation; treatment of acute bronchospasm (oral inhaler)

Warnings/Precautions

May cause hypercorticism or suppression of hypothalamic-pituitary-adrenal (HPA) axis, particularly in younger children or in patients receiving high doses for prolonged periods. HPA axis suppression may lead to adrenal crisis. Withdrawal and discontinuation of a corticosteroid should be done slowly and carefully. Particular care is required when patients are transferred from systemic corticosteroids to inhaled products due to possible adrenal insufficiency or withdrawal from steroids, including an increase in allergic symptoms. Patients receiving >20 mg per day of prednisone (or equivalent) may be most susceptible. Fatalities have occurred due to adrenal insufficiency in asthmatic patients during and after transfer from systemic corticosteroids to aerosol steroids; aerosol steroids do not provide the systemic steroid needed to treat patients having trauma, surgery, or infections. When transferring to oral inhaler, previously-suppressed allergic conditions (rhinitis, conjunctivitis, eczema) may be unmasked.

Bronchospasm may occur with wheezing after inhalation; if this occurs stop steroid and treat with a fast-acting bronchodilator. Supplemental steroids (oral or parenteral) may be needed during stress or severe asthma attacks. Not to be used in status asthmaticus or for the relief of acute bronchospasm. Corticosteroid use may cause psychiatric disturbances, including depression, euphoria, insomnia, mood swings, and personality changes. Pre-existing psychiatric conditions may be exacerbated by corticosteroid use. Prolonged use of corticosteroids may also increase the incidence of secondary infection, mask acute infection (including fungal infections), prolong or exacerbate viral infections, or limit response to vaccines. Exposure to chickenpox should be avoided; corticosteroids should not be used to treat ocular herpes simplex. Corticosteroids should not be used for cerebral malaria. Close observation is required in patients with latent tuberculosis and/or TB reactivity; restrict use in active TB

(Continued)

Mometasone Furoate *(Continued)*

(only in conjunction with antituberculosis treatment). Prolonged treatment with corticosteroids has been associated with the development of Kaposi's sarcoma (case reports); if noted, discontinuation of therapy should be considered.

Use with caution in patients with thyroid disease, hepatic impairment, renal impairment, cardiovascular disease, diabetes, glaucoma, cataracts, myasthenia gravis, patients at risk for osteoporosis, patients at risk for seizures, or GI diseases (diverticulitis, peptic ulcer, ulcerative colitis) due to perforation risk. Use caution following acute MI (corticosteroids have been associated with myocardial rupture). Because of the risk of adverse effects, systemic corticosteroids should be used cautiously in the elderly in the smallest possible effective dose for the shortest duration. Avoid nasal corticosteroid use in patients with recent nasal septal ulcers, nasal surgery or nasal trauma until healing has occurred.

Orally-inhaled and intranasal corticosteroids may cause a reduction in growth velocity in pediatric patients (~1 centimeter per year [range 0.3-1.8 cm per year] and related to dose and duration of exposure). To minimize the systemic effects of orally-inhaled and intranasal corticosteroids, each patient should be titrated to the lowest effective dose. Growth should be routinely monitored in pediatric patients. There have been reports of systemic corticosteroid withdrawal symptoms (eg, joint/muscle pain, lassitude, depression) when withdrawing oral inhalation therapy.

Drug Interactions
Cytochrome P450 Effect: Substrate of CYP3A4 (minor)
Increased Effect/Toxicity:
Concomittant use with ketoconazole may result in increased mometasone furoate plasma levels.
Dietary Considerations Asmanex® Twisthaler® contains lactose.
Pharmacodynamics/Kinetics
Absorption:
Nasal inhalation: Mometasone furoate monohydrate: Undetectable in plasma
Ointment: 0.7%; increased by occlusive dressings
Oral inhalation: <1%
Protein binding: Mometasone furoate: 98% to 99%
Metabolism: Mometasone furoate: Hepatic via CYP3A4; forms metabolite
Half-life elimination: Oral inhalation: 5 hours
Excretion: Feces, bile, urine
Pregnancy Risk Factor C
Dosage Forms
Cream, topical:
Elocon®: 0.1% (15 g, 45 g)
Lotion, topical:
Elocon®: 0.1% (30 mL, 60 mL)
Ointment, topical: 0.1% (15 g, 45 g)
Elocon®: 0.1% (15 g, 45 g)
Powder for oral inhalation:
Asmanex® Twisthaler®: 220 mcg (14 units, 30 units, 60 units, 120 units)
Suspension, intranasal [spray]:
Nasonex®: 50 mcg/spray (17 g)

MOM/Mineral Oil Emulsion *see* Magnesium Hydroxide and Mineral Oil *on page 1014*

Monacolin K *see* Lovastatin *on page 1007*

Monarc-M™ *see* Antihemophilic Factor (Human) *on page 131*

Monistat® 1 Combination Pack [OTC] *see* Miconazole *on page 1097*

Monistat® 3 [OTC] *see* Miconazole *on page 1097*

Monistat® 3 Combination Pack [OTC] *see* Miconazole *on page 1097*

Monistat® 7 [OTC] *see* Miconazole *on page 1097*

Monistat-Derm® [DSC] *see* Miconazole *on page 1097*

Monobenzone *(mon oh BEN zone)*

U.S. Brand Names Benoquin®
Generic Available No
Pharmacologic Category Topical Skin Product
Use Final depigmentation in extensive vitiligo
Local Anesthetic/Vasoconstrictor Precautions No information available to require special precautions
Effects on Dental Treatment No significant effects or complications reported
Common Adverse Effects Frequency not defined.

Local: Burning sensation, depigmentation of skin distant to application site, dermatitis, irritation

Mechanism of Action Increases excretion of melanin from melanocytes; causes melanocyte destruction and permanent depigmentation

Pharmacodynamics/Kinetics Onset of action: 1-4 months

Pregnancy Risk Factor C

Monocaps [OTC] *see* Vitamins (Multiple/Oral) *on page 1665*

Monoclate-P® *see* Antihemophilic Factor (Human) *on page 131*

Monoclonal Antibody *see* Muromonab-CD3 *on page 1133*

Monodox® *see* Doxycycline (Systemic) *on page 541*

Monoethanolamine *see* Ethanolamine Oleate *on page 621*

Monoket® *see* Isosorbide Mononitrate *on page 916*

MonoNessa™ *see* Ethinyl Estradiol and Norgestimate *on page 645*

Mononine® *see* Factor IX *on page 667*

Monopril® *see* Fosinopril *on page 748*

Monopril-HCT® *see* Fosinopril and Hydrochlorothiazide *on page 750*

Montelukast (mon te LOO kast)

Related Information
Respiratory Diseases *on page 1747*
U.S. Brand Names Singulair®
Canadian Brand Names Singulair®
Mexican Brand Names Singulair
Generic Available No
Index Terms Montelukast Sodium
Pharmacologic Category Leukotriene-Receptor Antagonist
Use Prophylaxis and chronic treatment of asthma; relief of symptoms of seasonal allergic rhinitis and perennial allergic rhinitis; prevention of exercise-induced bronchospasm
Unlabeled/Investigational Use Acute asthma
Local Anesthetic/Vasoconstrictor Precautions No information available to require special precautions
Effects on Dental Treatment Key adverse event(s) related to dental treatment: Dental pain.
Common Adverse Effects 1% to 10% (as reported in adults):
Central nervous system: Dizziness (2%), fatigue (2%), fever (2%)
Dermatologic: Rash (2%)
Gastrointestinal: Abdominal pain (3%), dyspepsia (2%), dental pain (2%), gastroenteritis (2%)
Hepatic: AST increased (2%)
Neuromuscular & skeletal: Weakness (2%)
Respiratory: Cough (3%), nasal congestion (2%)
Dosage Oral:
Children:
6-11 months: Asthma (unlabeled use): 4 mg (oral granules) once daily, taken in the evening
6-23 months: Perennial allergic rhinitis: 4 mg (oral granules) once daily
12-23 months: Asthma: 4 mg (oral granules) once daily, taken in the evening
2-5 years: Asthma, seasonal or perennial allergic rhinitis: 4 mg (chewable tablet or oral granules) once daily, taken in the evening
6-14 years: Asthma, seasonal or perennial allergic rhinitis: 5 mg (chewable tablet) once daily, taken in the evening
Children ≥15 years and Adults:
Asthma, seasonal or perennial allergic rhinitis: 10 mg/day, taken in the evening
Asthma, acute (unlabeled use): 10 mg as a single dose administered with first-line therapy
Bronchoconstriction, exercise-induced (prevention): 10 mg at least 2 hours prior to exercise; additional doses should not be administered within 24 hours. Daily administration to prevent exercise-induced bronchoconstriction has not been evaluated.
Dosing adjustment in renal impairment: No adjustment necessary
Dosing adjustment in hepatic impairment: Mild-to-moderate: No adjustment necessary. Patients with severe hepatic disease were **not** studied.
Mechanism of Action Selective leukotriene receptor antagonist that inhibits the cysteinyl leukotriene receptor. Cysteinyl leukotrienes and leukotriene receptor occupation have been correlated with the pathophysiology of asthma, including airway edema, smooth muscle contraction, and altered cellular activity associated with the inflammatory process, which contribute to the signs and symptoms of asthma. Cysteinyl leukotrienes are also released from the nasal
(Continued)

1121

Montelukast (Continued)

mucosa following allergen exposure leading to symptoms associated with allergic rhinitis.

Contraindications Hypersensitivity to montelukast or any component of the formulation

Warnings/Precautions Montelukast is not FDA approved for use in the reversal of bronchospasm in acute asthma attacks, including status asthmaticus; some clinicians, however, support its use (Cylly, 2003; Camargo, 2003; Ferreira, 2001). Advise patients to have appropriate rescue medication available. Appropriate clinical monitoring and caution are recommended when systemic corticosteroid reduction is considered in patients receiving montelukast. Inform phenylketonuric patients that the chewable tablet contains phenylalanine. Safety and efficacy in children <6 months of age have not been established.

In rare cases, patients on therapy with montelukast may present with systemic eosinophilia, sometimes presenting with clinical features of vasculitis consistent with Churg-Strauss syndrome, a condition which is often treated with systemic corticosteroid therapy. Healthcare providers should be alert to eosinophilia, vasculitic rash, worsening pulmonary symptoms, cardiac complications, and/or neuropathy presenting in their patients. A causal association between montelukast and these underlying conditions has not been established. Montelukast will not interrupt bronchoconstrictor response to aspirin or other NSAIDs; aspirin sensitive asthmatics should continue to avoid these agents.

Drug Interactions

Cytochrome P450 Effect: Substrate (major) of CYP2C9, 3A4; **Inhibits** CYP2C8 (weak), 2C9 (weak)

Increased Effect/Toxicity: CYP2C9 inhibitors may increase the levels/effects of montelukast; example inhibitors include delavirdine, fluconazole, flurbiprofen, gemfibrozil, ibuprofen, indomethacin, ketoconazole, mefenamic acid, miconazole, nicardipine, piroxicam, sulfadiazine, sulfisoxazole, and tolbutamide.

Decreased Effect: CYP2C9 inducers may decrease the levels/effects of montelukast; example inducers include carbamazepine, phenobarbital, phenytoin, rifampin, rifapentine, and secobarbital. CYP3A4 inducers may decrease the levels/effects of montelukast; example inducers include aminoglutethimide, carbamazepine, nafcillin, nevirapine, phenobarbital, phenytoin, and rifamycins.

Ethanol/Nutrition/Herb Interactions Herb/Nutraceutical: St John's wort may decrease montelukast levels.

Dietary Considerations Tablet, chewable: 4 mg strength contains phenylalanine 0.674 mg; 5 mg strength contains phenylalanine 0.842 mg

Pharmacodynamics/Kinetics

Duration: >24 hours

Absorption: Rapid

Distribution: V_d: 8-11 L

Protein binding, plasma: >99%

Metabolism: Extensively hepatic via CYP3A4 and 2C9

Bioavailability: Tablet: 10 mg: Mean: 64%; 5 mg: 63% to 73%

Half-life elimination, plasma: Mean: 2.7-5.5 hours

Time to peak, serum: Tablet: 10 mg: 3-4 hours; 5 mg: 2-2.5 hours; 4 mg: 2 hours

Excretion: Feces (86%); urine (<0.2%)

Pregnancy Risk Factor B

Dosage Forms

Granules:

Singulair®: 4 mg/packet

Tablet:

Singulair®: 10 mg

Tablet, chewable:

Singulair®: 4 mg, 5 mg

Montelukast Sodium see Montelukast on page 1121

Monurol™ see Fosfomycin on page 747

8-MOP see Methoxsalen on page 1074

8-MOP® see Methoxsalen on page 1074

More Attenuated Enders Strain see Measles Virus Vaccine (Live) on page 1021

MoreDophilus® [OTC] see Lactobacillus on page 942

Moricizine (mor I siz een)

Related Information
Cardiovascular Diseases *on page 1726*
U.S. Brand Names Ethmozine®
Canadian Brand Names Ethmozine®
Generic Available No
Index Terms Moricizine Hydrochloride
Pharmacologic Category Antiarrhythmic Agent, Class I
Use Treatment of ventricular tachycardia and life-threatening ventricular arrhythmias
Unlabeled/Investigational Use PVCs, complete and nonsustained ventricular tachycardia, atrial arrhythmias
Local Anesthetic/Vasoconstrictor Precautions No information available to require special precautions
Effects on Dental Treatment No significant effects or complications reported
Common Adverse Effects
>10%: Central nervous system: Dizziness
1% to 10%:
    Cardiovascular: Proarrhythmia, palpitation, cardiac death, ECG abnormalities, CHF
    Central nervous system: Headache, fatigue, insomnia
    Endocrine & metabolic: Decreased libido
    Gastrointestinal: Nausea, diarrhea, ileus
    Ocular: Blurred vision, periorbital edema
    Respiratory: Dyspnea
Mechanism of Action Class I antiarrhythmic agent; reduces the fast inward current carried by sodium ions, shortens Phase I and Phase II repolarization, resulting in decreased action potential duration and effective refractory period
Drug Interactions
  Cytochrome P450 Effect: Substrate of CYP3A4 (major); **Induces** CYP1A2 (weak), 3A4 (weak)
  Increased Effect/Toxicity: CYP3A4 inhibitors may increase the levels/effects of moricizine; example inhibitors include azole antifungals, clarithromycin, diclofenac, doxycycline, erythromycin, imatinib, isoniazid, nefazodone, nicardipine, propofol, protease inhibitors, quinidine, telithromycin, and verapamil. Moricizine levels may be increased by cimetidine and diltiazem. Digoxin may result in additive prolongation of the PR interval when combined with moricizine (but not rate of second- and third-degree AV block). Drugs which may prolong QT interval (including cisapride, erythromycin, phenothiazines, cyclic antidepressants, and some quinolones) are contraindicated with type Ia antiarrhythmics. Moricizine has some type Ia activity, and caution should be used.
  Decreased Effect: Moricizine may decrease levels of theophylline (50%) and diltiazem. CYP3A4 inducers may decrease the levels/effects of moricizine; example inducers include aminoglutethimide, carbamazepine, nafcillin, nevirapine, phenobarbital, phenytoin, and rifamycins.
Pharmacodynamics/Kinetics
  Protein binding, plasma: 95%
  Metabolism: Significant first-pass effect; some enterohepatic recycling
  Bioavailability: 38%
  Half-life elimination: Healthy volunteers: 3-4 hours; Cardiac disease: 6-13 hours
  Excretion: Feces (56%); urine (39%)
Pregnancy Risk Factor B

Moricizine Hydrochloride *see* Moricizine *on page 1123*
Morning After Pill *see* Ethinyl Estradiol and Norgestrel *on page 649*

Morphine Sulfate (MOR feen SUL fate)

Related Information
Oxymorphone *on page 1237*
U.S. Brand Names Astramorph/PF™; Avinza®; DepoDur™; Duramorph®; Infumorph®; Kadian®; MS Contin®; Oramorph SR®; RMS®; Roxanol™
Canadian Brand Names Kadian®; M-Eslon®; Morphine HP®; Morphine LP® Epidural; M.O.S.® 10; M.O.S.® 20; M.O.S.® 30; M.O.S.-SR®; M.O.S.-Sulfate®; MS Contin®; MS-IR®; PMS-Morphine Sulfate SR; ratio-Morphine SR; Statex®; Zomorph®
Mexican Brand Names Anafil - L.C.; Anafil - S.T.; Graten
Generic Available Yes: Excludes capsule, controlled release tablet, sustained release tablet, extended release liposomal suspension for injection
(Continued)

Morphine Sulfate *(Continued)*

Index Terms MSO₄ (error-prone abbreviation and should not be used)

Pharmacologic Category Analgesic, Opioid

Use Relief of moderate to severe acute and chronic pain; relief of pain of myocardial infarction; relief of dyspnea of acute left ventricular failure and pulmonary edema; preanesthetic medication

DepoDur™: Epidural (lumbar) single-dose management of surgical pain

Infumorph®: Used in microinfusion devices for intraspinal administration in treatment of intractable chronic pain

Local Anesthetic/Vasoconstrictor Precautions No information available to require special precautions

Effects on Dental Treatment Key adverse event(s) related to dental treatment: Xerostomia (normal salivary flow resumes upon discontinuation) and dysphagia. Anticholinergic side effects can cause a reduction of saliva production or secretion, contributing to discomfort and dental disease (ie, caries, oral candidiasis, and periodontal disease).

Common Adverse Effects Note: Individual patient differences are unpredictable, and percentage may differ in acute pain (surgical) treatment.

Frequency not defined: Flushing, CNS depression, sedation, antidiuretic hormone release, physical and psychological dependence, diaphoresis

>10%:

Cardiovascular: Palpitation, hypotension, bradycardia

Central nervous system: Drowsiness (48%, tolerance usually develops to drowsiness with regular dosing for 1-2 weeks); dizziness (20%), confusion, headache (following epidural or intrathecal use)

Dermatologic: Pruritus (may be secondary to histamine release)

Note: Pruritus may be dose-related, but not confined to the site of administration.

Gastrointestinal: Nausea (28%, tolerance usually develops to nausea and vomiting with chronic use); constipation (40%, tolerance develops very slowly if at all); xerostomia (78%)

Genitourinary: Urinary retention (16%; may be prolonged, up to 20 hours, following epidural or intrathecal use)

Local: Pain at injection site

Neuromuscular & skeletal: Weakness

Miscellaneous: Histamine release

1% to 10%:

Cardiovascular: Atrial fibrillation (<3%), chest pain (<3%), edema (<3%), syncope (<3%), tachycardia (<3%)

Central nervous system: Amnesia, anxiety, apathy, ataxia, chills, depression, euphoria, false feeling of well being, fever, headache, hypoesthesia, insomnia, lethargy, malaise, restlessness, seizure, vertigo

Endocrine & metabolic: Gynecomastia (<3%), hyponatremia (<3%)

Gastrointestinal: Anorexia, biliary colic, dyspepsia, dysphagia, GERD, GI irritation, paralytic ileus, vomiting (9%)

Genitourinary: Decreased urination

Hematologic: Anemia (<3%), leukopenia (<3%), thrombocytopenia (<3%)

Neuromuscular & skeletal: Arthralgia, back pain, bone pain, paresthesia, trembling

Ocular: Vision problems

Respiratory: Asthma, atelectasis, dyspnea, hiccups, hypoxia, noncardiogenic pulmonary edema, respiratory depression, rhinitis

Miscellaneous: Diaphoresis, flu-like syndrome, withdrawal syndrome

Restrictions C-II

Dosage Note: These are guidelines and do not represent the doses that may be required in all patients. Doses should be titrated to pain relief/prevention.

Children >6 months and <50 kg: Acute pain (moderate-to-severe):

Oral (prompt release): 0.15-0.3 mg/kg every 3-4 hours as needed

I.M.: 0.1 mg/kg every 3-4 hours as needed

I.V.: 0.05-0.1 mg/kg every 3-4 hours as needed

I.V. infusion: Range: 10-30 mcg/kg/hour

Adolescents >12 years: Sedation/analgesia for procedures: I.V.: 3-4 mg and repeat in 5 minutes if necessary

Adults:

Acute pain (moderate-to-severe):

Oral: Prompt release formulations: Opiate-naive: Initial: 10 mg every 3-4 hours as needed; patients with prior opiate exposure may require higher initial doses: usual dosage range: 10-30 mg every 3-4 hours as needed

I.M., SubQ: **Note:** Repeated SubQ administration causes local tissue irritation, pain, and induration.

Initial: Opiate-naive: 5-10 mg every 3-4 hours as needed; patients with prior opiate exposure may require higher initial doses; usual dosage range: 5-20 mg every 3-4 hours as needed

Rectal: 10-20 mg every 3-4 hours

I.V.: Initial: Opiate-naive: 2.5-5 mg every 3-4 hours; patients with prior opiate exposure may require higher initial doses. **Note:** Repeated doses (up to every 5 minutes if needed) in small increments (eg, 1-4 mg) may be preferred to larger and less frequent doses.

I.V., SubQ continuous infusion: 0.8-10 mg/hour; usual range: Up to 80 mg/hour

Mechanically-ventilated patients (based on 70 kg patient): 0.7-10 mg every 1-2 hours as needed; infusion: 5-35 mg/hour

Patient-controlled analgesia (PCA): (Opiate-naive: Consider lower end of dosing range):

Usual concentration: 1 mg/mL

Demand dose: Usual: 1 mg; range: 0.5-2.5 mg

Lockout interval: 5-10 minutes

Intrathecal (I.T.): **Note:** Administer with extreme caution and in reduced dosage to geriatric or debilitated patients.

Opioid-naive: 0.2-0.25 mg/dose (may provide adequate relief for 24 hours); repeat doses are **not** recommended.

Epidural: **Note:** Administer with extreme caution and in reduced dosage to geriatric or debilitated patients. Vigilant monitoring is particularly important in these patients.

Pain management:

Single-dose (Duramorph®): Initial: 3-5 mg

Infusion:

Bolus dose: 1-6 mg

Infusion rate: 0.1-0.2 mg/hour

Maximum dose: 10 mg/24 hours

Surgical anesthesia: Epidural: Single-dose (extended release, Depo-Dur™): Lumbar epidural only; not recommended in patients <18 years of age:

Cesarean section: 10 mg

Lower abdominal/pelvic surgery: 10-15 mg

Major orthopedic surgery of lower extremity: 15 mg

For Depo-Dur™: To minimize the pharmacokinetic interaction resulting in higher peak serum concentrations of morphine, administer the test dose of the local anesthetic at least 15 minutes prior to Depo-Dur™ administration. Use of Depo-Dur™ with epidural local anesthetics has not been studied. Other medications should not be administered into the epidural space for at least 48 hours after administration of DepoDur™.

Note: Some patients may benefit from a 20 mg dose, however, the incidence of adverse effects may be increased.

Chronic pain: Note: Patients taking opioids chronically may become tolerant and require doses higher than the usual dosage range to maintain the desired effect. Tolerance can be managed by appropriate dose titration. There is no optimal or maximal dose for morphine in chronic pain. The appropriate dose is one that relieves pain throughout its dosing interval without causing unmanageable side effects.

Oral: Controlled-, extended-, or sustained-release formulations: A patient's morphine requirement should be established using prompt-release formulations. Conversion to long-acting products may be considered when chronic, continuous treatment is required. Higher dosages should be reserved for use only in opioid-tolerant patients.

Capsules, extended release (Avinza™): Daily dose administered once daily (for best results, administer at same time each day)

Capsules, sustained release (Kadian®): Daily dose administered once daily or in 2 divided doses daily (every 12 hours)

Tablets, controlled release (MS Contin®), sustained release (Oramorph SR®), or extended release: Daily dose divided and administered every 8 or every 12 hours

Elderly or debilitated patients: Use with caution; may require dose reduction

Dosing adjustment in renal impairment:

Cl_{cr} 10-50 mL/minute: Administer at 75% of normal dose

Cl_{cr} <10 mL/minute: Administer at 50% of normal dose

Dosing adjustment/comments in hepatic disease: Unchanged in mild liver disease; substantial extrahepatic metabolism may occur; excessive sedation may occur in cirrhosis

Mechanism of Action Binds to opiate receptors in the CNS, causing inhibition of ascending pain pathways, altering the perception of and response to pain; produces generalized CNS depression

Contraindications Hypersensitivity to morphine sulfate or any component of the formulation; increased intracranial pressure; severe respiratory depression; acute or severe asthma; known or suspected paralytic ileus; sustained release (Continued)

Morphine Sulfate (Continued)

products are not recommended with gastrointestinal obstruction or in acute/postoperative pain; pregnancy (prolonged use or high doses at term)

Warnings/Precautions An opioid-containing analgesic regimen should be tailored to each patient's needs and based upon the type of pain being treated (acute versus chronic), the route of administration, degree of tolerance for opioids (naive versus chronic user), age, weight, and medical condition. The optimal analgesic dose varies widely among patients. Doses should be titrated to pain relief/prevention. When used as an epidural injection, monitor for delayed sedation.

May cause respiratory depression; use with caution in patients (particularly elderly or debilitated) with impaired respiratory function, morbid obesity, adrenal insufficiency, prostatic hyperplasia, urinary stricture, renal impairment, or severe hepatic dysfunction and in patients with hypersensitivity reactions to other phenanthrene derivative opioid agonists (codeine, hydrocodone, hydromorphone, levorphanol, oxycodone, oxymorphone). Use with caution in patients with biliary tract dysfunction; acute pancreatitis may cause constriction of sphincter of Oddi. Some preparations contain sulfites which may cause allergic reactions; infants <3 months of age are more susceptible to respiratory depression, use with caution and generally in reduced doses in this age group. May cause CNS depression, which may impair physical or mental abilities; patients must be cautioned about performing tasks which require mental alertness (eg, operating machinery or driving). Effects may be potentiated when used with other sedative drugs or ethanol. May cause hypotension in patients with acute myocardial infarction, volume depletion, or concurrent drug therapy which may exaggerate vasodilation. Use with extreme caution in patients with head injury, intracranial lesions, or elevated intracranial pressure; exaggerated elevation of ICP may occur. May obscure diagnosis or clinical course of patients with acute abdominal conditions. Tolerance or drug dependence may result from extended use. Concurrent use of agonist/antagonist analgesics may precipitate withdrawal symptoms and/or reduced analgesic efficacy in patients following prolonged therapy with mu opioid agonists. Abrupt discontinuation following prolonged use may also lead to withdrawal symptoms. Elderly may be particularly susceptible to adverse effects of narcotics.

Extended or sustained-release formulations:

[U.S. Boxed Warning]: Extended or sustained release dosage forms should not be crushed or chewed. Controlled-, extended-, or sustained-release products are not intended for "as needed (PRN)" use. MS Contin® 100 or 200 mg tablets are for use only in opioid-tolerant patients requiring >400 mg/day.

[U.S. Boxed Warning]: Avinza®: Do not administer with alcoholic beverages or ethanol-containing products, which may disrupt extended-release characteristic of product.

Injections: Note: Products are designed for administration by specific routes (I.V., intrathecal, epidural). Use caution when prescribing, dispensing, or administering to use formulations only by intended route(s).

[U.S. Boxed Warning]: Duramorph®: Due to the risk of severe and/or sustained cardiopulmonary depressant effects of Duramorph® must be administered in a fully equipped and staffed environment. Naloxone injection should be immediately available. Patient should remain in this environment for at least 24 hours following the initial dose.

Infumorph® solutions are **for use in microinfusion devices only**; not for I.V., I.M., or SubQ administration.

Depo-Dur™: **For epidural administration only.** Intrathecal administration has resulted in prolonged respiratory depression. Freezing may adversely affect modified-release mechanism of drug; check freeze indicator within carton prior to administration.

Drug Interactions

Cytochrome P450 Effect: Substrate of CYP2D6 (minor)

Increased Effect/Toxicity: Antipsychotic agents may increase the hypotensive effects of morphine. Use of selective serotonin reuptake inhibitors (SSRIs) or meperidine may lead to additive serotonergic effects with concomitant morphine, possibly precipitating serotonin syndrome. CNS depressants and tricyclic antidepressants may potentiate the effects of morphine. Concurrent use of MAO inhibitors and meperidine has been associated with significant adverse effects; use caution with morphine. Some manufacturers recommend avoiding use within 14 days of MAO inhibitors.

Decreased Effect: The therapeutic efficacy of pegvisomant may be decreased by concomitant opiates, possibly requiring dosage adjustment of pegvisomant. Rifamycin derivatives may decrease levels or effects of morphine.

Ethanol/Nutrition/Herb Interactions

Ethanol: Avoid ethanol (may increase CNS depression).

Avinza®: Alcoholic beverages or ethanol-containing products may disrupt extended-release formulation resulting in rapid release of entire morphine dose.

Food: Administration of oral morphine solution with food may increase bioavailability (ie, a report of 34% increase in morphine AUC when morphine oral solution followed a high-fat meal). The bioavailability of Oramorph SR® or Kadian® does not appear to be affected by food.

Herb/Nutraceutical: Avoid valerian, St John's wort, kava kava, gotu kola (may increase CNS depression).

Dietary Considerations Morphine may cause GI upset; take with food if GI upset occurs. Be consistent when taking morphine with or without meals.

Pharmacodynamics/Kinetics

Onset of action: Oral (immediate release): ~30 minutes; I.V.: 5-10 minutes

Duration: Pain relief:

Immediate release formulations: 4 hours

Extended release epidural injection (DepoDur™): >48 hours

Absorption: Variable

Distribution: V_d: 3-4 L/kg; binds to opioid receptors in the CNS and periphery (eg, GI tract)

Protein binding: 30% to 35%

Metabolism: Hepatic via conjugation with glucuronic acid to morphine-3-glucuronide (inactive), morphine-6-glucuronide (active), and in lesser amounts, morphine-3-6-diglucuronide; other minor metabolites include normorphine (active) and the 3-ethereal sulfate

Bioavailability: Oral: 17% to 33% (first-pass effect limits oral bioavailability; oral:parenteral effectiveness reportedly varies from 1:6 in opioid naive patients to 1:3 with chronic use)

Half-life elimination: Adults: 2-4 hours (immediate release forms)

Time to peak, plasma: Kadian®: ~10 hours

Excretion: Urine (primarily as morphine-3-glucuronide, ~2% to 12% excreted unchanged); feces (~7% to 10%). It has been suggested that accumulation of morphine-6-glucuronide might cause toxicity with renal insufficiency. All of the metabolites (ie, morphine-3-glucuronide, morphine-6-glucuronide, and normorphine) have been suggested as possible causes of neurotoxicity (eg, myoclonus).

Pregnancy Risk Factor C/D (prolonged use or high doses at term)

Dosage Forms

Capsule, extended release:

Avinza®: 30 mg, 60 mg, 90 mg, 120 mg

Capsule, sustained release:

Kadian®: 20 mg, 30 mg, 50 mg, 60 mg, 80 mg, 100 mg

Infusion [premixed in D_5W]: 1 mg/mL (100 mL, 250 mL)

Injection, extended release liposomal suspension [lumbar epidural injection, preservative free]:

DepoDur™: 10 mg/mL (1 mL, 1.5 mL, 2 mL)

Injection, solution: 2 mg/mL (1 mL); 4 mg/mL (1 mL); 5 mg/mL (1 mL); 8 mg/mL (1 mL); 10 mg/mL (1 mL, 10 mL); 15 mg/mL (1 mL, 20 mL); 25 mg/mL (4 mL, 10 mL, 20 mL, 40 mL, 50 mL, 100 mL, 250 mL); 50 mg/mL (20 mL, 40 mL)

Injection, solution [epidural, intrathecal, or I.V. infusion; preservative free]: 0.5 mg/mL (2 mL, 10 mL); 1 mg/mL (2 mL, 10 mL)

Astramorph/PF™: 0.5 mg/mL (2 mL, 10 mL); 1 mg/mL (2 mL, 10 mL)

Duramorph®: 0.5 mg/mL (10 mL); 1 mg/mL (10 mL)

Injection, solution [epidural or intrathecal infusion via microinfusion device; preservative free]: 10 mg/mL (20 mL); 25 mg/mL (20 mL)

Infumorph®: 10 mg/mL (20 mL); 25 mg/mL (20 mL)

Injection, solution [I.V. infusion via PCA pump]: 0.5 mg/mL (30 mL); 1 mg/mL (30 mL, 50 mL); 2 mg/mL (30 mL); 5 mg/mL (30 mL, 50 mL)

Injection, solution [preservative free]: 0.5 mg/mL (10 mL); 1 mg/mL (10 mL); 25 mg/mL (4 mL, 10 mL, 20 mL)

Solution, oral: 10 mg/5 mL, 20 mg/5 mL, 20 mg/mL

Roxanol™: 20 mg/mL

Suppository, rectal: 5 mg (12s), 10 mg (12s), 20 mg (12s), 30 mg (12s)

RMS®: 5 mg (12s), 10 mg (12s), 20 mg (12s), 30 mg (12s)

Tablet: 10 mg, 15 mg, 30 mg

Tablet, controlled release:

MS Contin®: 15 mg, 30 mg, 60 mg, 100 mg, 200 mg

Tablet, extended release: 15 mg, 30 mg, 60 mg, 100 mg, 200 mg

(Continued)

Morphine Sulfate *(Continued)*

Tablet, sustained release:
  Oramorph SR®: 15 mg, 30 mg, 60 mg, 100 mg

Morrhuate Sodium *(MOR yoo ate SOW dee um)*

U.S. Brand Names Scleromate®
Generic Available Yes
Pharmacologic Category Sclerosing Agent
Use Treatment of small, uncomplicated varicose veins of the lower extremities
Local Anesthetic/Vasoconstrictor Precautions No information available to require special precautions
Effects on Dental Treatment No significant effects or complications reported
Mechanism of Action Both varicose veins and esophageal varices are treated by the thrombotic action of morrhuate sodium. By causing inflammation of the vein's intima, a thrombus is formed. Occlusion secondary to the fibrous tissue and the thrombus results in the obliteration of the vein.
Pregnancy Risk Factor C

Mosco® Corn and Callus Remover [OTC] *see* Salicylic Acid *on page 1451*

Motofen® *see* Difenoxin and Atropine *on page 494*

Motrin® *see* Ibuprofen *on page 853*

Motrin® Children's [OTC] *see* Ibuprofen *on page 853*

Motrin® Cold and Sinus [OTC] *see* Pseudoephedrine and Ibuprofen *on page 1384*

Motrin® Cold, Children's [OTC] *see* Pseudoephedrine and Ibuprofen *on page 1384*

Motrin® IB [OTC] *see* Ibuprofen *on page 853*

Motrin® Infants' [OTC] *see* Ibuprofen *on page 853*

Motrin® Junior Strength [OTC] *see* Ibuprofen *on page 853*

Mouthkote® [OTC] *see* Saliva Substitute *on page 1452*

Mouthwash (Antiseptic) *(MOUTH wosh)*

Related Information
  Bacterial Infections *on page 1793*
  Dentin Hypersensitivity, High Caries Index, and Xerostomia *on page 1812*
  Oral Rinse Products *on page 1941*
  Periodontal Diseases *on page 1801*
  Ulcerative and Erosive Disorders *on page 1809*
Related Sample Prescriptions
  Antimicrobial Oral Rinse *on page 1840*
Index Terms Antiseptic Mouthwash
Pharmacologic Category Antimicrobial Mouth Rinse; Antiplaque Agent; Mouthwash
Dental Use Aid in prevention and reduction of plaque and gingivitis; halitosis
Local Anesthetic/Vasoconstrictor Precautions No information available to require special precautions
Effects on Dental Treatment No significant effects or complications reported (see Dental Comment)
Significant Adverse Effects No data reported
Dental Usual Dosing Plaque/gingivitis prevention: Adults: Oral: Rinse full strength for 30 seconds with 20 mL (²/₃ fluid ounce or 4 teaspoonfuls) morning and night
Dosage Rinse full strength for 30 seconds with 20 mL (²/₃ fluid ounce or 4 teaspoonfuls) morning and night
Contraindications Hypersensitivity to any component of the formulation
Dosage Forms Excipient information presented when available (limited, particularly for generics); consult specific product labeling.
  Rinse: 250 mL, 500 mL, 1000 mL
Dental Comment Active ingredients:
  Listerine® Antiseptic: Thymol 0.064%, eucalyptus 0.092%, methyl salicylate 0.060%, menthol 0.042%, alcohol 26.9%, water, benzoic acid, poloxamer 407, sodium benzoate, caramel
  Fresh Burst Listerine® Antiseptic: Thymol 0.064%, eucalyptus 0.092%, methyl salicylate 0.060%, menthol 0.042%, alcohol 26.9%, water, benzoic acid, poloxamer 407, sodium benzoate, flavoring, sodium, saccharin, sodium citrate, citric acid, D&C yellow #10, FD&C green #3
  Cool Mint Listerine® Antiseptic: Thymol 0.064%, eucalyptus 0.092%, methyl salicylate 0.060%, menthol 0.042%, alcohol 26.9%, water, benzoic acid,

poloxamer 407, sodium benzoate, flavoring, sodium, saccharin, sodium citrate, citric acid, FD&C green #3

The following information is endorsed on the label of the Listerine® products by the Council on Scientific Affairs, American Dental Association: "Listerine® Antiseptic has been shown to help prevent and reduce supragingival plaque accumulation and gingivitis when used in a conscientiously applied program of oral hygiene and regular professional care. Its effect on periodontitis has not been determined."

MoviPrep® *see* Polyethylene Glycol-Electrolyte Solution *on page 1321*

Moxifloxacin (moxs i FLOKS a sin)

Related Information
Bacterial Infections *on page 1793*
Respiratory Diseases *on page 1747*

U.S. Brand Names Avelox®; Avelox® I.V.; Vigamox™

Canadian Brand Names Avelox®; Avelox® I.V.; Vigamox™

Mexican Brand Names Avelox; Vigamoxi

Generic Available No

Index Terms Moxifloxacin Hydrochloride

Pharmacologic Category Antibiotic, Ophthalmic; Antibiotic, Quinolone

Use Treatment of mild-to-moderate community-acquired pneumonia, including multidrug-resistant *Streptococcus pneumoniae* (MDRSP); acute bacterial exacerbation of chronic bronchitis; acute bacterial sinusitis; complicated and uncomplicated skin and skin structure infections; complicated intra-abdominal infections; bacterial conjunctivitis (ophthalmic formulation)

Unlabeled/Investigational Use *Legionella*

Local Anesthetic/Vasoconstrictor Precautions Moxifloxacin is one of the drugs confirmed to prolong the QT interval and is accepted as having a risk of causing torsade de pointes. The risk of drug-induced torsade de pointes is extremely low when a single QT interval prolonging drug is prescribed. In terms of epinephrine, it is not known what effect vasoconstrictors in the local anesthetic regimen will have in patients with a known history of congenital prolonged QT interval or in patients taking any medication that prolongs the QT interval. Until more information is obtained, it is suggested that the clinician consult with the physician prior to the use of a vasoconstrictor in suspected patients, and that the vasoconstrictor (epinephrine, levonordefrin [Neo-Cobefrin®]) be used with caution.

Effects on Dental Treatment Key adverse event(s) related to dental treatment: Dry mouth, glossitis, stomatitis, and taste perversion.

Common Adverse Effects
Systemic:

3% to 10%: Gastrointestinal: Nausea (6%), diarrhea (5%)

0.1% to 3%:
Cardiovascular: Hypertension, palpitation, QT_c prolongation, tachycardia, vasodilation

Central nervous system: Anxiety, chills, dizziness, headache, insomnia, nervousness, pain, somnolence, tremor, vertigo

Dermatologic: Dry skin, pruritus, rash (maculopapular, purpuric, pustular)

Endocrine & metabolic: Serum chloride increased (≥2%), serum ionized calcium increased (≥2%), serum glucose decreased (≥2%)

Gastrointestinal: Abdominal pain, amylase increased, amylase decreased (≥2%), anorexia, constipation, dry mouth, dyspepsia, flatulence, glossitis, lactic dehydrogenase increased, stomatitis, taste perversion, vomiting

Genitourinary: Vaginal moniliasis, vaginitis

Hematologic: Eosinophilia, leukopenia, prothrombin time prolonged, increased INR, thrombocythemia

Increased serum levels of the following (≥2%): MCH, neutrophils, WBC

Decreased serum levels of the following (≥2%): Basophils, eosinophils, hemoglobin, RBC, neutrophils

Hepatic: Bilirubin decreased or increased (≥2%), GGTP increased, liver function test abnormal

Local: Injection site reaction

Neuromuscular & skeletal: Arthralgia, myalgia, weakness

Renal: Kidney function abnormal, serum albumin increased (≥2%)

Respiratory: Pharyngitis, pneumonia, rhinitis, sinusitis, pO_2 increased (≥2%)

Additional reactions with **ophthalmic** preparation: 1% to 6%: Conjunctivitis, dry eye, ocular discomfort, ocular hyperemia, ocular pain, ocular pruritus, subconjunctival hemorrhage, tearing, visual acuity decreased
(Continued)

Moxifloxacin *(Continued)*

Dosage

Usual dosage range:

Children ≥1 year and Adults: Ophthalmic: Instill 1 drop into affected eye(s) 3 times/day for 7 days

Adults: Oral, I.V.: 400 mg every 24 hours

Indication-specific dosing:

Children ≥1 year and Adults: Ophthalmic:

Bacterial conjunctivitis: Instill 1 drop into affected eye(s) 3 times/day for 7 days

Adults: Oral, I.V.:

Acute bacterial sinusitis: 400 mg every 24 hours for 10 days

Chronic bronchitis, acute bacterial exacerbation: 400 mg every 24 hours for 5 days

Intra-abdominal infections (complicated): 400 mg every 24 hours for 5-14 days (initiate with I.V.)

Pneumonia, community-acquired (including MDRSP): 400 mg every 24 hours for 7-14 days

Skin and skin structure infections:

Complicated: 400 mg every 24 hours for 7-21 days

Uncomplicated: 400 mg every 24 hours for 7 days

Elderly: No dosage adjustments are required based on age

Dosage adjustment in renal impairment: No dosage adjustment is required, including patients on hemodialysis or CAPD

Dosage adjustment in hepatic impairment: No dosage adjustment is required in mild to moderate hepatic insufficiency (Child-Pugh Class A and B). Not recommended in patients with severe hepatic insufficiency.

Mechanism of Action Moxifloxacin is a DNA gyrase inhibitor, and also inhibits topoisomerase IV. DNA gyrase (topoisomerase II) is an essential bacterial enzyme that maintains the superhelical structure of DNA. DNA gyrase is required for DNA replication and transcription, DNA repair, recombination, and transposition; inhibition is bactericidal.

Contraindications Hypersensitivity to moxifloxacin, other quinolone antibiotics, or any component of the formulation

Warnings/Precautions Use with caution in patients with significant bradycardia or acute myocardial ischemia. Moxifloxacin causes a concentration-dependent QT prolongation. Do not exceed recommended dose or infusion rate. Avoid use with uncorrected hypokalemia, with other drugs that prolong the QT interval or induce bradycardia, or with class IA or III antiarrhythmic agents. Use with caution in individuals at risk of seizures (CNS disorders or concurrent therapy with medications which may lower seizure threshold). Potential for seizures, although very rare, may be increased with concomitant NSAID therapy. Discontinue in patients who experience significant CNS adverse effects (dizziness, hallucinations, suicidal ideation or actions). Not recommended in patients with moderate to severe hepatic insufficiency. Use with caution in diabetes; glucose regulation may be altered. Tendon inflammation and/or rupture have been reported with quinolone antibiotics. Risk may be increased with concurrent corticosteroids, particularly in the elderly. Discontinue at first signs or symptoms of tendon pain.

Severe hypersensitivity reactions, including anaphylaxis, have occurred with quinolone therapy. If an allergic reaction occurs (itching, urticaria, dyspnea or facial edema, loss of consciousness, tingling, cardiovascular collapse) discontinue drug immediately. May cause photosensitivity. Prolonged use may result in fungal or bacterial superinfection, including *C. difficile*-associated diarrhea and pseudomembranous colitis. Quinolones may exacerbate myasthenia gravis. Peripheral neuropathy may rarely occur. Safety and efficacy of systemically administered moxifloxacin (oral, intravenous) in patients <18 years of age have not been established.

Ophthalmic: Eye drops should not be injected subconjunctivally or introduced directly into the anterior chamber of the eye. Contact lenses should not be worn during therapy.

Drug Interactions

Increased Effect/Toxicity: Moxifloxacin may increase the effects/toxicity of glyburide and warfarin. Concomitant use with corticosteroids may increase the risk of tendon rupture. Concomitant use with other QT$_c$-prolonging agents (eg, Class Ia and Class III antiarrhythmics, erythromycin, cisapride, antipsychotics, and cyclic antidepressants) may result in arrhythmias, such as torsade de pointes. Concomitant use with NSAIDs may rarely increase risk of seizure.

Decreased Effect: Concurrent administration of metal cations, including most antacids, oral electrolyte supplements, quinapril, sucralfate, some didanosine formulations (pediatric powder for oral suspension), and other higly-buffered oral drugs, may decrease quinolone levels; separate doses.

Ethanol/Nutrition/Herb Interactions Food: Absorption is not affected by administration with a high-fat meal or yogurt.

Dietary Considerations May be taken with or without food. Take 4 hours before or 8 hours after multiple vitamins, antacids, or other products containing magnesium, aluminum, iron, or zinc.

Pharmacodynamics/Kinetics

Absorption: Well absorbed; not affected by high fat meal or yogurt

Distribution: V_d: 1.7 to 2.7 L/kg; tissue concentrations often exceed plasma concentrations in respiratory tissues, alveolar macrophages, abdominal tissues/fluids, and sinus tissues

Protein binding: 30% to 50%

Metabolism: Hepatic (52% of dose) via glucuronide (14%) and sulfate (38%) conjugation

Bioavailability: 90%

Half-life elimination: Oral: 12 hours; I.V.: 15 hours

Excretion: Approximately 45% of a dose is excreted in feces (25%) and urine (20%) as unchanged drug

Metabolites: Sulfate conjugates in feces, glucuronide conjugates in urine

Pregnancy Risk Factor C

Dosage Forms

Infusion [premixed in sodium chloride 0.8%]:

Avelox® I.V.: 400 mg (250 mL)

Solution, ophthalmic:

Vigamox™: 0.5% (3 mL)

Tablet:

Avelox®: 400 mg

Avelox® ABC Pack [unit-dose pack]: 400 mg (5s)

Moxifloxacin Hydrochloride see Moxifloxacin on page 1129

4-MP see Fomepizole on page 739

MPA see MedroxyPROGESTERone on page 1026

MPA see Mycophenolate on page 1134

MPA and Estrogens (Conjugated) see Estrogens (Conjugated/Equine) and Medroxyprogesterone on page 612

6-MP (error-prone abbreviation) see Mercaptopurine on page 1051

MPSV4 see Meningococcal Polysaccharide Vaccine (Groups A, C, Y, and W-135) on page 1036

MS Contin® see Morphine Sulfate on page 1123

MSO₄ (error-prone abbreviation and should not be used) see Morphine Sulfate on page 1123

MTA see Pemetrexed on page 1264

MTC see Mitomycin on page 1112

M.T.E.-4® see Trace Metals on page 1595

M.T.E.-5® see Trace Metals on page 1595

M.T.E.-6® see Trace Metals on page 1595

M.T.E.-7® see Trace Metals on page 1595

MTX (error-prone abbreviation) see Methotrexate on page 1068

Mucinex® [OTC] see Guaifenesin on page 795

Mucinex®-D [OTC] see Guaifenesin and Pseudoephedrine on page 798

Mucinex®, Children's [OTC] see Guaifenesin on page 795

Mucinex® Children's Cough [OTC] see Guaifenesin and Dextromethorphan on page 796

Mucinex®, Children's Mini-Melts™ [OTC] see Guaifenesin on page 795

Mucinex® DM [OTC] see Guaifenesin and Dextromethorphan on page 796

Mucinex®, Junior Mini-Melts™ [OTC] see Guaifenesin on page 795

Mucomyst see Acetylcysteine on page 47

Multidex® [OTC] see Maltodextrin on page 1017

Multiple Vitamins see Vitamins (Multiple/Oral) on page 1665

Multiret Folic 500 see Vitamins (Multiple/Oral) on page 1665

Multitargeted Antifolate see Pemetrexed on page 1264

Multitrace™-4 see Trace Metals on page 1595

Multitrace™-4 Neonatal see Trace Metals on page 1595

Multitrace™-4 Pediatric see Trace Metals on page 1595

Multitrace™-5 see Trace Metals on page 1595

Multivitamins/Fluoride see Vitamins (Fluoride) on page 1665

Mumps, Measles and Rubella Vaccines, Combined see Measles, Mumps, and Rubella Vaccines (Combined) on page 1020

Mumps, Rubella, Varicella, and Measles Vaccine *see* Measles, Mumps, Rubella, and Varicella Virus Vaccine *on page 1021*

Mumpsvax® *see* Mumps Virus Vaccine (Live/Attenuated) *on page 1132*

Mumps Virus Vaccine (Live/Attenuated)
(mumpz VYE rus vak SEEN, live, a ten YOO ate ed)

Related Information
Immunizations (Vaccines) *on page 1886*

U.S. Brand Names Mumpsvax®

Generic Available No

Pharmacologic Category Vaccine

Use Mumps prophylaxis by promoting active immunity

Note: Trivalent measles-mumps-rubella (MMR) vaccine is the preferred agent for most children and many adults; persons born prior to 1957 are generally considered immune and need not be vaccinated

Local Anesthetic/Vasoconstrictor Precautions No information available to require special precautions

Effects on Dental Treatment No significant effects or complications reported

Common Adverse Effects All serious adverse reactions must be reported to the U.S. Department of Health and Human Services (DHHS) Vaccine Adverse Event Reporting System (VAERS) 1-800-822-7967.

Frequency not defined.
Cardiovascular: Syncope, vasculitis
Central nervous system: Encephalitis, febrile seizures, fever, Guillain-Barré syndrome, irritability
Dermatologic: Angioneurotic edema, erythema multiforme, purpura, Stevens-Johnson syndrome, urticaria
Endocrine & metabolic: Diabetes mellitus, parotitis
Gastrointestinal: Diarrhea, pancreatitis
Genitourinary: Orchitis
Hematologic: Leukocytosis, thrombocytopenia
Local: Burning/stinging at injection site, wheal and flare at injection site
Ocular: Conjunctivitis, ocular palsies, optic neuritis, papillitis, retrobulbar neuritis
Otic: Nerve deafness, otitis media
Respiratory: Bronchial spasm, cough, rhinitis
Miscellaneous: Anaphylaxis, anaphylactoid reactions, lymphadenopathy

Mechanism of Action Promotes active immunity to mumps virus by inducing specific antibodies.

Drug Interactions
Decreased Effect:
In patients receiving high doses of systemic corticosteroids for ≥14 days, wait at least 1 month between discontinuing steroid therapy and administering vaccine. Do not administer this vaccine with Immune globulin, whole blood, plasma; immune response may be compromised (defer vaccine administration for ≥3 months). The effect of the vaccine may be decreased with Immunosuppressant medications. Do not give within 1 month of other live virus vaccine.

Pregnancy Risk Factor C

Mupirocin (myoo PEER oh sin)

U.S. Brand Names Bactroban®; Bactroban® Nasal; Centany™

Canadian Brand Names Bactroban®

Mexican Brand Names Bactroban

Generic Available Yes: Topical ointment

Index Terms Mupirocin Calcium; Pseudomonic Acid A

Pharmacologic Category Antibiotic, Topical

Use
Intranasal: Eradication of nasal colonization with MRSA in adult patients and healthcare workers
Topical: Treatment of impetigo or secondary infected traumatic skin lesions due to *S. aureus* and *S. pyogenes*

Unlabeled/Investigational Use Intranasal: Surgical prophylaxis to prevent wound infections

Local Anesthetic/Vasoconstrictor Precautions No information available to require special precautions

Effects on Dental Treatment Key adverse event(s) related to dental treatment: Xerostomia (normal salivary flow resumes upon discontinuation) and taste perversion.

Common Adverse Effects Frequency not defined.

Central nervous system: Dizziness, headache

Dermatologic: Cellulitis, dermatitis, dry skin, erythema, hives, pruritus, rash, ulcerative stomatitis

Gastrointestinal: Abdominal pain, diarrhea, nausea, taste perversion, xerostomia

Local: Burning, edema, pain, stinging, tenderness

Ocular: Blepharitis

Otic: Ear pain

Respiratory: Cough, pharyngitis, rhinitis, upper respiratory tract congestion

Miscellaneous: Secondary wound infection

Mechanism of Action Binds to bacterial isoleucyl transfer-RNA synthetase resulting in the inhibition of protein synthesis

Pharmacodynamics/Kinetics

Absorption: Topical: Penetrates outer layers of skin; systemic absorption minimal through intact skin

Metabolism: Skin: 3% to monic acid (inactive)

Excretion: Urine

Pregnancy Risk Factor B

Mupirocin Calcium *see* Mupirocin *on page 1132*

Murine® Ear Wax Removal System [OTC] *see* Carbamide Peroxide *on page 276*

Murine® Tears [OTC] *see* Artificial Tears *on page 147*

Murine® Tears Plus [OTC] *see* Tetrahydrozoline *on page 1551*

Muro 128® [OTC] *see* Sodium Chloride *on page 1480*

Murocel® [OTC] *see* Artificial Tears *on page 147*

Murocoll-2® *see* Phenylephrine and Scopolamine *on page 1294*

Muromonab-CD3 (myoo roe MOE nab see dee three)

U.S. Brand Names Orthoclone OKT® 3

Canadian Brand Names Orthoclone OKT® 3

Mexican Brand Names Orthoclone OKT3

Generic Available No

Index Terms Monoclonal Antibody; OKT3

Pharmacologic Category Immunosuppressant Agent

Use Treatment of acute allograft rejection in renal transplant patients; treatment of acute hepatic, kidney, and pancreas rejection episodes resistant to conventional treatment. Acute graft-versus-host disease following bone marrow transplantation resistant to conventional treatment.

Local Anesthetic/Vasoconstrictor Precautions No information available to require special precautions

Effects on Dental Treatment No significant effects or complications reported

Common Adverse Effects Note: Signs and symptoms of Cytokine Release Syndrome (characterized by pyrexia, chills, dyspnea, nausea, vomiting, chest pain, diarrhea, tremor, wheezing, headache, tachycardia, rigor, hypertension, pulmonary edema and/or other cardiorespiratory manifestations) occurs in a significant proportion of patients following the first couple of doses of muromonab-CD3. Additionally, some patients have experienced immediate hypersensitivity reactions to muromonab-CD3 (characterized by cardiovascular collapse, cardiorespiratory arrest, loss of consciousness, hypotension/shock, tachycardia, tingling, angioedema (including laryngeal, pharyngeal, or facial edema), airway obstruction, bronchospasm, dyspnea, urticaria, and/or pruritus) upon initial exposure and re-exposure.

>10%:

Cardiovascular: Tachycardia (26%), hypotension (25%), hypertension (19%), edema (12%)

Central nervous system: Pyrexia (77%), chills (43%), headache (28%)

Dermatologic: Rash (14%; erythematous 2%)

Gastrointestinal: Diarrhea (37%), nausea (32%), vomiting (25%)

Respiratory: Dyspnea (16%)

1% to 10%:

Cardiovascular: Chest pain (9%), vasodilation (7%), arrhythmia (4%), bradycardia (4%), vascular occlusion (2%)

Central nervous system: Fatigue (9%), confusion (6%), dizziness (6%), lethargy (6%), pain trunk (6%), malaise (5%), nervousness (5%), depression (3%), somnolence (2%), meningitis (1%), seizure (1%)

Dermatologic: Pruritus (7%)

Gastrointestinal: Gastrointestinal pain (7%), abdominal pain (6%), anorexia (4%)

(Continued)

Muromonab-CD3 *(Continued)*

Hematologic: Leukopenia (7%), anemia (2%), thrombocytopenia (2%), leukocytosis (1%)

Neuromuscular & skeletal: Weakness (10%), arthralgia (7%), myalgia (1%), tremor (14%)

Ocular: Photophobia (1%)

Otic: Tinnitus (1%)

Renal: Renal dysfunction (3%)

Respiratory: Abnormal chest sound (10%), hyperventilation (7%), wheezing (6%), respiratory congestion (4%), pulmonary edema (2%), hypoxia (1%), pneumonia (1%)

Miscellaneous: Diaphoresis (7%), infections (various)

Mechanism of Action Reverses graft rejection by binding to T cells and interfering with their function by binding T-cell receptor-associated CD3 glycoprotein

Drug Interactions

Increased Effect/Toxicity: Recommend decreasing dose of prednisone to 0.5 mg/kg, azathioprine to 0.5 mg/kg (approximate 50% decrease in dose), and discontinuing cyclosporine while patient is receiving OKT3.

Decreased Effect: Decreased effect with immunosuppressive drugs.

Pharmacodynamics/Kinetics

Duration: 7 days after discontinuation

Time to peak: Steady-state: Trough: 3-14 days

Pregnancy Risk Factor C

Muse® *see* Alprostadil *on page 78*

Mutamycin® *see* Mitomycin *on page 1112*

Myambutol® *see* Ethambutol *on page 620*

Mycamine® *see* Micafungin *on page 1096*

Mycelex® *see* Clotrimazole *on page 398*

Mycelex®-7 [OTC] *see* Clotrimazole *on page 398*

Mycelex® Twin Pack [OTC] *see* Clotrimazole *on page 398*

Mycinaire™ [OTC] *see* Sodium Chloride *on page 1480*

Mycinettes® [OTC] *see* Benzocaine *on page 195*

Mycobutin® *see* Rifabutin *on page 1422*

Mycocide® NS [OTC] *see* Tolnaftate *on page 1587*

Mycolog®-II [DSC] *see* Nystatin and Triamcinolone *on page 1196*

Myco-Nail [OTC] *see* Triacetin *on page 1608*

Mycophenolate *(mye koe FEN oh late)*

U.S. Brand Names CellCept®; Myfortic®

Canadian Brand Names CellCept®; Myfortic®

Mexican Brand Names CellCept; Myfortic

Generic Available No

Index Terms MMF; MPA; Mycophenolate Mofetil; Mycophenolate Sodium; Mycophenolic Acid

Pharmacologic Category Immunosuppressant Agent

Use Prophylaxis of organ rejection concomitantly with cyclosporine and corticosteroids in patients receiving allogenic renal (CellCept®, Myfortic®), cardiac (CellCept®), or hepatic (CellCept®) transplants

Unlabeled/Investigational Use Treatment of rejection in liver transplant patients unable to tolerate tacrolimus or cyclosporine due to neurotoxicity; mild rejection in heart transplant patients; treatment of moderate-severe psoriasis; treatment of proliferative lupus nephritis; treatment of myasthenia gravis

Local Anesthetic/Vasoconstrictor Precautions No information available to require special precautions

Effects on Dental Treatment Key adverse event(s) related to dental treatment: Mouth ulceration, gum hyperplasia, gingivitis, dry mouth, dysphagia, oral moniliasis, and stomatitis.

Common Adverse Effects As reported in adults following oral dosing of CellCept® alone in renal, cardiac, and hepatic allograft rejection studies. In general, lower doses used in renal rejection patients had less adverse effects than higher doses. Rates of adverse effects were similar for each indication, except for those unique to the specific organ involved. The type of adverse effects observed in pediatric patients was similar to those seen in adults; abdominal pain, anemia, diarrhea, fever, hypertension, infection, pharyngitis, respiratory tract infection, sepsis, and vomiting were seen in higher proportion; lymphoproliferative disorder was the only type of malignancy observed. Percentages of adverse reactions were similar in studies comparing CellCept® to Myfortic® in patients following renal transplant.

>20%:

Cardiovascular: Hypertension (28% to 77%), hypotension (up to 33%), peripheral edema (27% to 64%), edema (27% to 28%), tachycardia (20% to 22%)

Central nervous system: Pain (31% to 76%), headache (16% to 54%), insomnia (41% to 52%), fever (21% to 52%), dizziness (up to 29%), anxiety (28%)

Dermatologic: Rash (up to 22%)

Endocrine & metabolic: Hyperglycemia (44% to 47%), hypercholesterolemia (41%), hypokalemia (32% to 37%), hypocalcemia (up to 30%), hypomagnesemia (up to 39%), hyperkalemia (up to 22%)

Gastrointestinal: Abdominal pain (25% to 62%), nausea (20% to 54%), diarrhea (31% to 52%), constipation (18% to 41%), vomiting (33% to 34%), anorexia (up to 25%), dyspepsia (22%)

Genitourinary: Urinary tract infection (37%)

Hematologic: Leukopenia (23% to 46%), leukocytosis (22% to 40%), hypochromic anemia (26% to 43%), thrombocytopenia (24% to 36%)

Hepatic: Liver function tests abnormal (up to 25%), ascites (24%)

Neuromuscular & skeletal: Back pain (35% to 47%), weakness (35% to 43%), tremor (24% to 34%), paresthesia (21%)

Renal: BUN increased (up to 35%), creatinine increased (up to 39%)

Respiratory: Dyspnea (31% to 37%), respiratory tract infection (22% to 37%), cough (31%), lung disorder (22% to 30%)

Miscellaneous: Infection (18% to 27%), *Candida* (11% to 22%), herpes simplex (10% to 21%)

3% to <20%:

Cardiovascular: Angina, arrhythmia, arterial thrombosis, atrial fibrillation, atrial flutter, bradycardia, cardiac arrest, cardiac failure, CHF, extrasystole, facial edema, hypervolemia, pallor, palpitation, pericardial effusion, peripheral vascular disorder, postural hypotension, supraventricular extrasystoles, supraventricular tachycardia, syncope, thrombosis, vasodilation, vasospasm, venous pressure increased, ventricular extrasystole, ventricular tachycardia

Central nervous system: Agitation, chills with fever, confusion, convulsion, delirium, depression, emotional lability, hallucinations, hypoesthesia, malaise, nervousness, psychosis, somnolence, thinking abnormal, vertigo

Dermatologic: Acne, alopecia, bruising, cellulitis, hirsutism, petechia, pruritus, skin carcinoma, skin hypertrophy, skin ulcer, vesiculobullous rash

Endocrine & metabolic: Acidosis, Cushing's syndrome, dehydration, diabetes mellitus, gout, hypercalcemia, hyperlipemia, hyperphosphatemia, hyperuricemia, hypochloremia, hypoglycemia, hyponatremia, hypoproteinemia, hypothyroidism, parathyroid disorder, weight gain/loss

Gastrointestinal: Abdomen enlarged, dry mouth, dysphagia, esophagitis, flatulence, gastritis, gastroenteritis, gastrointestinal hemorrhage, gastrointestinal moniliasis, gingivitis, gum hyperplasia, ileus, melena, mouth ulceration, oral moniliasis, stomach disorder, stomatitis

Genitourinary: Impotence, nocturia, pelvic pain, prostatic disorder, scrotal edema, urinary frequency, urinary incontinence, urinary retention, urinary tract disorder

Hematologic: Coagulation disorder, hemorrhage, neutropenia, pancytopenia, polycythemia, prothrombin time increased, thromboplastin increased

Hepatic: Alkaline phosphatase increased, alkalosis, bilirubinemia, cholangitis, cholestatic jaundice, GGT increased, hepatitis, jaundice, liver damage, transaminases increased

Local: Abscess

Neuromuscular & skeletal: Arthralgia, hypertonia, joint disorder, leg cramps, myalgia, myasthenia, neck pain, neuropathy, osteoporosis

Ocular: Amblyopia, cataract, conjunctivitis, eye hemorrhage, lacrimation disorder, vision abnormal

Otic: Deafness, ear disorder, ear pain, tinnitus

Renal: Albuminuria, creatinine increased, dysuria, hematuria, hydronephrosis, kidney failure, kidney tubular necrosis, oliguria

Respiratory: Apnea, asthma, atelectasis, bronchitis, epistaxis, hemoptysis, hiccup, hyperventilation, hypoxia, respiratory acidosis, lung edema, pharyngitis, pleural effusion, pneumonia, pneumothorax, pulmonary hypertension, respiratory moniliasis, rhinitis, sinusitis, sputum increased, voice alteration

Miscellaneous: *Candida* (mucocutaneous 15% to 18%), CMV viremia/syndrome (12% to 14%), CMV tissue invasive disease (6% to 11%), herpes zoster cutaneous disease (4% to 10%), cyst, diaphoresis, flu-like syndrome, fungal dermatitis, healing abnormal, hernia, ileus infection, lactic dehydrogenase increased, peritonitis, pyelonephritis, thirst

Mechanism of Action MPA exhibits a cytostatic effect on T and B lymphocytes. It is an inhibitor of inosine monophosphate dehydrogenase (IMPDH) which inhibits *de novo* guanosine nucleotide synthesis. T and B lymphocytes are dependent on this pathway for proliferation.

(Continued)

Mycophenolate *(Continued)*

Drug Interactions

Increased Effect/Toxicity: Acyclovir, valacyclovir, ganciclovir, and valganciclovir levels may increase due to competition for tubular secretion of these drugs. Probenecid may increase mycophenolate levels due to inhibition of tubular secretion. High doses of salicylates may increase free fraction of mycophenolic acid. Azathioprine's bone marrow suppression may be potentiated; do not administer together.

Decreased Effect: Antacids decrease serum levels (C_{max} and AUC); **do not administer together**. Cholestyramine resin decreases serum levels; **do not administer together**. Avoid use of live vaccines; vaccinations may be less effective. Influenza vaccine may be of value. During concurrent use of oral contraceptives, progesterone levels are not significantly affected, however, effect on estrogen component varies; an additional form of contraception should be used.

Pharmacodynamics/Kinetics

Onset of action: Peak effect: Correlation of toxicity or efficacy is still being developed, however, one study indicated that 12-hour AUCs >40 mcg/mL/hour were correlated with efficacy and decreased episodes of rejection

T_{max}: Oral: MPA:
   CellCept®: 1-1.5 hours
   Myfortic®: 1.5-2.5 hours

Absorption: AUC values for MPA are lower in the early post-transplant period versus later (>3 months) post-transplant period. The extent of absorption in pediatrics is similar to that seen in adults, although there was wide variability reported.
   Oral: Myfortic®: 93%

Distribution:
   CellCept®: MPA: Oral: 4 L/kg; I.V.: 3.6 L/kg
   Myfortic®: MPA: Oral: 54 L (at steady state); 112 L (elimination phase)

Protein binding: MPA: 97%, MPAG 82%

Metabolism: Hepatic and via GI tract; CellCept® is completely hydrolyzed in the liver to mycophenolic acid (MPA; active metabolite); enterohepatic recirculation of MPA may occur; MPA is glucuronidated to MPAG (inactive metabolite)

Bioavailability: Oral: CellCept®: 94%; Myfortic®: 72%

Half-life elimination:
   CellCept®: MPA: Oral: 18 hours; I.V.: 17 hours
   Myfortic®: MPA: Oral: 8-16 hours; MPAG: 13-17 hours

Excretion:
   CellCept®: MPA: Urine (<1%), feces (6%); MPAG: Urine (87%)
   Myfortic®: MPA: Urine (3%), feces; MPAG: Urine (>60%)

Pregnancy Risk Factor C (manufacturer)

Nabumetone (na BYOO me tone)

Related Information
Rheumatoid Arthritis, Osteoarthritis, and Osteoporosis *on page 1759*
Temporomandibular Dysfunction (TMD) *on page 1822*
U.S. Brand Names Relafen® [DSC]
Canadian Brand Names Apo-Nabumetone®; Gen-Nabumetone; Novo-Nabumetone; Relafen®; Rhoxal-nabumetone; Sandoz-Nabumetone
Mexican Brand Names Relifex
Generic Available Yes
Pharmacologic Category Nonsteroidal Anti-inflammatory Drug (NSAID), Oral
Use Management of osteoarthritis and rheumatoid arthritis
Unlabeled/Investigational Use Moderate pain
Local Anesthetic/Vasoconstrictor Precautions No information available to require special precautions
Effects on Dental Treatment Key adverse event(s) related to dental treatment: Xerostomia (normal salivary flow resumes upon discontinuation) and stomatitis. NSAID formulations are known to reversibly decrease platelet aggregation via mechanisms different than observed with aspirin. The dentist should be aware of the potential of abnormal coagulation. Caution should also be exercised in the use of NSAIDs in patients already on anticoagulant therapy with drugs such as warfarin (Coumadin®).
Common Adverse Effects
>10%: Gastrointestinal: Abdominal pain (12%), diarrhea (14%), dyspepsia (13%)
1% to 10%:
Cardiovascular: Edema (3% to 9%)
Central nervous system: Dizziness (3% to 9%), headache (3% to 9%), fatigue (1% to 3%), insomnia (1% to 3%), nervousness (1% to 3%), somnolence (1% to 3%)
Dermatologic: Pruritus (3% to 9%), rash (3% to 9%)
Gastrointestinal: Constipation (3% to 9%), flatulence (3% to 9%), guaic positive (3% to 9%), nausea (3% to 9%), gastritis (1% to 3%), stomatitis (1% to 3%), vomiting (1% to 3%), xerostomia (1% to 3%)
Otic: Tinnitus
Miscellaneous: Diaphoresis (1% to 3%)
Restrictions An FDA-approved medication guide must be distributed when dispensing an oral outpatient prescription (new or refill) where this medication is to be used without direct supervision of a healthcare provider. Medication guides are available at http://www.fda.gov/cder/Offices/ODS/medication_guides.htm.
Dosage Adults: Oral: 1000 mg/day; an additional 500-1000 mg may be needed in some patients to obtain more symptomatic relief; may be administered once or twice daily (maximum dose: 2000 mg/day)
Note: Patients <50 kg are less likely to require doses >1000 mg/day.
Dosage adjustment in renal impairment: In general, NSAIDs are not recommended for use in patients with advanced renal disease, but the manufacturer of nabumetone does provide some guidelines for adjustment in renal dysfunction:
Moderate impairment (Cl_{cr} 30-49 mL/minute): Initial dose: 750 mg/day; maximum dose: 1500 mg/day
Severe impairment (Cl_{cr} <30 mL/minute): Initial dose: 500 mg/day; maximum dose: 1000 mg/day
Mechanism of Action Nabumetone is a nonacidic NSAID that is rapidly metabolized after absorption to a major active metabolite, 6-methoxy-2-naphthylacetic acid. As found with previous NSAIDs, nabumetone's active metabolite inhibits the cyclooxygenase enzyme which is indirectly responsible for the production of inflammation and pain during arthritis by way of enhancing the production of endoperoxides and prostaglandins E_2 and I_2 (prostacyclin). The active metabolite of nabumetone is felt to be the compound primarily responsible for therapeutic effect. Comparatively, the parent drug is a poor inhibitor of prostaglandin synthesis.
(Continued)

Nabumetone *(Continued)*

Contraindications Hypersensitivity to nabumetone, aspirin, other NSAIDs, or any component of the formulation; perioperative pain in the setting of coronary artery bypass surgery (CABG); pregnancy (3rd trimester)

Warnings/Precautions [U.S. Boxed Warning]: NSAIDs are associated with an increased risk of adverse cardiovascular events, including MI, stroke, and new onset or worsening of pre-existing hypertension. Risk may be increased with duration of use or pre-existing cardiovascular risk factors or disease. Carefully evaluate individual cardiovascular risk profiles prior to prescribing. Use caution with fluid retention, CHF or hypertension. Concurrent administration of ibuprofen, and potentially other nonselective NSAIDs, may interfere with aspirin's cardioprotective effect.

Use of NSAIDs can compromise existing renal function. Renal toxicity can occur in patient with impaired renal function, dehydration, heart failure, liver dysfunction, those taking diuretics and ACEI and the elderly. Rehydrate patient before starting therapy. Monitor renal function closely. Not recommended for use in patients with advanced renal disease.

[U.S. Boxed Warning]: NSAIDs may increase risk of gastrointestinal irritation, ulceration, bleeding, and perforation. These events may occur at any time during therapy and without warning. Use caution with a history of GI disease (bleeding or ulcers), concurrent therapy with aspirin, anticoagulants and/or corticosteroids, smoking, use of alcohol, the elderly or debilitated patients.

Use the lowest effective dose for the shortest duration of time, consistent with individual patient goals, to reduce risk of cardiovascular or GI adverse events. Alternate therapies should be considered for patients at high risk.

NSAIDs may cause serious skin adverse events including exfoliative dermatitis, Stevens-Johnson syndrome (SJS) and toxic epidermal necrolysis (TEN). Anaphylactoid reactions may occur, even without prior exposure; patients with "aspirin triad" (bronchial asthma, aspirin intolerance, rhinitis) may be at increased risk. Do not use in patients who experience bronchospasm, asthma, rhinitis, or urticaria with NSAID or aspirin therapy. Use caution in other forms of asthma.

Use with caution in patients with decreased hepatic function. Closely monitor patients with any abnormal LFT. Severe hepatic reactions (eg, fulminant hepatitis, liver failure) have occurred with NSAID use, rarely; discontinue if signs or symptoms of liver disease develop, or if systemic manifestations occur.

The elderly are at increased risk for adverse effects (especially peptic ulceration, CNS effects, renal toxicity) from NSAIDs even at low doses.

Withhold for at least 4-6 half-lives prior to surgical or dental procedures. May cause photosensitivity reactions. Safety and efficacy have not been established in pediatric patients.

Drug Interactions

Increased Effect/Toxicity: NSAIDs may increase digoxin, methotrexate, and lithium serum concentrations. The renal adverse effects of ACE inhibitors may be potentiated by NSAIDs. Potential for bleeding may be increased with anticoagulants or antiplatelet agents. Concurrent use of corticosteroids may increase the risk of GI ulceration. Concomitant use with fluoroquinolones may rarely increase risk of seizure.

Decreased Effect: NSAIDs may decrease the effect of some antihypertensive agents, including ACE inhibitors, angiotensin receptor antagonists, beta-blockers, and hydralazine. The efficacy of diuretics (loop and/or thiazide) may be decreased. Cholestyramine (and other bile acid sequestrants) may decrease the absorption of NSAIDs; separate by at least 2 hours. Salicylates' antiplatelet effect may be reduced.

Ethanol/Nutrition/Herb Interactions

Ethanol: Avoid ethanol (may enhance gastric mucosal irritation).

Food: Nabumetone peak serum concentrations may be increased if taken with food or dairy products.

Herb/Nutraceutical: Avoid alfalfa, anise, bilberry, bladderwrack, bromelain, cat's claw, celery, coleus, cordyceps, dong quai, evening primrose, feverfew, fenugreek, garlic, ginger, ginkgo biloba, red clover, horse chestnut, grapeseed, green tea, ginseng, guggul, horse chestnut seed, horseradish, licorice, prickly ash, red clover, reishi, SAMe, sweet clover, turmeric, white willow (all have additional antiplatelet activity).

Pharmacodynamics/Kinetics

Onset of action: Several days

Distribution: Diffusion occurs readily into synovial fluid

V_d: 6MNA: 29-82 L

Protein binding: 6MNA: >99%

Metabolism: Prodrug, rapidly metabolized in the liver to an active metabolite [6-methoxy-2-naphthylacetic acid (6MNA)] and inactive metabolites; extensive first-pass effect

Half-life elimination: 6MNA: ~24 hours

Time to peak, serum: 6MNA: Oral: 2.5-4 hours; Synovial fluid: 4-12 hours

Excretion: 6MNA: Urine (80%) and feces (9%)

Pregnancy Risk Factor C/D (3rd trimester)

Dosage Forms Tablet: 500 mg, 750 mg

NAC *see* Acetylcysteine *on page 47*

N-Acetyl-L-cysteine *see* Acetylcysteine *on page 47*

N-Acetylcysteine *see* Acetylcysteine *on page 47*

N-Acetyl-P-Aminophenol *see* Acetaminophen *on page 31*

NaCl *see* Sodium Chloride *on page 1480*

Nadolol (NAY doe lol)

Related Information

Cardiovascular Diseases *on page 1726*

U.S. Brand Names Corgard®

Canadian Brand Names Alti-Nadolol; Apo-Nadol®; Corgard®; Novo-Nadolol

Mexican Brand Names Corgard

Generic Available Yes

Pharmacologic Category Beta-Adrenergic Blocker, Nonselective

Use Treatment of hypertension and angina pectoris; prophylaxis of migraine headaches

Local Anesthetic/Vasoconstrictor Precautions Use with caution; epinephrine has interacted with nonselective beta-blockers to result in initial hypertensive episode followed by bradycardia

Effects on Dental Treatment Nadolol is a nonselective beta-blocker and may enhance the pressor response to epinephrine, resulting in hypertension and bradycardia. Many nonsteroidal anti-inflammatory drugs, such as ibuprofen and indomethacin, can reduce the hypotensive effect of beta-blockers after 3 or more weeks of therapy with the NSAID. Short-term NSAID use (ie, 3 days) requires no special precautions in patients taking beta-blockers.

Common Adverse Effects

>10%:

Central nervous system: Drowsiness, insomnia

Endocrine & metabolic: Decreased sexual ability

1% to 10%:

Cardiovascular: Bradycardia, palpitation, edema, CHF, reduced peripheral circulation

Central nervous system: Mental depression

Gastrointestinal: Diarrhea or constipation, nausea, vomiting, stomach discomfort

Respiratory: Bronchospasm

Miscellaneous: Cold extremities

Mechanism of Action Competitively blocks response to beta$_1$- and beta$_2$-adrenergic stimulation; does not exhibit any membrane stabilizing or intrinsic sympathomimetic activity

Drug Interactions

Increased Effect/Toxicity: The heart rate lowering effects of nadolol are additive with other drugs which slow AV conduction (digoxin, verapamil, diltiazem). Concurrent use of alpha-blockers (prazosin, terazosin) with beta-blockers may increase risk of orthostasis. Nadolol may mask the tachycardia from hypoglycemia caused by insulin and oral hypoglycemics. In patients receiving concurrent therapy, the risk of hypertensive crisis is increased when either clonidine or the beta-blocker is withdrawn. Reserpine has been shown to enhance the effect of beta-blockers. Avoid using with alpha-adrenergic stimulants (phenylephrine, epinephrine, etc) which may have exaggerated hypertensive responses. Beta-blockers may affect the action or levels of ethanol, disopyramide, nondepolarizing muscle relaxants, and theophylline although the effects are difficult to predict. The vasoconstrictive effects of ergot alkaloids may be enhanced.

Decreased Effect: Decreased effect of beta-blockers with aluminum salts, barbiturates, calcium salts, cholestyramine, colestipol, NSAIDs, penicillins (ampicillin), rifampin, salicylates, and sulfinpyrazone due to decreased bioavailability and plasma levels. Beta-blockers may decrease the effect of sulfonylureas (possibly hyperglycemia). Nonselective beta-blockers blunt the effect of beta-2 adrenergic agonists (albuterol).

Pharmacodynamics/Kinetics

Duration: 17-24 hours

(Continued)

Nadolol *(Continued)*

Absorption: 30% to 40%

Distribution: Concentration in human breast milk is 4.6 times higher than serum

Protein binding: 28%

Half-life elimination: Adults: 10-24 hours; prolonged with renal impairment; End-stage renal disease: 45 hours

Time to peak, serum: 2-4 hours

Excretion: Urine (as unchanged drug)

Pregnancy Risk Factor C

Nadolol and Bendroflumethiazide

(NAY doe lol & ben droe floo meth EYE a zide)

Related Information

Nadolol *on page 1139*

U.S. Brand Names Corzide®

Generic Available No

Index Terms Bendroflumethiazide and Nadolol

Pharmacologic Category Antihypertensive Agent, Combination; Beta-Adrenergic Blocker, Nonselective; Diuretic, Thiazide

Use Treatment of hypertension; combination product should not be used for initial therapy

Local Anesthetic/Vasoconstrictor Precautions Use with caution; epinephrine has interacted with nonselective beta-blockers to result in initial hypertensive episode followed by bradycardia

Effects on Dental Treatment Nadolol is a nonselective beta-blocker and may enhance the pressor response to epinephrine, resulting in hypertension and bradycardia. Many nonsteroidal anti-inflammatory drugs, such as ibuprofen and indomethacin, can reduce the hypotensive effect of beta-blockers after 3 or more weeks of therapy with the NSAID. Short-term NSAID use (ie, 3 days) requires no special precautions in patients taking beta-blockers.

Common Adverse Effects See individual agents.

Mechanism of Action See individual agents.

Drug Interactions

Increased Effect/Toxicity: See individual agents.

Decreased Effect: See individual agents.

Pharmacodynamics/Kinetics Also see individual agents.

Bioavailability: Bendroflumethiazide: When used in this combination, bioavailability is increased 30% compared to single agent administration.

Pregnancy Risk Factor C

Nafarelin *(naf a REL in)*

U.S. Brand Names Synarel®

Canadian Brand Names Synarel®

Mexican Brand Names Synarel

Generic Available No

Index Terms Nafarelin Acetate

Pharmacologic Category Gonadotropin Releasing Hormone Agonist

Use Treatment of endometriosis, including pain and reduction of lesions; treatment of central precocious puberty (CPP; gonadotropin-dependent precocious puberty) in children of both sexes

Local Anesthetic/Vasoconstrictor Precautions No information available to require special precautions

Effects on Dental Treatment No significant effects or complications reported

Common Adverse Effects Note: Adverse events may be more frequent in the first 6 weeks of treatment due to stimulation of the pituitary-gonadal axis. Sensitivity reactions included chest pain, pruritus, shortness of breath, rash.

CPP: 1% to 10%:

Central nervous system: Emotional lability (6%)

Dermatologic: Acne (10%), seborrhea (3%)

Endocrine & metabolic: Breast enlargement (8%; transient), vaginal bleeding (8%), hot flashes (3%; transient), vaginal discharge (3%)

Respiratory: Rhinitis (5%)

Miscellaneous: Pubic hair increased (5%; transient), body odor (4%), sensitivity reactions (3%)

Endometriosis:

>10%:

Central nervous system: Headache, emotional lability

Dermatologic: Acne

Endocrine & metabolic: Hot flashes (90%), hyperphosphatemia, hypertriglyceridemia, hypocalcemia, libido decreased

Genitourinary: Vaginal dryness

Hematologic: Leukopenia

1% to 10%:

Cardiovascular: Edema

Central nervous system: Depression, insomnia

Dermatologic: Hirsutism, seborrhea

Endocrine & metabolic: Breast size reduced, cholesterol increased, hyperlipidemia, libido increased

Gastrointestinal: Weight gain/loss

Neuromuscular & skeletal: Bone mineral density decreased, myalgia

Respiratory: Nasal irritation

Mechanism of Action Potent synthetic decapeptide analogue of gonadotropin-releasing hormone (GnRH; LHRH) which is approximately 200 times more potent than GnRH in terms of pituitary release of luteinizing hormone (LH) and follicle-stimulating hormone (FSH). Effects on the pituitary gland and sex hormones are dependent upon its length of administration. After acute administration, an initial stimulation of the release of LH and FSH from the pituitary is observed; an increase in androgens and estrogens subsequently follows. Continued administration of nafarelin, however, suppresses gonadotrope responsiveness to endogenous GnRH resulting in reduced secretion of LH and FSH and, secondarily, decreased ovarian and testicular steroid production.

Pharmacodynamics/Kinetics

Protein binding, plasma: 80%

Metabolism: Degraded by peptidase; forms metabolites

Bioavailability: ~1% to 6%

Half-life elimination: ~3 hours; Metabolites: ~86 hours

Time to peak, serum: 10-45 minutes

Excretion: Urine (44% to 55%, ~3% as unchanged drug); feces (19% to 44%)

Pregnancy Risk Factor X

Nafarelin Acetate *see* Nafarelin *on page 1140*

Nafcillin (naf SIL in)

Canadian Brand Names Nallpen®; Unipen®

Generic Available Yes

Index Terms Ethoxynaphthamido Penicillin Sodium; Nafcillin Sodium; Nallpen; Sodium Nafcillin

Pharmacologic Category Antibiotic, Penicillin

Use Treatment of infections such as osteomyelitis, septicemia, endocarditis, and CNS infections caused by susceptible strains of staphylococci species

Local Anesthetic/Vasoconstrictor Precautions No information available to require special precautions

Effects on Dental Treatment Key adverse event(s) related to dental treatment: Prolonged use of penicillins may lead to the development of oral candidiasis.

Common Adverse Effects Frequency not defined.

Central nervous system: Pain, fever

Dermatologic: Rash

Gastrointestinal: Nausea, diarrhea, pseudomembranous colitis

Hematologic: Agranulocytosis, bone marrow depression, neutropenia

Local: Pain, swelling, inflammation, phlebitis, skin sloughing, and thrombophlebitis at the injection site; oxacillin (less likely to cause phlebitis) is often preferred in pediatric patients

Renal: Interstitial nephritis (acute)

Miscellaneous: Hypersensitivity reactions

Mechanism of Action Interferes with bacterial cell wall synthesis during active multiplication, causing cell wall death and resultant bactericidal activity against susceptible bacteria

Drug Interactions

Cytochrome P450 Effect: Induces CYP3A4 (strong)

Increased Effect/Toxicity: Probenecid may cause an increase in nafcillin levels. Penicillins may increase the exposure to methotrexate during concurrent therapy; monitor.

Decreased Effect: Nafcillin may decrease levels/effects of calcium channel blockers. If taken concomitantly with warfarin, nafcillin may inhibit the anticoagulant response to warfarin. This effect may persist for up to 30 days after nafcillin has been discontinued. Subtherapeutic cyclosporine levels may result when taken concomitantly with nafcillin. Although anecdotal reports suggest oral contraceptive efficacy could be reduced by penicillins, this has been refuted by more rigorous scientific and clinical data. Nafcillin may decrease

(Continued)

Nafcillin *(Continued)*

the levels/effects of benzodiazepines, calcium channel blockers, clarithro-mycin, cyclosporine, erythromycin, estrogens, mirtazapine, nateglinide, nefazodone, nevirapine, protease inhibitors, tacrolimus, venlafaxine, and other CYP3A4 substrates. Fusidic acid, tetracyclines may decrease the effects of penicillins. The effects of the typhoid vaccine may be decreased by nafcillin.

Pharmacodynamics/Kinetics
Distribution: Widely distributed; CSF penetration is poor but enhanced by meningeal inflammation; crosses placenta
Protein binding: 70% to 90%
Metabolism: Primarily hepatic; undergoes enterohepatic recirculation
Half-life elimination:
Neonates: <3 weeks: 2.2-5.5 hours; 4-9 weeks: 1.2-2.3 hours
Children 3 months to 14 years: 0.75-1.9 hours
Adults: 30 minutes to 1.5 hours with normal renal and hepatic function
Time to peak, serum: I.M.: 30-60 minutes
Excretion: Primarily feces; urine (10% to 30% as unchanged drug)
Pregnancy Risk Factor B

Nafcillin Sodium *see* Nafcillin *on page 1141*
Nafidimide *see* Amonafide *on page 106*

Naftifine *(NAF ti feen)*

U.S. Brand Names Naftin®
Generic Available No
Index Terms Naftifine Hydrochloride
Pharmacologic Category Antifungal Agent, Topical
Use Topical treatment of tinea cruris (jock itch), tinea corporis (ringworm), and tinea pedis (athlete's foot)
Local Anesthetic/Vasoconstrictor Precautions No information available to require special precautions
Effects on Dental Treatment No significant effects or complications reported
Common Adverse Effects
>10%: Local: Burning, stinging
1% to 10%:
Dermatologic: Erythema, itching
Local: Dryness, irritation
Mechanism of Action Synthetic, broad-spectrum antifungal agent in the allyla-mine class; appears to have both fungistatic and fungicidal activity. Exhibits antifungal activity by selectively inhibiting the enzyme squalene epoxidase in a dose-dependent manner which results in the primary sterol, ergosterol, within the fungal membrane not being synthesized.
Pharmacodynamics/Kinetics
Absorption: Systemic: Cream: 6%; Gel: ≤4%
Half-life elimination: 2-3 days
Excretion: Urine and feces (as metabolites)
Pregnancy Risk Factor B

Naftifine Hydrochloride *see* Naftifine *on page 1142*
Naftin® *see* Naftifine *on page 1142*
Naglazyme™ *see* Galsulfase *on page 763*
NaHCO₃ *see* Sodium Bicarbonate *on page 1480*

Nalbuphine *(NAL byoo feen)*

U.S. Brand Names Nubain®
Mexican Brand Names Bufigen; Nalcryn SP; Nubain SP
Generic Available Yes
Index Terms Nalbuphine Hydrochloride
Pharmacologic Category Analgesic, Opioid
Use Relief of moderate to severe pain; preoperative analgesia, postoperative and surgical anesthesia, and obstetrical analgesia during labor and delivery
Unlabeled/Investigational Use Opioid-induced pruritus
Local Anesthetic/Vasoconstrictor Precautions No information available to require special precautions
Effects on Dental Treatment Key adverse event(s) related to dental treatment: Xerostomia and changes in salivation (normal salivary flow resumes upon discontinuation). Anticholinergic side effects can cause a reduction of saliva

production or secretion, contributing to discomfort and dental disease (ie, caries, oral candidiasis, and periodontal disease).

Common Adverse Effects
>10%: Central nervous system: Sedation (36%)
1% to 10%:
  Central nervous system: Dizziness (5%), headache (3%)
  Gastrointestinal: Nausea/vomiting (6%), xerostomia (4%)
  Miscellaneous: Clamminess (9%)

Mechanism of Action Agonist of kappa opiate receptors and partial antagonist of mu opiate receptors in the CNS, causing inhibition of ascending pain pathways, altering the perception of and response to pain; produces generalized CNS depression

Drug Interactions
  Increased Effect/Toxicity: Barbiturate anesthetics may increase CNS depression.

Pharmacodynamics/Kinetics
  Onset of action: Peak effect: SubQ, I.M.: <15 minutes; I.V.: 2-3 minutes
  Metabolism: Hepatic
  Half-life elimination: 5 hours
  Excretion: Feces; urine (~7% as metabolites)

Pregnancy Risk Factor B/D (prolonged use or high doses at term)

Nalbuphine Hydrochloride see Nalbuphine on page 1142

Nalex®-A see Chlorpheniramine, Phenylephrine, and Phenyltoloxamine on page 343

Nalfon® see Fenoprofen on page 677

Nallpen see Nafcillin on page 1141

N-allylnoroxymorphine Hydrochloride see Naloxone on page 1144

Nalmefene (NAL me feen)

U.S. Brand Names Revex®
Generic Available No
Index Terms Nalmefene Hydrochloride
Pharmacologic Category Antidote
Use Complete or partial reversal of opioid drug effects, including respiratory depression induced by natural or synthetic opioids; reversal of postoperative opioid depression; management of known or suspected opioid overdose

Local Anesthetic/Vasoconstrictor Precautions No information available to require special precautions

Effects on Dental Treatment No significant effects or complications reported

Common Adverse Effects
>10%: Gastrointestinal: Nausea (18%)
1% to 10%:
  Cardiovascular: Tachycardia (5%), hypertension (5%), hypotension (1%), vasodilation (1%)
  Central nervous system: Fever (3%), dizziness (3%), headache (1%), chills (1%)
  Gastrointestinal: Vomiting (9%)
  Miscellaneous: Postoperative pain (4%)

Mechanism of Action As a 6-methylene analog of naltrexone, nalmefene acts as a competitive antagonist at opioid receptor sites, preventing or reversing the respiratory depression, sedation, and hypotension induced by opiates; no pharmacologic activity of its own (eg, opioid agonist activity) has been demonstrated

Drug Interactions
  Increased Effect/Toxicity: Potential increased risk of seizures may exist with use of flumazenil and nalmefene coadministration.

Pharmacodynamics/Kinetics
  Onset of action: I.M., SubQ: 5-15 minutes
  Distribution: V_d: 8.6 L/kg; rapid
  Protein binding: 45%
  Metabolism: Hepatic via glucuronide conjugation to metabolites with little or no activity
  Bioavailability: I.M., SubQ: 100%
  Half-life elimination: 10.8 hours
  Time to peak, serum: Serum: I.M.: 2.3 hours; I.V.: <2 minutes; SubQ: 1.5 hours
  Excretion: Feces (17%); urine (<5% as unchanged drug)
  Clearance: 0.8 L/hour/kg

Pregnancy Risk Factor B

Nalmefene Hydrochloride see Nalmefene on page 1143

Naloxone (nal OKS one)

Canadian Brand Names Naloxone Hydrochloride Injection®
Mexican Brand Names Narcanti
Generic Available Yes
Index Terms *N*-allylnoroxymorphine Hydrochloride; Naloxone Hydrochloride; Narcan
Pharmacologic Category Antidote
Dental Use Reverse overdose effects of the two narcotic agents, fentanyl and meperidine, used in the technique of I.V. conscious sedation
Use
Complete or partial reversal of opioid depression, including respiratory depression, induced by natural and synthetic opioids, including propoxyphene, methadone, and certain mixed agonist-antagonist analgesics: nalbuphine, pentazocine, and butorphanol
Diagnosis of suspected opioid tolerance or acute opioid overdose
Adjunctive agent to increase blood pressure in the management of septic shock
Unlabeled/Investigational Use PCP and ethanol ingestion; opioid-induced pruritus
Local Anesthetic/Vasoconstrictor Precautions No information available to require special precautions
Effects on Dental Treatment No significant effects or complications reported
Significant Adverse Effects Frequency not defined.
Cardiovascular: Hyper-/hypotension, tachycardia, ventricular arrhythmia, cardiac arrest
Central nervous system: Irritability, anxiety, narcotic withdrawal, restlessness, seizure
Gastrointestinal: Nausea, vomiting, diarrhea
Neuromuscular & skeletal: Tremulousness
Respiratory: Dyspnea, pulmonary edema, runny nose, sneezing
Miscellaneous: Diaphoresis
Dental Usual Dosing Narcotic overdose: Adults: I.V.: 0.4-2 mg every 2-3 minutes as needed; may need to repeat doses every 20-60 minutes, if no response is observed after 10 mg, question the diagnosis. **Note:** Use 0.1-0.2 mg increments in patients who are opioid dependent and in postoperative patients to avoid large cardiovascular changes.
Dosage I.M., I.V. (preferred), intratracheal, SubQ:
Postanesthesia narcotic reversal: Infants and Children: 0.01 mg/kg; may repeat every 2-3 minutes, as needed based on response
Opiate intoxication:
Children:
Birth (including premature infants) to 5 years or <20 kg: 0.1 mg/kg; repeat every 2-3 minutes if needed; may need to repeat doses every 20-60 minutes
>5 years or ≥20 kg: 2 mg/dose; if no response, repeat every 2-3 minutes; may need to repeat doses every 20-60 minutes
Children and Adults: Continuous infusion: I.V.: If continuous infusion is required, calculate dosage/hour based on effective intermittent dose used and duration of adequate response seen, titrate dose 0.04-0.16 mg/kg/hour for 2-5 days in children, adult dose typically 0.25-6.25 mg/hour (short-term infusions as high as 2.4 mg/kg/hour have been tolerated in adults during treatment for septic shock); alternatively, continuous infusion utilizes ⅔ of the initial naloxone bolus on an hourly basis; add 10 times this dose to each liter of D₅W and infuse at a rate of 100 mL/hour; ½ of the initial bolus dose should be readministered 15 minutes after initiation of the continuous infusion to prevent a drop in naloxone levels; increase infusion rate as needed to assure adequate ventilation
Narcotic overdose: Adults: I.V.: 0.4-2 mg every 2-3 minutes as needed; may need to repeat doses every 20-60 minutes, if no response is observed after 10 mg, question the diagnosis. **Note:** Use 0.1-0.2 mg increments in patients who are opioid dependent and in postoperative patients to avoid large cardiovascular changes.
Opioid-induced pruritus (unlabeled use): Adults: I.V. infusion: 0.25 mcg/kg/hour; **Note:** Monitor pain control; verify that the naloxone is not reversing analgesia.
Mechanism of Action Pure opioid antagonist that competes and displaces narcotics at opioid receptor sites
Contraindications Hypersensitivity to naloxone or any component of the formulation
Warnings/Precautions Due to an association between naloxone and acute pulmonary edema, use with caution in patients with cardiovascular disease or in patients receiving medications with potential adverse cardiovascular effects (eg, hypotension, pulmonary edema or arrhythmias). Excessive dosages should be

avoided after use of opiates in surgery. Abrupt postoperative reversal may result in nausea, vomiting, sweating, tachycardia, hypertension, seizures, and other cardiovascular events (including pulmonary edema and arrhythmias). May precipitate withdrawal symptoms in patients addicted to opiates, including pain, hypertension, sweating, agitation, irritability; in neonates: shrill cry, failure to feed. Recurrence of respiratory depression is possible if the opioid involved is long-acting; observe patients until there is no reasonable risk of recurrent respiratory depression.

Drug Interactions Opioid analgesics: Decreased effect of opioid analgesics; may precipitate acute withdrawal reaction in physically dependent patients

Pharmacodynamics/Kinetics
Onset of action: Endotracheal, I.M., SubQ: 2-5 minutes; I.V.: ~2 minutes
Duration: 20-60 minutes; since shorter than that of most opioids, repeated doses are usually needed
Distribution: Crosses placenta
Metabolism: Primarily hepatic via glucuronidation
Half-life elimination: Neonates: 1.2-3 hours; Adults: 1-1.5 hours
Excretion: Urine (as metabolites)

Pregnancy Risk Factor C

Lactation Excretion in breast milk unknown/not recommended

Breast-Feeding Considerations No data reported. Since naloxone is used for opiate reversal the concern should be on opiate drug levels in a breast-feeding mother and transfer to the infant rather than naloxone exposure. The safest approach would be **not** to breast-feed.

Dosage Forms Excipient information presented when available (limited, particularly for generics); consult specific product labeling.
Injection, solution, as hydrochloride: 0.4 mg/mL (1 mL, 10 mL); 1 mg/mL (2 mL)

Naloxone and Buprenorphine see Buprenorphine and Naloxone on page 240

Naloxone Hydrochloride see Naloxone on page 1144

Naloxone Hydrochloride and Pentazocine Hydrochloride see Pentazocine on page 1274

Naloxone Hydrochloride Dihydrate and Buprenorphine Hydrochloride see Buprenorphine and Naloxone on page 240

Naltrexone (nal TREKS one)

U.S. Brand Names Depade®; ReVia®; Vivitrol™
Canadian Brand Names ReVia®
Mexican Brand Names Re-Via
Generic Available Yes: Tablet
Index Terms Naltrexone Hydrochloride
Pharmacologic Category Antidote
Use Treatment of ethanol dependence; blockade of the effects of exogenously administered opioids
Local Anesthetic/Vasoconstrictor Precautions No information available to require special precautions
Effects on Dental Treatment Key adverse event(s) related to dental treatment: Dry mouth.
Common Adverse Effects Combined reporting of adverse events from oral and injectable formulations:
>10%:
Cardiovascular: Syncope (13%)
Central nervous system: Headache (25%), insomnia (14%), dizziness (13%), anxiety (12%), somnolence (4%), nervousness, fatigue
Gastrointestinal: Nausea (33%), vomiting (14%), appetite decreased (14%), diarrhea (13%), abdominal pain (11%), abdominal cramping
Local: Injection site reaction (69%)
Neuromuscular & skeletal: Arthralgia (12%), CPK increased (11%)
Respiratory: Upper respiratory tract infection (13%), pharyngitis (11%)
1% to 10%:
Central nervous system: Depression (8%), suicidal thoughts (1%), energy increased, feeling down
Dermatologic: Rash (6%)
Endocrine & metabolic: Polydipsia
Gastrointestinal: Dry mouth (5%)
Genitourinary: Delayed ejaculation, impotency
Hepatic: AST increased (2%)
Neuromuscular & skeletal: Muscle cramps (8%), back pain (6%)
Mechanism of Action Naltrexone (a pure opioid antagonist) is a cyclopropyl derivative of oxymorphone similar in structure to naloxone and nalorphine (a morphine derivative); it acts as a competitive antagonist at opioid receptor sites, showing the highest affinity for mu receptors.
(Continued)

Naltrexone *(Continued)*

Drug Interactions
Increased Effect/Toxicity: Lethargy and somnolence have been reported with the combination of naltrexone and thioridazine.

Decreased Effect: Naltrexone decreases effects of opioid-containing products.

Pharmacodynamics/Kinetics
Duration: Oral: 50 mg: 24 hours; 100 mg: 48 hours; 150 mg: 72 hours; I.M.: 4 weeks

Absorption: Oral: Almost complete

Distribution: V_d: 19 L/kg; widely throughout the body but considerable inter-individual variation exists

Protein binding: 21%

Metabolism: Noncytochrome-mediated dehydrogenase conversion to 6-β-naltrexol and related minor metabolites; Oral: Extensive first-pass effect

Half-life elimination: Oral: 4 hours; 6-β-naltrexol: 13 hours; I.M.: naltrexone and 6-β-naltrexol: 5-10 days

Time to peak, serum: Oral: ~60 minutes; I.M.: Biphasic: 2 hours (first peak), 2-3 days (second peak)

Excretion: Primarily urine (as metabolites and unchanged drug)

Pregnancy Risk Factor C

Naltrexone Hydrochloride *see* Naltrexone *on page 1145*

Namenda™ *see* Memantine *on page 1034*

Nandrolone *(NAN droe lone)*

Canadian Brand Names Deca-Durabolin®; Durabolin®

Mexican Brand Names Deca-Durabolin

Generic Available Yes

Index Terms Nandrolone Decanoate; Nandrolone Phenpropionate

Pharmacologic Category Androgen

Use Control of metastatic breast cancer; management of anemia of renal insufficiency

Local Anesthetic/Vasoconstrictor Precautions No information available to require special precautions

Effects on Dental Treatment No significant effects or complications reported

Common Adverse Effects
Male:
Postpubertal:
>10%:
Dermatologic: Acne
Endocrine & metabolic: Gynecomastia
Genitourinary: Bladder irritability, priapism
1% to 10%:
Central nervous system: Insomnia, chills
Endocrine & metabolic: Decreased libido, hepatic dysfunction
Gastrointestinal: Nausea, diarrhea
Genitourinary: Prostatic hyperplasia (elderly)
Hematologic: Iron deficiency anemia, suppression of clotting factors
Prepubertal:
>10%:
Dermatologic: Acne
Endocrine & metabolic: Virilism
1% to 10%:
Central nervous system: Chills, insomnia
Dermatologic: Hyperpigmentation
Gastrointestinal: Diarrhea, nausea
Hematologic: Iron deficiency anemia, suppression of clotting

Female:
>10%: Endocrine & metabolic: Virilism
1% to 10%:
Central nervous system: Chills, insomnia
Endocrine & metabolic: Hypercalcemia
Gastrointestinal: Nausea, diarrhea
Hematologic: Iron deficiency anemia, suppression of clotting factors
Hepatic: Hepatic dysfunction

Restrictions C-III

Mechanism of Action Promotes tissue-building processes, increases production of erythropoietin, causes protein anabolism; increases hemoglobin and red blood cell volume

Drug Interactions
  Increased Effect/Toxicity: Nandrolone may increase the effect of oral anti-coagulants, insulin, oral hypoglycemic agents, adrenal steroids, or ACTH when taken together.
Pharmacodynamics/Kinetics
  Onset of action: 3-6 months
  Duration: Up to 30 days
  Absorption: I.M.: 77%
  Metabolism: Hepatic
  Excretion: Urine
Pregnancy Risk Factor X

Nandrolone Decanoate *see* Nandrolone *on page 1146*
Nandrolone Phenpropionate *see* Nandrolone *on page 1146*

Naphazoline (naf AZ oh leen)

U.S. Brand Names AK-Con™; Albalon®; Clear eyes® for Dry Eyes and ACR Relief [OTC]; Clear eyes® for Dry Eyes and Redness Relief [OTC]; Clear eyes® Redness Relief [OTC]; Clear eyes® Seasonal Relief [OTC]; Naphcon® [OTC]; Privine® [OTC]
Canadian Brand Names Naphcon Forte®; Vasocon®
Mexican Brand Names Naphacel Ofteno
Generic Available No
Index Terms Naphazoline Hydrochloride
Pharmacologic Category Alpha₁ Agonist; Imidazoline Derivative; Ophthalmic Agent, Vasoconstrictor
Use Topical ocular vasoconstrictor; temporary relief of nasal congestion associated with the common cold, upper respiratory allergies or sinusitis; relief of redness of the eye due to minor irritation
Local Anesthetic/Vasoconstrictor Precautions No information available to require special precautions
Effects on Dental Treatment No significant effects or complications reported
Common Adverse Effects Frequency not defined.
  Cardiovascular: Cardiac irregularities, hypertension
  Central nervous system: Body temperature decreased, dizziness, drowsiness, headache, nervousness
  Endocrine & metabolic: Hyperglycemia
  Gastrointestinal: Nausea
  Local: Transient stinging, nasal mucosa irritation, dryness, rebound congestion
  Neuromuscular & skeletal: Weakness
  Ocular: Blurred vision, discomfort, intraocular pressure increased, irritation, lacrimation, mydriasis, punctuate keratitis, redness
  Respiratory: Sneezing
  Miscellaneous: Diaphoresis
Mechanism of Action Stimulates alpha-adrenergic receptors in the arterioles of the conjunctiva and the nasal mucosa to produce vasoconstriction
Drug Interactions
  Increased Effect/Toxicity: Guanadrel and methyldopa may enhance the therapeutic effect of alpha₁-agonists. MAO inhibitors may enhance the hypertensive effects of alpha₁-agonists (avoid use). TCAs may enhance the vasopressor effect of alpha₁-agonists (avoid use).
Pharmacodynamics/Kinetics
  Onset of action: Decongestant: Topical: ~10 minutes
  Duration: 2-6 hours
Pregnancy Risk Factor C

Naphazoline and Pheniramine (naf AZ oh leen & fen NIR a meen)

Related Information
  Naphazoline *on page 1147*
U.S. Brand Names Naphcon-A® [OTC]; Opcon-A® [OTC]; Visine-A® [OTC]
Canadian Brand Names Naphcon-A®; Visine® Advanced Allergy
Generic Available No
Index Terms Pheniramine and Naphazoline
Pharmacologic Category Ophthalmic Agent, Vasoconstrictor
Use Treatment of ocular congestion, irritation, and itching
Local Anesthetic/Vasoconstrictor Precautions No information available to require special precautions
Effects on Dental Treatment No significant effects or complications reported
Pregnancy Risk Factor C

Naproxen (na PROKS en)

Related Information
Oral Pain *on page 1788*
Rheumatoid Arthritis, Osteoarthritis, and Osteoporosis *on page 1759*
Temporomandibular Dysfunction (TMD) *on page 1822*

Related Sample Prescriptions
Mild/Moderate Oral Pain *on page 1834*

U.S. Brand Names Aleve® [OTC]; Anaprox®; Anaprox® DS; EC-Naprosyn®; Midol® Extended Relief; Naprelan®; Naprosyn®; Pamprin® Maximum Strength All Day Relief [OTC]

Canadian Brand Names Anaprox®; Anaprox® DS; Apo-Napro-Na®; Apo-Napro-Na DS®; Apo-Naproxen®; Apo-Naproxen EC®; Apo-Naproxen SR®; Gen-Naproxen EC; Naprosyn®; Naxen®; Naxen® EC; Novo-Naproc EC; Novo-Naprox; Novo-Naprox Sodium; Novo-Naprox Sodium DS; Novo-Naprox SR; Nu-Naprox; Riva-Naproxen

Mexican Brand Names Dafloxen; Deflamox; Diferbest; Flanax; Naxen

Generic Available Yes

Index Terms Naproxen Sodium

Pharmacologic Category Nonsteroidal Anti-inflammatory Drug (NSAID), Oral

Dental Use Management of pain and swelling

Use Management of ankylosing spondylitis, osteoarthritis, and rheumatoid disorders (including juvenile rheumatoid arthritis); acute gout; mild-to-moderate pain; tendonitis, bursitis; dysmenorrhea; fever

Local Anesthetic/Vasoconstrictor Precautions No information available to require special precautions

Effects on Dental Treatment Key adverse event(s) related to dental treatment: Stomatitis.

Naproxen and naproxen sodium have the potential to interfere with the antiplatelet effect of low-dose aspirin. One study of naproxen and low-dose aspirin has suggested that naproxen may interfere with aspirin's antiplatelet activity when they are coadministered (Steinhubl, 2005). However, naproxen 500 mg administered 2 hours before or after aspirin 100 mg did not interfere with aspirin's antiplatelet effect. The FDA stated that there is no data looking at doses of naproxen <500 mg. Naproxen over-the-counter strength is 220 mg tablets.

The FDA has warned that ibuprofen can interfere with the antiplatelet effect of low-dose aspirin (81 mg/day), potentially rendering aspirin less effective when used for cardioprotection and stroke protection. In situations where these drugs could be used concomitantly, the FDA has proved the following information: Patients who use immediate release aspirin (not enteric-coated aspirin) and take single doses of ibuprofen 400 mg, should dose the ibuprofen at least 30 minutes or longer after aspirin ingestion or more than 8 hours before aspirin ingestion to avoid attenuation of aspirin's effect. Similar recommendations may hold for concomitant may hold for concomitant naproxen and aspirin use.

Significant Adverse Effects
1% to 10%:
Cardiovascular: Edema (3% to 9%), palpitations (<3%)
Central nervous system: Dizziness (3% to 9%), drowsiness (3% to 9%), headache (3% to 9%), lightheadedness (<3%), vertigo (<3%)
Dermatologic: Pruritus (3% to 9%), skin eruption (3% to 9%), ecchymosis (3% to 9%), purpura (<3%), rash
Endocrine & metabolic: Fluid retention (3% to 9%)
Gastrointestinal: Abdominal pain (3% to 9%), constipation (3% to 9%), nausea (3% to 9%), heartburn (3% to 9%), diarrhea (<3%), dyspepsia (<3%), stomatitis (<3%), flatulence, gross bleeding/perforation, indigestion, ulcers, vomiting
Genitourinary: Abnormal renal function
Hematologic: Hemolysis (3% to 9%), ecchymosis (3% to 9%), anemia, bleeding time increased
Hepatic: LFTs increased
Ocular: Visual disturbances (<3%)
Otic: Tinnitus (3% to 9%), hearing disturbances (<3%)
Respiratory: Dyspnea (3% to 9%)

Miscellaneous: Diaphoresis (<3%), thirst (<3%)

<1% (Limited to important or life-threatening): Agranulocytosis, alopecia, anaphylactic/anaphylactoid reaction, angioneurotic edema, arrhythmia, aseptic meningitis, asthma, blurred vision, cognitive dysfunction, colitis, coma, confusion, CHF, conjunctivitis, cystitis, depression, dream abnormalities, dysuria, eosinophilia, eosinophilic pneumonitis, erythema multiforme, exfoliative dermatitis, glossitis, granulocytopenia, hallucinations, hematemesis, hepatitis, hyper-/hypoglycemia, hyper-/hypotension, infection, interstitial nephritis, melena, jaundice, leukopenia, liver failure, lymphadenopathy, menstrual disorders, malaise, MI, muscle weakness, myalgia, oliguria, pancreatitis, pancytopenia, paresthesia, photosensitivity, pneumonia, polyuria, proteinuria, pyrexia, rectal bleeding, renal failure, renal papillary necrosis, respiratory depression, sepsis, Stevens-Johnson syndrome, tachycardia, seizure, syncope, thrombocytopenia, toxic epidermal necrolysis ulcerative stomatitis, vasculitis

Restrictions An FDA-approved medication guide must be distributed when dispensing an oral outpatient prescription (new or refill) where this medication is to be used without direct supervision of a healthcare provider. Medication guides are available at http://www.fda.gov/cder/Offices/ODS/medication_guides.htm.

Dental Usual Dosing

Mild-to-moderate pain: Adults: Initial: 500 mg, then 250 mg every 6-8 hours; maximum: 1250 mg/day naproxen base

Pain/fever (OTC labeling):

Children ≥12 years and Adults ≤65 years: 200 mg naproxen base every 8-12 hours; if needed, may take 400 mg naproxen base for the initial dose; maximum: 600 mg naproxen base/24 hours

Adults >65 years: 200 mg naproxen base every 12 hours

Dosage Note: Dosage expressed as naproxen base; 200 mg naproxen base is equivalent to 220 mg naproxen sodium.

Oral:

Children >2 years: Juvenile arthritis: 10 mg/kg/day in 2 divided doses

Adults:

Gout, acute: Initial: 750 mg, followed by 250 mg every 8 hours until attack subsides. **Note:** EC-Naprosyn® is not recommended.

Migraine, acute (unlabeled use): Initial: 500-750 mg.; an additional 250-500 mg may be given if needed (maximum: 1250 mg in 24 hours). **Note:** EC-Naprosyn® is not recommended.

Pain (mild-to-moderate), dysmenorrhea, acute tendonitis, bursitis: Initial: 500 mg, then 250 mg every 6-8 hours; maximum: 1250 mg/day naproxen base

Rheumatoid arthritis, osteoarthritis, and ankylosing spondylitis: 500-1000 mg/day in 2 divided doses; may increase to 1.5 g/day of naproxen base for limited time period

OTC labeling: Pain/fever:

Children ≥12 years and Adults ≤65 years: 200 mg naproxen base every 8-12 hours; if needed, may take 400 mg naproxen base for the initial dose; maximum: 600 mg naproxen base/24 hours

Adults >65 years: 200 mg naproxen base every 12 hours

Dosing adjustment in renal impairment: Cl_{cr} <30 mL/minute: use is not recommended

Mechanism of Action Inhibits prostaglandin synthesis by decreasing the activity of the enzyme, cyclooxygenase, which results in decreased formation of prostaglandin precursors

Contraindications Hypersensitivity to naproxen, aspirin, other NSAIDs, or any component of the formulation; perioperative pain in the setting of coronary artery bypass surgery (CABG); pregnancy (3rd trimester)

Warnings/Precautions [U.S. Boxed Warning]: NSAIDs are associated with an increased risk of adverse cardiovascular events, including MI, stroke, and new onset or worsening of pre-existing hypertension. Risk may be increased with duration of use or pre-existing cardiovascular risk factors or disease. Carefully evaluate individual cardiovascular risk profiles prior to prescribing. Use caution with fluid retention, CHF or hypertension. Use the lowest effective dose for the shortest duration of time, consistent with individual patient goals, to reduce risk of cardiovascular or GI adverse events. Alternate therapies should be considered for patients at high risk. Concurrent administration of ibuprofen, and potentially other nonselective NSAIDs, may interfere with aspirin's cardioprotective effect.

[U.S. Boxed Warning]: NSAIDs may increase risk of gastrointestinal irritation, ulceration, bleeding, and perforation. These events may occur at any time during therapy and without warning. Use caution with a history of GI disease (bleeding or ulcers), concurrent therapy with aspirin, anticoagulants and/or corticosteroids, smoking, use of alcohol, the elderly or debilitated patients.

(Continued)

Naproxen *(Continued)*

Use of NSAIDs can compromise existing renal function. Renal toxicity can occur in patient with impaired renal function, dehydration, heart failure, liver dysfunction, those taking diuretics and ACEI and the elderly. Rehydrate patient before starting therapy. Monitor renal function closely. Naproxen is not recommended for patients with advanced renal disease.

NSAIDs may cause serious skin adverse events including exfoliative dermatitis, Stevens-Johnson Syndrome (SJS) and toxic epidermal necrolysis (TEN). Anaphylactoid reactions may occur, even without prior exposure; patients with "aspirin triad" (bronchial asthma, aspirin intolerance, rhinitis) may be at increased risk. Do not use in patients who experience bronchospasm, asthma, rhinitis, or urticaria with NSAID or aspirin therapy. Use caution in other forms of asthma.

Use with caution in patients with decreased hepatic function. Closely monitor patients with any abnormal LFT. Severe hepatic reactions (eg, fulminant hepatitis, liver failure) have occurred with NSAID use, rarely; discontinue if signs or symptoms of liver disease develop, or if systemic manifestations occur.

The elderly are at increased risk for adverse effects (especially peptic ulceration, CNS effects, renal toxicity) from NSAIDs even at low doses.

Withhold for at least 4-6 half-lives prior to surgical or dental procedures. Safety and efficacy have not been established in children <2 years of age.

OTC labeling: Prior to self-medication, patients should contact healthcare provider if they have had recurring stomach pain or upset, ulcers, bleeding problems, high blood pressure, heart or kidney disease, other serious medical problems, are currently taking a diuretic, or are ≥60 years of age. Recommended dosages should not be exceeded, due to an increased risk of GI bleeding. Consuming ≥3 alcoholic beverages/day or taking longer than recommended may increase the risk of GI bleeding. Not for self-medication (OTC use) in children <12 years of age.

Drug Interactions Substrate (minor) of CYP1A2, 2C9

ACE inhibitors: Antihypertensive effects may be decreased by concurrent therapy with NSAIDs; monitor blood pressure.

Angiotensin II antagonists: Antihypertensive effects may be decreased by concurrent therapy with NSAIDs; monitor blood pressure.

Anticoagulants (warfarin, heparin, LMWHs) in combination with NSAIDs can cause increased risk of bleeding.

Antiplatelet drugs (ticlopidine, clopidogrel, aspirin, abciximab, dipyridamole, eptifibatide, tirofiban) can cause an increased risk of bleeding.

Beta-blockers: NSAIDs may decrease the antihypertensive effect of beta-blockers. Monitor.

Cholestyramine (and other bile acid sequestrants): May decrease the absorption of NSAIDs. Separate by at least 2 hours.

Corticosteroids may increase the risk of GI ulceration; avoid concurrent use.

Cyclosporine: NSAIDs may increase serum creatinine, potassium, blood pressure, and cyclosporine levels; monitor cyclosporine levels and renal function carefully.

Fluoroquinolone antibiotics: Risk of seizures may be increased with concomitant quinolone use. Risk is considered quite low and may only be a factor with high serum levels of either agent and/or in patients with additional predisposing factors (eg, renal dysfunction, history of seizure or other neurological disorder).

Hydralazine's antihypertensive effect is decreased; avoid concurrent use.

Lithium levels can be increased; avoid concurrent use if possible or monitor lithium levels and adjust dose. Sulindac may have the least effect. When NSAID is stopped, lithium will need adjustment again.

Loop diuretics efficacy (diuretic and antihypertensive effect) is reduced. Indomethacin reduces this efficacy, however, it may be anticipated with any NSAID.

Methotrexate: Severe bone marrow suppression, aplastic anemia, and GI toxicity have been reported with concomitant NSAID therapy. Avoid use during moderate or high-dose methotrexate (increased and prolonged methotrexate levels). NSAID use during low-dose treatment of rheumatoid arthritis has not been fully evaluated; extreme caution is warranted.

Salicylates: NSAIDs (nonselective) may diminish the cardioprotective effect of acetylated salicylates. Avoid regular use of NSAIDs if possible; consider alternatives (eg, acetaminophen). Give salicylate before NSAID; for example ibuprofen should be given 30-120 minutes after aspirin (immediate release).

Thiazides antihypertensive effects are decreased; avoid concurrent use.

Warfarin's INRs may be increased by naproxen. Other NSAIDs may have the same effect depending on dose and duration. Monitor INR closely. Use the lowest dose of NSAIDs possible and for the briefest duration.

Ethanol/Nutrition/Herb Interactions

Ethanol: Avoid ethanol (may enhance gastric mucosal irritation).

Food: Naproxen absorption ratelevels may be decreased if taken with food.

Herb/Nutraceutical: Avoid alfalfa, anise, bilberry, bladderwrack, bromelain, cat's claw, celery, coleus, cordyceps, dong quai, evening primrose, feverfew, fenugreek, garlic, ginger, ginkgo biloba, red clover, horse chestnut, grapeseed, green tea, ginseng, guggul, horse chestnut seed, horseradish, licorice, prickly ash, red clover, reishi, SAMe, sweet clover, turmeric, white willow (all have additional antiplatelet activity).

Dietary Considerations Drug may cause GI upset, bleeding, ulceration, perforation; take with food or milk to minimize GI upset.

Pharmacodynamics/Kinetics

Onset of action: Analgesic: 1 hour; Anti-inflammatory: ~2 weeks

Peak effect: Anti-inflammatory: 2-4 weeks

Duration: Analgesic: ≤7 hours; Anti-inflammatory: ≤12 hours

Absorption: Almost 100%

Protein binding: >99%; increased free fraction in elderly

Half-life elimination: Normal renal function: 12-17 hours; End-stage renal disease: No change

Time to peak, serum: 1-4 hours

Excretion: Urine (95%)

Pregnancy Risk Factor C/D (3rd trimester)

Lactation Enters breast milk/not recommended (AAP rates "compatible")

Dosage Forms Excipient information presented when available (limited, particularly for generics); consult specific product labeling.

Caplet, as sodium (Aleve®, Midol® Extended Relief, Pamprin® Maximum Strength All Day Relief): 220 mg [equivalent to naproxen 200 mg and sodium 20 mg]

Gelcap, as sodium (Aleve®): 220 mg [equivalent to naproxen 200 mg and sodium 20 mg]

Suspension, oral (Naprosyn®): 125 mg/5 mL (480 mL) [contains sodium 0.3 mEq/mL; orange-pineapple flavor]

Tablet (Naprosyn®): 250 mg, 375 mg, 500 mg

Tablet, as sodium: 220 mg [equivalent to naproxen 200 mg and sodium 20 mg]; 275 mg [equivalent to naproxen 250 mg and sodium 25 mg]; 550 mg [equivalent to naproxen 500 mg and sodium 50 mg]

Aleve®: 220 mg [equivalent to naproxen 200 mg and sodium 20 mg]

Anaprox®: 275 mg [equivalent to naproxen 250 mg and sodium 25 mg]

Anaprox® DS: 550 mg [equivalent to naproxen 500 mg and sodium 50 mg]

Tablet, controlled release, as sodium: 550 mg [equivalent to naproxen 500 mg and sodium 50 mg]

Naprelan®: 421.5 mg [equivalent to naproxen 375 mg and sodium 37.5 mg]; 550 mg [equivalent to naproxen 500 mg and sodium 50 mg]

Tablet, delayed release (EC-Naprosyn®): 375 mg, 500 mg

Selected Readings

Ahmad N, Grad HA, Haas DA, et al, "The Efficacy of Nonopioid Analgesics for Postoperative Dental Pain: A Meta-Analysis," *Anesth Prog*, 1997, 44(4):119-26.

Brooks PM and Day RO, "Nonsteroidal Anti-inflammatory Drugs - Differences and Similarities," *N Engl J Med*, 1991, 324(24):1716-25.

Dionne R, "Additive Analgesia Without Opioid Side Effects," *Compend Contin Educ Dent*, 2000, 21(7):572-4, 576-7.

Dionne RA and Berthold CW, "Therapeutic Uses of Nonsteroidal Anti-inflammatory Drugs in Dentistry," *Crit Rev Oral Biol Med*, 2001, 12(4):315-30.

Forbes JA, Keller CK, Smith JW, et al, "Analgesic Effect of Naproxen Sodium, Codeine, a Naproxen-Codeine Combination and Aspirin on the Postoperative Pain of Oral Surgery," *Pharmacotherapy*, 1986, 6(5):211-8.

Nguyen AM, Graham DY, Gage T, et al, "Nonsteroidal Anti-inflammatory Drug Use in Dentistry: Gastrointestinal Implications," *Gen Dent*, 1999, 47(6):590-6.

Steinhubl SR, "The Use of Anti-Inflammatory Analgesics in the Patient With Cardiovascular Disease: What a Pain," *J Am Coll Cardiol*, 2005, 45(8):1302-3.

Naproxen and Lansoprazole *see* Lansoprazole and Naproxen *on page 949*

Naproxen and Pseudoephedrine
(na PROKS en & soo doe e FED rin)

Related Information

Naproxen *on page 1148*
Pseudoephedrine *on page 1381*

U.S. Brand Names Aleve® Cold & Sinus [OTC]; Aleve® Sinus & Headache [OTC]

Generic Available No

Index Terms Naproxen Sodium and Pseudoephedrine; Pseudoephedrine and Naproxen

(Continued)

Naproxen and Pseudoephedrine *(Continued)*

Pharmacologic Category Decongestant/Analgesic

Use Temporary relief of cold, sinus, and flu symptoms (including nasal congestion, sinus congestion/pressure, headache, minor body aches and pains, and fever)

Local Anesthetic/Vasoconstrictor Precautions Use with caution since pseudoephedrine is a sympathomimetic amine which could interact with epinephrine to cause a pressor response.

Effects on Dental Treatment Key adverse event(s) related to dental treatment: Pseudoephedrine: Xerostomia (normal salivary flow resumes upon discontinuation).

NSAID formulations are known to reversibly decrease platelet aggregation via mechanisms different than observed with aspirin. The dentist should be aware of the potential of abnormal coagulation.

Common Adverse Effects See individual agents.

Mechanism of Action

Naproxen: Inhibits prostaglandin synthesis by decreasing the activity of the enzyme, cyclooxygenase, which results in decreased formation of prostaglandin precursors

Pseudoephedrine: Directly stimulates alpha-adrenergic receptors of respiratory mucosa causing vasoconstriction; directly stimulates beta-adrenergic receptors causing bronchial relaxation

Drug Interactions

Cytochrome P450 Effect: Naproxen: **Substrate** (minor) of CYP1A2, 2C9

Pharmacodynamics/Kinetics See individual agents.

Naproxen Sodium *see* Naproxen *on page 1148*

Naproxen Sodium and Pseudoephedrine *see* Naproxen and Pseudoephedrine *on page 1151*

Naratriptan (NAR a trip tan)

U.S. Brand Names Amerge®
Canadian Brand Names Amerge®
Mexican Brand Names Naramig
Generic Available No
Index Terms Naratriptan Hydrochloride
Pharmacologic Category Antimigraine Agent; Serotonin 5-HT$_{1B, 1D}$ Receptor Agonist
Use Treatment of acute migraine headache with or without aura
Local Anesthetic/Vasoconstrictor Precautions No information available to require special precautions
Effects on Dental Treatment No significant effects or complications reported
Common Adverse Effects 1% to 10%:
Central nervous system: Dizziness, drowsiness, malaise/fatigue
Gastrointestinal: Nausea, vomiting
Neuromuscular & skeletal: Paresthesia
Miscellaneous: Pain or pressure in throat or neck
Mechanism of Action The therapeutic effect for migraine is due to serotonin agonist activity
Drug Interactions
Increased Effect/Toxicity: Ergot-containing drugs (dihydroergotamine or methysergide) may cause vasospastic reactions when taken with naratriptan. Avoid concomitant use with ergots; separate dose of naratriptan and ergots by at least 24 hours. Oral contraceptives taken with naratriptan reduced the clearance of naratriptan ~30% which may contribute to adverse effects. SSRIs/SNRIs may exhibit additive toxicity with naratriptan or other serotonin agonists (eg, antidepressants, dextromethorphan, tramadol) leading to serotonin syndrome.
Decreased Effect: Smoking increases the clearance of naratriptan.
Pharmacodynamics/Kinetics
Onset of action: 30 minutes
Absorption: Well absorbed
Protein binding, plasma: 28% to 31%
Metabolism: Hepatic via CYP
Bioavailability: 70%
Time to peak: 2-3 hours
Excretion: Urine
Pregnancy Risk Factor C

Naratriptan Hydrochloride *see* Naratriptan *on page 1152*
Narcan *see* Naloxone *on page 1144*

Natalizumab (na ta LIZ u mab)

U.S. Brand Names Tysabri®
Generic Available No
Index Terms AN100226; Anti-4 Alpha Integrin; IgG4-Kappa Monoclonal Antibody
Pharmacologic Category Monoclonal Antibody, Selective Adhesion-Molecule Inhibitor
Use Treatment of relapsing forms of multiple sclerosis
Unlabeled/Investigational Use Crohn's disease
Local Anesthetic/Vasoconstrictor Precautions No information available to require special precautions
Effects on Dental Treatment No significant effects or complications reported
Common Adverse Effects
>10%:
Central nervous system: Headache (38%), fatigue (27%), depression (19%)
Dermatologic: Rash (12%)
Gastrointestinal: Gastroenteritis (11%), abdominal discomfort (11%)
Genitourinary: Urinary tract infection (21%)
Neuromuscular & skeletal: Arthralgia (19%), extremity pain (16%)
Respiratory: Lower respiratory infection (17%)
Miscellaneous: Infusion-related reaction (24%)
1% to 10%:
Cardiovascular: Chest discomfort (5%), peripheral edema (5%)
Central nervous system: Vertigo (6%), syncope (2%), somnolence (2%)
Dermatologic: Dermatitis (7%), pruritus (4%), urticaria (2%)
Endocrine & metabolic: Menstrual irregularities (5%), dysmenorrhea (3%), amenorrhea (2%), ovarian cyst (2%)
Gastrointestinal: Diarrhea (10%), weight changes (2%), cholelithiasis (1%)
Genitourinary: Vaginitis (10%), urinary frequency (9%), urinary incontinence (4%)
Hepatic: Transaminase abnormal (5%)
Local: Bleeding at injection site (3%)
Neuromuscular & skeletal: Muscle cramp (5%), rigors (3%), tremor (3%), joint swelling (2%)
Respiratory: Tonsillitis (7%)
Miscellaneous: Tooth infection (9%), herpes (8%), hypersensitivity reactions (4% to 5%, anaphylaxis/anaphylactoid <1%), serious infection (3%), anaphylaxis (1%), night sweats (1%)
Restrictions Patients must be enrolled in the TOUCH Prescribing Program (800-456-2255) to receive natalizumab. Healthcare providers must also register with the program in order to prescribe, dispense or administer natalizumab. Medication guides are available at http://www.fda.gov/cder/Offices/ODS/MG/natalizumabMG.pdf and should be provided to every patient prior to initiation of therapy.
Mechanism of Action Natalizumab is a monoclonal antibody to the alpha-4 subunit of integrin molecules. These molecules are important to adhesion and migration of cells from the vasculature into inflamed tissue. Natalizumab blocks integrin association with vascular receptors, limiting adhesion and transmigration of leukocytes. Efficacy in specific disorders may be related to reduction in specific inflammatory cell populations in target tissues. In multiple sclerosis, efficacy may be related to blockade of T-lymphocyte migration into the central nervous system; treatment results in a decreased frequency of relapse.
Drug Interactions
Increased Effect/Toxicity: Concomitant immunosuppressant therapy may increase the risk of infection. Interferon beta-1a may increase the levels of natalizumab (no dosage adjustment necessary).
(Continued)

Natalizumab *(Continued)*

Pharmacodynamics/Kinetics
Distribution: 3.8-7.6 L
Half-life elimination: 7-15 days
Excretion: Clearance: 11-21 mL/hour
Pregnancy Risk Factor C

Natamycin (na ta MYE sin)

U.S. Brand Names Natacyn®
Canadian Brand Names Natacyn®
Mexican Brand Names Miconacina
Generic Available No
Index Terms Pimaricin
Pharmacologic Category Antifungal Agent, Ophthalmic
Use Treatment of blepharitis, conjunctivitis, and keratitis caused by susceptible fungi (*Aspergillus, Candida*), *Cephalosporium, Curvularia, Fusarium, Penicillium, Microsporum, Epidermophyton, Blastomyces dermatitidis, Coccidioides immitis, Cryptococcus neoformans, Histoplasma capsulatum, Sporothrix schenckii,* and *Trichomonas vaginalis*
Local Anesthetic/Vasoconstrictor Precautions No information available to require special precautions
Effects on Dental Treatment No significant effects or complications reported
Mechanism of Action Increases cell membrane permeability in susceptible fungi
Pregnancy Risk Factor C

Nateglinide (na te GLYE nide)

Related Information
Endocrine Disorders and Pregnancy *on page 1750*
U.S. Brand Names Starlix®
Canadian Brand Names Starlix®
Mexican Brand Names Starlix
Generic Available No
Pharmacologic Category Antidiabetic Agent, Meglitinide Derivative
Use Management of type 2 diabetes mellitus (noninsulin dependent, NIDDM) as monotherapy when hyperglycemia cannot be managed by diet and exercise alone; in combination with metformin or a thiazolidinedione to lower blood glucose in patients whose hyperglycemia cannot be controlled by exercise, diet, or a single agent alone
Local Anesthetic/Vasoconstrictor Precautions No information available to require special precautions
Effects on Dental Treatment No significant effects or complications reported
Common Adverse Effects As reported with nateglinide monotherapy: 1% to 10%:
Central nervous system: Dizziness (4%)
Endocrine & metabolic: Hypoglycemia (2%), increased uric acid
Gastrointestinal: Weight gain
Neuromuscular & skeletal: Arthropathy (3%)
Respiratory: Upper respiratory infection (10%)
Miscellaneous: Flu-like syndrome (4%)
Mechanism of Action A phenylalanine derivative, nonsulfonylurea hypoglycemic agent used in the management of type 2 diabetes mellitus (noninsulin dependent, NIDDM); stimulates insulin release from the pancreatic beta cells to reduce postprandial hyperglycemia; amount of insulin release is dependent upon existing glucose levels
Drug Interactions
Cytochrome P450 Effect: Substrate (major) of CYP2C9, 3A4; **Inhibits** CYP2C9 (weak)
Increased Effect/Toxicity: CYP2C9 inhibitors may increase the levels/effects of nateglinide; example inhibitors include delavirdine, fluconazole, gemfibrozil, ketoconazole, nicardipine, NSAIDs, sulfonamides, and tolbutamide. CYP3A4 inhibitors may increase the levels/effects of nateglinide; example inhibitors include azole antifungals, clarithromycin, diclofenac, doxycycline, erythromycin, imatinib, isoniazid, nefazodone, nicardipine, propofol, protease inhibitors, quinidine, telithromycin, and verapamil. Possible increased hypoglycemic effect may be seen with nonselective beta-adrenergic blocking agents, and pegvisomant; monitor glucose closely when agents are initiated, modified, or discontinued.

Decreased Effect: CYP2C9 inducers may decrease the levels/effects of nateglinide; example inducers include carbamazepine, phenobarbital, phenytoin, rifampin, rifapentine, and secobarbital. CYP3A4 inducers may decrease the levels/effects of nateglinide; example inducers include aminoglutethimide, carbamazepine, nafcillin, nevirapine, phenobarbital, phenytoin, and rifamycins. Possible decreased hypoglycemic effect may be seen with thiazides, corticosteroids; monitor glucose closely when agents are initiated, modified, or discontinued.

Pharmacodynamics/Kinetics
Onset of action: Insulin secretion: ~20 minutes
Peak effect: 1 hour
Duration: 4 hours
Absorption: Rapid
Distribution: 10 L
Protein binding: 98%, primarily to albumin
Metabolism: Hepatic via hydroxylation followed by glucuronide conjugation via CYP2C9 (70%) and CYP3A4 (30%) to metabolites
Bioavailability: 73%
Half-life elimination: 1.5 hours
Time to peak: ≤1 hour
Excretion: Urine (83%, 16% as unchanged drug); feces (10%)

Pregnancy Risk Factor C

Nedocromil (ne doe KROE mil)

Related Information
Respiratory Diseases *on page 1747*
U.S. Brand Names Alocril®; Tilade®
Canadian Brand Names Alocril®; Tilade®
Generic Available No
Index Terms Nedocromil Sodium
Pharmacologic Category Mast Cell Stabilizer
Use
Aerosol: Maintenance therapy in patients with mild to moderate bronchial asthma
Ophthalmic: Treatment of itching associated with allergic conjunctivitis
Local Anesthetic/Vasoconstrictor Precautions No information available to require special precautions
Effects on Dental Treatment Key adverse event(s) related to dental treatment: Unpleasant taste.
Common Adverse Effects
Inhalation aerosol:
>10%: Gastrointestinal: Unpleasant taste
1% to 10%:
Cardiovascular: Chest pain
Central nervous system: Dizziness, dysphonia, headache, fatigue
Dermatologic: Rash
Gastrointestinal: Nausea, vomiting, dyspepsia, diarrhea, abdominal pain, xerostomia, unpleasant taste
Hepatic: Increased ALT
Neuromuscular & skeletal: Arthritis, tremor
(Continued)

Nedocromil *(Continued)*

Respiratory: Cough, pharyngitis, rhinitis, bronchitis, upper respiratory infection, bronchospasm, increased sputum production

Ophthalmic solution:

>10%:

Central nervous system: Headache (40%)

Gastrointestinal: Unpleasant taste

Ocular: Burning, irritation, stinging

Respiratory: Nasal congestion

1% to 10%:

Ocular: Conjunctivitis, eye redness, photophobia

Respiratory: Asthma, rhinitis

Mechanism of Action Inhibits the activation of and mediator release from a variety of inflammatory cell types associated with asthma including eosinophils, neutrophils, macrophages, mast cells, monocytes, and platelets; it inhibits the release of histamine, leukotrienes, and slow-reacting substance of anaphylaxis; it inhibits the development of early and late bronchoconstriction responses to inhaled antigen

Pharmacodynamics/Kinetics

Duration: Therapeutic effect: 2 hours

Protein binding, plasma: 89%

Bioavailability: 7% to 9%

Half-life elimination: 1.5-2 hours

Excretion: Urine (as unchanged drug)

Pregnancy Risk Factor B

Nedocromil Sodium *see* Nedocromil *on page 1155*

Nefazodone *(nef AY zoe done)*

Generic Available Yes

Index Terms Nefazodone Hydrochloride; Serzone

Pharmacologic Category Antidepressant, Serotonin Reuptake Inhibitor/Antagonist

Use Treatment of depression

Unlabeled/Investigational Use Post-traumatic stress disorder

Local Anesthetic/Vasoconstrictor Precautions Nefazodone inhibits reuptake of both serotonin and norepinephrine and also blocks some serotonin receptors. No precautions with vasoconstrictors appear to be necessary.

Effects on Dental Treatment Key adverse event(s) related to dental treatment: Significant xerostomia (normal salivary flow resumes upon discontinuation) and taste perversion.

Common Adverse Effects

>10%:

Central nervous system: Headache, drowsiness, insomnia, agitation, dizziness

Gastrointestinal: Xerostomia, nausea, constipation

Neuromuscular & skeletal: Weakness

1% to 10%:

Cardiovascular: Bradycardia, hypotension, peripheral edema, postural hypotension, vasodilation

Central nervous system: Chills, fever, incoordination, lightheadedness, confusion, memory impairment, abnormal dreams, decreased concentration, ataxia, psychomotor retardation, tremor

Dermatologic: Pruritus, rash

Endocrine & metabolic: Breast pain, impotence, libido decreased

Gastrointestinal: Gastroenteritis, vomiting, dyspepsia, diarrhea, increased appetite, thirst, taste perversion

Genitourinary: Urinary frequency, urinary retention

Hematologic: Hematocrit decreased

Neuromuscular & skeletal: Arthralgia, hypertonia, paresthesia, neck rigidity, tremor

Ocular: Blurred vision (9%), abnormal vision (7%), eye pain, visual field defect

Otic: Tinnitus

Respiratory: Bronchitis, cough, dyspnea, pharyngitis

Miscellaneous: Flu syndrome, infection

Restrictions An FDA-approved medication guide concerning the use of antidepressants in children, adolescents, and young adults must be distributed when dispensing an outpatient prescription (new or refill) where this medication is to be used without direct supervision of a healthcare provider. Medication guides are available at http://www.fda.gov/cder/Offices/ODS/medication_guides.htm.

Dispense to parents or guardians of children and adolescents receiving this medication.

Mechanism of Action Inhibits neuronal reuptake of serotonin and norepinephrine; also blocks 5-HT$_2$ and alpha$_1$ receptors; has no significant affinity for alpha$_2$, beta-adrenergic, 5-HT$_{1A}$, cholinergic, dopaminergic, or benzodiazepine receptors

Drug Interactions

Cytochrome P450 Effect: Substrate (major) of CYP2D6, 3A4; **Inhibits** CYP1A2 (weak), 2B6 (weak), 2C8 (weak), 2D6 (weak), 3A4 (strong)

Increased Effect/Toxicity: Concurrent use of carbamazepine, cisapride, or pimozide is contraindicated. Concurrent therapy with triazolam or alprazolam is generally contraindicated (dosage must be reduced by 75% for triazolam and 50% for alprazolam; such reductions may not be possible with available dosage forms). Concurrent use of ergot alkaloids and/or selected HMG-CoA reductase inhibitors (lovastatin and simvastatin) is generally contraindicated with strong CYP3A4 inhibitors.

Concurrent use of MAO inhibitors may lead to serotonin syndrome; avoid concurrent use or use within 14 days (includes phenelzine, isocarboxazid, and linezolid). Selegiline may increase the risk of serotonin syndrome, particularly at higher doses (>10 mg/day, where selectivity for MAO type B is decreased). Theoretically, concurrent use of buspirone, meperidine, serotonin agonists (sumatriptan and rizatriptan), SSRIs, and venlafaxine may result in serotonin syndrome.

Nefazodone may increase the serum levels/effects of antiarrhythmics (amiodarone, lidocaine, propafenone, quinidine), some antipsychotics (clozapine, haloperidol, mesoridazine, quetiapine, and risperidone), some benzodiazepines (triazolam is contraindicated; decrease alprazolam dose by 50%), buspirone (limit buspirone dose to <2.5 mg/day), Nefazodone may increase the levels/effects of calcium channel blockers, cyclosporine, mirtazapine, nateglinide, nefazodone, quinidine, sildenafil (and other PDE-5 inhibitors), tacrolimus, venlafaxine, and other CYP3A4 substrates. When used with strong CYP3A4 inhibitors, dosage adjustment/limits are recommended for sildenafil and other PDE-5 inhibitors; refer to individual monographs.

The levels/effects of nefazodone may be increased by azole antifungals, chlorpromazine, clarithromycin, delavirdine, diclofenac, doxycycline, erythromycin, fluoxetine, imatinib, isoniazid, miconazole, nicardipine, paroxetine, pergolide, propofol, protease inhibitors, quinidine, quinine, ritonavir, ropinirole, telithromycin, verapamil, and other CYP2D6 or 3A4 inhibitors.

Decreased Effect: Carbamazepine may reduce serum concentrations of nefazodone; concurrent administration should be avoided. The levels/effects of nefazodone may be decreased by aminoglutethimide, nafcillin, nevirapine, phenobarbital, phenytoin, and rifamycins and other CYP3A4 inducers.

Pharmacodynamics/Kinetics

Onset of action: Therapeutic: Up to 6 weeks

Metabolism: Hepatic to three active metabolites: Triazoledione, hydroxynefazodone, and m-chlorophenylpiperazine (mCPP)

Bioavailability: 20% (variable)

Half-life elimination: Parent drug: 2-4 hours; active metabolites persist longer

Time to peak, serum: 1 hour, prolonged in presence of food

Excretion: Primarily urine (as metabolites); feces

Pregnancy Risk Factor C

Nefazodone Hydrochloride *see* Nefazodone *on page 1156*

Nelarabine (nel AY re been)

U.S. Brand Names Arranon®

Generic Available No

Index Terms 2-Amino-6-Methoxypurine Arabinoside; GW506U78; 506U78

Pharmacologic Category Antineoplastic Agent, Antimetabolite

Use Treatment of relapsed or refractory T-cell acute lymphoblastic leukemia (ALL) and T-cell lymphoblastic lymphoma

Unlabeled/Investigational Use CML (Philadelphia chromosome positive) T-Cell blast phase

Local Anesthetic/Vasoconstrictor Precautions No information available to require special precautions

Effects on Dental Treatment Key adverse event(s) related to dental treatment: Taste perversion and stomatitis.

Common Adverse Effects Note: Pediatric adverse reactions fell within a range similar to adults except where noted.

>10%:

Cardiovascular: Peripheral edema (15%), edema (11%)

(Continued)

Nelarabine *(Continued)*

Central nervous system: Fatigue (50%), fever (23%), somnolence (7% to 22%; grades 2-4: 3% to 6%), dizziness (21%; grade 2: 8% adults), headache (15% to 17%; grades 2-4: 4% to 8%), hypoesthesia (6% to 17%; grades 2-4: children 5%, adults 12%), pain (11%)

Dermatologic: Petechiae (12%)

Endocrine & metabolic: Hypokalemia (12%)

Gastrointestinal: Nausea (41%), diarrhea (22%), vomiting (10% to 22%), constipation (21%)

Hematologic: Anemia (95% to 99%; grade 4: 10% to 14%), neutropenia (81% to 94%; grade 4: children 62%, adults 49%), thrombocytopenia (86% to 88%; grade 4: 22% to 32%), leukopenia (38%; grade 4: 7%), febrile neutropenia (12%; grade 4: 1%)

Hepatic: Transaminases increased (12%)

Neuromuscular & skeletal: Peripheral neuropathy (12% to 21%; grades 2-4: 11% to 14%), weakness (6% to 17%; grade 4: 1%), paresthesia (4% to 15%; grades 2-4: 3% to 4%), myalgia (13%)

Respiratory: Cough (25%), dyspnea (7% to 20%)

1% to 10%:

Cardiovascular: Hypotension (8%), tachycardia (8%), chest pain (5%)

Central nervous system: Ataxia (2% to 9%; grades 2-4: children 1%, adults 8%), confusion (8%), insomnia (7%), depressed level of consciousness (6%; grades 2-4: 2%), depression (6%), seizure (grade 4: 6% children), motor dysfunction (4%; grades 2-4: 2%), amnesia (3%; grades 2-4: 1%), balance disorder (2%; grades 2-4: 1%), nerve paralysis (2%), sensory loss (1% to 2%), aphasia (1%), cerebral hemorrhage (1%), coma (1%), encephalopathy (1%), hemiparesis (1%), hydrocephalus (1%), lethargy (1%), leukoencephalopathy (1%), loss of consciousness (1%), mental impairment (1%), neuropathic pain (1%), nerve palsy (1%), nystagmus (1%), paralysis (1%), sciatica (1%), sensory disturbance (1%), speech disorder (1%), demyelination, ascending peripheral neuropathy

Endocrine & Metabolic: Hypocalcemia (8%), dehydration (7%), hyper-/hypoglycemia (6%), hypomagnesemia (6%)

Gastrointestinal: Abdominal pain (9%), anorexia (9%), stomatitis (8%), abdominal distension (6%), taste perversion (3%)

Hepatic: Albumin decreased (10%), bilirubin increased (10%), AST increased (6%)

Neuromuscular & skeletal: Arthralgia (9%), back pain (8%), muscle weakness (8%), rigors (8%), limb pain (7%), abnormal gait (6%), noncardiac chest pain (5%), tremor (4% to 5%; grades 2-4: 2% to 3%), dysarthria (1%), hyporeflexia (1%), hypertonia (1%), incoordination (1%)

Ocular: Blurred vision (4%)

Renal: Creatinine increased (6%)

Respiratory: Pleural effusion (10%), epistaxis (8%), pneumonia (8%), sinusitis (7%), wheezing (5%), sinus headache (1%)

Miscellaneous: Infection (5% to 9%)

Mechanism of Action Nelarabine is a prodrug of ara-G. It is demethylated by adenosine deaminase to ara-G and then converted to ara-GTP. Ara-GTP is incorporated into the DNA of the leukemic blasts, leading to inhibition of DNA synthesis and inducing apoptosis. Ara-GTP appears to accumulate at higher levels in T-cells, which correlates to clinical response.

Drug Interactions

Increased Effect/Toxicity: Vaccines: Avoid administration of live vaccines in immunosuppressive therapy.

Pharmacodynamics/Kinetics

Distribution: Nelarabine: 197-213 L/m^2; ara-G: 33-50 L/m^2

Protein binding: Nelarabine and ara-G: <25%

Metabolism: Hepatic; demethylated by adenosine deaminase to form ara-G (active); also hydrolyzed to form methylguanine. Both ara-G and methylguanine metabolized to guanine. Guanine is deaminated into xanthine, which is further oxidized to form uric acid, which is then oxidized to form allantoin.

Half-life elimination: Nelarabine: 30 minutes; ara-G: 3 hours

Excretion: Urine (nelarabine 7%, ara-G 27%) within 24 hours of infusion on day 1

Pregnancy Risk Factor D

Nelfinavir *(nel FIN a veer)*

Related Information

HIV Infection and AIDS *on page 1753*
Tuberculosis Treatment *on page 1909*

Viral Infections *on page 1806*
U.S. Brand Names Viracept®
Canadian Brand Names Viracept®
Mexican Brand Names Viracept
Generic Available No
Index Terms NFV
Pharmacologic Category Antiretroviral Agent, Protease Inhibitor
Use In combination with other antiretroviral therapy in the treatment of HIV infection
Local Anesthetic/Vasoconstrictor Precautions No information available to require special precautions
Effects on Dental Treatment Key adverse event(s) related to dental treatment: Mouth ulcers.
Common Adverse Effects Data presented on experience in adults, unless otherwise noted.

>10%: Gastrointestinal: Diarrhea (14% to 20%; children: 39% to 47%)

2% to 10%:
Dermatologic: Rash (1% to 3%)
Gastrointestinal: Nausea (3% to 7%), flatulence (1% to 5%)
Hematologic: Lymphocytes decreased (1% to 6%), neutrophils decreased (1% to 5%), hemoglobin decreased (2% to 3%), creatine kinase increased (2%)
Hepatic: Transaminases increased (1% to 2%)

Dosage Oral:
Children 2-13 years: 45-55 mg/kg twice daily **or** 25-35 mg/kg 3 times/day (maximum: 2500 mg/day). If tablets are unable to be taken, use oral powder in small amount of water, milk, formula, or dietary supplements; do not use acidic food/juice or store for >6 hours.
Adults: 750 mg 3 times/day or 1250 mg twice daily with meals in combination with other antiretroviral therapies
Dosing adjustment in renal impairment: No adjustment needed
Dosing adjustment in hepatic impairment: Insufficient data; use caution
Mechanism of Action Inhibits the HIV-1 protease; inhibition of the viral protease prevents cleavage of the gag-pol polyprotein resulting in the production of immature, noninfectious virus
Contraindications Hypersensitivity to nelfinavir or any component of the formulation; concurrent therapy with amiodarone, ergot derivatives, midazolam, pimozide, quinidine, triazolam
Warnings/Precautions Use with caution in patients taking strong CYP3A4 inhibitors, moderate or strong CYP3A4 inducers and major CYP3A4 substrates (see Drug Interactions); consider alternative agents that avoid or lessen the potential for CYP-mediated interactions. Not recommended for use with rifampin, St John's wort, lovastatin, simvastatin, or proton pump inhibitors (based on omeprazole data). Use caution with hepatic impairment. Warn patients that redistribution of body fat can occur. New onset diabetes mellitus, exacerbation of diabetes, and hyperglycemia have been reported in HIV-infected patients receiving protease inhibitors. Use with caution in patients with hemophilia A or B; increased bleeding during protease inhibitor therapy has been reported. Immune reconstitution syndrome has been reported; may require additional evaluation and treatment. The oral powder contains phenylalanine; use caution in patients with phenylketonuria. Safety and efficacy have not been established in children <2 years of age.
Drug Interactions
Cytochrome P450 Effect: Substrate of CYP2C9 (minor), 2C19 (major), 2D6 (minor), 3A4 (major); **Inhibits** CYP1A2 (weak), 2B6 (weak), 2C9 (weak), 2C19 (weak), 2D6 (weak), 3A4 (strong)
Increased Effect/Toxicity: Nelfinavir effects may be increased by azithromycin, azole antifungals, cimetidine, delavirdine, efavirenz, and protease inhibitors. Nelfinavir may increase the levels/effects of selected benzodiazepines, calcium channel blockers, clarithromycin, corticosteroids (eg, fluticasone), cyclosporine, eplerenone, fentanyl, mirtazapine, nateglinide, nefazodone, quinidine, sildenafil (and other PDE-5 inhibitors), tacrolimus, tenofovir, trazodone, tricyclic antidepressants, venlafaxine, and other CYP3A4 substrates. Selected benzodiazepines (midazolam, triazolam), cisapride, ergot alkaloids, selected HMG-CoA reductase inhibitors (lovastatin and simvastatin), and pimozide are generally contraindicated with strong CYP3A4 inhibitors. When used with strong CYP3A4 inhibitors, dosage adjustment/limits are recommended for sildenafil and other PDE-5 inhibitors; refer to individual monographs.
Decreased Effect: The levels/effects of nelfinavir may be decreased by aminoglutethimide, antacids, carbamazepine, nafcillin, nevirapine, omeprazole, phenobarbital, phenytoin, rifamycins, tenofovir, or other inducers of CYP2C19 or 3A4. Nelfinavir effects may be decreased by St John's wort.
(Continued)

Nelfinavir *(Continued)*

Nelfinavir may decrease the effects of delavirdine, methadone, hormonal contraceptives, and theophylline.

Ethanol/Nutrition/Herb Interactions

Food: Nelfinavir taken with food increases plasma concentration time curve (AUC) by two- to threefold. Do not administer with acidic food or juice (orange juice, apple juice, or applesauce) since the combination may have a bitter taste.

Herb/Nutraceutical: St John's wort may decrease nelfinavir serum concentrations; avoid concurrent use.

Dietary Considerations Should be taken as scheduled with food. Oral powder contains phenylalanine 11.2 mg/g.

Pharmacodynamics/Kinetics

Absorption: Food increases AUC of nelfinavir by two- to fivefold

Distribution: V_d: 2-7 L/kg

Protein binding: 98%

Metabolism: Hepatic via CYP2C19 and 3A4; major metabolite has activity comparable to parent drug

Half-life elimination: 3.5-5 hours

Time to peak, serum: 2-4 hours

Excretion: Feces (98% to 99%, 78% as metabolites, 22% as unchanged drug); urine (1% to 2%)

Pregnancy Risk Factor B

Dosage Forms

Powder, oral:

Viracept®: 50 mg/g

Tablet:

Viracept®: 250 mg, 625 mg

Nembutal® *see* Pentobarbital *on page 1276*

NeoCeuticals™ Acne Spot Treatment [OTC] *see* Salicylic Acid *on page 1451*

Neo DM *see* Chlorpheniramine, Phenylephrine, and Dextromethorphan *on page 342*

Neo-Fradin™ *see* Neomycin *on page 1160*

Neofrin™ *see* Phenylephrine *on page 1293*

Neomycin *(nee oh MYE sin)*

U.S. Brand Names Neo-Fradin™; Neo-Rx

Mexican Brand Names Gemicina

Generic Available Yes

Index Terms Neomycin Sulfate

Pharmacologic Category Ammonium Detoxicant; Antibiotic, Aminoglycoside; Antibiotic, Topical

Use Orally to prepare GI tract for surgery; topically to treat minor skin infections; treatment of diarrhea caused by *E. coli*; adjunct in the treatment of hepatic encephalopathy; bladder irrigation; ocular infections

Local Anesthetic/Vasoconstrictor Precautions No information available to require special precautions

Effects on Dental Treatment No significant effects or complications reported

Common Adverse Effects

Oral: >10%: Gastrointestinal: Nausea, diarrhea, vomiting, irritation or soreness of the mouth or rectal area

Topical: >10%: Dermatologic: Contact dermatitis

Mechanism of Action Interferes with bacterial protein synthesis by binding to 30S ribosomal subunits

Drug Interactions

Increased Effect/Toxicity: Oral neomycin may potentiate the effects of oral anticoagulants. Neomycin may increase the adverse effects with other neurotoxic, ototoxic, or nephrotoxic drugs.

Decreased Effect: May decrease GI absorption of digoxin and methotrexate.

Pharmacodynamics/Kinetics

Absorption: Oral, percutaneous: Poor (3%)

Distribution: 97% of an orally administered dose remains in the GI tract. Absorbed neomycin distributes to tissues and concentrates in the renal cortex. With repeated doses, accumulation also occurs in the inner ear.

V_d: 0.36 L/kg

Protein binding: 0% to 30%

Metabolism: Slightly hepatic

Half-life elimination (age and renal function dependent): 3 hours

Time to peak, serum: Oral: 1-4 hours

Excretion: Feces (97% of oral dose as unchanged drug); urine (30% to 50% of absorbed drug as unchanged drug)

Pregnancy Risk Factor D

Neomycin and Polymyxin B (nee oh MYE sin & pol i MIKS in bee)

Related Information
 Neomycin *on page 1160*
 Polymyxin B *on page 1322*

U.S. Brand Names Neosporin® G.U. Irrigant

Canadian Brand Names Neosporin® Irrigating Solution

Generic Available Yes: Irrigation solution 1 mL package size

Index Terms Polymyxin B and Neomycin

Pharmacologic Category Antibiotic, Topical; Genitourinary Irrigant

Use Short-term as a continuous irrigant or rinse in the urinary bladder to prevent bacteriuria and gram-negative rod septicemia associated with the use of indwelling catheters; to help prevent infection in minor cuts, scrapes, and burns

Local Anesthetic/Vasoconstrictor Precautions No information available to require special precautions

Effects on Dental Treatment No significant effects or complications reported

Common Adverse Effects Frequency not defined.
 Dermatologic: Contact dermatitis, erythema, rash, urticaria
 Genitourinary: Bladder irritation
 Local: Burning
 Neuromuscular & skeletal: Neuromuscular blockade
 Otic: Ototoxicity
 Renal: Nephrotoxicity

Mechanism of Action See individual agents.

Pharmacodynamics/Kinetics
 Absorption: Topical: Not absorbed following application to intact skin; absorbed through denuded or abraded skin, peritoneum, wounds, or ulcers
 See individual agents.

Pregnancy Risk Factor C/D (for G.U. irrigant)

Neomycin, Bacitracin, and Polymyxin B *see* Bacitracin, Neomycin, and Polymyxin B *on page 181*

Neomycin, Bacitracin, Polymyxin B, and Hydrocortisone *see* Bacitracin, Neomycin, Polymyxin B, and Hydrocortisone *on page 182*

Neomycin, Bacitracin, Polymyxin B, and Pramoxine *see* Bacitracin, Neomycin, Polymyxin B, and Pramoxine *on page 182*

Neomycin, Polymyxin B, and Dexamethasone
(nee oh MYE sin, pol i MIKS in bee, & deks a METH a sone)

Related Information
 Dexamethasone *on page 464*
 Neomycin *on page 1160*
 Polymyxin B *on page 1322*

U.S. Brand Names AK-Trol® [DSC]; Maxitrol®; Poly-Dex™

Canadian Brand Names Dioptrol®; Maxitrol®

Mexican Brand Names Maxitrol

Generic Available Yes

Index Terms Dexamethasone, Neomycin, and Polymyxin B; Polymyxin B, Neomycin, and Dexamethasone

Pharmacologic Category Antibiotic/Corticosteroid, Ophthalmic

Use Steroid-responsive inflammatory ocular conditions in which a corticosteroid is indicated and where bacterial infection or a risk of bacterial infection exists

Local Anesthetic/Vasoconstrictor Precautions No information available to require special precautions

Effects on Dental Treatment No significant effects or complications reported

Mechanism of Action See individual agents.

Pregnancy Risk Factor C

Neomycin, Polymyxin B, and Gramicidin
(nee oh MYE sin, pol i MIKS in bee, & gram i SYE din)

Related Information
 Neomycin *on page 1160*
 Polymyxin B *on page 1322*
 (Continued)

1161

Neomycin, Polymyxin B, and Gramicidin *(Continued)*

U.S. Brand Names Neosporin® Ophthalmic Solution
Canadian Brand Names Neosporin®; Optimyxin Plus®
Generic Available Yes
Index Terms Gramicidin, Neomycin, and Polymyxin B; Polymyxin B, Neomycin, and Gramicidin
Pharmacologic Category Antibiotic, Ophthalmic
Use Treatment of superficial ocular infection
Local Anesthetic/Vasoconstrictor Precautions No information available to require special precautions
Effects on Dental Treatment No significant effects or complications reported
Mechanism of Action Interferes with bacterial protein synthesis by binding to 30S ribosomal subunits; binds to phospholipids, alters permeability, and damages the bacterial cytoplasmic membrane permitting leakage of intracellular constituents
Pregnancy Risk Factor C

Neomycin, Polymyxin B, and Hydrocortisone
(nee oh MYE sin, pol i MIKS in bee, & hye droe KOR ti sone)

Related Information
Hydrocortisone *on page 836*
Neomycin *on page 1160*
Polymyxin B *on page 1322*
U.S. Brand Names Cortisporin® Cream; Cortisporin® Ophthalmic; Cortisporin® Otic; PediOtic®
Canadian Brand Names Cortimyxin®; Cortisporin® Otic
Generic Available Yes
Index Terms Hydrocortisone, Neomycin, and Polymyxin B; Polymyxin B, Neomycin, and Hydrocortisone
Pharmacologic Category Antibiotic/Corticosteroid, Ophthalmic; Antibiotic/Corticosteroid, Otic; Topical Skin Product
Use Steroid-responsive inflammatory condition for which a corticosteroid is indicated and where bacterial infection or a risk of bacterial infection exists
Local Anesthetic/Vasoconstrictor Precautions No information available to require special precautions
Effects on Dental Treatment No significant effects or complications reported
Common Adverse Effects Frequency not defined.
Dermatologic: Contact dermatitis, erythema, rash, urticaria
Local: Burning, itching, swelling, pain, stinging
Ocular: Intraocular pressure increased, glaucoma, cataracts, conjunctival erythema, transient irritation, burning, stinging, itching, inflammation, angioneurotic edema, urticaria, vesicular and maculopapular dermatitis
Otic: Ototoxicity
Miscellaneous: Hypersensitivity, sensitization to neomycin, secondary infection
Mechanism of Action See individual agents.
Drug Interactions
Cytochrome P450 Effect: Hydrocortisone: **Substrate** of CYP3A4 (minor); **Induces** CYP3A4 (weak)
Pharmacodynamics/Kinetics See individual agents.
Pregnancy Risk Factor C

Neomycin, Polymyxin B, and Prednisolone
(nee oh MYE sin, pol i MIKS in bee, & pred NIS oh lone)

Related Information
Neomycin *on page 1160*
Polymyxin B *on page 1322*
PrednisoLONE *on page 1339*
U.S. Brand Names Poly-Pred®
Generic Available No
Index Terms Polymyxin B, Neomycin, and Prednisolone; Prednisolone, Neomycin, and Polymyxin B
Pharmacologic Category Antibiotic/Corticosteroid, Ophthalmic
Use Steroid-responsive inflammatory ocular condition in which bacterial infection or a risk of bacterial ocular infection exists
Local Anesthetic/Vasoconstrictor Precautions No information available to require special precautions
Effects on Dental Treatment No significant effects or complications reported
Mechanism of Action See individual agents.
Pregnancy Risk Factor C

Nepafenac (ne pa FEN ak)

U.S. Brand Names Nevanac™
Generic Available No
Pharmacologic Category Nonsteroidal Anti-inflammatory Drug (NSAID), Ophthalmic
Use Treatment of pain and inflammation associated with cataract surgery
Local Anesthetic/Vasoconstrictor Precautions No information available to require special precautions
Effects on Dental Treatment No significant effects or complications reported
Mechanism of Action Nepafenac is a prodrug which once converted to amfenac inhibits prostaglandin synthesis by decreasing the activity of the enzyme, cyclooxygenase, which results in decreased formation of prostaglandin precursors.
Pregnancy Risk Factor C/D (3rd trimester)

Nesiritide (ni SIR i tide)

U.S. Brand Names Natrecor®
Generic Available No
Index Terms B-type Natriuretic Peptide (Human); hBNP; Natriuretic Peptide
Pharmacologic Category Natriuretic Peptide, B-Type, Human; Vasodilator
Use Treatment of acutely decompensated congestive heart failure (CHF) in patients with dyspnea at rest or with minimal activity
Local Anesthetic/Vasoconstrictor Precautions No information available to require special precautions
Effects on Dental Treatment No significant effects or complications reported
Common Adverse Effects Note: Frequencies cited below were recorded in VMAC trial at dosages similar to approved labeling. Higher frequencies have (Continued)

Nesiritide *(Continued)*

been observed in trials using higher dosages of nesiritide. The percentages marked with an asterisk (*) indicate frequency less than or equal to placebo or other standard therapy.

>10%:

Cardiovascular: Hypotension (total: 11%; symptomatic: 4% at recommended dose, up to 17% at higher doses)

Renal: Increased serum creatinine (28% with >0.5 mg/dL increase over baseline)

1% to 10%:

Cardiovascular: Ventricular tachycardia (3%)*, ventricular extrasystoles (3%)*, angina (2%)*, bradycardia (1%), tachycardia, atrial fibrillation, AV node conduction abnormalities

Central nervous system: Headache (8%)*, dizziness (3%)*, insomnia (2%)*, anxiety (3%), fever, confusion, paresthesia, somnolence, tremor

Dermatologic: Pruritus, rash

Gastrointestinal: Nausea (4%)*, abdominal pain (1%)*, vomiting (1%)*

Hematologic: Anemia

Local: Injection site reaction

Neuromuscular & skeletal: Back pain (4%), leg cramps

Ocular: Amblyopia

Respiratory: Cough (increased), hemoptysis, apnea

Miscellaneous: Increased diaphoresis

Mechanism of Action Binds to guanylate cyclase receptor on vascular smooth muscle and endothelial cells, increasing intracellular cyclic GMP, resulting in smooth muscle cell relaxation. Has been shown to produce dose-dependent reductions in pulmonary capillary wedge pressure (PCWP) and systemic arterial pressure.

Drug Interactions

Increased Effect/Toxicity: An increased frequency of symptomatic hypotension was observed with concurrent administration of ACE inhibitors. Other hypotensive agents (eg, diazoxide) are likely to have additive effects on hypotension. In patients receiving diuretic therapy leading to depletion of intravascular volume, the risk of hypotension and/or renal impairment may be increased.

Pharmacodynamics/Kinetics

Onset of action: 15 minutes (60% of 3-hour effect achieved)

Duration: >60 minutes (up to several hours) for systolic blood pressure; hemodynamic effects persist longer than serum half-life would predict

Distribution: V_{ss}: 0.19 L/kg

Metabolism: Proteolytic cleavage by vascular endopeptidases and proteolysis following receptor binding and cellular internalization

Half-life elimination: Initial (distribution) 2 minutes; Terminal: 18 minutes

Time to peak: 1 hour

Excretion: Urine

Pregnancy Risk Factor C

Neutrogena® On The Spot® Acne Treatment [OTC] *see* Benzoyl Peroxide *on page 200*

Neutrogena® T/Gel [OTC] *see* Coal Tar *on page 402*

Neutrogena® T/Gel Extra Strength [OTC] *see* Coal Tar *on page 402*

Neutrogena® T/Gel Stubborn Itch Control [OTC] *see* Coal Tar *on page 402*

Nevanac™ *see* Nepafenac *on page 1163*

Nevirapine (ne VYE ra peen)

Related Information
HIV Infection and AIDS *on page 1753*
Tuberculosis Treatment *on page 1909*
U.S. Brand Names Viramune®
Canadian Brand Names Viramune®
Generic Available No
Index Terms NVP
Pharmacologic Category Antiretroviral Agent, Reverse Transcriptase Inhibitor (Non-nucleoside)
Use In combination therapy with other antiretroviral agents for the treatment of HIV-1
Local Anesthetic/Vasoconstrictor Precautions No information available to require special precautions
Effects on Dental Treatment Key adverse event(s) related to dental treatment: Ulcerative stomatitis and oral lesions.
Common Adverse Effects Note: Potentially life-threatening nevirapine-associated adverse effects may present with the following symptoms: Abrupt onset of flu-like symptoms, abdominal pain, jaundice, or fever with or without rash; may progress to hepatic failure with encephalopathy. Skin rash is present in ~50% of cases.

Percentages of adverse effects vary by clinical trial:
>10%:
   Dermatologic: Rash (grade 1/2: 13%; grade 3/4: 1.5%) is the most common toxicity; occurs most frequently within the first 6 weeks of therapy; women may be at higher risk than men
   Hepatic: ALT >250 units/L (5% to 14%); symptomatic hepatic events (4%, range: up to 11%) are more common in women, women with $CD4^+$ cell counts >250 cells/mm^3, and men with $CD4^+$ cell counts >400 cells/mm^3
1% to 10%:
   Central nervous system: Headache (1% to 4%), fatigue (up to 5%)
   Gastrointestinal: Nausea (<1% to 9%), abdominal pain (<1% to 2%), diarrhea (up to 2%)
   Hepatic: AST >250 units/L (4% to 8%); coinfection with hepatitis B or C and/or increased liver function tests at the beginning of therapy are associated with a greater risk of asymptomatic transaminase elevations (ALT or AST >5 times ULN: 6%, range: up to 9%) or symptomatic events occurring ≥6 weeks after beginning treatment
Restrictions An FDA-approved medication guide must be distributed when dispensing an outpatient prescription (new or refill) where this medication is to be used without direct supervision of a healthcare provider. Medication guides are available at http://www.fda.gov/cder/Offices/ODS/medication_guides.htm.
Mechanism of Action As a non-nucleoside reverse transcriptase inhibitor, nevirapine has activity against HIV-1 by binding to reverse transcriptase. It consequently blocks the RNA-dependent and DNA-dependent DNA polymerase activities including HIV-1 replication. It does not require intracellular phosphorylation for antiviral activity.
Drug Interactions
Cytochrome P450 Effect: Substrate of CYP2B6 (minor), 2D6 (minor), 3A4 (major); **Inhibits** CYP1A2 (weak), 2D6 (weak), 3A4 (weak); **Induces** CYP2B6 (strong), 3A4 (strong)
Increased Effect/Toxicity: Cimetidine, itraconazole, ketoconazole, and some macrolide antibiotics may increase nevirapine plasma concentrations. Concurrent administration of prednisone for the first 14 days of nevirapine therapy was associated with an increased incidence and severity of rash. Rifabutin concentrations are increased by nevirapine.
Decreased Effect: The levels/effects of nevirapine may be decreased by aminoglutethimide, carbamazepine, nafcillin, nevirapine, phenobarbital, phenytoin, and rifamycins, and other CYP3A4 inducers; avoid concurrent use. Nevirapine may decrease the levels/effects of benzodiazepines, bupropion, calcium channel blockers, clarithromycin, cyclosporine, efavirenz, erythromycin, estrogens, mirtazapine, nateglinide, nefazodone, promethazine, selegiline, sertraline, tacrolimus, venlafaxine, and other CYP2B6 or 3A4 substrates.
(Continued)

Nevirapine *(Continued)*

Nevirapine may decrease serum concentrations of some protease inhibitors (AUC of indinavir, lopinavir, nelfinavir, and saquinavir may be decreased, however, no effect noted with ritonavir); specific dosage adjustments have not been recommended; no adjustment recommended for ritonavir, unless combined with lopinavir (Kaletra™). Nevirapine may decrease the effectiveness of oral contraceptives; suggest alternate method or additional form of birth control. Nevirapine also decreases the effect of ketoconazole and methadone.

Pharmacodynamics/Kinetics

Absorption: >90%

Distribution: Widely; V_d: 1.2-1.4 L/kg; CSF penetration approximates 40% to 50% of plasma

Protein binding, plasma: 60%

Metabolism: Extensively hepatic via CYP3A4 (hydroxylation to inactive compounds); may undergo enterohepatic recycling

Half-life elimination: Decreases over 2- to 4-week time with chronic dosing due to autoinduction (ie, half-life = 45 hours initially and decreases to 25-30 hours)

Time to peak, serum: 2-4 hours

Excretion: Urine (~81%, primarily as metabolites, <3% as unchanged drug); feces (~10%)

Pregnancy Risk Factor B

New-Fill® *see* Poly-L-Lactic Acid *on page 1321*

Nexavar® *see* Sorafenib *on page 1488*

Nexium® *see* Esomeprazole *on page 599*

Nexphen PD *see* Guaifenesin and Phenylephrine *on page 797*

NFV *see* Nelfinavir *on page 1158*

Niacin *(NYE a sin)*

U.S. Brand Names Niacor®; Niaspan®; Slo-Niacin® [OTC]

Canadian Brand Names Niaspan®

Mexican Brand Names Pepevit

Generic Available Yes

Index Terms Nicotinic Acid; Vitamin B_3

Pharmacologic Category Antilipemic Agent, Miscellaneous; Vitamin, Water Soluble

Use Adjunctive treatment of dyslipidemias (types IIa and IIb or primary hypercholesterolemia) to lower the risk of recurrent MI and/or slow progression of coronary artery disease, including combination therapy with other antidyslipidemic agents when additional triglyceride-lowering or HDL-increasing effects are desired; treatment of hypertriglyceridemia in patients at risk of pancreatitis; treatment of peripheral vascular disease and circulatory disorders; treatment of pellagra; dietary supplement

Local Anesthetic/Vasoconstrictor Precautions No information available to require special precautions

Effects on Dental Treatment No significant effects or complications reported

Common Adverse Effects Frequency not defined.

Cardiovascular: Arrhythmias, atrial fibrillation, edema, flushing, hypotension, orthostasis, palpitation, syncope (rare), tachycardia

Central nervous system: Chills, dizziness, headache, insomnia, migraine

Dermatologic: Acanthosis nigricans, dry skin, hyperpigmentation, maculopapular rash, pruritus, rash, urticaria

Endocrine & metabolic: Glucose tolerance decreased, gout, phosphorous levels decreased, uric acid level increased

Gastrointestinal: Abdominal pain, dyspepsia, eructation, flatulence, nausea, peptic ulcers, vomiting

Hematologic: Platelet counts decreased, prothrombin time increased

Hepatic: Hepatic necrosis (rare), jaundice, liver enzymes increased

Neuromuscular & skeletal: Leg cramps, myalgia, myasthenia, myopathy (with concurrent HMG-CoA reductase inhibitor), pain, rhabdomyolysis (with concurrent HMG-CoA reductase inhibitor; rare), weakness

Ocular: Cystoid macular edema, toxic amblyopia

Respiratory: Dyspnea

Miscellaneous: Diaphoresis, hypersensitivity reactions (rare)

Mechanism of Action Component of two coenzymes which is necessary for tissue respiration, lipid metabolism, and glycogenolysis; inhibits the synthesis of very low density lipoproteins

Drug Interactions

Decreased Effect: Bile acid sequestrants may decrease the absorption of niacin; separate administration by 4-6 hours.

Pharmacodynamics/Kinetics
Absorption: Rapid and extensive (60% to 76%)
Distribution: Mainly to hepatic, renal, and adipose tissue
Metabolism: Extensive first-pass effects; converted to nicotinamide adenine dinucleotide, nicotinuric acid, and other metabolites
Half-life elimination: 45 minutes
Time to peak, serum: Immediate release formulation: ~45 minutes; extended release formulation: 4-5 hours
Excretion: Urine 60% to 88% (unchanged drug and metabolites)
Pregnancy Risk Factor A/C (dose exceeding RDA recommendation)

Niacinamide (nye a SIN a mide)

U.S. Brand Names Nicomide-T™
Generic Available Yes: Tablet
Index Terms Nicotinamide; Nicotinic Acid Amide; Vitamin B$_3$
Pharmacologic Category Vitamin, Water Soluble
Use
Oral: Prophylaxis and treatment of pellagra
Topical: Improve the appearance of acne and decrease visible inflammation and irritation caused by acne medications
Local Anesthetic/Vasoconstrictor Precautions No information available to require special precautions
Effects on Dental Treatment No significant effects or complications reported
Common Adverse Effects Frequency not defined.
Cardiovascular: Tachycardia
Dermatologic: Increased sebaceous gland activity, rash
Endocrine & metabolic: Hyperglycemia, hyperuricemia
Gastrointestinal: Bloating, flatulence, nausea
Neuromuscular & skeletal: Paresthesia in extremities
Ocular: Blurred vision
Respiratory: Wheezing
Mechanism of Action Used by the body as a source of niacin; is a component of two coenzymes which is necessary for tissue respiration, lipid metabolism, and glycogenolysis; does not have hypolipidemia or vasodilating effects. Niacinamide has anti-inflammatory properties which are believed to help decrease inflammatory acne lesions.
Pharmacodynamics/Kinetics
Absorption: Oral: Rapid; Topical: Absorbed systemically
Metabolism: Hepatic
Half-life elimination: 45 minutes
Time to peak, serum: 20-70 minutes
Excretion: Urine (as metabolites)
Pregnancy Risk Factor A/C (dose exceeding RDA recommendation)

Niacin and Lovastatin (NYE a sin & LOE va sta tin)

Related Information
Lovastatin *on page 1007*
Niacin *on page 1166*
U.S. Brand Names Advicor®
Canadian Brand Names Advicor®
Generic Available No
Index Terms Lovastatin and Niacin
Pharmacologic Category Antilipemic Agent, HMG-CoA Reductase Inhibitor; Antilipemic Agent, Miscellaneous
Use Treatment of primary hypercholesterolemia (heterozygous familial and nonfamilial) and mixed dyslipidemia (Fredrickson types IIa and IIb) in patients previously treated with either agent alone (patients who require further lowering of triglycerides (TG) or increase in HDL-cholesterol (HDL-C) from addition of niacin or further lowering of LDL-cholesterol (LDL-C) from addition of lovastatin). Combination product; not intended for initial treatment.
Local Anesthetic/Vasoconstrictor Precautions No information available to require special precautions
Effects on Dental Treatment No significant effects or complications reported
Common Adverse Effects
>10%: Cardiovascular: Flushing (71%)
1% to 10%:
Central nervous system: Headache (9%), pain (8%)
Dermatologic: Pruritus (7%), rash (5%)
Endocrine & metabolic: Hyperglycemia (4%)
(Continued)

Niacin and Lovastatin *(Continued)*

Gastrointestinal: Nausea (7%), diarrhea (6%), abdominal pain (4%), dyspepsia (3%), vomiting (3%)

Neuromuscular & skeletal: Back pain (5%), weakness (5%), myalgia (3%)

Miscellaneous: Flu-like syndrome (6%)

Mechanism of Action Lovastatin acts by competitively inhibiting 3-hydroxyl-3-methylglutaryl-coenzyme A (HMG-CoA) reductase, the enzyme that catalyzes the rate-limiting step in cholesterol biosynthesis. Niacin is a component of two coenzymes which is necessary for tissue respiration, lipid metabolism, and glycogenolysis; inhibits the synthesis of very low density lipoproteins.

Drug Interactions

Cytochrome P450 Effect: Lovastatin: Substrate of CYP3A4 (major); **Inhibits** CYP2C9 (weak), 2D6 (weak), 3A4 (weak)

Increased Effect/Toxicity: See individual agents.

Decreased Effect: See individual agents.

Pharmacodynamics/Kinetics See individual agents.

Bioavailability: Tablet strengths (eg, two tablets of 500 mg/20 mg and one tablet of 1000 mg/40 mg) are not interchangeable; bioavailability varies.

Pregnancy Risk Factor X

Niacor® *see* Niacin *on page 1166*

Niaspan® *see* Niacin *on page 1166*

NiCARdipine *(nye KAR de peen)*

Related Information

Cardiovascular Diseases *on page 1726*

U.S. Brand Names Cardene®; Cardene® I.V.; Cardene® SR

Mexican Brand Names Ridene

Generic Available Yes: Capsule

Index Terms Nicardipine Hydrochloride

Pharmacologic Category Calcium Channel Blocker

Use Chronic stable angina (immediate-release product only); management of essential hypertension (immediate and sustained release; parenteral only for short time that oral treatment is not feasible)

Unlabeled/Investigational Use Congestive heart failure

Local Anesthetic/Vasoconstrictor Precautions No information available to require special precautions

Effects on Dental Treatment Key adverse event(s) related to dental treatment: Xerostomia (normal salivary flow resumes upon discontinuation). Other drugs of this class can cause gingival hyperplasia (ie, nifedipine). The first case of nicardipine-induced gingival hyperplasia has been reported in a child taking 40-50 mg daily for 20 months.

Common Adverse Effects

1% to 10%:

Cardiovascular: Flushing (6% to 10%), palpitation (3% to 4%), tachycardia (1% to 4%), peripheral edema (dose related 7% to 8%), increased angina (dose related 6%), hypotension (I.V. 6%), orthostasis (I.V. 1%)

Central nervous system: Headache (6% to 15%), dizziness (4% to 7%), somnolence (4% to 6%)

Dermatologic: Rash (1%)

Gastrointestinal: Nausea (2% to 5%), dry mouth (1%)

Genitourinary: Polyuria (1%)

Local: Injection site reaction (I.V. 1%)

Neuromuscular & skeletal: Weakness (4% to 6%), myalgia (1%), paresthesia (1%)

Miscellaneous: Diaphoresis

Mechanism of Action Inhibits calcium ion from entering the "slow channels" or select voltage-sensitive areas of vascular smooth muscle and myocardium during depolarization, producing a relaxation of coronary vascular smooth muscle and coronary vasodilation; increases myocardial oxygen delivery in patients with vasospastic angina

Drug Interactions

Cytochrome P450 Effect: Substrate of CYP1A2 (minor), 2C9 (minor), 2D6 (minor), 2E1 (minor), 3A4 (major); **Inhibits** CYP2C9 (strong), 2C19 (moderate), 2D6 (moderate), 3A4 (strong)

Increased Effect/Toxicity: H_2 blockers (cimetidine) may increase the bioavailability of nicardipine. The levels/effects of nicardipine may be increased by azole antifungals, clarithromycin, diclofenac, doxycycline, erythromycin, imatinib, isoniazid, nefazodone, propofol, protease inhibitors, quinidine, telithromycin, verapamil and other CYP3A4 inhibitors.

Nicardipine may increase the effect of vecuronium (reduce dose 25%). Nicardipine increase the levels/effects of amiodarone, amphetamines, selected benzodiazepines, selected beta-blockers, calcium channel blockers, cisapride, citalopram, cyclosporine, dextromethorphan, diazepam, ergot derivatives, fluoxetine, glimepiride, glipizide, HMG-CoA reductase inhibitors, lidocaine, methsuximide, mirtazapine, nateglinide, nefazodone, paroxetine, phenytoin, pioglitazone, propranolol, risperidone, ritonavir, rosiglitazone, sertraline, sildenafil (and other PDE-5 inhibitors), tacrolimus, thioridazine, tricyclic antidepressants, venlafaxine, warfarin, and other substrates of CYP2C9, 2C19, 2D6, or 3A4.

Decreased Effect: The levels/effects of nicardipine may be decreased by aminoglutethimide, carbamazepine, nafcillin, nevirapine, phenobarbital, phenytoin, rifamycins, and other CYP3A4 inducers. Nicardipine may decrease the levels/effects of CYP2D6 prodrug substrates (eg, codeine, hydrocodone, oxycodone, tramadol). Calcium may reduce the calcium channel blocker's effects, particularly hypotension.

Pharmacodynamics/Kinetics

Onset of action: Oral: 0.5-2 hours; I.V.: 10 minutes; Hypotension: ~20 minutes

Duration: ≤8 hours

Absorption: Oral: ~100%

Protein binding: >95%

Metabolism: Hepatic; CYP3A4 substrate (major); extensive first-pass effect (saturable)

Bioavailability: 35%

Half-life elimination: 2-4 hours

Time to peak, serum: 30-120 minutes

Excretion: Urine (60% as metabolites); feces (35%)

Pregnancy Risk Factor C

Nicotine (nik oh TEEN)

U.S. Brand Names Commit® [OTC]; NicoDerm® CQ® [OTC]; Nicorette® [OTC]; Nicotrol® Inhaler; Nicotrol® NS

Canadian Brand Names Habitrol®; Nicoderm®; Nicorette®; Nicorette® Plus; Nicotrol®

Mexican Brand Names Nicotinell TTS; Niquitin

Generic Available Yes: Transdermal patch and gum

Index Terms Habitrol

Pharmacologic Category Smoking Cessation Aid

Dental Use Treatment to aid smoking cessation for the relief of nicotine withdrawal symptoms (including nicotine craving)

Use Treatment to aid smoking cessation for the relief of nicotine withdrawal symptoms (including nicotine craving)

Unlabeled/Investigational Use Management of ulcerative colitis (transdermal)

Local Anesthetic/Vasoconstrictor Precautions No information available to require special precautions

Effects on Dental Treatment Key adverse event(s) related to dental treatment: Chewing gum: Excessive salivation, mouth/throat soreness, jaw muscle ache, hiccups, tachycardia, headache (mild), vomiting, belching, nausea, xerostomia (normal salivary flow resumes upon discontinuation), dizziness, nervousness, GI distress, hoarseness, and muscle pain.

Significant Adverse Effects

Nasal spray/inhaler:

>10%:

Central nervous system: Headache (18% to 26%)

Gastrointestinal: Inhaler: Mouth/throat irritation (66%), dyspepsia (18%)

Respiratory: Inhaler: Cough (32%), rhinitis (23%)

1% to 10%:

Dermatologic: Acne (3%)

Endocrine & metabolic: Dysmenorrhea (3%)

Gastrointestinal: Flatulence (4%), gum problems (4%), diarrhea, hiccup, nausea, taste disturbance, tooth disorder

Neuromuscular & skeletal: Back pain (6%), arthralgia (5%), jaw/neck pain

Respiratory: Sinusitis

Miscellaneous: Withdrawal symptoms

(Continued)

Nicotine (Continued)

<1% (Limited to important or life-threatening): Allergy, amnesia, aphasia, bronchitis, bronchospasm, edema, migraine, numbness, pain, purpura, rash, sputum increased, vision abnormalities, xerostomia

Adverse events previously reported in prescription labeling for chewing gum, lozenge and/or transdermal systems. Frequency not defined; may be product or dose specific:

Central nervous system: Concentration impaired, depression, dizziness, headache, insomnia, nervousness, pain

Gastrointestinal: Aphthous stomatitis, constipation, cough, diarrhea, dyspepsia, flatulence, gingival bleeding, glossitis, hiccups, jaw pain, nausea, salivation increased, stomatitis, taste perversion, tooth disorder, ulcerative stomatitis, xerostomia

Dermatologic: Rash

Local: Application site reaction, local edema, local erythema

Neuromuscular & skeletal: Arthralgia, myalgia, paresthesia

Respiratory: Cough, sinusitis

Miscellaneous: Allergic reaction, diaphoresis

Dental Usual Dosing

Tobacco cessation (patients should be advised to completely stop smoking upon initiation of therapy): Adults:

Gum: Chew 1 piece of gum when urge to smoke, up to 24 pieces/day. Patients who smoke <25 cigarettes/day should start with 2-mg strength; patients smoking ≥25 cigarettes/day should start with the 4-mg strength. Use according to the following 12-week dosing schedule:

Weeks 1-6: Chew 1 piece of gum every 1-2 hours; to increase chances of quitting, chew at least 9 pieces/day during the first 6 weeks

Weeks 7-9: Chew 1 piece of gum every 2-4 hours

Weeks 10-12: Chew 1 piece of gum every 4-8 hours

Inhaler: Oral: Usually 6 to 16 cartridges per day; best effect was achieved by frequent continuous puffing (20 minutes); recommended duration of treatment is 3 months, after which patients may be weaned from the inhaler by gradual reduction of the daily dose over 6-12 weeks

Lozenge: Oral: Patients who smoke their first cigarette within 30 minutes of waking should use the 4 mg strength; otherwise the 2 mg strength is recommended. Use according to the following 12-week dosing schedule:

Weeks 1-6: One lozenge every 1-2 hours

Weeks 7-9: One lozenge every 2-4 hours

Weeks 10-12: One lozenge every 4-8 hours

Note: Use at least 9 lozenges/day during first 6 weeks to improve chances of quitting; do not use more than one lozenge at a time (maximum: 5 lozenges every 6 hours, 20 lozenges/day)

Spray: Nasal: 1-2 sprays/hour; do not exceed more than 5 doses (10 sprays) per hour [maximum: 40 doses/day (80 sprays); each dose (2 sprays) contains 1 mg of nicotine

Transdermal patch: Topical: Apply new patch every 24 hours to nonhairy, clean, dry skin on the upper body or upper outer arm; each patch should be applied to a different site. **Note:** Adjustment may be required during initial treatment (move to higher dose if experiencing withdrawal symptoms; lower dose if side effects are experienced).

NicoDerm CQ®:

Patients smoking ≥10 cigarettes/day: Begin with step 1 (21 mg/day) for 4-6 weeks, **followed by** step 2 (14 mg/day) for 2 weeks; **finish with** step 3 (7 mg/day) for 2 weeks

Patients smoking <10 cigarettes/day: Begin with step 2 (14 mg/day) for 6 weeks, **followed by** step 3 (7 mg/day) for 2 weeks

Note: Initial starting dose for patients <100 pounds, history of cardiovascular disease: 14 mg/day for 4-6 weeks, **followed by** 7 mg/day for 2-4 weeks

Note: Patients who are receiving >600 mg/day of cimetidine: Decrease to the next lower patch size

Benefits of use of nicotine transdermal patches beyond 3 months have not been demonstrated

Dosage

Smoking deterrent: Patients should be advised to completely stop smoking upon initiation of therapy.

Oral:

Gum: Chew 1 piece of gum when urge to smoke, up to 24 pieces/day. Patients who smoke <25 cigarettes/day should start with 2-mg strength; patients smoking ≥25 cigarettes/day should start with the 4-mg strength. Use according to the following 12-week dosing schedule:

Weeks 1-6: Chew 1 piece of gum every 1-2 hours; to increase chances of quitting, chew at least 9 pieces/day during the first 6 weeks

Weeks 7-9: Chew 1 piece of gum every 2-4 hours

Weeks 10-12: Chew 1 piece of gum every 4-8 hours

Inhaler: Usually 6 to 16 cartridges per day; best effect was achieved by frequent continuous puffing (20 minutes); recommended duration of treatment is 3 months, after which patients may be weaned from the inhaler by gradual reduction of the daily dose over 6-12 weeks

Lozenge: Patients who smoke their first cigarette within 30 minutes of waking should use the 4 mg strength; otherwise the 2 mg strength is recommended. Use according to the following 12-week dosing schedule:

Weeks 1-6: One lozenge every 1-2 hours

Weeks 7-9: One lozenge every 2-4 hours

Weeks 10-12: One lozenge every 4-8 hours

Note: Use at least 9 lozenges/day during first 6 weeks to improve chances of quitting; do not use more than one lozenge at a time (maximum: 5 lozenges every 6 hours, 20 lozenges/day)

Topical:

Transdermal patch: Apply new patch every 24 hours to nonhairy, clean, dry skin on the upper body or upper outer arm; each patch should be applied to a different site. **Note:** Adjustment may be required during initial treatment (move to higher dose if experiencing withdrawal symptoms; lower dose if side effects are experienced).

NicoDerm CQ®:

Patients smoking ≥10 cigarettes/day: Begin with **step 1** (21 mg/day) for 4-6 weeks, followed by **step 2** (14 mg/day) for 2 weeks; finish with **step 3** (7 mg/day) for 2 weeks

Patients smoking <10 cigarettes/day: Begin with **step 2** (14 mg/day) for 6 weeks, followed by **step 3** (7 mg/day) for 2 weeks

Notes: Initial starting dose for patients <100 pounds, history of cardiovascular disease: 14 mg/day for 4-6 weeks, followed by 7 mg/day for 2-4 weeks

Note: Patients receiving >600 mg/day of cimetidine: Decrease to the next lower patch size

Note: Benefits of use of nicotine transdermal patches beyond 3 months have not been demonstrated.

Ulcerative colitis (unlabeled use): Transdermal: Titrated to 22-25 mg/day

Nasal: Spray: 1-2 sprays/hour; do not exceed more than 5 doses (10 sprays) per hour [maximum: 40 doses/day (80 sprays); each dose (2 sprays) contains 1 mg of nicotine

Mechanism of Action Nicotine is one of two naturally-occurring alkaloids which exhibit their primary effects via autonomic ganglia stimulation. The other alkaloid is lobeline which has many actions similar to those of nicotine but is less potent. Nicotine is a potent ganglionic and central nervous system stimulant, the actions of which are mediated via nicotine-specific receptors. Biphasic actions are observed depending upon the dose administered. The main effect of nicotine in small doses is stimulation of all autonomic ganglia; with larger doses, initial stimulation is followed by blockade of transmission. Biphasic effects are also evident in the adrenal medulla; discharge of catecholamines occurs with small doses, whereas prevention of catecholamines release is seen with higher doses as a response to splanchnic nerve stimulation. Stimulation of the central nervous system (CNS) is characterized by tremors and respiratory excitation. However, convulsions may occur with higher doses, along with respiratory failure secondary to both central paralysis and peripheral blockade to respiratory muscles.

Contraindications Hypersensitivity to nicotine or any component of the formulation; patients who are smoking during the postmyocardial infarction period; patients with life-threatening arrhythmias, or severe or worsening angina pectoris; active temporomandibular joint disease (gum); pregnancy; not for use in nonsmokers

Warnings/Precautions The risk versus the benefits must be weighed for each of these groups: patients with CAD, serious cardiac arrhythmias, vasospastic disease. Use caution in patients with hyperthyroidism, pheochromocytoma, or insulin-dependent diabetes. Use with caution in oropharyngeal inflammation and in patients with history of esophagitis, peptic ulcer, coronary artery disease, vasospastic disease, angina, hypertension, pheochromocytoma, severe renal dysfunction, and hepatic dysfunction. The inhaler should be used with caution in patients with bronchospastic disease (other forms of nicotine replacement may be preferred). Use of nasal product is not recommended with chronic nasal disorders (eg, allergy, rhinitis, nasal polyps, and sinusitis). Transdermal patch may contain conducting metal (eg, aluminum); remove patch prior to MRI. Cautious use of topical nicotine in patients with certain skin diseases. Hypersensitivity to the topical products can occur. Dental problems may be worsened (Continued)

Nicotine (Continued)

by chewing the gum. Urge patients to stop smoking completely when initiating therapy. Safety and efficacy have not been established in pediatric patients.

Drug Interactions Substrate (minor) of CYP1A2, 2A6, 2B6, 2C9, 2C19, 2D6, 2E1, 3A4; **Inhibits** CYP2A6 (weak), 2E1 (weak)

Adenosine: Nicotine increases the hemodynamic and AV blocking effects of adenosine; monitor

Bupropion: Monitor for treatment-emergent hypertension in patients treated with the combination of nicotine patch and bupropion

Cimetidine; May increases serum nicotine concentrations; therefore, may decrease amount of gum or patches needed

Ethanol/Nutrition/Herb Interactions Food: Lozenge: Acidic foods/beverages decrease absorption of nicotine.

Dietary Considerations

Commit®: Each lozenge contains phenylalanine 3.4 mg and sodium 18 mg.

Nicorette®: Fresh mint and fruit chill flavors: The 2-mg strength contains calcium 94 mg/gum and sodium 11 mg/gum. The 4-mg strength contains calcium 94 mg/gum and sodium 13 mg/gum.

Pharmacodynamics/Kinetics

Onset of action: Intranasal: More closely approximate the time course of plasma nicotine levels observed after cigarette smoking than other dosage forms

Duration: Transdermal: 24 hours

Absorption: Transdermal: Slow

Metabolism: Hepatic, primarily to cotinine ($\frac{1}{5}$ as active)

Half-life elimination: 4 hours

Time to peak, serum: Transdermal: 8-9 hours

Excretion: Urine

Clearance: Renal: pH dependent

Pregnancy Risk Factor D (nasal)

Lactation Excretion in breast milk unknown/use caution

Breast-Feeding Considerations Nicotine from cigarette smoke is found in breast milk at 1.5-3 times the maternal plasma concentrations. The amount from nicotine replacement products is not known. Women who are breast-feeding are encouraged not to smoke.

Dosage Forms Excipient information presented when available (limited, particularly for generics); consult specific product labeling.

Gum, chewing, as polacrilex: 2 mg (20s, 50s, 110s); 4 mg (20s, 50s, 110s)

Nicorette®:

2 mg (48s, 50s, 108s, 110s, 168s, 170s, 192s, 200s, 216s) [original and mint flavors]; (48s, 108s, 110s) [orange flavor]; (40s, 100s) [contains calcium 94 mg/gum and sodium 11 mg/gum; fresh mint and fruit chill flavors]

4 mg (48s, 50s, 108s, 110s, 168s, 170s, 192s, 200s, 216s) [original and mint flavors]; (48s, 108s, 110s) [orange flavor]; (40s, 100s) [contains calcium 94 mg/gum and sodium 13 mg/gum; fresh mint and fruit chill flavors]

Lozenge, as polacrilex:

Commit®:

2 mg (48s, 72s, 84s, 168s) [contains phenylalanine 3.4 mg/lozenge, sodium 18 mg/lozenge; mint flavor]; (108s) [contains phenylalanine 3.4 mg/lozenge, sodium 18 mg/lozenge; original flavor]

4 mg (48s, 72s, 84s, 168s, 192s) [contains phenylalanine 3.4 mg/lozenge, sodium 18 mg/lozenge; mint flavor]; (108s) [contains phenylalanine 3.4 mg/lozenge, sodium 18 mg/lozenge; original flavor]

Oral inhalation system:

Nicotrol® Inhaler: 10 mg cartridge (168s) [cartridge delivers nicotine 4 mg; each unit consists of 5 mouthpieces, 28 storage trays each containing 6 cartridges, and 1 storage case]

Patch, transdermal: 7 mg/24 (30s); 14 mg/24 hours (30s); 21 mg/24 hours (30s)

NicoDerm® CQ®: 7 mg/24 hours (14s) [step 3; available in tan or clear patch]; 14 mg/24 hours (14s) [step 2; available in tan or clear patch]; 21 mg/24 hours (7s, 14s) [step 1; available in tan or clear patch]

Solution, intranasal [spray]:

Nicotrol® NS: 10 mg/mL (10 mL) [delivers 0.5 mg/spray; 200 sprays]

Selected Readings

Christen AG and Christen JA, "The Prescription of Transdermal Nicotine Patches for Tobacco-Using Dental Patients: Current Status in Indiana," *J Indiana Dent Assoc*, 1992, 71(6):12-8.

Davies GM, Willner P, James DL, et al, "Influence of Nicotine Gum on Acute Cravings for Cigarettes," *J Psychopharmacol*, 2004, 18(1):83-7.

Li Wan Po A, "Transdermal Nicotine in Smoking Cessation. A Meta-Analysis," *Eur J Clin Pharmacol*, 1993, 45(6):519-28.

Stafne EE, "The Nicotine Transdermal Patch: Use in the Dental Office Tobacco Cessation Program," *Northwest Dent*, 1994, 73(3):19-22.

Tonstad S and Johnston JA, "Does Bupropion Have Advantages Over Other Medical Therapies in the Cessation of Smoking?" *Expert Opin Pharmacother*, 2004, 5(4):727-34.

Transdermal Nicotine Study Group, "Transdermal Nicotine for Smoking Cessation. Six-Month Results From Two Multicenter Controlled Clinical Trials," *JAMA*, 1991, 266(22):3133-8.

Westman EC, Levin ED, and Rose JE, "The Nicotine Patch in Smoking Cessation," *Arch Intern Med*, 1993, 153(16):1917-23.

Wynn RL, "Nicotine Patches in Smoking Cessation," *AGD Impact*, 1994, 22:14.

Nicotinic Acid *see* Niacin *on page 1166*

Nicotinic Acid Amide *see* Niacinamide *on page 1167*

Nicotrol® Inhaler *see* Nicotine *on page 1169*

Nicotrol® NS *see* Nicotine *on page 1169*

Nicoumalone *see* Acenocoumarol *on page 29*

Nifediac™ CC *see* NIFEdipine *on page 1173*

Nifedical™ XL *see* NIFEdipine *on page 1173*

NIFEdipine (nye FED i peen)

Related Information
Cardiovascular Diseases *on page 1726*

U.S. Brand Names Adalat® CC; Afeditab™ CR; Nifediac™ CC; Nifedical™ XL; Procardia®; Procardia XL®

Canadian Brand Names Adalat® XL®; Apo-Nifed®; Apo-Nifed PA®; Novo-Nifedin; Nu-Nifed; Procardia®

Mexican Brand Names Adalat; Adalat Oros; Adalat Retard

Generic Available Yes

Pharmacologic Category Calcium Channel Blocker

Use Angina and hypertension (sustained release only), pulmonary hypertension

Local Anesthetic/Vasoconstrictor Precautions No information available to require special precautions

Effects on Dental Treatment Nifedipine has been reported to cause 10% incidence of gingival hyperplasia; effects from 30-100 mg/day have appeared after 1-9 months. Discontinuance results in complete disappearance or marked regression of symptoms; symptoms will reappear upon remedication. Marked regression occurs after 1 week and complete disappearance of symptoms has occurred within 15 days. If a gingivectomy is performed and use of the drug is continued or resumed, hyperplasia usually will recur. The success of the gingivectomy usually requires that the medication be discontinued or that a switch to a noncalcium channel blocker be made. If for some reason nifedipine cannot be discontinued, hyperplasia has not recurred after gingivectomy when extensive plaque control was performed. If nifedipine is changed to another class of cardiovascular agent, the gingival hyperplasia will probably regress and resolve. Switching to another calcium channel blocker may result in continued hyperplasia.

Common Adverse Effects

>10%:

Cardiovascular: Flushing (10% to 25%), peripheral edema (dose related 7% to 10%; up to 50%)

Central nervous system: Dizziness/lightheadedness/giddiness (10% to 27%), headache (10% to 23%)

Gastrointestinal: Nausea/heartburn (10% to 11%)

Neuromuscular & skeletal: Weakness (10% to 12%)

≥1% to 10%:

Cardiovascular: Palpitation (≤2% to 7%), transient hypotension (dose related 5%), CHF (2%)

Central nervous system: Nervousness/mood changes (≤2% to 7%), shakiness (≤2%), jitteriness (≤2%), sleep disturbances (≤2%), difficulties in balance (≤2%), fever (≤2%), chills (≤2%)

Dermatologic: Dermatitis (≤2%), pruritus (≤2%), urticaria (≤2%)

Endocrine & metabolic: Sexual difficulties (≤2%)

Gastrointestinal: Diarrhea (≤2%), constipation (≤2%), cramps (≤2%), flatulence (≤2%), gingival hyperplasia (≤10%)

Neuromuscular & skeletal: Muscle cramps/tremor (≤2% to 8%), inflammation (≤2%), joint stiffness (≤2%)

Ocular: Blurred vision (≤2%)

Respiratory: Dyspnea/cough/wheezing (6%), nasal congestion/sore throat (≤2% to 6%), chest congestion (≤2%), dyspnea (≤2%)

Miscellaneous: Diaphoresis (≤2%)

Dosage Oral:

Children:

Hypertrophic cardiomyopathy: 0.6-0.9 mg/kg/24 hours in 3-4 divided doses

Hypertension: Children 1-17 years: Extended release tablet: Initial: 0.25-0.5 mg/kg/day once daily or in 2 divided doses; maximum: 3 mg/kg/day up to 120 mg/day

(Continued)

NIFEdipine *(Continued)*

Adults: (**Note:** When switching from immediate release to sustained release formulations, total daily dose will start the same)

Initial: 30 mg once daily as sustained release formulation, or if indicated, 10 mg 3 times/day as capsules

Usual dose: 10-30 mg 3 times/day as capsules or 30-60 mg once daily as sustained release

Maximum dose: 120-180 mg/day

Increase sustained release at 7- to 14-day intervals

Hemodialysis: Supplemental dose is not necessary.

Peritoneal dialysis effects: Supplemental dose is not necessary.

Dosing adjustment in hepatic impairment: Reduce oral dose by 50% to 60% in patients with cirrhosis.

Mechanism of Action Inhibits calcium ion from entering the "slow channels" or select voltage-sensitive areas of vascular smooth muscle and myocardium during depolarization, producing a relaxation of coronary vascular smooth muscle and coronary vasodilation; increases myocardial oxygen delivery in patients with vasospastic angina

Contraindications Hypersensitivity to nifedipine or any component of the formulation; immediate release preparation for treatment of urgent or emergent hypertension; acute MI

Warnings/Precautions Symptomatic hypotension with or without syncope can rarely occur; blood pressure must be lowered at a rate appropriate for the patient's clinical condition. **The use of sublingual short-acting nifedipine in hypertensive emergencies and urgencies is neither safe nor effective and SHOULD BE ABANDONED!** Serious adverse events (eg, cerebrovascular ischemia, syncope, stroke, acute myocardial infarction, and fetal distress) have been reported in relation to such use.

Severe hypotension may occur in patients taking immediate release concurrently with beta-blockers when undergoing CABG with high dose fentanyl anesthesia. When considering surgery with high dose fentanyl, may consider withdrawing nifedipine (>36 hours) before surgery if possible.

Increased angina may be seen upon starting or increasing doses; may increase frequency, duration, and severity of angina during initiation of therapy; use with caution in patients with CHF or aortic stenosis (especially with concomitant beta-adrenergic blocker); severe left ventricular dysfunction, hepatic or renal impairment, hypertrophic cardiomyopathy (especially obstructive), concomitant therapy with beta-blockers or digoxin, edema. The elderly may be more susceptible to adverse effects.

Mild and transient elevations in liver function enzymes may be apparent within 8 weeks of therapy initiation. The most common side effect is peripheral edema; occurs within 2-3 weeks of starting therapy. Reflex tachycardia may occur with use.

Avoid use of extended release tablets (Procardia XL®) in patients with known stricture/narrowing of the GI tract. Therapeutic potential of sustained-release formulation (elementary osmotic pump, gastrointestinal therapeutic system [GITS]) may be decreased in patients with certain GI disorders that accelerate intestinal transit time (eg, short bowel syndrome, inflammatory bowel disease, severe diarrhea).

Drug Interactions

Cytochrome P450 Effect: Substrate of CYP2D6 (minor), 3A4 (major); **Inhibits** CYP1A2 (moderate), 2C9 (weak), 2D6 (weak), 3A4 (weak)

Increased Effect/Toxicity: The levels/effects of nifedipine may be increased by alpha-1 blockers, azole antifungals, cisapride, clarithromycin, cyclosporine, diclofenac, doxycycline, erythromycin, grapefruit juice, imatinib, isoniazid, nefazodone, nicardipine, propofol, protease inhibitors, quinidine, quinupristin/dalfopristin, telithromycin, verapamil, and other CYP3A4 inhibitors. Cimetidine may also increase nifedipine levels. Nifedipine may increase the levels/effects of aminophylline, digoxin, fluvoxamine, mexiletine, mirtazapine, ropinirole, trifluoperazine, vincristine, and other CYP1A2 substrates. Digoxin, phenytoin, and vincristine levels may also be increased by nifedipine.

Blood pressure-lowering effects may be additive with sildenafil, tadalafil, and vardenafil (use caution). Concurrent use with magnesium salts may enhance the adverse/toxic effects of magnesium and enhance the hypotensive effects of the calcium channel blocker. Calcium channel blockers may enhance the neuromuscular blocking effect from nondepolarizing neuromuscular blockers. Calcium channel blocker (nondihydropyridine) may enhance the hypotensive effects of calcium channel blocker (dihydropyridine).

Decreased Effect: Nifedipine may decrease quinidine serum levels. Calcium may reduce the hypotension from of calcium channel blockers. The levels/effects of nifedipine may be decreased by aminoglutethimide, barbiturates, carbamazepine, nafcillin, nevirapine, phenobarbital, phenytoin, rifamycins, and other CYP3A4 inducers.

Ethanol/Nutrition/Herb Interactions

Ethanol: Avoid ethanol (may increase CNS depression and may increase the effects of nifedipine). Monitor.

Food: Nifedipine serum levels may be decreased if taken with food. Food may decrease the rate but not the extent of absorption of Procardia XL®. Increased therapeutic and vasodilator side effects, including severe hypotension and myocardial ischemia, may occur if nifedipine is taken by patients ingesting grapefruit.

Herb/Nutraceutical: St John's wort may decrease nifedipine levels. Avoid dong quai if using for hypertension (has estrogenic activity). Avoid ephedra, yohimbe, ginseng (may worsen hypertension). Avoid garlic (may have increased antihypertensive effect).

Dietary Considerations Capsule is rapidly absorbed orally if it is administered without food, but may result in vasodilator side effects; administration with low-fat meals may decrease flushing. Avoid grapefruit juice.

Pharmacodynamics/Kinetics

Onset of action: Immediate release: ~20 minutes

Protein binding (concentration dependent): 92% to 98%

Metabolism: Hepatic to inactive metabolites

Bioavailability: Capsule: 40% to 77%; Sustained release: 65% to 89% relative to immediate release capsules

Half-life elimination: Adults: Healthy: 2-5 hours, Cirrhosis: 7 hours; Elderly: 6.7 hours

Excretion: Urine (as metabolites)

Pregnancy Risk Factor C

Dosage Forms

Capsule, softgel: 10 mg, 20 mg

Procardia®: 10 mg

Tablet, extended release: 30 mg, 60 mg, 90 mg

Adalat® CC, Nifediac™ CC, Procardia XL®: 30 mg, 60 mg; 90 mg

Afeditab™ CR, Nifedical™ XL: 30 mg, 60 mg

Selected Readings

Deen-Duggins L, Fry HR, Clay JR, et al, "Nifedipine-Associated Gingival Overgrowth: A Survey of the Literature and Report of Four Cases," *Quintessence Int*, 1996, 27(3):163-70.

Desai P and Silver JG, "Drug-Induced Gingival Enlargements," *J Can Dent Assoc*, 1998, 64(4):263-8.

Harel-Raviv M, Eckler M, Lalani K, et al, "Nifedipine-Induced Gingival Hyperplasia. A Comprehensive Review and Analysis," *Oral Surg Oral Med Oral Pathol Oral Radiol Endod*, 1995, 79(6):715-22.

Lederman D, Lumerman H, Reuben S, et al, "Gingival Hyperplasia Associated With Nifedipine Therapy," *Oral Surg Oral Med Oral Pathol*, 1984, 57(6):620-2.

Lucas RM, Howell LP, and Wall BA, "Nifedipine-Induced Gingival Hyperplasia: A Histochemical and Ultrastructural Study," *J Periodontol*, 1985, 56(4):211-5.

Nery EB, Edson RG, Lee KK, et al, "Prevalence of Nifedipine-Induced Gingival Hyperplasia," *J Periodontol*, 1995, 66(7):572-8.

Nishikawa SJ, Tada H, Hamasaki A, et al, "Nifedipine-Induced Gingival Hyperplasia: A Clinical and In Vitro Study," *J Periodontol*, 1991, 62(1):30-5.

Pilloni A, Camargo PM, Carere M, et al, "Surgical Treatment of Cyclosporine A- and Nifedipine-Induced Gingival Enlargement: Gingivectomy Versus Periodontal Flap," *J Periodontol*, 1998, 69(7):791-7.

Saito K, Mori S, Iwakura M, et al, "Immunohistochemical Localization of Transforming Growth Factor Beta, Basic Fibroblast Growth Factor and Heparin Sulphate Glycosaminoglycan in Gingival Hyperplasia Induced by Nifedipine and Phenytoin," *J Periodontal Res*, 1996, 31(8):545-5.

Silverstein LH, Koch JP, Lefkove MD, et al, "Nifedipine-Induced Gingival Enlargement Around Dental Implants: A Clinical Report," *J Oral Implantol*, 1995, 21(2):116-20.

Westbrook P, Bednarczyk EM, Carlson M, et al, "Regression of Nifedipine-Induced Gingival Hyperplasia Following Switch to a Same Class Calcium Channel Blocker, Isradipine," *J Periodontol*, 1997, 68(7):645-50.

Wynn RL, "Calcium Channel Blockers and Gingival Hyperplasia," *Gen Dent*, 1991, 39(4):240-3.

Wynn RL, "Update on Calcium Channel Blocker-Induced Gingival Hyperplasia," *Gen Dent*, 1995, 43(3):218-22.

Niferex® [OTC] *see* Polysaccharide-Iron Complex *on page 1323*

Niftolid *see* Flutamide *on page 725*

Nilandron® *see* Nilutamide *on page 1175*

Nilutamide (ni LOO ta mide)

U.S. Brand Names Nilandron®
Canadian Brand Names Anandron®
Mexican Brand Names Anandron
Generic Available No
Index Terms NSC-684588; RU-23908
Pharmacologic Category Antiandrogen; Antineoplastic Agent, Antiandrogen
Use Treatment of metastatic prostate cancer

(Continued)

Nilutamide *(Continued)*

Local Anesthetic/Vasoconstrictor Precautions No information available to require special precautions

Effects on Dental Treatment Key adverse event(s) related to dental treatment: Xerostomia (normal salivary flow resumes upon discontinuation).

Common Adverse Effects

>10%:

Central nervous system: Headache, insomnia

Endocrine & metabolic: Hot flashes (30% to 67%), gynecomastia (10%)

Gastrointestinal: Nausea (mild - 10% to 32%), abdominal pain (10%), constipation, anorexia

Genitourinary: Testicular atrophy (16%), libido decreased

Hepatic: Transaminases increased (8% to 13%; transient)

Ocular: Impaired dark adaptation (13% to 57%), usually reversible with dose reduction, may require discontinuation of the drug in 1% to 2% of patients

Respiratory: Dyspnea (11%)

1% to 10%:

Cardiovascular: Chest pain, edema, heart failure, hypertension, syncope

Central nervous system: Dizziness, drowsiness, malaise, hypoesthesia, depression

Dermatologic: Pruritus, alopecia, dry skin, rash

Endocrine & metabolic: Disulfiram-like reaction (hot flashes, rash) (5%); Flu-like syndrome, fever

Gastrointestinal: Vomiting, diarrhea, dyspepsia, GI hemorrhage, melena, weight loss, xerostomia

Genitourinary: Hematuria, nocturia

Hematologic: Anemia

Hepatic: Hepatitis (1%)

Neuromuscular & skeletal: Arthritis, paresthesia

Ocular: Chromatopsia (9%), abnormal vision (6% to 7%), cataracts, photophobia

Respiratory: Interstitial pneumonitis (2% - typically exertional dyspnea, cough, chest pain, and fever; most often occurring within the first 3 months of treatment); rhinitis

Miscellaneous: Diaphoresis

Mechanism of Action Nonsteroidal antiandrogen that inhibits androgen uptake or inhibits binding of androgen in target tissues. It specifically blocks the action of androgens by interacting with cytosolic androgen receptor F sites in target tissue

Drug Interactions

Cytochrome P450 Effect: Substrate of CYP2C19 (major); Inhibits CYP2C19 (weak)

Increased Effect/Toxicity: CYP2C19 inhibitors may increase the levels/effects of nilutamide; example inhibitors include delavirdine, fluconazole, fluvoxamine, gemfibrozil, isoniazid, omeprazole, and ticlopidine.

Decreased Effect: CYP2C19 inducers may decrease the levels/effects of nilutamide; example inducers include aminoglutethimide, carbamazepine, phenytoin, and rifampin.

Pharmacodynamics/Kinetics

Absorption: Rapid and complete

Protein binding: 72% to 85%

Metabolism: Hepatic, forms active metabolites

Half-life elimination: Terminal: 23-87 hours; Metabolites: 35-137 hours

Excretion: Urine (up to 78% at 120 hours; <1% as unchanged drug); feces (1% to 7%)

Pregnancy Risk Factor C

Nimodipine *(nye MOE di peen)*

U.S. Brand Names Nimotop®

Canadian Brand Names Nimotop®

Mexican Brand Names Kenzolol; Nimotop

Generic Available No

Pharmacologic Category Calcium Channel Blocker

Use Spasm following subarachnoid hemorrhage from ruptured intracranial aneurysms regardless of the patients neurological condition postictus (Hunt and Hess grades I-V)

Local Anesthetic/Vasoconstrictor Precautions No information available to require special precautions

Effects on Dental Treatment Other drugs of this class can cause gingival hyperplasia (ie, nifedipine) but there have been no reports for nimodipine.

Common Adverse Effects 1% to 10%:
  Cardiovascular: Reductions in systemic blood pressure (1% to 8%)
  Central nervous system: Headache (1% to 4%)
  Dermatologic: Rash (1% to 2%)
  Gastrointestinal: Diarrhea (2% to 4%), abdominal discomfort (2%)

Mechanism of Action Nimodipine shares the pharmacology of other calcium channel blockers; animal studies indicate that nimodipine has a greater effect on cerebral arterials than other arterials; this increased specificity may be due to the drug's increased lipophilicity and cerebral distribution as compared to nifedipine; inhibits calcium ion from entering the "slow channels" or select voltage sensitive areas of vascular smooth muscle and myocardium during depolarization

Drug Interactions
  Cytochrome P450 Effect: Substrate of CYP3A4 (major)
  Increased Effect/Toxicity: Calcium channel blockers and nimodipine may result in enhanced cardiovascular effects of other calcium channel blockers. Cimetidine, omeprazole, and valproic acid may increase serum nimodipine levels. The effects of antihypertensive agents may be increased by nimodipine. Blood pressure-lowering effects may be additive with sildenafil, tadalafil, and vardenafil (use caution). CYP3A4 inhibitors may increase the levels/effects of nimodipine; example inhibitors include azole antifungals, clarithromycin, diclofenac, doxycycline, erythromycin, imatinib, isoniazid, nefazodone, nicardipine, propofol, protease inhibitors, quinidine, telithromycin, and verapamil.
  Decreased Effect: CYP3A4 inducers may decrease the levels/effects of nimodipine; example inducers include aminoglutethimide, carbamazepine, nafcillin, nevirapine, phenobarbital, phenytoin, and rifamycins.

Pharmacodynamics/Kinetics
  Protein binding: >95%
  Metabolism: Extensively hepatic
  Bioavailability: 13%
  Half-life elimination: 1-2 hours; prolonged with renal impairment
  Time to peak, serum: ~1 hour
  Excretion: Urine (50%) and feces (32%) within 4 days

Pregnancy Risk Factor C

Nimotop® see Nimodipine on page 1176
Nipent® see Pentostatin on page 1277
Niravam™ see Alprazolam on page 75

Nisoldipine (nye SOL di peen)

Related Information
  Cardiovascular Diseases on page 1726
U.S. Brand Names Sular®
Generic Available No
Pharmacologic Category Calcium Channel Blocker
Use Management of hypertension, alone or in combination with other antihypertensive agents
Local Anesthetic/Vasoconstrictor Precautions No information available to require special precautions
Effects on Dental Treatment Key adverse event(s) related to dental treatment: Xerostomia (normal salivary flow resumes upon discontinuation).
Common Adverse Effects
  >10%:
    Cardiovascular: Peripheral edema (dose related 7% to 29%)
    Central nervous system: Headache (22%)
  1% to 10%:
    Cardiovascular: Chest pain (2%), palpitation (3%), vasodilation (4%)
    Central nervous system: Dizziness (3% to 10%)
    Dermatologic: Rash (2%)
    Gastrointestinal: Nausea (3%)
    Respiratory: Pharyngitis (5%), sinusitis (3%), dyspnea (3%), cough (5%)

Mechanism of Action As a dihydropyridine calcium channel blocker, structurally similar to nifedipine, nisoldipine impedes the movement of calcium ions into vascular smooth muscle and cardiac muscle. Dihydropyridines are potent vasodilators and are not as likely to suppress cardiac contractility and slow cardiac conduction as other calcium antagonists such as verapamil and diltiazem; nisoldipine is 5-10 times as potent a vasodilator as nifedipine.

Drug Interactions
  Cytochrome P450 Effect: Substrate of CYP3A4 (major); **Inhibits** CYP1A2 (weak), 3A4 (weak)
  (Continued)

Nisoldipine (Continued)

Increased Effect/Toxicity: CYP3A4 inhibitors may increase the levels/effects of nisoldipine; example inhibitors include azole antifungals, clarithromycin, diclofenac, doxycycline, erythromycin, imatinib, isoniazid, nefazodone, nicardipine, propofol, protease inhibitors, quinidine, telithromycin, and verapamil. Calcium may reduce the calcium channel blocker's effects, particularly hypotension. Blood pressure-lowering effects may be additive with sildenafil, tadalafil, and vardenafil (use caution). Digoxin and nisoldipine may increase digoxin effect.

Decreased Effect: CYP3A4 inducers may decrease the levels/effects of nisoldipine; example inducers include aminoglutethimide, carbamazepine, nafcillin, nevirapine, phenobarbital, phenytoin, and rifamycins. Calcium may decrease the hypotension from calcium channel blockers.

Pharmacodynamics/Kinetics

Duration: >24 hours

Absorption: Well absorbed

Protein binding: >99%

Metabolism: Extensively hepatic; 1 active metabolite (10% of parent); first-pass effect

Bioavailability: 5%

Half-life elimination: 7-12 hours

Time to peak: 6-12 hours

Excretion: Urine (as metabolites)

Pregnancy Risk Factor C

Nitalapram see Citalopram on page 367

Nitazoxanide (nye ta ZOX a nide)

U.S. Brand Names Alinia®

Mexican Brand Names Daxon; Heliton

Generic Available No

Index Terms NTZ

Pharmacologic Category Antiprotozoal

Use Treatment of diarrhea caused by *Cryptosporidium parvum* or *Giardia lamblia*

Local Anesthetic/Vasoconstrictor Precautions No information available to require special precautions

Effects on Dental Treatment No significant effects or complications reported

Common Adverse Effects Rates of adverse effects were similar to those reported with placebo.

1% to 10%:

Central nervous system: Headache (1% to 3%)

Gastrointestinal: Abdominal pain (7% to 8%), diarrhea (2% to 4%), nausea (3%), vomiting (1%)

Mechanism of Action Nitazoxanide is rapidly metabolized to the active metabolite tizoxanide *in vivo*. Activity may be due to interference with the pyruvate:ferredoxin oxidoreductase (PFOR) enzyme-dependent electron transfer reaction which is essential to anaerobic metabolism. *In vitro*, nitazoxanide and tizoxanide inhibit the growth of sporozoites and oocysts of *Cryptosporidium parvum* and trophozoites of *Giardia lamblia*.

Pharmacodynamics/Kinetics

Protein binding: Tizoxanide: >99%

Bioavailability: Relative bioavailability of suspension compared to tablet: 70%

Metabolism: Hepatic, to an active metabolite, tizoxanide. Tizoxanide undergoes conjugation to form tizoxanide glucuronide. Nitazoxanide is not detectable in the serum following oral administration.

Time to peak, plasma: Tizoxanide and tizoxanide glucuronide: 1-4 hours

Excretion: Tizoxanide: Urine, bile, and feces; Tizoxanide glucuronide: Urine and bile

Pregnancy Risk Factor B

Nitisinone (ni TIS i known)

U.S. Brand Names Orfadin®

Generic Available No

Pharmacologic Category 4-Hydroxyphenylpyruvate Dioxygenase Inhibitor

Use Treatment of hereditary tyrosinemia type 1 (HT-1); to be used with dietary restriction of tyrosine and phenylalanine

Local Anesthetic/Vasoconstrictor Precautions No information available to require special precautions

Effects on Dental Treatment No significant effects or complications reported

Mechanism of Action In patients with HT-1, tyrosine metabolism is interrupted due to a lack of the enzyme (fumarylacetoacetate hydrolase) needed in the last step of tyrosine degradation. Toxic metabolites of tyrosine accumulate and cause liver and kidney toxicity. Nitisinone competitively inhibits 4-hydroxyphenyl-pyruvate dioxygenase, an enzyme needed earlier in the tyrosine degradation pathway, and therefore prevents the build-up of the damaging metabolites.

Pregnancy Risk Factor C

Nitrazepam (nye TRA ze pam)

Canadian Brand Names Apo-Nitrazepam®; Mogadon; Nitrazadon; Nitrazepam (Pro-Doc); Sandoz-Nitrazepam

Index Terms Nitrozepamum

Pharmacologic Category Benzodiazepine

Use Short-term management of insomnia; treatment of myoclonic seizures

Local Anesthetic/Vasoconstrictor Precautions No information available to require special precautions.

Effects on Dental Treatment Key adverse event(s) related to dental treatment: Excessive salivation has been reported. The mechanism of this effect is unknown, since many benzodiazepines cause xerostomia rather than salivation excess.

Common Adverse Effects Frequency not defined.

Cardiovascular: Hypotension, palpitation

Central nervous system: Agitation, aggressiveness, amnesia, ataxia, confusion, delusions, disorientation, dizziness, fatigue, hallucination, hangover, headache, irritability, nightmares, psychoses, rage, restlessness, sedation

Dermatologic: Rash

Endocrine & metabolic: Changes in libido

Gastrointestinal: Constipation, diarrhea, excessive salivation, heartburn, nausea, vomiting

Hematologic: Granulocytopenia, leukopenia

Neuromuscular & skeletal: Falling, muscle weakness

Ocular: Blurred vision, double vision

Otic: Tinnitus (associated with withdrawal)

Respiratory: Aspiration, bronchial hypersecretion, dyspnea

Restrictions CDSA IV; Not available in U.S.

Mechanism of Action Binds to stereospecific benzodiazepine receptors on the postsynaptic GABA neuron at several sites within the CNS, including the limbic system, reticular formation. Enhancement of the inhibitory effect of GABA on neuronal excitability results by increased neuronal membrane permeability to chloride ions. This shift in chloride ions results in hyperpolarization (a less excitable state) and stabilization.

Drug Interactions

Increased Effect/Toxicity: Sedative effects and/or respiratory depression may be additive with CNS depressants; includes ethanol, barbiturates, opioid analgesics, and other sedative agents; monitor for increased effect

Decreased Effect: Theophylline and/or caffeine may partially antagonize some of the effects of benzodiazepines; monitor for decreased response; may require higher doses for sedation

Pharmacodynamics/Kinetics

Onset: 20-50 minutes

Absorption: Rapid

Distribution: V_d: 2.4 L/kg, Elderly: 4.8 L/kg; also distributes into CSF, saliva, placenta

Protein binding: 87%

Metabolism: Hepatic: Nitroreduction, acetylation; no active metabolites

Bioavailability: ~80%

Half-life elimination: 30 hours, Elderly/ill patients: 40 hours

Time to peak, plasma: 2-3 hours

Excretion: Urine (65% to 70%, ~1% as unchanged drug); feces (14% to 20%)

Nitrek® see Nitroglycerin on page 1181

Nitric Oxide (NYE trik OKS ide)

U.S. Brand Names INOmax®
Canadian Brand Names INOmax®
Generic Available No
(Continued)

Nitric Oxide *(Continued)*

Pharmacologic Category Vasodilator, Pulmonary

Use Treatment of term and near-term (>34 weeks) neonates with hypoxic respiratory failure associated with pulmonary hypertension; used concurrently with ventilatory support and other agents

Unlabeled/Investigational Use Treatment of adult respiratory distress syndrome (ARDS)

Local Anesthetic/Vasoconstrictor Precautions No information available to require special precautions

Effects on Dental Treatment No significant effects or complications reported

Common Adverse Effects

>10%:
   Cardiovascular: Hypotension (13%)
   Miscellaneous: Withdrawal syndrome (12%)

1% to 10%:
   Dermatologic: Cellulitis (5%)
   Endocrine & metabolic: Hyperglycemia (8%)
   Genitourinary: Hematuria (8%)
   Respiratory: Atelectasis (9% - same as placebo), stridor (5%)
   Miscellaneous: Sepsis (7%), infection (6%)

Mechanism of Action In neonates with persistent pulmonary hypertension, nitric oxide improves oxygenation. Nitric oxide relaxes vascular smooth muscle by binding to the heme moiety of cytosolic guanylate cyclase, activating guanylate cyclase and increasing intracellular levels of cyclic guanosine 3',5'-monophosphate, which leads to vasodilation. When inhaled, pulmonary vasodilation occurs and an increase in the partial pressure of arterial oxygen results. Dilation of pulmonary vessels in well ventilated lung areas redistributes blood flow away from lung areas where ventilation/perfusion ratios are poor.

Drug Interactions

Increased Effect/Toxicity: Concurrent use of sodium nitroprusside, nitroglycerin, or prilocaine may result in an increased risk of developing methemoglobinemia.

Pharmacodynamics/Kinetics

Absorption: Systemic after inhalation

Metabolism: Nitric oxide combines with hemoglobin that is 60% to 100% oxygenated. Nitric oxide combines with oxyhemoglobin to produce methemoglobin and nitrate. Within the pulmonary system, nitric oxide can combine with oxygen and water to produce nitrogen dioxide and nitrite respectively, which interact with oxyhemoglobin and then produce methemoglobin and nitrate. At 80 ppm the methemoglobin percent is ~5% after 8 hours of administration. Methemoglobin levels >7% were attained only in patients receiving 80 ppm.

Excretion: Urine (as nitrate)

Clearance: Nitrate: At a rate approaching the glomerular filtration rate

Pregnancy Risk Factor C

Nitro-Bid® *see* Nitroglycerin *on page 1181*

Nitro-Dur® *see* Nitroglycerin *on page 1181*

Nitrofurantoin *(nye troe fyoor AN toyn)*

U.S. Brand Names Furadantin®; Macrobid®; Macrodantin®

Canadian Brand Names Apo-Nitrofurantoin®; Macrobid®; Macrodantin®; Novo-Furantoin

Mexican Brand Names Biofurin; Furadantina; Macrodantina

Generic Available Yes: Excludes suspension

Pharmacologic Category Antibiotic, Miscellaneous

Use Prevention and treatment of urinary tract infections caused by susceptible strains of *E. coli, S. aureus, Enterococcus, Klebsiella,* and *Enterobacter*

Local Anesthetic/Vasoconstrictor Precautions No information available to require special precautions

Effects on Dental Treatment No significant effects or complications reported

Common Adverse Effects Frequency not defined.

Cardiovascular: Chest pain, cyanosis, ECG changes

Central nervous system: Bulging fontanels (infants), chills, confusion, depression, dizziness, drowsiness, fever, headache, malaise, pseudotumor cerebri, psychotic reaction, vertigo

Dermatologic: Alopecia, angioedema, erythema multiforme, exfoliative dermatitis, pruritus, rash (eczematous, erythematous, maculopapular), Stevens-Johnson syndrome, urticaria

Gastrointestinal: Abdominal pain, *C. difficile* colitis, constipation, diarrhea, dyspepsia, flatulence, nausea, pancreatitis, sialadenitis, vomiting

Hematologic: Agranulocytosis, eosinophilia, granulocytopenia, hemolytic anemia, leukopenia, megaloblastic anemia, thrombocytopenia

Hepatic: Cholestasis, hepatitis, hepatic necrosis, transaminases increased, jaundice (cholestatic)

Neuromuscular & skeletal: Arthralgia, myalgia, numbness, paresthesia, peripheral neuropathy, weakness

Ocular: Amblyopia, nystagmus, optic neuritis

Respiratory: Cough, dyspnea, pneumonitis, pulmonary fibrosis (with long-term use), pulmonary infiltration

Miscellaneous: Anaphylaxis, hypersensitivity (including acute pulmonary hypersensitivity), lupus-like syndrome

Mechanism of Action Inhibits several bacterial enzyme systems including acetyl coenzyme A interfering with metabolism and possibly cell wall synthesis

Drug Interactions

Increased Effect/Toxicity: Probenecid and sulfinpyrazone decreases renal excretion of nitrofurantoin.

Decreased Effect: Antacids containing magnesium trisilicate may decrease absorption of nitrofurantoin.

Pharmacodynamics/Kinetics

Absorption: Well absorbed; macrocrystalline form absorbed more slowly due to slower dissolution (causes less GI distress)

Distribution: V_d: 0.8 L/kg; crosses placenta; enters breast milk

Protein binding: 60% to 90%

Metabolism: Body tissues (except plasma) metabolize 60% of drug to inactive metabolites

Bioavailability: Increased with food

Half-life elimination: 20-60 minutes; prolonged with renal impairment

Excretion:

Suspension: Urine (40%) and feces (small amounts) as metabolites and unchanged drug

Macrocrystals: Urine (20% to 25% as unchanged drug)

Pregnancy Risk Factor B (contraindicated at term)

Nitroglycerin (nye troe GLI ser in)

Related Information

Cardiovascular Diseases *on page 1726*

U.S. Brand Names Minitran™; Nitrek®; Nitro-Bid®; Nitro-Dur®; Nitrolingual®; NitroMist™; NitroQuick®; Nitrostat®; NitroTime®

Canadian Brand Names Gen-Nitro; Minitran™; Nitro-Dur®; Nitroglycerin Injection, USP; Nitrol®; Nitrostat™; Rho®-Nitro; Transderm-Nitro®; Trinipatch® 0.2; Trinipatch® 0.4; Trinipatch® 0.6

Mexican Brand Names Anglix; Cardinit; Nitradisc; Nitroderm TTS-5

Generic Available Yes: Capsule, injection, patch, tablet

Index Terms Glyceryl Trinitrate; Nitroglycerol; NTG

Pharmacologic Category Vasodilator

Use Treatment of angina pectoris; I.V. for congestive heart failure (especially when associated with acute myocardial infarction); pulmonary hypertension; hypertensive emergencies occurring perioperatively (especially during cardiovascular surgery)

Unlabeled/Investigational Use Esophageal spastic disorders (sublingual)

Local Anesthetic/Vasoconstrictor Precautions No information available to require special precautions

Effects on Dental Treatment Key adverse event(s) related to dental treatment: Xerostomia (normal salivary flow resumes upon discontinuation).

Dosage Note: Hemodynamic and antianginal tolerance often develop within 24-48 hours of continuous nitrate administration. Nitrate-free interval (10-12 hours/day) is recommended to avoid tolerance development; gradually decrease dose in patients receiving NTG for prolonged period to avoid withdrawal reaction.

Children: Pulmonary hypertension: Continuous infusion: Start 0.25-0.5 mcg/kg/minute and titrate by 1 mcg/kg/minute at 20- to 60-minute intervals to desired effect; usual dose: 1-3 mcg/kg/minute; maximum: 5 mcg/kg/minute

Adults:

Oral: 2.5-9 mg 2-4 times/day (up to 26 mg 4 times/day)

I.V.: 5 mcg/minute, increase by 5 mcg/minute every 3-5 minutes to 20 mcg/minute; if no response at 20 mcg/minute increase by 10 mcg/minute every 3-5 minutes, up to 200 mcg/minute

Ointment: 1/2" upon rising and 1/2" 6 hours later; the dose may be doubled and even doubled again as needed

(Continued)

Nitroglycerin *(Continued)*

Patch, transdermal: Initial: 0.2-0.4 mg/hour, titrate to doses of 0.4-0.8 mg/hour; tolerance is minimized by using a patch-on period of 12-14 hours and patch-off period of 10-12 hours

Sublingual: 0.2-0.6 mg every 5 minutes for maximum of 3 doses in 15 minutes; may also use prophylactically 5-10 minutes prior to activities which may provoke an attack

Esophageal spastic disorders (unlabeled use): 0.3-0.4 mg 5 minutes before meals

Translingual: 1-2 sprays into mouth under tongue every 5 minutes for maximum of 3 doses in 15 minutes, may also be used 5-10 minutes prior to activities which may provoke an attack prophylactically

Hemodialysis: Supplemental dose is not necessary

Peritoneal dialysis: Supplemental dose is not necessary

Elderly: In general, dose selection should be cautious, usually starting at the low end of the dosing range

Mechanism of Action Works by relaxation of smooth muscle, producing a vasodilator effect on the peripheral veins and arteries with more prominent effects on the veins. Primarily reduces cardiac oxygen demand by decreasing preload (left ventricular end-diastolic pressure); may modestly reduce afterload; dilates coronary arteries and improves collateral flow to ischemic regions

Contraindications Hypersensitivity to organic nitrates; hypersensitivity to isosorbide, nitroglycerin, or any component of the formulation; concurrent use with phosphodiesterase-5 (PDE-5) inhibitors (sildenafil, tadalafil, or vardenafil); angle-closure glaucoma (intraocular pressure may be increased); head trauma or cerebral hemorrhage (increase intracranial pressure); severe anemia; allergy to adhesive (transdermal product)

Additional contraindications for I.V. product: Hypotension; uncorrected hypovolemia; inadequate cerebral circulation; constrictive pericarditis; pericardial tamponade

Warnings/Precautions Severe hypotension can occur. Use with caution in volume depletion, hypotension, and right ventricular infarctions. Paradoxical bradycardia and increased angina pectoris can accompany hypotension. Orthostatic hypotension can also occur. Ethanol can accentuate this. Tolerance does develop to nitrates and appropriate dosing is needed to minimize this (drug-free interval). Avoid use of long-acting agents in acute MI or CHF; cannot easily reverse. Nitrate may aggravate angina caused by hypertrophic cardiomyopathy. Nitroglycerin transdermal patches should be removed prior to defibrillation or MRI study. Avoid concurrent use with PDE-5 inhibitors. Safety and efficacy have not been established in children.

Drug Interactions

Increased Effect/Toxicity: Significant reduction of systolic and diastolic blood pressure with concurrent use of sildenafil, tadalafil, or vardenafil (contraindicated); do not administer sildenafil, tadalafil, or vardenafil within 24 hours of a nitrate preparation.

Decreased Effect: I.V. nitroglycerin may antagonize the anticoagulant effect of heparin (possibly only at high nitroglycerin dosages); monitor closely. May need to decrease heparin dosage when nitroglycerin is discontinued. Ergot alkaloids may cause an increase in blood pressure and decrease in antianginal effects; avoid concurrent use.

Ethanol/Nutrition/Herb Interactions

Ethanol: Avoid ethanol (may increase the hypotensive effects of nitroglycerin). Monitor.

Herb/Nutraceutical: Avoid bayberry, blue cohosh, cayenne, ephedra, ginger, ginseng (american), kola, licorice (may worsen hypertension). Avoid black cohosh, California poppy, coleus, golden seal, hawthorn, mistletoe, periwinkle, quinine, shepherd's purse (may cause hypotension).

Pharmacodynamics/Kinetics

Onset of action: Sublingual tablet: 1-3 minutes; Translingual spray: 2 minutes; Sustained release: 20-45 minutes; Topical: 15-60 minutes; Transdermal: 40-60 minutes; I.V. drip: Immediate

Peak effect: Sublingual tablet: 4-8 minutes; Translingual spray: 4-10 minutes; Sustained release: 45-120 minutes; Topical: 30-120 minutes; Transdermal: 60-180 minutes; I.V. drip: Immediate

Duration: Sublingual tablet: 30-60 minutes; Translingual spray: 30-60 minutes; Sustained release: 4-8 hours; Topical: 2-12 hours; Transdermal: 18-24 hours; I.V. drip: 3-5 minutes

Protein binding: 60%

Metabolism: Extensive first-pass effect

Half-life elimination: 1-4 minutes

Excretion: Urine (as inactive metabolites)

Pregnancy Risk Factor C

Dosage Forms

Capsule, extended release: 2.5 mg, 6.5 mg, 9 mg

Nitro-Time®: 2.5 mg, 6.5 mg, 9 mg

Infusion [premixed in D$_5$W]: 25 mg (250 mL) [0.1 mg/mL]; 50 mg (250 mL) [0.2 mg/mL]; 50 mg (500 mL) [0.1 mg/mL]; 100 mg (250 mL) [0.4 mg/mL]; 200 mg (500 mL) [0.4 mg/mL]

Injection, solution: 5 mg/mL (5 mL, 10 mL)

Ointment, topical:

Nitro-Bid®: 2% [20 mg/g] (1 g, 30 g, 60 g)

Solution, translingual [spray]:

Nitrolingual®: 0.4 mg/metered spray (4.9 g, 12 g)

NitroMist™:0.4 mg/metered spray (8.5 g)

Tablet, sublingual: 0.3 mg, 0.4 mg, 0.6 mg

NitroQuick®, Nitrostat®, Nitro-Tab®: 0.3 mg, 0.4 mg, 0.6 mg

Transdermal system [once-daily patch]: 0.1 mg/hour (30s); 0.2 mg/hour (30s); 0.4 mg/hour (30s); 0.6 mg/hour (30s)

Minitran™: 0.1 mg/hour (30s); 0.2 mg/hour (30s); 0.4 mg/hour (30s); 0.6 mg/hour (30s)

Nitrek®: 0.2 mg/hour (30s); 0.4 mg/hour (30s); 0.6 mg/hour (30s)

Nitro-Dur®: 0.1 mg/hour (30s); 0.2 mg/hour (30s); 0.3 mg/hour (30s); 0.4 mg/hour (30s); 0.6 mg/hour (30s); 0.8 mg/hour (30s)

Nitroglycerol see Nitroglycerin on page 1181

Nitrolingual® see Nitroglycerin on page 1181

NitroMist™ see Nitroglycerin on page 1181

Nitropress® see Nitroprusside on page 1183

Nitroprusside (nye troe PRUS ide)

Related Information

Cardiovascular Diseases on page 1726

U.S. Brand Names Nitropress®

Mexican Brand Names Nitan

Generic Available Yes

Index Terms Nitroprusside Sodium; Sodium Nitroferricyanide; Sodium Nitroprusside

Pharmacologic Category Vasodilator

Use Management of hypertensive crises; congestive heart failure; used for controlled hypotension to reduce bleeding during surgery

Local Anesthetic/Vasoconstrictor Precautions No information available to require special precautions

Effects on Dental Treatment No significant effects or complications reported

Common Adverse Effects 1% to 10%:

Cardiovascular: Excessive hypotensive response, palpitation, substernal distress

Central nervous system: Disorientation, psychosis, headache, restlessness

Endocrine & metabolic: Thyroid suppression

Gastrointestinal: Nausea, vomiting

Neuromuscular & skeletal: Weakness, muscle spasm

Otic: Tinnitus

Respiratory: Hypoxia

Miscellaneous: Diaphoresis, thiocyanate toxicity

Mechanism of Action Causes peripheral vasodilation by direct action on venous and arteriolar smooth muscle, thus reducing peripheral resistance; will increase cardiac output by decreasing afterload; reduces aortal and left ventricular impedance

Pharmacodynamics/Kinetics

Onset of action: BP reduction <2 minutes

Duration: 1-10 minutes

Metabolism: Nitroprusside is converted to cyanide ions in the bloodstream; decomposes to prussic acid which in the presence of sulfur donor is converted to thiocyanate (hepatic and renal rhodanase systems)

Half-life elimination: Parent drug: <10 minutes; Thiocyanate: 2.7-7 days

Excretion: Urine (as thiocyanate)

Pregnancy Risk Factor C

Nitroprusside Sodium see Nitroprusside on page 1183

NitroQuick® see Nitroglycerin on page 1181

Nitrostat® see Nitroglycerin on page 1181

NitroTime® see Nitroglycerin on page 1181

4'-Nitro-3'-Trifluoromethylisobutyrantide see Flutamide on page 725

Nitrous Oxide (NYE trus OKS ide)

Related Information
Sedation *on page 1825*
Generic Available Yes
Pharmacologic Category Dental Gases; General Anesthetic
Dental Use Induction of sedation and analgesia in anxious dental patients
Use Produces sedation and analgesia; principal adjunct to inhalation and intravenous general anesthesia
Local Anesthetic/Vasoconstrictor Precautions No information available to require special precautions
Effects on Dental Treatment No significant effects or complications reported
Significant Adverse Effects Frequency not defined.
Cardiovascular: Hypotension
Central nervous system: Headache, dizziness, confusion, CNS excitation
Gastrointestinal: Possibly nausea and vomiting
Respiratory: Apnea
Miscellaneous: Personnel exposed to unscavenged nitrous oxide have an increased risk of renal and hepatic diseases and peripheral neuropathy similar to that of vitamin B_{12} deficiency. Female dental personnel who were exposed to unscavenged nitrous oxide for more than 5 hours/week were significantly less fertile than women who were not exposed, or who were exposed to lower levels of scavenged or unscavenged nitrous oxide.
Dental Usual Dosing
Sedation and analgesia: Children and Adults: Concentrations of 25% to 50% nitrous oxide with oxygen
Dosage Children and Adults:
Surgical: For sedation and analgesia: Concentrations of 25% to 50% nitrous oxide with oxygen. For general anesthesia, concentrations of 40% to 70% via mask or endotracheal tube. Minimal alveolar concentration (MAC), which can be considered the ED_{50} of inhalational anesthetics, is 105%; therefore delivery in a hyperbaric chamber is necessary to use as a complete anesthetic. When administered at 70%, reduces the MAC of other anesthetics by half.
Dental: For sedation and analgesia: Concentrations of 25% to 50% nitrous oxide with oxygen
Mechanism of Action General CNS depressant action; may act similarly as inhalant general anesthetics by stabilizing axonal membranes to partially inhibit action potentials leading to sedation; may partially act on opiate receptor systems to cause mild analgesia; central sympathetic stimulating action supports blood pressure, systemic vascular resistance, and cardiac output; it does not depress carbon dioxide drive to breath. Nitrous oxide increases cerebral blood flow and intracranial pressure while decreasing hepatic and renal blood flow; has analgesic action similar to morphine.
Contraindications Hypersensitivity to nitrous oxide or any component of the formulation; nitrous oxide should not be administered without oxygen; should not be given to patients after a full meal
Warnings/Precautions Nausea and vomiting occurs postoperatively in ~15% of patients. Prolonged use may produce bone marrow suppression and/or neurologic dysfunction. Oxygen should be briefly administered during emergence from prolonged anesthesia with nitrous oxide to prevent diffusion hypoxia. Patients with vitamin B_{12} deficiency (pernicious anemia) and those with other nutritional deficiencies (alcoholics) are at increased risk of developing neurologic disease and bone marrow suppression with exposure to nitrous oxide. May be addictive.
Drug Interactions No data reported
Pharmacodynamics/Kinetics
Onset of action: Inhalation: 2-5 minutes
Absorption: Rapid via lungs; blood/gas partition coefficient is 0.47
Metabolism: Body: <0.004%
Excretion: Primarily exhaled gases; skin (minimal amounts)
Pregnancy Risk Factor No data reported
Dosage Forms Excipient information presented when available (limited, particularly for generics); consult specific product labeling.
Supplied in blue cylinders

Nitrozepamum *see* Nitrazepam *on page 1179*
Nix® [OTC] *see* Permethrin *on page 1284*

Nizatidine (ni ZA ti deen)

Related Information
Gastrointestinal Disorders *on page 1745*

U.S. Brand Names Axid®; Axid® AR [OTC]
Canadian Brand Names Apo-Nizatidine®; Axid®; Gen-Nizatidine; Novo-Nizatidine; Nu-Nizatidine; PMS-Nizatidine
Mexican Brand Names Axid Pulvules
Generic Available Yes: Capsule
Pharmacologic Category Histamine H_2 Antagonist
Use Treatment and maintenance of duodenal ulcer; treatment of benign gastric ulcer; treatment of gastroesophageal reflux disease (GERD); OTC tablet used for the prevention of meal-induced heartburn, acid indigestion, and sour stomach
Unlabeled/Investigational Use Part of a multidrug regimen for *H. pylori* eradication to reduce the risk of duodenal ulcer recurrence
Local Anesthetic/Vasoconstrictor Precautions No information available to require special precautions
Effects on Dental Treatment Key adverse event(s) related to dental treatment: Xerostomia (normal salivary flow resumes upon discontinuation).
Common Adverse Effects
>10%: Central nervous system: Headache (16%)
1% to 10%:
Central nervous system: Anxiety, dizziness, fever (reported in children), insomnia, irritability (reported in children), somnolence, nervousness
Dermatologic: Pruritus, rash
Gastrointestinal: Abdominal pain, anorexia, constipation, diarrhea, dry mouth, flatulence, heartburn, nausea, vomiting
Respiratory: Reported in children: Cough, nasal congestion, nasopharyngitis
Mechanism of Action Competitive inhibition of histamine at H_2-receptors of the gastric parietal cells resulting in reduced gastric acid secretion, gastric volume and hydrogen ion concentration reduced. In healthy volunteers, nizatidine suppresses gastric acid secretion induced by pentagastrin infusion or food.
Drug Interactions
Cytochrome P450 Effect: Inhibits 3A4 (weak)
Decreased Effect: May decrease the absorption of itraconazole or ketoconazole.
Pharmacodynamics/Kinetics
Distribution: V_d: 0.8-1.5 L/kg
Protein binding: 35% to α_1-acid glycoprotein
Metabolism: Partially hepatic; forms metabolites
Bioavailability: >70%
Half-life elimination: 1-2 hours; prolonged with renal impairment
Time to peak, plasma: 0.5-3.0 hours
Excretion: Urine (90%; ~60% as unchanged drug); feces (<6%)
Pregnancy Risk Factor B

Nonoxynol 9 (non OKS i nole nine)

U.S. Brand Names Advantage-S™ [OTC]; Conceptrol® [OTC]; Delfen® [OTC]; Emko® [OTC] [DSC]; Encare® [OTC]; Gynol II® [OTC]; Shur-Seal® [OTC] [DSC]; Today® Sponge [OTC]; VCF™ [OTC]
Generic Available No
Index Terms N-9
Pharmacologic Category Contraceptive; Spermicide
Use Prevention of pregnancy
Local Anesthetic/Vasoconstrictor Precautions No information available to require special precautions
Effects on Dental Treatment No significant effects or complications reported
Common Adverse Effects Frequency not defined: Genitourinary: Irritation, burning, or itching of mucous membranes (including vaginal/urethral)
Mechanism of Action
Nonoxynol 9 is a surfactant which prevents pregnancy by damaging the cell membrane of sperm; some product formulations may also provide a physical barrier

Noradrenaline Acid Tartrate *see* Norepinephrine *on page 1186*

Norco® *see* Hydrocodone and Acetaminophen *on page 822*

Nordeoxyguanosine *see* Ganciclovir *on page 763*

Nordette® *see* Ethinyl Estradiol and Levonorgestrel *on page 633*

Norditropin® *see* Somatropin *on page 1486*

Norditropin® NordiFlex® *see* Somatropin *on page 1486*

norel® EX *see* Guaifenesin and Phenylephrine *on page 797*

Norelgestromin and Ethinyl Estradiol *see* Ethinyl Estradiol and Norelgestromin *on page 637*

Norepinephrine (nor ep i NEF rin)

U.S. Brand Names Levophed®
Canadian Brand Names Levophed®
Generic Available Yes
Index Terms Levarterenol Bitartrate; Noradrenaline; Noradrenaline Acid Tartrate; Norepinephrine Bitartrate
Pharmacologic Category Alpha/Beta Agonist
Use Treatment of shock which persists after adequate fluid volume replacement
Local Anesthetic/Vasoconstrictor Precautions No information available to require special precautions
Effects on Dental Treatment No significant effects or complications reported
Mechanism of Action Stimulates beta$_1$-adrenergic receptors and alpha-adrenergic receptors causing increased contractility and heart rate as well as vasoconstriction, thereby increasing systemic blood pressure and coronary blood flow; clinically alpha effects (vasoconstriction) are greater than beta effects (inotropic and chronotropic effects)
Pregnancy Risk Factor C

Norepinephrine Bitartrate *see* Norepinephrine *on page 1186*

Norethindrone (nor ETH in drone)

Related Information
  Endocrine Disorders and Pregnancy *on page 1750*
U.S. Brand Names Aygestin®; Camila™; Errin™; Jolivette™; Micronor®; Nora-BE™; Nor-QD®
Canadian Brand Names Micronor®; Norlutate®
Generic Available Yes
Index Terms Norethindrone Acetate; Norethisterone
Pharmacologic Category Contraceptive; Progestin
Use Treatment of amenorrhea; abnormal uterine bleeding; endometriosis, oral contraceptive; **higher rate of failure with progestin only contraceptives**
Local Anesthetic/Vasoconstrictor Precautions No information available to require special precautions
Effects on Dental Treatment Until we know more about the mechanism of interaction, caution is required in prescribing antibiotics to female dental patients taking progestin-only hormonal contraceptives.
Common Adverse Effects
  >10%:
    Cardiovascular: Edema
    Endocrine & metabolic: Breakthrough bleeding, spotting, changes in menstrual flow, amenorrhea
    Gastrointestinal: Anorexia
    Local: Pain at injection site
    Neuromuscular & skeletal: Weakness
  1% to 10%:
    Cardiovascular: Edema
    Central nervous system: Mental depression, fever, insomnia
    Dermatologic: Melasma or chloasma, allergic rash with or without pruritus
    Endocrine & metabolic: Increased breast tenderness
    Gastrointestinal: Weight gain/loss
    Genitourinary: Changes in cervical erosion and secretions
    Hepatic: Cholestatic jaundice
Mechanism of Action Inhibits secretion of pituitary gonadotropin (LH) which prevents follicular maturation and ovulation
Drug Interactions
  Cytochrome P450 Effect: Substrate of CYP3A4 (major); **Induces** CYP2C19 (weak)
  Decreased Effect: Nelfinavir decreases the pharmacologic effect of norethindrone. CYP3A4 inducers may decrease the levels/effects of norethindrone;

example inducers include aminoglutethimide, carbamazepine, nafcillin, nevirapine, phenobarbital, phenytoin, and rifamycins.

Pharmacodynamics/Kinetics

Absorption: Oral, transdermal: Rapidly absorbed

Distribution: V_d: 2-4 L/kg

Protein binding: 61% to albumin; 36% to sex hormone-binding globulin (SHBG); SHBG capacity affected by plasma ethinyl estradiol levels

Metabolism: Oral: Hepatic via reduction and conjugation; first-pass effect

Bioavailability: 64%

Half-life elimination: 5-14 hours

Time to peak: 1-2 hours

Excretion: Primarily urine (as metabolites)

Pregnancy Risk Factor X

Norethindrone Acetate *see* Norethindrone *on page 1186*

Norethindrone Acetate and Ethinyl Estradiol *see* Ethinyl Estradiol and Norethindrone *on page 640*

Norethindrone and Estradiol *see* Estradiol and Norethindrone *on page 603*

Norethindrone and Mestranol *see* Mestranol and Norethindrone *on page 1053*

Norethisterone *see* Norethindrone *on page 1186*

Norflex™ *see* Orphenadrine *on page 1212*

Norfloxacin (nor FLOKS a sin)

U.S. Brand Names Noroxin®

Canadian Brand Names Apo-Norflox®; CO Norfloxacin; Norfloxacine®; Noroxin®; Novo-Norfloxacin; PMS-Norfloxacin; Riva-Norfloxacin

Mexican Brand Names Floxacin; Noroxin; Noroxin Oftalmico; Oranor

Generic Available No

Pharmacologic Category Antibiotic, Quinolone

Use Uncomplicated and complicated urinary tract infections caused by susceptible gram-negative and gram-positive bacteria; sexually-transmitted disease (eg, uncomplicated urethral and cervical gonorrhea) caused by *N. gonorrhoeae*; prostatitis due to *E. coli*

Note: As of April 2007, the CDC no longer recommends the use of fluoroquinolones for the treatment of gonococcal disease.

Local Anesthetic/Vasoconstrictor Precautions Norfloxacin is one of the drugs confirmed to prolong the QT interval and is accepted as having a risk of causing torsade de pointes. The risk of drug-induced torsade de pointes is extremely low when a single QT interval prolonging drug is prescribed. In terms of epinephrine, it is not known what effect vasoconstrictors in the local anesthetic regimen will have in patients with a known history of congenital prolonged QT interval or in patients taking any medication that prolongs the QT interval. Until more information is obtained, it is suggested that the clinician consult with the physician prior to the use of a vasoconstrictor in suspected patients, and that the vasoconstrictor (epinephrine, levonordefrin [Neo-Cobefrin®]) be used with caution.

Effects on Dental Treatment No significant effects or complications reported

Common Adverse Effects 1% to 10%:

Central nervous system: Headache (3%), dizziness (3%)

Gastrointestinal: Nausea (4%), abdominal cramping (2%)

Neuromuscular & skeletal: Weakness (1%)

Mechanism of Action Norfloxacin is a DNA gyrase inhibitor. DNA gyrase is an essential bacterial enzyme that maintains the superhelical structure of DNA. DNA gyrase is required for DNA replication and transcription, DNA repair, recombination, and transposition; bactericidal

Drug Interactions

Cytochrome P450 Effect: Inhibits CYP1A2 (strong), 3A4 (moderate)

Increased Effect/Toxicity: Norfloxacin may increase the effects/toxicity of caffeine, cyclosporine, CYP1A2 substrates (eg, aminophylline, fluvoxamine, mexiletine, mirtazapine, ropinirole, and trifluoperazine), CYP3A4 substrates (such as benzodiazepines, calcium channel blockers, cisapride, ergot alkaloids, selected HMG-CoA reductase inhibitors, mirtazapine, nateglinide, nefazodone, pimozide, sildenafil (and other PDE-5 inhibitors), tacrolimus, and venlafaxine), glyburide, theophylline, and warfarin. Concomitant use with corticosteroids may increase the risk of tendon rupture. Concomitant use with other QT_c-prolonging agents (eg, Class Ia and Class III antiarrhythmics, erythromycin, cisapride, antipsychotics, and cyclic antidepressants) may result in arrhythmias such as torsade de pointes. Probenecid may increase norfloxacin levels. Concomitant use with NSAIDs may rarely increase risk of seizure.

Decreased Effect: Concurrent administration of metal cations, including most antacids, oral electrolyte supplements, quinapril, sucralfate, some didanosine *(Continued)*

Norfloxacin (Continued)

formulations (pediatric powder for oral suspension), and other highly-buffered oral drugs, may decrease quinolone levels; separate doses.

Pharmacodynamics/Kinetics

Absorption: Oral: Rapid, up to 40%

Distribution: Crosses placenta; small amounts enter breast milk

Protein binding: 10% to 15%

Metabolism: Hepatic

Half-life elimination: 3-4 hours; Renal impairment (Cl_{cr} ≤30 mL/minute): 6.5 hours; Elderly: 4 hours

Time to peak, serum: 1-2 hours

Excretion: Urine (26% to 32% as unchanged drug; 5% to 8% as metabolites); feces

Pregnancy Risk Factor C

Nortriptyline (nor TRIP ti leen)

U.S. Brand Names Pamelor®

Canadian Brand Names Alti-Nortriptyline; Apo-Nortriptyline®; Aventyl®; Gen-Nortriptyline; Norventyl; Novo-Nortriptyline; Nu-Nortriptyline; PMS-Nortriptyline

Generic Available Yes: Excludes solution

Index Terms Nortriptyline Hydrochloride

Pharmacologic Category Antidepressant, Tricyclic (Secondary Amine)

Dental Use Treatment of myofascial pain, neuralgia, burning mouth syndrome

Use Treatment of symptoms of depression

Unlabeled/Investigational Use Chronic pain, anxiety disorders, enuresis, attention-deficit/hyperactivity disorder (ADHD); adjunctive therapy for smoking cessation

Local Anesthetic/Vasoconstrictor Precautions Nortriptyline is one of the drugs confirmed to prolong the QT interval and is accepted as having a risk of causing torsade de pointes. In terms of epinephrine, it is not known what effect vasoconstrictors in the local anesthetic regimen will have in patients with a known history of congenital prolonged QT interval or in patients taking any medication that prolongs the QT interval. Until more information is obtained, it is suggested that the clinician consult with the physician prior to the use of a vasoconstrictor in suspected patients, and that the vasoconstrictor (epinephrine, levonordefrin [Neo-Cobefrin®]) be used with caution. See Dental Comment.

Effects on Dental Treatment Key adverse event(s) related to dental treatment: Xerostomia (normal salivary flow resumes upon discontinuation), black tongue, and unpleasant taste. Long-term treatment with TCAs, such as nortriptyline, increases the risk of caries by reducing salivation and salivary buffer capacity.

Significant Adverse Effects Frequency not defined.

Cardiovascular: Postural hypotension, arrhythmia, hypertension, heart block, tachycardia, palpitation, MI

Central nervous system: Confusion, delirium, hallucinations, restlessness, insomnia, disorientation, delusions, anxiety, agitation, panic, nightmares, hypomania, exacerbation of psychosis, incoordination, ataxia, extrapyramidal symptoms, seizure

Dermatologic: Alopecia, photosensitivity, rash, petechiae, urticaria, itching

Endocrine & metabolic: Sexual dysfunction, gynecomastia, breast enlargement, galactorrhea, increase or decrease in libido, increase in blood sugar, SIADH

Gastrointestinal: Xerostomia, constipation, vomiting, anorexia, diarrhea, abdominal cramps, black tongue, nausea, unpleasant taste, weight gain/loss

Genitourinary: Urinary retention, delayed micturition, impotence, testicular edema

Hematologic: Rarely agranulocytosis, eosinophilia, purpura, thrombocytopenia

Hepatic: Increased liver enzymes, cholestatic jaundice

Neuromuscular & skeletal: Tremor, numbness, tingling, paresthesia, peripheral neuropathy

Ocular: Blurred vision, eye pain, disturbances in accommodation, mydriasis

Otic: Tinnitus

Miscellaneous: Diaphoresis (excessive), allergic reactions

Restrictions An FDA-approved medication guide concerning the use of antidepressants in children, adolescents, and young adults must be distributed when dispensing an outpatient prescription (new or refill) where this medication is to be used without direct supervision of a healthcare provider. Medication guides are available at http://www.fda.gov/cder/Offices/ODS/medication_guides.htm. Dispense to parents or guardians of children and adolescents receiving this medication.

Dental Usual Dosing Myofascial pain, neuralgia, burning mouth syndrome: Adults: Initial: 10-25 mg at bedtime; dosage may be increased by 25 mg/day weekly, if tolerated; usual maintenance dose: 75 mg as a single bedtime dose or 2 divided doses

Dosage Oral:

Nocturnal enuresis: Children (unlabeled use): 10-20 mg/day; titrate to a maximum of 40 mg/day

Depression (unlabeled use): Children: 1-3 mg/kg/day

Depression:

Adults: 25 mg 3-4 times/day up to 150 mg/day

Elderly (**Note:** Nortriptyline is one of the best tolerated TCAs in the elderly)
Initial: 10-25 mg at bedtime
Dosage can be increased by 25 mg every 3 days for inpatients and weekly for outpatients if tolerated
Usual maintenance dose: 75 mg as a single bedtime dose or 2 divided doses; however, lower or higher doses may be required to stay within the therapeutic window

Myofascial pain, neuralgia, burning mouth syndrome (dental use): Initial: 10-25 mg at bedtime; dosage may be increased by 25 mg/day weekly, if tolerated; usual maintenance dose: 75 mg as a single bedtime dose or 2 divided doses

Chronic urticaria, angioedema, nocturnal pruritus (unlabeled use): Adults: Oral: 75 mg/day

Smoking cessation (unlabeled use): Adults: 25-75 mg/day beginning 10-14 days before "quit" day; continue therapy for ≥12 weeks after "quit" day

Dosing adjustment in hepatic impairment: Lower doses and slower titration dependent on individualization of dosage is recommended

Mechanism of Action Traditionally believed to increase the synaptic concentration of serotonin and/or norepinephrine in the central nervous system by inhibition of their reuptake by the presynaptic neuronal membrane. However, additional receptor effects have been found including desensitization of adenyl cyclase, down regulation of beta-adrenergic receptors, and down regulation of serotonin receptors.

Contraindications Hypersensitivity to nortriptyline and similar chemical class, or any component of the formulation; use of MAO inhibitors within 14 days; use in a patient during the acute recovery phase of MI; pregnancy

Warnings/Precautions [U.S. Boxed Warning]: Antidepressants increase the risk of suicidal thinking and behavior in children, adolescents, and young adults (18-24 years of age) with major depressive disorder (MDD) and other psychiatric disorders; consider risk prior to prescribing. Short-term studies did not show an increased risk in patients >24 years of age and showed a decreased risk in patients ≥65 years. Closely monitor for clinical worsening, suicidality, or unusual changes in behavior; the patient's family or caregiver should be instructed to closely observe the patient and communicate condition with healthcare provider. A medication guide should be dispensed with each prescription. **Nortriptyline is not FDA approved for use in children.**

The possibility of a suicide attempt is inherent in major depression and may persist until remission occurs. Monitor for worsening of depression or suicidality, especially during initiation of therapy (generally first 1-2 months) or with dose increases or decreases. Use caution in high-risk patients. Worsening depression and severe abrupt suicidality that are not part of the presenting symptoms may require discontinuation or modification of drug therapy. The patient's family or caregiver should be alerted to monitor patients for the emergence of (Continued)

Nortriptyline *(Continued)*

suicidality and associated behaviors (such as agitation, irritability, hostility, impulsivity, and hypomania) and call healthcare provider.

May worsen psychosis in some patients or precipitate a shift to mania or hypomania in patients with bipolar disorder. Patients presenting with depressive symptoms should be screened for bipolar disorder. Monotherapy in patients with bipolar disorder should be avoided. **Nortriptyline is not FDA approved for the treatment of bipolar depression.**

The risk of sedation and orthostatic effects are low relative to other antidepressants. However, nortriptyline may result in impaired performance of tasks requiring alertness (eg, operating machinery or driving). Sedative effects may be additive with other CNS depressants and/or ethanol. The degree of anticholinergic blockade produced by this agent is moderate relative to other cyclic antidepressants, however, caution should still be used in patients with urinary retention, benign prostatic hyperplasia, narrow-angle glaucoma, xerostomia, visual problems, constipation, or history of bowel obstruction. May cause orthostatic hypotension (risk is low relative to other antidepressants) or conduction disturbances. Use with caution in patients with a history of cardiovascular disease (including previous MI, stroke, tachycardia, or conduction abnormalities). The risk conduction abnormalities with this agent is moderate relative to other antidepressants.

Consider discontinuing, when possible, prior to elective surgery. Therapy should not be abruptly discontinued in patients receiving high doses for prolonged periods. May alter glucose regulation - use caution in patients with diabetes. Use caution in patients with a previous seizure disorder or condition predisposing to seizures such as brain damage, alcoholism, or concurrent therapy with other drugs which lower the seizure threshold. May increase the risks associated with electroconvulsive therapy. Use with caution in hyperthyroid patients or those receiving thyroid supplementation. Use with caution in patients with hepatic or renal dysfunction and in elderly patients.

Drug Interactions Substrate of CYP1A2 (minor), 2C19 (minor), 2D6 (major), 3A4 (minor); **Inhibits** CYP2D6 (weak), 2E1 (weak)

Altretamine: Concurrent use may cause orthostatic hypertension

Amphetamines: TCAs may enhance the effect of amphetamines; monitor for adverse CV effects

Anticholinergics: Combined use with TCAs may produce additive anticholinergic effects

Antihypertensives: TCAs may inhibit the antihypertensive response to bethanidine, clonidine, debrisoquin, guanadrel, guanethidine, guanabenz, guanfacine; monitor BP; consider alternate antihypertensive agent

Beta-agonists: When combined with TCAs may predispose patients to cardiac arrhythmias

Bupropion: May increase the levels of tricyclic antidepressants; based on limited information; monitor response

Carbamazepine: Tricyclic antidepressants may increase carbamazepine levels; monitor

Cholestyramine and colestipol: May bind TCAs and reduce their absorption; monitor for altered response

Clonidine: Abrupt discontinuation of clonidine may cause hypertensive crisis, amitriptyline may enhance the response

CNS depressants: Sedative effects may be additive with TCAs; monitor for increased effect; includes benzodiazepines, barbiturates, antipsychotics, ethanol and other sedative medications

CYP2D6 inhibitors: May increase the levels/effects of nortriptyline. Example inhibitors include chlorpromazine, delavirdine, fluoxetine, miconazole, paroxetine, pergolide, quinidine, quinine, ritonavir, and ropinirole.

Epinephrine (and other direct alpha-agonists): Pressor response to I.V. epinephrine, norepinephrine, and phenylephrine may be enhanced in patients receiving TCAs (**Note:** Effect is unlikely with epinephrine or levonordefrin dosages typically administered as infiltration in combination with local anesthetics)

Fenfluramine: May increase tricyclic antidepressant levels/effects

Hypoglycemic agents (including insulin): TCAs may enhance the hypoglycemic effects of tolazamide, chlorpropamide, or insulin; monitor for changes in blood glucose levels; reported with chlorpropamide, tolazamide, and insulin

Levodopa: Tricyclic antidepressants may decrease the absorption (bioavailability) of levodopa; rare hypertensive episodes have also been attributed to this combination

Linezolid: Hyperpyrexia, hypertension, tachycardia, confusion, seizures, and **deaths have been reported** with agents which inhibit MAO (serotonin syndrome); this combination should be avoided

Lithium: Concurrent use with a TCA may increase the risk for neurotoxicity

MAO inhibitors: Hyperpyrexia, hypertension, tachycardia, confusion, seizures, and **deaths have been reported** (serotonin syndrome); this combination should be avoided

Methylphenidate: Metabolism of TCAs may be decreased

Phenothiazines: Serum concentrations of some TCAs may be increased; in addition, TCAs may increase concentration of phenothiazines; monitor for altered clinical response

QT_c-prolonging agents: Concurrent use of tricyclic agents with other drugs which may prolong QT_c interval may increase the risk of potentially fatal arrhythmias; includes type Ia and type III antiarrhythmics agents, selected quinolones (sparfloxacin, gatifloxacin, moxifloxacin, grepafloxacin), cisapride, and other agents

Ritonavir: Combined use of high-dose tricyclic antidepressants with ritonavir may cause serotonin syndrome in HIV-positive patients; monitor

Sucralfate: Absorption of tricyclic antidepressants may be reduced with coadministration

Sympathomimetics, indirect-acting: Tricyclic antidepressants may result in a decreased sensitivity to indirect-acting sympathomimetics; includes dopamine and ephedrine; also see interaction with epinephrine (and direct-acting sympathomimetics)

Tramadol: Tramadol's risk of seizures may be increased with TCAs

Valproic acid: May increase serum concentrations/adverse effects of some tricyclic antidepressants

Warfarin (and other oral anticoagulants): TCAs may increase the anticoagulant effect in patients stabilized on warfarin; monitor INR

Ethanol/Nutrition/Herb Interactions

Ethanol: Avoid ethanol (may increase CNS depression).

Food: Grapefruit juice may inhibit the metabolism of some TCAs and clinical toxicity may result.

Herb/Nutraceutical: Avoid valerian, St John's wort, SAMe, kava kava (may increase risk of serotonin syndrome and/or excessive sedation).

Pharmacodynamics/Kinetics

Onset of action: Therapeutic: 1-3 weeks

Distribution: V_d: 21 L/kg

Protein binding: 93% to 95%

Metabolism: Primarily hepatic; extensive first-pass effect

Half-life elimination: 28-31 hours

Time to peak, serum: 7-8.5 hours

Excretion: Urine (as metabolites and small amounts of unchanged drug); feces (small amounts)

Pregnancy Risk Factor D

Lactation Enters breast milk/contraindicated (AAP rates "of concern")

Dosage Forms Excipient information presented when available (limited, particularly for generics); consult specific product labeling.

Capsule, as hydrochloride: 10 mg, 25 mg, 50 mg, 75 mg

Pamelor®: 10 mg, 25 mg, 50 mg, 75 mg [may contain benzyl alcohol; 50 mg may also contain sodium bisulfite]

Solution, as hydrochloride (Pamelor®): 10 mg/5 mL (473 mL) [contains alcohol 4% and benzoic acid]

Dental Comment Nortriptyline is known to prolong the QT interval. The QT interval is measured as the time and distance between the Q point of the QRS complex and the end of the T wave in the ECG tracing. After adjustment for heart rate, the QT interval is defined as prolonged if it is more than 450 msec in men and 460 msec in women. A long QT syndrome was first described in the 1950s and 60s as a congenital syndrome involving QT interval prolongation and syncope and sudden death. Some of the congenital long QT syndromes were characterized by a peculiar electrocardiographic appearance of the QRS complex involving a premature atria beat followed by a pause, then a subsequent sinus beat showing marked QT prolongation and deformity. This type of cardiac arrhythmia was originally termed "torsade de pointes" (translated from the French as "twisting of the points").

Prolongation of the QT interval is thought to result from delayed ventricular repolarization. The repolarization process within the myocardial cell is due to the efflux of intracellular potassium. The channels associated with this current can be blocked by many drugs and predispose the electrical propagation cycle to torsade de pointes.

Nortriptyline is considered as having a risk of causing torsade de pointes. The risk of drug-induced torsade de pointes is extremely low when a single QT interval prolonging drug is prescribed. It is not known what effect vasoconstrictors in the local anesthetic regimen will have in patients with a known history of congenital prolonged QT interval or in patients taking any medication that prolongs the QT interval. Until more information is obtained, it is suggested that the clinician consult with the physician prior to the use of a vasoconstrictor in (Continued)

Nortriptyline *(Continued)*

suspected patients, and that the vasoconstrictor (epinephrine, levonordefrin [Neo-Cobefrin®]) be used with caution.

Selected Readings

Friedlander AH and Mahler ME, "Major Depressive Disorder. Psychopathology, Medical Management, and Dental Implications," *J Am Dent Assoc,* 2001, 132(5):629-38.

Ganzberg S, "Psychoactive Drugs," *ADA Guide to Dental Therapeutics,* 2nd ed, Chicago, IL: ADA Publishing, a Division of ADA Business Enterprises, Inc, 2000, 376-405.

Jastak JT and Yagiela JA, "Vasoconstrictors and Local Anesthesia: A Review and Rationale for Use," *J Am Dent Assoc,* 1983, 107(4):623-30.

Rundegren J, van Dijken J, Mörnstad H, et al, "Oral Conditions in Patients Receiving Long-Term Treatment With Cyclic Antidepressant Drugs," *Swed Dent J,* 1985, 9(2):55-64.

Yagiela JA, "Adverse Drug Interactions in Dental Practice: Interactions Associated With Vasoconstrictors. Part V of a Series," *J Am Dent Assoc,* 1999, 130(5):701-9.

Nortriptyline Hydrochloride *see* Nortriptyline *on page 1188*

Norvasc® *see* Amlodipine *on page 101*

Norvir® *see* Ritonavir *on page 1436*

Nöstrilla® [OTC] *see* Oxymetazoline *on page 1236*

Novantrone® *see* Mitoxantrone *on page 1113*

Novarel® *see* Chorionic Gonadotropin (Human) *on page 352*

Novasal™ *see* Magnesium Salicylate *on page 1016*

Novocain® *see* Procaine *on page 1355*

Novolin® 70/30 *see* Insulin NPH and Insulin Regular *on page 888*

Novolin® N *see* Insulin NPH *on page 888*

Novolin® R *see* Insulin Regular *on page 889*

NovoLog® *see* Insulin Aspart *on page 883*

NovoLog® Mix 70/30 *see* Insulin Aspart Protamine and Insulin Aspart *on page 883*

NovoSeven® *see* Factor VIIa (Recombinant) *on page 666*

Noxafil® *see* Posaconazole *on page 1325*

NPH Insulin *see* Insulin NPH *on page 888*

NPH Insulin and Regular Insulin *see* Insulin NPH and Insulin Regular *on page 888*

NRP104 *see* Lisdexamfetamine *on page 989*

NRS® [OTC] *see* Oxymetazoline *on page 1236*

NSC-740 *see* Methotrexate *on page 1068*

NSC-750 *see* Busulfan *on page 246*

NSC-752 *see* Thioguanine *on page 1557*

NSC-755 *see* Mercaptopurine *on page 1051*

NSC-3053 *see* Dactinomycin *on page 437*

NSC-3088 *see* Chlorambucil *on page 329*

NSC-8806 *see* Melphalan *on page 1034*

NSC-13875 *see* Altretamine *on page 79*

NSC-15200 *see* Gallium Nitrate *on page 762*

NSC-26271 *see* Cyclophosphamide *on page 423*

NSC-26980 *see* Mitomycin *on page 1112*

NSC-27640 *see* Floxuridine *on page 696*

NSC-38721 *see* Mitotane *on page 1113*

NSC-49842 *see* VinBLAStine *on page 1658*

NSC-63878 *see* Cytarabine *on page 433*

NSC-66847 *see* Thalidomide *on page 1551*

NSC-67574 *see* VinCRIStine *on page 1659*

NSC-71423 *see* Megestrol *on page 1030*

NSC-77213 *see* Procarbazine *on page 1355*

NSC-79037 *see* Lomustine *on page 995*

NSC-82151 *see* DAUNOrubicin Hydrochloride *on page 450*

NSC-85998 *see* Streptozocin *on page 1497*

NSC-89199 *see* Estramustine *on page 605*

NSC-102816 *see* Azacitidine *on page 171*

NSC-105014 *see* Cladribine *on page 371*

NSC-106977 *(Erwinia) see* Asparaginase *on page 148*

NSC-109229 *(E. coli) see* Asparaginase *on page 148*

NSC-109724 *see* Ifosfamide *on page 861*

NSC-122758 *see* Tretinoin (Oral) *on page 1606*

NSC-123127 *see* DOXOrubicin *on page 536*

NSC-125066 *see* Bleomycin *on page 221*

NSC-125973 *see* Paclitaxel *on page 1240*

NSC-127716 *see* Decitabine *on page 451*

NSC-147834 *see* Flutamide *on page 725*

NSC-742319 *see* Panitumumab *on page 1248*

NTG *see* Nitroglycerin *on page 1181*

N-trifluoroacetyladriamycin-14-valerate *see* Valrubicin *on page 1642*

NTZ *see* Nitazoxanide *on page 1178*

Nubain® *see* Nalbuphine *on page 1142*

Nucofed® Expectorant [DSC] *see* Guaifenesin, Pseudoephedrine, and Codeine *on page 799*

Nucofed® Pediatric Expectorant [DSC] *see* Guaifenesin, Pseudoephedrine, and Codeine *on page 799*

Nu-Iron® 150 [OTC] *see* Polysaccharide-Iron Complex *on page 1323*

NuLev™ *see* Hyoscyamine *on page 847*

Nullo® [OTC] *see* Chlorophyll *on page 335*

NuLYTELY® *see* Polyethylene Glycol-Electrolyte Solution *on page 1321*

Numoisyn™ *see* Saliva Substitute *on page 1452*

Numorphan® *see* Oxymorphone *on page 1237*

Nupercainal® [OTC] *see* Dibucaine *on page 484*

Nupercainal® Hydrocortisone Cream [OTC] *see* Hydrocortisone *on page 836*

Nuquin HP® *see* Hydroquinone *on page 841*

Nu-Tears® [OTC] *see* Artificial Tears *on page 147*

Nu-Tears® II [OTC] *see* Artificial Tears *on page 147*

Nutracort® *see* Hydrocortisone *on page 836*

Nutralox® [OTC] *see* Calcium Carbonate *on page 260*

Nutraplus® [OTC] *see* Urea *on page 1632*

NutreStore™ *see* Glutamine *on page 786*

Nutropin® *see* Somatropin *on page 1486*

Nutropin AQ® *see* Somatropin *on page 1486*

NuvaRing® *see* Ethinyl Estradiol and Etonogestrel *on page 630*

NVB *see* Vinorelbine *on page 1661*

NVP *see* Nevirapine *on page 1165*

Nyamyc™ *see* Nystatin *on page 1194*

Nydrazid® [DSC] *see* Isoniazid *on page 912*

Nylidrin (NYE li drin)

Canadian Brand Names Arlidin®

Pharmacologic Category Vasodilator, Peripheral

Use Considered "possibly effective" for increasing blood supply to treat peripheral disease (arteriosclerosis obliterans, diabetic vascular disease, nocturnal leg cramps, Raynaud's disease, frost bite, ischemic ulcer, thrombophlebitis) and circulatory disturbances of the inner ear (cochlear ischemia, macular or ampullar ischemia, etc)

Local Anesthetic/Vasoconstrictor Precautions No information available to require special precautions

Effects on Dental Treatment No significant effects or complications reported

Common Adverse Effects
1% to 10%:
Central nervous system: Nervousness
Neuromuscular & skeletal: Trembling

Mechanism of Action Nylidrin is a peripheral vasodilator; this results from direct relaxation of vascular smooth muscle and beta-agonist action. Nylidrin does not appear to affect cutaneous blood flow; it reportedly increases heart rate and cardiac output; cutaneous blood flow is not enhanced to any appreciable extent.

Pregnancy Risk Factor C

Nystatin (nye STAT in)

Related Information
Fungal Infections *on page 1804*
Management of Patients Undergoing Cancer Therapy *on page 1826*
Treatment of Sexually-Transmitted Infections *on page 1920*

Related Sample Prescriptions
Topical Fungal Infections *on page 1841*

U.S. Brand Names Bio-Statin®; Mycostatin®; Nyamyc™; Nystat-Rx®; Nystop®; Pedi-Dri®

Canadian Brand Names Candistatin®; Nilstat; Nyaderm; PMS-Nystatin

Mexican Brand Names Mibesan-S; Micostatin

Generic Available Yes: Cream, ointment, powder, suspension, tablet

Pharmacologic Category Antifungal Agent, Oral Nonabsorbed; Antifungal Agent, Topical; Antifungal Agent, Vaginal

Dental Use Treatment of susceptible cutaneous, mucocutaneous, and oral cavity fungal infections normally caused by the *Candida* species

Use Treatment of susceptible cutaneous, mucocutaneous, and oral cavity fungal infections normally caused by the *Candida* species

Local Anesthetic/Vasoconstrictor Precautions No information available to require special precautions

Effects on Dental Treatment No significant effects or complications reported

Significant Adverse Effects

Frequency not defined: Dermatologic: Contact dermatitis, Stevens-Johnson syndrome

1% to 10%: Gastrointestinal: Nausea, vomiting, diarrhea, stomach pain

<1% (Limited to important or life-threatening): Hypersensitivity reactions

Dental Usual Dosing

Oral candidiasis:

Suspension (swish and swallow orally):

Premature infants: 100,000 units 4 times/day

Infants: 200,000 units 4 times/day or 100,000 units to each side of mouth 4 times/day

Children and Adults: 400,000-600,000 units 4 times/day

Mucocutaneous infections: Children and Adults: Topical: Apply 2-3 times/day to affected areas; very moist topical lesions are treated best with powder

Dosage

Oral candidiasis:

Suspension (swish and swallow orally):

Premature infants: 100,000 units 4 times/day

Infants: 200,000 units 4 times/day or 100,000 units to each side of mouth 4 times/day

Children and Adults: 400,000-600,000 units 4 times/day

Powder for compounding: Children and Adults: $1/_8$ teaspoon (500,000 units) to equal approximately $1/_2$ cup of water; give 4 times/day

Mucocutaneous infections: Children and Adults: Topical: Apply 2-3 times/day to affected areas; very moist topical lesions are treated best with powder

Intestinal infections: Adults: Oral: 500,000-1,000,000 units every 8 hours

Vaginal infections: Adults: Vaginal tablets: Insert 1 tablet/day at bedtime for 2 weeks

Mechanism of Action Binds to sterols in fungal cell membrane, changing the cell wall permeability allowing for leakage of cellular contents

Contraindications Hypersensitivity to nystatin or any component of the formulation

Drug Interactions No data reported

Pharmacodynamics/Kinetics

Onset of action: Symptomatic relief from candidiasis: 24-72 hours

Absorption: Topical: None through mucous membranes or intact skin; Oral: Poorly absorbed

Excretion: Feces (as unchanged drug)

Pregnancy Risk Factor B/C (oral)

Lactation Does not enter breast milk/compatible (not absorbed orally)

Dosage Forms Excipient information presented when available (limited, particularly for generics); consult specific product labeling.

Capsule:

Bio-Statin®: 500,000 units, 1 million units

Cream: 100,000 units/g (15 g, 30 g)

Mycostatin®: 100,000 units/g (30 g)

Ointment, topical: 100,000 units/g (15 g, 30 g)

Powder, for prescription compounding: 50 million units (10 g); 150 million units (30 g); 500 million units (100 g); 2 billion units (400 g)

Nystat-Rx®: 50 million units (10 g); 150 million units (30 g); 500 million units (100 g); 1 billion units (190 g); 2 billion units (350 g)

Powder, topical:

Mycostatin®: 100,000 units/g (15 g) [contains talc]

Nyamyc™: 100,000 units/g (15 g, 30 g) [contains talc]

Nystop®: 100,000 units/g (15 g, 30 g, 60 g) [contains talc]

Pedi-Dri®: 100,000 units/g (56.7 g) [contains talc]

Suspension, oral: 100,000 units/mL (5 mL, 60 mL, 480 mL)

Tablet: 500,000 units

Tablet, vaginal: 100,000 units (15s) [packaged with applicator]

Nystatin and Triamcinolone (nye STAT in & trye am SIN oh lone)

Related Information
Fungal Infections on page 1804
Nystatin on page 1194
Triamcinolone on page 1608

Related Sample Prescriptions
Angular Cheilitis on page 1842

U.S. Brand Names Mycolog®-II [DSC]

Generic Available Yes

Index Terms Triamcinolone and Nystatin

Pharmacologic Category Antifungal Agent, Topical; Corticosteroid, Topical

Dental Use Treatment of angular cheilitis and cutaneous candidiasis

Use Treatment of cutaneous candidiasis

Local Anesthetic/Vasoconstrictor Precautions No information available to require special precautions

Effects on Dental Treatment No significant effects or complications reported

Significant Adverse Effects 1% to 10%:
Dermatologic: Dryness, folliculitis, hypertrichosis, acne, hypopigmentation, allergic dermatitis, maceration of the skin, skin atrophy
Local: Burning, itching, irritation
Miscellaneous: Increased incidence of secondary infection

Dental Usual Dosing
Angular cheilitis and cutaneous candidiasis: Children and Adults: Topical: Apply sparingly 2-4 times/day. Therapy should be discontinued when control is achieved; if no improvement is seen, reassessment of diagnosis may be necessary.

Dosage Children and Adults: Topical: Apply sparingly 2-4 times/day. Therapy should be discontinued when control is achieved; if no improvement is seen, reassessment of diagnosis may be necessary.

Mechanism of Action Nystatin is an antifungal agent that binds to sterols in fungal cell membrane, changing the cell wall permeability allowing for leakage of cellular contents. Triamcinolone is a synthetic corticosteroid; it decreases inflammation by suppression of migration of polymorphonuclear leukocytes and reversal of increased capillary permeability. It suppresses the immune system reducing activity and volume of the lymphatic system. It suppresses adrenal function at high doses.

Contraindications Hypersensitivity to nystatin, triamcinolone, or any component of the formulation

Warnings/Precautions Avoid use of occlusive dressings; limit therapy to least amount necessary for effective therapy, pediatric patients may be more susceptible to HPA axis suppression due to larger BSA to weight ratio

Drug Interactions No data reported

Pharmacodynamics/Kinetics See individual agents.

Pregnancy Risk Factor C

Lactation Excretion in breast milk unknown

Breast-Feeding Considerations
Nystatin: Compatible
Triamcinolone: No data reported

Dosage Forms Excipient information presented when available (limited, particularly for generics); consult specific product labeling. [DSC] = Discontinued product
Cream (Mycolog®-II [DSC]): Nystatin 100,000 units and triamcinolone acetonide 0.1% (15 g, 30 g, 60 g)
Ointment: Nystatin 100,000 units and triamcinolone acetonide 0.1% (15 g, 30 g, 60 g)
Mycolog®-II: Nystatin 100,000 units and triamcinolone acetonide 0.1% (15 g, 30 g, 60 g) [DSC]

Nystat-Rx® see Nystatin on page 1194

Nystop® see Nystatin on page 1194

Nytol® Quick Caps [OTC] see DiphenhydrAMINE on page 510

Nytol® Quick Gels [OTC] see DiphenhydrAMINE on page 510

OCBZ see Oxcarbazepine on page 1221

Occlusal®-HP [OTC] see Salicylic Acid on page 1451

Ocean® [OTC] see Sodium Chloride on page 1480

Oceant® for Kids [OTC] see Sodium Chloride on page 1480

Octagam® see Immune Globulin (Intravenous) on page 870

Octreotide (ok TREE oh tide)

U.S. Brand Names Sandostatin®; Sandostatin LAR®

Canadian Brand Names Octreotide Acetate Injection; Octreotide Acetate Omega; Sandostatin®; Sandostatin LAR®

Mexican Brand Names Sandostatina; Sandostatina LAR

Generic Available Yes: Solution

Index Terms NSC-671663; Octreotide Acetate

Pharmacologic Category Antidiarrheal; Somatostatin Analog

Use Control of symptoms in patients with metastatic carcinoid and vasoactive intestinal peptide-secreting tumors (VIPomas); acromegaly

Unlabeled/Investigational Use AIDS-associated secretory diarrhea (including *Cryptosporidiosis*); control of bleeding of esophageal varices; breast cancer; cryptosporidiosis; Cushing's syndrome (ectopic); insulinomas; small bowel fistulas; pancreatic tumors; gastrinoma; postgastrectomy dumping syndrome; chemotherapy-induced diarrhea; graft-versus-host disease (GVHD) induced diarrhea; Zollinger-Ellison syndrome; congenital hyperinsulinism; hypothalamic obesity

Local Anesthetic/Vasoconstrictor Precautions Octreotide is one of the drugs confirmed to prolong the QT interval and is accepted as having a risk of causing torsade de pointes. The risk of drug-induced torsade de pointes is extremely low when a single QT interval prolonging drug is prescribed. In terms of epinephrine, it is not known what effect vasoconstrictors in the local anesthetic regimen will have in patients with a known history of congenital prolonged QT interval or in patients taking any medication that prolongs the QT interval. Until more information is obtained, it is suggested that the clinician consult with the physician prior to the use of a vasoconstrictor in suspected patients, and that the vasoconstrictor (epinephrine, levonordefrin [Neo-Cobefrin®]) be used with caution.

Effects on Dental Treatment Key adverse event(s) related to dental treatment: Xerostomia (normal salivary flow resumes upon discontinuation), gingivitis, glossitis, stomatitis, taste perversion, and dysphagia.

Common Adverse Effects Adverse reactions vary by route of administration. Frequency of cardiac, endocrine, and gastrointestinal adverse reactions was generally higher in acromegalics.

>16%:

  Cardiovascular: Sinus bradycardia (19% to 25%), chest pain (16% to 20%)

  Central nervous system: Fatigue (1% to 20%), malaise (16% to 20%), dizziness (5% to 20%), headache (6% to 20%), fever (16% to 20%)

  Endocrine & metabolic: Hyperglycemia (15% to 27%)

  Gastrointestinal: Diarrhea (36% to 58%), abdominal discomfort (5% to 61%), flatulence (<10% to 38%), constipation (9% to 21%), nausea (5% to 61%), cholelithiasis (27%; length of therapy dependent), biliary duct dilatation (12%), biliary sludge (24%; length of therapy dependent), loose stools (5% to 61%), vomiting (4% to 21%)

  Hematologic: Antibodies to octreotide (up to 25%; no efficacy change)

  Local: Injection pain (2% to 50%; dose and formulation related)

  Neuromuscular & skeletal: Backache (1% to 20%), arthropathy (16% to 20%)

  Respiratory: Dyspnea (16% to 20%), upper respiratory infection (16% to 20%)

  Miscellaneous: Flu symptoms (1% to 20%)

5% to 15%:

  Cardiovascular: Conduction abnormalities (9% to 10%), arrhythmia (3% to 9%), hypertension, palpitation, peripheral edema

  Central nervous system: Anxiety, confusion, depression, hypoesthesia, insomnia

  Dermatologic: Pruritus, rash

  Endocrine & metabolic: Hypothyroidism (2% to 12%), goiter (2% to 8%)

  Gastrointestinal: Abdominal pain, anorexia, cramping, dehydration, discomfort, hemorrhoids, tenesmus (4% to 15%), dyspepsia (4% to 15%), steatorrhea (4% to 6%), feces discoloration (4% to 6%), weight loss

  Genitourinary: UTI

  Hematologic: Anemia

  Hepatic: Hepatitis

  Neuromuscular & skeletal: Arthralgia, leg cramps, myalgia, paresthesia, rigors, weakness

  Otic: Earache, otitis media

  Renal: Renal calculus

  Respiratory: coughing, pharyngitis, sinusitis, rhinitis

  Miscellaneous: Allergy, diaphoresis

1% to 4%:

  Cardiovascular: Angina, cardiac failure, cerebral vascular disorder, edema, flushing, hematoma, phlebitis, tachycardia

(Continued)

Octreotide *(Continued)*

Central nervous system: Abnormal gait, amnesia, dysphonia, hallucinations, nervousness, neuralgia, neuropathy, somnolence, tremor, vertigo

Dermatologic: Acne, alopecia, bruising, cellulitis, urticaria

Endocrine & metabolic: Hypoglycemia (2% to 4%), hypokalemia, hypoproteinemia, gout, cachexia, menstrual irregularities, breast pain, impotence

Gastrointestinal: Colitis, diverticulitis, dysphagia, fat malabsorption, gastritis, gastroenteritis, gingivitis, glossitis, melena, rectal bleeding, stomatitis, taste perversion, xerostomia

Genitourinary: Incontinence

Hematologic: Epistaxis

Hepatic: Ascites, jaundice

Local: Injection hematoma

Neuromuscular & skeletal: Hyperkinesia, hypertonia, joint pain

Ocular: Blurred vision, visual disturbance

Otic: Tinnitus

Renal: Albuminuria, renal abscess

Respiratory: Bronchitis, pleural effusion, pneumonia, pulmonary embolism

Miscellaneous: Bacterial infection, cold symptoms, moniliasis

Mechanism of Action Mimics natural somatostatin by inhibiting serotonin release, and the secretion of gastrin, VIP, insulin, glucagon, secretin, motilin, and pancreatic polypeptide. Decreases growth hormone and IGF-1 in acromegaly.

Drug Interactions

Increased Effect/Toxicity: Bioavailability of bromocriptine may be increased by octreotide. Octreotide may enhance the adverse/toxic effects of other QT_c-prolonging agents.

Decreased Effect: Octreotide may lower cyclosporine serum levels (case reports of transplant rejection due to reduction of serum cyclosporine levels when cyclosporine was given orally in conjunction with a somatostatin analogue).

Pharmacodynamics/Kinetics

Duration: SubQ: 6-12 hours

Absorption: SubQ: Rapid

Distribution: V_d: 14 L (13-30 L in acromegaly)

Protein binding: 65%, mainly to lipoprotein (41% in acromegaly)

Metabolism: Extensively hepatic

Bioavailability: SubQ: 100%; I.M: 60% to 63% of SubQ dose

Half-life elimination: 1.7-1.9 hours; up to 3.7 hours with cirrhosis

Time to peak, plasma: SubQ: 0.4 hours (0.7 hours acromegaly); I.M.: 1 hour

Excretion: Urine (32%)

Pregnancy Risk Factor B

Octreotide Acetate *see* Octreotide *on page 1197*

OcuCoat® [OTC] *see* Artificial Tears *on page 147*

OcuCoat® PF [OTC] *see* Artificial Tears *on page 147*

Ocufen® *see* Flurbiprofen *on page 722*

Ocuflox® *see* Ofloxacin *on page 1198*

OcuNefrin™ [OTC] *see* Phenylephrine *on page 1293*

Ocupress® [DSC] *see* Carteolol *on page 290*

Ocuvite® [OTC] *see* Vitamins (Multiple/Oral) *on page 1665*

Ocuvite® Extra® [OTC] *see* Vitamins (Multiple/Oral) *on page 1665*

Ocuvite® Lutein [OTC] *see* Vitamins (Multiple/Oral) *on page 1665*

Ofloxacin *(oh FLOKS a sin)*

Related Information

Sexually-Transmitted Diseases *on page 1766*

Tuberculosis Treatment *on page 1909*

U.S. Brand Names Floxin®; Ocuflox®

Canadian Brand Names Apo-Oflox®; Apo-Ofloxacin®; Floxin®; Novo-Ofloxacin; Ocuflox®; PMS-Ofloxacin

Mexican Brand Names Bactocin; Floxil; Floxstat; Ocuflox

Generic Available Yes: Tablet, ophthalmic solution

Index Terms Floxin Otic Singles

Pharmacologic Category Antibiotic, Quinolone

Use Quinolone antibiotic for the treatment of acute exacerbations of chronic bronchitis, community-acquired pneumonia, skin and skin structure infections (uncomplicated), urethral and cervical gonorrhea (acute, uncomplicated), urethritis and cervicitis (nongonococcal), mixed infections of the urethra and cervix, pelvic inflammatory disease (acute), cystitis (uncomplicated), urinary tract infections (complicated), prostatitis

Note: As of April 2007, the CDC no longer recommends the use of fluoroquinolones for the treatment of gonococcal disease.

Ophthalmic: Treatment of superficial ocular infections involving the conjunctiva or cornea due to strains of susceptible organisms

Otic: Otitis externa, chronic suppurative otitis media, acute otitis media

Unlabeled/Investigational Use Epididymitis (nongonococcal), leprosy, Traveler's diarrhea

Local Anesthetic/Vasoconstrictor Precautions No information available to require special precautions

Effects on Dental Treatment Key adverse event(s) related to dental treatment: Xerostomia (normal salivary flow resumes upon discontinuation) and abnormal taste.

Common Adverse Effects

Systemic:

1% to 10%:

Cardiovascular: Chest pain (1% to 3%)

Central nervous system: Headache (1% to 9%), insomnia (3% to 7%), dizziness (1% to 5%), fatigue (1% to 3%), somnolence (1% to 3%), sleep disorders (1% to 3%), nervousness (1% to 3%), pyrexia (1% to 3%)

Dermatologic: Rash/pruritus (1% to 3%)

Gastrointestinal: Diarrhea (1% to 4%), vomiting (1% to 4%), GI distress (1% to 3%), abdominal cramps (1% to 3%), flatulence (1% to 3%), abnormal taste (1% to 3%), xerostomia (1% to 3%), appetite decreased (1% to 3%), nausea (3% to 10%), constipation (1% to 3%)

Genitourinary: Vaginitis (1% to 5%), external genital pruritus in women (1% to 3%)

Ocular: Visual disturbances (1% to 3%)

Respiratory: Pharyngitis (1% to 3%)

Miscellaneous: Trunk pain

Ophthalmic: Frequency not defined:

Central nervous system: Dizziness

Gastrointestinal: Nausea

Ocular: Blurred vision, burning, chemical conjunctivitis/keratitis, discomfort, dryness, edema, eye pain, foreign body sensation, itching, photophobia, redness, stinging, tearing

Otic:

>10%: Local: Application site reaction (<1% to 17%)

1% to 10%:

Central nervous system: Dizziness (≤1%), vertigo (≤1%)

Dermatologic: Pruritus (1% to 4%), rash (1%)

Gastrointestinal: Taste perversion (7%)

Neuromuscular & skeletal: Paresthesia (1%)

Mechanism of Action Ofloxacin is a DNA gyrase inhibitor. DNA gyrase is an essential bacterial enzyme that maintains the superhelical structure of DNA. DNA gyrase is required for DNA replication and transcription, DNA repair, recombination, and transposition; bactericidal

Drug Interactions

Cytochrome P450 Effect: Inhibits CYP1A2 (strong)

Increased Effect/Toxicity: Ofloxacin may increase the effects/toxicity of CYP1A2 substrates (eg, aminophylline, fluvoxamine, mexiletine, mirtazapine, ropinirole, and trifluoperazine), glyburide, theophylline, and warfarin. Concomitant use with corticosteroids may increase the risk of tendon rupture. Concomitant use with other QT$_c$-prolonging agents (eg, Class Ia and Class III antiarrhythmics, erythromycin, cisapride, antipsychotics, and cyclic antidepressants) may result in arrhythmias, such as torsade de pointes. Probenecid may increase ofloxacin levels. Concomitant use with NSAIDs may rarely increase risk of seizure.

Decreased Effect: Concurrent administration of metal cations, including most antacids, oral electrolyte supplements, quinapril, sucralfate, some didanosine formulations (pediatric powder for oral suspension), and other highly-buffered oral drugs, may decrease quinolone levels; separate doses.

Pharmacodynamics/Kinetics

Absorption: Well absorbed; food causes only minor alterations

Distribution: V$_d$: 2.4-3.5 L/kg

Protein binding: 20%

Bioavailability: Oral: 98%

Half-life elimination: Biphasic: 5-7.5 hours and 20-25 hours (accounts for <5%); prolonged with renal impairment

Excretion: Primarily urine (as unchanged drug)

Pregnancy Risk Factor C

Ogen® *see* Estropipate *on page 615*

Ogestrel® *see* Ethinyl Estradiol and Norgestrel *on page 649*

OGMT *see* Metyrosine *on page 1094*

OGT-918 *see* Miglustat *on page 1105*

9-OH-risperidone *see* Paliperidone *on page 1243*

OKT3 *see* Muromonab-CD3 *on page 1133*

Olanzapine (oh LAN za peen)

U.S. Brand Names Zyprexa®; Zyprexa® Zydis®

Canadian Brand Names Zyprexa®; Zyprexa® Zydis®

Mexican Brand Names Zyprexa

Generic Available No

Index Terms LY170053; Zyprexa Zydis

Pharmacologic Category Antipsychotic Agent, Atypical

Use Treatment of the manifestations of schizophrenia; treatment of acute or mixed mania episodes associated with Bipolar I Disorder (as monotherapy or in combination with lithium or valproate); maintenance treatment of bipolar disorder; acute agitation (patients with schizophrenia or bipolar mania)

Unlabeled/Investigational Use Treatment of psychosis/schizophrenia in children or adolescents; chronic pain

Local Anesthetic/Vasoconstrictor Precautions No information available to require special precautions

Effects on Dental Treatment No significant effects or complications reported

Common Adverse Effects

>10%:

Central nervous system: Somnolence (6% to 39% dose dependent), extrapyramidal symptoms (15% to 32% dose dependent), insomnia (up to 12%), dizziness (4% to 18%)

Gastrointestinal: Dyspepsia (7% to 11%), constipation (9% to 11%), weight gain (5% to 6%, has been reported as high as 40%), xerostomia (9% to 22% dose dependent)

Neuromuscular & skeletal: Weakness (2% to 20% dose dependent)

Miscellaneous: Accidental injury (12%)

1% to 10%:

Cardiovascular: Postural hypotension (1% to 5%), tachycardia (up to 3%), peripheral edema (up to 3%), chest pain (up to 3%), hyper-/hypotension (up to 2%)

Central nervous system: Personality changes (8%), speech disorder (7%), fever (up to 6%), abnormal dreams, euphoria, amnesia, delusions, emotional lability, mania, schizophrenia

Dermatologic: Bruising (up to 5%)

Endocrine & metabolic: Cholesterol increased, prolactin increased

Gastrointestinal: Nausea (up to 9% dose dependent), appetite increased (3% to 6%), vomiting (up to 4%), flatulence, salivation increased, thirst

Genitourinary: Incontinence (up to 2%), UTI (up to 2%), vaginitis

Hepatic: ALT increased (2%)

Local: Injection site pain (I.M. administration)

Neuromuscular & skeletal: Tremor (1% to 7% dose dependent), abnormal gait (6%), back pain (up to 5%), joint/extremity pain (up to 5%), akathisia (3% to 5% dose dependent), hypertonia (up to 3%), articulation impairment (up to 2%), falling (particularly in older patients), joint stiffness, paresthesia, twitching

Ocular: Amblyopia (up to 3%), conjunctivitis

Respiratory: Rhinitis (up to 7%), cough (up to 6%), pharyngitis (up to 4%), dyspnea

Miscellaneous: Dental pain, diaphoresis, flu-like syndrome

Dosage

Children: Schizophrenia/bipolar disorder (unlabeled use): Oral: Initial: 2.5 mg/day; titrate as necessary to 20 mg/day (0.12-0.29 mg/kg/day)

Adults:

Schizophrenia: Oral: Initial: 5-10 mg once daily (increase to 10 mg once daily within 5-7 days); thereafter, adjust by 5 mg/day at 1-week intervals, up to a recommended maximum of 20 mg/day. Maintenance: 10-20 mg once daily. **Note:** Doses of 30-50 mg/day have been used; however, doses >10 mg/day have not demonstrated better efficacy, and safety and efficacy of doses >20 mg/day have not been evaluated.

Bipolar I acute mixed or manic episodes: Oral:

Monotherapy: Initial: 10-15 mg once daily; increase by 5 mg/day at intervals of not less than 24 hours. Maintenance: 5-20 mg/day; recommended maximum dose: 20 mg/day.

Combination therapy (with lithium or valproate): Initial: 10 mg once daily; dosing range: 5-20 mg/day

Agitation (acute, associated with bipolar I mania or schizophrenia): I.M.: Initial dose: 5-10 mg (a lower dose of 2.5 mg may be considered when clinical factors warrant); additional doses (2.5-10 mg) may be considered; however, 2-4 hours should be allowed between doses to evaluate response (maximum total daily dose: 30 mg, per manufacturer's recommendation)

Elderly: Oral, I.M.: Consider lower starting dose of 2.5-5 mg/day for elderly or debilitated patients; may increase as clinically indicated and tolerated with close monitoring of orthostatic blood pressure

Dosage adjustment in renal impairment: No adjustment required. Not removed by dialysis.

Dosage adjustment in hepatic impairment: Dosage adjustment may be necessary, however, there are no specific recommendations. Monitor closely.

Mechanism of Action Olanzapine is a second generation thienobenzodiazepine antipsychotic which displays potent antagonist of serotonin 5-HT$_{2A}$ and 5-HT$_{2C}$, dopamine D$_{1-4}$, muscarinic M$_{1-5}$, histamine H$_1$- and alpha$_1$-adrenergic receptors. Olanzapine shows moderate antagonism of 5-HT$_3$ and muscarinic M$_{1-5}$ receptors, and weak binding to GABA-A, BZD, and beta-adrenergic receptors. Although the precise mechanism of action in schizophrenia and bipolar disorder is not known, the efficacy of olanzapine is thought to be mediated through combined antagonism of dopamine and serotonin type 2 receptor sites.

Contraindications Hypersensitivity to olanzapine or any component of the formulation

Warnings/Precautions [U.S. Boxed Warning]: Patients with dementia-related psychosis treated with atypical antipsychotics are at an increased risk of death compared to placebo. An increased incidence of cerebrovascular adverse events (including fatalities) has been reported in elderly patients with dementia-related psychosis. Risk may be increased by dehydration; use caution with concurrent diuretics. Olanzapine is not approved for this indication.

Moderate to highly sedating, use with caution in disorders where CNS depression is a feature; patients must be cautioned about performing tasks which require mental alertness (eg, operating machinery or driving). Use caution in patients with cardiac disease. Use with caution in Parkinson's disease, predisposition to seizures, or severe hepatic or renal disease. Life-threatening arrhythmias have occurred with therapeutic doses of some neuroleptics. May induce orthostatic hypotension; use caution with history of cardiovascular disease. Esophageal dysmotility and aspiration have been associated with antipsychotic use; use with caution in patients at risk of aspiration pneumonia. Caution in breast cancer or other prolactin-dependent tumors (elevates prolactin levels). Significant weight gain may occur; monitor waist circumference and BMI. Impaired core body temperature regulation may occur; caution with strenuous exercise, heat exposure, dehydration, and concomitant medication possessing anticholinergic effects.

May cause anticholinergic effects; use with caution in patients with decreased gastrointestinal motility, urinary retention, BPH, xerostomia, glaucoma, or myasthenia gravis. Relative to other neuroleptics, olanzapine has a moderate potency of cholinergic blockade. May cause extrapyramidal symptoms, although risk of these reactions is lower relative to other neuroleptics. May be associated with neuroleptic malignant syndrome (NMS). May cause extreme and life-threatening hyperglycemia; use with caution in patients with diabetes or other disorders of glucose regulation; monitor. Olanzapine levels may be lower in patients who smoke, requiring dosage adjustment.

The possibility of a suicide attempt is inherent in psychotic illness or bipolar disorder; use caution in high-risk patients during initiation of therapy. Prescriptions should be written for the smallest quantity consistent with good patient care. Safety and efficacy in pediatric patients have not been established.

Intramuscular administration: Patients should remain recumbent if drowsy/dizzy until hypotension, bradycardia and/or hypoventilation has been ruled out. Concurrent use of I.M./I.V. benzodiazepines is not recommended (fatalities have been reported, though causality not determined).

Drug Interactions

Cytochrome P450 Effect: Substrate of CYP1A2 (major), 2D6 (minor); **Inhibits** CYP1A2 (weak), 2C9 (weak), 2C19 (weak), 2D6 (weak), 3A4 (weak)

Increased Effect/Toxicity: Olanzapine levels may be increased by CYP1A2 inhibitors such as cimetidine and fluvoxamine. Sedation from olanzapine is increased with ethanol or other CNS depressants. Concomitant use with pramlintide and other anticholinergic agents may result in increased anticholinergic adverse effects. Concomitant use with ciprofloxacin may increase the levels/effects of olanzapine. Use of acetylcholinesterase inhibitors (central) or lithium may increase the risk of antipsychotic-related EPS. Concurrent use of (Continued)

Olanzapine (Continued)

intramuscular olanzapine and parenteral benzodiazepines may increase the risk of cardiopulmonary toxicity.

Decreased Effect: Olanzapine levels may be decreased by CYP1A2 inducers such as rifampin, omeprazole, and carbamazepine (also cigarette smoking).

Ethanol/Nutrition/Herb Interactions

Ethanol: Avoid ethanol (may increase CNS depression).

Herb/Nutraceutical: Avoid dong quai, St John's wort (may also cause photosensitization). Avoid kava kava, gotu kola, valerian, St John's wort (may increase CNS depression).

Dietary Considerations Tablets may be taken with or without food. Zyprexa® Zydis®: 5 mg tablet contains phenylalanine 0.34 mg; 10 mg tablet contains phenylalanine 0.45 mg; 15 mg tablet contains phenylalanine 0.67 mg; 20 mg tablet contains phenylalanine 0.9 mg.

Pharmacodynamics/Kinetics

Absorption:

I.M.: Rapidly absorbed

Oral: Well absorbed; not affected by food; tablets and orally-disintegrating tablets are bioequivalent

Distribution: V_d: Extensive, 1000 L

Protein binding, plasma: 93% bound to albumin and alpha$_1$-glycoprotein

Metabolism: Highly metabolized via direct glucuronidation and cytochrome P450 mediated oxidation (CYP1A2, CYP2D6); 40% removed via first pass metabolism

Bioavailability: >57%

Half-life elimination: 21-54 hours; ~1.5 times greater in elderly

Time to peak, plasma: Maximum plasma concentrations after I.M. administration are 5 times higher than maximum plasma concentrations produced by an oral dose.

I.M.: 15-45 minutes

Oral: ~6 hours

Excretion: Urine (57%, 7% as unchanged drug); feces (30%)

Clearance: 40% increase in olanzapine clearance in smokers; 30% decrease in females

Pregnancy Risk Factor C

Dosage Forms

Injection, powder for reconstitution:

Zyprexa® IntraMuscular: 10 mg

Tablet:

Zyprexa®: 2.5 mg, 5 mg, 7.5 mg, 10 mg, 15 mg, 20 mg

Tablet, orally disintegrating:

Zyprexa® Zydis®: 5 mg, 10 mg, 15 mg, 20 mg

Olanzapine and Fluoxetine (oh LAN za peen & floo OKS e teen)

Related Information

Fluoxetine *on page 714*

Olanzapine *on page 1200*

U.S. Brand Names Symbyax™

Generic Available No

Index Terms Fluoxetine and Olanzapine; Olanzapine and Fluoxetine Hydrochloride

Pharmacologic Category Antidepressant, Selective Serotonin Reuptake Inhibitor; Antipsychotic Agent, Atypical

Use Treatment of depressive episodes associated with bipolar disorder

Local Anesthetic/Vasoconstrictor Precautions No information available to require special precautions

Effects on Dental Treatment Key adverse event(s) related to dental treatment: Xerostomia or salivation increased (normal salivary flow resumes upon discontinuation), tooth disorder, and taste perversion.

Common Adverse Effects As reported with combination product (also see individual agents):

>10%:

Central nervous system: Somnolence (21% to 22%)

Gastrointestinal: Weight gain (17% to 21%), diarrhea (8% to 19%), appetite increased (13% to 16%), xerostomia (11% to 16%)

Neuromuscular & skeletal: Weakness (13% to 15%)

1% to 10%:

Cardiovascular: Peripheral edema (4% to 8%), edema (up to 5%), hypertension (2%), tachycardia (2%), vasodilation

Central nervous system: Thinking abnormal (6%), fever (3% to 4%), amnesia (1% to 3%), personality disorder (1% to 2%), sleep disorder (1% to 2%), speech disorder (up to 2%), chills, migraine

Dermatologic: Photosensitivity

Endocrine & metabolic: Ejaculation abnormal (2% to 7%), impotence (2% to 4%), libido decreased (2% to 4%), anorgasmia (1% to 3%), breast pain, menorrhagia

Gastrointestinal: Tooth disorder (1% to 2%), salivation increased, taste perversion, thirst, weight loss

Genitourinary: Urinary frequency, urinary incontinence, urinary tract infection

Neuromuscular & skeletal: Tremor (8% to 9%), twitching (2% to 6%), arthralgia (3% to 5%), hyperkinesias (1% to 2%), joint disorder (1% to 2%), bruising, neck pain/rigidity

Ocular: Amblyopia (4% to 5%), vision abnormal

Otic: Ear pain (1% to 2%), otitis media (up to 2%), tinnitus

Respiratory: Pharyngitis (4% to 6%), dyspnea (1% to 2%), bronchitis, lung disorder

Frequency not defined: Alkaline phosphate increased, cholesterol increased, GGT increased, hemoglobin decreased, prolactin increased, uric acid increased

Restrictions An FDA-approved medication guide concerning the use of antidepressants in children, adolescents, and young adults must be distributed when dispensing an outpatient prescription (new or refill) where this medication is to be used without direct supervision of a healthcare provider. Medication guides are available at http://www.fda.gov/cder/Offices/ODS/medication_guides.htm. Dispense to parents or guardians of children and adolescents receiving this medication.

Mechanism of Action Olanzapine is a thienobenzodiazepine antipsychotic (neuroleptic) which is thought to work by antagonizing dopamine and serotonin activities. It is a selective monoaminergic antagonist with high affinity binding to serotonin 5-HT$_{2A}$ and 5-HT$_{2C}$, dopamine D$_{1-4}$, muscarinic M$_{1-5}$, histamine H$_1$- and alpha$_1$-adrenergic receptor sites. Olanzapine binds weakly to GABA-A, BZD, and beta-adrenergic receptors. Fluoxetine inhibits CNS neuron serotonin reuptake; minimal or no effect on reuptake of norepinephrine or dopamine; does not significantly bind to alpha-adrenergic, histamine, or cholinergic receptors. The enhanced antidepressant effect of the combination may be due to synergistic increases in serotonin, norepinephrine, and dopamine.

Pharmacodynamics/Kinetics See individual agents.

Pregnancy Risk Factor C

Olmesartan (ole me SAR tan)

U.S. Brand Names Benicar®
Generic Available No
Index Terms Olmesartan Medoxomil
Pharmacologic Category Angiotensin II Receptor Blocker
Use Treatment of hypertension with or without concurrent use of other antihypertensive agents
Local Anesthetic/Vasoconstrictor Precautions No information available to require special precautions
Effects on Dental Treatment No significant effects or complications reported
Common Adverse Effects 1% to 10%:
Central nervous system: Dizziness (3%), headache
Endocrine & metabolic: Hyperglycemia, hypertriglyceridemia
Gastrointestinal: Diarrhea
Neuromuscular & skeletal: Back pain, CPK increased
Renal: Hematuria
Respiratory: Bronchitis, pharyngitis, rhinitis, sinusitis
Miscellaneous: Flu-like syndrome
(Continued)

Olmesartan *(Continued)*

Mechanism of Action As a selective and competitive, nonpeptide angiotensin II receptor antagonist, olmesartan blocks the vasoconstrictor and aldosterone-secreting effects of angiotensin II; olmesartan interacts reversibly at the AT1 and AT2 receptors of many tissues and has slow dissociation kinetics; its affinity for the AT1 receptor is 12,500 times greater than the AT2 receptor. Angiotensin II receptor antagonists may induce a more complete inhibition of the renin-angiotensin system than ACE inhibitors, they do not affect the response to bradykinin, and are less likely to be associated with nonrenin-angiotensin effects (eg, cough and angioedema). Olmesartan increases urinary flow rate and, in addition to being natriuretic and kaliuretic, increases excretion of chloride, magnesium, uric acid, calcium, and phosphate.

Drug Interactions

Increased Effect/Toxicity: The risk of hyperkalemia may be increased during concomitant use with potassium-sparing diuretics, potassium supplements, and trimethoprim; may increase risk of lithium toxicity.

Decreased Effect: NSAIDs may decrease the efficacy of olmesartan.

Pharmacodynamics/Kinetics

Distribution: 17 L; does not cross the blood-brain barrier (animal studies)

Protein binding: 99%

Metabolism: Olmesartan medoxomil is hydrolyzed in the GI tract to active olmesartan. No further metabolism occurs.

Bioavailability: 26%

Half-life elimination: Terminal: 13 hours

Time to peak: 1-2 hours

Excretion: All as unchanged drug: Feces (50% to 65%); urine (35% to 50%)

Pregnancy Risk Factor C/D (2nd and 3rd trimesters)

Olmesartan and Hydrochlorothiazide
(ole me SAR tan & hye droe klor oh THYE a zide)

Related Information

Hydrochlorothiazide *on page 819*

Olmesartan *on page 1203*

U.S. Brand Names Benicar HCT®

Generic Available No

Index Terms Hydrochlorothiazide and Olmesartan Medoxomil; Olmesartan Medoxomil and Hydrochlorothiazide

Pharmacologic Category Angiotensin II Receptor Blocker Combination; Antihypertensive Agent, Combination; Diuretic, Thiazide

Use Treatment of hypertension (not recommended for initial treatment)

Local Anesthetic/Vasoconstrictor Precautions No information available to require special precautions

Effects on Dental Treatment No significant effects or complications reported

Common Adverse Effects Frequencies reported with combination product. See individual monographs for additional adverse effects reported with each agent.

Cardiovascular: Chest pain, peripheral edema

Central nervous system: Dizziness (9%), vertigo

Dermatologic: Rash

Endocrine & metabolic: Hyperuricemia (4%), hyperglycemia

Gastrointestinal: Nausea (3%), abdominal pain, dyspepsia, gastroenteritis, diarrhea

Genitourinary: Hematuria

Hepatic: Transaminases increased

Neuromuscular & skeletal: Back pain, arthritis, arthralgia, myalgia

Respiratory: Upper respiratory infection (7%), cough

Miscellaneous: CPK increased

Angioedema and rhabdomyolysis have been reported with angiotensin-receptor blockers. Severe dermatologic reactions, hypokalemia, and pancreatitis have been reported with hydrochlorothiazide.

Mechanism of Action Olmesartan blocks the vasoconstrictor and aldosterone-secreting effects of angiotensin II. Hydrochlorothiazide inhibits sodium reabsorption in the distal tubules causing increased excretion of sodium and water as well as potassium and hydrogen ions.

Pharmacodynamics/Kinetics See individual agents.

Pregnancy Risk Factor C/D (2nd and 3rd trimesters)

Olmesartan Medoxomil *see* Olmesartan *on page 1203*

Olmesartan Medoxomil and Hydrochlorothiazide *see* Olmesartan and Hydrochlorothiazide *on page 1204*

Olopatadine (oh la PAT a deen)

U.S. Brand Names Pataday™; Patanol®
Canadian Brand Names Patanol®
Mexican Brand Names Patanol
Generic Available No
Pharmacologic Category Antihistamine; Ophthalmic Agent, Miscellaneous
Use Treatment of the signs and symptoms of allergic conjunctivitis
Local Anesthetic/Vasoconstrictor Precautions No information available to require special precautions
Effects on Dental Treatment Key adverse event(s) related to dental treatment: Taste perversion.
Pregnancy Risk Factor C

Olsalazine (ole SAL a zeen)

U.S. Brand Names Dipentum®
Canadian Brand Names Dipentum®
Generic Available No
Index Terms Olsalazine Sodium
Pharmacologic Category 5-Aminosalicylic Acid Derivative
Use Maintenance of remission of ulcerative colitis in patients intolerant to sulfasalazine
Local Anesthetic/Vasoconstrictor Precautions No information available to require special precautions
Effects on Dental Treatment No significant effects or complications reported
Common Adverse Effects
>10%: Gastrointestinal: Diarrhea, cramps, abdominal pain
1% to 10%:
Central nervous system: Headache, fatigue, depression
Dermatologic: Rash, itching
Gastrointestinal: Nausea, heartburn, bloating, anorexia
Neuromuscular & skeletal: Arthralgia
Mechanism of Action The mechanism of action appears to be topical rather than systemic
Drug Interactions
Increased Effect/Toxicity: Olsalazine has been reported to increase the prothrombin time in patients taking warfarin. Olsalazine may increase the risk of myelosuppression with azathioprine, mesalamine, or sulfasalazine.
Pharmacodynamics/Kinetics
Absorption: <3%; very little intact olsalazine is systemically absorbed
Protein binding, plasma: >99%
Metabolism: Primarily via colonic bacteria to active drug, 5-aminosalicylic acid
Half-life elimination: 56 minutes
Time to peak: ~1 hour
Excretion: Primarily feces
Pregnancy Risk Factor C

Olsalazine Sodium see Olsalazine on page 1205
Olux® see Clobetasol on page 383
Olux-E™ see Clobetasol on page 383

Omalizumab (oh mah lye ZOO mab)

U.S. Brand Names Xolair®
Canadian Brand Names Xolair®
Generic Available No
Index Terms rhuMAb-E25
Pharmacologic Category Monoclonal Antibody, Anti-Asthmatic
Use Treatment of moderate-to-severe, persistent allergic asthma not adequately controlled with inhaled corticosteroids
Local Anesthetic/Vasoconstrictor Precautions No information available to require special precautions
Effects on Dental Treatment No significant effects or complications reported
Common Adverse Effects
>10%:
Central nervous system: Headache (15%)
Local: Injection site reaction (45%; placebo 43%; severe 12%). Most reactions occurred within 1 hour, lasted <8 days, and decreased in frequency with additional dosing.
(Continued)

Omalizumab (Continued)

Respiratory: Upper respiratory tract infection (20%), sinusitis (16%), pharyngitis (11%)
Miscellaneous: Viral infection (23%)
1% to 10%:
Central nervous system: Pain (7%), fatigue (3%), dizziness (3%)
Dermatologic: Dermatitis (2%), pruritus (2%)
Neuromuscular & skeletal: Arthralgia (8%), leg pain (4%), arm pain (2%), fracture (2%)
Otic: Earache (2%)

Mechanism of Action Omalizumab is an IgG monoclonal antibody (recombinant DNA derived) which inhibits IgE binding to the high-affinity IgE receptor on mast cells and basophils. By decreasing bound IgE, the activation and release of mediators in the allergic response (early and late phase) is limited. Serum-free IgE levels and the number of high-affinity IgE receptors are decreased. Long-term treatment in patients with allergic asthma showed a decrease in asthma exacerbations and corticosteroid usage.

Pharmacodynamics/Kinetics
Absorption: Slow following SubQ injection
Distribution: V_d: 78 ± 32 mL/kg
Metabolism: Hepatic; IgG degradation by reticuloendothelial system and endothelial cells
Bioavailability: 62%
Half-life elimination: 26 days
Time to peak: 7-8 days
Excretion: Primarily via hepatic degradation; intact IgG may be secreted in bile
Pregnancy Risk Factor B

Omeprazole (oh MEP ra zole)

Related Information
Esomeprazole on page 599
Gastrointestinal Disorders on page 1745
U.S. Brand Names Prilosec®; Prilosec OTC™ [OTC]
Canadian Brand Names Apo-Omeprazole®; Losec®; Losec MUPS®
Mexican Brand Names Aleprozil; Azoran; Domer; Inhibitron; Losec; Mopral; Olexin; Ozoken; Prazidec; Suifac; Ulsen; Vulcasid
Generic Available Yes: Delayed release capsule
Pharmacologic Category Proton Pump Inhibitor; Substituted Benzimidazole
Use Short-term (4-8 weeks) treatment of active duodenal ulcer disease or active benign gastric ulcer; treatment of heartburn and other symptoms associated with gastroesophageal reflux disease (GERD); short-term (4-8 weeks) treatment of endoscopically-diagnosed erosive esophagitis; maintenance healing of erosive esophagitis; long-term treatment of pathological hypersecretory conditions; as part of a multidrug regimen for H. pylori eradication to reduce the risk of duodenal ulcer recurrence

OTC labeling: Short-term treatment of frequent, uncomplicated heartburn occurring ≥2 days/week
Unlabeled/Investigational Use Healing NSAID-induced ulcers; prevention of NSAID-induced ulcers
Local Anesthetic/Vasoconstrictor Precautions No information available to require special precautions
Effects on Dental Treatment Key adverse event(s) related to dental treatment: Taste perversion, dry mouth, esophageal candidiasis, and mucosal atrophy (tongue).
Common Adverse Effects 1% to 10%:
Central nervous system: Headache (3% to 7%), dizziness (2%)
Dermatologic: Rash (2%)
Gastrointestinal: Diarrhea (3% to 4%), abdominal pain (2% to 5%), nausea (2% to 4%), vomiting (2% to 3%), flatulence (3%), acid regurgitation (2%), constipation (1% to 2%), taste perversion
Neuromuscular & skeletal: Weakness (1%), back pain (1%)
Respiratory: Upper respiratory infection (2%), cough (1%)
Dosage Oral:
Children ≥2 years: GERD or other acid-related disorders:
<20 kg: 10 mg once daily
≥20 kg: 20 mg once daily
Adults:
Active duodenal ulcer: 20 mg/day for 4-8 weeks
Gastric ulcers: 40 mg/day for 4-8 weeks
Symptomatic GERD: 20 mg/day for up to 4 weeks

Erosive esophagitis: 20 mg/day for 4-8 weeks; maintenance of healing: 20 mg/day for up to 12 months total therapy (including treatment period of 4-8 weeks)

Helicobacter pylori eradication: Dose varies with regimen: 20 mg once daily **or** 40 mg/day as single dose or in 2 divided doses; requires combination therapy with antibiotics

Pathological hypersecretory conditions: Initial: 60 mg once daily; doses up to 120 mg 3 times/day have been administered; administer daily doses >80 mg in divided doses

Frequent heartburn (OTC labeling): 20 mg/day for 14 days; treatment may be repeated after 4 months if needed

Dosage adjustment in hepatic impairment: Specific guidelines are not available; bioavailability is increased with chronic liver disease

Mechanism of Action Suppresses gastric basal and stimulated acid secretion by inhibiting the parietal cell H+/K+ ATP pump

Contraindications Hypersensitivity to omeprazole, substituted benzimidazoles (ie, esomeprazole, lansoprazole, pantoprazole, rabeprazole), or any component of the formulation

Warnings/Precautions Relief of symptoms does not preclude the presence of a gastric malignancy. Atrophic gastritis (by biopsy) has been noted with long-term omeprazole therapy. In long-term (2-year) studies in rats, omeprazole produced a dose-related increase in gastric carcinoid tumors. While available endoscopic evaluations and histologic examinations of biopsy specimens from human stomachs have not detected a risk from short-term exposure to omeprazole, further human data on the effect of sustained hypochlorhydria and hypergastrinemia are needed to rule out the possibility of an increased risk for the development of tumors in humans receiving long-term therapy. Bioavailability may be increased in the elderly, Asian population, and with hepatic dysfunction. Safety and efficacy have not been established in children <2 years of age. When used for self-medication (OTC), do not use for >14 days. Treatment should not be repeated more often than every 4 months. OTC and oral suspension are not approved for use in children <18 years of age.

Drug Interactions

Cytochrome P450 Effect: Substrate of CYP2A6 (minor), 2C9 (minor), 2C19 (major), 2D6 (minor), 3A4 (minor); **Inhibits** CYP1A2 (weak), 2C9 (moderate), 2C19 (strong), 2D6 (weak), 3A4 (weak); **Induces** CYP1A2 (weak)

Increased Effect/Toxicity: Esomeprazole and omeprazole may increase the levels of benzodiazepines metabolized by oxidation (eg, diazepam, midazolam, triazolam), methotrexate, and carbamazepine. Elimination of phenytoin or warfarin may be prolonged when used concomitantly with omeprazole. Omeprazole may increase the levels/effects of amiodarone, citalopram, diazepam, fluoxetine, glimepiride, glipizide, methsuximide, nateglinide, phenytoin, pioglitazone, propranolol, rosiglitazone, sertraline, warfarin, and other CYP2C9 or 2C19 substrates. Omeprazole may alter the concentrations/effects of clozapine.

Decreased Effect: Proton pump inhibitors may decrease the absorption of atazanavir, indinavir, oral iron salts, itraconazole, and ketoconazole; avoid concurrent use. The levels/effects of omeprazole may be decreased by aminoglutethimide, carbamazepine, phenytoin, rifampin, and other CYP2C19 inducers. Omeprazole may alter the concentrations/effects of clozapine.

Ethanol/Nutrition/Herb Interactions

Ethanol: Avoid ethanol (may cause gastric mucosal irritation).

Food: Food delays absorption.

Herb/Nutraceutical: St John's wort may decrease omeprazole levels.

Dietary Considerations Should be taken on an empty stomach; best if taken before breakfast.

Pharmacodynamics/Kinetics

Onset of action: Antisecretory: ~1 hour

Peak effect: 2 hours

Duration: 72 hours

Protein binding: 95%

Metabolism: Extensively hepatic to inactive metabolites

Bioavailability: Oral: 30% to 40%; increased in Asian patients and patients with hepatic dysfunction

Half-life elimination: Delayed release capsule: 0.5-1 hour

Excretion: Urine (77% as metabolites, very small amount as unchanged drug); feces

Pregnancy Risk Factor C

Dosage Forms

Capsule, delayed release: 10 mg, 20 mg

Prilosec®: 10 mg, 20 mg, 40 mg

Tablet, delayed release:

Prilosec OTC™ [OTC]: 20 mg

Omeprazole and Sodium Bicarbonate
(oh MEP ra zole & SOW dee um bye KAR bun ate)

U.S. Brand Names Zegerid®
Generic Available No
Pharmacologic Category Proton Pump Inhibitor; Substituted Benzimidazole
Use Short-term (4-8 weeks) treatment of active duodenal ulcer disease or active benign gastric ulcer; treatment of heartburn and other symptoms associated with gastroesophageal reflux disease (GERD); short-term (4-8 weeks) treatment of endoscopically-diagnosed erosive esophagitis; maintenance healing of erosive esophagitis; reduction of risk of upper gastrointestinal bleeding in critically-ill patients
Local Anesthetic/Vasoconstrictor Precautions No information available to require special precautions
Effects on Dental Treatment Key adverse event(s) related to dental treatment: Oral candidiasis.
Common Adverse Effects
Frequency of adverse events reported for 40 mg dose of oral powder for suspension. **Note:** Asterisked (*) percentages indicate frequency reported from a controlled clinical trial of 359 critically-ill patients.
>10%:
Central nervous system: Pyrexia (20%*)
Endocrine & metabolic: Hypokalemia (12%*), hyperglycemia (11%*)
Respiratory: Nosocomial pneumonia (11%*)
1% to 10%:
Cardiovascular: Hypotension (10%*), hypertension (8%*), atrial fibrillation (6%*), ventricular tachycardia (5%*), bradycardia (4%*), tachycardia (3%*), supraventricular tachycardia (3%*), edema (3%*)
Central nervous system: Hyperpyrexia (5%), agitation (3%), headache (2%)
Dermatologic: Rash (6%*), decubitus ulcer (3%)
Endocrine & metabolic: Hypomagnesemia (10%*), hypocalcemia (6%*), hypophosphatemia (6%*), fluid overload (5%*), hypoglycemia (3%*), hyponatremia (4%*), hypernatremia (2%*), hyperkalemia (2%*)
Gastrointestinal: Constipation (5%*), diarrhea (4%*), hypomotility (2%*)
Genitourinary: Urinary tract infection (2%*)
Hematological: Thrombocytopenia (10%*), anemia (8%*), anemia increased (2%*)
Hepatic: LFTs increased (2%*)
Respiratory: ARDS (3%*), respiratory failure (2%*), URI (2%), cough (1%)
Miscellaneous: Sepsis (5%*), oral candidiasis (4%*), candidal infection (2%*)
Mechanism of Action Suppresses gastric basal and stimulated acid secretion by inhibiting the parietal cell H+/K+ ATP pump
Drug Interactions
Cytochrome P450 Effect: Substrate of CYP2A6 (minor), 2C9 (minor), 2C19 (major), 2D6 (minor), 3A4 (minor); **Inhibits** CYP1A2 (weak), 2C9 (moderate), 2C19 (strong), 2D6 (weak), 3A4 (weak); **Induces** CYP1A2 (weak)
Increased Effect/Toxicity: Esomeprazole and omeprazole may increase the levels of benzodiazepines metabolized by oxidation (eg, diazepam, midazolam, triazolam), methotrexate, and carbamazepine. Elimination of phenytoin or warfarin may be prolonged when used concomitantly with omeprazole. Omeprazole may increase the levels/effects of amiodarone, citalopram, diazepam, fluoxetine, glimepiride, glipizide, methsuximide, nateglinide, phenytoin, pioglitazone, propranolol, rosiglitazone, sertraline, warfarin, and other CYP2C9 or 2C19 substrates. Omeprazole may alter the concentrations/effects of clozapine.
Decreased Effect: Proton pump inhibitors may decrease the absorption of atazanavir, indinavir, itraconazole, and ketoconazole. The levels/effects of omeprazole may be decreased by aminoglutethimide, carbamazepine, phenytoin, rifampin, and other CYP2C19 inducers. Omeprazole may alter the concentrations/effects of clozapine.
Pharmacodynamics/Kinetics
Onset of action: Antisecretory: ~1 hour
Peak effect: 2 hours
Duration: 72 hours
Protein binding: 95%
Metabolism: Extensively hepatic to inactive metabolites
Bioavailability: Oral: 30% to 40%; increased in Asian patients and patients with hepatic dysfunction
Half-life elimination: 0.4-3.2 hours
Excretion: Urine (77% as metabolites, very small amount as unchanged drug); feces
Pregnancy Risk Factor C

Ondansetron (on DAN se tron)

U.S. Brand Names Zofran®; Zofran® ODT
Canadian Brand Names Apo-Ondansetron®; Zofran®; Zofran® ODT
Mexican Brand Names Zofran Zydis
Generic Available Yes
Index Terms GR38032R; Ondansetron Hydrochloride
Pharmacologic Category Antiemetic; Selective 5-HT$_3$ Receptor Antagonist
Use Prevention of nausea and vomiting associated with moderately- to highly-emetogenic cancer chemotherapy; radiotherapy in patients receiving total body irradiation or fractions to the abdomen; prevention of postoperative nausea and vomiting (PONV); treatment of PONV if no prophylactic dose received

Unlabeled/Investigational Use Treatment of early-onset alcoholism; hyperemesis gravidarum

Local Anesthetic/Vasoconstrictor Precautions No information available to require special precautions

Effects on Dental Treatment Key adverse event(s) related to dental treatment: Xerostomia (normal salivary flow resumes upon discontinuation).

Common Adverse Effects Note: Percentages reported in adult patients.
>10%:
   Central nervous system: Headache (9% to 27%), malaise/fatigue (9% to 13%)
   Gastrointestinal: Constipation (6% to 11%)
1% to 10%:
   Central nervous system: Drowsiness (8%), fever (2% to 8%), dizziness (4% to 7%), anxiety (6%), cold sensation (2%)
   Dermatologic: Pruritus (2% to 5%), rash (1%)
   Gastrointestinal: Diarrhea (2% to 7%)
   Genitourinary: Gynecological disorder (7%), urinary retention (5%)
   Hepatic: ALT/AST increased (1% to 5%)
   Local: Injection site reaction (4%; pain, redness, burning)
   Neuromuscular & skeletal: Paresthesia (2%)
   Respiratory: Hypoxia (9%)

Mechanism of Action Selective 5-HT$_3$-receptor antagonist, blocking serotonin, both peripherally on vagal nerve terminals and centrally in the chemoreceptor trigger zone

Drug Interactions
Cytochrome P450 Effect: Substrate of CYP1A2 (minor), 2C9 (minor), 2D6 (minor), 2E1 (minor), 3A4 (major); **Inhibits** CYP1A2 (weak), 2C9 (weak), 2D6 (weak)

Increased Effect/Toxicity: Ondansetron may enhance the hypotensive effect of apomorphine; concurrent use is contraindicated.

Decreased Effect: CYP3A4 inducers may decrease the levels/effects of ondansetron; example inducers include aminoglutethimide, carbamazepine, nafcillin, nevirapine, phenobarbital, phenytoin, and rifamycins. The manufacturer does not recommend dosage adjustment in patients receiving CYP3A4 inducers.

Pharmacodynamics/Kinetics
Onset of action: ~30 minutes
Distribution: V$_d$: Children: 1.7-3.7 L/kg; Adults: 2.2-2.5 L/kg
Protein binding, plasma: 70% to 76%
Metabolism: Extensively hepatic via hydroxylation, followed by glucuronide or sulfate conjugation; CYP1A2, CYP2D6, and CYP3A4 substrate; some demethylation occurs
Bioavailability: Oral: 56% to 71%; Rectal: 58% to 74%
Half-life elimination: Children <15 years: 2-7 hours; Adults: 3-6 hours
   Mild-to-moderate hepatic impairment: Adults: 12 hours
   Severe hepatic impairment (Child-Pugh C): Adults: 20 hours
Time to peak: Oral: ~2 hours
Excretion: Urine (44% to 60% as metabolites, 5% to 10% as unchanged drug); feces (~25%)

Pregnancy Risk Factor B

Opium Tincture (OH pee um TING chur)

Generic Available Yes
Index Terms DTO (error-prone abbreviation); Opium Tincture, Deodorized
Pharmacologic Category Analgesic, Opioid; Antidiarrheal
Use Treatment of diarrhea or relief of pain
Local Anesthetic/Vasoconstrictor Precautions No information available to require special precautions
Effects on Dental Treatment No significant effects or complications reported
Mechanism of Action Contains many narcotic alkaloids including morphine; its mechanism for gastric motility inhibition is primarily due to this morphine content; it results in a decrease in digestive secretions, an increase in GI muscle tone, and therefore a reduction in GI propulsion
Pregnancy Risk Factor B/D (prolonged use or high doses at term)

Opium Tincture, Deodorized *see* Opium Tincture *on page 1210*

Oprelvekin (oh PREL ve kin)

U.S. Brand Names Neumega®
Mexican Brand Names Neumega
Generic Available No
Index Terms IL-11; Interleukin-11; NSC-722848; Recombinant Human Interleukin-11; Recombinant Interleukin-11; rhIL-11; rIL-11
Pharmacologic Category Biological Response Modulator; Human Growth Factor
Use Prevention of severe thrombocytopenia; reduce the need for platelet transfusions following myelosuppressive chemotherapy
Local Anesthetic/Vasoconstrictor Precautions No information available to require special precautions
Effects on Dental Treatment Key adverse event(s) related to dental treatment: Oral moniliasis.
Common Adverse Effects
>10%:
Cardiovascular: Tachycardia (children 84%; adults 20%), edema (59%), palpitation (14%), cardiomegaly (children 21%), vasodilation (19%), syncope (13%), atrial arrhythmia (12%)
Central nervous system: Headache (41%), dizziness (38%), fever (36%), insomnia (33%), fatigue (30%)
Dermatologic: Rash (25%)
Endocrine & metabolic: Fluid retention

Gastrointestinal: Nausea/vomiting (77%), diarrhea (43%), oral moniliasis (14%)

Hematologic: Anemia (dilutional); appears within 3 days of initiation of therapy, resolves in about 1 week after cessation of oprelvekin

Neuromuscular & skeletal: Weakness (severe 14%), arthralgia, periostitis (children 11%)

Ocular: Conjunctival injection/redness/swelling (children 57%; adults 19%), papilledema (children 16%; adults 1%)

Respiratory: Dyspnea (48%), rhinitis (42%), cough (29%), pharyngitis (25%)

1% to 10%:

Gastrointestinal: Weight gain (5%)

Respiratory: Pleural effusion (10%)

Mechanism of Action Oprelvekin is a growth factor which stimulates multiple stages of megakaryocytopoiesis and thrombopoiesis, resulting in proliferation of megakaryocyte progenitors and megakaryocyte maturation, or increased platelet production.

Drug Interactions

Increased Effect/Toxicity: Hypokalemia may increase the risk of adverse cardiovascular events with oprelvekin; monitor.

Pharmacodynamics/Kinetics

Bioavailability: >80%

Half-life elimination: Terminal: 5-9 hours

Time to peak, serum: 1-6 hours

Excretion: Urine (primarily as metabolites)

Pregnancy Risk Factor C

Orlistat (OR li stat)

U.S. Brand Names Alli™ [OTC]; Xenical®
Canadian Brand Names Xenical®
Mexican Brand Names Xenical
Generic Available No
(Continued)

Orlistat (Continued)

Pharmacologic Category Lipase Inhibitor

Use Management of obesity, including weight loss and weight management, when used in conjunction with a reduced-calorie and low-fat diet; reduce the risk of weight regain after prior weight loss; indicated for obese patients with an initial body mass index (BMI) ≥30 kg/m² or ≥27 kg/m² in the presence of other risk factors

Local Anesthetic/Vasoconstrictor Precautions No information available to require special precautions

Effects on Dental Treatment No significant effects or complications reported

Common Adverse Effects

>10%:

Central nervous system: Headache (31%)

Gastrointestinal: Oily spotting (27%), abdominal pain/discomfort (26%), flatus with discharge (24%), fecal urgency (22%), fatty/oily stool (20%), oily evacuation (12%), defecation increased (11%)

Neuromuscular & skeletal: Back pain (14%)

Respiratory: Upper respiratory infection (38%)

1% to 10%:

Central nervous system: Fatigue (7%), anxiety (5%), sleep disorder (4%)

Dermatologic: Dry skin (2%)

Endocrine & metabolic: Menstrual irregularities (10%)

Gastrointestinal: Fecal incontinence (8%), nausea (8%), infectious diarrhea (5%), rectal pain/discomfort (5%), vomiting (4%)

Neuromuscular & skeletal: Arthritis (5%), myalgia (4%)

Otic: Otitis (4%)

Mechanism of Action A reversible inhibitor of gastric and pancreatic lipases, thus inhibiting absorption of dietary fats by 30% (at doses of 120 mg 3 times/day).

Drug Interactions

Decreased Effect: Orlistat may decrease amiodarone absorption (monitor). Coadministration with cyclosporine may decrease plasma levels of cyclosporine (administer cyclosporine 2 hours before or after orlistat and monitor). Orlistat does not alter the pharmacokinetics of warfarin, however, vitamin K absorption may be decreased during orlistat therapy (patients stabilized on warfarin should be monitored for changes in warfarin effects).

Pharmacodynamics/Kinetics

Onset: 24-48 hours

Duration of action: 48-72 hours

Absorption: Minimal

Metabolism: Metabolized within the gastrointestinal wall; forms inactive metabolites

Excretion: Feces (97%, 83% as unchanged drug); urine (<2%)

Pregnancy Risk Factor B

Ornex® [OTC] see Acetaminophen and Pseudoephedrine on page 38

Ornex® Maximum Strength [OTC] see Acetaminophen and Pseudoephedrine on page 38

Orphenadrine (or FEN a dreen)

Related Information

Temporomandibular Dysfunction (TMD) on page 1822

U.S. Brand Names Norflex™

Canadian Brand Names Norflex™; Orphenace®; Rhoxal-orphenadrine

Mexican Brand Names Norflex

Generic Available Yes

Index Terms Orphenadrine Citrate

Pharmacologic Category Anti-Parkinson's Agent, Anticholinergic; Skeletal Muscle Relaxant

Use Treatment of muscle spasm associated with acute painful musculoskeletal conditions

Local Anesthetic/Vasoconstrictor Precautions No information available to require special precautions

Effects on Dental Treatment The peripheral anticholinergic effects of orphenadrine may decrease or inhibit salivary flow; normal salivation will return with cessation of drug therapy.

Common Adverse Effects Frequency not defined.

Cardiovascular: Palpitation, tachycardia

Central nervous system: Agitation, drowsiness, dizziness, euphoria, hallucination, headache, mental confusion

Dermatologic: Pruritus, urticaria

Gastrointestinal: Constipation, gastric irritation, nausea, vomiting, xerostomia

Genitourinary: Urination hesitancy, urinary retention

Hematologic: Aplastic anemia (rare)

Neuromuscular & skeletal: Tremor, weakness

Ocular: Blurred vision, intraocular pressure increased, nystagmus, pupil dilation

Respiratory: Nasal congestion

Miscellaneous: Anaphylactic reaction (injection, rare), hypersensitivity

Dosage

Adults:

Oral: 100 mg twice daily

I.M., I.V.: 60 mg every 12 hours

Elderly: Use caution; generally not recommended for use in the elderly

Mechanism of Action Indirect skeletal muscle relaxant thought to work by central atropine-like effects; has some euphorigenic and analgesic properties

Contraindications Hypersensitivity to orphenadrine or any component of the formulation; glaucoma; GI obstruction, stenosing peptic ulcer; prostatic hypertrophy, bladder neck obstruction; cardiospasm; myasthenia gravis

Warnings/Precautions Use with caution in patients with CHF, cardiac decompensation, coronary insufficiency , tachycardia, or cardiac arrhythmias. May cause CNS depression, which may impair physical or mental abilities. Potential for abuse; use with caution in patients with history of drug abuse. Solution for injection contains sodium, bisulfite which may cause allergic reaction in some individuals. Has not been evaluated for continuous long-term use; monitor closely. Safety and efficacy in children have not been established.

Drug Interactions

Cytochrome P450 Effect: Substrate (minor) of CYP1A2, 2B6, 2D6, 3A4; **Inhibits** CYP1A2 (weak), 2A6 (weak), 2B6 (weak), 2C9 (weak), 2C19 (weak), 2D6 (weak), 2E1 (weak), 3A4 (weak)

Increased Effect/Toxicity: Orphenadrine may increase potential for anticholinergic adverse effects of anticholinergic agents; includes drugs with high anticholinergic activity (diphenhydramine, TCAs, phenothiazines). Pramlintide may enhance the gastrointestinal anticholinergic effect of orphenadrine. Sedative effects of may be additive in concurrent use of orphenadrine and CNS depressants (monitor).

Decreased Effect: Acetylcholinesterase inhibitors (donepezil, galantamine, rivastigmine, tacrine) may diminish the therapeutic effect of orphenadrine. Orphenadrine may diminish the therapeutic effect of acetylcholinesterase inhibitors.

Ethanol/Nutrition/Herb Interactions

Ethanol: Avoid ethanol (may increase CNS depression).

Herb/Nutraceutical: Avoid valerian, St John's wort, kava kava, gotu kola (may increase CNS depression).

Pharmacodynamics/Kinetics

Onset of effect: Peak effect: Oral: 2-4 hours

Duration: 4-6 hours

Protein binding: 20%

Metabolism: Extensively hepatic

Half-life elimination: 14-16 hours

Excretion: Primarily urine (8% as unchanged drug)

Pregnancy Risk Factor C

Dosage Forms

Injection, solution: 30 mg/mL (2 mL)

Norflex™: 30 mg/mL (2 mL)

Tablet, extended release: 100 mg

Norflex™: 100 mg

Orphenadrine, Aspirin, and Caffeine
(or FEN a dreen, AS pir in, & KAF een)

Related Information

Aspirin *on page 149*

Caffeine *on page 255*

Orphenadrine *on page 1212*

U.S. Brand Names Norgesic™ [DSC]; Norgesic™ Forte [DSC]; Orphengesic [DSC]; Orphengesic Forte [DSC]

Canadian Brand Names Norgesic™; Norgesic™ Forte

Generic Available Yes

Index Terms Aspirin, Orphenadrine, and Caffeine; Caffeine, Orphenadrine, and Aspirin

Pharmacologic Category Skeletal Muscle Relaxant

Use Relief of discomfort associated with skeletal muscular conditions

(Continued)

Orphenadrine, Aspirin, and Caffeine *(Continued)*

Local Anesthetic/Vasoconstrictor Precautions No information available to require special precautions

Effects on Dental Treatment Key adverse event(s) related to dental treatment: The peripheral anticholinergic effects of orphenadrine may decrease or inhibit salivary flow; normal salivation will return with cessation of drug therapy.

Aspirin: As with all drugs which may affect hemostasis, bleeding is associated with aspirin. Hemorrhage may occur at virtually any site; risk is dependent on multiple variables including dosage, concurrent use of multiple agents which alter hemostasis, and patient susceptibility. Many adverse effects of aspirin are dose related, and are rare at low dosages. Other serious reactions are idiosyncratic, related to allergy or individual sensitivity (see Dental Comment).

Drug Interactions

Cytochrome P450 Effect:

Orphenadrine: **Substrate** (minor) of CYP1A2, 2B6, 2D6, 3A4; **Inhibits** CYP1A2 (weak), 2A6 (weak), 2B6 (weak), 2C9 (weak), 2C19 (weak), 2D6 (weak), 2E1 (weak), 3A4 (weak)

Aspirin: **Substrate** of CYP2C9 (minor)

Caffeine: **Substrate** of CYP1A2 (major), 2C9 (minor), 2D6 (minor), 2E1 (minor), 3A4 (minor); **Inhibits** CYP1A2 (weak), 3A4 (moderate)

Pharmacodynamics/Kinetics See individual agents.

Pregnancy Risk Factor D

Dental Comment There is no scientific evidence to warrant discontinuance of aspirin prior to dental surgery. Patients taking one aspirin tablet daily as an antithrombotic and who require dental surgery should be given special consideration in consultation with the physician before removal of the aspirin relative to prevention of postoperative bleeding.

The Food and Drug Administration (FDA), has issued a letter updating information and considerations regarding the use of ibuprofen (400 mg doses) in patients who are taking low dose aspirin (81 mg, immediate release; not enteric coated) for cardioprotection and stroke prevention. Ibuprofen, at these doses, may interfere with aspirin's antiplatelet effect depending upon when it is administered. Patients initiated on aspirin first (for ~1 week) then ibuprofen (400 mg tid for 10 days) seem to maintain aspirin's platelet effect (Cryer B, 2005). Ibuprofen has the greatest impact on aspirin if administered less than 8 hours before aspirin (Catella-Lawson F, 2001).

Patients may require counseling about the appropriate timing of ibuprofen dosing in relationship to aspirin therapy. With occasional use of ibuprofen, a clinically-significant interaction with aspirin in unlikely. To avoid interference during chronic dosing, a single dose of ibuprofen should be taken 30-120 minutes after aspirin ingestion or at least 8 hours should elapse after ibuprofen dosing before giving aspirin (FDA, 2006; Catella-Lawson F, 2001).

The clinical implications of the interaction are unclear. There have not been any clinical endpoint studies conducted at this time. Avoidance of this interaction is potentially important because aspirin's vascular protection could be decreased or negated.

Other nonselective NSAIDs may have potential for a similar interaction with aspirin. Such has been described with naproxen (Capone ML, 2005). Acetaminophen does not appear to interfere with the antiplatelet effect of aspirin. Other clinical scenarios (use of smaller ibuprofen doses, other aspirin products, other doses of aspirin) have not been evaluated.

Additional information is available at: http://www.fda.gov/cder/drug/infopage/aspirin/default.htm.

Ortho-Novum® 1/50 *see* Mestranol and Norethindrone *on page 1053*

Ortho Prefest *see* Estradiol and Norgestimate *on page 604*

Ortho Tri Cyclen *see* Ethinyl Estradiol and Norgestimate *on page 645*

Ortho Tri-Cyclen® *see* Ethinyl Estradiol and Norgestimate *on page 645*

Ortho Tri-Cyclen® Lo *see* Ethinyl Estradiol and Norgestimate *on page 645*

Orthovisc® *see* Hyaluronate and Derivatives *on page 816*

Orudis® KT [OTC] [DSC] *see* Ketoprofen *on page 931*

Orvaten™ *see* Midodrine *on page 1102*

Os-Cal® 500 [OTC] [DSC] *see* Calcium Carbonate *on page 260*

Os-Cal® 500+D [OTC] *see* Calcium and Vitamin D *on page 259*

Oseltamivir (oh sel TAM i vir)

Related Information
  Systemic Viral Diseases *on page 1767*
U.S. Brand Names Tamiflu®
Canadian Brand Names Tamiflu®
Generic Available No
Pharmacologic Category Antiviral Agent; Neuraminidase Inhibitor
Use Treatment of uncomplicated acute illness due to influenza (A or B) infection in children ≥1 year of age and adults who have been symptomatic for no more than 2 days; prophylaxis against influenza (A or B) infection in children ≥1 year of age and adults
Local Anesthetic/Vasoconstrictor Precautions No information available to require special precautions
Effects on Dental Treatment No significant effects or complications reported
Common Adverse Effects
  >10%: Gastrointestinal: Vomiting (2% to 15%)
  1% to 10%: Gastrointestinal: Nausea (3% to 10%), abdominal pain (2% to 5%)
Mechanism of Action Oseltamivir, a prodrug, is hydrolyzed to the active form, oseltamivir carboxylate. It is thought to inhibit influenza virus neuraminidase, with the possibility of alteration of virus particle aggregation and release.
Drug Interactions
  Decreased Effect: Influenza virus vaccine nasal spray (fluMist™): Safety and efficacy for use with influenza virus vaccine nasal spray have not been established. Do not administer nasal spray until 48 hours after stopping antiviral; do not administer antiviral for 2 weeks after receiving influenza virus vaccine nasal spray.
Pharmacodynamics/Kinetics
  Absorption: Well absorbed
  Distribution: V_d: 23-26 L (oseltamivir carboxylate)
  Protein binding, plasma: Oseltamivir carboxylate: 3%; Oseltamivir: 42%
  Metabolism: Hepatic (90%) to oseltamivir carboxylate; neither the parent drug nor active metabolite has any effect on CYP
  Bioavailability: 75% as oseltamivir carboxylate
  Half-life elimination: Oseltamivir: 1-3 hours; Oseltamivir carboxylate: 6-10 hours
  Excretion: Urine (>90% as oseltamivir carboxylate); feces
Pregnancy Risk Factor C

OSI-774 *see* Erlotinib *on page 587*

Osmoglyn® [DSC] *see* Glycerin *on page 789*

OsmoPrep™ *see* Sodium Phosphates *on page 1484*

OTFC (Oral Transmucosal Fentanyl Citrate) *see* Fentanyl *on page 679*

Oticaine *see* Benzocaine *on page 195*

Otocaine™ *see* Benzocaine *on page 195*

Otrivin® [OTC] [DSC] *see* Xylometazoline *on page 1673*

Otrivin® Pediatric [OTC] [DSC] *see* Xylometazoline *on page 1673*

Outgro® [OTC] *see* Benzocaine *on page 195*

Ovace® *see* Sulfacetamide *on page 1502*

Ovace® Wash *see* Sulfacetamide *on page 1502*

Ovcon® *see* Ethinyl Estradiol and Norethindrone *on page 640*

Ovidrel® *see* Chorionic Gonadotropin (Recombinant) *on page 352*

Ovine Corticotropin-Releasing Hormone *see* Corticorelin *on page 414*

Oxacillin (oks a SIL in)

Generic Available Yes
(Continued)

Oxacillin (Continued)

Index Terms Methylphenyl Isoxazolyl Penicillin; Oxacillin Sodium

Pharmacologic Category Antibiotic, Penicillin

Use Treatment of infections such as osteomyelitis, septicemia, endocarditis, and CNS infections caused by susceptible strains of *Staphylococcus*

Local Anesthetic/Vasoconstrictor Precautions No information available to require special precautions

Effects on Dental Treatment Key adverse event(s) related to dental treatment: Prolonged use of penicillins may lead to development of oral candidiasis.

Common Adverse Effects Frequency not defined.

Central nervous system: Fever

Dermatologic: Rash

Gastrointestinal: Nausea, diarrhea, vomiting

Hematologic: Eosinophilia, leukopenia, neutropenia, thrombocytopenia, agranulocytosis

Hepatic: Hepatotoxicity, AST increased

Renal: Acute interstitial nephritis, hematuria

Miscellaneous: Serum sickness-like reactions

Mechanism of Action Inhibits bacterial cell wall synthesis by binding to one or more of the penicillin-binding proteins (PBPs); which in turn inhibits the final transpeptidation step of peptidoglycan synthesis in bacterial cell walls, thus inhibiting cell wall biosynthesis. Bacteria eventually lyse due to ongoing activity of cell wall autolytic enzymes (autolysins and murein hydrolases) while cell wall assembly is arrested.

Drug Interactions

Increased Effect/Toxicity: Probenecid increases penicillin levels. Penicillins and anticoagulants may increase the effect of anticoagulants. Penicillins may increase the exposure to methotrexate during concurrent therapy; monitor.

Decreased Effect: Although anecdotal reports suggest oral contraceptive efficacy could be reduced by penicillins, this has been refuted by more rigorous scientific and clinical data.

Pharmacodynamics/Kinetics

Distribution: Into bile, synovial and pleural fluids, bronchial secretions, peritoneal, and pericardial fluids; crosses placenta; enters breast milk; penetrates the blood-brain barrier only when meninges are inflamed

Protein binding: ~94%

Metabolism: Hepatic to active metabolites

Half-life elimination: Children 1 week to 2 years: 0.9-1.8 hours; Adults: 23-60 minutes; prolonged in neonates and with renal impairment

Time to peak, serum: I.M.: 30-60 minutes

Excretion: Urine and feces (small amounts as unchanged drug and metabolites)

Pregnancy Risk Factor B

Oxacillin Sodium *see* Oxacillin *on page 1215*

Oxaliplatin (ox AL i pla tin)

U.S. Brand Names Eloxatin®

Mexican Brand Names Eloxatin

Generic Available No

Index Terms Diaminocyclohexane Oxalatoplatinum; L-OHP; NSC-266046

Pharmacologic Category Antineoplastic Agent, Alkylating Agent

Use Treatment of stage III colon cancer and advanced colorectal cancer

Unlabeled/Investigational Use Head and neck cancer, nonsmall-cell lung cancer, non-Hodgkin's lymphoma, ovarian cancer

Local Anesthetic/Vasoconstrictor Precautions No information available to require special precautions

Effects on Dental Treatment Key adverse event(s) related to dental treatment: Stomatitis, dysphagia, mucositis, and taste perversion.

Common Adverse Effects Percentages reported with monotherapy.

>10%:

Central nervous system: Fatigue (61%), fever (25%), pain (14%), headache (13%), insomnia (11%)

Gastrointestinal: Nausea (64%), diarrhea (46%), vomiting (37%), abdominal pain (31%), constipation (31%), anorexia (20%), stomatitis (14%)

Hematologic: Anemia (64%), thrombocytopenia (30%), leukopenia (13%)

Hepatic: AST increased (54%; grades 3/4: 4%), ALT increased (36%; grades 3/4: 1%), total bilirubin increased (13%; grades 3/4: 5%)

Neuromuscular & skeletal: Peripheral neuropathy (may be dose limiting; 76%; acute 65%; grades 3/4: 5%; persistent 43%; grades 3/4: 3%), back pain (11%)

Respiratory: Dyspnea (13%), cough (11%)

1% to 10%:

Cardiovascular: Edema (10%), chest pain (5%), peripheral edema (5%), flushing (3%), thromboembolism (2%)

Central nervous system: Dizziness (7%)

Dermatologic: Rash (5%), alopecia (3%), hand-foot syndrome (1%)

Endocrine & metabolic: Dehydration (5%), hypokalemia (3%)

Gastrointestinal: Dyspepsia (7%), taste perversion (5%), flatulence (3%), mucositis (2%), gastroesophageal reflux (1%), dysphagia (acute 1% to 2%)

Genitourinary: Dysuria (1%)

Hematologic: Neutropenia (7%)

Local: Injection site reaction (9%; redness/swelling/pain)

Neuromuscular & skeletal: Rigors (9%), arthralgia (7%)

Ocular: Abnormal lacrimation (1%)

Renal: Serum creatinine increased (5% to 10%)

Respiratory: URI (7%), rhinitis (6%), epistaxis (2%), pharyngitis (2%), pharyngolaryngeal dysesthesia (grades 3/4: 1% to 2%)

Miscellaneous: Allergic reactions (3%); hypersensitivity (includes urticaria, pruritus, facial flushing, shortness of breath, bronchospasm, diaphoresis, hypotension, syncope: grades 3/4: 2% to 3%); hiccup (2%)

Mechanism of Action Oxaliplatin, a platinum derivative, is an alkylating agent. Following intracellular hydrolysis, the platinum compound binds to DNA forming cross-links which inhibit DNA replication and transcription, resulting in cell death. Cytotoxicity is cell-cycle nonspecific.

Drug Interactions

Increased Effect/Toxicity: Taxane derivatives may increase oxaliplatin toxicity if administered before the platin as a sequential infusion. Nephrotoxic agents may increase oxaliplatin toxicity.

Decreased Effect: Oxaliplatin may decrease plasma levels of digoxin.

Pharmacodynamics/Kinetics

Distribution: V_d: 440 L

Protein binding: >90% primarily albumin and gamma globulin (irreversible binding to platinum)

Metabolism: Nonenzymatic (rapid and extensive), forms active and inactive derivatives

Half-life elimination: Terminal: 391 hours; Distribution: Alpha phase: 0.4 hours, Beta phase: 16.8 hours

Excretion: Primarily urine (~54%); feces (~2%)

Pregnancy Risk Factor D

Oxandrin® *see* Oxandrolone *on page 1217*

Oxandrolone (oks AN droe lone)

U.S. Brand Names Oxandrin®

Generic Available Yes

Pharmacologic Category Androgen

Use Adjunctive therapy to promote weight gain after weight loss following extensive surgery, chronic infections, or severe trauma, and in some patients who, without definite pathophysiologic reasons, fail to gain or to maintain normal weight; to offset protein catabolism with prolonged corticosteroid administration; relief of bone pain associated with osteoporosis

Local Anesthetic/Vasoconstrictor Precautions No information available to require special precautions

Effects on Dental Treatment No significant effects or complications reported

Common Adverse Effects Frequency not defined.

Cardiovascular: Edema

Central nervous system: Depression, excitation, insomnia

Dermatologic: Acne (females and prepubertal males)

Also reported in females: Hirsutism, male-pattern baldness

Endocrine & metabolic: Electrolyte imbalances, glucose intolerance, gonadotropin secretion inhibited, gynecomastia, HDL decreased, LDL increased

Also reported in females: Clitoral enlargement, menstrual irregularities

Genitourinary:

Prepubertal males: Increased or persistent erections, penile enlargement

Postpubertal males: Bladder irritation, epididymitis, impotence, oligospermia, priapism (chronic), testicular atrophy, testicular function

Hepatic: Alkaline phosphatase increased, ALT/AST increased, bilirubin increased, cholestatic jaundice, hepatic necrosis (rare), hepatocellular neoplasms, peliosis hepatis (with long-term therapy)

Neuromuscular & skeletal: CPK increased, premature closure of epiphyses (in children)

Renal: Creatinine excretion increased

(Continued)

Oxandrolone *(Continued)*

Miscellaneous: Bromsulfophthalein retention, habituation, voice alteration (deepening, in females)

Restrictions C-III

Mechanism of Action Synthetic testosterone derivative with similar androgenic and anabolic actions

Drug Interactions

Increased Effect/Toxicity: ACTH, adrenal steroids may increase risk of edema and acne. Oxandrolone enhances the hypoprothrombinemic effects of oral anticoagulants, and enhances the hypoglycemic effects of insulin and sulfonylureas (oral hypoglycemics).

Pharmacodynamics/Kinetics Half-life elimination: 10-13 hours

Pregnancy Risk Factor X

Oxaprozin *(oks a PROE zin)*

Related Information

Rheumatoid Arthritis, Osteoarthritis, and Osteoporosis *on page 1759*
Temporomandibular Dysfunction (TMD) *on page 1822*

U.S. Brand Names Daypro®

Canadian Brand Names Apo-Oxaprozin®; Daypro®

Generic Available Yes

Pharmacologic Category Nonsteroidal Anti-inflammatory Drug (NSAID), Oral

Use Acute and long-term use in the management of signs and symptoms of osteoarthritis and rheumatoid arthritis; juvenile rheumatoid arthritis

Local Anesthetic/Vasoconstrictor Precautions No information available to require special precautions

Effects on Dental Treatment NSAID formulations are known to reversibly decrease platelet aggregation via mechanisms different than observed with aspirin. The dentist should be aware of the potential of abnormal coagulation. Caution should also be exercised in the use of NSAIDs in patients already on anticoagulant therapy with drugs such as warfarin (Coumadin®).

Common Adverse Effects

1% to 10%:

Cardiovascular: Edema

Central nervous system: Confusion, depression, dizziness, headache, sedation, sleep disturbance, somnolence

Dermatologic: Pruritus, rash

Gastrointestinal: Abdominal distress, abdominal pain, anorexia, constipation, diarrhea, flatulence, gastrointestinal ulcer, gross bleeding with perforation, heartburn, nausea, vomiting

Hematologic: Anemia, bleeding time increased

Hepatic: Liver enzyme elevation

Otic: Tinnitus

Renal: Dysuria, renal function abnormal, urinary frequency

Restrictions An FDA-approved medication guide must be distributed when dispensing an oral outpatient prescription (new or refill) where this medication is to be used without direct supervision of a healthcare provider. Medication guides are available at http://www.fda.gov/cder/Offices/ODS/medication_guides.htm.

Dosage Oral (individualize dosage to lowest effective dose to minimize adverse effects):

Children 6-16 years: Juvenile rheumatoid arthritis:

22-31 kg: 600 mg once daily

32-54 kg: 900 mg once daily

≥55 kg: 1200 mg once daily

Adults:

Osteoarthritis: 600-1200 mg once daily; patients should be titrated to lowest dose possible; patients with low body weight should start with 600 mg daily

Rheumatoid arthritis: 1200 mg once daily; a one-time loading dose of up to 1800 mg/day or 26 mg/kg (whichever is lower) may be given

Maximum doses:

Patient <50 kg: Maximum: 1200 mg/day

Patient >50 kg with normal renal/hepatic function and low risk of peptic ulcer: Maximum: 1800 mg or 26 mg/kg (whichever is lower) in divided doses

Dosing adjustment in renal impairment: In general, NSAIDs are not recommended for use in patients with advanced renal disease but the manufacturer of oxaprozin does provide some guidelines for adjustment in renal dysfunction.

Severe renal impairment or on dialysis: 600 mg once daily; may increase cautiously to 1200 mg/day with close monitoring

Dosing adjustment in hepatic impairment: Use caution in patients with severe dysfunction

Mechanism of Action Inhibits prostaglandin synthesis by decreasing the activity of the enzyme, cyclooxygenase, which results in decreased formation of prostaglandin precursors

Contraindications Hypersensitivity to oxaprozin, aspirin, other NSAIDs, or any component of the formulation; perioperative pain in the setting of coronary artery bypass surgery (CABG); pregnancy (3rd trimester)

Warnings/Precautions [U.S. Boxed Warning]: NSAIDs are associated with an increased risk of adverse cardiovascular events, including MI, stroke, and new onset or worsening of pre-existing hypertension. Risk may be increased with duration of use or pre-existing cardiovascular risk factors or disease. Carefully evaluate individual cardiovascular risk profiles prior to prescribing. Use caution with fluid retention, CHF, or hypertension. Concurrent administration of ibuprofen, and potentially other nonselective NSAIDs, may interfere with aspirin's cardioprotective effect.

Use of NSAIDs can compromise existing renal function. Renal toxicity can occur in patients with impaired renal function, dehydration, heart failure, liver dysfunction, those taking diuretics and ACEIs, and the elderly. Rehydrate patient before starting therapy. Monitor renal function closely. Oxaprozin is not recommended for patients with advanced renal disease.

[U.S. Boxed Warning]: NSAIDs may increase risk of gastrointestinal irritation, ulceration, bleeding, and perforation. These events may occur at any time during therapy and without warning. Use caution with a history of GI disease (bleeding or ulcers); concurrent therapy with aspirin, anticoagulants, and/or corticosteroids; smoking; use of alcohol; and the elderly or debilitated patients.

Use the lowest effective dose for the shortest duration of time, consistent with individual patient goals, to reduce risk of cardiovascular or GI adverse events. Alternate therapies should be considered for patients at high risk.

NSAIDs may cause serious skin adverse events including exfoliative dermatitis, Stevens-Johnson syndrome (SJS), and toxic epidermal necrolysis (TEN). Anaphylactoid reactions may occur, even without prior exposure; patients with "aspirin triad" (bronchial asthma, aspirin intolerance, rhinitis) may be at increased risk. Do not use in patients who experience bronchospasm, asthma, rhinitis, or urticaria with NSAID or aspirin therapy. Use caution in other forms of asthma.

Use with caution in patients with decreased hepatic function. Closely monitor patients with any abnormal LFT. Severe hepatic reactions (eg, fulminant hepatitis, liver failure) have occurred with NSAID use, rarely; discontinue if signs or symptoms of liver disease develop, or if systemic manifestations occur.

The elderly are at increased risk for adverse effects (especially peptic ulceration, CNS effects, renal toxicity) from NSAIDs even at low doses.

Withhold for at least 4-6 half-lives prior to surgical or dental procedures. May cause mild photosensitivity reactions. Safety and efficacy have not been established in children <6 years of age.

Drug Interactions

Increased Effect/Toxicity: Oxaprozin may increase cyclosporine, digoxin, lithium, and methotrexate serum concentrations. The renal adverse effects of ACE inhibitors may be potentiated by NSAIDs. Corticosteroids may increase the risk of GI ulceration. The risk of bleeding with anticoagulants (warfarin, antiplatelet agents, low molecular weight heparins) may be increased. Concomitant use with fluoroquinolones may rarely increase risk of seizure.

Decreased Effect: Oxaprozin may decrease the effect of some antihypertensive agents (including ACE inhibitors, beta-blockers, hydralazine, and angiotensin antagonists), diuretics. Cholestyramine (and other bile acid sequestrants) may decrease the absorption of NSAIDs; separate by at least 2 hours. Salicylates' antiplatelet effect may be reduced.

Ethanol/Nutrition/Herb Interactions

Ethanol: Avoid ethanol (may enhance gastric mucosal irritation).

Herb/Nutraceutical: Avoid alfalfa, anise, bilberry, bladderwrack, bromelain, cat's claw, celery, coleus, cordyceps, dong quai, evening primrose, feverfew, fenugreek, garlic, ginger, ginkgo biloba, red clover, horse chestnut, grapeseed, green tea, ginseng, guggul, horse chestnut seed, horseradish, licorice, prickly ash, red clover, reishi, SAMe, sweet clover, turmeric, white willow (all have additional antiplatelet activity).

Pharmacodynamics/Kinetics

Absorption: Almost complete

(Continued)

Oxaprozin *(Continued)*

Protein binding: >99%
Metabolism: Hepatic via oxidation and glucuronidation; no active metabolites
Half-life elimination: 40-50 hours
Time to peak: 2-4 hours
Excretion: Urine (5% unchanged, 65% as metabolites); feces (35% as metabolites)

Pregnancy Risk Factor C/D (3rd trimester)

Dosage Forms
  Tablet: 600 mg
    Daypro®: 600 mg

Oxazepam *(oks A ze pam)*

Related Information
  Sedation *on page 1825*

Related Sample Prescriptions
  Sedation (Prior to Dental Treatment) *on page 1846*

U.S. Brand Names Serax®

Canadian Brand Names Apo-Oxazepam®; Novoxapram®; Oxpam®; Oxpram®; PMS-Oxazepam; Riva-Oxazepam

Generic Available Yes: Capsule

Pharmacologic Category Benzodiazepine

Use Treatment of anxiety; management of ethanol withdrawal

Unlabeled/Investigational Use Anticonvulsant in management of simple partial seizures; hypnotic

Local Anesthetic/Vasoconstrictor Precautions No information available to require special precautions

Effects on Dental Treatment Key adverse event(s) related to dental treatment: Xerostomia (normal salivary flow resumes upon discontinuation).

Common Adverse Effects Frequency not defined.
  Cardiovascular: Syncope (rare), edema
  Central nervous system: Drowsiness, ataxia, dizziness, vertigo, memory impairment, headache, paradoxical reactions (excitement, stimulation of effect), lethargy, amnesia, euphoria
  Dermatologic: Rash
  Endocrine & metabolic: Decreased libido, menstrual irregularities
  Genitourinary: Incontinence
  Hematologic: Leukopenia, blood dyscrasias
  Hepatic: Jaundice
  Neuromuscular & skeletal: Dysarthria, tremor, reflex slowing
  Ocular: Blurred vision, diplopia
  Miscellaneous: Drug dependence

Restrictions C-IV

Dosage Oral:
  Adults:
    Anxiety: 10-30 mg 3-4 times/day
    Ethanol withdrawal: 15-30 mg 3-4 times/day
    Hypnotic: 15-30 mg
  Elderly: Oral: Anxiety: 10 mg 2-3 times/day; increase gradually as needed to a total of 30-45 mg/day. Dose titration should be slow to evaluate sensitivity.
  Hemodialysis: Not dialyzable (0% to 5%)

Mechanism of Action Binds to stereospecific benzodiazepine receptors on the postsynaptic GABA neuron at several sites within the central nervous system, including the limbic system, reticular formation. Enhancement of the inhibitory effect of GABA on neuronal excitability results by increased neuronal membrane permeability to chloride ions. This shift in chloride ions results in hyperpolarization (a less excitable state) and stabilization.

Contraindications Hypersensitivity to oxazepam or any component of the formulation (cross-sensitivity with other benzodiazepines may exist); narrow-angle glaucoma (not in product labeling, however, benzodiazepines are contraindicated); not indicated for use in the treatment of psychosis; pregnancy

Warnings/Precautions May cause hypotension (rare) - use with caution in patients with cardiovascular or cerebrovascular disease, or in patients who would not tolerate transient decreases in blood pressure. Serax® 15 contains tartrazine; Safety and efficacy in established in pediatric patients <6 years of age; dose has not been established between 6-12 years of age.

Use with caution in elderly or debilitated patients, patients with hepatic disease (including alcoholics), or renal impairment. Use with caution in patients with respiratory disease or impaired gag reflex. Avoid use in patients with sleep apnea.

Causes CNS depression (dose-related) resulting in sedation, dizziness, confusion, or ataxia which may impair physical and mental capabilities. Patients must be cautioned about performing tasks which require mental alertness (eg, operating machinery or driving). Use with caution in patients receiving other CNS depressants or psychoactive agents. Effects with other sedative drugs or ethanol may be potentiated. Benzodiazepines have been associated with falls and traumatic injury and should be used with extreme caution in patients who are at risk of these events (especially the elderly).

Use caution in patients with suicidal risk. Use with caution in patients with a history of drug dependence. Benzodiazepines have been associated with dependence and acute withdrawal symptoms on discontinuation or reduction in dose. Acute withdrawal, including seizures, may be precipitated after administration of flumazenil to patients receiving long-term benzodiazepine therapy.

Benzodiazepines have been associated with anterograde amnesia. Paradoxical reactions, including hyperactive or aggressive behavior have been reported with benzodiazepines, particularly in adolescent/pediatric or psychiatric patients. Does not have analgesic, antidepressant, or antipsychotic properties.

Drug Interactions
Increased Effect/Toxicity: Ethanol and other CNS depressants may increase the CNS effects of oxazepam. Oxazepam may decrease the antiparkinsonian efficacy of levodopa. Flumazenil may cause seizures if administered following long-term benzodiazepine treatment.

Decreased Effect: Oral contraceptives may increase the clearance of oxazepam. Theophylline and other CNS stimulants may antagonize the sedative effects of oxazepam. Phenytoin may increase the clearance of oxazepam.

Ethanol/Nutrition/Herb Interactions
Ethanol: Avoid ethanol (may increase CNS depression).
Herb/Nutraceutical: Avoid valerian, St John's wort, kava kava, gotu kola (may increase CNS depression).

Pharmacodynamics/Kinetics
Absorption: Almost complete
Protein binding: 86% to 99%
Metabolism: Hepatic to inactive compounds (primarily as glucuronides)
Half-life elimination: 2.8-5.7 hours
Time to peak, serum: 2-4 hours
Excretion: Urine (as unchanged drug (50%) and metabolites)

Pregnancy Risk Factor D

Dosage Forms
Capsule: 10 mg, 15 mg, 30 mg
Serax®: 10 mg, 15 mg, 30 mg
Tablet:
Serax®: 15 mg

Oxcarbazepine (ox car BAZ e peen)

U.S. Brand Names Trileptal®
Canadian Brand Names Trileptal®
Mexican Brand Names Trileptal
Generic Available No
Index Terms GP 47680; OCBZ
Pharmacologic Category Anticonvulsant, Miscellaneous
Use Monotherapy or adjunctive therapy in the treatment of partial seizures in adults and children ≥4 years of age with epilepsy; adjunctive therapy in the treatment of partial seizures in children ≥2 years of age with epilepsy
Unlabeled/Investigational Use Bipolar disorder; treatment of neuropathic pain

Local Anesthetic/Vasoconstrictor Precautions No information available to require special precautions
Effects on Dental Treatment No significant effects or complications reported
Common Adverse Effects As reported in adults with doses of up to 2400 mg/day (includes patients on monotherapy, adjunctive therapy, and those not previously on AEDs); incidence in children was similar.

>10%:
Central nervous system: Dizziness (22% to 49%), somnolence (20% to 36%), headache (13% to 32%, placebo 23%), ataxia (5% to 31%), fatigue (12% to 15%), vertigo (6% to 15%)
Gastrointestinal: Vomiting (7% to 36%), nausea (15% to 29%), abdominal pain (10% to 13%)
Neuromuscular & skeletal: Abnormal gait (5% to 17%), tremor (3% to 16%)
Ocular: Diplopia (14% to 40%), nystagmus (7% to 26%), abnormal vision (4% to 14%)
(Continued)

Oxcarbazepine *(Continued)*

1% to 10%:

Cardiovascular: Hypotension (1% to 2%), leg edema (1% to 2%, placebo 1%)

Central nervous system: Nervousness (2% to 5%, placebo 1% to 2%), amnesia (4%), abnormal thinking (2% to 4%), insomnia (2% to 4%), speech disorder (1% to 3%), EEG abnormalities (2%), abnormal feelings (1% to 2%), agitation (1% to 2%, placebo 1%), confusion (1% to 2%, placebo 1%)

Dermatologic: Rash (4%), acne (1% to 2%)

Endocrine & metabolic: Hyponatremia (1% to 3%, placebo 1%)

Gastrointestinal: Diarrhea (5% to 7%), dyspepsia (5% to 6%), constipation (2% to 6%, placebo 0% to 4%), gastritis (1% to 2%, placebo 1%), weight gain (1% to 2%, placebo 1%)

Neuromuscular & skeletal: Weakness (3% to 6%, placebo 5%), back pain (4%), falling down (4%), abnormal coordination (1% to 4%, placebo 1% to 2%), dysmetria (1% to 3%), sprains/strains (2%), muscle weakness (1% to 2%)

Ocular: Abnormal accommodation (2%)

Respiratory: Upper respiratory tract infection (7%), rhinitis (2% to 5%, placebo 4%), chest infection (4%), epistaxis (4%), sinusitis (4%)

Mechanism of Action Pharmacological activity results from both oxcarbazepine and its monohydroxy metabolite (MHD). Precise mechanism of anticonvulsant effect has not been defined. Oxcarbazepine and MHD block voltage-sensitive sodium channels, stabilizing hyperexcited neuronal membranes, inhibiting repetitive firing, and decreasing the propagation of synaptic impulses. These actions are believed to prevent the spread of seizures. Oxcarbazepine and MHD also increase potassium conductance and modulate the activity of high-voltage activated calcium channels.

Drug Interactions

Cytochrome P450 Effect: Inhibits CYP2C19 (weak); **Induces** CYP3A4 (strong)

Increased Effect/Toxicity: Serum concentrations of phenytoin and phenobarbital are increased by oxcarbazepine.

Decreased Effect: Oxcarbazepine serum concentrations may be reduced by carbamazepine, phenytoin, phenobarbital, valproic acid and verapamil (decreases levels of active oxcarbazepine metabolite). Oxcarbazepine reduces the serum concentrations of hormonal contraceptives; use alternative contraceptive measures. Oxcarbazepine may decrease the levels/effects of benzodiazepines, calcium channel blockers, clarithromycin, cyclosporine, erythromycin, estrogens, mirtazapine, nateglinide, nefazodone, nevirapine, protease inhibitors, tacrolimus, venlafaxine, and other CYP3A4 substrates.

Pharmacodynamics/Kinetics

Absorption: Complete; food has no affect on rate or extent

Distribution: MHD: V_d: 49 L

Protein binding, serum: MHD: 40%

Metabolism: Hepatic to 10-monohydroxy metabolite (MHD; active); MHD is further conjugated to DHD (inactive)

Bioavailability: Decreased in children <8 years; increased in elderly >60 years

Half-life elimination: Parent drug: 2 hours; MHD: 9 hours; renal impairment (Cl_{cr} 30 mL/minute): MHD: 19 hours

Clearance of MHD is increased in younger children (~80% in children 2-4 years of age) and approaches that of adults by ~13 years of age

Time to peak, serum: 4.5 hours (3-13 hours)

Excretion: Urine (95%, <1% as unchanged oxcarbazepine, 27% as unchanged MHD, 49% as MHD glucuronides); feces (<4%)

Pregnancy Risk Factor C

Oxiconazole *(oks i KON a zole)*

U.S. Brand Names Oxistat®

Canadian Brand Names Oxistat®

Mexican Brand Names Myfungar; Oxistat

Generic Available No

Index Terms Oxiconazole Nitrate

Pharmacologic Category Antifungal Agent, Topical

Use Treatment of tinea pedis (athlete's foot), tinea cruris (jock itch), and tinea corporis (ringworm)

Local Anesthetic/Vasoconstrictor Precautions No information available to require special precautions

Effects on Dental Treatment No significant effects or complications reported

Common Adverse Effects 1% to 10%:

Dermatologic: Itching, erythema

Local: Transient burning, local irritation, stinging, dryness

Mechanism of Action The cytoplasmic membrane integrity of fungi is destroyed by oxiconazole which exerts a fungicidal activity through inhibition of ergosterol synthesis. Effective for treatment of tinea pedis, tinea cruris, tinea corporis, and tinea versicolor. Active against *Trichophyton rubrum*, *Trichophyton mentagrophytes*, *Trichophyton violaceum*, *Microsporum canis*, *Microsporum audouinii*, *Microsporum gypseum*, *Epidermophyton floccosum*, *Candida albicans*, and *Malassezia furfur*.

Pharmacodynamics/Kinetics

Absorption: In each layer of the dermis; very little systemically after one topical dose

Distribution: To each layer of the dermis; enters breast milk

Excretion: Urine (<0.3%)

Pregnancy Risk Factor B

Oxiconazole Nitrate see Oxiconazole on page 1222

Oxidized Regenerated Cellulose see Cellulose (Oxidized/Regenerated) on page 316

Oxilapine Succinate see Loxapine on page 1009

Oxipor® VHC [OTC] see Coal Tar on page 402

Oxistat® see Oxiconazole on page 1222

Oxpentifylline see Pentoxifylline on page 1278

Oxprenolol (ox PREN oh lole)

Canadian Brand Names Slow-Trasicor®; Trasicor®

Generic Available No

Index Terms Oxprenolol Hydrochloride

Pharmacologic Category Antihypertensive; Beta Blocker, Nonselective

Use Treatment of mild or moderate hypertension

Unlabeled/Investigational Use Treatment of nonsevere hypertension in pregnancy (second-line agent)

Local Anesthetic/Vasoconstrictor Precautions No information available to require special precautions

Effects on Dental Treatment Nonselective beta-blockers may enhance the pressor response to epinephrine, resulting in hypertension and bradycardia. Many nonsteroidal anti-inflammatory drugs, such as ibuprofen and indomethacin, can reduce the hypotensive effect of beta-blockers after 3 or more weeks of therapy with the NSAID. Short-term NSAID use (ie, 3 days) requires no special precautions in patients taking beta-blockers.

Common Adverse Effects Frequency not defined.

Cardiovascular: CHF, pulmonary edema, cardiac enlargement, postural hypotension, severe bradycardia, lengthening of PR interval, second- and third-degree AV block, sinus arrest, palpitation, chest pain; peripheral vascular disorders, Raynaud's phenomenon, claudication, hot flashes, syncope

Central nervous system: Vertigo, lightheadedness, headache, dizziness, anxiety, mental depression, nervousness, irritability, hallucinations, sleep disturbances, nightmares, insomnia, weakness, sedation, vivid dreams, slurred speech

Dermatological: Dry skin, rash, pruritus

Endocrine & metabolic: Libido decreased, impotence, weight gain, hypoglycemia

Gastrointestinal: Diarrhea, constipation, flatulence, heartburn, anorexia, nausea, vomiting, abdominal pain, dry mouth

Hematological: Thrombocytopenia, leukopenia

Hepatic: Alkaline phosphatase increased, bilirubin increased, transaminases increased

Neuromuscular & skeletal: Paresthesia

Ocular: Keratoconjunctivitis, dry eyes, itching eyes, blurred vision

Otic: Tinnitus

Renal: BUN increased

Respiratory: Dyspnea, wheezing, bronchospasm, nasal congestion, status asthmaticus

Miscellaneous: Diaphoresis, exertional tiredness

Restrictions Not available in U.S.

Mechanism of Action Oxprenolol has a competitive ability to antagonize catecholamine-induced tachycardia at the beta-receptor sites in the heart, thus decreasing cardiac output; inhibits of renin release by the kidneys, and inhibits the vasomotor centers.

(Continued)

Oxprenolol *(Continued)*

Drug Interactions

Cytochrome P450 Effect: Inhibits CYP2D6 (weak)

Increased Effect/Toxicity: Oxprenolol may potentiate negative inotropic and negative dromotropic effect of antiarrhythmic agents (eg, quinidine, amiodarone). Concomitant use of I.V. calcium channel blockers with AV-blocking potential (eg, diltiazem and verapamil) may lead to severe hypotension; cardiac arrhythmias and cardiac arrest may occur. Catecholamine-depleting drugs (reserpine, guanethidine) may produce any excessive reduction of sympathetic activity, leading to severe bradycardia and hypotension.

Ergot alkaloids may cause deterioration in peripheral blood flow, leading to peripheral ischemia. Inhalational anesthetics may cause cardiodepressant effects in patients receiving oxprenolol. Oxprenolol may potentiate hypoglycemic effects of insulin and hypoglycemic agents. Concomitant use of MAO inhibitors may produce any excessive reduction of sympathetic activity. CNS depressants (opiate analgesics, antihistamines, ethanol, and psycho-active drugs) may potentiate CNS depressant effects of oxprenolol.

Decreased Effect: Concomitant use of NSAIDs (indomethacin) may decrease antihypertensive effect of oxprenolol. Concomitant use of sympathomimetic agents (eg, epinephrine) may cause hypertensive reactions.

Pharmacodynamics/Kinetics

Duration of beta-blocking effects: Immediate-release tablet: 8-12 hours; Slow-release tablet: Up to 24 hours

Absorption: 20% to 70%

Distribution: 1.3 L/kg

Protein binding: 80%

Metabolism: Hepatic first-pass effect

Half-life elimination: 1.3-1.5 hours

Time to peak, serum: Immediate-release tablet: 0.5-1.5 hours; Slow-release tablet: 2-4 hours

Excretion: Urine (as inactive metabolites, <5% as unchanged drug); major metabolite is glucuronide

Pregnancy Risk Factor Not assigned (similar agents rated C/D)

Oxybutynin *(oks i BYOO ti nin)*

U.S. Brand Names Ditropan®; Ditropan® XL; Oxytrol®

Canadian Brand Names Apo-Oxybutynin®; Ditropan®; Ditropan® XL; Gen-Oxybutynin; Novo-Oxybutynin; Nu-Oxybutyn; Oxytrol®; PMS-Oxybutynin; Uromax®

Mexican Brand Names Nefryl; Tavor

Generic Available Yes: Excludes transdermal patch

Index Terms Oxybutynin Chloride

Pharmacologic Category Antispasmodic Agent, Urinary

Use Antispasmodic for neurogenic bladder (urgency, frequency, urge incontinence) and uninhibited bladder

Local Anesthetic/Vasoconstrictor Precautions No information available to require special precautions

Effects on Dental Treatment Key adverse event(s) related to dental treatment: Xerostomia and changes in salivation (normal salivary flow resumes upon discontinuation), and taste perversion.

Common Adverse Effects

Oral:

>10%:

Central nervous system: Dizziness (6% to 16%), somnolence (12% to 13%)

Gastrointestinal: Xerostomia (61% to 71%), constipation (13%)

Genitourinary: Urination impaired (11%)

1% to 10%:

Cardiovascular: Palpitation (2% to <5%), peripheral edema (2% to <5%), hypertension (2% to <5%), vasodilation (2% to <5%)

Central nervous system: Headache (6% to 10%), pain (7%), confusion (2% to <5%), insomnia (2% to <5%), nervousness (2% to <5%)

Dermatologic: Dry skin (2% to <5%), skin rash (2% to <5%)

Gastrointestinal: Nausea (9% to 10%), dyspepsia (7%), abdominal pain (2% to 6%), diarrhea (5% to 9%), flatulence (2% to <5%), gastrointestinal reflux (2% to <5%), taste perversion (2% to <5%)

Genitourinary: Postvoid residuals increased (2% to 9%), urinary tract infection (5%)

Neuromuscular & skeletal: Weakness (2% to 7%)

Ocular: Blurred vision (8% to 9%), dry eyes (2% to 6%)

Respiratory: Rhinitis (6%), dry nasal and sinus membranes (2% to <5%)

Transdermal:

>10%: Local: Application site reaction (17%), pruritus (14%)

1% to 10%:

Gastrointestinal: Xerostomia (4% to 10%), diarrhea (3%), constipation (3%)

Genitourinary: Dysuria (2%)

Local: Erythema (6% to 8%), vesicles (3%), rash (3%)

Ocular: Vision changes (3%)

Mechanism of Action Direct antispasmodic effect on smooth muscle, also inhibits the action of acetylcholine on smooth muscle (exhibits 1/5 the anticholinergic activity of atropine, but is 4-10 times the antispasmodic activity); does not block effects at skeletal muscle or at autonomic ganglia; increases bladder capacity, decreases uninhibited contractions, and delays desire to void, therefore, decreases urgency and frequency

Drug Interactions

Cytochrome P450 Effect: Substrate of CYP3A4 (minor); **Inhibits** CYP2C8 (weak), 2D6 (weak), 3A4 (weak)

Increased Effect/Toxicity: Additive sedation with CNS depressants and ethanol. Additive anticholinergic effects with antihistamines and anticholinergic agents.

Pharmacodynamics/Kinetics

Onset of action: Oral: 30-60 minutes

Peak effect: 3-6 hours

Duration: 6-10 hours (up to 24 hours for extended release oral formulation)

Absorption: Oral: Rapid and well absorbed; Transdermal: High

Distribution: V_d: 193 L

Metabolism: Hepatic via CYP3A4; Oral: High first-pass metabolism (not with I.V. or transdermal use); forms active and inactive metabolites

Half-life elimination: I.V.: ~2 hours (parent drug), 7-8 hours (metabolites)

Time to peak, serum: Oral: ~60 minutes; Transdermal: 24-48 hours

Excretion: Urine, as metabolites (<0.1% as unchanged drug)

Pregnancy Risk Factor B

Oxybutynin Chloride *see* Oxybutynin *on page 1224*

Oxychlorosene (oks i KLOR oh seen)

U.S. Brand Names Clorpactin® WCS-90 [OTC]

Generic Available No

Index Terms Oxychlorosene Sodium

Pharmacologic Category Antibiotic, Topical

Use Treatment of localized infections

Local Anesthetic/Vasoconstrictor Precautions No information available to require special precautions

Effects on Dental Treatment No significant effects or complications reported

Oxychlorosene Sodium *see* Oxychlorosene *on page 1225*

Oxycodone (oks i KOE done)

Related Information

Oral Pain *on page 1788*

U.S. Brand Names ETH-Oxydose™; OxyContin®; OxyFast®; OxyIR®; Roxicodone®

Canadian Brand Names OxyContin®; Oxy.IR®; Supeudol®

Mexican Brand Names OxyContin

Generic Available Yes

Index Terms Dihydrohydroxycodeinone; Oxycodone Hydrochloride

Pharmacologic Category Analgesic, Opioid

Dental Use Treatment of postoperative pain

Use Management of moderate-to-severe pain, normally used in combination with nonopioid analgesics

(Continued)

Oxycodone *(Continued)*

OxyContin® is indicated for around-the-clock management of moderate-to-severe pain when an analgesic is needed for an extended period of time.

Local Anesthetic/Vasoconstrictor Precautions No information available to require special precautions

Effects on Dental Treatment Key adverse event(s) related to dental treatment: Xerostomia (normal salivary flow resumes upon discontinuation).

Significant Adverse Effects

>10%:

Central nervous system: Somnolence (23% to 24%), dizziness (13% to 16%)

Dermatologic: Pruritus (12% to 13%)

Gastrointestinal: Nausea (23% to 27%), constipation (23% to 26%), vomiting (12% to 14%)

1% to 10%:

Cardiovascular: Postural hypotension (1% to 5%)

Central nervous system: Headache (7% to 8%), abnormal dreams (1% to 5%), anxiety (1% to 5%), chills (1% to 5%), confusion (1% to 5%), euphoria (1% to 5%), fever (1% to 5%), insomnia (1% to 5%), nervousness (1% to 5%), thought abnormalities (1% to 5%)

Dermatologic: Rash (1% to 5%)

Gastrointestinal: Xerostomia (6% to 7%), abdominal pain (1% to 5%), anorexia (1% to 5%), diarrhea (1% to 5%), dyspepsia (1% to 5%), gastritis (1% to 5%)

Neuromuscular & skeletal: Weakness (6% to 7%), twitching (1% to 5%)

Respiratory: Dyspnea (1% to 5%), hiccups (1% to 5%)

Miscellaneous: Diaphoresis (5% to 6%)

<1% (Limited to important or life-threatening): Agitation, amenorrhea, amnesia, anaphylaxis, anaphylactoid reaction, appetite increased, chest pain, cough, dehydration, depression, dysphagia, dysuria, edema, emotional lability, eructation, exfoliative dermatitis, facial edema, hallucinations, hematuria, histamine release, hyperkinesia, hypoesthesia, hyponatremia, hypotonia, ileus, impotence, intracranial pressure increased, libido decreased, malaise, migraine, paradoxical CNS stimulation, paralytic ileus, paresthesia, pharyngitis, physical dependence, polyuria, psychological dependence, seizure, SIADH, speech disorder, ST segment depression, stomatitis, stupor, syncope, tablet in stool (OxyCodone®), taste perversion, thirst, tinnitus, tremor, urinary retention, urticaria, vasodilation, vertigo, vision change, voice alteration, withdrawal syndrome

Restrictions C-II

Dental Usual Dosing Postoperative pain: Adults: Oral: 5 mg every 6 hours as needed

Dosage Oral:

Children: Immediate release:

6-12 years: 1.25 mg every 6 hours as needed

>12 years: 2.5 mg every 6 hours as needed

Adults:

Immediate release: 5 mg every 6 hours as needed

Controlled release:

Opioid naive: 10 mg every 12 hours

Concurrent CNS depressants: Reduce usual dose by 1/3 to 1/2

Conversion from transdermal fentanyl: For each 25 mcg/hour transdermal dose, substitute 10 mg controlled release oxycodone every 12 hours; should be initiated 18 hours after the removal of the transdermal fentanyl patch

Currently on opioids: Use standard conversion chart to convert daily dose to oxycodone equivalent. Divide daily dose in 2 (for twice-daily dosing, usually every 12 hours) and round down to nearest dosage form.

Note: 60 mg, 80 mg, or 160 mg tablets are for use **only** in opioid-tolerant patients. Special safety considerations must be addressed when converting to OxyContin® doses ≥160 mg every 12 hours. Dietary caution must be taken when patients are initially titrated to 160 mg tablets. Using different strengths to obtain the same daily dose is equivalent (eg, four 40 mg tablets, two 80 mg tablets, one 160 mg tablet); all produce similar blood levels.

Multiplication factors for converting the daily dose of current oral opioid to the daily dose of oral oxycodone:

Current opioid mg/day dose x factor = Oxycodone mg/day dose

Codeine mg/day oral dose **x** 0.15 = Oxycodone mg/day dose

Hydrocodone mg/day oral dose **x** 0.9 = Oxycodone mg/day dose

Hydromorphone mg/day oral dose **x** 4 = Oxycodone mg/day dose

Levorphanol mg/day oral dose **x** 7.5 = Oxycodone mg/day dose

Meperidine mg/day oral dose **x** 0.1 = Oxycodone mg/day dose

Methadone mg/day oral dose **x** 1.5 = Oxycodone mg/day dose
Morphine mg/day oral dose **x** 0.5 = Oxycodone mg/day dose
Note: Divide the oxycodone mg/day dose into the appropriate dosing interval for the specific form being used.

Dosing adjustment in hepatic impairment: Reduce dosage in patients with severe liver disease

Mechanism of Action Binds to opiate receptors in the CNS, causing inhibition of ascending pain pathways, altering the perception of and response to pain; produces generalized CNS depression

Contraindications Hypersensitivity to oxycodone or any component of the formulation; significant respiratory depression; hypercarbia; acute or severe bronchial asthma; OxyContin® is also contraindicated in paralytic ileus (known or suspected); pregnancy (prolonged use or high doses at term)

Warnings/Precautions May cause CNS depression, which may impair physical or mental abilities; patients must be cautioned about performing tasks which require mental alertness (eg, operating machinery or driving). Effects may be potentiated when used with other sedative drugs or ethanol. Use with caution in patients with hypersensitivity reactions to other phenanthrene derivative opioid agonists (morphine, hydrocodone, hydromorphone, levorphanol, oxymorphone), respiratory diseases including asthma, emphysema, or COPD. Use with caution in pancreatitis or biliary tract disease, acute alcoholism (including delirium tremens), morbid obesity, adrenocortical insufficiency, history of seizure disorders, CNS depression/coma, kyphoscoliosis (or other skeletal disorder which may alter respiratory function), hypothyroidism (including myxedema), prostatic hyperplasia, urethral stricture, and toxic psychosis. May obscure diagnosis or clinical course of patients with acute abdominal conditions.

Use with caution in the elderly, debilitated, severe hepatic or renal function. Hemodynamic effects (hypotension, orthostasis) may be exaggerated in patients with hypovolemia, concurrent vasodilating drugs, or in patients with head injury. Respiratory depressant effects and capacity to elevate CSF pressure may be exaggerated in presence of head injury, other intracranial lesion, or pre-existing intracranial pressure.

Concurrent use of agonist/antagonist analgesics may precipitate withdrawal symptoms and/or reduced analgesic efficacy in patients following prolonged therapy with mu opioid agonists. Abrupt discontinuation following prolonged use may also lead to withdrawal symptoms.

[U.S. Boxed Warning]: Healthcare provider should be alert to problems of abuse, misuse, and diversion. Tolerance or drug dependence may result from extended use.

Controlled-release formulations:

[U.S. Boxed Warning]: OxyContin® is not intended for use as an "as needed" analgesic or for immediately-postoperative pain management (should be used postoperatively only if the patient has received it prior to surgery or if severe, persistent pain is anticipated). **[U.S. Boxed Warning]: Do NOT crush, break, or chew controlled-release tablets;** 60 mg, 80 mg, and 160 mg strengths are for use only in opioid-tolerant patients.

Drug Interactions Substrate of CYP2D6 (major)

Ammonium chloride: May increase the excretion of analgesics (opioid).

Antipsychotic agents (phenothiazines): May enhance the hypotensive effect of analgesics (opioid).

CNS depressants: May enhance the adverse/toxic effect of analgesics (opioids).

CYP2D6 inhibitors: May decrease the effects of oxycodone. Example inhibitors include chlorpromazine, delavirdine, fluoxetine, miconazole, paroxetine, pergolide, quinidine, quinine, ritonavir, and ropinirole.

Pegvisomant: Analgesics (opioid) may diminish the therapeutic effect of pegvisomant.

Selective serotonin reuptake inhibitors (SSRIs): Analgesics (opioid) may enhance the serotonergic effect of selective serotonin reuptake inhibitors. This may cause serotonin syndrome.

Ethanol/Nutrition/Herb Interactions

Ethanol: Avoid ethanol (may increase CNS depression).

Food: When taken with a high-fat meal, peak concentration is 25% greater following a single OxyContin® 160 mg tablet as compared to two 80 mg tablets.

Herb/Nutraceutical: Avoid valerian, St John's wort, kava kava, gotu kola (may increase CNS depression).

Dietary Considerations Instruct patient to avoid high-fat meals when taking OxyContin® 160 mg tablets.

Pharmacodynamics/Kinetics

Onset of action: Pain relief: 10-15 minutes
(Continued)

Oxycodone *(Continued)*

Peak effect: 0.5-1 hour

Duration: Immediate release: 3-6 hours; Controlled release: ≤12 hours

Distribution: V_d: 2.6 L/kg; distributed to skeletal muscle, liver, intestinal tract, lungs, spleen, brain, and breast milk

Protein binding: ~45%

Metabolism: Hepatically via CYP2D6 to various metabolites including noroxycodone (weak analgesic activity), oxymorphone (has analgesic activity; low concentrations in plasma) and their glucuronides

Bioavailability: Controlled release, immediate release: 60% to 87%

Half-life elimination: Immediate release: 2-3 hours; controlled release: ~5 hours

Excretion: Urine (~19% as parent; > 64% as metabolites)

Pregnancy Risk Factor B/D (prolonged use or high doses at term)

Lactation Enters breast milk/use caution

Dosage Forms Excipient information presented when available (limited, particularly for generics); consult specific product labeling.

Capsule, as hydrochloride: 5 mg

OxyIR®: 5 mg

Solution, oral, as hydrochloride: 5 mg/5 mL (500 mL)

Roxicodone®: 5 mg/5 mL (5 mL, 500 mL) [contains alcohol]

Solution, oral, as hydrochloride [concentrate]: 20 mg/mL (30 mL)

ETH-Oxydose™: 20 mg/mL (1 mL, 30 mL) [contains sodium benzoate; berry flavor]

OxyFast®: 20 mg/mL (30 mL) [contains sodium benzoate and dry natural rubber]

Roxicodone®: 20 mg/mL (30 mL) [contains sodium benzoate]

Tablet, as hydrochloride: 5 mg, 15 mg, 30 mg

Roxicodone®: 5 mg, 15 mg, 30 mg

Tablet, controlled release, as hydrochloride:

OxyContin®: 10 mg, 20 mg, 40 mg, 60 mg, 80 mg, 160 mg

Tablet, extended release, as hydrochloride: 10 mg, 20 mg, 40 mg, 80 mg

Selected Readings

Wynn RL, "Narcotic Analgesics for Dental Pain: Available Products, Strengths, and Formulations," *Gen Dent*, 2001, 49(2)126-36.

Oxycodone and Acetaminophen

(oks i KOE done & a seet a MIN oh fen)

Related Information

Acetaminophen *on page 31*

Oral Pain *on page 1788*

Oxycodone *on page 1225*

Related Sample Prescriptions

Severe Oral Pain *on page 1835*

U.S. Brand Names Endocet®; Percocet®; Roxicet™; Roxicet™ 5/500; Tylox®

Canadian Brand Names Endocet®; Oxycocet®; Percocet®; Percocet®-Demi; PMS-Oxycodone-Acetaminophen

Generic Available Yes: Excludes caplet and solution

Index Terms Acetaminophen and Oxycodone

Pharmacologic Category Analgesic, Opioid

Dental Use Treatment of postoperative pain

Use Management of moderate-to-severe pain

Local Anesthetic/Vasoconstrictor Precautions No information available to require special precautions

Effects on Dental Treatment Key adverse event(s) related to dental treatment: Nausea, sedation, constipation, and xerostomia (normal salivary flow resumes upon discontinuation). See Dental Comment.

Significant Adverse Effects Frequency not defined (also see individual agents): Allergic reaction, constipation, dizziness, dysphoria, euphoria, lightheadedness, nausea, pruritus, respiratory depression, sedation, skin rash, vomiting

Restrictions C-II

Dental Usual Dosing

Note: Initial dose is based on the **oxycodone** content; however, the maximum daily dose is based on the **acetaminophen** content.

Management of pain: Doses should be given every 4-6 hours as needed and titrated to appropriate analgesic effects.

Mild-to-moderate pain:

Children: Initial dose, **based on oxycodone content:** 0.05-0.1 mg/kg/dose

Maximum acetaminophen dose: Children <45 kg: 90 mg/kg/day; children >45 kg: 4 g/day

Adults: Initial dose, **based on oxycodone content:** 5 mg

Severe pain:

Children: Initial dose, **based on oxycodone content:** 0.3 mg/kg/dose

Adults: Initial dose, **based on oxycodone content:** 15-30 mg. Do not exceed acetaminophen 4 g/day.

Elderly: Doses should be titrated to appropriate analgesic effects: Initial dose, **based on oxycodone content:** 2.5-5 mg every 6 hours. Do not exceed acetaminophen 4 g/day.

Dosage adjustment in hepatic impairment: Dose should be reduced in patients with severe liver disease.

Dosage Oral: Doses should be given every 4-6 hours as needed and titrated to appropriate analgesic effects. **Note:** Initial dose is based on the **oxycodone** content; however, the maximum daily dose is based on the **acetaminophen** content.

Children: Maximum acetaminophen dose: Children <45 kg: 90 mg/kg/day; children >45 kg: 4 g/day

Mild-to-moderate pain: Initial dose, **based on oxycodone content:** 0.05-0.1 mg/kg/dose

Severe pain: Initial dose, **based on oxycodone content:** 0.3 mg/kg/dose

Adults:

Mild-to-moderate pain: Initial dose, **based on oxycodone content:** 5 mg

Severe pain: Initial dose, **based on oxycodone content:** 15-30 mg. Do not exceed acetaminophen 4 g/day.

Elderly: Doses should be titrated to appropriate analgesic effects: Initial dose, **based on oxycodone content:** 2.5-5 mg every 6 hours. Do not exceed acetaminophen 4 g/day.

Dosage adjustment in hepatic impairment: Dose should be reduced in patients with severe liver disease.

Mechanism of Action

Oxycodone, as with other narcotic (opiate) analgesics, blocks pain perception in the cerebral cortex by binding to specific receptor molecules (opiate receptors) within the neuronal membranes of synapses. This binding results in a decreased synaptic chemical transmission throughout the CNS thus inhibiting the flow of pain sensations into the higher centers. Mu and kappa are the two subtypes of the opiate receptor to which oxycodone binds to cause analgesia.

Acetaminophen inhibits the synthesis of prostaglandins in the CNS and peripherally blocks pain impulse generation; produces antipyresis from inhibition of hypothalamic heat-regulating center.

Contraindications Hypersensitivity to oxycodone, acetaminophen, or any component of the formulation; severe respiratory depression (in absence of resuscitative equipment or ventilatory support); pregnancy (prolonged periods or high doses at term)

Warnings/Precautions Use with caution in patients with hypersensitivity reactions to other phenanthrene-derivative opioid agonists (morphine, codeine, hydrocodone, hydromorphone, levorphanol, oxymorphone); respiratory diseases including asthma, emphysema, COPD; severe liver or renal insufficiency; hypothyroidism; Addison's disease; prostatic hyperplasia; or urethral stricture. Some preparations contain sulfites which may cause allergic reactions. May be habit-forming.

Use with caution in patients with head injury and increased intracranial pressure (respiratory depressant effects increased and may also elevate CSF pressure).

Enhanced analgesia has been seen in elderly patients on therapeutic doses of narcotics. Duration of action may be increased in the elderly. The elderly may be particularly susceptible to the CNS depressant and constipating effects of narcotics.

Drug Interactions Also see individual agents.

Oxycodone: **Substrate** of CYP2D6 (major).

Acetaminophen: **Substrate** (minor) of CYP1A2, 2A6, 2C9, 2D6, 2E1, 3A4.

Anesthetics, general: May have additive CNS depression; consider lowering dose of one or both agents.

Anticholinergics: Concomitant use may lead to paralytic ileus.

CNS depressants: May have additive CNS depression; consider lowering dose of one or both agents.

CYP2D6 inhibitors: May decrease the effects of oxycodone. Example inhibitors include chlorpromazine, delavirdine, fluoxetine, miconazole, paroxetine, pergolide, quinidine, quinine, ritonavir, and ropinirole.

Phenothiazines: May have additive CNS depression with phenothiazine and other tranquilizers; consider lowering dose of one or both agents.

Sedative hypnotics: May have additive CNS depression; consider lowering dose of one or both agents.

Ethanol/Nutrition/Herb Interactions Ethanol: May have additive CNS depression. In addition, excessive intake of ethanol may increase the risk of acetaminophen-induced hepatotoxicity. Avoid ethanol or limit to <3 drinks/day.

(Continued)

Oxycodone and Acetaminophen *(Continued)*

Pharmacodynamics/Kinetics See individual agents.

Pregnancy Risk Factor C/D (prolonged periods or high doses at term)

Lactation Enters breast milk/use caution

Breast-Feeding Considerations

Oxycodone: Excreted in breast milk. If occasional doses are used during breast-feeding, monitor infant for sedation, GI effects, and changes in feeding pattern.

Acetaminophen: May be taken while breast-feeding.

Dosage Forms Excipient information presented when available (limited, particularly for generics); consult specific product labeling.

Caplet:

Roxicet™ 5/500: Oxycodone hydrochloride 5 mg and acetaminophen 500 mg

Capsule: 5/500: Oxycodone hydrochloride 5 mg and acetaminophen 500 mg

Tylox®: 5/500: Oxycodone hydrochloride 5 mg and acetaminophen 500 mg [contains sodium benzoate and sodium metabisulfite]

Solution, oral:

Roxicet™: Oxycodone hydrochloride 5 mg and acetaminophen 325 mg per 5 mL (5 mL, 500 mL) [contains alcohol <0.5%]

Tablet: 5/325: Oxycodone hydrochloride 5 mg and acetaminophen 325 mg; 7.5/325: Oxycodone hydrochloride 7.5 mg and acetaminophen 325 mg; 7.5/500: Oxycodone hydrochloride 7.5 mg and acetaminophen 500 mg; 10/325: Oxycodone hydrochloride 10 mg and acetaminophen 325 mg; 10/650: Oxycodone hydrochloride 10 mg and acetaminophen 650 mg

Endocet® 5/325 [scored]: Oxycodone hydrochloride 5 mg and acetaminophen 325 mg

Endocet® 7.5/325: Oxycodone hydrochloride 7.5 mg and acetaminophen 325 mg

Endocet® 7.5/500: Oxycodone hydrochloride 7.5 mg and acetaminophen 500 mg

Endocet® 10/325: Oxycodone hydrochloride 10 mg and acetaminophen 325 mg

Endocet® 10/650: Oxycodone hydrochloride 10 mg and acetaminophen 650 mg

Percocet® 2.5/325: Oxycodone hydrochloride 2.5 mg and acetaminophen 325 mg

Percocet® 5/325 [scored]: Oxycodone hydrochloride 5 mg and acetaminophen 325 mg

Percocet® 7.5/325: Oxycodone hydrochloride 7.5 mg and acetaminophen 325 mg

Percocet® 7.5/500: Oxycodone hydrochloride 7.5 mg and acetaminophen 500 mg

Percocet® 10/325: Oxycodone hydrochloride 10 mg and acetaminophen 325 mg

Percocet® 10/650: Oxycodone hydrochloride 10 mg and acetaminophen 650 mg

Roxicet™ [scored]: Oxycodone hydrochloride 5 mg and acetaminophen 325 mg

Dental Comment Oxycodone, as with other narcotic analgesics, is recommended only for limited acute dosing (ie, 3 days or less). Oxycodone has an addictive liability, especially when given long-term. The acetaminophen component requires use with caution in patients with alcoholic liver disease.

Acetaminophen: A study by Hylek, et al, suggested that the combination of acetaminophen with warfarin (Coumadin®) may cause enhanced anticoagulation. The following recommendations have been made by Hylek, et al, and supported by an editorial in *JAMA* by Bell.

Dose and duration of acetaminophen should be as low as possible, individualized and monitored.

For patients who reported taking the equivalent of at least 4 regular strength (325 mg) tablets for longer than a week, the odds of having an INR >6.0 were increased 10-fold above those not taking acetaminophen. Risk decreased with lower intakes of acetaminophen reaching a background level of risk at a dose of 6 or fewer 325 mg tablets per week.

Selected Readings

Bell WR, "Acetaminophen and Warfarin: Undesirable Synergy," *JAMA*, 1998, 279(9):702-3.

Botting RM, "Mechanism of Action of Acetaminophen: Is There a Cyclooxygenase 3?" *Clin Infect Dis*, 2000, Suppl 5:S202-10.

Cooper SA, Precheur H, Rauch D, et al, "Evaluation of Oxycodone and Acetaminophen in Treatment of Postoperative Pain," *Oral Surg Oral Med Oral Pathol*, 1980, 50(6):496-501.

Dart RC, Kuffner EK, and Rumack BH, "Treatment of Pain or Fever With Paracetamol (Acetaminophen) in the Alcoholic Patient: A Systematic Review," *Am J Ther*, 2000, 7(2):123-34.

Dionne RA, "New Approaches to Preventing and Treating Postoperative Pain," *J Am Dent Assoc*, 1992, 123(6):26-34.

Gobetti JP, "Controlling Dental Pain," *J Am Dent Assoc*, 1992, 123(6):47-52.

Grant JA and Weiler JM, "A Report of a Rare Immediate Reaction After Ingestion of Acetaminophen," *Ann Allergy Asthma Immunol*, 2001, 87(3):227-9.

Hylek EM, Heiman H, Skates SJ, et al, "Acetaminophen and Other Risk Factors for Excessive Warfarin Anticoagulation 1998," *JAMA*, 1998, 279(9):702-3.

Kwan D, Bartle WR, and Walker SE, "The Effects of Acetaminophen on Pharmacokinetics and Pharmacodynamics of Warfarin," *J Clin Pharmacol*, 1999, 39(1):68-75.

McClain CJ, Price S, Barve S, et al, "Acetaminophen Hepatotoxicity: An Update," *Curr Gastroenterol Rep*, 1999, 1(1):42-9.

Shek KL, Chan LN, and Nutescu E, "Warfarin-Acetaminophen Drug Interaction Revisited," *Pharmacotherapy*, 1999, 19(10):1153-8.

Tanaka E, Yamazaki K, and Misawa S, "Update: The Clinical Importance of Acetaminophen Hepatotoxicity in Nonalcoholic and Alcoholic Subjects," *J Clin Pharm Ther*, 2000, 25(5):325-32.

Wynn RL, "Narcotic Analgesics for Dental Pain: Available Products, Strengths, and Formulations," *Gen Dent*, 2001, 49(2):126-8, 130, 132 passim.

Oxycodone and Aspirin (oks i KOE done & AS pir in)

Related Information

Aspirin *on page 149*
Oral Pain *on page 1788*
Oxycodone *on page 1225*

U.S. Brand Names Endodan®; Percodan®

Canadian Brand Names Endodan®; Oxycodan®; Percodan®

Generic Available Yes

Index Terms Aspirin and Oxycodone

Pharmacologic Category Analgesic, Opioid

Dental Use Treatment of postoperative pain

Use Management of moderate-to-severe pain

Local Anesthetic/Vasoconstrictor Precautions No information available to require special precautions

Effects on Dental Treatment Key adverse event(s) related to dental treatment: Nausea, sedation, constipation, and xerostomia (normal salivary flow resumes upon discontinuation). May have anticoagulant effects which may affect bleeding time. The elderly are a high-risk population for adverse effects from NSAIDs. As many as 60% of elderly patients with GI complications from NSAIDs can develop peptic ulceration and/or hemorrhage asymptomatically. Concomitant disease and drug use contribute to the risk of GI adverse effects. Enhanced analgesia has been seen with therapeutic doses of narcotics; duration of action may be increased. Elderly may also be particularly susceptible to the CNS depressant effects of narcotics. See Dental Comment.

Significant Adverse Effects Note: Also refer to individual agents

Common (frequency not defined):

Central nervous system: Dizziness, drowsiness, lightheadedness, sedation

Dermatologic: Pruritus

Gastrointestinal: Nausea, vomiting, constipation

<1%, postmarketing, and/or case reports (limited to important or life-threatening): Allergic reaction, anaphylaxis, anaphylactoid reaction, angioedema, apnea, asthma, bradycardia, bronchospasm, circulatory depression, confusion, duodenal ulcer, dysphoria, dyspnea, ecchymosis, euphoria, gastric ulcer, gastrointestinal bleeding, hallucination, hemorrhage, hepatitis, hepatotoxicity, hypotension, hypoglycemia, hyperglycemia, ileus, interstitial nephritis, intestinal obstruction, laryngeal edema, metabolic acidosis, pancreatitis, papillary necrosis, paresthesia, purpura, pulmonary edema, proteinuria, rash, renal failure, respiratory alkalosis, respiratory depression, Reye syndrome, rhabdomyolysis, seizure, shock, thrombocytopenia, tinnitus

Restrictions C-II

Dental Usual Dosing

Analgesic: Oral (based on oxycodone combined salts):

Children: Maximum oxycodone: 5 mg/dose; maximum aspirin dose should not exceed 4 g/day. Doses should be given every 6 hours as needed.

Mild-to-moderate pain: Initial dose, **based on oxycodone content:** 0.05-0.1 mg/kg/dose

Severe pain: Initial dose, **based on oxycodone content**: 0.3 mg/kg/dose

Adults: Percodan®: 1 tablet every 6 hours as needed for pain; maximum aspirin dose should not exceed 4 g/day.

Dosage Oral (based on oxycodone combined salts):

Children: Maximum oxycodone: 5 mg/dose; maximum aspirin dose should not exceed 4 g/day. Doses should be given every 6 hours as needed.

Mild-to-moderate pain: Initial dose, **based on oxycodone content**: 0.05-0.1 mg/kg/dose

Severe pain: Initial dose, **based on oxycodone content**: 0.3 mg/kg/dose

Adults: Percodan®: 1 tablet every 6 hours as needed for pain; maximum aspirin dose should not exceed 4 g/day.

Dosing adjustment in hepatic impairment: Dose should be reduced in patients with severe liver disease.

(Continued)

Oxycodone and Aspirin *(Continued)*

Mechanism of Action

Oxycodone, as with other narcotic (opiate) analgesics, blocks pain perception in the cerebral cortex by binding to specific receptor molecules (opiate receptors) within the neuronal membranes of synapses. This binding results in a decreased synaptic chemical transmission throughout the CNS, thus inhibiting the flow of pain sensations into the higher centers. Mu and kappa are the two subtypes of the opiate receptor to which oxycodone binds to cause analgesia.

Aspirin inhibits prostaglandin synthesis by decreasing the activity of the enzyme, cyclooxygenase, which results in decreased formation of prostaglandin precursors, acts on the hypothalamic heat-regulating center to reduce fever, blocks thromboxane synthetase action which prevents formation of the platelet-aggregating substance thromboxane A_2

Contraindications
Hypersensitivity to oxycodone, salicylates, other NSAIDs, or any component of the formulation; patients with the syndrome of asthma, rhinitis, and nasal polyps; inherited or acquired bleeding disorders (including factor VII and factor IX deficiency); do not use in children (<16 years of age) in the presence of viral infections (chickenpox or flu symptoms), with or without fever, due to a potential association with Reye's syndrome; significant respiratory depression; hypercarbia; known or suspected paralytic ileus; acute or severe bronchial asthma; pregnancy (3rd trimester)

Warnings/Precautions
Use with caution in patients with hypersensitivity reactions to other phenanthrene-derivative opioid agonists (morphine, hydrocodone, hydromorphone, levorphanol, oxycodone, oxymorphone), respiratory diseases including asthma, emphysema, or COPD. Use with caution in pancreatitis or biliary tract disease, acute alcoholism (including delirium tremens), adrenocortical insufficiency, CNS depression/coma, kyphoscoliosis (or other skeletal disorder which may alter respiratory function), hypothyroidism (including myxedema), prostatic hyperplasia, urethral stricture, and toxic psychosis.

Use with caution in the elderly, debilitated, severe hepatic or renal dysfunction. Hemodynamic effects (hypotension, orthostasis) may be exaggerated in patients with dehydration, hypovolemia, concurrent vasodilating drugs, or in patients with head injury. Respiratory depressant effects and capacity to elevate CSF pressure may be exaggerated in presence of head injury, other intracranial lesion, or pre-existing elevation of intracranial pressure. Tolerance or drug dependence may result from extended use. Healthcare provider should be alert to problems of abuse, misuse, and diversion. Taper dose gradually to avoid withdrawal symptoms in physically-dependent patients.

Use with caution in patients with platelet and bleeding disorders, erosive gastritis, or peptic ulcer disease. Heavy ethanol use (>3 drinks/day) can increase bleeding risks. Discontinue use if tinnitus or impaired hearing occurs. Patients with sensitivity to tartrazine dyes, nasal polyps, and asthma may have an increased risk of salicylate sensitivity. Surgical patients should avoid ASA if possible, for 1-2 weeks prior to surgery, to reduce the risk of excessive bleeding.

Drug Interactions

Oxycodone: **Substrate** of CYP2D6 (major)

Aspirin: **Substrate** of CYP2C9 (minor)

Also see individual agents.

CYP2D6 inhibitors: May decrease the effects of oxycodone. Example inhibitors include chlorpromazine, delavirdine, fluoxetine, miconazole, paroxetine, pergolide, quinidine, quinine, ritonavir, and ropinirole.

Increased effect/toxicity with CNS depressants, TCAs, dextroamphetamine

Dietary Considerations
May be taken with food or water.

Pharmacodynamics/Kinetics
See individual agents.

Pregnancy Risk Factor
D

Lactation
Enters breast milk/use caution

Breast-Feeding Considerations

Aspirin: Caution is suggested due to potential adverse effects in nursing infants.

Oxycodone: No data reported.

Dosage Forms
Excipient information presented when available (limited, particularly for generics); consult specific product labeling.

Tablet: Oxycodone hydrochloride 4.5 mg, oxycodone terephthalate 0.38 mg, and aspirin 325 mg

Endodan®, Percodan®: Oxycodone hydrochloride 4.8355 mg and aspirin 325 mg

Dental Comment
Oxycodone, as with other narcotic analgesics, is recommended only for limited acute dosing (ie, 3 days or less). Oxycodone has an addictive liability, especially when given long-term. The oxycodone with aspirin could have anticoagulant effects and could possibly affect bleeding times.

There is no scientific evidence to warrant discontinuance of aspirin prior to dental surgery. Patients taking one aspirin tablet daily as an antithrombotic and who require dental surgery should be given special consideration in consultation with the physician before removal of the aspirin relative to prevention of postoperative bleeding.

The Food and Drug Administration (FDA), has issued a letter updating information and considerations regarding the use of ibuprofen (400 mg doses) in patients who are taking low dose aspirin (81 mg, immediate release; not enteric coated) for cardioprotection and stroke prevention. Ibuprofen, at these doses, may interfere with aspirin's antiplatelet effect depending upon when it is administered. Patients initiated on aspirin first (for ~1 week) then ibuprofen (400 mg tid for 10 days) seem to maintain aspirin's platelet effect (Cryer B, 2005). Ibuprofen has the greatest impact on aspirin if administered less than 8 hours before aspirin (Catella-Lawson F, 2001).

Patients may require counseling about the appropriate timing of ibuprofen dosing in relationship to aspirin therapy. With occasional use of ibuprofen, a clinically-significant interaction with aspirin in unlikely. To avoid interference during chronic dosing, a single dose of ibuprofen should be taken 30-120 minutes after aspirin ingestion or at least 8 hours should elapse after ibuprofen dosing before giving aspirin (FDA, 2006; Catella-Lawson F, 2001).

The clinical implications of the interaction are unclear. There have not been any clinical endpoint studies conducted at this time. Avoidance of this interaction is potentially important because aspirin's vascular protection could be decreased or negated.

Other nonselective NSAIDs may have potential for a similar interaction with aspirin. Such has been described with naproxen (Capone ML, 2005). Acetaminophen does not appear to interfere with the antiplatelet effect of aspirin. Other clinical scenarios (use of smaller ibuprofen doses, other aspirin products, other doses of aspirin) have not been evaluated.

Additional information is available at: http://www.fda.gov/cder/drug/infopage/aspirin/default.htm.

Selected Readings

Dionne RA, "New Approaches to Preventing and Treating Postoperative Pain," *J Am Dent Assoc*, 1992, 123(6):26-34.

Gobetti JP, "Controlling Dental Pain," *J Am Dent Assoc*, 1992, 123(6):47-52.

Wynn RL, "Narcotic Analgesics for Dental Pain: Available Products, Strengths, and Formulations," *Gen Dent*, 2001, 49(2):126-8, 130, 132 passim.

Oxycodone and Ibuprofen (oks i KOE done & eye byoo PROE fen)

Related Information
Oral Pain *on page 1788*

Related Sample Prescriptions
Severe Oral Pain *on page 1835*

U.S. Brand Names Combunox™

Generic Available No

Index Terms Ibuprofen and Oxycodone

Pharmacologic Category Analgesic, Opioid; Nonsteroidal Anti-inflammatory Drug (NSAID), Oral

Dental Use Short-term (≤3-5 days) management of acute, moderate-to-severe pain

Use Short-term (≤7 days) management of acute, moderate-to-severe pain

Local Anesthetic/Vasoconstrictor Precautions No information available to require special precautions

Effects on Dental Treatment Key adverse event(s) related to dental treatment: Nausea, sedation, dizziness. See Dental Comment.

Significant Adverse Effects

>10%:
  Central nervous system: Dizziness (5% to 19%), somnolence (7% to 17%)
  Gastrointestinal: Nausea (9% to 25%)

2% to 10%:
  Cardiovascular: Vasodilation (<1% to 3%)
  Central nervous system: Headache (10%), fever (3%)
  Gastrointestinal: Constipation (<1% to 5%), vomiting (5%), diarrhea (2%), dyspepsia (<1% to 2%), flatulence (1%)
  Neuromuscular & skeletal: Weakness (3%)
  Miscellaneous: Diaphoresis (2%)

<2% (Limited to important or life-threatening): Abdominal enlargement/pain, anemia, amblyopia, anxiety, arthritis, back pain, chest pain, chills, edema, euphoria, hyperkinesias, hypertonia, hypokalemia, hypotension, hypoxia, (Continued)

Oxycodone and Ibuprofen *(Continued)*

ileus, infection, LFTs increased, lung disorder, pharyngitis, syncope, rash, tachycardia, taste perversion, thrombophlebitis, urinary retention

Restrictions C-II

A medication guide should be dispensed with each prescription for oral administration. A template for the required MedGuide can be found on the FDA website at http://www.fda.gov/cder/drug/infopage/COX2/NSAIDmedguide.htm.

Dental Usual Dosing Pain: Adults: Oral: Take 1 tablet every 6 hours as needed (maximum: 4 tablets/24 hours); do not take for longer than 7 days

Dosage Oral: Adults: Pain: Take 1 tablet every 6 hours as needed (maximum: 4 tablets/24 hours); do not take for longer than 7 days

Mechanism of Action

Based on **oxycodone** component: Binds to opiate receptors in the CNS, altering the perception of and response to pain; suppresses cough in medullary center; produces generalized CNS depression

Based on **ibuprofen** component: Inhibits prostaglandin synthesis by decreasing the activity of the enzyme, cyclooxygenase, which results in decreased formation of prostaglandin precursors

Contraindications Hypersensitivity to oxycodone, ibuprofen, aspirin, other NSAIDs, or any component of the formulation; patients with suspected paralytic ileus; perioperative pain in the setting of coronary artery bypass surgery (CABG); significant respiratory depression, hypercarbia, acute/severe bronchial asthma; pregnancy (3rd trimester)

Warnings/Precautions Use with caution in patients with hypersensitivity reactions to other phenanthrene-derivative opioid agonists (eg, morphine, hydrocodone, hydromorphone, levorphanol, oxycodone, oxymorphone) and in patients with respiratory diseases. Use with caution in pancreatitis or biliary tract disease, acute alcoholism, adrenocortical insufficiency, CNS depression/coma, kyphoscoliosis (or other skeletal disorder which may alter respiratory function), hypothyroidism, prostatic hyperplasia, urethral stricture, and toxic psychosis. Use with caution in the elderly, debilitated, severe hepatic or renal dysfunction. Hemodynamic effects (hypotension, orthostasis) may be exaggerated in patients with hypovolemia, concurrent vasodilating drugs, or in patients with head injury. Respiratory depressant effects and capacity to elevate CSF pressure may be exaggerated in presence of head injury, other intracranial lesion, or pre-existing increased intracranial pressure. Patients with acute abdominal condition should use this agent cautiously. Tolerance or drug dependence may result from extended use.

[U.S. Boxed Warnings]: NSAIDs are contraindicated for perioperative pain in the setting of coronary artery bypass surgery (CABG). NSAIDs are associated with an increased risk of adverse cardiovascular events, including MI and stroke. New onset or worsening of pre-existing hypertension may occur. Risk may be increased with duration of use or pre-existing cardiovascular risk factors or disease. Use caution with fluid retention, CHF, or hypertension. Use of NSAIDs can compromise existing renal function. Rehydrate patient before starting therapy. Monitor renal function closely. Ibuprofen is not recommended for patients with advanced renal disease. **[U.S. Boxed Warning]: NSAIDs may increase risk of gastrointestinal irritation, ulceration, bleeding, and perforation.** Use caution with a history of GI disease (bleeding or ulcers), concurrent therapy with aspirin, anticoagulants and/or corticosteroids, smoking, use of alcohol, the elderly or debilitated patients. NSAIDs may cause serious skin adverse events. Anaphylactoid reactions may occur, even without prior exposure. Do not use in patients who experience angioedema, bronchospasm, asthma, rhinitis, or urticaria with NSAID or aspirin therapy. Use caution with other forms of asthma. The elderly are at increased risk for adverse effects (especially peptic ulceration, CNS effects, renal toxicity) from NSAIDs even at low doses.

Safety and efficacy in pediatric patients have not been established.

Drug Interactions

Oxycodone: **Substrate** of CYP2D6

Ibuprofen: **Substrate** (minor) of CYP2C9, 2C19; **Inhibits** CYP2C9 (strong)

See individual agents.

Ethanol/Nutrition/Herb Interactions

Based on **oxycodone** component:

Ethanol: Avoid or limit ethanol (may increase CNS depression). Watch for sedation.

Based on **ibuprofen** component:

Ethanol: Avoid ethanol (may enhance gastric mucosal irritation).

Food: Food or milk are recommended to decrease gastric irritation.

Herb/Nutraceutical: Avoid alfalfa, anise, bilberry, bladderwrack, bromelain, cat's claw, celery, coleus, cordyceps, dong quai, evening primrose, feverfew, fenugreek, garlic, ginger, ginkgo biloba, red clover, horse chestnut, grapeseed, green tea, ginseng, guggul, horse chestnut seed, horseradish, licorice, prickly ash, red clover, reishi, SAMe, sweet clover, turmeric, white willow (all have additional antiplatelet activity).

Dietary Considerations Take with or without food.

Pharmacodynamics/Kinetics Also see individual agents.
Absorption: Ibuprofen, oxycodone: rapidly absorbed
Protein binding: Ibuprofen: 99%; Oxycodone: 45%
Metabolism: Oxycodone: Hepatic to metabolites, noroxycodone (major), and oxymorphone (minor)
Bioavailability: Oxycodone: increased with food (25%)
Half-life elimination: Ibuprofen: 1.8-2.6 hours; Oxycodone: 3.1-3.7 hours
Time to peak, serum: Ibuprofen: 1.6-3.1 hours; Oxycodone 1.3-2.1 hours
Excretion: Ibuprofen: Urine (<0.2% unchanged); Oxycodone: Urine (~4 % unchanged)

Pregnancy Risk Factor C/D (3rd trimester)

Lactation Enters breast milk/contraindicated

Breast-Feeding Considerations Ibuprofen is not transferred to milk in significant quantities and is considered compatible with breast-feeding by AAP. Oxycodone, however, is excreted in breast milk and withdrawal may occur in breast-fed infants when maternal opioid administration is discontinued. Discontinuation of either the opioid-containing medication (Combunox™) or breast-feeding is recommended.

Dosage Forms Excipient information presented when available (limited, particularly for generics); consult specific product labeling.
Tablet:
Combunox™: 5/400: Oxycodone 5 mg and ibuprofen 400 mg

Dental Comment The combination of oxycodone and ibuprofen in this dose form is appropriate for the management of moderate-to-severe pain when the concomitant anti-inflammatory action of ibuprofen is desired. Oxycodone is recommended only for limited acute dosing (ie, ≤3 days). Oxycodone has an addictive liability, especially when given long term.

Oxycodone Hydrochloride see Oxycodone on page 1225

OxyContin® see Oxycodone on page 1225

OxyFast® see Oxycodone on page 1225

Oxygen (OKS i jen)

Generic Available Yes

Pharmacologic Category Dental Gases

Dental Use Administered as a supplement with nitrous oxide to ensure adequate ventilation during sedation; a resuscitative agent for medical emergencies in dental office

Use Treatment of various clinical disorders, both respiratory and nonrespiratory; relief of arterial hypoxia and secondary complications; treatment of pulmonary hypertension, polycythemia secondary to hypoxemia, chronic disease states complicated by anemia, cancer, migraine headaches, coronary artery disease, seizure disorders, sickle-cell crisis, and sleep apnea

Local Anesthetic/Vasoconstrictor Precautions No information available to require special precautions

Effects on Dental Treatment No significant effects or complications reported

Significant Adverse Effects No data reported

Dental Usual Dosing Administered as a supplement with nitrous oxide to ensure adequate ventilation during sedation: Children and Adults: Average rate of 2 L/minute

Dosage Children and Adults: Average rate of 2 L/minute

Mechanism of Action Increased oxygen in tidal volume and oxygenation of tissues at molecular level

Contraindications No data reported

Warnings/Precautions Oxygen-induced hypoventilation is the greatest potential hazard of oxygen therapy. In patients with severe COPD, the respiratory drive results from hypoxic stimulation of the carotid chemoreceptors. If this hypoxic drive is diminished by excessive oxygen therapy, hypoventilation may occur and further carbon dioxide retention with possible cessation of ventilation.

Drug Interactions No data reported

Pregnancy Risk Factor No data reported

Dosage Forms Excipient information presented when available (limited, particularly for generics); consult specific product labeling.
(Continued)

Oxygen *(Continued)*

Liquid system with large reservoir holding 75-100 lb of liquid oxygen; compressed gas system consisting of high-pressure tank; tank sizes are "H" (6900 L of oxygen), "E" (622 L of oxygen) and "D" (356 L of oxygen)

OxyIR® *see* Oxycodone *on page 1225*

Oxymetazoline *(oks i met AZ oh leen)*

Related Information
Bacterial Infections *on page 1793*

Related Sample Prescriptions
Sinus Infection Treatment *on page 1839*

U.S. Brand Names Afrin® Extra Moisturizing [OTC]; Afrin® Original [OTC]; Afrin® Severe Congestion [OTC]; Afrin® Sinus [OTC]; Dristan™ 12-Hour [OTC]; Duramist® Plus [OTC]; Duration® [OTC]; Genasal [OTC]; Neo-Synephrine® 12 Hour [OTC]; Neo-Synephrine® 12 Hour Extra Moisturizing [OTC]; Nōstrilla® [OTC]; NRS® [OTC]; Vicks Sinex® 12 Hour [OTC]; Vicks Sinex® 12 Hour Ultrafine Mist [OTC]; Visine® L.R. [OTC]; 4-Way® 12 Hour [OTC]

Canadian Brand Names Claritin® Allergic Decongestant; Dristan® Long Lasting Nasal; Drixoral® Nasal

Generic Available Yes: Nasal spray

Index Terms Oxymetazoline Hydrochloride

Pharmacologic Category Adrenergic Agonist Agent; Imidazoline Derivative; Vasoconstrictor

Dental Use Symptomatic relief of nasal mucosal congestion

Use Adjunctive therapy of middle ear infections, associated with acute or chronic rhinitis, the common cold, sinusitis, hay fever, or other allergies
Ophthalmic: Relief of redness of eye due to minor eye irritations

Local Anesthetic/Vasoconstrictor Precautions No information available to require special precautions

Effects on Dental Treatment No significant effects or complications reported

Significant Adverse Effects Frequency not defined.
Cardiovascular: Hypertension, palpitation
Local: Transient burning, stinging
Respiratory: Dryness of the nasal mucosa, rebound congestion with prolonged use, sneezing

Dental Usual Dosing Symptomatic relief of nasal mucosal congestion: Children ≥6 years and Adults: Intranasal (therapy should not exceed 3 days): 0.05% solution: Instill 2-3 sprays into each nostril twice daily

Dosage
Intranasal (therapy should not exceed 3 days): Children ≥6 years and Adults: 0.05% solution: Instill 2-3 sprays into each nostril twice daily
Ophthalmic: Children ≥6 years and Adults: 0.025% solution: Instill 1-2 drops in affected eye(s) every 6 hours as needed or as directed by healthcare provider

Mechanism of Action Stimulates alpha-adrenergic receptors in the arterioles of the nasal mucosa to produce vasoconstriction

Contraindications Hypersensitivity to oxymetazoline or any component of the formulation

Warnings/Precautions
Nasal: Rebound congestion may occur with extended use (>3 days). Prior to self-medication (OTC use), contact healthcare provider in the presence of hypertension, diabetes, hyperthyroidism, heart disease, coronary artery disease, cerebral arteriosclerosis, or long-standing bronchial asthma.
Ophthalmic: Prior to OTC use, contact healthcare provider in the presence of glaucoma or if needed for >72 hours.

Drug Interactions Increased toxicity with MAO inhibitors.

Pharmacodynamics/Kinetics
Onset of action: Intranasal: 5-10 minutes
Duration: 5-6 hours

Dosage Forms Excipient information presented when available (limited, particularly for generics); consult specific product labeling.
Solution, intranasal, as hydrochloride [spray]: 0.05% (15 mL, 30 mL)
Afrin® Extra Moisturizing: 0.05% (15 mL) [contains benzyl alcohol and glycerin; regular or no drip formula]
Afrin® Original: 0.05% (15 mL, 30 mL) [contains benzalkonium chloride]
Afrin® Original: 0.05% (15 mL) [contains benzyl alcohol and benzalkonium chloride; no drip formula]
Afrin® Severe Congestion: 0.05% (15 mL) [contains benzyl alcohol and menthol; regular or no drip formula]
Afrin® Sinus: 0.05% (15 mL) [contains benzyl alcohol, benzalkonium chloride, camphor, phenol; regular or no drip formula]

Dristan™ 12-Hour: 0.05% (15 mL) [contains benzyl alcohol and benzalkonium chloride]

Duramist® Plus, Neo-Synephrine® 12 Hour, Nōstrilla®, Vicks Sinex® 12 Hour Ultrafine Mist, Vicks Sinex® 12 Hour, 4-Way® 12 Hour: 0.05% (15 mL) [contains benzalkonium chloride]

Duration®: 0.05% (30 mL) [contains benzalkonium chloride]

Genasal, NRS®: 0.05% (15 mL, 30 mL) [contains benzalkonium chloride]

Neo-Synephrine® 12 Hour Extra Moisturizing: 0.05% (15 mL) [contains glycerin]

Solution, ophthalmic, as hydrochloride (Visine® L.R.): 0.025% (15 mL, 30 mL) [contains benzalkonium chloride]

Oxymetazoline Hydrochloride *see* Oxymetazoline *on page 1236*

Oxymetholone (oks i METH oh lone)

U.S. Brand Names Anadrol®
Generic Available No
Pharmacologic Category Anabolic Steroid
Use Treatment of anemias caused by deficient red cell production
Local Anesthetic/Vasoconstrictor Precautions No information available to require special precautions
Effects on Dental Treatment No significant effects or complications reported
Common Adverse Effects Frequency not defined.
Cardiovascular: Coronary artery disease, peripheral edema
Central nervous system: Excitation, insomnia
Dermatologic: Acne (prepubertal males, women), hirsutism (women), hypercalcemia, hyperchloremia, hyperkalemia, hyperphosphatemia, hyperpigmentation, male-pattern baldness (postpubertal males, women)
Endocrine & metabolic: Amenorrhea, cholesterol increased, clitoromegaly, creatinine phosphokinase increased, glucose tolerance decreased, gynecomastia, HDL-cholesterol decreased, hoarseness (women), hypernatremia, impotence (postpubertal males), LDL-cholesterol decreased, libido increased/decreased, menstrual irregularities, oligospermia, phallic enlargement (prepubertal males), priapism (postpubertal males), testicular atrophy (postpubertal males), testicular dysfunction (postpubertal males); virilism (women, high dose); voice deepening (women)
Gastrointestinal: Diarrhea, nausea, vomiting
Genitourinary: Bladder irritability (postpubertal males), epididymitis (postpubertal males), prostatic hyperplasia (elderly males), seminal volume decreased (postpubertal males)
Hematologic: Iron-deficiency anemia, polycythemia, suppression of clotting factors
Hepatic: Cholestatic hepatitis, hepatic necrosis, hepatocellular carcinoma jaundice, liver cell tumors, peliosis hepatis, transaminases increased
Neuromuscular & skeletal: Premature closure of epiphysis (children)
Restrictions C-III
Mechanism of Action Enhances the production and urinary excretion of erythropoietin in patients with anemias due to bone marrow failure; stimulates erythropoiesis in anemias due to deficient red cell production.
Drug Interactions
Increased Effect/Toxicity: Androgens may enhance the hepatotoxic effect of cyclosporine; may enhance the anticoagulant effect of warfarin.
Pregnancy Risk Factor X

Oxymorphone (oks i MOR fone)

Related Information
Oral Pain *on page 1788*
U.S. Brand Names Numorphan®; Opana®; Opana® ER
Generic Available No
Index Terms Oxymorphone Hydrochloride
Pharmacologic Category Analgesic, Opioid
Use
Parenteral: Management of moderate-to-severe pain and preoperatively as a sedative and/or supplement to anesthesia
Oral, regular release: Management of moderate-to-severe pain
Oral, extended release: Management of moderate-to-severe pain in patients requiring around-the-clock opioid treatment for an extended period of time
Local Anesthetic/Vasoconstrictor Precautions No information available to require special precautions
(Continued)

Oxymorphone *(Continued)*

Effects on Dental Treatment Key adverse event(s) related to dental treatment: Xerostomia (normal salivary flow resumes upon discontinuation). Anticholinergic side effects can cause a reduction of saliva production or secretion, contributing to discomfort and dental disease (ie, caries, oral candidiasis, and periodontal disease).

Common Adverse Effects Frequency not defined.

Cardiovascular: Bradycardia, cardiac shock, flushing, hypotension, palpitation, peripheral vasodilation, shock, tachycardia

Central nervous system: Amnesia, anorexia, anxiety, CNS depression, coma, confusion, convulsion, drowsiness, dizziness, fatigue, fever, hallucinations, headache, insomnia, intracranial pressure increased, malaise, mental depression, nervousness, restlessness, paradoxical CNS stimulation

Dermatologic: Pruritus, urticaria, rash

Endocrine & metabolic: Antidiuretic hormone release, weight loss

Gastrointestinal: Abdominal pain, appetite depression, biliary tract spasm, constipation, dehydration, dry mouth, dyspepsia, flatulence, nausea, paralytic ileus, stomach cramps, vomiting, xerostomia

Genitourinary: Urination decreased, urinary retention, urinary tract spasm

Local: Pain at injection site

Neuromuscular & skeletal: Weakness

Ocular: Diplopia, miosis

Respiratory: Apnea, cyanosis, dyspnea, hypoventilation, respiratory depression

Miscellaneous: Diaphoresis, histamine release, physical and psychological dependence

Restrictions C-II

Mechanism of Action Oxymorphone hydrochloride (Numorphan®) is a potent narcotic analgesic with uses similar to those of morphine. The drug is a semisynthetic derivative of morphine (phenanthrene derivative) and is closely related to hydromorphone chemically (Dilaudid®).

Drug Interactions

Increased Effect/Toxicity: Increased effect/toxicity with CNS depressants (phenothiazines, tricyclic antidepressants, anxiolytics, sedatives, hypnotics, alcohol, and anesthetics). Dextroamphetamine may increase the analgesic effects of opiate agonists. Concurrent use with SSRIs may enhance serotonergic activity and may increase the risk of serotonin syndrome.

Pharmacodynamics/Kinetics

Onset of action: Analgesic: I.V., I.M., SubQ: 5-10 minutes

Duration: Analgesic: Parenteral: 3-4 hours

Protein binding: 10% to 12%

Metabolism: Hepatic via glucuronidation to active and inactive metabolites

Bioavailability: Oral: 10%

Half-life elimination: Oral: Immediate release: 7-9 hours; Extended release: 9-11 hours

Excretion: Urine

Pregnancy Risk Factor C/D (prolonged use or high doses at term)

Oxymorphone Hydrochloride *see* Oxymorphone *on page 1237*

Oxytetracycline *(oks i tet ra SYE kleen)*

U.S. Brand Names Terramycin® I.M. [DSC]

Canadian Brand Names Terramycin®

Mexican Brand Names Terramicina

Generic Available No

Index Terms Oxytetracycline Hydrochloride

Pharmacologic Category Antibiotic, Tetracycline Derivative

Use Treatment of susceptible bacterial infections; both gram-positive and gram-negative, as well as, *Rickettsia* and *Mycoplasma* organisms

Local Anesthetic/Vasoconstrictor Precautions No information available to require special precautions

Effects on Dental Treatment Key adverse event(s) related to dental treatment: Glossitis and dysphagia. Tetracyclines are not recommended for use during pregnancy or in children ≤8 years of age since they have been reported to cause enamel hypoplasia and permanent teeth discoloration. Tetracyclines should only be used in these patients if other agents are contraindicated or alternative antimicrobials will not eradicate the organism. Long-term use associated with oral candidiasis.

Common Adverse Effects Frequency not defined

Cardiovascular: Pericarditis

Central nervous system: Bulging fontanels (infants), intracranial hypertension (adults)

Dermatologic: Angioneurotic edema, erythematous rash, exfoliative dermatitis (uncommon), maculopapular rash, photosensitivity, urticaria

Gastrointestinal: Anogenital inflammatory lesions, diarrhea, dysphagia, enamel hypoplasia, enterocolitis, glossitis, nausea, tooth discoloration, vomiting

Hematologic: Anemia, eosinophilia, neutropenia, thrombocytopenia

Local: Irritation

Renal: BUN increased

Miscellaneous: Anaphylactoid purpura, anaphylaxis, hypersensitivity reaction, SLE exacerbation

Mechanism of Action Inhibits bacterial protein synthesis by binding with the 30S and possibly the 50S ribosomal subunit(s) of susceptible bacteria, cell wall synthesis is not affected

Drug Interactions

Increased Effect/Toxicity: Oral anticoagulant (warfarin) effects may be increased.

Decreased Effect: Barbiturates, phenytoin, and carbamazepine decrease serum levels of tetracyclines. Although anecdotal reports suggest oral contraceptive efficacy could be reduced by tetracyclines, this has been refuted by more rigorous scientific and clinical data.

Pharmacodynamics/Kinetics

Absorption: Poor

Metabolism: Hepatic (small amounts)

Half-life elimination: 8.5-9.6 hours; prolonged with renal impairment

Excretion: Urine; feces

Pregnancy Risk Factor D

Oxytetracycline Hydrochloride *see* Oxytetracycline *on page 1238*

Oxytocin (oks i TOE sin)

U.S. Brand Names Pitocin®

Canadian Brand Names Pitocin®; Syntocinon®

Mexican Brand Names Syntocinon INJ; Xitocin

Generic Available Yes

Index Terms Pit

Pharmacologic Category Oxytocic Agent

Use Induction of labor at term; control of postpartum bleeding; adjunctive therapy in management of abortion

Local Anesthetic/Vasoconstrictor Precautions No information available to require special precautions

Effects on Dental Treatment No significant effects or complications reported

Common Adverse Effects Frequency not defined.

Fetus or neonate:

Cardiovascular: Arrhythmias (including premature ventricular contractions), bradycardia

Central nervous system: Brain or CNS damage (permanent), neonatal seizure

Hepatic: Neonatal jaundice

Ocular: Neonatal retinal hemorrhage

Miscellaneous: Fetal death, low Apgar score (5 minute)

Mother:

Cardiovascular: Arrhythmias, hypertensive episodes, premature ventricular contractions

Gastrointestinal: Nausea, vomiting

Genitourinary: Pelvic hematoma, postpartum hemorrhage, uterine hypertonicity, tetanic contraction of the uterus, uterine rupture, uterine spasm

Hematologic: Afibrinogenemia (fatal)

Miscellaneous: Anaphylactic reaction, subarachnoid hemorrhage

Mechanism of Action Produces the rhythmic uterine contractions characteristic to delivery

Drug Interactions

Increased Effect/Toxicity: Dinoprostone and misoprostol may increase the effect of oxytocin; wait 6-12 hours after dinoprostone or misoprostol administration before initiating oxytocin.

Pharmacodynamics/Kinetics

Onset of action: Uterine contractions: I.M.: 3-5 minutes; I.V.: ~1 minute

Duration: I.M.: 2-3 hour; I.V.: 1 hour

Metabolism: Rapidly hepatic and via plasma (by oxytocinase) and to a smaller degree the mammary gland

Half-life elimination: 1-5 minutes

Excretion: Urine

Pregnancy Risk Factor X

Oxytrol® *see* Oxybutynin *on page 1224*

Paclitaxel (pac li TAKS el)

U.S. Brand Names Onxol™; Taxol®

Canadian Brand Names Apo-Paclitaxel®; Taxol®

Mexican Brand Names Asotax; Bristaxol; Ifaxol; Praxel

Generic Available Yes

Index Terms NSC-125973; NSC-673089

Pharmacologic Category Antineoplastic Agent, Antimicrotubular; Antineoplastic Agent, Natural Source (Plant) Derivative

Use Treatment of breast, nonsmall cell lung, and ovarian cancers; treatment of AIDS-related Kaposi's sarcoma (KS)

Unlabeled/Investigational Use Treatment of bladder, cervical, prostate, small cell lung, and head and neck cancers; treatment of (unknown primary) adenocarcinoma

Local Anesthetic/Vasoconstrictor Precautions No information available to require special precautions

Effects on Dental Treatment Key adverse event(s) related to dental treatment: Severe, potentially dose-limiting mucositis and stomatitis.

Common Adverse Effects Percentages reported with single-agent therapy. **Note:** Myelosuppression is dose related, schedule related, and infusion-rate dependent (increased incidences with higher doses, more frequent doses, and longer infusion times) and, in general, rapidly reversible upon discontinuation.

>10%:
  Cardiovascular: Flushing (28%), ECG abnormal (14% to 23%), edema (21%), hypotension (4% to 12%)

  Dermatologic: Alopecia (87%), rash (12%)

  Gastrointestinal: Nausea/vomiting (52%), diarrhea (38%), mucositis (17% to 35%; grades 3/4: up to 3%), stomatitis (15%; most common at doses >390 mg/m^2), abdominal pain (with intraperitoneal paclitaxel)

  Hematologic: Neutropenia (78% to 98%; grade 4: 14% to 75%; onset 8-10 days, median nadir 11 days, recovery 15-21 days), leukopenia (90%; grade 4: 17%), anemia (47% to 90%; grades 3/4: 2% to 16%), thrombocytopenia (4% to 20%; grades 3/4: 1% to 7%), bleeding (14%)

  Hepatic: Alkaline phosphatase increased (22%), AST increased (19%)

  Local: Injection site reaction (erythema, tenderness, skin discoloration, swelling: 13%)

  Neuromuscular & skeletal: Peripheral neuropathy (42% to 70%; grades 3/4: up to 7%), arthralgia/myalgia (60%), weakness (17%)

  Renal: Creatinine increased (observed in KS patients only: 18% to 34%; severe: 5% to 7%)

  Miscellaneous: Hypersensitivity reaction (31% to 45%; grades 3/4: up to 2%), infection (15% to 30%)

1% to 10%:
  Cardiovascular: Bradycardia (3%), tachycardia (2%), hypertension (1%), rhythm abnormalities (1%), syncope (1%), venous thrombosis (1%)

  Dermatologic: Nail changes (2%)

  Hematologic: Febrile neutropenia (2%)

  Hepatic: Bilirubin increased (7%)

  Respiratory: Dyspnea (2%)

Mechanism of Action Paclitaxel promotes microtubule assembly by enhancing the action of tubulin dimers, stabilizing existing microtubules, and inhibiting their disassembly, interfering with the late G$_2$ mitotic phase, and inhibiting cell replication. In addition, the drug can distort mitotic spindles, resulting in the breakage of chromosomes. Paclitaxel may also suppress cell proliferation and modulate immune response.

Drug Interactions

Cytochrome P450 Effect: Substrate (major) of CYP2C8, 3A4; **Induces** CYP3A4 (weak)

Increased Effect/Toxicity: CYP2C8 inhibitors may increase the levels/effects of paclitaxel; example inhibitors include gemfibrozil, ketoconazole, montelukast and ritonavir. CYP3A4 inhibitors may increase the levels/effects of paclitaxel; example inhibitors include azole antifungals, clarithromycin, diclofenac, doxycycline, erythromycin, imatinib, isoniazid, nefazodone, nicardipine, propofol, protease inhibitors, quinidine, telithromycin, and verapamil. Paclitaxel may increase anthracycline (doxorubicin, epirubicin) levels/toxicity. Concomitant therapy with taxane derivatives (docetaxel, paclitaxel) and platinum derivatives (carboplatin, cisplatin, oxaliplatin) may cause increased hematologic toxicity if the platinum agent is administered first (taxanes should be administered first).

Decreased Effect: CYP2C8 inducers may decrease the levels/effects of paclitaxel; example inducers include carbamazepine, phenobarbital, phenytoin, rifampin, rifapentine, and secobarbital. CYP3A4 inducers may decrease the levels/effects of paclitaxel; example inducers include aminoglutethimide, carbamazepine, nafcillin, nevirapine, phenobarbital, phenytoin, and rifamycins. Paclitaxel may decrease the absorption of digoxin (tablets).

Pharmacodynamics/Kinetics
Distribution:

V_d: Widely distributed into body fluids and tissues; affected by dose and duration of infusion

V_{dss}:
1- to 6-hour infusion: 67.1 L/m^2
24-hour infusion: 227-688 L/m^2

Protein binding: 89% to 98%

Metabolism: Hepatic via CYP2C8 and 3A4; forms metabolites (primarily 6α-hydroxypaclitaxel)

Half-life elimination:
1- to 6-hour infusion: Mean (beta): 6.4 hours
3-hour infusion: Mean (terminal): 13.1-20.2 hours
24-hour infusion: Mean (terminal): 15.7-52.7 hours

Excretion: Feces (~70%, 5% as unchanged drug); urine (14%)

Clearance: Mean: Total body: After 1- and 6-hour infusions: 5.8-16.3 L/hour/m^2; After 24-hour infusions: 14.2-17.2 L/hour/m^2

Pregnancy Risk Factor D

Paclitaxel (Protein Bound) (pac li TAKS el PROE teen bownd)

U.S. Brand Names Abraxane®

Generic Available No

Index Terms ABI-007; Albumin-Bound Paclitaxel; NAB-Paclitaxel; NSC-736631; Protein-Bound Paclitaxel

Pharmacologic Category Antineoplastic Agent, Antimicrotubular; Antineoplastic Agent, Natural Source (Plant) Derivative

Use Treatment of relapsed or refractory breast cancer

Local Anesthetic/Vasoconstrictor Precautions No information available to require special precautions

Effects on Dental Treatment Key adverse event(s) related to dental treatment: Mucositis.

Common Adverse Effects
>10%:

Cardiovascular: EKG abnormal (60%)

Dermatologic: Alopecia (90%)

Gastrointestinal: Nausea (30%; grades 3/4: 3%), diarrhea (27%; grades 3/4: <1%), vomiting (18%; grades 3/4: 4%)

Hematologic: Neutropenia (80%; grade 4: 9%), anemia (33%; grades 3/4: 1%)

Hepatic: AST increased (39%), alkaline phosphatase increased (36%), GGT increased (grades 3/4: 14%)

Neuromuscular & skeletal: Sensory neuropathy (71%; grades 3/4: 10%; dose dependent; may be cumulative), weakness (47%), myalgia/arthralgia (44%)

Ocular: Vision disturbance (13%; severe [keratitis, blurred vision]: 1%)

Respiratory: Dyspnea (12%)

Miscellaneous: Infections (24%; primarily included oral candidiasis, respiratory tract infection, and pneumonia)

1% to 10%:

Cardiovascular: Edema (10%), hypotension (5%), cardiovascular events (grades 3/4: 3%; included chest pain, cardiac arrest, supraventricular tachycardia, edema, thrombosis, pulmonary thromboembolism, pulmonary emboli, and hypertension)

Gastrointestinal: Mucositis (7%; grades 3/4: <1%)

Hematologic: Bleeding (2%), neutropenic fever (2%), thrombocytopenia (2%; grades 3/4: 1%)

Hepatic: Bilirubin increased (7%)

Neuromuscular and skeletal: Peripheral neuropathy (grade 3: 10%)

Renal: Creatinine increased (11%; severe 1%)

Respiratory: Cough (7%)

(Continued)

Paclitaxel (Protein Bound) *(Continued)*

Miscellaneous: Hypersensitivity reaction (4%)

Mechanism of Action Paclitaxel promotes microtubule assembly by enhancing the action of tubulin dimers, stabilizing existing microtubules, and inhibiting their disassembly, interfering with the late G_2 mitotic phase, and inhibiting cell replication. In addition, the drug can distort mitotic spindles, resulting in the breakage of chromosomes. Paclitaxel may also suppress cell proliferation and modulate immune response.

Drug Interactions

Cytochrome P450 Effect: Substrate (major) of CYP2C8, 2C9, 3A4; **Induces** CYP3A4 (weak)

Increased Effect/Toxicity: CYP2C8 Inhibitors may increase the levels/ effects of paclitaxel; example inhibitors include gemfibrozil, ketoconazole, montelukast, and ritonavir. CYP3A4 inhibitors may increase the levels/effects of paclitaxel; example inhibitors include azole antifungals, clarithromycin, diclofenac, doxycycline, erythromycin, imatinib, isoniazid, nefazodone, nicardipine, propofol, protease inhibitors, quinidine, telithromycin, and verapamil. Paclitaxel may increase anthracycline (doxorubicin, epirubicin) levels/toxicity. Concomitant therapy with taxane derivatives (docetaxel, paclitaxel) and platinum derivatives (carboplatin, cisplatin, oxaliplatin) may cause increased hematologic toxicity if the platinum agent is administered first (taxanes should be administered first).

Decreased Effect: CYP2C8 inducers may decrease the levels/effects of paclitaxel; example inducers include carbamazepine, phenobarbital, phenytoin, rifampin, rifapentine, and secobarbital. CYP3A4 inducers may decrease the levels/effects of paclitaxel; example inducers include aminoglutethimide, carbamazepine, nafcillin, nevirapine, phenobarbital, phenytoin, and rifamycins. Paclitaxel may decrease the absorption of digoxin (tablets).

Pharmacodynamics/Kinetics

Distribution: V_d: 632 L/m^2

Protein binding: 89% to 98%

Metabolism: Hepatic via CYP3A4 (to minor metabolites) and 2C8 (primarily to 6-alpha-hydroxypaclitaxel)

Half-life elimination: Terminal: 27 hours

Excretion: Urine (4% as unchanged drug, 1% as metabolites); feces (20%) Clearance 15 L/hour/m^2

Pregnancy Risk Factor D

Pain-A-Lay® [OTC] *see* Phenol *on page 1290*

Pain Eze [OTC] *see* Acetaminophen *on page 31*

Pain-Off [OTC] *see* Acetaminophen, Aspirin, and Caffeine *on page 41*

Palcaps *see* Pancrelipase *on page 1248*

Palgic® *see* Carbinoxamine *on page 281*

Palgic®-D [DSC] *see* Carbinoxamine and Pseudoephedrine *on page 282*

Palgic®-DS [DSC] *see* Carbinoxamine and Pseudoephedrine *on page 282*

Palifermin *(pal ee FER min)*

U.S. Brand Names Kepivance™

Generic Available No

Index Terms AMJ 9701; rHu-KGF

Pharmacologic Category Keratinocyte Growth Factor

Dental Use Decrease the incidence and severity of severe oral mucositis associated with hematologic malignancies in patients receiving myelotoxic therapy requiring hematopoietic stem cell support

Use Decrease the incidence and severity of severe oral mucositis associated with hematologic malignancies in patients receiving myelotoxic therapy requiring hematopoietic stem cell support

Local Anesthetic/Vasoconstrictor Precautions No information available to require special precautions

Effects on Dental Treatment Key adverse event(s) related to dental treatment: Taste alteration, mouth/tongue discoloration or thickness. See Dental Comment.

Significant Adverse Effects

>10%:

Cardiovascular: Edema (28%), hypertension (7% to 14%)

Central nervous system: Fever (39%), pain (16%), dysesthesia (12%)

Dermatologic: Rash (62%), pruritus (35%), erythema (32%)

Gastrointestinal: Mouth/tongue discoloration or thickness (17%), taste alteration (16%)

Miscellaneous: Serum amylase increased (grade 3/4, 38%); serum lipase increased (grade 3/4, 11%)

1% to 10%: Neuromuscular & skeletal: Arthralgia (10%)

Dental Usual Dosing Oral mucositis: Adults: I.V.: 60 mcg/kg/day for 3 consecutive days before and after myelotoxic therapy; total of 6 doses

Dosage I.V.: Adults: 60 mcg/kg/day for 3 consecutive days before and after myelotoxic therapy; total of 6 doses

Note: Administer first 3 doses prior to myelotoxic therapy, with the 3rd dose given 24-48 hours before therapy begins. The last 3 doses should be administered after myelotoxic therapy, with the first of these doses after but on the same day of hematopoietic stem cell infusion and at least 4 days after the most recent dose of palifermin.

Mechanism of Action Palifermin is a recombinant keratinocyte growth factor (KGF) produced in *E. coli*. Endogenous KGF is produced by mesenchymal cells in response to epithelial tissue injury. KGF binds to the KGF receptor resulting in proliferation, differentiation and migration of epithelial cells in multiple tissues, including (but not limited to) the tongue, buccal mucosa, esophagus, and salivary gland.

Contraindications Hypersensitivity to palifermin, *E. coli*-derived proteins, or any component of the formulation

Warnings/Precautions Safety and efficacy have not been established with nonhematologic malignancies; effect on the growth of nonhematopoietic human tumors is not known. Palifermin should be administered prior to and following, but not with, chemotherapy. If administered within 24 hours of chemotherapy, palifermin may increase the severity and duration of mucositis due to the increased sensitivity of rapidly-dividing epithelial cells. Safety and efficacy have not been established in children.

Drug Interactions Drug interaction studies have not been conducted.

Pharmacodynamics/Kinetics Half-life elimination: 4.5 hours (range: 3.3-5.7 hours)

Pregnancy Risk Factor C

Lactation Excretion in breast milk unknown/use caution

Dosage Forms Excipient information presented when available (limited, particularly for generics); consult specific product labeling.

Injection, powder for reconstitution [preservative free]: 6.25 mg [contains mannitol 50 mg, sucrose 25 mg]

Dental Comment Palifermin works at the cellular level by protecting the epithelial cells lining the mouth and throat from damage caused by chemotherapy and radiation and by stimulating the growth and development of new epithelial cells to build up the mucosal barrier.

Paliperidone (pal ee PER i done)

U.S. Brand Names Invega™
Generic Available No
Index Terms 9-hydroxy-risperidone; 9-OH-risperidone
Pharmacologic Category Antipsychotic Agent, Atypical
Use Treatment of schizophrenia
Local Anesthetic/Vasoconstrictor Precautions No information available to require special precautions
Effects on Dental Treatment Key adverse event(s) related to dental treatment: Significant xerostomia and changes in salivation (normal salivary flow resumes upon discontinuation).
Common Adverse Effects
>10%:
Cardiovascular: Tachycardia (12% to 14%)
Central nervous system: Headache (11% to 14%), somnolence (6% to 11% dose dependent)
1% to 10%:
Cardiovascular: QT$_c$ interval prolongation (3% to 5%), orthostatic hypotension (1% to 4% dose dependent), bundle branch block (<1% to 3%), AV block (first degree, up to 2%), arrhythmia (<1% to 2%), blood pressure increased (<1% to 2%), T-wave abnormality (1% to 2%), palpitation
Central nervous system: Akathisia (3% to 10% dose dependent), anxiety (5% to 9%), EPS (2% to 7% dose dependent), parkinsonism (up to 7% dose dependent), dizziness (4% to 6%), dystonia (1% to 5% dose dependent), hypertonia (1% to 4% dose dependent), fatigue (1% to 2%), fever (<1% to 2%)
Endocrine & metabolic: Weight gain (6% to 9% dose dependent), insulin increased (<1% to 2%)
(Continued)

Paliperidone *(Continued)*

Gastrointestinal: Nausea (4% to 6%), dyspepsia (2% to 5%), salivation increased (up to 4% dose dependent), xerostomia (2% to 3%), abdominal pain (1% to 3%)

Neuromuscular & skeletal: Hyperkinesia (3% to 10% dose dependent), dyskinesia (3% to 9% dose dependent), tremor (3% to 5%), back pain (1% to 2%), weakness (<1% to 2%), extremity pain (up to 2%)

Ocular: Vision blurred (up to 2%)

Respiratory: Cough (2% to 3%), dyspnea

Mechanism of Action Paliperidone is considered a benzisoxazole atypical antipsychotic as it is the primary active metabolite of risperidone. As with other atypical antipsychotics, it's therapeutic efficacy is believed to result from mixed central serotonergic and dopaminergic antagonism. The addition of serotonin antagonism to dopamine antagonism (classic neuroleptic mechanism) is thought to improve negative symptoms of psychoses and reduce the incidence of extrapyramidal side effects. Similar to risperidone, paliperidone demonstrates high affinity to α_1, D_2, H_1, and 5-HT$_{2C}$ receptors, and low affinity for muscarinic and 5-HT$_{1A}$ receptors. In contrast to risperidone, paliperidone displays nearly 10-fold lower affinity for α_2 and 5-HT$_{2A}$ receptors, and nearly three- to fivefold less affinity for 5-HT$_{1A}$ and 5-HT$_{1D}$, respectively.

Drug Interactions

Increased Effect/Toxicity: CNS depressants, centrally-acting acetylcholinesterase inhibitors, itraconazole, or lithium may increase adverse effects/toxicity of paliperidone.

Decreased Effect: Carbamazepine may decrease the levels/effects of paliperidone. Paliperidone may decrease effects of levodopa and other dopamine agonists.

Pharmacodynamics/Kinetics

Distribution: V_d: 487 L

Protein binding: 74%

Metabolism: Hepatic via CYP2D6 and 3A4

Bioavailability: 28%

Half-life elimination: 23 hours; 24-51 hours with renal impairment (Cl$_{cr}$ <80 mL/minute)

Time to peak, plasma: ~24 hours

Excretion: Urine (80%); feces (11%)

Pregnancy Risk Factor C

Palivizumab *(pah li VIZ u mab)*

U.S. Brand Names Synagis®
Canadian Brand Names Synagis®
Mexican Brand Names Synagis
Generic Available No
Pharmacologic Category Monoclonal Antibody
Use Prevention of serious lower respiratory tract disease caused by respiratory syncytial virus (RSV) in infants and children <2 years of age at high risk of RSV disease

Local Anesthetic/Vasoconstrictor Precautions No information available to require special precautions

Effects on Dental Treatment No significant effects or complications reported

Common Adverse Effects The incidence of adverse events was similar between the palivizumab and placebo groups.

>1%:

Central nervous system: Nervousness, fever

Dermatologic: Fungal dermatitis, eczema, seborrhea, rash

Gastrointestinal: Diarrhea, vomiting, gastroenteritis

Hematologic: Anemia

Hepatic: ALT increase, abnormal LFTs

Local: Injection site reaction, erythema, induration

Ocular: Conjunctivitis

Otic: Otitis media

Respiratory: Cough, wheezing, bronchiolitis, pneumonia, bronchitis, asthma, croup, dyspnea, sinusitis, apnea, upper respiratory infection, rhinitis

Miscellaneous: Oral moniliasis, failure to thrive, viral infection, flu syndrome

Postmarketing and/or case reports: Hypersensitivity reactions, anaphylaxis (very rare)

Mechanism of Action Exhibits neutralizing and fusion-inhibitory activity against RSV; these activities inhibit RSV replication in laboratory and clinical studies

Pharmacodynamics/Kinetics

Half-life elimination: Children <24 months: 20 days; Adults: 18 days

Time to peak, serum: 48 hours
Pregnancy Risk Factor C

Palmer's® Skin Success Acne [OTC] *see* Benzoyl Peroxide *on page 200*

Palmer's® Skin Success Acne Cleanser [OTC] *see* Salicylic Acid *on page 1451*

Palmer's® Skin Success Eventone® Fade Cream [OTC] *see* Hydroquinone *on page 841*

Palmitate-A® [OTC] *see* Vitamin A *on page 1663*

Palonosetron (pal oh NOE se tron)

U.S. Brand Names Aloxi®
Generic Available No
Index Terms Palonosetron Hydrochloride; RS-25259; RS-25259-197
Pharmacologic Category Antiemetic; Selective 5-HT$_3$ Receptor Antagonist
Use Prevention of acute (within 24 hours) and delayed (2-5 days) chemo-therapy-induced nausea and vomiting

Local Anesthetic/Vasoconstrictor Precautions No information available to require special precautions
Effects on Dental Treatment No significant effects or complications reported
Common Adverse Effects
>10%: Dermatologic: Pruritus (8% to 22%)
1% to 10%:
Cardiovascular: Bradycardia (1%), hypotension (1%), tachycardia (nonsustained) (1%)
Central nervous system: Headache (6% to 9%), anxiety (1% to 5%), dizziness (1%)
Endocrine & metabolic: Hyperkalemia (1%)
Gastrointestinal: Constipation (5% to 10%), diarrhea (1%)
Neuromuscular & skeletal: Weakness (1%)
Mechanism of Action Selective 5-HT$_3$ receptor antagonist, blocking serotonin, both peripherally on vagal nerve terminals and centrally in the chemoreceptor trigger zone
Drug Interactions
Cytochrome P450 Effect: Substrate (minor) of CYP1A2, 2D6, 3A4
Increased Effect/Toxicity: Palonosetron may enhance the hypotensive effect of apomorphine; concurrent use is contraindicated.
Pharmacodynamics/Kinetics
Distribution: V$_d$: 8.3 ± 2.5 L/kg
Protein binding: 62%
Metabolism: ~50% metabolized via CYP enzymes (and likely other pathways) to relatively inactive metabolites (N-oxide-palonosetron and 6-S-hydroxy-palonosetron); CYP1A2, 2D6, and 3A4 contribute to its metabolism
Half-life elimination: Terminal: 40 hours
Excretion: Urine (80%, 40% as unchanged drug)
Pregnancy Risk Factor B

Palonosetron Hydrochloride *see* Palonosetron *on page 1245*
Pamelor® *see* Nortriptyline *on page 1188*

Pamidronate (pa mi DROE nate)

Related Information
Management of Patients Undergoing Cancer Therapy *on page 1826*
U.S. Brand Names Aredia®
Canadian Brand Names Aredia®; Pamidronate Disodium®; Rhoxal-pamidronate
Mexican Brand Names Aredia
Generic Available Yes
Index Terms Pamidronate Disodium
Pharmacologic Category Antidote; Bisphosphonate Derivative
Use Treatment of hypercalcemia associated with malignancy; treatment of osteo-lytic bone lesions associated with multiple myeloma or metastatic breast cancer; moderate to severe Paget's disease of bone
Unlabeled/Investigational Use Treatment of pediatric osteoporosis, treatment of osteogenesis imperfecta
Local Anesthetic/Vasoconstrictor Precautions No information available to require special precautions
Effects on Dental Treatment Osteonecrosis of the jaw (ONJ), generally associated with local infection and/or tooth extraction and often with delayed healing,
(Continued)

Pamidronate *(Continued)*

has been reported in patients taking bisphosphonates. Most reported cases of bisphosphonate-associated osteonecrosis have been in cancer patients treated with intravenous bisphosphonates. However, some have occurred in patients with postmenopausal osteoporosis taking oral bisphosphonates. Dental surgery may exacerbate ONJ. For patients requiring dental procedures, there are no data available to suggest whether discontinuation of bisphosphonate treatment reduces the risk of ONJ. See Dental Comment.

Common Adverse Effects Percentage of adverse effect varies upon dose and duration of infusion.

>10%:

Central nervous system: Fatigue (12% to 40%), fever (18% to 39%), headache (24% to 27%), anxiety (8% to 18%), insomnia (1% to 25%), pain (13% to 15%)

Endocrine & metabolic: Hypophosphatemia (9% to 18%), hypokalemia (4% to 18%), hypomagnesemia (4% to 12%), hypocalcemia (1% to 12%)

Gastrointestinal: Nausea (4% to 64%), vomiting (4% to 46%), anorexia (1% to 31%), abdominal pain (1% to 24%), dyspepsia (4% to 23%)

Genitourinary: Urinary tract infection (15% to 20%)

Hematologic: Anemia (6% to 48%), leukopenia (4% to 21%)

Local: Infusion site reaction (4% to 18%)

Neuromuscular & skeletal: Weakness (16% to 26%), myalgia (1% to 26%), arthralgia (11% to 15%)

Renal: Serum creatinine increased (19%)

Respiratory: Dyspnea (22% to 35%), cough (25% to 26%), upper respiratory tract infection (3% to 20%), sinusitis (15% to 16%), pleural effusion (3% to 15%)

1% to 10%:

Cardiovascular: Atrial fibrillation (6%), hypertension (6%), syncope (6%), tachycardia (6%), atrial flutter (1%), cardiac failure (1%), edema (1%)

Central nervous system: Somnolence (1% to 6%), psychosis (4%)

Endocrine & metabolic: Hypothyroidism (6%)

Gastrointestinal: Constipation (4% to 6%), gastrointestinal hemorrhage (6%), diarrhea (1%), stomatitis (1%)

Hematologic: Neutropenia (1%), thrombocytopenia (1%)

Neuromuscular & skeletal: Back pain (5%), bone pain (5%)

Renal: Uremia (4%)

Respiratory: Rales (6%), rhinitis (6%)

Miscellaneous: Moniliasis (6%)

Mechanism of Action A bisphosphonate which inhibits bone resorption via actions on osteoclasts or on osteoclast precursors. Does not appear to produce any significant effects on renal tubular calcium handling and is poorly absorbed following oral administration (high oral doses have been reported effective); therefore, I.V. therapy is preferred.

Drug Interactions

Increased Effect/Toxicity: Aminoglycosides may lower serum calcium levels with prolonged administration; concomitant use may have an additive hypocalcemic effect. NSAIDs may enhance the gastrointestinal adverse/toxic effects (increased incidence of GI ulcers) of bisphosphonate derivatives. Bisphosphonate derivatives may enhance the hypocalcemic effect of phosphate supplements.

Decreased Effect: The following agents may decrease the absorption of oral bisphosphonate derivatives: Antacids (aluminum, calcium, magnesium), oral calcium salts, oral iron salts, and oral magnesium salts.

Pharmacodynamics/Kinetics

Onset of action: 24-48 hours

Peak effect: Maximum: 5-7 days

Absorption: Poor; pharmacokinetic studies lacking

Metabolism: Not metabolized

Half-life elimination: 21-35 hours

Excretion: Biphasic; urine (~50% as unchanged drug) within 120 hours

Pregnancy Risk Factor D

Dental Comment Novartis Pharmaceuticals Corporation has notified dental health professionals of the risk of **osteonecrosis of the jaw (ONJ)** and the use of the intravenous bisphosphonates, pamidronate (Zometa®) and zoledronic acid (Aredia®): *"Dear Dental Health Professional" Letter Issued for Intravenous Bisphosphonates, Pamidronate and Zoledronic Acid, Regarding the Risk of Osteonecrosis of the Jaw (ONJ) in Cancer Patients* - May 2005.

Often observed in patients receiving chemotherapy and corticosteroids, reports of ONJ (the majority being associated with dental procedures) have been documented in cancer patients. Dental exams and preventative dentistry should be performed prior to placing patients with risk factors (chemotherapy, corticosteroids, poor oral hygiene) on intravenous bisphosphonate therapy. Additionally, invasive dental procedures should be avoided during therapy; patients developing ONJ while on bisphosphonate therapy should not have invasive dental procedures because the condition may be exacerbated. It has not been determined whether the discontinuation of bisphosphonate therapy in patients requiring dental surgery decreases the risk of ONJ. The treating healthcare professional is encouraged to assess the benefits and risks.

Bisphosphonates are widely used in the management of metastatic bone disease to treat hypercalcemia associated with malignancies and to treat osteoporosis. It is suggested that because of the trend in the use of chronic bisphosphonate therapy, the observation of an associated risk of osteonecrosis of the jaw should alert practitioners to monitor for this previously unrecognized potential complication.

Additional information is available at http://www.fda.gov/medwatch/SAFETY/2005/safety05.htm#zometa2, or by contacting Novartis Oncology Medical Services at 1-888-669-6682.

Estimates of Percent Incidence of ONJ in Treated Cancer Patients

Two reports have attempted to assess the percent of cancer patients developing ONJ after bisphosphonate treatment. Maerevoet et al, reported that among 194 patients treated with Zometa® every 3-4 weeks, nine developed ONJ. Before receiving Zometa®, six had received Aredia® 90 mg every 3-4 weeks. The median duration of treatment with Aredia® was 39 months and for Zometa® 18 months. The incidence of ONJ in these patients was calculated to be 4.6%. Durie et al, described the results of a survey by the International Myeloma Foundation in 2004 to assess the risk factors of ONJ. Out of 1203 respondents, 904 had myeloma and 299 breast cancer. Of the myeloma patients, 62 developed ONJ and 54 had suspicious findings. Of the breast cancer patients, 13 had ONJ and 23 had suspicious findings. The total number of cases of either ONJ or suspicious findings was 152. ONJ developed in 10% of 211 patients receiving Zometa® compared to 4% of 413 receiving Aredia®. The mean time to onset of ONJ among patients taking Zometa® was 18 months; the mean time to onset after Aredia® was 6 years. It should be noted that an early report by authors from Novartis Pharmaceuticals Corporation (Tarassoff, 2003) stressed that Aredia® and Zometa® had been used in 2.5 million patients world wide and reports of ONJ during their extensive use had been rare. In addition, these authors stated that review of the reported cases revealed multiple risk factors for avascular necrosis. McMahon et al, followed up with a report that, along with other factors, bisphosphonates are additional stressors of bone health that can tip the balance to osteonecrosis. They suggested that the prevention of ONJ should be stressed such as the elimination of chronic dental infections prior to chemotherapy and bisphosphonate use in cancer patients.

Pamidronate Disodium *see* Pamidronate *on page 1245*

Pamine® *see* Methscopolamine *on page 1075*

Pamine® Forte *see* Methscopolamine *on page 1075*

p-Aminoclonidine *see* Apraclonidine *on page 136*

Pamprin® Maximum Strength All Day Relief [OTC] *see* Naproxen *on page 1148*

Pan-2400™ [OTC] *see* Pancreatin *on page 1247*

Panafil® *see* Chlorophyllin, Papain, and Urea *on page 335*

Panafil® SE *see* Chlorophyllin, Papain, and Urea *on page 335*

Pan-B Antibody *see* Rituximab *on page 1437*

Pancof® [DSC] *see* Pseudoephedrine, Dihydrocodeine, and Chlorpheniramine *on page 1385*

Pancof®-EXP *see* Dihydrocodeine, Pseudoephedrine, and Guaifenesin *on page 503*

Pancof-HC *see* Hydrocodone and Pseudoephedrine *on page 832*

Pancof®-PD *see* Dihydrocodeine, Chlorpheniramine, and Phenylephrine *on page 502*

Pancof-XP *see* Hydrocodone and Guaifenesin *on page 828*

Pancrease® [DSC] *see* Pancrelipase *on page 1248*

Pancrease® MT *see* Pancrelipase *on page 1248*

Pancreatin (PAN kree a tin)

U.S. Brand Names Dygase; Hi-Vegi-Lip [OTC]; kutrase®; ku-zyme®; Lapase; Pan-2400™ [OTC]; Pancreatin 4X [OTC]; Pancreatin 8X [OTC]; Veg-Pancreatin 4X [OTC]

Generic Available Yes

(Continued)

Pancreatin *(Continued)*

Pharmacologic Category Enzyme

Use Relief of functional indigestion due to enzyme deficiency or imbalance

Local Anesthetic/Vasoconstrictor Precautions No information available to require special precautions

Effects on Dental Treatment No significant effects or complications reported

Common Adverse Effects Frequency not defined.

Gastrointestinal: Loose stools (decrease dose)

Respiratory: Mucous membrane irritation or precipitation of asthma attack (due to inhalation of airborne powder)

Mechanism of Action An enzyme supplement, not a replacement, which contains a combination of lipase, amylase and protease. Enhances the digestion of proteins, starch and fat in the stomach and intestines.

Pregnancy Risk Factor C

Pancreatin 4X [OTC] *see* Pancreatin *on page 1247*

Pancreatin 8X [OTC] *see* Pancreatin *on page 1247*

Pancrecarb MS® *see* Pancrelipase *on page 1248*

Pancrelipase *(pan kre LYE pase)*

U.S. Brand Names Creon®; ku-zyme® HP; Lipram 4500; Lipram-CR; Lipram-PN; Lipram-UL; Palcaps; Pancrease® [DSC]; Pancrease® MT; Pancrecarb MS®; Pangestyme™ CN; Pangestyme™ EC; Pangestyme™ MT; Pangestyme™ UL; Panocaps; Panocaps MT; Panokase®; Panokase® 16; Plaretase® 8000; Ultracaps MT; Ultrase®; Ultrase® MT; Viokase®

Canadian Brand Names Cotazym®; Creon® 5; Creon® 10; Creon® 20; Creon® 25; Pancrease®; Pancrease® MT; Ultrase®; Ultrase® MT; Viokase®

Generic Available Yes: Excludes powder

Index Terms Lipancreatin

Pharmacologic Category Enzyme

Use Replacement therapy in symptomatic treatment of malabsorption syndrome caused by pancreatic insufficiency

Unlabeled/Investigational Use Treatment of occluded feeding tubes

Local Anesthetic/Vasoconstrictor Precautions No information available to require special precautions

Effects on Dental Treatment No significant effects or complications reported

Common Adverse Effects Frequency not defined; occurrence of events may be dose related.

Central nervous system: Pain

Dermatologic: Rash

Endocrine & metabolic: Hyperuricemia

Gastrointestinal: Nausea, cramps, constipation, diarrhea, perianal irritation/inflammation (large doses), irritation of the mouth, abdominal pain, intestinal obstruction, vomiting, flatulence, melena, weight loss, fibrotic strictures, greasy stools

Ocular: Lacrimation

Renal: Hyperuricosuria

Respiratory: Sneezing, dyspnea, bronchospasm

Miscellaneous: Allergic reactions

Mechanism of Action Pancrelipase is a natural product harvested from the hog pancreas. It contains a combination of lipase, amylase, and protease. Products are formulated to dissolve in the more basic pH of the duodenum so that they may act locally to break down fats, protein, and starch.

Pharmacodynamics/Kinetics

Absorption: None; acts locally in GI tract

Excretion: Feces

Pregnancy Risk Factor B/C (product specific)

Pandel® *see* Hydrocortisone *on page 836*

Pangestyme™ CN *see* Pancrelipase *on page 1248*

Pangestyme™ EC *see* Pancrelipase *on page 1248*

Pangestyme™ MT *see* Pancrelipase *on page 1248*

Pangestyme™ UL *see* Pancrelipase *on page 1248*

Panglobulin® NF *see* Immune Globulin (Intravenous) *on page 870*

Panhematin® *see* Hemin *on page 807*

Panitumumab *(pan i TOOM yoo mab)*

U.S. Brand Names Vectibix™

Generic Available No

Index Terms ABX-EGF; NSC-742319; rHuMAb-EGFr

Pharmacologic Category Antineoplastic Agent, Monoclonal Antibody; Epidermal Growth Factor Receptor (EGFR) Inhibitor

Use Treatment of refractory (EGFR positive) metastatic colorectal cancer

Local Anesthetic/Vasoconstrictor Precautions No information available to require special precautions

Effects on Dental Treatment Key adverse event(s) related to dental treatment: Stomatitis and mucositis.

Common Adverse Effects

>10%:

Cardiovascular: Peripheral edema (12%)

Central nervous system: Fatigue (28%)

Dermatologic: Skin toxicity (90%; grades 3/4: 16%), erythema (65%; grades 3/4: 5%), acneiform rash (57%; grades 3/4: 7%), pruritus (57%; grades 3/4: 2%), exfoliation (25%; grades 3/4: 2%), paronychia (25%), rash (22%; grades 3/4: 1%), fissures (20%; grades 3/4: 1%), acne (13%; grades 3/4: 1%)

Endocrine & metabolic: Hypomagnesemia (39%; grades 3/4: 4%)

Gastrointestinal: Abdominal pain (25%), nausea (23%), diarrhea (21%; grades 3/4: 2%), constipation (21%), vomiting (19%)

Respiratory: Cough (14%)

1% to 10%:

Dermatologic: Dry skin (10%), nail disorder (other than paronychia: 9%)

Gastrointestinal: Stomatitis (7%), mucositis (6%)

Ocular: Eyelash growth (6%), conjunctivitis (4%), ocular hyperemia (3%), lacrimation increased (2%), eye/eye lid irritation (1%)

Miscellaneous: Infusion reactions (3%; grades 3/4: 1%)

Mechanism of Action Recombinant human IgG2 monoclonal antibody which binds specifically to the epidermal growth factor receptor (EGFR, HER1, c-ErbB-1) and competitively inhibits the binding of epidermal growth factor (EGF) and other ligands. Binding to the EGFR blocks phosphorylation and activation of intracellular tyrosine kinases, resulting in inhibition of cell survival, growth, proliferation and transformation.

Pharmacodynamics/Kinetics Half-life elimination: ~7.5 days (range: 4-11 days)

Pregnancy Risk Factor C

Panixine DisperDose™ [DSC] *see* Cephalexin *on page 317*

Panlor® DC *see* Acetaminophen, Caffeine, and Dihydrocodeine *on page 42*

Panlor® SS *see* Acetaminophen, Caffeine, and Dihydrocodeine *on page 42*

Panocaps *see* Pancrelipase *on page 1248*

Panocaps MT *see* Pancrelipase *on page 1248*

Panokase® *see* Pancrelipase *on page 1248*

Panokase® 16 *see* Pancrelipase *on page 1248*

PanOxyl® *see* Benzoyl Peroxide *on page 200*

PanOxyl®-AQ *see* Benzoyl Peroxide *on page 200*

PanOxyl® Aqua Gel *see* Benzoyl Peroxide *on page 200*

PanOxyl® Bar [OTC] *see* Benzoyl Peroxide *on page 200*

Panretin® *see* Alitretinoin *on page 71*

Panthoderm® [OTC] *see* Dexpanthenol *on page 471*

Panto-250 *see* Pantothenic Acid *on page 1251*

Pantoprazole (pan TOE pra zole)

Related Information

Gastrointestinal Disorders *on page 1745*

U.S. Brand Names Protonix®

Canadian Brand Names Panto™ IV; Pantoloc®; Pantoloc® M; PMS-Pantoprazole; Protonix®

Mexican Brand Names Pantozol; Zurcal

Generic Available No

Pharmacologic Category Proton Pump Inhibitor; Substituted Benzimidazole

Use

Oral: Treatment and maintenance of healing of erosive esophagitis associated with GERD; reduction in relapse rates of daytime and nighttime heartburn symptoms in GERD; hypersecretory disorders associated with Zollinger-Ellison syndrome or other neoplastic disorders

I.V.: Short-term treatment (7-10 days) of patients with gastroesophageal reflux disease (GERD) and a history of erosive esophagitis; hypersecretory disorders associated with Zollinger-Ellison syndrome or other neoplastic disorders

(Continued)

Pantoprazole *(Continued)*

Unlabeled/Investigational Use Peptic ulcer disease, active ulcer bleeding (parenteral formulation); adjunct treatment with antibiotics for *Helicobacter pylori* eradication

Local Anesthetic/Vasoconstrictor Precautions No information available to require special precautions

Effects on Dental Treatment No significant effects or complications reported

Common Adverse Effects

≥1%:

Cardiovascular: Chest pain

Central nervous system: Headache (5% to 9%), insomnia (<1% to 1%), dizziness, migraine, anxiety

Dermatologic: Rash (<1% to 2%)

Endocrine and metabolic: Hyperglycemia (<1% to 1%), hyperlipidemia

Gastrointestinal: Diarrhea (4% to 6%), flatulence (2% to 4%), abdominal pain (1% to 4%), nausea (≤2%), vomiting (≤2%), eructation (≤1%), constipation, dyspepsia, gastroenteritis, rectal disorder

Genitourinary: Urinary frequency, UTI

Hepatic: Liver function abnormal (up to 2%)

Local: Injection site reaction (includes thrombophlebitis and abscess)

Neuromuscular & skeletal: Arthralgia, back pain, hypertonia, neck pain, weakness

Respiratory: Bronchitis, cough, dyspnea, pharyngitis, rhinitis, sinusitis, upper respiratory tract infection

Miscellaneous: Flu syndrome, infection, pain

Dosage Adults:

Oral:

Erosive esophagitis associated with GERD:

Treatment: 40 mg once daily for up to 8 weeks; an additional 8 weeks may be used in patients who have not healed after an 8-week course

Maintenance of healing: 40 mg once daily

Note: Lower doses (20 mg once daily) have been used successfully in mild GERD treatment and maintenance of healing

Hypersecretory disorders (including Zollinger-Ellison): Initial: 40 mg twice daily; adjust dose based on patient needs; doses up to 240 mg/day have been administered

Helicobacter pylori eradication (unlabeled use): Doses up to 40 mg twice daily have been used as part of combination therapy

I.V.:

Erosive esophagitis associated with GERD: 40 mg once daily for 7-10 days

Hypersecretory disorders: 80 mg twice daily; adjust dose based on acid output measurements; 160-240 mg/day in divided doses has been used for a limited period (up to 7 days)

Prevention of rebleeding in peptic ulcer bleed (unlabeled use): 80 mg, followed by 8 mg/hour infusion for 72 hours. **Note:** A daily infusion of 40 mg does not raise gastric pH sufficiently to enhance coagulation in active GI bleeds.

Elderly: Dosage adjustment not required

Dosage adjustment in renal impairment: Not required; pantoprazole is not removed by hemodialysis

Dosage adjustment in hepatic impairment: Not required

Mechanism of Action Suppresses gastric acid secretin by inhibiting the parietal cell H+/K+ ATP pump

Contraindications Hypersensitivity to pantoprazole, substituted benzamidazoles (ie, esomeprazole, lansoprazole, omeprazole, rabeprazole), or any component of the formulation

Warnings/Precautions Relief of symptoms does not preclude the presence of a gastric malignancy. Long-term omeprazole therapy has caused atrophic gastritis (by biopsy); this may also occur with pantoprazole. No reports of enterochromaffin-like (ECL) cell carcinoids, dysplasia, or neoplasia has occurred. Not indicated for maintenance therapy; safety and efficacy for use beyond 16 weeks have not been established. Prolonged treatment (typically >3 years) may lead to vitamin B_{12} malabsorption. Intravenous preparation contains edetate sodium (EDTA); use caution in patients who are risk for zinc deficiency if other EDTA-containing solutions are coadministered. Safety and efficacy in pediatric patients have not been established.

Drug Interactions

Cytochrome P450 Effect: Substrate of CYP2C19 (major), 3A4 (minor); **Inhibits** 2C9 (moderate); **Induces** CYP1A2 (weak), 3A4 (weak)

Increased Effect/Toxicity: Pantoprazole may increase the levels/effects of bosentan, dapsone, fluoxetine, glimepiride, glipizide, losartan, montelukast, nateglinide, paclitaxel, phenytoin, warfarin, zafirlukast, and other CYP2C9 substrates.

Decreased Effect: Proton pump inhibitors may decrease the absorption of atazanavir, indinavir, iron salts, itraconazole, and ketoconazole. The levels/effects of pantoprazole may be decreased by aminoglutethimide, carbamazepine, phenytoin, rifampin, and other CYP2C19 inducers.

Ethanol/Nutrition/Herb Interactions
Ethanol: Avoid ethanol (may cause gastric mucosal irritation).
Herb/Nutraceutical: Prolonged treatment (typically >3 years) may lead to vitamin B_{12} malabsorption.

Dietary Considerations
Oral: May be taken with or without food; best if taken before breakfast.
I.V.: Due to EDTA in preparation, zinc supplementation may be needed in patients prone to zinc deficiency.

Pharmacodynamics/Kinetics
Absorption: Well absorbed
Distribution: V_d: 11-24 L
Protein binding: 98%, primarily to albumin
Metabolism: Extensively hepatic; CYP2C19 (demethylation), CYP3A4; no evidence that metabolites have pharmacologic activity
Bioavailability: 77%
Half-life elimination: 1 hour; increased to 3.5-10 hours with CYP2C19 deficiency
Time to peak: Oral: 2.5 hours
Excretion: Urine (71%); feces (18%)

Pregnancy Risk Factor B

Dosage Forms
Injection, powder for reconstitution:
Protonix®: 40 mg
Tablet, delayed release:
Protonix®: 20 mg, 40 mg
Tablet, enteric coated, as magnesium:
Pantoloc® M [CAN]: 40 mg [not available in the U.S.]

Pantothenic Acid (pan toe THEN ik AS id)

U.S. Brand Names Panto-250
Generic Available Yes
Index Terms Calcium Pantothenate; Vitamin B_5
Pharmacologic Category Vitamin, Water Soluble
Use Pantothenic acid deficiency
Local Anesthetic/Vasoconstrictor Precautions No information available to require special precautions
Effects on Dental Treatment No significant effects or complications reported
Pregnancy Risk Factor A/C (dose exceeding RDA recommendation)

Pantothenyl Alcohol see Dexpanthenol on page 471

Papain and Urea (pa PAY in & yoor EE a)

U.S. Brand Names Accuzyme®; Allanzyme; Allanzyme 650; Ethezyme™; Ethezyme™ 830; Gladase®; Kovia®
Generic Available Yes: Ointment
Pharmacologic Category Enzyme, Topical Debridement
Use Debridement of necrotic tissue and liquefaction of slough in acute and chronic lesions such as pressure ulcers, varicose and diabetic ulcers, burns, postoperative wounds, pilonidal cyst wounds, carbuncles, and miscellaneous traumatic or infected wounds
Local Anesthetic/Vasoconstrictor Precautions No information available to require special precautions
Effects on Dental Treatment No significant effects or complications reported
Common Adverse Effects Frequency not defined: Local: Burning sensation, skin irritation

Mechanism of Action
Papain: Potent digestant of nonviable protein matter; harmless to viable tissue. Requires activation to exert its function.
Urea: Exposes papain activators (sulfhydryl groups) and denatures nonviable protein matter making it more susceptible to enzymatic digestion.

Drug Interactions
Decreased Effect: Heavy metals, hydrogen peroxide

Papain, Urea, and Chlorophyllin see Chlorophyllin, Papain, and Urea on page 335

Papaverine (pa PAV er een)

U.S. Brand Names Para-Time SR®
Generic Available Yes
Index Terms Papaverine Hydrochloride; Pavabid [DSC]
Pharmacologic Category Vasodilator
Use Oral: Relief of peripheral and cerebral ischemia associated with arterial spasm and myocardial ischemia complicated by arrhythmias
Unlabeled/Investigational Use Investigational: Parenteral: Various vascular spasms associated with muscle spasms as in myocardial infarction, angina, peripheral and pulmonary embolism, peripheral vascular disease, angiospastic states, and visceral spasm (ureteral, biliary, and GI colic); testing for impotence
Local Anesthetic/Vasoconstrictor Precautions No information available to require special precautions
Effects on Dental Treatment No significant effects or complications reported
Common Adverse Effects Frequency not defined.
Cardiovascular: Arrhythmias (with rapid I.V. use), flushing of the face, mild hypertension, tachycardia
Central nervous system: Drowsiness, headache, lethargy, sedation, vertigo
Gastrointestinal: Abdominal distress, anorexia, constipation, diarrhea, nausea
Hepatic: Chronic hepatitis, hepatic hypersensitivity
Respiratory: Apnea (with rapid I.V. use)
Mechanism of Action Smooth muscle spasmolytic producing a generalized smooth muscle relaxation including: vasodilatation, gastrointestinal sphincter relaxation, bronchiolar muscle relaxation, and potentially a depressed myocardium (with large doses); muscle relaxation may occur due to inhibition or cyclic nucleotide phosphodiesterase, increasing cyclic AMP; muscle relaxation is unrelated to nerve innervation; papaverine increases cerebral blood flow in normal subjects; oxygen uptake is unaltered
Drug Interactions
Decreased Effect: Papaverine decreases the effects of levodopa.
Pharmacodynamics/Kinetics
Onset of action: Oral: Rapid
Protein binding: 90%
Metabolism: Rapidly hepatic
Half-life elimination: 0.5-1.5 hours
Excretion: Primarily urine (as metabolites)
Pregnancy Risk Factor C

Papaverine Hydrochloride *see* Papaverine *on page 1252*

Papillomavirus (Types 6, 11, 16, 18) Recombinant Vaccine
(pap ih LO ma VYE rus typs six e LEV en SIX teen aye teen ree KOM be nant vak SEEN)

U.S. Brand Names Gardasil®
Generic Available No
Index Terms HPV Vaccine; Human Papillomavirus Vaccine; Papillomavirus Vaccine, Recombinant; Quadrivalent Human Papillomavirus Vaccine
Pharmacologic Category Vaccine
Use Females: Prevention of cervical cancer, genital warts, cervical adenocarcinoma *in situ*, and vulvar, vaginal, or cervical intraepithelial neoplasia caused by human papillomavirus (HPV) types 6, 11, 16, 18
Local Anesthetic/Vasoconstrictor Precautions No information available to require special precautions
Effects on Dental Treatment No significant effects or complications reported
Common Adverse Effects All serious adverse reactions must be reported to the U.S. Department of Health and Human Services (DHHS) Vaccine Adverse Event Reporting System (VAERS) 1-800-822-7967.
>10%:
Central nervous system: Fever (10% to 13%)
Local: Injection site: Pain (84%), swelling (25%), erythema (25%)
1% to 10%:
Central nervous system: Dizziness (4%), malaise (1%), insomnia (1%)
Gastrointestinal: Nausea (7%), diarrhea (4%), vomiting (2%), toothache (2%)
Local: Injection site pruritus (3%)
Neuromuscular & skeletal: Arthralgia (1%)
Respiratory: Cough (2%), nasal congestion (1%)
Mechanism of Action Contains inactive human papillomavirus (HPV) proteins HPV 6 L1, HPV 11 L1, HPV 16 L1, and HPV 18 L1 which produce neutralizing

antibodies to prevent cervical cancer, cervical adenocarcinoma, cervical, vaginal and vulvar neoplasia and genital warts caused by HPV.

Drug Interactions

Decreased Effect: Immunosuppressants may decrease the effect of vaccines.

Pregnancy Risk Factor B

Papillomavirus Vaccine, Recombinant *see* Papillomavirus (Types 6, 11, 16, 18) Recombinant Vaccine *on page 1252*

Para-Aminosalicylate Sodium *see* Aminosalicylic Acid *on page 91*

Paracetamol *see* Acetaminophen *on page 31*

Parafon Forte® DSC *see* Chlorzoxazone *on page 348*

Paraplatin® [DSC] *see* Carboplatin *on page 283*

Parathyroid Hormone (1-34) *see* Teriparatide *on page 1541*

Para-Time SR® *see* Papaverine *on page 1252*

Parcopa™ *see* Levodopa and Carbidopa *on page 964*

Paregoric (par e GOR ik)

Generic Available Yes

Index Terms Camphorated Tincture of Opium (error-prone synonym)

Pharmacologic Category Analgesic, Opioid

Use Treatment of diarrhea or relief of pain; neonatal opiate withdrawal

Local Anesthetic/Vasoconstrictor Precautions No information available to require special precautions

Effects on Dental Treatment No significant effects or complications reported

Mechanism of Action Increases smooth muscle tone in GI tract, decreases motility and peristalsis, diminishes digestive secretions

Pregnancy Risk Factor B/D (prolonged use or high doses)

Paremyd® *see* Hydroxyamphetamine and Tropicamide *on page 843*

Paricalcitol (pah ri KAL si tole)

U.S. Brand Names Zemplar®

Canadian Brand Names Zemplar®

Generic Available No

Pharmacologic Category Vitamin D Analog

Use

I.V.: Prevention and treatment of secondary hyperparathyroidism associated with stage 5 chronic kidney disease (CKD)

Oral: Prevention and treatment of secondary hyperparathyroidism associated with stage 3 and 4 CKD

Local Anesthetic/Vasoconstrictor Precautions No information available to require special precautions

Effects on Dental Treatment Key adverse event(s) related to dental treatment: Xerostomia (normal salivary flow resumes upon discontinuation).

Common Adverse Effects

>10%: Gastrointestinal: Nausea (6% to 13%)

1% to 10%:

Cardiovascular: Edema (7%), hypertension (7%), hypotension (5%), palpitation (3%), chest pain (3%), syncope (3%), cardiomyopathy (2%), MI (2%), postural hypotension (2%)

Central nervous system: Pain (8%), chills (5%), dizziness (5%), headache (5%), lightheadedness (5%), vertigo (5%), fever (3% to 5%), depression (3%), insomnia (2%)

Dermatologic: Rash (2% to 6%), skin ulcer (3%), pruritus (3%), skin hypertrophy (2%)

Endocrine & metabolic: Dehydration (3%), acidosis (2%), hypokalemia (2%)

Gastrointestinal: Vomiting (6% to 8%), diarrhea (7%), GI bleeding (5%), abdominal pain (4%), xerostomia (3%), constipation (4%), gastroenteritis (3%), dyspepsia (2%), gastritis (2%), rectal disorder (2%)

Genitourinary: Urinary tract infection (3%), kidney function abnormal (2%)

Neuromuscular & skeletal: Arthritis (5%), back pain (4%), leg cramps (3%), weakness (3%), neuropathy (2%)

Ocular: Amblyopia (2%), retinal disorder (2%)

Respiratory: Pneumonia (2% to 5%), rhinitis (5%), sinusitis (3%), bronchitis (3%), cough (3%), epistaxis (2%)

Miscellaneous: Infection (bacterial, fungal, viral: 2% to 8%); allergic reaction (6%), flu-like syndrome (2% to 5%), sepsis (5%), cyst (2%)

Mechanism of Action Decreased renal conversion of vitamin D to its primary active metabolite (1,25-hydroxyvitamin D) in chronic renal failure leads to (Continued)

Paricalcitol (Continued)

reduced activation of vitamin D receptor (VDR), which subsequently removes inhibitory suppression of parathyroid hormone (PTH) release; increased serum PTH (secondary hyperparathyroidism) reduces calcium excretion and enhances bone resorption. Paricalcitol is a synthetic vitamin D analog which binds to and activates the VDR in kidney, parathyroid gland, intestine and bone, thus reducing PTH levels and improving calcium and phosphate homeostasis.

Drug Interactions
Cytochrome P450 Effect: Substrate of CYP3A4 (major)
Increased Effect/Toxicity:
CYP3A4 inhibitors (strong) may increase the levels/effects of paricalcitol; example CYP3A4 inhibitors include azole antifungals, ciprofloxacin, clarithromycin, diclofenac, doxycycline, erythromycin, imatinib, isoniazid, nefazodone, nicardipine, propofol, protease inhibitors, quinidine, and verapamil. Ketoconazole may increase paricalcitol levels/effects.

Pharmacodynamics/Kinetics
Distribution: V_d:
Healthy subjects: Oral: 34 L; I.V.: 24 L
Stage 3 and 4 CKD: Oral: 44-46 L
Stage 5 CKD: I.V.: 31-35 L
Protein binding: >99%
Metabolism: Hydroxylation and glucuronidation via hepatic and nonhepatic enzymes, including CYP24, CYP3A4, UGT1A4; forms metabolites (at least one active)
Bioavailability: Oral: ~72% in healthy subjects
Half-life elimination:
Healthy subjects: Oral: 4-6 hours
Stage 3 and 4 CKD: Oral: 17-20 hours
Stage 5 CKD: I.V.: 14-15 hours
Excretion: Healthy subjects: Feces (oral: 70% to 74%; I.V.: 63%); urine (oral: 16% to 18%, I.V.: 19%); 51% to 59% as metabolites

Pregnancy Risk Factor C

Pariprazole see Rabeprazole on page 1401
Parlodel® see Bromocriptine on page 229
Parlodel® SnapTabs® see Bromocriptine on page 229
Parnate® see Tranylcypromine on page 1601

Paromomycin (par oh moe MYE sin)

U.S. Brand Names Humatin®
Canadian Brand Names Humatin®
Generic Available Yes
Index Terms Paromomycin Sulfate
Pharmacologic Category Amebicide
Use Treatment of acute and chronic intestinal amebiasis; hepatic coma
Unlabeled/Investigational Use Treatment of cryptosporidiosis
Local Anesthetic/Vasoconstrictor Precautions No information available to require special precautions
Effects on Dental Treatment No significant effects or complications reported
Common Adverse Effects
1% to 10%: Gastrointestinal: Diarrhea, abdominal cramps, nausea, vomiting, heartburn
Mechanism of Action Acts directly on ameba; has antibacterial activity against normal and pathogenic organisms in the GI tract; interferes with bacterial protein synthesis by binding to 30S ribosomal subunits
Pharmacodynamics/Kinetics
Absorption: None
Excretion: Feces (100% as unchanged drug)
Pregnancy Risk Factor C

Paromomycin Sulfate see Paromomycin on page 1254

Paroxetine (pa ROKS e teen)

Related Information
Sedation on page 1825
U.S. Brand Names Paxil®; Paxil CR®; Pexeva®
Canadian Brand Names Apo-Paroxetine®; CO Paroxetine; Gen-Paroxetine; Novo-Paroxetine; Paxil®; Paxil CR®; PMS-Paroxetine; ratio-Paroxetine; Rhoxal-paroxetine; Sandoz-Paroxetine

Mexican Brand Names Aropax 20; Paxil

Generic Available Yes: Tablet, as hydrochloride

Index Terms Paroxetine Hydrochloride; Paroxetine Mesylate

Pharmacologic Category Antidepressant, Selective Serotonin Reuptake Inhibitor

Use Treatment of major depressive disorder (MDD); treatment of panic disorder with or without agoraphobia; obsessive-compulsive disorder (OCD); social anxiety disorder (social phobia); generalized anxiety disorder (GAD); post-traumatic stress disorder (PTSD); premenstrual dysphoric disorder (PMDD)

Unlabeled/Investigational Use May be useful in eating disorders, impulse control disorders, self-injurious behavior; vasomotor symptoms of menopause; treatment of depression and obsessive-compulsive disorder (OCD) in children

Local Anesthetic/Vasoconstrictor Precautions Although caution should be used in patients taking tricyclic antidepressants, no interactions have been reported with vasoconstrictor and paroxetine, a nontricyclic antidepressant which acts to increase serotonin; no precautions appear to be needed

Effects on Dental Treatment Key adverse event(s) related to dental treatment: Xerostomia and changes in salivation (normal salivary flow resumes upon discontinuation), postural hypotension, and abnormal taste. Problems with SSRI-induced bruxism have been reported and may preclude their use; clinicians attempting to evaluate any patient with bruxism or involuntary muscle movement, who is simultaneously being treated with an SSRI drug, should be aware of the potential association. Prolonged use may decrease or inhibit salivary flow; normal salivation resumes upon discontinuation.

Common Adverse Effects Frequency varies by dose and indication. Adverse reactions reported as a composite of all indications.

>10%:

Central nervous system: Somnolence (15% to 24%), insomnia (11% to 24%), headache (17% to 18%), dizziness (6% to 14%)

Endocrine & metabolic: Libido decreased (3% to 15%)

Gastrointestinal: Nausea (19% to 26%), xerostomia (9% to 18%), constipation (5% to 16%), diarrhea (9% to 12%)

Genitourinary: Ejaculatory disturbances (10% to 28%)

Neuromuscular & skeletal: Weakness (12% to 22%), tremor (4% to 11%)

Miscellaneous: Diaphoresis (5% to 14%)

1% to 10%:

Cardiovascular: Vasodilation (2% to 4%), chest pain (3%), palpitation (2% to 3%), hypertension (≥1%), tachycardia (≥1%)

Central nervous system: Nervousness (4% to 9%), anxiety (5%), agitation (3% to 5%), abnormal dreams (3% to 4%), concentration impaired (3% to 4%), yawning (2% to 4%), depersonalization (up to 3%), amnesia (2%), emotional lability (≥1%), vertigo (≥1%), confusion (1%), chills (2%)

Dermatologic: Rash (2% to 3%), pruritus (≥1%)

Endocrine & metabolic: Orgasmic disturbance (2% to 9%), dysmenorrhea (5%)

Gastrointestinal: Anorexia, appetite decreased (5% to 9%), dyspepsia (2% to 5%), flatulence (4%), abdominal pain (4%), appetite increased (2% to 4%), vomiting (2% to 3%), taste perversion (2%), weight gain (≥1%)

Genitourinary: Impotence (2% to 9%), genital disorder (female 2% to 9%), urinary frequency (2% to 3%), urinary tract infection (2%)

Neuromuscular & skeletal: Paresthesia (4%), myalgia (2% to 4%), back pain (3%), myoclonus (2% to 3%), myopathy (2%), myasthenia (1%), arthralgia (≥1%)

Ocular: Blurred vision (4%), abnormal vision (2% to 4%)

Otic: Tinnitus (≥1%)

Respiratory: Respiratory disorder (up to 7%), pharyngitis (4%), sinusitis (up to 4%), rhinitis (3%)

Miscellaneous: Infection (5% to 6%)

Restrictions An FDA-approved medication guide concerning the use of antidepressants in children, adolescents, and young adults must be distributed when dispensing an outpatient prescription (new or refill) where this medication is to be used without direct supervision of a healthcare provider. Medication guides are available at http://www.fda.gov/cder/Offices/ODS/medication_guides.htm. Dispense to parents or guardians of children and adolescents receiving this medication.

Dosage Oral:

Children:

Depression (unlabeled use; not recommended by FDA): Initial: 10 mg/day and adjusted upward on an individual basis to 20 mg/day

OCD (unlabeled use): Initial: 10 mg/day and titrate up as necessary to 60 mg/day

Self-injurious behavior (unlabeled use): 20 mg/day

(Continued)

Paroxetine *(Continued)*

Social anxiety disorder (unlabeled use): 2.5-15 mg/day

Adults:

MDD:

Paxil®, Pexeva®: Initial: 20 mg once daily, preferably in the morning; increase if needed by 10 mg/day increments at intervals of at least 1 week; maximum dose: 50 mg/day

Paxil CR®: Initial: 25 mg once daily; increase if needed by 12.5 mg/day increments at intervals of at least 1 week; maximum dose: 62.5 mg/day

GAD (Paxil®, Pexeva®): Initial: 20 mg once daily, preferably in the morning (if dose is increased, adjust in increments of 10 mg/day at 1-week intervals); doses of 20-50 mg/day were used in clinical trials, however, no greater benefit was seen with doses >20 mg.

OCD (Paxil®, Pexeva™): Initial: 20 mg once daily, preferably in the morning; increase if needed by 10 mg/day increments at intervals of at least 1 week; recommended dose: 40 mg/day; range: 20-60 mg/day; maximum dose: 60 mg/day

Panic disorder:

Paxil®, Pexeva®: Initial: 10 mg once daily, preferably in the morning; increase if needed by 10 mg/day increments at intervals of at least 1 week; recommended dose: 40 mg/day; range: 10-60 mg/day; maximum dose: 60 mg/day

Paxil CR®: Initial: 12.5 mg once daily; increase if needed by 12.5 mg/day at intervals of at least 1 week; maximum dose: 75 mg/day

PMDD (Paxil CR®): Initial: 12.5 mg once daily in the morning; may be increased to 25 mg/day; dosing changes should occur at intervals of at least 1 week. May be given daily throughout the menstrual cycle or limited to the luteal phase.

PTSD (Paxil®): Initial: 20 mg once daily, preferably in the morning; increase if needed by 10 mg/day increments at intervals of at least 1 week; range: 20-50 mg. Limited data suggest doses of 40 mg/day were not more efficacious than 20 mg/day.

Social anxiety disorder:

Paxil®: Initial: 20 mg once daily, preferably in the morning; recommended dose: 20 mg/day; range: 20-60 mg/day; doses >20 mg may not have additional benefit

Paxil CR®: Initial: 12.5 mg once daily, preferably in the morning; may be increased by 12.5 mg/day at intervals of at least 1 week; maximum dose: 37.5 mg/day

Vasomotor symptoms of menopause (unlabeled use, Paxil CR®): 12.5-25 mg/day

Elderly:

Paxil®, Pexeva®: Initial: 10 mg/day; increase if needed by 10 mg/day increments at intervals of at least 1 week; maximum dose: 40 mg/day

Paxil CR®: Initial: 12.5 mg/day; increase if needed by 12.5 mg/day increments at intervals of at least 1 week; maximum dose: 50 mg/day

Note: Upon discontinuation of paroxetine therapy, gradually taper dose:

Paxil®, Pexeva®: 10 mg/day at weekly intervals; when 20 mg/day dose is reached, continue for 1 week before treatment is discontinued. Some patients may need to be titrated to 10 mg/day for 1 week before discontinuation.

Paxil CR®: Patients receiving 37.5 mg/day in clinical trials had their dose decreased by 12.5 mg/day to a dose of 25 mg/day and remained at a dose of 25 mg/day for 1 week before treatment was discontinued.

Dosage adjustment in renal impairment: Adults:

Cl_{cr} <30 mL/minute: Mean plasma concentration is ~4 times that seen in normal function.

Cl_{cr} 30-60 mL/minute: Plasma concentration is 2 times that seen in normal function.

Paxil®, Pexeva®: Initial: 10 mg/day; increase if needed by 10 mg/day increments at intervals of at least 1 week; maximum dose: 40 mg/day

Paxil CR®: Initial: 12.5 mg/day; increase if needed by 12.5 mg/day increments at intervals of at least 1 week; maximum dose: 50 mg/day

Dosage adjustment in severe hepatic impairment: Adults: In hepatic dysfunction, plasma concentration is 2 times that seen in normal function.

Paxil®, Pexeva®: Initial: 10 mg/day; increase if needed by 10 mg/day increments at intervals of at least 1 week; maximum dose: 40 mg/day

Paxil CR®: Initial: 12.5 mg/day; increase if needed by 12.5 mg/day increments at intervals of at least 1 week; maximum dose: 50 mg/day

Mechanism of Action Paroxetine is a selective serotonin reuptake inhibitor, chemically unrelated to tricyclic, tetracyclic, or other antidepressants; presumably, the inhibition of serotonin reuptake from brain synapse stimulated serotonin activity in the brain

Contraindications Hypersensitivity to paroxetine or any component of the formulation; use with or within 14 days of MAO inhibitors; concurrent use with thioridazine or pimozide

Warnings/Precautions [U.S. Boxed Warning]: **Antidepressants increase the risk of suicidal thinking and behavior in children, adolescents, and young adults (18-24 years of age) with major depressive disorder (MDD) and other psychiatric disorders;** consider risk prior to prescribing. Short-term studies did not show an increased risk in patients >24 years of age and showed a decreased risk in patients ≥65 years. Closely monitor patients for clinical worsening, suicidality, or unusual changes in behavior, particularly during the initial 1-2 months of therapy or during periods of dosage adjustments (increases or decreases); the patient's family or caregiver should be instructed to closely observe the patient and communicate condition with healthcare provider. A medication guide concerning the use of antidepressants should be dispensed with each prescription. **Paroxetine is not FDA approved for use in children.**

The possibility of a suicide attempt is inherent in major depression and may persist until remission occurs. Patients treated with antidepressants (for any indication) should be observed for clinical worsening and suicidality, especially during the initial few months of a course of drug therapy, or at times of dose changes, either increases or decreases. Use caution in high-risk patients. Worsening depression and severe abrupt suicidality that are not part of the presenting symptoms may require discontinuation or modification of drug therapy. The patient's family or caregiver should be alerted to monitor patients for the emergence of suicidality and associated behaviors (such as agitation, irritability, hostility, impulsivity, and hypomania) and call healthcare provider.

May worsen psychosis in some patients or precipitate a shift to mania or hypomania in patients with bipolar disorder. Patients presenting with depressive symptoms should be screened for bipolar disorder. Monotherapy in patients with bipolar disorder should be avoided. **Paroxetine is not FDA approved for the treatment of bipolar depression.**

Potential for severe reaction when used with MAO inhibitors, SSRIs/SNRIs or triptans; serotonin syndrome (hyperthermia, muscular rigidity, mental status changes/agitation, autonomic instability) may occur; concurrent use with MAO inhibitors contraindicated. May increase the risks associated with electroconvulsive therapy. Has a low potential to impair cognitive or motor performance - caution operating hazardous machinery or driving. Symptoms of agitation and/ or restlessness may occur during initial few weeks of therapy. Low potential for sedation or anticholinergic effects relative to cyclic antidepressants.

Use caution in patients with a previous seizure disorder or condition predisposing to seizures such as brain damage, alcoholism, or concurrent therapy with other drugs which lower the seizure threshold. Use with caution in patients with hepatic dysfunction and in elderly patients. May cause hyponatremia/ SIADH. Use with caution in patients at risk of bleeding or receiving anticoagulant therapy - may cause impairment in platelet aggregation. Use with caution in patients with renal insufficiency or other concurrent illness (due to limited experience); dose reduction recommended with severe renal impairment. May cause or exacerbate sexual dysfunction. Use caution in patients with narrow-angle glaucoma. Avoid use in the first trimester of pregnancy.

Upon discontinuation of paroxetine therapy, gradually taper dose and monitor for discontinuation symptoms (eg, dizziness, dysphoric mood, irritability, agitation, confusion, paresthesias). If intolerable symptoms occur following a decrease in dosage or upon discontinuation of therapy, then resuming the previous dose with a more gradual taper should be considered. Safety and efficacy in children have not been established.

Drug Interactions

    Cytochrome P450 Effect: Substrate of CYP2D6 (major); **Inhibits** CYP1A2 (weak), 2B6 (moderate), 2C9 (weak), 2C19 (weak), 2D6 (strong), 3A4 (weak)

    Increased Effect/Toxicity: Paroxetine should not be used with nonselective MAO inhibitors (phenelzine, isocarboxazid) or other drugs with MAO inhibition (linezolid); fatal reactions have been reported. Wait 2 weeks after stopping an MAO inhibitor before starting paroxetine. Concurrent selegiline has been associated with mania, hypertension, or serotonin syndrome (risk may be reduced relative to nonselective MAO inhibitors). Serum levels of atomoxetine, carbamazepine, duloxetine, galantamine, mexiletine, propafenone, and risperidone may be increased by paroxetine.

    Paroxetine may inhibit the metabolism of thioridazine or mesoridazine, resulting in increased plasma levels and increasing the risk of QT_c interval
(Continued)

Paroxetine *(Continued)*

prolongation. This may lead to serious ventricular arrhythmias, such as torsade de pointes-type arrhythmias and sudden death. Do not use together. Wait at least 5 weeks after discontinuing paroxetine prior to starting thioridazine.

The levels/effects of paroxetine may be increased by chlorpromazine, delavirdine, fluoxetine, miconazole, pergolide, quinidine, quinine, ritonavir, ropinirole, and other CYP2D6 inhibitors. Paroxetine may increase the levels/effects of amphetamines, selected beta-blockers, bupropion, dextromethorphan, fluoxetine, lidocaine, mirtazapine, nefazodone, promethazine, propofol, risperidone, ritonavir, sertraline, tricyclic antidepressants, venlafaxine, and other CYP2B6 or 2D6 substrates.

Concomitant use of paroxetine and NSAIDs, aspirin, or other drugs affecting coagulation has been associated with an increased risk of bleeding. Paroxetine may increase the hypoprothrombinemic response to warfarin. Paroxetine increases levels of procyclidine; this may result in increased anticholinergic effects; procyclidine dose reduction may be necessary. Concomitant use of paroxetine and beta-blockers may increase the risk of bradycardia. Concurrent use of paroxetine with CNS depressants may enhance the adverse effects/toxicity of CNS depressants.

Combined use of SSRIs and amphetamines, buspirone, meperidine, nefazodone, serotonin agonists (such as sumatriptan), sibutramine, other SSRIs/SNRIs, sympathomimetics, ritonavir, tramadol, and venlafaxine may increase the risk of serotonin syndrome. Combined use of sumatriptan (and other serotonin agonists) may result in toxicity; weakness, hyper-reflexia, and incoordination have been observed with sumatriptan and SSRIs. In addition, concurrent use may theoretically increase the risk of serotonin syndrome; includes sumatriptan, naratriptan, rizatriptan, and zolmitriptan. Concurrent lithium may increase risk of nephrotoxicity. Risk of hyponatremia may increase with concurrent use of loop diuretics (bumetanide, furosemide, torsemide).

Decreased Effect: Cyproheptadine, a serotonin antagonist, may inhibit the effects of serotonin reuptake inhibitors (paroxetine). Paroxetine may decrease the levels/effects of CYP2D6 prodrug substrates (eg, codeine, hydrocodone, oxycodone, tramadol).

Ethanol/Nutrition/Herb Interactions

Ethanol: Avoid ethanol (may increase CNS depression).

Food: Peak concentration is increased, but bioavailability is not significantly altered by food.

Herb/Nutraceutical: Avoid valerian, St John's wort, SAMe, kava kava.

Dietary Considerations May be taken with or without food.

Pharmacodynamics/Kinetics

Absorption: Completely absorbed following oral administration

Distribution: V_d: 8.7 L/kg (3-28 L/kg)

Protein binding: 93% to 95%

Metabolism: Extensively hepatic via CYP2D6 enzymes; primary metabolites are formed via oxidation and methylation of parent drug, with subsequent glucuronide/sulfate conjugation; nonlinear pharmacokinetics (via 2D6 saturation) may be seen with higher doses and longer duration of therapy. Metabolites exhibit ~2% potency of parent compound. C_{min} concentrations are 70% to 80% greater in the elderly compared to nonelderly patients; clearance is also decreased.

Half-life elimination: 21 hours (3-65 hours)

Time to peak: Immediate release: 5.2 hours; controlled release: 6-10 hours

Excretion: Urine (64%, 2% as unchanged drug); feces (36% primarily via bile, <1% as unchanged drug)

Pregnancy Risk Factor D

Dosage Forms Note: Strength expressed as base:

Suspension, oral:

Paxil®: 10 mg/5 mL (250 mL)

Tablet: 10 mg, 20 mg, 30 mg, 40 mg

Paxil®, Pexeva®: 10 mg, 20 mg, 30 mg, 40 mg

Tablet, controlled release:

Paxil CR®: 12.5 mg, 25 mg, 37.5 mg

Pavabid [DSC] see Papaverine on page 1252

Paxil® see Paroxetine on page 1254

Paxil CR® see Paroxetine on page 1254

PCA (error-prone abbreviation) see Procainamide on page 1354

PCE® see Erythromycin on page 589

PCEC see Rabies Virus Vaccine on page 1403

PCM see Chlorpheniramine, Phenylephrine, and Methscopolamine on page 342

PCM Allergy see Chlorpheniramine, Phenylephrine, and Methscopolamine on page 342

PCV7 see Pneumococcal Conjugate Vaccine (7-Valent) on page 1318

PD-Cof see Chlorpheniramine, Phenylephrine, and Dextromethorphan on page 342

PD-Hist-D see Chlorpheniramine and Phenylephrine on page 340

PediaCare® Children's Long Acting Cough Plus Cold [OTC] [DSC] see Pseudoephedrine and Dextromethorphan on page 1383

PediaCare® Children's Medicated Freezer Pops Long Acting Cough [OTC] [DSC] see Dextromethorphan on page 477

PediaCare® Cold and Allergy [OTC] [DSC] see Chlorpheniramine and Pseudoephedrine on page 340

PediaCare® Decongestant Infants [OTC] see Pseudoephedrine on page 1381

PediaCare® Infants' Decongestant & Cough [OTC] see Pseudoephedrine and Dextromethorphan on page 1383

PediaCare® Infants' Long-Acting Cough [OTC] see Dextromethorphan on page 477

Pediacof® [DSC] see Chlorpheniramine, Phenylephrine, Codeine, and Potassium Iodide on page 344

Pediaflor® [DSC] see Fluoride on page 710

Pediapred® see PrednisoLONE on page 1339

Pedia Relief Cough and Cold [OTC] see Pseudoephedrine and Dextromethorphan on page 1383

Pedia Relief Infants [OTC] see Pseudoephedrine and Dextromethorphan on page 1383

Pediarix® see Diphtheria, Tetanus Toxoids, Acellular Pertussis, Hepatitis B (Recombinant), and Poliovirus (Inactivated) Vaccine on page 515

PediaTan™ see Chlorpheniramine on page 338

PediaTan™D see Chlorpheniramine and Phenylephrine on page 340

Pediatex™-D [DSC] see Carbinoxamine and Pseudoephedrine on page 282

Pediatex™ DM [DSC] see Carbinoxamine, Pseudoephedrine, and Dextromethorphan on page 282

Pediazole® [DSC] see Erythromycin and Sulfisoxazole on page 595

Pedi-Boro® [OTC] see Aluminum Sulfate and Calcium Acetate on page 83

Pedi-Dri® see Nystatin on page 1194

PediOtic® see Neomycin, Polymyxin B, and Hydrocortisone on page 1162

Pedi-Pro® see Benzalkonium Chloride on page 194

Pedisilk™ [OTC] see Salicylic Acid on page 1451

Pedtrace-4® see Trace Metals on page 1595

PedvaxHIB® see Haemophilus b Conjugate Vaccine on page 802

PEG see Polyethylene Glycol 3350 on page 1321

PEG-L-asparaginase see Pegaspargase on page 1260

Pegademase Bovine (peg A de mase BOE vine)

U.S. Brand Names Adagen®
Canadian Brand Names Adagen®
Generic Available No
Pharmacologic Category Enzyme
Use Orphan drug: Enzyme replacement therapy for adenosine deaminase (ADA) deficiency in patients with severe combined immunodeficiency disease (SCID) who can not benefit from bone marrow transplant; not a cure for SCID, unlike bone marrow transplants, injections must be used the rest of the child's life, therefore is not really an alternative

Local Anesthetic/Vasoconstrictor Precautions No information available to require special precautions

Effects on Dental Treatment No significant effects or complications reported

Mechanism of Action Adenosine deaminase is an enzyme that catalyzes the deamination of both adenosine and deoxyadenosine. Hereditary lack of adenosine deaminase activity results in severe combined immunodeficiency disease, a fatal disorder of infancy characterized by profound defects of both cellular and humoral immunity. It is estimated that 25% of patients with the autosomal
(Continued)

Pegademase Bovine *(Continued)*

recessive form of severe combined immunodeficiency lack adenosine deaminase.

Pharmacodynamics/Kinetics
Absorption: Rapid
Half-life elimination: 48-72 hours
Time to peak: Plasma adenosine deaminase activity: 2-3 weeks

Pregnancy Risk Factor C

Peganone® *see* Ethotoin *on page 653*

Pegaptanib *(peg AP ta nib)*

U.S. Brand Names Macugen®
Canadian Brand Names Macugen®
Generic Available No
Index Terms EYE001; Pegaptanib Sodium
Pharmacologic Category Ophthalmic Agent; Vascular Endothelial Growth Factor (VEGF) Inhibitor
Use Treatment of neovascular (wet) age-related macular degeneration (AMD)

Local Anesthetic/Vasoconstrictor Precautions No information available to require special precautions

Effects on Dental Treatment No significant effects or complications reported

Common Adverse Effects
10% to 40%:
Cardiovascular: Hypertension
Ocular: Anterior chamber inflammation, blurred vision, cataract, conjunctival hemorrhage, corneal edema, eye discharge, eye irritation, eye pain, intraocular pressure increased, ocular discomfort, punctate keratitis, visual acuity decreased, visual disturbance, vitreous floaters, vitreous opacities

1% to 10%:
Cardiovascular: Carotid artery occlusion (1% to 5%), cerebrovascular accident (1% to 5%), chest pain (1% to 5%), transient ischemic attack (1% to 5%)
Central nervous system: Dizziness (6% to 10%), headache (6% to 10%), vertigo (1% to 5%)
Dermatologic: Contact dermatitis (1% to 5%)
Endocrine & metabolic: Diabetes mellitus (1% to 5%)
Gastrointestinal: Diarrhea (6% to 10%), nausea (6% to 10%), dyspepsia (1% to 5%), vomiting (1% to 5%)
Genitourinary: Urinary retention (1% to 5%)
Neuromuscular & skeletal: Arthritis (1% to 5%), bone spur (1% to 5%)
Ocular: Blepharitis (6% to 10%), conjunctivitis (6% to 10%), photopsia (6% to 10%), vitreous disorder (6% to 10%), allergic conjunctivitis (1% to 5%), conjunctival edema (1% to 5%), corneal abrasion (1% to 5%), corneal deposits (1% to 5%), corneal epithelium disorder (1% to 5%), endophthalmitis (1% to 5%), eye inflammation (1% to 5%), eye swelling (1% to 5%), eyelid irritation (1% to 5%), meibomianitis (1% to 5%), mydriasis (1% to 5%), periorbital hematoma (1% to 5%), retinal edema (1% to 5%), vitreous hemorrhage (1% to 5%)
Otic: Hearing loss (1% to 5%)
Renal: Urinary tract infection (6% to 10%)
Respiratory: Bronchitis (6% to 10%), pleural effusion (1% to 5%)
Miscellaneous: Contusion (1% to 5%)

Mechanism of Action Pegaptanib is an apatamer, an oligonucleotide covalently bound to polyethylene glycol, which can adopt a three-dimensional shape and bind to vascular endothelial growth factor (VEGF). Pegaptanib binds to extracellular VEGF, inhibiting VEGF from binding to its receptors and thereby suppressing neovascularization and slowing vision loss.

Pharmacodynamics/Kinetics
Absorption: Slow systemic absorption following intravitreous injection
Metabolism: Metabolized by endo- and exonucleases
Half-life elimination: Plasma: 6-14 days

Pregnancy Risk Factor B

Pegaptanib Sodium *see* Pegaptanib *on page 1260*

Pegaspargase *(peg AS par jase)*

Related Information
Asparaginase *on page 148*

U.S. Brand Names Oncaspar®
Generic Available No
Index Terms NSC-644954; PEG-L-asparaginase
Pharmacologic Category Antineoplastic Agent, Miscellaneous
Use Treatment of acute lymphocytic leukemia (ALL); treatment of ALL with previous hypersensitivity to native L-asparaginase
Local Anesthetic/Vasoconstrictor Precautions No information available to require special precautions
Effects on Dental Treatment No significant effects or complications reported
Common Adverse Effects In general, pegaspargase toxicities tend to be less frequent and appear somewhat later than comparable toxicities of asparaginase. Intramuscular rather than intravenous injection may decrease the incidence of coagulopathy; GI, hepatic, and renal toxicity. Except for hypersensitivity reactions, adults tend to have a higher incidence than children.
>5%:
  Cardiovascular: Edema
  Central nervous system: Fever, malaise
  Dermatologic: Rash (1% to >5%)
  Gastrointestinal: Nausea, vomiting
  Hematologic: Coagulopathy (7%; grades 3/4: 2%)
  Hepatic: Transaminases increased (11%; grades 3/4: 3%), ALT increased
  Miscellaneous: Allergic reactions (including bronchospasm, chills, dyspnea, edema, erythema, fever, rash, urticaria: 1% to 10%; 32% in patients with prior hypersensitivity to asparaginase products)
1% to 5%:
  Cardiovascular: Hypotension, peripheral edema, tachycardia, thrombosis (4%)
  Central nervous system: Chills, CNS thrombosis/hemorrhage (2%), headache, seizure
  Dermatologic: Lip edema, urticaria
  Endocrine & metabolic: Hyperglycemia (3% to 5%), hyperuricemia, hypoglycemia, hypoproteinemia
  Gastrointestinal: Abdominal pain, anorexia, diarrhea, pancreatitis (1% to 2%; grades 3/4: 2%)
  Hematologic: Anticoagulant effect decreased, disseminated intravascular coagulation (DIC), fibrinogen decreased, hemolytic anemia, leukopenia, pancytopenia, thrombocytopenia, thromboplastin increased, myelosuppression (mild to moderate; onset: 7 days; nadir: 14 days; recovery: 21 days)
  Hepatic: Liver function tests abnormal (5%), hyperbilirubinemia, jaundice, AST increased
  Local: Injection site hypersensitivity, pain or reaction
  Neuromuscular & skeletal: Arthralgia, limb pain, myalgia, paresthesia
  Respiratory: Dyspnea
  Miscellaneous: Anaphylactic reactions, night sweats
Mechanism of Action Pegaspargase is a modified version of asparaginase. Leukemic cells, especially lymphoblasts, require exogenous asparagine; normal cells can synthesize asparagine. Asparaginase contains L-asparaginase amidohydrolase type EC-2 which inhibits protein synthesis by deaminating asparagine to aspartic acid and ammonia in the plasma and extracellular fluid and therefore deprives tumor cells of the amino acid for protein synthesis. Asparaginase is cycle-specific for the G_1 phase of the cell cycle.
Pharmacodynamics/Kinetics
Duration: Asparaginase was measurable for at least 20 days following initial treatment with pegaspargase
Distribution: V_d: 4-5 L/kg; 70% to 80% of plasma volume; does not penetrate the CSF
Metabolism: Systemically degraded
Half-life elimination: 5.8 days; unaffected by age, renal or hepatic function; half life decreased to 3.2 days in patients with previous hypersensitivity to native L-asparaginase
Excretion: Urine (trace amounts)
Pregnancy Risk Factor C

Pegasys® *see* Peginterferon Alfa-2a *on page 1262*

Pegfilgrastim (peg fil GRA stim)

U.S. Brand Names Neulasta®
Canadian Brand Names Neulasta®
Generic Available No
Index Terms G-CSF (PEG Conjugate); Granulocyte Colony Stimulating Factor (PEG Conjugate); NSC-725961; SD/01
(Continued)

Pegfilgrastim (Continued)

Pharmacologic Category Colony Stimulating Factor

Use Decrease the incidence of infection, by stimulation of granulocyte production, in patients with nonmyeloid malignancies receiving myelosuppressive therapy associated with a significant risk of febrile neutropenia

Local Anesthetic/Vasoconstrictor Precautions No information available to require special precautions

Effects on Dental Treatment No significant effects or complications reported

Common Adverse Effects >10%:

Cardiovascular: Peripheral edema (12%)

Central nervous system: Headache (16%)

Gastrointestinal: Vomiting (13%), constipation (12%)

Neuromuscular & skeletal: Bone pain (31% to 57%), myalgia (21%), arthralgia (16%), weakness (13%)

Mechanism of Action Stimulates the production, maturation, and activation of neutrophils, pegfilgrastim activates neutrophils to increase both their migration and cytotoxicity. Pegfilgrastim has a prolonged duration of effect relative to filgrastim and a reduced renal clearance.

Drug Interactions

Increased Effect/Toxicity: No formal drug interactions studies have been conducted.

Pharmacodynamics/Kinetics Half-life elimination: SubQ: 15-80 hours

Pregnancy Risk Factor C

Peginterferon Alfa-2a (peg in ter FEER on AL fa too aye)

Related Information

Systemic Viral Diseases *on page 1767*

U.S. Brand Names Pegasys®

Canadian Brand Names Pegasys®

Mexican Brand Names Pegasys

Generic Available No

Index Terms Interferon Alfa-2a (PEG Conjugate); Pegylated Interferon Alfa-2a

Pharmacologic Category Interferon

Use Treatment of chronic hepatitis C (CHC), alone or in combination with ribavirin, in patients with compensated liver disease and histological evidence of cirrhosis (Child-Pugh class A) and patients with clinically-stable HIV disease; treatment of patients with HBeAg positive and HBeAg negative chronic hepatitis B with compensated liver disease and evidence of viral replication and liver inflammation

Local Anesthetic/Vasoconstrictor Precautions No information available to require special precautions

Effects on Dental Treatment Key adverse event(s) related to dental treatment: Xerostomia (normal salivary flow resumes upon discontinuation).

Common Adverse Effects Note: Percentages are reported for peginterferon alfa-2a in chronic hepatitis C (CHC) patients. Other percentages indicated as "with ribavirin" or "in HIV/CHC" are those which significantly exceed incidence reported for peginterferon monotherapy in CHC patients.

>10%:

Central nervous system: Headache (54%), fatigue (50%), pyrexia (37%; 41% with ribavirin; 54% in hepatitis B), insomnia (19%; 30% with ribavirin), depression (18%), dizziness (16%), irritability/anxiety/nervousness (19%; 33% with ribavirin), pain (11%)

Dermatologic: Alopecia (23%; 28% with ribavirin), pruritus (12%; 19% with ribavirin), dermatitis (16% with ribavirin)

Gastrointestinal: Nausea/vomiting (24%), anorexia (17%; 24% with ribavirin), diarrhea (16%), weight loss (16% in HIV/CHC), abdominal pain (15%)

Hematologic: Neutropenia (21%; 27% with ribavirin; 40% in HIV/CHC), lymphopenia (14% with ribavirin), anemia (11% with ribavirin; 14% in HIV/CHC)

Hepatic: ALT increases 5-10 x ULN during treatment (25% to 27% in hepatitis B); ALT increases >10 x ULN during treatment (12% to 18% in hepatitis B); ALT increases 5-10 x ULN after treatment (13% to 16% in hepatitis B); ALT increases >10 x ULN after treatment (7% to 12% in hepatitis B)

Local: Injection site reaction (22%)

Neuromuscular & skeletal: Weakness (56%; 65% with ribavirin), myalgia (37%), rigors (32%; 25% to 27% in hepatitis B), arthralgia (28%)

Respiratory: Dyspnea (13% with ribavirin)

1% to 10%:

Central nervous system: Concentration impaired (8%), memory impaired (5%), mood alteration (3%; 9% in HIV/CHC)

Dermatologic: Dermatitis (8%), rash (5%), dry skin (4%; 10% with ribavirin), eczema (5% with ribavirin)

Endocrine & metabolic: Hypothyroidism (4%), hyperthyroidism (1%)

Gastrointestinal: Xerostomia (6%), dyspepsia (6% with ribavirin), weight loss (4%; 10% with ribavirin)

Hematologic: Thrombocytopenia (5%), platelets decreased <50,000/mm^3 (5%), lymphopenia (3%), anemia (2%)

Hepatic: Hepatic decompensation (2% CHC/HIV patients)

Neuromuscular & skeletal: Back pain (9%)

Ocular: Blurred vision (4%)

Respiratory: Cough (4%; 10% with ribavirin), dyspnea (4%), exertional dyspnea (4% with ribavirin)

Miscellaneous: Diaphoresis (6%), bacterial infection (3%; 5% in HIV/CHC)

Restrictions An FDA-approved medication guide must be distributed when dispensing an outpatient prescription (new or refill) where this medication is to be used without direct supervision of a healthcare provider. Medication guides are available at http://www.fda.gov/cder/Offices/ODS/medication_guides.htm.

Mechanism of Action Alpha interferons are a family of proteins, produced by nucleated cells, that have antiviral, antiproliferative, and immune-regulating activity. There are 16 known subtypes of alpha interferons. Interferons interact with cells through high affinity cell surface receptors. Following activation, multiple effects can be detected including induction of gene transcription. Inhibits cellular growth, alters the state of cellular differentiation, interferes with oncogene expression, alters cell surface antigen expression, increases phagocytic activity of macrophages, and augments cytotoxicity of lymphocytes for target cells.

Drug Interactions

Cytochrome P450 Effect: Inhibits CYP1A2 (weak)

Increased Effect/Toxicity: Interferons may increase the risk of neutropenia when used with ACE inhibitors; fluorouracil concentrations doubled with interferon alfa-2b; interferon alfa may decrease the metabolism of theophylline and zidovudine; interferons may increase the anticoagulant effects of warfarin. Concurrent therapy with ribavirin may increase the risk of hemolytic anemia.

Decreased Effect: Prednisone may decrease the therapeutic effects of interferon alfa; interferon alfa may decrease the serum concentrations of melphalan

Pharmacodynamics/Kinetics

Half-life elimination: Terminal: 50-140 hours; increased with renal dysfunction

Time to peak, serum: 72-96 hours

Pregnancy Risk Factor C; X when used with ribavirin

Peginterferon Alfa-2b (peg in ter FEER on AL fa too bee)

Related Information

Systemic Viral Diseases *on page 1767*

U.S. Brand Names PEG-Intron®

Canadian Brand Names PEG-Intron®

Mexican Brand Names Pegtron

Generic Available No

Index Terms Interferon Alfa-2b (PEG Conjugate); Pegylated Interferon Alfa-2b

Pharmacologic Category Interferon

Use Treatment of chronic hepatitis C (as monotherapy or in combination with ribavirin) in adult patients who have never received interferon alpha and have compensated liver disease

Local Anesthetic/Vasoconstrictor Precautions No information available to require special precautions

Effects on Dental Treatment No significant effects or complications reported

Common Adverse Effects

>10%:

Central nervous system: Headache (56%), fatigue (52%), depression (16% to 29%), anxiety/emotional liability/irritability (28%), insomnia (23%), fever (22%), dizziness (12%), impaired concentration (5% to 12%), pain (12%)

Dermatologic: Alopecia (22%), pruritus (12%), dry skin (11%)

Gastrointestinal: Nausea (26%), anorexia (20%), diarrhea (18%), abdominal pain (15%), weight loss (11%)

Local: Injection site inflammation/reaction (47%)

Neuromuscular & skeletal: Musculoskeletal pain (56%), myalgia (38% to 42%), rigors (23% to 45%)

Respiratory: Epistaxis (14%), nasopharyngitis (11%)

Miscellaneous: Flu-like syndrome (46%), viral infection (11%)

(Continued)

Peginterferon Alfa-2b *(Continued)*

>1% to 10%:
Cardiovascular: Flushing (6%)
Central nervous system: Malaise (8%)
Dermatologic: Rash (6%), dermatitis (7%)
Endocrine & metabolic: Hypothyroidism (5%)
Gastrointestinal: Vomiting (7%), dyspepsia (6%), taste perversion
Hematologic: Neutropenia, thrombocytopenia
Hepatic: Hepatomegaly (6%), transaminases increased (10%; transient)
Local: Injection site pain (2%)
Neuromuscular & skeletal: Hypertonia (5%)
Respiratory: Pharyngitis (10%), sinusitis (7%), cough (6%)
Miscellaneous: Diaphoresis (6%)

Restrictions An FDA-approved medication guide must be distributed when dispensing an outpatient prescription (new or refill) where this medication is to be used without direct supervision of a healthcare provider. Medication guides are available at http://www.fda.gov/cder/Offices/ODS/medication_guides.htm.

Mechanism of Action Alpha interferons are a family of proteins, produced by nucleated cells, that have antiviral, antiproliferative, and immune-regulating activity. There are 16 known subtypes of alpha interferons. Interferons interact with cells through high affinity cell surface receptors. Following activation, multiple effects can be detected including induction of gene transcription. Inhibits cellular growth, alters the state of cellular differentiation, interferes with oncogene expression, alters cell surface antigen expression, increases phagocytic activity of macrophages, and augments cytotoxicity of lymphocytes for target cells.

Drug Interactions
Cytochrome P450 Effect: Inhibits CYP1A2 (weak)
Increased Effect/Toxicity: ACE inhibitors, clozapine, erythropoietin may increase risk of bone marrow suppression. Fluorouracil, theophylline, zidovudine concentrations may increase. Warfarin's anticoagulant effect may increase. Concurrent therapy with ribavirin may increase the risk of hemolytic anemia.
Decreased Effect: Melphalan concentrations may decrease. Prednisone may decrease effects of interferon alfa.

Pharmacodynamics/Kinetics
Bioavailability: Increases with chronic dosing
Half-life elimination: 40 hours
Time to peak: 15-44 hours
Excretion: Urine (30%)

Pregnancy Risk Factor C (manufacturer) as monotherapy; X in combination with ribavirin

PEG-Intron® *see* Peginterferon Alfa-2b *on page 1263*
Pegylated Interferon Alfa-2a *see* Peginterferon Alfa-2a *on page 1262*
Pegylated Interferon Alfa-2b *see* Peginterferon Alfa-2b *on page 1263*

Pemetrexed *(pem e TREKS ed)*

U.S. Brand Names Alimta®
Canadian Brand Names Alimta®
Generic Available No
Index Terms LY231514; MTA; Multitargeted Antifolate; NSC-698037; Pemetrexed Disodium
Pharmacologic Category Antineoplastic Agent, Antimetabolite; Antineoplastic Agent, Antimetabolite (Antifolate)
Use Treatment of malignant pleural mesothelioma; treatment of nonsmall cell lung cancer
Unlabeled/Investigational Use Bladder, breast, cervical, colorectal, esophageal, gastric, head and neck, ovarian, pancreatic, and renal cell cancers
Local Anesthetic/Vasoconstrictor Precautions No information available to require special precautions
Effects on Dental Treatment Key adverse event(s) related to dental treatment: Dysphagia, esophagitis, odynophagia, and stomatitis.
Common Adverse Effects Note: Percentages reported with single-agent therapy (in patients who received folate and B_{12} supplementation); dose limiting toxicities include myelosuppression (neutropenia, thrombocytopenia); fatigue and dermatitis.
>10%:
Cardiovascular: Chest pain (38%), edema (19%), hypertension (11%; grades 3/4 incidence higher in patients >65 years)

Central nervous system: Fatigue (87%; grade 3: 14%; grade 4: 2%), fever (26%), depression (11%)

Dermatologic: Rash/desquamation (17%), alopecia (11%)

Gastrointestinal: Anorexia (62%), nausea (39%), constipation (30%), vomiting (25%), diarrhea (21%), stomatitis (20%)

Hematologic: Anemia (33%; grade 4: 2%), leukopenia (13%), neutropenia (11%; grade 4: 2%; nadir: 8-10 days; recovery: 12-17 days)

Neuromuscular & skeletal: Neuropathy (29%), myalgia (13%)

Respiratory: Dyspnea (72%), pharyngitis (20%)

Miscellaneous: Infection (23%)

1% to 10%:

Cardiovascular: Thrombosis/embolism (4%), cardiac ischemia (3%)

Endocrine & metabolic: Dehydration (3%)

Gastrointestinal: Dysphagia/esophagitis/odynophagia (5%)

Hematologic: Thrombocytopenia (9%), febrile neutropenia (2% to 6%)

Hepatic: ALT increased (10%; grade 3: 2%; grade 4: 1%), AST increased (8%; grade 3: <1%; grade 4: 1%)

Neuromuscular & skeletal: Arthralgia (8%)

Renal: Creatinine clearance decreased (5%), serum creatinine increased (3%)

Miscellaneous: Allergic reaction/hypersensitivity (8%)

Mechanism of Action Inhibits thymidylate synthase (TS), dihydrofolate reductase (DHFR), glycinamide ribonucleotide formyltransferase (GARFT), and aminoimidazole carboxamide ribonucleotide formyltransferase (AICARFT), the enzymes involved in folate metabolism and DNA synthesis, resulting in inhibition of purine and thymidine nucleotide and protein synthesis.

Drug Interactions

Increased Effect/Toxicity: NSAIDs may increase the toxicity of pemetrexed.

Pharmacodynamics/Kinetics

Duration: V_{dss}: 16.1 L

Protein binding: ~73% to 81%

Metabolism: Minimal

Half-life elimination: Normal renal function: 3.5 hours; Cl_{cr} 40-59 mL/minute: 5.3-5.8 hours

Excretion: Urine (70% to 90% as unchanged drug)

Pregnancy Risk Factor D

Pemetrexed Disodium *see Pemetrexed on page 1264*

Pemirolast (pe MIR oh last)

U.S. Brand Names Alamast®

Canadian Brand Names Alamast®

Generic Available No

Pharmacologic Category Mast Cell Stabilizer; Ophthalmic Agent, Miscellaneous

Use Prevention of itching of the eye due to allergic conjunctivitis

Local Anesthetic/Vasoconstrictor Precautions No information available to require special precautions

Effects on Dental Treatment No significant effects or complications reported

Mechanism of Action Mast cell stabilizer that inhibits the *in vivo* type I immediate hypersensitivity reaction; in addition, inhibits chemotaxis of eosinophils into the ocular tissue and blocks their release of mediators; also reported to prevent calcium influx into mast cells following antigen stimulation

Pregnancy Risk Factor C

Penbutolol (pen BYOO toe lole)

Related Information

Cardiovascular Diseases *on page 1726*

U.S. Brand Names Levatol®

Canadian Brand Names Levatol®

Generic Available No

Index Terms Penbutolol Sulfate

Pharmacologic Category Beta Blocker With Intrinsic Sympathomimetic Activity

Use Treatment of mild to moderate arterial hypertension

Local Anesthetic/Vasoconstrictor Precautions No information available to require special precautions

Effects on Dental Treatment Key adverse event(s) related to dental treatment: Xerostomia (normal salivary flow resumes upon discontinuation). Penbutolol is a nonselective beta-blocker and may enhance the pressor (Continued)

Penbutolol *(Continued)*

response to epinephrine, resulting in hypertension and bradycardia. Many nonsteroidal anti-inflammatory drugs, such as ibuprofen and indomethacin, can reduce the hypotensive effect of beta-blockers after 3 or more weeks of therapy with the NSAID. Short-term NSAID use (ie, 3 days) requires no special precautions in patients taking beta-blockers.

Common Adverse Effects 1% to 10%:
Cardiovascular: CHF, arrhythmia
Central nervous system: Mental depression, headache, dizziness, fatigue
Gastrointestinal: Nausea, diarrhea, dyspepsia
Neuromuscular & skeletal: Arthralgia

Mechanism of Action Blocks both beta$_1$- and beta$_2$-receptors and has mild intrinsic sympathomimetic activity; has negative inotropic and chronotropic effects and can significantly slow AV nodal conduction

Drug Interactions
Increased Effect/Toxicity: The heart rate lowering effects of propranolol are beta-blockers are additive with other drugs which slow AV conduction (digoxin, verapamil, diltiazem). Concurrent use of beta-blockers may increase the effects of alpha-blockers (prazosin, terazosin), alpha-adrenergic stimulants (epinephrine, phenylephrine), and the vasoconstrictive effects of ergot alkaloids. Beta-blockers may mask the tachycardia from hypoglycemia caused by insulin and oral hypoglycemics. In patients receiving concurrent therapy, the risk of hypertensive crisis is increased when either clonidine or the beta-blocker is withdrawn. Beta-blockers may increase the action or levels of ethanol, disopyramide, nondepolarizing muscle relaxants, and theophylline although the effects are difficult to predict.

Beta-blocker effects may be enhanced by oral contraceptives, flecainide, haloperidol (hypotensive effects), H$_2$-antagonists (cimetidine, possibly ranitidine), hydralazine, loop diuretics, possibly MAO inhibitors, phenothiazines, propafenone, quinidine (in extensive metabolizers), ciprofloxacin, thyroid hormones (when hypothyroid patient is converted to euthyroid state). Beta-blockers may increase the effect/toxicity of flecainide, haloperidol (hypotensive effects), hydralazine, phenothiazines, acetaminophen, anticoagulants (warfarin), and benzodiazepines.

Decreased Effect: Aluminum salts, barbiturates, calcium salts, cholestyramine, colestipol, NSAIDs, penicillins (ampicillin), rifampin, salicylates, and sulfinpyrazone decrease effect of beta-blockers due to decreased bioavailability and plasma levels. Beta-blockers may decrease the effect of sulfonylureas. Nonselective beta-blockers blunt the response to beta-2 adrenergic agonists (albuterol).

Pharmacodynamics/Kinetics
Absorption: ~100%
Protein binding: 80% to 98%
Metabolism: Extensively hepatic (oxidation and conjugation)
Bioavailability: ~100%
Half-life elimination: 5 hours
Excretion: Urine

Pregnancy Risk Factor C (manufacturer); D (2nd and 3rd trimester - expert analysis)

Penbutolol Sulfate *see* Penbutolol *on page 1265*

Penciclovir *(pen SYE kloe veer)*

Related Information
Systemic Viral Diseases *on page 1767*
Viral Infections *on page 1806*
Related Sample Prescriptions
Herpes Simplex (Recurrent) *on page 1843*
U.S. Brand Names Denavir®
Generic Available No
Pharmacologic Category Antiviral Agent
Dental Use Topical treatment of herpes simplex labialis (cold sores)
Use Topical treatment of herpes simplex labialis (cold sores)
Local Anesthetic/Vasoconstrictor Precautions No information available to require special precautions
Effects on Dental Treatment No significant effects or complications reported
Significant Adverse Effects
>10%: Dermatologic: Mild erythema (50%)
1% to 10%: Central nervous system: Headache (5.3%)
<1%: Local anesthesia (0.9%)

Postmarketing and/or case reports: Application site reaction, local edema, urticaria, pain, pruritus, paresthesia, skin discoloration, erythematous rash, oropharyngeal edema, parosmia

Dental Usual Dosing Treatment of herpes simplex labialis (cold sores): Children ≥12 years and Adults: Topical: Apply cream at the first sign or symptom of cold sore (eg, tingling, swelling); apply every 2 hours during waking hours for 4 days

Dosage Children ≥12 years and Adults: Topical: Apply cream at the first sign or symptom of cold sore (eg, tingling, swelling); apply every 2 hours during waking hours for 4 days

Mechanism of Action In cells infected with HSV-1 or HSV-2, viral thymidine kinase phosphorylates penciclovir to a monophosphate form which, in turn, is converted to penciclovir triphosphate by cellular kinases. Penciclovir triphosphate inhibits HSV polymerase competitively with deoxyguanosine triphosphate. Consequently, herpes viral DNA synthesis and, therefore, replication are selectively inhibited

Contraindications Hypersensitivity to the penciclovir or any component of the formulation; previous and significant adverse reactions to famciclovir

Warnings/Precautions Apply only to herpes labialis on lips and face. Application to mucous membranes is not recommended. Effect has not been evaluated in immunocompromised patients.

Drug Interactions No data reported

Pharmacodynamics/Kinetics Absorption: Topical: None

Pregnancy Risk Factor B

Lactation Excretion in breast milk unknown

Dosage Forms Excipient information presented when available (limited, particularly for generics); consult specific product labeling.
Cream: 1% (1.5 g)

Pendex see Guaifenesin and Phenylephrine on page 797

Penicillamine (pen i SIL a meen)

U.S. Brand Names Cuprimine®; Depen®
Canadian Brand Names Cuprimine®; Depen®
Mexican Brand Names Adaleen
Generic Available No
Index Terms β,β-Dimethylcysteine; D-3-Mercaptovaline; D-Penicillamine
Pharmacologic Category Chelating Agent
Use Treatment of Wilson's disease, cystinuria; adjunctive treatment of rheumatoid arthritis
Unlabeled/Investigational Use Lead, mercury, copper, arsenic, and possibly gold poisoning (**Note:** Oral succimer [DMSA] is preferable for lead or mercury poisoning)
Local Anesthetic/Vasoconstrictor Precautions No information available to require special precautions
Effects on Dental Treatment Key adverse event(s) related to dental treatment: Oral ulcerations, glossitis, gingivostomatitis, and taste alteration.
Common Adverse Effects Frequency not defined, may vary by indication. Adverse effects requiring discontinuation of treatment have been reported in 20% to 30% of patients with Wilson's disease.
Cardiovascular: Vasculitis
Central nervous system: Anxiety, agitation, fever, hyperpyrexia, psychiatric disturbances; worsening neurologic symptoms (10% to 50% patients with Wilson's disease)
Dermatologic: Alopecia, cheilosis, dermatomyositis, exfoliative dermatitis, lichen planus, rash (early and late 5%), pemphigus, pruritus, skin friability increased, toxic epidermal necrolysis, urticaria, wrinkling (excessive), yellow nail syndrome
Endocrine & metabolic: Hypoglycemia, thyroiditis
Gastrointestinal: Anorexia, diarrhea (17%), epigastric pain, gingivostomatitis, glossitis, nausea, oral ulcerations, pancreatitis, peptic ulcer reactivation, taste alteration (12%), vomiting
Hematologic: Eosinophilia, hemolytic anemia, leukocytosis, leukopenia (2% to 5%), monocytosis, red cell aplasia, thrombocytopenia (4% to 5%), thrombotic thrombocytopenia purpura, thrombocytosis
Hepatic: Alkaline phosphatase increased, hepatic failure, intrahepatic cholestasis, toxic hepatitis
Local: Thrombophlebitis, white papules at venipuncture and surgical sites
Neuromuscular & skeletal: Arthralgia, dystonia, myasthenia gravis, muscle weakness, neuropathies, polyarthralgia (migratory, often with objective synovitis), polymyositis
(Continued)

Penicillamine *(Continued)*

Ocular: Diplopia, extraocular muscle weakness, optic neuritis, ptosis, visual disturbances

Otic: Tinnitus

Renal: Goodpasture's syndrome, hematuria, nephrotic syndrome, proteinuria (6%), renal failure, renal vasculitis

Respiratory: Asthma, interstitial pneumonitis, pulmonary fibrosis, obliterative bronchiolitis

Miscellaneous: Allergic alveolitis, anetoderma, elastosis perforans serpiginosa, lupus-like syndrome, lactic dehydrogenase increased, lymphadenopathy, mammary hyperplasia, positive ANA test

Mechanism of Action Chelates with lead, copper, mercury and other heavy metals to form stable, soluble complexes that are excreted in urine; depresses circulating IgM rheumatoid factor, depresses T-cell but not B-cell activity; combines with cystine to form a compound which is more soluble, thus cystine calculi are prevented

Drug Interactions

Decreased Effect: Antacids, iron salts may decrease the effects of penicillamine. Penicillamine may decrease the levels of digoxin.

Pharmacodynamics/Kinetics

Onset of action: Rheumatoid arthritis: 2-3 months; Wilson's disease: 1-3 months

Absorption: 40% to 70%

Protein binding: 80% to albumin

Metabolism: Hepatic (small amounts)

Half-life elimination: 1.7-3.2 hours

Time to peak, serum: ~2 hours

Excretion: Urine (30% to 60% as unchanged drug)

Pregnancy Risk Factor D

Penicillin G Benzathine *(pen i SIL in jee BENZ a theen)*

Related Information

Sexually-Transmitted Diseases *on page 1766*

U.S. Brand Names Bicillin® L-A

Canadian Brand Names Bicillin® L-A

Mexican Brand Names Benzanil Simple; Benzetacil; Lentopenil

Generic Available No

Index Terms Benzathine Benzylpenicillin; Benzathine Penicillin G; Benzylpenicillin Benzathine

Pharmacologic Category Antibiotic, Penicillin

Use Active against some gram-positive organisms, few gram-negative organisms such as *Neisseria gonorrhoeae*, and some anaerobes and spirochetes; used in the treatment of syphilis; used only for the treatment of mild to moderately severe infections caused by organisms susceptible to low concentrations of penicillin G or for prophylaxis of infections caused by these organisms

Local Anesthetic/Vasoconstrictor Precautions No information available to require special precautions

Effects on Dental Treatment No significant effects or complications reported

Common Adverse Effects Frequency not defined.

Central nervous system: Convulsions, confusion, drowsiness, myoclonus, fever

Dermatologic: Rash

Endocrine & metabolic: Electrolyte imbalance

Hematologic: Positive Coombs' reaction, hemolytic anemia

Local: Pain, thrombophlebitis

Renal: Acute interstitial nephritis

Miscellaneous: Anaphylaxis, hypersensitivity reactions, Jarisch-Herxheimer reaction

Mechanism of Action Interferes with bacterial cell wall synthesis during active multiplication, causing cell wall death and resultant bactericidal activity against susceptible bacteria

Drug Interactions

Increased Effect/Toxicity: Probenecid increases penicillin levels. Aminoglycosides may lead to synergistic efficacy. Penicillins may increase the exposure to methotrexate during concurrent therapy; monitor.

Decreased Effect: Tetracyclines may decrease penicillin effectiveness. Although anecdotal reports suggest oral contraceptive efficacy could be reduced by penicillins, this has been refuted by more rigorous scientific and clinical data.

Pharmacodynamics/Kinetics

Duration: 1-4 weeks (dose dependent); larger doses result in more sustained levels

Absorption: I.M.: Slow
Time to peak, serum: 12-24 hours
Pregnancy Risk Factor B

Penicillin G Benzathine and Penicillin G Procaine
(pen i SIL in jee BENZ a theen & pen i SIL in jee PROE kane)

Related Information
Penicillin G Benzathine *on page 1268*
Penicillin G Procaine *on page 1270*
U.S. Brand Names Bicillin® C-R; Bicillin® C-R 900/300
Generic Available No
Index Terms Penicillin G Procaine and Benzathine Combined
Pharmacologic Category Antibiotic, Penicillin
Use May be used in specific situations in the treatment of streptococcal infections
Local Anesthetic/Vasoconstrictor Precautions No information available to require special precautions
Effects on Dental Treatment No significant effects or complications reported
Common Adverse Effects Frequency not defined.
Central nervous system: CNS toxicity (convulsions, confusion, drowsiness, myoclonus)
Hematologic: Positive Coombs' reaction, hemolytic anemia
Renal: Interstitial nephritis
Miscellaneous: Hypersensitivity reactions, Jarisch-Herxheimer reaction
Mechanism of Action Inhibits bacterial cell wall synthesis by binding to one or more of the penicillin binding proteins (PBPs); which in turn inhibits the final transpeptidation step of peptidoglycan synthesis in bacterial cell walls, thus inhibiting cell wall biosynthesis. Bacteria eventually lyse due to ongoing activity of cell wall autolytic enzymes (autolysins and murein hydrolases) while cell wall assembly is arrested.
Drug Interactions
Increased Effect/Toxicity: Probenecid increases penicillin levels. Aminoglycosides may lead to synergistic efficacy. Warfarin effects may be increased. Penicillins may increase the exposure to methotrexate during concurrent therapy; monitor.
Decreased Effect: Tetracyclines may decrease penicillin effectiveness. Although anecdotal reports suggest oral contraceptive efficacy could be reduced by penicillins, this has been refuted by more rigorous scientific and clinical data.
Pregnancy Risk Factor B

Penicillin G (Parenteral/Aqueous)
(pen i SIL in jee, pa REN ter al, AYE kwee us)

Related Information
Sexually-Transmitted Diseases *on page 1766*
U.S. Brand Names Pfizerpen®
Canadian Brand Names Pfizerpen®
Mexican Brand Names Pengesod; Sodipen
Generic Available Yes
Index Terms Benzylpenicillin Potassium; Benzylpenicillin Sodium; Crystalline Penicillin; Penicillin G Potassium; Penicillin G Sodium
Pharmacologic Category Antibiotic, Penicillin
Use Active against some gram-positive organisms, generally not *Staphylococcus aureus*; some gram-negative organisms such as *Neisseria gonorrhoeae*, and some anaerobes and spirochetes
Local Anesthetic/Vasoconstrictor Precautions No information available to require special precautions
Effects on Dental Treatment No significant effects or complications reported
Common Adverse Effects Frequency not defined.
Central nervous system: Convulsions, confusion, drowsiness, myoclonus, fever
Dermatologic: Rash
Endocrine & metabolic: Electrolyte imbalance
Hematologic: Positive Coombs' reaction, hemolytic anemia
Local: Injection site reaction, thrombophlebitis
Renal: Acute interstitial nephritis
Miscellaneous: Anaphylaxis, hypersensitivity reactions, Jarisch-Herxheimer reaction
Mechanism of Action Interferes with bacterial cell wall synthesis during active multiplication, causing cell wall death and resultant bactericidal activity against susceptible bacteria
(Continued)

Penicillin G (Parenteral/Aqueous) *(Continued)*

Drug Interactions

Increased Effect/Toxicity: Probenecid increases penicillin levels. Aminoglycosides may lead to synergistic efficacy. Penicillins may increase the exposure to methotrexate during concurrent therapy; monitor.

Decreased Effect: Tetracyclines may decrease penicillin effectiveness. Although anecdotal reports suggest oral contraceptive efficacy could be reduced by penicillins, this has been refuted by more rigorous scientific and clinical data.

Pharmacodynamics/Kinetics

Distribution: Poor penetration across blood-brain barrier, despite inflamed meninges; crosses placenta; enters breast milk

Relative diffusion from blood into CSF: Good only with inflammation (exceeds usual MICs)

CSF:blood level ratio: Normal meninges: <1%; Inflamed meninges: 3% to 5%

Protein binding: 65%

Metabolism: Hepatic (30%) to penicilloic acid

Half-life elimination:

Neonates: <6 days old: 3.2-3.4 hours; 7-13 days old: 1.2-2.2 hours; >14 days old: 0.9-1.9 hours

Children and Adults: Normal renal function: 20-50 minutes

End-stage renal disease: 3.3-5.1 hours

Time to peak, serum: I.M.: ~30 minutes; I.V.: ~1 hour

Excretion: Urine

Pregnancy Risk Factor B

Penicillin G Potassium *see* Penicillin G (Parenteral/Aqueous) *on page 1269*

Penicillin G Procaine *(pen i SIL in jee PROE kane)*

Related Information

Treatment of Sexually-Transmitted Infections *on page 1920*

Canadian Brand Names Pfizerpen-AS®; Wycillin®

Generic Available Yes

Index Terms APPG; Aqueous Procaine Penicillin G; Procaine Benzylpenicillin; Procaine Penicillin G; Wycillin [DSC]

Pharmacologic Category Antibiotic, Penicillin

Use Moderately severe infections due to *Treponema pallidum* and other penicillin G-sensitive microorganisms that are susceptible to low, but prolonged serum penicillin concentrations; anthrax due to *Bacillus anthracis* (postexposure) to reduce the incidence or progression of disease following exposure to aerolized *Bacillus anthracis*

Local Anesthetic/Vasoconstrictor Precautions No information available to require special precautions

Effects on Dental Treatment No significant effects or complications reported

Common Adverse Effects Frequency not defined.

Cardiovascular: Myocardial depression, vasodilation, conduction disturbances

Central nervous system: Confusion, drowsiness, myoclonus, CNS stimulation, seizure

Hematologic: Positive Coombs' reaction, hemolytic anemia, neutropenia

Local: Pain at injection site, thrombophlebitis, sterile abscess at injection site

Renal: Interstitial nephritis

Miscellaneous: Pseudoanaphylactic reactions, hypersensitivity reactions, Jarisch-Herxheimer reaction, serum sickness

Mechanism of Action Inhibits bacterial cell wall synthesis by binding to one or more of the penicillin binding proteins (PBPs); which in turn inhibits the final transpeptidation step of peptidoglycan synthesis in bacterial cell walls, thus inhibiting cell wall biosynthesis. Bacteria eventually lyse due to ongoing activity of cell wall autolytic enzymes (autolysins and murein hydrolases) while cell wall assembly is arrested.

Drug Interactions

Increased Effect/Toxicity: Probenecid increases penicillin levels. Aminoglycosides may lead to synergistic efficacy. Penicillins may increase the exposure to methotrexate during concurrent therapy; monitor.

Decreased Effect: Tetracyclines may decrease penicillin effectiveness. Although anecdotal reports suggest oral contraceptive efficacy could be reduced by penicillins, this has been refuted by more rigorous scientific and clinical data.

Pharmacodynamics/Kinetics

Duration: Therapeutic: 15-24 hours

Absorption: I.M.: Slow

Distribution: Penetration across the blood-brain barrier is poor, despite inflamed meninges; enters breast milk

Protein binding: 65%

Metabolism: ~30% hepatically inactivated

Time to peak, serum: 1-4 hours

Excretion: Urine (60% to 90% as unchanged drug)

Clearance: Renal: Delayed in neonates, young infants, and with impaired renal function

Pregnancy Risk Factor B

Penicillin G Procaine and Benzathine Combined *see* Penicillin G Benzathine and Penicillin G Procaine *on page 1269*

Penicillin G Sodium *see* Penicillin G (Parenteral/Aqueous) *on page 1269*

Penicillin V Potassium (pen i SIL in vee poe TASS ee um)

Related Information
Antibiotic Prophylaxis *on page 1772*
Bacterial Infections *on page 1793*
Viral Infections *on page 1806*

Related Sample Prescriptions
Bacterial Infections and Periodontal Diseases *on page 1837*

Canadian Brand Names Apo-Pen VK®; Novo-Pen-VK; Nu-Pen-VK

Mexican Brand Names Anapenil; Kavipen; Pen-Vi-K

Generic Available Yes

Index Terms Pen VK; Phenoxymethyl Penicillin

Pharmacologic Category Antibiotic, Penicillin

Dental Use Antibiotic of first choice in treatment of common orofacial infections caused by aerobic gram-positive cocci and anaerobes. These orofacial infections include cellulitis, periapical abscess, periodontal abscess, acute suppurative pulpitis, oronasal fistula, pericoronitis, osteitis, osteomyelitis, postsurgical and post-traumatic infection. **Note: This agent is no longer recommended for dental procedure prophylaxis.**

Use Treatment of infections caused by susceptible organisms involving the respiratory tract, otitis media, sinusitis, skin, and urinary tract; prophylaxis in rheumatic fever

Local Anesthetic/Vasoconstrictor Precautions No information available to require special precautions

Effects on Dental Treatment Key adverse event(s) related to dental treatment: Oral candidiasis (prolonged use).

Significant Adverse Effects
>10%: Gastrointestinal: Mild diarrhea, vomiting, nausea, oral candidiasis
<1% (Limited to important or life-threatening): Acute interstitial nephritis, convulsions, hemolytic anemia, positive Coombs' reaction

Dental Usual Dosing Note: No longer recommended for dental procedure prophylaxis

Orofacial infections: Oral:

Children <12 years: 25-50 mg/kg/day in divided doses every 6-8 hours (maximum dose: 3 g/day)

Children ≥12 years and Adults: 125-500 mg every 6-8 hours

Dosage
Usual dosage range:
Children <12 years: Oral: 25-50 mg/kg/day in divided doses every 6-8 hours (maximum dose: 3 g/day)

Children ≥12 years and Adults: Oral: 125-500 mg every 6-8 hours

Indication-specific dosing:
Children: Oral:

Pharyngitis (streptococcal): 250 mg 2-3 times/day for 10 days

Prophylaxis of pneumococcal infections:
Children <5 years: 125 mg twice daily
Children ≥5 years: 250 mg twice daily

Prophylaxis of recurrent rheumatic fever:
Children <5 years: 125 mg twice daily
Children ≥5 years: 250 mg twice daily

Adults: Oral:

Acintomycosis:
Mild: 2-4 g/day in 4 divided doses for 8 weeks
Surgical: 2-4 g/day in 4 divided doses for 6-12 months (after I.V. penicillin G therapy of 4-6 weeks)

Erysipelas: 500 mg 4 times/day

Periodontal infections: 250-500 mg every 6 hours for 5-7 days

(Continued)

Penicillin V Potassium *(Continued)*

Note: Efficacy of antimicrobial therapy in periapical abscess is questionable; the American Academy of Periodontology recommends use of antibiotic therapy only when systemic symptoms (eg, fever, lymphadenopathy) are present or in immunocompromised patients.

Pharyngitis (streptococcal): 500 mg 3-4 times/day for 10 days

Prophylaxis of pneumococcal or recurrent rheumatic fever infections: 250 mg twice daily

Dosing interval in renal impairment: Cl_{cr} <10 mL/minute: Administer 250 mg every 6 hours

Mechanism of Action Inhibits bacterial cell wall synthesis by binding to one or more of the penicillin binding proteins (PBPs); which in turn inhibits the final transpeptidation step of peptidoglycan synthesis in bacterial cell walls, thus inhibiting cell wall biosynthesis. Bacteria eventually lyse due to ongoing activity of cell wall autolytic enzymes (autolysins and murein hydrolases) while cell wall assembly is arrested.

Contraindications Hypersensitivity to penicillin or any component of the formulation

Warnings/Precautions Use with caution in patients with severe renal impairment (modify dosage) or history of seizures. Serious and occasionally severe or fatal hypersensitivity (anaphylactoid) reactions have been reported in patients on penicillin therapy, especially with a history of beta-lactam hypersensitivity, history of sensitivity to multiple allergens, or previous IgE-mediated reactions (eg, anaphylaxis, angioedema, urticaria). Use with caution in asthmatic patients. Extended duration of therapy or use associated with high serum concentrations may be associated with an increased risk for some adverse reactions. Prolonged use may result in fungal or bacterial superinfection, including *C. difficile*-associated diarrhea and pseudomembranous colitis.

Drug Interactions

Aminoglycosides: May be synergistic against selected organisms

Methotrexate: Penicillins may increase the exposure to methotrexate during concurrent therapy; monitor.

Oral contraceptives: Anecdotal reports suggesting decreased contraceptive efficacy with penicillins have been refuted by more rigorous scientific and clinical data.

Probenecid, disulfiram: May increase penicillin levels

Tetracyclines: May decrease penicillin effectiveness

Warfarin: Effects of warfarin may be increased

Ethanol/Nutrition/Herb Interactions Food: Decreases drug absorption rate; decreases drug serum concentration.

Dietary Considerations Take on an empty stomach 1 hour before or 2 hours after meals.

Pharmacodynamics/Kinetics

Absorption: 60% to 73%

Distribution: Enters breast milk

Protein binding, plasma: 80%

Half-life elimination: 30 minutes; prolonged with renal impairment

Time to peak, serum: 0.5-1 hour

Excretion: Urine (as unchanged drug and metabolites)

Pregnancy Risk Factor B

Lactation Enters breast milk (other penicillins are compatible with breast-feeding)

Breast-Feeding Considerations No data reported; however, other penicillins may be taken while breast-feeding.

Dosage Forms Excipient information presented when available (limited, particularly for generics); consult specific product labeling.

Note: 250 mg = 400,000 units

Powder for oral solution: 125 mg/5 mL (100 mL, 200 mL); 250 mg/5 mL (100 mL, 200 mL)

Tablet: 250 mg, 500 mg

Selected Readings

Wynn RL and Bergman SA, "Antibiotics and Their Use in the Treatment of Orofacial Infections, Part I," *Gen Dent*, 1994, 42(5):398, 400, 402.

Wynn RL and Bergman SA, "Antibiotics and Their Use in the Treatment of Orofacial Infections, Part II," *Gen Dent*, 1994, 42(6):498-502.

Wynn RL, Bergman SA, Meiller TF, et al, "Antibiotics in Treating Oral-Facial Infections of Odontogenic Origin: An Update," *Gen Dent*, 2001, 49(3):238-40, 242, 244 passim.

Penicilloyl-polylysine *see* Benzylpenicilloyl-polylysine *on page 204*

Penlac® *see* Ciclopirox *on page 354*

Pentafluoropropane and Tetrafluoroethane
(pen ta flure oh PRO pane & tet ra flure oh ETH ane)

U.S. Brand Names Gebauer's Instant Ice™ [OTC]; Gebauer's Pain Ease®; Gebauer's Spray and Stretch®
Generic Available No
Index Terms Tetrafluoroethane and Pentafluoropropane
Pharmacologic Category Anesthetic, Topical
Use Treatment of myofascial pain, restricted motion due to muscle tension, muscle spasm and minor sports injuries (eg, bruises, contusions, swelling, minor sprains); pain associated with injections or minor surgical procedures
Local Anesthetic/Vasoconstrictor Precautions No information available to require special precautions
Effects on Dental Treatment No significant effects or complications reported
Common Adverse Effects
Frequency not defined.
Dermatologic: Skin irritation, skin pigmentation change, frostbite
Mechanism of Action Vapocoolant and counterirritant

Pentahydrate *see* Sodium Thiosulfate *on page 1484*

Pentam-300® *see* Pentamidine *on page 1273*

Pentamidine (pen TAM i deen)

U.S. Brand Names NebuPent®; Pentam-300®
Mexican Brand Names Pentam 300
Generic Available No
Index Terms Pentamidine Isethionate
Pharmacologic Category Antibiotic, Miscellaneous
Use Treatment and prevention of pneumonia caused by *Pneumocystis carinii* (PCP)
Unlabeled/Investigational Use Treatment of trypanosomiasis and visceral leishmaniasis
Local Anesthetic/Vasoconstrictor Precautions Pentamidine is one of the drugs confirmed to prolong the QT interval and is accepted as having a risk of causing torsade de pointes. The risk of drug-induced torsade de pointes is extremely low when a single QT interval prolonging drug is prescribed. In terms of epinephrine, it is not known what effect vasoconstrictors in the local anesthetic regimen will have in patients with a known history of congenital prolonged QT interval or in patients taking any medication that prolongs the QT interval. Until more information is obtained, it is suggested that the clinician consult with the physician prior to the use of a vasoconstrictor in suspected patients, and that the vasoconstrictor (epinephrine, levonordefrin [Neo-Cobefrin®]) be used with caution.
Effects on Dental Treatment No significant effects or complications reported
Common Adverse Effects Injection (I); Aerosol (A)
>10%:
Cardiovascular: Chest pain (A - 10% to 23%)
Central nervous system: Fatigue (A - 50% to 70%); dizziness (A - 31% to 47%)
Dermatologic: Rash (31% to 47%)
Endocrine & metabolic: Hyperkalemia
Gastrointestinal: Anorexia (A - 50% to 70%), nausea (A - 10% to 23%)
Local: Local reactions at injection site
Renal: Increased creatinine (I - 23%)
Respiratory: Wheezing (A - 10% to 23%), dyspnea (A - 50% to 70%), cough (A - 31% to 47%), pharyngitis (10% to 23%)
1% to 10%:
Cardiovascular: Hypotension (I - 4%)
Central nervous system: Confusion/hallucinations (1% to 2%), headache (A - 1% to 5%)
Dermatologic: Rash (I - 3.3%)
Endocrine & metabolic: Hypoglycemia <25 mg/dL (I - 2.4%)
Gastrointestinal: Nausea/anorexia (I - 6%), diarrhea (A - 1% to 5%), vomiting
Hematologic: Severe leukopenia (I - 2.8%), thrombocytopenia <20,000/mm^3 (I - 1.7%), anemia (A - 1% to 5%)
Hepatic: Increased LFTs (I - 8.7%)
(Continued)

Pentamidine (Continued)

Mechanism of Action Interferes with RNA/DNA, phospholipids and protein synthesis, through inhibition of oxidative phosphorylation and/or interference with incorporation of nucleotides and nucleic acids into RNA and DNA, in protozoa

Drug Interactions

Cytochrome P450 Effect: Substrate of CYP2C19 (major); **Inhibits** CYP2C8/9 (weak), 2C19 (weak), 2D6 (weak), 3A4 (weak)

Increased Effect/Toxicity: CYP2C19 inhibitors may increase the levels/ effects of pentamidine; example inhibitors include delavirdine, fluconazole, fluvoxamine, gemfibrozil, isoniazid, omeprazole, and ticlopidine. Pentamidine may potentiate the effect of other drugs which prolong QT interval (cisapride, sparfloxacin, gatifloxacin, moxifloxacin, pimozide, and type Ia and type III antiarrhythmics).

Decreased Effect: CYP2C19 inducers may decrease the levels/effects of pentamidine; example inducers include aminoglutethimide, carbamazepine, phenytoin, and rifampin.

Pharmacodynamics/Kinetics

Absorption: I.M.: Well absorbed; Inhalation: Limited systemic absorption

Half-life elimination: Terminal: 6.4-9.4 hours; may be prolonged with severe renal impairment

Excretion: Urine (33% to 66% as unchanged drug)

Pregnancy Risk Factor C

Pentamidine Isethionate *see* Pentamidine *on page 1273*

Pentasa® *see* Mesalamine *on page 1052*

Pentaspan® *see* Pentastarch *on page 1274*

Pentastarch (PEN ta starch)

U.S. Brand Names Pentaspan®
Canadian Brand Names Pentaspan®
Generic Available No
Pharmacologic Category Blood Modifiers
Use Orphan drug: Adjunct in leukapheresis to improve harvesting and increase yield of leukocytes by centrifugal means
Local Anesthetic/Vasoconstrictor Precautions No information available to require special precautions
Effects on Dental Treatment No significant effects or complications reported

Pentavalent Human-Bovine Reassortant Rotavirus Vaccine *see* Rotavirus Vaccine *on page 1449*

Pentazocine (pen TAZ oh seen)

U.S. Brand Names Talwin®; Talwin® NX
Canadian Brand Names Talwin®
Generic Available Yes: Tablet
Index Terms Naloxone Hydrochloride and Pentazocine Hydrochloride; Pentazocine Hydrochloride; Pentazocine Hydrochloride and Naloxone Hydrochloride; Pentazocine Lactate
Pharmacologic Category Analgesic, Opioid
Use Relief of moderate to severe pain; has also been used as a sedative prior to surgery and as a supplement to surgical anesthesia
Local Anesthetic/Vasoconstrictor Precautions No information available to require special precautions
Effects on Dental Treatment Key adverse event(s) related to dental treatment: Xerostomia (normal salivary flow resumes upon discontinuation).
Common Adverse Effects Frequency not defined.

Cardiovascular: Circulatory depression, facial edema, flushing, hypotension, shock, syncope, tachycardia

Central nervous system: Chills, CNS depression, confusion, disorientation, dizziness, drowsiness, euphoria, excitement, hallucinations, headache, insomnia, irritability, lightheadedness, malaise, nightmares, sedation

Dermatologic: dermatitis, erythema multiforme, pruritus, rash, Stevens-Johnson syndrome, toxic epidermal necrolysis, urticaria

Gastrointestinal: Abdominal distress, anorexia, constipation, diarrhea, nausea, vomiting, xerostomia

Genitourinary: Urinary retention

Hematologic: Decreased WBCs, eosinophilia

Local: Tissue damage and irritation with I.M./SubQ use

Neuromuscular & skeletal: Paresthesia, tremor, weakness

Ocular: Blurred vision, miosis

Otic: Tinnitus

Respiratory: Dyspnea, respiratory depression (rare)

Miscellaneous: Anaphylaxis, diaphoresis, physical and psychological dependence

Restrictions C-IV

Mechanism of Action Binds to opiate receptors in the CNS, causing inhibition of ascending pain pathways, altering the perception of and response to pain; produces generalized CNS depression; partial agonist-antagonist

Drug Interactions

Increased Effect/Toxicity: Increased effect/toxicity with tripelennamine (can be lethal), CNS depressants (eg, phenothiazines, tranquilizers, anxiolytics, sedatives, hypnotics, alcohol).

Decreased Effect: May potentiate or reduce analgesic effect of opiate agonist (eg, morphine) depending on patients tolerance to opiates; can precipitate withdrawal in narcotic addicts.

Pharmacodynamics/Kinetics

Onset of action: Oral, I.M., SubQ: 15-30 minutes; I.V.: 2-3 minutes

Duration: Oral: 4-5 hours; Parenteral: 2-3 hours

Protein binding: 60%

Metabolism: Hepatic via oxidative and glucuronide conjugation pathways; extensive first-pass effect

Bioavailability: Oral: ~20%; increased to 60% to 70% with cirrhosis

Half-life elimination: 2-3 hours; prolonged with hepatic impairment

Excretion: Urine (small amounts as unchanged drug)

Pregnancy Risk Factor C/D (prolonged use or high doses at term)

Pentazocine and Acetaminophen
(pen TAZ oh seen & a seet a MIN oh fen)

Related Information

Acetaminophen *on page 31*

Pentazocine *on page 1274*

U.S. Brand Names Talacen®

Generic Available Yes

Index Terms Acetaminophen and Pentazocine; Pentazocine Hydrochloride and Acetaminophen

Pharmacologic Category Analgesic Combination (Opioid)

Dental Use Relief of mild to moderate pain

Use Relief of mild to moderate pain

Local Anesthetic/Vasoconstrictor Precautions No information available to require special precautions

Effects on Dental Treatment No significant effects or complications reported

Significant Adverse Effects Frequency not defined.

Cardiovascular: Tachycardia, hypotension, syncope, flushing

Central nervous system: Headache, dizziness, drowsiness, lightheadedness, sedation, insomnia, hallucinations, euphoria, depression, confusion, disorientation, chills, irritability, excitement

Dermatologic: Rash, urticaria, erythema multiforme, Stevens-Johnson syndrome, toxic epidermal necrolysis

Gastrointestinal: Nausea, vomiting, biliary spasm, constipation, anorexia, diarrhea, abdominal distress

Genitourinary: Urinary retention

Hematologic: WBCs decreased, eosinophilia, thrombocytopenic purpura, hemolytic anemia, agranulocytosis

Neuromuscular & skeletal: Weakness, tremor, paresthesia

Ocular: Blurred vision

Otic: Tinnitus

Respiratory: Respiratory depression

Miscellaneous: Diaphoresis, facial edema, anaphylaxis

Restrictions C-IV

Dental Usual Dosing Analgesic: Adults: Oral: 1 caplet every 4 hours up to maximum of 6 caplets

Dosage Oral: Adults: Analgesic: 1 caplet every 4 hours, up to a maximum of 6 caplets

Mechanism of Action

Pentazocine: Binds to opiate receptors in the CNS, causing inhibition of ascending pain pathways, altering the perception of and response to pain; produces generalized CNS depression; partial agonist-antagonist

Acetaminophen: Inhibits the synthesis of prostaglandins in the central nervous system and peripherally blocks pain impulse generation

(Continued)

Pentazocine and Acetaminophen *(Continued)*

Contraindications Hypersensitivity to pentazocine, acetaminophen, or any component of the formulation; pregnancy (prolonged use or high doses at term)

Warnings/Precautions Contains sodium metasulfite; may cause allergic-type reactions; potential for elevating CSF pressure due to respiratory effects which may be exaggerated in presence of head injury, intracranial lesions, or pre-existing increase in intracranial lesions. May experience hallucinations, disorientation, and confusion. May cause psychological and physical dependence. Use with caution in patients with myocardial infarction who have nausea or vomiting, patients with respiratory depression, severely limited respiratory reserve, severe bronchial asthma, other obstructive respiratory conditions or cyanosis, impaired renal or hepatic function, patients prone to seizures. Abrupt discontinuation may result in withdrawal symptoms. Pentazocine may precipitate opiate withdrawal symptoms in patients who have been receiving opiates regularly.

Ethanol/Nutrition/Herb Interactions

Ethanol: Avoid ethanol (may increase CNS depression).

Herb/Nutraceutical: Avoid valerian, St John's wort, kava kava, gotu kola (may increase CNS depression).

Pharmacodynamics/Kinetics See individual agents.

Pregnancy Risk Factor C/D (prolonged use or high doses at term)

Lactation Excretion in breast milk unknown/use caution

Breast-Feeding Considerations Excretion of pentazocine in breast milk is unknown; acetaminophen is excreted in breast milk

Dosage Forms Excipient information presented when available (limited, particularly for generics); consult specific product labeling.

Caplet:

Talacen®: Pentazocine 25 mg and acetaminophen 650 mg [contains sodium metabisulfite]

Tablet: Pentazocine 25 mg and acetaminophen 650 mg

Pentazocine Hydrochloride *see* Pentazocine *on page 1274*

Pentazocine Hydrochloride and Acetaminophen *see* Pentazocine and Acetaminophen *on page 1275*

Pentazocine Hydrochloride and Naloxone Hydrochloride *see* Pentazocine *on page 1274*

Pentazocine Lactate *see* Pentazocine *on page 1274*

Pentetate Calcium Trisodium *see* Diethylene Triamine Penta-Acetic Acid *on page 493*

Pentetate Zinc Trisodium *see* Diethylene Triamine Penta-Acetic Acid *on page 493*

Pentobarbital (pen toe BAR bi tal)

U.S. Brand Names Nembutal®

Canadian Brand Names Nembutal® Sodium

Generic Available No

Index Terms Pentobarbital Sodium

Pharmacologic Category Anticonvulsant, Barbiturate; Barbiturate

Use Sedative/hypnotic; preanesthetic; high-dose barbiturate coma for treatment of increased intracranial pressure or status epilepticus unresponsive to other therapy

Local Anesthetic/Vasoconstrictor Precautions No information available to require special precautions

Effects on Dental Treatment No significant effects or complications reported

Mechanism of Action Short-acting barbiturate with sedative, hypnotic, and anticonvulsant properties. Barbiturates depress the sensory cortex, decrease motor activity, alter cerebellar function, and produce drowsiness, sedation, and hypnosis. In high doses, barbiturates exhibit anticonvulsant activity; barbiturates produce dose-dependent respiratory depression.

Pregnancy Risk Factor D

Pentobarbital Sodium *see* Pentobarbital *on page 1276*

Pentosan Polysulfate Sodium
(PEN toe san pol i SUL fate SOW dee um)

U.S. Brand Names Elmiron®

Canadian Brand Names Elmiron®

Generic Available No

Index Terms PPS

Pharmacologic Category Analgesic, Urinary

Use Orphan drug: Relief of bladder pain or discomfort due to interstitial cystitis

Local Anesthetic/Vasoconstrictor Precautions No information available to require special precautions

Effects on Dental Treatment No significant effects or complications reported

Common Adverse Effects 1% to 10%:

Central nervous system: Headache (3%), dizziness (1%)

Dermatologic: Alopecia (4%), rash (3%)

Gastrointestinal: Rectal hemorrhage (6%), diarrhea (4%), nausea (4%), dyspepsia (2%), abdominal pain (2%)

Hepatic: Liver function test abnormalities (1%)

Mechanism of Action Although pentosan polysulfate sodium is a low-molecular weight heparinoid, it is not known whether these properties play a role in its mechanism of action in treating interstitial cystitis; the drug appears to adhere to the bladder wall mucosa where it may act as a buffer to protect the tissues from irritating substances in the urine.

Drug Interactions

Increased Effect/Toxicity: Concomitant therapy with anticoagulants, anti-platelet agents, NSAIDs, or salicylates may increase the risk of bleeding.

Pharmacodynamics/Kinetics

Absorption: ~3%

Metabolism: Hepatic and via spleen; some metabolism occurs in renal parenchyma

Half-life elimination: 4.8 hours

Excretion: Urine (3% as unchanged drug)

Pregnancy Risk Factor B

Pentostatin (pen toe STAT in)

U.S. Brand Names Nipent®

Canadian Brand Names Nipent®

Generic Available No

Index Terms CL-825; Co-Vidarabine; dCF; Deoxycoformycin; NSC-218321; 2'-Deoxycoformycin

Pharmacologic Category Antineoplastic Agent, Antibiotic; Antineoplastic Agent, Antimetabolite (Purine Antagonist)

Use Treatment of hairy cell leukemia; non-Hodgkin's lymphoma, cutaneous T-cell lymphoma

Local Anesthetic/Vasoconstrictor Precautions No information available to require special precautions

Effects on Dental Treatment Key adverse event(s) related to dental treatment: Stomatitis.

Common Adverse Effects

>10%:

Central nervous system: Fever, chills, headache

Dermatologic: Skin rash (25% to 30%), alopecia (10%)

Gastrointestinal: Mild to moderate nausea, vomiting (60%), stomatitis, diarrhea (13%), anorexia

Genitourinary: Acute renal failure (35%)

Hematologic: Thrombocytopenia (50%), dose-limiting in 25% of patients; anemia (40% to 45%), neutropenia, mild to moderate, not dose-limiting (11%)

Nadir: 7 days

Recovery: 10-14 days

Hepatic: Transaminases increased, mild-moderate, usually transient (30%); hepatitis (19%), usually reversible

Respiratory: Pulmonary edema (15%), may be exacerbated by fludarabine

Miscellaneous: Infection (57%; 35% severe, life-threatening)

1% to 10%:

Cardiovascular: Chest pain, arrhythmia, peripheral edema

Central nervous system: Opportunistic infection (8%); anxiety, confusion, depression, dizziness, insomnia, nervousness, somnolence, myalgia, malaise

Dermatologic: Dry skin, eczema, pruritus

Gastrointestinal: Constipation, flatulence, weight loss

Neuromuscular & skeletal: Paresthesia, weakness

Ocular: Moderate to severe keratoconjunctivitis, abnormal vision, eye pain

Otic: Ear pain

Respiratory: Dyspnea, pneumonia, bronchitis, pharyngitis, rhinitis, epistaxis, sinusitis (3% to 7%)

(Continued)

Pentostatin *(Continued)*

Mechanism of Action Pentostatin is a purine antimetabolite that inhibits adenosine deaminase, preventing the deamination of adenosine to inosine. Accumulation of deoxyadenosine (dAdo) and deoxyadenosine 5'-triphosphate (dATP) results in a reduction of purine metabolism and DNA synthesis and cell death.

Drug Interactions
Increased Effect/Toxicity: Increased toxicity with vidarabine and allopurinol; combined use with fludarabine may lead to severe, even fatal, pulmonary toxicity

Pharmacodynamics/Kinetics
Distribution: I.V.: V_d: 36.1 L (20.1 L/m^2); rapidly to body tissues
Half-life elimination: Distribution half-life: 30-85 minutes; Terminal: 5-15 hours
Excretion: Urine (~50% to 96%) within 24 hours (30% to 90% as unchanged drug)

Pregnancy Risk Factor D

Pentothal® *see* Thiopental *on page 1557*

Pentoxifylline *(pen toks IF i lin)*

U.S. Brand Names Pentoxil®; Trental®
Canadian Brand Names Albert® Pentoxifylline; Apo-Pentoxifylline SR®; Nu-Pentoxifylline SR; ratio-Pentoxifylline; Trental®
Mexican Brand Names Fixoten; Kentadin; Peridane; Trental
Generic Available Yes
Index Terms Oxpentifylline
Pharmacologic Category Blood Viscosity Reducer Agent
Use Treatment of intermittent claudication on the basis of chronic occlusive arterial disease of the limbs; may improve function and symptoms, but not intended to replace more definitive therapy
Unlabeled/Investigational Use AIDS patients with increased TNF, CVA, cerebrovascular diseases, diabetic atherosclerosis, diabetic neuropathy, gangrene, hemodialysis shunt thrombosis, vascular impotence, cerebral malaria, septic shock, sickle cell syndromes, and vasculitis
Local Anesthetic/Vasoconstrictor Precautions No information available to require special precautions
Effects on Dental Treatment No significant effects or complications reported
Common Adverse Effects 1% to 10%: Gastrointestinal: Nausea (2%), vomiting (1%)
Mechanism of Action Reduces blood viscosity via increased leukocyte and erythrocyte deformability and decreased neutrophil adhesion/activation; improves peripheral tissue oxygenation presumably through enhanced blood flow.

Drug Interactions
Cytochrome P450 Effect: Inhibits CYP1A2 (weak)
Increased Effect/Toxicity:
Pentoxifylline may increase the serum levels of theophylline.

Pharmacodynamics/Kinetics
Absorption: Well absorbed
Metabolism: Hepatic and via erythrocytes; extensive first-pass effect
Half-life elimination: Parent drug: 24-48 minutes; Metabolites: 60-96 minutes
Time to peak, serum: 2-4 hours
Excretion: Primarily urine (active metabolites); feces (4%)

Pregnancy Risk Factor C

Pentoxil® *see* Pentoxifylline *on page 1278*

Pen VK *see* Penicillin V Potassium *on page 1271*

Pepcid® *see* Famotidine *on page 670*

Pepcid® AC [OTC] *see* Famotidine *on page 670*

Pepcid® Complete [OTC] *see* Famotidine, Calcium Carbonate, and Magnesium Hydroxide *on page 671*

Pepto-Bismol® [OTC] *see* Bismuth *on page 217*

Pepto-Bismol® Maximum Strength [OTC] *see* Bismuth *on page 217*

Perchloracap® [DSC] *see* Potassium Perchlorate *on page 1332*

Percocet® *see* Oxycodone and Acetaminophen *on page 1228*

Percodan® *see* Oxycodone and Aspirin *on page 1231*

Percogesic® [OTC] *see* Acetaminophen and Phenyltoloxamine *on page 38*

Percogesic® Extra Strength [OTC] *see* Acetaminophen and Diphenhydramine *on page 38*

Perdiem® Overnight Relief [OTC] *see* Senna *on page 1462*

Pergolide (PER go lide)

U.S. Brand Names Permax® [DSC]
Canadian Brand Names Permax®
Mexican Brand Names Permax
Generic Available Yes
Index Terms Pergolide Mesylate
Pharmacologic Category Anti-Parkinson's Agent, Dopamine Agonist; Ergot Derivative
Use Adjunctive treatment to levodopa/carbidopa in the management of Parkinson's disease
Unlabeled/Investigational Use Tourette's disorder, chronic motor or vocal tic disorder
Local Anesthetic/Vasoconstrictor Precautions No information available to require special precautions
Effects on Dental Treatment Key adverse event(s) related to dental treatment: Xerostomia (normal salivary flow resumes upon discontinuation). Prolonged use may decrease or inhibit salivary flow, contributing to discomfort and dental disease (ie, oral candidiasis and periodontal disease).
Common Adverse Effects
>10%:
 Central nervous system: Dizziness (19%), hallucinations (14%), dystonia (12%), somnolence (10%), confusion (10%)
 Gastrointestinal: Nausea (24%), constipation (11%)
 Neuromuscular & skeletal: Dyskinesia (62%)
 Respiratory: Rhinitis (12%)
1% to 10%:
 Cardiovascular: Hypotension or postural hypotension (10%), peripheral edema (7%), chest pain (4%), vasodilation (3%), palpitation (2%), syncope (2%), arrhythmia (1%), hypertension (2%), MI (1%)
 Central nervous system: Insomnia (8%), pain (7%), anxiety (6%), psychosis (2%), EPS (2%), incoordination (2%), chills (1%)
 Dermatologic: Rash (3%)
 Gastrointestinal: Diarrhea (6%), dyspepsia (6%), abdominal pain (6%), anorexia (5%), xerostomia (4%), vomiting (3%), dysphagia (1%), nausea (1%)
 Hematologic: Anemia (1%)
 Neuromuscular & skeletal: Myalgia (1%), neuralgia (1%)
 Ocular: Abnormal vision (6%), diplopia (2%)
 Respiratory: Dyspnea (5%), epistaxis (2%)
 Miscellaneous: Flu syndrome (3%), hiccups (1%)
Mechanism of Action Pergolide is a semisynthetic ergot alkaloid similar to bromocriptine but stated to be more potent (10-1000 times) and longer-acting; it is a centrally-active dopamine agonist stimulating both D_1 and D_2 receptors. Pergolide is believed to exert its therapeutic effect by directly stimulating postsynaptic dopamine receptors in the nigrostriatal system.
Drug Interactions
 Cytochrome P450 Effect: Substrate of CYP3A4 (major); **Inhibits** CYP2D6 (strong), 3A4 (weak)
 Increased Effect/Toxicity: Effects of pergolide may be increased by levodopa (hallucinations) and MAO inhibitors. Pergolide may increase the levels/effects of amphetamines, selected beta-blockers, dextromethorphan, fluoxetine, lidocaine, mirtazapine, nefazodone, paroxetine, risperidone, ritonavir, thioridazine, tricyclic antidepressants, venlafaxine, and other CYP2D6 substrates. Pergolide may increase the levels/effects of sibutramine and other serotonin agonists (serotonin syndrome). Macrolide antibiotics may increase the effects of pergolide. The levels/effects of pergolide may be increased by azole antifungals, clarithromycin, diclofenac, doxycycline, erythromycin, imatinib, isoniazid, nefazodone, nicardipine, propofol, protease inhibitors, quinidine, telithromycin, verapamil, and other CYP3A4 inhibitors.
 Decreased Effect: Effects of pergolide may be diminished by antipsychotics, metoclopramide. Pergolide may decrease the levels/effects of CYP2D6 prodrug substrates (eg, codeine, hydrocodone, oxycodone, tramadol).
Pharmacodynamics/Kinetics
 Absorption: Well absorbed
 Protein binding, plasma: 90%
 Metabolism: Extensively hepatic
 Half-life elimination: 27 hours
 Excretion: Urine (~50%); feces (50%)
Pregnancy Risk Factor B

Pergolide Mesylate see Pergolide on page 1279

Periactin *see* Cyproheptadine *on page 431*

Pericyazine (per ee CYE ah zeen)

Canadian Brand Names Neuleptil®

Pharmacologic Category Antipsychotic Agent, Typical, Phenothiazine, Piperidine

Use Adjunctive therapy in selected psychotic patients to control prevailing hostility, impulsivity, or aggression

Local Anesthetic/Vasoconstrictor Precautions Most pharmacology textbooks state that in presence of phenothiazines, systemic doses of epinephrine paradoxically decrease the blood pressure. This is the so called "epinephrine reversal" phenomenon. This has never been observed when epinephrine is given by infiltration as part of the anesthesia procedure. See Dental Comment.

Effects on Dental Treatment Key adverse event(s) related to dental treatment:

Significant hypotension may occur, especially when the drug is administered parenterally. Orthostatic hypotension is due to alpha-receptor blockade; elderly are at greater risk.

Tardive dyskinesia: Prevalence rate may be 40% in elderly; development of the syndrome and the irreversible nature are proportional to duration and total cumulative dose over time. Extrapyramidal reactions are more common in elderly with up to 50% developing these reactions after 60 years of age. Drug-induced Parkinson's syndrome occurs often; akathisia is the most common extrapyramidal reaction in elderly.

Increased confusion, memory loss, psychotic behavior, and agitation frequently occur as a consequence of anticholinergic effects. Antipsychotic-associated sedation in nonpsychotic patients is extremely unpleasant due to feelings of depersonalization, derealization, and dysphoria.

Common Adverse Effects Frequency not defined; listing includes adverse reactions reported with other agents from the phenothiazine class.

Cardiovascular: AV block, cardiac arrest, ECG changes, edema, hypotension, paroxysmal atrial tachycardia, QT_c prolongation, syncope, tachycardia

Central nervous system; Aggressive behavior, agitation, anxiety, bizarre dreams, cerebral edema, depression, dizziness, drowsiness, EEG changes, excitement; extrapyramidal symptoms (tremor, akathisia, dystonia, dyskinesia, oculogyric, opisthotonos, hyper-reflexia, pseudo-Parkinsonism, rigidity, sialorrhea); fatigue, fever, headache, insomnia, paradoxical psychosis, restlessness, seizures, sleep disturbance, tardive dyskinesia

Dermatologic: Angioedema, dermatitis, eczema, epithelial keratopathy, erythema, exfoliative dermatitis, photosensitivity, pruritus, rash, seborrhea, skin pigmentation (prolonged therapy), urticaria

Endocrine & metabolic: Anorexia, appetite increased, delayed ovulation, galactorrhea, gynecomastia, libido changes, menstrual irregularities, thirst, weight changes

Gastrointestinal: Adynamic ileus, constipation, fecal impaction, nausea, salivation, vomiting, xerostomia

Genitourinary: Bladder paralysis, impotence, incontinence, polyuria, urinary retention

Hematologic: Agranulocytosis, anemia, eosinophilia, leukopenia, pancytopenia, thrombocytopenia

Hepatic: Cholestasis, cholestatic jaundice, jaundice

Ocular: Blurred vision, corneal deposits (prolonged therapy), glaucoma, lenticular deposits, pigmentary retinopathy (prolonged therapy)

Respiratory: Nasal congestion, pneumonia, pneumonitis

Miscellaneous: Diaphoresis increased, Lupus-like syndrome

Restrictions Not available in U.S.

Dosage Oral:

Children >5 years: 2.5-10 mg in the morning, followed by 5-30 mg in the evening. In general, lower dosage should be used on initiation and gradually increased based on effect and tolerance.

Adults: 5-20 mg in the morning, followed by 10-40 mg in the evening. In dividing doses, it is suggested that the larger dose should be administered in the evening. In general, lower dosage should be used on initiation and gradually increased based on effect and tolerance.

Elderly: Initial daily dose should be ~5 mg/day. May be increased gradually based on effect and tolerance. Also see adult dosing.

Dosage adjustment in renal impairment: No dosage adjustment required.

Mechanism of Action Blocks postsynaptic mesolimbic dopaminergic receptors in the brain; depresses the release of hypothalamic and hypophyseal hormones.

Contraindications Hypersensitivity to pericyazine, phenothiazine derivatives, or any component of the formulation; severe CNS depression including acute intoxication with CNS depressant medications; subcortical brain damage; hepatic dysfunction; circulatory collapse; severely-depressed patients; bone marrow suppression; blood dyscrasias; coma; patients receiving spinal or regional anesthesia

Warnings/Precautions Cross-reactivity with other phenothiazine derivatives may occur. May be sedating; use with caution in disorders where CNS depression is a feature (risk may be lower than with other phenothiazines). Use with caution in Parkinson's disease, hemodynamic instability, predisposition to seizures, and severe disease. Esophageal dysmotility and aspiration have been associated with antipsychotic use; use with caution in patients at risk of pneumonia (eg, Alzheimer's disease). Caution in breast cancer or other prolactin-dependent tumors (may elevate prolactin levels). May alter temperature regulation or mask toxicity of other drugs due to antiemetic effects.

Use caution in cardiovascular disease (other piperidine phenothiazines have been associated with QT_c prolongation; relative risk with pericyazine has not been established, although rare cases of QT_c prolongation have been reported). May cause orthostatic hypotension; use with caution in patients at risk of this effect or those who would not tolerate transient hypotensive episodes (cerebrovascular disease, cardiovascular disease, or other medications which may predispose). Phenothiazines have been associated with worsening of pheochromocytoma and mitral valve prolapse; use caution.

Phenothiazines may cause anticholinergic effects (confusion, agitation, constipation, xerostomia, blurred vision, urinary retention; therefore, use with caution in patients with decreased gastrointestinal motility, urinary retention, BPH, xerostomia, or visual problems. Conditions which also may be exacerbated by cholinergic blockade include narrow-angle glaucoma (screening is recommended) and worsening of myasthenia gravis.

May cause extrapyramidal symptoms, including pseudoparkinsonism, acute dystonic reactions, akathisia, and tardive dyskinesia. May be associated with neuroleptic malignant syndrome (NMS). Prolonged therapy may cause pigmentary retinopathy, corneal deposits, and/or changes in skin pigmentation.

Drug Interactions

Cytochrome P450 Effect: No published data on CYP metabolism. Based on structural analysis, may be a substrate of CYP2D6 and 3A4.

Increased Effect/Toxicity: The levels/effects of pericyazine may be increased by azole antifungals, chlorpromazine, ciprofloxacin, clarithromycin, delavirdine, diclofenac, doxycycline, erythromycin, fluoxetine, imatinib, isoniazid, miconazole, nefazodone, nicardipine, paroxetine, pergolide, propofol, protease inhibitors, quinidine, quinine, ritonavir, ropinirole, verapamil and other CYP2D6 or 3A4 inhibitors.

Drugs which alter the QT_c interval may be additive with pericyazine, increasing the risk of malignant arrhythmias; includes type Ia antiarrhythmics, TCAs, and some quinolone antibiotics (sparfloxacin, moxifloxacin, and gatifloxacin). **These agents are contraindicated with other piperidine phenothiazines (thioridazine).** Potassium-depleting agents may increase the risk of serious arrhythmias with pericyazine (includes many diuretics, aminoglycosides, and amphotericin).

Phenothiazines inhibit the ability of bromocriptine to lower serum prolactin concentrations. The sedative effects of CNS depressants or ethanol may be additive with phenothiazines. Phenothiazines and trazodone may produce additive hypotensive effects. Metoclopramide may increase risk of extrapyramidal symptoms (EPS). Concurrent use of antihypertensives may result in additive hypotensive effects (particularly orthostasis).

Phenothiazines may produce neurotoxicity with lithium; this is a rare effect. Rare cases of respiratory paralysis have been reported with concurrent use of phenothiazines and polypeptide antibiotics (eg, bacitracin). Naltrexone in combination with some phenothiazines has been reported to cause lethargy and somnolence.

Decreased Effect:

Aluminum salts may decrease the absorption of phenothiazines. The efficacy of amphetamines may be diminished by antipsychotics; in addition, amphetamines may increase psychotic symptoms; avoid concurrent use. Anticholinergics may inhibit the therapeutic response to phenothiazines and excess anticholinergic effects may occur (includes benztropine, trihexyphenidyl, biperiden, and drugs with significant anticholinergic activity). Low potency antipsychotics (such as pericyazine) may diminish the pressor effects of epinephrine. The antihypertensive effects of guanethidine or guanadrel may be inhibited by phenothiazines. Phenothiazines may inhibit the antiparkinsonian effect of levodopa. Enzyme inducers may enhance the hepatic metabolism of phenothiazines; larger doses may be required; includes rifampin, rifabutin, barbiturates, and phenytoin.

(Continued)

Pericyazine *(Continued)*

Ethanol/Nutrition/Herb Interactions
Ethanol: Avoid ethanol (may increase CNS depression).

Herb/Nutraceutical: Avoid kava kava, valerian, St John's wort, gotu kola (may increase CNS depression). Avoid dong quai, St John's wort (may also cause photosensitization). Cigarette smoking may decrease the serum concentrations of pericyazine.

Dosage Forms [CAN] = Canadian brand name
Capsule:
Neuleptil® [CAN]: 5 mg, 10 mg, 20 mg [not available in the U.S.]
Solution, oral drops:
Neuleptil® [CAN]: 10 mg/mL [not available in the U.S.]

Dental Comment This drug is known to prolong the QT interval. The QT interval is measured as the time and distance between the Q point of the QRS complex and the end of the T wave in the ECG tracing. After adjustment for heart rate, the QT interval is defined as prolonged if it is more than 450 msec in men and 460 msec in women. A long QT syndrome was first described in the 1950s and 60s as a congenital syndrome involving QT interval prolongation and syncope and sudden death. Some of the congenital long QT syndromes were characterized by a peculiar electrocardiographic appearance of the QRS complex involving a premature atria beat followed by a pause, then a subsequent sinus beat showing marked QT prolongation and deformity. This type of cardiac arrhythmia was originally termed "torsade de pointes" (translated from the French as "twisting of the points").

Prolongation of the QT interval is thought to result from delayed ventricular repolarization. The repolarization process within the myocardial cell is due to the efflux of intracellular potassium. The channels associated with this current can be blocked by many drugs and predispose the electrical propagation cycle to torsade de pointes.

Periyazine is one of the drugs confirmed to prolong the QT interval and is accepted as having a risk of causing torsade de pointes. The risk of drug-induced torsade de pointes is extremely low when a single QT interval prolonging drug is prescribed. In terms of epinephrine, it is not known what effect vasoconstrictors in the local anesthetic regimen will have in patients with a known history of congenital prolonged QT interval or in patients taking any medication that prolongs the QT interval. Until more information is obtained, it is suggested that the clinician consult with the physician prior to the use of a vasoconstrictor in suspected patients, and that the vasoconstrictor (epinephrine, levonordefrin [Neo-Cobefrin®]) be used with caution.

Selected Readings
Buckley NA, Whyte IM, and Dawson AH, "Cardiotoxicity More Common in Thioridazine Overdose Than With Other Neuroleptics," *J Toxicol Clin Toxicol*, 1995, 33(3):199-204.

Jaworowsky S and Zamir S, "Cardiac Arrhythmia in a Child Receiving Pericyazine," *Isr J Psychiatry Relat Sci*, 1995, 32(4):299-300.

Johnson A, Giuffre RM, and O'Malley K, "ECG Changes in Pediatric Patients on Tricyclic Antidepressants, Desipramine, and Imipramine," *Can J Psychiatry*, 1996, 41(2):102-6.

Peridex® *see* Chlorhexidine Gluconate *on page 332*

Perindopril Erbumine *(per IN doe pril er BYOO meen)*

Related Information
Cardiovascular Diseases *on page 1726*
U.S. Brand Names Aceon®
Canadian Brand Names Apo-Perindopril®; Coversyl®
Mexican Brand Names Coversyl
Generic Available No
Pharmacologic Category Angiotensin-Converting Enzyme (ACE) Inhibitor
Use Treatment of essential hypertension; reduction of cardiovascular mortality or nonfatal myocardial infarction in patients with stable coronary artery disease
Unlabeled/Investigational Use As a class, ACE inhibitors are recommended in the treatment of congestive heart failure with left ventricular dysfunction.
Local Anesthetic/Vasoconstrictor Precautions No information available to require special precautions
Effects on Dental Treatment No significant effects or complications reported
Common Adverse Effects
>10%:
Central nervous system: Headache (24%)
Respiratory: Cough (incidence is higher in women, 3:1) (12%)
1% to 10%:
Cardiovascular: Edema (4%), chest pain (2%)), ECG abnormal (2%), palpitation (1%)

Central nervous system: Dizziness (8%, less than placebo), sleep disorders (3%), depression (2%), fever (2%), nervousness (1%), somnolence (1%)

Dermatologic: Rash (2%)

Endocrine & metabolic: Hyperkalemia (1%, less than placebo), triglycerides increased (1%), menstrual disorder (1%)

Gastrointestinal: Nausea (2%), diarrhea (4%), vomiting (2%), dyspepsia (2%), abdominal pain (3%), flatulence (1%)

Genitourinary: Urinary tract infection (3%), sexual dysfunction (male 1%)

Hepatic: Increased ALT (2%)

Neuromuscular & skeletal: Weakness (8%), back pain (6%), lower extremity pain (5%), upper extremity pain (3%), hypertonia (3%), paresthesia (2%), joint pain (1%), myalgia (1%), arthritis (1%), neck pain (1%)

Renal: Proteinuria (2%)

Respiratory: Upper respiratory tract infection (9%), sinusitis (5%), rhinitis (5%), pharyngitis (3%)

Otic: Tinnitus (2%), ear infection (1%)

Miscellaneous: Viral infection (3%), allergy (2%)

Note: Some reactions occurred at an incidence >1% but ≤ placebo.

Additional adverse effects that have been reported with **ACE inhibitors** include agranulocytosis (especially in patients with renal impairment or collagen vascular disease), neutropenia, anemia, bullous pemphigus, cardiac arrest, eosinophilic pneumonitis, exfoliative dermatitis, hepatic failure, hyponatremia, jaundice, pancreatitis (acute), pancytopenia, thrombocytopenia; decreases in creatinine clearance in some elderly hypertensive patients or those with chronic renal failure, and worsening of renal function in patients with bilateral renal artery stenosis or hypovolemic patients (diuretic therapy). In addition, a syndrome which may include fever, myalgia, arthralgia, interstitial nephritis, vasculitis, rash, eosinophilia and positive ANA, and elevated ESR has been reported with ACE inhibitors.

Mechanism of Action Perindopril is a prodrug for perindoprilat, which acts as a competitive inhibitor of angiotensin-converting enzyme (ACE); prevents conversion of angiotensin I to angiotensin II, a potent vasoconstrictor; results in lower levels of angiotensin II which, in turn, causes an increase in plasma renin activity and a reduction in aldosterone secretion

Drug Interactions

Increased Effect/Toxicity: Potassium supplements, co-trimoxazole (high dose), angiotensin II receptor antagonists (eg, candesartan, losartan, irbesartan), or potassium-sparing diuretics (amiloride, eplerenone, spironolactone, triamterene) may result in elevated serum potassium levels when combined with perindopril. ACE inhibitor effects may be increased by phenothiazines or probenecid (increases levels of captopril). ACE inhibitors may increase serum concentrations/effects of lithium. ACE inhibitors may enhance the adverse/toxic effects (nitritoid reaction) of gold sodium thiomalate.

Diuretics have additive hypotensive effects with ACE inhibitors, and hypovolemia increases the potential for adverse renal effects of ACE inhibitors. ACE inhibitors may increase nephrotoxicity of cyclosporine. In patients with compromised renal function, coadministration with NSAIDs may result in further deterioration of renal function. Allopurinol and ACE inhibitors may cause a higher risk of hypersensitivity reaction when taken concurrently.

Decreased Effect: Aspirin (high dose) may reduce the therapeutic effects of ACE inhibitors; at low dosages this does not appear to be significant. Rifampin may decrease the effect of ACE inhibitors. Antacids may decrease the bioavailability of ACE inhibitors (may be more likely to occur with captopril); separate administration times by 1-2 hours. NSAIDs, specifically indomethacin, may reduce the hypotensive effects of ACE inhibitors. More likely to occur in low renin or volume dependent hypertensive patients.

Pharmacodynamics/Kinetics

Onset of action: Peak effect: 1-2 hours

Distribution: Small amounts enter breast milk

Protein binding: Perindopril: 60%; Perindoprilat: 10% to 20%

Metabolism: Hepatically hydrolyzed to active metabolite, perindoprilat (~17% to 20% of a dose) and other inactive metabolites

Bioavailability: Perindopril: 75%; Perindoprilat ~25% (~16% with food)

Half-life elimination: Parent drug: 1.5-3 hours; Metabolite: Effective: 3-10 hours, Terminal: 30-120 hours

Time to peak: Chronic therapy: Perindopril: 1 hour; Perindoprilat: 3-7 hours (maximum perindoprilat serum levels are 2-3 times higher and T_{max} is shorter following chronic therapy); CHF: Perindoprilat: 6 hours

Excretion: Urine (75%, 4% to 12% as unchanged drug)

Pregnancy Risk Factor C (1st trimester) / D (2nd and 3rd trimesters)

PerioChip® see Chlorhexidine Gluconate on page 332
PerioGard® see Chlorhexidine Gluconate on page 332

PerioMed™ *see* Fluoride *on page 710*
Periostat® *see* Doxycycline (Subantimicrobial) *on page 540*
Permax® [DSC] *see* Pergolide *on page 1279*

Permethrin (per METH rin)

U.S. Brand Names A200® Lice [OTC]; Acticin®; Elimite®; Nix® [OTC]; Rid®
Spray [OTC]

Canadian Brand Names Kwellada-P™; Nix®

Mexican Brand Names Novo-Herklin 2000

Generic Available Yes: Excludes spray

Pharmacologic Category Antiparasitic Agent, Topical; Scabicidal Agent

Use Single-application treatment of infestation with *Pediculus humanus capitis*
(head louse) and its nits or *Sarcoptes scabiei* (scabies); indicated for prophylactic use during epidemics of lice

Local Anesthetic/Vasoconstrictor Precautions No information available to
require special precautions

Effects on Dental Treatment No significant effects or complications reported

Common Adverse Effects 1% to 10%:
Dermatologic: Pruritus, erythema, rash of the scalp
Local: Burning, stinging, tingling, numbness or scalp discomfort, edema

Mechanism of Action Inhibits sodium ion influx through nerve cell membrane
channels in parasites resulting in delayed repolarization and thus paralysis and
death of the pest

Pharmacodynamics/Kinetics
Absorption: <2%
Metabolism: Hepatic via ester hydrolysis to inactive metabolites
Excretion: Urine

Pregnancy Risk Factor B

Perphenazine (per FEN a zeen)

Canadian Brand Names Apo-Perphenazine®

Mexican Brand Names Leptopsique

Generic Available Yes

Pharmacologic Category Antipsychotic Agent, Typical, Phenothiazine

Use Treatment of schizophrenia; nausea and vomiting

Unlabeled/Investigational Use Ethanol withdrawal; behavioral symptoms
associated with dementia (elderly); Tourette's syndrome; Huntington's chorea;
spasmodic torticollis; Reye's syndrome; psychosis

Local Anesthetic/Vasoconstrictor Precautions Most pharmacology textbooks state that in presence of phenothiazines, systemic doses of epinephrine
paradoxically decrease the blood pressure. This is the so called "epinephrine
reversal" phenomenon. This has never been observed when epinephrine is
given by infiltration as part of the anesthesia procedure.

Effects on Dental Treatment Key adverse event(s) related to dental treatment:
Significant hypotension may occur, especially when the drug is administered
parenterally; orthostatic hypotension is due to alpha-receptor blockade, the
elderly are at greater risk for orthostatic hypotension.
Tardive dyskinesia: Prevalence rate may be 40% in elderly; development of the
syndrome and the irreversible nature are proportional to duration and total
cumulative dose over time. Extrapyramidal reactions are more common in
elderly with up to 50% developing these reactions after 60 years of age.
Drug-induced Parkinson's syndrome occurs often; akathisia is the most
common extrapyramidal reaction in elderly.

Common Adverse Effects Frequency not defined.
Cardiovascular: Hyper-/hypotension, orthostatic hypotension, tachycardia,
bradycardia, dizziness, cardiac arrest
Central nervous system: Extrapyramidal symptoms (pseudoparkinsonism,
akathisia, dystonias, tardive dyskinesia), dizziness, cerebral edema, seizure,
headache, drowsiness, paradoxical excitement, restlessness, hyperactivity,
insomnia, neuroleptic malignant syndrome (NMS), impairment of temperature
regulation
Dermatologic: Rash, discoloration of skin (blue-gray), photosensitivity
Endocrine & metabolic: Hypoglycemia, hyperglycemia, galactorrhea, lactation,
breast enlargement, gynecomastia, menstrual irregularity, amenorrhea,
SIADH, libido (changes in)
Gastrointestinal: Constipation, weight gain, vomiting, stomach pain, nausea,
xerostomia, salivation, diarrhea, anorexia, ileus

Genitourinary: Difficulty in urination, ejaculatory disturbances, incontinence, polyuria, ejaculating dysfunction, priapism

Hematologic: Agranulocytosis, leukopenia, eosinophilia, hemolytic anemia, thrombocytopenic purpura, pancytopenia

Hepatic: Cholestatic jaundice, hepatotoxicity

Neuromuscular & skeletal: Tremor

Ocular: Pigmentary retinopathy, blurred vision, cornea and lens changes

Respiratory: Nasal congestion

Miscellaneous: Diaphoresis

Mechanism of Action Perphenazine is a piperazine phenothiazine antipsychotic which blocks postsynaptic mesolimbic dopaminergic receptors in the brain; exhibits alpha-adrenergic blocking effect and depresses the release of hypothalamic and hypophyseal hormones

Drug Interactions

Cytochrome P450 Effect: Substrate of CYP1A2 (minor), 2C9 (minor), 2C19 (minor), 2D6 (major), 3A4 (minor); **Inhibits** CYP1A2 (weak), 2D6 (weak)

Increased Effect/Toxicity: CYP2D6 inhibitors may increase the levels/effects of perphenazine; example inhibitors include chlorpromazine, delavirdine, fluoxetine, miconazole, paroxetine, pergolide, quinidine, quinine, ritonavir, and ropinirole. Effects on CNS depression may be additive when perphenazine is combined with CNS depressants (opioid analgesics, ethanol, barbiturates, cyclic antidepressants, antihistamines, or sedative-hypnotics). Perphenazine may increase the effects/toxicity of anticholinergics, antihypertensives, lithium (rare neurotoxicity), trazodone, or valproic acid. Concurrent use with TCA may produce increased toxicity or altered therapeutic response. Chloroquine and propranolol may increase perphenazine concentrations. Hypotension may occur when perphenazine is combined with epinephrine. May increase the risk of arrhythmia when combined with antiarrhythmics, cisapride, pimozide, sparfloxacin, or other drugs which prolong QT interval. Metoclopramide may increase risk of extrapyramidal symptoms (EPS). Acetylcholinesterase inhibitors (central) may increase the risk of antipsychotic-related EPS.

Decreased Effect: Phenothiazines inhibit the ability of bromocriptine to lower serum prolactin concentrations. Benztropine (and other anticholinergics) may inhibit the therapeutic response to perphenazine and excess anticholinergic effects may occur. Cigarette smoking and barbiturates may enhance the hepatic metabolism of chlorpromazine. Antihypertensive effects of guanethidine and guanadrel may be inhibited by perphenazine. Perphenazine may inhibit the antiparkinsonian effect of levodopa. Perphenazine and possibly other low potency antipsychotics may reverse the pressor effects of epinephrine.

Pharmacodynamics/Kinetics

Absorption: Oral: Well absorbed

Distribution: Crosses placenta

Metabolism: Extensively hepatic to metabolites via sulfoxidation, hydroxylation, dealkylation, and glucuronidation

Half-life elimination: Perphenazine: 9-12 hours; 7-hydroxyperphenazine: 11.3 hours

Time to peak, serum: Perphenazine: 1-3 hours; 7-hydroxyperphenazine: 2-4 hours

Excretion: Urine and feces

Pregnancy Risk Factor C

Phenabid® *see* Chlorpheniramine and Phenylephrine *on page 340*

Phenabid DM® *see* Chlorpheniramine, Phenylephrine, and Dextromethorphan *on page 342*

Phenadoz™ *see* Promethazine *on page 1361*

Phenagesic [OTC] *see* Acetaminophen and Phenyltoloxamine *on page 38*

Phenaseptic [OTC] *see* Phenol *on page 1290*

PhenaVent™ *see* Guaifenesin and Phenylephrine *on page 797*

PhenaVent™ D *see* Guaifenesin and Phenylephrine *on page 797*

PhenaVent™ LA *see* Guaifenesin and Phenylephrine *on page 797*

PhenaVent™ Ped *see* Guaifenesin and Phenylephrine *on page 797*

Phenazopyridine (fen az oh PEER i deen)

U.S. Brand Names AZO-Gesic® [OTC]; AZO-Standard® [OTC]; Baridium® [OTC]; Prodium® [OTC]; Pyridium®; ReAzo [OTC]; Uristat® [OTC]; UTI Relief® [OTC]

Canadian Brand Names Phenazo™

Mexican Brand Names Pirimir

Generic Available Yes

Index Terms Phenazopyridine Hydrochloride; Phenylazo Diamino Pyridine Hydrochloride

Pharmacologic Category Analgesic, Urinary

Use Symptomatic relief of urinary burning, itching, frequency and urgency in association with urinary tract infection or following urologic procedures

Local Anesthetic/Vasoconstrictor Precautions No information available to require special precautions

Effects on Dental Treatment No significant effects or complications reported

Common Adverse Effects 1% to 10%:
Central nervous system: Headache, dizziness
Gastrointestinal: Stomach cramps

Mechanism of Action An azo dye which exerts local anesthetic or analgesic action on urinary tract mucosa through an unknown mechanism

Pharmacodynamics/Kinetics
Metabolism: Hepatic and via other tissues
Excretion: Urine (65% as unchanged drug)

Pregnancy Risk Factor B

Phenazopyridine Hydrochloride *see* Phenazopyridine *on page 1286*

Phencarb GG *see* Carbetapentane, Guaifenesin, and Phenylephrine *on page 279*

Phendimetrazine (fen dye ME tra zeen)

U.S. Brand Names Bontril PDM®; Bontril® Slow-Release; Melfiat® [DSC]

Canadian Brand Names Bontril®; Plegine®; Statobex®

Generic Available Yes

Index Terms Phendimetrazine Tartrate

Pharmacologic Category Anorexiant; Sympathomimetic

Use Short-term (few weeks) adjunct in exogenous obesity

Local Anesthetic/Vasoconstrictor Precautions Use vasoconstrictor with caution in patients taking phendimetrazine. Phendimetrazine can enhance the sympathomimetic response to epinephrine leading to potential hypertension and cardiotoxicity.

Effects on Dental Treatment Key adverse event(s) related to dental treatment: Xerostomia (normal salivary flow resumes upon discontinuation).

Common Adverse Effects Frequency not defined.
Cardiovascular: Flushing, hypertension, palpitation, tachycardia
Central nervous system: Agitation, dizziness, headache, insomnia, overstimulation, psychosis, restlessness
Endocrine & metabolic: Changes in libido
Gastrointestinal: Constipation, diarrhea, nausea, stomach pain, xerostomia
Genitourinary: Dysuria, urinary frequency
Neuromuscular & skeletal: Tremor
Ocular: Blurred vision, mydriasis
Miscellaneous: Diaphoresis, tachyphylaxis

Restrictions C-III

Pharmacotherapy for weight loss is recommended only for obese patients with a body mass index ≥30 kg/m², or ≥27 kg/m² in the presence of other risk factors such as hypertension, diabetes, and/or dyslipidemia or a high waist circumference; therapy should be used in conjunction with a comprehensive weight management program. Rule out organic causes of obesity (eg, untreated hypo-thyroidism) prior to use.

Note: Phendimetrazine is not approved for long-term use. The limited useful-ness of medications in this class should be weighed against possible risks associated with their use. Consult weight loss guidelines for current pharmaco-therapy recommendations.

Mechanism of Action Phendimetrazine is a sympathomimetic amine with pharmacologic properties similar to the amphetamines. The mechanism of action in reducing appetite appears to be secondary to CNS effects, including stimulation of the hypothalamus to release norepinephrine.

Drug Interactions

Increased Effect/Toxicity: Antacids and carbonic anhydrase inhibitors may decrease the excretion of phendimetrazine. Severe hypertensive episodes have occurred with amphetamine when used in patients receiving MAO inhibi-tors; concurrent use or use within 14 days is contraindicated. Due to MAO inhibition, use with linezolid should generally be avoided. Concomitant use with another sympathomimetic agent may increase the risk of related adverse effects, especially on the cardiovascular system (eg, increased blood pres-sure, tachycardia). Concomitant use with other CNS stimulants is contraindi-cated.

Pharmacodynamics/Kinetics

Metabolism: Forms 2 metabolites

Half-life elimination: Bontril® PDM: ~2 hours; Bontril® Slow Release: ~ 10 hours

Excretion: Urine

Pregnancy Risk Factor C

Phendimetrazine Tartrate *see* Phendimetrazine *on page 1286*

Phenelzine (FEN el zeen)

U.S. Brand Names Nardil®

Canadian Brand Names Nardil®

Generic Available No

Index Terms Phenelzine Sulfate

Pharmacologic Category Antidepressant, Monoamine Oxidase Inhibitor

Use Symptomatic treatment of atypical, nonendogenous, or neurotic depression

Unlabeled/Investigational Use Selective mutism

Local Anesthetic/Vasoconstrictor Precautions Attempts should be made to avoid use of vasoconstrictor due to possibility of hypertensive episodes with monoamine oxidase inhibitors

Effects on Dental Treatment Key adverse event(s) related to dental treat-ment: Orthostatic hypotension, xerostomia and changes in salivation (normal salivary flow resumes upon discontinuation). Avoid use as an analgesic due to toxic reactions with MAO inhibitors.

Mechanism of Action Thought to act by increasing endogenous concentra-tions of norepinephrine, dopamine, and serotonin through inhibition of the enzyme (monoamine oxidase) responsible for the breakdown of these neuro-transmitters

Pregnancy Risk Factor C

Phenelzine Sulfate *see* Phenelzine *on page 1287*

Phenergan® *see* Promethazine *on page 1361*

Phenindamine (fen IN dah meen)

U.S. Brand Names Nolahist® [OTC] [DSC]

Canadian Brand Names Nolahist®

Generic Available No

Index Terms Phenindamine Tartrate

Pharmacologic Category Antihistamine

Use Treatment of perennial and seasonal allergic rhinitis and chronic urticaria

Local Anesthetic/Vasoconstrictor Precautions No information available to require special precautions

Effects on Dental Treatment No significant effects or complications reported

Phenindamine Tartrate *see* Phenindamine *on page 1287*

Pheniramine and Naphazoline *see* Naphazoline and Pheniramine *on page 1147*

Phenobarbital (fee noe BAR bi tal)

U.S. Brand Names Luminal® Sodium
Canadian Brand Names PMS-Phenobarbital
Mexican Brand Names Alepsal
Generic Available Yes
Index Terms Phenobarbital Sodium; Phenobarbitone; Phenylethylmalonylurea
Pharmacologic Category Anticonvulsant, Barbiturate; Barbiturate
Use Management of generalized tonic-clonic (grand mal) and partial seizures; sedative
Unlabeled/Investigational Use Febrile seizures in children; may also be used for prevention and treatment of neonatal hyperbilirubinemia and lowering of bilirubin in chronic cholestasis; neonatal seizures; management of sedative/hypnotic withdrawal
Local Anesthetic/Vasoconstrictor Precautions No information available to require special precautions
Effects on Dental Treatment No significant effects or complications reported
Common Adverse Effects Frequency not defined.
　Cardiovascular: Bradycardia, hypotension, syncope
　Central nervous system: Drowsiness, lethargy, CNS excitation or depression, impaired judgment, "hangover" effect, confusion, somnolence, agitation, hyperkinesia, ataxia, nervousness, headache, insomnia, nightmares, hallucinations, anxiety, dizziness
　Dermatologic: Rash, exfoliative dermatitis, Stevens-Johnson syndrome
　Gastrointestinal: Nausea, vomiting, constipation
　Hematologic: Agranulocytosis, thrombocytopenia, megaloblastic anemia
　Local: Pain at injection site, thrombophlebitis with I.V. use
　Renal: Oliguria
　Respiratory: Laryngospasm, respiratory depression, apnea (especially with rapid I.V. use), hypoventilation
　Miscellaneous: Gangrene with inadvertent intra-arterial injection
Restrictions C-IV
Dosage
　Children:
　　Sedation: Oral: 2 mg/kg 3 times/day
　　Hypnotic: I.M., I.V., SubQ: 3-5 mg/kg at bedtime
　　Preoperative sedation: Oral, I.M., I.V.: 1-3 mg/kg 1-1.5 hours before procedure
　Adults:
　　Sedation: Oral, I.M.: 30-120 mg/day in 2-3 divided doses
　　Hypnotic: Oral, I.M., I.V., SubQ: 100-320 mg at bedtime
　　Preoperative sedation: I.M.: 100-200 mg 1-1.5 hours before procedure

　Anticonvulsant: Status epilepticus: Loading dose: I.V.:
　　Infants and Children: 10-20 mg/kg in a single or divided dose; in select patients may administer additional 5 mg/kg/dose every 15-30 minutes until seizure is controlled or a total dose of 40 mg/kg is reached
　　Adults: 300-800 mg initially followed by 120-240 mg/dose at 20-minute intervals until seizures are controlled or a total dose of 1-2 g
　Anticonvulsant maintenance dose: Oral, I.V.:
　　Infants: 5-8 mg/kg/day in 1-2 divided doses
　　Children:
　　　1-5 years: 6-8 mg/kg/day in 1-2 divided doses
　　　5-12 years: 4-6 mg/kg/day in 1-2 divided doses
　　Children >12 years and Adults: 1-3 mg/kg/day in divided doses or 50-100 mg 2-3 times/day
　Sedative/hypnotic withdrawal (unlabeled use): Initial daily requirement is determined by substituting phenobarbital 30 mg for every 100 mg pentobarbital used during tolerance testing; then daily requirement is decreased by 10% of initial dose

Dosing interval in renal impairment: Cl_{cr} <10 mL/minute: Administer every 12-16 hours
Hemodialysis: Moderately dialyzable (20% to 50%)
Dosing adjustment/comments in hepatic disease: Increased side effects may occur in severe liver disease; monitor plasma levels and adjust dose accordingly
Mechanism of Action Short-acting barbiturate with sedative, hypnotic, and anticonvulsant properties. Barbiturates depress the sensory cortex, decrease motor activity, alter cerebellar function, and produce drowsiness, sedation, and hypnosis. In high doses, barbiturates exhibit anticonvulsant activity; barbiturates produce dose-dependent respiratory depression.

Contraindications Hypersensitivity to barbiturates or any component of the formulation; marked hepatic impairment; dyspnea or airway obstruction; porphyria; pregnancy

Warnings/Precautions Use with caution in patients with hypovolemic shock, CHF, hepatic impairment, respiratory dysfunction or depression, previous addiction to the sedative/hypnotic group, chronic or acute pain, renal dysfunction, and the elderly, due to its long half-life and risk of dependence; phenobarbital is not recommended as a sedative in the elderly; tolerance or psychological and physical dependence may occur with prolonged use. Use with caution in patients with depression or suicidal tendencies, or in patients with a history of drug abuse. **Abrupt withdrawal in patients with epilepsy may precipitate status epilepticus.**

Drug Interactions

Cytochrome P450 Effect: Substrate of CYP2C9 (minor), 2C19 (major), 2E1 (minor); **Induces** CYP1A2 (strong), 2A6 (strong), 2B6 (strong), 2C8 (strong), 2C9 (strong), 3A4 (strong)

Increased Effect/Toxicity: When combined with other CNS depressants, ethanol, opioid analgesics, antidepressants, or benzodiazepines, additive respiratory and CNS depression may occur. Barbiturates may enhance the hepatotoxic potential of acetaminophen overdoses. Chloramphenicol, MAO inhibitors, valproic acid, and felbamate may inhibit barbiturate metabolism. Barbiturates may impair the absorption of griseofulvin, and may enhance the nephrotoxic effects of methoxyflurane. Concurrent use of phenobarbital with meperidine may result in increased CNS depression. Concurrent use of phenobarbital with primidone may result in elevated phenobarbital serum concentrations. The levels/effects of phenobarbital may be increased by delavirdine, fluconazole, fluvoxamine, gemfibrozil, isoniazid, omeprazole, ticlopidine, and other CYP2C19 inhibitors.

Decreased Effect: Barbiturates may increase the metabolism of estrogens and reduce the efficacy of oral contraceptives; an alternative method of contraception should be considered. Barbiturates inhibit the hypoprothrombinemic effects of oral anticoagulants via increased metabolism. Barbiturates may enhance the metabolism of methadone resulting in methadone withdrawal. The levels/effects of phenobarbital may be decreased by aminoglutethimide, carbamazepine, phenytoin, rifampin, and other CYP2C19 inducers.

Phenobarbital may decrease the levels/effects of aminophylline, amiodarone, benzodiazepines, bupropion, calcium channel blockers, carbamazepine, citalopram, clarithromycin, cyclosporine, diazepam, efavirenz, erythromycin, estrogens, fluoxetine, fluvoxamine, glimepiride, glipizide, ifosfamide, losartan, methsuximide, mirtazapine, nateglinide, nefazodone, nevirapine, phenytoin, pioglitazone, promethazine, propranolol, protease inhibitors, proton pump inhibitors, rifampin, ropinirole, rosiglitazone, selegiline, sertraline, sulfonamides, tacrolimus, theophylline, venlafaxine, voriconazole, warfarin, zafirlukast, and other CYP1A2, 2A6, 2B6, 2C8, 2C9, or 3A4 substrates.

Ethanol/Nutrition/Herb Interactions

Ethanol: Avoid ethanol (may increase CNS depression).

Food: May cause decrease in vitamin D and calcium.

Herb/Nutraceutical: Avoid evening primrose (seizure threshold decreased). Avoid valerian, St John's wort, kava kava, gotu kola (may increase CNS depression).

Dietary Considerations Vitamin D: Loss in vitamin D due to malabsorption; increase intake of foods rich in vitamin D. Supplementation of vitamin D and/or calcium may be necessary. Sodium content of injection (65 mg, 1 mL): 6 mg (0.3 mEq).

Pharmacodynamics/Kinetics

Onset of action: Oral: Hypnosis: 20-60 minutes; I.V.: ~5 minutes

Peak effect: I.V.: ~30 minutes

Duration: Oral: 6-10 hours; I.V.: 4-10 hours

Absorption: Oral: 70% to 90%

Protein binding: 20% to 45%; decreased in neonates

Metabolism: Hepatic via hydroxylation and glucuronide conjugation

Half-life elimination: Neonates: 45-500 hours; Infants: 20-133 hours; Children: 37-73 hours; Adults: 53-140 hours

Time to peak, serum: Oral: 1-6 hours

Excretion: Urine (20% to 50% as unchanged drug)

Pregnancy Risk Factor D

Dosage Forms

Elixir: 20 mg/5 mL

Injection, solution: 65 mg/mL (1 mL); 130 mg/mL (1 mL)

Luminal® Sodium: 60 mg/mL (1 mL); 130 mg/mL (1 mL)

Tablet: 15 mg, 30 mg, 60 mg, 100 mg

Phenobarbital, Belladonna, and Ergotamine Tartrate *see* Belladonna, Phenobarbital, and Ergotamine *on page 190*

Phenobarbital, Hyoscyamine, Atropine, and Scopolamine *see* Hyoscyamine, Atropine, Scopolamine, and Phenobarbital *on page 848*

Phenobarbital Sodium *see* Phenobarbital *on page 1288*

Phenobarbitone *see* Phenobarbital *on page 1288*

Phenol (FEE nol)

Related Information
Mouth Pain, Cold Sore, and Canker Sore Products *on page 1938*
U.S. Brand Names Castellani Paint Modified [OTC]; Cepastat® [OTC]; Cepastat® Extra Strength [OTC]; Cheracol® [OTC]; Chloraseptic® Gargle [OTC]; Chloraseptic® Mouth Pain [OTC]; Chloraseptic® Pocket Pump [OTC]; Chloraseptic® Spray [OTC]; Chloraseptic® Spray for Kids [OTC]; Pain-A-Lay® [OTC]; Phenaseptic® [OTC]; Phenol EZ® [OTC]; Ulcerease® [OTC]; Vicks® Formula 44® Sore Throat [OTC]
Canadian Brand Names P & S™ Liquid Phenol
Generic Available Yes: Oral spray
Index Terms Carbolic Acid
Pharmacologic Category Anesthetic, Topical
Use Relief of sore throat pain, mouth, gum, and throat irritations; antiseptic; topical anesthetic
Local Anesthetic/Vasoconstrictor Precautions No information available to require special precautions
Effects on Dental Treatment No significant effects or complications reported

Phenol and Camphor *see* Camphor and Phenol *on page 264*

Phenol EZ® [OTC] *see* Phenol *on page 1290*

Phenoxybenzamine (fen oks ee BEN za meen)

U.S. Brand Names Dibenzyline®
Canadian Brand Names Dibenzyline®
Generic Available No
Index Terms Phenoxybenzamine Hydrochloride
Pharmacologic Category Alpha₁ Blocker
Use Symptomatic management of pheochromocytoma; treatment of hypertensive crisis caused by sympathomimetic amines
Unlabeled/Investigational Use Micturition problems associated with neurogenic bladder, functional outlet obstruction, and partial prostate obstruction
Local Anesthetic/Vasoconstrictor Precautions No information available to require special precautions
Effects on Dental Treatment Key adverse event(s) related to dental treatment: Xerostomia (normal salivary flow resumes upon discontinuation).
Common Adverse Effects Frequency not defined.
Cardiovascular: Postural hypotension, shock, syncope, tachycardia
Central nervous system: Confusion, fatigue headache, lethargy
Gastrointestinal: Diarrhea, nausea, vomiting, xerostomia
Genitourinary: Inhibition of ejaculation
Neuromuscular & skeletal: Weakness
Ocular: Miosis
Respiratory: Nasal congestion
Mechanism of Action Produces long-lasting noncompetitive alpha-adrenergic blockade of postganglionic synapses in exocrine glands and smooth muscle; relaxes urethra and increases opening of the bladder
Drug Interactions
Increased Effect/Toxicity: Beta-blockers may result in increased toxicity (hypotension, tachycardia). Blood pressure-lowering effects are additive with sildenafil (use with extreme caution at a dose ≤25 mg), tadalafil (use is contraindicated by the manufacturer), and vardenafil (use is contraindicated by the manufacturer).
Decreased Effect: Alpha-adrenergic agonists decrease the effect of phenoxybenzamine.
Pharmacodynamics/Kinetics
Onset of action: ~2 hours
Peak effect: 4-6 hours
Duration: ≥4 days
Half-life elimination: 24 hours
Excretion: Primarily urine and feces
Pregnancy Risk Factor C

Phenoxybenzamine Hydrochloride *see* Phenoxybenzamine *on page 1290*
Phenoxymethyl Penicillin *see* Penicillin V Potassium *on page 1271*

Phentermine (FEN ter meen)

U.S. Brand Names Adipex-P®; Ionamin®
Canadian Brand Names Ionamin®
Mexican Brand Names Sinpet
Generic Available Yes: Capsule (excludes resin complex capsule), tablet
Index Terms Phentermine Hydrochloride
Pharmacologic Category Anorexiant; Sympathomimetic
Use Short-term (few weeks) adjunct in exogenous obesity
Local Anesthetic/Vasoconstrictor Precautions Use vasoconstrictor with caution in patients taking phentermine. Amphetamines enhance the sympathomimetic response of epinephrine and norepinephrine leading to potential hypertension and cardiotoxicity.
Effects on Dental Treatment Key adverse event(s) related to dental treatment: Xerostomia (normal salivary flow resumes upon discontinuation) and unpleasant taste. Up to 10% of patients may present with hypertension. The use of local anesthetic without vasoconstrictor is recommended in these patients. See Dental Comment.
Common Adverse Effects Frequency not defined.
Cardiovascular: Hypertension, palpitation, primary pulmonary hypertension and/or regurgitant cardiac valvular disease, tachycardia
Central nervous system: Dizziness, dysphoria, euphoria, headache, insomnia, overstimulation, psychosis, restlessness
Dermatologic: Urticaria
Endocrine & metabolic: Changes in libido
Gastrointestinal: Constipation, diarrhea, unpleasant taste, xerostomia
Genitourinary: Impotence
Neuromuscular & skeletal: Tremor
Restrictions C-IV

Pharmacotherapy for weight loss is recommended only for obese patients with a body mass index ≥ 30 kg/m^2, or ≥ 27 kg/m^2 in the presence of other risk factors such as hypertension, diabetes, and/or dyslipidemia or a high waist circumference; therapy should be used in conjunction with a comprehensive weight management program. Rule out organic causes of obesity (eg, untreated hypothyroidism) prior to use.

Note: Phentermine is not approved for long-term use. The limited usefulness of medications in this class should be weighed against possible risks associated with their use. Consult weight loss guidelines for current pharmacotherapy recommendations.
Mechanism of Action Phentermine is a sympathomimetic amine with pharmacologic properties similar to the amphetamines. The mechanism of action in reducing appetite appears to be secondary to CNS effects, including stimulation of the hypothalamus to release norepinephrine.
Drug Interactions
Increased Effect/Toxicity: Antacids and carbonic anhydrase inhibitors may decrease the excretion of phentermine. Severe hypertensive episodes have occurred with amphetamine when used in patients receiving MAO inhibitors; concurrent use or use within 14 days is contraindicated. Due to MAO inhibition, use with linezolid should generally be avoided. Concomitant use with another sympathomimetic agent may increase the risk of related adverse effects, especially on the cardiovascular system (eg, increased blood pressure, tachycardia). Concomitant use with other CNS stimulants is contraindicated.
Pharmacodynamics/Kinetics
Duration: Resin produces more prolonged clinical effects
Absorption: Well absorbed; resin absorbed slower
Excretion: Primarily urine
Pregnancy Risk Factor C
Dental Comment Many diet physicians have prescribed fenfluramine ("fen") and phentermine ("phen"). When taken together the combination is known as "fen-phen". The diet drug dexfenfluramine (Redux®) is chemically similar to fenfluramine (Pondimin®) and was also used in combination with phentermine called "Redux-phen". While each of the three drugs alone had approval from the FDA for sale in the treatment of obesity, neither combination had an official approval. The use of the combinations in the treatment of obesity was considered an "off-label" use. Reports in medical literature have been accumulating for some years about significant side effects associated with fenfluramine and dexfenfluramine. In 1997, the manufacturers, at the urging of the FDA, agreed
(Continued)

Phentermine *(Continued)*

to voluntarily withdraw the drugs from the market. The action was based on findings from physicians who evaluated patients taking fenfluramine and dexfenfluramine with echocardiograms. The findings indicated that approximately 30% of patients had abnormal echocardiograms, even though they had no symptoms. This was a much higher than expected percentage of abnormal test results. This conclusion was based on a sample of 291 patients examined by five different physicians. Under normal conditions, fewer than 1% of patients would be expected to show signs of heart valve disease. The findings suggested that fenfluramine and dexfenfluramine were the likely cause of heart valve problems of the type that promoted FDA's earlier warnings concerning "fen-phen". The earlier warning included the following: The mitral valve and other valves in the heart are damaged by a strange white coating and allow blood to flow back, causing heart muscle damage. In several cases, valve replacement surgery has been done. As a rule, the person must, thereafter for life, be on a blood thinner to prevent clots from the mechanical valve. This type of valve damage had only been seen before in persons who were exposed to large amounts of serotonin. The fenfluramine increases the availability of serotonin.

Phentermine Hydrochloride *see* Phentermine *on page 1291*

Phentolamine *(fen TOLE a meen)*

Canadian Brand Names Regitine®; Rogitine®
Generic Available Yes
Index Terms Phentolamine Mesylate; Regitine [DSC]
Pharmacologic Category Alpha$_1$ Blocker
Use Diagnosis of pheochromocytoma and treatment of hypertension associated with pheochromocytoma or other forms of hypertension caused by excess sympathomimetic amines; as treatment of dermal necrosis after extravasation of drugs with alpha-adrenergic effects (norepinephrine, dopamine, epinephrine)
Unlabeled/Investigational Use Treatment of pralidoxime-induced hypertension
Local Anesthetic/Vasoconstrictor Precautions Although the alpha-adrenergic blocking effects could antagonize epinephrine, there is no information available to require special precautions
Effects on Dental Treatment Key adverse event(s) related to dental treatment: Orthostatic hypotension.
Common Adverse Effects Frequency not defined.
  Cardiovascular: Hypotension, tachycardia, arrhythmia, flushing, orthostatic hypotension
  Central nervous system: Dizziness
  Gastrointestinal: Nausea, vomiting, diarrhea
  Neuromuscular & skeletal: Weakness
  Respiratory: Nasal congestion
  Case report: Pulmonary hypertension
Mechanism of Action Competitively blocks alpha-adrenergic receptors to produce brief antagonism of circulating epinephrine and norepinephrine to reduce hypertension caused by alpha effects of these catecholamines; also has a positive inotropic and chronotropic effect on the heart
Drug Interactions
  Increased Effect/Toxicity: Phentolamine's toxicity is increased with ethanol (disulfiram reaction). Blood pressure-lowering effects are additive with sildenafil (use with extreme caution at a dose ≤25 mg), tadalafil (use is contraindicated by the manufacturer), and vardenafil (use is contraindicated by the manufacturer).
  Decreased Effect: Decreased effect of phentolamine with epinephrine and ephedrine.
Pharmacodynamics/Kinetics
  Onset of action: I.M.: 15-20 minutes; I.V.: Immediate
  Duration: I.M.: 30-45 minutes; I.V.: 15-30 minutes
  Metabolism: Hepatic
  Half-life elimination: 19 minutes
  Excretion: Urine (10% as unchanged drug)
Pregnancy Risk Factor C

Phentolamine Mesylate *see* Phentolamine *on page 1292*
Phenylalanine Mustard *see* Melphalan *on page 1034*
Phenylazo Diamino Pyridine Hydrochloride *see* Phenazopyridine *on page 1286*

Phenylephrine (fen il EF rin)

U.S. Brand Names Ah-Chew D®; AK-Dilate®; Altafrin; Anu-Med [OTC]; Dimetapp® Toddler's [OTC]; Formulation R™ [OTC]; LuSonal™; Medicone® Suppositories [OTC]; Medi-Phenyl [OTC]; Mydfrin®; NāSop™; Neofrin™; Neo-Synephrine® Extra Strength [OTC]; Neo-Synephrine® Injection; Neo-Synephrine® Mild [OTC]; Neo-Synephrine® Regular Strength [OTC]; OcuNefrin™ [OTC]; Preparation H® [OTC]; Rectacaine [OTC]; Relief® [OTC]; Rhinall [OTC]; Sudafed PE™ [OTC]; Tronolane® Suppository [OTC]; Tur-bi-kal® [OTC]; Vicks® Sinex® Nasal Spray [OTC]; Vicks® Sinex® UltraFine Mist [OTC]; 4 Way® Fast Acting [OTC]; 4 Way® Menthol [OTC]; 4 Way® No Drip [OTC]

Canadian Brand Names Dionephrine®; Mydfrin®; Neo-Synephrine®

Generic Available Yes: Excludes cream, filmstrip, liquid, suspension

Index Terms Phenylephrine Hydrochloride; Phenylephrine Tannate

Pharmacologic Category Alpha/Beta Agonist; Ophthalmic Agent, Antiglaucoma; Ophthalmic Agent, Mydriatic

Use Treatment of hypotension, vascular failure in shock; as a vasoconstrictor in regional analgesia; as a mydriatic in ophthalmic procedures and treatment of wide-angle glaucoma; supraventricular tachycardia

For OTC use as symptomatic relief of nasal and nasopharyngeal mucosal congestion, treatment of hemorrhoids, relief of redness of the eye due to irritation

Local Anesthetic/Vasoconstrictor Precautions Use with caution since phenylephrine is a sympathomimetic amine which could interact with epinephrine to cause a pressor response

Effects on Dental Treatment Key adverse event(s) related to dental treatment: Tachycardia, palpitations (use vasoconstrictor with caution), and xerostomia (normal salivary flow resumes upon discontinuation).

Common Adverse Effects Frequency not defined.

Cardiovascular: Reflex bradycardia, excitability, restlessness, arrhythmia (rare), precordial pain or discomfort, pallor, hypertension, severe peripheral and visceral vasoconstriction, decreased cardiac output

Central nervous system: Headache, anxiety, dizziness, tremor, paresthesia, restlessness

Endocrine & metabolic: Metabolic acidosis

Local: I.V.: Extravasation which may lead to necrosis and sloughing of surrounding tissue, blanching of skin

Neuromuscular & skeletal: Pilomotor response, weakness

Renal: Decreased renal perfusion, reduced urine output, reduced urine output

Respiratory: Respiratory distress

Mechanism of Action Potent, direct-acting alpha-adrenergic stimulator with weak beta-adrenergic activity; causes vasoconstriction of the arterioles of the nasal mucosa and conjunctiva; activates the dilator muscle of the pupil to cause contraction; produces vasoconstriction of arterioles in the body; produces systemic arterial vasoconstriction

Drug Interactions

Increased Effect/Toxicity: Phenylephrine, taken with sympathomimetics, may induce tachycardia or arrhythmias. If taken with MAO inhibitors or oxytocic agents, actions may be potentiated. Nonselective beta-blockers may increase hypertensive effects; MAO inhibitors may potentiate hypertension and hypertensive crisis; TCAs may enhance vasopressor effect; avoid concurrent use with these agents. Methyldopa may increase pressor response.

Pharmacodynamics/Kinetics

Onset of action: I.M., SubQ: 10-15 minutes; I.V.: Immediate; Ophthalmic: 10-15 minutes

Duration: I.M.: 0.5-2 hours; I.V.: 15-30 minutes; SubQ: 1 hour; Ophthalmic: Maximal mydriasis: 1 hour, recover time: 3-6 hours

Metabolism: Hepatic, via intestinal monoamine oxidase to phenolic conjugates

Excretion: Urine (90%)

Pregnancy Risk Factor C

Phenylephrine CM *see* Chlorpheniramine, Phenylephrine, and Methscopolamine *on page 342*

Phenylephrine and Chlorpheniramine *see* Chlorpheniramine and Phenylephrine *on page 340*

Phenylephrine and Cyclopentolate *see* Cyclopentolate and Phenylephrine *on page 422*

Phenylephrine and Promethazine *see* Promethazine and Phenylephrine *on page 1363*

Phenylephrine and Scopolamine (fen il EF rin & skoe POL a meen)

Related Information
Phenylephrine *on page 1293*
Scopolamine *on page 1457*
U.S. Brand Names Murocoll-2®
Generic Available No
Index Terms Scopolamine and Phenylephrine
Pharmacologic Category Anticholinergic/Adrenergic Agonist
Use Mydriasis, cycloplegia, and to break posterior synechiae in iritis
Local Anesthetic/Vasoconstrictor Precautions Use with caution since phenylephrine is a sympathomimetic amine which could interact with epinephrine to cause a pressor response
Effects on Dental Treatment This form of phenylephrine will have no effect on dental treatment when given as eye drops.
Pharmacodynamics/Kinetics See individual agents.
Pregnancy Risk Factor C

Phenylephrine and Zinc Sulfate (fen il EF rin & zingk SUL fate)

Related Information
Phenylephrine *on page 1293*
Zinc Sulfate *on page 1683*
Canadian Brand Names Zincfrin®
Index Terms Zinc Sulfate and Phenylephrine
Pharmacologic Category Adrenergic Agonist Agent
Use Soothe, moisturize, and remove redness due to minor eye irritation
Local Anesthetic/Vasoconstrictor Precautions No information available to require special precautions
Effects on Dental Treatment No significant effects or complications reported
Restrictions Not available in the U.S.
Pharmacodynamics/Kinetics See individual agents.

Phenylephrine, Chlorpheniramine, and Dextromethorphan *see* Chlorpheniramine, Phenylephrine, and Dextromethorphan *on page 342*

Phenylephrine, Chlorpheniramine, and Dihydrocodeine *see* Dihydrocodeine, Chlorpheniramine, and Phenylephrine *on page 502*

Phenylephrine, Chlorpheniramine, and Phenyltoloxamine *see* Chlorpheniramine, Phenylephrine, and Phenyltoloxamine *on page 343*

Phenylephrine, Chlorpheniramine, Codeine, and Potassium Iodide *see* Chlorpheniramine, Phenylephrine, Codeine, and Potassium Iodide *on page 344*

Phenylephrine, Diphenhydramine, and Hydrocodone *see* Hydrocodone, Phenylephrine, and Diphenhydramine *on page 834*

Phenylephrine, Ephedrine, Chlorpheniramine, and Carbetapentane *see* Chlorpheniramine, Ephedrine, Phenylephrine, and Carbetapentane *on page 341*

Phenylephrine, Guaifenesin, and Hydrocodone *see* Hydrocodone, Phenylephrine, and Guaifenesin *on page 834*

Phenylephrine Hydrochloride *see* Phenylephrine *on page 1293*

Phenylephrine Hydrochloride and Guaifenesin *see* Guaifenesin and Phenylephrine *on page 797*

Phenylephrine Hydrochloride, Carbetapentane Citrate, and Guaifenesin *see* Carbetapentane, Guaifenesin, and Phenylephrine *on page 279*

Phenylephrine Hydrochloride, Guaifenesin, and Dextromethorphan Hydrobromide *see* Guaifenesin, Dextromethorphan, and Phenylephrine *on page 798*

Phenylephrine, Hydrocodone, Chlorpheniramine, Acetaminophen, and Caffeine *see* Hydrocodone, Chlorpheniramine, Phenylephrine, Acetaminophen, and Caffeine *on page 833*

Phenylephrine, Promethazine, and Codeine *see* Promethazine, Phenylephrine, and Codeine *on page 1364*

Phenylephrine Tannate *see* Phenylephrine *on page 1293*

Phenylephrine Tannate and Carbetapentane Tannate *see* Carbetapentane and Phenylephrine *on page 279*

Phenylephrine Tannate, Carbetapentane Tannate, and Pyrilamine Tannate *see* Carbetapentane, Phenylephrine, and Pyrilamine *on page 280*

Phenylephrine Tannate, Chlorpheniramine Tannate, and Methscopolamine Nitrate *see* Chlorpheniramine, Phenylephrine, and Methscopolamine *on page 342*

Phenylethylmalonylurea *see* Phenobarbital *on page 1288*

Phenylgesic [OTC] *see* Acetaminophen and Phenyltoloxamine *on page 38*

Phenyl Salicylate, Methenamine, Methylene Blue, Sodium Biphosphate, and Hyoscyamine *see* Methenamine, Sodium Biphosphate, Phenyl Salicylate, Methylene Blue, and Hyoscyamine *on page 1064*

Phenyltoloxamine, Chlorpheniramine, and Phenylephrine *see* Chlorpheniramine, Phenylephrine, and Phenyltoloxamine *on page 343*

Phenyltoloxamine Citrate and Acetaminophen *see* Acetaminophen and Phenyltoloxamine *on page 38*

Phenytek® *see* Phenytoin *on page 1295*

Phenytoin (FEN i toyn)

Related Information
Cardiovascular Diseases *on page 1726*
Fosphenytoin *on page 751*

U.S. Brand Names Dilantin®; Phenytek®

Canadian Brand Names Dilantin®

Mexican Brand Names Epamin (MX, MX); Nuctane

Generic Available Yes: Excludes chewable tablet

Index Terms Diphenylhydantoin; DPH; Phenytoin Sodium; Phenytoin Sodium, Extended; Phenytoin Sodium, Prompt

Pharmacologic Category Antiarrhythmic Agent, Class Ib; Anticonvulsant, Hydantoin

Use Management of generalized tonic-clonic (grand mal), complex partial seizures; prevention of seizures following head trauma/neurosurgery

Unlabeled/Investigational Use Ventricular arrhythmias, including those associated with digitalis intoxication, prolonged QT interval and surgical repair of congenital heart diseases in children; epidermolysis bullosa

Local Anesthetic/Vasoconstrictor Precautions No information available to require special precautions

Effects on Dental Treatment Gingival hyperplasia is a common problem observed during the first 6 months of phenytoin therapy appearing as gingivitis or gum inflammation. To minimize severity and growth rate of gingival tissue begin a program of professional cleaning and patient plaque control within 10 days of starting anticonvulsant therapy.

Common Adverse Effects I.V. effects: Hypotension, bradycardia, cardiac arrhythmia, cardiovascular collapse (especially with rapid I.V. use), venous irritation and pain, thrombophlebitis

Effects not related to plasma phenytoin concentrations: Hypertrichosis, gingival hypertrophy, thickening of facial features, carbohydrate intolerance, folic acid deficiency, peripheral neuropathy, vitamin D deficiency, osteomalacia, systemic lupus erythematosus

Concentration-related effects: Nystagmus, blurred vision, diplopia, ataxia, slurred speech, dizziness, drowsiness, lethargy, coma, rash, fever, nausea, vomiting, gum tenderness, confusion, mood changes, folic acid depletion, osteomalacia, hyperglycemia

Related to elevated concentrations:
>20 mcg/mL: Far lateral nystagmus
>30 mcg/mL: 45° lateral gaze nystagmus and ataxia
>40 mcg/mL: Decreased mentation
>100 mcg/mL: Death

Cardiovascular: Hypotension, bradycardia, cardiac arrhythmia, cardiovascular collapse

Central nervous system: Psychiatric changes, slurred speech, dizziness, drowsiness, headache, insomnia

Dermatologic: Rash

Gastrointestinal: Constipation, nausea, vomiting, gingival hyperplasia, enlargement of lips

Hematologic: Leukopenia, thrombocytopenia, agranulocytosis

Hepatic: Hepatitis

Local: Thrombophlebitis

Neuromuscular & skeletal: Tremor, peripheral neuropathy, paresthesia

Ocular: Diplopia, nystagmus, blurred vision

Rarely seen effects: SLE-like syndrome, lymphadenopathy, hepatitis, Stevens-Johnson syndrome, blood dyscrasias, dyskinesias, pseudolymphoma, lymphoma, venous irritation and pain, coarsening of the facial features, hypertrichosis

Dosage
Status epilepticus: I.V.:
Infants and Children: Loading dose: 15-20 mg/kg in a single or divided dose; maintenance dose: Initial: 5 mg/kg/day in 2 divided doses; usual doses:
6 months to 3 years: 8-10 mg/kg/day
4-6 years: 7.5-9 mg/kg/day

(Continued)

Phenytoin *(Continued)*

7-9 years: 7-8 mg/kg/day

10-16 years: 6-7 mg/kg/day, some patients may require every 8 hours dosing

Adults: Loading dose: Manufacturer recommends 10-15 mg/kg, however, 15-25 mg/kg has been used clinically; maintenance dose: 300 mg/day or 5-6 mg/kg/day in 3 divided doses or 1-2 divided doses using extended release

Anticonvulsant: Children and Adults: Oral:

Loading dose: 15-20 mg/kg; based on phenytoin serum concentrations and recent dosing history; administer oral loading dose in 3 divided doses given every 2-4 hours to decrease GI adverse effects and to ensure complete oral absorption; maintenance dose: same as I.V.

Neurosurgery (prophylactic): 100-200 mg at approximately 4-hour intervals during surgery and during the immediate postoperative period

Dosing adjustment/comments in renal impairment or hepatic disease: Safe in usual doses in mild liver disease; clearance may be substantially reduced in cirrhosis and plasma level monitoring with dose adjustment advisable. Free phenytoin levels should be monitored closely.

Mechanism of Action Stabilizes neuronal membranes and decreases seizure activity by increasing efflux or decreasing influx of sodium ions across cell membranes in the motor cortex during generation of nerve impulses; prolongs effective refractory period and suppresses ventricular pacemaker automaticity, shortens action potential in the heart

Contraindications Hypersensitivity to phenytoin, other hydantoins, or any component of the formulation; pregnancy

Warnings/Precautions May increase frequency of petit mal seizures; I.V. form may cause hypotension, skin necrosis at I.V. site; avoid I.V. administration in small veins; use with caution in patients with porphyria; discontinue if rash or lymphadenopathy occurs; a spectrum of hematologic effects have been reported with use (eg, neutropenia, leukopenia, thrombocytopenia, pancytopenia, and anemias); use with caution in patients with hepatic dysfunction, sinus bradycardia, S-A block, or AV block; use with caution in elderly or debilitated patients, or in any condition associated with low serum albumin levels, which will increase the free fraction of phenytoin in the serum and, therefore, the pharmacologic response. Sedation, confusional states, or cerebellar dysfunction (loss of motor coordination) may occur at higher total serum concentrations, or at lower total serum concentrations when the free fraction of phenytoin is increased. Effects with other sedative drugs or ethanol may be potentiated. Abrupt withdrawal may precipitate status epilepticus.

Drug Interactions

Cytochrome P450 Effect: Substrate of CYP2C9 (major), 2C19 (major), 3A4 (minor); **Induces** CYP2B6 (strong), 2C8 (strong), 2C9 (strong), 2C19 (strong), 3A4 (strong)

Increased Effect/Toxicity: The sedative effects of phenytoin may be additive with other CNS depressants including ethanol, barbiturates, sedatives, antidepressants, opioid analgesics, and benzodiazepines. Selected anticonvulsants (felbamate, gabapentin, and topiramate) have been reported to increase phenytoin levels/effects. In addition, serum phenytoin concentrations may be increased by allopurinol, amiodarone, calcium channel blockers (including diltiazem and nifedipine), cimetidine, disulfiram, methylphenidate, metronidazole, omeprazole, selective serotonin reuptake inhibitors (SSRIs), ticlopidine, tricyclic antidepressants, trazodone, and trimethoprim.

The levels/effects of phenytoin may be increased by delavirdine, fluconazole, fluvoxamine, gemfibrozil, isoniazid, ketoconazole, nicardipine, NSAIDs, omeprazole, sulfonamides, ticlopidine, tolbutamide, and other CYP2C9 or 2C19 inhibitors.

Phenytoin enhances the conversion of primidone to phenobarbital resulting in elevated phenobarbital serum concentrations. Concurrent use of acetazolamide with phenytoin may result in an increased risk of osteomalacia. Concurrent use of phenytoin and lithium has resulted in lithium intoxication. Valproic acid (and sulfisoxazole) may displace phenytoin from binding sites; valproic acid may increase, decrease, or have no effect on phenytoin serum concentrations. Phenytoin transiently increased the response to warfarin initially; this is followed by an inhibition of the hypoprothrombinemic response. Phenytoin may enhance the hepatotoxic potential of acetaminophen overdoses. Concurrent use of dopamine and intravenous phenytoin may lead to an increased risk of hypotension.

Decreased Effect: Phenytoin may enhance the metabolism of estrogen and/or oral contraceptives, decreasing their clinical effect; an alternative method of contraception should be considered. Phenytoin may increase the metabolism of anticonvulsants including barbiturates, carbamazepine, ethosuximide, felbamate, lamotrigine, tiagabine, topiramate, and zonisamide. Valproic acid may increase, decrease, or have no effect on phenytoin serum concentrations. Phenytoin may also decrease the serum concentrations/effects of some antiarrhythmics (disopyramide, propafenone, quinidine, quetiapine) and tricyclic antidepressants may be reduced by phenytoin. Phenytoin may enhance the metabolism of doxycycline, decreasing its clinical effect; higher dosages may be required. Phenytoin may increase the metabolism of chloramphenicol or itraconazole.

Phenytoin may decrease the levels/effects of amiodarone, benzodiazepines, bupropion, calcium channel blockers, carbamazepine, citalopram, clarithromycin, clozapine, cyclosporine, efavirenz, erythromycin, estrogens, fluoxetine, glimepiride, glipizide, losartan, methsuximide, mirtazapine, nateglinide, nefazodone, nevirapine, phenytoin, pioglitazone, promethazine, propranolol, protease inhibitors, proton pump inhibitors, rosiglitazone, selegiline, sertraline, sulfonamides, tacrolimus, venlafaxine. voriconazole, warfarin, zafirlukast, and other CYP2B6, 2C8, 2C9, 2C19, or 3A4 substrates.

The levels/effects of phenytoin may be decreased by aminoglutethimide, carbamazepine, phenobarbital, rifampin, rifapentine, secobarbital, and other CYP2C9 or 2C19 inducers. Clozapine and vigabatrin may reduce phenytoin serum concentrations. Ciprofloxacin may decrease serum phenytoin concentrations. Dexamethasone may decrease serum phenytoin concentrations. Replacement of folic acid has been reported to increase the metabolism of phenytoin, decreasing its serum concentrations and/or increasing seizures.

Initially, phenytoin increases the response to warfarin; this is followed by a decrease in response to warfarin. Phenytoin may inhibit the anti-Parkinson effect of levodopa. The duration of neuromuscular blockade from neuromuscular-blocking agents may be decreased by phenytoin. Phenytoin may enhance the metabolism of methadone resulting in methadone withdrawal. Phenytoin may decrease serum levels/effects of digitalis glycosides, theophylline, and thyroid hormones.

Several chemotherapeutic agents have been associated with a decrease in serum phenytoin levels; includes cisplatin, bleomycin, carmustine, methotrexate, and vinblastine. Enzyme-inducing anticonvulsant therapy may reduce the effectiveness of some chemotherapy regimens (specifically in ALL). Teniposide and methotrexate may be cleared more rapidly in these patients.

Ethanol/Nutrition/Herb Interactions

Ethanol:

Acute use: Avoid or limit ethanol (inhibits metabolism of phenytoin). Watch for sedation.

Chronic use: Avoid or limit ethanol (stimulates metabolism of phenytoin).

Food: Phenytoin serum concentrations may be altered if taken with food. If taken with enteral nutrition, phenytoin serum concentrations may be decreased. Tube feedings decrease bioavailability; hold tube feedings 1-2 hours before and 1-2 hours after phenytoin administration. May decrease calcium, folic acid, and vitamin D levels.

Herb/Nutraceutical: Avoid evening primrose (seizure threshold decreased). Avoid valerian, St John's wort, kava kava, gotu kola (may increase CNS depression).

Dietary Considerations

Folic acid: Phenytoin may decrease mucosal uptake of folic acid; to avoid folic acid deficiency and megaloblastic anemia, some clinicians recommend giving patients on anticonvulsants prophylactic doses of folic acid and cyanocobalamin. However, folate supplementation may increase seizures in some patients (dose dependent). Discuss with healthcare provider prior to using any supplements.

Calcium: Hypocalcemia has been reported in patients taking prolonged high-dose therapy with an anticonvulsant. Some clinicians have given an additional 4000 units/week of vitamin D (especially in those receiving poor nutrition and getting no sun exposure) to prevent hypocalcemia.

Vitamin D: Phenytoin interferes with vitamin D metabolism and osteomalacia may result; may need to supplement with vitamin D

Tube feedings: Tube feedings decrease phenytoin absorption. To avoid decreased serum levels with continuous NG feeds, hold feedings for 1-2 hours prior to and 1-2 hours after phenytoin administration, if possible. There is a variety of opinions on how to administer phenytoin with enteral feedings. Be **consistent** throughout therapy.

Sodium content of 1 g injection: 88 mg (3.8 mEq)

Pharmacodynamics/Kinetics

Onset of action: I.V.: ~0.5-1 hour

Absorption: Oral: Slow

(Continued)

Phenytoin (Continued)

Distribution: V_d:
  Neonates: Premature: 1-1.2 L/kg; Full-term: 0.8-0.9 L/kg
  Infants: 0.7-0.8 L/kg
  Children: 0.7 L/kg
  Adults: 0.6-0.7 L/kg
Protein binding:
  Neonates: ≥80% (≤20% free)
  Infants: ≥85% (≤15% free)
  Adults: 90% to 95%
  Others: Decreased protein binding
    Disease states resulting in a decrease in serum albumin concentration: Burns, hepatic cirrhosis, nephrotic syndrome, pregnancy, cystic fibrosis
    Disease states resulting in an apparent decrease in affinity of phenytoin for serum albumin: Renal failure, jaundice (severe), other drugs (displacers), hyperbilirubinemia (total bilirubin >15 mg/dL), Cl_{cr} <25 mL/minute (unbound fraction is increased two- to threefold in uremia)
Metabolism: Follows dose-dependent capacity-limited (Michaelis-Menten) pharmacokinetics with increased V_{max} in infants >6 months of age and children versus adults; major metabolite (via oxidation), HPPA, undergoes enterohepatic recirculation
Bioavailability: Form dependent
Half-life elimination: Oral: 22 hours (range: 7-42 hours)
Time to peak, serum (form dependent): Oral: Extended-release capsule: 4-12 hours; Immediate release preparation: 2-3 hours
Excretion: Urine (<5% as unchanged drug); as glucuronides
  Clearance: Highly variable, dependent upon intrinsic hepatic function and dose administered; increased clearance and decreased serum concentrations with febrile illness

Pregnancy Risk Factor D

Dosage Forms
  Capsule, extended release: 100 mg
    Dilantin®: 30 mg, 100 mg
    Phenytek®: 200 mg, 300 mg
  Capsule, prompt release: 100 mg
  Injection, solution: 50 mg/mL (2 mL, 5 mL)
  Suspension, oral: 100 mg/4 mL, 125 mg/5 mL
    Dilantin®: 125 mg/5 mL
  Tablet, chewable:
    Dilantin®: 50 mg

Selected Readings

Dooley G and Vasan N, "Dilantin® Hyperplasia: A Review of the Literature," *J N Z Soc Periodontol*, 1989, 68:19-22.

Iacopino AM, Doxey D, Cutler CW, et al, "Phenytoin and Cyclosporine A Specifically Regulate Macrophage Phenotype and Expression of Platelet-Derived Growth Factor and Interleukin-1 *In Vitro* and *In Vivo*: Possible Molecular Mechanism of Drug-Induced Gingival Hyperplasia," *J Periodontol*, 1997, 68(1):73-83.

Pihlstrom BL, "Prevention and Treatment of Dilantin®-Associated Gingival Enlargement," *Compendium*, 1990, 14:S506-10.

Saito K, Mori S, Iwakura M, et al, "Immunohistochemical Localization of Transforming Growth Factor Beta, Basic Fibroblast Growth Factor and Heparin Sulphate Glycosaminoglycan in Gingival Hyperplasia Induced by Nifedipine and Phenytoin," *J Periodontal Res*, 1996, 31(8):545-5.

Zhou LX, Pihlstrom B, Hardwick JP, et al, "Metabolism of Phenytoin by the Gingiva of Normal Humans: The Possible Role of Reactive Metabolites of Phenytoin in the Initiation of Gingival Hyperplasia," *Clin Pharmacol Ther*, 1996, 60(2):191-8.

Phenytoin Sodium *see* Phenytoin *on page 1295*

Phenytoin Sodium, Extended *see* Phenytoin *on page 1295*

Phenytoin Sodium, Prompt *see* Phenytoin *on page 1295*

Phillips'® M-O [OTC] *see* Magnesium Hydroxide and Mineral Oil *on page 1014*

Phillips'® Chews [OTC] *see* Magnesium Hydroxide *on page 1014*

Phillips'® Milk of Magnesia [OTC] *see* Magnesium Hydroxide *on page 1014*

Phillips'® Stool Softener Laxative [OTC] *see* Docusate *on page 522*

pHisoHex® *see* Hexachlorophene *on page 813*

Phlemex *see* Guaifenesin and Dextromethorphan *on page 796*

Phos-Flur® *see* Fluoride *on page 710*

Phos-Flur® Rinse [OTC] *see* Fluoride *on page 710*

PhosLo® *see* Calcium Acetate *on page 259*

Phos-NaK *see* Potassium Phosphate and Sodium Phosphate *on page 1332*

Phospha 250™ Neutral *see* Potassium Phosphate and Sodium Phosphate *on page 1332*

Phosphate, Potassium *see* Potassium Phosphate *on page 1332*

Phospholine Iodide® *see* Echothiophate Iodide *on page 553*

Phosphonoformate *see* Foscarnet *on page 744*

Phosphonoformic Acid *see* Foscarnet *on page 744*

Phosphorated Carbohydrate Solution *see* Fructose, Dextrose, and Phosphoric Acid *on page 754*

Phosphoric Acid, Levulose, and Dextrose *see* Fructose, Dextrose, and Phosphoric Acid *on page 754*

Photofrin® *see* Porfimer *on page 1324*

Phrenilin® *see* Butalbital and Acetaminophen *on page 249*

Phrenilin® Forte *see* Butalbital and Acetaminophen *on page 249*

p-Hydroxyampicillin *see* Amoxicillin *on page 108*

Phylloquinone *see* Phytonadione *on page 1299*

Physostigmine (fye zoe STIG meen)

Canadian Brand Names Eserine®; Isopto® Eserine
Generic Available Yes
Index Terms Eserine Salicylate; Physostigmine Salicylate; Physostigmine Sulfate
Pharmacologic Category Acetylcholinesterase Inhibitor
Use Reverse toxic CNS effects caused by anticholinergic drugs
Local Anesthetic/Vasoconstrictor Precautions No information available to require special precautions
Effects on Dental Treatment Key adverse event(s) related to dental treatment: Salivation.
Common Adverse Effects Frequency not defined.
Cardiovascular: Palpitation, bradycardia
Central nervous system: Restlessness, nervousness, hallucinations, seizure
Gastrointestinal: Nausea, salivation, diarrhea, stomach pain
Genitourinary: Frequent urge to urinate
Neuromuscular & skeletal: Muscle twitching
Ocular: Lacrimation, miosis
Respiratory: Dyspnea, bronchospasm, respiratory paralysis, pulmonary edema
Miscellaneous: Diaphoresis
Mechanism of Action Inhibits destruction of acetylcholine by acetylcholinesterase which facilitates transmission of impulses across myoneural junction and prolongs the central and peripheral effects of acetylcholine
Drug Interactions
Increased Effect/Toxicity: Increased toxicity with bethanechol, methacholine. Succinylcholine may increase neuromuscular blockade with systemic administration.
Pharmacodynamics/Kinetics
Onset of action: ~5 minutes
Duration: 0.5-5 hours
Absorption: I.M., SubQ: Readily absorbed
Distribution: Crosses blood-brain barrier readily and reverses both central and peripheral anticholinergic effects
Metabolism: Hepatic and via hydrolysis by cholinesterases
Half-life elimination: 15-40 minutes
Pregnancy Risk Factor C

Physostigmine Salicylate *see* Physostigmine *on page 1299*

Physostigmine Sulfate *see* Physostigmine *on page 1299*

Phytomenadione *see* Phytonadione *on page 1299*

Phytonadione (fye toe na DYE one)

U.S. Brand Names Mephyton®
Canadian Brand Names AquaMEPHYTON®; Konakion; Mephyton®
Mexican Brand Names Konakion (10 mg); Konakion MM Pediatric
Generic Available Yes
Index Terms Methylphytyl Napthoquinone; Phylloquinone; Phytomenadione; Vitamin K$_1$
Pharmacologic Category Vitamin, Fat Soluble
Use Prevention and treatment of hypoprothrombinemia caused by coumarin derivative-induced or other drug-induced vitamin K deficiency, hypoprothrombinemia caused by malabsorption or inability to synthesize vitamin K; hemorrhagic disease of the newborn
Local Anesthetic/Vasoconstrictor Precautions No information available to require special precautions
Effects on Dental Treatment Key adverse event(s) related to dental treatment: Abnormal taste.
(Continued)

Phytonadione *(Continued)*

Common Adverse Effects Parenteral administration: Frequency not defined.
Cardiovascular: Cyanosis, flushing, hypotension
Central nervous system: Dizziness
Dermatologic: Scleroderma-like lesions
Endocrine & metabolic: Hyperbilirubinemia (newborn; greater than recommended doses)
Gastrointestinal: Abnormal taste
Local: Injection site reactions
Respiratory: Dyspnea
Miscellaneous: Anaphylactoid reactions, diaphoresis, hypersensitivity reactions

Mechanism of Action Promotes liver synthesis of clotting factors (II, VII, IX, X); however, the exact mechanism as to this stimulation is unknown. Menadiol is a water soluble form of vitamin K; phytonadione has a more rapid and prolonged effect than menadione; menadiol sodium diphosphate (K_4) is half as potent as menadione (K_3).

Drug Interactions
Decreased Effect: Phytonadione may diminish the anticoagulant effect of coumarin derivatives (monitor INR). Phytonadione (oral) may not be properly absorbed when administered concurrently with orlistat (separate doses by at least 2 hours).

Pharmacodynamics/Kinetics
Onset of action: Increased coagulation factors: Oral: 6-10 hours; I.V.: 1-2 hours
Peak effect: INR values return to normal: Oral: 24-48 hours; I.V.: 12-14 hours
Absorption: Oral: From intestines in presence of bile; SubQ: Variable
Metabolism: Rapidly hepatic
Excretion: Urine and feces

Pregnancy Risk Factor C

α_1-PI *see* Alpha$_1$-Proteinase Inhibitor *on page 74*
Pidorubicin *see* Epirubicin *on page 577*
Pidorubicin Hydrochloride *see* Epirubicin *on page 577*
Pilocar® *see* Pilocarpine (Ophthalmic) *on page 1300*
Pilocarpine Hydrochloride *see* Pilocarpine (Ophthalmic) *on page 1300*
Pilocarpine Nitrate *see* Pilocarpine (Ophthalmic) *on page 1300*

Pilocarpine (Ophthalmic) *(pye loe KAR peen op THAL mik)*

U.S. Brand Names Isopto® Carpine; Pilocar®; Pilopine HS®; Piloptic®
Canadian Brand Names Diocarpine; Isopto® Carpine; Pilopine HS®
Mexican Brand Names Pilo Grin
Generic Available Yes: Hydrochloride solution
Index Terms Pilocarpine Hydrochloride; Pilocarpine Nitrate
Pharmacologic Category Cholinergic Agonist; Ophthalmic Agent, Antiglaucoma; Ophthalmic Agent, Miotic
Dental Use Treatment of xerostomia caused by radiation therapy in patients with head and neck cancer and from Sjögren's syndrome
Use Ophthalmic: Management of chronic simple glaucoma, chronic and acute angle-closure glaucoma
Unlabeled/Investigational Use Counter effects of cycloplegics
Local Anesthetic/Vasoconstrictor Precautions No information available to require special precautions
Effects on Dental Treatment No significant effects or complications reported
Significant Adverse Effects Ophthalmic (frequency not defined):
Gastrointestinal: Diarrhea
Ocular: Burning, ciliary spasm, conjunctival vascular congestion, corneal granularity (gel 10%), lacrimation, lens opacity, myopia, retinal detachment,
Respiratory: Pulmonary edema
Dental Usual Dosing Treatment of xerostomia: Adults: Oral: 1-2 tablets 3-4 times/day not to exceed 30 mg/day (minimum 90-day therapy required for optimum effects)
Dosage Adults:
Ophthalmic:
Glaucoma:
Solution: Instill 1-2 drops up to 6 times/day; adjust the concentration and frequency as required to control elevated intraocular pressure
Gel: Instill 0.5" ribbon into lower conjunctival sac once daily at bedtime.
Ocular systems: Systems are labeled in terms of mean rate of release of pilocarpine over 7 days; begin with 20 mcg/hour at night and adjust based on response.

To counteract the mydriatic effects of sympathomimetic agents (unlabeled use): Solution: Instill 1 drop of a 1% solution into the affected eye(s).

Mechanism of Action Directly stimulates cholinergic receptors in the eye causing miosis (by contraction of the iris sphincter), loss of accommodation (by constriction of ciliary muscle), and lowering of intraocular pressure (with decreased resistance to aqueous humor outflow)

Contraindications Hypersensitivity to pilocarpine or any component of the formulation; acute inflammatory disease of the anterior chamber of the eye

Warnings/Precautions May cause decreased visual acuity, especially at night or with reduced lighting.

Drug Interactions Inhibits CYP2A6 (weak), 2E1 (weak), 3A4 (weak)
Concurrent use with beta-blockers may cause conduction disturbances. Pilocarpine may antagonize the effects of anticholinergic drugs.

Ethanol/Nutrition/Herb Interactions Food: Avoid administering oral formulation with high-fat meal; fat decreases the rate of absorption, maximum concentration and increases the time it takes to reach maximum concentration.

Pharmacodynamics/Kinetics Ophthalmic:
Onset of action:
Miosis: 10-30 minutes
Intraocular pressure reduction: 1 hour
Duration:
Miosis: 4-8 hours
Intraocular pressure reduction: 4-12 hours

Pregnancy Risk Factor C

Lactation Excretion in breast milk unknown/not recommended

Breast-Feeding Considerations The excretion in breast milk is unknown; however, breast-feeding in women receiving this medication is not recommended.

Dosage Forms
Gel, ophthalmic, as hydrochloride (Pilopine HS®): 4% (3.5 g) [contains benzalkonium chloride]
Solution, ophthalmic, as hydrochloride: 1% (15 mL); 2% (15 mL); 4% (15 mL); 6% (15 mL) [may contain benzalkonium chloride]
Isopto® Carpine: 1% (15 mL); 2% (15 mL, 30 mL); 4% (15 mL, 30 mL); 6% (15 mL); 8% (15 mL) [contains benzalkonium chloride]
Pilocar®: 0.5% (15 mL); 1% (1 mL, 15 mL); 2% (1 mL, 15 mL); 3% (15 mL); 4% (1 mL, 15 mL); 6% (15 mL) [contains benzalkonium chloride]
Piloptic®: 0.5% (15 mL); 1% (15 mL); 2% (15 mL); 3% (15 mL); 4% (15 mL); 6% (15 mL) [contains benzalkonium chloride]

Dental Comment Pilocarpine may have potential as a salivary stimulant in individuals suffering from xerostomia induced by antidepressants and other medications. At the present time however, the FDA has not approved pilocarpine for use in drug-induced xerostomia (clinical studies required). In an attempt to discern the efficacy of pilocarpine as a salivary stimulant in patients suffering from Sjögren's syndrome (SS), Rhodus and Schuh studied 9 patients with SS given daily doses of pilocarpine over a 6-week period. A dose of 5 mg daily produced a significant overall increase in both whole unstimulated salivary flow and parotid stimulated salivary flow. These results support the use of pilocarpine to increase salivary flow in patients with SS.

Pilocarpine (Oral) (pye loe KAR peen OR al)

Related Information
Dentin Hypersensitivity, High Caries Index, and Xerostomia *on page 1812*
Management of Patients Undergoing Cancer Therapy *on page 1826*
Pilocarpine (Ophthalmic) *on page 1300*

U.S. Brand Names Salagen®

Canadian Brand Names Salagen®

Generic Available No

Pharmacologic Category Cholinergic Agonist

Dental Use Treatment of xerostomia caused by radiation therapy in patients with head and neck cancer and from Sjögren's syndrome

Use Treatment of xerostomia caused by radiation therapy in patients with head and neck cancer and from Sjögren's syndrome

Local Anesthetic/Vasoconstrictor Precautions No information available to require special precautions

Effects on Dental Treatment Key adverse event(s) related to dental treatment: Increased salivation (therapeutic effect). See Dental Comment.

Significant Adverse Effects Oral (frequency varies by indication and dose):
>10%: Genitourinary: Urinary frequency (9% to 12%)
1% to 10%:
Cardiovascular: Edema (<1% to 5%)
(Continued)

Pilocarpine (Oral) *(Continued)*

Dermatologic: Pruritus, rash

Gastrointestinal: Diarrhea (4% to 7%), constipation, flatulence

Genitourinary: Vaginitis, urinary incontinence

Neuromuscular & skeletal: Myalgias

Ocular: Lacrimation (6%), amblyopia (4%), conjunctivitis

Otic: Tinnitus

Miscellaneous: Allergic reaction, voice alteration

<1%: Abnormal dreams, abnormal thinking, alopecia, angina pectoris, anorexia, anxiety, aphasia, appetite increased, arrhythmia, arthralgia, arthritis, bilirubinemia, body odor, bone disorder, bradycardia, breast pain, bronchitis, cataract, cholelithiasis, colitis, confusion, contact dermatitis, cyst, deafness, depression, dry eyes, dry mouth, dry skin, dyspnea, dysuria, ear pain, ECG abnormality, eczema, emotional lability, eructation, erythema nodosum, esophagitis, exfoliative dermatitis, eye hemorrhage, eye pain, gastritis, gastroenteritis, gastrointestinal disorder, gingivitis, glaucoma, hematuria, hepatitis, herpes simplex, hiccup, hyperkinesias, hypesthesia, hypoglycemia, hypotension, hypothermia, insomnia, intracranial hemorrhage, laryngismus, laryngitis, leg cramps, leukopenia, liver function test abnormal, lymphadenopathy, mastitis, melena, menorrhagia, metrorrhagia, migraine, moniliasis, myasthenia, MI, neck pain, photosensitivity reaction, nervousness, ovarian disorder, pancreatitis, paresthesias, parotid gland enlargement, peripheral edema, platelet abnormality, pneumonia, pyuria, salivary gland enlargement, salpingitis, seborrhea, skin ulcer, speech disorder, sputum increased, stridor, syncope, taste loss, tendon disorder, tenosynovitis, thrombocythemia, thrombocytopenia, thrombosis, tongue disorder, twitching, urethral pain, urinary impairment, urinary urgency, vaginal hemorrhage, vaginal moniliasis, vesiculobullous rash, WBC abnormality, yawning

Dental Usual Dosing Treatment of xerostomia: Adults: Oral: 1-2 tablets 3-4 times/day not to exceed 30 mg/day (minimum 90-day therapy required for optimum effects)

Dosage Oral: Adults: 1-2 tablets 3-4 times/day not to exceed 30 mg/day (minimum 90-day therapy required for optimum effects)

Mechanism of Action Stimulates the muscarinic-type acetylcholine receptors in the salivary glands within the parasympathetic division of the autonomic nervous system to cause an increase in serous-type saliva

Contraindications Hypersensitivity to pilocarpine or any component of the formulation; uncontrolled asthma, angle-closure glaucoma, severe hepatic impairment

Warnings/Precautions Use caution with cardiovascular disease (patients may have difficulty compensating for transient changes in hemodynamics or rhythm induced by pilocarpine); controlled asthma, chronic bronchitis, or COPD (may increase airway resistance, bronchial smooth muscle tone, bronchial secretions); cholelithiasis, biliary tract disease, and nephrolithiasis. Adjust dose with moderate hepatic impairment.

Drug Interactions Increased Effect/Toxicity: Concurrent use with anticholinergics may cause antagonism of pilocarpine's cholinergic effect; medications with cholinergic actions may result in additive cholinergic effects. Beta-adrenergic receptor blocking drugs when used with pilocarpine may increase the possibility of myocardial conduction disturbances.

Pharmacodynamics/Kinetics

Onset of action: 20 minutes after single dose

Duration: 3-5 hours

Half-life, elimination: 0.76 hours

Time to peak: 1.25 hours

Pregnancy Risk Factor C

Breast-Feeding Considerations The excretion in breast milk is unknown; however, breast-feeding in women receiving this medication is not recommended.

Dosage Forms Tablet, as hydrochloride (Salagen®): 5 mg, 7.5 mg

Dental Comment Pilocarpine may have potential as a salivary stimulant in individuals suffering from xerostomia induced by antidepressants and other medications. At the present time however, the FDA has not approved pilocarpine for use in drug-induced xerostomia (clinical studies required). In an attempt to discern the efficacy of pilocarpine as a salivary stimulant in patients suffering from Sjögren's syndrome (SS), Rhodus and Schuh studied 9 patients with SS given daily doses of pilocarpine over a 6-week period. A dose of 5 mg daily produced a significant overall increase in both whole unstimulated salivary flow and parotid stimulated salivary flow. These results support the use of pilocarpine to increase salivary flow in patients with SS.

Selected Readings

Davies AN and Singer J, "A Comparison of Artificial Saliva and Pilocarpine in Radiation-Induced Xerostomia," *J Laryngol Otol*, 1994, 108(8):663-5.

Fox PC, "Management of Dry Mouth," *Dent Clin North Am*, 1997, 41(4):863-75.

Fox PC, Atkinson JC, Macynski AA, et al, "Pilocarpine Treatment of Salivary Gland Hypofunction and Dry Mouth (Xerostomia)," *Arch Intern Med*, 1991, 151(6):1149-52.

Fox PC, "Salivary Enhancement Therapies," *Caries Res*, 2004, 38(3):241-6.

Garg AK and Malo M, "Manifestations and Treatment of Xerostomia and Associated Oral Effects Secondary to Head and Neck Radiation Therapy," *J Am Dent Assoc*, 1997, 128(8):1128-33.

Gotrick B, Akerman S, Ericson D, et al, "Oral Pilocarpine for Treatment of Opioid-Induced Oral Dryness in Healthy Adults," *J Dent Res*, 2004, 83(5):393-7.

Hendrickson RG, Morocco AP, and Greenberg MI, "Pilocarpine Toxicity and the Treatment of Xerostomia," *J Emerg Med*, 2004, 26(4):429-32.

Johnson JT, Ferretti GA, Nethery WJ, et al, "Oral Pilocarpine for Postirradiation Xerostomia in Patients With Head and Neck Cancer," *N Engl J Med*, 1993, 329(6):390-5.

Mosqueda-Taylor A, Luna-Ortiz K, Irigoyen-Camacho ME, et al, "Effect of Pilocarpine Hydrochloride on Salivary Production in Previously Irradiated Head and Neck Cancer Patients," *Med Oral*, 2004, 9(3):204-11.

Nagler RM and Laufer D, "Protection Against Irradiation-Induced Damage to Salivary Glands by Adrenergic Agonist Administration," *Int J Radiat Oncol Biol Phys*, 1998, 40(2):477-81.

Nelson JD, Friedlaender M, Yeatts RP, et al, "Oral Pilocarpine for Symptomatic Relief of Keratocon-junctivitis Sicca in Patients With Sjögren's Syndrome. The MGI PHARMA Sjögren's Syndrome Study Group," *Adv Exp Med Biol*, 1998, 438:979-83.

Rhodus NL and Schuh MJ, "Effects of Pilocarpine on Salivary Flow in Patients With Sjögren's Syndrome," *Oral Surg Oral Med Oral Pathol*, 1991, 72(5):545-9.

Rieke JW, Hafermann MD, Johnson JT, et al, "Oral Pilocarpine for Radiation-Induced Xerostomia: Integrated Efficacy and Safety Results From Two Prospective Randomized Clinical Trials," *Int J Radiat Oncol Biol Phys*, 1995, 31(3):661-9.

Rousseau P, "Pilocarpine in Radiation-Induced Xerostomia," *Am J Hosp Palliat Care*, 1995, 12(2):38-9.

Schuller DE, Stevens P, Clausen KP, et al, "Treatment of Radiation Side Effects With Pilocarpine," *J Surg Oncol*, 1989, 42(4):272-6.

Singhal S, Mehta J, Rattenbury H, et al, "Oral Pilocarpine Hydrochloride for the Treatment of Refractory Xerostomia Associated With Chronic Graft-Versus-Host Disease," *Blood*, 1995, 85(4):1147-8.

Valdez IH, Wolff A, Atkinson JC, et al, "Use of Pilocarpine During Head and Neck Radiation Therapy to Reduce Xerostomia Salivary Dysfunction," *Cancer*, 1993, 71(5):1848-51.

Wiseman LR and Faulds D, "Oral Pilocarpine: A Review of Its Pharmacological Properties and Clinical Potential in Xerostomia," *Drugs*, 1995, 49(1):143-55.

Wynn RL, "Oral Pilocarpine (Salagen®) - A Recently Approved Salivary Stimulant," *Gen Dent*, 1996, 44(1):26,29-30.

Zimmerman RP, Mark RJ, Tran LM, et al, "Concomitant Pilocarpine During Head and Neck Irradia-tion Is Associated With Decreased Post-Treatment Xerostomia," *Int J Radiat Oncol Biol Phys*, 1997, 37(3):571-5.

Pilopine HS® *see* Pilocarpine (Ophthalmic) *on page 1300*

Piloptic® *see* Pilocarpine (Ophthalmic) *on page 1300*

Pima® *see* Potassium Iodide *on page 1330*

Pimaricin *see* Natamycin *on page 1154*

Pimecrolimus (pim e KROE li mus)

U.S. Brand Names Elidel®
Canadian Brand Names Elidel®
Mexican Brand Names Elidel
Generic Available No
Pharmacologic Category Immunosuppressant Agent; Topical Skin Product
Use Short-term and intermittent long-term treatment of mild to moderate atopic dermatitis in patients not responsive to conventional therapy or when conventional therapy is not appropriate

Local Anesthetic/Vasoconstrictor Precautions No information available to require special precautions

Effects on Dental Treatment No significant effects or complications reported

Common Adverse Effects
>10%:
   Central nervous system: Headache (7% to 25%), pyrexia (1% to 13%)
   Local: Burning at application site (2% to 26%; tends to resolve/improve as lesions resolve)
   Respiratory: Nasopharyngitis (8% to 27%), cough (2% to 16%), upper respiratory tract infection (4% to 19%), bronchitis (0.4% to 11%)
   Miscellaneous: Influenza (3% to 13%)
1% to 10%:
   Dermatologic: Skin papilloma (warts) (up to 3%), molluscum contagiosum (0.7% to 2%), herpes simplex dermatitis (up to 2%)
   Gastrointestinal: Diarrhea (0.6% to 8%), constipation (up to 4%)
   Local: Irritation at application site (0.4% to 6%), erythema at application site (0.4% to 2%), pruritus at application site (0.6% to 6%)
   Ocular: Eye infection (up to 1%)
   Otic: Ear infection (0.6% to 6%)
   Respiratory: Pharyngitis (0.7% to 8%), sinusitis (0.6% to 3%), nasal conges-tion (0.6% to 3%)
   Miscellaneous: Viral infection (up to 7%), herpes simplex infection (0.4% to 4%), tonsillitis (0.4% to 6%)
(Continued)

Pimecrolimus (Continued)

Restrictions An FDA-approved medication guide must be distributed when dispensing an outpatient prescription (new or refill) where this medication is to be used without direct supervision of a healthcare provider. Medication guides are available at http://www.fda.gov/cder/Offices/ODS/medication_guides.htm.

Dosage Children ≥2 years and Adults: Topical: Apply thin layer to affected area twice daily; rub in gently and completely. **Note:** Limit application to involved areas. Continue as long as signs and symptoms persist; discontinue if resolution occurs; re-evaluate if symptoms persist >6 weeks.

Mechanism of Action Penetrates inflamed epidermis to inhibit T cell activation by blocking transcription of proinflammatory cytokine genes such as interleukin-2, interferon gamma (Th1-type), interleukin-4, and interleukin-10 (Th2-type). Blocks catalytic function of calcineurin. Prevents release of inflammatory cytokines and mediators from mast cells *in vitro* after stimulation by antigen/IgE.

Contraindications Hypersensitivity to pimecrolimus or any component of the formulation; Netherton's syndrome

Warnings/Precautions [U.S. Boxed Warning]: Topical calcineurin inhibitors have been associated with rare cases of malignancy. Avoid use on malignant or premalignant skin conditions (eg, cutaneous T-cell lymphoma). Topical calcineurin agents are considered second-line therapies in the treatment of atopic dermatitis/eczema, and should be limited to use in patients who have failed treatment with other therapies. **[U.S. Boxed Warning]: They should be used for short-term and intermittent treatment using the minimum amount necessary for the control of symptoms should be used.** Application should be limited to involved areas. Safety of intermittent use for >1 year has not been established.

Should not be used in immunocompromised patients. Do not apply to areas of active viral infection; infections at the treatment site should be cleared prior to therapy. Patients with atopic dermatitis are predisposed to skin infections, and tacrolimus therapy has been associated with risk of developing eczema herpeticum, varicella zoster, and herpes simplex. May be associated with development of lymphadenopathy; possible infectious causes should be investigated. Discontinue use in patients with unknown cause of lymphadenopathy or acute infectious mononucleosis. Not recommended for use in patients with skin -disease which may increase systemic absorption (eg, Netherton's syndrome). Avoid artificial or natural sunlight exposure, even when Elidel® is not on the skin. Safety not established in patients with generalized erythroderma. **[U.S. Boxed Warning]: The use of Elidel® in children <2 years of age is not recommended,** particularly since the effect on immune system development is unknown.

Drug Interactions
Cytochrome P450 Effect: Substrate of CYP3A4 (minor)
Increased Effect/Toxicity: CYP3A inhibitors may increase pimecrolimus levels in patients where increased absorption expected.

Pharmacodynamics/Kinetics Absorption: Poor when applied to 13% to 62% body surface area for up to a year

Pregnancy Risk Factor C

Dosage Forms
Cream, topical:
Elidel®: 1% (30 g, 60 g, 100 g)

Pimozide (PI moe zide)

U.S. Brand Names Orap®
Canadian Brand Names Apo-Pimozide®; Orap®
Generic Available No
Pharmacologic Category Antipsychotic Agent, Typical
Use Suppression of severe motor and phonic tics in patients with Tourette's disorder who have failed to respond satisfactorily to standard treatment

Unlabeled/Investigational Use Psychosis; reported use in individuals with delusions focused on physical symptoms (ie, preoccupation with parasitic infestation); Huntington's chorea

Local Anesthetic/Vasoconstrictor Precautions Pimozide is one of the drugs confirmed to prolong the QT interval and is accepted as having a risk of causing torsade de pointes. The risk of drug-induced torsade de pointes is extremely low when a single QT interval prolonging drug is prescribed. In terms of epinephrine, it is not known what effect vasoconstrictors in the local anesthetic regimen will have in patients with a known history of congenital prolonged QT interval or in patients taking any medication that prolongs the QT interval. Until more information is obtained, it is suggested that the clinician consult with the physician prior to the use of a vasoconstrictor in suspected patients, and that the vasoconstrictor (epinephrine, levonordefrin [Neo-Cobefrin®]) be used with caution.

Effects on Dental Treatment Key adverse event(s) related to dental treatment: Tourette's disorder: Xerostomia and increased salivation (normal salivary flow resumes upon discontinuation), taste disturbance, and dysphagia.

Common Adverse Effects

Frequencies >1% reported in adults (limited data) and/or children with Tourette's disorder:

Cardiovascular: Abnormal ECG (3%)

Central nervous system: Somnolence (up to 28% in children), sedation (14%), akathisia (8%), drowsiness (7%), hyperkinesias (6%), insomnia (2%), depression (2%), headache (1%), nervousness (1% to 8%)

Dermatologic: Rash (8%)

Gastrointestinal: Xerostomia (25%), constipation (20%), increased salivation (14%), diarrhea (5%), thirst (5%), appetite increased (5%), taste disturbance (5%), dysphagia (3%)

Genitourinary: Impotence (15%)

Neuromuscular & skeletal: Weakness (22%), muscle tightness (15%), rigidity (10%), myalgia (3%), torticollis (3%), tremor (3%)

Ocular: Visual disturbance (6% to 20%), accommodation decreased (20%)

Miscellaneous: Speech disorder (10%)

Frequency not established (reported in disorders other than Tourette's disorder): Blood dyscrasias, breast edema, chest pain, dizziness, extrapyramidal symptoms (akathisia, akinesia, dystonia, pseudoparkinsonism, tardive dyskinesia); facial edema, gingival hyperplasia (case report), hyper-/hypotension, hyponatremia, jaundice, libido decreased, neuroleptic malignant syndrome, orthostatic hypotension, palpitation, periorbital edema, postural hypotension, QT_c prolongation, seizure, tachycardia, ventricular arrhythmia, vomiting, weight gain/loss

Mechanism of Action Pimozide, a diphenylbutylperidine antipsychotic, is a potent centrally-acting dopamine-receptor antagonist resulting in its characteristic neuroleptic effects

Drug Interactions

Cytochrome P450 Effect: Substrate (major) of CYP1A2, 3A4; **Inhibits** CYP2C19 (weak), 2D6 (weak), 2E1 (weak), 3A4 (weak)

Increased Effect/Toxicity: Concurrent use with QT_c-prolonging agents is contraindicated including Class Ia and Class III antiarrhythmics, arsenic trioxide, chlorpromazine, dolasetron, droperidol, levomethadyl, mefloquine, pentamidine, probucol, tacrolimus, ziprasidone, mesoridazine, thioridazine, tricyclic antidepressants, and some quinolone antibiotics (sparfloxacin, moxifloxacin, and gatifloxacin).

CYP1A2 inhibitors may increase the levels/effects of pimozide; example inhibitors include ciprofloxacin, fluvoxamine, ketoconazole, norfloxacin, ofloxacin, and rofecoxib. Chloroquine, propranolol, and sulfadoxine-pyrimethamine also may increase pimozide concentrations. Concurrent use with TCA may produce increased toxicity or altered therapeutic response. Pimozide plus lithium may (rarely) produce neurotoxicity. Pimozide and CNS depressants (ethanol, opioid analgesics) may produce additive CNS depressant effects. Pimozide with fluoxetine has been associated with the development of bradycardia (case report). Metoclopramide may increase risk of extrapyramidal symptoms (EPS). Acetylcholinesterase inhibitors (central) may increase the risk of antipsychotic-related EPS. Macrolide antibiotics may increase the effects of pimozide; **Note:** The manufacturer lists azithromycin and dirithromycin in its list of contraindicated macrolides; however, these drugs do not inhibit CYP3A4 and are not expected to interact with pimozide.

CYP3A4 inhibitors may increase the levels/effects of pimozide; example inhibitors include azole antifungals, clarithromycin, diclofenac, doxycycline, erythromycin, imatinib, isoniazid, nefazodone, nicardipine, propofol, protease inhibitors, quinidine, telithromycin, and verapamil. Concurrent use of strong CYP3A4 inhibitors with pimozide is contraindicated.

Decreased Effect: CYP1A2 inducers may decrease the levels/effects of pimozide; example inducers include aminoglutethimide, carbamazepine, phenobarbital, and rifampin. CYP3A4 inducers may decrease the levels/effects of pimozide; example inducers include aminoglutethimide, carbamazepine, nafcillin, nevirapine, phenobarbital, phenytoin, and rifamycins. Benztropine (and other anticholinergics) may inhibit the therapeutic response to pimozide. Antipsychotics such as pimozide inhibit the ability of bromocriptine to lower serum prolactin concentrations. The antihypertensive effects of guanethidine and guanadrel may be inhibited by pimozide. Pimozide may inhibit the antiparkinsonian effect of levodopa. Pimozide (and possibly other low potency antipsychotics) may reverse the pressor effects of epinephrine. (Continued)

Pimozide *(Continued)*

Pharmacodynamics/Kinetics
Absorption: 50%
Protein binding: 99%
Metabolism: Hepatic; significant first-pass effect
Half-life elimination: 50 hours
Time to peak, serum: 6-8 hours
Excretion: Urine

Pregnancy Risk Factor C

Pin-X® [OTC] *see Pyrantel Pamoate on page 1387*

Pindolol *(PIN doe lole)*

Related Information
Cardiovascular Diseases *on page 1726*

Canadian Brand Names Apo-Pindol®; Gen-Pindolol; Novo-Pindol; Nu-Pindol; PMS-Pindolol; Visken®

Mexican Brand Names Visken

Generic Available Yes

Pharmacologic Category Beta Blocker With Intrinsic Sympathomimetic Activity

Use Management of hypertension

Unlabeled/Investigational Use Potential augmenting agent for antidepressants; ventricular arrhythmias/tachycardia, antipsychotic-induced akathisia, situational anxiety; aggressive behavior associated with dementia

Local Anesthetic/Vasoconstrictor Precautions Use with caution; epinephrine has interacted with nonselective beta-blockers to result in initial hypertensive episode followed by bradycardia

Effects on Dental Treatment Pindolol is a nonselective beta-blocker and may enhance the pressor response to epinephrine, resulting in hypertension and bradycardia. Many nonsteroidal anti-inflammatory drugs, such as ibuprofen and indomethacin, can reduce the hypotensive effect of beta-blockers after 3 or more weeks of therapy with the NSAID. Short-term NSAID use (ie, 3 days) requires no special precautions in patients taking beta-blockers.

Common Adverse Effects 1% to 10%:
Cardiovascular: Chest pain (3%), edema (6%)
Central nervous system: Nightmares/vivid dreams (5%), dizziness (9%), insomnia (10%), fatigue (8%), nervousness (7%), anxiety (<2%)
Dermatologic: Rash, itching (4%)
Gastrointestinal: Nausea (5%), abdominal discomfort (4%)
Neuromuscular & skeletal: Weakness (4%), paresthesia (3%), arthralgia (7%), muscle pain (10%)
Respiratory: Dyspnea (5%)

Mechanism of Action Blocks both beta$_1$- and beta$_2$-receptors and has mild intrinsic sympathomimetic activity; pindolol has negative inotropic and chronotropic effects and can significantly slow AV nodal conduction. Augmentive action of antidepressants thought to be mediated via a serotonin 1A autoreceptor antagonism.

Drug Interactions
Cytochrome P450 Effect: Substrate of CYP2D6 (major); **Inhibits** CYP2D6 (weak)

Increased Effect/Toxicity: CYP2D6 inhibitors may increase the levels/effects of pindolol; example inhibitors include chlorpromazine, delavirdine, fluoxetine, miconazole, paroxetine, pergolide, quinidine, quinine, ritonavir, and ropinirole. Pindolol may increase the effects of other drugs which slow AV conduction (digoxin, verapamil, diltiazem), alpha-blockers (prazosin, terazosin), and alpha-adrenergic stimulants (epinephrine, phenylephrine). Pindolol may mask the tachycardia from hypoglycemia caused by insulin and oral hypoglycemics. In patients receiving concurrent therapy, the risk of hypertensive crisis is increased when either clonidine or the beta-blocker is withdrawn. Reserpine has been shown to enhance the effect of beta-blockers. Beta-blockers may increase the action or levels of ethanol, disopyramide, nondepolarizing muscle relaxants, and theophylline although the effects are difficult to predict.

Decreased Effect: Decreased levels/effect of pindolol with aluminum salts, barbiturates, calcium salts, cholestyramine, colestipol, NSAIDs, penicillins (ampicillin), rifampin, salicylates, and sulfinpyrazone due to decreased bioavailability and plasma levels. Beta-blockers may decrease the effect of sulfonylureas (possibly hyperglycemia). Nonselective beta-blockers blunt the effect of beta-2 adrenergic agonists (albuterol).

Pharmacodynamics/Kinetics

Absorption: Rapid, 50% to 95%

Protein binding: 50%

Metabolism: Hepatic (60% to 65%) to conjugates

Half-life elimination: 2.5-4 hours; prolonged with renal impairment, age, and cirrhosis

Time to peak, serum: 1-2 hours

Excretion: Urine (35% to 50% as unchanged drug)

Pregnancy Risk Factor B

Pink Bismuth *see* Bismuth *on page 217*

Pioglitazone (pye oh GLI ta zone)

U.S. Brand Names Actos®

Canadian Brand Names Actos®

Mexican Brand Names Zactos

Generic Available No

Pharmacologic Category Antidiabetic Agent, Thiazolidinedione

Use

Type 2 diabetes mellitus (noninsulin dependent, NIDDM), monotherapy: Adjunct to diet and exercise, to improve glycemic control

Type 2 diabetes mellitus (noninsulin dependent, NIDDM), combination therapy with sulfonylurea, metformin, or insulin: When diet, exercise, and a single agent alone does not result in adequate glycemic control

Unlabeled/Investigational Use

Polycystic ovary syndrome (PCOS)

Local Anesthetic/Vasoconstrictor Precautions No information available to require special precautions

Effects on Dental Treatment Key adverse event(s) related to dental treatment: Tooth disorder. Pioglitazone-dependent diabetics should be appointed for dental treatment in morning in order to minimize chance of stress-induced hypoglycemia.

Common Adverse Effects

>10%:

Cardiovascular: Edema (5%; in combination trials with sulfonlyureas or insulin, the incidence of edema was as high as 15%)

Respiratory: Upper respiratory tract infection (13%)

1% to 10%:

Cardiovascular: Heart failure (requiring hospitalization; up to 6% in patients with prior macrovascular disease)

Central nervous system: Headache (9%), fatigue (4%)

Gastrointestinal: Tooth disorder (5%)

Hematologic: Anemia (≤2%)

Neuromuscular & skeletal: Myalgia (5%)

Respiratory: Sinusitis (6%), pharyngitis (5%)

Frequency not defined: HDL-cholesterol increased, hypoglycemia (in combination trials with sulfonylureas or insulin), serum triglycerides decreased, weight gain/loss

Dosage Oral:

Adults:

Monotherapy: Initial: 15-30 mg once daily; if response is inadequate, the dosage may be increased in increments up to 45 mg once daily; maximum recommended dose: 45 mg once daily

Combination therapy: Maximum recommended dose: 45 mg/day

With sulfonylureas: Initial: 15-30 mg once daily; dose of sulfonylurea should be reduced if the patient reports hypoglycemia

With metformin: Initial: 15-30 mg once daily; it is unlikely that the dose of metformin will need to be reduced due to hypoglycemia

With insulin: Initial: 15-30 mg once daily; dose of insulin should be reduced by 10% to 25% if the patient reports hypoglycemia or if the plasma glucose falls to <100 mg/dL.

Dosage adjustment in patients with CHF (NYHA Class II) in mono- or combination therapy: Initial: 15 mg once daily; may be increased after several months of treatment, with close attention to heart failure symptoms

Elderly: No dosage adjustment is recommended in elderly patients.

Dosage adjustment in renal impairment: No dosage adjustment is required.

Dosage adjustment in hepatic impairment: Clearance is significantly lower in hepatic impairment (Child-Pugh Grade B/C). Therapy should not be initiated if the patient exhibits active liver disease or increased transaminases (>2.5 times ULN) at baseline. During treatment if ALT levels elevate >3 times ULN, the test should be repeated as soon as possible. If ALT levels remain >3 times ULN or if the patient is jaundiced, therapy should be discontinued.

(Continued)

Pioglitazone *(Continued)*

Mechanism of Action Thiazolidinedione antidiabetic agent that lowers blood glucose by improving target cell response to insulin, without increasing pancreatic insulin secretion. It has a mechanism of action that is dependent on the presence of insulin for activity. Pioglitazone is a potent and selective agonist for peroxisome proliferator-activated receptor-gamma (PPARgamma). Activation of nuclear PPARgamma receptors influences the production of a number of gene products involved in glucose and lipid metabolism. PPARgamma is abundant in the cells within the renal collecting tubules; fluid retention results from stimulation by thiazolidinediones which increases sodium reabsorption.

Contraindications Hypersensitivity to pioglitazone or any component of the formulation; active liver disease (transaminases >2.5 times the upper limit of normal at baseline); patients who have experienced jaundice during troglitazone therapy

Warnings/Precautions Should not be used in diabetic ketoacidosis. Mechanism requires the presence of insulin, therefore use in type 1 diabetes is not recommended. May potentiate hypoglycemia when used in combination with sulfonylureas or insulin. Use with caution in premenopausal, anovulatory women - may result in a resumption of ovulation, increasing the risk of pregnancy. Use with caution in patients with anemia (may reduce hemoglobin and hematocrit). Use with caution in patients with edema; may increase plasma volume and/or increase cardiac hypertrophy. Monitor closely for signs and symptoms of heart failure (including weight gain, edema, or dyspnea). Not recommended for use in patients with NYHA Class III or IV heart failure. In patients with NYHA class II (systolic) heart failure, initiate at lowest dosage and monitor closely. Discontinue if heart failure develops.

Use with caution in patients with minor elevations in transaminases (AST or ALT). Idiosyncratic hepatotoxicity has been reported with another thiazolidinedione agent (troglitazone) and postmarketing case reports of hepatitis (with rare hepatic failure) have been received for pioglitazone. Monitoring should include periodic determinations of liver function. Use caution with pre-existing macular edema or diabetic retinopathy. Postmarketing reports of new-onset or worsening diabetic macular edema with decreased visual acuity has been reported. Safety and efficacy have not been established in children.

Drug Interactions

Cytochrome P450 Effect: Substrate of CYP2C8 (major), 3A4 (minor); **Inhibits** CYP2C8 (moderate), 2C9 (weak), 2C19 (weak), 2D6 (moderate); **Induces** CYP3A4 (weak)

Increased Effect/Toxicity: Concomitant use with thioridazine is contraindicated, due to a risk of arrhythmias. The levels/effects of pioglitazone may be increased by atazanavir, gemfibrozil, ritonavir, and other CYP2C8 inhibitors. Pioglitazone level/effect may be increased if trimethoprim, and pioglitazone effect on fluid retention may be enhanced with pregabalin.

Pioglitazone may increase the levels/effects of amiodarone, amphetamines, selected beta-blockers, dextromethorphan, fluoxetine, lidocaine, mirtazapine, nefazodone, paclitaxel, paroxetine, risperidone, repaglinide, ritonavir, rosiglitazone, thioridazine, and other CYP2D6 or 2C8 substrates.

Decreased Effect: The levels/effects of pioglitazone may be decreased by carbamazepine, phenobarbital, phenytoin, rifampin, rifapentine, secobarbital, and other CYP2C8 inducers. Pioglitazone may decrease the levels/effects of CYP2D6 prodrug substrates (eg, codeine, hydrocodone, oxycodone, tramadol). Bile acid sequestrants may decrease pioglitazone levels.

Ethanol/Nutrition/Herb Interactions

Ethanol: Caution with ethanol (may cause hypoglycemia).

Food: Peak concentrations are delayed when administered with food, but the extent of absorption is not affected. Pioglitazone may be taken without regard to meals.

Herb/Nutraceutical: Caution with alfalfa, aloe, bilberry, bitter melon, burdock, celery, damiana, fenugreek, garcinia, garlic, ginger, ginseng (American), gymnema, marshmallow, and stinging nettle (may cause hypoglycemia).

Dietary Considerations Management of type 2 diabetes mellitus (noninsulin dependent, NIDDM) should include diet control. May be taken without regard to meals.

Pharmacodynamics/Kinetics

Onset of action: Delayed

Peak effect: Glucose control: Several weeks

Distribution: V_{ss} (apparent): 0.63 L/kg

Protein binding: 99.8%; primarily to albumin

Metabolism: Hepatic (99%) via CYP2C8 and 3A4 to both active and inactive metabolites

Half-life elimination: Parent drug: 3-7 hours; Total: 16-24 hours

Time to peak: ~2 hours; delayed with food

Excretion: Urine (15% to 30%) and feces as metabolites

Pregnancy Risk Factor C

Dosage Forms

Tablet:

Actos®: 15 mg, 30 mg, 45 mg

Pioglitazone and Glimepiride
(pye oh GLI ta zone & GLYE me pye ride)

U.S. Brand Names Duetact™

Generic Available No

Index Terms Glimepiride and Pioglitazone; Glimepiride and Pioglitazone Hydrochloride

Pharmacologic Category Antidiabetic Agent, Sulfonylurea; Antidiabetic Agent, Thiazolidinedione; Hypoglycemic Agent, Oral

Use Management of type 2 diabetes mellitus (noninsulin dependent, NIDDM) as an adjunct to diet and exercise

Local Anesthetic/Vasoconstrictor Precautions No information available to require special precautions

Effects on Dental Treatment Pioglitazone-dependent diabetics (noninsulin dependent, type 2) or glimepiride-dependent diabetics (noninsulin dependent, type 2) should be appointed for dental treatment in morning in order to minimize chance of stress-induced hypoglycemia.

Common Adverse Effects Also see individual agents.

>10%:

Cardiovascular: Peripheral edema (6% to 12%)

Endocrine & metabolic: Hypoglycemia (13 % to 16%)

Gastrointestinal: Weight gain (9% to 13%)

Respiratory: Upper respiratory tract infection (12% to 15%)

1% to 10%:

Central nervous system: Headache (4% to 7%)

Gastrointestinal: Diarrhea (4% to 6%), nausea (4% to 5%)

Genitourinary: Urinary tract infection (6% to 7%)

Hematologic: Anemia (≤2%)

Neuromuscular & skeletal: Limb pain (4% to 5%)

Mechanism of Action

Pioglitazone: A thiazolidinedione that lowers blood glucose by improving target cell response to insulin, without increasing pancreatic insulin secretion. It has a mechanism of action that is dependent on the presence of insulin for activity.

Glimepiride: A sulfonylurea that stimulates insulin release from the pancreatic beta cells; reduces glucose output from the liver; insulin sensitivity is increased at peripheral target sites.

Drug Interactions

Cytochrome P450 Effect:

Pioglitazone: **Substrate** of CYP2C8 (major), 3A4 (minor); **Inhibits** CYP2C8 (moderate), 2C9 (weak), 2C19 (weak), 2D6 (moderate); **Induces** CYP3A4 (weak)

Glimepiride: **Substrate** of CYP2C9 (major)

Also see individual agents.

Pharmacodynamics/Kinetics See individual agents.

Pregnancy Risk Factor C

Pioglitazone and Metformin (pye oh GLI ta zone & met FOR min)

U.S. Brand Names Actoplus Met™

Generic Available No

Index Terms Metformin Hydrochloride and Pioglitazone Hydrochloride

Pharmacologic Category Antidiabetic Agent, Biguanide; Antidiabetic Agent, Thiazolidinedione

Use Management of type 2 diabetes mellitus (noninsulin dependent, NIDDM)

Local Anesthetic/Vasoconstrictor Precautions No information available to require special precautions

Effects on Dental Treatment Pioglitazone-dependent diabetes (noninsulin dependent, type 2) or metformin-dependent diabetes (noninsulin dependent, type 2) should be appointed for dental treatment in morning in order to minimize chance of stress-induced hypoglycemia.

Common Adverse Effects Also see individual agents. Percentages of adverse effects as reported with the combination product.

>10%:

Cardiovascular: Edema (lower limb, 3% to 11%)

(Continued)

Pioglitazone and Metformin *(Continued)*

Respiratory: Upper respiratory infection (12% to 16%)

1% to 10%:

Central nervous system: Headache (2% to 6%), dizziness (5%)

Endocrine & metabolic: Weight gain (3% to 7%)

Gastrointestinal: Diarrhea (5% to 6%), nausea (4% to 6%)

Genitourinary: Urinary tract infection (5% to 6%)

Hematologic: Anemia (≤2%)

Respiratory: Sinusitis (4% to 5%)

Dosage Oral: Type 2 diabetes mellitus:

Adults: Initial dose should be based on current dose of pioglitazone and/or metformin; daily dose should be divided and given with meals

Patients inadequately controlled on **metformin alone**: Initial dose: Pioglitazone 15-30 mg/day plus current dose of metformin

Patients inadequately controlled on **pioglitazone alone**: Initial dose: Metformin 1000-1700 mg/day plus current dose of pioglitazone

Note: When switching from combination pioglitazone and metformin as separate tablets: Use current dose.

Dosing adjustment: Doses may be increased as increments of pioglitazone 15 mg and/or metformin 500-850 mg, up to the maximum dose; doses should be titrated gradually. Guidelines for frequency of adjustment (adapted from rosiglitazone/metformin combination labeling):

After a change in the **metformin** dosage, titration can be done after 1-2 weeks

After a change in the **pioglitazone** dosage, titration can be done after 8-12 weeks

Maximum dose: Pioglitazone 45 mg/metformin 2550 mg daily

Elderly: The initial and maintenance dosing should be conservative, due to the potential for decreased renal function (monitor). Generally, elderly patients should not be titrated to the maximum; do not use in patients ≥80 years of age unless normal renal function has been established.

Dosage adjustment in renal impairment: Do not use with renal disease or renal dysfunction (serum creatinine ≥1.5 mg/dL in males or ≥1.4 mg/dL in females or abnormal clearance).

Dosage adjustment in hepatic impairment: Do not initiate treatment with active liver disease or ALT >2.5 times ULN. During treatment if ALT levels elevate >3 times ULN, the test should be repeated as soon as possible. If ALT levels remain >3 times ULN or if the patient is jaundiced, therapy should be discontinued.

Mechanism of Action

Pioglitazone is a thiazolidinedione antidiabetic agent that lowers blood glucose by improving target cell response to insulin, without increasing pancreatic insulin secretion. It has a mechanism of action that is dependent on the presence of insulin for activity.

Metformin decreases hepatic glucose production, decreasing intestinal absorption of glucose, and improves insulin sensitivity (increases peripheral glucose uptake and utilization).

Contraindications Hypersensitivity to pioglitazone, metformin, or any component of the formulation; renal disease or renal dysfunction (serum creatinine ≥1.5 mg/dL in males or ≥1.4 mg/dL in females, or abnormal creatinine clearance which may also result from conditions such as cardiovascular collapse, acute myocardial infarction, and septicemia); acute or chronic metabolic acidosis with or without coma (including diabetic ketoacidosis). Metformin is also contraindicated in CHF requiring pharmacologic management (not included in labeling of the combination product).

Note: Temporarily discontinue in patients undergoing radiologic studies in which intravascular iodinated contrast materials are utilized.

Warnings/Precautions [U.S. Boxed Warning]: Lactic acidosis is a rare, but potentially severe consequence of therapy with metformin. Lactic acidosis should be suspected in any diabetic patient receiving metformin who has evidence of acidosis when evidence of ketoacidosis is lacking. Discontinue metformin in clinical situations predisposing to hypoxemia, including conditions such as cardiovascular collapse, respiratory failure, acute myocardial infarction, acute congestive heart failure, and septicemia.

Metformin is substantially excreted by the kidney. The risk of accumulation and lactic acidosis increases with the degree of impairment of renal function. Patients with renal function below the limit of normal for their age should not receive metformin. In elderly patients, renal function should be monitored regularly; should not be used in any patient ≥80 years of age unless measurement of creatinine clearance verifies normal renal function. Use of concomitant medications that may affect renal function (ie, affect tubular secretion) may also affect metformin disposition. Metformin should be suspended in patients with dehydration and/or prerenal azotemia. Therapy should be suspended for any surgical procedures (resume only after normal intake resumed and normal renal function is verified). Metformin should also be temporarily discontinued for 48 hours in patients undergoing radiologic studies involving the intravascular administration of iodinated contrast materials (potential for acute alteration in renal function).

Avoid use in patients with impaired liver function. Pioglitazone must be used with caution in patients with elevated transaminases (AST or ALT); avoid use in patients where hepatic dysfunction presents a risk of lactic acidosis. Idiosyncratic hepatotoxicity has been reported with another thiazolidinedione agent (troglitazone) and (rarely) with pioglitazone; discontinue if jaundice occurs. Monitoring should include periodic determinations of liver function. Patient must be instructed to avoid excessive acute or chronic ethanol use.

Pioglitazone may cause fluid retention which could exacerbate or lead to heart failure; monitor closely for signs and symptoms of heart failure; not recommended for use in patients with NYHA Class III or IV heart failure. May increase plasma volume and/or increase cardiac hypertrophy. Discontinue if heart failure develops. Use caution in patients with edema. Pioglitazone requires the presence of endogenous insulin to be active; therefore, use in type 1 diabetes (insulin dependent, IDDM) is not recommended. Use pioglitazone with caution in patients with anemia or depressed leukocyte counts (may reduce hemoglobin, hematocrit, and/or WBC). Use pioglitazone with caution in premenopausal, anovulatory women; may result in resumption of ovulation, increasing the risk of pregnancy. May result in hormonal imbalance; development of menstrual irregularities should prompt reconsideration of therapy. Use caution with pre-existing macular edema or diabetic retinopathy. New-onset or worsening diabetic macular edema with decreased visual acuity has been reported. Safety and efficacy of this combination have not been established in pediatric patients.

Drug Interactions
Cytochrome P450 Effect: Pioglitazone: **Substrate** of CYP2C8 (major), 3A4 (minor); **Inhibits** CYP2C8 (moderate), 2C9 (weak), 2C19 (weak), 2D6 (moderate); **Induces** CYP3A4 (weak)

Increased Effect/Toxicity: See individual agents.

Ethanol/Nutrition/Herb Interactions See individual agents.

Dietary Considerations Should be taken with meals. Avoid ethanol. Dietary modification based on ADA recommendations is a part of therapy. Monitor for signs and symptoms of vitamin B_{12} and/or folic acid deficiency; supplementation may be required.

Pharmacodynamics/Kinetics See individual agents.

Pregnancy Risk Factor C

Dosage Forms
Tablet:

Actoplus Met™: 15/500: Pioglitazone 15 mg and metformin 500 mg; 15/850: Pioglitazone 15 mg and metformin 850 mg

---

Piperacillin (pi PER a sil in)

Canadian Brand Names Piperacillin for Injection, USP

Generic Available Yes

Index Terms Piperacillin Sodium

Pharmacologic Category Antibiotic, Penicillin

Use Treatment of susceptible infections such as septicemia, acute and chronic respiratory tract infections, skin and soft tissue infections, and urinary tract infections due to susceptible strains of *Pseudomonas*, *Proteus*, and *Escherichia coli* and *Enterobacter*; active against some streptococci and some anaerobic bacteria; febrile neutropenia (as part of combination regimen)

Local Anesthetic/Vasoconstrictor Precautions No information available to require special precautions

Effects on Dental Treatment Key adverse event(s) related to dental treatment: Prolonged use of penicillins may lead to development of oral candidiasis.

Common Adverse Effects Frequency not defined.

Central nervous system: Confusion, convulsions, drowsiness, fever, Jarisch-Herxheimer reaction

Dermatologic: Rash, toxic epidermal necrolysis, urticaria

Endocrine & metabolic: Electrolyte imbalance, hypokalemia

Hematologic: Abnormal platelet aggregation and prolonged PT (high doses), agranulocytosis, Coombs' reaction (positive), hemolytic anemia, pancytopenia

Local: Thrombophlebitis

Neuromuscular & skeletal: Myoclonus

(Continued)

Piperacillin *(Continued)*

Renal: Acute interstitial nephritis, acute renal failure
Miscellaneous: Anaphylaxis, hypersensitivity reactions

Mechanism of Action Inhibits bacterial cell wall synthesis by binding to one or more of the penicillin binding proteins (PBPs); which in turn inhibits the final transpeptidation step of peptidoglycan synthesis in bacterial cell walls, thus inhibiting cell wall biosynthesis. Bacteria eventually lyse due to ongoing activity of cell wall autolytic enzymes (autolysins and murein hydrolases) while cell wall assembly is arrested.

Drug Interactions

Increased Effect/Toxicity: Probenecid may increase penicillin levels. Neuromuscular blockers may increase duration of blockade. Penicillins may increase the exposure to methotrexate during concurrent therapy; monitor.

Decreased Effect: Tetracyclines may decrease penicillin effectiveness. High concentrations of piperacillin may cause physical inactivation of aminoglycosides and lead to potential toxicity in patients with mild-moderate renal dysfunction. Although anecdotal reports suggest oral contraceptive efficacy could be reduced by penicillins, this has been refuted by more rigorous scientific and clinical data.

Pharmacodynamics/Kinetics

Absorption: I.M.: 70% to 80%
Distribution: Crosses placenta; low concentrations enter breast milk
Protein binding: 22%
Half-life elimination (dose dependent; prolonged with moderately severe renal or hepatic impairment):
Neonates: 1-5 days old: 3.6 hours; >6 days old: 2.1-2.7 hours
Children: 1-6 months: 0.79 hour; 6 months to 12 years: 0.39-0.5 hour
Adults: 36-80 minutes
Time to peak, serum: I.M.: 30-50 minutes
Excretion: Primarily urine; partially feces

Pregnancy Risk Factor B

Piperacillin and Tazobactam Sodium

(pi PER a sil in & ta zoe BAK tam SOW dee um)

Related Information
Piperacillin *on page 1311*
U.S. Brand Names Zosyn®
Canadian Brand Names Tazocin®
Mexican Brand Names Tazocin
Generic Available No
Index Terms Piperacillin Sodium and Tazobactam Sodium; Tazobactam and Piperacillin
Pharmacologic Category Antibiotic, Penicillin
Use Treatment of moderate-to-severe infections caused by susceptible organisms, including infections of the lower respiratory tract (community-acquired pneumonia, nosocomial pneumonia); urinary tract; uncomplicated and complicated skin and skin structures; gynecologic (endometritis, pelvic inflammatory disease); bone and joint infections; intra-abdominal infections (appendicitis with rupture/abscess, peritonitis); and septicemia. Tazobactam expands activity of piperacillin to include beta-lactamase producing strains of *S. aureus*, *H. influenzae*, *Bacteroides*, and other gram-negative bacteria.
Local Anesthetic/Vasoconstrictor Precautions No information available to require special precautions
Effects on Dental Treatment Key adverse event(s) related to dental treatment: Prolonged use of penicillins may lead to development of oral candidiasis.
Common Adverse Effects
>10%: Gastrointestinal: Diarrhea (7% to 11%)
>1% to 10%:
Cardiovascular: Hypertension (2%)
Central nervous system: Insomnia (7%), headache (8%), fever (2% to 5%), agitation (2%), pain (2%)
Dermatologic: Rash (4%), pruritus (3%)
Gastrointestinal: Constipation (1% to 8%), nausea (7%), vomiting (3% to 4%), dyspepsia (3%), stool changes (2%), abdominal pain (1% to 2%)
Hepatic: Transaminases increased
Local: Local reaction (3%), abscess (2%)
Respiratory: Pharyngitis (2%)
Miscellaneous: Moniliasis (2%), sepsis (2%), infection (2%)
Mechanism of Action Inhibits bacterial cell wall synthesis by binding to one or more of the penicillin binding proteins (PBPs); which in turn inhibits the final

transpeptidation step of peptidoglycan synthesis in bacterial cell walls, thus inhibiting cell wall biosynthesis. Bacteria eventually lyse due to ongoing activity of cell wall autolytic enzymes (autolysins and murein hydrolases) while cell wall assembly is arrested. Tazobactam inhibits many beta-lactamases, including staphylococcal penicillinase and Richmond and Sykes types II, III, IV, and V, including extended spectrum enzymes; it has only limited activity against class I beta-lactamases other than class Ic types.

Drug Interactions

Increased Effect/Toxicity: Probenecid may increase penicillin levels. Neuromuscular blockers may increase duration of blockade. Penicillins may increase methotrexate exposure; clinical significance has not been established.

Decreased Effect: Tetracyclines may decrease penicillin effectiveness. Aminoglycosides may cause physical inactivation of aminoglycosides in the presence of high concentrations of piperacillin and potential toxicity in patients with mild-moderate renal dysfunction. Although anecdotal reports suggest oral contraceptive efficacy could be reduced by penicillins, this has been refuted by more rigorous scientific and clinical data.

Pharmacodynamics/Kinetics Both AUC and peak concentrations are dose proportional; hepatic impairment does not affect kinetics

Distribution: Well into lungs, intestinal mucosa, skin, muscle, uterus, ovary, prostate, gallbladder, and bile; penetration into CSF is low in subject with noninflamed meninges

Protein binding: Piperacillin and tazobactam: ~30%

Metabolism:
Piperacillin: 6% to 9% to desethyl metabolite (weak activity)
Tazobactam: ~26% to inactive metabolite

Half-life elimination: Piperacillin and tazobactam: 0.7-1.2 hours

Time to peak, plasma: Immediately following infusion of 30 minutes

Excretion: Clearance of both piperacillin and tazobactam are directly proportional to renal function
Piperacillin: Urine (68% as unchanged drug); feces (10% to 20%)
Tazobactam: Urine (80% as inactive metabolite)

Pregnancy Risk Factor B

Piperacillin Sodium *see* Piperacillin *on page 1311*

Piperacillin Sodium and Tazobactam Sodium *see* Piperacillin and Tazobactam Sodium *on page 1312*

Piperazine (PI per a zeen)

Canadian Brand Names Entacyl®
Generic Available Yes
Index Terms Piperazine Citrate
Pharmacologic Category Anthelmintic
Use Treatment of pinworm and roundworm infections (used as an alternative to first-line agents, mebendazole, or pyrantel pamoate)
Local Anesthetic/Vasoconstrictor Precautions No information available to require special precautions
Effects on Dental Treatment No significant effects or complications reported
Mechanism of Action Causes muscle paralysis of the roundworm by blocking the effects of acetylcholine at the neuromuscular junction
Drug Interactions
Decreased Effect: Pyrantel pamoate (antagonistic mode of action).
Pharmacodynamics/Kinetics
Absorption: Well absorbed
Time to peak, serum: 1 hour
Excretion: Urine (as unchanged drug and metabolites)
Pregnancy Risk Factor B

Piperazine Citrate *see* Piperazine *on page 1313*

Piperazine Estrone Sulfate *see* Estropipate *on page 615*

Piperonyl Butoxide and Pyrethrins *see* Pyrethrins and Piperonyl Butoxide *on page 1388*

Pipotiazine (pip oh TYE a zeen)

Canadian Brand Names Piportil® L₄
Generic Available No
Index Terms Pipotiazine Palmitate
Pharmacologic Category Antipsychotic Agent, Typical, Phenothiazine, Piperidine
(Continued)

Pipotiazine *(Continued)*

Use Management of schizophrenia

Local Anesthetic/Vasoconstrictor Precautions No information available to require special precautions

Effects on Dental Treatment Key adverse event(s) related to dental treatment: Xerostomia and changes in salivation (normal salivary flow resumes upon discontinuation).

Common Adverse Effects Frequency not defined.

Cardiovascular: Tachycardia, hypotension, syncope, edema, ECG changes, QT_c prolongation, cardiac arrest

Central nervous system; Extrapyramidal symptoms (tremor, akathisia, dystonia, dyskinesia, oculogyric crisis, opisthotonos, hyper-reflexia, pseudo-Parkinsonism, rigidity, sialorrhea); tardive dyskinesia, sleep disturbance, dizziness, drowsiness, fatigue, insomnia, depression, agitation, anxiety, restlessness, excitement, bizarre dreams, fever, headache, cerebral edema, EEG changes, seizure, paradoxical psychosis

Dermatologic: Pruritus, dermatitis, rash, erythema, urticaria, seborrhea, eczema, exfoliative dermatitis, photosensitivity, skin pigmentation (prolonged therapy), epithelial keratopathy

Endocrine & metabolic: Anorexia, menstrual irregularities, thirst, weight changes, appetite increased, galactorrhea, gynecomastia, libido (changes in)

Gastrointestinal: Nausea, constipation, xerostomia, vomiting, salivation, adynamic ileus, fecal impaction, cholestasis, jaundice

Genitourinary: Urinary retention, bladder paralysis, incontinence, polyuria, impotence

Hematologic: Agranulocytosis, anemia, eosinophilia, leukopenia, pancytopenia, thrombocytopenia

Ocular: Blurred vision, glaucoma, corneal deposits (prolonged therapy), lenticular deposits, pigmentary retinopathy (prolonged therapy)

Respiratory: Nasal congestion, pneumonia, pneumonitis

Miscellaneous: Angioedema, diaphoresis increased, Lupus-like syndrome

Restrictions Not available in U.S.

Mechanism of Action Blocks postsynaptic mesolimbic dopaminergic receptors in the brain; depresses the release of hypothalamic and hypophyseal hormones. Relative to other piperidine phenothiazines, pipotiazine appears to be less sedating, with less potential to potentiate other CNS depressants, and may possess a lower propensity to cause hypotension. However, it has a relatively high propensity for cause extrapyramidal reactions.

Drug Interactions

Cytochrome P450 Effect: No published data on CYP metabolism. Based on structural analysis, pipotiazine may be a substrate of CYP2D6 and 3A4.

Increased Effect/Toxicity: The levels/effects of pipotiazine may be increased by azole antifungals, chlorpromazine, clarithromycin, delavirdine, diclofenac, doxycycline, erythromycin, fluoxetine, imatinib, isoniazid, miconazole, nefazodone, nicardipine, paroxetine, pergolide, propofol, protease inhibitors, quinidine, quinine, ritonavir, ropinirole, telithromycin, verapamil and other CYP2D6 or 3A4 inhibitors.

Drugs which alter the QT_c interval may be additive with pipotiazine, increasing the risk of malignant arrhythmias; includes type Ia antiarrhythmics, TCAs, and some quinolone antibiotics (sparfloxacin, moxifloxacin and gatifloxacin). **These agents are contraindicated with other piperadine phenothiazines (thioridazine)** Potassium depleting agents may increase the risk of serious arrhythmias with pipotiazine (includes many diuretics, aminoglycosides, and amphotericin).

Phenothiazines inhibit the ability of bromocriptine to lower serum prolactin concentrations. The sedative effects of CNS depressants or ethanol may be additive with phenothiazines. Phenothiazines and trazodone may produce additive hypotensive effects. Metoclopramide may increase risk of extrapyramidal symptoms (EPS). Concurrent use of antihypertensives may result in additive hypotensive effects (particularly orthostasis).

Phenothiazines may produce neurotoxicity with lithium; this is a rare effect. Rare cases of respiratory paralysis have been reported with concurrent use of phenothiazines and polypeptide antibiotics. Naltrexone in combination with pipotiazine has been reported to cause lethargy and somnolence. Phenylpropanolamine has been reported to result in cardiac arrhythmias when combined with some phenothiazines.

Decreased Effect: Aluminum salts may decrease the absorption of phenothiazines. The efficacy of amphetamines may be diminished by antipsychotics; in addition, amphetamines may increase psychotic symptoms; avoid concurrent use. Anticholinergics may inhibit the therapeutic response to phenothiazines and excess anticholinergic effects may occur (includes benztropine, trihexyphenidyl, biperiden, and drugs with significant anticholinergic activity). Low potency antipsychotics (such as pipotiazine) may diminish the pressor effects of epinephrine. The antihypertensive effects of guanethidine or guanadrel may be inhibited by phenothiazines. Phenothiazines may inhibit the antiparkinsonian effect of levodopa. Enzyme inducers may enhance the hepatic metabolism of phenothiazines; larger doses may be required; includes rifampin, rifabutin, barbiturates, phenytoin, and cigarette smoking.

Pharmacodynamics/Kinetics
Onset: I.M.: 2-3 days
Duration: 3-6 weeks

Pipotiazine Palmitate *see* Pipotiazine *on page 1313*

Pirbuterol (peer BYOO ter ole)

Related Information
Respiratory Diseases *on page 1747*
U.S. Brand Names Maxair™ Autohaler™
Generic Available No
Index Terms Pirbuterol Acetate
Pharmacologic Category Beta$_2$-Adrenergic Agonist
Use Prevention and treatment of reversible bronchospasm including asthma
Local Anesthetic/Vasoconstrictor Precautions No information available to require special precautions
Effects on Dental Treatment Key adverse event(s) related to dental treatment: Xerostomia (normal salivary flow resumes upon discontinuation) and taste changes.
Common Adverse Effects
>10%:
Central nervous system: Nervousness (7%)
Endocrine & metabolic: Serum glucose increased, serum potassium decreased
Neuromuscular & skeletal: Trembling (6%)
1% to 10%:
Cardiovascular: Palpitation (2%), tachycardia (1%)
Central nervous system: Headache (2%), dizziness (1%)
Gastrointestinal: Nausea (2%)
Respiratory: Cough (1%)
Mechanism of Action Pirbuterol is a beta$_2$-adrenergic agonist with a similar structure to albuterol, specifically a pyridine ring has been substituted for the benzene ring in albuterol. The increased beta$_2$ selectivity of pirbuterol results from the substitution of a tertiary butyl group on the nitrogen of the side chain, which additionally imparts resistance of pirbuterol to degradation by monoamine oxidase and provides a lengthened duration of action in comparison to the less selective previous beta-agonist agents.
Drug Interactions
Increased Effect/Toxicity: Increased toxicity with other beta-agonists, MAO inhibitors, tricyclic antidepressants.
Decreased Effect: Decreased effect with beta-blockers.
Pharmacodynamics/Kinetics
Onset of action: Peak effect: Therapeutic: Oral: 2-3 hours with peak serum concentration of 6.2-9.8 mcg/L; Inhalation: 0.5-1 hour
Half-life elimination: 2-3 hours
Metabolism: Hepatic
Excretion: Urine (10% as unchanged drug)
Pregnancy Risk Factor C

Pirbuterol Acetate *see* Pirbuterol *on page 1315*

Piroxicam (peer OKS i kam)

Related Information
Rheumatoid Arthritis, Osteoarthritis, and Osteoporosis *on page 1759*
Temporomandibular Dysfunction (TMD) *on page 1822*
U.S. Brand Names Feldene®
Canadian Brand Names Apo-Piroxicam®; Gen-Piroxicam; Novo-Pirocam; Nu-Pirox; Pexicam®
Mexican Brand Names Facicam; Feldene; Osteral; Piroxan
Generic Available Yes
Pharmacologic Category Nonsteroidal Anti-inflammatory Drug (NSAID), Oral
Use Symptomatic treatment of acute and chronic rheumatoid arthritis and osteoarthritis
(Continued)

Piroxicam *(Continued)*

Unlabeled/Investigational Use Ankylosing spondylitis

Local Anesthetic/Vasoconstrictor Precautions No information available to require special precautions

Effects on Dental Treatment NSAID formulations are known to reversibly decrease platelet aggregation via mechanisms different than observed with aspirin. The dentist should be aware of the potential of abnormal coagulation. Caution should also be exercised in the use of NSAIDs in patients already on anticoagulant therapy with drugs such as warfarin (Coumadin®).

Common Adverse Effects

>10%:
Central nervous system: Dizziness
Dermatologic: Rash
Gastrointestinal: Abdominal cramps, heartburn, indigestion, nausea

1% to 10%:
Central nervous system: Headache, nervousness
Dermatologic: Itching
Endocrine & metabolic: Fluid retention
Gastrointestinal: Vomiting
Otic: Tinnitus

Restrictions An FDA-approved medication guide must be distributed when dispensing an oral outpatient prescription (new or refill) where this medication is to be used without direct supervision of a healthcare provider. Medication guides are available at http://www.fda.gov/cder/Offices/ODS/medication_guides.htm.

Dosage Oral:
Children (unlabeled use): 0.2-0.3 mg/kg/day once daily; maximum dose: 15 mg/day
Adults: 10-20 mg/day once daily; although associated with increase in GI adverse effects, doses >20 mg/day have been used (ie, 30-40 mg/day)

Dosing adjustment in renal impairment: Not recommended in patients with advanced renal disease

Dosing adjustment in hepatic impairment: Reduction of dosage is necessary

Mechanism of Action Inhibits prostaglandin synthesis, acts on the hypothalamus heat-regulating center to reduce fever, blocks prostaglandin synthetase action which prevents formation of the platelet-aggregating substance thromboxane A_2; decreases pain receptor sensitivity. Other proposed mechanisms of action for salicylate anti-inflammatory action are lysosomal stabilization, kinin and leukotriene production, alteration of chemotactic factors, and inhibition of neutrophil activation. This latter mechanism may be the most significant pharmacologic action to reduce inflammation.

Contraindications Hypersensitivity to piroxicam, aspirin, other NSAIDs or any component of the formulation; perioperative pain in the setting of coronary artery bypass surgery (CABG); pregnancy (3rd trimester or near term)

Warnings/Precautions [U.S. Boxed Warning]: NSAIDs are associated with an increased risk of adverse cardiovascular events, including MI, stroke, and new onset or worsening of pre-existing hypertension. Risk may be increased with duration of use or pre-existing cardiovascular risk factors or disease. Carefully evaluate individual cardiovascular risk profiles prior to prescribing. Use caution with fluid retention, CHF or hypertension. Concurrent administration of ibuprofen, and potentially other nonselective NSAIDs, may interfere with aspirin's cardioprotective effect.

Use of NSAIDs can compromise existing renal function. Renal toxicity can occur in patient with impaired renal function, dehydration, heart failure, liver dysfunction, those taking diuretics and ACEI and the elderly. Rehydrate patient before starting therapy. Monitor renal function closely. Not recommended for use in patients with advanced renal disease.

[U.S. Boxed Warning]: NSAIDs may increase risk of gastrointestinal irritation, ulceration, bleeding, and perforation. These events may occur at any time during therapy and without warning. Use caution with a history of GI disease (bleeding or ulcers), concurrent therapy with aspirin, anticoagulants and/or corticosteroids, smoking, use of alcohol, the elderly or debilitated patients.

Use the lowest effective dose for the shortest duration of time, consistent with individual patient goals, to reduce risk of cardiovascular or GI adverse events. Alternate therapies should be considered for patients at high risk.

NSAIDs may cause serious skin adverse events including exfoliative dermatitis, Stevens-Johnson syndrome (SJS) and toxic epidermal necrolysis (TEN). Anaphylactoid reactions may occur, even without prior exposure; patients with "aspirin triad" (bronchial asthma, aspirin intolerance, rhinitis) may be at increased risk. Do not use in patients who experience bronchospasm, asthma, rhinitis, or urticaria with NSAID or aspirin therapy. Use caution with other forms of asthma. A serum sickness-like reaction can rarely occur; watch for arthralgias, pruritus, fever, fatigue, and rash.

Use with caution in patients with decreased hepatic function. Closely monitor patients with any abnormal LFT. Severe hepatic reactions (eg, fulminant hepatitis, liver failure) have occurred with NSAID use, rarely; discontinue if signs or symptoms of liver disease develop, or if systemic manifestations occur.

The elderly are at increased risk for adverse effects (especially peptic ulceration, CNS effects, renal toxicity) from NSAIDs even at low doses

Withhold for at least 4-6 half-lives prior to surgical or dental procedures. Safety and efficacy have not been established in children.

Drug Interactions
Cytochrome P450 Effect: Substrate of CYP2C9 (minor); **Inhibits** CYP2C9 (strong)

Increased Effect/Toxicity: Increased effect/toxicity of lithium and methotrexate (controversial). Piroxicam may increase the levels/effects of CYP2C9 substrates; example substrates include bosentan, dapsone, fluoxetine, glimepiride, glipizide, losartan, montelukast, nateglinide, paclitaxel, phenytoin, warfarin, and zafirlukast. Concomitant use with fluoroquinolones may rarely increase risk of seizure.

Decreased Effect: Decreased effect of diuretics, ACE inhibitors, angiotensin antagonists, beta-blockers, and hydralazine. Decreased effect with aspirin, antacids. Cholestyramine (and other bile acid sequestrants) may decrease the absorption of NSAIDs; separate by at least 2 hours. Salicylates' antiplatelet effect may be reduced.

Ethanol/Nutrition/Herb Interactions
Ethanol: Avoid ethanol (may enhance gastric mucosal irritation).
Food: Onset of effect may be delayed if piroxicam is taken with food.
Herb/Nutraceutical: Avoid alfalfa, anise, bilberry, bladderwrack, bromelain, cat's claw, celery, coleus, cordyceps, dong quai, evening primrose, feverfew, fenugreek, garlic, ginger, ginkgo biloba, red clover, horse chestnut, grapeseed, green tea, ginseng, guggul, horse chestnut seed, horseradish, licorice, prickly ash, red clover, reishi, SAMe, sweet clover, turmeric, white willow (all have additional antiplatelet activity).

Dietary Considerations May be taken with food to decrease GI adverse effect.

Pharmacodynamics/Kinetics
Onset of action: Analgesic: ~1 hour
Peak effect: 3-5 hours
Protein binding: 99%
Metabolism: Hepatic
Half-life elimination: 45-50 hours
Excretion: Primarily urine and feces (small amounts) as unchanged drug (5%) and metabolites

Pregnancy Risk Factor C/D (3rd trimester)

Dosage Forms
Capsule: 10 mg, 20 mg
Feldene®: 10 mg, 20 mg

p-Isobutylhydratropic Acid *see* Ibuprofen *on page 853*

Pit *see* Oxytocin *on page 1239*

Pitocin® *see* Oxytocin *on page 1239*

Pitressin® *see* Vasopressin *on page 1650*

Pivampicilin *see* Pivampicillin *on page 1317*

Pivampicillin (piv am pi SIL in)

Canadian Brand Names Pondocillin®
Generic Available No
Index Terms MK-191; Pivampicilin
Pharmacologic Category Antibiotic, Penicillin
Use Treatment of susceptible bacterial infections (nonbeta-lactamase-producing organisms); susceptible bacterial infections caused by streptococci, pneumococci, nonpenicillinase-producing staphylococci, *H. influenzae*, *N. gonorrhoeae*, *E. coli*, *P. mirabilis*, *Listeria*, *Salmonella*, *Shigella*, *Enterobacter*, and *Klebsiella*
Local Anesthetic/Vasoconstrictor Precautions No information available to require special precautions
Effects on Dental Treatment Key adverse event(s) related to dental treatment: Oral candidiasis, black "hairy" tongue, glossitis, and stomatitis.
Common Adverse Effects Frequency not defined; although some reactions may have not been reported with pivampicillin use, they are considered due to
(Continued)

Pivampicillin (Continued)

ampicillin component and events reported due to ampicillin, and therefore, may be expected to occur.

Central nervous system: Dizziness

Dermatologic: Erythema multiforme, exfoliative dermatitis, pruritus, rash (erythematous or macropapular), urticaria

Gastrointestinal: Black "hairy" tongue, diarrhea, enterocolitis, flatulence, glossitis, nausea, retrosternal pain, stomatitis, vomiting

Hematologic: Agranulocytosis, anemia, eosinophilia, leukopenia, thrombocytopenia, thrombocytopenic purpura

Hepatic: AST increased (transient)

Miscellaneous: Anaphylaxis

Restrictions Not available in the U.S.

Mechanism of Action Prodrug converted to microbiologically active component (ampicillin) which inhibits bacterial cell wall synthesis by binding to one or more of the penicillin-binding proteins (PBPs) which in turn inhibits the final transpeptidation step of peptidoglycan synthesis in bacterial cell walls, thus inhibiting cell wall biosynthesis. Bacteria eventually lyse due to ongoing activity of cell wall autolytic enzymes (autolysins and murein hydrolases) while cell wall assembly is arrested.

Drug Interactions

Increased Effect/Toxicity: Potential for increased risk of rash when ampicillin taken with allopurinol. Probenecid may increase penicillin levels. Ampicillin increases the effect of disulfiram and anticoagulants. Concurrent use of valproic acid, or other medications liberating pivalic acid, should be avoided.

Decreased Effect: Anecdotal reports suggesting decreased contraceptive efficacy with penicillins have been refuted by more rigorous scientific and clinical data.

Pharmacodynamics/Kinetics

Distribution: Bile, blister, and tissue fluids; penetration into CSF occurs with inflamed meninges only, good only with inflammation (exceeds usual MICs). Normal meninges: NIL; Inflamed meninges: 5% to 10%

Protein binding: 20% as ampicillin

Metabolism: Pivampicillin is converted to ampicillin within 15 minutes of absorption

Bioavailability: Amounts in excess of 99% absorbed

Half-life elimination: Children and Adults: 1-1.8 hours

Time to peak, plasma: 1 hour

Excretion: Urine (>70% as ampicillin); pivalic acid is excreted in urine in form of labile conjugates with glycine

Pregnancy Risk Factor B (based on ampicillin rating in the U.S.)

Pneumococcal Conjugate Vaccine (7-Valent)
(noo moe KOK al KON ju gate vak SEEN, seven vay lent)

Related Information

Immunizations (Vaccines) on page 1886

U.S. Brand Names Prevnar®

Canadian Brand Names Prevnar®

Generic Available No

Index Terms Diphtheria CRM$_{197}$ Protein; PCV7; Pneumococcal 7-Valent Conjugate Vaccine

Pharmacologic Category Vaccine

Use Immunization of infants and toddlers against *Streptococcus pneumoniae* infection caused by serotypes included in the vaccine

Advisory Committee on Immunization Practices (ACIP) guidelines also recommend PCV7 for use in:

All children 2-23 months

Children ≥2-59 months with cochlear implants

Children ages 24-59 months with: Sickle cell disease (including other sickle cell hemoglobinopathies, asplenia, splenic dysfunction), HIV infection, immunocompromising conditions (congenital immunodeficiencies, renal failure, nephrotic syndrome, diseases associated with immunosuppressive or radiation therapy, solid organ transplant), chronic illnesses (cardiac disease, cerebrospinal fluid leaks, diabetes mellitus, pulmonary disease excluding asthma unless on high dose corticosteroids)

Consider use in all children 24-59 months with priority given to:

Children 24-35 months

Children 24-59 months who are of Alaska native, American Indian, or African-American descent

Children 24-59 months who attend group day care centers

Local Anesthetic/Vasoconstrictor Precautions No information available to require special precautions

Effects on Dental Treatment No significant effects or complications reported

Common Adverse Effects All serious adverse reactions must be reported to the U.S. Department of Health and Human Services (DHHS) Vaccine Adverse Event Reporting System (VAERS) 1-800-822-7967.

>10%:

Central nervous system: Fever, irritability, drowsiness, restlessness

Dermatologic: Erythema

Gastrointestinal: Decreased appetite, vomiting, diarrhea

Local: Induration, tenderness, nodule

1% to 10%: Dermatologic: Rash

Mechanism of Action Promotes active immunization against invasive disease caused by *S. pneumoniae* capsular serotypes 4, 6B, 9V, 18C, 19F, and 23F, all which are individually conjugated to CRM197 protein

Drug Interactions

Decreased Effect: Immunosuppressants may decrease response to active immunizations.

Pregnancy Risk Factor C

Pneumotussin® *see* Hydrocodone and Guaifenesin *on page 828*

PNU-140690E *see* Tipranavir *on page 1575*

Podactin Cream [OTC] *see* Miconazole *on page 1097*

Podactin Powder [OTC] *see* Tolnaftate *on page 1587*

Podocon-25® *see* Podophyllum Resin *on page 1319*

Podofilox (poe DOF il oks)

U.S. Brand Names Condylox®

Canadian Brand Names Condyline™; Wartec®

Generic Available Yes: Topical solution

Pharmacologic Category Keratolytic Agent; Topical Skin Product

Use Treatment of external genital warts

Local Anesthetic/Vasoconstrictor Precautions No information available to require special precautions

Effects on Dental Treatment No significant effects or complications reported

Pregnancy Risk Factor C

Podophyllin *see* Podophyllum Resin *on page 1319*

Podophyllum Resin (po DOF fil um REZ in)

U.S. Brand Names Podocon-25®

Canadian Brand Names Podofilm®

Mexican Brand Names Podofilia No. 2

Generic Available No

Index Terms Mandrake; May Apple; Podophyllin

Pharmacologic Category Keratolytic Agent

Use Topical treatment of benign growths including external genital and perianal warts, papillomas, fibroids; compound benzoin tincture generally is used as the medium for topical application

Local Anesthetic/Vasoconstrictor Precautions No information available to require special precautions

Effects on Dental Treatment No significant effects or complications reported

Common Adverse Effects 1% to 10%:

Dermatologic: Pruritus

(Continued)

Podophyllum Resin *(Continued)*

Gastrointestinal: Nausea, vomiting, abdominal pain, diarrhea

Mechanism of Action Directly affects epithelial cell metabolism by arresting mitosis through binding to a protein subunit of spindle microtubules (tubulin)

Pregnancy Risk Factor X

Poliovirus Vaccine (Inactivated)

(POE lee oh VYE rus vak SEEN, in ak ti VAY ted)

Related Information

Immunizations (Vaccines) *on page 1886*

U.S. Brand Names IPOL®

Canadian Brand Names IPOL®

Generic Available No

Index Terms Enhanced-potency Inactivated Poliovirus Vaccine; IPV; Salk Vaccine

Pharmacologic Category Vaccine

Use Active immunization against poliomyelitis caused by poliovirus types 1, 2 and 3. Routine immunization of adults in the United States is generally not recommended. Adults with previous wild poliovirus disease, who have never been immunized, or those who are incompletely immunized may receive inactivated poliovirus vaccine if they fall into one of the following categories:

- Travelers to regions or countries where poliomyelitis is endemic or epidemic
- Healthcare workers in close contact with patients who may be excreting poliovirus
- Laboratory workers handling specimens that may contain poliovirus
- Members of communities or specific population groups with diseases caused by wild poliovirus
- Incompletely vaccinated or unvaccinated adults in a household or with other close contact with children receiving oral poliovirus (may be at increased risk of vaccine associated paralytic poliomyelitis)

Local Anesthetic/Vasoconstrictor Precautions No information available to require special precautions

Effects on Dental Treatment No significant effects or complications reported

Common Adverse Effects All serious adverse reactions must be reported to the U.S. Department of Health and Human Services (DHHS) Vaccine Adverse Event Reporting System (VAERS) 1-800-822-7967.

1% to 10%:

Percentages noted with concomitant administration of DTP or DTaP vaccine and observed within 48 hours of injection.

>10%:

Central nervous system: Irritability (7% to 65%), tiredness (4% to 61%), fever ≥39°C (≤38%)

Gastrointestinal: Anorexia (1% to 17%)

Local: Injection Site: Tenderness (≤29%), pain (13%), swelling (≤11%)

1% to 10%:

Gastrointestinal: Vomiting (1% to 3%)

Local: Injection site: Erythema (≤3%), induration (1%)

Miscellaneous: Persistent crying (up to 1% reported within 72 hours)

Drug Interactions

Decreased Effect:

The effect of the vaccine may be decreased when administered with immunosuppressant medications.

Pregnancy Risk Factor C

Polocaine® *see* Mepivacaine *on page 1042*

Polocaine® *see* Mepivacaine (Dental Anesthetic) *on page 1044*

Polocaine® Dental *see* Mepivacaine *on page 1042*

Polocaine® MPF *see* Mepivacaine *on page 1042*

Polycarbophil *(pol i KAR boe fil)*

U.S. Brand Names Equalactin® [OTC]; FiberCon® [OTC]; Fiber-Lax® [OTC]; Fiber-Tabs™ [OTC]; Konsyl® Fiber Caplets [OTC]

Generic Available Yes

Pharmacologic Category Antidiarrheal; Laxative, Bulk-Producing

Use Treatment of constipation or diarrhea

Local Anesthetic/Vasoconstrictor Precautions No information available to require special precautions

Effects on Dental Treatment Oral medication should be given at least 1 hour prior to taking the bulk-producing laxative in order to prevent decreased absorption of medication.

Mechanism of Action Restoring a more normal moisture level and providing bulk in the patient's intestinal tract

Pregnancy Risk Factor C

Polycitra® *see* Citric Acid, Sodium Citrate, and Potassium Citrate *on page 370*

Polycitra®-K *see* Potassium Citrate and Citric Acid *on page 1329*

Polycitra®-LC *see* Citric Acid, Sodium Citrate, and Potassium Citrate *on page 370*

Polycose® [OTC] *see* Glucose Polymers *on page 785*

Poly-Dex™ *see* Neomycin, Polymyxin B, and Dexamethasone *on page 1161*

Polyethylene Glycol 3350 (pol i ETH i leen GLY kol 3350)

U.S. Brand Names GlycoLax®; MiraLax® [OTC]
Generic Available Yes
Index Terms PEG
Pharmacologic Category Laxative, Osmotic
Use Treatment of occasional constipation in adults
Unlabeled/Investigational Use Treatment of constipation in children
Local Anesthetic/Vasoconstrictor Precautions No information available to require special precautions
Effects on Dental Treatment No significant effects or complications reported
Common Adverse Effects Frequency not defined.
Dermatologic: Urticaria
Gastrointestinal: Abdominal bloating, cramping, diarrhea, flatulence, nausea
Mechanism of Action An osmotic agent, polyethylene glycol 3350 causes water retention in the stool; increases stool frequency and consistency
Pharmacodynamics/Kinetics Onset of action: Oral: 48-96 hours
Pregnancy Risk Factor C

Polyethylene Glycol-Electrolyte Solution
(pol i ETH i leen GLY kol ee LEK troe lite soe LOO shun)

U.S. Brand Names Colyte®; GoLYTELY®; MoviPrep®; NuLYTELY®; TriLyte™
Canadian Brand Names Colyte™; Klean-Prep®; PegLyte®
Generic Available Yes
Index Terms Electrolyte Lavage Solution
Pharmacologic Category Laxative, Osmotic
Use Bowel cleansing prior to GI examination or following toxic ingestion
Local Anesthetic/Vasoconstrictor Precautions No information available to require special precautions
Effects on Dental Treatment No significant effects or complications reported
Common Adverse Effects
>10%:
Central nervous system: Malaise (18% to 27%)
Gastrointestinal: Abdominal distension (<60%), anal irritation (<52%), nausea (14% to 47%), abdominal pain (13% to 39%), vomiting (7% to 12%)
Neuromuscular & skeletal: Rigors (34%)
Miscellaneous: Thirst (<47%)
1% to 10%:
Central nervous system: Dizziness (7%), headache (2%)
Gastrointestinal: Dyspepsia (1% to 3%)
Frequency not defined, postmarketing, and/or case reports: Abdominal cramps, abdominal fullness, bloating, dermatitis, flatulence, rash, urticaria
Mechanism of Action Induces catharsis by strong electrolyte and osmotic effects
Pharmacodynamics/Kinetics Onset of effect: Oral: ~1-2 hours
Pregnancy Risk Factor C

Polygam® S/D *see* Immune Globulin (Intravenous) *on page 870*

Poly-L-Lactic Acid (POL i el LAK tik AS id)

U.S. Brand Names Sculptra®
Generic Available No
Index Terms New-Fill®; PLA
Pharmacologic Category Cosmetic Agent, Implant
Use Restoration and/or correction of facial lipoatrophy in patients with HIV
(Continued)

Poly-L-Lactic Acid *(Continued)*

Local Anesthetic/Vasoconstrictor Precautions No information available to require special precautions

Effects on Dental Treatment No significant effects or complications reported

Mechanism of Action Poly-L-lactic acid is an immunologically inert synthetic polymer. It increases dermal thickness by causing a local reaction leading to an increase in collagen deposits. It is eventually degraded and undergoes resorption.

Polymyxin B *(pol i MIKS in bee)*

U.S. Brand Names Poly-Rx

Generic Available Yes

Index Terms Polymyxin B Sulfate

Pharmacologic Category Antibiotic, Irrigation; Antibiotic, Miscellaneous

Use Treatment of acute infections caused by susceptible strains of *Pseudomonas aeruginosa*; used occasionally for gut decontamination; parenteral use of polymyxin B has mainly been replaced by less toxic antibiotics, reserved for life-threatening infections caused by organisms resistant to the preferred drugs (eg, pseudomonal meningitis - intrathecal administration)

Local Anesthetic/Vasoconstrictor Precautions No information available to require special precautions

Effects on Dental Treatment No significant effects or complications reported

Common Adverse Effects Frequency not defined.

Cardiovascular: Facial flushing

Central nervous system: Neurotoxicity (irritability, drowsiness, ataxia, perioral paresthesia, numbness of the extremities, and blurred vision); dizziness, drug fever, meningeal irritation with intrathecal administration

Dermatologic: Urticarial rash

Endocrine & metabolic: Hypocalcemia, hyponatremia, hypokalemia, hypochloremia

Local: Pain at injection site

Neuromuscular & skeletal: Neuromuscular blockade, weakness

Renal: Nephrotoxicity

Respiratory: Respiratory arrest

Miscellaneous: Anaphylactoid reaction

Mechanism of Action Binds to phospholipids, alters permeability, and damages the bacterial cytoplasmic membrane permitting leakage of intracellular constituents

Drug Interactions

Increased Effect/Toxicity: Increased/prolonged effect of neuromuscular blocking agents.

Pharmacodynamics/Kinetics

Absorption: Well absorbed from peritoneum; minimal from GI tract (except in neonates) from mucous membranes or intact skin

Distribution: Minimal into CSF; does not cross placenta

Half-life elimination: 4.5-6 hours; prolonged with renal impairment

Time to peak, serum: I.M.: ~2 hours

Excretion: Urine (>60% primarily as unchanged drug)

Pregnancy Risk Factor B (per expert opinion)

Polymyxin B and Bacitracin *see* Bacitracin and Polymyxin B *on page 181*

Polymyxin B and Neomycin *see* Neomycin and Polymyxin B *on page 1161*

Polymyxin B and Trimethoprim *see* Trimethoprim and Polymyxin B *on page 1621*

Polymyxin B, Bacitracin, and Neomycin *see* Bacitracin, Neomycin, and Polymyxin B *on page 181*

Polymyxin B, Bacitracin, Neomycin, and Hydrocortisone *see* Bacitracin, Neomycin, Polymyxin B, and Hydrocortisone *on page 182*

Polymyxin B, Neomycin, and Dexamethasone *see* Neomycin, Polymyxin B, and Dexamethasone *on page 1161*

Polymyxin B, Neomycin, and Gramicidin *see* Neomycin, Polymyxin B, and Gramicidin *on page 1161*

Polymyxin B, Neomycin, and Hydrocortisone *see* Neomycin, Polymyxin B, and Hydrocortisone *on page 1162*

Polymyxin B, Neomycin, and Prednisolone *see* Neomycin, Polymyxin B, and Prednisolone *on page 1162*

Polymyxin B, Neomycin, Bacitracin, and Pramoxine *see* Bacitracin, Neomycin, Polymyxin B, and Pramoxine *on page 182*

Polymyxin B Sulfate *see* Polymyxin B *on page 1322*

Poly-Pred® *see* Neomycin, Polymyxin B, and Prednisolone *on page 1162*

Poly-Rx see Polymyxin B on page 1322

Polysaccharide-Iron Complex
(pol i SAK a ride-EYE ern KOM pleks)

U.S. Brand Names Ferrex 150 [OTC]; Niferex® [OTC]; Nu-Iron® 150 [OTC]
Generic Available Yes: Capsule
Index Terms Iron-Polysaccharide Complex
Pharmacologic Category Iron Salt
Use Prevention and treatment of iron-deficiency anemias
Local Anesthetic/Vasoconstrictor Precautions No information available to require special precautions
Effects on Dental Treatment No significant effects or complications reported
Common Adverse Effects
  >10%: Gastrointestinal: Stomach cramping, constipation, nausea, vomiting, dark stools, GI irritation, epigastric pain, nausea
  1% to 10%:
    Gastrointestinal: Heartburn, diarrhea
    Genitourinary: Discolored urine
    Miscellaneous: Staining of teeth
Pregnancy Risk Factor A

Polysporin® [OTC] see Bacitracin and Polymyxin B on page 181
Polytar® [OTC] see Coal Tar on page 402

Polythiazide (pol i THYE a zide)

Related Information
  Cardiovascular Diseases on page 1726
U.S. Brand Names Renese®
Generic Available No
Pharmacologic Category Diuretic, Thiazide
Use Adjunctive therapy in treatment of edema and hypertension
Local Anesthetic/Vasoconstrictor Precautions No information available to require special precautions
Effects on Dental Treatment No significant effects or complications reported
Mechanism of Action The diuretic mechanism of action of the thiazides is primarily inhibition of sodium, chloride, and water reabsorption in the renal distal tubules, thereby producing diuresis with a resultant reduction in plasma volume. The antihypertensive mechanism of action of the thiazides is unknown. It is known that doses of thiazides produce greater reductions in blood pressure than equivalent diuretic doses of loop diuretics (eg, furosemide). There has been speculation that the thiazides may have some influence on vascular tone mediated through sodium depletion, but this remains to be proven.
Pregnancy Risk Factor D

Polythiazide and Prazosin see Prazosin and Polythiazide on page 1338
Polytrim® see Trimethoprim and Polymyxin B on page 1621
Poly-Vi-Flor® see Vitamins (Fluoride) on page 1665
Poly-Vi-Flor® With Iron see Vitamins (Fluoride) on page 1665
Polyvinyl Alcohol see Artificial Tears on page 147
Polyvinylpyrrolidone with Iodine see Povidone-Iodine on page 1332
Ponstel® see Mefenamic Acid on page 1028
Pontocaine® see Tetracaine on page 1546
Pontocaine® Niphanoid® see Tetracaine on page 1546

Poractant Alfa (por AKT ant AL fa)

U.S. Brand Names Curosurf®
Canadian Brand Names Curosurf®
Generic Available No
Pharmacologic Category Lung Surfactant
Use Orphan drug: Treatment and prevention of respiratory distress syndrome (RDS) in premature infants
Local Anesthetic/Vasoconstrictor Precautions No information available to require special precautions
Effects on Dental Treatment No significant effects or complications reported
Common Adverse Effects Frequency not defined.
  Cardiovascular: Bradycardia, hypotension
  Gastrointestinal: Endotracheal tube blockage
  Respiratory: Oxygen desaturation
  (Continued)

Poractant Alfa *(Continued)*

Mechanism of Action Endogenous pulmonary surfactant reduces surface tension at the air-liquid interface of the alveoli during ventilation and stabilizes the alveoli against collapse at resting transpulmonary pressures. A deficiency of pulmonary surfactant in preterm infants results in respiratory distress syndrome characterized by poor lung expansion, inadequate gas exchange, and atelectasis. Poractant alpha compensates for the surfactant deficiency and restores surface activity to the infant's lungs. It reduces mortality and pneumothoraces associated with RDS.

Pharmacodynamics/Kinetics Information limited to animal models. No human information about pharmacokinetics exists.

Porfimer *(POR fi mer)*

U.S. Brand Names Photofrin®
Canadian Brand Names Photofrin®
Generic Available No
Index Terms CL-184116; Dihematoporphyrin Ether; Porfimer Sodium
Pharmacologic Category Antineoplastic Agent, Miscellaneous
Use Adjunct to laser light therapy for obstructing esophageal cancer, obstructing endobronchial nonsmall cell lung cancer (NSCLC), ablation of high-grade dysplasia in Barrett's esophagus

Unlabeled/Investigational Use Transitional cell carcinoma *in situ* of the urinary bladder; gastric and rectal cancers

Local Anesthetic/Vasoconstrictor Precautions No information available to require special precautions

Effects on Dental Treatment Key adverse event(s) related to dental treatment: Dysphagia.

Common Adverse Effects
>10%:
  Cardiovascular: Chest pain (7% to 35%), edema (3% to 18%)
  Central nervous system: Fever (5% to 31%), pain (1% to 22%), insomnia (4% to 14%)
  Dermatologic: Photosensitivity reaction (4% to 37%, minor reactions may occur in up to 100%; severe: 10%)
  Endocrine & metabolic: Dehydration (7% to 11%)
  Gastrointestinal: Esophageal stricture (6% in esophageal cancer patients; up to 39% in Barrett's esophagus patients), nausea (24% to 39%), vomiting (17% to 34%), constipation (5% to 24%), dysphagia (10% to 24%), abdominal pain (12% to 20%)
  Genitourinary: Urinary tract irritation including frequency, urgency, nocturia, painful urination, or bladder spasm (~100% of bladder cancer patients)
  Hematologic: Anemia (32% in esophageal cancer patients)
  Neuromuscular & skeletal: Back pain (3% to 11%)
  Respiratory: Pleural effusion (32% in esophageal cancer patients; 11% in Barrett's esophagus patients), dyspnea (6% to 20%), pneumonia (6% to 18%), hemoptysis (7% to 16%), cough (6% to 15%), pharyngitis (11%)
  Miscellaneous: Mild-moderate allergic-type reactions (34% of lung cancer patients)
5% to 10%:
  Cardiovascular: Atrial fibrillation (10%), hyper-/hypotension (3% to 7%), cardiac failure (7% in esophageal cancer), tachycardia (6%), chest pain (substernal; 5%)
  Central nervous system: Confusion (7% to 8%), headache (6%), anxiety (3% to 7%), depression (3% to 5%)
  Dermatologic: Rash (7%), pruritus (4%)
  Gastrointestinal: Diarrhea (5% to 10%), weight loss (6% to 9%), esophageal edema (8%), esophageal tumor bleeding (8%), anorexia (4% to 8%), dyspepsia (1% to 6%), eructation (5%), esophagitis (5%), hematemesis (5%), melena (5%), odynophagia (5%)
  Genitourinary: Urinary tract infection (7%)
  Neuromuscular & skeletal: Weakness (6%), arthralgia (3% to 5%)
  Respiratory: Respiratory insufficiency (6% to 10%), bronchitis (4% to 10%), tracheoesophageal fistula (6%), sinusitis (4%)
  Miscellaneous: Moniliasis (9%), surgical complication (5% in esophageal cancer patients)

Mechanism of Action Porfimer's cytotoxic activity is dependent on light and oxygen. Following administration, the drug is selectively retained in neoplastic tissues. Exposure of the drug to laser light at wavelengths >630 nm results in the production of oxygen free-radicals. Release of thromboxane A_2, leading to vascular occlusion and ischemic necrosis, may also occur.

Drug Interactions
Increased Effect/Toxicity: Concomitant administration of other photosensitizing agents (eg, tetracyclines, sulfonamides, phenothiazines, sulfonylureas, thiazide diuretics, griseofulvin) could increase the photosensitivity reaction.

Decreased Effect: Compounds that quench active oxygen species or scavenge radicals (eg, dimethyl sulfoxide, beta-carotene, ethanol, mannitol) would be expected to decrease photodynamic therapy (PDT) activity. Allopurinol, calcium channel blockers, and some prostaglandin synthesis inhibitors could interfere with porfimer. Drugs that decrease clotting, vasoconstriction, or platelet aggregation could decrease the efficacy of PDT. Glucocorticoid hormones may decrease the efficacy of the treatment.

Pharmacodynamics/Kinetics
Distribution: V_{dss}: 0.49 L/kg
Protein binding, plasma: 90%
Half-life elimination: Mean: 21.5 days (range: 11-28 days)
Time to peak, serum: ~2 hours
Excretion: Feces; Clearance: Plasma: Total: 0.051 mL/minute/kg

Pregnancy Risk Factor C

Porfimer Sodium *see Porfimer on page 1324*

Portia™ *see Ethinyl Estradiol and Levonorgestrel on page 633*

Posaconazole (poe sa KON a zole)

Related Information
Fungal Infections *on page 1804*

Related Sample Prescriptions
Fungal Infections *on page 1841*

U.S. Brand Names Noxafil®

Generic Available No

Index Terms SCH 56592

Pharmacologic Category Antifungal Agent, Oral

Dental Use Treatment of oropharyngeal candidiasis (including patients refractory to itraconazole and/or fluconazole)

Use Prophylaxis of invasive *Aspergillus* and *Candida* infections in severely-immunocompromised patients [eg, hematopoietic stem cell transplant (HSCT) recipients with graft-versus-host disease (GVHD) or those with prolonged neutropenia secondary to chemotherapy for hematologic malignancies]; treatment of oropharyngeal candidiasis (including patients refractory to itraconazole and/or fluconazole)

Unlabeled/Investigational Use Salvage therapy of refractory invasive fungal infections

Local Anesthetic/Vasoconstrictor Precautions No information available to require special precautions

Effects on Dental Treatment Key adverse event(s) related to dental treatment: Xerostomia (normal salivary flow resumes upon discontinuation), abnormal taste, mucositis.

Significant Adverse Effects Note: A higher frequency of adverse reactions was observed in studies with refractory oropharyngeal candidiasis patients and percentages are included below.

>10%: Gastrointestinal: Diarrhea (3% to 11%)

1% to 10%:
Cardiovascular: QT_c prolongation (up to 4%), hypertension (1%)
Central nervous system: Headache (1% to 8%), dizziness (1% to 3%), fatigue (1% to 3%), insomnia (1% to 3%), fever (up to 3%), somnolence (1%)
Dermatologic: Rash (1% to 4%), pruritus (1% to 2%)
Endocrine & metabolic: Hypokalemia (3%)
Gastrointestinal: Nausea (5% to 8%), vomiting (4% to 7%), abdominal pain (1% to 5%), flatulence (1% to 5%), anorexia (1% to 3%), mucositis (2%), dyspepsia (1% to 2%), xerostoma (1% to 2%), taste perversion (1%), constipation (up to 1%)
Hematologic: Neutropenia (2% to 8%), anemia (up to 3%), thrombocytopenia (up to 2%)
Hepatic: Bilirubin increased (2% to 3%), ALT increased (2% to 3%), AST increased (2% to 3%), GGT increased (2% to 3%), alkaline phosphatase increased (2%), hepatocellular damage (1%)
Neuromuscular & skeletal: Weakness (1% to 3%), myalgia (up to 2%), tremor (1%)
Ocular: Blurred vision (1%)
Renal: Serum creatinine increased (2%)

<1% (Limited to important or life-threatening): Adrenal insufficiency, allergic/hypersensitivity reactions, cholestasis, hemolytic uremic syndrome, hepatic
(Continued)

Posaconazole *(Continued)*

failure, hepatitis, pulmonary embolus, thrombotic thrombocytopenic purpura, torsade de pointes

Dental Usual Dosing Children ≥13 years and Adults: Oral:

Oropharyngeal candidiasis: Initial: 100 mg twice daily for 1 day; maintenance dose: 100 mg once daily for 13 days

Refractory oropharyngeal candidiasis: 400 mg twice daily

Dosage Oral: Children ≥13 years and Adults:

Prophylaxis of invasive *Aspergillus* and *Candida* species: 200 mg 3 times/day

Treatment of oropharyngeal candidiasis: Initial: 100 mg twice daily for 1 day; maintenance: 100 mg once daily for 13 days

Treatment of refractory oropharyngeal candidiasis: 400 mg twice daily

Treatment of refractory invasive fungal infections (unlabeled use): 800 mg/day in divided doses

Dosage adjustment in renal impairment: No adjustment necessary; use caution in severe renal impairment and monitor for breakthrough fungal infections. Variability in posaconazole exposure observed with Cl_{cr}<20 mL/minute.

Dosage adjustment in hepatic impairment: No adjustment necessary; use with caution

Mechanism of Action Interferes with fungal cytochrome P450 activity, decreasing ergosterol synthesis (principal sterol in fungal cell membrane) and inhibiting fungal cell membrane formation.

Contraindications Hypersensitivity to posaconazole or any component of the formulation; coadministration of cisapride, pimozide, quinidine, or ergot alkaloids

Warnings/Precautions Use caution in hepatic impairment; hepatic dysfunction has occurred, ranging from mild/moderate increases of ALT/AST, alkaline phosphatase, and/or clinical hepatitis to severe reactions (cholestasis, hepatic failure including death). Use caution in patients with an increased risk of arrhythmia (concurrent QT_c-prolonging drugs, hypokalemia). Correct electrolyte abnormalities (eg, potassium, magnesium, and calcium) before initiating therapy.

Use caution in hypersensitivity with other azole antifungal agents; cross-reaction may occur, but has not been established. Alternative antifungal therapy should be considered in any patient unable to eat or tolerate an oral liquid nutritional supplement. Use caution in severe renal impairment; monitor for breakthrough fungal infections. Safety and efficacy have not been established in children <13 years of age.

Drug Interactions Inhibits CYP3A4 (moderate)

Calcium channel blockers: Posaconazole may increase the levels/effects of calcium channel blockers (applies to those agents metabolized by CYP3A4, including felodipine, nifedipine, and verapamil).

Cimetidine: May decrease the levels/effects of posaconazole. If needed, monitor for breakthrough fungal infections.

Cyclosporine: Posaconazole may increase the levels/effects of cyclosporine. Reduce cyclosporine dose to approximately 75% of original dose and monitor. Readjust dose when posaconazole is discontinued.

CYP3A4 substrates: Posaconazole may increase the levels/effects of CYP3A4 substrates. Examples substrates include benzodiazepines, calcium channel blockers, cyclosporine, mirtazapine, nateglinide, nefazodone, sildenafil (and other PDE-5 inhibitors), tacrolimus, and venlafaxine. Selected benzodiazepines (midazolam and triazolam), cisapride, ergot alkaloids, selected HMG-CoA reductase inhibitors (lovastatin and simvastatin), and pimozide are generally contraindicated with strong CYP3A4 inhibitors.

Ergot alkaloids: Posaconazole may increase the levels/effects of ergot alkaloids, leading to ergotism; concurrent use is contraindicated.

Glipizide: Posaconazole may increase level/effect of glipizide; monitor glucose concentrations.

HMG-CoA reductase inhibitors: Posaconazole may increase the levels/effects of HMG-CoA reductase inhibitors; consider reducing HMG-CoA dose.

Midazolam: Posaconazole may increase the levels/effects of midazolam. Monitor for midazolam adverse effects and/or consider reducing midazolam dose.

Phenytoin: Posaconazole may increase the levels/effects of phenytoin. Monitor phenytoin concentrations and/or consider reducing phenytoin dose. Phenytoin may decrease the levels/effects of posaconazole. Avoid concurrent use; if given, monitor for breakthrough fungal infections.

QT_c- prolonging agents: Risk of arrhythmia (torsade de pointes) may be increased. Posaconazole use with cisapride, pimozide or quinidine is contraindicated.

Rifabutin: Posaconazole may increase the levels/effects of rifabutin. If coadministered, monitor for rifabutin adverse effects (eg, uveitis, leukopenia).

Rifabutin may decrease the levels/effects of posaconazole. Avoid concurrent use; if given, monitor for breakthrough fungal infections.

Sirolimus: Posaconazole may increase the levels/effects of sirolimus. Monitor sirolimus concentrations and reduce dose accordingly.

Tacrolimus: Posaconazole may increase the levels/effects of tacrolimus. Reduce tacrolimus dose to approximately $1/3$ of original dose and monitor. Readjust dose when posaconazole is discontinued.

Vinca alkaloids: Posaconazole may increase the levels/effects of vinca alkaloids (eg, vincristine, vinblastine), leading to neurotoxicity; consider reducing vinca alkaloid dose.

Ethanol/Nutrition/Herb Interactions Food: Bioavailability increased ~3-4 times when posaconazole administered with a meal or an oral liquid nutritional supplement.

Dietary Considerations Give with meals. If alternative antifungal therapy can not be given to patients without food intake or severe diarrhea/vomiting, close monitoring for breakthrough fungal infections must be performed. Adequate posaconazole absorption from GI tract and subsequent plasma concentrations are dependent on food for efficacy. Lower average plasma concentrations have been associated with an increased risk of treatment failure.

Pharmacodynamics/Kinetics

Absorption: Food and/or liquid nutritional supplements increase absorption; fasting states do not provide sufficient absorption to ensure adequate plasma concentrations

Distribution: V_d: 465-1774 L

Protein binding: ≥97%; predominantly bound to albumin

Metabolism: Not significantly metabolized; ~15% to 17% undergoes non-CYP-mediated metabolism, primarily via hepatic glucuronidation into metabolites

Half-life elimination: 35 hours (range: 20-66 hours)

Time to peak, plasma: 3-5 hours

Excretion: Feces 71% to 77% (~66% as unchanged drug); urine 13% to 14% (<0.2% as unchanged drug)

Pregnancy Risk Factor C

Lactation Excretion in breast milk unknown/use caution

Breast-Feeding Considerations Excretion in breast milk has not been investigated; avoid breast-feeding until additional data is available

Dosage Forms Excipient information presented when available (limited, particularly for generics); consult specific product labeling.

Suspension, oral:

Noxafil®: 40 mg/mL (123 mL) [contains sodium benzoate; delivers 105 mL of suspension; cherry flavor; packaged with calibrated dosing spoon]

Dental Comment This drug is known to prolong the QT interval. The QT interval is measured as the time and distance between the Q point of the QRS complex and the end of the T wave in the ECG tracing. After adjustment for heart rate, the QT interval is defined as prolonged if it is more than 450 msec in men and 460 msec in women. A long QT syndrome was first described in the 1950s and 60s as a congenital syndrome involving QT interval prolongation and syncope and sudden death. Some of the congenital long QT syndromes were characterized by a peculiar electrocardiographic appearance of the QRS complex involving a premature atria beat followed by a pause, then a subsequent sinus beat showing marked QT prolongation and deformity. This type of cardiac arrhythmia was originally termed "torsade de pointes" (translated from the French as "twisting of the points").

Prolongation of the QT interval is thought to result from delayed ventricular repolarization. The repolarization process within the myocardial cell is due to the efflux of intracellular potassium. The channels associated with this current can be blocked by many drugs and predispose the electrical propagation cycle to torsade de pointes.

Posaconazole is one of the drugs confirmed to prolong the QT interval and is accepted as having a risk of causing torsade de pointes. The risk of drug-induced torsade de pointes is extremely low when a single QT interval prolonging drug is prescribed. In terms of epinephrine, it is not known what effect vasoconstrictors in the local anesthetic regimen will have in patients with a known history of congenital prolonged QT interval or in patients taking any medication that prolongs the QT interval. Until more information is obtained, it is suggested that the clinician consult with the physician prior to the use of a vasoconstrictor in suspected patients, and that the vasoconstrictor (epinephrine, levonordefrin [Neo-Cobefrin®]) be used with caution.

Selected Readings

Herbrecht R, "Posaconazole: A Potent, Extended-Spectrum Triazole Anti-Fungal for the Treatment of Serious Fungal Infections," *Int J Clin Pract*, 2004, 58(6): 612-24.

Keating G, "Posaconazole," *Drugs*, 2005, 65(11):1553-67.

(Continued)

Posaconazole *(Continued)*

Krieter P, Flannery B, Musick T, et al, "Disposition of Posaconazole Following Single-Dose Oral Administration in Healthy Subjects," *Antimicrob Agents Chemother*, 2004, 48(9):3543-51.

Raad II, Graybill JR, Bustamante AB, "Safety of Long-Term Oral Posaconazole Use in the Treatment of Refractory Invasive Fungal Infections," *Clin Infect Dis*, 2006, 42(12):1726-34.

Post Peel Healing Balm [OTC] *see* Hydrocortisone *on page 836*

Posture® [OTC] *see* Calcium Phosphate (Tribasic) *on page 263*

Potaba® *see* Potassium P-Aminobenzoate *on page 1331*

Potassium Acetate (poe TASS ee um AS e tate)

Generic Available Yes

Pharmacologic Category Electrolyte Supplement, Parenteral

Use Potassium deficiency; to avoid chloride when high concentration of potassium is needed, source of bicarbonate

Local Anesthetic/Vasoconstrictor Precautions No information available to require special precautions

Effects on Dental Treatment No significant effects or complications reported

Mechanism of Action Potassium is the major cation of intracellular fluid and is essential for the conduction of nerve impulses in heart, brain, and skeletal muscle; contraction of cardiac, skeletal and smooth muscles; maintenance of normal renal function, acid-base balance, carbohydrate metabolism, and gastric secretion

Pregnancy Risk Factor C

Potassium Acid Phosphate (poe TASS ee um AS id FOS fate)

U.S. Brand Names K-Phos® Original

Generic Available No

Pharmacologic Category Urinary Acidifying Agent

Use Acidifies urine and lowers urinary calcium concentration; reduces odor and rash caused by ammoniacal urine; increases the antibacterial activity of methenamine

Local Anesthetic/Vasoconstrictor Precautions No information available to require special precautions

Effects on Dental Treatment No significant effects or complications reported

Mechanism of Action The principal intracellular cation; involved in transmission of nerve impulses, muscle contractions, enzyme activity, and glucose utilization

Pregnancy Risk Factor C

Potassium Bicarbonate (poe TASS ee um bye KAR bun ate)

Generic Available Yes

Pharmacologic Category Electrolyte Supplement, Oral

Use Potassium deficiency, hypokalemia

Local Anesthetic/Vasoconstrictor Precautions No information available to require special precautions

Effects on Dental Treatment No significant effects or complications reported

Pregnancy Risk Factor C

Potassium Bicarbonate and Potassium Chloride
(poe TASS ee um bye KAR bun ate & poe TASS ee um KLOR ide)

Related Information

Potassium Bicarbonate *on page 1328*

Potassium Chloride *on page 1329*

U.S. Brand Names K-Lyte/Cl®

Generic Available Yes

Index Terms Potassium Bicarbonate and Potassium Chloride (Effervescent)

Pharmacologic Category Electrolyte Supplement, Oral

Use Treatment or prevention of hypokalemia

Local Anesthetic/Vasoconstrictor Precautions No information available to require special precautions

Effects on Dental Treatment No significant effects or complications reported

Pregnancy Risk Factor C

Potassium Bicarbonate and Potassium Chloride (Effervescent) *see* Potassium Bicarbonate and Potassium Chloride *on page 1328*

Potassium Bicarbonate and Potassium Citrate
(poe TASS ee um bye KAR bun ate & poe TASS ee um SIT rate)

Related Information
Potassium Bicarbonate *on page 1328*
Potassium Citrate *on page 1329*
U.S. Brand Names Effer-K™; Klor-Con®/EF; K-Lyte®; K-Lyte® DS
Generic Available Yes
Index Terms Potassium Bicarbonate and Potassium Citrate (Effervescent)
Pharmacologic Category Electrolyte Supplement, Oral
Use Treatment or prevention of hypokalemia
Local Anesthetic/Vasoconstrictor Precautions No information available to require special precautions
Effects on Dental Treatment No significant effects or complications reported
Mechanism of Action Needed for the conduction of nerve impulses in heart, brain, and skeletal muscle; contraction of cardiac, skeletal and smooth muscles; maintenance of normal renal function
Pregnancy Risk Factor C

Potassium Bicarbonate and Potassium Citrate (Effervescent) *see* Potassium Bicarbonate and Potassium Citrate *on page 1329*

Potassium Chloride (poe TASS ee um KLOR ide)

U.S. Brand Names Kaon-Cl-10®; Kaon-Cl® 20; Kay Ciel®; K-Dur® 10; K-Dur® 20; K-Lor®; Klor-Con®; Klor-Con® 8; Klor-Con® 10; Klor-Con®/25; Klor-Con® M; K+ Potassium; K-Tab®; microK®; microK® 10; Rum-K®
Canadian Brand Names Apo-K®; K-10®; K-Dur®; K-Lor®; K-Lyte®/Cl; Micro-K Extencaps®; Roychlor®; Slo-Pot; Slow-K®
Mexican Brand Names Clor-K-Zaf; Kaliolite
Generic Available Yes
Index Terms KCl
Pharmacologic Category Electrolyte Supplement, Oral; Electrolyte Supplement, Parenteral
Use Treatment or prevention of hypokalemia
Local Anesthetic/Vasoconstrictor Precautions No information available to require special precautions
Effects on Dental Treatment No significant effects or complications reported
Mechanism of Action Potassium is the major cation of intracellular fluid and is essential for the conduction of nerve impulses in heart, brain, and skeletal muscle; contraction of cardiac, skeletal and smooth muscles; maintenance of normal renal function, acid-base balance, carbohydrate metabolism, and gastric secretion
Pregnancy Risk Factor A

Potassium Citrate (poe TASS ee um SIT rate)

U.S. Brand Names Urocit®-K
Canadian Brand Names K-Citra®; K-Lyte®; Polycitra®-K
Generic Available Yes
Pharmacologic Category Alkalinizing Agent, Oral
Use Prevention of uric acid nephrolithiasis; prevention of calcium renal stones in patients with hypocitraturia; urinary alkalinizer when sodium citrate is contraindicated
Local Anesthetic/Vasoconstrictor Precautions No information available to require special precautions
Effects on Dental Treatment No significant effects or complications reported
Pregnancy Risk Factor Not available

Potassium Citrate and Citric Acid
(poe TASS ee um SIT rate & SI trik AS id)

Related Information
Potassium Citrate *on page 1329*
U.S. Brand Names Cytra-K; Polycitra®-K
Generic Available Yes
Index Terms Citric Acid and Potassium Citrate
Pharmacologic Category Alkalinizing Agent, Oral
Use Treatment of metabolic acidosis; alkalinizing agent in conditions where long-term maintenance of an alkaline urine is desirable
(Continued)

Potassium Citrate and Citric Acid *(Continued)*

Local Anesthetic/Vasoconstrictor Precautions No information available to require special precautions

Effects on Dental Treatment No significant effects or complications reported

Drug Interactions

Increased Effect/Toxicity: Concurrent administration with potassium-containing medications, potassium-sparing diuretics, ACE inhibitors, or cardiac glycosides could lead to toxicity.

Pharmacodynamics/Kinetics

Metabolism: To potassium bicarbonate; citric acid is metabolized to CO_2 and H_2O

Excretion: Urine

Pregnancy Risk Factor A

Potassium Citrate, Citric Acid, and Sodium Citrate *see* Citric Acid, Sodium Citrate, and Potassium Citrate *on page 370*

Potassium Gluconate *(poe TASS ee um GLOO coe nate)*

U.S. Brand Names Glu-K® [OTC]

Generic Available Yes

Pharmacologic Category Electrolyte Supplement, Oral

Use Treatment or prevention of hypokalemia

Local Anesthetic/Vasoconstrictor Precautions No information available to require special precautions

Effects on Dental Treatment No significant effects or complications reported

Mechanism of Action Potassium is the major cation of intracellular fluid and is essential for the conduction of nerve impulses in heart, brain, and skeletal muscle; contraction of cardiac, skeletal and smooth muscles; maintenance of normal renal function, acid-base balance, carbohydrate metabolism, and gastric secretion

Pregnancy Risk Factor A

Potassium Guaiacolsulfonate and Guaifenesin *see* Guaifenesin and Potassium Guaiacolsulfonate *on page 797*

Potassium Iodide *(poe TASS ee um EYE oh dide)*

Related Information

Endocrine Disorders and Pregnancy *on page 1750*

U.S. Brand Names Iosat™ [OTC]; Pima®; SSKI®; ThyroSafe™ [OTC]; ThyroShield™ [OTC]

Index Terms KI

Pharmacologic Category Antithyroid Agent; Expectorant

Use Expectorant for the symptomatic treatment of chronic pulmonary diseases complicated by mucous; reduce thyroid vascularity prior to thyroidectomy and management of thyrotoxic crisis; block thyroidal uptake of radioactive isotopes of iodine in a radiation emergency or other exposure to radioactive iodine

Unlabeled/Investigational Use Lymphocutaneous and cutaneous sporotrichosis

Local Anesthetic/Vasoconstrictor Precautions No information available to require special precautions

Effects on Dental Treatment Key adverse event(s) related to dental treatment: Metallic taste.

Common Adverse Effects Frequency not defined.

Cardiovascular: Irregular heart beat

Central nervous system: Confusion, tiredness, fever

Dermatologic: Skin rash

Endocrine & metabolic: Goiter, salivary gland swelling/tenderness, thyroid adenoma, swelling of neck/throat, myxedema, lymph node swelling, hyper-/hypothyroidism

Gastrointestinal: Diarrhea, gastrointestinal bleeding, metallic taste, nausea, stomach pain, stomach upset, vomiting

Neuromuscular & skeletal: Numbness, tingling, weakness, joint pain

Miscellaneous: Chronic iodine poisoning (with prolonged treatment/high doses); iodism, hypersensitivity reactions (angioedema, cutaneous and mucosal hemorrhage, serum sickness-like symptoms)

Mechanism of Action Reduces viscosity of mucus by increasing respiratory tract secretions; inhibits secretion of thyroid hormone, fosters colloid accumulation in thyroid follicles. Following radioactive iodine exposure, potassium iodide blocks uptake of radioiodine by the thyroid, reducing the risk of thyroid cancer.

Drug Interactions
Increased Effect/Toxicity: Lithium may cause additive hypothyroid effects; ACE inhibitors, potassium-sparing diuretics, and potassium/potassium-containing products may lead to hyperkalemia, cardiac arrhythmias, or cardiac arrest

Pharmacodynamics/Kinetics
Onset of action: Hyperthyroidism: 24-48 hours
Peak effect: 10-15 days after continuous therapy
Duration: Radioactive iodine exposure: ~ 24 hours
Pregnancy Risk Factor D

Potassium Iodide and Iodine
(poe TASS ee um EYE oh dide & EYE oh dine)

Generic Available Yes
Index Terms Lugol's Solution; Strong Iodine Solution
Pharmacologic Category Antithyroid Agent
Use Reduce thyroid vascularity prior to thyroidectomy and management of thyrotoxic crisis; block thyroidal uptake of radioactive isotopes of iodine in a radiation emergency or other exposure to radioactive iodine
Local Anesthetic/Vasoconstrictor Precautions No information available to require special precautions
Effects on Dental Treatment Key adverse event(s) related to dental treatment: Metallic taste.
Common Adverse Effects Frequency not defined.
Cardiovascular: Irregular heart beat
Central nervous system: Confusion, tiredness, fever
Dermatologic: Skin rash
Endocrine & metabolic: Goiter, salivary gland swelling/tenderness, thyroid adenoma, swelling of neck/throat, myxedema, lymph node swelling, hyper-/hypothyroidism
Gastrointestinal: Diarrhea, gastrointestinal bleeding, metallic taste, nausea, stomach pain, stomach upset, vomiting
Neuromuscular & skeletal: Numbness, tingling, weakness, joint pain
Miscellaneous: Chronic iodine poisoning (with prolonged treatment/high doses); iodism, hypersensitivity reactions (angioedema, cutaneous and mucosal hemorrhage, serum sickness-like symptoms)
Mechanism of Action Inhibits secretion of thyroid hormone, fosters colloid accumulation in thyroid follicles. Following radioactive iodine exposure, potassium iodide blocks uptake of radioiodine by the thyroid, reducing the risk of thyroid cancer.
Drug Interactions
Increased Effect/Toxicity: Concurrent use of ACE inhibitors, potassium-sparing diuretics, or potassium (and potassium-containing products) may lead to hyperkalemia, cardiac arrhythmias or cardiac arrest. Lithium may cause additive hypothyroid effects.
Pharmacodynamics/Kinetics
Onset of action: Hyperthyroidism: 24-48 hours
Peak effect: 10-15 days after continuous therapy
Pregnancy Risk Factor D (potassium iodide)

Potassium Iodide, Chlorpheniramine, Phenylephrine, and Codeine *see* Chlorpheniramine, Phenylephrine, Codeine, and Potassium Iodide *on page 344*

Potassium P-Aminobenzoate
(poe TASS ee um pe a mee noe BEN zoe ate)

U.S. Brand Names Potaba®
Generic Available Yes
Pharmacologic Category Vitamin, Water Soluble
Use Presently, all indications are classified by the FDA as "possibly effective." Treatment of scleroderma, dermatomyositis, morphea, linear scleroderma, pemphigus, Peyronie's disease
Local Anesthetic/Vasoconstrictor Precautions No information available to require special precautions
Effects on Dental Treatment No significant effects or complications reported
Mechanism of Action P-aminobenzoate is a member of the vitamin B complex family. It may have an antifibrotic effect due to increased oxygen uptake at the tissue level.

Potassium Perchlorate (poe TASS ee um per KLOR ate)

U.S. Brand Names Perchloracap® [DSC]
Generic Available No
Pharmacologic Category Diagnostic Agent
Use Minimizes accumulation of pertechnetate Tc 99m in imaging studies
Local Anesthetic/Vasoconstrictor Precautions No information available to require special precautions
Effects on Dental Treatment No significant effects or complications reported
Pregnancy Risk Factor C

Potassium Phosphate (poe TASS ee um FOS fate)

U.S. Brand Names Neutra-Phos®-K [OTC]
Generic Available Yes: Injection
Index Terms Phosphate, Potassium
Pharmacologic Category Electrolyte Supplement, Oral; Electrolyte Supplement, Parenteral
Use Treatment and prevention of hypophosphatemia or hypokalemia
Local Anesthetic/Vasoconstrictor Precautions No information available to require special precautions
Effects on Dental Treatment No significant effects or complications reported
Pregnancy Risk Factor C

Potassium Phosphate and Sodium Phosphate (poe TASS ee um FOS fate & SOW dee um FOS fate)

Related Information
Potassium Phosphate *on page 1332*
Sodium Phosphates *on page 1484*
U.S. Brand Names K-Phos® MF; K-Phos® Neutral; K-Phos® No. 2; Neutra-Phos® [OTC]; Phos-NaK; Phospha 250™ Neutral; Uro-KP-Neutral®
Generic Available Yes
Index Terms Sodium Phosphate and Potassium Phosphate
Pharmacologic Category Electrolyte Supplement, Oral
Use Treatment of conditions associated with excessive renal phosphate loss or inadequate GI absorption of phosphate; to acidify the urine to lower calcium concentrations; to increase the antibacterial activity of methenamine; reduce odor and rash caused by ammonia in urine
Local Anesthetic/Vasoconstrictor Precautions No information available to require special precautions
Effects on Dental Treatment No significant effects or complications reported
Pregnancy Risk Factor C

Povidine™ [OTC] *see* Povidone-Iodine *on page 1332*

Povidone-Iodine (POE vi done EYE oh dyne)

Related Information
Management of Patients Undergoing Cancer Therapy *on page 1826*
U.S. Brand Names Betadine® [OTC]; Betadine® Ophthalmic; Minidyne® [OTC]; Operand® [OTC]; Povidine™ [OTC]; Summer's Eve® Medicated Douche [OTC]; Vagi-Gard® [OTC]
Canadian Brand Names Betadine®; Proviodine
Generic Available Yes
Index Terms Polyvinylpyrrolidone with Iodine; PVP-I
Pharmacologic Category Antiseptic, Ophthalmic; Antiseptic, Topical; Antiseptic, Vaginal; Topical Skin Product
Use External antiseptic with broad microbicidal spectrum for the prevention or treatment of topical infections associated with surgery, burns, minor cuts/scrapes; relief of minor vaginal irritation
Local Anesthetic/Vasoconstrictor Precautions No information available to require special precautions
Effects on Dental Treatment No significant effects or complications reported
Common Adverse Effects Frequency not defined. Also refer to Iodine *on page 900*.
Local: Edema, irritation, pruritus, rash
Mechanism of Action Povidone-iodine is known to be a powerful broad spectrum germicidal agent effective against a wide range of bacteria, viruses, fungi, protozoa, and spores.

Pharmacodynamics/Kinetics Absorption: Topical: Absorbed systemically as iodine; amount depends upon concentration, route of administration, characteristics of skin

Pregnancy Risk Factor C (ophthalmic)

Pramipexole (pra mi PEKS ole)

U.S. Brand Names Mirapex®

Canadian Brand Names Apo-Pramipexole; Mirapex®; Novo-Pramipexole; PMS-Pramipexole

Mexican Brand Names Sifrol

Generic Available No

Pharmacologic Category Anti-Parkinson's Agent, Dopamine Agonist

Use Treatment of the signs and symptoms of idiopathic Parkinson's disease; treatment of moderate-to-severe primary Restless Legs Syndrome (RLS)

Unlabeled/Investigational Use Treatment of depression

Local Anesthetic/Vasoconstrictor Precautions No information available to require special precautions

Effects on Dental Treatment Key adverse event(s) related to dental treatment: Xerostomia (normal salivary flow resumes upon discontinuation) and dysphagia.

Common Adverse Effects Parkinson's disease (PD) unless identified as RLS:

>10%:

Cardiovascular: Postural hypotension (dose related; PD 53%)

Central nervous system: Dizziness (PD 25%), headache (RLS 16%), somnolence (dose related; RLS 6%; PD 9% to 22%), insomnia (RLS 13%; PD 17% to 27%), hallucinations (PD 9% to 17%), abnormal dreams (RLS up to 8%)

Gastrointestinal: Nausea (dose related; RLS: 5% to 27%; PD 28%), constipation (dose related; RLS: 4%; PD 10% to 14%)

Neuromuscular & skeletal: Weakness (PD 10% to 14%), dyskinesia (PD 47%), EPS

1% to 10%:

Cardiovascular: Edema, syncope, tachycardia, chest pain

Central nervous system: Malaise, confusion (PD 4% to 10%), amnesia (dose related), dystonias, akathisia, thinking abnormalities, myoclonus, hyperesthesia, paranoia, fever

Endocrine & metabolic: Decreased libido

Gastrointestinal: Anorexia, diarrhea (RLS 3% to7%), dysphagia, weight loss, xerostomia (up to 7%)

Genitourinary: Urinary frequency (PD 6%), impotence, urinary incontinence

Neuromuscular & skeletal: Muscle twitching, leg cramps, arthritis, bursitis, myasthenia, gait abnormalities, hypertonia

Ocular: Vision abnormalities

Respiratory: Dyspnea, nasal congestion (RLS up to 6%), rhinitis

Miscellaneous: Influenza (RLS 3%)

Mechanism of Action Pramipexole is a nonergot dopamine agonist with specificity for the D_2 subfamily dopamine receptor, and has also been shown to bind to D_3 and D_4 receptors. By binding to these receptors, it is thought that pramipexole can stimulate dopamine activity on the nerves of the striatum and substantia nigra.

Drug Interactions

Increased Effect/Toxicity: Cimetidine may increase level/effects of pramipexole. CNS depressants may enhance the adverse/toxic effect of pramipexole.

Decreased Effect: Dopamine antagonists (antipsychotics, metoclopramide) may decrease the efficiency of pramipexole.

Pharmacodynamics/Kinetics

Absorption: Rapid

Distribution: V_d: 500 L

Protein binding: 15%

Bioavailability: >90%

Half-life elimination: ~8 hours; Elderly: 12-14 hours

Time to peak, serum: ~2 hours

Excretion: Urine (90% as unchanged drug)

Pregnancy Risk Factor C

Pramlintide (PRAM lin tide)

U.S. Brand Names Symlin®
Generic Available No
Index Terms Pramlintide Acetate
Pharmacologic Category Amylinomimetic; Antidiabetic Agent
Use

Adjunctive treatment with mealtime insulin in type 1 diabetes mellitus (insulin dependent, IDDM) patients who have failed to achieve desired glucose control despite optimal insulin therapy

Adjunctive treatment with mealtime insulin in type 2 diabetes mellitus (noninsulin dependent, NIDDM) patients who have failed to achieve desired glucose control despite optimal insulin therapy, with or without concurrent sulfonylurea and/or metformin

Local Anesthetic/Vasoconstrictor Precautions No information available to require special precautions
Effects on Dental Treatment No significant effects or complications reported
Common Adverse Effects

>10%:
Central nervous system: Headache (5% to 13%)
Gastrointestinal: Nausea (28% to 48%), vomiting (7% to 11%), anorexia (<1% to 17%)
Endocrine & metabolic: Severe hypoglycemia (type 1 diabetes: <1% to 17%)
Miscellaneous: Inflicted injury (8% to 14%)

1% to 10%:
Central nervous system: Fatigue (3% to 7%), dizziness (2% to 6%)
Endocrine & metabolic: Severe hypoglycemia (type 2 diabetes: <1% to 8%)
Gastrointestinal: Abdominal pain (2% to 8%)
Respiratory: Pharyngitis (3% to 5%), cough (2% to 6%)
Neuromuscular & skeletal: Arthralgia (2% to 7%)
Miscellaneous: Allergic reaction (<1% to 6%)

Restrictions An FDA-approved medication guide must be distributed when dispensing an outpatient prescription (new or refill) where this medication is to be used without direct supervision of a healthcare provider. Medication guides are available at http://www.fda.gov/cder/Offices/ODS/medication_guides.htm.
Mechanism of Action Synthetic analog of human amylin cosecreted with insulin by pancreatic beta cells; reduces postprandial glucose increases via the following mechanisms: 1) prolongation of gastric emptying time, 2) reduction of postprandial glucagon secretion, and 3) reduction of caloric intake through centrally-mediated appetite suppression
Drug Interactions

Increased Effect/Toxicity: Medications which may induce or exacerbate hypoglycemia include ACE inhibitors, alcohol, alpha-blockers, anabolic steroids, beta-blockers, clofibrate, clonidine, disopyramide, fenfluramine, fibrates, fluoxetine, guanethidine, MAO inhibitors, pentamidine, pentoxifylline, phenylbutazone, propoxyphene, reserpine, salicylates, sulfinpyrazone, sulfonamides, and tetracyclines. Nonselective beta-blockers may delay recovery from hypoglycemic episodes and mask signs/symptoms of hypoglycemia. Anticholinergic agents may cause synergistic impairment of gastric motility.

Decreased Effect: Pramlintide may delay absorption of concomitantly administered medication due to increased gastric emptying time; coadministration with agents in which a rapid onset of action is desired (eg, analgesics) may delay drug response.

Pharmacodynamics/Kinetics
Duration: 3 hours
Protein binding: 60%
Metabolism: Primarily renal to des-lys[1] pramlintide (active metabolite)
Bioavailability: 30% to 40%
Half-life elimination: 48 minutes
Time to peak, plasma: 20 minutes
Excretion: Primarily urine
Pregnancy Risk Factor C

Pramlintide Acetate *see* Pramlintide *on page 1334*
Pramosone® *see* Pramoxine and Hydrocortisone *on page 1335*

Pramoxine (pra MOKS een)

U.S. Brand Names Anusol® Ointment [OTC]; Caladryl® Clear [OTC]; CalaMycin® Cool and Clear [OTC]; Callergy Clear [OTC]; Curasore® [OTC]; Itch-X® [OTC]; Prax® [OTC]; ProctoFoam® NS [OTC]; Sarna® Sensitive; Tronolane® Cream [OTC]; Tucks® Hemorrhoidal [OTC]

Generic Available Yes: Foam, lotion
Index Terms Pramoxine Hydrochloride
Pharmacologic Category Local Anesthetic
Use Temporary relief of pain and itching associated with anogenital pruritus or irritation; dermatosis, minor burns, or hemorrhoids
Local Anesthetic/Vasoconstrictor Precautions No information available to require special precautions
Effects on Dental Treatment No significant effects or complications reported
Common Adverse Effects 1% to 10%:
  Dermatologic: Angioedema
  Local: Contact dermatitis, burning, stinging
Mechanism of Action Pramoxine, like other anesthetics, decreases the neuronal membrane's permeability to sodium ions; both initiation and conduction of nerve impulses are blocked, thus depolarization of the neuron is inhibited
Pharmacodynamics/Kinetics
  Onset of action: Therapeutic: 2-5 minutes
    Peak effect: 3-5 minutes
  Duration: Several days
Pregnancy Risk Factor C

Pramoxine and Hydrocortisone
(pra MOKS een & hye droe KOR ti sone)

Related Information
  Hydrocortisone *on page 836*
  Pramoxine *on page 1334*
U.S. Brand Names Analpram-HC®; Enzone®; Epifoam®; Pramosone®; ProctoFoam®-HC; Zone-A®; Zone-A Forte®
Canadian Brand Names Pramox® HC; Proctofoam™-HC
Generic Available No
Index Terms Hydrocortisone and Pramoxine
Pharmacologic Category Anesthetic/Corticosteroid
Use Relief of inflammatory and pruritic manifestations of corticosteroid-responsive dermatoses
Local Anesthetic/Vasoconstrictor Precautions No information available to require special precautions
Effects on Dental Treatment No significant effects or complications reported
Common Adverse Effects See individual agents.
Drug Interactions
  Cytochrome P450 Effect: Hydrocortisone: **Substrate** of CYP3A4 (minor); **Induces** CYP3A4 (weak)
  Increased Effect/Toxicity: See individual agents.
  Decreased Effect: See individual agents.
Pharmacodynamics/Kinetics See individual agents.
Pregnancy Risk Factor C

Pramoxine Hydrochloride *see* Pramoxine *on page 1334*

Pramoxine, Neomycin, Bacitracin, and Polymyxin B *see* Bacitracin, Neomycin, Polymyxin B, and Pramoxine *on page 182*

Prandin® *see* Repaglinide *on page 1415*

Pravachol® *see* Pravastatin *on page 1335*

Pravastatin (prav a STAT in)

Related Information
  Cardiovascular Diseases *on page 1726*
U.S. Brand Names Pravachol®
Canadian Brand Names Apo-Pravastatin®; CO Pravastatin; Novo-Pravastatin; PMS-Pravastatin; Pravachol®; ratio-Pravastatin; Riva-Pravastatin; Sandoz-Pravastatin
Mexican Brand Names Astin; Kenstatin; Xipral
Generic Available Yes
Index Terms Pravastatin Sodium
Pharmacologic Category Antilipemic Agent, HMG-CoA Reductase Inhibitor
Use Use with dietary therapy for the following:
  Primary prevention of coronary events: In hypercholesterolemic patients without established coronary heart disease to reduce cardiovascular morbidity (myocardial infarction, coronary revascularization procedures) and mortality.
  Secondary prevention of cardiovascular events in patients with established coronary heart disease: To slow the progression of coronary atherosclerosis; to reduce cardiovascular morbidity (myocardial infarction, coronary vascular (Continued)

Pravastatin *(Continued)*

procedures) and to reduce mortality; to reduce the risk of stroke and transient ischemic attacks

Hyperlipidemias: Reduce elevations in total cholesterol, LDL-C, apolipoprotein B, and triglycerides (elevations of 1 or more components are present in Fredrickson type IIa, IIb, III, and IV hyperlipidemias)

Heterozygous familial hypercholesterolemia (HeFH): In pediatric patients, 8-18 years of age, with HeFH having LDL-C ≥190 mg/dL **or** LDL ≥160 mg/dL with positive family history of premature cardiovascular disease (CVD) or 2 or more CVD risk factors in the pediatric patient

Local Anesthetic/Vasoconstrictor Precautions No information available to require special precautions

Effects on Dental Treatment No significant effects or complications reported

Common Adverse Effects As reported in short-term trials; safety and tolerability with long-term use were similar to placebo

1% to 10%:

Cardiovascular: Chest pain (4%)

Central nervous system: Headache (2% to 6%), fatigue (4%), dizziness (1% to 3%)

Dermatologic: Rash (4%)

Gastrointestinal: Nausea/vomiting (7%), diarrhea (6%), heartburn (3%)

Hepatic: Transaminases increased (>3x normal on two occasions - 1%)

Neuromuscular & skeletal: Myalgia (2%)

Respiratory: Cough (3%)

Miscellaneous: Influenza (2%)

Additional class-related events or case reports (not necessarily reported with pravastatin therapy): Angioedema, cataracts, depression, dyspnea, eosinophilia, erectile dysfunction, facial paresis, hypersensitivity reaction, impaired extraocular muscle movement, impotence, leukopenia, malaise, memory loss, ophthalmoplegia, paresthesia, peripheral neuropathy, photosensitivity, psychic disturbance, skin discoloration, thrombocytopenia, thyroid dysfunction, toxic epidermal necrolysis, transaminases increased, vomiting

Dosage Oral: **Note:** Doses should be individualized according to the baseline LDL-cholesterol levels, the recommended goal of therapy, and patient response; adjustments should be made at intervals of 4 weeks or more; doses may need adjusted based on concomitant medications

Children: HeFH:

8-13 years: 20 mg/day

14-18 years: 40 mg/day

Dosage adjustment for pravastatin based on concomitant cyclosporine: Refer to adult dosing section

Adults: Hyperlipidemias, primary prevention of coronary events, secondary prevention of cardiovascular events: Initial: 40 mg once daily; titrate dosage to response; usual range: 10-80 mg; (maximum dose: 80 mg once daily)

Dosage adjustment for pravastatin based on concomitant cyclosporine: Initial: 10 mg/day, titrate with caution (maximum dose: 20 mg/day)

Elderly: No specific dosage recommendations. Clearance is reduced in the elderly, resulting in an increase in AUC between 25% to 50%. However, substantial accumulation is not expected.

Dosing adjustment in renal impairment: Initial: 10 mg/day

Dosing adjustment in hepatic impairment: Initial: 10 mg/day

Mechanism of Action Pravastatin is a competitive inhibitor of 3-hydroxy-3-methylglutaryl coenzyme A (HMG-CoA) reductase, which is the rate-limiting enzyme involved in *de novo* cholesterol synthesis.

Contraindications Hypersensitivity to pravastatin or any component of the formulation; active liver disease; unexplained persistent elevations of serum transaminases; pregnancy; breast-feeding

Warnings/Precautions Secondary causes of hyperlipidemia should be ruled out prior to therapy. Liver function must be monitored by periodic laboratory assessment. Rhabdomyolysis with acute renal failure has occurred. Risk may be increased with concurrent use of other drugs which may cause rhabdomyolysis (including gemfibrozil, fibric acid derivatives, or niacin at doses ≥1 g/day). Temporarily discontinue in any patient experiencing an acute or serious condition predisposing to renal failure secondary to rhabdomyolysis. Use with caution in patients with advanced age, these patients are predisposed to myopathy. Use caution in patients with previous liver disease or heavy ethanol use. Treatment in patients <8 years of age is not recommended.

Drug Interactions

Cytochrome P450 Effect: Substrate of CYP3A4 (minor); **Inhibits** CYP2C9 (weak), 2D6 (weak), 3A4 (weak)

Increased Effect/Toxicity: Clofibrate, cyclosporine, fenofibrate, gemfibrozil, and niacin may increase the risk of myopathy and rhabdomyolysis. Imidazole antifungals (itraconazole, ketoconazole), P-glycoprotein inhibitors may increase pravastatin concentrations.

Decreased Effect: Concurrent administration of cholestyramine or colestipol can decrease pravastatin absorption.

Ethanol/Nutrition/Herb Interactions

Ethanol: Consumption of large amounts of ethanol may increase the risk of liver damage with HMG-CoA reductase inhibitors.

Food: Red yeast rice contains an estimated 2.4 mg lovastatin per 600 mg rice.

Herb/Nutraceutical: St John's wort may decrease pravastatin levels.

Dietary Considerations May be taken without regard to meals. Before initiation of therapy, patients should be placed on a standard cholesterol-lowering diet for 6 weeks and the diet should be continued during drug therapy. Red yeast rice contains an estimated 2.4 mg lovastatin per 600 mg rice.

Pharmacodynamics/Kinetics

Onset of action: Several days

Peak effect: 4 weeks

Absorption: Rapidly absorbed; average absorption 34%

Protein binding: 50%

Metabolism: Hepatic to at least two metabolites

Bioavailability: 17%

Half-life elimination: ~2-3 hours

Time to peak, serum: 1-1.5 hours

Excretion: Feces (70%); urine (≤20%, 8% as unchanged drug)

Pregnancy Risk Factor X

Dosage Forms

Tablet: 10 mg, 20 mg, 40 mg, 80 mg

Pravachol®: 10 mg, 20 mg, 40 mg, 80 mg

Pravastatin and Aspirin *see* Aspirin and Pravastatin *on page 155*

Pravastatin Sodium *see* Pravastatin *on page 1335*

Pravigard™ PAC [DSC] *see* Aspirin and Pravastatin *on page 155*

Prax® [OTC] *see* Pramoxine *on page 1334*

Praziquantel (pray zi KWON tel)

U.S. Brand Names Biltricide®

Canadian Brand Names Biltricide®

Mexican Brand Names Cisticid

Generic Available No

Pharmacologic Category Anthelmintic

Use All stages of schistosomiasis caused by all *Schistosoma* species pathogenic to humans; clonorchiasis and opisthorchiasis

Unlabeled/Investigational Use Cysticercosis and many intestinal tapeworms

Local Anesthetic/Vasoconstrictor Precautions No information available to require special precautions

Effects on Dental Treatment No significant effects or complications reported

Common Adverse Effects 1% to 10%:

Central nervous system: Dizziness, drowsiness, headache, malaise, CSF reaction syndrome in patients being treated for neurocysticercosis

Gastrointestinal: Abdominal pain, loss of appetite, nausea, vomiting

Miscellaneous: Diaphoresis

Mechanism of Action Increases the cell permeability to calcium in schistosomes, causing strong contractions and paralysis of worm musculature leading to detachment of suckers from the blood vessel walls and to dislodgment

Drug Interactions

Cytochrome P450 Effect: Inhibits CYP2D6 (weak)

Pharmacodynamics/Kinetics

Absorption: Oral: ~80%

Distribution: CSF concentration is 14% to 20% of plasma concentration; enters breast milk

Protein binding: ~80%

Metabolism: Extensive first-pass effect

Half-life elimination: Parent drug: 0.8-1.5 hours; Metabolites: 4.5 hours

Time to peak, serum: 1-3 hours

Excretion: Urine (99% as metabolites)

Pregnancy Risk Factor B

Prazosin (PRAZ oh sin)

Related Information

Cardiovascular Diseases *on page 1726*

(Continued)

Prazosin *(Continued)*

U.S. Brand Names Minipress®
Canadian Brand Names Apo-Prazo®; Minipress®; Novo-Prazin; Nu-Prazo
Mexican Brand Names Minipres
Generic Available Yes
Index Terms Furazosin; Prazosin Hydrochloride
Pharmacologic Category Alpha₁ Blocker
Use Treatment of hypertension
Unlabeled/Investigational Use Post-traumatic stress disorder (PTSD); benign prostatic hyperplasia; Raynaud's syndrome
Local Anesthetic/Vasoconstrictor Precautions No information available to require special precautions
Effects on Dental Treatment Key adverse event(s) related to dental treatment: Significant xerostomia (normal salivary flow resumes upon discontinuation). Significant orthostatic hypotension is a possibility; monitor patient when getting out of dental chair.
Common Adverse Effects
>10%: Central nervous system: Dizziness (10%)
1% to 10%:
  Cardiovascular: Palpitation (5%), edema, orthostatic hypotension, syncope (1%)
  Central nervous system: Headache (8%), drowsiness (8%), weakness (7%), vertigo, depression, nervousness
  Dermatologic: Rash (1% to 4%)
  Endocrine & metabolic: Decreased energy (7%)
  Gastrointestinal: Nausea (5%), vomiting, diarrhea, constipation
  Genitourinary: Urinary frequency (1% to 5%)
  Ocular: Blurred vision, reddened sclera, xerostomia
  Respiratory: Dyspnea, epistaxis, nasal congestion
Mechanism of Action Competitively inhibits postsynaptic alpha-adrenergic receptors which results in vasodilation of veins and arterioles and a decrease in total peripheral resistance and blood pressure
Drug Interactions
  Increased Effect/Toxicity: Prazosin's hypotensive effect may be increased with beta-blockers, diuretics, ACE inhibitors, calcium channel blockers, other antihypertensive medications, sildenafil (use with extreme caution at a dose ≤25 mg), tadalafil (use is contraindicated by the manufacturer), and vardenafil (use is contraindicated by the manufacturer). Concurrent use with tricyclic antidepressants (TCAs) and low-potency antipsychotics may increase risk of orthostasis.
  Decreased Effect: Decreased antihypertensive effect if taken with NSAIDs.
Pharmacodynamics/Kinetics
Onset of action: BP reduction: ~2 hours
  Maximum decrease: 2-4 hours
Duration: 10-24 hours
Distribution: Hypertensive adults: V_d: 0.5 L/kg
Protein binding: 92% to 97%
Metabolism: Extensively hepatic
Bioavailability: 43% to 82%
Half-life elimination: 2-4 hours; prolonged with congestive heart failure
Excretion: Urine (6% to 10% as unchanged drug)
Pregnancy Risk Factor C

Prazosin and Polythiazide *(PRAZ oh sin & pol i THYE a zide)*

Related Information
  Polythiazide *on page 1323*
  Prazosin *on page 1337*
U.S. Brand Names Minizide® [DSC]
Generic Available No
Index Terms Polythiazide and Prazosin
Pharmacologic Category Antihypertensive Agent, Combination
Use Management of mild-to-moderate hypertension
Local Anesthetic/Vasoconstrictor Precautions No information available to require special precautions
Effects on Dental Treatment Key adverse event(s) related to dental treatment: Significant xerostomia (normal salivary flow resumes upon discontinuation). Significant orthostatic hypotension is a possibility; monitor patient when getting out of dental chair.
Common Adverse Effects See individual agents.
Pharmacodynamics/Kinetics See individual agents.
Pregnancy Risk Factor C

Prazosin Hydrochloride *see* Prazosin *on page 1337*

Precedex™ *see* Dexmedetomidine *on page 470*

Precose® *see* Acarbose *on page 27*

Pred Forte® *see* PrednisoLONE *on page 1339*

Pred-G® *see* Prednisolone and Gentamicin *on page 1342*

Pred Mild® *see* PrednisoLONE *on page 1339*

Prednicarbate (pred ni KAR bate)

U.S. Brand Names Dermatop®
Canadian Brand Names Dermatop®
Generic Available Yes: Cream
Pharmacologic Category Corticosteroid, Topical
Use Relief of the inflammatory and pruritic manifestations of corticosteroid-responsive dermatoses (medium potency topical corticosteroid)
Local Anesthetic/Vasoconstrictor Precautions No information available to require special precautions
Effects on Dental Treatment No significant effects or complications reported
Mechanism of Action Topical corticosteroids have anti-inflammatory, antipruritic, vasoconstrictive, and antiproliferative actions
Pregnancy Risk Factor C

PrednisoLONE (pred NISS oh lone)

Related Information
PredniSONE *on page 1342*
Respiratory Diseases *on page 1747*
U.S. Brand Names Econopred® Plus; Orapred®; Orapred ODT™; Pediapred®; Pred Forte®; Pred Mild®; Prelone®
Canadian Brand Names Diopred®; Hydeltra T.B.A.®; Inflamase® Mild; Novo-Prednisolone; Ophtho-Tate®; Pediapred®; Pred Forte®; Pred Mild®; Sab-Prenase
Mexican Brand Names Fisopred; Pred; Prednefrin SF; Pred Un
Generic Available Yes
Index Terms Deltahydrocortisone; Metacortandralone; Prednisolone Acetate; Prednisolone Acetate, Ophthalmic; Prednisolone Sodium Phosphate; Prednisolone Sodium Phosphate, Ophthalmic
Pharmacologic Category Corticosteroid, Ophthalmic; Corticosteroid, Systemic
Dental Use Treatment of a variety of oral diseases of allergic, inflammatory, or autoimmune origin
Use Treatment of palpebral and bulbar conjunctivitis; corneal injury from chemical, radiation, thermal burns, or foreign body penetration; endocrine disorders, rheumatic disorders, collagen diseases, dermatologic diseases, allergic states, ophthalmic diseases, respiratory diseases, hematologic disorders, neoplastic diseases, edematous states, and gastrointestinal diseases; resolution of acute exacerbations of multiple sclerosis; management of fulminating or disseminated tuberculosis and trichinosis; acute or chronic solid organ rejection
Local Anesthetic/Vasoconstrictor Precautions No information available to require special precautions
Effects on Dental Treatment Key adverse event(s) related to dental treatment: Ulcerative esophagitis.
Significant Adverse Effects Frequency not defined.
  Ophthalmic formulation:
    Endocrine & metabolic: Hypercorticoidism (rare)
    Ocular: Conjunctival hyperemia, conjunctivitis, corneal ulcers, delayed wound healing, glaucoma, intraocular pressure increased, keratitis, loss of accommodation, optic nerve damage, mydriasis, posterior subcapsular cataract formation, ptosis, secondary ocular infection
  Oral formulation:
    Cardiovascular: Cardiomyopathy, CHF, edema, facial edema, hypertension
    Central nervous system: Convulsions, headache, insomnia, malaise, nervousness, pseudotumor cerebri, psychic disorders, vertigo
    Dermatologic: Bruising, facial erythema, hirsutism, petechiae, skin test reaction suppression, thin fragile skin, urticaria
    Endocrine & metabolic: Carbohydrate tolerance decreased, Cushing's syndrome, diabetes mellitus, growth suppression, hyperglycemia, hypernatremia, hypokalemia, hypokalemic alkalosis, menstrual irregularities, negative nitrogen balance, pituitary adrenal axis suppression
(Continued)

PrednisoLONE (Continued)

Gastrointestinal: Abdominal distention, increased appetite, indigestion, nausea, pancreatitis, peptic ulcer, ulcerative esophagitis, weight gain

Hepatic: LFTs increased (usually reversible)

Neuromuscular & skeletal: Arthralgia, aseptic necrosis (humeral/femoral heads), fractures, muscle mass decreased, muscle weakness, osteoporosis, steroid myopathy, tendon rupture, weakness

Ocular: Cataracts, exophthalmus, eyelid edema, glaucoma, intraocular pressure increased, irritation

Respiratory: Epistaxis

Miscellaneous: Diaphoresis increased, impaired wound healing

Dental Usual Dosing Anti-inflammatory or immunosuppressive dose: Oral:

Children: 0.1-2 mg/kg/day in divided doses 1-4 times/day

Adults: Usual range: 5-60 mg/day

Dosage Dose depends upon condition being treated and response of patient; dosage for infants and children should be based on severity of the disease and response of the patient rather than on strict adherence to dosage indicated by age, weight, or body surface area. Consider alternate day therapy for long-term therapy. Discontinuation of long-term therapy requires gradual withdrawal by tapering the dose. Patients undergoing unusual stress while receiving corticosteroids, should receive increased doses prior to, during, and after the stressful situation.

Children: Oral:

Acute asthma: 1-2 mg/kg/day in divided doses 1-2 times/day for 3-5 days

Anti-inflammatory or immunosuppressive dose: 0.1-2 mg/kg/day in divided doses 1-4 times/day

Nephrotic syndrome:

Initial (first 3 episodes): 2 mg/kg/day **or** 60 mg/m^2/day (maximum: 80 mg/day) in divided doses 3-4 times/day until urine is protein free for 3 consecutive days (maximum: 28 days); followed by 1-1.5 mg/kg/dose **or** 40 mg/m^2/dose given every other day for 4 weeks

Maintenance (long-term maintenance dose for frequent relapses): 0.5-1 mg/kg/dose given every other day for 3-6 months

Adults: Oral:

Usual range: 5-60 mg/day

Multiple sclerosis: 200 mg/day for 1 week followed by 80 mg every other day for 1 month

Rheumatoid arthritis: Initial: 5-7.5 mg/day; adjust dose as necessary

Ophthalmic suspension/solution: Conjunctivitis, corneal injury: Children and Adults: Instill 1-2 drops into conjunctival sac every hour during day, every 2 hours at night until favorable response is obtained, then use 1 drop every 4 hours.

Elderly: Use lowest effective dose

Dosing adjustment in hyperthyroidism: Prednisolone dose may need to be increased to achieve adequate therapeutic effects

Hemodialysis: Slightly dialyzable (5% to 20%); administer dose posthemodialysis

Peritoneal dialysis: Supplemental dose is not necessary

Mechanism of Action Decreases inflammation by suppression of migration of polymorphonuclear leukocytes and reversal of increased capillary permeability; suppresses the immune system by reducing activity and volume of the lymphatic system

Contraindications Hypersensitivity to prednisolone or any component of the formulation; acute superficial herpes simplex keratitis; live or attenuated virus vaccines (with immunosuppressive doses of corticosteroids); systemic fungal infections; varicella

Warnings/Precautions May cause hypercorticism or suppression of hypothalamic-pituitary-adrenal (HPA) axis, particularly in younger children or in patients receiving high doses for prolonged periods. HPA axis suppression may lead to adrenal crisis. Withdrawal and discontinuation of a corticosteroid should be done slowly and carefully. Particular care is required when patients are transferred from systemic corticosteroids to inhaled products due to possible adrenal insufficiency or withdrawal from steroids, including an increase in allergic symptoms. Patients receiving >20 mg per day of prednisone (or equivalent) may be most susceptible. Fatalities have occurred due to adrenal insufficiency in asthmatic patients during and after transfer from systemic corticosteroids to aerosol steroids; aerosol steroids do **not** provide the systemic steroid needed to treat patients having trauma, surgery, or infections.

Acute myopathy has been reported with high dose corticosteroids, usually in patients with neuromuscular transmission disorders; may involve ocular and/or respiratory muscles; monitor creatine kinase; recovery may be delayed. Corticosteroid use may cause psychiatric disturbances, including depression, euphoria, insomnia, mood swings, and personality changes. Pre-existing psychiatric conditions may be exacerbated by corticosteroid use. Prolonged use of corticosteroids may also increase the incidence of secondary infection, mask acute infection (including fungal infections), prolong or exacerbate viral infections, or limit response to vaccines. Exposure to chickenpox should be avoided; corticosteroids should not be used to treat ocular herpes simplex. Corticosteroids should not be used for cerebral malaria. Close observation is required in patients with latent tuberculosis and/or TB reactivity; restrict use in active TB (only in conjunction with antituberculosis treatment). Prolonged use of corticosteroids may result in glaucoma; damage to the optic nerve (not indicated for treatment of optic neuritis); defects in visual acuity and fields of vision, and posterior subcapsular cataract formation may occur. Use following cataract surgery may delay healing or increase the incidence of bleb formation. Prolonged treatment with corticosteroids has been associated with the development of Kaposi's sarcoma (case reports); if noted, discontinuation of therapy should be considered.

Use with caution in patients with thyroid disease, hepatic impairment, renal impairment, cardiovascular disease, diabetes, glaucoma, cataracts, myasthenia gravis, patients at risk for osteoporosis, patients at risk for seizures, or GI diseases (diverticulitis, peptic ulcer, ulcerative colitis) due to perforation risk. Use caution following acute MI (corticosteroids have been associated with myocardial rupture). Because of the risk of adverse effects, systemic corticosteroids should be used cautiously in the elderly in the smallest possible effective dose for the shortest duration. Do not use occlusive dressings on weeping or exudative lesions and general caution with occlusive dressings should be observed; adverse effects may be increased. Discontinue if skin irritation or contact dermatitis should occur; do not use in patients with decreased skin circulation. Withdraw therapy with gradual tapering of dose. May affect growth velocity; growth should be routinely monitored in pediatric patients.

Drug Interactions **Substrate** of CYP3A4 (minor); **Inhibits** CYP3A4 (weak)

Aminoglutethimide: May reduce the serum levels/effects of prednisolone; likely via induction of microsomal isoenzymes.

Antacids: May increase the absorption of corticosteroids; separate administration by ≥2 hours.

Aprepitant: May increase effects of systemic corticosteroids.

Azole antifungals: May increase the serum levels of corticosteroids; monitor.

Barbiturates: May decrease prednisolone levels; monitor.

Bile acid sequestrants: May decrease the absorption of corticosteroids (oral).

Calcium channel blockers (nondihydropyridine): May increase the serum levels of corticosteroids; monitor.

Cyclosporine: Corticosteroids may increase the serum levels of cyclosporine. In addition, cyclosporine may increase levels of corticosteroids; monitor.

Estrogens: May increase the serum levels of corticosteroids; monitor.

Fluoroquinolones: Concurrent use may increase the risk of tendon rupture, particularly in elderly patients (overall incidence rare).

Isoniazid: Serum concentrations may be decreased by corticosteroids.

Ketoconazole: May decrease metabolism of certain corticosteroids leading to increased levels (up to 60%) and increased risk of adverse effects; monitor.

Macrolide antibiotics: May decrease the metabolism of corticosteroids.

Neuromuscular-blocking agents: Concurrent use with corticosteroids may increase the risk of myopathy.

Nonsteroidal anti-inflammatory drugs (NSAIDs), ophthalmic: Concurrent use with ophthalmic corticosteroids may lead to delayed healing.

Potassium-depleting agents (eg, diuretics, amphotericin B): Concurrent use increases risk of hypokalemia (especially if digitalized); monitor.

Primidone: May increase the metabolism of corticosteroids.

Rifampin: May decrease serum levels/effects of prednisolone; monitor.

Salicylates: Salicylates may increase the gastrointestinal adverse effects of corticosteroids.

Skin tests: Corticosteroids may suppress reactions to skin tests.

Vaccines (dead organisms): Immunosuppressants may diminish the effect of these vaccines.

Vaccines (live organisms): Immunosuppressants may enhance the adverse/toxic effects of these vaccines.

Ethanol/Nutrition/Herb Interactions

Ethanol: Avoid ethanol (may increase gastric mucosal irritation).

Food: Prednisolone interferes with calcium absorption. Limit caffeine.

Herb/Nutraceutical: St John's wort may decrease prednisolone levels. Avoid cat's claw, echinacea (have immunostimulant properties).

Dietary Considerations Should be taken after meals or with food or milk to decrease GI effects; increase dietary intake of pyridoxine, vitamin C, vitamin D, folate, calcium, and phosphorus.

(Continued)

PrednisoLONE *(Continued)*

Pharmacodynamics/Kinetics

Duration: 18-36 hours

Protein binding (concentration dependent): 65% to 91%; decreased in elderly

Metabolism: Primarily hepatic, but also metabolized in most tissues, to inactive compounds

Half-life elimination: 3.6 hours; End-stage renal disease: 3-5 hours

Excretion: Primarily urine (as glucuronides, sulfates, and unconjugated metabolites)

Pregnancy Risk Factor C

Lactation Enters breast milk/use caution (AAP rates "compatible")

Dosage Forms Excipient information presented when available (limited, particularly for generics); consult specific product labeling.

Solution, ophthalmic, as sodium phosphate: 1% (5 mL, 10 mL, 15 mL) [contains benzalkonium chloride]

Solution, oral, as sodium phosphate: Prednisolone base 5 mg/5 mL (120 mL)

Orapred®: 20 mg/5 mL (20 mL, 240 mL) [equivalent to prednisolone base 15 mg/5 mL; dye free; contains alcohol 2%, sodium benzoate; grape flavor]

Pediapred®: 6.7 mg/5 mL (120 mL) [equivalent to prednisolone base 5 mg/5 mL; dye free; raspberry flavor]

Suspension, ophthalmic, as acetate: 1% (5 mL, 10 mL, 15 mL)

Econopred® Plus: 1% (5 mL, 10 mL) [contains benzalkonium chloride]

Pred Forte®: 1% (1 mL, 5 mL, 10 mL, 15 mL) [contains benzalkonium chloride and sodium bisulfite]

Pred Mild®: 0.12% (5 mL, 10 mL) [contains benzalkonium chloride and sodium bisulfite]

Syrup, as base: 5 mg/5 mL (120 mL); 15 mg/5 mL (240 mL, 480 mL)

Prelone®: 15 mg/5 mL (240 mL, 480 mL) [contains alcohol 5%, benzoic acid; cherry flavor]

Tablet, as base: 5 mg

Tablet, orally disintegrating, as base:

Orapred ODT™: 10 mg, 15 mg, 30 mg [grape flavor]

Prednisolone Acetate *see* PrednisoLONE *on page 1339*

Prednisolone Acetate, Ophthalmic *see* PrednisoLONE *on page 1339*

Prednisolone and Gentamicin
(pred NIS oh lone & jen ta MYE sin)

Related Information

Gentamicin *on page 776*
PrednisoLONE *on page 1339*

U.S. Brand Names Pred-G®

Generic Available No

Index Terms Gentamicin and Prednisolone

Pharmacologic Category Antibiotic/Corticosteroid, Ophthalmic

Use Treatment of steroid responsive inflammatory conditions and superficial ocular infections due to microorganisms susceptible to gentamicin

Local Anesthetic/Vasoconstrictor Precautions No information available to require special precautions

Effects on Dental Treatment No significant effects or complications reported

Pregnancy Risk Factor C

Prednisolone and Sulfacetamide *see* Sulfacetamide and Prednisolone *on page 1503*

Prednisolone, Neomycin, and Polymyxin B *see* Neomycin, Polymyxin B, and Prednisolone *on page 1162*

Prednisolone Sodium Phosphate *see* PrednisoLONE *on page 1339*

Prednisolone Sodium Phosphate, Ophthalmic *see* PrednisoLONE *on page 1339*

PredniSONE *(PRED ni sone)*

Related Information

PrednisoLONE *on page 1339*
Respiratory Diseases *on page 1747*
Rheumatoid Arthritis, Osteoarthritis, and Osteoporosis *on page 1759*
Ulcerative and Erosive Disorders *on page 1809*

Related Sample Prescriptions

Erosive Lichen Planus and Major Aphthae *on page 1845*

U.S. Brand Names Prednisone Intensol™; Sterapred®; Sterapred® DS
Canadian Brand Names Apo-Prednisone®; Novo-Prednisone; Winpred™
Mexican Brand Names Meticorten
Generic Available Yes
Index Terms Deltacortisone; Deltadehydrocortisone
Pharmacologic Category Corticosteroid, Systemic
Dental Use Treatment of a variety of oral diseases of allergic, inflammatory, or autoimmune origin
Use Treatment of a variety of diseases including adrenocortical insufficiency, hypercalcemia, rheumatic, and collagen disorders; dermatologic, ocular, respiratory, gastrointestinal, and neoplastic diseases; organ transplantation and a variety of diseases including those of hematologic, allergic, inflammatory, and autoimmune in origin; not available in injectable form, prednisolone must be used
Unlabeled/Investigational Use Investigational: Prevention of postherpetic neuralgia and relief of acute pain in the early stages
Local Anesthetic/Vasoconstrictor Precautions No information available to require special precautions
Effects on Dental Treatment No significant effects or complications reported
Significant Adverse Effects
>10%:
Central nervous system: Insomnia, nervousness
Gastrointestinal: Increased appetite, indigestion
1% to 10%:
Central nervous system: Dizziness or lightheadedness, headache
Dermatologic: Hirsutism, hypopigmentation
Endocrine & metabolic: Diabetes mellitus, glucose intolerance, hyperglycemia
Neuromuscular & skeletal: Arthralgia
Ocular: Cataracts, glaucoma
Respiratory: Epistaxis
Miscellaneous: Diaphoresis
<1% (Limited to important or life-threatening): Cushing's syndrome, edema, fractures, hallucinations, hypertension, muscle-wasting, osteoporosis, pancreatitis, pituitary-adrenal axis suppression, seizure
Dental Usual Dosing
Anti-inflammatory or immunosuppressive dose: Children: Oral: 0.05-2 mg/kg/day divided 1-4 times/day
Immunosuppression/chemotherapy adjunct: Adults: Oral: Range: 5-60 mg/day in divided doses 1-4 times/day
Dosage Oral: Dose depends upon condition being treated and response of patient; dosage for infants and children should be based on severity of the disease and response of the patient rather than on strict adherence to dosage indicated by age, weight, or body surface area. Consider alternate day therapy for long-term therapy. Discontinuation of long-term therapy requires gradual withdrawal by tapering the dose.

Children:
Anti-inflammatory or immunosuppressive dose: 0.05-2 mg/kg/day divided 1-4 times/day
Acute asthma: 1-2 mg/kg/day in divided doses 1-2 times/day for 3-5 days
Alternatively (for 3- to 5-day "burst"):
<1 year: 10 mg every 12 hours
1-4 years: 20 mg every 12 hours
5-13 years: 30 mg every 12 hours
>13 years: 40 mg every 12 hours
Asthma long-term therapy (alternative dosing by age):
<1 year: 10 mg every other day
1-4 years: 20 mg every other day
5-13 years: 30 mg every other day
>13 years: 40 mg every other day
Nephrotic syndrome:
Initial (first 3 episodes): 2 mg/kg/day or 60 mg/m²/day (maximum: 80 mg/day) in divided doses 3-4 times/day until urine is protein free for 3 consecutive days (maximum: 28 days); followed by 1-1.5 mg/kg/dose or 40 mg/m²/dose given every other day for 4 weeks
Maintenance dose (long-term maintenance dose for frequent relapses): 0.5-1 mg/kg/dose given every other day for 3-6 months
Children and Adults: Physiologic replacement: 4-5 mg/m²/day
Children ≥5 years and Adults: Asthma:
Moderate persistent: Inhaled corticosteroid (medium dose) or inhaled corticosteroid (low-medium dose) with a long-acting bronchodilator
Severe persistent: Inhaled corticosteroid (high dose) and corticosteroid tablets or syrup long term: 2 mg/kg/day, generally not to exceed 60 mg/day
(Continued)

PredniSONE *(Continued)*

Adults:

Immunosuppression/chemotherapy adjunct: Range: 5-60 mg/day in divided doses 1-4 times/day

Allergic reaction (contact dermatitis):

Day 1: 30 mg divided as 10 mg before breakfast, 5 mg at lunch, 5 mg at dinner, 10 mg at bedtime

Day 2: 5 mg at breakfast, 5 mg at lunch, 5 mg at dinner, 10 mg at bedtime

Day 3: 5 mg 4 times/day (with meals and at bedtime)

Day 4: 5 mg 3 times/day (breakfast, lunch, bedtime)

Day 5: 5 mg 2 times/day (breakfast, bedtime)

Day 6: 5 mg before breakfast

Pneumocystis carinii pneumonia (PCP):

40 mg twice daily for 5 days **followed by**

40 mg once daily for 5 days **followed by**

20 mg once daily for 11 days or until antimicrobial regimen is completed

Thyrotoxicosis: Oral: 60 mg/day

Chemotherapy (refer to individual protocols): Oral: Range: 20 mg/day to 100 mg/m²/day

Rheumatoid arthritis: Oral: Use lowest possible daily dose (often ≤7.5 mg/day)

Idiopathic thrombocytopenia purpura (ITP): Oral: 60 mg daily for 4-6 weeks, gradually tapered over several weeks

Systemic lupus erythematosus (SLE): Oral:

Acute: 1-2 mg/kg/day in 2-3 divided doses

Maintenance: Reduce to lowest possible dose, usually <1 mg/kg/day as single dose (morning)

Elderly: Use the lowest effective dose

Dosing adjustment in hepatic impairment: Prednisone is inactive and must be metabolized by the liver to prednisolone. This conversion may be impaired in patients with liver disease, however, prednisolone levels are observed to be higher in patients with severe liver failure than in normal patients. Therefore, compensation for the inadequate conversion of prednisone to prednisolone occurs.

Dosing adjustment in hyperthyroidism: Prednisone dose may need to be increased to achieve adequate therapeutic effects

Hemodialysis: Supplemental dose is not necessary

Peritoneal dialysis: Supplemental dose is not necessary

Mechanism of Action Decreases inflammation by suppression of migration of polymorphonuclear leukocytes and reversal of increased capillary permeability; suppresses the immune system by reducing activity and volume of the lymphatic system; suppresses adrenal function at high doses. Antitumor effects may be related to inhibition of glucose transport, phosphorylation, or induction of cell death in immature lymphocytes. Antiemetic effects are thought to occur due to blockade of cerebral innervation of the emetic center via inhibition of prostaglandin synthesis.

Contraindications Hypersensitivity to prednisone or any component of the formulation; serious infections, except tuberculous meningitis; systemic fungal infections; varicella

Warnings/Precautions May cause hypercorticism or suppression of hypothalamic-pituitary-adrenal (HPA) axis, particularly in younger children or in patients receiving high doses for prolonged periods. HPA axis suppression may lead to adrenal crisis. Withdrawal and discontinuation of a corticosteroid should be done slowly and carefully. Particular care is required when patients are transferred from systemic corticosteroids to inhaled products due to possible adrenal insufficiency or withdrawal from steroids, including an increase in allergic symptoms. Patients receiving >20 mg per day of prednisone (or equivalent) may be most susceptible. Fatalities have occurred due to adrenal insufficiency in asthmatic patients during and after transfer from systemic corticosteroids to aerosol steroids; aerosol steroids do **not** provide the systemic steroid needed to treat patients having trauma, surgery, or infections.

Acute myopathy has been reported with high dose corticosteroids, usually in patients with neuromuscular transmission disorders; may involve ocular and/or respiratory muscles; monitor creatine kinase; recovery may be delayed. Corticosteroid use may cause psychiatric disturbances, including depression, euphoria, insomnia, mood swings, and personality changes. Pre-existing psychiatric conditions may be exacerbated by corticosteroid use. Prolonged use of corticosteroids may also increase the incidence of secondary infection, mask acute infection (including fungal infections), prolong or exacerbate viral infections, or limit response to vaccines. Exposure to chickenpox should be avoided; corticosteroids should not be used to treat ocular herpes simplex. Corticosteroids should not be used for cerebral malaria. Close observation is required in patients with latent tuberculosis and/or TB reactivity; restrict use in active TB (only in conjunction with antituberculosis treatment). Prolonged treatment with corticosteroids has been associated with the development of Kaposi's sarcoma (case reports); if noted, discontinuation of therapy should be considered.

Use with caution in patients with thyroid disease, hepatic impairment, renal impairment, cardiovascular disease, diabetes, glaucoma, cataracts, myasthenia gravis, patients at risk for osteoporosis, patients at risk for seizures, or GI diseases (diverticulitis, peptic ulcer, ulcerative colitis) due to perforation risk. Use caution following acute MI (corticosteroids have been associated with myocardial rupture). Because of the risk of adverse effects, systemic corticosteroids should be used cautiously in the elderly in the smallest possible effective dose for the shortest duration. Withdraw therapy with gradual tapering of dose. May affect growth velocity; growth should be routinely monitored in pediatric patients.

Drug Interactions Substrate of CYP3A4 (minor); **Induces** CYP2C19 (weak), 3A4 (weak)
Decreased effect:
  Barbiturates, phenytoin, rifampin decrease corticosteroid effectiveness
  Decreases salicylates
  Decreases vaccines
  Decreases toxoids effectiveness
Increased effect/toxicity: NSAIDs: Concurrent use of prednisone may increase the risk of GI ulceration

Ethanol/Nutrition/Herb Interactions
  Ethanol: Avoid ethanol (may increase gastric mucosal irritation)
  Food: Prednisone interferes with calcium absorption, Limit caffeine.
  Herb/Nutraceutical: St John's wort may decrease prednisone levels. Avoid cat's claw, echinacea (have immunostimulant properties).

Dietary Considerations Should be taken after meals or with food or milk; increase dietary intake of pyridoxine, vitamin C, vitamin D, folate, calcium, and phosphorus.

Pharmacodynamics/Kinetics
  Protein binding (concentration dependent): 65% to 91%
  Metabolism: Hepatically converted from prednisone (inactive) to prednisolone (active); may be impaired with hepatic dysfunction
  Half-life elimination: Normal renal function: 2.5-3.5 hours
  See Prednisolone monograph for complete information.

Pregnancy Risk Factor B

Lactation Enters breast milk/compatible

Breast-Feeding Considerations Crosses into breast milk. No data on clinical effects on the infant. AAP considers **compatible** with breast-feeding.

Dosage Forms Excipient information presented when available (limited, particularly for generics); consult specific product labeling.
  Solution, oral: 1 mg/mL (5 mL, 120 mL, 500 mL) [contains alcohol 5%, sodium benzoate; vanilla flavor]
  Solution, oral concentrate (Prednisone Intensol™): 5 mg/mL (30 mL) [contains alcohol 30%]
  Tablet: 1 mg, 2.5 mg, 5 mg, 10 mg, 20 mg, 50 mg
    Sterapred®: 5 mg [supplied as 21 tablet 6-day unit-dose package or 48 tablet 12-day unit-dose package]
    Sterapred® DS: 10 mg [supplied as 21 tablet 6-day unit-dose package or 48 tablet 12-day unit-dose package]

Prednisone Intensol™ *see* PredniSONE *on page 1342*

Prefest™ *see* Estradiol and Norgestimate *on page 604*

Pregabalin (pre GAB a lin)

U.S. Brand Names Lyrica®
Canadian Brand Names Lyrica®
Mexican Brand Names Lyrica
Generic Available No
Index Terms CI-1008; S-(+)-3-isobutylgaba
Pharmacologic Category Analgesic, Miscellaneous; Anticonvulsant, Miscellaneous
Use Management of pain associated with diabetic peripheral neuropathy; management of postherpetic neuralgia; adjunctive therapy for partial-onset seizure disorder in adults
Local Anesthetic/Vasoconstrictor Precautions No information available to require special precautions
Effects on Dental Treatment Key adverse event(s) related to dental treatment: Xerostomia and changes in salivation (normal salivary flow resumes upon discontinuation).
(Continued)

Pregabalin *(Continued)*

Common Adverse Effects Note: Frequency of adverse effects may be influenced by dose or concurrent therapy. In add-on trials in epilepsy, frequency of CNS and visual adverse effects were higher than those reported in pain management trials. Range noted below is inclusive of all trials.

>10%:
Cardiovascular: Peripheral edema (up to 16%)
Central nervous system: Dizziness (8% to 38%), somnolence (4% to 28%), ataxia (1% to 20%)
Gastrointestinal: Weight gain (up to 16%), xerostomia (1% to 15%)
Neuromuscular & skeletal: Tremor (1% to 11%)
Ocular: Blurred vision (1% to 12%), diplopia (up to 12%)
Miscellaneous: Infection (up to 14%), accidental injury (2% to 11%)

1% to 10%:
Cardiovascular: Chest pain (up to 4%), edema (up to 6%)
Central nervous system: Neuropathy (up to 9%), headache (up to 9%), thinking abnormal (up to 9%), confusion (up to 7%), speech disorder (up to 7%), incoordination (up to 6%), amnesia (up to 6%), pain (up to 5%), vertigo (up to 4%), nervousness (>2%), euphoria (up to 3%), fever (≥1%), anxiety (≥1%), depersonalization (≥1%), hypertonia (≥1%), hypoesthesia (≥1%), stupor (≥1%)
Dermatologic: Facial edema (up to 3%), ecchymosis (≥1%), pruritus (≥1%)
Endocrine & metabolic: Appetite increased (up to 6%), hypoglycemia (up to 3%), libido decreased (≥1%)
Gastrointestinal: Constipation (up to 7%), flatulence (up to 3%), vomiting (up to 3%), abdominal pain (≥1%), gastroenteritis (≥1%)
Genitourinary: Anorgasmia (≥1%), impotence (≥1%), urinary frequency (≥1%), incontinence (≥1%)
Hematologic: Thrombocytopenia (3%)
Neuromuscular & skeletal: Abnormal gait (up to 8%), weakness (up to 7%), twitching (up to 5%), myoclonus (up to 4%), back pain (up to 2%), paresthesia (>2%), CPK increased (2%), arthralgia (≥1%), leg cramps (≥1%), myalgia (≥1%), myasthenia (≥1%)
Ocular: Visual abnormalities (up to 5%), visual field defect (≥2%), eye disorder (up to 2%), nystagmus (>2%), conjunctivitis (≥1%)
Otic: Otitis media (≥1%), tinnitus (≥1%)
Respiratory: Dyspnea (up to 3%), bronchitis (up to 3%)
Miscellaneous: Flu-like syndrome (up to 2%), allergic reaction (≥1%)

Restrictions C-V

Dosage Oral: Adults:
Neuropathic pain (diabetes-associated): Initial: 150 mg/day in divided doses (50 mg 3 times/day); may be increased within 1 week based on tolerability and effect; maximum dose: 300 mg/day (dosages up to 600 mg/day were evaluated with no significant additional benefit and an increase in adverse effects)
Postherpetic neuralgia: Initial: 150 mg/day in divided doses (75 mg 2 times/day or 50 mg 3 times/day); may be increased to 300 mg/day within 1 week based on tolerability and effect; further titration (to 600 mg/day) after 2-4 weeks may be considered in patients who do not experience sufficient relief of pain provided they are able to tolerate pregabalin. Maximum dose: 600 mg/day
Partial-onset seizures (adjunctive therapy): Initial: 150 mg per day in divided doses (75 mg 2 times/day or 50 mg 3 times/day); may be increased based on tolerability and effect (optimal titration schedule has not been defined). Maximum dose: 600 mg/day
Discontinuing therapy: Pregabalin should not be abruptly discontinued; taper dosage over at least 1 week

Dosage adjustment in renal impairment: Cl$_{cr}$ ≥60 mL/minute: No dosage adjustment required. In renally-impaired patients, dosage adjustment depends on renal function and daily dosage:

Cl$_{cr}$ 30-60 mL/minute: Total daily dose:
  75 mg in 2-3 divided doses **or**
  150 mg in 2-3 divided doses **or**
  300 mg in 2-3 divided doses
Cl$_{cr}$ 15-30 mL/minute: Total daily dose:
  25-50 mg in once daily or in 2 divided doses **or**
  75 mg once daily or in 2 divided doses **or**
  150 mg once daily or in 2 divided doses
Cl$_{cr}$ <15 mL/minute: Total daily dose:
  25 mg once daily **or**
  25-50 mg once daily **or**
  75 mg once daily
Hemodialysis: Total daily dose:
  25 mg: Single supplementary dose of 25 mg **or** 50 mg

25-50 mg: Single supplementary dose of 50 mg **or** 75 mg

75 mg: Single supplementary dose of 100 mg **or** 150 mg

Mechanism of Action Binds to alpha$_2$-delta subunit of voltage-gated calcium channels within the CNS, inhibiting excitatory neurotransmitter release. Although structurally related to GABA, it does not bind to GABA or benzodiazepine receptors. Exerts antinociceptive and anticonvulsant activity. Decreases symptoms of painful peripheral neuropathies and, as adjunctive therapy in partial seizures, decreases the frequency of seizures.

Contraindications Hypersensitivity to pregabalin or any component of the formulation

Warnings/Precautions May cause CNS depression and/or dizziness, which may impair physical or mental abilities. Patients must be cautioned about performing tasks which require mental alertness (eg, operating machinery or driving). Effects with other sedative drugs or ethanol may be potentiated. Visual disturbances (blurred vision, decreased acuity and visual field changes) have been associated with pregabalin therapy; patients should be instructed to notify their physician if these effects are noted.

Pregabalin has been associated with increases in CPK and rare cases of rhabdomyolysis. Patients should be instructed to notify their prescriber if unexplained muscle pain, tenderness, or weakness, particularly if fever and/or malaise are associated with these symptoms. Use may be associated with weight gain and peripheral edema; use caution in patients with congestive heart failure, hypertension, or diabetes. Effect on weight gain/edema may be additive to thiazolidinedione antidiabetic agent; particularly in patients with prior cardiovascular disease. May decrease platelet count or prolong PR interval.

Has been noted to be tumorigenic (increased incidence of hemangiosarcoma) in animal studies; significance of these findings in humans is unknown. Pregabalin has been associated with discontinuation symptoms following abrupt cessation, and increases in seizure frequency (when used as an antiepileptic) may occur. Should not be discontinued abruptly; dosage tapering over at least 1 week is recommended. Use caution in renal impairment; dosage adjustment required. Safety and efficacy have not been established in pediatric patients.

Drug Interactions

Increased Effect/Toxicity: Sedative effects may be additive with CNS depressants (includes ethanol, barbiturates, opioid analgesics, and other sedative agents). Pregabalin's effect on weight gain/edema may be additive with thiazolidinedione antidiabetic agents (includes pioglitazone, rosiglitazone).

Ethanol/Nutrition/Herb Interactions

Ethanol: Avoid ethanol (may increase CNS depression).

Herb/Nutraceutical: Avoid valerian, St John's wort, kava kava, gotu kola (may increase CNS depression).

Dietary Considerations May be taken with or without food.

Pharmacodynamics/Kinetics

Onset: Pain management: Effects may be noted as early as the first week of therapy.

Distribution: V$_d$: 0.5 L/kg

Protein binding: 0%

Metabolism: Negligible

Bioavailability: >90%

Half-life elimination: 6.3 hours

Time to peak, plasma: 1.5 hours (3 hours with food)

Excretion: Urine (90% as unchanged drug; minor metabolites)

Pregnancy Risk Factor C

Dosage Forms

Capsule:

Lyrica®: 25 mg, 50 mg, 75 mg, 100 mg, 150 mg, 200 mg, 225 mg, 300 mg

Selected Readings

Hill CM, Balkenohl M, Thomas DW, et al, "Pregabalin in Patients With Postoperative Dental Pain," *Eur J Pain*, 2001, 5(2):119-24.

Prilocaine (PRIL oh kane)

Related Information
  Oral Pain *on page 1788*
U.S. Brand Names Citanest® Plain
Canadian Brand Names Citanest® Plain
Generic Available No
Pharmacologic Category Local Anesthetic
Dental Use Amide-type anesthetic used for local infiltration anesthesia; injection near nerve trunks to produce nerve block
Local Anesthetic/Vasoconstrictor Precautions No information available to require special precautions
Effects on Dental Treatment It is common to misinterpret psychogenic responses to local anesthetic injection as an allergic reaction. Intraoral injections are perceived by many patients as a stressful procedure in dentistry. Common symptoms to this stress are diaphoresis, palpitations, hyperventilation, generalized pallor and a fainting feeling.

Degree of adverse effects in the CNS and cardiovascular system is directly related to blood levels of prilocaine (frequency not defined; more likely to occur after systemic administration rather than infiltration): Bradycardia and reduction in cardiac output, hypersensitivity reactions (may be manifest as dermatologic reactions and edema at injection site), asthmatic syndromes

High blood levels: Anxiety, restlessness, disorientation, confusion, dizziness, tremors, and seizures, followed by CNS depression, resulting in somnolence, unconsciousness and possible respiratory arrest; nausea and vomiting

In some cases, symptoms of CNS stimulation may be absent and the primary CNS effects are somnolence and unconsciousness.

Significant Adverse Effects
  1% to 10%: Cardiovascular: Hypotension
  <1% (Limited to important or life-threatening): Anaphylactoid reaction, aseptic meningitis resulting in paralysis, chills, CNS stimulation followed by CNS depression, miosis, nausea, skin discoloration, tinnitus, vomiting

Prilocaine

# of Cartridges (1.8 mL)	mg Prilocaine (4%)
1	72
2	144
3	216
4	288
5	360
6	432
7	504
8	576

Dental Usual Dosing

Children <10 years: Doses >40 mg (1 mL) as a 4% solution per procedure rarely needed

Children >10 years and Adults: Dental anesthesia, infiltration, or conduction block: Initial: 40-80 mg (1-2 mL) as a 4% solution; up to a maximum of 400 mg (10 mL) as a 4% solution within a 2-hour period. Manufacturer's maximum recommended dose is not more than 600 mg to normal healthy adults. The effective anesthetic dose varies with procedure, intensity of anesthesia needed, duration of anesthesia required and physical condition of the patient. Always use the lowest effective dose along with careful aspiration.

The following numbers of dental carpules (1.8 mL) provide the indicated amounts of prilocaine hydrochloride 4%. See table on previous page.

Note: Adult and children doses of prilocaine hydrochloride cited from USP Dispensing Information (USP DI), 17th ed, The United States Pharmacopeial Convention, Inc, Rockville, MD, 1997, 139.

Dosage

Children <10 years: Doses >40 mg (1 mL) as a 4% solution per procedure rarely needed

Children >10 years and Adults: Dental anesthesia, infiltration, or conduction block: Initial: 40-80 mg (1-2 mL) as a 4% solution; up to a maximum of 400 mg (10 mL) as a 4% solution within a 2-hour period. Manufacturer's maximum recommended dose is not more than 600 mg to normal healthy adults. The effective anesthetic dose varies with procedure, intensity of anesthesia needed, duration of anesthesia required and physical condition of the patient. Always use the lowest effective dose along with careful aspiration.

Note: Adult and children doses of prilocaine hydrochloride cited from USP Dispensing Information (USP DI), 17th ed, The United States Pharmacopeial Convention, Inc, Rockville, MD, 1997, 139.

Mechanism of Action Local anesthetics bind selectively to the intracellular surface of sodium channels to block influx of sodium into the axon. As a result, depolarization necessary for action potential propagation and subsequent nerve function is prevented. The block at the sodium channel is reversible. When drug diffuses away from the axon, sodium channel function is restored and nerve propagation returns.

Contraindications Hypersensitivity to local anesthetics of the amide type or any component of the formulation

Warnings/Precautions Aspirate the syringe after tissue penetration and before injection to minimize chance of direct vascular injection.

Drug Interactions No data reported

Pharmacodynamics/Kinetics

Onset of action: Infiltration: ~2 minutes; Inferior alveolar nerve block: ~3 minutes

Duration: Infiltration: Complete anesthesia for procedures lasting 20 minutes; Inferior alveolar nerve block: ~2.5 hours

Distribution: V_d: 0.7-4.4 L/kg; crosses blood-brain barrier

Protein binding: 55%

Metabolism: Hepatic and renal

Half-life elimination: 10-150 minutes; prolonged with hepatic or renal impairment

Pregnancy Risk Factor B

Breast-Feeding Considerations Usual infiltration doses of prilocaine given to nursing mothers has not been shown to affect the health of the nursing infant.

Dosage Forms Excipient information presented when available (limited, particularly for generics); consult specific product labeling.

Injection, solution: Prilocaine hydrochloride 4% (1.8 mL) [prefilled cartridge]

Selected Readings

Budenz AW, "Local Anesthetics in Dentistry: Then and Now," *J Calif Dent Assoc*, 2003, 31(5):388-96.

Dower JS Jr, "A Review of Paresthesia in Association With Administration of Local Anesthesia," *Dent Today*, 2003, 22(2):64-9.

Finder RL and Moore PA, "Adverse Drug Reactions to Local Anesthesia," *Dent Clin North Am*, 2002, 46(4):747-57, x.

Haas DA, "An Update on Local Anesthetics in Dentistry," *J Can Dent Assoc*, 2002, 68(9):546-51.

Hawkins JM and Moore PA, "Local Anesthesia: Advances in Agents and Techniques," *Dent Clin North Am*, 2002, 46(4):719-32, ix.

"Injectable Local Anesthetics," *J Am Dent Assoc*, 2003, 134(5):628-9.

Jastak JT and Yagiela JA, "Vasoconstrictors and Local Anesthesia: A Review and Rationale for Use," *J Am Dent Assoc*, 1983, 107(4):623-30.

MacKenzie TA and Young ER, "Local Anesthetic Update," *Anesth Prog*, 1993, 40(2):29-34.

Malamed SF, "Allergy and Toxic Reactions to Local Anesthetics," *Dent Today*, 2003, 22(4):114-6, 118-21.

Wahl MJ, Schmitt MM, Overton DA, et al, "Injection Pain of Bupivacaine With Epinephrine vs. Prilocaine Plain," *J Am Dent Assoc*, 2002, 133(12):1652-6.

Wynn RL, "Epinephrine Interactions With Beta-Blockers," *Gen Dent*, 1994, 42(1):16, 18.

Yagiela JA, "Local Anesthetics," *Anesth Prog*, 1991, 38(4-5):128-41.

Prilocaine and Epinephrine (PRIL oh kane & ep i NEF rin)

Related Information
Epinephrine *on page 572*
Oral Pain *on page 1788*
Prilocaine *on page 1348*

U.S. Brand Names Citanest® Forte Dental
Canadian Brand Names Citanest® Forte
Generic Available No
Index Terms Epinephrine and Prilocaine (Dental)
Pharmacologic Category Local Anesthetic
Dental Use Amide-type anesthetic used for local infiltration anesthesia; injection near nerve trunks to produce nerve block
Local Anesthetic/Vasoconstrictor Precautions No information available to require special precautions
Effects on Dental Treatment It is common to misinterpret psychogenic responses to local anesthetic injection as an allergic reaction. Intraoral injections are perceived by many patients as a stressful procedure in dentistry. Common symptoms to this stress are diaphoresis, palpitations, hyperventilation, generalized pallor and a fainting feeling. Patients may exhibit hypersensitivity to bisulfites contained in local anesthetic solution to prevent oxidation of epinephrine. In general, patients reacting to bisulfites have a history of asthma and their airways are hyper-reactive to asthmatic syndrome.

Degree of adverse effects in the CNS and cardiovascular system is directly related to blood levels of prilocaine (frequency not defined; more likely to occur after systemic administration rather than infiltration): Bradycardia and reduction in cardiac output, hypersensitivity reactions (extremely rare; may be manifest as dermatologic reactions and edema at injection site), asthmatic syndromes

High blood levels: Anxiety, restlessness, disorientation, confusion, dizziness, tremors, and seizures, followed by CNS depression, resulting in somnolence, unconsciousness and possible respiratory arrest; nausea and vomiting

In some cases, symptoms of CNS stimulation may be absent and the primary CNS effects are somnolence and unconsciousness.

Significant Adverse Effects Degree of adverse effects in the CNS and cardiovascular system are directly related to the blood levels of prilocaine. The effects below are more likely to occur after systemic administration rather than infiltration.

Cardiovascular: Myocardial effects include a decrease in contraction force as well as a decrease in electrical excitability and myocardial conduction rate resulting in bradycardia and reduction in cardiac output.

Central nervous system: High blood levels result in anxiety, restlessness, disorientation, confusion, dizziness, tremor and seizure. This is followed by depression of CNS resulting in somnolence, unconsciousness and possible respiratory arrest. Nausea and vomiting may also occur. In some cases, symptoms of CNS stimulation may be absent and the primary CNS effects are somnolence and unconsciousness.

Hypersensitivity reactions: Extremely rare, but may be manifest as dermatologic reactions and edema at injection site. Asthmatic syndromes have occurred. Patients may exhibit hypersensitivity to bisulfites contained in local anesthetic solution to prevent oxidation of epinephrine. In general, patients reacting to bisulfites have a history of asthma and their airways are hyper-reactive to asthmatic syndrome.

Psychogenic reactions: It is common to misinterpret psychogenic responses to local anesthetic injection as an allergic reaction. Intraoral injections are perceived by many patients as a stressful procedure in dentistry. Common symptoms to this stress are diaphoresis, palpitation, hyperventilation, generalized pallor, and a fainting feeling.

Dental Usual Dosing
Children <10 years: Doses >40 mg (1 mL) of prilocaine hydrochloride as a 4% solution with epinephrine 1:200,000 are rarely needed

Children >10 years and Adults: Dental anesthesia, infiltration, or conduction block: Initial: 40-80 mg (1-2 mL) of prilocaine hydrochloride as a 4% solution with epinephrine 1:200,000; up to a maximum of 400 mg (10 mL) of prilocaine hydrochloride within a 2-hour period. The effective anesthetic dose varies with procedure, intensity of anesthesia needed, duration of anesthesia required, and physical condition of the patient. Always use the lowest effective dose along with careful aspiration.

The following numbers of dental carpules (1.8 mL) provide the indicated amounts of prilocaine hydrochloride 4% and epinephrine 1:200,000. See table on next page.

Prilocaine With Epinephrine

# of Cartridges (1.8 mL)	mg Prilocaine (4%)	mg Vasoconstrictor (Epinephrine 1:200,000)
1	72	0.009
2	144	0.018
3	216	0.027
4	288	0.036
5	360	0.045
6	432	0.054
7	504	0.063
8	576	0.072

Note: Adult and pediatric doses of prilocaine hydrochloride with epinephrine cited from USP Dispensing Information (USP DI), 17th ed, The United States Pharmacopeial Convention, Inc, Rockville, MD, 1997, 140.

Dosage

Children <10 years: Doses >40 mg (1 mL) of prilocaine hydrochloride as a 4% solution with epinephrine 1:200,000 are rarely needed

Children >10 years and Adults: Dental anesthesia, infiltration, or conduction block: Initial: 40-80 mg (1-2 mL) of prilocaine hydrochloride as a 4% solution with epinephrine 1:200,000; up to a maximum of 400 mg (10 mL) of prilocaine hydrochloride within a 2-hour period. The effective anesthetic dose varies with procedure, intensity of anesthesia needed, duration of anesthesia required, and physical condition of the patient. Always use the lowest effective dose along with careful aspiration.

Note: Adult and pediatric doses of prilocaine hydrochloride with epinephrine cited from USP Dispensing Information (USP DI), 17th ed, The United States Pharmacopeial Convention, Inc, Rockville, MD, 1997, 140.

Mechanism of Action Local anesthetics bind selectively to the intracellular surface of sodium channels to block influx of sodium into the axon. As a result, depolarization necessary for action potential propagation and subsequent nerve function is prevented. The block at the sodium channel is reversible. When drug diffuses away from the axon, sodium channel function is restored and nerve propagation returns.

Epinephrine prolongs the duration of the anesthetic actions of prilocaine by causing vasoconstriction (alpha-adrenergic receptor agonist) of the vasculature surrounding the nerve axons. This prevents the diffusion of prilocaine away from the nerves resulting in a longer retention in the axon.

Contraindications Hypersensitivity to local anesthetics of the amide-type or any component of the formulation

Warnings/Precautions Should be avoided in patients with uncontrolled hyperthyroidism. Should be used in minimal amounts in patients with significant cardiovascular problems (because of epinephrine component). Aspirate the syringe after tissue penetration and before injection to minimize chance of direct vascular injection

Drug Interactions

Beta-blockers, nonselective (ie, propranolol): Concurrent use could result in serious hypertension and reflex bradycardia

MAO inhibitors: Administration of local anesthetic solutions containing epinephrine may produce severe, prolonged hypertension

Tricyclic antidepressants: Pressor response to I.V. epinephrine, norepinephrine, and phenylephrine may be enhanced in patients receiving TCAs (**Note:** Effect is unlikely with epinephrine or levonordefrin dosages typically administered as infiltration in combination with local anesthetics)

Pharmacodynamics/Kinetics

Onset of action: Infiltration: <2 minutes; Inferior alveolar nerve block: <3 minutes

Duration: Infiltration: 2.25 hours; Inferior alveolar nerve block: 3 hours

Pregnancy Risk Factor C

Breast-Feeding Considerations Usual infiltration doses of prilocaine with epinephrine given to nursing mothers has not been shown to affect the health of the nursing infant.

Dosage Forms Excipient information presented when available (limited, particularly for generics); consult specific product labeling.

Injection, solution: Prilocaine hydrochloride 4% and epinephrine bitartrate 1:200,000 (1.8 mL)

Selected Readings

Ayoub ST and Coleman AE, "A Review of Local Anesthetics," *Gen Dent*, 1992, 40(4):285-7, 289-90.
Blanton PL and Roda RS, "The Anatomy of Local Anesthesia," *J Calif Dent Assoc*, 1995, 23(4):55-65.

(Continued)

Prilocaine and Epinephrine *(Continued)*

Budenz AW, "Local Anesthetics in Dentistry: Then and Now," *J Calif Dent Assoc*, 2003, 31(5):388-96.

Dower JS Jr, "A Review of Paresthesia in Association With Administration of Local Anesthesia," *Dent Today*, 2003, 22(2):64-9.

Finder RL and Moore PA, "Adverse Drug Reactions to Local Anesthesia," *Dent Clin North Am*, 2002, 46(4):747-57, x.

Haas DA, "An Update on Local Anesthetics in Dentistry," *J Can Dent Assoc*, 2002, 68(9):546-51.

Hawkins JM and Moore PA, "Local Anesthesia: Advances in Agents and Techniques," *Dent Clin North Am*, 2002, 46(4):719-32, ix.

"Injectable Local Anesthetics," *J Am Dent Assoc*, 2003, 134(5):628-9.

Jastak JT and Yagiela JA, "Vasoconstrictors and Local Anesthesia: A Review and Rationale for Use," *J Am Dent Assoc*, 1983, 107(4):623-30.

MacKenzie TA and Young ER, "Local Anesthetic Update," *Anesth Prog*, 1993, 40(2):29-34.

Malamed SF, "Allergy and Toxic Reactions to Local Anesthetics," *Dent Today*, 2003, 22(4):114-6, 118-21.

Wynn RL, "Epinephrine Interactions With Beta-Blockers," *Gen Dent*, 1994, 42(1):16, 18.

Yagiela JA, "Local Anesthetics," *Anesth Prog*, 1991, 38(4-5):128-41.

Yagiela JA, "Vasoconstrictor Agents for Local Anesthesia," *Anesth Prog*, 1995, 42(3-4):116-20.

Prilocaine and Lidocaine *see* Lidocaine and Prilocaine *on page 981*

Prilosec® *see* Omeprazole *on page 1206*

Prilosec OTC™ [OTC] *see* Omeprazole *on page 1206*

Primaclone *see* Primidone *on page 1352*

Primacor® *see* Milrinone *on page 1106*

Primaquine *(PRIM a kween)*

Generic Available Yes

Index Terms Primaquine Phosphate; Prymaccone

Pharmacologic Category Aminoquinoline (Antimalarial)

Use Treatment of malaria

Unlabeled/Investigational Use Prevention of malaria; treatment *Pneumocystis carinii* pneumonia

Local Anesthetic/Vasoconstrictor Precautions No information available to require special precautions

Effects on Dental Treatment No significant effects or complications reported

Common Adverse Effects Frequency not defined.

Cardiovascular: Arrhythmias

Central nervous system: Headache

Dermatologic: Pruritus

Gastrointestinal: Abdominal pain, nausea, vomiting

Hematologic: Agranulocytosis, hemolytic anemia in G6PD deficiency, leukopenia, leukocytosis, methemoglobinemia in NADH-methemoglobin reductase-deficient individuals

Ocular: Interference with visual accommodation

Mechanism of Action Eliminates the primary tissue exoerythrocytic forms of *P. falciparum*; disrupts mitochondria and binds to DNA

Drug Interactions

Cytochrome P450 Effect: Substrate of CYP3A4 (major); **Inhibits** CYP1A2 (strong), 2D6 (weak), 3A4 (weak); **Induces** CYP1A2 (weak)

Increased Effect/Toxicity: Increased toxicity/levels with quinacrine. Primaquine may increase the levels/effects of aminophylline, fluvoxamine, mexiletine, mirtazapine, ropinirole, theophylline, trifluoperazine, and other CYP1A2 substrates.

Decreased Effect: The levels/effects of primaquine may be decreased by aminoglutethimide, carbamazepine, nafcillin, nevirapine, phenobarbital, phenytoin, rifamycins, and other CYP3A4 inducers.

Pharmacodynamics/Kinetics

Absorption: Well absorbed

Metabolism: Hepatic to carboxyprimaquine (active)

Half-life elimination: 3.7-9.6 hours

Time to peak, serum: 1-2 hours

Excretion: Urine (small amounts as unchanged drug)

Pregnancy Risk Factor C

Primaquine Phosphate *see* Primaquine *on page 1352*

Primatene® Mist [OTC] *see* Epinephrine *on page 572*

Primaxin® *see* Imipenem and Cilastatin *on page 865*

Primidone *(PRI mi done)*

U.S. Brand Names Mysoline®

Canadian Brand Names Apo-Primidone®

Generic Available Yes

Index Terms Desoxyphenobarbital; Primaclone
Pharmacologic Category Anticonvulsant, Miscellaneous; Barbiturate
Use Management of grand mal, psychomotor, and focal seizures
Unlabeled/Investigational Use Benign familial tremor (essential tremor)
Local Anesthetic/Vasoconstrictor Precautions No information available to require special precautions
Effects on Dental Treatment No significant effects or complications reported
Common Adverse Effects Frequency not defined.

Central nervous system: Drowsiness, vertigo, ataxia, lethargy, behavior change, fatigue, hyperirritability

Dermatologic: Rash

Gastrointestinal: Nausea, vomiting, anorexia

Genitourinary: Impotence

Hematologic: Agranulocytopenia, agranulocytosis, anemia

Ocular: Diplopia, nystagmus

Mechanism of Action Decreases neuron excitability, raises seizure threshold similar to phenobarbital; primidone has two active metabolites, phenobarbital and phenylethylmalonamide (PEMA); PEMA may enhance the activity of phenobarbital

Drug Interactions

Cytochrome P450 Effect: Metabolized to phenobarbital; **Induces** CYP1A2 (strong), 2B6 (strong), 2C8 (strong), 2C9 (strong), 3A4 (strong)

Increased Effect/Toxicity: When combined with other CNS depressants, ethanol, opioid analgesics, antidepressants, or benzodiazepines, additive respiratory and CNS depression may occur. Barbiturates may enhance the hepatotoxic potential of acetaminophen overdoses. Chloramphenicol, MAO inhibitors, valproic acid, and felbamate may inhibit barbiturate metabolism. Barbiturates may impair the absorption of griseofulvin, and may enhance the nephrotoxic effects of methoxyflurane. Concurrent use of phenobarbital with meperidine may result in increased CNS depression. Concurrent use of phenobarbital with primidone may result in elevated phenobarbital serum concentrations. CYP2C19 inhibitors may increase the levels/effects of primidone; example inhibitors include delavirdine, fluconazole, fluvoxamine, gemfibrozil, isoniazid, omeprazole, and ticlopidine.

Decreased Effect: Barbiturates may increase the metabolism of estrogens and reduce the efficacy of oral contraceptives; an alternative method of contraception should be considered. Barbiturates inhibit the hypoprothrombinemic effects of oral anticoagulants via increased metabolism. Barbiturates may enhance the metabolism of methadone resulting in methadone withdrawal. The levels/effects of primidone may be decreased by aminoglutethimide, carbamazepine, phenytoin, rifampin, and other CYP2C19 inducers.

Primidone may decrease the levels/effects of aminophylline, amiodarone, benzodiazepines, bupropion, calcium channel blockers, carbamazepine, citalopram, clarithromycin, cyclosporine, diazepam, efavirenz, erythromycin, estrogens, fluoxetine, fluvoxamine, glimepiride, glipizide, ifosfamide, losartan, methsuximide, mirtazapine, nateglinide, nefazodone, nevirapine, phenytoin, pioglitazone, promethazine, propranolol, protease inhibitors, proton pump inhibitors, rifampin, ropinirole, rosiglitazone, selegiline, sertraline, sulfonamides, tacrolimus, theophylline, venlafaxine. voriconazole, warfarin, zafirlukast, and other CYP1A2, 2A6, 2B6, 2C8, 2C9, or 3A4 substrates.

Pharmacodynamics/Kinetics

Distribution: Adults: V_d: 2-3 L/kg

Protein binding: 99%

Metabolism: Hepatic to phenobarbital (active) and phenylethylmalonamide (PEMA)

Bioavailability: 60% to 80%

Half-life elimination (age dependent): Primidone: 10-12 hours; PEMA: 16 hours; Phenobarbital: 52-118 hours

Time to peak, serum: ~4 hours

Excretion: Urine (15% to 25% as unchanged drug and active metabolites)

Pregnancy Risk Factor D

Probenecid (proe BEN e sid)

Related Information
Treatment of Sexually-Transmitted Infections *on page 1920*
Canadian Brand Names Benuryl™
Mexican Brand Names Benecid
Generic Available Yes
Index Terms Benemid [DSC]
Pharmacologic Category Uricosuric Agent
Use Prevention of hyperuricemia associated with gout or gouty arthritis; prolongation and elevation of beta-lactam plasma levels
Local Anesthetic/Vasoconstrictor Precautions No information available to require special precautions
Effects on Dental Treatment Key adverse event(s) related to dental treatment: Sore gums.
Common Adverse Effects Frequency not defined.
Cardiovascular: Flushing
Central nervous system: Dizziness, fever, headache
Dermatologic: Alopecia, dermatitis, pruritus, rash
Gastrointestinal: Anorexia, nausea, sore gums, vomiting
Genitourinary: Hematuria, polyuria
Hematologic: Anemia, aplastic anemia, hemolytic anemia, leukopenia
Hepatic: Hepatic necrosis
Neuromuscular & skeletal: Costovertebral pain, gouty arthritis (acute)
Renal: Nephrotic syndrome, renal colic
Miscellaneous: Anaphylaxis, hypersensitivity
Mechanism of Action Competitively inhibits the reabsorption of uric acid at the proximal convoluted tubule, thereby promoting its excretion and reducing serum uric acid levels; increases plasma levels of weak organic acids (penicillins, cephalosporins, or other beta-lactam antibiotics) by competitively inhibiting their renal tubular secretion
Drug Interactions
Cytochrome P450 Effect: Inhibits CYP2C19 (weak)
Increased Effect/Toxicity: Probenecid may decrease the excretion of carbapenems, cephalosporins, dapsone, methotrexate, and penicillins. Concomitant use with methotrexate should be avoided. Probenecid may increase the serum concentration of NSAIDs; the manufacturer of ketorolac contraindicates concomitant use. Probenecid may enhance the therapeutic effect of thiopental. Probenecid may decrease the metabolism of zidovudine.
Decreased Effect: Salicylates may diminish the therapeutic effect of probenecid.
Pharmacodynamics/Kinetics
Onset of action: Effect on penicillin levels: 2 hours
Absorption: Rapid and complete
Metabolism: Hepatic
Half-life elimination (dose dependent): Normal renal function: 6-12 hours
Time to peak, serum: 2-4 hours
Excretion: Urine

Probenecid and Colchicine *see* Colchicine and Probenecid *on page 407*

Procainamide (pro KANE a mide)

Related Information
Cardiovascular Diseases *on page 1726*
U.S. Brand Names Procanbid®
Canadian Brand Names Apo-Procainamide®; Procainamide Hydrochloride Injection, USP; Procan® SR; Pronestyl®-SR
Generic Available Yes
Index Terms PCA (error-prone abbreviation); Procainamide Hydrochloride; Procaine Amide Hydrochloride
Pharmacologic Category Antiarrhythmic Agent, Class Ia
Use Treatment of ventricular tachycardia (VT), premature ventricular contractions, paroxysmal atrial tachycardia (PSVT), and atrial fibrillation (AF); prevent recurrence of ventricular tachycardia, paroxysmal supraventricular tachycardia, atrial fibrillation or flutter
Unlabeled/Investigational Use ACLS guidelines:
Stable monomorphic VT (EF >40%, no CHF)
Stable wide complex tachycardia, likely VT (EF >40%, no CHF, patient stable)
Atrial fibrillation or flutter, including pre-excitation syndrome (EF >40%, no CHF)

AV reentrant, narrow complex tachycardia (eg, reentrant SVT) [preserved ventricular function]

PALS guidelines: Tachycardia with pulses and poor perfusion (possible VT)

Local Anesthetic/Vasoconstrictor Precautions Procainamide is one of the drugs confirmed to prolong the QT interval and is accepted as having a risk of causing torsade de pointes. The risk of drug-induced torsade de pointes is extremely low when a single QT interval prolonging drug is prescribed. In terms of epinephrine, it is not known what effect vasoconstrictors in the local anesthetic regimen will have in patients with a known history of congenital prolonged QT interval or in patients taking any medication that prolongs the QT interval. Until more information is obtained, it is suggested that the clinician consult with the physician prior to the use of a vasoconstrictor in suspected patients, and that the vasoconstrictor (epinephrine, levonordefrin [Neo-Cobefrin®]) be used with caution.

Effects on Dental Treatment Key adverse event(s) related to dental treatment: Taste disorder.

Mechanism of Action Decreases myocardial excitability and conduction velocity and may depress myocardial contractility, by increasing the electrical stimulation threshold of ventricle, His-Purkinje system and through direct cardiac effects

Pregnancy Risk Factor C

Procainamide Hydrochloride *see* Procainamide *on page 1354*

Procaine (PROE kane)

U.S. Brand Names Novocain®
Generic Available No
Index Terms Procaine Hydrochloride
Pharmacologic Category Local Anesthetic
Use Produces spinal anesthesia and epidural and peripheral nerve block by injection and infiltration methods
Local Anesthetic/Vasoconstrictor Precautions No information available to require special precautions
Effects on Dental Treatment This is no longer a useful anesthetic in dentistry due to high incidence of allergic reactions.
Mechanism of Action Blocks both the initiation and conduction of nerve impulses by decreasing the neuronal membrane's permeability to sodium ions, which results in inhibition of depolarization with resultant blockade of conduction
Pregnancy Risk Factor C

Procaine Amide Hydrochloride *see* Procainamide *on page 1354*
Procaine Benzylpenicillin *see* Penicillin G Procaine *on page 1270*
Procaine Hydrochloride *see* Procaine *on page 1355*
Procaine Penicillin G *see* Penicillin G Procaine *on page 1270*
Procanbid® *see* Procainamide *on page 1354*

Procarbazine (proe KAR ba zeen)

U.S. Brand Names Matulane®
Canadian Brand Names Matulane®; Natulan®
Generic Available No
Index Terms Benzmethyzin; N-Methylhydrazine; NSC-77213; Procarbazine Hydrochloride
Pharmacologic Category Antineoplastic Agent, Alkylating Agent
Use Treatment of Hodgkin's disease
Unlabeled/Investigational Use Treatment of non-Hodgkin's lymphoma, brain tumors, melanoma, lung cancer, multiple myeloma
Local Anesthetic/Vasoconstrictor Precautions No information available to require special precautions
Effects on Dental Treatment Key adverse event(s) related to dental treatment: Xerostomia (normal salivary flow resumes upon discontinuation), stomatitis, and dysphagia.
Common Adverse Effects Most frequencies not defined.
Cardiovascular: Edema, flushing, hypotension, syncope, tachycardia
Central nervous system: Apprehension, ataxia, chills, coma, confusion, depression, dizziness, drowsiness, fatigue, fever, hallucination, headache, insomnia, lethargy, nervousness, nightmares, pain, seizure, slurred speech
Dermatologic: Alopecia, dermatitis, hyperpigmentation, petechiae, pruritus, purpura, rash, urticaria
Endocrine & metabolic: Gynecomastia (in prepubertal and early pubertal males)
(Continued)

Procarbazine *(Continued)*

Hematologic: Eosinophilia; hemolysis (in patients with G6PD deficiency); hemolytic anemia; myelosuppression (leukopenia, anemia, thrombocytopenia); pancytopenia

Gastrointestinal: Abdominal pain, anorexia, constipation, diarrhea, dysphagia, hematemesis, melena; nausea and vomiting ([60% to 90%], increasing the dose in a stepwise fashion over several days may minimize); stomatitis, xerostomia

Genitourinary: Azoospermia (reported with combination chemotherapy), hematuria, nocturia, polyuria, reproductive dysfunction (>10%)

Hepatic: Hepatic dysfunction, jaundice

Neuromuscular & skeletal: Arthralgia, falling, foot drop, myalgia, neuropathy, paresthesia, reflex diminished, tremor, unsteadiness, weakness

Ocular: Diplopia, inability to focus, nystagmus, papilledema, photophobia, retinal hemorrhage

Otic: Hearing loss

Respiratory: Cough, epistaxis, hemoptysis, hoarseness, pleural effusion, pneumonitis, pulmonary toxicity (<1%)

Miscellaneous: Allergic reaction, diaphoresis, herpes, infection, secondary malignancies (2% to 15%; reported with combination therapy)

Mechanism of Action Mechanism of action is not clear, methylating of nucleic acids; inhibits DNA, RNA, and protein synthesis; may damage DNA directly and suppresses mitosis; metabolic activation required by host

Drug Interactions

Increased Effect/Toxicity: Procarbazine may enhance the vasopressor effect of direct-acting alpha-/beta-agonists. Procarbazine may enhance the hypertensive effect of indirect-acting alpha-/beta-agonists, $alpha_1$-agonists, $alpha_2$-agonists (ophthalmic), amphetamines, dexmethylphenidate, and methylphenidate. Procarbazine may enhance the serotonergic effect of serotonin/norepinephrine reuptake inhibitors, cyclobenzaprine, dextromethorphan, meperidine, selective serotonin reuptake inhibitors, serotonin modulators, and tricyclic antidepressants. Procarbazine may enhance the neurotoxic (central) effect of atomoxetine, bupropion, lithium and mirtazapine. Procarbazine may enhance the adverse/toxic effect of disulfiram and rauwolfia alkaloids. Procarbazine may increase the levels/effects of serotonin $5-HT_{1D}$ receptor agonists. Altretamine may enhance the orthostatic effect of procarbazine. Buspirone may enhance the adverse/toxic effect of procarbazine. COMT Inhibitors may enhance the cardiovascular adverse/toxic effects of procarbazine. Levodopa may enhance the hypertensive effect of procarbazine. Sibutramine may enhance the serotonergic effect of procarbazine. Tramadol may enhance the neurotoxic effects of procarbazine.

Decreased Effect: Procarbazine may decrease the absorption of digoxin tablets. Procarbazine may diminish the antihypertensive effect of false neurotransmitters.

Pharmacodynamics/Kinetics

Absorption: Rapid and complete

Distribution: Crosses blood-brain barrier; equilibrates between plasma and CSF

Metabolism: Hepatic and renal

Half-life elimination: 1 hour

Time to peak, plasma: 1 hour

Excretion: Urine and respiratory tract (<5% as unchanged drug, 70% as metabolites)

Pregnancy Risk Factor D

Procarbazine Hydrochloride *see* Procarbazine *on page 1355*

Procardia® *see* NIFEdipine *on page 1173*

Procardia XL® *see* NIFEdipine *on page 1173*

Procetofene *see* Fenofibrate *on page 674*

Prochieve® *see* Progesterone *on page 1360*

Prochlorperazine *(proe klor PER a zeen)*

Related Information

Sedation *on page 1825*

U.S. Brand Names Compro™

Canadian Brand Names Apo-Prochlorperazine®; Compazine®; Nu-Prochlor; Stemetil®

Generic Available Yes: Injection, tablet, suppository

Index Terms Chlormeprazine; Compazine; Prochlorperazine Edisylate; Prochlorperazine Maleate

Pharmacologic Category Antiemetic; Antipsychotic Agent, Typical, Phenothiazine

Use Management of nausea and vomiting; psychotic disorders including schizophrenia; anxiety

Unlabeled/Investigational Use Behavioral syndromes in dementia

Local Anesthetic/Vasoconstrictor Precautions Most pharmacology textbooks state that in presence of phenothiazines, systemic doses of epinephrine paradoxically decrease the blood pressure. This is the so called "epinephrine reversal" phenomenon. This has never been observed when epinephrine is given by infiltration as part of the anesthesia procedure.

Effects on Dental Treatment Key adverse event(s) related to dental treatment: Xerostomia and changes in salivation (normal salivary flow resumes upon discontinuation). Significant hypotension may occur, especially when the drug is administered parenterally; orthostatic hypotension is due to alpha-receptor blockade, the elderly are at greater risk for orthostatic hypotension.

Tardive dyskinesia: Prevalence rate may be 40% in elderly; development of the syndrome and the irreversible nature are proportional to duration and total cumulative dose over time. Extrapyramidal reactions are more common in elderly with up to 50% developing these reactions after 60 years of age. Drug-induced Parkinson's syndrome occurs often; akathisia is the most common extrapyramidal reaction in elderly.

Common Adverse Effects Reported with prochlorperazine or other phenothiazines. Frequency not defined

Cardiovascular: Cardiac arrest, hypotension, peripheral edema, Q-wave distortions, T-wave distortions

Central nervous system: Agitation, catatonia, cerebral edema, cough reflex suppressed, dizziness, drowsiness, fever (mild - I.M.), headache, hyperactivity, hyperpyrexia, impairment of temperature regulation, insomnia, neuroleptic malignant syndrome (NMS), paradoxical excitement, restlessness, seizure

Dermatologic: Angioedema, contact dermatitis, discoloration of skin (blue-gray), epithelial keratopathy, erythema, eczema, exfoliative dermatitis (injectable), itching, photosensitivity, rash, skin pigmentation, urticaria

Endocrine & metabolic: Amenorrhea, breast enlargement, galactorrhea, gynecomastia, glucosuria, hyperglycemia, hypoglycemia, lactation, libido (changes in), menstrual irregularity, SIADH

Gastrointestinal: Appetite increased, atonic colon, constipation, ileus, nausea, weight gain, xerostomia

Genitourinary: Ejaculating dysfunction, ejaculatory disturbances, impotence, incontinence, polyuria, priapism, urinary retention, urination difficulty

Hematologic: Agranulocytosis, aplastic anemia, eosinophilia, hemolytic anemia, leukopenia, pancytopenia, thrombocytopenic purpura

Hepatic: Biliary stasis, cholestatic jaundice, hepatotoxicity

Neuromuscular & skeletal: Dystonias (torticollis, opisthotonos, carpopedal spasm, trismus, oculogyric crisis, protusion of tongue); extrapyramidal symptoms (pseudoparkinsonism, akathisia, dystonias, tardive dyskinesia); SLE-like syndrome, tremor

Ocular: blurred vision, cornea and lens changes, lenticular/corneal deposits, miosis, mydriasis, pigmentary retinopathy

Respiratory: Asthma, laryngeal edema, nasal congestion

Miscellaneous: Allergic reactions, diaphoresis

Dosage

Antiemetic: Children (therapy >1 day usually not required): **Note:** Not recommended for use in children <9 kg or <2 years:

Oral, rectal: >9 kg: 0.4 mg/kg/24 hours in 3-4 divided doses; **or**
9-13 kg: 2.5 mg every 12-24 hours as needed; maximum: 7.5 mg/day
13.1-17 kg: 2.5 mg every 8-12 hours as needed; maximum: 10 mg/day
17.1-37 kg: 2.5 mg every 8 hours or 5 mg every 12 hours as needed; maximum: 15 mg/day

I.M.: 0.13 mg/kg/dose; change to oral as soon as possible

Antiemetic: Adults:

Oral (tablet): 5-10 mg 3-4 times/day; usual maximum: 40 mg/day; larger doses may rarely be required

I.M. (deep): 5-10 mg every 3-4 hours; usual maximum: 40 mg/day

I.V.: 2.5-10 mg; maximum 10 mg/dose or 40 mg/day; may repeat dose every 3-4 hours as needed

Rectal: 25 mg twice daily

Surgical nausea/vomiting: Adults: **Note:** Should not exceed 40 mg/day

I.M.: 5-10 mg 1-2 hours before induction or to control symptoms during or after surgery; may repeat once if necessary

I.V. (administer slow IVP <5 mg/minute): 5-10 mg 15-30 minutes before induction or to control symptoms during or after surgery; may repeat once if necessary

Rectal (unlabeled use): 25 mg

(Continued)

Prochlorperazine *(Continued)*

Antipsychotic:

Children 2-12 years (not recommended in children <9 kg or <2 years):

Oral, rectal: 2.5 mg 2-3 times/day; do not give more than 10 mg the first day; increase dosage as needed to maximum daily dose of 20 mg for 2-5 years and 25 mg for 6-12 years

I.M.: 0.13 mg/kg/dose; change to oral as soon as possible

Adults:

Oral: 5-10 mg 3-4 times/day; titrate dose slowly every 2-3 days; doses up to 150 mg/day may be required in some patients for treatment of severe disturbances

I.M.: Initial: 10-20 mg; if necessary repeat initial dose every 1-4 hours to gain control; more than 3-4 doses are rarely needed. If parenteral administration is still required; give 10-20 mg every 4-6 hours; change to oral as soon as possible.

Nonpsychotic anxiety: Oral (tablet): Adults: Usual dose: 15-20 mg/day in divided doses; do not give doses >20 mg/day or for longer than 12 weeks

Elderly: Behavioral symptoms associated with dementia (unlabeled use): Initial: 2.5-5 mg 1-2 times/day; increase dose at 4- to 7-day intervals by 2.5-5 mg/day; increase dosing intervals (twice daily, 3 times/day, etc) as necessary to control response or side effects; maximum daily dose should probably not exceed 75 mg in elderly; gradual increases (titration) may prevent some side effects or decrease their severity

Mechanism of Action Prochlorperazine is a piperazine phenothiazine antipsychotic which blocks postsynaptic mesolimbic dopaminergic D_1 and D_2 receptors in the brain, including the chemoreceptor trigger zone; exhibits a strong alpha-adrenergic and anticholinergic blocking effect and depresses the release of hypothalamic and hypophyseal hormones; believed to depress the reticular activating system, thus affecting basal metabolism, body temperature, wakefulness, vasomotor tone and emesis

Contraindications Hypersensitivity to prochlorperazine or any component of the formulation (cross-reactivity between phenothiazines may occur); severe CNS depression; coma; pediatric surgery; Reye's syndrome; should not be used in children <2 years of age or <9 kg

Warnings/Precautions May be sedating; use with caution in disorders where CNS depression is a feature. May obscure intestinal obstruction or brain tumor. May impair physical or mental abilities. Effects with other sedative drugs or ethanol may be potentiated. Use with caution in Parkinson's disease; hemodynamic instability; bone marrow suppression; predisposition to seizures; subcortical brain damage; and in severe cardiac, hepatic, renal or respiratory disease. Caution in breast cancer or other prolactin-dependent tumors. May alter temperature regulation or mask toxicity of other drugs. Use caution with exposure to heat. May alter cardiac conduction. May cause orthostatic hypotension. Hypotension may occur following administration, particularly when parenteral form is used or in high dosages.

Phenothiazines may cause anticholinergic effects; therefore, they should be used with caution in patients with decreased gastrointestinal motility, urinary retention, BPH, xerostomia, or visual problems. Conditions which also may be exacerbated by cholinergic blockade include narrow-angle glaucoma (screening is recommended) and worsening of myasthenia gravis. May cause extrapyramidal symptoms. Use caution in the elderly. Children with acute illness or dehydration are more susceptible to neuromuscular reactions; use cautiously. May be associated with neuroleptic malignant syndrome (NMS).

Drug Interactions

Increased Effect/Toxicity: Prochlorperazine plus lithium may rarely produce neurotoxicity. Prochlorperazing may produce additive CNS depressant effects with other CNS depressants. Acetylcholinesterase inhibitors may increase the risk of EPS. Alpha-/beta-agonists, antihistamines, QT_c-prolonging agents may enhance the arrhythmogenic effects of phenothiazines. Concurrent use may enhance the hypotensive effects of narcotics and beta-blockers. SSRIs may increase risk of hypotension. Antimalarials and beta-blockers may increase serum levels of prochlorperazine.Pramlintide may increase anticholinergic effects of prochlorperazine.

Decreased Effect: The antihypertensive effects of methyldopa and guanadrel may be inhibited by prochlorperazine. Prochlorperazine may inhibit the antiparkinsonian effect of levodopa. Prochlorperazine may reverse the pressor effects of epinephrine. Antacids and attapulgite may decreased absorption of phenothiazines. Anticholinertics may decrease the therapeutic response to phenothiazines.

Ethanol/Nutrition/Herb Interactions

Ethanol: Avoid ethanol (may increase CNS depression).

Food: Limit caffeine.

Herb/Nutraceutical: Avoid dong quai, St John's wort (may also cause photosensitization). Avoid kava kava, gotu kola, valerian, St John's wort (may increase CNS depression).

Dietary Considerations Increase dietary intake of riboflavin; should be administered with food or water. Rectal suppositories may contain coconut and palm oil.

Pharmacodynamics/Kinetics

Onset of action: Oral: 30-40 minutes; I.M.: 10-20 minutes; Rectal: ~60 minutes
Peak antiemetic effect: I.V.: 30-60 minutes

Duration: Rectal: 12 hours; Oral: 3-4 hours; I.M., I.V.: Adults: 4-6 hours; I.M.: Children: 12 hours

Distribution: V_d: 1400-1548 L; crosses placenta; enters breast milk

Metabolism: Primarily hepatic; N-desmethyl prochlorperazine (major active metabolite)

Bioavailability: Oral: 12.5%

Half-life elimination: Oral: 3-5 hours; I.V.: ~7 hours

Dosage Forms

Injection, solution: 5 mg/mL (2 mL, 10 mL)

Suppository, rectal: 2.5 mg (12s), 5 mg (12s), 25 mg (12s)
Compro™: 25 mg (12s)

Tablet: 5 mg, 10 mg

Procyclidine (proe SYE kli deen)

U.S. Brand Names Kemadrin®

Canadian Brand Names PMS-Procyclidine

Generic Available No

Index Terms Procyclidine Hydrochloride

Pharmacologic Category Anti-Parkinson's Agent, Anticholinergic; Anticholinergic Agent

Use Relieves symptoms of parkinsonian syndrome and drug-induced extrapyramidal symptoms

Local Anesthetic/Vasoconstrictor Precautions No information available to require special precautions

Effects on Dental Treatment Key adverse event(s) related to dental treatment: Xerostomia (normal salivary flow resumes upon discontinuation) and dry throat and nose. Prolonged use of antidyskinetics may decrease or inhibit salivary flow, contributing to discomfort and dental disease (ie, caries, oral candidiasis, and periodontal disease).

Common Adverse Effects Frequency not defined.

Cardiovascular: Palpitation, tachycardia

Central nervous system: Ataxia, confusion, drowsiness, fatigue, giddiness, headache, lightheadedness, loss of memory

Dermatologic: Dry skin, photosensitivity, rash

Gastrointestinal: Constipation, dry throat, epigastric distress, nausea, vomiting, xerostomia

Genitourinary: Difficult urination

Neuromuscular & skeletal: Weakness

Ocular: Blurred vision, increased intraocular pain, mydriasis

Respiratory: Dry nose

Miscellaneous: Diaphoresis decreased

Mechanism of Action Thought to act by blocking excess acetylcholine at cerebral synapses; many of its effects are due to its pharmacologic similarities with atropine; it exerts an antispasmodic effect on smooth muscle, is a potent mydriatic; inhibits salivation

(Continued)

Procyclidine (Continued)

Drug Interactions

Increased Effect/Toxicity: Central and/or peripheral anticholinergic syndrome can occur when administered with amantadine, rimantadine, opioid analgesics, phenothiazines and other antipsychotics (especially with high anticholinergic activity), tricyclic antidepressants, quinidine and some other antiarrhythmics, and antihistamines.

Decreased Effect: May increase gastric degradation of levodopa and decrease the amount of levodopa absorbed by delaying gastric emptying; the opposite may be true for digoxin. Therapeutic effects of cholinergic agents (tacrine, donepezil) and neuroleptics may be antagonized.

Pharmacodynamics/Kinetics
Onset of action: 30-40 minutes
Duration: 4-6 hours

Pregnancy Risk Factor C

Procyclidine Hydrochloride see Procyclidine on page 1359

Prodium® [OTC] see Phenazopyridine on page 1286

Profen II DM® see Guaifenesin, Pseudoephedrine, and Dextromethorphan on page 800

Profen Forte™ DM see Guaifenesin, Pseudoephedrine, and Dextromethorphan on page 800

Profilnine® SD see Factor IX Complex (Human) on page 667

Progesterone (proe JES ter one)

U.S. Brand Names Crinone®; Prochieve®; Prometrium®
Canadian Brand Names Crinone®; Prometrium®
Mexican Brand Names Gepromi; Geslutin; Utrogestan
Generic Available Yes: Injection
Index Terms Pregnenedione; Progestin
Pharmacologic Category Progestin

Use
Oral: Prevention of endometrial hyperplasia in nonhysterectomized, postmenopausal women who are receiving conjugated estrogen tablets; secondary amenorrhea

I.M.: Amenorrhea; abnormal uterine bleeding due to hormonal imbalance

Intravaginal gel: Part of assisted reproductive technology (ART) for infertile women with progesterone deficiency; secondary amenorrhea

Local Anesthetic/Vasoconstrictor Precautions No information available to require special precautions

Effects on Dental Treatment Key adverse event(s) related to dental treatment: Progestins may predispose the patient to gingival bleeding.

Common Adverse Effects

Injection (I.M.):
Cardiovascular: Cerebral edema, cerebral thrombosis, edema
Central nervous system: Depression, fever, insomnia, somnolence
Dermatologic: Acne, allergic rash (rare), alopecia, hirsutism, pruritus, rash, urticaria
Endocrine & metabolic: Amenorrhea, breakthrough bleeding, breast tenderness, galactorrhea, menstrual flow changes, spotting
Gastrointestinal: Nausea, weight gain/loss
Genitourinary: Cervical erosion changes, cervical secretion changes
Hepatic: Cholestatic jaundice
Local: Injection site: Irritation, pain, redness
Ocular: Optic neuritis, retinal thrombosis
Respiratory: Pulmonary embolism
Miscellaneous: Anaphylactoid reactions

Oral capsule (percentages reported when used in combination with or cycled with conjugated estrogens):
>10%:
Central nervous system: Headache (10% to 31%), dizziness (15% to 24%), depression (19%)
Endocrine & metabolic: Breast tenderness (27%), breast pain (6% to 16%)
Gastrointestinal: Abdominal pain (6% to 12%), abdominal bloating (10% to 20%)
Genitourinary: Urinary problems (11%)
Neuromuscular & skeletal: Joint pain (20%), musculoskeletal pain (6% to 12%)
Miscellaneous: Viral infection (7% to 12%)
5% to 10%:
Cardiovascular: Chest pain (7%)

Central nervous system: Fatigue (8% to 9%), emotional lability (6%), irritability (5% to 8%), worry (8%)

Gastrointestinal: Nausea/vomiting (8%), diarrhea (8%)

Respiratory: Upper respiratory tract infection (5%), cough (8%)

Miscellaneous: Night sweats (7%)

Vaginal gel (percentages reported with ART); also refer to oral capsule reactions listing for additional effects noted with progesterone:

>10%:

Central nervous system: Somnolence (27%), headache (13% to 17%), nervousness (16%), depression (11%)

Endocrine & metabolic: Breast enlargement (40%), breast pain (13%), libido decreased (11%)

Gastrointestinal: Constipation (27%), nausea (7% to 22%), cramps (15%), abdominal pain (12%)

Genitourinary: Perineal pain (17%), nocturia (13%)

5% to 10%:

Central nervous system: Pain (8%), dizziness (5%)

Gastrointestinal: Diarrhea (8%), bloating (7%), vomiting (5%)

Genitourinary: Vaginal discharge (7%), dyspareunia (6%), genital moniliasis (5%), genital pruritus (5%)

Neuromuscular & skeletal: Arthralgia (8%)

Mechanism of Action Natural steroid hormone that induces secretory changes in the endometrium, promotes mammary gland development, relaxes uterine smooth muscle, blocks follicular maturation and ovulation, and maintains pregnancy

Drug Interactions

Cytochrome P450 Effect: Substrate of CYP1A2 (minor), 2A6 (minor), 2C9 (minor), 2C19 (major), 2D6 (minor), 3A4 (major); **Inhibits** CYP2C9 (weak), 2C19 (weak), 3A4 (weak)

Increased Effect/Toxicity: Progesterone may increase concentrations of estrogenic compounds during concurrent therapy with conjugated estrogens. Progestins may enhance the hepatotoxic effects of cyclosporine.

Decreased Effect: CYP2C19 inducers may decrease the levels/effects of progesterone; example inducers include aminoglutethimide, carbamazepine, phenytoin, and rifampin. CYP3A4 inducers may decrease the levels/effects of progesterone; example inducers include aminoglutethimide, carbamazepine, nafcillin, nevirapine, phenobarbital, phenytoin, and rifamycins.

Pharmacodynamics/Kinetics

Absorption: Vaginal gel: Prolonged

Absorption half-life: 25-50 hours

Protein binding: Albumin (50% to 54%) and cortisol-binding protein (43% to 48%)

Metabolism: Hepatic to metabolites

Half-life elimination: Vaginal gel: 5-20 minutes

Time to peak: Oral: Within 3 hours; I.M.: ~8 hours

Excretion: Urine, bile, feces

Pregnancy Risk Factor B (Prometrium®, per manufacturer); none established for vaginal gel or injection (contraindicated)

Promethazine (proe METH a zeen)

U.S. Brand Names Phenadoz™; Phenergan®; Promethegan™

Canadian Brand Names Phenergan®

Generic Available Yes

Index Terms Promethazine Hydrochloride

Pharmacologic Category Antiemetic; Antihistamine; Phenothiazine Derivative; Sedative

(Continued)

Promethazine (Continued)

Use Symptomatic treatment of various allergic conditions; antiemetic; motion sickness; sedative; postoperative pain (adjunctive therapy); anesthetic (adjunctive therapy); anaphylactic reactions (adjunctive therapy)

Local Anesthetic/Vasoconstrictor Precautions Most pharmacology textbooks state that in presence of phenothiazines, systemic doses of epinephrine paradoxically decrease the blood pressure. This is the so called "epinephrine reversal" phenomenon. This has never been observed when epinephrine is given by infiltration as part of the anesthesia procedure.

Effects on Dental Treatment Key adverse event(s) related to dental treatment: Xerostomia (normal salivary flow resumes upon discontinuation). Significant hypotension may occur, especially when the drug is administered parenterally; orthostatic hypotension is due to alpha-receptor blockade, the elderly are at greater risk for orthostatic hypotension.

Tardive dyskinesia: Prevalence rate may be 40% in elderly; development of the syndrome and the irreversible nature are proportional to duration and total cumulative dose over time. Extrapyramidal reactions are more common in elderly with up to 50% developing these reactions after 60 years of age. Drug-induced Parkinson's syndrome occurs often; akathisia is the most common extrapyramidal reaction in elderly.

Increased confusion, memory loss, psychotic behavior, and agitation frequently occur as a consequence of anticholinergic effects. Antipsychotic associated sedation in nonpsychotic patients is extremely unpleasant due to feelings of depersonalization, derealization, and dysphoria.

Common Adverse Effects

Cardiovascular: Bradycardia, hypertension, nonspecific QT changes, postural hypotension, tachycardia

Central nervous system: Akathisia, catatonic states, confusion, delirium, disorientation, dizziness, drowsiness, dystonias, euphoria, excitation, extrapyramidal symptoms, fatigue, hallucinations, hysteria, insomnia, lassitude, nervousness, neuroleptic malignant syndrome, nightmares, pseudoparkinsonism, sedation, seizure, somnolence, tardive dyskinesia

Dermatologic: Angioneurotic edema, dermatitis, photosensitivity, skin pigmentation (slate gray), urticaria

Endocrine & metabolic: Amenorrhea, breast engorgement, gynecomastia, hyper-/hypoglycemia, lactation

Gastrointestinal: Constipation, nausea, vomiting, xerostomia

Genitourinary: Ejaculatory disorder, impotence, urinary retention

Hematologic: Agranulocytosis, aplastic anemia, eosinophilia, hemolytic anemia, leukopenia, thrombocytopenia, thrombocytopenic purpura

Hepatic: Jaundice

Local: Venous thrombosis; injection site reactions (burning, erythema, pain, edema)

Neuromuscular & skeletal: Incoordination, tremor

Ocular: Blurred vision, corneal and lenticular changes, diplopia, epithelial keratopathy, pigmentary retinopathy

Otic: Tinnitus

Respiratory: Apnea, asthma, nasal congestion, respiratory depression

Mechanism of Action Blocks postsynaptic mesolimbic dopaminergic receptors in the brain; exhibits a strong alpha-adrenergic blocking effect and depresses the release of hypothalamic and hypophyseal hormones; competes with histamine for the H_1-receptor; reduces stimuli to the brainstem reticular system

Drug Interactions

Cytochrome P450 Effect: Substrate (major) of CYP2B6, 2D6; **Inhibits** CYP2D6 (weak)

Increased Effect/Toxicity: CYP2B6 inhibitors may increase the levels/effects of promethazine; example inhibitors include desipramine, paroxetine, and sertraline. CYP2D6 inhibitors may increase the levels/effects of promethazine; example inhibitors include chlorpromazine, delavirdine, fluoxetine, miconazole, paroxetine, pergolide, quinidine, quinine, ritonavir, and ropinirole. Pramlintide may enhance the gastrointestinal anticholinergic effects of promethazine.

Decreased Effect: Acetylcholinesterase inhibitors (centrally-acting) may diminish the effects of promethazine. CYP2B6 inducers may decrease the levels/effects of promethazine; example inducers include carbamazepine, nevirapine, phenobarbital, phenytoin, and rifampin. Benztropine (and other anticholinergics) may inhibit the therapeutic response to promethazine. Promethazine may diminish the effect of centrally-acting acetylcholinesterase inhibitors.

Pharmacodynamics/Kinetics

Onset of action: I.M.: ~20 minutes; I.V.: 3-5 minutes

Peak effect: C_{max}: 9.04 ng/mL (suppository); 19.3 ng/mL (syrup)

Duration: 2-6 hours

Absorption:

I.M.: Bioavailability may be greater than with oral or rectal administration

Oral: Rapid and complete; large first pass effect limits systemic bioavailability

Distribution: V_d: 171 L

Protein binding: 93%

Metabolism: Hepatic; primarily oxidation; forms metabolites

Half-life elimination: 9-16 hours

Time to maximum serum concentration: 4.4 hours (syrup); 6.7-8.6 hours (suppositories)

Excretion: Primarily urine and feces (as inactive metabolites)

Pregnancy Risk Factor C

Promethazine and Codeine (proe METH a zeen & KOE deen)

Related Information
Codeine on page 404
Promethazine on page 1361

Generic Available Yes

Index Terms Codeine and Promethazine

Pharmacologic Category Antihistamine/Antitussive

Use Temporary relief of coughs and upper respiratory symptoms associated with allergy or the common cold

Local Anesthetic/Vasoconstrictor Precautions No information available to require special precautions

Effects on Dental Treatment Although promethazine is a phenothiazine derivative, extrapyramidal reactions or tardive dyskinesias are not seen with the use of this drug.

Common Adverse Effects See individual agents.

Restrictions C-V

Drug Interactions
Cytochrome P450 Effect: Promethazine: **Substrate** (major) of CYP2B6, 2D6; **Inhibits** CYP2D6 (weak)

Pharmacodynamics/Kinetics See individual agents.

Pregnancy Risk Factor C

Promethazine and Dextromethorphan
(proe METH a zeen & deks troe meth OR fan)

Related Information
Dextromethorphan on page 477
Promethazine on page 1361

Generic Available Yes

Index Terms Dextromethorphan and Promethazine

Pharmacologic Category Antihistamine/Antitussive

Use Temporary relief of coughs and upper respiratory symptoms associated with allergy or the common cold

Local Anesthetic/Vasoconstrictor Precautions No information available to require special precautions

Effects on Dental Treatment Although promethazine is a phenothiazine derivative, extrapyramidal reactions or tardive dyskinesias are not seen with the use of this drug.

Drug Interactions
Cytochrome P450 Effect:
Promethazine: **Substrate** (major) of CYP2B6, 2D6; **Inhibits** CYP2D6 (weak)
Dextromethorphan: **Substrate** of CYP2B6 (minor), 2C9 (minor), 2C19 (minor), 2D6 (major), 2E1 (minor), 3A4 (minor); **Inhibits** CYP2D6 (weak)

Pharmacodynamics/Kinetics See individual agents.

Pregnancy Risk Factor C

Promethazine and Meperidine see Meperidine and Promethazine on page 1041

Promethazine and Phenylephrine
(proe METH a zeen & fen il EF rin)

Related Information
Phenylephrine on page 1293
Promethazine on page 1361

Generic Available Yes

(Continued)

Promethazine and Phenylephrine *(Continued)*

Index Terms Phenylephrine and Promethazine

Pharmacologic Category Antihistamine/Decongestant Combination

Use Temporary relief of upper respiratory symptoms associated with allergy or the common cold

Local Anesthetic/Vasoconstrictor Precautions

Phenylephrine: Use with caution since phenylephrine is a sympathomimetic amine which could interact with epinephrine to cause a pressor response

Promethazine: No information available to require special precautions

Effects on Dental Treatment Key adverse event(s) related to dental treatment: Phenylephrine: Tachycardia, palpitations, xerostomia (normal salivary flow resumes upon discontinuation); use vasoconstrictor with caution. Although promethazine is a phenothiazine derivative, extrapyramidal reactions or tardive dyskinesias are not seen with the use of this drug.

Drug Interactions

Cytochrome P450 Effect: Promethazine: **Substrate** (major) of CYP2B6, 2D6; **Inhibits** CYP2D6 (weak)

Pharmacodynamics/Kinetics See individual agents.

Pregnancy Risk Factor C

Promethazine Hydrochloride *see* Promethazine *on page 1361*

Promethazine, Phenylephrine, and Codeine
(proe METH a zeen, fen il EF rin, & KOE deen)

Related Information
Codeine *on page 404*
Phenylephrine *on page 1293*
Promethazine *on page 1361*

Generic Available Yes

Index Terms Codeine, Promethazine, and Phenylephrine; Phenylephrine, Promethazine, and Codeine

Pharmacologic Category Antihistamine/Decongestant/Antitussive

Use Temporary relief of coughs and upper respiratory symptoms including nasal congestion associated with allergy or the common cold

Local Anesthetic/Vasoconstrictor Precautions

Phenylephrine: Use with caution since phenylephrine is a sympathomimetic amine which could interact with epinephrine to cause a pressor response

Promethazine: No information available to require special precautions

Effects on Dental Treatment Key adverse event(s) related to dental treatment: Phenylephrine: Tachycardia, palpitations, xerostomia (normal salivary flow resumes upon discontinuation); use vasoconstrictor with caution. Although promethazine is a phenothiazine derivative, extrapyramidal reactions or tardive dyskinesias are not seen with the use of this drug.

Common Adverse Effects See individual agents.

Restrictions C-V

Drug Interactions

Cytochrome P450 Effect:

Promethazine: **Substrate** (major) of CYP2B6, 2D6; **Inhibits** CYP2D6 (weak)

Codeine: **Substrate** of CYP2D6 (major), 3A4 (minor); **Inhibits** CYP2D6 (weak)

Pharmacodynamics/Kinetics See individual agents.

Pregnancy Risk Factor C

Promethegan™ *see* Promethazine *on page 1361*

Prometrium® *see* Progesterone *on page 1360*

Promit® [DSC] *see* Dextran 1 *on page 473*

Pronap-100® *see* Propoxyphene and Acetaminophen *on page 1369*

Pronto® Complete Lice Killing Kit [OTC] *see* Pyrethrins and Piperonyl Butoxide *on page 1388*

Pronto® Plus Hair and Scalp Masque [OTC] *see* Pyrethrins and Piperonyl Butoxide *on page 1388*

Pronto® Plus Lice Egg Remover Kit [OTC] *see* Benzalkonium Chloride *on page 194*

Pronto® Plus Mousse [OTC] *see* Pyrethrins and Piperonyl Butoxide *on page 1388*

Pronto® Plus Warm Oil Treatment and Conditioner [OTC] *see* Pyrethrins and Piperonyl Butoxide *on page 1388*

Pronto® Plus with Natural Extracts and Oils [OTC] *see* Pyrethrins and Piperonyl Butoxide *on page 1388*

Propafenone (pro PAF en one)

Related Information
Cardiovascular Diseases *on page 1726*

U.S. Brand Names Rythmol®; Rythmol® SR

Canadian Brand Names Apo-Propafenone®; Rythmol® Gen-Propafenone

Mexican Brand Names Nistaken; Norfenon

Generic Available Yes: Tablet

Index Terms Propafenone Hydrochloride

Pharmacologic Category Antiarrhythmic Agent, Class Ic

Use Treatment of life-threatening ventricular arrhythmias

Rythmol® SR: Maintenance of normal sinus rhythm in patients with symptomatic atrial fibrillation

Unlabeled/Investigational Use Supraventricular tachycardias, including those patients with Wolff-Parkinson-White syndrome

Local Anesthetic/Vasoconstrictor Precautions In some patients, propafenone has been reported to induce new or worsened arrhythmias (proarrhythmic effect). It is suggested that vasoconstrictors be used with caution since epinephrine has the potential to stimulate the heart rate when given in the anesthetic regimen. Propafenone is one of the drugs confirmed to prolong the QT interval and is accepted as having a risk of causing torsade de pointes. The risk of drug-induced torsade de pointes is extremely low when a single QT interval prolonging drug is prescribed. In terms of epinephrine, it is not known what effect vasoconstrictors in the local anesthetic regimen will have in patients with a known history of congenital prolonged QT interval or in patients taking any medication that prolongs the QT interval. Until more information is obtained, it is suggested that the clinician consult with the physician prior to the use of a vasoconstrictor in suspected patients, and that the vasoconstrictor (epinephrine, levonordefrin [Neo-Cobefrin®]) be used with caution.

Effects on Dental Treatment Key adverse event(s) related to dental treatment: Unusual taste and significant xerostomia (normal salivary flow resumes upon discontinuation).

Common Adverse Effects 1% to 10%:

Cardiovascular: New or worsened arrhythmia (proarrhythmic effect) (2% to 10%), angina (2% to 5%), CHF (1% to 4%), ventricular tachycardia (1% to 3%), palpitation (1% to 3%), AV block (first-degree) (1% to 3%), syncope (1% to 2%), increased QRS interval (1% to 2%), chest pain (1% to 2%), PVCs (1% to 2%), bradycardia (1% to 2%), edema (0% to 1%), bundle branch block (0% to 1%), atrial fibrillation (1%), hypotension (0% to 1%), intraventricular conduction delay (0% to 1%)

Central nervous system: Dizziness (4% to 15%), fatigue (2% to 6%), headache (2% to 5%), ataxia (0% to 2%), insomnia (0% to 2%), anxiety (1% to 2%), drowsiness (1%)

Dermatologic: Rash (1% to 3%)

Gastrointestinal: Nausea/vomiting (2% to 11%), unusual taste (3% to 23%), constipation (2% to 7%), dyspepsia (1% to 3%), diarrhea (1% to 3%), xerostomia (1% to 2%), anorexia (1% to 2%), abdominal pain (1% to 2%), flatulence (0% to 1%)

Neuromuscular & skeletal: Tremor (0% to 1%), arthralgia (0% to 1%), weakness (1% to 2%)

Ocular: Blurred vision (1% to 6%)

Respiratory: Dyspnea (2% to 5%)

Miscellaneous: Diaphoresis (1%)

Mechanism of Action Propafenone is a class 1c antiarrhythmic agent which possesses local anesthetic properties, blocks the fast inward sodium current, and slows the rate of increase of the action potential. Prolongs conduction and refractoriness in all areas of the myocardium, with a slightly more pronounced effect on intraventricular conduction; it prolongs effective refractory period, reduces spontaneous automaticity and exhibits some beta-blockade activity.

Drug Interactions

Cytochrome P450 Effect: Substrate of CYP1A2 (minor), 2D6 (major), 3A4 (minor); **Inhibits** CYP1A2 (weak), 2D6 (weak)

Increased Effect/Toxicity: Cimetidine and quinidine may increase propafenone levels. Ritonavir may increase propafenone levels; concurrent use is contraindicated. CYP2D6 inhibitors may increase the levels/effects of propafenone; example inhibitors include chlorpromazine, delavirdine, fluoxetine, miconazole, paroxetine, pergolide, quinine, and ropinirole. Digoxin (reduce dose by 25%), metoprolol, propranolol, theophylline, and warfarin blood levels are increased by propafenone. Use caution with Class Ia and Class III antiarrhythmics, erythromycin, cisapride, antipsychotics, and cyclic antidepressants; QT_c-prolonging effects may be additive with propafenone.

(Continued)

Propafenone *(Continued)*

Decreased Effect: Enzyme inducers (phenobarbital, phenytoin, rifabutin, rifampin) may decrease propafenone blood levels.

Pharmacodynamics/Kinetics

Absorption: Well absorbed

Metabolism: Hepatic; two genetically determined metabolism groups exist: fast or slow metabolizers; 10% of Caucasians are slow metabolizers; exhibits nonlinear pharmacokinetics; when dose is increased from 300-900 mg/day, serum concentrations increase tenfold; this nonlinearity is thought to be due to saturable first-pass effect

Bioavailability: 150 mg: 3.4%; 300 mg: 10.6%

Half-life elimination: Single dose (100-300 mg): 2-8 hours; Chronic dosing: 10-32 hours

Time to peak: 150 mg dose: 2 hours, 300 mg dose: 3 hours

Pregnancy Risk Factor C

Propafenone Hydrochloride *see* Propafenone *on page 1365*

Propantheline *(proe PAN the leen)*

Generic Available Yes

Index Terms Propantheline Bromide

Pharmacologic Category Anticholinergic Agent

Dental Use Induce dry field (xerostomia) in oral cavity

Use Adjunctive treatment of peptic ulcer, irritable bowel syndrome, pancreatitis, ureteral and urinary bladder spasm; reduce duodenal motility during diagnostic radiologic procedures

Local Anesthetic/Vasoconstrictor Precautions No information available to require special precautions

Effects on Dental Treatment Key adverse event(s) related to dental treatment: Significant xerostomia (therapeutic effect; normal salivary flow resumes upon discontinuation), dry throat, nasal dryness, and dysphagia.

Significant Adverse Effects Frequency not defined.

Dermatologic: Dry skin

Gastrointestinal: Constipation, dry mouth and throat, dysphagia

Respiratory: Dry nose

Miscellaneous: Diaphoresis (decreased)

Dental Usual Dosing Antisecretory: Oral:

Children: 1-2 mg/kg/day in 3-4 divided doses

Adults: 15 mg 3 times/day before meals or food and 30 mg at bedtime

Elderly: 7.5 mg 3 times/day before meals and at bedtime

Dosage Oral:

Antisecretory:

Children: 1-2 mg/kg/day in 3-4 divided doses

Adults: 15 mg 3 times/day before meals or food and 30 mg at bedtime

Elderly: 7.5 mg 3 times/day before meals and at bedtime

Antispasmodic:

Children: 2-3 mg/kg/day in divided doses every 4-6 hours and at bedtime

Adults: 15 mg 3 times/day before meals or food and 30 mg at bedtime

Mechanism of Action Competitively blocks the action of acetylcholine at postganglionic parasympathetic receptor sites

Contraindications Hypersensitivity to propantheline or any component of the formulation; ulcerative colitis, toxic megacolon, obstructive disease of the GI or urinary tract; narrow-angle glaucoma; myasthenia gravis

Warnings/Precautions Use with caution in patients with hyperthyroidism, hepatic, cardiac, or renal disease, hypertension, GI infections, or other endocrine diseases.

Drug Interactions

Decreased effect with antacids (decreased absorption); decreased effect of sustained release dosage forms (decreased absorption)

Increased effect/toxicity with anticholinergics, disopyramide, opioid analgesics, bretylium, type I antiarrhythmics, antihistamines, phenothiazines, TCAs, corticosteroids (increased IOP), CNS depressants (sedation), adenosine, amiodarone, beta-blockers, amoxapine

Dietary Considerations Should be taken 30 minutes before meals so that the drug's peak effect occurs at the proper time. The tablet (15 mg) contains lactose 23.2 mg.

Pharmacodynamics/Kinetics

Onset of action: 30-45 minutes

Duration: 4-6 hours

Half-life elimination, serum: Average: 1.6 hours

Pregnancy Risk Factor C

Lactation Excretion in breast milk unknown

Breast-Feeding Considerations No data reported; however, atropine may be taken while breast-feeding.

Dosage Forms Excipient information presented when available (limited, particularly for generics); consult specific product labeling.

Tablet, as bromide: 15 mg [contains lactose 23.2 mg]

Propantheline Bromide *see* Propantheline *on page 1366*

Propa pH [OTC] *see* Salicylic Acid *on page 1451*

Proparacaine (proe PAR a kane)

U.S. Brand Names Alcaine®; Ophthetic®

Canadian Brand Names Alcaine®; Diocaine®

Generic Available Yes

Index Terms Proparacaine Hydrochloride; Proxymetacaine

Pharmacologic Category Local Anesthetic, Ophthalmic

Use Anesthesia for tonometry, gonioscopy; suture removal from cornea; removal of corneal foreign body; cataract extraction, glaucoma surgery; short operative procedure involving the cornea and conjunctiva

Local Anesthetic/Vasoconstrictor Precautions No information available to require special precautions

Effects on Dental Treatment No significant effects or complications reported

Mechanism of Action Prevents initiation and transmission of impulse at the nerve cell membrane by decreasing ion permeability through stabilizing

Pregnancy Risk Factor C

Proparacaine and Fluorescein
(proe PAR a kane & FLURE e seen)

Related Information

Proparacaine *on page 1367*

U.S. Brand Names Flucaine®; Fluoracaine®

Generic Available Yes

Index Terms Fluorescein and Proparacaine

Pharmacologic Category Diagnostic Agent; Local Anesthetic

Use Anesthesia for tonometry, gonioscopy; suture removal from cornea; removal of corneal foreign body; cataract extraction, glaucoma surgery

Local Anesthetic/Vasoconstrictor Precautions No information available to require special precautions

Effects on Dental Treatment No significant effects or complications reported

Common Adverse Effects 1% to 10%: Local: Burning, stinging of eye

Mechanism of Action Prevents initiation and transmission of impulse at the nerve cell membrane by decreasing ion permeability through stabilizing

Pharmacodynamics/Kinetics

Onset of action: ~20 seconds

Duration: 15-20 minutes

Pregnancy Risk Factor C

Proparacaine Hydrochloride *see* Proparacaine *on page 1367*

Propecia® *see* Finasteride *on page 691*

Propine® *see* Dipivefrin *on page 516*

Proplex® T [DSC] *see* Factor IX Complex (Human) *on page 667*

Propofol (PROE po fole)

U.S. Brand Names Diprivan®

Canadian Brand Names Diprivan®

Mexican Brand Names Cryotol; Diprivan; Propocam; Recofol

Generic Available Yes

Pharmacologic Category General Anesthetic

Use Induction of anesthesia for inpatient or outpatient surgery in patients ≥3 years of age; maintenance of anesthesia for inpatient or outpatient surgery in patients >2 months of age; in adults, for the induction and maintenance of monitored anesthesia care sedation during diagnostic procedures; treatment of agitation in intubated, mechanically-ventilated ICU patients

Unlabeled/Investigational Use Postoperative antiemetic; refractory delirium tremens (case reports); moderate sedation (conscious sedation)

Local Anesthetic/Vasoconstrictor Precautions No information available to require special precautions

Effects on Dental Treatment No significant effects or complications reported

(Continued)

Propofol *(Continued)*

Common Adverse Effects

>10%:
Cardiovascular: Hypotension (children 17%; adults 26%)
Central nervous system: Movement (children 17%; adults 3% to 10%)
Local: Injection site burning, stinging, or pain (children 10%; adults 18%)
Respiratory: Apnea lasting 30-60 seconds (children 10%; adults 24%), apnea lasting >60 seconds (children 5%; adults 12%)

1% to 10%:
Cardiovascular: Hypertension (children 8%), arrhythmia, bradycardia, cardiac output decreased, tachycardia
Dermatologic: Pruritus (children 2%), rash (children 5%)
Endocrine & metabolic: Hyperlipidemia
Respiratory: Respiratory acidosis during weaning

Note: A "propofol infusion syndrome" resulting in fatalities has been described in patients receiving high-dose, prolonged infusion; symptoms include severe metabolic acidosis, hyperkalemia, lipemia, rhabdomyolysis, hepatomegaly, and cardiac and renal failure.

Mechanism of Action Propofol is a sterically hindered, alkyl-phenolic compound with intravenous general anesthetic properties. The drug is unrelated to any of the currently used barbiturate, opioid, benzodiazepine, arylcyclohexylamine, or imidazole intravenous anesthetic agents.

Drug Interactions

Cytochrome P450 Effect: Substrate of CYP1A2 (minor), 2A6 (minor), 2B6 (major), 2C9 (major), 2C19 (minor), 2D6 (minor), 2E1 (minor), 3A4 (minor); **Inhibits** CYP1A2 (moderate), 2C9 (weak), 2C19 (moderate), 2D6 (weak), 2E1 (weak), 3A4 (strong)

Increased Effect/Toxicity: Additive CNS depression and respiratory depression may necessitate dosage reduction when used with anesthetics, benzodiazepines, opiates, ethanol, narcotics, phenothiazines. The levels/effects of propofol may be increased by delavirdine, desipramine, fluconazole, gemfibrozil, ketoconazole, nicardipine, NSAIDs, paroxetine, sertraline, sulfonamides, tolbutamide, and other inhibitors of CYP2B6 or 2C9.

Propofol may increase the levels/effects of aminophylline, benzodiazepines, calcium channel blockers, cyclosporine, fluvoxamine, selected HMG-CoA reductase inhibitors, mexiletine, mirtazapine, nateglinide, nefazodone, ropinirole, ropivacaine, sildenafil (and other PDE-5 inhibitors) tacrolimus, theophylline, trifluoperazine, venlafaxine, and other CYP1A2 or 3A4 substrates. Selected benzodiazepines (midazolam and triazolam), cisapride, ergot alkaloids, selected HMG-CoA reductase inhibitors (lovastatin and simvastatin), and pimozide are generally contraindicated with strong CYP3A4 inhibitors.

Decreased Effect: CYP2C9 inducers may cause decrease in propofol levels by increasing the metabolism, via CYP isoenzymes, of propofol; example inducers include bosentan, carbamazepine, fosphenytoin, phenobarbital, phenytoin,primidone, rifampin, rifapentine, and secobarbital.

Pharmacodynamics/Kinetics

Onset of action: Anesthetic: Bolus infusion (dose dependent): 9-51 seconds (average 30 seconds)
Duration (dose and rate dependent): 3-10 minutes
Distribution: V_d: 2-10 L/kg; highly lipophilic
Protein binding: 97% to 99%
Metabolism: Hepatic to water-soluble sulfate and glucuronide conjugates
Half-life elimination: Biphasic: Initial: 40 minutes; Terminal: 4-7 hours (up to 1-3 days)
Excretion: Urine (~88% as metabolites, 40% as glucuronide metabolite); feces (<2%)
Clearance: 23-50 mL/kg/minute; total body clearance exceeds liver blood flow

Pregnancy Risk Factor B

Propoxyphene *(proe POKS i feen)*

U.S. Brand Names Darvon®; Darvon-N®
Canadian Brand Names Darvon-N®; 642® Tablet
Generic Available Yes: Capsule
Index Terms Dextropropoxyphene; Propoxyphene Hydrochloride; Propoxyphene Napsylate
Pharmacologic Category Analgesic, Opioid
Use Management of mild to moderate pain
Local Anesthetic/Vasoconstrictor Precautions No information available to require special precautions

Effects on Dental Treatment Key adverse event(s) related to dental treatment: Xerostomia (normal salivary flow resumes upon discontinuation).

Common Adverse Effects Frequency not defined.

Cardiovascular: Bundle branch block, hypotension

Central nervous system: Confusion, dizziness, dysphoria, drowsiness, fatigue, hallucinations, headache, increased intracranial pressure, lightheadedness, malaise, mental depression, nervousness, paradoxical CNS stimulation, paradoxical excitement and insomnia, restlessness, sedation, vertigo

Dermatologic: Rash, urticaria

Endocrine & metabolic: Decreased urinary 17-OHCS, hypoglycemia

Gastrointestinal: Abdominal pain, anorexia, biliary spasm, constipation, nausea, paralytic ileus, stomach cramps, vomiting, xerostomia

Genitourinary: Decreased urination, ureteral spasms

Hepatic: LFTs increased, jaundice

Neuromuscular & skeletal: Weakness

Ocular: Visual disturbances

Respiratory: Dyspnea

Miscellaneous: Histamine release, hypersensitivity reaction psychologic and physical dependence with prolonged use

Restrictions C-IV

Mechanism of Action Propoxyphene is a weak narcotic analgesic which acts through binding to opiate receptors to inhibit ascending pain pathways. Propoxyphene, as with other narcotic (opiate) analgesics, blocks pain perception in the cerebral cortex by binding to specific receptor molecules (opiate receptors) within the neuronal membranes of synapses. This binding results in a decreased synaptic chemical transmission throughout the CNS thus inhibiting the flow of pain sensations into the higher centers. Mu and kappa are the two subtypes of the opiate receptor which propoxyphene binds to cause analgesia.

Drug Interactions

Cytochrome P450 Effect: Inhibits CYP2C9 (weak), 2D6 (weak), 3A4 (weak)

Increased Effect/Toxicity: CNS depressants (phenothiazines, tranquilizers, anxiolytics, sedatives, hypnotics, or alcohol) may potentiate pharmacologic effects. Propoxyphene may inhibit the metabolism and increase the serum concentrations of carbamazepine, phenobarbital, MAO inhibitors, tricyclic antidepressants, and warfarin.

Decreased Effect: Decreased effect with cigarette smoking.

Pharmacodynamics/Kinetics

Onset of action: 0.5-1 hour

Duration: 4-6 hours

Metabolism: Hepatic to active metabolite (norpropoxyphene) and inactive metabolites; first-pass effect

Half-life elimination: Adults: Parent drug: 6-12 hours; Norpropoxyphene: 30-36 hours

Excretion: Urine (primarily as metabolites)

Pregnancy Risk Factor C/D (prolonged use)

Propoxyphene and Acetaminophen

(proe POKS i feen & a seet a MIN oh fen)

Related Information

Acetaminophen *on page 31*

Propoxyphene *on page 1368*

Related Sample Prescriptions

Moderate/Moderately Severe Oral Pain *on page 1834*

U.S. Brand Names Balacet 325™; Darvocet A500™; Darvocet-N® 50; Darvocet-N® 100; Pronap-100®

Canadian Brand Names Darvocet-N® 50; Darvocet-N® 100

Generic Available Yes

Index Terms Acetaminophen and Propoxyphene; Propoxyphene Hydrochloride and Acetaminophen; Propoxyphene Napsylate and Acetaminophen

Pharmacologic Category Analgesic Combination (Opioid)

Dental Use Management of postoperative pain

Use Management of mild to moderate pain

Local Anesthetic/Vasoconstrictor Precautions No information available to require special precautions

Effects on Dental Treatment Key adverse event(s) related to dental treatment: Xerostomia (normal salivary flow resumes upon discontinuation). See Dental Comment.

Significant Adverse Effects See individual agents.

Restrictions C-IV

(Continued)

Propoxyphene and Acetaminophen *(Continued)*

Dental Usual Dosing Postoperative pain: Adults: Oral:

Darvocet A500™, Darvocet-N® 100: 1 tablet every 4 hours as needed; maximum: 600 mg propoxyphene napsylate/day

Darvocet-N® 50: 1-2 tablets every 4 hours as needed; maximum: 600 mg propoxyphene napsylate/day

Note: Dosage of acetaminophen should not exceed 4 g/day (6 tablets of Darvocet-N® 100); possibly less in patients with ethanol

Dosage Oral: Adults:

Darvocet A500™, Darvocet-N® 100: 1 tablet every 4 hours as needed; maximum: 600 mg propoxyphene napsylate/day

Darvocet-N® 50: 1-2 tablets every 4 hours as needed; maximum: 600 mg propoxyphene napsylate/day

Propoxyphene hydrochloride 65 mg and acetaminophen 650 mg: 1 tablet every 4 hours as needed; maximum: 390 mg/day propoxyphene hydrochloride, 4 g/day acetaminophen)

Note: Dosage of acetaminophen should not exceed 4 g/day (6 tablets of Darvocet-N® 100); possibly less in patients with ethanol

Elderly: Refer to adult dosing

Dosing adjustment in renal/hepatic impairment: Serum concentrations of propoxyphene may be increased or elimination may be delayed; specific dosing recommendations not available.

Mechanism of Action

Propoxyphene is a weak narcotic analgesic which acts through binding to opiate receptors to inhibit ascending pain pathways

Propoxyphene, as with other narcotic (opiate) analgesics, blocks pain perception in the cerebral cortex by binding to specific receptor molecules (opiate receptors) within the neuronal membranes of synapses. This binding results in a decreased synaptic chemical transmission throughout the CNS thus inhibiting the flow of pain sensations into the higher centers. Mu and kappa are the two subtypes of the opiate receptor to which propoxyphene binds to cause analgesia.

Acetaminophen inhibits the synthesis of prostaglandins in the CNS and peripherally blocks pain impulse generation; produces antipyresis from inhibition of hypothalamic heat-regulating center

Contraindications Hypersensitivity to propoxyphene, acetaminophen, or any component of the formulation

Warnings/Precautions [U.S. Boxed Warning]: When given in excessive doses, either alone or in combination with other CNS depressants (including alcohol), propoxyphene is a major cause of drug-related deaths; recommended dosage must not be exceeded and alcohol intake should be limited. Avoid use in severely depressed or suicidal patients. Should not be prescribed in patients who are addiction prone or suicidal. Use caution in patients taking CNS depressant medications or antidepressants, and in patients who use alcohol in excess.

Use caution in patients dependent on opiates, substitution may result in acute opiate withdrawal symptoms. Tolerance or drug dependence may result from extended use. Propoxyphene should be used with caution in patients with renal or hepatic dysfunction or in the elderly; consider dosing adjustment.

Propoxyphene should be used with caution in patients with renal or hepatic dysfunction or in the elderly; consider dosing adjustment. Acetaminophen should be used with caution in patients with liver disease; consuming ≥3 alcoholic drinks/day may increase risk of liver damage. Use caution in patients with known G6PD deficiency. Safety and efficacy of this combination have not been established in pediatric patients.

Drug Interactions

Propoxyphene: **Inhibits** CYP2C9 (weak), 2D6 (weak), 3A4 (weak)

Acetaminophen: **Substrate** (minor) of CYP1A2, 2A6, 2C9, 2D6, 2E1, 3A4; **Inhibits** CYP3A4 (weak)

Also see individual agents.

Ethanol/Nutrition/Herb Interactions

Based on **propoxyphene** component:

Ethanol: Avoid or limit ethanol (may increase CNS depression). Watch for sedation.

Food: May decrease rate of absorption, but may slightly increase bioavailability.

Based on **acetaminophen** component:

Ethanol: Excessive intake of ethanol may increase the risk of acetaminophen-induced hepatotoxicity. Avoid ethanol or limit to <3 drinks/day.

Food: Rate of absorption may be decreased when given with food.

Herb/Nutraceutical: St John's wort may decrease acetaminophen levels.

Dietary Considerations May be taken with food if gastrointestinal distress occurs.

Pharmacodynamics/Kinetics See individual agents.

Pregnancy Risk Factor C

Lactation Enters breast milk/compatible

Breast-Feeding Considerations Propoxyphene, norpropoxyphene and acetaminophen are excreted in breast milk. The AAP considers propoxyphene and acetaminophen to be "compatible" with breast-feeding.

Dosage Forms Excipient information presented when available (limited, particularly for generics); consult specific product labeling.

> Tablet: Propoxyphene hydrochloride 65 mg and acetaminophen 650 mg, propoxyphene napsylate 100 mg, and acetaminophen 650 mg
>
> Balacet 325™: Propoxyphene napsylate 100 mg and acetaminophen 325 mg
>
> Darvocet A500™: Propoxyphene napsylate 100 mg and acetaminophen 500 mg [contains lactose]
>
> Darvocet-N® 50: Propoxyphene napsylate 50 mg and acetaminophen 325 mg
>
> Darvocet-N® 100, Pronap-100®: Propoxyphene napsylate 100 mg and acetaminophen 650 mg

Dental Comment Propoxyphene is a narcotic analgesic and shares many properties including addiction liability. The acetaminophen component requires use with caution in patients with alcoholic liver disease.

Selected Readings

Botting RM, "Mechanism of Action of Acetaminophen: Is There a Cyclooxygenase 3?" *Clin Infect Dis*, 2000, Suppl 5:S202-10.

Dart RC, Kuffner EK, and Rumack BH, "Treatment of Pain or Fever with Paracetamol (Acetaminophen) in the Alcoholic Patient: A Systematic Review," *Am J Ther*, 2000, 7(2):123-34.

Grant JA and Weiler JM, "A Report of a Rare Immediate Reaction After Ingestion of Acetaminophen," *Ann Allergy Asthma Immunol*, 2001, 87(3):227-9.

Kwan D, Bartle WR, and Walker SE, "The Effects of Acetaminophen on Pharmacokinetics and Pharmacodynamics of Warfarin," *J Clin Pharmacol*, 1999, 39(1):68-75.

McClain CJ, Price S, Barve S, et al, "Acetaminophen Hepatotoxicity: An Update," *Curr Gastroenterol Rep*, 1999, 1(1):42-9.

Shek KL, Chan LN, and Nutescu E, "Warfarin-Acetaminophen Drug Interaction Revisited," *Pharmacotherapy*, 1999, 19(10):1153-8.

Tanaka E, Yamazaki K, and Misawa S, "Update: The Clinical Importance of Acetaminophen Hepatotoxicity in Nonalcoholic and Alcoholic Subjects," *J Clin Pharm Ther*, 2000, 25(5):325-32.

Propoxyphene, Aspirin, and Caffeine
(proe POKS i feen, AS pir in, & KAF een)

Related Information

Aspirin *on page 149*
Caffeine *on page 255*
Propoxyphene *on page 1368*

U.S. Brand Names Darvon® Compound [DSC]

Generic Available No

Index Terms Aspirin, Caffeine, and Propoxyphene; Caffeine, Propoxyphene, and Aspirin; Propoxyphene Hydrochloride, Aspirin, and Caffeine

Pharmacologic Category Analgesic Combination (Opioid)

Dental Use Treatment of mild-to-moderate pain

Use Treatment of mild-to-moderate pain

Local Anesthetic/Vasoconstrictor Precautions No information available to require special precautions

Effects on Dental Treatment Key adverse event(s) related to dental treatment: As with all drugs which may affect hemostasis, bleeding is associated with aspirin. Hemorrhage may occur at virtually any site; risk is dependent on multiple variables including dosage, concurrent use of multiple agents which alter hemostasis, and patient susceptibility. Many adverse effects of aspirin are dose-related, and are rare at low dosages. Other serious reactions are idiosyncratic, related to allergy or individual sensitivity. See Dental Comment.

Elderly are a high-risk population for adverse effects from nonsteroidal anti-inflammatory agents. As many as 60% of elderly patients with GI complications from NSAIDs can develop peptic ulceration and/or hemorrhage asymptomatically. Concomitant disease and drug use contribute to the risk of GI adverse effects. Use lowest effective dose for shortest period possible. Consider renal function decline with age.

Significant Adverse Effects See individual agents.

Restrictions C-IV

Dental Usual Dosing

Pain: Adults: Oral: One capsule (providing propoxyphene 65 mg) every 4 hours as needed; maximum propoxyphene 390 mg/day. This will also provide aspirin 389 mg and caffeine 32.4 mg per capsule.

(Continued)

Propoxyphene, Aspirin, and Caffeine *(Continued)*

Dosage Oral: Adults: Pain: One capsule (providing propoxyphene 65 mg) every 4 hours as needed; maximum propoxyphene 390 mg/day. This will also provide aspirin 389 mg and caffeine 32.4 mg per capsule.

Elderly: Refer to adult dosing; consider increasing dosing interval

Dosage adjustment in renal impairment: Serum concentrations of propoxyphene may be increased or elimination may be delayed; specific dosing recommendations not available. Avoid use with Cl_{cr} <10 mL/minute.

Dosage adjustment in hepatic impairment: Serum concentrations or propoxyphene may be increased or elimination may be delayed; specific dosing recommendations not available.

Mechanism of Action Propoxyphene is a weak narcotic analgesic which acts through binding to opiate receptors to inhibit ascending pain pathways. Propoxyphene, as with other narcotic (opiate) analgesics, blocks pain perception in the cerebral cortex by binding to specific receptor molecules (opiate receptors) within the neuronal membranes of synapses. This binding results in a decreased synaptic chemical transmission throughout the CNS thus inhibiting the flow of pain sensations into the higher centers. Mu and kappa are the two subtypes of the opiate receptor to which propoxyphene binds to cause analgesia.

Aspirin inhibits prostaglandin synthesis, acts on the hypothalamus heat-regulating center to reduce fever, blocks prostaglandin synthetase action which prevents formation of the platelet-aggregating substance thromboxane A_2.

Caffeine is a CNS stimulant; use with propoxyphene and aspirin increases the level of analgesia provided by each agent.

Contraindications Hypersensitivity to propoxyphene, aspirin, caffeine, or any component of the formulation

Warnings/Precautions [U.S. Boxed Warning]: When given in excessive doses, either alone or in combination with other CNS depressants (including alcohol), propoxyphene is a major cause of drug-related deaths; recommended dosage must not be exceeded and alcohol intake should be limited. Avoid use in severely depressed or suicidal patients. Should not be prescribed in patients who are addiction prone or suicidal. Use caution in patients taking CNS depressant medications or antidepressants, and in patients who use alcohol in excess.

Use caution in patients dependent on opiates, substitution may result in acute opiate withdrawal symptoms. Tolerance or drug dependence may result from extended use. Propoxyphene should be used with caution in patients with renal or hepatic dysfunction or in the elderly; consider dosing adjustment.

Aspirin should be used with caution in patients with ulcers or coagulation abnormalities. Patients with sensitivity to tartrazine dyes, nasal polyps and asthma may have an increased risk of salicylate sensitivity. Surgical patients should avoid ASA if possible, for 1-2 weeks prior to surgery, to reduce the risk of excessive bleeding. Heavy ethanol use (≥3 drinks/day) can increase bleeding risks. Aspirin should be avoided in children (<16 years of age) with viral infections (chickenpox or flu symptoms), with or without fever, due to a potential association with Reye's syndrome. Safety and efficacy of this combination product in children have not been established.

Drug Interactions See individual agents for Propoxyphene and Aspirin.

Ethanol/Nutrition/Herb Interactions Based on **propoxyphene** component:
Ethanol: Avoid or limit ethanol (may increase CNS depression). Watch for sedation.
Food: May decrease rate of absorption, but may slightly increase bioavailability.

Pharmacodynamics/Kinetics See individual agents.

Pregnancy Risk Factor C

Lactation Enters breast milk/use caution

Breast-Feeding Considerations Propoxyphene, norpropoxyphene, aspirin, and caffeine are excreted in breast milk. The AAP recommends that aspirin be used "with caution" during breast-feeding; propoxyphene and caffeine (moderate intake) are considered "compatible."

Dosage Forms Excipient information presented when available (limited, particularly for generics); consult specific product labeling. [DSC] = Discontinued product
Capsule (Darvon® Compound 65): Propoxyphene hydrochloride 65 mg, aspirin 389 mg, and caffeine 32.4 mg [DSC]

Dental Comment Propoxyphene is a narcotic analgesic and shares many properties including addiction liability. The aspirin component could have anticoagulant effects and could possibly affect bleeding times.

There is no scientific evidence to warrant discontinuance of aspirin prior to dental surgery. Patients taking one aspirin tablet daily as an antithrombotic and who require dental surgery should be given special consideration in consultation with the physician before removal of the aspirin relative to prevention of postoperative bleeding.

The Food and Drug Administration (FDA), has issued a letter updating information and considerations regarding the use of ibuprofen (400 mg doses) in patients who are taking low dose aspirin (81 mg, immediate release; not enteric coated) for cardioprotection and stroke prevention. Ibuprofen, at these doses, may interfere with aspirin's antiplatelet effect depending upon when it is administered. Patients initiated on aspirin first (for ~1 week) then ibuprofen (400 mg tid for 10 days) seem to maintain aspirin's platelet effect (Cryer B, 2005). Ibuprofen has the greatest impact on aspirin if administered less than 8 hours before aspirin (Catella-Lawson F, 2001).

Patients may require counseling about the appropriate timing of ibuprofen dosing in relationship to aspirin therapy. With occasional use of ibuprofen, a clinically-significant interaction with aspirin in unlikely. To avoid interference during chronic dosing, a single dose of ibuprofen should be taken 30-120 minutes after aspirin ingestion or at least 8 hours should elapse after ibuprofen dosing before giving aspirin (FDA, 2006; Catella-Lawson F, 2001).

The clinical implications of the interaction are unclear. There have not been any clinical endpoint studies conducted at this time. Avoidance of this interaction is potentially important because aspirin's vascular protection could be decreased or negated.

Other nonselective NSAIDs may have potential for a similar interaction with aspirin. Such has been described with naproxen (Capone ML, 2005). Acetaminophen does not appear to interfere with the antiplatelet effect of aspirin. Other clinical scenarios (use of smaller ibuprofen doses, other aspirin products, other doses of aspirin) have not been evaluated.

Additional information is available at: http://www.fda.gov/cder/drug/infopage/aspirin/default.htm.

Propoxyphene Hydrochloride see Propoxyphene on page 1368

Propoxyphene Hydrochloride and Acetaminophen see Propoxyphene and Acetaminophen on page 1369

Propoxyphene Hydrochloride, Aspirin, and Caffeine see Propoxyphene, Aspirin, and Caffeine on page 1371

Propoxyphene Napsylate see Propoxyphene on page 1368

Propoxyphene Napsylate and Acetaminophen see Propoxyphene and Acetaminophen on page 1369

Propranolol (proe PRAN oh lole)

Related Information
Cardiovascular Diseases on page 1726
Endocrine Disorders and Pregnancy on page 1750

U.S. Brand Names Inderal®; Inderal® LA; InnoPran XL™

Canadian Brand Names Apo-Propranolol®; Inderal®; Inderal®-LA; Novo-Pranol; Nu-Propranolol; Propranolol Hydrochloride Injection, USP

Mexican Brand Names Acifol

Generic Available Yes

Index Terms Propranolol Hydrochloride

Pharmacologic Category Antiarrhythmic Agent, Class II; Beta-Adrenergic Blocker, Nonselective

Use Management of hypertension; angina pectoris; pheochromocytoma; essential tremor; supraventricular arrhythmias (such as atrial fibrillation and flutter, AV nodal re-entrant tachycardias), ventricular tachycardias (catecholamine-induced arrhythmias, digoxin toxicity); prevention of myocardial infarction; migraine headache prophylaxis; symptomatic treatment of hypertrophic subaortic stenosis

Unlabeled/Investigational Use Tremor due to Parkinson's disease; ethanol withdrawal; aggressive behavior; antipsychotic-induced akathisia; prevention of bleeding esophageal varices; anxiety; schizophrenia; acute panic; gastric bleeding in portal hypertension; thyrotoxicosis; tetralogy of Fallot (TOF) hypercyanotic spells

Local Anesthetic/Vasoconstrictor Precautions Use with caution; epinephrine has interacted with nonselective beta-blockers to result in initial hypertensive episode followed by bradycardia

Effects on Dental Treatment Propranolol is a nonselective beta-blocker and may enhance the pressor response to epinephrine, resulting in hypertension and bradycardia. Many nonsteroidal anti-inflammatory drugs, such as ibuprofen (Continued)

Propranolol *(Continued)*

and indomethacin, can reduce the hypotensive effect of beta-blockers after 3 or more weeks of therapy with the NSAID. Short-term NSAID use (ie, 3 days) requires no special precautions in patients taking beta-blockers.

Common Adverse Effects Frequency not defined.

Cardiovascular: Arterial insufficiency, AV conduction disturbance increased, bradycardia, cardiogenic shock, CHF, chest pain, hypotension, impaired myocardial contractility, mesenteric thrombosis (rare), Raynaud's syndrome, syncope

Central nervous system: Amnesia, cognitive dysfunction, cold extremities, confusion, depression, dizziness, emotional lability, fatigue, hallucinations, hypersomnolence, insomnia, lethargy, lightheadedness, memory loss (short-term), psychosis, vertigo, vivid dreams

Dermatologic: Alopecia, contact dermatitis, eczematous eruptions, erythema multiforme, exfoliative dermatitis, hyperkeratosis, nail changes, oculomucocutaneous reactions, pruritus, psoriasiform eruptions, rash, Stevens-Johnson syndrome, toxic epidermal necrolysis, ulcers, ulcerative lichenoid, urticaria

Endocrine & metabolic: Hyper-/hypoglycemia, hyperkalemia, hyperlipidemia

Gastrointestinal: Anorexia, cramping, constipation, diarrhea, ischemic colitis, mesenteric arterial thrombosis, nausea, stomach discomfort, vomiting

Genitourinary: Impotence, interstitial nephritis (rare), oliguria (rare), Peyronie's disease, proteinuria (rare)

Hematologic: Agranulocytosis, nonthrombocytopenic purpura, thrombocytopenia, thrombocytopenic purpura

Neuromuscular & skeletal: Arthropathy, carpal tunnel syndrome (rare), myotonus, paresthesia, polyarthritis, weakness

Ocular: Hyperemia of the conjunctiva, mydriasis, tear production decreased, visual acuity decreased

Respiratory: Bronchospasm, laryngospasm, pharyngitis, pulmonary edema, respiratory distress, wheezing

Miscellaneous: Anaphylactic/anaphylactoid allergic reaction, lupus-like syndrome (rare)

Dosage

Akathisia (unlabeled use): Oral: Adults: 30-120 mg/day in 2-3 divided doses

Essential tremor: Oral: Adults: 20-40 mg twice daily initially; maintenance doses: usually 120-320 mg/day

Hypertension:

Oral:

Children (unlabeled use): Initial: 0.5-1 mg/kg/day in divided doses every 6-12 hours; increase gradually every 5-7 days; maximum: 16 mg/kg/24 hours

Adults: Initial: 40 mg twice daily; increase dosage every 3-7 days; usual dose: ≤320 mg divided in 2-3 doses/day; maximum daily dose: 640 mg; usual dosage range (JNC 7): 40-160 mg/day in 2 divided doses

Long-acting formulation: Initial: 80 mg once daily; usual maintenance: 120-160 mg once daily; maximum daily dose: 640 mg; usual dosage range (JNC 7): 60-180 mg/day once daily

I.V.: Children (unlabeled use): 0.01-0.05 mg/kg over 1 hour; maximum dose: 10 mg

Hypertrophic subaortic stenosis: Oral: Adults: 20-40 mg 3-4 times/day

Long-acting formulation: 80-160 mg once daily

Migraine headache prophylaxis: Oral:

Children (unlabeled use): Initial: 2-4 mg/kg/day **or**

≤35 kg: 10-20 mg 3 times/day

>35 kg: 20-40 mg 3 times/day

Adults: Initial: 80 mg/day divided every 6-8 hours; increase by 20-40 mg/dose every 3-4 weeks to a maximum of 160-240 mg/day given in divided doses every 6-8 hours; if satisfactory response not achieved within 6 weeks of starting therapy, drug should be withdrawn gradually over several weeks

Long-acting formulation: 80 mg once daily; effective dose range: 160-240 mg once daily

Post-MI mortality reduction: Oral: Adults: 180-240 mg/day in 3-4 divided doses

Pheochromocytoma: Oral: Adults: 30-60 mg/day in divided doses

Stable angina: Oral: Adults: 80-320 mg/day in doses divided 2-4 times/day

Long-acting formulation: Initial: 80 mg once daily; maximum dose: 320 mg once daily

Tachyarrhythmias:

Oral:

Children (unlabeled use): Initial: 0.5-1 mg/kg/day in divided doses every 6-8 hours; titrate dosage upward every 3-7 days; usual dose: 2-6 mg/kg/day; higher doses may be needed; do not exceed 16 mg/kg/day or 60 mg/day

Adults: 10-30 mg/dose every 6-8 hours

Elderly: Initial: 10 mg twice daily; increase dosage every 3-7 days; usual dosage range: 10-320 mg given in 2 divided doses

I.V.:

Children (unlabeled use): 0.01-0.1 mg/kg/dose slow IVP over 10 minutes; maximum dose: 1 mg for infants; 3 mg for children

Adults (in patients having nonfunctional GI tract): 1 mg/dose slow IVP; repeat every 5 minutes up to a total of 5 mg; titrate initial dose to desired response

Elderly: Use caution; initiate at lower end of the dosing range.

Hypercyanotic spells (TOF) (unlabeled use): Children:

Oral: Palliation: Initial: 1 mg/kg/day every 6 hours; if ineffective, may increase dose after 1 week by 1 mg/kg/day to a maximum of 5 mg/kg/day; if patient becomes refractory, may increase slowly to a maximum of 10-15 mg/kg/day. Allow 24 hours between dosing changes.

I.V.: 0.01-0.2 mg/kg/dose infused over 10 minutes; maximum initial dose: 1 mg

Thyrotoxicosis (unlabeled use):

Oral:

Children: 2 mg/kg/day, divided every 6-8 hours, titrate to effective dose

Adolescents and Adults: Oral: 10-40 mg/dose every 6 hours

I.V.: Adults: 1-3 mg/dose slow IVP as a single dose

Dosing adjustment in renal impairment:
Not dialyzable (0% to 5%); supplemental dose is not necessary.
Peritoneal dialysis effects: Supplemental dose is not necessary.

Dosing adjustment in hepatic disease: Marked slowing of heart rate may occur in chronic liver disease with conventional doses; low initial dose and regular heart rate monitoring

Mechanism of Action Nonselective beta-adrenergic blocker (class II antiarrhythmic); competitively blocks response to beta$_1$- and beta$_2$-adrenergic stimulation which results in decreases in heart rate, myocardial contractility, blood pressure, and myocardial oxygen demand

Contraindications Hypersensitivity to propranolol, beta-blockers, or any component of the formulation; uncompensated congestive heart failure (unless the failure is due to tachyarrhythmias being treated with propranolol), cardiogenic shock, bradycardia or heart block (2nd or 3rd degree); pulmonary edema, severe hyperactive airway disease (asthma or COPD), Raynaud's disease; pregnancy (2nd and 3rd trimesters)

Warnings/Precautions Consider pre-existing conditions such as sick sinus syndrome before initiating. Administer cautiously in compensated heart failure and monitor for a worsening of the condition (efficacy of propranolol in CHF has not been demonstrated). Beta-blocker therapy should not be withdrawn abruptly (particularly in patients with CAD), but gradually tapered to avoid acute tachycardia, hypertension, and/or ischemia. Use caution in patient with peripheral vascular disease (PVD). Use caution with concurrent use of beta-blockers and either verapamil or diltiazem; bradycardia or heart block can occur. Avoid concurrent I.V. use of both agents. Use cautiously in diabetics because it can mask prominent hypoglycemic symptoms. Use with caution in myasthenia gravis or psychiatric disease (may cause CNS depression). Use cautiously in renal and hepatic dysfunction; dosage adjustment required in hepatic impairment. Use care with anesthetic agents which decrease myocardial function. In general, patients with bronchospastic disease should not receive beta-blockers; if used at all, should be used cautiously with close monitoring. Not indicated for hypertensive emergencies. Adequate alpha-blockade is required prior to use of any beta-blocker for patients with untreated pheochromocytoma. Safety and efficacy in children have not been established.

Drug Interactions

Cytochrome P450 Effect: Substrate of CYP1A2 (major), 2C19 (minor), 2D6 (major), 3A4 (minor); **Inhibits** CYP1A2 (weak), 2D6 (weak)

Increased Effect/Toxicity: Beta-blockers may enhance the vasopressor effect of alpha-/beta-agonists (direct-acting). Concurrent use of alpha$_1$-blockers may increase risk of orthostasis. Beta-blockers may increase the rebound hypertensive effect when alpha$_2$-agonists are abruptly withdrawn.

CYP1A2 inhibitors (eg, rifamycin derivatives) may increase the levels/effects of propranolol. CYP2D6 inhibitors may increase the levels/effects of propranolol. Aminoquinolines (antimalarial), propoxyphene, propafenone, quinidine, and zileuton may increase levels/effects of beta-blockers. Propafenone possesses some beta-blocking activity and can contribute to bradycardia. The negative chronotropic effects of propranolol are enhanced with other drugs including: acetylcholinesterase inhibitors, amiodarone, digoxin, diltiazem, dipyridamole, disopyramide, SSRIs, and verapamil. Beta-blockers may mask the tachycardia from hypoglycemia caused by insulin and sulfonylureas; the hypoglycemic effect may be enhanced. Beta-blockers may increase the

(Continued)

Propranolol *(Continued)*

levels/effects of antipsychotics (phenothiazines), lidocaine, rizatriptan, and warfarin.

Decreased Effect: CYP1A2 inducers may decrease the levels/effects of propranolol. Nonselective beta-blockers blunt the response to beta₂-agonists and theophylline. NSAIDs may blunt the antihypertensive effect of beta-blockers.

Ethanol/Nutrition/Herb Interactions

Ethanol: Ethanol may increase or decrease plasma levels of propranolol. Reports are variable and have shown both enhanced as well as inhibited hepatic metabolism (of propranolol). Caution advised with consumption of alcohol and monitor for heart rate and/or blood pressure changes.

Food: Propranolol serum levels may be increased if taken with food. Protein-rich foods may increase bioavailability; a change in diet from high carbohydrate/low protein to low carbohydrate/high protein may result in increased oral clearance.

Cigarette: Smoking may decrease plasma levels of propranolol by increasing metabolism.

Herb/Nutraceutical: Avoid dong quai if using for hypertension (has estrogenic activity). Avoid bayberry, blue cohosh, cayenne, ephedra, ginger, ginseng (american), gotu kola, licorice, yohimbe (may worsen hypertension). Avoid black cohosh, california poppy, coleus, garlic, golden seal, hawthorn, mistletoe, periwinkle, quinine, shepherd's purse (have antihypertensive activity, may cause hypotension).

Dietary Considerations
Tablets should be taken on an empty stomach; capsules may be taken with or without food, but should always be taken consistently (with food or on an empty stomach)

Pharmacodynamics/Kinetics

Onset of action: Beta-blockade: Oral: 1-2 hours

Duration: ~6 hours

Distribution: V_d: 3.9 L/kg in adults; crosses placenta; small amounts enter breast milk

Protein binding: Newborns: 68%; Adults: 93%

Metabolism: Hepatic to active and inactive compounds; extensive first-pass effect

Bioavailability: 30% to 40%; may be increased in Down syndrome

Half-life elimination: Neonates and Infants: Possible increased half-life; Children: 3.9-6.4 hours; Adults: 4-6 hours

Excretion: Urine (96% to 99%)

Pregnancy Risk Factor
C (manufacturer); D (2nd and 3rd trimesters - expert analysis)

Dosage Forms

Capsule, extended release: 60 mg, 80 mg, 120 mg, 160 mg
  InnoPran XL™: 80 mg, 120 mg

Capsule, sustained release:
  Inderal® LA: 60 mg, 80 mg, 120 mg, 160 mg

Injection, solution: 1 mg/mL (1 mL)
  Inderal®: 1 mg/mL (1 mL)

Solution, oral: 4 mg/mL, 8 mg/mL

Tablet: 10 mg, 20 mg, 40 mg, 80 mg
  Inderal®: 40 mg, 60 mg, 80 mg

Selected Readings

Foster CA and Aston SJ, "Propranolol-Epinephrine Interaction: A Potential Disaster," *Plast Reconstr Surg*, 1983, 72(1):74-8.

Wong DG, Spence JD, Lamki L, et al, "Effect of Nonsteroidal Anti-inflammatory Drugs on Control of Hypertension of Beta-Blockers and Diuretics," *Lancet*, 1986, 1(8488):997-1001.

Wynn RL, "Dental Nonsteroidal Anti-inflammatory Drugs and Prostaglandin-Based Drug Interactions, Part Two," *Gen Dent*, 1992, 40(2):104, 106, 108.

Wynn RL, "Epinephrine Interactions With Beta-Blockers," *Gen Dent*, 1994, 42(1):16, 18.

Propranolol and Hydrochlorothiazide
(proe PRAN oh lole & hye droe klor oh THYE a zide)

Related Information
Hydrochlorothiazide *on page 819*
Propranolol *on page 1373*

U.S. Brand Names Inderide®

Generic Available Yes

Index Terms Hydrochlorothiazide and Propranolol

Pharmacologic Category Antihypertensive Agent, Combination

Use Management of hypertension

Local Anesthetic/Vasoconstrictor Precautions Use with caution; epinephrine has interacted with nonselective beta-blockers to result in initial hypertensive episode followed by bradycardia

Effects on Dental Treatment Noncardioselective beta-blockers (ie, propranolol, nadolol) enhance the pressor response to epinephrine, resulting in hypertension and bradycardia. Many nonsteroidal anti-inflammatory drugs, such as
ibuprofen and indomethacin, can reduce the hypotensive effect of beta-blockers
after 3 or more weeks of therapy with the NSAID. Short-term NSAID use (ie, 3
days) requires no special precautions in patients taking beta-blockers.

Common Adverse Effects See individual agents.

Drug Interactions
Cytochrome P450 Effect: Propranolol: **Substrate** of CYP1A2 (major), 2C19
(major), 2D6 (major), 3A4 (minor); **Inhibits** CYP1A2 (weak), 2D6 (weak)

Pharmacodynamics/Kinetics See individual agents.

Pregnancy Risk Factor C

Propranolol Hydrochloride *see* Propranolol *on page 1373*

Proprinal [OTC] *see* Ibuprofen *on page 853*

Proprinal® Cold and Sinus [OTC] *see* Pseudoephedrine and Ibuprofen *on
page 1384*

Propulsid® *see* Cisapride *on page 365*

Propylene Glycol Diacetate, Acetic Acid, and Hydrocortisone *see* Acetic Acid,
Propylene Glycol Diacetate, and Hydrocortisone *on page 45*

Propylhexedrine (proe pil HEKS e dreen)

U.S. Brand Names Benzedrex® [OTC]
Generic Available No
Pharmacologic Category Adrenergic Agonist Agent
Use Topical nasal decongestant
Local Anesthetic/Vasoconstrictor Precautions No information available to
require special precautions
Effects on Dental Treatment No significant effects or complications reported

2-Propylpentanoic Acid *see* Valproic Acid and Derivatives *on page 1638*

Propylthiouracil (proe pil thye oh YOOR a sil)

Related Information
Endocrine Disorders and Pregnancy *on page 1750*
Canadian Brand Names Propyl-Thyracil®
Generic Available Yes
Index Terms PTU (error-prone abbreviation)
Pharmacologic Category Antithyroid Agent
Use Palliative treatment of hyperthyroidism as an adjunct to ameliorate hyperthy-
roidism in preparation for surgical treatment or radioactive iodine therapy;
management of thyrotoxic crisis
Local Anesthetic/Vasoconstrictor Precautions No information available to
require special precautions
Effects on Dental Treatment Key adverse event(s) related to dental treat-
ment: Loss of taste perception.

Common Adverse Effects Frequency not defined.
Cardiovascular: ANCA-positive vasculitis, cutaneous vasculitis, edema, leuko-
cytoclastic vasculitis
Central nervous system: Dizziness, drowsiness, drug fever, fever, headache,
neuritis, vertigo
Dermatologic: Alopecia, erythema nodosum, exfoliative dermatitis, pruritus, skin
rash, urticaria
Endocrine & metabolic: Goiter, swollen salivary glands, weight gain
Gastrointestinal: Constipation, loss of taste perception, nausea, stomach pain,
vomiting
Hematologic: Agranulocytosis, aplastic anemia, bleeding, leukopenia, thrombo-
cytopenia
Hepatic: Cholestatic jaundice, hepatitis
Neuromuscular & skeletal: Arthralgia, paresthesia
Renal: Acute renal failure, glomerulonephritis, nephritis
Respiratory: Alveolar hemorrhage, interstitial pneumonitis
Miscellaneous: SLE-like syndrome
Mechanism of Action Inhibits the synthesis of thyroid hormones by blocking
the oxidation of iodine in the thyroid gland; blocks synthesis of thyroxine and
triiodothyronine
(Continued)

Propylthiouracil (Continued)

Drug Interactions

Increased Effect/Toxicity: Propylthiouracil may increase the anticoagulant activity of warfarin.

Decreased Effect: Oral anticoagulant activity is increased only until metabolic effect stabilizes. Anticoagulants may be potentiated by antivitamin K effect of propylthiouracil. Correction of hyperthyroidism may alter disposition of beta-blockers, digoxin, and theophylline, necessitating a dose reduction of these agents.

Pharmacodynamics/Kinetics

Onset of action: Therapeutic: 24-36 hours
 Peak effect: Remission: 4 months of continued therapy
Duration: 2-3 hours
Distribution: Concentrated in the thyroid gland
Protein binding: 75% to 80%
Metabolism: Hepatic
Bioavailability: 80% to 95%
Half-life elimination: 1.5-5 hours; End-stage renal disease: 8.5 hours
Time to peak, serum: ~1 hour
Excretion: Urine (35%)

Pregnancy Risk Factor D

2-Propylvaleric Acid *see* Valproic Acid and Derivatives *on page 1638*

ProQuad® *see* Measles, Mumps, Rubella, and Varicella Virus Vaccine *on page 1021*

Proquin® XR *see* Ciprofloxacin *on page 359*

Proscar® *see* Finasteride *on page 691*

ProSom® *see* Estazolam *on page 601*

Prostacyclin *see* Epoprostenol *on page 579*

Prostacyclin PGI₂ *see* Iloprost *on page 862*

Prostaglandin E₁ *see* Alprostadil *on page 78*

Prostaglandin E₂ *see* Dinoprostone *on page 509*

Prostaglandin F₂ *see* Carboprost Tromethamine *on page 284*

Prostin E₂ *see* Dinoprostone *on page 509*

Prostin VR Pediatric® *see* Alprostadil *on page 78*

Protamine Sulfate (PROE ta meen SUL fate)

Generic Available Yes

Pharmacologic Category Antidote

Use Treatment of heparin overdosage; neutralize heparin during surgery or dialysis procedures

Unlabeled/Investigational Use Treatment of low molecular weight heparin (LMWH) overdose

Local Anesthetic/Vasoconstrictor Precautions No information available to require special precautions

Effects on Dental Treatment No significant effects or complications reported

Common Adverse Effects Frequency not defined.

Cardiovascular: Sudden fall in blood pressure, bradycardia, flushing, hypotension
Central nervous system: Lassitude
Gastrointestinal: Nausea, vomiting
Hematologic: Hemorrhage
Respiratory: Dyspnea, pulmonary hypertension
Miscellaneous: Hypersensitivity reactions

Mechanism of Action Combines with strongly acidic heparin to form a stable complex (salt) neutralizing the anticoagulant activity of both drugs

Pharmacodynamics/Kinetics Onset of action: I.V.: Heparin neutralization: ~5 minutes

Pregnancy Risk Factor C

Protein C *see* Protein C Concentrate (Human) *on page 1378*

Protein C (Activated), Human, Recombinant *see* Drotrecogin Alfa *on page 548*

Protein-Bound Paclitaxel *see* Paclitaxel (Protein Bound) *on page 1241*

Protein C Concentrate (Human)
(PROE teen cee KON suhn trate HYU man)

U.S. Brand Names Ceprotin

Generic Available No

Index Terms Protein C

Pharmacologic Category Anticoagulant

Use Enzyme replacement therapy for the prevention and treatment of venous thrombosis and purpura fulminans in patients with severe congenital protein C deficiency

Local Anesthetic/Vasoconstrictor Precautions No information available to require special precautions

Effects on Dental Treatment No significant effects or complications reported

Common Adverse Effects As with all drugs which may affect hemostasis, bleeding may be associated with protein C. Hemorrhage may occur at virtually any site. Risk is dependent on multiple variables, including the concurrent use of multiple agents which alter hemostasis and patient susceptibility. Frequency not defined.

Central nervous system: Lightheadedness

Hematologic: Bleeding (concurrent anticoagulant also administered)

Miscellaneous: Hypersensitivity reactions (itching and rash)

Postmarketing and/or case reports: Fever, hemothorax, hypotension, hyperhydrosis, restlessness

Mechanism of Action Converted to activated protein C (APC). APC is a serine protease which inactivates factors Va and VIIIa, limiting thrombotic effects. In vitro data also suggest inhibition of plasminogen activator inhibitor-1 (PAF-1) resulting in profibrinolytic activity, inhibition of macrophage production of tumor necrosis factor, blocking of leukocyte adhesion, and limitation of thrombin-induced inflammatory responses.

Drug Interactions

Increased Effect/Toxicity: Concurrent use of heparin, antiplatelet agents, thrombolytic agents, and/or warfarin may increase the risk of bleeding.

Pharmacodynamics/Kinetics

Distribution: V_d: 0.074L/kg

Metabolism: Activated protein C (APC) inactivated by plasma protease inhibitors

Half-life elimination: 4.9-14.7 hours

Time to peak, plasma: T_{max}: 0.5 hours

Pregnancy Risk Factor C

Prothrombin Complex Concentrate see Factor IX Complex (Human) on page 667

Protirelin (proe TYE re lin)

U.S. Brand Names Thyrel® TRH [DSC]

Canadian Brand Names Relefact® TRH

Generic Available No

Index Terms Lopremone; Thyrotropin Releasing Hormone; TRH

Pharmacologic Category Diagnostic Agent

Use Adjunct in the diagnostic assessment of thyroid function, and an adjunct to other diagnostic procedures in patients with pituitary or hypothalamic dysfunction; also causes release of prolactin from the pituitary and is used to detect defective control of prolactin secretion

Local Anesthetic/Vasoconstrictor Precautions No information available to require special precautions

Effects on Dental Treatment Key adverse event(s) related to dental treatment: Xerostomia (normal salivary flow resumes upon discontinuation) and unpleasant taste.

Common Adverse Effects

>10%:

Central nervous system: Headache, lightheadedness

Dermatologic: Flushing of face

Gastrointestinal: Nausea, xerostomia

Genitourinary: Urge to urinate

1% to 10%:

Central nervous system: Anxiety

Endocrine & metabolic: Breast enlargement and leaking in lactating women

Gastrointestinal: Bad taste in mouth, abdominal discomfort

Neuromuscular & skeletal: Tingling

Miscellaneous: Diaphoresis

Mechanism of Action Increase release of thyroid stimulating hormone from the anterior pituitary

Drug Interactions

Decreased Effect: Aspirin, levodopa, thyroid hormones, adrenocorticoid drugs

(Continued)

Protirelin (Continued)

Pharmacodynamics/Kinetics
Onset of action: Peak effect: TSH: 20-30 minutes
Duration: TSH returns to baseline after ~3 hours
Half-life elimination, serum: Mean plasma: 5 minutes

Pregnancy Risk Factor C

Protonix® see Pantoprazole on page 1249
Protopic® see Tacrolimus on page 1516

Protriptyline (proe TRIP ti leen)

U.S. Brand Names Vivactil®
Generic Available No
Index Terms Protriptyline Hydrochloride
Pharmacologic Category Antidepressant, Tricyclic (Secondary Amine)
Use Treatment of depression

Local Anesthetic/Vasoconstrictor Precautions Use with caution; epinephrine and levonordefrin have been shown to have an increased pressor response in combination with TCAs. Protriptyline is one of the drugs confirmed to prolong the QT interval and is accepted as having a risk of causing torsade de pointes. The risk of drug-induced torsade de pointes is extremely low when a single QT interval prolonging drug is prescribed. In terms of epinephrine, it is not known what effect vasoconstrictors in the local anesthetic regimen will have in patients with a known history of congenital prolonged QT interval or in patients taking any medication that prolongs the QT interval. Until more information is obtained, it is suggested that the clinician consult with the physician prior to the use of a vasoconstrictor in suspected patients, and that the vasoconstrictor (epinephrine, levonordefrin [Neo-Cobefrin®]) be used with caution.

Effects on Dental Treatment Key adverse event(s) related to dental treatment: Xerostomia and changes in salivation (normal salivary flow resumes upon discontinuation), unpleasant taste, and trouble with gums. Long-term treatment with TCAs, such as protriptyline, increases the risk of caries by reducing salivation and salivary buffer capacity.

Common Adverse Effects Frequency not defined.
Cardiovascular: Arrhythmias, heart block, hyper-/hypotension, MI, palpitation, stroke, tachycardia
Central nervous system: agitation, anxiety, ataxia, confusion, delirium, delusions, dizziness, drowsiness, EPS, exacerbation of psychosis, fatigue, hallucinations, headache, hypomania, incoordination, insomnia, nightmares, panic, restlessness, seizure
Dermatologic: Alopecia, itching, petechiae, photosensitivity, rash, urticaria
Endocrine & metabolic: Breast enlargement, galactorrhea, gynecomastia, increased or decreased libido, syndrome of inappropriate ADH secretion (SIADH)
Gastrointestinal: Anorexia, constipation, decreased lower esophageal sphincter tone may cause GE reflux, diarrhea, heartburn, increased appetite, nausea, trouble with gums, unpleasant taste, vomiting, weight gain/loss, xerostomia
Genitourinary: Difficult urination, impotence, testicular edema
Hematologic: Agranulocytosis, eosinophilia, leukopenia, purpura, thrombocytopenia
Hepatic: Cholestatic jaundice, increased liver enzymes
Neuromuscular & skeletal: Fine muscle tremor, numbness, tingling, tremor, weakness
Ocular: Blurred vision, eye pain, increased intraocular pressure
Otic: Tinnitus
Miscellaneous: Allergic reactions, excessive diaphoresis

Restrictions An FDA-approved medication guide concerning the use of antidepressants in children, adolescents, and young adults must be distributed when dispensing an outpatient prescription (new or refill) where this medication is to be used without direct supervision of a healthcare provider. Medication guides are available at http://www.fda.gov/cder/Offices/ODS/medication_guides.htm. Dispense to parents or guardians of children and adolescents receiving this medication.

Mechanism of Action Increases the synaptic concentration of serotonin and/or norepinephrine in the central nervous system by inhibition of their reuptake by the presynaptic neuronal membrane

Drug Interactions
Cytochrome P450 Effect: Substrate of CYP2D6 (major)
Increased Effect/Toxicity: Protriptyline increases the effects of amphetamines, anticholinergics, other CNS depressants (sedatives, hypnotics, or ethanol), chlorpropamide, tolazamide, and warfarin. When used with MAO

inhibitors, hyperpyrexia, hypertension, tachycardia, confusion, seizures, and **deaths have been reported** (serotonin syndrome). The SSRIs (to varying degrees), cimetidine, grapefruit juice, indinavir, methylphenidate, ritonavir, quinidine, diltiazem, and verapamil inhibit the metabolism of TCAs. Levels/ effects of protriptyline may be increased by chlorpromazine, delavirdine, fluoxetine, miconazole, paroxetine, pergolide, quinidine, quinine, ritonavir, ropinirole, and other CYP2D6 inhibitors. Use of lithium with a TCA may increase the risk for neurotoxicity. Phenothiazines may increase concentration of some TCAs and TCAs may increase concentration of phenothiazines. Pressor response to I.V. epinephrine, norepinephrine, and phenylephrine may be enhanced in patients receiving TCAs (**Note:** Effect is unlikely with epinephrine or levonordefrin dosages typically administered as infiltration in combination with local anesthetics). Combined use of beta-agonists or drugs which prolong QT$_c$ (including quinidine, procainamide, disopyramide, cisapride, sparfloxacin, gatifloxacin, moxifloxacin) with TCAs may predispose patients to cardiac arrhythmias.

Decreased Effect: Carbamazepine, phenobarbital, and rifampin may increase the metabolism of protriptyline, decreasing its effects. Protriptyline inhibits the antihypertensive response to bethanidine, clonidine, debrisoquin, guanadrel, guanethidine, guanabenz, guanfacine. Cimetidine and methylphenidate may decrease the metabolism of protriptyline. Cholestyramine and colestipol may bind TCAs and reduce their absorption.

Pharmacodynamics/Kinetics
Distribution: Crosses placenta
Protein binding: 92%
Metabolism: Extensively hepatic via N-oxidation, hydroxylation, and glucuronidation; first-pass effect (10% to 25%)
Half-life elimination: 54-92 hours (average: 74 hours)
Time to peak, serum: 24-30 hours
Excretion: Urine

Pregnancy Risk Factor C

Pseudoephedrine (soo doe e FED rin)

Related Information
Bacterial Infections on page 1793
Related Sample Prescriptions
Sinus Infection Treatment on page 1839
U.S. Brand Names Contac® Cold [OTC] [DSC]; Dimetapp® 12-Hour Non-Drowsy Extentabs® [OTC] [DSC]; Dimetapp® Decongestant Infant [OTC] [DSC]; Genaphed® [OTC]; Kidkare Decongestant [OTC]; Kodet SE [OTC]; Oranyl [OTC]; PediaCare® Decongestant Infants [OTC]; Silfedrine Children's [OTC]; Simply Stuffy™ [OTC] [DSC]; Sudafed® 12 Hour [OTC]; Sudafed® 24 Hour [OTC]; Sudafed® Children's [OTC]; Sudafed® Maximum Strength Nasal Decongestant [OTC]; Sudodrin [OTC]; SudoGest [OTC]; Sudo-Tab® [OTC]
Canadian Brand Names Balminil Decongestant; Benylin® D for Infants; Contac® Cold 12 Hour Relief Non Drowsy; Drixoral® ND; Eltor®; PMS-Pseudoephedrine; Pseudofrin; Robidrine®; Sudafed® Decongestant
Mexican Brand Names Sudafed
Generic Available Yes: Liquid, tablet
Index Terms d-Isoephedrine Hydrochloride; Pseudoephedrine Hydrochloride; Pseudoephedrine Sulfate
(Continued)

Pseudoephedrine (Continued)

Pharmacologic Category Alpha/Beta Agonist

Dental Use Temporary symptomatic relief of nasal congestion due to common cold, upper respiratory allergies, and sinusitis; also promotes nasal or sinus drainage

Use Temporary symptomatic relief of nasal congestion due to common cold, upper respiratory allergies, and sinusitis; also promotes nasal or sinus drainage

Local Anesthetic/Vasoconstrictor Precautions Use with caution since pseudoephedrine is a sympathomimetic amine which could interact with epinephrine to cause a pressor response

Effects on Dental Treatment Key adverse event(s) related to dental treatment: Xerostomia (normal salivary flow resumes upon discontinuation).

Significant Adverse Effects Frequency not defined.

Cardiovascular: Arrhythmia, palpitaion, tachycardia

Central nervous system: Convulsion, dizziness, drowsiness, excitability, hallucination, headache, insomnia, nervousness, transient stimulation

Gastrointestinal: Nausea, vomiting

Genitourinary: Dysuria

Neuromuscular & skeletal: Tremor, weakness

Respiratory: Dyspnea

Miscellaneous: Diaphoresis

Dosage Oral: General dosing guidelines:

Children:

<2 years: 4 mg/kg/day in divided doses every 6 hours

2-5 years: 15 mg every 4-6 hours; maximum: 60 mg/24 hours

6-12 years: 30 mg every 4-6 hours; maximum: 120 mg/24 hours

Adults: 30-60 mg every 4-6 hours, sustained release: 120 mg every 12 hours; maximum: 240 mg/24 hours

Dosing adjustment in renal impairment: Reduce dose

Mechanism of Action Directly stimulates alpha-adrenergic receptors of respiratory mucosa causing vasoconstriction; directly stimulates beta-adrenergic receptors causing bronchial relaxation, increased heart rate and contractility

Contraindications Hypersensitivity to pseudoephedrine or any component of the formulation; with or within 14 days of MAO inhibitor therapy

Warnings/Precautions Use with caution in patients >60 years of age. Administer with caution to patients with hypertension, hyperthyroidism, diabetes mellitus, cardiovascular disease, ischemic heart disease, increased intraocular pressure, or prostatic hyperplasia. Elderly patients are more likely to experience adverse reactions to sympathomimetics. Overdosage may cause hallucinations, seizures, CNS depression, and death. When used for self-medication (OTC), notify prescriber if symptoms do not improve within 7 days or are accompanied by fever.

Drug Interactions

Decreased effect of methyldopa, reserpine

Increased toxicity: MAO inhibitors may increase blood pressure effects of pseudoephedrine; propranolol, sympathomimetic agents may increase toxicity

Ethanol/Nutrition/Herb Interactions

Food: Onset of effect may be delayed if pseudoephedrine is taken with food.

Herb/Nutraceutical: Avoid ephedra, yohimbe (may cause hypertension).

Dietary Considerations Should be taken with water or milk to decrease GI distress.

Pharmacodynamics/Kinetics

Onset of action: Decongestant: Oral: 15-30 minutes

Duration: Immediate release tablet: 4-6 hours; Extended release: ≤12 hours

Absorption: Rapid

Metabolism: Partially hepatic

Half-life elimination: 9-16 hours

Excretion: Urine (70% to 90% as unchanged drug, 1% to 6% as active norpseudoephedrine); dependent on urine pH and flow rate; alkaline urine decreases renal elimination of pseudoephedrine

Pregnancy Risk Factor C

Lactation Enters breast milk/use caution (AAP rates "compatible")

Dosage Forms Excipient information presented when available (limited, particularly for generics); consult specific product labeling. [DSC] = Discontinued product

Caplet, extended release, as hydrochloride:

Contac® Cold [DSC], Sudafed® 12 Hour: 120 mg

Liquid, as hydrochloride: 30 mg/5 mL (120 mL, 480 mL)

Silfedrine Children's: 15 mg/5 mL (120 mL, 480 mL) [alcohol and sugar free; grape flavor]

Simply Stuffy™: 15 mg/5 mL (120 mL) [alcohol free; contains sodium benzoate; cherry berry flavor] [DSC]

Sudafed® Children's: 15 mg/5 mL (120 mL) [alcohol and sugar free; contains sodium benzoate; grape flavor]

Liquid, oral, as hydrochloride [drops]:
Dimetapp® Decongestant Infant Drops: 7.5 mg/0.8 mL (15 mL) [alcohol free; contains sodium benzoate; grape flavor] [DSC]
Kidkare Decongestant: 7.5 mg/0.8 mL (30 mL) [alcohol free; contains benzoic acid and sodium benzoate; cherry flavor]
PediaCare® Decongestant: 7.5 mg/0.8 mL (15 mL) [alcohol free, dye free; contains benzoic acid, sodium benzoate; fruit flavor]

Tablet, as hydrochloride: 30 mg, 60 mg
Genaphed®, Kodet SE, Oranyl, Sudafed®, Sudodrin, Sudo-Tab®: 30 mg
SudoGest: 30 mg, 60 mg

Tablet, chewable, as hydrochloride:
Sudafed® Children's: 15 mg [sugar free; contains phenylalanine 0.78 mg/tablet; orange flavor]

Tablet, extended release, as hydrochloride:
Dimetapp® 12-Hour Non-Drowsy Extentabs®: 120 mg [DSC]
Sudafed® 24 Hour: 240 mg

Pseudoephedrine, Acetaminophen, and Chlorpheniramine see Acetaminophen, Chlorpheniramine, and Pseudoephedrine on page 43

Pseudoephedrine, Acetaminophen, and Dextromethorphan see Acetaminophen, Dextromethorphan, and Pseudoephedrine on page 44

Pseudoephedrine and Acetaminophen see Acetaminophen and Pseudoephedrine on page 38

Pseudoephedrine and Brompheniramine see Brompheniramine and Pseudoephedrine on page 231

Pseudoephedrine and Carbinoxamine see Carbinoxamine and Pseudoephedrine on page 282

Pseudoephedrine and Chlorpheniramine see Chlorpheniramine and Pseudoephedrine on page 340

Pseudoephedrine and Desloratadine see Desloratadine and Pseudoephedrine on page 461

Pseudoephedrine and Dexbrompheniramine see Dexbrompheniramine and Pseudoephedrine on page 468

Pseudoephedrine and Dextromethorphan
(soo doe e FED rin & deks troe meth OR fan)

Related Information
Dextromethorphan on page 477
Pseudoephedrine on page 1381

U.S. Brand Names Dimetapp® Infant Decongestant Plus Cough [OTC] [DSC]; PediaCare® Children's Long Acting Cough Plus Cold [OTC] [DSC]; PediaCare® Infants' Decongestant & Cough [OTC]; Pedia Relief Cough and Cold [OTC]; Pedia Relief Infants [OTC]; Robitussin® Maximum Strength Cough & Cold [OTC] [DSC]; Robitussin® Pediatric Cough & Cold [OTC] [DSC]; Sudafed® Children's Cold & Cough [OTC]; SudoGest Children's [OTC]; Triaminic® Cough [OTC] [DSC]; Triaminic® Cough & Nasal Congestion [OTC] [DSC]; Vicks® 44D Cough & Head Congestion [OTC] [DSC]

Canadian Brand Names Balminil DM D; Benylin® DM-D; Koffex DM-D; Novahistex® DM Decongestant; Novahistine® DM Decongestant; Robitussin® Childrens Cough & Cold

Generic Available Yes: Liquid drops, syrup

Index Terms Dextromethorphan and Pseudoephedrine

Pharmacologic Category Antitussive/Decongestant

Use Temporary symptomatic relief of nasal congestion and cough due to common cold, hay fever, upper respiratory allergies

Local Anesthetic/Vasoconstrictor Precautions Use with caution since pseudoephedrine is a sympathomimetic amine which could interact with epinephrine to cause a pressor response

Effects on Dental Treatment Key adverse event(s) related to dental treatment: Pseudoephedrine: Xerostomia (normal salivary flow resumes upon discontinuation).

Common Adverse Effects See individual agents.

Drug Interactions
Cytochrome P450 Effect: Dextromethorphan: **Substrate** of CYP2B6 (minor), 2C9 (minor), 2C19 (minor), 2D6 (major), 2E1 (minor), 3A4 (minor); **Inhibits** CYP2D6 (weak)

Increased Effect/Toxicity: Based on **pseudoephedrine** component: MAO inhibitors may increase blood pressure effects of pseudoephedrine. Sympathomimetic agents may increase toxicity.

(Continued)

Pseudoephedrine and Dextromethorphan *(Continued)*

Decreased Effect: Based on **pseudoephedrine** component: Decreased effect of methyldopa, reserpine.

Pharmacodynamics/Kinetics See individual agents.

Pseudoephedrine and Diphenhydramine *see* Diphenhydramine and Pseudoephedrine *on page 514*

Pseudoephedrine and Fexofenadine *see* Fexofenadine and Pseudoephedrine *on page 690*

Pseudoephedrine and Guaifenesin *see* Guaifenesin and Pseudoephedrine *on page 798*

Pseudoephedrine and Hydrocodone *see* Hydrocodone and Pseudoephedrine *on page 832*

Pseudoephedrine and Ibuprofen
(soo doe e FED rin & eye byoo PROE fen)

Related Information
Ibuprofen *on page 853*
Pseudoephedrine *on page 1381*

U.S. Brand Names Advil® Cold & Sinus [OTC]; Advil® Cold, Children's [OTC]; Motrin® Cold and Sinus [OTC]; Motrin® Cold, Children's [OTC]; Proprinal® Cold and Sinus [OTC]

Canadian Brand Names Advil® Cold & Sinus; Children's Advil® Cold; Sudafed® Sinus Advance

Generic Available Yes: Caplet

Index Terms Ibuprofen and Pseudoephedrine

Pharmacologic Category Decongestant/Analgesic

Use For temporary relief of cold, sinus and flu symptoms (including nasal congestion, headache, sore throat, minor body aches and pains, and fever)

Local Anesthetic/Vasoconstrictor Precautions Use with caution since pseudoephedrine is a sympathomimetic amine which could interact with epinephrine to cause a pressor response

Effects on Dental Treatment Key adverse event(s) related to dental treatment: Pseudoephedrine: Xerostomia (normal salivary flow resumes upon discontinuation).

Common Adverse Effects See individual agents.

Drug Interactions
Cytochrome P450 Effect: Ibuprofen: **Substrate** (minor) of CYP2C9, 2C19; **Inhibits** CYP2C9 (strong)
Increased Effect/Toxicity: See individual agents.
Decreased Effect: See individual agents.

Pharmacodynamics/Kinetics See individual agents.

Pregnancy Risk Factor Ibuprofen: B/D (3rd trimester)

Pseudoephedrine and Loratadine *see* Loratadine and Pseudoephedrine *on page 1000*

Pseudoephedrine and Methscopolamine
(soo doe e FED rin & meth skoe POL a meen)

U.S. Brand Names AlleRx™-D; Amdry-D; Extendryl PSE

Generic Available Yes

Index Terms Methscopolamine and Pseudoephedrine; Pseudoephedrine hydrochloride and Methscopolamine Nitrate

Pharmacologic Category Decongestant/Anticholingeric Combination

Use Relief of symptoms of allergic rhinitis, vasomotor rhinitis, sinusitis, and the common cold

Local Anesthetic/Vasoconstrictor Precautions Use with caution since pseudoephedrine is a sympathomimetic amine which could interact with epinephrine to cause a pressor response

Effects on Dental Treatment Key adverse event(s) related to dental treatment:
Pseudoephedrine: Xerostomia (normal salivary flow resumes upon discontinuation).
Methscopolamine: Xerostomia and changes in salivation (normal salivary flow resumes upon discontinuation), and dry throat and nose. Anticholinergic side effects can cause a reduction of saliva production or secretion, contributing to discomfort and dental disease (ie, caries, oral candidiasis and periodontal disease).

Common Adverse Effects Frequency not defined.

Cardiovascular: Arrhythmias, bradycardia, cardiovascular collapse, flushing, hypotension, pallor, palpitation, tachycardia

Central nervous system: Anxiety, convulsions, CNS depression, dizziness, drowsiness, excitability, fear, giddiness, hallucination, headache, insomnia, irritability, lassitude, nervousness, restlessness

Gastrointestinal: Gastric irritation, nausea, xerostomia

Genitourinary: Dysuria, urinary retention

Neuromuscular & skeletal: Tremor, weakness

Ocular: Blurred vision

Respiratory: Respiratory difficulty

Mechanism of Action

Pseudoephedrine: Acts as a decongestant in respiratory tract mucous membranes.

Methscopolamine nitrate: Derivative of scopolamine; a peripheral anticholinergic agent

Pharmacodynamics/Kinetics See individual agents.

Pregnancy Risk Factor C

Pseudoephedrine and Naproxen *see* Naproxen and Pseudoephedrine *on page 1151*

Pseudoephedrine and Triprolidine *see* Triprolidine and Pseudoephedrine *on page 1624*

Pseudoephedrine, Carbinoxamine, and Dextromethorphan *see* Carbinoxamine, Pseudoephedrine, and Dextromethorphan *on page 282*

Pseudoephedrine, Chlorpheniramine, and Acetaminophen *see* Acetaminophen, Chlorpheniramine, and Pseudoephedrine *on page 43*

Pseudoephedrine, Chlorpheniramine, and Codeine *see* Chlorpheniramine, Pseudoephedrine, and Codeine *on page 344*

Pseudoephedrine, Chlorpheniramine, and Dihydrocodeine *see* Pseudoephedrine, Dihydrocodeine, and Chlorpheniramine *on page 1385*

Pseudoephedrine, Codeine, and Triprolidine *see* Triprolidine, Pseudoephedrine, and Codeine *on page 1624*

Pseudoephedrine, Dextromethorphan, and Acetaminophen *see* Acetaminophen, Dextromethorphan, and Pseudoephedrine *on page 44*

Pseudoephedrine, Dextromethorphan, and Carbinoxamine *see* Carbinoxamine, Pseudoephedrine, and Dextromethorphan *on page 282*

Pseudoephedrine, Dextromethorphan, and Guaifenesin *see* Guaifenesin, Pseudoephedrine, and Dextromethorphan *on page 800*

Pseudoephedrine, Dihydrocodeine, and Chlorpheniramine

(soo doe e FED rin, dye hye droe KOE deen, & klor fen IR a meen)

Related Information

Chlorpheniramine *on page 338*

Pseudoephedrine *on page 1381*

U.S. Brand Names Coldcough; DiHydro-CP; Hydro-Tussin™ DHC; Pancof® [DSC]; Uni-Cof [DSC]

Generic Available Yes

Index Terms Chlorpheniramine, Pseudoephedrine, and Dihydrocodeine; Dihydrocodeine Bitartrate, Pseudoephedrine Hydrochloride, and Chlorpheniramine Maleate; Pseudoephedrine, Chlorpheniramine, and Dihydrocodeine

Pharmacologic Category Antihistamine/Decongestant/Antitussive

Use Temporary relief of cough, congestion, and sneezing due to colds, respiratory infections, or hay fever

Local Anesthetic/Vasoconstrictor Precautions Use with caution since pseudoephedrine is a sympathomimetic amine which could interact with epinephrine to cause a pressor response

Effects on Dental Treatment Key adverse event(s) related to dental treatment:

Chlorpheniramine: Prolonged use will cause significant xerostomia (normal salivary flow resumes upon discontinuation).

Pseudoephedrine: Xerostomia (prolonged use worsens; normal salivary flow resumes upon discontinuation).

Common Adverse Effects See individual agents.

Restrictions C-III

Mechanism of Action

Pseudoephedrine: Directly stimulates alpha-adrenergic receptors of respiratory mucosa causing vasoconstriction; directly stimulates beta-adrenergic receptors causing bronchial relaxation

Dihydrocodeine: Binds to opiate receptors in the CNS; suppresses cough in medullary center

(Continued)

Pseudoephedrine, Dihydrocodeine, and
Chlorpheniramine *(Continued)*

Chlorpheniramine: Competes with histamine for H_1-receptor sites on effector cells in the gastrointestinal tract, blood vessels, and respiratory tract

Drug Interactions

Cytochrome P450 Effect:

Dihydrocodeine: **Substrate** of CYP2D6 (major)

Chlorpheniramine: **Substrate** of CYP2D6 (minor), 3A4 (major); Inhibits CYP2D6 (weak).

Increased Effect/Toxicity: Also see individual agents. CYP3A4 inhibitors may increase the levels/effects of chlorpheniramine (example inhibitors include azole antifungals, clarithromycin, diclofenac, doxycycline, erythromycin, imatinib, isoniazid, nefazodone, nicardipine, propofol, protease inhibitors, quinidine, telithromycin, and verapamil).

Decreased Effect: Also see individual agents. CYP2D6 inhibitors may decrease the effects of dihydrocodeine (example inhibitors include chlorpromazine, delavirdine, fluoxetine, miconazole, paroxetine, pergolide, quinidine, quinine, ritonavir, and ropinirole).

Pharmacodynamics/Kinetics See individual agents.

Pregnancy Risk Factor C

Psyllium (SIL i yum)

U.S. Brand Names Fiberall®; Fibro-Lax [OTC]; Fibro-XL [OTC]; Genfiber® [OTC]; Hydrocil® Instant [OTC]; Konsyl® [OTC]; Konsyl-D® [OTC]; Konsyl® Easy Mix [OTC]; Konsyl® Orange [OTC]; Metamucil® [OTC]; Metamucil® Plus Calcium [OTC]; Metamucil® Smooth Texture [OTC]; Modane® Bulk [OTC]; Natural Fiber Therapy [OTC]; Reguloid® [OTC]; Serutan® [OTC]

Canadian Brand Names Metamucil®

Generic Available Yes: Capsule, powder

Index Terms Plantago Seed; Plantain Seed; Psyllium Hydrophilic Mucilloid

Pharmacologic Category Antidiarrheal; Laxative, Bulk-Producing

Use Treatment of chronic atonic or spastic constipation and in constipation associated with rectal disorders; management of irritable bowel syndrome; labeled for OTC use as fiber supplement, treatment of constipation

Local Anesthetic/Vasoconstrictor Precautions No information available to require special precautions

Effects on Dental Treatment No significant effects or complications reported

Common Adverse Effects Frequency not defined.

Gastrointestinal: Abdominal cramps, constipation, diarrhea, esophageal or bowel obstruction

Respiratory: Bronchospasm

Miscellaneous: Anaphylaxis upon inhalation in susceptible individuals, rhinoconjunctivitis

Mechanism of Action Adsorbs water in the intestine to form a viscous liquid which promotes peristalsis and reduces transit time

Drug Interactions

Decreased Effect: Decreased effect of warfarin, digitalis, potassium-sparing diuretics, salicylates, tetracyclines, nitrofurantoin when taken together. Separate administration times to reduce potential for drug-drug interaction.

Pharmacodynamics/Kinetics

Onset of action: 12-24 hours

Peak effect: 2-3 days

Absorption: None; small amounts of grain extracts present in the preparation have been reportedly absorbed following colonic hydrolysis

Pregnancy Risk Factor B

Pyrantel Pamoate (pi RAN tel PAM oh ate)

U.S. Brand Names Pin-X® [OTC]; Reese's® Pinworm Medicine [OTC]

Canadian Brand Names Combantrin™

Generic Available No

Pharmacologic Category Anthelmintic

Use Treatment of pinworms (Enterobius vermicularis) and roundworms (Ascaris lumbricoides)

Unlabeled/Investigational Use Treatment of whipworms (Trichuris trichiura) and hookworms (Ancylostoma duodenale)

Local Anesthetic/Vasoconstrictor Precautions No information available to require special precautions

Effects on Dental Treatment No significant effects or complications reported

Common Adverse Effects Frequency not defined.

Central nervous system: Dizziness, drowsiness, insomnia, headache

Dermatologic: Rash

Gastrointestinal: Abdominal cramps, anorexia, diarrhea, nausea, vomiting, tenesmus

Hepatic: Liver enzymes increased

Neuromuscular & skeletal: Weakness

Mechanism of Action Causes the release of acetylcholine and inhibits cholinesterase; acts as a depolarizing neuromuscular blocker, paralyzing the helminths

Drug Interactions

Decreased Effect: Decreased effect with piperazine

Pharmacodynamics/Kinetics

Absorption: Oral: Poor

Metabolism: Partially hepatic

Time to peak, serum: 1-3 hours

Excretion: Feces (50% as unchanged drug); urine (7% as unchanged drug)

Pregnancy Risk Factor C

Pyrazinamide (peer a ZIN a mide)

Related Information
Tuberculosis *on page 1765*
Canadian Brand Names Tebrazid™
Generic Available Yes
Index Terms Pyrazinoic Acid Amide
Pharmacologic Category Antitubercular Agent
Use Adjunctive treatment of tuberculosis in combination with other anti-tuberculosis agents
Local Anesthetic/Vasoconstrictor Precautions No information available to require special precautions
Effects on Dental Treatment No significant effects or complications reported
Common Adverse Effects 1% to 10%:
Central nervous system: Malaise
Gastrointestinal: Anorexia, nausea, vomiting
Neuromuscular & skeletal: Arthralgia, myalgia
Mechanism of Action Converted to pyrazinoic acid in susceptible strains of *Mycobacterium* which lowers the pH of the environment; exact mechanism of action has not been elucidated
Drug Interactions
Increased Effect/Toxicity: Combination therapy with rifampin and pyrazinamide has been associated with severe and fatal hepatotoxic reactions.
Pharmacodynamics/Kinetics Bacteriostatic or bactericidal depending on drug's concentration at infection site

Absorption: Well absorbed
Distribution: Widely into body tissues and fluids including liver, lung, and CSF
Relative diffusion from blood into CSF: Adequate with or without inflammation (exceeds usual MICs)
CSF:blood level ratio: Inflamed meninges: 100%
Protein binding: 50%
Metabolism: Hepatic
Half-life elimination: 9-10 hours
Time to peak, serum: Within 2 hours
Excretion: Urine (4% as unchanged drug)
Pregnancy Risk Factor C

Pyrazinamide, Rifampin, and Isoniazid *see* Rifampin, Isoniazid, and Pyrazinamide *on page 1425*
Pyrazinoic Acid Amide *see* Pyrazinamide *on page 1388*

Pyrethrins and Piperonyl Butoxide
(pye RE thrins & pi PER oh nil byo TOKS ide)

U.S. Brand Names A-200® Maximum Strength [OTC]; Lice-Aid [OTC]; Licide® [OTC]; Pronto® Complete Lice Killing Kit [OTC]; Pronto® Plus Hair and Scalp Masque [OTC]; Pronto® Plus Mousse [OTC]; Pronto® Plus Warm Oil Treatment and Conditioner [OTC]; Pronto® Plus with Natural Extracts and Oils [OTC]; Pyrinyl Plus® [OTC]; RID® Maximum Strength [OTC]; Tisit® [OTC]; Tisit® Blue Gel [OTC]
Canadian Brand Names Pronto® Lice Control; R & C™ II; R & C™ Shampoo/Conditioner; RID® Mousse
Generic Available Yes: Shampoo
Index Terms Piperonyl Butoxide and Pyrethrins
Pharmacologic Category Antiparasitic Agent, Topical; Pediculocide; Shampoo, Pediculocide
Use Treatment of *Pediculus humanus* infestations (head lice, body lice, pubic lice and their eggs)
Local Anesthetic/Vasoconstrictor Precautions No information available to require special precautions
Effects on Dental Treatment No significant effects or complications reported
Common Adverse Effects Frequency not defined.
Dermatologic: Pruritus
Local: Burning, stinging, irritation with repeat use
Mechanism of Action Pyrethrins are derived from flowers that belong to the chrysanthemum family. The mechanism of action on the neuronal membranes of lice is similar to that of DDT. Piperonyl butoxide is usually added to pyrethrin to enhance the product's activity by decreasing the metabolism of pyrethrins in arthropods.
Pharmacodynamics/Kinetics
Onset of action: ~30 minutes

Absorption: Minimal
Metabolism: Via ester hydrolysis and hydroxylation
Pregnancy Risk Factor C

Pyridium® *see* Phenazopyridine *on page 1286*

Pyridostigmine (peer id oh STIG meen)

U.S. Brand Names Mestinon®; Mestinon® Timespan®; Regonol®
Canadian Brand Names Mestinon®; Mestinon®-SR
Mexican Brand Names Mestinon
Generic Available Yes: Tablet
Index Terms Pyridostigmine Bromide
Pharmacologic Category Acetylcholinesterase Inhibitor
Use Symptomatic treatment of myasthenia gravis; antidote for nondepolarizing neuromuscular blockers
Military use: Pretreatment for Soman nerve gas exposure
Local Anesthetic/Vasoconstrictor Precautions No information available to require special precautions
Effects on Dental Treatment Key adverse event(s) related to dental treatment: Dysphagia.
Common Adverse Effects Frequency not defined.
Cardiovascular: Arrhythmias (especially bradycardia), AV block, cardiac arrest, decreased carbon monoxide, flushing, hypotension, nodal rhythm, nonspecific ECG changes, syncope, tachycardia
Central nervous system: Convulsions, dizziness, drowsiness, dysphonia, headache, loss of consciousness
Dermatologic: Skin rash, thrombophlebitis (I.V.), urticaria
Gastrointestinal: Abdominal pain, diarrhea, dysphagia, flatulence, hyperperistalsis, nausea, salivation, stomach cramps, vomiting
Genitourinary: Urinary urgency
Neuromuscular & skeletal: Arthralgia, dysarthria, fasciculations, muscle cramps, myalgia, spasms, weakness
Ocular: Amblyopia, lacrimation, small pupils
Respiratory: Bronchial secretions increased, bronchiolar constriction, bronchospasm, dyspnea, laryngospasm, respiratory arrest, respiratory depression, respiratory muscle paralysis
Miscellaneous: Allergic reactions, anaphylaxis, diaphoresis increased
Mechanism of Action Inhibits destruction of acetylcholine by acetylcholinesterase which facilitates transmission of impulses across myoneural junction
Drug Interactions
Increased Effect/Toxicity: Increased effect of depolarizing neuromuscular blockers (succinylcholine). Increased toxicity with edrophonium. Increased bradycardia/hypotension with beta-blockers.
Decreased Effect: Neuromuscular blockade reversal effect of pyridostigmine may be decreased by aminoglycosides, quinolones, tetracyclines, bacitracin, colistin, polymyxin B, sodium colistimethate, quinidine, elevated serum magnesium concentrations.
Pharmacodynamics/Kinetics
Onset of action: Oral, I.M.: 15-30 minutes; I.V. injection: 2-5 minutes
Duration: Oral: Up to 6-8 hours (due to slow absorption); I.V.: 2-3 hours
Absorption: Oral: Very poor
Distribution: 19 ± 12 L
Metabolism: Hepatic
Bioavailability: 10% to 20%
Half-life elimination: 1-2 hours; Renal failure: ≤6 hours
Excretion: Urine (80% to 90% as unchanged drug)
Pregnancy Risk Factor B

Pyridostigmine Bromide *see* Pyridostigmine *on page 1389*

Pyridoxine (peer i DOKS een)

U.S. Brand Names Aminoxin® [OTC]
Generic Available Yes
Index Terms Pyridoxine Hydrochloride; Vitamin B_6
Pharmacologic Category Vitamin, Water Soluble
Use Prevention and treatment of vitamin B_6 deficiency, pyridoxine-dependent seizures in infants; adjunct to treatment of acute toxicity from isoniazid, cycloserine, or hydrazine overdose
Local Anesthetic/Vasoconstrictor Precautions No information available to require special precautions
(Continued)

Pyridoxine *(Continued)*

Effects on Dental Treatment No significant effects or complications reported

Common Adverse Effects Frequency not defined.

Central nervous system: Headache, seizure (following very large I.V. doses), sensory neuropathy

Endocrine & metabolic: Decreased serum folic acid secretions

Gastrointestinal: Nausea

Hepatic: Increased AST

Neuromuscular & skeletal: Paresthesia

Miscellaneous: Allergic reactions

Mechanism of Action Precursor to pyridoxal, which functions in the metabolism of proteins, carbohydrates, and fats; pyridoxal also aids in the release of liver and muscle-stored glycogen and in the synthesis of GABA (within the central nervous system) and heme

Drug Interactions

Decreased Effect: Pyridoxine may decrease serum levels of levodopa, phenobarbital, and phenytoin (patients taking levodopa without carbidopa should avoid supplemental vitamin B_6 >5 mg per day, which includes multivitamin preparations).

Pharmacodynamics/Kinetics

Absorption: Enteral, parenteral: Well absorbed

Metabolism: Via 4-pyridoxic acid (active form) and other metabolites

Half-life elimination: 15-20 days

Excretion: Urine

Pregnancy Risk Factor A/C (dose exceeding RDA recommendation)

Pyridoxine, Folic Acid, and Cyanocobalamin *see* Folic Acid, Cyanocobalamin, and Pyridoxine *on page 738*

Pyridoxine Hydrochloride *see* Pyridoxine *on page 1389*

Pyrilamine, Phenylephrine, and Carbetapentane *see* Carbetapentane, Phenylephrine, and Pyrilamine *on page 280*

Pyrimethamine *(peer i METH a meen)*

U.S. Brand Names Daraprim®
Canadian Brand Names Daraprim®
Mexican Brand Names Daraprim
Generic Available No
Pharmacologic Category Antimalarial Agent

Use Prophylaxis of malaria due to susceptible strains of plasmodia; used in conjunction with quinine and sulfadiazine for the treatment of uncomplicated attacks of chloroquine-resistant *P. falciparum* malaria; used in conjunction with fast-acting schizonticide to initiate transmission control and suppression cure; synergistic combination with sulfonamide in treatment of toxoplasmosis

Local Anesthetic/Vasoconstrictor Precautions No information available to require special precautions

Effects on Dental Treatment Key adverse event(s) related to dental treatment: Xerostomia (normal salivary flow resumes upon discontinuation). Atrophic glossitis has been reported.

Common Adverse Effects Frequency not defined.

Cardiovascular: Arrhythmias (large doses)

Central nervous system: Depression, fever, insomnia, lightheadedness, malaise, seizure

Dermatologic: Abnormal skin pigmentation, dermatitis, erythema multiforme, rash, Stevens-Johnson syndrome, toxic epidermal necrolysis

Gastrointestinal: Anorexia, abdominal cramps, vomiting, diarrhea, xerostomia, atrophic glossitis

Genitourinary: Hematuria

Hematologic: Megaloblastic anemia, leukopenia, pancytopenia, thrombocytopenia, pulmonary eosinophilia

Miscellaneous: Anaphylaxis

Mechanism of Action Inhibits parasitic dihydrofolate reductase, resulting in inhibition of vital tetrahydrofolic acid synthesis

Drug Interactions

Cytochrome P450 Effect: Inhibits CYP2C9 (moderate), 2D6 (moderate)

Increased Effect/Toxicity: Serum levels of antipsychotic agents may be increased by pyrimethamine. Sulfonamides (synergy), methotrexate, TMP/SMZ, and zidovudine may increase the risk of bone marrow suppression. Pyrimethamine may increase the levels/effects of amphetamines, selected beta-blockers, bosentan, dapsone, dextromethorphan, fluoxetine, glimepiride, glipizide, lidocaine, losartan, mirtazapine, montelukast, nateglinide, nefazodone, paclitaxel, paroxetine, phenytoin, risperidone, ritonavir, thiorida-zine, tricyclic antidepressants, venlafaxine, warfarin, zafirlukast, and other CYP2C9 and 2D6 substrates.

Decreased Effect: Pyrimethamine may decrease the levels/effects of CYP2D6 prodrug substrates (eg, codeine, hydrocodone, oxycodone, tram-adol).

Pharmacodynamics/Kinetics
Onset of action: ~1 hour
Absorption: Well absorbed
Distribution: Widely, mainly in blood cells, kidneys, lungs, liver, and spleen; crosses into CSF; crosses placenta; enters breast milk
Protein binding: 80% to 87%
Metabolism: Hepatic
Half-life elimination: 80-95 hours
Time to peak, serum: 1.5-8 hours
Excretion: Urine (20% to 30% as unchanged drug)

Pregnancy Risk Factor C

Pyrimethamine and Sulfadoxine *see* Sulfadoxine and Pyrimethamine *on page 1503*

Pyrinyl Plus® [OTC] *see* Pyrethrins and Piperonyl Butoxide *on page 1388*

Pyrithione Zinc (peer i THYE one zingk)

U.S. Brand Names BetaMed [OTC]; DermaZinc™ [OTC]; DHS™ Zinc [OTC]; Head & Shoulders® Citrus Breeze [OTC]; Head & Shoulders® Classic Clean [OTC]; Head & Shoulders® Classic Clean 2-In-1 [OTC]; Head & Shoulders® Dry Scalp Care [OTC]; Head & Shoulders® Extra Volume [OTC]; Head & Shoul-ders® Leave-in Treatment [OTC]; Head & Shoulders® Refresh [OTC]; Head & Shoulders® Sensitive Care [OTC]; Head & Shoulders® Smooth & Silky 2-In-1 [OTC]; Skin Care™ [OTC]; Zincon® [OTC]; ZNP® Bar [OTC]

Generic Available No
Pharmacologic Category Topical Skin Product
Use Relieves the itching, irritation and scalp flaking associated with dandruff and/or seborrheal dermatitis

Local Anesthetic/Vasoconstrictor Precautions No information available to require special precautions

Effects on Dental Treatment No significant effects or complications reported

QDALL® *see* Chlorpheniramine and Pseudoephedrine *on page 340*

QDALL® AR *see* Chlorpheniramine *on page 338*

Q-Naftate [OTC] *see* Tolnaftate *on page 1587*

Quadrivalent Human Papillomavirus Vaccine *see* Papillomavirus (Types 6, 11, 16, 18) Recombinant Vaccine *on page 1252*

Quadrivalent Meningococcal Conjugate Vaccine *see* Meningococcal Polysac-charide (Groups A / C / Y and W-135) Diphtheria Toxoid Conjugate Vaccine *on page 1035*

Quadrivalent Meningococcal Conjugate Vaccine *see* Meningococcal Polysac-charide Vaccine (Groups A, C, Y, and W-135) *on page 1036*

Qualaquin™ *see* Quinine *on page 1399*

Quasense™ *see* Ethinyl Estradiol and Levonorgestrel *on page 633*

Quaternium-18 Bentonite *see* Bentoquatam *on page 193*

Quazepam (KWAZ e pam)

U.S. Brand Names Doral®
Canadian Brand Names Doral®
Generic Available No
Pharmacologic Category Benzodiazepine
Use Treatment of insomnia

Local Anesthetic/Vasoconstrictor Precautions No information available to require special precautions

Effects on Dental Treatment Key adverse event(s) related to dental treat-ment: Xerostomia (normal salivary flow resumes upon discontinuation) and abnormal taste perception.

Common Adverse Effects Frequency not defined.
Cardiovascular: Palpitation
Central nervous system: Abnormal thinking, agitation, anxiety, ataxia, confu-sion, depression, dizziness, drowsiness, euphoria, fatigue, headache, hyper-/hypokinesia, incoordination, memory impairment, nervousness, nightmare, paranoid reaction
Dermatologic: Dermatitis, pruritus, rash
(Continued)

Quazepam *(Continued)*

Endocrine & metabolic: Libido decreased, menstrual irregularities
Gastrointestinal: Abdominal pain, abnormal taste perception, anorexia, appetite increased/decreased, constipation, diarrhea, dyspepsia, nausea, xerostomia
Genitourinary: Impotence, incontinence
Hematologic: Blood dyscrasias
Neuromuscular & skeletal: Dysarthria, muscle cramps, reflex slowing, rigidity, tremor
Ocular: Blurred vision
Miscellaneous: Drug dependence

Restrictions C-IV

Mechanism of Action Binds to stereospecific benzodiazepine receptors on the postsynaptic GABA neuron at several sites within the central nervous system, including the limbic system, reticular formation. Enhancement of the inhibitory effect of GABA on neuronal excitability results by increased neuronal membrane permeability to chloride ions. This shift in chloride ions results in hyperpolarization (a less excitable state) and stabilization.

Drug Interactions

Cytochrome P450 Effect: Substrate of CYP3A4 (minor)

Increased Effect/Toxicity: Serum levels and/or toxicity of quazepam may be increased by cimetidine, ciprofloxacin, clarithromycin, clozapine, CNS depressants, diltiazem, disulfiram, digoxin, erythromycin, ethanol, fluconazole, fluoxetine, fluvoxamine, grapefruit juice, isoniazid, itraconazole, ketoconazole, labetalol, levodopa, loxapine, metoprolol, metronidazole, miconazole, nefazodone, omeprazole, phenytoin, rifabutin, rifampin, troleandomycin, valproic acid, and verapamil.

Pharmacodynamics/Kinetics

Absorption: Rapid
Protein binding: 95%
Half-life elimination, serum: Parent drug: 25-41 hours; Active metabolite: 40-114 hours

Pregnancy Risk Factor X

Quelicin® *see* Succinylcholine *on page 1498*

Questran® *see* Cholestyramine Resin *on page 349*

Questran® Light *see* Cholestyramine Resin *on page 349*

Quetiapine *(kwe TYE a peen)*

U.S. Brand Names Seroquel®
Canadian Brand Names Seroquel®
Mexican Brand Names Seroquel
Generic Available No
Index Terms Quetiapine Fumarate
Pharmacologic Category Antipsychotic Agent, Atypical
Use Treatment of schizophrenia; treatment of acute manic episodes associated with bipolar disorder (as monotherapy or in combination with lithium or valproate); treatment of depressive episodes associated with bipolar disorder
Unlabeled/Investigational Use Autism, psychosis (children)
Local Anesthetic/Vasoconstrictor Precautions Quetiapine is one of the drugs confirmed to prolong the QT interval and is accepted as having a risk of causing torsade de pointes. The risk of drug-induced torsade de pointes is extremely low when a single QT interval prolonging drug is prescribed. In terms of epinephrine, it is not known what effect vasoconstrictors in the local anesthetic regimen will have in patients with a known history of congenital prolonged QT interval or in patients taking any medication that prolongs the QT interval. Until more information is obtained, it is suggested that the clinician consult with the physician prior to the use of a vasoconstrictor in suspected patients, and that the vasoconstrictor (epinephrine, levonordefrin [Neo-Cobefrin®]) be used with caution.
Effects on Dental Treatment Key adverse event(s) related to dental treatment: Xerostomia (normal salivary flow resumes upon discontinuation).
Common Adverse Effects
>10%:
Central nervous system: Agitation, dizziness, headache, somnolence
Endocrine & metabolic: Cholesterol increased (11%), triglycerides increased (17%)
Gastrointestinal: Weight gain (≥7% body weight, dose related), xerostomia
1% to 10%:
Cardiovascular: Palpitation, peripheral edema, postural hypotension, tachycardia
Central nervous system: Anxiety, fever, pain

Dermatologic: Rash

Gastrointestinal: Abdominal pain (dose related), anorexia, constipation, dyspepsia (dose related), gastroenteritis, vomiting

Hematologic: Leukopenia

Hepatic: AST increased, ALT increased, GGT increased

Neuromuscular & skeletal: Back pain, dysarthria, hypertonia, tremor, weakness

Ocular: Amblyopia

Respiratory: Cough, dyspnea, pharyngitis, rhinitis

Miscellaneous: Diaphoresis, flu-like syndrome

Restrictions An FDA-approved medication guide concerning the use of antidepressants in children, adolescents, and young adults must be distributed when dispensing an outpatient prescription (new or refill) where this medication is to be used without direct supervision of a healthcare provider. Medication guides are available at http://www.fda.gov/cder/drug/antidepressants/MG_template.pdf. Dispense to parents or guardians of children and adolescents receiving this medication.

Dosage Oral:

Children and Adolescents:

Autism (unlabeled use): 100-350 mg/day (1.6-5.2 mg/kg/day)

Psychosis and mania (unlabeled use): Initial: 25 mg twice daily; titrate as necessary to 450 mg/day

Adults:

Bipolar depression: Initial: 50 mg/day the first day; increase to 100 mg/day on day 2, further increasing by 100 mg/day each day to a target of 300 mg/day by day 4. Further increases up to 600 mg/day by day 8 have been evaluated in clinical trials, but no additional antidepressant efficacy was noted.

Bipolar mania: Initial: 50 mg twice daily on day 1, increase dose in increments of 100 mg/day to 200 mg twice daily on day 4; may increase to a target dose of 800 mg/day by day 6 at increments ≤200 mg/day. Usual dosage range: 400-800 mg/day.

Schizophrenia/psychoses: Initial: 25 mg twice daily; increase in increments of 25-50 mg 2-3 times/day on the second and third day, if tolerated, to a target dose of 300-400 mg/day in 2-3 divided doses by day 4. Make further adjustments as needed at intervals of at least 2 days in adjustments of 25-50 mg twice daily. Usual maintenance range: 300-800 mg/day.

Note: Dose reductions should be attempted periodically to establish lowest effective dose in patients with psychosis. Patients being restarted after 1 week of no drug need to be titrated as above.

Elderly: 40% lower mean oral clearance of quetiapine in adults >65 years of age; higher plasma levels expected and, therefore, dosage adjustment may be needed; elderly patients usually require 50-200 mg/day with a slower titration schedule. See "Note" in adult dosing.

Dosing comments in renal insufficiency: 25% lower mean oral clearance of quetiapine than normal subjects; however, plasma concentrations similar to normal subjects receiving the same dose; no dosage adjustment required

Dosing comments in hepatic insufficiency: 30% lower mean oral clearance of quetiapine than normal subjects; higher plasma levels expected in hepatically impaired subjects; dosage adjustment may be needed

Initial: 25 mg/day, increase dose by 25-50 mg/day to effective dose, based on clinical response and tolerability to patient

Mechanism of Action Quetiapine is a dibenzothiazepine atypical antipsychotic. It has been proposed that this drug's antipsychotic activity is mediated through a combination of dopamine type 2 (D_2) and serotonin type 2 (5-HT_2) antagonism. It is an antagonist at multiple neurotransmitter receptors in the brain: serotonin 5-HT_{1A} and 5-HT_2, dopamine D_1 and D_2, histamine H_1, and adrenergic alpha$_1$- and alpha$_2$- receptors; but appears to have no appreciable affinity at cholinergic muscarinic and benzodiazepine receptors.

Antagonism at receptors other than dopamine and 5-HT_2 with similar receptor affinities may explain some of the other effects of quetiapine. The drug's antagonism of histamine H_1-receptors may explain the somnolence observed with it. The drug's antagonism of adrenergic alpha$_1$-receptors may explain the orthostatic hypotension observed with it.

Contraindications Hypersensitivity to quetiapine or any component of the formulation; severe CNS depression; bone marrow suppression; blood dyscrasias; severe hepatic disease; coma

Warnings/Precautions [U.S. Boxed Warning]: Antidepressants increase the risk of suicidal thinking and behavior in children, adolescents, and young adults (18-24 years of age) with major depressive disorder (MDD) and other psychiatric disorders; consider risk prior to prescribing. Short-term studies did not show an increased risk in patients >24 years of age and showed a decreased risk in patients ≥65 years. Closely monitor all patients for clinical worsening, suicidality, or unusual changes in behavior; particularly during the (Continued)

Quetiapine *(Continued)*

initial 1-2 months of therapy or during periods of dosage adjustments (increased or decreases); the patient's family or caregiver should be instructed to closely observe the patient and communicate condition with healthcare provider. A medication guide concerning the use of antidepressants should be dispensed with each prescription. **Quetiapine is not FDA approved for use in children.**

May be sedating, use with caution in disorders where CNS depression is a feature. Use with caution in Parkinson's disease. May induce orthostatic hypotension associated with dizziness, tachycardia, and, in some cases, syncope, especially during the initial dose titration period. Should be used with particular caution in patients with known cardiovascular disease (history of MI or ischemic heart disease, heart failure, or conduction abnormalities), cerebrovascular disease, or conditions that predispose to hypotension. Esophageal dysmotility and aspiration have been associated with antipsychotic use; use with caution in patients at risk of aspiration pneumonia (eg, Alzheimer's disease). Development of cataracts has been observed in animal studies, therefore, lens examinations should be made upon initiation of therapy and every 6 months thereafter.

Due to anticholinergic effects, use with caution in patients with decreased gastrointestinal motility, urinary retention, BPH, xerostomia, visual problems, narrow-angle glaucoma (screening is recommended), and myasthenia gravis. Relative to other antipsychotics, quetiapine has a moderate potency of cholinergic blockade. May cause extrapyramidal symptoms, pseudoparkinsonism, and/or tardive dyskinesia. Impaired core body temperature regulation may occur; caution with strenuous exercise, heat exposure, dehydration, and concomitant medication possessing anticholinergic effects. Neuroleptic malignant syndrome (NMS) is a potentially fatal symptom complex that has been reported in association with administration of antipsychotic drugs. Clinical manifestations of NMS are hyperpyrexia, muscle rigidity, altered mental status, and evidence of autonomic instability (irregular pulse or blood pressure, tachycardia, diaphoresis, and cardiac dysrhythmia). Management of NMS should include immediate discontinuation of antipsychotic drugs and other drugs not essential to concurrent therapy, intensive symptomatic treatment and medication monitoring, and treatment of any concomitant medical problems for which specific treatment are available.

Use caution in patients with a history of seizures. May cause decreases in total free thyroxine, elevations of liver enzymes, cholesterol levels, and/or triglyceride increases.

May cause hyperglycemia; in some cases may be extreme and associated with ketoacidosis, hyperosmolar coma, or death. Use with caution in patients with diabetes or other disorders of glucose regulation; monitor for worsening of glucose control. Significant weight gain has been observed with antipsychotic therapy; incidence varies with product. Monitor waist circumference and BMI.

Drug Interactions

Cytochrome P450 Effect: Substrate of CYP2D6 (minor), 3A4 (major)

Increased Effect/Toxicity: Quetiapine increases levels of lorazepam. The effects of other centrally-acting drugs, sedatives, or ethanol may be potentiated by quetiapine. Quetiapine may enhance the effects of antihypertensive agents. CYP3A4 inhibitors may increase the levels/effects of quetiapine; example inhibitors include azole antifungals, clarithromycin, diclofenac, doxycycline, erythromycin, imatinib, isoniazid, nefazodone, nicardipine, propofol, protease inhibitors, quinidine, telithromycin, and verapamil; ketoconazole increased serum concentrations of quetiapine by 335%. Cimetidine increases blood levels of quetiapine. Acetylcholinesterase inhibitors (central) may increase the risk of antipsychotic-related EPS. Concurrent use with other QT$_c$-prolonging agents may increase risk of serious arrhythmias.

Decreased Effect: Thioridazine increases quetiapine's clearance (by 65%), decreasing serum levels. CYP3A4 inducers may decrease the levels/effects of quetiapine. Example inducers include aminoglutethimide, carbamazepine, nafcillin, nevirapine, phenobarbital, phenytoin, and rifamycins.

Ethanol/Nutrition/Herb Interactions

Ethanol: Avoid ethanol (may cause excessive impairment in cognition/motor function).

Food: In healthy volunteers, administration of quetiapine with food resulted in an increase in the peak serum concentration and AUC (each by ~15%) compared to the fasting state.

Herb/Nutraceutical: St John's wort may decrease quetiapine levels. Avoid valerian, St John's wort, kava kava, gotu kola (may increase CNS depression).

Dietary Considerations May be taken with or without food.

Pharmacodynamics/Kinetics

Absorption: Rapidly absorbed following oral administration

Distribution: V_d: 10 ± 4 L/kg; V_{dss}: ~2 days

Protein binding, plasma: 83%

Metabolism: Primarily hepatic; via CYP3A4; forms two inactive metabolites

Bioavailability: 9% ± 4%; tablet is 100% bioavailable relative to solution

Half-life elimination: Mean: Terminal: ~6 hours

Time to peak, plasma: 1.5 hours

Excretion: Urine (73% as metabolites, <1% as unchanged drug); feces (20%)

Pregnancy Risk Factor C

Dosage Forms

Tablet:

Seroquel®: 25 mg, 50 mg, 100 mg, 200 mg, 300 mg, 400 mg

Quetiapine Fumarate *see* Quetiapine *on page 1392*

Quibron® [DSC] *see* Theophylline and Guaifenesin *on page 1555*

Quibron®-T [DSC] *see* Theophylline *on page 1554*

Quibron®-T/SR [DSC] *see* Theophylline *on page 1554*

Quinalbarbitone Sodium *see* Secobarbital *on page 1459*

Quinapril (KWIN a pril)

Related Information

Cardiovascular Diseases *on page 1726*

U.S. Brand Names Accupril®

Canadian Brand Names Accupril®; GD-Quinapril

Mexican Brand Names Acupril

Generic Available Yes

Index Terms Quinapril Hydrochloride

Pharmacologic Category Angiotensin-Converting Enzyme (ACE) Inhibitor

Use Management of hypertension; treatment of congestive heart failure

Unlabeled/Investigational Use Treatment of left ventricular dysfunction after myocardial infarction; pediatric hypertension

Local Anesthetic/Vasoconstrictor Precautions No information available to require special precautions

Effects on Dental Treatment No significant effects or complications reported

Common Adverse Effects Note: Frequency ranges include data from hypertension and heart failure trials. Higher rates of adverse reactions have generally been noted in patients with CHF. However, the frequency of adverse effects associated with placebo is also increased in this population.

1% to 10%:

Cardiovascular: Hypotension (3%), chest pain (2%), first-dose hypotension (up to 3%)

Central nervous system: Dizziness (4% to 8%), headache (2% to 6%), fatigue (3%)

Dermatologic: Rash (1%)

Endocrine & metabolic: Hyperkalemia (2%)

Gastrointestinal: Vomiting/nausea (1% to 2%), diarrhea (2%)

Neuromuscular & skeletal: Myalgias (2% to 5%), back pain (1%)

Renal: BUN/serum creatinine increased (2%, transient elevations may occur with a higher frequency), worsening of renal function (in patients with bilateral renal artery stenosis or hypovolemia)

Respiratory: Upper respiratory symptoms, cough (2% to 4%; up to 13% in some studies), dyspnea (2%)

Dosage Oral:

Children (unlabeled use): Hypertension: Initial 5-10 mg once daily; maximum: 80 mg/day

Adults:

Hypertension: Initial: 10-20 mg once daily, adjust according to blood pressure response at peak and trough blood levels; initial dose may be reduced to 5 mg in patients receiving diuretic therapy if the diuretic is continued; usual dose range (JNC 7): 10-40 mg once daily

Congestive heart failure or post-MI: Initial: 5 mg once or twice daily, titrated at weekly intervals to 20-40 mg daily in 2 divided doses; target dose (heart failure): 20 mg twice daily (ACC/AHA 2005 Heart Failure Guidelines)

Elderly: Initial: 2.5-5 mg/day; increase dosage at increments of 2.5-5 mg at 1- to 2-week intervals.

Dosing adjustment in renal impairment: Lower initial doses should be used; after initial dose (if tolerated), administer initial dose twice daily; may be increased at weekly intervals to optimal response:

Hypertension: Initial:

Cl$_{cr}$ >60 mL/minute: Administer 10 mg/day

Cl$_{cr}$ 30-60 mL/minute: Administer 5 mg/day

Cl$_{cr}$ 10-30 mL/minute: Administer 2.5 mg/day

(Continued)

Quinapril *(Continued)*

Congestive heart failure: Initial:

Cl$_{cr}$ >30 mL/minute: Administer 5 mg/day

Cl$_{cr}$ 10-30 mL/minute: Administer 2.5 mg/day

Dosing comments in hepatic impairment: In patients with alcoholic cirrhosis, hydrolysis of quinapril to quinaprilat is impaired; however, the subsequent elimination of quinaprilat is unaltered.

Mechanism of Action Competitive inhibitor of angiotensin-converting enzyme (ACE); prevents conversion of angiotensin I to angiotensin II, a potent vasoconstrictor; results in lower levels of angiotensin II which causes an increase in plasma renin activity and a reduction in aldosterone secretion; a CNS mechanism may also be involved in hypotensive effect as angiotensin II increases adrenergic outflow from CNS; vasoactive kallikreins may be decreased in conversion to active hormones by ACE inhibitors, thus reducing blood pressure

Contraindications Hypersensitivity to quinapril or any component of the formulation; angioedema related to previous treatment with an ACE inhibitor; bilateral renal artery stenosis; patients with idiopathic or hereditary angioedema; pregnancy (2nd and 3rd trimesters)

Warnings/Precautions Anaphylactic reactions can occur. Use with caution in patients with renal insufficiency, autoimmune disease, renal artery stenosis; excessive hypotension may be more likely in volume-depleted patients, the elderly, and following the first dose (first dose phenomenon); quinapril should be discontinued if laryngeal stridor or angioedema is observed. Angioedema can occur at any time during treatment (especially following first dose). It may involve head and neck (potentially affecting the airway) or the intestine (presenting with abdominal pain). Prolonged monitoring may be required, especially if tongue, glottis, or larynx are involved as they are associated with airway obstruction. Those with a history of airway surgery in this situation have a higher risk. **[U.S. Boxed Warning]: Based on human data, ACEIs can cause injury and death to the developing fetus when used in the second and third trimesters. ACEIs should be discontinued as soon as possible once pregnancy is detected.** Rare toxicities associated with ACE inhibitors include cholestatic jaundice (which may progress to hepatic necrosis) and neutropenia/agranulocytosis with myeloid hyperplasia. Hyperkalemia may rarely occur. May be associated with deterioration of renal function and/or increases in serum creatinine, particularly in patients dependent on renin-angiotensin-aldosterone system. Use with caution in unilateral renal artery stenosis and pre-existing renal insufficiency; if patient has renal impairment, then a baseline WBC with differential and serum creatinine should be evaluated and monitored closely during the first 3 months of therapy. Hypersensitivity reactions may be seen during hemodialysis with high-flux dialysis membranes (eg, AN69). Safety and efficacy have not been established in children.

Drug Interactions

Increased Effect/Toxicity: Potassium supplements, co-trimoxazole (high dose), angiotensin II receptor antagonists (eg, candesartan, losartan, irbesartan), or potassium-sparing diuretics (amiloride, spironolactone, triamterene) may result in elevated serum potassium levels when combined with quinapril. ACE inhibitor effects may be increased by phenothiazines or probenecid (increases levels of captopril). ACE inhibitors may increase serum concentrations/effects of lithium. ACE inhibitors may enhance the adverse/toxic effects (nitritoid reaction) of gold sodium thiomalate.

Diuretics have additive hypotensive effects with ACE inhibitors, and hypovolemia increases the potential for adverse renal effects of ACE inhibitors. In patients with compromised renal function, coadministration with NSAIDs may result in further deterioration of renal function. Allopurinol and ACE inhibitors may cause a higher risk of hypersensitivity reaction when taken concurrently.

Decreased Effect: Quinapril may reduce the absorption of quinolones and tetracycline antibiotics. Aspirin (high dose) may reduce the therapeutic effects of ACE inhibitors; at low dosages this does not appear to be significant. Rifampin may decrease the effect of ACE inhibitors. Antacids may decrease the bioavailability of ACE inhibitors (may be more likely to occur with captopril); separate administration times by 1-2 hours. NSAIDs, specifically indomethacin, may reduce the hypotensive effects of ACE inhibitors.

Ethanol/Nutrition/Herb Interactions Herb/Nutraceutical: Avoid dong quai if using for hypertension (has estrogenic activity). Avoid ephedra, yohimbe, ginseng (may worsen hypertension). Avoid garlic (may have increased antihypertensive effect).

Pharmacodynamics/Kinetics

Onset of action: 1 hour

Duration: 24 hours

Absorption: Quinapril: ≥60%

Protein binding: Quinapril: 97%; Quinaprilat: 97%

Metabolism: Rapidly hydrolyzed to quinaprilat, the active metabolite
Half-life elimination: Quinapril: 0.8 hours; Quinaprilat: 3 hours; increases as Cl_{cr} decreases
Time to peak, serum: Quinapril: 1 hour; Quinaprilat: ~2 hours
Excretion: Urine (50% to 60% primarily as quinaprilat)
Pregnancy Risk Factor C (1st trimester)/D (2nd and 3rd trimesters)
Dosage Forms
Tablet: 5 mg, 10 mg, 20 mg, 40 mg
Accupril®: 5 mg, 10 mg, 20 mg, 40 mg

Quinapril and Hydrochlorothiazide
(KWIN a pril & hye droe klor oh THYE a zide)

Related Information
Hydrochlorothiazide *on page 819*
Quinapril *on page 1395*
U.S. Brand Names Accuretic®; Quinaretic
Canadian Brand Names Accuretic®
Generic Available Yes
Index Terms Hydrochlorothiazide and Quinapril
Pharmacologic Category Angiotensin-Converting Enzyme (ACE) Inhibitor; Antihypertensive; Diuretic, Thiazide
Use Treatment of hypertension (not for initial therapy)
Local Anesthetic/Vasoconstrictor Precautions No information available to require special precautions
Effects on Dental Treatment No significant effects or complications reported
Common Adverse Effects
1% to 10%:
Central nervous system: Dizziness (5%), somnolence (1%)
Neuromuscular & skeletal: Weakness (1%)
Renal: Serum creatinine increased (3%), blood urea nitrogen increased (4%)
Respiratory: Cough (3%), bronchitis (1%)
Drug Interactions
Increased Effect/Toxicity: See individual agents.
Decreased Effect: See individual agents.
Pharmacodynamics/Kinetics See individual agents.
Pregnancy Risk Factor C (1st trimester); D (2nd and 3rd trimesters)

Quinapril Hydrochloride *see* Quinapril *on page 1395*
Quinaretic *see* Quinapril and Hydrochlorothiazide *on page 1397*
Quin B Strong [OTC] *see* Vitamin B Complex Combinations *on page 1664*

Quinidine (KWIN i deen)

Related Information
Cardiovascular Diseases *on page 1726*
Canadian Brand Names Apo-Quinidine®; BioQuin® Durules™; Novo-Quinidin; Quinate®
Generic Available Yes
Index Terms Quinidine Gluconate; Quinidine Polygalacturonate; Quinidine Sulfate
Pharmacologic Category Antiarrhythmic Agent, Class Ia
Use Prophylaxis after cardioversion of atrial fibrillation and/or flutter to maintain normal sinus rhythm; prevent recurrence of paroxysmal supraventricular tachycardia, paroxysmal AV junctional rhythm, paroxysmal ventricular tachycardia, paroxysmal atrial fibrillation, and atrial or ventricular premature contractions; has activity against *Plasmodium falciparum* malaria
Local Anesthetic/Vasoconstrictor Precautions Quinidine is one of the drugs confirmed to prolong the QT interval and is accepted as having a risk of causing torsade de pointes. The risk of drug-induced torsade de pointes is extremely low when a single QT interval prolonging drug is prescribed. In terms of epinephrine, it is not known what effect vasoconstrictors in the local anesthetic regimen will have in patients with a known history of congenital prolonged QT interval or in patients taking any medication that prolongs the QT interval. Until more information is obtained, it is suggested that the clinician consult with the physician prior to the use of a vasoconstrictor in suspected patients, and that the vasoconstrictor (epinephrine, levonordefrin [Neo-Cobefrin®]) be used with caution.
Effects on Dental Treatment When taken over a long period of time, the anticholinergic side effects from quinidine can cause a reduction of saliva production or secretion contributing to discomfort and dental disease (ie, caries, oral candidiasis, and periodontal disease).
(Continued)

Quinidine *(Continued)*

Common Adverse Effects

Frequency not defined: Hypotension, syncope

>10%:

Cardiovascular: QT_c prolongation (modest prolongation is common, however, excessive prolongation is rare and indicates toxicity)

Central nervous system: Lightheadedness (15%)

Gastrointestinal: Diarrhea (35%), upper GI distress, bitter taste, diarrhea, anorexia, nausea, vomiting, stomach cramping (22%)

1% to 10%:

Cardiovascular: Angina (6%), palpitation (7%), new or worsened arrhythmia (proarrhythmic effect)

Central nervous system: Syncope (1% to 8%), headache (7%), fatigue (7%), sleep disturbance (3%), tremor (2%), nervousness (2%), incoordination (1%)

Dermatologic: Rash (5%)

Neuromuscular & skeletal: Weakness (5%)

Ocular: Blurred vision

Otic: Tinnitus

Respiratory: Wheezing

Note: Cinchonism, a syndrome which may include tinnitus, high-frequency hearing loss, deafness, vertigo, blurred vision, diplopia, photophobia, headache, confusion, and delirium has been associated with quinidine use. Usually associated with chronic toxicity, this syndrome has also been described after brief exposure to a moderate dose in sensitive patients. Vomiting and diarrhea may also occur as isolated reactions to therapeutic quinidine levels.

Mechanism of Action Class Ia antiarrhythmic agent; depresses phase O of the action potential; decreases myocardial excitability and conduction velocity, and myocardial contractility by decreasing sodium influx during depolarization and potassium efflux in repolarization; also reduces calcium transport across cell membrane

Drug Interactions

Cytochrome P450 Effect: Substrate of CYP2C9 (minor), 2E1 (minor), 3A4 (major); **Inhibits** CYP2C9 (weak), 2D6 (strong), 3A4 (strong)

Increased Effect/Toxicity: Effects may be additive with drugs which prolong the QT interval, including amiodarone, amitriptyline, bepridil, cisapride (use is contraindicated), disopyramide, erythromycin, haloperidol, imipramine, pimozide, procainamide, sotalol, thioridazine, and some quinolones (sparfloxacin, gatifloxacin, moxifloxacin - concurrent use is contraindicated). Concurrent use of amprenavir or ritonavir is contraindicated. Quinidine increases digoxin serum concentrations; digoxin dosage may need to be reduced (by 50%) when quinidine is initiated; new steady-state digoxin plasma concentrations occur in 5-7 days.

Quinidine may increase the levels/effects of amphetamines, selected beta-blockers, selected benzodiazepines, calcium channel blockers, cisapride, cyclosporine, dextromethorphan, ergot alkaloids, fluoxetine, selected HMG-CoA reductase inhibitors, lidocaine, mesoridazine, mirtazapine, nateglinide, nefazodone, paroxetine, risperidone, ritonavir, sildenafil (and other PDE-5 inhibitors), tacrolimus, thioridazine, tricyclic antidepressants, venlafaxine, and other substrates of CYP2D6 or 3A4. Selected benzodiazepines (midazolam and triazolam), cisapride, ergot alkaloids, selected HMG-CoA reductase inhibitors (lovastatin and simvastatin), mesoridazine, pimozide, and thioridazine are generally contraindicated with strong CYP3A4 inhibitors. When used with strong CYP3A4 inhibitors, dosage adjustment/limits are recommended for sildenafil and other PDE-5 inhibitors; refer to individual monographs.

The levels/effects of quinidine may be increased by azole antifungals, clarithromycin, diclofenac, doxycycline, erythromycin, imatinib, isoniazid, nefazodone, nicardipine, propofol, protease inhibitors (amprenavir and ritonavir are contraindicated), telithromycin, verapamil, and other CYP3A4 inhibitors. Quinidine potentiates nondepolarizing and depolarizing muscle relaxants. When combined with quinidine, amiloride may cause prolonged ventricular conduction leading to arrhythmias. Urinary alkalinizers (antacids, sodium bicarbonate, acetazolamide) increase quinidine blood levels. Warfarin effects may be increased by quinidine.

Decreased Effect: The levels/effects of quinidine may be decreased by aminoglutethimide, carbamazepine, nafcillin, nevirapine, phenobarbital, phenytoin, rifamycins, and other CYP3A4 inducers. Quinidine may decrease the levels/effects of CYP2D6 prodrug substrates (eg, codeine, hydrocodone, oxycodone, tramadol).

Pharmacodynamics/Kinetics

Distribution: V_d: Adults: 2-3.5 L/kg, decreased with congestive heart failure, malaria; increased with cirrhosis; crosses placenta; enters breast milk

Protein binding:

Newborns: 60% to 70%; decreased protein binding with cyanotic congenital heart disease, cirrhosis, or acute myocardial infarction

Adults: 80% to 90%

Metabolism: Extensively hepatic (50% to 90%) to inactive compounds

Bioavailability: Sulfate: 80%; Gluconate: 70%

Half-life elimination, plasma: Children: 2.5-6.7 hours; Adults: 6-8 hours; prolonged with elderly, cirrhosis, and congestive heart failure

Excretion: Urine (15% to 25% as unchanged drug)

Pregnancy Risk Factor C

Quinidine Gluconate see Quinidine on page 1397

Quinidine Polygalacturonate see Quinidine on page 1397

Quinidine Sulfate see Quinidine on page 1397

Quinine (KWYE nine)

U.S. Brand Names Qualaquin™

Canadian Brand Names Apo-Quinine®; Novo-Quinine; Quinine-Odan™

Generic Available No

Index Terms Quinine Sulfate

Pharmacologic Category Antimalarial Agent

Use In conjunction with other antimalarial agents, treatment of uncomplicated chloroquine-resistant *P. falciparum* malaria

Unlabeled/Investigational Use Treatment of *Babesia microti* infection in conjunction with clindamycin

Note: Prevention/treatment of nocturnal leg cramps (unapproved) removed following FDA-issued warning regarding severe adverse events (eg, cardiac arrhythmias, thrombocytopenia, and severe hypersensitivity reactions) and potentially serious drug interactions associated with quinine; use not justified in this condition.

Local Anesthetic/Vasoconstrictor Precautions No information available to require special precautions

Effects on Dental Treatment No significant effects or complications reported

Common Adverse Effects

Frequency not defined.

Cardiovascular: Atrial fibrillation, atrioventricular block, bradycardia, cardiac arrest, chest pain, hypotension, irregular rhythm, nodal escape beats, palpitation, postural hypotension, QT prolongation, syncope, tachycardia, torsade de pointes, unifocal premature ventricular contractions, U waves, vasodilation, ventricular fibrillation, ventricular tachycardia

Central nervous system: Aphasia, ataxia, chills, coma, confusion, disorientation, dizziness, dystonic reaction, fever, flushing, headache, mental status altered, restlessness, seizure, suicide, vertigo

Dermatologic: Acral necrosis, allergic contact dermatitis, bullous dermatitis, bruising, cutaneous rash (urticaria, papular, scarlatinal), cutaneous vasculitis, diaphoresis, exfoliative dermatitis, erythema multiforme, petechiae, photosensitivity, pruritus, Stevens-Johnson syndrome, toxic epidermal necrolysis

Endocrine & metabolic: Hypoglycemia

Gastrointestinal: Abdominal pain, anorexia, diarrhea, esophagitis, gastric irritation, nausea, vomiting

Hematologic: Agranulocytosis, aplastic anemia, coagulopathy, disseminated intravascular coagulation, hemolytic anemia, hemolytic uremic syndrome, hemorrhage, hypoprothrombinemia, leukopenia, neutropenia, pancytopenia, thrombocytopenia, thrombotic thrombocytopenic purpura

Hepatic: Granulomatous hepatitis, hepatitis, jaundice, liver function test abnormalities

Neuromuscular & skeletal: Myalgia, tremor, weakness

Ocular: Blindness, blurred vision (with or without scotomata), color vision disturbance, diminished visual fields, diplopia, night blindness, optic neuritis, photophobia, pupillary dilation, vision loss (sudden)

Otic: Deafness, hearing impaired, tinnitus

Respiratory: Asthma, dyspnea, pulmonary edema

Renal: Acute interstitial nephritis, hemoglobinuria, renal failure, renal impairment

Miscellaneous: Black water fever, hypersensitivity syndrome, lupus anticoagulant, lupus-like syndrome

(Continued)

Quinine *(Continued)*

Mechanism of Action Depresses oxygen uptake and carbohydrate metabolism; intercalates into DNA, disrupting the parasite's replication and transcription; cardiovascular effects similar to quinidine

Drug Interactions

  Cytochrome P450 Effect: Substrate of CYP1A2 (minor), 2C19 (minor), 3A4 (major); **Inhibits** CYP2C8 (moderate), 2C9 (moderate), 2D6 (strong), 3A4 (weak)

  Increased Effect/Toxicity: Antacids products containing aluminum or magnesium may decrease absorption of quinine; avoid concurrent administration. Quinine may increase the serum concentration of cardiac glycosides. Quinine may increase the levels/effects of CYP2C8 substrates (example substrates include amiodarone, paclitaxel, pioglitazone, repaglinide, and rosiglitazone). Quinine may increase the levels/effects of CYP2C9 substrates (example substrates include bosentan, dapsone, fluoxetine, glimepiride, glipizide, losartan, montelukast, nateglinide, paclitaxel, phenytoin, warfarin, and zafirlukast). Quinine may increase the levels/effects of CYP2D6 substrates (example substrates include amphetamines, selected beta-blockers, dextromethorphan, fluoxetine, lidocaine, mirtazapine, nefazodone, paroxetine, risperidone, ritonavir, thioridazine, tricyclic antidepressants, and venlafaxine).

  Quinine may increase the serum concentration of phenothiazine antipsychotic agents. QT_c-prolonging agents (eg, amiodarone, amitriptyline, bepridil, disopyramide, erythromycin, haloperidol, imipramine, pimozide, procainamide, sotalol, thioridazine) may have additive effects; use with caution. Urinary alkalinizers (sodium bicarbonate, acetazolamide) may increase quinine blood levels.

  Decreased Effect: Phenobarbital, phenytoin, and rifampin may decrease quinine serum concentrations. Quinine may decrease the levels/effects of CYP2D6 prodrug substrates (eg, codeine, hydrocodone, oxycodone, tramadol). CYP3A4 inducers may decrease the levels/effects of quinine (example inducers include aminoglutethimide, carbamazepine, nafcillin, nevirapine, phenobarbital, phenytoin, and rifamycins).

Pharmacodynamics/Kinetics

  Absorption: Readily, mainly from upper small intestine

  Distribution: 2.5-7.1 L/kg; varies with severity of infection

    Intraerythrocytic levels are ~30% to 50% of the plasma concentration; distributes poorly to the CSF (~2% to 7% of plasma concentration)

  Protein binding: 69% to 92% in healthy subjects; 78% to 95% with malaria

  Metabolism: Primarily hepatic via CYP450 enzymes, including CYP3A4 and 2C19; forms metabolites

  Bioavailability: 76% to 88% in healthy subjects; increased with malaria

  Half-life elimination:

    Children: ~3 hours in healthy subjects; ~12 hours with malaria

    Healthy adults: 10-13 hours

  Time to peak, serum:

    Children: 2 hours in healthy subjects; 4 hours with malaria

    Adults: 1-3 hours in healthy subjects; 1.2-11 hours with malaria

  Excretion: Urine (<20% as unchanged drug)

Pregnancy Risk Factor C

Quinine Sulfate *see* Quinine *on page 1399*

Quinol *see* Hydroquinone *on page 841*

Quintabs [OTC] *see* Vitamins (Multiple/Oral) *on page 1665*

Quintabs-M [OTC] *see* Vitamins (Multiple/Oral) *on page 1665*

Quinupristin and Dalfopristin

  (kwi NYOO pris tin & dal FOE pris tin)

U.S. Brand Names Synercid®

Canadian Brand Names Synercid®

Generic Available No

Index Terms Pristinamycin; RP-59500

Pharmacologic Category Antibiotic, Streptogramin

Use Treatment of serious or life-threatening infections associated with vancomycin-resistant *Enterococcus faecium* bacteremia; treatment of complicated skin and skin structure infections caused by methcillin-susceptible *Staphylococcus aureus* or *Streptococcus pyogenes*

Has been studied in the treatment of a variety of infections caused by *Enterococcus faecium* (not *E. fecalis*) including vancomycin-resistant strains. May also be effective in the treatment of serious infections caused by *Staphylococcus* species including those resistant to methicillin.

Local Anesthetic/Vasoconstrictor Precautions No information available to require special precautions

Effects on Dental Treatment No significant effects or complications reported

Common Adverse Effects

>10%:
- Hepatic: Hyperbilirubinemia (3% to 35%)
- Local: Inflammation at infusion site (38% to 42%), local pain (40% to 44%), local edema (17% to 18%), infusion site reaction (12% to 13%)
- Neuromuscular & skeletal: Arthralgia (up to 47%), myalgia (up to 47%)

1% to 10%:
- Central nervous system: Pain (2% to 3%), headache (2%)
- Dermatologic: Pruritus (2%), rash (3%)
- Endocrine & metabolic: Hyperglycemia (1%)
- Gastrointestinal: Nausea (3% to 5%), diarrhea (3%), vomiting (3% to 4%)
- Hematologic: Anemia (3%)
- Hepatic: GGT increased (2%), LDH increased (3%)
- Local: Thrombophlebitis (2%)
- Neuromuscular & skeletal: CPK increased (2%)

Mechanism of Action Quinupristin/dalfopristin inhibits bacterial protein synthesis by binding to different sites on the 50S bacterial ribosomal subunit thereby inhibiting protein synthesis

Drug Interactions

Cytochrome P450 Effect: Quinupristin: **Inhibits** CYP3A4 (weak)

Increased Effect/Toxicity: The manufacturer states that quinupristin/dalfopristin may increase cisapride concentrations and cause QT_c prolongation, and recommends to avoid concurrent use with cisapride. Quinupristin/dalfopristin may increase cyclosporine concentrations; monitor.

Pharmacodynamics/Kinetics

Distribution: Quinupristin: 0.45 L/kg; Dalfopristin: 0.24 L/kg

Protein binding: Moderate

Metabolism: To active metabolites via nonenzymatic reactions

Half-life elimination: Quinupristin: 0.85 hour; Dalfopristin: 0.7 hour (mean elimination half-lives, including metabolites: 3 and 1 hours, respectively)

Excretion: Feces (75% to 77% as unchanged drug and metabolites); urine (15% to 19%)

Pregnancy Risk Factor B

Quixin™ see Levofloxacin on page 965

QVAR® see Beclomethasone on page 188

R 14-15 see Erlotinib on page 587

R-3827 see Abarelix on page 24

RabAvert® see Rabies Virus Vaccine on page 1403

Rabeprazole (ra BEP ra zole)

U.S. Brand Names AcipHex®

Canadian Brand Names AcipHex®; Pariet®

Mexican Brand Names Pariet

Generic Available No

Index Terms Pariprazole

Pharmacologic Category Proton Pump Inhibitor; Substituted Benzimidazole

Use Short-term (4-8 weeks) treatment and maintenance of erosive or ulcerative gastroesophageal reflux disease (GERD); symptomatic GERD; short-term (up to 4 weeks) treatment of duodenal ulcers; long-term treatment of pathological hypersecretory conditions, including Zollinger-Ellison syndrome; H. pylori eradication (in combination with amoxicillin and clarithromycin)

Unlabeled/Investigational Use Maintenance of duodenal ulcer

Local Anesthetic/Vasoconstrictor Precautions No information available to require special precautions

Effects on Dental Treatment No significant effects or complications reported

Common Adverse Effects 1% to 10%: Central nervous system: Headache

Dosage Oral: Adults >18 years and Elderly:

GERD: 20 mg once daily for 4-8 weeks; maintenance: 20 mg once daily

Duodenal ulcer: 20 mg/day before breakfast for 4 weeks

H. pylori eradication: 20 mg twice daily for 7 days; to be administered with amoxicillin 1000 mg and clarithromycin 500 mg, also given twice daily for 7 days.

Hypersecretory conditions: 60 mg once daily; dose may need to be adjusted as necessary. Doses as high as 100 mg once daily and 60 mg twice daily have been used.

Dosage adjustment in renal impairment: No dosage adjustment required

(Continued)

Rabeprazole *(Continued)*

Dosage adjustment in hepatic impairment:
Mild to moderate: Elimination decreased; no dosage adjustment required
Severe: Use caution

Mechanism of Action Potent proton pump inhibitor; suppresses gastric acid secretion by inhibiting the parietal cell $H+/K+$ ATP pump

Contraindications Hypersensitivity to rabeprazole, substituted benzimidazoles (ie, esomeprazole, lansoprazole, omeprazole, pantoprazole), or any component of the formulation

Warnings/Precautions Use caution in severe hepatic impairment; relief of symptoms with rabeprazole does not preclude the presence of a gastric malignancy

Drug Interactions
Cytochrome P450 Effect: Substrate (major) of CYP2C19, 3A4; **Inhibits** CYP2C8 (moderate), 2C19 (moderate), 2DC (weak), 3A4 (weak)

Increased Effect/Toxicity: Rabeprazole may increase the levels/effects of citalopram, diazepam, methsuximide, phenytoin, propranolol, sertraline, and other CYP2C19 substrates. Rabeprazole may increase the levels/effects of amiodarone, paclitaxel, pioglitazone, repaglinide, rosiglitazone, and other CYP2C8 substrates.

Decreased Effect: Proton pump inhibitors may decrease the absorption of atazanavir, indinavir, oral iron salts, itraconazole, and ketoconazole. The levels/effects of rabeprazole may be decreased by aminoglutethimide, carbamazepine, nafcillin, nevirapine, phenobarbital, phenytoin, rifampin, and other CYP2C19 or 3A4 inducers.

Ethanol/Nutrition/Herb Interactions
Ethanol: Avoid ethanol (may cause gastric mucosal irritation).
Food: High-fat meals may delay absorption, but C_{max} and AUC are not altered.

Dietary Considerations May be taken with or without food; best if taken before breakfast.

Pharmacodynamics/Kinetics
Onset of action: 1 hour
Duration: 24 hours
Absorption: Oral: Well absorbed within 1 hour
Distribution: 96.3%
Protein binding, serum: 94.8% to 97.5%
Metabolism: Hepatic via CYP3A and 2C19 to inactive metabolites
Bioavailability: Oral: 52%
Half-life elimination (dose dependent): 0.85-2 hours
Time to peak, plasma: 2-5 hours
Excretion: Urine (90% primarily as thioether carboxylic acid); remainder in feces

Pregnancy Risk Factor B

Dosage Forms
Tablet, delayed release, enteric coated:
AcipHex®: 20 mg

Rabies Immune Globulin (Human)
(RAY beez i MYUN GLOB yoo lin, HYU man)

Related Information
Immunizations (Vaccines) *on page 1886*
U.S. Brand Names BayRab® [DSC]; HyperRAB™ S/D; Imogam® Rabies-HT
Canadian Brand Names BayRab™; Imogam® Rabies Pasteurized
Generic Available No
Index Terms RIG
Pharmacologic Category Immune Globulin
Use Part of postexposure prophylaxis of persons with rabies exposure who lack a history of pre-exposure or postexposure prophylaxis with rabies vaccine or a recently documented neutralizing antibody response to previous rabies vaccination; although it is preferable to administer RIG with the first dose of vaccine, it can be given up to 8 days after vaccination

Local Anesthetic/Vasoconstrictor Precautions No information available to require special precautions

Effects on Dental Treatment No significant effects or complications reported

Common Adverse Effects 1% to 10%:
Central nervous system: Fever (mild)
Local: Soreness at injection site

Mechanism of Action Rabies immune globulin is a solution of globulins dried from the plasma or serum of selected adult human donors who have been immunized with rabies vaccine and have developed high titers of rabies antibody. It generally contains 10% to 18% of protein of which not less than 80% is monomeric immunoglobulin G.

Pregnancy Risk Factor C

Rabies Virus Vaccine (RAY beez VYE rus vak SEEN)

Related Information
Immunizations (Vaccines) *on page 1886*

U.S. Brand Names Imovax® Rabies; RabAvert®

Canadian Brand Names Imovax® Rabies; RabAvert®

Generic Available No

Index Terms HDCV; Human Diploid Cell Cultures Rabies Vaccine; PCEC; Purified Chick Embryo Cell

Pharmacologic Category Vaccine

Use Pre-exposure immunization: Vaccinate persons with greater than usual risk due to occupation or avocation including veterinarians, rangers, animal handlers, certain laboratory workers, and persons living in or visiting countries for longer than 1 month where rabies is a constant threat.

Postexposure prophylaxis: If a bite from a carrier animal is unprovoked, if it is not captured and rabies is present in that species and area, administer rabies immune globulin (RIG) and the vaccine as indicated

Local Anesthetic/Vasoconstrictor Precautions No information available to require special precautions

Effects on Dental Treatment No significant effects or complications reported

Common Adverse Effects All serious adverse reactions must be reported to the U.S. Department of Health and Human Services (DHHS) Vaccine Adverse Event Reporting System (VAERS) 1-800-822-7967.

Frequency not defined.

Cardiovascular: Edema

Central nervous system: Dizziness, malaise, encephalomyelitis, transverse myelitis, fever, pain, headache, neuroparalytic reactions

Gastrointestinal: Nausea, abdominal pain

Local: Local discomfort, pain at injection site, itching, erythema, swelling or pain

Neuromuscular & skeletal: Myalgia

Mechanism of Action Rabies vaccine is an inactivated virus vaccine which promotes immunity by inducing an active immune response. The production of specific antibodies requires about 7-10 days to develop. Rabies immune globulin or antirabies serum, equine (ARS) is given in conjunction with rabies vaccine to provide immune protection until an antibody response can occur.

Pharmacodynamics/Kinetics
Onset of action: I.M.: Rabies antibody: ~7-10 days
Peak effect: ~30-60 days
Duration: ≥1 year

Pregnancy Risk Factor C

Racepinephrine *see* Epinephrine *on page 572*

Radiogardase™ *see* Ferric Hexacyanoferrate *on page 687*

rAHF *see* Antihemophilic Factor (Recombinant) *on page 132*

R-albuterol *see* Levalbuterol *on page 959*

Ralix *see* Chlorpheniramine, Phenylephrine, and Methscopolamine *on page 342*

Raloxifene (ral OKS i feen)

Related Information
Endocrine Disorders and Pregnancy *on page 1750*
Rheumatoid Arthritis, Osteoarthritis, and Osteoporosis *on page 1759*

U.S. Brand Names Evista®

Canadian Brand Names Evista®

Mexican Brand Names Evista

Generic Available No

Index Terms Keoxifene Hydrochloride; NSC-706725; Raloxifene Hydrochloride

Pharmacologic Category Selective Estrogen Receptor Modulator (SERM)

Use Prevention and treatment of osteoporosis in postmenopausal women

Unlabeled/Investigational Use Risk reduction for invasive breast cancer in postmenopausal women at increased risk for breast cancer

Local Anesthetic/Vasoconstrictor Precautions No information available to require special precautions

Effects on Dental Treatment No significant effects or complications reported (Continued)

Raloxifene *(Continued)*

Common Adverse Effects Note: Raloxifene has been associated with increased risk of thromboembolism (DVT, PE) and superficial thrombophlebitis; risk is similar to reported risk of HRT

>10%:

Endocrine & metabolic: Hot flashes (10% to 29%)

Neuromuscular & skeletal: Arthralgia (11% to 16%)

Miscellaneous: Flu syndrome (14% to 15%), infection (11% to 15%)

1% to 10%:

Cardiovascular: Peripheral edema (3% to 5%), chest pain (3% to 4%), syncope (2%), varicose vein (2%)

Central nervous system: Headache (9%), depression (6%), insomnia (6%), vertigo (4%), fever (3% to 4%), migraine (3%)

Dermatologic: Rash (6%)

Endocrine & metabolic: Breast pain (4%)

Gastrointestinal: Nausea (8% to 9%), weight gain (9%), abdominal pain (7%), diarrhea (7%), dyspepsia (6%), vomiting (3% to 5%), flatulence (2% to 3%), gastroenteritis (≤3%)

Genitourinary: Vaginal bleeding (6%), cystitis (3% to 5%), urinary tract infection (4%), vaginitis (4%), leukorrhea (3%), urinary tract disorder (3%), uterine disorder (3%), vaginal hemorrhage (3%), endometrial disorder (≤3%)

Neuromuscular & skeletal: Myalgia (7%), leg cramps (6% to 7%), arthritis (4%), tendon disorder (4%), hypoesthesia (≤2%), neuralgia (≤2%)

Ocular: Conjunctivitis (2%)

Respiratory: Bronchitis (10%), rhinitis (10%), sinusitis (8% to 10%), cough (6% to 9%), pharyngitis (5% to 8%), pneumonia (3%), laryngitis (≤2%)

Miscellaneous: Diaphoresis (3%)

Dosage Adults: Female: Oral:

Osteoporosis: 60 mg/day

Invasive breast cancer risk reduction (investigational use): 60 mg/day for 5 years

Dosage adjustment in hepatic impairment: Child-Pugh class A: Plasma concentrations were higher and correlated with total bilirubin. Safety and efficacy in hepatic insufficiency have not been established.

Mechanism of Action A selective estrogen receptor modulator, meaning that it affects some of the same receptors that estrogen does, but not all, and in some instances, it antagonizes or blocks estrogen; it acts like estrogen to prevent bone loss and improve lipid profiles (decreases total and LDL-cholesterol but does not raise triglycerides), but it has the potential to block some estrogen effects such as those that lead to breast cancer and uterine cancer

Contraindications Hypersensitivity to raloxifene or any component of the formulation; active or history of venous thromboembolic events; pregnancy; breast-feeding

Warnings/Precautions Use caution in patients at high risk for venous thromboembolism (deep vein thrombosis, pulmonary embolism); patients with cardiovascular disease; history of cervical/uterine carcinoma; renal/hepatic insufficiency (however, pharmacokinetic data are lacking); concurrent use of estrogens; women with a history of elevated triglycerides in response to treatment with oral estrogens (or estrogen/progestin). Safety and efficacy in premenopausal women or men have not been established.

Drug Interactions

Decreased Effect: Cholestyramine decreases raloxifene absorption; raloxifene decreases levothyroxine absorption

Ethanol/Nutrition/Herb Interactions Ethanol: Avoid ethanol (may increase risk of osteoporosis).

Dietary Considerations Supplemental calcium or vitamin D may be required if dietary intake is not adequate.

Pharmacodynamics/Kinetics

Onset of action: 8 weeks

Absorption: ~60%

Distribution: 2348 L/kg

Protein binding: >95% to albumin and α-glycoprotein

Metabolism: Hepatic, extensive first-pass effect; metabolized to glucuronide conjugates

Bioavailability: ~2%

Half-life elimination: 27.7-32.5 hours

Excretion: Primarily feces; urine (0.2%)

Pregnancy Risk Factor X

Dosage Forms

Tablet:

Evista®: 60 mg

Raloxifene Hydrochloride *see* Raloxifene *on page 1403*

Ramelteon (ra MEL tee on)

U.S. Brand Names Rozerem™
Generic Available No
Index Terms TAK-375
Pharmacologic Category Hypnotic, Nonbenzodiazepine
Use Treatment of insomnia characterized by difficulty with sleep onset
Local Anesthetic/Vasoconstrictor Precautions No information available to require special precautions
Effects on Dental Treatment Key adverse event(s) related to dental treatment: Taste perversion.
Common Adverse Effects 1% to 10%:
Central nervous system: Headache (7%, same as placebo), somnolence (5%), dizziness (5%), fatigue (4%), insomnia worsened (3%), depression (2%)
Endocrine & metabolic: Serum cortisol decreased (1%)
Gastrointestinal: Nausea (3%), diarrhea (2%, same as placebo), taste perversion (2%)
Neuromuscular & skeletal: Myalgia (2%), arthralgia (2%)
Respiratory: Upper respiratory infection (3%; 2 % with placebo)
Miscellaneous: Influenza (1%)
Dosage
Oral: Adults: One 8 mg tablet within 30 minutes of bedtime
Dosage adjustment in renal impairment: No dosage adjustment required
Dosage adjustment in hepatic impairment: No adjustment required for mild-to-moderate impairment. Avoid use with severe impairment.
Mechanism of Action Potent, selective agonist of melatonin receptors MT_1 and MT_2 (with little affinity for MT_3) within the suprachiasmic nucleus of the hypothalamus, an area responsible for determination of circadian rhythms and synchronization of the sleep-wake cycle. Agonism of MT_1 is thought to preferentially induce sleepiness, while MT_2 receptor activation preferentially influences regulation of circadian rhythms. Ramelteon is eightfold more selective for MT_1 than MT_2 and exhibits nearly sixfold higher affinity for MT_1 than melatonin, presumably allowing for enhanced effects on sleep induction.
Contraindications Hypersensitivity to ramelteon or any component of the formulation; severe hepatic impairment; concurrent use with fluvoxamine
Warnings/Precautions
Symptomatic treatment of insomnia should be initiated only after careful evaluation of potential causes of sleep disturbance. Failure of sleep disturbance to resolve after a reasonable period of treatment may indicate psychiatric and/or medical illness. Because of the rapid onset of action, administer immediately prior to bedtime or after the patient has gone to bed and is having difficulty falling asleep. Hypnotics/sedatives have been associated with abnormal thinking and behavior changes including decreased inhibition, aggression, bizarre behavior, agitation, hallucinations, and depersonalization. These changes may occur unpredictably and may indicate previously unrecognized psychiatric disorders; evaluate appropriately. Postmarketing studies have indicated that the use of hypnotic/sedative agents for sleep has been associated with hypersensitivity reactions including anaphylaxis as well as angioedema. An increased risk for hazardous sleep-related activities such as sleep-driving; cooking and eating food, and making phone calls while asleep have also been noted. Use caution with pre-existing depression or other psychiatric conditions. Caution when using with other CNS depressants; avoid engaging in hazardous activities or activities requiring mental alertness. Not recommended for use in patients with severe sleep apnea or COPD. Use caution with moderate hepatic impairment. May cause disturbances of hormonal regulation. Use caution when administered concomitantly with strong CYP1A2 inhibitors. Safety and efficacy in pediatric patients have not been established.
Drug Interactions
Cytochrome P450 Effect: Substrate of CYP1A2 (major), CYP3A4 (minor), CYP2C family (minor)
Increased Effect/Toxicity: The following agents may increase the levels/effects of ramelteon: CNS depressants, CYP1A2 inhibitors (example inhibitors include ciprofloxacin, fluvoxamine (concomitant use not recommended), ketoconazole, norfloxacin, ofloxacin, and rofecoxib), fluvoxamine, fluconazole, and ketoconazole.
Decreased Effect: Rifampin may decrease the levels/effects of ramelteon.
Ethanol/Nutrition/Herb Interactions
Ethanol: Avoid ethanol (may increase CNS depression).
Food: Taking with high-fat meal delays T_{max} and increases AUC (~31%); do not take with high-fat meal.
(Continued)

Ramelteon *(Continued)*

Dietary Considerations Taking with high-fat meal delays T_{max} and increases AUC (~31%); do not take with high-fat meal.

Pharmacodynamics/Kinetics

Onset of action: 30 minutes

Absorption: Rapid; high-fat meal delays T_{max} and increases AUC (~31%)

Distribution: 74 L

Protein binding: 82%

Metabolism: Extensive first-pass effect; oxidative metabolism primarily through CYP1A2 and to a lesser extent through CYP2C and CYP3A4; forms active metabolite (M-II)

Bioavailability: Absolute: 1.8%

Half-life elimination: Ramelteon: 1-2.6 hours; M-II: 2-5 hours

Time to peak, plasma: Median: 0.5-1.5 hours

Excretion: Primarily as metabolites: Urine (84%); feces (4%)

Pregnancy Risk Factor C

Dosage Forms

Tablet:

Rozerem™: 8 mg

Selected Readings

Kato K, Hirai K, Nishiyama K, et al, "Neurochemical Properties of Ramelteon (TAK-375), A Selective MT1/MT2 Receptor Agonist," *Neuropharmacology,* 2005, 48(2):301-10.

Nguyen NN, Uy SS, and Song JC, "Ramelteon: A Novel Melatonin Receptor Agonist for the Treatment of Insomnia," *Formulary,* 2005, 40:146-55.

Ramipril *(RA mi pril)*

Related Information

Cardiovascular Diseases *on page 1726*

U.S. Brand Names Altace®

Canadian Brand Names Altace®; Apo-Ramipril®

Mexican Brand Names Tritace

Generic Available No

Pharmacologic Category Angiotensin-Converting Enzyme (ACE) Inhibitor

Use Treatment of hypertension, alone or in combination with thiazide diuretics; treatment of left ventricular dysfunction after myocardial infarction; to reduce risk of heart attack, stroke, and death in patients at increased risk for these problems

Unlabeled/Investigational Use Treatment of heart failure

Local Anesthetic/Vasoconstrictor Precautions No information available to require special precautions

Effects on Dental Treatment No significant effects or complications reported

Common Adverse Effects Note: Frequency ranges include data from hypertension and heart failure trials. Higher rates of adverse reactions have generally been noted in patients with CHF. However, the frequency of adverse effects associated with placebo is also increased in this population.

>10%: Respiratory: Cough (increased) (7% to 12%)

1% to 10%:

Cardiovascular: Hypotension (11%), angina (3%), postural hypotension (2%), syncope (2%)

Central nervous system: Headache (1% to 5%), dizziness (2% to 4%), fatigue (2%), vertigo (2%)

Endocrine & metabolic: Hyperkalemia (1% to 10%)

Gastrointestinal: Nausea/vomiting (1% to 2%)

Neuromuscular & skeletal: Chest pain (noncardiac) (1%)

Renal: Renal dysfunction (1%), elevation in serum creatinine (1% to 2%), increased BUN (<1% to 3%); transient elevations of creatinine and/or BUN may occur more frequently

Respiratory: Cough (estimated 1% to 10%)

Worsening of renal function may occur in patients with bilateral renal artery stenosis or in hypovolemia. In addition, a syndrome which may include fever, myalgia, arthralgia, interstitial nephritis, vasculitis, rash, eosinophilia and positive ANA, and elevated ESR has been reported with ACE inhibitors. Risk of pancreatitis and agranulocytosis may be increased in patients with collagen vascular disease or renal impairment.

Dosage Adults: Oral:

Hypertension: 2.5-5 mg once daily, maximum: 20 mg/day

Reduction in risk of MI, stroke, and death from cardiovascular causes: Initial: 2.5 mg once daily for 1 week, then 5 mg once daily for the next 3 weeks, then increase as tolerated to 10 mg once daily (may be given as divided dose)

Heart failure postmyocardial infarction: Initial: 2.5 mg twice daily titrated upward, if possible, to 5 mg twice daily.

Heart failure (unlabeled use): Initial: 1.25-2.5 mg once daily; target dose: 10 mg once daily (ACC/AHA 2005 Heart Failure Guidelines)

Note: The dose of any concomitant diuretic should be reduced. If the diuretic cannot be discontinued, initiate therapy with 1.25 mg. After the initial dose, the patient should be monitored carefully until blood pressure has stabilized.

Dosing adjustment in renal impairment:

Cl_{cr} <40 mL/minute: Administer 25% of normal dose.

Renal failure and hypertension: Administer 1.25 mg once daily, titrated upward as possible.

Renal failure and heart failure: Administer 1.25 mg once daily, increasing to 1.25 mg twice daily up to 2.5 mg twice daily as tolerated.

Mechanism of Action Ramipril is an ACE inhibitor which prevents the formation of angiotensin II from angiotensin I and exhibits pharmacologic effects that are similar to captopril. Ramipril must undergo enzymatic saponification by esterases in the liver to its biologically active metabolite, ramiprilat. The pharmacodynamic effects of ramipril result from the high-affinity, competitive, reversible binding of ramiprilat to angiotensin-converting enzyme thus preventing the formation of the potent vasoconstrictor angiotensin II. This isomerized enzyme-inhibitor complex has a slow rate of dissociation, which results in high potency and a long duration of action; a CNS mechanism may also be involved in the hypotensive effect as angiotensin II increases adrenergic outflow from CNS; vasoactive kallikreins may be decreased in conversion to active hormones by ACE inhibitors, thus reducing blood pressure

Contraindications Hypersensitivity to ramipril or any component of the formulation; prior hypersensitivity (including angioedema) to ACE inhibitors; bilateral renal artery stenosis; pregnancy (2nd and 3rd trimesters)

Warnings/Precautions Anaphylactic or anaphylactoid reactions can occur. Use with caution and modify dosage in patients with renal impairment (especially renal artery stenosis), severe CHF. Severe hypotension may occur in the elderly and patients who are sodium and/or volume depleted, initiate lower doses and monitor closely when starting therapy in these patients. Angioedema can occur at any time during treatment (especially following first dose). It may involve head and neck (potentially affecting the airway) or the intestine (presenting with abdominal pain). Prolonged monitoring may be required especially if tongue, glottis, or larynx are involved as they are associated with airway obstruction. Those with a history of airway surgery in this situation have a higher risk. **[U.S. Boxed Warning]: Based on human data, ACEIs can cause injury and death to the developing fetus when used in the second and third trimesters. ACEIs should be discontinued as soon as possible once pregnancy is detected.** Careful blood pressure monitoring with first dose (hypotension can occur especially in volume-depleted patients). Use with caution in hypovolemia; collagen vascular diseases; valvular stenosis (particularly aortic stenosis); hyperkalemia; or before, during, or immediately after anesthesia. Avoid rapid dosage escalation, which may lead to renal insufficiency. Hyperkalemia may rarely occur. Rare toxicities associated with ACE inhibitors include cholestatic jaundice (which may progress to hepatic necrosis) and neutropenia/agranulocytosis with myeloid hyperplasia. May be associated with deterioration of renal function and/or increases in serum creatinine, particularly in patients dependent on renin-angiotensin-aldosterone system. Use with caution in unilateral renal artery stenosis and pre-existing renal insufficiency; if patient has renal impairment then a baseline WBC with differential and serum creatinine should be evaluated and monitored closely during the first 3 months of therapy. Hypersensitivity reactions may be seen during hemodialysis with high-flux dialysis membranes (eg, AN69). Safety and efficacy have not been established in children.

Drug Interactions

Increased Effect/Toxicity: Potassium supplements, co-trimoxazole (high dose), angiotensin II receptor antagonists (eg, candesartan, losartan, irbesartan), or potassium-sparing diuretics (amiloride, spironolactone, triamterene) may result in elevated serum potassium levels when combined with ramipril. ACE inhibitor effects may be increased by phenothiazines or probenecid (increases levels of captopril). ACE inhibitors may increase serum concentrations/effects of lithium. ACE inhibitors may enhance the adverse/toxic effects (nitritoid reaction) of gold sodium thiomalate.

Diuretics have additive hypotensive effects with ACE inhibitors, and hypovolemia increases the potential for adverse renal effects of ACE inhibitors. In patients with compromised renal function, coadministration with NSAIDs may result in further deterioration of renal function. Allopurinol and ACE inhibitors may cause a higher risk of hypersensitivity reaction when taken concurrently.

Decreased Effect: Aspirin (high dose) may reduce the therapeutic effects of ACE inhibitors; at low dosages this does not appear to be significant. Rifampin may decrease the effect of ACE inhibitors. Antacids may decrease

(Continued)

Ramipril *(Continued)*

the bioavailability of ACE inhibitors (may be more likely to occur with capto-pril); separate administration times by 1-2 hours. NSAIDs, specifically indo-methacin, may reduce the hypotensive effects of ACE inhibitors. More likely to occur in low renin or volume dependent hypertensive patients.

Ethanol/Nutrition/Herb Interactions Herb/Nutraceutical: Avoid dong quai if using for hypertension (has estrogenic activity). Avoid ephedra, yohimbe, ginseng (may worsen hypertension). Avoid garlic (may have increased antihy-pertensive effect).

Pharmacodynamics/Kinetics

Onset of action: 1-2 hours

Duration: 24 hours

Absorption: Well absorbed (50% to 60%)

Distribution: Plasma levels decline in a triphasic fashion; rapid decline is a distribution phase to peripheral compartment, plasma protein and tissue ACE (half-life 2-4 hours); 2nd phase is an apparent elimination phase representing the clearance of free ramiprilat (half-life: 9-18 hours); and final phase is the terminal elimination phase representing the equilibrium phase between tissue binding and dissociation

Metabolism: Hepatic to the active form, ramiprilat

Half-life elimination: Ramiprilat: Effective: 13-17 hours; Terminal: >50 hours

Time to peak, serum: ~1 hour

Excretion: Urine (60%) and feces (40%) as parent drug and metabolites

Pregnancy Risk Factor C (1st trimester)/D (2nd and 3rd trimesters)

Dosage Forms

Capsule:

Altace®: 1.25 mg, 2.5 mg, 5 mg, 10 mg

Ranexa™ *see* Ranolazine *on page 1411*

Ranibizumab *(ra nib i ZUE mab)*

U.S. Brand Names Lucentis®

Generic Available No

Index Terms rhuFabV2

Pharmacologic Category Monoclonal Antibody; Ophthalmic Agent; Vascular Endothelial Growth Factor (VEGF) Inhibitor

Use Treatment of neovascular (wet) age-related macular degeneration (AMD)

Local Anesthetic/Vasoconstrictor Precautions No information available to require special precautions

Effects on Dental Treatment No significant effects or complications reported

Common Adverse Effects Note: Rates of ocular adverse reactions reported for control group when percentages overlapped with treatment group.

>10%:

Central nervous system: Headache (2% to 15%)

Neuromuscular & skeletal: Arthralgia (3% to 11%)

Ocular: Conjunctival hemorrhage (43% to 77%; control: 29% to 66%), eye pain (17% to 37%; control 11% to 33%), vitreous floaters (3% to 32%), retinal hemorrhage (15% to 26%; control 37% to 56%), intraocular pressure increased (8% to 24%), vitreous detachment (7% to 22%; control 13% to 18%), intraocular inflammation (5% to 18%; control 3% to 11%), eye irrita-tion (4% to 19%; control 6% to 20%), visual disturbance (up to 14%), blepharitis (3% to 13%)

Note: Cataract, foreign body sensation, lacrimation increased, pruritus, and subretinal fibrosis occurred in >10% of patients, but also occurred in similar percentages to the control; visual acuity blurred/decreased occurred more often in the control.

Respiratory: Nasopharyngitis (5% to 16%), upper respiratory tract infection (2% to 15%)

1% to 10%:

Cardiovascular: Arterial thromboembolic events (up to 5%; stroke up to 3%)

Gastrointestinal: Nausea (2% to 9%)

Ocular: Conjunctival hyperemia (up to 9%), posterior capsule opacification (up to 8%)

Note: Ocular hyperemia, maculopathy, dry eye, and ocular discomfort occurred in 1% to 10% of patients, but also occurred in similar percent-ages to the control; retinal exudates occurred more often in the control.

Respiratory: Bronchitis (3% to 10%), cough (3% to 10%), sinusitis (2% to 8%)

Miscellaneous: Influenza (2% to 10%), ranibizumab antibodies (1% to 6%)

Mechanism of Action Ranibizumab is a recombinant humanized monoclonal antibody fragment which binds to and inhibits human vascular endothelial growth factor A (VEGF-A). Ranibizumab inhibits VEGF from binding to its receptors and thereby suppressing neovascularization and slowing vision loss.

Pharmacodynamics/Kinetics

Absorption: Low levels are detected in the serum following intravitreal injection
Half-life elimination: Vitreous: 9 days

Pregnancy Risk Factor C

Raniclor™ *see Cefaclor on page 295*

Ranitidine (ra NI ti deen)

Related Information
Gastrointestinal Disorders *on page 1745*

U.S. Brand Names Zantac®; Zantac 75® [OTC]; Zantac 150™ [OTC]; Zantac® EFFERdose®

Canadian Brand Names Alti-Ranitidine; Apo-Ranitidine®; BCI-Ranitidine; CO Ranitidine; Gen-Ranidine; Novo-Ranidine; Nu-Ranit; PMS-Ranitidine; Ranitidine Injection, USP; Rhoxal-ranitidine; Sandoz-Ranitidine; Zantac®; Zantac 75®

Mexican Brand Names Acloral; Anistal; Azantac; Galidrin; Iqfadina; Microtid; Ranisen

Generic Available Yes: Excludes effervescent tablet

Index Terms Ranitidine Hydrochloride

Pharmacologic Category Histamine H_2 Antagonist

Use
Zantac®: Short-term and maintenance therapy of duodenal ulcer, gastric ulcer, gastroesophageal reflux, active benign ulcer, erosive esophagitis, and pathological hypersecretory conditions; as part of a multidrug regimen for *H. pylori* eradication to reduce the risk of duodenal ulcer recurrence
Zantac® 75 [OTC]: Relief of heartburn, acid indigestion, and sour stomach

Unlabeled/Investigational Use Recurrent postoperative ulcer, upper GI bleeding, prevention of acid-aspiration pneumonitis during surgery, and prevention of stress-induced ulcers

Local Anesthetic/Vasoconstrictor Precautions No information available to require special precautions

Effects on Dental Treatment No significant effects or complications reported

Common Adverse Effects Frequency not defined.
Cardiovascular: Atrioventricular block, bradycardia, premature ventricular beats, tachycardia, vasculitis
Central nervous system: Agitation, dizziness, depression, hallucinations, headache, insomnia, malaise, mental confusion, somnolence, vertigo
Dermatologic: Alopecia, erythema multiforme, rash
Endocrine & metabolic: Increased prolactin levels
Gastrointestinal: Abdominal discomfort/pain, constipation, diarrhea, nausea, pancreatitis, vomiting
Hematologic: Acquired hemolytic anemia, agranulocytosis, aplastic anemia, granulocytopenia, leukopenia, pancytopenia, thrombocytopenia
Hepatic: Hepatic failure, hepatitis
Local: Transient pain, burning or itching at the injection site
Neuromuscular & skeletal: Arthralgia, involuntary motor disturbance, myalgia
Ocular: Blurred vision
Renal: Increased serum creatinine
Respiratory: Pneumonia (causal relationship not established)
Miscellaneous: Anaphylaxis, angioneurotic edema, hypersensitivity reactions

Dosage
Children 1 month to 16 years:
Duodenal and gastric ulcer:
Oral:
Treatment: 2-4 mg/kg/day divided twice daily; maximum treatment dose: 300 mg/day
Maintenance: 2-4 mg/kg once daily; maximum maintenance dose: 150 mg/day
I.V.: 2-4 mg/kg/day divided every 6-8 hours; maximum: 200 mg/day
GERD and erosive esophagitis:
Oral: 5-10 mg/kg/day divided twice daily; maximum: GERD: 300 mg/day, erosive esophagitis: 600 mg/day
I.V. (unlabeled): 2-4 mg/kg/day divided every 6-8 hours; maximum: 200 mg/day **or as an alternative**
Continuous infusion: Initial: 1 mg/kg/dose for one dose followed by infusion of 0.08-0.17 mg/kg/hour or 2-4 mg/kg/day
Children ≥12 years: Prevention of heartburn: Oral: Zantac® 75 [OTC]: 75 mg 30-60 minutes before eating food or drinking beverages which cause heartburn; maximum: 150 mg/24 hours; do not use for more than 14 days
(Continued)

Ranitidine *(Continued)*

Adults:

    Duodenal ulcer: Oral: Treatment: 150 mg twice daily, or 300 mg once daily after the evening meal or at bedtime; maintenance: 150 mg once daily at bedtime

    Helicobacter pylori eradication: 150 mg twice daily; requires combination therapy

    Pathological hypersecretory conditions:

      Oral: 150 mg twice daily; adjust dose or frequency as clinically indicated; doses of up to 6 g/day have been used

      I.V.: Continuous infusion for Zollinger-Ellison: 1 mg/kg/hour; measure gastric acid output at 4 hours, if >10 mEq or if patient is symptomatic, increase dose in increments of 0.5 mg/kg/hour; doses of up to 2.5 mg/kg/hour have been used

    Gastric ulcer, benign: Oral: 150 mg twice daily; maintenance: 150 mg once daily at bedtime

    Erosive esophagitis: Oral: Treatment: 150 mg 4 times/day; maintenance: 150 mg twice daily

    Prevention of heartburn: Oral: Zantac® 75 [OTC]: 75 mg 30-60 minutes before eating food or drinking beverages which cause heartburn; maximum: 150 mg in 24 hours; do not use for more than 14 days

    Patients not able to take oral medication:

      I.M.: 50 mg every 6-8 hours

      I.V.: Intermittent bolus or infusion: 50 mg every 6-8 hours

      Continuous I.V. infusion: 6.25 mg/hour

Elderly: Ulcer healing rates and incidence of adverse effects are similar in the elderly, when compared to younger patients; dosing adjustments not necessary based on age alone

Dosing adjustment in renal impairment: Adults: Cl_{cr} <50 mL/minute:

    Oral: 150 mg every 24 hours; adjust dose cautiously if needed

    I.V.: 50 mg every 18-24 hours; adjust dose cautiously if needed

    Hemodialysis: Adjust dosing schedule so that dose coincides with the end of hemodialysis

Dosing adjustment/comments in hepatic disease: Patients with hepatic impairment may have minor changes in ranitidine half-life, distribution, clearance, and bioavailability; dosing adjustments not necessary, monitor

Mechanism of Action Competitive inhibition of histamine at H_2-receptors of the gastric parietal cells, which inhibits gastric acid secretion, gastric volume, and hydrogen ion concentration are reduced. Does not affect pepsin secretion, pentagastrin-stimulated intrinsic factor secretion, or serum gastrin.

Contraindications Hypersensitivity to ranitidine or any component of the formulation

Warnings/Precautions Ranitidine has been associated with confusional states (rare). Use with caution in patients with hepatic impairment; use with caution in renal impairment, dosage modification required. Avoid use in patients with history of acute porphyria (may precipitate attacks); long-term therapy may be associated with vitamin B_{12} deficiency. Symptoms of GI distress may be associated with a variety of conditions; symptomatic response to H_2 antagonists does not rule out the potential for significant pathology (eg, malignancy). EFFERdose® formulations contain phenylalanine. Safety and efficacy of ranitidine have not been established for pediatric patients <1 month of age

Drug Interactions

    Cytochrome P450 Effect: Substrate (minor) of CYP1A2, 2C19, 2D6; **Inhibits** CYP1A2 (weak), 2D6 (weak)

    Increased Effect/Toxicity: Increased the effect/toxicity of cyclosporine (increased serum creatinine).

    Decreased Effect: Ranitidine may have variable effects on warfarin (monitor INR closely). The absorption/efficacy of ketoconazole and itraconazole are decreased by ranitidine; avoid concurrent therapy. The absorption of some cephalosporins (cefuroxime, cefpodoxime) may be reduced by ranitidine (separate administrations times by at least 2 hours). The absorption of atazanavir and cyanocobalamin may be decreased by ranitidine.

Ethanol/Nutrition/Herb Interactions

    Ethanol: Avoid ethanol (may cause gastric mucosal irritation).

    Food: Does not interfere with absorption of ranitidine.

Dietary Considerations Oral dosage forms may be taken with or without food.

    Zantac® EFFERdose®:

      Effervescent tablet 25 mg contains sodium 1.33 mEq/tablet and phenylalanine 2.81 mg/tablet

      Effervescent tablet 150 mg contains sodium 7.96 mEq/tablet and phenylalanine 16.84 mg/tablet

Pharmacodynamics/Kinetics

Absorption: Oral: 50%

Distribution: Normal renal function: V_d: 1.7 L/kg; Cl_{cr} 25-35 mL/minute: 1.76 L/kg minimally penetrates the blood-brain barrier; enters breast milk

Protein binding: 15%

Metabolism: Hepatic to N-oxide, S-oxide, and N-desmethyl metabolites

Bioavailability: Oral: 48%

Half-life elimination:

Oral: Normal renal function: 2.5-3 hours; Cl_{cr} 25-35 mL/minute: 4.8 hours

I.V.: Normal renal function: 2-2.5 hours

Time to peak, serum: Oral: 2-3 hours; I.M.: ≤15 minutes

Excretion: Urine: Oral: 30%, I.V.: 70% (as unchanged drug); feces (as metabolites)

Pregnancy Risk Factor B

Dosage Forms

Capsule: 150 mg, 300 mg

Infusion [premixed in NaCl 0.45%; preservative free]: 50 mg (50 mL)
Zantac®: 50 mg (50 mL)

Injection, solution: 25 mg/mL (2 mL, 6 mL)
Zantac®: 25 mg/mL (2 mL, 6 mL, 40 mL)

Syrup: 15 mg/mL
Zantac®: 15 mg/mL

Tablet: 75 mg [OTC], 150 mg, 300 mg
Zantac®: 150 mg, 300 mg
Zantac 75® [OTC]: 75 mg
Zantac 150™ [OTC]: 150 mg

Tablet, effervescent:
Zantac® EFFERdose®: 25 mg, 150 mg

Ranitidine Hydrochloride *see* Ranitidine *on page 1409*

Ranolazine (ra NOE la zeen)

U.S. Brand Names Ranexa™
Generic Available No
Pharmacologic Category Cardiovascular Agent, Miscellaneous
Use Treatment of chronic angina in combination with amlodipine, beta-blockers, or nitrates

Local Anesthetic/Vasoconstrictor Precautions Ranolazine is one of the drugs confirmed to prolong the QT interval and is accepted as having a risk of causing torsade de pointes. The risk of drug-induced torsade de pointes is extremely low when a single QT interval prolonging drug is prescribed. In terms of epinephrine, it is not known what effect vasoconstrictors in the local anesthetic regimen will have in patients with a known history of congenital prolonged QT interval or in patients taking any medication that prolongs the QT interval. Until more information is obtained, it is suggested that the clinician consult with the physician prior to the use of a vasoconstrictor in suspected patients, and that the vasoconstrictor (epinephrine, levonordefrin [Neo-Cobefrin®]) be used with caution.

Effects on Dental Treatment Key adverse event(s) related to dental treatment: Xerostomia (normal salivary flow resumes upon discontinuation).

Common Adverse Effects

>10%: Gastrointestinal: Constipation (5% to 8%; 19% in the elderly)

>0.5% to 10%:

Cardiovascular: Syncope (0.7%), palpitation, peripheral edema

Central nervous system: Dizziness (5% to 6%), headache (3% to 6%), vertigo

Gastrointestinal: Nausea (4% to 6%), abdominal pain, vomiting, xerostomia

Hematologic: Hematocrit decreased

Neuromuscular & skeletal: Weakness

Respiratory: Dyspnea

Mechanism of Action A proposed mechanism suggests ranolazine is a partial fatty acid oxidation inhibitor; may change myocardial energy metabolism from fatty acids to glucose, increasing the efficiency of ATP production under hypoxic conditions. Exerts antianginal and anti-ischemic effects without changing hemodynamic parameters. In addition, it is a late sodium channel inhibitor.

Drug Interactions

Cytochrome P450 Effect: Substrate of CYP3A4 (major), 2D6 (minor); **Inhibits** CYP3A4 (weak), 2D6 (weak)

Increased Effect/Toxicity: CYP3A4 inhibitors (eg, diltiazem, ketoconazole, verapamil) may increase the effects of ranolazine. Ranolazine may increase the effects of simvastatin and digoxin. Concurrent use of QT_c-prolonging agents may further increase QT interval.

(Continued)

Ranolazine *(Continued)*

Decreased Effect: CYP3A4 inducers may decrease the effect of ranolazine.

Pharmacodynamics/Kinetics

Absorption: Highly variable; ranolazine is a substrate of P-glycoprotein; concurrent use of P-glycoprotein inhibitors may increase absorption

Protein binding: 62%

Metabolism: Hepatic via CYP3A (major) and 2D6 (minor)

Half-life elimination: Terminal: 7 hours

Time to peak, plasma: 2-5 hours

Excretion: Primarily urine (75% mostly as metabolites, <5% to 7% excreted unchanged); feces (25% mostly as metabolites)

Rapamune® *see* Sirolimus *on page 1475*

Raphon [OTC] *see* Epinephrine *on page 572*

Raptiva® *see* Efalizumab *on page 557*

Rasagiline (ra SA ji leen)

U.S. Brand Names Azilect®

Generic Available No

Index Terms AGN 1135; Rasagiline Mesylate; TVP-1012

Pharmacologic Category Anti-Parkinson's Agent, MAO Type B Inhibitor

Use Initial monotherapy or as adjunct to levodopa in the treatment of idiopathic Parkinson's disease

Local Anesthetic/Vasoconstrictor Precautions Rasagiline in approved doses of 0.5-1 mg daily should not inhibit type-A MAO; however, the possibility exists of nonselective MAO inhibition at higher doses and/or in certain sensitive individuals. Therefore, attempts should be made to avoid use of vasoconstrictors due to possibility of hypertensive episodes.

Effects on Dental Treatment Key adverse event(s) related to dental treatment: Xerostomia and changes in salivation (normal salivary flow resumes upon discontinuation). Anticholinergic side effects can cause a reduction of saliva production or secretion, contributing to discomfort and dental disease (ie, caries, oral candidiasis, and periodontal disease). May cause orthostatic hypotension particularly during the first 2 months of therapy.

Common Adverse Effects Unless otherwise noted, the following adverse reactions are as reported for monotherapy. Spectrum of adverse events was generally similar with adjunctive (levodopa) therapy, though the incidence tended to be higher.

>10%:

Central nervous system: Dyskinesia (18% adjunct therapy), headache (14%)

Gastrointestinal: Nausea (10% to 12% adjunct therapy)

1% to 10%:

Cardiovascular: Postural hypotension (6% to 9% adjunct therapy; dose dependent), bundle branch block angina, chest pain, syncope

Central nervous system: Depression (5%), hallucinations (4% to 5% adjunct therapy), fever (3%), malaise (2%), vertigo (2%), anxiety, dizziness

Dermatologic: Bruising (2%), alopecia, skin carcinoma, vesiculobullous rash

Endocrine & metabolic: Impotence, libido decreased

Gastrointestinal: Constipation (4% to 9% adjunct therapy), weight loss (2% to 9% adjunct therapy; dose dependent), dyspepsia (7%), xerostomia (2% to 6% adjunct therapy; dose dependent), gastroenteritis (3%), anorexia, diarrhea, gastrointestinal hemorrhage, vomiting

Genitourinary: Hematuria, urinary incontinence

Hematologic: Leukopenia

Hepatic: Liver function tests increased

Neuromuscular & skeletal: Arthralgia (7%), neck pain (2%), arthritis (2%), paresthesia (2%), abnormal gait, hyperkinesias, hypertonia, neuropathy, tremor, weakness

Ocular: Conjunctivitis (3%)

Renal: Albuminuria

Respiratory: Rhinitis (3%), asthma, cough increased

Miscellaneous: Fall (5%), flu-like syndrome (5%), allergic reaction

Mechanism of Action Potent, irreversible and selective inhibitor of brain monoamine oxidase (MAO) type B, which plays a major role in the catabolism of dopamine. Inhibition of dopamine depletion in the striatal region of the brain reduces the symptomatic motor deficits of Parkinson's disease. There is also experimental evidence of rasagiline conferring neuroprotective effects (antioxidant, antiapoptotic), which may delay onset of symptoms and progression of neuronal deterioration.

Drug Interactions

Cytochrome P450 Effect: Substrate of CYP1A2 (major)

Increased Effect/Toxicity: CYP1A2 inhibitors may increase the levels/effects of rasagiline (example inhibitors include amiodarone, ciprofloxacin, fluvoxamine, ketoconazole, norfloxacin, and ofloxacin). Concurrent use of rasagiline in combination with amphetamines, methylphenidate, dextromethorphan, meperidine, methadone, mirtazapine, propoxyphene, tramadol, tricyclic or tetracyclic antidepressants may result in serotonin syndrome; these combinations are contraindicated. Concurrent use of rasagiline with an SSRI or SNRI may result in mania or hypertension; it is generally best to avoid these combinations.

Decreased Effect: CYP1A2 Inducers may decrease the levels/effects of rasagiline (example inducers include aminoglutethimide, carbamazepine, phenobarbital, and rifampin).

Pharmacodynamics/Kinetics

Onset of action: Therapeutic: Within 1 hour

Duration: ~1 week (irreversible inhibition); may require ~14-40 days for complete restoration of (brain) MAO-B activity

Absorption: Rapid

Protein binding: 88% to 94%

Metabolism: Hepatic N-dealkylation and/or hydroxylation via CYP1A2 to multiple inactive metabolites (nonamphetamine derivatives)

Distribution: V_{dss}: 87 L

Bioavailability: 36%

Half-life elimination: ~1.3-3 hours (no correlation with biologic effect due to irreversible inhibition)

Time to peak, plasma: 30 minutes to 1 hour

Excretion: Urine (62%, >99% as metabolites); feces (7%)

Pregnancy Risk Factor C

Rasagiline Mesylate *see* Rasagiline *on page 1412*

Rasburicase (ras BYOOR i kayse)

U.S. Brand Names Elitek™

Canadian Brand Names Fasturtec®

Generic Available No

Index Terms NSC-721631; Recombinant Urate Oxidase

Pharmacologic Category Enzyme; Enzyme, Urate-Oxidase (Recombinant)

Use Initial management of uric acid levels in pediatric patients with leukemia, lymphoma, and solid tumor malignancies receiving anticancer therapy expected to result in tumor lysis and elevation of plasma uric acid

Unlabeled/Investigational Use Prevention and treatment of malignancy-associated hyperuricemia in adults

Local Anesthetic/Vasoconstrictor Precautions No information available to require special precautions

Effects on Dental Treatment Key adverse event(s) related to dental treatment: Mucositis.

Common Adverse Effects As reported in patients receiving rasburicase with antitumor therapy versus active-control:

>10%:

Central nervous system: Fever (5% to 46%), headache (26%)

Dermatologic: Rash (13%)

Gastrointestinal: Vomiting (50%), nausea (27%), abdominal pain (20%), constipation (20%), mucositis (2% to 15%), diarrhea (≤1% to 20%)

1% to 10%:

Hematologic: Neutropenia with fever (4%), neutropenia (2%)

Respiratory: Respiratory distress (3%)

Miscellaneous: Sepsis (3%)

Mechanism of Action Rasburicase is a recombinant urate-oxidase enzyme, which converts uric acid to allantoin (an inactive and soluble metabolite of uric acid); it does not inhibit the formation of uric acid.

Pharmacodynamics/Kinetics

Distribution: Pediatric patients: 110-127 mL/kg

Half-life elimination: Pediatric patients: 18 hours

Pregnancy Risk Factor C

Razadyne™ *see* Galantamine *on page 762*

Razadyne™ ER *see* Galantamine *on page 762*

Readi-Cat® *see* Barium *on page 185*

Readi-Cat® 2 *see* Barium *on page 185*

Rea-Lo® [OTC] *see* Urea *on page 1632*

ReAzo [OTC] *see* Phenazopyridine *on page 1286*

Rebetol® *see* Ribavirin *on page 1420*

Rebetron® *see* Interferon Alfa-2b and Ribavirin *on page 895*

Rebif® *see* Interferon Beta-1a *on page 897*

Reclast® *see* Zoledronic Acid *on page 1685*

Reclipsen™ *see* Ethinyl Estradiol and Desogestrel *on page 621*

Recombinant α-L-Iduronidase (Glycosaminoglycan α-L-Iduronohydrolase) *see* Laronidase *on page 951*

Recombinant Hirudin *see* Lepirudin *on page 956*

Recombinant Human Deoxyribonuclease *see* Dornase Alfa *on page 527*

Recombinant Human Insulin-Like Growth Factor-1 *see* Mecasermin *on page 1023*

Recombinant Human Interleukin-11 *see* Oprelvekin *on page 1210*

Recombinant Human Luteinizing Hormone *see* Lutropin Alfa *on page 1011*

Recombinant Human Parathyroid Hormone (1-34) *see* Teriparatide *on page 1541*

Recombinant Human Platelet-Derived Growth Factor B *see* Becaplermin *on page 187*

Recombinant Interleukin-11 *see* Oprelvekin *on page 1210*

Recombinant N-Acetylgalactosamine 4-Sulfatase *see* Galsulfase *on page 763*

Recombinant Plasminogen Activator *see* Reteplase *on page 1417*

Recombinant Urate Oxidase *see* Rasburicase *on page 1413*

Recombinate *see* Antihemophilic Factor (Recombinant) *on page 132*

Recombivax HB® *see* Hepatitis B Vaccine *on page 811*

Rectacaine [OTC] *see* Phenylephrine *on page 1293*

Red Cross™ Canker Sore [OTC] *see* Benzocaine *on page 195*

Reese's® Pinworm Medicine [OTC] *see* Pyrantel Pamoate *on page 1387*

ReFacto® *see* Antihemophilic Factor (Recombinant) *on page 132*

Refenesen Plus [OTC] *see* Guaifenesin and Pseudoephedrine *on page 798*

Refludan® *see* Lepirudin *on page 956*

Refresh® [OTC] *see* Artificial Tears *on page 147*

Refresh Liquigel™ [OTC] *see* Carboxymethylcellulose *on page 285*

Refresh Plus® [OTC] *see* Artificial Tears *on page 147*

Refresh Plus® [OTC] *see* Carboxymethylcellulose *on page 285*

Refresh Tears® [OTC] *see* Artificial Tears *on page 147*

Refresh Tears® [OTC] *see* Carboxymethylcellulose *on page 285*

Regitine [DSC] *see* Phentolamine *on page 1292*

Reglan® *see* Metoclopramide *on page 1086*

Regonol® *see* Pyridostigmine *on page 1389*

Regranex® *see* Becaplermin *on page 187*

Regular Insulin *see* Insulin Regular *on page 889*

Reguloid® [OTC] *see* Psyllium *on page 1386*

Relacon-DM NR *see* Guaifenesin, Pseudoephedrine, and Dextromethorphan *on page 800*

Relafen® [DSC] *see* Nabumetone *on page 1137*

Relenza® *see* Zanamivir *on page 1677*

Relera *see* Chlorpheniramine and Phenylephrine *on page 340*

Relief® [OTC] *see* Phenylephrine *on page 1293*

Relpax® *see* Eletriptan *on page 561*

Remeron® *see* Mirtazapine *on page 1110*

Remeron SolTab® *see* Mirtazapine *on page 1110*

Reme-T™ [OTC] *see* Coal Tar *on page 402*

Remicade® *see* Infliximab *on page 879*

Remifentanil (rem i FEN ta nil)

U.S. Brand Names Ultiva®

Canadian Brand Names Ultiva®

Generic Available No

Index Terms GI87084B

Pharmacologic Category Analgesic, Opioid

Use Analgesic for use during the induction and maintenance of general anesthesia; for continued analgesia into the immediate postoperative period; analgesic component of monitored anesthesia

Unlabeled/Investigational Use Management of pain in mechanically-ventilated patients

Local Anesthetic/Vasoconstrictor Precautions No information available to require special precautions

Effects on Dental Treatment No significant effects or complications reported

Common Adverse Effects
>10%: Gastrointestinal: Nausea, vomiting
1% to 10%:
Cardiovascular: Hypotension (dose dependent), bradycardia (dose dependent), tachycardia, hypertension
Central nervous system: Dizziness, headache, agitation, fever
Dermatologic: Pruritus
Neuromuscular & skeletal: Muscle rigidity (dose dependent)
Ocular: Visual disturbances
Respiratory: Respiratory depression, apnea, hypoxia
Miscellaneous: Shivering, postoperative pain

Restrictions C-II

Mechanism of Action Binds with stereospecific mu-opioid receptors at many sites within the CNS, increases pain threshold, alters pain reception, inhibits ascending pain pathways

Drug Interactions
Increased Effect/Toxicity: Additive effects with other CNS depressants. Synergistic with other anesthetics, may need to decrease thiopental, propofol, isoflurane, and midazolam by up to 75%.

Pharmacodynamics/Kinetics
Onset of action: I.V.: 1-3 minutes
Distribution: V_d: 100 mL/kg; increased in children
Protein binding: ~70% (primarily alpha$_1$ acid glycoprotein)
Metabolism: Rapid via blood and tissue esterases
Half-life elimination (dose dependent): Terminal: 10-20 minutes; effective: 3-10 minutes
Excretion: Urine

Pregnancy Risk Factor C

Repaglinide (re PAG li nide)

Related Information
Endocrine Disorders and Pregnancy on page 1750
U.S. Brand Names Prandin®
Canadian Brand Names GlucoNorm®; Prandin®
Mexican Brand Names NovoNorm
Generic Available No
Pharmacologic Category Antidiabetic Agent, Meglitinide Derivative
Use Management of type 2 diabetes mellitus (noninsulin dependent, NIDDM); may be used in combination with metformin or thiazolidinediones
Local Anesthetic/Vasoconstrictor Precautions No information available to require special precautions
Effects on Dental Treatment Key adverse event(s) related to dental treatment: Tooth disorder.
Common Adverse Effects
>10%:
Central nervous system: Headache (9% to 11%)
Endocrine & metabolic: Hypoglycemia (16% to 31%)
Respiratory: Upper respiratory tract infection (10% to 16%)
1% to 10%:
Cardiovascular: Ischemia (4%), chest pain (2% to 3%)
(Continued)

Repaglinide *(Continued)*

Gastrointestinal: Diarrhea (4% to 5%), constipation (2% to 3%), tooth disorder (<1% to 2%)

Genitourinary: Urinary tract infection (2% to 3%)

Neuromuscular & skeletal: Arthralgia (3% to 6%), back pain (5% to 6%)

Respiratory: Sinusitis (3% to 6%), bronchitis (2% to 6%)

Miscellaneous: Allergy (1% to 2%)

Mechanism of Action Nonsulfonylurea hypoglycemic agent of the meglitinide class (the nonsulfonylurea moiety of glyburide) used in the management of type 2 diabetes mellitus; stimulates insulin release from the pancreatic beta cells

Drug Interactions

Cytochrome P450 Effect: Substrate of CYP2C8 (major), 3A4 (major)

Increased Effect/Toxicity: Concurrent use of other hypoglycemic agents may increase risk of hypoglycemia. Gemfibrozil may increase the serum concentration of repaglinide (resulting in severe, prolonged hypoglycemia), and the addition of itraconazole may augment the effects of gemfibrozil on repaglinide. Macrolide antibiotics or trimethoprim may increase the effects of repaglinide. CYP2C8 Inhibitors may increase the levels/effects of repaglinide; example inhibitors include atazanavir, gemfibrozil, and ritonavir. CYP3A4 inhibitors may increase the levels/effects of repaglinide; example inhibitors include azole antifungals, clarithromycin, diclofenac, doxycycline, erythromycin, imatinib, isoniazid, nefazodone, nicardipine, propofol, protease inhibitors, quinidine, telithromycin, and verapamil.

Decreased Effect: CYP2C8 inducers may decrease the levels/effects of repaglinide; example inducers include carbamazepine, phenobarbital, phenytoin, rifampin, rifapentine, and secobarbital. CYP3A4 inducers may decrease the levels/effects of repaglinide; example inducers include aminoglutethimide, carbamazepine, nafcillin, nevirapine, phenobarbital, phenytoin, and rifamycins.

Pharmacodynamics/Kinetics

Onset of action: Single dose: Increased insulin levels: ~15-60 minutes

Duration: 4-6 hours

Absorption: Rapid and complete

Distribution: V_d: 31 L

Protein binding, plasma: >98%

Metabolism: Hepatic via CYP3A4 isoenzyme and glucuronidation to inactive metabolites

Bioavailability: Mean absolute: ~56%

Half-life elimination: 1 hour

Time to peak, plasma: ~1 hour

Excretion: Within 96 hours: Feces (~90%, <2% as parent drug); Urine (~8%)

Pregnancy Risk Factor C

Repan® *see* Butalbital, Acetaminophen, and Caffeine *on page 247*

Replace [OTC] *see* Vitamins (Multiple/Oral) *on page 1665*

Replace with Iron [OTC] *see* Vitamins (Multiple/Oral) *on page 1665*

Repliva 21/7™ *see* Vitamins (Multiple/Oral) *on page 1665*

Reprexain™ *see* Hydrocodone and Ibuprofen *on page 830*

Repronex® *see* Menotropins *on page 1037*

Requip® *see* Ropinirole *on page 1442*

Rescon® *see* Chlorpheniramine, Phenylephrine, and Methscopolamine *on page 342*

Rescon® MX *see* Chlorpheniramine, Phenylephrine, and Methscopolamine *on page 342*

Rescon GG *see* Guaifenesin and Phenylephrine *on page 797*

Rescon-Jr *see* Chlorpheniramine and Phenylephrine *on page 340*

Rescriptor® *see* Delavirdine *on page 453*

Reserpine *(re SER peen)*

Related Information

Cardiovascular Diseases *on page 1726*

Generic Available Yes

Pharmacologic Category Central Monoamine-Depleting Agent; Rauwolfia Alkaloid

Use Management of mild-to-moderate hypertension; treatment of agitated psychotic states (schizophrenia)

Unlabeled/Investigational Use Management of tardive dyskinesia

Local Anesthetic/Vasoconstrictor Precautions No information available to require special precautions

Effects on Dental Treatment Key adverse event(s) related to dental treatment: Xerostomia and changes in salivation (normal salivary flow resumes upon discontinuation).

Mechanism of Action Reduces blood pressure via depletion of sympathetic biogenic amines (norepinephrine and dopamine); this also commonly results in sedative effects

Pregnancy Risk Factor C

Retapamulin (re te PAM ue lin)

U.S. Brand Names Altabax™
Generic Available No
Pharmacologic Category Antibiotic, Pleuromutilin; Antibiotic, Topical
Use Treatment of impetigo caused by susceptible strains of *S. pyogenes* or methicillin-susceptible *S. aureus*
Local Anesthetic/Vasoconstrictor Precautions No information available to require special precautions
Effects on Dental Treatment No significant effects or complications reported
Common Adverse Effects 1% to 10%:
Central nervous system: Headache (1% to 2%), pyrexia (1%)
Dermatologic: Pruritus (2%), eczema (1%)
Gastrointestinal: Diarrhea (1% to 2%), nausea (1%)
Local: Application site irritation (2%), application site pruritus (2%)
Respiratory: Nasopharyngitis (1% to 2%)
Mechanism of Action Primarily bacteriostatic. Inhibits normal bacterial protein biosynthesis by binding at a unique site (protein L3) on the ribosomal 50S subunit; prevents formation of active 50S ribosomal subunits by inhibiting peptidyl transfer and blocking P-site interactions at this site
Pharmacodynamics/Kinetics
Absorption: Topical: Low; increased when applied to abraded skin
Protein binding: 94%
Metabolism: Hepatic via CYP 3A4; extensively metabolized by mono-oxygenation and di-oxygenation to multiple metabolites
Pregnancy Risk Factor B

Reteplase (RE ta plase)

Related Information
Cardiovascular Diseases *on page 1726*
U.S. Brand Names Retavase®
Canadian Brand Names Retavase®
Generic Available No
Index Terms Recombinant Plasminogen Activator; r-PA
Pharmacologic Category Thrombolytic Agent
Use Management of acute myocardial infarction (AMI); improvement of ventricular function; reduction of the incidence of CHF and the reduction of mortality following AMI
Local Anesthetic/Vasoconstrictor Precautions No information available to require special precautions
Effects on Dental Treatment No significant effects or complications reported
Common Adverse Effects Bleeding is the most frequent adverse effect associated with reteplase. Heparin and aspirin have been administered concurrently with reteplase in clinical trials. The incidence of adverse events is a reflection of these combined therapies, and are comparable with comparison thrombolytics.

>10%: Local: Injection site bleeding (4.6% to 48.6%)
1% to 10%:
Gastrointestinal: Bleeding (1.8% to 9.0%)
Genitourinary: Bleeding (0.9% to 9.5%)
Hematologic: Anemia (0.9% to 2.6%)
(Continued)

Reteplase *(Continued)*

Other adverse effects noted are frequently associated with MI (and therefore may or may not be attributable to Retavase®) and include arrhythmia, hypotension, cardiogenic shock, pulmonary edema, cardiac arrest, reinfarction, pericarditis, tamponade, thrombosis, and embolism.

Mechanism of Action Reteplase is a nonglycosylated form of tPA produced by recombinant DNA technology using *E. coli*; it initiates local fibrinolysis by binding to fibrin in a thrombus (clot) and converts entrapped plasminogen to plasmin

Drug Interactions

Increased Effect/Toxicity: The risk of bleeding associated with reteplase may be increased by oral anticoagulants (warfarin), heparin, low molecular weight heparins, and drugs which affect platelet function (eg, NSAIDs, dipyridamole, ticlopidine, clopidogrel, IIb/IIIa antagonists). Concurrent use with aspirin and heparin may increase the risk of bleeding; however, aspirin and heparin were used concomitantly with reteplase in the majority of patients in clinical studies.

Decreased Effect: Aminocaproic acid (antifibrinolytic agent) may decrease effectiveness of thrombolytic agents.

Pharmacodynamics/Kinetics

Onset of action: Thrombolysis: 30-90 minutes

Half-life elimination: 13-16 minutes

Excretion: Feces and urine

Clearance: Plasma: 250-450 mL/minute

Pregnancy Risk Factor C

Retin-A® *see* Tretinoin (Topical) *on page 1607*

Retin-A® Micro *see* Tretinoin (Topical) *on page 1607*

Retinoic Acid *see* Tretinoin (Topical) *on page 1607*

Retisert™ *see* Fluocinolone *on page 706*

Retrovir® *see* Zidovudine *on page 1680*

Revatio™ *see* Sildenafil *on page 1468*

Reversol® *see* Edrophonium *on page 556*

Revex® *see* Nalmefene *on page 1143*

Rēv-Eyes™ *see* Dapiprazole *on page 441*

ReVia® *see* Naltrexone *on page 1145*

Revlimid® *see* Lenalidomide *on page 954*

Reyataz® *see* Atazanavir *on page 156*

rFSH-alpha *see* Follitropin Alfa *on page 738*

rFSH-beta *see* Follitropin Beta *on page 739*

rFVIIa *see* Factor VIIa (Recombinant) *on page 666*

R-Gene® *see* Arginine *on page 141*

rGM-CSF *see* Sargramostim *on page 1456*

rhASB *see* Galsulfase *on page 763*

r-hCG *see* Chorionic Gonadotropin (Recombinant) *on page 352*

Rhenaphro *see* Vitamin B Complex Combinations *on page 1664*

Rheumatrex® *see* Methotrexate *on page 1068*

rhFSH-alpha *see* Follitropin Alfa *on page 738*

rhFSH-beta *see* Follitropin Beta *on page 739*

r-h α-GAL *see* Agalsidase Beta *on page 56*

RhIG *see* Rh$_0$(D) Immune Globulin *on page 1418*

rhIGF-1 *see* Mecasermin *on page 1023*

rhIGF-1/rhIGFBP-3 *see* Mecasermin *on page 1023*

rhIL-11 *see* Oprelvekin *on page 1210*

Rhinall [OTC] *see* Phenylephrine *on page 1293*

Rhinocort® Aqua® *see* Budesonide *on page 232*

RhinoFlex™ *see* Acetaminophen and Phenyltoloxamine *on page 38*

RhinoFlex 650 *see* Acetaminophen and Phenyltoloxamine *on page 38*

r-hLH *see* Lutropin Alfa *on page 1011*

Rh$_0$(D) Immune Globulin (Human) *see* Rh$_0$(D) Immune Globulin *on page 1418*

Rh$_0$(D) Immune Globulin (ar aych oh (dee) i MYUN GLOB yoo lin)

Related Information

Immunizations (Vaccines) *on page 1886*

U.S. Brand Names HyperRHO™ S/D Full Dose; HyperRHO™ S/D Mini Dose; MICRhoGAM®; RhoGAM®; Rhophylac®; WinRho® SDF

Canadian Brand Names WinRho® SDF
Mexican Brand Names Probi RHO (D)
Generic Available No
Index Terms RhIG; Rho(D) Immune Globulin (Human); RhoIGIV; RhoIVIM
Pharmacologic Category Immune Globulin

Use

Suppression of Rh isoimmunization: Use in the following situations when an $Rh_o(D)$-negative individual is exposed to $Rh_o(D)$-positive blood: During delivery of an $Rh_o(D)$-positive infant; abortion; amniocentesis; chorionic villus sampling; ruptured tubal pregnancy; abdominal trauma; hydatidiform mole; transplacental hemorrhage. Used when the mother is $Rh_o(D)$ negative, the father of the child is either $Rh_o(D)$ positive or $Rh_o(D)$ unknown, the baby is either $Rh_o(D)$ positive or $Rh_o(D)$ unknown.

Transfusion: Suppression of Rh isoimmunization in $Rh_o(D)$-negative individuals transfused with $Rh_o(D)$ antigen-positive RBCs or blood components containing $Rh_o(D)$ antigen-positive RBCs

Treatment of idiopathic thrombocytopenic purpura (ITP): Used in the following nonsplenectomized $Rh_o(D)$ positive individuals: Children with acute or chronic ITP, adults with chronic ITP, children and adults with ITP secondary to HIV infection

Local Anesthetic/Vasoconstrictor Precautions No information available to require special precautions

Effects on Dental Treatment No significant effects or complications reported

Common Adverse Effects Frequency not defined.

Cardiovascular: Hyper-/hypotension, pallor, tachycardia, vasodilation

Central nervous system: Chills, dizziness, fever, headache, malaise, somnolence

Dermatologic: Pruritus, rash

Gastrointestinal: Abdominal pain, diarrhea, nausea, vomiting

Hematologic: Haptoglobin decreased, hemoglobin decreased (patients with ITP), intravascular hemolysis (patients with ITP)

Hepatic: Bilirubin increased, LDH increased

Local: Injection site reaction: Discomfort, induration, mild pain, redness, swelling

Neuromuscular & skeletal: Arthralgia, back pain, hyperkinesia, myalgia, weakness

Renal: Acute renal insufficiency

Miscellaneous: Anaphylaxis, diaphoresis, infusion-related reactions, positive anti-C antibody test (transient), shivering

Mechanism of Action

Rh suppression: Prevents isoimmunization by suppressing the immune response and antibody formation by $Rh_o(D)$ negative individuals to $Rh_o(D)$ positive red blood cells.

ITP: Not completely characterized; $Rh_o(D)$ immune globulin is thought to form anti-D-coated red blood cell complexes which bind to macrophage Fc receptors within the spleen; blocking or saturating the spleens ability to clear antibody-coated cells, including platelets. In this manner, platelets are spared from destruction.

Drug Interactions

Decreased Effect: $Rh_o(D)$ immune globulin may interfere with the response of live vaccines; vaccines should not be administered within 3 months after $Rh_o(D)$

Pharmacodynamics/Kinetics

Onset of platelet increase: ITP: Platelets should rise within 1-2 days
Peak effect: In 7-14 days

Duration: Suppression of Rh isoimmunization: ~12 weeks; Treatment of ITP: 30 days (variable)

Distribution: V_d: I.M.: 8.59 L

Bioavailability: I.M.: Rhophylac®: 69%

Half-life elimination: 12-30 days

Time to peak, plasma: I.M.: 5-10 days; I.V. (WinRho® SDF): ≤2 hours

Pregnancy Risk Factor C

Ribavirin (rye ba VYE rin)

Related Information
Systemic Viral Diseases *on page 1767*
U.S. Brand Names Copegus®; Rebetol®; RibaPak™; Ribasphere™; Virazole®
Canadian Brand Names Virazole®
Mexican Brand Names Desiken; Vilona; Virazide
Generic Available Yes: Capsule, tablet
Index Terms RTCA; Tribavirin
Pharmacologic Category Antiviral Agent
Use
Inhalation: Treatment of patients with respiratory syncytial virus (RSV) infections; specially indicated for treatment of severe lower respiratory tract RSV infections in patients with an underlying compromising condition (prematurity, bronchopulmonary dysplasia and other chronic lung conditions, congenital heart disease, immunodeficiency, immunosuppression), and recent transplant recipients

Oral capsule:
In combination with interferon alfa-2b (Intron® A) injection for the treatment of chronic hepatitis C in patients with compensated liver disease who have relapsed after alpha interferon therapy or were previously untreated with alpha interferons

In combination with peginterferon alfa-2b (PEG-Intron®) injection for the treatment of chronic hepatitis C in patients with compensated liver disease who were previously untreated with alpha interferons

Oral solution: In combination with interferon alfa 2b (Intron® A) injection for the treatment of chronic hepatitis C in patients ≥3 years of age with compensated liver disease who were previously untreated with alpha interferons or patients ≥18 years of age who have relapsed after alpha interferon therapy

Oral tablet: In combination with peginterferon alfa-2a (Pegasys®) injection for the treatment of chronic hepatitis C in patients with compensated liver disease who were previously untreated with alpha interferons (includes patients with histological evidence of cirrhosis [Child-Pugh class A] and patients with clinically-stable HIV disease)

Unlabeled/Investigational Use Used in other viral infections including influenza A and B and adenovirus

Local Anesthetic/Vasoconstrictor Precautions No information available to require special precautions

Effects on Dental Treatment Key adverse event(s) related to dental treatment: Xerostomia (normal salivary flow resumes upon discontinuation) and taste perversion.

Common Adverse Effects
Inhalation:
1% to 10%:
Central nervous system: Fatigue, headache, insomnia
Gastrointestinal: Nausea, anorexia
Hematologic: Anemia

Note: Incidence of adverse effects (approximate) in healthcare workers: Headache (51%); conjunctivitis (32%); rhinitis, nausea, rash, dizziness, pharyngitis, and lacrimation (10% to 20%)

Oral (all adverse reactions are documented while receiving combination therapy with interferon alpha-2b or interferon alpha-2a; percentages as reported in adults):
>10%:
Central nervous system: Fatigue (60% to 70%)*, headache (43% to 66%)*, fever (32% to 46%)*, insomnia (26% to 41%), depression (20% to 36%)*, irritability (23% to 32%), dizziness (14% to 26%), impaired concentration (10% to 14%)*, emotional lability (7% to 12%)*
Dermatologic: Alopecia (27% to 36%), pruritus (13% to 29%), dry skin (13% to 24%), rash (5% to 28%), dermatitis (up to 16%)
Gastrointestinal: Nausea (33% to 47%), anorexia (21% to 32%), weight decrease (10% to 29%), diarrhea (10% to 22%), dyspepsia (8% to 16%), vomiting (9% to 14%)*, abdominal pain (8% to 13%), xerostomia (up to 12%), RUQ pain (up to 12%)
Hematologic: Neutropenia (8% to 27%; 40% with HIV coinfection), hemoglobin decreased (25% to 36%), hyperbilirubinemia (24% to 34%), anemia (11% to 17%), lymphopenia (12% to 14%), absolute neutrophil count <0.5 x

10^9/L (5% to 11%), thrombocytopenia (<1% to 14%), hemolytic anemia (10% to 13%), WBC decreased

Neuromuscular & skeletal: Myalgia (40% to 64%)*, rigors (40% to 48%), arthralgia (22% to 34%)*, musculoskeletal pain (19% to 28%)

Respiratory: Dyspnea (13% to 26%), cough (7% to 23%), pharyngitis (up to 13%), sinusitis (up to 12%)*, nasal congestion

Miscellaneous: Flu-like syndrome (13% to 18%)*, viral infection (up to 12%), diaphoresis increased (up to 11%)

*Similar to interferon alone

1% to 10%:

Cardiovascular: Chest pain (5% to 9%)*, flushing (up to 4%)

Central nervous system: Mood alteration (up to 6%; 9% with HIV coinfection), memory impairment (up to 6%), malaise (up to 6%), nervousness (~5%)*

Dermatologic: Eczema (4% to 5%)

Endocrine & metabolic: Hypothyroidism (up to 5%)

Gastrointestinal: Taste perversion (4% to 9%), constipation (up to 5%)

Genitourinary: Menstrual disorder (up to 7%)

Hepatic: Hepatomegaly (up to 4%)

Neuromuscular & skeletal: Weakness (9% to 10%), back pain (5%)

Ocular: Conjunctivitis (up to 6%), blurred vision (up to 5%)

Respiratory: Rhinitis (up to 8%), exertional dyspnea (up to 7%)

Miscellaneous: Fungal infection (up to 6%)

*Similar to interferon alone

Note: Incidence of anorexia, headache, fever, suicidal ideation, and vomiting are higher in children.

Restrictions An FDA-approved medication guide must be distributed when dispensing an outpatient prescription (new or refill) for treatment of hepatitis C where this medication is to be used without direct supervision of a healthcare provider. Medication guides are available at http://www.fda.gov/cder/Offices/ODS/medication_guides.htm.

Mechanism of Action Inhibits replication of RNA and DNA viruses; inhibits influenza virus RNA polymerase activity and inhibits the initiation and elongation of RNA fragments resulting in inhibition of viral protein synthesis

Drug Interactions

Increased Effect/Toxicity: Concomitant use of ribavirin and nucleoside analogues may increase the risk of developing lactic acidosis (includes adefovir, didanosine, lamivudine, stavudine, zalcitabine, zidovudine). Concurrent therapy of zidovudine with ribavirin/interferon alfa-2a may cause increased risk of severe anemia and/or severe neutropenia. Concurrent use with didanosine has been noted to increase the risk of pancreatitis and/or peripheral neuropathy in addition to lactic acidosis. Suspend therapy if signs/symptoms of toxicity are present. Concurrent therapy with Interferons (alfa) may increase the risk of hemolytic anemia.

Decreased Effect: Decreased effect of lamivudine, stavudine, and zidovudine (*in vitro*).

Pharmacodynamics/Kinetics

Absorption: Inhalation: Systemic; dependent upon respiratory factors and method of drug delivery; maximal absorption occurs with the use of aerosol generator via endotracheal tube; highest concentrations in respiratory tract and erythrocytes

Distribution: Oral capsule: Single dose; V$_d$ 2825 L; distribution significantly prolonged in the erythrocyte (16-40 days), which can be used as a marker for intracellular metabolism

Protein binding: Oral: None

Metabolism: Hepatically and intracellularly (forms active metabolites); may be necessary for drug action

Bioavailability: Oral: 64%

Half-life elimination, plasma:

Children: Inhalation: 6.5-11 hours

Adults: Oral:

Capsule, single dose (Rebetol®, Ribasphere™): 24 hours in healthy adults, 44 hours with chronic hepatitis C infection (increases to ~298 hours at steady state)

Tablet, single dose (Copegus®): 120-170 hours

Time to peak, serum: Inhalation: At end of inhalation period; Oral capsule: Multiple doses: 3 hours; Tablet: 2 hours

Excretion: Inhalation: Urine (40% as unchanged drug and metabolites); Oral capsule: Urine (61%), feces (12%)

Pregnancy Risk Factor X

Ribavirin and Interferon Alfa-2b Combination Pack *see* Interferon Alfa-2b and Ribavirin *on page 895*

Ribo-100 *see* Riboflavin *on page 1422*

Riboflavin (RYE boe flay vin)

U.S. Brand Names Ribo-100
Generic Available Yes
Index Terms Lactoflavin; Vitamin B_2; Vitamin G
Pharmacologic Category Vitamin, Water Soluble
Use Prevention of riboflavin deficiency and treatment of ariboflavinosis
Local Anesthetic/Vasoconstrictor Precautions No information available to require special precautions
Effects on Dental Treatment No significant effects or complications reported
Significant Adverse Effects Frequency not defined: Genitourinary: Discoloration of urine (yellow-orange)
Dosage Oral:
Riboflavin deficiency:
Children: 2.5-10 mg/day in divided doses
Adults: 5-30 mg/day in divided doses
Recommended daily allowance:
Children: 0.4-1.8 mg
Adults: 1.2-1.7 mg
Mechanism of Action Component of flavoprotein enzymes that work together, which are necessary for normal tissue respiration; also needed for activation of pyridoxine and conversion of tryptophan to niacin
Warnings/Precautions Riboflavin deficiency often occurs in the presence of other B vitamin deficiencies.
Drug Interactions Decreased absorption with probenecid
Pharmacodynamics/Kinetics
Absorption: Readily via GI tract, however, food increases extent; decreased with hepatitis, cirrhosis, or biliary obstruction
Metabolism: None
Half-life elimination: Biologic: 66-84 minutes
Excretion: Urine (9%) as unchanged drug
Pregnancy Risk Factor A/C (dose exceeding RDA recommendation)
Lactation Enters breast milk/compatible
Dosage Forms Excipient information presented when available; consult specific product labeling.
Tablet: 25 mg, 50 mg, 100 mg
Ribo-100: 100 mg

Rid-A-Pain Dental Drops [OTC] see Benzocaine on page 195

Ridaura® see Auranofin on page 170

RID® Maximum Strength [OTC] see Pyrethrins and Piperonyl Butoxide on page 1388

Rid® Spray [OTC] see Permethrin on page 1284

Rifabutin (rif a BYOO tin)

Related Information
Systemic Viral Diseases on page 1767
Tuberculosis on page 1765
U.S. Brand Names Mycobutin®
Canadian Brand Names Mycobutin®
Generic Available No
Index Terms Ansamycin
Pharmacologic Category Antibiotic, Miscellaneous; Antitubercular Agent
Use Prevention of disseminated *Mycobacterium avium* complex (MAC) in patients with advanced HIV infection
Unlabeled/Investigational Use Utilized in multidrug regimens for treatment of MAC
Local Anesthetic/Vasoconstrictor Precautions No information available to require special precautions
Effects on Dental Treatment Key adverse event(s) related to dental treatment: Saliva (reddish orange).
Common Adverse Effects
>10%:
Dermatologic: Rash (11%)
Genitourinary: Discoloration of urine (30%)
Hematologic: Neutropenia (25%), leukopenia (17%)
1% to 10%:
Central nervous system: Headache (3%)
Gastrointestinal: Vomiting/nausea (3%), abdominal pain (4%), diarrhea (3%), anorexia (2%), flatulence (2%), eructation (3%)

Hematologic: Anemia, thrombocytopenia (5%)

Hepatic: Increased AST/ALT (7% to 9%)

Neuromuscular & skeletal: Myalgia

Mechanism of Action Inhibits DNA-dependent RNA polymerase at the beta subunit which prevents chain initiation

Drug Interactions

Cytochrome P450 Effect: Substrate of CYP3A4 (major); **Induces** CYP3A4 (strong)

Increased Effect/Toxicity: Rifabutin may increase the therapeutic effect of clopidogrel; concurrent use with isoniazid may increase risk of hepatotoxicity; the levels/toxicity of rifabutin may be increased by imidazole antifungals, macrolide antibiotics, and protease inhibitors

Decreased Effect: Rifabutin may decrease the levels/effects of alfentanil, amiodarone, angiotensin II receptor blockers (irbesartan, losartan), CYP3A4 substrates (eg, clarithromycin, erythromycin, mirtazapine, nefazodone, venlafaxine), $5-HT_3$ antagonists, imidazole antifungals, aprepitant, barbiturates, benzodiazepines (metabolized by oxidation), beta blockers, buspirone, calcium channel blockers, chloramphenicol, corticosteroids, cyclosporine, dapsone, disopyramide, estrogen and progestin contraceptives, fluconazole, gefitinib, HMG-CoA reductase inhibitors, methadone, morphine, phenytoin, propafenone, protease inhibitors, quinidine, repaglinide, reverse transcriptase inhibitors (non-nucleoside), tacrolimus, tamoxifen, terbinafine, tocainide, tricyclic antidepressants, warfarin, zaleplon, zolpidem. The effects of rifabutin may be decreased by CYP3A4 inducers (eg, aminoglutethimide, carbamazepine, nafcillin, nevirapine, phenobarbital, phenytoin).

Pharmacodynamics/Kinetics

Absorption: Readily, 53%

Distribution: V_d: 9.32 L/kg; distributes to body tissues including the lungs, liver, spleen, eyes, and kidneys

Protein binding: 85%

Metabolism: To active and inactive metabolites

Bioavailability: Absolute: HIV: 20%

Half-life elimination: Terminal: 45 hours (range: 16-69 hours)

Time to peak, serum: 2-4 hours

Excretion: Urine (10% as unchanged drug, 53% as metabolites); feces (10% as unchanged drug, 30% as metabolites)

Pregnancy Risk Factor B

Rifadin® *see* Rifampin *on page 1423*

Rifamate® *see* Rifampin and Isoniazid *on page 1424*

Rifampicin *see* Rifampin *on page 1423*

Rifampin (rif AM pin)

Related Information

Rifapentine *on page 1425*

Tuberculosis *on page 1765*

U.S. Brand Names Rifadin®

Canadian Brand Names Rifadin®; Rofact™

Mexican Brand Names Rifadin; Rimactan

Generic Available Yes

Index Terms Rifampicin

Pharmacologic Category Antibiotic, Miscellaneous; Antitubercular Agent

Use Management of active tuberculosis in combination with other agents; elimination of meningococci from the nasopharynx in asymptomatic carriers

Unlabeled/Investigational Use Prophylaxis of *Haemophilus influenzae* type b infection; *Legionella* pneumonia; used in combination with other anti-infectives in the treatment of staphylococcal infections; treatment of *M. leprae* infections

Local Anesthetic/Vasoconstrictor Precautions No information available to require special precautions

Effects on Dental Treatment No significant effects or complications reported

Common Adverse Effects

Frequency not defined:

Cardiovascular: Edema, flushing

Central nervous system: Ataxia, behavioral changes, concentration impaired, confusion, dizziness, drowsiness, fatigue, fever, headache, numbness, psychosis

Dermatologic: Pemphigoid reaction, pruritus, urticaria

Endocrine & metabolic: Adrenal insufficiency, menstrual disorders

Hematologic: Agranulocytosis (rare), DIC, eosinophilia, hemoglobin decreased, hemolysis, hemolytic anemia, leukopenia, thrombocytopenia (especially with high-dose therapy)

(Continued)

Rifampin (Continued)

Hepatic: Hepatitis (rare), jaundice

Neuromuscular & skeletal: Myalgia, osteomalacia, weakness

Ocular: Exudative conjunctivitis, visual changes

Renal: Acute renal failure, BUN increased, hemoglobinuria, hematuria, interstitial nephritis, uric acid increased

Miscellaneous: Flu-like syndrome

1% to 10%:

Dermatologic: Rash (1% to 5%)

Gastrointestinal (1% to 2%): Anorexia, cramps, diarrhea, epigastric distress, flatulence, heartburn, nausea, pseudomembranous colitis, pancreatitis vomiting

Hepatic: LFTs increased (up to 14%)

Mechanism of Action Inhibits bacterial RNA synthesis by binding to the beta subunit of DNA-dependent RNA polymerase, blocking RNA transcription

Drug Interactions

Cytochrome P450 Effect: Induces CYP1A2 (strong), 2A6 (strong), 2B6 (strong), 2C8 (strong), 2C9 (strong), 2C19 (strong), 3A4 (strong)

Increased Effect/Toxicity: Rifampin may increase the therapeutic effect of clopidogrel; concurrent use with isoniazid, pyrazinamide, or protease inhibitors (amprenavir, saquinavir/ritonavir) may increase risk of hepatotoxicity; macrolide antibiotics may increase levels/toxicity of rifampin

Decreased Effect: Rifampin may decrease the levels/effects of the following drugs: Acetaminophen, alfentanil, amiodarone, angiotensin II receptor blockers (irbesartan and losartan), 5-HT$_3$ antagonists, imidazole antifungals, aprepitant, barbiturates, benzodiazepines (metabolized by oxidation), beta blockers, buspirone, calcium channel blockers, chloramphenicol, corticosteroids, cyclosporine; CYP1A2, 2A6, 2B6, 2C8, 2C9, 2C19, and 3A4 substrates (eg, aminophylline, amiodarone, bupropion, fluoxetine, fluvoxamine, ifosfamide, methsuximide, mirtazapine, nateglinide, pioglitazone, promethazine, proton pump inhibitors, ropinirole, rosiglitazone, selegiline, sertraline, theophylline, venlafaxine, and zafirlukast); dapsone, disopyramide, estrogen and progestin contraceptives, fexofenadine, fluconazole, fusidic acid, gefitinib, HMG-CoA reductase inhibitors, methadone, morphine, phenytoin, propafenone, protease inhibitors, quinidine, repaglinide, reverse transcriptase inhibitors (non-nucleoside), sulfonylureas, tacrolimus, tamoxifen, terbinafine, tocainide, tricyclic antidepressants, warfarin, zaleplon, zidovudine, zolpidem.

Pharmacodynamics/Kinetics

Duration: ≤24 hours

Absorption: Oral: Well absorbed; food may delay or slightly reduce peak

Distribution: Highly lipophilic; crosses blood-brain barrier well

Relative diffusion from blood into CSF: Adequate with or without inflammation (exceeds usual MICs)

CSF:blood level ratio: Inflamed meninges: 25%

Protein binding: 80%

Metabolism: Hepatic; undergoes enterohepatic recirculation

Half-life elimination: 3-4 hours; prolonged with hepatic impairment; End-stage renal disease: 1.8-11 hours

Time to peak, serum: Oral: 2-4 hours

Excretion: Feces (60% to 65%) and urine (~30%) as unchanged drug

Pregnancy Risk Factor C

Rifampin and Isoniazid (rif AM pin & eye soe NYE a zid)

Related Information

Isoniazid on page 912

Rifampin on page 1423

U.S. Brand Names IsonaRif™; Rifamate®

Canadian Brand Names Rifamate®

Mexican Brand Names Rifinah

Generic Available Yes

Index Terms Isoniazid and Rifampin

Pharmacologic Category Antibiotic, Miscellaneous

Use Management of active tuberculosis; see individual agents for additional information

Local Anesthetic/Vasoconstrictor Precautions No information available to require special precautions

Effects on Dental Treatment No significant effects or complications reported

Drug Interactions
Cytochrome P450 Effect:
Rifampin: **Induces** CYP1A2 (strong), 2A6 (strong), 2B6 (strong), 2C8 (strong), 2C9 (strong), 2C19 (strong), 3A4 (strong)
Isoniazid: **Substrate** of CYP2E1 (major); **Inhibits** CYP1A2 (weak), 2A6 (moderate), 2C9 (weak), 2C19 (strong), 2D6 (moderate), 2E1 (moderate), 3A4 (strong); **Induces** CYP2E1 (after discontinuation) (weak)
Pharmacodynamics/Kinetics See individual agents.
Pregnancy Risk Factor C

Rifampin, Isoniazid, and Pyrazinamide
(rif AM pin, eye soe NYE a zid, & peer a ZIN a mide)

Related Information
Isoniazid on page 912
Pyrazinamide on page 1388
Rifampin on page 1423
U.S. Brand Names Rifater®
Canadian Brand Names Rifater®
Generic Available No
Index Terms Isoniazid, Rifampin, and Pyrazinamide; Pyrazinamide, Rifampin, and Isoniazid
Pharmacologic Category Antibiotic, Miscellaneous
Use Initial phase, short-course treatment of pulmonary tuberculosis; see individual agents for additional information
Local Anesthetic/Vasoconstrictor Precautions No information available to require special precautions
Effects on Dental Treatment No significant effects or complications reported
Common Adverse Effects Note: During clinical trial evaluation, the frequency of cardiorespiratory events (eg, chest pain, hemoptysis, palpitation, chest tightness, and pneumothorax) was higher with the combination product (7%) that that reported with individual agents (2%). Also see individual agents.
Drug Interactions
Cytochrome P450 Effect:
Rifampin: **Induces** CYP1A2 (strong), 2A6 (strong), 2B6 (strong), 2C8 (strong), 2C9 (strong), 2C19 (strong), 3A4 (strong)
Isoniazid: **Substrate** of CYP2E1 (major); **Inhibits** CYP1A2 (weak), 2A6 (moderate), 2C9 (weak), 2C19 (strong), 2D6 (moderate), 2E1 (moderate), 3A4 (strong); CYP2E1 (after discontinuation) (weak)
Increased Effect/Toxicity: Increased effect/toxicity: Combination therapy with rifampin and pyrazinamide has been associated with severe and fatal hepatotoxic reactions.
Based on **rifampin** component: Rifampin levels may be increased when given with co-trimoxazole, probenecid, or ritonavir. Rifampin given with halothane or isoniazid increases the potential for hepatotoxicity.
Pharmacodynamics/Kinetics See individual agents.
Pregnancy Risk Factor C

Rifapentine (rif a PEN teen)

Related Information
Rifampin on page 1423
U.S. Brand Names Priftin®
Canadian Brand Names Priftin®
Generic Available No
Pharmacologic Category Antitubercular Agent
Use Treatment of pulmonary tuberculosis; rifapentine must always be used in conjunction with at least one other antituberculosis drug to which the isolate is susceptible; it may also be necessary to add a third agent (either streptomycin or ethambutol) until susceptibility is known.
Local Anesthetic/Vasoconstrictor Precautions No information available to require special precautions
Effects on Dental Treatment No significant effects or complications reported
Common Adverse Effects
>10%: Endocrine & metabolic: Hyperuricemia (most likely due to pyrazinamide from initiation phase combination therapy)
1% to 10%:
Cardiovascular: Hypertension
Central nervous system: Headache, dizziness
Dermatologic: Rash, pruritus, acne
Gastrointestinal: Anorexia, nausea, vomiting, dyspepsia, diarrhea
(Continued)

Rifapentine *(Continued)*

Hematologic: Neutropenia, lymphopenia, anemia, leukopenia, thrombocytosis
Hepatic: Increased ALT/AST
Neuromuscular & skeletal: Arthralgia, pain
Renal: Pyuria, proteinuria, hematuria, urinary casts
Respiratory: Hemoptysis

Mechanism of Action Inhibits DNA-dependent RNA polymerase in susceptible strains of *Mycobacterium tuberculosis* (but not in mammalian cells). Rifapentine is bactericidal against both intracellular and extracellular MTB organisms. MTB resistant to other rifamycins including rifampin are likely to be resistant to rifapentine. Cross-resistance does not appear between rifapentine and other nonrifamycin antimycobacterial agents.

Drug Interactions

Cytochrome P450 Effect: Induces CYP2C8 (strong), 2C9 (strong), 3A4 (strong)

Increased Effect/Toxicity: Rifapentine may increase the therapeutic effect of clopidogrel; concurrent use with isoniazid may increase risk of hepatotoxicity

Decreased Effect: Rifapentine may decrease the levels/effects of the following drugs: alfentanil, amiodarone, angiotensin II receptor blockers (irbesartan, losartan), 5-HT$_3$ antagonists, imidazole antifungals, aprepitant, barbiturates, benzodiazepines (metabolized by oxidation), beta blockers, buspirone, calcium channel blockers, corticosteroids, cyclosporine; CYP2C8, 2C9 and 3A4 substrates (eg, amiodarone, clarithromycin, erythromycin, fluoxetine, mirtazapine, nateglinide, nefazodone, nevirapine, pioglitazone, rosiglitazone, sertraline, venlafaxine, and zafirlukast); dapsone, disopyramide, estrogen and progestin contraceptives, fluconazole, gefitinib, HMG-CoA reductase inhibitors, methadone, morphine, phenytoin, propafenone, protease inhibitors, quinidine, repaglinide, reverse transcriptase inhibitors (non-nucleoside), tacrolimus, tamoxifen, terbinafine, tocainide, tricyclic antidepressants, warfarin, zaleplon, zidovudine, and zolpidem.

Pharmacodynamics/Kinetics

Absorption: Food increases AUC and C$_{max}$ by 43% and 44% respectively.
Distribution: V$_d$: ~70.2 L; rifapentine and metabolite accumulate in human monocyte-derived macrophages with intracellular/extracellular ratios of 24:1 and 7:1 respectively
Protein binding: Rifapentine and 25-desacetyl metabolite: 97.7% and 93.2%, primarily to albumin
Metabolism: Hepatic; hydrolyzed by an esterase and esterase enzyme to form the active metabolite 25-desacetyl rifapentine
Bioavailability: ~70%
Half-life elimination: Rifapentine: 14-17 hours; 25-desacetyl rifapentine: 13 hours
Time to peak, serum: 5-6 hours
Excretion: Urine (17% primarily as metabolites)

Pregnancy Risk Factor C

Rifater® *see Rifampin, Isoniazid, and Pyrazinamide on page 1425*

Rifaximin *(rif AX i min)*

U.S. Brand Names Xifaxan™
Mexican Brand Names Flonorm; Redactiv
Generic Available No
Pharmacologic Category Antibiotic, Miscellaneous
Use Treatment of travelers' diarrhea caused by noninvasive strains of *E. coli*
Local Anesthetic/Vasoconstrictor Precautions No information available to require special precautions
Effects on Dental Treatment No significant effects or complications reported
Common Adverse Effects Incidence of adverse effects reported as ≥2% occurred more in the placebo group than the rifaximin group except for headache.
2% to 10%: Central nervous system: Headache (10%; placebo 9%)
Mechanism of Action Rifaximin inhibits bacterial RNA synthesis by binding to bacterial DNA-dependent RNA polymerase.

Drug Interactions

Cytochrome P450 Effect: Induces CYP3A4 (minor)

Pharmacodynamics/Kinetics

Absorption: Oral: <0.4%
Distribution: 80% to 90% in the gut
Half-life elimination: ~6 hours
Excretion: Feces (~97% as unchanged drug); urine (<1%)

Pregnancy Risk Factor C

Riluzole (RIL yoo zole)

U.S. Brand Names Rilutek®
Canadian Brand Names Rilutek®
Mexican Brand Names Rilutek
Generic Available No
Index Terms 2-Amino-6-Trifluoromethoxy-benzothiazole; RP-54274
Pharmacologic Category Glutamate Inhibitor
Use Treatment of amyotrophic lateral sclerosis (ALS); riluzole can extend survival or time to tracheostomy
Local Anesthetic/Vasoconstrictor Precautions No information available to require special precautions
Effects on Dental Treatment Key adverse event(s) related to dental treatment: Oral moniliasis and stomatitis.
Common Adverse Effects
>10%:
  Gastrointestinal: Nausea (12% to 21%)
  Neuromuscular & skeletal: Weakness (15% to 20%)
  Respiratory: Lung function decreased (10% to 16%)
1% to 10%:
  Cardiovascular: Edema, hypertension, tachycardia
  Central nervous system: Agitation, circumoral paresthesia, depression, dizziness, headache, insomnia, malaise, somnolence, tremor, vertigo
  Dermatologic: Alopecia, eczema, pruritus
  Gastrointestinal: Abdominal pain, anorexia, diarrhea, dyspepsia, flatulence, oral moniliasis, stomatitis, vomiting
  Hepatic: Liver function tests increased
  Neuromuscular & skeletal: Arthralgia, back pain
  Respiratory: Cough increased, rhinitis, sinusitis
  Miscellaneous: Aggravation reaction
Mechanism of Action Mechanism of action is not known. Pharmacologic properties include inhibitory effect on glutamate release, inactivation of voltage-dependent sodium channels; and ability to interfere with intracellular events that follow transmitter binding at excitatory amino acid receptors
Drug Interactions
  Cytochrome P450 Effect: Substrate of CYP1A2 (major)
  Increased Effect/Toxicity: CYP1A2 inhibitors may increase the levels/effects of riluzole; example inhibitors include amiodarone, ciprofloxacin, fluvoxamine, ketoconazole, norfloxacin, ofloxacin, and rofecoxib.
  Decreased Effect: CYP1A2 inducers may decrease the levels/effects of riluzole; example inducers include aminoglutethimide, carbamazepine, phenobarbital, and rifampin.
Pharmacodynamics/Kinetics
  Absorption: 90%; high-fat meal decreases AUC by 20% and peak blood levels by 45%
  Protein binding, plasma: 96%, primarily to albumin and lipoproteins
  Metabolism: Extensively hepatic to six major and a number of minor metabolites via CYP1A2 dependent hydroxylation and glucuronidation
  Bioavailability: Oral: Absolute: 60%
  Half-life elimination: 12 hours
  Excretion: Urine (90%; 85% as metabolites, 2% as unchanged drug) and feces (5%) within 7 days
Pregnancy Risk Factor C

Rimantadine (ri MAN ta deen)

Related Information
  Systemic Viral Diseases *on page 1767*
U.S. Brand Names Flumadine®
Canadian Brand Names Flumadine®
Mexican Brand Names Gabirol
Generic Available Yes: Tablet
(Continued)

RIMEXOLONE

Rimantadine *(Continued)*

Index Terms Rimantadine Hydrochloride

Pharmacologic Category Antiviral Agent, Adamantane

Use Prophylaxis (adults and children >1 year of age) and treatment (adults) of influenza A viral infection (per manufacturer labeling; also refer to current CDC guidelines for recommendations during current flu season)

Local Anesthetic/Vasoconstrictor Precautions No information available to require special precautions

Effects on Dental Treatment Key adverse event(s) related to dental treatment: Xerostomia (normal salivary flow resumes upon discontinuation).

Common Adverse Effects 1% to 10%:

Central nervous system: Dizziness (1% to 2%), insomnia (2% to 3%), concentration impaired (2%), anxiety (1%), fatigue (1%), headache (1%), nervousness (1% to 2%)

Gastrointestinal: Nausea (3%), anorexia (2%), vomiting (2%), xerostomia (2%), abdominal pain (1%)

Neuromuscular & skeletal: Weakness (1%)

Mechanism of Action Exerts its inhibitory effect on three antigenic subtypes of influenza A virus (H1N1, H2N2, H3N2) early in the viral replicative cycle, possibly inhibiting the uncoating process; it has no activity against influenza B virus and is two- to eightfold more active than amantadine

Drug Interactions

Decreased Effect: Rimantadine may decrease the efficacy of the influenza live virus vaccine. Administer vaccine at least 48 hours after rimantadine. Do not give rimantadine within 2 weeks of live virus vaccine.

Pharmacodynamics/Kinetics

Onset of action: Antiviral activity: No data exist establishing a correlation between plasma concentration and antiviral effect

Absorption: Tablet and syrup formulations are equally absorbed

Metabolism: Extensively hepatic

Half-life elimination: 25.4 hours; prolonged in elderly

Time to peak: 6 hours

Excretion: Urine (<25% as unchanged drug)

Clearance: Hemodialysis does not contribute to clearance

Pregnancy Risk Factor C

Rimantadine Hydrochloride *see* Rimantadine *on page 1427*

Rimexolone *(ri MEKS oh lone)*

U.S. Brand Names Vexol®

Canadian Brand Names Vexol®

Mexican Brand Names Vexol

Generic Available No

Pharmacologic Category Corticosteroid, Ophthalmic

Use Treatment of inflammation after ocular surgery and the treatment of anterior uveitis

Local Anesthetic/Vasoconstrictor Precautions No information available to require special precautions

Effects on Dental Treatment No significant effects or complications reported

Mechanism of Action Decreases inflammation by suppression of migration of polymorphonuclear leukocytes and reversal of increased capillary permeability

Pregnancy Risk Factor C

Rindal HPD *see* Hydrocodone, Phenylephrine, and Diphenhydramine *on page 834*

Riomet™ *see* Metformin *on page 1056*

Riopan Plus® [OTC] [DSC] *see* Magaldrate and Simethicone *on page 1013*

Riopan Plus® Double Strength [OTC] [DSC] *see* Magaldrate and Simethicone *on page 1013*

Risedronate *(ris ED roe nate)*

Related Information

Rheumatoid Arthritis, Osteoarthritis, and Osteoporosis *on page 1759*

U.S. Brand Names Actonel®

Canadian Brand Names Actonel®

Mexican Brand Names Actonel

Generic Available No

Index Terms Risedronate Sodium

Pharmacologic Category Bisphosphonate Derivative

Use Paget's disease of the bone; treatment and prevention of glucocorticoid-induced osteoporosis; treatment and prevention of osteoporosis in postmenopausal women; treatment of osteoporosis in men

Local Anesthetic/Vasoconstrictor Precautions No information available to require special precautions

Effects on Dental Treatment Osteonecrosis of the jaw (ONJ), generally associated with local infection and/or tooth extraction and often with delayed healing, has been reported in patients taking bisphosphonates. Symptoms included nonhealing extraction socket or an exposed jawbone. Most reported cases of bisphosphonate-associated osteonecrosis have been in cancer patients treated with intravenous bisphosphonates. However, some have occurred in patients with postmenopausal osteoporosis taking oral bisphosphonates. Dental surgery may exacerbate ONJ. For patients requiring dental procedures, there are no data available to suggest whether discontinuation of bisphosphonate treatment reduces the risk of ONJ. Patients who develop ONJ while on bisphosphonate therapy should receive care by an oral surgeon. See Dental Comment.

Common Adverse Effects Frequency may vary with dose and indication.

>10%:
  Central nervous system: Headache (18%), pain (14%)
  Dermatologic: Rash (8% to 12%)
  Gastrointestinal: Diarrhea (11% to 20%), abdominal pain (12%)
  Genitourinary: Urinary tract infection (11%)
  Neuromuscular & skeletal: Arthralgia (14% to 33%), back pain (26%)

1% to 10%:
  Cardiovascular: Hypertension (10%), peripheral edema (8%), chest pain (5% to 7%), cardiovascular disorder (3%), angina (3%), arrhythmia (2%)
  Central nervous system: Depression (7%), dizziness (6% to 7%), insomnia (5%), anxiety (4%)
  Dermatologic: Pruritus (3%)
  Endocrine & metabolic: Hypophosphatemia (<3%)
  Gastrointestinal: Constipation (7%), nausea (7%), flatulence (5%), belching (3%), colitis (3%), gastritis (3%)
  Genitourinary: Prostatic hyperplasia (5%), cystitis (4%), nephrolithiasis (3%)
  Hematologic: Anemia (2%)
  Neuromuscular & skeletal: Joint disorder (7%), myalgia (5% to 7%), neck pain (5%), bone pain (5%), weakness (5%), neuralgia (4%), leg cramps (4%), myasthenia (3%), tendon disorder (3%)
  Ocular: Cataract (6%), dry eyes (3%)
  Respiratory: Pharyngitis (6%), rhinitis (6%), sinusitis (5%), dyspnea (4%), bronchitis (3%)
  Miscellaneous: Flu symptoms (10%), neoplasm (3%), hernia (3%)

Dosage Oral: Adults:
  Paget's disease of bone: 30 mg once daily for 2 months
    Retreatment may be considered (following post-treatment observation of at least 2 months) if relapse occurs, or if treatment fails to normalize serum alkaline phosphatase. For retreatment, the dose and duration of therapy are the same as for initial treatment. No data are available on more than one course of retreatment.
  Osteoporosis (postmenopausal) prevention and treatment: 5 mg once daily **or** 35 mg once weekly **or** one 75 mg tablet taken on 2 consecutive days once a month (total of 2 tablets/month)
  Osteoporosis (male) treatment: 35 mg once weekly
  Osteoporosis (glucocorticoid-induced) prevention and treatment: 5 mg once daily

Dosage adjustment in renal impairment: Cl_{cr} <30 mL/minute: **Not** recommended for use

Mechanism of Action A bisphosphonate which inhibits bone resorption via actions on osteoclasts or on osteoclast precursors; decreases the rate of bone resorption, leading to an indirect increase in bone mineral density. In Paget's disease, characterized by disordered resorption and formation of bone, inhibition of resorption leads to an indirect decrease in bone formation; but the newly-formed bone has a more normal architecture.

Contraindications Hypersensitivity to risedronate, bisphosphonates, or any component of the formulation; hypocalcemia; abnormalities of the esophagus which delay esophageal emptying such as stricture or achalasia; inability to stand or sit upright for at least 30 minutes; severe renal impairment (Cl_{cr} <30 mL/minute)

Warnings/Precautions Bisphosphonates may cause upper gastrointestinal disorders such as dysphagia, esophagitis, esophageal ulcer, and gastric ulcer. Use caution in patients with renal impairment (not recommended in patients with a Cl_{cr} <30 mL/minute). Hypocalcemia must be corrected before therapy (Continued)

Risedronate *(Continued)*

initiation with risedronate. Ensure adequate calcium and vitamin D intake, especially for patients with Paget's disease in whom the pretreatment rate of bone turnover may be greatly elevated.

Bisphosphonate therapy has been associated with osteonecrosis, primarily of the jaw; this has been observed mostly in cancer patients, but also in patients with postmenopausal osteoporosis and other diagnoses. Dental exams and preventative dentistry should be performed prior to placing patients with risk factors on chronic bisphosphonate therapy. Invasive dental procedures should be avoided during treatment.

Infrequently, severe (and occasionally debilitating) bone, joint, and/or muscle pain have been reported during bisphosphonate treatment. The onset of pain ranged from a single day to several months. Symptoms usually resolve upon discontinuation. Some patients experienced recurrence when rechallenged with same drug or another bisphosphonate; avoid use in patients with a history of these symptoms in association with bisphosphonate therapy.

Safety and efficacy in pediatric patients have not been established.

Drug Interactions

Increased Effect/Toxicity:
Aminoglycosides may lower serum calcium levels with prolonged administration; concomitant use may have an additive hypocalcemic effect. NSAIDs may enhance the gastrointestinal adverse/toxic effects (increased incidence of GI ulcers) of bisphosphonate derivatives. Bisphosphonate derivatives may enhance the hypocalcemic effect of phosphate supplements.

Decreased Effect: The following agents may decrease the absorption of oral bisphosphonate derivatives: Antacids (aluminum, calcium, magnesium), oral calcium salts, oral iron salts, and oral magnesium salts

Ethanol/Nutrition/Herb Interactions
Ethanol: Avoid ethanol (may increase risk of osteoporosis).

Food: Food reduces absorption (similar to other bisphosphonates); mean oral bioavailability is decreased when given with food.

Dietary Considerations Take ≥30 minutes before the first food or drink of the day other than water. Supplemental calcium or vitamin D may be required if dietary intake is not adequate.

Pharmacodynamics/Kinetics
Onset of action: May require weeks

Absorption: Rapid

Distribution: V_d: 6.3 L/kg

Protein binding: ~24%

Metabolism: None

Bioavailability: Poor, ~0.54% to 0.75%

Half-life elimination: Initial: 1.5 hours; Terminal: 480 hours

Time to peak, serum: 1 hour

Excretion: Urine (up to 85%); feces (as unabsorbed drug)

Pregnancy Risk Factor C

Dosage Forms
Tablet:

Actonel®: 5 mg, 30 mg, 35 mg, 75 mg

Dental Comment Cases of oral bisphosphonate-associated ONJ have been reported. A report by the Council of Scientific Affairs of the American Dental Association (accessed at: http://www.ada.org/prof/resources/topics/osteonecrosis.asp) as of July 2006 gave an estimated incidence of 0.7 cases for every 100,000 person-years of exposure to alendronate (Fosamax®). This translates to one case for every 142,857 person-years exposure. This figure from the ADA report was based on information received from Merck & Co citing 170 worldwide cases for alendronate (Fosamax®). In addition, Procter & Gamble Pharmaceuticals has cited 20 cases for risedronate (Actonel®) and Roche Laboratories has cited one case for ibandronate (Boniva®).

Consumer Reports On Health stated that the risk of jaw bone osteoporosis due to alendronate (Fosamax®), risedronate (Actonel®), or ibandronate (Boniva®) taken to prevent osteoporosis is very low and is estimated to be one out of every 20,000 users. That report mentioned that tooth extraction or implants increase the risk of developing osteonecrosis in patients taking any of these drugs for osteoporosis. The report also recommended that patients should stop taking any of these oral drugs 1-2 months before and after such dental treatment. No evidence was presented to support this statement.

In terms of length of exposure to oral bisphosphonates prior to onset of ONJ, data from large population studies or controlled studies is lacking. A report by Marx et al, observed that of three cases of ONJ associated with Fosamax® exposure, one patient had been taking 10 mg/day by mouth for 6 years and the other two patients 10 mg/day by mouth for 3 and 2 years respectively. In contrast, they observed that in cancer patients receiving intravenous bisphosphonates, the time period between the first doses of the bisphosphonate to first recognition of exposed bone either by the patients or by the clinician, was 9.4 months for zoledronate (Zometa®), 14.3 months for pamidronate (Aredia®), and 12.1 months for pamidronate then to zoledronate.

Selected Readings

Author Unknown, "Safety Update: Bone-Building Drugs: Risks Explained," *Consumer Reports on Health*, 2006, 18(5):3.

Marx RE, Sawatari Y, Fortin M, et al, "Bisphosphonate-Induced Exposed Bone (Osteonecrosis/ Osteopetrosis) of the Jaws: Risk Factors, Recognition, Prevention, and Treatment," *J Oral Maxillofac Surg*, 2005, 63(11):1567-75.

Risedronate and Calcium (ris ED roe nate & KAL see um)

U.S. Brand Names Actonel® and Calcium

Generic Available No

Index Terms Calcium and Risedronate; Risedronate Sodium and Calcium Carbonate

Pharmacologic Category Bisphosphonate Derivative; Calcium Salt

Use Treatment and prevention of osteoporosis in postmenopausal women

Local Anesthetic/Vasoconstrictor Precautions No information available to require special precautions

Effects on Dental Treatment Osteonecrosis of the jaw (ONJ), generally associated with local infection and/or tooth extraction and often with delayed healing, has been reported in patients taking bisphosphonates. Symptoms included nonhealing extraction socket or an exposed jawbone. Most reported cases of bisphosphonate-associated osteonecrosis have been in cancer patients treated with intravenous bisphosphonates. However, some have occurred in patients with postmenopausal osteoporosis taking oral bisphosphonates. Dental surgery may exacerbate ONJ. For patients requiring dental procedures, there are no data available to suggest whether discontinuation of bisphosphonate treatment reduces the risk of ONJ. Patients who develop ONJ while on bisphosphonate therapy should receive care by an oral surgeon. See Dental Comment in Risedronate monograph.

Common Adverse Effects See individual agents.

Dosage

Oral: Adults: Osteoporosis in postmenopausal females:

Risedronate: 35 mg once weekly on day 1 of 7-day treatment cycle

Calcium carbonate: 1250 mg (elemental calcium 500 mg) once daily on days 2 through 7 of 7-day treatment cycle

Dosage adjustment in renal impairment: Cl$_{cr}$ <30 mL/minute: Not recommended for use

Mechanism of Action

Risedronate inhibits bone resorption via actions on osteoclasts or on osteoclast precursors; decreases the rate of bone resorption, leading to an indirect increase in bone mineral density.

Calcium helps to prevent or decrease the rate of bone loss.

Contraindications Hypersensitivity to risedronate, bisphosphonates, or any component of the formulation; hypocalcemia, hypercalcemia; abnormalities of the esophagus which delay esophageal emptying (eg, stricture or achalasia); inability to stand or sit upright for at least 30 minutes; severe renal impairment (Cl$_{cr}$ <30 mL/minute)

Warnings/Precautions Bisphosphonates may cause upper gastrointestinal disorders such as dysphagia, esophageal ulcer, and gastric ulcer. Use caution in patients with renal impairment (not recommended in patients with a Cl$_{cr}$ <30 mL/minute). Hypocalcemia must be corrected before therapy initiation. Ensure adequate vitamin D intake. Severe bone pain has been reported (rare) with the use of bisphosphonates; onset varied from 1 day to several months following the onset of therapy.

Bisphosphonate therapy has been associated with osteonecrosis, primarily of the jaw; this has been observed mostly in cancer patients, but also in patients with postmenopausal osteoporosis and other diagnoses. Dental exams and preventative dentistry should be performed prior to placing patients with risk factors on chronic bisphosphonate therapy. Invasive dental procedures should be avoided during treatment.

Infrequently, severe (and occasionally debilitating) bone, joint, and/or muscle pain have been reported during bisphosphonate treatment. The onset of pain ranged from a single day to several months. Symptoms usually resolve upon discontinuation. Some patients experienced recurrence when rechallenged with same drug or another bisphosphonate; avoid use in patients with a history of these symptoms in association with bisphosphonate therapy.

(Continued)

Risedronate and Calcium *(Continued)*

Calcium carbonate absorption is impaired in achlorhydria (common in elderly); administer calcium component with food. Calcium should be used with caution in patients with a history of kidney stones or hypercalciuria.

Safety and efficacy using the combination as packaged have not been established in pediatric patients or for the treatment of primary osteoporosis in men.

Drug Interactions
Increased Effect/Toxicity: See individual agents.

Ethanol/Nutrition/Herb Interactions
Ethanol: Avoid ethanol (may increase risk of osteoporosis).
Food:
Risedronate: Food may reduce absorption (similar to other bisphosphonates); mean oral bioavailability is decreased when given with food.
Calcium: Food increases absorption. Calcium may decrease iron absorption. Bran, foods high in oxalates, or whole grain cereals may decrease calcium absorption

Dietary Considerations Take risedronate ≥30 minutes before the first food or drink of the day other than water. Calcium should be taken with food. Vitamin D supplementation may be needed.

Pharmacodynamics/Kinetics See individual agents.

Pregnancy Risk Factor C

Dosage Forms
Combination package [each package contains]:
Actonel® and Calcium:
Tablet (Actonel®): Risedronate 35 mg (4s)
Tablet: Calcium 1250 mg (24s)

Dental Comment See Risedronate monograph.

Selected Readings
Ruggiero SL, Mehrotra B, Rosenberg TJ, et al, "Osteonecrosis of the Jaws Associated With the Use of Bisphosphonates: A Review of 63 Cases," *J Oral Maxillofac Surg*, 2004, 62(5):527-34.

Risedronate Sodium *see* Risedronate *on page 1428*

Risedronate Sodium and Calcium Carbonate *see* Risedronate and Calcium *on page 1431*

Risperdal® *see* Risperidone *on page 1432*

Risperdal M-Tab *see* Risperidone *on page 1432*

Risperdal® M-Tab® *see* Risperidone *on page 1432*

Risperdal® Consta® *see* Risperidone *on page 1432*

Risperidone *(ris PER i done)*

U.S. Brand Names Risperdal®; Risperdal® Consta®; Risperdal® M-Tab®

Canadian Brand Names Apo-Risperidone®; PMS-Risperidone ODT; Risperdal®; Risperdal® Consta®; Risperdal® M-Tab®; Sandoz Risperidone

Mexican Brand Names Risperdal

Generic Available No

Index Terms Risperdal M-Tab

Pharmacologic Category Antipsychotic Agent, Atypical

Use Treatment of schizophrenia; treatment of acute mania or mixed episodes associated with bipolar I disorder (as monotherapy or in combination with lithium or valproate); treatment of irritability/aggression associated with autistic disorder

Unlabeled/Investigational Use Behavioral symptoms associated with dementia in elderly; treatment of Tourette's disorder; treatment of pervasive developmental disorder

Local Anesthetic/Vasoconstrictor Precautions No information available to require special precautions

Effects on Dental Treatment Key adverse event(s) related to dental treatment: Significant xerostomia (normal salivary flow resumes upon discontinuation) and toothache.

Common Adverse Effects
The frequency of adverse effects is reported as absolute percentages and is not based upon net frequencies as compared to placebo. Unless otherwise noted, frequency of adverse effects is reported for the oral formulation in adults.
>10%:
Central nervous system: Fatigue (adults 4%; children 42%), extrapyramidal symptoms (adults 17% to 34%; children 28%), somnolence (adults 3% to 28%; children 67%), insomnia (23% to 26%), agitation (8% to 26%), anxiety (4% to 20%), dystonia (adults 18%; children 12%), akathisia (16%), headache (12% to 14%), dizziness (4% to 11%)

Gastrointestinal: Appetite increased (children 49%), salivation increased (adults up to 5%; children 22%), weight gain (adults 2% to 18%; children 5%), constipation (adults 7% to 13%; children 21%), xerostomia (adults 3% to ≥5%; children 13%), dyspepsia (5% to 11%), nausea (4% to 11%)

Neuromuscular & skeletal: Tremor (children 12%)

Respiratory: Upper respiratory infection (adults 3%; children 34%)

1% to 10%:

Cardiovascular: Tachycardia (adults 3% to 5%; children 7%), hypertension (3%), chest pain (2% to 3%), hypotension (2%; especially orthostatic)

Central nervous system: Mania (8%), automatism (children 7%), pseudoparkinsonism (adults 6%; children 7%), dreaming increased (≥5%), sleep prolonged (≥5%), confusion (children 5%), pain (5%), fever (2% to 3%), aggressiveness (1% to 3%), concentration impaired (2%), hypoesthesia (2%), tardive dyskinesia, neuroleptic malignant syndrome, altered central temperature regulation, nervousness, sleep duration increased

Dermatologic: Rash (2% to 5%), dry skin (2% to 4%), acne (2%), pruritus (2%), seborrhea (up to 1%), pigmentation increased, photosensitivity

Endocrine & metabolic: Sexual dysfunction (3%), menorrhagia (≥5%), galactorrhea (children 1%), gynecomastia (children 2%)

Gastrointestinal: Vomiting (5% to 7%), diarrhea (≥5%), abdominal pain (1% to 4%), toothache (up to 2%), anorexia

Genitourinary: Micturition disturbances (≥5%)

Hematologic: Anemia (≥1% I.M. injection)

Hepatic: Transaminases increased (≥1% I.M. injection)

Neuromuscular & skeletal: Dyskinesia (children 7%), myalgia (5%), arthralgia (2% to 3%), skeletal pain (2%), back pain (up to 2%)

Ocular: Abnormal vision (1% to 6%), accommodation disturbances (≥5%)

Renal: Polydipsia, polyuria

Respiratory: Rhinitis (3% to 10%), sinusitis (1% to 4%), cough (2% to 3%), pharyngitis (2% to 3%), dyspnea (up to 1%)

Miscellaneous: Injury (2%)

Dosage

Oral:

Children ≥5 years and Adolescents: Autism:

<15 kg: Use with caution; specific dosing recommendations not available

<20 kg: Initial: 0.25 mg/day; may increase dose to 0.5 mg/day after ≥4 days, maintain dose for ≥14 days. In patients not achieving sufficient clinical response, may increase dose by 0.25 mg/day in ≥2-week intervals. Therapeutic effect reached plateau at 1 mg/day in clinical trials. Following clinical response, consider gradually lowering dose. May be administered once daily or in divided doses twice daily.

≥20 kg: Initial: 0.5 mg/day; may increase dose to 1 mg/day after ≥4 days, maintain dose for ≥14 days. In patients not achieving sufficient clinical response, may increase dose by 0.5 mg/day in ≥2-week intervals. Therapeutic effect reached plateau at 2.5 mg/day (3 mg/day in children >45 kg) in clinical trials. Following clinical response, consider gradually lowering dose. May be administered once daily or in divided doses twice daily.

Children and Adolescents:

Pervasive developmental disorder (unlabeled use): Initial: 0.25 mg twice daily; titrate up 0.25 mg/day every 5-7 days; optimal dose range: 0.75-3 mg/day

Schizophrenia (unlabeled use): Initial: 0.5 mg once or twice daily; titrate as necessary up to 2-6 mg/day

Bipolar disorder (unlabeled use): Initial: 0.5 mg; titrate to 0.5-3 mg/day

Tourette's disorder (unlabeled use): Initial: 0.5 mg; titrate to 2-4 mg/day

Adults:

Schizophrenia:

Initial: 1 mg twice daily; may be increased by 2 mg/day to a target dose of 6 mg/day; usual range: 4-8 mg/day; may be given as a single daily dose once maintenance dose is achieved; daily dosages >6 mg do not appear to confer any additional benefit, and the incidence of extrapyramidal symptoms is higher than with lower doses. Further dose adjustments should be made in increments/decrements of 1-2 mg/day on a weekly basis. Dose range studied in clinical trials: 4-16 mg/day.

Maintenance: Target dose: 4 mg once daily (range 2-8 mg/day)

Bipolar mania:

Initial: 2-3 mg once daily; if needed, adjust dose by 1 mg/day in intervals ≥24 hours; dosing range: 1-6 mg/day

Maintenance: No dosing recommendation available for treatment >3 weeks duration.

Elderly: A starting dose of 0.5 mg twice daily, and titration should progress slowly in increments of no more than 0.5 mg twice daily; increases to dosages >1.5 mg twice daily should occur at intervals of ≥1 week.

(Continued)

Risperidone *(Continued)*

Additional monitoring of renal function and orthostatic blood pressure may be warranted. If once-a-day dosing in the elderly or debilitated patient is considered, a twice daily regimen should be used to titrate to the target dose, and this dose should be maintained for 2-3 days prior to attempts to switch to a once-daily regimen.

I.M.: Adults: Schizophrenia (Risperdal® Consta®): 25 mg every 2 weeks; some patients may benefit from larger doses; maximum dose not to exceed 50 mg every 2 weeks. Dosage adjustments should not be made more frequently than every 4 weeks. A lower initial dose of 12.5 mg may be appropriate in some patients.

Note: Oral risperidone (or other antipsychotic) should be administered with the initial injection of Risperdal® Consta® and continued for 3 weeks (then discontinued) to maintain adequate therapeutic plasma concentrations prior to main release phase of risperidone from injection site. When switching from depot administration to a short-acting formulation, administer short-acting agent in place of the next regularly-scheduled depot injection.

Dosing adjustment in renal impairment:

Oral: Starting dose of 0.5 mg twice daily; clearance of the active moiety is decreased by 60% in patients with moderate to severe renal disease compared to healthy subjects.

I.M.: An initial dose of 12.5 mg may be considered

Dosing adjustment in hepatic impairment:

Oral: Starting dose of 0.5 mg twice daily; the mean free fraction of risperidone in plasma was increased by 35% compared to healthy subjects.

I.M.: An initial dose of 12.5 mg may be considered

Mechanism of Action Risperidone is a benzisoxazole atypical antipsychotic with mixed serotonin-dopamine antagonist activity that binds to 5-HT$_2$-receptors in the CNS and in the periphery with a very high affinity; binds to dopamine-D$_2$ receptors with less affinity. The binding affinity to the dopamine-D$_2$ receptor is 20 times lower than the 5-HT$_2$ affinity. The addition of serotonin antagonism to dopamine antagonism (classic neuroleptic mechanism) is thought to improve negative symptoms of psychoses and reduce the incidence of extrapyramidal side effects. Alpha$_1$, alpha$_2$ adrenergic, and histaminergic receptors are also antagonized with high affinity. Risperidone has low to moderate affinity for 5-HT$_{1C}$, 5-HT$_{1D}$, and 5-HT$_{1A}$ receptors, weak affinity for D$_1$ and no affinity for muscarinics or beta$_1$ and beta$_2$ receptors

Contraindications Hypersensitivity to risperidone or any component of the formulation

Warnings/Precautions [U.S. Boxed Warning]: Patients with dementia-related psychosis treated with atypical antipsychotics are at an increased risk of death compared to placebo. An increased incidence of cerebrovascular adverse events (including fatalities) has been reported in elderly patients with dementia-related psychosis. Risk may be increased by dehydration; use caution with concurrent diuretics. Risperidone is not approved for the treatment of dementia-related psychosis.

Low- to moderately-sedating, use with caution in disorders where CNS depression is a feature. Use with caution in Parkinson's disease. Caution in patients with predisposition to seizures; or severe cardiac disease. Use with caution in renal or hepatic dysfunction; dose reduction recommended. Esophageal dysmotility and aspiration have been associated with antipsychotic use; use with caution in patients at risk of aspiration pneumonia (eg, Alzheimer's disease). Elevates prolactin levels; effects seen in adults and children. Use with caution in breast cancer or other prolactin-dependent tumors. May alter temperature regulation. May mask toxicity of other drugs or conditions (eg intestinal obstruction, Reyes syndrome, brain tumor) due to antiemetic effects.

Use with caution in patients with cardiovascular diseases (eg, heart failure, history of myocardial infarction or ischemia, cerebrovascular disease, conduction abnormalities). May cause orthostatic hypotension; use with caution in patients at risk of this effect (eg, concurrent medication use which may predispose to hypotension/bradycardia or presence of hypovolemia) or in those who would not tolerate transient hypotensive episodes. May alter cardiac conduction (low risk relative to other neuroleptics); life-threatening arrhythmias have occurred with therapeutic doses of neuroleptics.

May cause anticholinergic effects (confusion, agitation, constipation, xerostomia, blurred vision, urinary retention); therefore, they should be used with caution in patients with decreased gastrointestinal motility, urinary retention, BPH, xerostomia, or visual problems. Conditions which also may be exacerbated by cholinergic blockade include narrow-angle glaucoma (screening is recommended) and worsening of myasthenia gravis. Relative to other neuroleptics, risperidone has a low potency of cholinergic blockade.

May cause extrapyramidal symptoms, including pseudoparkinsonism, acute dystonic reactions, akathisia, and tardive dyskinesia (risk of these reactions is low relative to other neuroleptics, and is dose dependent). Risk of neuroleptic malignant syndrome (NMS) may be increased in patients with Parkinson's disease or Lewy body dementia; monitor for symptoms of confusion, obtundation, postural instability and extrapyramidal symptoms. May cause hyperglycemia; in some cases may be extreme and associated with ketoacidosis, hyperosmolar coma, or death. Use with caution in patients with diabetes or other disorders of glucose regulation; monitor for worsening of glucose control. Significant weight gain has been observed with antipsychotic therapy; incidence varies with product. Monitor waist circumference and BMI.

The possibility of a suicide attempt is inherent in psychotic illness or bipolar disorder; use caution in high-risk patients during initiation of therapy. Prescriptions should be written for the smallest quantity consistent with good patient care. Safety and efficacy have not been established in children for schizophrenia or bipolar disorder. Long-term effects on growth or sexual maturation have not been evaluated.

Drug Interactions
  Cytochrome P450 Effect: Substrate of CYP2D6 (major), 3A4 (minor); **Inhibits** CYP2D6 (weak), 3A4 (weak)
  Increased Effect/Toxicity: CNS depressants and valproic acid may increase adverse effects/toxicity of risperidone. CYP2D6 inhibitors may increase the levels/effects of risperidone; example inhibitors include chlorpromazine, delavirdine, fluoxetine, miconazole, paroxetine, pergolide, quinidine, quinine, ritonavir, and ropinirole. Clozapine decreases clearance of risperidone. Acetylcholinesterase inhibitors (central) may increase the risk of antipsychotic-related EPS. Pramlintide may increase anticholinergic effects of risperidone on the GI tract. Verapamil, SSRIs, and lithium may increase the levels and effects of risperidone. May enhance the effects of other anticholinergics.
  Decreased Effect: Carbamazepine decreases risperidone serum concentrations.

Ethanol/Nutrition/Herb Interactions
  Ethanol: Avoid ethanol (may increase CNS depression).
  Herb/Nutraceutical: Avoid kava kava, gotu kola, valerian, St John's wort (may increase CNS depression).

Dietary Considerations May be taken with or without food. Risperdal® M-Tabs® contain phenylalanine.

Pharmacodynamics/Kinetics
  Absorption:
    Oral: Rapid and well absorbed; food does not affect rate or extent
    Injection: <1% absorbed initially; main release occurs at ~3 weeks and is maintained from 4-6 weeks
  Distribution: V_d: 1-2 L/kg
  Protein binding, plasma: Risperidone 90%; 9-hydroxyrisperidone: 77%
  Metabolism: Extensively hepatic via CYP2D6 to 9-hydroxyrisperidone (similar pharmacological activity as risperidone); N-dealkylation is a second minor pathway
  Bioavailability: Solution: 70%; Tablet: 66%; orally-disintegrating tablets and oral solution are bioequivalent to tablets
  Half-life elimination: Active moiety (risperidone and its active metabolite 9-hydroxyrisperidone)
    Oral: 20 hours (mean)
      Extensive metabolizers: Risperidone: 3 hours; 9-hydroxyrisperidone: 21 hours
      Poor metabolizers: Risperidone: 20 hours; 9-hydroxyrisperidone: 30 hours
    Injection: 3-6 days; related to microsphere erosion and subsequent absorption of risperidone
  Time to peak, plasma: Oral: Risperidone: Within 1 hour; 9-hydroxyrisperidone: Extensive metabolizers: 3 hours; Poor metabolizers: 17 hours
  Excretion: Urine (70%); feces (15%)

Pregnancy Risk Factor C

Dosage Forms
  Injection, microspheres for reconstitution, extended release:
    Risperdal® Consta®: 12.5 mg, 25 mg, 37.5 mg, 50 mg
  Solution, oral:
    Risperdal®: 1 mg/mL
  Tablet:
    Risperdal®: 0.25 mg, 0.5 mg, 1 mg, 2 mg, 3 mg, 4 mg
  Tablet, orally disintegrating:
    Risperdal® M-Tabs®: 0.5 mg, 1 mg, 2 mg, 3 mg, 4 mg

Ritalin® *see* Methylphenidate *on page 1079*
Ritalin® LA *see* Methylphenidate *on page 1079*

Ritalin-SR® see Methylphenidate on page 1079

Ritonavir (ri TOE na veer)

Related Information
HIV Infection and AIDS on page 1753
Tuberculosis Treatment on page 1909
U.S. Brand Names Norvir®
Canadian Brand Names Norvir®; Norvir® SEC
Mexican Brand Names Norvir
Generic Available No
Pharmacologic Category Antiretroviral Agent, Protease Inhibitor
Use Treatment of HIV infection; should always be used as part of a multidrug regimen (at least three antiretroviral agents); may be used as a pharmacokinetic "booster" for other protease inhibitors
Local Anesthetic/Vasoconstrictor Precautions No information available to require special precautions
Effects on Dental Treatment Key adverse event(s) related to dental treatment: Xerostomia (normal salivary flow resumes upon discontinuation) and taste perversion.
Common Adverse Effects Protease inhibitors cause dyslipidemia which includes elevated cholesterol and triglycerides and a redistribution of body fat centrally to cause increased abdominal girth, buffalo hump, facial atrophy, and breast enlargement. These agents also cause hyperglycemia. Percentages as reported in adults:

>10%:
Endocrine & metabolic: Hypercholesterolemia (>240 mg/dL: 37% to 45%), triglycerides increased (>800 mg/dL: 17% to 34%; >1500 mg/dL: 1% to 13%)
Gastrointestinal: Nausea (26% to 30%), diarrhea (15% to 23%), vomiting (14% to 17%), taste perversion (7% to 11%)
Hematologic: WBCs decreased
Hepatic: GGT increased (5% to 20%)
Neuromuscular & skeletal: Weakness (10% to 15%), creatine phosphokinase increased (9% to 12%)

2% to 10%:
Cardiovascular: Syncope (<1% to 2%), vasodilation (2%)
Central nervous system: Fever (4% to 5%), dizziness (3% to 4%), insomnia (2% to 3%), somnolence (2% to 3%), anxiety (2%),
Dermatologic: Rash
Endocrine & metabolic: Uric acid increased (up to 4%)
Gastrointestinal: Abdominal pain (6% to 8%), anorexia (2% to 8%), dyspepsia (up to 6%), local throat irritation (2% to 3%)
Hematologic: Eosinophilia, neutropenia, neutrophilia
Hepatic: LFTs increased (6% to 10%)
Neuromuscular & skeletal: Paresthesia (3% to 7%), arthralgia (up to 2%), myalgia (2%)
Respiratory: Pharyngitis
Miscellaneous: Circumoral paresthesia, diaphoresis (2% to 3%)

Mechanism of Action Ritonavir inhibits HIV protease and renders the enzyme incapable of processing of polyprotein precursor which leads to production of noninfectious immature HIV particles

Drug Interactions
Cytochrome P450 Effect: Substrate of CYP1A2 (minor), 2B6 (minor), 2D6 (major), 3A4 (major); **Inhibits** CYP2C8 (strong), 2C9 (weak), 2C19 (weak), 2D6 (strong), 2E1 (weak), 3A4 (strong); **Induces** CYP1A2 (weak), 2C8 (weak), 2C9 (weak), 3A4 (weak)
Increased Effect/Toxicity: Concurrent use of alfuzosin, amiodarone, cisapride, ergot alkaloids (including dihydroergotamine, ergonovine, methylergonovine), flecainide, midazolam, pimozide, propafenone, quinidine, and triazolam is contraindicated.

Saquinavir's serum concentrations are increased by ritonavir; the dosage of both agents should be reduced to 400 mg twice daily. Concurrent therapy with amprenavir may result in increased serum concentrations: dosage adjustment is recommended. Metronidazole or disulfiram may cause disulfiram reaction (oral solution contains 43% ethanol). Serum levels/effects of corticosteroids (eg, budesonide, fluticasone) and immunosuppressants (cyclosporine, sirolimus, tacrolimus; monitor) may be increased by ritonavir. Serum concentrations of the parent drug and/or metabolite(s) of several analgesics (eg, tramadol, meperidine, propoxyphene) may be increased by ritonavir; increased levels of normeperidine may increase the risk of CNS toxicity/

seizures. Rifabutin and rifabutin metabolite serum concentrations may be increased by ritonavir; reduce rifabutin dose to 150 mg every other day.

Ritonavir may increase the levels/effects of amiodarone, amphetamines, selected beta-blockers, selected benzodiazepines (midazolam and triazolam contraindicated), calcium channel blockers, bupropion, carbamazepine, cisapride (contraindicated), delavirdine, dextromethorphan, digoxin, eplerenone, ergot alkaloids (contraindicated), ethosuximide, fentanyl, fluoxetine, lidocaine, HMG-CoA reductase inhibitors, mirtazapine, nateglinide, nefazodone, paclitaxel, paroxetine, perphenazine, pimozide (contraindicated), propafenone (contraindicated), repaglinide, risperidone, rosiglitazone, sildenafil (and other PDE-5 inhibitors), thioridazine, trazodone, tricyclic antidepressants, venlafaxine, zolpidem, and other substrates of CYP2D6 or 3A4. Thioridazine is generally contraindicated with strong CYP2D6 inhibitors. When used with strong CYP3A4 inhibitors, dosage adjustment/limits are recommended for sildenafil and other PDE-5 inhibitors; refer to individual monographs.

Decreased Effect: The administration of didanosine (buffered formulation) should be separated from ritonavir by 2.5 hours to limit interaction with ritonavir. Concurrent use of rifampin, rifabutin, dexamethasone, and many anticonvulsants may lower serum concentration of ritonavir. Ritonavir may reduce the concentration of ethinyl estradiol which may result in loss of contraception (including combination products). Theophylline concentrations may be reduced in concurrent therapy. Levels of didanosine and zidovudine may be decreased by ritonavir, however, no dosage adjustment is necessary. Voriconazole serum levels are reduced by ritonavir. In addition, ritonavir may decrease the serum concentrations of the following drugs: Atovaquone, divalproex, lamotrigine, methadone, phenytoin. The levels/effects of ritonavir may be decreased by aminoglutethimide, carbamazepine, nafcillin, nevirapine, phenobarbital, phenytoin, rifamycins, and other CYP3A4 inducers. Ritonavir may decrease the levels/effects of CYP2D6 prodrug substrates (eg, codeine, hydrocodone, oxycodone, tramadol).

Pharmacodynamics/Kinetics
Absorption: Variable; increased with food
Distribution: High concentrations in serum and lymph nodes
Protein binding: 98% to 99%
Metabolism: Hepatic via CYP3A4 and 2D6; five metabolites, low concentration of an active metabolite achieved in plasma (oxidative)
Half-life elimination: 3-5 hours
Time to peak, plasma: 2 hours (fasted); 4 hours (nonfasted)
Excretion: Urine (~11%); feces (~86%)

Pregnancy Risk Factor B

Ritonavir and Lopinavir *see* Lopinavir and Ritonavir *on page 997*
Rituxan® *see* Rituximab *on page 1437*

Rituximab (ri TUK si mab)

U.S. Brand Names Rituxan®
Canadian Brand Names Rituxan®
Mexican Brand Names Mabthera
Generic Available No
Index Terms Anti-CD20 Monoclonal Antibody; C2B8; C2B8 Monoclonal Antibody; IDEC-C2B8; NSC-687451; Pan-B Antibody
Pharmacologic Category Antineoplastic Agent, Monoclonal Antibody; Monoclonal Antibody
Use Treatment of low-grade or follicular CD20-positive, B-cell non-Hodgkin's lymphoma (NHL); treatment of diffuse large B-cell CD20-positive NHL; treatment of rheumatoid arthritis (RA) in combination with methotrexate
Unlabeled/Investigational Use Treatment of autoimmune hemolytic anemia (AIHA) in children; chronic immune thrombocytopenic purpura (ITP); chronic lymphocytic leukemia (CLL); small lymphocytic lymphoma (SLL); pemphigus vulgaris, Waldenström's macroglobulinemia (WM); treatment of systemic autoimmune diseases (other than rheumatoid arthritis); treatment of refractory chronic graft-versus-host disease (GVHD)
Local Anesthetic/Vasoconstrictor Precautions No information available to require special precautions
Effects on Dental Treatment No significant effects or complications reported
Common Adverse Effects Note: Patients treated with rituximab for rheumatoid arthritis (RA) may experience fewer adverse reactions.
>10%:
Central nervous system: Fever (5% to 53%), chills (3% to 33%), headache (19%), pain (12%)
(Continued)

Rituximab *(Continued)*

Dermatologic: Rash (15%), pruritus (5% to 14%), angioedema (11%)

Gastrointestinal: Nausea (8% to 23%), abdominal pain (2% to 14%)

Hematologic: Lymphopenia (48%; grade 3/4: 40%; median duration 14 days), leukopenia (14%; grade 3/4: 4%), neutropenia (14%; grade 3/4: 6%; median duration 13 days), thrombocytopenia (12%; grade 3/4: 2%)

Neuromuscular & skeletal: Weakness (2% to 26%)

Respiratory: Cough (13%), rhinitis (3% to 12%)

Miscellaneous: Infection (31%; grade 3/4: 2%; bacterial: 19%; viral 10%; fungal: 1%), night sweats (15%)

Mild-to-moderate infusion-related reactions: Chills, fever, rigors, dizziness, hypertension, myalgia, nausea, pruritus, rash, and vomiting (lymphoma: first dose 77%; fourth dose 30%; eighth dose 14%); infusion-related reactions reported are lower in RA

1% to 10%:

Cardiovascular: Hypotension (10%), peripheral edema (8%), hypertension (6% to 8%), flushing (5%), edema (<5%)

Central nervous system: Dizziness (10%), anxiety (2% to 5%), agitation (<5%), depression (<5%), hypoesthesia (<5%), insomnia (<5%), malaise (<5%), nervousness (<5%), neuritis (<5%), somnolence (<5%), vertigo (<5%), migraine (RA: 2%)

Dermatologic: Urticaria (2% to 8%)

Endocrine & metabolic: Hyperglycemia (9%), hypoglycemia (<5%), hypercholesterolemia (2%)

Gastrointestinal: Diarrhea (10%), vomiting (10%), dyspepsia (3% to 5%), anorexia (<5%), weight loss (<5%)

Hematologic: Anemia (8%; grade 3/4: 3%)

Local: Pain at the injection site (<5%)

Neuromuscular & skeletal: Back pain (10%), myalgia (10%), arthralgia (6% to 10%), paresthesia (2% to 5%), arthritis (<5%), hyperkinesia (<5%), hypertonia (<5%), neuropathy (<5%)

Ocular: Conjunctivitis (<5%), lacrimation disorder (<5%)

Respiratory: Throat irritation (2% to 9%), bronchospasm (8%), dyspnea (7%), upper respiratory tract infection (RA: 7%), sinusitis (6%)

Miscellaneous: LDH increased (7%)

Restrictions An FDA-approved medication guide is available; distribute to each patient to whom this medication is dispensed.

Mechanism of Action Rituximab is a monoclonal antibody directed against the CD20 antigen on B-lymphocytes. CD20 regulates cell cycle initiation; and, possibly, functions as a calcium channel. Rituximab binds to the antigen on the cell surface, activating complement-dependent cytotoxicity; and to human Fc receptors, mediating cell killing through an antibody-dependent cellular toxicity. B-cells are believed to play a role in the development and progression of rheumatoid arthritis. Signs and symptoms of RA are reduced by targeting B-cells.

Drug Interactions

Increased Effect/Toxicity: Monoclonal antibodies may increase the risk for allergic reactions to rituximab due to the presence of HACA antibody. Antihypertensive medications may exacerbate hypotension.

Decreased Effect: Currently recommended not to administer live vaccines during rituximab treatment.

Pharmacodynamics/Kinetics

Duration: Detectable in serum 3-6 months after completion of treatment; B-cell recovery begins ~6 months following completion of treatment; median B-cell levels return to normal by 12 months following completion of treatment

Absorption: I.V.: Immediate and results in a rapid and sustained depletion of circulating and tissue-based B cells

Distribution: 4.3 L (following two 1000 mg doses for rheumatoid arthritis)

Half-life elimination:

Cancer: Proportional to dose; wide ranges reflect variable tumor burden and changes in CD20 positive B-cell populations with repeated doses:

>100 mg/m^2: 4.4 days (range 1.6-10.5 days)

375 mg/m^2:

Following first dose: Mean half-life: 3.2 days (range 1.3-6.4 days)

Following fourth dose: Mean half-life: 8.6 days (range 3.5-17 days)

RA: Mean terminal half-life: 19 days

Excretion: Uncertain; may undergo phagocytosis and catabolism in the reticuloendothelial system (RES)

Pregnancy Risk Factor C

Rivastigmine (ri va STIG meen)

U.S. Brand Names Exelon®
Canadian Brand Names Exelon®
Mexican Brand Names Exelon
Generic Available No
Index Terms ENA 713; Rivastigmine Tartrate; SDZ ENA 713
Pharmacologic Category Acetylcholinesterase Inhibitor (Central)
Use Treatment of mild-to-moderate dementia associated with Alzheimer's disease and Parkinson's disease
Local Anesthetic/Vasoconstrictor Precautions No information available to require special precautions
Effects on Dental Treatment No significant effects or complications reported
Common Adverse Effects
>10%:
Central nervous system: Dizziness (6% to 21%), headache (4% to 17%)
Gastrointestinal: Nausea (29% to 47%), vomiting (17% to 31%), diarrhea (7% to 19%), anorexia (6% to 17%), abdominal pain (4% to 13%)
2% to 10%:
Cardiovascular: Syncope (3%), hypertension (3%)
Central nervous system: Fatigue (4% to 9%), insomnia (9%), confusion (8%), depression (6%), anxiety (5%), malaise (5%), somnolence (4% to 5%), hallucinations (4%), aggressiveness (3%), parkinsonism symptoms worsening (2% to 3%)
Gastrointestinal: Dyspepsia (9%), constipation (5%), flatulence (4%), weight loss (3%), eructation (2%), dehydration (2%)
Genitourinary: Urinary tract infection (7%)
Neuromuscular & skeletal: Weakness (2% to 6%), tremor (4%; up to 10% in Parkinson's patients)
Respiratory: Rhinitis (4%)
Miscellaneous: Diaphoresis (4%), flu-like syndrome (3%)
≥1% (Drug causality indeterminate; frequency most often similar to placebo): Accidental trauma, agitation, allergy, anemia, angina, arthralgia, arthritis, ataxia, atrial fibrillation, back pain, bone fracture, bradycardia, bronchitis, cardiac failure, cataract, chest pain, confusion, cough, delusion, depression, dyspnea, dyskinesia, edema, epistaxis, fecal incontinence, fever, gait abnormal, gastritis, hematuria, hot flushes, hypokalemia, hypotension (including postural), infection, leg cramps, MI, myalgia, nervousness, pain, palpitation, paranoid reaction, paresthesia, peripheral edema, pharyngitis, rash, restlessness, rigors, salivation increased, seizure, tinnitus, transient ischemic attack, upper respiratory tract infection, urinary incontinence, vertigo
Mechanism of Action A deficiency of cortical acetylcholine is thought to account for some of the symptoms of Alzheimer's disease and the dementia of Parkinson's disease; rivastigmine increases acetylcholine in the central nervous system through reversible inhibition of its hydrolysis by cholinesterase
Drug Interactions
Increased Effect/Toxicity: Acetylcholinesterase inhibitors (central) may increase the risk of antipsychotic-related extrapyramidal symptoms. Beta-blockers without ISA activity may increase risk of bradycardia. Calcium channel blockers (diltiazem or verapamil) may increase risk of bradycardia. Cholinergic agonists effects may be increased with rivastigmine. Depolarizing neuromuscular blocking agents effects may be increased with rivastigmine. Digoxin may increase risk of bradycardia.
Decreased Effect: Anticholinergic agents effects may be reduced with rivastigmine.
Pharmacodynamics/Kinetics
Duration: Anticholinesterase activity (CSF): ~10 hours (6 mg dose)
Absorption: Fasting: Rapid and complete within 1 hour
Distribution: V_d: 1.8-2.7 L/kg
Protein binding: 40%
Metabolism: Extensively via cholinesterase-mediated hydrolysis in the brain; metabolite undergoes N-demethylation and/or sulfate conjugation hepatically; CYP minimally involved; linear kinetics at 3 mg twice daily, but nonlinear at higher doses
Bioavailability: 36% to 40%
Half-life elimination: 1.5 hours
Time to peak: 1 hour
Excretion: Urine (97% as metabolites); feces (0.4%)
Pregnancy Risk Factor B

Rivastigmine Tartrate see Rivastigmine *on page 1439*

Rizatriptan (rye za TRIP tan)

Related Information
Temporomandibular Dysfunction (TMD) *on page 1822*
U.S. Brand Names Maxalt®; Maxalt-MLT®
Canadian Brand Names Maxalt™; Maxalt RPD™
Mexican Brand Names Maxalt
Generic Available No
Index Terms MK462
Pharmacologic Category Antimigraine Agent; Serotonin 5-HT$_{1B, 1D}$ Receptor Agonist
Use Acute treatment of migraine with or without aura
Local Anesthetic/Vasoconstrictor Precautions No information available to require special precautions
Effects on Dental Treatment Key adverse event(s) related to dental treatment: Xerostomia (normal salivary flow resumes upon discontinuation).
Common Adverse Effects 1% to 10%:
Cardiovascular: Systolic/diastolic blood pressure increases (5-10 mm Hg), chest pain (5%), palpitation
Central nervous system: Dizziness, drowsiness, fatigue (13% to 30%, dose related)
Dermatologic: Skin flushing
Endocrine & metabolic: Mild increase in growth hormone, hot flashes
Gastrointestinal: Abdominal pain, dry mouth (<5%), nausea
Respiratory: Dyspnea
Dosage Note: In patients with risk factors for coronary artery disease, following adequate evaluation to establish the absence of coronary artery disease, the initial dose should be administered in a setting where response may be evaluated (physician's office or similarly staffed setting). ECG monitoring may be considered.
Oral: 5-10 mg, repeat after 2 hours if significant relief is not attained; maximum: 30 mg in a 24-hour period (use 5 mg dose in patients receiving propranolol with a maximum of 15 mg in 24 hours)
Note: For orally-disintegrating tablets (Maxalt-MLT®): Patient should be instructed to place tablet on tongue and allow to dissolve. Dissolved tablet will be swallowed with saliva.
Mechanism of Action Selective agonist for serotonin (5-HT$_{1D}$ receptor) in cranial arteries to cause vasoconstriction and reduce sterile inflammation associated with antidromic neuronal transmission correlating with relief of migraine
Contraindications Hypersensitivity to rizatriptan or any component of the formulation; documented ischemic heart disease or Prinzmetal's angina; uncontrolled hypertension; basilar or hemiplegic migraine; during or within 2 weeks of MAO inhibitors; during or within 24 hours of treatment with another 5-HT$_1$ agonist, or an ergot-containing or ergot-type medication (eg, methysergide, dihydroergotamine)
Warnings/Precautions Use only in patients with a clear diagnosis of migraine. May cause vasospastic reactions resulting in colonic, peripheral, or coronary ischemia. Use with caution in elderly or patients with hepatic or renal impairment (including dialysis patients); history of hypersensitivity to sumatriptan or adverse effects from sumatriptan, and in patients at risk of coronary artery disease (as predicted by presence of risk factors) unless cardiovascular evaluation provides evidence that the patient is free of cardiovascular disease. In patients with risk factors for coronary artery disease, following adequate evaluation to establish the absence of coronary artery disease, the initial dose should be administered in a setting where response may be evaluated (physician's office or similarly staffed setting). ECG monitoring may be considered. May increase blood pressure transiently; may cause coronary vasospasm (less than sumatriptan); avoid in patients with signs/symptoms suggestive of reduced arterial flow (ischemic bowel, Raynaud's) which could be exacerbated by vasospasm. Cerebral/subarachnoid hemorrhage and stroke have been reported with 5-HT$_1$ agonist administration.

Patients who experience sensations of chest pain/pressure/tightness or symptoms suggestive of angina following dosing should be evaluated for coronary artery disease or Prinzmetal's angina before receiving additional doses. Symptoms of agitation, confusion, hallucinations, hyper-reflexia, myoclonus, shivering, and tachycardia (serotonin syndrome) may occur with concomitant proserotonergic drugs (ie, SSRIs/SNRIs or triptans) or agents which reduce rizatriptan's metabolism. Concurrent use of serotonin precursors (eg, tryptophan) is not recommended.

Reconsider diagnosis of migraine if no response to initial dose. Long-term effects on vision have not been evaluated. Safety and efficacy have not been established in children <18 years of age. Maxalt-MLT® tablets contain phenylalanine.

Drug Interactions

Increased Effect/Toxicity: Use within 24 hours of another selective 5-HT₁ antagonist or ergot-containing drug should be avoided due to possible additive vasoconstriction. Use with propranolol increased plasma concentration of rizatriptan by 70%. SSRIs/SNRIs may exhibit additive toxicity with rizatriptan or other serotonin agonists (eg, antidepressants, dextromethorphan, tramadol) leading to serotonin syndrome. MAO inhibitors and nonselective MAO inhibitors increase concentration of rizatriptan.

Ethanol/Nutrition/Herb Interactions Food: Food delays absorption.

Dietary Considerations Orally-disintegrating tablet contains phenylalanine (1.05 mg per 5 mg tablet, 2.10 mg per 10 mg tablet).

Pharmacodynamics/Kinetics

Onset of action: ~30 minutes

Duration: 14-16 hours

Protein binding: 14%

Metabolism: Via monoamine oxidase-A; first-pass effect

Bioavailability: 40% to 50%

Half-life elimination: 2-3 hours

Time to peak: 1-1.5 hours

Excretion: Urine (82%, 8% to 16% as unchanged drug); feces (12%)

Pregnancy Risk Factor C

Dosage Forms

Tablet:

Maxalt®: 5 mg, 10 mg

Tablet, orally disintegrating:

Maxalt-MLT®: 5 mg, 10 mg

rLFN-α2 *see* Interferon Alfa-2b *on page 891*

RMS® *see* Morphine Sulfate *on page 1123*

Ro 5488 *see* Tretinoin (Oral) *on page 1606*

Robafen® AC *see* Guaifenesin and Codeine *on page 795*

Robafen DM [OTC] *see* Guaifenesin and Dextromethorphan *on page 796*

Robafen DM Clear [OTC] *see* Guaifenesin and Dextromethorphan *on page 796*

Robaxin® *see* Methocarbamol *on page 1065*

Robinul® *see* Glycopyrrolate *on page 790*

Robinul® Forte *see* Glycopyrrolate *on page 790*

Robitussin® [OTC] *see* Guaifenesin *on page 795*

Robitussin® Cough and Cold [OTC] *see* Guaifenesin, Pseudoephedrine, and Dextromethorphan *on page 800*

Robitussin® Cough and Cold CF [OTC] *see* Guaifenesin, Pseudoephedrine, and Dextromethorphan *on page 800*

Robitussin® Cough and Cold Infant CF [OTC] *see* Guaifenesin, Pseudoephedrine, and Dextromethorphan *on page 800*

Robitussin® Cough and Congestion [OTC] *see* Guaifenesin and Dextromethorphan *on page 796*

Robitussin® CoughGels™ [OTC] *see* Dextromethorphan *on page 477*

Robitussin® DM [OTC] *see* Guaifenesin and Dextromethorphan *on page 796*

Robitussin® DM Infant [OTC] *see* Guaifenesin and Dextromethorphan *on page 796*

Robitussin® Maximum Strength Cough [OTC] *see* Dextromethorphan *on page 477*

Robitussin® Maximum Strength Cough & Cold [OTC] [DSC] *see* Pseudoephedrine and Dextromethorphan *on page 1383*

Robitussin®-PE® [OTC] [DSC] *see* Guaifenesin and Pseudoephedrine *on page 798*

Robitussin® Pediatric Cough [OTC] *see* Dextromethorphan *on page 477*

Robitussin® Pediatric Cough & Cold [OTC] [DSC] *see* Pseudoephedrine and Dextromethorphan *on page 1383*

Robitussin® Severe Congestion [OTC] [DSC] *see* Guaifenesin and Pseudoephedrine *on page 798*

Robitussin® Sugar Free Cough [OTC] *see* Guaifenesin and Dextromethorphan *on page 796*

Rocaltrol® *see* Calcitriol *on page 258*

Rocephin® *see* Ceftriaxone *on page 309*

Roferon®-A *see* Interferon Alfa-2a *on page 890*

Rogaine® Extra Strength for Men [OTC] *see* Minoxidil *on page 1109*

Rogaine® for Men [OTC] *see* Minoxidil *on page 1109*

Rogaine® for Women [OTC] *see* Minoxidil *on page 1109*

Rolaids® [OTC] *see* Calcium Carbonate and Magnesium Hydroxide *on page 261*

Ropinirole (roe PIN i role)

U.S. Brand Names Requip®
Canadian Brand Names Requip®
Generic Available No
Index Terms Ropinirole Hydrochloride
Pharmacologic Category Anti-Parkinson's Agent, Dopamine Agonist
Use Treatment of idiopathic Parkinson's disease; in patients with early Parkinson's disease who were not receiving concomitant levodopa therapy as well as in patients with advanced disease on concomitant levodopa; treatment of moderate-to-severe primary Restless Legs Syndrome (RLS)
Local Anesthetic/Vasoconstrictor Precautions No information available to require special precautions
Effects on Dental Treatment Key adverse event(s) related to dental treatment: Xerostomia and increased salivation (normal salivary flow resumes upon discontinuation) and dysphagia.
Common Adverse Effects
Data inclusive of trials in early Parkinson's disease (without levodopa) and Restless Legs Syndrome:
>10%:
Cardiovascular: Syncope (1% to 12%)
Central nervous system: Somnolence (12% to 40%), dizziness (11% to 40%), fatigue (8% to 11%)
Gastrointestinal: Nausea (40% to 60%), vomiting (12%)
Miscellaneous: Viral infection (11%)
1% to 10%:
Cardiovascular: Dependent/leg edema (2% to 7%), orthostasis (1% to 6%), hypertension (5%), chest pain (4%), flushing (3%), palpitation (3%), peripheral ischemia (3%), hypotension (2%), tachycardia (2%)
Central nervous system: Pain (3% to 8%), confusion (5%), hallucinations (up to 5%, dose related), hypoesthesia (4%), amnesia (3%), malaise (3%), paresthesia (3%), vertigo (2%), yawning (3%)
Gastrointestinal: Constipation (>5%), dyspepsia (4% to 10%), abdominal pain (3% to 6%), xerostomia (3% to 5%), diarrhea (5%), anorexia (4%), flatulence (3%)
Genitourinary: Urinary tract infection (5%), impotence (3%)
Hepatic: Alkaline phosphatase increased (3%)
Neuromuscular & skeletal: Weakness (6%), arthralgia (4%), muscle cramps (3%)
Ocular: Abnormal vision (6%), xerophthalmia (2%)
Respiratory: Pharyngitis (6% to 9%), rhinitis (4%), sinusitis (4%), dyspnea (3%), influenza (3%), cough (3%), nasal congestion (2%)
Miscellaneous: Diaphoresis increased (3% to 6%)

Advanced Parkinson's disease (with levodopa):
>10%:
Central nervous system: Dizziness (26%), somnolence (20%), headache (17%)
Gastrointestinal: Nausea (30%)
Neuromuscular & skeletal: Dyskinesias (34%)
1% to 10%:
Cardiovascular: Syncope (3%), hypotension (2%)
Central nervous system: Hallucinations (10%, dose related), aggravated parkinsonism, confusion (9%), pain (5%), paresis (3%), amnesia (5%), anxiety (6%), abnormal dreaming (3%), insomnia
Gastrointestinal: Abdominal pain (9%), vomiting (7%), constipation (6%), diarrhea (5%), dysphagia (2%), flatulence (2%), increased salivation (2%), xerostomia, weight loss (2%)
Genitourinary: Urinary tract infection
Hematologic: Anemia (2%)
Neuromuscular & skeletal: Falls (10%), arthralgia (7%), tremor (6%), hypokinesia (5%), paresthesia (5%), arthritis (3%)
Respiratory: Upper respiratory tract infection (9%), dyspnea (3%)

Miscellaneous: Injury, diaphoresis increased (7%), viral infection, increased drug level (7%)

Other adverse effects (all phase 2/3 trials):
1% to 10%:
Central nervous system: Neuralgia (>1%)
Renal: BUN increased (>1%)

Mechanism of Action Ropinirole has a high relative *in vitro* specificity and full intrinsic activity at the D_2 and D_3 dopamine receptor subtypes, binding with higher affinity to D_3 than to D_2 or D_4 receptor subtypes; relevance of D_3 receptor binding in Parkinson's disease is unknown. Ropinirole has moderate *in vitro* affinity for opioid receptors. Ropinirole and its metabolites have negligible *in vitro* affinity for dopamine D_1, 5-HT$_1$, 5-HT$_2$, benzodiazepine, GABA, muscarinic, alpha$_1$-, alpha$_2$-, and beta-adrenoreceptors. Although precise mechanism of action of ropinirole is unknown, it is believed to be due to stimulation of postsynaptic dopamine D_2-type receptors within the caudate putamen in the brain. Ropinirole caused decreases in systolic and diastolic blood pressure at doses >0.25 mg. The mechanism of ropinirole-induced postural hypotension is believed to be due to D_2-mediated blunting of the noradrenergic response to standing and subsequent decrease in peripheral vascular resistance.

Drug Interactions

Cytochrome P450 Effect: Substrate of CYP1A2 (major), 3A4 (minor); **Inhibits** CYP1A2 (weak), 2D6 (strong)

Increased Effect/Toxicity: The levels/effects of ropinirole may be increased by ciprofloxacin, fluvoxamine, ketoconazole, norfloxacin, ofloxacin, rofecoxib, and other CYP1A2 inhibitors. Estrogens may also reduce the metabolism of ropinirole; dosage adjustments may be needed. Ropinirole may increase the levels/effects of amphetamines, selected beta-blockers, dextromethorphan, fluoxetine, lidocaine, mirtazapine, nefazodone, paroxetine, risperidone, ritonavir, thioridazine, tricyclic antidepressants, venlafaxine, and other CYP2D6 substrates.

Decreased Effect: The levels/effects of ropinirole may be decreased by aminoglutethimide, carbamazepine, phenobarbital, rifampin, and other CYP1A2 inducers. Antipsychotics, cigarette smoking, and metoclopramide may reduce the effect or serum concentrations of ropinirole. Ropinirole may decrease the levels/effects of CYP2D6 prodrug substrates (eg, codeine, hydrocodone, oxycodone, tramadol).

Pharmacodynamics/Kinetics

Absorption: Not affected by food

Distribution: V_d: 525 L

Metabolism: Extensively hepatic via CYP1A2 to inactive metabolites; first-pass effect

Bioavailability: Absolute: 55%

Half-life elimination: ~6 hours

Time to peak: ~1-2 hours; T_{max} increased by 2.5 hours when drug taken with food

Excretion: Clearance: Reduced by 30% in patients >65 years of age

Pregnancy Risk Factor C

Ropinirole Hydrochloride *see* Ropinirole *on page 1442*

Ropivacaine (roe PIV a kane)

Related Information
Oral Pain *on page 1788*

U.S. Brand Names Naropin®

Canadian Brand Names Naropin®

Mexican Brand Names Naropin

Generic Available No

Index Terms Ropivacaine Hydrochloride

Pharmacologic Category Local Anesthetic

Use Local anesthetic for use in surgery, postoperative pain management, and obstetrical procedures when local or regional anesthesia is needed

Local Anesthetic/Vasoconstrictor Precautions No information available to require special precautions (see Dental Comment)

Effects on Dental Treatment No significant effects or complications reported

Common Adverse Effects
>10%:
Cardiovascular: Hypotension (dose-related and age-related: 32% to 69%), bradycardia (6% to 20%)
Gastrointestinal: Nausea (11% to 29%), vomiting (7% to 14%)
Neuromuscular & skeletal: Back pain (7% to 16%)
(Continued)

Ropivacaine (Continued)

1% to 10%:
Cardiovascular: Hypertension, tachycardia, chest pain (1% to 5%)
Central nervous system: Fever (3% to 9%), headache (5% to 8%), dizziness (3%), chills (2% to 3%), anxiety (1%), lightheadedness
Dermatologic: Pruritus (1% to 5%)
Endocrine & metabolic: Hypokalemia
Genitourinary: Urinary retention (1% to 5%), urinary tract infection (1% to 5%)
Hematologic: Anemia (6%)
Neuromuscular & skeletal: Paresthesia (2% to 6%), hypoesthesia, rigors, circumoral paresthesia
Renal: Oliguria
Respiratory: Dyspnea
Miscellaneous: Shivering

Mechanism of Action Blocks both the initiation and conduction of nerve impulses by decreasing the neuronal membrane's permeability to sodium ions, which results in inhibition of depolarization with resultant blockade of conduction

Drug Interactions
Cytochrome P450 Effect: Substrate of CYP1A2 (major), 2B6 (minor), 2D6 (minor), 3A4 (minor; may be major in cases of 1A2 inhibition/deficiency)
Increased Effect/Toxicity: Cardiac effects may be additive with amiodarone and other class III antiarrhythmics. Amiodarone, ciprofloxacin, fluvoxamine, and propofol may increase ropivacaine levels/effects (monitor). Other CYP1A2 inhibitors may increase the levels/effects of ropivacaine; example inhibitors include ketoconazole, norfloxacin, ofloxacin, and rofecoxib.

Pharmacodynamics/Kinetics
Onset of action: Anesthesia (route dependent): 3-15 minutes
Duration (dose and route dependent): 3-15 hours
Metabolism: Hepatic, via CYP1A2 to metabolites
Half-life elimination: Epidural: 5-7 hours
Excretion: Urine (86% as metabolites)

Pregnancy Risk Factor B

Dental Comment Not available with vasoconstrictor (epinephrine) and not available in dental (1.8 mL) carpules

Ropivacaine Hydrochloride see Ropivacaine on page 1443

Rosiglitazone (roh si GLI ta zone)

U.S. Brand Names Avandia®
Canadian Brand Names Avandia®
Mexican Brand Names Avandia
Generic Available No
Pharmacologic Category Antidiabetic Agent, Thiazolidinedione
Use Type 2 diabetes mellitus (noninsulin dependent, NIDDM):
Monotherapy: Improve glycemic control as an adjunct to diet and exercise
Combination therapy: In combination with a sulfonylurea, metformin, or insulin, or sulfonylurea plus metformin when diet, exercise, and a single agent do not result in adequate glycemic control
Unlabeled/Investigational Use Polycystic ovary syndrome (PCOS)
Local Anesthetic/Vasoconstrictor Precautions No information available to require special precautions
Effects on Dental Treatment Rosiglitazone-dependent diabetics should be appointed for dental treatment in morning in order to minimize chance of stress-induced hypoglycemia.
Common Adverse Effects Rare cases of hepatocellular injury have been reported in men in their 60s within 2-3 weeks after initiation of rosiglitazone therapy. LFTs in these patients revealed severe hepatocellular injury which responded with rapid improvement of liver function and resolution of symptoms upon discontinuation of rosiglitazone. Patients were also receiving other potentially hepatotoxic medications (*Ann Intern Med*, 2000, 132:121-4; 132:164-6). The rate of certain adverse reactions (eg, anemia, edema, hypoglycemia) may be higher with some combination therapies. Patients with Class I or II heart failure (EF ≤45%) have a higher frequency of cardiovascular adverse events (edema, dyspnea in ≥25%).

>10%: Endocrine & metabolic: Weight gain, increase in total cholesterol, increased LDL-cholesterol, increased HDL-cholesterol
1% to 10%:
Cardiovascular: Edema (5%), heart failure/CHF (up to 2% to 3% in patients receiving insulin; incidence likely higher in patients with pre-existing CHF or macrovascular disease)
Central nervous system: Headache (6%), fatigue (4%)

Endocrine & metabolic: Hyperglycemia (4%), hypoglycemia (1%; increased with insulin to 12% to 14%)

Gastrointestinal: Diarrhea (2%)

Hematologic: Anemia (2%)

Neuromuscular & skeletal: Back pain (4%)

Respiratory: Upper respiratory tract infection (10%), sinusitis (3%)

Miscellaneous: Injury (8%)

Dosage Oral:

Adults: **Note:** All patients should be initiated at the lowest recommended dose.

Monotherapy: Initial: 4 mg daily as a single daily dose or in divided doses twice daily. If response is inadequate after 8-12 weeks of treatment, the dosage may be increased to 8 mg daily as a single daily dose or in divided doses twice daily. In clinical trials, the 4 mg twice-daily regimen resulted in the greatest reduction in fasting plasma glucose and Hb A_{1c}.

Combination therapy: When adding rosiglitazone to existing therapy, continue current dose(s) of previous agents:

With sulfonylureas or metformin (or sulfonylurea plus metformin): Initial: 4 mg daily as a single daily dose or in divided doses twice daily. If response is inadequate after 8-12 weeks of treatment, the dosage may be increased to 8 mg daily as a single daily dose or in divided doses twice daily. Reduce dose of sulfonylurea if hypoglycemia occurs. It is unlikely that the dose of metformin will need to be reduced to hypoglycemia.

With insulin: Initial: 4 mg daily as a single daily dose or in divided doses twice daily. Dose of insulin should be reduced by 10% to 25% if the patient reports hypoglycemia or if the plasma glucose falls to <100 mg/dL. Doses of rosiglitazone >4 mg/day are not indicated in combination with insulin.

Elderly: No dosage adjustment is recommended

Dosage adjustment in renal impairment: No dosage adjustment is required

Dosage comment in hepatic impairment: Clearance is significantly lower in hepatic impairment. Therapy should not be initiated if the patient exhibits active liver disease of increased transaminases (>2.5 times the upper limit of normal) at baseline.

Mechanism of Action Thiazolidinedione antidiabetic agent that lowers blood glucose by improving target cell response to insulin, without increasing pancreatic insulin secretion. It has a mechanism of action that is dependent on the presence of insulin for activity. Rosiglitazone is an agonist for peroxisome proliferator-activated receptor-gamma (PPARgamma). Activation of nuclear PPARgamma receptors influences the production of a number of gene products involved in glucose and lipid metabolism. Thiazolidinedione antidiabetic agent that lowers blood glucose by improving target cell response to insulin, without increasing pancreatic insulin secretion. It has a mechanism of action that is dependent on the presence of insulin for activity. PPARgamma is abundant in the cells within the renal collecting tubules; fluid retention results from stimulation by thiazolidinediones which increases sodium reabsorption.

Contraindications Hypersensitivity to rosiglitazone or any component of the formulation; active liver disease (transaminases >2.5 times the upper limit of normal at baseline); contraindicated in patients who previously experienced jaundice during troglitazone therapy

Warnings/Precautions Should not be used in diabetic ketoacidosis. Mechanism requires the presence of insulin; therefore, use in type 1 diabetes (insulin dependent, IDDM) is not recommended.

May increase plasma volume and/or increase cardiac hypertrophy. Use with caution in patients with edema. Assess for fluid accumulation in patients with unusually rapid weight gain. Monitor closely for signs and symptoms of heart failure. Drug discontinuation is recommended if cardiovascular status worsens. A higher frequency of cardiovascular events has been noted in patients with NYHA Class I or II heart failure; up to 33% require adjustment of medications. Not recommended for use in patients with NYHA class III or IV heart failure. In patients with NYHA class II (systolic) heart failure, initiate at lowest dosage and monitor closely. Discontinue if heart failure develops. Use with caution in patients with anemia or depressed leukocyte counts (may reduce hemoglobin, hematocrit, and/or WBC).

Use with caution in patients with elevated transaminases (AST or ALT). Idiosyncratic hepatotoxicity has been reported with another thiazolidinedione agent (troglitazone) and (rarely) with rosiglitazone; discontinue if jaundice occurs. Monitoring should include periodic determinations of liver function. Rosiglitazone has been associated with new onset and/or worsening of macular edema in diabetic patients. Rosiglitazone should be used with caution in patients with a pre-existing macular edema or diabetic retinopathy. Discontinuation of rosiglitazone should be considered in any patient who reports visual deterioration. In addition, ophthalmological consultation should be initiated in these patients. May result in hormonal imbalance; development of menstrual irregularities should prompt reconsideration of therapy. Use with caution in (Continued)

Rosiglitazone *(Continued)*

premenopausal, anovulatory women; may result in resumption of ovulation, increasing the risk of pregnancy. Safety and efficacy in pediatric patients have not been established.

Drug Interactions

Cytochrome P450 Effect: Substrate of CYP2C8 (major), 2C9 (minor); **Inhibits** CYP2C8 (moderate), 2C9 (weak), 2C19 (weak), 2D6 (weak)

Increased Effect/Toxicity: The levels/effects of rosiglitazone may be increased by atazanavir, ritonavir, and other CYP2C8 inhibitors. Gemfibrozil may increase rosiglitazone levels; severe hypoglycemic episodes have been reported. Rosiglitazone may increase the levels/effects of amiodarone, paclitaxel, pioglitazone, repaglinide, rosiglitazone, and other CYP2C8 substrates.

Decreased Effect: The levels/effects of rosiglitazone may be decreased by carbamazepine, phenobarbital, phenytoin, rifampin, rifapentine, and secobarbital, and other CYP2C8 inducers. Bile acid sequestrants may decrease rosiglitazone levels.

Ethanol/Nutrition/Herb Interactions

Ethanol: Avoid ethanol (may cause hypoglycemia).

Food: Peak concentrations are lower by 28% and delayed when administered with food, but these effects are not believed to be clinically significant.

Herb/Nutraceutical: Avoid garlic, gymnema (may cause hypoglycemia).

Dietary Considerations Management of type 2 diabetes mellitus (noninsulin dependent, NIDDM) should include diet control. May be taken without regard to meals.

Pharmacodynamics/Kinetics

Onset of action: Delayed; Maximum effect: Up to 12 weeks

Distribution: V_{dss} (apparent): 17.6 L

Protein binding: 99.8%; primarily albumin

Metabolism: Hepatic (99%) via CYP2C8; minor metabolism via CYP2C9

Bioavailability: 99%

Half-life elimination: 3-4 hours

Time to peak, plasma: 1 hour; delayed with food

Excretion: Urine (64%) and feces (23%) as metabolites

Pregnancy Risk Factor C

Dosage Forms

Tablet:

Avandia®: 2 mg, 4 mg, 8 mg

Rosiglitazone and Glimepiride

(roh si GLI ta zone & GLYE me pye ride)

Related Information

Glimepiride *on page 780*

Rosiglitazone *on page 1444*

U.S. Brand Names Avandaryl™

Generic Available No

Index Terms Glimepiride and Rosiglitazone Maleate

Pharmacologic Category Antidiabetic Agent, Sulfonylurea; Antidiabetic Agent, Thiazolidinedione

Use Management of type 2 diabetes mellitus (noninsulin dependent, NIDDM) as an adjunct to diet and exercise

Local Anesthetic/Vasoconstrictor Precautions No information available to require special precautions

Effects on Dental Treatment Dependent diabetics (noninsulin dependent, type 2) should be appointed for dental treatment in the morning in order to minimize chance of stress-induced hypoglycemia.

Common Adverse Effects Percentages below refer to combination Avandaryl™. Also see individual agents.

1% to 10%:

Cardiovascular: Edema (3%), hypertension (2% to 3%)

Central nervous system: Headache (3% to 6%)

Endocrine & metabolic: Hypoglycemia (4% to 6%)

Respiratory: Nasopharyngitis (4% to 5%)

Mechanism of Action

Rosiglitazone is a thiazolidinedione antidiabetic agent that lowers blood glucose by improving target cell response to insulin, without increasing pancreatic insulin secretion. It has a mechanism of action that is dependent on the presence of insulin for activity.

Glimepiride stimulates insulin release from the pancreatic beta cells; reduces glucose output from the liver; insulin sensitivity is increased at peripheral target sites.

Drug Interactions
Cytochrome P450 Effect:
Rosiglitazone: **Substrate** of CYP2C8 (major), 2C9 (minor); **Inhibits** CYP2C8 (moderate), 2C9 (weak), 2C19 (weak), 2D6 (weak)
Glimepiride: **Substrate** of CYP2C9 (major)

Increased Effect/Toxicity: See individual agents.

Decreased Effect: See individual agents.

Pharmacodynamics/Kinetics See individual agents.

Pregnancy Risk Factor C

Rosiglitazone and Metformin (roh si GLI ta zone & met FOR min)

Related Information
Metformin *on page 1056*
Rosiglitazone *on page 1444*

U.S. Brand Names Avandamet®

Canadian Brand Names Avandamet®

Generic Available No

Index Terms Metformin and Rosiglitazone; Metformin Hydrochloride and Rosiglitazone Maleate; Rosiglitazone Maleate and Metformin Hydrochloride

Pharmacologic Category Antidiabetic Agent, Biguanide; Antidiabetic Agent, Thiazolidinedione

Use Management of type 2 diabetes mellitus (noninsulin dependent, NIDDM) as an adjunct to diet and exercise in patients where dual rosiglitazone and metformin therapy is appropriate

Local Anesthetic/Vasoconstrictor Precautions No information available to require special precautions

Effects on Dental Treatment Dependent diabetics (noninsulin dependent, type 2) should be appointed for dental treatment in the morning in order to minimize chance of stress-induced hypoglycemia.

Common Adverse Effects Also see individual agents. Percentages of adverse effects as reported with the combination product.
>10%:
Gastrointestinal: Nausea/vomiting (16%), diarrhea (13% to 14%)
Respiratory: Upper respiratory tract infection (9% to 16%)
1% to 10%:
Cardiovascular: Edema (6%)
Central nervous system: Headache (7% to 11%), dizziness (8%), fatigue (6%)
Endocrine & metabolic: Hypoglycemia (3%), hyperglycemia (2%)
Gastrointestinal: Dyspepsia (10%), abdominal pain (5%), loose stools (5%), constipation (5%)
Hematologic: Anemia (4% to 7%)
Neuromuscular & skeletal: Arthralgia (5%), back pain (5%)
Respiratory: Sinusitis (6%), nasopharyngitis (6%)
Miscellaneous: Injury (8%), viral infection (5%), flu-like syndrome (1%)

Mechanism of Action Rosiglitazone is a thiazolidinedione antidiabetic agent that lowers blood glucose by improving target cell response to insulin, without increasing pancreatic insulin secretion. It has a mechanism of action that is dependent on the presence of insulin for activity. Metformin decreases hepatic glucose production, decreases intestinal absorption of glucose, and improves insulin sensitivity (increases peripheral glucose uptake and utilization).

Drug Interactions
Cytochrome P450 Effect: Rosiglitazone: **Substrate** of CYP2C8 (major), 2C9 (minor); **Inhibits** CYP2C8 (moderate), 2C9 (weak), 2C19 (weak), 2D6 (weak)

Increased Effect/Toxicity: See individual agents.

Decreased Effect: See individual agents.

Pharmacodynamics/Kinetics See individual agents.

Pregnancy Risk Factor C

Rosiglitazone Maleate and Metformin Hydrochloride *see* Rosiglitazone and Metformin *on page 1447*

Rosula® NS *see* Sulfacetamide *on page 1502*

Rosuvastatin (roe soo va STAT in)

U.S. Brand Names Crestor®
Canadian Brand Names Crestor®
Mexican Brand Names Crestor
Generic Available No
Index Terms Rosuvastatin Calcium
Pharmacologic Category Antilipemic Agent, HMG-CoA Reductase Inhibitor
Use Used with dietary therapy for hyperlipidemias to reduce elevations in total cholesterol (TC), LDL-C, apolipoprotein B, and triglycerides (TG) in patients with primary hypercholesterolemia (elevations of 1 or more components are present in Fredrickson type IIa, IIb, and IV hyperlipidemias); treatment of homozygous familial hypercholesterolemia (FH)
Local Anesthetic/Vasoconstrictor Precautions No information available to require special precautions
Effects on Dental Treatment No significant effects or complications reported
Common Adverse Effects
1% to 10%:
Cardiovascular: Chest pain, hypertension, palpitation, peripheral edema
Central nervous system: Headache (6%), anxiety, depression, dizziness, insomnia, neuralgia, pain, vertigo
Dermatologic: Rash
Gastrointestinal: Pharyngitis (9%), abdominal pain, constipation, diarrhea, dyspepsia, gastroenteritis, nausea, vomiting
Hematologic: Anemia, bruising
Neuromuscular & skeletal: Myalgia (3%), arthralgia, arthritis, back pain, hypertonia, paresthesia, weakness
Respiratory: Bronchitis, cough, rhinitis, sinusitis
Miscellaneous: Flu-like syndrome
Adverse reactions reported with other HMG-CoA reductase inhibitors include a hypersensitivity syndrome (symptoms may include anaphylaxis, angioedema, arthralgia, erythema multiforme, eosinophilia, hemolytic anemia, lupus syndrome, photosensitivity, polymyalgia rheumatica, positive ANA, purpura, Stevens-Johnson syndrome, toxic epidermal necrolysis, urticaria, vasculitis)
Mechanism of Action Inhibitor of 3-hydroxy-3-methylglutaryl coenzyme A (HMG-CoA) reductase, the rate-limiting enzyme in cholesterol synthesis (reduces the production of mevalonic acid from HMG-CoA); this then results in a compensatory increase in the expression of LDL receptors on hepatocyte membranes and a stimulation of LDL catabolism
Drug Interactions
Cytochrome P450 Effect: Substrate (minor) of CYP2C9, 3A4
Increased Effect/Toxicity: Cyclosporine may increase serum concentrations of rosuvastatin (up to 10-fold); limit dose to 5 mg/day. Serum concentrations of rosuvastatin may be increased (doubled) during concurrent administration of gemfibrozil; combination should be avoided; limit dose to 10 mg/day. Clofibrate, fenofibrate, or niacin may increase the risk of myopathy and rhabdomyolysis with HMG-CoA reductase inhibitors; the effects on lipids may be additive. The anticoagulant effects of warfarin may be increased by rosuvastatin (monitor). Rosuvastatin increases serum concentrations of hormonal contraceptives (ethinyl estradiol and norgestrel).
Decreased Effect: Plasma concentrations of rosuvastatin may be decreased when given with magnesium/aluminum hydroxide-containing antacids; antacids should be administered at least 2 hours after rosuvastatin. Cholestyramine and colestipol (bile acid sequestrants) may reduce absorption of several HMG-CoA reductase inhibitors; separate administration times by at least 4 hours; cholesterol-lowering effects are additive.
Pharmacodynamics/Kinetics
Onset: Within 1 week; maximal at 4 weeks
Distribution: V_d: 134 L
Protein binding: 90%
Metabolism: Hepatic (10%), via CYP2C9 (1 active metabolite identified)
Bioavailability: 20% (high first-pass extraction by liver)
Asian patients have been noted to have increased bioavailability.
Half-life elimination: 19 hours
Time to peak, plasma: 3-5 hours
Excretion: Feces (90%), primarily as unchanged drug
Pregnancy Risk Factor X

Rosuvastatin Calcium see Rosuvastatin on page 1448
RotaTeq® see Rotavirus Vaccine on page 1449

Rotavirus Vaccine (ROE ta vye rus vak SEEN)

U.S. Brand Names RotaTeq®
Mexican Brand Names Rotarix
Generic Available No
Index Terms Pentavalent Human-Bovine Reassortant Rotavirus Vaccine; Rotavirus Vaccine, Pentavalent
Pharmacologic Category Vaccine
Use Prevention of rotavirus gastroenteritis in infants and children
Local Anesthetic/Vasoconstrictor Precautions No information available to require special precautions
Effects on Dental Treatment No significant effects or complications reported
Common Adverse Effects All serious adverse reactions must be reported to the U.S. Department of Health and Human Services (DHHS) Vaccine Adverse Event Reporting System (VAERS) 1-800-822-7967.

>10%:
Central nervous system: Fever >38.1°C (17% to 20% , equal to placebo)
Gastrointestinal: Diarrhea (3% to 24%), vomiting (3% to 15%)
Otic: Otitis media (15%)
1% to 10%:
Central nervous system: Irritability (3% to 8%)
Respiratory: Nasopharyngitis (7%), bronchospasm (1%)

Mechanism of Action A live vaccine obtained from human and bovine sources; replicates in the small intestine and promotes active immunity to rotavirus gastroenteritis caused by serotypes G1, G2, G3, and G4.

Drug Interactions
Increased Effect/Toxicity: In clinical trials, rotavirus vaccine was administered with DTaP, IPV, HiB, hepatitis B vaccine, and pneumococcal conjugate vaccine. Antibody response was not decreased, with the exception of pertussis (insufficient data). Infants needing oral polio vaccine were excluded from clinical studies.
Decreased Effect: In clinical trials, rotavirus vaccine was administered with DTaP, IPV, HiB, hepatitis B vaccine and pneumococcal conjugate vaccine. Antibody response was not decreased, with the exception of pertussis (insufficient data). Infants needing oral polio vaccine were excluded from clinical studies.

Pharmacodynamics/Kinetics
Onset of action: A threefold increase in antirotavirus IgA was noted following completion of the 3-dose regimen in 93% to 100% of infants.
Duration: At least 2 years

Rubella Virus Vaccine (Live) (rue BEL a VYE rus vak SEEN, live)

Related Information
Immunizations (Vaccines) *on page 1886*
U.S. Brand Names Meruvax® II
Generic Available No
Index Terms German Measles Vaccine
Pharmacologic Category Vaccine
Use Selective active immunization against rubella
Note: Trivalent measles - mumps - rubella (MMR) vaccine is the preferred immunizing agent for most children and many adults.
Local Anesthetic/Vasoconstrictor Precautions No information available to require special precautions
Effects on Dental Treatment No significant effects or complications reported
Common Adverse Effects All serious adverse reactions must be reported to the U.S. Department of Health and Human Services (DHHS) Vaccine Adverse Event Reporting System (VAERS) 1-800-822-7967.
Frequency not defined.
Cardiovascular: Syncope, vasculitis
Central nervous system: Dizziness, encephalitis, fever, Guillain-Barré syndrome, headache, irritability, malaise, polyneuritis, polyneuropathy
Dermatologic: Angioneurotic edema, erythema multiforme, pruritus, purpura, rash, Stevens-Johnson syndrome, urticaria
Gastrointestinal: Diarrhea, nausea, sore throat, vomiting
Hematologic: Leukocytosis, thrombocytopenia
Local: Injection site reactions which include burning, induration, pain, redness, stinging, wheal and flare
Neuromuscular & skeletal: Arthralgia/arthritis (variable; highest rates in women, 12% to 26% versus children, up to 3%), myalgia, paresthesia
Ocular: Conjunctivitis, optic neuritis, papillitis, retrobulbar neuritis
Otic: Nerve deafness, otitis media
Respiratory: Bronchial spasm, cough, rhinitis
Miscellaneous: Anaphylactoid reactions, anaphylaxis, regional lymphadenopathy
Mechanism of Action Rubella vaccine is a live attenuated vaccine that contains the Wistar Institute RA 27/3 strain, which is adapted to and propagated in human diploid cell culture. Promotes active immunity by inducing rubella hemagglutination-inhibiting antibodies.
Drug Interactions
Decreased Effect: The effect of the vaccine may be decreased in individuals who are receiving immunosuppressant drugs (including high-dose systemic corticosteroids). Effect of vaccine may be decreased in given with immune globulin, whole blood or plasma; do not administer with vaccine.
Pharmacodynamics/Kinetics Onset of action: Antibodies to vaccine: 2-4 weeks
Pregnancy Risk Factor C

Saccharomyces boulardii (sak roe MYE sees boo LAR dee)

U.S. Brand Names Florastor® [OTC]; Florastor® Kids [OTC]
Generic Available No
Index Terms Saccharomyces boulardii lyo; S. boulardii
Pharmacologic Category Dietary Supplement; Probiotic
Use Promote maintenance of normal microflora in the gastrointestinal tract; used in management of bloating, gas, and diarrhea, particularly to decrease the incidence of diarrhea associated with antibiotic use
Local Anesthetic/Vasoconstrictor Precautions No information available to require special precautions
Effects on Dental Treatment No significant effects or complications reported
Common Adverse Effects Frequency not defined.
Gastrointestinal: Constipation, flatulence
Miscellaneous: Thirst
Mechanism of Action S. boulardii, a nonpathogenic live yeast probiotic, acts as temporary flora to help re-establish the normal gastrointestinal microflora. May also modulate the immune system by inducing cytokines and suppress pathogenic bacteria growth.
Drug Interactions
Decreased Effect: S. boulardii effect may be decreased by systemic antifungals.
Pharmacodynamics/Kinetics
Onset of action: Yeast cell release from capsules/powder: 30 minutes
Duration: Yeast cells cleared in 5-7 days

Saccharomyces boulardii lyo see Saccharomyces boulardii on page 1451

Sacrosidase (sak ROE si dase)

U.S. Brand Names Sucraid®
Canadian Brand Names Sucraid®
Generic Available No
Pharmacologic Category Enzyme, Gastrointestinal
Use Orphan drug: Oral replacement therapy in sucrase deficiency, as seen in congenital sucrase-isomaltase deficiency (CSID)
Local Anesthetic/Vasoconstrictor Precautions No information available to require special precautions
Effects on Dental Treatment No significant effects or complications reported
Common Adverse Effects 1% to 10%: Gastrointestinal: Abdominal pain, vomiting, nausea, diarrhea, constipation
Mechanism of Action Sacrosidase is a naturally-occurring gastrointestinal enzyme which breaks down the disaccharide sucrose to its monosaccharide components. Hydrolysis is necessary to allow absorption of these nutrients.
Drug Interactions
Increased Effect/Toxicity: Drug-drug interactions have not been evaluated.
Pharmacodynamics/Kinetics
Absorption: Amino acids
Metabolism: GI tract to individual amino acids
Pregnancy Risk Factor C

Safe Tussin® [OTC] see Guaifenesin and Dextromethorphan on page 796

SAHA see Vorinostat on page 1668

Saizen® see Somatropin on page 1486

SalAc® [OTC] see Salicylic Acid on page 1451

Sal-Acid® [OTC] see Salicylic Acid on page 1451

Salactic® [OTC] see Salicylic Acid on page 1451

Salagen® see Pilocarpine (Oral) on page 1301

Salbutamol see Albuterol on page 58

Salbutamol and Ipratropium see Ipratropium and Albuterol on page 905

Salicylazosulfapyridine see Sulfasalazine on page 1507

Salicylic Acid (sal i SIL ik AS id)

U.S. Brand Names Compound W® [OTC]; Compound W® One Step Wart Remover [OTC]; DHS™ Sal [OTC]; Dr. Scholl's® Callus Remover [OTC]; Dr. Scholl's® Clear Away [OTC]; DuoFilm® [OTC]; DuoPlant® [DSC] [OTC]; Freezone® [OTC]; Fung-O® [OTC]; Gordofilm® [OTC]; Hydrisalic™ [OTC]; Ionil® [OTC]; Ionil® Plus [OTC]; Keralyt® [OTC]; LupiCare™ Dandruff [OTC]; Lupi-Care™ II Psoriasis [OTC]; LupiCare™ Psoriasis [OTC]; Mediplast® [OTC]; (Continued)

Salicylic Acid *(Continued)*

MG217 Sal-Acid® [OTC]; Mosco® Corn and Callus Remover [OTC]; NeoCeuticals™ Acne Spot Treatment [OTC]; Neutrogena® Acne Wash [OTC]; Neutrogena® Body Clear™ [OTC]; Neutrogena® Clear Pore [OTC]; Neutrogena® Clear Pore Shine Control [OTC]; Neutrogena® Healthy Scalp [OTC]; Neutrogena® Maximum Strength T/Sal® [OTC]; Neutrogena® On The Spot® Acne Patch [OTC]; Occlusal®-HP [OTC]; Oxy Balance® [OTC]; Oxy Balance® Deep Pore [OTC]; Palmer's® Skin Success Acne Cleanser [OTC]; Pedisilk® [OTC]; Propa pH [OTC]; SalAc® [OTC]; Sal-Acid® [OTC]; Salactic® [OTC]; Sal-Plant® [OTC]; Stri-dex® [OTC]; Stri-dex® Body Focus [OTC]; Stri-dex® Facewipes To Go™ [OTC]; Stri-dex® Maximum Strength [OTC]; Tinamed® [OTC]; Tiseb® [OTC]; Trans-Ver-Sal® [OTC]; Wart-Off® Maximum Strength [OTC]; Zapzyt® Acne Wash [OTC]; Zapzyt® Pore Treatment [OTC]

Canadian Brand Names Duofilm®; Duoforte® 27; Occlusal™-HP; Sebcur®; Soluver®; Soluver® Plus; Trans-Plantar®; Trans-Ver-Sal®

Generic Available Yes: Gel, soap

Pharmacologic Category Acne Products; Keratolytic Agent; Topical Skin Product, Acne

Use Topically for its keratolytic effect in controlling seborrheic dermatitis or psoriasis of body and scalp, dandruff, and other scaling dermatoses; also used to remove warts, corns, and calluses; acne

Local Anesthetic/Vasoconstrictor Precautions No information available to require special precautions

Effects on Dental Treatment No significant effects or complications reported

Mechanism of Action Produces desquamation of hyperkeratotic epithelium via dissolution of the intercellular cement which causes the cornified tissue to swell, soften, macerate, and desquamate. Salicylic acid is keratolytic at concentrations of 3% to 6%; it becomes destructive to tissue at concentrations >6%. Concentrations of 6% to 60% are used to remove corns and warts and in the treatment of psoriasis and other hyperkeratotic disorders.

Pregnancy Risk Factor C

Salicylic Acid and Coal Tar *see* Coal Tar and Salicylic Acid *on page 402*

Salicylsalicylic Acid *see* Salsalate *on page 1454*

SalineX® [OTC] *see* Sodium Chloride *on page 1480*

Salivart® [OTC] *see* Saliva Substitute *on page 1452*

Saliva Substitute *(sa LYE va SUB stee tute)*

Related Information
Management of Patients Undergoing Cancer Therapy *on page 1826*

Related Sample Prescriptions
Mild/Moderate Oral Pain *on page 1834*

U.S. Brand Names Aquoral™; Caphasol; Entertainer's Secret® [OTC]; Moi-Stir® [OTC]; Mouthkote® [OTC]; Numoisyn™; Salivart® [OTC]; Saliva Substitute™ [OTC]; SalivaSure™ [OTC]

Generic Available No

Pharmacologic Category Gastrointestinal Agent, Miscellaneous

Dental Use Relief of dry mouth and throat in xerostomia

Use Relief of dry mouth and throat in xerostomia

Local Anesthetic/Vasoconstrictor Precautions No information available to require special precautions

Effects on Dental Treatment No significant effects or complications reported

Dosage Use as needed

Dosage Forms Excipient information presented when available (limited, particularly for generics); consult specific product labeling. [DSC] = Discontinued product

Liquid:
Numoisyn™: Water, sorbitol, linseed extract, *Chondrus crispus*, methylparaben, sodium benzoate, potassium sorbate, dipotassium phosphate, propylparaben (300 mL)

Lozenge:
Numoisyn™: Sorbitol 0.3 g/lozenge, polyethylene glycol, malic acid, sodium citrate, calcium phosphate dibasic, hydrogenated cottonseed oil, citric acid, magnesium stearate, silicon dioxide (100s)

SalivaSure™: Xylitol, citric acid, apple acid, sodium citrate dihydrate, sodium carboxymethylcellulose, dibasic calcium phosphate, silica colloidal, magnesium stearate, stearic acid (90s)

Solution, oral:
Caphosol: Dibasic sodium phosphate 0.032%, monobasic sodium phosphate 0.009%, calcium chloride 0.052%, sodium chloride 0.569%, purified water

(30 mL) [packaged in two 15 mL ampuls when mixed together provide one 30 mL dose]

Entertainer's Secret®: Sodium carboxymethylcellulose, aloe vera gel, glycerin (60 mL) [honey-apple flavor]

Saliva Substitute®: Sorbitol, sodium carboxymethylcellulose, methylparaben (120 mL)

Solution, oral [spray]:

Aquoral™: Oxidized glycerol triesters and silicon dioxide (40 mL) [contains aspartame; delivers 400 sprays]

Moi-Stir®: Water, sorbitol, sodium carboxymethylcellulose, methylparaben, propylparaben, potassium chloride, dibasic sodium phosphate, calcium chloride, magnesium chloride, sodium chloride (120 mL)

Mouthkote®: Water, xylitol, sorbitol, yerba santa, citric acid, ascorbic acid, sodium saccharin, sodium benzoate (5 mL, 60 mL, 240 mL) [alcohol free, sugar free; lemon-lime flavor]

Salivart®: Water, sodium carboxymethylcellulose, sorbitol, sodium chloride, potassium chloride, calcium chloride, magnesium chloride, potassium phosphate (70 mL) [alcohol free]

Saliva Substitute™ [OTC] *see* Saliva Substitute *on page 1452*

SalivaSure™ [OTC] *see* Saliva Substitute *on page 1452*

Salk Vaccine *see* Poliovirus Vaccine (Inactivated) *on page 1320*

Salmeterol (sal ME te role)

Related Information
Respiratory Diseases *on page 1747*

U.S. Brand Names Serevent® Diskus®

Canadian Brand Names Serevent®

Mexican Brand Names Serevent

Generic Available No

Index Terms Salmeterol Xinafoate

Pharmacologic Category Beta$_2$-Adrenergic Agonist

Use Maintenance treatment of asthma and in prevention of bronchospasm with reversible obstructive airway disease, including patients with symptoms of nocturnal asthma; prevention of exercise-induced bronchospasm; maintenance treatment of bronchospasm associated with COPD

Local Anesthetic/Vasoconstrictor Precautions No information available to require special precautions

Effects on Dental Treatment Key adverse event(s) related to dental treatment: Xerostomia (normal salivary flow resumes upon discontinuation), dental pain, and oropharyngeal candidiasis.

Common Adverse Effects

>10%:
Central nervous system: Headache (13% to 17%)
Neuromuscular & skeletal: Pain (1% to 12%)

1% to 10%:
Cardiovascular: Hypertension (4%), edema (1% to <3%)
Central nervous system: Dizziness (4%), sleep disturbance (1% to 3%), fever (1% to 3%), anxiety (1% to <3%), migraine (1% to <3%)
Dermatologic: Rash (1% to 4%), contact dermatitis (1% to 3%), eczema (1% to 3%), urticaria (3%), photodermatitis (1% to 2%)
Endocrine & metabolic: Hyperglycemia (1% to <3%)
Gastrointestinal: Nausea (1% to 3%), dyspepsia (1% to <3%), dental pain (1% to <3%), infections (1% to <3%), oropharyngeal candidiasis (1% to <3%), xerostomia (1% to <3%)
Neuromuscular & skeletal: Muscular cramps/spasm (3%), paresthesia (1% to 3%), arthralgia (1% to <3%), muscular stiffness, rigidity (1% to <3%)
Ocular: Keratitis/conjunctivitis (1% to <3%)
Respiratory: Tracheitis/bronchitis (7%), pharyngitis (up to 6%), cough (5%), influenza (5%), infection (5%), sinusitis (4% to 5%), rhinitis (4% to 5%), nasal congestion (4%), asthma (3% to 4%)

Restrictions An FDA-approved medication guide must be distributed when dispensing an outpatient prescription (new or refill) where this medication is to be used without direct supervision of a healthcare provider. Medication guides are available at http://www.fda.gov/cder/Offices/ODS/medication_guides.htm.

Mechanism of Action Relaxes bronchial smooth muscle by selective action on beta$_2$-receptors with little effect on heart rate; because salmeterol acts locally in the lung, therapeutic effect is not predicted by plasma levels
(Continued)

Salmeterol (Continued)

Drug Interactions

Cytochrome P450 Effect: Substrate of CYP3A4 (major)

Increased Effect/Toxicity: Atomoxetine may enhance the tachycardia effect of beta$_2$-agonists. Sympathomimetics may enhance the adverse/toxic effect of salmeterol.

Decreased Effect: Beta$_2$-agonists may diminish the bradycardia effect of beta-blockers (beta$_1$ selective). Beta-blockers (nonselective) may diminish the bronchodilator effect of beta$_2$-agonists.

Pharmacodynamics/Kinetics

Onset of action: Asthma: 30-48 minutes, COPD: 2 hours

Peak effect: 2-4 hours, COPD: 3.27-4.75 hours

Duration: 12 hours

Absorption: Systemic: Inhalation: Undetectable to poor

Protein binding: 96%

Metabolism: Hepatically hydroxylated via CYP3A4

Half-life elimination: 5.5 hours

Excretion: Feces (60%), urine (25%)

Pregnancy Risk Factor C

Salmeterol and Fluticasone see Fluticasone and Salmeterol on page 729

Salmeterol Xinafoate see Salmeterol on page 1453

Sal-Plant® [OTC] see Salicylic Acid on page 1451

Salsalate (SAL sa late)

Related Information

Rheumatoid Arthritis, Osteoarthritis, and Osteoporosis on page 1759

Temporomandibular Dysfunction (TMD) on page 1822

U.S. Brand Names Amigesic®

Canadian Brand Names Amigesic®; Salflex®

Generic Available Yes

Index Terms Disalicylic Acid; Salicylsalicylic Acid

Pharmacologic Category Salicylate

Use Treatment of minor pain or fever; arthritis

Local Anesthetic/Vasoconstrictor Precautions No information available to require special precautions

Effects on Dental Treatment NSAID formulations are known to reversibly decrease platelet aggregation via mechanisms different than observed with aspirin. The dentist should be aware of the potential of abnormal coagulation. Caution should also be exercised in the use of NSAIDs in patients already on anticoagulant therapy with drugs such as warfarin (Coumadin®).

Common Adverse Effects

>10%: Gastrointestinal: Nausea, heartburn, stomach pain, dyspepsia

1% to 10%:

Central nervous system: Fatigue

Dermatologic: Rash

Gastrointestinal: Gastrointestinal ulceration

Hematologic: Hemolytic anemia

Neuromuscular & skeletal: Weakness

Respiratory: Dyspnea

Miscellaneous: Anaphylactic shock

Dosage Adults: Oral: 3 g/day in 2-3 divided doses

Dosing comments in renal impairment: In patients with end-stage renal disease undergoing hemodialysis: 750 mg twice daily with an additional 500 mg after dialysis

Mechanism of Action Inhibits prostaglandin synthesis, acts on the hypothalamus heat-regulating center to reduce fever, blocks prostaglandin synthetase action which prevents formation of the platelet-aggregating substance thromboxane A$_2$

Contraindications Hypersensitivity to salsalate or any component of the formulation; GI ulcer or bleeding; pregnancy (3rd trimester)

Warnings/Precautions Use with caution in patients with platelet and bleeding disorders, dehydration, renal dysfunction, erosive gastritis, or peptic ulcer disease; patients with sensitivity to tartrazine dyes, nasal polyps, and asthma may have an increased risk of salicylate sensitivity, previous nonreaction does not guarantee future safe taking of medication; children and teenagers who have or are recovering from chickenpox or flu-like symptoms should not use this product. Changes in behavior (along with nausea and vomiting) may be an early sign of Reye's syndrome; patients should be instructed to contact their healthcare provider if these occur.

Drug Interactions
  Increased Effect/Toxicity: Increased effect/toxicity of oral anticoagulants, hypoglycemics, and methotrexate.
  Decreased Effect: Decreased effect with urinary alkalinizers, antacids, and corticosteroids. Decreased effect of uricosurics and spironolactone.
Ethanol/Nutrition/Herb Interactions
  Ethanol: Avoid ethanol (may enhance gastric mucosal irritation).
  Food: Salsalate peak serum levels may be delayed if taken with food.
  Herb/Nutraceutical: Avoid cat's claw, dong quai, evening primrose, feverfew, garlic, ginger, ginkgo, red clover, horse chestnut, green tea, ginseng (all have additional antiplatelet activity).
Dietary Considerations May be taken with food to decrease GI distress.
Pharmacodynamics/Kinetics
  Onset of action: Therapeutic: 3-4 days of continuous dosing
  Absorption: Complete from small intestine
  Metabolism: Hepatically hydrolyzed to two moles of salicylic acid (active)
  Half-life elimination: 7-8 hours
  Excretion: Primarily urine
Pregnancy Risk Factor C/D (3rd trimester)
Dosage Forms
  Tablet: 500 mg, 750 mg
    Amigesic®: 500 mg, 750 mg

Saquinavir (sa KWIN a veer)

Related Information
  HIV Infection and AIDS *on page 1753*
  Tuberculosis Treatment *on page 1909*
U.S. Brand Names Fortovase® [DSC]; Invirase®
Canadian Brand Names Fortovase®; Invirase®
Mexican Brand Names Fortovase
Generic Available No
Index Terms Saquinavir Mesylate
Pharmacologic Category Antiretroviral Agent, Protease Inhibitor
Use Treatment of HIV infection; used in combination with at least two other antiretroviral agents
Local Anesthetic/Vasoconstrictor Precautions No information available to require special precautions
Effects on Dental Treatment Key adverse event(s) related to dental treatment: Buccal mucosa ulceration and taste alteration.
Common Adverse Effects Protease inhibitors cause dyslipidemia which includes elevated cholesterol and triglycerides and a redistribution of body fat centrally to cause increased abdominal girth, buffalo hump, facial atrophy, and breast enlargement. These agents also cause hyperglycemia.

10%: Gastrointestinal: Diarrhea, nausea
1% to 10%:
  Cardiovascular: Chest pain
  Central nervous system: Anxiety, depression, fatigue, headache, insomnia, pain
  Dermatologic: Rash, verruca
  Endocrine & metabolic: Hyper-/hypoglycemia, hyperkalemia, libido disorder, serum amylase increased
  Gastrointestinal: Abdominal discomfort, abdominal pain, appetite decreased, buccal mucosa ulceration, constipation, dyspepsia, flatulence, taste alteration, vomiting
  Hepatic: AST increased, ALT increased, bilirubin increased
  Neuromuscular & skeletal: CPK increased, paresthesia, weakness
  Renal: Creatinine kinase increased
Mechanism of Action As an inhibitor of HIV protease, saquinavir prevents the cleavage of viral polyprotein precursors which are needed to generate functional proteins in and maturation of HIV-infected cells
(Continued)

Saquinavir *(Continued)*

Drug Interactions

Cytochrome P450 Effect: Substrate of CYP2D6 (minor), 3A4 (major); **Inhibits** CYP2C9 (weak), 2C19 (weak), 2D6 (weak), 3A4 (moderate)

Increased Effect/Toxicity: Concurrent use of amiodarone, bepridil, cisapride, flecainide, midazolam, pimozide, propafenone, quinidine, rifampin, triazolam, or ergot derivatives is contraindicated.

Saquinavir may increase the levels/effects of selected benzodiazepines, calcium channel blockers, cisapride, cyclosporine, ergot alkaloids, selected HMG-CoA reductase inhibitors, mirtazapine, nateglinide, nefazodone, pimozide, quinidine, sildenafil (and other PDE-5 inhibitors), tacrolimus, venlafaxine, and other CYP3A4 substrates. The effects of warfarin may also be increased.

Serum concentrations of saquinavir may be increased by azole antifungals (itraconazole, ketoconazole); dose adjustment was not needed at the study dose when used for a limited time (ketoconazole 400 mg once daily and Fortovase® 1200 mg 3 times/day). Saquinavir serum concentrations may be increased by delavirdine. Atazanavir, indinavir, and ritonavir may increase serum levels of saquinavir. Serum levels of saquinavir and nelfinavir may be increased with concurrent use. Lopinavir/ritonavir (combination product) may increase serum levels of saquinavir. Refer to Dosage (dosage adjustment recommendations with atazanavir have not been established).

Serum concentrations of saquinavir and clarithromycin may both be increased. Dose adjustment not was not needed at the study dose when used for 7 days (clarithromycin 500 mg twice daily and Fortovase® 1200 mg 3 times/day); dosage adjustment of clarithromycin is recommended in patients with renal impairment.

Serum concentrations of saquinavir are decreased and levels of rifabutin are increased when used together. Saquinavir should not be used as the sole protease inhibitor when given with rifabutin.

Decreased Effect: The levels/effects of saquinavir may be reduced by amino-glutethimide, carbamazepine, nafcillin, nevirapine, phenobarbital, phenytoin, rifamycins, and other CYP3A4 inducers. Loss of efficacy and potential resistance may occur. Concurrent use with rifampin is contraindicated.

Serum concentrations of methadone may be decreased; an increased dose may be needed when administered with saquinavir. Serum levels of the hormones in oral contraceptives may decrease significantly with administration of saquinavir. Patients should use alternative methods of contraceptives during saquinavir therapy.

Serum levels of saquinavir and efavirenz may be decreased with concurrent use; saquinavir should not be used as the sole protease inhibitor with efavirenz or nevirapine.

Dexamethasone may decrease serum concentrations of saquinavir; use with caution. Serum concentrations of saquinavir are decreased and levels of rifabutin are increased when used together. Saquinavir should not be used as the sole protease inhibitor when given with rifabutin.

Pharmacodynamics/Kinetics

Absorption: Poor; increased with high fat meal; Fortovase® has improved absorption over Invirase®

Distribution: V_d: 700 L; does not distribute into CSF

Protein binding, plasma: ~98%

Metabolism: Extensively hepatic via CYP3A4; extensive first-pass effect

Bioavailability: Invirase®: ~4%; Fortovase®: 12% to 15%

Excretion: Feces (81% to 88%), urine (1% to 3%) within 5 days

Pregnancy Risk Factor B

Sargramostim *(sar GRAM oh stim)*

U.S. Brand Names Leukine®

Canadian Brand Names Leukine®

Generic Available No

Index Terms GM-CSF; Granulocyte-Macrophage Colony Stimulating Factor; NSC-613795; rGM-CSF

Pharmacologic Category Colony Stimulating Factor

Use

Acute myelogenous leukemia (AML) following induction chemotherapy in older adults (≥55 years of age) to shorten time to neutrophil recovery and to reduce the incidence of severe and life-threatening infections and infections resulting in death

Bone marrow transplant (allogeneic or autologous) failure or engraftment delay

Myeloid reconstitution after allogeneic bone marrow transplantation

Myeloid reconstitution after autologous bone marrow transplantation: Non-Hodgkin's lymphoma (NHL), acute lymphoblastic leukemia (ALL), Hodgkin's lymphoma

Peripheral stem cell transplantation: Mobilization and myeloid reconstitution following peripheral stem cell transplantation

Local Anesthetic/Vasoconstrictor Precautions No information available to require special precautions

Effects on Dental Treatment Key adverse event(s) related to dental treatment: Dysphagia.

Common Adverse Effects
>10%:
Cardiovascular: Hypertension (34%), pericardial effusion (4% to 25%), edema (13% to 25%), chest pain (15%), peripheral edema (11%), tachycardia (11%)

Central nervous system: Fever (81%), malaise (57%), headache (26%), chills (25%), anxiety (11%), insomnia (11%)

Dermatologic: Rash (44%), pruritus (23%)

Endocrine & metabolic: Hyperglycemia (25%), hypercholesterolemia (17%)

Gastrointestinal: Diarrhea (52% to 89%), nausea (58% to 70%), vomiting (46% to 70%), abdominal pain (38%), weight loss (37%), hematemesis (13%), dysphagia (11%), gastrointestinal hemorrhage (11%)

Genitourinary: Urinary tract disorder (14%)

Hepatic: Hyperbilirubinemia (30%)

Neuromuscular & skeletal: Weakness (66%), bone pain (21%), arthralgia (11% to 21%) myalgia (18%)

Ocular: Eye hemorrhage (11%)

Renal: BUN increased (23%), serum creatinine increased (15%)

Respiratory: Pharyngitis (23%), epistaxis (17%), dyspnea (15%)

1% to 10%: Respiratory: Pleural effusion (1%)

Mechanism of Action Stimulates proliferation, differentiation and functional activity of neutrophils, eosinophils, monocytes, and macrophages, as indicated.

Pharmacodynamics/Kinetics
Onset of action: Increase in WBC: 7-14 days
Duration: WBCs return to baseline within 1 week of discontinuing drug
Half-life elimination: I.V.: 60 minutes; SubQ: 2.7 hours
Time to peak, serum: SubQ: 1-2 hours

Pregnancy Risk Factor C

Scopolamine (skoe POL a meen)

U.S. Brand Names Isopto® Hyoscine; Maldemar™; Scopace™; Transderm Scōp®

Canadian Brand Names Buscopan®; Transderm-V®

Generic Available Yes: Injection

Index Terms Hyoscine Butylbromide; Hyoscine Hydrobromide; Scopolamine Base; Scopolamine Butylbromide; Scopolamine Hydrobromide

Pharmacologic Category Anticholinergic Agent

Use
Scopolamine base:
Transdermal: Prevention of nausea/vomiting associated with motion sickness and recovery from anesthesia and surgery

Scopolamine hydrobromide:
Injection: Preoperative medication to produce amnesia, sedation, tranquilization, antiemetic effects, and decrease salivary and respiratory secretions
(Continued)

Scopolamine *(Continued)*

Ophthalmic: Produce cycloplegia and mydriasis; treatment of iridocyclitis

Oral: Symptomatic treatment of postencephalitic parkinsonism and paralysis agitans; in spastic states; inhibits excessive motility and hypertonus of the gastrointestinal tract in such conditions as the irritable colon syndrome, mild dysentery, diverticulitis, pylorospasm, and cardiospasm

Scopolamine butylbromide [not available in the U.S.]:

Oral/injection: Treatment of smooth muscle spasm of the genitourinary or gastrointestinal tract; injection may also be used to prior to radiological/diagnostic procedures to prevent spasm

Local Anesthetic/Vasoconstrictor Precautions No information available to require special precautions

Effects on Dental Treatment Key adverse event(s) related to dental treatment: Significant xerostomia (normal salivary flow resumes upon discontinuation), dry throat (transdermal), and dysphagia.

Common Adverse Effects Frequency not defined.

Ophthalmic: Note: Systemic adverse effects have been reported following ophthalmic administration.

Cardiovascular: Vascular congestion, edema

Central nervous system: Drowsiness

Dermatologic: Eczematoid dermatitis

Ocular: Blurred vision, photophobia, local irritation, increased intraocular pressure, follicular conjunctivitis, exudate

Respiratory: Congestion

Systemic:

Cardiovascular: Orthostatic hypotension, ventricular fibrillation, tachycardia, palpitation

Central nervous system: Confusion, drowsiness, headache, loss of memory, ataxia, fatigue

Dermatologic: Dry skin, increased sensitivity to light, rash

Endocrine & metabolic: Decreased flow of breast milk

Gastrointestinal: Constipation, xerostomia, dry throat, dysphagia, bloated feeling, nausea, vomiting

Genitourinary: Dysuria

Local: Irritation at injection site

Neuromuscular & skeletal: Weakness

Ocular: Increased intraocular pain, blurred vision

Respiratory: Dry nose

Miscellaneous: Diaphoresis (decreased)

Mechanism of Action Blocks the action of acetylcholine at parasympathetic sites in smooth muscle, secretory glands and the CNS; increases cardiac output, dries secretions, antagonizes histamine and serotonin; dilates pupils

Drug Interactions

Increased Effect/Toxicity: Adverse anticholinergic effects may be additive with other anticholinergic agents (includes tricyclic antidepressants, antihistamines, and phenothiazines). Pramlintide may enhance the gastrointestinal anticholinergic effect of scopolamine. Sedative effects of other CNS depressants may be additive with scopolamine.

Decreased Effect: Acetylcholinesterase inhibitors (donepezil, galantamine, rivastigmine, tacrine) may diminish the therapeutic effect of scopolamine. Scopolamine may diminish the therapeutic effect of acetylcholinesterase inhibitors.

Pharmacodynamics/Kinetics

Onset of action: Oral, I.M.: 0.5-1 hour; I.V.: 10 minutes

Peak effect: 20-60 minutes; may take 3-7 days for full recovery; transdermal: 24 hours

Duration: Oral, I.M.: 4-6 hours; I.V.: 2 hours

Absorption: Tertiary salts (hydrobromide) are well absorbed; quaternary salts (butylbromide) are poorly absorbed (local concentrations in the GI tract following oral dosing may be high)

Metabolism: Hepatic

Half-life elimination: 4.8 hours

Excretion: Urine (<10%, as parent drug and metabolites)

Pregnancy Risk Factor C

Scopolamine and Phenylephrine *see* Phenylephrine and Scopolamine *on page 1294*

Scopolamine Base *see* Scopolamine *on page 1457*

Scopolamine Butylbromide *see* Scopolamine *on page 1457*

Scopolamine Hydrobromide *see* Scopolamine *on page 1457*

Scopolamine, Hyoscyamine, Atropine, and Phenobarbital *see* Hyoscyamine, Atropine, Scopolamine, and Phenobarbital *on page 848*

Secobarbital (see koe BAR bi tal)

U.S. Brand Names Seconal®
Generic Available No
Index Terms Quinalbarbitone Sodium; Secobarbital Sodium
Pharmacologic Category Barbiturate
Use Preanesthetic agent; short-term treatment of insomnia
Local Anesthetic/Vasoconstrictor Precautions No information available to require special precautions
Effects on Dental Treatment No significant effects or complications reported
Mechanism of Action Depresses CNS activity by binding to barbiturate site at GABA-receptor complex enhancing GABA activity, depressing reticular activity system; higher doses may be gabamimetic
Pregnancy Risk Factor D

Secretin (SEE kre tin)

U.S. Brand Names ChiRhoStim™; SecreFlo™
Generic Available No
Index Terms Secretin, Human; Secretin, Porcine
Pharmacologic Category Diagnostic Agent
Use Secretin-stimulation testing to aid in diagnosis of pancreatic exocrine dysfunction; diagnosis of gastrinoma (Zollinger-Ellison syndrome); facilitation of ERCP visualization
Local Anesthetic/Vasoconstrictor Precautions No information available to require special precautions
Effects on Dental Treatment No significant effects or complications reported
Common Adverse Effects 1% to 10%:
Cardiovascular: Flushing (1%)
Gastrointestinal: Abdominal discomfort (1%), nausea (1%)
Miscellaneous: Bleeding (sphincterectomy, 1%)
Mechanism of Action Human and porcine secretin are both synthetically derived products and are equally potent on an osmolar basis. Secretin is a hormone which is normally secreted by duodenal mucosa and upper jejunal mucosa. It increases the volume and bicarbonate content of pancreatic juice; stimulates the flow of hepatic bile with a high bicarbonate concentration; stimulates gastrin release in patients with Zollinger-Ellison syndrome.
Drug Interactions
Decreased Effect: The response to secretin stimulation may be blunted by drugs with high anticholinergic activity such as tricyclic antidepressants, phenothiazines, and antihistamines as well as anticholinergic agents (ie, atropine, benztropine, biperiden).
Pharmacodynamics/Kinetics
Peak output of pancreatic secretions: ~30 minutes
Duration: At least 2 hours
Distribution: V_d: Human: 2.7 L; Porcine: 2 L
Half-life elimination: Human: 45 minutes; Porcine: 27 minutes
Pregnancy Risk Factor C

Selegiline (se LE ji leen)

U.S. Brand Names Eldepryl®; Emsam®; Zelapar™
Canadian Brand Names Apo-Selegiline®; Gen-Selegiline; Novo-Selegiline; Nu-Selegiline
Mexican Brand Names Niar
Generic Available Yes: Capsule, tablet
Index Terms Deprenyl; L-Deprenyl; Selegiline Hydrochloride
Pharmacologic Category Anti-Parkinson's Agent, MAO Type B Inhibitor; Antidepressant, Monoamine Oxidase Inhibitor
Use Adjunct in the management of parkinsonian patients in which levodopa/carbidopa therapy is deteriorating (oral products); treatment of major depressive disorder (transdermal product)
Unlabeled/Investigational Use Early Parkinson's disease; attention-deficit/hyperactivity disorder (ADHD); negative symptoms of schizophrenia; extrapyramidal symptoms; Alzheimer's disease (studies have shown some improvement in behavioral and cognitive performance)
Local Anesthetic/Vasoconstrictor Precautions Selegiline in doses of 10 mg a day or less does not inhibit type-A MAO. Therefore, there are no precautions with the use of vasoconstrictors.
Effects on Dental Treatment Key adverse event(s) related to dental treatment: Xerostomia and changes in salivation (normal salivary flow resumes upon discontinuation). Anticholinergic side effects can cause a reduction of saliva production or secretion, contributing to discomfort and dental disease (ie, caries, oral candidiasis, and periodontal disease).
Orally disintegrating tablet: Dysphagia, tooth disorder, stomatitis, and taste perversion.
Common Adverse Effects Unless otherwise noted, the percentage of adverse events is reported for the transdermal patch (**Note:** ODT = orally disintegrating tablet, Oral = capsule/tablet)
>10%:
  Central nervous system: Headache (18%; ODT 7%; oral 2%), insomnia (12%; ODT 7%), dizziness (ODT 11%; oral 7%)
  Gastrointestinal: Nausea (ODT 11%; oral 10%)
  Local: Application site reaction (24%)
1% to 10%:
  Cardiovascular: Hypotension (including postural 3% to 10%), chest pain (≥1%; ODT 2%), hypertension (≥1%), peripheral edema (≥1%)
  Central nervous system: Pain (ODT 8%), hallucinations (ODT 4%; oral 3%), confusion (ODT 4%; oral 3%), headache (ODT 7%; oral 2%), ataxia (ODT 3%), somnolence (ODT 3%), agitation (≥1%), amnesia (≥1%), paresthesia (≥1%), thinking abnormal (≥1%), depression (<1%; ODT 2%)
  Dermatologic: Rash (4%), ecchymosis (ODT 2%), bruising (≥1%), pruritus (≥1%), acne (≥1%)
  Endocrine and metabolic: Weight loss (5%), hypokalemia (ODT 2%), sexual side effects (≤1%)
  Gastrointestinal: Diarrhea (9%; ODT 2%), xerostomia (8%; ODT 4%), stomatitis (ODT 5%), abdominal pain (oral 4%), dyspepsia (4%; ODT 5%), constipation (≥1%; ODT 4%), flatulence (≥1%; ODT 2%), anorexia (≥1%), gastroenteritis (≥1%), taste perversion (≥1%; ODT 2%), vomiting (≥1%; ODT 3%), tooth disorder (ODT 2%), dysphagia (ODT 2%)
  Genitourinary: Dysmenorrhea (≥1%), metrorrhagia (≥1%), UTI (≥1%), urinary frequency (≥1%)
  Neuromuscular & skeletal: Dyskinesia (ODT 6%), back pain (ODT 5%), ataxia (<1%; ODT 3%), leg cramps (ODT 3%), myalgia (≥1%; ODT 3%), neck pain (≥1%), tremor (<1%; ODT 3%)
  Otic: Tinnitus (≥1%)
  Respiratory: Rhinitis (ODT 7%), pharyngitis (3%; ODT 4%), sinusitis (3%), cough (≥1%), bronchitis (≥1%), dyspnea (<1%; ODT 3%)
  Miscellaneous: Diaphoresis (≥1%)
Restrictions An FDA-approved medication guide concerning the use of antidepressants in children, adolescents, and young adults must be distributed when dispensing a transdermal selegiline outpatient prescription (new or refill) where this medication is to be used without direct supervision of a healthcare provider. Medication guides are available at http://www.fda.gov/cder/Offices/ODS/medication_guides.htm. Dispense to parents or guardians of children and adolescents receiving this medication.
Mechanism of Action Potent, irreversible inhibitor of monoamine oxidase (MAO). Plasma concentrations achieved via administration of oral dosage forms in recommended doses confer selective inhibition of MAO type B, which plays a major role in the metabolism of dopamine; selegiline may also increase dopaminergic activity by interfering with dopamine reuptake at the synapse. When

administered transdermally in recommended doses, selegiline achieves higher blood levels and effectively inhibits both MAO-A and MAO-B, which blocks catabolism of other centrally-active biogenic amine neurotransmitters.

Drug Interactions

Cytochrome P450 Effect: Substrate of CYP1A2 (minor), 2A6 (minor), 2B6 (major), 2C8 (minor), 2C19 (minor), 2D6 (minor), 3A4 (minor); **Inhibits** CYP1A2 (weak), 2A6 (weak), 2C9 (weak), 2C19 (weak), 2D6 (weak), 2E1 (weak), 3A4 (weak)

Increased Effect/Toxicity: CYP2B6 inhibitors may increase the levels/ effects of selegiline; example inhibitors include desipramine, paroxetine, and sertraline. Concurrent use of oral selegiline (high dose) in combination with amphetamines, methylphenidate, dextromethorphan, fenfluramine, meperidine, nefazodone, sibutramine, tramadol, trazodone, tricyclic antidepressants, and venlafaxine may result in serotonin syndrome; these combinations are best avoided. Concurrent use of selegiline with an SSRI or SNRI may result in mania or hypertension; it is generally best to avoid these combinations. Transdermal selegiline is contraindicated with amphetamines, sympathomimetics or other CNS stimulants, dextromethorphan, meperidine, methadone, mirtazapine, propoxyphene, SSRIs/SNRIs, tramadol, tricyclic antidepressants. The toxicity of levodopa (hypertension), lithium (hyperpyrexia), and reserpine may be increased by MAO inhibitors.

Decreased Effect: CYP2B6 inducers may decrease the levels/effects of selegiline; example inducers include carbamazepine, nevirapine, phenobarbital, phenytoin, and rifampin.

Pharmacodynamics/Kinetics
Onset of action: Therapeutic: Oral: Within 1 hour
Duration: Oral: 24-72 hours
Absorption:
Orally disintegrating tablet: Rapid; greater bioavailability than capsule/tablet
Transdermal: 25% to 30% (of total selegiline content) over 24 hours
Protein binding: ~90%
Metabolism: Hepatic, primarily via CYP2B6 to active (N-desmethylselegiline, amphetamine, methamphetamine) and inactive metabolites
Half-life elimination: Oral: 10 hours; Transdermal: 18-25 hours
Excretion: Urine (primarily metabolites); feces

Pregnancy Risk Factor C

Selegiline Hydrochloride *see* Selegiline *on page 1460*
Selenicaps [OTC] *see* Selenium *on page 1461*
Selenimin [OTC] *see* Selenium *on page 1461*

Selenium *(se LEE nee um)*

Related Information
Trace Metals *on page 1595*
U.S. Brand Names Selenicaps [OTC]; Selenimin [OTC]; Selepen®
Generic Available Yes
Pharmacologic Category Trace Element, Parenteral
Use Trace metal supplement
Local Anesthetic/Vasoconstrictor Precautions No information available to require special precautions
Effects on Dental Treatment No significant effects or complications reported
Common Adverse Effects Frequency not defined.
Central nervous system: Lethargy
Dermatologic: Alopecia or hair discoloration
Gastrointestinal: Vomiting following long-term use on damaged skin; abdominal pain, garlic breath
Local: Irritation
Neuromuscular & skeletal: Tremor
Miscellaneous: Diaphoresis
Mechanism of Action Part of glutathione peroxidase which protects cell components from oxidative damage due to peroxidases produced in cellular metabolism
Pharmacodynamics/Kinetics Excretion: Urine, feces, lungs, skin
Pregnancy Risk Factor C

Selenium *see* Trace Metals *on page 1595*
Selepen® *see* Selenium *on page 1461*
Selepen® *see* Trace Metals *on page 1595*
Semprex®-D *see* Acrivastine and Pseudoephedrine *on page 48*
Senexon [OTC] *see* Senna *on page 1462*
Senilezol *see* Vitamin B Complex Combinations *on page 1664*

Senna (SEN na)

U.S. Brand Names Black-Draught Tablets [OTC]; Evac-U-Gen [OTC]; ex-lax®
[OTC]; ex-lax® Maximum Strength [OTC]; Fletcher's® [OTC]; Perdiem® Over-
night Relief [OTC]; Senexon [OTC]; Senna-Gen® [OTC]; Sennatural™ [OTC];
Senokot® [OTC]; SenokotXTRA® [OTC]; Uni-Senna [OTC]

Generic Available Yes

Pharmacologic Category Laxative, Stimulant

Use Short-term treatment of constipation; evacuate the colon for bowel or rectal
examinations

Local Anesthetic/Vasoconstrictor Precautions No information available to
require special precautions

Effects on Dental Treatment No significant effects or complications reported

Common Adverse Effects Frequency not defined: Gastrointestinal: Nausea,
vomiting, diarrhea, abdominal cramps

Senna-Gen® [OTC] see Senna on page 1462

Sennatural™ [OTC] see Senna on page 1462

Senokot® [OTC] see Senna on page 1462

SenokotXTRA® [OTC] see Senna on page 1462

Sensipar™ see Cinacalcet on page 359

Sensorcaine® see Bupivacaine on page 236

Sensorcaine®-MPF see Bupivacaine on page 236

Sensorcaine®-MPF Spinal see Bupivacaine on page 236

Sensorcaine®-MPF with Epinephrine see Bupivacaine and Epinephrine on
page 237

Sensorcaine® with Epinephrine see Bupivacaine and Epinephrine on
page 237

Septocaine® with epinephrine 1:100,000 see Articaine and Epinephrine on
page 143

Septocaine® with epinephrine 1:200,000 see Articaine and Epinephrine on
page 143

Septra® see Sulfamethoxazole and Trimethoprim on page 1504

Septra® DS see Sulfamethoxazole and Trimethoprim on page 1504

Serax® see Oxazepam on page 1220

Serevent® Diskus® see Salmeterol on page 1453

Sermorelin Acetate (ser moe REL in AS e tate)

U.S. Brand Names Geref® Diagnostic

Generic Available No

Pharmacologic Category Diagnostic Agent; Growth Hormone

Use
Geref® Diagnostic: For evaluation of the ability of the pituitary gland to secrete
growth hormone (GH)

Local Anesthetic/Vasoconstrictor Precautions No information available to
require special precautions

Effects on Dental Treatment Key adverse event(s) related to dental treatment: Dysphagia.

Common Adverse Effects Frequency not defined.
Cardiovascular: Tightness in the chest
Central nervous system: Headache, dizziness, hyperactivity, somnolence
Dermatologic: Transient flushing of the face, urticaria
Gastrointestinal: Dysphagia, nausea, vomiting
Local: Pain, redness, and/or swelling at the injection site

Drug Interactions
Decreased Effect: The test should not be conducted in the presence of drugs
that directly affect the pituitary secretion of somatotropin. These include preparations that contain or release somatostatin, insulin, glucocorticoids, or
cyclooxygenase inhibitors such as ASA or indomethacin. Somatotropin levels
may be transiently elevated by clonidine, levodopa, and insulin-induced hypoglycemia. Response to sermorelin may be blunted in patients who are
receiving muscarinic antagonists (atropine) or who are hypothyroid or being
treated with antithyroid medications such as propylthiouracil. Obesity, hyperglycemia, and elevated plasma fatty acids generally are associated with
subnormal GH responses to sermorelin. Exogenous growth hormone therapy
should be discontinued at least 1 week before administering the test.

Pharmacodynamics/Kinetics Onset of action: Peak response: Diagnostic:
Children 30 ± 27 minutes; Adults: 35 ± 29 minutes

Pregnancy Risk Factor C

Seromycin® *see* CycloSERINE *on page 425*
Serophene® *see* ClomiPHENE *on page 388*
Seroquel® *see* Quetiapine *on page 1392*
Serostim® *see* Somatropin *on page 1486*

Sertaconazole (ser ta KOE na zole)

U.S. Brand Names Ertaczo™
Generic Available No
Index Terms Sertaconazole Nitrate
Pharmacologic Category Antifungal Agent, Topical
Use Topical treatment of tinea pedis (athlete's foot)
Local Anesthetic/Vasoconstrictor Precautions No information available to require special precautions
Effects on Dental Treatment No significant effects or complications reported
Common Adverse Effects 1% to 10%: Dermatologic: Burning, contact dermatitis, dry skin, tenderness
Mechanism of Action Alters fungal cell wall membrane permeability; inhibits the CYP450-dependent synthesis of ergosterol
Pharmacodynamics/Kinetics
 Absorption: Topical: Minimal
Pregnancy Risk Factor C

Sertaconazole Nitrate *see* Sertaconazole *on page 1463*

Sertraline (SER tra leen)

Related Information
 Sedation *on page 1825*
U.S. Brand Names Zoloft®
Canadian Brand Names Apo-Sertraline®; Gen-Sertraline; GMD-Sertraline; Novo-Sertraline; Nu-Sertraline; PMS-Sertraline; ratio-Sertraline; Rhoxal-sertraline; Sandoz-Sertraline; Zoloft®
Mexican Brand Names Altruline
Generic Available Yes
Index Terms Sertraline Hydrochloride
Pharmacologic Category Antidepressant, Selective Serotonin Reuptake Inhibitor
Use Treatment of major depression; obsessive-compulsive disorder (OCD); panic disorder; post-traumatic stress disorder (PTSD); premenstrual dysphoric disorder (PMDD); social anxiety disorder
Unlabeled/Investigational Use Eating disorders; generalized anxiety disorder (GAD); impulse control disorders
Local Anesthetic/Vasoconstrictor Precautions Although caution should be used in patients taking tricyclic antidepressants, no interactions have been reported with vasoconstrictor and sertraline, a nontricyclic antidepressant which acts to increase serotonin; no precautions appear to be needed
Effects on Dental Treatment Key adverse event(s) related to dental treatment: Xerostomia (normal salivary flow resumes upon discontinuation) (see Dental Comment).
Common Adverse Effects
 >10%:
  Central nervous system: Dizziness, fatigue, headache, insomnia, somnolence
  Endocrine & metabolic: Libido decreased
  Gastrointestinal: Anorexia, diarrhea, nausea, xerostomia
  Genitourinary: Ejaculatory disturbances
  Neuromuscular & skeletal: Tremors
  Miscellaneous: Diaphoresis
 1% to 10%:
  Cardiovascular: Chest pain, palpitation
  Central nervous system: Agitation, anxiety, hypoesthesia, malaise, nervousness, pain
  Dermatologic: Rash
  Endocrine & metabolic: Impotence
  Gastrointestinal: Appetite increased, constipation, dyspepsia, flatulence, vomiting, weight gain
  Neuromuscular & skeletal: Back pain, hypertonia, myalgia, paresthesia, weakness
  Ocular: Visual difficulty, abnormal vision
  Otic: Tinnitus
  Respiratory: Rhinitis
  Miscellaneous: Yawning
(Continued)

Sertraline *(Continued)*

Additional adverse reactions reported in pediatric patients (frequency >2%): Aggressiveness, epistaxis, hyperkinesia, purpura, sinusitis, urinary incontinence

Restrictions An FDA-approved medication guide concerning the use of antidepressants in children, adolescents, and young adults must be distributed when dispensing an outpatient prescription (new or refill) where this medication is to be used without direct supervision of a healthcare provider. Medication guides are available at http://www.fda.gov/cder/Offices/ODS/medication_guides.htm. Dispense to parents or guardians of children and adolescents receiving this medication.

Dosage Oral:

Children and Adolescents: OCD:

6-12 years: Initial: 25 mg once daily

13-17 years: Initial: 50 mg once daily

Note: May increase daily dose, at intervals of not less than 1 week, to a maximum of 200 mg/day. If somnolence is noted, give at bedtime.

Adults:

Depression/OCD: Oral: Initial: 50 mg/day (see "Note" above)

Panic disorder, PTSD, social anxiety disorder: Initial: 25 mg once daily; increase to 50 mg once daily after 1 week (see "Note" above)

PMDD: 50 mg/day either daily throughout menstrual cycle **or** limited to the luteal phase of menstrual cycle, depending on physician assessment. Patients not responding to 50 mg/day may benefit from dose increases (50 mg increments per menstrual cycle) up to 150 mg/day when dosing throughout menstrual cycle **or** up to 100 mg day when dosing during luteal phase only. If a 100 mg/day dose has been established with luteal phase dosing, a 50 mg/day titration step for 3 days should be utilized at the beginning of each luteal phase dosing period.

Elderly: Depression/OCD: Start treatment with 25 mg/day in the morning and increase by 25 mg/day increments every 2-3 days if tolerated to 50-100 mg/day; additional increases may be necessary; maximum dose: 200 mg/day

Dosage adjustment/comment in renal impairment: Multiple-dose pharmacokinetics are unaffected by renal impairment.

Hemodialysis: Not removed by hemodialysis

Dosage adjustment/comment in hepatic impairment: Sertraline is extensively metabolized by the liver; caution should be used in patients with hepatic impairment; a lower dose or less frequent dosing should be used.

Mechanism of Action Antidepressant with selective inhibitory effects on presynaptic serotonin (5-HT) reuptake and only very weak effects on norepinephrine and dopamine neuronal uptake. *In vitro* studies demonstrate no significant affinity for adrenergic, cholinergic, GABA, dopaminergic, histaminergic, serotonergic, or benzodiazepine receptors.

Contraindications Hypersensitivity to sertraline or any component of the formulation; use of MAO inhibitors within 14 days; concurrent use of pimozide; concurrent use of sertraline oral concentrate with disulfiram

Warnings/Precautions [U.S. Boxed Warning]: Antidepressants increase the risk of suicidal thinking and behavior in children, adolescents, and young adults (18-24 years of age) with major depressive disorder (MDD) and other psychiatric disorders; consider risk prior to prescribing. Short-term studies did not show an increased risk in patients >24 years of age and showed a decreased risk in patients ≥65 years. Closely monitor patients for clinical worsening, suicidality, or unusual changes in behavior, particularly during the initial 1-2 months of therapy or during periods of dosage adjustments (increases or decreases); the patient's family or caregiver should be instructed to closely observe the patient and communicate condition with healthcare provider. A medication guide concerning the use of antidepressants should be dispensed with each prescription. **Sertraline is not FDA approved for use in children with major depressive disorder (MDD). However, it is approved for the treatment of obsessive-compulsive disorder (OCD) in children ≥6 years of age.**

The possibility of a suicide attempt is inherent in major depression and may persist until remission occurs. Use caution in high-risk patients. Worsening depression and severe abrupt suicidality that are not part of the presenting symptoms may require discontinuation or modification of drug therapy. The patient's family or caregiver should be alerted to monitor patients for the emergence of suicidality and associated behaviors (such as agitation, irritability, hostility, impulsivity, and hypomania) and call healthcare provider.

May worsen psychosis in some patients or precipitate a shift to mania or hypomania in patients with bipolar disorder. Patients presenting with depressive symptoms should be screened for bipolar disorder. Monotherapy in patients with bipolar disorder should be avoided. **Sertraline is not FDA approved for the treatment of bipolar depression.**

The potential for severe reaction exists when used with MAO inhibitors, SSRIs/ SNRIs or triptans; serotonin syndrome (hyperthermia, muscular rigidity, mental status changes/agitation, autonomic instability) may occur; concomitant use with MAO inhibitors is contraindicated. Has a very low potential to impair cognitive or motor performance. However, caution patients regarding activities requiring alertness until response to sertraline is known. Does not appear to potentiate the effects of alcohol, however, ethanol use is not advised.

Use caution in patients with a previous seizure disorder or condition predisposing to seizures such as brain damage, alcoholism, or concurrent therapy with other drugs which lower the seizure threshold. May increase the risks associated with electroconvulsive therapy. Use with caution in patients with hepatic or renal dysfunction and in elderly patients. May cause hyponatremia/ SIADH. Use with caution in patients with renal insufficiency or other concurrent illness (due to limited experience). Sertraline acts as a mild uricosuric; use with caution in patients at risk of uric acid nephropathy. Use with caution in patients at risk of bleeding or receiving anticoagulant therapy; may cause impairment in platelet aggregation. Use with caution in patients where weight loss is undesirable. May cause or exacerbate sexual dysfunction.

Use oral concentrate formulation with caution in patients with latex sensitivity; dropper dispenser contains dry natural rubber. Monitor growth in pediatric patients. Discontinuation symptoms (eg, dysphoric mood, irritability, agitation, confusion, anxiety, insomnia, hypomania) may occur upon abrupt discontinuation. Taper dose when discontinuing therapy.

Drug Interactions

Cytochrome P450 Effect: Substrate of CYP2B6 (minor), 2C9 (minor), 2C19 (major), 2D6 (major), 3A4 (minor); **Inhibits** CYP1A2 (weak), 2B6 (moderate), 2C8 (weak), 2C9 (weak), 2C19 (moderate), 2D6 (moderate), 3A4 (moderate)

Increased Effect/Toxicity: Sertraline should not be used with nonselective MAO inhibitors (phenelzine, isocarboxazid) or other drugs with MAO inhibition (linezolid); fatal reactions have been reported. Wait 2 weeks after stopping an MAO inhibitor before starting sertraline. Concurrent selegiline has been associated with mania, hypertension, or serotonin syndrome (risk may be reduced relative to nonselective MAO inhibitors). Sertraline may increase serum concentrations of pimozide; concurrent use is contraindicated. Avoid use of oral concentrate with disulfiram.

Sertraline may inhibit the metabolism of thioridazine or mesoridazine, resulting in increased plasma levels and increasing the risk of QT_c interval prolongation. This may lead to serious ventricular arrhythmias, such as torsade de pointes-type arrhythmias and sudden death. Do not use together. Wait at least 5 weeks after discontinuing sertraline prior to starting thioridazine.

Sertraline may increase the levels/effects of amphetamines, selected beta-blockers, bupropion, selected benzodiazepines, calcium channel blockers, cisapride, cyclosporine, dextromethorphan, ergot alkaloids, fluoxetine, selected HMG-CoA reductase inhibitors, lidocaine, mesoridazine, mirtazapine, nateglinide, nefazodone, paroxetine, phenytoin, promethazine, propofol, risperidone, ritonavir, selegiline, sildenafil (and other PDE-5 inhibitors), tacrolimus, thioridazine, tricyclic antidepressants, venlafaxine, and other substrates of CYP2B6, 2D6 or 3A4. Sertraline may increase the hypoprothrombinemic response to warfarin.

The levels/effects of sertraline may be increased by chlorpromazine, delavirdine, fluconazole, fluoxetine, fluvoxamine, gemfibrozil, isoniazid, miconazole, omeprazole, paroxetine, pergolide, quinidine, quinine, ritonavir, ropinirole, ticlopidine, and other CYP2C19 or 2D6 inhibitors.

Combined use of SSRIs and amphetamines, buspirone, meperidine, nefazodone, serotonin agonists (such as sumatriptan), sibutramine, other SSRIs/SNRIs, sympathomimetics, ritonavir, tramadol, and venlafaxine may increase the risk of serotonin syndrome. Combined use of sumatriptan (and other serotonin agonists) may result in toxicity; weakness, hyper-reflexia, and incoordination have been observed with sumatriptan and SSRIs. In addition, concurrent use may theoretically increase the risk of serotonin syndrome; includes sumatriptan, naratriptan, rizatriptan, and zolmitriptan.

Concurrent lithium may increase risk of nephrotoxicity. Risk of hyponatremia may increase with concurrent use of loop diuretics (bumetanide, furosemide, torsemide). Concomitant use of sertraline and NSAIDs, aspirin, or other drugs affecting coagulation has been associated with an increased risk of bleeding; monitor.

Decreased Effect: The levels/effects of sertraline may be decreased by aminoglutethimide, carbamazepine, phenytoin, rifampin, and other CYP2C19 inducers. Sertraline may decrease the metabolism of tolbutamide; monitor for changes in glucose control. Sertraline may decrease the levels/effects of (Continued)

Sertraline *(Continued)*

CYP2D6 prodrug substrates (eg, codeine, hydrocodone, oxycodone, tramadol).

Ethanol/Nutrition/Herb Interactions

Ethanol: Avoid ethanol (may increase CNS depression).

Food: Sertraline average peak serum levels may be increased if taken with food.

Herb/Nutraceutical: Avoid valerian, St John's wort, kava kava, gotu kola (may increase CNS depression).

Pharmacodynamics/Kinetics

Absorption: Slow

Protein binding: 98%

Metabolism: Hepatic; may involve CYP2C19 and CYP2D6; extensive first pass metabolism; forms metabolite N-desmethylsertraline

Bioavailability: Bioavailability of tablets and solution are equivalent

Half-life elimination: Sertraline: 26 hours; N-desmethylsertraline: 66 hours (range: 62-104 hours)

Time to peak, plasma: Sertraline: 4.5-8.4 hours

Excretion: Urine and feces

Pregnancy Risk Factor C

Dosage Forms

Solution, oral [concentrate]: 20 mg/mL (60 mL)

Zoloft®: 20 mg/mL

Tablet: 25 mg, 50 mg, 100 mg

Zoloft®: 25 mg, 50 mg, 100 mg

Dental Comment Problems with SSRI-induced bruxism have been reported and may preclude their use; clinicians attempting to evaluate any patient with bruxism or involuntary muscle movement, who is simultaneously being treated with an SSRI drug, should be aware of the potential association.

Selected Readings

Gerber PE and Lynd LD, "Selective Serotonin Reuptake Inhibitor-Induced Movement Disorders," *Ann Pharmacother*, 1998, 32(6):692-8.

Sertraline Hydrochloride *see* Sertraline *on page 1463*

Serutan® [OTC] *see* Psyllium *on page 1386*

Serzone *see* Nefazodone *on page 1156*

Sevelamer *(se VEL a mer)*

U.S. Brand Names Renagel®

Canadian Brand Names Renagel®

Generic Available No

Index Terms Sevelamer Hydrochloride

Pharmacologic Category Phosphate Binder

Use Reduction of serum phosphorous in patients with chronic kidney disease on hemodialysis

Local Anesthetic/Vasoconstrictor Precautions No information available to require special precautions

Effects on Dental Treatment No significant effects or complications reported

Common Adverse Effects

>10%:

Dermatologic: Rash (13%)

Gastrointestinal: Vomiting (22%), nausea (7% to 20%), diarrhea (4% to 19%), dyspepsia (5% to 16%)

Neuromuscular & skeletal: Limb pain (13%), arthralgia (12%)

Respiratory: Nasopharyngitis (14%), bronchitis (11%)

1% to 10%:

Cardiovascular: Hypertension (10%)

Central nervous system: Headache (9%), pyrexia (5%)

Gastrointestinal: Constipation (2% to 8%), flatulence (4%)

Neuromuscular & skeletal: Back pain (4%)

Respiratory: Dyspnea (10%), cough (7%), upper respiratory tract infection (5%)

Postmarketing and/or case reports: Abdominal pain

Mechanism of Action Sevelamer (a polymeric compound) binds phosphate within the intestinal lumen, limiting absorption and decreasing serum phosphate concentrations without altering calcium, aluminum, or bicarbonate concentrations

Drug Interactions

Decreased Effect: Sevelamer may bind to some drugs in the gastrointestinal tract and decrease their absorption. When changes in absorption of oral medications may have significant clinical consequences (such as antiarrhythmic and antiseizure medications), these medications should be taken at least 1 hour before or 3 hours after a dose of sevelamer. Sevelamer may decrease the bioavailability of ciprofloxacin by 50%.

Pharmacodynamics/Kinetics
Absorption: None
Excretion: Feces

Pregnancy Risk Factor C

Sevelamer Hydrochloride *see* Sevelamer *on page 1466*
Shingles Vaccine *see* Zoster Vaccine *on page 1693*
Shur-Seal® [OTC] [DSC] *see* Nonoxynol 9 *on page 1185*

Sibutramine (si BYOO tra meen)

U.S. Brand Names Meridia®
Canadian Brand Names Meridia®
Mexican Brand Names Ectiva; Raductil; Reductil
Generic Available No
Index Terms Sibutramine Hydrochloride Monohydrate
Pharmacologic Category Anorexiant; Sympathomimetic
Use Management of obesity
Local Anesthetic/Vasoconstrictor Precautions No information available to require special precautions
Effects on Dental Treatment Key adverse event(s) related to dental treatment: Xerostomia (normal salivary flow resumes upon discontinuation) and taste perversion (see Dental Comment).
Common Adverse Effects
>10%:
  Central nervous system: Headache (30%), insomnia (11%)
  Gastrointestinal: Xerostomia (17%), anorexia (13%), constipation (12%)
1% to 10%:
  Cardiovascular: Tachycardia (3%), vasodilation (2%), hypertension (2%), palpitation (2%), chest pain (2%)
  Central nervous system: Dizziness (7%), nervousness (5%), anxiety (5%), depression (4%), somnolence (2%), CNS stimulation (2%), emotional lability (1%)
  Dermatologic: Rash (4%)
  Endocrine & metabolic: Dysmenorrhea (4%)
  Gastrointestinal: Appetite increased (9%), nausea (6%), abdominal pain (5%), dyspepsia (5%), gastritis (2%), taste perversion (2%)
  Genitourinary: Vaginal *Monilia* (1%)
  Hepatic: Abnormal LFTs (2%)
  Neuromuscular & skeletal: Back pain (8%), weakness (6%), arthralgia (6%), neck pain (2%), myalgia (2%), paresthesia (2%), tenosynovitis (1%), joint disorder (1%)
  Otic: Ear disorder (2%)
  Respiratory: Pharyngitis (10%), rhinitis (10%), sinusitis (5%), cough (4%)
  Miscellaneous: Flu-like syndrome (8%), diaphoresis (3%), allergic reactions (2%), thirst (2%)

Frequency not defined:
  Cardiovascular: Peripheral edema
  Central nervous system: Thinking abnormal, agitation, fever
  Dermatologic: Pruritus
  Endocrine & metabolic: Menstrual disorders/irregularities
  Gastrointestinal: Diarrhea, flatulence, gastroenteritis, tooth disorder
  Neuromuscular & skeletal: Arthritis, hypertonia, leg cramps
  Ocular: Amblyopia
  Respiratory: Bronchitis, dyspnea
Restrictions C-IV

Pharmacotherapy for weight loss is recommended only for obese patients with a body mass index ≥30 kg/m², or ≥27 kg/m² in the presence of other risk factors such as hypertension, diabetes, and/or dyslipidemia or a high waist circumference; therapy should be used in conjunction with a comprehensive weight management program. Rule out organic causes of obesity (eg, untreated hypothyroidism) prior to use.

Mechanism of Action Sibutramine and its two primary metabolites block the neuronal uptake of norepinephrine, serotonin, and (to a lesser extent) dopamine. There is no monoamine-releasing (or depleting) activity.
(Continued)

Sibutramine (Continued)

Drug Interactions

Cytochrome P450 Effect: Substrate of CYP3A4 (major)

Increased Effect/Toxicity: Serotonergic agents such as buspirone, selective serotonin reuptake inhibitors (eg, citalopram, fluoxetine, fluvoxamine, paroxetine, sertraline), sumatriptan (and similar serotonin agonists), ergot derivatives, lithium, tryptophan, some opioid/analgesics (eg, fentanyl, meperidine, tramadol), and venlafaxine, when combined with sibutramine may result in serotonin syndrome. Dextromethorphan, MAO inhibitors and other drugs that can raise the blood pressure (eg decongestants, centrally-acting weight loss products, amphetamines, and amphetamine-like compounds) can increase the possibility of sibutramine-associated cardiovascular complications. Sibutramine may increase serum levels of tricyclic antidepressants. CYP3A4 inhibitors may increase the levels/effects of sibutramine; example inhibitors include azole antifungals, clarithromycin, diclofenac, doxycycline, erythromycin, imatinib, isoniazid, nefazodone, nicardipine, propofol, protease inhibitors, quinidine, telithromycin, and verapamil.

Decreased Effect: Inducers of CYP3A4 (including phenytoin, phenobarbital, carbamazepine, and rifampin) theoretically may reduce sibutramine serum concentrations.

Pharmacodynamics/Kinetics

Absorption: 77%; rapid

Protein binding, plasma: Parent drug and metabolites: >94%

Metabolism: Hepatic; undergoes first-pass metabolism via CYP3A4; forms two primary metabolites (M_1 and M_2; active)

Half-life elimination: Sibutramine: 1 hour; Metabolites: M_1: 14 hours; M_2: 16 hours

Time to peak: Sibutramine: 1.2 hours; Metabolites (M_1 and M_2): 3-4 hours

Excretion: Primarily urine (77% as inactive metabolites); feces

Pregnancy Risk Factor C

Dental Comment The mechanism of action is thought to be different from the "fen" drugs. Sibutramine works to suppress the appetite by inhibiting the reuptake of norepinephrine and serotonin. Unlike dexfenfluramine and fenfluramine, it is not a serotonin releaser. Sibutramine is closer chemically to the widely used antidepressants such as fluoxetine (Prozac®). The FDA approved sibutramine over the objections of its own advisory panel, who called the drug too risky. FDA reported that the drug causes blood pressure to increase, generally by a small amount, though in some patients the increases were higher. It is now recommended that patients taking sibutramine have their blood pressure evaluated regularly.

Sildenafil (sil DEN a fil)

U.S. Brand Names GD-Sildenafil; Revatio™; Viagra®

Canadian Brand Names Viagra®

Mexican Brand Names Viagra

Generic Available No

Index Terms UK92480

Pharmacologic Category Phosphodiesterase-5 Enzyme Inhibitor

Use Treatment of erectile dysfunction; treatment of pulmonary arterial hypertension

Unlabeled/Investigational Use Psychotropic-induced sexual dysfunction; pulmonary arterial hypertension in children

Local Anesthetic/Vasoconstrictor Precautions No information available to require special precautions

Effects on Dental Treatment No significant effects or complications reported

Common Adverse Effects Based upon normal doses. (Adverse effects such as flushing, diarrhea, myalgia, and visual disturbances may be increased with doses >100 mg/24 hours.)

>10%:

Central nervous system: Headache (16% to 46%)

Gastrointestinal: Dyspepsia (7% to 17%)

1% to 10%:

Cardiovascular: Flushing (10%)

Central nervous system: Dizziness, insomnia, pyrexia

Dermatologic: Erythema, rash

Gastrointestinal: Diarrhea (3% to 9%), gastritis

Genitourinary: Urinary tract infection

Hematologic: Anemia, leukopenia

Hepatic: LFTs increased

Neuromuscular & skeletal: Myalgia, paresthesia

Ocular: Abnormal vision (color changes, blurred or increased sensitivity to light 3%; up to 11% with doses >100 mg)

Respiratory: Dyspnea exacerbated, epistaxis, nasal congestion, rhinitis, sinusitis

Dosage Adults: Oral:

Erectile dysfunction (Viagra®): For most patients, the recommended dose is 25-50 mg taken as needed, approximately 1 hour before sexual activity. However, sildenafil may be taken anywhere from 30 minutes to 4 hours before sexual activity. Based on effectiveness and tolerance, the dose may be increased to a maximum recommended dose of 100 mg or decreased to 25 mg. The maximum recommended dosing frequency is once daily.

Pulmonary arterial hypertension (Revatio™): 20 mg 3 times/day, taken 4-6 hours apart

Dosage adjustment for patients >65 years of age: Hepatic impairment (cirrhosis), severe renal impairment (creatinine clearance <30 mL/minute): Higher plasma levels have been associated which may result in increase in efficacy and adverse effects; Viagra®: Starting dose of 25 mg should be considered

Dosage considerations for patients stable on alpha-blockers: Viagra®: Initial 25 mg

Dosage adjustment for concomitant use of potent CYP34A inhibitors:

Revatio™:

Erythromycin, saquinavir: No dosage adjustment

Itraconazole, ketoconazole, ritonavir: Not recommended

Viagra®:

Erythromycin, itraconazole, ketoconazole, saquinavir: Starting dose of 25 mg should be considered

Ritonavir: Maximum: 25 mg every 48 hours

Mechanism of Action

Erectile dysfunction: Does not directly cause penile erections, but affects the response to sexual stimulation. The physiologic mechanism of erection of the penis involves release of nitric oxide (NO) in the corpus cavernosum during sexual stimulation. NO then activates the enzyme guanylate cyclase, which results in increased levels of cyclic guanosine monophosphate (cGMP), producing smooth muscle relaxation and inflow of blood to the corpus cavernosum. Sildenafil enhances the effect of NO by inhibiting phosphodiesterase type 5 (PDE-5), which is responsible for degradation of cGMP in the corpus cavernosum; when sexual stimulation causes local release of NO, inhibition of PDE-5 by sildenafil causes increased levels of cGMP in the corpus cavernosum, resulting in smooth muscle relaxation and inflow of blood to the corpus cavernosum; at recommended doses, it has no effect in the absence of sexual stimulation.

Pulmonary arterial hypertension (PAH): Inhibits phosphodiesterase type 5 (PDE-5) in smooth muscle of pulmonary vasculature where PDE-5 is responsible for the degradation of cyclic guanosine monophosphate (cGMP). Increased cGMP concentration results in pulmonary vasculature relaxation; vasodilation in the pulmonary bed and the systemic circulation (to a lesser degree) may occur.

Contraindications Hypersensitivity to sildenafil or any component of the formulation; concurrent use of organic nitrates (nitroglycerin) in any form (potentiates the hypotensive effects)

Warnings/Precautions Decreases in blood pressure may occur due to vasodilator effects; use caution in patients with resting hypotension (BP <90/50), hypertension (BP >170/110), fluid depletion, severe left ventricular outflow obstruction, or autonomic dysfunction, and patients receiving alpha-blockers or other antihypertensive medication. Not recommended for use with pulmonary veno-occlusive disease.

(Continued)

Sildenafil *(Continued)*

Use caution in patients with cardiovascular disease, including cardiac failure, unstable angina, or a recent history (within the last 6 months) of myocardial infarction, stroke, or life-threatening arrhythmia. Use caution in patients receiving concurrent bosentan. Use caution in patients with bleeding disorders or with active peptic ulcer disease; safety and efficacy have not been established.

There is a degree of cardiac risk associated with sexual activity; therefore, physicians may wish to consider the cardiovascular status of their patients prior to initiating any treatment for erectile dysfunction. Sildenafil should be used with caution in patients with anatomical deformation of the penis (angulation, cavernosal fibrosis, or Peyronie's disease), or in patients who have conditions which may predispose them to priapism (sickle cell anemia, multiple myeloma, leukemia).

Rare cases of nonarteritic ischemic optic neuropathy (NAION) have been reported; risk may be increased with history of vision loss. Other risk factors for NAION include low cup-to-disc ratio ("crowded disc"), coronary artery disease, diabetes, hypertension, hyperlipidemia, smoking, and age >50 years.

The safety and efficacy of sildenafil with other treatments for erectile dysfunction have not been established; use is not recommended. May cause dose-related impairment of color discrimination. Use caution in patients with retinitis pigmentosa; a minority have genetic disorders of retinal phosphodiesterases (no safety information available). Use with caution in patients taking strong CYP3A4 inhibitors. All patients should be instructed to seek medical attention if erection persists >4 hours. Safety and efficacy in pediatric patients have not been established.

Drug Interactions

Cytochrome P450 Effect: Substrate of CYP2C9 (minor), 3A4 (major); **Inhibits** CYP1A2 (weak), 2C9 (weak), 2C19 (weak), 2D6 (weak), 2E1 (weak), 3A4 (weak)

Increased Effect/Toxicity: Sildenafil potentiates the hypotensive effects of nitrates (amyl nitrate, isosorbide dinitrate, isosorbide mononitrate, nitroglycerin); severe reactions have occurred and concurrent use is contraindicated. Concomitant use of alpha-blockers (doxazosin) may lead to symptomatic hypotension. Macrolide antibiotics may increase the effects of sildenafil.

CYP3A4 inhibitors may increase the levels/effects of sildenafil; example inhibitors include azole antifungals, clarithromycin, diclofenac, doxycycline, erythromycin, imatinib, isoniazid, nefazodone, nicardipine, propofol, protease inhibitors, quinidine, telithromycin, and verapamil. Sildenafil may potentiate the effect of other antihypertensives. Reduce sildenafil dose to 25 mg/24 hours in patients receiving azole antifungals or protease inhibitors (use of Revatio™ with concurrent protease inhibitors is not recommended).

Decreased Effect: Enzyme inducers (including phenytoin, carbamazepine, phenobarbital, rifampin) may decrease the serum concentration and efficacy of sildenafil. Bosentan may decrease serum concentration and effect of sildenafil.

Ethanol/Nutrition/Herb Interactions

Food: Amount and rate of absorption of sildenafil is reduced when taken with a high-fat meal. Serum concentrations/toxicity may be increased with grapefruit juice; avoid concurrent use.

Herb/Nutraceutical: St John's wort may decrease sildenafil levels.

Pharmacodynamics/Kinetics

Onset of action: ~60 minutes

Duration: 2-4 hours

Absorption: Rapid; slower with a high-fat meal

Distribution: V_{dss}: 105 L

Protein binding, plasma: ~96%

Metabolism: Hepatic via CYP3A4 (major) and CYP2C9 (minor route)

Bioavailability: 40%

Half-life elimination: 4 hours

Time to peak: 30-120 minutes; delayed by 60 minutes with a high-fat meal

Excretion: Feces (80%); urine (13%)

Pregnancy Risk Factor B

Dosage Forms

Tablet:

Revatio™: 20 mg

Viagra®: 25 mg, 50 mg, 100 mg

Silexin [OTC] *see* Guaifenesin and Dextromethorphan *on page 796*

Silfedrine Children's [OTC] *see* Pseudoephedrine *on page 1381*

Silphen® [OTC] *see* DiphenhydrAMINE *on page 510*

Silphen DM® [OTC] *see* Dextromethorphan *on page 477*
Sil-Tex *see* Guaifenesin and Phenylephrine *on page 797*
Siltussin DAS [OTC] *see* Guaifenesin *on page 795*
Siltussin DM [OTC] *see* Guaifenesin and Dextromethorphan *on page 796*
Siltussin DM DAS [OTC] *see* Guaifenesin and Dextromethorphan *on page 796*
Siltussin SA [OTC] *see* Guaifenesin *on page 795*
Silvadene® *see* Silver Sulfadiazine *on page 1471*

Silver Nitrate (SIL ver NYE trate)

Generic Available Yes
Index Terms AgNO$_3$
Pharmacologic Category Antibiotic, Topical; Cauterizing Agent, Topical; Topical Skin Product, Antibacterial
Use Cauterization of wounds and sluggish ulcers, removal of granulation tissue and warts; aseptic prophylaxis of burns
Local Anesthetic/Vasoconstrictor Precautions No information available to require special precautions
Effects on Dental Treatment No significant effects or complications reported
Common Adverse Effects Frequency not defined.
Dermatologic: Burning and skin irritation, staining of the skin
Endocrine & metabolic: Hyponatremia
Hematologic: Methemoglobinemia
Dosage Children and Adults:
Sticks: Apply to mucous membranes and other moist skin surfaces only on area to be treated 2-3 times/week for 2-3 weeks
Topical solution: Apply a cotton applicator dipped in solution on the affected area 2-3 times/week for 2-3 weeks
Mechanism of Action Free silver ions precipitate bacterial proteins by combining with chloride in tissue forming silver chloride; coagulates cellular protein to form an eschar; silver ions or salts or colloidal silver preparations can inhibit the growth of both gram-positive and gram-negative bacteria. This germicidal action is attributed to the precipitation of bacterial proteins by liberated silver ions. Silver nitrate coagulates cellular protein to form an eschar, and this mode of action is the postulated mechanism for control of benign hematuria, rhinitis, and recurrent pneumothorax.
Contraindications Hypersensitivity to silver nitrate or any component of the formulation; not for use on broken skin, cuts, or wounds
Warnings/Precautions Do not use applicator sticks on the eyes. Prolonged use may result in skin discoloration.
Pharmacodynamics/Kinetics
Absorption: Because silver ions readily combine with protein, there is minimal GI and cutaneous absorption of the 0.5% and 1% preparations
Excretion: Highest amounts of silver noted on autopsy have been in kidneys, excretion in urine is minimal
Pregnancy Risk Factor C
Dosage Forms
Applicator sticks, topical: Silver nitrate 75% and potassium 25% (6", 12", 18")
Solution, topical: 10% (30 mL); 25% (30 mL); 50% (30 mL)
Selected Readings
Cushing AH and Smith S, "Methemoglobinemia With Silver Nitrate Therapy of a Burn: Report of a Case," *J Pediatr*, 1969, 74(4):613-5.
Hammerschlag MR, Cummings C, Roblin PM, et al, "Efficacy of Neonatal Ocular Prophylaxis for the Prevention of Chlamydial and Gonococcal Conjunctivitis," *N Engl J Med*, 1989, 320(12):769-72.
U.S. Department of Health and Human Services, "1993 Sexually Transmitted Diseases Treatment Guidelines," *MMWR Recomm Rep*, 1993, 42(RR-14).

Silver Sulfadiazine (SIL ver sul fa DYE a zeen)

U.S. Brand Names Silvadene®; SSD®; SSD® AF; Thermazene®
Canadian Brand Names Flamazine®
Mexican Brand Names Silvadene
Generic Available Yes
Pharmacologic Category Antibiotic, Topical
Use Prevention and treatment of infection in second and third degree burns
Local Anesthetic/Vasoconstrictor Precautions No information available to require special precautions
Effects on Dental Treatment No significant effects or complications reported
Common Adverse Effects Frequency not defined.
Dermatologic: Itching, rash, erythema multiforme, discoloration of skin, photosensitivity
Hematologic: Hemolytic anemia, leukopenia, agranulocytosis, aplastic anemia
(Continued)

Silver Sulfadiazine (Continued)

Hepatic: Hepatitis
Renal: Interstitial nephritis
Miscellaneous: Allergic reactions may be related to sulfa component

Mechanism of Action Acts upon the bacterial cell wall and cell membrane. Bactericidal for many gram-negative and gram-positive bacteria and is effective against yeast. Active against *Pseudomonas aeruginosa*, *Pseudomonas maltophilia*, *Enterobacter* species, *Klebsiella* species, *Serratia* species, *Escherichia coli*, *Proteus mirabilis*, *Morganella morganii*, *Providencia rettgeri*, *Proteus vulgaris*, *Providencia* species, *Citrobacter* species, *Acinetobacter calcoaceticus*, *Staphylococcus aureus*, *Staphylococcus epidermidis*, *Enterococcus* species, *Candida albicans*, *Corynebacterium diphtheriae*, and *Clostridium perfringens*

Drug Interactions
Decreased Effect: Topical proteolytic enzymes are inactivated by silver sulfadiazine.

Pharmacodynamics/Kinetics
Absorption: Significant percutaneous absorption of silver sulfadiazine can occur especially when applied to extensive burns
Half-life elimination: 10 hours; prolonged with renal impairment
Time to peak, serum: 3-11 days of continuous therapy
Excretion: Urine (~50% as unchanged drug)

Pregnancy Risk Factor B

Simethicone (sye METH i kone)

U.S. Brand Names Equalizer Gas Relief [OTC]; GasAid [OTC]; Gas-X® [OTC]; Gas-X® Extra Strength [OTC]; Gas-X® Maximum Strength [OTC]; Genasyme® [OTC]; Infantaire Gas Drops [OTC]; Mylanta® Gas [OTC]; Mylanta® Gas Maximum Strength [OTC]; Mylicon® Infants [OTC]; Phazyme® Quick Dissolve [OTC]; Phazyme® Ultra Strength [OTC]

Canadian Brand Names Ovol®; Phazyme™

Generic Available Yes

Index Terms Activated Dimethicone; Activated Methylpolysiloxane

Pharmacologic Category Antiflatulent

Use Relieves flatulence and functional gastric bloating, and postoperative gas pains

Local Anesthetic/Vasoconstrictor Precautions No information available to require special precautions

Effects on Dental Treatment No significant effects or complications reported

Common Adverse Effects No data reported

Mechanism of Action Decreases the surface tension of gas bubbles thereby disperses and prevents gas pockets in the GI system

Pregnancy Risk Factor C

Simethicone, Aluminum Hydroxide, and Magnesium Hydroxide see Aluminum Hydroxide, Magnesium Hydroxide, and Simethicone on page 82

Simethicone and Calcium Carbonate see Calcium Carbonate and Simethicone on page 261

Simethicone and Loperamide Hydrochloride see Loperamide and Simethicone on page 996

Simethicone and Magaldrate see Magaldrate and Simethicone on page 1013

Similac® Glucose see Dextrose on page 478

Simply Cough® [OTC] [DSC] see Dextromethorphan on page 477

Simply Saline® [OTC] see Sodium Chloride on page 1480

Simply Saline® Baby [OTC] see Sodium Chloride on page 1480

Simply Saline® Nasal Moist® [OTC] see Sodium Chloride on page 1480

Simply Sleep® [OTC] see DiphenhydrAMINE on page 510

Simply Stuffy™ [OTC] [DSC] see Pseudoephedrine on page 1381

Simuc see Guaifenesin and Phenylephrine on page 797

Simuc-DM see Guaifenesin and Dextromethorphan on page 796

Simulect® see Basiliximab on page 185

Simvastatin (sim va STAT in)

Related Information
Cardiovascular Diseases on page 1726

U.S. Brand Names Zocor®

Canadian Brand Names Apo-Simvastatin®; BCI-Simvastatin; CO Simvastatin; Gen-Simvastatin; Novo-Simvastatin; PMS-Simvastatin; ratio-Simvastatin; Riva-Simvastatin; Sandoz-Simvastatin; Taro-Simvastatin; Zocor®

Mexican Brand Names Zocor

Generic Available Yes

Pharmacologic Category Antilipemic Agent, HMG-CoA Reductase Inhibitor

Use Used with dietary therapy for the following:

Secondary prevention of cardiovascular events in hypercholesterolemic patients with established coronary heart disease (CHD) or at high risk for CHD: To reduce cardiovascular morbidity (myocardial infarction, coronary revascularization procedures) and mortality; to reduce the risk of stroke and transient ischemic attacks

Hyperlipidemias: To reduce elevations in total cholesterol, LDL-C, apolipoprotein B, and triglycerides in patients with primary hypercholesterolemia (elevations of 1 or more components are present in Fredrickson type IIa, IIb, III, and IV hyperlipidemias); treatment of homozygous familial hypercholesterolemia

Heterozygous familial hypercholesterolemia (HeFH): In adolescent patients (10-17 years of age, females >1 year postmenarche) with HeFH having LDL-C ≥190 mg/dL **or** LDL ≥160 mg/dL with positive family history of premature cardiovascular disease (CVD), or 2 or more CVD risk factors in the adolescent patient

Local Anesthetic/Vasoconstrictor Precautions No information available to require special precautions

Effects on Dental Treatment No significant effects or complications reported

Common Adverse Effects 1% to 10%:

Gastrointestinal: Constipation (2%), dyspepsia (1%), flatulence (2%)

Neuromuscular & skeletal: CPK elevation (>3x normal on one or more occasions - 5%)

Respiratory: Upper respiratory infection (2%)

Additional class-related events or case reports (not necessarily reported with simvastatin therapy): Alopecia, alteration in taste, anaphylaxis, angioedema, anorexia, anxiety, arthritis, cataracts, chills, cholestatic jaundice, cirrhosis, decreased libido, depression, dermatomyositis, dryness of skin/mucous membranes, dyspnea, elevated transaminases, eosinophilia, erectile dysfunction/impotence, erythema multiforme, facial paresis, fatty liver, fever, flushing, fulminant hepatic necrosis, gynecomastia, hemolytic anemia, hepatitis, hepatoma, hyperbilirubinemia, hypersensitivity reaction, impaired extraocular muscle movement, increased alkaline phosphatase, increased CPK (>10x normal), increased ESR, increased GGT, leukopenia, malaise, memory loss, myopathy, nail changes, nodules, ophthalmoplegia, pancreatitis, paresthesia, peripheral nerve palsy, peripheral neuropathy, photosensitivity, polymyalgia rheumatica, positive ANA, pruritus, psychic disturbance, purpura, rash, renal failure (secondary to rhabdomyolysis), rhabdomyolysis, skin discoloration, Stevens-Johnson syndrome, systemic lupus erythematosus-like syndrome, thrombocytopenia, thyroid dysfunction, toxic epidermal necrolysis, tremor, urticaria, vasculitis, vertigo, vomiting

Dosage Oral: **Note:** Doses should be individualized according to the baseline LDL-cholesterol levels, the recommended goal of therapy, and the patient's response; adjustments should be made at intervals of 4 weeks or more; doses may need adjusted based on concomitant medications

Children 10-17 years (females >1 year postmenarche): HeFH: 10 mg once daily in the evening; range: 10-40 mg/day (maximum: 40 mg/day)

Dosage adjustment for simvastatin with concomitant cyclosporine, danazol, fibrates, niacin, amiodarone, or verapamil: Refer to drug-specific dosing in adult dosing section

Adults:

Homozygous familial hypercholesterolemia: 40 mg once daily in the evening **or** 80 mg/day (given as 20 mg, 20 mg, and 40 mg evening dose)

Prevention of cardiovascular events, hyperlipidemias: 20-40 mg once daily in the evening; range: 5-80 mg/day

Patients requiring only moderate reduction of LDL-cholesterol may be started at 10 mg once daily

Patients requiring reduction of >45% in low-density lipoprotein (LDL) cholesterol may be started at 40 mg once daily in the evening

Patients with CHD or at high risk for CHD: Dosing should be started at 40 mg once daily in the evening; simvastatin may be started simultaneously with diet

Dosage adjustment with concomitant medications:

Cyclosporine or danazol (patient must first demonstrate tolerance to simvastatin ≥5 mg once daily): Initial: 5 mg simvastatin, should **not** exceed 10 mg/day

Fibrates or niacin: Simvastatin dose should **not** exceed 10 mg/day

Amiodarone or verapamil: Simvastatin dose should **not** exceed 20 mg/day

Dosing adjustment/comments in renal impairment: Because simvastatin does not undergo significant renal excretion, modification of dose should not be necessary in patients with mild to moderate renal insufficiency.

(Continued)

Simvastatin *(Continued)*

Severe renal impairment: Cl_{cr} <10 mL/minute: Initial: 5 mg/day with close monitoring.

Mechanism of Action Simvastatin is a methylated derivative of lovastatin that acts by competitively inhibiting 3-hydroxy-3-methylglutaryl-coenzyme A (HMG-CoA) reductase, the enzyme that catalyzes the rate-limiting step in cholesterol biosynthesis

Contraindications Hypersensitivity to simvastatin or any component of the formulation; acute liver disease; unexplained persistent elevations of serum transaminases; pregnancy; breast-feeding

Warnings/Precautions Secondary causes of hyperlipidemia should be ruled out prior to therapy. Liver function must be monitored by laboratory assessment. Rhabdomyolysis with acute renal failure has occurred. Risk is dose-related and is increased with concurrent use of lipid-lowering agents which may cause rhabdomyolysis (gemfibrozil, fibric acid derivatives, or niacin at doses ≥1 g/day), during concurrent use with danazol or strong CYP3A4 inhibitors (including amiodarone, clarithromycin, cyclosporine, erythromycin, telithromycin, itraconazole, ketoconazole, nefazodone, grapefruit juice in large quantities, verapamil, or protease inhibitors such as indinavir, nelfinavir, or ritonavir). Weigh the risk versus benefit when combining any of these drugs with simvastatin. Do not initiate simvastatin-containing treatment in a patient with pre-existing therapy of cyclosporine or danazol, unless the patient has previously demonstrated tolerance to ≥5 mg/day simvastatin. Temporarily discontinue in any patient experiencing an acute or serious major medical or surgical condition which may increase the risk of rhabdomyolysis. Discontinue temporarily for elective surgical procedures. Use caution in patients with renal insufficiency. Use with caution in patients with advanced age, these patients are predisposed to myopathy. Use with caution in patients who consume large amounts of ethanol or have a history of liver disease. Safety and efficacy have not been established in patients <10 years of age or in premenarcheal girls.

Drug Interactions

Cytochrome P450 Effect: Substrate of CYP3A4 (major); **Inhibits** CYP2C8 (weak), 2C9 (weak), 2D6 (weak)

Increased Effect/Toxicity: Risk of myopathy/rhabdomyolysis may be increased by concurrent use of lipid-lowering agents which may cause rhabdomyolysis (gemfibrozil, fibric acid derivatives, or niacin at doses ≥1 g/day), or during concurrent use of strong CYP3A4 inhibitors.

CYP3A4 inhibitors may increase the levels/effects of simvastatin; example inhibitors include azole antifungals, clarithromycin, diclofenac, diltiazem, doxycycline, erythromycin, imatinib, isoniazid, nefazodone, nicardipine, propofol, protease inhibitors, quinidine, telithromycin, and verapamil. In large quantities (ie, >1 quart/day), grapefruit juice may also increase simvastatin serum concentrations, increasing the risk of rhabdomyolysis. In general, concurrent use with CYP3A4 inhibitors is not recommended; manufacturer recommends limiting simvastatin dose to 20 mg/day when used with amiodarone or verapamil, and 10 mg/day when used with cyclosporine, gemfibrozil, or fibric acid derivatives.

The anticoagulant effect of warfarin may be increased by simvastatin. Cholesterol-lowering effects are additive with bile-acid sequestrants (colestipol and cholestyramine).

Decreased Effect: When taken within 1 before or up to 2 hours after cholestyramine, a decrease in absorption of simvastatin can occur.

Ethanol/Nutrition/Herb Interactions

Ethanol: Avoid excessive ethanol consumption (due to potential hepatic effects).

Food: Simvastatin serum concentration may be increased when taken with grapefruit juice; avoid concurrent intake of large quantities (>1 quart/day). Red yeast rice contains an estimated 2.4 mg lovastatin per 600 mg rice.

Herb/Nutraceutical: St John's wort may decrease simvastatin levels.

Dietary Considerations Red yeast rice contains an estimated 2.4 mg lovastatin per 600 mg rice.

Pharmacodynamics/Kinetics

Onset of action: >3 days

Peak effect: 2 weeks

Absorption: 85%

Protein binding: ~95%

Metabolism: Hepatic via CYP3A4; extensive first-pass effect

Bioavailability: <5%

Half-life elimination: Unknown

Time to peak: 1.3-2.4 hours

Excretion: Feces (60%); urine (13%)

Pregnancy Risk Factor X

Dosage Forms
  Tablet: 5 mg, 10 mg, 20 mg, 40 mg
    Zocor®: 5 mg, 10 mg, 20 mg, 40 mg, 80 mg

Sina-12X *see* Guaifenesin and Phenylephrine *on page 797*

Sincalide (SIN ka lide)

U.S. Brand Names Kinevac®
Generic Available No
Index Terms C8-CCK; OP-CCK
Pharmacologic Category Diagnostic Agent
Use Postevacuation cholecystography; gallbladder bile sampling; stimulate pancreatic secretion for analysis; accelerate the transit of barium through the small bowel
Local Anesthetic/Vasoconstrictor Precautions No information available to require special precautions
Effects on Dental Treatment No significant effects or complications reported
Mechanism of Action Stimulates contraction of the gallbladder; inhibits gastric emptying by causing pyloric contraction, and increases intestinal motility; stimulates pancreatic secretion; causes smooth muscle contraction
Pregnancy Risk Factor B

Sinemet® *see* Levodopa and Carbidopa *on page 964*

Sinemet® CR *see* Levodopa and Carbidopa *on page 964*

Sinequan® [DSC] *see* Doxepin *on page 531*

Singulair® *see* Montelukast *on page 1121*

Sinografin® *see* Diatrizoate Meglumine and Iodipamide Meglumine *on page 480*

Sinus-Relief [OTC] [DSC] *see* Acetaminophen and Pseudoephedrine *on page 38*

Sinutab® Non-Drying [OTC] *see* Guaifenesin and Pseudoephedrine *on page 798*

Sinutab® Sinus Allergy Maximum Strength [OTC] *see* Acetaminophen, Chlorpheniramine, and Pseudoephedrine *on page 43*

SINUtuss® DM *see* Guaifenesin, Dextromethorphan, and Phenylephrine *on page 798*

SINUvent® PE *see* Guaifenesin and Phenylephrine *on page 797*

Sirdalud® *see* Tizanidine *on page 1577*

Sirolimus (sir OH li mus)

U.S. Brand Names Rapamune®
Canadian Brand Names Rapamune®
Mexican Brand Names Rapamune
Generic Available No
Pharmacologic Category Immunosuppressant Agent
Use Prophylaxis of organ rejection in patients receiving renal transplants, in combination with corticosteroids and cyclosporine (cyclosporine may be withdrawn in low-to-moderate immunological risk patients after 2-4 months, in conjunction with an increase in sirolimus dosage)
Unlabeled/Investigational Use Investigational: Immunosuppression in peripheral stem cell/bone marrow transplantation
Local Anesthetic/Vasoconstrictor Precautions No information available to require special precautions
Effects on Dental Treatment Key adverse event(s) related to dental treatment: Mouth ulceration, oral moniliasis, stomatitis, gingival hyperplasia, gingivitis, and dysphagia.
Common Adverse Effects Incidence of many adverse effects is dose related
  >20%:
    Cardiovascular: Peripheral edema (54% to 64%), hypertension (39% to 49%), edema (16% to 24%), chest pain (16% to 24%)
    Central nervous system: Fever (23% to 34%), headache (23% to 34%), pain (24% to 33%), insomnia (13% to 22%)
    Dermatologic: Acne (20% to 31%), rash (10% to 20%)
    Endocrine & metabolic: Hyperlipidemia (38% to 57%), hypercholesterolemia (38% to 46%), hypophosphatemia (15% to 23%), hypokalemia (11% to 21%)
    Gastrointestinal: Diarrhea (25% to 42%), constipation (28% to 38%), abdominal pain (28% to 36%), nausea (25% to 36%), vomiting (19% to 25%), dyspepsia (17% to 25%), weight gain (8% to 21%)
    Genitourinary: Urinary tract infection (20% to 33%)
    Hematologic: Anemia (23% to 37%), thrombocytopenia (13% to 30%)
(Continued)

Sirolimus *(Continued)*

Neuromuscular & skeletal: Weakness (22% to 40%), arthralgia (25% to 31%), tremor (21% to 31%), back pain (16% to 26%)

Renal: Serum creatinine increased (35% to 40%)

Respiratory: Dyspnea (22% to 30%), upper respiratory infection (20% to 26%), pharyngitis (16% to 21%)

3% to 20%:

Cardiovascular: Atrial fibrillation, CHF, facial edema, hypervolemia, hypotension, palpitation, peripheral vascular disorder, postural hypotension, syncope, tachycardia, thrombosis, vasodilation, venous thromboembolism

Central nervous system: Chills, malaise, anxiety, confusion, depression, dizziness, emotional lability, hypoesthesia, hypotonia, neuropathy, somnolence

Dermatologic: Dermatitis (fungal), hirsutism, pruritus, skin hypertrophy, dermal ulcer, ecchymosis, cellulitis, skin carcinoma (up to 3%)

Endocrine & metabolic: Cushing's syndrome, diabetes mellitus, glycosuria, acidosis, dehydration, hypercalcemia, hyperglycemia, hyperphosphatemia, hypocalcemia, hypoglycemia, hypomagnesemia, hyponatremia, hyperkalemia (12% to 17%)

Gastrointestinal: Enlarged abdomen, anorexia, dysphagia, eructation, esophagitis, flatulence, gastritis, gastroenteritis, gingivitis, gingival hyperplasia, ileus, mouth ulceration, oral moniliasis, stomatitis, weight loss

Genitourinary: Pelvic pain, scrotal edema, testis disorder, impotence

Hematologic: Leukocytosis, polycythemia, TTP, hemolytic-uremic syndrome, hemorrhage, leukopenia (9% to 15%)

Hepatic: Abnormal liver function tests, alkaline phosphatase increased, ascites, LDH increased, transaminases increased

Local: Thrombophlebitis

Neuromuscular & skeletal: Arthrosis, bone necrosis, CPK increased, leg cramps, myalgia, osteoporosis, tetany, hypertonia, paresthesia

Ocular: Abnormal vision, cataract, conjunctivitis

Otic: Ear pain, deafness, otitis media, tinnitus

Renal: Albuminuria, bladder pain, BUN increased, dysuria, hematuria, hydronephrosis, kidney pain, tubular necrosis, nocturia, oliguria, pyelonephritis, pyuria, nephropathy (toxic), urinary frequency, urinary incontinence, urinary retention

Respiratory: Asthma, atelectasis, bronchitis, cough, epistaxis, hypoxia, lung edema, pleural effusion, pneumonia, rhinitis, sinusitis

Miscellaneous: Abscess, diaphoresis, flu-like syndrome, herpesvirus infection, hernia, infection, lymphadenopathy, lymphoma (1% to 3%), lymphocele, lymphoproliferative disease, peritonitis, sepsis

Dosage Oral:

Combination therapy with cyclosporine: Doses should be taken 4 hours after cyclosporine, and should be taken consistently either with or without food.

Low- to moderate-risk renal transplant patients: Children ≥13 years and Adults: Dosing by body weight:

<40 kg: Loading dose: Loading dose: 3 mg/m^2 on day 1, followed by maintenance dosing of 1 mg/m^2 once daily

≥40 kg: Loading dose: 6 mg on day 1; maintenance: 2 mg once daily

High-risk renal transplant patients: Adults: Loading dose: Up to 15 mg on day 1; maintenance: 5 mg/day; obtain trough concentration between days 5-7. Continue concurrent cyclosporine/sirolimus therapy for 1 year following transplantation. Further adjustment of the regimen must be based on clinical status.

Dosage adjustment: Sirolimus dosages should be adjusted to maintain trough concentrations within desired range based on risk and concomitant therapy. Maximum daily dose: 40 mg. Dosage should be adjusted at intervals of 7-14 days to account for the long half-life of sirolimus. In general, dose proportionality may be assumed. New sirolimus dose **equals** current dose **multiplied by** (target concentration/current concentration). **Note:** If large dose increase is required, consider loading dose calculated as:

Loading dose **equals** (new maintenance dose **minus** current maintenance dose) **multiplied by** 3

Doses >40 mg (with inclusion of loading dose) may be administered over 2 days. Serum concentrations should not be used as the sole basis for dosage adjustment (monitor clinical signs/symptoms, tissue biopsy, and laboratory parameters).

Maintenance therapy after withdrawal of cyclosporine: Cyclosporine withdrawal is not recommended in high immunological risk patients. Following 2-4 months of combined therapy, withdrawal of cyclosporine may be considered in low-to-moderate risk patients. Cyclosporine should be discontinued over

4-8 weeks, and a necessary increase in the dosage of sirolimus (up to four-fold) should be anticipated due to removal of metabolic inhibition by cyclosporine and to maintain adequate immunosuppressive effects. Dose-adjusted trough target concentrations are typically 16-24 ng/mL for the first year post-transplant and 12-20 ng/mL thereafter (measured by chromatographic methodology).

Dosage adjustment in renal impairment: No dosage adjustment is necessary in renal impairment. However, adjustment of regimen (including discontinuation of therapy) should be considered when used concurrently with cyclosporine and elevated or increasing serum creatinine is noted.

Dosage adjustment in hepatic impairment: Reduce maintenance dose by approximately 33% in hepatic impairment. Loading dose is unchanged.

Mechanism of Action Sirolimus inhibits T-lymphocyte activation and proliferation via mTOR in response to antigenic and cytokine stimulation and inhibits antibody production. Its mechanism differs from other immunosuppressants. It inhibits acute rejection of allografts and prolongs graft survival.

Contraindications Hypersensitivity to sirolimus or any component of the formulation

Warnings/Precautions [U.S. Boxed Warning]: Immunosuppressive agents, including sirolimus, increase the risk of infection and may be associated with the development of lymphoma. Immune suppression may also increase the risk of opportunistic infections and sepsis. Prophylactic treatment for *Pneumocystis jirovec* pneumonia (PCP) should be administered for 1 year post-transplant; prophylaxis for cytomegalovirus (CMV) should be taken for 3 months in patients at risk for CMV.

In renal transplant patients, *de novo* use without cyclosporine has been associated with higher rates of acute rejection. May increase serum lipids (cholesterol and triglycerides). Use with caution in patients with hyperlipidemia. May increase serum creatinine and decrease GFR. Use caution in patients with renal impairment, or when used concurrently with medications which may alter renal function. Monitor renal function closely when combined with cyclosporine; consider dosage adjustment or discontinue in patients with increasing serum creatinine.

Use caution with hepatic impairment; reduced dosage is recommended. Has been associated with an increased risk of lymphocele. Cases of interstitial lung disease (eg, pneumonitis, bronchiolitis obliterans organizing pneumonia, pulmonary fibrosis) have been observed; risk may be increased with higher trough levels. Avoid concurrent use of strong CYP3A4 inhibitors or strong inducers of either CYP3A4 or P-glycoprotein. Concurrent use with a calcineurin inhibitor (cyclosporine, tacrolimus) may increase the risk of calcineurin inhibitor-induced hemolytic uremic syndrome/thrombotic thrombocytopenic purpura/thrombotic microangiopathy (HUS/TTP/TMA). Anaphylactic reactions, angioedema and hypersensitivity vasculitis have been reported. Concurrent use with other drugs known to cause angioedema (eg, ACE inhibitors) may increase risk. May increase sensitivity to UV light; use appropriate sun protection.

Sirolimus is not recommended for use in liver transplant patients; studies indicate an association with an increase risk of hepatic artery thrombosis and graft failure in these patients. Cases of bronchial anastomotic dehiscence have been reported in lung transplant patients when sirolimus was used as part of an immunosuppressive regimen; most of these reactions were fatal. Use in patients with lung transplants is not recommended. Safety and efficacy of cyclosporine withdrawal in high-risk patients has not been established and is not currently recommended. Safety and efficacy in children <13 years of age, or in adolescent patients <18 years of age considered at high immunological risk, have not been established.

Drug Interactions

Cytochrome P450 Effect: Substrate of CYP3A4 (major); **Inhibits** CYP3A4 (weak)

Increased Effect/Toxicity: Cyclosporine increases sirolimus concentrations during concurrent therapy, and cyclosporine levels may be increased; sirolimus should be taken 4 hours after cyclosporine oral solution (modified) and/or cyclosporine capsules (modified). CYP3A4 inhibitors may increase the levels/effects of sirolimus; example inhibitors include azole antifungals, clarithromycin, diclofenac, diltiazem, doxycycline, erythromycin, imatinib, isoniazid, nefazodone, nicardipine, propofol, protease inhibitors, quinidine, telithromycin, and verapamil; avoid concurrent use. Concurrent use of ACE inhibitors may increase the risk of angioedema. Concurrent live organism vaccines may increase the adverse/toxic effect of the vaccine; vaccinial infections are possible (avoid concurrent use). Concurrent therapy with calcineurin inhibitors (cyclosporine, tacrolimus) may increase the risk of HUS/TTP/TMA.

Decreased Effect: CYP3A4 inducers may decrease the levels/effects of sirolimus; example inducers include aminoglutethimide, carbamazepine, (Continued)

Sirolimus *(Continued)*

nafcillin, nevirapine, phenobarbital, phenytoin, and rifamycins. Vaccination (dead organisms) may be less effective with concurrent sirolimus (monitor).

Ethanol/Nutrition/Herb Interactions

Food: Do not administer with grapefruit juice; may decrease clearance of sirolimus. Ingestion with high-fat meals decreases peak concentrations but increases AUC by 35%. Sirolimus should be taken consistently either with or without food to minimize variability.

Herb/Nutraceutical: St John's wort may decrease sirolimus levels; avoid concurrent use. Avoid cat's claw, echinacea (have immunostimulant properties; consider therapy modifications). Herbs with hypoglycemic properties may increase the risk of sirolimus-induced hypoglycemia; includes alfalfa, aloe, bilberry, bitter melon, burdock, celery, damiana, fenugreek, garcinia, garlic, ginger, ginseng (American), gymnema, marshmallow, stinging nettle.

Dietary Considerations Take consistently, with or without food, to minimize variability of absorption.

Pharmacodynamics/Kinetics

Absorption: Rapid

Distribution: 12 L/kg (range: 4-20 L/kg)

Protein binding: 92%, primarily to albumin

Metabolism: Extensively hepatic via CYP3A4; to 7 major metabolites

Bioavailability: Oral solution: 14%; Oral tablet: 18%

Half-life elimination: Mean: 62 hours (range: 46-78 hours); extended in hepatic impairment (Child-Pugh class A or B) to 113 hours

Time to peak: 1-2 hours

Excretion: Feces (91% due to P-glycoprotein-mediated efflux into gut lumen); urine (2%)

Pregnancy Risk Factor C

Dosage Forms

Solution, oral [bottle]:

Rapamune®: 1 mg/mL

Tablet:

Rapamune®: 1 mg, 2 mg

Sitagliptin *(sit a GLIP tin)*

U.S. Brand Names Januvia™

Generic Available No

Index Terms MK-0431; Sitagliptin Phosphate

Pharmacologic Category Antidiabetic Agent, Dipeptidyl Peptidase IV (DPP-IV) Inhibitor

Use Management of type 2 diabetes mellitus (noninsulin dependent, NIDDM) as an adjunct to diet and exercise as monotherapy or in combination therapy with metformin or a peroxisome proliferator-actived receptor (PPAR) gamma agonist (eg, a thiazolidinedione)

Local Anesthetic/Vasoconstrictor Precautions No information available to require special precautions

Effects on Dental Treatment Sitagliptin-dependent diabetics should be appointed for dental treatment in morning in order to minimize chance of stress-induced hypoglycemia.

Common Adverse Effects

1% to 10%:

Central nervous system: Headache (5%)

Gastrointestinal: Diarrhea (3%)

Respiratory: Upper respiratory tract infection (6%), nasopharyngitis (5%)

Incidence less than or equal to placebo: Abdominal pain (2%), hypoglycemia (1%), nausea (1%), neutrophils increased, serum creatinine increased

Dosage Oral: Adults: Type 2 diabetes: 100 mg once daily

Dosage adjustment in renal impairment:

Cl_{cr} ≥30 to <50 mL/minute: 50 mg once daily

S_{cr}: Males: >1.7 to ≤3.0 mg/dL; Females: >1.5 to ≤2.5 mg/dL: 50 mg once daily

Cl_{cr}<30 mL/minute: 25 mg once daily

S_{cr}: Males: >3.0 mg/dL; Females: >2.5 mg/dL: 25 mg once daily

ESRD requiring hemodialysis or peritoneal dialysis: 25 mg once daily; administered without regard to timing of hemodialysis

Dosage adjustment in hepatic impairment:

Mild-to-moderate impairment (Child-Pugh score 7-9): No dosage adjustment required

Severe impairment (Child-Pugh score >9): Not studied

Mechanism of Action Sitagliptin inhibits dipeptidyl peptidase IV (DPP-IV) enzyme resulting in prolonged active incretin levels. Incretin hormones [eg, glucagon-like peptide-1 (GLP-1) and glucose-dependent insulinotropic polypeptide (GIP)] regulate glucose homeostasis by increasing insulin synthesis and release from pancreatic beta cells and decreasing glucagon secretion from pancreatic alpha cells. Decreased glucagon secretion results in decreased hepatic glucose production. Under normal physiologic circumstances, incretin hormones are released by the intestine throughout the day and levels are increased in response to a meal; incretin hormones are rapidly inactivated by the DPP-IV enzyme.

Contraindications Hypersensitivity to sitagliptin or any component of the formulation; type 1 diabetes mellitus (insulin dependent, IDDM), diabetic ketoacidosis

Warnings/Precautions Use with caution in patients with moderate-to-severe renal dysfunction and end-stage renal disease (ESRD) requiring hemodialysis or peritoneal dialysis; dosing adjustment required. Safety and efficacy have not been established in children <18 years of age.

Drug Interactions
Cytochrome P450 Effect: Substrate (minor) of CYP2C8, 3A4

Pharmacodynamics/Kinetics
Absorption: Rapid
Distribution: 198 L
Protein binding: 38%
Metabolism: Not extensively metabolized; minor metabolism via CYP3A4 and 2C8 to metabolites (inactive) suggested by *in vitro* studies
Bioavailability: 87%
Half-life elimination: 12 hours
Time to peak, plasma: 1-4 hours
Excretion: Urine 87% (79% as unchanged drug, 16% as metabolites); feces 13%

Pregnancy Risk Factor B
Dosage Forms
Tablet:
Januvia™: 25 mg, 50 mg, 100 mg

Sitagliptin and Metformin (sit a GLIP tin & met FOR min)

U.S. Brand Names Janumet™
Generic Available No
Index Terms Metformin and Sitagliptin; Sitagliptin Phosphate and Metformin Hydrochloride
Pharmacologic Category Antidiabetic Agent, Biguanide; Antidiabetic Agent, Dipeptidyl Peptidase IV (DPP-IV) Inhibitor; Hypoglycemic Agent, Oral
Use Management of type 2 diabetes mellitus (noninsulin dependent, NIDDM) as an adjunct to diet and exercise
Local Anesthetic/Vasoconstrictor Precautions No information available to require special precautions
Effects on Dental Treatment Sitagliptin and metformin-dependent diabetics (noninsulin dependent, Type 2) should be appointed for dental treatment in morning in order to minimize chance of stress-induced hypoglycemia.
Common Adverse Effects See individual agents.
Mechanism of Action Sitagliptin inhibits dipeptidyl peptidase IV (DPP-IV) enzymes resulting in prolonged active incretin levels. Incretin hormones [eg, glucagon-like peptide-1 (GLP-1) and glucose-dependent insulinotropic polypeptide (GIP)] regulate glucose homeostasis by increasing insulin synthesis and release from pancreatic beta cells and decreasing glucagon secretion from pancreatic alpha cells. Decreased glucagon secretion results in decreased hepatic glucose production. Under normal physiologic circumstances, incretin hormones are released by the intestine throughout the day and levels are increased in response to a meal; incretin hormones are rapidly inactivated by DPP-IV enzymes.
Metformin decreases hepatic glucose production, decreasing intestinal absorption of glucose, and improves insulin sensitivity (increases peripheral glucose uptake and utilization).
Pharmacodynamics/Kinetics See individual agents.
Pregnancy Risk Factor B

SODIUM BICARBONATE

Sodium Bicarbonate (SOW dee um bye KAR bun ate)

U.S. Brand Names Brioschi® [OTC]; Neut®
Mexican Brand Names Betsol "Z"
Generic Available Yes
Index Terms Baking Soda; $NaHCO_3$; Sodium Acid Carbonate; Sodium Hydrogen Carbonate
Pharmacologic Category Alkalinizing Agent; Antacid; Electrolyte Supplement, Oral; Electrolyte Supplement, Parenteral
Use Management of metabolic acidosis; gastric hyperacidity; as an alkalinization agent for the urine; treatment of hyperkalemia; management of overdose of certain drugs, including tricyclic antidepressants and aspirin
Local Anesthetic/Vasoconstrictor Precautions No information available to require special precautions
Effects on Dental Treatment No significant effects or complications reported
Common Adverse Effects Frequency not defined.
Cardiovascular: Cerebral hemorrhage, CHF (aggravated), edema
Central nervous system: Tetany
Gastrointestinal: Belching, flatulence (with oral), gastric distension
Endocrine & metabolic: Hypernatremia, hyperosmolality, hypocalcemia, hypokalemia, increased affinity of hemoglobin for oxygen-reduced pH in myocardial tissue necrosis when extravasated, intracranial acidosis, metabolic alkalosis, milk-alkali syndrome (especially with renal dysfunction)
Respiratory: Pulmonary edema
Mechanism of Action Dissociates to provide bicarbonate ion which neutralizes hydrogen ion concentration and raises blood and urinary pH
Drug Interactions
Increased Effect/Toxicity: Increased toxicity/levels of amphetamines, ephedrine, pseudoephedrine, flecainide, quinidine, and quinine due to urinary alkalinization.
Decreased Effect: Decreased effect/levels of lithium, chlorpropamide, and salicylates due to urinary alkalinization.
Pharmacodynamics/Kinetics
Onset of action: Oral: Rapid; I.V.: 15 minutes
Duration: Oral: 8-10 minutes; I.V.: 1-2 hours
Absorption: Oral: Well absorbed
Excretion: Urine (<1%)
Pregnancy Risk Factor C

Sodium Chloride (SOW dee um KLOR ide)

U.S. Brand Names Altachlore [OTC]; Altamist [OTC]; Ayr® Baby Saline [OTC]; Ayr® Saline [OTC]; Ayr® Saline No-Drip [OTC]; Breathe Right® Saline [OTC]; Broncho Saline® [OTC] [DSC]; Deep Sea [OTC]; Entsol® [OTC]; Muro 128® [OTC]; Mycinaire™ [OTC]; NaSal™ [OTC]; Nasal Moist® [OTC]; Na-Zone® [OTC]; Ocean® [OTC]; Oceant® for Kids [OTC]; Pretz® [OTC]; SalineX® [OTC]; Simply Saline® [OTC]; Simply Saline® Baby [OTC]; Simply Saline® Nasal Moist®

[OTC]; Syrex; 4-Way® Saline Moisturizing Mist [OTC]; Wound Wash Saline™ [OTC]

Generic Available Yes

Index Terms NaCl; Normal Saline; Salt

Pharmacologic Category Electrolyte Supplement, Parenteral; Genitourinary Irrigant; Irrigant; Lubricant, Ocular; Sodium Salt

Use

Parenteral: Restores sodium ion in patients with restricted oral intake (especially hyponatremia states or low salt syndrome). In general, parenteral saline uses:

Bacteriostatic sodium chloride: Dilution or dissolving drugs for I.M., I.V., or SubQ injections

Concentrated sodium chloride: Additive for parenteral fluid therapy

Hypertonic sodium chloride: For severe hyponatremia and hypochloremia

Hypotonic sodium chloride: Hydrating solution

Normal saline: Restores water/sodium losses

Pharmaceutical aid/diluent for infusion of compatible drug additives

Ophthalmic: Reduces corneal edema

Inhalation: Restores moisture to pulmonary system; loosens and thins congestion caused by colds or allergies; diluent for bronchodilator solutions that require dilution before inhalation

Intranasal: Restores moisture to nasal membranes

Irrigation: Wound cleansing, irrigation, and flushing

Unlabeled/Investigational Use Traumatic brain injury (hypertonic sodium chloride)

Local Anesthetic/Vasoconstrictor Precautions No information available to require special precautions

Effects on Dental Treatment No significant effects or complications reported

Common Adverse Effects Frequency not defined.

Cardiovascular: Congestive conditions

Endocrine & metabolic: Extravasation, hypervolemia, hypernatremia, dilution of serum electrolytes, overhydration, hypokalemia

Local: Thrombosis, phlebitis, extravasation

Respiratory: Pulmonary edema

Mechanism of Action Principal extracellular cation; functions in fluid and electrolyte balance, osmotic pressure control, and water distribution

Drug Interactions

Decreased Effect: Lithium levels/effects may be decreased.

Pharmacodynamics/Kinetics

Absorption: Oral, I.V.: Rapid

Distribution: Widely distributed

Excretion: Primarily urine; also sweat, tears, saliva

Pregnancy Risk Factor C

Sodium Chondroitin Sulfate and Sodium Hyaluronate *see* Chondroitin Sulfate and Sodium Hyaluronate *on page 351*

Sodium Citrate and Citric Acid
(SOW dee um SIT rate & SI trik AS id)

U.S. Brand Names Bicitra®; Cytra-2; Oracit®

Canadian Brand Names PMS-Dicitrate

Generic Available Yes

Index Terms Modified Shohl's Solution

Pharmacologic Category Alkalinizing Agent, Oral

Use Treatment of metabolic acidosis; alkalinizing agent in conditions where long-term maintenance of an alkaline urine is desirable

Local Anesthetic/Vasoconstrictor Precautions No information available to require special precautions

Effects on Dental Treatment No significant effects or complications reported

Common Adverse Effects Frequency not defined. Generally well tolerated with normal renal function.

Central nervous system: Tetany

Endocrine & metabolic: Metabolic alkalosis, hyperkalemia

Gastrointestinal: Diarrhea, nausea, vomiting

Drug Interactions

Increased Effect/Toxicity: Increased toxicity/levels of amphetamines, ephedrine, pseudoephedrine, flecainide, quinidine, and quinine due to urinary alkalinization.

Decreased Effect: Decreased effect/levels of lithium, chlorpropamide, and salicylates due to urinary alkalinization.

(Continued)

Sodium Citrate and Citric Acid *(Continued)*

Pharmacodynamics/Kinetics
Metabolism: Oxidized to sodium bicarbonate
Excretion: Urine (<5% as sodium citrate)

Pregnancy Risk Factor Not established

Sodium Citrate, Citric Acid, and Potassium Citrate *see* Citric Acid, Sodium Citrate, and Potassium Citrate *on page 370*

Sodium Edetate *see* Edetate Disodium *on page 555*

Sodium Etidronate *see* Etidronate Disodium *on page 654*

Sodium Ferric Gluconate *see* Ferric Gluconate *on page 686*

Sodium Fluoride *see* Fluoride *on page 710*

Sodium Hyaluronate *see* Hyaluronate and Derivatives *on page 816*

Sodium Hyaluronate and Chondroitin Sulfate *see* Chondroitin Sulfate and Sodium Hyaluronate *on page 351*

Sodium Hydrogen Carbonate *see* Sodium Bicarbonate *on page 1480*

Sodium Hypochlorite Solution
(SOW dee um hye poe KLOR ite soe LOO shun)

U.S. Brand Names Dakin's Solution; Di-Dak-Sol
Generic Available No
Index Terms Modified Dakin's Solution
Pharmacologic Category Disinfectant, Antibacterial (Topical)
Use Treatment of athlete's foot (0.5%); wound irrigation (0.5%); disinfection of utensils and equipment (5%)
Local Anesthetic/Vasoconstrictor Precautions No information available to require special precautions
Effects on Dental Treatment No significant effects or complications reported
Common Adverse Effects Frequency not defined.
Dermatologic: Irritating to skin
Hematologic: Dissolves blood clots, delays clotting
Pregnancy Risk Factor C

Sodium Hyposulfate *see* Sodium Thiosulfate *on page 1484*

Sodium Nafcillin *see* Nafcillin *on page 1141*

Sodium Nitroferricyanide *see* Nitroprusside *on page 1183*

Sodium Nitroprusside *see* Nitroprusside *on page 1183*

Sodium Oxybate (SOW dee um ox i BATE)

U.S. Brand Names Xyrem®
Canadian Brand Names Xyrem®
Generic Available No
Index Terms Gamma Hydroxybutyric Acid; GHB; 4-Hydroxybutyrate; Sodium 4-Hydroxybutyrate
Pharmacologic Category Central Nervous System Depressant
Use Treatment of cataplexy and daytime sleepiness in patients with narcolepsy
Local Anesthetic/Vasoconstrictor Precautions No information available to require special precautions
Effects on Dental Treatment Key adverse event(s) related to dental treatment: Tooth ache (see Dental Comment).
Common Adverse Effects
>10%:
Central nervous system: Dizziness (8% to 37%), headache (9% to 37%), pain (9% to 20%), somnolence (1% to 14%), confusion (3% to 17%), sleep disorder (6% to 14%)
Gastrointestinal: Nausea (8% to 40%), vomiting (2% to 23%), abdominal pain (3% to 11%)
Genitourinary: Urinary incontinence (<1% to 14%, usually nocturnal), enuresis (3% to 17%), cystitis, metrorrhagia, urinary frequency
Miscellaneous: Diaphoresis (3% to 11%)
1% to 10%:
Cardiovascular: Hypertension (6%), chest pain, edema
Central nervous system: Disorientation (up to 9%), inebriation (up to 9%), concentration decreased (3% to 9%), dream abnormality (3% to 9%), sleepwalking (4% to 7%), depression (3% to 6%), amnesia (3% to 6%), anxiety (3% to 6%), thinking abnormality (3% to 6%), lethargy (up to 6%), insomnia (5%), agitation, ataxia, chills, fatigue, malaise, memory impairment, nervousness, pyrexia, seizure, stupor, tremor, vertigo
Dermatologic: Hyperhidrosis (3% to 6%), pruritus, rash

Endocrine & metabolic: Dysmenorrhea (3% to 6%)

Gastrointestinal: Dyspepsia (6% to 9%), diarrhea (6%·to 8%), abdominal pain (6%), nausea and vomiting (6%), anorexia, constipation, tooth ache, weight gain

Hepatic: Alkaline phosphatase increased, hypercholesteremia, hypocalcemia

Neuromuscular & skeletal: Hypoesthesia (6%), weakness (6% to 8%), myasthenia (3% to 6%), pain (3% to 6%), arthritis, leg cramps, myalgia

Ocular: Amblyopia (6%), blurred vision (6%)

Otic: Tinnitus (6%), ear pain

Renal: Albuminuria, hematuria

Respiratory: Pharyngitis (6% to 8%), rhinitis (8%), nasopharyngitis (3% to 8%), infection (3% to 6%), bronchitis, cough, dyspnea

Miscellaneous: Infection (3% to 6%), viral infection (3% to 9%), allergic reaction, flu-like syndrome

Restrictions C-I (illicit use); C-III (medical use)

Sodium oxybate oral solution will be available only to prescribers enrolled in the Xyrem® Patient Success Program® and dispensed to the patient through the designated centralized pharmacy (1-866-997-3688). Prior to dispensing the first prescription, prescribers will be sent educational materials to be reviewed with the patient and enrollment forms for the postmarketing surveillance program. Patients must be seen at least every 3 months; prescriptions can be written for a maximum of 3 months (the first prescription may only be written for a 1-month supply).

An FDA-approved medication guide must be distributed when dispensing an outpatient prescription (new or refill) where this medication is to be used without direct supervision of a healthcare provider. Medication guides are available at http://www.fda.gov/cder/Offices/ODS/medication_guides.htm.

Mechanism of Action Sodium oxybate is derived from gamma aminobutyric acid (GABA) and acts as an inhibitory chemical transmitter in the brain. May function through specific receptors for gamma hydroxybutyrate (GHB) and GABA (B).

Drug Interactions

Increased Effect/Toxicity: CNS depressants: CNS depressant effects are potentiated; concomitant use with sodium oxybate is contraindicated.

Pharmacodynamics/Kinetics

Absorption: Rapid

Distribution: 190-384 mL/kg

Protein binding: <1%

Metabolism: Primarily via the Krebs cycle to form water and carbon dioxide; secondarily via beta oxidation; significant first-pass effect; no active metabolites; metabolic pathways are saturable

Bioavailability: 25%

Half-life elimination: 30-60 minutes

Time to peak: 30-75 minutes

Excretion: Primarily pulmonary (as carbon dioxide); urine (<5% unchanged drug)

Pregnancy Risk Factor B

Dental Comment Sodium oxybate is a known substance of abuse. When used illegally, it has been referred to as a "date-rape drug". The dentist should be aware of patients showing signs of CNS depression, as with all other drugs in this class.

Sodium PAS see Aminosalicylic Acid on page 91

Sodium-PCA and Lactic Acid see Lactic Acid on page 941

Sodium Phenylbutyrate (SOW dee um fen il BYOO ti rate)

U.S. Brand Names Buphenyl®

Generic Available No

Index Terms Ammonapse

Pharmacologic Category Urea Cycle Disorder (UCD) Treatment Agent

Use Orphan drug: Adjunctive therapy in the chronic management of patients with urea cycle disorder involving deficiencies of carbamoylphosphate synthetase, ornithine transcarbamylase, or argininosuccinic acid synthetase

Local Anesthetic/Vasoconstrictor Precautions No information available to require special precautions

Effects on Dental Treatment Key adverse event(s) related to dental treatment: Abnormal taste.

Common Adverse Effects

>10%: Endocrine & metabolic: Amenorrhea, menstrual dysfunction

1% to 10%:

Gastrointestinal: Anorexia, abnormal taste

(Continued)

Sodium Phenylbutyrate *(Continued)*

Miscellaneous: Offensive body odor

Mechanism of Action Sodium phenylbutyrate is a prodrug that, when given orally, is rapidly converted to phenylacetate, which is in turn conjugated with glutamine to form the active compound phenylacetylglutamine; phenylacetylglutamine serves as a substitute for urea and is excreted in the urine whereby it carries with it 2 moles of nitrogen per mole of phenylacetylglutamine and can thereby assist in the clearance of nitrogenous waste in patients with urea cycle disorders

Pregnancy Risk Factor C

Sodium Phosphate and Potassium Phosphate *see* Potassium Phosphate and Sodium Phosphate *on page 1332*

Sodium Phosphates (SOW dee um FOS fates)

U.S. Brand Names Fleet® Accu-Prep® [OTC]; Fleet® Enema [OTC]; Fleet® Phospho-Soda® [OTC]; OsmoPrep™; Visicol®
Canadian Brand Names Fleet Enema®; Fleet® Phospho-Soda® Oral Laxative
Generic Available Yes: Enema, injection
Pharmacologic Category Cathartic; Electrolyte Supplement, Oral; Electrolyte Supplement, Parenteral; Laxative, Bowel Evacuant
Use
Oral, rectal: Short-term treatment of constipation and to evacuate the colon for rectal and bowel exams
I.V.: Source of phosphate in large volume I.V. fluids and parenteral nutrition; treatment and prevention of hypophosphatemia
Local Anesthetic/Vasoconstrictor Precautions No information available to require special precautions
Effects on Dental Treatment No significant effects or complications reported
Mechanism of Action As a laxative, exerts osmotic effect in the small intestine by drawing water into the lumen of the gut, producing distention and promoting peristalsis and evacuation of the bowel; phosphorous participates in bone deposition, calcium metabolism, utilization of B complex vitamins, and as a buffer in acid-base equilibrium
Pregnancy Risk Factor C

Sodium Sulfacetamide *see* Sulfacetamide *on page 1502*

Sodium Tetradecyl (SOW dee um tetra DEK il)

U.S. Brand Names Sotradecol®
Canadian Brand Names Trombovar®
Generic Available No
Index Terms Sodium Tetradecyl Sulfate
Pharmacologic Category Sclerosing Agent
Use Treatment of small, uncomplicated varicose veins of the lower extremities
Local Anesthetic/Vasoconstrictor Precautions No information available to require special precautions
Effects on Dental Treatment No significant effects or complications reported
Common Adverse Effects Frequency not defined.
Central nervous system: Headache
Dermatologic: Discoloration at site of injection, sloughing and tissue necrosis following extravasation
Gastrointestinal: Nausea, vomiting
Local: Pain, itching, or ulceration at injection site
Miscellaneous: Allergic reaction (including hives, asthma, hay fever); anaphylactic shock
Mechanism of Action Acts by irritation of the vein intimal endothelium and causes thrombosis formation leading to occlusion of the injected vein
Pregnancy Risk Factor C

Sodium Tetradecyl Sulfate *see* Sodium Tetradecyl *on page 1484*

Sodium Thiosulfate (SOW dee um thye oh SUL fate)

U.S. Brand Names Versiclear™
Generic Available Yes: Injection
Index Terms Disodium Thiosulfate Pentahydrate; Pentahydrate; Sodium Hyposulfate; Sodium Thiosulphate; Thiosulfuric Acid Disodium Salt

Pharmacologic Category Antidote
Use
Parenteral: Used alone or with sodium nitrite or amyl nitrite in cyanide poisoning; reduce the risk of nephrotoxicity associated with cisplatin therapy
Topical: Treatment of tinea versicolor
Unlabeled/Investigational Use Management of I.V. extravasation
Local Anesthetic/Vasoconstrictor Precautions No information available to require special precautions
Effects on Dental Treatment No significant effects or complications reported
Common Adverse Effects 1% to 10%:
Cardiovascular: Hypotension
Central nervous system: Coma, CNS depression secondary to thiocyanate intoxication, psychosis, confusion
Dermatologic: Contact dermatitis, local irritation
Neuromuscular & skeletal: Weakness
Otic: Tinnitus
Mechanism of Action
Cyanide toxicity: Increases the rate of detoxification of cyanide by the enzyme rhodanese by providing an extra sulfur
Cisplatin toxicity: Complexes with cisplatin to form a compound that is nontoxic to either normal or cancerous cells
Pharmacodynamics/Kinetics
Absorption: Oral: Poor
Distribution: Extracellular fluid
Half-life elimination: 0.65 hour
Excretion: Urine (28.5% as unchanged drug)
Pregnancy Risk Factor C

Solifenacin (sol i FEN a sin)

U.S. Brand Names VESIcare®
Generic Available No
Index Terms Solifenacin Succinate
Pharmacologic Category Anticholinergic Agent
Use Treatment of overactive bladder with symptoms of urinary frequency, urgency, or urge incontinence
Local Anesthetic/Vasoconstrictor Precautions No information available to require special precautions
Effects on Dental Treatment Key adverse event(s) related to dental treatment: Xerostomia (normal salivary flow resumes upon discontinuation). Prolonged xerostomia may contribute to discomfort and dental disease (eg, caries, periodontal disease, and oral candidiasis).
Common Adverse Effects Adverse reactions are dose related.
>10%: Gastrointestinal: Xerostomia (11% to 28%), constipation (5% to 13%)
1% to 10%:
Cardiovascular: Edema (up to 1%), hypertension (up to 1%)
Central nervous system: Dizziness (2%), fatigue (1% to 2%), depression (up to 1%)
Gastrointestinal: Nausea (2% to 3%), dyspepsia (1% to 4%), upper abdominal pain (1% to 2%), vomiting (up to 1%)
Genitourinary: Urinary tract infection (3% to 5%), urinary retention (up to 1%)
Ocular: Blurred vision (4% to 5%), dry eyes (up to 2%)
Respiratory: Cough (up to 1%), pharyngitis (up to 1%)
Miscellaneous: Influenza (1% to 2%)
Mechanism of Action Inhibits muscarinic receptors resulting in decreased urinary bladder contraction, increased residual urine volume, and decreased detrusor muscle pressure.
Drug Interactions
Cytochrome P450 Effect: Substrate of CYP3A4 (major)
Increased Effect/Toxicity: CYP3A4 inhibitors may increase the levels/effects of solifenacin; example inhibitors include azole antifungals, clarithromycin, diclofenac, doxycycline, erythromycin, ketoconazole, imatinib, isoniazid, nefazodone, nicardipine, propofol, protease inhibitors, quinidine, telithromycin, and verapamil; solifenacin dose should not exceed 5 mg/day.
(Continued)

Solifenacin *(Continued)*

Decreased Effect: CYP3A4 inducers may decrease the levels/effects of solifenacin; example inducers include aminoglutethimide, carbamazepine, nafcillin, nevirapine, phenobarbital, and phenytoin.

Pharmacodynamics/Kinetics

Distribution: V_d: 600 L

Protein binding: 98% bound to alpha$_1$-acid glycoprotein

Metabolism: Extensively hepatic; via N-oxidation and 4 R-hydroxylation, forms one active and three inactive metabolites; primary pathway for elimination is via CYP3A4 route

Bioavailability: 90%

Half-life elimination: 45-68 hours following chronic dosing

Time to peak, plasma: 3-8 hours

Excretion: Urine 69% (<15% as unchanged drug); feces 23%

Pregnancy Risk Factor C

Solifenacin Succinate *see Solifenacin on page 1485*

Soliris™ *see Eculizumab on page 554*

Solodyn™ *see Minocycline on page 1107*

Soltamox™ *see Tamoxifen on page 1522*

Solu-Cortef® *see Hydrocortisone on page 836*

Solu-Medrol® *see MethylPREDNISolone on page 1083*

Soluvite-F *see Vitamins (Fluoride) on page 1665*

Soma® *see Carisoprodol on page 285*

Soma® Compound *see Carisoprodol and Aspirin on page 286*

Soma® Compound w/Codeine *see Carisoprodol, Aspirin, and Codeine on page 287*

Somatrem *see Somatropin on page 1486*

Somatropin *(soe ma TROE pin)*

U.S. Brand Names Genotropin®; Genotropin Miniquick®; Humatrope®; Norditropin®; Norditropin® NordiFlex®; Nutropin®; Nutropin AQ®; Omnitrope™; Saizen®; Serostim®; Tev-Tropin®; Zorbtive®

Canadian Brand Names Humatrope®; Nutropin® AQ; Nutropine®; Saizen®; Serostim®

Mexican Brand Names Humatrope; Saizen; Serostim

Generic Available No

Index Terms hGH; Human Growth Hormone; Somatrem

Pharmacologic Category Growth Hormone

Use

Children:

Treatment of growth failure due to inadequate endogenous growth hormone secretion (Genotropin®, Humatrope®, Norditropin®, Nutropin®, Nutropin AQ®, Omnitrope™, Saizen®, Tev-Tropin®)

Treatment of short stature associated with Turner syndrome (Genotropin®, Humatrope®, Nutropin®, Nutropin AQ®)

Treatment of Prader-Willi syndrome (Genotropin®)

Treatment of growth failure associated with chronic renal insufficiency (CRI) up until the time of renal transplantation (Nutropin®, Nutropin AQ®)

Treatment of growth failure in children born small for gestational age who fail to manifest catch-up growth by 2 years of age (Genotropin®)

Treatment of idiopathic short stature (nongrowth hormone-deficient short stature) defined by height standard deviation score (SDS) less than or equal to -2.25 and growth rate not likely to attain normal adult height (Humatrope®, Nutropin®, Nutropin AQ®)

Treatment of short stature or growth failure associated with short stature homeobox gene (SHOX) deficiency (Humatrope®)

Adults:

HIV patients with wasting or cachexia with concomitant antiviral therapy (Serostim®)

Replacement of endogenous growth hormone in patients with adult growth hormone deficiency who meet both of the following criteria (Genotropin®, Humatrope®, Norditropin®, Nutropin®, Nutropin AQ®, Omnitrope™, Saizen®):

Biochemical diagnosis of adult growth hormone deficiency by means of a subnormal response to a standard growth hormone stimulation test (peak growth hormone ≤5 mcg/L). Confirmatory testing may not be required in patients with congenital/genetic growth hormone deficiency or multiple pituitary hormone deficiencies due to organic diseases.

and

Adult-onset: Patients who have adult growth hormone deficiency whether alone or with multiple hormone deficiencies (hypopituitarism) as a result of pituitary disease, hypothalamic disease, surgery, radiation therapy, or trauma

or

Childhood-onset: Patients who were growth hormone deficient during childhood, confirmed as an adult before replacement therapy is initiated

Treatment of short-bowel syndrome (Zorbtive®)

Unlabeled/Investigational Use Investigational: Congestive heart failure; pediatric HIV patients with wasting/cachexia (Serostim®)

Local Anesthetic/Vasoconstrictor Precautions No information available to require special precautions

Effects on Dental Treatment No significant effects or complications reported

Common Adverse Effects

Growth hormone deficiency: Adverse reactions reported with growth hormone deficiency vary greatly by age. Generally, percentages are less in pediatric patients than adults, and many of the reactions reported in adults are dose related. Percentages reported also vary by product. Below is a listing by age group; events reported more commonly overall are noted with an asterisk (*).

Children: Antibodies development, arthralgia, edema, eosinophilia, glycosuria, Hb A_{1c} increased, headache, hematoma, hematuria, hyperglycemia (mild), hypertriglyceridemia, hypoglycemia, hypothyroidism, injection site reaction, leg pain, lipoatrophy, muscle pain, rash, weakness

Adults: Arthralgia*, bronchitis, carpal tunnel syndrome, chest pain, depression, diaphoresis, dizziness, edema*, fatigue, flu-like syndrome*, glucose intolerance, glucosuria, headache*, hyperglycemia (mild), hypertension, hypoesthesia, hypothyroidism, infection, insomnia, leg edema, muscle pain, myalgia*, nausea, pain in extremities, paresthesia*, peripheral edema*, rhinitis, skeletal pain*, stiffness in extremities, upper respiratory tract infection, weakness

Additional/postmarketing reactions observed with growth hormone deficiency: Gynecomastia, increased growth of pre-existing nevi, pancreatitis

Idiopathic short stature: Percentages reported using Humatrope® versus placebo: Myalgia (24%), scoliosis (19%), otitis media (16%), arthralgia (11%), arthrosis (11%), hyperlipidemia (8%), gynecomastia (5%), hip pain (3%), hypertension (3%). Additional adverse reactions listed as reported using other products from ISS NCGS Cohort (frequencies <1%): Aggressiveness, benign intracranial hypertension, diabetes, edema, hair loss, headache, injection site reaction

Prader-Willi syndrome: Genotropin® (frequency not defined): Aggressiveness, arthralgia, edema, hair loss, headache, benign intracranial hypertension, myalgia; fatalities associated with use in this population have been reported

Turner syndrome: Percentages reported using Humatrope® compared to untreated patients. Additional adverse reactions reported from other products, frequency not specified: Surgical procedures (45%), otitis media (43%), ear disorders (18%), hypothyroidism (14%), nevi increased (11%), peripheral edema (7%), joint pain, respiratory illness, urinary tract infection

HIV patients with wasting or cachexia: Serostim® (limited to ≥5%): Musculoskeletal disorders (arthralgia, arthrosis, myalgia: 78%), peripheral edema (26%), headache (13%), nausea (9%), paresthesia (8%), edema (6%), gynecomastia (6%), hypoesthesia (5%)

Short-bowel syndrome: Zorbtive® (limited to >10%): Peripheral edema (69% to 81%), facial edema (44% to 50%), arthralgia (31% to 44%), nausea (13% to 31%), injection site pain (up to 31%), flatulence (25%), injection site reaction (19% to 25%), abdominal pain (13% to 25%), vomiting (19%), pain (6% to 19%), chest pain (up to 19%), dehydration (up to 19%), infection (up to 19%), rhinitis (up to 19%), hearing symptoms (13%), dizziness (6% to 13%), rash (6% to 13%), diaphoresis (up to 13%), generalized edema (up to 13%), malaise (up to 13%), moniliasis (up to 13%), myalgia (up to 13%)

SHOX deficiency: Humatrope®: Arthralgia (11%), gynecomastia (8%), excessive cutaneous nevi (7%), scoliosis (4%)

Small for gestational age: Genotropin® (frequency not defined): Mild, transient hyperglycemia; benign intracranial hypertension (rare); central precocious puberty; jaw prominence (rare); aggravation of pre-existing scoliosis (rare); injection site reactions; progression of pigmented nevi

Mechanism of Action Somatropin is a purified polypeptide hormones of recombinant DNA origin; somatropin contains the identical sequence of amino acids found in human growth hormone; human growth hormone stimulates growth of linear bone, skeletal muscle, and organs; stimulates erythropoietin which increases red blood cell mass; exerts both insulin-like and diabetogenic effects; enhances the transmucosal transport of water, electrolytes, and nutrients across the gut

(Continued)

Somatropin *(Continued)*

Drug Interactions
Increased Effect/Toxicity: Larger doses of somatropin may be needed for women taking oral estrogen replacement products; dosing not affected by topical products.

Decreased Effect: Glucocorticoid therapy may inhibit growth-promoting effects. Growth hormone may induce insulin resistance in patients with diabetes mellitus; monitor glucose and adjust insulin dose as necessary.

Pharmacodynamics/Kinetics
Duration: Maintains supraphysiologic levels for 18-20 hours
Absorption: I.M., SubQ: Well absorbed
Distribution: ~1 L/kg
Metabolism: Hepatic and renal (~90%)
Bioavailability: SubQ: ~70% to 90%
Half-life elimination: Preparation and route of administration dependent; SubQ: ~2-4 hours
Excretion: Urine

Pregnancy Risk Factor B/C (depending upon manufacturer)

Sominex® [OTC] *see* DiphenhydrAMINE *on page 510*
Sominex® Maximum Strength [OTC] *see* DiphenhydrAMINE *on page 510*
Somnote™ *see* Chloral Hydrate *on page 327*
Sonata® *see* Zaleplon *on page 1676*
Soothe® [OTC] *see* Artificial Tears *on page 147*

Sorafenib *(sor AF e nib)*

U.S. Brand Names Nexavar®
Generic Available No
Index Terms BAY 43-9006; NSC-724772; Sorafenib Tosylate
Pharmacologic Category Antineoplastic Agent, Tyrosine Kinase Inhibitor; Vascular Endothelial Growth Factor (VEGF) Inhibitor
Use Treatment of advanced renal cell cancer
Unlabeled/Investigational Use Treatment of hepatocellular, breast, colon, colorectal, nonsmall cell lung, ovarian, pancreatic and thyroid cancers; melanoma, sarcoma
Local Anesthetic/Vasoconstrictor Precautions Sorafenib may cause hypertension; monitor blood pressure prior to vasoconstrictor use
Effects on Dental Treatment Key adverse event(s) related to dental treatment: Mouth pain, mucositis, stomatitis, xerostomia (normal salivary flow resumes upon discontinuation), and dysphagia.
Common Adverse Effects Note: Dose-limiting toxicities (diarrhea, fatigue, and hand-foot syndrome) were reversible upon discontinuation; rash and hand-foot syndrome are dose related; percentages not always reported.
>10%:
Cardiovascular: Hypertension (17% to 60%; grade 3: 3% to 31%; grade 4: <1%; onset: ~3 weeks)
Central nervous system: Fatigue (32% to 33%; grade 3/4: 5% to <6%), sensory neuropathy (13%)
Dermatologic: Rash (38% to 40%), hand-foot syndrome (30% to 35%; grade 3: 6%), alopecia (27%), pruritus (19%), dry skin (11%), erythema &
Endocrine & metabolic: Hypophosphatemia (45%; grade 3: 13%)
Gastrointestinal: Diarrhea (37% to 43%; grade 3: 2%), lipase increased (41%), amylase increased (30%), nausea (23%), anorexia (16%), vomiting (16%), constipation (15%), abdominal pain (11%), mouth pain
Hematologic: Lymphopenia (23%; grades 3/4: 13%), neutropenia (<10% to 18%; grades 3/4: 5%), hemorrhage (15%; grade 3: 2%), thrombocytopenia (<10% to 12%; grades 3/4: 1%), leukopenia
Neuromuscular & skeletal: Bone pain, muscle pain, weakness
Respiratory: Dyspnea (14%), cough (13%)
1% to 10%:
Cardiovascular: Flushing
Central nervous system: Headache (10%), depression, fever
Dermatologic: Acne, exfoliative dermatitis
Gastrointestinal: Weight loss (10%), appetite decreased, dyspepsia, dysphagia, glossodynia, mucositis, stomatitis, xerostomia
Genitourinary: Erectile dysfunction
Hematologic: Anemia (8%; grades 3/4: 3%)
Hepatic: Transaminases increased
Neuromuscular & skeletal: Joint pain (10%), arthralgia, myalgia
Respiratory: Hoarseness
Miscellaneous: Influenza-like symptoms

Mechanism of Action Multikinase inhibitor; inhibits tumor growth and angiogenesis by inhibiting intracellular Raf kinases (CRAF, BRAF, and mutant BRAF), and cell surface kinase receptors (VEGFR-2, VEGFR-3, PDGFR-beta, cKIT, and FLT-3)

Drug Interactions

Cytochrome P450 Effect: Substrate of CYP3A4 (minor); **Inhibits** CYP2B6 (weak) and 2C8 (weak)

Increased Effect/Toxicity: Sorafenib may increase the levels/effects of doxorubicin.

Decreased Effect: Sorafenib may decrease the absorption of digoxin tablets.

Pharmacodynamics/Kinetics

Absorption: Bioavailability decreased 29% with a high-fat meal (bioavailability similar to fasting state when administered with a moderate-fat meal).

Protein binding: 99.5%

Metabolism: Hepatic, via CYP3A4 (primarily oxidated to the pyridine N-oxide; active, minor) and UGT1A9 (glucuronidation)

Bioavailability: 38% to 49%

Half-life elimination: 25-48 hours

Time to peak, plasma: 3 hours

Excretion: Feces (77%, 51% as unchanged drug); urine (19%, as metabolites)

Pregnancy Risk Factor D

Sorafenib Tosylate *see* Sorafenib *on page 1488*

Sorbitol (SOR bi tole)

Generic Available Yes

Pharmacologic Category Genitourinary Irrigant; Laxative, Osmotic

Use Genitourinary irrigant in transurethral prostatic resection or other transurethral resection or other transurethral surgical procedures; diuretic; humectant; sweetening agent; hyperosmotic laxative; facilitate the passage of sodium polystyrene sulfonate through the intestinal tract

Local Anesthetic/Vasoconstrictor Precautions No information available to require special precautions

Effects on Dental Treatment Key adverse event(s) related to dental treatment: Xerostomia (normal salivary flow resumes upon discontinuation).

Common Adverse Effects Frequency not defined.

Cardiovascular: Edema

Endocrine & metabolic: Fluid and electrolyte losses, hyperglycemia, lactic acidosis

Gastrointestinal: Diarrhea, nausea, vomiting, abdominal discomfort, xerostomia

Mechanism of Action A polyalcoholic sugar with osmotic cathartic actions

Pharmacodynamics/Kinetics

Onset of action: 0.25-1 hour

Absorption: Oral, rectal: Poor

Metabolism: Primarily hepatic to fructose

Pregnancy Risk Factor C

Sorine® *see* Sotalol *on page 1489*

Sotalol (SOE ta lole)

Related Information

Cardiovascular Diseases *on page 1726*

U.S. Brand Names Betapace®; Betapace AF®; Sorine®

Canadian Brand Names Alti-Sotalol; Apo-Sotalol®; Betapace AF®; CO Sotalol; Gen-Sotalol; Lin-Sotalol; Novo-Sotalol; Nu-Sotalol; PMS-Sotalol; Rho®-Sotalol; Riva-Sotalol; Rylosol; Sotacor®

Generic Available Yes

Index Terms Sotalol Hydrochloride

Pharmacologic Category Antiarrhythmic Agent, Class II; Antiarrhythmic Agent, Class III; Beta-Adrenergic Blocker, Nonselective

Use Treatment of documented ventricular arrhythmias (ie, sustained ventricular tachycardia), that in the judgment of the physician are life-threatening; maintenance of normal sinus rhythm in patients with symptomatic atrial fibrillation and atrial flutter who are currently in sinus rhythm. Manufacturer states substitutions should not be made for Betapace AF® since Betapace AF® is distributed with a patient package insert specific for atrial fibrillation/flutter.

Local Anesthetic/Vasoconstrictor Precautions Use with caution; epinephrine has interacted with nonselective beta-blockers to result in initial hypertensive episode followed by bradycardia. Sotalol is one of the drugs confirmed to prolong the QT interval and is accepted as having a risk of causing torsade de pointes. The risk of drug-induced torsade de pointes is extremely low when a

(Continued)

Sotalol *(Continued)*

single QT interval prolonging drug is prescribed. In terms of epinephrine, it is not known what effect vasoconstrictors in the local anesthetic regimen will have in patients with a known history of congenital prolonged QT interval or in patients taking any medication that prolongs the QT interval. Until more information is obtained, it is suggested that the clinician consult with the physician prior to the use of a vasoconstrictor in suspected patients, and that the vasoconstrictor (epinephrine, levonordefrin [Neo-Cobefrin®]) be used with caution.

Effects on Dental Treatment Sotalol is a nonselective beta-blocker and may enhance the pressor response to epinephrine, resulting in hypertension and bradycardia. Many nonsteroidal anti-inflammatory drugs, such as ibuprofen and indomethacin, can reduce the hypotensive effect of beta-blockers after 3 or more weeks of therapy with the NSAID. Short-term NSAID use (ie, 3 days) requires no special precautions in patients taking beta-blockers.

Common Adverse Effects
>10%:
  Cardiovascular: Bradycardia (16%), chest pain (16%), palpitation (14%)
  Central nervous system: Fatigue (20%), dizziness (20%), lightheadedness (12%)
  Neuromuscular & skeletal: Weakness (13%)
  Respiratory: Dyspnea (21%)
1% to 10%:
  Cardiovascular: CHF (5%), peripheral vascular disorders (3%), edema (8%), abnormal ECG (7%), hypotension (6%), proarrhythmia (5%), syncope (5%)
  Central nervous system: Mental confusion (6%), anxiety (4%), headache (8%), sleep problems (8%), depression (4%)
  Dermatologic: Itching/rash (5%)
  Endocrine & metabolic: Sexual ability decreased (3%)
  Gastrointestinal: Diarrhea (7%), nausea/vomiting (10%), stomach discomfort (3% to 6%), flatulence (2%)
  Genitourinary: Impotence (2%)
  Hematologic: Bleeding (2%)
  Neuromuscular & skeletal: Paresthesia (4%), extremity pain (7%), back pain (3%)
  Ocular: Visual problems (5%)
  Respiratory: Upper respiratory problems (5% to 8%), asthma (2%)

Mechanism of Action
Beta-blocker which contains both beta-adrenoreceptor-blocking (Vaughan Williams Class II) and cardiac action potential duration prolongation (Vaughan Williams Class III) properties
Class II effects: Increased sinus cycle length, slowed heart rate, decreased AV nodal conduction, and increased AV nodal refractoriness
Class III effects: Prolongation of the atrial and ventricular monophasic action potentials, and effective refractory prolongation of atrial muscle, ventricular muscle, and atrioventricular accessory pathways in both the antegrade and retrograde directions
Sotalol is a racemic mixture of *d*- and *l*-sotalol; both isomers have similar Class III antiarrhythmic effects while the *l*-isomer is responsible for virtually all of the beta-blocking activity
Sotalol has both beta$_1$- and beta$_2$-receptor blocking activity
The beta-blocking effect of sotalol is a noncardioselective [half maximal at about 80 mg/day and maximal at doses of 320-640 mg/day]. Significant beta-blockade occurs at oral doses as low as 25 mg/day.
The Class III effects are seen only at oral doses ≥160 mg/day

Drug Interactions
Increased Effect/Toxicity: Increased effect/toxicity of beta-blockers with calcium blockers since there may be additive effects on AV conduction or ventricular function. Other agents which prolong QT interval, including Class I antiarrhythmic agents, bepridil, cisapride, erythromycin, haloperidol, pimozide, phenothiazines, tricyclic antidepressants, and specific quinolones (including sparfloxacin, gatifloxacin, moxifloxacin) may increase the effect of sotalol on the prolongation of QT interval. Amiodarone may cause additive effects on QT$_c$ prolongation as well as decreased heart rate, and has been associated with cardiac arrest in patients receiving some beta-blockers. When used concurrently with clonidine, sotalol may increase the risk of rebound hypertension after or during withdrawal of either agent. Beta-blocker and catecholamine depleting agents (reserpine or guanethidine) may result in additive hypotension or bradycardia. Beta-blockers may increase the action or levels of ethanol, nondepolarizing muscle relaxants, and theophylline although the effects are difficult to predict.

Decreased Effect: Decreased effect of sotalol may occur with aluminum-magnesium antacids (if taken within 2 hours), aluminum salts, barbiturates, calcium salts, cholestyramine, colestipol, NSAIDs, penicillins (ampicillin), rifampin, salicylates, and sulfinpyrazone due to decreased bioavailability and plasma levels. Beta-blockers may decrease the effect of sulfonylureas. Beta-agonists such as albuterol, terbutaline may have less of a therapeutic effect when administered concomitantly.

Pharmacodynamics/Kinetics
Onset of action: Rapid, 1-2 hours
Peak effect: 2.5-4 hours
Duration: 8-16 hours
Absorption: Decreased 20% to 30% by meals compared to fasting
Distribution: Low lipid solubility; enters milk of laboratory animals and is reported to be present in human milk
Protein binding: None
Metabolism: None
Bioavailability: 90% to 100%
Half-life elimination: 12 hours; Children: 9.5 hours; terminal half-life decreases with age <2 years (may by ≥1 week in neonates)
Excretion: Urine (as unchanged drug)
Pregnancy Risk Factor B

Spectinomycin (spek ti noe MYE sin)

Related Information
Sexually-Transmitted Diseases *on page 1766*
U.S. Brand Names Trobicin® [DSC]
Generic Available No
Index Terms Spectinomycin Hydrochloride
Pharmacologic Category Antibiotic, Miscellaneous
Use Treatment of uncomplicated gonorrhea
Local Anesthetic/Vasoconstrictor Precautions No information available to require special precautions
Effects on Dental Treatment No significant effects or complications reported
Mechanism of Action A bacteriostatic antibiotic that selectively binds to the 30s subunits of ribosomes, and thereby inhibiting bacterial protein synthesis
Pharmacodynamics/Kinetics
Duration: Up to 8 hours
Absorption: I.M.: Rapid and almost complete
Distribution: Concentrates in urine; does not distribute well into the saliva
Half-life elimination: 1.7 hours
Time to peak: ~1 hour
Excretion: Urine (70% to 100% as unchanged drug)
Pregnancy Risk Factor B

Spiramycin (speer a MYE sin)

Canadian Brand Names Rovamycine®
Generic Available No
Pharmacologic Category Antibiotic, Macrolide
Use Treatment of infections of the respiratory tract, buccal cavity, skin and soft tissues due to susceptible organisms. *N. gonorrhoeae*: as an alternate choice of treatment for gonorrhea in patients allergic to the penicillins. Before treatment of gonorrhea, the possibility of concomitant infection due to *T. pallidum* should be excluded.
Unlabeled/Investigational Use Treatment of *Toxoplasma gondii* to prevent transmission from mother to fetus
Local Anesthetic/Vasoconstrictor Precautions No information available to require special precautions
Effects on Dental Treatment No significant effects or complications reported
(Continued)

Spiramycin *(Continued)*

Common Adverse Effects Frequency not defined.
Dermatologic: Rash, urticaria, pruritus, angioedema (rare)
Gastrointestinal: Nausea, vomiting, diarrhea, pseudomembranous colitis (rare)
Hepatic: Transaminases increased
Neuromuscular & skeletal: Paresthesia (rare)
Miscellaneous: Anaphylactic shock (rare)

Restrictions Not available in U.S.

Mechanism of Action Inhibits growth of susceptible organisms; mechanism not established.

Drug Interactions
Cytochrome P450 Effect: Substrate of CYP3A4 (major)
Increased Effect/Toxicity: CYP3A4 inhibitors may increase the levels/effects of spiramycin; example inhibitors include azole antifungals, clarithromycin, diclofenac, doxycycline, erythromycin, imatinib, isoniazid, nefazodone, nicardipine, propofol, protease inhibitors, quinidine, telithromycin, and verapamil.
Decreased Effect: Spiramycin has been reported to decrease carbidopa absorption and decrease levodopa concentrations. CYP3A4 inducers may decrease the levels/effects of spiramycin; example inducers include aminoglutethimide, carbamazepine, nafcillin, nevirapine, phenobarbital, phenytoin, and rifamycins.

Pregnancy Risk Factor Not assigned (other macrolides rated B); C per expert analysis

Spiriva® see Tiotropium *on page 1574*

Spironolactone *(speer on oh LAK tone)*

Related Information
Cardiovascular Diseases *on page 1726*
U.S. Brand Names Aldactone®
Canadian Brand Names Aldactone®; Novo-Spiroton
Mexican Brand Names Aldactone
Generic Available Yes
Pharmacologic Category Diuretic, Potassium-Sparing; Selective Aldosterone Blocker
Use Management of edema associated with excessive aldosterone excretion; hypertension; congestive heart failure; primary hyperaldosteronism; hypokalemia; cirrhosis of liver accompanied by edema or ascites
Unlabeled/Investigational Use Female acne (adjunctive therapy); hirsutism; hypertension (pediatric); diuretic (pediatric)
Local Anesthetic/Vasoconstrictor Precautions No information available to require special precautions
Effects on Dental Treatment No significant effects or complications reported
Common Adverse Effects Incidence of adverse events is not always reported. (Mean daily dose: 26 mg)

Cardiovascular: Edema (2%, placebo 2%)
Central nervous system: Disorders (23%, placebo 21%) which may include drowsiness, lethargy, headache, mental confusion, drug fever, ataxia, fatigue
Dermatologic: Maculopapular, erythematous cutaneous eruptions, urticaria, hirsutism, eosinophilia
Endocrine & metabolic: Gynecomastia (men 9%; placebo 1%), breast pain (men 2%; placebo 0.1%), serious hyperkalemia (2%, placebo 1%), hyponatremia, dehydration, hyperchloremic metabolic acidosis in decompensated hepatic cirrhosis, inability to achieve or maintain an erection, irregular menses, amenorrhea, postmenopausal bleeding
Gastrointestinal: Disorders (29%, placebo 29%) which may include anorexia, nausea, cramping, diarrhea, gastric bleeding, ulceration, gastritis, vomiting
Genitourinary: Disorders (12%, placebo 11%)
Hematologic: Agranulocytosis
Hepatic: Cholestatic/hepatocellular toxicity
Renal: Increased BUN concentration
Respiratory: Disorders (32%, placebo 34%)
Miscellaneous: Deepening of the voice, anaphylactic reaction, breast cancer

Dosage To reduce delay in onset of effect, a loading dose of 2 or 3 times the daily dose may be administered on the first day of therapy. Oral:
Children:
Diuretic, hypertension (unlabeled use): Children 1-17 years: Initial: 1 mg/kg/day divided every 12-24 hours (maximum dose: 3.3 mg/kg/day, up to 100 mg/day)

Diagnosis of primary aldosteronism (unlabeled use): 125-375 mg/m²/day in divided doses

Adults:

Edema, hypokalemia: 25-200 mg/day in 1-2 divided doses

Hypertension (JNC 7): 25-50 mg/day in 1-2 divided doses

Diagnosis of primary aldosteronism: 100-400 mg/day in 1-2 divided doses

Acne in women (unlabeled use): 25-200 mg once daily

Hirsutism in women (unlabeled use): 50-200 mg/day in 1-2 divided doses

CHF, severe (with ACE inhibitor and a loop diuretic ± digoxin): 12.5-25 mg/day; maximum daily dose: 50 mg (higher doses may occasionally be used). In the RALES trial, 25 mg every other day was the lowest maintenance dose possible.

Note: If potassium >5.4 mEq/L, consider dosage reduction.

Elderly: Initial: 25-50 mg/day in 1-2 divided doses, increasing by 25-50 mg every 5 days as needed.

Dosing interval in renal impairment:

Cl$_{cr}$ 10-50 mL/minute: Administer every 12-24 hours.

Cl$_{cr}$ <10 mL/minute: Avoid use.

Mechanism of Action Competes with aldosterone for receptor sites in the distal renal tubules, increasing sodium chloride and water excretion while conserving potassium and hydrogen ions; may block the effect of aldosterone on arteriolar smooth muscle as well

Contraindications Hypersensitivity to spironolactone or any component of the formulation; anuria; acute renal insufficiency; significant impairment of renal excretory function; hyperkalemia; pregnancy (pregnancy-induced hypertension - per expert analysis)

Warnings/Precautions Avoid potassium supplements, potassium-containing salt substitutes, a diet rich in potassium, or other drugs that can cause hyperkalemia. Excess amounts can lead to profound diuresis with fluid and electrolyte loss; close medical supervision and dose evaluation are required. Watch for and correct electrolyte disturbances; adjust dose to avoid dehydration. In cirrhosis, avoid electrolyte and acid/base imbalances that might lead to hepatic encephalopathy. Gynecomastia is related to dose and duration of therapy. Discontinue use prior to adrenal vein catheterization. When evaluating a heart failure patient for spironolactone treatment, creatinine should be ≤2.5 mg/dL in men or ≤2 mg/dL in women and potassium <5 mEq/L. **[U.S. Boxed Warning]: Shown to be a tumorigen in chronic toxicity animal studies. Avoid unnecessary use.**

Drug Interactions

Increased Effect/Toxicity: Concurrent use of spironolactone with other potassium-sparing diuretics, potassium supplements, angiotensin receptor antagonists, co-trimoxazole (high dose), and ACE inhibitors can increase the risk of hyperkalemia, especially in patients with renal impairment. Cholestyramine can cause hyperchloremic acidosis in cirrhotic patients; avoid concurrent use.

Decreased Effect: The effects of digoxin (loss of positive inotropic effect) and mitotane may be reduced by spironolactone. Salicylates and NSAIDs (indomethacin) may decrease the natriuretic effect of spironolactone.

Ethanol/Nutrition/Herb Interactions

Food: Food increases absorption.

Herb/Nutraceutical: Avoid natural licorice (due to mineralocorticoid activity)

Dietary Considerations Should be taken with food to decrease gastrointestinal irritation and to increase absorption. Excessive potassium intake (eg, salt substitutes, low-salt foods, bananas, nuts) should be avoided.

Pharmacodynamics/Kinetics

Duration of action: 2-3 days

Protein binding: 91% to 98%

Metabolism: Hepatic to multiple metabolites, including canrenone (active)

Half-life elimination: 78-84 minutes

Time to peak, serum: 1-3 hours (primarily as the active metabolite)

Excretion: Urine and feces

Pregnancy Risk Factor C/D in pregnancy-induced hypertension (per expert analysis)

Dosage Forms

Tablet: 25 mg, 50 mg, 100 mg

Aldactone®: 25 mg, 50 mg, 100 mg

Sronyx™ *see* Ethinyl Estradiol and Levonorgestrel *on page 633*

SSD® *see* Silver Sulfadiazine *on page 1471*

SSD® AF *see* Silver Sulfadiazine *on page 1471*

SSKI® *see* Potassium Iodide *on page 1330*

S.T. 37® [OTC] *see* Hexylresorcinol *on page 814*

Stadol® *see* Butorphanol *on page 254*

Staflex *see* Acetaminophen and Phenyltoloxamine *on page 38*

Stagesic® *see* Hydrocodone and Acetaminophen *on page 822*

Stalevo™ *see* Levodopa, Carbidopa, and Entacapone *on page 965*

StanGard® *see* Fluoride *on page 710*

StanGard® Perio *see* Fluoride *on page 710*

Stannous Fluoride *see* Fluoride *on page 710*

Stanozolol (stan OH zoe lole)

U.S. Brand Names Winstrol®

Generic Available No

Pharmacologic Category Anabolic Steroid

Use Prophylactic use against hereditary angioedema

Local Anesthetic/Vasoconstrictor Precautions No information available to require special precautions

Effects on Dental Treatment No significant effects or complications reported

Common Adverse Effects

Male:

Postpubertal:

>10%:

Dermatologic: Acne

Endocrine & metabolic: Gynecomastia

Genitourinary: Bladder irritability, priapism

1% to 10%:

Central nervous system: Insomnia, chills

Endocrine & metabolic: Decreased libido, hepatic dysfunction

Gastrointestinal: Nausea, diarrhea

Genitourinary: Prostatic hyperplasia (elderly)

Hematologic: Iron deficiency anemia, suppression of clotting factors

Prepubertal:

>10%:

Dermatologic: Acne

Endocrine & metabolic: Virilism

1% to 10%:

Central nervous system: Chills, insomnia, factors

Dermatologic: Hyperpigmentation

Gastrointestinal: Diarrhea, nausea

Hematologic: Iron deficiency anemia, suppression of clotting

Female:

>10%: Endocrine & metabolic: Virilism

1% to 10%:

Central nervous system: Chills, insomnia

Endocrine & metabolic: Hypercalcemia

Gastrointestinal: Nausea, diarrhea

Hematologic: Iron deficiency anemia, suppression of clotting factors

Hepatic: Hepatic dysfunction

Restrictions C-III

Mechanism of Action Synthetic testosterone derivative with similar androgenic and anabolic actions

Drug Interactions

Increased Effect/Toxicity: ACTH, adrenal steroids may increase risk of edema and acne. Stanozolol enhances the hypoprothrombinemic effects of oral anticoagulants and enhances the hypoglycemic effects of insulin and sulfonylureas (oral hypoglycemics).

Pharmacodynamics/Kinetics

Metabolism: Hepatic

Excretion: Urine (90%); feces (6%)

Pregnancy Risk Factor X

Starlix® *see* Nateglinide *on page 1154*

Statuss™ DM *see* Chlorpheniramine, Phenylephrine, and Dextromethorphan *on page 342*

Stavudine (STAV yoo deen)

Related Information
HIV Infection and AIDS *on page 1753*
U.S. Brand Names Zerit®
Canadian Brand Names Zerit®
Mexican Brand Names Zerit
Generic Available No
Index Terms d4T
Pharmacologic Category Antiretroviral Agent, Reverse Transcriptase Inhibitor (Nucleoside)
Use Treatment of HIV infection in combination with other antiretroviral agents
Local Anesthetic/Vasoconstrictor Precautions No information available to require special precautions
Effects on Dental Treatment No significant effects or complications reported
Common Adverse Effects All adverse reactions reported below were similar to comparative agent, zidovudine, except for peripheral neuropathy, which was greater for stavudine. Selected adverse events reported as monotherapy or in combination therapy include:

>10%:
Central nervous system: Headache
Dermatologic: Rash
Gastrointestinal: Nausea, vomiting, diarrhea
Hepatic: Hepatic transaminases increased
Neuromuscular & skeletal: Peripheral neuropathy
Miscellaneous: Amylase increased
1% to 10%: Hepatic: Bilirubin increased

Mechanism of Action Stavudine is a thymidine analog which interferes with HIV viral DNA dependent DNA polymerase resulting in inhibition of viral replication; nucleoside reverse transcriptase inhibitor

Drug Interactions
Increased Effect/Toxicity: Risk of pancreatitis may be increased with concurrent didanosine use; cases of fatal lactic acidosis have been reported with this combination when used during pregnancy (use only if clearly needed). Risk of hepatotoxicity or pancreatitis may be increased with concurrent hydroxyurea use. Zalcitabine may increase risk of peripheral neuropathy; concurrent use not recommended. Concomitant use of ribavirin with or without interferon alfa and nucleoside analogues may increase the risk of developing hepatic decompensation or other signs of mitochondrial toxicity, including pancreatitis or lactic acidosis.
Decreased Effect: Zidovudine inhibits intracellular phosphorylation of stavudine; concurrent use not recommended. Doxorubicin may inhibit intracellular phosphorylation of stavudine; use with caution. Ribavirin may inhibit intracellular phosphorylation of stavudine; use with caution.

Pharmacodynamics/Kinetics
Distribution: V_d: 0.5 L/kg
Bioavailability: 86.4%
Metabolism: Undergoes intracellular phosphorylation to an active metabolite
Half-life elimination: 1-1.6 hours
Time to peak, serum: 1 hour
Excretion: Urine (40% as unchanged drug)

Pregnancy Risk Factor C

Sterapred® *see* PredniSONE *on page 1342*
Sterapred® DS *see* PredniSONE *on page 1342*
STI571 *see* Imatinib *on page 863*
Stimate™ *see* Desmopressin *on page 462*
Sting-Kill [OTC] *see* Benzocaine *on page 195*
St. Joseph® Adult Aspirin [OTC] *see* Aspirin *on page 149*
Stop® *see* Fluoride *on page 710*
Strattera® *see* Atomoxetine *on page 160*
Streptase® *see* Streptokinase *on page 1495*

Streptokinase (strep toe KYE nase)

Related Information
Cardiovascular Diseases *on page 1726*
(Continued)

Streptokinase (Continued)

U.S. Brand Names Streptase®

Canadian Brand Names Streptase®

Mexican Brand Names Streptase

Generic Available No

Index Terms SK

Pharmacologic Category Thrombolytic Agent

Use Thrombolytic agent used in treatment of recent severe or massive deep vein thrombosis, pulmonary emboli, myocardial infarction, and occluded arteriovenous cannulas

Local Anesthetic/Vasoconstrictor Precautions No information available to require special precautions

Effects on Dental Treatment No significant effects or complications reported

Common Adverse Effects As with all drugs which may affect hemostasis, bleeding is the major adverse effect associated with streptokinase. Hemorrhage may occur at virtually any site. Risk is dependent on multiple variables, including the dosage administered, concurrent use of multiple agents which alter hemostasis, and patient predisposition (including hypertension). Rapid lysis of coronary artery thrombi by thrombolytic agents may be associated with reperfusion-related atrial and/or ventricular arrhythmia.

>10%:

Cardiovascular: Hypotension

Local: Injection site bleeding

1% to 10%:

Central nervous system: Fever (1% to 4%)

Dermatologic: Bruising, rash, pruritus

Gastrointestinal: Gastrointestinal hemorrhage, nausea, vomiting

Genitourinary: Genitourinary hemorrhage

Hematologic: Anemia

Neuromuscular & skeletal: Muscle pain

Ocular: Eye hemorrhage, periorbital edema

Respiratory: Bronchospasm, epistaxis

Miscellaneous: Diaphoresis hemorrhage, gingival hemorrhage

Additional cardiovascular events associated with use in MI: Asystole, AV block, cardiac arrest, cardiac tamponade, cardiogenic shock, electromechanical dissociation, heart failure, mitral regurgitation, myocardial rupture, pericardial effusion, pericarditis, pulmonary edema, recurrent ischemia/infarction, thromboembolism, ventricular tachycardia

Mechanism of Action Activates the conversion of plasminogen to plasmin by forming a complex, exposing plasminogen-activating site, and cleaving a peptide bond that converts plasminogen to plasmin; plasmin degrades fibrin, fibrinogen and other procoagulant proteins into soluble fragments; effective both outside and within the formed thrombus/embolus

Drug Interactions

Increased Effect/Toxicity: The risk of bleeding with streptokinase is increased by oral anticoagulants (warfarin), heparin, low molecular weight heparins, and drugs which affect platelet function (eg, NSAIDs, dipyridamole, ticlopidine, clopidogrel, IIb/IIIa antagonists). Although concurrent use with aspirin and heparin may increase the risk of bleeding. Aspirin and heparin were used concomitantly with streptokinase in the majority of patients in clinical studies of MI.

Decreased Effect: Antifibrinolytic agents (aminocaproic acid) may decrease effectiveness to thrombolytic agents.

Pharmacodynamics/Kinetics

Onset of action: Activation of plasminogen occurs almost immediately

Duration: Fibrinolytic effect: Several hours; Anticoagulant effect: 12-24 hours

Half-life elimination: 83 minutes

Excretion: By circulating antibodies and the reticuloendothelial system

Pregnancy Risk Factor C

Streptomycin (strep toe MYE sin)

Related Information

Tuberculosis on page 1765

Mexican Brand Names Estrepto-Monaxin

Generic Available Yes

Index Terms Streptomycin Sulfate

Pharmacologic Category Antibiotic, Aminoglycoside; Antitubercular Agent

Use Part of combination therapy of active tuberculosis; used in combination with other agents for treatment of streptococcal or enterococcal endocarditis, mycobacterial infections, plague, tularemia, and brucellosis

Local Anesthetic/Vasoconstrictor Precautions No information available to require special precautions

Effects on Dental Treatment No significant effects or complications reported

Common Adverse Effects Frequency not defined.

Cardiovascular: Hypotension

Central nervous system: Neurotoxicity, drowsiness, headache, drug fever, paresthesia

Dermatologic: Skin rash

Gastrointestinal: Nausea, vomiting

Hematologic: Eosinophilia, anemia

Neuromuscular & skeletal: Arthralgia, weakness, tremor

Otic: Ototoxicity (auditory), ototoxicity (vestibular)

Renal: Nephrotoxicity

Respiratory: Difficulty in breathing

Mechanism of Action Inhibits bacterial protein synthesis by binding directly to the 30S ribosomal subunits causing faulty peptide sequence to form in the protein chain

Drug Interactions

Increased Effect/Toxicity: Increased/prolonged effect with depolarizing and nondepolarizing neuromuscular blocking agents. Concurrent use with amphotericin or loop diuretics may increase nephrotoxicity.

Pharmacodynamics/Kinetics

Absorption:

Oral: Poorly absorbed

I.M.: Well absorbed

Distribution: To extracellular fluid including serum, abscesses, ascitic, pericardial, pleural, synovial, lymphatic, and peritoneal fluids; poorly distributed into CSF

Protein binding: 34%

Half-life elimination: Newborns: 4-10 hours; Adults: 2-4.7 hours, prolonged with renal impairment

Time to peak: I.M.: Within 1 hour

Excretion: Urine (90% as unchanged drug); feces, saliva, sweat, and tears (<1%)

Pregnancy Risk Factor D

Streptomycin Sulfate *see* Streptomycin *on page 1496*

Streptozocin (strep toe ZOE sin)

U.S. Brand Names Zanosar®

Canadian Brand Names Zanosar®

Generic Available No

Index Terms NSC-85998

Pharmacologic Category Antineoplastic Agent, Alkylating Agent

Use Treatment of metastatic islet cell carcinoma of the pancreas, carcinoid tumor and syndrome, Hodgkin's disease, palliative treatment of colorectal cancer

Local Anesthetic/Vasoconstrictor Precautions No information available to require special precautions

Effects on Dental Treatment No significant effects or complications reported

Common Adverse Effects

>10%:

Gastrointestinal: Nausea and vomiting (100%)

Hepatic: Increased LFTs

Miscellaneous: Hypoalbuminemia

Renal: BUN increased, Cl_{cr} decreased, hypophosphatemia, nephrotoxicity (25% to 75%), proteinuria, renal dysfunction (65%), renal tubular acidosis

1% to 10%:

Endocrine & metabolic: Hypoglycemia (6%)

Gastrointestinal: Diarrhea (10%)

Local: Pain at injection site

Mechanism of Action Interferes with the normal function of DNA by alkylation and cross-linking the strands of DNA, and by possible protein modification

Drug Interactions

Increased Effect/Toxicity: Doxorubicin toxicity may be increased with concurrent use of streptozocin. Manufacturer recommends doxorubicin dosage adjustment be considered.

(Continued)

Streptozocin *(Continued)*

Decreased Effect: Phenytoin results in negation of streptozocin cytotoxicity.

Pharmacodynamics/Kinetics

Duration: Disappears from serum in 4 hours

Distribution: Concentrates in liver, intestine, pancreas, and kidney

Metabolism: Rapidly hepatic

Half-life elimination: 35-40 minutes

Excretion: Urine (60% to 70% as metabolites); exhaled gases (5%); feces (1%)

Pregnancy Risk Factor D

Stresstabs® High Potency Advanced [OTC] *see* Vitamin B Complex Combinations *on page 1664*

Stresstabs® High Potency Energy [OTC] *see* Vitamin B Complex Combinations *on page 1664*

Stresstabs® High Potency Weight [OTC] *see* Vitamin B Complex Combinations *on page 1664*

Striant® *see* Testosterone *on page 1543*

Stri-dex® [OTC] *see* Salicylic Acid *on page 1451*

Stri-dex® Body Focus [OTC] *see* Salicylic Acid *on page 1451*

Stri-dex® Facewipes To Go™ [OTC] *see* Salicylic Acid *on page 1451*

Stri-dex® Maximum Strength [OTC] *see* Salicylic Acid *on page 1451*

Stromectol® *see* Ivermectin *on page 924*

Strong Iodine Solution *see* Potassium Iodide and Iodine *on page 1331*

Strovite *see* Vitamin B Complex Combinations *on page 1664*

Strovite® Forte *see* Vitamins (Multiple/Oral) *on page 1665*

SU11248 *see* Sunitinib *on page 1513*

Suberoylanilide Hydroxamic Acid *see* Vorinostat *on page 1668*

Sublimaze® *see* Fentanyl *on page 679*

Suboxone® *see* Buprenorphine and Naloxone *on page 240*

Subutex® *see* Buprenorphine *on page 239*

Succinylcholine *(suks in il KOE leen)*

U.S. Brand Names Quelicin®

Canadian Brand Names Quelicin®

Mexican Brand Names Anectine

Generic Available No

Index Terms Succinylcholine Chloride; Suxamethonium Chloride

Pharmacologic Category Neuromuscular Blocker Agent, Depolarizing

Use Adjunct to general anesthesia to facilitate both rapid sequence and routine endotracheal intubation and to relax skeletal muscles during surgery; to reduce the intensity of muscle contractions of pharmacologically- or electrically-induced convulsions; does not relieve pain or produce sedation

Local Anesthetic/Vasoconstrictor Precautions No information available to require special precautions

Effects on Dental Treatment No significant effects or complications reported

Common Adverse Effects

>10%:

Ocular: Increased intraocular pressure

Miscellaneous: Postoperative stiffness

1% to 10%:

Cardiovascular: Bradycardia, hypotension, cardiac arrhythmia, tachycardia

Gastrointestinal: Intragastric pressure, salivation

Causes of prolonged neuromuscular blockade: Excessive drug administration; cumulative drug effect; decreased metabolism/excretion (hepatic and/or renal impairment); accumulation of active metabolites; electrolyte imbalance (hypokalemia, hypocalcemia, hypermagnesemia, hypernatremia); hypothermia; drug interactions; increased sensitivity to muscle relaxants (eg, neuromuscular disorders such as myasthenia gravis or polymyositis)

Mechanism of Action Acts similar to acetylcholine, produces depolarization of the motor endplate at the myoneural junction which causes sustained flaccid skeletal muscle paralysis produced by state of accommodation that develops in adjacent excitable muscle membranes

Drug Interactions

Increased Effect/Toxicity:

Increased toxicity: Anticholinesterase drugs (neostigmine, physostigmine, or pyridostigmine) in combination with succinylcholine can cause cardiorespiratory collapse; cyclophosphamide, oral contraceptives, lidocaine, thiotepa, pancuronium, lithium, magnesium salts, aprotinin, chloroquine, metoclopramide, terbutaline, and procaine enhance and prolong the effects of succinylcholine

Prolonged neuromuscular blockade: Inhaled anesthetics, local anesthetics, calcium channel blockers, antiarrhythmics (eg, quinidine or procainamide), antibiotics (eg, aminoglycosides, tetracyclines, vancomycin, clindamycin), immunosuppressants (eg, cyclosporine)

Pharmacodynamics/Kinetics
Onset of action: I.M.: 2-3 minutes; I.V.: Complete muscular relaxation: 30-60 seconds
Duration: I.M.: 10-30 minutes; I.V.: 4-6 minutes with single administration
Metabolism: Rapidly hydrolyzed by plasma pseudocholinesterase
Pregnancy Risk Factor C

Succinylcholine Chloride see Succinylcholine on page 1498
Sucraid® see Sacrosidase on page 1451

Sucralfate (soo KRAL fate)

Related Information
Management of Patients Undergoing Cancer Therapy on page 1826
U.S. Brand Names Carafate®
Canadian Brand Names Novo-Sucralate; Nu-Sucralate; PMS-Sucralate; Sulcrate®; Sulcrate® Suspension Plus
Mexican Brand Names Unival
Generic Available Yes
Index Terms Aluminum Sucrose Sulfate, Basic
Pharmacologic Category Gastrointestinal Agent, Miscellaneous
Use Short-term management of duodenal ulcers; maintenance of duodenal ulcers
Unlabeled/Investigational Use Gastric ulcers; suspension may be used topically for treatment of stomatitis due to cancer chemotherapy and other causes of esophageal and gastric erosions; GERD, esophagitis; treatment of NSAID mucosal damage; prevention of stress ulcers; postsclerotherapy for esophageal variceal bleeding
Local Anesthetic/Vasoconstrictor Precautions No information available to require special precautions
Effects on Dental Treatment No significant effects or complications reported
Common Adverse Effects 1% to 10%: Gastrointestinal: Constipation
Dosage Oral:
Children: Dose not established, doses of 40-80 mg/kg/day divided every 6 hours have been used
Stomatitis (unlabeled use): 2.5-5 mL (1 g/10 mL suspension), swish and spit or swish and swallow 4 times/day
Adults:
Stress ulcer prophylaxis: 1 g 4 times/day
Stress ulcer treatment: 1 g every 4 hours
Duodenal ulcer:
Treatment: 1 g 4 times/day on an empty stomach and at bedtime for 4-8 weeks, or alternatively 2 g twice daily; treatment is recommended for 4-8 weeks in adults, the elderly may require 12 weeks
Maintenance: Prophylaxis: 1 g twice daily
Stomatitis (unlabeled use): 1 g/10 mL suspension, swish and spit or swish and swallow 4 times/day
Dosage comment in renal impairment: Aluminum salt is minimally absorbed (<5%), however, may accumulate in renal failure
Mechanism of Action Forms a complex by binding with positively charged proteins in exudates, forming a viscous paste-like, adhesive substance. This selectively forms a protective coating that protects the lining against peptic acid, pepsin, and bile salts.
Contraindications Hypersensitivity to sucralfate or any component of the formulation
Warnings/Precautions Successful therapy with sucralfate should not be expected to alter the posthealing frequency of recurrence or the severity of duodenal ulceration; use with caution in patients with chronic renal failure who have an impaired excretion of absorbed aluminum. Because of the potential for sucralfate to alter the absorption of some drugs, separate administration (take other medication 2 hours before sucralfate) should be considered when alterations in bioavailability are believed to be critical
Drug Interactions
Decreased Effect: Sucralfate may alter the absorption of digoxin, phenytoin (hydantoins), warfarin, ketoconazole, quinidine, quinolones, tetracycline, (Continued)

Sucralfate *(Continued)*

theophylline. Because of the potential for sucralfate to alter the absorption of some drugs; separate administration (take other medications at least 2 hours before sucralfate). The potential for decreased absorption should be considered when alterations in bioavailability are believed to be critical.

Ethanol/Nutrition/Herb Interactions Food: Sucralfate may interfere with absorption of vitamin A, vitamin D, vitamin E, and vitamin K.

Dietary Considerations Administer with water on an empty stomach.

Pharmacodynamics/Kinetics
Onset of action: Paste formation and ulcer adhesion: 1-2 hours
Duration: Up to 6 hours
Absorption: Oral: <5%
Distribution: Acts locally at ulcer sites; unbound in GI tract to aluminum and sucrose octasulfate
Metabolism: None
Excretion: Urine (small amounts as unchanged compounds)

Pregnancy Risk Factor B

Dosage Forms
Suspension, oral: 1 g/10 mL (10 mL)
Carafate®: 1 g/10 mL
Tablet: 1 g
Carafate®: 1 g

Sucrets® [OTC] *see* Dyclonine *on page 552*

Sucrets® Original [OTC] *see* Hexylresorcinol *on page 814*

Sudafed® 12 Hour [OTC] *see* Pseudoephedrine *on page 1381*

Sudafed® 24 Hour [OTC] *see* Pseudoephedrine *on page 1381*

Sudafed® Children's [OTC] *see* Pseudoephedrine *on page 1381*

Sudafed® Children's Cold & Cough [OTC] *see* Pseudoephedrine and Dextromethorphan *on page 1383*

Sudafed® Maximum Strength Nasal Decongestant [OTC] *see* Pseudoephedrine *on page 1381*

Sudafed® Maximum Strength Sinus Nighttime [OTC] [DSC] *see* Triprolidine and Pseudoephedrine *on page 1624*

Sudafed® Multi-Symptom Sinus and Cold [OTC] *see* Acetaminophen and Pseudoephedrine *on page 38*

Sudafed® Non-Drying Sinus [OTC] [DSC] *see* Guaifenesin and Pseudoephedrine *on page 798*

Sudafed PE™ [OTC] *see* Phenylephrine *on page 1293*

Sudafed® Severe Cold [OTC] *see* Acetaminophen, Dextromethorphan, and Pseudoephedrine *on page 44*

Sudafed® Sinus & Allergy [OTC] *see* Chlorpheniramine and Pseudoephedrine *on page 340*

Sudal® 12 *see* Chlorpheniramine and Pseudoephedrine *on page 340*

Sudodrin [OTC] *see* Pseudoephedrine *on page 1381*

SudoGest [OTC] *see* Pseudoephedrine *on page 1381*

SudoGest Children's [OTC] *see* Pseudoephedrine and Dextromethorphan *on page 1383*

Sudo-Tab® [OTC] *see* Pseudoephedrine *on page 1381*

Sufenta® *see* Sufentanil *on page 1500*

Sufentanil *(soo FEN ta nil)*

U.S. Brand Names Sufenta®
Canadian Brand Names Sufenta®; Sufentanil Citrate Injection, USP
Generic Available Yes
Index Terms Sufentanil Citrate
Pharmacologic Category Analgesic, Opioid; General Anesthetic
Use Analgesic supplement in maintenance of balanced general anesthesia
Local Anesthetic/Vasoconstrictor Precautions No information available to require special precautions
Effects on Dental Treatment Key adverse event(s) related to dental treatment: Orthostatic hypotension.
Common Adverse Effects
>10%:
Cardiovascular: Bradycardia, hypotension
Central nervous system: Somnolence
Gastrointestinal: Nausea, vomiting
Respiratory: Respiratory depression
1% to 10%:
Cardiovascular: Cardiac arrhythmia, orthostatic hypotension

Central nervous system: CNS depression, confusion
Gastrointestinal: Biliary spasm
Ocular: Blurred vision

Restrictions C-II

Mechanism of Action Binds to opioid receptors throughout the CNS. Once receptor binding occurs, effects are exerted by opening K+ channels and inhibiting Ca++ channels. These mechanisms increase pain threshold, alter pain perception, inhibit ascending pain pathways; short-acting narcotic

Drug Interactions
Cytochrome P450 Effect: Substrate of CYP3A4 (major)
Increased Effect/Toxicity: Additive effect/toxicity with CNS depressants or beta-blockers. May increase response to neuromuscular-blocking agents. CYP3A4 inhibitors may increase the levels/effects of sufentanil; example inhibitors include azole antifungals, clarithromycin, diclofenac, doxycycline, erythromycin, imatinib, isoniazid, nefazodone, nicardipine, propofol, protease inhibitors, quinidine, telithromycin, and verapamil.

Pharmacodynamics/Kinetics
Onset of action: 1-3 minutes
Duration: Dose dependent
Metabolism: Primarily hepatic

Pregnancy Risk Factor C

Sufentanil Citrate *see* Sufentanil *on page 1500*
Sular® *see* Nisoldipine *on page 1177*
Sulbactam and Ampicillin *see* Ampicillin and Sulbactam *on page 122*

Sulconazole (sul KON a zole)

U.S. Brand Names Exelderm®
Canadian Brand Names Exelderm®
Generic Available No
Index Terms Sulconazole Nitrate
Pharmacologic Category Antifungal Agent, Topical
Use Treatment of superficial fungal infections of the skin, including tinea cruris (jock itch), tinea corporis (ringworm), tinea versicolor, and possibly tinea pedis (athlete's foot, cream only)
Local Anesthetic/Vasoconstrictor Precautions No information available to require special precautions
Effects on Dental Treatment No significant effects or complications reported
Common Adverse Effects 1% to 10%:
Dermatologic: Itching
Local: Burning, stinging, redness
Mechanism of Action Substituted imidazole derivative which inhibits metabolic reactions necessary for the synthesis of ergosterol, an essential membrane component. The end result is usually fungistatic; however, sulconazole may act as a fungicide in *Candida albicans* and *Candida parapsilosis* during certain growth phases.
Drug Interactions
Cytochrome P450 Effect: Inhibits CYP1A2 (weak), 2A6 (weak), 2C9 (weak), 2C19 (weak), 2D6 (weak), 2E1 (weak), 3A4 (weak)
Pharmacodynamics/Kinetics
Absorption: Topical: ~8.7% percutaneously
Excretion: Primarily urine
Pregnancy Risk Factor C

Sulconazole Nitrate *see* Sulconazole *on page 1501*

Sulfabenzamide, Sulfacetamide, and Sulfathiazole
(sul fa BENZ a mide, sul fa SEE ta mide, & sul fa THYE a zole)

Related Information
Sulfacetamide *on page 1502*
U.S. Brand Names V.V.S.®
Generic Available Yes
Index Terms Triple Sulfa
Pharmacologic Category Antibiotic, Vaginal
Use Treatment of *Haemophilus vaginalis* vaginitis
Local Anesthetic/Vasoconstrictor Precautions No information available to require special precautions
Effects on Dental Treatment No significant effects or complications reported
Common Adverse Effects Frequency not defined.
Dermatologic: Pruritus, urticaria, Stevens-Johnson syndrome
(Continued)

Sulfabenzamide, Sulfacetamide, and Sulfathiazole
(Continued)

Local: Local irritation

Miscellaneous: Allergic reactions

Mechanism of Action Interferes with microbial folic acid synthesis and growth via inhibition of para-aminobenzoic acid metabolism

Pharmacodynamics/Kinetics

Absorption: Absorption from vagina is variable and unreliable

Metabolism: Primarily via acetylation

Excretion: Urine

Pregnancy Risk Factor C (avoid if near term)

Sulfacetamide (sul fa SEE ta mide)

U.S. Brand Names Bleph®-10; Carmol® Scalp; Klaron®; Mexar™ Wash; Ovace®; Ovace® Wash; Rosula® NS

Canadian Brand Names Cetamide™; Diosulf™

Mexican Brand Names Blef 10 con Lagrifilm; Sul 10

Generic Available Yes: Ointment, solution, suspension

Index Terms Sodium Sulfacetamide; Sulfacetamide Sodium

Pharmacologic Category Acne Products; Antibiotic, Ophthalmic; Antibiotic, Sulfonamide Derivative; Topical Skin Product, Acne

Use

Ophthalmic: Treatment and prophylaxis of conjunctivitis due to susceptible organisms; corneal ulcers; adjunctive treatment with systemic sulfonamides for therapy of trachoma

Dermatologic: Scaling dermatosis (seborrheic); bacterial infections of the skin; acne vulgaris

Local Anesthetic/Vasoconstrictor Precautions No information available to require special precautions

Effects on Dental Treatment No significant effects or complications reported

Common Adverse Effects Frequency not defined.

Cardiovascular: Edema

Dermatologic: Burning, erythema, irritation, itching, stinging, Stevens-Johnson syndrome

Ocular (following ophthalmic application): Burning, conjunctivitis, conjunctival hyperemia, corneal ulcers, irritation, stinging

Miscellaneous: Allergic reactions, systemic lupus erythematosus

Mechanism of Action Interferes with bacterial growth by inhibiting bacterial folic acid synthesis through competitive antagonism of PABA

Drug Interactions

Decreased Effect: Silver containing products are incompatible with sulfacetamide solutions.

Pharmacodynamics/Kinetics

Half-life elimination: 7-13 hours

Excretion: When absorbed, primarily urine (as unchanged drug)

Pregnancy Risk Factor C

Sulfacetamide and Fluorometholone
(sul fa SEE ta mide & flure oh METH oh lone)

Related Information

Fluorometholone on page 712

Sulfacetamide on page 1502

U.S. Brand Names FML-S®

Generic Available No

Index Terms Fluorometholone and Sulfacetamide

Pharmacologic Category Antibiotic/Corticosteroid, Ophthalmic

Use Steroid-responsive inflammatory ocular conditions where infection is present or there is a risk of infection

Local Anesthetic/Vasoconstrictor Precautions No information available to require special precautions

Effects on Dental Treatment No significant effects or complications reported

Mechanism of Action

See individual agents.

Pregnancy Risk Factor C

Sulfacetamide and Prednisolone
(sul fa SEE ta mide & pred NIS oh lone)

Related Information
PrednisoLONE *on page 1339*
Sulfacetamide *on page 1502*
U.S. Brand Names Blephamide®
Canadian Brand Names Blephamide®; Dioptimyd®
Generic Available Yes: Solution
Index Terms Prednisolone and Sulfacetamide
Pharmacologic Category Antibiotic/Corticosteroid, Ophthalmic
Use Steroid-responsive inflammatory ocular conditions where infection is present or there is a risk of infection; ophthalmic suspension may be used as an otic preparation
Local Anesthetic/Vasoconstrictor Precautions No information available to require special precautions
Effects on Dental Treatment No significant effects or complications reported
Mechanism of Action Interferes with bacterial growth by inhibiting bacterial folic acid synthesis through competitive antagonism of PABA; decreases inflammation by suppression of migration of polymorphonuclear leukocytes and reversal of increased capillary permeability; suppresses the immune system by reducing activity and volume of the lymphatic system
Pregnancy Risk Factor C

Sulfacetamide Sodium *see* Sulfacetamide *on page 1502*

SulfaDIAZINE (sul fa DYE a zeen)

Generic Available Yes
Pharmacologic Category Antibiotic, Sulfonamide Derivative
Use Treatment of urinary tract infections and nocardiosis; adjunctive treatment in toxoplasmosis; uncomplicated attack of malaria
Unlabeled/Investigational Use Rheumatic fever prophylaxis
Local Anesthetic/Vasoconstrictor Precautions No information available to require special precautions
Effects on Dental Treatment No significant effects or complications reported
Mechanism of Action Interferes with bacterial growth by inhibiting bacterial folic acid synthesis through competitive antagonism of PABA
Pregnancy Risk Factor B/D (at term)

Sulfadoxine and Pyrimethamine
(sul fa DOKS een & peer i METH a meen)

Related Information
Pyrimethamine *on page 1390*
U.S. Brand Names Fansidar®
Generic Available No
Index Terms Pyrimethamine and Sulfadoxine
Pharmacologic Category Antimalarial Agent
Use Treatment of *Plasmodium falciparum* malaria in patients in whom chloroquine resistance is suspected; malaria prophylaxis for travelers to areas where chloroquine-resistant malaria is endemic
Local Anesthetic/Vasoconstrictor Precautions No information available to require special precautions
Effects on Dental Treatment Key adverse event(s) related to dental treatment: Atrophic glossitis.
Common Adverse Effects Frequency not defined.
Cardiovascular: Myocarditis (allergic), pericarditis (allergic), periorbital edema
Central nervous system: Ataxia, hallucinations, headache, polyneuritis, seizure
Dermatologic: Photosensitivity, Stevens-Johnson syndrome, erythema multiforme, toxic epidermal necrolysis, rash
Endocrine & metabolic: Thyroid function dysfunction
Gastrointestinal: Anorexia, atrophic glossitis, gastritis, pancreatitis, vomiting
Genitourinary: Crystalluria
Hematologic: Megaloblastic anemia, leukopenia, thrombocytopenia, pancytopenia
Hepatic: Hepatic necrosis, hepatitis
Neuromuscular & skeletal: Tremors
Renal: BUN increased, interstitial nephritis, renal failure, serum creatinine increased
Respiratory: Respiratory failure, alveolitis (resembling eosinophilic or allergic)
(Continued)

Sulfadoxine and Pyrimethamine *(Continued)*

Miscellaneous: Anaphylactoid reaction, drug fever, hypersensitivity, Lupus-like syndrome, periarteritis nodosum

Mechanism of Action Sulfadoxine interferes with bacterial folic acid synthesis and growth via competitive inhibition of para-aminiobenzoic acid; pyrimethamine inhibits microbial dihydrofolate reductase, resulting in inhibition of tetrahydrofolic acid synthesis

Drug Interactions

Cytochrome P450 Effect: Pyrimethamine: **Inhibits** CYP2C8/9 (moderate), 2D6 (moderate)

Increased Effect/Toxicity: Effect of oral hypoglycemics (rare, but severe) may occur. Combination with methenamine may result in crystalluria; avoid use. May increase methotrexate-induced bone marrow suppression. NSAIDs and salicylates may increase sulfonamide concentrations. Pyrimethamine may increase the levels/effects of amiodarone, amphetamines, selected beta-blockers, dextromethorphan, fluoxetine, glimepiride, glipizide, lidocaine, mirtazapine, nateglinide, nefazodone, paroxetine, phenytoin, pioglitazone, risperidone, ritonavir, rosiglitazone, sertraline, thioridazine, tricyclic antidepressants, venlafaxine, warfarin, and other CYP2C8/9 and 2D6 substrates.

Decreased Effect: Cyclosporine concentrations may be decreased; monitor levels and renal function. PABA (para-aminobenzoic acid - may be found in some vitamin supplements): interferes with the antibacterial activity of sulfonamides; avoid concurrent use. Pyrimethamine may decrease the levels/effects of CYP2D6 prodrug substrates (eg, codeine, hydrocodone, oxycodone, tramadol).

Pharmacodynamics/Kinetics

Absorption: Well absorbed

Distribution: Sulfadoxine: Well distributed like other sulfonamides; Pyrimethamine: Widely distributed, mainly in blood cells, kidneys, lungs, liver, and spleen

Metabolism: Pyrimethamine: Hepatic; Sulfadoxine: None

Half-life elimination: Pyrimethamine: 80-95 hours; Sulfadoxine: 5-8 days

Time to peak, serum: 2-8 hours

Excretion: Urine (as unchanged drug and several unidentified metabolites)

Pregnancy Risk Factor C/D (at term)

Sulfamethoxazole and Trimethoprim

(sul fa meth OKS a zole & trye METH oh prim)

Related Information

Trimethoprim *on page 1620*

U.S. Brand Names Bactrim™; Bactrim™ DS; Septra®; Septra® DS

Canadian Brand Names Apo-Sulfatrim®; Apo-Sulfatrim® DS; Apo-Sulfatrim® Pediatric; Novo-Trimel; Novo-Trimel D.S.; Nu-Cotrimox; Septra® Injection

Mexican Brand Names Anitrix; Bactrim; Ectaprim; Septrin Familia; Servitrim; Trimetox

Generic Available Yes

Index Terms Co-Trimoxazole; SMZ-TMP; Sulfatrim; TMP-SMZ; Trimethoprim and Sulfamethoxazole

Pharmacologic Category Antibiotic, Miscellaneous; Antibiotic, Sulfonamide Derivative

Use

Oral treatment of urinary tract infections due to *E. coli*, *Klebsiella* and *Enterobacter* sp, *M. morganii*, *P. mirabilis* and *P. vulgaris*; acute otitis media in children; acute exacerbations of chronic bronchitis in adults due to susceptible strains of *H. influenzae* or *S. pneumoniae*; treatment and prophylaxis of *Pneumocystis jiroveci* pneumonitis (PCP); traveler's diarrhea due to enterotoxigenic *E. coli*; treatment of enteritis caused by *Shigella flexneri* or *Shigella sonnei*

I.V. treatment or severe or complicated infections when oral therapy is not feasible, for documented PCP, empiric treatment of PCP in immune compromised patients; treatment of documented or suspected shigellosis, typhoid fever, *Nocardia asteroides* infection, or other infections caused by susceptible bacteria

Unlabeled/Investigational Use Cholera and *Salmonella*-type infections and nocardiosis; chronic prostatitis; as prophylaxis in neutropenic patients with *P. jiroveci* infections, in leukemics, and in patients following renal transplantation, to decrease incidence of PCP; treatment of *Cyclospora* infection, typhoid fever, *Nocardia asteroides* infection

Local Anesthetic/Vasoconstrictor Precautions No information available to require special precautions

Effects on Dental Treatment Key adverse event(s) related to dental treatment: Stomatitis.

Common Adverse Effects The most common adverse reactions include gastrointestinal upset (nausea, vomiting, anorexia) and dermatologic reactions (rash or urticaria). Rare, life-threatening reactions have been associated with co-trimoxazole, including severe dermatologic reactions and hepatotoxic reactions. Most other reactions listed are rare, however, frequency cannot be accurately estimated.

Cardiovascular: Allergic myocarditis

Central nervous system: Confusion, depression, hallucinations, seizure, aseptic meningitis, peripheral neuritis, fever, ataxia, kernicterus in neonates

Dermatologic: Rashes, pruritus, urticaria, photosensitivity; rare reactions include erythema multiforme, Stevens-Johnson syndrome, toxic epidermal necrolysis, exfoliative dermatitis, and Henoch-Schönlein purpura

Endocrine & metabolic: Hyperkalemia (generally at high dosages), hypoglycemia

Gastrointestinal: Nausea, vomiting, anorexia, stomatitis, diarrhea, pseudomembranous colitis, pancreatitis

Hematologic: Thrombocytopenia, megaloblastic anemia, granulocytopenia, eosinophilia, pancytopenia, aplastic anemia, methemoglobinemia, hemolysis (with G6PD deficiency), agranulocytosis

Hepatic: Hepatotoxicity (including hepatitis, cholestasis, and hepatic necrosis), hyperbilirubinemia, transaminases increased

Neuromuscular & skeletal: Arthralgia, myalgia, rhabdomyolysis

Renal: Interstitial nephritis, crystalluria, renal failure, nephrotoxicity (in association with cyclosporine), diuresis

Respiratory: Cough, dyspnea, pulmonary infiltrates

Miscellaneous: Serum sickness, angioedema, periarteritis nodosa (rare), systemic lupus erythematosus (rare)

Dosage Dosage recommendations are based on the trimethoprim component. Double-strength tablets are equivalent to sulfamethoxazole 800 mg and trimethoprim 160 mg.

Children >2 months:

General dosing guidelines:

Mild-to-moderate infections: Oral: 8-12 mg TMP/kg/day in divided doses every 12 hours

Serious infection:

Oral: 20 mg TMP/kg/day in divided doses every 6 hours

I.V.: 8-12 mg TMP/kg/day in divided doses every 6 hours

Acute otitis media: Oral: 8 mg TMP/kg/day in divided doses every 12 hours for 10 days

Urinary tract infection:

Treatment:

Oral: 6-12 mg TMP/kg/day in divided doses every 12 hours

I.V.: 8-10 mg TMP/kg/day in divided doses every 6, 8, or 12 hours for up to 4 days with serious infections

Prophylaxis: Oral: 2 mg TMP/kg/dose daily or 5 mg TMP/kg/dose twice weekly

Pneumocystis:

Treatment: Oral, I.V.: 15-20 mg TMP/kg/day in divided doses every 6-8 hours

Prophylaxis: Oral, 150 mg TMP/m^2/day in divided doses every 12 hours for 3 days/week; dose should not exceed trimethoprim 320 mg and sulfamethoxazole 1600 mg daily

Alternative prophylaxis dosing schedules include:

150 mg TMP/m^2/day as a single daily dose 3 times/week on consecutive days

or

150 mg TMP/m^2/day in divided doses every 12 hours administered 7 days/week

or

150 mg TMP/m^2/day in divided doses every 12 hours administered 3 times/week on alternate days

Shigellosis:

Oral: 8 mg TMP/kg/day in divided doses every 12 hours for 5 days

I.V.: 8-10 mg TMP/kg/day in divided doses every 6, 8, or 12 hours for up to 5 days

Cyclospora (unlabeled use): Oral, I.V.: 5 mg TMP/kg twice daily for 7-10 days

Adults:

Urinary tract infection:

Oral: One double-strength tablet every 12 hours

Duration of therapy: Uncomplicated: 3-5 days; Complicated: 7-10 days

Pyelonephritis: 14 days

(Continued)

Sulfamethoxazole and Trimethoprim *(Continued)*

Prostatitis: Acute: 2 weeks; Chronic: 2-3 months

I.V.: 8-10 mg TMP/kg/day in divided doses every 6, 8, or 12 hours for up to 14 days with severe infections

Chronic bronchitis: Oral: One double-strength tablet every 12 hours for 10-14 days

Meningitis (bacterial): I.V.: 10-20 mg TMP/kg/day in divided doses every 6-12 hours

Shigellosis:

Oral: One double strength tablet every 12 hours for 5 days

I.V.: 8-10 mg TMP/kg/day in divided doses every 6, 8, or 12 hours for up to 5 days

Travelers' diarrhea: Oral: One double strength tablet every 12 hours for 5 days

Sepsis: I.V.: 20 TMP/kg/day divided every 6 hours

Pneumocystis jiroveci:

Prophylaxis: Oral: 1 double strength tablet daily or 3 times/week

Treatment: Oral, I.V.: 15-20 mg TMP/kg/day in 3-4 divided doses

Cyclospora (unlabeled use): Oral, I.V.: 160 mg TMP twice daily for 7-10 days

Nocardia (unlabeled use): Oral, I.V.:

Cutaneous infections: 5 mg TMP/kg/day in 2 divided doses

Severe infections (pulmonary/cerebral): 10-15 mg TMP/kg/day in 2-3 divided doses. Treatment duration is controversial; an average of 7 months has been reported.

Note: Therapy for severe infection may be initiated I.V. and converted to oral therapy (frequently converted to approximate dosages of oral solid dosage forms: 2 DS tablets every 8-12 hours). Although not widely available, sulfonamide levels should be considered in patients with questionable absorption, at risk for dose-related toxicity, or those with poor therapeutic response.

Dosing adjustment in renal impairment: Oral, I.V.:

Cl_{cr} 15-30 mL/minute: Administer 50% of recommended dose

Cl_{cr} <15 mL/minute: Use is not recommended

Mechanism of Action Sulfamethoxazole interferes with bacterial folic acid synthesis and growth via inhibition of dihydrofolic acid formation from para-aminobenzoic acid; trimethoprim inhibits dihydrofolic acid reduction to tetrahydrofolate resulting in sequential inhibition of enzymes of the folic acid pathway

Contraindications Hypersensitivity to any sulfa drug, trimethoprim, or any component of the formulation; porphyria; megaloblastic anemia due to folate deficiency; infants <2 months of age; marked hepatic damage; severe renal disease; pregnancy (at term)

Warnings/Precautions Use with caution in patients with G6PD deficiency, impaired renal or hepatic function or potential folate deficiency (malnourished, chronic anticonvulsant therapy, or elderly); maintain adequate hydration to prevent crystalluria; adjust dosage in patients with renal impairment. Injection vehicle contains benzyl alcohol and sodium metabisulfite.

Chemical similarities are present among sulfonamides, sulfonylureas, carbonic anhydrase inhibitors, thiazides, and loop diuretics (except ethacrynic acid). Use in patients with sulfonamide allergy is specifically contraindicated in product labeling, however, a risk of cross-reaction exists in patients with allergy to any of these compounds; avoid use when previous reaction has been severe.

Fatalities associated with severe reactions including Stevens-Johnson syndrome, toxic epidermal necrolysis, hepatic necrosis, agranulocytosis, aplastic anemia and other blood dyscrasias; discontinue use at first sign of rash. Elderly patients appear at greater risk for more severe adverse reactions. May cause hypoglycemia, particularly in malnourished, or patients with renal or hepatic impairment. Use with caution in patients with porphyria or thyroid dysfunction. Slow acetylators may be more prone to adverse reactions. Caution in patients with allergies or asthma. May cause hyperkalemia (associated with high doses of trimethoprim). Incidence of adverse effects appears to be increased in patients with AIDS.

Drug Interactions

Cytochrome P450 Effect:

Sulfamethoxazole: **Substrate** of CYP2C9 (major), 3A4 (minor); **Inhibits** CYP2C9 (moderate)

Trimethoprim: **Substrate** (major) of CYP2C9, 3A4; **Inhibits** CYP2C8 (moderate), 2C9 (moderate)

Increased Effect/Toxicity: Sulfamethoxazole/trimethoprim may increase toxicity of methotrexate. Sulfamethoxazole/trimethoprim may increase the serum levels of procainamide. Concurrent therapy with pyrimethamine (in doses >25 mg/week) may increase the risk of megaloblastic anemia. Sulfamethoxazole/trimethoprim may increase the levels/effects of amiodarone, fluoxetine, glimepiride, glipizide, nateglinide, phenytoin, pioglitazone, rosiglitazone, sertraline, warfarin, and other CYP2C8 and 2C9 substrates.

ACE Inhibitors, angiotensin receptor antagonists, or potassium-sparing diuretics may increase the risk of hyperkalemia. Concurrent use with cyclosporine may result in an increased risk of nephrotoxicity when used with sulfamethoxazole/trimethoprim. Trimethoprim may increase the serum concentration of dapsone.

Decreased Effect: The levels/effects of sulfamethoxazole may be decreased by carbamazepine, phenobarbital, phenytoin, rifampin, rifapentine, secobarbital, and other CYP2C9 inducers. Although occasionally recommended to limit or reverse hematologic toxicity of high-dose sulfamethoxazole/trimethoprim, concurrent use has been associated with a decreased effectiveness in treating *Pneumocystis carinii.*

Ethanol/Nutrition/Herb Interactions Herb/Nutraceutical: Avoid dong quai, St John's wort (may also cause photosensitization).

Dietary Considerations Should be taken with 8 oz of water.

Pharmacodynamics/Kinetics

Absorption: Oral: Almost completely, 90% to 100%

Protein binding: SMX: 68%, TMP: 45%

Metabolism: SMX: N-acetylated and glucuronidated; TMP: Metabolized to oxide and hydroxylated metabolites

Half-life elimination: SMX: 9 hours, TMP: 6-17 hours; both are prolonged in renal failure

Time to peak, serum: Within 1-4 hours

Excretion: Both are excreted in urine as metabolites and unchanged drug

Effects of aging on the pharmacokinetics of both agents has been variable; increase in half-life and decreases in clearance have been associated with reduced creatinine clearance

Pregnancy Risk Factor C/D (at term - expert analysis)

Dosage Forms The 5:1 ratio (SMX:TMP) remains constant in all dosage forms.

Injection, solution: Sulfamethoxazole 80 mg and trimethoprim 16 mg per mL (5 mL, 10 mL, 30 mL)

Suspension, oral: Sulfamethoxazole 200 mg and trimethoprim 40 mg per 5 mL

Tablet: Sulfamethoxazole 400 mg and trimethoprim 80 mg

Bactrim™, Septra®: Sulfamethoxazole 400 mg and trimethoprim 80 mg

Tablet, double strength: Sulfamethoxazole 800 mg and trimethoprim 160 mg

Bactrim™ DS, Septra® DS: Sulfamethoxazole 800 mg and trimethoprim 160 mg

Sulfamylon® *see* Mafenide *on page 1012*

Sulfasalazine (sul fa SAL a zeen)

U.S. Brand Names Azulfidine®; Azulfidine® EN-tabs®; Sulfazine; Sulfazine EC

Canadian Brand Names Alti-Sulfasalazine; Salazopyrin®; Salazopyrin En-Tabs®

Mexican Brand Names Azulfidina

Generic Available Yes

Index Terms Salicylazosulfapyridine

Pharmacologic Category 5-Aminosalicylic Acid Derivative

Use Management of ulcerative colitis; enteric coated tablets are also used for rheumatoid arthritis (including juvenile rheumatoid arthritis) in patients who inadequately respond to analgesics and NSAIDs

Unlabeled/Investigational Use Ankylosing spondylitis, collagenous colitis, Crohn's disease, psoriasis, psoriatic arthritis, juvenile chronic arthritis

Local Anesthetic/Vasoconstrictor Precautions No information available to require special precautions

Effects on Dental Treatment No significant effects or complications reported

Common Adverse Effects

>10%:

Central nervous system: Headache (33%)

Dermatologic: Photosensitivity

Gastrointestinal: Anorexia, nausea, vomiting, diarrhea (33%), gastric distress

Genitourinary: Reversible oligospermia (33%)

<3%:

Dermatologic: Urticaria/pruritus (<3%)

Hematologic: Hemolytic anemia (<3%), Heinz body anemia (<3%)

(Continued)

Sulfasalazine *(Continued)*

Additional events reported with sulfonamides and/or 5-ASA derivatives: Cholestatic jaundice, eosinophilia pneumonitis, erythema multiforme, fibrosing alveolitis, hepatic necrosis, Kawasaki-like syndrome, SLE-like syndrome, pericarditis, seizure, transverse myelitis

Mechanism of Action Acts locally in the colon to decrease the inflammatory response and systemically interferes with secretion by inhibiting prostaglandin synthesis

Drug Interactions

Increased Effect/Toxicity: Sulfasalazine may increase hydantoin levels. Effects of thiopental, oral hypoglycemics, and oral anticoagulants may be increased. Sulfasalazine may increase the risk of myelosuppression with azathioprine, mercaptopurine, or thioguanine (due to TPMT inhibition); may also increase the toxicity of methotrexate. Risk of thrombocytopenia may be increased with thiazide diuretics. Concurrent methenamine may increase risk of crystalluria.

Decreased Effect: Decreased effect with iron, digoxin and PABA or PABA metabolites of drugs (eg, procaine, proparacaine, tetracaine). Sulfasalazine may decrease serum cyclosporine concentrations.

Pharmacodynamics/Kinetics

Absorption: 10% to 15% as unchanged drug from small intestine

Distribution: Small amounts enter feces and breast milk

Metabolism: Via colonic intestinal flora to sulfapyridine and 5-aminosalicylic acid (5-ASA); following absorption, sulfapyridine undergoes N-acetylation and ring hydroxylation while 5-ASA undergoes N-acetylation

Half-life elimination: 5.7-10 hours

Excretion: Primarily urine (as unchanged drug, components, and acetylated metabolites)

Pregnancy Risk Factor B/D (at term)

Sulfatrim *see* Sulfamethoxazole and Trimethoprim *on page 1504*

Sulfazine *see* Sulfasalazine *on page 1507*

Sulfazine EC *see* Sulfasalazine *on page 1507*

SulfiSOXAZOLE *(sul fi SOKS a zole)*

U.S. Brand Names Gantrisin®
Canadian Brand Names Novo-Soxazole; Sulfizole®
Generic Available Yes: Tablet
Index Terms Sulfisoxazole Acetyl; Sulphafurazole
Pharmacologic Category Antibiotic, Sulfonamide Derivative
Use Treatment of urinary tract infections, otitis media, *Chlamydia*; nocardiosis
Local Anesthetic/Vasoconstrictor Precautions No information available to require special precautions
Effects on Dental Treatment No significant effects or complications reported
Mechanism of Action Interferes with bacterial growth by inhibiting bacterial folic acid synthesis through competitive antagonism of PABA
Pregnancy Risk Factor B/D (near term)

Sulfisoxazole Acetyl *see* SulfiSOXAZOLE *on page 1508*

Sulfisoxazole and Erythromycin *see* Erythromycin and Sulfisoxazole *on page 595*

Sulfonated Phenolics in Aqueous Solution
(SUL fo NATE ed fe NOL iks in AYE kwee us so LU shun)

Related Information
Ulcerative and Erosive Disorders *on page 1809*
U.S. Brand Names Debacterol®
Generic Available No
Pharmacologic Category Aphthous Ulcer Treatment Agent
Dental Use Therapeutic cauterization in the treatment of oral mucosal lesions (aphthous stomatitis, gingivitis, moderate to severe periodontitis)
Local Anesthetic/Vasoconstrictor Precautions No information available to require special precautions
Effects on Dental Treatment No significant effects or complications reported
Significant Adverse Effects Frequency not defined: Local: Irritation upon administration
Dental Usual Dosing Apply applicator tip to the lesion as directed (see Dental Comment)

Mechanism of Action Semiviscous, chemical cautery agent which provides controlled, focal debridement and sterilization of necrotic tissues; relieving pain, sealing damaged tissue, and providing local antiseptic action

Contraindications For external use only

Warnings/Precautions For topical use only. Debacterol® is not intended for the treatment of cold sores and fever blisters. Prolonged use of Debacterol® on normal tissue should be avoided. If ingested, do not induce vomiting; immediately dilute with milk or water and get medical help or contact a Poison Control Center. If eye exposure occurs, immediately remove contact lenses, irrigate eyes for at least 15 minutes with lukewarm water, and contact a physician. Safety and efficacy in children <12 years have not been established.

Pregnancy Risk Factor C

Breast-Feeding Considerations Unknown if excreted in breast milk; use with caution

Dosage Forms Excipient information presented when available (limited, particularly for generics); consult specific product labeling.

Debacterol® single-use applicator package: Prefilled cotton swab applicator and drying cotton swab: 0.2 mL (30% sulfuric acid, 22% sulfonated phenolics in aqueous solution) [also supplied as one box of 12 single-use applicator packages]

Dental Comment Prior to application/treatment, the ulcerated mucosal area should be thoroughly dried using the drying swab. After drying lesion, hold applicator "swab" with the colored ring end up. Bend the colored ring tip gently to the side until it snaps to release liquid inside. Liquid flows down into the white tip applicator. Apply the Debacterol® coated applicator tip to the dried ulcer area for at least 5 seconds, but no more than 10 seconds. Use rolling motion to completely cover the entire ulcer bed and ulcer rim. A "stinging" sensation is experienced immediately upon application. Debacterol® will not harm normal mucosa when used as directed. Thoroughly rinse out the mouth with water and spit out the rinse water. If the ulcer pain returns shortly after rinsing with water, it is an indication that some part of the ulcer was not covered. Repeat application one more time following directions above. One application per ulcer is usually sufficient. If excess irritation occurs during use, a rinse with sodium bicarbonate (baking soda) solution will neutralize the reaction (use 0.5 teaspoon in 120 mL water). It is not recommended that more than one Debacterol® treatment session be performed on an individual ulcer.

Selected Readings

Rhodus NL and Bereuter J, "An Evaluation of a Chemical Cautery Agent and an Anti-inflammatory Ointment for the Treatment of Recurrent Aphthous Stomatitis: A Pilot Study," *Quintessence Int*, 1998, 29(12):769-73.

Sulindac (SUL in dak)

Related Information

Rheumatoid Arthritis, Osteoarthritis, and Osteoporosis *on page 1759*
Temporomandibular Dysfunction (TMD) *on page 1822*

U.S. Brand Names Clinoril®

Canadian Brand Names Apo-Sulin®; Novo-Sundac; Nu-Sundac

Mexican Brand Names Clinoril; Copal

Generic Available Yes

Pharmacologic Category Nonsteroidal Anti-inflammatory Drug (NSAID), Oral

Use Management of inflammatory disease, osteoarthritis, rheumatoid disorders, acute gouty arthritis, ankylosing spondylitis, bursitis/tendonitis of shoulder

Local Anesthetic/Vasoconstrictor Precautions No information available to require special precautions

Effects on Dental Treatment NSAID formulations are known to reversibly decrease platelet aggregation via mechanisms different than observed with aspirin. The dentist should be aware of the potential of abnormal coagulation. Caution should also be exercised in the use of NSAIDs in patients already on anticoagulant therapy with drugs such as warfarin (Coumadin®).

Common Adverse Effects 1% to 10%:

Cardiovascular: Edema (1% to 3%)

Central nervous system: Dizziness (3% to 9%), headache (3% to 9%), nervousness (1% to 3%)

Dermatologic: Rash (3% to 9%), pruritus (1% to 3%)

Gastrointestinal: GI pain (10%), constipation (3% to 9%), diarrhea (3% to 9%), dyspepsia (3% to 9%), nausea (3% to 9%), abdominal cramps (1% to 3%), anorexia (1% to 3%), flatulence (1% to 3%), vomiting (1% to 3%)

Otic: Tinnitus (1% to 3%)

Restrictions An FDA-approved medication guide must be distributed when dispensing an oral outpatient prescription (new or refill) where this medication is to be used without direct supervision of a healthcare provider. Medication (Continued)

Sulindac *(Continued)*

guides are available at http://www.fda.gov/cder/Offices/ODS/medication_guides.htm.

Dosage Oral:

Children: Dose not established

Adults: **Note:** Maximum daily dose: 400 mg

Osteoarthritis, rheumatoid arthritis, ankylosing spondylitis: 150 mg twice/daily

Bursitis/tendonitis: 200 mg twice daily; usual treatment: 7-14 days

Acute gouty arthritis: 200 mg twice daily; usual treatment: 7 days

Dosing adjustment in renal impairment: Not recommended with advanced renal impairment; if required, decrease dose and monitor closely

Dosing adjustment in hepatic impairment: Dose reduction is necessary; discontinue if abnormal liver function tests occur

Mechanism of Action Inhibits prostaglandin synthesis by decreasing the activity of the enzyme, cyclooxygenase, which results in decreased formation of prostaglandin precursors

Contraindications Hypersensitivity to sulindac, aspirin, other NSAIDs, or any component of the formulation; perioperative pain in the setting of coronary artery bypass surgery (CABG); pregnancy (3rd trimester)

Warnings/Precautions [U.S. Boxed Warning]: NSAIDs are associated with an increased risk of adverse cardiovascular events, including MI, stroke, and new onset or worsening of pre-existing hypertension. Use caution with fluid retention, CHF or hypertension. Concurrent administration of ibuprofen, and potentially other nonselective NSAIDs, may interfere with aspirin's cardioprotective effect. Use of NSAIDs can compromise existing renal function. Sulindac is not recommended for patients with advanced renal disease. Use caution in patients with renal lithiasis; sulindac metabolites have been reported as components of renal stones. Use hydration in patients with a history of renal stones. Use with caution in patients with decreased hepatic function. May require dosage adjustment in hepatic dysfunction; sulfide and sulfone metabolites may accumulate.

[U.S. Boxed Warning]: NSAIDs may increase risk of gastrointestinal irritation, ulceration, bleeding, and perforation. Use the lowest effective dose for the shortest duration of time, consistent with individual patient goals, to reduce risk of cardiovascular or GI adverse events.

NSAIDs may cause serious skin adverse events including exfoliative dermatitis, Stevens-Johnson syndrome (SJS) and toxic epidermal necrolysis (TEN). Anaphylactoid reactions may occur. Do not use in patients who experience bronchospasm, asthma, rhinitis, or urticaria with NSAID or aspirin therapy. Use caution in other forms of asthma.

Withhold for at least 4-6 half-lives prior to surgical or dental procedures.

Drug Interactions

Increased Effect/Toxicity: Sulindac may increase effect/toxicity of anticoagulants (bleeding), antiplatelet agents (bleeding), aminoglycosides, bisphosphonates (GI irritation), corticosteroids (GI irritation), cyclosporine (nephrotoxicity), lithium, methotrexate, pemetrexed, treprostinil (bleeding), vancomycin. Concomitant use with fluoroquinolones may rarely increase risk of seizure.

Decreased Effect: May reduce effect of some diuretics and antihypertensive effect of beta-blockers, ACE inhibitors, angiotensin II inhibitors, and hydralazine. Dimethyl sulfoxide may decrease active metabolite of sulindac; combination may cause peripheral neuropathy. Cholestyramine (and other bile acid sequestrants) may decrease the absorption of NSAIDs; separate by at least 2 hours. Salicylates' antiplatelet effect may be reduced.

Ethanol/Nutrition/Herb Interactions

Ethanol: Avoid ethanol (may enhance gastric mucosal irritation).

Food: Food may decrease the rate but not the extent of oral absorption. The therapeutic effect of sulindac may be decreased if taken with food.

Herb/Nutraceutical: Avoid alfalfa, anise, bilberry, bladderwrack, bromelain, cat's claw, celery, coleus, cordyceps, dong quai, evening primrose, feverfew, fenugreek, garlic, ginger, ginkgo biloba, red clover, horse chestnut, grapeseed, green tea, ginseng, guggul, horse chestnut seed, horseradish, licorice, prickly ash, red clover, reishi, SAMe, sweet clover, turmeric, white willow (all have additional antiplatelet activity).

Dietary Considerations Drug may cause GI upset, bleeding, ulceration, perforation; take with food or milk to minimize GI upset.

Pharmacodynamics/Kinetics

Onset of action: Analgesic: ~1 hour

Duration: 12-24 hours

Absorption: 90%

Protein binding: Parent, sulfide metabolite (active): 93% to 98% primarily to albumin

Distribution: Crosses blood-brain barrier and placental barriers

Metabolism: Hepatic; prodrug metabolized to sulfide metabolite (active) for therapeutic effects and to sulfone metabolites (inactive); parent and inactive sulfone metabolite undergo extensive enterohepatic recirculation

Half-life elimination: Parent drug: ~8 hours; Active metabolite: ~16 hours

Excretion: Urine (50%, primarily as inactive metabolites); feces (25%, primarily as metabolites)

Pregnancy Risk Factor C/D (3rd trimester)

Dosage Forms
  Tablet: 150 mg, 200 mg
  Clinoril®: 200 mg

Sulphafurazole *see* SulfiSOXAZOLE *on page 1508*

Sumatriptan (soo ma TRIP tan)

U.S. Brand Names Imitrex®
Canadian Brand Names Apo-Sumatriptan®; CO Sumatriptan; Dom-Sumatriptan; Gen-Sumatriptan; Imitrex®; Imitrex® DF; Imitrex® Nasal Spray; Novo-Sumatriptan; PHL-Sumatriptan; PMS-Sumatriptan; ratio-Sumatriptan; Rhoxal-sumatriptan; Riva-Sumatriptan; Sandoz-Sumatriptan; Sumatryx
Mexican Brand Names Imigran
Generic Available No
Index Terms Sumatriptan Succinate
Pharmacologic Category Antimigraine Agent; Serotonin 5-HT$_{1B, 1D}$ Receptor Agonist
Use
  Oral, SubQ: Acute treatment of migraine with or without aura
  SubQ: Acute treatment of cluster headache episodes
Local Anesthetic/Vasoconstrictor Precautions No information available to require special precautions
Effects on Dental Treatment Key adverse event(s) related to dental treatment: Bad taste, dysphagia, hyposalivation (tablet), mouth/tongue discomfort (injection).
Common Adverse Effects
  Injection:
  >10%:
    Central nervous system: Dizziness (12%), warm/hot sensation (11%)
    Local: Pain at injection site (59%)
    Neuromuscular & skeletal: Paresthesia (14%)
  1% to 10%:
    Cardiovascular: Chest pain/tightness/heaviness/pressure (2% to 3%), hyper-/hypotension (1%)
    Central nervous system: Burning (7%), feeling of heaviness (7%), flushing (7%), pressure sensation (7%), feeling of tightness (5%), drowsiness (3%), malaise/fatigue (1%), feeling strange (2%), headache (2%), tight feeling in head (2%), cold sensation (1%), anxiety (1%)
    Gastrointestinal: Abdominal discomfort (1%), dysphagia (1%)
    Neuromuscular & skeletal: Neck, throat, and jaw pain/tightness/pressure (2% to 5%), mouth/tongue discomfort (5%), weakness (5%), myalgia (2%); muscle cramps (1%), numbness (5%)
    Ocular: Vision alterations (1%)
    Respiratory: Throat discomfort (3%), nasal disorder/discomfort (2%)
    Miscellaneous: Diaphoresis (2%)

  Nasal spray:
  >10%: Gastrointestinal: Bad taste (13% to 24%), nausea (11% to 13%), vomiting (11% to 13%)
  1% to 10%:
    Central nervous system: Dizziness (1% to 2%)
    Respiratory: Nasal disorder/discomfort (2% to 4%), throat discomfort (1% to 2%)

  Tablet:
  1% to 10%:
    Cardiovascular: Chest pain/tightness/heaviness/pressure (1% to 2%), hyper-/hypotension (1%), palpitation (1%), syncope (1%)
    Central nervous system: Burning (1%), dizziness (>1%), drowsiness (>1%), malaise/fatigue (2% to 3%), headache (>1%), nonspecified pain (1% to 2%, placebo 1%), vertigo (<1% to 2%), migraine (>1%), sleepiness (>1%)
(Continued)

Sumatriptan *(Continued)*

Gastrointestinal: Diarrhea (1%), nausea (>1%), vomiting (>1%), hyposalivation (>1%)

Genitourinary: Hematuria (1%)

Hematologic: Hemolytic anemia (1%)

Neuromuscular & skeletal: Neck, throat, and jaw pain/tightness/pressure (2%
to 3%), paresthesia (3% to 5%), myalgia (1%), numbness (1%)

Otic: Ear hemorrhage (1%), hearing loss (1%), sensitivity to noise (1%),
tinnitus (1%)

Respiratory: Allergic rhinitis (1%), dyspnea (1%), nasal inflammation (1%),
nose/throat hemorrhage (1%), sinusitis (1%), upper respiratory inflammation
(1%)

Miscellaneous: Hypersensitivity reactions (1%), nonspecified pressure/tight-
ness/heaviness (1% to 3%, placebo 2%); warm/cold sensation (2% to 3%,
placebo 2%)

Dosage Adults:

Oral: A single dose of 25 mg, 50 mg, or 100 mg (taken with fluids). If a
satisfactory response has not been obtained at 2 hours, a second dose may
be administered. Results from clinical trials show that initial doses of 50 mg
and 100 mg are more effective than doses of 25 mg, and that 100 mg doses
do not provide a greater effect than 50 mg and may have increased incidence
of side effects. Although doses of up to 300 mg/day have been studied, the
total daily dose should not exceed 200 mg. The safety of treating an average
of >4 headaches in a 30-day period have not been established.

Intranasal: A single dose of 5 mg, 10 mg, or 20 mg administered in one nostril. A
10 mg dose may be achieved by administering a single 5 mg dose in each
nostril. If headache returns, the dose may be repeated once after 2 hours, not
to exceed a total daily dose of 40 mg. The safety of treating an average of >4
headaches in a 30-day period has not been established.

SubQ: Up to 6 mg; if side effects are dose-limiting, lower doses may be used. A
second injection may be administered at least 1 hour after the initial dose, but
not more than 2 injections in a 24-hour period.

Dosage adjustment in renal impairment: Dosage adjustment not necessary

Dosage adjustment in hepatic impairment: Bioavailability of oral sumatriptan
is increased with liver disease. If treatment is needed, do not exceed single
doses of 50 mg. The nasal spray has not been studied in patients with hepatic
impairment, however, because the spray does not undergo first-pass metabolism, levels would not be expected to alter. Use of all dosage forms is contraindicated with severe hepatic impairment.

Mechanism of Action Selective agonist for serotonin (5-HT$_{1D}$ receptor) in
cranial arteries to cause vasoconstriction and reduces sterile inflammation
associated with antidromic neuronal transmission correlating with relief of
migraine

Contraindications Hypersensitivity to sumatriptan or any component of the
formulation; patients with ischemic heart disease or signs or symptoms of
ischemic heart disease (including Prinzmetal's angina, angina pectoris, myocardial infarction, silent myocardial ischemia); cerebrovascular syndromes
(including strokes, transient ischemic attacks); peripheral vascular syndromes
(including ischemic bowel disease); uncontrolled hypertension; use within 24
hours of ergotamine derivatives; use within 24 hours of another 5-HT$_1$ agonist;
concurrent administration or within 2 weeks of discontinuing an MAO inhibitor,
specifically MAO type A inhibitors; management of hemiplegic or basilar
migraine; prophylactic treatment of migraine; severe hepatic impairment; not for
I.V. administration

Warnings/Precautions Sumatriptan is indicated only in patients ≥18 years of
age with a clear diagnosis of migraine or cluster headache. Cardiac events
(coronary artery vasospasm, transient ischemia, myocardial infarction, ventricular tachycardia/fibrillation, cardiac arrest and death), cerebral/subarachnoid
hemorrhage, and stroke have been reported with 5-HT$_1$ agonist administration.
Do not give to patients with risk factors for CAD until a cardiovascular evaluation
has been performed; if evaluation is satisfactory, the healthcare provider should
administer the first dose and cardiovascular status should be periodically evaluated.

Significant elevation in blood pressure, including hypertensive crisis, has also
been reported on rare occasions in patients with and without a history of hypertension. Vasospasm-related reactions have been reported other than coronary
artery vasospasm. Peripheral vascular ischemia and colonic ischemia with
abdominal pain and bloody diarrhea have occurred. Use with caution in patients
with a history of seizure disorder or in patients with a lowered seizure threshold.
Use with caution in patients with hepatic impairment. Symptoms of agitation,
confusion, hallucinations, hyper-reflexia, myoclonus, shivering, and tachycardia
(serotonin syndrome) may occur with concomitant proserotonergic drugs (ie,

SSRIs/SNRIs or triptans) or agents which reduce sumatriptan's metabolism. Concurrent use of serotonin precursors (eg, tryptophan) is not recommended. Safety and efficacy in pediatric patients have not been established.

Drug Interactions

Increased Effect/Toxicity: Increased toxicity with ergot-containing drugs, avoid use, wait 24 hours from last ergot containing drug (dihydroergotamine, or methysergide) before administering sumatriptan. MAO inhibitors decrease clearance of sumatriptan increasing the risk of systemic sumatriptan toxic effects. SSRIs/SNRIs or other serotonin agonists may increase symptoms of hyper-reflexia, weakness, and incoordination. **Note:** Use cautiously in patients receiving concomitant medications that can lower the seizure threshold.

Pharmacodynamics/Kinetics

Onset of action: ~30 minutes

Distribution: V_d: 2.4 L/kg

Protein binding: 14% to 21%

Metabolism: Hepatic, primarily via MAO-A isoenzyme

Bioavailability: SubQ: 97% ± 16% of that following I.V. injection; Oral: 15%

Half-life elimination: Injection, tablet: 2.5 hours; Nasal spray: 2 hours

Time to peak, serum: 5-20 minutes

Excretion:

Injection: Urine (38% as indole acetic acid metabolite, 22% as unchanged drug)

Nasal spray: Urine (42% as indole acetic acid metabolite, 3% as unchanged drug)

Tablet: Urine (60% as indole acetic acid metabolite, 3% as unchanged drug); feces (40%)

Pregnancy Risk Factor C

Dosage Forms

Injection, solution:

Imitrex®: 8 mg/mL (0.5 mL); 12 mg/mL (0.5 mL)

Solution, intranasal spray:

Imitrex®: 5 mg (100 µL unit dose spray device); 20 mg (100 µL unit dose spray device)

Tablet:

Imitrex®: 25 mg, 50 mg, 100 mg

Sumatriptan Succinate *see* Sumatriptan *on page 1511*

Summer's Eve® Medicated Douche [OTC] *see* Povidone-Iodine *on page 1332*

Summer's Eve® SpecialCare™ Medicated Anti-Itch Cream [OTC] *see* Hydrocortisone *on page 836*

Sumycin® [DSC] *see* Tetracycline *on page 1548*

Sunitinib (su NIT e nib)

U.S. Brand Names Sutent®

Generic Available No

Index Terms NSC736511; SU11248; Sunitinib Maleate

Pharmacologic Category Antineoplastic Agent, Tyrosine Kinase Inhibitor; Vascular Endothelial Growth Factor (VEGF) Inhibitor

Use Treatment of gastrointestinal stromal tumor (GIST) following failure of or intolerance to imatinib; treatment of advanced renal cell cancer (RCC)

Local Anesthetic/Vasoconstrictor Precautions No information available to require special precautions

Effects on Dental Treatment Key adverse event(s) related to dental treatment: Xerostomia (normal salivary flow resumes upon discontinuation), mucositis/stomatitis, taste perversion, and oral pain.

Common Adverse Effects

>10%:

Cardiovascular: Hypertension (15% to 30%; grades 3/4: 4% to 10%), LVEF decreased (11% to 21%; grades 3/4: 1%), peripheral edema (11%)

Central nervous system: Fatigue (42% to 58%), fever (17% to 18%), headache (13% to 18%), chills (11%), insomnia (11%)

Dermatologic: Hyperpigmentation (19% to 33%), skin discoloration (19% to 30%), rash (14% to 27%), hand-foot syndrome (12% to 21%), dry skin (17% to 18%), hair color changes (7% to 16%)

Endocrine & metabolic: Hyperuricemia (15% to 41%), hypophosphatemia (9% to 36%), hypocalcemia (35%), hypoglycemia (19%), hypoalbuminemia (18%), hyperglycemia (15%), hyponatremia (6% to 14%), hypokalemia (12%), hyperkalemia (6% to 11%), hypernatremia (10% to 11%)

Gastrointestinal: Diarrhea (40% to 58%), lipase increased (25% to 52%), nausea (31% to 49%), taste perversion (21% to 44%), mucositis/stomatitis

(Continued)

Sunitinib (Continued)

(29% to 43%), anorexia (31% to 38%), constipation (16% to 34%), abdominal pain (22% to 33%), dyspepsia (28%), vomiting (24% to 28%), amylase increased (5% to 17%), weight loss (12%), xerostomia (12%), GERD/reflux (11%)

Hematologic: Leukopenia (up to 78%; grades 3/4: 5%), neutropenia (53% to 72%; grades 3/4: 10% to 12%), anemia (26% to 72%; grades 3/4: 3% to 7%), thrombocytopenia (38% to 65%; grades 3/4: 5% to 8%), lymphopenia (38% to 59%; grades 3/4: up to 59%), hemorrhage/bleeding (18% to 30%)

Hepatic: AST increased (39% to 52%), ALT increased (39% to 46%), alkaline phosphatase increased (24% to 42%), hyperbilirubinemia (10% to 19%)

Neuromuscular & skeletal: Creatine kinase increased (41%), weakness (21% to 22%), back pain (11% to 19%), arthralgia (12% to 18%), limb pain (14% to 17%), myalgia (14%)

Renal: Creatinine increased (12% to 66%)

Respiratory: Dyspnea (10% to 28%), cough (8% to 17%)

1% to 10%:

Cardiovascular: Venous thrombotic events (2% to 3%), DVT (1% to 3%), myocardial ischemia (1%)

Central nervous system: Depression (8%), dizziness (7%)

Dermatologic: Skin blistering (7%), alopecia (5%)

Endocrine & metabolic: Dehydration (8%), hypothyroidism (3% to 7%)

Gastrointestinal: Flatulence (10%), glossodynia (10%), oral pain (6% to 10%), appetite disturbance (9%), pancreatitis (1%)

Neuromuscular & skeletal: Peripheral neuropathy (10%)

Ocular: Periorbital edema (7%), lacrimation increased (6%)

Respiratory: Pulmonary embolism (1%)

Restrictions Pharmacies must obtain an Order Authorization Number (OAN) from McKesson Specialty at 1-800-496-6540 prior to ordering sunitinib.

Mechanism of Action Exhibits antitumor and antiangiogenic properties by inhibiting multiple receptor tyrosine kinases, including platelet-derived growth factors (PDGFRα and PDGFRβ), vascular endothelial growth factors (VEGFR1, VEGFR2, and VEGFR3), FMS-like tyrosine kinase-3 (FLT3), colony-stimulating factor type 1 (CSF-1R), and glial cell-line-derived neurotrophic factor receptor (RET).

Drug Interactions

Cytochrome P450 Effect: Substrate of CYP3A4 (major)

Increased Effect/Toxicity: CYP3A4 inhibitors may increase the levels/effects of sunitinib (example inhibitors include azole antifungals, clarithromycin, diclofenac, doxycycline, erythromycin, imatinib, isoniazid, nefazodone, nicardipine, propofol, protease inhibitors, quinidine, telithromycin, and verapamil). Ketoconazole may increase the effects of sunitinib. Concurrent use of sunitinib with other drugs which may prolong QT$_c$ interval may increase the risk of potentially-fatal arrhythmias; includes type Ia and type III antiarrhythmic agents, selected quinolones (eg, moxifloxacin), cisapride, dolasetron, palonosetron, thioridazine, and other agents.

Decreased Effect: CYP3A4 inducers may decrease the levels/effects of sunitinib (example inducers include aminoglutethimide, carbamazepine, dexamethasone, nafcillin, nevirapine, phenobarbital, and phenytoin. Rifamycins may decrease the effects of sunitinib.

Pharmacodynamics/Kinetics

Distribution: V$_d$/F: 2230 L

Protein binding: Sunitinib: 95%; SU12662: 90%

Metabolism: Hepatic; primarily metabolized by CYP3A4 to the N-desethyl metabolite SU12662 (active)

Half-life elimination: Sunitinib: 40-60 hours; SU12662: 80-110 hours

Time to peak, plasma: 6-12 hours

Excretion: Feces (61%); urine (16%)

Pregnancy Risk Factor D

Tacrine (TAK reen)

U.S. Brand Names Cognex®
Generic Available No
Index Terms Tacrine Hydrochloride; Tetrahydroaminoacrine; THA
Pharmacologic Category Acetylcholinesterase Inhibitor (Central)
Use Treatment of mild to moderate dementia of the Alzheimer's type
Local Anesthetic/Vasoconstrictor Precautions No information available to require special precautions
Effects on Dental Treatment No significant effects or complications reported
Common Adverse Effects
>10%:
 Central nervous system: Dizziness, headache
 Gastrointestinal: Diarrhea, nausea, vomiting
 Miscellaneous: Transaminases increased
1% to 10%:
 Cardiovascular: Flushing
 Central nervous system: Ataxia, confusion, depression, fatigue, insomnia, somnolence
 Dermatologic: Rash
 Gastrointestinal: Abdominal pain, anorexia, constipation, dyspepsia, flatulence, weight loss
 Neuromuscular & skeletal: Myalgia, tremor
 Respiratory: Rhinitis
Mechanism of Action Centrally-acting cholinesterase inhibitor. It elevates acetylcholine in cerebral cortex by slowing the degradation of acetylcholine.
Drug Interactions
 Cytochrome P450 Effect: Substrate of CYP1A2 (major); **Inhibits** CYP1A2 (weak)
 Increased Effect/Toxicity: CYP1A2 inhibitors may increase the levels/effects of tacrine; example inhibitors include ciprofloxacin, fluvoxamine, ketoconazole, norfloxacin, ofloxacin, and rofecoxib. Tacrine in combination with
(Continued)

Tacrine *(Continued)*

other cholinergic agents (eg, ambenonium, edrophonium, neostigmine, pyridostigmine, bethanechol), will likely produce additive cholinergic effects. Tacrine in combination with beta-blockers may produce additive bradycardia. Tacrine may increase the levels/effect of succinylcholine and theophylline. in elevated plasma levels. Fluvoxamine, enoxacin, and cimetidine increase tacrine concentrations via enzyme inhibition (CYP1A2). Acetylcholinesterase inhibitors (central) may increase the risk of antipsychotic-related extrapyramidal symptoms.

Decreased Effect: CYP1A2 inducers may decrease the levels/effects of tacrine; example inducers include aminoglutethimide, carbamazepine, phenobarbital, rifampin, and cigarette smoking, Tacrine may worsen Parkinson's disease and inhibit the effects of levodopa. Tacrine may antagonize the therapeutic effect of anticholinergic agents (benztropine, trihexyphenidyl).

Pharmacodynamics/Kinetics
Absorption: Oral: Rapid
Distribution: V_d: Mean: 349 L; reduced by food
Protein binding, plasma: 55%
Metabolism: Extensively by CYP450 to multiple metabolites; first pass effect
Bioavailability: Absolute: 17%
Half-life elimination, serum: 2-4 hours; Steady-state: 24-36 hours
Time to peak, plasma: 1-2 hours

Pregnancy Risk Factor C

Tacrine Hydrochloride *see* Tacrine *on page 1515* '

Tacrolimus *(ta KROE li mus)*

U.S. Brand Names Prograf®; Protopic®
Canadian Brand Names Prograf®; Protopic®
Mexican Brand Names Prograf
Generic Available No
Index Terms FK506
Pharmacologic Category Immunosuppressant Agent; Topical Skin Product
Dental Use Topical: Treatment of severe ulcerative or vesicobullous lesions (usually in consult with patient's physician)
Use
Oral/injection: Potent immunosuppressive drug used in heart, kidney, or liver transplant recipients
Topical: Moderate-to-severe atopic dermatitis in patients not responsive to conventional therapy or when conventional therapy is not appropriate

Unlabeled/Investigational Use Potent immunosuppressive drug used in lung, small bowel transplant recipients; immunosuppressive drug for peripheral stem cell/bone marrow transplantation

Local Anesthetic/Vasoconstrictor Precautions No information available to require special precautions

Effects on Dental Treatment Key adverse event(s) related to dental treatment: Stomatitis, oral moniliasis, dysphagia, and esophagitis (including ulcerative).

Significant Adverse Effects
Oral, I.V.:
≥15%:
Cardiovascular: Chest pain, hypertension, pericardial effusion (heart transplant)
Central nervous system: Dizziness, headache, insomnia, tremor (headache and tremor are associated with high whole blood concentrations and may respond to decreased dosage)
Dermatologic: Pruritus, rash
Endocrine & metabolic: Diabetes mellitus, hyperglycemia, hyper-/hypokalemia, hyperlipemia, hypomagnesemia, hypophosphatemia
Gastrointestinal: Abdominal pain, constipation, diarrhea, dyspepsia, nausea, vomiting
Genitourinary: Urinary tract infection
Hematologic: Anemia, leukocytosis, leukopenia, thrombocytopenia
Hepatic: Ascites
Neuromuscular & skeletal: Arthralgia, back pain, paresthesia, tremor, weakness
Renal: Abnormal kidney function, BUN increased, creatinine increased, oliguria, urinary tract infection
Respiratory: Atelectasis, bronchitis, dyspnea, increased cough, pleural effusion
Miscellaneous: CMV infection, infection

<15%:

Cardiovascular: Abnormal ECG (QRS or ST segment abnormal), angina pectoris, cardiopulmonary failure, deep thrombophlebitis, heart rate decreased, hemorrhage, hemorrhagic stroke, hypervolemia, hypotension, generalized edema, peripheral vascular disorder, phlebitis, postural hypotension, tachycardia, thrombosis, vasodilation

Central nervous system: Abnormal dreams, abnormal thinking, agitation, amnesia, anxiety, chills, confusion, depression, dizziness, elevated mood, emotional lability, encephalopathy, hallucinations, nervousness, paralysis, psychosis, quadriparesis, seizure, somnolence

Dermatologic: Acne, alopecia, cellulitis, exfoliative dermatitis, fungal dermatitis, hirsutism, increased diaphoresis, photosensitivity reaction, skin discoloration, skin disorder, skin ulcer

Endocrine & metabolic: Acidosis, alkalosis, Cushing's syndrome, decreased bicarbonate, decreased serum iron, diabetes mellitus, hypercalcemia, hypercholesterolemia, hyperphosphatemia, hypoproteinemia, increased alkaline phosphatase

Gastrointestinal: Anorexia, appetite increased, cramps, duodenitis, dysphagia, enlarged abdomen, esophagitis (including ulcerative), flatulence, gastritis, gastroesophagitis, GI perforation/hemorrhage, ileus, oral moniliasis, pancreatic pseudocyst, rectal disorder, stomatitis, weight gain

Genitourinary: Bladder spasm, cystitis, dysuria, nocturia, oliguria, urge incontinence, urinary frequency, urinary incontinence, urinary retention, vaginitis

Hematologic: Bruising, coagulation disorder, decreased prothrombin, hypochromic anemia, polycythemia

Hepatic: Abnormal liver function tests, ALT/AST increased, bilirubinemia, cholangitis, cholestatic jaundice, GGT increased, hepatitis (including granulomatous), jaundice, liver damage, increase LDH

Neuromuscular & skeletal: Hypertonia, incoordination, joint disorder, leg cramps, myalgia, myasthenia, myoclonus, nerve compression, neuropathy, osteoporosis

Ocular: Abnormal vision, amblyopia

Otic: Ear pain, otitis media, tinnitus

Renal: Albuminuria, renal tubular necrosis, toxic nephropathy

Respiratory: Asthma, lung disorder, pharyngitis, pneumonia, pneumothorax, pulmonary edema, respiratory disorder, rhinitis, sinusitis, voice alteration

Miscellaneous: Abscess, abnormal healing, allergic reaction, crying, flu-like syndrome, generalized spasm, hernia, herpes simplex, peritonitis, sepsis, writing impaired

Topical:

>10%:

Central nervous system: Headache (5% to 20%), fever (1% to 21%)

Dermatologic: Skin burning (43% to 58%; tends to improve as lesions resolve), pruritus (41% to 46%), erythema (12% to 28%)

Respiratory: Increased cough (18% children)

Miscellaneous: Flu-like syndrome (23% to 28%), allergic reaction (4% to 12%)

Oral, I.V., topical: Postmarketing and/or case reports (limited to important or life-threatening): Acute renal failure, alopecia, anaphylaxis, anaphylactoid reaction, angioedema, ARDS, arrhythmia, atrial fibrillation, atrial flutter, bile duct stenosis, blindness, cardiac arrest, cerebral infarction, cerebrovascular accident, deafness, delirium, depression, DIC, hemiparesis, hemolytic-uremic syndrome, hemorrhagic cystitis, hepatic necrosis, hepatotoxicity, hyperglycemia, leukoencephalopathy, lymphoproliferative disorder (related to EBV), myocardial hypertrophy (associated with ventricular dysfunction; reversible upon discontinuation), MI, neutropenia, pancreatitis (hemorrhagic and necrotizing), pancytopenia, paresthesia, photosensitivity reaction (topical), quadriplegia, QT_c prolongation, respiratory failure, seizure, skin discoloration (topical), Stevens-Johnson syndrome, syncope, toxic epidermal necrolysis, thrombocytopenic purpura, torsade de pointes, TTP, veno-occlusive hepatic disease, venous thrombosis, ventricular fibrillation

Note: Calcineurin inhibitor-induced hemolytic uremic syndrome/thrombotic thrombocytopenic purpura/thrombotic microangiopathy (HUS/TTP/TMA) have been reported (with concurrent sirolimus).

Restrictions An FDA-approved medication guide must be distributed when dispensing the outpatient prescription (new or refill) for tacrolimus ointment where this medication is to be used without direct supervision of a healthcare provider. Medication guides are available at http://www.fda.gov/cder/Offices/ODS/medication_guides.htm.

Dosage

Oral:

Children: **Notes:** Patients without pre-existing renal or hepatic dysfunction have required (and tolerated) higher doses than adults to achieve similar

(Continued)

Tacrolimus *(Continued)*

blood concentrations. It is recommended that therapy be initiated at high end of the recommended adult I.V. and oral dosing ranges; dosage adjustments may be required. If switching from I.V. to oral, the oral dose should be started 8-12 hours after stopping the infusion. Adjunctive therapy with corticosteroids is recommended early post-transplant.

Liver transplant: Initial dose: 0.15-0.20 mg/kg/day in 2 divided doses, given every 12 hours; begin oral dose no sooner than 6 hours post-transplant

Adults: **Notes:** If switching from I.V. to oral, the oral dose should be started 8-12 hours after stopping the infusion. Adjunctive therapy with corticosteroids is recommended early post-transplant.

Heart transplant: Initial dose: 0.075 mg/kg/day in 2 divided doses, given every 12 hours; begin oral dose no sooner than 6 hours post-transplant

Kidney transplant: Initial dose: 0.2 mg/kg/day in 2 divided doses, given every 12 hours; initial dose may be given within 24 hours of transplant, but should be delayed until renal function has recovered; African-American patients may require larger doses to maintain trough concentration

Liver transplant: Initial dose: 0.1-0.15 mg/kg/day in 2 divided doses, given every 12 hours; begin oral dose no sooner than 6 hours post-transplant

I.V.: Children and Adults: Note: I.V. route should only be used in patients not able to take oral medications and continued only until oral medication can be tolerated; anaphylaxis has been reported. Begin no sooner than 6 hours post-transplant; adjunctive therapy with corticosteroids is recommended.

Heart transplant: Initial dose: 0.01 mg/kg/day as a continuous infusion

Kidney, liver transplant: Initial dose: 0.03-0.05 mg/kg/day as a continuous infusion

Prevention of graft-vs-host disease: 0.03 mg/kg/day as continuous infusion

Topical: Children ≥2 years and Adults: Atopic dermatitis (moderate to severe): Apply minimum amount of 0.03% or 0.1% ointment to affected area twice daily; rub in gently and completely. Discontinue use when symptoms have cleared. If no improvement within 6 weeks, patients should be re-examined to confirm diagnosis.

Dosing adjustment in renal impairment: Evidence suggests that lower doses should be used; patients should receive doses at the lowest value of the recommended I.V. and oral dosing ranges; further reductions in dose below these ranges may be required.

Tacrolimus therapy should usually be delayed up to 48 hours or longer in patients with postoperative oliguria.

Hemodialysis: Not removed by hemodialysis; supplemental dose is not necessary.

Peritoneal dialysis: Significant drug removal is unlikely based on physiochemical characteristics.

Dosing adjustment in hepatic impairment: Use of tacrolimus in liver transplant recipients experiencing post-transplant hepatic impairment may be associated with increased risk of developing renal insufficiency related to high whole blood levels of tacrolimus. The presence of moderate-to-severe hepatic dysfunction (serum bilirubin >2 mg/dL; Child-Pugh score ≥10) appears to affect the metabolism of tacrolimus. The half-life of the drug was prolonged and the clearance reduced after I.V. administration. The bioavailability of tacrolimus was also increased after oral administration. The higher plasma concentrations as determined by ELISA, in patients with severe hepatic dysfunction are probably due to the accumulation of metabolites of lower activity. These patients should be monitored closely and dosage adjustments should be considered. Some evidence indicates that lower doses could be used in these patients.

Mechanism of Action Suppresses cellular immunity (inhibits T-lymphocyte activation), possibly by binding to an intracellular protein, FKBP-12

Contraindications Hypersensitivity to tacrolimus or any component of the formulation

Warnings/Precautions

Oral/injection: Insulin-dependent post-transplant diabetes mellitus (PTDM) has been reported (1% to 20%); risk increases in African-American and Hispanic kidney transplant patients. **[U.S. Boxed Warning]: Increased susceptibility to infection and the possible development of lymphoma may occur after administration of tacrolimus.** Nephrotoxicity and neurotoxicity have been reported, especially with higher doses; to avoid excess nephrotoxicity do not administer simultaneously with cyclosporine; monitoring of serum concentrations (trough for oral therapy) is essential to prevent organ rejection and reduce drug-related toxicity; tonic clonic seizures may have been triggered by tacrolimus. A period of 24 hours should elapse between discontinuation of cyclosporine and the initiation of tacrolimus. Use caution in renal or hepatic dysfunction, dosing adjustments may be required. Delay initiation if postoperative oliguria occurs. Use may be associated with the development of hypertension (common). Myocardial hypertrophy has been reported (rare). Each mL of injection contains polyoxyl 60 hydrogenated castor oil (HCO-60) (200 mg) and dehydrated alcohol USP 80% v/v. Anaphylaxis has been reported with the injection, use should be reserved for those patients not able to take oral medications.

Topical: [U.S. Boxed Warning]: Topical calcineurin inhibitors have been associated with rare cases of malignancy. Avoid use on malignant or premalignant skin conditions (eg cutaneous T-cell lymphoma). Topical calcineurin agents are considered second-line therapies in the treatment of atopic dermatitis/eczema, and should be limited to use in patients who have failed treatment with other therapies. **[U.S. Boxed Warning]: They should be used for short-term and intermittent treatment using the minimum amount necessary for the control of symptoms should be used.** Application should be limited to involved areas. Safety of intermittent use for >1 year has not been established.

Should not be used in immunocompromised patients. Do not apply to areas of active viral infection; infections at the treatment site should be cleared prior to therapy. Patients with atopic dermatitis are predisposed to skin infections, and tacrolimus therapy has been associated with risk of developing eczema herpeticum, varicella zoster, and herpes simplex. May be associated with development of lymphadenopathy; possible infectious causes should be investigated. Discontinue use in patients with unknown cause of lymphadenopathy or acute infectious mononucleosis. Not recommended for use in patients with skin disease which may increase systemic absorption (eg, Netherton's syndrome). Avoid artificial or natural sunlight exposure, even when Protopic® is not on the skin. Safety not established in patients with generalized erythroderma. **[U.S. Boxed Warning]: The use of Protopic® in children <2 years of age is not recommended,** particularly since the effect on immune system development is unknown.

Drug Interactions Substrate of CYP3A4 (major); Inhibits CYP3A4 (weak)

Antacids: Separate administration by at least 2 hours

Anticonvulsants: Carbamazepine, phenobarbital, phenytoin: May decrease tacrolimus blood levels.

Calcium channel blockers: May increase tacrolimus serum concentrations; monitor.

Caspofungin: May decrease tacrolimus serum concentrations.

Cisapride (and metoclopramide): May increase serum concentration of tacrolimus

Cyclosporine: Concomitant use is associated with synergistic immunosuppression and increased nephrotoxicity; give first dose of tacrolimus no sooner than 24 hours after last cyclosporine dose. In the presence of elevated tacrolimus or cyclosporine concentration, dosing of the other usually should be delayed longer.

CYP3A4 inducers: CYP3A4 inducers may decrease the levels/effects of tacrolimus. Example inducers include aminoglutethimide, carbamazepine, nafcillin, nevirapine, phenobarbital, phenytoin, and rifamycins.

CYP3A4 inhibitors: May increase the levels/effects of tacrolimus. Example inhibitors include azole antifungals, clarithromycin, diclofenac, doxycycline, erythromycin, imatinib, isoniazid, nefazodone, nicardipine, propofol, protease inhibitors, quinidine, telithromycin, and verapamil.

Ganciclovir: Nephrotoxicity may be additive with tacrolimus; use caution.

Macrolides: May increase tacrolimus serum concentrations (limited documentation); monitor.

Potassium-sparing diuretics: Tacrolimus use may lead to hyperkalemia; avoid concomitant use

Rifabutin, rifampin: May decrease serum levels of tacrolimus.

Sirolimus: May decrease tacrolimus serum concentrations. Concurrent therapy may increase the risk of HUS/TTP/TMA.

St John's wort: May decrease tacrolimus serum concentrations; avoid concurrent use.

Sucralfate: Separate administration by at least 2 hours

Vaccines (live): Vaccine may be less effective; avoid vaccination during treatment if possible

Voriconazole: Tacrolimus serum concentrations may be increased; monitor serum concentrations and renal function. Decrease tacrolimus dosage by 66% when initiating voriconazole.

Ethanol/Nutrition/Herb Interactions

Ethanol: Localized flushing (redness, warm sensation) may occur at application site of topical tacrolimus following ethanol consumption.

Food: Decreases rate and extent of absorption. High-fat meals have most pronounced effect (35% decrease in AUC, 77% decrease in C_{max}). Grapefruit

(Continued)

Tacrolimus *(Continued)*

juice, CYP3A4 inhibitor, may increase serum level and/or toxicity of tacrolimus; avoid concurrent use.

Herb/Nutraceutical: St John's wort: May reduce tacrolimus serum concentrations (avoid concurrent use).

Dietary Considerations Capsule: Take on an empty stomach; be consistent with timing and composition of meals if GI intolerance occurs (per manufacturer).

Pharmacodynamics/Kinetics

Absorption: Better in resected patients with a closed stoma; unlike cyclosporine, clamping of the T-tube in liver transplant patients does not alter trough concentrations or AUC

Oral: Incomplete and variable; food within 15 minutes of administration decreases absorption (27%)

Topical: Serum concentrations range from undetectable to 20 ng/mL (<5 ng/mL in majority of adult patients studied)

Protein binding: 99%

Metabolism: Extensively hepatic via CYP3A4 to eight possible metabolites (major metabolite, 31-demethyl tacrolimus, shows same activity as tacrolimus *in vitro*)

Bioavailability: Oral: Adults: 7% to 28%, Children: 10% to 52%; Topical: <0.5%; Absolute: Unknown

Half-life elimination: Variable, 21-61 hours in healthy volunteers

Time to peak: 0.5-4 hours

Excretion: Feces (~92%); feces/urine (<1% as unchanged drug)

Pregnancy Risk Factor C

Lactation Enters breast milk/contraindicated

Breast-Feeding Considerations Concentrations in breast milk are equivalent to plasma concentrations; breast-feeding is not advised.

Dosage Forms Excipient information presented when available (limited, particularly for generics); consult specific product labeling.

Capsule (Prograf®): 0.5 mg, 1 mg, 5 mg

Injection, solution (Prograf®): 5 mg/mL (1 mL) [contains dehydrated alcohol 80% and polyoxyl 60 hydrogenated castor oil]

Ointment, topical (Protopic®): 0.03% (30 g, 60 g, 100 g); 0.1% (30 g, 60 g, 100 g)

Tadalafil *(tah DA la fil)*

U.S. Brand Names Cialis®

Canadian Brand Names Cialis®

Mexican Brand Names Cialis

Generic Available No

Index Terms GF196960

Pharmacologic Category Phosphodiesterase-5 Enzyme Inhibitor

Use Treatment of erectile dysfunction

Local Anesthetic/Vasoconstrictor Precautions No information available to require special precautions

Effects on Dental Treatment No significant effects or complications reported

Common Adverse Effects

>10%: Central nervous system: Headache (11% to 15%)

2% to 10%:

Cardiovascular: Flushing (2% to 3%)

Gastrointestinal: Dyspepsia (4% to 10%)

Neuromuscular & skeletal: CPK increased (2%), back pain (3% to 6%), myalgia (1% to 4%), limb pain (1% to 3%)

Respiratory: Nasal congestion (2% to 3%)

Dosage Oral: Adults: Erectile dysfunction: 10 mg prior to anticipated sexual activity (dosing range: 5-20 mg); to be given as one single dose and not given more than once daily. **Note:** Erectile function may be improved for up to 36 hours following a single dose; adjust dose.

Elderly: Dosage is based on renal function; refer to "Dosage adjustment in renal impairment"

Dosing adjustment with concomitant medications:

Alpha$_1$-blockers: If stabilized on either alpha-blockers or tadalafil therapy, initiate new therapy with the other agent at the lowest possible dose.

CYP3A4 inhibitors: Dose reduction of tadalafil is recommended with strong CYP3A4 inhibitors. The dose of tadalafil should not exceed 10 mg, and tadalafil should not be taken more frequently than once every 72 hours. Examples of such inhibitors include amprenavir, atazanavir, clarithromycin, conivaptan, delavirdine, diclofenac, fosamprenavir, imatinib, indinavir, isoniazid, itraconazole, ketoconazole, miconazole, nefazodone, nelfinavir, nicardipine, propofol, quinidine, ritonavir, and telithromycin.

Dosage adjustment in renal impairment:
Cl_{cr} 31-50 mL/minute: Initial dose 5 mg once daily; maximum dose 10 mg not to be given more frequently than every 48 hours.
Cl_{cr} <30 mL/minute or hemodialysis: Maximum dose 5 mg.

Dosage adjustment in hepatic impairment:
Mild-to-moderate hepatic impairment (Child-Pugh class A or B): Dose should not exceed 10 mg once daily
Severe hepatic impairment: Use is not recommended

Mechanism of Action Does not directly cause penile erections, but affects the response to sexual stimulation. The physiologic mechanism of erection of the penis involves release of nitric oxide (NO) in the corpus cavernosum during sexual stimulation. NO then activates the enzyme guanylate cyclase, which results in increased levels of cyclic guanosine monophosphate (cGMP), producing smooth muscle relaxation and inflow of blood to the corpus cavernosum. Tadalafil enhances the effect of NO by inhibiting phosphodiesterase type 5 (PDE-5), which is responsible for degradation of cGMP in the corpus cavernosum; when sexual stimulation causes local release of NO, inhibition of PDE-5 by tadalafil causes increased levels of cGMP in the corpus cavernosum, resulting in smooth muscle relaxation and inflow of blood to the corpus cavernosum. At recommended doses, it has no effect in the absence of sexual stimulation.

Contraindications Hypersensitivity to tadalafil or any component of the formulation; concurrent use of organic nitrates (nitroglycerin) in any form

Warnings/Precautions There is a degree of cardiac risk associated with sexual activity; therefore, physicians may wish to consider the cardiovascular status of their patients prior to initiating any treatment for erectile dysfunction. Use caution in patients with left ventricular outflow obstruction (aortic stenosis or IHSS); may be more sensitive to hypotensive actions. Concurrent use with alpha-adrenergic antagonist therapy may cause symptomatic hypotension; patients should be hemodynamically stable prior to initiating tadalafil therapy at the lowest possible dose. Use caution in patients receiving strong CYP3A4 inhibitors, the elderly, or those with hepatic impairment or renal impairment; dosage adjustment/limitation is needed. Use caution in patients with peptic ulcer disease.

Agents for the treatment of erectile dysfunction should be used with caution in patients with anatomical deformation of the penis (angulation, cavernosal fibrosis, or Peyronie's disease), or in patients who have conditions which may predispose them to priapism (sickle cell anemia, multiple myeloma, leukemia). All patients should be instructed to seek medical attention if erection persists >4 hours. The safety and efficacy of tadalafil with other treatments for erectile dysfunction have not been studied and are, therefore, not recommended as combination therapy.

Rare cases of nonarteritic ischemic optic neuropathy (NAION) have been reported; risk may be increased with history of vision loss. Other risk factors for NAION include heart disease, diabetes, hypertension, smoking, age >50 years, or history of certain eye problems.

Safety and efficacy have not been studied in patients with the following conditions, therefore, use in these patients is not recommended: Arrhythmias, hypotension, uncontrolled hypertension, unstable angina or angina during intercourse, cardiac failure (NYHA Class II or greater), myocardial infarction within the last 3 months, or stroke within the last 6 months. A minority of patients with retinitis pigmentosa have genetic disorders of retinal phosphodiesterases; use is not recommended. Safety and efficacy in children have not been established.

Drug Interactions
Cytochrome P450 Effect: Substrate of CYP3A4 (major)
Increased Effect/Toxicity:
Tadalafil increases the hypotensive effects of alpha$_1$-blockers. Concurrent use with organic nitrates may cause severe hypotension. Antifungals agents (imidazole), macrolide antibiotics (clarithromycin, erythromycin, telithromycin, troleandomycin), protease inhibitors (amprenavir, atazanavir, fosamprenavir, indinavir, lopinavir, nelfinavir, ritonavir, saquinavir), and other CYP3A4 inhibitors may increase tadalafil levels.

Ethanol/Nutrition/Herb Interactions
Ethanol: Substantial consumption of ethanol may increase the risk of hypotension and orthostasis. Lower ethanol consumption has not been associated with significant changes in blood pressure or increase in orthostatic symptoms.
(Continued)

Tadalafil *(Continued)*

Food: Rate and extent of absorption are not affected by food. Grapefruit juice may increase serum levels/toxicity of tadalafil. Do not give more than a single 10 mg dose of tadalafil more frequently than every 72 hours in patients who regularly consume grapefruit juice.

Dietary Considerations May be taken with or without food.

Pharmacodynamics/Kinetics

Onset: Within 1 hour

Duration: Up to 36 hours

Distribution: V_d: 63 L

Protein binding: 94%

Metabolism: Hepatic, via CYP3A4 to metabolites (inactive)

Half-life elimination: 17.5 hours

Time to peak, plasma: 2 hours

Excretion: Feces (61%, as metabolites); urine (36%, as metabolites)

Pregnancy Risk Factor B

Dosage Forms

Tablet:

Cialis®: 5 mg, 10 mg, 20 mg

Tagamet® [DSC] *see* Cimetidine *on page 358*

Tagamet® HB 200 [OTC] *see* Cimetidine *on page 358*

TAK-375 *see* Ramelteon *on page 1405*

Talacen® *see* Pentazocine and Acetaminophen *on page 1275*

Talwin® *see* Pentazocine *on page 1274*

Talwin® NX *see* Pentazocine *on page 1274*

TAM *see* Tamoxifen *on page 1522*

Tambocor™ *see* Flecainide *on page 694*

Tamiflu® *see* Oseltamivir *on page 1215*

Tamoxifen (ta MOKS i fen)

U.S. Brand Names Nolvadex® [DSC]; Soltamox™

Canadian Brand Names Apo-Tamox®; Gen-Tamoxifen; Nolvadex®; Nolvadex®-D; Novo-Tamoxifen; Tamofen®

Mexican Brand Names Nolvadex; Tecnofen

Generic Available Yes: Tablet

Index Terms ICI-46474; NSC-180973; TAM; Tamoxifen Citrate

Pharmacologic Category Antineoplastic Agent, Estrogen Receptor Antagonist

Use Palliative or adjunctive treatment of advanced breast cancer; reduce the incidence of breast cancer in women at high risk; reduce risk of invasive breast cancer in women with ductal carcinoma *in situ* (DCIS); metastatic female and male breast cancer

Unlabeled/Investigational Use Treatment of mastalgia, gynecomastia, pancreatic carcinoma, melanoma and desmoid tumors; induction of ovulation; treatment of precocious puberty in females, secondary to McCune-Albright syndrome

Local Anesthetic/Vasoconstrictor Precautions No information available to require special precautions

Effects on Dental Treatment No significant effects or complications reported

Common Adverse Effects

>10%:

Cardiovascular: Flushing (33% to 41%), hypertension (11%), peripheral edema (11%)

Central nervous system: Pain (3% to 16%), mood changes (12% to 18%), depression (2% to 12%)

Dermatologic: Skin changes (6% to 19%), rash (13%)

Endocrine & metabolic: Hot flashes (3% to 80%), fluid retention (32%), altered menses (13% to 25%), amenorrhea (16%)

Gastrointestinal: Nausea (5% to 26%), weight loss (23%)

Genitourinary: Vaginal bleeding (2% to 23%), vaginal discharge (13% to 55%)

Neuromuscular & skeletal: Weakness (19%), arthritis (14%), arthralgia (11%)

Respiratory: Pharyngitis (14%)

1% to 10%:

Cardiovascular: Chest pain (5%), venous thrombotic events (5%), edema (4%), cardiovascular ischemia (3%), cerebrovascular ischemia (3%), angina (2%), deep venous thrombus (2%), MI (1%)

Central nervous system: Insomnia (9%), dizziness (8%), headache (8%), anxiety (6%), fatigue (4%)

Dermatologic: Alopecia (<1% to 5%)

Endocrine & metabolic: Oligomenorrhea (9%), breast pain (6%), menstrual disorder (6%), breast neoplasm (5%), hypercholesterolemia (4%)

Gastrointestinal: Abdominal pain (9%), weight gain (9%), throat irritation (oral solution 5%), constipation (4% to 8%), diarrhea (7%), dyspepsia (6%), abdominal cramps (1%), anorexia (1%)

Genitourinary: Urinary tract infection (10%), leukorrhea (9%), vaginal hemorrhage (6%), vaginitis (5%), ovarian cyst (3%)

Hematologic: Thrombocytopenia (<1% to 10%), anemia (5%)

Hepatic: AST increased (5%), serum bilirubin increased (2%)

Neuromuscular & skeletal: Bone pain (6% to 10%), osteoporosis (7%), fracture (7%), arthrosis (5%), myalgia (5%), paresthesia (5%), musculoskeletal pain (3%)

Ocular: Cataract (7%)

Renal: Serum creatinine increased (up to 2%)

Respiratory: Cough (4% to 9%), dyspnea (8%), bronchitis (5%), sinusitis (5%)

Miscellaneous: Infection/sepsis (up to 9%), diaphoresis (6%), flu-like syndrome (6%), allergic reaction (3%)

Restrictions An FDA-approved medication guide must be distributed when dispensing the outpatient prescription (new or refill) to females for breast cancer prevention or treatment of ductal carcinoma *in situ* where this medication is to be used without direct supervision of a healthcare provider. Medication guides are available at http://www.fda.gov/cder/Offices/ODS/medication_guides.htm.

Dosage Oral (refer to individual protocols):

Children: Female: Precocious puberty and McCune-Albright syndrome (unlabeled use): A dose of 20 mg/day has been reported in patients 2-10 years of age; safety and efficacy have not been established for treatment of longer than 1 year duration

Adults:

Breast cancer:

Metastatic (males and females) or adjuvant therapy (females): 20-40 mg/day; daily doses >20 mg should be given in 2 divided doses (morning and evening)

Prevention (high-risk females): 20 mg/day for 5 years

DCIS (females): 20 mg once daily for 5 years

Note: Higher dosages (up to 700 mg/day) have been investigated for use in modulation of multidrug resistance (MDR), but are not routinely used in clinical practice

Induction of ovulation (unlabeled use): 5-40 mg twice daily for 4 days

Mechanism of Action Competitively binds to estrogen receptors on tumors and other tissue targets, producing a nuclear complex that decreases DNA synthesis and inhibits estrogen effects; nonsteroidal agent with potent antiestrogenic properties which compete with estrogen for binding sites in breast and other tissues; cells accumulate in the G_0 and G_1 phases; therefore, tamoxifen is cytostatic rather than cytocidal.

Contraindications Hypersensitivity to tamoxifen or any component of the formulation; concurrent warfarin therapy or history of deep vein thrombosis or pulmonary embolism (when tamoxifen is used for cancer risk reduction); pregnancy

Warnings/Precautions Hazardous agent - use appropriate precautions for handling and disposal. **[U.S. Boxed Warning]: Serious and life-threatening events (including stroke, pulmonary emboli, and uterine malignancy) have occurred at an incidence greater than placebo during use for cancer risk reduction;** these events are rare, but require consideration in risk:benefit evaluation. An increased incidence of thromboembolic events has been associated with use for breast cancer; risk may increase with chemotherapy addition; use caution in individuals with a history of thromboembolic events. Use with caution in patients with leukopenia, thrombocytopenia, or hyperlipidemias. Decreased visual acuity, retinopathy, corneal changes, and increased incidence of cataracts have been reported. Hypercalcemia has occurred in patients with bone metastasis. Significant bone loss of the lumbar spine and hip was associated with use in premenopausal women. Liver abnormalities such as cholestasis, fatty liver, hepatitis, and hepatic necrosis have occurred. Hepatocellular carcinomas have been reported in some studies; relationship to treatment is unclear. Endometrial hyperplasia, polyps, endometriosis, uterine fibroids, and ovarian cysts have occurred. Increased risk of uterine or endometrial cancer; monitor. Safety and efficacy in children <2 years of age, or for treatment durations >1 year in children 2-10 years, have not been established.

Drug Interactions

Cytochrome P450 Effect: Substrate of CYP2A6 (minor), 2B6 (minor), 2C9 (major), 2D6 (major), 2E1 (minor), 3A4 (major); **Inhibits** CYP2B6 (weak), 2C8 (moderate), 2C9 (weak), 3A4 (weak)

(Continued)

Tamoxifen *(Continued)*

Increased Effect/Toxicity: Concomitant use of warfarin is contraindicated when used for risk reduction; results in significant enhancement of the anticoagulant effects of warfarin. Tamoxifen may increase the levels/effects of CYP2C8 substrates; example substrates include amiodarone, paclitaxel, pioglitazone, repaglinide, and rosiglitazone. CYP2C9 inhibitors may increase the levels/effects of tamoxifen; example inhibitors include delavirdine, fluconazole, gemfibrozil, ketoconazole, nicardipine, NSAIDs, sulfonamides, and tolbutamide. CYP2D6 inhibitors may increase the levels/effects of tamoxifen; example inhibitors include chlorpromazine, delavirdine, fluoxetine, miconazole, paroxetine, pergolide, quinidine, quinine, ritonavir, and ropinirole. CYP3A4 inhibitors may increase the levels/effects of tamoxifen; example inhibitors include azole antifungals, clarithromycin, diclofenac, doxycycline, erythromycin, imatinib, isoniazid, nefazodone, nicardipine, propofol, protease inhibitors, quinidine, telithromycin, and verapamil. Rifamycin derivatives may increase the metabolism (via CYP isoenzymes) of tamoxifen.

Decreased Effect: CYP2C9 inducers may decrease the levels/effects of tamoxifen; example inducers include carbamazepine, phenobarbital, phenytoin, rifampin, rifapentine, and secobarbital. CYP3A4 inducers may decrease the levels/effects of tamoxifen; example inducers include aminoglutethimide, carbamazepine, nafcillin, nevirapine, phenobarbital, phenytoin, and rifamycins. Tamoxifen may reduce the levels/effects of anastrozole (concurrent therapy is not recommended per manufacturer).

Ethanol/Nutrition/Herb Interactions Herb/Nutraceutical: Avoid black cohosh, dong quai in estrogen-dependent tumors. Avoid St John's wort (may decrease levels/effects of tamoxifen).

Pharmacodynamics/Kinetics

Absorption: Well absorbed; tablet and oral solution are bioequivalent

Distribution: High concentrations found in uterus, endometrial and breast tissue

Protein binding: 99%

Metabolism: Hepatic (via CYP3A4) to major metabolites, N-desmethyl tamoxifen (major) and 4-hydroxytamoxifen (minor), and a tamoxifen derivative (minor); undergoes enterohepatic recirculation

Half-life elimination: Distribution: 7-14 hours; Elimination: 5-7 days; Metabolites: 14 days

Time to peak, serum: 5 hours

Excretion: Feces (26% to 51%); urine (9% to 13%)

Pregnancy Risk Factor D

Dosage Forms

Solution, oral:

Soltamox™: 10 mg/5 mL

Tablet: 10 mg, 20 mg

Tamoxifen Citrate *see* Tamoxifen *on page 1522*

Tamsulosin *(tam SOO loe sin)*

U.S. Brand Names Flomax®

Canadian Brand Names Flomax®; Flomax® CR

Mexican Brand Names Secotex

Generic Available No

Index Terms Tamsulosin Hydrochloride

Pharmacologic Category Alpha₁ Blocker

Use Treatment of signs and symptoms of benign prostatic hyperplasia (BPH)

Unlabeled/Investigational Use Symptomatic treatment of bladder outlet obstruction or dysfunction

Local Anesthetic/Vasoconstrictor Precautions No information available to require special precautions

Effects on Dental Treatment Key adverse event(s) related to dental treatment: Orthostatic hypotension and tooth disorder.

Common Adverse Effects

>10%:

Cardiovascular: Orthostatic hypotension (6 % to 19%)

Central nervous system: Headache (19% to 21%), dizziness (15% to 17%)

Genitourinary: Abnormal ejaculation (8% to 18%)

Respiratory: Rhinitis (13% to 18%)

Miscellaneous: Infection (9% to 11%)

1% to 10%:

Cardiovascular: Chest pain (4%)

Central nervous system: Somnolence (3% to 4%), insomnia (1% to 2%), vertigo (≤1%)

Endocrine & metabolic: Libido decreased (1% to 2%)

Gastrointestinal: Diarrhea (4% to 6%), nausea (3% to 4%), tooth disorder (1% to 2%)

Neuromuscular & skeletal: Weakness (8% to 9%), back pain (7% to 8%)

Ocular: Blurred vision (up to 2%)

Respiratory: Pharyngitis (5% to 6%), cough (3% to 5%), sinusitis (2% to 4%)

Dosage Oral: Adults:

BPH: 0.4 mg once daily ~30 minutes after the same meal each day; dose may be increased after 2-4 weeks to 0.8 mg once daily in patients who fail to respond. If therapy is interrupted for several days, restart with 0.4 mg once daily.

Bladder outlet obstruction (unlabeled use): 0.4 mg once daily ~30 minutes after the same meal each day

Dosage adjustment in renal impairment:

Cl_{cr} ≥10 mL/minute: No adjustment needed

Cl_{cr} <10 mL/minute: Not studied

Mechanism of Action Tamsulosin is an antagonist of alpha$_{1A}$-adrenoreceptors in the prostate. Smooth muscle tone in the prostate is mediated by alpha$_{1A}$-adrenoreceptors; blocking them leads to relaxation of smooth muscle in the bladder neck and prostate causing an improvement of urine flow and decreased symptoms of BPH. Approximately 75% of the alpha$_1$-receptors in the prostate are of the alpha$_{1A}$ subtype.

Contraindications Hypersensitivity to tamsulosin or any component of the formulation; concurrent use with phosphodiesterase-5 (PDE-5) inhibitors including sildenafil (>25 mg), tadalafil (if tamsulosin dose >0.4 mg/day), or vardenafil

Warnings/Precautions Not intended for use as an antihypertensive drug. May cause significant orthostatic hypotension and syncope, especially with first dose; anticipate a similar effect if therapy is interrupted for a few days, if dosage is rapidly increased, or if another antihypertensive drug (particularly vasodilators) or a PDE-5 inhibitor is introduced. "First-dose" orthostatic hypotension may occur 4-8 hours after dosing; may be dose related. Patients should be cautioned about performing hazardous tasks when starting new therapy or adjusting dosage upward. Discontinue if symptoms of angina occur or worsen. Rule out prostatic carcinoma before beginning therapy with tamsulosin. Intraoperative floppy iris syndrome has been observed in cataract surgery patients who were on or were previously treated with alpha$_1$-blockers; causality has not been established and there appears to be no benefit in discontinuing alpha-blocker therapy prior to surgery. Priapism has been associated with use (rarely). Rarely, patients with a sulfa allergy have also developed an allergic reaction to tamsulosin; avoid use when previous reaction has been severe. Safety and efficacy have not been established in children.

Drug Interactions

Cytochrome P450 Effect: Substrate (major) of CYP2D6, 3A4

Increased Effect/Toxicity: Alpha-adrenergic blockers and calcium channel blockers may increase risk of hypotension. Risk of first-dose orthostatic hypotension may increase with beta-blockers. Cimetidine may decrease tamsulosin clearance. Blood pressure-lowering effects are additive with phosphodiesterase-5 inhibitors; sildenafil (use with extreme caution), tadalafil (may be used when tamsulosin dose is ≤0.4 mg/day), and vardenafil (use is contraindicated by the manufacturer).

CYP2D6 inhibitors may increase the levels/effects of tamsulosin; example inhibitors include chlorpromazine, delavirdine, fluoxetine, miconazole, paroxetine, pergolide, quinidine, quinine, ritonavir, and ropinirole. CYP3A4 inhibitors may increase the levels/effects of tamsulosin; example inhibitors include azole antifungals, clarithromycin, diclofenac, doxycycline, erythromycin, imatinib, isoniazid, nefazodone, nicardipine, propofol, protease inhibitors, quinidine, telithromycin, and verapamil.

Decreased Effect: CYP3A4 inducers may decrease the levels/effects of tamsulosin; example inducers include aminoglutethimide, carbamazepine, nafcillin, nevirapine, phenobarbital, phenytoin, and rifamycins.

Ethanol/Nutrition/Herb Interactions

Food: Fasting increases bioavailability by 30% and peak concentration 40% to 70%.

Herb/Nutraceutical: St John's wort: May decrease the levels/effects of tamsulosin. Avoid herbs with hypotensive properties (black cohosh, California poppy, coleus, golden seal, hawthorn, mistletoe, periwinkle, quinine, Shepherd's purse); may enhance the hypotensive effect of tamsulosin. Avoid saw palmetto (due to limited experience with this combination).

Dietary Considerations Take once daily, 30 minutes after the same meal each day.

Pharmacodynamics/Kinetics

Absorption: >90%

Protein binding: 94% to 99%, primarily to alpha$_1$ acid glycoprotein (AAG)

(Continued)

Tamsulosin *(Continued)*

Metabolism: Hepatic via CYP3A4 and 2D6; metabolites undergo extensive conjugation to glucuronide or sulfate

Bioavailability: Fasting: 30% increase

Distribution: V_d: 16 L

Steady-state: By the fifth day of once-daily dosing

Half-life elimination: Healthy volunteers: 9-13 hours; Target population: 14-15 hours

Time to peak: Fasting: 4-5 hours; With food: 6-7 hours

Excretion: Urine (76%, <10% as unchanged drug); feces (21%)

Pregnancy Risk Factor B

Dosage Forms

Capsule:

Flomax®: 0.4 mg

Tamsulosin Hydrochloride *see* Tamsulosin *on page 1524*

Tanac® [OTC] *see* Benzocaine *on page 195*

TanaCof-XR *see* Brompheniramine *on page 230*

Tanafed DP™ *see* Dexchlorpheniramine and Pseudoephedrine *on page 469*

Tannate 12 S *see* Carbetapentane and Chlorpheniramine *on page 278*

Tannic-12 *see* Carbetapentane and Chlorpheniramine *on page 278*

Tannic-12 S *see* Carbetapentane and Chlorpheniramine *on page 278*

Tannihist-12 RF *see* Carbetapentane and Chlorpheniramine *on page 278*

TAP-144 *see* Leuprolide *on page 958*

Tapazole® *see* Methimazole *on page 1064*

Tarceva® *see* Erlotinib *on page 587*

Targretin® *see* Bexarotene *on page 213*

Tarka® *see* Trandolapril and Verapamil *on page 1599*

Tarsum® [OTC] *see* Coal Tar and Salicylic Acid *on page 402*

Tasmar® *see* Tolcapone *on page 1584*

Tavist® Allergy [OTC] *see* Clemastine *on page 376*

Tavist® ND [OTC] *see* Loratadine *on page 999*

Taxol® *see* Paclitaxel *on page 1240*

Taxotere® *see* Docetaxel *on page 521*

Tazarotene *(taz AR oh teen)*

U.S. Brand Names Avage™; Tazorac®

Canadian Brand Names Tazorac®

Mexican Brand Names Suretin

Generic Available No

Pharmacologic Category Acne Products; Keratolytic Agent; Topical Skin Product, Acne

Use Topical treatment of facial acne vulgaris; topical treatment of stable plaque psoriasis of up to 20% body surface area involvement; mitigation (palliation) of facial skin wrinkling, facial mottled hyper-/hypopigmentation, and benign facial lentigines

Local Anesthetic/Vasoconstrictor Precautions No information available to require special precautions

Effects on Dental Treatment No significant effects or complications reported

Common Adverse Effects Percentage of incidence varies with formulation and/or strength:

>10%: Dermatologic: Burning/stinging, desquamation, dry skin, erythema, pruritus, skin pain, worsening of psoriasis

1% to 10%: Dermatologic: Contact dermatitis, discoloration, fissuring, hypertriglyceridemia, inflammation, irritation, localized bleeding, rash

Frequency not defined:

Dermatologic: Photosensitization

Neuromuscular & skeletal: Peripheral neuropathy

Mechanism of Action Synthetic, acetylenic retinoid which modulates differentiation and proliferation of epithelial tissue and exerts some degree of anti-inflammatory and immunological activity

Drug Interactions

Increased Effect/Toxicity: Increased toxicity may occur with sulfur, benzoyl peroxide, salicylic acid, resorcinol, or any product with strong drying effects (including alcohol-containing compounds) due to increased drying actions. May augment phototoxicity of sensitizing medications (thiazides, tetracyclines, fluoroquinolones, phenothiazines, sulfonamides).

Pharmacodynamics/Kinetics

Duration: Therapeutic: Psoriasis: Effects have been observed for up to 3 months after a 3-month course of topical treatment

Absorption: Minimal following cutaneous application (≤6% of dose)

Distribution: Retained in skin for prolonged periods after topical application.

Protein binding: >99%

Metabolism: Prodrug, rapidly metabolized via esterases to an active metabolite (tazarotenic acid) following topical application and systemic absorption; tazarotenic acid undergoes further hepatic metabolism

Half-life elimination: 18 hours

Excretion: Urine and feces (as metabolites)

Pregnancy Risk Factor X

Tegaserod (teg a SER od)

U.S. Brand Names Zelnorm® [DSC]

Canadian Brand Names Zelnorm® [DSC]

Mexican Brand Names Zelmac

Generic Available No

Index Terms HTF919; Tegaserod Maleate

Pharmacologic Category Serotonin 5-HT$_4$ Receptor Agonist

Use Short-term treatment of constipation-predominate irritable bowel syndrome (IBS) in women; treatment of chronic idiopathic constipation

Local Anesthetic/Vasoconstrictor Precautions No information available to require special precautions

Effects on Dental Treatment No significant effects or complications reported

Common Adverse Effects

>10%:

Central nervous system: Headache (15%)

Gastrointestinal: Abdominal pain (12%)

1% to 10%:

Central nervous system: Dizziness (4%), migraine (2%)

Gastrointestinal: Diarrhea (9%; severe <1%), nausea (8%), flatulence (6%)

Neuromuscular & skeletal: Back pain (5%), arthropathy (2%), leg pain (1%)

Mechanism of Action Tegaserod is a partial neuronal 5-HT$_4$ receptor agonist. Its action at the receptor site leads to stimulation of the peristaltic reflex and intestinal secretion, and moderation of visceral sensitivity.

Pharmacodynamics/Kinetics

Distribution: V_d: 368 ± 223 L

Protein binding: 98% primarily to α_1-acid glycoprotein

(Continued)

Tegaserod *(Continued)*

Metabolism: GI: Hydrolysis in the stomach; Hepatic: Oxidation, conjugation, and glucuronidation; metabolite (negligible activity); significant first-pass effect

Bioavailability: Fasting: 10%

Half-life elimination: I.V.: 11 ± 5 hours

Time to peak: 1 hour

Excretion: Feces (~66% as unchanged drug); urine (~33% as metabolites)

Pregnancy Risk Factor B

Tegaserod Maleate *see* Tegaserod *on page 1527*

Tegretol® *see* Carbamazepine *on page 272*

Tegretol®-XR *see* Carbamazepine *on page 272*

Tekturna® *see* Aliskiren *on page 70*

Telbivudine *(tel BI vyoo deen)*

U.S. Brand Names Tyzeka™

Canadian Brand Names Sebivo™

Generic Available No

Index Terms L-Deoxythymidine

Pharmacologic Category Antiretroviral Agent, Reverse Transcriptase Inhibitor (Nucleoside)

Use Treatment of chronic hepatitis B with evidence of viral replication and either persistent transaminase elevations or histologically-active disease

Local Anesthetic/Vasoconstrictor Precautions No information available to require special precautions

Effects on Dental Treatment No significant effects or complications reported

Common Adverse Effects

>10%:

Central nervous system: Fatigue (12%), malaise (12%), headache (11%)

Gastrointestinal: Abdominal pain (12%)

Neuromuscular & skeletal: CPK increased (72%; grades 3/4: 9%)

Respiratory: Upper respiratory tract infection (14%), nasopharyngitis (11%)

1% to 10%:

Central nervous system: Dizziness (4%), fever (4%), insomnia (3%)

Dermatologic: Rash (4%)

Endocrine & metabolic: Lipase increased (2%)

Gastrointestinal: Nausea (7%), vomiting (7%), diarrhea (7%), dyspepsia (3%)

Hematologic: Neutropenia (2%)

Hepatic: ALT increased (grades 3/4: 3% to 4%), AST increased (grades 3/4: 3%)

Neuromuscular & skeletal: Arthralgia (4%), back pain (4%), myalgia (3%)

Respiratory: Cough (7%), pharyngolaryngeal pain (5%)

Miscellaneous: Flu-like syndrome (7%), postprocedural pain (7%)

Mechanism of Action Telbivudine, a synthetic thymidine nucleoside analogue, is intracellularly phosphorylated to the active triphosphate form, which competes with the natural substrate, thymidine 5'-triphosphate, to inhibit hepatitis B viral DNA polymerase; enzyme inhibition blocks reverse transcriptase activity thereby reducing viral DNA replication.

Drug Interactions

Increased Effect/Toxicity: No interactions identified.

Pharmacodynamics/Kinetics

Distribution: V_d > total body water

Protein binding: 3%

Metabolism: No metabolites detected

Half-life elimination: Terminal: 40-49 hours

Time to peak, plasma: 1-4 hours

Excretion: Urine (as unchanged drug)

Pregnancy Risk Factor B

Teldrin® HBP [OTC] *see* Chlorpheniramine *on page 338*

Telithromycin *(tel ith roe MYE sin)*

U.S. Brand Names Ketek®

Canadian Brand Names Ketek®

Mexican Brand Names Ketek

Generic Available No

Index Terms HMR 3647

Pharmacologic Category Antibiotic, Ketolide

Use Treatment of community-acquired pneumonia (mild-to-moderate) caused by susceptible strains of *Streptococcus pneumoniae* (including multidrug-resistant isolates), *Haemophilus influenzae*, *Chlamydophila pneumoniae*, *Moraxella catarrhalis*, and *Mycoplasma pneumoniae*

Unlabeled/Investigational Use Approved in Canada for use in the treatment of tonsillitis/pharyngitis due to *S. pyogenes* (as an alternative to beta-lactam antibiotics when necessary/appropriate)

Local Anesthetic/Vasoconstrictor Precautions Telithromycin is one of the drugs confirmed to prolong the QT interval and is accepted as having a risk of causing torsade de pointes. The risk of drug-induced torsade de pointes is extremely low when a single QT interval prolonging drug is prescribed. In terms of epinephrine, it is not known what effect vasoconstrictors in the local anesthetic regimen will have in patients with a known history of congenital prolonged QT interval or in patients taking any medication that prolongs the QT interval. Until more information is obtained, it is suggested that the clinician consult with the physician prior to the use of a vasoconstrictor in suspected patients, and that the vasoconstrictor (epinephrine, levonordefrin [Neo-Cobefrin®]) be used with caution.

Effects on Dental Treatment Key adverse event(s) related to dental treatment: Xerostomia (normal salivary flow resumes upon discontinuation), glossitis, stomatitis, and tooth discoloration.

Common Adverse Effects

>10%: Gastrointestinal: Diarrhea (10% to 11%)

2% to 10%:
Central nervous system: Headache (2% to 6%), dizziness (3% to 4%)
Gastrointestinal: Nausea (7% to 8%), vomiting (2% to 3%), loose stools (2%), dysgeusia (2%)

≥0.2% to <2%:
Central nervous system: Vertigo, fatigue, somnolence, insomnia
Dermatologic: Rash
Gastrointestinal: Abdominal distension, abdominal pain, anorexia, constipation, dyspepsia, flatulence, gastritis, gastroenteritis, GI upset, glossitis, stomatitis, watery stools, xerostomia
Genitourinary: Vaginal candidiasis
Hematologic: Platelets increased
Hepatic: Transaminases increased
Ocular: Blurred vision, accommodation delayed, diplopia
Miscellaneous: Candidiasis, diaphoresis increased

Restrictions

An FDA-approved Medication Guide is available and must be dispensed with every prescription. Copies may be found at: http://www.fda.gov/cder/foi/label/2007/021144s012medg.pdf.

Dosage Oral:

Children ≥13 years and Adults: Tonsillitis/pharyngitis (unlabeled use; Canadian indication): 800 mg once daily for 5 days

Adults:
Community-acquired pneumonia: 800 mg once daily for 7-10 days

Dosage adjustment in renal impairment:
U.S. product labeling: Cl_{cr} <30 mL/minute, including dialysis: 600 mg once daily; when renal impairment is accompanied by hepatic impairment, reduce dosage to 400 mg once daily
Canadian product labeling: Cl_{cr} <30 mL/minute: Reduce dose to 400 mg once daily
Hemodialysis: Administer following dialysis

Dosage adjustment in hepatic impairment: No adjustment recommended, unless concurrent severe renal impairment is present

Mechanism of Action Inhibits bacterial protein synthesis by binding to two sites on the 50S ribosomal subunit. Telithromycin has also been demonstrated to alter secretion of IL-1alpha and TNF-alpha; the clinical significance of this immunomodulatory effect has not been evaluated.

Contraindications Hypersensitivity to telithromycin, macrolide antibiotics, or any component of the formulation; myasthenia gravis; history of hepatitis and/or jaundice associated with telithromycin or other macrolide antibiotic use; concurrent use of cisapride or pimozide

Warnings/Precautions Acute hepatic failure and severe liver injury, including hepatitis and hepatic necrosis (leading to some fatalities) have been reported, in some cases after only a few doses; if signs/symptoms of hepatitis or liver damage occur, discontinue therapy and initiate liver function tests. **[U.S. Boxed Warning]: Life-threatening (including fatal) respiratory failure has occurred in patients with myasthenia gravis;** use in these patients is contraindicated. May prolong QT_c interval, leading to a risk of ventricular arrhythmias; closely-related antibiotics have been associated with malignant ventricular arrhythmias and torsade de pointes. Avoid in patients with prolongation of QTc interval due to congenital causes, history of long QT syndrome, uncorrected (Continued)

Telithromycin *(Continued)*

electrolyte disturbances (hypokalemia or hypomagnesemia), significant brady-cardia (<50 bpm), or concurrent therapy with QT_c-prolonging drugs (eg, class Ia and class III antiarrhythmics). Avoid use in patients with a prior history of confirmed cardiogenic syncope or ventricular arrhythmias while receiving macrolide antibiotics or other QT_c-prolonging drugs. May cause severe visual disturbances (eg, changes in accommodation ability, diplopia, blurred vision). May cause loss of consciousness (possibly vagal-related); caution patients that these events may interfere with ability to operate machinery or drive, and to use caution until effects are known. Use caution in renal impairment; severe impairment (Cl_{cr} <30 mL/minute) requires dosage adjustment. Pseudomembranous colitis has been reported. Safety and efficacy not established in pediatric patients <13 years of age per Canadian approved labeling and <18 years of age per U.S. approved labeling.

Drug Interactions

Cytochrome P450 Effect: Substrate of CYP1A2 (minor), 3A4 (major); **Inhibits** CYP2D6 (weak), 3A4 (strong)

Increased Effect/Toxicity: Concurrent use of cisapride or pimozide is contraindicated. Concurrent use with antiarrhythmics (eg, class Ia and class III) or other drugs which prolong QT_c (eg, disopyramide, moxifloxacin, pimozide, thioridazine) may be additive; serious arrhythmias may occur. Neuromuscular-blocking agents may be potentiated by telithromycin.

Telithromycin may increase the levels/effects of alfentanil, selected benzodiazepines, buspirone, calcium channel blockers, cilostazol, clozapine, corticosteroids, cyclosporine, eletriptan, eplerenone, ergot alkaloids, selected HMG-CoA reductase inhibitors, mirtazapine, nateglinide, nefazodone, pimozide, repaglinide, quinidine, sildenafil (and other PDE-5 inhibitors), SSRIs, tacrolimus, venlafaxine, warfarin (monitor), and other CYP3A4 substrates. Selected benzodiazepines (midazolam, triazolam), and selected HMG-CoA reductase inhibitors (atorvastatin, lovastatin and simvastatin) are generally contraindicated with strong CYP3A4 inhibitors. When used with strong CYP3A4 inhibitors, dosage adjustment/limits are recommended for sildenafil and other PDE-5 inhibitors; refer to individual monographs.

The levels/effects of telithromycin may be increased by azole antifungals, clarithromycin, diclofenac, doxycycline, erythromycin, imatinib, isoniazid, nefazodone, nicardipine, propofol, protease inhibitors, quinidine, verapamil, and other CYP3A4 inhibitors.

Decreased Effect: The levels/effects of telithromycin may be decreased by aminoglutethimide, carbamazepine, nafcillin, nevirapine, phenobarbital, phenytoin, rifamycins, and other CYP3A4 inducers; avoid concurrent use. Telithromycin may decrease the levels/effects of clopidogrel, or the live, attenuated Ty21a strain of typhoid vaccine.

Ethanol/Nutrition/Herb Interactions Herb/nutraceutical: St John's wort: May decrease the levels/effects of telithromycin.

Dietary Considerations May be taken with or without food.

Pharmacodynamics/Kinetics

Absorption: Rapid

Distribution: 2.9 L/kg

Protein binding: 60% to 70%

Metabolism: Hepatic, via CYP3A4 (50%) and non-CYP-mediated pathways

Bioavailability: 57% (significant first-pass metabolism)

Half-life elimination: 10 hours

Time to peak, plasma: 1 hour

Excretion: Urine (13% unchanged drug, remainder as metabolites); feces (7%)

Pregnancy Risk Factor C

Dosage Forms

Tablet:

Ketek®: 300 mg [not available in Canada], 400 mg

Ketek Pak™ [blister pack]: 400 mg (10s)

Selected Readings

Araujo FG, Slifer TL, and Remington JS, "Inhibition of Secretion of Interleukin-1alpha and Tumor Necrosis Factor Alpha by the Ketolide Antibiotic Telithromycin," *Antimicrob Agents Chemother*, 2002, 46(10):3327-30.

Bhargava V, Lenfant B, Perret C, et al, "Lack of Effect of Food on the Bioavailability of a New Ketolide Antibacterial, Telithromycin," *Scand J Infect Dis*, 2002, 34(11):823-6.

Cantalloube C, Bhargava V, Sultan E, et al, "Pharmacokinetics of the Ketolide Telithromycin After Single and Repeated Doses in Patients With Hepatic Impairment," *Int J Antimicrob Agents*, 2003, 22(2):112-21.

Canton R, Morosini M, Enright MC, et al, "Worldwide Incidence, Molecular Epidemiology and Mutations Implicated in Fluoroquinolone-resistant *Streptococcus pneumoniae*: Data From the Global PROTEKT Surveillance Programme," *J Antimicrob Chemother*, 2003, 52(6):944-52.

Carbon C, "A Pooled Analysis of Telithromycin in the Treatment of Community-Acquired Respiratory Tract Infections in Adults," *Infection*, 2003, 31(5):308-17.

Demolis JL, Vacheron F, Cardus S, et al, "Effect of Single and Repeated Oral Doses of Telithromycin on Cardiac QT Interval in Healthy Subjects," *Clin Pharmacol Ther*, 2003, 73(3):242-52.

Perret C, Lenfant B, Weinling E, et al, "Pharmacokinetics and Absolute Oral Bioavailability of an 800-mg Oral Dose of Telithromycin in Healthy Young and Elderly Volunteers," *Chemotherapy*, 2002, 48(5):217-23.

Nieman RB, Sharma K, Edelberg H, et al, "Telithromycin and Myasthenia Gravis," *Clin Infect Dis*, 2003, 37(11):1579.

Quinn J, Ruoff GE, and Ziter PS, "Efficacy and tolerability of 5-day, once-daily telithromycin compared with 10-day, twice-daily clarithromycin for the treatment of group A beta-hemolytic streptococcal tonsillitis/pharyngitis: a multicenter, randomized, double-blind, parallel-group study," *Clin Ther*, 2003, 25(2):422-43.

Ubukata K, Iwata S, and Sunakawa K, "*In vitro* Activities of New Ketolide, Telithromycin, and Eight Other Macrolide Antibiotics Against *Streptococcus pneumoniae* Having mefA and ermB Genes That Mediate Macrolide Resistance," *J Infect Chemother*, 2003, 9(3):221-6.

Zervos MJ, Heyder AM, and Leroy B, "Oral Telithromycin 800 mg Once Daily for 5 Days Versus Cefuroxime Axetil 500 mg Twice Daily for 10 Days in Adults With Acute Exacerbations of Chronic Bronchitis," *J Int Med Res*, 2003, 31(3):157-69.

Telisartan (tel mi SAR tan)

Related Information
Cardiovascular Diseases *on page 1726*

U.S. Brand Names Micardis®
Canadian Brand Names Micardis®
Mexican Brand Names Micardis; Predxal
Generic Available No
Pharmacologic Category Angiotensin II Receptor Blocker
Use Treatment of hypertension; may be used alone or in combination with other antihypertensive agents
Local Anesthetic/Vasoconstrictor Precautions No information available to require special precautions
Effects on Dental Treatment No significant effects or complications reported
Common Adverse Effects May be associated with worsening of renal function in patients dependent on renin-angiotensin-aldosterone system.

1% to 10%:
Cardiovascular: Hypertension (1%), chest pain (1%), peripheral edema (1%)
Central nervous system: Headache (1%), dizziness (1%), pain (1%), fatigue (1%)
Gastrointestinal: Diarrhea (3%), dyspepsia (1%), nausea (1%), abdominal pain (1%)
Genitourinary: Urinary tract infection (1%)
Neuromuscular & skeletal: Back pain (3%), myalgia (1%)
Respiratory: Upper respiratory infection (7%), sinusitis (3%), pharyngitis (1%), cough (2%)
Miscellaneous: Flu-like syndrome (1%)

Dosage Adults: Oral: Initial: 40 mg once daily; usual maintenance dose range: 20-80 mg/day. Patients with volume depletion should be initiated on the lower dosage with close supervision.
Dosage adjustment in renal impairment: No adjustment required; hemodialysis patients are more susceptible to orthostatic hypotension
Dosage adjustment in hepatic impairment: Supervise patients closely.
Mechanism of Action Angiotensin II acts as a vasoconstrictor. In addition to causing direct vasoconstriction, angiotensin II also stimulates the release of aldosterone. Once aldosterone is released, sodium as well as water are reabsorbed. The end result is an elevation in blood pressure. Telmisartan is a nonpeptide AT1 angiotensin II receptor antagonist. This binding prevents angiotensin II from binding to the receptor thereby blocking the vasoconstriction and the aldosterone secreting effects of angiotensin II.
Contraindications Hypersensitivity to telmisartan or any component of the formulation; hypersensitivity to other A-II receptor antagonists; bilateral renal artery stenosis; pregnancy
Warnings/Precautions [U.S. Boxed Warning]: Based on human data, drugs that act on the angiotensin system can cause injury and death to the developing fetus when used in the second and third trimesters. Angiotensin receptor blockers should be discontinued as soon as possible once pregnancy is detected. May cause hyperkalemia; avoid potassium supplementation unless specifically required by healthcare provider. Avoid use or use a smaller dose in patients who are volume depleted; correct depletion first. May be associated with deterioration of renal function and/or increases in serum creatinine, particularly in patients dependent on renin-angiotensin-aldosterone system. Use with caution in unilateral renal artery stenosis and pre-existing renal insufficiency; significant aortic/mitral stenosis. Use with caution in patients who have biliary obstructive disorders or hepatic dysfunction. Safety and efficacy have not been established in children.
(Continued)

Telmisartan *(Continued)*

Drug Interactions

Cytochrome P450 Effect: Inhibits CYP2C19 (weak)

Increased Effect/Toxicity: Telmisartan may increase serum digoxin concentrations. Potassium salts/supplements, co-trimoxazole (high dose), ACE inhibitors, eplerenone, and potassium-sparing diuretics (amiloride, spironolactone, triamterene) may increase the risk of hyperkalemia with telmisartan.

Ethanol/Nutrition/Herb Interactions Herb/Nutraceutical: Avoid dong quai if using for hypertension (has estrogenic activity). Avoid ephedra, yohimbe, ginseng (may worsen hypertension). Avoid garlic (may have increased antihypertensive effect).

Dietary Considerations May be taken without regard to food.

Pharmacodynamics/Kinetics Orally active, not a prodrug

Onset of action: 1-2 hours

Peak effect: 0.5-1 hours

Duration: Up to 24 hours

Protein binding: >99.5%

Metabolism: Hepatic via conjugation to inactive metabolites; not metabolized via CYP

Bioavailability (dose dependent): 42% to 58%

Half-life elimination: Terminal: 24 hours

Excretion: Feces (97%)

Clearance: Total body: 800 mL/minute

Pregnancy Risk Factor C (1st trimester); D (2nd and 3rd trimesters)

Dosage Forms

Tablet:

Micardis®: 20 mg, 40 mg, 80 mg

Telmisartan and Hydrochlorothiazide
(tel mi SAR tan & hye droe klor oh THYE a zide)

Related Information

Hydrochlorothiazide *on page 819*

Telmisartan *on page 1531*

U.S. Brand Names Micardis® HCT

Canadian Brand Names Micardis® Plus

Generic Available No

Index Terms Hydrochlorothiazide and Telmisartan

Pharmacologic Category Angiotensin II Receptor Blocker Combination; Antihypertensive Agent, Combination; Diuretic, Thiazide

Use Treatment of hypertension; combination product should not be used for initial therapy

Local Anesthetic/Vasoconstrictor Precautions No information available to require special precautions

Effects on Dental Treatment No significant effects or complications reported

Common Adverse Effects The following reactions have been reported with the combination product; see individual agents for additional adverse reactions that may be expected from each agent.

2% to 10%:

Central nervous system: Dizziness (5%)

Gastrointestinal: Diarrhea (3%), nausea (2%)

Renal: BUN increased (3%)

Respiratory: Upper respiratory tract infection (8%), sinusitis (4%)

Miscellaneous: Flu-like syndrome (2%)

<2%: Abdominal pain, back pain, bilirubin increased, bronchitis, dyspepsia, hematocrit decreased, hemoglobin decreased, hypokalemia, liver enzymes increased, pharyngitis, postural hypotension, rash, serum creatinine increased, tachycardia, vomiting; rhabdomyolysis has been reported (rarely) with angiotensin-receptor antagonists

Mechanism of Action

Telmisartan: Telmisartan is an angiotensin receptor antagonist. Angiotensin II acts as a vasoconstrictor. In addition to causing direct vasoconstriction, angiotensin II also stimulates the release of aldosterone. Once aldosterone is released, sodium as well as water are reabsorbed. The end result is an elevation in blood pressure. Telmisartan binds to the AT1 angiotensin II receptor. This binding prevents angiotensin II from binding to the receptor thereby blocking the vasoconstriction and the aldosterone secreting effects of angiotensin II.

Hydrochlorothiazide: Inhibits sodium reabsorption in the distal tubules causing increased excretion of sodium and water as well as potassium and hydrogen ions

Drug Interactions
  Cytochrome P450 Effect: Telmisartan: **Inhibits** CYP2C19 (weak)
  Increased Effect/Toxicity: See individual agents.
  Decreased Effect: See individual agents.
Pharmacodynamics/Kinetics See individual agents.
Pregnancy Risk Factor C (1st trimester); D (2nd and 3rd trimesters)

Temazepam (te MAZ e pam)

U.S. Brand Names Restoril®
Canadian Brand Names Apo-Temazepam®; CO Temazepam;
Gen-Temazepam; Novo-Temazepam; Nu-Temazepam; PMS-Temazepam;
ratio-Temazepam; Restoril®
Generic Available Yes
Pharmacologic Category Hypnotic, Benzodiazepine
Use Short-term treatment of insomnia
Unlabeled/Investigational Use Treatment of anxiety; adjunct in the treatment
of depression; management of panic attacks
Local Anesthetic/Vasoconstrictor Precautions No information available to
require special precautions
Effects on Dental Treatment Key adverse event(s) related to dental treat-
ment: Significant xerostomia (normal salivary flow resumes upon discontinua-
tion).
Common Adverse Effects
  1% to 10%:
    Central nervous system: Confusion, dizziness, drowsiness, fatigue, anxiety,
      headache, lethargy, hangover, euphoria, vertigo
    Dermatologic: Rash
    Endocrine & metabolic: Decreased libido
    Gastrointestinal: Diarrhea
    Neuromuscular & skeletal: Dysarthria, weakness
    Ocular: Blurred vision
    Miscellaneous: Diaphoresis
Restrictions C-IV
Dosage Oral:
  Adults: 15-30 mg at bedtime
  Elderly or debilitated patients: 15 mg
Mechanism of Action Binds to stereospecific benzodiazepine receptors on the
postsynaptic GABA neuron at several sites within the central nervous system,
including the limbic system, reticular formation. Enhancement of the inhibitory
effect of GABA on neuronal excitability results by increased neuronal
membrane permeability to chloride ions. This shift in chloride ions results in
hyperpolarization (a less excitable state) and stabilization.
Contraindications Hypersensitivity to temazepam or any component of the
formulation (cross-sensitivity with other benzodiazepines may exist);
narrow-angle glaucoma (not in product labeling, however, benzodiazepines are
contraindicated); pregnancy
Warnings/Precautions Should be used only after evaluation of potential
causes of sleep disturbance. Failure of sleep disturbance to resolve after 7-10
days may indicate psychiatric or medical illness. A worsening of insomnia or the
emergence of new abnormalities of thought or behavior may represent unrecognized psychiatric or medical illness and requires immediate and careful evaluation.

Use with caution in elderly or debilitated patients, patients with hepatic disease
(including alcoholics), or renal impairment. Use with caution in patients with
respiratory disease, or impaired gag reflex. Avoid use inpatients with sleep
apnea.

Causes CNS depression (dose-related) resulting in sedation, dizziness, confusion, or ataxia which may impair physical and mental capabilities. Patients must
be cautioned about performing tasks which require mental alertness (eg, operating machinery or driving). Use with caution in patients receiving other CNS
depressants or psychoactive agents. Postmarketing studies have indicated that
the use of hypnotic/sedative agents for sleep has been associated with hypersensitivity reactions including anaphylaxis as well as angioedema. An increased
risk for hazardous sleep-related activities such as sleep-driving; cooking and
eating food, and making phone calls while asleep have also been noted. Effects
with other sedative drugs or ethanol may be potentiated. Benzodiazepines have
been associated with falls and traumatic injury and should be used with extreme
caution in patients who are at risk of these events (especially the elderly).

Use caution in patients with suicidal risk. Use with caution in patients with a
history of drug dependence. Benzodiazepines have been associated with
(Continued)

Temazepam *(Continued)*

dependence and acute withdrawal symptoms on discontinuation or reduction in dose (may occur after as little as 10 days). Acute withdrawal, including seizures, may be precipitated after administration of flumazenil to patients receiving long-term benzodiazepine therapy.

Benzodiazepines have been associated with anterograde amnesia. Paradoxical reactions, including hyperactive or aggressive behavior, have been reported with benzodiazepines, particularly in adolescent/pediatric or psychiatric patients. Does not have analgesic, antidepressant, or antipsychotic properties.

Drug Interactions

Cytochrome P450 Effect: Substrate (minor) of CYP2B6, 2C9, 2C19, 3A4

Increased Effect/Toxicity: Temazepam potentiates the CNS depressant effects of opioid analgesics, barbiturates, phenothiazines, ethanol, antihistamines, MAO inhibitors, sedative-hypnotics, and cyclic antidepressants. Serum levels of temazepam may be increased by inhibitors of CYP3A4, including cimetidine, ciprofloxacin, clarithromycin, clozapine, diltiazem, disulfiram, digoxin, erythromycin, ethanol, fluconazole, fluoxetine, fluvoxamine, grapefruit juice, isoniazid, itraconazole, ketoconazole, labetalol, levodopa, loxapine, metoprolol, metronidazole, miconazole, nefazodone, omeprazole, phenytoin, rifabutin, rifampin, troleandomycin, valproic acid, and verapamil.

Decreased Effect: Oral contraceptives may increase the clearance of temazepam. Temazepam may decrease the antiparkinsonian efficacy of levodopa. Theophylline and other CNS stimulants may antagonize the sedative effects of temazepam. Carbamazepine, rifampin, rifabutin may enhance the metabolism of temazepam and decrease its therapeutic effect.

Ethanol/Nutrition/Herb Interactions

Ethanol: Avoid ethanol (may increase CNS depression).

Food: Serum levels may be increased by grapefruit juice.

Herb/Nutraceutical: St John's wort may decrease temazepam levels. Avoid valerian, St John's wort, kava kava, gotu kola (may increase CNS depression).

Pharmacodynamics/Kinetics

Distribution: V_d: 1.4 L/kg

Protein binding: 96%

Metabolism: Hepatic

Half-life elimination: 9.5-12.4 hours

Time to peak, serum: 2-3 hours

Excretion: Urine (80% to 90% as inactive metabolites)

Pregnancy Risk Factor X

Dosage Forms

Capsule: 15 mg, 30 mg

Restoril®: 7.5 mg, 15 mg, 30 mg

Temodar® *see* Temozolomide *on page 1534*

Temovate® *see* Clobetasol *on page 383*

Temovate E® *see* Clobetasol *on page 383*

Temozolomide *(te moe ZOE loe mide)*

U.S. Brand Names Temodar®

Canadian Brand Names Temodal®; Temodar®

Mexican Brand Names Temodal

Generic Available No

Index Terms NSC-362856; TMZ

Pharmacologic Category Antineoplastic Agent, Alkylating Agent (Triazene)

Use Treatment of adult patients with refractory anaplastic astrocytoma; newly-diagnosed glioblastoma multiforme

Unlabeled/Investigational Use Metastatic melanoma

Local Anesthetic/Vasoconstrictor Precautions No information available to require special precautions

Effects on Dental Treatment Key adverse event(s) related to dental treatment: Stomatitis, dysphagia, and taste perversion.

Common Adverse Effects Note: With CNS malignancies, it is difficult to distinguish between CNS adverse events caused by temozolomide versus the effects of progressive disease.

>10%:

Cardiovascular: Peripheral edema (11%)

Central nervous system: Fatigue (34% to 61%), headache (23% to 41%), seizure (6% to 23%), hemiparesis (18%), fever (13%), dizziness (5% to 12%), coordination abnormality (11%)

Dermatologic: Alopecia (55%), rash (8% to 13%)

Gastrointestinal: Nausea (49% to 53%; grades 3/4: 1% to 10%), vomiting (29% to 42%; grades 3/4: 2% to 6%), constipation (22% to 33%), anorexia (9% to 27%), diarrhea (10% to 16%)

Hematologic: Lymphopenia (grades 3/4: 55%), thrombocytopenia (grades 3/4: adults: 4% to 19%; children: 25%), neutropenia (grades 3/4: adults: 8% to 14%; children: 20%), leukopenia (grades 3/4: 11%)

Neuromuscular & skeletal: Weakness (7% to 13%)

Miscellaneous: Viral infection (11%)

1% to 10%:

Central nervous system: Amnesia (10%), insomnia (4% to 10%), somnolence (9%), ataxia (8%), paresis (8%), anxiety (7%), memory impairment (7%), depression (6%), confusion (5%)

Dermatologic: Pruritus (5% to 8%), dry skin (5%), radiation injury (2% maintenance phase after radiotherapy), erythema (1%)

Endocrine & metabolic: Hypercorticism (8%), breast pain (females 6%)

Gastrointestinal: Stomatitis (9%), abdominal pain (5% to 9%), dysphagia (7%), taste perversion (5%), weight gain (5%)

Genitourinary: Incontinence (8%), urinary tract infection (8%), urinary frequency (6%)

Hematologic: Anemia (grades 3/4: 4%)

Neuromuscular & skeletal: Paresthesia (9%), back pain (8%), abnormal gait (6%), arthralgia (6%), myalgia (5%)

Ocular: Blurred vision (5% to 8%), diplopia (5%), vision abnormality (visual deficit/vision changes 5%)

Respiratory: Pharyngitis (8%), upper respiratory tract infection (8%), cough (5% to 8%), sinusitis (6%), dyspnea (5%)

Miscellaneous: Allergic reaction (up to 3%)

Mechanism of Action Like dacarbazine, temozolomide is converted to the active alkylating metabolite MTIC [(methyl-triazene-1-yl)-imidazole-4-carboxamide]. Unlike dacarbazine, however, this conversion is spontaneous, nonenzymatic, and occurs under physiologic conditions in all tissues to which the drug distributes.

Pharmacodynamics/Kinetics

Absorption: Rapid and complete

Distribution: V_d: Parent drug: 0.4 L/kg; penetrates blood brain barrier; CSF levels are ~35% to 39% of plasma levels

Protein binding: 15%

Metabolism: Prodrug, hydrolyzed to the active form, MTIC; MTIC is eventually eliminated as CO_2 and 5-aminoimidazole-4-carboxamide (AIC), a natural constituent in urine

Bioavailability: 100%

Half-life elimination: Mean: Parent drug: 1.8 hours

Time to peak: Empty stomach: 1 hour

Excretion: Urine (~38%; parent drug 6%); feces 0.8%

Pregnancy Risk Factor D

Tenecteplase (ten EK te plase)

Related Information

Cardiovascular Diseases *on page 1726*

U.S. Brand Names TNKase™

Canadian Brand Names TNKase™

Mexican Brand Names Metalyse

Generic Available No

Pharmacologic Category Thrombolytic Agent

Use Thrombolytic agent used in the management of acute myocardial infarction for the lysis of thrombi in the coronary vasculature to restore perfusion and reduce mortality.

Unlabeled/Investigational Use Acute MI - combination regimen of tenecteplase (unlabeled dose), abciximab, and heparin (unlabeled dose)

Local Anesthetic/Vasoconstrictor Precautions No information available to require special precautions

Effects on Dental Treatment No significant effects or complications reported

Common Adverse Effects As with all drugs which may affect hemostasis, bleeding is the major adverse effect associated with tenecteplase. Hemorrhage may occur at virtually any site. Risk is dependent on multiple variables, including the dosage administered, concurrent use of multiple agents which alter hemostasis, and patient predisposition. Rapid lysis of coronary artery thrombi by thrombolytic agents may be associated with reperfusion-related arterial and/or ventricular arrhythmia. The incidence of stroke and bleeding increase in patients >65 years.

(Continued)

Tenecteplase *(Continued)*

>10%:
    Hematologic: Bleeding (22% minor: ASSENT-2 trial)
    Local: Hematoma (12% minor)
1% to 10%:
    Central nervous system: Stroke (2%)
    Gastrointestinal: GI hemorrhage (1% major, 2% minor), epistaxis (2% minor)
    Genitourinary: GU bleeding (4% minor)
    Hematologic: Bleeding (5% major: ASSENT-2 trial)
    Local: Bleeding at catheter puncture site (4% minor), hematoma (2% major)
    Respiratory: Pharyngeal bleeding (3% minor)
Additional cardiovascular events associated with use in MI: Cardiogenic shock, arrhythmia, AV block, pulmonary edema, heart failure, cardiac arrest, recurrent myocardial ischemia, myocardial reinfarction, myocardial rupture, cardiac tamponade, pericarditis, pericardial effusion, mitral regurgitation, thrombosis, embolism, electromechanical dissociation, hypotension, fever, nausea, vomiting

Mechanism of Action Initiates fibrinolysis by binding to fibrin and converting plasminogen to plasmin.

Drug Interactions
  Increased Effect/Toxicity: Drugs which affect platelet function (eg, NSAIDs, dipyridamole, ticlopidine, clopidogrel, IIb/IIIa antagonists) may potentiate the risk of hemorrhage; use with caution.
    Heparin and aspirin: Use with aspirin and heparin may increase bleeding. However, aspirin and heparin were used concomitantly with tenecteplase in the majority of patients in clinical studies.
    Warfarin or oral anticoagulants: Risk of bleeding may be increased during concurrent therapy.
  Decreased Effect: Aminocaproic acid (antifibrinolytic agent) may decrease effectiveness.

Pharmacodynamics/Kinetics
Distribution: V_d is weight related and approximates plasma volume
Metabolism: Primarily hepatic
Half-life elimination: 90-130 minutes
Excretion: Clearance: Plasma: 99-119 mL/minute

Pregnancy Risk Factor C

Tenex® *see Guanfacine on page 801*

Teniposide *(ten i POE side)*

U.S. Brand Names Vumon®
Canadian Brand Names Vumon®
Mexican Brand Names Vumon
Generic Available No
Index Terms EPT; VM-26
Pharmacologic Category Antineoplastic Agent, Miscellaneous
Use Treatment of acute lymphocytic leukemia, small cell lung cancer
Local Anesthetic/Vasoconstrictor Precautions No information available to require special precautions
Effects on Dental Treatment Key adverse event(s) related to dental treatment: Mucositis.

Common Adverse Effects
>10%:
    Gastrointestinal: Mucositis (75%); diarrhea, nausea, vomiting (20% to 30%); anorexia
    Hematologic: Myelosuppression, leukopenia, neutropenia (95%), thrombocytopenia (65% to 80%), anemia
      Onset: 5-7 days
      Nadir: 7-10 days
      Recovery: 21-28 days
1% to 10%:
    Cardiovascular: Hypotension (2%), associated with rapid (<30 minutes) infusions
    Dermatologic: Alopecia (9%), rash (3%)
    Miscellaneous: Anaphylactoid reactions (5%) (fever, rash, hyper-/hypotension, dyspnea, bronchospasm), usually seen with rapid (<30 minutes) infusions

Mechanism of Action Teniposide does not inhibit microtubular assembly; it has been shown to delay transit of cells through the S phase and arrest cells in late S or early G_2 phase. Teniposide is a topoisomerase II inhibitor, and appears to cause DNA strand breaks by inhibition of strand-passing and DNA ligase action.

Drug Interactions

Cytochrome P450 Effect: Substrate of CYP3A4 (major); **Inhibits** CYP2C9 (weak), 3A4 (weak)

Increased Effect/Toxicity: May increase toxicity of methotrexate. Sodium salicylate, sulfamethizole, and tolbutamide displace teniposide from protein-binding sites which could cause substantial increases in free drug levels, resulting in potentiation of toxicity. Concurrent use of vincristine may increase the incidence of peripheral neuropathy. CYP3A4 inhibitors may increase the levels/effects of teniposide; example inhibitors include azole antifungals, clarithromycin, diclofenac, doxycycline, erythromycin, imatinib, isoniazid, nefazodone, nicardipine, propofol, protease inhibitors, quinidine, telithromycin, and verapamil.

Decreased Effect: CYP3A4 inducers may decrease the levels/effects of teniposide; example inducers include aminoglutethimide, carbamazepine, nafcillin, nevirapine, phenobarbital, phenytoin, and rifamycins.

Pharmacodynamics/Kinetics

Distribution: V_d: 0.28 L/kg; Adults: 8-44 L; Children: 3-11 L; mainly into liver, kidneys, small intestine, and adrenals; crosses blood-brain barrier to a limited extent

Protein binding: 99.4%

Metabolism: Extensively hepatic

Half-life elimination: 5 hours

Excretion: Urine (44%, 21% as unchanged drug); feces (≤10%)

Pregnancy Risk Factor D

Tenofovir (te NOE fo veer)

Related Information

HIV Infection and AIDS *on page 1753*

U.S. Brand Names Viread®

Canadian Brand Names Viread®

Generic Available No

Index Terms PMPA; TDF; Tenofovir Disoproxil Fumarate

Pharmacologic Category Antiretroviral Agent, Reverse Transcriptase Inhibitor (Nucleotide)

Use Management of HIV infections in combination with at least two other antiretroviral agents

Local Anesthetic/Vasoconstrictor Precautions No information available to require special precautions

Effects on Dental Treatment No significant effects or complications reported

Common Adverse Effects

>10%:

Central nervous system: Pain (7% to 12%)

Gastrointestinal: Diarrhea (11% to 16%), nausea (8% to 11%),

Neuromuscular & skeletal: Weakness (7% to 11%)

1% to 10%:

Central nervous system: Headache (5% to 8%), depression (4% to 8%; treatment naïve 11%), insomnia (3% to 4%), fever (2% to 4%; treatment naïve 8%), dizziness (1% to 3%)

Dermatologic: Rash event (maculopapular, pustular, or vesiculobullous rash, pruritus or urticaria 5% to 7%; treatment naïve 18%)

Endocrine & metabolic: Amylase increased (9%, treatment naïve)

Gastrointestinal: Vomiting (4% to 7%), abdominal pain (4% to 7%), dyspepsia (3% to 4%), flatulence (3% to 4%), anorexia (3% to 4%), weight loss (2% to 4%)

Hematologic: Neutropenia (1% to 2%)

Hepatic: Transaminases increased (2% to 4%)

Neuromuscular & skeletal: Back pain (3% to 4%; treatment naïve 9%), myalgia (3% to 4%), neuropathy (peripheral 1% to 3%)

Respiratory: Pneumonia (2% to 3%)

Miscellaneous: Diaphoresis (3%)

Mechanism of Action Tenofovir disoproxil fumarate (TDF) is an analog of adenosine 5'-monophosphate; it interferes with the HIV viral RNA dependent DNA polymerase resulting in inhibition of viral replication. TDF is first converted intracellularly by hydrolysis to tenofovir and subsequently phosphorylated to the active tenofovir diphosphate; nucleotide reverse transcriptase inhibitor.

Drug Interactions

Cytochrome P450 Effect: Inhibits CYP1A2 (weak)

Increased Effect/Toxicity: Concurrent use has been noted to increase serum concentrations/exposure to didanosine and its metabolites, potentially
(Continued)

Tenofovir *(Continued)*

increasing the risk of didanosine toxicity (hyperglycemia, pancreatitis, peripheral neuropathy, or lactic acidosis); decreased CD4 cell counts and
decreased virologic response have been reported. Use caution and monitor
closely; suspend therapy if signs/symptoms of toxicity are present. Drugs
which may compete for renal tubule secretion (including acyclovir, cidofovir,
ganciclovir, valacyclovir, valganciclovir) may increase the serum concentrations of tenofovir. Drugs causing nephrotoxicity may reduce elimination of
tenofovir. Protease inhibitors (especially ritonavir and combinations with
ritonavir) may increase serum concentrations of tenofovir.

Decreased Effect: Tenofovir may decrease serum concentrations of
atazanavir and other protease inhibitors, resulting in a loss of virologic
response (specific atazanavir dosing recommendations provided by manufacturer).

Pharmacodynamics/Kinetics

Distribution: 1.2-1.3 L/kg

Protein binding: 7% to serum proteins

Metabolism: Tenofovir disoproxil fumarate (TDF) is converted intracellularly by
hydrolysis (by non-CYP enzymes) to tenofovir, then phosphorylated to the
active tenofovir diphosphate

Bioavailability: 25% (fasting); increases ~40% with high-fat meal

Half-life elimination: 17 hours

Time to peak, serum: Fasting: 36-84 minutes; With food: 96-144 minutes

Excretion: Urine (70% to 80%) via filtration and active secretion, primarily as
unchanged tenofovir

Pregnancy Risk Factor B

Tenofovir and Emtricitabine *see* Emtricitabine and Tenofovir *on page 563*

Tenofovir Disoproxil Fumarate *see* Tenofovir *on page 1537*

Tenofovir Disoproxil Fumarate, Efavirenz, and Emtricitabine *see* Efavirenz,
Emtricitabine, and Tenofovir *on page 559*

Tenoretic® *see* Atenolol and Chlorthalidone *on page 160*

Tenormin® *see* Atenolol *on page 158*

Tenuate® [DSC] *see* Diethylpropion *on page 493*

Tenuate® Dospan® [DSC] *see* Diethylpropion *on page 493*

Tequin® [DSC] *see* Gatifloxacin *on page 766*

Tera-Gel™ [OTC] *see* Coal Tar *on page 402*

Terazol® 3 *see* Terconazole *on page 1541*

Terazol® 7 *see* Terconazole *on page 1541*

Terazosin *(ter AY zoe sin)*

Related Information

Cardiovascular Diseases *on page 1726*

U.S. Brand Names Hytrin® [DSC]

Canadian Brand Names Alti-Terazosin; Apo-Terazosin®; Hytrin®;
Novo-Terazosin; Nu-Terazosin; PMS-Terazosin

Mexican Brand Names Adecur; Hytrin

Generic Available Yes

Pharmacologic Category Alpha₁ Blocker

Use Management of mild to moderate hypertension; alone or in combination with
other agents such as diuretics or beta-blockers; benign prostate hyperplasia
(BPH)

Unlabeled/Investigational Use Pediatric hypertension

Local Anesthetic/Vasoconstrictor Precautions No information available to
require special precautions

Effects on Dental Treatment Key adverse event(s) related to dental treatment: Xerostomia (normal salivary flow resumes upon discontinuation) and
orthostatic hypotension.

Common Adverse Effects Asthenia, postural hypotension, dizziness, somnolence, nasal congestion/rhinitis, and impotence were the only events noted in
clinical trials to occur at a frequency significantly greater than placebo (p <0.05).

>10%:
Central nervous system: Dizziness, headache
Neuromuscular & skeletal: Muscle weakness

1% to 10%:
Cardiovascular: Edema, palpitation, chest pain, peripheral edema (3%),
orthostatic hypotension (3% to 4%), tachycardia
Central nervous system: Fatigue, nervousness, drowsiness
Gastrointestinal: Dry mouth
Genitourinary: Urinary incontinence

Ocular: Blurred vision

Respiratory: Dyspnea, nasal congestion

Dosage Oral:

Hypertension:

Children (unlabeled use): Initial: 1 mg once daily; gradually increase dose as necessary, up to maximum of 20 mg/day

Adults: Initial: 1 mg at bedtime; slowly increase dose to achieve desired blood pressure, up to 20 mg/day; usual dose range (JNC 7): 1-20 mg once daily

Dosage reduction may be needed when adding a diuretic or other antihypertensive agent; if drug is discontinued for greater than several days, consider beginning with initial dose and retitrate as needed; dosage may be given on a twice daily regimen if response is diminished at 24 hours and hypotensive is observed at 2-4 hours following a dose

Benign prostatic hyperplasia: Adults: Initial: 1 mg at bedtime, increasing as needed; most patients require 10 mg day; if no response after 4-6 weeks of 10 mg/day, may increase to 20 mg/day

Mechanism of Action Alpha$_1$-specific blocking agent with minimal alpha$_2$ effects; this allows peripheral postsynaptic blockade, with the resultant decrease in arterial tone, while preserving the negative feedback loop which is mediated by the peripheral presynaptic alpha$_2$-receptors; terazosin relaxes the smooth muscle of the bladder neck, thus reducing bladder outlet obstruction

Contraindications Hypersensitivity to quinazolines (doxazosin, prazosin, terazosin) or any component of the formulation; concurrent use with phosphodiesterase-5 (PDE-5) inhibitors including sildenafil (>25 mg), tadalafil, or vardenafil

Warnings/Precautions Can cause significant orthostatic hypotension and syncope, especially with first dose; anticipate a similar effect if therapy is interrupted for a few days, if dosage is rapidly increased, or if another antihypertensive drug (particularly vasodilators) or a PDE5 inhibitor is introduced. Discontinue if symptoms of angina occur or worsen. Patients should be cautioned about performing hazardous tasks when starting new therapy or adjusting dosage upward. Prostate cancer should be ruled out before starting for BPH. Use with caution in hepatic impairment. Intraoperative floppy iris syndrome has been observed in cataract surgery patients who were on or were previously treated with alpha$_1$-blockers. Causality has not been established and there appears to be no benefit in discontinuing alpha-blocker therapy prior to surgery. Safety and efficacy in children have not been established.

Drug Interactions

Increased Effect/Toxicity: Terazosin's hypotensive effect is increased with beta-blockers, diuretics, ACE inhibitors, calcium channel blockers, other antihypertensive medications, sildenafil (use with extreme caution at a dose ≤25 mg), tadalafil (use is contraindicated by the manufacturer), and vardenafil (use is contraindicated by the manufacturer).

Decreased Effect: Decreased antihypertensive response with NSAIDs. Alpha-blockers reduce the response to pressor agents (norepinephrine).

Ethanol/Nutrition/Herb Interactions Herb/Nutraceutical: Avoid dong quai if using for hypertension (has estrogenic activity). Avoid ephedra, yohimbe, ginseng (may worsen hypertension). Avoid saw palmetto. Avoid garlic (may have increased antihypertensive effect).

Dietary Considerations May be taken without regard to meals at the same time each day.

Pharmacodynamics/Kinetics

Onset of action: 1-2 hours

Absorption: Rapid

Protein binding: 90% to 95%

Metabolism: Extensively hepatic

Half-life elimination: 9.2-12 hours

Time to peak, serum: ~1 hour

Excretion: Feces (60%); urine (40%)

Pregnancy Risk Factor C

Dosage Forms

Capsule: 1 mg, 2 mg, 5 mg, 10 mg

Terbinafine (TER bin a feen)

U.S. Brand Names Lamisil®; Lamisil® AT™ [OTC]

Canadian Brand Names Apo-Terbinafine®; CO Terbinafine; Gen-Terbinafine; Lamisil®; Novo-Terbinafine; PMS-Terbinafine

Mexican Brand Names Lamisil

Generic Available No

(Continued)

Terbinafine (Continued)

Index Terms Terbinafine Hydrochloride

Pharmacologic Category Antifungal Agent, Oral; Antifungal Agent, Topical

Use Active against most strains of *Trichophyton mentagrophytes*, *Trichophyton rubrum*; may be effective for infections of *Microsporum gypseum* and *M. nanum*, *Trichophyton verrucosum*, *Epidermophyton floccosum*, *Candida albicans*, and *Scopulariopsis brevicaulis*

Oral: Onychomycosis of the toenail or fingernail due to susceptible dermatophytes

Topical: Antifungal for the treatment of tinea pedis (athlete's foot), tinea cruris (jock itch), and tinea corporis (ringworm) [OTC/prescription formulations]; tinea versicolor [prescription formulations]

Local Anesthetic/Vasoconstrictor Precautions No information available to require special precautions

Effects on Dental Treatment Key adverse event(s) related to dental treatment: Taste disturbance.

Common Adverse Effects

Oral: 1% to 10%:

Central nervous system: Headache, dizziness, vertigo

Dermatologic: Rash, pruritus, urticaria

Gastrointestinal: Diarrhea, dyspepsia, abdominal pain, appetite decrease, taste disturbance

Hematologic: Lymphocytopenia

Hepatic: Liver enzymes increased

Ocular: Visual disturbance

Topical: 1% to 10%:

Dermatologic: Pruritus, contact dermatitis, irritation, burning, dryness

Local: Irritation, stinging

Mechanism of Action Synthetic allylamine derivative which inhibits squalene epoxidase, a key enzyme in sterol biosynthesis in fungi. This results in a deficiency in ergosterol within the fungal cell wall and results in fungal cell death.

Drug Interactions

Cytochrome P450 Effect: Substrate (minor) of 1A2, 2C9, 2C19, 3A4; **Inhibits** CYP2D6 (strong); **Induces** CYP3A4 (weak)

Increased Effect/Toxicity: Terbinafine may increase the levels/effects of amphetamines, beta-blockers, dextromethorphan, fluoxetine, lidocaine, mirtazapine, nefazodone, paroxetine, risperidone, ritonavir, thioridazine, tricyclic antidepressants, venlafaxine, and other CYP2D6 substrates. The effects of warfarin may be increased.

Decreased Effect: Terbinafine may decrease the levels/effects of CYP2D6 prodrug substrates (eg, codeine, hydrocodone, oxycodone, tramadol).

Pharmacodynamics/Kinetics

Absorption: Topical: Limited (<5%); Oral: >70%

Distribution: V_d: 2000 L; distributed to sebum and skin predominantly

Protein binding, plasma: >99%

Metabolism: Hepatic; no active metabolites; first-pass effect; little effect on CYP

Bioavailability: Oral: 40%

Half-life elimination:

Topical: 22-26 hours

Oral: Terminal half-life: 200-400 hours; very slow release of drug from skin and adipose tissues occurs; effective half-life: ~36 hours

Time to peak, plasma: 1-2 hours

Excretion: Urine (70% to 75%)

Pregnancy Risk Factor B

Terbinafine Hydrochloride *see* Terbinafine *on page 1539*

Terbutaline (ter BYOO ta leen)

Related Information

Respiratory Diseases *on page 1747*

Canadian Brand Names Bricanyl®

Generic Available Yes

Index Terms Brethaire [DSC]; Bricanyl [DSC]

Pharmacologic Category Beta₂-Adrenergic Agonist

Use Bronchodilator in reversible airway obstruction and bronchial asthma

Unlabeled/Investigational Use Tocolytic agent (management of preterm labor)

Local Anesthetic/Vasoconstrictor Precautions No information available to require special precautions

Effects on Dental Treatment Key adverse event(s) related to dental treatment: Xerostomia (normal salivary flow resumes upon discontinuation) and bad taste in mouth.

Common Adverse Effects
>10%:
Central nervous system: Nervousness, restlessness
Endocrine & metabolic: Serum glucose increased, serum potassium decreased
Neuromuscular & skeletal: Trembling
1% to 10%:
Cardiovascular: Tachycardia, hypertension
Central nervous system: Dizziness, drowsiness, headache, insomnia
Gastrointestinal: Xerostomia, nausea, vomiting, bad taste in mouth
Neuromuscular & skeletal: Muscle cramps, weakness
Miscellaneous: Diaphoresis

Mechanism of Action Relaxes bronchial smooth muscle by action on beta$_2$-receptors with less effect on heart rate

Drug Interactions
Increased Effect/Toxicity: Increased toxicity with MAO inhibitors, tricyclic antidepressants.
Decreased Effect: Decreased effect with beta-blockers.

Pharmacodynamics/Kinetics
Onset of action: Oral: 30-45 minutes; SubQ: 6-15 minutes
Protein binding: 25%
Metabolism: Hepatic to inactive sulfate conjugates
Bioavailability: SubQ doses are more bioavailable than oral
Half-life elimination: 11-16 hours
Excretion: Urine

Pregnancy Risk Factor B

Terconazole (ter KONE a zole)

Related Information
Treatment of Sexually-Transmitted Infections *on page 1920*
U.S. Brand Names Terazol® 3; Terazol® 7
Canadian Brand Names Terazol®
Mexican Brand Names Fungistat
Generic Available Yes: Cream
Index Terms Triaconazole
Pharmacologic Category Antifungal Agent, Vaginal
Use Local treatment of vulvovaginal candidiasis
Local Anesthetic/Vasoconstrictor Precautions No information available to require special precautions
Effects on Dental Treatment No significant effects or complications reported
Common Adverse Effects 1% to 10%:
Central nervous system; Fever, chills
Gastrointestinal: Abdominal pain
Genitourinary: Vulvar/vaginal burning, dysmenorrhea
Mechanism of Action Triazole ketal antifungal agent; involves inhibition of fungal cytochrome P450. Specifically, terconazole inhibits cytochrome P450-dependent 14-alpha-demethylase which results in accumulation of membrane disturbing 14-alpha-demethylsterols and ergosterol depletion.
Pharmacodynamics/Kinetics Absorption: Extent of systemic absorption after vaginal administration may be dependent on presence of a uterus; 5% to 8% in women who had a hysterectomy versus 12% to 16% in nonhysterectomy women
Pregnancy Risk Factor C

Teriparatide (ter i PAR a tide)

U.S. Brand Names Forteo™
Canadian Brand Names Forteo™
Generic Available No
Index Terms Parathyroid Hormone (1-34); Recombinant Human Parathyroid Hormone (1-34); rhPTH(1-34)
Pharmacologic Category Parathyroid Hormone Analog
Use Treatment of osteoporosis in postmenopausal women at high risk of fracture; treatment of primary or hypogonadal osteoporosis in men at high risk of fracture
Local Anesthetic/Vasoconstrictor Precautions No information available to require special precautions
(Continued)

Teriparatide *(Continued)*

Effects on Dental Treatment Key adverse event(s) related to dental treatment: Tooth disorder.

Common Adverse Effects 1% to 10%:

Cardiovascular: Chest pain (3%), syncope (3%)

Central nervous system: Dizziness (8%), depression (4%), vertigo (4%)

Dermatologic: Rash (5%)

Endocrine & metabolic: Hypercalcemia (transient increases noted 4-6 hours postdose in 11% of women and 6% of men)

Gastrointestinal: Nausea (9%), dyspepsia (5%), vomiting (3%), tooth disorder (2%)

Genitourinary: Hyperuricemia (3%)

Neuromuscular & skeletal: Arthralgia (10%), weakness (9%), leg cramps (3%)

Respiratory: Rhinitis (10%), pharyngitis (6%), dyspnea (4%), pneumonia (4%)

Miscellaneous: Antibodies to teriparatide (3% of women in long-term treatment; hypersensitivity reactions or decreased efficacy were not associated in preclinical trials)

Restrictions An FDA-approved medication guide must be distributed when dispensing an outpatient prescription (new or refill) where this medication is to be used without direct supervision of a healthcare provider. Medication guides are available at http://www.fda.gov/cder/Offices/ODS/medication_guides.htm.

Mechanism of Action Teriparatide is a recombinant formulation of endogenous parathyroid hormone (PTH), containing a 34-amino-acid sequence which is identical to the N-terminal portion of this hormone. The pharmacologic activity of teriparatide is similar to the physiologic activity of PTH, stimulating osteoblast function, increasing gastrointestinal calcium absorption, increasing renal tubular reabsorption of calcium. Treatment with teriparatide increases bone mineral density, bone mass, and strength. In postmenopausal women, it has been shown to decrease osteoporosis-related fractures.

Drug Interactions

Increased Effect/Toxicity: Digitalis serum concentrations are not affected, however, transient hypercalcemia may increase risk of digitalis toxicity (case reports).

Pharmacodynamics/Kinetics

Distribution: V_d: 0.12 L/kg

Metabolism: Hepatic (nonspecific proteolysis)

Bioavailability: 95%

Half-life elimination: Serum: I.V.: 5 minutes; SubQ: 1 hour

Excretion: Urine (as metabolites)

Pregnancy Risk Factor C

Terramycin® I.M. [DSC] *see* Oxytetracycline *on page 1238*

Teslac® *see* Testolactone *on page 1542*

TESPA *see* Thiotepa *on page 1559*

Tessalon® *see* Benzonatate *on page 200*

Testim® *see* Testosterone *on page 1543*

Testolactone *(tes toe LAK tone)*

U.S. Brand Names Teslac®

Canadian Brand Names Teslac®

Generic Available No

Pharmacologic Category Androgen

Use Palliative treatment of advanced or disseminated breast carcinoma

Local Anesthetic/Vasoconstrictor Precautions No information available to require special precautions

Effects on Dental Treatment Key adverse event(s) related to dental treatment: Tongue edema.

Common Adverse Effects Frequency not defined.

Cardiovascular: Blood pressure increased, edema

Central nervous system: Malaise

Dermatologic: Alopecia (rare), maculopapular rash

Endocrine & metabolic: Hypercalcemia

Gastrointestinal: Anorexia, diarrhea, nausea, tongue edema

Neuromuscular & skeletal: Paresthesia, peripheral neuropathies

Miscellaneous: Nail growth disturbance (rare)

Restrictions C-III

Mechanism of Action Testolactone is a synthetic testosterone derivative without significant androgen activity. The drug inhibits steroid aromatase activity, thereby blocking the production of estradiol and estrone from androgen precursors such as testosterone and androstenedione. Unfortunately, the enzymatic block provided by testolactone is transient and is usually limited to a period of 3 months.

Drug Interactions
Increased Effect/Toxicity: Increased effects of oral anticoagulants.
Pharmacodynamics/Kinetics
Absorption: Well absorbed
Metabolism: Hepatic (forms metabolites)
Excretion: Urine
Pregnancy Risk Factor C

Testopel® see Testosterone on page 1543

Testosterone (tes TOS ter one)

U.S. Brand Names Androderm®; AndroGel®; Delatestryl®; Depo®-Testosterone; First® Testosterone; First® Testosterone MC; Striant®; Testim®; Testopel®
Canadian Brand Names Andriol®; Androderm®; AndroGel®; Andropository; Delatestryl®; Depotest® 100; Everone® 200; Virilon® IM
Generic Available Yes: Injection
Index Terms Testosterone Cypionate; Testosterone Enanthate
Pharmacologic Category Androgen
Use

Injection: Androgen replacement therapy in the treatment of delayed male puberty; male hypogonadism (primary or hypogonadotropic); inoperable metastatic female breast cancer (enanthate only)

Pellet: Androgen replacement therapy in the treatment of delayed male puberty; male hypogonadism (primary or hypogonadotropic)

Topical (buccal system, gel, transdermal system): Male hypogonadism (primary or hypogonadotropic)

Capsule (not available in U.S.): Androgen replacement therapy in the treatment of delayed male puberty; male hypogonadism (primary or hypogonadotropic); replacement therapy in impotence or for male climacteric symptoms due to androgen deficiency

Unlabeled/Investigational Use Androgen deficiency in men with AIDS wasting; postmenopausal women with decreased sexual desire (in combination with estrogen therapy)

Local Anesthetic/Vasoconstrictor Precautions No information available to require special precautions

Effects on Dental Treatment Key adverse event(s) related to dental treatment: Buccal administration: Bitter taste, gum edema, gum or mouth irritation, gum tenderness, and taste perversion

Common Adverse Effects Frequency rarely defined.
Cardiovascular: Edema, hypertension, vasodilation
Central nervous system: Aggressive behavior, amnesia, anxiety, dizziness, emotional lability, excitation, headache, mental depression, nervousness, sleeplessness
Dermatologic: Acne, alopecia, dry skin, hirsutism (increase in pubic hair growth), pruritus, rash, seborrhea
Endocrine & metabolic: Breast soreness, gonadotropin secretion decreased, growth acceleration, gynecomastia, hot flashes, hypercalcemia, hyperchloremia, hypercholesterolemia, hyper-/hypokalemia, hyperlipidemia, hypernatremia, hypoglycemia, inorganic phosphate retention, libido changes, menstrual problems (including amenorrhea), virilism, water retention
Gastrointestinal: GI bleeding, GI irritation, nausea, taste disorder, vomiting
Following buccal administration (most common): Bitter taste, gum edema, gum or mouth irritation, gum pain, gum tenderness, taste perversion
Genitourinary: Bladder irritability, epididymitis, impotence, oligospermia, priapism, prostatic carcinoma, prostatic hyperplasia, PSA increased, testicular atrophy, urination impaired
Hepatic: Bilirubin increased, cholestatic hepatitis, cholestatic jaundice, hepatic dysfunction, hepatic necrosis, hepatocellular neoplasms, liver function test changes, peliosis hepatis
Hematologic: Bleeding, hematocrit/hemoglobin increased, leukopenia, polycythemia, suppression of clotting factors
Local: Application site reaction (gel), injection site pain
Transdermal system: Pruritus at application site (37%), burn-like blisters under system (12%), erythema at application site (7%), vesicles at application site (6%), allergic contact dermatitis to system (4%), burning at application site (3%), induration at application site (3%)
Neuromuscular & skeletal: Paresthesia, weakness
Ocular: Lacrimation increased
(Continued)

Testosterone *(Continued)*

Renal: Creatinine increased
Miscellaneous: Anaphylactoid reactions, diaphoresis, hypersensitivity reactions, smell disorder

Restrictions C-III

Mechanism of Action Principal endogenous androgen responsible for promoting the growth and development of the male sex organs and maintaining secondary sex characteristics in androgen-deficient males

Drug Interactions

Cytochrome P450 Effect: Substrate (minor) of CYP2B6, 2C9, 2C19, 3A4; **Inhibits** CYP3A4 (weak)

Increased Effect/Toxicity: Androgens may enhance the anticoagulant effect of coumarin derivatives and the serum concentration and hepatotoxic effect of cyclosporine.

Pharmacodynamics/Kinetics

Duration (route and ester dependent): I.M.: Cypionate and enanthate esters have longest duration, ≤2-4 weeks; gel: 24-48 hours

Absorption: Transdermal gel: ~10% of applied dose

Protein binding: 98%; bound to sex hormone-binding globulin (40%) and albumin

Metabolism: Hepatic; forms metabolites, including dihydrotestosterone (DHT) and estradiol (both active)

Half-life elimination: 10-100 minutes

Excretion: Urine (90%); feces (6%)

Pregnancy Risk Factor X

Testosterone Cypionate *see* Testosterone *on page 1543*

Testosterone Enanthate *see* Testosterone *on page 1543*

Testred® *see* MethylTESTOSTERone *on page 1085*

Tetanus Immune Globulin (Human)
(TET a nus i MYUN GLOB yoo lin HYU man)

U.S. Brand Names BayTet™ [DSC]; HyperTET™ S/D
Canadian Brand Names BayTet™
Mexican Brand Names BayTet; Tetanogamma P
Generic Available No
Index Terms TIG
Pharmacologic Category Immune Globulin
Use Passive immunization against tetanus; tetanus immune globulin is preferred over tetanus antitoxin for treatment of active tetanus; part of the management of an unclean, wound in a person whose history of previous receipt of tetanus toxoid is unknown or who has received less than three doses of tetanus toxoid; elderly may require TIG more often than younger patients with tetanus infection due to declining antibody titers with age
Local Anesthetic/Vasoconstrictor Precautions No information available to require special precautions
Effects on Dental Treatment No significant effects or complications reported
Common Adverse Effects
>10%: Local: Pain, tenderness, erythema at injection site
1% to 10%:
Central nervous system: Fever (mild)
Dermatologic: Urticaria, angioedema
Neuromuscular & skeletal: Muscle stiffness
Miscellaneous: Anaphylaxis reaction
Mechanism of Action Passive immunity toward tetanus
Pharmacodynamics/Kinetics Absorption: Well absorbed
Pregnancy Risk Factor C

Tetanus Toxoid (Adsorbed) (TET a nus TOKS oyd, ad SORBED)

Generic Available No
Pharmacologic Category Toxoid
Use Active immunization against tetanus when combination antigen preparations are not indicated. **Note:** Tetanus and diphtheria toxoids for adult use (Td) is the preferred immunizing agent for most adults and for children after their seventh birthday. Young children should receive trivalent DTaP (diphtheria/tetanus/acellular pertussis), as part of their childhood immunization program, unless pertussis is contraindicated, then TD is warranted.
Local Anesthetic/Vasoconstrictor Precautions No information available to require special precautions

Effects on Dental Treatment No significant effects or complications reported

Common Adverse Effects All serious adverse reactions must be reported to the U.S. Department of Health and Human Services (DHHS) Vaccine Adverse Event Reporting System (VAERS) 1-800-822-7967.

Frequency not defined.

Cardiovascular: Hypotension

Central nervous system: Brachial neuritis, fever, malaise, pain

Gastrointestinal: Nausea

Local: Edema, induration (with or without tenderness), rash, redness, urticaria, warmth

Neuromuscular: Arthralgia, Guillain-Barré syndrome

Miscellaneous: Anaphylactic reaction, Arthus-type hypersensitivity reaction

Mechanism of Action Tetanus toxoid preparations contain the toxin produced by virulent tetanus bacilli (detoxified growth products of *Clostridium tetani*). The toxin has been modified by treatment with formaldehyde so that it has lost toxicity but still retains ability to act as antigen and produce active immunity; the aluminum salt, a mineral adjuvant, delays the rate of absorption and prolongs and enhances its properties; duration ~10 years.

Drug Interactions
Decreased Effect: When used in greater than physiologic doses, corticosteroids lead to decreased effect of vaccine (consider deferring immunization for 1 month after steroid is discontinued). Consider deferring immunization for 1 month after immunosuppressive agent is discontinued (decreased response to vaccine).

Pharmacodynamics/Kinetics Duration: Primary immunization: ~10 years

Pregnancy Risk Factor C

Tetanus Toxoid (Fluid) (TET a nus TOKS oyd FLOO id)

Mexican Brand Names Tetanol

Generic Available No

Index Terms Tetanus Toxoid Plain

Pharmacologic Category Toxoid

Use Indicated as booster dose in the active immunization against tetanus in the rare adult or child who is allergic to the aluminum adjuvant (a product containing adsorbed tetanus toxoid is preferred); not indicated for primary immunization

Unlabeled/Investigational Use Anergy testing (no longer recommended)

Local Anesthetic/Vasoconstrictor Precautions No information available to require special precautions

Effects on Dental Treatment No significant effects or complications reported

Common Adverse Effects All serious adverse reactions must be reported to the U.S. Department of Health and Human Services (DHHS) Vaccine Adverse Event Reporting System (VAERS) 1-800-822-7967.

Frequency not defined.

Cardiovascular: Hypotension

Central nervous system: Brachial neuritis, fever, Guillain-Barré syndrome, malaise

Dermatologic: Rash, urticaria

Gastrointestinal: Nausea

Local: Edema, induration (with or without tenderness), redness, warmth

Neuromuscular & skeletal: Arthralgia

Miscellaneous: Anaphylaxis, Arthus-type hypersensitivity reactions (severe local reaction developing 2-8 hours following injection)

Mechanism of Action Tetanus toxoid preparations contain the toxin produced by virulent tetanus bacilli (detoxified growth products of *Clostridium tetani*). The toxin has been modified by treatment with formaldehyde so that is has lost toxicity but still retains ability to act as antigen and produce active immunity.

Drug Interactions
Increased Effect/Toxicity: Increased bleeding and bruising may occur from I.M. injection in patients on anticoagulants.

Decreased Effect: Decreased effect of vaccine may occur with corticosteroids (greater than physiologic doses) or immunosuppressive agents

Pregnancy Risk Factor C

Tetanus Toxoid Plain *see* Tetanus Toxoid (Fluid) *on page 1545*

Tetrabenazine (tet ra BEN a zeen)

Canadian Brand Names Nitoman™

Pharmacologic Category Central Monoamine-Depleting Agent

Use Treatment of hyperkinetic movement disorders, including Huntington's chorea, hemiballismus, senile chorea, Tourette syndrome, and tardive dyskinesia

Local Anesthetic/Vasoconstrictor Precautions No information available to require special precautions

Effects on Dental Treatment

Key adverse event(s) related to dental treatment: Orthostatic hypotension has been reported; monitor patient during erect posture from dental chair and dysphagia.

Common Adverse Effects Note: Many adverse effects are dose-related and may resolve at lower dosages.

>10%: Central nervous system: Drowsiness (37%), parkinsonism (29%), depression (15%), insomnia (11%)

1% to 10%:

Cardiovascular: Orthostasis (2%)

Central nervous system: Nervousness (10%), anxiety (10%), akathisia (10%), dystonic reaction (3%), confusion (2%), memory impairment (2%), dizziness (1%), headache (1%), hallucination (1%), panic attack (1%), paranoia (1%)

Gastrointestinal: Nausea (5%), vomiting (5%), diarrhea (1%), dysphagia (1%), drooling, epigastric pain

Neuromuscular & skeletal: Tremor (3%), gait disturbance (1%), paresthesia (1%)

Ocular: Blurred vision (1%)

Respiratory: Pharyngeal spasm (1%), pharyngeal pain (1%)

Frequency not defined: Disorientation, fatigue, irritability, neuroleptic malignant syndrome, restlessness, weakness

Restrictions Not available in U.S.

Mechanism of Action Within basal ganglia, interferes with storage of neurotransmitters (including dopamine, serotonin, and norepinephrine) in presynaptic vesicles (likely through actions on vesicle monoamine transporter) resulting in depletion of these neurotransmitters. Tetrabenazine inhibits presynaptic dopamine release and also blocks CNS dopamine receptors. The effects resemble reserpine but with less peripheral activity and a shorter duration of action. Treatment results in symptomatic improvement of hyperkinetic movement disorders, including Huntington's chorea, hemiballismus, senile chorea, Tic and Hille's de la Tourette syndrome, and tardive dyskinesia.

Drug Interactions

Increased Effect/Toxicity: Tetrabenazine may increase the toxicity of cyclic antidepressants; CNS excitation and hypertension may occur during concurrent therapy. Concurrent use of tetrabenazine with antipsychotic agents may result in severe manifestations of dopamine deficiency. Neuroleptic malignant syndrome has been reported. CNS depressants may increase the adverse effects of tetrabenazine.

Tetrabenazine may increase the toxicity of MAO inhibitors; CNS excitation and hypertension may occur during concurrent therapy. Tetrabenazine should not be administered within 14 days of an MAO inhibitor. Concurrent therapy with reserpine may increase the effect/toxicity of both agents (due to similarities in mechanism of action). In the management of movement disorders, lithium may be additive with tetrabenazine, allowing management at lower dosages of both agents (limited data).

Decreased Effect: Tetrabenazine may reduce the anti-Parkinsonian effect of levodopa; avoid concurrent use.

Pharmacodynamics/Kinetics

Duration of action: 16-24 hours

Metabolism: Hepatic, to hydroxytetrabenazine (primary active moiety)

Bioavailability: Low and erratic (due to extensive first-pass effects)

Excretion: Urine (40% as metabolites); feces (2.5%)

Tetracaine (TET ra kane)

Related Information

Mouth Pain, Cold Sore, and Canker Sore Products *on page 1938*

Oral Pain *on page 1788*

Ulcerative and Erosive Disorders *on page 1809*

U.S. Brand Names Pontocaine®; Pontocaine® Niphanoid®

Canadian Brand Names Ametop™; Pontocaine®

Generic Available Yes: Ophthalmic solution, solution for injection

Index Terms Amethocaine Hydrochloride; Tetracaine Hydrochloride

Pharmacologic Category Local Anesthetic

Dental Use Ester-type local anesthetic; applied topically to throat for various diagnostic procedures and on cold sores and fever blisters for pain

Use Spinal anesthesia; local anesthesia in the eye for various diagnostic and examination purposes; topically applied to nose and throat for various diagnostic procedures

Local Anesthetic/Vasoconstrictor Precautions No information available to require special precautions

Effects on Dental Treatment No significant effects or complications reported

Significant Adverse Effects Frequency not defined.

> **Injection: Note:** Adverse effects listed are those characteristics of local anesthetics.
>
> > Cardiovascular: Cardiac arrest, hypotension
> > Central nervous system: Chills, convulsions, dizziness, drowsiness, nervousness, unconsciousness
> > Gastrointestinal: Nausea, vomiting
> > Neuromuscular & skeletal: Tremors
> > Ocular: Blurred vision, pupil constriction
> > Otic: Tinnitus
> > Respiratory: Respiratory arrest
> > Miscellaneous: Allergic reaction
>
> **Ophthalmic:** Ocular: Chemosis, lacrimation, photophobia, transient stinging
> > With chronic use: Corneal erosions, corneal healing retardation, corneal opacification (permanent), corneal scarring, keratitis (severe)

Dental Usual Dosing

> Topical mucous membranes (rhinolaryngology): Adults: Used as a 0.25% or 0.5% solution by direct application or nebulization; total dose should not exceed 20 mg

Dosage Adults:

> Ophthalmic: Short-term anesthesia of the eye: 0.5% solution: Instill 1-2 drops; prolonged use (especially for at-home self-medication) is not recommended
> Injection: Spinal anesthesia: **Note:** Dosage varies with the anesthetic procedure, the degree of anesthesia required, and the individual patient response; it is administered by subarachnoid injection for spinal anesthesia.
> > Perineal anesthesia: 5 mg
> > Perineal and lower extremities: 10 mg
> > Anesthesia extending up to costal margin: 15 mg; doses up to 20 mg may be given, but are reserved for exceptional cases
> > Low spinal anesthesia (saddle block): 2-5 mg
>
> Topical mucous membranes (rhinolaryngology): Used as a 0.25% or 0.5% solution by direct application or nebulization; total dose should not exceed 20 mg

Mechanism of Action Ester local anesthetic blocks both the initiation and conduction of nerve impulses by decreasing the neuronal membrane's permeability to sodium ions, which results in inhibition of depolarization with resultant blockade of conduction

Contraindications Hypersensitivity to tetracaine, ester-type anesthetics, aminobenzoic acid, or any component of the formulation; injection should not be used when spinal anesthesia is contraindicated

Warnings/Precautions Use with caution in patients with cardiac disease, hyperthyroidism, abnormal or decreased levels of plasma esterases. Use of the lowest effective dose is recommended. Acutely ill, elderly, debilitated, obstetric patients, or patients with increased intra-abdominal pressure may require decreased doses. Products may contain sodium bisulfite which may cause allergic reactions in some individuals.

> Ophthalmic: May delay wound healing. Prolonged use is not recommended. The anesthetized eye should be protected from irritation, foreign bodies, and rubbing to prevent inadvertent damage.

Pharmacodynamics/Kinetics

> Onset of action: Anesthetic: Rhinolaryngology: 5-10 minutes
> Duration: Rhinolaryngology: ~30 minutes
> Metabolism: Hepatic; detoxified by plasma esterases to aminobenzoic acid
> Excretion: Urine

Pregnancy Risk Factor C

Lactation Excretion in breast milk unknown/use caution

Dosage Forms Excipient information presented when available (limited, particularly for generics); consult specific product labeling.

> Injection, solution, as hydrochloride [preservative free] (Pontocaine®): 1% [10 mg/mL] (2 mL) [contains sodium bisulfite]
> Injection, powder for reconstitution, as hydrochloride [preservative free] (Pontocaine® Niphanoid®): 20 mg
> Solution, ophthalmic, as hydrochloride: 0.5% [5 mg/mL] (15 mL)
> Solution, topical, as hydrochloride (Pontocaine®): 2% [20 mg/mL] (30 mL, 118 mL) [for rhinolaryngology]

Tetracaine and Lidocaine *see* Lidocaine and Tetracaine *on page 983*

Tetracaine, Benzocaine, and Butamben *see* Benzocaine, Butamben, and Tetracaine *on page 198*

Tetracaine Hydrochloride *see* Tetracaine *on page 1546*

Tetracosactide *see* Cosyntropin *on page 416*

Tetracycline (tet ra SYE kleen)

Related Information
Bacterial Infections *on page 1793*
Gastrointestinal Disorders *on page 1745*
Periodontal Diseases *on page 1801*
Treatment of Sexually-Transmitted Infections *on page 1920*
Ulcerative and Erosive Disorders *on page 1809*

U.S. Brand Names Sumycin® [DSC]

Canadian Brand Names Apo-Tetra®; Nu-Tetra

Mexican Brand Names Acromicina; Ofticlin; Quimocyclar; Tetra-Atlantis; Tetrex

Generic Available Yes: Capsule

Index Terms Achromycin; TCN; Tetracycline Hydrochloride

Pharmacologic Category Antibiotic, Tetracycline Derivative

Dental Use Treatment of periodontitis associated with presence of *Actinobacillus actinomycetemcomitans* (AA); as adjunctive therapy in recurrent aphthous ulcers

Use Treatment of susceptible bacterial infections of both gram-positive and gram-negative organisms; also infections due to *Mycoplasma*, *Chlamydia*, and *Rickettsia*; indicated for acne, exacerbations of chronic bronchitis, and treatment of gonorrhea and syphilis in patients who are allergic to penicillin; as part of a multidrug regimen for *H. pylori* eradication to reduce the risk of duodenal ulcer recurrence

Local Anesthetic/Vasoconstrictor Precautions No information available to require special precautions

Effects on Dental Treatment Key adverse event(s) related to dental treatment: Esophagitis, superinfections, and candidal superinfection. Opportunistic "superinfection" with *Candida albicans*; tetracyclines are not recommended for use during pregnancy or in children ≤8 years of age since they have been reported to cause enamel hypoplasia and permanent teeth discoloration. The use of tetracyclines should only be used in these patients if other agents are contraindicated or alternative antimicrobials will not eradicate the organism. Long-term use associated with oral candidiasis.

Significant Adverse Effects Frequency not defined.
Cardiovascular: Pericarditis
Central nervous system: Intracranial pressure increased, bulging fontanels in infants, pseudotumor cerebri, paresthesia
Dermatologic: Photosensitivity, pruritus, pigmentation of nails, exfoliative dermatitis
Endocrine & metabolic: Diabetes insipidus syndrome
Gastrointestinal: Discoloration of teeth and enamel hypoplasia (young children), nausea, diarrhea, vomiting, esophagitis, anorexia, abdominal cramps, antibiotic-associated pseudomembranous colitis, staphylococcal enterocolitis, pancreatitis
Hematologic: Thrombophlebitis
Hepatic: Hepatotoxicity
Renal: Acute renal failure, azotemia, renal damage
Miscellaneous: Superinfection, anaphylaxis, hypersensitivity reactions, candidal superinfection

Dental Usual Dosing Periodontitis: Adults: Oral: 250 mg every 6 hours until improvement (usually 10 days)

Dosage
Usual dosage range:
Children >8 years: Oral: 25-50 mg/kg/day in divided doses every 6 hours
Adults: Oral: 250-500 mg/dose every 6 hours
Indication-specific dosing:
Adults: Oral:
Acne: 250-500 twice daily
Chronic bronchitis, acute exacerbation: 500 mg 4 times/day
Erlichiosis: 500 mg 4 times/day for 7-14 days

Peptic ulcer disease: Eradication of *Helicobacter pylori:* 500 mg 2-4 times/day depending on regimen; requires combination therapy with at least one other antibiotic and an acid-suppressing agent (proton pump inhibitor or H₂ blocker)

Periodontitis: 250 mg every 6 hours until improvement (usually 10 days)

Vibrio cholerae: 500 mg 4 times/day for 3 days

Dosing interval in renal impairment:

Cl_cr 50-80 mL/minute: Administer every 8-12 hours

Cl_cr 10-50 mL/minute: Administer every 12-24 hours

Cl_cr <10 mL/minute: Administer every 24 hours

Dialysis: Slightly dialyzable (5% to 20%) via hemo- and peritoneal dialysis or via continuous arteriovenous or venovenous hemofiltration; no supplemental dosage necessary

Dosing adjustment in hepatic impairment: Avoid use or maximum dose is 1 g/day

Mechanism of Action Inhibits bacterial protein synthesis by binding with the 30S and possibly the 50S ribosomal subunit(s) of susceptible bacteria; may also cause alterations in the cytoplasmic membrane

Contraindications Hypersensitivity to tetracycline or any component of the formulation; do not administer to children ≤8 years of age; pregnancy

Warnings/Precautions Use of tetracyclines during tooth development may cause permanent discoloration of the teeth and enamel, hypoplasia and retardation of skeletal development and bone growth with risk being the greatest for children <4 years and those receiving high doses; use with caution in patients with renal or hepatic impairment (eg, elderly); dosage modification required in patients with renal impairment since it may increase BUN as an antianabolic agent; pseudotumor cerebri has been reported with tetracycline use (usually resolves with discontinuation); outdated drug can cause nephropathy; use protective measure to avoid photosensitivity. Prolonged use may result in fungal or bacterial superinfection, including *C. difficile*-associated diarrhea and pseudomembranous colitis.

Drug Interactions Substrate of CYP3A4 (major); **Inhibits** CYP3A4 (moderate)

Antacids: May decrease tetracycline absorption; separate doses.

Calcium supplements (oral): May decrease tetracycline absorption; separate doses.

CYP3A4 inducers: CYP3A4 inducers may decrease the levels/effects of tetracycline. Example inducers include aminoglutethimide, carbamazepine, nafcillin, nevirapine, phenobarbital, phenytoin, and rifamycins.

CYP3A4 substrates: Tetracycline may increase the levels/effects of CYP3A4 substrates. Example substrates include benzodiazepines, calcium channel blockers, cyclosporine, mirtazapine, nateglinide, nefazodone, sildenafil (and other PDE-5 inhibitors), tacrolimus, and venlafaxine. Selected benzodiazepines (midazolam and triazolam), cisapride, ergot alkaloids, selected HMG-CoA reductase inhibitors (lovastatin and simvastatin), and pimozide are generally contraindicated with strong CYP3A4 inhibitors.

Didanosine: May decrease tetracycline absorption; separate doses.

Digoxin: Tetracyclines may rarely increase digoxin serum levels.

Iron: May decrease tetracycline absorption; separate doses.

Methoxyflurane anesthesia when concurrent with tetracycline may cause fatal nephrotoxicity.

Oral contraceptives: Anecdotal reports suggesting decreased contraceptive efficacy with tetracyclines have been refuted by more rigorous scientific and clinical data.

Quinapril: May decrease tetracycline absorption; separate doses.

Warfarin with tetracyclines may result in increased anticoagulation.

Ethanol/Nutrition/Herb Interactions

Food: Tetracycline serum concentrations may be decreased if taken with dairy products.

Herb/Nutraceutical: Avoid dong quai, St John's wort (may also cause photosensitization)

Pharmacodynamics/Kinetics

Absorption: Oral: 75%

Distribution: Small amount appears in bile

Relative diffusion from blood into CSF: Good only with inflammation (exceeds usual MICs)

CSF:blood level ratio: Inflamed meninges: 25%

Protein binding: ~65%

Half-life elimination: Normal renal function: 8-11 hours; End-stage renal disease: 57-108 hours

Time to peak, serum: Oral: 2-4 hours

Excretion: Urine (60% as unchanged drug); feces (as active form)

Pregnancy Risk Factor D

Lactation Enters breast milk/not recommended (AAP rates "compatible")

(Continued)

Tetracycline *(Continued)*

Breast-Feeding Considerations Tetracyclines are excreted in breast milk. Breast-feeding is not recommended by the manufacturer.

Tetracycline binds to calcium. The calcium in the maternal milk will decrease the amount of tetracycline absorbed by the breast-feeding infant. Because of this "negligible absorption by the neonate", the American Academy of Pediatrics considers tetracycline to be "usually compatible with breast-feeding." Nondose-related effects could include modification of bowel flora.

Tetracycline is generally considered compatible (low risk to fetus) during breast-feeding [human data].

Dosage Forms Excipient information presented when available (limited, particularly for generics); consult specific product labeling.

Capsule, as hydrochloride: 250 mg, 500 mg

Suspension, oral, as hydrochloride:

Sumycin®: 125 mg/5 mL (480 mL) [contains sodium benzoate and sodium metabisulfite; fruit flavor] [DSC]

Tablet, as hydrochloride:

Sumycin®: 250 mg, 500 mg [DSC]

Selected Readings

Gordon JM and Walker CB, "Current Status of Systemic Antibiotic Usage in Destructive Periodontal Disease," *J Periodontol*, 1993, 64(8 Suppl): 760-71.

Rams TE and Slots J, "Antibiotics in Periodontal Therapy: An Update," *Compendium*, 1992, 13(12):1130, 1132, 1134.

Seymour RA and Heasman PA, "Tetracyclines in the Management of Periodontal Diseases. A Review," *J Clin Periodontol*, 1995, 22(1):22-35.

Seymour RA and Heasman PA, "Pharmacological Control of Periodontal Disease. II. Antimicrobial Agents," *J Dent*, 1995, 23(1):5-14

Tetracycline Hydrochloride *see* Tetracycline *on page 1548*

Tetracycline, Metronidazole, and Bismuth Subsalicylate *see* Bismuth Subsalicylate, Metronidazole, and Tetracycline *on page 218*

Tetrafluoroethane and Pentafluoropropane *see* Pentafluoropropane and Tetrafluoroethane *on page 1273*

Tetrahydroaminoacrine *see* Tacrine *on page 1515*

Tetrahydrocannabinol *see* Dronabinol *on page 545*

Tetrahydrocannabinol and Cannabidiol

(TET ra hye droe can NAB e nol & can nab e DYE ol)

Canadian Brand Names Sativex®

Generic Available No

Index Terms Cannabidiol and Tetrahydrocannabinol; Delta-9-Tetrahydrocannabinol and Cannabinol; GW-1000-02; THC and CBD

Pharmacologic Category Analgesic, Miscellaneous

Use Adjunctive treatment of neuropathic pain in multiple sclerosis

Local Anesthetic/Vasoconstrictor Precautions No information available to require special precautions

Effects on Dental Treatment Key adverse event(s) related to dental treatment: Xerostomia and changes in salivation (normal salivary flow resumes upon discontinuation), abnormal taste, oral pain, orthostatic hypotension; administered as buccal spray, associated with irritation to the buccal (oral) mucosa.

Common Adverse Effects

>10%:

Central nervous system: Dizziness (41%), fatigue (11%)

Gastrointestinal: Oral application site events (20% to 25%)

1% to 10%:

Cardiovascular: Tachycardia, orthostatic hypotension, syncope

Central nervous system: Headache (9%), somnolence (8%), impaired balance (5%), euphoria (5%), depression (4% to 5%), memory impairment (4%), disorientation (4%), dissociation (3%), vertigo (3%), lethargy (3%)

Endocrine & metabolic: Appetite increased (4%), thirst (3%)

Gastrointestinal: Nausea (10%), xerostomia (8%), application site pain (8%), oral pain (7%), abnormal taste (4%), mucosal irritation/ulceration (3%), vomiting (2%)

Hepatic: ALT increased (2.6%)

Neuromuscular & skeletal: Weakness (4%)

Respiratory: Pharyngitis (4%)

Miscellaneous: Feeling drunk (7%), falls (3%), sensation of heaviness (2%)

Restrictions Not available in U.S.; CDSA-II

Mechanism of Action Stimulates cannabinoid receptors CB1 and CB2 in the CNS and dorsal root ganglia as well as other sites in the body. Cannabinoid receptors in the pain pathways of the brain and spinal cord mediate cannabinoid-induced analgesia. Peripheral CB2 receptors modulate immune function through cytokine release.

Drug Interactions
  Cytochrome P450 Effect: Substrate (minor) of CYP2C9, 2C19, 2D6, 3A4; **Inhibits** (weak) CYP1A2, 2C19, 2D6, 3A4
  Increased Effect/Toxicity: CNS depressants: The depressant effects may be additive/synergistic with cannabinoids (includes ethanol, barbiturates, and benzodiazepines).

Pharmacodynamics/Kinetics
  Absorption: Rapidly absorbed from the buccal mucosa
  Distribution: Widely distributed, particularly to fatty tissues
  Protein binding: Extensive
  Metabolism: Hepatic, via CYP isoenzymes (2C9, 2C19, 2D6 and 3A4)
  Half-life elimination: Initial: 1.3-2.2 hours; terminal half-life may require 24-36 hours (or longer) due to redistribution from fatty tissue
  Time to peak, plasma: 2-4 hours
  Excretion: As metabolites, urine and feces

Tetrahydrozoline (tet ra hye DROZ a leen)

U.S. Brand Names Eye-Sine™ [OTC]; Geneye® [OTC]; Murine® Tears Plus [OTC]; Optigene® 3 [OTC]; Tyzine®; Tyzine® Pediatric; Visine® Advanced Relief [OTC]; Visine® Original [OTC]
Generic Available Yes: Ophthalmic solution
Index Terms Tetrahydrozoline Hydrochloride; Tetryzoline
Pharmacologic Category Adrenergic Agonist Agent; Imidazoline Derivative; Ophthalmic Agent, Vasoconstrictor
Use Symptomatic relief of nasal congestion and conjunctival congestion
Local Anesthetic/Vasoconstrictor Precautions No information available to require special precautions
Effects on Dental Treatment No significant effects or complications reported
Common Adverse Effects
  >10%:
    Local: Transient stinging
    Respiratory: Sneezing
  1% to 10%:
    Cardiovascular: Tachycardia, palpitation, hypertension, heart rate
    Central nervous system: Headache
    Neuromuscular & skeletal: Tremor
    Ocular: Blurred vision
Mechanism of Action Stimulates alpha-adrenergic receptors in the arterioles of the conjunctiva and the nasal mucosa to produce vasoconstriction
Pharmacodynamics/Kinetics
  Onset of action: Decongestant: Intranasal: 4-8 hours
  Duration: Ophthalmic vasoconstriction: 2-3 hours
Pregnancy Risk Factor C

Tetrahydrozoline Hydrochloride see Tetrahydrozoline *on page 1551*

Tetra Tannate Pediatric see Chlorpheniramine, Ephedrine, Phenylephrine, and Carbetapentane *on page 341*

Tetryzoline see Tetrahydrozoline *on page 1551*

Teveten® see Eprosartan *on page 580*

Teveten® HCT see Eprosartan and Hydrochlorothiazide *on page 581*

Tev-Tropin® see Somatropin *on page 1486*

Texacort® see Hydrocortisone *on page 836*

TG see Thioguanine *on page 1557*

6-TG (error-prone abbreviation) see Thioguanine *on page 1557*

THA see Tacrine *on page 1515*

Thalidomide (tha LI doe mide)

Related Information
  HIV Infection and AIDS *on page 1753*
  Ulcerative and Erosive Disorders *on page 1809*
U.S. Brand Names Thalomid®
Canadian Brand Names Thalomid®
Generic Available No
Index Terms NSC-66847
Pharmacologic Category Angiogenesis Inhibitor; Immunosuppressant Agent; Tumor Necrosis Factor (TNF) Blocking Agent
(Continued)

Thalidomide *(Continued)*

Use Treatment of multiple myeloma; treatment and maintenance of cutaneous manifestations of erythema nodosum leprosum (ENL)

Unlabeled/Investigational Use Treatment of Crohn's disease; graft-versus-host reactions after bone marrow transplantation; AIDS-related aphthous stomatitis; Behçet's syndrome; Waldenström's macroglobulinemia; Langerhans cell histiocytosis; may be effective in rheumatoid arthritis, discoid lupus erythematosus, and erythema multiforme

Local Anesthetic/Vasoconstrictor Precautions No information available to require special precautions

Effects on Dental Treatment Key adverse event(s) related to dental treatment: Oral moniliasis (HIV-seropositive patients), toothache, xerostomia (normal salivary flow resumes upon discontinuation), and aphthous stomatitis.

Common Adverse Effects

>10%:

Cardiovascular: Edema (57%), thrombosis/embolism (23%; grade 3: 13%, grade 4: 9%), hypotension (16%)

Central nervous system: Fatigue (79%; grade 3: 3%, grade 4: 1%), somnolence (36% to 38%), dizziness (4% to 20%), sensory neuropathy (54%), confusion (28%), anxiety/agitation (9% to 26%), fever (19% to 23%), motor neuropathy (22%), headache (13% to 19%)

Dermatologic: Rash (21% to 31%), rash/desquamation (30%; grade 3: 4%), dry skin (21%), maculopapular rash (4% to 19%), acne (3% to 11%)

Endocrine & metabolic: Hypocalcemia (72%)

Gastrointestinal: Constipation (3% to 55%), anorexia (3% to 28%), nausea (4% to 24%), weight loss (23%), weight gain (22%), diarrhea (4% to 19%), oral moniliasis (4% to 11%)

Hematologic: Leukopenia (17% to 35%), neutropenia (31%), anemia (6% to 13%), lymphadenopathy (6% to 13%)

Hepatic: AST increased (3% to 25%), bilirubin increased (14%)

Neuromuscular & skeletal: Muscle weakness (40%), tremor (4% to 26%), weakness (6% to 22%), myalgia (17%), paresthesia (6% to 16%), arthralgia (13%)

Renal: Hematuria (11%)

Respiratory: Dyspnea (42%)

Miscellaneous: Diaphoresis (13%)

1% to 10%:

Cardiovascular: Facial edema (4%), peripheral edema (3% to 8%)

Central nervous system: Insomnia (9%), nervousness (3% to 9%), malaise (8%), vertigo (8%), pain (3% to 8%)

Dermatologic: Dermatitis (fungal 4% to 9%), pruritus (3% to 8%), nail disorder (3% to 4%)

Endocrine & metabolic: Hyperlipemia (6% to 9%)

Gastrointestinal: Xerostomia (8% to 9%), flatulence (8%), tooth pain (4%)

Genitourinary: Impotence (3% to 8%)

Hepatic: LFTs abnormal (9%)

Neuromuscular & skeletal: Neuropathy (8%), back pain (4% to 6%), neck pain (4%), neck rigidity (4%)

Renal: Albuminuria (3% to 8%)

Respiratory: Pharyngitis (4% to 8%), rhinitis (4%), sinusitis (4% to 8%)

Miscellaneous: Infection (6% to 8%)

Restrictions Thalidomide is approved for marketing only under a special distribution program. This program, called the "System for Thalidomide Education and Prescribing Safety" (STEPS® 1-888-423-5436), has been approved by the FDA. Prescribers and pharmacists must be registered with the program. No more than a 4-week supply should be dispensed. Blister packs should be dispensed intact (do not repackage capsules). Prescriptions must be filled within 7 days. Subsequent prescriptions may be filled only if fewer than 7 days of therapy remain on the previous prescription. A new prescription is required for further dispensing (a telephone prescription may not be accepted.)

Dosage Oral:

Multiple myeloma: 200 mg once daily (with dexamethasone 40 mg daily on days 1-4, 9-12, and 17-20 of a 28-day treatment cycle)

Cutaneous ENL:

Initial: 100-300 mg/day taken once daily at bedtime with water (at least 1 hour after evening meal)

Patients weighing <50 kg: Initiate at lower end of the dosing range

Severe cutaneous reaction or patients previously requiring high dose may be initiated at 400 mg/day; doses may be divided, but taken 1 hour after meals

Maintenance: Dosing should continue until active reaction subsides (usually at least 2 weeks), then tapered in 50 mg decrements every 2-4 weeks

Patients who flare during tapering or with a history or requiring prolonged maintenance should be maintained on the minimum dosage necessary to control the reaction. Efforts to taper should be repeated every 3-6 months, in increments of 50 mg every 2-4 weeks.

Behçet's syndrome (unlabeled use): 100-400 mg/day

Graft-vs-host reactions (unlabeled use): 100-1600 mg/day; usual initial dose: 200 mg 4 times/day for use up to 700 days

AIDS-related aphthous stomatitis (unlabeled use): 200 mg twice daily for 5 days, then 200 mg/day for up to 8 weeks

Discoid lupus erythematosus (unlabeled use): 100-400 mg/day; maintenance dose: 25-50 mg

Mechanism of Action Has immunomodulatory and antiangiogenic characteristics. Immunologic effects may vary based on conditions; may suppress excessive tumor necrosis factor-alpha production in patients with ENL, yet may increase plasma tumor necrosis factor-alpha levels in HIV-positive patients. In multiple myeloma, thalidomide is associated with an increase in natural killer cells and increased levels of interleukin-2 and interferon gamma. Other proposed mechanisms of action include suppression of angiogenesis, prevention of free-radical-mediated DNA damage, increased cell mediated cytotoxic effects, and altered expression of cellular.

Contraindications Hypersensitivity to thalidomide or any component of the formulation; neuropathy (peripheral); patient unable to comply with STEPS® program (including males); women of childbearing potential unless alternative therapies are inappropriate and adequate precautions are taken to avoid pregnancy; pregnancy

Warnings/Precautions Hazardous agent - use appropriate precautions for handling and disposal. **[U.S. Boxed Warning]: Thalidomide is a known teratogen; effective contraception must be used for at least 4 weeks before initiating therapy, during therapy, and for 4 weeks following discontinuation of thalidomide for women of childbearing potential.** Use caution with drugs which may decrease the efficacy of hormonal contraceptives.

[U.S. Boxed Warning]: Thrombotic events have been reported, generally in patients with other risk factors for thrombosis (neoplastic disease, inflammatory disease, or concurrent therapy with combination chemotherapy. Use in combination with dexamethasone is associated with increased risk for deep vein thrombosis (DVT) and pulmonary embolism (PE), monitor for signs and symptoms of thromboembolism; patients at risk may benefit from prophylactic anticoagulation or aspirin.

May cause sedation; patients must be warned to use caution when performing tasks which require alertness. Use caution in patients with renal or hepatic impairment, neurological disorders, or constipation. Thalidomide has been associated with the development of peripheral neuropathy, which may be irreversible; use caution with other medications which may cause peripheral neuropathy. Consider immediate discontinuation (if clinically appropriate) in patients who develop neuropathy. May cause seizures; use caution in patients with a history of seizures, concurrent therapy with drugs which alter seizure threshold, or conditions which predispose to seizures. May cause neutropenia; discontinue therapy if absolute neutrophil count decreases to <750/mm^3. Use caution in patients with HIV infection; has been associated with increased viral loads. May cause orthostasis and/or bradycardia; use with caution in patients with cardiovascular disease or in patients who would not tolerate transient hypotensive episodes. Hypersensitivity, Stevens-Johnson syndrome (SJS) and toxic epidermal necrolysis (TEN) have been reported; withhold therapy and evaluate with skin rashes; permanently discontinue if rash is exfoliative, purpuric, bullous or if SJS or TEN is suspected. Safety and efficacy have not been established in children <12 years of age.

Drug Interactions

Increased Effect/Toxicity: Thalidomide may enhance the sedative activity of other drugs such as ethanol, barbiturates, reserpine, and chlorpromazine. Thalidomide may be associated with increased risk of serious infection when used in combination with abatacept or anakinra. Thalidomide may increase the risk of vaccinal infection with vaccine (live attenuated).

Decreased Effect: Thalidomide may decrease the effect of vaccines (killed).

Ethanol/Nutrition/Herb Interactions

Ethanol: Avoid ethanol (may increase sedation).

Herb/Nutraceutical: Avoid cat's claw and echinacea (have immunostimulant properties; consider therapy modifications).

Dietary Considerations Should be taken at least 1 hour after the evening meal.

Pharmacodynamics/Kinetics

Distribution: V_d: 120 L

Protein binding: 55% to 66%

(Continued)

Thalidomide *(Continued)*

Metabolism: Nonenzymatic hydrolysis in plasma; forms multiple metabolites

Half-life elimination: 5-7 hours

Time to peak, plasma: 3-6 hours

Excretion: Urine (<1% as unchanged drug)

Pregnancy Risk Factor X

Dosage Forms

Capsule:

Thalomid®: 50 mg, 100 mg, 200 mg

Selected Readings

Beckman DA and Brent RL, "Mechanism of Known Environmental Teratogens: Drugs and Chemicals," *Clin Perinatol*, 1986, 13(3):649-87.

Gunzler V, "Thalidomide in Human Immunodeficiency Virus (HIV) Patients. A Review of Safety Considerations," *Drug Saf*, 1992, 7(2):116-34.

Hamuryudan V, Mat C, Saip S, et al, "Thalidomide in the Treatment of the Mucocutaneous Lesions of the Behçet Syndrome. A Randomized, Double-Blind, Placebo-Controlled Trial," *Ann Intern Med*, 1998, 128(6):443-50.

Jacobson JM, Greenspan JS, Spritzler J, et al, "Thalidomide for the Treatment of Oral Aphthous Ulcers in Patients With Human Immunodeficiency Virus Infection. National Institute of Allergy and Infectious Diseases AIDS Clinical Trials Group," *N Engl J Med*, 1997, 336(21):1487-93.

Levien T, Baker DE, and Ballasiotes AA, "Reviews of Dexrazoxane and Thalidomide," *Hosp Pharm*, 1996, 31(5):487-8, 493-4, 499-500, 504, 508, 510.

Schuler U and Ehninger G, "Thalidomide: Rationale for Renewed Use in Immunological Disorders," *Drug Saf*, 1995, 12(6):364-9.

"Thalidomide," *Med Lett Drugs Ther*, 1998, 40(1038):103-4.

Thalitone® *see* Chlorthalidone *on page 347*

Thalomid® *see* Thalidomide *on page 1551*

THAM® *see* Tromethamine *on page 1626*

THC *see* Dronabinol *on page 545*

THC and CBD *see* Tetrahydrocannabinol and Cannabidiol *on page 1550*

Theo-24® *see* Theophylline *on page 1554*

TheoCap™ *see* Theophylline *on page 1554*

Theochron® *see* Theophylline *on page 1554*

Theophylline (thee OFF i lin)

Related Information

Aminophylline *on page 90*

Respiratory Diseases *on page 1747*

U.S. Brand Names Elixophyllin®; Quibron®-T [DSC]; Quibron®-T/SR [DSC]; Theo-24®; TheoCap™; Theochron®; Uniphyl®

Canadian Brand Names Apo-Theo LA®; Novo-Theophyl SR; PMS-Theophylline; Pulmophylline; ratio-Theo-Bronc; Theochron® SR; Theolair™; Uniphyl® SRT

Mexican Brand Names Slo-Bid; Uni-Dur

Generic Available Yes: Extended release capsule and tablet, infusion

Index Terms Theophylline Anhydrous

Pharmacologic Category Theophylline Derivative

Use Treatment of symptoms and reversible airway obstruction due to chronic asthma, chronic bronchitis, or COPD

Local Anesthetic/Vasoconstrictor Precautions No information available to require special precautions

Effects on Dental Treatment Prescribe erythromycin products with caution to patients taking theophylline products. Erythromycin will delay the normal metabolic inactivation of theophyllines leading to increased blood levels; this has resulted in nausea, vomiting, and CNS restlessness. Azithromycin does not cause these effects in combination with theophylline products.

Common Adverse Effects

Adverse reactions/theophylline serum level: (Adverse effects do not necessarily occur according to serum levels. Arrhythmia and seizure can occur without seeing the other adverse effects).

15-25 mcg/mL: GI upset, diarrhea, nausea/vomiting, abdominal pain, nervousness, headache, insomnia, agitation, dizziness, muscle cramp, tremor

25-35 mcg/mL: Tachycardia, occasional PVC

>35 mcg/mL: Ventricular tachycardia, frequent PVC, seizure

Uncommon at serum theophylline concentrations ≤20 mcg/mL:

1% to 10%:

Cardiovascular: Tachycardia

Central nervous system: Nervousness, restlessness

Gastrointestinal: Nausea, vomiting

Mechanism of Action Causes bronchodilatation, diuresis, CNS and cardiac stimulation, and gastric acid secretion by blocking phosphodiesterase which increases tissue concentrations of cyclic adenine monophosphate (cAMP) which in turn promotes catecholamine stimulation of lipolysis, glycogenolysis, and gluconeogenesis and induces release of epinephrine from adrenal medulla cells

Drug Interactions

Cytochrome P450 Effect: Substrate of CYP1A2 (major), 2C9 (minor), 2D6 (minor), 2E1 (major), 3A4 (major); **Inhibits** CYP1A2 (weak)

Increased Effect/Toxicity: CYP1A2 inhibitors may increase the levels/ effects of theophylline; example inhibitors include ciprofloxacin, fluvoxamine, ketoconazole, norfloxacin, ofloxacin, and rofecoxib. CYP2E1 inhibitors may increase the levels/effects of theophylline; example inhibitors include disulfiram, isoniazid, and miconazole. Changes in diet may affect the elimination of theophylline. CYP3A4 inhibitors may increase the levels/effects of theophylline; example inhibitors include azole antifungals, clarithromycin, diclofenac, doxycycline, erythromycin, imatinib, isoniazid, nefazodone, nicardipine, propofol, protease inhibitors, quinidine, telithromycin, and verapamil.

Decreased Effect: CYP1A2 inducers may decrease the levels/effects of theophylline; example inducers include aminoglutethimide, carbamazepine, phenobarbital, and rifampin. CYP3A4 inducers may decrease the levels/ effects of theophylline; example inducers include aminoglutethimide, carbamazepine, nafcillin, nevirapine, phenobarbital, phenytoin, and rifamycins.

Pharmacodynamics/Kinetics

Absorption: Oral: Dosage form dependent

Distribution: 0.45 L/kg based on ideal body weight

Metabolism: Children >1 year and Adults: Hepatic; involves CYP1A2, 2E1 and 3A4; forms active metabolites (caffeine and 3-methylxanthine)

Half-life elimination: Highly variable and dependent upon age, liver function, cardiac function, lung disease, and smoking history

Time to peak, serum:

Oral: Liquid: 1 hour; Tablet, enteric-coated: 5 hours; Tablet, uncoated: 2 hours
I.V.: Within 30 minutes

Excretion: Urine

Neonates: 50% unchanged
Children >3 months and Adults: 10% unchanged

Pregnancy Risk Factor C

Theophylline and Guaifenesin (thee OFF i lin & gwye FEN e sin)

Related Information

Guaifenesin on page 795
Theophylline on page 1554

U.S. Brand Names Elixophyllin-GG®; Quibron® [DSC]

Generic Available No

Index Terms Guaifenesin and Theophylline

Pharmacologic Category Theophylline Derivative

Use Symptomatic treatment of bronchospasm associated with bronchial asthma, chronic bronchitis, and pulmonary emphysema

Local Anesthetic/Vasoconstrictor Precautions No information available to require special precautions

Effects on Dental Treatment Prescribe erythromycin products with caution to patients taking theophylline products. Erythromycin will delay the normal metabolic inactivation of theophyllines leading to increased blood levels; this has resulted in nausea, vomiting, and CNS restlessness.

Drug Interactions

Cytochrome P450 Effect: Theophylline: **Substrate** of CYP1A2 (major), 2C9 (minor), 2D6 (minor), 2E1 (major), 3A4 (major); **Inhibits** CYP1A2 (weak)

Pharmacodynamics/Kinetics See individual agents.

Pregnancy Risk Factor C

Thiabendazole (thye a BEN da zole)

U.S. Brand Names Mintezol®
Generic Available No
Index Terms Tiabendazole
Pharmacologic Category Anthelmintic
Use Treatment of strongyloidiasis, cutaneous larva migrans, visceral larva migrans, dracunculiasis, trichinosis, and mixed helminthic infections
Unlabeled/Investigational Use Cutaneous larva migrans (topical application)
Local Anesthetic/Vasoconstrictor Precautions No information available to require special precautions
Effects on Dental Treatment Key adverse event(s) related to dental treatment: Drying of mucous membranes.
Common Adverse Effects Frequency not defined.
Central nervous system: Chills, delirium, dizziness, drowsiness, hallucinations, headache, seizure
Dermatologic: Angioedema, pruritus, rash, Stevens-Johnson syndrome
Endocrine & metabolic: Hyperglycemia
Gastrointestinal: Abdominal pain, anorexia, diarrhea, drying of mucous membranes, nausea, vomiting
Genitourinary: Crystalluria, enuresis, hematuria, malodor of urine
Hematologic: Leukopenia
Hepatic: Cholestasis, hepatic failure, hepatotoxicity, jaundice
Neuromuscular & skeletal: Incoordination, numbness
Ocular: Abnormal sensation in eyes, blurred vision, dry eyes, Sicca syndrome, vision decreased, xanthopsia
Otic: Tinnitus
Renal: Nephrotoxicity
Miscellaneous: Anaphylaxis, hypersensitivity reactions, lymphadenopathy
Mechanism of Action Inhibits helminth-specific mitochondrial fumarate reductase
Drug Interactions
Cytochrome P450 Effect: Substrate of CYP1A2 (minor); **Inhibits** CYP1A2 (strong)
Increased Effect/Toxicity: Thiabendazole may increase the levels/effects of aminophylline, fluvoxamine, mexiletine, mirtazapine, ropinirole, theophylline, trifluoperazine, and other CYP1A2 substrates.
Pharmacodynamics/Kinetics
Absorption: Rapid and well absorbed
Metabolism: Rapidly hepatic; metabolized to 5-hydroxy form
Half-life elimination: 1.2 hours
Time to peak, plasma: Oral suspension: Within 1-2 hours
Excretion: Urine (90%) and feces (5%) primarily as conjugated metabolites
Pregnancy Risk Factor C

Thiamazole see Methimazole on page 1064
Thiamin see Thiamine on page 1556

Thiamine (THYE a min)

Canadian Brand Names Betaxin®
Mexican Brand Names Benerva
Generic Available Yes
Index Terms Aneurine Hydrochloride; Thiamin; Thiamine Hydrochloride; Thiaminium Chloride Hydrochloride; Vitamin B_1
Pharmacologic Category Vitamin, Water Soluble
Use Treatment of thiamine deficiency including beriberi, Wernicke's encephalopathy, Korsakoff's syndrome, neuritis associated with pregnancy, or in alcoholic patients; dietary supplement
Local Anesthetic/Vasoconstrictor Precautions No information available to require special precautions
Effects on Dental Treatment Key adverse event(s) related to dental treatment: Tightness of the throat.
Common Adverse Effects Adverse reactions reported with injection. Frequency not defined.
Cardiovascular: Cyanosis
Central nervous system: Restlessness
Dermatologic: Angioneurotic edema, pruritus, urticaria
Gastrointestinal: Hemorrharge into GI tract, nausea, tightness of the throat
Local: Induration and/or tenderness at the injection site (following I.M. administration)

Neuromuscular & skeletal: Weakness

Respiratory: Pulmonary edema

Miscellaneous: Anaphylactic/hypersensitivity reactions (following I.V. administration), diaphoresis, warmth

Mechanism of Action An essential coenzyme in carbohydrate metabolism by combining with adenosine triphosphate to form thiamine pyrophosphate

Pharmacodynamics/Kinetics

Absorption: Oral: Adequate; I.M.: Rapid and complete

Distribution: Highest concentrations found in brain, heart, kidney, liver; crosses the placenta, enters breast milk

Excretion: Urine (as unchanged drug and as pyrimidine after body storage sites become saturated)

Pregnancy Risk Factor A/C (dose exceeding RDA recommendation)

Thiamine Hydrochloride *see* Thiamine *on page 1556*

Thiaminium Chloride Hydrochloride *see* Thiamine *on page 1556*

Thioguanine (thye oh GWAH neen)

U.S. Brand Names Tabloid®

Canadian Brand Names Lanvis®

Generic Available No

Index Terms 2-Amino-6-Mercaptopurine; NSC-752; TG; 6-TG (error-prone abbreviation); 6-Thioguanine (error-prone abbreviation); Tioguanine

Pharmacologic Category Antineoplastic Agent, Antimetabolite (Purine Antagonist)

Use Treatment of acute myelogenous (nonlymphocytic) leukemia; treatment of chronic myelogenous leukemia and granulocytic leukemia

Local Anesthetic/Vasoconstrictor Precautions No information available to require special precautions

Effects on Dental Treatment Key adverse event(s) related to dental treatment: Stomatitis.

Common Adverse Effects

>10%: Hematologic: Myelosuppressive:

WBC: Moderate

Platelets: Moderate

Onset (days): 7-10

Nadir (days): 14

Recovery (days): 21

1% to 10%:

Dermatologic: Skin rash

Endocrine & metabolic: Hyperuricemia

Gastrointestinal: Mild nausea or vomiting, anorexia, stomatitis, diarrhea

Neuromuscular & skeletal: Unsteady gait

Restrictions The I.V. formulation is not available in U.S.

Mechanism of Action Purine analog that is incorporated into DNA and RNA resulting in the blockage of synthesis and metabolism of purine nucleotides

Drug Interactions

Increased Effect/Toxicity: Allopurinol can be used in full doses with thioguanine unlike mercaptopurine. Use with busulfan may cause hepatotoxicity and esophageal varices. Aminosalicylates (olsalazine, mesalamine, sulfasalazine) may inhibit TPMT, increasing toxicity/myelosuppression of thioguanine.

Pharmacodynamics/Kinetics

Absorption: 30% (highly variable)

Distribution: Crosses placenta

Metabolism: Hepatic; rapidly and extensively via TPMT to 2-amino-6-methylthioguanine (active) and inactive compounds

Half-life elimination: Terminal: 11 hours

Time to peak, serum: Within 8 hours

Excretion: Urine

Pregnancy Risk Factor D

6-Thioguanine (error-prone abbreviation) *see* Thioguanine *on page 1557*

Thiola® *see* Tiopronin *on page 1574*

Thiopental (thye oh PEN tal)

U.S. Brand Names Pentothal®

Canadian Brand Names Pentothal®

Generic Available No

(Continued)

Thiopental (Continued)

Index Terms Thiopental Sodium

Pharmacologic Category Anticonvulsant, Barbiturate; Barbiturate; General Anesthetic

Use Induction of anesthesia; adjunct for intubation in head injury patients; control of convulsive states; treatment of elevated intracranial pressure

Local Anesthetic/Vasoconstrictor Precautions No information available to require special precautions

Effects on Dental Treatment No significant effects or complications reported

Mechanism of Action Short-acting barbiturate with sedative, hypnotic, and anticonvulsant properties. Barbiturates depress the sensory cortex, decrease motor activity, alter cerebellar function, and produce drowsiness, sedation, and hypnosis. In high doses, barbiturates exhibit anticonvulsant activity; barbiturates produce dose-dependent respiratory depression.

Pregnancy Risk Factor C

Thiopental Sodium see Thiopental on page 1557

Thiophosphoramide see Thiotepa on page 1559

Thioridazine (thye oh RID a zeen)

Canadian Brand Names Mellaril®

Mexican Brand Names Melleril

Generic Available Yes

Index Terms Thioridazine Hydrochloride

Pharmacologic Category Antipsychotic Agent, Typical, Phenothiazine

Use Management of schizophrenic patients who fail to respond adequately to treatment with other antipsychotic drugs, either because of insufficient effectiveness or the inability to achieve an effective dose due to intolerable adverse effects from those medications

Unlabeled/Investigational Use Behavior problems (children); severe psychoses (children); schizophrenia/psychoses (children); depressive disorders/dementia (children and adults); behavioral symptoms associated with dementia (elderly)

Local Anesthetic/Vasoconstrictor Precautions Most pharmacology textbooks state that in presence of phenothiazines, systemic doses of epinephrine paradoxically decrease the blood pressure. This is the so called "epinephrine reversal" phenomenon. This has never been observed when epinephrine is given by infiltration as part of the anesthesia procedure. Thioridazine is one of the drugs confirmed to prolong the QT interval and is accepted as having a risk of causing torsade de pointes. The risk of drug-induced torsade de pointes is extremely low when a single QT interval prolonging drug is prescribed. In terms of epinephrine, it is not known what effect vasoconstrictors in the local anesthetic regimen will have in patients with a known history of congenital prolonged QT interval or in patients taking any medication that prolongs the QT interval. Until more information is obtained, it is suggested that the clinician consult with the physician prior to the use of a vasoconstrictor in suspected patients, and that the vasoconstrictor (epinephrine, levonordefrin [Neo-Cobefrin®]) be used with caution.

Effects on Dental Treatment Key adverse event(s) related to dental treatment: Xerostomia and changes in salivation (normal salivary flow resumes upon discontinuation). Significant hypotension may occur, especially when the drug is administered parenterally; orthostatic hypotension is due to alpha-receptor blockade, the elderly are at greater risk for orthostatic hypotension.

Tardive dyskinesia; Prevalence rate may be 40% in elderly; development of the syndrome and the irreversible nature are proportional to duration and total cumulative dose over time. Extrapyramidal reactions are more common in elderly with up to 50% developing these reactions after 60 years of age. Drug-induced Parkinson's syndrome occurs often; akathisia is the most common extrapyramidal reaction in elderly.

Common Adverse Effects Frequency not defined.

Cardiovascular: Hypotension, orthostatic hypotension, peripheral edema, ECG changes

Central nervous system: EPS (pseudoparkinsonism, akathisia, dystonias, tardive dyskinesia), dizziness, drowsiness, neuroleptic malignant syndrome (NMS), impairment of temperature regulation, lowering of seizure threshold, seizure

Dermatologic: Increased sensitivity to sun, rash, discoloration of skin (blue-gray)

Endocrine & metabolic: Changes in menstrual cycle, libido (changes in), breast pain, galactorrhea, amenorrhea

Gastrointestinal: Constipation, weight gain, nausea, vomiting, stomach pain, xerostomia, nausea, vomiting, diarrhea

Genitourinary: Difficulty in urination, ejaculatory disturbances, urinary retention, priapism

Hematologic: Agranulocytosis, leukopenia

Hepatic: Cholestatic jaundice, hepatotoxicity

Neuromuscular & skeletal: Tremor

Ocular: Pigmentary retinopathy, blurred vision, cornea and lens changes

Respiratory: Nasal congestion

Mechanism of Action Thioridazine is a piperidine phenothiazine which blocks postsynaptic mesolimbic dopaminergic receptors in the brain; exhibits a strong alpha-adrenergic blocking effect and depresses the release of hypothalamic and hypophyseal hormones

Drug Interactions

Cytochrome P450 Effect: Substrate of CYP2C19 (minor), 2D6 (major); **Inhibits** CYP1A2 (weak), 2C9 (weak), 2D6 (moderate), 2E1 (weak)

Increased Effect/Toxicity: Concurrent use fluvoxamine, propranolol, and pindolol. The levels/effects of thioridazine may be increased by chlorpromazine, delavirdine, fluoxetine, miconazole, paroxetine, pergolide, quinidine, quinine, ritonavir, ropinirole, and other CYP2D6 inhibitors. **Thioridazine is contraindicated with strong inhibitors of this enzyme.**

Drugs which alter the QT_c interval may be additive with thioridazine, increasing the risk of malignant arrhythmias; includes type Ia antiarrhythmics, TCAs, and some quinolone antibiotics (sparfloxacin, moxifloxacin and gatifloxacin). **These agents are contraindicated with thioridazine.** Potassium depleting agents may increase the risk of serious arrhythmias with thioridazine (includes many diuretics, aminoglycosides, and amphotericin).

Phenothiazines inhibit the ability of bromocriptine to lower serum prolactin concentrations. The sedative effects of CNS depressants or ethanol may be additive with phenothiazines. Phenothiazines and trazodone may produce additive hypotensive effects. Metoclopramide may increase risk of extrapyramidal symptoms (EPS). Acetylcholinesterase inhibitors (central) may increase the risk of antipsychotic-related EPS. Concurrent use of antihypertensives may result in additive hypotensive effects (particularly orthostasis).

Thioridazine may increase the levels/effects of amphetamines, beta-blockers, dextromethorphan, fluoxetine, lidocaine, mirtazapine, nefazodone, paroxetine, risperidone, ritonavir, tricyclic antidepressants, venlafaxine, and other CYP2D6 substrates. **Concurrent use with fluvoxamine is contraindicated.**

Phenothiazines may produce neurotoxicity with lithium; this is a rare effect. Rare cases of respiratory paralysis have been reported with concurrent use of phenothiazines and polypeptide antibiotics. Naltrexone in combination with thioridazine has been reported to cause lethargy and somnolence. Phenylpropanolamine has been reported to result in cardiac arrhythmias when combined with thioridazine.

Decreased Effect: Aluminum salts may decrease the absorption of phenothiazines. The efficacy of amphetamines may be diminished by antipsychotics; in addition, amphetamines may increase psychotic symptoms; avoid concurrent use. Anticholinergics may inhibit the therapeutic response to phenothiazines and excess anticholinergic effects may occur (includes benztropine, trihexyphenidyl, biperiden, and drugs with significant anticholinergic activity). Chlorpromazine (and possibly other low potency antipsychotics) may diminish the pressor effects of epinephrine. The antihypertensive effects of guanethidine or guanadrel may be inhibited by phenothiazines. Phenothiazines may inhibit the antiparkinsonian effect of levodopa. Enzyme inducers may enhance the hepatic metabolism of phenothiazines; larger doses may be required; includes rifampin, rifabutin, barbiturates, phenytoin, and cigarette smoking. Thioridazine may decrease the levels/effects of CYP2D6 prodrug substrates (eg, codeine, hydrocodone, oxycodone, tramadol).

Pharmacodynamics/Kinetics

Duration: 4-5 days

Half-life elimination: 21-25 hours

Time to peak, serum: ~1 hour

Pregnancy Risk Factor C

Thiotepa (thye oh TEP a)

Generic Available Yes

(Continued)

Thiotepa *(Continued)*

Index Terms TESPA; Thiophosphoramide; Triethylenethiophosphoramide; TSPA

Pharmacologic Category Antineoplastic Agent, Alkylating Agent

Use Treatment of superficial tumors of the bladder; palliative treatment of adenocarcinoma of breast or ovary; lymphomas and sarcomas; controlling intracavitary effusions caused by metastatic tumors; I.T. use: CNS leukemia/lymphoma, CNS metastases

Local Anesthetic/Vasoconstrictor Precautions No information available to require special precautions

Effects on Dental Treatment No significant effects or complications reported

Common Adverse Effects

>10%:

Hematopoietic: Dose-limiting toxicity which is dose related and cumulative; moderate to severe leukopenia and severe thrombocytopenia have occurred. Anemia and pancytopenia may become fatal, so careful hematologic monitoring is required; intravesical administration may cause bone marrow suppression as well.

Hematologic: Myelosuppression (WBC: moderate; platelets: severe; onset: 7-10 days, nadir: 14 days, recovery: 28 days)

Local: Injection site pain

1% to 10%:

Central nervous system: Dizziness, fatigue, fever, headache

Dermatologic: Alopecia, depigmentation (with topical treatment), hyperpigmentation (with high-dose therapy), pruritus, rash, urticaria

Endocrine & metabolic: Amenorrhea, hyperuricemia

Gastrointestinal: Anorexia, nausea and vomiting rarely occur

Emetic potential: Low (<10%)

Genitourinary: Dysuria, hemorrhagic cystitis (intravesicular administration: rare), urinary retention

Neuromuscular & skeletal: Weakness

Ocular: Conjunctivitis

Renal: Hematuria

Miscellaneous: Tightness of the throat, allergic reactions

Mechanism of Action Alkylating agent that reacts with DNA phosphate groups to produce cross-linking of DNA strands leading to inhibition of DNA, RNA, and protein synthesis; mechanism of action has not been explored as thoroughly as the other alkylating agents, it is presumed that the aziridine rings open and react as nitrogen mustard; reactivity is enhanced at a lower pH

Drug Interactions

Cytochrome P450 Effect: Inhibits CYP2B6 (strong)

Increased Effect/Toxicity: Phenytoin may increase the levels/effects of TEPA (active metabolite). Thiotepa may increase the levels/effects of CYP2B6 substrates; example substrates include bupropion, promethazine, propofol, selegiline, and sertraline.

Decreased Effect: Phenytoin may decrease the levels/effects of thiotepa.

Pharmacodynamics/Kinetics

Absorption: Intracavitary instillation: Unreliable (10% to 100%) through bladder mucosa; I.M.: variable

Metabolism: Extensively hepatic; major metabolite (active): TEPA

Half-life elimination: Terminal (dose-dependent clearance): 109 minutes

Excretion: Urine (as metabolites and unchanged drug)

Pregnancy Risk Factor D

Thiothixene *(thye oh THIKS een)*

U.S. Brand Names Navane®

Canadian Brand Names Navane®

Generic Available Yes

Index Terms Tiotixene

Pharmacologic Category Antipsychotic Agent, Typical

Use Management of schizophrenia

Unlabeled/Investigational Use Psychotic disorders (children); rapid tranquilization of the agitated patient (children); nonpsychotic patient, dementia behavior (elderly)

Local Anesthetic/Vasoconstrictor Precautions Most pharmacology textbooks state that in presence of phenothiazines, systemic doses of epinephrine paradoxically decrease the blood pressure. This is the so called "epinephrine reversal" phenomenon. This has never been observed when epinephrine is given by infiltration as part of the anesthesia procedure. Thiothixene is one of the drugs confirmed to prolong the QT interval and is accepted as having a risk of causing torsade de pointes. The risk of drug-induced torsade de pointes is extremely low when a single QT interval prolonging drug is prescribed. In terms of epinephrine, it is not known what effect vasoconstrictors in the local anesthetic regimen will have in patients with a known history of congenital prolonged QT interval or in patients taking any medication that prolongs the QT interval. Until more information is obtained, it is suggested that the clinician consult with the physician prior to the use of a vasoconstrictor in suspected patients, and that the vasoconstrictor (epinephrine, levonordefrin [Neo-Cobefrin®]) be used with caution.

Effects on Dental Treatment Key adverse event(s) related to dental treatment: Xerostomia and changes in salivation (normal salivary flow resumes upon discontinuation), significant hypotension may occur, especially when the drug is administered parenterally; orthostatic hypotension is due to alpha-receptor blockade, the elderly are at greater risk for orthostatic hypotension.

Tardive dyskinesia: Prevalence rate may be 40% in elderly; development of the syndrome and the irreversible nature are proportional to duration and total cumulative dose over time. Extrapyramidal reactions are more common in elderly with up to 50% developing these reactions after 60 years of age. Drug-induced Parkinson's syndrome occurs often; akathisia is the most common extrapyramidal reaction in elderly.

Common Adverse Effects Frequency not defined.

Cardiovascular: Hypotension, nonspecific ECG changes, syncope, tachycardia

Central nervous system: Agitation, dizziness, drowsiness, extrapyramidal symptoms (akathisia, dystonias, lightheadedness, pseudoparkinsonism, tardive dyskinesia), insomnia restlessness

Dermatologic: Discoloration of skin (blue-gray), photosensitivity, pruritus, rash, urticaria

Endocrine & metabolic: Amenorrhea, breast pain, libido (changes in), changes in menstrual cycle, galactorrhea, gynecomastia, hyper-/hypoglycemia, lactation

Gastrointestinal: Constipation, nausea, salivation increased, stomach pain, vomiting, weight gain, xerostomia

Genitourinary: Difficulty in urination, ejaculatory disturbances, impotence

Hematologic: Leukocytes, leukopenia

Neuromuscular & skeletal: Tremors

Ocular: Blurred vision, pigmentary retinopathy

Respiratory: Nasal congestion

Miscellaneous: Diaphoresis

Mechanism of Action Thiothixene is a thioxanthene antipsychotic which elicits antipsychotic activity by postsynaptic blockade of CNS dopamine receptors resulting in inhibition of dopamine-mediated effects; also has alpha-adrenergic blocking activity

Drug Interactions

Cytochrome P450 Effect: Substrate of CYP1A2 (major); **Inhibits** CYP2D6 (weak)

Increased Effect/Toxicity: CYP1A2 inhibitors may increase the levels/ effects of thiothixene; example inhibitors include ciprofloxacin, fluvoxamine, ketoconazole, norfloxacin, ofloxacin, and rofecoxib. Thiothixene and CNS depressants (ethanol, opioid analgesics) may produce additive CNS depressant effects. Thiothixene may increase the effect/toxicity of antihypertensives, benztropine (and other anticholinergic agents), lithium, trazodone, and TCAs. Thiothixene's concentrations may be increased by chloroquine, sulfadoxine-pyrimethamine, and propranolol. Metoclopramide may increase risk of extrapyramidal symptoms (EPS). Acetylcholinesterase inhibitors (central) may increase the risk of antipsychotic-related EPS.

Decreased Effect: CYP1A2 inducers may decrease the levels/effects of thiothixene; example inducers include aminoglutethimide, carbamazepine, phenobarbital, and rifampin. Thiothixene inhibits the activity of guanadrel, guanethidine, levodopa, and bromocriptine. Benztropine (and other anticholinergics) may inhibit the therapeutic response to thiothixene. Thiothixene and low potency antipsychotics may reverse the pressor effects of epinephrine.

Pharmacodynamics/Kinetics

Metabolism: Extensively hepatic

Half-life elimination: >24 hours with chronic use

Pregnancy Risk Factor C

Thrombin (Topical) (THROM bin, TOP i kal)

U.S. Brand Names Thrombin-JMI®
Generic Available No
Pharmacologic Category Hemostatic Agent
Dental Use Hemostasis whenever minor bleeding from capillaries and small venules is accessible
Use Hemostasis whenever minor bleeding from capillaries and small venules is accessible
Local Anesthetic/Vasoconstrictor Precautions No information available to require special precautions
Effects on Dental Treatment No significant effects or complications reported
Significant Adverse Effects 1% to 10%:
Central nervous system: Fever
Miscellaneous: Allergic type reaction
Dental Usual Dosing Bleeding: Adults: Topical: Use 1000-2000 units/mL of solution where bleeding is profuse; apply powder directly to the site of bleeding or on oozing surfaces; use 100 units/mL for bleeding from skin or mucosal surfaces
Dosage Use 1000-2000 units/mL of solution where bleeding is profuse; apply powder directly to the site of bleeding or on oozing surfaces; use 100 units/mL for bleeding from skin or mucosal surfaces
Mechanism of Action Catalyzes the conversion of fibrinogen to fibrin
Contraindications Hypersensitivity to thrombin or any component of the formulation
Warnings/Precautions Do not inject, for topical use only.

[U.S. Boxed Warning]: Bovine-source topical thrombin may be associated with abnormal hemostasis, ranging from asymptomatic laboratory alterations to severe bleeding and/or thrombosis. Abnormalities appear to be immunologically mediated; repeated applications increase risk. Consult expert in coagulation disorders if laboratory evidence and/or signs and symptoms of bleeding are noted. Re-exposure of patients who develop antibodies to bovine thrombin preparations should be avoided.
Drug Interactions No data reported
Pregnancy Risk Factor C
Dosage Forms Excipient information presented when available (limited, particularly for generics); consult specific product labeling.
Powder for reconstitution, topical:
Thrombin-JMI®: 5000 units, 20,000 units [packaged with diluent]
Thrombin-JMI® Spray Kit: 20,000 units [packaged with diluent and spray pump]
Thrombin-JMI® Syringe Spray Kit: 20,000 units [packaged with diluent, spray tip, and syringe]

Thymocyte Stimulating Factor *see* Aldesleukin *on page 62*
Thyrel® TRH [DSC] *see* Protirelin *on page 1379*
Thyrogen® *see* Thyrotropin Alpha *on page 1563*

Thyroid (THYE roid)

Related Information
Endocrine Disorders and Pregnancy *on page 1750*
U.S. Brand Names Armour® Thyroid; Nature-Throid® NT; Westhroid®
Generic Available Yes
Index Terms Desiccated Thyroid; Thyroid Extract; Thyroid USP
Pharmacologic Category Thyroid Product
Use Replacement or supplemental therapy in hypothyroidism; pituitary TSH suppressants (thyroid nodules, thyroiditis, multinodular goiter, thyroid cancer), thyrotoxicosis, diagnostic suppression tests
Local Anesthetic/Vasoconstrictor Precautions No precautions with vasoconstrictor are necessary if patient is well controlled with thyroid preparations
Effects on Dental Treatment No significant effects or complications reported
Mechanism of Action The primary active compound is T_3 (triiodothyronine), which may be converted from T_4 (thyroxine) and then circulates throughout the body to influence growth and maturation of various tissues; exact mechanism of action is unknown; however, it is believed the thyroid hormone exerts its many metabolic effects through control of DNA transcription and protein synthesis; involved in normal metabolism, growth, and development; promotes gluconeogenesis, increases utilization and mobilization of glycogen stores and stimulates protein synthesis, increases basal metabolic rate

Drug Interactions

Increased Effect/Toxicity: Thyroid may potentiate the hypoprothrombinemic effect of oral anticoagulants. Tricyclic antidepressants (TAD) coadministered with thyroid hormone may increase potential for toxicity of both drugs.

Decreased Effect: Thyroid hormones increase the therapeutic need for oral hypoglycemics or insulin. Cholestyramine can bind thyroid and reduce its absorption. Phenytoin may decrease thyroxine serum levels. Thyroid hormone may decrease effect of oral sulfonylureas.

Pharmacodynamics/Kinetics

Absorption: T_4: 48% to 79%; T_3: 95%; desiccated thyroid contains thyroxine, liothyronine, and iodine (primarily bound)

Metabolism: Thyroxine: Largely converted to liothyronine

Half-life elimination, serum: Liothyronine: 1-2 days; Thyroxine: 6-7 days

Pregnancy Risk Factor A

Thyrotropin Alpha (thye roe TROH pin AL fa)

U.S. Brand Names Thyrogen®

Canadian Brand Names Thyrogen®

Generic Available No

Index Terms Human Thyroid Stimulating Hormone; TSH

Pharmacologic Category Diagnostic Agent

Use As an adjunctive diagnostic tool for serum thyroglobulin (Tg) testing with or without radioiodine imaging in the follow-up of patients with well-differentiated thyroid cancer

Potential clinical use:

1. Patients with an undetectable Tg on thyroid hormone suppressive therapy to exclude the diagnosis of residual or recurrent thyroid cancer
2. Patients requiring serum Tg testing and radioiodine imaging who are unwilling to undergo thyroid hormone withdrawal testing and whose treating physician believes that use of a less sensitive test is justified
3. Patients who are either unable to mount an adequate endogenous TSH response to thyroid hormone withdrawal or in whom withdrawal is medically contraindicated

Local Anesthetic/Vasoconstrictor Precautions No information available to require special precautions

Effects on Dental Treatment No significant effects or complications reported

Common Adverse Effects

>10 %: Gastrointestinal: Nausea (11%)

1% to 10%:

Central nervous system: Headache (7%), dizziness (2%), chills (1%), fever (1%)

Gastrointestinal: Vomiting (2%)

Neuromuscular & skeletal: Weakness (3%), paresthesia (2%)

Miscellaneous: Flu-like syndrome (1%)

Adverse reactions which may be related to local edema or hemorrhage at metastatic sites: Acute visual loss, enlargement of locally-recurring papillary carcinoma, laryngeal edema with respiratory distress, stridor

Mechanism of Action A recombinant DNA source of human TSH that serves as an additional diagnostic tool in the follow-up of patients with a history of well-differentiated thyroid cancer. Binding of thyrotropin alpha to TSH receptors on normal thyroid epithelial cells or on well-differentiated thyroid cancer tissue stimulates iodine uptake and organification, and synthesis and secretion of thyroglobulin, triiodothyronine, and thyroxine. In thyroid cancer patients with near total thyroidectomy, thyrotropin is used to stimulate thyroglobulin from residual or remnant thyroid cancer tissue, which prevents the need for thyroid hormone therapy withdrawal.

Pharmacodynamics/Kinetics

Half-life elimination: 25 ± 10 hours

Time to peak: Median: 10 hours (range: 3-24 hours)

Pregnancy Risk Factor C

Tiagabine (tye AG a been)

U.S. Brand Names Gabitril®
Canadian Brand Names Gabitril®
Generic Available No
Index Terms Tiagabine Hydrochloride
Pharmacologic Category Anticonvulsant, Miscellaneous
Use Adjunctive therapy in adults and children ≥12 years of age in the treatment of partial seizures
Local Anesthetic/Vasoconstrictor Precautions No information available to require special precautions
Effects on Dental Treatment Key adverse event(s) related to dental treatment: Stomatitis, gingivitis, and mouth ulceration.
Common Adverse Effects
>10%:
    Central nervous system: Concentration decreased, dizziness, nervousness, somnolence
    Gastrointestinal: Nausea
    Neuromuscular & skeletal: Weakness, tremor
1% to 10%:
    Cardiovascular: Chest pain, edema, hypertension, palpitation, peripheral edema, syncope, tachycardia, vasodilation
    Central nervous system: Agitation, ataxia, chills, confusion, difficulty with memory, confusion, depersonalization, depression, euphoria, hallucination, hostility, insomnia, malaise, migraine, paranoid reaction, personality disorder, speech disorder
    Dermatologic: Alopecia, bruising, dry skin, pruritus, rash
    Gastrointestinal: Abdominal pain, diarrhea, gingivitis, increased appetite, mouth ulceration, stomatitis, vomiting, weight gain/loss
    Neuromuscular & skeletal: Abnormal gait, arthralgia, dysarthria, hyper-/hypokinesia, hyper-/hypotonia, myasthenia, myalgia, myoclonus, neck pain, paresthesia, reflexes decreased, stupor, twitching, vertigo
    Ocular: Abnormal vision, amblyopia, nystagmus
    Otic: Ear pain, hearing impairment, otitis media, tinnitus
    Respiratory: Bronchitis, cough, dyspnea, epistaxis, pneumonia
    Miscellaneous: Allergic reaction, cyst, diaphoresis, flu-like syndrome, lymphadenopathy
Mechanism of Action The exact mechanism by which tiagabine exerts antiseizure activity is not definitively known; however, *in vitro* experiments demonstrate that it enhances the activity of gamma aminobutyric acid (GABA), the major neuroinhibitory transmitter in the nervous system; it is thought that binding to the GABA uptake carrier inhibits the uptake of GABA into presynaptic neurons, allowing an increased amount of GABA to be available to postsynaptic neurons; based on *in vitro* studies, tiagabine does not inhibit the uptake of dopamine, norepinephrine, serotonin, glutamate, or choline
Drug Interactions
    Cytochrome P450 Effect: Substrate of 3A4 (major)
    Increased Effect/Toxicity: Sedative effects may be additive with other CNS depressants. CYP3A4 inhibitors may increase the levels/effects of tiagabine; example inhibitors include azole antifungals, clarithromycin, diclofenac, doxycycline, erythromycin, imatinib, isoniazid, nefazodone, nicardipine, propofol, protease inhibitors, quinidine, telithromycin, and verapamil. Valproate increased free tiagabine concentrations (*in vitro*) by 40%.
    Decreased Effect: CYP3A4 inducers may decrease the levels/effects of tiagabine; example inducers include aminoglutethimide, carbamazepine, nafcillin, nevirapine, phenobarbital, phenytoin, and rifamycins.
Pharmacodynamics/Kinetics
    Absorption: Rapid (45 minutes); prolonged with food
    Protein binding: 96%, primarily to albumin and α_1-acid glycoprotein
    Metabolism: Hepatic via CYP (primarily 3A4)
    Bioavailability: Oral: Absolute: 90%
    Half-life elimination: 2-5 hours when administered with enzyme inducers; 7-9 hours when administered without enzyme inducers
    Time to peak, plasma: 45 minutes
    Excretion: Feces (63%); urine (25%); 2% as unchanged drug; primarily as metabolites
Pregnancy Risk Factor C

Tiagabine Hydrochloride see Tiagabine on page 1564

Tiazac® see Diltiazem on page 505

Ticar® see Ticarcillin on page 1565

Ticarcillin (tye kar SIL in)

U.S. Brand Names Ticar®
Generic Available No
Index Terms Ticarcillin Disodium
Pharmacologic Category Antibiotic, Penicillin
Use Treatment of susceptible infections such as septicemia, acute and chronic respiratory tract infections, skin and soft tissue infections, and urinary tract infections due to susceptible strains of *Pseudomonas*, and other gram-negative bacteria
Local Anesthetic/Vasoconstrictor Precautions No information available to require special precautions
Effects on Dental Treatment Key adverse event(s) related to dental treatment: Prolonged use of penicillins may lead to development of oral candidiasis.
Common Adverse Effects Frequency not defined.
Central nervous system: Confusion, convulsions, drowsiness, fever, Jarisch-Herxheimer reaction
Dermatologic: Rash
Endocrine & metabolic: Electrolyte imbalance
Gastrointestinal: *Clostridium difficile* colitis
Hematologic: Bleeding, eosinophilia, hemolytic anemia, leukopenia, neutropenia, positive Coombs' reaction, thrombocytopenia
Hepatic: Hepatotoxicity, jaundice
Local: Thrombophlebitis
Neuromuscular & skeletal: Myoclonus
Renal: Interstitial nephritis (acute)
Miscellaneous: Anaphylaxis, hypersensitivity reactions
Mechanism of Action Inhibits bacterial cell wall synthesis by binding to one or more of the penicillin binding proteins (PBPs); which in turn inhibits the final transpeptidation step of peptidoglycan synthesis in bacterial cell walls, thus inhibiting cell wall biosynthesis. Bacteria eventually lyse due to ongoing activity of cell wall autolytic enzymes (autolysins and murein hydrolases) while cell wall assembly is arrested.
Drug Interactions
Increased Effect/Toxicity: Probenecid may increase penicillin levels. Neuromuscular blockers may have an increased duration of action (neuromuscular blockade). Penicillins may increase the exposure to methotrexate during concurrent therapy; monitor.
Decreased Effect: Tetracyclines may decrease penicillin effectiveness. Aminoglycosides may cause physical inactivation of aminoglycosides in the presence of high concentrations of ticarcillin and potential toxicity in patients with mild-moderate renal dysfunction. Although anecdotal reports suggest oral contraceptive efficacy could be reduced by penicillins, this has been refuted by more rigorous scientific and clinical data.
Pharmacodynamics/Kinetics
Absorption: I.M.: 86%
Distribution: Blister fluid, lymph tissue, and gallbladder; low concentrations into CSF increasing with inflamed meninges, otherwise widely distributed; crosses placenta; enters breast milk (low concentrations)
Protein binding: 45% to 65%
Half-life elimination:
Neonates: <1 week old: 3.5-5.6 hours; 1-8 weeks old: 1.3-2.2 hours
Children 5-13 years: 0.9 hour
Adults: 66-72 minutes; prolonged with renal and/or hepatic impairment
Time to peak, serum: I.M.: 30-75 minutes
Excretion: Almost entirely urine (as unchanged drug and metabolites); feces (3.5%)
Pregnancy Risk Factor B

Ticarcillin and Clavulanate Potassium
(tye kar SIL in & klav yoo LAN ate poe TASS ee um)

Related Information
Ticarcillin *on page 1565*
U.S. Brand Names Timentin®
Canadian Brand Names Timentin®
Mexican Brand Names Timentin
Generic Available No
(Continued)

Ticarcillin and Clavulanate Potassium (Continued)

Index Terms Ticarcillin and Clavulanic Acid

Pharmacologic Category Antibiotic, Penicillin

Use Treatment of infections of lower respiratory tract, urinary tract, skin and skin structures, bone and joint, and septicemia caused by susceptible organisms. Clavulanate expands activity of ticarcillin to include beta-lactamase producing strains of *S. aureus*, *H. influenzae*, *Bacteroides* species, and some other gram-negative bacilli

Local Anesthetic/Vasoconstrictor Precautions No information available to require special precautions

Effects on Dental Treatment Key adverse event(s) related to dental treatment: Prolonged use of penicillins may lead to development of oral candidiasis.

Common Adverse Effects Frequency not defined.

Central nervous system: Confusion, convulsions, drowsiness, fever, Jarisch-Herxheimer reaction

Dermatologic: Rash, erythema multiforme, toxic epidermal necrolysis, Stevens-Johnson syndrome

Endocrine & metabolic: Electrolyte imbalance

Gastrointestinal: *Clostridium difficile* colitis

Hematologic: Bleeding, hemolytic anemia, leukopenia, neutropenia, positive Coombs' reaction, thrombocytopenia

Hepatic: Hepatotoxicity, jaundice

Local: Thrombophlebitis

Neuromuscular & skeletal: Myoclonus

Renal: Interstitial nephritis (acute)

Miscellaneous: Anaphylaxis, hypersensitivity reactions

Mechanism of Action Inhibits bacterial cell wall synthesis by binding to one or more of the penicillin binding proteins (PBPs); which in turn inhibits the final transpeptidation step of peptidoglycan synthesis in bacterial cell walls, thus inhibiting cell wall biosynthesis. Bacteria eventually lyse due to ongoing activity of cell wall autolytic enzymes (autolysins and murein hydrolases) while cell wall assembly is arrested.

Drug Interactions

Increased Effect/Toxicity: Probenecid may increase penicillin levels. Neuromuscular blockers may have an increased duration of action (neuromuscular blockade). Penicillins may increase the exposure to methotrexate during concurrent therapy; monitor.

Decreased Effect: Tetracyclines may decrease penicillin effectiveness. Aminoglycosides may cause physical inactivation of aminoglycosides in the presence of high concentrations of ticarcillin and potential toxicity in patients with mild-moderate renal dysfunction. Although anecdotal reports suggest oral contraceptive efficacy could be reduced by penicillins, this has been refuted by more rigorous scientific and clinical data.

Pharmacodynamics/Kinetics

Ticarcillin: See Ticarcillin monograph.

Clavulanic acid:

Protein binding: 9% to 30%

Metabolism: Hepatic

Half-life elimination: 66-90 minutes

Excretion: Urine (45% as unchanged drug)

Clearance: Does not affect clearance of ticarcillin

Pregnancy Risk Factor B

Ticarcillin and Clavulanic Acid see Ticarcillin and Clavulanate Potassium on page 1565

Ticarcillin Disodium see Ticarcillin on page 1565

TICE® BCG see BCG Vaccine on page 186

Ticlid® see Ticlopidine on page 1566

Ticlopidine (tye KLOE pi deen)

Related Information

Cardiovascular Diseases on page 1726

U.S. Brand Names Ticlid®

Canadian Brand Names Alti-Ticlopidine; Apo-Ticlopidine®; Gen-Ticlopidine; Novo-Ticlopidine; Nu-Ticlopidine; Rhoxal-ticlopidine; Sandoz-Ticlopidine; Ticlid®

Mexican Brand Names Ticlid

Generic Available Yes

Index Terms Ticlopidine Hydrochloride

Pharmacologic Category Antiplatelet Agent

Use Platelet aggregation inhibitor that reduces the risk of thrombotic stroke in patients who have had a stroke or stroke precursors. **Note:** Due to its association with life-threatening hematologic disorders, ticlopidine should be reserved for patients who are intolerant to aspirin, or who have failed aspirin therapy. Adjunctive therapy (with aspirin) following successful coronary stent implantation to reduce the incidence of subacute stent thrombosis.

Unlabeled/Investigational Use Protection of aortocoronary bypass grafts, diabetic microangiopathy, ischemic heart disease, prevention of postoperative DVT, reduction of graft loss following renal transplant

Local Anesthetic/Vasoconstrictor Precautions No information available to require special precautions

Effects on Dental Treatment No significant effects or complications reported; if a patient is to undergo elective surgery and an antiplatelet effect is not desired, ticlopidine should be discontinued at least 7 days prior to surgery.

Common Adverse Effects As with all drugs which may affect hemostasis, bleeding is associated with ticlopidine. Hemorrhage may occur at virtually any site. Risk is dependent on multiple variables, including the use of multiple agents which alter hemostasis and patient susceptibility.

>10%:
   Endocrine & metabolic: Increased total cholesterol (increases of ~8% to 10% within 1 month of therapy)
   Gastrointestinal: Diarrhea (13%)
1% to 10%:
   Central nervous system: Dizziness (1%)
   Dermatologic: Rash (5%), purpura (2%), pruritus (1%)
   Gastrointestinal: Nausea (7%), dyspepsia (7%), gastrointestinal pain (4%), vomiting (2%), flatulence (2%), anorexia (1%)
   Hematologic: Neutropenia (2%)
   Hepatic: Abnormal liver function test (1%)

Mechanism of Action Ticlopidine is an inhibitor of platelet function with a mechanism which is different from other antiplatelet drugs. The drug significantly increases bleeding time. This effect may not be solely related to ticlopidine's effect on platelets. The prolongation of the bleeding time caused by ticlopidine is further increased by the addition of aspirin in *ex vivo* experiments. Although many metabolites of ticlopidine have been found, none have been shown to account for *in vivo* activity.

Drug Interactions
   Cytochrome P450 Effect: Substrate of CYP3A4 (major); **Inhibits** CYP1A2 (weak), 2C9 (weak), 2C19 (strong), 2D6 (moderate), 2E1 (weak), 3A4 (weak)
   Increased Effect/Toxicity: Ticlopidine may increase effect/toxicity of aspirin, anticoagulants, theophylline, and NSAIDs. Cimetidine may increase ticlopidine blood levels. Ticlopidine may increase the levels/effects of amphetamines, selected beta-blockers, citalopram, dextromethorphan, diazepam, fluoxetine, lidocaine, methsuximide, mirtazapine, nefazodone, paroxetine, phenytoin, sertraline, risperidone, ritonavir, thioridazine, tricyclic antidepressants, venlafaxine, and other CYP2C19 or 2D6 substrates.
   Decreased Effect: Decreased effect of ticlopidine with antacids (decreased absorption). Ticlopidine may decrease the effect of digoxin or cyclosporine. The levels/effects of ticlopidine may be decreased by aminoglutethimide, carbamazepine, nafcillin, nevirapine, phenobarbital, phenytoin, rifamycins, and other CYP3A4 inducers. Ticlopidine may decrease the levels/effects of CYP2D6 prodrug substrates (eg, codeine, hydrocodone, oxycodone, tramadol).

Pharmacodynamics/Kinetics
   Onset of action: ~6 hours
      Peak effect: 3-5 days; serum levels do not correlate with clinical antiplatelet activity
   Metabolism: Extensively hepatic; has at least one active metabolite
   Half-life elimination: 24 hours

Pregnancy Risk Factor B

Tigecycline (tye ge SYE kleen)

U.S. Brand Names Tygacil™

Generic Available No

(Continued)

Tigecycline *(Continued)*

Index Terms GAR-936
Pharmacologic Category Antibiotic, Glycylcycline
Use Treatment of complicated skin and skin structure infections caused by susceptible organisms, including methicillin-resistant *Staphylococcus aureus* and vancomycin-sensitive *Enterococcus faecalis*; treatment of complicated intra-abdominal infections

Local Anesthetic/Vasoconstrictor Precautions No information available to require special precautions

Effects on Dental Treatment Key adverse events(s) related to dental treatment: Tigecycline is structurally similar to tetracycline. Therefore, tigecycline is not recommended for use in pregnancy or in children ≤8 years of age. Permanent discoloration of the teeth may occur if used during tooth development.

Common Adverse Effects Note: Frequencies relative to placebo are not available; some frequencies are lower than those experienced with comparator drugs.

>10%: Gastrointestinal: Nausea (25% to 30%; severe in 1%), vomiting (20%; severe in 1%), diarrhea (13%)

2% to 10%:
Cardiovascular: Hypertension (5%), peripheral edema (3%), hypotension (2%), phlebitis (2%)
Central nervous system: Fever (7%), headache (6%), dizziness (4%), pain (4%), insomnia (2%)
Dermatologic: Pruritus (3%), rash (2%)
Endocrine & metabolic: Hypoproteinemia (5%), hyperglycemia (2%), hypokalemia (2%)
Gastrointestinal: Abdominal pain (7%), constipation (3%), dyspepsia (3%)
Hematologic: Thrombocythemia (6%), anemia (4%), leukocytosis (4%)
Hepatic: ALT increased (6%), AST increased (4%), alkaline phosphatase increased (4%), amylase increased (3%), bilirubin increased (2%), LDH increased (4%)
Local: Reaction to procedure (9%)
Neuromuscular & skeletal: Weakness (3%)
Renal: BUN increased (2%)
Respiratory: Cough increased (4%), dyspnea (3%), pulmonary physical finding (2%)
Miscellaneous: Abnormal healing (4%), infection (8%), abscess (3%), diaphoresis increased (2%)

Mechanism of Action Binds to the 30S ribosomal subunit of susceptible bacteria, inhibiting protein synthesis.

Drug Interactions
Increased Effect/Toxicity: Retinoic acid derivatives may increase risk of pseudotumor cerebri (reported with tetracyclines). Hypoprothrombinemic response of warfarin may be increased with tigecycline; monitor INR closely during initiation or discontinuation.

Decreased Effect: Anecdotal reports of oral contraceptives suggesting decreased contraceptive efficacy with tetracyclines have been refuted by more rigorous scientific and clinical data.

Pharmacodynamics/Kinetics Note: Systemic clearance is reduced by 55% and half-life increased by 43% in moderate hepatic impairment.
Distribution: V_d: 7-9 L/kg; extensive tissue distribution
Protein binding: 71% to 89%
Metabolism: Hepatic, via glucuronidation, N-acetylation, and epimerization to several metabolites, each <10% of the dose
Half-life elimination: Single dose: 27 hours; following multiple doses: 42 hours
Excretion: Urine (33%; with 22% as unchanged drug); feces (59%; primarily as unchanged drug)

Pregnancy Risk Factor D

Tikosyn® *see* Dofetilide *on page 523*
Tilade® *see* Nedocromil *on page 1155*

Tiludronate *(tye LOO droe nate)*

Related Information
Rheumatoid Arthritis, Osteoarthritis, and Osteoporosis *on page 1759*
U.S. Brand Names Skelid®
Generic Available No
Index Terms Tiludronate Disodium
Pharmacologic Category Bisphosphonate Derivative
Use Treatment of Paget's disease of the bone (osteitis deformans) in patients who have a level of serum alkaline phosphatase (SAP) at least twice the upper

limit of normal, or who are symptomatic, or who are at risk for future complications of their disease

Local Anesthetic/Vasoconstrictor Precautions No information available to require special precautions

Effects on Dental Treatment Osteonecrosis of the jaw (ONJ), generally associated with local infection and/or tooth extraction and often with delayed healing, has been reported in patients taking bisphosphonates. Symptoms included nonhealing extraction socket or an exposed jawbone. Most reported cases of bisphosphonate-associated osteonecrosis have been in cancer patients treated with intravenous bisphosphonates. However, some have occurred in patients with postmenopausal osteoporosis taking oral bisphosphonates. Dental surgery may exacerbate ONJ. For patients requiring dental procedures, there are no data available to suggest whether discontinuation of bisphosphonate treatment reduces the risk of ONJ. Patients who develop ONJ while on bisphosphonate therapy should receive care by an oral surgeon. See Dental Comment.

Common Adverse Effects The following events occurred >2% and at a frequency greater than placebo:

1% to 10%:
Cardiovascular: Chest pain (3%), edema (3%)
Central nervous system: Dizziness (4%), paresthesia (4%)
Dermatologic: Rash (3%), skin disorder (3%)
Gastrointestinal: Nausea (9%), diarrhea (9%), heartburn (5%), vomiting (4%), flatulence (3%)
Neuromuscular & skeletal: Arthrosis (3%)
Ocular: cataract (3%), conjunctivitis (3%), glaucoma (3%)
Respiratory: Rhinitis (5%), sinusitis (5%), cough (3%), pharyngitis (3%)

Mechanism of Action Inhibition of normal and abnormal bone resorption. Inhibits osteoclasts through at least two mechanisms: disruption of the cytoskeletal ring structure, possibly by inhibition of protein-tyrosine-phosphatase, thus leading to the detachment of osteoclasts from the bone surface area and the inhibition of the osteoclast proton pump.

Drug Interactions
Increased Effect/Toxicity: Aminoglycosides may lower serum calcium levels with prolonged administration; concomitant use may have an additive hypocalcemic effect. NSAIDs may enhance the gastrointestinal adverse/toxic effects (increased incidence of GI ulcers) of bisphosphonate derivatives. Bisphosphonate derivatives may enhance the hypocalcemic effect of phosphate supplements.

Decreased Effect: The following agents may decrease the absorption of oral bisphosphonate derivatives: Antacids (aluminum, calcium, magnesium), oral calcium salts, oral iron salts, and oral magnesium salts.

Pharmacodynamics/Kinetics
Onset of action: Delayed, may require several weeks
Absorption: Rapid
Distribution: Widely to bone and soft tissue
Protein binding: 90%, primarily to albumin
Metabolism: Little, if any
Bioavailability: 6%; reduced by food
Half-life elimination: Healthy volunteers: 50 hours; Pagetic patients: 150 hours
Time to peak, plasma: ~2 hours
Excretion: Urine (60% as unchanged drug) within 13 days

Pregnancy Risk Factor C

Dental Comment There is no data on the incidence of ONJ associated with use of tiludronate. A report by the Council of Scientific Affairs of the American Dental Association (accessed at: http://www.ada.org/prof/resources/topics/osteonecrosis.asp) as of July 2006 gave an estimated incidence of 0.7 cases for every 100,000 person-years of exposure to alendronate (Fosamax®). This translates to one case for every 142,857 person-years exposure. This figure from the ADA report was based on information received from Merck & Co citing 170 worldwide cases for alendronate (Fosamax®). In addition, Procter & Gamble Pharmaceuticals has cited 20 cases for risedronate (Actonel®) and Roche Laboratories has cited one case for ibandronate (Boniva®).

Consumer Reports On Health stated that the risk of jaw bone osteoporosis due to alendronate (Fosamax®), risedronate (Actonel®), or ibandronate (Boniva®) taken to prevent osteoporosis is very low and is estimated to be one out of every 20,000 users. That report mentioned that tooth extraction or implants increase the risk of developing osteonecrosis in patients taking any of these drugs for osteoporosis. The report also recommended that patients should stop taking any of these oral drugs 1-2 months before and after such dental treatment. No evidence was presented to support this statement.

In terms of length of exposure to oral bisphosphonates prior to onset of ONJ, data from large population studies or controlled studies is lacking. A report by
(Continued)

Tiludronate *(Continued)*

Marx et al, observed that of three cases of ONJ associated with Fosamax® exposure, one patient had been taking 10 mg/day by mouth for 6 years and the other two patients 10 mg/day by mouth for 3 and 2 years respectively. In contrast, they observed that in cancer patients receiving intravenous bisphosphonates, the time period between the first doses of the bisphosphonate to first recognition of exposed bone either by the patients or by the clinician, was 9.4 months for zoledronate (Zometa®), 14.3 months for pamidronate (Aredia®), and 12.1 months for pamidronate then to zoledronate.

Tiludronate Disodium *see* Tiludronate *on page 1568*

Timentin® *see* Ticarcillin and Clavulanate Potassium *on page 1565*

Timolol *(TIM oh lol)*

Related Information
Cardiovascular Diseases *on page 1726*

U.S. Brand Names Betimol®; Blocadren®; Istalol™; Timoptic®; Timoptic® in OcuDose®; Timoptic-XE®

Canadian Brand Names Alti-Timolol; Apo-Timol®; Apo-Timop®; Gen-Timolol; Nu-Timolol; Phoxal-timolol; PMS-Timolol; Sandoz-Timolol; Tim-AK; Timoptic®; Timoptic-XE®

Mexican Brand Names Nyolol; Timoptol; Timoptol-XE; Timozzard

Generic Available Yes: Excludes hemihydrate ophthalmic solutions

Index Terms Timolol Hemihydrate; Timolol Maleate

Pharmacologic Category Beta-Adrenergic Blocker, Nonselective; Ophthalmic Agent, Antiglaucoma

Use
Ophthalmic: Treatment of elevated intraocular pressure such as glaucoma or ocular hypertension

Oral: Treatment of hypertension and angina; to reduce mortality following myocardial infarction; prophylaxis of migraine

Local Anesthetic/Vasoconstrictor Precautions Epinephrine has interacted with nonselective beta-blockers such as propranolol to result in initial hypertensive episode followed by bradycardia. Timolol is also a nonselective beta-blocker. Timolol is available as an eye drop and oral dose form. When administered as an eye drop, the significance of a potential systemic interaction with epinephrine is unknown. However, it is suggested that cautionary procedures be used, particularly if vasoconstrictor is used immediately following an ophthalmic dose of timolol taken by the patient. If patients are taking the oral form of timolol, then the significance of a potential systemic interaction is well known and cautionary use of epinephrine is advised.

Effects on Dental Treatment Key adverse event(s) related to dental treatment: Xerostomia (normal salivary flow resumes upon discontinuation).

Timolol is a nonselective beta-blocker and may enhance the pressor response to epinephrine, resulting in hypertension and bradycardia. Many nonsteroidal anti-inflammatory drugs, such as ibuprofen and indomethacin, can reduce the hypotensive effect of beta-blockers after 3 or more weeks of therapy with the NSAID. Short-term NSAID use (ie, 3 days) requires no special precautions in patients taking beta-blockers.

Common Adverse Effects
Ophthalmic:
>10%: Ocular: Burning, stinging
1% to 10%:
Cardiovascular: Hypertension
Central nervous system: Headache
Ocular: Blurred vision, cataract, conjunctival injection, itching, visual acuity decreased
Miscellaneous: Infection

Systemic:
1% to 10%:
Cardiovascular: Bradycardia
Central nervous system: Fatigue, dizziness
Respiratory: Dyspnea

Frequency not defined (reported with any dosage form):
Cardiovascular: Angina pectoris, arrhythmia, bradycardia, cardiac failure, cardiac arrest, cerebral vascular accident, cerebral ischemia, edema, hypotension, heart block, palpitation, Raynaud's phenomenon
Central nervous system: Anxiety, confusion, depression, disorientation, dizziness, hallucinations, insomnia, memory loss, nervousness, nightmares, somnolence

Dermatologic: Alopecia, angioedema, pseudopemphigoid, psoriasiform rash, psoriasis exacerbation, rash, urticaria

Endocrine & metabolic: Hypoglycemia masked, libido decreased

Gastrointestinal: Anorexia, diarrhea, dyspepsia, nausea, xerostomia

Genitourinary: Impotence, retoperitoneal fibrosis

Hematologic: Claudication

Neuromuscular & skeletal: Myasthenia gravis exacerbation, paresthesia

Ocular: Blepharitis, conjunctivitis, corneal sensitivity decreased, cystoid macular edema, diplopia, dry eyes, foreign body sensation, keratitis, ocular discharge, ocular pain, ptosis, refractive changes, tearing, visual disturbances

Otic: Tinnitus

Respiratory: Bronchospasm, cough, dyspnea, nasal congestion, pulmonary edema, respiratory failure

Miscellaneous: Allergic reactions, cold hands/feet, Peyronie's disease, systemic lupus erythematosus

Mechanism of Action Blocks both beta$_1$- and beta$_2$-adrenergic receptors, reduces intraocular pressure by reducing aqueous humor production or possibly outflow; reduces blood pressure by blocking adrenergic receptors and decreasing sympathetic outflow, produces a negative chronotropic and inotropic activity through an unknown mechanism

Drug Interactions

Cytochrome P450 Effect: Substrate of CYP2D6 (major); **Inhibits** CYP2D6 (weak)

Increased Effect/Toxicity: CYP2D6 inhibitors may increase the levels/effects of timolol; example inhibitors include chlorpromazine, delavirdine, fluoxetine, miconazole, paroxetine, pergolide, quinidine, quinine, ritonavir, and ropinirole. The heart rate-lowering effects of timolol are additive with other drugs which slow AV conduction (digoxin, verapamil, diltiazem). Reserpine increases the effects of timolol. Concurrent use of timolol may increase the effects of alpha-blockers (prazosin, terazosin), alpha-adrenergic stimulants (epinephrine, phenylephrine), and the vasoconstrictive effects of ergot alkaloids. Timolol may mask the tachycardia from hypoglycemia caused by insulin and oral hypoglycemics. In patients receiving concurrent therapy, the risk of hypertensive crisis is increased when either clonidine or the beta-blocker is withdrawn. Beta-blockers may increase the action or levels of ethanol, disopyramide, nondepolarizing muscle relaxants, and theophylline although the effects are difficult to predict.

Decreased Effect: Decreased effect of timolol with aluminum salts, barbiturates, calcium salts, cholestyramine, colestipol, NSAIDs, penicillins (ampicillin), rifampin, salicylates, and sulfinpyrazone due to decreased bioavailability and plasma levels. Beta-blockers may decrease the effect of sulfonylureas. Beta-blockers may affect the action or levels of ethanol, disopyramide, nondepolarizing muscle relaxants, and theophylline, although the effects are difficult to predict.

Pharmacodynamics/Kinetics

Onset of action:

Hypotensive: Oral: 15-45 minutes

Peak effect: 0.5-2.5 hours

Intraocular pressure reduction: Ophthalmic: 30 minutes

Peak effect: 1-2 hours

Duration: ~4 hours; Ophthalmic: Intraocular: 24 hours

Protein binding: 60%

Metabolism: Extensively hepatic; extensive first-pass effect

Half-life elimination: 2-2.7 hours; prolonged with renal impairment

Excretion: Urine (15% to 20% as unchanged drug)

Pregnancy Risk Factor C (manufacturer); D (2nd and 3rd trimesters - expert analysis)

Ting® Spray Liquid [OTC] *see* Tolnaftate *on page 1587*

Tinidazole (tye NI da zole)

U.S. Brand Names Tindamax™
Mexican Brand Names Estovit-T; Fasigyn; Induken
Generic Available No
Pharmacologic Category Amebicide; Antibiotic, Miscellaneous; Antiprotozoal, Nitroimidazole
Use Treatment of trichomoniasis caused by *T. vaginalis*; treatment of giardiasis caused by *G. duodenalis* (*G. lamblia*); treatment of intestinal amebiasis and amebic liver abscess caused by *E. histolytica*
Local Anesthetic/Vasoconstrictor Precautions No information available to require special precautions
Effects on Dental Treatment Key adverse event(s) related to dental treatment: Xerostomia and changes in salivation (normal salivary flow resumes upon discontinuation), metallic/bitter taste, oral candidiasis, tongue discoloration, stomatitis, furry tongue. See Dental Comment.
Common Adverse Effects
1% to 10%:
   Central nervous system: Fatigue/malaise (1% to 2%), dizziness (≤1%), headache (≤1%)
   Gastrointestinal: Metallic/bitter taste (4% to 6%), nausea (3% to 5%), anorexia (2% to 3%), dyspepsia/cramps/epigastric discomfort (1% to 2%), vomiting (1% to 2%), constipation (≤1%)
   Neuromuscular & skeletal: Weakness (1% to 2%)
Frequency not defined.
   Cardiovascular: Flushing, palpitation
   Central nervous system: Ataxia, coma, confusion, convulsions, depression, drowsiness, fever, giddiness, insomnia, vertigo
   Dermatologic: Angioedema, pruritus, rash, urticaria
   Gastrointestinal: Diarrhea, furry tongue, oral candidiasis, salivation, stomatitis, thirst, tongue discoloration, xerostomia
   Genitourinary: Urine darkened, vaginal discharge increased
   Hematologic: Leukopenia (transient), neutropenia (transient), thrombocytopenia (reversible)
   Hepatic: Transaminases increased
   Neuromuscular & skeletal: Arthralgia, arthritis, myalgia, peripheral neuropathy (transient, includes numbness and paresthesia)
   Respiratory: Bronchospasm, dyspnea, pharyngitis
   Miscellaneous: Burning sensation, *Candida* overgrowth, diaphoresis
Mechanism of Action After diffusing into the organism, it is proposed that tinidazole causes cytotoxicity by damaging DNA and preventing further DNA synthesis.
Drug Interactions
   Cytochrome P450 Effect: Substrate of CYP3A4 (minor)
   Increased Effect/Toxicity: Specific interaction studies have not been conducted. Refer to Metronidazole monograph *on page 1091*.
   Decreased Effect: Specific interaction studies have not been conducted. Refer to Metronidazole monograph *on page 1091*.
Pharmacodynamics/Kinetics
   Absorption: Rapid and complete
   Distribution: V_d: 50 L
   Protein binding: 12%
   Metabolism: Hepatic via CYP3A4 (primarily); undergoes oxidation, hydroxylation and conjugation; forms a metabolite
   Half-life elimination: 13 hours
   Excretion: Urine (20% to 25%); feces (12%)
Pregnancy Risk Factor C
Dental Comment Although this drug is a member of the metronidazole family, there is no specific dental indication for its use. Just as with metronidazole, alcohol in any form is contraindicated while the patient is on this medication because of the danger of a disulfiram-type reaction.

Tinzaparin (tin ZA pa rin)

Related Information
   Cardiovascular Diseases *on page 1726*
U.S. Brand Names Innohep®
Canadian Brand Names Innohep®
Generic Available No

Index Terms Tinzaparin Sodium

Pharmacologic Category Low Molecular Weight Heparin

Use Treatment of acute symptomatic deep vein thrombosis, with or without pulmonary embolism, in conjunction with warfarin sodium

Local Anesthetic/Vasoconstrictor Precautions No information available to require special precautions

Effects on Dental Treatment No significant effects or complications reported

Common Adverse Effects As with all anticoagulants, bleeding is the major adverse effect of tinzaparin. Hemorrhage may occur at virtually any site. Risk is dependent on multiple variables.

>10%:

Hepatic: Increased ALT (13%)

Local: Injection site hematoma (16%)

1% to 10%:

Cardiovascular: Angina pectoris, chest pain (2%), hyper-/hypotension, tachycardia

Central nervous system: Confusion, dizziness, fever (2%), headache (2%), insomnia, pain (2%)

Dermatologic: Bullous eruption, pruritus, rash (1%), skin disorder

Gastrointestinal: Constipation (1%), dyspepsia, flatulence, nausea (2%), nonspecified gastrointestinal disorder, vomiting (1%)

Genitourinary: Dysuria, urinary retention, urinary tract infection (4%)

Hematologic: Anemia, hematoma, hemorrhage (2%), thrombocytopenia (1%)

Hepatic: Increased AST (9%)

Local: Thrombophlebitis (deep)

Neuromuscular & skeletal: Back pain (2%)

Renal: Hematuria (1%)

Respiratory: Dyspnea (1%), epistaxis (2%), pneumonia, pulmonary embolism (2%), respiratory disorder

Miscellaneous: Impaired healing, infection, unclassified reactions

Mechanism of Action Standard heparin consists of components with molecular weights ranging from 4000-30,000 daltons with a mean of 16,000 daltons. Heparin acts as an anticoagulant by enhancing the inhibition rate of clotting proteases by antithrombin III, impairing normal hemostasis and inhibition of factor Xa. Low molecular weight heparins have a small effect on the activated partial thromboplastin time and strongly inhibit factor Xa. The primary inhibitory activity of tinzaparin is through antithrombin. Tinzaparin is derived from porcine heparin that undergoes controlled enzymatic depolymerization. The average molecular weight of tinzaparin ranges between 5500 and 7500 daltons which is distributed as (<10%) 2000 daltons (60% to 72%) 2000-8000 daltons, and (22% to 36%) >8000 daltons. The antifactor Xa activity is approximately 100 int. units/mg.

Drug Interactions

Increased Effect/Toxicity: Drugs which affect platelet function (eg, aspirin, NSAIDs, dipyridamole, ticlopidine, clopidogrel, sulfinpyrazone, dextran) may potentiate the risk of hemorrhage. Thrombolytic agents increase the risk of hemorrhage.

Warfarin: Risk of bleeding may be increased during concurrent therapy. Tinzaparin is commonly continued during the initiation of warfarin therapy to assure anticoagulation and to protect against possible transient hypercoagulability

Pharmacodynamics/Kinetics

Onset of action: 2-3 hours

Distribution: 3-5 L

Half-life elimination: 3-4 hours

Metabolism: Partially metabolized by desulphation and depolymerization

Bioavailability: 87%

Time to peak: 4-5 hours

Excretion: Urine

Pregnancy Risk Factor B

Tinzaparin Sodium *see* Tinzaparin *on page 1572*

Tioconazole (tye oh KONE a zole)

U.S. Brand Names 1-Day™ [OTC]; Vagistat®-1 [OTC]

Generic Available No

Pharmacologic Category Antifungal Agent, Vaginal

Use Local treatment of vulvovaginal candidiasis

Local Anesthetic/Vasoconstrictor Precautions No information available to require special precautions

Effects on Dental Treatment No significant effects or complications reported

Common Adverse Effects Frequency not defined.

(Continued)

Tioconazole *(Continued)*

Central nervous system: Headache

Gastrointestinal: Abdominal pain

Dermatologic: Burning, desquamation

Genitourinary: Discharge, dyspareunia, dysuria, irritation, itching, nocturia, vaginal pain, vaginitis, vulvar swelling

Mechanism of Action A 1-substituted imidazole derivative with a broad antifungal spectrum against a wide variety of dermatophytes and yeasts, including *Trichophyton mentagrophytes, T. rubrum, T. erinacei, T. tonsurans, Microsporum canis, Microsporum gypseum,* and *Candida albicans.* Both agents appear to be similarly effective against *Epidermophyton floccosum.*

Drug Interactions

Cytochrome P450 Effect: Inhibits CYP1A2 (weak), 2A6 (weak), 2C9 (weak), 2C19 (weak), 2D6 (weak), 2E1 (weak)

Pharmacodynamics/Kinetics

Onset of action: Some improvement: Within 24 hours; Complete relief: Within 7 days

Absorption: Intravaginal: Systemic (small amounts)

Distribution: Vaginal fluid: 24-72 hours

Excretion: Urine and feces

Pregnancy Risk Factor C

Tioguanine *see* Thioguanine *on page 1557*

Tiopronin *(tye oh PROE nin)*

U.S. Brand Names Thiola®

Canadian Brand Names Thiola®

Generic Available No

Pharmacologic Category Urinary Tract Product

Use Prevention of kidney stone (cystine) formation in patients with severe homozygous cystinuric who have urinary cystine >500 mg/day who are resistant to treatment with high fluid intake, alkali, and diet modification, or who have had adverse reactions to penicillamine

Local Anesthetic/Vasoconstrictor Precautions No information available to require special precautions

Effects on Dental Treatment No significant effects or complications reported

Pregnancy Risk Factor C

Tiotixene *see* Thiothixene *on page 1560*

Tiotropium *(ty oh TRO pee um)*

U.S. Brand Names Spiriva®

Canadian Brand Names Spiriva®

Mexican Brand Names Spiriva

Index Terms Tiotropium Bromide Monohydrate

Pharmacologic Category Anticholinergic Agent

Use Maintenance treatment of bronchospasm associated with COPD (bronchitis and emphysema)

Local Anesthetic/Vasoconstrictor Precautions No information available to require special precautions

Effects on Dental Treatment Key adverse event(s) related to dental treatment: Xerostomia (normal salivary flow resumes upon discontinuation) and ulcerative stomatitis.

Common Adverse Effects

>10%:

Gastrointestinal: Xerostomia (16%)

Respiratory: Upper respiratory tract infection (41% vs 37% with placebo), sinusitis (11% vs 9% with placebo), pharyngeal irritation (frequency not specified)

1% to 10%:

Cardiovascular: Angina, edema (dependent, 5%)

Central nervous system: Paresthesia, depression

Dermatologic: Rash (4%)

Endocrine & metabolic: Hypercholesterolemia, hyperglycemia

Gastrointestinal: Dyspepsia (6%), abdominal pain (5%), constipation (4%), vomiting (4%), reflux, ulcerative stomatitis

Genitourinary: Urinary tract infection (7%)

Neuromuscular & skeletal: Myalgia (4%), leg pain, skeletal pain

Ocular: Cataract

Respiratory: Pharyngitis (9%), rhinitis (6%), epistaxis (4%), dysphonia, laryngitis

Miscellaneous: Infection (4%), moniliasis (4%), allergic reaction, herpes zoster

Mechanism of Action Blocks the action of acetylcholine at parasympathetic sites in bronchial smooth muscle causing bronchodilation

Drug Interactions

Cytochrome P450 Effect: Substrate (minor) of CYP2D6, 3A4

Increased Effect/Toxicity: Increased toxicity with anticholinergics or drugs with anticholinergic properties.

Decreased Effect:

Acetylcholinesterase inhibitors (central) may diminish the therapeutic effect of anticholinergics; anticholinergics may diminish the therapeutic effect of acetylcholinesterase inhibitors (central).

Pharmacodynamics/Kinetics

Absorption: Poorly absorbed from GI tract, systemic absorption may occur from lung

Distribution: V_d: 32 L/kg

Protein binding: 72%

Metabolism: Hepatic (minimal), via CYP2D6 and CYP3A4

Bioavailability: Following inhalation, 19.5%; oral solution: 2% to 3%

Half-life elimination: 5-6 days

Time to peak, plasma: 5 minutes (following inhalation)

Excretion: Urine (14% of an inhaled dose); feces (primarily nonabsorbed drug)

Pregnancy Risk Factor C

Tiotropium Bromide Monohydrate *see* Tiotropium *on page 1574*

Tipranavir (tip RA na veer)

U.S. Brand Names Aptivus®
Canadian Brand Names Aptivus®
Generic Available No
Index Terms PNU-140690E; TPV
Pharmacologic Category Antiretroviral Agent, Protease Inhibitor
Use Treatment of HIV-1 infections in combination with ritonavir and other antiretroviral agents; limited to highly treatment-experienced or multiprotease inhibitor-resistant patients.
Local Anesthetic/Vasoconstrictor Precautions No information available to require special precautions
Effects on Dental Treatment No significant effects or complications reported
Common Adverse Effects

>10%:

Dermatologic: Rash (2% to 14%)

Endocrine & metabolic: Hypercholesterolemia (>300 mg/dL: 11%), hypertriglyceridemia (>400 mg/dL: 26%)

Gastrointestinal: Diarrhea (11%)

Hepatic: Transaminases increased (>2.5 x ULN: 24%; grade 3/4: 6%)

2% to 10%:

Central nervous system: Fever (5%), fatigue (4%), headache (3%), depression (2%)

Gastrointestinal: Nausea (7%), vomiting (3%), abdominal pain (3%), amylase increased (grades 3/4: 3%)

Hematologic: WBC decreased (grades 3/4: 4%)

Neuromuscular & skeletal: Weakness (2%)

Respiratory: Bronchitis (3%)

Mechanism of Action Tipranavir is a nonpeptide inhibitor of HIV-1 protease. It binds to the protease activity site and inhibits the activity of the enzyme. HIV protease is required for the cleavage of viral polyprotein precursors into individual functional proteins found in infectious HIV. Inhibition prevents cleavage of these polyproteins, resulting in the formation of immature, noninfectious viral particles.

Drug Interactions

Cytochrome P450 Effect: Substrate of CYP3A4 (major; minimal metabolism when coadministered with ritonavir)

Increased Effect/Toxicity: Note: Listed interactions include interactions resulting from coadministration with ritonavir. Refer to Ritonavir monograph *on page 1436* for additional interaction concerns. The serum concentration of tipranavir may be increased by ritonavir. This combination is recommended to enhance the effect ("boost") tipranavir.

Tipranavir/ritonavir may increase the levels/effects of CYP3A4 substrates. Tipranavir/ritonavir may increase the toxicity of benzodiazepines; concurrent

(Continued)

Tipranavir *(Continued)*

use of midazolam and triazolam is specifically contraindicated. Tipranavir may increase serum concentrations of cisapride, increasing the risk of malignant arrhythmias; use is contraindicated. Toxicity of pimozide is significantly increased by tipranavir/ritonavir; concurrent use is contraindicated. Tipranavir/ritonavir may increase serum concentrations/toxicity of several antiarrhythmic agents; contraindicated with amiodarone, flecainide, propafenone, and quinidine (use extreme caution with lidocaine). Tipranavir/ritonavir may also increase serum concentrations/effects of imidazole antifungal agents, calcium channel blockers, orally-inhaled corticosteroids (eg, fluticasone), immunosuppressants (eg, cyclosporine, sirolimus, tacrolimus), and trazodone.

Serum concentrations of HMG-CoA reductase inhibitors (atorvastatin, lovastatin, simvastatin) may be increased by tipranavir/ritonavir, increasing the risk of myopathy/rhabdomyolysis. Lovastatin and simvastatin are not recommended. Use lowest possible dose of atorvastatin. Fluvastatin and pravastatin may be safer alternatives. Serum concentrations of rifabutin may be increased by tipranavir/ritonavir; dosage adjustment of rifabutin is required.

The toxicity of ergot derivatives (dihydroergotamine, ergotamine, ergonovine, methylergonovine) is increased by tipranavir; concurrent use is contraindicated. Effects of hypoglycemic agents may be altered by tipranavir/ritonavir. Concurrent therapy with tipranavir may increase serum concentrations of normeperidine, and decrease serum concentrations of meperidine. The serum concentrations of sildenafil, tadalafil, and vardenafil may be increased by tipranavir/ritonavir; dose adjustment and limitations related to ritonavir coadministration must be recognized.

Concurrent use of disulfiram with tipranavir oral solution is contraindicated due to risk of adverse reaction (due to alcohol content of formulation). Clarithromycin may increase serum concentrations of tipranavir. Tipranavir/ritonavir may increase serum concentrations of clarithromycin. Use with caution and adjust dose of clarithromycin during concurrent therapy in renally impaired patients.

Decreased Effect: CYP3A4 inducers may decrease the levels/effects of tipranavir. Example inducers include aminoglutethimide, carbamazepine, nafcillin, nevirapine, phenobarbital, phenytoin, and rifamycins. When coadministered with ritonavir, reduction of tipranavir serum concentrations is unlikely. Rifampin may decrease serum concentrations of tipranavir. Concurrent use of rifampin is not recommended. The effect of methadone may be reduced by tipranavir (methadone dosage increase may be required).

Serum concentrations of protease inhibitors may be decreased by tipranavir. Concurrent therapy with amprenavir, lopinavir, or saquinavir is not recommended. Tipranavir/ritonavir may decrease serum concentrations of nucleoside reverse transcriptase inhibitors (NRTIs, including abacavir, didanosine, and zidovudine); administer tipranavir/ritonavir 2 hours before or after didanosine.

Pharmacodynamics/Kinetics

Absorption: Incomplete (percentage not established)

Distribution: V_d: 7.7-10 L

Protein binding: 99%

Metabolism: Hepatic, via CYP3A4 (minimal when coadministered with ritonavir)

Bioavailability: Not established

Half-life elimination: 6 hours

Time to peak, plasma: 3 hours

Excretion: Feces (82%); urine (4%); primarily as unchanged drug (when coadministered with ritonavir)

Pregnancy Risk Factor C

Tirofiban *(tye roe FYE ban)*

Related Information

Cardiovascular Diseases *on page 1726*

U.S. Brand Names Aggrastat®

Canadian Brand Names Aggrastat®

Mexican Brand Names Agrastat

Generic Available No

Index Terms MK383; Tirofiban Hydrochloride

Pharmacologic Category Antiplatelet Agent, Glycoprotein IIb/IIIa Inhibitor

Use In combination with heparin, is indicated for the treatment of acute coronary syndrome, including patients who are to be managed medically and those undergoing PTCA or atherectomy. In this setting, it has been shown to decrease the rate of a combined endpoint of death, new myocardial infarction or refractory ischemia/repeat cardiac procedure.

Local Anesthetic/Vasoconstrictor Precautions No information available to require special precautions

Effects on Dental Treatment No significant effects or complications reported

Common Adverse Effects Bleeding is the major drug-related adverse effect. Patients received background treatment with aspirin and heparin. Major bleeding was reported in 1.4% to 2.2%; minor bleeding in 10.5% to 12%; transfusion was required in 4% to 4.3%.

>1% (nonbleeding adverse events):

Cardiovascular: Bradycardia (4%), coronary artery dissection (5%), edema (2%)

Central nervous system: Dizziness (3%), fever (>1%), headache (>1%), vaso-vagal reaction (2%)

Gastrointestinal: Nausea (>1%)

Genitourinary: Pelvic pain (6%)

Hematologic: Thrombocytopenia: <90,000/mm^3 (1.5%), <50,000/mm^3 (0.3%)

Neuromuscular & skeletal: Leg pain (3%)

Miscellaneous: Diaphoresis (2%)

Mechanism of Action A reversible antagonist of fibrinogen binding to the GP IIb/IIIa receptor, the major platelet surface receptor involved in platelet aggregation. When administered intravenously, it inhibits *ex vivo* platelet aggregation in a dose- and concentration-dependent manner. When given according to the recommended regimen, >90% inhibition is attained by the end of the 30-minute infusion. Platelet aggregation inhibition is reversible following cessation of the infusion.

Drug Interactions

Increased Effect/Toxicity: Use of tirofiban with aspirin and heparin is associated with an increase in bleeding over aspirin and heparin alone; however, efficacy of tirofiban is improved. Risk of bleeding is increased when used with thrombolytics, oral anticoagulants, NSAIDs, dipyridamole, ticlopidine, and clopidogrel. Avoid concomitant use of other IIb/IIIa antagonists. Cephalosporins which contain the MTT side chain may theoretically increase the risk of hemorrhage.

Decreased Effect: Levothyroxine and omeprazole decrease tirofiban levels; however, the clinical significance of this interaction remains to be demonstrated.

Pharmacodynamics/Kinetics

Distribution: 35% unbound

Metabolism: Minimally hepatic

Half-life elimination: 2 hours

Excretion: Urine (65%) and feces (25%) primarily as unchanged drug

Clearance: Elderly: Reduced by 19% to 26%

Pregnancy Risk Factor B

Tizanidine (tye ZAN i deen)

U.S. Brand Names Zanaflex®

Canadian Brand Names Apo-Tizanidine®; Gen-Tizanidine; Zanaflex®

Mexican Brand Names Sirdalud

Generic Available Yes: Tablet

Index Terms Sirdalud®

Pharmacologic Category Alpha$_2$-Adrenergic Agonist

Use Skeletal muscle relaxant used for treatment of muscle spasticity

Unlabeled/Investigational Use Tension headaches, low back pain, and trigeminal neuralgia

Local Anesthetic/Vasoconstrictor Precautions No information available to require special precautions

Effects on Dental Treatment Key adverse event(s) related to dental treatment: Significant xerostomia (normal salivary flow resumes upon discontinuation).

Common Adverse Effects

>10%:

Cardiovascular: Hypotension (16% to 33%)

(Continued)

Tizanidine *(Continued)*

    Central nervous system: Somnolence (48%), dizziness (16%)
    Gastrointestinal: Xerostomia (49%)
    Neuromuscular & skeletal: Weakness (41%)
  1% to 10%:
    Cardiovascular: Bradycardia (2% to 10%)
    Central nervous system: Nervousness (3%), speech disorder (3%), visual
      hallucinations/delusions (3%; occurring in first 6 weeks of therapy)
    Gastrointestinal: Constipation (4%), vomiting (3%), pharyngitis (3%)
    Genitourinary: UTI (10%), urinary frequency (3%)
    Hepatic: Liver enzymes increased (3% to 5%)
    Neuromuscular & skeletal: Dyskinesia (3%)
    Ocular: Blurred vision (3%)
    Respiratory: Rhinitis (3%)
    Miscellaneous: Infection (6%), flu-like syndrome (3%)

Dosage Adults: 2-4 mg 3 times/day
  Usual initial dose: 4 mg, may increase by 2-4 mg as needed for satisfactory
    reduction of muscle tone every 6-8 hours to a maximum of three doses in any
    24-hour period
  Maximum dose: 36 mg/day
  Dosing adjustment in renal impairment: May require dose reductions or less
    frequent dosing
  Dosing adjustment in hepatic impairment: Avoid use in hepatic impairment;
    if used, lowest possible dose should be used initially with close monitoring for
    adverse effects (eg, hypotension).

Mechanism of Action An alpha$_2$-adrenergic agonist agent which decreases
excitatory input to alpha motor neurons; an imidazole derivative chemi-
cally-related to clonidine, which acts as a centrally acting muscle relaxant with
alpha$_2$-adrenergic agonist properties; acts on the level of the spinal cord

Contraindications Hypersensitivity to tizanidine or any component of the
formulation; concomitant therapy with ciprofloxacin or fluvoxamine

Warnings/Precautions Significant hypotension (possibly with bradycardia or
orthostatic hypotension) and sedation may occur; use caution in patients with
cardiac disease or those at risk for severe hypotensive or sedative effects.
Avoid concomitant administration with CYP1A2 inhibitors; increased tizanidine
levels/effects (severe hypotension and sedation) may occur. These effects may
also be increased with concomitant administration with other CNS depressants
and/or antihypertensives; use caution. Elderly patients are particularly at risk;
clearance is reduced by >50% in elderly patients with renal insufficiency (Cl$_{cr}$
<25 mL/minute) compared to healthy elderly subjects; this may lead to a longer
duration of effects. Use caution in any patient with renal impairment; consider
dose reductions or increased dosing intervals. Use with extreme caution in
hepatic impairment due to extensive hepatic metabolism and potential hepatotoxicity; AST/ALT elevations (≥2 baseline) and rarely hepatic failure have
occurred. Use has been associated with visual hallucinations or delusions in
first 6 weeks of therapy; use caution in patients with psychiatric disorders.
Withdrawal resulting in rebound hypertension, tachycardia, and hypertonia may
occur upon discontinuation; doses should be decreased slowly, particularly in
patients receiving high doses for prolonged periods. Safety and efficacy have
not been established in children.

Drug Interactions
  Cytochrome P450 Effect:
    Substrate of CYP1A2 (major)
  Increased Effect/Toxicity: Additive hypotensive effects may be seen with
    diuretics, clonidine and other alpha-adrenergic agonists, or antihypertensives;
    CNS depression with baclofen or other CNS depressants; hormonal contra-
    ceptives, CYP1A2 inhibitors may increase the levels/effects of tizanidine;
    example inhibitors include amiodarone, ciprofloxacin (contraindicated), fluvox-
    amine (contraindicated), ketoconazole, norfloxacin, ofloxacin, and rofecoxib.
    Beta-blockers may increase bradycardia and increase rebound hypertension
    with tizanidine withdrawal.
  Decreased Effect: Mirtazapine may decrease the alpha-agonist effects of
    tizanidine.

Ethanol/Nutrition/Herb Interactions
  Ethanol: Avoid ethanol (may increase CNS depression).
  Food: The tablet and capsule dosage forms are not bioequivalent when admin-
    istered with food. Food increases both the time to peak concentration and the
    extent of absorption for both the tablet and capsule. However, maximal
    concentrations of tizanidine achieved when administered with food were
    increased by 30% for the tablet, but decreased by 20% for the capsule. Under
    fed conditions, the capsule is approximately 80% bioavailable relative to the
    tablet.

Herb/Nutraceutical: Avoid valerian, St John's wort, kava kava, gotu kola (may increase CNS depression). Avoid black cohosh, California poppy, coleus, golden seal, hawthorn, mistletoe, periwinkle, quinine, shepherd's purse (may increase hypotensive effects).

Dietary Considerations Administration with food compared to administration in the fasting state results in clinically-significant differences in absorption and other pharmacokinetic parameters. Patients should be consistent and should not switch administration of the tablets or the capsules between the fasting and nonfasting state. In addition, switching between the capsules and the tablets in the fed state will also result in significant differences. Opening capsule contents to sprinkle on applesauce compared to swallowing intact capsules whole will also result in significant absorption differences. Patients should be consistent with regards to administration.

Pharmacodynamics/Kinetics

Duration: 3-6 hours

Absorption: Tablets and capsules are bioequivalent under fasting conditions, but not under nonfasting conditions.

Tablets administered with food: Peak plasma concentration is increased by ~30%; time to peak increased by 25 minutes; extent of absorption increased by ~30%.

Capsules administered with food: Peak plasma concentration decreased by 20%; time to peak increased by 2-3 hours; extent of absorption increased by ~10%.

Capsules opened and sprinkled on applesauce are not bioequivalent to administration of intact capsules under fasting conditions. Peak plasma concentration and AUC are increased by 15% to 20%.

Metabolism: Extensively hepatic

Half-life elimination: 2 hours

Time to peak, serum:

Fasting state: Capsule, tablet: 1 hour

Fed state: Capsule: 3-4 hours, Tablet: 1.5 hours

Excretion: Urine (60%); feces (20%)

Pregnancy Risk Factor C

Dosage Forms

Capsule:

Zanaflex®: 2 mg, 4 mg, 6 mg

Tablet: 2 mg, 4 mg

Zanaflex®: 4 mg

TMC-114 see Darunavir on page 446

TMP see Trimethoprim on page 1620

TMP-SMZ see Sulfamethoxazole and Trimethoprim on page 1504

TMZ see Temozolomide on page 1534

TNKase™ see Tenecteplase on page 1535

TOBI® see Tobramycin on page 1579

TobraDex® see Tobramycin and Dexamethasone on page 1580

Tobramycin (toe bra MYE sin)

U.S. Brand Names AKTob®; TOBI®; Tobrex®

Canadian Brand Names PMS-Tobramycin; Sandoz-Tobramycin; TOBI®; Tobramycin Injection, USP; Tobrex®

Mexican Brand Names Eyebrex; Obry; Tobra; Trazil ofteno

Generic Available Yes: Excludes ophthalmic ointment, solution for nebulization

Index Terms Tobramycin Sulfate

Pharmacologic Category Antibiotic, Aminoglycoside; Antibiotic, Ophthalmic

Use Treatment of documented or suspected infections caused by susceptible gram-negative bacilli including *Pseudomonas aeruginosa*; topically used to treat superficial ophthalmic infections caused by susceptible bacteria. Tobramycin solution for inhalation is indicated for the management of cystic fibrosis patients (>6 years of age) with *Pseudomonas aeruginosa*.

Local Anesthetic/Vasoconstrictor Precautions No information available to require special precautions

Effects on Dental Treatment No significant effects or complications reported

Common Adverse Effects

Injection: Frequency not defined:

Central nervous system: Confusion, disorientation, dizziness, fever, headache, lethargy, vertigo

Dermatologic: Exfoliative dermatitis, itching, rash, urticaria

Endocrine & metabolic: Serum calcium, magnesium, potassium, and/or sodium decreased

Gastrointestinal: Diarrhea, nausea, vomiting

(Continued)

Tobramycin *(Continued)*

Hematologic: Anemia, eosinophilia, granulocytopenia, leukocytosis, leukopenia, thrombocytopenia

Hepatic: ALT, AST, bilirubin, and/or LDH increased

Local: Pain at the injection site

Otic: Hearing loss, tinnitus, ototoxicity (auditory), ototoxicity (vestibular), roaring in the ears

Renal: BUN increased, cylindruria, serum creatinine increased, oliguria, proteinuria

Inhalation:
>10%:
Gastrointestinal: Sputum discoloration (21%)
Respiratory: Voice alteration (13%)
1% to 10%:
Central nervous system: Malaise (6%)
Otic: Tinnitus (3%)

Mechanism of Action Interferes with bacterial protein synthesis by binding to 30S and 50S ribosomal subunits resulting in a defective bacterial cell membrane

Drug Interactions

Increased Effect/Toxicity: Increased antimicrobial effect of tobramycin with extended spectrum penicillins (synergistic). Neuromuscular blockers may have an increased duration of action (neuromuscular blockade). Amphotericin B, cephalosporins, and loop diuretics may increase the risk of nephrotoxicity.

Pharmacodynamics/Kinetics

Absorption:
Oral: Poorly absorbed
I.M.: Rapid and complete
Inhalation: Peak serum concentrations are ~1 mcg/mL following a 300 mg dose

Distribution: V_d: 0.2-0.3 L/kg; Pediatrics: 0.2-0.7 L/kg; to extracellular fluid including serum, abscesses, ascitic, pericardial, pleural, synovial, lymphatic, and peritoneal fluids; poor penetration into CSF, eye, bone, prostate
Inhalation: Tobramycin remains concentrated primarily in the airways

Protein binding: <30%

Half-life elimination:
Neonates: ≤1200 g: 11 hours; >1200 g: 2-9 hours
Adults: 2-3 hours; directly dependent upon glomerular filtration rate
Adults with impaired renal function: 5-70 hours

Time to peak, serum: I.M.: 30-60 minutes; I.V.: ~30 minutes

Excretion: Normal renal function: Urine (~90% to 95%) within 24 hours

Pregnancy Risk Factor D (injection, inhalation); B (ophthalmic)

Tobramycin and Dexamethasone

(toe bra MYE sin & deks a METH a sone)

Related Information
Dexamethasone *on page 464*
Tobramycin *on page 1579*

U.S. Brand Names TobraDex®

Canadian Brand Names Tobradex®

Mexican Brand Names Obrydex; Tobradex

Generic Available No

Index Terms Dexamethasone and Tobramycin

Pharmacologic Category Antibiotic/Corticosteroid, Ophthalmic

Use Treatment of external ocular infection caused by susceptible gram-negative bacteria and steroid responsive inflammatory conditions of the palpebral and bulbar conjunctiva, lid, cornea, and anterior segment of the globe

Local Anesthetic/Vasoconstrictor Precautions No information available to require special precautions

Effects on Dental Treatment No significant effects or complications reported

Common Adverse Effects Unless otherwise noted, frequency not defined.
Dermatologic: Allergic contact dermatitis, delayed wound healing
Ocular: Cataract formation, conjunctival erythema (<4%), glaucoma, intraocular pressure increased, keratitis, lacrimation, lid itching (<4%), lid swelling (<4%), optic nerve damage, secondary infection

Mechanism of Action Refer to individual monographs for Dexamethasone and Tobramycin

Drug Interactions

Cytochrome P450 Effect: Dexamethasone: **Substrate** of CYP3A4 (minor); **Induces** CYP2A6 (weak), 2B6 (weak), 2C8 (weak), 2C9 (weak), 3A4 (weak)

Increased Effect/Toxicity: See individual agents.
Decreased Effect: See individual agents.
Pharmacodynamics/Kinetics
Absorption: Into aqueous humor
Time to peak, serum: 1-2 hours in the cornea and aqueous humor
Pregnancy Risk Factor C

Tobramycin and Loteprednol Etabonate *see* Loteprednol and Tobramycin *on page 1006*
Tobramycin Sulfate *see* Tobramycin *on page 1579*
Tobrex® *see* Tobramycin *on page 1579*

Tocainide (TOE kay nide)

U.S. Brand Names Tonocard® [DSC]
Generic Available No
Index Terms Tocainide Hydrochloride
Pharmacologic Category Antiarrhythmic Agent, Class Ib
Use Suppression and prevention of symptomatic life-threatening ventricular arrhythmias
Unlabeled/Investigational Use Trigeminal neuralgia
Local Anesthetic/Vasoconstrictor Precautions No information available to require special precautions
Effects on Dental Treatment Key adverse event(s) related to dental treatment: Loss of taste.
Common Adverse Effects
>10%:
Central nervous system: Dizziness (8% to 15%)
Gastrointestinal: Nausea (14% to 15%)
1% to 10%:
Cardiovascular: Tachycardia (3%), bradycardia/angina/palpitation (0.5% to 1.8%), hypotension (3%)
Central nervous system: Nervousness (0.5% to 1.5%), confusion (2% to 3%), headache (4.6%), anxiety, incoordination, giddiness, vertigo
Dermatologic: Rash (0.5% to 8.4%)
Gastrointestinal: Vomiting (4.5%), diarrhea (4% to 5%), anorexia (1% to 2%), loss of taste
Neuromuscular & skeletal: Paresthesia (3.5% to 9%), tremor (dose related: 2.9% to 8.4%), ataxia (dose related: 2.9% to 8.4%), hot and cold sensations
Ocular: Blurred vision (~1.5%), nystagmus (1%)

Note: Rare, potentially severe hematologic reactions, have occurred (generally within the first 12 weeks of therapy). These may include agranulocytosis, bone marrow depression, aplastic anemia, hypoplastic anemia, hemolytic anemia, anemia, leukopenia, neutropenia, thrombocytopenia, and eosinophilia.
Mechanism of Action Class 1B antiarrhythmic agent; suppresses automaticity of conduction tissue, by increasing electrical stimulation threshold of ventricle, His-Purkinje system, and spontaneous depolarization of the ventricles during diastole by a direct action on the tissues; blocks both the initiation and conduction of nerve impulses by decreasing the neuronal membrane's permeability to sodium ions, which results in inhibition of depolarization with resultant blockade of conduction
Drug Interactions
Cytochrome P450 Effect: Inhibits CYP1A2 (weak)
Increased Effect/Toxicity: Tocainide may increase serum levels of caffeine and theophylline.
Decreased Effect: Decreased tocainide plasma levels with cimetidine, phenobarbital, phenytoin, rifampin, and other hepatic enzyme inducers.
Pharmacodynamics/Kinetics
Absorption: Oral: 99% to 100%
Distribution: V_d: 1.62-3.2 L/kg
Protein binding: 10% to 20%
Metabolism: Hepatic to inactive metabolites; negligible first-pass effect
Half-life elimination: 11-14 hours; Renal and hepatic impairment: 23-27 hours
Time to peak, serum: 30-160 minutes
Excretion: Urine (40% to 50% as unchanged drug)
Pregnancy Risk Factor C

Tocainide Hydrochloride *see* Tocainide *on page 1581*
Today® Sponge [OTC] *see* Nonoxynol 9 *on page 1185*
Tofranil® *see* Imipramine *on page 866*
Tofranil-PM® *see* Imipramine *on page 866*

TOLAZamide (tole AZ a mide)

Related Information
Endocrine Disorders and Pregnancy *on page 1750*
Canadian Brand Names Tolinase®
Generic Available Yes
Pharmacologic Category Antidiabetic Agent, Sulfonylurea
Use Adjunct to diet for the management of mild to moderately severe, stable, type 2 diabetes mellitus (noninsulin dependent, NIDDM)
Local Anesthetic/Vasoconstrictor Precautions No information available to require special precautions
Effects on Dental Treatment Use salicylates with caution in patients taking tolazamide due to potential increased hypoglycemia; NSAIDs such as ibuprofen and naproxen may be safely used. Tolazamide-dependent diabetics (noninsulin dependent, type 2) should be appointed for dental treatment in morning in order to minimize chance of stress-induced hypoglycemia.
Common Adverse Effects Frequency not defined.
Central nervous system: Dizziness, fatigue, headache, malaise, vertigo
Dermatologic: Maculopapular eruptions, morbilliform eruptions, photosensitivity, pruritus, rash, urticaria
Endocrine & metabolic: Disulfiram-like reaction, hypoglycemia, hyponatremia, SIADH
Gastrointestinal: Anorexia, constipation, diarrhea, epigastric fullness, heartburn, nausea, vomiting
Hematologic: Agranulocytosis, aplastic anemia, hemolytic anemia, leukopenia, pancytopenia, porphyria cutanea tarda, thrombocytopenia
Hepatic: Cholestatic jaundice, hepatic porphyria
Neuromuscular & skeletal: Weakness
Renal: Diuretic effect
Mechanism of Action Stimulates insulin release from the pancreatic beta cells; reduces glucose output from the liver; insulin sensitivity is increased at peripheral target sites
Drug Interactions
Increased Effect/Toxicity: Cyclic antidepressants, fibric acid derivatives, pegvisomant, salicylates (higher doses, not sporadic, low doses), and sulfonamide derivatives (except sulfacetamide) may enhance the hypoglycemic effect of tolazamide. Beta-blockers may enhance the hypoglycemic effect of tolazamide and mask tachycardia as an initial symptom of hypoglycemia. Chloramphenicol and cimetidine may decrease the metabolism of tolazamide. Fluconazole may increase the serum concentration of tolazamide. Tolazamide may increase the serum concentration of cyclosporine.
Decreased Effect: Rifampin may increase the metabolism of tolazamide.
Pharmacodynamics/Kinetics
Onset of hypoglycemic effect: 20 minutes
Peak hypoglycemic effect: 4-6 hours
Duration: 10-24 hours
Absorption: Rapid
Protein binding: 94%
Metabolism: Extensively hepatic to 5 metabolites (activity 0% to 70%)
Half-life elimination: 7 hours
Time to peak, serum: 3-4 hours
Excretion: Urine (85%); feces (7%)
Pregnancy Risk Factor C

Tolazoline (tole AZ oh leen)

U.S. Brand Names Priscoline® [DSC]
Generic Available No
Index Terms Benzazoline Hydrochloride; Tolazoline Hydrochloride
Pharmacologic Category Vasodilator
Use Treatment of persistent pulmonary vasoconstriction and hypertension of the newborn (persistent fetal circulation), peripheral vasospastic disorders
Local Anesthetic/Vasoconstrictor Precautions No information available to require special precautions
Effects on Dental Treatment No significant effects or complications reported
Common Adverse Effects Frequency not defined.
Cardiovascular: Arrhythmia, hyper-/hypotension, peripheral vasodilation, tachycardia
Endocrine & metabolic: Hypochloremic alkalosis
Gastrointestinal: Abdominal pain, diarrhea, GI bleeding, nausea
Hematologic: Agranulocytosis increased, pancytopenia, thrombocytopenia

Local: Burning at injection site
Neuromuscular & skeletal: Pilomotor activity increased
Ocular: Mydriasis
Renal: Acute renal failure, oliguria
Respiratory: Pulmonary hemorrhage
Miscellaneous: Increased secretions

Mechanism of Action Competitively blocks alpha-adrenergic receptors to produce brief antagonism of circulating epinephrine and norepinephrine; reduces hypertension caused by catecholamines and causes vascular smooth muscle relaxation (direct action); results in peripheral vasodilation and decreased peripheral resistance

Drug Interactions
  Increased Effect/Toxicity: Disulfiram reaction may possibly be seen with concomitant ethanol use.
  Decreased Effect: Decreased effect (vasopressor) of epinephrine followed by a rebound increase in blood pressure.

Pharmacodynamics/Kinetics
  Half-life elimination: Neonates: 3-10 hours; prolonged with renal impairment
  Time to peak, serum: Within 30 minutes
  Excretion: Urine (primarily as unchanged drug)

Pregnancy Risk Factor C

Tolazoline Hydrochloride *see* Tolazoline *on page 1582*

TOLBUTamide (tole BYOO ta mide)

Related Information
  Endocrine Disorders and Pregnancy *on page 1750*
Canadian Brand Names Apo-Tolbutamide®
Mexican Brand Names Artosin; Rastinon
Generic Available Yes
Index Terms Tolbutamide Sodium
Pharmacologic Category Antidiabetic Agent, Sulfonylurea
Use Adjunct to diet for the management of type 2 diabetes mellitus (noninsulin dependent, NIDDM)
Local Anesthetic/Vasoconstrictor Precautions No information available to require special precautions
Effects on Dental Treatment Key adverse event(s) related to dental treatment: Taste alteration.
  Use salicylates with caution in patients taking tolazamide due to potential increased hypoglycemia; NSAIDs such as ibuprofen and naproxen may be safely used. Tolbutamide-dependent diabetics (noninsulin dependent, type 2) should be appointed for dental treatment in morning in order to minimize chance of stress-induced hypoglycemia.
Common Adverse Effects Frequency not defined.
  Central nervous system: Headache
  Dermatologic: Erythema, maculopapular rash, morbilliform rash, pruritus, urticaria, photosensitivity
  Endocrine & metabolic: Disulfiram-like reactions, hypoglycemia, hyponatremia, SIADH
  Gastrointestinal: Epigastric fullness, heartburn, nausea, taste alteration
  Hematologic: Agranulocytosis, aplastic anemia, hemolytic anemia, leukopenia, pancytopenia, thrombocytopenia
  Hepatic: Cholestatic jaundice, hepatic porphyria, porphyria cutanea tarda
  Miscellaneous: Hypersensitivity reaction
Mechanism of Action Stimulates insulin release from the pancreatic beta cells; reduces glucose output from the liver; insulin sensitivity is increased at peripheral target sites, suppression of glucagon may also contribute
Drug Interactions
  Cytochrome P450 Effect: Substrate of CYP2C9 (major), 2C19 (minor); **Inhibits** CYP2C8 (weak), 2C9 (strong)
  Increased Effect/Toxicity: CYP2C9 Inhibitors may increase the levels/effects of tolbutamide; example inhibitors include delavirdine, fluconazole, gemfibrozil, ketoconazole, nicardipine, NSAIDs, and sulfonamides. Cyclic antidepressants, fibric acid derivatives, pegvisomant, salicylates (higher doses, not sporadic, low doses), and sulfonamide derivatives (except sulfacetamide) may enhance the hypoglycemic effect of tolbutamide. Beta-blockers may enhance the hypoglycemic effect of tolbutamide and mask tachycardia as an initial symptom of hypoglycemia. Chloramphenicol and cimetidine may decrease the metabolism of tolbutamide. Fluconazole may increase the serum concentration of tolbutamide.
  (Continued)

TOLBUTamide (Continued)

Tolbutamide may increase the levels/effects of CYP2C9 substrates; example substrates include bosentan, dapsone, fluoxetine, glimepiride, glipizide, losartan, montelukast, nateglinide, paclitaxel, phenytoin, warfarin, and zafirlukast. Tolbutamide may increase the serum concentration of cyclosporine.

Decreased Effect: CYP2C9 inducers may decrease the levels/effects of tolbutamide; example inducers include carbamazepine, phenobarbital, phenytoin, rifampin, rifapentine, and secobarbital.

Pharmacodynamics/Kinetics

Onset of action: 1 hour
Duration: Oral: 6-24 hours
Absorption: Oral: Rapid
Distribution: V_d: 0.15 L/kg
Protein binding: ~95% (concentration dependent)
Metabolism: Hepatic via CYP2C9 to hydroxymethyltolbutamide (mildly active) and carboxytolbutamide (inactive); metabolism does not appear to be affected by age
Half-life elimination: 4.5-6.5 hours (range: 4-25 hours)
Time to peak, serum: 3-4 hours
Excretion: Urine (75% to 85% primarily as metabolites); feces

Pregnancy Risk Factor C

Tolbutamide Sodium see TOLBUTamide on page 1583

Tolcapone (TOLE ka pone)

U.S. Brand Names Tasmar®
Generic Available No
Pharmacologic Category Anti-Parkinson's Agent, COMT Inhibitor
Use Adjunct to levodopa and carbidopa for the treatment of signs and symptoms of idiopathic Parkinson's disease in patients with motor fluctuations not responsive to other therapies

Local Anesthetic/Vasoconstrictor Precautions No information available to require special precautions

Effects on Dental Treatment Key adverse event(s) related to dental treatment: Significant xerostomia (normal salivary flow resumes upon discontinuation) and tooth disorder.

Dopaminergic therapy in Parkinson's disease (ie, treatment with levodopa) is associated with orthostatic hypotension. Tolcapone enhances levodopa bioavailability and may increase the occurrence of hypotension/syncope in the dental patient. The patient should be carefully assisted from the chair and observed for signs of orthostatic hypotension.

Common Adverse Effects

>10%:
Cardiovascular: Orthostatic hypotension (17%)
Central nervous system: Sleep disorder (24% to 25%), excessive dreaming (16% to 21%), somnolence (14% to 32%), hallucinations (8% to 24%) dizziness (6% to 13%), headache (10% to 11%), confusion (10% to 11%)
Gastrointestinal: Nausea (28% to 50%), anorexia (19% to 23%), diarrhea (16% to 34%; approximately 3% to 4% severe)
Neuromuscular & skeletal: Dyskinesia (42% to 51%), dystonia (19% to 22%), muscle cramps (17% to 18%)

1% to 10%:
Cardiovascular: Syncope (4% to 5%), chest pain (1% to 3%), hypotension (2%), palpitation
Central nervous system: Fatigue (3% to 7%), loss of balance (2% to 3%), agitation (1%), euphoria (1%), hyperactivity (1%), malaise (1%), panic reaction (1%), irritability (1%), mental deficiency (1%), fever (1%), depression, hypoesthesia, tremor, speech disorder, vertigo, emotional lability, hyperkinesia
Dermatologic: Alopecia (1%), bleeding (1%), tumor (1%), rash
Gastrointestinal: Vomiting (8% to 10%), constipation (6% to 8%), xerostomia (5% to 6%), abdominal pain (5% to 6%), dyspepsia (3% to 4%), flatulence (2% to 4%), tooth disorder
Genitourinary: UTI (5%), hematuria (4% to 5%), urine discoloration (2% to 3%), urination disorder (1% to 2%), uterine tumor (1%), incontinence, impotence
Hepatic: Transaminases increased (1% to 3%; 3 times ULN, usually with first 6 months of therapy)
Neuromuscular & skeletal: Paresthesia (1% to 3%), hyper-/hypokinesia (1% to 3%), arthritis (1% to 2%), neck pain (2%), stiffness (2%), myalgia, rhabdomyolysis

Ocular: Cataract (1%), eye inflammation (1%)

Otic: Tinnitus

Respiratory: Upper respiratory infection (5% to 7%), dyspnea (3%), sinus congestion (1% to 2%), bronchitis, pharyngitis

Miscellaneous: Diaphoresis (4% to 7%), influenza (3% to 4%), burning (1% to 2%), flank pain, injury, infection

Restrictions A patient signed consent form acknowledging the risks of hepatic injury should be obtained by the treating physician.

Mechanism of Action Tolcapone is a selective and reversible inhibitor of catechol-o-methyltransferase (COMT). In the presence of a decarboxylase inhibitor (eg, carbidopa), COMT is the major degradation pathway for levodopa. Inhibition of COMT leads to more sustained plasma levels of levodopa and enhanced central dopaminergic activity.

Drug Interactions

Cytochrome P450 Effect: Inhibits CYP2C9 (weak)

Increased Effect/Toxicity: Tolcapone may decrease the metabolism and increase the side effects of COMT substrates (eg, apomorphine, bitolterol, dobutamine, dopamine, epinephrine, norepinephrine, isoproterenol, isoetharine, and methyldopa). Effects on mental status may be additive with other CNS depressants; includes barbiturates, benzodiazepines, TCAs, antipsychotics, ethanol, opioid analgesics, and other sedative-hypnotics. Concurrent use of nonselective MAO inhibitors with tolcapone may increase the risk of cardiovascular side effects; selective MAO inhibitors (eg, selegiline ≤10 mg/day) appear to pose limited risk.

Pharmacodynamics/Kinetics

Absorption: Rapid

Distribution: 9 L

Protein binding: >99.0%

Metabolism: Hepatic, via glucuronidation, to inactive metabolite (>99%)

Bioavailability: 65%

Half-life elimination: 2-3 hours

Time to peak: ~2 hours

Excretion: Urine (60% as metabolites, 0.5% as unchanged drug); feces (40%)

Pregnancy Risk Factor C

Tolectin® see Tolmetin on page 1585

Tolmetin (TOLE met in)

Related Information

Rheumatoid Arthritis, Osteoarthritis, and Osteoporosis on page 1759
Temporomandibular Dysfunction (TMD) on page 1822

U.S. Brand Names Tolectin®

Generic Available Yes

Index Terms Tolmetin Sodium

Pharmacologic Category Nonsteroidal Anti-inflammatory Drug (NSAID), Oral

Use Treatment of rheumatoid arthritis and osteoarthritis, juvenile rheumatoid arthritis

Local Anesthetic/Vasoconstrictor Precautions No information available to require special precautions

Effects on Dental Treatment NSAID formulations are known to reversibly decrease platelet aggregation via mechanisms different than observed with aspirin. The dentist should be aware of the potential of abnormal coagulation. Caution should also be exercised in the use of NSAIDs in patients already on anticoagulant therapy with drugs such as warfarin (Coumadin®).

Common Adverse Effects 1% to 10%:

Cardiovascular: Chest pain, hypertension, edema

Central nervous system: Headache, dizziness, drowsiness, depression

Dermatologic: Skin irritation

Endocrine & metabolic: Weight gain/loss

Gastrointestinal: Heartburn, abdominal pain, diarrhea, flatulence, vomiting, constipation, gastritis, peptic ulcer, nausea

Genitourinary: Urinary Tract Infection

Hematologic: Elevated BUN, transient decreases in hemoglobin/hematocrit

Ocular: Visual disturbances

Otic: Tinnitus

Restrictions An FDA-approved medication guide must be distributed when dispensing an oral outpatient prescription (new or refill) where this medication is to be used without direct supervision of a healthcare provider. Medication guides are available at http://www.fda.gov/cder/Offices/ODS/medication_guides.htm.

(Continued)

Tolmetin *(Continued)*

Dosage Oral:

Children ≥2 years:

Anti-inflammatory: Initial: 20 mg/kg/day in 3 divided doses, then 15-30 mg/kg/day in 3 divided doses

Analgesic: 5-7 mg/kg/dose every 6-8 hours

Adults: 400 mg 3 times/day; usual dose: 600 mg to 1.8 g/day; maximum: 2 g/day

Mechanism of Action Inhibits prostaglandin synthesis by decreasing the activity of the enzyme, cyclooxygenase, which results in decreased formation of prostaglandin precursors

Contraindications Hypersensitivity to tolmetin, aspirin, other NSAIDs, or any component of the formulation; perioperative pain in the setting of coronary artery bypass surgery (CABG); pregnancy (3rd trimester or near term)

Warnings/Precautions [U.S. Boxed Warning]: NSAIDs are associated with an increased risk of adverse cardiovascular events, including MI, stroke, and new onset or worsening of pre-existing hypertension. Risk may be increased with duration of use or pre-existing cardiovascular risk factors or disease. Carefully evaluate individual cardiovascular risk profiles prior to prescribing. Use caution with fluid retention, CHF or hypertension. Concurrent administration of ibuprofen, and potentially other nonselective NSAIDs, may interfere with aspirin's cardioprotective effect.

Use of NSAIDs can compromise existing renal function. Renal toxicity can occur in patient with impaired renal function, dehydration, heart failure, liver dysfunction, those taking diuretics and ACEI and the elderly. Rehydrate patient before starting therapy. Monitor renal function closely. Use caution in patients with advanced renal disease.

[U.S. Boxed Warning]: NSAIDs may increase risk of gastrointestinal irritation, ulceration, bleeding, and perforation. These events may occur at any time during therapy and without warning. Use caution with a history of GI disease (bleeding or ulcers), concurrent therapy with aspirin, anticoagulants and/or corticosteroids, smoking, use of alcohol, the elderly or debilitated patients.

Use the lowest effective dose for the shortest duration of time, consistent with individual patient goals, to reduce risk of cardiovascular or GI adverse events. Alternate therapies should be considered for patients at high risk.

NSAIDs may cause serious skin adverse events including exfoliative dermatitis, Stevens-Johnson syndrome (SJS) and toxic epidermal necrolysis (TEN). Anaphylactoid reactions may occur, even without prior exposure; patients with "aspirin triad" (bronchial asthma, aspirin intolerance, rhinitis) may be at increased risk. Do not use in patients who experience bronchospasm, asthma, rhinitis, or urticaria with NSAID or aspirin therapy.

Use with caution in patients with decreased hepatic function. Closely monitor patients with any abnormal LFT. Severe hepatic reactions (eg, fulminant hepatitis, liver failure) have occurred with NSAID use, rarely; discontinue if signs or symptoms of liver disease develop, or if systemic manifestations occur.

The elderly are at increased risk for adverse effects (especially peptic ulceration, CNS effects, renal toxicity) from NSAIDs even at low doses.

Withhold for at least 4-6 half-lives prior to surgical or dental procedures. Safety and efficacy have not been established in children <2 years of age.

Drug Interactions

Increased Effect/Toxicity: Increased toxicity of digoxin, methotrexate, cyclosporine, lithium, insulin, sulfonylureas, potassium-sparing diuretics, and aspirin. Concomitant use with fluoroquinolones may rarely increase risk of seizure.

Decreased Effect: Decreased effect with aspirin. Salicylates' antiplatelet effect may be reduced. Decreased effect of thiazides and furosemide. NSAIDs may decrease the antihypertensive effect of ACE inhibitors, beta-blockers, hydralazine, and angiotensin antagonists. Cholestyramine (and other bile acid sequestrants) may decrease the absorption of NSAIDs; separate by at least 2 hours.

Ethanol/Nutrition/Herb Interactions

Ethanol: Avoid ethanol (may enhance gastric mucosal irritation).

Food: Tolmetin peak serum concentrations may be decreased if taken with food or milk.

Herb/Nutraceutical: Avoid alfalfa, anise, bilberry, bladderwrack, bromelain, cat's claw, celery, coleus, cordyceps, dong quai, evening primrose, feverfew, fenugreek, garlic, ginger, ginkgo biloba, red clover, horse chestnut, grapeseed, green tea, ginseng, guggul, horse chestnut seed, horseradish, licorice, prickly ash, red clover, reishi, SAMe, sweet clover, turmeric, white willow (all have additional antiplatelet activity).

Dietary Considerations Should be taken with food, milk, or antacids to decrease GI adverse effects. Sodium content of 200 mg: 0.8 mEq.

Pharmacodynamics/Kinetics
Onset of action: Analgesic: 1-2 hours; Anti-inflammatory: Days to weeks
Absorption: Well absorbed
Bioavailability: Reduced 16% with food or milk
Half-life elimination: Biphasic: Rapid: 1-2 hours; Slow: 5 hours
Time to peak, serum: 30-60 minutes
Excretion: Urine (as inactive metabolites or conjugates) within 24 hours

Pregnancy Risk Factor C/D (3rd trimester)

Dosage Forms
Capsule: 400 mg
Tablet: 200 mg, 600 mg
Tolectin®: 600 mg

Tolmetin Sodium *see* Tolmetin *on page 1585*

Tolnaftate (tole NAF tate)

U.S. Brand Names Blis-To-Sol® [OTC]; Fungi-Guard [OTC]; Gold Bond® Antifungal [OTC] [DSC]; Mycocide® NS [OTC]; Podactin Powder [OTC]; Q-Naftate [OTC]; Tinactin® Antifungal [OTC]; Tinactin® Antifungal Jock Itch [OTC]; Tinaderm [OTC]; Ting® Cream [OTC]; Ting® Spray Liquid [OTC]

Canadian Brand Names Pitrex

Generic Available Yes: Cream, powder, solution

Pharmacologic Category Antifungal Agent, Topical

Use Treatment of tinea pedis, tinea cruris, tinea corporis

Local Anesthetic/Vasoconstrictor Precautions No information available to require special precautions

Effects on Dental Treatment No significant effects or complications reported

Common Adverse Effects Frequency not defined.
Dermatologic: Pruritus, contact dermatitis
Local: Irritation, stinging

Mechanism of Action Distorts the hyphae and stunts mycelial growth in susceptible fungi

Pharmacodynamics/Kinetics Onset of action: 24-72 hours

Pregnancy Risk Factor C

Tolterodine (tole TER oh deen)

U.S. Brand Names Detrol®; Detrol® LA

Canadian Brand Names Detrol®; Detrol® LA; Unidet®

Mexican Brand Names Detrusitol

Generic Available No

Index Terms Tolterodine Tartrate

Pharmacologic Category Anticholinergic Agent

Use Treatment of patients with an overactive bladder with symptoms of urinary frequency, urgency, or urge incontinence

Local Anesthetic/Vasoconstrictor Precautions No information available to require special precautions

Effects on Dental Treatment The anticholinergic effects of tolterodine are selective for the urinary bladder rather than salivary glands; xerostomia and changes in salivation (normal salivary flow resumes upon discontinuation).

Common Adverse Effects As reported with immediate release tablet, unless otherwise specified
>10%: Gastrointestinal: Dry mouth (35%; extended release capsules 23%)
1% to 10%:
Cardiovascular: Chest pain (2%)
Central nervous system: Headache (7%; extended release capsules 6%), somnolence (3%; extended release capsules 3%), fatigue (4%; extended release capsules 2%), dizziness (5%; extended release capsules 2%), anxiety (extended release capsules 1%)
Dermatologic: Dry skin (1%)
Gastrointestinal: Abdominal pain (5%; extended release capsules 4%), constipation (7%; extended release capsules 6%), dyspepsia (4%; extended release capsules 3%), diarrhea (4%), weight gain (1%)
Genitourinary: Dysuria (2%; extended release capsules 1%)
Neuromuscular & skeletal: Arthralgia (2%)
Ocular: Abnormal vision (2%; extended release capsules 1%), dry eyes (3%; extended release capsules 3%)
(Continued)

Tolterodine *(Continued)*

Respiratory: Bronchitis (2%), sinusitis (extended release capsules 2%)
Miscellaneous: Flu-like syndrome (3%), infection (1%)

Dosage

Oral: Adults: Treatment of overactive bladder:

Immediate release tablet: 2 mg twice daily; the dose may be lowered to 1 mg twice daily based on individual response and tolerability

Dosing adjustment in patients concurrently taking CYP3A4 inhibitors: 1 mg twice daily

Extended release capsule: 4 mg once a day; dose may be lowered to 2 mg daily based on individual response and tolerability

Dosing adjustment in patients concurrently taking CYP3A4 inhibitors: 2 mg daily

Elderly: Safety and efficacy in patients >64 years was found to be similar to that in younger patients; no dosage adjustment is needed based on age

Dosing adjustment in renal impairment: Use with caution (studies conducted in patients with Cl_{cr} 10-30 mL/minute):
Immediate release tablet: 1 mg twice daily
Extended release capsule: 2 mg daily

Dosing adjustment in hepatic impairment:
Immediate release tablet: 1 mg twice daily
Extended release capsule: 2 mg daily

Mechanism of Action Tolterodine is a competitive antagonist of muscarinic receptors. In animal models, tolterodine demonstrates selectivity for urinary bladder receptors over salivary receptors. Urinary bladder contraction is mediated by muscarinic receptors. Tolterodine increases residual urine volume and decreases detrusor muscle pressure.

Contraindications Hypersensitivity to tolterodine or any component of the formulation; urinary retention; gastric retention; uncontrolled narrow-angle glaucoma; myasthenia gravis

Warnings/Precautions Use with caution in patients with bladder flow obstruction, may increase the risk of urinary retention. Use with caution in patients with gastrointestinal obstructive disorders (ie, pyloric stenosis), may increase the risk of gastric retention. Use with caution in patients with controlled (treated) narrow-angle glaucoma; metabolized in the liver and excreted in the urine and feces, dosage adjustment is required for patients with renal or hepatic impairment. Tolterodine has been associated with QT_c prolongation at high (supratherapeutic) doses. The manufacturer recommends caution in patients with congenital prolonged QT or in patients receiving concurrent therapy with QT_c-prolonging drugs (class Ia or III antiarrhythmics). However, the mean change in QT_c even at supratherapeutic dosages was less than 15 msec. Individuals who are poor metabolizers via CYP2D6 or in the presence of inhibitors of CYP2D6 and CYP3A4 may be more likely to exhibit prolongation. Dosage adjustment is recommended in patients receiving CYP3A4 inhibitors (a lower dose of tolterodine is recommended). Safety and efficacy in pediatric patients have not been established.

Drug Interactions

Cytochrome P450 Effect: Substrate of CYP2C9 (minor), 2C19 (minor), 2D6 (major), 3A4 (major)

Increased Effect/Toxicity: CYP2D6 inhibitors may increase the levels/effects of tolterodine, which may include QT_c prolongation; example inhibitors include chlorpromazine, delavirdine, fluoxetine, miconazole, paroxetine, pergolide, quinidine, quinine, ritonavir, and ropinirole. No dosage adjustment was needed in patients coadministered tolterodine and fluoxetine. CYP3A4 inhibitors may increase the levels/effects of tolterodine, which may include QT_c prolongation; example inhibitors include azole antifungals, clarithromycin, diclofenac, doxycycline, erythromycin, imatinib, isoniazid, nefazodone, nicardipine, propofol, protease inhibitors, quinidine, telithromycin, and verapamil. Concomitant use with systemic anticholinergic agents may increase the risk of anticholinergic side effects. Use with pramlintide may result in increased slowing of gut motility. Additive effects on QT_c prolongation may occur with concurrent therapy with QT_c prolonging agents. Tolterodine may increase the effects of warfarin.

Decreased Effect: CYP3A4 inducers may decrease the levels/effects of tolterodine; example inducers include aminoglutethimide, carbamazepine, nafcillin, nevirapine, phenobarbital, phenytoin, and rifamycins. Use with acetylcholinesterase inhibitors may result in reduced therapeutic efficacy.

Ethanol/Nutrition/Herb Interactions

Food: Increases bioavailability (~53% increase) of tolterodine tablets, but does not affect the pharmacokinetics of tolterodine extended release capsules; adjustment of dose is not needed. As a CYP3A4 inhibitor, grapefruit juice may increase the serum level and/or toxicity of tolterodine, but unlikely secondary to high oral bioavailability.

Herb/Nutraceutical: St John's wort (*Hypericum*) appears to induce CYP3A enzymes.

Pharmacodynamics/Kinetics

Absorption: Immediate release tablet: Rapid; ≥77%

Distribution: I.V.: V_d: 113 ± 27 L

Protein binding: >96% (primarily to alpha$_1$-acid glycoprotein)

Metabolism: Extensively hepatic, primarily via CYP2D6 (some metabolites share activity) and 3A4 usually (minor pathway). In patients with a genetic deficiency of CYP2D6, metabolism via 3A4 predominates. Forms three active metabolites.

Bioavailability: Immediate release tablet: Increased 53% with food

Half-life elimination:

Immediate release tablet: Extensive metabolizers: ~2 hours; Poor metabolizers: ~10 hours

Extended release capsule: Extensive metabolizers: ~7 hours; Poor metabolizers: ~18 hours

Time to peak: Immediate release tablet: 1-2 hours; Extended release tablet: 2-6 hours

Excretion: Urine (77%); feces (17%); excreted primarily as metabolites (<1% unchanged drug) of which the active 5-hydroxymethyl metabolite accounts for 5% to 14% (<1% in poor metabolizers)

Pregnancy Risk Factor C

Dosage Forms

Capsule, extended release:

Detrol® LA: 2 mg, 4 mg

Tablet:

Detrol®: 1 mg, 2 mg

Topiramate (toe PYRE a mate)

U.S. Brand Names Topamax®

Canadian Brand Names Dom-Topiramate; Gen-Topiramate; Novo-Topiramate; PHL-Topiramate; PMS-Topiramate; ratio-Topiramate; Rhoxal-topiramate; Sandoz-Topiramate; Topamax®

Mexican Brand Names Topamax

Generic Available No

Pharmacologic Category Anticonvulsant, Miscellaneous

Use Monotherapy or adjunctive therapy for partial onset seizures and primary generalized tonic-clonic seizures; adjunctive treatment of seizures associated with Lennox-Gastaut syndrome; prophylaxis of migraine headache

Unlabeled/Investigational Use Infantile spasms, neuropathic pain, cluster headache

Local Anesthetic/Vasoconstrictor Precautions No information available to require special precautions

Effects on Dental Treatment Key adverse event(s) related to dental treatment: Gingivitis, dysphagia, glossitis, gum hyperplasia, and xerostomia (normal salivary flow resumes upon discontinuation).

Common Adverse Effects Adverse events are reported for placebo-controlled trials of adjunctive therapy in adult and pediatric patients. Unless otherwise noted, the percentages refer to incidence in epilepsy trials. Note: A wide range of dosages were studied; incidence of adverse events was frequently lower in the pediatric population studied.

>10%:

Central nervous system: Dizziness (4% to 32%), ataxia (6% to 16%), somnolence (15% to 29%), psychomotor slowing (3% to 21%), nervousness (9% to 19%), memory difficulties (2% to 14%), speech problems (2% to 13%), (Continued)

Topiramate *(Continued)*

fatigue (9% to 30%), difficulty concentrating (5% to 14%), depression (9% to 13%), confusion (4% to 14%)

Endocrine & metabolic: Serum bicarbonate decreased (dose-related: 7% to 67%; marked reductions [to <17 mEq/L] 1% to 11%)

Gastrointestinal: Nausea (6% to 12%; migraine trial: 14%), weight loss (8% to 13%), anorexia (4% to 24%)

Neuromuscular & skeletal: Paresthesia (1% to 19%; migraine trial: 35% to 51%)

Ocular: Nystagmus (10% to 11%), abnormal vision (<1% to 13%)

Respiratory: Upper respiratory infection (migraine trial: 12% to 13%)

Miscellaneous: Injury (6% to 14%)

1% to 10%:

Cardiovascular: Chest pain (2% to 4%), edema (1% to 2%), bradycardia (1%), pallor (up to 1%), hypertension (1% to 2%)

Central nervous system: Abnormal coordination (4%), hypoesthesia (1% to 2%; migraine trial: 8%), convulsions (1%), depersonalization (1% to 2%), apathy (1% to 3%), cognitive problems (3%), emotional lability (3%), agitation (3%), aggressive reactions (2% to 9%), tremor (3% to 9%), stupor (1% to 2%), mood problems (4% to 9%), anxiety (2% to 10%), insomnia (4% to 8%), neurosis (1%), vertigo (1% to 2%)

Dermatologic: Pruritus (migraine trial: 2% to 4%), skin disorder (1% to 3%), alopecia (2%), dermatitis (up to 2%), hypertrichosis (up to 2%), rash erythematous (up to 2%), eczema (up to 1%), seborrhea (up to 1%), skin discoloration (up to 1%)

Endocrine & metabolic: Hot flashes (1% to 2%); metabolic acidosis (hyperchloremia, nonanion gap), dehydration, breast pain (up to 4%), menstrual irregularities (1% to 2%), hypoglycemia (1%), libido decreased (<1% to 2%)

Gastrointestinal: Dyspepsia (2% to 7%), abdominal pain (5% to 7%), constipation (3% to 5%), xerostomia (2% to 4%), fecal incontinence (1%), gingivitis (1%), diarrhea (2%; migraine trial: 11%), vomiting (1% to 3%), gastroenteritis (1% to 3%), appetite increased (1%), GI disorder (1%), dysgeusia (2% to 4%; migraine trial: 12% to 15%), dysphagia (1%), flatulence (1%), GERD (1%), glossitis (1%), gum hyperplasia (1%), weight increase (1%)

Genitourinary: Impotence, dysuria/incontinence (<1% to 4%), prostatic disorder (2%), UTI (2% to 3%), premature ejaculation (migraine trial: 3%), cystitis (2%)

Hematologic: Leukopenia (1% to 2%), purpura (8%), hematoma (1%), prothrombin time increased (1%), thrombocytopenia (1%)

Neuromuscular & skeletal: Myalgia (2%), weakness (3% to 6%), back pain (1% to 5%), leg pain (2% to 4%), rigors (1%), hypertonia, arthralgia (1% to 7%), gait abnormal (2% to 8%), involuntary muscle contractions (2%; migraine trial: 4%), skeletal pain (1%), hyperkinesia (up to 5%), hyporeflexia (up to 2%)

Ocular: Conjunctivitis (1%), diplopia (2% to 10%), myopia (up to 1%)

Otic: Hearing decreased (1% to 2%), tinnitus (1% to 2%), otitis media (migraine trial: 1% to 2%)

Renal: Nephrolithiasis, renal calculus (migraine trial: 2%), hematuria (<1% to 2%)

Respiratory: Pharyngitis (3% to 6%), sinusitis (4% to 6%; migraine trial: 8% to 10%), epistaxis (1% to 4%), rhinitis (4% to 7%), dyspnea (1% to 2%), pneumonia (5%), coughing (migraine trial: 2% to 3%), bronchitis (migraine trial: 3%)

Miscellaneous: Flu-like syndrome (3% to 7%), allergy (2% to 3%), body odor (up to 1%), fever (migraine trial: 1% to 2%), viral infection (migraine trial: 3% to 4%), infection (<1% to 2%), diaphoresis (≤1%), thirst (2%)

Dosage Oral: **Note:** Do not abruptly discontinue therapy; taper dosage gradually to prevent rebound seizure.

Monotherapy: Children ≥10 years and Adults: Partial onset seizure and primary generalized tonic-clonic seizure: Initial: 25 mg twice daily; may increase weekly by 50 mg/day up to 100 mg twice daily (week 4 dose); thereafter, may further increase weekly by 100 mg/day up to the recommended maximum of 200 mg twice daily.

Adjunctive therapy:

Children 2-16 years:

Partial onset seizure or seizure associated with Lennox-Gastaut syndrome: Initial dose titration should begin at 25 mg (or less, based on a range of 1-3 mg/kg/day) nightly for the first week; dosage may be increased in increments of 1-3 mg/kg/day (administered in 2 divided doses) at 1- or 2-week intervals to a total daily dose of 5-9 mg/kg/day

Primary generalized tonic-clonic seizure: Use initial dose listed above, but use slower initial titration rate; titrate to recommended maintenance dose by the end of 8 weeks

Adolescents ≥17 years and Adults:

Partial onset seizures: Initial: 25-50 mg/day (given in 2 divided doses) for 1 week; increase at weekly intervals by 25-50 mg/day until response; usual maintenance dose: 100-200 mg twice daily. Doses >1600 mg/day have not been studied.

Primary generalized tonic-clonic seizures: Use initial dose as listed above for partial onset seizures, but use slower initial titration rate; titrate upwards to recommended dose by the end of 8 weeks; usual maintenance dose: 200 mg twice daily. Doses >1600 mg/day have not been studied.

Adults:

Migraine prophylaxis: Initial: 25 mg/day (in the evening), titrated at weekly intervals in 25 mg increments, up to the recommended total daily dose of 100 mg/day given in 2 divided doses

Cluster headache (unlabeled use): Initial: 25 mg/day, titrated at weekly intervals in 25 mg increments, up to 200 mg/day

Neuropathic pain (unlabeled use): Initial: 25 mg/day, titrated at weekly intervals in 25-50 mg increments to target dose of 400 mg daily in 2 divided doses. Reported dosage range studied: 25-800 mg/day

Dosing adjustment in renal impairment: Cl$_{cr}$ <70 mL/minute: Administer 50% dose and titrate more slowly

Hemodialysis: Supplemental dose may be needed during hemodialysis

Dosing adjustment in hepatic impairment: Clearance may be reduced

Mechanism of Action Anticonvulsant activity may be due to a combination of potential mechanisms: Blocks neuronal voltage-dependent sodium channels, enhances GABA(A) activity, antagonizes AMPA/kainate glutamate receptors, and weakly inhibits carbonic anhydrase.

Contraindications Hypersensitivity to topiramate or any component of the formulation

Warnings/Precautions Use with caution in patients with hepatic, respiratory, or renal impairment. Topiramate may decrease serum bicarbonate concentrations (up to 67% of patients); treatment-emergent metabolic acidosis is less common. Risk may be increased in patients with a predisposing condition (organ dysfunction, ketogenic diet, or concurrent treatment with other drugs which may cause acidosis). Metabolic acidosis may occur at dosages as low as 50 mg/day. Monitor serum bicarbonate as well as potential complications of chronic acidosis (nephrolithiasis, osteomalacia, and reduced growth rates in children). The risk of kidney stones is about 2-4 times that of the untreated population, the risk of this event may be reduced by increasing fluid intake.

Cognitive dysfunction, psychiatric disturbances (mood disorders), and sedation (somnolence or fatigue) may occur with topiramate use; incidence may be related to rapid titration and higher doses. Topiramate may also cause paresthesia and ataxia. Topiramate has been associated with secondary angle-closure glaucoma in adults and children, typically within 1 month of initiation; discontinue in patients with acute onset of decreased visual acuity or ocular pain. Hyperammonemia with or without encephalopathy may occur with concomitant valproate administration; use with caution in patients with inborn errors of metabolism or decreased hepatic mitochondrial activity. Topiramate may be associated (rarely) with severe oligohydrosis and hyperthermia, most frequently in children; use caution and monitor closely during strenuous exercise, during exposure to high environmental temperature, or in patients receiving drugs with anticholinergic activity.

Avoid abrupt withdrawal of topiramate therapy, it should be withdrawn/tapered slowly to minimize the potential of increased seizure frequency. Effects with other sedative drugs or ethanol may be potentiated. Safety and efficacy have not been established in children <2 years of age for adjunctive treatment and <10 years of age for monotherapy.

Drug Interactions

Cytochrome P450 Effect: Inhibits CYP2C19 (weak); **Induces** CYP3A4 (weak)

Increased Effect/Toxicity: Concomitant administration with other CNS depressants will increase its sedative effects. Coadministration with acetazolamide: may increase the chance of nephrolithiasis and/or hyperthermia. Topiramate may increase phenytoin concentration by 25%. Concurrent administration with anticholinergic drugs may increase the risk of oligohydrosis and/or hyperthermia (includes drugs with high anticholinergic activity such as antihistamines, cyclic antidepressants, and antipsychotics); use caution.

(Continued)

Topiramate (Continued)

Decreased Effect: Phenytoin can decrease topiramate levels by as much as 48%, carbamazepine reduces it by 40%. Digoxin levels and ethinyl estradiol blood levels are decreased when coadministered with topiramate. Hyperammonemia (with or without encephalopathy) has been reported in patients who tolerated valproic acid or topiramate alone; these drugs may modestly decrease the serum concentrations of the other drug.

Ethanol/Nutrition/Herb Interactions

Ethanol: Avoid ethanol (may increase CNS depression).

Food: Ketogenic diet may increase the possibility of acidosis.

Herb/Nutraceutical: Avoid evening primrose (seizure threshold decreased).

Pharmacodynamics/Kinetics

Absorption: Good, rapid; unaffected by food

Protein binding: 15% to 41% (inversely related to plasma concentrations)

Metabolism: Hepatic via P450 enzymes

Bioavailability: 80%

Half-life elimination: Mean: Adults: Normal renal function: 21 hours; shorter in pediatric patients; clearance is 50% higher in pediatric patients

Time to peak, serum: ~2-4 hours

Excretion: Urine (~70% to 80% as unchanged drug)

Dialyzable: ~30%

Pregnancy Risk Factor C

Dosage Forms

Capsule, sprinkle:

Topamax®: 15 mg, 25 mg

Tablet:

Topamax®: 25 mg, 50 mg, 100 mg, 200 mg

TOPO see Topotecan on page 1592

Toposar® see Etoposide on page 660

Topotecan (toe poe TEE kan)

U.S. Brand Names Hycamtin®

Canadian Brand Names Hycamtin®

Generic Available No

Index Terms Hycamptamine; NSC-609699; SK and F 104864; SKF 104864; SKF 104864-A; TOPO; Topotecan Hydrochloride; TPT

Pharmacologic Category Antineoplastic Agent, Natural Source (Plant) Derivative

Use Treatment of ovarian cancer and small cell lung cancer; cervical cancer (in combination with cisplatin)

Unlabeled/Investigational Use Investigational: Treatment of nonsmall cell lung cancer, sarcoma (pediatrics)

Local Anesthetic/Vasoconstrictor Precautions No information available to require special precautions

Effects on Dental Treatment Key adverse event(s) related to dental treatment: Stomatitis.

Common Adverse Effects

>10%:

Central nervous system: Fatigue (29%), fever (28%), pain (23%), headache (18%)

Dermatologic: Alopecia (31% to 49%), rash (16%)

Gastrointestinal: Nausea (64%), vomiting (45%), diarrhea (32%), constipation (29%), abdominal pain (22%)anorexia (19%), stomatitis (18%)

Hematologic: Neutropenia (97%; grade 4: 70% to 80%; nadir 8-11 days; recovery <21 days), leukopenia (97%), anemia (89%), thrombocytopenia (69%; grade 4: 27% to 29%), neutropenic fever/sepsis (43%; grade 4: 23% to 28%)

Neuromuscular & skeletal: Weakness (25%)

Respiratory: Dyspnea (22%), cough (15%)

1% to 10%:

Hepatic: Transient increases in liver enzymes (8%)

Neuromuscular & skeletal: Paresthesia (7%)

Miscellaneous: Sepsis (grades 3/4: 5%)

Mechanism of Action Binds to topoisomerase I and stabilizes the cleavable complex so that religation of the cleaved DNA strand cannot occur. This results in the accumulation of cleavable complexes and single-strand DNA breaks. Topotecan acts in S phase.

Drug Interactions

Increased Effect/Toxicity: Myelosuppression was more severe when given in combination with cisplatin. Filgrastim may cause prolonged and severe neutropenia and thrombocytopenia if administered concurrently with topotecan; initiate filgrastim at least 24 hours after topotecan.

Pharmacodynamics/Kinetics

Absorption: Oral: ~30%

Distribution: V_{dss} of the lactone is high (mean: 87.3 L/mm^2; range: 25.6-186 L/mm^2), suggesting wide distribution and/or tissue sequestering

Protein binding: 35%

Metabolism: Undergoes a rapid, pH-dependent opening of the lactone ring to yield a relatively inactive hydroxy acid in plasma; metabolized in the liver to N-demethylated metabolite

Half-life elimination: 2-3 hours; renal impairment: 5 hours

Excretion: Urine (51%; 3% as desmethyl topotecan); feces (18%; 2% as desmethyl topotecan)

Pregnancy Risk Factor D

Topotecan Hydrochloride see Topotecan on page 1592

Toprol-XL® see Metoprolol on page 1088

Toradol® see Ketorolac on page 934

Toremifene (tore EM i feen)

U.S. Brand Names Fareston®

Canadian Brand Names Fareston®

Mexican Brand Names Fareston

Generic Available No

Index Terms FC1157a; Toremifene Citrate

Pharmacologic Category Antineoplastic Agent, Estrogen Receptor Antagonist

Use Treatment of advanced breast cancer; management of desmoid tumors and endometrial carcinoma

Local Anesthetic/Vasoconstrictor Precautions No information available to require special precautions

Effects on Dental Treatment No significant effects or complications reported

Common Adverse Effects

>10%:

Endocrine & metabolic: Vaginal discharge, hot flashes

Gastrointestinal: Nausea, vomiting

Miscellaneous: Diaphoresis

1% to 10%:

Cardiovascular: Thromboembolism: Toremifene has been associated with the occurrence of venous thrombosis and pulmonary embolism; arterial thrombosis has also been described in a few case reports; cardiac failure, MI, edema

Central nervous system: Dizziness

Endocrine & metabolic: Hypercalcemia may occur in patients with bone metastases; galactorrhea and vitamin deficiency, menstrual irregularities

Genitourinary: Vaginal bleeding or discharge, endometriosis, priapism, possible endometrial cancer

Ocular: Ophthalmologic effects (visual acuity changes, cataracts, or retinopathy), corneal opacities, dry eyes

Mechanism of Action Nonsteroidal, triphenylethylene derivative. Competitively binds to estrogen receptors on tumors and other tissue targets, producing a nuclear complex that decreases DNA synthesis and inhibits estrogen effects. Nonsteroidal agent with potent antiestrogenic properties which compete with estrogen for binding sites in breast and other tissues; cells accumulate in the G_0 and G_1 phases; therefore, toremifene is cytostatic rather than cytocidal.

Drug Interactions

Cytochrome P450 Effect: Substrate of CYP1A2 (minor), 3A4 (major)

Increased Effect/Toxicity: Concurrent therapy with warfarin results in significant enhancement of anticoagulant effects; has been speculated that a decrease in antitumor effect of tamoxifen may also occur due to alterations in the percentage of active tamoxifen metabolites.

Decreased Effect: CYP3A4 inducers may decrease the levels/effects of toremifene; example inducers include aminoglutethimide, carbamazepine, nafcillin, nevirapine, phenobarbital, phenytoin, and rifamycins.

Pharmacodynamics/Kinetics

Absorption: Well absorbed

Distribution: V_d: 580 L

Protein binding, plasma: >99.5%, primarily to albumin

Metabolism: Extensively hepatic, principally by CYP3A4 to N-demethyl-toremifene, which is also antiestrogenic but with weak *in vivo* antitumor potency

(Continued)

Toremifene (Continued)

Half-life elimination: ~5 days
Time to peak, serum: ~3 hours
Excretion: Primarily feces; urine (10%) during a 1-week period

Pregnancy Risk Factor D

Toremifene Citrate see Toremifene on page 1593

Torsemide (TORE se mide)

Related Information
Cardiovascular Diseases on page 1726

U.S. Brand Names Demadex®

Generic Available Yes: Tablet

Pharmacologic Category Diuretic, Loop

Use Management of edema associated with congestive heart failure and hepatic or renal disease; used alone or in combination with antihypertensives in treatment of hypertension; I.V. form is indicated when rapid onset is desired

Local Anesthetic/Vasoconstrictor Precautions No information available to require special precautions

Effects on Dental Treatment No significant effects or complications reported

Common Adverse Effects 1% to 10%:
Cardiovascular: Edema (1.1%), ECG abnormality (2%), chest pain (1.2%)
Central nervous system: Headache (7.3%), dizziness (3.2%), insomnia (1.2%), nervousness (1%)
Endocrine & metabolic: Hyperglycemia, hyperuricemia, hypokalemia
Gastrointestinal: Diarrhea (2%), constipation (1.8%), nausea (1.8%), dyspepsia (1.6%), sore throat (1.6%)
Genitourinary: Excessive urination (6.7%)
Neuromuscular & skeletal: Weakness (2%), arthralgia (1.8%), myalgia (1.6%)
Respiratory: Rhinitis (2.8%), cough increase (2%)

Mechanism of Action Inhibits reabsorption of sodium and chloride in the ascending loop of Henle and distal renal tubule, interfering with the chloride-binding cotransport system, thus causing increased excretion of water, sodium, chloride, magnesium, and calcium; does not alter GFR, renal plasma flow, or acid-base balance

Drug Interactions
Cytochrome P450 Effect: Substrate of CYP2C8 (miinor), 2C9 (major); **Inhibits** CYP2C19 (weak)

Increased Effect/Toxicity: Torsemide-induced hypokalemia may predispose to digoxin toxicity and may increase the risk of arrhythmia with drugs which may prolong QT interval, including type Ia and type III antiarrhythmic agents, cisapride, and some quinolones (sparfloxacin, gatifloxacin, and moxifloxacin). The risk of toxicity from lithium and salicylates (high dose) may be increased by loop diuretics. Hypotensive effects and/or adverse renal effects of ACE inhibitors and NSAIDs are potentiated by bumetanide-induced hypovolemia. The effects of peripheral adrenergic-blocking drugs or ganglionic blockers may be increased by bumetanide.

Torsemide may increase the risk of ototoxicity with other ototoxic agents (aminoglycosides, cis-platinum), especially in patients with renal dysfunction. Synergistic diuretic effects occur with thiazide-type diuretics. Diuretics tend to be synergistic with other antihypertensive agents, and hypotension may occur.

Decreased Effect: Torsemide action may be reduced with probenecid. Diuretic action may be impaired in patients with cirrhosis and ascites if used with salicylates. Glucose tolerance may be decreased when used with sulfonylureas. CYP2C9 inducers may decrease the levels/effects of torsemide; example inducers include carbamazepine, phenobarbital, phenytoin, rifampin, rifapentine, and secobarbital. Torsemide efficacy may be decreased with NSAIDs.

Pharmacodynamics/Kinetics
Onset of action: Diuresis: 30-60 minutes
Peak effect: 1-4 hours
Duration: ~6 hours
Absorption: Oral: Rapid
Protein binding, plasma: ~97% to 99%
Metabolism: Hepatic (80%) via CYP
Bioavailability: 80% to 90%
Half-life elimination: 2-4; Cirrhosis: 7-8 hours
Excretion: Urine (20% as unchanged drug)

Pregnancy Risk Factor B

Touro® CC *see* Guaifenesin, Pseudoephedrine, and Dextromethorphan *on page 800*

Touro® CC-LD *see* Guaifenesin, Pseudoephedrine, and Dextromethorphan *on page 800*

Touro® Allergy *see* Brompheniramine and Pseudoephedrine *on page 231*

Touro® DM *see* Guaifenesin and Dextromethorphan *on page 796*

Touro® HC *see* Hydrocodone and Guaifenesin *on page 828*

Touro LA® *see* Guaifenesin and Pseudoephedrine *on page 798*

tPA *see* Alteplase *on page 78*

TPT *see* Topotecan *on page 1592*

TPV *see* Tipranavir *on page 1575*

tRA *see* Tretinoin (Oral) *on page 1606*

Trace Metals (trase MET als)

Related Information
Chromium *on page 1705*
Iodine *on page 900*
Selenium *on page 1461*

U.S. Brand Names Iodopen®; Molypen®; M.T.E.-4®; M.T.E.-5®; M.T.E.-6®; M.T.E.-7®; Multitrace™-4; Multitrace™-4 Neonatal; Multitrace™-4 Pediatric; Multitrace™-5; Neotrace-4®; Pedtrace-4®; P.T.E.-4®; P.T.E.-5®; Selepen®

Generic Available Yes

Index Terms Chromium; Copper; Iodine; Manganese; Molybdenum; Neonatal Trace Metals; Selenium; Zinc

Pharmacologic Category Trace Element, Parenteral

Use Prevention and correction of trace metal deficiencies

Local Anesthetic/Vasoconstrictor Precautions No information available to require special precautions

Effects on Dental Treatment No significant effects or complications reported

Pregnancy Risk Factor C

Tracleer® *see* Bosentan *on page 223*

Tramadol (TRA ma dole)

Related Sample Prescriptions
Moderate/Moderately Severe Oral Pain *on page 1834*

U.S. Brand Names Ultram®; Ultram® ER

Canadian Brand Names Ultram®; Zytram® XL

Mexican Brand Names Tradol; Trexol

Generic Available Yes: Excludes extended release tablet

Index Terms Tramadol Hydrochloride

Pharmacologic Category Analgesic, Nonopioid

Dental Use Relief of moderate to moderately-severe dental pain

Use Relief of moderate to moderately-severe pain

Local Anesthetic/Vasoconstrictor Precautions No information available to require special precautions

Effects on Dental Treatment Key adverse event(s) related to dental treatment: Xerostomia and changes in salivation (normal salivary flow resumes upon discontinuation). See Dental Comment.

Significant Adverse Effects
>10%:
  Cardiovascular: Flushing (8% to 16%)
  Central nervous system: Dizziness (16% to 33%), headache (8% to 32%), insomnia (7% to 11%), somnolence (7% to 25%)
  Dermatologic: Pruritus (6% to 12%)
  Gastrointestinal: Constipation (12% to 46%), nausea (15% to 40%)
  Neuromuscular & skeletal: Weakness (4% to 12%)
1% to 10%:
  Cardiovascular: Chest pain (1% to <5%), postural hypotension (2% to 5%), vasodilation (1% to <5%)
  Central nervous system: Agitation, anxiety (1% to <5%), confusion (1% to <5%), coordination impaired (1% to <5%), depression (1% to <5%), emotional lability, euphoria, hallucinations, hypoesthesia, lethargy, malaise, nervousness (1% to <5%), pain, pyrexia, restlessness
  Dermatologic: Dermatitis, rash
  Endocrine & metabolic: Hot flashes (2% to 9%), menopausal symptoms (1% to <5%)
  Gastrointestinal: Abdominal pain, anorexia (<6%), diarrhea (5% to 10%), dry mouth (5% to 10%), dyspepsia, flatulence, vomiting (5% to 9%), weight loss
(Continued)

Tramadol *(Continued)*

Genitourinary: Urinary frequency (1% to <5%), urinary retention (1% to <5%), urinary tract infection (1% to <5%)

Neuromuscular & skeletal: Arthralgia (1% to <5%), hypertonia (1% to <5%), rigors (<4%), paresthesia (1% to <5%), spasticity (1% to <5%), tremor (1% to <5%), creatinine phosphokinase increased

Ocular: Blurred vision (1% to <5%), miosis (1% to <5%)

Respiratory: Bronchitis (1% to <5%), cough (1% to <5%), dyspnea (1% to <5%), pharyngitis (1% to <5%), rhinorrhea (1% to <5%), sinusitis (1% to <5%)

Miscellaneous: Diaphoresis (2% to 6%), flu-like syndrome (<2%)

<1% (Limited to important or life-threatening): Allergic reaction, amnesia, anaphylactoid reactions, anaphylaxis, angioedema, bronchospasm, cataracts, cholecystitis, cholelithiasis, cognitive dysfunction, concentration difficulty, creatinine increased, deafness, gastrointestinal bleeding, hepatitis, hyper-/hypotension, liver failure, MI, migraine, myocardial ischemia, night sweats, pancreatitis, peripheral ischemia, pulmonary edema, pulmonary embolism, seizure, serotonin syndrome, Stevens-Johnson syndrome, suicidal tendency, syncope, toxic epidermal necrolysis, vertigo

A withdrawal syndrome may occur with abrupt discontinuation; includes anxiety, diarrhea, hallucinations (rare), nausea, pain, piloerection, rigors, sweating, and tremor. Uncommon discontinuation symptoms may include severe anxiety, panic attacks, or paresthesia.

Dental Usual Dosing Moderate-to-severe chronic pain: Oral:

Adults:

Immediate release formulation: 50-100 mg every 4-6 hours (not to exceed 400 mg/day)

For patients not requiring rapid onset of effect, tolerability may be improved by starting dose at 25 mg/day and titrating dose by 25 mg every 3 days, until reaching 25 mg 4 times/day. Dose may then be increased by 50 mg every 3 days as tolerated, to reach dose of 50 mg 4 times/day.

Extended release formulations:

Ultram® ER: 100 mg once daily; titrate every 5 days (maximum: 300 mg/day)

Zytram® XL [Per Canadian labeling: Not available in U.S.]: 150 mg once daily; if pain relief is not achieved may titrate by increasing dosage incrementally, with sufficient time to evaluate effect of increased dosage; generally not more often than every 7 days (maximum: 400 mg/day)

Elderly >75 years:

Immediate release: 50 mg every 6 hours (not to exceed 300 mg/day); see dosing adjustments for renal and hepatic impairment.

Extended release formulation: Use with great caution. See adult dosing.

Dosage Moderate-to-severe chronic pain: Oral:

Adults:

Immediate release formulation: 50-100 mg every 4-6 hours (not to exceed 400 mg/day)

For patients not requiring rapid onset of effect, tolerability may be improved by starting dose at 25 mg/day and titrating dose by 25 mg every 3 days, until reaching 25 mg 4 times/day. Dose may then be increased by 50 mg every 3 days as tolerated, to reach dose of 50 mg 4 times/day.

Extended release formulations:

Ultram® ER: 100 mg once daily; titrate every 5 days (maximum: 300 mg/day)

Zytram® XL [per Canadian labeling: Not available in U.S.]: 150 mg once daily; if pain relief is not achieved may titrate by increasing dosage incrementally, with sufficient time to evaluate effect of increased dosage; generally not more often than every 7 days (maximum: 400 mg/day)

Elderly >75 years:

Immediate release: 50 mg every 6 hours (not to exceed 300 mg/day); see dosing adjustments for renal and hepatic impairment.

Extended release formulation: Use with great caution. See adult dosing.

Dosing adjustment in renal impairment:

Immediate release: Cl$_{cr}$ <30 mL/minute: Administer 50-100 mg dose every 12 hours (maximum: 200 mg/day)

Extended release: Should not be used in patients with Cl$_{cr}$ <30 mL/minute

Dosing adjustment in hepatic impairment:

Immediate release: Cirrhosis: Recommended dose: 50 mg every 12 hours

Extended release: Should not be used in patients with severe (Child-Pugh Class C) hepatic dysfunction

Mechanism of Action Binds to μ-opiate receptors in the CNS causing inhibition of ascending pain pathways, altering the perception of and response to pain; also inhibits the reuptake of norepinephrine and serotonin, which also modifies the ascending pain pathway

Contraindications Hypersensitivity to tramadol, opioids, or any component of the formulation; opioid-dependent patients; acute intoxication with alcohol, hypnotics, centrally-acting analgesics, opioids, or psychotropic drugs

Extended release formulations (Ultram® ER and Zytram® XL [CAN]): Additional contraindications: Severe (Cl_{cr} <30 mL/minute) renal dysfunction, severe (Child-Pugh Class C) hepatic dysfunction

Note: Based on Canadian product labeling, tramadol is contraindicated during or within 14 days following MAO inhibitor therapy

Warnings/Precautions May cause CNS depression, which may impair physical or mental abilities; patients must be cautioned about performing tasks which require mental alertness (eg, operating machinery or driving). Should be used only with extreme caution in patients receiving MAO inhibitors. May cause CNS depression and/or respiratory depression, particularly when combined with other CNS depressants. Use with caution and reduce dosage when administered to patients receiving other CNS depressants. An increased risk of seizures may occur in patients receiving serotonin reuptake inhibitors (SSRIs or anorectics), tricyclic antidepressants, other cyclic compounds (including cyclobenzaprine, promethazine), neuroleptics, MAO inhibitors (contraindicated in Canadian product labeling), or drugs which may lower seizure threshold. Patients with a history of seizures, or with a risk of seizures (head trauma, metabolic disorders, CNS infection, or malignancy, or during ethanol/drug withdrawal) are also at increased risk.

Elderly, debilitated patients and patients with chronic respiratory disorders may be at greater risk of adverse events. Use with caution in patients with increased intracranial pressure or head injury. Avoid use in patients who are suicidal or addiction prone. Use caution in heavy alcohol users. Use caution in treatment of acute abdominal conditions; may mask pain. Use tramadol with caution and reduce dosage in patients with liver disease or renal dysfunction. Tolerance or drug dependence may result from extended use (withdrawal symptoms have been reported); abrupt discontinuation should be avoided. Tapering of dose at the time of discontinuation limits the risk of withdrawal symptoms. Safety and efficacy in pediatric patients <18 years of age have not been established.

Drug Interactions **Substrate** of CYP2B6 (minor), 2D6 (major), 3A4 (minor)

Carbamazepine: Tramadol metabolism is increased by carbamazepine. Avoid concurrent use; increases risk of seizures.

Cyclobenzaprine: May enhance the neuroexcitatory and/or seizure-potentiating effect of tramadol.

CYP2D6 inhibitors: May decrease the effects of tramadol. Example inhibitors include chlorpromazine, delavirdine, fluoxetine, miconazole, paroxetine, pergolide, quinidine, quinine, ritonavir, and ropinirole.

Ethanol: Tramadol may enhance the CNS depressant effect of ethanol.

MAO inhibitors: May increase the neuroexcitatory effects or risk of seizures. Examples of inhibitors include isocarboxazid, linezolid, phenelzine, selegiline, and tranylcypromine.

Naloxone: May increase the risk of seizures (if administered in tramadol overdose).

Quinidine: May increase the tramadol serum concentrations and decrease serum concentrations of M1

SSRIs: May increase the neuroexcitatory effects or risk of seizures with tramadol. Examples of SSRIs include citalopram, escitalopram, fluoxetine, fluvoxamine, paroxetine, sertraline.

Serotonin modulators: May enhance the adverse/toxic effects of tramadol. The development of serotonin syndrome may occur.

Sibutramine: May enhance the serotonergic effects of tramadol. Avoid concurrent use.

Tricyclic antidepressants: May increase the risk of seizures.

Ethanol/Nutrition/Herb Interactions

Ethanol: Avoid ethanol (may increase CNS depression).

Food:

Immediate release: Does not affect the rate or extent of absorption.

Extended release: Reduced C_{max} and AUC and T_{max} occurred 3 hours earlier when taken with a high-fat meal.

Herb/Nutraceutical: Avoid valerian, St John's wort, kava kava, gotu kola (may increase CNS depression).

Dietary Considerations May be taken with or without food. Extended release formulation: Be consistent; always give with food or always give on an empty stomach.

Pharmacodynamics/Kinetics

Onset of action: ~1 hour

Duration of action: 9 hours

Absorption: Rapid and complete

Distribution: V_d: 2.5-3 L/kg

Protein binding, plasma: 20%

(Continued)

Tramadol *(Continued)*

Metabolism: Extensively hepatic via demethylation, glucuronidation, and sulfation; has pharmacologically active metabolite formed by CYP2D6 (M1; O-desmethyl tramadol)

Bioavailability: Immediate release: 75%; Extended release: 85% to 90% as compared to immediate release (Zytram® XL: 70%)

Half-life elimination: Tramadol: ~6-8 hours; Active metabolite: 7-9 hours; prolonged in elderly, hepatic or renal impairment; Zytram® XL: ~16 hours

Time to peak: Immediate release: 2 hours; Extended release: 12 hours

Excretion: Urine (30% as unchanged drug; 60% as metabolites)

Pregnancy Risk Factor C

Lactation Enters breast milk/contraindicated

Breast-Feeding Considerations Not recommended for postdelivery analgesia in nursing mothers.

Dosage Forms Excipient information presented when available (limited, particularly for generics); consult specific product labeling. [CAN] = Canadian brand name

Tablet, as hydrochloride: 50 mg

Ultram®: 50 mg

Tablet, extended release, as hydrochloride:

Ultram® ER: 100 mg, 200 mg, 300 mg

Zytram® XL [CAN]: 150 mg, 200 mg, 300 mg, 400 mg [not available in the U.S.]

Dental Comment Literature reports suggest that the efficacy of tramadol in oral surgery pain is equivalent to the combination of aspirin and codeine. One study (Olson et al 1990) showed acetaminophen and dextropropoxyphene combination to be superior to tramadol and another study showed tramadol to be superior to acetaminophen and dextropropoxyphene combination. Tramadol appears to be at least equal to if not better than codeine alone. Seizures have been reported with the use of tramadol.

Selected Readings

Collins M, Young I, Sweeney P, et al, "The Effect of Tramadol on Dento-Alveolar Surgical Pain," *Br J Oral Maxillofac Surg*, 1997, 35(1):54-8.

Doroschak AM, Bowles WR, and Hargreaves KM, "Evaluation of the Combination of Flurbiprofen and Tramadol for Management of Endodontic Pain," *J Endod*, 1999, 25(10):660-3.

Kahn LH, Alderfer RJ, and Graham DJ, "Seizures Reported With Tramadol," *JAMA*, 1997, 278(20):1661.

Lewis KS and Han NH, "Tramadol: A New Centrally Acting Analgesic," *Am J Health Syst Pharm*, 1997, 54(6):643-52.

Moore PA, "Pain Management in Dental Practice: Tramadol vs. Codeine Combinations," *J Am Dent Assoc*, 1999, 130(7):1075-9.

Moore PA, Crout RJ, Jackson DL, et al, "Tramadol Hydrochloride: Analgesic Efficacy Compared With Codeine, Aspirin With Codeine, and Placebo After Dental Extraction," *J Clin Pharmacol*, 1998, 38(6):554-60.

Roelofse JA and Payne KA, "Oral Tramadol: Analgesic Efficacy in Children Following Multiple Dental Extractions," *Eur J Anaesthesiol*, 1999, 16(7):441-7.

Sunshine A, "New Clinical Experience With Tramadol," *Drugs*, 1994, 47(Suppl 1):8-18.

Sunshine A, Olson NZ, Zighelboim I, et al, "Analgesic Oral Efficacy of Tramadol Hydrochloride in Postoperative Pain," *Clin Pharmacol Ther*, 1992; 51(6):740-6.

Wynn RL, "Tramadol (Ultram) - A New Kind of Analgesic," *Gen Dent*, 1996, 44(3):216-8,220.

Tramadol Hydrochloride *see* Tramadol *on page 1595*

Tramadol Hydrochloride and Acetaminophen *see* Acetaminophen and Tramadol *on page 39*

Trandate® *see* Labetalol *on page 940*

Trandolapril *(tran DOE la pril)*

Related Information

Cardiovascular Diseases *on page 1726*

U.S. Brand Names Mavik®

Canadian Brand Names Mavik™

Mexican Brand Names Gopten

Generic Available Yes

Pharmacologic Category Angiotensin-Converting Enzyme (ACE) Inhibitor

Use Management of hypertension alone or in combination with other antihypertensive agents; treatment of left ventricular dysfunction after myocardial infarction

Unlabeled/Investigational Use As a class, ACE inhibitors are recommended in the treatment of systolic congestive heart failure

Local Anesthetic/Vasoconstrictor Precautions No information available to require special precautions

Effects on Dental Treatment No significant effects or complications reported

Common Adverse Effects Note: Frequency ranges include data from hypertension and heart failure trials. Higher rates of adverse reactions have generally been noted in patients with CHF. However, the frequency of adverse effects associated with placebo is also increased in this population.

>1%:
Cardiovascular: Hypotension (<1% to 11%), bradycardia (<1% to 4.7%), intermittent claudication (3.8%), stroke (3.3%)

Central nervous system: Dizziness (1.3% to 23%), syncope (5.9%), asthenia (3.3%)

Endocrine & metabolic: Elevated uric acid (15%), hyperkalemia (5.3%), hypocalcemia (4.7%)

Gastrointestinal: Dyspepsia (6.4%), gastritis (4.2%)

Neuromuscular & skeletal: Myalgia (4.7%)

Renal: Elevated BUN (9%), elevated serum creatinine (1.1% to 4.7%) Respiratory: Cough (1.9% to 35%)

Mechanism of Action Trandolapril is an ACE inhibitor which prevents the formation of angiotensin II from angiotensin I. Trandolapril must undergo enzymatic hydrolysis, mainly in liver, to its biologically active metabolite, trandolaprilat. A CNS mechanism may also be involved in the hypotensive effect as angiotensin II increases adrenergic outflow from the CNS. Vasoactive kallikrein's may be decreased in conversion to active hormones by ACE inhibitors, thus reducing blood pressure.

Drug Interactions

Increased Effect/Toxicity: Potassium supplements, co-trimoxazole (high dose), angiotensin II receptor antagonists (eg, candesartan, losartan, irbesartan), or potassium-sparing diuretics (amiloride, spironolactone, triamterene) may result in elevated serum potassium levels when combined with trandolapril. ACE inhibitor effects may be increased by phenothiazines or probenecid (increases levels of captopril). ACE inhibitors may increase serum concentrations/effects of lithium. ACE inhibitors may enhance the adverse/toxic effects (nitritoid reaction) of gold sodium thiomalate.

Diuretics have additive hypotensive effects with ACE inhibitors, and hypovolemia increases the potential for adverse renal effects of ACE inhibitors. In patients with compromised renal function, coadministration with NSAIDs may result in further deterioration of renal function. Allopurinol and ACE inhibitors may cause a higher risk of hypersensitivity reaction when taken concurrently.

Decreased Effect: Aspirin (high dose) may reduce the therapeutic effects of ACE inhibitors; at low dosages this does not appear to be significant. Rifampin may decrease the effect of ACE inhibitors. Antacids may decrease the bioavailability of ACE inhibitors (may be more likely to occur with captopril); separate administration times by 1-2 hours. NSAIDs, specifically indomethacin, may reduce the hypotensive effects of ACE inhibitors. More likely to occur in low renin or volume dependent hypertensive patients.

Pharmacodynamics/Kinetics

Onset of action: 1-2 hours

Peak effect: Reduction in blood pressure: 6 hours

Duration: Prolonged; 72 hours after single dose

Absorption: Rapid

Distribution: Trandolaprilat (active metabolite) is very lipophilic in comparison to other ACE inhibitors

Protein binding: 80%

Metabolism: Hepatically hydrolyzed to active metabolite, trandolaprilat

Half-life elimination:

Trandolapril: 6 hours; Trandolaprilat: Effective: 10 hours, Terminal: 24 hours

Time to peak: Parent: 1 hour; Active metabolite trandolaprilat: 4-10 hours

Excretion: Urine (as metabolites)

Clearance: Reduce dose in renal failure; creatinine clearances ≤30 mL/minute result in accumulation of active metabolite

Pregnancy Risk Factor C (1st trimester)/D (2nd and 3rd trimesters)

Trandolapril and Verapamil (tran DOE la pril & ver AP a mil)

Related Information

Trandolapril *on page 1598*

Verapamil *on page 1654*

U.S. Brand Names Tarka®

Canadian Brand Names Tarka®

Generic Available No

Index Terms Verapamil and Trandolapril

Pharmacologic Category Antihypertensive Agent, Combination

Use Combination drug for the treatment of hypertension, however, not indicated for initial treatment of hypertension; replacement therapy in patients receiving separate dosage forms (for patient convenience); when monotherapy with one (Continued)

Trandolapril and Verapamil *(Continued)*

component fails to achieve desired antihypertensive effect, or when dose-limiting adverse effects limit upward titration of monotherapy

Local Anesthetic/Vasoconstrictor Precautions No information available to require special precautions

Effects on Dental Treatment No significant effects or complications reported

Common Adverse Effects See individual agents.

Drug Interactions

Cytochrome P450 Effect: Verapamil: **Substrate** of CYP1A2 (major), 2B6 (minor), 2C8/9 (minor), 2C19 (minor), 2E1 (minor), 3A4 (major); **Inhibits** CYP1A2 (weak), 2C8/9 (weak), 2D6 (weak), 3A4 (moderate)

Pharmacodynamics/Kinetics See individual agents.

Pregnancy Risk Factor C/D (2nd and 3rd trimesters)

Tranexamic Acid *(tran eks AM ik AS id)*

U.S. Brand Names Cyklokapron®

Canadian Brand Names Cyklokapron®; Tranexamic Acid Injection BP

Generic Available No

Pharmacologic Category Antihemophilic Agent

Use Short-term use (2-8 days) in hemophilia patients during and following tooth extraction to reduce or prevent hemorrhage

Unlabeled/Investigational Use Has been used as an alternative to aminocaproic acid for subarachnoid hemorrhage

Local Anesthetic/Vasoconstrictor Precautions No information available to require special precautions

Effects on Dental Treatment No significant effects or complications reported (see Dental Comment)

Common Adverse Effects

>10%: Gastrointestinal: Nausea, diarrhea, vomiting

1% to 10%:

Cardiovascular: Hypotension, thrombosis

Ocular: Blurred vision

Mechanism of Action Forms a reversible complex that displaces plasminogen from fibrin resulting in inhibition of fibrinolysis; it also inhibits the proteolytic activity of plasmin

Drug Interactions

Increased Effect/Toxicity: Chlorpromazine may increase cerebral vasospasm and ischemia. Coadministrations of Factor IX complex or anti-inhibitor coagulant concentrates may increase risk of thrombosis.

Pharmacodynamics/Kinetics

Half-life elimination: 2-10 hours

Excretion: Urine (>90% as unchanged drug)

Pregnancy Risk Factor B

Dental Comment Antifibrinolytic drugs are useful for the control of bleeding after dental extractions in patients with hemophilia because the oral mucosa and saliva are rich in plasminogen activators. In a clinical trial, tranexamic acid reduced recurrent bleeding and the amount of clotting-factor-replacement therapy needed. In adults, the oral dose was 20-25 mg/kg tranexamic acid every 8 hours until the dental sockets were completely healed. Mouthwashes containing tranexamic acid are effective for preventing oral bleeding in patients with hemophilia and in patients requiring dental extraction while receiving long-term oral anticoagulant therapy.

Immediately before dental extraction in hemophilic patients, administer 10 mg/kg tranexamic acid I.V. together with replacement therapy. Following surgery, a dose of 25 mg/kg may be given orally 3-4 times/day for 2-8 days.

Tranylcypromine (tran il SIP roe meen)

U.S. Brand Names Parnate®
Canadian Brand Names Parnate®
Generic Available No
Index Terms Transamine Sulphate; Tranylcypromine Sulfate
Pharmacologic Category Antidepressant, Monoamine Oxidase Inhibitor
Use Treatment of major depressive episode without melancholia
Unlabeled/Investigational Use Post-traumatic stress disorder
Local Anesthetic/Vasoconstrictor Precautions Attempts should be made to avoid use of vasoconstrictor due to possibility of hypertensive episodes with monoamine oxidase inhibitors
Effects on Dental Treatment Key adverse event(s) related to dental treatment: Orthostatic hypotension. Avoid use as an analgesic due to toxic reactions with MAO inhibitors. Xerostomia (normal salivary flow resumes upon discontinuation).
Common Adverse Effects Frequency not defined.
Cardiovascular: Edema, orthostatic hypotension, palpitation, tachycardia
Central nervous system: Agitation, akinesia, anxiety, ataxia, chills, confusion, disorientation, dizziness, drowsiness, fatigue, headache, hyper-reflexia, insomnia, mania, memory loss, restlessness, sleep disturbances, twitching
Dermatologic: Alopecia, cystic acne (flare), pruritus, rash, urticaria, scleroderma (localized)
Endocrine & metabolic: Hypernatremia, hypermetabolic syndrome; sexual dysfunction (anorgasmia, ejaculatory disturbances, impotence); SIADH
Gastrointestinal: Abdominal pain, anorexia, constipation, diarrhea, nausea, vomiting, weight gain, xerostomia
Genitourinary: Incontinence, urinary retention
Hematologic: Agranulocytosis, anemia, leukopenia, thrombocytopenia
Hepatic: Hepatitis
Neuromuscular & skeletal: Akinesis, muscle spasm, myoclonus, numbness, paresthesia, tremor, weakness
Ocular: Blurred vision, glaucoma
Otic: Tinnitus
Miscellaneous: Diaphoresis
Restrictions An FDA-approved medication guide concerning the use of antidepressants in children, adolescents, and young adults must be distributed when dispensing an outpatient prescription (new or refill) where this medication is to be used without direct supervision of a healthcare provider. Medication guides are available at http://www.fda.gov/cder/Offices/ODS/medication_guides.htm. Dispense to parents or guardians of children and adolescents receiving this medication.
Mechanism of Action Tranylcypromine is a nonhydrazine monoamine oxidase inhibitor. It increases endogenous concentrations of epinephrine, norepinephrine, dopamine, and serotonin through inhibition of the enzyme (monoamine oxidase) responsible for the breakdown of these neurotransmitters.
Drug Interactions
Cytochrome P450 Effect: Inhibits CYP1A2 (moderate), 2A6 (strong), 2C8 (weak), 2C9 (weak), 2C19 (moderate), 2D6 (moderate), 2E1 (weak), 3A4 (weak)
Increased Effect/Toxicity: Tranylcypromine may enhance the adverse effects of ethanol (CNS depression), amphetamines (hypertension), general anesthetics (hypotension), atomoxetine (CNS toxicity), buspirone (hypertension), CYP1A2 substrates, CYP2A6 substrates, CYP2C19 substrates, CYP2D6 substrates, dexmethylphenidate (hypertension), disulfiram (delirium), levodopa (hypertension), lithium (CNS toxicity), methylphenidate (hypertension), mirtazapine (CNS toxicity), rauwolfia alkaloids, and thioridazine. Tranylcypromine may enhance the vasopressor effects of alpha-/beta-agonists and enhance the hypertensive effects of alpha$_1$-agonists. Altretamine may enhance the orthostatic effects of tranylcypromine. Anticholinergics may enhance the side effects of tranylcypromine. Concurrent use of anorexiants, cyclobenzaprine, dextromethorphan, meperidine, SSRIs/SNRIs, serotonin 5-HT$_{1D}$ receptor agonist, sibutramine, and tricyclic antidepressants may result in a serotonin syndrome. Concurrent use of bupropion may lead to hypertensive crisis. COMT inhibitors may cause adverse/toxic effects. Pramlintide may increase anticholinergic effects of tranylcypromine. Serotonin modulators may enhance the adverse/toxic effects of tranylcypromine. Tramadol may increase the neuroexcitatory and seizure-potentiating effects of tranylcypromine.
Decreased Effect: Acetylcholinesterase inhibitors decrease tranylcypromine's anticholinergic side effects. Tranylcypromine may decrease the effects (Continued)

Tranylcypromine *(Continued)*

of CYP2D6 prodrug substrates, and false neurotransmitters (guanadrel, methyldopa).

Pharmacodynamics/Kinetics
Onset of action: Therapeutic: 2 days to 3 weeks continued dosing
Half-life elimination: 90-190 minutes
Time to peak, serum: ~2 hours
Excretion: Urine

Pregnancy Risk Factor C

Tranylcypromine Sulfate *see* Tranylcypromine *on page 1601*

Trastuzumab *(tras TU zoo mab)*

U.S. Brand Names Herceptin®
Canadian Brand Names Herceptin®
Mexican Brand Names Herceptin
Generic Available No
Index Terms NSC-688097
Pharmacologic Category Antineoplastic Agent, Monoclonal Antibody; Monoclonal Antibody
Use Treatment of HER-2/*neu* overexpressing metastatic breast cancer; adjuvant treatment of HER-2/*neu* overexpressing node- positive breast cancer
Unlabeled/Investigational Use Treatment of ovarian, gastric, colorectal, endometrial, lung, bladder, prostate, and salivary gland tumors
Local Anesthetic/Vasoconstrictor Precautions No information available to require special precautions
Effects on Dental Treatment No significant effects or complications reported
Common Adverse Effects Note: Percentages reported with single-agent therapy.

>10%:
Central nervous system: Pain (47%), fever (36%), chills (32%), headache (26%), insomnia (14%), dizziness (13%)
Dermatologic: Rash (18%)
Gastrointestinal: Nausea (8% to 33%), diarrhea (25%), vomiting (8% to 23%), abdominal pain (22%), anorexia (14%)
Neuromuscular & skeletal: Weakness (42%), back pain (22%)
Respiratory: Cough (26%), dyspnea (22%), rhinitis (14%), pharyngitis (12%)
Miscellaneous: Infusion reaction (21% to 40%, chills and fever most common; severe: 1%), infection (20%)

1% to 10%:
Cardiovascular: Peripheral edema (10%), edema (8%), CHF (7%), tachycardia (5%)
Central nervous system: Depression (6%)
Dermatologic: Acne (2%)
Genitourinary: Urinary tract infection (5%)
Hematologic: Anemia (4%), leukopenia (3%)
Neuromuscular & skeletal: Paresthesia (9%), bone pain (7%), arthralgia (6%), peripheral neuritis (2%), neuropathy (1%)
Respiratory: Sinusitis (9%)
Miscellaneous: Flu syndrome (10%), accidental injury (6%), allergic reaction (3%), herpes simplex (2%)

Mechanism of Action Trastuzumab is a monoclonal antibody which binds to the extracellular domain of the human epidermal growth factor receptor 2 protein (HER-2); it mediates antibody-dependent cellular cytotoxicity against cells which overproduce HER-2

Drug Interactions
Increased Effect/Toxicity: Paclitaxel may result in a decrease in clearance of trastuzumab, increasing serum concentrations. Combined use with anthracyclines may increase the incidence/severity of cardiac dysfunction. Monoclonal antibodies may increase the risk for allergic reactions to trastuzumab due to the presence of HACA antibodies. Trastuzumab may increase the incidence of neutropenia and/or febrile neutropenia when used in combination with myelosuppressive chemotherapy.

Pharmacodynamics/Kinetics
Distribution: V_d: 44 mL/kg
Half-life elimination: Mean: 5.8 days (range: 1-32 days)

Pregnancy Risk Factor B

Trasylol® *see* Aprotinin *on page 138*
Travatan® *see* Travoprost *on page 1603*
Travatan® Z *see* Travoprost *on page 1603*

Travoprost (TRA voe prost)

U.S. Brand Names Travatan®; Travatan® Z
Canadian Brand Names Travatan®
Mexican Brand Names Travatan
Generic Available No
Pharmacologic Category Ophthalmic Agent, Antiglaucoma; Prostaglandin, Ophthalmic
Use Reduction of elevated intraocular pressure in patients with open-angle glaucoma or ocular hypertension who are intolerant of the other IOP-lowering medications or insufficiently responsive (failed to achieve target IOP determined after multiple measurements over time) to another IOP-lowering medication
Local Anesthetic/Vasoconstrictor Precautions No significant effects or complications reported
Effects on Dental Treatment No information available to require special precautions
Mechanism of Action A selective FP prostanoid receptor agonist which lowers intraocular pressure by increasing trabecular meshwork and outflow
Pregnancy Risk Factor C

Trazodone (TRAZ oh done)

Related Information
Sedation *on page 1825*
U.S. Brand Names Desyrel® [DSC]
Canadian Brand Names Alti-Trazodone; Apo-Trazodone®; Apo-Trazodone D®; Desyrel®; Gen-Trazodone; Novo-Trazodone; Nu-Trazodone; PMS-Trazodone; ratio-Trazodone; Trazorel®
Generic Available Yes
Index Terms Trazodone Hydrochloride
Pharmacologic Category Antidepressant, Serotonin Reuptake Inhibitor/Antagonist
Use Treatment of depression
Unlabeled/Investigational Use Potential augmenting agent for antidepressants, hypnotic
Local Anesthetic/Vasoconstrictor Precautions Trazodone inhibits reuptake of both serotonin and norepinephrine and also blocks some serotonin receptors. No precautions with vasoconstrictors appear to be necessary.
Effects on Dental Treatment Key adverse event(s) related to dental treatment: Significant xerostomia (normal salivary flow resumes upon discontinuation).
Common Adverse Effects
>10%:
  Central nervous system: Dizziness, headache, sedation
  Gastrointestinal: Nausea, xerostomia
  Ocular: Blurred vision
1% to 10%:
  Cardiovascular: Syncope, hyper-/hypotension, edema
  Central nervous system: Confusion, decreased concentration, fatigue, incoordination
  Gastrointestinal: Diarrhea, constipation, weight gain/loss
  Neuromuscular & skeletal: Tremor, myalgia
  Respiratory: Nasal congestion
Restrictions An FDA-approved medication guide concerning the use of antidepressants in children, adolescents, and young adults must be distributed when dispensing an outpatient prescription (new or refill) where this medication is to be used without direct supervision of a healthcare provider. Medication guides are available at http://www.fda.gov/cder/Offices/ODS/medication_guides.htm. Dispense to parents or guardians of children and adolescents receiving this medication.
Dosage Oral: Therapeutic effects may take up to 6 weeks to occur; therapy is normally maintained for 6-12 months after optimum response is reached to prevent recurrence of depression

Children 6-12 years: Depression (unlabeled use): Initial: 1.5-2 mg/kg/day in divided doses; increase gradually every 3-4 days as needed; maximum: 6 mg/kg/day in 3 divided doses
Adolescents: Depression (unlabeled use): Initial: 25-50 mg/day; increase to 100-150 mg/day in divided doses
(Continued)

Trazodone *(Continued)*

Adults:

Depression: Initial: 150 mg/day in 3 divided doses (may increase by 50 mg/day every 3-7 days); maximum: 600 mg/day

Sedation/hypnotic (unlabeled use): 25-50 mg at bedtime (often in combination with daytime SSRIs); may increase up to 200 mg at bedtime

Elderly: 25-50 mg at bedtime with 25-50 mg/day dose increase every 3 days for inpatients and weekly for outpatients, if tolerated; usual dose: 75-150 mg/day

Mechanism of Action Inhibits reuptake of serotonin, causes adrenoreceptor subsensitivity, and induces significant changes in 5-HT presynaptic receptor adrenoreceptors. Trazodone also significantly blocks histamine (H_1) and alpha$_1$-adrenergic receptors.

Contraindications Hypersensitivity to trazodone or any component of the formulation

Warnings/Precautions [U.S. Boxed Warning]: Antidepressants increase the risk of suicidal thinking and behavior in children, adolescents, and young adults (18-24 years of age) with major depressive disorder (MDD) and other psychiatric disorders; consider risk prior to prescribing. Short-term studies did not show an increased risk in patients >24 years of age and showed a decreased risk in patients ≥65 years. Closely monitor for clinical worsening, suicidality, or unusual changes in behavior; the patient's family or caregiver should be instructed to closely observe the patient and communicate condition with healthcare provider. A medication guide should be dispensed with each prescription. **Trazodone is not FDA approved for use in children.**

The possibility of a suicide attempt is inherent in major depression and may persist until remission occurs. Monitor for worsening of depression or suicidality, especially during initiation of therapy (generally first 1-2 months) or with dose increases or decreases. Use caution in high-risk patients. Worsening depression and severe abrupt suicidality that are not part of the presenting symptoms may require discontinuation or modification of drug therapy. The patient's family or caregiver should be alerted to monitor patients for the emergence of suicidality and associated behaviors (such as agitation, irritability, hostility, impulsivity, and hypomania) and call healthcare provider.

May worsen psychosis in some patients or precipitate a shift to mania or hypomania in patients with bipolar disorder. Patients presenting with depressive symptoms should be screened for bipolar disorder. Monotherapy in patients with bipolar disorder should be avoided. **Trazodone is not FDA approved for the treatment of bipolar depression.**

Priapism, including cases resulting in permanent dysfunction, has occurred with the use of trazodone. Not recommended for use in a patient during the acute recovery phase of MI. Trazodone should be initiated with caution in patients who are receiving concurrent or recent therapy with a MAO inhibitor.

The risks of sedation and/or postural hypotension are high relative to other antidepressants. Trazodone frequently causes sedation, which may result in impaired performance of tasks requiring alertness (eg, operating machinery or driving). Sedative effects may be additive with other CNS depressants and ethanol. Use with caution in patients with a history of cardiovascular disease (including previous MI, stroke, tachycardia, or conduction abnormalities). The risk of conduction abnormalities with this agent is low relative to other antidepressants.

Consider discontinuing, when possible, prior to elective surgery. Therapy should not be abruptly discontinued in patients receiving high doses for prolonged periods. Use caution in patients with a previous seizure disorder or condition predisposing to seizures such as brain damage, alcoholism, or concurrent therapy with other drugs which lower the seizure threshold. Use with caution in patients with hepatic or renal dysfunction and in elderly patients.

Drug Interactions

Cytochrome P450 Effect: Substrate of CYP2D6 (minor), 3A4 (major); **Inhibits** CYP2D6 (moderate), 3A4 (weak)

Increased Effect/Toxicity: Sedative effects may be additive with other CNS depressants. Trazodone, in combination with other serotonergic agents (buspirone, MAO inhibitors), may produce additive serotonergic effects, including serotonin syndrome. Trazodone, in combination with other psychotropics (low potency antipsychotics), may result in additional hypotension. Fluoxetine may inhibit the metabolism of trazodone resulting in elevated plasma levels.

Trazodone may increase the levels/effects of amphetamines, beta-blockers, dextromethorphan, fluoxetine, lidocaine, mirtazapine, nefazodone, paroxetine, risperidone, ritonavir, thioridazine, tricyclic antidepressants, venlafaxine, and other CYP2D6 substrates. The levels/effects of trazodone may be increased by azole antifungals, clarithromycin, diclofenac, doxycycline, erythromycin, imatinib, isoniazid, nefazodone, nicardipine, propofol, protease inhibitors, quinidine, telithromycin, verapamil, and other CYP3A4 inhibitors.

Decreased Effect: Trazodone inhibits the hypotensive response to clonidine. The levels/effects of trazodone may be decreased by aminoglutethimide, carbamazepine, nafcillin, nevirapine, phenobarbital, phenytoin, rifamycins, and other CYP3A4 inducers. Trazodone may decrease the levels/effects of CYP2D6 prodrug substrates (eg, codeine, hydrocodone, oxycodone, tramadol).

Ethanol/Nutrition/Herb Interactions
Ethanol: Avoid ethanol (may increase CNS depression).
Food: Time to peak serum levels may be increased if trazodone is taken with food.
Herb/Nutraceutical: Avoid valerian, St John's wort, SAMe, kava kava (may increase risk of serotonin syndrome and/or excessive sedation).

Pharmacodynamics/Kinetics
Onset of action: Therapeutic (antidepressant): 1-3 weeks; sleep aid: 1-3 hours
Protein binding: 85% to 95%
Metabolism: Hepatic via CYP3A4 to an active metabolite (mCPP)
Half-life elimination: 7-8 hours, two compartment kinetics
Time to peak, serum: 30-100 minutes; delayed with food (up to 2.5 hours)
Excretion: Primarily urine; secondarily feces

Pregnancy Risk Factor C
Dosage Forms Tablet: 50 mg, 100 mg, 150 mg, 300 mg

Treprostinil (tre PROST in il)

U.S. Brand Names Remodulin®
Canadian Brand Names Remodulin®
Generic Available No
Index Terms Treprostinil Sodium
Pharmacologic Category Vasodilator
Use Treatment of pulmonary arterial hypertension (PAH) in patients with NYHA Class II-IV symptoms to decrease exercise-associated symptoms; to diminish clinical deterioration when transitioning from epoprostenol (I.V.)
Local Anesthetic/Vasoconstrictor Precautions No information available to require special precautions
Effects on Dental Treatment No significant effects or complications reported
Common Adverse Effects
>10%:
Cardiovascular: Vasodilation (11%)
Central nervous system: Headache (27%)
Dermatologic: Rash (14%)
Gastrointestinal: Diarrhea (25%), nausea (22%)
Local: Infusion site pain (SubQ 85%, may improve after several months of therapy); infusion site reaction (SubQ 83%)
Miscellaneous: Jaw pain (13%)
1% to 10%:
Cardiovascular: Edema (9%), hypotension (4%)
Central nervous system: Dizziness (9%)
Dermatologic: Pruritus (8%)
Mechanism of Action Treprostinil is a direct dilator of both pulmonary and systemic arterial vascular beds; also inhibits platelet aggregation.
Drug Interactions
Increased Effect/Toxicity: Concomitant use of treprostinil with other agents that inhibit platelet aggregation (eg, NSAIDs, ASA, antiplatelet agents, salicylates) or promote anticoagulation (eg, warfarin) may increase the risk of bleeding.
Pharmacodynamics/Kinetics
Absorption: SubQ: Rapidly and completely
Distribution: 14 L/70 kg lean body weight
Protein binding: 91%
Metabolism: Hepatic (enzymes unknown); forms metabolites
Bioavailability: 100%
Half-life elimination: Terminal: 2-4 hours
(Continued)

Treprostinil *(Continued)*

Excretion: Urine (79% - 4% as unchanged drug, 64% as metabolites); feces (13%)

Pregnancy Risk Factor B

Treprostinil Sodium *see* Treprostinil *on page 1605*

Tretinoin and Clindamycin *see* Clindamycin and Tretinoin *on page 382*

Tretinoin and Mequinol *see* Mequinol and Tretinoin *on page 1050*

Tretinoin, Fluocinolone Acetonide, and Hydroquinone *see* Fluocinolone, Hydroquinone, and Tretinoin *on page 708*

Tretinoin (Oral) (TRET i noyn, oral)

U.S. Brand Names Vesanoid®
Canadian Brand Names Vesanoid®
Generic Available No
Index Terms All-*trans*-Retinoic Acid; ATRA; NSC-122758; Ro 5488; tRA; *trans*-Retinoic Acid
Pharmacologic Category Antineoplastic Agent, Miscellaneous
Use Induction of remission in patients with acute promyelocytic leukemia (APL), French American British (FAB) classification M3 (including the M3 variant)
Local Anesthetic/Vasoconstrictor Precautions No information available to require special precautions
Effects on Dental Treatment Key adverse event(s) related to dental treatment: Xerostomia (normal salivary flow resumes upon discontinuation).
Common Adverse Effects Virtually all patients experience some drug-related toxicity, especially headache, fever, weakness and fatigue. These adverse effects are seldom permanent or irreversible nor do they usually require therapy interruption.

>10%:
Cardiovascular: Peripheral edema (52%), chest discomfort (32%), edema (29%), arrhythmias (23%), flushing (23%), hypotension (14%), hypertension (11%)

Central nervous system: Headache (86%), fever (83%), malaise (66%), pain (37%), dizziness (20%), anxiety (17%), insomnia (14%), depression (14%), confusion (11%)

Dermatologic: Skin/mucous membrane dryness (77%), pruritus (20%), rash (54%), alopecia (14%)

Endocrine & metabolic: Hypercholesterolemia and/or hypertriglyceridemia (60%)

Gastrointestinal: Nausea/vomiting (57%), liver function tests increased (50% to 60%), GI hemorrhage (34%), abdominal pain (31%), mucositis (26%), diarrhea (23%), constipation (17%), dyspepsia (14%), abdominal distention (11%), weight gain (23%), weight loss (17%), xerostomia, anorexia (17%)

Hematologic: Hemorrhage (60%), leukocytosis (40%), disseminated intravascular coagulation (DIC) (26%)

Local: Phlebitis (11%), injection site reactions (17%)

Neuromuscular & skeletal: Bone pain (77%), myalgia (14%), paresthesia (17%)

Ocular: Visual disturbances (17%)

Otic: Earache/ear fullness (23%)

Renal: Renal insufficiency (11%)

Respiratory: Upper respiratory tract disorders (63%), dyspnea (60%), respiratory insufficiency (26%), pleural effusion (20%), pneumonia (14%), rales (14%), expiratory wheezing (14%), dry nose

Miscellaneous: Infection (58%), shivering (63%), retinoic acid-acute promyelocytic leukemia syndrome (25%), diaphoresis increased (20%)

1% to 10%:
Cardiovascular: Cerebral hemorrhage (9%), pallor (6%), cardiac failure (6%), cardiac arrest (3%), MI (3%), enlarged heart (3%), heart murmur (3%), ischemia, stroke (3%), myocarditis (3%), pericarditis (3%), pulmonary hypertension (3%), secondary cardiomyopathy (3%)

Central nervous system: Intracranial hypertension (9%), agitation (9%), hallucination (6%), agnosia (3%), aphasia (3%), cerebellar edema (3%), cerebral hemorrhage (9%), seizure (3%), coma (3%), CNS depression (3%), dysarthria (3%), encephalopathy (3%), hypotaxia (3%), light reflex absent (3%), spinal cord disorder (3%), unconsciousness (3%), dementia (3%), forgetfulness (3%), somnolence (3%), slow speech (3%), hypothermia (3%)

Dermatologic: Cellulitis (8%), photosensitivity

Endocrine & metabolic: Acidosis (3%)

Gastrointestinal: Hepatosplenomegaly (9%), hepatitis (3%), ulcer (3%)

Genitourinary: Dysuria (9%), acute renal failure (3%), micturition frequency (3%), renal tubular necrosis (3%), enlarged prostate (3%)

Hepatic: Ascites (3%), hepatitis

Neuromuscular & skeletal: Tremor (3%), leg weakness (3%), hyporeflexia, dysarthria, facial paralysis, hemiplegia, flank pain, asterixis, abnormal gait (3%), bone inflammation (3%)

Ocular: Dry eyes, visual acuity change (6%), visual field deficit (3%)

Otic: Hearing loss

Renal: Acute renal failure, renal tubular necrosis

Respiratory: Lower respiratory tract disorders (9%), pulmonary infiltration (6%), bronchial asthma (3%), pulmonary/larynx edema

Miscellaneous: Face edema

Mechanism of Action Tretinoin appears to bind one or more nuclear receptors and inhibits clonal proliferation and/or granulocyte differentiation

Drug Interactions

Cytochrome P450 Effect: Substrate (minor) of CYP2A6 (minor), 2B6 (minor), 2C8 (major), 2C9 (minor); **Inhibits** CYP2C9 (weak); **Induces** CYP2E1 (weak)

Increased Effect/Toxicity: Ketoconazole increases the mean plasma AUC of tretinoin. Concurrent use with antifibrinolytic agents (eg, aminocaproic acid, aprotinin, tranexamic acid) may increase risk of thrombosis. Concurrent use with tetracyclines may increase risk of pseudotumor cerebri. CYP2C8 Inhibitors may increase the levels/effects of tretinoin; example inhibitors include atazanavir, gemfibrozil, and ritonavir.

Pharmacodynamics/Kinetics

Protein binding: >95%

Metabolism: Hepatic via CYP; primary metabolite: 4-oxo-all-*trans*-retinoic acid

Half-life elimination: Terminal: Parent drug: 0.5-2 hours

Time to peak, serum: 1-2 hours

Excretion: Urine (63%); feces (30%)

Pregnancy Risk Factor D

Tretinoin (Topical) (TRET i noyn, TOP i kal)

U.S. Brand Names Avita®; Renova®; Retin-A®; Retin-A® Micro

Canadian Brand Names Rejuva-A®; Retin-A®; Retin-A® Micro; Retinova®

Generic Available Yes: Cream, gel

Index Terms Retinoic Acid; *trans*-Retinoic Acid; Vitamin A Acid

Pharmacologic Category Acne Products; Retinoic Acid Derivative; Topical Skin Product, Acne

Use Treatment of acne vulgaris; photodamaged skin; palliation of fine wrinkles, mottled hyperpigmentation, and tactile roughness of facial skin as part of a comprehensive skin care and sun avoidance program

Unlabeled/Investigational Use Some skin cancers

Local Anesthetic/Vasoconstrictor Precautions No information available to require special precautions

Effects on Dental Treatment No significant effects or complications reported

Common Adverse Effects

>10%: Dermatologic: Excessive dryness, erythema, scaling of the skin, pruritus

1% to 10%:

Dermatologic: Hyperpigmentation or hypopigmentation, photosensitivity, initial acne flare-up

Local: Edema, blistering, stinging

Mechanism of Action Keratinocytes in the sebaceous follicle become less adherent which allows for easy removal; inhibits microcomedone formation and eliminates lesions already present

Drug Interactions

Cytochrome P450 Effect: Substrate of CYP2A6 (minor), 2B6 (minor), 2C8 (major), 2C9 (minor); **Inhibits** CYP2C9 (weak); **Induces** CYP2E1 (weak)

Increased Effect/Toxicity: Topical application of sulfur, benzoyl peroxide, salicylic acid, resorcinol, or any product with strong drying effects potentiates adverse reactions with tretinoin.

Photosensitizing medications (thiazides, tetracyclines, fluoroquinolones, phenothiazines, sulfonamides) augment phototoxicity and should not be used when treating palliation of fine wrinkles, mottled hyperpigmentation, and tactile roughness of facial skin.

Pharmacodynamics/Kinetics

Absorption: Minimal

Metabolism: Hepatic for the small amount absorbed

Excretion: Urine and feces

Pregnancy Risk Factor C

Trexall™ *see* Methotrexate *on page 1068*
TRH *see* Protirelin *on page 1379*

Triacetin (trye a SEE tin)

U.S. Brand Names Myco-Nail [OTC]
Generic Available No
Index Terms Glycerol Triacetate
Pharmacologic Category Antifungal Agent, Topical
Use Fungistat for athlete's foot and other superficial fungal infections
Local Anesthetic/Vasoconstrictor Precautions No information available to require special precautions
Effects on Dental Treatment No significant effects or complications reported

Triacin-C® [DSC] *see* Triprolidine, Pseudoephedrine, and Codeine *on page 1624*
Triaconazole *see* Terconazole *on page 1541*

Triamcinolone (trye am SIN oh lone)

Related Information
  Respiratory Diseases *on page 1747*
  Ulcerative and Erosive Disorders *on page 1809*
Related Sample Prescriptions
  Mild Lichen Planus *on page 1845*
  Recurrent Aphthous Stomatitis *on page 1844*
U.S. Brand Names Aristocort® [DSC]; Aristocort® A [DSC]; Aristospan®; Azmacort®; Kenalog®; Kenalog-10®; Kenalog-40®; Nasacort® AQ; Triderm®; Tri-Nasal®
Canadian Brand Names Aristospan®; Kenalog®; Kenalog® in Orabase; Nasacort® AQ; Oracort; Triaderm; Trinasal®
Generic Available Yes: Cream, lotion, ointment, paste
Index Terms Triamcinolone Acetonide, Aerosol; Triamcinolone Acetonide, Parenteral; Triamcinolone Diacetate, Oral; Triamcinolone Diacetate, Parenteral; Triamcinolone Hexacetonide; Triamcinolone, Oral
Pharmacologic Category Corticosteroid, Adrenal; Corticosteroid, Inhalant (Oral); Corticosteroid, Nasal; Corticosteroid, Systemic; Corticosteroid, Topical
Dental Use Oral, topical: Adjunctive treatment and temporary relief of symptoms associated with oral inflammatory lesions and ulcerative lesions resulting from trauma
Use
  Nasal inhalation: Management of seasonal and perennial allergic rhinitis in patients ≥6 years of age
  Oral inhalation: Control of bronchial asthma and related bronchospastic conditions
  Oral topical: Adjunctive treatment and temporary relief of symptoms associated with oral inflammatory lesions and ulcerative lesions resulting from trauma
  Systemic: Adrenocortical insufficiency, rheumatic disorders, allergic states, respiratory diseases, systemic lupus erythematosus (SLE), and other diseases requiring anti-inflammatory or immunosuppressive effects
  Topical: Inflammatory dermatoses responsive to steroids
Local Anesthetic/Vasoconstrictor Precautions No information available to require special precautions
Effects on Dental Treatment Key adverse event(s) related to dental treatment: Ulcerative esophagitis, perioral dermatitis, atrophy of oral mucosa, burning, irritation, and oral monilia (oral inhaler).
Significant Adverse Effects
  Systemic: Frequency not defined:
    Cardiovascular: Angioedema, bradycardia, CHF, hypertension, myocardial rupture (following recent MI), thrombophlebitis, vasculitis
    Central nervous system: Convulsions, depression, emotional instability, fever, headache, intracranial pressure increased, neuropathy, paresthesia, personality changes, vertigo
    Dermatologic: Acne, allergic dermatitis, bruising, cutaneous atrophy, dry/scaly skin, ecchymoses, facial erythema, petechiae, photosensitivity, rash, striae, thin/fragile skin, wound healing impaired
    Endocrine & metabolic: Adrenocortical/pituitary unresponsiveness (particularly during stress), carbohydrate tolerance decreased, cushingoid state, diabetes mellitus (manifestations of latent disease), fluid retention, growth suppression (children), hirsutism, hypokalemic alkalosis, menstrual irregularities, negative nitrogen balance, potassium loss, sodium retention

Gastrointestinal: Abdominal distention, bowel perforation, diarrhea, dyspepsia, nausea, oral *Monilia* (oral inhaler), pancreatitis, peptic ulcer, ulcerative esophagitis, weight gain

Hepatic: Hepatomegaly

Local: Skin atrophy (at the injection site)

Neuromuscular & skeletal: Calcinosis (following intra-articular or intralesional injection), Charcot-like arthropathy, femoral/humeral head aseptic necrosis, muscle mass decreased, muscle weakness, osteoporosis, pathologic fracture of long bones, steroid myopathy, tendon rupture, vertebral compression fractures

Ocular: Blindness (periocular injections), cataracts, intraocular pressure increased, exophthalmos, glaucoma, subcapsular cataract

Respiratory: Cough increased (nasal spray), epistaxis (nasal inhaler/spray), pharyngitis (nasal spray/oral inhaler), sinusitis (oral inhaler), voice alteration (oral inhaler)

Miscellaneous: Abnormal fat deposition (moon face), anaphylactoid reaction, anaphylaxis, diaphoresis increased, suppression to skin tests

Topical: Frequency not defined:

Dermatologic: Itching, allergic contact dermatitis, dryness, folliculitis, skin infection (secondary), itching, hypertrichosis, acneiform eruptions, hypopigmentation, skin maceration, skin atrophy, striae, miliaria, perioral dermatitis, atrophy of oral mucosa

Local: Burning, irritation

Dental Usual Dosing Oral inflammatory lesions/ulcers: Adults: Oral topical: Press a small dab (about 1/4 inch) to the lesion until a thin film develops; a larger quantity may be required for coverage of some lesions. For optimal results, use only enough to coat the lesion with a thin film; do not rub in.

Dosage The lowest possible dose should be used to control the condition; when dose reduction is possible, the dose should be reduced gradually. Parenteral dose is usually 1/3 to 1/2 the oral dose given every 12 hours. In life-threatening situations, parenteral doses larger than the oral dose may be needed.

Injection:

Acetonide:

Intra-articular, intrabursal, tendon sheaths: Adults: Initial: Smaller joints: 2.5-5 mg, larger joints: 5-15 mg

Intradermal: Adults: Initial: 1 mg

I.M.: Range: 2.5-60 mg/day

Children 6-12 years: Initial: 40 mg

Children >12 years and Adults: Initial: 60 mg

Hexacetonide: Adults:

Intralesional, sublesional: Up to 0.5 mg/square inch of affected skin

Intra-articular: Range: 2-20 mg

Triamcinolone Dosing

	Acetonide	Hexacetonide
Intrasynovial	5-40 mg	
Intralesional	1-30 mg (usually 1 mg per injection site); 10 mg/mL suspension usually used	Up to 0.5 mg/sq inch affected area
Sublesional	1-30 mg	
Systemic I.M.	2.5-60 mg/dose (usual adult dose: 60 mg; may repeat with 20-100 mg dose when symptoms recur)	
Intra-articular	2.5-40 mg	2-20 mg average
large joints	5-15 mg	10-20 mg
small joints	2.5-5 mg	2-6 mg
Tendon sheaths	2.5-10 mg	
Intradermal	1 mg/site	

Intranasal: Perennial allergic rhinitis, seasonal allergic rhinitis:

Nasal spray:

Children 6-11 years: 110 mcg/day as 1 spray in each nostril once daily.

Children ≥12 years and Adults: 220 mcg/day as 2 sprays in each nostril once daily

(Continued)

Triamcinolone *(Continued)*

Nasal inhaler:
Children 6-11 years: Initial: 220 mcg/day as 2 sprays in each nostril once daily

Children ≥12 years and Adults: Initial: 220 mcg/day as 2 sprays in each nostril once daily; may increase dose to 440 mcg/day (given once daily or divided and given 2 or 4 times/day)

Oral: Adults:
Acute rheumatic carditis: Initial: 20-60 mg/day; reduce dose during maintenance therapy

Acute seasonal or perennial allergic rhinitis: 8-12 mg/day

Adrenocortical insufficiency: Range 4-12 mg/day

Bronchial asthma: 8-16 mg/day

Dermatological disorders, contact/atopic dermatitis: Initial: 8-16 mg/day

Ophthalmic disorders: 12-40 mg/day

Rheumatic disorders: Range: 8-16 mg/day

SLE: Initial: 20-32 mg/day, some patients may need initial doses ≥48 mg; reduce dose during maintenance therapy

Oral inhalation: Asthma:
Children 6-12 years: 100-200 mcg 3-4 times/day **or** 200-400 mcg twice daily; maximum dose: 1200 mcg/day

Children >12 years and Adults: 200 mcg 3-4 times/day **or** 400 mcg twice daily; maximum dose: 1600 mcg/day

Oral topical: Oral inflammatory lesions/ulcers: Press a small dab (about ¼ inch) to the lesion until a thin film develops. A larger quantity may be required for coverage of some lesions. For optimal results use only enough to coat the lesion with a thin film; do not rub in.

Topical:
Cream, Ointment: Apply thin film to affected areas 2-4 times/day
Spray: Apply to affected area 3-4 times/day

Mechanism of Action Decreases inflammation by suppression of migration of polymorphonuclear leukocytes and reversal of increased capillary permeability; suppresses the immune system by reducing activity and volume of the lymphatic system; suppresses adrenal function at high doses

Contraindications Hypersensitivity to triamcinolone or any component of the formulation; systemic fungal infections; serious infections (except septic shock or tuberculous meningitis); primary treatment of status asthmaticus; fungal, viral, or bacterial infections of the mouth or throat (oral topical formulation)

Warnings/Precautions May cause hypercorticism or suppression of hypothalamic-pituitary-adrenal (HPA) axis, particularly in younger children or in patients receiving high doses for prolonged periods. HPA axis suppression may lead to adrenal crisis. Withdrawal and discontinuation of a corticosteroid should be done slowly and carefully. Particular care is required when patients are transferred from systemic corticosteroids to inhaled products due to possible adrenal insufficiency or withdrawal from steroids, including an increase in allergic symptoms. Patients receiving >20 mg per day of prednisone (or equivalent) may be most susceptible. Fatalities have occurred due to adrenal insufficiency in asthmatic patients during and after transfer from systemic corticosteroids to aerosol steroids; aerosol steroids do not provide the systemic steroid needed to treat patients having trauma, surgery, or infections.

Bronchospasm may occur with wheezing after inhalation; if this occurs stop steroid and treat with a fast-acting bronchodilator. Supplemental steroids (oral or parenteral) may be needed during stress or severe asthma attacks. Not to be used in status asthmaticus or for the relief of acute bronchospasm. Acute myopathy has been reported with high dose corticosteroids, usually in patients with neuromuscular transmission disorders; may involve ocular and/or respiratory muscles; monitor creatine kinase; recovery may be delayed. Corticosteroid use may cause psychiatric disturbances, including depression, euphoria, insomnia, mood swings, and personality changes. Pre-existing psychiatric conditions may be exacerbated by corticosteroid use. Prolonged use of corticosteroids may also increase the incidence of secondary infection, mask acute infection (including fungal infections), prolong or exacerbate viral infections, or limit response to vaccines. Exposure to chickenpox should be avoided; corticosteroids should not be used to treat ocular herpes simplex. Corticosteroids should not be used for cerebral malaria. Close observation is required in patients with latent tuberculosis and/or TB reactivity; restrict use in active TB (only in conjunction with antituberculosis treatment). Prolonged treatment with corticosteroids has been associated with the development of Kaposi's sarcoma (case reports); if noted, discontinuation of therapy should be considered.

Use with caution in patients with thyroid disease, hepatic impairment, renal impairment, cardiovascular disease, diabetes, glaucoma, cataracts, myasthenia gravis, patients at risk for osteoporosis, patients at risk for seizures, or GI diseases (diverticulitis, peptic ulcer, ulcerative colitis) due to perforation risk. Use caution following acute MI (corticosteroids have been associated with myocardial rupture). Because of the risk of adverse effects, systemic corticosteroids should be used cautiously in the elderly in the smallest possible effective dose for the shortest duration. Azmacort® (metered dose inhaler) comes with its own spacer device attached and may be easier to use in older patients. Avoid nasal corticosteroid use in patients with recent nasal septal ulcers, nasal surgery or nasal trauma until healing has occurred. Do not use occlusive dressings on weeping or exudative lesions and general caution with occlusive dressings should be observed; discontinue if skin irritation or contact dermatitis should occur; do not use in patients with decreased skin circulation; avoid the use of high potency steroids on the face.

Intravitreal injection has been associated with endophthalmitis and visual disturbances. Blindness has been reported following injection into nasal turbinates and intralesional injections into the head. Safety of intraturbinal, subconjunctival, subtenons, retrobulbar, or intravitreal injection has not been demonstrated.

Orally-inhaled and intranasal corticosteroids may cause a reduction in growth velocity in pediatric patients (~1 centimeter per year [range 0.3-1.8 cm per year] and related to dose and duration of exposure). To minimize the systemic effects of orally-inhaled and intranasal corticosteroids, each patient should be titrated to the lowest effective dose. Growth should be routinely monitored in pediatric patients. Withdraw systemic therapy with gradual tapering of dose. There have been reports of systemic corticosteroid withdrawal symptoms (eg, joint/muscle pain, lassitude, depression) when withdrawing oral inhalation therapy. Injection suspension contains benzyl alcohol; benzyl alcohol has been associated with the "gasping syndrome" in neonates and low-birth-weight infants.

Oral topical: Discontinue if local irritation or sensitization should develop. If significant regeneration or repair of oral tissues has not occurred in seven days, re-evaluation of the etiology of the oral lesion is advised.

Drug Interactions

Decreased effect: Barbiturates, phenytoin, rifampin increase metabolism of triamcinolone; vaccine and toxoid effects may be reduced

Increased effect: Salmeterol: The addition of salmeterol has been demonstrated to improve response to inhaled corticosteroids (as compared to increasing steroid dosage).

Increased toxicity: Salicylates may increase risk of GI ulceration

Ethanol/Nutrition/Herb Interactions

Ethanol: Avoid ethanol (may enhance gastric mucosal irritation).

Food: Triamcinolone interferes with calcium absorption.

Herb/Nutraceutical: Avoid cat's claw, echinacea (have immunostimulant properties).

Dietary Considerations May be taken with food to decrease GI distress.

Pharmacodynamics/Kinetics

Duration: Oral: 8-12 hours

Absorption: Topical: Systemic

Time to peak: I.M.: 8-10 hours

Half-life elimination: Biologic: 18-36 hours

Pregnancy Risk Factor C

Lactation Excretion in breast milk unknown/use caution

Breast-Feeding Considerations It is not known if triamcinolone is excreted in breast milk, however, other corticosteroids are excreted. Prednisone and prednisolone are excreted in breast milk; the AAP considers them to be "usually compatible" with breast-feeding. Hypertension was reported in a nursing infant when a topical corticosteroid was applied to the nipples of the mother.

Dosage Forms Excipient information presented when available (limited, particularly for generics); consult specific product labeling. [DSC] = Discontinued product

Aerosol for oral inhalation, as acetonide:

Azmacort®: 100 mcg per actuation (20 g) [240 actuations]

Aerosol, topical, as acetonide:

Kenalog®: 0.2 mg/2-second spray (63 g)

Cream, as acetonide: 0.025% (15 g, 80 g, 454 g); 0.1% (15 g, 80 g, 454 g, 2270 g); 0.5% (15 g)

Aristocort® A: 0.025% (15 g, 60 g); 0.1% (15 g, 60 g); 0.5% (15 g) [DSC]

Triderm®: 0.1% (30 g, 85 g)

Injection, suspension, as acetonide:

Kenalog-10®: 10 mg/mL (5 mL) [contains benzyl alcohol; not for I.V. or I.M. use]

Kenalog-40®: 40 mg/mL (1 mL, 5 mL, 10 mL) [contains benzyl alcohol; not for I.V. or intradermal use]

(Continued)

Triamcinolone *(Continued)*

Injection, suspension, as hexacetonide:
Aristospan®: 5 mg/mL (5 mL); 20 mg/mL (1 mL, 5 mL) [contains benzyl alcohol; not for I.V. use]
Lotion, as acetonide: 0.025% (60 mL); 0.1% (60 mL)
Ointment, topical, as acetonide: 0.025% (15 g, 80 g, 454 g); 0.1% (15 g, 80 g, 454 g); 0.5% (15 g)
Aristocort® A: 0.1% (15 g, 60 g) [DSC]
Paste, oral, topical, as acetonide: 0.1% (5 g)
Solution, intranasal, as acetonide [spray]:
Tri-Nasal®: 50 mcg/inhalation (15 mL) [120 actuations]
Suspension, intranasal, as acetonide [spray]:
Nasacort® AQ: 55 mcg/inhalation (16.5 g) [120 actuations]
Tablet:
Aristocort®: 4 mg [DSC]

Triamcinolone Acetonide, Aerosol *see* Triamcinolone *on page 1608*

Triamcinolone Acetonide (Dental Paste)
(trye am SIN oh lone a SEE toe nide paste)

Related Information
Triamcinolone *on page 1608*
Canadian Brand Names Oracort®
Generic Available Yes
Pharmacologic Category Anti-inflammatory Agent; Corticosteroid, Topical
Dental Use For adjunctive treatment and for the temporary relief of symptoms associated with oral inflammatory lesions and ulcerative lesions resulting from trauma
Local Anesthetic/Vasoconstrictor Precautions No information available to require special precautions
Effects on Dental Treatment No significant effects or complications reported
Significant Adverse Effects No data reported
Dental Usual Dosing Oral inflammatory lesions/ulcers: Adults: Topical: Press a small dab (about 1/4 inch) to the lesion until a thin film develops. A larger quantity may be required for coverage of some lesions. For optimal results use only enough to coat the lesion with a thin film.
Dosage Press a small dab (about 1/4 inch) to the lesion until a thin film develops. A larger quantity may be required for coverage of some lesions. For optimal results use only enough to coat the lesion with a thin film.
Mechanism of Action Decreases inflammation by suppression of migration of polymorphonuclear leukocytes and reversal of increased capillary permeability; suppresses the immune system by reducing activity and volume of the lymphatic system; suppresses adrenal function at high doses
Contraindications Hypersensitivity to triamcinolone or any component of the formulation; contraindicated in the presence of fungal, viral, or bacterial infections of the mouth or throat
Warnings/Precautions Patients with tuberculosis, peptic ulcer or diabetes mellitus should not be treated with any corticosteroid preparation without the advice of the patient's physician. Normal immune responses of the oral tissues are depressed in patients receiving topical corticosteroid therapy. Virulent strains of oral microorganisms may multiply without producing the usual warning symptoms of oral infections. The small amount of steroid released from the topical preparation makes systemic effects very unlikely. If local irritation or sensitization should develop, the preparation should be discontinued. If significant regeneration or repair of oral tissues has not occurred in seven days, re-evaluation of the etiology of the oral lesion is advised.
Drug Interactions No data reported
Pharmacodynamics/Kinetics
Absorption: Systemic
Half-life elimination, serum: Biological: 18-36 hours
Pregnancy Risk Factor C
Dosage Forms Excipient information presented when available (limited, particularly for generics); consult specific product labeling.
Paste, oral, topical, as acetonide: 0.1% (5 g)

Triamcinolone Acetonide, Parenteral *see* Triamcinolone *on page 1608*
Triamcinolone and Nystatin *see* Nystatin and Triamcinolone *on page 1196*
Triamcinolone Diacetate, Oral *see* Triamcinolone *on page 1608*
Triamcinolone Diacetate, Parenteral *see* Triamcinolone *on page 1608*
Triamcinolone Hexacetonide *see* Triamcinolone *on page 1608*
Triamcinolone, Oral *see* Triamcinolone *on page 1608*

Triamterene (trye AM ter een)

Related Information
Cardiovascular Diseases *on page 1726*
U.S. Brand Names Dyrenium®
Generic Available No
Pharmacologic Category Diuretic, Potassium-Sparing
Use Alone or in combination with other diuretics in treatment of edema and hypertension; decreases potassium excretion caused by kaliuretic diuretics
Local Anesthetic/Vasoconstrictor Precautions No information available to require special precautions
Effects on Dental Treatment No significant effects or complications reported
Common Adverse Effects 1% to 10%:
Cardiovascular: Hypotension, edema, CHF, bradycardia
Central nervous system: Dizziness, headache, fatigue
Gastrointestinal: Constipation, nausea
Respiratory: Dyspnea
Mechanism of Action Interferes with potassium/sodium exchange (active transport) in the distal tubule, cortical collecting tubule and collecting duct by inhibiting sodium, potassium-ATPase; decreases calcium excretion; increases magnesium loss
Drug Interactions
Increased Effect/Toxicity: ACE inhibitors or spironolactone can cause hyperkalemia, especially in patients with renal impairment, potassium-rich diets, or on other drugs causing hyperkalemia; avoid concurrent use or monitor closely. Potassium supplements may further increase potassium retention and cause hyperkalemia; avoid concurrent use.
Pharmacodynamics/Kinetics
Onset of action: Diuresis: 2-4 hours
Duration: 7-9 hours
Absorption: Unreliable
Pregnancy Risk Factor B (manufacturer); D (expert analysis)

Triazolam (trye AY zoe lam)

Related Information
Sedation *on page 1825*
Related Sample Prescriptions
Sedation (Prior to Dental Treatment) *on page 1846*
U.S. Brand Names Halcion® [DSC]
Canadian Brand Names Apo-Triazo®; Gen-Triazolam; Halcion®
Mexican Brand Names Halcion
Generic Available Yes
Pharmacologic Category Hypnotic, Benzodiazepine
Dental Use Oral premedication before dental procedures
Use Short-term treatment of insomnia
Local Anesthetic/Vasoconstrictor Precautions No information available to require special precautions
Effects on Dental Treatment No significant effects or complications reported (see Dental Comment)
Significant Adverse Effects
>10%: Central nervous system: Drowsiness, anteriograde amnesia
(Continued)

Triazolam *(Continued)*

1% to 10%:

Central nervous system: Headache, dizziness, nervousness, lightheadedness, ataxia

Gastrointestinal: Nausea, vomiting

<1% (Limited to important or life-threatening): Anaphylaxis, angioedema, complex sleep-related behavior (sleep-driving, cooking or eating food, making phone calls), confusion, depression, euphoria, memory impairment

Restrictions C-IV

Dental Usual Dosing Note: Onset of action is rapid, patient should be in bed when taking medication

Preprocedure sedation: Adults: Oral: 0.25 mg taken the evening before oral surgery; or 0.25 mg 1 hour before procedure

Dosage Oral (onset of action is rapid, patient should be in bed when taking medication):

Children <18 years: Dosage not established

Adults:

Hypnotic: 0.125-0.25 mg at bedtime (maximum dose: 0.5 mg/day)

Preprocedure sedation (dental): 0.25 mg taken the evening before oral surgery; or 0.25 mg 1 hour before procedure

Elderly: Insomnia (short-term use): 0.0625-0.125 mg at bedtime; maximum dose: 0.25 mg/day

Dosing adjustment/comments in hepatic impairment: Reduce dose or avoid use in cirrhosis

Mechanism of Action Binds to stereospecific benzodiazepine receptors on the postsynaptic GABA neuron at several sites within the central nervous system, including the limbic system, reticular formation. Enhancement of the inhibitory effect of GABA on neuronal excitability results by increased neuronal membrane permeability to chloride ions. This shift in chloride ions results in hyperpolarization (a less excitable state) and stabilization.

Contraindications Hypersensitivity to triazolam or any component of the formulation (cross-sensitivity with other benzodiazepines may exist); concurrent therapy with atazanavir, ketoconazole, itraconazole, nefazodone, and ritonavir; pregnancy

Warnings/Precautions As a hypnotic, should be used only after evaluation of potential causes of sleep disturbance. Failure of sleep disturbance to resolve after 7-10 days may indicate psychiatric or medical illness. Prescription should be written for a maximum of 7-10 days and should not be prescribed in quantities exceeding a 1-month supply. Abrupt discontinuation after sustained use (generally >10 days) may cause withdrawal symptoms. Use is not recommended in patients with depressive disorders or psychoses. Avoid use in patients with sleep apnea. Use with caution in elderly or debilitated patients, patients with hepatic disease (including alcoholics), renal impairment, respiratory disease, impaired gag reflex, or obese patients. Use caution with potent CYP3A4 inhibitors, as they may significantly decreased the clearance of triazolam.

Causes CNS depression (dose-related) which may impair physical and mental capabilities. Use with caution in patients receiving other CNS depressants or psychoactive agents. Postmarketing studies have indicated that the use of hypnotic/sedative agents for sleep has been associated with hypersensitivity reactions including anaphylaxis as well as angioedema. An increased risk for hazardous sleep-related activities such as sleep-driving; cooking and eating food, and making phone calls while asleep have also been noted. Benzodiazepines have been associated with falls and traumatic injury and should be used with extreme caution in patients who are at risk of these events (especially the elderly). May cause physical or psychological dependence - use with caution in patients with a history of drug dependence.

Benzodiazepines have been associated with anterograde amnesia. Paradoxical reactions, including hyperactive or aggressive behavior, have been reported with benzodiazepines, particularly in adolescent/pediatric or psychiatric patients. Does not have analgesic, antidepressant, or antipsychotic properties.

Drug Interactions Substrate of CYP3A4 (major); **Inhibits** CYP2C8 (weak), 2C9 (weak)

Clozapine: Benzodiazepines may enhance the adverse/toxic effect of clozapine.

CNS depressants: Sedative effects and/or respiratory depression may be additive with CNS depressants; includes ethanol, barbiturates, opioid analgesics, and other sedative agents; monitor for increased effect

CYP3A4 inducers: CYP3A4 inducers may decrease the levels/effects of triazolam. Example inducers include aminoglutethimide, carbamazepine, nafcillin, nevirapine, phenobarbital, phenytoin, and rifamycins.

CYP3A4 inhibitors: May increase the levels/effects of triazolam. Example inhibitors include azole antifungals, clarithromycin, diclofenac, doxycycline, erythromycin, imatinib, isoniazid, nefazodone, nicardipine, propofol, protease inhibitors, quinidine, telithromycin, and verapamil.

Disulfiram: May decrease the metabolism, via CYP isoenzymes, of triazolam.

Isoniazid: Isoniazid may increase triazolam levels.

Oral contraceptives: May decrease the clearance and increase the half-life of triazolam; monitor for increased triazolam effect

Proton Pump Inhibitors: May increase the serum concentration of triazolam.

Theophylline: May partially antagonize some of the effects of benzodiazepines; monitor for decreased response; may require higher doses for sedation

Ethanol/Nutrition/Herb Interactions

Ethanol: Avoid ethanol (may increase CNS depression).

Food: Food may decrease the rate of absorption. Triazolam serum concentration may be increased by grapefruit juice; avoid concurrent use.

Herb/Nutraceutical: St John's wort may decrease levels. Avoid valerian, St John's wort, kava kava, gotu kola (may increase CNS depression).

Pharmacodynamics/Kinetics

Onset of action: Hypnotic: 15-30 minutes

Duration: 6-7 hours

Distribution: V_d: 0.8-1.8 L/kg

Protein binding: 89%

Metabolism: Extensively hepatic

Half-life elimination: 1.7-5 hours

Excretion: Urine as unchanged drug and metabolites

Pregnancy Risk Factor X

Lactation Excretion in breast milk unknown/not recommended

Breast-Feeding Considerations It is not known if triazolam is excreted in breast milk; however, other benzodiazepines are known to be excreted in breast milk. The AAP rates use of related agents as "of concern" and breast-feeding is not recommended.

Dosage Forms Excipient information presented when available (limited, particularly for generics); consult specific product labeling.

Tablet: 0.125 mg, 0.25 mg

Halcion®: 0.125 mg, 0.25 mg [DSC]

Dental Comment Triazolam (0.25 mg) 1 hour prior to dental procedure has been used as an oral preop sedative.

Triazolam is a benzodiazepine and is being used in dentistry as a preprocedural oral sedative. There has been recent interest in its use as an orally titratable sedative to render anxious patients at ease during difficult dental procedures. This technique has been referred to as enteral conscious sedation (ECS) and oral conscious sedation (OCS).

Triazolam has the shortest half-life of all the orally administered benzodiazepines. Although midazolam is shorter, it is used parenterally, not orally. The relatively fast onset of action (15-30 minutes) of triazolam offers an advantage in its use as an oral sedative. The clinician is reminded that no kinetic data has been reported with multiple titration doses of triazolam, a technique often used in the ECS/OCS regimen.

Selected Readings

Berthold CW, Dionne RA, and Corey SE, "Comparison of Sublingually and Orally Administered Triazolam for Premedication Before Oral Surgery," *Oral Surg Oral Med Oral Pathol Oral Radiol Endod*, 1997, 84(2):119-24.

Berthold CW, Schneider A, and Dionne RA, "Using Triazolam to Reduce Dental Anxiety," *J Am Dent Assoc*, 1993, 124(11):58-64.

Dionne R, "Oral Sedation," *Compend Contin Educ Dent*, 1998, 19(9):868-70.

Flanagan D, "Oral Triazolam Sedation in Implant Dentistry," *J Oral Implantol*, 2004, 30(2):93-7.

Goodchild JH, Feck AS, and Silverman MD, "Anxiolysis in General Dental Practice," *Dent Today*, 2003, 22(3):106-11.

Kaufman E, Hargreaves KM, and Dionne RA, "Comparison of Oral Triazolam and Nitrous Oxide With Placebo and Intravenous Diazepam for Outpatient Premedication," *Oral Surg Oral Med Oral Pathol*, 1993, 75(2):156-64.

Kurzrock M, "Triazolam and Dental Anxiety," *J Am Dent Assoc*, 1994, 125(4):358, 360.

Lieblich SE and Horswell B, "Attenuation of Anxiety in Ambulatory Oral Surgery Patients With Oral Triazolam," *J Oral Maxillofac Surg*, 1991, 49(8):792-7.

Matear DW and Clarke D, "Considerations for the Use of Oral Sedation in the Institutionalized Geriatric Patient During Dental Interventions: A Review of the Literature," *Spec Care Dentist*, 1999, 19(2):56-63.

Milgrom P, Quarnstrom FC, Longley A, et al, "The Efficacy and Memory Effects of Oral Triazolam Premedication in Highly Anxious Dental Patients," *Anesth Prog*, 1994, 41(3):70-6.

Quarnstrom F, "Should Dentists Do Oral Sedation?" *Dent Today*, 2004, 23(3):16-8.

Tri-Chlor® *see* Trichloroacetic Acid *on page 1616*
Trichlor Fresh Pac™ *see* Trichloroacetic Acid *on page 1616*
Trichloroacetaldehyde Monohydrate *see* Chloral Hydrate *on page 327*

Trichloroacetic Acid (trye klor oh a SEE tik AS id)

U.S. Brand Names Tri-Chlor®; Trichlor Fresh Pac™
Generic Available Yes
Pharmacologic Category Keratolytic Agent
Use Chemical used in compounding agents for the treatment of warts, skin resurfacing (chemical peels)
Local Anesthetic/Vasoconstrictor Precautions No information available to require special precautions
Effects on Dental Treatment No significant effects or complications reported

Trichloromonofluoromethane and Dichlorodifluoromethane *see* Dichlorodifluoromethane and Trichloromonofluoromethane *on page 485*

Triclosan and Fluoride (trye KLOE san & FLOR ide)

Related Information
Fluoride *on page 710*
Periodontal Diseases *on page 1801*
U.S. Brand Names Colgate Total®
Generic Available No
Index Terms Fluoride and Triclosan (Dental)
Pharmacologic Category Antibacterial, Dental; Mineral, Oral (Topical)
Dental Use Anticavity, antigingivitis, antiplaque toothpaste
Use Used exclusively in dental applications
Local Anesthetic/Vasoconstrictor Precautions No information available to require special precautions
Effects on Dental Treatment No significant effects or complications reported (see Dental Comment)
Significant Adverse Effects No data reported
Dental Usual Dosing
Prevention of dental caries and gingivitis: Adults: Oral: Brush teeth thoroughly after each meal or at least twice daily
Dosage Brush teeth thoroughly after each meal or at least twice daily
Mechanism of Action Triclosan is an antibacterial agent which helps to prevent gingivitis with regular use. Fluoride promotes remineralization of decalcified enamel, inhibits the cariogenic microbial process in dental plaque, and increases tooth resistance to acid dissolution
Warnings/Precautions Antigingivitis and antiplaque effects have not been determined in children <6 years of age. If an amount greater than used for brushing is swallowed, seek professional assistance of contact a poison control center immediately
Pregnancy Risk Factor No data reported
Dosage Forms Excipient information presented when available (limited, particularly for generics); consult specific product labeling.
Gel, oral [toothpaste]: Triclosan 0.30% and sodium fluoride 0.24% (119 g, 170 g, 221 g)
Paste, oral [toothpaste]: Triclosan 0.30% and sodium fluoride 0.24% (119 g, 170 g, 221 g)
Dental Comment It has been shown that stannous fluoride and triclosan when formulated into a toothpaste vehicle provide plaque inhibitory effects. To provide a longer retention time of the triclosan in plaque, a polymer has been added to the toothpaste vehicle. The polymer is known as PVM/MA which stands for polyvinylmethyl ether/maleic acid copolymer, and is listed as an inactive ingredient (PVM/MA Copolymer) on the manufacturer's label. Studies have reported that the retention of triclosan in plaque (exceeding the minimal inhibitory concentration) after polymer application was 14 hours after brushing. Ongoing studies are evaluating the effects of triclosan/copolymer on alveolar bone loss. Rosling et al. have reported that the daily use of Colgate Total® reduced (1) the frequency of deep periodontal pockets and (2) the number of sites that exhibited additional probing attachment and bone loss.

Selected Readings
Binney A, Addy M, Owens J, et al, "A Comparison of Triclosan and Stannous Fluoride Toothpastes for Inhibition of Plaque Regrowth. A Crossover Study Designed to Access Carry Over," *J Clin Periodontol*, 1997, 24(3):166-70.
Ellwood RP, Worthington HV, Blinkhorn AS, et al, "Effect of a Triclosan/Copolymer Dentifrice on the Incidence of Periodontal Attachment Loss in Adolescents," *J Clin Periodontol*, 1998, 25(5):363-7.
Mandel ID, "The New Toothpastes," *J Calif Dent Assoc*, 1998, 26(3):186-90.
Rosling B, Wannfors B, Volpe AR, et al, "The Use of a Triclosan/Copolymer Dentifrice May Retard the Progression of Periodontitis," *J Clin Periodontol*, 1997, 24(12):873-80.

TriCor® *see* Fenofibrate *on page 674*

Tricosal *see* Choline Magnesium Trisalicylate *on page 350*

Triderm® *see* Triamcinolone *on page 1608*

Tridione® *see* Trimethadione *on page 1620*

Triethanolamine Polypeptide Oleate-Condensate
(trye eth a NOLE a meen pol i PEP tide OH lee ate-KON den sate)

U.S. Brand Names Cerumenex® [DSC]
Canadian Brand Names Cerumenex®
Generic Available No
Pharmacologic Category Otic Agent, Cerumenolytic
Use Removal of ear wax (cerumen)
Local Anesthetic/Vasoconstrictor Precautions No information available to require special precautions
Effects on Dental Treatment No significant effects or complications reported
Mechanism of Action Emulsifies and disperses accumulated cerumen
Pregnancy Risk Factor C

Triethanolamine Salicylate (TROLE a meen)

U.S. Brand Names Aspercreme® [OTC]; Flex-Power [OTC]; Mobisyl® [OTC]; Myoflex® [OTC]; Sportscreme® [OTC]
Canadian Brand Names Antiphlogistine Rub A-535 No Odour; Myoflex®
Generic Available Yes: Cream
Index Terms TEAS; Triethanolamine Salicylate; Trolamine Salicylate
Pharmacologic Category Analgesic, Topical; Salicylate; Topical Skin Product
Use Relief of pain of muscular aches, rheumatism, neuralgia, sprains, arthritis on intact skin
Local Anesthetic/Vasoconstrictor Precautions No information available to require special precautions
Effects on Dental Treatment No significant effects or complications reported
Common Adverse Effects 1% to 10%:
Central nervous system: Confusion, drowsiness
Gastrointestinal: Nausea, vomiting, diarrhea
Respiratory: Hyperventilation

Triethanolamine Salicylate *see* Triethanolamine Salicylate *on page 1617*

Triethylenethiophosphoramide *see* Thiotepa *on page 1559*

Trifluoperazine (trye floo oh PER a zeen)

Canadian Brand Names Apo-Trifluoperazine®; Novo-Trifluzine; PMS-Trifluoperazine; Terfluzine
Mexican Brand Names Stelazine
Generic Available Yes
Index Terms Trifluoperazine Hydrochloride
Pharmacologic Category Antipsychotic Agent, Typical, Phenothiazine
Use Treatment of schizophrenia
Unlabeled/Investigational Use Management of psychotic disorders; behavioral symptoms associated with dementia behavior (elderly)
Local Anesthetic/Vasoconstrictor Precautions Most pharmacology textbooks state that in presence of phenothiazines, systemic doses of epinephrine paradoxically decrease the blood pressure. This is the so called "epinephrine reversal" phenomenon. This has never been observed when epinephrine is given by infiltration as part of the anesthesia procedure.
Effects on Dental Treatment Key adverse event(s) related to dental treatment: Significant hypotension may occur, especially when the drug is administered parenterally; orthostatic hypotension is due to alpha-receptor blockade, the elderly are at greater risk for orthostatic hypotension. Xerostomia (normal salivary flow resumes upon discontinuation).

Tardive dyskinesia: Prevalence rate may be 40% in elderly; development of the syndrome and the irreversible nature are proportional to duration and total cumulative dose over time. Extrapyramidal reactions are more common in elderly with up to 50% developing these reactions after 60 years of age. Drug-induced Parkinson's syndrome occurs often; akathisia is the most common extrapyramidal reaction in elderly.
(Continued)

Trifluoperazine *(Continued)*

Common Adverse Effects Frequency not defined.

Cardiovascular: Hypotension, orthostatic hypotension, cardiac arrest

Central nervous system: Extrapyramidal signs (pseudoparkinsonism, akathisia, dystonias, tardive dyskinesia), dizziness, headache, neuroleptic malignant syndrome (NMS), impairment of temperature regulation, lowering of seizure threshold

Dermatologic: Increased sensitivity to sun, rash, discoloration of skin (blue-gray), photosensitivity

Endocrine & metabolic: Changes in menstrual cycle, libido (changes in), breast pain, hyperglycemia, hypoglycemia, gynecomastia, lactation, galactorrhea

Gastrointestinal: Constipation, weight gain, nausea, vomiting, stomach pain, xerostomia

Genitourinary: Difficulty in urination, ejaculatory disturbances, urinary retention, priapism

Hematologic: Agranulocytosis, leukopenia, pancytopenia, thrombocytopenic purpura, eosinophilia, hemolytic anemia, aplastic anemia

Hepatic: Cholestatic jaundice, hepatotoxicity

Neuromuscular & skeletal: Tremor

Ocular: Pigmentary retinopathy, cornea and lens changes

Respiratory: Nasal congestion

Mechanism of Action Trifluoperazine is a piperazine phenothiazine antipsychotic which blocks postsynaptic mesolimbic dopaminergic receptors in the brain; exhibits alpha-adrenergic blocking effect and depresses the release of hypothalamic and hypophyseal hormones

Drug Interactions

Cytochrome P450 Effect: Substrate of CYP1A2 (major)

Increased Effect/Toxicity: CYP1A2 inhibitors may increase the levels/effects of trifluoperazine; example inhibitors include ciprofloxacin, fluvoxamine, ketoconazole, norfloxacin, ofloxacin, and rofecoxib. Trifluoperazine's effects on CNS depression may be additive when trifluoperazine is combined with CNS depressants (opioid analgesics, ethanol, barbiturates, cyclic antidepressants, antihistamines, or sedative-hypnotics). Trifluoperazine may increase the effects/toxicity of anticholinergics, antihypertensives, lithium (rare neurotoxicity), trazodone, or valproic acid. Concurrent use with TCA may produce increased toxicity or altered therapeutic response. Chloroquine and propranolol may increase trifluoperazine concentrations. Hypotension may occur when trifluoperazine is combined with epinephrine. May increase the risk of arrhythmia when combined with antiarrhythmics, cisapride, pimozide, sparfloxacin, or other drugs which prolong QT interval. Metoclopramide may increase risk of extrapyramidal symptoms (EPS). Acetylcholinesterase inhibitors (central) may increase the risk of antipsychotic-related EPS.

Decreased Effect: CYP1A2 inducers may decrease the levels/effects of trifluoperazine; example inducers include aminoglutethimide, carbamazepine, phenobarbital, and rifampin. Phenothiazines inhibit the effects of levodopa, guanadrel, guanethidine, and bromocriptine. Benztropine (and other anticholinergics) may inhibit the therapeutic response to trifluoperazine and excess anticholinergic effects may occur. Cigarette smoking may enhance the hepatic metabolism of trifluoperazine. Trifluoperazine and possibly other low potency antipsychotics may reverse the pressor effects of epinephrine.

Pharmacodynamics/Kinetics

Metabolism: Extensively hepatic

Half-life elimination: >24 hours with chronic use

Pregnancy Risk Factor C

Trifluoperazine Hydrochloride *see* Trifluoperazine *on page 1617*

Trifluorothymidine *see* Trifluridine *on page 1618*

Trifluridine *(trye FLURE i deen)*

Related Information

Systemic Viral Diseases *on page 1767*

U.S. Brand Names Viroptic®

Canadian Brand Names SAB-Trifluridine; Sandoz-Trifluridine; Viroptic®

Generic Available Yes

Index Terms F_3T; Trifluorothymidine

Pharmacologic Category Antiviral Agent, Ophthalmic

Use Treatment of primary keratoconjunctivitis and recurrent epithelial keratitis caused by herpes simplex virus types I and II

Local Anesthetic/Vasoconstrictor Precautions No information available to require special precautions

Effects on Dental Treatment No significant effects or complications reported

Mechanism of Action Interferes with viral replication by incorporating into viral DNA in place of thymidine, inhibiting thymidylate synthetase resulting in the formation of defective proteins

Pregnancy Risk Factor C

Triglide™ *see* Fenofibrate *on page 674*

Triglycerides, Medium Chain *see* Medium Chain Triglycerides *on page 1026*

Trihexyphenidyl (trye heks ee FEN i dil)

Canadian Brand Names Apo-Trihex®
Mexican Brand Names Artane
Generic Available Yes
Index Terms Artane; Benzhexol Hydrochloride; Trihexyphenidyl Hydrochloride
Pharmacologic Category Anti-Parkinson's Agent, Anticholinergic; Anticholinergic Agent

Use Adjunctive treatment of Parkinson's disease; treatment of drug-induced extrapyramidal symptoms

Local Anesthetic/Vasoconstrictor Precautions No information available to require special precautions

Effects on Dental Treatment Key adverse event(s) related to dental treatment: Xerostomia, dry throat (normal salivary flow resumes upon discontinuation). Prolonged xerostomia may contribute to discomfort and dental disease (ie, caries, periodontal disease, and oral candidiasis).

Common Adverse Effects Frequency not defined.

Cardiovascular: Tachycardia

Central nervous system: Confusion, agitation, euphoria, drowsiness, headache, dizziness, nervousness, delusions, hallucinations, paranoia

Dermatologic: Dry skin, increased sensitivity to light, rash

Gastrointestinal: Constipation, xerostomia, dry throat, ileus, nausea, vomiting, parotitis

Genitourinary: Urinary retention

Neuromuscular & skeletal: Weakness

Ocular: Blurred vision, mydriasis, increase in intraocular pressure, glaucoma, blindness (long-term use in narrow-angle glaucoma)

Respiratory: Dry nose

Miscellaneous: Diaphoresis (decreased)

Mechanism of Action Exerts a direct inhibitory effect on the parasympathetic nervous system. It also has a relaxing effect on smooth musculature; exerted both directly on the muscle itself and indirectly through parasympathetic nervous system (inhibitory effect)

Drug Interactions

Increased Effect/Toxicity: Central and/or peripheral anticholinergic syndrome can occur when administered with amantadine, rimantadine, opioid analgesics, phenothiazines and other antipsychotics (especially with high anticholinergic activity), tricyclic antidepressants, MAO inhibitors, quinidine and some other antiarrhythmics, and antihistamines. CNS depressants (cannabinoids, ethanol, barbiturates, and opioid analgesics) may have additive effects with trihexyphenidyl; an abuse potential exits.

Decreased Effect: May increase gastric degradation of levodopa and decrease the amount of levodopa absorbed by delaying gastric emptying; the opposite may be true for digoxin. Therapeutic effects of cholinergic agents (tacrine, donepezil, rivastigmine, galantamine) and neuroleptics may be antagonized.

Pharmacodynamics/Kinetics

Onset of action: Peak effect: ~1 hour

Half-life elimination: 3.3-4.1 hours

Time to peak, serum: 1-1.5 hours

Excretion: Primarily urine

Pregnancy Risk Factor C

Trihexyphenidyl Hydrochloride *see* Trihexyphenidyl *on page 1619*

Trileptal® *see* Oxcarbazepine *on page 1221*

Tri-Levlen® *see* Ethinyl Estradiol and Levonorgestrel *on page 633*

Trilisate® [DSC] *see* Choline Magnesium Trisalicylate *on page 350*

Tri-Luma™ *see* Fluocinolone, Hydroquinone, and Tretinoin *on page 708*

TriLyte™ *see* Polyethylene Glycol-Electrolyte Solution *on page 1321*

Trimethadione (trye meth a DYE one)

U.S. Brand Names Tridione®
Generic Available No
Index Terms Troxidone
Pharmacologic Category Anticonvulsant, Oxazolidinedione
Use Control absence (petit mal) seizures refractory to other drugs
Local Anesthetic/Vasoconstrictor Precautions No information available to require special precautions
Effects on Dental Treatment No significant effects or complications reported
Mechanism of Action An oxazolidinedione with anticonvulsant sedative properties; elevates the cortical and basal seizure thresholds, and reduces the synaptic response to low frequency impulses
Pregnancy Risk Factor D

Trimethobenzamide (trye meth oh BEN za mide)

U.S. Brand Names Tigan®
Canadian Brand Names Tigan®
Generic Available Yes: Injection
Index Terms Trimethobenzamide Hydrochloride
Pharmacologic Category Anticholinergic Agent; Antiemetic
Use Treatment of nausea and vomiting
Local Anesthetic/Vasoconstrictor Precautions No information available to require special precautions
Effects on Dental Treatment No significant effects or complications reported
Common Adverse Effects Frequency not defined.
   Cardiovascular: Hypotension
   Central nervous system: Coma, depression, disorientation, dizziness, drowsiness, EPS, headache, opisthotonos, Parkinson-like syndrome, seizure
   Gastrointestinal: Diarrhea
   Hematologic: Blood dyscrasias
   Hepatic: Jaundice
   Neuromuscular & skeletal: Muscle cramps
   Ocular: Blurred vision
   Miscellaneous: Hypersensitivity reactions
Mechanism of Action Acts centrally to inhibit the medullary chemoreceptor trigger zone
Pharmacodynamics/Kinetics
   Onset of action: Antiemetic: Oral: 10-40 minutes; I.M.: 15-35 minutes
   Duration: 3-4 hours
   Bioavailability: Oral: 60% to 100%
   Half-life elimination: 7-9 hours
   Time to peak: Oral: 45 minutes; I.M.: 30 minutes
   Excretion: Urine (30% to 50%)
Pregnancy Risk Factor C

Trimethobenzamide Hydrochloride *see* Trimethobenzamide *on page 1620*

Trimethoprim (trye METH oh prim)

U.S. Brand Names Primsol®; Proloprim®
Canadian Brand Names Apo-Trimethoprim®
Generic Available Yes: Tablet
Index Terms TMP
Pharmacologic Category Antibiotic, Miscellaneous
Use Treatment of urinary tract infections due to susceptible strains of *E. coli*, *P. mirabilis*, *K. pneumoniae*, *Enterobacter* sp and coagulase-negative *Staphylococcus* including *S. saprophyticus*; acute otitis media in children; acute exacerbations of chronic bronchitis in adults; in combination with other agents for treatment of toxoplasmosis, *Pneumocystis carinii*; treatment of superficial ocular infections involving the conjunctiva and cornea
Local Anesthetic/Vasoconstrictor Precautions No information available to require special precautions
Effects on Dental Treatment Key adverse event(s) related to dental treatment: Glossitis.
Common Adverse Effects Frequency not defined.
   Central nervous system: Aseptic meningitis (rare), fever
   Dermatologic: Maculopapular rash (3% to 7% at 200 mg/day; incidence higher with larger daily doses), erythema multiforme (rare), exfoliative dermatitis

(rare), pruritus (common), phototoxic skin eruptions, Stevens-Johnson syndrome (rare), toxic epidermal necrolysis (rare)

Endocrine & metabolic: Hyperkalemia, hyponatremia

Gastrointestinal: Epigastric distress, glossitis, nausea, vomiting

Hematologic: Leukopenia, megaloblastic anemia, methemoglobinemia, neutropenia, thrombocytopenia

Hepatic: Liver enzyme elevation, cholestatic jaundice (rare)

Renal: BUN and creatinine increased

Miscellaneous: Anaphylaxis, hypersensitivity reactions

Mechanism of Action Inhibits folic acid reduction to tetrahydrofolate, and thereby inhibits microbial growth

Drug Interactions

Cytochrome P450 Effect: Substrate (major) of CYP2C9, 3A4; **Inhibits** CYP2C8 (moderate), 2C9 (moderate)

Increased Effect/Toxicity: Increased effect/toxicity/levels of phenytoin. Concurrent use with ACE inhibitors increases risk of hyperkalemia. Increased myelosuppression with methotrexate. May increase levels of digoxin. Concurrent use with dapsone may increase levels of dapsone and trimethoprim. Concurrent use with procainamide may increase levels of procainamide and trimethoprim. Trimethoprim may increase the levels/effects of amiodarone, fluoxetine, glimepiride, glipizide, nateglinide, phenytoin, pioglitazone, rosiglitazone, sertraline, warfarin, and other CYP2C8 and 2C9 substrates.

Decreased Effect: The levels/effects of trimethoprim may be decreased by aminoglutethimide, carbamazepine, nafcillin, nevirapine, phenobarbital, phenytoin, rifampin, rifapentine, secobarbital, and other CYP2C9 or 3A4 inducers.

Pharmacodynamics/Kinetics

Absorption: Readily and extensive

Distribution: Widely into body tissues and fluids (middle ear, prostate, bile, aqueous humor, CSF); crosses placenta; enters breast milk

Protein binding: 42% to 46%

Metabolism: Partially hepatic

Half-life elimination: 8-14 hours; prolonged with renal impairment

Time to peak, serum: 1-4 hours

Excretion: Urine (60% to 80%) as unchanged drug

Pregnancy Risk Factor C

Trimethoprim and Polymyxin B
(trye METH oh prim & pol i MIKS in bee)

Related Information
Polymyxin B *on page 1322*
Trimethoprim *on page 1620*

U.S. Brand Names Polytrim®

Canadian Brand Names PMS-Polytrimethoprim; Polytrim™

Generic Available Yes

Index Terms Polymyxin B and Trimethoprim

Pharmacologic Category Antibiotic, Ophthalmic

Use Treatment of surface ocular bacterial conjunctivitis and blepharoconjunctivitis

Local Anesthetic/Vasoconstrictor Precautions No information available to require special precautions

Effects on Dental Treatment No significant effects or complications reported

Pregnancy Risk Factor C

Trimethoprim and Sulfamethoxazole *see* Sulfamethoxazole and Trimethoprim *on page 1504*

Trimetrexate (tri me TREKS ate)

U.S. Brand Names NeuTrexin® [DSC]

Generic Available No

Index Terms NSC-352122; Trimetrexate Glucuronate

Pharmacologic Category Antineoplastic Agent, Miscellaneous

Use Alternative therapy for the treatment of moderate-to-severe *Pneumocystis jiroveci* pneumonia (PCP) in immunocompromised patients, including patients with acquired immunodeficiency syndrome (AIDS), who are intolerant of, are refractory to, sulfamethoxazole/trimethoprim therapy or for whom sulfamethoxazole/trimethoprim and pentamidine are contraindicated

Unlabeled/Investigational Use Treatment of nonsmall cell lung cancer, metastatic colorectal cancer, metastatic head and neck cancer, pancreatic adenocarcinoma, cutaneous T-cell lymphoma

(Continued)

Trimetrexate *(Continued)*

No information available to require special precautions

Key adverse event(s) related to dental treatment: Stomatitis.

Common Adverse Effects

>10%:
Hematologic: Neutropenia (30%)
Hepatic: AST increased (14%), ALT increased (11%)

1% to 10%:
Central nervous system: Fever (8%), confusion (3%), fatigue (2%)
Dermatologic: Rash/pruritus (6%)
Endocrine & metabolic: Hyponatremia (5%), hypocalcemia (2%)
Gastrointestinal: Nausea/vomiting (5%), stomatitis
Hematologic: Thrombocytopenia (10%), anemia (7%)
Hepatic: Alkaline phosphatase increased (5%), bilirubin increased (2%)
Neuromuscular & skeletal: Peripheral neuropathy
Miscellaneous: Flu-like illness; hypersensitivity/allergic reactions (chills, rigors); anaphylactoid reactions (acute hypotension, loss of consciousness)

Mechanism of Action Trimetrexate is a folate antimetabolite that inhibits DNA synthesis by inhibition of dihydrofolate reductase (DHFR); DHFR inhibition reduces the formation of reduced folates and thymidylate synthetase, resulting in inhibition of purine and thymidylic acid synthesis.

Drug Interactions

Increased Effect/Toxicity: Zidovudine may increase the myelotoxicity of trimetrexate; discontinue zidovudine during trimetrexate treatment. Trimetrexate may increase toxicity (infections) of live virus vaccines.

Pharmacodynamics/Kinetics

Distribution: V_d: 0.62 L/kg
Protein binding: 80% to 90% (concentration dependent)
Metabolism: Extensively hepatic: O-demethylation followed by conjugation to glucuronide or sulfate (major); N-demethylation and oxidation (minor)
Half-life elimination: 9-18 hours (11 hours with leucovorin)
Excretion: Urine (10% to 40% as unchanged drug); feces (<1% to 8%)

Pregnancy Risk Factor D

Trimetrexate Glucuronate *see* Trimetrexate *on page 1621*

Trimipramine *(trye MI pra meen)*

U.S. Brand Names Surmontil®
Canadian Brand Names Apo-Trimip®; Nu-Trimipramine; Rhotrimine®; Surmontil®
Generic Available No
Index Terms Trimipramine Maleate
Pharmacologic Category Antidepressant, Tricyclic (Tertiary Amine)
Use Treatment of depression

Use with caution; epinephrine and levonordefrin have been shown to have an increased pressor response in combination with TCAs. Trimipramine is one of the drugs confirmed to prolong the QT interval and is accepted as having a risk of causing torsade de pointes. The risk of drug-induced torsade de pointes is extremely low when a single QT interval prolonging drug is prescribed. In terms of epinephrine, it is not known what effect vasoconstrictors in the local anesthetic regimen will have in patients with a known history of congenital prolonged QT interval or in patients taking any medication that prolongs the QT interval. Until more information is obtained, it is suggested that the clinician consult with the physician prior to the use of a vasoconstrictor in suspected patients, and that the vasoconstrictor (epinephrine, levonordefrin [Neo-Cobefrin®]) be used with caution.

Key adverse event(s) related to dental treatment: Xerostomia (normal salivary flow resumes upon discontinuation) and unpleasant taste. Long-term treatment with TCAs, such as trimipramine, increases the risk of caries by reducing salivation and salivary buffer capacity.

Common Adverse Effects Frequency not defined.
Cardiovascular: Arrhythmias, hyper-/hypotension, tachycardia, palpitation, heart block, stroke, MI
Central nervous system: Headache, exacerbation of psychosis, confusion, delirium, hallucinations, nervousness, restlessness, delusions, agitation, insomnia, nightmares, anxiety, seizure, drowsiness
Dermatologic: Photosensitivity, rash, petechiae, itching
Endocrine & metabolic: Sexual dysfunction, breast enlargement, galactorrhea, SIADH

Gastrointestinal: Xerostomia, constipation, increased appetite, nausea, unpleasant taste, weight gain, diarrhea, heartburn, vomiting, anorexia, trouble with gums, decreased lower esophageal sphincter tone may cause GE reflux

Genitourinary: Difficult urination, urinary retention, testicular edema

Hematologic: Agranulocytosis, eosinophilia, purpura, thrombocytopenia

Hepatic: Cholestatic jaundice, increased liver enzymes

Neuromuscular & skeletal: Tremors, numbness, tingling, paresthesia, incoordination, ataxia, peripheral neuropathy, extrapyramidal symptoms

Ocular: Blurred vision, eye pain, disturbances in accommodation, mydriasis, increased intraocular pressure

Otic: Tinnitus

Miscellaneous: Allergic reactions

Restrictions An FDA-approved medication guide concerning the use of antidepressants in children, adolescents, and young adults must be distributed when dispensing an outpatient prescription (new or refill) where this medication is to be used without direct supervision of a healthcare provider. Medication guides are available at http://www.fda.gov/cder/Offices/ODS/medication_guides.htm. Dispense to parents or guardians of children and adolescents receiving this medication.

Mechanism of Action Increases the synaptic concentration of serotonin and/or norepinephrine in the central nervous system by inhibition of their reuptake by the presynaptic neuronal membrane

Drug Interactions

Cytochrome P450 Effect: Substrate (major) of CYP2C19, 2D6, 3A4

Increased Effect/Toxicity: Pressor response to I.V. epinephrine, norepinephrine, and phenylephrine may be enhanced in patients receiving TCAs (**Note:** Effect is unlikely with epinephrine or levonordefrin dosages typically administered as infiltration in combination with local anesthetics). Trimipramine increases the effects of amphetamines, anticholinergics, other CNS depressants (sedatives, hypnotics, or ethanol), chlorpropamide, tolazamide, and warfarin. When used with MAO inhibitors, hyperpyrexia, hypertension, tachycardia, confusion, seizures, and **deaths have been reported** (serotonin syndrome). Serotonin syndrome has also been reported with ritonavir (rare).

CYP2C19 inhibitors may increase the levels/effects of trimipramine; example inhibitors include delavirdine, fluconazole, fluvoxamine, gemfibrozil, isoniazid, omeprazole, and ticlopidine. CYP2D6 inhibitors may increase the levels/effects of trimipramine; example inhibitors include chlorpromazine, delavirdine, fluoxetine, miconazole, paroxetine, pergolide, quinidine, quinine, ritonavir, and ropinirole. CYP3A4 inhibitors may increase the levels/effects of trimipramine; example inhibitors include azole antifungals, clarithromycin, diclofenac, doxycycline, erythromycin, imatinib, isoniazid, nefazodone, nicardipine, propofol, protease inhibitors, quinidine, telithromycin, and verapamil. Use of lithium with a TCA may increase the risk for neurotoxicity. Phenothiazines may increase concentration of some TCAs and TCAs may increase concentration of phenothiazines. Combined use of beta-agonists or drugs which prolong QT$_c$ (including quinidine, procainamide, disopyramide, cisapride, sparfloxacin, gatifloxacin, moxifloxacin) with TCAs may predispose patients to cardiac arrhythmias.

Decreased Effect: CYP2C19 inducers may decrease the levels/effects of trimipramine; example inducers include aminoglutethimide, carbamazepine, phenytoin, and rifampin. Trimipramine inhibits the antihypertensive response to bethanidine, clonidine, debrisoquin, guanadrel, guanethidine, guanabenz, and guanfacine. Cholestyramine and colestipol may bind TCAs and reduce their absorption; monitor for altered response. CYP3A4 inducers may decrease the levels/effects of trimipramine; example inducers include aminoglutethimide, carbamazepine, nafcillin, nevirapine, phenobarbital, phenytoin, and rifamycins.

Pharmacodynamics/Kinetics

Distribution: V$_d$: 17-48 L/kg

Protein binding: 95%; free drug: 3% to 7%

Metabolism: Hepatic; significant first-pass effect

Bioavailability: 18% to 63%

Half-life elimination: 16-40 hours

Excretion: Urine

Pregnancy Risk Factor C

Triple Antibiotic *see* Bacitracin, Neomycin, and Polymyxin B *on page 181*

Triple Sulfa *see* Sulfabenzamide, Sulfacetamide, and Sulfathiazole *on page 1501*

Tri-Previfem™ *see* Ethinyl Estradiol and Norgestimate *on page 645*

Triprolidine and Pseudoephedrine
(trye PROE li deen & soo doe e FED rin)

Related Information
Pseudoephedrine *on page 1381*

U.S. Brand Names Actifed® Cold and Allergy [OTC] [DSC]; Allerfrim® [OTC]; Aprodine® [OTC]; Genac® [OTC]; Silafed® [OTC]; Sudafed® Maximum Strength Sinus Nighttime [OTC] [DSC]; Tri-Sudo® [OTC] [DSC]; Zymine®-D

Canadian Brand Names Actifed®

Generic Available Yes

Index Terms Pseudoephedrine and Triprolidine

Pharmacologic Category Alpha/Beta Agonist; Antihistamine

Use Temporary relief of nasal congestion, decongest sinus openings, running nose, sneezing, itching of nose or throat and itchy, watery eyes due to common cold, hay fever, or other upper respiratory allergies

Local Anesthetic/Vasoconstrictor Precautions Use with caution since pseudoephedrine is a sympathomimetic amine which could interact with epinephrine to cause a pressor response

Effects on Dental Treatment Key adverse event(s) related to dental treatment: Pseudoephedrine: Xerostomia (normal salivary flow resumes upon discontinuation). Chronic use of antihistamines will inhibit salivary flow, particularly in elderly patients; this may contribute to periodontal disease and oral discomfort.

Common Adverse Effects Frequency not defined.

Cardiovascular: Tachycardia

Central nervous system: Drowsiness, nervousness, insomnia, transient stimulation, headache, fatigue, dizziness

Respiratory: Thickening of bronchial secretions, pharyngitis

Gastrointestinal: Appetite increase, weight gain, nausea, diarrhea, abdominal pain, xerostomia

Genitourinary: Dysuria

Neuromuscular & skeletal: Arthralgia, weakness

Miscellaneous: Diaphoresis

Mechanism of Action Refer to Pseudoephedrine monograph.

Triprolidine is a member of the propylamine (alkylamine) chemical class of H_1-antagonist antihistamines. As such, it is considered to be relatively less sedating than traditional antihistamines of the ethanolamine, phenothiazine, and ethylenediamine classes of antihistamines. Triprolidine has a shorter half-life and duration of action than most of the other alkylamine antihistamines. Like all H_1-antagonist antihistamines, the mechanism of action of triprolidine is believed to involve competitive blockade of H_1-receptor sites resulting in the inability of histamine to combine with its receptor sites and exert its usual effects on target cells. Antihistamines do not interrupt any effects of histamine which have already occurred. Therefore, these agents are used more successfully in the prevention rather than the treatment of histamine-induced reactions.

Drug Interactions

Cytochrome P450 Effect: Triprolidine: **Inhibits** CYP2D6 (weak)

Increased Effect/Toxicity: Increased toxicity with MAO inhibitors or drugs with MAO inhibiting activity such as linezolid or furazolidone (hypertensive crisis). May increase toxicity of sympathomimetics, CNS depressants, and alcohol.

Decreased Effect: Decreased effect of guanethidine, reserpine, methyldopa.

Pharmacodynamics/Kinetics See Pseudoephedrine monograph.

Pregnancy Risk Factor C

Triprolidine, Codeine, and Pseudoephedrine *see* Triprolidine, Pseudoephedrine, and Codeine *on page 1624*

Triprolidine, Pseudoephedrine, and Codeine
(trye PROE li deen, soo doe e FED rin, & KOE deen)

Related Information
Codeine *on page 404*

Pseudoephedrine *on page 1381*

U.S. Brand Names Triacin-C® [DSC]

Canadian Brand Names CoActifed®; Covan®; ratio-Cotridin

Generic Available No

Index Terms Codeine, Pseudoephedrine, and Triprolidine; Codeine, Triprolidine, and Pseudoephedrine; Pseudoephedrine, Codeine, and Triprolidine; Pseudoephedrine, Triprolidine, and Codeine; Triprolidine, Codeine, and Pseudoephedrine

Pharmacologic Category Antihistamine/Decongestant/Antitussive

Use Symptomatic relief of upper respiratory symptoms and cough

Local Anesthetic/Vasoconstrictor Precautions Use with caution since pseudoephedrine is a sympathomimetic amine which could interact with epinephrine to cause a pressor response

Effects on Dental Treatment Key adverse event(s) related to dental treatment: Pseudoephedrine: Xerostomia (normal salivary flow resumes upon discontinuation) and taste disturbance.

Common Adverse Effects Frequency not defined.

Cardiovascular: Hypotension

Central nervous system: Sedation, dizziness, drowsiness, increased ICP, lightheadedness, dysphoria, euphoria, headache, agitation, hallucinations, seizure, respiratory depression

Dermatologic: Pruritus, rash

Gastrointestinal: Constipation, nausea, vomiting, anorexia, xerostomia, taste disturbance, biliary tract spasm

Genitourinary: Urinary retention, urinary tract spasm

Neuromuscular & skeletal: Muscle tremor, paresthesia, muscular rigidity (rare)

Ocular: Blurred vision, nystagmus

Miscellaneous: Diaphoresis, physical or psychological dependence with continued use, withdrawal syndrome

Restrictions C-V (CDSA-I)

Drug Interactions

Cytochrome P450 Effect:

Triprolidine: **Inhibits** CYP2D6 (weak)

Codeine: **Substrate** of CYP2D6 (major), 3A4 (minor); **Inhibits** CYP2D6 (weak)

Pharmacodynamics/Kinetics See Pseudoephedrine and Codeine monographs.

Pregnancy Risk Factor C

TripTone® [OTC] [DSC] *see* DimenhyDRINATE *on page 508*

Triptoraline *see* Triptorelin *on page 1625*

Triptorelin (trip toe REL in)

U.S. Brand Names Trelstar™ Depot; Trelstar™ LA

Canadian Brand Names Trelstar™; Trelstar™ Depot; Trelstar™ LA

Generic Available No

Index Terms AY-25650; CL-118,532; D-Trp(6)-LHRH; Triptoraline; Triptorelin Pamoate; Tryptoreline

Pharmacologic Category Gonadotropin Releasing Hormone Agonist

Use Palliative treatment of advanced prostate cancer as an alternative to orchiectomy or estrogen administration

Unlabeled/Investigational Use Treatment of endometriosis, growth hormone deficiency, hyperandrogenism, *in vitro* fertilization, ovarian carcinoma, pancreatic carcinoma, precocious puberty, uterine leiomyomata

Local Anesthetic/Vasoconstrictor Precautions No information available to require special precautions

Effects on Dental Treatment No significant effects or complications reported

Common Adverse Effects As reported with Trelstar™ Depot and Trelstar™ LA; frequency of effect may vary by product:

>10%:

Central nervous system: Headache (30% to 60%)

Endocrine & metabolic: Hot flashes (95% to 100%), glucose increased

Hematologic: Hemoglobin decreased, RBC count decreased

Hepatic: Alkaline phosphatase increased, ALT increased, AST increased

Neuromuscular & skeletal: Skeletal pain (12% to 13%)

Renal: BUN increased

1% to 10%:

Cardiovascular: Leg edema (6%), hypertension (4%), chest pain (2%), peripheral edema (1%)

Central nervous system: Dizziness (1% to 3%), pain (2% to 3%), emotional lability (1%), fatigue (2%), insomnia (2%)

Dermatologic: Rash (2%), pruritus (1%)

Endocrine & metabolic: Alkaline phosphatase increased (2%), breast pain (2%), gynecomastia (2%), libido decreased (2%), tumor flare (8%)

(Continued)

Triptorelin *(Continued)*

Gastrointestinal: Nausea (3%), anorexia (2%), constipation (2%), dyspepsia (2%), vomiting (2%), abdominal pain (1%), diarrhea (1%)

Genitourinary: Dysuria (5%), impotence (2% to 7%), urinary retention (1%), urinary tract infection (1%)

Hematologic: Anemia (1%)

Local: Injection site pain (4%)

Neuromuscular & skeletal: Leg pain (2% to 5%), back pain (3%), arthralgia (2%), leg cramps (2%), myalgia (1%), weakness (1%)

Ocular: Conjunctivitis (1%), eye pain (1%)

Respiratory: Cough (2%), dyspnea (1%), pharyngitis (1%)

Postmarketing and/or case reports: Anaphylaxis, angioedema, hypersensitivity reactions, spinal cord compression, renal dysfunction

Mechanism of Action Causes suppression of ovarian and testicular steroidogenesis due to decreased levels of LH and FSH with subsequent decrease in testosterone (male) and estrogen (female) levels. After chronic and continuous administration, usually 2-4 weeks after initiation, a sustained decrease in LH and FSH secretion occurs.

Drug Interactions

Increased Effect/Toxicity: Not studied. Hyperprolactinemic drugs (dopamine antagonists such as antipsychotics, and metoclopramide) are contraindicated.

Decreased Effect: Not studied. Hyperprolactinemic drugs (dopamine antagonists such as antipsychotics, and metoclopramide) are contraindicated.

Pharmacodynamics/Kinetics

Absorption: Oral: Not active

Distribution: V_d: 30-33 L

Protein binding: None

Metabolism: Unknown; unlikely to involve CYP; no known metabolites

Half-life elimination: 2.8 ± 1.2 hours

    Moderate to severe renal impairment: 6.5-7.7 hours

    Hepatic impairment: 7.6 hours

Time to peak: 1-3 hours

Excretion: Urine (42% as intact peptide); hepatic

Pregnancy Risk Factor X

Triptorelin Pamoate *see* Triptorelin *on page 1625*

Tris Buffer *see* Tromethamine *on page 1626*

Tris(hydroxymethyl)aminomethane *see* Tromethamine *on page 1626*

Trisodium Calcium Diethylenetriaminepentaacetate (Ca-DTPA) *see* Diethylene Triamine Penta-Acetic Acid *on page 493*

Tri-Sprintec™ *see* Ethinyl Estradiol and Norgestimate *on page 645*

Tri-Sudo® [OTC] [DSC] *see* Triprolidine and Pseudoephedrine *on page 1624*

TriTuss® *see* Guaifenesin, Dextromethorphan, and Phenylephrine *on page 798*

TriTuss® ER *see* Guaifenesin, Dextromethorphan, and Phenylephrine *on page 798*

Trivalent Inactivated Influenza Vaccine (TIV) *see* Influenza Virus Vaccine *on page 880*

Tri-Vent™ DM *see* Guaifenesin, Pseudoephedrine, and Dextromethorphan *on page 800*

Tri-Vent™ DPC *see* Chlorpheniramine, Phenylephrine, and Dextromethorphan *on page 342*

Tri-Vent™ HC *see* Hydrocodone, Carbinoxamine, and Pseudoephedrine *on page 832*

Tri-Vi-Flor® *see* Vitamins (Fluoride) *on page 1665*

Tri-Vi-Flor® with Iron *see* Vitamins (Fluoride) *on page 1665*

Trivora® *see* Ethinyl Estradiol and Levonorgestrel *on page 633*

Trizivir® *see* Abacavir, Lamivudine, and Zidovudine *on page 23*

Trobicin® [DSC] *see* Spectinomycin *on page 1491*

Trocaine® [OTC] *see* Benzocaine *on page 195*

Trolamine Salicylate *see* Triethanolamine Salicylate *on page 1617*

Tromethamine *(troe METH a meen)*

U.S. Brand Names THAM®

Generic Available No

Index Terms Tris Buffer; Tris(hydroxymethyl)aminomethane

Pharmacologic Category Alkalinizing Agent, Parenteral

Use Correction of metabolic acidosis associated with cardiac bypass surgery or cardiac arrest; to correct excess acidity of stored blood that is preserved with acid citrate dextrose (ACD); indicated in infants needing alkalinization after receiving maximum sodium bicarbonate (8-10 mEq/kg/24 hours)

Local Anesthetic/Vasoconstrictor Precautions No information available to require special precautions

Effects on Dental Treatment No significant effects or complications reported

Common Adverse Effects Frequency not defined.

Cardiovascular: Hypervolemia, venospasm

Endocrine and Metabolic: Hyperkalemia, hypoglycemia (usually doses >500 mg/kg administered over <1 hour)

Hepatic: Hepatic necrosis (resulted during delivery via umbilical venous catheter)

Local: Necrosis with extravasation, phlebitis, tissue irritation

Respiratory: Apnea, pulmonary edema, respiratory depression

Mechanism of Action Acts as a proton acceptor, which combines with hydrogen ions, liberating bicarbonate buffer, to correct acidosis. It buffers both metabolic and respiratory acids, limiting carbon dioxide generation. Also an osmotic diuretic.

Pharmacodynamics/Kinetics

Distribution: Distributes quickly into extracellular space; at steady state distributes into a volume slightly greater than total body water; penetrates slowly intracellularly

Half-life elimination: 5.6 hours

Excretion: Urine (>75%) within 8 hours

Pregnancy Risk Factor C

Tronolane® Cream [OTC] *see* Pramoxine *on page 1334*

Tronolane® Suppository [OTC] *see* Phenylephrine *on page 1293*

Tropicacyl® *see* Tropicamide *on page 1627*

Tropicamide (troe PIK a mide)

U.S. Brand Names Mydral™; Mydriacyl®; Tropicacyl®

Canadian Brand Names Diotrope®; Mydriacyl®

Generic Available Yes

Index Terms Bistropamide

Pharmacologic Category Ophthalmic Agent, Mydriatic

Use Short-acting mydriatic used in diagnostic procedures; as well as preoperatively and postoperatively; treatment of some cases of acute iritis, iridocyclitis, and keratitis

Local Anesthetic/Vasoconstrictor Precautions No information available to require special precautions

Effects on Dental Treatment Key adverse event(s) related to dental treatment: Dryness of mouth.

Mechanism of Action Prevents the sphincter muscle of the iris and the muscle of the ciliary body from responding to cholinergic stimulation

Pregnancy Risk Factor C

Tropicamide and Hydroxyamphetamine *see* Hydroxyamphetamine and Tropicamide *on page 843*

Trospium (TROSE pee um)

U.S. Brand Names Sanctura®

Canadian Brand Names Trosec

Generic Available No

Index Terms Trospium Chloride

Pharmacologic Category Anticholinergic Agent

Use Treatment of overactive bladder with symptoms of urgency, incontinence, and urinary frequency

Local Anesthetic/Vasoconstrictor Precautions No information available to require special precautions

Effects on Dental Treatment Key adverse event(s) related to dental treatment: Significant xerostomia and changes in salivation (normal salivary flow resumes upon discontinuation).

Common Adverse Effects

>10%: Gastrointestinal: Xerostomia (20%)

1% to 10%:

Cardiovascular: Tachycardia, heart rate increase

Central nervous system: Headache (4%), fatigue (2%)

Dermatologic: Dry skin

Gastrointestinal: Constipation (10%), abdominal pain (2%), dyspepsia (1%), flatulence (1%), abdominal distention, vomiting, dysgeusia

(Continued)

Trospium *(Continued)*

Genitourinary: Urinary retention (1%)

Ocular: Dry eyes (1%), blurred vision

Mechanism of Action Trospium antagonizes the effects of acetylcholine on muscarinic receptors in cholinergically innervated organs. It reduces the smooth muscle tone of the bladder.

Drug Interactions

Increased Effect/Toxicity: Trospium anticholinergic effects may be increased when administered with other anticholinergics and pramlintide.

Decreased Effect: Trospium anticholinergic effect may be decreased when administered with acetylcholinesterase inhibitors (central).

Pharmacodynamics/Kinetics

Absorption: <10%; decreased with food

Distribution: V_d: 395 L, primarily in plasma

Protein binding: 50% to 85% *in vitro*

Metabolism: Hypothesized to be via esterase hydrolysis and conjugation; forms metabolites

Bioavailability: ~10%

Half-life elimination: 20 hours; severe renal insufficiency (Cl_{cr} <30 mL/minute): ~33 hours

Time to peak, plasma: 5-6 hours

Excretion: Feces (85%); urine (~6%; mostly as unchanged drug) primarily via active tubular secretion

Pregnancy Risk Factor C

Trospium Chloride *see* Trospium *on page 1627*

Troxidone *see* Trimethadione *on page 1620*

Trusopt® *see* Dorzolamide *on page 528*

Truvada® *see* Emtricitabine and Tenofovir *on page 563*

Trypsin, Balsam Peru, and Castor Oil
(TRIP sin, BAL sam pe RUE, & KAS tor oyl)

Related Information

Castor Oil *on page 295*

U.S. Brand Names Granulex®; Optase™; Xenaderm™

Generic Available Yes: Aerosol

Index Terms Balsam Peru, Trypsin, and Castor Oil; Castor Oil, Trypsin, and Balsam Peru

Pharmacologic Category Protectant, Topical

Use Treatment of decubitus ulcers, varicose ulcers, debridement of eschar, dehiscent wounds and sunburn; promote wound healing; reduce odor from necrotic wounds

Local Anesthetic/Vasoconstrictor Precautions No information available to require special precautions

Effects on Dental Treatment No significant effects or complications reported

Common Adverse Effects Frequency not defined: Local: Temporary stinging at application site

Mechanism of Action Trypsin is used to debride necrotic tissue; balsam peru stimulates circulation at the wound site and may be mildly bactericidal; castor oil improves epithelialization, acts as a protectant covering and helps reduce pain

Tryptoreline *see* Triptorelin *on page 1625*

TSH *see* Thyrotropin Alpha *on page 1563*

TSPA *see* Thiotepa *on page 1559*

TST *see* Tuberculin Tests *on page 1628*

Tuberculin Purified Protein Derivative *see* Tuberculin Tests *on page 1628*

Tuberculin Skin Test *see* Tuberculin Tests *on page 1628*

Tuberculin Tests (too BER kyoo lin tests)

U.S. Brand Names Aplisol®; Tubersol®

Generic Available No

Index Terms Mantoux; PPD; TB Skin Test; TST; Tuberculin Purified Protein Derivative; Tuberculin Skin Test

Pharmacologic Category Diagnostic Agent

Use Skin test in diagnosis of tuberculosis

Local Anesthetic/Vasoconstrictor Precautions No information available to require special precautions

Effects on Dental Treatment No significant effects or complications reported

Common Adverse Effects Suspected adverse reactions should be reported to the Food and Drug Administration (FDA) MedWatch Program at 1-800-332-1088

Frequency not defined:

Dermatologic: Rash

Local: Injection site reactions: Bleeding, bruising, discomfort, erythematous reaction, hematoma, necrosis, pain, pruritus, redness, scarring, ulceration, vesiculation

Miscellaneous: Anaphylaxis

Mechanism of Action Tuberculosis results in individuals becoming sensitized to certain antigenic components of the *M. tuberculosis* organism. Culture extracts called tuberculins are contained in tuberculin skin test preparations. Upon intracutaneous injection of these culture extracts, a classic delayed (cellular) hypersensitivity reaction occurs. This reaction is characteristic of a delayed course (peak occurs >24 hours after injection, induration of the skin secondary to cell infiltration, and occasional vesiculation and necrosis). Delayed hypersensitivity reactions to tuberculin may indicate infection with a variety of nontuberculosis mycobacteria, or vaccination with the live attenuated mycobacterial strain of *M. bovis* vaccine, BCG, in addition to previous natural infection with *M. tuberculosis*.

Drug Interactions

Decreased Effect: Reaction may be depressed or suppressed in patients receiving systemic corticosteroids, immunosuppressants, live viral vaccines.

Pharmacodynamics/Kinetics

Onset of action: Delayed hypersensitivity reactions: 5-6 hours

Peak effect: 48-72 hours

Duration: Reactions subside over a few days

Pregnancy Risk Factor C

Tubersol® *see* Tuberculin Tests *on page 1628*

Tucks® Anti-Itch [OTC] *see* Hydrocortisone *on page 836*

Tucks® Hemorrhoidal [OTC] *see* Pramoxine *on page 1334*

Tuinal® [DSC] *see* Amobarbital and Secobarbital *on page 106*

Tums® [OTC] *see* Calcium Carbonate *on page 260*

Tums® E-X [OTC] *see* Calcium Carbonate *on page 260*

Tums® Extra Strength Sugar Free [OTC] *see* Calcium Carbonate *on page 260*

Tums® Smoothies™ [OTC] *see* Calcium Carbonate *on page 260*

Tums® Ultra [OTC] *see* Calcium Carbonate *on page 260*

Tur-bi-kal® [OTC] *see* Phenylephrine *on page 1293*

Tusnel Pediatric® *see* Guaifenesin, Pseudoephedrine, and Dextromethorphan *on page 800*

Tussafed® [DSC] *see* Carbinoxamine, Pseudoephedrine, and Dextromethorphan *on page 282*

Tussafed® HC *see* Hydrocodone, Phenylephrine, and Guaifenesin *on page 834*

Tussafed® HCG *see* Hydrocodone, Phenylephrine, and Guaifenesin *on page 834*

Tussend® Expectorant [DSC] *see* Hydrocodone, Pseudoephedrine, and Guaifenesin *on page 835*

Tussi-12® *see* Carbetapentane and Chlorpheniramine *on page 278*

Tussi-12® D *see* Carbetapentane, Phenylephrine, and Pyrilamine *on page 280*

Tussi-12® DS *see* Carbetapentane, Phenylephrine, and Pyrilamine *on page 280*

Tussi-12 S™ *see* Carbetapentane and Chlorpheniramine *on page 278*

Tussigon® *see* Hydrocodone and Homatropine *on page 829*

TussiNate™ *see* Hydrocodone, Phenylephrine, and Diphenhydramine *on page 834*

Tussionex® *see* Hydrocodone and Chlorpheniramine *on page 827*

Tussi-Organidin® DM NR *see* Guaifenesin and Dextromethorphan *on page 796*

Tussi-Organidin® DM-S NR *see* Guaifenesin and Dextromethorphan *on page 796*

Tussi-Organidin® NR *see* Guaifenesin and Codeine *on page 795*

Tussi-Organidin® S-NR *see* Guaifenesin and Codeine *on page 795*

Tussizone-12 RF™ *see* Carbetapentane and Chlorpheniramine *on page 278*

Tusso-DF® *see* Hydrocodone and Guaifenesin *on page 828*

T-Vites [OTC] *see* Vitamins (Multiple/Oral) *on page 1665*

TVP-1012 *see* Rasagiline *on page 1412*

Twelve Resin-K *see* Cyanocobalamin *on page 418*

Twilite® [OTC] *see* DiphenhydrAMINE *on page 510*

Twinject™ *see* Epinephrine *on page 572*

Twinrix® *see* Hepatitis A Inactivated and Hepatitis B (Recombinant) Vaccine *on page 808*

Typhoid Vaccine (TYE foid vak SEEN)

Related Information
Immunizations (Vaccines) *on page 1886*

U.S. Brand Names Typhim Vi®; Vivotif®

Generic Available No

Index Terms Ty21a Vaccine; Typhoid Vaccine Live Oral Ty21a; Vi Vaccine

Pharmacologic Category Vaccine

Use Active immunization against typhoid fever caused by *Salmonella typhi*
Not for routine vaccination. In the United States, use should be limited to:
— Travelers to areas with risk of exposure to *S. typhi*
— Persons with intimate exposure to a *S. typhi* carrier
— Laboratory technicians with exposure to *S. typhi*

Local Anesthetic/Vasoconstrictor Precautions No information available to require special precautions

Effects on Dental Treatment No significant effects or complications reported

Common Adverse Effects All serious adverse reactions must be reported to the U.S. Department of Health and Human Services (DHHS) Vaccine Adverse Event Reporting System (VAERS) 1-800-822-7967.

Oral:
1% to 10%:
Central nervous system: Headache (5%), fever (3%)
Dermatologic: Rash (1%)
Gastrointestinal: Abdominal pain (6%), diarrhea (3%), nausea (6%), vomiting (2%)

Injection:
>10%:
Central nervous system: Headache (16% to 20%), fever <100°F (3% to 11%), malaise (4% to 24%)
Local: Tenderness (97% to 98%), induration (5% to 15%), pain at injection site (27% to 41%)
1% to 10%:
Central nervous system: Fever ≥100°F (2%)
Gastrointestinal: Nausea (2% to 8%), vomiting (2%)
Local: Erythema at injection site (4% to 5%)
Neuromuscular & skeletal: Myalgia (3% to 7%)

Mechanism of Action Virulent strains of *Salmonella typhi* cause disease by penetrating the intestinal mucosa and entering the systemic circulation via the lymphatic vasculature. One possible mechanism of conferring immunity may be the provocation of a local immune response in the intestinal tract induced by oral ingesting of a live strain with subsequent aborted infection. The ability of *Salmonella typhi* to produce clinical disease (and to elicit an immune response) is dependent on the bacteria having a complete lipopolysaccharide. The live attenuate Ty21a strain lacks the enzyme UDP-4-galactose epimerase so that lipopolysaccharide is only synthesized under conditions that induce bacterial autolysis. Thus, the strain remains avirulent despite the production of sufficient lipopolysaccharide to evoke a protective immune response. Despite low levels of lipopolysaccharide synthesis, cells lyse before gaining a virulent phenotype due to the intracellular accumulation of metabolic intermediates.

Drug Interactions

Increased Effect/Toxicity: Immunosuppressants may enhance the adverse/ toxic effect of live vaccines; vaccinial infections may develop.

Decreased Effect: Antibiotics (systemic) may decrease the effect of oral live attenuated Ty21a vaccine (Vivotif®); delay vaccine administration for at least 24 hours after administration of these drugs. Mefloquine may decrease the effect of oral live attenuated Ty21a vaccine (Vivotif®); the CDC recommends delaying vaccine administration for at least 24 hours after administration of mefloquine (the manufacturer notes that no delay is needed). Proguanil may decrease the effect of oral live attenuated Ty21a vaccine (Vivotif®); separate dosing by at least 10 days. Immune globulins may diminish the therapeutic effect of live vaccines.

Pharmacodynamics/Kinetics

Onset of action: Immunity to *Salmonella typhi*: Oral: ~1 week

Duration: Immunity: Oral: ~4-7 years; Parenteral: >17-21 months

Pregnancy Risk Factor C

Undecylenic Acid and Derivatives

(un de sil EN ik AS id & dah RIV ah tivs)

U.S. Brand Names Fungi-Nail® [OTC]

Generic Available No

Index Terms Zinc Undecylenate

Pharmacologic Category Antifungal Agent, Topical

Use Treatment of athlete's foot (tinea pedis); ringworm (except nails and scalp)

Local Anesthetic/Vasoconstrictor Precautions No information available to require special precautions

Effects on Dental Treatment No significant effects or complications reported

Unicap M® [OTC] *see* Vitamins (Multiple/Oral) *on page 1665*

Unicap Sr® [OTC] *see* Vitamins (Multiple/Oral) *on page 1665*

Unicap T™ [OTC] *see* Vitamins (Multiple/Oral) *on page 1665*

Uni-Cof [DSC] *see* Pseudoephedrine, Dihydrocodeine, and Chlorpheniramine *on page 1385*

Uniphyl® *see* Theophylline *on page 1554*

Uniretic® *see* Moexipril and Hydrochlorothiazide *on page 1117*

Uni-Senna [OTC] *see* Senna *on page 1462*

Unisom® Maximum Strength SleepGels® [OTC] *see* DiphenhydrAMINE *on page 510*

Unisom® SleepTabs® [OTC] *see* Doxylamine *on page 544*

Unithroid® *see* Levothyroxine *on page 970*

Univasc® *see* Moexipril *on page 1116*

Unna's Boot *see* Zinc Gelatin *on page 1682*

Unna's Paste *see* Zinc Gelatin *on page 1682*

Unoprostone (yoo noe PROS tone)

Canadian Brand Names Rescula®
Mexican Brand Names Rescula
Generic Available No
Index Terms Unoprostone Isopropyl
Pharmacologic Category Ophthalmic Agent, Antiglaucoma; Prostaglandin, Ophthalmic
Use To lower intraocular pressure (IOP) in patients with open-angle glaucoma or ocular hypertension; should be used in patients who are not tolerant of, or failed treatment with other IOP-lowering medications
Local Anesthetic/Vasoconstrictor Precautions No information available to require special precautions
Effects on Dental Treatment No significant effects or complications reported
Mechanism of Action The exact mechanism of action is unknown; however, unoprostone decreases IOP by increasing the outflow of aqueous humor. Cardiovascular and pulmonary function were not affected in clinical studies. IOP was decreased by 3-4 mm Hg in patients with a mean baseline IOP of 23 mm Hg.
Pregnancy Risk Factor C

Unoprostone Isopropyl *see* Unoprostone *on page 1632*

Urea (yoor EE a)

U.S. Brand Names Amino-Cerv™; Aquacare® [OTC]; Aquaphilic® With Carbamide [OTC]; Carmol® 10 [OTC]; Carmol® 20 [OTC]; Carmol® 40; Carmol® Deep Cleaning; Cerovel™; DPM™ [OTC]; Gormel® [OTC]; Keralac™; Keralac™ Nailstik; Lanaphilic® [OTC]; Nutraplus® [OTC]; Rea-Lo® [OTC]; Ultra Mide® [OTC]; Umecta®; Ureacin® [OTC]; Vanamide™
Canadian Brand Names UltraMide 25™; Uremol®; Urisec®
Mexican Brand Names Nutraplus
Generic Available Yes: Excludes ointment, shampoo
Index Terms Carbamide
Pharmacologic Category Diuretic, Osmotic; Keratolytic Agent; Topical Skin Product
Use
Topical: Keratolytic agent to soften nails or skin; OTC: Moisturizer for dry, rough skin
Vaginal: Treatment of cervicitis
Local Anesthetic/Vasoconstrictor Precautions No information available to require special precautions
Effects on Dental Treatment No significant effects or complications reported
Common Adverse Effects Frequency not defined: Topical: Local: Transient stinging, local irritation
Mechanism of Action
Topical: Urea softens hyperkeratotic areas by dissolving the intracellular matrix, resulting in loosening the horny layer of the skin, or softening and debridement of the nail plate
Vaginal: Urea aids in debridement, promotes epithelialization, and prevents excessive tissue formation
Pregnancy Risk Factor C

Urea and Hydrocortisone (yoor EE a & hye droe KOR ti sone)

Related Information
Hydrocortisone *on page 836*
Urea *on page 1632*
U.S. Brand Names Carmol-HC®
Canadian Brand Names Ti-U-Lac® H; Uremol® HC
Generic Available No
Index Terms Hydrocortisone and Urea
Pharmacologic Category Corticosteroid, Topical
Use Inflammation of corticosteroid-responsive dermatoses
Local Anesthetic/Vasoconstrictor Precautions No information available to require special precautions
Effects on Dental Treatment No significant effects or complications reported
Drug Interactions
Cytochrome P450 Effect: Hydrocortisone: **Substrate** of CYP3A4 (minor); **Induces** CYP3A4 (weak)
Pharmacodynamics/Kinetics See individual agents.
Pregnancy Risk Factor C

Urea, Chlorophyllin, and Papain *see Chlorophyllin, Papain, and Urea on page 335*

Ureacin® [OTC] *see Urea on page 1632*

Urea Peroxide *see Carbamide Peroxide on page 276*

Urecholine® *see Bethanechol on page 211*

Urelle® *see Methenamine, Sodium Biphosphate, Phenyl Salicylate, Methylene Blue, and Hyoscyamine on page 1064*

Urex® *see Methenamine on page 1063*

Urimar-T *see Methenamine, Sodium Biphosphate, Phenyl Salicylate, Methylene Blue, and Hyoscyamine on page 1064*

Urispas® *see Flavoxate on page 693*

Uristat® [OTC] *see Phenazopyridine on page 1286*

Urocit®-K *see Potassium Citrate on page 1329*

Urofollitropin (yoor oh fol li TROE pin)

U.S. Brand Names Bravelle®
Canadian Brand Names Bravelle®; Fertinorm® H.P.
Index Terms Follicle-Stimulating Hormone, Human; FSH; hFSH
Pharmacologic Category Gonadotropin; Ovulation Stimulator
Use Ovulation induction in patients who previously received pituitary suppression; development of multiple follicles with Assisted Reproductive Technologies (ART)
Local Anesthetic/Vasoconstrictor Precautions No information available to require special precautions
Effects on Dental Treatment No significant effects or complications reported
Common Adverse Effects Percentage may vary by indication, route of administration.
>10%:
Central nervous system: Headache
Endocrine & metabolic: Ovarian enlargement, ovarian hyperstimulation syndrome
Gastrointestinal: Abdominal cramps
1% to 10%:
Cardiovascular: Hypertension
Central nervous system: Depression, emotional lability, fever, pain
Dermatologic: Acne, exfoliative dermatitis, rash
Endocrine & metabolic: Breast tenderness, hot flashes, ovarian disorder (pain, cyst)
Gastrointestinal: Abdomen enlarged, abdominal pain, constipation, diarrhea, dehydration, nausea, vomiting, weight gain
Genitourinary: Cervical disorder, urinary tract infection, pelvic pain/cramps, uterine spasms, vaginal discharge, vaginal hemorrhage, vaginal spotting
Local: Injection site reaction
Neuromuscular & skeletal: Neck pain
Respiratory: Respiratory disorder, sinusitis
Miscellaneous: Infection, post retrieval pain
Mechanism of Action Urofollitropin is a preparation of highly purified follicle-stimulating hormone (FSH) extracted from the urine of postmenopausal women. Follitropins stimulate ovarian follicular growth in women who do not (Continued)

Urofollitropin (Continued)

have primary ovarian failure. FSH is required for normal follicular growth, maturation, gonadal steroid production, and spermatogenesis.

Pharmacodynamics/Kinetics

Half-life elimination

I.M.: 37 hours, 15 hours following multiple doses

SubQ: 32 hours, 21 hours following multiple doses

Time to peak, plasma:

I.M.: 17 hours, 11 hours following multiple doses

SubQ: 21 hours, 10 hours following multiple doses

Pregnancy Risk Factor X

Uro-KP-Neutral® *see* Potassium Phosphate and Sodium Phosphate *on page 1332*

Uro-Mag® [OTC] *see* Magnesium Oxide *on page 1015*

Uroxatral® *see* Alfuzosin *on page 69*

Urso 250™ *see* Ursodiol *on page 1634*

Ursodeoxycholic Acid *see* Ursodiol *on page 1634*

Ursodiol (ur soe DYE ol)

U.S. Brand Names Actigall®; Urso 250™; Urso Forte™

Canadian Brand Names Urso®; Urso® DS

Mexican Brand Names Ursofalk

Generic Available Yes: Capsule

Index Terms Ursodeoxycholic Acid

Pharmacologic Category Gallstone Dissolution Agent

Use Actigall®: Gallbladder stone dissolution; prevention of gallstones in obese patients experiencing rapid weight loss; Urso®: Primary biliary cirrhosis

Unlabeled/Investigational Use Liver transplantation

Local Anesthetic/Vasoconstrictor Precautions No information available to require special precautions

Effects on Dental Treatment No significant effects or complications reported

Common Adverse Effects

>10%:

Central nervous system: Headache (up to 25%), dizziness (up to 17%)

Gastrointestinal: In treatment of primary biliary cirrhosis: Constipation (up to 26%)

1% to 10%:

Dermatologic: Rash (<1% to 3%), alopecia (<1% to 5%)

Gastrointestinal:

In gallstone dissolution: Most GI events (diarrhea, nausea, vomiting) are similar to placebo and attributable to gallstone disease.

In treatment of primary biliary cirrhosis: Diarrhea (1%)

Hematologic: Leukopenia (3%)

Miscellaneous: Allergy (5%)

Mechanism of Action Decreases the cholesterol content of bile and bile stones by reducing the secretion of cholesterol from the liver and the fractional reabsorption of cholesterol by the intestines. Mechanism of action in primary biliary cirrhosis is not clearly defined.

Drug Interactions

Decreased Effect: Decreased effect with aluminum-containing antacids, cholestyramine, colestipol, clofibrate, and oral contraceptives (estrogens).

Pharmacodynamics/Kinetics

Metabolism: Undergoes extensive enterohepatic recycling; following hepatic conjugation and biliary secretion, the drug is hydrolyzed to active ursodiol, where it is recycled or transformed to lithocholic acid by colonic microbial flora

Half-life elimination: 100 hours

Excretion: Feces

Pregnancy Risk Factor B

Urso Forte™ *see* Ursodiol *on page 1634*

UTI Relief® [OTC] *see* Phenazopyridine *on page 1286*

Uvadex® *see* Methoxsalen *on page 1074*

Vaccinia Immune Globulin (Intravenous)
(vax IN ee a i MYUN GLOB yoo lin IN tra VEE nus)

U.S. Brand Names CNJ-016™

Generic Available No

Index Terms VIGIV

Pharmacologic Category Immune Globulin

Use Treatment of infectious complications of smallpox (vaccinia virus) vaccination, such as eczema vaccinatum, progressive vaccinia, and severe generalized vaccinia; treatment of vaccinia infections in individuals with concurrent skin conditions or accidental virus exposure to eyes (except vaccinia keratitis), mouth, or other areas where viral infection would pose significant risk

Local Anesthetic/Vasoconstrictor Precautions No information available to require special precautions

Effects on Dental Treatment No significant effects or complications reported

Common Adverse Effects Note: Actual frequency varies by dose, rate of infusion, and specific product used

Cardiovascular: Flushing

Central nervous system: Cold or hot feeling, dizziness, fatigue, headache, pain, pallor, pyrexia

Dermatologic: Erythema, urticaria

Gastrointestinal: Abdominal pain, appetite decreased, nausea, vomiting

Local: Injection site reaction

Neuromuscular & skeletal: Arthralgia, back pain, paraesthesia, muscle cramp, rigors, tremor, weakness

Miscellaneous: Diaphoresis

Mechanism of Action Antibodies obtained from pooled human plasma of individuals immunized with the smallpox vaccine provide passive immunity

Drug Interactions

Decreased Effect: Vaccina immune globulin may interfere with immune response to live virus vaccines (eg, polio, measles, mumps, and rubella); live virus vaccinations should be deferred until 6 months after administration of VIGIV. If given shortly before receiving VIGIV, revaccination with the live virus may be necessary (consult individual products for guidance).

Pharmacodynamics/Kinetics

Distribution: V_d: CNJ-016™ (Cangene product): 6630 L

Half-life elimination:

CNJ-016™ (Cangene product): 30 days (range 13-67 days)

DynPort product: 22 days

Pregnancy Risk Factor C

Vagifem® *see* Estradiol *on page 602*

Vagi-Gard® [OTC] *see* Povidone-Iodine *on page 1332*

Vagistat®-1 [OTC] *see* Tioconazole *on page 1573*

Valacyclovir (val ay SYE kloe veer)

Related Information

Acyclovir *on page 49*

Systemic Viral Diseases *on page 1767*

Treatment of Sexually-Transmitted Infections *on page 1920*

Viral Infections *on page 1806*

Related Sample Prescriptions

Herpes Simplex (Recurrent) *on page 1843*

Shingles (Varicella-Zoster Virus) *on page 1843*

U.S. Brand Names Valtrex®

Canadian Brand Names Valtrex®

Mexican Brand Names Rapivir

Generic Available No

Index Terms Valacyclovir Hydrochloride

Pharmacologic Category Antiviral Agent, Oral

Dental Use Treatment of herpes labialis (cold sores)

Use Treatment of herpes zoster (shingles) in immunocompetent patients; treatment of first-episode genital herpes; episodic treatment of recurrent genital herpes; suppression of recurrent genital herpes and reduction of heterosexual transmission of genital herpes in immunocompetent patients; suppression of genital herpes in HIV-infected individuals; treatment of herpes labialis (cold sores)

Local Anesthetic/Vasoconstrictor Precautions No information available to require special precautions

Effects on Dental Treatment No significant effects or complications reported

Significant Adverse Effects

>10%: Central nervous system: Headache (14% to 35%)

1% to 10%:

Central nervous system: Dizziness (2% to 4%), depression (0% to 7%)

Endocrine: Dysmenorrhea (≤1% to 8%)

(Continued)

Valacyclovir *(Continued)*

Gastrointestinal: Abdominal pain (2% to 11%), vomiting (<1% to 6%), nausea (6% to 15%)

Hematologic: Leukopenia (≤1%), thrombocytopenia (≤1%)

Hepatic: AST increased (1% to 4%)

Neuromuscular & skeletal: Arthralgia (≤1 to 6%)

<1% (Limited to important or life-threatening): Acute hypersensitivity reactions (angioedema, anaphylaxis, dyspnea, pruritus, rash, urticaria), aggression, agitation, alopecia, aplastic anemia, ataxia, coma, confusion, dysarthria, encephalopathy, erythema multiforme, hallucinations (auditory and visual), hemolytic uremic syndrome (HUS), hepatitis, leukocytoclastic vasculitis, mania, photosensitivity reaction, psychosis, rash, renal failure, seizure, thrombotic thrombocytopenic purpura/hemolytic uremic syndrome, tremor

Dental Usual Dosing

Herpes labialis (cold sores): Adolescents and Adults: Oral: 2 g twice daily for 1 day (separate doses by ~12 hours)

Dosage Oral:

Adolescents and Adults: Herpes labialis (cold sores): 2 g twice daily for 1 day (separate doses by ~12 hours)

Adults:

Herpes zoster (shingles): 1 g 3 times/day for 7 days

Genital herpes:

Initial episode: 1 g twice daily for 10 days

Recurrent episode: 500 mg twice daily for 3 days

Reduction of transmission: 500 mg once daily (source partner)

Suppressive therapy:

Immunocompetent patients: 1000 mg once daily (500 mg once daily in patients with <9 recurrences per year)

HIV-infected patients (CD4 ≥100 cells/mm^3): 500 mg twice daily

Dosing interval in renal impairment:

Herpes zoster: Adults:

Cl_{cr} 30-49 mL/minute: 1 g every 12 hours

Cl_{cr} 10-29 mL/minute: 1 g every 24 hours

Cl_{cr} <10 mL/minute: 500 mg every 24 hours

Genital herpes: Adults:

Initial episode:

Cl_{cr} 10-29 mL/minute: 1 g every 24 hours

Cl_{cr} <10 mL/minute: 500 mg every 24 hours

Recurrent episode: Cl_{cr} <10-29 mL/minute: 500 mg every 24 hours

Suppressive therapy: Cl_{cr} <10-29 mL/minute:

For usual dose of 1 g every 24 hours, decrease dose to 500 mg every 24 hours

For usual dose of 500 mg every 24 hours, decrease dose to 500 mg every 48 hours

HIV-infected patients: 500 mg every 24 hours

Herpes labialis: Adolescents and Adults:

Cl_{cr} 30-49 mL/minute: 1 g every 12 hours for 2 doses

Cl_{cr} 10-29 mL/minute: 500 mg every 12 hours for 2 doses

Cl_{cr} <10 mL/minute: 500 mg as a single dose

Hemodialysis: Dialyzable (~33% removed during 4-hour session); administer dose postdialysis

Chronic ambulatory peritoneal dialysis/continuous arteriovenous hemofiltration dialysis: Pharmacokinetic parameters are similar to those in patients with ESRD; supplemental dose not needed following dialysis

Mechanism of Action Valacyclovir is rapidly and nearly completely converted to acyclovir by intestinal and hepatic metabolism. Acyclovir is converted to acyclovir monophosphate by virus-specific thymidine kinase then further converted to acyclovir triphosphate by other cellular enzymes. Acyclovir triphosphate inhibits DNA synthesis and viral replication by competing with deoxyguanosine triphosphate for viral DNA polymerase and being incorporated into viral DNA.

Contraindications Hypersensitivity to valacyclovir, acyclovir, or any component of the formulation

Warnings/Precautions Hazardous agent - use appropriate precautions for handling and disposal. Thrombotic thrombocytopenic purpura/hemolytic uremic syndrome has occurred in immunocompromised patients (at doses of 8 g/day); use caution and adjust the dose in elderly patients or those with renal insufficiency and in patients receiving concurrent nephrotoxic agents. For genital herpes, treatment should begin as soon as possible after the first signs and symptoms (within 72 hours of onset of first diagnosis or within 24 hours of onset of recurrent episodes). For herpes zoster, treatment should begin within 72 hours of onset of rash. For cold sores, treatment should begin at with earliest symptom (tingling, itching, burning). Safety and efficacy in prepubertal patients have not been established.

Drug Interactions

Cimetidine: Decreased renal clearance of acyclovir; no dosage adjustment needed in patients with normal renal function.

Probenecid: Decreased renal clearance of acyclovir; no dosage adjustment needed in patients with normal renal function.

Dietary Considerations May be taken with or without food.

Pharmacodynamics/Kinetics

Absorption: Rapid

Distribution: Acyclovir is widely distributed throughout the body including brain, kidney, lungs, liver, spleen, muscle, uterus, vagina, and CSF

Protein binding: 13.5% to 17.9%

Metabolism: Hepatic; valacyclovir is rapidly and nearly completely converted to acyclovir and L-valine by first-pass effect; acyclovir is hepatically metabolized to a very small extent by aldehyde oxidase and by alcohol and aldehyde dehydrogenase (inactive metabolites)

Bioavailability: ~55% once converted to acyclovir

Half-life elimination: Normal renal function: Adults: Acyclovir: 2.5-3.3 hours, Valacyclovir: ~30 minutes; End-stage renal disease: Acyclovir: 14-20 hours

Excretion: Urine, primarily as acyclovir (88%); **Note:** Following oral administration of radiolabeled valacyclovir, 46% of the label is eliminated in the feces (corresponding to nonabsorbed drug), while 47% of the radiolabel is eliminated in the urine.

Pregnancy Risk Factor B

Lactation Enters breast milk/use caution

Breast-Feeding Considerations Peak concentrations in breast milk range from 0.5-2.3 times the corresponding maternal acyclovir serum concentration. This is expected to provide a nursing infant with a dose of acyclovir equivalent to ~0.6 mg/kg/day following ingestion of valacyclovir 500 mg twice daily by the mother. Use with caution while breast-feeding.

Dosage Forms Excipient information presented when available (limited, particularly for generics); consult specific product labeling.

Caplet: 500 mg, 1000 mg

Valacyclovir Hydrochloride *see* Valacyclovir *on page 1635*

Valcyte™ *see* Valganciclovir *on page 1637*

Valganciclovir (val gan SYE kloh veer)

Related Information

Ganciclovir *on page 763*

U.S. Brand Names Valcyte™

Canadian Brand Names Valcyte™

Mexican Brand Names Valcyte

Generic Available No

Index Terms Valganciclovir Hydrochloride

Pharmacologic Category Antiviral Agent

Use Treatment of cytomegalovirus (CMV) retinitis in patients with acquired immunodeficiency syndrome (AIDS); prevention of CMV disease in high-risk patients (donor CMV positive/recipient CMV negative) undergoing kidney, heart, or kidney/pancreas transplantation

Local Anesthetic/Vasoconstrictor Precautions No information available to require special precautions

Effects on Dental Treatment No significant effects or complications reported

Common Adverse Effects

>10%:

Central nervous system: Fever (31%), headache (9% to 22%), insomnia (16%)

Gastrointestinal: Diarrhea (16% to 41%), nausea (8% to 30%), vomiting (21%), abdominal pain (15%)

Hematologic: Granulocytopenia (11% to 27%), anemia (8% to 26%)

Ocular: Retinal detachment (15%)

1% to 10%:

Central nervous system: Peripheral neuropathy (9%), paresthesia (8%), seizure (<5%), psychosis, hallucinations (<5%), confusion (<5%), agitation (<5%)

Hematologic: Thrombocytopenia (8%), pancytopenia (<5%), bone marrow depression (<5%), aplastic anemia (<5%), bleeding (potentially life-threatening due to thrombocytopenia <5%)

Renal: Renal function decreased (<5%)

Miscellaneous: Local and systemic infection, including sepsis (<5%); allergic reaction (<5%)

(Continued)

Valganciclovir (Continued)

Mechanism of Action Valganciclovir is rapidly converted to ganciclovir in the body. The bioavailability of ganciclovir from valganciclovir is increased 10-fold compared to oral ganciclovir. A dose of 900 mg achieved systemic exposure of ganciclovir comparable to that achieved with the recommended doses of intravenous ganciclovir of 5 mg/kg. Ganciclovir is phosphorylated to a substrate which competitively inhibits the binding of deoxyguanosine triphosphate to DNA polymerase resulting in inhibition of viral DNA synthesis.

Drug Interactions

Increased Effect/Toxicity: Reported for ganciclovir: Immunosuppressive agents may increase hematologic toxicity of ganciclovir. Imipenem/cilastatin may increase seizure potential. Oral ganciclovir increases blood levels of zidovudine, although zidovudine decreases steady-state levels of ganciclovir. Since both drugs have the potential to cause neutropenia and anemia, some patients may not tolerate concomitant therapy with these drugs at full dosage. Didanosine levels are increased with concurrent ganciclovir. Other nephrotoxic drugs (eg, amphotericin and cyclosporine) may have additive nephrotoxicity with ganciclovir.

Decreased Effect: Reported for ganciclovir: A decrease in blood levels of ganciclovir AUC may occur when used with didanosine.

Pharmacodynamics/Kinetics

Absorption: Well absorbed; high-fat meal increases AUC by 30%

Distribution: Ganciclovir: V_d: 15.26 L/1.73 m^2; widely to all tissue including CSF and ocular tissue

Protein binding: 1% to 2%

Metabolism: Converted to ganciclovir by intestinal mucosal cells and hepatocytes

Bioavailability: With food: 60%

Half-life elimination: Ganciclovir: 4.08 hours; prolonged with renal impairment; Severe renal impairment: Up to 68 hours

Excretion: Urine (primarily as ganciclovir)

Pregnancy Risk Factor C

Valganciclovir Hydrochloride see Valganciclovir on page 1637

Valium® see Diazepam on page 480

Valorin [OTC] see Acetaminophen on page 31

Valorin Extra [OTC] see Acetaminophen on page 31

Valproate Semisodium see Valproic Acid and Derivatives on page 1638

Valproate Sodium see Valproic Acid and Derivatives on page 1638

Valproic Acid see Valproic Acid and Derivatives on page 1638

Valproic Acid and Derivatives
(val PROE ik AS id & dah RIV ah tives)

U.S. Brand Names Depacon®; Depakene®; Depakote®; Depakote® ER; Depakote® Sprinkle

Canadian Brand Names Alti-Divalproex; Apo-Divalproex®; Apo-Valproic®; Depakene®; Epival® I.V.; Gen-Divalproex; Novo-Divalproex; Nu-Divalproex; PMS-Valproic Acid; PMS-Valproic Acid E.C.; Rhoxal-valproic; Sandoz-Valproic

Mexican Brand Names Depakene; Epival; Leptilan

Generic Available Yes: Capsule (excluding sprinkle), injection, syrup

Index Terms Dipropylacetic Acid; Divalproex Sodium; DPA; 2-Propylpentanoic Acid; 2-Propylvaleric Acid; Valproate Semisodium; Valproate Sodium; Valproic Acid

Pharmacologic Category Anticonvulsant, Miscellaneous

Use

Depacon®, Depakene®, Depakote®, Depakote® ER, Depakote® Sprinkle: Monotherapy and adjunctive therapy in the treatment of patients with complex partial seizures; monotherapy and adjunctive therapy of simple and complex absence seizures; adjunctive therapy in patients with multiple seizure types that include absence seizures

Depakote®, Depakote® ER: Mania associated with bipolar disorder; migraine prophylaxis

Unlabeled/Investigational Use Status epilepticus

Local Anesthetic/Vasoconstrictor Precautions No information available to require special precautions

Effects on Dental Treatment Key adverse event(s) related to dental treatment: Periodontal abscess and taste perversion.

Common Adverse Effects

Adverse reactions reported when used as monotherapy for complex partial seizure:

>10%:

Central nervous system: Somnolence (18% to 30%), dizziness (13% to 18%), insomnia (9% to 15%), nervousness (7% to 11%)

Dermatologic: Alopecia (13% to 24%)

Gastrointestinal: Nausea (26% to 34%), vomiting (15% to 23%), diarrhea (19% to 23%), abdominal pain (9% to 12%), dyspepsia (10% to 11%), anorexia (4% to 11%)

Hematologic: Thrombocytopenia (1% to 24%)

Neuromuscular & skeletal: Tremor (19% to 57%), weakness (10% to 21%)

Miscellaneous: Infection (13% to 20%)

1% to 10%:

Cardiovascular: Chest pain, hypertension, palpitation, peripheral edema, tachycardia

Central nervous system: Abnormal dreams, amnesia, anxiety, confusion, coordination abnormal, depression, headache, malaise, personality disorder

Dermatologic: Bruising, dry skin, petechia, pruritus, rash

Endocrine & metabolic: Amenorrhea, dysmenorrhea

Gastrointestinal: Appetite increased, eructation, flatulence, hematemesis, pancreatitis, periodontal abscess, taste perversion, weight gain

Genitourinary: Urinary frequency, urinary incontinence, vaginitis

Hepatic: AST/ALT increased

Neuromuscular & skeletal: Abnormal gait, arthralgia, back pain, hypertonia, leg cramps, myalgia, myasthenia, paresthesia, twitching

Ocular: Abnormal vision, amblyopia/blurred vision, nystagmus

Otic: Deafness, otitis media, tinnitus

Respiratory: Cough increased, dyspnea, epistaxis, pharyngitis, pneumonia, sinusitis

Additional adverse effects: Frequency not defined:

Cardiovascular: Bradycardia, edema

Central nervous system: Aggression, ataxia, behavioral deterioration, cerebral atrophy (reversible), coma (rare), dementia, encephalopathy (rare), fever, hallucinations, hostility, hyperactivity, hypoesthesia, hypothermia, parkinsonism, psychosis, sedation, vertigo

Dermatologic: Cutaneous vasculitis, erythema multiforme, photosensitivity, Stevens-Johnson syndrome, toxic epidermal necrolysis (rare)

Endocrine & metabolic: Breast enlargement, galactorrhea, hyperammonemia, hyponatremia, inappropriate ADH secretion, parotid gland swelling, polycystic ovary disease (rare), abnormal thyroid function tests

Gastrointestinal: Abdominal cramps, constipation, indigestion, weight loss

Genitourinary: Enuresis, urinary tract infection

Hematologic: Agranulocytosis, anemia, aplastic anemia, bone marrow suppression, eosinophilia, hematoma formation, hemorrhage, hypofibrinogenemia, intermittent porphyria, leukopenia, lymphocytosis, macrocytosis, pancytopenia

Hepatic: Bilirubin increased, hyperammonemic encephalopathy (in patients with UCD)

Neuromuscular & skeletal: Asterixis, bone pain, dysarthria

Ocular: Diplopia, seeing "spots before the eyes"

Otic: Ear pain

Renal: Fanconi-like syndrome (rare, in children)

Miscellaneous: Allergic reaction, anaphylaxis, carnitine decreased, hyperglycinemia, lupus

Dosage

Seizure disorders: **Note:** Administer doses >250 mg/day in divided doses.

Oral:

Simple and complex absence seizures: Children and Adults: Initial: 15 mg/kg/day; increase by 5-10 mg/kg/day at weekly intervals until therapeutic levels are achieved; maximum: 60 mg/kg/day. Larger maintenance doses may be required in younger children.

Complex partial seizures: Children ≥10 years and Adults: Initial: 10-15 mg/kg/day; increase by 5-10 mg/kg/day at weekly intervals until therapeutic levels are achieved; maximum: 60 mg/kg/day. Larger maintenance doses may be required in younger children.

Note: Regular release and delayed release formulations are usually given in 2-4 divided doses/day; extended release formulation (Depakote® ER) is usually given once daily. Conversion to Depakote® ER from a stable dose of Depakote® may require an increase in the total daily dose between 8% and 20% to maintain similar serum concentrations.

I.V.: Administer as a 60-minute infusion (≤20 mg/minute) with the same frequency as oral products; switch patient to oral products as soon as (Continued)

Valproic Acid and Derivatives *(Continued)*

possible. Rapid infusions ≤15 mg/kg over 5-10 minutes (1.5-3 mg/kg/minute) were generally well tolerated in a clinical trial.

Rectal (unlabeled): Dilute syrup 1:1 with water for use as a retention enema; loading dose: 17-20 mg/kg one time; maintenance: 10-15 mg/kg/dose every 8 hours

Status epilepticus (unlabeled use): Adults:
Loading dose: I.V.: 15-25 mg/kg administered at 3 mg/kg/minute.
Maintenance dose: I.V. infusion: 1-4 mg/kg/hour; titrate dose as needed based upon patient response and evaluation of drug-drug interactions

Mania: Adults: Oral: Initial: 750 mg/day in divided doses; dose should be adjusted as rapidly as possible to desired clinical effect; maximum recommended dosage: 60 mg/kg/day
Depakote® ER: Initial: 25 mg/kg/day given once daily; dose should be adjusted as rapidly as possible to desired clinical effect; maximum recommended dose: 60 mg/kg/day.

Migraine prophylaxis: Children ≥16 years and Adults: Oral:
Depakote® ER: 500 mg once daily for 7 days, then increase to 1000 mg once daily; adjust dose based on patient response; usual dosage range 500-1000 mg/day
Depakote® tablet: 250 mg twice daily; adjust dose based on patient response, up to 1000 mg/day

Elderly: Elimination is decreased in the elderly. Studies of elderly patients with dementia show a high incidence of somnolence. In some patients, this was associated with weight loss. Starting doses should be lower and increases should be slow, with careful monitoring of nutritional intake and dehydration. Safety and efficacy for use in patients >65 years have not been studied for migraine prophylaxis.

Dosing adjustment in renal impairment: A 27% reduction in clearance of unbound valproate is seen in patients with Cl_{cr} <10 mL/minute. Hemodialysis reduces valproate concentrations by 20%, therefore no dose adjustment is needed in patients with renal failure. Protein binding is reduced, monitoring only total valproate concentrations may be misleading.

Dosing adjustment/comments in hepatic impairment: Reduce dose. Clearance is decreased with liver impairment. Hepatic disease is also associated with decreased albumin concentrations and 2- to 2.6-fold increase in the unbound fraction. Free concentrations of valproate may be elevated while total concentrations appear normal.

Mechanism of Action Causes increased availability of gamma-aminobutyric acid (GABA), an inhibitory neurotransmitter, to brain neurons or may enhance the action of GABA or mimic its action at postsynaptic receptor sites

Contraindications Hypersensitivity to valproic acid, derivatives, or any component of the formulation; hepatic dysfunction; urea cycle disorders

Warnings/Precautions
[U.S. Boxed Warning]: **Hepatic failure resulting in fatalities has occurred in patients; children <2 years of age are at considerable risk.** Other risk factors include organic brain disease, mental retardation with severe seizure disorders, congenital metabolic disorders, and patients on multiple anticonvulsants. Hepatotoxicity has been reported within 6 months of therapy. Monitor patients closely for appearance of malaise, weakness, facial edema, anorexia, jaundice, and vomiting.

[U.S. Boxed Warning]: **Cases of life-threatening pancreatitis, occurring at the start of therapy or following years of use, have been reported in adults and children.** Some cases have been hemorrhagic with rapid progression of initial symptoms to death. Evaluate symptoms of abdominal pain, nausea, vomiting, and/or anorexia.

[U.S. Boxed Warning]: **May cause teratogenic effects such as neural tube defects (eg, spina bifida).** Use in women of childbearing potential requires that benefits of use in mother be weighed against the potential risk to fetus, especially when used for conditions not associated with permanent injury or risk of death (eg, migraine).

May cause severe thrombocytopenia, inhibition of platelet aggregation, and bleeding. Tremors may indicate overdosage; use with caution in patients receiving other anticonvulsants. Hypersensitivity reactions affecting multiple organs have been reported in association with valproic acid use; may include dermatologic and/or hematologic changes (eosinophilia, neutropenia, thrombocytopenia) or symptoms of organ dysfunction.

Hyperammonemia and/or encephalopathy, sometimes fatal, have been reported following the initiation of valproic acid therapy and may be present with normal transaminase levels. Ammonia levels should be measured in patients who develop unexplained lethargy and vomiting, or changes in mental status. Discontinue therapy if ammonia levels are increased and evaluate for possible urea cycle disorder (UCD). Although rare genetic disorders, UCD evaluation should be considered for the following patients prior to the start of therapy: History of unexplained encephalopathy or coma; encephalopathy associated with protein load; pregnancy or postpartum encephalopathy; unexplained mental retardation; history of elevated plasma ammonia or glutamine; history of cyclical vomiting and lethargy; episodic extreme irritability, ataxia; low BUN or protein avoidance; family history of UCD or unexplained infant deaths (particularly male); or signs or symptoms of UCD (hyperammonemia, encephalopathy, respiratory alkalosis).

In vitro studies have suggested valproic acid stimulates the replication of HIV and CMV viruses under experimental conditions. The clinical consequence of this is unknown, but should be considered when monitoring affected patients.

Use of Depacon® injection is not recommended for post-traumatic seizure prophylaxis following acute head trauma. Anticonvulsants should not be discontinued abruptly because of the possibility of increasing seizure frequency; valproic acid should be withdrawn gradually to minimize the potential of increased seizure frequency, unless safety concerns require a more rapid withdrawal. Concomitant use with clonazepam may induce absence status. Patients treated for bipolar disorder should be monitored closely for clinical worsening or suicidality; prescriptions should be written for the smallest quantity consistent with good patient care.

CNS depression may occur with valproic acid use. Patients must be cautioned about performing tasks which require mental alertness (operating machinery or driving). Effects with other sedative drugs or ethanol may be potentiated. Use with caution in the elderly.

Drug Interactions

Cytochrome P450 Effect: For valproic acid: **Substrate** (minor) of CYP2A6, 2B6, 2C9, 2C19, 2E1; **Inhibits** CYP2C9 (weak), 2C19 (weak), 2D6 (weak), 3A4 (weak); **Induces** CYP2A6 (weak)

Increased Effect/Toxicity: Absence seizures have been reported in patients receiving VPA and clonazepam. Valproic acid may increase, decrease, or have no effect on carbamazepine and phenytoin levels. Valproic acid may increase serum concentrations of carbamazepine - epoxide (active metabolite). Valproic acid may increase serum concentrations of lamotrigine, phenobarbital, tricyclic antidepressants, and zidovudine. Macrolide antibiotics (clarithromycin, erythromycin, troleandomycin), felbamate, and isoniazid may inhibit the metabolism of valproic acid. Aspirin or other salicylates may displace valproic acid from protein-binding sites, leading to acute toxicity. When combined with topiramate, hyperammonemia with or without encephalopathy has been reported in patients who tolerated either drug alone. Valproic acid may enhance the adverse/toxic effect of risperidone; monitor for the development of peripheral edema.

Decreased Effect: Carbapenem antibiotics (ertapenem, imipenem, meropenem) may decrease valproic acid concentrations to subtherapeutic levels; monitor. Valproic acid may decrease the serum concentration of oxcarbazepine.

Ethanol/Nutrition/Herb Interactions

Ethanol: Avoid ethanol (may increase CNS depression).

Food: Food may delay but does not affect the extent of absorption. Valproic acid serum concentrations may be decreased if taken with food. Milk has no effect on absorption.

Herb/Nutraceutical: Avoid evening primrose (seizure threshold decreased).

Dietary Considerations Valproic acid may cause GI upset; take with large amount of water or food to decrease GI upset. May need to split doses to avoid GI upset.

Depakote® Sprinkle capsule contents may be mixed with semisolid food (eg, applesauce or pudding) in patients having difficulty swallowing; particles should be swallowed and not chewed.

Valproate sodium oral solution will generate valproic acid in carbonated beverages and may cause mouth and throat irritation; do not mix valproate sodium oral solution with carbonated beverages.

Pharmacodynamics/Kinetics

Distribution: Total valproate: 11 L/1.73 m²; free valproate 92 L/1.73 m²

Protein binding (dose dependent): 80% to 90%; decreased in the elderly and with hepatic or renal dysfunction

Metabolism: Extensively hepatic via glucuronide conjugation and mitochondrial beta-oxidation. The relationship between dose and total valproate concentration is nonlinear; concentration does not increase proportionally with the dose, (Continued)

Valproic Acid and Derivatives *(Continued)*

but increases to a lesser extent due to saturable plasma protein binding. The kinetics of unbound drug are linear.

Bioavailability: Depakote® ER: 90% of I.V. dose and ~89% of delayed release formulation

Half-life elimination (increased in neonates and with liver disease): Children >2 months: 7-13 hours; Adults: 9-16 hours

Time to peak, serum: Depakote® tablet: ~4 hours; Depakote® ER: 4-17 hours

Excretion: Urine (30% to 50% as glucuronide conjugate, 3% as unchanged drug)

Pregnancy Risk Factor D

Dosage Forms Strength expressed as valproic acid.

Capsule: 250 mg

Depakene®: 250 mg

Capsule, sprinkles:

Depakote® Sprinkle: 125 mg

Injection, solution: 100 mg/mL (5 mL)

Depacon®: 100 mg/mL (5 mL)

Syrup: 250 mg/5 mL

Depakene®: 250 mg/5 mL

Tablet, delayed release:

Depakote®: 125 mg, 250 mg, 500 mg

Tablet, extended release:

Depakote® ER: 250 mg, 500 mg

Selected Readings

Redington K, Wells C, and Petito F, "Erythromycin and Valproic Acid Interaction," *Ann Intern Med*, 1992, 116(10):877-8.

Valrubicin *(val ROO bi sin)*

U.S. Brand Names Valstar® [DSC]

Canadian Brand Names Valstar®; Valtaxin®

Generic Available No

Index Terms AD3L; *N*-trifluoroacetyladriamycin-14-valerate

Pharmacologic Category Antineoplastic Agent, Anthracycline

Use Intravesical therapy of BCG-refractory carcinoma *in situ* of the urinary bladder

Local Anesthetic/Vasoconstrictor Precautions No information available to require special precautions

Effects on Dental Treatment No significant effects or complications reported

Common Adverse Effects

>10%: Genitourinary: Frequency (61%), dysuria (56%), urgency (57%), bladder spasm (31%), hematuria (29%), bladder pain (28%), urinary incontinence (22%), cystitis (15%), urinary tract infection (15%)

1% to 10%:

Cardiovascular: Chest pain (2%), vasodilation (2%), peripheral edema (1%)

Central nervous system: Headache (4%), malaise (4%), dizziness (3%), fever (2%)

Dermatologic: Rash (3%)

Endocrine & metabolic: Hyperglycemia (1%)

Gastrointestinal: Abdominal pain (5%), nausea (5%), diarrhea (3%), vomiting (2%), flatulence (1%)

Genitourinary: Nocturia (7%), burning symptoms (5%), urinary retention (4%), urethral pain (3%), pelvic pain (1%), hematuria (microscopic) (3%)

Hematologic: Anemia (2%)

Neuromuscular & skeletal: Weakness (4%), back pain (3%), myalgia (1%)

Respiratory: Pneumonia (1%)

Mechanism of Action Blocks function of DNA topoisomerase II; inhibits DNA synthesis, causes extensive chromosomal damage, and arrests cell development; unlike other anthracyclines, does not appear to intercalate DNA

Drug Interactions

Increased Effect/Toxicity: No specific drug interactions studies have been performed. Systemic exposure to valrubicin is negligible, and interactions are unlikely.

Decreased Effect: No specific drug interactions studies have been performed. Systemic exposure to valrubicin is negligible, and interactions are unlikely.

Pharmacodynamics/Kinetics

Absorption: Well absorbed into bladder tissue, negligible systemic absorption. Trauma to mucosa may increase absorption, and perforation greatly increases absorption with significant systemic myelotoxicity.

Metabolism: Negligible after intravesical instillation and 2-hour retention

Excretion: Urine when expelled from urinary bladder (98.6% as intact drug; 0.4% as *N*-trifluoroacetyladriamycin)

Pregnancy Risk Factor C

Valsartan (val SAR tan)

Related Information
Cardiovascular Diseases *on page 1726*

U.S. Brand Names Diovan®

Canadian Brand Names Diovan®

Mexican Brand Names Diovan

Generic Available No

Pharmacologic Category Angiotensin II Receptor Blocker

Use Alone or in combination with other antihypertensive agents in the treatment of essential hypertension; treatment of heart failure (NYHA Class II-IV); reduction of cardiovascular mortality in patients with left ventricular dysfunction post-myocardial infarction

Local Anesthetic/Vasoconstrictor Precautions No information available to require special precautions

Effects on Dental Treatment No significant effects or complications reported

Common Adverse Effects

>10%:
Central nervous system: Dizziness (heart failure 17%)
Renal: Bun increased >50% (heart failure 17%)

1% to 10%:
Cardiovascular: Hypotension (1% to 7%), postural hypotension (2%), syncope (up to >1%)
Central nervous system: Fatigue (2% to 3%), headache (heart failure >1%)
Endocrine & metabolic: Serum potassium increased by >20% (4% to 10%), hyperkalemia (heart failure 2%)
Gastrointestinal: Diarrhea (heart failure 5%), abdominal pain (2%), nausea (>1%)
Hematologic: Neutropenia (2%)
Neuromuscular & skeletal: Arthralgia (3%), back pain (up to 3%)
Ocular: Blurred vision (heart failure >1%)
Otic: Vertigo (up to >1%)
Renal: Creatinine doubled (MI 4%), creatinine increased >50% (heart failure 4%), renal dysfunction (up to >1%)
Respiratory: Cough (1% to 3%)
Miscellaneous: Viral infection (3%)

Dosage Adults: Oral:
Hypertension: Initial: 80 mg or 160 mg once daily (in patients who are not volume depleted); dose may be increased to achieve desired effect; maximum recommended dose: 320 mg/day
Heart failure: Initial: 40 mg twice daily; titrate dose to 80-160 mg twice daily, as tolerated; maximum daily dose: 320 mg
Left ventricular dysfunction after MI: Initial: 20 mg twice daily; titrate dose to target of 160 mg twice daily as tolerated; may initiate ≥12 hours following MI

Dosing adjustment in renal impairment: No dosage adjustment necessary if Cl_{cr} >10 mL/minute.
Dialysis: Not significantly removed.

Dosing adjustment in hepatic impairment In mild-to-moderate liver disease no adjustment is needed. Use caution in patients with liver disease. Patients with mild to moderate chronic disease have twice the exposure as healthy volunteers.

Mechanism of Action Valsartan produces direct antagonism of the angiotensin II (AT2) receptors, unlike the ACE inhibitors. It displaces angiotensin II from the AT1 receptor and produces its blood pressure-lowering effects by antagonizing AT1-induced vasoconstriction, aldosterone release, catecholamine release, arginine vasopressin release, water intake, and hypertrophic responses. This action results in more efficient blockade of the cardiovascular effects of angiotensin II and fewer side effects than the ACE inhibitors.

Contraindications Hypersensitivity to valsartan or any component of the formulation; hypersensitivity to other A-II receptor antagonists; bilateral renal artery stenosis; pregnancy

Warnings/Precautions [U.S. Boxed Warning]: Based on human data, drugs that act on the angiotensin system can cause injury and death to the developing fetus when used in the second and third trimesters. Angiotensin receptor blockers should be discontinued as soon as possible once pregnancy is detected. May cause hyperkalemia; avoid potassium supplementation unless specifically required by healthcare provider. During the initiation of therapy, hypotension may occur, particularly in patients with heart
(Continued)

Valsartan *(Continued)*

failure or post-MI patients. Use extreme caution with concurrent administration of potassium-sparing diuretics or potassium supplements, in patients with mild-to-moderate hepatic dysfunction (adjust dose), in those who may be sodium/water depleted (eg, on high-dose diuretics), and in the elderly. Avoid use in patients with CHF, unilateral renal artery stenosis, aortic/mitral valve stenosis, coronary artery disease, or hypertrophic cardiomyopathy, if possible. May be associated with deterioration of renal function and/or increases in serum creatinine, particularly in patients dependent on renin-angiotensin-aldosterone system. Safety and efficacy have not been established in children.

Drug Interactions

Cytochrome P450 Effect: Inhibits CYP2C9 (weak)

Increased Effect/Toxicity: Lithium toxicity may be increased by valsartan. Concurrent use of eplerenone, potassium salts/supplements, and potassium-sparing diuretics (amiloride, spironolactone, triamterene) may increase the risk of hyperkalemia.

Decreased Effect: NSAIDs may decrease the efficacy of valsartan

Ethanol/Nutrition/Herb Interactions

Food: Decreases rate and extent of absorption by 50% and 40%, respectively.

Herb/Nutraceutical: Avoid dong quai if using for hypertension (has estrogenic activity). Avoid ephedra, yohimbe, ginseng (may worsen hypertension). Avoid garlic (may have increased antihypertensive effect).

Dietary Considerations Avoid salt substitutes which contain potassium. May be taken with or without food.

Pharmacodynamics/Kinetics

Onset of antihypertensive effect: 2 weeks (maximal: 4 weeks)

Distribution: V_d: 17 L (adults)

Protein binding: 95%, primarily albumin

Metabolism: To inactive metabolite

Bioavailability: 25% (range 10% to 35%)

Half-life elimination: 6 hours

Time to peak, serum: 2-4 hours

Excretion: Feces (83%) and urine (13%) as unchanged drug

Pregnancy Risk Factor C/D (2nd and 3rd trimesters)

Dosage Forms

Tablet:

Diovan®: 40 mg, 80 mg, 160 mg, 320 mg

Valsartan and Hydrochlorothiazide

(val SAR tan & hye droe klor oh THYE a zide)

Related Information

Cardiovascular Diseases *on page 1726*

Hydrochlorothiazide *on page 819*

Valsartan *on page 1643*

U.S. Brand Names Diovan HCT®

Canadian Brand Names Diovan HCT®

Mexican Brand Names CoDiovan

Generic Available No

Index Terms Hydrochlorothiazide and Valsartan

Pharmacologic Category Angiotensin II Receptor Blocker Combination; Antihypertensive Agent, Combination; Diuretic, Thiazide

Use Treatment of hypertension (not indicated for initial therapy)

Local Anesthetic/Vasoconstrictor Precautions No information available to require special precautions

Effects on Dental Treatment No significant effects or complications reported

Common Adverse Effects Percentages reported with combination product; other reactions have been reported (see individual agents for additional information)

1% to 10%:

Central nervous system: Dizziness (9%; dose related), fatigue (5%)

Endocrine & metabolic: Hypokalemia (3%)

Gastrointestinal: Diarrhea (3%)

Respiratory: Cough (3%), nasopharyngitis (3%)

Drug Interactions

Cytochrome P450 Effect: Valsartan: **Inhibits** CYP2C9 (weak)

Increased Effect/Toxicity: See individual agents.

Decreased Effect: See individual agents.

Pharmacodynamics/Kinetics See individual agents.

Pregnancy Risk Factor C/D (2nd and 3rd trimester)

Valstar® [DSC] *see* Valrubicin *on page 1642*

Valtrex® *see Valacyclovir on page 1635*
Vanamide™ *see Urea on page 1632*
Vancocin® *see Vancomycin on page 1645*

Vancomycin (van koe MYE sin)

U.S. Brand Names Vancocin®
Canadian Brand Names Vancocin®
Mexican Brand Names Vancocin CP; Vancox
Generic Available Yes: Injection
Index Terms Vancomycin Hydrochloride
Pharmacologic Category Antibiotic, Miscellaneous
Use Treatment of patients with infections caused by staphylococcal species and streptococcal species; used orally for staphylococcal enterocolitis or for antibiotic-associated pseudomembranous colitis produced by *C. difficile*
Local Anesthetic/Vasoconstrictor Precautions No information available to require special precautions
Effects on Dental Treatment Key adverse event(s) related to dental treatment: Bitter taste. "Red man syndrome", characterized by skin rash and hypotension, is not an allergic reaction but rather is associated with too rapid infusion of the drug. To alleviate or prevent the reaction, infuse vancomycin at a rate of ≥30 minutes for each 500 mg of drug being administered (eg, 1 g over ≥60 minutes); 1.5 g over ≥90 minutes.
Common Adverse Effects
Oral:
>10%: Gastrointestinal: Bitter taste, nausea, vomiting
1% to 10%:
Central nervous system: Chills, drug fever
Hematologic: Eosinophilia
Parenteral:
>10%:
Cardiovascular: Hypotension accompanied by flushing
Dermatologic: Erythematous rash on face and upper body (red neck or red man syndrome - infusion rate related)
1% to 10%:
Central nervous system: Chills, drug fever
Dermatologic: Rash
Hematologic: Eosinophilia, reversible neutropenia
Dosage Initial dosage recommendation:
Neonates: I.V.:
Postnatal age ≤7 days:
<1200 g: 15 mg/kg/dose every 24 hours
1200-2000 g: 10 mg/kg/dose every 12 hours
>2000 g: 15 mg/kg/dose every 12 hours
Postnatal age >7 days:
<1200 g: 15 mg/kg/dose every 24 hours
≥1200 g: 10 mg/kg/dose every 8 hours
Infants >1 month and Children: I.V.:
40 mg/kg/day in divided doses every 6 hours
Prophylaxis for bacterial endocarditis:
Dental, oral, or upper respiratory tract surgery: 20 mg/kg 1 hour prior to the procedure
GI/GU procedure: 20 mg/kg plus gentamicin 2 mg/kg 1 hour prior to surgery
Infants >1 month and Children with staphylococcal central nervous system infection: I.V.: 60 mg/kg/day in divided doses every 6 hours
Adults: I.V.:
With normal renal function: 1 g **or** 10-15 mg/kg/dose every 12 hours
Hospital-acquired pneumonia (HAP): 15 mg/kg/dose every 12 hours (American Thoracic Society (ATS) guidelines)
Meningitis *(Pneumococcus* or *Staphylococcus)*: 30-45 mg/kg/day in divided doses every 8-12 hours **or** 500-750 mg every 6 hours (with third-generation cephalosporin for PCN-resistant *Streptococcus pneumoniae*); maximum dose: 2-3 g/day
Prophylaxis for bacterial endocarditis:
Dental, oral, or upper respiratory tract surgery: 1 g 1 hour before surgery
GI/GU procedure: 1 g plus 1.5 mg/kg gentamicin 1 hour prior to surgery
Antibiotic lock technique (for catheter infections): 2 mg/mL in SWI/NS or D_5W; instill 3-5 mL into catheter port as a flush solution instead of heparin lock (**Note:** Do not mix with any other solutions)
Intrathecal: Vancomycin is available as a powder for injection and may be diluted to 1-5 mg/mL concentration in preservative-free 0.9% sodium chloride for administration into the CSF
(Continued)

Vancomycin (Continued)

  Neonates: 5-10 mg/day
  Children: 5-20 mg/day
  Adults: Up to 20 mg/day

Oral: Pseudomembranous colitis produced by *C. difficile*:
  Neonates: 10 mg/kg/day in divided doses
  Children: 40 mg/kg/day in divided doses, added to fluids
  Adults: 125 mg 4 times/day for 10 days

Dosing interval in renal impairment (vancomycin levels should be monitored in patients with any renal impairment):
  Cl_{cr} >60 mL/minute: Start with 1 g or 10-15 mg/kg/dose every 12 hours
  Cl_{cr} 40-60 mL/minute: Start with 1 g or 10-15 mg/kg/dose every 24 hours
  Cl_{cr} <40 mL/minute: Will need longer intervals; determine by serum concentration monitoring

  Hemodialysis: Not dialyzable (0% to 5%); generally not removed; exception minimal-to-moderate removal by some of the newer high-flux filters; dose may need to be administered more frequently; monitor serum concentrations
  Continuous ambulatory peritoneal dialysis (CAPD): Not significantly removed; administration via CAPD fluid: 15-30 mg/L (15-30 mcg/mL) of CAPD fluid
  Continuous arteriovenous hemofiltration: Dose as for Cl_{cr} 10-40 mL/minute

Mechanism of Action Inhibits bacterial cell wall synthesis by blocking glycopeptide polymerization through binding tightly to D-alanyl-D-alanine portion of cell wall precursor

Contraindications Hypersensitivity to vancomycin or any component of the formulation; avoid in patients with previous severe hearing loss

Warnings/Precautions May cause nephrotoxicity; usual risk factors include pre-existing renal impairment, concomitant nephrotoxic medications, advanced age, and dehydration. Discontinue treatment if signs of nephrotoxicity occur; renal damage is usually reversible. May cause neurotoxicity; usual risk factors include pre-existing renal impairment, concomitant neuro-/nephrotoxic medications, advanced age, and dehydration. Ototoxicity is proportional to the amount of drug given and the duration of treatment. Tinnitus or vertigo may be indications of vestibular injury and impending bilateral irreversible damage. Discontinue treatment if signs of ototoxicity occur. Prolonged therapy (>1 week) or total doses exceeding 25 g may increase the risk of neutropenia; prompt reversal of neutropenia is expected after discontinuation of therapy. Prolonged use may result in fungal or bacterial superinfection, including *C. difficile*-associated diarrhea and pseudomembranous colitis. Use with caution in patients with renal impairment or those receiving other nephrotoxic or ototoxic drugs; dosage modification required in patients with impaired renal function (especially elderly). Rapid I.V. administration may result in hypotension, flushing, erythema, urticaria, and/or pruritus; rate of infusion should be ≥60 minutes.

Drug Interactions
  Increased Effect/Toxicity: Increased toxicity with other ototoxic or nephrotoxic drugs. Increased neuromuscular blockade with most neuromuscular blocking agents.

Dietary Considerations May be taken with food.

Pharmacodynamics/Kinetics
  Absorption: Oral: Poor; I.M.: Erratic; Intraperitoneal: ~38%
  Distribution: Widely in body tissue and fluids. except for CSF
    Relative diffusion from blood into CSF: Good only with inflammation (exceeds usual MICs)
    CSF:blood level ratio: Normal meninges: Nil; Inflamed meninges: 20% to 30%
  Protein binding: 10% to 50%
  Half-life elimination: Biphasic: Terminal:
    Newborns: 6-10 hours
    Infants and Children 3 months to 4 years: 4 hours
    Children >3 years: 2.2-3 hours
    Adults: 5-11 hours; significantly prolonged with renal impairment
    End-stage renal disease: 200-250 hours
  Time to peak, serum: I.V.: 45-65 minutes
  Excretion: I.V.: Urine (80% to 90% as unchanged drug); Oral: Primarily feces

Pregnancy Risk Factor C

Dosage Forms
  Capsule:
    Vancocin®: 125 mg, 250 mg
  Infusion [premixed in iso-osmotic dextrose]:
    Vancocin®: 500 mg (100 mL); 1 g (200 mL)
  Injection, powder for reconstitution: 500 mg, 1 g, 5 g, 10 g

Vancomycin Hydrochloride see Vancomycin on page 1645
Vandazole™ see Metronidazole on page 1091

Vardenafil (var DEN a fil)

U.S. Brand Names Levitra®
Canadian Brand Names Levitra®
Mexican Brand Names Levitra
Generic Available No
Index Terms Vardenafil Hydrochloride
Pharmacologic Category Phosphodiesterase-5 Enzyme Inhibitor
Use Treatment of erectile dysfunction
Local Anesthetic/Vasoconstrictor Precautions No information available to require special precautions
Effects on Dental Treatment No significant effects or complications reported
Common Adverse Effects
>10%:
  Cardiovascular: Flushing (11%)
  Central nervous system: Headache (15%)
2% to 10%:
  Central nervous system: Dizziness (2%)
  Gastrointestinal: Dyspepsia (4%), nausea (2%)
  Neuromuscular & skeletal: CPK increased (2%)
  Respiratory: Rhinitis (9%), sinusitis (3%)
  Miscellaneous: Flu-like syndrome (3%)
Dosage Oral: Adults: Erectile dysfunction: 10 mg 60 minutes prior to sexual activity; dosing range: 5-20 mg; to be given as one single dose and not given more than once daily
Dosing adjustment with concomitant medications:
  Alpha-blocker (dose should be stable at time of vardenafil initiation): Initial vardenafil dose: 5 mg/24 hours; if an alpha-blocker is added to vardenafil therapy, it should be initiated at the smallest possible dose, and titrated carefully.
  Atazanavir: Maximum vardenafil dose: 2.5 mg/24 hours
  Clarithromycin: Maximum vardenafil dose: 2.5 mg/24 hours
  Erythromycin: Maximum vardenafil dose: 5 mg/24 hours
  Indinavir: Maximum vardenafil dose: 2.5 mg/24 hours
  Itraconazole:
    200 mg/day: Maximum vardenafil dose: 5 mg/24 hours
    400 mg/day: Maximum vardenafil dose: 2.5 mg/24 hours
  Ketoconazole:
    200 mg/day: Maximum vardenafil dose: 5 mg/24 hours
    400 mg/day: Maximum vardenafil dose: 2.5 mg/24 hours
  Ritonavir: Maximum vardenafil dose: 2.5 mg/72 hours
  Saquinavir: Maximum vardenafil dose: 2.5 mg/24 hours
Elderly ≥65 years: Initial: 5 mg 60 minutes prior to sexual activity; to be given as one single dose and not given more than once daily
Dosage adjustment in renal impairment: Dose adjustment not needed for mild, moderate, or severe impairment; use has not been studied in patients on renal dialysis
Dosage adjustment in hepatic impairment: Child-Pugh class B: Initial: 5 mg 60 minutes prior to sexual activity (maximum dose: 10 mg); to be given as one single dose and not given more than once daily
Mechanism of Action Does not directly cause penile erections, but affects the response to sexual stimulation. The physiologic mechanism of erection of the penis involves release of nitric oxide (NO) in the corpus cavernosum during sexual stimulation. NO then activates the enzyme guanylate cyclase, which results in increased levels of cyclic guanosine monophosphate (cGMP), producing smooth muscle relaxation and inflow of blood to the corpus cavernosum. Vardenafil enhances the effect of NO by inhibiting phosphodiesterase type 5 (PDE-5), which is responsible for degradation of cGMP in the corpus cavernosum; when sexual stimulation causes local release of NO, inhibition of (Continued)

Vardenafil *(Continued)*

PDE-5 by vardenafil causes increased levels of cGMP in the corpus cavernosum, resulting in smooth muscle relaxation and inflow of blood to the corpus cavernosum; at recommended doses, it has no effect in the absence of sexual stimulation.

Contraindications Hypersensitivity to vardenafil or any component of the formulation; concurrent use of organic nitrates (nitroglycerin; scheduled dosing or as needed)

Warnings/Precautions There is a degree of cardiac risk associated with sexual activity; therefore, physicians may wish to consider the patient's cardiovascular status prior to initiating any treatment for erectile dysfunction. Use caution in patients with anatomical deformation of the penis (angulation, cavernosal fibrosis, or Peyronie's disease) and in patients who have conditions which may predispose them to priapism (sickle cell anemia, multiple myeloma, leukemia). Patients should be instructed to seek medical attention if erection persists >4 hours.

Not recommended for use in patients with congenital QT prolongation or those taking Class Ia or III antiarrhythmics. Concomitant use with alpha-blockers may cause hypotension; safety of this combination may be affected by other antihypertensives and intravascular volume depletion. Patients should be hemodynamically stable prior to initiating therapy. Use caution with alpha-blockers, effective CYP3A4 inhibitors, the elderly, or those with hepatic impairment (Child-Pugh class B); dosage adjustment is needed.

Rare cases of nonarteritic ischemic optic neuropathy (NAION) have been reported; risk may be increased with history of vision loss. Other risk factors for NAION include heart disease, diabetes, hypertension, smoking, age >50 years, or history of certain eye problems.

Safety and efficacy have not been studied in patients with the following conditions, therefore, use in these patients is not recommended at this time: Hypotension, uncontrolled hypertension, unstable angina, severe cardiac failure; a life-threatening arrhythmia, myocardial infarction, or stroke within the last 6 months; severe hepatic impairment (Child-Pugh class C); end-stage renal disease requiring dialysis; retinitis pigmentosa or other degenerative retinal disorders. The safety and efficacy of vardenafil with other treatments for erectile dysfunction have not been studied and are not recommended as combination therapy. Safety and efficacy have not been established in children.

Drug Interactions

Cytochrome P450 Effect: Substrate of CYP2C (minor), 3A5 (minor), 3A4 (major)

Increased Effect/Toxicity: CYP3A4 inhibitors may increase the levels/effects of vardenafil; example inhibitors include azole antifungals, clarithromycin, diclofenac, doxycycline, erythromycin, imatinib, isoniazid, nefazodone, nicardipine, propofol, protease inhibitors, quinidine, telithromycin, and verapamil. Nitroglycerin may lead to excessive hypotension; concomitant use is contraindicated. Alpha-blockers may also lead to excessive hypotension; initiate vardenafil at lowest possible dose if patient is stabilized on alpha-blocker; initiate alpha-blocker at lowest possible dose and titrate cautiously in patients on a stable dose of vardenafil.

Ethanol/Nutrition/Herb Interactions Food: High-fat meals decrease maximum serum concentration 18% to 50%. Serum concentrations/toxicity may be increased with grapefruit juice; avoid concurrent use.

Dietary Considerations May take with or without food.

Pharmacodynamics/Kinetics

Absorption: Rapid

Distribution: V_d: 208 L; <0.01% found in semen 1.5 hours after dose

Metabolism: Hepatic via CYP3A4 (major), CYP2C and 3A5 (minor); forms metabolite (active)

Bioavailability: 15%; Elderly (≥65 years): 52%; Hepatic impairment (Child-Pugh class B): 160%

Half-life elimination: Terminal: Vardenafil and metabolite: 4-5 hours

Time to peak, plasma: 0.5-2 hours

Excretion: Feces (91% to 95% as metabolites); urine (2% to 6%)

Clearance: 56 L/hour

Pregnancy Risk Factor B

Dosage Forms

Tablet:

Levitra®: 2.5 mg, 5 mg, 10 mg, 20 mg

Vardenafil Hydrochloride *see* Vardenafil *on page 1647*

Varenicline (var e NI kleen)

U.S. Brand Names Chantix™
Canadian Brand Names Champix®
Generic Available No
Index Terms Varenicline Tartrate
Pharmacologic Category Partial Nicotine Agonist; Smoking Cessation Aid
Use Treatment to aid in smoking cessation
Local Anesthetic/Vasoconstrictor Precautions No information available to require special precautions
Effects on Dental Treatment Key adverse event(s) related to dental treatment: Xerostomia (normal salivary flow resumes upon discontinuation).
Common Adverse Effects
>10%:
Central nervous system: Insomnia (18% to 19%), headache (15% to 19%), abnormal dreams (9% to 13%)
Gastrointestinal: Nausea (16% to 40%; dose related)
1% to 10%:
Central nervous system: Somnolence (3%), nightmares (1% to 2%), lethargy (1% to 2%), malaise (≤7%)
Dermatologic: Rash (≤3%)
Gastrointestinal: Flatulence (6% to 9%), abdominal pain (6% to 7%), constipation (5% to 8%), dysgeusia (5% to 8%), xerostomia (5% to 6%), dyspepsia (5%), vomiting (1% to 5%), appetite increased (3% to 4%), anorexia (≤2%), gastroesophageal reflux (1%)
Respiratory: Dyspnea (≤2%), rhinorrhea (≤1%)
Dosage Oral: Adults:
Initial:
Days 1-3: 0.5 mg once daily
Days 4-7: 0.5 mg twice daily
Maintenance (week 2-12): 1 mg twice daily
Note: Start 1 week before target quit date. Patients who cannot tolerate adverse events may require temporary reduction in dose. If patient successfully quits smoking during the 12 weeks, may continue for another 12 weeks to help maintain success. If not successful in first 12 weeks, then stop medication and reassess factors contributing to failure.
Dosage adjustment for toxicity: Lower dose for a period of time, then increase again
Dosage adjustment in renal impairment:
Cl_{cr} ≥30 mL/minute: No adjustment required
Cl_{cr} <30 mL/minute: Initial: 0.5 mg once daily; maximum dose: 0.5 mg twice daily
Hemodialysis: Maximum dose: 0.5 mg once daily
Dosage adjustment in hepatic impairment: No adjustment required
Mechanism of Action Partial neuronal alpha$_4$ β$_2$ nicotinic receptor agonist; prevents nicotine stimulation of mesolimbic dopamine system associated with nicotine addiction. Also binds to 5 HT$_3$ receptor (significance not determined) with moderate affinity. Varenicline stimulates dopamine activity but to a much smaller degree than nicotine does, resulting in decreased craving and withdrawal symptoms.
Contraindications Hypersensitivity to varenicline tartrate or any component of the formulation
Warnings/Precautions Use caution in renal dysfunction; dosage adjustment required. Safety and efficacy of varenicline with other smoking cessation therapies have not been established; increased adverse events when used concurrently with nicotine replacement therapy. Safety and efficacy have not been established in children.
Drug Interactions
Increased Effect/Toxicity: Successful cessation of smoking may alter pharmacokinetic properties of other medications (eg, theophylline, warfarin, insulin).
Dietary Considerations Should be given with food and a full glass of water to decrease gastric upset.
Pharmacodynamics/Kinetics
Absorption: Well absorbed; unaffected by food
Protein binding: ≤20%
Half-life elimination: 24 hours
Time to peak, plasma: 3-4 hours
Excretion: Primarily urine (92% as unchanged drug)
Dosage Forms
Tablet, as tartrate:
Chantix™: 0.5 mg, 1 mg

Vasopressin (vay soe PRES in)

U.S. Brand Names Pitressin®

Canadian Brand Names Pressyn®; Pressyn® AR

Generic Available Yes

Index Terms ADH; Antidiuretic Hormone; 8-Arginine Vasopressin

Pharmacologic Category Antidiuretic Hormone Analog; Hormone, Posterior Pituitary

Use Treatment of diabetes insipidus; prevention and treatment of postoperative abdominal distention; differential diagnosis of diabetes insipidus

Unlabeled/Investigational Use Adjunct in the treatment of GI hemorrhage and esophageal varices; pulseless arrest (ventricular tachycardia [VT]/ventricular fibrillation [VF], asystole/pulseless electrical activity [PEA]); vasodilatory shock (septic shock)

Local Anesthetic/Vasoconstrictor Precautions No information available to require special precautions

Effects on Dental Treatment No significant effects or complications reported

Common Adverse Effects Frequency not defined.

Cardiovascular: Arrhythmia, asystole (>0.4 units/minute), blood pressure increased, cardiac output decreased (>0.4 units/minute), chest pain, MI, vasoconstriction (with higher doses), venous thrombosis

Central nervous system: Pounding in the head, fever, vertigo

Dermatologic: Ischemic skin lesions, circumoral pallor, urticaria

Gastrointestinal: Abdominal cramps, flatulence, mesenteric ischemia, nausea, vomiting

Genitourinary: Uterine contraction

Neuromuscular & skeletal: Tremor

Respiratory: Bronchial constriction

Miscellaneous: Diaphoresis

Mechanism of Action Increases cyclic adenosine monophosphate (cAMP) which increases water permeability at the renal tubule resulting in decreased urine volume and increased osmolality; causes peristalsis by directly stimulating the smooth muscle in the GI tract; direct vasoconstrictor without inotropic or chronotropic effects

Drug Interactions

Increased Effect/Toxicity: Chlorpropamide, urea, clofibrate, carbamazepine, and fludrocortisone potentiate antidiuretic response.

Decreased Effect: Lithium, epinephrine, demeclocycline, heparin, and ethanol block antidiuretic activity to varying degrees.

Pharmacodynamics/Kinetics

Onset of action: Nasal: 1 hour

Duration: Nasal: 3-8 hours; I.M., SubQ: 2-8 hours

Metabolism: Nasal/Parenteral: Hepatic, renal

Half-life elimination: Nasal: 15 minutes; Parenteral: 10-20 minutes

Excretion: Nasal: Urine; SubQ: Urine (5% as unchanged drug) after 4 hours

Pregnancy Risk Factor C

Venlafaxine (ven la FAX een)

U.S. Brand Names Effexor®; Effexor® XR
Canadian Brand Names Effexor® XR; Novo-Venlafaxine XR
Mexican Brand Names Efexor XR
Generic Available Yes: Tablet
Pharmacologic Category Antidepressant, Serotonin/Norepinephrine Reuptake Inhibitor
Use Treatment of major depressive disorder, generalized anxiety disorder (GAD), social anxiety disorder (social phobia), panic disorder
Unlabeled/Investigational Use Obsessive-compulsive disorder (OCD); hot flashes; neuropathic pain; attention-deficit/hyperactivity disorder (ADHD)
Local Anesthetic/Vasoconstrictor Precautions Although venlafaxine is not a tricyclic antidepressant, it does block norepinephrine reuptake within CNS synapses as part of its mechanisms. It has been suggested that vasoconstrictor be administered with caution and to monitor vital signs in dental patients taking antidepressants that affect norepinephrine in this way. This is particularly important in patients taking venlafaxine, which has been noted to produce a sustained increase in diastolic blood pressure and heart rate as a side effect.
Effects on Dental Treatment Key adverse event(s) related to dental treatment: Significant xerostomia (normal salivary flow resumes upon discontinuation); may contribute to oral discomfort, especially in the elderly; taste perversion
Common Adverse Effects
>10%:
  Central nervous system: Headache (25% to 34%), insomnia (15% to 23%), somnolence (12% to 23%), nervousness (6% to 21%), dizziness (11% to 20%)
  Gastrointestinal: Nausea (21% to 58%), xerostomia (12% to 22%), anorexia (8% to 20%), constipation (8% to 15%)
  Genitourinary: Abnormal ejaculation/orgasm (2% to 16%)
  Neuromuscular & skeletal: Weakness (8% to 17%)
  Miscellaneous: Diaphoresis (10% to 14%)
1% to 10%:
  Cardiovascular: Hypertension (dose related; 3% in patients receiving <100 mg/day, up to 13% in patients receiving >300 mg/day), vasodilation (3% to 4%), palpitation (3%), tachycardia (2%), chest pain (2%), postural hypotension (1%), edema
  Central nervous system: Abnormal dreams (3% to 7%), anxiety (5% to 6%), yawning (3% to 5%), agitation (2% to 4%), chills (3%), confusion (2%), abnormal thinking (2%), depersonalization (1%), depression (1% to 3%), chills, fever, migraine, amnesia, hypoesthesia, trismus, vertigo
  Dermatologic: Rash (3%), pruritus (1%), bruising
  Endocrine & metabolic: Libido decreased (3% to 9%)
  Gastrointestinal: Diarrhea (6% to 8%), vomiting (3% to 6%), dyspepsia (5%), abdominal pain (4%), flatulence (3% to 4%), taste perversion (2%), weight loss (1% to 4%), appetite increased, weight gain
  Genitourinary: Impotence (4% to 10%), urinary frequency (3%), urination impaired (2%), urinary retention (1%), prostatic disorder
  Neuromuscular & skeletal: Tremor (4% to 10%), hypertonia (3%), paresthesia (2% to 3%), twitching (1% to 2%), neck pain, arthralgia
  Ocular: Abnormal or blurred vision (4% to 6%), mydriasis (2%
  Otic: Tinnitus (2%)
  Respiratory: Pharyngitis (7%), sinusitis (2%), cough increased, dyspnea
  Miscellaneous: Infection (6%), flu-like syndrome (6%), trauma (2%)
Restrictions An FDA-approved medication guide concerning the use of antidepressants in children, adolescents, and young adults must be distributed when dispensing an outpatient prescription (new or refill) where this medication is to be used without direct supervision of a healthcare provider. Medication guides are available at http://www.fda.gov/cder/Offices/ODS/medication_guides.htm. Dispense to parents or guardians of children and adolescents receiving this medication.
Dosage Oral:
Children and Adolescents:
  ADHD (unlabeled use): Initial: 12.5 mg/day
    Children <40 kg: Increase by 12.5 mg/week to maximum of 50 mg/day in 2 divided doses
    Children ≥40 kg: Increase by 25 mg/week to maximum of 75 mg/day in 3 divided doses.
    Mean dose: 60 mg or 1.4 mg/kg administered in 2-3 divided doses
(Continued)

Venlafaxine *(Continued)*

Adults:

Depression:

Immediate-release tablets: 75 mg/day, administered in 2 or 3 divided doses, taken with food; dose may be increased in 75 mg/day increments at intervals of at least 4 days, up to 225-375 mg/day

Extended-release capsules: 75 mg once daily taken with food; for some new patients, it may be desirable to start at 37.5 mg/day for 4-7 days before increasing to 75 mg once daily; dose may be increased by up to 75 mg/day increments every 4 days as tolerated, up to a recommended maximum of 225 mg/day

GAD, social anxiety disorder: Extended-release capsules: 75 mg once daily taken with food; for some new patients, it may be desirable to start at 37.5 mg/day for 4-7 days before increasing to 75 mg once daily; dose may be increased by up to 75 mg/day increments every 4 days as tolerated, up to a maximum of 225 mg/day

Panic disorder: Extended-release capsules: 37.5 mg once daily for 1 week; may increase to 75 mg daily, with subsequent weekly increases of 75 mg/day up to a maximum of 225 mg/day.

Obsessive-compulsive disorder (unlabeled use): Titrate to usual dosage range of 150-300 mg/day; however, doses up to 375 mg daily have been used; response may be seen in 4 weeks

Neuropathic pain (unlabeled use): Dosages evaluated varied considerably based on etiology of chronic pain, but efficacy has been shown for many conditions in the range of 75-225 mg/day; onset of relief may occur in 1-2 weeks, or take up to 6 weeks for full benefit.

Hot flashes (unlabeled use): Doses of 37.5-75 mg/day have demonstrated significant improvement of vasomotor symptoms after 4-8 weeks of treatment; in one study, doses >75 mg/day offered no additional benefit; however, higher doses (225 mg/day) may be beneficial in patients with perimenopausal depression.

Attention-deficit disorder (unlabeled use): Initial: Doses vary between 18.75 to 75 mg/day; may increase after 4 weeks to 150 mg/day; if tolerated, doses up to 225 mg/day have been used

Note: When discontinuing this medication after more than 1 week of treatment, it is generally recommended that the dose be tapered. If venlafaxine is used for 6 weeks or longer, the dose should be tapered over 2 weeks when discontinuing its use.

Dosing adjustment in renal impairment: Cl_{cr} 10-70 mL/minute: Decrease dose by 25%; decrease total daily dose by 50% if dialysis patients; dialysis patients should receive dosing after completion of dialysis

Dosing adjustment in moderate hepatic impairment: Reduce total daily dosage by 50%

Mechanism of Action Venlafaxine and its active metabolite, o-desmethylvenlafaxine (ODV), are potent inhibitors of neuronal serotonin and norepinephrine reuptake and weak inhibitors of dopamine reuptake. Venlafaxine and ODV have no significant activity for muscarinic cholinergic, H_1-histaminergic, or alpha$_2$-adrenergic receptors. Venlafaxine and ODV do not possess MAO-inhibitory activity.

Contraindications Hypersensitivity to venlafaxine or any component of the formulation; use of MAO inhibitors within 14 days; should not initiate MAO inhibitor within 7 days of discontinuing venlafaxine

Warnings/Precautions [U.S. Boxed Warning]: **Antidepressants increase the risk of suicidal thinking and behavior in children, adolescents, and young adults (18-24 years of age) with major depressive disorder (MDD) and other psychiatric disorders;** consider risk prior to prescribing. Short-term studies did not show an increased risk in patients >24 years of age and showed a decreased risk in patients ≥65 years. Closely monitor for clinical worsening, suicidality, or unusual changes in behavior; the patient's family or caregiver should be instructed to closely observe the patient and communicate condition with healthcare provider. Reduced growth rate has been observed with venlafaxine therapy in children. A medication guide should be dispensed with each prescription. **Venlafaxine is not FDA approved for use in children.**

The possibility of a suicide attempt is inherent in major depression and may persist until remission occurs. Monitor for worsening of depression or suicidality, especially during initiation of therapy (generally first 1-2 months) or with dose increases or decreases. Use caution in high-risk patients. Worsening depression and severe abrupt suicidality that are not part of the presenting symptoms may require discontinuation or modification of drug therapy. The patient's family or caregiver should be alerted to monitor patients for the emergence of suicidality and associated behaviors (such as agitation, irritability, hostility, impulsivity, and hypomania) and call healthcare provider.

May worsen psychosis in some patients or precipitate a shift to mania or hypomania in patients with bipolar disorder. Patients presenting with depressive symptoms should be screened for bipolar disorder. Monotherapy in patients with bipolar disorder should be avoided. **Venlafaxine is not FDA approved for the treatment of bipolar depression.**

The potential for severe reactions exists when used with MAO inhibitors, SSRIs/SNRIs or triptans (myoclonus, diaphoresis, hyperthermia, NMS features, seizures, and death). May cause sustained increase in blood pressure or tachycardia; dose related and increases are generally modest (12-15 mm Hg diastolic). Control pre-existing hypertension prior to initiation of venlafaxine. Use caution in patients with recent history of MI, unstable heart disease, or hyperthyroidism; may cause increase in anxiety, nervousness, insomnia; may cause weight loss (use with caution in patients where weight loss is undesirable); may cause increases in serum cholesterol. Use caution with hepatic or renal impairment. Venlafaxine has been associated with the development of SIADH and hyponatremia.

Interstitial lung disease and eosinophilic pneumonia have been rarely reported; may present as progressive dyspnea, cough, and/or chest pain. Prompt evaluation and possible discontinuation of therapy may be necessary. Venlafaxine may increase the risks associated with electroconvulsive therapy. Use cautiously in patients with a history of seizures. The risks of cognitive or motor impairment, as well as the potential for anticholinergic effects are very low. May cause or exacerbate sexual dysfunction. May impair platelet aggregation, resulting in bleeding.

Abrupt discontinuation or dosage reduction after extended (≥6 weeks) therapy may lead to agitation, dysphoria, nervousness, anxiety, and other symptoms. When discontinuing therapy, dosage should be tapered gradually over at least a 2-week period. If intolerable symptoms occur following a decrease in dosage or upon discontinuation of therapy, then resuming the previous dose with a more gradual taper should be considered. Use caution in patients with increased intraocular pressure or at risk of acute narrow-angle glaucoma.

Drug Interactions

Cytochrome P450 Effect: Substrate of CYP2C9 (minor), 2C19 (minor), 2D6 (major), 3A4 (major); **Inhibits** CYP2B6 (weak), 2D6 (weak), 3A4 (weak)

Increased Effect/Toxicity: Concurrent use of MAO inhibitors (phenelzine, isocarboxazid), or drugs with MAO inhibitor activity (linezolid) may result in serotonin syndrome; should not be used within 2 weeks of each other. Selegiline may have a lower risk of this effect, particularly at low dosages, due to selectivity for MAO type B. In addition, concurrent use of buspirone, lithium, meperidine, nefazodone, selegiline, serotonin agonists (sumatriptan, naratriptan), sibutramine, SSRIs/SNRIs, trazodone, or tricyclic antidepressants may increase the risk of serotonin syndrome. Serum levels of haloperidol may be increased by venlafaxine. CYP2D6 inhibitors may increase the levels/effects of venlafaxine; example inhibitors include chlorpromazine, delavirdine, fluoxetine, miconazole, paroxetine, pergolide, quinidine, quinine, ritonavir, and ropinirole. CYP3A4 inhibitors may increase the levels/effects of venlafaxine; example inhibitors include azole antifungals, clarithromycin, diclofenac, doxycycline, erythromycin, imatinib, isoniazid, nefazodone, nicardipine, propofol, protease inhibitors, quinidine, telithromycin, and verapamil. Concomitant use with other CNS depressants may enhance the CNS depressant effects of venlafaxine.

Decreased Effect: Serum levels of indinavir may be reduced be venlafaxine (AUC reduced by 28%); clinical significance not determined. CYP3A4 inducers may decrease the levels/effects of venlafaxine; example inducers include aminoglutethimide, carbamazepine, nafcillin, nevirapine, phenobarbital, phenytoin, and rifamycins.

Ethanol/Nutrition/Herb Interactions

Ethanol: Avoid ethanol (may increase CNS effects).

Herb/Nutraceutical: Avoid valerian, St John's wort, SAMe, kava kava, tryptophan (may increase risk of serotonin syndrome and/or excessive sedation).

Dietary Considerations Should be taken with food.

Pharmacodynamics/Kinetics

Absorption: Oral: 92% to 100%; food has no significant effect on the absorption of venlafaxine or formation of the active metabolite O-desmethylvenlafaxine (ODV)

Distribution: At steady state: Venlafaxine 7.5 ± 3.7 L/kg, ODV 5.7 ± 1.8 L/Kg

Protein binding: Bound to human plasma protein: Venlafaxine 27%, ODV 30%

Metabolism: Hepatic via CYP2D6 to active metabolite, O-desmethylvenlafaxine (ODV); other metabolites include N-desmethylvenlafaxine and N,O-didesmethylvenlafaxine

Bioavailability: Absolute: ~45%

(Continued)

Venlafaxine *(Continued)*

Half-life elimination: Venlafaxine: 3-7 hours; ODV: 9-13 hours; Steady-state, plasma: Venlafaxine/ODV: Within 3 days of multiple-dose therapy; prolonged with cirrhosis (Adults: Venlafaxine: ~30%, ODV: ~60%) and with dialysis (Adults: Venlafaxine: ~180%, ODV: ~142%)

Time to peak:

Immediate release: Venlafaxine: 2 hours, ODV: 3 hours

Extended release: Venlafaxine: 5.5 hours, ODV: 9 hours

Excretion: Urine (~87%, 5% as unchanged drug, 29% as unconjugated ODV, 26% as conjugated ODV, 27% as minor inactive metabolites) within 48 hours

Clearance at steady state: Venlafaxine: 1.3 ± 0.6 L/hour/kg, ODV: 0.4 ± 0.2 L/hour/kg

Clearance decreased with:

Cirrhosis: Adults: Venlafaxine: ~50%, ODV: ~30%

Severe cirrhosis: Adults: Venlafaxine: ~90%

Renal impairment (Cl_{cr} 10-70 mL/minute): Adults: Venlafaxine: ~24%

Dialysis: Adults: Venlafaxine: ~57%, ODV: ~56%; due to large volume of distribution, a significant amount of drug is not likely to be removed.

Pregnancy Risk Factor C

Dosage Forms

Capsule, extended release:

Effexor® XR: 37.5 mg, 75 mg, 150 mg

Tablet: 25 mg, 37.5 mg, 50 mg, 75 mg, 100 mg

Effexor®: 25 mg, 37.5 mg, 50 mg, 75 mg, 100 mg

Selected Readings

Ganzber S, "Psychoactive Drugs," *ADA Guide to Dental Therapeutics*, 2nd edition, Chapter 21, Chicago, IL: ADA Publishing, 2000, 381.

Venofer® *see* Iron Sucrose *on page 911*

Ventavis™ *see* Iloprost *on page 862*

Ventolin® HFA *see* Albuterol *on page 58*

VePesid® *see* Etoposide *on page 660*

Veracolate [OTC] *see* Bisacodyl *on page 216*

Verapamil *(ver AP a mil)*

Related Information

Cardiovascular Diseases *on page 1726*

U.S. Brand Names Calan®; Calan® SR; Covera-HS®; Isoptin® SR; Verelan®; Verelan® PM

Canadian Brand Names Alti-Verapamil; Apo-Verap®; Apo-Verap® SR; Calan®; Chronovera®; Covera®; Covera-HS®; Gen-Verapamil; Gen-Verapamil SR; Isoptin® SR; Novo-Veramil SR; Nu-Verap; Riva-Verapamil SR; Verapamil Hydrochloride Injection, USP

Mexican Brand Names Dilacoran; Dilacoran HTA

Generic Available Yes: Excludes controlled onset products

Index Terms Iproveratril Hydrochloride; Verapamil Hydrochloride

Pharmacologic Category Antiarrhythmic Agent, Class IV; Calcium Channel Blocker

Use Orally for treatment of angina pectoris (vasospastic, chronic stable, unstable) and hypertension; I.V. for supraventricular tachyarrhythmias (PSVT, atrial fibrillation, atrial flutter)

Unlabeled/Investigational Use Migraine; hypertrophic cardiomyopathy; bipolar disorder (manic manifestations)

Local Anesthetic/Vasoconstrictor Precautions No information available to require special precautions

Effects on Dental Treatment Key adverse event(s) related to dental treatment: Gingival hyperplasia. Calcium channel blockers (CCB) have been reported to cause gingival hyperplasia (GH). Verapamil-induced GH has appeared 11 months or more after subjects took daily doses of 240-360 mg. The severity of hyperplastic syndrome does not seem to be dose dependent. Gingivectomy is only successful if CCB therapy is discontinued. GH regresses markedly 1 week after CCB discontinuance with all symptoms resolving in 2 months. If a patient must continue CCB therapy, begin a program of professional cleaning and patient plaque control to minimize severity and growth rate of gingival tissue.

Common Adverse Effects

>10%: Gastrointestinal: Gingival hyperplasia (19%)

1% to 10%:
  Cardiovascular: Bradycardia (1.4% oral, 1.2% I.V.); first-, second-, or third-degree AV block (1.2% oral, unknown I.V.); CHF (1.8% oral); hypotension (2.5% oral, 3% I.V.); peripheral edema (1.9% oral); symptomatic hypotension (1.5% I.V.); severe tachycardia (1% I.V.)
  Central nervous system: Dizziness (3.3% oral, 1.2% I.V.), fatigue (1.7% oral), headache (2.2% oral, 1.2% I.V.)
  Dermatologic: Rash (1.2% oral)
  Gastrointestinal: Constipation (12% up to 42% in clinical trials), nausea (2.7% oral, 0.9% I.V.)
  Respiratory: Dyspnea (1.4% oral)

Dosage
  Children: SVT:
    I.V.:
      <1 year: 0.1-0.2 mg/kg over 2 minutes; repeat every 30 minutes as needed
      1-15 years: 0.1-0.3 mg/kg over 2 minutes; maximum: 5 mg/dose, may repeat dose in 15 minutes if adequate response not achieved; maximum for second dose: 10 mg/dose
    Oral (dose not well established):
      1-5 years: 4-8 mg/kg/day in 3 divided doses **or** 40-80 mg every 8 hours
      >5 years: 80 mg every 6-8 hours
  Adults:
    SVT: I.V.: 2.5-5 mg (over 2 minutes); second dose of 5-10 mg (~0.15 mg/kg) may be given 15-30 minutes after the initial dose if patient tolerates, but does not respond to initial dose; maximum total dose: 20 mg
    Angina: Oral: Initial dose: 80-120 mg 3 times/day (elderly or small stature: 40 mg 3 times/day); range: 240-480 mg/day in 3-4 divided doses
    Hypertension: Oral:
      Immediate release: 80 mg 3 times/day; usual dose range (JNC 7): 80-320 mg/day in 2 divided doses
      Sustained release: 240 mg/day; usual dose range (JNC 7): 120-360 mg/day in 1-2 divided doses; 120 mg/day in the elderly or small patients (no evidence of additional benefit in doses >360 mg/day).
      Extended release:
        Covera-HS®: Usual dose range (JNC 7): 120-360 mg once daily (once-daily dosing is recommended at bedtime)
        Verelan® PM: Usual dose range: 200-400 mg once daily at bedtime
  Dosing adjustment in renal impairment: Cl$_{cr}$ <10 mL/minute: Administer at 50% to 75% of normal dose.
  Dialysis: Not dialyzable (0% to 5%) via hemo- or peritoneal dialysis; supplemental dose is not necessary.
  Dosing adjustment/comments in hepatic disease: Reduce dose in cirrhosis, reduce dose to 20% to 50% of normal and monitor ECG.

Mechanism of Action Inhibits calcium ion from entering the "slow channels" or select voltage-sensitive areas of vascular smooth muscle and myocardium during depolarization; produces a relaxation of coronary vascular smooth muscle and coronary vasodilation; increases myocardial oxygen delivery in patients with vasospastic angina; slows automaticity and conduction of AV node.

Contraindications Hypersensitivity to verapamil or any component of the formulation; severe left ventricular dysfunction; hypotension (systolic pressure <90 mm Hg) or cardiogenic shock; sick sinus syndrome (except in patients with a functioning artificial pacemaker); second- or third-degree AV block (except in patients with a functioning artificial pacemaker); atrial flutter or fibrillation and an accessory bypass tract (WPW, Lown-Ganong-Levine syndrome)

Warnings/Precautions Use with caution in sick-sinus syndrome, severe left ventricular dysfunction, hepatic or renal impairment, and hypertrophic cardiomyopathy (especially obstructive). Abrupt withdrawal may cause increased duration and frequency of chest pain. Avoid I.V. use in neonates and young infants due to severe apnea, bradycardia, or hypotensive reactions. Elderly may experience more constipation and hypotension. Monitor ECG and blood pressure closely in patients receiving I.V. therapy particularly in patients with supraventricular tachycardia. May prolong recovery from nondepolarizing neuromuscular-blocking agents.

Drug Interactions
  Cytochrome P450 Effect: Substrate of CYP1A2 (minor), 2B6 (minor), 2C9 (minor), 2C18 (minor), 2E1 (minor), 3A4 (major); **Inhibits** CYP1A2 (weak), 2C9 (weak), 2D6 (weak), 3A4 (moderate)
  Increased Effect/Toxicity: Use of verapamil with amiodarone, beta-blockers, or flecainide may lead to bradycardia and decreased cardiac output. Aspirin and concurrent verapamil use may increase bleeding times. Lithium neurotoxicity may result when verapamil is added. Effect of nondepolarizing neuromuscular blocker is prolonged by verapamil. Grapefruit juice
  (Continued)

Verapamil *(Continued)*

may increase verapamil serum concentrations. Blood pressure-lowering effects may be additive with sildenafil, tadalafil, and vardenafil (use caution).

Cisapride levels may be increased by verapamil, potentially resulting in life-threatening arrhythmias; avoid concurrent use. Verapamil may increase the levels/effects of selected benzodiazepines, other calcium channel blockers, cyclosporine, ergot alkaloids, selected HMG-CoA reductase inhibitors, mirtazapine, nateglinide, nefazodone, pimozide, quinidine, risperidone, sildenafil (and other PDE-5 inhibitors), tacrolimus, telithromycin, venlafaxine, and other CYP3A4 substrates. In addition, serum concentrations of the following drugs may be increased by verapamil: Alfentanil, digoxin, doxorubicin, ethanol, prazosin, and theophylline. Verapamil may increase colchicine toxicity (especially nephrotoxicity).

The levels/effects of verapamil may be increased by azole antifungals, clarithromycin, diclofenac, doxycycline, erythromycin, imatinib, isoniazid, nefazodone, nicardipine, propofol, protease inhibitors, quinidine, telithromycin, and other CYP3A4 inhibitors.

Decreased Effect: The levels/effects of verapamil may be decreased by aminoglutethimide, carbamazepine, nafcillin, nevirapine, phenobarbital, phenytoin, rifamycins, and other CYP3A4 inducers. Lithium levels may be decreased by verapamil. Nafcillin decreases plasma concentration of verapamil.

Ethanol/Nutrition/Herb Interactions

Ethanol: Avoid or limit ethanol (may increase ethanol levels).

Food: Grapefruit juice may increase the serum concentration of verapamil; avoid concurrent use.

Herb/Nutraceutical: St John's wort may decrease levels. Avoid dong quai if using for hypertension (has estrogenic activity). Avoid ephedra, yohimbe, ginseng (may worsen arrhythmia or hypertension). Avoid garlic (may have increased antihypertensive effect).

Dietary Considerations Calan® SR and Isoptin® SR products may be taken with food or milk, other formulations may be administered without regard to meals; sprinkling contents of Verelan® or Verelan® PM capsule onto applesauce does not affect oral absorption.

Pharmacodynamics/Kinetics

Onset of action: Peak effect: Oral: Immediate release: 1-2 hours; I.V.: 1-5 minutes

Duration: Oral: Immediate release tablets: 6-8 hours; I.V.: 10-20 minutes

Protein binding: 90%

Metabolism: Hepatic via multiple CYP isoenzymes; extensive first-pass effect

Bioavailability: Oral: 20% to 35%

Half-life elimination: Infants: 4.4-6.9 hours; Adults: Single dose: 2-8 hours, Multiple doses: 4.5-12 hours; prolonged with hepatic cirrhosis

Excretion: Urine (70%, 3% to 4% as unchanged drug); feces (16%)

Pregnancy Risk Factor C

Dosage Forms

Caplet, sustained release: 120 mg, 180 mg, 240 mg
Calan® SR: 120 mg, 180 mg, 240 mg

Capsule, extended release, controlled onset:
Verelan® PM: 100 mg, 200 mg, 300 mg

Capsule, sustained release: 120 mg, 180 mg, 240 mg, 360 mg
Verelan®: 120 mg, 180 mg, 240 mg, 360 mg

Injection, solution: 2.5 mg/mL (2 mL, 4 mL)

Tablet: 80 mg, 120 mg
Calan®: 40 mg, 80 mg, 120 mg

Tablet, extended release: 120 mg, 180 mg, 240 mg

Tablet, extended release, controlled onset:
Covera-HS®: 180 mg, 240 mg

Tablet, sustained release: 120 mg, 180 mg, 240 mg
Isoptin® SR: 120 mg, 180 mg, 240 mg

Selected Readings

Wynn RL, "Update on Calcium Channel Blocker Induced Gingival Hyperplasia," *Gen Dent*, 1995, 43(3):218-22.

Verteporfin (ver te POR fin)

U.S. Brand Names Visudyne®
Canadian Brand Names Visudyne®
Generic Available No
Pharmacologic Category Ophthalmic Agent
Use Treatment of predominantly classic subfoveal choroidal neovascularization due to macular degeneration, presumed ocular histoplasmosis, or pathologic myopia
Unlabeled/Investigational Use Predominantly **occult** subfoveal choroidal neovascularization
Local Anesthetic/Vasoconstrictor Precautions No information available to require special precautions
Effects on Dental Treatment No significant effects or complications reported
Mechanism of Action Following intravenous administration, verteporfin is transported by lipoproteins to the neovascular endothelium in the affected eye(s), including choroidal neovasculature and the retina. Verteporfin then needs to be activated by nonthermal red light, which results in local damage to the endothelium, leading to temporary choroidal vessel occlusion.
Pregnancy Risk Factor C

Vesanoid® *see* Tretinoin (Oral) *on page 1606*

VESIcare® *see* Solifenacin *on page 1485*

Vexol® *see* Rimexolone *on page 1428*

VFEND® *see* Voriconazole *on page 1666*

Viactiv® Multivitamin [OTC] *see* Vitamins (Multiple/Oral) *on page 1665*

Viadur® *see* Leuprolide *on page 958*

Viagra® *see* Sildenafil *on page 1468*

Vibramycin® *see* Doxycycline (Systemic) *on page 541*

Vibra-Tabs® *see* Doxycycline (Systemic) *on page 541*

Vicks® 44® Cough Relief [OTC] *see* Dextromethorphan *on page 477*

Vicks® 44D Cough & Head Congestion [OTC] [DSC] *see* Pseudoephedrine and Dextromethorphan *on page 1383*

Vicks® 44E [OTC] *see* Guaifenesin and Dextromethorphan *on page 796*

Vicks® Casero™ Chest Congestion Relief [OTC] *see* Guaifenesin *on page 795*

Vicks® DayQuil® Multi-Symptom Cold and Flu [OTC] [DSC] *see* Acetaminophen, Dextromethorphan, and Pseudoephedrine *on page 44*

Vicks® Formula 44® Sore Throat [OTC] *see* Phenol *on page 1290*

Vicks® Pediatric Formula 44E [OTC] *see* Guaifenesin and Dextromethorphan *on page 796*

Vicks Sinex® 12 Hour [OTC] *see* Oxymetazoline *on page 1236*

Vicks Sinex® 12 Hour Ultrafine Mist [OTC] *see* Oxymetazoline *on page 1236*

Vicks® Sinex® Nasal Spray [OTC] *see* Phenylephrine *on page 1293*

Vicks® Sinex® UltraFine Mist [OTC] *see* Phenylephrine *on page 1293*

Vicodin® *see* Hydrocodone and Acetaminophen *on page 822*

Vicodin® ES *see* Hydrocodone and Acetaminophen *on page 822*

Vicodin® HP *see* Hydrocodone and Acetaminophen *on page 822*

Vicon Forte® *see* Vitamins (Multiple/Oral) *on page 1665*

Vicoprofen® *see* Hydrocodone and Ibuprofen *on page 830*

Vi-Daylin®/F [DSC] *see* Vitamins (Fluoride) *on page 1665*

Vi-Daylin®/F ADC [DSC] *see* Vitamins (Fluoride) *on page 1665*

Vi-Daylin®/F ADC + Iron [DSC] *see* Vitamins (Fluoride) *on page 1665*

Vi-Daylin®/F + Iron [DSC] *see* Vitamins (Fluoride) *on page 1665*

Vi-Daylin® + Iron Liquid [OTC] [DSC] *see* Vitamins (Multiple/Oral) *on page 1665*

Vi-Daylin® Liquid [OTC] [DSC] *see* Vitamins (Multiple/Oral) *on page 1665*

Vidaza® *see* Azacitidine *on page 171*

Videx® *see* Didanosine *on page 492*

Videx® EC *see* Didanosine *on page 492*

Vigabatrin (vye GA ba trin)

Canadian Brand Names Sabril®
Generic Available No
Pharmacologic Category Anticonvulsant, Miscellaneous
Use Active management of partial or secondary generalized seizures not controlled by usual treatments; treatment of infantile spasms
(Continued)

Vigabatrin *(Continued)*

Unlabeled/Investigational Use Spasticity, tardive dyskinesias

Local Anesthetic/Vasoconstrictor Precautions No information available to require special precautions

Effects on Dental Treatment No significant effects or complications reported

Common Adverse Effects

>10%:

Central nervous system: Fatigue (27%), headache (26%), drowsiness (22%), dizziness (19%), depression (13%), tremor (11%), agitation (11%). **Note:** In pediatric use, hyperactivity (hyperkinesia, agitation, excitation, or restlessness) was reported in 11% of patients.

Endocrine & metabolic: Weight gain (12%)

Ocular: Visual field defects (33%), abnormal vision (11%)

1% to 10%:

Cardiovascular: Chest pain, edema (dependent)

Central nervous system: Abnormal thinking, aggression, amnesia, anxiety, ataxia, concentration impaired, confusion, emotional lability, insomnia, personality disorder, speech disorder, vertigo, nervousness

Dermatologic: Rash (5%, similar to placebo), skin disorder

Endocrine & metabolic: Dysmenorrhea, menstrual disorder

Gastrointestinal: Abdominal pain, appetite increased, constipation, diarrhea, nausea, vomiting

Genitourinary: Urinary tract infection

Hematologic: Purpura

Neuromuscular & skeletal: Abnormal coordination, abnormal gait, arthralgia, arthrosis, back pain, hyporeflexia, paresthesia, weakness

Ocular: Diplopia, eye pain, nystagmus

Otic: Ear pain

Respiratory: Nasal congestion, sinusitis, throat irritation, upper respiratory tract infection

Restrictions Not available in U.S.

Mechanism of Action Irreversibly inhibits gamma-aminobutyric acid transaminase (GABA-T), increasing the levels of the inhibitory compound gamma amino butyric acid (GABA) within the brain. Duration of effect is dependent upon rate of GABA-T resynthesis.

Drug Interactions

Decreased Effect: Serum concentrations of phenytoin and phenobarbital may be decreased by vigabatrin.

Pharmacodynamics/Kinetics

Duration (rate of GABA-T resynthesis dependent): Variable (not strictly correlated to serum concentrations)

Absorption: Rapid

Metabolism: Minimal

Half-life elimination: 5-8 hours; Elderly: Up to 13 hours

Time to peak: 2 hours

Excretion: Urine (70%, as unchanged drug)

Pregnancy Risk Factor Not assigned; contraindicated per manufacturer

Vigamox™ *see* Moxifloxacin *on page 1129*

VIGIV *see* Vaccinia Immune Globulin (Intravenous) *on page 1634*

VinBLAStine *(vin BLAS teen)*

Mexican Brand Names Lemblastine

Generic Available Yes

Index Terms NSC-49842; Vinblastine Sulfate; VLB

Pharmacologic Category Antineoplastic Agent, Natural Source (Plant) Derivative; Antineoplastic Agent, Vinca Alkaloid

Use Treatment of Hodgkin's and non-Hodgkin's lymphoma; testicular, lung, head and neck, breast, and renal carcinomas; Mycosis fungoides; Kaposi's sarcoma; histiocytosis; choriocarcinoma; and idiopathic thrombocytopenic purpura

Local Anesthetic/Vasoconstrictor Precautions No information available to require special precautions

Effects on Dental Treatment Key adverse event(s) related to dental treatment: Stomatitis, metallic taste, and jaw pain.

Common Adverse Effects

>10%:

Dermatologic: Alopecia

Endocrine & metabolic: SIADH

Gastrointestinal: Diarrhea (less common), stomatitis, anorexia, metallic taste

Hematologic: May cause severe bone marrow suppression and is the dose-limiting toxicity of vinblastine (unlike vincristine); severe granulocytopenia and thrombocytopenia may occur following the administration of vinblastine and nadir 5-10 days after treatment

Myelosuppression (primarily leukopenia, may be dose limiting)

Onset: 4-7 days

Nadir: 5-10 days

Recovery: 4-21 days

1% to 10%:

Cardiovascular: Hypertension, Raynaud's phenomenon

Central nervous system: Depression, malaise, headache, seizure

Dermatologic: Rash, photosensitivity, dermatitis

Endocrine & metabolic: Hyperuricemia

Gastrointestinal: Constipation, abdominal pain, nausea (mild), vomiting (mild), paralytic ileus, stomatitis

Genitourinary: Urinary retention

Neuromuscular & skeletal: Jaw pain, myalgia, paresthesia

Respiratory: Bronchospasm

Mechanism of Action Vinblastine binds to tubulin and inhibits microtubule formation, therefore, arresting the cell at metaphase by disrupting the formation of the mitotic spindle; it is specific for the M and S phases. Vinblastine may also interfere with nucleic acid and protein synthesis by blocking glutamic acid utilization.

Drug Interactions

Cytochrome P450 Effect: Substrate of CYP2D6 (minor), 3A4 (major); **Inhibits** CYP2D6 (weak), 3A4 (weak)

Increased Effect/Toxicity: CYP3A4 inhibitors may increase the levels/effects of vinblastine; example inhibitors include azole antifungals, clarithromycin, diclofenac, doxycycline, erythromycin, imatinib, isoniazid, nefazodone, nicardipine, propofol, protease inhibitors, quinidine, telithromycin, and verapamil.

Previous or simultaneous use with mitomycin-C has resulted in acute shortness of breath and severe bronchospasm within minutes or several hours after vinca alkaloid injection and may occur up to 2 weeks after the dose of mitomycin. Mitomycin-C, in combination with administration of vinblastine, may cause acute shortness of breath and severe bronchospasm. Onset may be within minutes or several hours after vinblastine injection.

Decreased Effect: CYP3A4 inducers may decrease the levels/effects of vinblastine; example inducers include aminoglutethimide, carbamazepine, nafcillin, nevirapine, phenobarbital, phenytoin (may reduce vinblastine serum concentrations), and rifamycins.

Pharmacodynamics/Kinetics

Distribution: V_d: 27.3 L/kg; binds extensively to tissues; does not penetrate CNS or other fatty tissues; distributes to liver

Protein binding: 99%

Metabolism: Hepatic to active metabolite

Half-life elimination: Biphasic: Initial: 0.164 hours; Terminal: 25 hours

Excretion: Feces (95%); urine (<1% as unchanged drug)

Pregnancy Risk Factor D

Vinblastine Sulfate *see* VinBLAStine *on page 1658*

Vincasar PFS® *see* VinCRIStine *on page 1659*

VinCRIStine (vin KRIS teen)

U.S. Brand Names Vincasar PFS®

Canadian Brand Names Vincasar® PFS®

Mexican Brand Names Citomid RU; Vintec

Generic Available Yes

Index Terms LCR; Leurocristine Sulfate; NSC-67574; VCR; Vincristine Sulfate

Pharmacologic Category Antineoplastic Agent, Natural Source (Plant) Derivative; Antineoplastic Agent, Vinca Alkaloid

Use Treatment of leukemias, Hodgkin's disease, non-Hodgkin's lymphomas, Wilms' tumor, neuroblastoma, rhabdomyosarcoma

Local Anesthetic/Vasoconstrictor Precautions No information available to require special precautions

Effects on Dental Treatment Key adverse event(s) related to dental treatment: Oral ulceration, metallic taste, orthostatic hypotension or hypertension.

Common Adverse Effects

>10%: Dermatologic: Alopecia (20% to 70%)

1% to 10%:

Cardiovascular: Orthostatic hypotension or hypertension, hyper-/hypotension

(Continued)

VinCRIStine (Continued)

Central nervous system: CNS depression, confusion, cranial nerve paralysis, fever, headache, insomnia, motor difficulties, seizure

Intrathecal administration of vincristine has uniformly caused death; vincristine should never be administered by this route. Neurologic effects of vincristine may be additive with those of other neurotoxic agents and spinal cord irradiation.

Dermatologic: Rash

Endocrine & metabolic: Hyperuricemia

Gastrointestinal: Abdominal cramps, anorexia, bloating, constipation (and possible paralytic ileus secondary to neurologic toxicity), diarrhea, metallic taste, nausea (mild), oral ulceration, vomiting, weight loss

Genitourinary: Bladder atony (related to neurotoxicity), dysuria, polyuria, urinary retention

Hematologic: Leukopenia (mild), thrombocytopenia, myelosuppression (onset: 7 days; nadir: 10 days; recovery: 21 days)

Local: Phlebitis, tissue irritation and necrosis if infiltrated

Neuromuscular & skeletal: Cramping, jaw pain, leg pain, myalgia, numbness, weakness

Peripheral neuropathy: Frequently the dose-limiting toxicity of vincristine. Most frequent in patients >40 years of age; occurs usually after an average of 3 weekly doses, but may occur after just one dose. Manifested as loss of the deep tendon reflexes in the lower extremities, numbness, tingling, pain, paresthesia of the fingers and toes (stocking glove sensation), and "foot drop" or "wrist drop."

Ocular: Optic atrophy, photophobia

Mechanism of Action Binds to tubulin and inhibits microtubule formation, therefore, arresting the cell at metaphase by disrupting the formation of the mitotic spindle; it is specific for the M and S phases. Vincristine may also interfere with nucleic acid and protein synthesis by blocking glutamic acid utilization.

Drug Interactions

Cytochrome P450 Effect: Substrate of CYP3A4 (major); **Inhibits** CYP3A4 (weak)

Increased Effect/Toxicity: Vincristine should be given 12-24 hours before asparaginase to minimize toxicity (may decrease the hepatic clearance of vincristine). Acute pulmonary reactions may occur with mitomycin-C. Previous or simultaneous use with mitomycin-C has resulted in acute shortness of breath and severe bronchospasm within minutes or several hours after vinca alkaloid injection and may occur up to 2 weeks after the dose of mitomycin. Itraconazole may enhance the neurotoxicity of vincristine.

CYP3A4 inhibitors may increase the levels/effects of vincristine. Example inhibitors include azole antifungals, clarithromycin, diclofenac, doxycycline, erythromycin, imatinib, isoniazid, nefazodone, nicardipine, propofol, protease inhibitors, quinidine, telithromycin, and verapamil. Digoxin plasma levels and renal excretion may decrease with combination chemotherapy including vincristine. Nifedipine may increase the levels/effects of vincristine.

Decreased Effect: Digoxin levels may decrease with combination chemotherapy. CYP3A4 inducers may decrease the levels/effects of vincristine; example inducers include aminoglutethimide, carbamazepine, nafcillin, nevirapine, phenobarbital, phenytoin, and rifamycins.

Pharmacodynamics/Kinetics

Absorption: Oral: Poor

Distribution: V_d: 163-165 L/m^2; poor penetration into CSF; rapidly removed from bloodstream and tightly bound to tissues; penetrates blood-brain barrier poorly

Protein binding: 75%

Metabolism: Extensively hepatic

Half-life elimination: Terminal: 24 hours

Excretion: Feces (~80%); urine (<1% as unchanged drug)

Pregnancy Risk Factor D

Vincristine Sulfate *see* VinCRIStine *on page 1659*

Vindesine (VIN de seen)

Generic Available No

Index Terms DAVA; Deacetyl Vinblastine Carboxamide; Desacetyl Vinblastine Amide Sulfate; DVA; Eldisine Lilly 99094; Lilly CT-3231; NSC-245467; Vindesine Sulfate

Pharmacologic Category Antineoplastic Agent, Vinca Alkaloid

Unlabeled/Investigational Use Investigational: Management of acute lympho-cytic leukemia, chronic myelogenous leukemia; breast, head, neck, and lung cancers; lymphomas (Hodgkin's and non-Hodgkin's)

Local Anesthetic/Vasoconstrictor Precautions No information available to require special precautions

Effects on Dental Treatment Key adverse event(s) related to dental treatment: Loss of taste and facial paralysis.

Common Adverse Effects

>10%:

Central nervous system: Pyrexia, malaise (up to 60%)

Dermatologic: Alopecia (6% to 92%)

Gastrointestinal: Mild nausea and vomiting (7% to 27%), constipation (10% to 17%) - related to the neurotoxicity

Hematologic: Leukopenia (50%) and thrombocytopenia (14% to 26%), may be dose limiting; thrombocytosis (20% to 28%)

Nadir: 6-12 days

Recovery: Days 14-18

Neuromuscular & skeletal: Paresthesia (40% to 70%); loss of deep tendon reflexes (35% to 60%, may be dose limiting); myalgia (up to 60%)

1% to 10%:

Dermatologic: Rashes

Gastrointestinal: Loss of taste

Hematologic: Anemia

Local: Phlebitis

Neuromuscular & skeletal: Facial paralysis

Restrictions Not available in U.S./Investigational

Mechanism of Action Vindesine is a semisynthetic vinca alkaloid, having a mechanism of action similar to the other vinca derivatives. It arrests cell division in metaphase through inhibition of microtubular formation of the mitotic spindle. The drug is cell-cycle specific for the S phase.

Pharmacodynamics/Kinetics

Distribution: V_d: 8 L/kg; minimal distribution to adipose tissue or CNS

Metabolism: Hepatic

Half-life elimination:

Triphasic; Alpha: 2 minutes; Beta: 1 hour

Terminal: 24 hours

Excretion: Feces; urine (~3% to 25% of dose as unchanged drug)

Vindesine Sulfate *see* Vindesine *on page 1660*

Vinorelbine (vi NOR el been)

U.S. Brand Names Navelbine®

Canadian Brand Names Navelbine®; Vinorelbine Injection, USP; Vinorelbine Tartrate for Injection

Mexican Brand Names Navelbine

Generic Available Yes

Index Terms Dihydroxydeoxynorvinkaleukoblastine; NVB; Vinorelbine Tartrate

Pharmacologic Category Antineoplastic Agent, Natural Source (Plant) Derivative; Antineoplastic Agent, Vinca Alkaloid

Use Treatment of nonsmall-cell lung cancer

Unlabeled/Investigational Use Treatment of breast cancer, ovarian carcinoma, Hodgkin's disease, non-Hodgkin's lymphoma

Local Anesthetic/Vasoconstrictor Precautions No information available to require special precautions

Effects on Dental Treatment No significant effects or complications reported

Common Adverse Effects

>10%:

Central nervous system: Fatigue (27%)

Dermatologic: Alopecia (12%)

Gastrointestinal: Nausea (44%, severe <2%) and vomiting (20%) are most common and are easily controlled with standard antiemetics; constipation (35%), diarrhea (17%)

Emetic potential: Moderate (30% to 60%)

Hematologic: May cause severe bone marrow suppression and is the dose-limiting toxicity of vinorelbine; severe granulocytopenia (90%) may occur following the administration of vinorelbine; leukopenia (92%), anemia (83%)

Myelosuppressive:

WBC: Moderate - severe

Onset: 4-7 days

Nadir: 7-10 days

(Continued)

Vinorelbine *(Continued)*

Recovery: 14-21 days
Hepatic: AST (67%) increased, total bilirubin increased (13%)
Local: Injection site reaction (28%), injection site pain (16%)
Neuromuscular & skeletal: Weakness (36%), peripheral neuropathy (20% to 25%)
1% to 10%:
Cardiovascular: Chest pain (5%)
Gastrointestinal: Paralytic ileus (1%)
Hematologic: Thrombocytopenia (5%)
Local: Phlebitis (7%)
Neuromuscular & skeletal: Mild-to-moderate peripheral neuropathy manifested by paresthesia and hyperesthesia, loss of deep tendon reflexes (<5%); myalgia (<5%), arthralgia (<5%), jaw pain (<5%)
Respiratory: Dyspnea (3% to 7%)

Mechanism of Action Semisynthetic vinca alkaloid which binds to tubulin and inhibits microtubule formation, therefore, arresting the cell at metaphase by disrupting the formation of the mitotic spindle; it is specific for the M and S phases. Vinorelbine may also interfere with nucleic acid and protein synthesis by blocking glutamic acid utilization.

Drug Interactions

Cytochrome P450 Effect: Substrate of CYP2D6 (minor), 3A4 (major); **Inhibits** CYP2D6 (weak), 3A4 (weak)

Increased Effect/Toxicity: Previous or simultaneous use with mitomycin-C has resulted in acute shortness of breath and severe bronchospasm within minutes or several hours after vinca alkaloid injection and may occur up to 2 weeks after the dose of mitomycin. CYP3A4 inhibitors may increase the levels/effects of vinorelbine; example inhibitors include azole antifungals, clarithromycin, diclofenac, doxycycline, erythromycin, imatinib, isoniazid, nefazodone, nicardipine, propofol, protease inhibitors, quinidine, telithromycin, and verapamil. Incidence of granulocytopenia is significantly higher in cisplatin/vinorelbine combination therapy than with single-agent vinorelbine.

Decreased Effect: CYP3A4 inducers may decrease the levels/effects of vinorelbine; example inducers include aminoglutethimide, carbamazepine, nafcillin, nevirapine, phenobarbital, phenytoin, and rifamycins.

Pharmacodynamics/Kinetics

Absorption: Unreliable; must be given I.V.
Distribution: V_d: 25.4-40.1 L/kg; binds extensively to human platelets and lymphocytes (79.6% to 91.2%)
Protein binding: 80% to 90%
Metabolism: Extensively hepatic to two metabolites, deacetylvinorelbine (active) and vinorelbine N-oxide
Bioavailability: Oral: 26% to 45%
Half-life elimination: Triphasic: Terminal: 27.7-43.6 hours
Excretion: Feces (46%); urine (18%, 10% to 12% as unchanged drug)
Clearance: Plasma: Mean: 0.97-1.26 L/hour/kg

Pregnancy Risk Factor D

Vitafol *see* Vitamin B Complex Combinations *on page 1664*

Vitamin C *see* Ascorbic Acid *on page 148*

Vitamin D₂ *see* Ergocalciferol *on page 583*

Vitamin D₃ *see* Alendronate and Cholecalciferol *on page 67*

Vitamin D and Calcium Carbonate *see* Calcium and Vitamin D *on page 259*

Vitamin A (VYE ta min aye)

U.S. Brand Names Aquasol A®; Palmitate-A® [OTC]

Generic Available Yes: Capsule

Index Terms Oleovitamin A

Pharmacologic Category Vitamin, Fat Soluble

Use Treatment and prevention of vitamin A deficiency; parenteral (I.M.) route is indicated when oral administration is not feasible or when absorption is insufficient (malabsorption syndrome)

Local Anesthetic/Vasoconstrictor Precautions No information available to require special precautions

Effects on Dental Treatment No significant effects or complications reported

Common Adverse Effects 1% to 10%:

Central nervous system: Fever, headache, irritability, lethargy, malaise, vertigo

Dermatologic: Drying or cracking of skin

Endocrine & metabolic: Hypercalcemia

Gastrointestinal: Weight loss

Ocular: Visual changes

Miscellaneous: Hypervitaminosis A

Mechanism of Action Needed for bone development, growth, visual adaptation to darkness, testicular and ovarian function, and as a cofactor in many biochemical processes

Drug Interactions

Increased Effect/Toxicity: Retinoids may have additive adverse effects.

Decreased Effect: Cholestyramine resin decreases absorption of vitamin A. Neomycin and mineral oil may also interfere with vitamin A absorption.

Pharmacodynamics/Kinetics

Absorption: Vitamin A in dosages **not** exceeding physiologic replacement is well absorbed after oral administration; water miscible preparations are absorbed more rapidly than oil preparations; large oral doses, conditions of fat malabsorption, low protein intake, or hepatic or pancreatic disease reduces oral absorption

Distribution: Large amounts concentrate for storage in the liver; enters breast milk

Metabolism: Conjugated with glucuronide; undergoes enterohepatic recirculation

Excretion: Feces

Pregnancy Risk Factor A/X (dose exceeding RDA recommendation)

Vitamin A Acid *see* Tretinoin (Topical) *on page 1607*

Vitamin A and Vitamin D (VYE ta min aye & VYE ta min dee)

Related Information

Vitamin A *on page 1663*

U.S. Brand Names A and D® Original [OTC]; Baza® Clear [OTC]; Sween Cream® [OTC]

Generic Available Yes: Capsule, ointment

Index Terms Cod Liver Oil

Pharmacologic Category Topical Skin Product

Use Temporary relief of discomfort due to chapped skin, diaper rash, minor burns, abrasions, as well as irritations associated with ostomy skin care

Local Anesthetic/Vasoconstrictor Precautions No information available to require special precautions

Effects on Dental Treatment No significant effects or complications reported

Common Adverse Effects Frequency not defined: Local: Irritation

Pregnancy Risk Factor B

Vitamin B₁ *see* Thiamine *on page 1556*

Vitamin B₂ *see* Riboflavin *on page 1422*

Vitamin B₃ *see* Niacin *on page 1166*

Vitamin B₃ *see* Niacinamide *on page 1167*

Vitamin B₅ *see* Pantothenic Acid *on page 1251*

Vitamin B₆ *see* Pyridoxine *on page 1389*

Vitamin B₁₂ *see* Cyanocobalamin *on page 418*

Vitamin B₁₂ₐ *see* Hydroxocobalamin *on page 842*

Vitamin B Complex Combinations
(VYE ta min bee KOM pleks kom bi NAY shuns)

U.S. Brand Names Allbee® C-800 [OTC]; Allbee® C-800 + Iron [OTC]; Allbee® with C [OTC]; Apatate® [OTC]; DexFol™; Diatx™; Gevrabon® [OTC]; Kobee [OTC]; NephPlex® Rx; Nephrocaps®; Nephronex®; Nephron FA®; Nephro-Vite®; Nephro-Vite® Rx; Quin B Strong [OTC]; Rena-Vite [OTC]; Rena-Vite RX; Rhenaphro; Senilezol; Stresstabs® High Potency Advanced [OTC]; Stresstabs® High Potency Energy [OTC]; Stresstabs® High Potency Weight [OTC]; Strovite; Super Quints 50 [OTC]; Surbex-T® [OTC]; Trinsicon® [DSC]; Vitafol; Z-Bec® [OTC]

Generic Available Yes

Index Terms B Complex Combinations; B Vitamin Combinations

Pharmacologic Category Vitamin

Use Supplement for use in the wasting syndrome in chronic renal failure, uremia, impaired metabolic functions of the kidney, dialysis; labeled for OTC use as a dietary supplement

Local Anesthetic/Vasoconstrictor Precautions No information available to require special precautions

Effects on Dental Treatment No significant effects or complications reported

Common Adverse Effects Frequency not defined.
Central nervous system: Somnolence
Dermatologic: Itching
Gastrointestinal: Bloating, constipation, diarrhea, flatulence, nausea, vomiting
Hematologic: Peripheral vascular thrombosis, polycythemia vera
Neuromuscular & skeletal: Paresthesia
Miscellaneous: Allergic reaction

Pregnancy Risk Factor A (RDA recommended doses)

Vitamin E (VYE ta min ee)

U.S. Brand Names Alph-E [OTC]; Alph-E-Mixed [OTC]; Aquasol E® [OTC]; Aquavit-E [OTC]; d-Alpha-Gems™ [OTC]; E-Gems® [OTC]; E-Gems Elite® [OTC]; E-Gems Plus® [OTC]; Ester-E™ [OTC]; Gamma E-Gems® [OTC]; Gamma-E Plus [OTC]; High Gamma Vitamin E Complete™ [OTC]; Key-E® [OTC]; Key-E® Kaps [OTC]

Generic Available Yes

Index Terms *d*-Alpha Tocopherol; *dl*-Alpha Tocopherol

Pharmacologic Category Vitamin, Fat Soluble

Use Dietary supplement

Unlabeled/Investigational Use To reduce the risk of bronchopulmonary dysplasia or retrolental fibroplasia in infants exposed to high concentrations of oxygen; prevention and treatment of tardive dyskinesia and Alzheimer's disease; prevention and treatment of hemolytic anemia secondary to vitamin E deficiency

Local Anesthetic/Vasoconstrictor Precautions No information available to require special precautions

Effects on Dental Treatment No significant effects or complications reported

Common Adverse Effects Frequency not defined.
Central nervous system: Fatigue, headache, weakness
Dermatologic: Contact dermatitis with topical preparation
Endocrine & metabolic: Gonadal dysfunction
Gastrointestinal: Diarrhea, intestinal cramps, nausea
Neuromuscular & skeletal: Weakness
Ocular: Blurred vision

Mechanism of Action Prevents oxidation of vitamin A and C; protects polyunsaturated fatty acids in membranes from attack by free radicals and protects red blood cells against hemolysis

Drug Interactions
Increased Effect/Toxicity: Vitamin E may alter the effect of vitamin K actions on clotting factors resulting in an increase hypoprothrombinemic response to warfarin; monitor.
Decreased Effect: Vitamin E may impair the hematologic response to iron in children with iron-deficiency anemia; monitor.

Pharmacodynamics/Kinetics
Absorption: Oral: Depends on presence of bile; reduced in conditions of malabsorption, in low birth weight premature infants, and as dosage increases; water miscible preparations are better absorbed than oil preparations
Distribution: To all body tissues, especially adipose tissue, where it is stored

Metabolism: Hepatic to glucuronides
Excretion: Feces
Pregnancy Risk Factor A/C (dose exceeding RDA recommendation)

Vitamin G *see* Riboflavin *on page 1422*
Vitamin K₁ *see* Phytonadione *on page 1299*

Vitamins (Fluoride) (VYE ta mins, FLOOR ide)

U.S. Brand Names Poly-Vi-Flor®; Poly-Vi-Flor® With Iron; Soluvite-F; Tri-Vi-Flor®; Tri-Vi-Flor® with Iron; Vi-Daylin®/F [DSC]; Vi-Daylin®/F ADC [DSC]; Vi-Daylin®/F + Iron [DSC]
Index Terms Multivitamins/Fluoride
Pharmacologic Category Vitamin
Use Prevention/treatment of vitamin deficiency; products containing fluoride are used to prevent dental caries; labeled for OTC use as a dietary supplement
Local Anesthetic/Vasoconstrictor Precautions No information available to require special precautions
Effects on Dental Treatment No significant effects or complications reported
Dosage Daily dose varies by product; refer to package insert for specific product labeling
Contraindications Hypersensitivity to any component of the formulation; pre-existing hypervitaminosis
Dietary Considerations May take with food to decrease stomach upset.
Dosage Forms Content varies depending on product used. For more detailed information on ingredients in these and other multivitamins, please refer to package labeling.
Dental Comment Chronic overdose of fluoride may result in mottling of tooth enamel and osseous changes.

Vitamins (Multiple/Oral) (VYE ta mins, MUL ti pul/OR al)

U.S. Brand Names Centrum® [OTC]; Centrum® Performance™ [OTC]; Centrum® Silver® [OTC]; Geriation [OTC]; Geritol Complete® [OTC]; Geritol Extend® [OTC]; Geritol® Tonic [OTC]; Glutofac®-MX; Glutofac®-ZX; Gynovite® Plus [OTC]; Hemocyte Plus®; Hi-Kovite [OTC]; Iberet® [OTC]; Iberet®-500 [OTC]; Monocaps [OTC]; Multiret Folic 500; Ocuvite® [OTC]; Ocuvite® Extra® [OTC]; Ocuvite® Lutein [OTC]; Olay® Vitamins Complete Women's [OTC]; Olay® Vitamins Complete Women's 50+[OTC]; Olay® Vitamins Even Complexion [OTC]; One-A-Day® 50 Plus Formula [OTC]; One-A-Day® Active Formula [OTC]; One-A-Day® Carb Smart [OTC]; One-A-Day® Cholesterol Plus™ [OTC]; One-A-Day® Essential Formula [OTC]; One-A-Day® Maximum Formula [OTC]; One-A-Day® Men's Formula [OTC]; One-A-Day® Today [OTC]; One-A-Day® Weight Smart [OTC]; One-A-Day® Women's Formula [OTC]; Optivite® P.M.T. [OTC]; PreserVision® AREDS [OTC]; PreserVision® Lutein [OTC]; Quintabs [OTC]; Quintabs-M [OTC]; Replace [OTC]; Replace with Iron [OTC]; Repliva 21/7™; Strovite® Forte; Theragran® Heart Right™ [OTC] [DSC]; Theragran-M® Advanced Formula [OTC] [DSC]; T-Vites [OTC]; Ultra Freeda Iron Free [OTC]; Ultra Freeda with Iron [OTC]; Unicap M® [OTC]; Unicap Sr® [OTC]; Unicap T™ [OTC]; Viactiv® Multivitamin [OTC]; Vicon Forte®; Vi-Daylin® + Iron Liquid [OTC] [DSC]; Vi-Daylin® Liquid [OTC] [DSC]; Vitacon Forte; Xtramins [OTC]
Generic Available Yes
Index Terms Multiple Vitamins; Therapeutic Multivitamins; Vitamins, Multiple (Oral); Vitamins, Multiple (Therapeutic); Vitamins, Multiple With Iron
Pharmacologic Category Vitamin
Use Prevention/treatment of vitamin and mineral deficiencies; labeled for OTC use as a dietary supplement
Local Anesthetic/Vasoconstrictor Precautions No information available to require special precautions
Effects on Dental Treatment No significant effects or complications reported
Common Adverse Effects Refer to individual vitamin monographs.
Pregnancy Risk Factor A (at RDA recommended dose)

Vitamins, Multiple (Oral) *see* Vitamins (Multiple/Oral) *on page 1665*
Vitamins, Multiple (Therapeutic) *see* Vitamins (Multiple/Oral) *on page 1665*
Vitamins, Multiple With Iron *see* Vitamins (Multiple/Oral) *on page 1665*
Vitelle™ Irospan® [OTC] [DSC] *see* Ferrous Sulfate and Ascorbic Acid *on page 688*
Vitrase® *see* Hyaluronidase *on page 817*
Vitrasert® *see* Ganciclovir *on page 763*
Vitravene™ [DSC] *see* Fomivirsen *on page 740*

Voriconazole (vor i KOE na zole)

Related Information
Fungal Infections *on page 1841*
U.S. Brand Names VFEND®
Canadian Brand Names VFEND®
Mexican Brand Names VFEND
Generic Available No
Index Terms UK109496
Pharmacologic Category Antifungal Agent, Oral; Antifungal Agent, Parenteral
Use Treatment of invasive aspergillosis; treatment of esophageal candidiasis; treatment of candidemia (in non-neutropenic patients); treatment of disseminated *Candida* infections of the skin and viscera; treatment of serious fungal infections caused by *Scedosporium apiospermum* and *Fusarium* spp (including *Fusarium solani*) in patients intolerant of, or refractory to, other therapy

Local Anesthetic/Vasoconstrictor Precautions Voriconazole is one of the drugs confirmed to prolong the QT interval and is accepted as having a risk of causing torsade de pointes. The risk of drug-induced torsade de pointes is extremely low when a single QT interval prolonging drug is prescribed. In terms of epinephrine, it is not known what effect vasoconstrictors in the local anesthetic regimen will have in patients with a known history of congenital prolonged QT interval or in patients taking any medication that prolongs the QT interval. Until more information is obtained, it is suggested that the clinician consult with the physician prior to the use of a vasoconstrictor in suspected patients, and that the vasoconstrictor (epinephrine, levonordefrin [Neo-Cobefrin®]) be used with caution.

Effects on Dental Treatment Key adverse event(s) related to dental treatment: Xerostomia (normal salivary flow resumes upon discontinuation).

Common Adverse Effects
>10%: Ocular: Visual changes (dose dependent — photophobia, color changes, increased or decreased visual acuity, or blurred vision occur in ~21%)

2% to 10%:
Cardiovascular: Tachycardia (up to 2%), hyper-/hypotension (2%), vasodilation (2%)

Central nervous system: Fever (up to 6%), chills (up to 4%), headache (up to 3%), hallucinations (up to 3%)

Dermatologic: Rash (up to 7%)

Endocrine & metabolic: Hypokalemia (up to 2%)

Gastrointestinal: Nausea (1% to 5%), vomiting (1% to 4%), abdominal pain (2%)

Hepatic: Alkaline phosphatase increased (4% to 5%), AST increased (2% to 4%), ALT increased (2% to 3%), cholestatic jaundice (1% to 2%)

Ocular: Photophobia (2% to 3%)

Dosage
Usual dosage ranges:
Children <12 years: Dosage not established
Children ≥12 years and Adults:
Oral: 100-300 mg every 12 hours
I.V.: 6 mg/kg every 12 hours for 2 doses; followed by maintenance dose of 4 mg/kg every 12 hours

Indication-specific dosing: Children ≥12 years and Adults:

Aspergillosis (invasive), scedosporiosis, fusariosis: I.V.: Initial: Loading dose: 6 mg/kg every 12 hours for 2 doses; followed by maintenance dose of 4 mg/kg every 12 hours

Candidemia and other deep tissue *Candida* infections: I.V.: Initial: Loading dose 6 mg/kg every 12 hours for 2 doses; followed by maintenance dose of 3-4 mg/kg every 12 hours

Endophthalmitis, fungal: I.V.: 6 mg/kg every 12 hours for 2 doses, then 200 mg orally twice daily

Esophageal candidiasis: Oral:

Patients <40 kg: 100 mg every 12 hours; maximum: 300 mg/day

Patients ≥40 kg: 200 mg every 12 hours; maximum: 600 mg/day

Note: Treatment should continue for a minimum of 14 days, and for at least 7 days following resolution of symptoms.

Conversion to oral dosing:

Patients <40 kg: 100 mg every 12 hours; increase to 150 mg every 12 hours in patients who fail to respond adequately

Patients ≥40 kg: 200 mg every 12 hours; increase to 300 mg every 12 hours in patients who fail to respond adequately

Dosage adjustment in patients unable to tolerate treatment:

I.V.: Dose may be reduced to 3 mg/kg every 12 hours

Oral: Dose may be reduced in 50 mg increments to a minimum dosage of 200 mg every 12 hours in patients weighing ≥40 kg (100 mg every 12 hours in patients <40 kg)

Dosage adjustment in patients receiving concomitant CYP450 enzyme inducers or substrates:

Cyclosporine: Reduce cyclosporine dose by $1/2$ and monitor closely.

Efavirenz: Oral: Increase maintenance dose of voriconazole to 400 mg every 12 hours and reduce efavirenz dose to 300 mg once daily

Phenytoin:

I.V.: Increase maintenance dosage to 5 mg/kg every 12 hours

Oral: Increase dose to 400 mg every 12 hours in patients ≥40 kg (200 mg every 12 hours in patients <40 kg)

Dosage adjustment in renal impairment: In patients with Cl$_{cr}$ <50 mL/minute, accumulation of the intravenous vehicle (SBECD) occurs. After initial loading dose, oral voriconazole should be administered to these patients, unless an assessment of the benefit:risk to the patient justifies the use of I.V. voriconazole. Monitor serum creatinine and change to oral voriconazole therapy when possible.

Hemodialysis: Oral dosage adjustment not required; for I.V. dosing, see dosage adjustment in renal impairment

Dosage adjustment in hepatic impairment:

Mild-to-moderate hepatic dysfunction (Child-Pugh Class A and B): Following standard loading dose, reduce maintenance dosage by 50%

Severe hepatic impairment: Should only be used if benefit outweighs risk; monitor closely for toxicity

Mechanism of Action Interferes with fungal cytochrome P450 activity, decreasing ergosterol synthesis (principal sterol in fungal cell membrane) and inhibiting fungal cell membrane formation.

Contraindications Hypersensitivity to voriconazole or any component of the formulation (cross-reaction with other azole antifungal agents may occur but has not been established, use caution); coadministration of CYP3A4 substrates which may lead to QT$_c$ prolongation (cisapride, pimozide, or quinidine); coadministration with barbiturates (long acting), carbamazepine, efavirenz (with standard [eg, not adjusted] voriconazole and efavirenz doses), ergot alkaloids, rifampin, rifabutin, ritonavir (≥800 mg/day), and sirolimus; pregnancy (unless risk:benefit justifies use)

Warnings/Precautions Visual changes are commonly associated with treatment. Patients should be warned to avoid tasks which depend on vision, including operating machinery or driving. Changes are reversible on discontinuation following brief exposure/treatment regimens (≤28 days).

Serious hepatic reactions (including hepatitis, cholestasis, and fulminant hepatic failure) have occurred during treatment, primarily in patients with serious concomitant medical conditions. However, hepatotoxicity has occurred in patients with no identifiable risk factors. Use caution in patients with pre-existing hepatic impairment (dose adjustment required).

Voriconazole tablets contain lactose; avoid administration in hereditary galactose intolerance, Lapp lactase deficiency, or glucose-galactose malabsorption. Suspension contains sucrose; use caution with fructose intolerance, sucrose-isomaltase deficiency, or glucose-galactose malabsorption. Avoid/limit use of intravenous formulation in patients with renal impairment; intravenous formulation contains excipient sulfobutyl ether beta-cyclodextrin (SBECD), (Continued)

Voriconazole *(Continued)*

which may accumulate in renal insufficiency. Infusion-related reactions may occur with intravenous dosing. Consider discontinuation of infusion if reaction is severe.

Use caution in patients with an increased risk of arrhythmia (concurrent QT_c-prolonging drugs, hypokalemia, cardiomyopathy, or prior cardiotoxic therapy). Correct electrolyte abnormalities before initiating therapy. Use caution in patients receiving concurrent non-nucleoside reverse transcriptase inhibitors (efavirenz is contraindicated).

Safety and efficacy have not been established in children <12 years of age.

Drug Interactions

Cytochrome P450 Effect: Substrate of CYP2C9 (major), 2C19 (major), 3A4 (minor); **Inhibits** CYP2C9 (weak), 2C19 (weak), 3A4 (moderate)

Increased Effect/Toxicity: Voriconazole increases serum levels/effects of efavirenz, ergot alkaloids, pimozide, quinidine, rifabutin, and sirolimus; concurrent use is contraindicated (adjusted doses of efavirenz and voriconazole may be used together). Voriconazole increases serum levels/effects of benzodiazepines (metabolized by oxidation; eg, alprazolam, diazepam, triazolam, midazolam), buspirone, busulfan, calcium channel blockers (eg, felodipine, nifedipine, verapamil), cisapride, CYP2C9 substrates, CYP3A4 substrates, cyclosporine, HMG-CoA reductase inhibitors (except pravastatin and fluvastatin), methadone, omeprazole, phenytoin, tacrolimus, warfarin, and vinca alkaloids. Voriconazole may increase the levels of ethinyl estradiol and/or norethindrone; conversely, hormonal contraceptive agents may increase the levels/effects of voriconazole. Use with QT_c-prolonging agents may increase risk of malignant arrhythmia.

Decreased Effect: Barbiturates (phenobarbital, secobarbital), carbamazepine, efavirenz, rifampin, and ritonavir (≥800 mg/day) decrease serum levels/effects of voriconazole; concurrent use is contraindicated. Use caution with smaller doses (<800 mg/day) of ritonavir. CYP2C9 inducers, CYP2C19 inducers, and phenytoin decrease serum levels/effects of voriconazole.

Ethanol/Nutrition/Herb Interactions

Food: May decrease voriconazole absorption. Voriconazole should be taken 1 hour before or 1 hour after a meal.

Herb/Nutraceutical: St John's wort may decrease voriconazole levels.

Dietary Considerations Oral: Should be taken 1 hour before or 1 hour after a meal. Voriconazole tablets contain lactose; avoid administration in hereditary galactose intolerance, Lapp lactase deficiency, or glucose-galactose malabsorption. Suspension contains sucrose; use caution with fructose intolerance, sucrose-isomaltase deficiency, or glucose-galactose malabsorption.

Pharmacodynamics/Kinetics

Absorption: Well absorbed after oral administration; administration of crushed tablets is considered bioequivalent to whole tablets

Distribution: V_d: 4.6 L/kg

Protein binding: 58%

Metabolism: Hepatic, via CYP2C19 (major pathway) and CYP2C9 and CYP3A4 (less significant); saturable (may demonstrate nonlinearity)

Bioavailability: 96%

Half-life elimination: Variable, dose-dependent

Time to peak: Oral: 1-2 hours; 0.5 hours (crushed tablet)

Excretion: Urine (as inactive metabolites)

Pregnancy Risk Factor D

Dosage Forms

Injection, powder for reconstitution:
VFEND®: 200 mg

Powder for oral suspension:
VFEND®: 200 mg/5 mL

Tablet:
VFEND®: 50 mg, 200 mg

Vorinostat *(vor IN oh stat)*

U.S. Brand Names Zolinza™

Generic Available No

Index Terms NSC-701852; SAHA; Suberoylanilide Hydroxamic Acid

Pharmacologic Category Antineoplastic Agent, Histone Deacetylase Inhibitor

Use Treatment of relapsed or refractory cutaneous T-cell lymphoma (CTCL)

Local Anesthetic/Vasoconstrictor Precautions No information available to require special precautions

Effects on Dental Treatment Key adverse event(s) related to dental treatment: High incidence of xerostomia (normal salivary flow resumes upon discontinuation) and taste perversion.

Common Adverse Effects

>10%:

Cardiovascular: Peripheral edema (13%)

Central nervous system: Fatigue (52% to 73%), chills (16%), dizziness (15%), headache (12%), fever (11%)

Dermatologic: Alopecia (19%), pruritus (12%)

Endocrine & metabolic: Hyperglycemia (8% to 69%; grade 3: 5%), dehydration (16%)

Gastrointestinal: Diarrhea (49% to 52%), nausea (41% to 49%), taste perversion (28% to 46%), xerostomia (16% to 35%), weight loss (21% to 27%), anorexia (22% to 24%), vomiting (15% to 24%), appetite decreased (14% to 22%), constipation (15%)

Hematologic: Thrombocytopenia (26% to 54%; grades 3/4: 6% to 19%), anemia (2% to 14%; grades 3/4: 2% to 3%)

Neuromuscular & skeletal: Muscle spasm (20%)

Renal: Proteinuria (51%), creatinine increased (16% to 47%)

Respiratory: Dyspnea (34%), cough (11%), upper respiratory infection (11%)

1% to 10%:

Cardiovascular: QT_c prolongation (3% to 6%)

Dermatologic: Squamous cell carcinoma (4%)

Respiratory: Pulmonary embolism (5%)

Mechanism of Action Inhibition of histone deacetylase enzymes, HDAC1, HDAC2, HDAC3, and HDAC6, which catalyze acetyl group removal from protein lysine residues (including histones and transcription factors). Inhibition of histone deacetylase results in accumulation of acetyl groups, leading to alterations in chromatin structure and transcription factor activation causing termination of cell growth leading to cell death.

Drug Interactions

Increased Effect/Toxicity:

Concomitant QT_c prolonging agents may increase the risk of arrhythmia. Valproic acid may enhance thrombocytopenia or gastrointestinal bleeding. Vorinostat may enhance the anticoagulant effect of warfarin.

Pharmacodynamics/Kinetics

Protein binding: ~71%

Metabolism: Glucuronidated and hydrolyzed (followed by beta-oxidation) to inactive metabolites

Bioavailability: Fasting: ~43%

Half-life elimination: ~2 hours

Time to peak, plasma: With high-fat meal: ~4 hours

Excretion: Urine: 52% (<1% as unchanged drug, ~52% as inactive metabolites)

Pregnancy Risk Factor D

Dental Comment This drug is known to prolong the QT interval. The QT interval is measured as the time and distance between the Q point of the QRS complex and the end of the T wave in the ECG tracing. After adjustment for heart rate, the QT interval is defined as prolonged if it is more than 450 msec in men and 460 msec in women. A long QT syndrome was first described in the 1950s and 60s as a congenital syndrome involving QT interval prolongation and syncope and sudden death. Some of the congenital long QT syndromes were characterized by a peculiar electrocardiographic appearance of the QRS complex involving a premature atria beat followed by a pause, then a subsequent sinus beat showing marked QT prolongation and deformity. This type of cardiac arrhythmia was originally termed "torsade de pointes" (translated from the French as "twisting of the points").

Prolongation of the QT interval is thought to result from delayed ventricular repolarization. The repolarization process within the myocardial cell is due to the efflux of intracellular potassium. The channels associated with this current can be blocked by many drugs and predispose the electrical propagation cycle to torsade de pointes.

Vorinostat is one of the drugs confirmed to prolong the QT interval and is accepted as having a risk of causing torsade de pointes. The risk of drug-induced torsade de pointes is extremely low when a single QT interval prolonging drug is prescribed. In terms of epinephrine, it is not known what effect vasoconstrictors in the local anesthetic regimen will have in patients with a known history of congenital prolonged QT interval or in patients taking any medication that prolongs the QT interval. Until more information is obtained, it is suggested that the clinician consult with the physician prior to the use of a vasoconstrictor in suspected patients, and that the vasoconstrictor (epinephrine, levonordefrin [Neo-Cobefrin®]) be used with caution.

Warfarin (WAR far in)

Related Information
Cardiovascular Diseases *on page 1726*

U.S. Brand Names Coumadin®; Jantoven™

Canadian Brand Names Apo-Warfarin®; Coumadin®; Gen-Warfarin; Novo-Warfarin; Taro-Warfarin

Generic Available Yes: Tablet

Index Terms Warfarin Sodium

Pharmacologic Category Anticoagulant, Coumarin Derivative

Use Prophylaxis and treatment of venous thrombosis, pulmonary embolism, and thromboembolic disorders; atrial fibrillation with risk of embolism; adjunct in the prophylaxis of systemic embolism after myocardial infarction; reduce risk of recurrent myocardial infarction

Unlabeled/Investigational Use Prevention of recurrent transient ischemic attacks

Local Anesthetic/Vasoconstrictor Precautions No information available to require special precautions

Effects on Dental Treatment Key adverse event(s) related to dental treatment: Mouth ulcers and taste disturbance.

Signs of warfarin overdose may first appear as bleeding from gingival tissue; consultation with prescribing physician is advisable prior to surgery to determine temporary dose reduction or withdrawal of medication.

Common Adverse Effects Bleeding is the major adverse effect of warfarin. Hemorrhage may occur at virtually any site. Risk is dependent on multiple variables, including the intensity of anticoagulation and patient susceptibility.

Cardiovascular: Angina, edema, hemorrhagic shock, hypotension, pallor, syncope, vasculitis

Central nervous system: Asthenia, dizziness, fever, headache, lethargy, malaise, pain, stroke

Dermatologic: Alopecia, bullous eruptions, dermatitis, rash, pruritus, urticaria

Gastrointestinal: Abdominal cramps, abdominal pain, anorexia, diarrhea, flatulence, gastrointestinal bleeding, mouth ulcers, nausea, taste disturbance, vomiting

Genitourinary: Hematuria, priapism

Hematologic: Agranulocytosis, anemia, hemorrhage, leukopenia, retroperitoneal hematoma, unrecognized bleeding sites (eg, colon cancer) may be uncovered by anticoagulation

Hepatic: Hepatic injury, hepatitis, jaundice, transaminases increased

Neuromuscular & skeletal: Osteoporosis, paresthesia, weakness

Respiratory: Epistaxis, hemoptysis, pulmonary hemorrhage, tracheobronchial calcification

Miscellaneous: Hypersensitivity/allergic reactions

Skin necrosis/gangrene (<0.1%), due to paradoxical local thrombosis, is a known but rare risk of warfarin therapy. Its onset is usually within the first few days of therapy and is frequently localized to the limbs, breast, or penis. The risk of this effect is increased in patients with protein C or S deficiency.

"Purple toes syndrome," caused by cholesterol microembolization, also occurs rarely. Typically, this occurs after several weeks of therapy, and may present as a dark, purplish, mottled discoloration of the plantar and lateral surfaces. Other manifestations of cholesterol microembolization may include rash; livedo reticularis; gangrene; abrupt and intense pain in lower extremities; abdominal, flank, or back pain; hematuria, renal insufficiency; hypertension; cerebral ischemia; spinal cord infarction; or other symptoms of vascular compromise.

Restrictions An FDA-approved medication guide must be distributed when dispensing an outpatient prescription (new or refill) where this medication is to be used without direct supervision of a healthcare provider. Medication guides are available at http://www.fda.gov/cder/Offices/ODS/medication_guides.htm.

Dosage

Oral:

Infants and Children (unlabeled use): Initial loading dose (if baseline INR is 1.0-1.3): 0.2 mg/kg (maximum: 10 mg/dose); adjust dose based on INR (reported ranges to maintain INR of 2-3: 0.09-0.33 mg/kg/day). Infants <12 months of age may require doses at or near the high end of this range; consistent anticoagulation may be difficult to maintain in children <5 years of age.

Adults: Initial dosing must be individualized. Consider the patient (hepatic function, cardiac function, age, nutritional status, concurrent therapy, risk of bleeding) in addition to prior dose response (if available) and the clinical situation. Start 5-10 mg daily for 2 days. Adjust dose according to INR results; usual maintenance dose ranges from 2-10 mg daily (individual patients may require loading and maintenance doses outside these general guidelines).

Note: Lower starting doses may be required for patients with hepatic impairment, poor nutrition, CHF, elderly, high risk of bleeding, or patients who are debilitated. Higher initial doses may be reasonable in selected patients (ie, receiving enzyme-inducing agents and with low risk of bleeding).

I.V.: Adults: 2-5 mg/day administered as a slow bolus injection

Dosing adjustment in renal disease: No adjustment required, however, patients with renal failure have an increased risk of bleeding complications. Monitor closely.

Dosing adjustment in hepatic disease: Monitor effect at usual doses; the response to oral anticoagulants may be markedly enhanced in obstructive jaundice (due to reduced vitamin K absorption) and also in hepatitis and cirrhosis (due to decreased production of vitamin K-dependent clotting factors); INR should be closely monitored

Mechanism of Action Interferes with hepatic synthesis of vitamin K-dependent coagulation factors (II, VII, IX, X)

Contraindications Hypersensitivity to warfarin or any component of the formulation; hemorrhagic tendencies; hemophilia; thrombocytopenia purpura; leukemia; recent or potential surgery of the eye or CNS; major regional lumbar block anesthesia or surgery resulting in large, open surfaces; patients bleeding from the GI, respiratory, or GU tract; threatened abortion; aneurysm; ascorbic acid deficiency; history of bleeding diathesis; prostatectomy; continuous tube drainage of the small intestine; polyarthritis; diverticulitis; emaciation; malnutrition; cerebrovascular hemorrhage; eclampsia/pre-eclampsia; blood dyscrasias; severe uncontrolled or malignant hypertension; severe hepatic disease; pericarditis or pericardial effusion; subacute bacterial endocarditis; visceral carcinoma; following spinal puncture and other diagnostic or therapeutic procedures with potential for significant bleeding; history of warfarin-induced necrosis; an unreliable, noncompliant patient; alcoholism; patient who has a history of falls or is a significant fall risk; unsupervised senile or psychotic patient; pregnancy

Warnings/Precautions Use care in the selection of patients appropriate for this treatment. Ensure patient cooperation especially from the alcoholic, illicit drug user, demented, or psychotic patient. Use with caution in trauma, acute infection, moderate-severe renal insufficiency, prolonged dietary insufficiencies, moderate-severe hypertension, polycythemia vera, vasculitis, open wound, active TB, history of PUD, anaphylactic disorders, indwelling catheters, severe diabetes, thyroid disease, and menstruating and postpartum women. Use with caution in protein C deficiency. Use with caution in patients with heparin-induced thrombocytopenia and DVT. Warfarin monotherapy is contraindicated in the initial treatment of active HIT.

[U.S. Boxed Warning]: May cause major or fatal bleeding. Risk factors for bleeding include high intensity anticoagulation, age, variable INRs, history of GI bleeding, hypertension, cerebrovascular disease, serious heart disease, anemia, malignancy, trauma, renal insufficiency, drug-drug interactions, and long duration of therapy. Patient must be instructed to report bleeding, accidents, or falls. Patient must also report any new or discontinued medications, herbal or alternative products used, or significant changes in smoking or dietary habits. Necrosis or gangrene of the skin and other tissue can occur. "Purple toes syndrome" may rarely occur. Women may be at risk of developing ovarian hemorrhage at the time of ovulation. The elderly may be more sensitive to anticoagulant therapy. Safety and efficacy have not been established in children; monitor closely.
(Continued)

Warfarin *(Continued)*

Drug Interactions

Cytochrome P450 Effect: Substrate of CYP1A2 (minor), 2C9 (major), 2C19 (minor), 3A4 (minor); **Inhibits** CYP2C9 (moderate), 2C19 (weak)

Increased Effect/Toxicity: Serum levels/effects of warfarin may be increased by acetaminophen (>1.3 g for >1 week), allopurinol, amiodarone, androgens, other anticoagulants, antifungal agents (imidazole), antiplatelet agents, capecitabine, cephalosporins, cimetidine, CYP2C9 inhibitors, disulfiram, drotrecogin alfa, etoposide, fibric acid derivatives, fluconazole, fluorouracil, gefitinib, glucagon, HMG-CoA reductase inhibitors, ifosfamide, leflunomide, macrolide antibiotics, mefloquine, metronidazole, NSAIDs (COX-2 inhibitors and nonselective), omega-3-acids, orlistat, phenytoin, propafenone, propoxyphene, proton pump inhibitors (omeprazole), quinidine, quinolone antibiotics, ropinirole, salicylates, SSRIs, sulfinpyrazone, sulfonamide derivatives, tetracycline derivatives, thyroid products, tigecycline, tolterodine, treprostinil, tricyclic antidepressants, vitamin A, vitamin E, voriconazole, zafirlukast, and zileuton.

Decreased Effect: Serum levels/effects of warfarin may be decreased by aminoglutethimide, antithyroid agents, aprepitant, azathioprine, barbiturates, bile acid sequestrants, bosentan, carbamazepine, CYP2C9 inducers, dicloxacillin, griseofulvin, hormonal contraceptives (estrogens and progestins), mercaptopurine, mitotane, nafcillin, phytonadione, rifamycin derivatives, and sulfasalazine.

Ethanol/Nutrition/Herb Interactions

Ethanol: Avoid ethanol. Acute ethanol ingestion (binge drinking) decreases the metabolism of warfarin and increases PT/INR. Chronic daily ethanol use increases the metabolism of warfarin and decreases PT/INR.

Food: The anticoagulant effects of warfarin may be decreased if taken with foods rich in vitamin K. Vitamin E may increase warfarin effect. Cranberry juice may increase warfarin effect.

Herb/Nutraceutical: Cranberry, fenugreek, ginkgo biloba, glucosamine, may enhance bleeding or increase warfarin's effect. Ginseng (American), coenzyme Q$_{10}$, and St John's wort may decrease warfarin levels and effects. Avoid alfalfa, anise, bilberry, bladderwrack, bromelain, cat's claw, celery, coleus, cordyceps, dong quai, evening primrose oil, fenugreek, feverfew, garlic, ginger, ginkgo biloba, ginseng (American), ginseng (Panax), ginseng (Siberian), grapeseed, green tea, guggul, horse chestnut seed, horseradish, licorice, omega-3-acids, prickly ash, red clover, reishi, same (s-adenosylmethionine), sweet clover, turmeric, and white willow (all have additional antiplatelet activity).

Dietary Considerations Foods high in vitamin K (eg, beef liver, pork liver, green tea, and leafy green vegetables) inhibit anticoagulant effect. Do not change dietary habits once stabilized on warfarin therapy. A balanced diet with a consistent intake of vitamin K is essential. Avoid large amounts of alfalfa, asparagus, broccoli, Brussels sprouts, cabbage, cauliflower, green teas, kale, lettuce, spinach, turnip greens, and watercress; decreased efficacy of warfarin. It is recommended that the diet contain a CONSISTENT vitamin K content of 70-140 mcg/day. Check with healthcare provider before changing diet.

Pharmacodynamics/Kinetics

Onset of action: Anticoagulation: Oral: 36-72 hours

Peak effect: Full therapeutic effect: 5-7 days; INR may increase in 36-72 hours

Duration: 2-5 days

Absorption: Oral: Rapid, complete

Distribution: 0.14 L/kg

Protein binding: 99%

Metabolism: Hepatic, primarily via CYP2C9; minor pathways include CYP2C19, 1A2, and 3A4

Half-life elimination: 20-60 hours; Mean: 40 hours; highly variable among individuals

Pregnancy Risk Factor X

Dosage Forms

Injection, powder for reconstitution:

Coumadin®: 5 mg

Tablet: 1 mg, 2 mg, 2.5 mg, 3 mg, 4 mg, 5 mg, 6 mg, 7.5 mg, 10 mg

Coumadin®, Jantoven™: 1 mg, 2 mg, 2.5 mg, 3 mg, 4 mg, 5 mg, 6 mg, 7.5 mg, 10 mg

Selected Readings

Jeske AH, Suchko GD, ADA Council on Scientific Affairs and Division of Science, et al, "Lack of a Scientific Basis for Routine Discontinuation of Oral Anticoagulation Therapy Before Dental Treatment," *J Am Dent Assoc*, 2003, 134(11):1492-7.

Little JW, Miller CS, Henry RG, et al, "Antithrombotic Agents: Implications in Dentistry," *Oral Surg Oral Med Oral Pathol Oral Radiol Endod*, 2002, 93(5):544-51.

Scully C and Wolff A, "Oral Surgery in Patients on Anticoagulant Therapy," *Oral Surg Oral Med Oral Pathol Oral Radiol Endod*, 2002, 94(1):57-64.

Warfarin Sodium *see* Warfarin *on page 1670*
Wart-Off® Maximum Strength [OTC] *see* Salicylic Acid *on page 1451*
4-Way® 12 Hour [OTC] *see* Oxymetazoline *on page 1236*
4 Way® Fast Acting [OTC] *see* Phenylephrine *on page 1293*
4 Way® Menthol [OTC] *see* Phenylephrine *on page 1293*
4 Way® No Drip [OTC] *see* Phenylephrine *on page 1293*
4-Way® Saline Moisturizing Mist [OTC] *see* Sodium Chloride *on page 1480*
WelChol® *see* Colesevelam *on page 408*
Wellbutrin® *see* BuPROPion *on page 241*
Wellbutrin XL™ *see* BuPROPion *on page 241*
Wellbutrin SR® *see* BuPROPion *on page 241*
Westcort® *see* Hydrocortisone *on page 836*
Westhroid® *see* Thyroid *on page 1562*
WinRho® SDF *see* Rh$_o$(D) Immune Globulin *on page 1418*
Winstrol® *see* Stanozolol *on page 1494*
Wound Wash Saline™ [OTC] *see* Sodium Chloride *on page 1480*
WR-2721 *see* Amifostine *on page 85*
WR-139007 *see* Dacarbazine *on page 435*
WR-139013 *see* Chlorambucil *on page 329*
WR-139021 *see* Carmustine *on page 288*
Wycillin [DSC] *see* Penicillin G Procaine *on page 1270*
Xalatan® *see* Latanoprost *on page 952*
Xanax® *see* Alprazolam *on page 75*
Xanax XR® *see* Alprazolam *on page 75*
Xeloda® *see* Capecitabine *on page 267*
Xenaderm™ *see* Trypsin, Balsam Peru, and Castor Oil *on page 1628*
Xenical® *see* Orlistat *on page 1211*
Xibrom™ *see* Bromfenac *on page 228*
Xifaxan™ *see* Rifaximin *on page 1426*
Xigris® *see* Drotrecogin Alfa *on page 548*
Xodol® *see* Hydrocodone and Acetaminophen *on page 822*
Xodol® 5/300 *see* Hydrocodone and Acetaminophen *on page 822*
Xolair® *see* Omalizumab *on page 1205*
Xolegel™ *see* Ketoconazole *on page 928*
Xopenex® *see* Levalbuterol *on page 959*
Xopenex HFA™ *see* Levalbuterol *on page 959*
XPECT™ [OTC] *see* Guaifenesin *on page 795*
Xpect-HC™ *see* Hydrocodone and Guaifenesin *on page 828*
XPECT-PE™ *see* Guaifenesin and Phenylephrine *on page 797*
X-Seb T® Pearl [OTC] *see* Coal Tar and Salicylic Acid *on page 402*
X-Seb T® Plus [OTC] *see* Coal Tar and Salicylic Acid *on page 402*
Xtramins [OTC] *see* Vitamins (Multiple/Oral) *on page 1665*
Xylocaine® *see* Lidocaine *on page 972*
Xylocaine® MPF *see* Lidocaine *on page 972*
Xylocaine® MPF With Epinephrine *see* Lidocaine and Epinephrine *on page 977*
Xylocaine® Viscous *see* Lidocaine *on page 972*
Xylocaine® With Epinephrine *see* Lidocaine and Epinephrine *on page 977*

Xylometazoline (zye loe met AZ oh leen)

U.S. Brand Names Otrivin® [OTC] [DSC]; Otrivin® Pediatric [OTC] [DSC]
Canadian Brand Names Balminil
Generic Available No
Index Terms Xylometazoline Hydrochloride
Pharmacologic Category Imidazoline Derivative; Vasoconstrictor, Nasal
Use Symptomatic relief of nasal and nasopharyngeal mucosal congestion
Local Anesthetic/Vasoconstrictor Precautions No information available to require special precautions
Effects on Dental Treatment No significant effects or complications reported
Common Adverse Effects Frequency not defined.
  Cardiovascular: Palpitation
  Central nervous system: Dizziness, drowsiness, headache, seizure
  Ocular: Blurred vision, ocular irritation, photophobia
  Miscellaneous: Diaphoresis
  (Continued)

Xylometazoline (Continued)

Mechanism of Action Stimulates alpha-adrenergic receptors in the arterioles of the conjunctiva and the nasal mucosa to produce vasoconstriction

Pharmacodynamics/Kinetics

Onset of action: Intranasal: Local vasoconstriction: 5-10 minutes

Duration: 5-6 hours

Pregnancy Risk Factor C

Yohimbine (yo HIM bine)

Related Information

Yohimbe *on page 1724*

U.S. Brand Names Aphrodyne®; Yocon®

Canadian Brand Names PMS-Yohimbine; Yocon®

Generic Available Yes

Index Terms Yohimbine Hydrochloride

Pharmacologic Category Miscellaneous Product

Unlabeled/Investigational Use Treatment of SSRI-induced sexual dysfunction; weight loss; impotence; sympathicolytic and mydriatic; may have activity as an aphrodisiac

Local Anesthetic/Vasoconstrictor Precautions No information available to require special precautions

Effects on Dental Treatment No significant effects or complications reported

Common Adverse Effects Frequency not defined.

Cardiovascular: Tachycardia, hypertension, hypotension (orthostatic), flushing

Central nervous system: Anxiety, mania, hallucinations, irritability, dizziness, psychosis, insomnia, headache, panic attacks

Gastrointestinal: Nausea, vomiting, anorexia, salivation

Neuromuscular & skeletal: Tremors

Miscellaneous: Antidiuretic action, diaphoresis

Mechanism of Action Derived from the bark of the yohimbe tree (*Corynanthe yohimbe*), this indole alkaloid produces a presynaptic alpha$_2$-adrenergic blockade. Peripheral autonomic effect is to increase cholinergic and decrease adrenergic activity; yohimbine exerts a stimulating effect on the mood and a mild antidiuretic effect.

Drug Interactions

Cytochrome P450 Effect: **Substrate** of CYP2D6 (minor); **Inhibits** CYP2D6 (weak)

Increased Effect/Toxicity: Caution with other CNS acting drugs. When used in combination with CYP3A4 inhibitors, serum level and/or toxicity of yohimbine may be increased. Inhibitors include amiodarone, cimetidine, clarithromycin, erythromycin, delavirdine, diltiazem, dirithromycin, disulfiram, fluoxetine, fluvoxamine, grapefruit juice, indinavir, itraconazole, ketoconazole, metronidazole, nefazodone, nevirapine, propoxyphene, quinupristin-dalfopristin, ritonavir, saquinavir, verapamil, zafirlukast, and zileuton; monitor for altered response. MAO inhibitors or drugs with MAO inhibition (linezolid, furazolidone) theoretically may increase toxicity or adverse effects.

Pharmacodynamics/Kinetics

Duration of action: Usually 3-4 hours, but may last 36 hours

Absorption: 33%

Distribution: V_d: 0.3-3 L/kg

Half-life elimination: 0.6 hour

Zafirlukast (za FIR loo kast)

Related Information
Respiratory Diseases *on page 1747*
U.S. Brand Names Accolate®
Canadian Brand Names Accolate®
Mexican Brand Names Accolate
Generic Available No
Index Terms ICI-204,219
Pharmacologic Category Leukotriene-Receptor Antagonist
Use Prophylaxis and chronic treatment of asthma in adults and children ≥5 years of age
Local Anesthetic/Vasoconstrictor Precautions No information available to require special precautions
Effects on Dental Treatment No significant effects or complications reported
Common Adverse Effects
>10%: Central nervous system: Headache (13%)
1% to 10%:
Central nervous system: Dizziness (2%), pain (2%), fever (2%)
Gastrointestinal: Nausea (3%), diarrhea (3%), abdominal pain (2%), vomiting (2%), dyspepsia (1%)
Hepatic: ALT increased (2%)
Neuromuscular & skeletal: Back pain (2%), myalgia (2%), weakness (2%)
Miscellaneous: Infection (4%)
Mechanism of Action Zafirlukast is a selectively and competitive leukotriene-receptor antagonist (LTRA) of leukotriene D4 and E4 (LTD4 and LTE4), components of slow-reacting substance of anaphylaxis (SRSA). Cysteinyl leukotriene production and receptor occupation have been correlated with the pathophysiology of asthma, including airway edema, smooth muscle constriction, and altered cellular activity associated with the inflammatory process, which contribute to the signs and symptoms of asthma.
Drug Interactions
Cytochrome P450 Effect: Substrate of CYP2C9 (major); **Inhibits** CYP1A2 (weak), 2C8 (weak), 2C9 (moderate), 2C19 (weak), 2D6 (weak), 3A4 (weak)
Increased Effect/Toxicity: Zafirlukast concentrations are increased by aspirin. Zafirlukast may increase theophylline levels. Zafirlukast may increase the levels/effects of bosentan, dapsone, fluoxetine, glimepiride, glipizide, losartan, montelukast, nateglinide, paclitaxel, phenytoin, warfarin, zafirlukast, and other CYP2C9 substrates.
Decreased Effect: The levels/effects of zafirlukast may be decreased by carbamazepine, phenobarbital, phenytoin, rifampin, rifapentine, secobarbital, and other CYP2C9 inducers. Zafirlukast concentrations may be reduced by erythromycin.
Pharmacodynamics/Kinetics
Protein binding: >99%, primarily to albumin
Metabolism: Extensively hepatic via CYP2C9
Bioavailability: Reduced 40% with food
Half-life elimination: 10 hours
Time to peak, serum: 3 hours
Excretion: Urine (10%); feces
Pregnancy Risk Factor B

Zalcitabine (zal SITE a been)

Related Information
HIV Infection and AIDS *on page 1753*
U.S. Brand Names Hivid® [DSC]
Canadian Brand Names Hivid®
Mexican Brand Names Hivid
Generic Available No
Index Terms ddC; Dideoxycytidine
Pharmacologic Category Antiretroviral Agent, Reverse Transcriptase Inhibitor (Nucleoside)
Use In combination with at least two other antiretrovirals in the treatment of patients with HIV infection; it is not recommended that zalcitabine be given in combination with didanosine, stavudine, or lamivudine due to overlapping toxicities, virologic interactions, or lack of clinical data
Local Anesthetic/Vasoconstrictor Precautions No information available to require special precautions
(Continued)

Zalcitabine *(Continued)*

Effects on Dental Treatment Key adverse event(s) related to dental treatment: Oral ulcerations and dysphagia.

Common Adverse Effects

>10%:

Central nervous system: Fever (5% to 17%), malaise (2% to 13%)

Neuromuscular & skeletal: Peripheral neuropathy (28%)

1% to 10%:

Central nervous system: Headache (2%), dizziness (1%), fatigue (4%), seizure (1.3%)

Dermatologic: Rash (2% to 11%), pruritus (3% to 5%)

Endocrine & metabolic: Hypoglycemia (2% to 6%), hyponatremia (4%), hyperglycemia (1% to 6%)

Gastrointestinal: Nausea (3%), dysphagia (1% to 4%), anorexia (4%), abdominal pain (3% to 8%), vomiting (1% to 3%), diarrhea (<1% to 10%), weight loss, oral ulcers (3% to 7%), amylase increased (3% to 8%)

Hematologic: Anemia (occurs as early as 2-4 weeks), granulocytopenia (usually after 6-8 weeks)

Hepatic: Abnormal hepatic function (9%), hyperbilirubinemia (2% to 5%)

Neuromuscular & skeletal: Myalgia (1% to 6%), foot pain

Respiratory: Pharyngitis (2%), cough (6%), nasal discharge (4%)

Mechanism of Action Purine nucleoside (cytosine) analog, zalcitabine or 2′,3′-dideoxycytidine (ddC) is converted to active metabolite ddCTP; lack the presence of the 3′-hydroxyl group necessary for phosphodiester linkages during DNA replication. As a result, viral replication is prematurely terminated. ddCTP acts as a competitor for binding sites on the HIV-RNA dependent DNA polymerase (reverse transcriptase) to further contribute to inhibition of viral replication.

Drug Interactions

Increased Effect/Toxicity: Amphotericin, foscarnet, and aminoglycosides may potentiate the risk of developing peripheral neuropathy or other toxicities associated with zalcitabine by interfering with the renal elimination of zalcitabine. Other drugs associated with peripheral neuropathy include chloramphenicol, cisplatin, dapsone, disulfiram, ethionamide, gold, hydralazine, iodoquinol, isoniazid, metronidazole, nitrofurantoin, phenytoin, ribavirin, and vincristine. Concomitant use with zalcitabine may increase risk of peripheral neuropathy. Concomitant use of zalcitabine with didanosine is not recommended. Concomitant use of ribavirin with or without interferon alfa and nucleoside analogues may increase the risk of developing hepatic decompensation or other signs of mitochondrial toxicity, including pancreatitis or lactic acidosis.

Decreased Effect: It is not recommended that zalcitabine be given in combination with didanosine, stavudine, or lamivudine due to overlapping toxicities, virologic interactions, and lack of clinical data. Doxorubicin and lamivudine have been shown *in vitro* to decrease zalcitabine phosphorylation. Magnesium-/aluminum-containing antacids and metoclopramide may decrease the absorption of zalcitabine.

Pharmacodynamics/Kinetics

Absorption: Well, but variable; decreased 39% with food

Distribution: Minimal data available; variable CSF penetration

Protein binding: <4%

Metabolism: Intracellularly to active triphosphorylated agent

Bioavailability: >80%

Half-life elimination: 2.9 hours; Renal impairment: ≤8.5 hours

Excretion: Urine (>70% as unchanged drug)

Pregnancy Risk Factor C

Zaleplon *(ZAL e plon)*

U.S. Brand Names Sonata®

Canadian Brand Names Sonata®; Starnoc®

Mexican Brand Names Sonata

Generic Available No

Pharmacologic Category Hypnotic, Nonbenzodiazepine

Dental Use Has not be established

Use Short-term (7-10 days) treatment of insomnia (has been demonstrated to be effective for up to 5 weeks in controlled trial)

Local Anesthetic/Vasoconstrictor Precautions No information available to require special precautions

Effects on Dental Treatment Key adverse event(s) related to dental treatment: Xerostomia (normal salivary flow resumes upon discontinuation).

Common Adverse Effects

1% to 10%:

Cardiovascular: Chest pain, peripheral edema

Central nervous system: Amnesia, anxiety, coordination impaired, depersonalization, depression, dizziness, fever, hallucination, hypoesthesia, lightheadedness, malaise, migraine, somnolence, vertigo

Dermatologic: Photosensitivity reaction, pruritus, rash

Gastrointestinal: Abdominal pain, anorexia, colitis, constipation, dyspepsia, nausea, xerostomia

Genitourinary: Dysmenorrhea

Neuromuscular & skeletal: Arthralgia, back pain, myalgia, paresthesia, tremor, weakness

Ocular: Abnormal vision, eye pain

Otic: Hyperacusis

Miscellaneous: Parosmia

Restrictions C-IV

Mechanism of Action Zaleplon is unrelated to benzodiazepines, barbiturates, or other hypnotics. However, it interacts with the benzodiazepine GABA receptor complex. Nonclinical studies have shown that it binds selectively to the brain omega-1 receptor situated on the alpha subunit of the GABA-A receptor complex.

Drug Interactions

Cytochrome P450 Effect: Substrate of CYP3A4 (minor)

Increased Effect/Toxicity: Zaleplon potentiates the CNS effects of CNS depressants, including anticonvulsants, antipsychotics, barbiturates, benzodiazepines, opioid agonists, and other sedative agents. Cimetidine increases concentrations of zaleplon; Use or use 5 mg zaleplon as starting dose in patient receiving cimetidine.

Decreased Effect:

Flumazenil and rifamycin derivatives may decrease the effect of zaleplon.

Pharmacodynamics/Kinetics

Onset of action: Rapid

Peak effect: ~1 hour

Duration: 6-8 hours

Absorption: Rapid and almost complete

Distribution: V_d: 1.4 L/kg

Protein binding: 60% ± 15%

Metabolism: Extensive, primarily via aldehyde oxidase to form 5-oxo-zaleplon and, to a lesser extent, by CYP3A4 to desethylzaleplon; all metabolites are pharmacologically inactive

Bioavailability: 30%

Half-life elimination: 1 hour

Time to peak, serum: 1 hour

Excretion: Urine (primarily metabolites, <1% as unchanged drug)

Clearance: Plasma: Oral: 3 L/hour/kg

Pregnancy Risk Factor C

Zanaflex® see Tizanidine on page 1577

Zanamivir (za NA mi veer)

Related Information

Systemic Viral Diseases on page 1767

U.S. Brand Names Relenza®

Canadian Brand Names Relenza®

Mexican Brand Names Relenza

Generic Available No

Pharmacologic Category Antiviral Agent; Neuraminidase Inhibitor

Use Treatment of uncomplicated acute illness due to influenza virus A and B in patients who have been symptomatic for no more than 2 days; prophylaxis against influenza virus A and B

Local Anesthetic/Vasoconstrictor Precautions No information available to require special precautions

Effects on Dental Treatment No significant effects or complications reported

Common Adverse Effects Most adverse reactions occurred at a frequency which was less than or equal to the control (lactose vehicle).

>10%:

Central nervous system: Headache (prophylaxis 13% to 24%; treatment 2%)

Gastrointestinal: Throat/tonsil discomfort/pain (prophylaxis 8% to 19%)

Respiratory: Cough (prophylaxis 7% to 17%; treatment ≤2%), nasal signs and symptoms (prophylaxis 12%; treatment 2%)

Miscellaneous: Viral infection (prophylaxis 3% to 13%)

(Continued)

Zanamivir *(Continued)*

1% to 10%:

Central nervous system: Fever/chills (prophylaxis 5% to 9%; treatment <1.5%), fatigue (prophylaxis 5% to 8%; treatment <1.5%), malaise (prophylaxis 5% to 8%; treatment <1.5%), dizziness (treatment 1% to 2%)

Dermatologic: Urticaria (treatment <1.5%)

Gastrointestinal: Anorexia/appetite decreased (prophylaxis 2% to 4%), nausea (prophylaxis 1% to 2%; treatment ≤3%), diarrhea (prophylaxis 2%; treatment 2% to 3%), vomiting (prophylaxis 1% to 2%; treatment 1% to 2%), abdominal pain (treatment <1.5%)

Neuromuscular & skeletal: Muscle pain (prophylaxis 3% to 8%), musculoskeletal pain (prophylaxis 6%), arthralgia/articular rheumatism (prophylaxis 2%), arthralgia (treatment <1.5%), myalgia (treatment <1.5%)

Respiratory: Infection (ear/nose/throat; prophylaxis 2%; treatment 2% to 5%), sinusitis (treatment 3%), bronchitis (treatment 2%), nasal inflammation (prophylaxis 1%)

Mechanism of Action Zanamivir inhibits influenza virus neuraminidase enzymes, potentially altering virus particle aggregation and release.

Drug Interactions

Decreased Effect: Zanamivir may diminish the therapeutic effect of live, attentuated influenza virus vaccine (FluMist™). The manufacturer of FluMist™ recommends that the administration of anti-influenza virus medications be avoided during the period beginning 48 hours prior to vaccine administration and ending 2 weeks after vaccine.

Pharmacodynamics/Kinetics

Absorption: Inhalation: 4% to 17%

Protein binding, plasma: <10%

Metabolism: None

Half-life elimination, serum: 2.5-5.1 hours

Excretion: Urine (as unchanged drug); feces (unabsorbed drug)

Pregnancy Risk Factor C

Zestril® *see* Lisinopril *on page 990*
Zetar® [OTC] *see* Coal Tar *on page 402*
Zetia™ *see* Ezetimibe *on page 665*
Zevalin® *see* Ibritumomab *on page 851*
Ziac® *see* Bisoprolol and Hydrochlorothiazide *on page 219*
Ziagen® *see* Abacavir *on page 22*
Ziana™ *see* Clindamycin and Tretinoin *on page 382*

Ziconotide (zi KOE no tide)

U.S. Brand Names Prialt®
Generic Available No
Pharmacologic Category Analgesic, Nonopioid; Calcium Channel Blocker, N-Type
Use Management of severe chronic pain in patients requiring intrathecal (I.T.) therapy and who are intolerant or refractory to other therapies
Local Anesthetic/Vasoconstrictor Precautions No information available to require special precautions
Effects on Dental Treatment Key adverse event(s) related to dental treatment: Xerostomia (normal salivary flow resumes upon discontinuation) and taste perversion.
Common Adverse Effects Percentages reported when using the slow (21-day) titration schedule; frequencies may be higher with faster titration.
>10%:
 Central nervous system: Dizziness (47%), somnolence (22%), confusion (18%), ataxia (16%), headache (15%), memory impairment (12%), pain (11%)
 Gastrointestinal: Nausea (41%), diarrhea (19%), vomiting (15%)
 Neuromuscular & skeletal: Weakness (22%), gait disturbances (15%), hypertonia (11%)
2% to 10%:
 Cardiovascular: Chest pain, edema, hyper-/hypotension, postural hypotension, tachycardia, vasodilation
 Central nervous system: Anxiety (9%), speech disorder (9%), aphasia (8%), dysesthesia (7%), fever (7%), hallucinations (7%), nervousness (7%), vertigo (7%), agitation, chills, depression, dreams abnormal, emotional lability, hostility, hyperesthesia, insomnia, malaise, meningitis, paranoid reaction, stupor
 Dermatologic: Bruising, cellulitis, dry skin, pruritus, rash
 Endocrine & metabolic: Hypokalemia
 Gastrointestinal: Anorexia (10%), abdominal pain, constipation, dehydration, dyspepsia, taste perversion, weight loss, xerostomia
 Genitourinary: Urinary retention (9%), dysuria, urinary incontinence, urinary tract infection, urination impaired
 Hematologic: Anemia
 Local: Catheter complication, catheter site pain, pump site complication, pump site mass, pump site pain
 Neuromuscular & skeletal: Paresthesia (7%), arthralgia, arthritis, back pain, incoordination, leg cramps, myalgia, myasthenia, neck pain, neck rigidity, neuralgia, reflexes decreased, tremor
 Ocular: Vision abnormal (10%), nystagmus (8%), diplopia, photophobia
 Otic: Tinnitus
 Respiratory: Bronchitis, cough, dyspnea, pharyngitis, pneumonia, rhinitis, sinusitis
 Miscellaneous: CSF abnormalities, diaphoresis, flu-like syndrome, infection
Mechanism of Action Ziconotide selectively binds to N-type voltage-sensitive calcium channels located on the afferent nerves of the dorsal horn in the spinal cord. This binding is thought to block N-type calcium channels, leading to a blockade of excitatory neurotransmitter release and reducing sensitivity to painful stimuli.
Drug Interactions
 Increased Effect/Toxicity: May enhance the adverse/toxic effects of other CNS depressants
Pharmacodynamics/Kinetics
 Distribution: I.T.: V_d: ~140 mL
 Protein binding: 50%
 Metabolism: Metabolized via endopeptidases and exopeptidases present on multiple organs including kidney, liver, lung; degraded to peptide fragments and free amino acids
 Half-life elimination: I.V.: 1-1.6 hours (plasma); I.T.: 2.9-6.5 hours (CSF)
 Excretion: I.V.: Urine (<1%)
Pregnancy Risk Factor C

Zidovudine (zye DOE vyoo deen)

Related Information
HIV Infection and AIDS *on page 1753*
Systemic Viral Diseases *on page 1767*
U.S. Brand Names Retrovir®
Canadian Brand Names Apo-Zidovudine®; AZT™; Retrovir®
Mexican Brand Names Pranadox; Retrovir-AZT
Generic Available Yes: Tablet
Index Terms Azidothymidine; AZT (error-prone abbreviation); Compound S; ZDV
Pharmacologic Category Antiretroviral Agent, Reverse Transcriptase Inhibitor (Nucleoside)
Use Treatment of HIV infection in combination with at least two other antiretroviral agents; prevention of maternal/fetal HIV transmission as monotherapy
Unlabeled/Investigational Use Postexposure prophylaxis for HIV exposure as part of a multidrug regimen
Local Anesthetic/Vasoconstrictor Precautions No information available to require special precautions
Effects on Dental Treatment Key adverse event(s) related to dental treatment: Taste perversion, oral mucosa pigmentation, dysphagia, and mouth ulcer.
Common Adverse Effects As reported in adult patients with asymptomatic HIV infection. Frequency and severity may increase with advanced disease.
>10%:
  Central nervous system: Headache (63%), malaise (53%)
  Gastrointestinal: Nausea (51%), anorexia (20%), vomiting (17%)
1% to 10%:
  Gastrointestinal: Constipation (6%)
  Hematologic: Granulocytopenia (2%; onset 6-8 weeks), anemia (1%; onset 2-4 weeks)
  Hepatic: Transaminases increased (1% to 3%)
  Neuromuscular & skeletal: Weakness (9%)

Frequency not defined:
  Cardiovascular: Cardiomyopathy, chest pain, syncope, vasculitis
  Central nervous system: Anxiety, chills, confusion, depression, dizziness, fatigue, insomnia, loss of mental acuity, mania, seizure, somnolence, vertigo
  Dermatologic: Pruritus, rash, skin/nail pigmentation changes, Stevens-Johnson syndrome, toxic epidermal necrolysis, urticaria
  Endocrine & metabolic: Body fat redistribution, gynecomastia
  Gastrointestinal: Abdominal cramps, abdominal pain, dyspepsia, dysphagia, flatulence, mouth ulcer, oral mucosa pigmentation, pancreatitis, taste perversion
  Genitourinary: Urinary frequency, urinary hesitancy
  Hematologic: Aplastic anemia, hemolytic anemia, leukopenia, lymphadenopathy, pancytopenia with marrow hypoplasia, pure red cell aplasia
  Hepatic: Hepatitis, hepatomegaly with steatosis, hyperbilirubinemia, jaundice, lactic acidosis
  Neuromuscular & skeletal: Arthralgia, back pain, CPK increased, LDH increased, musculoskeletal pain, myalgia, neuropathy, muscle spasm, myopathy, myositis, paresthesia, rhabdomyolysis, tremor
  Ocular: Amblyopia, macular edema, photophobia
  Otic: Hearing loss
  Respiratory: Cough, dyspnea, rhinitis, sinusitis
  Miscellaneous: Allergic reactions, anaphylaxis, angioedema, diaphoresis, flu-like syndrome, immune reconstitution syndrome
Mechanism of Action Zidovudine is a thymidine analog which interferes with the HIV viral RNA-dependent DNA polymerase resulting in inhibition of viral replication; nucleoside reverse transcriptase inhibitor
Drug Interactions
  Cytochrome P450 Effect: Substrate (minor) of CYP2A6, 2C9, 2C19, 3A4
  Increased Effect/Toxicity: Concomitant use with myelosuppressive or cytotoxic agents (eg, doxorubicin, dapsone, ganciclovir/valganciclovir, vincristine) may increase the risk of hematologic toxicity. Fluconazole, methadone, probenecid and valproic acid may increase the levels/effects of zidovudine; monitor.

  Zidovudine may increase the myelosuppressive effects of trimetrexate; concurrent use not recommended. Acyclovir/valacyclovir may increase the CNS-depressant effects of zidovudine. Concomitant use of ribavirin, with or without interferon alfa and nucleoside analogues, may increase the risk of developing hepatic decompensation or other signs of mitochondrial toxicity, including pancreatitis or lactic acidosis.

Decreased Effect: Based on *in vitro* data, doxorubicin and ribavirin may decrease the phosphorylation of zidovudine; similarly, zidovudine may reduce the phosphorylation of stavudine; avoid concurrent use of these pairs. Rifampin and nelfinavir may decrease levels/effects of zidovudine; monitor.

Pharmacodynamics/Kinetics

Distribution: Significant penetration into the CSF; crosses placenta

V_d: 1-2.2 L/kg

Relative diffusion from blood into CSF: Adequate with or without inflammation (exceeds usual MICs)

CSF:blood level ratio: Normal meninges: ~60%

Protein binding: 25% to 38%

Metabolism: Hepatic via glucuronidation to inactive metabolites; extensive first-pass effect

Bioavailability: 54% to 74%

Half-life elimination: Terminal: 0.5-3 hours

Time to peak, serum: 30-90 minutes

Excretion:

Oral: Urine (72% to 74% as metabolites, 14% to 18% as unchanged drug)

I.V.: Urine (45% to 60% as metabolites, 18% to 29% as unchanged drug)

Pregnancy Risk Factor C

Zidovudine, Abacavir, and Lamivudine *see* Abacavir, Lamivudine, and Zidovudine *on page 23*

Zidovudine and Lamivudine
(zye DOE vyoo deen & la MI vyoo deen)

Related Information

HIV Infection and AIDS *on page 1753*

Lamivudine *on page 944*

Zidovudine *on page 1680*

U.S. Brand Names Combivir®

Canadian Brand Names Combivir®

Generic Available No

Index Terms AZT + 3TC (error-prone abbreviation); Lamivudine and Zidovudine

Pharmacologic Category Antiretroviral Agent, Reverse Transcriptase Inhibitor (Nucleoside)

Use Treatment of HIV infection when therapy is warranted based on clinical and/ or immunological evidence of disease progression

Local Anesthetic/Vasoconstrictor Precautions No information available to require special precautions

Effects on Dental Treatment No significant effects or complications reported

Common Adverse Effects See individual agents.

Mechanism of Action The combination of zidovudine and lamivudine is believed to act synergistically to inhibit reverse transcriptase via DNA chain termination after incorporation of the nucleoside analogue as well as to delay the emergence of mutations conferring resistance

Drug Interactions

Cytochrome P450 Effect: Zidovudine: **Substrate** (minor) of CYP2A6, 2C9, 2C19, 3A4

Increased Effect/Toxicity: See individual agents.

Decreased Effect: See individual agents.

Pharmacodynamics/Kinetics See individual agents.

Pregnancy Risk Factor C

Zilactin-L® [OTC] *see* Lidocaine *on page 972*

Zilactin®-B [OTC] *see* Benzocaine *on page 195*

Zilactin Toothache and Gum Pain® [OTC] *see* Benzocaine *on page 195*

Zileuton (zye LOO ton)

Related Information

Respiratory Diseases *on page 1747*

U.S. Brand Names Zyflo®

Generic Available No

Pharmacologic Category 5-Lipoxygenase Inhibitor

Use Prophylaxis and chronic treatment of asthma in children ≥12 years of age and adults

Local Anesthetic/Vasoconstrictor Precautions No information available to require special precautions

(Continued)

Zileuton *(Continued)*

Effects on Dental Treatment No significant effects or complications reported

Common Adverse Effects

>10%: Central nervous system: Headache (25%)

1% to 10%:

Central nervous system: Pain (8%)

Gastrointestinal: Dyspepsia (8%), nausea (6%), abdominal pain (5%)

Hematologic: Leukopenia (1%)

Hepatic: ALT increased (2%)

Neuromuscular & skeletal: Asthenia (4%), myalgia (3%)

Frequency not defined:

Cardiovascular: Chest pain

Central nervous system: Dizziness, fever, insomnia, malaise, nervousness, somnolence

Dermatologic: Pruritus

Gastrointestinal: Constipation, flatulence, vomiting

Genitourinary: Urinary tract infection, vaginitis

Neuromuscular & skeletal: Arthralgia, hypertonia, neck pain/rigidity

Ocular: Conjunctivitis

Miscellaneous: Lymphadenopathy

Mechanism of Action Specific 5-lipoxygenase inhibitor which inhibits leukotriene formation. Leukotrienes augment neutrophil and eosinophil migration, neutrophil and monocyte aggregation, leukocyte adhesion, increased capillary permeability, and smooth muscle contraction (which contribute to inflammation, edema, mucous secretion, and bronchoconstriction in the airway of the asthmatic.)

Drug Interactions

Cytochrome P450 Effect: Substrate (minor) of CYP1A2, 2C9, 3A4; **Inhibits** CYP1A2 (moderate)

Increased Effect/Toxicity: Zileuton may increase the serum concentration/effects of theophylline, propranolol, and warfarin; monitor and reduce doses accordingly. Zileuton may increase the levels/effects of CYP1A2 substrates; example substrates include aminophylline, fluvoxamine, mexiletine, mirtazapine, ropinirole, and trifluoperazine.

Pharmacodynamics/Kinetics

Absorption: Rapid

Distribution: 1.2 L/kg

Protein binding: 93%

Metabolism: Several metabolites in plasma and urine; metabolized by CYP1A2, 2C9, and 3A4

Bioavailability: Unknown

Half-life elimination: 2.5 hours

Time to peak, serum: 1.7 hours

Excretion: Urine (~95% primarily as metabolites); feces (~2%)

Pregnancy Risk Factor C

Zinacef® *see* Cefuroxime *on page 310*

Zinc *see* Trace Metals *on page 1595*

Zincate® *see* Zinc Sulfate *on page 1683*

Zinc Chloride *(zink KLOR ide)*

Generic Available Yes

Pharmacologic Category Trace Element

Use Cofactor for replacement therapy to different enzymes; helps maintain normal growth rates, normal skin hydration, and senses of taste and smell

Local Anesthetic/Vasoconstrictor Precautions No information available to require special precautions

Effects on Dental Treatment No significant effects or complications reported

Pregnancy Risk Factor C

Zinc Diethylenetriaminepentaacetate (Zn-DTPA) *see* Diethylene Triamine Penta-Acetic Acid *on page 493*

Zinc Gelatin *(zink JEL ah tin)*

U.S. Brand Names Gelucast®

Generic Available Yes

Index Terms Dome Paste Bandage; Unna's Boot; Unna's Paste; Zinc Gelatin Boot

Pharmacologic Category Topical Skin Product
Use As a protectant and to support varicosities and similar lesions of the lower limbs
Local Anesthetic/Vasoconstrictor Precautions No information available to require special precautions
Effects on Dental Treatment No significant effects or complications reported
Common Adverse Effects 1% to 10%: Local: Irritation

Zinc Gelatin Boot see Zinc Gelatin on page 1682
Zincon® [OTC] see Pyrithione Zinc on page 1391

Zinc Oxide (zink OKS ide)

U.S. Brand Names Ammens® Medicated Deodorant [OTC]; Balmex® [OTC]; Boudreaux's® Butt Paste [OTC]; Critic-Aid Skin Care® [OTC]; Desitin® [OTC]; Desitin® Creamy [OTC]
Canadian Brand Names Zincofax®
Generic Available Yes: Ointment
Index Terms Base Ointment; Lassar's Zinc Paste
Pharmacologic Category Topical Skin Product
Use Protective coating for mild skin irritations and abrasions; soothing and protective ointment to promote healing of chapped skin, diaper rash
Local Anesthetic/Vasoconstrictor Precautions No information available to require special precautions
Effects on Dental Treatment No significant effects or complications reported
Common Adverse Effects 1% to 10%: Local: Skin sensitivity, irritation
Mechanism of Action Mild astringent with weak antiseptic properties

Zinc Oxide and Miconazole Nitrate see Miconazole and Zinc Oxide on page 1098

Zinc Sulfate (zink SUL fate)

U.S. Brand Names Orazinc® [OTC]; Zincate®
Canadian Brand Names Anuzinc; Rivasol
Generic Available Yes
Index Terms ZnSO$_4$ (error-prone abbreviation)
Pharmacologic Category Trace Element
Use Zinc supplement (oral and parenteral); may improve wound healing in those who are deficient
Local Anesthetic/Vasoconstrictor Precautions No information available to require special precautions
Effects on Dental Treatment No significant effects or complications reported
Pregnancy Risk Factor C

Zinc Sulfate and Phenylephrine see Phenylephrine and Zinc Sulfate on page 1294
Zinc Undecylenate see Undecylenic Acid and Derivatives on page 1631
Zinecard® see Dexrazoxane on page 472
Ziox™ [DSC] see Chlorophyllin, Papain, and Urea on page 335
Ziox 405™ see Chlorophyllin, Papain, and Urea on page 335

Ziprasidone (zi PRAS i done)

U.S. Brand Names Geodon®
Mexican Brand Names Geodon
Generic Available No
Index Terms Zeldox; Ziprasidone Hydrochloride; Ziprasidone Mesylate
Pharmacologic Category Antipsychotic Agent, Atypical
Use Treatment of schizophrenia; treatment of acute manic or mixed episodes associated with bipolar disorder with or without psychosis; acute agitation in patients with schizophrenia
Unlabeled/Investigational Use Tourette's syndrome
Local Anesthetic/Vasoconstrictor Precautions Ziprasidone is one of the drugs confirmed to prolong the QT interval and is accepted as having a risk of causing torsade de pointes. The risk of drug-induced torsade de pointes is extremely low when a single QT interval prolonging drug is prescribed. In terms of epinephrine, it is not known what effect vasoconstrictors in the local anesthetic regimen will have in patients with a known history of congenital prolonged QT interval or in patients taking any medication that prolongs the QT interval. Until more information is obtained, it is suggested that the clinician consult with the physician prior to the use of a vasoconstrictor in suspected patients, and (Continued)

Ziprasidone *(Continued)*

that the vasoconstrictor (epinephrine, levonordefrin [Neo-Cobefrin®]) be used with caution.

Effects on Dental Treatment Key adverse event(s) related to dental treatment: Xerostomia and changes in salivation (normal salivary flow resumes upon discontinuation), orthostatic hypotension, tongue edema, dysphagia, and tooth disorder.

Common Adverse Effects Note: Although minor QT$_c$ prolongation (mean 10 msec at 160 mg/day) may occur more frequently (incidence not specified), clinically-relevant prolongation (>500 msec) was rare (0.06%) and less than placebo (0.23%).

>10%:

Central nervous system: Extrapyramidal symptoms (2% to 31%), somnolence (8% to 31%), headache (3% to 18%), dizziness (3% to 16%)

Gastrointestinal: Nausea (4% to 12%)

1% to 10%:

Cardiovascular: Chest pain (5%), postural hypotension (5%), hypertension (2% to 3%), bradycardia (2%), tachycardia (2%), vasodilation (1%), facial edema, orthostatic hypotension

Central nervous system: Akathisia (2% to 10%), anxiety (2% to 5%), insomnia (3%), agitation (2%), speech disorder (2%), personality disorder (2%), psychosis (1%), akinesia, amnesia, ataxia, chills, confusion, coordination abnormal, delirium, dystonia, fever, hostility, hypothermia, oculogyric crisis, vertigo

Dermatologic: Rash (4%), fungal dermatitis (2%)

Endocrine & metabolic: Dysmenorrhea (2%)

Gastrointestinal: Weight gain (10%), constipation (2% to 9%), dyspepsia (1% to 8%), diarrhea (3% to 5%), vomiting (3% to 5%), salivation increased (4%), xerostomia (1% to 5%), tongue edema (3%), abdominal pain (2%), anorexia (2%), dysphagia (2%), rectal hemorrhage (2%), tooth disorder (1%), buccoglossal syndrome

Genitourinary: Priapism (1%)

Local: Injection site pain (7% to 9%)

Neuromuscular & skeletal: Weakness (2% to 6%), hypoesthesia (2%), myalgia (2%), paresthesia (2%), back pain (1%), cogwheel rigidity (1%), hypertonia (1%), abnormal gait, choreoathetosis, dysarthria, dyskinesia, hyper-/hypokinesia, hypotonia, neuropathy, tremor, twitching

Ocular: Vision abnormal (3% to 6%), diplopia

Respiratory: Infection (8%), rhinitis (1% to 4%), cough (3%), pharyngitis (3%), dyspnea (2%)

Miscellaneous: Diaphoresis (2%), furunculosis (2%), flu-like syndrome (1%), photosensitivity reaction, withdrawal syndrome

Mechanism of Action Ziprasidone is a benzylisothiazolylpiperazine antipsychotic. The exact mechanism of action is unknown. However, *in vitro* radioligand studies show that ziprasidone has high affinity for D$_2$, D$_3$, 5-HT$_{2A}$, 5-HT$_{1A}$, 5-HT$_{2C}$, 5-HT$_{1D}$, and alpha$_1$-adrenergic; moderate affinity for histamine H$_1$ receptors; and no appreciable affinity for alpha$_2$-adrenergic receptors, beta-adrenergic, 5-HT$_3$, 5-HT$_4$, cholinergic, mu, sigma, or benzodiazepine receptors. Ziprasidone functions as an antagonist at the D$_2$, 5-HT$_{2A}$, and 5-HT$_{1D}$ receptors and as an agonist at the 5-HT$_{1A}$ receptor. Ziprasidone moderately inhibits the reuptake of serotonin and norepinephrine.

Drug Interactions

Cytochrome P450 Effect: Substrate (minor) of CYP1A2, 3A4; **Inhibits** CYP2D6 (weak), 3A4 (weak)

Increased Effect/Toxicity:

Ketoconazole may increase serum concentrations of ziprasidone. Other CYP3A4 inhibitors may share this potential.

Concurrent use with QT$_c$-prolonging agents may result in additive effects on cardiac conduction, potentially resulting in malignant or lethal arrhythmias. Concurrent use is contraindicated; includes amiodarone, arsenic trioxide, bretylium, chlorpromazine, cisapride, class Ia antiarrhythmics (quinidine, procainamide), dofetilide, dolasetron, droperidol, ibutilide, levomethadyl, mefloquine, mesoridazine, pentamidine, pimozide, probucol, some quinolone antibiotics (moxifloxacin, sparfloxacin, gatifloxacin), sotalol, tacrolimus, and thioridazine. Potassium- or magnesium-depleting agents (diuretics, aminoglycosides, cyclosporine, and amphotericin B) may increase the risk of QT$_c$ prolongation. Antihypertensive agents may increase the risk of orthostatic hypotension. CNS depressants may increase the degree of sedation caused by ziprasidone. Metoclopramide may increase risk of extrapyramidal symptoms (EPS). Acetylcholinesterase inhibitors (central) may increase the risk of antipsychotic-related EPS.

Decreased Effect: Carbamazepine may decrease serum concentrations of ziprasidone. Other enzyme-inducing agents may share this potential. Amphetamines may decrease the efficacy of ziprasidone. Ziprasidone may inhibit the efficacy of levodopa.

Pharmacodynamics/Kinetics

Absorption: Well absorbed

Distribution: V_d: 1.5 L/kg

Protein binding: 99%, primarily to albumin and alpha$_1$-acid glycoprotein

Metabolism: Extensively hepatic, primarily via aldehyde oxidase; less than $1/3$ of total metabolism via CYP3A4 and CYP1A2 (minor)

Bioavailability: Oral (with food): 60% (up to twofold increase with food); I.M.: 100%

Half-life elimination: Oral: 7 hours; I.M.: 2-5 hours

Time to peak: Oral: 6-8 hours; I.M.: ≤60 minutes

Excretion: Feces (66%) and urine (20%) as metabolites; little as unchanged drug (1% urine, 4% feces)

Clearance: 7.5 mL/minute/kg

Pregnancy Risk Factor C

Zoledronic Acid (zoe le DRON ik AS id)

Related Information

Management of Patients Undergoing Cancer Therapy *on page 1826*

U.S. Brand Names Reclast®; Zometa®

Canadian Brand Names Aclasta®; Zometa®

Generic Available No

Index Terms CGP-42446; NSC-721517; Zoledronate

Pharmacologic Category Antidote; Bisphosphonate Derivative

Use Treatment of hypercalcemia of malignancy, multiple myeloma, bone metastases of solid tumors, Paget's disease of bone

Unlabeled/Investigational Use Prevention of bone loss associated with aromatase inhibitor therapy in postmenopausal women with breast cancer; prevention of bone loss associated with androgen deprivation therapy in prostate cancer; treatment of postmenopausal osteoporosis

Local Anesthetic/Vasoconstrictor Precautions No information available to require special precautions

Effects on Dental Treatment Key adverse event(s) related to dental treatment: Mucositis, dysphagia, stomatitis, and sore throat.

Osteonecrosis of the jaw (ONJ), generally associated with local infection and/or tooth extraction and often with delayed healing, has been reported in patients taking bisphosphonates. Most reported cases of bisphosphonate-associated osteonecrosis have been in cancer patients treated with intravenous bisphosphonates. However, some have occurred in patients with postmenopausal osteoporosis taking oral bisphosphonates. Dental surgery may exacerbate ONJ. For patients requiring dental procedures, there are no data available to suggest whether discontinuation of bisphosphonate treatment reduces the risk of ONJ. See Dental Comment.

Common Adverse Effects Note: Percentages reported with Zometa®. In general, the rates of adverse reactions were decreased with Reclast® when used for Paget's disease of the bone.

>10%:

Cardiovascular: Leg edema (5% to 21%), hypotension (11%)

Central nervous system: Fatigue (39%), fever (32% to 44%), headache (5% to 19%), dizziness (18%), insomnia (15% to 16%), anxiety (11% to 14%),

(Continued)

Zoledronic Acid *(Continued)*

depression (14%), agitation (13%), confusion (7% to 13%), hypoesthesia (12%)

Dermatologic: Alopecia (12%), dermatitis (11%)

Endocrine & metabolic: Dehydration (5% to 14%), hypophosphatemia (12% to 13%), hypokalemia (12%), hypomagnesemia (11%)

Gastrointestinal: Nausea (29% to 46%), constipation (27% to 31%), vomiting (14% to 32%), diarrhea (17% to 24%), anorexia (9% to 22%), abdominal pain (14% to 16%), weight loss (16%), appetite decreased (13%)

Genitourinary: Urinary tract infection (12% to 14%)

Hematologic: Anemia (22% to 33%), neutropenia (12%)

Neuromuscular & skeletal: Bone pain (55%), weakness (5% to 24%), myalgia (23%), arthralgia (5% to 21%), back pain (15%), paresthesia (15%), limb pain (14%), skeletal pain (12%), rigors (11%)

Renal: Renal deterioration (8% to 17%; up to 40% in patients with abnormal baseline creatinine)

Respiratory: Dyspnea (22% to 27%), cough (12% to 22%)

Miscellaneous: Cancer progression (16%), moniliasis (12%)

1% to 10%:

Cardiovascular: Chest pain (5% to 10%)

Central nervous system: Somnolence (5% to 10%)

Endocrine & metabolic: Hypocalcemia (1% to 10%), hypermagnesemia (2%)

Gastrointestinal: Dysphagia (10%), dyspepsia (10%), mucositis (5% to 10%), stomatitis (8%), sore throat (8%)

Hematologic: Thrombocytopenia (5% to 10%), pancytopenia (5% to 10%), granulocytopenia (5% to 10%)

Renal: Serum creatinine increased (grades 3/4: 2%)

Respiratory: Pleural effusion, upper respiratory tract infection (10%)

Miscellaneous: Metastases (5% to 10%), nonspecific infection (5% to 10%)

Dosage I.V.: Adults:

Hypercalcemia of malignancy (albumin-corrected serum calcium ≥12 mg/dL) (Zometa®): 4 mg (maximum) given as a single dose. Wait at least 7 days before considering retreatment. Dosage adjustment may be needed in patients with decreased renal function following treatment.

Multiple myeloma or metastatic bone lesions from solid tumors (Zometa®): 4 mg every 3-4 weeks

Note: Patients should receive a daily calcium supplement and multivitamin containing vitamin D

Paget's disease (Reclast®, Aclasta® [not available in U.S.]): 5 mg infused over at least 15 minutes. **Note:** Data concerning retreatment is not available, but may be considered. Patients should receive a daily calcium supplement and multivitamin containing vitamin D.

Postmenopausal osteoporosis (unlabeled use): 5 mg every 12 months

Prevention of aromatase inhibitor-induced bone loss in breast cancer (unlabeled use): 4 mg every 6 months

Prevention of androgen deprivation-induced bone loss in nonmetastatic prostate cancer (unlabeled use): 4 mg every 3-12 months

Dosage adjustment in renal impairment (at treatment initiation):

Reclast®: Cl_{cr} <35 mL/minute: Not recommended

Zometa®: Multiple myeloma and bone metastases:

Cl_{cr} >60 mL/minute: 4 mg

Cl_{cr} 50-60 mL/minute: 3.5 mg

Cl_{cr} 40-49 mL/minute: 3.3 mg

Cl_{cr} 30-39 mL/minute: 3 mg

Cl_{cr} <30 mL/minute: Not recommended

Zometa®: Hypercalcemia of malignancy:

Mild-to-moderate impairment: No adjustment necessary

Severe impairment (serum creatinine >4.5 mg/dL): Evaluate risk versus benefit

Aclasta® [not available in U.S.]: Cl_{cr} >30 mL/minute: No adjustment recommended

Dosage adjustment for renal toxicity (during treatment):

Hypercalcemia of malignancy: Evidence of renal deterioration: Evaluate risk versus benefit.

Multiple myeloma and bone metastases: Evidence of renal deterioration: Withhold dose until renal function returns to within 10% of baseline; renal deterioration defined as follows:

Normal baseline creatinine: Increase of 0.5 mg/dL

Abnormal baseline creatinine: Increase of 1 mg/dL

Reinitiate dose at the same dose administered prior to treatment interruption.

Dosage adjustment in hepatic impairment: Specific guidelines are not available.

Mechanism of Action A bisphosphonate which inhibits bone resorption via actions on osteoclasts or on osteoclast precursors; inhibits osteoclastic activity and skeletal calcium release induced by tumors. Decreases serum calcium and phosphorus, and increases their elimination.

Contraindications Hypersensitivity to zoledronic acid, other bisphosphonates, or any component of the formulation; pregnancy; breast-feeding

Warnings/Precautions Bisphosphonate therapy has been associated with osteonecrosis, primarily of the jaw; this has been observed mostly in cancer patients, but also in patients with postmenopausal osteoporosis and other diagnoses. Dental exams and preventative dentistry should be performed prior to placing patients with risk factors on chronic bisphosphonate therapy. Invasive dental procedures should be avoided during treatment.

Infrequently, severe (and occasionally debilitating) bone, joint, and/or muscle pain have been reported during bisphosphonate treatment. The onset of pain ranged from a single day to several months. Symptoms usually resolve upon discontinuation. Some patients experienced recurrence when rechallenged with same drug or another bisphosphonate; avoid use in patients with a history of these symptoms in association with bisphosphonate therapy.

May cause hypocalcemia in patients with Paget's disease, in whom the pretreatment rate of bone turnover may be greatly elevated. Hypocalcemia must be corrected before initiation of therapy. Ensure adequate calcium and vitamin D intake during therapy. Use caution in patients with disturbances of calcium and mineral metabolism (eg, hypoparathyroidism, thyroid surgery, malabsorption syndromes).

Adequate hydration is required during treatment (urine output ~2 L/day); avoid overhydration, especially in patients with heart failure.

Reclast®: Use is not recommended in patients with severe renal impairment (Cl_{cr} <35 mL/minute). When used in the treatment of Paget's disease significant renal deterioration has not been observed with the usual 5 mg dose administered over at least 15 minutes.

Zometa®: Use caution in renal dysfunction; dosage adjustment required. In cancer patients, renal toxicity has been reported with doses >4 mg or infusions administered over 15 minutes. Risk factors for renal deterioration include pre-existing renal insufficiency and repeated doses of zoledronic acid and other bisphosphonates. Dehydration and the use of other nephrotoxic drugs which may contribute to renal deterioration should be identified and managed. Use is not recommended in patients with severe renal impairment (serum creatinine >3 mg/dL) and bone metastases (limited data); use in patients with hypercalcemia of malignancy and severe renal impairment should only be done if the benefits outweigh the risks. Renal function should be assessed prior to treatment; if decreased after treatment, additional treatments should be withheld until renal function returns to within 10% of baseline. Diuretics should not be used before correcting hypovolemia. Renal deterioration, resulting in renal failure and dialysis has occurred in patients treated with zoledronic acid after single and multiple infusions at recommended doses of 4 mg over 15 minutes.

Use caution in patients with aspirin-sensitive asthma (may cause bronchoconstriction), hepatic dysfunction, and the elderly. Women of childbearing age should be advised against becoming pregnant. Safety and efficacy in pediatric patients have not been established.

Drug Interactions

Increased Effect/Toxicity: Aminoglycosides may lower serum calcium levels with prolonged administration; concomitant use may have an additive hypocalcemic effect. NSAIDs may enhance the gastrointestinal adverse/toxic effects (increased incidence of GI ulcers) of bisphosphonate derivatives. Bisphosphonate derivatives may enhance the hypocalcemic effect of phosphate supplements.

Dietary Considerations

Multiple myeloma or metastatic bone lesions from solid tumors: Take daily calcium supplement (500 mg) and daily multivitamin (with 400 int. units vitamin D).

Paget's disease: Take calcium 1500 mg/day and vitamin D 800 units/day, particularly during the first 2 weeks after administration.

Pharmacodynamics/Kinetics

Distribution: Binds to bone

Protein binding: ~22%

Half-life elimination: Triphasic; Terminal: 146 hours

Excretion: Urine (39% ± 16% as unchanged drug) within 24 hours; feces (<3%)

Pregnancy Risk Factor D

Dosage Forms [CAN] = Canadian brand name

Infusion, solution [premixed]:

Aclasta® [CAN]): 5 mg (100 mL) [not available in the U.S.]

Relcast®: 5 mg (100 mL)

(Continued)

Zoledronic Acid (Continued)

Injection, solution:
Zometa®: 4 mg/5 mL (5 mL)

Dental Comment Novartis Pharmaceuticals Corporation has notified dental health professionals of the risk of **osteonecrosis of the jaw (ONJ)** and the use of the intravenous bisphosphonates, pamidrate (Zometa®) and zoledronic acid (Aredia®): *"Dear Dental Health Professional Letter" Issued for Intravenous Bisphosphonates, Pamidronate and Zoledronic Acid, Regarding the Risk of Osteonecrosis of the Jaw (ONJ) in Cancer Patients* — May 2005.

Often observed in patients receiving chemotherapy and corticosteroids, reports of ONJ (the majority being associated with dental procedures) have been documented in cancer patients. Dental exams and preventative dentistry should be performed prior to placing patients with risk factors (chemotherapy, corticosteroids, poor oral hygiene) on intravenous bisphosphonate therapy. Additionally, invasive dental procedures should be avoided during therapy; patients developing ONJ while on bisphosphonate therapy should not have invasive dental procedures because the condition may be exacerbated. It has not been determined whether the discontinuation of bisphosphonate therapy in patients requiring dental surgery decreases the risk of ONJ. The treating healthcare professional is encouraged to assess the benefits and risks.

Bisphosphonates are widely used in the management of metastatic bone disease to treat hypercalcemia associated with malignancies and to treat osteoporosis. It is suggested that because of the trend in the use of chronic bisphosphonate therapy, the observation of an associated risk of osteonecrosis of the jaw should alert practitioners to monitor for this previously unrecognized potential complication.

Additional information is available at http://www.fda.gov/medwatch/SAFETY/2005/safety05.htm#zometa2, or by contacting Novartis Oncology Medical Services at 1-888-669-6682.

Estimates of Percent Incidence of ONJ in Treated Cancer Patients

Two reports have attempted to assess the percent of cancer patients developing ONJ after bisphosphonate treatment. Maerevoet et al, reported that among 194 patients treated with Zometa® every 3-4 weeks, nine developed ONJ. Before receiving Zometa®, six had received Aredia® 90 mg every 3-4 weeks. The median duration of treatment with Aredia® was 39 months and for Zometa® 18 months. The incidence of ONJ in these patients was calculated to be 4.6%. Durie et al, described the results of a survey by the International Myeloma Foundation in 2004 to assess the risk factors of ONJ. Out of 1203 respondents, 904 had myeloma and 299 breast cancer. Of the myeloma patients, 62 developed ONJ and 54 had suspicious findings. Of the breast cancer patients, 13 had ONJ and 23 had suspicious findings. The total number of cases of either ONJ or suspicious findings was 152. ONJ developed in 10% of 211 patients receiving Zometa® compared to 4% of 413 receiving Aredia®. The mean time to onset of ONJ among patients taking Zometa® was 18 months; the mean time to onset after Aredia® was 6 years. It should be noted that an early report by authors from Novartis Pharmaceuticals Corporation (Tarassoff, 2003) stressed that Aredia® and Zometa® had been used in 2.5 million patients world wide and reports of ONJ during their extensive use had been rare. In addition, these authors stated that review of the reported cases revealed multiple risk factors for avascular necrosis. McMahon et al, followed up with a report that, along with other factors, bisphosphonates are additional stressors of bone health that can tip the balance to osteonecrosis. They suggested that the prevention of ONJ should be stressed such as the elimination of chronic dental infections prior to chemotherapy and bisphosphonate use in cancer patients.

Selected Readings

American Dental Association Council on Scientific Affairs, "Dental Management of Patients Receiving Oral Bisphosphonate Therapy," *JADA*, 2006, 137(8):1144-50. Available at: http://www.ada.org/prof/resources/pubs/jada/reports/report bisphosphonate.pdf.

Durie BG, Katz M, and Crowley J, "Osteonecrosis of the Jaw and Bisphosphonates," *N Engl J Med*, 2005, 353(1):99-102.

Maerevoet M, Martin C, and Duck L, "Osteonecrosis of the Jaw and Bisphosphonates," *N Engl J Med*, 2005, 353(1):99-102.

McMahon RE, Bouquot JE, Glueck CJ, et al, "Osteonecrosis: A Multifactorial Etiology," *J Oral Maxillofac Surg*, 2004, 62(7):904-5.

Ruggiero S, Gralow J, Marx RE, et al, "Practical Guidelines for the Prevention, Diagnosis, and Treatment of Osteonecrosis of the Jaw in Patients With Cancer," *J Clin Oncol*, 2006, 2(1):7-14.

Tarassoff P and Csermak K, "Avascular Necrosis of the Jaws: Risk Factors in Metastatic Cancer Patients," *J Oral Maxillofac Surg*, 2003, 61(10):1238-9.

Zolinza™ *see* Vorinostat *on page 1668*

Zolmitriptan (zohl mi TRIP tan)

U.S. Brand Names Zomig®; Zomig-ZMT™
Canadian Brand Names Zomig®; Zomig® Nasal Spray; Zomig® Rapimelt
Mexican Brand Names Zomig
Generic Available No
Index Terms 311C90
Pharmacologic Category Antimigraine Agent; Serotonin 5-HT$_{1B, 1D}$ Receptor Agonist
Use Acute treatment of migraine with or without aura
Local Anesthetic/Vasoconstrictor Precautions No information available to require special precautions
Effects on Dental Treatment Key adverse event(s) related to dental treatment: Xerostomia (normal salivary flow resumes upon discontinuation) and dysphagia.
Common Adverse Effects Percentages noted from oral preparations.
1% to 10%:
Cardiovascular: Chest pain (2% to 4%), palpitation (up to 2%)
Central nervous system: Dizziness (6% to 10%), somnolence (5% to 8%), pain (2% to 3%), vertigo (≤2%)
Gastrointestinal: Nausea (4% to 9%), xerostomia (3% to 5%), dyspepsia (1% to 3%), dysphagia (≤2%)
Neuromuscular & skeletal: Paresthesia (5% to 9%), weakness (3% to 9%), warm/cold sensation (5% to 7%), hypoesthesia (1% to 2%), myalgia (1% to 2%), myasthenia (up to 2%)
Miscellaneous: Neck/throat/jaw pain (4% to 10%), diaphoresis (up to 3%), allergic reaction (up to 1%)
Mechanism of Action Selective agonist for serotonin (5-HT$_{1B}$ and 5-HT$_{1D}$ receptors) in cranial arteries to cause vasoconstriction and reduce sterile inflammation associated with antidromic neuronal transmission correlating with relief of migraine
Drug Interactions
Cytochrome P450 Effect: Substrate of CYP1A2 (minor)
Increased Effect/Toxicity: Ergot-containing drugs may lead to vasospasm; cimetidine, MAO inhibitors, oral contraceptives, propranolol increase levels of zolmitriptan; concurrent use with sibutramine, SSRIs/SNRIs, or other serotonin agonists may lead to serotonin syndrome.
Pharmacodynamics/Kinetics
Onset of action: 0.5-1 hour
Absorption: Well absorbed
Distribution: V$_d$: 7 L/kg
Protein binding: 25%
Metabolism: Converted to an active N-desmethyl metabolite (2-6 times more potent than zolmitriptan)
Bioavailability: 40%
Half-life elimination: 2.8-3.7 hours
Time to peak, serum: Tablet: 1.5 hours; Orally-disintegrating tablet and nasal spray: 3 hours
Excretion: Urine (~60% to 65% total dose); feces (30% to 40%)
Pregnancy Risk Factor C

Zoloft® see Sertraline on page 1463

Zolpidem (zole PI dem)

U.S. Brand Names Ambien®; Ambien CR™
Mexican Brand Names Stilnox
Generic Available No
Index Terms Zolpidem Tartrate
Pharmacologic Category Hypnotic, Nonbenzodiazepine
Dental Use Has not been established
Use
Ambien®: Short-term treatment of insomnia (with difficulty of sleep onset)
Ambien CR™: Short-term treatment of insomnia (with difficulty of sleep onset and/or sleep maintenance)
Local Anesthetic/Vasoconstrictor Precautions No information available to require special precautions
Effects on Dental Treatment Key adverse event(s) related to dental treatment: Xerostomia (normal salivary flow resumes upon discontinuation).
Common Adverse Effects Actual frequency may be dosage form, dose, and/or age dependent
(Continued)

Zolpidem (Continued)

>10%: Central nervous system: Dizziness, headache, somnolence

1% to 10%:

Cardiovascular: Blood pressure increased, chest discomfort/pain, palpitation

Central nervous system: Abnormal dreams, anxiety, apathy, amnesia, ataxia, attention disturbance, body temperature increased, confusion, depersonalization, depression, disinhibition, disorientation, drowsiness, drugged feeling, euphoria, fatigue, fever, hallucinations, hypoesthesia, insomnia, memory disorder, lethargy, lightheadedness, mood swings, sleep disorder, stress

Dermatologic: Rash, urticaria, wrinkling

Endocrine & metabolic: Menorrhagia

Gastrointestinal: Abdominal discomfort, abdominal pain, abdominal tenderness, appetite disorder, constipation, diarrhea, dyspepsia, flatulence, gastroenteritis, gastroesophageal reflux, hiccup, nausea, vomiting, xerostomia

Genitourinary: Urinary tract infection

Neuromuscular & skeletal: Arthralgia, back pain, balance disorder, myalgia, neck pain, paresthesia, psychomotor retardation, tremor, weakness

Ocular: Asthenopia, blurred vision, depth perception altered, diplopia, visual disturbance, red eye

Otic: Labyrinthitis, tinnitus, vertigo

Renal: Dysuria

Respiratory: Pharyngitis, sinusitis, upper respiratory tract infection, throat irritation

Miscellaneous: Allergy, binge eating, flu-like syndrome

Restrictions C-IV

Dosage Oral:

Adults:

Ambien®: 10 mg immediately before bedtime; maximum dose: 10 mg

Ambien CR™: 12.5 mg immediately before bedtime

Elderly:

Ambien®: 5 mg immediately before bedtime

Ambien CR™: 6.25 mg immediately before bedtime

Dosing adjustment in renal impairment: Dose adjustment not required; monitor closely

Hemodialysis: Not dialyzable

Dosing adjustment in hepatic impairment:

Ambien®: 5 mg

Ambien CR™: 6.25 mg

Mechanism of Action Structurally dissimilar to benzodiazepines. Selective hypnotic effects (with minor anxiolytic, myorelaxant, and anticonvulsant properties) mediated through selective affinity for the alpha-1 subunit of the omega-1 (benzodiazepine) receptor located on the GABA$_A$ receptor complex. Agonism at this site enhances GABA-ergic chloride conductance hyperpolarizing neuronal membranes thereby reducing the responsiveness to excitatory signals.

Contraindications Hypersensitivity to zolpidem or any component of the formulation

Warnings/Precautions Should be used only after evaluation of potential causes of sleep disturbance. Failure of sleep disturbance to resolve after 7-10 days may indicate psychiatric or medical illness. Hypnotics/sedatives have been associated with abnormal thinking and behavior changes including decreased inhibition, aggression, bizarre behavior, agitation, hallucinations, and depersonalization. These changes may occur unpredictably and may indicate previously unrecognized psychiatric disorders; evaluate appropriately. Sedative/hypnotics may produce withdrawal symptoms following abrupt discontinuation. Use with caution in patients with depression; worsening of depression, including suicidal ideation has been reported with the use of hypnotics. Intentional overdose may be an issue in this population. The minimum dose that will effectively treat the individual patient should be used. Prescriptions should be written for the smallest quantity consistent with good patient care. Causes CNS depression, which may impair physical and mental capabilities. Effects with other sedative drugs or ethanol may be potentiated. Use caution in the elderly; dose adjustment recommended. Closely monitor elderly or debilitated patients for impaired cognitive or motor performance. Avoid use in patients with sleep apnea or a history of sedative-hypnotic abuse. Postmarketing studies have indicated that the use of hypnotic/sedative agents for sleep has been associated with hypersensitivity reactions including anaphylaxis as well as angioedema. An increased risk for hazardous sleep-related activities such as sleep-driving; cooking and eating food, and making phone calls while asleep have also been noted. Discontinue treatment in patients who report a sleep-driving episode.

Use caution with respiratory disease. Use caution with hepatic impairment; dose adjustment required. Because of the rapid onset of action, administer immediately prior to bedtime or after the patient has gone to bed and is having difficulty falling asleep. Safety and efficacy have not been established in pediatric patients.

Drug Interactions

Cytochrome P450 Effect: Substrate of CYP1A2 (minor), 2C9 (minor), 2C19 (minor), 2D6 (minor), 3A4 (major)

Increased Effect/Toxicity: Use of zolpidem in combination with other centrally-acting drugs may produce additive CNS depression. CYP3A4 inhibitors may increase the levels/effects of zolpidem; example inhibitors include azole antifungals, clarithromycin, diclofenac, doxycycline, erythromycin, imatinib, isoniazid, nefazodone, nicardipine, propofol, protease inhibitors, quinidine, telithromycin, troleandomycin, and verapamil. Antifungal agents (itraconazole and ketoconazole) may decrease the metabolism of zolpidem; consider using lower dose of zolpidem; monitor closely.

Decreased Effect: CYP3A4 inducers may decrease the levels/effects of zolpidem; example inducers include aminoglutethimide, carbamazepine, nafcillin, nevirapine, phenobarbital, phenytoin, and rifamycins.

Ethanol/Nutrition/Herb Interactions

Ethanol: Avoid ethanol (may increase CNS depression).

Food: Maximum plasma concentration and bioavailability are decreased with food; time to peak plasma concentration is increased; half-life remains unchanged. Grapefruit juice may decrease the metabolism of zolpidem.

Herb/Nutraceutical: St John's wort may decrease zolpidem levels. Avoid valerian, St John's wort, kava kava, gotu kola (may increase CNS depression).

Dietary Considerations For faster sleep onset, do not administer with (or immediately after) a meal.

Pharmacodynamics/Kinetics

Onset of action: 30 minutes

Duration: 6-8 hours

Absorption: Rapid

Protein binding: 92%

Metabolism: Hepatic, primarily via CYP3A4 (~60%), to inactive metabolites

Half-life elimination: 2.5-2.8 hours (range 1.4-4.5 hours); Cirrhosis: Up to 9.9 hours

Time to peak, plasma: 2 hours; 4 hours with food

Excretion: As metabolites in urine, bile, feces

Pregnancy Risk Factor C

Dosage Forms

Tablet:

Ambien®: 5 mg, 10 mg

Ambien® PAK™ [dose pack]: 5 mg (30s)

Tablet, extended release:

Ambien CR™: 6.25 mg, 12.5 mg

Selected Readings

Garnier R, Guerault E, Muzard D, et al, "Acute Zolpidem Poisoning - Analysis of 344 Cases," *J Toxicol Clin Toxicol*, 1994, 32(4):391-404.

Holm KJ and Goa KL, "Zolpidem: An Update of Its Pharmacology, Therapeutic Efficacy and Tolerability in the Treatment of Insomnia," *Drugs*, 2000, 59(4):865-89.

Lange CL, "Medication-Associated Somnambulism," *J Am Acad Child Adolesc Psychiatry*, 2005, 44(3):211-2.

Langtry HD and Benfield P, "Zolpidem: A Review of Its Pharmacodynamic and Pharmacokinetic Properties and Therapeutic Potential," *Drugs*, 1990, 40(2):291-313.

Lheureux P, Debailleul G, De Witte O, et al, "Zolpidem Intoxication Mimicking Narcotic Overdose: Response to Flumazenil," *Hum Exp Toxicol*, 1990, 9(2):105-7.

Meram D and Descotes J, "Acute Poisoning By Zolpidem," *Rev Med Interne*, 1989, 10(5):466.

Mercurio M, De Roos F, and Hoffman RS, "Zolpidem (Ambien®): Exposure Assessment of a New Nonbenzodiazepine GABA Agonist," *Vet Hum Toxicol*, 1994, 36:371.

Pacifici GM, Viani A, Rizzo G, et al, "Plasma Protein Binding of Zolpidem in Liver and Renal Insufficiency," *Int J Clin Pharmacol Ther Toxicol*, 1988, 26(9):439-43.

Queneau PE, Koch S, Hrusovsky S, et al, "Cytolytic Hepatitis Related to Zolpidem," 1st International Symposium on Hepatology and Clinical Pharmacology Liver and Drugs, Abstract, 1994, 39.

Salva P and Costa J, "Clinical Pharmacokinetics and Pharmacodynamics of Zolpidem. Therapeutic Implications," *Clin Pharmacokinet*, 1995, 29(3):142-53.

Sanger DJ, "The Pharmacology and Mechanisms of Action of New Generation, Non-Benzodiazepine Hypnotic Agents," *CNS Drugs*, 2004, 18 (Suppl 1):9-15.

Simcox DA, "Zolpidem-Associated Falls," *Consult Pharm*, 1995, 10:1378-80.

Zonisamide (zoe NIS a mide)

U.S. Brand Names Zonegran®
Canadian Brand Names Zonegran®
Generic Available Yes
Pharmacologic Category Anticonvulsant, Miscellaneous
Use Adjunct treatment of partial seizures in children >16 years of age and adults with epilepsy
Unlabeled/Investigational Use Bipolar disorder
Local Anesthetic/Vasoconstrictor Precautions No information available to require special precautions
Effects on Dental Treatment Key adverse event(s) related to dental treatment: Xerostomia (normal salivary flow resumes upon discontinuation) and abnormal taste.
Common Adverse Effects Adjunctive Therapy: Frequencies noted in patients receiving other anticonvulsants:

>10%:
Central nervous system: Somnolence (17%), dizziness (13%)
Gastrointestinal: Anorexia (13%)
1% to 10%:
Central nervous system: Headache (10%), agitation/irritability (9%), fatigue (8%), tiredness (7%), ataxia (6%), confusion (6%), concentration decreased (6%), memory impairment (6%), depression (6%), insomnia (6%), speech disorders (5%), mental slowing (4%), anxiety (3%), nervousness (2%), schizophrenic/schizophreniform behavior (2%), difficulty in verbal expression (2%), status epilepticus (1%), tremor (1%), convulsion (1%), hyperesthesia (1%), incoordination (1%)
Dermatologic: Rash (3%), bruising (2%), pruritus (1%)
Gastrointestinal: Nausea (9%), abdominal pain (6%), diarrhea (5%), dyspepsia (3%), weight loss (3%), constipation (2%), dry mouth (2%), taste perversion (2%), vomiting (1%)
Neuromuscular & skeletal: Paresthesia (4%), weakness (1%), abnormal gait (1%)
Ocular: Diplopia (6%), nystagmus (4%), amblyopia (1%)
Otic: Tinnitus (1%)
Respiratory: Rhinitis (2%), pharyngitis (1%), increased cough (1%)
Miscellaneous: Flu-like syndrome (4%) accidental injury (1%)
Mechanism of Action The exact mechanism of action is not known. May stabilize neuronal membranes and suppress neuronal hypersynchronization through action at sodium and calcium channels. Does not affect GABA activity.
Drug Interactions
Cytochrome P450 Effect: Substrate of CYP2C19 (minor), 3A4 (major)
Increased Effect/Toxicity: Sedative effects may be additive with other CNS depressants; monitor for increased effect (includes barbiturates, benzodiazepines, opioid analgesics, ethanol, and other sedative agents). CYP3A4 inhibitors may increase the levels/effects of zonisamide; example inhibitors include azole antifungals, clarithromycin, diclofenac, doxycycline, erythromycin, imatinib, isoniazid, nefazodone, nicardipine, propofol, protease inhibitors, quinidine, telithromycin, and verapamil.
Decreased Effect: CYP3A4 inducers may decrease the levels/effects of zonisamide; example inducers include aminoglutethimide, carbamazepine, nafcillin, nevirapine, phenobarbital, phenytoin, and rifamycins.
Pharmacodynamics/Kinetics
Distribution: V_d: 1.45 L/kg
Protein binding: 40%
Metabolism: Hepatic via CYP3A4; forms N-acetyl zonisamide and 2-sulfamoylacetyl phenol (SMAP)
Half-life elimination: 63 hours
Time to peak: 2-6 hours
Excretion: Urine (62%, 35% as unchanged drug, 65% as metabolites); feces (3%)
Pregnancy Risk Factor C

Zopiclone (ZOE pi clone)

Canadian Brand Names Alti-Zopiclone; Apo-Zopiclone®; CO Zopiclone; Gen-Zopiclone; Imovane®; Novo-Zopiclone; Nu-Zopiclone; PMS-Zopiclone; RAN™-Zopiclone; Rhovane®; Rhoxal-zopiclone; Riva-Zopiclone; Sandoz-Zopiclone
Generic Available Yes

Pharmacologic Category Hypnotic, Nonbenzodiazepine
Dental Use Has not been established
Use Symptomatic relief of transient and short-term insomnia
Local Anesthetic/Vasoconstrictor Precautions No information available to require special precautions
Effects on Dental Treatment Key adverse event(s) related to dental treatment: Coated tongue, dry mouth, halitosis, taste alteration (bitter taste, common).
Common Adverse Effects Frequency not defined.
Cardiovascular: Palpitations
Central nervous system: Agitation, anterograde amnesia, anxiety, asthenia, chills, confusion, depression, dizziness, drowsiness, euphoria, headache, hostility, memory impairment, nervousness, nightmares, somnolence, speech abnormalities
Dermatological: Rash, spots on skin
Endocrine & metabolic: Anorexia; libido decreased; alkaline phosphatase, ALT, and AST increased; appetite increased
Gastrointestinal: Constipation, coated tongue, diarrhea, dry mouth, dyspepsia, halitosis, nausea, taste alteration (bitter taste, common), vomiting
Neuromuscular & skeletal: Coordination impaired, hypotonia, limb heaviness, muscle spasms, paresthesia, tremor
Ocular: Amblyopia
Respiratory: Dyspnea
Miscellaneous: Diaphoresis
Restrictions Not available in U.S.
Mechanism of Action Zopiclone is a cyclopyrrolone derivative and has a pharmacological profile similar to benzodiazepines. Zopiclone reduces sleep latency, increases duration of sleep, and decreases the number of nocturnal awakenings.
Drug Interactions
Cytochrome P450 Effect: Substrate (major) of CYP2C9, 3A4
Increased Effect/Toxicity: Zopiclone may produce additive CNS depressant effects when coadministered with ethanol, sedatives, antihistamines, anticonvulsants, or psychotropic medications. CYP2C9 inhibitors may increase the levels/effects of zopiclone; example inhibitors include delavirdine, fluconazole, gemfibrozil, ketoconazole, nicardipine, NSAIDs, sulfonamides, and tolbutamide. CYP3A4 inhibitors may increase the levels/effects of zopiclone; example inhibitors include azole antifungals, clarithromycin, diclofenac, doxycycline, erythromycin, imatinib, isoniazid, nefazodone, nicardipine, propofol, protease inhibitors, quinidine, telithromycin, and verapamil.
Decreased Effect: CYP2C9 inducers may decrease the levels/effects of zopiclone; example inducers include carbamazepine, phenobarbital, phenytoin, rifampin, rifapentine, and secobarbital. CYP3A4 inducers may decrease the levels/effects of zopiclone; example inducers include aminoglutethimide, carbamazepine, nafcillin, nevirapine, phenobarbital, phenytoin, and rifamycins.
Pharmacodynamics/Kinetics
Absorption: Elderly: 75% to 94%
Distribution: Rapidly from vascular compartment
Protein binding: ~45%
Metabolism: Extensively hepatic
Half-life elimination: 5 hours; Elderly: 7 hours; Hepatic impairment: 11.9 hours
Time to peak, serum: <2 hours; Hepatic impairment: 3.5 hours
Excretion: Urine (75%); feces (16%)
Pregnancy Risk Factor Not assigned; similar agents rated D

Zorbtive® see Somatropin on page 1486
Zorcaine™ see Articaine and Epinephrine on page 143
ZORprin® see Aspirin on page 149
Zostavax® see Zoster Vaccine on page 1693

Zoster Vaccine (ZOS ter vak SEEN)

U.S. Brand Names Zostavax®
Generic Available No
Index Terms Shingles Vaccine; Varicella-Zoster (VZV) Vaccine (Zoster); VZV Vaccine (Zoster)
Pharmacologic Category Vaccine
Use Prevention of herpes zoster (shingles) in patients ≥60 years of age
Local Anesthetic/Vasoconstrictor Precautions No information available to require special precautions
Effects on Dental Treatment No significant effects or complications reported
(Continued)

Zoster Vaccine *(Continued)*

Common Adverse Effects All serious adverse reactions must be reported to the U.S. Department of Health and Human Services (DHHS) Vaccine Adverse Event Reporting System (VAERS) 1-800-822-7967.

>10%: Local: Injection site reaction (48%; includes erythema, tenderness, swelling, hematoma, pruritus, and/or warmth)

1% to 10%:
Central nervous system: Fever (2%), headache (1%)
Dermatologic: Skin disorder (1%)
Gastrointestinal: Diarrhea (2%)
Neuromuscular & skeletal: Weakness (1%)
Respiratory: Respiratory tract infection (2%), rhinitis (1%)
Miscellaneous: Flu-like syndrome (2%)

Mechanism of Action As a live, attenuated vaccine (Oka/Merck strain of varicella-zoster virus), zoster virus vaccine stimulates active immunity to disease caused by the varicella-zoster virus. Administration has been demonstrated to protect against the development of herpes zoster, with the highest efficacy in patients 60-69 years of age. It may also reduce the severity of complications, including postherpetic neuralgia, in patients who develop zoster following vaccination.

Drug Interactions

Decreased Effect: The effect of the vaccine may be decreased and the risk of varicella disease in individuals who are receiving immunosuppressant drugs (including high-dose systemic corticosteroids) may be increased. Effect of vaccine may be decreased if given within 5 months of immune globulins.

Pharmacodynamics/Kinetics

Onset of action: Seroconversion: ~6 weeks
Duration: Not established; protection has been demonstrated for at least 4 years

Pregnancy Risk Factor C

Zostrix® [OTC] *see* Capsaicin *on page 268*

Zostrix®-HP [OTC] *see* Capsaicin *on page 268*

Zosyn® *see* Piperacillin and Tazobactam Sodium *on page 1312*

Zovia™ *see* Ethinyl Estradiol and Ethynodiol Diacetate *on page 628*

Zovirax® *see* Acyclovir *on page 49*

Ztuss™ Tablet *see* Hydrocodone, Pseudoephedrine, and Guaifenesin *on page 835*

Ztuss™ ZT *see* Hydrocodone and Guaifenesin *on page 828*

Zyban® *see* BuPROPion *on page 241*

Zydone® *see* Hydrocodone and Acetaminophen *on page 822*

Zyflo® *see* Zileuton *on page 1681*

Zylet™ *see* Loteprednol and Tobramycin *on page 1006*

Zyloprim® *see* Allopurinol *on page 71*

Zymar™ *see* Gatifloxacin *on page 766*

Zymine®-D *see* Triprolidine and Pseudoephedrine *on page 1624*

Zyprexa® *see* Olanzapine *on page 1200*

Zyprexa Zydis *see* Olanzapine *on page 1200*

Zyprexa® Zydis® *see* Olanzapine *on page 1200*

Zyrtec® *see* Cetirizine *on page 321*

Zyrtec-D 12 Hour™ *see* Cetirizine and Pseudoephedrine *on page 322*

Zyvox® *see* Linezolid *on page 986*

NATURAL PRODUCTS: HERBAL AND DIETARY SUPPLEMENTS

Medical problem: " I have a toothache."
2000 BC response: "Here, eat this root."
1000 AD: "That root is heathen; here, say this prayer."
1850 AD: "That prayer is superstitious; here, drink this potion."
1940 AD: "That potion is snake oil; here, swallow this pill."
1985 AD: "That pill is ineffective; here, take this new antibiotic."
2000 AD: "That antibiotic is artificial; here, eat this root."

Adapted from an anonymous Internet communication.

INTRODUCTION

For centuries, Eastern and Western civilizations have attributed a large number of medical uses to plants and herbs. Over time, modern scientific methodologies have emerged from some of these remedies. Conversely, some of these agents have fallen into less popularity as more medical knowledge has evolved. In spite of this dichotomy, herbal and natural therapies for treatment of common medical ailments have become exceedingly popular. In America, people consistently seek out natural products that may be able to offset some perceived ailment or assist in the prevention of an ailment. One area of particular interest to those individuals using herbal or natural remedies has commonly been weight loss. There are numerous systemic considerations when some of the natural products that have been attributed weight loss powers are utilized. Many of these products are sold under the blanket of dietary supplements and, therefore, have avoided some of the more stringent Food and Drug Administration legislation. However, in 1994, that legislation was modified to include herbs, vitamins, minerals, and amino acids that may be taken as dietary supplements and the federal guidelines were further modified in 1999. This information must be made available to patients taking these types of products.

The real concern lies in the fact that health claims need not be approved by the FDA, but advertisements must include a disclaimer saying that the product has not yet been fully evaluated. Claims of medicinal use/value are often drawn from popular use, not necessarily from scientific studies. Safety is a concern when these agents are taken in combination with other prescription drugs due to the medical risk which might result. Many of these natural products may have real medicinal value but caution on the part of the dental clinician is prudent. It is impossible to cover all of the natural products, therefore, this chapter has been limited to some of the most popular dietary and herbal supplements and natural remedies used by patients you might treat and what we know about the effects of some of these agents on the body's various systems.

EFFECTS ON VARIOUS SYSTEMS

CARDIOVASCULAR SYSTEM

CONGESTIVE HEART FAILURE

(Diuretics, Xanthine derivatives, Licorice, Ginseng, Aconite)

Alisma plantago, bearberry (*Arctostaphylos uva-ursi*), buchu (*Barosma betulina*), couch grass, dandelion, horsetail rush, juniper, licorice, and xanthine derivatives exert varying degrees of diuretic action. Many patients with congestive heart failure (CHF) are already taking a diuretic medication. By taking products containing one or more of these components, patients already on diuretic medications may increase their risk for dehydration.

Ginseng and licorice can potentially worsen congestive heart failure and edema by causing fluid retention. Aconite has varying effects on the heart that itself could lead to heart failure. Patients with CHF should be advised to consult with their healthcare provider before using products containing any of these components.

HYPERTENSION/HYPOTENSION

(Diuretics, Ginkgo biloba, Ginseng, Hawthorn, Ma-huang, Xanthine derivatives)

The stimulant properties of ginseng and ma-huang could worsen pre-existing hypertension. Elevated blood pressure has been reported as a side effect of ginseng. Although ma-huang contains ephedrine, a known vasoconstrictor, ma-huang's effect on blood pressure varies between individuals. Ma-huang can cause hypotension or hypertension. Due to its unpredictable effects, patients with pre-existing hypertension should use caution when using natural products containing ma-huang. Providers should caution patients with labile hypertension against the use of ginseng.

The diuretic effect of xanthine derivatives and other diuretic components could increase the effects of antihypertensive medications, increasing the risk for hypotension. Hawthorn and ginkgo biloba can cause vasodilation increasing the hypotensive effects of antihypertensive medication. Patients susceptible to hypotension or patients taking antihypertensive medication should use caution when taking products containing xanthine derivatives or diuretics. Patients with pre-existing hypertension or hypotension who wish to use products containing these components should be closely monitored by a healthcare professional for changes in blood pressure control.

ARRHYTHMIAS

(Ginseng)

It has been reported that ginseng may increase the risk of arrhythmias, although it is unclear whether this effect is due to the actual ingredient (ginseng) or other possible impurities. Patients at risk for arrhythmias should be cautioned against the use of products containing ginseng without first consulting with their healthcare provider.

CENTRAL NERVOUS SYSTEM

(Aconite, Ginseng, Xanthine derivatives)

Aconite and hawthorn have potentially sedating effects, and aconite also contains various alkaloids and traces of ephedrine. Some documented central nervous system (CNS) effects of aconite include sedation, vertigo, and incoordination. Hawthorn has been reported to exert a depressive effect on the CNS leading to sedation.

Ginseng, ma-huang, and xanthine derivatives can exert a stimulant effect on the central nervous system. Some of the CNS effects of ginseng include nervousness, insomnia, and euphoria. The action of ma-huang is due to the presence of ephedrine and pseudoephedrine. Ma-huang exerts a stimulant action on the CNS similar to decongestant/weight loss products (Dexatrim®, etc) thus causing nervousness, insomnia, and anxiety. Kola nut, green tea, guarana, and yerba mate contain varying amounts of caffeine, a xanthine derivative. Stimulant properties exerted by these herbs are expected to be comparable to those of caffeine, including insomnia, nervousness, and anxiety.

Products containing aconite and hawthorn should be used with caution in patients with known history of depression, vertigo, or syncope. Ginseng or xanthine derivatives should be avoided in patients with history of insomnia or anxiety. Use of natural products with these components may contribute to a worsening of a patient's pre-existing medical condition. Patients taking CNS-active medications should avoid or use extreme caution when using preparations containing any of the above components. These components may interact directly or indirectly with CNS-active medications causing an increase or decrease in overall effect.

ENDOCRINE SYSTEM

DIABETES MELLITUS

(Chromium, Glucomannan, Ginseng, Hawthorn, Ma-huang, Periploca, Spirulina)

Ma-huang and spirulina both may increase glucose levels. This could cause a decrease in glucose control, thereby, increasing a patient's risk for hyperglycemia. Patients with diabetes or glucose intolerance should avoid using ma-huang and spirulina containing products.

Chromium, ginseng, glucomannan, periploca (*gymneme sylvestre*), and hawthorn should be used with caution in patients being treated for diabetes. These ingredients may reduce glucose levels increasing the risk for hypoglycemia in patients who are already taking a hypoglycemic agent. Patients with diabetes who wish to use products containing these ingredients should be closely monitored for fluctuations in blood glucose levels.

GASTROINTESTINAL SYSTEM

PEPTIC ULCER DISEASE

(Betaine Hydrochloride, White Willow)

Betaine hydrochloride is a source of hydrochloric acid. The acid released from betaine hydrochloride could aggravate an existing ulcer. White willow, like aspirin, contains salicylates.

Aspirin has been known to induce gastric damage by direct irritation on the gastric mucosa and by an indirect systemic effect. As a result, patients with a history of peptic ulcer disease or gastritis are informed to avoid use of aspirin and other salicylate derivatives. These precautions should also apply to white willow. Patients with a history of peptic ulcer disease or gastritis should not use products containing white willow or betaine hydrochloride as either could exacerbate ulcers.

INFLAMMATORY BOWEL DISEASE

(Cascara Sagrada, Senna, Dandelion)

Cascara sagrada and senna are stimulant laxatives. Their laxative effect is exerted by stimulation of peristalsis in the colon and by inhibition of water and electrolyte secretion. The laxative effect produced by these herbs could induce an exacerbation of inflammatory bowel disease. Patients with a history of inflammatory bowel disease should avoid using products containing cascara sagrada or senna, and use caution when taking products containing dandelion which may also have a laxative effect.

OBSTRUCTION/ILEUS

(Glucomannan, Kelp, Psyllium)

Glucomannan, kelp, and psyllium act as bulk laxatives. In the presence of water, bulk laxatives swell or form a viscous solution adding extra bulk in the gastrointestinal tract. The resulting mass is thought to stimulate peristalsis. In the presence of an ileus, these laxatives could cause an obstruction.

If sufficient water is not consumed when taking a bulk laxative, a semisolid mass can form resulting in an obstruction. Any patient who wishes to take a natural product containing kelp, psyllium, or glucomannan should drink sufficient water to decrease the risk of obstruction. This may be of concern in particular disease states such as CHF or other cases where excess fluid intake may influence the existing disease presentation. Patients with a suspected obstruction or ileus should avoid using products containing kelp, psyllium, or glucomannan without consent of their primary healthcare provider.

HEMATOLOGIC SYSTEM

ANTICOAGULATION THERAPY & COAGULATION DISORDERS

(Horsetail Rush, Ginseng, Ginkgo Biloba, Guarana, White Willow)

Horsetail rush, ginseng, ginkgo biloba, guarana, and white willow can potentially affect platelet aggregation and bleeding time. Ginkgo biloba, ginseng, guarana, and white willow inhibit platelet aggregation resulting in an increase in bleeding time. Horsetail rush, on the other hand, may decrease bleeding time. Patients with coagulation disorders or patients on anticoagulation therapy may be sensitive to the effects on coagulation by these components and should, therefore, avoid use of products containing any of these components.

EFFECTS ON VARIOUS SYSTEMS *(Continued)*

OTHER

PHENYLKETONURIA

(Aspartame, Spirulina)

Patients with phenylketonuria should not use products containing aspartame or spirulina. Aspartame, a common artificial sweetener, is metabolized to phenylalanine, while spirulina contains phenylalanine.

GOUT

(Diuretics, White Willow)

Patients with a history of gout should avoid using natural products containing components with diuretic action or white willow. By increasing urine output, ingredients with diuretic action may concentrate uric acid in the blood increasing the risk of gout in these patients. White willow, like aspirin, may inhibit excretion of urate resulting in an increase in uric acid concentration. The increase in urate levels could cause precipitation of uric acid resulting in an exacerbation of gout.

ALPHABETICAL LISTING OF NATURAL PRODUCTS

Aloe

Index Terms Aloe Barbadensis; Aloe Capensis; Aloe vera; Cape
Pharmacologic Category Herb; Topical Skin Product
Use Aloe has been used as an analgesic, antibacterial, antifungal, antiviral, anti-inflammatory, emollient/moisturizer, laxative, wound-healing, and hypoglycemic agent. Topical treatment of minor burns, cuts, and skin irritations, including irritant and roentgen dermatitis. Aloe has been used as an oral rinse for gums and soft tissue. Aloe has been used to reduce discomfort following oral and periodontal surgery and in reducing pain from mouth ulcers. Aloe has been shown to reduce bleeding times after dental surgery and to accelerate the healing process after surgeries. When placed over an extraction site immediately after a tooth has been removed, the application of aloe resulted in significant reduction in postoperative pain, swelling, and bleeding. Aloe promotes wound healing and shows tremendous therapeutic value in a wide variety of soft tissue injuries including tissue insults within the oral cavity. Juice may be taken internally for digestive disorders (eg, constipation, peptic ulcers, irritable bowel syndrome) and as a blood purifier; root ingested for colic. Gel used in many cosmetic and pharmaceutical formulations.
Local Anesthetic/Vasoconstrictor Precautions No information available to require special precautions
Effects on Bleeding None reported
Warnings/Precautions Use with caution in diabetics and those taking hypoglycemic agents or insulin; may lower blood sugar. Some juice products may have high sodium content. Some wound healing may be delayed when administered topically. May alter GI absorption of other herbs or drugs. Avoid other herbs with hypoglycemic or laxative properties. Chronic ingestion of juice may lead to electrolyte abnormalities, especially potassium (if not using as laxative, look for juice products that do not contain the chemical anthranoids responsible for laxative properties); should not be used as a laxative for >2 weeks.

Alpha-Lipoic Acid

Index Terms Alpha-lipoate; Lipoic Acid; Thioctic acid
Pharmacologic Category Nutritional Supplement
Use Antioxidant; treatment of diabetes, diabetic neuropathy, glaucoma; prevention of cataracts and neurologic disorders including stroke
Local Anesthetic/Vasoconstrictor Precautions No information available to require special precautions
Effects on Bleeding None reported
Warnings/Precautions Use with caution in individuals predisposed to hypoglycemia including those receiving antidiabetic agents.

Androstenedione

Index Terms Andro
Pharmacologic Category Nutraceutical
Use Androgenic, anabolic; Athletic performance and libido enhancement; believed to facilitate faster recovery from exercise, increase strength, and promote muscle development in response to training (studies inconclusive)
Local Anesthetic/Vasoconstrictor Precautions No information available to require special precautions
Effects on Bleeding None reported
Warnings/Precautions Use with caution in individuals with CHF, prostate conditions, or hormone-sensitive tumors. The FDA requires specific labeling

noting that it "contains steroid hormones that may cause breast enlargement, testicular shrinkage, and infertility in males, and increased facial/body hair, voice-deepening, and clitoral enlargement in females." Avoid herbs with hypertensive properties. Increased cancer risk, decrease in HDL cholesterol.

Angelica sinensis see Dong Quai *on page 1707*
Arctostaphylos uva-ursi see Uva Ursi *on page 1723*

Arnica

Index Terms *Arnica chamissonis*; *Arnica cordifolia*; *Arnica fulgens*; *Arnica latifolia*; *Arnica sororia*; Leopard's Bane; Mountain Daisy; Mountain Tobacco; Wolf's Bane
Pharmacologic Category Herb
Use Bruising, coagulation, diabetic retinopathy, osteoarthritis, trauma
Local Anesthetic/Vasoconstrictor Precautions May cause serious interactions with anesthetic drugs
Effects on Bleeding May see increased bleeding due to inhibition of platelet aggregation
Warnings/Precautions Avoid full strength arnica tinctures on hypersensitive or broken skin. Use with caution in individuals with a history of bleeding, hemostatic disorders, or drug-related hemostatic problems. Use with caution in individuals taking anticoagulant medications, including warfarin, aspirin, aspirin-containing products, NSAIDs, or antiplatelet agents (eg, ticlopidine, clopidogrel, dipyridamole). Discontinue use prior to dental or surgical procedures (generally at least 14 days before). Use with caution in individuals taking lipid-lowering agents. Use with caution in individuals taking anesthetic drugs.

Arnica chamissonis see Arnica *on page 1701*
Arnica cordifolia see Arnica *on page 1701*
Arnica fulgens see Arnica *on page 1701*
Arnica latifolia see Arnica *on page 1701*
Arnica sororia see Arnica *on page 1701*
Asian Ginseng see Ginseng, Panax *on page 1711*

Astragalus

Index Terms *Astragalus membranaceus*; Milk Vetch
Pharmacologic Category Herb
Use Adaptogen, antibacterial, diuretic, immunostimulant/immunosupportive, radioprotective, vasodilator; treatment of cancer (adjunct to chemotherapy/radiation), hepatitis, peripheral vascular diseases, respiratory infections; disease resistance, stamina, tissue oxygenation; promotes adrenal cortical function
Unlabeled/Investigational: Treatment of HIV/AIDS; antiaging
Local Anesthetic/Vasoconstrictor Precautions No information available to require special precautions
Effects on Bleeding Astragalus may increase the risk of bleeding.
Warnings/Precautions Use with caution in individuals with acute infection, especially when fever is present.

Astragalus membranaceus see Astragalus *on page 1701*
Awa see Kava *on page 1715*
Bachelor's Button see Feverfew *on page 1708*

Barberry

Index Terms *Berberis dumetorum*; *Berberis vulgaris*; Berberry; Pipperidge Bush
Pharmacologic Category Herb
Use Sore throat, bladder infection, bronchitis, yeast infection
Local Anesthetic/Vasoconstrictor Precautions No information available to require special precautions
Effects on Bleeding May see increased bleeding due to inhibition of platelet aggregation
Warnings/Precautions Avoid in women who are pregnant or lactating. Barberry has exhibited uterine stimulant properties, and berberine has been shown to have antifertility activity. Use with caution in individuals with cardiovascular disease; has been shown to cause hypotension and bradycardia. Use with caution in individuals with gastrointestinal disease; may irritate the gastrointestinal tract. Use with caution in individuals with kidney disease; may cause kidney irritation and nephritis.

Use with caution in individuals with a history of bleeding, hemostatic disorders, or drug-related hemostatic problems. Use with caution in individuals taking (Continued)

Barberry *(Continued)*

anticoagulant medications, including warfarin, aspirin, aspirin-containing products, NSAIDs, or antiplatelet agents (eg, ticlopidine, clopidogrel, dipyridamole). Discontinue use prior to dental or surgical procedures (generally at least 14 days before).

Bearberry *see* Uva Ursi *on page 1723*

Berberis dumetorum *see* Barberry *on page 1701*

Berberis vulgaris *see* Barberry *on page 1701*

Berberry *see* Barberry *on page 1701*

Bifidobacterium bifidum / Lactobacillus acidophilus

Related Information
Lactobacillus on page 942

Pharmacologic Category Antidiarrheal; Gastrointestinal Agent, Miscellaneous

Use Antidiarrheal, digestive aid; treatment of GI complaints.

B. bifidum: Maintenance of anaerobic microflora in the colon; treatment of Crohn's disease, diarrhea, ulcerative colitis

L. acidophilus: Recolonization of the GI tract with beneficial bacteria during and after antibiotic use; treatment of constipation, infant diarrhea, lactose intolerance

Local Anesthetic/Vasoconstrictor Precautions No information available to require special precautions

Effects on Bleeding None reported

Warnings/Precautions There are no warnings or reports of toxicity.

Bilberry

Index Terms *Vaccinium myrtillus*

Pharmacologic Category Herb

Use Anticoagulant, antioxidant; treatment of ophthalmic disorders (cataracts, diabetic retinopathy, day/night blindness, diminished visual acuity, macular degeneration, myopia) and vascular disorders (phlebitis, varicose veins); helps maintain capillary integrity and reduce hyperpermeability

Local Anesthetic/Vasoconstrictor Precautions No information available to require special precautions

Effects on Bleeding May see increased bleeding due to inhibition of platelet aggregation

Warnings/Precautions Use with caution in diabetics (may lower blood sugar), individuals with a history of bleeding, hemostatic or drug-related hemostatic disorders, those taking anticoagulants (eg, aspirin or aspirin-containing products, NSAIDs, and warfarin) or antiplatelet agents (eg, ticlopidine, clopidogrel, and dipyridamole), hypoglycemic agents or insulin. Avoid other herbs with anticoagulant/antiplatelet and/or hypoglycemic properties. May alter absorption of calcium, copper, magnesium, and zinc due to tannins. Discontinue at least 14 days prior to dental or surgical procedures.

Black Cohosh

Index Terms *Cimicifuga racemosa*

Pharmacologic Category Herb

Use Analgesic, anti-inflammatory, phytoestrogenic; treatment of rheumatoid arthritis, mild depression, vasomotor symptoms of menopause and premenstrual syndrome (PMS)

Local Anesthetic/Vasoconstrictor Precautions No information available to require special precautions

Effects on Bleeding None reported

Warnings/Precautions Use with caution in individuals taking hormonal contraceptives or receiving hormone replacement therapy (HRT), those with endometrial cancer, history of estrogen-dependent tumors, hypotension, thromboembolic disease, stroke, or salicylate allergy (unknown whether amount of salicylic acid may affect platelet aggregation or have other effects associated with salicylates). Monitor serum hormone levels after 6 months of therapy. Avoid other hypotensive or phytoestrogenic herbs.

Black Susans *see* Echinacea *on page 1707*

Bladderwrack

Index Terms *Fucus vesiculosus*
Pharmacologic Category Herb
Use Rich source of iodine, potassium, magnesium, calcium, and iron; hypothyroidism; fibrocystic breast disease (Bradley, 1992)
Effects on Bleeding May see increased bleeding due to anticoagulant properties.
Warnings/Precautions Use all herbal supplements with extreme caution in children <2 years of age and in pregnancy or lactation. Some herbs are contraindicated in pregnancy or lactation; make sure to observe warnings. Use with caution in individuals on medication and with pre-existing medical conditions. Always review for potential herb-drug interactions (HDIs) and other warnings. Large and prolonged doses may increase the potential for adverse effects. Herbs may cause transient adverse effects such as nausea, vomiting, and GI distress due to a variety of chemical constituents. Caution should be used in individuals having known allergies to plants.

Blue-Green Algae *see* Spirulina *on page 1722*

BN-52063 *see* Ginkgo Biloba *on page 1710*

Bromelain

Index Terms *Anas comosus*
Pharmacologic Category Herb
Use Anticoagulant, anti-inflammatory, digestive aid; treatment of arthritis, dyspepsia, sinusitis
Local Anesthetic/Vasoconstrictor Precautions No information available to require special precautions
Effects on Bleeding May cause increased bleeding due to inhibition of platelet aggregation
Warnings/Precautions Use with caution in individuals with cardiovascular disease (eg, CHF, hypertension), GI ulceration, history of bleeding, hemostatic or drug-related hemostatic disorders, those taking anticoagulants (eg, aspirin or aspirin-containing products, NSAIDs, warfarin), or antiplatelet agents (eg, ticlopidine, clopidogrel, dipyridamole). Avoid other herbs with anticoagulant/antiplatelet properties. Discontinue at least 14 days prior to dental or surgical procedures.

Calendula

Index Terms *Calendula officinalis*
Pharmacologic Category Herb
Use Analgesic, anti-inflammatory, antimicrobial (antibacterial, antifungal, antiviral), antiprotozoal, antiseptic, antispasmodic, immunostimulant, wound-healing agent; treatment of minor burns, cuts, and other skin irritation
Local Anesthetic/Vasoconstrictor Precautions No information available to require special precautions
Effects on Bleeding None reported
Warnings/Precautions Use with caution in individuals with plant allergies.

Calendula officinalis see Calendula *on page 1703*

Camellia sinensis see Green Tea *on page 1713*

Cape *see* Aloe *on page 1700*

Capsicum annuum see Cayenne *on page 1704*

Capsicum frutescens see Cayenne *on page 1704*

Carnitine

Index Terms L-Carnitine
Pharmacologic Category Amino Acid
Use Treatment of CHF, hyperlipidemia, male infertility; athletic performance enhancement, weight loss
Local Anesthetic/Vasoconstrictor Precautions No information available to require special precautions
Effects on Bleeding None reported
Warnings/Precautions L-carnitine appears to be safe; there are no reports of toxicity due to overdosing. Avoid D- or D,L-carnitine since this form can interfere (Continued)

Carnitine *(Continued)*

with the body's own production of L-carnitine and can produce a relative carnitine deficiency. Carnitine should not be used by people with cardiovascular diseases.

Cascara

Index Terms Cascara Sagrada

Pharmacologic Category Laxative

Use Temporary relief of constipation; sometimes used with milk of magnesia ("black and white" mixture)

Local Anesthetic/Vasoconstrictor Precautions No information available to require special precautions

Effects on Bleeding None reported

Warnings/Precautions Excessive use can lead to electrolyte imbalance, fluid imbalance, vitamin deficiency, steatorrhea, osteomalacia, cathartic colon, and dependence; should be avoided during nursing because it may have a laxative effect on the infant

Cascara Sagrada *see* Cascara *on page 1704*

Cat's Claw

Index Terms *Uncaria tomentosa*

Pharmacologic Category Herb

Use Anticoagulant, anti-inflammatory, antimicrobial (antibacterial, antifungal, antiviral), antiplatelet, antioxidant, immunosupportive; treatment of allergies and minor infections or inflammatory conditions

Local Anesthetic/Vasoconstrictor Precautions No information available to require special precautions

Effects on Bleeding May cause increased bleeding due to inhibition of platelet aggregation

Warnings/Precautions Use with caution in individuals taking anticoagulants (eg, aspirin or aspirin-containing products, NSAIDs, warfarin) or antiplatelet agents (eg, clopidogrel, dipyridamole, ticlopidine), therapeutic immunosuppression or I.V. immunoglobulin therapy (eg, transplant recipients), those with a history of bleeding, and hemostatic or drug-related hemostatic disorders. Avoid other herbs with anticoagulant/antiplatelet properties. Discontinue at least 14 days prior to dental or surgical procedures.

Cayenne

Related Information

Capsaicin *on page 268*

Index Terms *Capsicum annuum*; *Capsicum frutescens*

Pharmacologic Category Herb

Use Analgesic, anti-inflammatory, digestive stimulant, sympathomimetic; treatment of arthritis (osteo and rheumatoid), diabetic neuropathy, postmastectomy pain syndrome, postherpetic neuralgia, pruritus, psoriasis; appetite suppressant, bronchial relaxation, cardiovascular circulatory support, decongestant

Local Anesthetic/Vasoconstrictor Precautions No information available to require special precautions

Effects on Bleeding None reported

Warnings/Precautions Use with caution in individuals with GI ulceration, hypertension, and those taking MAO inhibitors. May alter GI absorption of other herbs or drugs; avoid other herbs with hypertensive or sympathomimetic properties.

Centella asiatica see Gotu Kola *on page 1712*

Chamomile

Index Terms *Matricaria chamomilla*; *Matricaria recutita*

Pharmacologic Category Herb

Use Antibacterial, anti-inflammatory, antispasmodic, antiulcer agent, anxiolytic, appetite stimulant, carminative, digestive aid, sedative (mild); treatment of eczema and psoriasis, hemorrhoids, inflammatory skin conditions, indigestion and irritable bowel syndrome (IBS), insomnia, leg ulcers, mastitis, premenstrual syndrome (PMS)

Local Anesthetic/Vasoconstrictor Precautions No information available to require special precautions

Effects on Bleeding None reported

Warnings/Precautions Use with caution in individuals with allergies and asthma (cross sensitivity may occur in those with allergies to asters, chrysanthemums, daisies, feverfew, sunflowers, or ragweed), and those taking anticoagulants, antiplatelets, and sedatives. Avoid other herbs with allergenic, anticoagulant, or antiplatelet properties.

Chasteberry

Index Terms Chastetree; *Vitex agnus-castus*

Pharmacologic Category Herb

Use Treatment of acne vulgaris, amenorrhea, corpus luteum insufficiency, endometriosis, hyperprolactinemia, lactation insufficiency, menopausal symptoms, premenstrual syndrome [PMS]

Local Anesthetic/Vasoconstrictor Precautions No information available to require special precautions

Effects on Bleeding None reported

Warnings/Precautions Use with caution in individuals taking hormonal contraceptives or receiving hormone replacement therapy (HRT). Avoid other phytoprogestogenic herbs.

Chastetree *see* Chasteberry *on page 1705*

Chinese angelica *see* Dong Quai *on page 1707*

Chondroitin Sulfate

Pharmacologic Category Nutraceutical

Use Treatment of osteoarthritis

Local Anesthetic/Vasoconstrictor Precautions No information available to require special precautions

Effects on Bleeding None reported

Warnings/Precautions No known toxicity or serious side effects

Chromium

Related Information
Trace Metals *on page 1595*

Pharmacologic Category Nutraceutical

Use Treatment of hyper- and hypoglycemia, hyperlipidemia, hypercholesterolemia, obesity

Local Anesthetic/Vasoconstrictor Precautions No information available to require special precautions

Effects on Bleeding None reported

Warnings/Precautions There are no warnings or reports of toxicity when taken according to manufacturer's labeled instructions.

Cimicifuga racemosa see Black Cohosh *on page 1702*

Citrus paradisi see Grapefruit Seed *on page 1712*

Cloud Mushroom *see* Maitake *on page 1716*

Coenzyme 1 *see* Nicotinamide Adenine Dinucleotide *on page 1718*

Coenzyme Q₁₀

Index Terms CoQ₁₀; Ubiquinone

Pharmacologic Category Nutraceutical

Use Antioxidant; treatment of angina, breast cancer, cardiovascular diseases (eg, CHF), chronic fatigue syndrome, diabetes, hypertension, muscular dystrophy, obesity, periodontal disease

Local Anesthetic/Vasoconstrictor Precautions No information available to require special precautions

Effects on Bleeding None reported

Warnings/Precautions Avoid other agents with hypoglycemic properties.

Comb Flower *see* Echinacea *on page 1707*

Comphor of the Poor *see* Garlic *on page 1709*

CoQ₁₀ *see* Coenzyme Q₁₀ *on page 1705*

Cranberry

Index Terms *Vaccinium macrocarpon*
Pharmacologic Category Herb
Use Treatment of urinary tract infection and prevention of nephrolithiasis
Local Anesthetic/Vasoconstrictor Precautions No information available to require special precautions
Effects on Bleeding None reported
Warnings/Precautions There are no warnings or reports of toxicity.

Crataegus laevigata see Hawthorn *on page 1713*
Crataegus monogyna see Hawthorn *on page 1713*
Crataegus oxyacantha see Hawthorn *on page 1713*
Crataegus pinnatifida see Hawthorn *on page 1713*

Creatine

Pharmacologic Category Nutraceutical
Use Athletic performance enhancement, energy production, and protein synthesis for muscle building
Local Anesthetic/Vasoconstrictor Precautions No information available to require special precautions
Effects on Bleeding None reported
Warnings/Precautions There are no warnings or reports of toxicity when taken according to manufacturer's labeled instructions.

Curcuma longa see Turmeric *on page 1723*
Cyanobacteria *see* Spirulina *on page 1722*

Damiana

Index Terms Herba de la Pastora; Mexican Damiana; Mizibcoc; Old Woman's Broom; *Turnera aphrodisiaca*; *Turnera diffusa*
Pharmacologic Category Herb
Use Female sexual dysfunction, weight loss/obesity
Local Anesthetic/Vasoconstrictor Precautions No information available to require special precautions
Effects on Bleeding None reported
Warnings/Precautions Avoid in individuals with Alzheimer's disease or Parkinson's disease; ethanol extracts of the leaves and stem have exhibited CNS depressant activity. Use with caution in individuals with a history of breast cancer; may interact with progesterone receptors on cells. Use with caution in individuals with psychiatric disorders; may cause hallucinations and mood changes. Use with caution in individuals with diabetes or in those taking medications to control blood sugar levels; may affect blood sugar levels.

Dancing Mushroom *see* Maitake *on page 1716*

Dehydroepiandrosterone

Index Terms DHEA
Pharmacologic Category Nutraceutical
Use Antiaging; treatment of depression, diabetes, fatigue, lupus
Local Anesthetic/Vasoconstrictor Precautions No information available to require special precautions
Effects on Bleeding None reported
Warnings/Precautions Use with caution in individuals with diabetes, hepatic dysfunction, or those predisposed to hypoglycemia (monitor blood glucose and dosage of antidiabetic agents). Avoid other agents with hypoglycemic properties.

Devil's Claw

Index Terms *Harpagophytum procumbens*
Pharmacologic Category Herb
Use Anti-inflammatory, cardiotonic; treatment of back pain, gout, osteoarthritis, and other inflammatory conditions
Local Anesthetic/Vasoconstrictor Precautions No information available to require special precautions

Effects on Bleeding May see increased bleeding due to inhibition of platelet aggregation

Warnings/Precautions Use with caution in individuals with history of bleeding, hemostatic or drug-related hemostatic disorders, and those taking anticoagulants (eg, aspirin or aspirin-containing products, NSAIDs, warfarin) or antiplatelet agents (eg, clopidogrel, dipyridamole, ticlopidine), antiarrhythmic agents, or cardiac glycosides (eg, digoxin). Avoid herbs with anticoagulant/antiplatelet properties. Discontinue at least 14 days prior to dental or surgical procedures.

DHA *see* Docosahexaenoic Acid *on page 1707*

DHEA *see* Dehydroepiandrosterone *on page 1706*

Dimethyl Sulfone *see* Methyl Sulfonyl Methane *on page 1717*

Dioscorea villosa see Wild Yam *on page 1724*

DMSO₂ *see* Methyl Sulfonyl Methane *on page 1717*

Docosahexaenoic Acid

Index Terms DHA

Pharmacologic Category Nutraceutical

Use Treatment of Alzheimer's disease, attention deficit disorder (ADD) and attention deficit hyperactivity disorder (ADHD), Crohn's disease, diabetes, eczema and psoriasis, hypertension, hypertriglyceridemia, and rheumatoid arthritis; coronary heart disease risk reduction

Local Anesthetic/Vasoconstrictor Precautions No information available to require special precautions

Effects on Bleeding None reported

Warnings/Precautions Use caution with individuals taking anticoagulants (eg, aspirin or aspirin-containing products, NSAIDs, warfarin) or antiplatelet agents (eg, clopidogrel, dipyridamole, ticlopidine), insulin or oral hypoglycemics. Avoid herbs with anticoagulant/antiplatelet properties; may intensify the blood-thinning effect

Dong Quai

Index Terms *Angelica sinensis*; Chinese angelica

Pharmacologic Category Herb

Use Anabolic, anticoagulant; treatment of amenorrhea, anemia, dysmenorrhea, hypertension, menopausal symptoms, premenstrual syndrome (PMS); female vitality

Local Anesthetic/Vasoconstrictor Precautions No information available to require special precautions

Effects on Bleeding Has potential for decreasing platelet aggregation and may increase bleeding

Warnings/Precautions May alter hemostasis, potentiate effects of warfarin, and/or cause photosensitization; use with caution in lactation, pregnancy, cardiovascular or cerebrovascular disease, endometrial cancer, estrogen-dependent tumors, hemostatic or drug-related hemostatic disorders, history of bleeding, hypotension, stroke, thromboembolic disease, and individuals taking anticoagulants (eg, aspirin or aspirin-containing products, NSAIDs, warfarin), antiplatelet agents (eg, clopidogrel, dipyridamole, ticlopidine), antihypertensive medications, hormonal contraceptives or hormone replacement therapy (HRT), or steroids. Avoid other herbs with anabolic, anticoagulant, or antiplatelet properties. Discontinue at least 14 days prior to dental or surgical procedures.

Echinacea

Index Terms American Coneflower; Black Susans; Comb Flower; *Echinacea angustifolia*; *Echinacea purpurea*; Indian Head; Purple Coneflower; Scury Root; Snakeroot

Pharmacologic Category Herb

Use Antibacterial, antihyaluronidase, anti-infective, anti-inflammatory, antiviral, immunostimulant, wound-healing agent; treatment of arthritis, chronic skin complaints, cold, flu, sore throat, tonsillitis, minor upper respiratory tract infections, urinary tract infections

Local Anesthetic/Vasoconstrictor Precautions No information available to require special precautions

Effects on Bleeding None reported

Warnings/Precautions Use as a preventative treatment should be discouraged; may alter immunosuppression; long-term use may cause immunosuppression. Individuals allergic to asters, chamomile, chrysanthemums, daisies, (Continued)

Echinacea (Continued)

feverfew, sunflowers, or ragweed may display cross-allergy potential (rare but severe); avoid other allergenic herbs. Use with caution in individuals with renal impairment.

Evening Primrose

Index Terms Evening Primrose Oil; *Oenothera biennis*

Pharmacologic Category Herb

Use Anticoagulant, anti-inflammatory, hormone stimulant; treatment of atopic eczema and psoriasis, attention deficit disorder (ADD) and attention deficit hyperactivity disorder (ADHD), dermatitis, diabetic neuropathy, endometriosis, hyperglycemia, irritable bowel syndrome (IBS), multiple sclerosis (MS), omega-6 fatty acid supplementation, premenstrual syndrome (PMS), menopausal symptoms, rheumatoid arthritis

Local Anesthetic/Vasoconstrictor Precautions No information available to require special precautions

Effects on Bleeding May see increased bleeding due to inhibition of platelet aggregation

Warnings/Precautions Use with caution in individuals with a history of bleeding, hemostatic or drug-related hemostatic disorders, those taking anticoagulants (eg, aspirin or aspirin-containing products, NSAIDs, warfarin) or antiplatelet agents (eg, clopidogrel, dipyridamole, ticlopidine). Avoid other herbs with anticoagulant/antiplatelet properties. Discontinue at least 14 days prior to dental or surgical procedures.

Fennel

Index Terms Fenkel; *Foeniculum officinale*; *Foeniculum vulgare* Mill.; Sweet Fennel; Wild Fennel

Pharmacologic Category Herb

Use ACE inhibitor-associated cough; colic, infantile; dysmenorrhea; ultraviolet skin protection

Local Anesthetic/Vasoconstrictor Precautions No information available to require special precautions

Effects on Bleeding May see increased bleeding

Warnings/Precautions Use with caution in individuals with diabetes or in those taking antidiabetic agents. Fennel preparations, other than fennel seed infusions and fennel honey, should be avoided in infants and toddlers. Use with caution in individuals with a history of bleeding, hemostatic disorders, or drug-related hemostatic problems. Use with caution in individuals taking anticoagulant medications, including warfarin, aspirin, aspirin-containing products, NSAIDs, or antiplatelet agents (eg, ticlopidine, clopidogrel, dipyridamole). Discontinue use prior to dental or surgical procedures (generally at least 14 days before).

Feverfew

Index Terms Altamisa; Bachelor's Button; Featherfew; Featherfoil; Nosebleed; *Tanacetum parthenium*; Wild Quinine

Pharmacologic Category Herb

Use Anticoagulant/anti-inflammatory, antiprostaglandin, antispasmodic, digestive aid, emmenagogue, sedative; prophylaxis and treatment of migraine headaches and rheumatoid arthritis; treatment of fever, hypertension, premenstrual syndrome (PMS), tinnitus

Local Anesthetic/Vasoconstrictor Precautions No information available to require special precautions

Effects on Bleeding May see increased bleeding due to inhibition of platelet aggregation

Warnings/Precautions Use with caution in individuals with a history of bleeding, hemostatic disorders or drug-related hemostatic problems, and those taking anticoagulants (eg, aspirin or aspirin-containing products, NSAIDs, warfarin), antiplatelet agents (eg, clopidogrel, dipyridamole, ticlopidine), or medications with serotonergic properties. Abrupt discontinuation may increase migraine frequency. May alter absorption of calcium, copper, magnesium, and zinc due to tannins. Avoid other herbs with allergenic, anticoagulant, or anti-platelet properties. Discontinue at least 14 days prior to dental or surgical procedures.

Fish Oil *see* Omega-3-Acid Ethyl Esters *on page 1718*

Flaxseed Oil

Index Terms ALA; Alpha-linolenic Acid
Pharmacologic Category Nutraceutical
Use Antioxidant, antiatherogenic; treatment of eczema and psoriasis, hypertension, hypercholesterolemia, hypertriglyceridemia; contains 3 times more omega-3 than omega-6 and may be used to help reverse the imbalance between omega-3 and omega-6 (estimated optimal ratio between omega-3 and omega-6 fatty acids is about 1:4 and ratio for many in U.S. is 1:20 to 1:30)

Local Anesthetic/Vasoconstrictor Precautions No information available to require special precautions

Effects on Bleeding None reported

Warnings/Precautions Use with caution in individuals with plant allergies, those taking anticoagulants (eg, aspirin or aspirin-containing products, NSAIDs, warfarin) or antiplatelet agents (eg, clopidogrel, dipyridamole, ticlopidine), insulin or oral hypoglycemics. Avoid herbs with allergenic, anticoagulant, or antiplatelet properties; may intensify the blood-thinning effect.

Foeniculum officinale *see* Fennel *on page 1708*
Foeniculum vulgare Mill. *see* Fennel *on page 1708*
French Maritime Pine Bark Extract *see* Pycnogenol *on page 1719*
Fucus vesiculosus *see* Bladderwrack *on page 1703*

Gamma Linolenic Acid

Index Terms GLA; Omega-6 Fatty Acids
Pharmacologic Category Nutraceutical
Use Acute respiratory distress syndrome, atopic dermatitis, attention-deficit hyperactivity disorder, blood pressure control, cancer treatment, diabetic neuropathy, immune enhancement, mastalgia, menopausal hot flashes, migraine, osteoporosis, pre-eclampsia, premenstrual syndrome, pruritus, rheumatoid arthritis, Sjogren's syndrome, ulcerative colitis

Local Anesthetic/Vasoconstrictor Precautions No information available to require special precautions

Effects on Bleeding None reported

Warnings/Precautions Contraindicated in individuals with active bleeding (eg, peptic ulcer, intracranial bleeding). Use with caution in individuals with a history of bleeding, hemostatic disorders, or drug-related hemostatic problems. Use with caution in individuals taking anticoagulant medications, including warfarin, aspirin, aspirin-containing products, NSAIDs, or antiplatelet agents (eg, ticlopidine, clopidogrel, dipyridamole). Discontinue use prior to dental or surgical procedures (generally at least 14 days before.)

Garlic

Index Terms *Allium savitum*; Comphor of the Poor; Nectar of the Gods; Poor Mans Treacle; Rustic Treacle; Stinking Rose
Pharmacologic Category Herb
Use Antibiotic, anticoagulant/antiplatelet (potent), anti-inflammatory, antioxidant (aged extract improves benefits), antitumor agent, immunosupportive; treatment of hypercholesterolemia, hypertension, hypertriglyceridemia, hypoglycemia; may decrease thrombosis

Local Anesthetic/Vasoconstrictor Precautions No information available to require special precautions

Effects on Bleeding May see increased bleeding due to potent platelet inhibition

(Continued)

Garlic *(Continued)*

Warnings/Precautions Use with caution in diabetics (may lower blood sugar), individuals taking anticoagulants (eg, aspirin or aspirin-containing products, NSAIDs, warfarin), antihypertensives, antiplatelet agents (eg, clopidogrel, dipyridamole, ticlopidine), hypoglycemic agents or insulin, hypolipidemic agents, and those with a history of bleeding, hemostatic or drug-related hemostatic disorders; may cause GI distress in sensitive individuals. Avoid other herbs with allergenic, anticoagulant/antiplatelet, hypoglycemic, or hypolipidemic properties. Discontinue at least 14 days prior to dental or surgical procedures.

GBE *see* Ginkgo Biloba *on page 1710*

Ge-gen *see* Kudzu *on page 1715*

Giant Hyssop Herb *see* Hyssop *on page 1714*

Ginger

Index Terms *Zingiber officinale*

Pharmacologic Category Herb

Use Analgesic, anticoagulant, antiemetic (lack of sedative effects is advantageous over other antiemetics), anti-inflammatory (musculoskeletal), digestive aid; treatment of amenorrhea (Chinese remedy), arthritis, colds, culinary herb, dyspepsia, flu, headaches, motion sickness, nausea/vomiting (eg, from chemotherapy/radiation)

Local Anesthetic/Vasoconstrictor Precautions No information available to require special precautions

Effects on Bleeding Very high doses may inhibit platelet aggregation.

Warnings/Precautions Use with caution in diabetics, individuals with a history of bleeding, hemostatic or drug-related hemostatic disorders, those taking anticoagulants (eg, aspirin or aspirin-containing products, NSAIDs, warfarin), antiplatelet agents (eg, clopidogrel, dipyridamole, ticlopidine), cardiac glycosides (eg, digoxin), hypolipidemic agents, hypoglycemic agents, or insulin. Has cardioactive constituents; avoid large and/or prolonged doses. Avoid other herbs with anticoagulant/antiplatelet, hypertensive, hyperlipidemic, or hypoglycemic properties. Discontinue at least 14 days prior to dental or surgical procedures.

Ginkgo Biloba

Index Terms BN-52063; EGb; GBE; ginkgold; Ginkgopowder; Ginkogink; Kaveri; Kew Tree; Maidenhair Tree; Oriental Plum Tree; Rökan; Silver Apricot; Superginkgo; Tanakan; Tanakene; Tebonin; Tramisal; Valverde; Vasan; Vital

Pharmacologic Category Herb

Use Anticoagulant/antiplatelet, antioxidant

Per Commission E: Treatment of primary degenerative dementia, vascular dementia, and demential syndromes (eg, memory deficit), depressive emotional conditions, headache, and tinnitus

Treatment of Alzheimer's disease, arterial insufficiency and intermittent claudication (European remedy), cerebral vascular disease (dementia), macular degeneration, resistant depression, traumatic brain injury, tinnitus, visual disorders, vertigo of vascular origin

Local Anesthetic/Vasoconstrictor Precautions No information available to require special precautions

Effects on Bleeding May see increased bleeding due to inhibition of platelet aggregation; antagonizes platelet activating factor (PAF)

Warnings/Precautions Use with caution in individuals with a history of bleeding, hemostatic drug-related hemostatic disorders, those taking anticoagulants (eg, aspirin or aspirin-containing products, NSAIDs, warfarin) or antiplatelet agents (eg, clopidogrel, dipyridamole, ticlopidine), and MAO inhibitors. Cross reactivity for contact dermatitis (due to fruit pulp) exists with poison ivy and poison oak; may last for 10 days (washing skin within 10 minutes may prevent reaction or topical corticosteroids may be helpful). Fruit pulp contains ginkolic acids which are allergens (seeds are not sensitizing). Admit individuals with neurologic abnormalities after ingestion or ingestions >2 pieces of fruit; pyridoxine may be useful after ingestion of ginkgo seeds or kernels. Avoid other herbs with anticoagulant/antiplatelet properties. Discontinue at least 2-3 weeks prior to surgery; use with caution following recent surgery or trauma.

ginkgold *see* Ginkgo Biloba *on page 1710*

Ginkgopowder *see* Ginkgo Biloba *on page 1710*

Ginkogink *see* Ginkgo Biloba *on page 1710*

Ginseng, Panax

Index Terms Asian Ginseng; *Panax ginseng*
Pharmacologic Category Herb
Use Adaptogen, adrenal tonic, anticoagulant, cardiotonic, hormone stimulant, immunostimulant; support in chemotherapy and radiation (decreases weight loss), postsurgical recovery (stabilize white blood cell counts), endurance
Local Anesthetic/Vasoconstrictor Precautions Has potential to interact with epinephrine and levonordefrin to result in increased BP; use vasoconstrictor with caution
Effects on Bleeding May have antiplatelet effects
Warnings/Precautions Use with caution in elderly or individuals with cardiovascular disease (eg, hypertension), history of bleeding, hemostatic or drug-related hemostatic disorders, and those receiving anticoagulants (eg, aspirin or aspirin-containing products, NSAIDs, warfarin) or antiplatelet agents (eg, clopidogrel, dipyridamole, ticlopidine), hormonal contraceptives, MAO inhibitors, stimulants (eg, OTC decongestants, caffeine), and those receiving hormonal replacement therapy (HRT). May cause "Ginseng Abuse Syndrome"; monitor for signs/symptoms. Avoid other herbs with allergenic, anticoagulant/antiplatelet or hypertensive properties. Discontinue at least 14 days prior to dental or surgical procedures.

Ginseng, Siberian

Index Terms *Eleutherococcus senticosus*; Siberian Ginseng
Pharmacologic Category Herb
Use Adaptogen, anticoagulant, antiviral, immunosupportive; treatment of arteriosclerosis, chronic inflammatory disease, diabetes, hypertension; adaptation to stress, athletic performance enhancement, energy production
Local Anesthetic/Vasoconstrictor Precautions Has potential to interact with epinephrine and levonordefrin to result in increased BP; use vasoconstrictor with caution
Effects on Bleeding May have antiplatelet effects
Warnings/Precautions Use with caution in the elderly or individuals with cardiovascular disease (eg, CHF, hypertension), history of bleeding, hemostatic or drug-related hemostatic disorders, those taking anticoagulants (eg, aspirin or aspirin-containing products, NSAIDs, warfarin) or antiplatelet agents (eg, clopidogrel, dipyridamole, ticlopidine), antihypertensive agents, digoxin, hexobarbital, hypoglycemic agents or insulin, and steroids. Extensive or prolonged use may heighten estrogenic activity. Avoid other herbs with allergenic, anabolic, anticoagulant/antiplatelet, or hypertensive properties. Discontinue at least 14 days prior to dental or surgical procedures.

GLA *see* Gamma Linolenic Acid *on page 1709*

Glucosamine

Index Terms Glucosamine Hydrochloride; Glucosamine Sulfate
Pharmacologic Category Nutraceutical
Use Treatment of bursitis, gout, osteoarthritis, rheumatoid arthritis, tendonitis
Local Anesthetic/Vasoconstrictor Precautions No information available to require special precautions
Effects on Bleeding None reported
Warnings/Precautions Use with caution in diabetics (may cause insulin resistance) and those taking oral anticoagulants (may increase effect). Avoid other herbs with hyperglycemic properties.

Glucosamine Hydrochloride *see* Glucosamine *on page 1711*
Glucosamine Sulfate *see* Glucosamine *on page 1711*

Glutathione

Index Terms L-Glutathione
Pharmacologic Category Nutraceutical
Use Peptic ulcer diseases; support of immune function; hepatoprotection
Local Anesthetic/Vasoconstrictor Precautions No information available to require special precautions
Effects on Bleeding None reported
Warnings/Precautions There are no warnings or reports of toxicity.

Glycocome *see* Licorice *on page 1716*

Glycyrrhiza glabra *see* Licorice *on page 1716*

Goatweed *see* St John's Wort *on page 1722*

Golden Seal

Index Terms Eye Balm; Eye Root; *Hydrastis canadensis*; Indian Eye; Jaundice Root; Orange Root; Turmeric Root; Yellow Indian Paint; Yellow Root

Pharmacologic Category Herb

Use Antibacterial, antifungal, anti-inflammatory, coagulant; treatment of bronchitis, cystitis, gastritis, infectious diarrhea, inflammation of mucosal membranes, hemorrhoids, postpartum hemorrhage

Local Anesthetic/Vasoconstrictor Precautions No information available to require special precautions

Effects on Bleeding None reported

Warnings/Precautions Efficacy not established in clinical studies. High doses (2-3 g) may cause hypotension or GI distress; toxic doses (18 g) reported to induce CNS depression. Overdose associated with myocardial damage and respiratory failure; extended use of high doses associated with delirium, GI disorders, hallucinations, and neuroexcitation. May alter liver enzymes. Use with caution in individuals with history of bleeding, hemostatic or drug-related hemostatic disorders, hypotension, those taking anticoagulants (aspirin or aspirin-containing products, NSAIDs, and warfarin) or antiplatelet agents (ticlopidine, clopidogrel, and dipyridamole). Avoid other herbs with coagulant or hypotensive properties.

Gotu Kola

Index Terms *Centella asiatica*

Pharmacologic Category Herb

Use Diuretic (mild), sedative (high doses), thermogenic, thyroid-stimulant, wound-healing agent; treatment of hemorrhoids, hypertension, poor circulation, psoriasis, tumors, varicose veins, venous insufficiency, and wounds from infection, inflammation, trauma, or surgery (scar reduction); memory enhancement; modulation/support of connective tissue synthesis; Ayurvedic medicine uses for revitalizing nerves and brain cells; Eastern healers use for emotional disorders (eg, depression) thought to be rooted in physical problems; alcoholic extract was used to treat leprosy in Western medicine

Local Anesthetic/Vasoconstrictor Precautions No information available to require special precautions

Effects on Bleeding None reported

Warnings/Precautions Advise caution when driving or operating machinery; large doses may be sedating. Use with caution in individuals taking sedatives (eg, anxiolytics, benzodiazepines); effects may be additive with other CNS depressants. Topical administration may cause contact dermatitis in sensitive individuals. High or prolonged doses may elevate cholesterol levels. Avoid other allergenic, hyperglycemic, or thyroid-stimulating herbs.

Grapefruit Seed

Index Terms *Citrus paradisi*; GSE

Pharmacologic Category Herb

Use Antibiotic, antimycotic, antiparasitic, antiprotozoan, antimicrobial (antibacterial, antifungal, antiviral), disinfectant, immunostimulant; treatment of GI complaints, herpes, various bacterial and fungal infections (eg, *Candida albicans*, *Salmonella*), inflammatory conditions of the gums, parasites; facial cleanser, water disinfectant; used topically for antifungal and antibiotic effects

Local Anesthetic/Vasoconstrictor Precautions No information available to require special precautions

Effects on Bleeding None reported

Warnings/Precautions GSE is not the equivalent of grapefruit juice but since grapefruit juice/pulp has been associated with the inhibition of drug metabolism via cytochrome P450 isoenzyme 3A4 (CYP3A4), resulting in a number of drug interactions, it is reasonable to avoid the concurrent use of grapefruit seed extract in individuals receiving astemizole, cisapride, terfenadine and other medications metabolized by this pathway.

Grape Seed

Index Terms *Vitis vinifera*
Pharmacologic Category Herb
Use Anticoagulant/antiplatelet, anti-inflammatory, antioxidant (potent), and source of potent free radical scavengers; treatment of allergies and asthma, arterial/venous insufficiency (capillary fragility, intermittent claudication, poor circulation, varicose veins); improves peripheral circulation; treatment of gingivitis
Local Anesthetic/Vasoconstrictor Precautions No information available to require special precautions
Effects on Bleeding May see increase in bleeding due to inhibition of platelet aggregation
Warnings/Precautions Use with caution in individuals with history of bleeding, hemostatic or drug-related hemostatic problems, those taking anticoagulants (eg, aspirin or aspirin-containing products, NSAIDs, warfarin) or antiplatelet agents (eg, clopidogrel, dipyridamole, ticlopidine). Avoid other herbs with anticoagulant/antiplatelet properties. May alter absorption of calcium, copper, magnesium, and zinc due to tannins. Discontinue use at least 14 days before dental or surgical procedures.

Grape Skin

Index Terms Resveratrol
Pharmacologic Category Herb
Use Antioxidant; cardioprotectant; antiplatelet
Local Anesthetic/Vasoconstrictor Precautions No information available to require special precautions
Effects on Bleeding May see increased bleeding due to inhibition of platelet aggregation
Warnings/Precautions None reported

Green Tea

Index Terms *Camellia sinensis*
Pharmacologic Category Herb
Use Antibacterial, anticarcinogen, antioxidant, astringent, anticoagulant/antiplatelet, antifungal, antiviral, diuretic, immunosupportive; prophylaxis and treatment of cancer, cardiovascular disease, hypercholesterolemia
Local Anesthetic/Vasoconstrictor Precautions No information available to require special precautions
Effects on Bleeding May see increased bleeding due to inhibition of platelet aggregation
Warnings/Precautions Use caffeinated products with caution in individuals with cardiovascular disease, peptic ulcer, and those taking other stimulants (eg, decongestants). Use with caution in individuals with a history of bleeding, hemostatic or drug-related hemostatic disorders, those taking anticoagulants (aspirin or aspirin-containing products, NSAIDs, warfarin) or antiplatelet agents (eg, ticlopidine, clopidogrel, dipyridamole). Addition of milk to any tea may significantly lower antioxidant potential. May alter absorption of calcium, copper, magnesium, and zinc due to tannins. Avoid other herbs with anticoagulant/antiplatelet properties. Discontinue at least 14 days prior to dental or surgical procedures.

Grey Elm *see* Slippery Elm *on page 1721*
Grifola frondosa see Maitake *on page 1716*
GSE *see* Grapefruit Seed *on page 1712*
Harpagophytum procumbens see Devil's Claw *on page 1706*
Haw *see* Hawthorn *on page 1713*

Hawthorn

Index Terms *Crataegus laevigata*; *Crataegus monogyna*; *Crataegus oxyacantha*; *Crataegus pinnatifida*; English Hawthorn; Haw; Maybush; Whitehorn
Pharmacologic Category Herb
Use Cardiotonic, sedative, vasodilator; treatment of cardiovascular abnormalities (eg, arrhythmia, angina, CHF, hyper- or hypotension, peripheral vascular diseases, tachycardia); used synergistically with digoxin (Europe)
Local Anesthetic/Vasoconstrictor Precautions No information available to require special precautions
(Continued)

Hawthorn *(Continued)*

Effects on Bleeding None reported

Warnings/Precautions Use with caution in individuals taking ACE inhibitors and antihypertensive agents (may lower BP further). Avoid other herbs with hypotensive properties.

Herba de la Pastora *see* Damiana *on page 1706*

Holy Herb *see* Hyssop *on page 1714*

Horse Chestnut

Index Terms *Aesculus hippocastanum*

Pharmacologic Category Herb

Use Analgesic, anticoagulant/antiplatelet, anti-inflammatory, cardiotonic, sedative, wound-healing agent; treatment of varicose veins, hemorrhoids, other venous insufficiencies, deep vein thrombosis, lower extremity edema

Local Anesthetic/Vasoconstrictor Precautions No information available to require special precautions

Effects on Bleeding Inhibits platelet aggregation; may see increased bleeding

Warnings/Precautions Use with caution in individuals with a history of bleeding, hemostatic or drug-related hemostatic disorders, hepatic or renal impairment, and those taking anticoagulants (eg, aspirin or aspirin-containing products, NSAIDs, warfarin) or antiplatelets (eg, clopidogrel, dipyridamole, ticlopidine). Avoid other herbs with anticoagulant/antiplatelet or parasympathomimetic properties. May alter GI absorption of other herbs, minerals, or drugs (especially calcium, copper, magnesium, and zinc) due to tannins. Discontinue at least 14 days prior to dental or surgical procedures.

Huperzia serrata *see* HuperzineA *on page 1714*

HuperzineA

Index Terms *Huperzia serrata*

Pharmacologic Category Herb

Use Acetylcholinesterase inhibitor; treatment of senile dementia and Alzheimer's disease

Local Anesthetic/Vasoconstrictor Precautions No information available to require special precautions

Effects on Bleeding None reported

Warnings/Precautions Use with caution in individuals taking AChE inhibitors (eg, donepezil or tacrine). Avoid cholinergic drugs and other herbs with parasympathomimetic properties.

Hydrastis canadensis *see* Golden Seal *on page 1712*

Hypercium perforatum *see* St John's Wort *on page 1722*

Hyssop

Index Terms Giant Hyssop Herb; Holy Herb; *Hyssopus officinalis*; *Origanum aegypticum*; *Origanum syriacum*

Pharmacologic Category Herb

Use Kidney inflammation

Local Anesthetic/Vasoconstrictor Precautions No information available to require special precautions

Effects on Bleeding None reported

Warnings/Precautions Avoid in individuals with epilepsy, fever, hypertension, or pregnancy. Children should avoid hyssop; may cause seizures. Use with caution in individuals taking antidiabetic agents or in those who have diabetes; may lower blood sugar levels. Due to the possible immunomodulatory activity, hyssop may interact with immunosuppressant medications.

Hyssopus officinalis *see* Hyssop *on page 1714*

Indian Elm *see* Slippery Elm *on page 1721*

Indian Eye *see* Golden Seal *on page 1712*

Indian Head *see* Echinacea *on page 1707*

Isoflavones *see* Soy Isoflavones *on page 1722*

Jaundice Root *see* Golden Seal *on page 1712*

Johimbe *see* Yohimbe *on page 1724*

Kakkonto *see* Kudzu *on page 1715*

Kava

Index Terms Awa; Kava Kava; Kew; *Piper methysticum*; Tonga
Pharmacologic Category Herb
Use Anxiolytic, diuretic, sedative; treatment of insomnia, nervous anxiety, postischemic episodes, stress; skeletal muscle relaxation
Local Anesthetic/Vasoconstrictor Precautions No information available to require special precautions
Effects on Bleeding None reported
Warnings/Precautions The FDA Center for Food Safety and Applied Nutrition (CFSAN) notified healthcare professionals and consumers of the potential risk of severe liver associated with the use of kava-containing dietary supplements. Recently, more than 20 cases of hepatitis, cirrhosis, and liver failure have been reported in Europe, with at least one individual requiring a liver transplant. Given these reports, individuals with hepatic impairment or those taking drugs which can affect the liver, should consult a physician before using supplements containing kava. Physicians are urged to closely evaluate these individuals for potential liver complications. Discontinue if yellow discoloration of skin, hair, or nails occurs (temporary; caused by extended continuous use). Accommodative disturbances (eg, enlargement of the pupils and disturbances of the oculomotor equilibrium) have been described.

Use with caution in individuals taking antianxiety or antidepressant agents, diuretics, hypnotic or sedative agents, alprazolam, or alcohol. May cause sedation; advise caution when driving or operating heavy machinery. Long-term use has resulted in rash. Avoid other herbs with diuretic properties. Discontinue if depression occurs (per Commission E, should not be used >3 months without medical supervision).

Kava Kava *see* Kava *on page 1715*
Kaveri *see* Ginkgo Biloba *on page 1710*
Kew *see* Kava *on page 1715*
Kew Tree *see* Ginkgo Biloba *on page 1710*
King of Mushroom *see* Maitake *on page 1716*
Klamath Weed *see* St John's Wort *on page 1722*

Kudzu

Index Terms Ge-gen; Kakkonto; NPI-028; *Pueraria lobata*
Pharmacologic Category Herb
Use Alcoholism, cardiovascular disease/angina, deafness, diabetes, diabetic retinopathy, glaucoma, menopausal symptoms
Local Anesthetic/Vasoconstrictor Precautions No information available to require special precautions
Effects on Bleeding May see increased bleeding due to inhibition of platelet aggregation
Warnings/Precautions Use with caution in individuals taking antiarrhythmic agents; the kudzu constituent, daidzein, may have antiarrhythmic properties. Use with caution in individuals with a history of bleeding, hemostatic disorders, or drug-related hemostatic problems. Use with caution in individuals taking anticoagulant medications, including warfarin, aspirin, aspirin-containing products, NSAIDs, or antiplatelet agents (eg, ticlopidine, clopidogrel, dipyridamole). Use with caution in individuals with diabetes or who are taking antidiabetic drugs; kudzu may lower blood glucose levels and have additive effects. Use with caution in individuals using agents with estrogenic activity; kudzu may competitively inhibit the effects of estrogen therapy.

Lakriment Neu *see* Licorice *on page 1716*
Laurus Sassafras *see* Sassafras Oil *on page 1721*
L-Carnitine *see* Carnitine *on page 1703*

Lemon Balm/Melissa

Index Terms *Melissa officinalis*
Pharmacologic Category Herb
Use Antiviral (oral herpes virus)
Local Anesthetic/Vasoconstrictor Precautions No information available to require special precautions
Effects on Bleeding None reported
Warnings/Precautions There are no warnings or reports of toxicity.

Lentisk *see* Mastic *on page 1717*

Leopard's Bane *see* Arnica *on page 1701*

L-Glutathione *see* Glutathione *on page 1711*

Licorice

Index Terms Glycocome; Glycyrrhiza glabra; Lakriment Neu; Liquorice; Sweet Root; Ulgastrin Neo

Pharmacologic Category Herb

Use Adaptogen, adrenocorticotropic, antidote, anti-inflammatory, antimicrobial (antibacterial, antifungal, antiviral), antioxidant, antispasmodic, antitussive, detoxification agent, emollient, emmenagogue (high doses), expectorant, immunostimulant, laxative (mild), phytoestrogenic; treatment of abdominal pain, Addison's disease, adrenal insufficiency, age spots, arthritis, asthma, atherosclerosis, benign prostatic hyperplasia (BPH), bronchitis, burns, cancer, candidiasis, carbuncle, chronic gastritis, circulatory disorders, colic, colitis, cold/flu, constipation, contact dermatitis, cough, debility, diabetes, diphtheria, diverticulosis, dizziness, dropsy, duodenal ulcer, dyspepsia, excessive thirst, fever, gastric ulcer, gastritis, hay fever, heart palpitation, heartburn, hemorrhoids, hypercholesterolemia, hyperglycemia, hypotension, inflammation, irritable bowel syndrome (IBS), laryngitis, liver disorders, malaria, menopausal symptoms, menstrual cramps, nausea, peptic ulcer, poisoning (eg, ethanol, atropine, chloral hydrate, cocaine, snakebite), pharyngitis, polyuria, rheumatism, rash, sore throat, stress, tetanus, vertigo; adjunct in long-term cortisone treatment

Per Commission E: GI ulceration, upper/lower respiratory tract infections; foodstuff in candy, chewing gum, chewing tobacco, and cough preparations

Local Anesthetic/Vasoconstrictor Precautions No information available to require special precautions

Effects on Bleeding None reported

Warnings/Precautions Use caution in diabetics, individuals with plant allergies, hypertension, and those taking antihypertensive agents, cardiac glycosides, corticosteroids, diuretics, hormonal contraceptives, laxatives, nitrofurantoin, or receiving hormone replacement therapy (HRT). Avoid other herbs that may be aldosterone synergistic (eg, horehound), hypertensive, or phytoestrogenic.

Lipoic Acid *see* Alpha-Lipoic Acid *on page 1700*

Liquorice *see* Licorice *on page 1716*

Lutein

Pharmacologic Category Nutraceutical

Use Antioxidant; treatment of cataracts and macular degeneration

Local Anesthetic/Vasoconstrictor Precautions No information available to require special precautions

Effects on Bleeding None reported

Warnings/Precautions There are no warnings or reports of toxicity.

Lycopene

Pharmacologic Category Nutraceutical

Use Treatment of atherosclerosis, macular degeneration; prevention of cancer (especially prostate)

Local Anesthetic/Vasoconstrictor Precautions No information available to require special precautions

Effects on Bleeding None reported

Warnings/Precautions There are no warnings or reports of toxicity.

Maidenhair Tree *see* Ginkgo Biloba *on page 1710*

Maitake

Index Terms Cloud Mushroom; Dancing Mushroom; *Grifola frondosa*; King of Mushroom; Maitake Mushroom

Pharmacologic Category Herb

Use Cancer, diabetes, immune stimulation

Local Anesthetic/Vasoconstrictor Precautions No information available to require special precautions

Effects on Bleeding None reported

Warnings/Precautions Use with caution in individuals taking hypotensive/hypertensive agents; may decrease blood pressure. Use with caution in individuals taking hypoglycemic agents; research suggests maitake has hypoglycemic properties

Maitake Mushroom see Maitake on page 1716

Mastic

Index Terms Lentisk; Mastic Gum; Mastix; *Pistacia lentiscus*
Pharmacologic Category Herb
Use Dental plaque, *H. pylori* inhibitor, peptic ulcer disease
Local Anesthetic/Vasoconstrictor Precautions No information available to require special precautions
Effects on Bleeding None reported
Warnings/Precautions Use with caution in individuals taking hypotensive/hypertensive agents; may decrease blood pressure.

Mastic Gum see Mastic on page 1717
Mastix see Mastic on page 1717
Matricaria chamomilla see Chamomile on page 1704
Matricaria recutita see Chamomile on page 1704
Maybush see Hawthorn on page 1713
Melaleuca alternifolia see Melaleuca Oil on page 1717

Melaleuca Oil

Index Terms *Melaleuca alternifolia*; Tea Tree Oil
Pharmacologic Category Herb
Use Analgesic, anti-inflammatory, antibacterial, antifungal, antiseptic, antiviral, disinfectant, immunosupportive, wound-healing agent; treatment of acne, allergy and cold symptoms, minor bruises/burns/cuts, dental plaque, gum inflammation, insect bites, eczema and psoriasis, fungal infections (eg, athlete's foot, oral thrush), hair lice, herpes, muscle pain, respiratory tract infections (eg, bronchitis), toothache, warts; aromatherapy, facial skin toner, household disinfectant (to remove dust mites and lice from laundry), insect repellent, massage oil
Local Anesthetic/Vasoconstrictor Precautions No information available to require special precautions
Effects on Bleeding None reported
Warnings/Precautions Contains cineole; may cause rash in sensitive individuals if applied directly to skin undiluted. Store in dark glass bottle; may react badly with some polymer plastics.

Melatonin

Index Terms N-Acetyl-5-methoxytryptamine
Pharmacologic Category Nutraceutical
Use Antioxidant; treatment of sleep disorders (eg, jet lag, insomnia, neurologic problems, shift work), aging, cancer; supports immune system
Local Anesthetic/Vasoconstrictor Precautions No information available to require special precautions
Effects on Bleeding None reported
Warnings/Precautions Avoid agents that may cause additional CNS depression.

Melissa officinalis see Lemon Balm/Melissa on page 1715

Methyl Sulfonyl Methane

Index Terms Dimethyl Sulfone; $DMSO_2$; MSM
Pharmacologic Category Nutraceutical
Use Analgesic, anti-inflammatory; treatment of interstitial cystitis, lupus, and osteoarthritis
Local Anesthetic/Vasoconstrictor Precautions No information available to require special precautions
Effects on Bleeding None reported
Warnings/Precautions There are no warnings or reports of toxicity when taken according to manufacturer's labeled instructions.

Mexican Damiana see Damiana on page 1706
Microcystis aeruginosa see Spirulina on page 1722

Microcystis wesenbergii see Spirulina *on page 1722*

Milk Thistle

Index Terms *Silybum marianum*

Pharmacologic Category Herb

Use Antidote (Death Cap mushroom), antioxidant (hepatoprotective, including drug toxicities); treatment of acute/chronic hepatitis, jaundice, and stimulation of bile secretion/cholagogue

Local Anesthetic/Vasoconstrictor Precautions No information available to require special precautions

Effects on Bleeding None reported

Warnings/Precautions There are no warnings or reports of toxicity when taken according to manufacturer's labeled instructions.

Milk Vetch *see* Astragalus *on page 1701*

Mizibcoc *see* Damiana *on page 1706*

Monascus purpureus see Red Yeast Rice *on page 1720*

Moose Elm *see* Slippery Elm *on page 1721*

Mountain Daisy *see* Arnica *on page 1701*

Mountain Tobacco *see* Arnica *on page 1701*

MSM *see* Methyl Sulfonyl Methane *on page 1717*

N-Acetyl-5-methoxytryptamine *see* Melatonin *on page 1717*

NADH *see* Nicotinamide Adenine Dinucleotide *on page 1718*

Nectar of the Gods *see* Garlic *on page 1709*

Nicotinamide Adenine Dinucleotide

Index Terms Coenzyme 1; NADH

Pharmacologic Category Nutraceutical

Use Treatment of chronic fatigue, Parkinson's disease; increases stamina and energy

Local Anesthetic/Vasoconstrictor Precautions No information available to require special precautions

Effects on Bleeding None reported

Warnings/Precautions There are no warnings or reports of toxicity when taken according to manufacturer's labeled instructions.

Nosebleed *see* Feverfew *on page 1708*

Nostoc spp see Spirulina *on page 1722*

NPI-028 *see* Kudzu *on page 1715*

Octacosanol *see* Policosanol *on page 1719*

Oenothera biennis see Evening Primrose *on page 1708*

Old Woman's Broom *see* Damiana *on page 1706*

Oligomeric Proanthocyanidin Complexes *see* Pycnogenol *on page 1719*

Omega-3-Acid Ethyl Esters

Index Terms Ethyl Esters of Omega-3 Fatty Acids; Fish Oil

Pharmacologic Category Nutraceutical

Use Antiatherogenic, anticoagulant/antiplatelet, anti-inflammatory; prevention and treatment of cardiovascular diseases; treatment of arteriosclerosis, arthritis, Crohn's disease, diabetes, dyslipidemia, dysmenorrhea, eczema and psoriasis, glaucoma, hypercholesterolemia, hypertension, hypertriglyceridemia; memory enhancement

Local Anesthetic/Vasoconstrictor Precautions No information available to require special precautions

Effects on Bleeding None reported

Warnings/Precautions Use caution with individuals taking anticoagulants (eg, aspirin or aspirin-containing products, NSAIDs, warfarin) or antiplatelet agents (eg, clopidogrel, dipyridamole, ticlopidine), insulin or oral hypoglycemics. Avoid herbs with anticoagulant/antiplatelet properties; may intensify the blood-thinning effect.

Omega-6 Fatty Acids *see* Gamma Linolenic Acid *on page 1709*

OPCs *see* Pycnogenol *on page 1719*

Orange Root *see* Golden Seal *on page 1712*

Oriental Plum Tree *see* Ginkgo Biloba *on page 1710*

Origanum aegypticum see Hyssop *on page 1714*

Origanum syriacum see Hyssop *on page 1714*

Palmetto Scrub *see* Saw Palmetto *on page 1721*
Panax ginseng see Ginseng, Panax *on page 1711*

Parsley

Index Terms *Petroselinum crispum*
Pharmacologic Category Herb
Use Halitosis; antibacterial, antifungal
Local Anesthetic/Vasoconstrictor Precautions No information available to require special precautions
Effects on Bleeding None reported
Warnings/Precautions There are no warnings or reports of toxicity.

Passiflora spp *see* Passion Flower *on page 1719*

Passion Flower

Index Terms *Passiflora* spp
Pharmacologic Category Herb
Use Sedative
Local Anesthetic/Vasoconstrictor Precautions No information available to require special precautions
Effects on Bleeding None reported
Warnings/Precautions Advise caution when driving or operating heavy machinery. Use with caution in individuals taking antianxiety agents or antidepressants and other sedatives; reported in animal studies to increase sleeping time induced by hexobarbital.

Pausinystalia yohimbe see Yohimbe *on page 1724*
Petroselinum crispum see Parsley *on page 1719*
Pinus maritime see Pycnogenol *on page 1719*
Pinus pinaster see Pycnogenol *on page 1719*
Piper methysticum see Kava *on page 1715*
Pipperidge Bush *see* Barberry *on page 1701*
Pistacia lentiscus see Mastic *on page 1717*

Policosanol

Index Terms Octacosanol; Sugar Cane Policosanol; Sunflower Seed Policosanols; Triacontanol; Wheat Germ Policosanol
Pharmacologic Category Nutraceutical
Use Coronary heart disease, hypercholesterolemia, intermittent claudication, platelet aggregation inhibition, reactivity/brain activity
Local Anesthetic/Vasoconstrictor Precautions No information available to require special precautions
Effects on Bleeding May see increased bleeding due to inhibition of platelet aggregation
Warnings/Precautions Use with caution in individuals currently receiving other cholesterol-lowering medications. Use with caution in individuals with a history of bleeding, hemostatic disorders, or drug-related hemostatic problems. Use with caution in individuals taking anticoagulant medications, including warfarin, aspirin, aspirin-containing products, NSAIDs, or antiplatelet agents (eg, ticlopidine, clopidogrel, dipyridamole). Discontinue use prior to dental or surgical procedures (generally at least 14 days before).

Poor Mans Treacle *see* Garlic *on page 1709*
Pueraria lobata see Kudzu *on page 1715*
Purple Coneflower *see* Echinacea *on page 1707*

Pycnogenol

Index Terms French Maritime Pine Bark Extract; Oligomeric Proanthocyanidin Complexes; OPCs; *Pinus maritime*; *Pinus pinaster*; Pygenol
Pharmacologic Category Nutraceutical
Use Asthma, attention-deficit hyperactivity disorder (ADHD), chronic venous insufficiency, diabetes (type 2), diabetic microangiopathy, erectile dysfunction, gingival bleeding/plaque, hypertension, platelet aggregation, prevention of blood clots during long airplane flights, retinopathy, systemic lupus erythematosus (SLE), venous leg ulcers
Local Anesthetic/Vasoconstrictor Precautions No information available to require special precautions
(Continued)

Pycnogenol *(Continued)*

Effects on Bleeding May see increased bleeding due to inhibition of platelet aggregation

Warnings/Precautions Use with caution in individuals with diabetes or hypoglycemia; poor theoretical potential for blood glucose lowering. Use with caution in individuals using hypolipidemics; may significantly decrease serum cholesterol and LDL. Use with caution in individuals with a history of bleeding, hemostatic disorders, or drug-related hemostatic problems. Use with caution in individuals taking anticoagulant medications, including warfarin, aspirin, aspirin-containing products, NSAIDs, or antiplatelet agents (eg, ticlopidine, clopidogrel, dipyridamole). Discontinue use prior to dental or surgical procedures (generally at least 14 days before). Use with caution in individuals taking hypertensive medications; potential for additive hypotensive effects. Use with caution in individuals using immune-stimulating or -inhibiting drugs; potential for immune modulating effects.

Pygenol *see* Pycnogenol *on page 1719*

Quercetin

Pharmacologic Category Nutraceutical

Use Antioxidant

Local Anesthetic/Vasoconstrictor Precautions No information available to require special precautions

Effects on Bleeding None reported

Warnings/Precautions There are no warnings or reports of toxicity.

Radix *see* Valerian *on page 1723*

Red Elm *see* Slippery Elm *on page 1721*

Red Valerian *see* Valerian *on page 1723*

Red Yeast Rice

Index Terms *Monascus purpureus*

Pharmacologic Category Herb

Use Antibiotic, anti-inflammatory, antioxidant, HMG-CoA reductase inhibitor; treatment of hypercholesterolemia, hypertension, hypertriglyceridemia

Local Anesthetic/Vasoconstrictor Precautions No information available to require special precautions

Effects on Bleeding None reported

Warnings/Precautions Use with caution in individuals with a history of bleeding, hemostatic or drug-related hemostatic disorders, and those taking anticoagulants (eg, aspirin or aspirin-containing products, NSAIDs, warfarin) or antiplatelet agents (eg, clopidogrel, dipyridamole, ticlopidine), cyclosporine, erythromycin, itraconazole, niacin, HMG-CoA reductase inhibitors (associated with rare but serious adverse effects, including hepatic and skeletal muscle disorders), and other hyperlipidemic agents. Avoid other herbs with hyperlipidemic properties. Discontinue at the first sign of hepatic dysfunction; discontinue at least 14 days prior to dental or surgical procedures.

Resveratrol *see* Grape Skin *on page 1713*

Rökan *see* Ginkgo Biloba *on page 1710*

Rosin Rose *see* St John's Wort *on page 1722*

Rustic Treacle *see* Garlic *on page 1709*

Sabal serrulata *see* Saw Palmetto *on page 1721*

Sabasilis serrulatae *see* Saw Palmetto *on page 1721*

S-adenosylmethionine *see* SAMe *on page 1720*

SAMe

Index Terms S-adenosylmethionine

Pharmacologic Category Nutritional Supplement

Use Treatment of depression

Local Anesthetic/Vasoconstrictor Precautions No information available to require special precautions

Effects on Bleeding None reported

Warnings/Precautions Use caution when combining with other antidepressants, tryptophan, or 5-HTP; ineffective in the treatment of depressive symptoms associated with bipolar disorder

Sassafras albidum *see* Sassafras Oil *on page 1721*

Sassafras Oil

Index Terms *Laurus Sassafras*; *Sassafras albidum*; *Sassafras radix*; *Sassafras varifolium*; *Sassafrax*

Pharmacologic Category Herb

Use Demulcent; treatment of inflammation of the eyes, insect bites, rheumatic pain; used in the past as a flavoring for beer, sauces, and tea

Local Anesthetic/Vasoconstrictor Precautions No information available to require special precautions

Effects on Bleeding None reported

Warnings/Precautions Ingestion can result in poisoning or death (dose-dependent). Sassafras tea can contain as much as 200 mg (3 mg/kg) of safrole; emesis (within 30 minutes) can be considered for ingestion >5 mL (considered lethal).

Saw Palmetto

Index Terms Palmetto Scrub; *Sabal serrulata*; *Sabasilis serrulatae*; *Serenoa repens*

Pharmacologic Category Herb

Use Antiandrogen, anti-inflammatory; treatment of benign prostatic hyperplasia (BPH)

Local Anesthetic/Vasoconstrictor Precautions No information available to require special precautions

Effects on Bleeding None reported

Warnings/Precautions Not FDA approved; use with caution in individuals on alpha-adrenergic blocking agents and finasteride.

Schisandra

Index Terms *Schizandra chinensis*

Pharmacologic Category Herb

Use Adaptogen, anti-inflammatory, antioxidant, antitussive, hepatoprotective, immunostimulant; treatment of cancer, chronic diarrhea, cough, diabetes, diaphoresis, fatigue, hepatitis; adjunct support for chemotherapy and radiation, detoxification, energy production, health tonic

Local Anesthetic/Vasoconstrictor Precautions No information available to require special precautions

Effects on Bleeding None reported

Warnings/Precautions May alter metabolism of many drugs; use with caution in individuals taking calcium channel blockers.

Shark Cartilage

Pharmacologic Category Nutraceutical

Use Treatment of cancer, osteoarthritis, and rheumatoid arthritis

Local Anesthetic/Vasoconstrictor Precautions No information available to require special precautions

Effects on Bleeding None reported

Warnings/Precautions There are no warnings or reports of toxicity.

Slippery Elm

Index Terms Grey Elm; Indian Elm; Moose Elm; Red Elm; Sweet Elm; *Ulmus fulva*; *Ulmus rubra*; Winged Elm

Pharmacologic Category Herb

Use Cancer, diarrhea, gastrointestinal disorders, sore throat

(Continued)

Slippery Elm *(Continued)*

Local Anesthetic/Vasoconstrictor Precautions No information available to require special precautions

Effects on Bleeding None reported

Warnings/Precautions Avoid during pregnancy due to risk of contamination with slippery elm whole bark; may have abortifacient properties.

Snakeroot *see Echinacea on page 1707*

Soy Isoflavones

Index Terms Isoflavones

Pharmacologic Category Nutraceutical

Use Estrogenic (weak); treatment of bone loss, hypercholesterolemia, menopausal symptoms

Local Anesthetic/Vasoconstrictor Precautions No information available to require special precautions

Effects on Bleeding None reported

Warnings/Precautions May alter response to hormone replacement therapy; use with caution in individuals with history of thromboembolism or stroke

Spirulina

Index Terms Blue-Green Algae; Cyanobacteria; *Microcystis aeruginosa*; *Microcystis wesenbergii*; *Nostoc* spp; *Spirulina fusiformis*; *Spirulina maxima*; *Spirulina platensis*; Tecuitatl

Pharmacologic Category Dietary Supplement; Probiotic

Use Diabetes (type 2), hypercholesterolemia, oral leukoplakia, weight loss

Local Anesthetic/Vasoconstrictor Precautions No information available to require special precautions

Effects on Bleeding None reported

Warnings/Precautions Use with caution in individuals with phenylketonuria; content in blue-green algae theoretically may exacerbate this condition.

Spirulina fusiformis see Spirulina *on page 1722*

Spirulina maxima see Spirulina *on page 1722*

Spirulina platensis see Spirulina *on page 1722*

Stinking Rose *see Garlic on page 1709*

St John's Wort

Index Terms Amber Touch-and-Feel; Goatweed; *Hypercium perforatum*; Klamath Weed; Rosin Rose

Pharmacologic Category Herb

Use Antibacterial, anti-inflammatory, antiviral (high doses), anxiolytic, wound-healing agent; treatment of AIDS (popular due to possible antiretroviral activity), anxiety and stress, insomnia; mild to moderate depression; bruises, muscle soreness, and sprains; vitiligo

Per Commission E: Psychovegetative disorders, depressive moods, anxiety and/or nervous unrest; oily preparations for dyspeptic complaints; oily preparations externally for treatment of post-therapy of acute and contused injuries, myalgia, first degree burns

Local Anesthetic/Vasoconstrictor Precautions No information available to require special precautions

Effects on Bleeding None reported

Warnings/Precautions May be photosensitizing; use caution with drugs metabolized by CYP3A3/4 and tyramine-containing foods (eg, cheese, wine). Use with caution in individuals taking antidepressants, cardiac glycosides, MAO inhibitors, narcotics, reserpine, stimulants, and SSRIs. High does may elevate LFTs (reversible). May alter absorption of calcium, copper, magnesium, and zinc due to tannins. Interacts with many drugs.

Sugar Cane Policosanol *see Policosanol on page 1719*

Sunflower Seed Policosanols *see Policosanol on page 1719*

Superginkgo *see Ginkgo Biloba on page 1710*

Sweet Elm *see Slippery Elm on page 1721*

Sweet Fennel *see Fennel on page 1708*

Sweet Root *see Licorice on page 1716*

Tanacetum parthenium see Feverfew on page 1708

Tanakan *see Ginkgo Biloba on page 1710*

Tanakene *see* Ginkgo Biloba *on page 1710*

Tea Tree Oil *see* Melaleuca Oil *on page 1717*

Tebonin *see* Ginkgo Biloba *on page 1710*

Tecuitatl *see* Spirulina *on page 1722*

Thioctic acid *see* Alpha-Lipoic Acid *on page 1700*

Tonga *see* Kava *on page 1715*

Tramisal *see* Ginkgo Biloba *on page 1710*

Triacontanol *see* Policosanol *on page 1719*

Turmeric

Index Terms *Curcuma longa*
Pharmacologic Category Herb
Use Anti-inflammatory, antioxidant, antiplatelet, antirheumatic; treatment of rheumatoid arthritis and other inflammatory conditions, hypercholesterolemia, and hyperlipidemia
Local Anesthetic/Vasoconstrictor Precautions No information available to require special precautions
Effects on Bleeding May see increased bleeding due to inhibition of platelet aggregation
Warnings/Precautions Use with caution in individuals with history of bleeding, hemostatic or drug-related hemostatic disorders, and those taking anticoagulants (eg, aspirin or aspirin-containing products, NSAIDs, warfarin) or antiplatelet agents (eg, clopidogrel, dipyridamole, ticlopidine). Discontinue at least 14 days prior to dental or surgical procedures.

Turmeric Root *see* Golden Seal *on page 1712*

Turnera aphrodisiaca see Damiana *on page 1706*

Turnera diffusa see Damiana *on page 1706*

Ubiquinone *see* Coenzyme Q$_{10}$ *on page 1705*

Ulgastrin Neo *see* Licorice *on page 1716*

Ulmus fulva see Slippery Elm *on page 1721*

Ulmus rubra see Slippery Elm *on page 1721*

Uncaria tomentosa see Cat's Claw *on page 1704*

Uva Ursi

Index Terms *Arctostaphylos uva-ursi*; Bearberry
Pharmacologic Category Herb
Use Analgesic, antiseptic, astringent, diuretic; treatment and prevention of urinary tract infections; prevention of kidney stones; treatment of bladder infections, urethritis, and a variety of renal disorders (eg, cystitis, nephritis, nephrolithiasis)
Local Anesthetic/Vasoconstrictor Precautions No information available to require special precautions
Effects on Bleeding None reported
Warnings/Precautions May cause green-brown discoloration of urine; may alter GI absorption of other herbs, minerals, or drugs (especially calcium, copper, magnesium, and zinc) due to tannins. Use caution with individuals taking diuretics; avoid other herbs with diuretic properties.

Vaccinium macrocarpon see Cranberry *on page 1706*

Vaccinium myrtillus see Bilberry *on page 1702*

Valerian

Index Terms Radix; Red Valerian; *Valeriana edulis*; *Valeriana wallichi*
Pharmacologic Category Herb
Use Antispasmotic, anxiolytic, sedative (mild); treatment of anxiety and panic attacks, headache, intestinal cramps, nervous tension during PMS and menopause, restless motor syndrome and muscle spasms, sleep disorders (eg, insomnia, jet lag)

Per Commission E: Treatment of sleep disorders based on nervous conditions, restlessness
Local Anesthetic/Vasoconstrictor Precautions No information available to require special precautions
Effects on Bleeding None reported
Warnings/Precautions Advise caution when driving or operating heavy machinery. Use only valepotriate and baldrinal-free supplements in children <12
(Continued)

Valerian *(Continued)*

years of age due to potential mutagenic properties. Use with caution in individuals taking antianxiety or antidepressant agents, antipsychotics, histamines, and hypnotics/sedatives. Avoid herbs with sedative properties.

Valeriana edulis see Valerian *on page 1723*

Valeriana wallichi see Valerian *on page 1723*

Valverde *see* Ginkgo Biloba *on page 1710*

Vanadium

Pharmacologic Category Mineral

Use Treatment of type 1 and type 2 diabetes

Local Anesthetic/Vasoconstrictor Precautions No information available to require special precautions

Effects on Bleeding None reported

Warnings/Precautions May alter glucose regulation; use with caution in diabetics, those predisposed to hypoglycemia, or taking hypoglycemic agents (eg, insulin). Monitor blood sugar and dosage of these agents; may require adjustment (should be carefully coordinated among the individual's healthcare providers).

Vasan *see* Ginkgo Biloba *on page 1710*

Vital *see* Ginkgo Biloba *on page 1710*

Vitex agnus-castus see Chasteberry *on page 1705*

Vitis vinifera see Grape Seed *on page 1713*

Wheat Germ Policosanol *see* Policosanol *on page 1719*

Whitehorn *see* Hawthorn *on page 1713*

Wild Fennel *see* Fennel *on page 1708*

Wild Quinine *see* Feverfew *on page 1708*

Wild Yam

Index Terms *Dioscorea villosa*

Pharmacologic Category Herb

Use Anti-inflammatory, antispasmodic, cholagogue, diuretic (high doses), expectorant (high doses); treatment of diverticulitis, dysmenorrhea, intestinal colic, menopausal symptoms, nausea, premenstrual syndrome (PMS), rheumatic and other inflammatory conditions; female vitality

Local Anesthetic/Vasoconstrictor Precautions No information available to require special precautions

Effects on Bleeding None reported

Warnings/Precautions Use with caution in individuals with a history of stroke or thromboembolic disease and those taking steroids, hormonal contraceptives, or receiving hormone replacement therapy (HRT). Use in children, or women during lactation or pregnancy is not recommended. Overdose may result in poisoning. Avoid other anabolic herbs.

Winged Elm *see* Slippery Elm *on page 1721*

Wolf's Bane *see* Arnica *on page 1701*

Yellow Indian Paint *see* Golden Seal *on page 1712*

Yellow Root *see* Golden Seal *on page 1712*

Yohimbe

Related Information

Yohimbine *on page 1674*

Index Terms Johimbe; *Pausinystalia yohimbe*; Yohimbehe cortex

Pharmacologic Category Herb

Use Anesthetic (local), antiatherogenic, antiviral, aphrodesiac, stimulant, sympathomimetic, thermogenic, vasodilator, vasopressomimetic; treatment of angina pectoris, arteriosclerosis, exhaustion, male erectile dysfunction

Local Anesthetic/Vasoconstrictor Precautions Has potential to interact with epinephrine and levonordefrin to result in increased BP; use vasoconstrictor with caution

Effects on Bleeding None reported

Warnings/Precautions Toxic doses may trigger cardiac failure, hypotension, and psychosis. Use with caution in individuals with diabetes, GI ulceration, or osteoporosis. Avoid other herbs with hypertensive, parasympathomimetic, sympathomimetic, thyroid-stimulating, or vasopressomimetic properties.

Yohimbehe cortex *see* Yohimbe *on page 1724*

Zingiber officinale see Ginger *on page 1710*

ORAL MEDICINE TOPICS

PART I:

DENTAL MANAGEMENT
AND THERAPEUTIC CONSIDERATIONS
IN MEDICALLY-COMPROMISED PATIENTS

This first part of the chapter focuses on common medical conditions and
their associated drug therapies with which the dentist must be familiar.
Patient profiles with commonly associated drug regimens are described.

TABLE OF CONTENTS

CARDIOVASCULAR DISEASES

Cardiovascular disease is the most prevalent human disease affecting over 60 million Americans and this group of diseases accounts >50% of all deaths in the United States. Surgical and pharmacological therapy have resulted in many cardiovascular patients living healthy and profitable lives. Consequently, patients presenting to the dental office may require treatment planning modifications related to the medical management of their cardiovascular disease. For the purposes of this text, we will cover coronary artery disease (CAD) including angina pectoris and myocardial infarction, cardiac arrhythmias, heart failure, and hypertension.

CARDIOVASCULAR DRUGS AND DENTAL CONSIDERATIONS

Some of the drug listings are redundant because the drugs are used to treat more than one cardiovascular disorder. As a convenience to the reader, each table has been constructed as a stand alone listing of drugs for the given disorder. The dental implications of these cardiovascular drugs are listed in Tables 8 and 9. Each of these 2 tables is a consolidation of the drugs from Tables 1-7. The more frequent cardiovascular, respiratory, and central nervous system adverse reactions which you may see in the dental patient are described in Table 8. Table 9 describes the effects on dental treatment reported for these drugs. It is suggested that the reader use Tables 8 and 9 to check for potential effects which could occur in the medicated cardiovascular dental patients.

CORONARY ARTERY DISEASE

Any long-term decrease in the delivery of oxygen to the heart muscle can lead to the condition ischemic heart disease. Often arteriosclerosis and atherosclerosis result in a narrowing of the coronary vessels' lumina and are the most common causes of vascular ischemic heart disease. Other causes such as previous infarct, mitral valve regurgitation, and ruptured septa may also lead to ischemia in the heart muscle. The two most common major conditions that result from ischemic heart disease are angina pectoris and myocardial infarction. Sudden death, a third category, can likewise result from ischemia.

To the physician, the most common presenting sign or symptom of ischemic heart disease is chest pain. This chest pain can be of a transient nature as in angina pectoris or the result of a myocardial infarction. It is now believed that sudden death represents a separate occurrence that essentially involves the development of a lethal cardiac arrhythmia or coronary artery spasm leading to an acute shutdown of the heart muscle blood supply. Risk factors in patients for coronary atherosclerosis include cigarette smoking, elevated blood lipids, hypertension, as well as diabetes mellitus, age, and gender (male).

Coronary artery disease (CAD) is the cause of about half of all deaths in the United States. CAD has been shown to be correlated with the levels of plasma cholesterol and/or triacylglycerol-containing lipoprotein particles. Primary prevention focuses on averting the development of CAD. In contrast, secondary prevention of CAD focuses on therapies to reduce morbidity and mortality in patients with clinically documented CAD.

Lipid-lowering and cardioprotective drugs provide significant risk-reducing benefits in the secondary prevention of CAD. By reducing the levels of total and low density cholesterol through the inhibition of hydroxymethylglutaryl coenzyme A (HMG-CoA) reductase, statin drugs significantly improve survival. Cardioprotective drug therapy includes antiplatelet/anticoagulant agents to inhibit platelet adhesion, aggregation and blood coagulation; beta-blockers to lower heart rate, contractility and blood pressure; and the angiotensin-converting enzyme (ACE) inhibitors to lower peripheral resistance and workload. For a listing of these drugs, see Table 1.

Table 1.
DRUGS USED IN THE TREATMENT OF CAD

Reduction of Total and Low-Density Cholesterol Levels
  Bile Acid Sequestrant
    Colesevelam *on page 408*
  HMG-CoA Reductase Inhibitors
    Fluvastatin *on page 733*
    Lovastatin *on page 1007*
    Pravastatin *on page 1335*
    Simvastatin *on page 1472*
    Atorvastatin *on page 162*

  Fibrate Group
    Fenofibrate *on page 674*
    Gemfibrozil *on page 772*
  Bile Acid Resins
    Cholestyramine Resin *on page 349*
    Colestipol *on page 409*
  Nicotinic Acid

Cardioprotective Therapy
  Antiplatelet / Anticoagulant Agents
    Aspirin *on page 149*
    Clopidogrel *on page 395*
    Ticlopidine *on page 1566*
    Warfarin *on page 1670*
  Beta-Adrenergic Receptor Blockers
    Atenolol *on page 158*
    Metoprolol *on page 1088*
    Propranolol *on page 1373*
  Angiotensin-Converting Enzyme (ACE) Inhibitors
    Captopril *on page 269*
    Enalapril *on page 564*
    Fosinopril *on page 748*
    Lisinopril *on page 990*
    Ramipril *on page 1406*

ANGINA PECTORIS
(EMPHASIS ON UNSTABLE ANGINA)

Numerous physiologic triggers can initiate the rupture of plaque in coronary blood vessels. Rupture leads to the activation, adhesion, and aggregation of platelets, and the activation of the clotting cascade, resulting in the formation of occlusive thrombus. If this process leads to the complete occlusion of the artery, acute myocardial infarction with ST-segment elevation occurs. Alternatively, if the process leads to severe stenosis and the artery remains patent, unstable angina occurs. Triggers which induce unstable angina include physical exertion, mechanical stress due to an increase in cardiac contractility, pulse rate, blood pressure, and vasoconstriction.

Unstable angina accounts for more than 1 million hospital admissions annually. In 1989, Braunwald devised a classification system according to the severity of the clinical manifestations of angina. These manifestations are defined as acute angina while at rest (within the 48 hours before presentation), subacute angina while at rest (within the previous month but not within the 48 hours before presentation), or new onset of accelerated (progressively more severe) angina. The system also classifies angina according to the clinical circumstances in which unstable angina develops, defined as either angina in the presence or absence of other conditions (ie, fever, hypoxia, tachycardia, thyrotoxicosis) and whether or not ECG abnormalities are present. Recently, the term "acute coronary syndrome" has been used to describe the range of conditions that includes unstable angina, non-Q-wave myocardial infarction, and Q-wave myocardial infarction.

Pharmacologic therapy to treat unstable angina includes antiplatelet drugs, antithrombin therapy, and conventional antianginal therapy with beta-blockers, nitrates, and calcium channel blockers. These drug groups and selected agents are listed in Table 3.

CARDIOVASCULAR DISEASES *(Continued)*

Antiplatelet Drugs

Aspirin reduces platelet aggregation by blocking platelet cyclo-oxygenase through irreversible acetylation. This action prevents the formation of thromboxane A_2. A number of studies have confirmed that aspirin reduces the risk of death from cardiac causes and fatal and nonfatal myocardial infarction by approximately 50% to 70% in patients presenting with unstable angina. Ticlopidine is a second-line alternative to aspirin in the treatment of unstable angina and is also used as adjunctive therapy with aspirin to prevent thrombosis after placement of intracoronary stents. Ticlopidine blocks ADP-mediated platelet aggregation. Clopidogrel inhibits platelet aggregation by affecting the ADP-dependent activation of the glycoprotein IIb/IIIa complex. Clopidogrel is chemically related to ticlopidine, but has fewer side effects.

Platelet Glycoprotein IIb / IIIa Receptor Antagonists

Antagonists of glycoprotein IIb/IIIa, a receptor on the platelet for adhesive proteins, inhibit the final common pathway involved in adhesion, activation, and aggregation. Presently, there exist three classes of inhibitors. One class is murine-human chimeric antibodies of which abciximab is the prototype. The other two classes are the synthetic peptide forms (eg, eptifibatide) and the synthetic nonpeptide forms (eg, tirofiban). These agents, in combination with heparin and aspirin, have been used to treat unstable angina, significantly reducing the incidence of death or myocardial infarction.

Antithrombin Drugs

Unfractionated heparin, in combination with aspirin, is used to treat unstable angina. Unfractionated heparin consists of polysaccharide chains which bind to antithrombin III, causing a conformational change that accelerates the inhibition of thrombin and factor Xa. Unfractionated heparin is therefore an indirect thrombin inhibitor. Unfractionated heparin can only be administered intravenously. Low-molecular-weight heparins (LMWH) have a more predictable pharmacokinetic profile than the unfractionated heparin and can be administered subcutaneously. These heparins have a mechanism of action and use similar to unfractionated heparin.

The direct antithrombins decrease thrombin activity in a manner independent of any actions on antithrombin III. Two such direct antithrombins are lepirudin (also known as recombinant hirudin) and argatroban. These agents are highly specific, direct thrombin inhibitor with each molecule capable of binding to one molecule of thrombin and inhibiting its thrombogenic activity. Direct antithrombins are used for the prevention or reduction of ischemic complications associated with unstable angina.

Warfarin (Coumadin®) elicits its anticoagulant effect by interfering with the hepatic synthesis of vitamin K-dependent coagulation factors II, VII, IX, and X. Although warfarin appears to be somewhat effective after myocardial infarction in preventing death or recurrent myocardial infarction, its effectiveness in the treatment of acute coronary syndrome is questionable. Combination therapy with aspirin and heparin followed by warfarin has resulted in reduced incidence of recurrent angina, myocardial infarction, death, or all three at 14 days as compared with aspirin alone. In contrast, another study failed to show any additional benefit in the treatment of acute coronary syndrome using a combination of aspirin and warfarin compared to aspirin alone.

Conventional Antianginal Therapy: Beta-Blockers, Nitrates, Calcium Channel Blockers

Current thinking is that there is a definite link between unstable angina and acute myocardial infarction. In this regard, beta-blockers are currently recommended as first-line agents in all acute coronary syndromes. A meta-analysis of studies involving 4700 patients with unstable angina demonstrated a 13% reduction in the risk of myocardial infarction among patients treated with beta-blockers. The various preparations of beta-blockers appear to have equal efficacy. The effects of beta-blockers are thought to be due to their ability to decrease myocardial oxygen demand.

Nitrates, such as nitroglycerin, are widely used in the management of unstable angina. Nitrates elicit a number of effects including a reduction in oxygen demand, arteriolar vasodilation, augmentation of collateral coronary blood flow and frequency of coronary vasospasm. Intravenous nitroglycerin is one of the first line therapies for unstable angina because of the ease of dose titration and the rapid resolution of effects. Continuous nitrate therapy with oral and transdermal patch preparations has resulted in tolerance to the beneficial effects of nitrates. A 6- to 8-hour daily nitrate-free interval will minimize the tolerance phenomenon. Also, supplemental use of vitamin C appears to prevent nitrate tolerance.

Calcium channel blockers such as nifedipine, verapamil, and diltiazem cause coronary vasodilation and reduced blood pressure. Because of these actions, the calcium channel blockers were thought to be a drug group which could be effective in the treatment of unstable angina. However, a meta-analysis of studies in which patients with unstable angina were treated with calcium channel blockers found no effect of the drugs on the incidence of death or myocardial infarction. More recently, it has been shown that treatment with diltiazem and verapamil may result in increased survival and reduced rates of reinfarction in patients with acute coronary syndrome. Current thinking suggests that calcium channel blockers should be used in patients in whom beta-blockers are contraindicated or in those with refractory symptoms after treatments with aspirin, nitrates, or beta-blockers.

Dental Management

The dental management of the patient with angina pectoris may include sedation techniques for complicated procedures (see "Sedation" *on page 1825*), to limit the extent of procedures, and to limit the use of local anesthesia containing 1:100,000 epinephrine to two capsules. Anesthesia without a vasoconstrictor might also be selected. The appropriate use of a vasoconstrictor in anesthesia, however, should be weighed against the necessity to maximize anesthesia. Complete history and appropriate referral and consultation with the patient's physician for those patients who are known to be at risk for angina pectoris is recommended.

MYOCARDIAL INFARCTION

Myocardial infarction is the leading cause of death in the United States. It is an acute irreversible ischemic event that produces an area of myocardial necrosis in the heart tissue. If a patient has a previous history of myocardial infarction, he/she may be taking a variety of drugs (ie, antihypertensives, lipid lowering drugs, ACE inhibitors, and antianginal medications) to not only prevent a second infarct, but to treat the long-term associated ischemic heart disease. Postmyocardial infarction patients are often taking anticoagulants such as warfarin and antiplatelet agents such as aspirin. Consultation with the prescribing physician by the dentist is necessary prior to invasive procedures. Temporary dose reduction may allow the dentist to proceed with very invasive procedures. Most procedures, however, can be accomplished without changing the anticoagulant therapy at all, using local hemostasis techniques.

Aspirin   *on page 149*
Warfarin   *on page 1670*

Thrombolytic drugs, which might dissolve hemostatic plugs, may also be given on a short-term basis immediately following an infarct and include:

Alteplase   *on page 78*
Reteplase   *on page 1417*
Streptokinase   *on page 1495*
Tenecteplase   *on page 1535*

Alteplase [tissue plasminogen activator (TPA)] is also currently in use for acute myocardial infarction. Following myocardial infarction and rehabilitation, outpatients may be placed on anticoagulants (such as Coumadin®), diuretics, beta-adrenergic blockers, ACE inhibitors to reduce blood pressure, and calcium channel blockers. Depending on the presence or absence of continued angina pectoris, patients may also be taking nitrates, beta-blockers, or calcium channel blockers as indicated for treatment of angina.

BETA-ADRENERGIC BLOCKING AGENTS CATEGORIZED ACCORDING TO SPECIFIC PROPERTIES

Alpha-Adrenergic Blocking Activity
Labetalol   *on page 940*

Intrinsic Sympathomimetic Activity
Acebutolol   *on page 28*
Pindolol   *on page 1306*

Long Duration of Action and Fewer CNS Effects
Acebutolol   *on page 28*
Atenolol   *on page 158*
Betaxolol   *on page 210*
Nadolol   *on page 1139*

Beta$_1$-Receptor Selectivity
Acebutolol   *on page 28*
Atenolol   *on page 158*
Metoprolol   *on page 1088*

Nonselective (blocks both beta$_1$- and beta$_2$-receptors)
Betaxolol   *on page 210*
Labetalol   *on page 940*
Nadolol   *on page 1139*
Pindolol   *on page 1306*
Propranolol   *on page 1373*
Timolol   *on page 1570*

CARDIOVASCULAR DISEASES *(Continued)*

ARRHYTHMIAS

Abnormal cardiac rhythm can develop spontaneously and survivors of a myocardial infarction are often left with an arrhythmia. An arrhythmia is any alteration or disturbance in the normal rate, rhythm, or conduction through the cardiac tissue. This is known as a cardiac arrhythmia. Abnormalities in rhythm can occur in either the atria or the ventricles. Various valvular deformities, drug effects, and chemical derangements can initiate arrhythmias. These arrhythmias can be a slowing of the heart rate (<60 beats/minute) as defined in bradycardia or tachycardia resulting in a rapid heart beat (usually >150 beats/minute). The dentist will encounter a variety of treatments for management of arrhythmias. Usually, underlying causes such as reduced cardiac output, hypertension, and irregular ventricular beats will require treatment. Pacemaker therapy is also sometimes used. Indwelling pacemakers may require supplementation with antibiotics, and consultation with the physician is certainly appropriate. Sinus tachycardia is often treated with drugs such as:

Propranolol *on page 1373*

Quinidine *on page 1397*

Beta-blockers are often used to slow cardiac rate and diazepam may be helpful when anxiety is a contributing factor in arrhythmia. When atrial flutter and atrial fibrillation are diagnosed, drug therapy is usually required.

Digoxin *on page 497*

Atrial fibrillation (AF) is an arrhythmia characterized by multiple electrical activations in the atria resulting in scattered and disorganized depolarization and repolarization of the myocardium. Atrial contraction can lead to an irregular and rapid rate of ventricular contraction. The prevalence of atrial fibrillation within the US population ranges between 1% and 4%, with the incidence increasing with age. It is often associated with rheumatic valvular disease and nonvalvular conditions including coronary artery disease and hypertension. Coronary artery disease is present in about one-half of the patients with atrial fibrillation. Atrial fibrillation is a major risk factor for systemic and cerebral embolism. It is thought that thrombi develop as a result of stasis in the dilated left atrium and is dislodged by sudden changes in cardiac rhythm. About 10% of all strokes in patients >60 years of age are caused by atrial fibrillation.

The cornerstones of drug therapy for atrial fibrillation are the restoration and maintenance of a normal sinus rhythm through the use of antiarrhythmic drugs, ventricular rate control through the use of beta-blockers, digitalis drugs or calcium channel blockers, and stroke prevention through the use of anticoagulants.

Antiarrhythmic Drugs

Cardiac rhythm is conducted through the sinoatrial (SA) and atrioventricular (AV) nodes, bundle branches, and Purkinje fibers. Electrical impulses are transmitted within this system by the opening and closing of sodium and potassium channels. Antiarrhythmic drugs are classified by which channel they act upon, a classification known as Vaughan Williams after the author of the published paper. The Class I agents act primarily on sodium channels, and the Class III agents act on potassium channels. In addition, there are subclassifications within the Class I agents according to effects of the drug on conduction and refractoriness within the Purkinje and ventricular tissues. Class IA agents show moderate depression of conduction and prolongation of repolarization. Class IB agents show modest depression of conduction and shortening of repolarization. Class IC agents show marked depression of conduction and mild or no effect on repolarization. Class IA and IC agents are effective in the treatment of atrial fibrillation. Class IB agents (ie, lidocaine, phenytoin) are not used to treat atrial fibrillation, but are effective in treating ventricular arrhythmias. Class II drugs are the beta-adrenergic blocking drugs and Class IV are the calcium channel blockers. Table 2 lists the drugs and the categories used to treat atrial fibrillation.

Table 2.
DRUGS USED IN THE TREATMENT OF ATRIAL FIBRILLATION

Class I Antiarrhythmic Agents	
Disopyramide *on page 518*	
Flecainide *on page 694*	
Moricizine *on page 1123*	
Procainamide *on page 1354*	
Propafenone *on page 1365*	
Quinidine *on page 1397*	
Class II Antiarrhythmic Agents (Beta-Adrenergic Blockers)	
Cardioselective (Beta₁-Receptor Block only)	
Acebutolol *on page 28*	
Atenolol *on page 158*	
Betaxolol *on page 210*	
Metoprolol *on page 1088*	
Noncardioselective (Beta₁- and Beta₂-Receptor Block)	
Nadolol *on page 1139*	
Penbutolol *on page 1265*	
Pindolol *on page 1306*	
Propranolol *on page 1373*	
Timolol *on page 1570*	
Class III Antiarrhythmic Agents	
Amiodarone *on page 92*	
Dofetilide *on page 523*	
Ibutilide *on page 858*	
Sotalol *on page 1489*	
Class IV Antiarrhythmic Agents (Calcium Channel Blockers)	
Diltiazem *on page 505*	
Verapamil *on page 1654*	
Anticoagulant Agents	
Aspirin *on page 149*	
Warfarin *on page 1670*	

Source: USP DI, Volumes I and II, Update, April, 1998.

Restoring and Maintaining Normal Sinus Rhythm

Cardioversion induced by drugs can usually restore sinus rhythm in patients with atrial fibrillation. Class I drugs (moricizine), Class IA drugs (disopyramide, procainamide, quinidine), Class IC drugs (flecainide, propafenone), and Class III antiarrhythmics (amiodarone, sotalol) are all effective in restoring normal sinus rhythm. Success rates may vary greatly and are complicated by the high rate of spontaneous conversion. The drugs used for pharmacologic conversion are also used to maintain sinus rhythm.

Ventricular Rate Control

It is accepted practice to treat patients with medication when the resting ventricular rate is >110 beats/minute. Digoxin, calcium channel blockers, and beta-adrenergic blockers are used in the regulation of ventricular rate. Digoxin increases the vagal tone to the AV node, calcium channel blockers slow the AV nodal conduction, and the beta-adrenergic blocking drugs decrease the sympathetic activation of the AV nodal conduction.

ANTICOAGULANT THERAPY

Over the last thirty years, there has been an increasing use of drugs that relate to the clotting mechanisms in patients. These drugs have included the wide spread use of aspirin as well as an increasing use of anticoagulants found in warfarin as well as synthetic drugs that also have anticoagulation effects. Many patients with ischemic heart disease, atherosclerosis, those with atrial fibrillation and in patients at high risk for stroke, we find the increased use of these anticoagulants. Large numbers of these patients are receiving oral anticoagulation therapy as out patients. The dental clinician is often faced with the decision as to how to manage these patients prior to dental procedures. Key factors regarding the patient receiving anticoagulation therapy include:

- What is the thromboembolytic risk for this patient?

- What is the bleeding risk of the dental procedure planned?

- If an invasive procedure is planned in the face of a high thromboembolytic risk, what is the managing physician's opinion on altering the dosage of anticoagulation therapy?

Often times, to access these factors, consultation with a patient's physician is necessary. However, recent reviews have suggested by Jeske, 2003 and others in our suggested readings list have argued that inappropriate adjustments in anticoagulation therapy create far greater risk for the patient than the risk of hemorrhage during most dental

CARDIOVASCULAR DISEASES *(Continued)*

procedures. Therefore, the scientific evidence does not support changing regimens of anticoagulation therapy in many, perhaps even most instances. However, this decision can only be determined by weighing the factors described above and discussing the situation with the patient's physician.

Table 3.
DRUGS USED TO MANAGE UNSTABLE ANGINA

Antiplatelet Drugs
    Aspirin *on page 149*
    Clopidogrel *on page 395*
    Ticlopidine *on page 1566*
    Glycoprotein IIb / IIIa Receptor Antagonists
        Abciximab *on page 26*
        Eptifibatide *on page 582*
        Tirofiban *on page 1576*

Antithrombin Drugs
    Indirect Thrombin Inhibitors
        Heparin (unfractionated) *on page 807*
        Low molecular weight heparins
            Dalteparin *on page 438*
            Enoxaparin *on page 568*
            Tinzaparin *on page 1572*
    Direct Thrombin Inhibitors
        Lepirudin *on page 956*
        Argatroban *on page 139*
    Dicumarols
        Warfarin *on page 1670*

Conventional Antianginal Drugs
    Beta-Blockers
        Atenolol *on page 158*
        Bisoprolol *on page 218*
        Carteolol *on page 290*
        Nadolol *on page 1139*
        Propranolol *on page 1373*
    Nitrates
        Isosorbide Dinitrate *on page 914*
        Isosorbide Mononitrate *on page 916*
        Nitroglycerin *on page 1181*
    Calcium Channel Blockers
        Diltiazem *on page 505*
        Nifedipine *on page 1173*
        Verapamil *on page 1654*

Evaluating Antiplatelet Response

Partial thromboplastin time and bleeding time (IVY) are appropriate measures for platelet dysfunction. Aspirin, ticlopidine (Ticlid®), and other new drugs, such as Clopidogrel (Plavix®), are actually considered antiplatelet drugs, whereas oral Coumadin® is considered an oral anticoagulant. Aspirin works by inhibiting cyclo-oxygenase which is an enzyme involved in the platelet system associated with clot formation. As little as one aspirin (300 mg dose) can result in an alteration in this enzyme pathway. Although aspirin is cleared from the circulation very quickly (within 15-30 minutes), the effect on the life of the platelet may last up to 7-10 days. Most routine dental procedures can be accomplished with no change in these medications using aggressive local hemostasis efforts and prudent treatment planning.

Evaluating Coumadin® Response

The effects of Coumadin® on the coagulation within patients occur by way of the vitamin K-dependent clotting mechanism and are generally monitored by measuring the prothrombin time known as the PT. Often to prevent venous thrombosis, a patient will be maintained at approximately 1.5 times their normal prothrombin time. Other anticoagulant goals such as prevention of arterial thromboembolism, as in patients with artificial heart valves, may require 2-2.5 times the normal prothrombin time. It is important for the clinician to obtain not only the accurate PT but also the International Normalized Ratio (INR) for the patient. This ratio is calculated by dividing the patient's PT by the mean normal PT for the laboratory, which is determined by using the International Sensitivity Index (ISI) to adjust for the lab's reagents.

The response to oral anticoagulants varies greatly in patients and should be monitored regularly. The dental clinician planning an invasive procedure should consider not only what the patient can tell them from a historical point-of-view, but also when the last monitoring test was performed. In general, most dental procedures can be performed in patients that are 1.5-2.5 times normal or less. Most researchers further suggest that 2.5-3 times normal pose little risk in most dental patients and procedures, but these values may be misleading unless the INR is also determined. When in doubt, the prudent dental clinician would consult with the patient's physician and obtain current prothrombin time and INR in order to evaluate fully and plan for his patients.

Coumadin®-Like Anticoagulants

Dicumarol
Warfarin *on page 1670*

Platelet Aggregation Inhibitors

Aspirin *on page 149*
Clopidogrel *on page 395*
Eptifibatide *on page 582*
Ticlopidine *on page 1566*
Tirofiban *on page 1576*

Anticoagulant, Other

Lepirudin *on page 956*

Antiplatelet Agent

Aspirin and Dipyridamole *on page 154*

Regarding dental management patients that are already taking warfarin, the use of analgesics is implicated as a potential source of drug interaction. In an article by Hayek in *JAMA*, it was found that patients taking warfarin for anticoagulation identified the use of dangerously elevated INRs and the fact was discovered that they concomitantly had been taking acetaminophen (not necessarily with their physician's recommendation). The study of the international normalized ratio (INR) in these patients has indicated that additional factors independently influence the INR, as well as the potential interaction with acetaminophen. Potential effects on the INR are greatest in patients taking acetaminophen at high doses over a protracted time period. Short-term pain management with acetaminophen poses little risk. These factors included advanced malignancy, patients who did not take their warfarin properly (therefore, took more than was necessary), changes in oral intake of liquids or solids, acute diarrhea leading to dehydration, alcohol consumption, and vitamin K intake.

The mechanisms of these augmenting factors for enhancement of the INR are that the cytochrome P450 system, present in the liver, is also affected by changes in metabolism associated with these factors. For instance, the metabolism of alcohol in the liver alters its ability to manage the CYP450 enzyme system necessary for warfarin, therefore, enhancing its presence and potentially increasing the half-life of warfarin. As oral intake of nutrients declines in patients with either diarrhea or reduced intake of liquids and/or solids, absorption of vitamin K is reduced and the vitamin K dependent system of metabolism of warfarin changes, therefore increasing warfarin blood levels. These factors, along with the liver metabolism of acetaminophen, have resulted in the increased concern that patients, who may be taking acetaminophen as an analgesic or for other reasons, may be at risk for enhancing or elevating, inadvertently, their anticoagulation effect of warfarin. The dentist should be aware of this potential interaction in prescribing any drug containing acetaminophen or in recommending that a patient use an analgesic for relief of even mild pain on a prolonged basis. Therefore, the dentist must be concerned with these factors and is referred to the discussion in the Oral Pain section *on page 1788* for more consideration (adapted from *JAMA*, March 4, 1998, Vol 279, No 9).

Acetaminophen *on page 31*

Although not used specifically for this purpose, numerous herbal medicines and natural dietary supplements have been associated with inhibition of platelet aggregation or other anticoagulation effects, and therefore may lead to increased bleeding during invasive dental procedures. Current reports include bilberry, bromelain, cat's claw, devil's claw, dong quai, evening primrose, feverfew, garlic (irreversible inhibition), ginger (only at very high doses), ginkgo biloba, ginseng, grape seed, green tea, horse chestnut, and turmeric.

References

Jeske AH, Suchko GD, ADA Council on Scientific Affairs and Division of Science, et al, "Lack of a Scientific Basis for Routine Discontinuation of Oral Anticoagulation Therapy Before Dental Treatment,"*J Am Dent Assoc*, 2003, 134(11):1492-7.

Lockhart PB, Gibson J, Pond SH, et al, "Dental Management Considerations for the Patient With an Acquired Coagulopathy. Part 2: Coagulopathies From Drugs," *Br Dent J*, 2003, 195(9):495-501.

Carter G, Goss AN, Lloyd J, et al, "Current Concepts of the Management of Dental Extractions for Patients Taking Warfarin," *Aust Dent J*, 2003, 48(2):89-96.

Little JW, Miller CS, Henry RG, et al, "Antithrombotic Agents: Implications in Dentistry," *Oral Surg Oral Med Oral Pathol Oral Radiol Endod*, 2002, 93(5):544-51.

CARDIOVASCULAR DISEASES *(Continued)*

HEART FAILURE

Heart failure is a condition in which the heart is unable to pump sufficient blood to meet the needs of the body. It is caused by impaired ability of the cardiac muscle to contract or by an increased workload imposed on the heart. Most frequently, the underlying cause of heart failure is coronary artery disease. Other contributory causes include hypertension, diabetes, idiopathic dilated cardiomyopathy, and valvular heart disease. It is estimated that heart failure affects approximately 5 million Americans. The New York Heart Association functional classification is regarded as the standard measure to describe the severity of a patient's symptom. Class I is characterized by having no limitation of physical activity. There is no dyspnea, fatigue, palpitations, or angina with ordinary physical activity. There is no objective evidence of cardiovascular dysfunction. Class II includes those patients having slight limitation of physical activity. These patients experience fatigue, palpitations, dyspnea, or angina with ordinary physical activity, but are comfortable at rest. There is evidence of minimal cardiovascular dysfunction. Class III is characterized by marked limitation of activity. Less than ordinary physical activity causes fatigue, palpitations, dyspnea, or angina, but patients are comfortable at rest. There is objective evidence of moderately severe cardiovascular dysfunction. Class IV is characterized by the inability to carry out any physical activity without discomfort. Symptoms of heart failure or anginal syndrome may be present even at rest, and any physical activity undertaken increases discomfort. There is objective evidence of severe cardiovascular dysfunction. Drug classes and the specific agents used to treat heart failure are listed in Table 4.

Table 4.
DRUGS USED IN THE TREATMENT OF HEART FAILURE

Angiotensin-Converting Enzyme Inhibitors (ACE)[1]

    Benazepril *on page 191*
    Captopril *on page 269*
    Enalapril *on page 564*
    Fosinopril *on page 748*
    Lisinopril *on page 990*
    Perindopril Erhumine *on page 1282*
    Quinapril *on page 1395*
    Ramipril *on page 1406*
    Trandolapril *on page 1598*

Diuretics

    Thiazides
        Hydrochlorothiazide *on page 819*
    Loop Diuretics
        Furosemide *on page 756*
    Potassium-Sparing Agents
        Spironolactone *on page 1492*

Digitalis Glycosides

    Digoxin *on page 497*

Beta-Adrenergic Receptor Blockers

    Bisoprolol *on page 218*
    Carvedilol *on page 291*
    Metoprolol *on page 1088*

Catecholamines

    Dobutamine *on page 520*
    Dopamine

Supplemental Agents

    Direct-Acting Vasodilators
        Hydralazine *on page 817*
        Nitroglycerin *on page 1181*
        Nitroprusside *on page 1183*
    Phosphodiesterase Inhibitors
        Inamrinone *on page 874*
        Milrinone *on page 1106*

[1]Regarded as the cornerstone of treatment of heart failure and should be used routinely and early in all patients.

From USP DI, Volumes I and II, Update, December 1998.

Drug Classes and Specific Agents Used to Treat Heart Failure

Angiotensin-converting enzyme (ACE) inhibitors reduce left ventricular volume and filling pressure while decreasing total peripheral resistance. They induce cardiac output (modestly) and natriuresis. ACE inhibitors are usually used in all patients with heart failure if no contraindication or intolerance exists. This group of drugs is considered the cornerstone of treatment and are used routinely and early if pharmacologic treatment is indicated.

Diuretics increase sodium chloride and water excretion resulting in reduction of preload, thus relieving the symptoms of pulmonary congestion associated with heart failure. They may also reduce myocardial oxygen demand. The thiazides, loop diuretics, and potassium-sparing agents are all useful in reducing preload by way of their diuretic actions.

Digitalis glycosides have been used in the treatment of heart failure for more than 200 years. Digitalis drugs increase cardiac output by a direct positive inotropic action on the myocardium. This increased cardiac output results in decreased venous pressure, reduced heart size, and diminished compensatory tachycardia.

Beta-adrenergic receptor blocking drugs (beta-blockers) are used in the treatment of heart failure because of their beneficial effect in reducing mortality. A meta-analysis of randomized clinical trials showed that the beta-blockers significantly reduced all causes of cardiac-related deaths, with carvedilol (Coreg®) showing the greatest efficacy. The overall risk of death was reduced by over 30%.

Other drugs used in the treatment of heart failure are referred to as supplemental agents. The direct-acting vasodilators reduce excessive vasoconstriction and reduce workload of the failing heart. The catecholamines and phosphodiesterase inhibitors are alternative agents with positive inotropic effects, are effective for short-term therapy, and have not been demonstrated to prolong life during long-term therapy.

Treatment of arrhythmias often can result in oral manifestations including oral ulcerations with drugs such as procainamide, lupus-like lesions, as well as xerostomia.

HYPERTENSION

In the United States, almost 50 million adults, 25-74 years of age, have hypertension. Hypertension is defined as systolic blood pressure ≥140 mm Hg, and/or diastolic pressure >90 mm Hg. People with blood pressure above normal are considered at increased risk of developing damage to the heart, kidney, brain, and eyes, resulting in premature morbidity and mortality.

Recently, the Joint National Committee on Prevention, Detection, Evaluation, and Treatment of High Blood Pressure, released its 7th Report in the summer of 2003. The highlights of the new report are that several of the categories have been renamed to connote changes in philosophy towards earlier treatment and intervention for patients with elevated blood pressure.

Also, there is an increased importance in the elevation of systolic blood pressure for people >50 years of age. The category of high normal blood pressure has now been replaced with the term prehypertension for those patients with systolic blood pressure of 120-139 mm Hg and for those with diastolic blood pressure of 80-89 mm Hg. The remaining stages of hypertension have been broken into simply two categories: Stage 1 and Stage 2. Stage 1 diastolic pressure is 90-99 mm Hg and systolic pressure is 140-159 mm Hg, whereas in Stage 2, diastolic pressure >100 mm Hg or systolic pressure >160 mm Hg are the respective cut-off for treatment decisions. This greatly simplifies the classification of blood pressure.

In addition, the 7th Joint National Committee Report highlights the importance of life style modifications in controlling blood pressure along with pharmacologic intervention. Thiazide diuretics have again been considered one of the most important treatments in uncomplicated hypertension and their benefits of lowering blood pressure have been greatly emphasized. The role of dentistry in detection as well as assisting in compliance for patients, has been clearly emphasized in this report.

The suggested initial goals of drug therapy are the maintenance of an arterial pressure of ≤140/90 mm Hg with concurrent control of other modifiable cardiovascular risk factors. Further reduction to 130/85 mm Hg should be pursued if cardiovascular and cerebrovascular function is not compromised. The Hypertension Optimal Treatment (HOT) randomized trial using patients 50-80 years of age found that the lowest incidence of major cardiovascular events and the lowest risk of cardiovascular mortality occurred at a mean diastolic blood pressure of 82.6 and 86.5 mm Hg respectively.

CARDIOVASCULAR DISEASES *(Continued)*

Table 5.
CLASSIFICATION OF BLOOD PRESSURE
FOR ADULTS ≥18 YEARS OF AGE

BP Classification	Systolic BP (mm Hg)	Diastolic BP (mm Hg)
Normotensive	<120	<80
Prehypertension[1]	120-139	80-89
Stage 1 hypertension[2]	140-159	90-99
Stage 2 hypertension[3]	≥160	≥100

[1]Not taking antihypertensive drugs and not acutely ill. When systolic and diastolic blood pressures fall into different categories, the higher category should be selected to classify the individual's blood pressure status. In addition to classifying stages of hypertension on the basis of average blood pressure levels, clinicians should specify presence or absence of target organ disease and additional risk factors. The specificity is important for risk classification and treatment.

[2]Optimal blood pressure with respect to cardiovascular risk is below 120/80 mm Hg. However, unusually low readings should be evaluated for clinical significance.

[3]Based on the average of two or more readings taken at each of two or more visits after an initial screening.

Adapted from Chobanian AV, Bakris GL, Black HR, et al, Joint National Committee on Prevention, Detection, Evaluation, and Treatment of High Blood Pressure. National Heart, Lung, and Blood Institute; National High Blood Pressure Education Program Coordinating Committee. Seventh Report of the Joint National Committee on Prevention, Detection, Evaluation, and Treatment of High Blood Pressure, *Hypertension*, 2003, 42(6):1206-52.

Table 6.
LIFESTYLE MODIFICATIONS TO MANAGE HYPERTENSION[1-3]

Modification	Recommendation	Approximate Systolic Reduction (Range)
Weight reduction	Maintain normal body weight (body mass index 18.5-24.9 kg/m^2)	5-20 mm of mercury/ 10 kg weight loss[4]
Adopt DASH[5] eating plan	Consume a diet rich in fruits, vegetables, and low fat dairy products with a reduced content of saturated and total fat	8-14 mm Hg[6]
Dietary sodium reduction	Reduce dietary sodium intake to ≤100 mmol/day (2.4 g sodium or 6 g sodium chloride)	2-8 mm Hg[7]
Physical activity	Engage in regular aerobic physical activity such as brisk walking (≥30 minutes/day, most days of the week)	4-9 mm Hg[8]
Moderation of alcohol consumption	Limit consumption to ≤2 drinks (1 oz or 30 mL ethanol); (eg, 24 oz beer, 10 oz wine, or 3 oz 80-proof whiskey) per day in most men and to ≤1 drink/day in women and lighter weight people	2-4 mm Hg[9]

[1]Adapted from U.S. Department of Health and Human Services; National Institutes of Health; National Heart, Lung, and Blood Institute; National High Blood Pressure Education Program

[2]Overall cardiovascular risk education can be achieved by cessation of smoking

[3]The effects of implementing these modifications are dose- and time-dependent and could be greater for some people

[4]The trials of Hypertension Prevention Collaborative Research Group; He and colleagues

[5]DASH: Dietary Approaches to Stop Hypertension

[6]Sacks and colleagues; Vollmer and colleagues

[7]Sacks and colleagues; Vollmer and colleagues; Chobanian and Hill

[8]Kelley and Kelley; Whelton and colleagues

[9]Xin and colleagues

CLASSES OF DRUGS USED IN THE TREATMENT OF HYPERTENSION

Diuretics

Beta-adrenergic receptor blocking agents (beta-blockers)

Alpha$_1$-adrenergic receptor blocking agents (alpha$_1$-blockers)

Agents which have both alpha- and beta-adrenergic blocking properties (alpha-/beta-blockers)

Angiotensin-converting enzyme (ACE) inhibitors

Angiotensin II receptor blockers

Calcium channel blocking agents

Supplemental agents such as central-acting alpha$_2$-adrenergic receptor agonists and direct-acting peripheral vasodilators.

Table 7 lists the drug categories and representative agents used to treat hypertension. Combination drugs are now available to supply several classes of these drugs.

Table 7.
DRUG CATEGORIES AND REPRESENTATIVE AGENTS USED IN THE TREATMENT OF HYPERTENSION[1]

Diuretics

    Thiazide Types

        Chlorothiazide *on page 337*

        Chlorthalidone *on page 347*

        Hydrochlorothiazide *on page 819*

        Indapamide *on page 874*

        Methyclothiazide *on page 1077*

        Metolazone *on page 1087*

        Polythiazide *on page 1323*

    Loops

        Bumetanide *on page 235*

        Ethacrynic Acid *on page 619*

        Furosemide *on page 756*

        Torsemide *on page 1594*

    Potassium-Sparing

        Amiloride *on page 86*

        Spironolactone *on page 1492*

        Triamterene *on page 1613*

    Potassium-Sparing Combinations

        Hydrochlorothiazide and Spironolactone *on page 820*

        Hydrochlorothiazide and Triamterene *on page 821*

Beta-Blockers

    Cardioselective

        Acebutolol *on page 28*

        Atenolol *on page 158*

        Betaxolol *on page 210*

        Bisoprolol *on page 218*

        Metoprolol *on page 1088*

        Sotalol *on page 1489*

    Noncardioselective

        Carteolol *on page 290*

        Carvedilol *on page 291*

        Nadolol *on page 1139*

        Penbutolol *on page 1265*

        Pindolol *on page 1306*

        Propranolol *on page 1373*

        Timolol *on page 1570*

Alpha₁-Blocker

    Doxazosin *on page 529*

    Prazosin *on page 1337*

    Reserpine *on page 1416*

    Terazosin *on page 1538*

Alpha- / Beta-Blocker

    Carvedilol *on page 291*

    Labetalol *on page 940*

Angiotensin-Converting Enzyme (ACE) Inhibitors

    Benazepril *on page 191*

    Captopril *on page 269*

    Enalapril *on page 564*

    Fosinopril *on page 748*

    Lisinopril *on page 990*

    Moexipril *on page 1116*

    Quinapril *on page 1395*

    Ramipril *on page 1406*

    Trandolapril *on page 1598*

Angiotensin-Converting Enzyme (ACE) Inhibitor / Diuretic Combination

    Captopril and Hydrochlorothiazide *on page 271*

    Enalapril and Hydrochlorothiazide *on page 567*

    Lisinopril and Hydrochlorothiazide *on page 992*

Angiotensin II Receptor Blockers

    Candesartan *on page 264*

    Eprosartan *on page 580*

    Irbesartan *on page 907*

    Losartan *on page 1003*

    Telmisartan *on page 1531*

    Valsartan *on page 1643*

Angiotensin II Receptor Blocker / Diuretic Combination

    Candesartan + Hydrochlorothiazide *on page 265*

    Irbesartan + Hydrochlorothiazide *on page 908*

    Valsartan + Hydrochlorothiazide *on page 1644*

CARDIOVASCULAR DISEASES (Continued)

(continued)

Calcium Channel Blockers

    Amlodipine *on page 101*

    Diltiazem *on page 505*

    Felodipine *on page 673*

    Isradipine *on page 919*

    Nicardipine *on page 1168*

    Nifedipine *on page 1173*

    Nisoldipine *on page 1177*

    Verapamil *on page 1654*

Supplemental Agents

    Central-Acting Alpha₂-Agonist

        Clonidine *on page 392*

        Guanabenz *on page 800*

        Guanfacine *on page 801*

        Methyldopa *on page 1077*

    Direct-Acting Peripheral Vasodilator

        Hydralazine *on page 817*

        Minoxidil *on page 1109*

---

[1]Source: USP DI, Volumes I and II, Update, November 1998.

Current Thinking Regarding Antihypertensive Drug Selection

Medications in the first eight categories in Table 7 were held to be equally effective in two large-scale studies reported in the *New England Journal of Medicine* and the *Journal of the American Medical Association*, and that any of the medications could be used initially for monotherapy. According to the Seventh Report of the Joint National Committee on Prevention, Detection, Evaluation, and Treatment of High Blood Pressure (JNC VI), diuretics or beta-blockers are recommended as initial therapy for uncomplicated hypertension. If a diuretic is selected as initial therapy, a thiazide diuretic is preferred in patients with normal renal function. If necessary, potassium replacement or concurrent treatment with a potassium-sparing agent may prevent hypokalemia. Loop diuretics are used in patients with impaired renal function or who cannot tolerate thiazides. Diuretics are well tolerated and inexpensive. They are considered the drugs of choice for treating isolated systolic hypertension in the elderly.

Beta-blockers are the agents of choice in patients with coronary artery disease or supraventricular arrhythmia, and in young patients with hyperdynamic circulation. Beta-blockers are alternatives for initial therapy and are more effective in Caucasian patients than in African-American patients. Beta-blockers are not considered first choice drugs in elderly patients with uncomplicated hypertension. The beta-blocking drug carvedilol also selectively blocks alpha₁ receptors and has been shown to reduce mortality in hypertensive patients.

Alpha₁-adrenergic blocking agents can be used as initial therapy. The alpha₁-blocking agent prazosin and related drugs have an added advantage in treating hypertensive patients with coexisting hyperlipidemia since these medications seem to have beneficial effects on lipid levels. Selective blockade of the post-synaptic alpha₁-receptors by prazosin and related agents reduces peripheral vascular resistance and systemic blood pressure. In addition, all alpha₁-adrenergic blocking agents relieve symptoms of benign prostatic hyperplasia.

ACE inhibitors are the preferred drugs for patients with coexisting heart failure. They are useful as initial therapy in hypertensive patients with kidney damage or diabetes mellitus with proteinuria, and in Caucasian patients. No clinically relevant differences have been found among the available ACE inhibitors. The ACE inhibitors are well tolerated by young, physically active patients, and the elderly. The most common adverse effect of the ACE inhibitors is dry cough. Angiotensin II receptor blockers produce hemodynamic effects similar to ACE inhibitors while avoiding dry cough. These agents are similar to the ACE inhibitors in potency and are useful for initial therapy.

Calcium channel blocking agents are effective as initial therapy in both African-American and Caucasian patients, and are well tolerated by the elderly. These agents inhibit entry of calcium ion into cardiac cells and smooth muscle cells of the coronary and systemic vasculature. Nifedipine (Procardia®) and amlodipine (Norvasc®) are more potent as peripheral vasodilators than diltiazem (Cardizem®). Long-acting formulations of the calcium channel blockers have been shown to be very safe despite some earlier reports that short-acting calcium channel blockers were associated with a 60% increase in heart attacks among hypertensive patients given a short-acting calcium antagonist.

Supplemental antihypertensive agents include the central-acting alpha₂ agonists and direct-acting vasodilators. These agents are less commonly prescribed for initial therapy because of the impressive effectiveness of the other drug groups. Clonidine (Catapres®) lowers blood pressure by activating inhibitory alpha₂ receptors in the CNS, thus reducing sympathetic outflow. It lowers both supine and standing blood pressure by reducing total peripheral resistance. Hydralazine reduces blood pressure by directly relaxing arteriolar smooth muscle. Hydralazine is given orally for the management of chronic hypertension, usually with a diuretic and a beta-blocker.

The most common oral side effects of the management of the hypertensive patient are related to the antihypertensive drug therapy. A dry sore mouth can be caused by diuretics and central-acting adrenergic inhibitors. Occasionally, lichenoid reactions can occur in patients taking quinidine and methyldopa. The thiazides are occasionally also implicated. Lupus-like face rashes can be seen in patients taking calcium channel blockers as well.

Table 8.
CARDIOVASCULAR / RESPIRATORY / NERVOUS SYSTEM EFFECTS CAUSED BY DRUGS USED FOR CARDIOVASCULAR DISORDERS[1]

Agent	Incidence	Adverse Effect
Alpha₁-Blocker		
Prazosin (Minipress®)	More frequent	Orthostatic hypotension, dizziness
	Less frequent	Heart Palpitations
	Rare	Angina
Alpha-/ Beta-Blocker		
Carvedilol (Coreg®)	More frequent	Bradycardia, postural hypotension, dizziness
	Rare	A-V block, hypertension, hypotension, palpitations, vertigo, nervousness, asthma
Angiotensin-Converting Enzyme (ACE) Inhibitors		
Benazepril (Lotensin®)	Less frequent	Dizziness, insomnia, headache
	Rare	Hypotension, bronchitis
Captopril (Capoten®)	Less frequent	Tachycardia, insomnia, transient cough, dizziness, headache
	Rare	Hypotension
Enalapril (Vasotec®)	Less frequent	Chest pain, palpitations, tachycardia, syncope, dizziness, dyspnea
	Rare	Angina pectoris, asthma
Fosinopril (Monopril®)	Less frequent	Orthostatic hypotension, dizziness, cough, headache
	Rare	Syncope, insomnia
Lisinopril (Prinivil®)	Less frequent	Hypotension, dizziness
	Rare	Angina pectoris, orthostatic hypotension, rhythm disturbances, tachycardia
Moexipril (Univasc®)	Less frequent	Hypotension, peripheral edema, headache, dizziness, fatigue, cough, pharyngitis, upper respiratory infection, sinusitis
	Rare	Chest pain, myocardial infarction, palpitations, arrhythmias, syncope, CVA, orthostatic hypotension, dyspnea, bronchospasm
Perindopril Erbumine (Aceon®)	Less frequent	Headache, dizziness, cough[2]
	Rare	Hypotension
Quinapril (Accupril®)	Less frequent	Hypotension, dizziness, headache, cough
	Rare	Orthostatic hypotension, angina, insomnia
Ramipril (Altace®)	Less frequent	Tachycardia, dizziness, headache, cough
	Rare	Hypotension
Trandolapril (Mavik®)	Less frequent	Tachycardia, headache, dizziness, cough[3]
	Rare	Hypotension
Angiotensin-Converting Enzyme Inhibitor / Diuretic Combination		
Captopril/HCTZ (Capozide®)	Less frequent	Tachycardia, palpitations, chest pain, dizziness
	Rare	Hypotension
Angiotensin II Receptor Blockers		
Candesartan (Atacand®)	Less frequent	Chest pain, flushing
	Rare	Myocardial infarction, tachycardia, angina, palpitations, dyspnea
Losartan (Cozaar®)	Less frequent	Hypotension without reflex tachycardia, dizziness
	Rare	Orthostatic hypotension, angina, A-V block (second degree), CVA, palpitations, tachycardia, sinus bradycardia, flushing, dyspnea
Angiotensin II Receptor Blocker / Diuretic Combination		
Candesartan (Atacand HCT™) + HCTZ	Less frequent	Chest pain, flushing
	Rare	Myocardial infarction, tachycardia, angina, palpitations, dyspnea
Irbesartan/HCTZ (Avalide®)		Effects unavailable
Valsartan/HCTZ (Diovan HCT®)		Effects unavailable

CARDIOVASCULAR DISEASES *(Continued)*

Agent	Incidence	Adverse Effect
Antiplatelet / Anticoagulant Agents		
Abciximab (ReoPro®)	More frequent Less frequent	Hypotension, pain Bradycardia
Aspirin	Less frequent or Rare	Anaphylactoid reaction, bronchospastic allergic reaction
Clopidogrel (Plavix®)	Less frequent	Chest pain, edema, hypertension, headache, dizziness, depression, fatigue, dyspnea, rhinitis, bronchitis, coughing, upper respiratory infection, syncope, palpitations, cardiac failure, paresthesia, vertigo, atrial fibrillation, neuralgia
Eptifibatide (Integrilin®)	More frequent	Hypotension, bleeding
Ticlopidine (Ticlid®)	Less frequent Rare	Dizziness Peripheral neuropathy, angioedema, vasculitis, allergic pneumonitis
Tirofiban (Aggrastat®)	More frequent Less frequent	Bleeding Bradycardia, dizziness, headache
Warfarin (Coumadin®)	Less frequent Rare	Hemoptysis Fever, purple toes syndrome
Beta-Blockers		
Acebutolol (Sectral®)	Less frequent Rare	Chest pain, bradycardia, hypotension, dizziness, dyspepsia, dyspnea Ventricular arrhythmias
Atenolol (Tenormin®)	Less frequent Rare	Bradycardia, hypotension, chest pain, dizziness, dyspepsia, dyspnea Ventricular arrhythmias
Betaxolol (Kerlone®)	Less frequent Rare	Bradycardia, palpitations, dizziness Chest pain
Bisoprolol (Zebeta®)	More frequent Less frequent	Lethargy Hypotension, chest pain, bradycardia, headache, dizziness, insomnia, cough
Labetalol (Trandate®)	Less frequent Rare	Orthostatic hypotension, dizziness, nasal congestion Bradycardia, chest pain
Metoprolol (Lopressor®)	More frequent Less frequent Rare	Dizziness Bradycardia, heartburn, wheezing Chest pain, confusion
Nadolol (Corgard®)	More frequent Less frequent Rare	Bradycardia Dizziness, dyspepsia, wheezing Congestive heart failure, orthostatic hypotension, confusion, paresthesia
Penbutolol (Levatol®)	Less frequent Rare	Congestive heart failure, dizziness Bradycardia, chest pain, hypotension, confusion
Pindolol	More frequent Less frequent	Dizziness Congestive heart failure, dyspnea
Propranolol (Inderal®)	More frequent Less frequent Rare	Bradycardia Congestive heart failure, dizziness, wheezing Chest pain, hypotension, bronchospasm
Timolol (Blocadren®)	Less frequent Rare	Bradycardia, dizziness, dyspnea Chest pain, congestive heart failure
Calcium Channel Blockers		
Amlodipine (Norvasc®)	Less frequent Rare	Palpitations, dizziness, dyspnea Hypotension, bradycardia, arrhythmias
Diltiazem (Cardizem®)	Less frequent Rare	Bradycardia, dizziness Dyspepsia, paresthesia, tremor
Nifedipine (Procardia®)	More frequent Less frequent Rare	Flushing, dizziness Palpitations, hypotension, dyspnea Tachycardia, syncope
Verapamil (Calan®)	Less frequent Rare	Bradycardia, congestive heart failure, hypotension Chest pain, hypotension (excessive)
Class I Antiarrhythmics		
Disopyramide (Norpace®)	More frequent Less frequent Rare	Exacerbation of angina pectoris, dizziness Hypotension, hypertension, tachycardia, dyspnea Syncope, flushing, hyperventilation
Flecainide (Tambocor™)	More frequent Less frequent Rare	Dizziness, dyspnea Palpitations, chest pain, tachycardia, tremor Bradycardia, nervousness, paresthesia
Procainimide (Procanbid®)	Less frequent Rare	Tachycardia, dizziness, lightheadedness Hypotension, confusion, disorientation
Propafenone (Rythmol®)	More frequent Less frequent Rare	Dizziness Palpitations, angina, bradycardia, loss of balance, dyspepsia, dyspnea Paresthesia
Quinidine	Less frequent Rare	Hypotension, syncope, lightheadedness, wheezing Confusion, vertigo, angina, edema

Agent	Incidence	Adverse Effect
Class III Antiarrhythmics		
Amiodarone (Cordarone®)	*More frequent*	Dizziness, tremor, paresthesia, dyspnea
	Less frequent	Congestive heart failure, bradycardia, tachycardia
	Rare	Hypotension
Sotalol (Betapace®)	*More frequent*	Bradycardia, chest pain, palpitations, fatigue, dizziness, lightheadedness, dyspnea
	Less frequent	CHF, hypotension, proarrhythmia, syncope, reduced peripheral circulation, edema, asthma, upper respiratory problems
	Rare	Diaphoresis, clouded sensorium, fever, lack of coordination
Digitalis Glycosides		
Digoxin (Lanoxicaps®, Lanoxin®)	*Rare*	Atrial tachycardia, sinus bradycardia, ventricular fibrillation, vertigo
Diuretics		
Thiazide type	*Rare*	Hypotension
Loops	*More frequent*	Orthostatic hypotension, dizziness
Potassium-sparing	*Less frequent*	Hypotension, bradycardia, dizziness
	Rare	Flushing
Potassium-sparing combination	*Rare*	Dizziness
HMG-CoA Reductase Inhibitors		
Atorvastatin Fluvastatin Lovastatin Pravastatin Simvastatin	*Less frequent*	Headache, dizziness
Nitrates		
Nitroglycerins	*More frequent*	Postural hypotension, flushing, headache, dizziness
	Rare	Reflex tachycardia, bradycardia, arrhythmia
Supplemental Drugs for Heart Failure		
Inamrinone	*Less frequent*	Arrhythmia, chest pain
Dobutamine	*Less frequent*	Tachycardia, chest pain
	Rare	Headache, dyspnea
Hydralazine	*More frequent*	Tachycardia, headache
	Less frequent	Hypotension, nasal congestion
	Rare	Edema, dizziness
Milrinone (Primacor®)	*More frequent*	Arrhythmias
	Less frequent	Chest pain
Nitroprusside sodium (Nitropress®)	*Less frequent*	Palpitations, headache
Supplemental Drugs for Hypertension		
Central-Acting Alpha$_2$-Agonists		
Clonidine (Catapres®)	*More frequent*	Dizziness
	Less frequent	Orthostatic hypotension, nervousness/agitation
	Rare	Palpitations, tachycardia, bradycardia, congestive heart failure
Direct-Acting		
Hydralazine	*More frequent*	Tachycardia, headache
	Less frequent	Hypotension, nasal congestion
	Rare	Edema, dizziness

Legend: % of incidence: More frequent = >10%, less frequent = 1% to 10%, rare = <1%.

[1]Source: Professional package insert for individual agents or United States Pharmacopeial Dispensing Information. *Drug Information for the Health Care Professional*, Vol I, 19th ed, Rockville, MD: The United States Pharmacopeial Convention, Inc, 1999.

[2]Incidence greater in women 3:1.

[3]More frequent in women.

CARDIOVASCULAR DISEASES *(Continued)*

Table 9.
CARDIOVASCULAR DRUGS
DENTAL DRUG INTERACTIONS
AND EFFECTS ON DENTAL TREATMENT

Alpha₁-Blocker	
Prazosin (Minipress®)	Significant orthostatic hypotension a possibility; monitor patient when getting out of dental chair; significant dry mouth in up to 10% of patients.
Alpha- / Beta-Blocker	
Carvedilol (Coreg®)	See Nonselective Beta-Blockers
ACE Inhibitors	The NSAID indomethacin reduces the hypotensive effects of ACE inhibitors. Effects of other NSAIDs such as ibuprofen not considered significant.
Angiotensin-Converting Enzyme Inhibitor / Diuretic Combination	
Captopril/HCTZ (Capozide®)	No effect or complications on dental treatment reported.
Angiotensin II Receptor Blockers	
Candesartan (Atacand®)	No effect or complications on dental treatment reported.
Losartan (Cozaar®)	
Antiplatelet / Anticoagulant Agents	
Aspirin	May cause a reduction in the serum levels of NSAIDs if they are used to manage post-operative pain.
Clopidogrel (Plavix®)	If a patient is to undergo elective surgery and an antiplatelet effect is not desired, clopidogrel should be discontinued 7 days prior to surgery.
Eptifibatide (Integrilin®)	Bleeding may occur while patient is medicated with eptifibatide; platelet function is restored in about 4 hours following discontinuation.
Warfarin (Coumadin®)	Signs of warfarin overdose may first appear as bleeding from gingival tissue; consultation with prescribing physician is advisable prior to surgery to determine temporary dose reduction or withdrawal of medication.
Beta-Blockers	
Cardioselective	Cardioselective beta-blockers (ie, atenolol) have no effect or complications on dental treatment reported.
Noncardioselective	Any of the noncardioselective beta-blockers (ie, nadolol, penbutolol, pindolol, propranolol, timolol) may enhance the pressor response to vasoconstrictor epinephrine resulting in hypertension and reflex bradycardia. Although not reported, it is assumed that similar effects could be caused with levonordefrin (Neo-Cobefrin®). Use either vasoconstrictor with caution in hypertensive patients medicated with noncardioselective beta-adrenergic blockers.
Calcium Channel Blockers	Cause gingival hyperplasia in approximately 1% of the general population taking these drugs. There have been fewer reports with diltiazem and amlodipine than with other CBs such as nifedipine. The hyperplasia will usually disappear with cessation of drug therapy. Consultation with the physician is suggested
Class I Antiarrhythmics	
Disopyramide (Norpace®)	Increased serum levels and toxicity with erythromycin. High incidence of anticholinergic effect manifested as dry mouth and throat.
Flecainide (Tambocor™)	No effects or complications on dental treatment reported.
Procainamide (Procanbid®)	Systemic lupus-like syndrome has been reported resulting in joint pain and swelling, pains with breathing, skin rash.
Propafenone (Rythmol®)	Greater than 10 % experience significantly reduced salivary flow; taste disturbance, bitter or metallic taste
Quinidine	Secondary anticholinergic effects may decrease salivary flow, especially in middle-aged and elderly patients; known to contribute to caries, periodontal disease, and oral candidiasis.
Class III Antiarrhythmics	
Amiodarone	Bitter or metallic taste has been reported.
Digitalis Glycosides	Use vasoconstrictor with caution due to risk of cardiac arrhythmias. Sensitive gag reflex induced by digitalis drugs may cause difficulty in taking dental impressions.
Diuretics	
Thiazide type	No effects or complications on dental treatment reported.
Loops	NSAIDs may increase chloride and tubular water reuptake to counter-act loop type diuretics.
Potassium-sparing	No effects or complications on dental treatment reported.
Potassium-sparing combination	No effects or complications on dental treatment reported.

HMG-CoA Reductase Inhibitors	Concurrent use of erythromycin, clarithromycin, and some of the statin drugs may result in rhabdomyolysis.
Nitrates	No effects or complications on dental treatment reported.
Supplemental Drugs for Heart Failure	
Inamrinone Milrinone (Primacor®)	No effects or complications on dental treatment reported
Supplemental Drugs for Hypertension	
Central-Acting Alpha₂-Agonists	
Clonidine (Catapres®)	Greater than 10% of patients experience significant dry mouth.
Direct-Acting	
Hydralazine	No effect or complications on dental treatment reported.

References

Chobanian AV, Bakris GL, Black HR, et al, "The Seventh Report of the Joint National Committee on Prevention, Detection, Evaluation, and Treatment of High Blood Pressure: The JNC 7 Report," *JAMA*, 2003, 289(19):2560-72.

Chobanian AV and Hill M, "National Heart, Lung, and Blood Institute Workshop on Sodium and Blood Pressure: A Critical Review of Current Scientific Evidence," *Hypertension*, 2000, 35(4):858-63.

"Effects of Weight Loss and Sodium Reduction Intervention on Blood Pressure and Hypertension Incidence in Overweight People With High-Normal Blood Pressure. The Trials of Hypertension Prevention, Phase II. The Trials of Hypertension Prevention Collaborative Research Group," *Arch Intern Med*, 1997, 157(6):657-67.

He J, Whelton PK, Appel LJ, et al, "Long-Term Effects of Weight Loss and Dietary Sodium Reduction on Incidence of Hypertension," *Hypertension*, 2000, 35(2):544-9.

Kelley GA and Kelley KS, "Progressive Resistance Exercise and Resting Blood Pressure: A Meta-Analysis of Randomized Controlled Trials," *Hypertension*, 2000, 35(3):838-43.

Sacks FM, Svetkey LP, Vollmer WM, et al, "Effects on Blood Pressure of Reduced Dietary Sodium and the Dietary Approaches to Stop Hypertension (DASH) Diet. DASH-Sodium Collaborative Research Group," *N Engl J Med*, 2001, 344(1):3-10.

Vollmer WM, Sacks FM, Ard J, et al, "Effects of Diet and Sodium Intake on Blood Pressure: Subgroup Analysis of the DASH-Sodium Trial," *Ann Intern Med*, 2001, 135(12):1019-28.

Whelton SP, Chin A, Xin X, et al, "Effect of Aerobic Exercise on Blood Pressure: A Meta-Analysis of Randomized, Controlled Trials," *Ann Intern Med*, 2002, 136(7):493-503.

Xin X, He J, Frontini MG, et al, "Effects of Alcohol Reduction on Blood Pressure: A Meta-Analysis of Randomized Controlled Trials," *Hypertension*, 2001, 38(5):1112-7.

ADDITIONAL CLINICAL RISK RELATED TO DRUGS PROLONGING QT INTERVAL

The QT interval is measured as the time and distance between the Q point of the QRS complex and the end of the T wave in the ECG tracing. After adjustment for heart rate, the QT interval is defined as prolonged if it is more than 450 msec in men and 460 msec in women. A long QT syndrome was first described in the 1950s and 60s as a congenital syndrome involving QT interval prolongation, syncope, and sudden death. Some of the congenital long QT syndromes were characterized by a peculiar electrocardiographic appearance of the QRS complex involving a premature atria beat followed by a pause, then a subsequent sinus beat showing marked QT prolongation and deformity. This type of cardiac arrhythmia was originally termed "torsade de pointes" (translated from the French as "twisting of the points").

Prolongation of the QT interval is thought to result from delayed ventricular repolarization. The repolarization process within the myocardial cell is due to the efflux of intracellular potassium. The channels associated with this current can be blocked by many drugs and predispose the electrical propagation cycle to torsade de pointes.

Erythromycin, a drug often associated with dental antibiotics, is considered as having a risk of causing torsade de pointes. The risk of drug-induced torsade de pointes is extremely low when a single QT interval prolonging drug is prescribed. It is not known what effect vasoconstrictors in the local anesthetic regimen will have in patients with a known history of congenital prolonged QT interval or in patients taking any medication that prolongs the QT interval. Until more information is obtained, it is suggested that the clinician consult with the physician prior to the use of a vasoconstrictor in suspected patients, and that the vasoconstrictor (epinephrine, levonordefrin [Neo-Cobefrin®]) be used with caution.

Thioridazine is another one of the drugs confirmed to prolong the QT interval and is accepted as having a risk of causing torsade de pointes. The risk of drug-induced torsade de pointes is extremely low when a single QT interval prolonging drug is prescribed. In terms of epinephrine, it is not known what effect vasoconstrictors in the local anesthetic regimen will have in patients with a known history of congenital prolonged QT interval or in patients taking any medication that prolongs the QT interval. Until more information is obtained, it is suggested that the clinician consult with the physician prior to the use of a vasoconstrictor in suspected patients, and that the vasoconstrictor (epinephrine, levonordefrin [Neo-Cobefrin®]) be used with caution.

CARDIOVASCULAR DISEASES *(Continued)*

Table 10.
DRUGS GENERALLY ACCEPTED AS HAVING A RISK OF CAUSING TORSADES DE POINTES

Generic Name	Brand Name	Use
Amiodarone	Cordarone®	Antiarrhythmic
Arsenic Trioxide	Trisenox®	Antileukemic agent
Chloroquine	Aralen®	Antimalarial
Chlorpromazine	–	Antipsychotic
Clarithromycin	**Biaxin®**	Antibiotic
Disopyramide	Norpace®	Antiarrhythmic
Dofetilide	Tikosyn®	Antiarrhythmic
Droperidol	Inapsine®	Antiemetic
Erythromycin	**Various brand names available**	**Antibiotic**
Haloperidol	Haldol®	Antipsychotic
Ibutilide	Corvert®	Antiarrhythmic
Mesoridazine	–	Antipsychotic
Methadone	Various brand names available	Analgesic, Opioid
Pentamidine	NebuPent®	Antibiotic
Pimozide	Orap®	Antipsychotic
Posaconazole	**Noxafil®**	**Antifungal**
Procainamide	Procanbid®	Antiarrhythmic
Quinidine	–	Antiarrhythmic
Sotalol	Betapace®	Antiarrhythmic
Thioridazine	–	Antipsychotic

Note: Dental drugs are identified by bold print. Adapted from: http://www.torsades.org.

GASTROINTESTINAL DISORDERS

The oral cavity and related structures comprise the first part of the gastrointestinal tract. Diseases affecting the oral cavity are often reflected in GI disturbances. In addition, the oral cavity may indeed reflect diseases of the GI tract, including ulcers, polyps, and liver and gallbladder diseases. The first oral condition that may reflect or be reflected in GI disturbances is that of taste. Typically, complaints of taste abnormalities are presented to the dentist. The sweet, saline, sour, and bitter taste sensations all vary in quality and intensity and are affected by the olfactory system. Often, anemic conditions are reflected in changes in the tongue, resulting in taste aberrations.

Gastric and duodenal ulcers represent the primary diseases that can reflect themselves in the oral cavity. Gastric reflux and problems with food metabolism often present as acid erosions to the teeth and occasionally, changes in the mucosal surface as well. Patients may be encountered that may be identified, upon diagnosis, as harboring the organism *Helicobacter pylori*. Treatment with antibiotics can oftentimes aid in correcting the ulcerative disease.

Proton Pump and Gastric Acid Secretion Inhibitors

Lansoprazole *on page 947*

Lansoprazole, Amoxicillin, and Clarithromycin *on page 948*

Lansoprazole and Naproxen *on page 949*

Omeprazole *on page 1206*

Pantoprazole *on page 1249*

Histamine H₂ Antagonist

Cimetidine *on page 358*

Famotidine *on page 670*

Nizatidine *on page 1184*

Ranitidine *on page 1409*

The oral aspects of gastrointestinal disease are often nonspecific and are related to the patient's gastric reflux problems. Intestinal polyps occasionally present as part of the "Peutz-Jeghers Syndrome", resulting in pigmented areas of the peri-oral region that resemble freckles. The astute dentist will need to differentiate these from melanin pigmentation, while at the same time encouraging the patient to perhaps seek evaluation for an intestinal disorder.

Diseases of the liver and gallbladder system are complex. Most of the disorders that the dentist is interested in are covered in the section Systemic Viral Diseases *on page 1767*. All of the new drugs, including interferons, are mentioned in this section.

GASTROINTESTINAL DISORDERS *(Continued)*

Multiple Drug Regimens for the Treatment of *H. pylori* Infection

Drug	Dosages	Duration of Therapy
H₂-receptor antagonist[1]	Any one given at appropriate dose	4 weeks
plus		
Bismuth *on page 217*	525 mg 4 times/day	2 weeks
plus		
Metronidazole *on page 1091*	250 mg 4 times/day	2 weeks
plus		
Tetracycline *on page 1548*	500 mg 4 times/day	2 weeks
Proton pump inhibitor[1]	Esomeprazole 40 mg once daily	10 days
plus		
Clarithromycin *on page 371*	500 mg twice daily	10 days
plus		
Amoxicillin *on page 108*	1000 mg twice daily	10 days
Proton pump inhibitor[1]	Lansoprazole 30 mg twice daily or Omeprazole 20 mg twice daily	10-14 days
plus		
Clarithromycin *on page 371*	500 mg twice daily	10-14 days
plus		
Amoxicillin *on page 108*	1000 mg twice daily	10-14 days
Proton pump inhibitor[1]	Rabeprazole 20 mg twice daily	7 days
plus		
Clarithromycin *on page 371*	500 mg twice daily	7 days
plus		
Amoxicillin *on page 108*	1000 mg twice daily	7 days
Proton pump inhibitor	Lansoprazole 30 mg twice daily or Omeprazole 20 mg twice daily	2 weeks
plus		
Clarithromycin *on page 371*	500 mg twice daily	2 weeks
plus		
Metronidazole *on page 1091*	500 mg twice daily	2 weeks
Proton pump inhibitor	Lansoprazole 30 mg once daily or Omeprazole 20 mg once daily	2 weeks
plus		
Bismuth *on page 217*	525 mg 4 times/day	2 weeks
plus		
Metronidazole *on page 1091*	500 mg 3 times/day	2 weeks
plus		
Tetracycline *on page 1548*	500 mg 4 times/day	2 weeks

[1]FDA-approved regimen

Modified from Howden CS and Hunt RH, "Guidelines for the Management of *Helicobacter pylori* Infection," *AJG*, 1998, 93:2336.

RESPIRATORY DISEASES

Diseases of the respiratory system put dental patients at increased risk in the dental office because of their decreased pulmonary reserve, the medications they may be taking, drug interactions between these medications, medications the dentist may prescribe, and in some patients with infectious respiratory diseases, a risk of disease transmission.

The respiratory system consists of the nasal cavity, the nasopharynx, the trachea, and the components of the lung including, of course, the bronchi, the bronchioles, and the alveoli. The diseases that affect the lungs and the respiratory system can be separated by location of affected tissue. Diseases that affect the lower respiratory tract are often chronic, although infections can also occur. Three major diseases that affect the lower respiratory tract are often encountered in the medical history for dental patients. These include chronic bronchitis, emphysema, and asthma. Diseases that affect the upper respiratory tract are usually of the infectious nature and include sinusitis and the common cold. The upper respiratory tract infections may also include a wide variety of nonspecific infections, most of which are also caused by viruses. Influenza produces upper respiratory type symptoms and is often caused by orthomyxoviruses. Herpangina is caused by the Coxsackie type viruses and results in upper respiratory infections in addition to pharyngitis or sore throat. One serious condition, known as croup, has been associated with *Haemophilus influenzae* infections. Other more serious infections might include respiratory syncytial virus, adenoviruses, and parainfluenza viruses.

The respiratory symptoms that are often encountered in both upper respiratory and lower respiratory disorders include cough, dyspnea (difficulty in breathing), the production of sputum, hemoptysis (coughing up blood), a wheeze, and occasionally chest pain. One additional symptom, orthopnea (difficulty in breathing when lying down), is often used by the dentist to assist in evaluating the patient with the condition, pulmonary edema. This condition results from either respiratory disease or congestive heart failure.

No effective drug treatments are available for the management of many of the upper respiratory tract viral infections. However, amantadine (sold under the brand name Symmetrel®) is a synthetic drug given orally (200 mg/day) and has been found to be effective against some strains of influenza. Treatment other than for influenza includes supportive care products, available over-the-counter. These might include antihistamines for symptomatic relief of the upper respiratory congestion, antibiotics to combat secondary bacterial infections, and in severe cases, fluids, when patients have become dehydrated during the illness (see Pharmacologic Category Index for selection). The treatment of herpangina may include management of the painful ulcerations of the oropharynx. The dentist may become involved in managing these lesions in a similar way to those seen in other acute viral infections (see Systemic Viral Diseases *on page 1767*).

SINUSITIS

Sinusitis also represents an upper respiratory infection that often comes under the purview of the practicing dentist. Acute sinusitis, characterized by nasal obstruction, fever, chills, and midface head pain, may be encountered by the dentist and discovered as part of a differential workup for other facial or dental pain. Chronic sinusitis may likewise produce similar dental symptoms. Dental drugs of choice may include ephedrine or nasal drops, antihistamines, and analgesics. These drugs sometimes require supplementation with antibiotics. Most commonly, broad spectrum antibiotics such as ampicillin are prescribed. These are often combined with antral lavage to re-establish drainage from the sinus area. Surgical intervention, such as a Caldwell-Luc procedure opening into the sinus, is rarely necessary and many of the second generation antibiotics, such as cephalosporins, are used successfully in treating the acute and chronic sinusitis patient (see Antibiotic Prophylaxis *on page 1772*).

> Gatifloxacin *on page 766*
> Moxifloxacin *on page 1129*

LOWER RESPIRATORY DISEASES

Lower respiratory tract diseases, including asthma, chronic bronchitis, and emphysema are often identified in dental patients. Asthma is an intermittent respiratory disorder that produces recurrent bronchial smooth muscle spasm, inflammation of the bronchial mucosa, and hypersecretion of mucus. The incidence of childhood asthma appears to be increasing and may be related to the presence of pollutants such as sulfur dioxide and indoor cigarette smoke. The end result is widespread narrowing of the airways and decreased ventilation with increased airway resistance, especially to expiration. Asthmatic patients often suffer from asthmatic attacks when stimulated by respiratory tract infections, exercise, and cold air. Medications such as aspirin and some NSAIDs, as well as cholinergic and beta-adrenergic blocking drugs, can also trigger asthmatic attacks in addition to chemicals, smoke, and emotional anxiety.

RESPIRATORY DISEASES *(Continued)*

The classical chronic obstructive pulmonary diseases (COPD) of chronic bronchitis and emphysema are both characterized by chronic airflow obstructions during normal ventilatory efforts. They often occur in combination in the same patient and their treatment is similar. One common finding is that the patient is often a smoker. The dentist can play a role in reinforcement of smoking cessation in patients with chronic respiratory diseases.

Treatments include a variety of drugs depending on the severity of the symptoms and the respiratory compromise upon full respiratory evaluation. Patients who are having acute and chronic obstructive pulmonary attacks may be susceptible to infection and antibiotics such as penicillin, ampicillin, tetracycline, or sulfamethoxazole-trimethoprim are often used to eradicate susceptible infective organisms. Corticosteroids, as well as a wide variety of respiratory stimulants, are available in inhalant and/or oral forms. In patients using inhalant medication, oral candidiasis is occasionally encountered.

Amantadine *on page 83*
Analgesics
Antibiotics
Antihistamines
Decongestants
Epinephrine *on page 572*
Gatifloxacin *on page 766*
Moxifloxacin *on page 1129*

SPECIFIC DRUGS USED IN THE TREATMENT OF CHRONIC RESPIRATORY CONDITIONS

Beta$_2$-Selective Agonists

Albuterol *on page 58*
Metaproterenol *on page 1055*
Pirbuterol *on page 1315*
Salmeterol *on page 1453*
Terbutaline *on page 1540*

Methylxanthines

Aminophylline *on page 90*
Theophylline *on page 1554*

Mast Cell Stabilizer

Cromolyn *on page 417*
Nedocromil *on page 1155*

Corticosteroids

Beclomethasone *on page 188*
Dexamethasone *on page 464*
Flunisolide *on page 705*
Fluticasone *on page 725*
Mometasone Furoate *on page 1118*
Prednisone *on page 1342*
Triamcinolone *on page 1608*

Anticholinergics

Ipratropium *on page 905*

Leukotriene Receptor Antagonists

Montelukast *on page 1121*
Zafirlukast *on page 1675*

5-Lipoxygenase Inhibitors

Zileuton *on page 1681*

Other respiratory diseases include tuberculosis and sarcoidosis which are considered to be restrictive granulomatous respiratory diseases (see Tuberculosis *on page 1765*). Sarcoidosis is a condition that at one time was thought to be similar to tuberculosis, however, it is a multisystem disorder of unknown origin which has as a characteristic lymphocytic and mononuclear phagocytic accumulation in epithelioid granulomas within the lung. It occurs worldwide but shows a slight increased prevalence in temperate climates. The treatment of sarcoidosis is usually one that corresponds to its usually benign course, however, many patients are placed on corticosteroids at the level of 40-60 mg of prednisone daily. This treatment is continued for a protracted period of time. As in any disease requiring steroid therapy, consideration of adrenal suppression is necessary. Alteration of steroid dosage prior to stressful dental procedures may be necessary, usually increasing the steroid dosage prior to and during the stressful procedures and then gradually returning the patient to the original dosage over several days. Many dentists prefer to use the Medrol® Dosepak®, however, consultation with the patient's physician regarding dose selection is always advised. Even in the absence of evidence of adrenal suppression, consultation with the prescribing physician for appropriate dosing and timing of procedures is advisable.

Prednisone *on page 1342*

RELATIVE POTENCY OF ENDOGENOUS AND SYNTHETIC CORTICOSTEROIDS

Agent	Equivalent Dose (mg)
Short-Acting (8-12 h)	
Cortisol	20
Cortisone acetate	25
Intermediate-Acting (18-36 h)	
Prednisolone	5
Prednisone	5
Methylprednisolone	4
Triamcinolone	4
Long-Acting (36-54 h)	
Betamethasone	0.75
Dexamethasone	0.75

Potential drug interactions for the respiratory disease patient exist. An acute sensitivity to aspirin-containing drugs and some of the nonsteroidal anti-inflammatory drugs is a threat for the asthmatic patient. Barbiturates and narcotics may occasionally precipitate asthmatic attacks as well. Erythromycin, clarithromycin, and ketoconazole are contraindicated in patients who are taking theophylline due to potential enhancement of theophylline toxicity. Patients that are taking steroid preparations as part of their respiratory therapy may require alteration in dosing prior to stressful dental procedures. The physician should be consulted.

Barbiturates
Clarithromycin *on page 371*
Erythromycin *on page 589*
Ketoconazole *on page 928*

ENDOCRINE DISORDERS AND PREGNANCY

The human endocrine system manages metabolism and homeostasis. Numerous glandular tissues produce hormones that act in broad reactions with tissues throughout the body. Cells in various organ systems may be sensitive to the hormone, or they release, in reaction to the hormone, a second hormone that acts directly on another organ. Diseases of the endocrine system may have importance in dentistry. For the purposes of this section, we will limit our discussion to diseases of the thyroid tissues, diabetes mellitus, and conditions requiring the administration of synthetic hormones, and pregnancy.

THYROID

Thyroid diseases can be classified into conditions that cause the thyroid to be overactive (hyperthyroidism) and those that cause the thyroid to be underactive (hypothyroidism). Clinical signs and symptoms associated with hyperthyroidism may include goiter, heat intolerance, tremor, weight loss, diarrhea, and hyperactivity. Thyroid hormone production can be tested by TSH levels and additional screens may include radioactive iodine uptake or a pre-T_4 (tetraiodothyronine, thyroxine) assay or iodine index or total serum T_3 (triiodothyronine). The results of thyroid function tests may be altered by ingestion of antithyroid drugs such as propylthiouracil, estrogen-containing drugs, and organic and inorganic iodides. When a diagnosis of hyperthyroidism has been made, treatment usually begins with antithyroid drugs which may include propranolol coupled with radioactive iodides as well as surgical procedures to reduce thyroid tissue. Generally, the beta-blockers are used to control cardiovascular effects of excessive T_4. Propylthiouracil or methimazole are the most common antithyroid drugs used. The dentist should be aware that epinephrine is definitely contraindicated in patients with uncontrolled hyperthyroidism.

Diseases and conditions associated with hypothyroidism may include bradycardia, drowsiness, cold intolerance, thick dry skin, and constipation. Generally, hypothyroidism is treated with replacement thyroid hormone until a euthyroid state is achieved. Various preparations are available, the most common is levothyroxine, commonly known as Synthroid® or Levothroid®, and is generally the drug of choice for thyroid replacement therapy.

Drugs to Treat Hypothyroidism

Drugs to Treat Hyperthyroidism

DIABETES

Diabetes mellitus refers to a condition of prolonged hyperglycemia associated with either abnormal production or lack of production of insulin. Commonly known as Type 1 diabetes, insulin-dependent diabetes (IDDM) is a condition where there are absent or deficient levels of circulating insulin therefore triggering tissue reactions associated with prolonged hyperglycemia. The kidney's attempt to excrete the excess glucose and the organs that do not receive adequate glucose essentially are damaged. Small vessels and arterial vessels in the eye, kidney, and brain are usually at the greatest risk. Generally, blood sugar levels between 70-120 mg/dL are considered to be normal. Inadequate insulin levels allow glucose to rise to greater than the renal threshold which is 180 mg/dL, and such elevations prolonged lead to organ damage.

The goals of treatment of the diabetic are to maintain metabolic control of the blood glucose levels and to reduce the morbid effects of periodic hyperglycemia. Insulin therapy is the primary mechanism to attain management of consistent insulin levels. Insulin preparations are categorized according to their duration of action. Generally, NPH or intermediate-acting insulin and long-acting insulin can be used in combination with short-acting or regular insulin to maintain levels consistent throughout the day.

In Type 2 or noninsulin-dependent diabetes (NIDDM), the receptor for insulin in the tissues is generally down regulated and the glucose, therefore, is not utilized at an appropriate rate. There is perhaps a stronger genetic basis for noninsulin-dependent diabetes than for Type 1. Treatment of the diabetes Type 2 patient is generally directed toward early nonpharmacologic intervention, mainly weight reduction, moderate exercise, and lower plasma-glucose concentrations. Oral hypoglycemic agents as seen in the list below are often used to maintain blood sugar levels. Thirty percent of Type 2 diabetics require insulin, as well as, oral hypoglycemics in order to manage their diabetes. Generally, the two classes of oral hypoglycemics are the sulfonylureas and the biguanides. The sulfonylureas are prescribed more frequently and they stimulate beta cell production of insulin, increase glucose utilization, and tend to normalize glucose metabolism in the liver. The uncontrolled diabetic may represent a challenge to the dental practitioner.

Glycosylated hemoglobin or glycol-hemoglobin assays have emerged as a "gold standard" by which glycemic control is measured in diabetic patients. The test does not rely on the patient's ability to monitor their daily blood glucose levels and is not influenced by acute changes in blood glucose or by the interval since the last meal. Glycohemoglobin is formed when glucose reacts with hemoglobin A in the blood and is composed of several fractions. Numerous assay methods have been developed, however, they vary in their precision. Dental clinicians are advised to be aware of the laboratory's particular standardization procedures when requesting glycosylated hemoglobin values. One major advantage of the glycosylated hemoglobin assay is that it provides an overview of the level of glucose in the life span of the red blood cell population in the patient, and therefore is a measure of overall glycemic control for the previous six to twelve weeks. Thus, clinicians use glycosylated hemoglobin values to determine whether their patient is under good control, on average. These assays have less value in medication dosing decisions. Blood glucose monitoring methods are actually better in that respect. The values of glycosylated hemoglobin are expressed as a percentage of the total hemoglobin in the red blood cell population and a normal value is considered to be <6%. The goal is generally for diabetic patients to remain at <7% and values >8% would constitute a worrisome signal. Medical conditions such as anemias or any red blood cell disease, numerous levels of myelosuppression, or pregnancy can artificially lower glycosylated hemoglobin values.

See Insulin Regular *on page 889*

Oral Hypoglycemic Agents

Acarbose *on page 27*

Chlorpropamide *on page 346*

Glimepiride *on page 780*

Glipizide *on page 782*

Glyburide *on page 786*

Glyburide and Metformin *on page 787*

Metformin *on page 1056*

Miglitol *on page 1104*

Nateglinide *on page 1154*

Repaglinide *on page 1415*

Tolazamide *on page 1582*

Tolbutamide *on page 1583*

Adjunct Therapy

Metoclopramide *on page 1086*

Oral manifestations of uncontrolled diabetes might include abnormal neutrophil function resulting in a poor response to periodontal pathogens. Increased risk of gingivitis and periodontitis in these patients is common. Candidiasis is also a frequent occurrence. Denture-sore mouth may be more prominent. Poor wound-healing following extractions may be one of the complications encountered.

HORMONAL THERAPY

Two uses of hormonal supplementation include oral contraceptives and estrogen replacement therapy. Drugs used for contraception interfere with fertility by inhibiting release of follicle stimulating hormone, luteinizing hormone, and by preventing ovulation. There are few oral side effects; however, moderate gingivitis, similar to that seen during pregnancy, has been reported. The dentist should be aware that decreased effect of oral contraceptives has been reported with most antibiotics (see individual monographs for specific details). It is therefore recommended that dental professionals, when prescribing antibiotics to oral contraceptive users, advise them of this interaction and suggest consulting their physician for additional barrier contraception during antibiotic therapy.

The combination estradiol cypionate and medroxyprogesterone acetate has recently been approved. It is a single monthly injection and has similar warnings and guidelines. However, it's use with antibiotics have not been firmly established. Therefore, discussion/consultation with the patient's OB/GYN physician is indicated.

ENDOCRINE DISORDERS AND PREGNANCY *(Continued)*

Drugs commonly encountered include:

Estradiol *on page 602*
Medroxyprogesterone *on page 1026*
Mestranol and Norethindrone *on page 1053*
Norethindrone *on page 1186*

Estrogens or derivatives are usually prescribed as replacement therapy following menopause or cyclic irregularities and to inhibit osteoporosis. The following list of drugs may interact with antidepressants and barbiturates. New tissue-specific estrogens like Evista® may help with the problem of osteoporosis.

Estrogens (Conjugated/Equine) *on page 609*
Estrogens (Conjugated A/Synthetic) *on page 606*
Estrogens (Esterified) *on page 613*
Estrogens (Conjugated/Equine) and Medroxyprogesterone *on page 612*
Estrogens (Esterified) and Methyltestosterone *on page 614*
Estropipate *on page 615*
Raloxifene *on page 1403*

PREGNANCY

Normal endocrine and physiologic functions are altered during pregnancy. Endogenous estrogens and progesterone increase and placental hormones are secreted. Thyroid stimulating hormone and growth hormone also increase. Cardiovascular changes can result and increased blood volume can lead to blood pressure elevations and transient heart murmurs. Generally, in a normal pregnancy, oral gingival changes will be limited to gingivitis. Alteration of treatment plans might include limiting administration of all drugs to emergency procedures only during the first and third trimesters and medical consultation regarding the patients' status for all elective procedures. Limiting dental care throughout pregnancy to preventive procedures is not unreasonable. The effects on dental treatment of the "morning after pill" (Plan B® and PREVEN®) and the abortifacient, mifepristone *on page 1103*, have not been documented at this time.

HIV INFECTION AND AIDS

Human immunodeficiency virus (HIV) represents agents HIV-1 and HIV-2 that produce a devastating systemic disease. The virus causes disease by leading to elevated risk of infections in patients and, from our experience over the last 18 years, there clearly are oral manifestations associated with these patients. Also, there has been a revolution in infection control in our dental offices over the last two decades due to our expanding knowledge of this infectious agent. Infection control practices have been elevated to include all of the infectious agents with which dentists often come into contact. These might include, in addition to HIV, hepatitis viruses (of which the serotypes include A, B, C, D, E, F, and G; see Occupational Exposure to Bloodborne Pathogens (Standard/Universal Precautions) *on page 1871*); the herpes viruses (see Systemic Viral Diseases *on page 1767*); STDs such as syphilis, gonorrhea, and papillomavirus (see Sexually-Transmitted Diseases *on page 1766*).

Acquired immunodeficiency syndrome (AIDS) has been recognized since early 1981 as a unique clinical syndrome manifest by opportunistic infections or by neoplasms complicating the underlying defect in the cellular immune system. These defects are now known to be brought on by infection and pathogenesis with human immunodeficiency virus 1 or 2 (HIV-1 is the predominant serotype identified). The major cellular defect brought on by infection with HIV is a depletion of T-cells, primarily the sub-type, T-helper cells, known as CD4+ cells. Over these years, our knowledge regarding HIV infection and the oral manifestations often associated with patients with HIV or AIDS, has increased dramatically. Populations of individuals known to be at high risk of HIV transmission include homosexuals, intravenous drug abuse patients, transfusion recipients, patients with other sexually transmitted diseases, and patients practicing promiscuous sex.

The definitions of AIDS have also evolved over this period of time. The natural history of HIV infection along with some of the oral manifestations can be reviewed in Table 1. The risk of developing these opportunistic infections increases as the patient progresses to AIDS.

Table 1.
NATURAL HISTORY OF HIV INFECTION/ORAL MANIFESTATIONS

Time From Transmission (Average)	Observation	CD4 Cell Count
0	Viral transmissions	Normal: 1000 ($\pm$500/mm^3)
2-4 weeks	Self-limited infectious mononucleosis-like illness with fever, rash, leukopenia, mucocutaneous ulcerations (mouth, genitals, etc), thrush	Transient decrease
6-12 weeks	Seroconversion (rarely requires $\geq$3 months for seroconversion)	Normal
0-8 years	Healthy/asymptomatic HIV infection; peripheral/persistent generalized lymphadenopathy; HPV, thrush, OHL; RAU, periodontal diseases, salivary gland diseases; dermatitis	$\geq$500/mm^3 gradual reduction with average decrease of 50-80/mm^3/year
4-8 years	Early symptomatic HIV infection previously called (AIDS-related complex): Thrush, vaginal candidiasis (persistent, frequent and/or severe), cervical dysplasia/CA Hodgkin's lymphoma, B-cell lymphoma, oral hairy leukoplakia, salivary gland diseases, ITP, xerostomia, dermatitis, shingles; RAU, herpes simplex, HPV, bacterial infections, periodontal diseases, molluscum contagiosum, other physical symptoms: fever, weight loss, fatigue	$\geq$300-500/mm^3
6-10 years	AIDS: Wasting syndrome, *Candida* esophagitis, Kaposi's sarcoma, HIV-associated dementia, disseminated *M. avium*, Hodgkin's or B-cell lymphoma, herpes simplex >30 days; PCP; cryptococcal meningitis, other systemic fungal infections; CMV	<200/mm^3

Natural history indicates course of HIV infection in absence of antiretroviral treatment. Adapted from Bartlett JG, "A Guide to HIV Care from the AIDS Care Program of the Johns Hopkins Medical Institutions," 2nd ed.

PCP -*Pneumocystis carinii* pneumonia; ITP -idiopathic thrombocytopenia purpura; HPV - human papilloma virus; OHL - oral hairy leukoplakia; RAU - recurrent aphthous ulcer

Patients with HIV infection and/or AIDS are seen in dental offices throughout the country. In general, it is the dentist's obligation to treat HIV individuals including patients of record and other patients who may seek treatment when the office is accepting new patients. These patients are protected under the Americans with Disabilities Act and the dentist has an obligation as described. Two excellent publications, one by the American Dental Association and the other by the American Academy of Oral Medicine, outline the dentist's responsibility as well as a very detailed explanation of dental management protocols for HIV patients. These protocols, however, are evolving just as our knowledge of HIV has evolved. New drugs and their interactions present the dentist with continuous

HIV INFECTION AND AIDS (Continued)

need for updates regarding the appropriate management of HIV patients. Diagnostic tests, including determining viral load in combination with the CD4 status, now are used to modify a patient's treatment in ways that allow them to remain relatively illness-free for longer periods of time. This places more of a responsibility on the dental practice team to be aware of drug changes, of new drugs, and of the appropriate oral management in such patients.

Our knowledge of AIDS allows us to properly treat these patients while protecting ourselves, our staff, and other patients in the office. All types of infectious disease require consistent practices in our dental offices known as Standard/Universal Precautions (see Occupational Exposure to Bloodborne Pathogens Standard/Universal Precautions *on page 1871*). The office team that utilizes these precautions appropriately is well protected against passage of infectious agents. These agents include sexually transmitted disease agents, the highly virulent hepatitis viruses, and the less virulent but always worrisome HIV. In general, an office that is practicing standard/universal precautions is one that is considered safe for patients and staff. Throughout this spectrum, HIV is placed somewhere in the middle, in terms of infection risk in the dental office. Other sexually transmitted diseases and infectious diseases such as tuberculosis represent a greater threat to the dentist than HIV itself. However, due to the grave danger of HIV infection, many of our precautions have been instituted to assist the dentist in protecting himself, his staff, and other patients in situations where the office may be involved in treating a patient that is HIV positive.

As in the management of all medically compromised patients, the appropriate care of HIV patients begins with a complete and thorough history. This history must allow the dentist to identify risk factors in the development of HIV, as well as, identify those patients known to be HIV positive. Knowledge of all medications prescribed to patients at risk is also important.

The current antiretroviral therapy used to treat patients with HIV infection and/or AIDS includes three primary classifications of drugs. These are the nucleoside analogs, protease inhibitors, and the non-nucleoside/nucleotide analogs (analogs refers to chemicals that can substitute competitively for naturally produced cell components such as found in DNA, RNA, or proteins). The newest drugs include several nucleoside analogs, abacavir (Ziagen®), subprotease inhibitors, amprenavir, and several non-nucleoside analogs, efavirenz (Sustiva®), and adefovir. Finding the perfect "cocktail" of anti-HIV medications still eludes clinicians. This is partly due to the fact that therapies are still too novel and the patient's years too few to study. Numerous recently-published studies have indicated that combinations of drugs are far better than individual drug therapy. Several of these studies have looked at two drug combinations, particularly between nucleoside analogs, in combination with protease inhibitors. The newer drugs (non-nucleoside analogs) have added the possibility of a triple "cocktail". Recently several studies indicated that this three-drug combination may be the best in managing HIV infection.

When HIV was first discovered, the efforts for monitoring HIV infection focused on the CD4 blood levels and the ratios between the helper cells, suppressor cells within the patient's immune system. These markers were used to indicate success or failure of drug therapies as patients moved through HIV pathogenesis toward AIDS. More recently, however, the advent of protease inhibitors has allowed clinicians to monitor the actual presence of viral RNA within the patient and the term viral load has become the focus of therapy monitoring. The availability of better therapies and our rapidly expanding knowledge of molecular biology of the HIV virus have created new opportunities to control the AIDS epidemic. Cases can be monitored quite closely looking at the number of copy units or virions within the patient's bloodstream as an indication in combination with other infections and/or declining or increasing CD4 numbers to establish prognostic values for the patient's success. Long-term survival of patients infected with HIV has been accomplished by monitoring and adjusting therapy to these numbers.

Comprehensive coordinated approaches, that have been advocated by researchers, have sought to establish national standards for HIV reporting, greater access to effective newly approved medications, improved access to individual physicians treating HIV patients, and continued protection of patient's privacy. These goals allow the reporting of studies that suggest that combination therapies, some of which have been tried in less controlled individual patient treatments, may prove useful in larger populations of HIV-infected individuals. As these studies are reported, the dental clinician should be aware that patients' drug therapies change rapidly, various combinations may be tried, and the side effects and interactions as described in the chapter on drug interactions and the CYP system will also emerge. The dentist must be aware of these potential interactions with seemingly innocuous drugs such as clarithromycin, erythromycin, and some of the sedative drugs that a dentist may utilize in their practice as well as some of the analgesics. These drug interactions may be the most important part of monitoring that the dentist provides in helping to manage a situation. Some of the antiviral drugs more commonly used for HIV, AIDS, Asymptomatic, CD4 <500, and the newer drugs (ie, protease inhibitors, nucleoside analogs, and non-nucleoside nucleotide analogs) are listed in Table 2.

Table 2. EXAMPLES OF DRUGS

Nucleoside Analogs	Protease Inhibitors	Non-nucleoside / Nucleotide Analogs
Zidovudine (Retrovir®, AZT, SDV)	Saquinavir (Invirase®)	Nevirapine (Viramune®)
Didanosine (Videx®, ddi)	Ritonavir (Norvir®)	Delavirdine (Rescriptor®)
Zalcitabine (Hivid® [DSC], ddc)	Indinavir (Crixivan®)	Efavirenz (Sustiva®)
Stavudine (Zerit®, d4T)	Nelfinavir (Viracept®)	Adefovir (Hepsera™)
Lamivudine (Epivir®)	Amprenavir (Agenerase®)	
Abacavir (Ziagen®)	Fosamprenavir (Lexiva™)	

The presence of other infections is an important part of the health history. Appropriate medical consultation may be mandated after a health history in order to accomplish a complete evaluation of the patients at risk. Uniformity in the taking of a history from a patient is the dentist's best plan for all patients so that no selectivity or discrimination can be implicated.

An appropriate review of symptoms may also identify oral and systemic conditions that may be present in aggressive HIV disease. Medical physical examination may reveal pre-existing or developing intra- or extra-oral signs/symptoms of progressive disease. Aggressive herpes simplex, herpes zoster, papillomavirus, Kaposi's sarcoma or lymphoma are among the disorders that might be identified. In addition to these, intra-oral examination may raise suspicion regarding fungal infections, angular cheilitis, squamous cell carcinoma, and recurrent aphthous ulcers. The dentist should be vigilant in all patients regardless of HIV risk.

It will always be up to the dental practitioner to determine whether testing for HIV should be recommended following the history and physical examination of a new patient. Because of the severe psychological implications of learning of HIV positivity for a patient, the dentist should be aware that there are appropriate referral sites where psychological counseling and appropriate discrete testing for the patient is available. The dentist's office should have these sites available for referral should the patient be interested. Candid discussions, however, with the patient regarding risk factors and/or other signs or symptoms in their history and physical condition that may indicate a higher HIV risk than the normal population, should be an area the dentist feels comfortable in broaching with any new patient. Oftentimes, it is appropriate to recommend testing for other infectious diseases should risk factors be present. For example, testing for hepatitis B may be appropriate for the patient and along with this the dentist could recommend that the patient consider HIV testing. Because of the legal issues involved, anonymity for HIV testing may be appropriate and it is always up to the patient to follow the doctor's recommendations.

When a patient has either given a positive history of knowing that they are HIV positive or it has been determined after referral for consultation, the dentist should be aware of the AIDS-defining illnesses. Of course, current medical status and drug therapy that the patient may be undergoing is of equal importance. The dentist, through medical consultation and regular follow-up with the patient's physician, should be made aware of the CD4 count (Table 3), the viral load, and the drugs that the patient is taking. The presence of other AIDS-defining illnesses as well as complications, such as higher risk of endocarditis and the risk of other systemic infections such as tuberculosis, are extremely important for the dentist. These may make an impact on the dental treatment plan in terms of the selection of preprocedural antibiotics or the use of oral medications to treat opportunistic infections in or around the oral cavity.

HIV INFECTION AND AIDS *(Continued)*

Table 3. CD4+ LYMPHOCYTE COUNT AND PERCENTAGE AS RELATED TO THE RISK OF OPPORTUNISTIC INFECTION

CD4+ Cells/mm³	CD4+ Percentage[1]	Risk of Opportunistic Infection
>600	32-60	No increased risk
400-500	<29	Initial immune suppression
200-400	14-28	Appearance of opportunistic infections, some may be major
<200	<14	Severe immune suppression. AIDS diagnosis. Major opportunistic infections. Although variable, prognosis for surviving greater than 3 years is poor
<50	—	Although variable, prognosis for surviving greater than 1 year is poor

[1]Several studies have suggested that the CD4+ percentage demonstrates less variability between measurements, as compared to the absolute CD4+ cell count. CD4+ percentages may therefore give a clearer impression of the course of disease.

Adapted from Glick M and Silverman S, "Dental Management of HIV-Infected Patients," *J Am Dent Assoc* (Supplement to Reviewers), 1995.

AIDS-defining illnesses such as candidiasis, recurrent pneumonia, or lymphoma are clearly important to the dentist. Chemotherapy that might be being given to the patient for treatment for any or all of these disorders can have implications in terms of the patient's response to simple dental procedures.

Drug therapies have become complex in the treatment of HIV/AIDS. Because of the moderate successes with protease inhibitors and the drug combination therapies, more patients are living longer and receiving more dental care throughout their lives. Drug therapies are often tailored to the current CD4 count in combination with the viral load. In general, patients with high CD4 counts are usually at lower risk for complications in the dental office than patients with low CD4 counts. However, the presence of a high viral load with or without a stable CD4 count may be indicative or a more rapid progression of the HIV/AIDS disease process than had previously been thought. Patients with a high viral load and a declining CD4 count are considered to have the greatest risk and the poorest prognosis of all the groups.

Other organ damage, such as liver compromise potentially leading to bleeding disorders, can be found as the disease progresses to AIDS. Liver dysfunction may be related to pre-existing hepatic diseases due to previous infection with a hepatitis virus such as hepatitis B or other drug toxicities associated with the treatment of AIDS. The dentist must have available current prothrombin and partial thromboplastin times (PT and PTT) in order to accurately evaluate any risk of bleeding abnormality. Platelet count and liver function studies are also important. Potential drug interactions include some antibiotics, as well as any anticoagulating drugs, which may be contraindicated in such patients. It may be necessary to avoid NSAIDs, as well as aspirin. (See Pharmacology of Drug Metabolism and Interactions *on page 1855*).

The use of preprocedural antibiotics is another issue in the HIV patient. As the absolute neutrophil count declines during the progression of AIDS, the use of antibiotics as a preprocedural step prior to dental care may be necessary. If protracted treatment plans are necessary, the dentist should receive updated information as the patient receives such from their physician. It is always important that the dentist have current CD4 counts, viral load assay, as well as liver function studies, AST and ALT, and bleeding indicators including platelet count, PT, and PTT. If any other existing conditions such as cardiac involvement or joint prostheses are involved, antibiotic coverage may also be necessary. However, these determinations are no different than in the non-HIV population and this subject is covered in Antibiotic Prophylaxis - Preprocedural Guidelines for Dental Patients *on page 1772*. Use the table of Normal Blood Values *on page 1923* as a general guideline for provision of dental care.

The consideration of current blood values is important in long-term care of any medically compromised patient and in particular the HIV-positive patient. Preventive dental care is likewise valuable in these patients, however, the dentist's approach should be no different than as with all patients. See Table 4 for oral lesions commonly associated with HIV disease and a brief description of their usual treatment (see Part II of this Oral Medicine chapter for more detailed descriptions of these common oral lesions).

The clinician should be aware that several of the protease inhibitors have now been associated with drug interactions. Some of these drug interactions include therapies that the dentist may be utilizing. The basis for these drug interactions with protease inhibitors is the inhibition of cytochrome P450 isoforms, which are important in normal liver function and metabolism of drugs. A detailed description of the mechanisms of inhibition can be found in Pharmacology of Drug Metabolism and Interactions *on page 1855*, as well as a table illustrating some known drug interactions with antiviral therapy and drugs commonly prescribed in the dental office. The metabolism of these drugs could be affected by the patient's antiviral therapy.

The dentist should also review office protocol for Occupational Exposure to Bloodborne Pathogens (Standard/Universal Precautions) *on page 1871* and the answers to "Frequently Asked Questions" at the end of this section.

Table 4. ORAL LESIONS COMMONLY SEEN IN HIV/AIDS

Condition	Management
Oral candidiasis Angular cheilitis	See "Fungal Infections" *on page 1804*
Oral hairy leukoplakia	See "Systemic Viral Diseases" *on page 1767*
Periodontal diseases 　Linear gingivitis 　Ulcerative periodontitis	See "Bacterial Infections" *on page 1793*
Herpes simplex Herpes zoster	Acyclovir - see "Systemic Viral Diseases" *on page 1767*
Chronic aphthous ulceration	Palliation / Thalidomide (Thalomid®)
Salivary gland disease	Referral
Human papillomavirus	Laser / Surgical excision
Kaposi's sarcoma	See "Antibiotic Prophylaxis" *on page 1772*; Biopsy / Laser
Non-Hodgkin's lymphoma	Biopsy / Referral
Tuberculosis	Referral

Dapsone *on page 441*
Delavirdine *on page 453*
Didanosine *on page 492*
Indinavir *on page 875*
Lamivudine *on page 944*
Lopinavir and Ritonavir *on page 997*
Nelfinavir *on page 1158*
Ritonavir *on page 1436*
Stavudine *on page 1495*
Tenofovir *on page 1537*
Thalidomide *on page 1551*
Zalcitabine *on page 1675*
Zidovudine *on page 1680*
Zidovudine and Lamivudine *on page 1681*

FREQUENTLY ASKED QUESTIONS

How does one get AIDS, aside from having unprotected sex?

Our current knowledge about the immunodeficiency virus is that it is carried via semen, contaminated needles, blood products, transfusion products not tested, and potentially in other fluids of the body. Patients at highest risk include I.V. drug-abusers, those receiving multiple transfusions with blood that has not been screened for HIV, or patients practicing unprotected sex with multiple partners, where the history of the partner may not be as clear as the patient would like.

Are patients safe from AIDS or HIV infection when they present to the dentist office?

Our current knowledge indicates that the answer is an unequivocal "yes". The patient is protected because dental offices are practicing standard/universal precautions, using antimicrobial handwashing agents, gloves, face masks, eye protection, special clothing, aerosol control, and instrument soaking and autoclaving. All of these procedures stop potential transmission to a new patient, as well as, allow for easy disposal of contaminated office supplies for elimination of microbes by an antimicrobial technique, should they be contaminated through treatment of another patient. These precautions are mandated by OSHA requirements (see Occupational Exposure to Bloodborne Pathogens Standard/Universal Precautions *on page 1871*).

What is the most common opportunistic infection that HIV-positive patients suffer that may be important in dentistry?

The most common opportunistic infection important to dentistry is oral candidiasis. This disease can present as white plaques, red areas, or angular cheilitis occurring at the corners of the mouth. Management of such lesions is appropriate by the dentist and is described in this handbook (see Fungal Infections *on page 1804*). Other oral complications include HIV-associated periodontal disease, as well as the other conditions outlined in Table 4. Of great concern to the dentist is the risk of tuberculosis. In many HIV-positive patients, tuberculosis has become a serious, life-threatening opportunistic infection. The dentist should be aware that appropriate referral for anyone showing such respiratory signs and symptoms would be prudent.

HIV INFECTION AND AIDS *(Continued)*

Can one patient infect another through unprotected sex if the other patient has tested negative for HIV?

Yes, there is always the possibility that a sexual partner may be in the early window of time when plasma viremia is not at a detectable level. The antibody response to plasma viremia may be slightly delayed and diagnostic testing may not indicate HIV positivity. This window of time represents a period when the patient may be infectious but not show up yet on normal diagnostic testing.

Can HIV be passed by oral fluids?

As our knowledge about HIV has evolved, we have thought that HIV is inactivated in saliva by an agent possibly associated with secretory leukocyte protease inhibitors known as SLPI. There is, however, a current resurgence in our interest in oral transmission because some research indicates that in moderate to advanced periodontal lesions or other oral lesions where there is tissue damage, the presence of a serous exudate may increase the risk of transmission. The dentist should be aware of this ongoing research and attempt to renew knowledge regularly so that any future breakthroughs will be noted.

RHEUMATOID ARTHRITIS, OSTEOARTHRITIS, AND OSTEOPOROSIS

RA AND OSTEOARTHRITIS MANAGEMENT

Arthritis and its variations represent the most common chronic musculoskeletal disorders of man. The conditions can essentially be divided into rheumatoid, osteoarthritic, and polyarthritic presentations. Differences in age of onset and joint involvement exist and it is now currently believed that the diagnosis of each may be less clear than previously thought. These autoinflammatory diseases have now been shown to affect young and old alike. Criteria for a diagnosis of rheumatoid arthritis include a positive serologic test for rheumatoid factor, subcutaneous nodules, affected joints on opposite sides of the body, and clear radiographic changes. The hematologic picture includes moderate normocytic hypochromic anemia, mild leukocytosis, and mild thrombocytopenia. During acute inflammatory periods, C-reactive protein is elevated and IgG and IgM (rheumatoid factors) can be detected. Osteoarthritis lacks these diagnostic features.

Other systemic conditions, such as systemic lupus erythematosus and Sjögren's syndrome, are often found simultaneously with some of the arthritic conditions. The treatment of arthritis includes the use of slow-acting and rapid-acting anti-inflammatory agents ranging from the gold salts to aspirin (see following listings). Long-term usage of these drugs can lead to numerous adverse effects including bone marrow suppression, platelet suppression, and oral ulcerations. The dentist should be aware that steroids (usually prednisone) are often prescribed along with the listed drugs and are often used in dosages sufficient to induce adrenal suppression. Adjustment of dosing prior to invasive dental procedures may be indicated along with consultation with the managing physician. Alteration of steroid dosage prior to stressful dental procedures may be necessary, usually increasing the steroid dosage prior to and during the stressful procedures and then gradually returning the patient to the original dosage over several days. Even in the absence of evidence of adrenal suppression, consultation with the prescribing physician for appropriate dosing and timing of procedures is advisable.

Antirheumatic, Disease Modifying

Gold Salts

Metabolic Inhibitor

Immunomodulator

Nonsteroidal Anti-inflammatory Agents

RHEUMATOID ARTHRITIS, OSTEOARTHRITIS, AND OSTEOPOROSIS *(Continued)*

COX-2 Inhibitor NSAID

Celecoxib *on page 311*

Combination NSAID Product to Prevent GI Distress

Diclofenac and Misoprostol *on page 489*

Salicylates

Aspirin *on page 149*
Choline Magnesium Trisalicylate *on page 350*
Salsalate *on page 1454*

Other

Hydroxychloroquine *on page 843*
Prednisone *on page 1342*

ANTI-INFLAMMATORY AGENTS USED IN THE TREATMENT OF RA AND OSTEOARTHRITIS

Drug	Adverse Effects
SLOW-ACTING	
Gold Salts	
Aurothioglucose; Auranofin; Gold Sodium Thiomalate	GI intolerance, diarrhea; leukopenia, thrombocytopenia, and/or anemia; skin and oral eruptions; possible nephrotoxicity and hepatotoxicity
Metabolic Inhibitor	
Leflunomide (Arava™)	Diarrhea, respiratory tract infection
Methotrexate	Oral ulcerations, leukopenia
Immunomodulator	
Etanercept (Enbrel®)	Headache, respiratory tract infection, positive ANA
Other	
Hydroxychloroquine (Plaquenil®)	Usually mild and reversible; ophthalmic complications
Prednisone	Insomnia, nervousness, indigestion, increased appetite
RAPID-ACTING	
Salicylates	
Aspirin	Inhibition of platelet aggregation; gastrointestinal (GI) irritation, ulceration, and bleeding; tinnitus; teratogenicity
Choline magnesium trisalicylate (Trilisate®)	GI irritation and ulceration, weakness, skin rash, hemolytic anemia, troubled breathing
Salsalate	
Other Nonsteroidal Anti-inflammatory Drugs	
Diclofenac (Cataflam®, Voltaren®); Diflunisal (Dolobid®); Etodolac (Lodine®); Fenoprofen calcium (Nalfon®); Flurbiprofen (Ansaid®); Ibuprofen (Motrin®); Indomethacin (Indocin®); Ketoprofen; Ketorolac (Toradol®); Meclofenamate; Nabumetone (Relafen®); Naproxen (Naprosyn®); Oxaprozin (Daypro®); Piroxicam (Feldene®); Salsalate (Mono-Gesic®, Salflex®); Sulindac (Clinoril®); Tolmetin (Tolectin®)	GI irritation, ulceration, and bleeding; inhibition of platelet aggregation; displacement of protein-bound drugs (eg, oral anticoagulants, sulfonamides, and sulfonylureas); headache; vertigo; mucocutaneous rash or ulceration; parotid enlargement
COX-2 Inhibitor NSAID	
Celecoxib (Celebrex®) Rofecoxib (Vioxx®) Valdecoxib (Bextra®)	Headache, dyspepsia, upper respiratory tract infection, sinusitis
COMBINATION NSAID PRODUCT TO PREVENT GI DISTRESS	
Diclofenac and Misoprostol (Arthrotec®)	Inhibition of platelet aggregation; displacement of protein-bound drugs (eg, oral anticoagulants, sulfonamides, and sulfonylureas); headache; vertigo; mucocutaneous rash or ulceration; parotid enlargement; diarrhea

OSTEOPOROSIS MANAGEMENT

PREVALENCE

Osteoporosis effects 25 million Americans of which 80% are women; 27% of American women >80 years of age have osteopenia and 70% of American women >80 years of age have osteoporosis.

CONSEQUENCES

1.3 million bone fractures annually (low impact/nontraumatic) and pain, pulmonary insufficiency, decreased quality of life, and economic costs; >250,000 hip fractures per year with a 20% mortality rate.

RISK FACTORS

Advanced age, female, chronic renal disease, hyperparathyroidism, Cushing's disease, hypogonadism/anorexia, hyperprolactinemia, cancer, large and prolonged dose heparin or glucocorticoids, anticonvulsants, hyperthyroidism (current or history, or excessive thyroid supplements), sedentary, excessive exercise, early menopause, oophorectomy without hormone replacement, excessive aluminum-containing antacid, smoking, methotrexate.

DIAGNOSIS/MONITORING

DXA bone density, history of fracture (low impact or nontraumatic), compressed vertebrae, decreased height, hump-back appearance. Osteomark™ urine assay measures bone breakdown fragments and may help assess therapy response earlier than DXA but diagnostic value is uncertain as Osteomark™ does not reveal extent of bone loss. Bone markers may be tested to evaluate effectiveness of antiresorptive urine therapy.

PREVENTION

1. Adequate dietary calcium (eg, dairy products)

2. Vitamin D (eg, fortified dairy products, cod, fatty fish)

3. Weight-bearing exercise (eg, walking) as tolerated

4. Calcium supplement of 1000-1500 mg <u>elemental</u> calcium daily (divided in 500 mg increments); women >65 years on estrogen replacement therapy supplement 1000 mg <u>elemental</u> calcium; women >65 not receiving estrogens and men >55 years supplement 1500 mg <u>elemental</u> calcium. To minimize constipation add fiber and start with 500 mg/day for several months, then increase to 500 mg twice daily taken at different times than fiber. Chewable and liquid products are available. Calcium carbonate is given with food to enhance bioavailability. Calcium citrate may be given without regards to meals.

   - Contraindications: Hypercalcemia, ventricular fibrillation
   - Side effects: Constipation, anorexia
   - Drug interactions: Fiber, tetracycline, iron supplement, minerals

5. Vitamin D Supplement: 400-800 units daily (often satisfied by 1-2 multivitamins or fortified milk) in addition to calcium or a combined calcium and vitamin D supplement and/or >15 minutes direct sunlight/day. Some elderly, especially with significant renal or liver disease cannot metabolize (activate) vitamin D and require calcitriol 0.25 mcg orally twice daily or adjusted per serum calcium level, the active form of vitamin D; can check 1,25 OH vitamin D level to confirm need for calcitriol.

   - Contraindications: Hypercalcemia (weakness, headache, drowsiness, nausea, diarrhea), hypercalciuria and renal stones
   - Side effects (uncommon): Hypercalcemia (see above)
   - Monitor 24-hour urine and serum calcium if using >1000 units/day

6. Estrogen: Especially useful if bone density <80% of average plus symptoms of estrogen deficiency or cardiac disease. Bone density increases over 1-2 years then plateaus. This is considered 1st line therapy unless contraindicated due to medicinal history (see below) or risk:benefit assessment which leads to decision to avoid HRT (hormone replacement therapy). **Note:** Estrogens should not be used to prevent coronary heart disease.

   - Contraindications: Pregnancy, breast or estrogen-dependent cancer, undiagnosed abnormal genital bleeding, active thrombophlebitis, or history of thromboembolism during previous estrogen or oral contraceptive therapy or pregnancy. Pretreatment mammogram, gynecological exam are advised along with routine breast exam because of an increased risk of breast cancer with long-term use.

   - Dose: Conjugated estrogen of 0.625 mg/day or its equivalent (continuous therapy preferred).

RHEUMATOID ARTHRITIS, OSTEOARTHRITIS, AND OSTEOPOROSIS *(Continued)*

- Side effects: Vaginal spotting/bleeding, nausea, vomiting, breast tenderness/enlargement, amenorrheic with extended use.
  Initiate therapy slowly (side effects are more common and severe in women without estrogen for many years). Administer with medroxyprogesterone acetate (MPA) 2.5-5 mg daily, or another oral progesterone, in women with uterus (unopposed estrogen can cause endometrial cancer). MPA can increase vaginal bleeding, increase weight, edema, mood changes.

- Drug interactions: May increase corticosteroid effect, monitor for need to decrease corticosteroid dose.

7. Selective estrogen receptor modulators: Selective-estrogen receptor modulators (SERMs) are nonsteroidal modulators of estrogen-receptor mediated reactions. The key difference between these agents and estrogen replacement therapies is the potential to exert tissue specific effects. Due to their chemical differences, these agents retain some of estrogen's beneficial effects on bone metabolism and lipid levels, but differ in their actions on breast and endometrial tissues, potentially limiting adverse effects related to nonspecific hormone stimulation. Among the SERMs, tamoxifen retains stimulatory effects in endometrial tissue, while raloxifene does not stimulate endometrial or breast tissue, limiting the potential for endometrial or breast cancer related to this agent. Raloxifene is the only SERM which has been approved by the FDA for osteoporosis prevention.

   It should be noted that the effects on bone observed with SERMs appear to be less than that observed with estrogen replacement. In one study, the effect of raloxifene on hip bone mineral density was approximately half of that observed with conjugated estrogens. In addition, the effects on lipid profiles are less than with estrogen replacement. Finally, SERMs do not block the vasomotor effects observed with menopause, which may limit compliance with therapy. As with estrogen replacement, raloxifene has been associated with an increased risk of thromboembolism and is contraindicated in patients with a history of thromboembolic disease.

8. Estradiol, as well as various combination therapies, including ethinyl estradiol with norethindrone (Femhrt®) and estradiol with norgestimate (Ortho-Prefest™), have been approved for the prevention of osteoporosis (see Estradiol *on page 602*).

TREATMENT

1. Calcium, vitamin D, exercise, and estrogen: As above

2. Bisphosphonates:

   Consider if patient is intolerant of, or refuses estrogen or it is contraindicated, especially if severe osteoporosis (ie, ≥2.5 standard deviations below average young adult bone density, T-score, or history of low impact or nontraumatic fracture). Increasing bone density of hip and spine observed for at least 3 years (ie, no plateau as seen with estrogen).

   Contraindications: Hypocalcemia, not advised if existing gastrointestinal disorders (eg, esophageal disorders such as reflux, sensitive stomach).

   - Alendronate (Fosamax®) *on page 65*: Dose: 10 mg once daily or 70 mg/week (treatment dose for osteoporosis; not recommended if creatinine clearance <35 mL/minute). Osteopenia: 5 mg per day or 35 mg/week for prevention.

   - Risedronate (Actonel®) *on page 1428*: Dose: 5 mg daily or 35 mg/week for treatment or prevention

   Take before breakfast on an empty stomach with 6-8 ounces tap water (not mineral water, coffee, or juice) and remain upright or raise head of bed for bedridden patients at least 30 degree angle for at least 30 minutes (otherwise may cause ulcerative esophagitis) before eating or drinking.

   Therapy with calcium and vitamin D is advised, but must be given at a different time of day than alendronate.

   - Side effects (well tolerated): Difficulty swallowing, heartburn, abdominal discomfort, nausea (GI side effects increase with aspirin products), arthralgia/myalgia, constipation, diarrhea, headache, esophagitis.

   - Drug interactions: None known to date.

   Osteonecrosis of the jaw (ONJ) is an uncommon condition that results in exposure of bone in the oral cavity along with other signs and symptoms that may be associated with changes in bone metabolism and/or poor wound healing, but also can develop spontaneously, such as along the myelohyoid ridge, away from teeth, or any site where obvious trauma could have occurred. Cases of ONJ began to emerge in approximately 2003 and were linked primarily with patients with cancer and those receiving the drugs zoledronic acid (Zometa®) and/or pamidronate

(Aredia®) which are bisphosphonates administered by an intravenous route. A third intravenous bisphosphonate, clodronate (Bonefos®) is encountered much less commonly. Other bisphosphonates have been used for many years in the treatment of osteoporosis, Paget's disease, and other bone mineralization diseases. These include a group of bisphosphonates that are administered orally.

Bone disease occurs in many patients with cancer, particularly those with multiple myeloma and metastatic lesions associated with breast cancer, prostate cancer, and other cancers. These changes are often associated with pain and pathologic fractures. This bone destruction often results from changes in the osteoclast and osteoblast activities related to bone remodeling and healing following trauma. Bisphosphonates act at sites of active bone remodeling, changing the activity of the cells necessary for osteoclastic activity. There are no data that indicate that bisphosphonates directly change mineralization of the bone, however, these drugs do result in changes in the vascularity of the bone and cell activity.

Since the emergence of numerous cases of ONJ and their documentation, the American Dental Association through its Council on Scientific Affairs has released various news reports and position statements related to the state of the current knowledge and recommendations for the practicing dental professionals to manage patients who may be at risk for ONJ. Most of the data that exist are related to the use of intravenous bisphosphonates in cancer patients. Only recently, data has begun to emerge related to oral bisphosphonates and the risk of ONJ in this much larger population of patients who are receiving a significantly lower dosage of bisphosphonate via the oral route. Also refer to Management of Patients Undergoing Cancer Therapy *on page 1826*

A panel of experts convened by the American Dental Association believes that dental patients who are taking oral bisphosphonates should discuss the risks that they face when undergoing procedures that involve the jaw bone, such as tooth extraction or placement of implants with their dentist. The ADA recommends that a comprehensive oral evaluation be carried out on all patients and if they are about to begin oral bisphosphonates, patients should be made aware of the potential long-term risks. However, the ADA notes that dentists generally will not need to modify dental treatments based solely on bisphosphonate therapy. Furthermore, patients must understand that the risk for developing osteonecrosis of the jaw is considered very small and the vast majority of patients taking oral bisphosphonates will never develop any particular oral complication.

Orally Administered Bisphosphonates

Alendronate (Fosamax®) *on page 65*

Etidronate Disodium (Didronel®) *on page 654*

Ibandronate (Boniva®) *on page 849*

Risedronate (Actonel®) *on page 1428*

Tiludronate (Skelid®) *on page 1568*

The current dental management recommendations for patients on oral bisphosphonates recently comprised by the American Dental Association's Council on Scientific Affairs was released, June 2006. The risk of developing ONJ is very low, however, millions of patients take these drugs; therefore, the recommendations must be disseminated to the dental community. The Panel's recommendations focus on conservative dental procedures, proper sterile technique, appropriate use of oral disinfectants, and principles of effective antibiotic therapy. There are currently no data from clinical trials evaluating dental management of patients on oral bisphosphonates and therefore these recommendations are based on expert opinion only.

Obviously, the dentist must always carry out a comprehensive oral evaluation and should stay active in reviewing the literature as new data emerge. The reference list below refers primarily to intravenous bisphosphonate therapy since this is where most of the data have been accumulated. The various drug manufacturers have placed precautionary statements in their product inserts and the dentist should be familiar with reviewing these precaution statements since the wording is very carefully based on the data that are available.

The latest reference on the management treatment of patients with osteonecrosis of the jaw has been published in the *Journal of Oncology Practice*. All of the information contained in these recommendations is available through the drug companies' precautionary statements as well as doctor letters which have been disseminated to every practicing dentist in the world. In addition, new information is emerging as data develop.

3. Etidronate Disodium: Not FDA approved for postmenopausal osteoporosis and can decrease the quality of bone formation, therefore, change to alendronate.

4. Calcitonin (nasal; Miacalcin®): Indicated if estrogen refused, intolerant, or contraindicated. Potential analgesic effect.

RHEUMATOID ARTHRITIS, OSTEOARTHRITIS, AND OSTEOPOROSIS *(Continued)*

- Contraindications: Hypersensitivity to salmon protein or gelatin diluent; 1 spray (200 units) into 1 nostril daily (alternate right and left nostril daily); 5 days on and 2 days off is also effective; alternate day administration not effective. If used only for pain, can decrease dose once pain is controlled.

- Side effects (few): Nasal dryness and irritation (periodically inspect); adequate dietary or supplemental calcium + vitamin D is essential.

Subcutaneous route (100 units daily): Many side effects (eg, nausea, flushing, anorexia) and the discomfort/inconvenience of injection.

5. Fall prevention: Minimize psychoactive and cardiovascular drugs (monitor BP for orthostasis), give diuretics early in the day, environmental safety check.

	% Elemental Calcium	Elemental Calcium
Calcium gluconate (various)	9	500 mg = 45 mg
Calcium glubionate (Calcionate)	6.5	1.8 g = 115 g/5 mL
Calcium lactate (various)	13	325 mg = 42.25 mg
Calcium citrate (Citrical®)	21	950 mg = 200 mg
Effervescent tabs (Citrical Liquitab®)		2376 mg = 500 mg
Calcium acetate		
Phos-Ex 250®	25	1000 mg = 250 mg
Phos-Lo®		667 mg = 169 mg
Calcium phosphate, tribasic (Posture®)	39	1565.2 mg = 600 mg
Calcium carbonate		
Tums®	40	1.2 g = 500 mg
Oscal-500® oral suspension		1.2 g/5 mL = 500 mg
Caltrate 600®		1.5 g = 600 mg

References

ADA Council on Scientific Affairs. Expert Panel Recommendations: Dental Management of Patients on Oral Bisphosphonate Therapy, June 2006. Available at: http://www.ada.org/prof/resources/pubs/jada/reports/report_bisphosphonate.pdf.

Ashworth L, "Focus on Alendronate. A Nonhormonal Option for the Treatment of Osteoporosis in Postmenopausal Women," *Formulary*, 1996, 31:23-30.

Johnson SR, "Should Older Women Use Estrogen Replacement," *J Am Geriatr Soc*, 1996, 44:89-90.

Badros A, Weikel D, Salama A, et al, "Osteonecrosis of the Jaw in Multiple Myeloma Patients: Clinical Features and Risk Factors," *J Clin Oncol*, 2006, 24(6):945-52.

Expert Panel Recommendations for the Prevention, Diagnosis, and Treatment of Osteonecrosis of the Jaws, June 2004. Available at: http://www.ada.org/prof/resources/topics/topics_osteonecrosis_whitepaper.pdf.

Liberman UA, Weiss SR, and Brool J, "Effect of Oral Alendronate on Bone-Mineral Density and the Incidence of Fracture in Postmenopausal Osteoporosis," *N Engl J Med*, 1995, 333:1437-43.

Migliorati CA, Casiglia J, Epstein J, et al, "Managing the Care of Patients With Bisphosphonate-Associated Osteonecrosis: An American Academy of Oral Medicine Position Paper," *J Am Dent Assoc*, 2005, 136(12):1658-68.

"New Drugs for Osteoporosis," *Med Lett Drugs Ther*, 1996, 38:1-3.

NIH Consensus Development Panel on Optimal Calcium Intake, *JAMA*, 1994, 272:1942-8.

Ott SM, "Long-Term Safety of Bisphosphonates," *J Clin Endocrinol Metab*, 2005, 90(3):1294-301.

Ruggiero S, Gralow J, Marx RE, et al, "Practical Guidelines for the Prevention, Diagnosis, and Treatment of Osteonecrosis of the Jaw in Patients With Cancer," *Journal of Oncology Practice*, 2006, 2(1):7-14.

Ruggiero SL, Mehrotra B, Rosenberg TJ, et al, "Osteonecrosis of the Jaws Associated With the Use of Bisphosphonates: A Review of 63 Cases," *J Oral Maxillofac Surg*, 2004, 62(5):527-34.

Woo SB, Hande K, and Richardson PG, "Osteonecrosis of the Jaw and Bisphosphonates," *N Engl J Med*, 2005, 353(1):99-102.

TUBERCULOSIS

Tuberculosis is caused by the organism *Mycobacterium tuberculosis* as well as a variety of other mycobacteria including *M. bovis*, *M. avium-intracellulare*, and *M. kansasii*. Diagnosis of tuberculosis can be made from a skin test and a positive chest x-ray as well as acid-fast smears of cultures from respiratory secretions. Nucleic acid probes and polymerase chain reaction (PCR) to identify nucleic acid of *M. tuberculosis* have recently become useful.

The treatment of tuberculosis is based on the general principle that multiple drugs should reduce infectivity within 2 weeks and that failures in therapy may be due to noncompliance with the long-term regimens necessary. General treatment regimens last 6-12 months.

Isoniazid-resistant and multidrug-resistant mycobacterial infections have become an increasingly significant problem in recent years. TB as an opportunistic disease in HIV-positive patients has also risen. Combination drug therapy has always been popular in TB management and the advent of new antibiotics has not diminished this need.

ANTITUBERCULOSIS DRUGS

Bactericidal Agents

Capreomycin *on page 268*
*Isoniazid *on page 912*
Kanamycin *on page 926*
*Pyrazinamide *on page 1388*
Rifabutin *on page 1422*
*Rifampin *on page 1423*
*Streptomycin *on page 1496*

Bacteriostatic Agents

Cycloserine *on page 425*
*Ethambutol *on page 620*
Ethionamide *on page 651*
Aminosalicylic Acid *on page 91*

*Drugs of choice.

SEXUALLY-TRANSMITTED DISEASES

Sexually transmitted diseases (STDs) represent a group of infectious diseases that include bacterial, fungal, and viral etiologies. Several related infections are covered elsewhere. Gonorrhea and syphilis will be covered here.

The management of a patient with a STD begins with identification. Paramount to the correct management of patients with a history of gonorrhea or syphilis is when the condition was diagnosed, how and with what agent it was treated, did the condition recur, and are there any residual signs and symptoms potentially indicating active or recurrent disease. With standard/universal precautions, the patient with *Neisseria gonorrhoea* or *Treponema pallidum* infection poses little threat to the dentist; however, diagnosis of oral lesions may be problematic. Gonococcal pharyngitis, primary syphilitic lesions (chancre), secondary syphilitic lesions (mucous patch), and tertiary lesions (gumma) may be identified by the dentist.

Drugs used in treatment of gonorrhea/syphilis include:

> Cefixime *on page 303*
> Ceftriaxone *on page 309*
> Ciprofloxacin *on page 359*
> Doxycycline (Systemic) *on page 541*
> Ofloxacin *on page 1198*
> Penicillin G Benzathine *on page 1268*
> Penicillin G (Parenteral/Aqueous) *on page 1269*
> Spectinomycin (alternate) *on page 1491*

The drugs listed above are often used alone or in stepped regimens, particularly when there is concomitant *Chlamydia* infection or when there is evidence of disseminated disease. The proper treatment for syphilis depends on the state of the disease.

SYSTEMIC VIRAL DISEASES

HEPATITIS

The hepatitis viruses are a group of DNA and RNA viruses that produce symptoms associated with inflammation of the liver. Currently, hepatitis A through G have been identified by immunological testing; however, hepatitis A through E have received most attention in terms of disease identification. Recently, however, there has been increased interest in hepatitis viruses F and G, particularly as relate to healthcare professionals. Our knowledge is expanding rapidly in this area and the clinician should be alert to changes in the literature that might update their knowledge. Hepatitis F, for instance, remains a diagnosis of exclusion effectively being non-A, B, C, D, E, or G. Whereas, hepatitis G has serologic testing available, however, not commercially at this time. Research evaluations of various antibody and RT-PCR tests for hepatitis G are under development at this time.

Signs and symptoms of viral hepatitis in general are quite variable. Patients infected may range from asymptomatic to experiencing flu-like symptoms only. In addition, fever, nausea, joint muscle pain, jaundice, and hepatomegaly along with abdominal pain can result from infection with one of the hepatitis viruses. The virus also can create an acute or chronic infection. Usually following these early symptoms or the asymptomatic period, the patient may recover or may go on to develop chronic liver dysfunction. Liver dysfunction may be represented primarily by changes in liver function tests known as LFTs and these primarily include aspartate aminotransferase known as AST and alanine aminotransferase known as ALT. In addition, for A, B, C, D, and E there are serologic tests for either antigen, antibody, or both. Of hepatitis A through G, five forms have both acute and chronic forms whereas A and E appear to only create acute disease. There are differences in the way clinicians may approach a known postexposure to one of the hepatitis viruses. In many instances, gamma globulin may be used, however, the indications for gamma globulin as a drug limit their use to several of the viruses only. The dental clinician should be aware that the gastroenterologist may choose to give gamma globulin off-label.

Hepatitis A

Hepatitis A virus is an enteric virus that is a member of the Picornavirus family along with Coxsackie viruses and poliovirus. Previously known as infectious hepatitis, hepatitis A has been detected in humans for centuries. It causes acute hepatitis, often transmitted by oral-fecal contamination and having an incubation period of approximately 30 days. Typically, constitutional symptoms are present and jaundice may occur. Drug therapy that the dentist may encounter in a patient being treated for hepatitis A would primarily include immunoglobulin. Hepatitis A vaccine (inactivated) is an FDA-approved vaccine indicated in the prevention of contracting hepatitis A in exposed or high-risk individuals. Candidates at high-risk for HAV infection include persons traveling internationally to highly endemic areas, individuals with chronic liver disease, individuals engaging in high-risk sexual behavior, illicit drug-users, persons with high-risk occupational exposure, hemophiliacs or other persons receiving blood products, pediatric populations, and food handlers in high-risk environments. Two formulations of hepatitis A vaccine are available, Havrix® and VAQTA®. Each is administered as an injection in the deltoid region and both are available in pediatric and adult dosages.

Hepatitis B

Hepatitis B virus is previously known as serum hepatitis and has particular trophism for liver cells. Hepatitis B virus causes both acute and chronic disease in susceptible patients. The incubation period is often long and the diagnosis might be made by serologic markers even in the absence of symptoms. No drug therapy for acute hepatitis B is known; however, chronic hepatitis has recently been successfully-treated with Interferon Alfa-2b.

Hepatitis C

Hepatitis C virus was described in 1988 and has been formerly classified as non-A/non-B. It is clear that hepatitis C represents a high percentage of the transfusion-associated hepatitis that is seen. Treatment of acute hepatitis C infection is generally supportive. Interferon Alfa-2a therapy has been used with some success recently and interferon-alfa may be beneficial with hepatitis C-related chronic hepatitis.

SYSTEMIC VIRAL DISEASES *(Continued)*

Hepatitis D

Hepatitis D, previously known as the delta agent, is a virus that is incomplete in that it requires previous infection with hepatitis B in order to be manifested. In the past, no antiviral therapy has been effective, however, Interferon Alfa-2b is currently being investigated for unlabeled use in hepatitis D.

Hepatitis E

Hepatitis E virus is an RNA virus that represents a proportion of the previously classified non-A/non-B diagnoses. There is currently no antiviral therapy against hepatitis E.

Hepatitis F

Hepatitis F, as was mentioned, remains a diagnosis of exclusion. There are no known immunological tests available for identification of hepatitis F at present and currently the Centers for Disease Control have not come out with specific guidelines or recommendations. It is thought, however, that hepatitis F is a bloodborne virus and it has been used as a diagnosis in several cases of post-transfusion hepatitis.

Hepatitis G

Hepatitis G virus (HGV) is the newest hepatitis and is also assumed to be a bloodborne virus. Similar in family to hepatitis C, it is thought to occur concomitantly with hepatitis C and appears to be even more prevalent in some blood donors than hepatitis C. Occupational transmission of HGV is currently under study (see the references for updated information) and currently there are no specific CDC recommendations for postexposure to an HGV individual as the testing for identification remains experimental.

For further information, refer to the following:

Occupational Exposure to Bloodborne Pathogens *on page 1871*

Immunizations (Vaccines) *on page 1886*

Hepatitis A Vaccine *on page 809*

Hepatitis A (Inactivated) and Hepatitis B (Recombinant) Vaccine *on page 808*

Hepatitis B Immune Globulin *on page 810*

Hepatitis B Vaccine *on page 811*

Immune Globulin, Intramuscular *on page 869*

Immune Globulin, Intravenous *on page 870*

Interferon Alfa-2a *on page 890*

Interferon Alfa-2b *on page 891*

Interferon Alfa-2b and Ribavirin *on page 895*

Peginterferon Alfa-2a *on page 1262*

Peginterferon Alfa-2b *on page 1263*

TYPES OF HEPATITIS VIRUS

Features	A	B	C	D	E	F	G
Incubation Period	2-6 wks	8-24 wks	2-52 wks	3-13 wks	3-6 wks	Unknown	Unknown
Onset	Abrupt	Insidious	Insidious	Abrupt	Abrupt	Insidious	Insidious
Symptoms							
Jaundice	Adults: 70% to 80%; Children: 10%	25%	25%	Varies	Unknown	Unknown	Unknown
Asymptomatic patients	Adults: 50%; Children: Most	~75%	~75%	Rare	Rare	Common	Common
Routes of Transmission							
Fecal/Oral	Yes	No	No	No	Yes	Unknown	Unknown
Parenteral	Rare	Yes	Yes	Yes	No		
Sexual	No	Yes	Possible	Yes	No		
Perinatal	No	Yes	Possible	Possible	No		
Water/Food	Yes	No	No	No	Yes		
Sequelae (% of patients)							
Chronic state	No	Adults: 6% to 10%; Children: 25% to 50%; Infants: 70% to 90%	>75%	10% to 15%	No	Unknown	Likely
Case-Fatality Rate	0.6%	1.4%	1% to 2%	30%	1% to 2% Pregnant women: 20%	Unknown	Unknown

PRE-EXPOSURE RISK FACTORS FOR HEPATITIS B

Healthcare factors:

Healthcare workers[1]

Special patient groups (eg, adolescents, infants born to HB$_s$Ag–positive mothers, military personnel, etc)

Hemodialysis patients[2]

Recipients of certain blood products[3]

Lifestyle factors:

Homosexual and bisexual men

Intravenous drug-abusers

Heterosexually active persons with multiple sexual partners or recently acquired sexually transmitted diseases

Environmental factors:

Household and sexual contacts of HBV carriers

Prison inmates

Clients and staff of institutions for the mentally handicapped

Residents, immigrants, and refugees from areas with endemic HBV infection

International travelers at increased risk of acquiring HBV infection

[1]The risk of hepatitis B virus (HBV) infection for healthcare workers varies both between hospitals and within hospitals. Hepatitis B vaccination is recommended for all healthcare workers with blood exposure.

[2]Hemodialysis patients often respond poorly to hepatitis B vaccination; higher vaccine doses or increased number of doses are required. A special formulation of one vaccine is now available for such persons (Recombivax HB®, 40 mcg/mL). The anti-HB$_s$ (antibody to hepatitis B surface antigen) response of such persons should be tested after they are vaccinated, and those who have not responded should be revaccinated with 1-3 additional doses.

Patients with chronic renal disease should be vaccinated as early as possible, ideally before they require hemodialysis. In addition, their anti- HB$_s$ levels should be monitored at 6- to 12-month intervals to assess the need for revaccination.

[3]Patients with hemophilia should be immunized subcutaneously, not intramuscularly.

POSTEXPOSURE PROPHYLAXIS FOR HEPATITIS B[1]

Exposure	Hepatitis B Immune Globulin	Hepatitis B Vaccine
Perinatal	0.5 mL I.M. within 12 hours of birth	0.5 mL[2] I.M. within 12 hours of birth (no later than 7 days), and at 1 and 6 months[3]; test for HB$_s$Ag and anti-HB$_s$ at 12-15 months
Sexual	0.06 mL/kg I.M. within 14 days of sexual contact; a second dose should be given if the index patient remains HB$_s$Ag-positive after 3 months and hepatitis B vaccine was not given initially	1 mL I.M. at 0, 1, and 6 months for homosexual and bisexual men and regular sexual contacts of persons with acute and chronic hepatitis B
Percutaneous; exposed person unvaccinated		
Source known HB$_s$Ag-positive	0.06 mL/kg I.M. within 24 hours	1 mL I.M. within 7 days, and at 1 and 6 months[4]
Source known, HB$_s$Ag status unknown	Test source for HB$_s$Ag; if source is positive, give exposed person 0.06 mL/kg I.M. once within 7 days	1 mL I.M. within 7 days, and at 1 and 6 months[4]
Source not tested or unknown	Nothing required	1 mL I.M. within 7 days, and at 1 and 6 months
Percutaneous; exposed person vaccinated		
Source known HB$_s$Ag-positive	Test exposed person for anti-HB$_s$.[5] If titer is protective, nothing is required; if titer is not protective, give 0.06 mL/kg within 24 hours	Review vaccination status[6]
Source known, HB$_s$Ag status unknown	Test source for HB$_s$Ag and exposed person for anti-HB$_s$. If source is HB$_s$Ag-negative, or if source is HB$_s$Ag-positive but anti-HB$_s$ titer is protective, nothing is required. If source is HB$_s$Ag-positive and anti-HB$_s$ titer is not protective or if exposed person is a known nonresponder, give 0.06 mL/kg I.M. within 24 hours. A second dose of hepatitis B immune globulin can be given 1 month later if a booster dose of hepatitis B vaccine is not given.	Review vaccination status[6]

Table continued on next page

SYSTEMIC VIRAL DISEASES *(Continued)*

POSTEXPOSURE PROPHYLAXIS FOR HEPATITIS B[1] *(continued)*

Exposure	Hepatitis B Immune Globulin	Hepatitis B Vaccine
Source not tested or unknown	Test exposed person for anti-HB$_s$. If anti-HB$_s$ titer is protective, nothing is required. If anti-HB$_s$ titer is not protective, 0.06 mL/kg may be given along with a booster dose of hepatitis B vaccine.	Review vaccination status[6]

[1]HB$_s$Ag = hepatitis B surface antigen; anti-HB$_s$ = antibody to hepatitis B surface antigen; I.M. = intramuscularly; SRU = standard ratio units.

[2]Each 0.5 mL dose of plasma-derived hepatitis B vaccine contains 10 mcg of HB$_s$Ag; each 0.5 mL dose of recombinant hepatitis B vaccine contains 5 mcg or 10 mcg of HB$_s$Ag.

[3]If hepatitis B immune globulin and hepatitis B vaccine are given simultaneously, they should be given at separate sites.

[4]If hepatitis B vaccine is not given, a second dose of hepatitis B immune globulin should be given 1 month later.

[5]Anti-HB$_s$ titers <10 SRU by radioimmunoassay or negative by enzyme immunoassay indicate lack of protection. Testing the exposed person for anti-HB$_s$ is not necessary if a protective level of antibody has been shown within the previous 24 months.

[6]If the exposed person has not completed a three-dose series of hepatitis B vaccine, the series should be completed. Test the exposed person for anti-HB$_s$. If the antibody level is protective, nothing is required. If an adequate antibody response in the past is shown on retesting to have declined to an inadequate level, a booster dose (1 mL) of hepatitis B vaccine should be given. If the exposed person has inadequate antibody or is a known nonresponder to vaccination, a booster dose can be given along with one dose of hepatitis B immune globulin.

HERPES

The herpes viruses not only represent a topic of specific interest to the dentist due to oral manifestations, but are widespread as systemic infections. Herpes simplex virus is also of interest because of its central nervous system infections and its relationship as one of the viral infections commonly found in AIDS patients. Oral herpes infections will be covered elsewhere. Treatment of herpes simplex primary infection includes acyclovir. Ganciclovir is an alternative drug and foscarnet is also occasionally used. Epstein-Barr virus is a member of the herpesvirus family and produces syndromes important in dentistry, including infectious mononucleosis with the commonly found oral pharyngitis and petechial hemorrhages, as well as being the causative agent of Burkitt's lymphoma. The relationship between Epstein-Barr virus to oral hairy leukoplakia in AIDS patients has not been shown to be one of cause and effect; however, the presence of Epstein-Barr in these lesions is consistent. Currently, there is no accepted treatment for Epstein-Barr virus, although acyclovir has been shown in *in vitro* studies to have some efficacy. Varicella-zoster virus is another member of the herpesvirus family and is the causative agent of two clinical entities, chickenpox and shingles, or herpes zoster. Oral manifestations of both chickenpox and herpes zoster include vesicular eruptions often leading to confluent mucosal ulcerations. Acyclovir is the drug of choice for treatment of herpes zoster infections.

There are other herpes viruses that produce disease in man and animals. These viruses have no specific treatment, therefore, incidence is thought to be less common than those mentioned and the specific treatment is not determined at present. The role of some of these viruses in concomitant infection with the HIV and other coinfection viruses is still under study.

ANTIVIRALS

AGENTS OF ESTABLISHED EFFECTIVENESS

Viral Infection	Drug
Cytomegalovirus	
Retinitis	Ganciclovir, Foscarnet
Pneumonia	Ganciclovir
Hepatitis viruses	
Chronic hepatitis A & B	Hepatitis A (Inactivated) and Hepatitis B (Recombinant) Vaccine
Chronic hepatitis C	Interferon Alfa-2a, Interferon Alfa-2b, Interferon Alfa-2b and Ribavirin, Peginterferon Alfa-2a, Peginterferon Alfa-2b
Chronic hepatitis B	Interferon Alfa-2b
Herpes simplex virus	
Orofacial herpes	
First episode	Acyclovir[1], Valacyclovir
Recurrence	Acyclovir[1], Penciclovir[1], Valacyclovir
Genital herpes	
First episode, recurrence, suppression	Acyclovir, Valacyclovir
Encephalitis	Acyclovir
Mucocutaneous disease in immunocompromised	Acyclovir
Neonatal	Acyclovir
Keratoconjunctivitis	Trifluridine Vidarabine
Influenza A virus	Amantadine, Oseltamivir, Rimantadine, Zanamivir
Papillomavirus	
Condyloma acuminatum	Interferon Alfa-2b, Imiquimod (Aldara™): (use for oral lesions is under study)
Respiratory syncytial virus	Ribavirin
Varicella-zoster virus	
Varicella in normal children	Acyclovir
Varicella in immunocompromised	Acyclovir
Herpes zoster in immunocompromised	Acyclovir
Herpes zoster in normal hosts	Acyclovir, Famciclovir, Valacyclovir

[1]Although acyclovir is often used for these infections, penciclovir and valacyclovir are specifically approved for herpes labialis. The clinician is referred to the monographs.

ANTIBIOTIC PROPHYLAXIS

PREPROCEDURAL GUIDELINES FOR DENTAL PATIENTS

INTRODUCTION

In dental practice, the clinician is often confronted with a decision to prescribe antibiotics. The focus of this section is on the use of antibiotics as a preprocedural treatment in the prevention of adverse infectious sequelae in two commonly encountered situations: prevention of infective endocarditis and prevention of late infections of prosthetic implants.

The criteria for preprocedural decisions begins with patient evaluation. An accurate and complete medical history is always the initial basis for any prescriptive treatments on the part of the dentist. These prescriptive treatments can include ordering appropriate laboratory tests, referral to the patient's physician for consultation, or immediate decision to prescribe preprocedural antibiotics. The dentist should also be aware that antibiotic coverage of the patient might be appropriate due to diseases that are covered elsewhere in this text, such as human immunodeficiency virus, cavernous thrombosis, undiagnosed or uncontrolled diabetes, lupus, renal failure, and periods of neutropenia as are often associated with cancer chemotherapy. In these instances, medical consultation is almost always necessary in making antibiotic decisions in order to tailor the treatment and dosing to the individual patient's needs. When in doubt regarding a patient's medical status communicating with the physician is always an appropriate and prudent step.

Note: The ADA Council on Scientific Affairs recently restated the dentist's responsibility when prescribing antibiotics to oral contraceptive users (*JADA*, 2002, 133:880). It is recommended that dental professionals advise these patients to consult their physician for additional barrier contraception due to potential reduction in the efficacy of oral contraceptives from antibiotic interaction.

PREVENTION OF INFECTIVE ENDOCARDITIS

In one of the most significant examples of Evidence Based Science, the American Heart Association (AHA) in conjunction with the American Dental Association (ADA) and other experts in both medicine and dentistry reviewed the evidence regarding the use of antibiotic prophylaxis to prevent infective endocarditis (IE) prior to dental appointments. The reviewers concluded that IE is more frequently caused by a patient's susceptibility to bacteremias associated with normal activities rather than bacteremia caused by dental procedures. Therefore, maintaining oral health to reduce bacteremia is more effective in reducing the risk of IE than the use of prophylactic antiobiotics before dental procedures. Since the mid-1950s, patients at risk for IE from a variety of conditions have been routinely premedicated with antibiotics prior to dental and other procedures. After a review of the evidence, it has been concluded that the majority of patients did not benefit from this prophylaxis. The incidence of IE was not changed when compared to patients who received IE prophylaxis and those who did not and the risk for adverse effects from antibiotic use exceeds the benefit of therapy. Therefore, based on the evidence, a change in the Guidelines has been recommended by AHA, the ADA as well as the Infectious Disease Society. The AHA/ADA recommends that most patients no longer need short-term antibiotics as a preventive measure before their dental treatment. Only those patients with the highest risk should receive prophylaxis.

Antibiotic prophylaxis with dental procedures is recommended for patients at high risk of adverse effects due to specific cardiac conditions (ie, prosthetic cardiac valve) or a prior incidence of IE. Prophylaxis is also required for heart transplant patients who develop cardiac valvulopathy. Patients with congenital heart disease (CHD) are only required prophylaxis with the following conditions: 1) Unrepaired cyanotic CHD, including palliative shunts and conduits; 2) CHD repaired by prosthetic material or device (for first 6 months after procedure); 3) or if there are residual defects after repair (inhibiting endothelialization). These patients with high risk cardiac conditions are recommended for **prophylaxis for all dental procedures involving manipulation of gingival tissue or the periapical region of teeth or perforation of the oral mucosa. Dental procedures that do not require prophylaxis include routine anesthetic injection into noninfected tissue, taking dental radiographs, placement of removable prosthodontic or orthodontic appliances, adjustment of orthodontic appliances, placement of orthodontic brackets, shedding of deciduous teeth, and bleeding for trauma to the lips or oral mucosa.**

ANTIBIOTIC SELECTION

For examples of sample prescriptions see Infective Endocarditis (Prevention) *on page 1832*. The dentist should be vigilant in reviewing literature for updates.

Amoxicillin is an amino-type penicillin with an extended spectrum of antibacterial action compared to penicillin VK. The pharmacology of amoxicillin as a dental antibiotic has been reviewed previously in *General Dentistry*. The suggested regimen for standard general prophylaxis is a dose of 2 g 30-60 minutes before the procedure. A follow-up dose is no longer necessary. The pediatric dose is 50 mg/kg orally 30-60 minutes before the procedure and not to exceed the adult dose. Amoxicillin is available in capsules (250 mg and 500 mg), chewable tablets (125 mg, 200 mg, 250 mg, 400 mg), tablets (500 mg, 875 mg) and liquid suspension (125 mg/5 mL, 200 mg/5 mL, 250 mg/5 mL, 400 mg/5 mL).

For individuals unable to take oral medications, intramuscular or intravenous ampicillin is recommended for both adults and children. It is to be given at the same doses used for the oral amoxicillin medication. Ampicillin is also an amino-type penicillin having an antibacterial spectrum similar to amoxicillin. Ampicillin is not absorbed from the GI tract as effectively as amoxicillin and, therefore, is not recommended for oral use. Cefazolin or ceftriaxone are alternatives.

Table 1.
PROPHYLACTIC REGIMENS FOR INFECTIVE ENDOCARDITIS
FOR DENTAL PROCEDURES

Situation	Drug	Single Dosage 30-60 minutes prior to procedure
Oral	Amoxicillin *on page 108*	Children: 50 mg/kg Adults: 2 g
Unable to take oral medications	Ampicillin *on page 119* **or**	Children: 50 mg/kg I.M. or I.V. Adults: 2 g I.M. or I.V.
	Cefazolin *on page 297* **or** Ceftriaxone *on page 309*	Children: 50 mg/kg I.M. or I.V. Adults: 1 g I.M. or I.V.
Allergic to penicillins or ampicillin (oral)	Cephalexin *on page 317*[1,2] **or**	Children: 50 mg/kg Adults: 2 g
	Clindamycin *on page 378* **or**	Children: 20 mg/kg Adults: 600 mg
	Azithromycin *on page 176* **or** Clarithromycin *on page 371*	Children: 15 mg/kg Adults: 500 mg
Allergic to penicillins or ampicillin and unable to take oral medications	Cefazolin *on page 297* **or** Ceftriaxone *on page 309*[2]	Children: 50 mg/kg I.M. or I.V. Adults: 1 g I.M. or I.V.
	Clindamycin *on page 378*	Children: 20 mg/kg I.M. or I.V. Adults: 600 mg I.M. or I.V.

Note: Intramuscular injections should be avoided in patients receiving anticoagulant therapy.

[1]Can use first- or second-generation oral cephalosporins in equivalent doses.

[2]Cephalosporins should not be used in individuals with immediate-type hypersensitivity reaction (urticaria, angioedema, or anaphylaxis) to penicillins.

Individuals who are allergic to the penicillins, such as amoxicillin or ampicillin, should be treated with an alternate antibiotic. The new guidelines have suggested a number of alternate agents including clindamycin, cephalosporins, azithromycin, and clarithromycin. Clindamycin (Cleocin®) occupies an important niche in dentistry as a useful and effective antibiotic and it was a recommended alternative agent for the prevention of bacterial endocarditis in the previous guidelines. In the new guidelines, the oral adult dose is 600 mg 30-60 minutes before the procedure. A follow-up dose is not necessary. Clindamycin is available as 300 mg capsules; thus 2 capsules will provide the recommended dose. The children's oral dose for clindamycin is 20 mg/kg 30-60 minutes before the procedure. Clindamycin is also available as flavored granules for oral solution. When reconstituted with water, each bottle yields a solution containing 75 mg/5 mL. Intravenous clindamycin is recommended in adults and children who are allergic to penicillin and unable to take oral medications.

Clindamycin was developed in the 1960s as a semisynthetic derivative of lincomycin which was found in the soil organism, *Streptomyces lincolnensis*, near Lincoln, Nebraska. It is commercially available as the hydrochloride salt to improve solubility in the GI tract. Clindamycin is antibacterial against most aerobic Gram-positive cocci including staphylococci and streptococci, and against many types of anaerobic Gram-negative and Gram-positive organisms. It has been used over the years in dentistry as an alternative to penicillin and erythromycins for the treatment of oral-facial infections.

The mechanism of antibacterial action of clindamycin is the same as erythromycin. It inhibits protein synthesis in susceptible bacteria resulting in the inhibition of bacterial growth and replication. Following oral administration of a single dose of clindamycin (150 mg, 300 mg, or 600 mg) on an empty stomach, 90% of the dose is rapidly absorbed into the bloodstream and peak serum concentrations are attained within 45-80 minutes. Administration with food does not markedly impair absorption into the bloodstream.

ANTIBIOTIC PROPHYLAXIS *(Continued)*

Clindamycin serum levels exceed the minimum inhibitory concentration (MIC) for bacterial growth for at least 6 hours after the recommended dose of 600 mg. The serum half-life is 2-3 hours.

Adverse effects of clindamycin after a single dose are virtually nonexistent. Although it is estimated that 1% of patients taking clindamycin will develop symptoms of pseudomembranous colitis, these symptoms usually develop after 9-14 days of clindamycin therapy. These symptoms are rare and only one case has been reported in a patient taking an acute dose for the prevention of endocarditis.

In lieu of clindamycin, penicillin-allergic individuals may receive cephalexin (Keflex®) provided that they have not had an immediate-type sensitivity reaction such as anaphylaxis, urticaria, or angioedema to penicillins. These antibiotics are first-generation cephalosporins having an antibacterial spectrum of action similar to amoxicillin and ampicillin. They elicit a bactericidal action by inhibiting cell wall synthesis in susceptible bacteria. The recommended adult prophylactic dose for either of these drugs is 2 g 30-60 minutes before the procedure. Again, no follow-up dose is needed. The children's oral dose for cephalexin is 50 mg/kg 30-60 minutes before the procedure. Cephalexin is supplied as capsules (250 mg, 500 mg, 750 mg) and is available in the form of powder for oral suspension at concentrations of 125 mg/5 mL and 250 mg/5 mL.

For those individuals (adults and children) allergic to penicillin and unable to take oral medicines, parenteral cefazolin (Ancef®) may be used, provided that they do not have the sensitivities described previously. Cefazolin is also a first-generation cephalosporin. Please note that the parenteral cefazolin can be given I.M. or I.V. (refer to Table 1, for the adult and children's doses of parenteral cefazolin).

Azithromycin (Zithromax®) and clarithromycin (Biaxin®) are members of the class of antibiotics known as the macrolides. The pharmacology of these drugs has been reviewed previously in *General Dentistry*. The erythromycins have been available for use in dentistry and medicine since the mid 1950s. Azithromycin and clarithromycin represent the first additions to this class in >40 years. The adult prophylactic dose for either drug is 500 mg 30-60 minutes before the procedure with no follow-up dose. The pediatric prophylactic dose of azithromycin and clarithromycin is 15 mg/kg orally 30-60 minutes before the procedure. Although the erythromycin family of drugs are known to inhibit the hepatic metabolism of theophylline and carbamazepine to enhance their effects, azithromycin has not been shown to affect the liver metabolism of these drugs.

Azithromycin is well absorbed from the gastrointestinal tract and is extensively taken up from the circulation into tissues with a slow release from those tissues. It reaches peak serum levels in 2-4 hours and serum half-life is 68 hours. Zithromax® is supplied as 250 mg, 500 mg, and 600 mg tablets. It is also available for oral suspension at concentrations of 100 mg/5 mL, 200 mg/5 mL, and single-dose packets containing 1 g.

Clarithromycin (Biaxin®) achieves peak plasma concentrations in 3 hours and maintains effective serum concentrations over a 12-hour period. Reports indicate that it probably interacts with theophylline and carbamazepine by elevating the plasma concentrations of the two drugs. Biaxin® is supplied as 250 mg and 500 mg tablets and 500 mg extended release tablets. It is also available as granules for oral suspension at concentrations of 125 mg/5 mL and 250 mg/5 mL.

Clinical Considerations for Dentistry

See Figure 1 on page 1779.

Patients with a suspicious history of one of the high risk cardiac conditions who are in need of an immediate dental procedure should be prophylaxed with an appropriate antibiotic prior to the procedure(s) until medical evaluation has been completed and the risk level determined. If unanticipated dental risk develops during a procedure in a cardiac at-risk patient, appropriate antibiotics should be given immediately.

If a series of dental procedures is planned, the clinician must judge whether an interval between procedures, requiring prophylaxis, should be scheduled. The literature supports 9- to 14-day intervals as ideal to minimize the risk of emergence of resistant organisms. Since serum levels of the standard amoxicillin dose may be adequate for 6-14 hours depending on the specific organism challenge, the clinician may have to consider the efficacy of a second dose if multiple procedures are planned over the course of a single day.

PREPROCEDURAL ANTIBIOTICS FOR PROSTHETIC IMPLANTS

To date there have not been any recommended changes in these guidelines but the clinicin should be aware that in light of the new IE prevention guidelines, changes in the prosthetic implant guidelines may occur.

A significant number of dental patients have had total joint replacements or other implanted prosthetic devices. Prior to performing dental procedures that might induce bacteremia, the dentist must consider the use of antibiotic prophylaxis in these patients. Until recently, only the American Heart Association had taken a formal stance on implanted devices by suggesting guidelines for the use of antibiotic prophylaxis in patients with prosthetic heart valves. These guidelines and the recent guidelines for prevention of bacterial endocarditis have been published in *General Dentistry*.

The use of antibiotics in patients with other prosthetic devices, including total joint replacements has remained controversial because of several issues. Late infections of implanted prosthetic devices have rarely been associated with microbial organisms of oral origin. Secondly, since late infections in such patients are often not reported, data is lacking to substantiate or refute this potential. Also, there is general acceptance that patients with acute infections at distant sites such as the oral cavity may be at greater risk of infection of an implanted prosthetic device. Periodontal disease has been implicated as a distant site infection. Since antibiotics are associated with allergies and other adverse reactions, and because the frequent use of antibiotics may lead to emergence of resistant organisms, any perceived benefit of antibiotic prophylaxis must always be weighed against known risks of toxicity, allergy, or potential microbial resistance.

Recently, an advisory group made up of representatives from the American Dental Association and the American Academy of Orthopaedic Surgeons published a statement in the *Journal of the American Dental Association* on the use of antibiotics prior to dental procedures in patients with total joint replacements. The statement concluded that antibiotic prophylaxis should not be prescribed routinely for most dental patients with total joint replacements or for any patients with pins, plates, and screws. However, in an attempt to base the guidelines on available scientific evidence, the advisory group stated that certain patients may be potential risks for joint infection thus justifying the use of prophylactic antibiotics. Those conditions considered by the advisory group to be associated with potential elevated risk of joint infections are listed in Table 2. The dentist should carefully review the patient's history to ensure identification of those medical problems leading to potential elevated risks of joint infections as listed in Table 2. Where appropriate, medical consultation with the patient's internist or orthopedist may be prudent to assist in this determination. The orthopedist should be queried specifically, as to the status of the joint prosthesis itself.

Table 2.
PATIENTS WITH POTENTIAL ELEVATED RISK OF JOINT INFECTION

Inflammatory arthropathies: Rheumatoid arthritis, systemic lupus erythematosus
Disease-, drug-, or radiation-induced immunosuppression
Insulin-dependent diabetes
First 2 years following joint replacement
Previous prosthetic joint infections
Patients with acute infections at a distant site
Hemophilia
Malnourishment[1]
Patients with malignancies[1]
Patients with HIV infection[1]

[1]Source: American Dental Association; American Academy of Orthopedic Surgeons, "Antibiotic Prophylaxis for Dental Patients With Total Joint Replacements," *J Am Dent Assoc*, 2003, 134(7):895-9.

ANTIBIOTIC PROPHYLAXIS *(Continued)*

Patients who present with elevated risks of joint infections, in which the dentist is going to perform any procedures associated with a high risk, need to receive preprocedural antibiotics. Patients undergoing dental procedures involving low risk, probably do not require premedication even though the patient may be in the category of elevated risk of joint infections. The listing of low bacteremia risks may need to be reconsidered, depending on the patient's oral health.

For examples of sample prescriptions see Prosthetic Joint Late Infections (Prevention) *on page 1833*

ANTIBIOTIC REGIMENS

The antibiotic prophylaxis regimens as suggested by the advisory panel are listed in Table 3. These regimens are not exactly the same as those listed in Table 1 (for prevention of endocarditis) and must be reviewed carefully to avoid confusion. Cephalexin, cephradine, or amoxicillin may be used in patients not allergic to penicillin. The selected antibiotic is given as a single 2 g dose 1 hour before the procedure. A follow-up dose is not recommended. Cephalexin (Keflex®) and amoxicillin were described earlier in this section. Cephradine (Velosef®) is a first-generation cephalosporin-type antibiotic, effective against anaerobic bacteria and aerobic Gram-positive bacteria. It is predominantly used to treat infections of the bones and joints, lower respiratory tract, urinary tract, skin, and soft tissues.

Parenteral cefazolin (Ancef®) or ampicillin are the recommended antibiotics for patients unable to take oral medications (see Table 3 for doses). Cefazolin is a first-generation cephalosporin, effective against anaerobes and aerobic Gram-positive bacteria. Ampicillin is an aminopenicillin (described earlier). For patients allergic to penicillin, clindamycin is the recommended antibiotic of choice. Clindamycin is active against aerobic and anaerobic streptococci, most staphylococci, the *Bacteroides*, and the *Actinomyces* families of bacteria. The recommended oral and parenteral doses of clindamycin in the joint prosthetic patient are listed in Table 3 below.

Table 3.
ANTIBIOTIC REGIMENS FOR PATIENTS WITH PROSTHETIC IMPLANTS

Patients not allergic to penicillin:	Cephalexin, cephradine, or amoxicillin:	2 g orally 1 hour prior to the procedure
Patients not allergic to penicillin and unable to take oral medications:	Cefazolin: or Ampicillin:	1 g I.M. or I.V. 1 hour prior to the procedure 2 g I.M. or I.V. 1 hour prior to the procedure
Patients allergic to penicillin:	Clindamycin:	600 mg orally 1 hour prior to dental procedure
Patients allergic to penicillin and unable to take oral medications:	Clindamycin:	600 mg I.V. 1 hour prior to the procedure

Amoxicillin *on page 108*
Ampicillin *on page 119*
Cefazolin *on page 297*
Cephalexin *on page 317*
Cephradine *on page 319*
Clindamycin *on page 378*

Clinical Considerations for Dentistry

See Figure 2 on page 1780.

The frequency of postinsertion infections in patients who have undergone total joint replacement or prosthetic device placement is variable. The most common cause of infection with all devices is found to be from contamination at the time of surgical insertions. The presence of an acute distant infection at a site other than the joint, however, appears to be a risk factor for late infection of these devices. The rationale by the American Dental Association and the American Academy of Orthopedic Surgeons in their advisory statement has been to provide guidelines to minimize the use of antibiotics to the first 2 years following total joint replacement. As more data are collected, these recommendations may be revised. However, it is thought to be prudent for the dental clinician to fully evaluate all patients with respect to history and or physical findings prior to determining the risk.

If a dental procedure considered to be low risk is performed in a patient at risk for joint complications, and inadvertent bleeding occurs, then an appropriate antibiotic should be given immediately. Although this is not ideal, animal studies suggest that it may be useful. Likewise, in patients where concern exists over joint complications and a medical consultation cannot be immediately obtained, the patient should be treated as though antibiotic coverage is necessary until such time that an appropriate consultation can be completed. The presence of an acute oral infection, in addition to any pre-existing dental conditions, may increase the risk of late infection at the prosthetic joint. Even though most late joint infections are caused by *Staphylococcus* sp, the risk of bacteremia involving another organism, predominant in an acute infection, may increase the risk of joint infection.

The dentist may also need to consider the question of multiple procedures over a period of time. Procedures planned over a period of several days would best be rescheduled at intervals of 9-14 days. The risk of emergence of resistant organisms in patients receiving multiple short-term doses of antibiotics has been shown to be greater than those receiving antibiotics over longer intervals of time.

FREQUENTLY ASKED QUESTIONS FOR INFECTIVE ENDOCARDITIS (IE) AND PROSTHETIC IMPLANTS

When should we start following the new prevention of IE guidelines?

Immediately

What should we do for patients who have been premedicated in the past?

Most patients will no longer require premedication. If the patient does not fall into one of the highest risk groups, premedication should be discontinued. If it cannot be clearly determined if the patient is in the highest risk group, a medical consultation should be sent to determine if prophylaxis should be continued.

Are there different drugs and regimens?

The drugs have undergone minor revisions (see Table 1) and the dosing regimens for all drugs has been changed from 1 hour prior to 30-60 minutes prior to procedure.

Should I just premedicate to be safe?

No, the new guidelines are based on evidence which documents that the risk of adverse side effects from the antibiotics (allergy, GI upset, development of microbial resistance, etc) outweigh the benefits in most patients who previously received SBE/IE prophylaxis. The new Guidelines clearly recommend the use of prophylactic antibiotics only for those with the highest risk.

Has there been any change in the Guidelines for prophylaxis for patients with prosthetic joint replacements?

No, continue to use the published Guidelines.

What if a pateint did not meet the new high risk criteria outlined in the new Guidelines and the patient's physician still recommends IE prophylaxis?

Please contact the physician to see if there are compelling medical reasons for continuing IE prophylaxis.

What if a patient who has received IE prophylaxis in the past for a condition that is now deemed as NOT being high risk for IE prophylaxis still insists on being premedicate?

Contact the physician to see if there are compelling medical reasons for continuing IE prophylaxis.

If the patient is presently taking antibiotics for some other ailment, is prophylaxis still necessary?

If a patient is already taking antibiotics for another condition, prophylaxis should be accomplished with a drug from another class. For example, in the patient who is not allergic to penicillin who is taking a macrolide antibiotic for a medical condition such as mycoplasma infection, amoxicillin would be the drug of choice for prophylaxis. Also, in the penicillin-allergic patient taking clindamycin, prophylaxis would best be accomplished with azithromycin or clarithromycin.

Can clindamycin be used safely in patients with gastrointestinal disorders?

If a patient has a history of inflammatory bowel disease and is allergic to penicillin, azithromycin or clarithromycin should be selected over clindamycin. In patients with a negative history of inflammatory bowel disease, clindamycin has not been shown to induce colitis following a single-dose administration.

Why do the suggested drug regimens for patients with joint prostheses resemble so closely the regimens for the prevention of endocarditis?

Bacteremia is the predisposing risk factor for the development of endocarditis in those patients at high risk due to a cardiac condition. Likewise, the potential of bacteremia during dental procedures is considered to be the risk factor in some late joint prostheses infections, even though this risk is presumed to be much lower.

ANTIBIOTIC PROPHYLAXIS *(Continued)*

How do we determine those patients who have had joint replacement complications?

Patients who have had complications during the initial placement of a total joint would be those who had infection following placement, those with recurrent pain, or those who have had previous joint replacement failures. If the patient reports even minor complications, a medical consultation with the orthopedist would be the most appropriate action for the dentist.

Is prophylaxis required in patients with pins, screws, or plates often used in orthopedic repairs?

There is currently no evidence supporting use of antibiotics following the placement of pins, plates, or screws. Breast implants, dental implants, and implanted lenses in the eye following cataract surgery are also all thought to be at minimal risk for infection following dental procedures. Therefore, no antibiotic prophylaxis is recommended in these situations. There is, however, some evidence indicating elevated risk of infection following some types of penile implants and some vascular access devices, used during chemotherapy. It is recommended that the dentist discuss such patients with the physician prior to determining the need for antibiotics.

What should I do if medical consultation results in a recommendation that differs from the published guidelines endorsed by the American Dental Association?

The dentist is ultimately responsible for treatment recommendations. Ideally, by communicating with the physician, a consensus can be achieved that is either in agreement with the guidelines or is based on other established medical reasoning.

What is the best antibiotic modality for treating dental infections?

Penicillin is still the drug of choice for treatment of infections in and around the oral cavity. Phenoxy-methyl penicillin (Pen VK®) has long been the most commonly-selected antibiotic. In penicillin-allergic individuals, erythromycin may be an appropriate consideration. If another drug is sought, clindamycin prescribed 300 mg as a loading dose followed by 150 mg 4 times/day would be an appropriate regimen for a dental infection. In general, if there is no response to Pen VK®, then Augmentin® may be a good alternative in the nonpenicillin-allergic patient because of its slightly altered spectrum. Recommendations would include that the patient should take the drug with food.

Is there cross-allergenicity between the cephalosporins and penicillin?

The incidence of cross-allergenicity is 5% to 8% in the overall population. If a patient has demonstrated a Type I hypersensitivity reaction to penicillin, namely urticaria or anaphylaxis, then this incidence would increase to 20%.

Is there definitely an interaction between contraception agents and antibiotics?

There are well founded interactions between contraceptives and antibiotics. The best instructions that a patient could be given by their dentist are that should an antibiotic be necessary and the dentist is aware that the patient is on contraceptives, and if the patient is using chemical contraceptives, the patient should seriously consider additional means of contraception during the antibiotic management.

Are antibiotics necessary in diabetic patients?

In the management of diabetes, control of the diabetic status is the key factor relative to all morbidity issues. If a patient is well controlled, then antibiotics will likely not be necessary. However, in patients where the control is questionable or where they have recently been given a different drug regimen for their diabetes or if they are being titrated to an appropriate level of either insulin or oral hypoglycemic agents during these periods of time, the dentist might consider preprocedural antibiotics to be efficacious.

Do nonsteroidal anti-inflammatory drugs interfere with blood pressure medication?

At the current time there is no clear evidence that NSAIDs interfere with any of the blood pressure medications that are currently in use.

Some materials in this chapter were adapted from the newly released guidelines Wilson W, Taubert KA, Gewitz M, et al, "Prevention of Infective Endocarditis. Guidelines From the American Heart Association," *Circulation*, April 2007 [Epub ahead of print].

Figure 1
Preprocedural Dental Action Plan for Patients With a History
Indicative of Elevated Endocarditis Risk

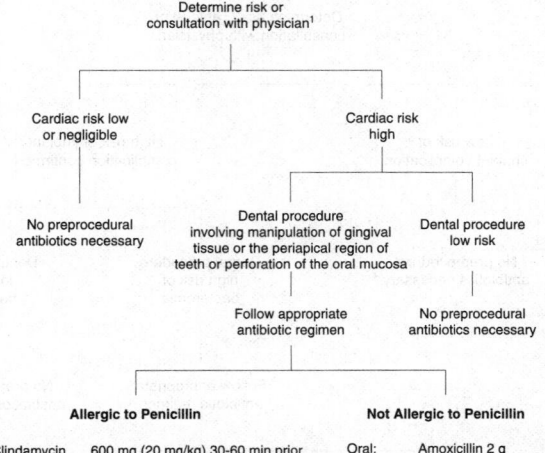

Allergic to Penicillin

Oral:	Clindamycin	600 mg (20 mg/kg) 30-60 min prior
	Cephalexin	2 g (50 mg/kg) 30-60 min prior
	Azithromycin	500 mg (15 mg/kg) 30-60 min prior
	Clarithromycin	500 mg (15 mg/kg) 30-60 min prior
I.V.:	Clindamycin	600 mg (20 mg/kg) 30-60 min prior
I.M. or I.V.:	Cefazolin	1 g (25 mg/kg) 30-60 min prior
	Ceftriaxone	1 g (25 mg/kg) 30-60 min prior

Not Allergic to Penicillin

Oral:	Amoxicillin 2 g	(50 mg/kg) 30-60 min prior
I.M. or I.V.:	Ampicillin 2 g	(50 mg/kg) 30-60 min prior

Dosages for children are in parentheses and should never exceed adult dose. Cephalosporins should be avoided in patients with previous Type I hypersensitivity reactions to penicillin due to some evidence of cross-allergenicity.

[1]For Emergency Dental Care, the clinician should attempt phone consultation. If unable to contact patient's physician or determine risk, the patient should be treated as though there is a high risk of cardiac complication and follow the algorithm.

ANTIBIOTIC PROPHYLAXIS *(Continued)*

Figure 2
Preprocedural Dental Action Plan for
Patients With Prosthetic Implants

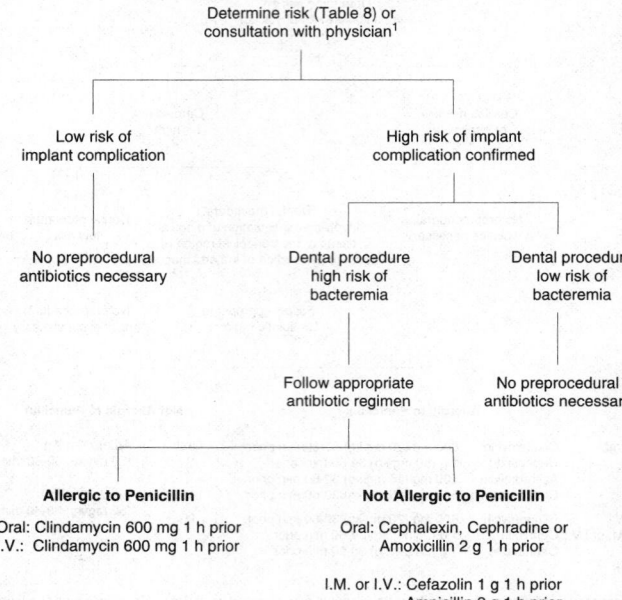

Cephalosporins should be avoided in patients with previous Type I hypersensitivity reactions to penicillin due to some evidence of cross allergenicity.

[1]For Emergency Dental Care the clinician should attempt phone consultation. If unable to contact patient's physician or determine risk, the patient should be treated as though there is high risk of implant complication and follow the algorithm.

MANAGEMENT OF THE CHEMICALLY DEPENDENT PATIENT

INTRODUCTION

As long as history has been recorded, man has used drugs to alter mood, thought, and feeling. The financial and emotional cost to society due to the abuse and addiction of these substances is staggering. Some reports place the cost to society of alcoholism and alcohol abuse as high as $185 billion dollars annually. Increased on-the-job accidents, absenteeism, welfare costs, and alcohol related auto fatalities contribute to this cost.

In 1986, the American Dental Association (ADA) passed a policy statement recognizing chemical dependency as a disease. In recognizing this disease, the Association mandated that dentists have a responsibility to include questions relating to a history of chemical dependency, or more broadly, substance abuse in their health history question-naire. This policy statement included patients who are actively abusing drugs as well as patients who are in recovery. An affirmative response was an alert to the dentist and dental team to use caution with certain medications and that the treatment plan may have to be altered. This policy statement was revised in 1989 and 1991 with minor changes. In October 2005 at the annual ADA session, the House of Delegates passed several resolutions encompassing the use of opioids in management of dental pain, alcohol, and other substance use by pregnant and postpartum patients, and guidelines related to alcohol, nicotine, and/or drug use by child or adolescent patients. The House of Delegates in 2005 reaffirmed the disease concept of alcoholism and other substance use disorders and provided a more current statement on provision of dental treatment for patients with substance use disorders. For an in-depth review of these resolutions, refer to www.ada.org. At the minimum, the patient's past medical history questionnaire should include a question asking if there is a history of chemical dependency and if so, how long they have been in recovery. The dental office should have a list available of local resources for drug counseling in the event the patient admits drug use and seeks some help.

This chapter reviews substances of abuse, where they come from, signs and symptoms of the substance abuser, and some of the dental implications of treating patients actively using or in recovery from these substances. There are many books and articles devoted to this topic that provide greater detail. The intent of this chapter is to provide an overview of some of the most prevalent drugs, how abuse of these substances by patients may influence dental treatment, and how to recognize some signs and symptoms of substance abuse and withdrawal.

Substances of abuse originate from many sources. They may be naturally occurring, semisynthetic, synthetic, over-the-counter, or prescription drugs. There is a paucity of information in the dental literature correlating substance abuse with dental manifesta-tions for a simple reason. Most substance abusers do not seek routine dental care because obtaining their drug of choice is their top priority. Most often they will be episodic patients. In fact, that is one of the cardinal signs of addiction, a preoccupation with obtaining the drug or sex or gambling or whatever the addiction. Again, it is not the intent of this chapter to explore addiction or abuse in detail. The reader is referred to several comprehensive texts on this disease.

As a general rule, the stimulant (uppers) abusing dental patient will not be going to the dentist while under the influence of the drug because the upper will increase their already existing anxiety. It is more likely that a patient will use or abuse a depressant (downer) substance to self-medicate anxiety. This is important to the dentist because uppers such as cocaine, methamphetamine, and ecstasy are sympathomimetics and in combination with vasoconstrictor could result in a hypertensive crisis (stroke). **Plain local anesthetic without vasoconstrictor is not contraindicated in that patient.** Patients who self-medicate with depressant drugs such as alcohol, opiates, barbiturates, or marijuana are generally more compliant while in the dental chair, and the drug combination does not pose a serious threat.

ALCOHOL

Ethyl alcohol (referred to as alcohol) is the most abused drug in the United States today and the number one most abused drug by dentists. As mentioned above, the cost to society for the treatment of alcoholism and alcohol abuse is billions of dollars annually. Alcohol is a depressant drug (downer) and not a stimulant as many people (particularly the adolescent population) believe. Its effect on the central nervous system is dose-dependent and correlated with the rising blood alcohol concentration rather than the falling concentration. Cognitive ability, reaction time, memory, psychomotor, and perceptual ability are impaired to varying degrees.

The majority of consumed alcohol is absorbed from the small intestine and is, therefore, affected by the gastric emptying time and the consumption of food. Alcohol is metabo-lized by the liver and excess consumption of alcohol can result in hepatic damage that may affect the patient's ability to metabolize medications. Doses of medications that are

MANAGEMENT OF THE CHEMICALLY DEPENDENT PATIENT
(Continued)

metabolized by the liver, such as acetaminophen, may have to be reduced when treating a patient with confirmed hepatic damage from alcohol or other substance abuse. Alcohol readily crosses the placental barrier and has the potential of producing fetal alcohol syndrome (FAS) resulting in mental retardation, supernumerary teeth, and facial deformities to name a few. There are many resources that provide greater detail about this preventable syndrome and the reader is referred to those sources.

Excessive alcohol use has been associated with an increased incidence of periodontal disease, poor wound healing, chronic orofacial infections, iatrogenic injury, and an increased incidence of oral cancer. Since alcohol is a depressant drug, any medication that causes respiratory depression should be prescribed or administered with caution or not at all. Patients who present to the dental office and are obviously intoxicated should not be provided dental treatment. The major concern with the intoxicated patient is a failure to follow directions while in the chair, and the inability to follow postoperative instructions. An additional concern is the aggressive, combative behavior exhibited by some that are intoxicated.

Signs and Symptoms of Alcohol Use or Abuse	
Lethargic, slow to respond	Odor on breath and/or clothes
Slurred speech	Inability to respond to commands
Telangiectasia	Psychomotor impairment

MARIJUANA

The most abused illegal drug by high school students today is marijuana. Marijuana is a plant that grows throughout the world, but is particularly suited for a warm, humid environment. There are three species of plants but the two most frequently cited are *Cannabis sativa* and *Cannabis indica*. All species possess a female and male plant. Although approximately 450 chemicals have been isolated from the plant, the major psychoactive ingredient is delta-9-tetrahydrocannabinol (THC). Of these 450 chemicals, there are approximately 23 psychoactive chemicals, THC being the most abundant. The highest concentration of THC is found in the bud of the female plant (hashish). The concentration of THC varies according to growing conditions and the part of the plant but has increased from approximately 2% to 3% in marijuana sold in the 1950s to approximately 40% sold on the streets today. Marijuana can be smoked in cigarettes (joints), pipes, water pipes (bongs), or baked in brownies, cakes, etc, and then ingested. However, smoking marijuana is more efficient and the "high" has a quicker onset. Marijuana is a Schedule I drug but has been promoted as medicinal for the treatment of glaucoma, for increasing appetite in patients who have HIV disease, to prevent the nausea associated with cancer chemotherapy, and as an analgesic for chronic pain. In response to this request, the FDA approved dronabinol (Marinol®), a synthetic THC, and placed this drug in Schedule III to be prescribed by physicians for the indicated medical conditions. The synthetic THC does not produce a "high" and in fact is not well absorbed from the gastrointestinal tract.

An individual under the influence of marijuana may exhibit no signs or symptoms of intoxication. The pharmacologic effects are dose-dependent and depend to a large extent on the set and setting of the intoxicated individual. As the dose of THC increases, the person experiences euphoria or a state of well-being, often referred to as "mellowing out". Everything becomes comical, problems disappear, and their appetite for snack foods increases. This is called the "munchies". Additionally, marijuana produces time and spatial distortion, which contribute, as the dose increases, to a dysphoria characterized by paranoia and fear. Although there has never been a death reported from marijuana overdose, certainly the higher doses may produce such bizarre circumstances as to increase the chances of accidental death. THC is fat soluble. Daily consumption of marijuana will result in THC being stored in body fat which will result in detectable amounts of THC being found in the urine for as long as 60 days in some cases.

Because of anxiety associated with dental visits, marijuana would be the most likely drug, after alcohol, to be used when coming to the dental office. But, unlike alcohol, marijuana may not produce any detectable odor on the breath nor signs of intoxication. Fortunately, local anesthetics, analgesics, and antibiotics used by the general dentist do not interact with marijuana. The major concern with the marijuana-intoxicated patient, similar to the alcohol-intoxicated patient, is a failure to follow directions while in the chair, and the inability to follow postoperative instructions.

Signs and Symptoms of Marijuana Use	
Blood shot eyes	Odor on breath and clothes
Lethargic, slow to respond	Inability to respond to commands
Slurred speech	Memory impairment

OPIATES

The opiates are most often called narcotics. The word "narcosis" means sleep. These drugs are referred to on the street as "downers", the most common being heroin. Heroin is the diacetyl derivative of morphine which is extracted from opium. Although commercial production of morphine involves extraction from the dried opium plant which grows in many parts of the world, some areas still harvest opium by making slits in the unripened seed pod. The pod secretes a white, viscous material which upon contact with the air turns a blackish-brown color. It is this off-white material that is called opium. The opium is then dried and smoked or processed to yield morphine and codeine. Actually, the raw opium contains several chemicals that are used medicinally or commercially. Much (approximately 50%) of morphine is converted chemically into heroin which finds its way into the United States and then on the street. Heroin is a Schedule I drug and has no acceptable use in the United States today. In fact, possession is a violation of the Controlled Substances Act of 1970. The majority of the heroin found on the streets in the United States is from Colombia, South America (65%) and can be as pure as 50% to 60%.

The heroin user goes through many phases once the drug has been administered. When administered intravenously, the user initially feels a "rush" often described as an "orgasmic rush". This initial feeling is most likely due to the release of histamine resulting in cutaneous vasodilation, itching, and a flushed appearance. Shortly after this "rush" the user becomes euphoric. This euphoric stage often called "stoned" or being "high" lasts approximately 3-4 hours. During this stage, the user is lethargic, slow to react to stimuli, speech is slurred, pain reaction threshold is elevated, exhibits xerostomia, experiences slowed heart rate, and his/hers pupils may be constricted. Following the "high", the abuser is "straight" for about 2 hours, with no tell-tale signs of abuse. Approximately 6-8 hours following the last injection of heroin, the user begins to experience a runny nose, lacrimation, and abdominal muscle cramps as the withdrawal from the drug begins. During this stage and the one that follows, the person may become agitated as he/she develops anxiety about where the next "hit" will come from. The withdrawal signs and symptoms become more intense. For the next 3 days, the abuser begins to sweat profusely in combination with cutaneous vasoconstriction. The skin becomes cold and clammy, hence the term "cold turkey". Tachycardia, pupillary dilation, diarrhea, and salivation occur for 3 days following the last injection. Withdrawal signs and symptoms may last longer than the average of 3 days or they may be more abrupt.

Many patients who have been abusing opiates will exhibit multiple carious lesions, particularly class V lesions. This increased caries rate is probably a result of the heroin-induced xerostomia, high intake of sweets, and lack of daily oral hygiene. Patients who are recovering from heroin or any opiate addiction should not be given any kind of opiate analgesic, whether it is for sedation or as a postoperative analgesic because of the increased chance of relapse. Nonsteroidal anti-inflammatory drugs (NSAIDs) should be used to control any postoperative discomfort. Patients who admit to a past history of intravenous heroin use, or any intravenous drug for that matter, are at higher risk for subacute bacterial endocarditis (SBE), HIV disease, and hepatitis, with the exception of postoperative analgesia should present no special problem for dental care.

Signs and Symptoms of Narcotic Use	
Pin point pupils	Glazed eyes
Lethargic, slow to respond	Inability to respond to commands
Slurred speech	Xerostomia

METHAMPHETAMINE

Methamphetamine has been available clinically for 45 years as a medication to curb appetite. Today it is one of the most widely abused drugs on the street. Methamphetamine can be smoked in the form of "ice", snorted, injected, or consumed orally. The onset of action varies with the route of administration, smoking providing the most rapid onset of action. Clandestine methamphetamine is usually synthesized from pseudoephedrine or ephedrine. The methamphetamine molecule can exist in either the "D" isomer or the "L" isomer. The latter isomer has its greatest effect on the cardiovascular system and, in fact, is available commercially over-the-counter as a nasal decongestant. The "D" isomer has its principle effects on the central nervous system as a stimulant (upper) and can not be converted from the "L" form. It is a sympathomimetic and as such raises blood pressure. This effect on the autonomic nervous system results in increased basal metabolic rate (BMR) and increased body temperature resulting in the "sweats". Methamphetamine users crave sweets possibly as a source of energy to fuel the increased BMR. As a consequence of the increased sweating the individual becomes dehydrated and thirsty. The sympathetic stimulation produces a thick, ropey saliva. This lack of saliva, increased consumption of sweets in the form of soda pop, and lack of routine dental care no doubt is the primary cause of "meth mouth". Initially the meth user experiences a feeling of exhileration, alertness, and incredible energy. With successive uses, tolerance occurs

MANAGEMENT OF THE CHEMICALLY DEPENDENT PATIENT
(Continued)

and the user abuses increasing amounts of methamphetamine looking for the same high they experienced on the first time. They never quite attain it. This has been referred to on the street as "chasing the monkey". As a substitute, the user continues their high for several hours or days in some cases. This is called bingeing. A binge may last for 5 or 6 days. The user becomes very paranoid, develops psychotic episodes, and has the potential of becoming violent. Sterotypical behavior develops such as rocking back and forth in a chair, picking their fingernails, or other behavior. During this stage the user begins "tweaking", using small amounts to stay high, and begins to hallucinate. Characteristically, they will describe the feeling that bugs are crawling under their skin and they scratch their arms, face, and any other exposed part of their body. The street term for this hallucination is called "coke bugs". Usually, the user will collapse from the physical exhaustion. Withdrawal can take weeks after the last use. As mentioned above, vasoconstrictor is contraindicated if there has been methamphetamine use within the last 24 hours.

Methamphetamine Signs and Symptoms in the Dental Office	
Dilated pupils	Jittery, irritable behavior
Rapid speech	Unable to sit still, twitching
Tremendous anxiety	Difficult to anesthetize

BENZODIAZEPINES AND OTHER NONALCOHOL SEDATIVES

These drugs are used mainly for treatment of anxiety disorders and, in some instances, insomnia. These drugs are commonly abused, either by themselves or as adjunct to the opiates. They have the ability to produce a strong physical dependency on the use of the medication. As tolerance builds up to the drug, the physical dependency increases dramatically. Unlike street drugs, where addiction is a primary consideration, the overuse of benzodiazepine lies in their ability to induce physical dependency. When these drugs are taken for several weeks, there is relatively little tolerance induced. However, after several months, the proportion of patients who become tolerant increases and reducing the dose or stopping the medication produces severe withdrawal symptoms often resulting in death.

It is extremely difficult for the physician to distinguish between the withdrawal symptoms and the reappearance of the myriad anxiety symptoms that cause the drug to be prescribed initially. Many patients increase their dose over time because tolerance develops to at least the sedative effects of the drug. The antianxiety benefits of the benzodiazepines continue to occur long after tolerance to the sedating effects. Patients often take these drugs for many years with relatively few ill effects other than the risk of withdrawal. The dentist should be keenly aware of the signs and symptoms and the historical pattern in patients taking benzodiazepines.

NICOTINE

Cigarette (nicotine) addiction is influenced by multiple variables. Nicotine itself produces reinforcement; users compare nicotine to stimulants such as cocaine or amphetamine, although its effects are of lower magnitude.

Nicotine is absorbed readily through the skin, mucous membranes, and of course, through the lungs. The pulmonary route produces discernible central nervous system effects in as little as 7 seconds. Thus, each puff produces some discrete reinforcement. With 10 puffs per cigarette, the 1 pack per day smoker reinforces the habit 200 times daily. The timing, setting, situation, and preparation all become associated repetitively with the effects of nicotine.

Nicotine has both stimulant and depressant actions. The smoker feels alert, yet there is some muscle relaxation. Nicotine activates the nucleus accumbens reward system in the brain. Increased extracellular dopamine has been found in this region after nicotine injections in rats. Nicotine affects other systems as well, including the release of endogenous opioids and glucocorticoids.

Nicotine Withdrawal Syndrome Signs and Symptoms	
Irritability, impatience, hostility	Restlessness
Anxiety	Decreased heart rate
Dysphoric or depressed mood	Increased appetite or weight gain
Difficulty concentrating	

SMOKING CESSATION PRODUCTS

Several years ago, the journal, *Science*, stated that approximately 80% of smokers say they want to quit, but each year <1 in 10 actually succeed. Nicotine transdermal delivery preparations (or nicotine patches) were approved by the U.S. Food and Drug Administration in 1992 as aids to smoking cessation for the relief of nicotine withdrawal symptoms. Four preparations were approved simultaneously: Habitrol®, Nicoderm®, Nicotrol®, and ProStep®. These products differ in how much nicotine is released and whether they provide a 24- or 16-hour release time.

Studies are still being reported on the effectiveness of nicotine patches on tobacco cessation. Most previous studies had good entry criteria including definition of the Fagerstrom score. Dr Fred Cowan of Oregon Health Sciences University described these Fagerstrom criteria in a previous report on nicotine substitutes in AGD *Impact*. Abstinence of smoking cessation has usually been assessed by self-report, measurement of carbon monoxide in breath, and plasma or urine nicotine products.

In numerous protocols, percentages of study subjects who abstained from smoking after 3-10 weeks of patch treatment with nicotine compared to placebo, have never exceeded 40%. After the initial assessment, six studies continued to follow the study subjects through 24-52 weeks of patch treatment. The results were even poorer with <25% sustained success. A review of these and additional studies, reveals some general conclusions regarding the effectiveness of nicotine patches in tobacco cessation. In every study, many smokers abstained after treatment with placebo patches; nicotine treatment was initially more effective than placebo; and improved abstinence rates were more marked in the short term (10 weeks) than in the long term (52 weeks). Subjects undergoing tobacco cessation trials tended to gain weight irrespective of whether placebo or nicotine patches were worn. Patients often favor the nicotine polacrilex gum (Nicorette®) which releases nicotine into the blood stream via the oral mucosa.

Data are now available from tobacco cessation studies carried out in general medical practices. The effectiveness of nicotine patch substitution under these conditions is similar to the results described previous. Most patch systems and gum are now available as over-the-counter products; only Habitrol® remains prescription. Buproprion (Zyban®) is another approach to the treatment of tobacco cessation. This drug is a norepinephrine/serotonin/dopamine reuptake inhibitor and its action directly affects the craving for tobacco. Another new product just introduced is varenicline (Chantix®). This product targets certain nicotine receptors to prevent nicotine access and diminishes the mesolimbic dopamine reward associated with nicotine use. The reader is referred to more comprehensive information about these products and the treatment of tobacco cessation. In addition, the reader should familiarize themselves with the supportive ADA posture on the role of the dental team in tobacco cessation treatment.

COCAINE

Cocaine, referred to on the street as "snow", "nose candy", "girl", and many other euphemisms, has created an epidemic. This drug is like no other local anesthetic. Known for about the last 2000 years, cocaine has been used and abused by politicians, scientists, farmers, warriors, and of course, on the street. Cocaine is derived from the leaves of a plant called *Erythroxylon coca* which grows in South America. Ninety percent of the world's supply of cocaine originates in Peru, Bolivia, and Colombia. At last estimate, the United States consumes 75% of the world's supply. The plant grows to a height of approximately 4 feet and produces a red berry. Farmers go through the fields stripping the leaves from the plant three times a year. During the working day, the farmers chew the coca leaves to suppress appetite and fight the fatigue of working the fields. The leaves are transported to a laboratory site where the cocaine is extracted by a process called maceration. It takes approximately 7-8 pounds of leaves to produce 1 ounce of cocaine.

On the streets of the United States, cocaine can be found in two forms – one is the hydrochloride salt which can be "snorted" or dissolved in water and injected intravenously, the other is the free base form which can be smoked and is sometimes referred to as "crack", "rock", or "free base". It is called crack because it cracks or pops when large pieces are smoked. It is called rock because it is hard and difficult to break into smaller pieces. The most popular method of administration of cocaine is "snorting" in which small amounts of cocaine hydrochloride are divided into segments or "lines" and any straw-like device can be used to inhale one or more lines of the cocaine into the nose. Although cocaine does not reach the lungs, enough cocaine is absorbed through nasal mucosa to provide a "high" within 3-5 minutes. Rock or crack, on the other hand, is heated and inhaled from any device available. This form of cocaine does reach the lungs and provides a much faster onset of action as well as a more intense stimulation. There are dangers to the user with any form of cocaine. Undoubtedly, the most dangerous form is the intravenous route.

MANAGEMENT OF THE CHEMICALLY DEPENDENT PATIENT
(Continued)

Signs and Symptoms of Cocaine Use	
Dilated pupils	Tremors
Jitteriness	Talkative
Irritability	Increased blood pressure

The cocaine user, regardless of how the cocaine was administered, presents a potential life-threatening situation in the dental operatory. The patient under the influence of cocaine could be compared to a car going 100 miles per hour. Blood pressure is elevated and heart rate is likely increased. Use of a local anesthetic with epinephrine in such a patient may result in a medical emergency. Such patients can be identified by jitteriness, irritability, talkativeness, tremors, and short abrupt speech patterns. These same signs and symptoms may also be seen in a normal dental patient with preoperative dental anxiety; therefore, the dentist must be particularly alert to identify the potential cocaine abuser. If a patient is suspected, they should never be given a local anesthetic with vasoconstrictor for fear of exacerbating cocaine-induced sympathetic response. Life-threatening episodes of cardiac arrhythmias and hypertensive crises have been reported when local anesthetic with vasoconstrictor was administered to a patient under the influence of cocaine. No local anesthetic used by any dentist can interfere with, nor test positive for cocaine in any urine testing screen. Therefore, the dentist need not be concerned with any false drug use accusations associated with dental anesthesia.

CLUB DRUGS

Perceptual distortions that include hallucinations, illusions, and disorders of thinking such as paranoia can be produced by toxic doses of many drugs. These phenomena also may be seen during toxic withdrawal from sedatives such as alcohol. There are, however, certain drugs that have as their primary effect the production of perception, thought, or mood disturbances at low doses with minimal effects on memory and orientation. These are commonly called *hallucinogenic drugs*, but their use does not always result in frank hallucinations.

Ecstasy (MDMA) and Phenylethylamines (MDA): MDA and MDMA have stimulant, as well as, psychedelic effects and produce degeneration of serotonergic nerve cells and axons. While nerve degeneration has not been well-demonstrated in human beings, the potential remains. Thus, there is possible neurotoxicity with overuse of these drugs. Ecstasy became popular during the 1980s on college campuses and it is still recommended by some psychotherapists as an aid to the process of therapy, although very little controlled data is available. Acute effects are dose-dependent and include dry mouth, jaw clinching, muscle aches, and tachycardia. At higher doses, effects include agitation, hyperthermia, panic attacks, and visual hallucinations. Frequent, repeated use of psychedelic drugs is unusual and, therefore, tolerance is not commonly seen. However, tolerance does develop to the behavioral effects of various psychedelic drugs, and after numerous doses, the tendency towards behavioral tolerance can be observed.

Lysergic Acid Diethylamide (LSD): LSD is the most potent hallucinogenic drug and produces significant psychedelic effects with a total dose of as little as 25-50 mcg. This drug is over 3000 times more potent than mescaline. It is sold on the illicit market in a variety of forms, as a tablet, capsule, sugar cube, or on blotting paper, a popular contemporary system involving postage stamp-sized papers impregnated with varying doses of LSD (50-300 mcg). A majority of street samples sold as LSD actually do contain LSD, while mushrooms and other botanicals sold as sources of psilocybin and other psychedelics have a low probability of containing the advertised hallucinogenics. Adverse effects which may affect treatment include visual and auditory hallucinations, tachycardia, psychosis, fear, tremors, delirium, hyperglycemia, fever, sweating, flushing, euphoria, hypertonia, nausea, vomiting, coma, seizures, tachypnea, and respiratory arrest.

INHALANTS

Anesthetic gases such as nitrous oxide or halothane are sometimes used as intoxicants by medical personnel. Nitrous oxide also is abused by food service employees because it is supplied for use as a propellant in disposable aluminum minitanks for whipping cream canisters. Nitrous oxide produces euphoria and analgesia and then loss of consciousness. Compulsive use and chronic toxicity rarely are reported, but there are obvious risks of overdose associated with the abuse of this anesthetic. Chronic use has been reported to cause peripheral neuropathy. Glue, correction fluid, gasoline, aerosol key board cleaners, model paint, in fact, any volatile substance has the potential to cause a "high" and like all of the above can become very addictive and deadly.

The dental team should be alert to the signs and symptoms of drug abuse and withdrawal. Further reading is recommended.

ORAL MEDICINE TOPICS

PART II:

DENTAL MANAGEMENT AND THERAPEUTIC CONSIDERATIONS IN PATIENTS WITH SPECIFIC ORAL CONDITIONS AND OTHER MEDICINE TOPICS

This second part of the chapter focuses on therapies the dentist may choose to prescribe for patients suffering from oral disease or who are in need of special care. Some overlap between these sections has resulted from systemic conditions that have oral manifestations and vice-versa. Cross-references to the descriptions and the monographs for individual drugs described elsewhere in this handbook allow for easy retrieval of information. Example prescriptions of selected drug therapies for each condition are presented so that the clinician can evaluate alternate approaches to treatment, since there is seldom a single drug of choice.

Drug prescriptions shown represent prototype drugs and popular prescriptions and are examples only. The pharmacologic category index is available for cross-referencing if alternatives and additional drugs are sought.

TABLE OF CONTENTS

ORAL PAIN

PAIN PREVENTION

For the dental patient, the prevention of pain aids in relieving anxiety and reduces the probability of stress during dental care. For the practitioner, dental procedures can be accomplished more efficiently in a "painless" situation. Appropriate selection and use of local anesthetics is one of the foundations for success in this arena. Local anesthetics listed below include drugs for the most commonly confronted dental procedures. Ester anesthetics are no longer available in dose form for dental injections, and historically had a higher incidence of allergic manifestations due to the formation of the metabolic byproduct, para-aminobenzoic acid. Articaine, which has an ester side chain, is rapidly metabolized to a non-PABA acid and, hence, functions as an amide and has a low allergic potential. The amides, in general, have an almost negligible allergic rate, and only one well-documented case of amide allergy has been reported by Seng, et al. Although injectable diphenhydramine (Benadryl®) has been used in an attempt to provide anesthesia in patients allergic to all the local anesthetics, it is no longer recommended in this context. The vehicle for injectable diphenhydramine can cause tissue necrosis.

The potential interaction between acetaminophen and warfarin has been recently raised in the literature. The cytochrome P450 system of drug metabolism for these vitamin K dependent metabolic pathways has raised the possibility that prolonged use of acetaminophen may inadvertently enhance, to dangerous levels, the anticoagulation effect of warfarin. As monitored by the INR, the effects of these drugs may be one and one-half to two times greater than as expected from the warfarin dosage alone. This potential interaction could be of importance in selecting an analgesic/antipyretic drug for the dental patient.

LOCAL ANESTHETICS

Articaine and Epinephrine [U.S.] *on page 143*

Bupivacaine *on page 236*

Bupivacaine and Epinephrine *on page 237*

Chloroprocaine *on page 335*

Levobupivacaine *on page 961*

Lidocaine and Epinephrine *on page 977*

Lidocaine *on page 972*

Lidocaine (Transoral) *on page 984*

Mepivacaine Dental Anesthetic *on page 1044*

Mepivacaine and Levonordefrin *on page 1045*

Prilocaine *on page 1348*

Prilocaine and Epinephrine *on page 1350*

Ropivacaine *on page 1443*

Tetracaine *on page 1546*

The selection of a vasoconstrictor with the local anesthetic must be based on the length of the procedure to be performed, the patient's medical status (epinephrine is contraindicated in patients with uncontrolled hyperthyroidism), and the need for hemorrhage control. The following table lists some of the common drugs with their duration of action. Transoral patches with lidocaine are now available (DentiPatch®) and the new long-acting amide injectable, Ropivacaine (Naropin®) may be useful for postoperative pain management.

DENTAL ANESTHETICS
(Average Duration by Route)

Product	Infiltration	Inferior Alveolar Block
Articaine HCl 4% and epinephrine 1:100,000	60 minutes	~60 minutes
Articaine HCl 4% and epinephrine 1:200,000	40 minutes	50 minutes
Carbocaine® HCl 2% with Neo-Cobefrin® 1:20,000 (mepivacaine HCl and levonordefrin)	50 minutes	60-75 minutes
Citanest® Plain 4% (prilocaine)	20 minutes	2.5 hours
Citanest Forte® with Epinephrine 1:200,000 (prilocaine with epinephrine)	2.25 hours	3 hours
Lidocaine HCl 2% and epinephrine 1:100,000	60 minutes	90 minutes
Marcaine® HCl 0.5% with epinephrine 1:200,000 (bupivacaine and epinephrine)	60 minutes	5-7 hours

The use of articaine 4% with epinephrine 1:100,000 solution for mandibular blocks has been associated occasionally with paresthesia (*J Am Dent Assoc*, 2001, 132(2):177-85).

The use of preinjection topical anesthetics can assist in pain prevention (see also Viral Infections *on page 1806* and Ulcerative and Erosive Disorders *on page 1809*). It should be noted that the FDA recently warned healthcare professionals regarding potential risks associated with unsupervised patient cutaneous use of topical anesthetic products. Life-threatening adverse events such as arrhythmias, seizures, coma, and allowed or stopped breathing have been reported. Thus, healthcare professionals are advised to prescribe FDA-approved topical anesthetics in the lowest concentration consistent with pain relief goals. It is not known if oral mucosa misuse may pose the same risk factors.

Clinicians are also using a eutectic mixture of 2.5% lidocaine with 2.5% prilocaine in a periodontal gel form (Oraquix®) in adults who require localized anesthesia in periodontal pockets during scaling and/or root planing. However, the same mixture available as a skin patch (EMLA®) from Astra is not currently approved for oral use.

Benzocaine *on page 195*

Lidocaine *on page 972*

Lidocaine Transoral *on page 984*

Tetracaine *on page 1546*

PAIN MANAGEMENT

The patient with existing acute or chronic oral pain requires appropriate treatment and sensitivity on the part of the dentist, all for the purpose of achieving relief from the oral source of pain. Pain can be divided into mild, moderate, and severe levels and requires a subjective assessment by the dentist based on knowledge of the dental procedures to be performed, the presenting signs and symptoms of the patient, and the realization that most dental procedures are invasive often leading to pain once the patient has left the dental office. The practitioner must be aware that the treatment of the source of the pain is usually the best management. If infection is present, treatment of the infection will directly alleviate the patient's discomfort. However, a patient who is not in pain tends to heal better and it is wise to adequately cover the patient for any residual or recurrent discomfort suffered. Likewise, many of the procedures that the dentist performs have pain associated with them. Much of this pain occurs after leaving the dentist office due to an inflammatory process or a healing process that has been initiated. It is difficult to assign specific pain levels (mild, moderate, or severe) for specific procedures; however, the dentist should use his or her prescribing capacity judiciously so that overmedication is avoided.

The following categories of drugs and appropriate example prescriptions for each follow. These include management of mild pain with aspirin products, acetaminophen, and some of the nonsteroidal noninflammatory agents (eg, ibuprofen). Management of moderate pain includes codeine, Toradol®, Vicodin®, Vicodin ES®, Lorcet® 10/650, Opana®, and Motrin® in the 800 mg dosage. Severe pain may require treatment with Percodan®, Percocet®, or Demerol®. All prescription pain preparations should be closely monitored for efficacy and discontinued if the pain persists or requires a higher level formulation. Combination drugs such as the recently released Combunox™ containing 5 mg of oxycodone and 400 mg of ibuprofen have proven usefulness in acute moderately severe to severe pain management.

The chronic pain patient represents a particular challenge for the practitioner. Some additional drugs that may be useful in managing the patient with chronic pain of neuropathic origin are covered in the temporomandibular dysfunction section *on page 1822*. It is always incumbent on the practitioner to reevaluate the diagnosis, source of pain, and

ORAL PAIN *(Continued)*

treatment, whenever prolonged use of analgesics (narcotic or non-narcotic) is contemplated. Drugs such as Dilaudid® are not recommended for management of dental pain in most states.

Narcotic analgesics can be used on a short-term basis or intermittently in combination with non-narcotic therapy in the chronic pain patient. Judicious prescribing, monitoring, and maintenance by the practitioner are imperative, particularly whenever considering the use of a narcotic analgesic due to the abuse and addiction liabilities.

MILD PAIN

MODERATE / MODERATELY SEVERE PAIN

An additional class of NSAIDs has been approved and indicated in the treatment of arthritis, COX-2 inhibitors. Celecoxib (Celebrex®) has been approved for use in oral pain management.

The following is a guideline to use when prescribing codeine with either aspirin or acetaminophen (Tylenol®):

Codeine No. 2 = codeine 15 mg

Codeine No. 3 = codeine 30 mg

Codeine No. 4 = codeine 60 mg

Example: ASA No. 3 = aspirin 325 mg + codeine 30 mg

HYDROCODONE PRODUCTS

Available hydrocodone oral products are listed in the following table and are scheduled as C-III controlled substances, indicating that prescriptions may either be oral or written. Thus, the prescriber may call–in a prescription to the pharmacy for any of these hydrocodone products. All the formulations are combined with acetaminophen except for Vicoprofen®, which contains ibuprofen, and Lortab® ASA and Damason–P®, which all contain aspirin. Most of these brand name drugs are available generically and the pharmacist will dispense the generic equivalent if available, unless the prescriber indicates otherwise.

HYDROCODONE ANALGESIC COMBINATION ORAL PRODUCTS
(All Products DEA Schedule C-III)

Hydrocodone is available under numerous brand names with varying dosages and in combination with aspirin or ibuprofen.					
Hydrocodone Bitartrate	Acetaminophen (APAP[1])	Other	Brand Name	Generic Available	Form
2.5 mg	500 mg	–	Lortab® 2.5/500	Yes	Tablet
5 mg	400 mg	–	Zydone®	No	Tablet
5 mg	500 mg	–	Vicodin®; Dolagesic®; Hy-Phen®; Hydrocet®; Anexsia® 5/500; Lortab®5/500	Yes	Tablet
5 mg	500 mg	–	Polygesic®; Lorcet-HD®	Yes	Capsule
7.5 mg	400 mg	–	Zydone®	No	Tablet
7.5 mg	500 mg	–	Lortab® 7.5/500	Yes	Tablet
7.5 mg	650 mg	–	Anexsia® 7.5/650; Lorcet Plus®	Yes	Tablet
7.5 mg	750 mg	–	Vicodin ES®	Yes	Tablet
10 mg	400 mg	–	Zydone®	No	Tablet
10 mg	325 mg	–	Norco®	Yes	Tablet
10 mg	500 mg	–	Lortab® 10/500	Yes	Tablet
10 mg	650 mg	–	Lorcet®	Yes	Tablet
10 mg	660 mg	–	Vicodin HP®; Anexsia® 10/660	Yes	Tablet
10 mg	750 mg	–	Maxidone™	Yes	Tablet
7.5 mg/15 mL	500 mg/15 mL	–	Lortab® Elixir	Yes	Elixir
5 mg	–	Aspirin 500 mg	Lortab® ASA; Damason–P®	Yes	Tablet
7.5 mg	–	Ibuprofen 200 mg	Vicoprofen®	Yes	Tablet

[1]APAP is the common acronym for acetaminophen and is the abbreviation of the chemical name N-acetylparaminophenol.

The following are the usual adult doses of the hydrocodone oral products as listed by the most recent edition of the Drug Information for the Health Care Professional (USPDI).

1 or 2 tablets containing 2.5 mg of hydrocodone and 500 mg of acetaminophen every 4-6 hours; or

1 tablet containing 5 mg of hydrocodone and 500 mg acetaminophen every 4-6 hours as needed, with dosage being increased to 2 tablets every 6 hours, if necessary; or

1 capsule containing 5 mg of hydrocodone and 500 mg of acetaminophen every 4-6 hours as needed, with dosage being increased to 2 capsules every 6 hours if necessary; or

1 tablet containing 7.5 mg hydrocodone and 650 mg of acetaminophen every 4-6 hours as needed, with dosage being increased to 2 tablets every 6 hours if necessary; or

1 tablet containing 7.5 mg hydrocodone and 750 mg of acetaminophen every 4-6 hours as needed; or

1 tablet containing 10 mg of hydrocodone and 650 mg acetaminophen every 4-6 hours as needed.

For the elixir (Lortab®), the recommended dose is 1 tablespoonful every 4-6 hours when necessary for pain.

For the aspirin products (Lortab® ASA and Damason-P®), the recommended dose is 1 or 2 tablets every 4-6 hours as needed.

For the ibuprofen product (Vicoprofen®), the recommended dose is 1 or 2 tablets every 4-6 hours as needed. The manufacturer recommends that the maximum dose of Vicoprofen® should not exceed 5 tablets in 24 hours.

The usual adult prescribing limits for the combination hydrocodone-acetaminophen products is up to 40 mg of hydrocodone and up to 4000 mg (4 g) of acetaminophen in a 24-hour period.

ORAL PAIN *(Continued)*

SEVERE PAIN

Hydromorphone *on page 840*
Meperidine *on page 1038*
Oxycodone *on page 1225*
Oxycodone and Acetaminophen *on page 1228*
Oxycodone and Aspirin *on page 1231*
Oxycodone and Ibuprofen *on page 1233*

Oxycodone is available in a variety of dosages and combinations under numerous brand names.

SAMPLE PRESCRIPTIONS

Rx:

Ibuprofen 800 mg tablets
Disp: 16 tablets
Sig: Take 1 tablet 3 times/day as needed for pain

Note: For severe pain can be given up to 4 times/day. Also available as 600 mg tablets

Rx:

Lortab® 5 mg
Disp: 16 tablets
Sig: Take 1 or 2 tablets every 4 hours as needed for pain; not to exceed 8 tablets in 24 hours

Note: Restrictions: C-III; no refills
Ingredients: Hydrocodone 5 mg and acetaminophen 500 mg; available as generic equivalent

For additional sample prescriptions see Oral Pain *on page 1834*

BACTERIAL INFECTIONS

Dental infection can occur for any number of reasons, primarily involving pulpal and periodontal infections. Secondary infections of the soft tissues as well as sinus infections pose special treatment challenges. The drugs of choice in treating most oral infections have been selected because of their efficacy in providing adequate blood levels for delivery to the oral tissues and their proven usefulness in managing dental infections. Penicillin remains the primary drug for treatment of dental infections of pulpal origin. The management of soft tissue infections may require the use of additional drugs.

OROFACIAL INFECTIONS

The basis of all infections is the successful multiplication of a microbial pathogen on or within a host. The pathogen is usually defined as any microorganism that has the capacity to cause disease. If the pathogen is bacterial in nature, antibiotic therapy is often indicated.

DIFFERENTIAL DIAGNOSIS OF ODONTOGENIC INFECTIONS

In choosing the appropriate antibiotic for therapy of a given infection, a number of important factors must be considered. First, the identity of the organism must be known. In odontogenic infections involving dental or periodontal structures, this is seldom the case. Secondly, accurate information regarding antibiotic susceptibility is required. Again, unless the organism has been identified, this is not possible. And thirdly, host factors must be taken into account, in terms of ability to absorb an antibiotic, to achieve appropriate host response. When clinical evidence of cellulitis or odontogenic infection has been found and the cardinal signs of swelling, inflammation, pain, and perhaps fever are present, the selection by the clinician of the appropriate antibiotic agent may lead to eradication.

CAUSES OF ODONTOGENIC INFECTIONS

Most acute orofacial infections are of odontogenic origin. Dental caries, resulting in infection of dental pulp, is the leading cause of odontogenic infection.

The major causative organisms involved in dental caries have been identified as members of the viridans (alpha-hemolytic) streptococci and include *Streptococcus mutans, Streptococcus sobrinus,* and *Streptococcus milleri.* Once the bacteria have breached the enamel they invade the dentin and eventually the dental pulp. An inflammatory reaction occurs in the pulp tissue resulting in necrosis and a lower tissue oxidation-reduction potential. At this point, the bacterial flora changes from predominantly aerobic to a more obligate anaerobic flora. The anaerobic gram-positive cocci *(Peptostreptococcus* species), and the anaerobic gram-negative rods, including *Bacteroides, Prevotella, Porphyromonas,* and *Fusobacterium* are most frequently present. An abscess usually forms at the apex of the involved tooth resulting in destruction of bone. Depending on the effectiveness of the host resistance and the virulence of the bacteria, the infection may spread through the marrow spaces, perforate the cortical plate, and enter the surrounding soft tissues.

The other major source of odontogenic infection arises from the anaerobic bacterial flora that inhabits the periodontal and supporting structures of the teeth. The most important potential pathogenic anaerobes within these structures are *Actinobacillus actinomycetemcomitans, Prevotella intermedius, Porphyromonas gingivalis, Fusobacterium nucleatum,* and *Eikenella corrodens.*

Most odontogenic infections (70%) have mixed aerobic and anaerobic flora. Pure aerobic infections are much less common and comprise ~5% incidence. Pure anaerobic infections make up the remaining 25% of odontogenic infections. Clinical correlates suggest that early odontogenic infections are characterized by rapid spreading and cellulitis with the absence of abscess formation. The bacteria are predominantly aerobic with gram-positive, alpha-hemolytic streptococci *(S. viridans)* the predominant pathogen. As the infection matures and becomes more severe, the microbial flora becomes a mix of aerobes and anaerobes. The anaerobes present are determined by the characteristic flora associated with the site of origin, whether it is pulpal or periodontal. Finally, as the infectious process becomes controlled by host defenses, the flora becomes primarily anaerobic. For example, Lewis and MacFarlane found a predominance of facultative oral streptococci in the early infections (<3 days of symptoms) with the later predominance of obligate anaerobes.

In a review of severe odontogenic infections, it was reported that Brook, et al, observed that 50% of odontogenic deep facial space infections yielded anaerobic bacteria only. Also, 44% of these infections yielded a mix of aerobic and anaerobic flora. The results of a study published in 1998 by Sakamoto, et al, were also described in the review. The study confirmed that odontogenic infections usually result from a synergistic interaction among several bacterial species and usually consist of an oral streptococcus and an oral anaerobic gram-negative rod. Sakamoto and his group reported a high level of the

BACTERIAL INFECTIONS (Continued)

Streptococcus milleri group of aerobic gram-positive cocci, and high levels of oral anaerobes, including the *Peptostreptococcus* species and the *Prevotella, Porphyromonas,* and *Fusobacterium* species.

Oral streptococci, especially of the *Streptococcus milleri* group, can invade soft tissues initially, thus preparing an environment conducive to growth of anaerobic bacteria. Obligate oral anaerobes are dependent on nutrients synthesized by the aerobes. Thus the anaerobes appear approximately 3 days after onset of symptoms. Early infections are thus caused primarily by the aerobic streptococci (exquisitely sensitive to penicillin) and late infections are caused by the anaerobes (frequently resistant to penicillin).

It appears logical, as Flynn has noted, to separate infections presenting early in their course from those presenting later when selecting empiric antibiotics of choice for odontogenic infections.

If the patient is not allergic to penicillin, penicillin VK still remains the empiric antibiotic of first choice to treat mild or early odontogenic infections (see Table 1). In patients allergic to penicillin, clindamycin clearly remains the alternative antibiotic for treatment of mild or early infections. Secondary alternative antibiotics still recognized as useful in these conditions are cephalexin (Keflex®), or other first generation cephalosporins available in oral dose forms. The first generation cephalosporins can be used in both penicillin-allergic and nonallergic patients, providing that the penicillin allergy is not the anaphylactoid type.

PENICILLIN VK

The spectrum of antibacterial action of penicillin VK is consistent with most of the organisms identified in odontogenic infections (see Table 2). Penicillin VK is a beta-lactam antibiotic, as are all the penicillins and cephalosporins, and is bactericidal against gram-positive cocci and the major pathogens of mixed anaerobic infections. It elicits virtually no adverse effects in the absence of allergy and is relatively low in cost. Adverse drug reactions occurring in >10% of patients include mild diarrhea, nausea, and oral candidiasis. To treat odontogenic infections and other orofacial infections, the usual dose for adults and children >12 years of age is 500 mg every 6 hours for at least 7 days (see Table 4). The daily dose for children ≤12 years of age is 25-50 mg/kg of body weight in divided doses every 6-8 hours (see Table 4). The patient must be instructed to take the penicillin continuously for the duration of therapy.

After oral dosing, penicillin VK achieves peak serum levels within 1 hour. Penicillin VK may be given with meals, however, blood concentrations may be slightly higher when penicillin is given on an empty stomach. The preferred dosing is 1 hour before meals or 2 hours after meals to ensure maximum serum levels. Penicillin VK diffuses into most body tissues, including oral tissues, soon after dosing. Hepatic metabolism accounts for <30% of the elimination of penicillins. Elimination is primarily renal. The nonmetabolized penicillin is excreted largely unchanged in the urine by glomerular filtration and active tubular secretion. Penicillins cross the placenta and are distributed in breast milk. Penicillin VK, like all beta-lactam antibiotics, causes death of bacteria by inhibiting synthesis of the bacterial cell wall during cell division. This action is dependent on the ability of penicillins to reach and bind to penicillin-binding proteins (PBPs) located on the inner membrane of the bacterial cell wall. PBPs (which include transpeptidases, carboxypeptidases, and endopeptidases) are enzymes that are involved in the terminal stages of assembling and reshaping the bacterial cell wall during growth. Penicillins and beta-lactams bind to and inactivate PBPs resulting in lysis of the cell due to weakening of the cell wall.

Penicillin VK is considered a "narrow spectrum" antibiotic. This class of antibiotics produces less alteration of normal microflora thereby reducing the incidence of superinfection. Also, its bactericidal action will reduce the numbers of microorganisms resulting in less reliance on host-phagocyte mechanisms for eradication of the pathogen.

Among patients, 0.7% to 10% are allergic to penicillins. There is no evidence that any single penicillin derivative differs from others in terms of incidence or severity when administered orally. About 85% of allergic reactions associated with penicillin VK are delayed and take >2 days to develop. This allergic response manifests as skin rashes characterized as erythema and bullous eruptions. This type of allergic reaction is mild, reversible, and usually responds to concurrent antihistamine therapy, such as diphenhydramine (Benadryl®). Severe reactions of angioedema have occurred, characterized by marked swelling of the lips, tongue, face, and periorbital tissues. Patients with a history of penicillin allergy must never be given penicillin VK for treatment of infections. The alternative antibiotic is clindamycin. If the allergy is the delayed type and not the anaphylactoid type, a first generation cephalosporin may be used as an alternate antibiotic.

CLINDAMYCIN

In the event of penicillin allergy, clindamycin is clearly an alternative of choice in treating mild or early odontogenic infections (see Table 1). It is highly effective against almost all oral pathogens. Clindamycin is active against most aerobic gram-positive cocci, including staphylococci, *S. pneumoniae*, other streptococci, and anaerobic gram-negative and gram-positive organisms, including *Bacteroides* sp (see Table 3). Clindamycin is not effective against mycoplasma or gram-negative aerobes. It inhibits protein synthesis in bacteria through binding to the 50 S subunit of bacterial ribosomes. Clindamycin has bacteriostatic actions at low concentrations, but is known to elicit bactericidal effects against susceptible bacteria at higher concentrations of drug at the site of infection.

The usual adult oral dose of clindamycin to treat orofacial infections of odontogenic origin is 150-450 mg every 6 hours for 7-10 days. The usual daily oral dose for children is 8-25 mg/kg in 3-4 equally divided doses (see Table 4).

Following oral administration of a 150 mg or a 300 mg dose on an empty stomach, 90% of the dose is rapidly absorbed into the bloodstream and peak serum concentrations are attained in 45-60 minutes. Administration with food does not markedly impair absorption into the bloodstream. Clindamycin serum levels exceed the minimum inhibitory concentration for bacterial growth for at least 6 hours after the recommended doses. The serum half-life is 2-3 hours. Clindamycin is distributed effectively to most body tissues, including saliva and bone. Its small molecular weight enables it to more readily enter bacterial cytoplasm and to penetrate bone. It is partially metabolized in the liver to active and inactive metabolites and is excreted in the urine, bile, and feces.

Adverse effects caused by clindamycin can include abdominal pain, nausea, vomiting, and diarrhea. Hypersensitivity reactions are rare, but have resulted in skin rash. Approximately 1% of clindamycin users develop pseudomembranous colitis characterized by severe diarrhea, abdominal cramps, and excretion of blood or mucus in the stools. The mechanism is disruption of normal bacterial flora of the colon, which leads to colonization of the bacterium *Clostridium difficile*. This bacterium releases endotoxins that cause mucosal damage and inflammation. Symptoms usually develop 2-9 days after initiation of therapy, but may not occur until several weeks after taking the drug. If significant diarrhea develops, clindamycin therapy should be discontinued immediately. Theoretically, any antibiotic can cause antibiotic-associated colitis and clindamycin probably has an undeserved reputation associated with this condition.

Sandor, et al, also notes that odontogenic infections are typically polymicrobial and that anaerobes outnumber aerobes by at least four-fold. The penicillins have historically been used as the first-line therapy in these cases, but increasing rates of resistance have lowered their usefulness. Bacterial resistance to penicillins is predominantly achieved through production of beta-lactamases. Clindamycin, because of its relatively broad spectrum of activity and resistance to beta-lactamase degradation, is an attractive first-line therapy in treatment of odontogenic infections. Recently, researchers have established a causal link between exposure to antibiotics and antibiotic resistance and they also have established evidence that the development of resistance to one class of antibiotic may confer persistent increased resistance to other antibiotic classes.

FIRST GENERATION CEPHALOSPORINS

Antibiotics of this class, which are available in oral dosage forms, include cefadroxil (Duricef®), cephalexin (Keflex®), and cephradine (Velosef®). The first generation cephalosporins are alternates to penicillin VK in the treatment of odontogenic infections based on bactericidal effectiveness against the oral streptococci. These drugs are most active against gram-positive cocci, but are not very active against many anaerobes. First generation cephalosporins are indicated as alternatives in early infections because they are effective in killing the aerobes. First generation cephalosporins are active against gram-positive staphylococci and streptococci, but not enterococci. They are active against many gram-negative aerobic bacilli, including *E. coli*, *Klebsiella*, and *Proteus mirabilis*. They are inactive against methicillin-resistant *S. aureus* and penicillin-resistant *S. pneumoniae*. The gram-negative aerobic cocci, *Moraxella catarrhalis*, portrays variable sensitivity to first generation cephalosporins.

Cephalexin (Keflex®) is the first generation cephalosporin often used to treat odontogenic infections. The usual adult dose is 250-1000 mg every 6 hours with a maximum of 4 g/day. Children's dose is 25-50 mg/kg/day in divided doses every 6 hours; for severe infections: 50-100 mg/kg/day in divided doses every 6 hours with a maximum dose of 3 g/day (see Table 4).

Cephalexin (Keflex®) causes diarrhea in about 1% to 10% of patients. About 90% of the cephalexin is excreted unchanged in urine.

BACTERIAL INFECTIONS *(Continued)*

SECOND GENERATION CEPHALOSPORINS

The second generation cephalosporins such as cefaclor (Ceclor®) have better activity against some of the anaerobes including some *Bacteroides, Peptococcus,* and *Peptostreptococcus* species. Cefaclor (Ceclor®) and cefuroxime (Ceftin®) have been used to treat early stage infections. These antibiotics have the advantage of twice-a-day dosing. The usual oral adult dose of cefaclor is 250-500 mg every 8 hours (or daily dose can be given in 2 divided doses) for at least 7 days. Children's dose is 20-40 mg/kg/day divided every 8-12 hours with a maximum dose of 2 g/day. The usual adult oral dose of cefuroxime is 250-500 mg twice daily. Children's dose is 20 mg/kg/day (maximum 500 mg/day) in 2 divided doses.

The cephalosporins inhibit bacterial cell wall synthesis by binding to one or more of the penicillin-binding proteins (PBPs), which in turn inhibit the final transpeptidation step of peptidoglycan synthesis in bacterial cell walls, thus inhibiting cell wall biosynthesis. Bacteria eventually lyse due to ongoing activity of cell wall autolytic enzymes while cell wall assembly is arrested.

BACTERIAL RESISTANCE TO ANTIBIOTICS

If a patient with an early stage odontogenic infection does not respond to penicillin VK within 24-36 hours, it is evidence of the presence of resistant bacteria. Bacterial resistance to the penicillins is predominantly achieved through the production of beta-lactamase. A switch to beta-lactamase-stable antibiotics should be made. For example, Kuriyama, et al, reported that past beta-lactam administration increases the emergence of beta-lactamase-producing bacteria and that beta-lactamase-stable antibiotics should be prescribed to patients with unresolved infections who have received beta-lactams. These include either clindamycin or amoxicillin/clavulanic acid (Augmentin®). Doses are listed in Table 4.

In the past, all *S. viridans* species were uniformly susceptible to beta-lactam antibiotics. However, over the years, there has been a significant increase in resistant strains. Resistance may also be due to alteration of penicillin-binding proteins. Consequently, drugs which combine a beta-lactam antibiotic with a beta-lactamase inhibitor, such as amoxicillin/clavulanic acid (Augmentin®), may no longer be more effective than the penicillin VK alone. In these situations, clindamycin is the recommended alternate antibiotic.

Evidence suggests that empirical use of penicillin VK as the first-line drug in treating early odontogenic infections is still the best way to ensure the minimal production of resistant bacteria to other classes of antibiotics, since any overuse of clindamycin or amoxicillin/clavulanic acid (Augmentin®) is minimized in these situations. There is concern that overuse of clindamycin could contribute to development of clindamycin-resistant pathogens.

In late odontogenic infections, it is suggested that clindamycin be considered the first-line antibiotic to treat these infections. The dose of clindamycin would be the same as that used to treat early infections (see Table 4). In these infections, anaerobic bacteria usually predominate. Since penicillin spectrum includes anaerobes, penicillin VK is also useful as an empiric drug of first choice in these infections. It has been reported, however, that the penicillin resistance rate among patients with serious and late infections is in the 35% to 50% range. Therefore, if penicillin is the drug of first choice and the patient does not respond within 24-36 hours, a resistant pathogen should be suspected and a switch to clindamycin be made. Clindamycin, because of its relatively broad spectrum of activity and resistance to beta-lactamase degradation, is an attractive first-line therapy in the treatment of these infections. Another alternative is to add a second drug to the penicillin (eg, metronidazole [Flagyl®]). Consequently, for those infections not responding to treatment with penicillin, the addition of a second drug (eg, metronidazole), not a beta-lactam or macrolide, is likely to be more effective. Bacterial resistance to metronidazole is very rare. The metronidazole dose is listed in Table 4.

Nonionized metronidazole is readily taken up by anaerobic organisms. Its selectivity for anaerobic bacteria is a result of the ability of these organisms to reduce metronidazole to its active form within the bacterial cell. The electron transport proteins necessary for this reaction are found only in anaerobic bacteria. Reduced metronidazole then disrupts DNA's helical structure, thereby inhibiting bacterial nucleic acid synthesis leading to death of the organism. Consequently, metronidazole is not effective against gram-positive aerobic cocci and most *Actinomyces, Lactobacillus,* and *Proprionibacterium* species. Since most odontogenic infections are mixed aerobic and anaerobic, metronidazole should rarely be used as a single agent. Alternatively, one can switch to a beta-lactamase resistant drug (eg, amoxicillin/clavulanic acid [Augmentin®]). The beta-lactamase resistant penicillins including methicillin, oxacillin, cloxacillin, dicloxacillin, and nafcillin, are only effective against gram-positive cocci and have no activity against anaerobes, hence, should not be used to treat the late stage odontogenic infections.

RESISTANCE IN ODONTOGENIC INFECTIONS

Recently, there has been an alarming increase in the incidence of resistant bacterial isolates in odontogenic infections. Many anaerobic bacteria have developed resistance to beta-lactam antibiotics via production of beta-lactamase enzymes. These include several species of *Prevotella, Porphyromonas, Fusobacterium nucleatum,* and *Campylobacter gracilus. Fusobacterium,* especially in combination with *S. viridans* species, has been associated with severe odontogenic infections. Often, they are resistant to macrolides. Clindamycin is the empiric drug of first choice in these patients.

SEVERE INFECTIONS

In patients hospitalized for severe odontogenic infections, I.V. antibiotics are indicated and clindamycin is the clear empiric drug of choice. Alternative antibiotics include an I.V. combination of penicillin and metronidazole or I.V. ampicillin-sulbactam (Unasyn®). Clindamycin, I.V. cephalosporins (if penicillin allergy is not the anaphylactoid type), and ciprofloxacin have been used in patients allergic to penicillins. Flynn notes that *Eikenella corrodens,* an occasional oral pathogen, is resistant to clindamycin. Ciprofloxacin is an excellent antibiotic for this organism.

ERYTHROMYCIN, CLARITHROMYCIN, AND AZITHROMYCIN

In the past, erythromycins were considered highly effective antibiotics for treating odontogenic infections, especially in penicillin allergy. At the present time, however, the current high resistance rates of both oral streptococci and oral anaerobes have rendered the entire macrolide family of antibiotics obsolete for odontogenic infections. Montgomery has noted that resistance develops rapidly to macrolides and there may be cross-resistance between erythromycin and newer macrolides, particularly among streptococci and staphylococci. Hardee has stated that erythromycin is no longer very useful because of resistant pathogens. The antibacterial spectrum of the erythromycin family is similar to penicillin VK. Erythromycins are effective against streptococcus, staphylococcus, and gram-negative aerobes, such as *H. influenzae, M. catarrhalis, N. gonorrhoeae, Bordetella pertussis,* and *Legionella pneumophilia.* Erythromycins are considered narrow spectrum antibiotics.

Both azithromycin and clarithromycin have been used to treat acute odontogenic infections. This is because of the following spectrum of actions: Clarithromycin shows good activity against many gram-positive and gram-negative aerobic and anaerobic organisms. It is active against methicillin-sensitive *S. aureus* and most streptococcus species. *S. aureus* strains resistant to erythromycin are resistant to clarithromycin. Clarithromycin is active against *H. influenzae.* It is similar to erythromycin in effectiveness against anaerobic gram-positive cocci and *Bacteroides* sp. Clarithromycin has been suggested as an alternative antibiotic if the prescriber wants to give an antibiotic from the macrolide family (see Table 3). The recommended oral adult dose is 500 mg twice daily for 7 days.

Azithromycin is active against staphylococci, including *S. aureus* and *S. epidermidis,* as well as streptococci, such as *S. pyogenes* and *S. pneumoniae.* Erythromycin-resistant strains of staphylococcus, enterococcus, and streptococcus, including methicillin-resistant *S. aureus,* are also resistant to azithromycin. It has excellent activity against *H. influenzae.* Inhibition of anaerobes, such as *Clostridium perfringens,* is better with azithromycin than with erythromycin. Inhibition of *Bacteroides fragilis* and other *bacteroides* species by azithromycin is comparable to erythromycin. Both azithromycin and clarithromycin are presently recommended as alternatives in the prophylactic regimen for prevention of bacterial endocarditis.

AMOXICILLIN

Some clinicians select amoxicillin over penicillin VK as the penicillin of choice to empirically treat odontogenic infections. Except for coverage of *Haemophilus influenzae* in acute sinus and otitis media infections, amoxicillin does not offer any advantage over penicillin VK for treatment of odontogenic infections. It is less effective than penicillin VK for aerobic gram-positive cocci, and similar to penicillin for coverage of anaerobes. Although it does provide coverage against gram-negative enteric bacteria, this is not needed to treat odontogenic infections, except in immunosuppressed patients where these organisms may be present. If one adheres to the principle of using the most effective narrow spectrum antibiotic, amoxicillin should not be favored over penicillin VK.

Note: The ADA Council on Scientific Affairs has published a review on the subject of antibiotic interaction with oral contraceptives in which a clear statement of the dental professional's responsibility was made. In essence, it was concluded that in any situation where a dentist is planning to prescribe a course of antibiotics, alternative/additional means of contraception should be recommended to the oral contraceptive users. Specifically, patients should be told about the potential for antibiotics to lower the usefulness of oral contraceptives and advised to consult their physician about nonhormonal contraceptive techniques while continuing their oral contraceptive regimen. Even though there is minimal scientific data supporting this position, the risk of possible unwanted pregnancies warrants this simple approach for professionals licensed to prescribe antibiotics (*JADA,* 2002, 133:880).

BACTERIAL INFECTIONS *(Continued)*

The following tables have been adapted from Wynn RL, Bergman SA, Meiller TF, et al. "Antibiotics in Treating Orofacial Infections of Odontogenic Origin," *Gen Dent*, 2001, 47(3):238-52.

Table 1.
EMPIRIC ANTIBIOTICS OF CHOICE FOR ODONTOGENIC INFECTIONS

Type of Infection	Antibiotic of Choice
Early (first 3 days of symptoms)	Penicillin VK, amoxicillin Clindamycin Cephalexin (or other first generation cephalosporin)[1]
No improvement in 24-36 hours	Beta-lactamase-stable antibiotic: Clindamycin or amoxicillin / clavulanic acid
Penicillin allergy	Clindamycin Cephalexin (if penicillin allergy is not anaphylactoid type) Clarithromycin (Biaxin®)[2]
Late (>3 days)	Clindamycin Penicillin VK-metronidazole, amoxicillin-metronidazole
Penicillin allergy	Clindamycin

[1]For better patient compliance, second generation cephalosporins (cefaclor; cefuroxime) at twice daily dosing have been used; see text.

[2]A macrolide useful in patients allergic to penicillin, given as twice daily dosing for better patient compliance; see text.

Table 2.
PENICILLIN VK: ANTIBACTERIAL SPECTRUM

Gram-Positive Cocci	Oral Anaerobes
Streptococci	*Bacteroides*
Nonresistant staphylococci[1]	*Porphyromonas*
Pneumococci	*Prevotella*
	Peptococci
Gram-Negative Cocci	Peptostreptococci
Neisseria meningitides	*Actinomyces*
Neisseria gonorrhoeae	*Veillonella*
	Eubacterium
Gram-Positive Rods	*Eikenella*
Bacillus	*Capnocytophaga*
Corynebacterium	*Campylobacter*
Clostridium	*Fusobacterium*
	Others

[1]Nonresistant staphylococcus represents a small portion of community-acquired strains of *S. aureus* (5% to 15%). Most strains of *S. aureus* and *S. epidermidis* produce beta-lactamases, which destroy penicillins.

Table 3.
CLINDAMYCIN: ANTIBACTERIAL SPECTRUM[1]

Gram-Positive Cocci	Anaerobes[2]
Streptococci[3]	**Gram-Negative Bacilli**
S. aureus[4]	*Bacteroides* species including *B. fragilis*
Penicillinase and nonpenicillinase-producing staphylococcus	*B. melaninogenicus* *Fusobacterium species*
S. epidermidis	**Gram-Positive Nonsporeforming Bacilli**
Pneumococci	*Propionibacterium*
	Eubacterium
	Actinomyces species
	Gram-Positive Cocci
	Peptococcus
	Peptostreptococcus
	Microaerophilic streptococci

[1]*In vitro* activity against isolates; information from manufacturer's package insert

[2]*Clostridia* are more resistant than most anaerobes to clindamycin. Most *Clostridium perfringens* are susceptible but *C. sporogens* and *C. tertium* are frequently resistant.

[3]Except *S. faecalis*

[4]Some staph strains originally resistant to erythromycin rapidly develop resistance to clindamycin.

Table 4.
ORAL DOSE RANGES OF ANTIBIOTICS USEFUL IN TREATING ODONTOGENIC INFECTIONS[1]

Clinicians must select specific dose and regimen from ranges available to be prescribed based on clinical judgment		
Antibiotic	**Dosage**	
	Children	**Adults**
Penicillin VK	≤12 years: 25-50 mg/kg body weight in equally divided doses q6-8h for at least 7 days; maximum dose: 3 g/day	>12 years: 500 mg q6h for at least 7 days
Clindamycin	8-25 mg/kg in 3-4 equally divided doses	150-450 mg q6h for at least 7 days; maximum dose: 1.8 g/day
Cephalexin (Keflex®)	25-50 mg/kg/d in divided doses q6h severe infection: 50-100 mg/kg/d in divided doses q6h; maximum dose: 3 g/24 h	250-1000 mg q6h; maximum dose: 4 g/day
Amoxicillin	<40 kg: 20-40 mg (amoxicillin)/kg/d in divided doses q8h >40 kg: 250-500 mg q8h or 875 mg q12h for at least 7 days; maximum dose 2 g/day	>40 kg: 250-500 mg q8h or 875 mg q12h for at least 7 days; maximum dose: 2 g/day
Amoxicillin/ clavulanic acid (Augmentin®)	<40 kg: 20-40 mg (amoxicillin)/kg/d in divided doses q8h >40 kg: 250-500 mg q8h or 875 mg q12h for at least 7 days; maximum dose 2 g/day	>40 kg: 250-500 mg q8h or 875 mg q12h for at least 7 days; maximum dose: 2 g/day
Metronidazole (Flagyl®)		500 mg q6-8h for 7-10 days; maximum dose: 4 g/day

[1]For doses of other antibiotics, see monographs

SAMPLE PRESCRIPTIONS

Rx:

Penicillin V potassium 500 mg
Disp: 40 tablets
Sig: Take 1 tablet 4 times/day for 7-10 days (consider a loading dose of 1 g for acute infection)

Rx:

Clindamycin 300 mg
Disp: 40 capsules
Sig: Take 1 capsule 4 times/day for 7-10 days

Note: Prescription for patients allergic to penicillin

Rx:

Amoxicillin 500 mg
Disp: 30 capsules or tablets
Sig: Take 1 capsule or tablet 3 times/day for 7-10 days

For additional sample prescriptions see Bacterial Infections and Periodontal Diseases *on page 1837*

BACTERIAL INFECTIONS *(Continued)*

SINUS INFECTION TREATMENT

Sinus infections represent a common condition which may present with confounding dental complaints. Treatment is sometimes instituted by the dentist, but due to the often chronic and recurrent nature of sinus infections, early involvement of an otolaryngologist is advised. These infections may require antibiotics of varying spectrum as well as requiring the management of sinus congestion. Although amoxicillin is usually adequate, many otolaryngologists initially prescribe Augmentin®. Second-generation cephalosporins and clarithromycin are sometimes used depending on the chronicity of the problem.

For examples of sample prescriptions see Sinus Infection Treatment *on page 1839*

FREQUENTLY ASKED QUESTIONS

What is the best antibiotic modality for treating dental infections?

Penicillin is still the drug of choice for treatment of infections in and around the oral cavity. Phenoxy-methyl penicillin (Pen VK) long has been the most commonly selected antibiotic. In penicillin-allergic individuals, clindamycin may be an appropriate consideration, prescribing 300 mg as a loading dose followed by 150 mg 4 times/day would be an appropriate regimen for a dental infection. In general, if there is no response to Pen VK, then Augmentin® may be a good alternative in the nonpenicillin-allergic patient because of its slightly altered spectrum. Recommendations would include that the patient should take the drug with food.

Is there cross-allergenicity between the cephalosporins and penicillin?

The incidence of cross-allergenicity is 5% to 8% in the overall population. If a patient has demonstrated a Type I hypersensitivity reaction to penicillin, namely urticaria or anaphylaxis, then this incidence would increase to 20%.

Is there definitely an interaction between contraception agents and antibiotics?

There are well founded interactions between contraceptives and antibiotics. The best instructions that a patient could be given by their dentist are that should an antibiotic be necessary and the dentist is aware that the patient is on contraceptives, and if the patient is using chemical contraceptives, the patient should seriously consider additional means of contraception during the antibiotic management.

Are antibiotics necessary in diabetic mellitus patients?

In the management of diabetes, control of the diabetic status is the key factor relative to all morbidity issues. If a patient is well controlled, then antibiotics will likely not be necessary. However, in patients where the control is questionable or where they have recently been given a different drug regimen for their diabetes or if they are being titrated to an appropriate level of either insulin or oral hypoglycemic agents during these periods of time, the dentist might consider preprocedural antibiotics to be efficacious.

Do nonsteroidal anti-inflammatory drugs interfere with blood pressure medication?

At the current time there is no clear evidence that NSAIDs interfere with any of the blood pressure medications that are currently in usage.

PERIODONTAL DISEASES

Periodontal diseases are common to mankind affecting, according to some epidemiologic studies, greater than 80% of the worldwide population. The conditions refer primarily to diseases that are caused by accumulations of dental plaque and the subsequent immune response of the host to the bacteria and toxins present in this plaque. Although most of the organisms that have been implicated in advanced periodontal diseases are anaerobic in nature, some aerobes contribute by either coaggregation with the anaerobic species or direct involvement with specific disease types.

Periodontal condition, as a group of diseases, affects the soft tissues supporting the teeth (ie, gingiva) leading to the term gingivitis or inflammation of gingival structures and those conditions that affect the bone and ligament supporting the teeth (ie, periodontitis) resulting from the infection and/or inflammation of these structures. Diseases of the periodontia can be further subdivided into various types including chronic periodontitis (localized and generalized, mainly in adults), aggressive periodontitis (localized and generalized, including previously classified), early onset periodontitis, prepubertal periodontitis, and rapidly progressing periodontitis. In addition, periodontitis as a manifestation of systemic diseases (hematologic, genetic disorders, not otherwise specified) as well as a necrotizing type due to specific conditions associated with predisposing immunodeficiency disease, such as those found in HIV-infected patients, create further subclassifications of the periodontal diseases, some of which are covered in those chapters associated with those conditions.

It is well accepted that control of most periodontal diseases requires, at the very minimum, appropriate mechanical cleansing of the dentition and the supporting structures by the patient. These efforts include brushing, some type of interdental cleaning, preferably with either floss or other aids, as well as appropriate sulcular cleaning usually with a brush.

Following appropriate dental treatment by the general dental practitioner and/or the periodontist, aids to these efforts by the patient might include the use of chemical agents to assist in the control of the periodontal diseases, or to prevent periodontal diseases. There are many available chemical agents on the market, only some of which are approved by the American Dental Association. Several have been tested utilizing guidelines published in 1986 by the American Dental Association for assessment of agents that claim efficacy in the management of periodontal diseases. These chemical agents include chlorhexidine (Peridex®, PerioGard®), which are bisbiguanides and benzalkonium chloride, which is a quarternary compound. Chlorhexidine, in various concentrations, has shown efficacy in reducing plaque and gingivitis in patients with short-term utilization. Some side effects include staining of the dentition which is reversible by dental prophylaxis. Chlorhexidine demonstrates the concept of substantivity, indicating that after its use, it has a continued effect in reducing the ability of plaque to form. It has been shown to be useful in a variety of periodontal conditions including acute necrotizing ulcerative gingivitis and healing studies. Some disturbances in taste and accumulation of calculus have been reported, however, chlorhexidine is the most applicable chemical agent of the bisbiguanides that has been studied to date.

Other chemical agents available as mouthwashes include the phenol compound Listerine Antiseptic®. These compounds are primarily restricted to prototype agents; the first to be approved by the ADA being Listerine Antiseptic®. Listerine Antiseptic® has been shown to be effective against plaque and gingivitis in long-term studies and comparable to chlorhexidine in these long-term investigations. However, chlorhexidine performs better than Listerine Antiseptic® in short-term investigations. Triclosan, the chemical agent found in the toothpaste Total®, has been recently approved by the FDA and is an aid in the prevention of gingivitis. Antiplaque activity of triclosan is enhanced with the addition of zinc citrate and there are no serious side effects to the use of triclosan. Sanguinarine is a principle herbal extract used for antiplaque activity. It is an alkaloid from the plant Sanguinaria canadensis and has some antimicrobial properties perhaps due to its enzyme activity although a relationship was found between epithelial mucosa premalignant changes and sanguinarine use in mouth rinse. Zinc citrate and zinc chloride have often been added to toothpastes as well as enzymes such as mucinase, mutanase, and dextrinase which have demonstrated varying results in studies. Some commercial anionic surfactants are available on the market which include aminoalcohols and the agent Plax® which essentially is comprised of sodium thiosulfate as a surfactant. Recent studies have shown Plax® to have some efficacy when it is added to triclosan.

Long-term use of prescription medications, including antibiotics, is seldom recommended and is not in any way a substitute for general dental/periodontal therapies. As adjunctive therapy, however, benefit has been shown and the new formulations of doxycycline (Periostat® and Atridox™), are recommended for long-term or repetitive treatments. It should be noted that the manufacturer's claims indicate that Periostat® functions as a collagenase inhibitor not as an antibiotic at recommended low doses for long-term therapy. Atridox™, however, functions as an antibiotic and is not recommended for constant long-term therapy, but rather in repetitive applications as necessary. Prescription medications used in efforts to treat periodontal diseases have historically included the use of antibiotics such as tetracycline although complications with use with young patients (ie, teeth intrinsic staining) have often precluded their prescription. Doxycycline

PERIODONTAL DISEASES *(Continued)*

is often preferred to tetracycline in low doses. This broad-spectrum bacteriostatic agent has shown efficacy against a wide variety of bacterial organisms found in periodontal disease. Minocycline slow-release (Arestin™) has recently been approved.

The drug metronidazole is a nitromidazole. It is an agent that was originally used in treatment of protozoan infections and some anaerobic bacteria. It is bactericidal and has a good absorption and distribution throughout the body. The studies using metronidazole have suggested that it has a variety of uses in periodontal treatment and can be used as adjunct in both acute necrotizing ulcerative gingivitis and has specific efficacy against spirochetes, bacteria, and some *Porphyromonas* species. Clindamycin is a derivative of vancomycin and has been useful in treatment of suppurative periodontal lesions. Long-term use is precluded by its complicating toxicities associated with colitis and gastrointestinal problems; however, recent studies have shown that a variety of antibiotics can result in colitis, thus, clindamycin should not be singled out as the sole or main culprit of this reported complication.

Research has also shown that various combination therapies of metronidazole and tetracycline for localized aggressive periodontitis and metronidazole with amoxicillin for rapidly progressive disease can be useful. The use of other prescription drugs including nonsteroidal anti-inflammatory, as well as other antibacterial agents, have been under study. Effects on prostaglandins of NSAIDs may indirectly slow periodontal disease progression. New research is currently underway in this regard. Perhaps, in combination therapy with some of the antibiotics, these drugs may assist in reducing the patient's immune response or inflammatory response to the presence of disease-causing bacteria.

Of greatest interest has been the improvement in technology for delivery of chemical agents to the periodontally-diseased site. These systems include biodegradable gelatins and biodegradable chips that can be placed under the gingiva and deliver antibacterial agents directly to the site as an adjunct to periodontal treatment. The initial therapy of mechanical debridement by the periodontal therapist is essential prior to using any chemical agent, and the dentist should be aware that the development of newer agents does not substitute for appropriate periodontal therapy and maintenance. The trade names of the gelatin chips and subgingival delivery systems include Periochip®, Atridox®, and Periostat®.

In addition to the periodontal therapy, consideration of the patient's pre-existing or developing medical conditions are important in the management of the periodontal patient. Several diseases illustrate these points most acutely. The reader is referred to the chapters on Diabetes, Cardiovascular Disease, Pregnancy, Respiratory Disease, HIV, and Cancer Chemotherapy. It has long been accepted that uncontrolled diabetes mellitus may predispose to periodontal lesions. Now, under current investigation is the hypothesis that pre-existing periodontal diseases may make it more difficult for a diabetic patient to come under control. In addition, the inflammatory response and immune challenge that is ongoing in periodontal disease appears to be implicated in the development of coronary artery disease as well as an increased risk of myocardial infarction and/or stroke. The accumulation of intra-arterial plaques appears enhanced by the presence of the inflammatory response often seen systemically in patients suffering with periodontal disease. In addition, the clinician is referred to the section on preprocedural antibiotics in the text for a consideration of antibiotic usage in patients that may be at risk for infective endocarditis. Other conditions including pregnancy and respiratory diseases such as COPD, HIV, and cancer therapy must be considered in the overall view of periodontal diseases. The reader is referred to the sections within the text.

Amoxicillin *on page 108*

Benzalkonium Chloride *on page 194*

Chlorhexidine Gluconate *on page 332*

Ciprofloxacin *on page 359*

Clindamycin *on page 378*

Doxycycline Hyclate (Periodontal) *on page 539*

Listerine Antiseptic® *on page 1128*

Metronidazole *on page 1091*

Minocycline Hydrochloride (Periodontal) *on page 1108*

NSAIDs see Oral Pain section *on page 1788*

Tetracycline *on page 1548*

Triclosan and Fluoride *on page 1616*

For examples of sample prescriptions see Bacterial Infections and Periodontal Diseases *on page 1837*

Pharmacologic Management of Periodontal Diseases

Antibiotic	Adult Dosage
Azithromycin	500 mg once daily for 4-7 days
Ciprofloxacin	500 mg bid for 8 days
Clindamycin	300 mg tid for 8 days
Doxycycline or minocycline	100-200 mg once daily for 21 days
Metronidazole	500 mg tid for 8 days
Metronidazole + amoxicillin	250 mg tid for 8 days of each drug
Metronidazole + ciprofloxacin	500 mg bid for 8 days of each drug

Adapted from: Recommendations from the American Academy of Periodontology.
Available at: www.perio.org

FUNGAL INFECTIONS

Oral fungal infections can result from alteration in oral flora, immunosuppression, and underlying systemic diseases that may allow the overgrowth of these opportunistic organisms. These systemic conditions might include diabetes mellitus, long-term xerostomia, adrenal suppression, anemia, and chemotherapy-induced myelosuppression for the management of cancer. The inappropriate use of oral inhalers that include steroids, such as Advair™ Diskus®, have been implicated in the enhancing of the risk of fungal overgrowth. Drugs of choice in treating fungal infections are amphotericin B, caspofungin, ciclopirox olamine, clotrimazole, itraconazole, ketoconazole, fluconazole, naftifine hydrochloride, nystatin, and oxiconazole. Patients being treated for fungal skin infections may also be using topical antifungal preparations coupled with a steroid such as triamcinolone. Clinical presentation might include pseudomembranous, erythematous, and hyperkeratotic forms. Fungus has also been implicated in denture stomatitis, angular cheilitis, and symptomatic geographic tongue.

Nystatin (Mycostatin®) is effective topically in the treatment of candidal infections of the skin and mucous membrane. The drug is extremely well tolerated and appears to be nonsensitizing although gastrointestinal upset and nausea are fairly common side effects. Clotrimazole troches are also useful as a topical therapy. Due to the significant sugar content in nystatin, patients with salivary gland hypofunction should be prescribed an alternative medication such as clotrimazole in order to lessen the caries risk. Clotrimazole is also available as an over-the-counter product in vaginal suppository formulations. In persons with denture stomatitis in which *Candida albicans* plays at least a contributory role, it is important to soak the prosthesis (laden with organisms) overnight in a nystatin liquid suspension besides treatment of the affected oral mucosa. Nystatin ointment can be placed in the denture during the daytime much like a denture adhesive.

Antifungal medication should be continued for at least 14 days in order to prevent relapse and the patient must be re-evaluated. Predisposing systemic factors must be reconsidered if the oral fungal infection persists. Topical applications rely on contact of the drug with the organism within the lesions. Therefore, 4-5 times daily with a dissolving troche or pastille is appropriate.

MANAGEMENT OF FUNGAL INFECTIONS REQUIRING SYSTEMIC MEDICATION

If the patient is refractory to topical treatment, consideration of a systemic route might include Diflucan® or Nizoral®. Also, when the patient cannot tolerate topical therapy, ketoconazole (Nizoral®) is an effective, well tolerated, systematic drug for mucocutaneous candidiasis. Concern over liver function and possible drug interactions must be considered.

In patients that appear to be refractory to itraconazole or fluconazole related to the treatment of oropharyngeal candidiasis, posaconazole has been approved for usage. Caspofungin (Cancidas®) or voriconazole (VFEND®) are also indicated for treatment of serious fungal infections in patients intolerant of, or refractory to, other therapy.

Amphotericin B (Conventional) *on page 115*
Caspofungin *on page 294*
Clotrimazole *on page 398*
Fluconazole *on page 697*
Ketoconazole *on page 928*
Nystatin *on page 1194*
Nystatin and Triamcinolone *on page 1196*
Posaconazole *on page 1325*
Voriconazole *on page 1666*

Note: Consider Peridex® oral rinse, or Listerine® antiseptic oral rinse for long-term control in immunosuppressed patients.

SAMPLE PRESCRIPTIONS FOR SYSTEMIC TREATMENT

Rx:

Diflucan® 100 mg tablets
Disp: 16 tablets
Sig: Take 2 tablets day 1, then 1 tablet/day until gone

Note: Sometimes a shorter course is adequate. However, oral infections commonly are more difficult to eradicate and even a second course may be necessary.

Ingredient: Fluconazole

Rx:

> Nizoral® 200 mg
> Disp: 14 tablets
> Sig: Take 1 tablet daily, with a meal for 2 weeks
>
> **Note:** May cause irreversible liver damage; liver function should be monitored with long-term use (ie, >3 weeks)
>
> Ingredient: Ketoconazole

SAMPLE PRESCRIPTIONS FOR TOPICAL TREATMENT

Rx:

> Nystatin 100,000 units/mL oral suspension
> Disp: 300 mL
> Sig: Rinse with 1 teaspoon (5 mL) for 2 minutes 4-5 times/day and expectorate

Rx:

> Mycelex® 10 mg troches
> Disp: 70 troches
> Sig: Dissolve 1 troche in mouth 5 times/day until gone; leave any prosthesis out during treatment and soak prosthesis in nystatin liquid suspension overnight
>
> Ingredient: Clotrimazole

For additional sample prescriptions see Fungal Infections *on page 1841*

MANAGEMENT OF ANGULAR CHEILITIS

Angular cheilitis may represent the clinical manifestation of a multitude of etiologic factors. Cheilitis-like lesions may result from local habits, from a decrease in the intermaxillary space, or from nutritional deficiency. More commonly, angular cheilitis represents a mixed infection coupled with an inflammatory response involving *Candida albicans* and other organisms (most frequently *Staphylococcus aureus*). The drug of choice is now formulated to contain nystatin and triamcinolone and the effect is excellent. In addition, an off-label use of iodoquinol and hydrocortisone has also been reported to be effective in the treatment of angular cheilitis.

VIRAL INFECTIONS

Oropharyngeal viral infections are most commonly caused by herpes simplex viruses and Coxsackie viruses. Infections of the oropharynx and upper respiratory infections are commonly caused by the Coxsackie group A viruses. Oral cavity proper soft tissue viral infections, on the other hand, are most often caused by the herpes simplex viruses. Herpes zoster or varicella-zoster virus, which is one of the herpes family of viruses, can likewise cause similar viral eruptions involving the oral mucosa.

The diagnosis of an acute viral infection is one that begins by ruling out bacterial etiology and having an awareness of the presenting signs and symptoms associated with viral infection. Acute onset and vesicular eruption on the soft tissues generally favors a diagnosis of viral infection. Unfortunately, vesicles do not remain for a great length of time in the oral cavity; therefore, the short-lived vesicles rupture leaving ulcerated bases as the only indication of their presence. These ulcers, however, are generally small in size and only when left unmanaged, coalesce to form larger, irregular ulcerations. Distinction must be made between the commonly recurring intraoral atraumatic ulcers (aphthous ulcerations) which do not have a viral etiology and the lesions associated with intraoral recurrent herpes since their effective treatment is distinctly different. The management of an oral viral infection may be palliative for the most part; however, with the advent of improved antiviral prescription medications there now exists a family of drugs that can assist in managing primary and secondary infection. Human *Papillomavirus* is causative in a number of oral lesions, the most common of which are *Condyloma acuminatum* and Verruca vulgaris. Within the past few years certain subtypes of human *Papillomavirus* already proven to cause uterine cervical carcinoma are suspected of also being responsible for some posterior oral squamous cell carcinomas. Aldara® has been approved for treatment of genital warts (superficial basal cell carcinomas and actinic keratosis); oral mucosa use is still under study.

It should be noted that herpes can present as a primary infection (gingivostomatitis or pharyngostomatitis), recurrent lip lesions (herpes labialis of the skin and adjacent vermilion border), and intraoral ulcers (recurrent intraoral herpes), involving the oral and perioral tissues. Primary infection is a systemic infection that leads to acute gingivostomatitis that may involve all moveable and nonmovable sites of the oral cavity (buccal mucosa, lips, tongue, floor of the mouth, palate, and the gingiva). Treatment of primary infections utilizes prescription antivirals such as acyclovir in combination with supportive care. Topical anesthetics, such as lidocaine 1% or dyclonine HCl 1%, used in combination with Benadryl® 0.5% in a saline vehicle was found to be an effective oral rinse in the symptomatic treatment of primary herpetic gingivostomatitis. Other agents for symptomatic and supportive treatment include commercially available elixir of Benadryl®, Xylocaine® viscous, Orajel® (OTC), and antibiotics to prevent secondary infections. Systemic supportive therapy should include forced fluids, high concentration protein, vitamin and mineral food supplements, and rest.

Antivirals

Abreva™(OTC) *on page 522*

Acyclovir *on page 49*

Famciclovir *on page 668*

Imiquimod *on page 867*

L-Lysine *on page 1012*

Nelfinavir *on page 1158*

Penciclovir *on page 1266*

Valacyclovir *on page 1635*

Viroxyn® *on page 194*

Supportive Therapy

Diphenhydramine *on page 510*

Lidocaine *on page 972*

Prevention of Secondary Bacterial Infection

Penicillin V Potassium *on page 1271*

SUPPORTIVE CARE FOR PAIN AND PREVENTION OF SECONDARY INFECTION

Primary infections often become secondarily infected with bacteria, requiring antibiotics. Dietary supplement may be necessary. Options are presented due to variability in patient compliance and response.

RECURRENT HERPETIC INFECTIONS

Following the primary herpetic infection, the herpesvirus remains latent until such time as it has the opportunity to recur. The etiology of this latent period and the degree of viral shedding present during latency is currently under study; however, it is thought that some trigger in the mucosa or the skin causes the virus to begin to replicate. This process may involve Langerhans cells which are immunocompetent antigen-presenting cells resident in all epidermal and epithelial surfaces. The virus replication then leads to physical movement of the virus along the sensory axon leading to eruptions in innervated tissues surrounding the mouth or within. The most common form of recurrence is the lip lesion or herpes labialis, however, intraoral recurrent herpes also occurs with some frequency (attached gingival and hard palate only). Prevention of recurrences has been attempted with lysine (OTC) 500-1000 mg/day and acylovir but response has been variable. Herpes zoster outbreaks can also involve the oral and facial tissues although this is uncommon. Valacyclovir or famciclovir are the drugs of choice. Of the two medications, famciclovir is reported to be more effective against postherpetic neuralgia. Valacyclovir HCl in 500 mg and 1 g tablets has recently been approved by the FDA for first time generic formulations.

Water-soluble bioflavonoid-ascorbic acid complex, now available as Peridin-C®, may be helpful in reducing the signs and symptoms associated with recurrent herpes simplex virus infections. As with all agents used, the therapy is more effective when instituted in the early prodromal stage of the disease process.

PREVENTATIVE SAMPLE PRESCRIPTIONS

Rx:

L-Lysine (OTC) 500 mg
Sig: Take 2 tablets/day as preventive; increase to 4 tablets/day if prodrome or recurrence begins

Rx:

Citrus bioflavonoids and ascorbic acid tablets 400 mg (Peridin-C®)
Disp: 10 tablets
Sig: Take 2 tablets at once, then 1 tablet 3 times/day for 3 days

Where a recurrence is usually precipitated by exposure to sunlight, the lesion may be prevented by the application to the area of a sunscreen, with a high skin protection factor (SPF) in the range of ≥25.

SUPPORTIVE CARE FOR PAIN AND MAINTENANCE OF NUTRITION DURING ORAL VIRAL INFECTIONS

Rx:

Benadryl® liquid 12.5 mg/5mL
Disp: 4 oz bottle
Sig: Rinse with 1-2 teaspoonfuls every 2 hours and expectorate

Note: Benadryl® is available as a generic diphenhydramine liquid.

Rx:

Benadryl® liquid 12.5 mg/5 mL (mix 50/50) with Kaopectate®
Disp: 8 oz total
Sig: Rinse with 1-2 teaspoonfuls every 2 hours and expectorate.

Note: Maalox® can be used in place of Kaopectate® if constipation is a problem. Benadryl® is available as a generic diphenhydramine liquid.

Rx:

Xylocaine® viscous 2%
Disp: 450 mL bottle
Sig: Swish with 1 tablespoon 4 times/day and spit out

Ingredient: Lidocaine

Rx:

Meritene®
Disp: 1 lb can (plain, chocolate, eggnog flavors)
Sig: Take 3 servings daly; prepare as indicated on can

Ingredient: Protein-vitamin-mineral food supplement

VIRAL INFECTIONS *(Continued)*

PRESCRIPTIVE TREATMENT

Acyclovir (Zovirax®) possesses antiviral activity against herpes simplex types 1 and 2. Historically, ophthalmic ointments were used topically to treat recurrent mucosal and skin lesions. These do not penetrate well on the skin lesions, thereby providing questionable relief of symptoms. If recommended, use should be closely monitored. Penciclovir, an active metabolite of famciclovir, has been specifically approved in a cream for treatment of recurrent herpes lesions. Valacyclovir and famciclovir have also been approved for treatment of herpes labialis (see monograph for dosing). The FDA has also approved acyclovir cream 5% for treatment of herpes labialis in adults and adolescents. Recently, in addition to docosanol (Abreva®), another over-the-counter preparation for treatment of recurrent herpes labialis has been approved. Benzalkonium chloride and isopropyl alcohol (Viroxyn®) is an alcohol/benzalkonium chloride medication in a single dose applicator kit (3 pack) that is marketed to reduce the duration and symptoms of cold sores. Other over-the-counter preparations include 2% tetracaine gel and L-lysine 500 mg tablets.

SAMPLE PRESCRIPTIONS

Rx:

    Zovirax 200 mg capsules
    Disp: 50 or 60 capsules
    Sig: Take 1 capsule 5 times/day for 10 days or 2 capsules 3 times/day for 10 days

    Ingredient: Acyclovir

Rx:

    Valtrex® 500 mg caplets
    Disp: 42 caplets
    Sig: Take 2 caplets 3 times/day for 7 days without regard to meals

    Ingredient: Valacyclovir

Rx:

    Famvir® 500 mg tablets
    Disp: 3 tablets
    Sig: Take 1500 mg as a single dose

    Ingredient: Famciclovir

Rx:

    Denavir® topical ointment 5%
    Disp: 1.5 g tube
    Sig: Apply locally as directed to lesion every 2 hours during waking hours (begin when symptoms first occur)

    Ingredient: Penciclovir

For additional sample prescriptions see Viral Infections *on page 1843*

ULCERATIVE AND EROSIVE DISORDERS

RECURRENT APHTHOUS STOMATITIS - MINOR, MAJOR, AND HERPETIFORM TYPES

Recurrent aphthous stomatitis is thought to be caused by a temporary glitch in the immune system with subsequent self destruction in a localized manner of the oral mucosa's epithelium. No definitive organism has been proven to cause the disease process. It is known that different subsets of patients have different triggering factors (eg, stress, hormonal, sunlight) and thus no one product or technique is universally effective in all patients. For minor or major aphthous ulcers that severely affect daily living and quality of life, corticosteroids seem to be the mainstay drug. It is believed that the immunomodulating effect of a short-term regimen of corticosteroids in an immunocompetent sufferer is effective without creating the well known side effects of long-term or high-dose corticosteroid therapy. Sufferers of the herpetiform type of aphthae, in which as many as a hundred small ulcers appear per crop, may also obtain relief from an oral suspension form of corticosteroid.

Triamcinolone (Kenalog® in Orabase) paste is indicated for the temporary relief of minor symptoms associated with infrequent recurrences of minor aphthous lesions and ulcerative lesions resulting from trauma. Some clinicians have pharmacists compound a soothing rinse containing corticosteroid (eg, dexamethasone), an antifungal agent (eg, nystatin), a topical anesthetic (eg, viscous lidocaine), an antihistamine (eg, diphenhydramine), an antimicrobial/antibiotic (chlorhexidine), and/or coating agent such as attapulgite creating a so-called "magic elixir". More severe forms of recurrent aphthous stomatitis may be treated with topical corticosteroids of high strength (eg, fluconazole, clobetasol) alone or mixed with Orabase®; an oral suspension of tetracycline may be prescribed for avoidance of secondary infection. Tetracycline use is contraindicated during the last half of pregnancy, infancy, and childhood to the age of 8 years due to intrinsic staining of teeth. *Lactobacillus acidophilus* preparations (Bacid®, Lactinex®) are occasionally effective for reducing the frequency and severity of the minor lesions. A cauterizing agent, such as Debacterol® with professional oversight may markedly decrease the pain associated with the aphthous ulcer. Clinician and patient must be extremely careful in using cauterizing agents within the oral cavity. Patients with long-standing history of recurrent aphthous stomatitis should be evaluated for iron, folic acid, and vitamin B_{12} deficiencies; one subset of recurrent aphthous stomatitis sufferers markedly improve when tooth dentifrices lacking sodium lauryl sulfate are used.

A noncorticosteroid prescription medication, 5% aphthasol paste, has been approved for recurrent aphthous stomatitis and published studies indicate it hastens the healing of these lesions by more than a day. In patients with medical contraindications for corticosteroid use and aphthasol has not been effective, alternatives (eg, colchicine, dapsone, immune globulin (intravenous), methotrexate, misoprostol, mycophenolate mofetil, pentoxifylline, tacrolimus, and tretinoin) have had reports of effectiveness. These alternative drugs should be used in consultation with the patient's physician. Regular use of Listerine® antiseptic has been shown in clinical trials to reduce the severity, duration, and frequency of aphthous stomatitis. An antimicrobial such as chlorhexidine oral rinses (20 mL for 30 seconds 2-3 times/day) have also demonstrated efficacy in reducing the duration of aphthae. With both of these products, however, patient intolerance of the burning from the alcohol content is of concern. Viractin® has been approved for symptomatic relief although it is primarily intended for relief in recurrent herpes labialis. Immunocompromised patients such as those with AIDS may have severe ulcer recurrences and the drug thalidomide has been approved for these patients on an FDA orphan drug approved basis.

ULCERATIVE AND EROSIVE DISORDERS *(Continued)*

EROSIVE LICHEN PLANUS AND OTHER VESICULOEROSIVE DISEASES

Elixir of dexamethasone (Decadron®), a potent anti-inflammatory agent, is used topically (as a 2 minute rinse and expectorate) in the management of acute episodes of erosive lichen planus and other vesiculoerosive disease processes such as benign mucous membrane pemphigoid and pemphigus vulgaris. Some patients will not achieve relief from topical agents and systemic delivery either by swish and swallow or tablets may be necessary. Prednisone corticosteroid tablet is a popular and often effective starting point with a regimen consisting of burst therapy (eg, 6-80 mg) for several days followed by 7-10 days of a maintenance and tapering dose. Continued supervision of the patient during treatment is essential and the dentist must be aware that treatment of any secondary infections such as fungal overgrowth may be essential in gaining control of the erosive lesions. Also, patients should be counseled that maximum benefit of the medication will be achieved when oral hygiene is maintained at excellent levels.

For examples of sample prescriptions see Ulcerative and Erosive Disorders *on page 1844*

NECROTIZING ULCERATING PERIODONTITIS (HIV Periodontal Disease)

Initial Treatment *(In-Office)*

Gentle debridement

Note: Ensure patient has no iodine allergies

Betadine® rinse *on page 1332*

At-Home Treatment

Listerine® antiseptic rinse (20 mL for 30 seconds twice daily)

Peridex® rinse *on page 332*

Metronidazole (Flagyl®) 7-10 days *on page 1091*

Follow-Up Therapy

Proper dental cleaning, including scaling and root planing (repeat as needed)

Continue Peridex® and Listerine® rinse (indefinitely)

BURNING TONGUE SYNDROME

Burning mouth syndrome is extremely difficult to both diagnose and treat. Initially, systemic factors, including changes in patient's medication, control of diabetes mellitus (if the disease is present), concomitant xerostomia, and the presence of fungal infections often complicate the diagnosis and management of burning mouth syndrome. Once these systemic and/or local factors have been eliminated, oftentimes the patient presents with none or minimal clinically-visible changes and only the subjective complaint of burning mouth. In these instances, a variety of drugs, including clonazepam 0.25-3 mg/day is sometimes used; also the drugs amitriptyline 25-100 mg/day, nortriptyline 10-50 mg/day, gabapentin 900-1500 mg/day, and doxepin as a cream, applied to the lateral borders of the tongue and the areas affected, are sometimes utilized. These drugs should be selected and managed in collaboration with the patient's physician, particularly since many of these patients suffering with burning mouth syndrome have complicated medical histories including the use of additional medications that could be affected.

SYMPTOMATIC GEOGRAPHIC TONGUE (BENIGN MIGRATORY GLOSSITIS, ERYTHEMA MIGRANS)

Geographic tongue is a localized, transitory loss of the tongue's filiform papillae. Although disconcerting in appearance to patients, it usually is asymptomatic; however, occasionally patients will report a burning sensation.

Benadryl® elixir, a potent antihistamine, is used in the oral cavity primarily as a mild topical anesthetic agent for the symptomatic relief of certain allergic deficiencies which should be ruled out as possible etiologies for the oral condition under treatment. It is often used alone as well as in solutions with agents such as Kaopectate® or Maalox® to assist in coating the oral mucosa. Benadryl® can also be used in capsule form. Frequently, Benadryl® alone or in combination with the above agents, will be very effective in the relief of symptomatic geographic tongue.

When Benadryl® is ineffective, patients often achieve relief with prednisolone syrup used in a 2-minute rinse and expectorate regimen, several times a day.

MILD-TO-MODERATE FORMS OF ULCERATIONS AND EROSIONS

In addition to the medications listed above there are several over-the-counter preparations that may give the patient some or total relief. Examples include Ulcerease®, BetaCell oral rinse®, Cankermelts-GX®, Gelclair Bioadherent Oral Gel®, Orabase Sooth-N-Seal®, OraPatch®, Ricinol P.R.N.®, and Zilactin® gel.

DENTIN HYPERSENSITIVITY, HIGH CARIES INDEX, AND XEROSTOMIA

DENTIN HYPERSENSITIVITY

Suggested steps in resolving dentin hypersensitivity when a thorough exam has ruled-out any other source for the problem:

Treatment Steps

- Home treatment with a desensitizing toothpaste containing potassium nitrate (used to brush teeth as well as a thin layer applied, each night for 2 weeks)
- If needed, in office potassium oxalate (Protect® by Butler) and/or in office fluoride iontophoresis
- If sensitivity is still not tolerable to the patient, consider pumice then dentin adhesive and unfilled resin or composite restoration overlaying a glass ionomer base

Home Products (all contain nitrate as active ingredient):

Promise®
Denquel®
Sensodyne®
THERADENT™

Dentifrice Products *on page 1924*

Other major brand name companies have added ingredients to their dentifrice product lines that also make hypersensitivity claims.

ANTICARIES AGENTS

Fluoride (Gel 0.4%, Rinse 0.05%) *on page 710*

Toothpastes with triclosan such as Colgate Total® show promise for combined treatment/prevention of caries, plaque, and gingivitis. The use of 5% sodium fluoride varnishes (Duraflor® and Duraphat®) have been encouraged for the prevention of decay in persons of high-risk populations.

FLUORIDES

Used for the prevention of demineralization of the tooth structure secondary to xerostomia. For patients with long-term or permanent xerostomia, daily application is accomplished using custom applicator trays, such as omnivac. Patients with porcelain crowns should use a neutral pH fluoride (see Fluoride monograph *on page 710*). Final selection of a fluoride product and/or saliva replacement/stimulant product must be based on patient comfort, taste, and ultimately, compliance. Experience has demonstrated that, often times, patients must try various combinations to achieve the greatest effect and their highest comfort levels. The presence of mucositis during cancer management complicates the clinician's selection of products.

See also Oral Rinse Products *on page 1941*

OVER-THE-COUNTER (OTC) PRODUCTS

Form	Brand Name	Strength / Size
Gel, topical (stannous fluoride)	Gel-Kam® (cinnamon, fruit, mint flavors)	0.4% [0.1%] (65 g, 105 g, 122 g)
	Gel-Tin® (lime, grape, cinnamon, raspberry, mint, orange flavors)	0.4% [0.1%] (60 g, 120 g)
	Stop® (grape, cinnamon, bubblegum, piña colada, mint flavors)	0.4% [0.1%] (60 g, 120 g)
Rinse, topical (as sodium)	ACT®, Fluorigard®	0.05% [0.02%] (90 mL, 180 mL, 300 mL, 360 mL, 480 mL)
	Listermint® with Fluoride	0.02% [0.01%] (180 mL, 300 mL, 360 mL, 480 mL, 540 mL, 720 mL, 960 mL, 1740 mL)

PRESCRIPTION ONLY (Rx) PRODUCTS

Form	Brand Name	Strength / Size
Drops, oral (as sodium)		0.275 mg/drop [0.125 mg/drop]
	Fluoritab®, Flura-Drops®	0.55 mg/drop [0.25 mg/drop] (22.8 mL, 24 mL)
	Karidium®, Luride®	0.275 mg/drop [0.125 mg/drop] (30 mL, 60 mL)
	Pediaflor®	1.1 mg/mL [0.5 mg/mL] (50 mL)
Gel-Drops	Thera-Flur® (lime flavor), Thera-Flur-N®	1.1% [0.55%] (24 mL)
Gel, topical	Minute-Gel® (spearmint, strawberry, grape, apple-cinnamon, cherry cola, bubblegum flavors)	
Acidulated phosphate fluoride	FluoroCare® Fluoridex Maximum Uptake™	1.23% (480 mL)
Sodium fluoride	Karigel® (orange flavor)	1.1% [0.5%]
	Karigel®-N	1.1% [0.5%]
	PreviDent® (mint, berry, cherry, fruit sherbet flavors)	1.1% [0.5%] (24 g, 30 g, 60 g, 120 g, 130 g, 250 g)
Lozenge (as sodium)	Flura-Loz® (raspberry flavor)	2.2 mg [1 mg]
Rinse, topical (as sodium)	Fluorinse®, Point-Two®	0.2% [0.09%] (240 mL, 480 mL, 3780 mL)
Solution, oral (as sodium)	Phos-Flur® (cherry, cinnamon, grape, wintergreen flavors)	0.44 mg/mL [0.2 mg/mL] (250 mL, 500 mL, 3780 mL)
Tablet (as sodium)		1.1 mg [0.5 mg]; 2.2 mg [1 mg]
Chewable	Fluor-A-Day®	0.55 mg [0.25 mg]
	Fluor-A-Day®, Fluoritab®, Luride® Lozi-Tab®, Pharmaflur®	1.1 mg [0.5 mg]
	Fluor-A-Day®, Fluoritab®, Karidium®, Luride® Lozi-Tab®, Luride®-SF Lozi-Tab®, Pharmaflur®	2.2 mg [1 mg]
Oral	Flura®, Karidium®	2.2 mg [1 mg]
Varnish	Duraflor®, Duraphat®	5% [50 mg/mL] (10 mL)

Tables used with permission from Newland JR, Meiller TF, Wynn RL, et al, *Oral Soft Tissue Diseases*, 2nd ed, Hudson (Cleveland), OH: Lexi-Comp, Inc, 2002.

ANTIMICROBIAL ORAL RINSE

Chlorhexidine Gluconate (Peridex®) *on page 332*

Chlorhexidine Gluconate alcohol-free (CHX®)

Mouthwash (Antiseptic) (Listerine®) *on page 1128*

For examples of sample prescriptions see Antimicrobial Rinses *on page 1840*

MANAGEMENT OF SIALORRHEA

In patients suffering with medical conditions that result in hypersalivation, the dentist may determine that it is appropriate to use an atropine sulfate medication to achieve a dry field for dental procedures or to reduce excessive drooling. Currently there is one ADA approved medication sold under the name of Sal-Tropine™. Pro-Banthine® (propantheline bromide), an antimuscarinic used for excessive stomach acid production is advocated by some for off-label use. See Atropine Sulfate Dental Tablets *on page 169*

XEROSTOMIA

Xerostomia refers to the subjective sensation of a dry mouth while salivary gland hypofunction can be objectively measured. Numerous factors can play a role in the patient's perception of xerostomia. Changes in salivary function caused by drugs, surgical intervention, or treatment of cancer are among the leading causes of xerostomia. Other factors including aging, smoking, mouth breathing, and autoimmune disorders such as Sjögren's syndrome, can also be implicated in a patient's perception of xerostomia. Human immunodeficiency virus (HIV) may produce xerostomia when viral changes in salivary glands are present. Xerostomia affects women more frequently than men and is also more common in older individuals. Some alteration in salivary function naturally occurs with age, but it is extremely difficult to quantify the effects. Xerostomia and

DENTIN HYPERSENSITIVITY, HIGH CARIES INDEX, AND XEROSTOMIA *(Continued)*

salivary gland hypofunction in the elderly population are contributory to deterioration in the quality of life.

Once a diagnosis of xerostomia or salivary gland hypofunction is made and possible causes confirmed, treatment for the condition usually involves management of the underlying disease and avoidance of unnecessary medications. In addition, good hydration is essential and water is the drink of choice. Also, the use of artificial saliva substitutes, selected chewing gums, and/or toothpastes formulated to treat xerostomia, is often warranted. In more difficult cases, such as patients receiving radiotherapy for cancer of the head and neck regions or patients with Sjögren's syndrome, systemic cholinergic stimulants may be administered if no contraindications exist.

CLINICAL PRODUCT USE

Because of the complex nature of xerostomia, management by the dental clinician is difficult. Treatment success is also difficult to assess and is often unsatisfactory. The salivary stimulants, pilocarpine and cevimeline, may aid in some conditions but are only approved for use as sialogogues in patients receiving radiotherapy and in Sjögren's patients, specifically as described above. Artificial salivas are available as over-the-counter products and represent the potential for continuous application by the patient to achieve comfort for their xerostomic condition.

The role of the clinician in attempting treatment of dry mouth is to first achieve a differential diagnosis and to ensure that other conditions are not simultaneously present. For example, many patients suffer burning mouth syndrome or painful oral tissues with no obvious etiology accompanying dry mouth. Also, higher caries incidence may be associated with changes in salivary flow. As previously mentioned, Sjögren's syndrome represents an immune complex of disorders that can affect the eyes, oral tissues, and other organ systems. The reader is referred to current oral pathology or oral medicine textbooks for review of signs and symptoms of Sjögren's syndrome.

Treatment of cancer often leads to dry mouth. Surgical intervention removing salivary tissue due to the presence of a salivary gland tumor results in loss of salivary function. Also, many of the chemotherapeutic agents produce transitory changes in salivary flow, such that the patient may perceive a dry mouth during chemotherapy. Most notably related to salivary dysfunction is the use of radiation regimens to head and neck tissues. Tumors in or about salivary gland tissue, the oral cavity, and oropharynx are most notably sensitive to radiation therapy and subsequent dry mouth. In the head and neck, therapeutic radiation is commonly used in treatment of squamous cell carcinomas and lymphomas. The radiation level necessary to destroy malignant cells ranges from 40-70 Gy. Salivary tissue is extremely sensitive to radiation changes. Radiation dosages >70 Gy are sufficient to permanently change salivary function. In addition to the mucositis and subsequent secondary infection by fungal colonization or viral exacerbation, oral tissues can become exceptionally dry due to the effects of radiation on salivary glands. In fact, permanent damage to salivary gland tissue within the beam path produces significant levels of xerostomia in most patients. Some recovery may be noted by the patient. Most often, the effects are permanent and even progressive as the radiation dosage increases.

Artificial salivas do not produce any protectant or stimulation of the salivary gland. The use of pilocarpine and cevimeline as salivary stimulants in pre-emptive treatment, as well as postradiation treatment, have been shown to have some efficacy in management of dry mouth. The success rate, however, still is often unsatisfactory and post-treatment management by the dentist usually requires fluoride supplements to prevent radiation-induced caries due to dry mouth. Also, management of dry mouth through patient use of the artificial salivary gel, solutions and sprays, or other over-the-counter products for dry mouth (eg, chewing gum, toothpaste, mouthwash, swab-sticks, sugar-free candy) is highly recommended. The use of pilocarpine or cevimeline should only be considered by the dentist in consultation with the managing physician. The oftentimes severe and widespread cholinergic side effects of pilocarpine and cevimeline mandate close monitoring of the patient and certain medical conditions contraindicated their use.

The use of artificial salivary substitutes is less problematic for the dentist. The dentist should, in considering selection of a drug, base his or her decision on patient compliance and comfort. Salivary substitutes presently on the market may have some benefit in terms of electrolyte balance and salivary consistency. However, the ultimate decision needs to be based on patients' taste, their willingness to use the medication ad libitum, and improvement in their comfort related to dry mouth. Many of the drugs are pH balanced to reduce additional risk of dental demineralization or caries. Oftentimes, the dentist must try numerous medications, one at a time, prior to finding one which gives the patient some comfort. Another gauge of acceptability is to investigate whether the artificial saliva substitute has the American Dental Association's seal of approval. Most of the currently accepted saliva substitute products have been evaluated by the ADA.

In general, considerations that the clinician might use in a prescribed regimen would be that saliva substitutes are meant to be used regularly throughout the day by the patient to achieve comfort during meals, reduce tissue abrasion, and prevent salivary stagnation on teeth. Other than these, there are no specific recommendations for patients. Recommendations by the dentist need to be tailored to the patient's acceptance. Salivary substitutes may provide an allergic potential in patients who are sensitive to some of the preservatives present in artificial saliva products. In addition to this allergic potential, there is a risk of microbial contamination by placement of the salivary substitute container in close contact with the oral cavity.

Patient education regarding the use of saliva substitutes is also part of the clinical approach. The patient with chronic xerostomia should be educated about regular professional care, high performance in dental hygiene, the need to re-evaluate oral soft tissue pathology, and any changes that might occur long term. In patients with severe xerostomia, artificial salivary medications should be given in combination with topical fluoride treatment programs designed by the dentist to reduce caries.

DENTIN HYPERSENSITIVITY, HIGH CARIES INDEX, AND XEROSTOMIA *(Continued)*

PRODUCTS AND DRUGS TO TREAT DRY MOUTH

Medication	Manufacturer and Phone Number	Product Type	Manufacturer's Description	Indication	Ingredients	Directions for Use	Form and Availability
Artificial Salivas (OTC)							
Biotene® OralBalance® Mouth Moisturizing Gel	Laclede Professional Products, Inc (800) 922-5856	Gel	Sugar-free oral lubricant; relieves dry mouth symptoms up to 8 hours; soothes and protects oral tissue to promote healing; helps to inhibit harmful bacteria; improves retention under dentures	Relieves symptoms of dry mouth: burning, itching, cotton palate, sore tissue swallowing difficulties	Contains the "Biotene®" protective salivary enzyme system Active: Glucose oxidase (2000 units), lactoperoxidase (3000 units), lysozyme (5 mg), lactoferrin (5 mg) Other: Hydrogenated starch, xylitol, hydroxyethyl cellulose, glycerate polyhydrate, aloe vera	Using a clean fingertip, apply a 1" ribbon of gel on tongue; add additional amount of gel on other dry; use as needed	1.4 oz tube; available at mass merchandise stores, food stores, and drugstores
BreathTech™ Plaque Fighter Mouth Spray	Omnii Oral Pharmaceuticals (800) 445-3386	Pump dispenser	Plaque inhibitor in vanilla-mint flavor for breath malodor or reduced salivary flow	Treats the discomfort of oral dryness	Microdent® patented plaque-inhibitor formula	Spray directly into mouth; spread over teeth and tissue with tongue	18 mL pump dispenser; order directly from manufacturer
Moi-Stir® Moistening Solution	Kingswood Laboratories, Inc (800) 968-7772	Pump spray	Saliva supplement for moistening of mouth and mucosal area	Nontherapeutic treatment of dry mouth; intended for comfort only	Water, sorbitol, sodium carboxymethylcellulose, methylparaben, propylparaben, potassium chloride, sodium chloride, flavoring	Spray directly into mouth as necessary to treat drying conditions	4 oz spray bottle; order directly from manufacturer or various distributors
MouthKote® Oral Moisturizer	Parnell Pharmaceuticals, Inc (800) 457-4276	Aqueous solution	Pleasant lemon-lime flavored oral moisturizer to lubricate and protect oral tissue	Treats the discomfort of oral dryness caused by medications, disease, surgery, irradiation, aging	Water, xylitol, sorbitol, yerba santa, citric acid, ascorbic acid, flavor, sodium benzoate, sodium saccharin	Swirl 1 or 2 teaspoonfuls in mouth for 8-10 seconds; swallow or spit out; shake well before using	2 oz and 8 oz bottles; available at drugstores or order directly from manufacturer

PRODUCTS AND DRUGS TO TREAT DRY MOUTH *(continued)*

Medication	Manufacturer and Phone Number	Product Type	Manufacturer's Description	Indication	Ingredients	Directions for Use	Form and Availability
Oasis® Moisturizing Mouthwash	GlaxoSmithKline (800) 777-2500	Oral moisturizer, aqueous solution	Moisturizing mouthwash for a dry mouth indication	Moisturizes mouth and helps it from drying out	**Active:** Glycerin. **Other:** Water, sorbitol, poloxamer 338, PEG-60 hydrogenated castor oil, cellulose gum, cetylpyridinium chloride, copovidone, disodium phosphate, flavor, methylparaben, propylparaben, sodium benzoate, sodium phosphate, sodium saccharin, xanthan gum, FD&C blue #1	Rinse for 30 seconds with 1 ounce of mouthwash first thing in the morning and before going to bed or as needed; do not swallow; use as part of an effective oral hygiene program	16 oz bottle
Optimoist™ Oral Moisturizer	Colgate Oral Pharmaceuticals (800) 225-3756	Oral moisturizer, aqueous solution	Pleasant tasting saliva substitute for instant relief of dry mouth and throat without demineralizing tooth enamel	Treats the discomfort of oral dryness	Deionized water, xylitol, calcium phosphate monobasic, citric acid, sodium hydroxide, sodium benzoate, flavoring, acesulfame potassium, hydroxyethylcellulose, polysorbate 20 and sodium monofluorophosphate (fluoride concentration is 2 parts per million)	Spray directly into mouth to relieve dry mouth discomfort; may be swallowed or expectorated; use as needed	2 oz and 12 oz bottles; available at mass merchandise stores, food stores, and drugstores
Salivart® Synthetic Saliva, Aqueous Solution	Gebauer Co (800) 321-9348	Aerosol aqueous spray	Oral moisturizer for patients with reduced salivary flow	Replacement therapy for patients complaining of xerostomia	Sodium carboxymethylcellulose, sorbitol, sodium chloride, potassium chloride, calcium chloride dihydrate, magnesium chloride hexahydrate, potassium phosphate dibasic, purified water, nitrogen (propellant)	Spray directly into mouth or throat for 1-2 seconds; use as needed	2.48 fl oz (75 g); available at most drugstores or directly from manufacturer
Other Dry Mouth Products (OTC)							
Biotene® Dry Mouth Gum	Laclede Professional Products, Inc (800) 922-9348	Chewing gum	Sugar-free; helps stimulate saliva flow; fights cause/ effect of bad breath; reduces plaque	Treats oral dryness	**Active:** Lactoperoxidase (0.11 Units), glucose oxidase (0.15 Units). **Other:** Sorbitol, gum base, xylitol, hydrogenated glucose, potassium thiocyanate	Chew 1 or 2 pieces; use as needed	Each package contains 17 pieces; available at drugstores or directly from manufacturer

DENTIN HYPERSENSITIVITY, HIGH CARIES INDEX, AND XEROSTOMIA *(Continued)*

PRODUCTS AND DRUGS TO TREAT DRY MOUTH *(continued)*

Medication	Manufacturer and Phone Number	Product Type	Manufacturer's Description	Indication	Ingredients	Directions for Use	Form and Availability
Biotene® Dry Mouth Toothpaste	Laclede Professional Products, Inc (800) 922-9348	Toothpaste	Reduces harmful bacteria which cause cavities, periodontal disease, and oral infections	Use in place of regular toothpaste for dry mouth	Active: Lactoperoxidase (15,000 Units), glucose oxidase (10,000 Units), lysozyme (16 mg), sodium monofluorophosphate Other: Sorbitol, glycerin, calcium pyrophosphate, hydrated silica, xylitol, isoceteth-20, cellulose gum, flavoring, sodium benzoate, beta-d-glucose, potassium thiocyanate	Use in place of regular toothpaste; rinse toothbrush before applying; brush for 2 minutes; rinse lightly	4.5 oz tube; available at drugstores or directly from manufacturer
Biotene® Gentle Mouthwash	Laclede Professional Products, Inc (800) 922-9348	Mouthwash	Alcohol-free; strong antibacterial formula neutralizes mouth odors; soothes as it cleans to protect teeth and oral tissue	Treats dry mouth or oral irritations	Lysozyme, lactoferrin, glucose oxidase, lactoperoxidase	Use 15 mL (1 tablespoonful); swish thoroughly for 30 seconds and spit out; for dry throat, sip 1 tablespoonful of mouthwash 2-3 times/day	Available at drugstores or directly from manufacturer
Moi-Stir® Oral Swabsticks	Kingswood Laboratories, Inc (800) 968-7772	Swabsticks	Lubricates and moistens mouth and mucosal area	Lubricates and moistens mouth and mucosal area	Water, sorbitol, sodium carboxymethylcellulose, methylparaben, propylparaben, potassium chloride, sodium chloride, flavoring	Gently swab all intraoral surfaces of mouth, gums, tongue, palate, buccal mucosa, gingival, teeth, and lips where uncomfortable dryness exists	3 swabsticks/packet, 100 packets/case; order directly from manufacturer or from various distributors.
Oasis® Moisturizing Mouth Spray	GlaxoSmithKline (800) 777-2500	Oral moisturizer	Moisturizing mouth spray for a dry mouth indication	Moisturizes mouth and helps it from drying out	Active: Glycerin 35% (prediluted) Other: Cetylpyridinium chloride, copovidone, flavor, methylparaben, PEG-60 hydrogenated castor oil, propylparaben, sodium benzoate, sodium saccharin, water, xanthan gum, xylitol	Use as required up to a maximum of 30 times or 60 sprays a day; spray 1-2 times into the affected area of mouth; do not rinse out	1 oz bottle

PRODUCTS AND DRUGS TO TREAT DRY MOUTH (continued)

Medication	Manufacturer and Phone Number	Product Type	Manufacturer's Description	Indication	Ingredients	Directions for Use	Form and Availability
				Cholinergic Salivary Stimulants (Rx)			
Cevimeline (Evoxac®)	Daiichi Sankyo, Inc (877) 437-7763			Treats symptoms of dry mouth in patients with Sjögren's syndrome	Active: Cevimeline 30 mg Other: Lactose monohydrate, hydroxypropyl cellulose, magnesium stearate	1 capsule (30 mg) 3 times/day	30 mg capsules
Pilocarpine (Salagen®)	MGI Pharmaceuticals, Inc (800) 562-5580			Treats xerostomia caused by radiation therapy in patients with head/neck cancer, Sjögren's syndrome	Active: Pilocarpine 5 mg and 7.5 mg Other: Carnauba wax, hydroxypropyl methylcellulose, iron oxide, microcrystalline cellulose, stearic acid, titanium dioxide	1-2 tablets (5 mg) 3-4 times/day, not to exceed 30 mg/day	5 mg tablets

DENTIN HYPERSENSITIVITY, HIGH CARIES INDEX, AND XEROSTOMIA *(Continued)*

CHOLINERGIC SALIVARY STIMULANTS (PRESCRIPTION ONLY)

Pilocarpine (Dental)(Salagen® *on page 1301*), approved in 1994, and cevimeline (Evoxac® *on page 325*), approved in 2000, are cholinergic drugs which stimulate salivary flow. They stimulate muscarinic-type acetylcholine receptors in salivary glands within the parasympathetic division of the autonomic nervous system, causing an increase in serous-type saliva. Thus, they are considered cholinergic, muscarinic-type (parasympathomimetic) drugs. Due to significant side effects caused by these drugs, they are available by prescription only.

Pilocarpine (Salagen®) is indicated for the treatment of xerostomia caused by radiation therapy in patients with head and neck cancer and xerostomia in patients suffering from Sjögren's syndrome. The usual adult dosage is 1-2 tablets (5 mg or 7.5 mg) 3-4 times/ day, not to exceed 30 mg/day. Patients should be treated for a minimum of 90 days for optimum effect. The most frequent adverse side effect is perspiration, which occurs in about 30% of patients who use 5 mg 3 times/day. Other adverse effects (in about 10% of patients) are nausea, rhinitis, chills, frequent urination, dizziness, headache, lacrimation, and pharyngitis. Salagen® is contraindicated for patients with uncontrolled asthma and narrow-angle glaucoma.

The salivary-stimulative effects of oral pilocarpine have been documented since the late 1960s and 1970s. Pilocarpine has been documented to overcome xerostomia from different causes. More recent studies confirm its effectiveness in improving salivary flow in patients undergoing irradiation therapy for head and neck cancer. A capstone study by Johnson, et al, reported the effects of pilocarpine in 208 irradiation patients at 39 different treatment sites. Salagen®, at a dose of 5 mg 3 times/day, improved salivation in 44% of patients, compared with 25% in the placebo group. They concluded that treatment with pilocarpine (Salagen®) produced the best overall outcome with respect to saliva production and relief of symptoms of xerostomia in patients undergoing irradiation therapy.

Additional studies have been published showing the effectiveness of pilocarpine (Salagen®) in stimulating salivary flow in patients suffering from Sjögren's syndrome and the FDA has approved the use of Salagen® for this indication.

Recent reports suggest that pre-emptive use of pilocarpine may be effective in protecting salivary glands during therapeutic irradiation; further studies are needed to confirm this. As of this publication date, the use of pilocarpine has not been approved to treat xerostomia induced by chronic medication. Pilocarpine could be used as a sialagogue for individuals with xerostomia induced by antidepressants and other medications. However, the potential for serious drug interactions is a concern and more studies are needed to clarify the safety and effectiveness of pilocarpine when given in the presence of other medications.

Cevimeline (Evoxac®) is indicated for treatment of symptoms of dry mouth in patients with Sjögren's syndrome. The usual dosage in adults is 1 capsule (30 mg) 3 times/day. Cevimeline (Evoxac®) is supplied in 30 mg capsules. Some adverse effects reported for Evoxac® include increased sweating (19%), nausea (14%), rhinitis (11%), sinusitis (12%), and upper respiratory infection (11%). Evoxac® is contraindicated for patients with uncontrolled asthma, narrow-angle glaucoma, acute iritis, and other conditions where miosis is undesirable. Cevimeline's half-life elimination is significantly slower than pilocarpines (0.76 hours versus 5 hours).

OTHER DRUGS IMPLICATED IN XEROSTOMIA

>10%	1% to 10%
Alprazolam	Acrivastine and Pseudoephedrine
Amitriptyline hydrochloride	Albuterol
Amoxapine	Amantadine hydrochloride
Anisotropine methylbromide	Amphetamine sulfate
Atropine sulfate	Astemizole (withdrawn from market)
Belladonna and Opium	Azatadine maleate
Benztropine mesylate	Beclomethasone dipropionate
Bupropion	Bepridil hydrochloride
Chlordiazepoxide	Bitolterol mesylate
Clomipramine hydrochloride	Brompheniramine maleate
Clonazepam	Carbinoxamine and Pseudoephedrine
Clonidine	Chlorpheniramine maleate
Clorazepate dipotassium	Clemastine fumarate
Cyclobenzaprine	Clozapine
Desipramine hydrochloride	Cromolyn sodium
Diazepam	Cyproheptadine hydrochloride
Dicyclomine hydrochloride	Dexchlorpheniramine maleate
Diphenoxylate and Atropine	Dextroamphetamine sulfate
Doxepin hydrochloride	Dimenhydrinate
Ergotamine	Diphenhydramine hydrochloride
Estazolam	Disopyramide phosphate
Flavoxate	Doxazosin
Flurazepam hydrochloride	Dronabinol
Glycopyrrolate	Ephedrine sulfate
Guanabenz acetate	Flumazenil
Guanfacine hydrochloride	Fluvoxamine
Hyoscyamine sulfate	Gabapentin
Interferon alfa-2a	Guaifenesin and Codeine
Interferon alfa-2b	Guanadrel sulfate
Interferon alfa-N3	Guanethidine sulfate
Ipratropium bromide	Hydroxyzine
Isoproterenol	Hyoscyamine, Atropine, Scopolamine, and Phenobarbital
Isotretinoin	Imipramine
Loratadine	Isoetharine
Lorazepam	Levocabastine hydrochloride
Loxapine	Levodopa
Maprotiline hydrochloride	Levodopa and Carbidopa
Methscopolamine bromide	Levorphanol tartrate
Molindone hydrochloride	Meclizine hydrochloride
Nabilone	Meperidine hydrochloride
Nefazodone	Methadone hydrochloride
Oxybutynin chloride	Methamphetamine hydrochloride
Oxazepam	Methyldopa
Paroxetine	Metoclopramide
Phenelzine sulfate	Morphine sulfate
Prochlorperazine	Nortriptyline hydrochloride
Propafenone hydrochloride	Ondansetron
Protriptyline hydrochloride	Oxycodone and Acetaminophen
Quazepam	Oxycodone and Aspirin
Reserpine	Pentazocine
Selegiline hydrochloride	Phenylpropanolamine hydrochloride
Temazepam	Prazosin hydrochloride
Thiethylperazine maleate	Promethazine hydrochloride
Trihexyphenidyl hydrochloride	Propoxyphene
Trimipramine maleate	Pseudoephedrine
Venlafaxine	Risperidone
	Sertraline hydrochloride
	Terazosin
	Terbutaline sulfate

TEMPOROMANDIBULAR DYSFUNCTION (TMD)

Temporomandibular dysfunction comprises a broad spectrum of signs and symptoms. Although TMD presents in patterns, diagnosis is often difficult. Evaluation and treatment is time-intensive and no single therapy or drug regimen has been shown to be universally beneficial.

The thorough diagnostician should perform a screening examination for the temporomandibular joint on all patients. Ideally, a baseline maximum mandibular opening along with lateral and protrusive movement evaluation should be performed. Secondly, the joint area should be palpated and an adequate exam of the muscles of mastication and the muscles of the neck and shoulders should be made. These muscle would include the elevators of the mandible (masseter, internal pterygoid, and temporalis); the depressors of the mandible (including the external pterygoid and digastric); extrusive muscles (including the temporalis and digastric), and protrusive muscles (including the external and internal pterygoids). These muscles also account for lateral movement of the mandible. The clinician should also be alert to indicators of dysfunction, primarily a history of pain with jaw function, chronic history of joint noise (although this can often be misinterpreted), pain in the muscles of the neck, limited jaw movement, pain in the actual muscles of mastication, and headache or even earache. The signs and symptoms are extremely variable and the clinician should be alert for any or all of these areas of interest. Because of the complexity of both evaluation and diagnosis, the general dentist often finds it too time consuming to spend the countless hours evaluating and treating the temporomandibular dysfunction patient. Therefore, oral medicine specialists trained in temporomandibular evaluation and treatment often accept referrals for the management of these complicated patients.

The oral medicine specialist in TMD management, the physical therapist interested in head and neck pain, and the oral and maxillofacial surgeon will all work together with the referring general dentist to accomplish successful patient treatment. Table 1 lists the wide variety of treatment alternatives available to the team. Depending on the diagnosis, one or more of the therapies might be selected. For organic diseases of the joint not responding to nonsurgical approaches, a wide variety of surgical techniques are available (Table 2).

ACUTE TMD

Acute TMD oftentimes presents alone or as an episode during a chronic pattern of signs and symptoms. Trauma, such as a blow to the chin or the side of the face, can result in acute TMD. Occasionally, similar symptoms will follow a lengthy wide open mouth dental procedure.

The condition usually presents as continuous deep pain in the TMJ. If edema is present in the joint, the condyle sometimes can be displaced which will cause abnormal occlusion of the posterior teeth on the affected side. The diagnosis is usually based on the history and clinical presentation. Management of the patient includes:

1. Restriction of all mandibular movement to function in a pain-free range of motion

2. Soft diet

3. NSAIDs (eg, Anaprox® DS 1 tablet every 12 hours for 7-10 days)

4. Moist heat applications to the affected area for 15-20 minutes, 4-6 times/day

5. Consideration of a muscle relaxant, such as Methocarbamol (Robaxin®) *on page 1065*, adult patient of average height/weight, two (500 mg) tablets at bedtime; daytime dose can be tailored to patient

Additional therapies could include referral to a physical therapist for ultrasound therapy 2-4 times/week and a single injection of steroid in the joint space. A team approach with an oral maxillofacial surgeon for this procedure may be helpful. Spray and stretch with Fluori-Methane® is often helpful for rapid relief of trismus.

Dichlorodifluoromethane and Trichloromonofluoromethane *on page 485*

CHRONIC TMD

Following diagnosis which is often problematic, the most common therapeutic modalities include:

- Explaining the problem to the patient
- Recommending a soft diet:

    Diet should consist of soft foods (eg, eggs, yogurt, casseroles, soup, ground meat).

    Avoid chewing gum, salads, large sandwiches, and hard fruit.
- Reducing stress; moist heat application 4-6 times/day for 15-20 minutes coupled with a monitored exercise program will be beneficial. Usually, working with a physical therapist is ideal.
- Medications include analgesics, anti-inflammatories, tranquilizers, and muscle relaxants

MEDICATION OPTIONS

Most commonly used medication (NSAIDs)

Tranquilizers and muscle relaxants, when used appropriately, can provide excellent adjunctive therapy. These drugs should be primarily used for a short period of time to manage acute pain. In low dosages, amitriptyline is often used to treat chronic pain and occasionally migraine headache. Two drugs similar to the prototype drug, amitriptyline, have been approved for use in adults only, for treatment of acute migraine with or without aura: Almotriptan malate (Axert™ [tablets]; Pharmacia Corp) and frovatriptan succinate (Frova™ [tablets]; Endo Pharmaceuticals). Other approved abortive (but not preventative) antimigraine triptan drugs include eletriptan (Relpax®), naratriptan (Amerge®), rizatriptan (Maxalt®), sumatriptan (Imitrex®), and zolmitriptan (Zomig®). Selective serotonin reuptake inhibitors (SSRIs) are sometimes used in the management of chronic neuropathic pain, particularly in patients not responding to amitriptyline. Recently, gabapentin (Neurontin®) has been approved for chronic pain. Problems of inducing bruxism with SSRIs, however, have been reported and may preclude their use. Clinicians attempting to evaluate any patient with bruxism or involuntary muscle movement, who is simultaneously being treated with an SSRI, should be aware of this potential association.

See individual monographs for dosing instructions.

Common minor tranquilizers include:

Chronic neuropathic pain management:

Acute migraine management:

TEMPOROMANDIBULAR DYSFUNCTION (TMD) *(Continued)*

Common muscle relaxants include:
>Chlorzoxazone *on page 348*
>Cyclobenzaprine *on page 421*
>Methocarbamol *on page 1065*
>Orphenadrine *on page 1212*

Note: Muscle relaxants and tranquilizers should generally be prescribed with an analgesic or NSAID to relieve pain as well.

Narcotic analgesics can be used on a short-term basis or intermittently in combination with non-narcotic therapy in the chronic pain patient. Judicious prescribing, monitoring, and maintenance by the practitioner is imperative whenever considering the use of narcotic analgesics due to the abuse and addiction liabilities.

Table 1.
TMD - NONSURGICAL THERAPIES

1. Moist heat and cold spray
2. Injections in muscle trigger areas (procaine)
3. Exercises (passive, active)
4. Medications
   a. Muscle relaxants
   b. Minerals (magnesium, glucosamine, chondroitin)
   c. Multiple vitamins (Ca, B_6, B_{12})
   d. NSAIDs, opioid combinations, antidepressants
5. Orthopedic craniomandibular repositioning appliance (splints)
6. Biofeedback, acupuncture
7. Physiotherapy: TMJ muscle therapy
8. Myofunctional therapy (occasionally)
9. TENS (transcutaneous electrical neural stimulation), Myo-Monitor (occasionally)
10. Dental therapy
    a. Equilibration (coronoplasty) (occasionally)
    b. Restoring occlusion to proper vertical dimension of maxilla to mandible by orthodontics, dental restorative procedures, orthognathic surgery, permanent splint, or any combination of these

Table 2.
TMD – SURGICAL THERAPIES

1. Cortisone injection into joint (with local anesthetic)
2. Bony and/or fibrous ankylosis: requires surgery (osteoarthrotomy with prosthetic appliance)
3. Chronic subluxation: requires surgery, depending on problem (possibly eminectomy and/or prosthetic implant)
4. Osteoarthritis: requires surgery (arthroscopy), depending on problem
   a. Arthroplasty
   b. Meniscectomy
   c. Arthroplasty with repair of disc
   d. Arthrocentesis
5. Rheumatoid arthritis
   a. Arthroplasty
   b. "Total" TMJ replacement
6. Tumors: require osteoarthrotomy – removal of tumor and restoring of joint when possible
7. Chronic disc displacement: Arthroscopy with arthrocentesis; possible removal of bone from condyle

SEDATION

Anxiety constitutes the most frequently found psychiatric problem in the general population. Anxiety can range from simple phobias to severe debilitating anxiety disorders. Functional results of this anxiety can, therefore, range from simple avoidance of dental procedures to panic attacks when confronting stressful situations such as seen in some patients regarding dental visits. Many patients claim to be anxious over dental care when in reality they simply have not been managed with modern techniques of local anesthesia, the availability of sedation, or the caring dental practitioner.

The dentist may detect anxiety in patients during the treatment planning evaluation phase of the care. The anxious person may appear overly alert, may lean forward in the dental chair during conversation or may appear concerned over time, possibly using this as a guise to require that they cut short their dental visit. Anxious persons may also show signs of being nervous by demonstrating sweating, tension in their muscles including their temporomandibular musculature, or they may complain of being tired due to an inability to obtain an adequate night's sleep.

The management of such patients requires a methodical approach to relaxing the patient, discussing their dental needs, and then planning, along with the patient the best way to accomplish dental treatment in the presence of their fears, either real or imagined. Consideration may be given to sedation to assist with managing the patient. This sedation can be oral or parenteral, or inhalation in the case of nitrous oxide. The dentist must be adequately trained in administering the sedative of choice, as well as in monitoring the patient during the sedated procedures. Numerous medications are available to achieve the level of sedation usually necessary in the dental office: Valium®, Ativan®, Xanax®, Vistaril®, Serax®, and BuSpar® represent a few. These oral sedatives can be given prior to dental visits as outlined in the following prescriptions. They have the advantage of allowing the patient a good night's sleep prior to the day of the procedures and providing on-the-spot sedation during the procedures. Nitrous oxide represents an in the office administered sedative that is relatively safe, but requires additional training and carefully planned monitoring protocols of any auxiliary personnel during the inhalation procedures. Both the oral and the inhalation techniques can, however, be applied in a very useful manner to manage the anxious patient in the dental office.

It is recommended that patients not drive themselves to or from dental appointments following use of these medications. Also, these medications should not be prescribed during pregnancy.

Alprazolam *on page 75*
Buspirone *on page 244*
Diazepam *on page 480*
Hydroxyzine *on page 846*
Lorazepam *on page 1001*
Nitrous Oxide *on page 1184*
Oxazepam *on page 1220*
Prochlorperazine *on page 1356*
Triazolam *on page 1613*

Note: Although various antidepressants have been used for preprocedure sedation, no specific regimens or protocols have been established. Guidelines for use are still under study.

Doxepin *on page 531*
Fluoxetine *on page 714*
Fluvoxamine *on page 734*
Paroxetine *on page 1254*
Sertraline *on page 1463*
Trazodone *on page 1603*

For examples of sample prescriptions see Sedation (Prior to Dental Treatment) *on page 1846*

MANAGEMENT OF PATIENTS UNDERGOING CANCER THERAPY

CANCER PATIENT DENTAL PROTOCOL

The objective in treatment of a patient with cancer is eradication of the disease. Oral complications, such as mucosal ulceration, xerostomia, bleeding, and infections can cause significant morbidity and may compromise systemic treatment of the patient. With proper oral evaluation before systemic treatment, many of the complications can be minimized or prevented.

MUCOSITIS

Normal oral mucosa acts as a barrier against chemical and food irritants and oral microorganisms. Disruption of the mucosal barrier can therefore lead to secondary infection, increased pain, delayed healing, and decreased nutritional intake.

Mucositis is inflammation of the mucous membranes. It is a common reaction to chemotherapy and radiation therapy. It is first seen as an erythematous patch. The mucosal epithelium becomes thin as a result of the killing of the rapidly dividing basal layer mucosal cells. Seven to ten days after cytoreduction chemotherapy and between 1000 cGy and 3000 cGy of radiation to the head and neck, mucosal tissues begin to desquamate and eventually develop into frank ulcerations. The mucosal integrity is broken and is secondarily infected by normal oral flora. The resultant ulcerations can also act as a portal of entry for pathogenic organisms into the patient's bloodstream and may lead to systemic infections. These ulcerations often force interruption of therapy.

Prevention of radiation mucositis is difficult. Stents can be constructed to prevent irradiation of uninvolved tissues. The use of multiple ports and fractionation of therapy into smaller doses over a longer period of time can reduce the severity. Fractured restorations, sharp teeth, and ill-fitted prostheses can damage soft tissues and lead to additional interruption of mucosal barriers. Correction of these problems before radiation therapy can diminish these complications.

CHEMOTHERAPY

Chemotherapy for neoplasia also frequently results in oral complications. Infections and mucositis are the most common complications seen in patients receiving chemotherapy. Also occurring frequently are pain, altered nutrition, and xerostomia, which can significantly affect the quality of life.

Certain chemotherapeutic agents, such as 5-fluorouracil, methotrexate, and doxorubicin, are more commonly associated with the development of oral mucositis. Treatment of oral mucositis is mainly palliative, but steps should be taken to minimize secondary pathogenic infections. Culture and sensitivity data should be obtained to select appropriate therapy for the bacterial, viral, or fungal organisms found.

RADIATION CARIES

Dental caries that sometimes follows radiation therapy is called radiation caries. It usually develops in the cervical smooth surface region of the teeth adjacent to the gingiva, often affecting many teeth. It is secondary to the irreversible damage done to the salivary glands and is initiated by dental plaque, but its rapid progress is due to changes in saliva. In addition to the diminution in the amount of saliva, both the salivary pH and buffering capacity are diminished, which decreases anticaries activity of saliva. Oral bacterial flora also change with xerostomia leading to the increase in caries activity. Typically patients that receive a cumulative radiation dose of 30 Gy or more will suffer significant loss of saliva production.

SALIVARY CHANGES

Chemotherapy is not thought to directly alter salivary flow, but alterations in taste and subjective sensations of dry mouth are relatively common complaints. Patients with mucositis and graft-vs-host disease following bone marrow or stem cell transplantation often demonstrate signs and symptoms of xerostomia. Radiation does directly affect salivary production. Radiation to the salivary glands produces fibrosis and alters the production of saliva. If all the major salivary glands are in the field, the decrease in saliva can be dramatic and the serous portion of the glands seems to be most severely affected. The saliva produced is increased in viscosity, which contributes to food retention and increased plaque formation. These xerostomic patients have difficulty in managing a normal diet. Normal saliva also has bacteriostatic properties that are diminished in these patients.

The dental management recommendations for patients undergoing chemotherapy, bone marrow transplantation, and/or radiation therapy for the treatment of cancer are based primarily on clinical observations. The following protocols will provide a conservative, consistent approach to the dental management of patients undergoing chemotherapy or bone marrow transplantation. Many of the cancer chemotherapy drugs produce oral side effects including mucositis, oral ulceration, dry mouth, acute infections, and taste aberrations. Cancer drugs include antibiotics, alkylating agents, antimetabolites, DNA inhibitors, hormones, and cytokines.

All patients undergoing chemotherapy or bone marrow transplantation for malignant disease should have the following baseline:

A. Panoramic radiograph

B. Dental consultation and examination

C. Dental prophylaxis and cleaning (if the neutrophil count is >1500/mm^3 and the platelet count is >50,000/mm^3)

    –   Prophylaxis and cleaning will be deferred if the patient's neutrophil count is <1500 and the platelet count is <50,000. Oral hygiene recommendations will be made. These levels are arbitrary guidelines and the dentist should consider the patient's oral condition and planned procedure relative to hemorrhage and level of bacteremia.

D. Oral Hygiene: Patients should be encouraged to follow normal hygiene procedures. Addition of a chlorhexidine mouth rinse such as Peridex® or PerioGard® *on page 332* is usually helpful. If the patient develops oral mucositis, tolerance of such alcohol-based products may be limited. Recently, a nonalcohol-containing chlorhexidine mouth rinse CHX® is also available.

E. If the patient develops mucositis, bacterial, viral, and fungal cultures should be obtained. Sucralfate suspension in a pharmacy-prepared form or Carafate® suspension, as well as Benadryl® *on page 510* or Xylocaine® viscous *on page 972* can assist in helping the patient to tolerate food. Patients may also require systemic and topical analgesics for pain relief depending on the presence of mucositis. Positive fungal cultures may require a nystatin swish-and-swallow prescription or the selection of another antifungal agent (see Fungal Infections *on page 1804*).

F. The determination of performing dental procedures must be based on the goal of preventing infection during periods of neutropenia. Timing of procedures must be coordinated with the patient's hematologic status.

G. If oral surgery is required, at least 7-10 days of healing should be allowed before the anticipated date of bone marrow suppression (eg, ANC <1000/mm^3 and/or platelet count of 50,000/mm^3).

H. Daily use of topical fluorides is recommended for those who have received radiation therapy to the head and neck region involving salivary glands. Any patients with prolonged xerostomia subsequent to graft-vs-host disease and/or chemotherapy can also be considered for fluoride supplement. Use the fluoride-containing mouthwashes (Act®, Fluorigard®, etc) each night before going to sleep; swish, hold 1-2 minutes, spit out or use prescription fluorides (gels or rinses); apply daily for 1-4 minutes as directed; if mouth is sore (mucositis), use flavorless/colorless gels (Thera-Flur®, Gel-Kam®). Custom trays for fluoride applications can be produced by the clinician for the patient's home use using heat-formed materials such as omnivan. Improvement in salivary flow following radiation therapy to the head and neck has been noted with prescription sialogogues Salagen® *on page 1301* or Evoxac® *on page 325*.

> Benzonatate *on page 200*
> Cevimeline *on page 325*
> Chlorhexidine Gluconate *on page 332*
> Diphenhydramine *on page 510*
> Lidocaine *on page 972*
> MuGard™
> Pilocarpine (Oral) *on page 1301*
> Povidone-Iodine *on page 1332*
> Sucralfate *on page 1499*

OSTEONECROSIS OF THE JAW

Osteonecrosis of the jaw (ONJ) is an uncommon condition that results in exposure of bone in the oral cavity along with other signs and symptoms that may be associated with changes in bone metabolism and/or poor wound healing, but also can develop spontaneously, such as along the myelohyoid ridge, away from teeth, or any site where obvious trauma could have occurred. Cases of ONJ began to emerge in approximately 2003 and were linked primarily with patients with cancer and those receiving the drugs zoledronic acid (Zometa®) *on page 1685* and/or pamidronate (Aredia®) *on page 1245* which are bisphosphonates administered by an intravenous route. A third intravenous bisphosphonate, clodronate (Bonefos®) is encountered much less commonly. Other bisphosphonates have been used for many years in the treatment of osteoporosis, Paget's disease, and other bone mineralization diseases. These include a group of bisphosphonates that are administered orally.

Bone disease occurs in many patients with cancer, particularly those with multiple myeloma and metastatic lesions associated with breast cancer, prostate cancer, and other cancers. These changes are often associated with pain and pathologic fractures. This bone destruction often results from changes in the osteoclast and osteoblast activities related to bone remodeling and healing following trauma. Bisphosphonates act at sites of active bone remodeling, changing the activity of the cells necessary for osteoclastic activity. There are no data that indicate that bisphosphonates directly change

MANAGEMENT OF PATIENTS UNDERGOING CANCER
THERAPY *(Continued)*

mineralization of the bone, however, these drugs do result in changes in the vascularity of the bone and cell activity.

Since the emergence of numerous cases of ONJ and their documentation, the American Dental Association through its Council on Scientific Affairs has released various news reports and position statements related to the state of the current knowledge and recommendations for the practicing dental professionals to manage patients who may be at risk for ONJ. Most of the data that exist are related to the use of intravenous bisphosphonates in cancer patients.

Related to patients receiving intravenous bisphosphonate therapy, invasive dental procedures should be avoided in patients receiving these drugs and, if possible, the dentist should carry out invasive procedures for those patients who are planning to begin treatment with I.V. bisphosphonates and should carry out those treatments prior to the beginning of the periodic infusions with the intravenous drugs. Clinical judgment by the treating physician should guide the management plan with each patient based on communication with the dentist. For patients requiring dental procedures, there are no data available to suggest whether discontinuation of bisphosphonate treatment reduces the risk of ONJ. Clinical judgment of the treating physician should guide the management plan of each patient based on individual benefit:risk assessment. If a patient requires invasive therapy while on bisphosphonate therapy, consultation, advisement of the patient, and judicious use of other dental options would be appropriate.

There are five primary actions in this management plan:

1. Patients should be educated on maintaining excellent oral hygiene to reduce the risk of need for invasive procedures in the future.

2. Patients should check and adjust removable appliances such as prostheses to avoid soft tissue injury.

3. Routine cleaning should be performed with care, attempting to reduce any soft tissue injury; however, since hygiene is important, the normal recall planning and treatment should continue.

4. Dental infection should be managed aggressively and nonsurgically when possible. Alternatives such as endodontic therapy or over extraction may be advisable.

5. Endodontic therapy is preferable to extractions and even treatment with endodontics followed coronal amputation and root canal therapy on the retained roots may be necessary to avoid an intra-boney such as surgery.

The latest reference on the management treatment of patients with osteonecrosis of the jaw has been published in the *Journal of Oncology Practice*. All of the information contained in these recommendations is available through the drug companies' precautionary statements as well as doctor letters which have been disseminated to every practicing dentist in the world. In addition, new information is emerging as data develop.

ORAL CARE PRODUCTS

BACTERIAL PLAQUE CONTROL

Patients should use an extra soft bristle toothbrush and dental floss for removal of plaque. Sponge/foam sticks and lemon-glycerine swabs do not adequately remove bacterial plaque.

CHOLINERGIC AGENTS

See Products for Xerostomia *on page 1812*

Used for the treatment of xerostomia caused by radiation therapy in patients with head and neck cancer and from Sjögren's syndrome

Cevimeline *on page 325*
Pilocarpine (Oral) *on page 1301*

FLUORIDES

See Fluorides in the Dentin Hypersensitivity, High Caries Index, and Xerostomia section.

Used for the prevention of demineralization of the tooth structure secondary to xerostomia. For patients with long-term or permanent xerostomia, daily application is accomplished using custom gel applicator trays, such as omnivac. Patients with porcelain crowns should use a neutral pH fluoride (see Fluoride monograph *on page 710*). Final selection of a fluoride product and/or saliva replacement/stimulant product must be based on patient comfort, taste, and ultimately, compliance. Experience has demonstrated that, often times, patients must try various combinations to achieve the greatest effect and their highest comfort levels. The presence of mucositis during cancer management complicates the clinician's selection of products.

SALIVA SUBSTITUTES

See Products for Xerostomia *on page 1812*

ORAL AND LIP MOISTURIZERS/LUBRICANTS

See Mouth Pain, Cold Sore, and Canker Sore Products *on page 1938*

Note: Water-based gels should first be used to provide moisture to dry oral tissues.

Surgi-Lube®
K-Y Jelly®
Oral Balance®
Mouth Moisturizer®
Caphosol®

PALLIATION OF PAIN

See Mouth Pain, Cold Sore, and Canker Sore Products *on page 1938*

Note: Palliative pain preparations should be monitored for efficacy.

- For relief of pain associated with isolated ulcerations, topical anesthetic and protective preparations may be used.

  Orabase-B® with 20% benzocaine *on page 195*
  Zilactin-B® gel with 10% benzocaine

- For generalized oral pain:

  Chloraseptic Spray® (OTC) anesthetic spray without alcohol *on page 1290*
  Ulcer-Ease® anesthetic/analgesic mouthrinse
  BetaCell® oral rinse
  Xylocaine® 2% viscous *on page 972*

  Note: May anesthetize swallowing mechanism and cause aspiration of food; caution patient against using too close to eating; lack of sensation may also allow patient to damage intact mucosa

  Tantum Mouthrinse® (benzydamine hydrochloride); may be diluted as required

  Note: Available only in Canada and Europe

PATIENT PREPARED PALLIATIVE MIXTURES

Coating agents:

Maalox® *on page 81*
Mylanta® *on page 82*
Kaopectate® *on page 170*

These products can be mixed with Benadryl® elixir (50:50):

Diphenhydramine (Benadryl®) *on page 510*

Mouth Pain, Cold Sore, and Canker Sore Products *on page 1938*

Topical anesthetics (diphenhydramine chloride):

Benadryl® elixir or Benylin® cough syrup *on page 510*

Note: Choose product with lowest alcohol and sucrose content; ask pharmacist for assistance
Mucotrol gel wafer

PHARMACY PREPARATIONS

A pharmacist may also prepare the following solutions for relief of generalized oral pain:

Benadryl-Lidocaine Solution

Diphenhydramine injectable 1.5 mL (50 mg/mL) *on page 510*
Xylocaine viscous 2% (45 mL) *on page 972*
Magnesium aluminum hydroxide solution (45 mL)
Swish and hold 1 teaspoonful in mouth for 30 seconds; do not use too close to eating

MANAGEMENT OF PATIENTS UNDERGOING CANCER THERAPY *(Continued)*

References

ADA Council on Scientific Affairs. Expert Panel Recommendations: Dental Management of Patients on Oral Bisphosphonate Therapy, June 2006. Available at: http://www.ada.org/prof/resources/pubs/jada/reports/report_bisphosphonate.pdf.

Badros A, Weikel D, Salama A, et al, "Osteonecrosis of the Jaw in Multiple Myeloma Patients: Clinical Features and Risk Factors," *J Clin Oncol*, 2006, 24(6):945-52.

Expert Panel Recommendations for the Prevention, Diagnosis, and Treatment of Osteonecrosis of the Jaws, June 2004. Available at: http://www.ada.org/prof/resources/topics/topics_osteonecrosis_whitepaper.pdf.

Migliorati CA, Casiglia J, Epstein J, et al, "Managing the Care of Patients With Bisphosphonate-Associated Osteonecrosis: An American Academy of Oral Medicine Position Paper," *J Am Dent Assoc*, 2005, 136(12):1658-68.

Ott SM, "Long-Term Safety of Bisphosphonates," *J Clin Endocrinol Metab*, 2005, 90(3):1294-301.

Ruggiero S, Gralow J, Marx RE, et al, "Practical Guidelines for the Prevention, Diagnosis, and Treatment of Osteonecrosis of the Jaw in Patients With Cancer," *Journal of Oncology Practice*, 2006, 2(1):7-14.

Ruggiero SL, Mehrotra B, Rosenberg TJ, et al, "Osteonecrosis of the Jaws Associated With the Use of Bisphosphonates: A Review of 63 Cases," *J Oral Maxillofac Surg*, 2004, 62(5):527-34.

Woo SB, Hande K, and Richardson PG, "Osteonecrosis of the Jaw and Bisphosphonates," *N Engl J Med*, 2005, 353(1):99-102.

ORAL MEDICINE TOPICS

PART III:

SAMPLE PRESCRIPTIONS

Drug prescriptions shown represent prototype drugs and popular prescriptions and are examples only. The pharmacologic category index is available for cross-referencing if alternatives and additional drugs are sought.

TABLE OF CONTENTS

INFECTIVE ENDOCARDITIS (PREVENTION)

General Prescription Comments

Prescriptions dispense amounts are for 3 visits. These numbers can be adjusted for each patient treatment plan.

Sample Prescriptions

Rx:

Amoxicillin 500 mg
Disp: 12 tablets
Sig: 4 tablets (2 g) 30-60 minutes prior to dental visit and repeat at each appointment

Rx:

Clindamycin 150 mg
Disp: 12 capsules
Sig: 4 capsules (600 mg) 30-60 minutes prior to dental visit and repeat at each appointment

Rx:

Cephalexin 500 mg
Disp: 12 tablets
Sig: 4 tablets (2 g) 30-60 minutes prior to dental visit and repeat at each appointment

Rx:

Azithromycin 500 mg
Disp: 3 tablets
Sig: 1 tablet 30-60 minutes prior to dental visit and repeat at each appointment

PROSTHETIC JOINT LATE INFECTIONS (PREVENTION)

General Prescription Comments

Prescriptions dispense amounts are for 3 visits. These numbers can be adjusted for each patient treatment plan.

Sample Prescriptions

Rx:

Amoxicillin 500 mg
Disp: 12 tablets
Sig: 4 tablets (2 g) 1 hour prior to dental visit and repeat at each appointment

Rx:

Clindamycin 150 mg
Disp: 12 capsules
Sig: 4 capsules (600 mg) 1 hour prior to dental visit and repeat at each appointment

Rx:

Cephalexin 500 mg
Disp: 12 tablets
Sig: 4 tablets (2 g) 1 hour prior to dental visit and repeat at each appointment

ORAL PAIN

Mild / Moderate Oral Pain

General Prescription Comments

Closely monitor and re-evaluate response at least every 2 weeks. If response is inadequate, re-evaluate diagnosis, medication choice, and dosage.

Sample Prescriptions

Rx:

Acetaminophen 325 mg tablets
Disp: To be determined by practitioner
Sig: Take 2-3 tablets every 4 hours

Note: Products include Tylenol® and others.
Note: Acetaminophen can be given if patient has allergies, bleeding problems, or stomach upset secondary to aspirin or NSAIDs.

Rx:

Ibuprofen 200 mg tablets
Disp: To be determined by practitioner
Sig: Take 1-2 tablets every 4 hours

Note: Ibuprofen is an available OTC as Advil®, Motrin® IB, Nuprin®, and many store brand generic names. NSAIDs should not be combined with aspirin. NSAIDs may increase post-treatment bleeding. Use with caution in patients receiving anticoagulants or antiplatelet drugs.

Rx:

Naproxen sodium 220 mg tablets
Disp: To be determined by practitioner
Sig: Take 1-2 tablets every 8 hours

Note: Naproxen sodium is an available OTC as Aleve® and many store brand generic names.

Rx:

Ibuprofen 400 mg tablets
Disp: 20 tablets
Sig: Take 1 tablet every 4-6 hours as needed for pain

Note: Prescription strength ibuprofen is available as the brand name Motrin®.

Rx:

Dolobid® 500 mg tablets
Disp: 16 tablets
Sig: Take 2 tablets initially, then 1 tablet every 8-12 hours as needed for pain
Ingredient: Diflunisal

Rx:

Belcalir bioadherent oral gel
Disp: 15 mL per single-dose packet; one box contains 21 single dose packets
Sig: 3 times/day or as often as needed, pour entire contents of single-dose packet into glass and add 1 tablespoon of water. Stir mixture and immediately rinse for at least 1 minute and expectorate. Avoid eating or drinking for at least 1 hour after use.

Rx:

Caphasol® neutral calcium/phosphate rinse
Disp: 30 mL
Sig: Rinse with 30 mL of solution 4 times/day following topical application of neutral 2% sodium fluoride gel administered by tray

Moderate / Moderately Severe Oral Pain

General Prescription Comments

Closely monitor and re-evaluate response at least every 2 weeks. If response is inadequate, re-evaluate diagnosis, medication choice, and dosage.

Sample Prescriptions

Rx:

Ibuprofen 800 mg tablets
Disp: 16 tablets
Sig: Take 1 tablet 3 times/day as needed for pain

Note: For severe pain can be given up to 4 times/day. Also available as 600 mg tablets.

Rx:

Tramadol 50 mg tablets
Disp: 36 tablets
Sig: Take 1-2 tablets every 4-6 hours as needed for pain

Note: Also available as the brand name Ultram®.

Rx:

Ultracet™ tablets
Disp: 36 tablets
Sig: Take 2 tablets every 4-6 hours as needed for pain, not to exceed 8 tablets in 24 hours

Ingredients: Acetaminophen 325 mg and tramadol 37.5 mg

Rx:

Darvocet-N® 100 tablets
Disp: 36 tablets
Sig: Take 1 tablet every 4 hours as needed for pain, not to exceed 6 tablets in 24 hours

Ingredients: Propoxyphene napsylate 100 mg and acetaminophen 650 mg

Rx:

Vicoprofen® tablets
Disp: 16 tablets
Sig: Take 1-2 tablets every 4-6 hours as needed for pain

Note: Restrictions: C-III; no refills
Ingredients: Hydrocodone 7.5 mg and ibuprofen 200 mg; available as generic equivalent

Rx:

Vicodin® ES tablets
Disp: 16 tablets
Sig: Take 1 tablet every 4-6 hours as needed for pain

Note: Restrictions: C-III; no refills
Ingredients: Hydrocodone bitartrate 7.5 mg and acetaminophen 750 mg; available as generic equivalent. Also available as Vicodin® tablets: Ingredients: Hydrocodone bitartrate 5 mg and acetaminophen 500 mg; take 1 tablet every 4 hours as needed for pain.

Rx:

Lortab® 5 mg
Disp: 16 tablets
Sig: Take 1 or 2 tablets every 4 hours as needed for pain; not to exceed 8 tablets in 24 hours

Note: Restrictions: C-III; no refills
Ingredients: Hydrocodone 5 mg and acetaminophen 500 mg; available as generic equivalent

Rx:

Tylenol® #3
Disp: 16 tablets
Sig: Take 1 tablet every 4 hours as needed for pain

Note: Restrictions: C-III; no refills
Ingredients: Codeine 30 mg and acetaminophen 300 mg; available as generic equivalent

Rx:

Naproxen 275 mg tablets
Disp: 16 tablets
Sig: Take 2 tablets initially, then one tablet 3 times/day as needed for pain

Severe Oral Pain

General Prescription Comments

Closely monitor and re-evaluate response at least every 2 weeks. If response is inadequate, re-evaluate diagnosis, medication choice, and dosage.

Liquid volumes are suggested for a typical 2-week course. Check with pharmacist for available sizes.

Cream and ointment tube sizes may vary based on availability. Refer to individual monograph or check with pharmacist for available sizes.

Sample Prescriptions

Rx:

Percocet® tablets or Tylox® capsules
Disp: 16 tablets or capsules
Sig: Take 1 tablet or capsule every 6 hours as needed for pain

Note: Restrictions: C-II; no refills
Ingredients: Oxycodone 5 mg and acetaminophen 325 mg (Tylox® contains acetaminophen 500 mg); available as generic equivalent; triplicate prescription required in some states

ORAL PAIN *(Continued)*

Rx:

Combunox™ tablets
Disp: 16 tablets
Sig: Take 1 tablet every 6 hours as needed for pain

Note: Restrictions: C-II; no refills
Ingredients: Oxycodone 5 mg and ibuprofen 400 mg; not available as generic
    equivalent; triplicate prescription required in some states

Rx:

Demerol® 50 mg tablets
Disp: 16 tablets
Sig: Take 1 tablet every 4 hours as needed for pain

Note: Restrictions: C-II; no refills
Ingredients: Meperidine; triplicate prescription required in some states

BACTERIAL INFECTIONS AND PERIODONTAL DISEASES

General Prescription Comments

Closely monitor and re-evaluate response at least every 2 weeks. If response is inadequate, re-evaluate diagnosis, medication choice, and dosage.

Sample Prescriptions

Rx:

Penicillin V potassium 500 mg
Disp: 40 tablets
Sig: Take 1 tablet 4 times/day for 7-10 days (consider a loading dose of 1 g for acute infection)

Rx:

Clindamycin 150 mg
Disp: 40 capsules
Sig: Take 1 capsule 4 times/day for 7-10 days

Note: Prescription for patients allergic to penicillin

Rx:

Clindamycin 300 mg
Disp: 40 capsules
Sig: Take 1 capsule 4 times/day for 7-10 days

Note: Prescription for patients allergic to penicillin

Rx:

Azithromycin 250 mg
Disp: 1 Z-Pak®
Sig: 2 tablets day 1, then 1 tablet/day until gone

OTHER ANTIBIOTICS:

Rx:

Amoxicillin 250 mg
Disp: 30 capsules
Sig: Take 1 capsule 3 times/day for 7-10 days

Rx:

Amoxicillin 500 mg
Disp: 30 capsules or tablets
Sig: Take 1 capsule or tablet 3 times/day for 7-10 days

Rx:

Amoxicillin 875 mg
Disp: 20 tablets
Sig: Take 1 tablet twice daily

Rx:

Augmentin® 250 mg
Disp: 30 tablets
Sig: Take 1 tablet 3 times/day for 7-10 days

Rx:

Augmentin® 500 mg
Disp: 30 tablets
Sig: Take 1 tablet 3 times/day for 7-10 days

Rx:

Augmentin® 875 mg
Disp: 20 tablets
Sig: Take 1 tablet twice daily for 7-10 days

Rx:

Augmentin XR™ 1000 mg
Disp: 20 tablets
Sig: Take 1 tablet twice daily for 7-10 days

Rx:

Cephalexin 250 mg
Disp: 40 capsules
Sig: Take 1 capsule 4 times/day for 7-10 days

Rx:

Metronidazole 500 mg
Disp: 40 tablets
Sig: Take 1 tablet 4 times/day for 7-10 days

Rx:

Erythromycin 250 mg
Disp: 40 tablets
Sig: Take 1 tablet 4 times/day for 7-10 days

Note: Prescription for patients allergic to penicillin

BACTERIAL INFECTIONS AND PERIODONTAL DISEASES
(Continued)

Rx:
Zithromax® TRI-PAK™ 500 mg
Disp: 1 PAK
Sig: Follow package insert directions until gone

Ingredient: Azithromycin

Rx:
Levaquin® 500 mg
Disp: 10 tablets
Sig: Take 1 tablet/day until gone

PERIODONTAL DISEASE

Note: Sample prescriptions based on dosing suggestions from the American Academy of Periodontology

Rx:
Azithromycin 500 mg tablets
Disp: Dispense a dose pack
Sig: Take 1 tablet daily for 4-7 days as directed

Rx:
Ciprofloxacin 100 mg tablets
Disp: 16 tablets
Sig: Take 1 tablet 2 times/day for 8 days

Rx:
Clindamycin 300 mg tablets
Disp: 24 tablets
Sig: Take 1 tablet 3 times/day for 8 days

Rx:
Doxycycline or minocycline 100-200 mg tablets
Disp: 21 tablets of selected dose
Sig: Take 1 tablet daily for 21 days

Rx:
Metronidazole 500 mg
Disp: 24 tablets
Sig: Take 1 tablet 3 times/day for 8 days

Rx:
Metronidazole and amoxicillin 250 mg tablets
Disp: 24 tablets of each drug
Sig: Take 1 tablet of each drug 3 times/day for 8 days

Rx:
Metronidazole and ciprofloxacin 500 mg tablets
Disp: 16 tablets of each drug
Sig: Take 1 tablet of each drug 2 times/day for 8 days

SINUS INFECTION TREATMENT

General Prescription Comments

Closely monitor and re-evaluate response at least every 2 weeks. If response is inadequate, re-evaluate diagnosis, medication choice, and dosage.

Sinus infections are not usually true infections. Some clinicians however, couple the medications listed below with antibiotics such as amoxicillin or Augmentin®. when they are uncertain.

Sample Prescriptions

Rx:

Afrin® nasal spray [OTC]
Disp: 15 mg
Sig: Spray once in each nostril every 6-8 hours for no more than 3 days

Ingredient: Oxymetazoline

Rx:

Sudafed® 60 mg tablets [OTC]
Disp: 30 tablets
Sig: Take 1 tablet every 4-6 hours as needed for congestion

Ingredient: Pseudoephedrine

Rx:

Chlor-Trimeton® 4 mg [OTC]
Disp: 14 tablets
Sig: Take 1 tablet twice daily

Ingredient: Chlorpheniramine

ANTIMICROBIAL ORAL RINSES

General Prescription Comments

Closely monitor and re-evaluate response at least every 2 weeks. If response is inadequate, re-evaluate diagnosis, medication choice, and dosage.

Liquid volumes for antimicrobial rinses are suggested for a typical 1 month course. Check with pharmacist for available sizes.

Sample Prescriptions

Rx:

Chlorhexidine gluconate 0.12% oral rinse
Disp: 32 oz bottle
Sig: Rinse with ½ oz twice daily for 30 seconds and expectorate

Note: Chlorhexidine gluconate available as the following brands: Peridex®, Perio-Gard®

Rx:

Listerine® antiseptic mouthwash [OTC]
Disp: Bottle
Sig: 20 mL, swish for 30 seconds twice daily

FUNGAL INFECTIONS

Topical Fungal Infections

General Prescription Comments

Closely monitor and re-evaluate response at least every 2 weeks. If response is inadequate, re-evaluate diagnosis, medication choice, and dosage.

Liquid volumes are suggested for a typical 2-week course. Check with pharmacist for available sizes.

Cream and ointment tube sizes may vary based on availability. Refer to individual monograph or check with pharmacist for available sizes.

Sample Prescriptions

Rx:

Nystatin 100,000 units/mL oral suspension
Disp: 300 mL
Sig: Rinse with 1 teaspoon (5 mL) for 2 minutes 4-5 times/day and expectorate

Rx:

Nystatin ointment
Disp: 45 g tube
Sig: Apply locally as directed with a thin coat to inner surface of denture and the affected area 4-5 times/day

Rx:

Mycelex® 10 mg troches
Disp: 70 troches
Sig: Dissolve 1 troche in mouth 5 times/day until gone; leave any prosthesis out during treatment and soak prosthesis in nystatin liquid suspension overnight

Ingredient: Clotrimazole

Rx:

Nizoral® 2% cream
Disp: 45 g tube
Sig: Apply locally as directed with a thin coat to inner surface of denture and affected areas after meals

Ingredient: Ketoconazole

Systemic Fungal Infections

General Prescription Comments

Note: Decision to use systemic antifungals should be based on diagnostic culture results or positive smear.

Closely monitor and re-evaluate response at least every 2 weeks. If response is inadequate, re-evaluate diagnosis, medication choice, and dosage.

Sample Prescriptions

Rx:

Nizoral® 200 mg tablets
Disp: 14 tablets
Sig: Take 1 tablet daily, with a meal for 2 weeks

Note: May cause irreversible liver damage; liver function should be monitored with long-term use (ie, >3 weeks)

Ingredient: Ketoconazole

Rx:

Diflucan® 100 mg tablets
Disp: 16 tablets
Sig: Take 2 tablets day 1, then 1 tablet/day until gone

Note: Sometimes a shorter course is adequate. However, oral infections commonly are more difficult to eradicate and even a second course may be necessary.
Ingredient: Fluconazole

Rx:

Posaconazole 100 mg tablets
Disp: 14 tablets
Sig: Take 2 tablets the first day, followed by 1 tablet each day for 13 days

Note: Posaconazole has been recently approved for use in patients refractory to itraconazole or fluconazole

FUNGAL INFECTIONS *(Continued)*

Angular Cheilitis

General Prescription Comments

Closely monitor and re-evaluate response at least every 2 weeks. If response is inadequate, re-evaluate diagnosis, medication choice, and dosage.

Cream and ointment tube sizes may vary based on availability. Refer to individual monograph or check with pharmacist for available sizes.

Sample Prescriptions

Rx:

Iodoquinol and hydrocortisone cream
Disp: 45 g tube
Sig: Apply locally as directed 3-4 times/day for 10 days to 2 weeks and then re-evaluate

Note: Available sizes may include 15 g, 30 g, 45 g, and 60 g tubes. Other associated etiologies for angular cheilitis must also be considered such as loss of vertical dimension, trauma, and vitamin deficiencies.

Rx:

Nystatin and triamcinolone acetonide ointment
Disp: 45 g tube
Sig: Apply locally as directed to affected area 4 times/day for 10 days to 2 weeks and then re-evaluate

Note: Available sizes may include 15 g, 30 g, 45 g, and 60 g tubes. Other associated etiologies for angular cheilitis must also be considered such as loss of vertical dimension, trauma, and vitamin deficiencies.

VIRAL INFECTIONS

Herpes Simplex (Primary)

General Prescription Comments

Closely monitor and re-evaluate response at least every 2 weeks. If response is inadequate, re-evaluate diagnosis, medication choice, and dosage.

Sample Prescriptions

Rx:

Zovirax 200 mg capsules
Disp: 50 or 60 capsules
Sig: Take 1 capsule 5 times/day for 10 days or 2 capsules 3 times/day for 10 days

Ingredient: Acyclovir

Herpes Simplex (Recurrent)

General Prescription Comments

Closely monitor and re-evaluate response at least every 2 weeks. If response is inadequate, re-evaluate diagnosis, medication choice, and dosage.

Cream and ointment tube sizes may vary based on availability. Refer to individual monograph or check with pharmacist for available sizes.

Sample Prescriptions

Rx:

Denavir® topical ointment 5%
Disp: 1.5 g tube
Sig: Apply locally as directed to lesion every 2 hours during waking hours (begin when symptoms first occur)

Ingredient: Penciclovir

Rx:

Famciclovir 125 mg
Disp: 10 tablets
Sig: 1 tablet twice daily for 5 days

Rx:

Valacyclovir 500 mg
Disp: 8 caplets
Sig: 4 caplets twice daily for 1 day (separate doses by 12 hours)

Rx:

Abreva® cream [OTC]
Disp: 2 g tube
Sig: Apply to lesion 5 times/day during waking hours for 4 days (begin when symptoms first occur)

Ingredient: Docosanol

Rx:

Viroxyn® [OTC]
Disp: 1 pack of 3 individual swab kits
Sig: Apply locally as directed at first symptoms of recurrence

Ingredient: Benzalkonium 0.13% in isopropyl alcohol

Shingles (Varicella-Zoster Virus)

General Prescription Comments

Closely monitor and re-evaluate response at least every 2 weeks. If response is inadequate, re-evaluate diagnosis, medication choice, and dosage.

Sample Prescriptions

Rx:

Zovirax® 200 mg capsules
Disp: 200 capsules
Sig: Take 4 capsules 5 times/day for 10 days

Ingredient: Acyclovir

Rx:

Famciclovir 500 mg
Disp: 21 tablets
Sig: 1 tablet 3 times/day for 7 days

ULCERATIVE AND EROSIVE DISORDERS

Recurrent Aphthous Stomatitis

General Prescription Comments

Some intraoral uses are off-label. Write directions as "use locally as directed" and closely monitor and re-evaluate response at least every 2 weeks. If response is inadequate, re-evaluate diagnosis, medication choice, and dosage.

Liquid volumes are suggested for a typical 2-week course. Check with pharmacist for available sizes.

Cream and ointment tube sizes may vary based on availability. Refer to individual monograph or check with pharmacist for available sizes.

Sample Prescriptions

Rx:

Amlexanox oral paste 5%
Disp: 5 g tube
Sig: Apply locally as directed, 4 times/day until area heals

Rx:

Orabase® Protective Barrier [OTC]
Disp: 1 package
Sig: Apply locally as directed, every 6 hours as needed

Rx:

Benadryl® liquid 12.5 mg/5 mL (mix 50/50) with Kaopectate®
Disp: 8 oz total
Sig: Rinse with 1-2 teaspoonfuls every 2 hours and expectorate.

Note: Maalox® can be used in place of Kaopectate® if constipation is a problem. Benadryl® is available as a generic diphenhydramine liquid.

Rx:

Benadryl® liquid 12.5 mg/5mL / Kaopectate® / Lidocaine viscous (mix 1/3, 1/3, 1/3)
Disp: 8 oz total
Sig: Rinse with 1-2 teaspoonfuls every 2 hours and expectorate

Note: Maalox® can be used in place of Kaopectate® if constipation is a problem. Benadryl® is available as a generic diphenhydramine liquid. Lidocaine viscous is available as a prescription only.

Rx:

Benadryl® liquid 12.5 mg/5mL
Disp: 4 oz bottle
Sig: Rinse with 1-2 teaspoonfuls every 2 hours and expectorate

Note: Benadryl® is available as a generic diphenhydramine liquid.

Rx:

Kenalog® in Orabase 0.1%
Disp: 5 g tube
Sig: Apply locally as directed to the lesion after each meal and at bedtime

Ingredient: Triamcinolone acetonide

Rx:

Lidex® 0.05% gel
Disp: 45 g tube
Sig: Apply locally as directed to lesion 4 times daily

Ingredient: Fluocinonide 0.05%

Rx:

Temovate® 0.05%
Disp: 45 g tube
Sig: Apply locally as directed a small quantity with a Q-tip to affected area 3-4 times/ day

Ingredient: Clobetasol propionate

Rx:

Valisone® 0.1%
Disp: 45 g tube
Sig: Apply locally as directed a small quantity with a Q-tip to affected area 3-4 times/ day

Ingredient: Betamethasone valerate

Rx:

Decadron® elixir 0.5 mg/5 mL
Disp: 300 mL
Sig: Rinse with 1 teaspoon for 2 minutes 4 times/day and expectorate

Ingredient: Dexamethasone

Note: Depending on severity of ulceration, instructions can be tailored to include swallowing initial doses and then tapering to every other dose eventually over 4-7 days to no swallowing. See Erosive Lichen Planus and Major Aphthae for more examples.

Mild Lichen Planus

General Prescription Comments

Some intraoral uses are off-label. Write directions as "use locally as directed" and closely monitor and re-evaluate response at least every 2 weeks. If response is inadequate, re-evaluate diagnosis, medication choice, and dosage.

Cream and ointment tube sizes may vary based on availability. Refer to individual monograph or check with pharmacist for available sizes.

Sample Prescriptions

Rx:

Kenalog® in Orabase 0.1%
Disp: 5 g tube
Sig: Apply locally as directed by coating the lesion with a thin film after each meal and at bedtime

Ingredient: Triamcinolone 0.1%

Rx:

Lidex® 0.05% gel
Disp: 45 g tube
Sig: Apply locally as directed to lesion 4 times daily

Ingredient: Fluocinonide 0.05%

Erosive Lichen Planus and Major Aphthae

General Prescription Comments

Some intraoral uses are off-label. Write directions as "use locally as directed" and closely monitor and re-evaluate response at least every 2 weeks. If response is inadequate, re-evaluate diagnosis, medication choice, and dosage.

Liquid volumes are suggested for a typical 2-week course. Check with pharmacist for available sizes.

Cream and ointment tube sizes may vary based on availability. Refer to individual monograph or check with pharmacist for available sizes.

Sample Prescriptions

Rx:

Decadron® 0.5 mg/5 mL elixir
Disp: 400 mL bottle
Sig: For 3 days, rinse with 1 tablespoonful (15 mL) 4 times/day and swallow; then for 3 days, rinse with 1 teaspoonful (5 mL) 4 times/day and swallow; then for 3 days, rinse with 1 teaspoonful (5 mL) 4 times/day and swallow every other time. Then for 3 days rinse with 1 teaspoonful (5 mL) 4 times/day and expectorate. Continue the rinse and expectorate mode for 2 minutes but discontinue medication when mouth becomes completely comfortable.

Ingredient: Dexamethasone; the practitioner can tailor this rinse, hold expectorate and/or swallow prescription to the severity and lesion location for each individual patient.

Rx:

Temovate® 0.05% cream
Disp: 15 g tube
Sig: Apply locally as directed 4-5 times/day

Ingredient: Clobetasol; high potency topical steroid

Rx:

Prednisone 5 mg tablets
Disp: 40 tablets
Sig: Take 5 tablets in the morning for 5 days, then 5 tablets in the morning every other day until gone

Rx:

Prednisone 10 mg tablets
Disp: 50 tablets
Sig: Take 4 tablets in the morning for 5 days, then decrease by 1 tablet on each successive series of 5 days

Rx:

Medrol® Dose Pak
Disp: 1 Pack
Sig: Follow package insert directions until gone

Ingredient: Methylprednisolone

SEDATION
(PRIOR TO DENTAL TREATMENT)

General Prescription Comments

Closely monitor and re-evaluate response at least every 2 weeks. If response is inadequate, re-evaluate diagnosis, medication choice, and dosage.

Sample Prescriptions

Rx:

> Valium® 5 mg
> Disp: 6 tablets
> Sig: Take 1 tablet in evening before going to bed and 1 tablet 1 hour before appointment
>
> **Note:** Also available as 2 mg and 10 mg.
> Ingredient: Diazepam

Rx:

> Ativan® 1 mg
> Disp: 4 tablets
> Sig: Take 2 tablets in evening before going to bed and 2 tablets 1 hour before appointment
>
> **Note:** Also available as 0.5 mg and 2 mg.
> Ingredient: Lorazepam

Rx:

> Xanax® 0.5 mg
> Disp: 4 tablets
> Sig: Take 1 tablet in evening before going to bed and 1 tablet 1 hour before appointment
>
> Ingredient: Alprazolam

Rx:

> Vistaril® 25 mg
> Disp: 16 capsules
> Sig: Take 2 capsules in evening before going to bed and 2 capsules 1 hour before appointment
>
> Ingredient: Hydroxyzine

Rx:

> Halcion® 0.25 mg
> Disp: 4 tablets
> Sig: Take 1 tablet in evening before going to bed and 1 tablet 1 hour before appointment
>
> Ingredient: Triazolam

Rx:

> Serax 10 mg
> Disp: 2 capsules
> Sig: Take 1 capsule before bed and 1 capsule 30 minutes before appointment
>
> Ingredient: Oxazepam

APPENDIX

TABLE OF CONTENTS

ABBREVIATIONS, ACRONYMS, AND SYMBOLS

Abbreviation	Meaning
<	less than
>	greater than
≤	less than or equal to
≥	greater than or equal to
a̅a̅, aa	of each
AA	Alcoholics Anonymous
ABG	arterial blood gases
ac	before meals or food
ACA	Adult Children of Alcoholics
ACLS	advanced cardiac life support
ad	to, up to
a.d.	right ear
ADHD	attention-deficit/hyperactivity disorder
ADLs	activities of daily living
ad lib	at pleasure
AIDS	acquired immune deficiency syndrome
AIMS	Abnormal Involuntary Movement Scale
a.l.	left ear
ALS	amyotrophic lateral sclerosis
AM	morning
AMA	against medical advice
amp	ampul
amt	amount
aq	water
aq. dest.	distilled water
ARC	AIDS-related complex
ARDS	adult respiratory distress syndrome
ARF	acute renal failure
a.s.	left ear
ASAP	as soon as possible
ASA-PS	American Society of Anesthesiologists - Physical Status P1: Normal, healthy patient P2: Patient having mild systemic disease P3: Patient having severe systemic disease P4: Patient having severe systemic disease which is a constant threat to life P5: Moribund patient; not expected to survive without the procedure P6: Patient declared brain-dead; organs being removed for donor purposes
a.u.	each ear
AUC	area under the curve
BDI	Beck Depression Inventory
bid	twice daily
BLS	basic life support
bm	bowel movement
BMI	body mass index
bp	blood pressure
BPH	benign prostatic hyperplasia
BPRS	Brief Psychiatric Rating Scale
BSA	body surface area
c	a gallon
c̄	with
CA	cancer
CABG	coronary artery bypass graft
CAD	coronary artery disease
cal	calorie
cap	capsule
CBT	cognitive behavioral therapy

Abbreviation	Meaning
cc	cubic centimeter
CCL	creatinine clearance
CF	cystic fibrosis
CGI	Clinical Global Impression
CIE	chemotherapy-induced emesis
cm	centimeter
CIV	continuous I.V. infusion
CNS	central nervous system
comp	compound
cont	continue
COPD	chronic obstructive pulmonary disease
CRF	chronic renal failure
CT	computed tomography
d	day
DBP	diastolic blood pressure
d/c	discontinue
dil	dilute
disp	dispense
div	divide
DOE	dyspnea on exertion
DSC	discontinued
DSM-IV	Diagnostic and Statistical Manual
DTs	delirium tremens
dtd	give of such a dose
DVT	deep vein thrombosis
Dx	diagnosis
ECG	electrocardiogram
ECT	electroconvulsive therapy
EEG	electroencephalogram
elix, el	elixir
emp	as directed
EPS	extrapyramidal side effects
ESRD	end stage renal disease
et	and
EtOH	alcohol
ex aq	in water
f, ft	make, let be made
FDA	Food and Drug Administration
FMS	fibromyalgia syndrome
g	gram
GA	Gamblers Anonymous
GAD	generalized anxiety disorder
GAF	Global Assessment of Functioning Scale
GABA	gamma-aminobutyric acid
GERD	gastroesophageal reflux disease
GFR	glomerular filtration rate
GITS	gastrointestinal therapeutic system
gr	grain
gtt	a drop
GVHD	graft versus host disease
h	hour
HAM-A	Hamilton Anxiety Scale
HAM-D	Hamilton Depression Scale
hs	at bedtime
HSV	herpes simplex virus
HTN	hypertension
IBD	inflammatory bowel disease
IBS	irritable bowel syndrome
ICH	intracranial hemorrhage
IHSS	idiopathic hypertrophic subaortic stenosis

ABBREVIATIONS, ACRONYMS, AND SYMBOLS *(Continued)*

Abbreviation	Meaning
I.M.	intramuscular
IOP	intraocular pressure
IU	international unit
I.V.	intravenous
kcal	kilocalorie
kg	kilogram
KIU	kallikrein inhibitor unit
L	liter
LAMM	L-α-acetyl methadol
liq	a liquor, solution
LVH	left ventricular hypertrophy
M.	mix; Molar
MADRS	Montgomery Asbery Depression Rating Scale
MAOIs	monamine oxidase inhibitors
mcg	microgram
MDEA	3,4-methylene-dioxy amphetamine
m. dict	as directed
MDMA	3,4-methylene-dioxy methamphetamine
mEq	milliequivalent
mg	milligram
mixt	a mixture
mL	milliliter
mm	millimeter
mM	millimolar
MMSE	mini mental status examination
MPPP	l-methyl-4-proprionoxy-4-phenyl pyridine
MR	mental retardation
MRI	magnetic resonance imaging
MS	multiple sclerosis
NF	National Formulary
NKA	no known allergies
NMS	neuroleptic malignant syndrome
no.	number
noc	in the night
non rep	do not repeat, no refills
NPO	nothing by mouth
NSAID	nonsteroidal anti-inflammatory drug
NV	nausea and vomiting
O, Oct	a pint
OA	osteoarthritis
OCD	obsessive-compulsive disorder
o.d.	right eye
o.l.	left eye
o.s.	left eye
o.u.	each eye
PANSS	Positive and Negative Symptom Scale
PAT	paroxysmal artrial tachycardia
pc, post cib	after meals
PCP	phencyclidine
PD	Parkinson's disease
PE	pulmonary embolus
per	through or by
PID	pelvic inflammatory disease
PM	afternoon or evening
P.O.	by mouth
PONV	postoperative nausea and vomiting
P.R.	rectally
prn	as needed

Abbreviation	Meaning
PSVT	paroxysmal supraventricular tachycardia
PTA	prior to admission
PTSD	post-traumatic stress disorder
PUD	peptic ulcer disease
pulv	a powder
PVD	peripheral vascular disease
q	every
qad	every other day
qd	every day, daily
qh	every hour
qid	four times a day
qod	every other day
qs	a sufficient quantity
qs ad	a sufficient quantity to make
qty	quantity
qv	as much as you wish
RA	rheumatoid arthritis
REM	rapid eye movement
Rx	take, a recipe
rep	let it be repeated
$\bar{s}$	without
sa	according to art
SAH	subarachnoid hemorrhage
sat	saturated
SBE	subacute bacterial endocarditis
SBP	systolic blood pressure
SIADH	syndrome of inappropriate antidiuretic hormone secretion
sig	label, or let it be printed
SL	sublingual
SLE	systemic lupus erythematosus
SOB	shortness of breath
sol	solution
solv	dissolve
$\overline{ss}$	one-half
sos	if there is need
SSKI	saturated solution of potassium iodide
SSRIs	selective serotonin reuptake inhibitors
stat	at once, immediately
STD	sexually transmitted disease
SubQ	subcutaneous
supp	suppository
SVT	supraventricular tachycardia
Sx	symptom
syr	syrup
tab	tablet
tal	such
TCA	tricyclic antidepressant
TD	tardive dyskinesia
tid	three times a day
TKO	to keep open
TPN	total parenteral nutrition
tr, tinct	tincture
trit	triturate
tsp	teaspoonful
Tx	treatment
ULN	upper limits of normal
ung	ointment
URI	upper respiratory infection
USAN	United States Adopted Names
USP	United States Pharmacopeia

ABBREVIATIONS, ACRONYMS, AND SYMBOLS *(Continued)*

Abbreviation	Meaning
UTI	urinary tract infection
u.d., ut dict	as directed
v.o.	verbal order
VTE	venous thromboembolism
VZV	varicella zoster virus
w.a.	while awake
x3	3 times
x4	4 times
YBOC	Yale Brown Obsessive-Compulsive Scale
YMRS	Young Mania Rating Scale

STANDARD CONVERSIONS

APOTHECARY / METRIC EQUIVALENTS

Approximate Liquid Measures

Basic equivalent: 1 fluid ounce = 30 mL

Examples:

1 gallon	3800 mL	15 minims	1 mL
1 quart	960 mL	10 minims	0.6 mL
1 pint	480 mL	1 gallon	128 fluid ounces
8 fluid ounces	240 mL	1 quart	32 fluid ounces
4 fluid ounces	120 mL	1 pint	16 fluid ounces

Approximate Household Equivalents

1 teaspoonful .... 5 mL   1 tablespoonful .... 15 mL

Weights

Basic equivalents:

1 ounce = 30 g   15 grains = 1 g

Examples:

4 ounces	120 g	1/100 grain	600 mcg
2 ounces	60 g	1/150 grain	400 mcg
10 grains	600 mg	1/200 grain	300 mcg
7 1/2 grains	500 mg	16 ounces	1 pound
1 grain	60 mg		

Metric Conversions

Basic equivalents:

1 g .... 1000 mg   1 mg .... 1000 mcg

Examples:

5 g	5000 mg	5 mg	5000 mcg
0.5 g	500 mg	0.5 mg	500 mcg
0.05 g	50 mg	0.05 mg	50 mcg

Exact Equivalents

1 g	=	15.43 grains (gr)		0.1 mg	=	1/600 gr
1 mL	=	16.23 minims		0.12 mg	=	1/500 gr
1 minim	=	0.06 mL		0.15 mg	=	1/400 gr
1 gr	=	64.8 mg		0.2 mg	=	1/300 gr
1 pint (pt)	=	473.2 mL		0.3 mg	=	1/200 gr
1 oz	=	28.35 g		0.4 mg	=	1/150 gr
1 lb	=	453.6 g		0.5 mg	=	1/120 gr
1 kg	=	2.2 lb		0.6 mg	=	1/100 gr
1 qt	=	946.4 mL		0.8 mg	=	1/80 gr
				1 mg	=	1/65 gr

Solids[1]

1/4 grain	=	15 mg
1/2 grain	=	30 mg
1 grain	=	60 mg
1 1/2 grains	=	90 mg
5 grains	=	300 mg
10 grains	=	600 mg

[1]Use exact equivalents for compounding and calculations requiring a high degree of accuracy.

STANDARD CONVERSIONS (Continued)

POUNDS / KILOGRAMS CONVERSION

1 pound = 0.45359 kilograms
1 kilogram = 2.2 pounds

lb	=	kg	lb	=	kg	lb	=	kg
1		0.45	70		31.75	140		63.50
5		2.27	75		34.02	145		65.77
10		4.54	80		36.29	150		68.04
15		6.80	85		38.56	155		70.31
20		9.07	90		40.82	160		72.58
25		11.34	95		43.09	165		74.84
30		13.61	100		45.36	170		77.11
35		15.88	105		47.63	175		79.38
40		18.14	110		49.90	180		81.65
45		20.41	115		52.16	185		83.92
50		22.68	120		54.43	190		86.18
55		24.95	125		56.70	195		88.45
60		27.22	130		58.91	200		90.72
65		29.48	135		61.24			

PHARMACOLOGY OF DRUG METABOLISM AND INTERACTIONS

Most drugs are eliminated from the body, at least in part, by being chemically altered to less lipid-soluble products (ie, metabolized), and thus are more likely to be excreted via the kidneys or the bile. Phase I metabolism includes drug hydrolysis, oxidation, and reduction, and results in drugs that are more polar in their chemical structure, while Phase II metabolism involves the attachment of an additional molecule onto the drug (or partially metabolized drug) in order to create an inactive and/or more water soluble compound. Phase II processes include (primarily) glucuronidation, sulfation, glutathione conjugation, acetylation, and methylation.

Virtually any of the Phase I and II enzymes can be inhibited by some xenobiotic or drug. Some of the Phase I and II enzymes can be induced. Inhibition of the activity of metabolic enzymes will result in increased concentrations of the substrate (drug), whereas induction of the activity of metabolic enzymes will result in decreased concentrations of the substrate. For example, the well-documented enzyme-inducing effects of phenobarbital may include a combination of Phase I and II enzymes. Phase II glucuronidation may be increased via induced UDP-glucuronosyltransferase (UGT) activity, whereas Phase I oxidation may be increased via induced cytochrome P450 (CYP) activity. However, for most drugs, the primary route of metabolism (and the primary focus of drug-drug interaction) is Phase I oxidation, and specifically, metabolism.

CYP enzymes may be responsible for the metabolism (at least partial metabolism) of approximately 75% of all drugs, with the CYP3A subfamily responsible for nearly half of this activity. Found throughout plant, animal, and bacterial species, CYP enzymes represent a superfamily of xenobiotic metabolizing proteins. There have been several hundred CYP enzymes identified in nature, each of which has been assigned to a family (1, 2, 3, etc), subfamily (A, B, C, etc), and given a specific enzyme number (1, 2, 3, etc) according to the similarity in amino acid sequence that it shares with other enzymes. Of these many enzymes, only a few are found in humans, and even fewer appear to be involved in the metabolism of xenobiotics (eg, drugs). The key human enzyme subfamilies include CYP1A, CYP2A, CYP2B, CYP2C, CYP2D, CYP2E, and CYP3A.

CYP enzymes are found in the endoplasmic reticulum of cells in a variety of human tissues (eg, skin, kidneys, brain, lungs), but their predominant sites of concentration and activity are the liver and intestine. Though the abundance of CYP enzymes throughout the body is relatively equally distributed among the various subfamilies, the relative contribution to drug metabolism is (in decreasing order of magnitude) CYP3A4 (nearly 50%), CYP2D6 (nearly 25%), CYP2C8/9 (nearly 15%), then CYP1A2, CYP2C19, CYP2A6, and CYP2E1. Owing to their potential for numerous drug-drug interactions, those drugs that are identified in preclinical studies as substrates of CYP3A enzymes are often given a lower priority for continued research and development in favor of drugs that appear to be less affected by (or less likely to affect) this enzyme subfamily.

Each enzyme subfamily possesses unique selectivity toward potential substrates. For example, CYP1A2 preferentially binds medium-sized, planar, lipophilic molecules, while CYP2D6 preferentially binds molecules that possess a basic nitrogen atom. Some CYP subfamilies exhibit polymorphism (ie, multiple allelic variants that manifest differing catalytic properties). The best described polymorphisms involve CYP2C9, CYP2C19, and CYP2D6. Individuals possessing "wild type" gene alleles exhibit normal functioning CYP capacity. Others, however, possess allelic variants that leave the person with a subnormal level of catalytic potential (so called "poor metabolizers"). Poor metabolizers would be more likely to experience toxicity from drugs metabolized by the affected enzymes (or less effects if the enzyme is responsible for converting a prodrug to it's active form as in the case of codeine). The percentage of people classified as poor metabolizers varies by enzyme and population group. As an example, approximately 7% of Caucasians and only about 1% of Orientals appear to be CYP2D6 poor metabolizers.

CYP enzymes can be both inhibited and induced by other drugs, leading to increased or decreased serum concentrations (along with the associated effects), respectively. Induction occurs when a drug causes an increase in the amount of smooth endoplasmic reticulum, secondary to increasing the amount of the affected CYP enzymes in the tissues. This "revving up" of the CYP enzyme system may take several days to reach peak activity, and likewise, may take several days, even months, to return to normal following discontinuation of the inducing agent.

CYP inhibition occurs via several potential mechanisms. Most commonly, a CYP inhibitor competitively (and reversibly) binds to the active site on the enzyme, thus preventing the substrate from binding to the same site, and preventing the substrate from being metabolized. The affinity of an inhibitor for an enzyme may be expressed by an inhibition constant (Ki) or IC50 (defined as the concentration of the inhibitor required to cause 50% inhibition under a given set of conditions). In addition to reversible competition for an enzyme site, drugs may inhibit enzyme activity by binding to sites on the enzyme other than that to which the substrate would bind, and thereby cause a change in the functionality or physical structure of the enzyme. A drug may also bind to the enzyme in an irreversible (ie, "suicide") fashion. In such a case, it is not the concentration of drug at the enzyme site that is important (constantly binding and releasing), but the number of molecules available for binding (once bound, always bound).

Although an inhibitor or inducer may be known to affect a variety of CYP subfamilies, it may only inhibit one or two in a clinically important fashion. Likewise, although a substrate is

PHARMACOLOGY OF DRUG METABOLISM AND INTERACTIONS (Continued)

known to be at least partially metabolized by a variety of CYP enzymes, only one or two enzymes may contribute significantly enough to its overall metabolism to warrant concern when used with potential inducers or inhibitors. Therefore, when attempting to predict the level of risk of using two drugs that may affect each other via altered CYP function, it is important to identify the relative effectiveness of the inhibiting/inducing drug on the CYP subfamilies that significantly contribute to the metabolism of the substrate. The contribution of a specific CYP pathway to substrate metabolism should be considered not only in light of other known CYP pathways, but also other nonoxidative pathways for substrate metabolism (eg, glucuronidation) and transporter proteins (eg, P-glycoprotein) that may affect the presentation of a substrate to a metabolic pathway.

SMOKING AND DRUG METABOLISM

Another area of intense interest involves smoking effects on drug metabolism, as well as, the effects of smoking cessation drugs. A review of the literature suggests that at least a dozen drugs interact with cigarette smoke in a clinically significant manner. Polycyclic aromatic hydrocarbons (PAHs) are largely responsible for enhancing drug metabolism. Cigarette smoke induces an increase in the concentration of CYP1A2, the isoenzyme responsible for metabolism of theophylline. Theophylline is, therefore, eliminated more quickly in smokers than in nonsmokers. As a result of hepatic induction of CYP1A2, serum concentrations of theophylline have been shown to be reduced in smokers. Cigarette smoking may substantially reduce tacrine plasma concentrations. The manufacturer states that mean plasma tacrine concentrations in smokers are about one-third of the concentration in nonsmokers (presumably after multiple doses of tacrine).

Patients with insulin-dependent diabetes who smoke heavily may require a higher dosage of insulin than nonsmokers. Cigarette smoking may also reduce serum concentrations of flecainide. Although the mechanism of this interaction is unknown, enhanced hepatic metabolism is possible. Propoxyphene, a pain reliever, has been found to be less effective in heavy smokers than in nonsmokers. The mechanism for the inefficacy of propoxyphene in smokers compared with nonsmokers may be enhanced biotransformation.

Frankl and Soloff reported in a study of five young, healthy, chronic smokers that propranolol, followed by smoking, significantly decreased cardiac output and significantly increased blood pressure and peripheral resistance compared with smoking alone. Steady-state concentrations of propranolol were found to be lower in smokers than in nonsmokers. Lastly, the incidence of drowsiness associated with the use of diazepam and chlordiazepoxide showed that drowsiness was less likely to occur in smokers than in nonsmokers. Smoking probably acts by producing arousal of the central nervous system rather than by accelerating metabolism and reducing concentrations of these drugs in the brain. Finally, the interaction between smoking and oral contraceptives is complex and may be deadly. Women >35 years of age who smoke >15 cigarettes daily may be at increased risk of myocardial infarction.

The norepinephrine and serotonin reuptake inhibitors, as a new class of smoking cessation drugs, have also received attention relative to metabolic interactions. In vitro studies indicate that bupropion is primarily metabolized to hydroxybupropion by the CYP2B6 isoenzyme. Therefore, the potential exists for a drug interaction between Zyban® and drugs that affect the CYP2B6 isoenzyme metabolism (eg, orphenadrine and cyclophosphamide). The hydroxybupropion metabolite of bupropion does not appear to be metabolized by the cytochrome P450 isoenzymes. No systemic data have been collected on the metabolism of Zyban® following concomitant administration with other drugs, or alternatively, the effect of concomitant administration of Zyban® on the metabolism of other drugs.

Animal data, however, indicated that bupropion may be an inducer of drug-metabolizing enzymes in humans. However, following chronic administration of bupropion, 100 mg 3 times/day, to 8 healthy male volunteers for 14 days, there was no evidence of induction of its own metabolism. Because bupropion is extensively metabolized, coadministration of other drugs may affect its clinical activity. Certain drugs may induce the metabolism of bupropion (eg, carbamazepine, phenobarbital, phenytoin), while other drugs may inhibit its metabolism (eg, cimetidine). Studies in animals demonstrated that the acute toxicity of bupropion is enhanced by the MAO inhibitor, phenelzine.

Limited clinical data suggest a higher incidence of adverse experiences in patients receiving concurrent administration of bupropion and levodopa. Administration of Zyban® to patients receiving levodopa concurrently should be undertaken with caution, using small initial doses and gradual dosage increases. Concurrent administration of Zyban® and agents that lower the seizure threshold should be undertaken only with extreme caution. Physiological changes resulting from smoking cessation itself, with or without treatment with Zyban®, may alter the pharmacokinetics of some concomitant medications, which may require dosage adjustment.

INTERACTIONS BETWEEN CIGARETTE SMOKE AND DRUGS

Drug	Mechanism	Effect on Cigarette Smokers
Theophylline	Induction of the CYP1A2 isoenzyme	May lead to reduced theophylline serum concentrations and decreased clinical effect; elimination of theophylline is considerably more rapid
Tacrine	Induction of the CYP1A2 isoenzyme	Effectiveness of tacrine may be decreased
Insulin	Decreased insulin absorption; may be related to peripheral vasoconstriction	Insulin-dependent diabetics who smoke heavily may require a 15% to 30% higher dose of insulin than nonsmokers
Flecainide	Unknown	May reduce flecainide serum concentrations
Propoxyphene	Unknown	May require higher dosage of propoxyphene to achieve analgesic effects
Propranolol	Increased release of catacholamines (eg, epinephrine) in smokers	May have increased blood pressure and heart rate relative to nonsmokers; consider effects on prevention of angina pectoris and stroke
Diazepam	Unclear as to whether pharmacokinetics are altered or end-organ responsiveness is decreased	May require larger doses of diazepam and chlordiazepoxide to achieve sedative effects

Adapted from Schein, JR, "Cigarette Smoking and Clinically Significant Drug Interactions," *Ann Pharmacother*, 1995, 29(11):1139-47.

SUMMARY

Once a drug has been metabolized in the liver, it is eliminated through several different mechanisms. One is directly through bile, into the intestine, and eventually excreted in feces. More commonly, the metabolites and the original drug pass back into the liver from the general circulation and are carried to other organs and tissues. Eventually, these metabolites are excreted through the kidney. In the kidney, the drug and its metabolites may be filtered by the glomerulus or secreted by the renal tubules into the urine. From the kidney, some of the drug may be reabsorbed and pass back into the blood. The drug may also be carried to the lung. If the drug or its metabolite is volatile, it can pass from the blood into the alveolar air and be eliminated in the breath. To a minor extent, drugs and metabolites can be excreted by sweat and saliva. In nursing mothers, drugs are also excreted in mother's milk.

The clinical considerations of drug metabolism may affect which other drugs can and should be administered. Drug tolerance may be a consideration, in that larger doses of a drug may be necessary to obtain effect in patients in which the metabolism is extremely rapid. These interactions, via cytochrome P450 or its isoforms, can occasionally be used beneficially to increase/maintain blood levels of one drug by administering a second drug. Dental clinicians should attempt to stay current on this topic of drug interactions as knowledge evolves.

HOW TO USE THE TABLES

The following CYP SUBSTRATES, INHIBITORS, and INDUCERS tables provide a clinically relevant perspective on drugs that are affected by, or affect, cytochrome P450 (CYP) enzymes. Not all human, drug-metabolizing CYP enzymes are specifically (or separately) included in the tables. Some enzymes have been excluded because they do not appear to significantly contribute to the metabolism of marketed drugs (eg, CYP2C18). Others have been combined in recognition of the difficulty in distinguishing their metabolic activity one from another, or the clinical practicality of doing so (eg, CYP2C8/9, CYP3A4). In the case of CYP3A4, the industry routinely uses this single enzyme designation to represent all enzymes in the CYP3A subfamily. CYP3A7 is present in fetal livers. It is effectively absent from adult livers. CYP3A4 (adult) and CYP3A7 (fetal) appear to share similar properties in their respective hosts. The impact of CYP3A7 in fetal and neonatal drug interactions has not been investigated.

The **CYP Substrates table** contains a list of drugs reported to be metabolized, at least in part, by one or more CYP enzymes. An enzyme that appears to play a clinically significant (major) role in a drug's metabolism is indicated by "●", and an enzyme whose role appears to be clinically insignificant (minor) is indicated by "○". A clinically significant designation is the result of a two-phase review. The first phase considered the contribution of each CYP enzyme to the overall metabolism of the drug. The enzyme pathway was considered potentially clinically relevant if it was responsible for at least 30% of the metabolism of the drug. If so, the drug was subjected to a second phase. The second phase considered the clinical relevance of a substrate's concentration being increased twofold, or decreased by one-half (such as might be observed if combined with an effective CYP inhibitor or inducer, respectively). If either of these changes was considered to present a clinically significant concern, the CYP pathway for the drug was designated "major." If neither change would appear to

PHARMACOLOGY OF DRUG METABOLISM AND INTERACTIONS (Continued)

present a clinically significant concern, or if the CYP enzyme was responsible for a smaller portion of the overall metabolism (ie, <30%), the pathway was designated "minor."

The **CYP Inhibitors table** contains a list of drugs that are reported to inhibit one or more CYP enzymes. Enzymes that are strongly inhibited by a drug are indicated by "●". Enzymes that are moderately inhibited are indicated by "◐". Enzymes that are weakly inhibited are indicated by "○". The designations are the result of a review of published clinical reports, available Ki data, and assessments published by other experts in the field. As it pertains to Ki values set in a ratio with achievable serum drug concentrations ([I]) under normal dosing conditions, the following parameters were employed: [I]/Ki ≥1 = strong; [I]/Ki 0.1-1 = moderate; [I]/Ki <0.1 = weak.

The **CYP Inducers table** contains a list of drugs that are reported to induce one or more CYP enzymes. Enzymes that appear to be effectively induced by a drug are indicated by "●", and enzymes that do not appear to be effectively induced are indicated by "○". The designations are the result of a review of published clinical reports and assessments published by experts in the field.

In general, clinically significant interactions are more likely to occur between substrates and either inhibitors or inducers of the same enzyme(s), all of which have been indicated by "●". However, these assessments possess a degree of subjectivity, at times based on limited indications regarding the significance of CYP effects of particular agents. An attempt has been made to balance a conservative, clinically-sensitive presentation of the data with a desire to avoid the numbing effect of a "beware of everything" approach. Even so, other potential interactions (ie, those involving enzymes indicated by "○") may warrant consideration in some cases. It is important to note that information related to CYP metabolism of drugs is expanding at a rapid pace, and thus, the contents of this table should only be considered to represent a "snapshot" of the information available at the time of publication.

Selected Readings

Bjornsson TD, Callaghan JT, Einolf HJ, et al, "The Conduct of *in vitro* and *in vivo* Drug-Drug Interaction Studies: A PhRMA Perspective," *J Clin Pharmacol*, 2003, 43(5):443-69.

Drug-Drug Interactions, Rodrigues AD, ed, New York, NY: Marcel Dekker, Inc, 2002.

Hersh EV and Moore PA, "Drug Interactions in Dentistry: The Importance of Knowing Your CYP's," *J Am Dent Assoc*, 2004, 135(3):298-311.

Levy RH, Thummel KE, Trager WF, et al, eds, *Metabolic Drug Interactions*, Philadelphia, PA: Lippincott Williams & Wilkins, 2000.

Michalets EL, "Update: Clinically Significant Cytochrome P-450 Drug Interactions," *Pharmacotherapy*, 1998, 18(1):84-112.

Thummel KE and Wilkinson GR, "*In vitro* and *in vivo* Drug Interactions Involving Human CYP3A," *Annu Rev Pharmacol Toxicol*, 1998, 38:389-430.

Wynn RL and Meiller TF, "CYP Enzymes and Adverse Drug Reactions," *Gen Dent*, 1998, 46(5):436-8.

Zhang Y and Benet LZ, "The Gut as a Barrier to Drug Absorption: Combined Role of Cytochrome P450 3A and P-Glycoprotein," *Clin Pharmacokinet*, 2001, 40(3):159-68.

Selected Websites

http://www.gentest.com
http://www.imm.ki.se/CYPalleles
http://medicine.iupui.edu/flockhart
http://www.mhc.com/Cytochromes

CYP Substrates

● = major substrate
○ = minor substrate

Drug	1A2	2A6	2B6	2C8	2C9	2C19	2D6	2E1	3A4
Acenocoumarol	●				●	○			
Acetaminophen	○	○			○		○	○	○
Albendazole	○								●
Albuterol									●
Alfentanil									●
Almotriptan							○		○
Alosetron	○				●				○
Alprazolam									●
Aminophylline	●							○	○
Amiodarone	○			●		○	○		●
Amitriptyline	○		○		○	○	●		○
Amlodipine									●
Amoxapine							●		
Amphetamine							○		
Amprenavir					○				●
Aprepitant	○					○			●
Argatroban									○
Aripiprazole							●		●
Aspirin					○				
Atazanavir									●
Atomoxetine						○	●		
Atorvastatin									●
Azelastine	○					○	○		○
Azithromycin									○
Benzphetamine			○						●
Benztropine							○		
Betaxolol	●						●		
Bexarotene									○
Bezafibrate									○
Bisoprolol							○		●
Bortezomib	○				○	○	○		●
Bosentan					●				●
Brinzolamide									○
Bromazepam									●
Bromocriptine									●
Budesonide									●
Bupivacaine	○					○	○		○
Buprenorphine									●
BuPROPion	○	○	●		○		○	○	○
BusPIRone							○		●
Busulfan									●
Caffeine	●				○		○	○	○
Candesartan					○				
Capsaicin								○	
Captopril							●		
Carbamazepine				○					●
Carisoprodol						●			
Carteolol							○		
Carvedilol	○				●		●	○	○
Celecoxib					●				○
Cerivastatin									●
Cetirizine									○
Cevimeline							○		○
Chlordiazepoxide									●
Chloroquine							●		●
Chlorpheniramine							○		●
ChlorproMAZINE	○						●		○
ChlorproPAMIDE					○				
Chlorzoxazone	○	○					○	●	○
Cilostazol	○					●	○		●
Cinacalcet	○						○		○
Cisapride	○	○	○		○	○			●
Citalopram						●	○		●
Clarithromycin									●
Clobazam						●			●
Clofibrate									○
ClomiPRAMINE	●					●	●		○

PHARMACOLOGY OF DRUG METABOLISM AND INTERACTIONS (Continued)

CYP Substrates (continued)

Drug	1A2	2A6	2B6	2C8	2C9	2C19	2D6	2E1	3A4
Clonazepam									●
Clopidogrel	○								○
Clorazepate									●
Clozapine	●	○			○	○	○		○
Cocaine									●
Codeine[1]							●		○
Colchicine									●
Conivaptan									●
Cyclobenzaprine	●						○		○
Cyclophosphamide[2]		○	●		○	○			●
CycloSPORINE									●
Dacarbazine	●							●	
Dantrolene									●
Dapsone				○	●	○		○	●
Delavirdine							○		●
Desipramine	○						●		
Desogestrel						●			
Dexamethasone									○
Dexmedetomidine		●							
Dextroamphetamine							●		
Dextromethorphan		○			○	○	●	○	○
Diazepam	○		○		○	●			●
Diclofenac	○		○	○	○	○	○		○
Digoxin									○
Dihydrocodeine[1]							●		
Dihydroergotamine									●
Diltiazem					○		○		●
Dirithromycin									○
Disopyramide									●
Disulfiram	○	○	○				○	○	○
Docetaxel									●
Dofetilide									○
Dolasetron						○			○
Domperidone									○
Donepezil							○		○
Dorzolamide					○				○
Doxepin	●						●		●
DOXOrubicin							●		●
Doxycycline									●
Drospirenone									○
Duloxetine	●						●		
Dutasteride									○
Efavirenz			●						●
Eletriptan									●
Enalapril									●
Enflurane								●	
Eplerenone									●
Ergoloid mesylates									●
Ergonovine									●
Ergotamine									●
Erythromycin			○						●
Escitalopram						●			●
Esomeprazole						●			○
Estazolam									○
Estradiol	●	○	○		○	○	○	○	●
Estrogens, conjugated A/synthetic	●	○	○		○	○	○	○	●
Estrogens, conjugated equine	●	○	○		○	○	○	○	●
Estrogens, conjugated esterified	●		○		○			○	●
Estrone	●		○		○			○	●
Estropipate	●		○		○			○	●
Ethinyl estradiol					○				●
Ethosuximide									●
Etonogestrel									○
Etoposide	○							○	●
Exemestane									●

CYP Substrates *(continued)*

Drug	1A2	2A6	2B6	2C8	2C9	2C19	2D6	2E1	3A4
Felbamate								○	
Felodipine									●
Fenofibrate									○
Fentanyl									●
Fexofenadine									○
Finasteride									○
Flecainide	○						●		
Fluoxetine	○		○		●	○	●	○	○
Fluphenazine							●		
Flurazepam									●
Flurbiprofen					○				
Flutamide	●								●
Fluticasone									●
Fluvastatin					○		○		○
Fluvoxamine	●						●		
Formoterol		○			○	○	○		
Fosamprenavir (as amprenavir)					○				●
Fosphenytoin (as phenytoin)					●	●			○
Frovatriptan	○								
Fulvestrant									○
Galantamine							○		○
Gefitinib									●
Gemfibrozil									○
Glimepiride					●				
GlipiZIDE					●				
Granisetron									○
Guanabenz	●								
Halazepam									○
Haloperidol	○						●		●
Halothane		○	○		○		○	●	○
Hydrocodone[1]							●		
Hydrocortisone									○
Ibuprofen					○	○			
Ifosfamide[3]		○	○	○	○	○			●
Imatinib	○				○	○	○		●
Imipramine	○		○		●		●		○
Imiquimod	○								○
Indinavir							○		●
Indomethacin					○	○			
Irbesartan					○				
Irinotecan			●						●
Isoflurane								●	
Isoniazid								●	
Isosorbide									●
Isosorbide dinitrate									●
Isosorbide mononitrate									●
Isradipine									●
Itraconazole									●
Ivermectin									○
Ketamine			●		●				●
Ketoconazole									●
Labetalol							●		
Lansoprazole					○	●			●
Letrozole		○							●
Levobupivacaine	○								○
Levonorgestrel									●
Lidocaine	○	○	○		○		●		●
Lomustine							●		
Lopinavir									○
Loratadine							○		○
Losartan					●				●
Lovastatin									●
Maprotiline							●		
MedroxyPROGESTERone									●
Mefenamic acid					○				
Mefloquine									●
Meloxicam					○				○
Mephobarbital			○		○	●			
Mestranol[4]					●				●

PHARMACOLOGY OF DRUG METABOLISM AND INTERACTIONS (Continued)

CYP Substrates (continued)

Drug	1A2	2A6	2B6	2C8	2C9	2C19	2D6	2E1	3A4
Methadone					○	○	○		●
Methamphetamine							●		
Methoxsalen		○							
Methsuximide						●			
Methylergonovine									●
Methylphenidate							●		
MethylPREDNISolone									○
Metoclopramide	○						○		
Metoprolol						○	●		
Mexiletine	●						●		
Miconazole									●
Midazolam			○						●
Mifepristone									○
Miglustat									●
Mirtazapine	●				○		●		●
Moclobemide						●	●		
Modafinil									●
Mometasone furoate									○
Montelukast					●				●
Moricizine									●
Morphine sulfate							○		
Naproxen	○				○				
Nateglinide					●				●
Nefazodone							●		●
Nelfinavir					○	●	○		●
Nevirapine			○				○		●
NiCARdipine	○				○	○	○	○	○
Nicotine	○	○	○		○	○	○	○	○
NIFEdipine							○		●
Nilutamide						●			
Nimodipine									●
Nisoldipine									●
Norelgestromin									○
Norethindrone									●
Norgestrel									●
Nortriptyline	○					○	●		○
Olanzapine	○						○		
Omeprazole		○			○	●			○
Ondansetron	○					○	○	○	●
Orphenadrine	○		○				○		○
Oxybutynin									○
Oxycodone[1]							●		
Paclitaxel				●	●				●
Palonosetron	○						○		○
Pantoprazole						●			○
Paroxetine							●		
Pentamidine						●			
Pergolide									●
Perphenazine	○				○	○	●		○
Phencyclidine									●
Phenobarbital					○	●		○	
Phenytoin					●	●			○
Pimecrolimus									○
Pimozide	●								●
Pindolol							●		
Pioglitazone				●					○
Pipotiazine							●		●
Piroxicam					○				
Pravastatin									○
PrednisoLONE									○
PredniSONE									○
Primaquine									●
Procainamide							●		
Progesterone	○	○			○	●	○		●
Proguanil	○					○			○
Promethazine			●				●		
Propafenone	○						●		○

CYP Substrates (continued)

Drug	1A2	2A6	2B6	2C8	2C9	2C19	2D6	2E1	3A4
Propofol	○	○	●		●	○	○	○	○
Propranolol	●					○	●		○
Protriptyline							●		
Quazepam									○
Quetiapine							○		●
Quinidine					○		○		●
Quinine	○					○			○
Rabeprazole						●			●
Ranitidine	○					○	○		
Ranolazine							○		●
Repaglinide				●					●
Rifabutin									●
Riluzole	●								
Risperidone							●		○
Ritonavir	○		○				○		●
Rofecoxib					○				
Ropinirole	●								○
Ropivacaine	○		○				○		○
Rosiglitazone				●	○				
Rosuvastatin					○				○
Salmeterol									●
Saquinavir									●
Selegiline	○	○	●	○		○	○		○
Sertraline			○		○	●	●		○
Sevoflurane		○	○					●	○
Sibutramine									●
Sildenafil					○				●
Simvastatin									●
Sirolimus									●
Sorafenib									○
Spiramycin									●
Sufentanil									●
SulfaDIAZINE					●			○	○
Sulfamethoxazole					●				○
Sulfinpyrazone					●				○
SulfiSOXAZOLE					●				
Sunitinib									●
Tacrine	●								
Tacrolimus									●
Tamoxifen		○	○		●		●	○	●
Tamsulosin							●		●
Telithromycin	○								●
Temazepam			○		○	○			○
Teniposide									●
Terbinafine	○				○	○			○
Testosterone			○		○	○			○
Tetracycline									●
Theophylline	●				○		○	●	●
Thiabendazole	○								
Thioridazine						○	●		
Thiothixene	●								
Tiagabine									●
Ticlopidine									●
Timolol							●		
Tinidazole									○
Tiotropium							○		○
Tipranavir									●
TOLBUTamide					●	○			
Tolcapone		○							○
Tolterodine					○	○	●		●
Toremifene	○								●
Torsemide				○	●				
Tramadol[1]			○				●		○
Trazodone							○		●
Tretinoin		○	○	●	○				
Triazolam									●
Trifluoperazine	●								
Trimethadione					○	○		●	○
Trimethoprim					●				●
Trimipramine						●	●		●

PHARMACOLOGY OF DRUG METABOLISM AND INTERACTIONS *(Continued)*

CYP Substrates *(continued)*

Drug	1A2	2A6	2B6	2C8	2C9	2C19	2D6	2E1	3A4
Troleandomycin									●
Valdecoxib					○				○
Valproic acid		○	○		○	○		○	
Vardenafil									●
Venlafaxine					○	○	●		●
Verapamil	○		○		○			○	●
VinBLAStine							○		●
VinCRIStine									●
Vinorelbine							○		●
Voriconazole					●	●			○
Warfarin	○				●	○			○
Yohimbine							○		
Zafirlukast					●				
Zaleplon									○
Zidovudine		○			○	○			○
Zileuton	○				○				○
Ziprasidone	○								○
Zolmitriptan	○								
Zolpidem	○				○	○	○		●
Zonisamide						○			●
Zopiclone					●				●
Zuclopenthixol							●		

[1]This opioid analgesic is bioactivated *in vivo* via CYP2D6. Inhibiting this enzyme would decrease the effects of the analgesic. The active metabolite might also affect, or be affected by, CYP enzymes.
[2]Cyclophosphamide is bioactivated *in vivo* to acrolein via CYP2B6 and 3A4. Inhibiting these enzymes would decrease the effects of cyclophosphamide.
[3]Ifosfamide is bioactivated *in vivo* to acrolein via CYP3A4. Inhibiting this enzyme would decrease the effects of ifosfamide.
[4]Mestranol is bioactivated *in vivo* to ethinyl estradiol via CYP2C8/9. See Ethinyl Estradiol for additional CYP information.

CYP Inhibitors

● = strong inhibitor
◐ = moderate inhibitor
○ = weak inhibitor

Drug	1A2	2A6	2B6	2C8	2C9	2C19	2D6	2E1	3A4
Acebutolol							○		
Acetaminophen									○
AcetaZOLAMIDE									○
Albendazole	○								
Alosetron	○							○	
Amiodarone	○	◐	○		◐	○	◐		◐
Amitriptyline	○				○	○	○	○	
Amlodipine	◐	○	○	○	○		○		○
Amphetamine							○		
Amprenavir						○			●
Anastrozole	○			○	○				○
Aprepitant					○	○			◐
Atazanavir	○			●	○				●
Atorvastatin									○
Azelastine			○		○	○	○		○
Azithromycin									○
Bepridil							○		
Betamethasone									○
Betaxolol							○		
Biperiden							○		
Bortezomib	○				○	◐	○		○
Bromazepam							○		
Bromocriptine	○								○
Buprenorphine	○	○				○	○		
BuPROPion							○		
Caffeine	●								◐
Candesartan				○	○				
Celecoxib				◐			○		
Cerivastatin									○
Chloramphenicol					○				○
Chloroquine							◐		
Chlorpheniramine							○		
ChlorproMAZINE							●	○	
Chlorzoxazone							○		○
Cholecalciferol					○	○			
Cimetidine	◐				○	◐	◐	○	◐
Cinacalcet							○		
Ciprofloxacin	●								○
Cisapride							○		○
Citalopram	○		○			○	○		
Clarithromycin	○								●
Clemastine							○		○
Clofazimine									○
Clofibrate		○							
ClomiPRAMINE							◐		
Clopidogrel					○				
Clotrimazole	○	○	○	○	○	○	○	○	◐
Clozapine	○				○	○	◐	○	○
Cocaine							●		○
Codeine							○		
Conivaptan									●
Cyclophosphamide									○
CycloSPORINE					○				◐
Danazol									○
Delavirdine	○				●	●	●		●
Desipramine		◐	◐				◐	○	◐
Dexmedetomidine	○				○		●		○
Dextromethorphan							○		
Diazepam						○			○
Diclofenac	◐				○			○	○
Dihydroergotamine									○
Diltiazem					○		○		◐
Dimethyl sulfoxide					○	○			
DiphenhydrAMINE							◐		
Disulfiram	○	○	○		○		○	●	○
Docetaxel									○

PHARMACOLOGY OF DRUG METABOLISM AND INTERACTIONS (Continued)

CYP Inhibitors (continued)

Drug	1A2	2A6	2B6	2C8	2C9	2C19	2D6	2E1	3A4
Dolasetron							○		
DOXOrubicin			◐				○		○
Doxycycline									◐
Drospirenone	○				○	○			○
Duloxetine							◐		
Econazole								○	
Efavirenz					○	○			○
Enoxacin	●								●
Entacapone	○	○			○	○	○	○	○
Eprosartan					○				
Ergotamine									○
Erythromycin	○								◐
Escitalopram							○		
Estradiol	○			○					
Estrogens, conjugated A/synthetic	○								
Estrogens, conjugated equine	○								
Ethinyl estradiol	○		○	○		○			○
Ethotoin						○			
Etoposide					○				○
Felbamate						○			
Felodipine				◐	○		○		○
Fenofibrate		○		◐	◐	○			
Fentanyl									○
Fexofenadine							○		
Flecainide							○		
Fluconazole	○				●	●			◐
Fluoxetine	◐		○		○	◐	●		○
Fluphenazine	○				○		○	○	
Flurazepam								○	
Flurbiprofen					●				
Flutamide	○								
Fluvastatin	○			○	◐		○		○
Fluvoxamine	●		○		○	●	○		○
Fosamprenavir (as amprenavir)						○			●
Gefitinib						○	○		
Gemfibrozil	◐			●	●	●			
Glyburide				○					○
Grapefruit juice									◐
Haloperidol							◐		◐
HydrALAZINE									○
HydrOXYzine							○		
Ibuprofen					●				
Ifosfamide									○
Imatinib					○		○		●
Imipramine	○					○	◐	○	
Indinavir					○	○	○		●
Indomethacin					●	○			
Interferon alfa-2a	○								
Interferon alfa-2b	○								
Interferon gamma-1b	○							○	
Irbesartan				◐	◐		○		○
Isoflurane			○						
Isoniazid	○	◐			○	●	◐	◐	●
Isradipine									○
Itraconazole									●
Ketoconazole	●	◐	○	○	●	◐	◐		●
Ketoprofen					○				
Labetalol							○		
Lansoprazole					○	◐	○		○
Leflunomide					○				
Letrozole		●				○			
Lidocaine	●						◐		◐
Lomefloxacin	○								
Lomustine							○		○
Loratadine				○		◐	○		

CYP Inhibitors *(continued)*

Drug	1A2	2A6	2B6	2C8	2C9	2C19	2D6	2E1	3A4
Losartan	○			◐	◐	○			○
Lovastatin					○		○		○
Mefenamic acid					●				
Mefloquine							○		○
Meloxicam					○				
Mephobarbital						○			
Mestranol	○		○			○			○
Methadone							◐		○
Methimazole	○	○	○		○	○	◐	○	
Methotrimeprazine							○		
Methoxsalen	●	●			○	○	○	○	○
Methsuximide						○			
Methylphenidate							○		
MethylPREDNISolone				○					○
Metoclopramide							○		
Metoprolol							○		
Metronidazole					○				◐
Metyrapone		○							
Mexiletine	●								
Miconazole	◐	●	○		●	●	●	◐	●
Midazolam				○	○				○
Mifepristone							○		○
Mirtazapine	○								○
Mitoxantrone									○
Moclobemide	○					○	○		
Modafinil	○	○			○	●		○	○
Montelukast				○	○				
Nalidixic acid	○								
Nateglinide					○				
Nefazodone	○		○	○			○		●
Nelfinavir	○		○		○	○	○		●
Nevirapine	○						○		○
NiCARdipine					●	◐	◐		●
Nicotine		○						○	
NIFEdipine	◐				○		○		○
Nilutamide						○			
Nisoldipine	○								○
Nizatidine									○
Norfloxacin	●								◐
Nortriptyline							○	○	
Ofloxacin	●								
Olanzapine	○				○	○	○		○
Omeprazole	○				◐	●	○		○
Ondansetron	○					○			○
Orphenadrine	○	○	○		○	○	○	○	○
Oxcarbazepine						○			
Oxprenolol							○		
Oxybutynin				○			○		○
Pantoprazole					◐				
Paroxetine	○		◐		○	○	●		○
Peginterferon alfa-2a	○								
Peginterferon alfa-2b	○								
Pentamidine					○	○	○		○
Pentoxifylline	○								
Pergolide							●		○
Perphenazine	○						○		
Phencyclidine									○
Pilocarpine		○						○	○
Pimozide						○	○	○	○
Pindolol							○		
Pioglitazone				◐	○	○	◐		
Piroxicam					●				
Pravastatin					○				○
Praziquantel							○		
PrednisoLONE									○
Primaquine	●						○		○
Probenecid						○			
Progesterone					○	○			○
Promethazine							○		
Propafenone	○						○		

PHARMACOLOGY OF DRUG METABOLISM AND INTERACTIONS (Continued)

CYP Inhibitors (continued)

Drug	1A2	2A6	2B6	2C8	2C9	2C19	2D6	2E1	3A4
Propofol	◐				○	◐	○	○	●
Propoxyphene					○		○		○
Propranolol	○						○		
Pyrimethamine					◐		◐		
Quinidine					○		●		●
Quinine				◐	◐		●		○
Quinupristin									○
Rabeprazole				◐		◐	○		○
Ranitidine	○						○		
Ranolazine							○		○
Risperidone							○		○
Ritonavir				●	○	○	●	○	●
Rofecoxib	○								
Ropinirole	○						●		
Rosiglitazone				◐	○	○	○		
Saquinavir					○	○	○		◐
Selegiline	○	○			○	○	○	○	○
Sertraline	○		◐	○	○	◐	◐		◐
Sildenafil	○				○	○	○	○	○
Simvastatin				○	○		○		
Sirolimus									○
Sorafenib			○	○					
Sulconazole	○	○			○	○	○	○	○
SulfaDIAZINE					●				
Sulfamethoxazole					◐				
Sulfinpyrazone					◐				
SulfiSOXAZOLE					●				
Tacrine	○								
Tacrolimus									○
Tamoxifen			○	◐	○				○
Telithromycin							○		●
Telmisartan						○			
Teniposide					○				○
Tenofovir	○								
Terbinafine							●		
Testosterone									○
Tetracycline									◐
Theophylline	○								
Thiabendazole	●								
Thioridazine	○				○		◐	○	
Thiotepa			○						
Thiothixene							○		
Ticlopidine	○				○	●	◐	○	○
Timolol							○		
Tioconazole	○	○			○	○	○	○	
Tocainide	○								
TOLBUTamide				○	●				
Tolcapone					○				
Topiramate							○		
Torsemide						○			
Tranylcypromine	◐	●			○	○	◐	◐	○
Trazodone							◐		○
Tretinoin					○				
Triazolam				○	○				
Trimethoprim				◐	◐				
Tripelennamine							◐		
Triprolidine							○		
Troleandomycin									◐
Valdecoxib				○	○	○			
Valproic acid					○	○	○		○
Valsartan					○				
Venlafaxine			○				○		○
Verapamil	○				○		○		◐
VinBLAStine							○		○
VinCRIStine									○
Vinorelbine							○		○
Voriconazole					○	○			◐

CYP Inhibitors *(continued)*

Drug	1A2	2A6	2B6	2C8	2C9	2C19	2D6	2E1	3A4
Warfarin					◑	○			
Yohimbine							○		
Zafirlukast	○			○	◑	○	○		○
Zileuton	◑								
Ziprasidone							○		○

PHARMACOLOGY OF DRUG METABOLISM AND INTERACTIONS (Continued)

CYP Inducers

● = effectively induced
○ = not effectively induced

Drug	1A2	2A6	2B6	2C8	2C9	2C19	2D6	2E1	3A4
Aminoglutethimide	●					●			●
Amobarbital		●							
Aprepitant					○				○
Bexarotene									○
Bosentan					○				○
Calcitriol									○
Carbamazepine	●		●	●	●	●			●
Clofibrate			○					○	○
Colchicine				○	○			○	○
Cyclophosphamide			○	○	○				
Dexamethasone		○	○	○	○				○
Dicloxacillin									○
Efavirenz (in liver only)			○						○
Estradiol									○
Estrogens, conjugated A/synthetic									○
Estrogens, conjugated equine									○
Exemestane									○
Felbamate									○
Fosphenytoin (as phenytoin)			●	●	●	●			●
Griseofulvin	○				○	○			○
Hydrocortisone									○
Ifosfamide				○	○				
Insulin preparations	○								
Isoniazid (after D/C)								○	
Lansoprazole	○								
MedroxyPROGESTERone									○
Mephobarbital		○							
Metyrapone									○
Modafinil	○		○						○
Moricizine	○								○
Nafcillin									●
Nevirapine			●						●
Norethindrone						○			
Omeprazole	○								
Oxcarbazepine									●
Paclitaxel									○
Pantoprazole	○								○
Pentobarbital		●							●
Phenobarbital	●	●	●	●	●				●
Phenytoin			●	●	●	●			●
Pioglitazone									○
PredniSONE						○			○
Primaquine	○								
Primidone[1]	●		●	●	●				●
Rifabutin									●
Rifampin	●	●	●	●	●	●			●
Rifapentine				●	●				●
Ritonavir (long-term)	○			○	○				○
Rofecoxib									○
Secobarbital		●		●	●				
Sulfinpyrazone									○
Terbinafine									○
Topiramate									○
Tretinoin								○	
Troglitazone									○
Valproic acid		○							

[1]Primidone is partially metabolized to phenobarbital. See Phenobarbital for additional CYP information.

OCCUPATIONAL EXPOSURE TO BLOODBORNE PATHOGENS (STANDARD / UNIVERSAL PRECAUTIONS)

OVERVIEW AND REGULATORY CONSIDERATIONS

Every healthcare employee, from nurse to housekeeper, has some (albeit small) risk of exposure to HIV and other viral agents such as hepatitis B and Jakob-Creutzfeldt agent. The incidence of HIV-1 transmission associated with a percutaneous exposure to blood from an HIV-1 infected patient is approximately 0.3% per exposure.[1] In 1989, it was estimated that 12,000 United States healthcare workers acquired hepatitis B annually.[2] An understanding of the appropriate procedures, responsibilities, and risks inherent in the collection and handling of patient specimens is necessary for safe practice and is required by Occupational Safety and Health Administration (OSHA) regulations.

The Occupational Safety and Health Administration published its "Final Rule on Occupational Exposure to Bloodborne Pathogens" in the Federal Register on December 6, 1991. OSHA has chosen to follow the Center for Disease Control (CDC) definition of universal precautions. The Final Rule provides full legal force to universal precautions and requires employers and employees to treat blood and certain body fluids as if they were infectious. The Final Rule mandates that healthcare workers must avoid parenteral contact and must avoid splattering blood or other potentially infectious material on their skin, hair, eyes, mouth, mucous membranes, or on their personal clothing. Hazard abatement strategies must be used to protect the workers. Such plans typically include, but are not limited to, the following:

- safe handling of sharp items ("sharps") and disposal of such into puncture resistant containers
- gloves required for employees handling items soiled with blood or equipment contaminated by blood or other body fluids
- provisions of protective clothing when more extensive contact with blood or body fluids may be anticipated (eg, surgery, autopsy, or deliveries)
- resuscitation equipment to reduce necessity for mouth to mouth resuscitation
- restriction of HIV- or hepatitis B-exposed employees to noninvasive procedures

OSHA has specifically defined the following terms: **Occupational exposure** means reasonably anticipated skin, eye mucous membrane, or parenteral contact with blood or other potentially infectious materials that may result from the performance of an employee's duties. **Other potentially infectious materials** are human body fluids including semen, vaginal secretions, cerebrospinal fluid, synovial fluid, pleural fluid, pericardial fluid, peritoneal fluid, amniotic fluid, saliva in dental procedures, and body fluids that are visibly contaminated with blood, and all body fluids in situations where it is difficult or impossible to differentiate between body fluids; any unfixed tissue or organ (other than intact skin) from a human (living or dead); and HIV-containing cell or tissue cultures, organ cultures, and HIV- or HBV-containing culture medium or other solutions, and blood, organs, or other tissues from experimental animals infected with HIV or HBV. An **exposure incident** involves specific eye, mouth, other mucous membrane, nonintact skin, or parenteral contact with blood or other potentially infectious materials that results from the performance of an employee's duties.[3] It is important to understand that some exposures may go unrecognized despite the strictest precautions.

A written Exposure Control Plan is required. Employers must provide copies of the plan to employees and to OSHA upon request. Compliance with OSHA rules may be accomplished by the following methods.

- **Universal precautions (UPs)** means that all human blood and certain body fluids are treated as if known to be infectious for HIV, HBV, and other bloodborne pathogens. UPs do not apply to feces, nasal secretions, saliva, sputum, sweat, tears, urine, or vomitus unless they contain visible blood.
- **Engineering controls (ECs)** are physical devices which reduce or remove hazards from the workplace by eliminating or minimizing hazards or by isolating the worker from exposure. Engineering control devices include sharps disposal containers, self-resheathing syringes, etc.
- **Work practice controls (WPCs)** are practices and procedures that reduce the likelihood of exposure to hazards by altering the way in which a task is performed. Specific examples are the prohibition of two-handed recapping of needles, prohibition of storing food alongside potentially contaminated material, discouragement of pipetting fluids by mouth, encouraging handwashing after removal of gloves, safe handling of contaminated sharps, and appropriate use of sharps containers.
- **Personal protective equipment (PPE)** is specialized clothing or equipment worn to provide protection from occupational exposure. PPE includes gloves, gowns, laboratory coats (the type and characteristics will depend upon the task and degree of exposure anticipated), face shields or masks, and eye protection. Surgical caps or hoods and/or shoe covers or boots are required in instances in which gross contamination can reasonably be anticipated (eg, autopsies, orthopedic surgery). If PPE is penetrated by blood or any contaminated material, the item must be removed immediately or as soon as feasible. **The employer must provide and launder or dispose of all PPE at no cost to the employee.** Gloves must be worn when there is a reasonable anticipation of hand contact with potentially infectious material, including a patient's mucous membranes or nonintact skin. Disposable

OCCUPATIONAL EXPOSURE TO BLOODBORNE PATHOGENS (STANDARD / UNIVERSAL PRECAUTIONS) *(Continued)*

gloves must be changed as soon as possible after they become torn or punctured. Hands must be washed after gloves are removed. OSHA has revised the PPE standards, effective July 5, 1994, to include the requirement that the employer certify in writing that it has conducted a hazard assessment of the workplace to determine whether hazards are present that will necessitate the use of PPE. Also, verification that the employee has received and understood the PPE training is required.[4]

Housekeeping protocols: OSHA requires that all bins, cans, and similar receptacles, intended for reuse which have a reasonable likelihood for becoming contaminated, be inspected and decontaminated immediately or as soon as feasible upon visible contamination and on a regularly scheduled basis. Broken glass that may be contaminated must not be picked up directly with the hands. Mechanical means (eg, brush, dust pan, tongs, or forceps) must be used. Broken glass must be placed in a proper sharps container.

Employers are responsible for teaching appropriate clean-up procedures for the work area and personal protective equipment. A 1:10 dilution of household bleach is a popular and effective disinfectant. It is prudent for employers to maintain signatures or initials of employees who have been properly educated. If one does not have written proof of education of universal precautions teaching, then by OSHA standards, such education never happened.

Pre-exposure and postexposure protocols: OSHA's Final Rule includes the provision that employees, who are exposed to contamination, be offered the hepatitis B vaccine at no cost to the employee. Employees may decline; however, a declination form must be signed. The employee must be offered free vaccine if he/she changes his/her mind. Vaccination to prevent the transmission of hepatitis B in the healthcare setting is widely regarded as sound practice.[5] In the event of exposure, a confidential medical evaluation and follow-up must be offered at no cost to the employee. Follow-up must include collection and testing of blood from the source individual for HBV and HIV if permitted by state law if a blood sample is available. If a postexposure specimen must be specially drawn, the individual's consent is usually required. Some states may not require consent for testing of patient blood after accidental exposure. One must refer to state and/or local guidelines for proper guidance.

The employee follow-up must also include appropriate postexposure prophylaxis, counseling, and evaluation of reported illnesses. The employee has the right to decline baseline blood collection and/or testing. If the employee gives consent for the collection but not the testing, the sample must be preserved for 90 days in the event that the employee changes his/her mind within that time. Confidentiality related to blood testing must be ensured. **The employer does not have the right to know the results** of the testing of either the source individual or the exposed employee.

MANAGEMENT OF HEALTHCARE WORKER EXPOSURES TO HBV, HCV, AND HIV

Adapted from Updated U.S. Public Health Service Guidelines for the Management of Occupational Exposures to HIV and Recommendations for Postexposure Prophylaxis, "Recommended HIV Postexposure Prophylaxis (PEP) for Percutaneous Injuries," *MMWR Recomm Rep*, 2005, 54(RR-9):3-17.

Likelihood of transmission of HIV-1 from occupational exposure is 0.2% per parenteral exposure (eg, needlestick) to blood from HIV infected patients. Factors that increase risk for occupational transmission include advanced stages of HIV in source patient, hollow bore needle puncture, a poor state of health or inexperience of healthcare worker (HCW). After first aid is initiated, the healthcare worker should report exposure to a supervisor and to the institution's occupational medical service for evaluation. All parenteral exposures should be treated equally until they can be evaluated by the occupational medicine service, who will then determine the actual risk of exposure. Counselling regarding risk of exposure, antiviral prophylaxis, plans for follow up, exposure prevention, sexual activity, and providing emotional support and response to concerns are necessary to support the exposed healthcare worker. Additional information should be provided to healthcare workers who are pregnant or planning to become pregnant.

Immediate actions include aggressive first aid at the puncture site (eg, scrubbing site with povidone-iodine solution or soap and water for 10 minutes) or at mucus membrane site (eg, saline irrigation of eye for 15 minutes), followed by immediate reporting to the hospital's occupational medical service where a thorough investigation should be performed, including identification of the source, type of exposure, volume of inoculum, timing of exposure, extent of injury, appropriateness of first aid, as well as psychological status of the healthcare worker. HIV serologies should be performed on the healthcare worker and HIV risk counselling should begin at this point. Although the data are not clear, antiviral prophylaxis may be offered to healthcare workers who are parenterally or mucous membrane exposed. If used, antiretroviral prophylaxis should be initiated within 1-2 hours after exposure.

Factors to Consider in Assessing the Need for Follow-up of Occupational Exposures

- **Type of exposure**
  - Percutaneous injury
  - Mucous membrane exposure
  - Nonintact skin exposure
  - Bites resulting in blood exposure to either person involved
- **Type and amount of fluid/tissue**
  - Blood
  - Fluids containing blood
  - Potentially infectious fluid or tissue (semen; vaginal secretions; and cerebro-spinal, synovial, pleural, peritoneal, pericardial, and amniotic fluids)
  - Direct contact with concentrated virus
- **Infectious status of source**
  - Presence of HB_sAg
  - Presence of HCV antibody
  - Presence of HIV antibody
- **Susceptibility of exposed person**
  - Hepatitis B vaccine and vaccine response status
  - HBV, HCV, HIV immune status

Evaluation of Occupational Exposure Sources

Known sources

- Test known sources for HB_sAg, anti-HCV, and HIV antibody
  - Direct virus assays for routine screening of source patients are **not** recommended
  - Consider using a rapid HIV-antibody test
  - If the source person is **not** infected with a bloodborne pathogen, baseline testing or further follow-up of the exposed person is **not** necessary
- For sources whose infection status remains unknown (eg, the source person refuses testing), consider medical diagnoses, clinical symptoms, and history of risk behaviors
- Do not test discarded needles for bloodborne pathogens

Unknown sources

- For unknown sources, evaluate the likelihood of exposure to a source at high risk for infection
  - Consider the likelihood of bloodborne pathogen infection among patients in the exposure setting

OCCUPATIONAL EXPOSURE TO BLOODBORNE PATHOGENS (STANDARD / UNIVERSAL PRECAUTIONS) *(Continued)*

Recommended Postexposure Prophylaxis for Exposure to Hepatitis B Virus

Vaccination and Antibody Response Status of Exposed Workers[1]	Treatment		
	Source HB$_s$Ag[2]-Positive	Source HB$_s$Ag[2]-Negative	Source Unknown or Not Available for Testing
Unvaccinated	HBIG[3] x 1 and initiate HB vaccine series[4]	Initiate HB vaccine series	Initiate HB vaccine series
Previously vaccinated			
Known responder[5]	No treatment	No treatment	No treatment
Known nonresponder[6]	HBIG x 1 and initiate revaccination or HBIG x 2[7]	No treatment	If known high risk source, treat as if source was HB$_s$Ag-positive
Antibody response unknown	Test exposed person for anti-HB$_s$[8] 1. If adequate,[5] no treatment is necessary 2. If inadequate,[6] administer HBIG x 1 and vaccine booster	No treatment	Test exposed person for anti-HB$_s$ 1. If adequate,[4] no treatment is necessary 2. If inadequate,[4] administer vaccine booster and recheck titer in 1-2 months

[1]Persons who have previously been infected with HBV are immune to reinfection and do not require postexposure prophylaxis.

[2]Hepatitis B surface antigen.

[3]Hepatitis B immune globulin; dose is 0.06 mL/kg intramuscularly.

[4]Hepatitis B vaccine.

[5]A responder is a person with adequate levels of serum antibody to HB$_s$Ag (ie, anti-HB$_s$ $\geq$10 mIU/mL).

[6]A nonresponder is a person with inadequate response to vaccination (ie, serum anti-HB$_s$ <10 mIU/mL).

[7]The option of giving one dose of HBIG and reinitiating the vaccine series is preferred for nonresponders who have not completed a second 3-dose vaccine series. For persons who previously completed a second vaccine series but failed to respond, two doses of HBIG are preferred.

[8]Antibody to HB$_s$Ag.

Recommended HIV Postexposure Prophylaxis (PEP) for Percutaneous Injuries

Exposure Type	HIV-Positive, Class 1[1]	HIV-Positive, Class 2[1]	Infection Status of Source		HIV-Negative
			Source of Unknown HIV Status[2]	Unknown Source[3]	
Less severe[4]	Recommend basic 2-drug PEP	Recommend expanded ≥3-drug PEP	Generally, no PEP warranted; however, consider basic 2-drug PEP[5] for source with HIV risk factors[6]	Generally, no PEP warranted; however, consider basic 2-drug PEP[5] in settings in which exposure to HIV-infected persons is likely	No PEP warranted
More severe[7]	Recommend expanded 3-drug PEP	Recommend expanded ≥3-drug PEP	Generally, no PEP warranted; however consider basic 2-drug PEP[5] for source with HIV risk factors[6]	Generally, no PEP warranted; however, consider basic 2-drug PEP[5] in settings in which exposure to HIV-infected persons is likely	No PEP warranted

[1]HIV-positive, class 1 – asymptomatic HIV infection or known low viral load (eg, <1500 ribonucleic acid copies/mL). HIV-positive, class 2 – symptomatic HIV infection, AIDS, acute seroconversion, or known high viral load. If drug resistance is a concern, obtain expert consultation. Initiation of PEP should not be delayed pending expert consultation, and, because expert consultation alone cannot substitute for face-to-face counseling, resources should be available to provide immediate evaluation and follow-up care for all exposures.

[2]For example, deceased source person with no samples available for HIV testing.

[3]For example, a needle from a sharps disposal container.

[4]For example, solid needle or superficial injury.

[5]The recommendation "consider PEP" indicates that PEP is optional; a decision to initiate PEP should be based on a discussion between the exposed person and the treating clinician regarding the risks versus benefits of PEP.

[6]If PEP is offered and administered and the source is later determined to be HIV-negative, PEP should be discontinued.

[7]For example, large-bore hollow needle, deep puncture, visible blood on device, or needle used in patient's artery or vein.

OCCUPATIONAL EXPOSURE TO BLOODBORNE PATHOGENS (STANDARD / UNIVERSAL PRECAUTIONS) *(Continued)*

Recommended HIV Postexposure Prophylaxis (PEP) for Mucous Membrane Exposures and Nonintact Skin[1] Exposures

Exposure Type	HIV-Positive, Class 1[2]	HIV-Positive, Class 2[2]	Source of Unknown HIV Status[3]	Unknown Source[4]	HIV-Negative
			Infection Status of Source		
Small volume[5]	Consider basic 2-drug PEP[6]	Recommend basic 2-drug PEP	Generally, no PEP warranted[7]	Generally, no PEP warranted	No PEP warranted
Large volume[8]	Recommend basic 2-drug PEP	Recommend expanded ≥3-drug PEP	Generally, no PEP warranted; however, consider basic 2-drug PEP[6] for source with HIV risk factors[7]	Generally, no PEP warranted; however, consider basic 2-drug PEP[6] in settings in which exposure to HIV-infected persons is likely	No PEP warranted

[1]For skin exposures, follow-up is indicated only if evidence exists of compromised skin integrity (eg, dermatitis, abrasion, or open wound).

[2]HIV-positive, class 1 – asymptomatic HIV infection or known low viral load (eg, <1500 ribonucleic acid copies/mL). HIV-positive, class 2 – symptomatic HIV infection, AIDS, acute seroconversion, or known high viral load. If drug resistance is a concern, obtain expert consultation. Initiation of PEP should not be delayed pending expert consultation, and, because expert consultation alone cannot substitute for face-to-face counseling, resources should be available to provide immediate evaluation and follow-up care for all exposures.

[3]For example, deceased source person with no samples available for HIV testing.

[4]For example, splash from inappropriately disposed blood.

[5]For example, a few drops.

[6]The recommendation "consider PEP" indicates that PEP is optional; a decision to initiate PEP should be based on a discussion between the exposed person and the treating clinician regarding the risks versus benefits of PEP.

[7]If PEP is offered and administered and the source is later determined to be HIV-negative, PEP should be discontinued.

[8]For example, a major blood splash.

Situations for Which Expert[1] Consultation for HIV Postexposure Prophylaxis Is Advised

- **Delayed (ie, later than 24-36 hours) exposure report**
  - The interval after which there is no benefit from postexposure prophylaxis (PEP) is undefined

- **Unknown source (eg, needle in sharps disposal container or laundry)**
  - Decide use of PEP on a case-by-case basis
  - Consider the severity of the exposure and the epidemiologic likelihood of HIV exposure
  - Do not test needles or sharp instruments for HIV

- **Known or suspected pregnancy in the exposed person**
  - Does not preclude the use of optimal PEP regimens
  - Do not deny PEP solely on the basis of pregnancy

- **Breast-feeding in the exposed person**
  - Use of optimal PEP regimen not precluded
  - PEP should not be denied solely on the basis of breast-feeding

- **Resistance of the source virus to antiretroviral agents**
  - Influence of drug resistance on transmission risk is unknown
  - Selection of drugs to which the source person's virus is unlikely to be resistant is recommended, if the source person's virus is unknown or suspected to be resistant to ≥1 of the drugs considered for the PEP regimen
  - Resistance testing of the source person's virus at the time of the exposure is not recommended
  - Initiation of PEP not to be delayed while awaiting results of resistance testing

- **Toxicity of the initial PEP regimen**
  - Adverse symptoms, such as nausea and diarrhea, are common with PEP
  - Symptoms can often be managed without changing the PEP regimen by prescribing antimotility and/or antiemetic agents
  - Modification of dose intervals (ie, administering a lower dose of drug more frequently throughout the day, as recommended by the manufacturer), in other situations, might help alleviate symptoms

[1]Local experts and/or the National Clinicians' Postexposure Prophylaxis Hotline (PEPline 1-888-448-4911).

OCCUPATIONAL EXPOSURE TO BLOODBORNE PATHOGENS (STANDARD / UNIVERSAL PRECAUTIONS) *(Continued)*

Occupational Exposure Management Resources

National Clinicians' Postexposure Prophylaxis Hotline (PEPline)
Run by University of California-San Francisco/San Francisco General Hospital staff; supported by the Health Resources and Services Administration Ryan White CARE Act, HIV/AIDS Bureau, AIDS Education and Training Centers, and CDC

Phone: (888) 448-4911
Internet: http://www.ucsf.edu/hivcntr

Needlestick!
A website to help clinicians manage and document occupational blood and body fluid exposures. Developed and maintained by the University of California, Los Angeles (UCLA), Emergency Medicine Center, UCLA School of Medicine, and funded in part by CDC and the Agency for Healthcare Research and Quality.

Internet: http://
www.needlestick.mednet.ucla.edu

Hepatitis Hotline

Phone: (888) 443-7232
Internet: http://www.cdc.gov/hepatitis

Reporting to CDC:
Occupationally acquired HIV infections and failures of PEP

Phone: (800) 893-0485

HIV Antiretroviral Pregnancy Registry

Phone: (800) 258-4263
Fax: (800) 800-1052
Address: 1410 Commonwealth Drive, Suite 215
Wilmington, NC 28405
Internet: http://www.glaxowellcome.com/
preg_reg/antiretroviral

Food and Drug Administration
Report unusual or severe toxicity to antiretroviral agents

Phone: (800) 332-1088
Address: MedWatch
HF-2, FDA
5600 Fishers Lane
Rockville, MD 20857
Internet: http://www.fda.gov/medwatch

HIV/AIDS Treatment Information Service

Internet: http://www.aidsinfo.nih.gov

Management of Occupational Blood Exposures

Provide immediate care to the exposure site

- Wash wounds and skin with soap and water
- Flush mucous membranes with water

Determine risk associated with exposure by:

- Type of fluid (eg, blood, visibly bloody fluid, other potentially infectious fluid or tissue, and concentrated virus)
- Type of exposure (ie, percutaneous injury, mucous membrane or nonintact skin exposure, and bites resulting in blood exposure)

Evaluate exposure source

- Assess the risk of infection using available information
- Test known sources for HB$_s$Ag, anti-HCV, and HIV antibody (consider using rapid testing)
- For unknown sources, assess risk of exposure to HBV, HCV, or HIV infection
- Do not test discarded needle or syringes for virus contamination

Evaluate the exposed person

- Assess immune status for HBV infection (ie, by history of hepatitis B vaccination and vaccine response)

Give PEP for exposures posing risk of infection transmission

- HBV: See Recommended Postexposure Prophylaxis for Exposure to Hepatitis B Virus Table
- HCV: PEP not recommended
- HIV: See Recommended HIV Postexposure Prophylaxis for Percutaneous Injuries Table and Recommended HIV Postexposure Prophylaxis for Mucous Membrane Exposures and Nonintact Skin Exposures Table
  - Initiate PEP as soon as possible, preferably within hours of exposure
  - Offer pregnancy testing to all women of childbearing age not known to be pregnant
  - Seek expert consultation if viral resistance is suspected
  - Administer PEP for 4 weeks if tolerated

Perform follow-up testing and provide counseling

- Advise exposed persons to seek medical evaluation for any acute illness occurring during follow-up

HBV exposures

- Perform follow-up anti-HB$_s$ testing in persons who receive hepatitis B vaccine
  - Test for anti-HB$_s$ 1-2 months after last dose of vaccine
  - Anti-HB$_s$ response to vaccine cannot be ascertained if HBIG was received in the previous 3-4 months

HCV exposures

- Perform baseline and follow-up testing for anti-HCV and alanine amino-transferase (ALT) 4-6 months after exposures
- Perform HCV RNA at 4-6 months if earlier diagnosis of HCV infection is desired
- Confirm repeatedly reactive anti-HCV enzyme immunoassays (EIAs) with supplemental tests

HIV exposures

- Perform HIV antibody testing for at least 6 months postexposure (eg, at baseline, 6 weeks, 3 months, and 6 months)
- Perform HIV antibody testing if illness compatible with an acute retroviral syndrome occurs
- Advise exposed persons to use precautions to prevent secondary transmission during the follow-up period
- Evaluate exposed persons taking PEP within 72 hours after exposure and monitor for drug toxicity for at least 2 weeks

OCCUPATIONAL EXPOSURE TO BLOODBORNE PATHOGENS (STANDARD / UNIVERSAL PRECAUTIONS) *(Continued)*

Basic and Expanded HIV Postexposure Prophylaxis Regimens

BASIC REGIMENS

Zidovudine (Retrovir®; ZDV; AZT) + lamivudine (Epivir®; 3TC); available as Combivir®

Preferred dosing
- ZDV: 300 mg twice daily or 200 mg three times daily, with food; total: 600 mg daily
- 3TC: 300 mg once daily or 150 mg twice daily
- Combivir®: One tablet twice daily

Advantages
- ZDV associated with decreased risk for HIV transmission
- ZDV used more often than other drugs for PEP for healthcare personnel (HCP)
- Serious toxicity rare when used for PEP
- Side effects predictable and manageable with antimotility and antiemetic agents
- Can be used by pregnant HCP
- Can be given as a single tablet (Combivir®) twice daily

Disadvantages
- Side effects (especially nausea and fatigue) common and might result in low adherence
- Source-patient virus resistance to this regimen possible
- Potential for delayed toxicity (oncogenic/teratogenic) unknown

Zidovudine (Retrovir®; ZDV; AZT) + emtricitabine (Emtriva®; FTC)

Preferred dosing
- ZDV: 300 mg twice daily or 200 mg three times daily, with food; total: 600 mg/day, in 2-3 divided doses
- FTC: 200 mg (one capsule) once daily

Advantages
- ZDV: See above
- FTC
  - Convenient (once daily)
  - Well tolerated
  - Long intracellular half-life (~40 hours)

Disadvantages
- ZDV: See above
- FTC
  - Rash perhaps more frequent than with 3TC
  - No long-term experience with this drug
  - Cross resistance to 3TC
  - Hyperpigmentation among non-Caucasians with long-term use: 3%

Tenofovir DF (Viread®; TDF) + lamivudine (Epivir®; 3TC)

Preferred dosing
- TDF: 300 mg once daily
- 3TC: 300 mg once daily or 150 mg twice daily

Advantages
- 3TC: See above
- TDF
  - Convenient dosing (single pill once daily)
  - Resistance profile activity against certain thymidine analogue mutations
  - Well tolerated

Disadvantages
- TDF
  - Same class warnings as nucleoside reverse transcriptase inhibitors (NRTIs)
  - Drug interactions
  - Increased TDF concentrations among persons taking atazanavir and lopinavir/ritonavir; need to monitor patients for TDF-associated toxicities
- Preferred dosage of atazanavir if used with TDF: 300 mg + ritonavir 100 mg once daily + TDF 300 mg once daily

Tenofovir DF (Viread®; TDF) + emtricitabine (Emtriva®; FTC); available as Truvada®

Preferred dosing
- TDF: 300 mg once daily
- FTC: 200 mg once daily
- As Truvada®: One tablet daily

Advantages
- FTC: See above
- TDF
  - Convenient dosing (single pill once daily)
  - Resistance profile activity against certain thymidine analogue mutations
  - Well tolerated

Disadvantages
- TDF
  - Same class warnings as NRTIs
  - Drug interactions
  - Increased TDF concentrations among persons taking atazanavir and lopinavir/ritonavir; need to monitor patients for TDF-associated toxicities
  - Preferred dosing of atazanavir if used with TDF: 300 mg + ritonavir 100 mg once daily + TDF 300 mg once daily

ALTERNATE BASIC REGIMENS

Lamivudine (Epivir®; 3TC) + stavudine (Zerit®; d4T)
Preferred dosing
- 3TC: 300 mg once daily or 150 mg twice daily
- d4T: 40 mg twice daily (can use lower doses of 20-30 mg twice daily if toxicity occurs; equally effective but less toxic among HIV-infected patients with peripheral neuropathy); 30 mg twice daily if body weight is <60 kg

Advantages
- 3TC: See above
- d4T: Gastrointestinal (GI) side effects rare

Disadvantages
- Possibility that source-patient virus is resistant to this regimen
- Potential for delayed toxicity (oncogenic/teratogenic) unknown

Emtricitabine (Emtriva®; FTC) + stavudine (Zerit®; d4T)
Preferred dosing
- FTC: 200 mg daily
- d4T: 40 mg twice daily (can use lower doses of 20-30 mg twice daily if toxicity occurs; equally effective but less toxic among HIV-infected patients who developed peripheral neuropathy); if body weight is <60 kg, 30 mg twice daily

Advantages
- 3TC and FTC: See above; d4T's GI side effects rare

Disadvantages
- Potential that source-patient virus is resistant to this regimen
- Unknown potential for delayed toxicity (oncogenic/teratogenic) unknown

Lamivudine (Epivir®; 3TC) + didanosine (Videx®; ddI)
Preferred dosing
- 3TC: 300 mg once daily or 150 mg twice daily
- ddI: Videx® chewable/dispersible buffered tablets can be administered on an empty stomach as either 200 mg twice daily or 400 mg once daily. Patients must take at least two of the appropriate strength tablets at each dose to provide adequate buffering and prevent gastric acid degradation of ddI. Because of the need for adequate buffering, the 200 mg strength tablet should be used only as a component of a once-daily regimen. The dose is either 200 mg twice daily or 400 mg once daily for patients weighing >60 kg and 125 mg twice daily or 250 mg once daily for patients weighing >60 kg.

Advantages
- ddI: Once-daily dosing option
- 3TC: See above

Disadvantages
- Tolerability: Diarrhea more common with buffered preparation than with enteric-coated preparation
- Associated with toxicity: Peripheral neuropathy, pancreatitis, and lactic acidosis
- Must be taken on empty stomach except with TDF
- Drug interactions
- 3TC: See above

Emtricitabine (Emtriva®; FTC) + didanosine (Videx®; ddI)
Preferred dosing
- FTC: 200 mg once daily
- ddI: See above

OCCUPATIONAL EXPOSURE TO BLOODBORNE PATHOGENS (STANDARD / UNIVERSAL PRECAUTIONS) *(Continued)*

Advantages
- ddI: See above
- FTC: See above

Disadvantages
- Tolerability: Diarrhea more common with buffered than with enteric-coated preparation
- Associated with toxicity: Peripheral neuropathy, pancreatitis, and lactic acidosis
- Must be taken on empty stomach except with TDF
- Drug interactions
- FTC: See above

PREFERRED EXPANDED REGIMEN

Basic regimen plus:

Lopinavir / Ritonavir (Kaletra®; LPV/RTV)
Preferred dosing
- LPV/RTV: 400 mg/100 mg = twice daily with food

Advantages
- Potent HIV protease inhibitor
- Generally well-tolerated

Disadvantages
- Potential for serious or life-threatening drug interactions
- Might accelerate clearance of certain drugs, including oral contraceptives (requiring alternative or additional contraceptive measures for women taking these drugs)
- Can cause severe hyperlipidemia, especially hypertriglyceridemia
- GI (eg, diarrhea) events common

ALTERNATE EXPANDED REGIMEN

Basic regimen plus one of the following:

Atazanavir (Reyataz®; ATV) ± ritonavir (Norvir®; RTV)
Preferred dosing
- ATV: 400 mg once daily, unless used in combination with TDF, in which case ATV should be boosted with RTV, preferred dosing of ATV 300 mg + RTV: 100 mg once daily

Advantages
- Potent HIV protease inhibitor
- Convenient dosing – once daily
- Generally well tolerated

Disadvantages
- Hyperbilirubinemia and jaundice common
- Potential for serious or life-threatening drug interactions
- Avoid coadministration with proton pump inhibitors
- Separate antacids and buffered medications by 2 hours and H$_2$-receptor antagonists by 12 hours to avoid decreasing ATV levels
- Caution should be used with ATV and products known to induce PR prolongation (eg, diltiazem)

Fosamprenavir (Lexiva™; FOSAPV) ± ritonavir (Norvir®; RTV)
Preferred dosing
- FOSAPV: 1400 mg twice daily (without RTV)
- FOSAPV: 1400 mg once daily + RTV 200 mg once daily
- FOSAPV: 700 mg twice daily + RTV 100 mg twice daily

Advantages
- Once daily dosing when given with ritonavir

Disadvantages
- Tolerability: GI side effects common
- Multiple drug interactions. Oral contraceptives decrease fosamprenavir concentrations.
- Incidence of rash in healthy volunteers, especially when used with low doses of ritonavir. Differentiating between early drug-associated rash and acute seroconversion can be difficult and cause extraordinary concern for the exposed person.

Indinavir (Crixivan®; IDV) ± ritonavir (Norvir®; RTV)
Preferred dosing
- IDV 800 mg + RTV 100 mg twice daily without regard to food

Alternative dosing
- IDV: 800 mg every 8 hours, on an empty stomach

Advantages
- Potent HIV inhibitor

Disadvantages
- Potential for serious or life-threatening drug interactions
- Serious toxicity (eg, nephrolithiasis) possible; consumption of 8 glasses of fluid/day required
- Hyperbilirubinemia common; must avoid this drug during late pregnancy
- Requires acid for absorption and cannot be taken simultaneously with ddl, chewable/dispersible buffered tablet formulation (doses must be separated by ≥1 hour)

Saquinavir (Invirase®; SQV) + ritonavir (Norvir®; RTV)

Preferred dosing
- SQV: 1000 mg (given as Invirase®) + RTV 100 mg, twice daily
- SQV: Five capsules twice daily + RTV: One capsule twice daily

Advantages
- Generally well-tolerated, although GI events common

Disadvantages
- Potential for serious or life-threatening drug interactions
- Substantial pill burden

Nelfinavir (Viracept®; NFV)

Preferred dosing
- NFV: 1250 mg (2 x 625 mg or 5 x 250 mg tablets), twice daily with a meal

Advantages
- Generally well-tolerated

Disadvantages
- Diarrhea or other GI events common
- Potential for serious and/or life-threatening drug interactions

Efavirenz (Sustiva®; EFV)

Preferred dosing
- EFV: 600 mg daily, at bedtime

Advantages
- Does not require phosphorylation before activation and might be active earlier than other antiretroviral agents (a theoretic advantage of no demonstrated clinical benefit)
- Once daily dosing

Disadvantages
- Drug associated with rash (early onset) that can be severe and might rarely progress to Stevens-Johnson syndrome
- Differentiating between early drug-associated rash and acute seroconversion can be difficult and cause extraordinary concern for the exposed person
- Central nervous system side effects (eg, dizziness, somnolence, insomnia, or abnormal dreaming) common; severe psychiatric symptoms possible (dosing before bedtime might minimize these side effects)
- Teratogen; should not be used during pregnancy
- Potential for serious or life-threatening drug interactions

ANTIRETROVIRAL AGENTS GENERALLY NOT RECOMMENDED FOR USE AS PEP

Nevirapine (Viramune®; NVP)

Disadvantages
- Associated with severe hepatotoxicity (including at least one case of liver failure requiring liver transplantation in an exposed person taking PEP)
- Associated with rash (early onset) that can be severe and progress to Stevens-Johnson syndrome
- Differentiating between early drug-associated rash and acute seroconversion can be difficult and cause extraordinary concern for the exposed person
- Drug interactions: Can lower effectiveness of certain antiretroviral agents and other commonly used medicines

Delavirdine (Rescriptor®; DLV)

Disadvantages
- Drug associated with rash (early onset) that can be severe and progress to Stevens-Johnson syndrome
- Multiple drug interactions

OCCUPATIONAL EXPOSURE TO BLOODBORNE PATHOGENS (STANDARD / UNIVERSAL PRECAUTIONS) *(Continued)*

Abacavir (Ziagen®; ABC)

Disadvantages

- – Severe hypersensitivity reactions can occur, usually within the first 6 weeks
- – Differentiating between early drug-associated rash/hypersensitivity and acute seroconversion can be difficult

Zalcitabine (Hivid®; ddC)

Disadvantages

- – Three times a day dosing
- – Tolerability
- – Weakest antiretroviral agent

ANTIRETROVIRAL AGENT FOR USE AS PEP ONLY WITH EXPERT CONSULTATION

Enfuvirtide (Fuzeon™; T20)

Preferred dosing

- – T20: 90 mg (1 mL) twice daily by subcutaneous injection

Advantages

- – New class
- – Unique viral target; to block cell entry
- – Prevalence of resistance low

Disadvantages

- – Twice-daily injection
- – Safety profile: Local injection site reactions
- – Never studied among antiretroviral-naive or HIV-negative patients
- – False-positive EIA HIV antibody tests might result from formation of anti-T20 antibodies that cross-react with anti-gp41 antibodies

HAZARDOUS COMMUNICATION

Communication regarding the dangers of bloodborne infections through the use of labels, signs, information, and education is required. Storage locations (eg, refrigerators and freezers, waste containers) that are used to store, dispose of, transport, or ship blood or other potentially infectious materials require labels. The label background must be red or bright orange with the biohazard design and the word biohazard in a contrasting color. The label must be part of the container or affixed to the container by permanent means.

Education provided by a qualified and knowledgeable instructor is mandated. The sessions for employees must include:

- • accessible copies of the regulation
- • general epidemiology of bloodborne diseases
- • modes of bloodborne pathogen transmission
- • an explanation of the exposure control plan and a means to obtain copies of the written plan
- • an explanation of the tasks and activities that may involve exposure
- • the use of exposure prevention methods and their limitations (eg, engineering controls, work practices, personal protective equipment)
- • information on the types, proper use, location, removal, handling, decontamination, and disposal of personal protective equipment
- • an explanation of the basis for selection of personal protective equipment
- • information on the HBV vaccine, including information on its efficacy, safety, and method of administration and the benefits of being vaccinated (ie, the employee must understand that the vaccine and vaccination will be offered free of charge)
- • information on the appropriate actions to take and persons to contact in an emergency involving exposure to blood or other potentially infectious materials
- • an explanation of the procedure to follow if an exposure incident occurs, including the method of reporting the incident
- • information on the postexposure evaluation and follow-up that the employer is required to provide for the employee following an exposure incident
- • an explanation of the signs, labels, and color coding
- • an interactive question-and-answer period

RECORD KEEPING

The OSHA Final Rule requires that the employer maintain both education and medical records. The medical records must be kept confidential and be maintained for the duration of employment plus 30 years. They must contain a copy of the employee's HBV vaccination status and postexposure incident information. Education records must be maintained for 3 years from the date the program was given.

OSHA has the authority to conduct inspections without notice. Penalties for cited violation may be assessed as follows:

Serious violations. In this situation, there is a substantial probability of death or serious physical harm, and the employer knew, or should have known, of the hazard. A violation of this type carries a mandatory penalty of up to $7000 for each violation.

Other-than-serious violations. The violation is unlikely to result in death or serious physical harm. This type of violation carries a discretionary penalty of up to $7000 for each violation.

Willful violations. These are violations committed knowingly or intentionally by the employer and have penalties of up to $70,000 per violation with a minimum of $5000 per violation. If an employee dies as a result of a willful violation, the responsible party, if convicted, may receive a personal fine of up to $250,000 and/or a 6-month jail term. A corporation may be fined $500,000.

Large fines frequently follow visits to laboratories, physicians' offices, and healthcare facilities by OSHA Compliance Safety and Health Offices (CSHOS). Regulations are vigorously enforced. A working knowledge of the final rule and implementation of appropriate policies and practices is imperative for all those involved in the collection and analysis of medical specimens.

Effectiveness of universal precautions in averting exposure to potentially infectious materials has been documented.[7] Compliance with appropriate rules, procedures, and policies, including reporting exposure incidents, is a matter of personal professionalism and prudent self-preservation.

Footnotes

1. Henderson DK, Fahey BJ, Willy M, et al, "Risk for Occupational Transmission of Human Immunodeficiency Virus Type 1 (HIV-1) Associated With Clinical Exposures. A Prospective Evaluation," *Ann Intern Med*, 1990, 113(10):740-6.
2. Niu MT and Margolis HS, "Moving Into a New Era of Government Regulation: Provisions for Hepatitis B Vaccine in the Workplace, *Clin Lab Manage Rev*, 1989, 3:336-40.
3. Bruning LM, "The Bloodborne Pathogens Final Rule — Understanding the Regulation," *AORN Journal*, 1993, 57(2):439-40.
4. "Rules and Regulations," *Federal Register*, 1994, 59(66):16360-3.
5. Schaffner W, Gardner P, and Gross PA, "Hepatitis B Immunization Strategies: Expanding the Target," *Ann Intern Med*, 1993, 118(4):308-9.
6. Fahey BJ, Beekmann SE, Schmitt JM, et al, "Managing Occupational Exposures to HIV-1 in the Healthcare Workplace," *Infect Control Hosp Epidemiol*, 1993, 14(7):405-12.
7. Wong ES, Stotka JL, Chinchilli VM, et al, "Are Universal Precautions Effective in Reducing the Number of Occupational Exposures Among Healthcare Workers?" *JAMA*, 1991, 265(9):1123-8.

References

Buehler JW and Ward JW, "A New Definition for AIDS Surveillance," *Ann Intern Med*, 1993, 118(5):390-2.

Brown JW and Blackwell H, "Complying With the New OSHA Regs, Part 1: Teaching Your Staff About Biosafety," *MLO*, 1992, 24(4)24-8. Part 2: "Safety Protocols No Lab Can Ignore," 1992, 24(5):27-9. Part 3: "Compiling Employee Safety Records That Will Satisfy OSHA," 1992, 24(6):45-8.

Department of Labor, Occupational Safety and Health Administration, "Occupational Exposure to Bloodborne Pathogens; Final Rule (29 CFR Part 1910.1030), "*Federal Register*, December 6, 1991, 64004-182.

Gold JW, "HIV-1 Infection: Diagnosis and Management," *Med Clin North Am*, 1992, 76(1):1-18.

"Hepatitis B Virus: A Comprehensive Strategy for Eliminating Transmission in the United States Through Universal Childhood Vaccination," Recommendations of the Immunization Practices Advisory Committee (ACIP), *MMWR Morb Mortal Wkly Rep*, 1991, 40(RR-13):1-25.

"Mortality Attributable to HIV Infection/AIDS — United States", *MMWR Morb Mortal Wkly Rep*, 1991, 40(3):41-4.

National Committee for Clinical Laboratory Standards, "Protection of Laboratory Workers From Infectious Disease Transmitted by Blood, Body Fluids, and Tissue," NCCLS Document M29-T, Villanova, PA: NCCLS, 1989, 9(1).

"Nosocomial Transmission of Hepatitis B Virus Associated With a Spring-Loaded Fingerstick Device — California," *MMWR Morb Mortal Wkly Rep*, 1990, 39(35):610-3.

Polish LB, Shapiro CN, Bauer F, et al, "Nosocomial Transmission of Hepatitis B Virus Associated With the Use of a Spring-Loaded Fingerstick Device," *N Engl J Med*, 1992, 326(11):721-5.

"Recommendations for Preventing Transmission of Human Immunodeficiency Virus and Hepatitis B Virus to Patients During Exposure-Prone Invasive Procedures," *MMWR Morb Mortal Wkly Rep*, 1991, 40(RR-8):1-9.

"Update: Acquired Immunodeficiency Syndrome — United States," *MMWR Morb Mortal Wkly Rep*, 1992, 41(26):463-8.

"Update: Transmission of HIV Infection During an Invasive Dental Procedure — Florida," *MMWR Morb Mortal Wkly Rep*, 1991, 40(2):21-7, 33.

"Update: Universal Precautions for Prevention of Transmission of Human Immunodeficiency Virus, Hepatitis B Virus, and Other Bloodborne Pathogens in Healthcare Settings," *MMWR Morb Mortal Wkly Rep*, 1988, 37(24):377-82, 387-8.

"U.S. Public Health Service Guidelines for the Management of Occupational Exposures to HBV, HCV, and HIV and Recommendations for Postexposure Prophylaxis," *MMWR Morb Mortal Wkly Rep*, 2001, 50(RR-11).

IMMUNIZATIONS[1] (VACCINES[2])

Anthrax Vaccine Adsorbed[2]

U.S. Brand Name: BioThrax™

Use: Immunization against *Bacillus anthracis*. Recommended for individuals who may come in contact with animal products which come from anthrax endemic areas and may be contaminated with *Bacillus anthracis* spores; recommended for high-risk persons such as veterinarians and other handling potentially infected animals. Routine immunization for the general population is not recommended.

The Department of Defense is implementing an anthrax vaccination program against the biological warfare agent anthrax, which will be administered to all active duty and reserve personnel.

Use: Unlabeled/Investigational: Postexposure prophylaxis in combination with antibiotics

Stability: Store under refrigeration at 2°C to 8°C (36°F to 46°F); do not freeze.

Dosage: SubQ:

Children <18 years: Safety and efficacy have not been established

Children ≥18 years and Adults:

Primary immunization: Three injections of 0.5 mL each given 2 weeks apart, followed by three additional injections given at 6, 12, and 18 months; it is not necessary to restart the series if a dose is not given on time; resume as soon as practical

Subsequent booster injections: 0.5 mL at 1-year intervals are recommended for immunity to be maintained

Elderly: Safety and efficacy have not been established for patients >65 years of age

Administration: Administer SubQ; shake well before use. Do not use if discolored or contains particulate matter. Do not use the same site for more than one injection. Do not mix with other injections. After administration, massage injection site to disperse the vaccine.

Antithymocyte Globulin (Rabbit)

U.S. Brand Name: Thymoglobulin®

Use: Treatment of renal transplant acute rejection in conjunction with concomitant immunosuppression

Stability: Store powder under refrigeration at 2°C to 8°C (36°F to 46°F); do not freeze. Protect from light. Allow vials to reach room temperature, then reconstitute using provided diluent. Rotate vial gently until dissolved. Prior to administration, further dilute one vial in 50 mL saline or dextrose (total volume is usually 50-500 mL depending on total number of vials needed per dose). Mix by gently inverting infusion bag once or twice. Reconstituted vials should be used within 4 hours. Use immediately following dilution for infusion.

Dosage: I.V.: 1.5 mg/kg/day for 7-14 days

Dosage adjustment for toxicity:

WBC count 2000-3000 cells/mm³ or platelet count 50,000-75,000 cells/mm³: Reduce dose by 50%

WBC count <2000 cells/mm³ or platelet count <50,000 cells/mm³: Consider discontinuing treatment

Administration: The first dose should be infused over at least 6 hours through a high-flow vein. Subsequent doses should be administered over at least 4 hours. Administer through an in-line 0.22 micron filter. Premedication with corticosteroids, acetaminophen, and/or an antihistamine may reduce infusion-related reactions.

BCG Vaccine[3]

U.S. Brand Name: TheraCys®, TICE® BCG

Use: Immunization against tuberculosis and immunotherapy for cancer; treatment and prophylaxis of carcinoma *in situ* of the bladder; prophylaxis of primary or recurrent superficial papillary tumors following transurethral resection

Stability: Store vials under refrigeration at 2°C to 8°C (36°F to 46°F); protect from light. Use within 2 hours of mixing.

TheraCys®: Reconstitute with 3 mL of diluent provided and shake gently. Withdraw contents and add 50 mL of 0.9% NaCl (preservative free).

TICE® BCG: Reconstitute with 1 mL 0.9% NaCl (preservative free) using a 3 mL syringe. Mix by drawing and expelling solution into ampul three times. Add to a catheter tip syringe containing 49 mL of 0.9% NaCl (preservative free). Use within 2 hours of mixing.

BCG Vaccine U.S.P.: Reconstitute with 1 mL of SWFI; swirl gently, do not vigorously shake. For children <1 month, reconstitute with 2 mL SWFI.

Dosage:

Immunization against tuberculosis: Percutaneous: **Note:** Initial lesion usually appears after 10-14 days consisting of small, red papule at injection site and reaches maximum diameter of 3 mm in 4-6 weeks.

Children <1 month: 0.2-0.3 mL (half-strength dilution). Administer tuberculin test (5 TU) after 2-3 months; repeat vaccination after 1 year of age for negative tuberculin test if indications persist.

Children >1 month and Adults: 0.2-0.3 mL (full strength dilution); conduct postvaccinal tuberculin test (5 TU of PPD) in 2-3 months; if test is negative, repeat vaccination.

Immunotherapy for bladder cancer: Intravesicular: Adults:

TheraCys®: One dose instilled into bladder (for 2 hours) once weekly for 6 weeks followed by one treatment at 3, 6, 12, 18, and 24 months after initial treatment

TICE® BCG: One dose instilled into the bladder (for 2 hours) once weekly for 6 weeks followed by once monthly for 6-12 months

Administration: Should only be given intravesicularly (bladder irrigation) or percutaneously; **do not administer I.V., SubQ, or intradermally.**

Intravesicular: Empty or drain bladder. Instill BCG vaccine; retain for up to 2 hours. Patient should lie prone, rotating positions every 15 minutes to maximize bladder surface exposure.

Percutaneous: Apply vaccine with syringe and needle by dropping onto 1-2 inch area of horizontally positioned surface of cleansed, dry site (deltoid region of arm preferred); pulling skin tight, puncture skin with multiple puncture device centered over the vaccine; apply pressure for 5 seconds; spread vaccine evenly over puncture area. Apply loose covering and keep dry for 24 hours.

Botulinum Pentavalent (ABCDE) Toxoid

Use: Investigational: Prophylaxis for *C. botulinum* exposure (high-risk research laboratory personnel actively working with, or expect to work with, known cultures and purified botulinum toxin)

Dosage: Do not inject intracutaneously or into superficial structures.

Initial vaccination series: 0.5 mL deep SubQ at 0, 2, and 12 weeks

First booster: 0.5 mL deep SubQ 12 months after first injection of the initial series

Subsequent boosters: 0.5 mL deep SubQ at 2-year intervals based on antitoxin titers as checked by CDC

Botulism Immune Globulin (Intravenous-Human)

U.S. Brand Name: BabyBIG®

Use: Treatment of infant botulism caused by toxin type A or B

Stability: Prior to reconstitution, store between 2°C to 8°C (35.6°F to 46.4°F). Infusion should begin within 2 hours of reconstitution and be completed within 4 hours of reconstitution. Reconstitute with SWFI 2 mL. Swirl gently to wet powder; do not shake. Powder should dissolve in ~30 minutes.

Dosage: I.V.: Children <1 year: Infant botulism: 1 mL/kg (50 mg/kg) as a single dose; infuse at 0.5 mL/kg/hour (25 mg/kg/hour) for the first 15 minutes; if well tolerated, may increase to 1 mL/kg/hour (50 mg/kg/hour)

Administration: For I.V. infusion only. Do not administer if solution is turbid. Epinephrine should be available for the treatment of acute allergic reaction. Administer using low volume tubing and infusion pump with an in-line or syringe tip 18 μm filter. Infuse at 0.5 mL/kg/hour (25 mg/kg/hour) for the first 15 minutes; if well tolerated, may increase to 1 mL/kg/hour (50 mg/kg/hour). Infusion should take ~67.5 minutes. Infusion should be slowed or temporarily interrupted for minor side effects; discontinue in case of hypotension or anaphylaxis.

Cytomegalovirus Immune Globulin (Intravenous-Human)

U.S. Brand Name: CytoGam®

Use: Prophylaxis of cytomegalovirus (CMV) disease associated with kidney, lung, liver, pancreas, and heart transplants; concomitant use with ganciclovir should be considered in organ transplants (other than kidney) from CMV seropositive donors to CMV seronegative recipients

Use: Unlabeled/Investigational: Adjunct therapy in the treatment of CMV disease in immunocompromised patients

Stability: Store between 2°C and 8°C (35.6°F and 46.4°F). Use reconstituted product within 6 hours; do not admix with other medications; do not use if turbid. Do not shake vials. Dilution is not recommended. Infusion with other products is not recommended.

Dosage: I.V.: Adults:

Kidney transplant:

Initial dose (within 72 hours of transplant): 150 mg/kg/dose

2, 4, 6, and 8 weeks after transplant: 100 mg/kg/dose

12 and 16 weeks after transplant: 50 mg/kg/dose

Liver, lung, pancreas, or heart transplant:

Initial dose (within 72 hours of transplant): 150 mg/kg/dose

2, 4, 6, and 8 weeks after transplant: 150 mg/kg/dose

12 and 16 weeks after transplant: 100 mg/kg/dose

Severe CMV pneumonia (unlabeled): Various regimens have been used, including 400 mg/kg CMV-IGIV in combination with ganciclovir on days 1, 2, 7, or 8, followed by 200 mg/kg CMV-IGIV on days 14 and 21

Elderly: Use with caution in patients >65 years of age, may be at increased risk of renal insufficiency

IMMUNIZATIONS[1] (VACCINES[2]) *(Continued)*

Dosage adjustment in renal impairment: Use with caution; specific dosing adjustments are not available. Infusion rate should be the minimum practical; do not exceed 180 mg/kg/hour

Administration: Administer through an I.V. line containing an in-line filter (pore size 15 micron) using an infusion pump. Do not mix with other infusions; do not use if turbid. Begin infusion within 6 hours of entering vial, complete infusion within 12 hours.

Infuse at 15 mg/kg/hour. If no adverse reactions occur within 30 minutes, may increase rate to 30 mg/kg/hour. If no adverse reactions occur within the second 30 minutes, may increase rate to 60 mg/kg/hour; maximum rate of infusion: 75 mL/hour. When infusing subsequent doses, may decrease titration interval from 30 minutes to 15 minutes. If patient develops nausea, back pain, or flushing during infusion, slow the rate or temporarily stop the infusion. Discontinue if blood pressure drops or in case of anaphylactic reaction.

Diphtheria and Tetanus Toxoid[3,4]

U.S. Brand Name: Decavac™

Use:

Diphtheria and tetanus toxoids adsorbed for pediatric use (DT): Infants and children through 6 years of age: Active immunity against diphtheria and tetanus when pertussis vaccine is contraindicated

Tetanus and diphtheria toxoids adsorbed for adult use (Td) (Decavac™): Children ≥7 years of age and Adults: Active immunity against diphtheria and tetanus; tetanus prophylaxis in wound management

Stability: Store at 2°C to 8°C (35°F to 46°F); do not freeze. Discard if product has been frozen.

Dosage: I.M.:

Infants and Children ≤6 years (DT): Primary immunization:

6 weeks to 1 year: Three 0.5 mL doses at least 4 weeks apart; administer a reinforcing dose 6-12 months after the third injection

1-6 years: Two 0.5 mL doses at least 4 weeks apart; reinforcing dose 6-12 months after second injection; if final dose is given after seventh birthday, use adult preparation

4-6 years (booster immunization): 0.5 mL; not necessary if the fourth dose was given after fourth birthday; routinely administer booster doses at 10-year intervals with the adult preparation

Children ≥7 years and Adults (Td):

Primary immunization: Patients previously not immunized should receive 2 primary doses of 0.5 mL each, given at an interval of 4-6 weeks; third (reinforcing) dose of 0.5 mL 6-12 months later

Booster immunization: 0.5 mL every 10 years; to be given to children 11-12 years of age if at least 5 years have elapsed since last dose of toxoid containing vaccine. Subsequent routine doses are not recommended more often than every 10 years. The ACIP prefers Tdap for use in adolescents 11-18 years; refer to Diphtheria and Tetanus Toxoids and Acellular Pertussis Vaccine monograph for additional information.

Tetanus prophylaxis in wound management; use of tetanus toxoid (Td) and/or tetanus immune globulin (TIG) depends upon the number of prior tetanus toxoid doses and type of wound: See table.

Tetanus Prophylaxis in Wound Management

Number of Prior Tetanus Toxoid Doses	Clean, Minor Wounds		All Other Wounds	
	Td[1]	TIG[2]	Td[1]	TIG[2]
Unknown or <3	Yes	No	Yes	Yes
≥3[3]	No[4]	No	No[5]	No

[1]Adult tetanus and diphtheria toxoids; use pediatric preparations (DT or DTP) if the patient is <7 years old.

[2]Tetanus immune globulin.

[3]If only three doses of fluid tetanus toxoid have been received, a fourth dose of toxoid, preferably an adsorbed toxoid, should be given.

[4]Yes, if >10 years since last dose.

[5]Yes, if >5 years since last dose.

Adapted from Report of the Committee on Infectious Diseases, American Academy of Pediatrics, Elk Grove Village, IL: American Academy of Pediatrics, 1986.

Administration: For I.M. administration; prior to use, shake suspension well

Td: Administer in the deltoid muscle; do not inject in the gluteal area

DT: Administer in the anterolateral aspect of the thigh or the deltoid muscle; do not inject in the gluteal area

Diphtheria, Tetanus Toxoids, Acellular Pertussis, Hepatitis B (Recombinant), and Poliovirus (Inactivated) Vaccine[3,4]

U.S. Brand Name: Pediarix®

Use: Combination vaccine for the active immunization against diphtheria, tetanus, pertussis, hepatitis B virus (all known subtypes), and poliomyelitis (caused by poliovirus types 1, 2, and 3)

Stability: Store under refrigeration at 2°C to 8°C (36°F to 46°F); do not freeze. Discard if frozen.

Dosage: I.M.: Children 6 weeks to <7 years:

Immunization: 0.5 mL; repeat in 6-8 week intervals (preferably 8-week intervals) for a total of 3 doses. Vaccination usually begins at 2 months, but may be started as early as 6 weeks of age.

Use in children previously vaccinated with one or more component, and who are also scheduled to receive all vaccine components:

Hepatitis B vaccine: Infants born of HB$_s$Ag-negative mothers who received 1 dose of hepatitis B vaccine at birth may be given Pediarix® (safety data limited); use in infants who received more than 1 dose of hepatitis B vaccine has not been studied. Infants who received 1 or more doses of hepatitis B vaccine (recombinant) may be given Pediarix® to complete the hepatitis B series (safety and efficacy not established).

Diphtheria and tetanus toxoids, and acellular pertussis vaccine (DTaP): Infants previously vaccinated with 1 or 2 doses of Infanrix® may use Pediarix® to complete the first 3 doses of the series (safety and efficacy not established); use of Pediarix® to complete DTaP vaccination started with products other than Infanrix® is not recommended.

Inactivated polio vaccine (IPV): Infants previously vaccinated with 1 or 2 doses of IPV may use Pediarix® to complete the first 3 doses of the series (safety and efficacy not established).

Administration: For I.M. use only; do not administer I.V. or SubQ. Shake well prior to use; do not use unless a homogeneous, turbid, white suspension forms. Administer in the anterolateral aspects of the thigh or the deltoid muscle of the upper arm. Do not inject in the gluteal area (suboptimal hepatitis B immune response) or where there may be a major nerve trunk. Do not administer additional vaccines or immunoglobulins at the same site, or using the same syringe.

Diphtheria, Tetanus Toxoids, and Acellular Pertussis Vaccine[3,4]

U.S. Brand Name: Adacel™, Boostrix®, Daptacel®, Infanrix®, Tripedia®

Use:

Daptacel®, Infanrix®, Tripedia® (DTaP): Active immunization against diphtheria, tetanus, and pertussis from age 6 weeks through 6 years of age (prior to seventh birthday)

Adacel™, Boostrix® (Tdap): Active booster immunization against diphtheria, tetanus, and pertussis

Stability: Refrigerate at 2°C to 8°C (35°F to 46°F); do not freeze.

Dosage:

Primary immunization: Children 6 weeks to <7 years: I.M.: **Note:** Whenever possible, the same product should be used for all doses. Interruption of recommended schedule does not require starting the series over; a delay between doses should not interfere with final immunity.

Daptacel®: 0.5 mL per dose, total of 4 doses administered as follows (data insufficient to recommend a fifth dose):

Three doses, usually given at 2, 4, and 6 months of age; may be given as early as 6 weeks of age and repeated every 6-8 weeks

Fourth dose: Given at ~15-20 months of age, but at least 6 months after third dose

Infanrix®, Tripedia®: 0.5 mL per dose, total of 5 doses administered as follows:

Three doses, usually given at 2, 4, and 6 months of age; may be given as early as 6 weeks of age and repeated every 4-8 weeks

Fourth dose: Given at ~15-20 months of age, but at least 6 months after third dose

Fifth dose: Given at 5-6 years of age, prior to starting school or kindergarten; if the fourth dose is given at ≥4 years of age, the fifth dose may be omitted

Booster immunization:

ACIP recommendations:

Adolescents 11-18 years: I.M.: 0.5 mL. A single dose of Tdap should be given instead of Td in adolescents who have completed the recommended childhood DTP/DTaP series and have not received Td or Tdap; preferred age of vaccination with Tdap is 11-12 years. Adolescents who received Td but not Tdap and who have completed the recommended childhood DTP/DTaP series are encouraged to receive Tdap; an interval of at least 5 years between Td and Tdap is recommended, but lesser intervals may be used if the benefit outweighs the risk.

IMMUNIZATIONS[1] (VACCINES[2]) *(Continued)*

Adults 19-64 years (Adacel™): I.M.: 0.5 mL. A single dose should be given instead of Td in adults if they received their last dose of Td ≥10 years previous. Shorter intervals (as short as 2 years) may used among healthcare providers, adults in contact with infants, or others in settings with increased risk for pertussis, including during pertussis outbreaks. Adacel™ should only be used to replace a single booster dose of Td.

Manufacturer's labeling:

Children 10-18 years (Boostrix®): I.M.: 0.5 mL as a single dose, administered 5 years after last dose of DTwP or DTaP vaccine.

Children ≥11 years and Adults ≤64 years (Adacel™): I.M.: 0.5 mL as a single dose, administered 5 years after last dose of DTwP or DTaP vaccine.

Wound management: Adacel™ (in patients 11-64 years of age) or Boostrix® (in patients 10-18 years of age) may be used as an alternative to Td vaccine when a tetanus toxoid-containing vaccine is needed for wound management, and in whom the pertussis component is also indicated. Td vaccine is the preferred agent in children ≥7 years and adults.

ACIP recommendations: ACIP prefers Tdap for adolescents 11-18 years requiring a tetanus toxoid product and who were vaccinated against tetanus ≥5 years earlier. Adolescents who completed the primary 3 dose series containing tetanus toxoid <5 years earlier are protected against tetanus and do not need a tetanus toxoid vaccine as part of wound management. The ACIP prefers Adacel™ for use in adults <65 years requiring a tetanus toxoid product and who were vaccinated against tetanus ≥5 years earlier if they have not previously received Tdap.

Administration: Shake suspension well.

Adacel™, Boostrix®: Administer only I.M. in deltoid muscle of upper arm.

Daptacel®, Infanrix®, Tripedia®: Administer only I.M. in anterolateral aspect of thigh or deltoid muscle of upper arm.

Diphtheria, Tetanus Toxoids, and Acellular Pertussis Vaccine and *Haemophilus influenzae* B Conjugate Vaccine[4]

U.S. Brand Name: TriHIBit®

Use: Active immunization of children 15-18 months of age for prevention of diphtheria, tetanus, pertussis, and invasive disease caused by *H. influenzae* type b

Dosage: Children >15 months of age: I.M.: 0.5 mL (as part of a general vaccination schedule; see individual vaccines). Vaccine should be used within 30 minutes of reconstitution.

Haemophilus B Conjugate and Hepatitis B Vaccine[3,4]

U.S. Brand Name: Comvax®

Use:

Immunization against invasive disease caused by *H. influenzae* type b and against infection caused by all known subtypes of hepatitis B virus in infants 6 weeks to 15 months of age born of hepatitis B surface antigen (HB$_s$Ag) negative mothers

Infants born of HB$_s$Ag-positive mothers or mothers of unknown HB$_s$Ag status should receive hepatitis B immune globulin and hepatitis B vaccine (recombinant) at birth and should complete the hepatitis B vaccination series given according to a particular schedule

Stability: Store at 2°C to 8°C (36°F to 48°F); do not freeze.

Dosage: Infants: I.M.: 0.5 mL at 2, 4, and 12-15 months of age (total of 3 doses)

If the recommended schedule cannot be followed, the interval between the first two doses should be at least 6 weeks and the interval between the second and third dose should be as close as possible to 8-11 months. Minimum age for first dose is 6 weeks.

Modified Schedule: Children who receive one dose of hepatitis B vaccine at or shortly after birth may receive Comvax® on a schedule of 2, 4, and 12-15 months of age

Administration: Shake well prior to use. Administer 0.5 mL I.M. into anterolateral thigh [data suggests that injections given in the buttocks frequently are given into fatty tissue instead of into muscle to result in lower seroconversion rates]; **do not administer intravenously, intradermally, or subcutaneously**. May be administered with DTP, DTaP, OPV, IPV, MMR-II and varicella virus vaccines, using separate injection sites and syringes (for the injectable vaccines).

Haemophilus B Conjugate Vaccine[3,4]

U.S. Brand Name: ActHIB®, HibTITER®, PedvaxHIB®

Use: Routine immunization of children 2 months to 5 years of age against invasive disease caused by *H. influenzae* type b

Unimmunized children ≥5 years of age with a chronic illness known to be associated with increased risk of *Haemophilus influenzae* type b disease, specifically, persons with anatomic or functional asplenia or sickle cell anemia or those who have undergone splenectomy, should receive *H. influenzae* type b (Hib) vaccine.

Haemophilus b conjugate vaccines are not indicated for prevention of bronchitis or other infections due to *H. influenzae* in adults; adults with specific dysfunction or certain complement deficiencies who are at especially high risk of *H. influenzae* type b infection (HIV-infected adults); patients with Hodgkin's disease (vaccinated at least 2 weeks before the initiation of chemotherapy or 3 months after the end of chemotherapy)

Stability: Store under refrigeration at 2°C to 8°C (36°F to 46°F); do not freeze.

ActHIB®: Use within 24 hours following reconstitution with saline. Use within 30 minutes following reconstitution with Tripedia®.

Dosage: Children: I.M.: 0.5 mL as a single dose should be administered according to one of the following "brand-specific" schedules; do not inject I.V. (see table)

Vaccination Schedule for *Haemophilus* B Conjugate Vaccines

Age at 1st Dose (mo)	ActHIB®, HibTITER®		PedvaxHIB®	
	Primary Series	**Booster**	**Primary Series**	**Booster**
2-6	3 doses, 2 months apart	15 mo[1]	2 doses, 2 months apart	12-15 mo[1]
7-11	2 doses, 2 months apart	15 mo[1]	2 doses, 2 months apart	12-15 mo[1]
12-14	1 dose	15 mo[1]	1 dose	15 mo[1]
15-71	1 dose	–	1 dose	–

[1]At least 2 months after previous dose.

Note: DTaP/Hib combination vaccines should not be used for infants at ages 2, 4, or 6 months, but can be used as boosters following any Hib vaccine.

Hepatitis A Inactivated and Hepatitis B (Recombinant) Vaccine[3,4]

U.S. Brand Name: Twinrix®

Use: Active immunization against disease caused by hepatitis A virus and hepatitis B virus (all known subtypes) in populations desiring protection against or at high risk of exposure to these viruses.

Populations include travelers to areas of intermediate/high endemicity for **both** HAV and HBV; those at increased risk of HBV infection due to behavioral or occupational factors; patients with chronic liver disease; laboratory workers who handle live HAV and HBV; healthcare workers, police, and other personnel who render first-aid or medical assistance; workers who come in contact with sewage; employees of day care centers and correctional facilities; patients/staff of hemodialysis units; male homosexuals; patients frequently receiving blood products; military personnel; users of injectable illicit drugs; close household contacts of patients with hepatitis A and hepatitis B infection; residents of drug and alcohol treatment centers

Stability: Store in refrigerator at 2°C to 8°C (36°F to 46°F); do not freeze (discard if frozen).

Dosage: I.M.: Adults: Primary immunization: Three doses (1 mL each) given on a 0-, 1-, and 6-month schedule

Alternative regimen: Accelerated regimen (1 mL doses at day 0, 7, and 21-30, followed by a booster at 12 months) has demonstrated similar safety, tolerability, and immunogenicity to the standard regimen.

Administration: I.M.: Shake well prior to use. Do not dilute prior to administration. Administer in the deltoid region; do not administer in the gluteal region (may give suboptimal response). Do not administer at the same site, or using the same syringe, as additional vaccines or immunoglobulins.

Hepatitis A Vaccine[3,4]

U.S. Brand Name: Havrix®, VAQTA®

Use:

Active immunization against disease caused by hepatitis A virus in populations desiring protection against or at high risk of exposure

Populations at high risk of exposure to hepatitis A virus may include children and adolescents in selected states and regions, travelers to developing countries, household and sexual contacts of persons infected with hepatitis A, child day care employees, patients with chronic liver disease, illicit drug users, male homosexuals, institutional workers (eg, institutions for the mentally and physically handicapped persons, prisons), and healthcare workers who may be exposed to hepatitis A virus (eg, laboratory employees)

Stability: Store under refrigeration at 2°C to 8°C (36°F to 46°F); do not freeze.

IMMUNIZATIONS[1] (VACCINES[2]) *(Continued)*

Dosage: I.M.:

Havrix®:

Children 12 months to 18 years: 720 ELISA units (0.5 mL) with a booster dose of 720 ELISA units 6-12 months following primary immunization

Adults: 1440 ELISA units (1 mL) with a booster dose of 1440 ELISA units 6-12 months following primary immunization

VAQTA®:

Children 12 months to 18 years: 25 units (0.5 mL) with 25 units (0.5 mL) booster dose of 25 units to be given 6-18 months after primary immunization (6-12 months if initial dose was with Havrix®)

Adults: 50 units (1 mL) with 50 units (1 mL) booster dose of 50 units to be given 6-18 months after primary immunization (6-12 months if initial dose was with Havrix®)

Administration: The deltoid muscle is the preferred site for injection. Shake well prior to use. For optimal protection, travelers should receive 1st dose at least 4 weeks prior to departure.

Hepatitis B Immune Globulin

U.S. Brand Name: HepaGam B™, HyperHEP B™ S/D, Nabi-HB®

Use: Passive prophylactic immunity to hepatitis B following: Acute exposure to blood containing hepatitis B surface antigen (HB_sAg); perinatal exposure of infants born to HB_sAg-positive mothers; sexual exposure to HB_sAg-positive persons; household exposure to persons with acute HBV infection

Prevention of hepatitis B virus recurrence after liver transplantation in HBsAg-positive transplant patients

Note: Hepatitis B immune globulin is not indicated for treatment of active hepatitis B infection and is ineffective in the treatment of chronic active hepatitis B infection.

Stability: Refrigerate at 2°C to 8°C (36°F to 46°F); do not freeze. Use within 6 hours of entering vial. Do not shake vial; avoid foaming.

Dosage:

I.M.:

Newborns: Perinatal exposure of infants born to HBsAg-positive mothers: 0.5 mL as soon after birth as possible (within 12 hours); active vaccination with hepatitis B vaccine may begin at the same time in a different site (if not contraindicated). If first dose of hepatitis B vaccine is delayed for as long as 3 months, dose may be repeated. If hepatitis B vaccine is refused, dose may be repeated at 3 and 6 months.

Infants <12 months: Household exposure prophylaxis: 0.5 mL (to be administered if mother or primary caregiver has acute HBV infection)

Children ≥12 months and Adults: Postexposure prophylaxis: 0.06 mL/kg as soon as possible after exposure (ie, within 24 hours of needlestick, ocular, or mucosal exposure or within 14 days of sexual exposure); usual dose: 3-5 mL; repeat at 28-30 days after exposure in nonresponders to hepatitis B vaccine or in patients who refuse vaccination

Note: HBIG may be administered at the same time (but at a different site) or up to 1 month preceding hepatitis B vaccination without impairing the active immune response

I.V. : Adults: Prevention of hepatitis B virus recurrence after liver transplantation (HepaGam B™): 20,000 int. units/dose according to the following schedule:

Anhepatic phase (Initial dose): One dose given with the liver transplant

Week 1 postop: One dose daily for 7 days (days 1-7)

Weeks 2-12 postop: One dose every 2 weeks starting day 14

Month 4 onward: One dose monthly starting on month 4

Dose adjustment: Adjust dose to reach anti-HBs levels of 500 int. units/L within the first week after transplantation. In patients with surgical bleeding, abdominal fluid drainage >500 mL or those undergoing plasmapheresis, administer 10,000 int. units/dose every 6 hours until target anti-HBs levels are reached.

Administration:

I.M.: Postexposure prophylaxis: I.M. injection only in anterolateral aspect of upper thigh and deltoid muscle of upper arm; to prevent injury from injection, care should be taken when giving to patients with thrombocytopenia or bleeding disorders

I.V.:

HepaGam B™: Liver transplant: Administer at 2 mL/minute. Decrease infusion to ≤1 mL/minute for patient discomfort or infusion-related adverse events. Actual volume of infusion is dependant upon potency labeled on each individual vial.

Nabi-HB®: Although not an FDA-approved for this purpose, Nabi-HB® has been administered intravenously in hepatitis B-positive liver transplant patients

Hepatitis B Vaccine[2,3,4]

U.S. Brand Name: Engerix-B®, Recombivax HB®

Use: Immunization against infection caused by all known subtypes of hepatitis B virus (HBV), in individuals seeking protection from HBV infection and/or in the following individuals considered at high risk of potential exposure to hepatitis B virus or HB_sAg-positive materials:

Workplace Exposure

- Healthcare workers[1] (including students, custodial staff, lab personnel, etc)
- Police and fire personnel
- Military personnel
- Morticians and embalmers
- Clients/staff of institutions for the developmentally disabled

Lifestyle Factors

- Homosexual men
- Heterosexually-active persons with multiple partners in a 6-month period or those with recently acquired sexually-transmitted disease
- Intravenous drug users

Specific Patient Groups

- Those on hemodialysis,[2] receiving transfusions,[3] or in hematology/oncology units
- Adolescents
- Infants born of HB_sAG-positive mothers
- Individuals with chronic liver disease
- Individual with HIV infection

Others

- Prison inmates and staff of correctional facilities
- Household and sexual contacts of HBV carriers
- Residents, immigrants, adoptees, and refugees from areas with endemic HBV infection (eg, Alaskan Eskimos, Pacific Islanders, Indochinese, and Haitian descent)
- International travelers to areas of endemic HBV
- Children born after 11/21/1991

[1]The risk of hepatitis B virus (HBV) infection for healthcare workers varies both between hospitals and within hospitals. Hepatitis B vaccination is recommended for all healthcare workers with blood exposure.

[2]Hemodialysis patients often respond poorly to hepatitis B vaccination; higher vaccine doses or increased number of doses are required. A special formulation of one vaccine is now available for such persons (Recombivax HB®, 40 mcg/mL). The anti-HB_s (antibody to hepatitis B surface antigen) response of such persons should be tested after they are vaccinated, and those who have not responded should be revaccinated with 1-3 additional doses. Patients with chronic renal disease should be vaccinated as early as possible, ideally before they require hemodialysis. In addition, their anti-HB_s levels should be monitored at 6- to 12-month intervals to assess the need for revaccination.

[3]Patients with hemophilia should be immunized subcutaneously, not intramuscularly.

Stability: Refrigerate at 2°C to 8°C (36°F to 46°F); do not freeze.

Dosage: I.M.:

> Immunization regimen: Regimen consists of 3 doses (0, 1, and 6 months): First dose given on the elected date, second dose given 1 month later, third dose given 6 months after the first dose; see table.

> **Note:**

>> Infants born to mothers whose HB_sAg status is unknown should follow the regimen for HB_sAg-positive mothers, omitting the dose of HBIG.

>> Preterm infants <2000 g and born to HB_sAg-negative mothers should have the first dose delayed until 1 month after birth or hospital discharge due to decreased immune response in underweight infants.

IMMUNIZATIONS[1] (VACCINES[2]) *(Continued)*

Routine Immunization Regimen of Three I.M. Hepatitis B Vaccine Doses

Age	Initial		1 mo		2 mo		6 mo[1]	
	Recombivax HB® (mL)	Engerix-B® (mL)	Recombivax HB® (mL)	Engerix-B® (mL)	Recombivax HB® (mL)	Engerix-B® (mL)	Recombivax HB® (mL)	Engerix-B® (mL)
Birth[2] to 19 y	0.5[3]	0.5[4]	0.5[3]	0.5[4]	–	–	0.5[3]	0.5[4]
≥20 y[5]	1[6]	1[7]	1[6]	1[7]	–	–	1[6]	1[7]
Dialysis or immunocompromised patients[8]	1[9]	2[10]	1[9]	2[10]	2[10]	2[10]	1[9]	2[10]

[1]Final dose in series should not be administered before age of 24 weeks.

[2]Infants born of HB$_s$Ag negative mothers.

[3]5 mcg/0.5 mL pediatric/adolescent formulation.

[4]10 mcg/0.5 mL formulation.

[5]Alternately, doses may be administered at 0, 1, and 4 months or at 0, 2, and 4 months.

[6]10 mcg/mL adult formulation.

[7]20 mcg/mL formulation.

[8]Revaccinate if anti-HB$_s$ <10 mIU/mL ≥1-2 months after third dose.

[9]40 mcg/mL dialysis formulation.

[10]Two 1 mL doses given at different sites using the 20 mcg/mL formulation.

Alternative dosing schedule for **Recombivax HB®**:

Children 11-15 years (10 mcg/mL adult formulation): First dose of 1 mL given on the elected date, second dose given 4-6 months later

Adults ≥20 years: Doses may be administered at 0, 1, and 4 months **or** at 0, 2, and 4 months

Alternative dosing schedules for **Engerix-B®**:

Children ≤10 years (10 mcg/0.5 mL formulation): High-risk children: 0.5 mL at 0, 1, 2, and 12 months; lower-risk children ages 5-10 who are candidates for an extended administration schedule may receive an alternative regimen of 0.5 mL at 0, 12, and 24 months. If booster dose is needed, revaccinate with 0.5 mL.

Adolescents 11-19 years (20 mcg/mL formulation): 1 mL at 0, 1, and 6 months. High-risk adolescents: 1 mL at 0, 1, 2, and 12 months; lower-risk adolescents 11-16 years who are candidates for an extended administration schedule may receive an alternative regimen of 0.5 mL (using the 10 mcg/0.5 mL) formulation at 0, 12, and 24 months. If booster dose is needed, revaccinate with 20 mcg.

Adults ≥20 years: Doses may be administered at 0, 1, and 4 months or at 0, 2, and 4 months

High-risk adults (20 mcg/mL formulation): 1 mL at 0, 1, 2, and 12 months. If booster dose is needed, revaccinate with 1 mL.

Postexposure prophylaxis: **Note:** High-risk individuals may include children born of hepatitis B-infected mothers, those who have been or might be exposed or those who have traveled to high-risk areas. See table.

Postexposure Prophylaxis Recommended Dosage for Infants Born to HB$_s$Ag-Positive Mothers

Treatment	Birth ≤12 h	1 mo	6 mo
Engerix-B® (pediatric formulation 10 mcg/0.5 mL)[1]	0.5 mL[2]	0.5 mL	0.5 mL
Recombivax HB® (pediatric/adolescent formulation 5 mcg/0.5 mL)	0.5 mL[2]	0.5 mL	0.5 mL
Hepatitis B immune globulin	0.5 mL[2]	–	–

[1]An alternate regimen is administration of the vaccine at birth, and 1, 2, and 12 months later.

[2]The first dose of vaccine may be given at birth at the same time as HBIG, but give in the opposite anterolateral thigh. This may better ensure vaccine absorption. HBIG should be given immediately if mother is determined to be HB$_s$Ag-positive within 7 days of birth.

Administration: It is possible to interchange the vaccines for completion of a series or for booster doses; the antibody produced in response to each type of vaccine is comparable, however, the quantity of the vaccine will vary

I.M. injection only; in adults, the deltoid muscle is the preferred site; the anterolateral thigh is the recommended site in infants and young children. Not for gluteal administration. Shake well prior to withdrawal and use.

Immune Globulin (Intramuscular)[4]

U.S. Brand Name: BayGam® [DSC], GammaSTAN™ S/D

Use: To provide passive immunity in susceptible individuals under the following circumstances:

Hepatitis A: Within 14 days of exposure and prior to manifestation of disease

Measles: For use within 6 days of exposure in an unvaccinated person, who has not previously had measles

Varicella: When varicella zoster immune globulin is not available

Rubella: Postexposure prophylaxis (within 72 hours) to reduce the risk of infection in exposed pregnant women who will not consider therapeutic abortion

Immunoglobulin deficiency: To help prevent serious infections

Stability: Store under refrigeration at 2°C to 8°C (36°F to 46°F).

Dosage: I.M.: Children and Adults:

Hepatitis A

Pre-exposure prophylaxis upon travel into endemic areas (hepatitis A vaccine preferred):

0.02 mL/kg for anticipated risk of exposure <3 months

0.06 mL/kg for anticipated risk of exposure ≥3 months

Repeat approximate dose every 5 months if exposure continues

Postexposure prophylaxis: 0.02 mL/kg given within 14 days of exposure. IG is not needed if at least 1 dose of hepatitis A vaccine was given at ≥1 month before exposure

Measles:

Prophylaxis, immunocompetent: 0.25 mL/kg/dose (maximum dose: 15 mL) given within 6 days of exposure followed by live attenuated measles vaccine in 5-6 months when indicated

Prophylaxis, immunocompromised: 0.5 mL/kg (maximum dose: 15 mL) immediately following exposure

IMMUNIZATIONS[1] (VACCINES[2]) *(Continued)*

Rubella: Prophylaxis during pregnancy: 0.55 mL/kg/dose within 72 hours of exposure

Varicella: Prophylaxis: 0.6-1.2 mL/kg (varicella zoster immune globulin preferred) within 72 hours of exposure

IgG deficiency: 0.66 mL/kg/dose every 3-4 weeks. A double dose may be given at onset of therapy; some patients may require more frequent injections.

Administration: Not for I.V. administration

Administer I.M. in the anterolateral aspects of the upper thigh or deltoid muscle of the upper arm. Avoid gluteal region due to risk of injury to sciatic nerve; use upper outer quadrant only. Divide doses >10 mL.

Influenza Virus Vaccine[3,4]

U.S. Brand Name: Fluarix®, FluLaval™, fluMist®, Fluvirin®, Fluzone®

Use: Provide active immunity to influenza virus strains contained in the vaccine

Groups at Increased Risk for Influenza-Related Complications: Advisory Committee on Immunization Practices (ACIP) recommendations for vaccination:

- Persons ≥50 years of age
- Residents of nursing homes and other chronic-care facilities that house persons of any age with chronic medical conditions
- Adults and children with chronic disorders of the pulmonary or cardiovascular systems, including asthma
- Adults and children who have required regular medical follow-up or hospitalization during the preceding year because of chronic metabolic diseases (including diabetes mellitus), renal dysfunction, hemoglobinopathies, or immunosuppression (including immunosuppression caused by medications or HIV)
- Adults and children with conditions which may compromise respiratory function, the handling of respiratory secretions, or that can increase the risk of aspiration (eg, cognitive dysfunction, spinal; cord injuries, seizure disorders, other neuromuscular disorders)
- Children and adolescents (6 months to 18 years of age) who are receiving long-term aspirin therapy and therefore, may be at risk for developing Reye's syndrome after influenza
- Women who will be pregnant during the influenza season
- Children 6-59 months of age

Vaccination is also recommended for close contacts of children 0-59 months of age, healthy persons who may transmit influenza to those at risk, and all healthcare workers.

Stability:

Injection: Store between 2°C to 8°C (36°F to 46°F). Potency is destroyed by freezing; do not use if product has been frozen.

Fluarix®: Protect from light.

FluLaval™: Discard 28 days after initial entry. Protect from light.

Nasal spray: Store in a freezer at or below -15°C (5°F). May thaw in refrigerator and store at 2°C to 8°C (36°F to 46°F) ≤60 hours. Do not refreeze after thawing.

Dosage: Optimal time to receive vaccine is October-November, prior to exposure to influenza; however, vaccination can continue into December and throughout the influenza season as long as vaccine is available.

I.M.:

Fluzone®:

Children 6-35 months: 0.25 mL/dose (1 or 2 doses per season; see **Note**)

Children 3-8 years: 0.5 mL/dose (1 or 2 doses per season; see **Note**)

Children ≥9 years and Adults: 0.5 mL/dose (1 dose per season)

Fluvirin®:

Children 4-8 years: 0.5 mL/dose (1 or 2 doses per season; see **Note**)

Children ≥9 years and Adults: 0.5 mL/dose (1 dose per season)

Note: Previously unvaccinated children <9 years should receive 2 doses, given >1 month apart in order to achieve satisfactory antibody response.

Fluarix®, FluLaval™: Adults: 0.5 mL/dose (1 dose per season)

Intranasal (fluMist®):

Children 5-8 years, previously **not vaccinated** with influenza vaccine: Initial season: Two 0.5 mL doses separated by 6-10 weeks

Children 5-8 years, previously **vaccinated** with influenza vaccine: 0.5 mL/dose (1 dose per season)

Children ≥9 years and Adults ≤49 years: 0.5 mL/dose (1 dose per season)

Administration:

Injection: For I.M. administration only. Inspect for particulate matter and discoloration prior to administration. Adults and older children should be vaccinated in the deltoid muscle using a ≥1 inch needle length. Infants and young children <12 months of age should be vaccinated in the anterolateral aspect of the thigh using a $7/8$ inch to 1 inch needle length. Young children with adequate deltoid muscle mass should be vaccinated using a $7/8$ inch to 1.25 inch needle. Suspensions should be shaken well prior to use.

Intranasal: Must be thawed prior to administration. May thaw in refrigerator and store at 2°C to 8°C (36°F to 46°F) ≤60 hours. May also be thawed by holding sprayer in the palm of the hand and supporting the plunger rod with thumb; use immediately. Half the dose (0.25 mL) is administered to each nostril; patient should be in upright position. A dose divider clip is provided. Severely-immunocompromised persons should not administer the live vaccine. If recipient sneezes following administration, the dose should not be repeated.

Influenza Virus Vaccine (H5N1)[4]

Use: Active immunization of adults at increased risk of exposure to the H5N1 viral subtype of influenza

Stability: Store between 2°C to 8°C (36°F to 46°F). Potency is destroyed by freezing; do not use if product has been frozen. Protect from light.

Dosage: I.M.: Adults 18-64 years: 1 mL, followed by second 1 mL dose given 28 days later (acceptable range: 21-35 days)

Administration: For I.M. administration only. Inspect for particulate matter and discoloration prior to administration. Vaccinate in the deltoid muscle using a ≥1 inch needle length. Suspension should be shaken well prior to use.

Japanese Encephalitis Virus Vaccine (Inactivated)[3]

U.S. Brand Name: JE-VAX®

Use: Active immunization against Japanese encephalitis

Stability: Prior to and following reconstitution, store under refrigeration at 2°C to 8°C (35°F to 46°F). Reconstitute with 1.3 mL of provided diluent. Shake well. Discard 8 hours after reconstitution. Do not freeze.

Dosage: U.S. recommended primary immunization schedule:
Children 1-3 years: SubQ: Three 0.5 mL doses given on days 0, 7, and 30
Children 1-3 years: SubQ: Three 0.5 mL doses given on days 0, 7, and 30
Children >3 years and Adults: SubQ: Three 1 mL doses given on days 0, 7, and 30
Booster dose: Give after 2 years, or according to current recommendation
Abbreviated dosing schedule: Three recommended doses, given on days 0, 7, and 14 with the last dose given at least 10 days before travel. Alternately, two doses given 1 week apart provide immunity in ~80% of patients. Abbreviated schedules should be used only when necessary due to time constraints.
Elderly: Refer to adult dosing. Elderly may be at increased risk of developing neuroinvasive disease if infected with Japanese encephalitis virus.

Administration: The single-dose vial should only be reconstituted with the full 1.3 mL of diluent supplied. Administer 1 mL of the resulting liquid as one standard adult dose; discard the unused portion.

Measles, Mumps, and Rubella Vaccines (Combined)[2,3]

U.S. Brand Name: M-M-R® II

Use: Measles, mumps, and rubella prophylaxis

Stability: Prior to reconstitution, store the powder at 2°C to 8°C (36°F to 46°F) or colder (freezing does not affect potency). Protect from light. Diluent may be stored with powder or at room temperature. Use entire contents of the provided diluent to reconstitute vaccine. Gently agitate to mix thoroughly. Discard if powder does not dissolve. Use as soon as possible following reconstitution (may be stored at 2°C to 8°C/36°F to 46°F; protect from light); discard if not used within 8 hours.

Dosage: SubQ:
Infants <12 months: If there is risk of exposure to measles, single-antigen measles vaccine should be administered at 6-11 months of age with a second dose (of MMR) at >12 months of age.
Children ≥12 months:
Primary immunization: 0.5 mL at 12-15 months
Revaccination: 0.5 mL at 4-6 years of age; revaccination is recommended prior to elementary school. If the second dose was not received, the schedule should be completed by the 11- to 12-year old visit. During a mumps outbreak, children ages 1-4 should consider a second dose of a live mumps virus vaccine. (Minimum interval between doses is 28 days.)
Adults:
Birth year ≥1957 without evidence of immunity (also see Additional Information): 1 or 2 doses (0.5 mL/dose); minimum interval between doses is 28 days
Routine vaccination of healthcare workers:
Birth year ≥1957 without evidence of immunity: 2 doses of a live mumps virus vaccine; minimum interval between doses is 28 days
Birth year <1957 without evidence of immunity: 1 dose of a live mumps virus vaccine.
Mumps outbreak:
Healthcare workers born <1957 without other evidence of immunity: Consider 2 doses of a live mumps virus vaccine; minimum interval between doses is 28 days

IMMUNIZATIONS[1] (VACCINES[2]) *(Continued)*

Low-risk adults: A second dose of a live mumps virus vaccine should be considered
in adults who previously received 1 dose; minimum interval between doses is
28 days

Administration: Administer SubQ in outer aspect of the upper arm. **Not for I.V. administration.**

Measles, Mumps, Rubella, and Varicella Virus Vaccine[3]

U.S. Brand Name: ProQuad®

Use: To provide simultaneous active immunization against measles, mumps, rubella,
and varicella

Stability:

Vaccine: During shipment, powder should be stored at or below -20°C (-4°F). Prior
to reconstitution, may be stored in a freezer for up to 18 months at temperatures at or below -15°C (-5°F). Do not store in refrigerator; discard if refrigerated. Protect from light. Following reconstitution, use within 30 minutes.

Diluent: Store at under refrigeration at 2°C to 8°C (36°F to 46°F) or at room
temperature of 20°C to 25°C (68°F to 77°F). When reconstituting, use only
diluent provided. Gently agitate to dissolve powder. Use only sterile syringes
that are free of preservatives, antiseptics, detergents, or other antiviral
substances.

Dosage: SubQ: Children 12 months to 12 years: One dose (0.5 mL)

Allow at least 1 month between administering a dose of a measles containing
vaccine (eg, M-M-R® II) and ProQuad®.

Allow at least 3 months between administering a varicella containing vaccine (eg,
Varivax®and ProQuad®.

Administration: For SubQ injection only; inject in the outer aspect of the deltoid region
of the upper arm or in the higher anterolateral area of the thigh. Administer immediately following reconstitution.

Measles Virus Vaccine (Live)[3]

U.S. Brand Name: Attenuvax®

Use: Active immunization against measles (rubeola)

Note: Trivalent measles-mumps-rubella (MMR) is the vaccine of choice if recipients
are likely to be susceptible to rubella and/or mumps as well as to measles.

Stability: During shipment, store at ≤10°C (50°F). Prior to and following reconstitution,
refrigerate at 2°C to 8°C (36°F to 46°). Protect from light at all times. Following
reconstitution, use within 8 hours.

Dosage: Note: Trivalent measles-mumps-rubella (MMR) vaccine should be used unless
contraindicated in adults and children ≥12 months of age.

Children ≥6 months and Adults: SubQ: 0.5 mL in outer aspect of the upper arm

Primary vaccination recommended at 12-15 months of age and repeated at 4-6
years of age. Children requiring vaccination with measles virus vaccine prior to
12 months of age (eg, during local outbreak, international travel to endemic
area) should receive another dose between 12-15 months and again prior to
elementary school.

Adults born in or after 1957 without documentation of live vaccine on or after first
birthday, without physician-diagnosed measles, or without laboratory evidence
of immunity should be vaccinated, ideally with 2 doses of vaccine separated by
no less than 1 month. For those previously vaccinated with 1 dose of measles
vaccine, revaccination is recommended for students entering colleges and
other institutions of higher education, for healthcare workers at the time of
employment, and for international travelers who visit endemic areas. Persons
vaccinated between 1963 and 1967 with a killed measles vaccine, followed by
live vaccine within 3 months, or with a vaccine of unknown type should be
revaccinated with live measles virus vaccine.

Administration: Vaccine should not be administered I.V.; SubQ injection preferred with
a 25-gauge ⅝" needle.

Meningococcal Polysaccharide (Groups A / C / Y and W-135) Diphtheria Toxoid Conjugate Vaccine[3,4]

U.S. Brand Name: Menactra®

Use: Provide active immunization of adolescents and adults (11-55 years of age) against
invasive meningococcal disease caused by *N. meningitidis* serogroups A, C, Y and
W-135

The ACIP recommends routine vaccination of all adolescents at age 11-12 years.
For adolescents not previously vaccinated, vaccine should be administered
prior to high school entry (~15 years of age).

The ACIP also recommends routine vaccination for persons at increased risk for
meningococcal disease. (MCV4 is preferred for persons aged 11-55 years;
MPSV4 may be used if MCV4 is not available). Persons at increased risk
include:

• College freshmen living in dormitories
• Microbiologists routinely exposed to isolates of *N. meningitides*

- Military recruits
- Persons traveling to or who reside in countries where *N. meningitides* is hyperendemic or epidemic, particularly if contact with local population will be prolonged
- Persons with terminal complement component deficiencies
- Persons with anatomic or functional asplenia

Use is also recommended during meningococcal outbreaks caused by vaccine preventable serogroups.

Stability: Store between 2°C to 8°C (35°F to 46°F); do not freeze. Discard product exposed to freezing. Do not mix with other vaccines in the same syringe.

Dosage: I.M.:

Adolescents 11-18 years and Adults ≤55 years: 0.5 mL. **Note:** Revaccination: May be indicated in patients previously vaccinated with MPSV4 who remain at increased risk for infection. The ACIP recommends the use of MCV4 for revaccination in patients 11-55 years, however use of MPSV4 is also acceptable. Consider revaccination after 3-5 years. The need for revaccination in patients previously vaccinated with MCV4 is currently under study.

Elderly: Safety and efficacy not established in patients >55 years

Administration: Administer by I.M. route, preferably into the upper deltoid region. Do not administer via I.V., SubQ or I.D. route. Based on limited data, inadvertent SubQ administration provides a lower serologic response, however the response is still considered to be protective. If inadvertently administered by the SubQ route, revaccination is not necessary.

Meningococcal Polysaccharide Vaccine (Groups A / C / Y and W-135)[3]

U.S. Brand Name: Menomune®-A/C/Y/W-135

Use: Provide active immunity to meningococcal serogroups contained in the vaccine.

The ACIP recommends routine vaccination for persons at increased risk for meningococcal disease. (Use of MPSV4 is recommended in children 2-10 years and adults >55 years. MCV4 is preferred for persons aged 11-55 years; MPSV4 may be used if MCV4 is not available). Persons at increased risk include:

- College freshmen living in dormitories
- Microbiologists routinely exposed to isolates of *N. meningitides*
- Military recruits
- Persons traveling to or who reside in countries where *N. meningitides* is hyperendemic or epidemic, particularly if contact with local population will be prolonged
- Persons with terminal complement component deficiencies
- Persons with anatomic or functional asplenia

Use is also recommended during meningococcal outbreaks caused by vaccine preventable serogroups.

Stability: Prior to and following reconstitution, store at 2°C to 8°C (35°F to 46°F). Reconstitute using provided diluent; shake well. Use single-dose vial within 30 minutes of reconstitution. Use multidose vial within 35 days of reconstitution.

Dosage: SubQ:

Children <2 years: Not usually recommended. Two doses (0.5 mL/dose), 3 months apart, may be considered in children 3-18 months to elicit short-term protection against serogroup A disease. A single dose may be considered in children 19-23 months.

Children ≥2 years and Adults: 0.5 mL

Note: Revaccination: May be indicated in patients previously vaccinated with MPSV4 who remain at increased risk for infection. The ACIP recommends the use of MCV4 for revaccination in patients 11-55 years, however use of MPSV4 is also acceptable.

Children first vaccinated at <4 years: Revaccinate after 2-3 years.

Adults: Not determined, consider revaccination after 3-5 years.

Administration: Administer by SubQ injection; do not administer intradermally, I.M., or I.V.

Mumps Virus Vaccine (Live/Attenuated)[3]

U.S. Brand Name: Mumpsvax®

Use: Mumps prophylaxis by promoting active immunity

Note: Trivalent measles-mumps-rubella (MMR) vaccine is the preferred agent for most children and many adults; persons born prior to 1957 are generally considered immune and need not be vaccinated

Stability: Product is shipped at ≤10°C (50°F). Prior to reconstitution, vaccine must be stored at ≤2°C to 8°C (36°F to 46°F). Reconstitute using entire contents of one vial of provided preservative free diluent. Following reconstitution, use as soon as possible, but may be stored at 2°C to 8°C (36°F to 46°F) for up to 8 hours. Protect from light prior to and after reconstitution.

Dosage: Children ≥12-15 months and Adults: SubQ: 0.5 mL as a single dose

Administration: For SubQ administration in outer aspect of the upper arm using a 25-gauge ⁵/₈" needle

IMMUNIZATIONS[1] (VACCINES[2]) *(Continued)*

Papillomavirus (Types 6, 11, 16, 18) Recombinant Vaccine[3]

U.S. Brand Name: Gardasil®

Use: Females: Prevention of cervical cancer, genital warts, cervical adenocarcinoma *in situ*, and vulvar, vaginal, or cervical intraepithelial neoplasia caused by human papillomavirus (HPV) types 6, 11, 16, 18

Stability: Store at 2°C to 8°C (36°F to 46°F); do not freeze. Protect from light.

Dosage: I.M.: Females: Children ≥9 years and Adults ≤26 years: 0.5 mL followed by 0.5 mL at 2 and 6 months after initial dose CDC recommended immunization schedule: Administer first dose to females at age 11-12 years; begin series in females aged 13-26 years if not previously vaccinated

Administration: Shake suspension well before use. Inject I.M. into the deltoid region of the upper arm or higher anterolateral thigh area.

Pneumococcal Conjugate Vaccine (7-Valent)[3,4]

U.S. Brand Name: Prevnar®

Use: Immunization of infants and toddlers against *Streptococcus pneumoniae* infection caused by serotypes included in the vaccine

Advisory Committee on Immunization Practices (ACIP) guidelines also recommend PCV7 for use in:

All children 2-23 months

Children ≥2-59 months with cochlear implants

Children ages 24-59 months with: Sickle cell disease (including other sickle cell hemoglobinopathies, asplenia, splenic dysfunction), HIV infection, immunocompromising conditions (congenital immunodeficiencies, renal failure, nephrotic syndrome, diseases associated with immunosuppressive or radiation therapy, solid organ transplant), chronic illnesses (cardiac disease, cerebrospinal fluid leaks, diabetes mellitus, pulmonary disease excluding asthma unless on high dose corticosteroids)

Consider use in all children 24-59 months with priority given to:

Children 24-35 months

Children 24-59 months who are of Alaska native, American Indian, or African-American descent

Children 24-59 months who attend group day care centers

Stability: Store refrigerated at 2°C to 8°C (36°F to 46°F).

Dosage: I.M.:

Infants: 2-6 months: 0.5 mL at approximately 2-month intervals for 3 consecutive doses, followed by a fourth dose of 0.5 mL at 12-15 months of age; first dose may be given as young as 6 weeks of age, but is typically given at 2 months of age. In case of a moderate shortage of vaccine, defer the fourth dose until shortage is resolved; in case of a severe shortage of vaccine, defer third and fourth doses until shortage is resolved.

Previously Unvaccinated Older Infants and Children:

7-11 months: 0.5 mL for a total of 3 doses; 2 doses at least 4 weeks apart, followed by a third dose after the 1-year birthday (12-15 months), separated from the second dose by at least 2 months. In case of a severe shortage of vaccine, defer the third dose until shortage is resolved.

12-23 months: 0.5 mL for a total of 2 doses, separated by at least 2 months. In case of a severe shortage of vaccine, defer the second dose until shortage is resolved.

24-59 months:

Healthy Children: 0.5 mL as a single dose. In case of a severe shortage of vaccine, defer dosing until shortage is resolved.

Children with sickle cell disease, asplenia, HIV infection, chronic illness or immunocompromising conditions (not including bone marrow transplants – results pending; use PPV23 [pneumococcal polysaccharide vaccine, polyvalent] at 12 and 24 months until studies are complete): 0.5 mL for a total of 2 doses, separated by 2 months

Previously Vaccinated Children With a Lapse in Vaccine Administration:

7-11 months: Previously received 1 or 2 doses PCV7: 0.5 mL dose at 7-11 months of age, followed by a second dose ≥2 months later at 12-15 months of age

12-23 months:

Previously received 1 dose before 12 months of age: 0.5 mL dose, followed by a second dose ≥2 months later

Previously received 2 doses before age 12 months: 0.5 mL dose ≥2 months after the most recent dose

24-59 months: Any incomplete schedule: 0.5 mL as a single dose. **Note:** Patients with chronic diseases or immunosuppressing conditions should receive 2 doses ≥2 months apart

Administration: Shake well prior to use. Do not inject I.V.; avoid intradermal route; administer I.M. (deltoid muscle for toddlers and young children or lateral midthigh in infants)

Pneumococcal Polysaccharide Vaccine (Polyvalent)[3,4]

U.S. Brand Name: Pneumovax® 23

Use: Children ≥2 years of age and adults who are at increased risk of pneumococcal disease and its complications because of underlying health conditions (including patients with cochlear implants); routine use in older adults >50 years of age, including all those ≥65 years

Current Advisory Committee on Immunization Practices (ACIP) guidelines recommend **pneumococcal 7-valent conjugate vaccine (PCV7)** be used for children 2-23 months of age and, in certain situations, children up to 59 months of age

Stability: Store under refrigeration at 2°C to 8°C (36°F to 46°F).

Dosage: I.M., SubQ:

Children >2 years and Adults: 0.5 mL

Previously vaccinated with PCV7 vaccine: Children ≥2 years and Adults:

With sickle cell disease, asplenia, immunocompromised or HIV infection: 0.5 mL at ≥2 years of age and ≥2 months after last dose of PCV7; revaccination with PPV23 should be given ≥5 years for children >10 years of age and every 3-5 years for children ≤10 years of age; revaccination should not be administered <3 years after the previous PPV23 dose

With chronic illness: 0.5 mL at ≥2 years of age and ≥2 months after last dose of PCV7; revaccination with PPV23 is not recommended

Following bone marrow transplant (use of PCV7 under study): Administer one dose PPV23 at 12 and 24 months following BMT

Revaccination should be considered:

1. If ≥6 years since initial vaccination has elapsed, or
2. In patients who received 14-valent pneumococcal vaccine and are at highest risk (asplenic) for fatal infection or
3. At ≥6 years in patients with nephrotic syndrome, renal failure, or transplant recipients, or
4. 3-5 years in children with nephrotic syndrome, asplenia, or sickle cell disease

Administration: Do not inject I.V., avoid intradermal, administer SubQ or I.M. (deltoid muscle or lateral midthigh)

Poliovirus Vaccine (Inactivated)[3]

U.S. Brand Name: IPOL®

Use: Active immunization against poliomyelitis caused by poliovirus types 1, 2, and 3. Routine immunization of adults in the United States is generally not recommended. Adults with previous wild poliovirus disease, who have never been immunized, or those who are incompletely immunized may receive inactivated poliovirus vaccine if they fall into one of the following categories:

- Travelers to regions or countries where poliomyelitis is endemic or epidemic
- Healthcare workers in close contact with patients who may be excreting poliovirus
- Laboratory workers handling specimens that may contain poliovirus
- Members of communities or specific population groups with diseases caused by wild poliovirus
- Incompletely vaccinated or unvaccinated adults in a household or with other close contact with children receiving oral poliovirus (may be at increased risk of vaccine associated paralytic poliomyelitis)

Stability: Store under refrigeration 2°C to 8°C (35°F to 46°F); do not freeze.

Dosage: I.M., SubQ:

Children:

Primary immunization: Administer three 0.5 mL doses, preferably 8 or more weeks apart, at 2, 4, and 6-18 months of age. First dose may be given as early as 6 weeks of age. Do not administer more frequently than 4 weeks apart.

Booster dose: 0.5 mL at 4-6 years of age

Adults:

Previously unvaccinated: Two 0.5 mL doses administered at 1- to 2-month intervals, followed by a third dose 6-12 months later. If <3 months, but at least 2 months are available before protection is needed, 3 doses may be administered at least 1 month apart. If administration must be completed within 1-2 months, give 2 doses at least 1 month apart. If <1 month is available, give 1 dose.

Incompletely vaccinated: Adults with at least 1 previous dose of OPV, <3 doses of IPV, or a combination of OPV and IPV equaling <3 doses, administer at least one 0.5 mL dose of IPV. Additional doses to complete the series may be given if time permits.

Completely vaccinated: One 0.5 mL dose

Administration: Do not administer I.V.; for I.M. or SubQ administration. Administer to midlateral aspect of the thigh in infants and small children. Administer in the deltoid area to adults or older children.

IMMUNIZATIONS[1] (VACCINES[2]) *(Continued)*

Rabies Immune Globulin (Human)

U.S. Brand Name: BayRab® [DSC], HyperRAB™ S/D, Imogam® Rabies-HT

Use: Part of postexposure prophylaxis of persons with rabies exposure who lack a history of pre-exposure or postexposure prophylaxis with rabies vaccine or a recently documented neutralizing antibody response to previous rabies vaccination; although it is preferable to administer RIG with the first dose of vaccine, it can be given up to 8 days after vaccination

Stability: Refrigerate

Dosage: Children and Adults: Postexposure prophylaxis: Local wound infiltration: 20 units/kg in a single dose, RIG should always be administered as part of rabies vaccine (HDCV) regimen as soon as possible (after the first dose of vaccine, up to 8 days). If anatomically feasible, the full rabies immune globulin dose should be infiltrated around and into the wound(s); remaining volume should be administered I.M. at a site distant from the vaccine administration site. If rabies vaccine was initiated without rabies immune globulin, rabies immune globulin may be administered through the seventh day after the first vaccine dose.

> **Note:** Persons known to have an adequate titer or who have been completely immunized with rabies vaccine should not receive RIG, only booster doses of HDCV

Administration: Do not administer I.V. Do not administer vaccine with or at same site as RIG administration. Postexposure wound infiltration: If anatomically feasible, the full rabies immune globulin dose should be infiltrated around and into the wound(s); remaining volume should be administered I.M. at a site distant from the vaccine administration site.

Rabies Virus Vaccine[3,4]

U.S. Brand Name: Imovax® Rabies, RabAvert®

Use:

> Pre-exposure immunization: Vaccinate persons with greater than usual risk due to occupation or avocation including veterinarians, rangers, animal handlers, certain laboratory workers, and persons living in or visiting countries for longer than 1 month where rabies is a constant threat.

> Postexposure prophylaxis: If a bite from a carrier animal is unprovoked, if it is not captured and rabies is present in that species and area, administer rabies immune globulin (RIG) and the vaccine as indicated

Stability: Store under refrigeration at 2°C to 8°C (36°F to 46°F); do not freeze. Protect from light.

Dosage:

> **Pre-exposure prophylaxis:** 1 mL I.M. on days 0, 7, and 21-28. **Note:** Prolonging the interval between doses does not interfere with immunity achieved after the concluding dose of the basic series.

> **Postexposure prophylaxis:** All postexposure treatment should begin with immediate cleansing of the wound with soap and water

> > Persons not previously immunized as above: I.M.: 5 doses (1 mL each) on days 0, 3, 7, 14, 28. In addition, patients should receive rabies immune globulin 20 units/kg body weight, half infiltrated at bite site if possible, remainder I.M.)

> > Persons who have previously received postexposure prophylaxis with rabies vaccine, received a recommended I.M. pre-exposure series of rabies vaccine or have a previously documented rabies antibody titer considered adequate: 1 mL of either vaccine I.M. only on days 0 and 3; do not administer RIG

> > Booster (for occupational or other continuing risk): 1 mL I.M. every 2-5 years or based on antibody titers

Administration: For I.M. administration only; this rabies vaccine product must not be administered intradermally; in adults and children, administer I.M. injections in the deltoid muscle, not the gluteal; for younger children, use the outer aspect of the thigh.

Rh$_o$(D) Immune Globulin

U.S. Brand Name: HyperRHO™ S/D Full Dose, HyperRHO™ S/D Mini Dose, MICRhoGAM®, RhoGAM®, Rhophylac®, WinRho® SDF

Use:

> Suppression of Rh isoimmunization: Use in the following situations when an Rh$_o$(D)-negative individual is exposed to Rh$_o$(D)-positive blood: During delivery of an Rh$_o$(D)-positive infant; abortion; amniocentesis; chorionic villus sampling; ruptured tubal pregnancy; abdominal trauma; hydatidiform mole; transplacental hemorrhage. Used when the mother is Rh$_o$(D) negative, the father of the child is either Rh$_o$(D) positive or Rh$_o$(D) unknown, the baby is either Rh$_o$(D) positive or Rh$_o$(D) unknown.

> Transfusion: Suppression of Rh isoimmunization in Rh$_o$(D)-negative individuals transfused with Rh$_o$(D) antigen-positive RBCs or blood components containing Rh$_o$(D) antigen-positive RBCs

Treatment of idiopathic thrombocytopenic purpura (ITP): Used in the following nonsplenectomized $Rh_o(D)$ positive individuals: Children with acute or chronic ITP, adults with chronic ITP, children and adults with ITP secondary to HIV infection

Stability: Store at 2°C to 8°C (35°F to 46°F); do not freeze.

Rhophylac®: Protect from light.

Dosage:

ITP: Children and Adults:

Rhophylac®: I.V.: 50 mcg/kg

WinRho® SDF: I.V.:

Initial: 50 mcg/kg as a single injection, or can be given as a divided dose on separate days. If hemoglobin is <10 g/dL: Dose should be reduced to 25-40 mcg/kg.

Subsequent dosing: 25-60 mcg/kg can be used if required to elevate platelet count

Maintenance dosing if patient **did respond** to initial dosing: 25-60 mcg/kg based on platelet and hemoglobin levels

Maintenance dosing if patient **did not respond** to initial dosing:

Hemoglobin 8-10 g/dL: Redose between 25-40 mcg/kg

Hemoglobin >10 g/dL: Redose between 50-60 mcg/kg

Hemoglobin <8 g/dL: Use with caution

$Rh_o(D)$ suppression: Adults: **Note:** One "full dose" (300 mcg) provides enough antibody to prevent Rh sensitization if the volume of RBC entering the circulation is ≤15 mL. When >15 mL is suspected, a fetal red cell count should be performed to determine the appropriate dose.

Pregnancy:

Antepartum prophylaxis: In general, dose is given at 28 weeks. If given early in pregnancy, administer every 12 weeks to ensure adequate levels of passively acquired anti-Rh

HyperRHO™ S/D Full Dose, RhoGAM®: I.M.: 300 mcg

Rhophylac®, WinRho® SDF: I.M., I.V.: 300 mcg

Postpartum prophylaxis: In general, dose is administered as soon as possible after delivery, preferably within 72 hours. Can be given up to 28 days following delivery

HyperRHO™ S/D Full Dose, RhoGAM®: I.M.: 300 mcg

Rhophylac®: I.M., I.V.: 300 mcg

WinRho® SDF: I.M., I.V.: 120 mcg

Threatened abortion, any time during pregnancy (with continuation of pregnancy):

HyperRHO™ S/D Full Dose, RhoGAM®: I.M.: 300 mcg; administer as soon as possible

Rhophylac®, WinRho® SDF: I.M., I.V.: 300 mcg; administer as soon as possible

Abortion, miscarriage, termination of ectopic pregnancy:

RhoGAM®: I.M.: ≥13 weeks gestation: 300 mcg

HyperRHO™ S/D Mini Dose, MICRhoGAM®: <13 weeks gestation: I.M.: 50 mcg

Rhophylac®: I.M., I.V.: 300 mcg

WinRho® SDF: I.M., I.V.: After 34 weeks gestation: 120 mcg; administer immediately or within 72 hours

Amniocentesis, chorionic villus sampling:

HyperRHO™ S/D Full Dose, RhoGAM®: I.M.: At 15-18 weeks gestation or during the 3rd trimester: 300 mcg. If dose is given between 13-18 weeks, repeat at 26-28 weeks and within 72 hours of delivery.

Rhophylac®: I.M., I.V.: 300 mcg

WinRho® SDF: I.M., I.V.: Before 34 weeks gestation: 300 mcg; administer immediately, repeat dose every 12 weeks during pregnancy. After 34 weeks gestation: 120 mcg, administered immediately or within 72 hours.

Excessive fetomaternal hemorrhage (>15 mL): Rhophylac®: I.M., I.V.: 300 mcg within 72 hours plus 20 mcg/mL fetal RBCs in excess of 15 mL if excess transplacental bleeding is quantified or 300 mcg/dose if bleeding cannot be quantified

Abdominal trauma, manipulation:

HyperRHO™ S/D Full Dose, RhoGAM®: I.M.: 2nd or 3rd trimester: 300 mcg. If dose is given between 13-18 weeks, repeat at 26-28 weeks and within 72 hours of delivery

Rhophylac®: I.M., I.V.: 300 mcg within 72 hours

WinRho® SDF: I.M./I.V.: After 34 weeks gestation: 120 mcg; administer immediately or within 72 hours

IMMUNIZATIONS[1] (VACCINES[2]) *(Continued)*

Transfusion:

Children and Adults: WinRho® SDF: Administer within 72 hours after exposure of incompatible blood transfusions or massive fetal hemorrhage.

I.V.: Calculate dose as follows; administer 600 mcg every 8 hours until the total dose is administered:

Exposure to $Rh_o(D)$ positive whole blood: 9 mcg/mL blood

Exposure to $Rh_o(D)$ positive red blood cells: 18 mcg/mL cells

I.M.: Calculate dose as follows; administer 1200 mcg every 12 hours until the total dose is administered:

Exposure to $Rh_o(D)$ positive whole blood: 12 mcg/mL blood

Exposure to $Rh_o(D)$ positive red blood cells: 24 mcg/mL cells

Adults

HyperRHO™ S/D Full Dose, RhoGAM®: I.M.: Multiply the volume of Rh positive whole blood administered by the hematocrit of the donor unit to equal the volume of RBCs transfused. The volume of RBCs is then divided by 15 mL, providing the number of 300 mcg doses (vials/syringes) to administer. If the dose calculated results in a fraction, round up to the next higher whole 300 mcg dose (vial/syringe).

Rhophylac®: I.M., I.V.: 20 mcg/2 mL transfused blood or 20 mcg/mL erythrocyte concentrate

Dosage adjustment in renal impairment: I.V. infusion: Use caution; may require infusion rate reduction or discontinuation.

Administration: The total volume can be administered in divided doses at different sites at one time or may be divided and given at intervals, provided the total dosage is given within 72 hours of the fetomaternal hemorrhage or transfusion.

I.M.: Administer into the deltoid muscle of the upper arm or anterolateral aspect of the upper thigh; avoid gluteal region due to risk of sciatic nerve injury. If large doses (>5 mL) are needed, administration in divided doses at different sites is recommended. **Note:** Do not administer I.M. $Rh_o(D)$ immune globulin for ITP.

I.V.: WinRho® SDF: Infuse over at least 3-5 minutes; do not administer with other medications

Note: If preparing dose using liquid formulation, withdraw the entire contents of the vial to ensure accurate calculation of the dosage requirement.

Rotavirus Vaccine[3]

U.S. Brand Name: RotaTeq®

Use: Prevention of rotavirus gastroenteritis in infants and children

Stability: Store and transport under refrigeration at 2°C to 8°C (36°F to 46°F). Use as soon as possible once removed from refrigerator. Protect from light.

Dosage: Oral: Children 6-32 weeks: Three 2 mL doses at 2, 4, and 6 months of age, the first given at 6-12 weeks of age, followed by subsequent doses at 4- to 10-week intervals. Routine administration of the first dose at >12 weeks of age is not recommended (insufficient data). Administer all doses by 32 weeks of age. Infants who have had rotavirus gastroenteritis before getting the full course of vaccine should still initiate or complete the 3-dose schedule; initial infection provides only partial immunity.

Administration: Gently squeeze dose from ready-to-use dosing tube. If infant spits or regurgitates vaccine, a replacement dose is not recommended. In general, vaccine administration should be deferred for 42 days following an antibody-containing product. However, if deferral causes first dose of vaccine to be scheduled at ≥13 weeks of age, a shorter deferral interval should be used. After use, dispose of the empty tube and cap in a biologic waste container.

Rubella Virus Vaccine (Live)[3]

U.S. Brand Name: Meruvax® II

Use: Selective active immunization against rubella

Note: Trivalent measles-mumps-rubella (MMR) vaccine is the preferred immunizing agent for most children and many adults.

Stability: Vaccine is to be shipped at 10°C (50°F). May use dry ice. Protect from light at all times. Prior to reconstitution, store at 2°C to 8°C (36°F to 46°F) or colder. Discard reconstituted vaccine after 8 hours.

Dosage: Children ≥12 months and Adults: SubQ: 0.5 mL

Primary immunization is recommended at 12-15 months; revaccination with MMR-II at 4-6 years of age is recommended prior to elementary school. Previously unvaccinated children of susceptible pregnant women should be vaccinated.

Adults without documentation of immunity: Vaccination is recommended for students entering colleges and other institutions of higher education, for military personal, for healthcare workers, for international travelers who visit endemic areas, and to women of childbearing potential. Do not administer to women who may become pregnant within 4 weeks of receiving vaccine; administer following completion or termination of pregnancy

Administration: SubQ injection only in outer aspect of upper arm; avoid injection into blood vessel. **Not for I.V. administration.**

Smallpox Vaccine[3]

U.S. Brand Name: Dryvax®

Use: Active immunization against vaccinia virus, the causative agent of smallpox in persons determined to be at risk for smallpox infection. The ACIP recommends vaccination of laboratory workers at risk of exposure from cultures or contaminated animals which may be a source of vaccinia or related Orthopoxviruses capable of causing infections in humans (monkeypox, cowpox, or variola). The ACIP also recommends that consideration be given for vaccination in healthcare workers having contact with clinical specimens, contaminated material, or patients receiving vaccinia or recombinant vaccinia viruses. Revaccination is recommended every 10 years. The Armed Forces recommend vaccination of certain personnel categories. Recommendations for use in response to bioterrorism are regularly updated by the CDC, and may be found at www.cdc.gov.

Stability: Store at 2°C to 8°C (36°F to 46°F); do not freeze. Following reconstitution, stable for up to 90 days when refrigerated at 2°C to 8°C (36°F to 46°F).

Release vacuum in vial prior to reconstitution by inserting a sterile 21-gauge needle (or smaller) through the stopper. Do not use this needle to reconstitute vaccine. Use the vented needle (provided with kit) to reconstitute solution. Solution should be reconstituted with the diluent provided (to reduce viscosity, this solution may require warming in hands prior to drawing into the syringe). Reconstitute with entire volume of diluent. Following reconstitution, allow to stand for 3-5 minutes, then swirl gently (if necessary) to effect complete reconstitution.

Dosage: Not for I.M., I.V., or SubQ injection: Vaccination by scarification (multiple-puncture technique) only: **Note:** A trace of blood should appear at vaccination site after 15-20 seconds; if no trace of blood is visible, an additional 3 insertions should be made using the same needle, without reinserting the needle into the vaccine bottle.

Adults (children ≥12 months in emergency conditions only):

> Primary vaccination: Use a single drop of vaccine suspension and 2 or 3 needle punctures (using the same needle) into the superficial skin

> Revaccination: Use a single drop of vaccine suspension and 15 needle punctures (using the same needle) into the superficial skin

> **Dosage adjustment in renal impairment:** No dosage adjustment required

Administration: Using a bifurcated needle, 1 drop of vaccine is introduced into the superficial layers of the skin using a multiple-puncture technique. The skin over the insertion of the deltoid muscle or the posterior aspect of the arm over the triceps are the preferred sites for vaccination.

A single-use bifurcated needle should be dipped carefully into the reconstituted vaccine (following removal of rubber stopper). Visually confirm that the needle picks up a drop of vaccine solution. Deposit the drop of vaccine onto clean, dry skin at the vaccination site. Holding the bifurcated needle perpendicular to the skin, punctures are to be made rapidly into the superficial skin of the vaccination site. The puncture strokes should be vigorous enough to allow a trace of blood to appear after approximately 15-20 seconds. Wipe off any remaining vaccine with dry sterile gauze. Dispose of all materials in a biohazard waste container. All materials must be burned, boiled, or autoclaved. If no evidence of vaccine take is apparent after 7 days, the individual may be vaccinated again.

To prevent transmission of the virus, cover vaccination site with gauze and cover gauze with a semipermeable barrier or clothing. Good handwashing prevents inadvertent inoculation. Vaccinees should change bandages away from others and launder their own linens to prevent transmission.

Tetanus Immune Globulin (Human)

U.S. Brand Name: BayTet™ [DSC], HyperTET™ S/D

Use: Passive immunization against tetanus; tetanus immune globulin is preferred over tetanus antitoxin for treatment of active tetanus; part of the management of an unclean, wound in a person whose history of previous receipt of tetanus toxoid is unknown or who has received less than three doses of tetanus toxoid; elderly may require TIG more often than younger patients with tetanus infection due to declining antibody titers with age

Stability: Refrigerate

Dosage: I.M.:

Prophylaxis of tetanus:

> Children: 4 units/kg; some recommend administering 250 units to small children

> Adults: 250 units

Treatment of tetanus:

> Children: 500-3000 units; some should infiltrate locally around the wound

> Adults: 3000-6000 units

Administration: Do not administer I.V.; I.M. use only

IMMUNIZATIONS[1] (VACCINES[2]) *(Continued)*

Tetanus Toxoid (Adsorbed)[3,4]

Use: Active immunization against tetanus when combination antigen preparations are not indicated. **Note:** Tetanus and diphtheria toxoids for adult use (Td) is the preferred immunizing agent for most adults and for children after their seventh birthday. Young children should receive trivalent DTaP (diphtheria/tetanus/acellular pertussis), as part of their childhood immunization program, unless pertussis is contraindicated, then TD is warranted.

Stability: Refrigerate; do not freeze.

Dosage: Children ≥7 years and Adults: I.M.:

Primary immunization: 0.5 mL; repeat 0.5 mL at 4-8 weeks after first dose and at 6-12 months after second dose

Routine booster dose: Recommended every 10 years

Note: In most patients, Td is the recommended product for primary immunization, booster doses, and tetanus immunization in wound management (refer to Diphtheria and Tetanus Toxoid monograph)

Administration: Inject intramuscularly in the area of the vastus lateralis (midthigh laterally) or deltoid. Do not inject into gluteal area. Shake well prior to withdrawing dose; do not use if product does not form a suspension.

Tetanus Toxoid (Fluid)[3,4]

Use: Indicated as booster dose in the active immunization against tetanus in the rare adult or child who is allergic to the aluminum adjuvant (a product containing adsorbed tetanus toxoid is preferred); not indicated for primary immunization

Use: Unlabeled/Investigational: Anergy testing (no longer recommended)

Stability: Refrigerate 2°C to 8°C (35°F to 46°F); do not freeze.

Dosage:

Primary immunization: Not indicated for this use.

Booster doses: I.M., SubQ: 0.5 mL every 10 years

Anergy testing (unlabeled use; no longer recommended for this indication): Intradermal: 0.1 mL; doses that have been used range from 0.1 mL of a 1:10 dilution to 0.1 mL of the undiluted product

Administration:

I.M. Shake well prior to use. Administer I.M. in lateral aspect of midthigh or deltoid muscle of upper arm

SubQ: Shake well prior to use. Administer in area of the lateral aspect of midthigh or deltoid. SubQ route may be preferred in patients with thrombocytopenia or coagulation disorders.

Travelers' Diarrhea and Cholera Vaccine[5]

Use: Protection against travelers' diarrhea and/or cholera in adults and children ≥2 years of age who will be visiting areas where there is a risk of contacting travelers' diarrhea caused by enterotoxigenic *E. coli* (ETEC) or cholera caused by *V. cholerae* 01 (classical and El Tor biotypes)

Stability: The effervescent granules contained in the sachet, should be dissolved in a glass with 150 mL of water resulting in a buffer solution; do not use juice milk or other beverages. For children 2-6 years, half the amount of the buffer solution is poured away. The vial containing the vaccine should be shaken and the entire contents should be added to the buffer solution and mixed.

Reconstituted solution may be stored at room temperature (<27°C) for up to 2 hours. Vial should be stored between 2°C to 8°C (35°F to 46°F), and may be stored at room temperature up to 2 weeks on one occasion only. The sachet may be stored with the vial between 2°C to 8°C (35°F to 46°F) or separately at room temperature (<27°C). Use reconstituted solution within 2 hours of mixing.

Dosage: Oral:

Cholera:

Primary immunization:

Children 2-6 years: 3 doses given at intervals of ≥1 week and completed at least 1 week prior to trip to endemic/epidemic areas; restart treatment if interval between doses >6 weeks

Children ≥6 years and Adults: 2 doses given at intervals of ≥1 week and completed at least 1 week prior to trip to endemic/epidemic areas; restart treatment if interval between doses >6 weeks

Booster:

Children 2-6 years: 1 dose after 6 months have elapsed since vaccination

Children ≥6 years and Adults: 1 dose after 2 years have elapsed since vaccination

ETEC:

Primary immunization: Children ≥2 years and Adults: 2 doses given at intervals of ≥ 1 week; restart treatment if interval between doses >6 weeks

Booster: Children ≥2 years and Adults:

Continued risk: 1 dose every 3 months

Renewed protection: 1 dose may be given if last booster or original immunization was <5 years ago (if >5 years, revaccinate)

Administration: For oral use only; do no administer I.M., I.V., or SubQ. Food should be avoided 1 hour before and 1 hour following vaccine administration. Use reconstituted solution within 2 hours of mixing.

Typhoid Vaccine[3,4]

U.S. Brand Name: Typhim Vi®, Vivotif®

Use: Active immunization against typhoid fever caused by *Salmonella typhi*. Not for routine vaccination. In the United States, use should be limited to:

- Travelers to areas with risk of exposure to *S. typhi*
- Persons with intimate exposure to a *S. typhi* carrier
- Laboratory technicians with exposure to *S. typhi*

Stability:
Typhim Vi®: Store between 2°C to 8°C (35°F to 46°F); do not freeze.
Vivotif®: Store between 2°C to 8°C (35°F to 46°F).

Dosage: Immunization:
Oral: Children ≥6 years and Adults:
Primary immunization: One capsule on alternate days (day 1, 3, 5, and 7) for a total of 4 doses; all doses should be complete at least 1 week prior to potential exposure
Booster immunization: Repeat full course of primary immunization every 5 years
I.M.: Children ≥2 years and Adults: 0.5 mL given at least 2 weeks prior to expected exposure
Reimmunization: 0.5 mL; optimal schedule has not been established; a single dose every 2 years is currently recommended for repeated or continued exposure

Administration:
Injection: Typhim Vi® may be given I.M. and is indicated for children ≥2 years of age; administer as a single 0.5 mL (25 mcg) injection in deltoid muscle.
Oral: Swallow capsule whole soon after placing into mouth; do not chew or open capsule. Capsule should be taken with a cold or lukewarm beverage (≤37°C/ 98.6°F). Take one hour prior to a meal. Avoid alcohol within 2 hours of administration.

Vaccinia Immune Globulin (Intravenous)

U.S. Brand Name: CNJ-016™

Use: Treatment of infectious complications of smallpox (vaccinia virus) vaccination, such as eczema vaccinatum, progressive vaccinia, and severe generalized vaccinia; treatment of vaccinia infections in individuals with concurrent skin conditions or accidental virus exposure to eyes (except vaccinia keratitis), mouth, or other areas where viral infection would pose significant risk

Stability: Store between 2°C and 8°C (35.6°F to 46.4°F).
CNJ-016™ (Cangene product): If frozen, use within 60 days of thawing at 2°C and 8°C. Infusion should begin within 4 hours after entering vial.
DynPort product: Use within 6 hours of piercing vial stopper; complete infusion within 12 hours of spiking vial.

Dosage: I.V.:
Adults:
CNJ-016™ (Cangene product): 6000 units/kg; 9000 units/kg may be considered if patient does not respond to initial dose.
DynPort product: Total dose: 2 mL/kg (100 mg/kg); higher doses (200-500 mg/ kg) may be considered if patient does not respond to initial recommended dose (sucrose-related renal impairment is worsened at doses ≥400 mg/ kg)
Elderly: Safety and efficacy have not been established

Dosage adjustment in renal impairment: Use caution. Doses ≥400 mg/kg of the DynPort product are not recommended.

Administration: Do not shake; avoid foaming. For intravenous use only. Predilution is not recommended. If dedicated line is not available, flush with NS prior to administration of VIGIV. Do not exceed recommended rates of infusion.
CNJ-016™ (Cangene product): Patients ≥50 kg: Infuse at ≤2 mL/minute; Patients <50 kg: Infuse at 0.04 mL/kg/minute. Maximum assessed rate of infusion: 4 mL/minute. Decrease rate of infusion if minor adverse reactions develop in patients with risk factors for thrombosis/thromboembolism and/or renal insufficiency.
DynPort product: Infuse at 1 mL/kg/hour for 30 minutes, then 2 mL/kg/hour for 30 minutes, then 3 mL/kg/hour until complete. Administer through 0.22 micron filtered set; use of infusion pump is recommended.

Varicella Virus Vaccine[3]

U.S. Brand Name: Varivax®

Use: Immunization against varicella in children ≥12 months of age and adults

Stability: Store powder in freezer at -15°C (5°F) or colder; protect from light. Store diluent separately at room temperature or in refrigerator. Powder may be stored under refrigeration for up to 72 continuous hours prior to reconstitution; if not used

IMMUNIZATIONS[1] (VACCINES[2]) *(Continued)*

within 72 hours, vaccine should be discarded. Use 0.7 mL of the provided diluent to reconstitute vaccine. Gently agitate to mix thoroughly. (Total volume of reconstituted vaccine will be ~0.5 mL.) Following reconstitution, discard reconstituted vaccine if not used within 30 minutes.

Canadian formulations: **Note:** Varicella vaccine has been reformulated to produce a refrigerator-stable preparation. Previously, the product required storage in a freezer prior to reconstitution. The new Canadian formulation may be stored in a freezer, but if transferred to a refrigerator, may not be refrozen. Individual product labeling should be consulted to confirm proper conditions.

Dosage: SubQ:

Children 12 months to 12 years: 0.5 mL; a second dose may be administered ≥3 months later

Children ≥13 years to Adults: 2 doses of 0.5 mL separated by 4-8 weeks

Administration: Do not administer I.V. Inject immediately after reconstitution. Inject SubQ into the outer aspect of the upper arm, if possible. Federal law requires that the date of administration, the vaccine manufacturer, lot number of vaccine, and the administering person's name, title and address be entered into the patient's permanent medical record.

Yellow Fever Vaccine[3]

U.S. Brand Name: YF-VAX®

Use: Induction of active immunity against yellow fever virus, primarily among persons traveling or living in areas where yellow fever infection exists

Stability: Yellow fever vaccine is shipped with dry ice. Do not use vaccine unless shipping case contains some dry ice on arrival. Maintain vaccine continuously at a temperature between 0°C to 5°C (32°F to 41°F); do not freeze. Reconstitute only with diluent provided. Inject diluent slowly into vial and allow to stand for 1-2 minutes. Gently swirl until a uniform suspension forms; swirl well before withdrawing dose. Avoid vigorous shaking to prevent foaming of suspension. Vaccine must be used within 60 minutes of reconstitution. Keep suspension refrigerated until used.

Dosage: Children ≥9 months and Adults: SubQ: One dose (0.5 mL) ≥10 days before travel. Booster: Every 10 years

Administration: For SubQ injection only. Do not administer I.M. or I.V.

Zoster Vaccine[2,3]

U.S. Brand Name: Zostavax®

Use: Prevention of herpes zoster (shingles) in patients ≥60 years of age

Stability: During shipment, should be maintained at -20°C (-4°F) or colder. Store powder in freezer at -15°C (5°F). Protect from light. Store diluent separately at room temperature or in refrigerator. Withdraw entire contents of the vial containing the provided diluent to reconstitute vaccine. Gently agitate to mix thoroughly. Withdraw entire contents of reconstituted vaccine vial for administration. Discard if reconstituted vaccine is not used within 30 minutes. Do not freeze reconstituted vaccine.

Dosage: SubQ: Adults ≥65 years: 0.65 mL administered as a single dose; there is no data to support readministration of the vaccine

Dosage adjustment in renal impairment: No adjustment required

Administration: Do not administer I.V.; inject immediately after reconstitution. Inject SubQ into the outer aspect of the upper arm, if possible.

Footnotes

[1] Contact Poison Control Center.

[2] Federal law requires that date of administration, name of vaccine manufacturer, lot number of vaccine, and administering person's name, title, and address be entered into the patient's permanent medical record.

[3] All serious adverse reactions must be reported to the U.S. Department of Health and Human Services (DHHS) Vaccine Adverse Event Reporting System (VAERS), 1-800-822-7967.

[4] For patients at risk of hemorrhage following intramuscular injection, the ACIP recommends "it should be administered intramuscularly if, in the opinion of the physician familiar with the patients bleeding risk, the vaccine can be administered with reasonable safety by this route. If the patient receives antihemophilia or other similar therapy, intramuscular vaccination can be scheduled shortly after such therapy is administered. A fine needle (23 gauge or smaller) can be used for the vaccination and firm pressure applied to the site (without rubbing) for at least 2 minutes. The patient should be instructed concerning the risk of hematoma from the injection."

[5] All serious adverse reactions related to the administration of the product should be reported in accordance with local requirements and to the Senior Product Safety Officer, Pharmacovigilance Department, Aventis Pasteur Limited, 1755 Steeles Avenue West, Toronto, ON, M2R2T4, Canada. 1-888-621-1146 (phone) or 416-667-2435 (fax).

TUBERCULOSIS TREATMENT

Tuberculin Skin Test Recommendations[1]

Children for whom immediate skin testing is indicated:

- Contacts of persons with confirmed or suspected infectious tuberculosis (TB) (contact investigation); this includes children identified as contacts of family members or associates in jail or prison in the last 5 years

- Children with radiographic or clinical findings suggesting tuberculosis

- Children immigrating from endemic countries (eg, Asia, Middle East, Africa, Latin America)

- Children with travel histories to endemic countries and/or significant contact with indigenous persons from such countries

Children who should be tested annually for tuberculosis[2]:

- Children infected with human immunodeficiency virus (HIV) or living in household with HIV-infected persons

- Incarcerated adolescents

Children who should be tested every 2-3 years[2]:

- Children exposed to the following individuals: HIV-infected, homeless, residents of nursing homes, institutionalized adolescents or adults, users of illicit drugs, incarcerated adolescents or adults, and migrant farm workers. Foster children with exposure to adults in the preceding high-risk groups are included.

Children who should be considered for tuberculin skin testing at ages 4-6 and 11-16 years:

- Children whose parents immigrated (with unknown tuberculin skin test status) from regions of the world with high prevalence of tuberculosis; continued potential exposure by travel to the endemic areas and/or household contact with persons from the endemic areas (with unknown tuberculin skin test status) should be an indication for repeat tuberculin skin testing

- Children without specific risk factors who reside in high-prevalence areas; in general, a high-risk neighborhood or community does not mean an entire city is at high risk; rates in any area of the city may vary by neighborhood, or even from block to block; physicians should be aware of these patterns in determining the likelihood of exposure; public health officials or local tuberculosis experts should help clinicians identify areas that have appreciable tuberculosis rates

Children at increased risk of progression of infection to disease: Those with other medical risk factors, including diabetes mellitus, chronic renal failure, malnutrition, and congenital or acquired immunodeficiencies deserve special consideration. Without recent exposure, these persons are not at increased risk of acquiring tuberculosis infection. Underlying immune deficiencies associated with these conditions theoretically would enhance the possibility for progression to severe disease. Initial histories of potential exposure to tuberculosis should be included on all of these patients. If these histories or local epidemiologic factors suggest a possibility of exposure, immediate and periodic tuberculin skin testing should be considered. An initial Mantoux tuberculin skin test should be performed before initiation of immunosuppressive therapy in any child with an underlying condition that necessitates immunosuppressive therapy.

---

[1]BCG immunization is not a contraindication to tuberculin skin testing.

[2]Initial tuberculin skin testing is at the time of diagnosis or circumstance, beginning as early as at age 3 months.

Adapted from "Report of the Committee on Infectious Diseases," *2003 Red Book*®, 26th ed, 646.

TUBERCULOSIS TREATMENT *(Continued)*

Table 1. Tuberculosis Prophylaxis
Infection Without Disease (Positive Tuberculin Test)[1]

Specific Circumstances/ Organism	Comments	Regimen
Regardless of age (see INH Preventive Therapy)	Rx indicated	INH (5 mg/kg/d, maximum: 300 mg/d for adults, 10 mg/kg/d not to exceed 300 mg/d for children). Results with 6 months of treatment are nearly as effective as 12 months (65% vs 75% reduction in disease). *Am Thoracic Society* (6 months), *Am Acad Pediatrics*, 1991 (9 months). If CXR is abnormal, treat for 12 months. In HIV-positive patient, treatment for a minimum of 12 months, some suggest longer. Monitor transaminases monthly (*MMWR Morb Mortal Wkly Rep* 1989, 38:247).
Age <35 y	Rx indicated	Reanalysis of earlier studies favors INH prophylaxis for 6 months (if INH-related hepatitis case fatality rate is <1% and TB case fatality is ≥6.7%, which appears to be the case, monitor transaminases monthly (*Arch Int Med*, 1990, 150:2517).
INH-resistant organisms likely	Rx indicated	Data on efficacy of alternative regimens is currently lacking. Regimens include ETB + RIF daily for 6 months. PZA + RIF daily for 2 months, then INH + RIF daily until sensitivities from index case (if available) known, then if INH-CR, discontinue INH and continue RIF for 9 months, otherwise INH + RIF for 9 months (this latter is *Am Acad Pediatrics*, 1991 recommendation).
INH + RIF resistant organisms likely	Rx indicated	Efficacy of alternative regimens is unknown; PZA (25-30 mg/kg/d P.O.) + ETB (15-25 mg/kg/d P.O.) (at 25 mg/kg ETB, monitoring for retrobulbar neuritis required), for 6 months unless HIV-positive, then 12 months; PZA + ciprofloxacin (750 mg P.O. bid) or ofloxacin (400 mg P.O. bid) for 6-12 months (*MMWR Morb Mortal Wkly Rep*, 1992, 41(RR11):68).

INH = isoniazid; RIF = rifampin; KM = kanamycin; ETB = ethambutol
SM = streptomycin; PZA = pyrazinamide; CXR = chest x-ray; Rx = treatment
See also guidelines for interpreting PPD in "Skin Testing for Delayed Hypersensitivity."
[1]Tuberculin test (TBnT). The standard is the Mantoux test, 5 TU PPD in 0.1 mL diluent stabilized with Tween 80. Read at 48-72 hours measuring maximum diameter of induration. A reaction ≥5 mm is defined as positive in the following: positive HIV or risk factors, recent close case contacts, CXR consistent with healed TBc. A reaction ≥10 mm is positive in foreign-born in countries of high prevalence, injection drug users, low income populations, nursing home residents, patients with medical conditions which increase risk (see above, preventive treatment). A reaction ≥15 mm is positive in all others (*Am Rev Resp Dis*, 1990, 142:725). Two-stage TBnT: Use in individuals to be tested regularly (ie, healthcare workers). TBn reactivity may decrease over time but be boosted by skin testing. If unrecognized, individual may be incorrectly diagnosed as recent converter. If first TBnT is reactive but <10 mm, repeat 5 TU in 1 week, if then ≥10 mm = positive, not recent conversion (*Am Rev Resp Dis*, 1979, 119:587).

Changes From Prior Recommendations on Tuberculin Testing and Treatment of Latent Tuberculosis Infection (LTBI)

Tuberculin Testing

- Emphasis on targeted tuberculin testing among persons at high risk for recent LTBI or with clinical conditions that increase the risk for TB, regardless of age; testing is discouraged among persons at lower risk

- For patients with organ transplants and other immunosuppressed patients (eg, persons receiving the equivalent of ≥15 mg/day prednisone for 1 month or more), 5 mm of induration rather than 10 mm of induration rather than 10 mm of induration as a cut-off level for tuberculin positivity

- A tuberculin skin test conversion is defined as in increase of ≥10 mm of induration within a 2-year period, regardless of age

Treatment of Latent Tuberculosis Infection

- For HIV-negative persons, isoniazid given for 9 months is preferred over 6-month regimens

- For HIV-positive persons and those with fibrotic lesions on chest x-ray consistent with previous TB, isoniazid should be given for 9 months instead of 12 months

- For HIV-negative and HIV-positive persons, rifampin and pyrazinamide should be given for 2 months

- For HIV-negative and HIV-positive persons, rifampin should be given for 4 months

Clinical and Laboratory Monitoring

- Routine baseline and follow-up laboratory monitoring can be eliminated in most persons with LTBI, except for those with HIV infection, pregnant women (or those in the immediate postpartum period), and persons with chronic liver disease or those who use alcohol regularly

- Emphasis on clinical monitoring for signs and symptoms of possible adverse effects, with prompt evaluation and changes in treatment, as indicated

Adapted from *MMWR*, 2000, 49(RR-6).

TUBERCULOSIS TREATMENT *(Continued)*

Table 2. Recommended Treatment Regimens for Drug-Susceptible Tuberculosis in Infants, Children, and Adolescents

Infection or Disease Category	Regimen	Remarks
Latent tuberculosis infection (positive tuberculin skin test, no disease):		
• Isoniazid-susceptible	9 months of isoniazid once a day	If daily therapy is not possible, directly observed therapy twice a week may be used for 9 months.
• Isoniazid-resistant	6 months of rifampin once a day	
• Isoniazid-rifampin-resistant[1]	Consult a tuberculosis specialist	
Pulmonary and extrapulmonary (except meningitis)	2 months of isoniazid, rifampin, and pyrazinamide daily, followed by 4 months of isoniazid and rifampin[2]	If possible drug resistance is a concern, another drug (ethambutol or aminoglycoside) is added to the initial 3-drug therapy until drug susceptibilities are determined. Directly observed therapy is highly desirable.
		If hilar adenopathy only, a 6-month course of isoniazid and rifampin is sufficient.
		Drugs can be given 2 or 3 times/week under directly observed therapy in the initial phase if nonadherence is likely.
Meningitis	2 months of isoniazid, rifampin, pyrazinamide, and aminoglycoside or ethionamide, once a day, followed by 7-10 months of isoniazid and rifampin once a day or twice a week (9-12 months total)	A fourth drug, usually an aminoglycoside, is given with initial therapy until drug susceptibility is known.
		For patients who may have acquired tuberculosis in geographic areas where resistance to streptomycin is common, capreomycin, kanamycin, or amikacin may be used instead of streptomycin.

[1]Duration of therapy is longer for human immunodeficiency virus (HIV)-infected people, and additional drugs may be indicated.

[2]Medications should be administered daily for the first 2 weeks to 2 months of treatment and then can be administered 2-3 times/week by directly observed therapy.

Adapted from "Report of the Committee on Infectious Diseases," *2003 Red Book®*, 26th ed, 649.

Table 3. Recommended Drug Regimens for Treatment of Latent Tuberculosis Infection in Children

Drug	Interval and Duration	Comments
Isoniazid	Daily for 9 mo Twice weekly for 9 mo	This includes treatment for any child <5 years of age who is exposed to household members or other close contacts who are potentially infectious even if skin test is negative
Rifampin	Daily for 4-9 mo	No controlled trials; only to be used in INH intolerant or resistant
Rifampin-pyrazinamide	Daily for 3 mo	No controlled trials; only to be used in INH intolerant or resistant

Modified from *MMWR*, 2000, 14(RR-6).

Table 4. Recommended Drug Regimens for Treatment of Latent Tuberculosis Infection in Adults

Drug	Interval and Duration	Comments	Rating[1] (Evidence)[2] HIV−	Rating[1] (Evidence)[2] HIV+
Isoniazid	Daily for 9 months[3,4]	In HIV-infected patients, isoniazid may be administered concurrently with nucleoside reverse transcriptase inhibitors (NRTIs), protease inhibitors (PIs), or non-nucleoside reverse transcriptase inhibitors (NNRTIs)	A (II)	A (II)
	Twice weekly for 9 months[3,4]	Directly-observed therapy (DOT) must be used with twice-weekly dosing	B (II)	B (II)
Isoniazid	Daily for 6 months[4]	Not indicated for HIV-infected persons, those with fibrotic lesions on chest radiographs, or children	B (I)	C (I)
	Twice weekly for 6 months[4]	DOT must be used with twice-weekly dosing	B (II)	C (I)
Rifampin	Daily for 4 months	For persons who cannot tolerate pyrazinamide For persons who are contacts of patients with isoniazid-resistant, rifampin-susceptible TB who cannot tolerate pyrazinamide	B (II)	B (III)
Rifampin plus pyrazinamide	Daily for 2 months	May also be offered to persons who are contacts of pyrazinamide patients with isoniazid-resistant, rifampin-susceptible TB In HIV-infected patients, protease inhibitors or NNRTIs should generally not be administered concurrently with rifampin. Rifabutin can be used as an alternative for patients treated with indinavir, nelfinavir, amprenavir, ritonavir, or efavirenz, and possibly with nevirapine or soft-gel saquinavir[5]	B (II)	A (I)
	Twice weekly for 2-3 months	DOT must be used with twice-weekly dosing	C (II)	C (I)

[1]Strength of recommendation: A = preferred; B = acceptable alternative; C = offer when A and B cannot be given.

[2]Quality of evidence: I = randomized clinical trial data; II = data from clinical trials that are not randomized or were conducted in other populations; III = expert opinion.

[3]Recommended regimen for children <18 years of age.

[4]Recommended regimens for pregnant women. Some experts would use rifampin and pyrazinamide for 2 months as an alternative regimen in HIV-infected pregnant women, although pyrazinamide should be avoided during the first trimester.

[5]Rifabutin should not be used with hard-gel saquinavir or delavirdine. When used with other protease inhibitors or NNRTIs, dose adjustment of rifabutin may be required.

Adapted from *MMWR Recomm Rep*, 2000, 49(RR6).

TUBERCULOSIS TREATMENT *(Continued)*

Table 5. TB Drugs in Special Situations

Drug	Pregnancy[1]	CNS TB Disease	Renal Insufficiency
Isoniazid	Safe	Good penetration	Normal clearance
Rifampin	Safe	Fair penetration Penetrates inflamed meninges (10% to 20%)	Normal clearance
Pyrazinamide	Avoid	Good penetration	Clearance reduced Decrease dose or prolong interval
Ethambutol	Safe	Penetrates inflamed meninges only (4% to 64%)	Clearance reduced Decrease dose or prolong interval
Streptomycin	Avoid	Penetrates inflamed meninges only	Clearance reduced Decrease dose or prolong interval
Capreomycin	Avoid	Penetrates inflamed meninges only	Clearance reduced Decrease dose or prolong interval
Kanamycin	Avoid	Penetrates inflamed meninges only	Clearance reduced Decrease dose or prolong interval
Ethionamide	Do not use	Good penetration	Normal clearance
Para-amino-salicylic acid	Safe	Penetrates inflamed meninges only (10% to 50%)	Incomplete data on clearance
Cycloserine	Avoid	Good penetration	Clearance reduced Decrease dose or prolong interval
Ciprofloxacin	Do not use	Fair penetration (5% to 10%) Penetrates inflamed meninges (50% to 90%)	Clearance reduced Decrease dose or prolong interval
Ofloxacin	Do not use	Fair penetration (5% to 10%) Penetrates inflamed meninges (50% to 90%)	Clearance reduced Decrease dose or prolong interval
Amikacin	Avoid	Penetrates inflamed meninges only	Clearance reduced Decrease dose or prolong interval
Clofazimine	Avoid	Penetration unknown	Clearance probably normal

[1]Safe = the drug has not been demonstrated to have teratogenic effects.

Avoid = data on the drug's safety are limited, or the drug is associated with mild malformations (as in the aminoglycosides).

Do not use = studies show an association between the drug and premature labor, congenital malformations, or teratogenicity.

Table 6. Recommendations for Coadministering Different Antiretroviral Drugs With the Antimycobacterial Drugs Rifabutin and Rifampin

Antiretroviral	Use in Combination with Rifabutin	Use in Combination with Rifampin	Comments
Saquinavir[1]			
Hard-gel capsules (HGC)	Possibly[2], if antiretroviral regimen also includes ritonavir	Possibly, if antiretroviral regimen also includes ritonavir	Coadministration of saquinavir SGC with usual-dose rifabutin (300 mg/day or 2-3 times/week) is a possibility. However, the pharmacokinetic data and clinical experience for this combination are limited.
Soft-gel capsules (SGC)	Probably[3]	Possibly, if antiretroviral regimen also includes ritonavir	The combination of saquinavir SGC or saquinavir HGC and ritonavir, coadministered with 1) usual-dose rifampin (600 mg/day or 2-3 times/ week), or 2) reduced-dose rifabutin (150 mg 2-3 times/week) is a possibility. However, the pharmacokinetic data and clinical experience for these combinations are limited. Coadministration of saquinavir or saquinavir SGC with rifampin is not recommended because rifampin markedly decreases concentrations of saquinavir.
Ritonavir	Probably	Probably	If the combination of ritonavir and rifabutin is used, then a substantially reduced-dose rifabutin regimen (150 mg 2-3 times/week) is recommended. Coadministration of ritonavir with usual-dose rifampin (600 mg/day or 2-3 times/week) is a possibility, though pharmacokinetic data and clinical experience are limited.
Indinavir	Yes	No	There is limited, but favorable, clinical experience with coadministration of indinavir[4] with a reduced daily dose of rifabutin (150 mg) or with the usual dose of rifabutin (300 mg 2-3 times/ week). Coadministration of indinavir with rifampin is not recommended because rifampin markedly decreases concentrations of indinavir.
Nelfinavir	Yes	No	There is limited, but favorable, clinical experience with coadministration of nelfinavir[5] with a reduced daily dose of rifabutin (150 mg) or with the usual dose of rifabutin (300 mg 2-3 times/ week). Coadministration of nelfinavir with rifampin is not recommended because rifampin markedly decreases concentrations of nelfinavir.
Amprenavir	Yes	No	Coadministration of amprenavir with a reduced daily dose of rifabutin (150 mg) or with the usual dose of rifabutin (300 mg 2-3 times/week) is a possibility, but there is no published clinical experience. Coadministration of amprenavir with rifampin is not recommended because rifampin markedly decreases concentrations of amprenavir.
Nevirapine	Yes	Possibly	Coadministration of nevirapine with usual-dose rifabutin (300 mg/day or 2-3 times/week) is a possibility based on pharmacokinetic study data. However, there is no published clinical experience for this combination. Data are insufficient to assess whether dose adjustments are necessary when rifampin is coadministered with nevirapine. Therefore, rifampin and nevirapine should be used only in combination if clearly indicated and with careful monitoring.
Delavirdine	No	No	Contraindicated because of the marked decrease in concentrations of delavirdine when administered with either rifabutin or rifampin.

TUBERCULOSIS TREATMENT *(Continued)*

Table 6. Recommendations for Coadministering Different Antiretroviral Drugs With the Antimycobacterial Drugs Rifabutin and Rifampin *(continued)*

Antiretroviral	Use in Combination with Rifabutin	Use in Combination with Rifampin	Comments
Efavirenz	Probably	Probably	Coadministration of efavirenz with increased-dose rifabutin (450 mg/day or 600 mg/day, or 600 mg 2-3 times/week) is a possibility, though there is no published clinical experience. Coadministration of efavirenz[6] with usual-dose rifampin (600 mg/day or 2-3 times/week) is a possibility, though there is no published clinical experience.

[1]Usual recommended doses are 400 mg twice daily for each of these protease inhibitors and 400 mg of ritonavir.

[2]Despite limited data and clinical experience, the use of this combination is potentially successful.

[3]Based on available data and clinical experience, the successful use of this combination is likely.

[4] Usual recommended dose is 800 mg every 8 hours; some experts recommend increasing the indinavir dose to 1000 mg every 8 hours if indinavir is used in combination with rifabutin.

[5]Usual recommended dose is 750 mg 3 times/day or 1250 mg twice daily; some experts recommend increasing the nelfinavir dose to 1000 mg if the 3-times/day dosing is used and nelfinavir is used in combination with rifabutin.

[6]Usual recommended dose is 600 mg/day; some experts recommend increasing the efavirenz dose to 800 mg/day if efavirenz is used in combination with rifampin.

Updated March 2000 from www.aidsinfo.nih.gov -"Updated Guidelines for the Use of Rifabutin or Rifampin for the Treatment and Prevention of Tuberculosis Among HIV-Infected Patients Taking Protease Inhibitors or Non-nucleoside Reverse Transcriptase Inhibitors," *MMWR,* March 10, 2000, 49(09):185-9.

Table 7. Criteria for Tuberculin Positivity, by Risk Group

Reaction ≥5 mm of Induration	Reaction ≥10 mm of Induration	Reaction ≥15 mm of Induration
HIV-positive persons	Recent immigrants (ie, within the last 5 years) from high prevalence countries	Persons with no risk factors for TB
Recent contacts of tuberculosis (TB) case patients	Injection drug users	
Fibrotic changes on chest radiograph consistent with prior TB	Residents and employees[1] of the following high risk congregate settings: prisons and jails, nursing homes and other long-term facilities for the elderly, hospitals and other healthcare facilities, residential facilities for patients with AIDS, and homeless shelters	
Patients with organ transplant and other immunosuppressed patients (receiving the equivalent of ≥15 mg/day of prednisone for 1 month)[2]	Mycobacteriology laboratory personnel	
	Persons with the following clinical conditions that place them at high risk: Silicosis, diabetes mellitus, chronic renal failure, some hematologic disorders (eg, leukemias and lymphomas), other specific malignancies (eg, carcinoma of the head or neck and lung), weight loss of ≥10% of ideal body weight, gastrectomy, and jejunoileal bypass	
	Children <4 years of age or infants, children, and adolescents exposed to adults at high-risk	

[1]For persons who are otherwise at low risk and are tested at the start of employment, a reaction of ≥15 mm induration is considered positive.

[2]Risk of TB in patients treated with corticosteroids increases with higher dose and longer duration.

Modified from *MMWR Morb Mortal Wkly Rep*, 2000, 49(RR-6).

Table 8. Recommendations, Rankings, and Performance Indicators for Treatment of Patients With Tuberculosis (TB)

Recommendation	Ranking[1] (Evidence)[2]	Performance Indicator
Obtain bacteriologic confirmation and susceptibility testing for patients with TB or suspected of having TB	A (II)	90% of adults with or suspected of having TB have 3 cultures for mycobacteria obtained before initiation of antituberculosis therapy (50% of children 0-12 y)
Place persons with suspected or confirmed smear-positive pulmonary or laryngeal TB in respiratory isolation until noninfectious	A (II)	90% of persons with sputum smear-positive TB remain in respiratory isolation until smear converts to negative
Begin treatment of patients with confirmed or suspected TB disease with one of the following drug combinations, depending on local resistance patterns: INH + RIF + PZA **or** INH + RIF + PZA + EMB **or** INH + RIF + PZA + SM	A (III)	90% of all patients with TB are started on INH + RIF + PZA + EMB or SM in geographic areas where >4% of TB isolates are resistant to INH
Report each case of TB promptly to the local public health department	A (III)	100% of persons with active TB are reported to the local public health department within 1 week of diagnosis
Perform HIV testing for all patients with TB	A (III)	80% of all patients with TB have HIV status determined within 2 months of a diagnosis of TB
Treat patients with TB caused by a susceptible organism for 6 months, using an ATS/CDC-approved regimen	A (I)	90% of all patients with TB complete 6 months of therapy with 12 months of beginning treatment
Re-evaluate patients with TB who are smear positive at 3 months for possible nonadherence or infection with drug-resistant bacilli	A (III)	90% of all patients with TB who are smear positive at 3 months have sputum culture/susceptibility testing performed within 1 month of the 3-month visit
Add ≥2 new antituberculosis agents when TB treatment failure is suspected	A (II)	100% of patients with TB with suspected treatment failure are prescribed ≥2 new antituberculosis agents
Perform tuberculin skin testing on all patients with a history of ≥1 of the following: HIV infection, I.V. drug use, homelessness, incarceration, or contact with a person with pulmonary TB	A (II)	80% of persons in the indicated population groups receive tuberculin skin test and return for reading
Administer treatment for latent TB infection to all persons with latent TB infection, unless it can be documented that they received such treatment previously	A (I)	75% of patients with positive tuberculin skin tests who are candidates for treatment for latent TB infection complete a course of therapy within 12 months of initiation

Note: ATS/CDC = American Thoracic Society and Centers for Disease Control and Prevention; EMB = ethambutol; INH = isoniazid; PZA = pyrazinamide; RIF = rifampin; SM = streptomycin.

[1]Strength of recommendation: A = preferred; B = acceptable alternative; C = offer when A and B cannot be given.

[2]Quality of evidence: I = randomized clinical trial data; II = data from clinical trials that are not randomized or were conducted in other populations; III = expert opinion.

Adapted from the Infectious Diseases Society of America, *Clinical Infectious Diseases*, 2000, 31:633-9.

TUBERCULOSIS TREATMENT *(Continued)*

Table 9. Drug Regimens for Culture-Positive Pulmonary Tuberculosis Caused by Drug-Susceptible Organisms

Initial Phase			Continuation Phase			Range of Total Doses (minimal duration)	Rating[1] (Evidence)[2]	
Regimen	Drugs	Interval and Doses[3] (minimal duration)	Regimen	Drugs	Interval and Doses[3,4] (minimal duration)		HIV−	HIV+
1	INH RIF PZA EMB	Seven days per week for 56 doses (8 wk) or 5 d/wk for 40 doses (8 wk)[5]	1a	INH/RIF	Seven days per week for 126 doses (18 wk) or 5 d/wk for 90 doses (18 wk)[5]	182-130 (26 wk)	A (I)	A (II)
			1b	INH/RIF	Twice weekly for 36 doses (18 wk)	92-76 (26 wk)	A (I)	A (II)[6]
			1c[7]	INH/RPT	Once weekly for 18 doses (18 wk)	74-58 (26 wk)	B (I)	E (I)
2	INH RIF PZA EMB	Seven days per week for 14 doses (2 wk), then twice weekly for 12 doses (6 wk) or 5 d/wk for 10 doses (2 wk)[5] then twice weekly for 12 doses (6 wk)	2a	INH/RIF	Twice weekly for 36 doses (18 wk)	62-58 (26 wk)	A (II)	B (II)[6]
			2b[7]	INH/RPT	Once weekly for 18 doses (18 wk)	44-40 (26 wk)	B (I)	E (I)
3	INH RIF PZA EMB	Three times weekly for 24 doses (8 wk)	3a	INH/RIF	Three times weekly for 54 doses (18 wk)	78 (26 wk)	B (I)	B (II)
4	INH RIF EMB	Seven days per week for 56 doses (8 wk) or 5 d/wk for 40 doses (8 wk)[5]	4a	INH/RIF	Seven days per week for 217 doses (31 wk) or 5 d/wk for 155 doses (31 wk)[5]	273-195 (39 wk)	C (I)	C (II)
			4b	INH/RIF	Twice weekly for 62 doses (31 wk)	118-102 (39 wk)	C (I)	C (II)

Definition of abbreviations: EMB = ethambutol; INH = isoniazid; PZA = pyrazinamide; RIF = rifampin; RPT = rifapentine.

[1]Definitions of evidence ratings: A = preferred; B = acceptable alternative; C = offer when A and B cannot be given; E = should never be given.

[2]Definitions of evidence ratings: I = randomized clinical trial; II = data from clinical trials that were not randomized or were conducted in other populations; III = expert opinion.

[3]When directly observed therapy (DOT) is used, drugs may be given 5 days/week and the necessary number of doses adjusted accordingly. Although there are no studies that compare five with seven daily doses, extensive experience indicates this would be an effective practice.

[4]Patients with cavitation on initial chest radiograph and positive cultures at completion of 2 months of therapy should receive a 7-month (31-week; either 217 doses daily] or 62 doses [twice weekly]) continuation phase.

[5]Five-day/week administration is always given by DOT. Rating for 5 day/week regimens is AIII.

[6]Not recommended for HIV-infected patients with CD4+ cell counts <100 cells/μL.

[7]Options 1c and 2b should be used only in HIV-negative patients who have negative sputum smears at the time of completion of 2 months of therapy and who do not have cavitation on initial chest radiograph. For patients started on this regimen and found to have a positive culture from the 2-month specimen, treatment should be extended an extra 3 months.

Adapted from *MMWR*, 2003, 52[RR11].

**Table 10. Suggested Pyrazinamide Doses, Using Whole Tablets,
for Adults Weighing 40-90 kg**

	Weight (kg)[1]		
	40-55	56-75	76-90
Daily, mg (mg/kg)	1000 (18.2-25)	1500 (20-26.8)	2000[2] (22.2-26.3)
Thrice weekly, mg (mg/kg)	1500 (27.3-37.5)	2500 (33.3-44.6)	3000[2] (33.3-39.5)
Twice weekly, mg (mg/kg)	2000 (36.4-50)	3000 (40-53.6)	4000[2] (44.4-52.6)

[1]Based on estimated lean body weight

[2]Maximum dose regardless of weight.

**Table 11. Suggested Ethambutol Doses, Using Whole Tablets,
for Adults Weighing 40-90 kg**

	Weight (kg)[1]		
	40-55	56-75	76-90
Daily, mg (mg/kg)	800 (14.5-20)	1200 (16-21.4)	1600[2] (17.8-21.1)
Thrice weekly, mg (mg/kg)	1200 (21.8-30)	2000 (26.7-35.7)	2400[2] (26.7-31.6)
Twice weekly, mg (mg/kg)	2000 (36.4-50)	2800 (37.3-50)	4000[2] (44.4-52.6)

[1]Based on estimated lean body weight

[2]Maximum dose regardless of weight.

TREATMENT OF SEXUALLY TRANSMITTED INFECTIONS

Type or Stage	Drugs of Choice / Dosage	Alternatives
CHLAMYDIAL INFECTION AND RELATED CLINICAL SYNDROMES[1]		
Urethritis, cervicitis, conjunctivitis, or proctitis (except lymphogranuloma venereum)		
	Azithromycin 1 g oral once **or** Doxycycline[2,3] 100 mg oral bid x 7 d	Ofloxacin[3] 300 mg oral bid x 7 d **or** Levofloxacin[3] 500 mg oral once daily x 7 d **or** Erythromycin[4] 500 mg oral qid x 7 d
Infection in pregnancy		
	Azithromycin 1 g oral once **or** Amoxicillin 500 mg oral tid x 7 d	Erythromycin[4] 500 mg oral qid x 7 d
Neonatal ophthalmia or pneumonia		
	Azithromycin 20 mg/kg oral once daily x 3 d	Erythromycin 12.5 mg/kg oral qid x 14 d[5]
Lymphogranuloma venereum		
	Doxycycline[2,3] 100 mg oral bid x 21 d	Erythromycin[4] 500 mg oral qid x 21 d
EPIDIDYMITIS		
	Ceftriaxone 250 mg I.M. once **plus** doxycycline[2] 100 mg oral bid x 10 d	Only if negative for gonococcal organism: Ofloxacin 300 mg bid x 10 d **or** Levofloxacin 500 mg oral once daily x 10 d
GONORRHEA[6]		
Disseminated gonococcal infection		
	Ceftriaxone 1 g I.M. or I.V. q24h	Cefotaxime 1 g I.V. q8h **or** Ceftizoxime 1 g I.V. q8h **or** **For persons allergic to β-lactam drugs:** Ciprofloxacin 400 mg I.V. q12h **or** Levofloxacin 250 mg I.V. once daily **or** Ofloxacin 400 mg I.V. q12h **or** Spectinomycin 2 g I.M. q12h[7]
		All regimens should be continued for 24-48 hours after improvement begins, at which time therapy may be switched to one of the following regimens to complete a full week of antimicrobial therapy:
		Cefixime suspension 500 mg oral bid **or** Cefpodoxime 400 mg bid
Gonococcal meningitis and endocarditis		
	Ceftriaxone 1-2 g I.V. q12h	
Uncomplicated urethral, cervical, or rectal		
	Cefixime 400 mg oral once **or** Ceftriaxone 125 mg I.M. once	Cefpodoxime 400 mg or cefuroxime axetil 1 g orally once **or** Cefotaxime 500 mg I.M. **or** Ceftizoxime 500 mg I.M. **or** Cefoxitin 2 g I.M. (with 1 g probenecid orally) **or** Spectinomycin 2 g I.M. once[7]
Uncomplicated pharyngeal:		
	Ceftriaxone 125 mg I.M. once	
PELVIC INFLAMMATORY DISEASE		
– parenteral	Cefoxitin 2 g I.V. q6h **plus** doxycycline[3] 100 mg oral or I.V. q12h, until improved **followed by** doxycycline[3] 100 mg oral bid to complete 14 d[10] **or** Clindamycin 900 mg I.V. q8h **plus** gentamicin 2 mg/kg I.V. once, then 1.5 mg/kg I.V. q8h,[11] until improved **followed by** doxycycline[3] 100 mg oral bid to complete 14 d[10]	Ampicillin/sulbactam 3 g I.V. q6h **plus** doxycycline[3] 100 mg oral or I.V. q12h; continue until improved, then doxycycline[3] 100 mg oral bid to complete 14 d[10]

Type or Stage	Drugs of Choice / Dosage	Alternatives
– oral	Cefoxitin 2 g once **plus** probenecid 1 g oral once **plus** doxyxycline[3,12] 100 mg bid ± metronidazole x 14 d **or** Ceftriaxone 250 mg I.M. once (or other perenteral third generation cephalosporin) **plus** doxycycline[3,12] 100 mg bid ± metronidazole x 14 d	Ofloxacin[3] 400 mg bid x 14 d **or** Levofloxacin[3] 500 mg once daily x 14 d ± metronidazole[9] 500 mg bid x 14 d **Note:** Only if community prevalence (of quinolone-resistant organisms) and individual patient risk is low and quinolone susceptibility can be established.

TRICHOMONIASIS

	Metronidazole 2 g oral once **or** Tinidazole 2 g oral once	Metronidazole 375 or 500 mg oral bid x 7 d

BACTERIAL VAGINOSIS

	Metronidazole 500 mg oral bid x 7 d **or** Metronidazole gel 0.75%[14] 5 g intravaginally once or twice daily x 5 d **or** Clindamycin 2% cream[14] 5 g intravaginally qhs x 3-7 d	Metronidazole 2 g oral once[13] or Flagyl ER® 750 mg once daily x 7 d **or** Clindamycin 300 mg oral bid x 7 d **or** Clindamycin ovules[14] 100 mg intravaginally once daily x 3 d

VULVOVAGINAL CANDIDIASIS

	Intravaginal butoconazole, clotrimazole, miconazole, terconazole, or tioconazole[15] **or** Fluconazole 150 mg oral once	Nystatin 100,000 unit vaginal tablet once daily x 14 d

SYPHILIS

Early (primary, secondary, or latent <1 y)

	Penicillin G benzathine 2.4 million units I.M. once[16]	Doxycycline[3] 100 mg oral bid x 14 d

Late (>1 year's duration, cardiovascular, gumma, late-latent)

	Penicillin G benzathine 2.4 million units I.M. weekly x 3 wk	Doxycycline[3] 100 mg oral bid x 4 wk

Neurosyphilis[17]

	Penicillin G 3-4 million units I.V. q4h or 24 million units continuous I.V. infusion x 10-14 d	Penicillin G procaine 2.4 million units I.M. daily **plus** probenecid 500 mg qid oral, both x 10-14 d **or** Ceftriaxone 2 g I.V. once daily x 10-14 d

Congenital

	Penicillin G 50,000 units/kg I.V. q8-12h for 10-14 d **or** Penicillin G procaine 50,000 units/kg I.M. daily for 10-14 d	

CHANCROID[18]

	Azithromycin 1 g oral once **or** Ceftriaxone 250 mg I.M. once	Ciprofloxacin[3] 500 mg oral bid x 3 d **or** Erythromycin[4] 500 mg oral qid x 7 d

GENITAL WARTS[19]

	Trichloroacetic or bichloroacetic acid, or podophyllin[3] or liquid nitrogen 1-2 times/wk until resolved **or** Imiquimod 5% 3 times/wk x 16 wk **or** Podofilox 0.5% bid x 3 d, 4 days rest, then repeated up to 4 times	Surgical removal **or** Laser surgery **or** Intralesional interferon

GENITAL HERPES

First episode

	Acyclovir 400 mg oral tid x 7-10 d **or** Famciclovir 250 mg oral tid x 7-10 d **or** Valacyclovir 1 g oral bid x 7-10 d	Acyclovir 200 mg oral 5 times/d x 7-10 d

Severe (hospitalized patients)

	Acyclovir 5-10 mg/kg I.V. q8h x 5-7 d	

Suppression of recurrences[20]

	Acyclovir 400 mg oral bid **or** Famciclovir 250 mg oral bid **or** Valacyclovir 500 mg - 1 g once daily[21]	Acyclovir 200 mg oral, 2-5 times/d

Episodic treatment of recurrences[22]

	Acyclovir 800 mg oral tid x 2 d or 400 mg oral tid x 3-5 d[23] **or** Famciclovir 125 mg oral bid x 3-5 d[23] **or** Valacyclovir 500 mg oral bid x 3 d	

TREATMENT OF SEXUALLY TRANSMITTED INFECTIONS
(Continued)

Type or Stage	Drugs of Choice / Dosage	Alternatives
GRANULOMA INGUINALE		
	TMP-SMZ 1 double-strength tablet oral bid for a minimum of 3 wk **or** Doxycycline 100 oral bid for a minimum of 3 wk	Ciprofloxacin 750 mg oral bid for a minimum of 3 wk **or** Erythromycin base 500 mg oral qid for a minimum of 3 wk **or** Azithromycin 1 g oral once per week for a minimum of 3 weeks

[1]Related clinical syndromes include nonchlamydial nongonococcal urethritis and cervicitis.

[2]Or oral tetracycline 500 mg qid.

[3]Not recommended in pregnancy.

[4]Erythromycin ethylsuccinate 800 mg may be substituted for erythromycin base 500 mg; erythromycin estolate is contraindicated in pregnancy.

[5]Pyloric stenosis has been associated with use of erythromycin in newborns.

[6]All patients should also receive a course of treatment effective for *Chlamydia*.

[7]Not available in the United States

[8]Recommended only for use during pregnancy in patients allergic to β-lactams.

[9]Some clinicians believe the addition of metronidazole is not required.

[10]Or clindamycin 450 mg oral qid to complete 14 days.

[11]A single daily dose of 3 mg/kg is likely to be effective, but has not been studied in pelvic inflammatory disease.

[12]Some experts would add metronidazole 500 mg bid.

[13]Higher relapse rate with single dose, but useful for patients who may not comply with multiple-dose therapy.

[14]In pregnancy, topical preparations have not been effective in preventing premature delivery; oral metronidazole has been effective in some studies.

[15]For preparations and dosage of topical products, see *Med Lett Drugs Ther*, 1994, 36:81; single-dose therapy is not recommended.

[16]Some experts recommend a repeat dose after 7 days, especially in patients with HIV infection or pregnant women.

[17]Patients allergic to penicillin should be desensitized and treated with penicillin.

[18]All regimens, especially single-dose ceftriaxone, are less effective in HIV-infected patients.

[19]Recommendations for external genital warts. Liquid nitrogen can also be used for vaginal, urethral, and oral warts. Podofilox or imiquimod can be used for urethral meatus warts. Trichloroacetic or bichloroacetic acid can be used for anal warts.

[20]Some Medical Letter consultants discontinue preventive treatment for 1-2 months once a year to reassess the frequency of recurrence.

[21]Use 500 mg once daily in patients with <10 recurrences per year and 500 mg bid or 1 g daily in patients with <10 recurrences per year.

[22]Antiviral therapy is variably effective for episodic treatment of recurrences; only effective if started early.

[23]No published data are available to support 3 days' use.

Adapted from "Sexually Transmitted Diseases Treatment Guidelines 2002," *MMWR*, 2002, 51(RR-6).

Adapted from "Drugs for Sexually Transmitted Infections," *Treatment Guidelines From The Medical Letter®*, 2004, 2(26):70-2.

Adapted from "Update to CDC's Sexually Transmitted Diseases Treatment Guidelines, 2006: Fluoroquinolones No Longer Recommended for Treatment of Gonococcal Infections," *MMWR*, 2007, 56(14):332-6.

NORMAL BLOOD VALUES

Test	Range of Normal Values
Complete Blood Count (CBC)	
White blood cells	4,500-11,000
Red blood cells (male)	4.6-6.2 x 10^6 μL
Red blood cells (female)	4.2-5.4 x 10^6 μL
Platelets	150,000-450,000
Hematocrit (male)	40% to 54%
Hematocrit (female)	38% to 47%
Hemoglobin (male)	13.5-18 g/dL
Hemoglobin (female)	12-16 g/dL
Mean corpuscular volume (MCV)	80-96 μm³
Mean corpuscular hemoglobin (MCH)	27-31 pg
Mean corpuscular hemoglobin concentration (MCHC)	32% to 36%
Differential White Blood Cell Count (%)	
Segmented neutrophils	56
Bands	3.0
Eosinophils	2.7
Basophils	0.3
Lymphocytes	34.0
Monocytes	4.0
Hemostasis	
Bleeding time (BT)	2-8 minutes
Prothrombin time (PT)	10-13 seconds
Activated partial thromboplastin time (aPTT)	25-35 seconds
Serum Chemistry	
Glucose (fasting)	70-110 mg/dL
Blood urea nitrogen (BUN)	8-23 mg/dL
Creatinine (male)	0.1-0.4 mg/dL
Creatinine (female)	0.2-0.7 mg/dL
Bilirubin, indirect (unconjugated)	0.3 mg/dL
Bilirubin, direct (conjugated)	0.1-1 mg/dL
Calcium	9.2-11 mg/dL
Magnesium	1.8-3 mg/dL
Phosphorus	2.3-4.7 mg/dL
Serum Electrolytes	
Sodium (Na^+)	136-142 mEq/L
Potassium (K^+)	3.8-5 mEq/L
Chloride (Cl^-)	95-103 mEq/L
Bicarbonate (HCO_3^-)	21-28 mmol/L
Serum Enzymes	
Alkaline phosphatase	20-130 IU/L
Alanine aminotransferase (ALT) (formerly called SGPT)	4-36 units/L
Aspartate aminotransferase (AST) (formerly called SGOT)	8-33 units/L
Amylase	16-120 Somogyi units/dL
Creatine kinase (CK) (male)	55-170 units/L
Creatine kinase (CK) (female)	30-135 units/L

DENTIFRICE PRODUCTS

Brand Name	Abrasive Ingredient	Therapeutic Ingredient	Foaming Agent
Aim® Baking Soda Gel	Hydrated silica, sodium bicarbonate	Sodium monofluorophosphate 0.7% (fluoride 0.14%)	Sodium lauryl sulfate
	Other Ingredients: Sorbitol and related polyols, water, glycerin, SD alcohol 38B, flavor, cellulose gum, sodium saccharin, blue no. 1, yellow no. 10		
Aim® Extra Strength Gel	Hydrated silica	Sodium monofluorophosphate 1.2%	Sodium lauryl sulfate
	Other Ingredients: Sorbitol, water, PEG-32, SD alcohol 38B, flavor, cellulose gum, sodium saccharin, sodium benzoate, blue no. 1, yellow no. 10		
Aim® Regular Strength	Hydrated silica	Sodium monofluorophosphate 0.8% (fluoride 0.14%)	Sodium lauryl sulfate
	Other Ingredients: Sorbitol and other related polyols, water, glycerin, SD alcohol 38B, flavor, cellulose gum, sodium saccharin, blue no. 1, yellow no. 10		
Aim® Tartar Control Gel	Hydrated silica	Sodium monofluorophosphate 0.8% (fluoride 0.14%)	Sodium lauryl sulfate
	Other Ingredients: Sorbitol and related polyols, water, glycerin, zinc citrate trihydrate, SD alcohol 38B, flavor, cellulose gum, sodium saccharin, blue no. 1, yellow no. 10		
Aquafresh® Baking Soda Toothpaste	Calcium carbonate, hydrated silica, sodium bicarbonate	Sodium monofluorophosphate	Sodium lauryl sulfate
	Other Ingredients: Calcium carrageenan, cellulose gum, colors, flavor, glycerin, PEG-8, sodium benzoate, sodium saccharin, sorbitol, titanium dioxide, water		
Aquafresh® Extra Fresh Toothpaste[1]	Hydrated silica, calcium carbonate	Sodium monofluorophosphate	Sodium lauryl sulfate
	Other Ingredients: Sorbitol, water, glycerin, PEG-8, titanium dioxide, cellulose gum, flavor, sodium saccharin, sodium benzoate, calcium carrageenan, colors		
Aquafresh® Extreme Clean® Arctic Cool	Precipitated silica	Sodium fluoride 0.15%	Sodium lauryl sulfate
	Other Ingredients: Cocamidopropyl betaine, D&C red no. 30, flavor, glycerin, PEG-8, sodium saccharin, sorbitol, synthetic iron oxide, titanium dioxide, water, xanthan gum		
Aquafresh® Extreme Clean® Original Experience	Precipitated silica	Sodium fluoride 0.15%	Sodium lauryl sulfate
	Other Ingredients: Cocamidopropyl betaine, D&C red no. 30, flavor, PEG-8, sodium saccharin, sorbitol, iron oxide, titanium dioxide, water, xanthan gum		
Aquafresh® Extreme Clean® EMPOWERMINT	Precipitated silica	Sodium fluoride 0.15%	Sodium lauryl sulfate
	Other Ingredients: Cocamidopropyl betaine, D&C red no. 30, flavor, glycerin, PEG-8, sodium saccharin, sorbitol, synthetic iron oxide, titanium dioxide, water, xanthan gum		
Aquafresh® Extreme Clean® Whitening	Precipitated silica	Sodium fluoride 0.15%	Sodium lauryl sulfate
	Other Ingredients: Cocamidopropyl betaine, D&C red no. 30, flavor, glycerin, PEG-8, sodium saccharin, sorbitol, synthetic iron oxide, titanium dioxide, water, xanthan gum		
Aquafresh® for Kids Toothpaste[1]	Hydrated silica, calcium carbonate	Sodium monofluorophosphate	Sodium lauryl sulfate
	Other Ingredients: Sorbitol, water, glycerin, PEG-8, titanium dioxide, cellulose gum, flavor, sodium saccharin, calcium carrageenan, sodium benzoate, colors		
Aquafresh® Gum Care Toothpaste	Hydrated silica, calcium carbonate	Sodium monofluorophosphate	Sodium lauryl sulfate
	Other Ingredients: Calcium carrageenan, cellulose gum, colors, flavor, PEG-8, sodium benzoate, sodium saccharin, sorbitol, titanium dioxide, water		
Aquafresh® Multi-Action Whitening	Hydrated silica	Sodium fluoride 0.15%	Sodium lauryl sulfate
	Other Ingredients: D&C red no. 30 lake, D&C yellow no. 10 lake, FD&C blue no. 1 lake, flavor, glycerin, PEG-8, povidone K30, sodium benzoate, sodium hydroxide, sodium saccharin, sodium tripolyphosphate, sorbitol, titanium dioxide, water, xanthan gum		

Brand Name	Abrasive Ingredient	Therapeutic Ingredient	Foaming Agent
Aquafresh® Multi-Action Whitening with Triclene® Stain & Tartar Defense™	Hydrated silica	Sodium fluoride 0.15%	Sodium lauryl sulfate
	Other Ingredients: D&C red no. 30 lake, D&C yellow no. 10 lake, FD&C blue no. 1 lake, flavor, glycerin, PEG-8, povidone K30, sodium benzoate, sodium hydroxide, sodium saccharin, sodium tripolyphosphate, sorbitol, titanium dioxide, water, xanthan gum		
Aquafresh® Sensitive Toothpaste	Hydrated silica	Potassium nitrate, sodium fluoride	Sodium lauryl sulfate
	Other Ingredients: Colors, flavor, glycerin, sodium benzoate, sodium saccharin, sorbitol, titanium dioxide, water, xanthan gum		
Aquafresh® Sensitive® Maximum Strength	Hydrated silica	Sodium fluoride 0.15%, potassium nitrate 5%	Sodium lauryl sulfate
	Other Ingredients: D&C red no. 30 lake, FD&C blue no. 1 lake, flavor, glycerin, sodium benzoate, sodium hydroxide, sodium saccharin, sorbitol, titanium dioxide, water, xanthan gum		
Aquafresh® Tartar Control Toothpaste[1]	Hydrated silica	Sodium fluoride	Sodium lauryl sulfate
	Other Ingredients: Tetrapotassium pyrophosphate, tetrasodium pyrophosphate, sorbitol, glycerin, PEG-8, flavor, xanthan gum, sodium saccharin, sodium benzoate, colors, titanium dioxide, water		
Aquafresh® Triple Protection Toothpaste[1]	Hydrated silica, calcium carbonate	Sodium monofluorophosphate	Sodium lauryl sulfate
	Other Ingredients: PEG-8, sorbitol, cellulose gum, sodium benzoate, titanium dioxide, calcium carrageenan, flavor, sodium saccharin, colors, water		
Aquafresh® Ultimate White	Hydrated silica	Sodium fluoride 0.15%	Sodium lauryl sulfate
	Other Ingredients: D&C red no. 30 lake, FD&C blue no. 1 lake, flavor, glycerin, PEG-8, sodium benzoate, sodium hydroxide, sodium saccharin, sodium tripolyphosphate, sorbitol, titanium dioxide, water, xanthan gum		
Aquafresh® White and Shine™[1]	Hydrated silica, mica	Sodium fluoride 0.15%	Sodium lauryl sulfate
	Other Ingredients: Disodium phosphate, flavor, PEG-8, sodium saccharin, sodium sulfite, sorbitol, titanium dioxide, water, xanthan gum		
Aquafresh® Whitening Gel or Toothpaste	Hydrated silica	Sodium fluoride	Sodium lauryl sulfate
	Other Ingredients: Colors, flavor, glycerin, PEG-8, sodium benzoate, sodium hydroxide, sodium saccharin, sodium tripolyphosphate, sorbitol, titanium dioxide, water, xanthan gum		
Arm & Hammer Advance Breath Care™ Cool Fresh Toothpaste	Calcium carbonate poloxamer 407, sodium bicarbonate	Sodium monofluorophosphate 0.76%	
	Other Ingredients: Water, glycerin, sodium citrate dihydrate, flavor, cellulose gum, cocamidopropyl betaine, zinc, citrate trihydrate, sodium saccharin, titanium dioxide		
Arm & Hammer Advance White™ Toothpaste for Sensitive Teeth	Silica, sodium bicarbonate	Sodium fluoride 0.243%, potassium nitrate 5%	
	Other Ingredients: Cellulose gum, cocamidopropyl betaine, flavor, glycerin, sorbitol, titanium dioxide, water		
Arm & Hammer Advance White™ with Baking Soda & Peroxide	Sodium bicarbonate, silica	Sodium fluoride	Sodium lauryl sulfate
	Other Ingredients: Flavor, PEG-8, poloxapol 1220, sodium carbonate peroxide, sodium lauroyl sarcosinate, sodium saccharin, tetrasodium pyrophosphate, water		
Arm & Hammer Advance White™ with Baking Soda Tartar Control	Sodium bicarbonate, hydrated silica	Sodium fluoride	Sodium lauryl sulfate
	Other Ingredients: Cellulose gum, flavor, glycerin, sodium lauroyl sarcosinate, sodium saccharin, sorbitol, tetrasodium pyrophosphate, titanium dioxide, water		

DENTIFRICE PRODUCTS (Continued)

Brand Name	Abrasive Ingredient	Therapeutic Ingredient	Foaming Agent
Arm & Hammer Advance White™ with Gel Micro-Polishers Gel	Sodium bicarbonate, hydrated silica	Sodium fluoride 0.24%	Sodium lauryl sulfate
	Other Ingredients: Cellulose gum, FD&C blue no. 1, FD&C yellow no. 5, flavor, glycerin, sodium lauroyl sarcosinate, sodium saccharin, sorbitol, tetrasodium pyrophosphate, water		
Arm & Hammer Complete Care™ Extra Whitening	Silica, sodium bicarbonate	Sodium fluoride 0.24%	Sodium lauryl sulfate
	Other Ingredients: PEG-8, PEG/PPG-116/66 copolymer, sodium carbonate peroxide, sodium lauroyl sarcosinate, sodium saccharin, flavor, zinc citrate trihydrate, water		
Arm & Hammer Dental Care Tartar Control	Sodium bicarbonate	Sodium fluoride 0.24%	Sodium lauryl sulfate
	Other Ingredients: Water, glycerin, tetrasodium pyrophosphate, PEG-8, sodium saccharin, flavors, cellulose gum, sodium lauroyl sarcosinate		
Arm & Hammer Enamel Care™	Hydrated silica	Sodium fluoride 0.24%	Sodium lauryl sulfate
	Other Ingredients: Glycerin, sodium bicarbonate, water, sorbitol, calcium sulfate, sodium sulfate, flavor, dipotassium phosphate, sodium carbonate, sodium saccharin, cellulose gum, xanthan gum, methylparaben, propylparaben, blue 1, may contain sodium lauroyl sarcosinate		
Arm & Hammer Multi-Benefit PeroxiCare Baking Soda & Peroxide Toothpaste	Sodium bicarbonate, sodium carbonate peroxide, silica	Sodium fluoride 0.24%	Sodium lauryl sulfate
	Other Ingredients: PEG/PPG-38/8 copolymer, PEG/PPG-116/66 copolymer, water, flavor, sodium saccharin, sodium lauroyl sarcosinate, hydrogenated starch hydrolysate, gum Arabic, D&C green no. 5		
Arm & Hammer PeroxiCare®	Sodium bicarbonate, silica	Sodium fluoride 0.24%	Sodium lauryl sulfate, sodium lauroyl sarcosinate
	Other Ingredients: PEG/PPG-38/8 copolymer, PEG/PPG-116/66 copolymer, sodium carbonate peroxide, sodium saccharin, flavor, water		
Arm & Hammer P.M.™ Bold Mint	Sodium bicarbonate, silica	Sodium fluoride	Sodium lauryl sulfate
	Other Ingredients: Flavor, PEG-B, poloxapol 1220, sodium percarbonate, sodium lauroyl sarcosinate, sodium saccharin, water, zinc citrate trihydrate		
Arm & Hammer P.M.™ Fresh Mint	Aluminum oxide, hydrated silica	Sodium monofluorophosphate	Sodium lauryl sulfate
	Other Ingredients: Cellulose gum, flavor, glycerin, sodium saccharin, sorbital, water, zinc citrate trihydrate		
Biotene® Antibacterial Dry Mouth Toothpaste	Hydrated silica, calcium pyrophosphate	Lactoperoxidase, glucose oxidase, lysozyme, sodium monofluorophosphate (0.76%)	
	Other Ingredients: Sorbitol, glycerin, xylitol, isoceteth-20, cellulose gum, flavor, sodium benzoate, beta-d-glucose, potassium thiocyanate		
Close-Up® Baking Soda Toothpaste (mint)	Hydrated silica, sodium bicarbonate	Sodium monofluorophosphate 0.79% (fluoride 0.15%)	Sodium lauryl sulfate
	Other Ingredients: Sorbitol and related polyols, water, glycerin, SD alcohol 38B, flavor, cellulose gum, sodium saccharin, sodium benzoate, red no. 33, red no. 40, titanium dioxide		
Close-Up® Classic Red Gel	Hydrated silica	Sodium monofluorophosphate 0.8% (fluoride 0.14%)	Sodium lauryl sulfate
	Other Ingredients: Sorbitol and related polyols, water, glycerin, SD alcohol 38B, flavor, cellulose gum, sodium saccharin, sodium chloride, red no. 33, red no. 40		
Close-Up® Cool Mint Gel	Hydrated silica	Sodium monofluorophosphate 0.79% (fluoride 0.15%)	Sodium lauryl sulfate
	Other Ingredients: Sorbitol, water, glycerin, SD alcohol 38B, flavor, cellulose gum, sodium saccharin, polysorbate 20, blue no. 1, mica, red no. 33, titanium dioxide		

Brand Name	Abrasive Ingredient	Therapeutic Ingredient	Foaming Agent
Close-Up® Original Red Whitening Toothpaste	Hydrated silica	Sodium monofluorophosphate 0.8% (fluoride 0.14%)	Sodium lauryl sulfate
	Other Ingredients: Sorbitol and related polyols, water, glycerin, SD alcohol 38B, flavor, cellulose gum, sodium saccharin, sodium chloride, red no. 30 lake, titanium dioxide, blue no. 1		
Close-Up® Tartar Control Gel (mint)	Hydrated silica	Sodium monofluorophosphate 0.79% (fluoride 0.15%)	Sodium lauryl sulfate
	Other Ingredients: Sorbitol and related polyols, water, glycerin, zinc citrate trihydrate, SD alcohol 38B, flavor, cellulose gum, sodium saccharin, red no. 33, red no. 40, **caffeine free**		
Close-Up® Tartar Control Whitening Toothpaste	Hydrated silica	Sodium monofluorophosphate 0.8% (fluoride 0.14%)	Sodium lauryl sulfate
	Other Ingredients: Sorbitol and related polypols, water, glycerin, SD alcohol 38B, flavor, zinc citrate trihydrate, cellulose gum, sodium saccharin, titanium dioxide, blue no. 1, yellow no. 10		
Colgate® Baking Soda & Peroxide Tartar Control Toothpaste[1]	Hydrated silica, sodium bicarbonate	Sodium monofluorophosphate 0.76%	Sodium lauryl sulfate
	Other Ingredients: Glycerin, propylene glycol, water, pentasodium triphosphate, tetrasodium pyrophosphate, titanium dioxide, flavor, sodium hydroxide, calcium peroxide, sodium saccharin, carrageenan, cellulose gum, FD&C blue no. 1, D&C yellow no. 10		
Colgate® Baking Soda & Peroxide Whitening Toothpaste[1]	Hydrated silica, sodium bicarbonate, aluminum oxide	Sodium monofluorophosphate 0.76%	Sodium lauryl sulfate
	Other Ingredients: Glycerin, polypylene glycol, water, pentasodium triphosphate, tetrasodium pyrophosphate, titanium dioxide, flavor, sodium hydroxide, calcium peroxide, sodium saccharin, carrageenan, cellulose gum, **dietetically sucrose free**		
Colgate® Baking Soda Tartar Control Gel or Toothpaste	Hydrated silica, sodium bicarbonate	Sodium fluoride 0.243%	Sodium lauryl sulfate
	Other Ingredients: Glycerin, tetrasodium pyrophosphate, PVM/MA copolymer, cellulose gum, flavor, sodium saccharin, sodium hydroxide, titanium dioxide (paste), FD&C blue no. 1, D&C yellow no. 10 (gel), **dietetically sucrose free**		
Colgate® Cavity Protection Toothpaste	Dicalcium phosphate dihydrate	Sodium monofluorophosphate 0.15%	Sodium lauryl sulfate
	Other Ingredients: Water, glycerin, sorbitol, cellulose gum, flavor, tetrapotassium pyrophosphate, sodium saccharin		
Colgate® Herbal White	Hydrated silica	Sodium monofluorophosphate 0.76%	Sodium lauryl sulfate
	Other Ingredients: Calcium carbonate, water, sorbitol, flavor, sodium carbonate, sodium hydroxide, cellulose gum, sodium saccharin, carrageenan, xanthan gum, parabens, balm mint extract, fennel extract, FD&C blue no. 1, D&C yellow no. 10		
Colgate® Icy Blast® Whitening	Hydrated silica, mica	Sodium fluoride 0.24%	Sodium lauryl sulfate
	Other Ingredients: Water, sorbitol, glycerin, PVM/MA copolymer, tetrasodium pyrophosphate, polyethylene, sodium saccharin, cocoamidopropyl betaine, cellulose gum, sodium hydroxide, carrageenan, titanium dioxide, FD&C blue no. 1		
Colgate® Luminous™ Paradise Fresh	Hydrated silica	Sodium fluoride 0.24%	Sodium lauryl sulfate
	Other Ingredients: Sorbitol, water, PEG-12, flavor, cellulose gum, tetrasodium pyrophosphate, cocoamidopropyl betaine, sodium saccharin, mica, titanium dioxide, FD&C red no. 40, FD&C blue no. 1		
Colgate® Junior Gel[1]	Hydrated silica	Sodium fluoride 0.243%	Sodium lauryl sulfate
	Other Ingredients: Sorbitol, water, PEG-12, flavor, tetrasodium pyrophosphate, cellulose gum, sodium saccharin, mica, titanium dioxide, colorants, **dietetically sucrose free**		
Colgate® MaxFresh® Spearmint Burst	Hydrated silica	Sodium fluoride 0.24%	Sodium lauryl sulfate
	Other Ingredients: Sorbitol, water, PEG-12, flavor, cellulose gum, tetrasodium pyrophosphate, sodium saccharin, cocoamidopropyl betaine, methylcellulose, FD&C blue no. 1, FD&C yellow no. 5		
Colgate® Platinum™ Whitening Toothpaste[1]	Silica, aluminum oxide	Sodium monofluorophosphate	Sodium lauryl sulfate
	Other Ingredients: Water, hydrated silica, sorbitol, glycerin, PEG-12, tetrapotassium pyrophosphate, PVM/MA copolymer, flavor, sodium hydroxide, sodium saccharin, titanium dioxide		

DENTIFRICE PRODUCTS *(Continued)*

Brand Name	Abrasive Ingredient	Therapeutic Ingredient	Foaming Agent
Colgate® Platinum™ Whitening with Baking Soda Toothpaste[1]	Sodium bicarbonate, aluminum oxide	Sodium monofluorophosphate 0.76%	Sodium lauryl sulfate
Other Ingredients: Water, glycerin, PEG-12, tetrapotassium pyrophosphate, PVM/MA copolymer, flavor, sodium hydroxide, sodium saccharin, titanium dioxide, cellulose gum			
Colgate® Sensitive Maximum Strength Toothpaste	Hydrated silica, sodium bicarbonate	Potassium nitrate 5%, stannous fluoride 0.45%	Sodium lauryl sulfate
Other Ingredients: Glycerin and/or sorbitol, water, PEG-40 castor oil, PEG-12, poloxamer 407, sodium citrate, flavor, titanium dioxide, sodium hydroxide, cellulose gum, xanthan gum, sodium saccharin, stannous chloride, citric acid, tetrasodium pyrophosphate, FD&C blue no. 1			
Colgate® Sensitive Plus Whitening	Hydrated silica, Sodium bicarbonate	Potassium nitrate 5% antisensitivity (FDA required amount), Stannous Fluoride 0.45% (0.15% w/v fluoride ion)	Sodium lauryl sulfate
Other Ingredients: Glycerin and/or sorbitol, water, PEG-40 castor oil, PEG-12, poloxamer 405, sodium citrate, flavor, titanium dioxide, sodium hydroxide, cellulose gum, xanthan gum, sodium saccharin, stannous chloride, citric acid, tetrasodium pyrophosphate, mica, FD&C blue no. 1, D&C yellow no. 10			
Colgate® Simply White®	Silica	Sodium fluoride 0.24%	Sodium lauryl sulfate
Other Ingredients: Water, glycerin, sorbitol, PEG-12, pentasodium triphosphate, flavor, carbomer, hydrogen peroxide, sodium hydroxide, tetrasodium pyrophosphate, PVM/MA copolymer, cellulose gum, sodium saccharin, sodium magnesium silicate, xanthan gum, carrageenan, phosphoric acid, manganese gluconate, butylated hydroxytoluene, titanium dioxide, FD&C blue no. 1			
Colgate® Simply White®	Silica	Sodium fluoride 0.24%	Sodium lauryl sulfate
Other Ingredients: Water, glycerin, sorbitol, PEG-12, pentasodium triphosphate, flavor, carbomer, hydrogen peroxide, sodium hydroxide, tetrasodium pyrophosphate, PVM/MA copolymer, cellulose gum, sodium saccharin, sodium magnesium silicate, xanthan gum, carrageenan, phosphoric acid, manganese gluconate, butylated hydroxytoluene, titanium dioxide, FD&C blue no. 1			
Colgate® Sparkling White™ Vanilla Mint	Hydrated silica, mica	Sodium fluoride 0.24%	Sodium lauryl sulfate
Other Ingredients: Sorbitol, water, PEG-12, flavor, cellulose gum, tetrasodium pyrophosphate, cocoamidopropyl betaine, sodium saccharin, FD&C yellow no. 6			
Colgate® Tartar Control Plus Whitening	Hydrated silica, aluminum oxide	Sodium monofluorophosphate 0.76%	Sodium lauryl sulfate
Other Ingredients: Water, sorbitol, glycerin, pentasodium triphosphate, tetrasodium pyrophosphate, PVM/MA copolymer, cellulose gum, flavor, sodium hydroxide, titanium dioxide, sodium saccharin, carrageenan			
Colgate® Toothpaste[1]	Dicalcium phosphate dihydrate	Sodium monofluorophosphate 0.76%	Sodium lauryl sulfate
Other Ingredients: Glycerin, cellulose gum, tetrasodium pyrophosphate, sodium saccharin, flavor, **dietetically sucrose free**			
Colgate® Total® Advanced Clean Plus Whitening	Hydrated silica, mica	Sodium fluoride 0.24%, triclosan 0.3%	Sodium lauryl sulfate
Other Ingredients: Water, glycerin, sorbitol, PVM/MA copolymer, flavor, cellulose gum, sodium hydroxide, propylene glycol, carrageenan, sodium saccharin, titanium dioxide			
Colgate® Total® Advanced Fresh Gel	Hydrated silica	Sodium fluoride 0.24%, triclosan 0.3%	Sodium lauryl sulfate
Other Ingredients: Water, glycerin, sorbitol, PVM/MA copolymer, flavor, cellulose gum, sodium hydroxide, propylene glycol, carrageenan, sodium saccharin, FD&C blue no. 1, D&C yellow no. 10			
Colgate® Total® Toothpaste	Hydrated silica	Sodium fluoride 0.243%, triclosan 0.3%	Sodium lauryl sulfate
Other Ingredients: Water, glycerin, sorbitol, PVM/MA copolymer, cellulose gum, flavor, sodium hydroxide, propylene glycol, carrageenan, sodium saccharin, titanium dioxide			

Brand Name	Abrasive Ingredient	Therapeutic Ingredient	Foaming Agent
Colgate® Total® Clean Mint Paste[1]	Hydrated silica	Triclosan 0.30%, sodium fluoride 0.24%	Sodium lauryl sulfate
	Other Ingredients: Water, glycerin, sorbitol, PVM/MA copolymer, cellulose gum, flavor, sodium hydroxide, propylene glycol, carrageenan, sodium saccharin, titanium dioxide		
Colgate® Total® Mint Stripe™ Gel[1]	Hydrated silica, mica	Triclosan 0.30%, sodium fluoride 0.24%	Sodium lauryl sulfate
	Other Ingredients: Water, glycerin, sorbitol, PVM/MA copolymer, cellulose gum, flavor, sodium saccharin, titanium dioxide, FD&C blue no. 1, D&C yellow no. 10		
Colgate® Total® Fresh Stripe Toothpaste	Hydrated silica	Sodium fluoride 0.243%, triclosan 0.3%	Sodium lauryl sulfate
	Other Ingredients: Water, glycerin, sorbitol, PVM/MA copolymer, cellulose gum, flavor, sodium hydroxide, propylene glycol, carrageenan, sodium saccharin, mica, titanium dioxide, FD&C blue no. 1, D&C yellow no. 10		
Colgate® Total® Whitening Gel[1]	Hydrated silica, mica	Triclosan 0.30%, sodium fluoride 0.24%	Sodium lauryl sulfate
	Other Ingredients: Water, glycerin, sorbitol, PVM/MA copolymer, cellulose gum, flavor, sodium hydroxide, propylene glycol, carrageenan, sodium saccharin, titanium dioxide, FD&C blue no. 1		
Colgate® Total® Whitening Paste[1]	Hydrated silica	Triclosan 0.30%, sodium fluoride 0.24%	Sodium lauryl sulfate
	Other Ingredients: Water, glycerin, sorbitol, PVM/MA copolymer, cellulose gum, flavor, sodium hydroxide, propylene glycol, carrageenan, sodium saccharin, titanium dioxide		
Colgate® Winterfresh Gel[1]	Hydrated silica	Sodium fluoride 0.243%	Sodium lauryl sulfate
	Other Ingredients: Sorbitol, water, PEG-12, flavor, tetrasodium pyrophosphate, cellulose gum, sodium saccharin, FD&C blue no. 1, **dietetically sucrose free**		
Colgate® Whitening Oxygen Bubbles Brisk Mint®	Hydrated silica, sodium bicarbonate	Sodium fluoride 0.24%	Sodium lauryl sulfate
	Other Ingredients: Glycerin, sorbitol, propylene glycol, aluminum oxide, water, pentasodium triphosphate, tetrasodium pyrophosphate, flavor, sodium hydroxide, calcium peroxide, sodium saccharin, carrageenan, cellulose gum, titanium dioxide		
Crest® Baking Soda Tartar Protection Gel or Toothpaste (mint)[1]	Hydrated silica, sodium bicarbonate	Sodium fluoride 0.243%	Sodium lauryl sulfate
	Other Ingredients: Water, glycerin, sorbitol, tetrasodium pyrophosphate, PEG-6, flavor, cellulose gum, sodium saccharin, titanium dioxide (paste), FD&C blue no. 1 (gel), disodium pyrophosphate, tetrapotassium pyrophosphate, carbomer 956, xanthan gum, FD&C yellow no. 5 (gel)		
Crest® Baking Soda & Peroxide Whitening with Tarter Protection	Hydrated silica, sodium bicarbonate	Sodium fluoride 0.24%	Sodium lauryl sulfate
	Other Ingredients: Glycerin, water, propylene glycol, sorbitol, tetrasodium pyrophosphate, sorbitol, PEG-12, flavor, sodium hydroxide, sodium saccharin, poloxamer 407, xanthan gum, calcium peroxide, titanium dioxide, blue no. 1		
Crest® Cavity Protection with Baking Soda Gel or Toothpaste[1] (mint)	Hydrated silica, sodium bicarbonate	Sodium fluoride 0.243%	Sodium lauryl sulfate
	Other Ingredients: Sorbitol, water, glycerin, sodium carbonate, flavor, cellulose gum, sodium saccharin, titanium dioxide (paste), FD&C blue no. 1 (gel)		
Crest® Cavity Protection Gel (cool mint)[1]	Hydrated silica	Sodium fluoride 0.243%	Sodium lauryl sulfate
	Other Ingredients: Sorbitol, water, trisodium phosphate, flavor, sodium phosphate, xanthan gum, sodium saccharin, carbomer 956, FD&C blue no. 1, carbomer 940A		
Crest® Cavity Protection Toothpaste[1] (icy mint or regular)	Hydrated silica	Sodium fluoride 0.243%	Sodium lauryl sulfate
	Other Ingredients: Sorbitol, water, glycerin (mint), trisodium phosphate, flavor, sodium phosphate, cellulose gum (mint), xanthan gum (regular), sodium saccharin, carbomer 956, titanium dioxide, FD&C blue 1, carbomer 940A		

DENTIFRICE PRODUCTS *(Continued)*

Brand Name	Abrasive Ingredient	Therapeutic Ingredient	Foaming Agent
Crest® Extra Whitening Gel or Toothpaste	Hydrated silica	Sodium fluoride 0.15%	Sodium lauryl sulfate, poloxamer 407
	Other Ingredients: Sorbitol, water, glycerin, tetrasodium pyrophosphate, sodium carbonate, carboxymethylcellulose sodium, titanium dioxide, carnauba wax, sodium saccharin, flavor, FD&C blue no. 1, FD&C yellow no. 5, PEG-6, sodium bicarbonate²		
Crest® for Kids Cavity Protection Gel	Hydrated silica	Sodium fluoride 0.243%	Sodium lauryl sulfate
	Other Ingredients: Sorbitol, water, trisodium phosphate, sodium phosphate, xanthan gum, flavor, sodium saccharin, carbomer 956, mica, titanium dioxide, FD&C blue no. 1		
Crest® Gum Care Gel or Toothpaste	Hydrated silica	Stannous fluoride 0.454%	Sodium lauryl sulfate
	Other Ingredients: Sorbitol, water, stannous chloride, titanium dioxide (paste), flavor, sodium hydroxide, sodium saccharin, sodium carrageenan, FD&C blue no. 1 (gel), sodium gluconate, hydroxyethylcellulose		
Crest® Multicare Gel or Toothpaste (cool mint, fresh mint)	Hydrated silica, sodium bicarbonate	Sodium fluoride 0.243%	Sodium lauryl sulfate
	Other Ingredients: Tetrasodium pyrophosphate, xylitol, water, glycerin, PEG-6, poloxamer 407, sodium carbonate, flavor, cellulose gum, xanthan gum, sodium saccharin, titanium dioxide, FD&C blue no. 1, FD&C yellow no. 5 (cool mint)		
Crest® Nature's Expressions Mint + Green Tea Extract	Hydrated silica	Sodium fluoride 0.243%	Sodium lauryl sulfate
	Other Ingredients: Sorbitol, water, tetrasodium pyrophosphate, disodium pyrophosphate, flavor (peppermint oil, anise oil, menthol, and green tea extract), xanthan gum, sodium saccharin, carbomer 956, poloxamer 407, polyethylene, iron oxide, blue no. 1 aluminum lake, yellow no. 10 aluminum lake		
Crest® Sensitivity Protection Toothpaste¹ (mild mint)	Hydrated silica	Potassium nitrate 5%, sodium fluoride 0.15%	Sodium lauryl sulfate
	Other Ingredients: Water, glycerin, sorbitol, trisodium phosphate, cellulose gum, flavor, xanthan gum, sodium saccharin, titanium dioxide, **dye free**		
Crest® Sensitivity Whitening Plus Scope	Hydrated silica	Potassium nitrate 5%, sodium fluoride 0.24%	Sodium lauryl sulfate
	Other Ingredients: Water, glycerin, sorbitol, trisodium phosphate, flavor, cellulose guym, alcohol (1.09%), xanthan gum, sodium saccharin, sucralose, polysorbate 80, sodium benzoate, cetylpyridinium chloride, benzoic acid, polyethylene, iron oxides, titanium dioxide, blue no. 1 aluminum lake, yellow no. 10 aluminum lake, blue no. 1, yellow no. 5		
Crest® Tartar Protection Gel¹ (fresh mint, smooth mint)		Sodium fluoride 0.243%	Sodium lauryl sulfate
	Other Ingredients: Water, sorbitol, glycerin, tetrapotassium pyrophosphate, PEG-6, disodium pyrophosphate, tetrasodium pyrophosphate, flavor, xanthan gum, sodium saccharin, carbomer 956, FD&C blue no. 1, FD&C yellow no. 5 (smooth mint)		
Crest® Tartar Protection Toothpaste¹ (original flavor)	Silica	Sodium fluoride 0.243%	Sodium lauryl sulfate
	Other Ingredients: Water, sorbitol, glycerin, tetrapotassium pyrophosphate, PEG-6, disodium pyrophosphate, tetrasodium pyrophosphate, flavor, xanthan gum, sodium saccharin, carbomer 956, titanium dioxide, FD&C blue no. 1		
Crest® Vivid White™	Hydrated silica	Sodium fluoride 0.243%	Sodium lauryl sulfate
	Other ingredients: Glycerin, water, sorbitol, sodium hexametaphosphate, propylene glycol, flavor, PEG-12, cocamidopropyl betaine, carbomer 956, sodium saccharin, poloxamer 407, polyethylene oxide, xanthan gum, sodium hydroxide, cellulose gum, titanium dioxide		
Crest® Whitening Expressions Extreme Herbal Mint	Hydrated silica	Sodium fluoride 0.243%	Sodium lauryl sulfate
	Other ingredients: Sorbitol, water, glycerin, tetrasodium pyrophosphate, PEG-6, flavor, disodium pyrophosphate, xanthan gum, sodium saccharin, carbomer 956, sucralose, polyethylene, titanium dioxide, blue 1 aluminum lake, yellow 11 aluminum lake		

Brand Name	Abrasive Ingredient	Therapeutic Ingredient	Foaming Agent
Crest® Whitening Expressions Fresh Citrus Breeze	Hydrated silica	Sodium fluoride 0.243%	Sodium lauryl sulfate
	Other ingredients: Sorbitol, water, glycerin, tetrasodium pyrophosphate, PEG-6, flavor, disodium pyrophosphate, xanthan gum, sodium saccharin, carnuba wax, carbomer 956, sucralose, titanium dioxide, yellow 6		
Crest® Whitening Plus Scope®	Hydrated silica	Sodium fluoride 0.243% (0.15% w/v fluoride ion)	Sodium lauryl sulfate
	Other ingredients: Water, sorbitol, glycerin, tetrapotassium pyrophosphate, PEG-6, disodium pyrophosphate, tetrasodium pyrophosphate, flavor, alcohol (1.14%), xanthan gum, sodium saccharin, carbomer 956, polysorbate 80, sodium benzoate, cetylpyridinium chloride, benzoic acid, domiphen bromide (.0002 w/v%)		
Dr. Tichenor's Toothpaste	Hydrated silica	Sodium fluoride	Sodium lauryl sulfate
	Other Ingredients: Water, glycerin, sorbitol, insoluble sodium metaphosphate, peppermint oil, cellulose gum, sodium saccharin, sodium phosphate, titanium dioxide, magnesium aluminum silicate, **dye free**		
Enamelon® All-Family Toothpaste	Hydrated silica	Sodium fluoride (fluoride 0.14%)	Sodium lauryl sulfate
	Other Ingredients: Water, glycerin, sorbitol, monoammonium phosphate, calcium sulfate, xanthan gum, flavor, PEG-60 hydrogenated castor oil, sodium saccharin, ammonium chloride, cellulose gum, titanium dioxide, magnesium chloride, methylparaben, propylparaben, FD&C blue no. 1		
First Teeth™ Baby Gel		Lactoperoxidase 0.7 units/g, lactoferrin, glucose oxidase	Sodium lauryl sulfate
	Other Ingredients: Water, glycerin, sorbitol, pectin, xylitol, flavor, aloe vera, propylene glycol		
Fluoride Foam™[1,3]	**Ingredients:** Fluoride 1.23% (from sodium fluoride and hydrogen fluoride), water, phosphoric acid, poloxamer, sodium saccharin, flavor		
Fluorigard® Anti-Cavity Liquid [1,3]	**Ingredients:** Sodium fluoride 0.05%, ethyl alcohol, pluronic F108 and F127, sweetener, flavor, glycerin, sorbitol, preservatives, **dye free**, **gluten free**		
Gleem® Toothpaste	Hydrated silica	Sodium fluoride 0.243%	Sodium lauryl sulfate
	Other Ingredients: Sorbitol, water, trisodium phosphate, flavors, sodium phosphate, xanthan gum, sodium saccharin, carbomer 956, titanium dioxide, **dye free**		
Listerine® Essential Care Gel	Hydrated silica	Anticavity: Sodium monofluorophosphate 0.76% (0.13% W/V fluoride ion Antiplaque/ Antigingivitis: Eucalyptol 0.738%, menthol 0.340%, methyl salicylate 0.480%, thymol 0.511%	Sodium lauryl sulfate
	Other Ingredients: Water, sorbitol, glycerin, flavors, cellulose gum, sodium saccharin, phosphoric acid, FD&C blue no. 1, D&C yellow no. 10, sodium phosphate, benzoic acid, PEG-32, and xanthan gum		
Listerine® Gel or Toothpaste (cool mint)	Hydrated silica	Sodium monofluorophosphate	Sodium lauryl sulfate
	Other Ingredients: Water, sorbitol, glycerin, flavors, cellulose gum, sodium saccharin, phosphoric acid, FD&C blue no. 1, D&C yellow no. 10, sodium phosphate, benzoic acid, titanium dioxide (paste), xanthan gum		
Listerine® Tartar Control Gel or Toothpaste (cool mint)	Hydrated silica	Sodium fluoride	Sodium lauryl sulfate
	Other Ingredients: Water, sorbitol, glycerin, PEG-32, flavor, cellulose gum, sodium saccharin, tetrapotassium pyrophosphate, FD&C blue no. 1, D&C yellow no. 10, titanium dioxide (paste)		
Mentadent® Advanced Whitening Gel or Toothpaste	Hydrated silica, sodium bicarbonate	Sodium fluoride 0.15%	Sodium lauryl sulfate, hydrogen peroxide
	Other Ingredients: Zinc citrate trihydrate, water, sorbitol, glycerin, poloxamer 407, PEG-32, SD alcohol 38B, flavor, cellulose gum, sodium saccharin, phosphoric acid, blue no. 1, titanium dioxide		

DENTIFRICE PRODUCTS *(Continued)*

Brand Name	Abrasive Ingredient	Therapeutic Ingredient	Foaming Agent
Mentadent® Gum Care Gel or Toothpaste	Hydrated silica, sodium bicarbonate	Sodium fluoride 0.24% (fluoride 0.15%)	Sodium lauryl sulfate, hydrogen peroxide
	Other Ingredients: Zinc citrate trihydrate (1.8%), water, sorbitol, glycerin, poloxamer 407, PEG-32, SD alcohol 38B, flavor, cellulose gum, sodium saccharin, menthol, methyl salicylate, phosphoric acid, green no. 3, titanium dioxide		
Mentadent® Sensitive Plus™	Hydrated silica, sodium bicarbonate	Potassium nitrate (5%), sodium fluoride	Sodium lauryl sulfate, hydrogen peroxide
	Other Ingredients: Water, glycerin, sorbitol, poloxamer 407, PEG-32, SD alcohol, cellulose gum, sodium saccharin, phosphoric acid, blue no. 1, titanium dioxide		
Mentadent® Tartar Control Gel or Toothpaste	Hydrated silica, sodium bicarbonate	Sodium fluoride 0.24%	Sodium lauryl sulfate, hydrogen peroxide
	Other Ingredients: Water, sorbitol, glycerin, poloxamer 407, PEG-32, zinc citrate, SD alcohol 38B, flavor, cellulose gum, sodium saccharin, phosphoric acid, blue no. 1, titanium dioxide, menthol		
Mentadent® with Baking Soda & Peroxide Gel or Toothpaste[1]	Hydrated silica, sodium bicarbonate	Sodium fluoride 0.24% (fluoride 0.15%)	Sodium lauryl sulfate, hydrogen peroxide
	Other Ingredients: Water, sorbitol, glycerin, poloxamer 407, PEG-32, SD alcohol 38B, flavor, cellulose gum, sodium saccharin, phosphoric acid, blue no. 1, titanium dioxide		
My First Colgate® Gel[1]	Hydrated silica	Sodium fluoride 0.243%	Sodium lauryl sulfate
	Other Ingredients: Water, sorbitol, PEG-12, flavor, tetrasodium pyrophosphate, cellulose gum, sodium saccharin, FD&C red no. 40, D&C red no. 33, **dietetically sucrose free**		
Natural Dentist™ Herbal Toothpaste & Gum Therapy, Cinnamon Flavored	Calcium carbonate	Sodium monofluorophosphate	Sodium lauryl sulfate
	Other Ingredients: Vegetable glycerin, aloe vera gel, sodium carrageenan, echinacea, goldenseal, calendula, bloodroot, bee propolis, grapefruit seed extract, sodium bicarbonate[2], cinnamon oil		
Natural Dentist™ Herbal Toothpaste & Gum Therapy, Mint Flavored	Calcium carbonate	Sodium monofluorophosphate	Sodium lauryl sulfate
	Other Ingredients: Vegetable glycerin, aloe vera gel, sodium carrageenan, echinacea, goldenseal, calendula, bloodroot, bee propolis, grapefruit seed extract, sodium bicarbonate[2], spearmint and peppermint oils		
Natural White® Toothpaste	Hydrated silica	Sodium fluoride	Sodium lauryl sulfate
	Other Ingredients: Sorbitol, water, glycerin, sodium benzoate, titanium dioxide, flavor, cellulose gum, **dietetically sucrose free**		
Natural White® Baking Soda Toothpaste	Calcium carbonate	Sodium monofluorophosphate	Sodium lauryl sulfate
	Other Ingredients: Sorbitol, water, glycerin, sodium bicarbonate[2], carrageenan, natural flavor, **dietetically sucrose free**		
Natural White® Fights Plaque Toothpaste	Hydrated silica	Sodium fluoride	Sodium lauryl sulfate
	Other Ingredients: Sorbitol, water, glycerin, sodium benzoate, titanium dioxide, flavor, cellulose gum, **dietetically sucrose free**		
Natural White® Sensitive Toothpaste	Hydrated silica	Sodium monofluorophosphate, potassium nitrate	Sodium lauryl sulfate
	Other Ingredients: Sorbitol, water, glycerin, flavor, FD&C red no. 40, sodium benzoate, titanium dioxide, sodium saccharin, **dietetically sucrose free**		
Natural White® Tartar Control Toothpaste	Hydrated silica	Sodium fluoride	Sodium lauryl sulfate
	Other Ingredients: Sorbitol, water, glycerin, xanthan gum, tetrapotassium pyrophosphate, titanium dioxide, cellulose gum, flavor, sodium benzoate, FD&C blue no. 1, D&C yellow no. 10, **dietetically sucrose free**		
Natural White® with Peroxide Gel		Hydrogen peroxide	
	Other Ingredients: Water, glycerin, flavor, dipotassium phosphate, sodium saccharin, phosphoric acid, poloxamer, **dietetically sucrose free**		

Brand Name	Abrasive Ingredient	Therapeutic Ingredient	Foaming Agent
Oxyfresh Toothpaste	Fine chalk	Oxygene® (stabilized chlorine dioxide)	Sodium lauryl sulfate
	Other Ingredients: Purified deionized water, sorbitol, glycerin, carrageenan, natural flavors, sodium saccharin		
Orajel® Baby Tooth & Gum Cleanser Gel			
	Other Ingredients: Poloxamer 407 (2%), simethicone (0.12%), Microdent, carboxymethylcellulose, sodium, citric acid, flavor, glycerin, methylparaben, potassium sorbate, propylene glycol, propylparaben, water, sodium saccharin, sorbitol, **fluoride free**		
Orajel® Gold Sensitive Teeth Gel for Adults	Hydrated silica	Potassium nitrate 5%, sodium monofluorophosphate 0.2%	Sodium lauryl sulfate
	Other Ingredients: FD&C blue no. 1, flavor, glycerin, sodium lauroyl sarcosinate, sodium saccharin, sorbitol, xanthan gum		
Pearl Drops® Toothpolish Paste	Hydrated silica, calcium pyrophosphate, dicalcium phosphate, aluminum hydroxide	Sodium monofluorophosphate	Sodium lauryl sulfate
	Other Ingredients: Water, sorbitol, glycerin, PEG-12, flavor, cellulose gum, trisodium phosphate, sodium phosphate, sodium saccharin, **dietetically sucrose free, dye free**		
Pearl Drops® Toothpolish Gel	Hydrated silica	Sodium monofluorophosphate	Sodium lauryl sulfate
	Other Ingredients: Sorbitol, water, glycerin, PEG-12, flavor, cellulose gum, sodium saccharin, FD&C blue no. 1, FD&C yellow no. 10, **dietetically sucrose free**		
Pearl Drops® Whitening Extra Strength Paste	Hydrated silica, calcium pyrophosphate, dicalcium phosphate	Sodium monofluorophosphate	Sodium lauryl sulfate
	Other Ingredients: Water, sorbitol, glycerin, PEG-12, flavor, cellulose gum, trisodium phosphate, sodium phosphate, sodium saccharin, titanium dioxide, **dietetically sucrose free, dye free**		
Pearl Drops® Whitening Gel (icy cool mint)	Hydrated silica	Sodium monofluorophosphate	Sodium lauryl sulfate
	Other Ingredients: Sorbitol, water, glycerin, PEG-12, flavor, cellulose gum, sodium saccharin, FD&C blue no. 1, FD&C yellow no. 10, **dietetically sucrose free**		
Pepsodent® Baking Soda Toothpaste	Hydrated silica	Sodium monofluorophosphate 0.8% (fluoride (0.14%)	Sodium lauryl sulfate
	Other Ingredients: Sorbitol, water, sodium bicarbonate[2], PEG-32, SD alcohol 38B, flavor, cellulose gum, sodium saccharin, titanium dioxide		
Pepsodent® Original Toothpaste	Hydrated silica	Sodium monofluorophosphate 0.8% (fluoride 0.14%)	Sodium lauryl sulfate
	Other Ingredients: Sorbitol and related polyols, water, glycerin, SD alcohol 38B, flavor, cellulose gum, sodium saccharin, titanium dioxide		
Pepsodent® Tartar Control Toothpaste	Hydrated silica	Sodium monofluorophosphate 0.8% (fluoride 0.14%)	Sodium lauryl sulfate
	Other Ingredients: Sorbitol and related polyols, water, glycerin, SD alcohol 38B, zinc citrate trihydrate, flavor, cellulose gum, sodium saccharin, titanium dioxide, blue no. 1, yellow no. 1		
Pete & Pam™ Gel (premeasured strips)	Hydrated silica	Sodium monofluorophosphate 0.76%	Sodium lauroyl sarcosinate
	Other Ingredients: Sorbitol, water, glycerin, xanthan gum, polysorbate 20, sodium benzoate, pluronic P84, FD&C blue no. 1, FD&C red no. 33, FD&C yellow no. 5, flavor, xylitol		
Promise® Toothpaste	Dicalcium phosphate	Potassium nitrate, sodium monofluorophosphate	Sodium lauryl sulfate
	Other Ingredients: Water, hydroxyethylcellulose, flavor, sodium saccharin, methylparaben, propylparaben, D&C yellow no. 10, FD&C blue no. 1, glycerin, sorbitol, silicon dioxide, **dietetically sucrose free**		
Q-Dent – The Antioxidant Toothpaste	Silica	Sodium fluoride 0.15%	Sodium lauryl sulfate
	Other Ingredients: Sorbitol, water, glycerin, tetrasodium pyrophosphate, tetrapotassium pyrophosphate, PEG-300, flavor, coenzyme Q_{10}, cellulose gum, titanium dioxide, sodium saccharin, FD&C blue no. 1		

DENTIFRICE PRODUCTS (Continued)

Brand Name	Abrasive Ingredient	Therapeutic Ingredient	Foaming Agent
Q-Dent – The Coenzyme Q₁₀ Toothpaste	Silica	Sodium fluoride 0.15%	Sodium lauryl sulfate
	Other Ingredients: Sorbitol, water, glycerin, tetrasodium pyrophosphate, tetrapotassium pyrophosphate, PEG-300, flavor, coenzyme Q₁₀, cellulose gum, sodium saccharin, FD&C blue no. 1		
Reach Act Adult Anti-Cavity Treatment Liquid (cinnamon, mint)[3]	**Ingredients:** Sodium fluoride 0.05%, cetylpyridinium chloride, D&C red no. 33 (cinnamon), EDTA calcium disodium, FD&C yellow no. 5, flavor, glycerin, monobasic sodium phosphate, dibasic sodium phosphate, poloxamer 407, polysorbate 80 (cinnamon), polysorbate 20 (mint), propylene glycol, sodium benzoate, sodium saccharin, water, FD&C green no. 3 (mint), menthol (mint), methyl salicylate (mint), potassium sorbate (mint), **alcohol free**		
Reach Act for Kids[1,3]	**Ingredients:** Sodium fluoride 0.05%, cetylpyridinium chloride, D&C red no. 33, EDTA calcium disodium, flavor, glycerin, monobasic sodium phosphate, dibasic sodium phosphate, poloxamer 407, polysorbate 80, propylene glycol, sodium benzoate, sodium saccharin, water, **alcohol free**		
Rembrandt® Age-Defying Adult Toothpaste (original or mint)	Dicalcium orthophosphate, soft silica	Sodium monofluorophosphate (fluoride 0.15%)	
	Other Ingredients: Trihydroxy propane, perhydrol urea, aluminum oxide, acetylated pectins, sodium citrate, iridium, papain, carboxyl polymethylene, saccharin, propylene glycol, flavor		
Rembrandt® Age-Defying™ Whitening Toothpaste	Silica	Sodium fluoride 0.15%	Sodium lauryl sulfate
	Other Ingredients: Glycerin, dicalcium phosphate, acylated amylopectins, alumina oxide, carbamide peroxide, sodium citrate, flavor, papain, citric acid, EDTA, sodium saccharin		
Rembrandt® Age-Defying Adult Formula Mouthwash[3]	**Ingredients:** Sodium fluoride 0.05%, water, glycerin, hydrogen peroxide solution, sodium citrate, polyoxyl 40 hydrogenated castor oil, flavor, cocamidopropyl betaine, citric acid, sodium benzoate, sodium saccharin, sodium hydroxide, **alcohol free**		
Rembrandt® Daily Whitening Gel	Silica	Sodium monofluorophosphate (fluoride 0.15%)	Carbamide peroxide, sodium lauryl sulfate
	Other Ingredients: Glycerin, sodium citrate, carbopol, triethanolamine, flavor		
Rembrandt® Extra Whitening Fluoride Toothpaste for Canker Sore Sufferers	Silica	Sodium fluoride 0.15%	
	Other Ingredients: Dicalcium phosphate, glycerin, water, xylitol, alumina, sodium citrate, natural flavors, cocamidopropyl betaine, sodium carrageenan, papain, citric acid, sodium saccharin		
Rembrandt® Intense Stain Removal with Alumasil®	Silica	Sodium fluoride 0.15%	Sodium lauryl sulfate
	Other Ingredients: Dicalcium phosphate, glycerin, sorbitol, water, alumina, sodium citrate, cocamidopropyl betaine, flavor, papain, sodium carrageenan, citric acid, sodium saccharin, methylparaben, vitamin E, FD&C blue no. 1, FD&C yellow no. 5		
Rembrandt® Naturals Toothpaste	Silica	0.15% fluoride ion from sodium monofluorophosphate wt/vol%	None
	Other ingredients: Water (artesian springs), dicalcium phosphate (from monetite, a mineral), glycerine (by-product of vegetable soap), xylitol (from birch trees), cocamidopropyl betaine (from coconut), flavor (spearmint, peppermint, other natural sources), sodium citrate (from citrus fruit), stevia (from stevia plant), papain (from papaya plant), sodium carrageenan (from seaweed), citric acid and vitamin C (from citrus fruit), ginkgo extract, raspberry leaf extract. Also available containing aloe vera and echinacea or papaya and ginseng.		
Rembrandt® Plus with Active Dental Peroxide Superior Whitening Toothpaste Minty Fresh Flavor	Silica	Sodium fluoride 0.15%	Sodium lauryl sulfate
	Other Ingredients: Glycerin, carbamide peroxide, alumina, acylated amylopectins, flavors, sodium citrate, propylene glycol, cocamidopropyl betaine, papain, carbomer, sodium saccharin, EDTA		

Brand Name	Abrasive Ingredient	Therapeutic Ingredient	Foaming Agent
Rembrandt® Whitening Baking Soda Toothpaste	Sodium bicarbonate, silica	Sodium monofluorophosphate (fluoride 0.15%)	Sodium lauryl sulfate
	Other Ingredients: Glycerin, sorbitol, alumina, water, sodium citrate, sodium carrageenan, papain, flavor, sodium hydroxide, FD&C blue no. 1, sodium saccharin		
Rembrandt® Whitening Canker Sore Prevention Toothpaste	Dicalcium phosphate, silica	Sodium monofluorophosphate (fluoride 0.15%)	
	Other Ingredients: Water, glycerin, xylitol, sodium citrate, natural flavors, sodium carrageenan, papain, citric acid, **dye free**		
Rembrandt® Whitening Natural Toothpaste	Dicalcium phosphate, silica	Sodium monofluorophosphate	
	Other Ingredients: Water, glycerin, xylitol, sodium citrate, natural flavors, sodium carrageenan, papain, citric acid, **dye free**		
Rembrandt® Whitening Sensitive Toothpaste	Dicalcium phosphate dihydrate	Potassium nitrate 5%, sodium monofluorophosphate 0.76%	Sodium lauryl sulfate
	Other Ingredients: Glycerin, sorbitol, water, alumina, papain, sodium citrate, flavor, carboxymethylcellulose sodium, sodium saccharin, methylparaben, FD&C red no. 40, citric acid		
Rembrandt® Whitening Toothpaste (mint or original)	Dicalcium phosphate dihydrate	Sodium monofluorophosphate 0.76%	Sodium lauryl sulfate
	Other Ingredients: Glycerin, sorbitol, water, alumina, sodium citrate, flavor, sodium carrageenan, papain, sodium saccharin, methylparaben, citric acid, FD&C blue no. 1, FD&C yellow no. 5		
Revelation® Toothpowder	Calcium carbonate		Vegetable soap powder
	Other Ingredients: Methyl salicylate, menthol, **dye free**		
Sensodyne® Baking Soda Toothpaste	Sodium bicarbonate, silica	Potassium nitrate, sodium fluoride	Sodium lauryl sulfate
	Other Ingredients: Water, glycerin, flavor, hydroxyethylcellulose, titanium dioxide, sodium saccharin, **dietetically sucrose free**, **dye free**		
Sensodyne® Cool Gel	Silica	Potassium nitrate, sodium fluoride	Sodium methyl cocoyl taurate
	Other Ingredients: Water, sorbitol, glycerin, sodium carboxymethylcellulose, flavor, sodium saccharin, FD&C blue no. 1, trisodium phosphate, **dietetically sucrose free**		
Sensodyne® Extra Whitening Toothpaste	Silica	Potassium nitrate, sodium monofluorophosphate	Sodium lauryl sulfate
	Other Ingredients: Water, flavor, glycerin, PEG-12, PEG-75, sodium carbonate, sodium saccharin, titanium dioxide, calcium peroxide, **dietetically sucrose free**		
Sensodyne® Full Protection™	Silica	Potassium nitrate 5%, sodium fluoride 0.145%	
	Other Ingredients: Cellulose gum, flavor, glycerin, polyethylene glycol, sodium saccharin, tetrapotassium pyrophosphate, titanium dioxide, water		
Sensodyne® Tartar Control Toothpaste	Hydrated silica, silica, sodium bicarbonate	Potassium nitrate, sodium fluoride	Cocamidopropyl betaine
	Other Ingredients: Cellulose gum, flavor, glycerin, sodium saccharin, tetrasodium pyrophosphate, titanium dioxide, water		
Sensodyne® Toothpaste[1] (fresh mint)	Dicalcium phosphate	Potassium nitrate, sodium monofluorophosphate	Sodium lauryl sulfate
	Other Ingredients: Water, glycerin, sorbitol, hydroxymethylcellulose, flavor, sodium saccharin, methylparaben, propylparaben, D&C yellow no. 10, FD&C blue no. 1, silicon dioxide, **dietetically sucrose free**		
Sensodyne® Toothpaste (original)	Silica	Potassium nitrate, sodium fluoride	Sodium methyl cocoyl taurate
	Other Ingredients: Water, glycerin, sorbitol, cellulose gum, titanium dioxide, sodium saccharin, flavor, D&C red no. 28, trisodium phosphate		
Slimer® Gel[1]	Hydrated silica	Sodium fluoride 0.15%	
	Other Ingredients: Sorbitol, water, glycerin, PEG-32, flavor, ethyl alcohol, propylene glycol, glyceryl triacetate, cellulose gum, sodium saccharin, sodium benzoate, FD&C blue no. 1, FD&C red no. 33, **dietetically sucrose free**		
Thermodent Toothpaste	Diatomaceous earth, silica	Strontium chloride hexahydrate	Sodium methyl cocoyl taurate
	Other Ingredients: Sorbitol, glycerin, titanium dioxide, guar gum, PEG-40 stearate, hydroxyethylcellulose, flavor, preservative, water		

DENTIFRICE PRODUCTS *(Continued)*

Brand Name	Abrasive Ingredient	Therapeutic Ingredient	Foaming Agent
Tom's® Natural Baking Soda with Propolis & Myrrh Toothpaste	Calcium carbonate, sodium bicarbonate		Sodium lauryl sulfate
Other Ingredients: Glycerin, water, carrageenan, peppermint oil, myrrh, propolis, **fluoride free**			
Tom's® Natural Baking Soda, Calcium, and Fluoride Toothpaste	Calcium carbonate, sodium bicarbonate	Sodium monofluorophosphate	Sodium lauryl sulfate
Other Ingredients: Glycerin, water, carrageenan, peppermint oil, xylitol			
Tom's® Natural Calcium and Fluoride Toothpaste[1]	Calcium carbonate	Sodium monofluorophosphate	Sodium lauryl sulfate
Other Ingredients: Glycerin; water; carrageenan; xylitol (spearmint); cinnamon, fennel oil, or spearmint; peppermint oil (cinnamon, spearmint)			
Tom's® Natural Calcium and Fluoride Toothpaste	Calcium carbonate, hydrated silica	Sodium monofluorophosphate	Sodium lauryl sulfate
Other Ingredients: Glycerin, water, carrageenan, xylitol, natural wintergreen oil			
Tom's® Natural for Children with Calcium and Fluoride Toothpaste	Calcium carbonate, hydrated silica	Sodium monofluorophosphate	Sodium lauryl sulfate
Other Ingredients: Glycerin, fruit extracts, carrageenan, water			
Tom's® Natural with Propolis and Myrrh Toothpaste	Calcium carbonate		Sodium lauryl sulfate
Other Ingredients: Glycerin; water; carrageenan; spearmint, peppermint, cassia, or fennel oil; propolis; myrrh, **fluoride free**			
Topol® Plus Whitening Gel with Calcium Toothpaste	Hydrated silicas	Sodium monofluorophosphate	Sodium lauryl sulfate
Other Ingredients: Water, sorbitol and glycerin, calcium carbonate, PEG-6, disodium phosphate, flavor, xanthan gum, sodium saccharin, methylparaben and propylparaben, FD&C blue no. 1			
Topol® Plus Whitening Toothpaste with Baking Soda	Hydrated silicas, sodium bicarbonate	Sodium monofluorophosphate	Sodium lauryl sulfate
Other Ingredients: Water, glycerin, sorbitol, PEG-6, disodium phosphate, flavor, xanthan gum, sodium saccharin, titanium dioxide, methylparaben, propylparaben			
Topol® Plus Whitening Toothpaste with Natural Papain	Hydrated silicas, calcium carbonate	Sodium monofluorophosphate	Sodium lauryl sulfate
Other Ingredients: Water, sorbitol, glycerin, PEG-6, disodium phosphate, flavor, xanthan gum, sodium saccharin, methylparaben, propylparaben, FD&C blue no. 1			
Topol® Smoker's Toothpaste	Hydrated silicas	Sodium monofluorophosphate	Sodium lauryl sulfate
Other Ingredients: Sorbitol, deionized water, glycerin, PEG-6, flavor, xanthan gum, titanium dioxide, sodium saccharin, methylparaben, propylparaben zirconium silicate			
Topol® Smoker's Peppermint Toothpaste		Sodium monofluorophosphate	
Ultra Brite® Baking Soda & Peroxide Toothpaste	Hydrated silica, sodium bicarbonate	Sodium monofluorophosphate 0.76%	Sodium lauryl sulfate
Other Ingredients: Glycerin, water, propylene glycol, cellulose gum, flavor, sodium saccharin, titanium dioxide, sodium hydroxide, calcium peroxide, carrageenan, **dietetically sucrose free**			
Ultra Brite® Gel	Hydrated silica	Sodium monofluorophosphate 0.76%	Sodium lauryl sulfate
Other Ingredients: Sorbitol, water, PEG-12, flavor, cellulose gum, sodium saccharin, FD&C blue no. 1, D&C red no. 33			
Ultra Brite® Toothpaste	Hydrated silica, alumina	Sodium monofluorophosphate 0.76%	Sodium lauryl sulfate
Other Ingredients: Glycerin, cellulose gum, sorbitol, carrageenan gum, titanium dioxide, sodium saccharin, flavor, tetrasodium pyrophosphate, **dietetically sucrose free**			

Brand Name	Abrasive Ingredient	Therapeutic Ingredient	Foaming Agent
Viadent® Fluoride Gel	Hydrated silica	Sodium monofluorophosphate 0.8%	Sodium lauryl sulfate
	Other Ingredients: Sodium saccharin, zinc chloride, teaberry flavor, sodium carboxymethylcellulose, sorbitol, sanguinaria extract		
Viadent® Fluoride Toothpaste	Hydrated silica	Sodium monofluorophosphate 0.8%	Sodium lauryl sulfate
	Other Ingredients: Sorbitol, titanium dioxide, carboxymethylcellulose, flavor, sodium saccharin, citric acid, zinc chloride, anhydrous sanguinaria extract, citric acid		
Viadent® Original Toothpaste	Dicalcium phosphate		Sodium lauryl sulfate
	Other Ingredients: Glycerin, sorbitol, titanium dioxide, zinc chloride, carrageenan, flavor, sodium saccharin, citric acid, sanguinaria extract, **fluoride free**		
Vince Tooth Powder	Calcium carbonate, sodium carbonate, tricalcium phosphate		
	Other Ingredients: Sodium alum, sodium perborate monohydrate, magnesium trisilicate, sodium saccharin, flavor, D&C red no. 28		

[1]Carries American Dental Association (ADA) seal indicating safety and efficacy.

[2]Sodium bicarbonate can also be considered an abrasive.

[3]Topical fluoride product

Adapted with permission from *Nonprescription Products: Formulations & Features, Companion to the Handbook of Nonprescription Drugs,* 11th ed,, Washington, DC, American Pharmaceutical Association, 1998, 344-58.

MOUTH PAIN, COLD SORE, AND CANKER SORE PRODUCTS

Brand Name	Anesthetic / Analgesic	Other Ingredients
Abreva™ [OTC]		**Cream:** Docosanol 10%, benzyl alcohol, light mineral oil, propylene glycol, purified water, sucrose distearate, sucrose stearate
Anbesol® Baby Gel (grape, original)	Benzocaine 7.5%	Benzoic acid (grape), carbomer 934P, D&C red #33, EDTA disodium, FD&C blue #1 (grape), flavor (grape), glycerin, methylparaben (grape), PEG, propylparaben (grape), saccharin, purified water, clove oil (original)
Anbesol® Gel or Liquid	Benzocaine 6.3% (gel), 6.4% (liquid); phenol 0.5%	**Gel:** Alcohol 70%, glycerin, carbomer 934P, D&C red #33, D&C yellow #10, FD&C blue #1, FD&C yellow #6, flavor, camphor **Liquid:** Alcohol 70%, potassium iodide, povidone iodine, camphor, menthol, glycerin
Anbesol® Maximum Strength Gel or Liquid	Benzocaine 20%	Alcohol 60%, carbomer 934P (gel), D&C yellow #10, FD&C blue #1, FD&C red #40, flavor, PEG, saccharin
Aveeno® Active Naturals™		White petrolatum, alcohol, lanolin oil, mineral oil, propolis extract, water
Baby® Gumz	Benzocaine 10%	PEG 8 and 32, **alcohol free**, **dietetically sucrose free**
Banadyne-3	Benzocaine 5%	Dimethicone, methol, propylene glycol, SD alcohol
Benzodent® Denture Analgesic Ointment[1]	Benzocaine 20%	8-hydroxyquinoline sulfate, petrolatum, sodium carboxymethylcellulose, color, eugenol
Blistex® Lip Medex Ointment	Camphor 1%, menthol 1%, phenol 0.5%	Petrolatum, cocoa butter, flavor, lanolin, mixed waxes, oil of cloves
Blistex® Medicated Ointment	Menthol 0.6%, camphor 0.5%, phenol 0.5%	Water, mixed waxes, mineral oil, petrolatum, lanolin
Campho-Phenique® Cold Sore Gel[2]	Camphor 10.8%, phenol 4.7%	Eucalyptus oil, colloidal silicon dioxide, glycerin, light mineral oil, **alcohol free**
Cankaid® Liquid		Carbamide peroxide 10%[3], citric acid monohydrate, sodium citrate, dihydrate, EDTA disodium
Carmex Lip Balm Ointment	Menthol, camphor, salicylic acid, phenol	Alum, fragrance, petrolatum, lanolin, cocoa butter, wax, **alcohol free**, **dye free**, **gluten free**, **dietetically sucrose free**
Cepacol® Viractin®	Tetracaine 2%	Water, ethoxydiglycol, hydroxyethyl cellulose, maleated soybean oil, sodium lauryl sulfate, methylparaben, propylparaben, eucalyptus oil
Chap Stick® Medicated Lip Balm (stick, ointment)	Camphor 1%, menthol 0.6%, phenol 0.5%	**Stick:** Petrolatum 41%, paraffin wax, mineral oil, cocoa butter, 2-octyl dodecanol, arachidyl propionate, polyphenylmethylsiloxane 556, white wax, isopropyl lanolate, carnauba wax, isopropyl myristate, lanolin, fragrance, methylparaben, propylparaben, oleyl alcohol, cetyl alcohol **Ointment:** Petrolatum (jar 60%, tube 67%), microcrystalline wax, mineral oil, cocoa butter, lanolin, paraffin war (jar), fragrance, methylparaben, propylparaben
Dent's® Double-Action Kit (tablets, drops)	Benzocaine 20% (drops), acetaminophen 325 mg (tablet)	**Drops:** Denatured alcohol 74%, chlorobutanol anhydrous 0.09%, propylene glycol, FD&C red #40, eugenol
Dent's® Extra Strength Toothache Gum	Benzocaine 20%	Petrolatum, cotton and wax base, beeswax, FD&C red #40 aluminum lake, eugenol
Dent's® Maxi-Strength Toothache Treatment Drops	Benzocaine 20%	Denatured alcohol 74%, chlorobutanol anhydrous 0.09%, propylene glycol, FD&C red #40, eugenol
Dent-Zel-Ite® Oral Mucosal Analgesic Liquid	Benzocaine 5%, camphor	Alcohol 81%, wintergreen, glycerin, **dye free**
Dent-Zel-Ite® Temporary Dental Filling Liquid	Camphor	Alcohol 56.18%, sandarac gum, methyl salicylate
Dent-Zel-Ite® Toothache Relief Drops	Eugenol 85%, camphor	Alcohol 13.5%, wintergreen
Dentapaine® Gel	Benzocaine 20%	Glycerin, oil of cloves, sodium saccharin, methylparaben, PEG 400 and 4000, water, **alcohol free**, **dye free**, **gluten free**, **dietetically sucrose free**
Dr. Hand's® Teething Gel or Lotion	Menthol	SD alcohol 38B (gel 10%, lotion 11%), sterilized water, carbomer 940, witch hazel, polysorbate 80, sodium hydroxide, simethicone, D&C red #33, FD&C red #3

Brand Name	Anesthetic / Analgesic	Other Ingredients
Gly-Oxide® Liquid		Carbamide peroxide 10%[3], citric acid, flavor, glycerin, propylene glycol, sodium stannate, water
Herpecin-L®		Octinoxate, oxybenzone, meradimate, octisalate, dimethacone, sunflower oil, petrolatum, ozokerite, mineral oil, microcrystalline wax, talc, titanium dioxide, beeswax, mellissa extract, cetyl lactate, glyceryl laurate, flavor, lysine, ascorbyl palmitate, tocopheryl acetate, pyridoxine HCl, panthenol, BHT (244-014)
Herpecin-L® Cold Sore Lip Balm Stick[2]		Padimate O 7%, allantoin 0.5%, titanium dioxide, beeswax, cetyl esters, flavor, octyldodecanol, paraffin, petrolatum, sesame oil, vitamins B₆, C, and E
Hurricaine® Aerosol[1] (wild cherry)	Benzocaine 20%	PEG, saccharin, flavor, alcohol, **dye free, gluten free, sulfite free**
Hurricaine® Gel[1] (wild cherry, pina colada, watermelon)	Benzocaine 20%	PEG, saccharin, flavor, **alcohol free, dye free, gluten free, sulfite free**
Hurricaine® Liquid[1] (wild cherry, pina colada)	Benzocaine 20%	PEG, saccharin, flavor, **alcohol free, dye free, gluten free, dietetically sucrose free**
Kank-A® Professional Strength Liquid[1]	Benzocaine 20%	Benzoin tincture compound, cetylpyridinium chloride, ethylcellulose, SD alcohol 24%, dimethyl isosorbide, castor oil, flavor, tannic acid, propylene glycol, saccharin, benzyl alcohol
Lipclear™ Lysine Plus™		Zinc oxide, l-lysine, vitamin A, vitamin D, vitamin E, olive oil, yellow beeswax, goldenseal extract, propolis extract, calendula extract, echinacea extract, cajeput oil, tea tree oil, gum benzoin tincture, honey, lithium carbonate (3x)
Lip-Ex® Ointment	Phenol, camphor, salicylic acid, menthol	Petrolatum, cherry flavor
Lipmagik® Liquid	Benzocaine 6.3%, phenol 0.5%	Alcohol 70%, **dye free, sulfite free, gluten free**
Little Teethers® Oral Pain Relief Gel	Benzocaine 7.5%	Carbomer, glycerin, flavor, potassium sorbate, acesulfame K, PEGs, **alcohol free, dye free, dietetically sodium free, dietetically sucrose free**
Medadyne® Liquid	Benzocaine 10%, menthol, camphor, benzyl alcohol	Benzalkonium chloride, tannic acid, flavor, SD alcohol, thymol
Novitra™		Zincum oxydatum (2x), HPUS, alpha tocopherol, benzalkonium chloride, setyl alcohol, cocoa butter, glyceryl monostearate, glycine, modified lanolin, methylparaben, PEG 8000, propylparaben, water, sodium lauryl sulfate
Numzident® Adult Strength Gel	Benzocaine 10%	PEG-8, glycerin, PEG-75, sodium saccharin, purified water, flavor
Numzit® Teething Gel	Benzocaine 7.5%	PEG-8, PEG-75, sodium saccharin, clove oil, peppermint oil, purified water
Orabase® Baby Gel[1]	Benzocaine 7.5%	Glycerin, PEG, carbopol, preservative, sweetener, flavor, **alcohol free**
Orabase® Gel	Benzocaine 15%	Ethanol, propylene glycol, ethylcellulose, tannic acid, salicylic acid, flavor, sodium saccharin
Orabase® Lip Cream	Benzocaine 5%, menthol 0.5%, camphor, phenol	Allantoin 1%, carboxymethylcellulose sodium, veegum, Tween 80, phenonip, PEG, biopure, talc, kaolin, lanolin, petrolatum, oil of clove, hydrated silica, **alcohol free**
Orabase® Plain Paste[1]		Pectin, gelatin, carboxymethylcellulose sodium, polyethylene, mineral oil, flavor, preservative, guar, tragacanth, **alcohol free**
Orabase-B® with Benzocaine Paste[1]	Benzocaine 20%	Plasticized hydrocarbon gel, guar, carboxymethylcellulose, tragacanth, pectin, preservatives, flavor, **alcohol free**
Oragesic Solution	Benzyl alcohol 2%, menthol	Water, sorbitol, polysorbate 20, sodium chloride, yerba santa, saccharin, flavor, **sulfite free**
Orajel® Baby Gel or Liquid	Benzocaine 7.5%	**Gel:** FD&C red #40, flavor, glycerin, PEGs, sodium saccharin, sorbic acid, sorbitol, **alcohol free** **Liquid:** Not applicable
Orajel® Baby Nighttime Gel	Benzocaine 10%	FD&C red #40, flavor, glycerin, PEGs, sodium saccharin, sorbic acid, sorbitol, **alcohol free**
Orajel® CoverMed Cream (tinted light, medium)	Dyclonine HCl 1%	Allantoin 0.5%
Orajel® Denture Gel	Benzocaine 20%	Cellulose gum, gelatin, menthol, methyl salicylate, pectin, plasticized hydrocarbon gel, PEG, sodium saccharin

MOUTH PAIN, COLD SORE, AND CANKER SORE PRODUCTS *(Continued)*

Brand Name	Anesthetic / Analgesic	Other Ingredients
Orajel® Maximum Strength Gel	Benzocaine 20%	Clove oil, flavor, PEGs, sodium saccharin, sorbic acid
Orajel® Mouth-Aid Gel or Liquid	Benzocaine 20%	**Gel:** Zinc chloride 0.1%, benzalkonium chloride 0.02%. allantoin, carbomer, EDTA disodium, peppermint oil, PEG, polysorbate 60, propyl gallate, propylene glycol, purified water, povidone, sodium saccharin, sorbic acid, stearyl alcohol **Liquid:** Ethyl alcohol 44.2%
Orajel® PM Cream	Benzocaine 20%	
Orajel® Periostatic Spot Treatment Oral Cleanser		Carbamide peroxide 15%[3], citric acid, EDTA disodium, flavor, methylparaben, PEG, purified water, sodium chloride, sodium saccharin
Orajel® Periostatic Super Cleaning Oral Rinse		Hydrogen peroxide 1.5%[3], ethyl alcohol 4%
Orajel® Regular Strength Gel	Benzocaine 10%	Clove oil, flavor, PEGs, sodium saccharin, sorbic acid
Peroxyl® Hygienic Dental Rinse		Hydrogen peroxide 1.5%[3], alcohol 5%, pluronic F108, sorbitol, sodium saccharin, dye, polysorbate 20, mint flavor, **gluten free, sulfite free**
Peroxyl® Oral Spot Treatment Gel		Hydrogen peroxide 1.5%[3], ethyl alcohol 5%, pluronic F108, sorbitol, sodium saccharin, dye, polysorbate 20, mint flavor, dye, pluronic F127, **gluten free, dietetically sucrose free**
Proxigel® Gel[2]	Menthol	Carbamide peroxide 10%[3], glycerin, carbomer, phosphoric acid, triethanolamine, flavor, **dye free, gluten free, dietetically sucrose free**
Red Cross® Canker Sore Medication Ointment[2]	Benzocaine 20%, phenol	Carbomer 974P, mineral oil, petrolatum, propylparaben
Red Cross® Toothache Medication Drops	Eugenol 85%	Sesame oil
Retre-Gel®[2]	Benzocaine 5%, menthol 1%	Glycerin 20%
Tanac® Medicated Gel	Dyclonine HCl 1%	Allantoin 0.5%
Tanac® No Sting Liquid	Benzocaine 10%	Benzalkonium chloride 0.125%, saccharin
Zilactin® Gel	Benzyl alcohol 10%	**Gluten free**
Zilactin® Baby Gel	Benzocaine 10%	**Alcohol free, dye free, gluten free**
Zilactin®-B Gel	Benzocaine 10%	**Gluten free**
Zilactin®-L Liquid	Lidocaine 2.5%	Boric acid, propylene glycol, water, salicylic acid, SD alcohol 37, tannic acid

[1]Carries American Dental Association (ADA) seal indicating safety and efficacy

[2]Agent for cold sore treatment only

[3]Agent for debridement or wound cleansing

Adapted with permission from *Nonprescription Products: Formulations & Features, Companion to the Handbook of Nonprescription Drugs*, 11th ed,, Washington, DC, American Pharmaceutical Association, 1998, 338-40.

ORAL RINSE PRODUCTS

Brand Name	Active Ingredients	Other Ingredients
ACT® Anticavity Fluoride Rinse, Bubble Gum Blowout™	Cetylpyridinium chloride	Sodium fluoride 0.05%, D&C red no. 33, calcium EDTA, flavor, glycerin, monobasic and dibasic sodium phosphates, poloxamer 407, polysorbate 80, propylene glycol, sodium benzoate, water, sodium saccharin, **alcohol free**
ACT® Anticavity Fluoride Treatment Rinse, Mint	Cetylpyridinium chloride	Sodium fluoride 0.05%, D&C red no. 33, calcium EDTA, FD&C yellow no. 5, flavor, glycerin, monobasic and dibasic sodium phosphates, poloxamer 407, polysorbate 80, propylene glycol, sodium benzoate, sodium saccharin, water, **alcohol free**
Arm & Hammer Advance Breath Care™ Cool Fresh Mint Mouthwash	Alcohol 15%, cetylpyridinium chloride, zinc citrate	Water, glycerin and/or sorbitol, sodium bicarbonate, sodium citrate, poloxamer 407, flavor, sucrose and/or sodium saccharin, D&C green no. 5, FD&C yellow no. 5
Arm & Hammer Advance Breath Care™ Icy Fresh Mint Mouthwash	Alcohol 15%, cetylpyridinium chloride, zinc citrate	Water, glycerin and/or sorbitol, sodium bicarbonate, sodium citrate, poloxamer 407, flavor, sucrose and/or sodium saccharin, D&C green no. 5
Astring-O-Sol® Liquid	SD alcohol 38B 75.6%, methyl salicylate	Water, myrrh extract, zinc chloride, citric acid
Betadine® Mouthwash Gargle	Alcohol 8%	Povidone-iodine 0.5%, glycerin, sodium saccharin, flavor
Biotene® Alcohol-Free Mouthwash	Lysozyme (40 mg), lactoferrin (15 mg), glucose oxidase (2500 units), lactoperoxidase (2500 units)	Water, xylitol, hydrogenated starch, propylene glycol, hydroxyethylcellulose, aloe vera, peppermint, poloxamer 407, sodium benzoate, **alcohol free**
Biotene® Mouthwash	Lysozyme (6 mg), lactoferrin (6 mg), glucose oxidase (4000 units), zinc gluconate	Water, xylitol, hydrogenated starch, propylene glycol, hydroxy ethylcellulose, aloe vera, natural peppermint, poloxamer 407, calcium lactate, sodium benzoate, benzoic acid
Cepacol® Mouthwash/Gargle	Alcohol 14%, cetylpyridinium chloride 0.05%	EDTA disodium, color, flavor, glycerin, polysorbate 80, saccharin, sodium biphosphate, sodium phosphate, water, **gluten free, dietetically sucrose free**
Cepacol® Mouthwash/Gargle (mint)	Alcohol 14.5%, cetylpyridinium chloride 0.5%	Color, flavor, glucono delta-lactone, glycerin, poloxamer 407, sodium saccharin, sodium gluconate, water, **gluten free, dietetically sucrose free**
Crest® Pro-Health™ Rinse	Cetylpyridinium chloride 0.07%	Water, glycerin, flavor, poloxamer 407, sodium saccharin, blue no. 1
Crest® Whitening Rinse	Hydrogen peroxide	Water, glycerin, propylene glycol, sodium hexametaphosphate, poloxamer 407, sodium citrate, flavor, sodium saccharin, citric acid
Dr. Tichenor's® Antiseptic Liquid	SDA alcohol 38B 70%	Oil of peppermint, extract of arnica, water, **dye free, gluten free**
Lavoris Crystal Fresh	SD alcohol 38-B, zantrate (citric acid, zinc oxide, sodium hydroxide)	Purified spring water, glycerin, poloxamer 407, saccharin, polysorbate 80, flavors
Lavoris Mint Mouthwash	Zinc chloride and/or zinc oxide, aromatic oils	Glycerin
Lavoris Original Cinnamon Mouthwash	Zinc chloride and/or zinc oxide, aromatic oils	Glycerin
Lavoris Original Mouthwash	SD alcohol 38-B, zinc chloride (zinc oxide, sodium hydroxide, citric acid)	Water, glycerin, poloxamer 407, saccharin, clove oil, polysorbate 80, flavor, D&C red no. 6 and no. 33
Lavoris Peppermint Mouthwash	SD alcohol 38-B, zantrate (sodium hydroxide, citric acid, zinc oxide)	Water, glycerin, poloxamer 407, polysorbate 80, peppermint oil, saccharin, FD&C blue no. 4

ORAL RINSE PRODUCTS *(Continued)*

Brand Name	Active Ingredients	Other Ingredients
Listerine®	Eucalyptol 0.092%, menthol 0.042%, methyl salicylate 0.06%, thymol 0.064%	Water, alcohol (21.6%), sorbitol solution, flavoring, poloxamer 407, benzoic acid, zinc chloride, sodium benzoate, sucralose, sodium saccharin, FD&C blue no. 1
Listerine®¹ Liquid	Alcohol 26.9%, eucalyptol 0.092%, thymol 0.064%, methyl salicylate 0.06%, menthol 0.042%	Benzoic acid, poloxamer 407, caramel, water, sodium benzoate
Listerine®¹ Liquid (freshburst, cool mint)	Alcohol 21.6%, eucalyptol 0.092%, thymol 0.064%, methyl salicylate 0.06%, menthol 0.042%	Water, sorbitol solution, poloxamer 407, benzoic acid, flavor, sodium saccharin, sodium citrate, citric acid, FD&C green no. 3, D&C yellow no. 10 (freshburst)
Listerine® Tooth Defense™ Anticavity Rinse	Alcohol 21.6%, sodium fluoride 0.01%	Water, sorbitol solution, flavors, poloxamer 407, sodium lauryl sulfate, phosphoric acid, dibasic sodium phosphate, FD&C red no. 33, FD&C blue no. 1
Listerine® Vanilla Mint Antiseptic	Eucalyptol 0.92%, menthol 0.042%, methyl salicylate 0.06%, thymol 0.64%	Not listed
Listerine® Whitening Pre-Brush	Alcohol 8%, hydrogen peroxide	Water, glycerin, alcohol (8%), flavor, poloxamer 407, sodium lauryl sulfate, sodium citrate, sodium saccharin, sucralose
Mentadent® Mouthwash (cool mint, fresh mint)	Alcohol 10%	Water, sorbitol, sodium bicarbonate, hydrogen peroxide, poloxamer 407, sodium lauryl sulfate, flavor, polysorbate 20, methyl salicylate (cool mint), sodium saccharin, phosphoric acid, blue no. 1, yellow no. 5 (cool mint)
Oasis® Moisturizing Mouthwash	Glycerin	Water, sorbitol, poloxamer 338, PEG-60 hydrogenated castor oil, cellulose gum, cetylpyridinium chloride, copovidone, disodium phosphate, flavor, methylparaben, propylparaben, sodium benzoate, sodium phosphate, sodium saccharin, xanthan gum, FD&C blue no. 1
Oasis® Moisturizing Mouth Spray	Glycerin 35% (prediluted)	Cetylpyridinium chloride, copovidone, flavor, methylparaben, PEG-60 hydrogenated castor oil, propylparaben, sodium benzoate, sodium saccharin, water, xanthan gum, xylitol
Oxyfresh Fresh Mint Mouthrinse	Oxygene® (stabilized chlorine dioxide)	Purified deionized water, xylitol, mint oils, sodium benzoate, **alcohol free**
Oxyfresh Fresh Mint with Fluoride Mouthrinse	Oxygene® (stabilized chlorine dioxide)	Sodium fluoride (0.05%), purified deionized water, xylitol, mint oils, sodium benzoate, **alcohol free**
Oxyfresh Fresh Mint with Zinc Mouthrinse	Oxygene® (stabilized chlorine dioxide), zinc acetate	Purified deionized water, xylitol, sodium citrate, peppermint oil, **alcohol free**
Oxyfresh Original Mint Mouthrinse	Oxygene® (stabilized chlorine dioxide)	Purified deionized water, mint oils, sodium benzoate, **alcohol free**
Oxyfresh Professional Strength Zinc Mouthrinse	Oxygene® (stabilized chlorine dioxide), zinc acetate	Purified deionized water, xylitol, sodium citrate, peppermint oil, **alcohol free**
Oxyfresh Unflavored Mouthrinse	Oxygene® (stabilized chlorine dioxide)	Purified deionized water, sodium benzoate, **alcohol free**
Plax® Advanced Formula (mint sensation)	Alcohol 8.7%	Water, sorbitol solution, tetrasodium pyrophosphate, benzoic acid, flavor, poloxamer 407, sodium benzoate, sodium lauryl sulfate, sodium saccharin, xanthan gum, FD&C blue no. 1

Brand Name	Active Ingredients	Other Ingredients
Plax® Advanced Formula (original, SoftMINT)	Alcohol 8.7%	Sodium lauryl sulfate, water, sorbitol solution, sodium benzoate, tetrasodium pyrophosphate, benzoic acid, poloxamer 407, sodium saccharin, flavor (SoftMINT), xanthan gum (SoftMINT), flavor enhancer (SoftMINT), FD&C blue no. 1 (SoftMINT), FD&C yellow no. 5 (SoftMINT)
Rembrandt® Naturals Mouthwash		Spring water, glycerin, xylitol, sodium citrate, vitamin C, stevia, citric acid, dicalcium phosphate, cocamidopropyl betain, flavor, ginkgo extract, raspberry leaf extract, alcohol free. Also available with papaya and ginseng or aloe and echinacea
S.T. 37® Solution	Hexylresorcinol 0.1%	Glycerin, propylene glycol, citric acid, EDTA disodium, sodium bisulfite, sodium citrate
Scope® Baking Soda	SD alcohol 38F 9.9%, cetylpyridinium chloride, domiphen bromide	Sorbitol, sodium bicarbonate, sodium saccharin, flavor
Scope® (cool peppermint)	SD alcohol 38F 14%, cetylpyridinium chloride, domiphen bromide	Purified water, glycerin, poloxamer 407, sodium saccharin, sodium benzoate, N-ethylmethylcarboxamide, benzoic acid, FD&C blue no. 1, flavor
Targon® Smokers' Mouthwash (clean taste)	SDA alcohol 38B 15.6%	Water, glycerin, polyoxyl 40 hydrogenated castor oil, sodium lauryl sulfate, dibasic sodium phosphate, benzoic acid, sodium saccharin, caramel powder, **dietetically sucrose free**
Targon® Smokers' Mouthwash (original)	SDA alcohol 38B 16%	Water, sodium saccharin, sodium benzoate, glycerin, sodium lauryl sulfate, FD&C green no. 3, FD&C yellow no. 5, polyoxyl 40 hydrogenated castor oil, **dietetically sucrose free**
Tom's of Maine® Natural Mouthwash (cinnamon, original)	Menthol	Water, glycerin, aloe vera juice, witch hazel, poloxamer 335, spearmint oil, ascorbic acid, **alcohol free**
Viadent Advanced Care Oral Rinse	Cetylpyridium chloride 0.05%	Purified water, sorbitol, ethyl alcohol (5.5% w/w), glycerin, propylene glycol, PEG-40 sorbitan diisostearate, flavor, sodium benzoate, sodium saccharin, FD&C yellow No. 6

[1]Carries American Dental Association (ADA) seal indicating safety and efficacy

Note: SD alcohol refers to "specially denatured" alcohol

Adapted with permission from *Nonprescription Products: Formulations & Features, Companion to the Handbook of Nonprescription Drugs,* 11th ed,, Washington, DC, American Pharmaceutical Association, 1998, 341-2.

TOP 200 MOST PRESCRIBED DRUGS IN 2006*

1.	Hydrocodone and Acetaminophen	53.	Amitriptyline
2.	Lipitor®	54.	Lovastatin
3.	Lisinopril	55.	Lotrel®
4.	Amoxicillin	56.	Levaquin®
5.	Hydrochlorothiazide	57.	Premarin® (tablet)
6.	Atenolol	58.	Simvastatin
7.	Levothyroxine	59.	Enalapril
8.	Alprazolam	60.	Omeprazole
9.	Toprol-XL®	61.	Naproxen
10.	Furosemide (oral)	62.	Trimethoprim and Sulfamethoxazole
11.	Azithromycin	63.	Diazepam
12.	Metformin	64.	Zetia™
13.	Norvasc®	65.	Wellbutrin XL™
14.	Albuterol (aerosol)	66.	Ranitidine
15.	Synthroid®	67.	Citalopram
16.	Lexapro®	68.	Klor-Con®
17.	Nexium®	69.	Fluconazole
18.	Metoprolol	70.	Diovan HCT®
19.	Singulair®	71.	Crestor®
20.	Ibuprofen	72.	Avandia®
21.	Cephalexin	73.	Actos®
22.	Prednisone (oral)	74.	Altace®
23.	Triamterene and Hydrochlorothiazide	75.	Fluticasone (nasal)
24.	Propoxyphene-N and Acetaminophen	76.	Celebrex®
		77.	Allopurinol
25.	Fluoxetine	78.	Doxycycline
26.	Prevacid®	79.	Carisoprodol
27.	Ambien®	80.	Viagra®
28.	Lorazepam	81.	Levoxyl®
29.	Warfarin	82.	Clonidine
30.	Oxycodone and Acetaminophen	83.	Coreg®
31.	Zoloft®	84.	Yasmin® 28
32.	Amoxicillin and Clavulanate Potassium	85.	Methylprednisolone (tablet)
		86.	Nasonex®
33.	Advair Diskus®	87.	Seroquel®
34.	Clonazepam	88.	Tricor®
35.	Zyrtec®	89.	Lantus®
36.	Cyclobenzaprine	90.	Flomax®
37.	Effexor® XR	91.	Sertraline
38.	Fosamax®	92.	Isosorbide Mononitrate
39.	Potassium Chloride	93.	Actonel®
40.	Plavix®	94.	Promethazine (tablet)
41.	Paroxetine	95.	Adderall XR®
42.	Fexofenadine	96.	Verapamil SR
43.	Gabapentin	97.	Glyburide
44.	Protonix®	98.	Cymbalta®
45.	Tramadol	99.	Cozaar®
46.	Ciprofloxacin	100.	Oxycodone
47.	Vytorin®	101.	Omnicef®
48.	Acetaminophen and Codeine	102.	Folic Acid
49.	Zocor®	103.	Penicillin VK
50.	Trazodone	104.	Concerta®
51.	Diovan®	105.	Digitek®
52.	Lisinopril and Hydrochlorothiazide	106.	Spironolactone

107.	Risperdal®	155.	Endocet®
108.	Temazepam	156.	Coumadin® (tablet)
109.	Ortho Tri-Cyclen® Lo	157.	Propranolol
110.	Valtrex®	158.	Imitrex® (oral)
111.	Albuterol (solution for oral inhalation)	159.	Cialis®
112.	Glipizide (extended release)	160.	Ortho Evra®
113.	AcipHex®	161.	Pravastatin
114.	Glimepiride	162.	Acyclovir
115.	Quinapril	163.	Minocycline
116.	Clindamycin (systemic)	164.	Flovent® HFA
117.	Topamax®	165.	Butalbital, Acetaminophen, and Caffeine
118.	Metformin (extended release)	166.	Tramadol Hydrochloride and Acetaminophen
119.	Hyzaar®		
120.	Xalatan®	167.	Niaspan®
121.	Triamcinolone Acetonide Paste (topical)	168.	Promethazine and Codeine
		169.	Buspirone
122.	Glipizide	170.	Methotrexate
123.	Benazepril	171.	Allegra-D® 12 Hour
124.	Ambien CR™	172.	Bupropion SR
125.	Metronidazole (tablet)	173.	Avalide®
126.	Metoclopramide	174.	Cartia XT™
127.	Avapro®	175.	Zyprexa®
128.	Hydroxyzine	176.	Pravachol®
129.	Lunesta™	177.	Terazosin
130.	Estradiol (oral)	178.	Clotrimazole and Betamethasone
131.	Diclofenac	179.	Amphetamine and Dextroamphetamine
132.	Gemfibrozil		
133.	Clopidogrel	180.	Zyrtec® (syrup)
134.	Benicar®	181.	Quinine
135.	Lyrica®	182.	Nasacort® AQ
136.	Lamictal®	183.	Mobic®
137.	Doxazosin	184.	Strattera®
138.	Combivent®	185.	Fentanyl
139.	Detrol® LA	186.	NuvaRing®
140.	Diltiazem CD	187.	Clarinex®
141.	Meclizine	188.	Skelaxin®
142.	Glyburide and Metformin	189.	Sulfamethoxazole and Trimethoprim
143.	Benicar HCT®		
144.	TriNessa™	190.	Patanol®
145.	Nitrofurantoin	191.	Depakote®
146.	Aricept®	192.	Nifedipine ER
147.	Evista®	193.	Abilify®
148.	Mirtazapine	194.	Flonase®
149.	Nabumetone	195.	Famotidine
150.	Spiriva®	196.	Phenytoin
151.	Zithromax® (suspension)	197.	Digoxin
152.	GlycoLax®	198.	Avelox®
153.	Bisoprolol and Hydrochlorothiazide	199.	Ferrous Sulfate
154.	Tri-Sprintec™	200.	Humalog®

*Based on units dispensed in U.S.
Source: Verispan Scott-Levin, SPA

DENTAL DRUG USE IN PREGNANCY AND BREAST-FEEDING[1]

Drug	FDA Pregnancy Category	Use During Pregnancy	Use During Breast-Feeding
Acetaminophen	B	Yes	Yes
Acetaminophen and codeine	C	Low dose for short duration	Yes (with caution)
Acetaminophen and tramadol	C	No information	No information
Acyclovir	B	No information	No information
Alclometasone	C	Yes	No information
Alprazolam	D	Avoid	Avoid
Amitriptyline	C	Yes	Avoid
Amlexanox	B	Yes	Yes
Ammonia spirit (aromatic)	C	No information	No information
Amoxicillin	B	Yes	Yes
Amoxicillin and clavulanate potassium	B	Yes	Yes
Ampicillin	B	Yes	Yes
Ampicillin and sulbactam	B	Yes	Yes
Articaine hydrochloride and epinephrine (U.S.)	C	Yes	Yes
Aspirin	C/D	Not in third trimester	Avoid
Aspirin and codeine	D	Not in third trimester	Avoid
Atropine sulfate (dental tablets)	C	Yes	Avoid
Azithromycin	B	Yes	Yes
Beclomethasone	C	Yes	Avoid
Benzocaine	C	Yes	Yes
Betamethasone and clotrimazole	C	Yes	No information
Bupivacaine	C	Yes	Yes
Bupivacaine and epinephrine	C	Yes	Yes
Butalbital, acetaminophen, caffeine, and codeine	C/D	Not in third trimester	Avoid
Carbamazepine	D	Avoid	Avoid
Carbamide peroxide	C	Yes	Yes
Carisoprodol	C	Yes	Avoid
Carisoprodol and aspirin	C/D	Not in third trimester	Avoid
Carisoprodol, aspirin, and codeine	C/D	Not in third trimester	Avoid
Cefaclor	B	Yes	Yes
Cefadroxil	B	Yes	Yes
Cefazolin	B	Yes	Yes
Cefditoren	B	Yes	Yes
Celecoxib[2]	C/D	No information	No information
Cephalexin	B	Yes	Yes
Cephradine	B	Yes	Yes
Cevimeline	C	No information	No information
Ciprofloxacin	C	Yes	Avoid
Clarithromycin	C	Yes	Yes
Clindamycin	B	Yes	Yes
Clobetasol	C	Yes	Yes
Clonazepam	D	Avoid	Avoid
Clotrimazole	C (troches)	Yes	Yes
Cloxacillin	B	Yes	Yes
Codeine	C	Low dose for short duration	Yes (with caution)
Cyclobenzaprine	B	Yes	No information
Dexamethasone	C	Yes	No information
Diazepam	D	Avoid	Avoid
Dibucaine	C	Yes	Yes
Diclofenac[2]	B/D	Not in third trimester	Yes
Dicloxacillin	B	Yes	Yes
Diflunisal	C/D	Not in third trimester	Yes
Diphenhydramine	B	Yes	Yes
Doxycycline hyclate (periodontal)	D	Avoid	Avoid
Doxycycline (subantimicrobial)	D	Avoid	Avoid

Drug	FDA Pregnancy Category	Use During Pregnancy	Use During Breast-Feeding
Epinephrine	C	Yes	Yes
Erythromycin	B	Yes (avoid estolate)	Yes
Eszopiclone	C	Yes	No information
Etidocaine and epinephrine	B	Yes	Yes
Etodolac	C/D	Not in third trimester	Yes
Famciclovir	B	Yes	No information
Fentanyl	C/D	Yes (with caution)	Yes
Fluocinolone	C	Yes	No information
Fluocinonide	C	Yes	No information
Fluconazole	C	Yes	Yes
Flurbiprofen	C/D	Not in third trimester	Yes
Gabapentin	C	Yes	Avoid
Halobetasol	C	Yes (with caution)	Yes (with caution)
Hydrocodone and acetaminophen	C	Low dose for short term	Yes (with caution)
Hydrocodone and aspirin	D	Not in third trimester	Avoid
Hydrocodone and ibuprofen	C/D	Not in third trimester	Yes (with caution)
Hydrocortisone	C	Yes	No information
Ibuprofen[2]	B/D	Not in third trimester	Yes
Iodoquinol and hydrocortisone	C	Yes	No information
Ketoconazole	C	Yes	Yes
Ketoprofen	B/D	Not in third trimester	Yes
Ketorolac	C/D	Not in third trimester	Yes
Lidocaine	B	Yes	Yes
Lidocaine and epinephrine	B	Yes	Yes
Lidocaine and prilocaine	B	Yes	Yes
Lorazepam	D	Avoid	Avoid
Meperidine	B/D	Low dose for short duration	Yes (with caution)
Mepivacaine	C	Yes	Yes
Mepivacaine (dental anesthetic)	C	Yes	Yes
Mepivacaine and levonordefrin	C	Yes	Yes
Methocarbamol	C	Yes	No information
Methohexital	C	Yes	Yes
Methylprednisolone	C	Yes	No information
Metronidazole	B	Yes (with caution)	Yes (with caution)
Midazolam	D	Avoid	Avoid
Minocycline	D	Avoid	Avoid
Minocycline hydrochloride (periodontal)	D	Avoid	Avoid
Naloxone	C	Yes	Yes
Naproxen[2]	B/D	Not in third trimester	Yes
Nicotine	D	Avoid	Avoid
Nitrous oxide[3]	None reported	Acute use in patients: Yes (with caution)	Acute use in patients: Yes
Nortriptyline	D	Avoid	Avoid
Nystatin	B/C	Yes	Yes
Nystatin and triamcinolone	C	Yes	No information
Oxycodone	B/D	Low dose for short duration	Yes
Oxycodone and acetaminophen	C/D	Low dose for short duration	Yes
Oxycodone and aspirin	D	Not in third trimester	Avoid
Oxycodone and ibuprofen	C/D	Not in third trimester	Yes (with caution)
Oxygen	None reported	Yes	Yes
Palifermin	C	Yes	No information
Penciclovir	B	Yes	Yes
Penicillin V potassium	B	Yes	Yes

DENTAL DRUG USE IN PREGNANCY AND BREAST-FEEDING[1]
(Continued)

Drug	FDA Pregnancy Category	Use During Pregnancy	Use During Breast-Feeding
Pentazocine and acetaminophen	C	Low dose for short duration	Yes (with caution)
Pilocarpine (dental)	C	Yes	Avoid
Pimecrolimus	C	Yes	No information
Posaconazole	C	Avoid	Yes (with caution)
Prednisolone	C	Yes	Yes (with caution)
Prednisone	B	Yes	Yes
Prilocaine	B	Yes	Yes
Prilocaine and epinephrine	C	Yes	Yes
Propantheline	C	Yes	Yes
Propoxyphene and acetaminophen	C	Low dose for short duration	Yes (with caution)
Propoxyphene, aspirin, and caffeine	D	Not in third trimester	Avoid
Sulfonated phenolics in aqueous solution	C	Yes	Yes
Telithromycin	C	Yes	Yes (with caution)
Tetracaine	C	Yes	Yes
Tetracycline	D	Avoid	Avoid
Tetracycline (periodontal)	C	Avoid	Avoid
Tramadol	C	No (labor and delivery)	No
Triamcinolone acetonide paste	C	Yes	No information
Triazolam	X	Avoid	Avoid
Valacyclovir	B	Yes	Yes
Valdecoxib	C/D	No information	No information
Zaleplon	C	Yes	Avoid
Zolpidem	B	Yes	Yes (with caution)

[1]Pregnant or breast-feeding women should be encouraged to consult a physician prior to the use of any prescription or nonprescription medication. Additional information concerning other medications may be found in individual drug monographs.

[2]A study from Quebec Canada has shown that women who take prescribed nonsteroidal anti-inflammatory drugs (NSAIDs) in early pregnancy may increase their risk of giving birth to a child with congenital anomalies, especially cardiac septal anomalies, compared with women who do not take NSAIDs during this period. The NSAIDs involved included ibuprofen, naproxen, rofecoxib, diclofenac, and celecoxib. Of the 1056 women who took NSAIDs before giving birth, there were 93 (8.8%) live births of children with congenital anomalies. Of 35,331 women not taking any NSAID during pregnancy, there were 2478 (7%) live births of children with congenital anomalies. Further, the proportion of infants with one or more congenital defects who were born to women taking NSAIDs in the first trimester was 16.1% and the proportion of infants who were born to women not taking NSAIDs was 14.2%. Women who took NSAIDs during early pregnancy may be at greater risk of having children with congenital anomalies, specifically cardiac septal defects.

[3]Female dental personnel to avoid chronic exposure to unscavenged nitrous oxide.

References:

Della-Giustina K and Chow G, "Medications in Pregnancy and Lactation," *Emerg Med Clin North Am*, 2003, 21(3):585-613.

Drug Information for the Health Care Professional, 20th ed, Vol 1, Rockville, MD: Medical Economics Company, 2000.

Haas DA, Pynn BR, and Sands TD, "Drug Use for the Pregnant or Lactating Patient," *Gen Dent*, 2000, 48(1):54-60.

Mariotti AJ, "Agents That Affect the Fetus and Nursing Infant," *ADA Guide to Dental Therapeutics*, 2nd ed, Chicago IL: ADA Publishing, 2000, 594-5.

Ofori B, Oraichi D, Blais L, et al, "Risk of Congenital Anomalies in Pregnant Users of Nonsteroidal Anti-Inflammatory Drugs: A Nested Case-Control Study," *Birth Defects Res B Dev Reprod Toxicol*, 2006, 77(4):268-79.

VASOCONSTRICTOR INTERACTIONS WITH ANTIDEPRESSANTS

Antidepressant	Effects with Epinephrine, Levonordefrin	Contraindicated	Recommendation
Tricyclics			
Amitriptyline (Elavil® [DSC])	Epinephrine = increased pressor response; cardiac dysrhythmias Levonordefrin = increased pressor response	No	Potentially dangerous; use minimal amounts with caution in local anesthetics
Amoxapine			
Clomipramine (Anafranil®)			
Desipramine (Norpramin®)			
Doxepin (Prudoxin™, Sinequan®, Zonalon®)			
Imipramine (Tofranil-PM®, Tofranil®)			
Nortriptyline (Pamelor®)			
Protriptyline (Vivactil®)			
Trimipramine (Surmontil®)			
Serotonin / Norepinephrine Reuptake Inhibitor			
Venlafaxine (Effexor® XR, Effexor®)	No adverse interactions reported	No	Suggest caution since venlafaxine blocks norepinephrine uptake in CNS
Serotonin Only Reuptake Inhibitors			
Citalopram (Celexa™)	No adverse interactions reported	No	No precautions appear to be necessary
Escitalopram (Lexapro™)			
Fluoxetine (Prozac® Weekly™, Prozac®, Sarafem™)			
Fluvoxamine			
Paroxetine (Paxil CR™, Paxil®, Pexeva™)			
Sertraline (Zoloft®)			
Central Alpha-2 Antagonist			
Mirtazapine (Remeron SolTab®, Remeron®)	No adverse interactions reported	No	Suggest caution since mirtazapine increases release of norepinephrine
Dopamine Reuptake Inhibitor			
Bupropion (Wellbutrin SR®, Wellbutrin XL™, Wellbutrin®, Zyban®)	No adverse interactions reported	No	Part of the mechanism of bupropion is to block norepinephrine reuptake within CNS; it has been suggested that vasoconstrictor be administered with caution
Others			
Duloxetine (Cymbalta®)	No adverse interactions reported	No	Part of the mechanism of duloxetine is to block norepinephrine reuptake within CNS; it has been suggested that vasoconstrictor be administered with caution
Maprotiline	Potential for increased pressor response	No	Potentially dangerous; use minimal amounts with caution in local anesthetics
MAO Inhibitors			
Isocarboxazid (Marplan®)	No effects on blood pressure or heart rate reported; however, potential exists for slight increase in pressor response	No	Use vasoconstrictor with caution
Phenelzine (Nardil®)			
Tranylcypromine (Parnate®)			

VASOCONSTRICTOR INTERACTIONS WITH ANTIDEPRESSANTS *(Continued)*

Antidepressant	Effects with Epinephrine, Levonordefrin	Contraindicated	Recommendation
Serotonin Reuptake Inhibitor / Serotonin Antagonist			
Nefazodone (Serzone® [DSC])	No adverse interactions reported	No	No precautions appear to be necessary
Trazodone (Desyrel®)			

Naftalin LW and Yagiela JA, "Vasoconstrictors: Indications and Precautions," *Dent Clin North Am*, 2002, 46(4):733-46.

Wynn RL, "Antidepressant Medications," *Gen Dent*, 1992, 40(3):192-7.

Yagiela JA, "Adverse Drug Interactions in Dental Practice: Interactions Associated With Vasoconstrictors. Part V of a Series," *J Am Dent Assoc*, 1999, 130(5):701-9.

Yagiela JA, "Injectable and Topical Local Anesthetics," *ADA Guide to Dental Therapeutics*, 2nd ed, Chicago, IL: ADA Publishing, 2000, 1-16.

PHARMACOLOGIC CATEGORY INDEX

ALPHABETICAL INDEX

Other Products Offered by Lexi-Comp®

Employee Embezzlement and Fraud in the Dental Office
by Donald P Lewis, Jr., DDS, CFE

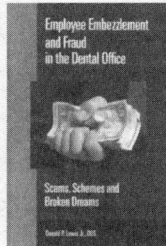

Incidents of fraud and embezzlement are on the rise in the Untied States, and dental offices are a particular target. This book by a dentist in private practice gives inside information on prevention fraud and embezzlement from occurring in your office. After discovering that one of his own employees was embezzling money from his practice, author Donald P. Lewis Jr, DDS wants other dentists and spouses to avoid such a devastating experience. In order to equip you with strong preventive measures, he shares all he has learned - from the criminal investigation and interrogation, to prosecution and restitution processes - in this comprehensive guide. This book shows you how to: Discover if your practice is a target for theft; Recognize the profile of an embezzler; Enact policies and procedures to protect yourself and avoid hiring embezzlers; Conduct background checks and testing of potential employees; Establish internal controls to prevent thefts; Identify some of the common scams and schemes used by embezzlers in dentistry; A must have for every dental office, this book should save your practice thousands of dollars.

Illustrated Handbook of Clinical Dentistry
by Richard A. Lehman, DMD, MPH

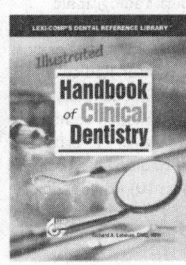

The *Illustrated Handbook of Clinical Dentistry* is an invaluable manual for dentists and dental students that concisely summarizes the major disciplines of clinical dentistry. This handbook is written as an aid for transition into clinical practice, or as a refresher for a seasoned dental professional. It offers a quick reference for basic clinical principles and procedures encountered on a daily basis.

Manual of Clinical Periodontics
by Francis G. Serio, DMD, MS and Charles E. Hawley, DDS, PhD

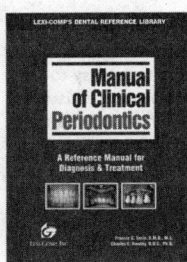

A reference manual for diagnosis and treatment including sample treatment plans. It is organized by basic principles and is visually-cued with over 220 high quality color photos. The presentation is in a "question & answer" format. There are 12 chapters tabbed for easy access: 1) Problem-based Periodontal Diagnosis; 2) Anatomy, Histology, and Physiology; 3) Etiology and Disease Classification; 4) Assessment, Diagnosis, and Treatment Planning; 5) Prevention and Maintenance; 6) Nonsurgical Treatment; 7) Surgical Treatment: Principles; 8) Repair, Resection, and Regeneration; 9) Periodontal Plastic Surgery; 10) Periodontal Emergencies; 11) Implant Considerations; 12) Appendix

Other Products Offered by Lexi-Comp®

Manual Of Dental Implants
by David P. Sarment, DDS, MS and Beth Peshman, RDH

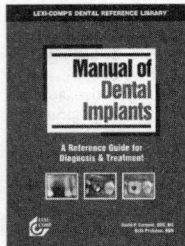

Contains over 220 quality color photos, plus diagrams and decision trees. The diagnosis and treatment plans are explained in detail. Restorative step-by-step illustrations are included for each case type. Hygiene techniques and protocols are also included as well as assistant and staff training guidelines.

8 Tabbed Sections for Ease-of-Use:

- Basic Principles
- Diagnosis
- Treatment Planning
- Restoration Sequences
- Maintenance
- Implants and Your Practice
- Appendix
- Index

Oral Hard Tissue Diseases
by J. Robert Newland, Dds, Ms

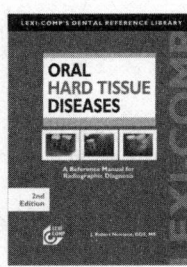

A reference manual for radiographic diagnosis, visually-cued with over 130 high quality radiographs is designed to require little more than visual recognition to make an accurate diagnosis. Each lesion is illustrated by one or more photographs depicting the typical radiographic features and common variations. There are 12 chapters tabbed for easy access: 1) Periapical Radiolucent Lesions; 2) Pericoronal Radiolucent Lesions; 3) Inter-Radicular Radiolucent Lesions; 4) Periodontal Radiolucent Lesions; 5) Radiolucent Lesions Not Associated With Teeth; 6) Radiolucent Lesions With Irregular Margins; 7) Periapical Radiopaque Lesions; 8) Periocoronal Radiopaque Lesions; 9) Inter-Radicular Radiopaque Lesions; 10) Radiopaque Lesions Not Associated With Teeth; 11) Radiopaque Lesions With Irregular Margins; 12) Selected Readings / Alphabetical Index

Oral Soft Tissue Diseases
by J. Robert Newland, DDS, MS; Timothy F. Meiller, DDS, PhD; Richard L. Wynn, BSPharm, PhD; and Harold L.Crossley, DDS, PhD

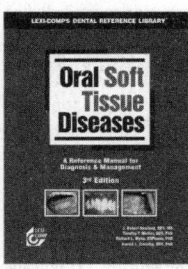

Designed for all dental professionals, a pictorial reference to assist in the diagnosis and management of oral soft tissue diseases (over 160 photos). Easy-to-use, sections include: Diagnosis process: obtaining a history, examining the patient, establishing a differential diagnosis, selecting appropriate diagnostic tests, interpreting the results, etc.; white lesions; red lesions; blistering-sloughing lesions; ulcerated lesions; pigmented lesions; papillary lesions; soft tissue swelling (each lesion is illustrated with a color representative photograph); specific medications to treat oral soft tissue diseases; sample prescriptions; and special topics.

Other Products Offered by Lexi-Comp®

Oral Surgery for the General Dentist
by Lawrence I. Gaum, DDS, FADSA, FICD

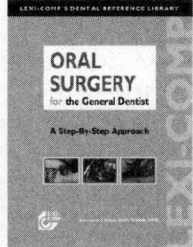

Oral Surgery for the General Dentist literally leads the practitioner through numerous surgical procedures in a well organized fashion. Utilizing a step-by-step approach for a variety of surgical techniques accompanied by detailed color photographs, this manual is filled with fantastic tips and suggestions that have been kept secret from the general dentist for many years. This manual will show how to achieve success, avoid failures, and perform surgery with confidence and expertise.

The Little Dental Drug Booklet
by Peter L. Jacobsen, PhD, DDS

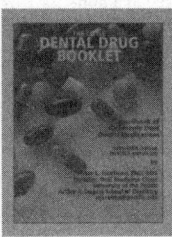

A quick reference for drugs most commonly used in dental practice.

Features
- Prescription Writing Information
- Common Abbreviations
- Pain Management
- Infection Management
- Prophylactic Antibiotic Coverage

Your Roadmap to Financial Integrity in the Dental Practice
by Donald P. Lewis, Jr., DDS, CFE

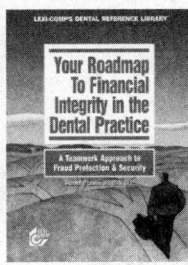

A Teamwork Approach to Fraud Protection & Security Ideal practice management reference, designed and written by a dentist in private practice. Covers four basic areas of financial security. Utilizes tabbed paging system with 8 major tabs for quick reference. Part I: Financial Transactions Incoming: Financial Arrangements, Billing, Accounts Receivable, Banking, Cash, Checks, and Credit Cards; Part II: Financial Transactions Outgoing: Accounts Payable, Supplies, Cash-on-hand, Payroll; Part III: Internal Controls: Banking, General Office Management, Human Resource (H/R) issues; Part IV: Employees: Employee Related Issues and Employees Manual Topics Part V: Report Checklist: Daily, Weekly, Monthly, Quarterly, Semi-annually, Annually; Additional Features: Glossary terms for clarification, alphabetical index for quick reference, 1600 bulleted points of interest, over 180 checklist options, 12 real-life stories (names changed to protect the innocent!), 80-boxed topics of special interest for quick review.

Other Products Offered by Lexi-Comp®

A Patient Guide to Dental Implants

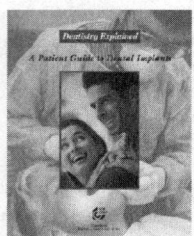

A highly illustrative description of the options available for various types of implants, including a frequently asked question-and-answer section. The flip-chart format allows for display on a desk, if required.

Tabbed sections include:
- Single Tooth Replacement
- Replacement of Several Teeth
- Four-Implant Retained Overdenture
- Two-Implant Retained Overdenture
- Screw-Retained Denture

Additional Features:
- Over 1600 bulleted points of interest
- Over 180 checklist options
- 13 real-life stories
- Over 80 boxed topics of special interest

A Patient Guide to Dental Implants Booklet

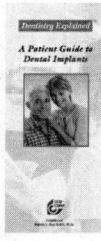

This simplified guide to dental implants will help your patients understand the different options for this procedure. Easy to read and illustrated in a non-frightening way, the diagrams show how single or multiple implants can be achieved.

Useful for reception areas, these leaflets can be supplied in bulk quantities.

A Patient Guide to Periodontal Disease

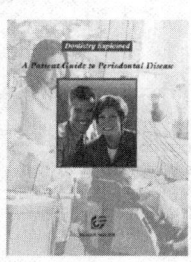

This informative patient guide provides a colorful visual overview of the procedures involved with the treatment of Periodontal Disease. The flip-chart format allows for display on a desk, if required.

Tabbed sections include:
- Healthy Gums
- Gingivitis
- Mild to Moderate Periodontitis
- Advanced Periodontitis
- Treatment Options
- If Left Untreated
- Oral Hygiene Instruction
- Prevention

Patient Guide to Root Canal Therapy

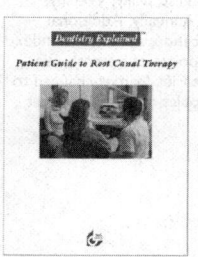

An illustrated, detailed explanation of Root Canal Therapy including a frequently asked question-and-answer section. The flip-chart format allows for display on a desk, if required.

Tabbed sections include:
- What is Root Canal Therapy?
- Access Opening
- Cleaning & Shaping the Root Canal System
- Filling the Root Canal System
- Temporary Restoration
- Permanent Restoration
- Crown Restoration

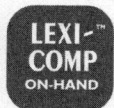
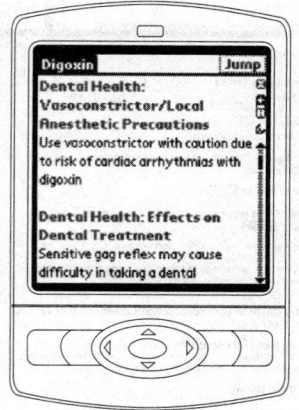

Other Products Offered by Lexi-Comp®

Lexi-Comp ONLINE for Dentistry

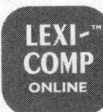

This powerful Internet-based application provides **real-time** access to all Lexi-Comp dentistry knowledge areas. Simply enter a user name and password on a computer with Internet connectivity and navigate to any content area within three mouse clicks! Drug monographs can be accessed directly from a condition or procedure using built-in links. Detailed photographs and radiographs are included.

- Obtain instant DENTAL ALERTS warning of medications that will influence treatment or cause harmful effects to the patient
    - o Effects on Dental Treatment
    - o Effects on Bleeding
    - o Vasoconstrictor/Local Anesthetic Precautions
    - o Dental Comment
- Easily implement Drug Interaction Analysis into your office workflow
    - o Supplemental Patient Drug Form provided (English/Spanish)
- Compare therapeutic categories to your patient drug regimens to select the most appropriate medication
- Access over 1,000 color photographs and radiographs
- Review nearly 12,000 drugs in the Drug ID module
- Print medication leaflets for your patients in 18 languages
- Utilize Web Search and expand your search capabilities to other qualified health web sites

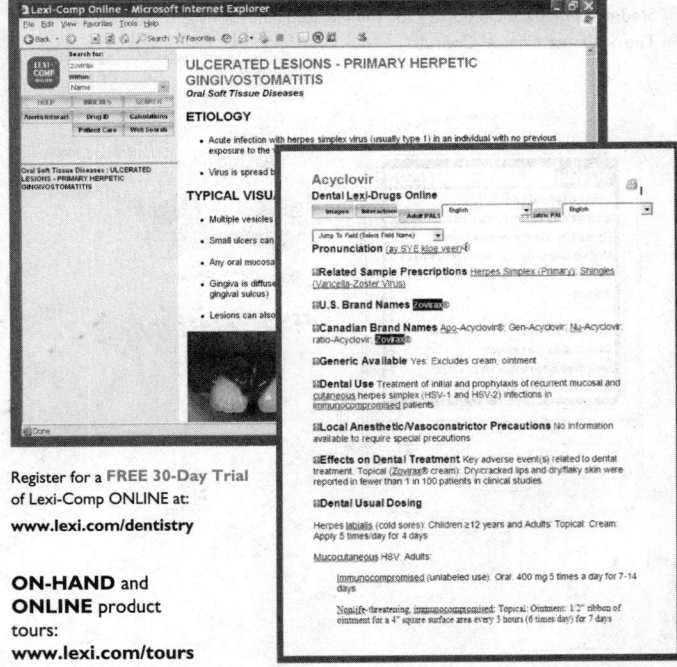

Register for a FREE 30-Day Trial of Lexi-Comp ONLINE at:

www.lexi.com/dentistry

ON-HAND and **ONLINE** product tours:

www.lexi.com/tours

Call or visit our web site to register for a live Internet demonstration.

www.lexi.com/dentistry • 1-800-837-5394